CONTRIBUTORS

JO ANN ALBERS, R.N., B.S.N., M.S.N.

Training Director, St. Joseph's General Hospital, Bellingham, Washington

JUDITH ATWOOD, R.N., M.N.

CCU-ICU Clinical Nurse Specialist, Harborview Medical Center, Seattle, Washington

MARIE JEANETTE COWAN, R.N., B.S.N., M.S.

Instructor, Pathophysiology, Basic Nursing and Medical-Surgical Nursing, Seattle University, Seattle Washington

SHIRLEY JEAN HARLOW, R.N., B.S.N., B.A., M.A.

Corporate Director of Nursing for Royal Care Centers, Seattle, Washington

ROSEMARY JEANNE PITTMAN, R.N., B.S.N., M.S.

Associate Professor, Department of Family and Community Nursing, University of Washington School of Nursing, Seattle, Washington

JOYCE V. ZERWEKH, R.N., B.S.N., M.A.

Assistant Professor, School of Nursing, Pacific Lutheran University, Tacoma, Washington

MEDICAL–SURGICAL NURSING

A Psychophysiologic Approach

JOAN LUCKMANN, R.N., B.S., M.A.

Formerly Instructor of Nursing, University of Washington, Seattle, Washington;
Instructor of Nursing at Highline College, Seattle, Washington,
Oakland City College, and Providence Hospital College of Nursing,
Oakland, California

KAREN CREASON SORENSEN, R.N., B.S., M.N.

Formerly Lecturer in Nursing, University of Washington, Seattle;
Instructor of Nursing at Highline College, Seattle,
Nurse Clinical Specialist, University Hospital and Firland Sanatorium,
Seattle, Washington

W. B. SAUNDERS COMPANY / PHILADELPHIA / LONDON / TORONTO

W. B. Saunders Company: West Washington Square
Philadelphia, Pa. 19105

1 St. Anne's Road
Eastbourne, East Sussex BN21 3UN, England

833 Oxford Street
Toronto, M8Z 5T9, Canada

Medical-Surgical Nursing—A Psychophysiologic Approach ISBN 0-7216-5805-9

 Library of Congress catalog card number 73-88262.

Last digit is the print No: 9 8 7 6 5

Preface

One outstanding hallmark of a profession is the willingness of its members to help one another learn and, thereby, improve the services that the profession performs. A textbook is one means of communicating nursing knowledge, both to the student of nursing and the practicing professional nurse.

The body of knowledge required to practice medical-surgical nursing is rapidly growing as the nursing profession continues to evolve. The fact that nursing knowledge is increasing is reflected in the size of this text. Modern patient care is based upon the holistic intertwining of information from a variety of disciplines, from the physical and social sciences as well as the arts. The professions of nursing and medicine are especially closely interrelated. Increasingly nurses are performing activities that were formerly carried out by physicians. For example, nurses are assuming enlarging responsibilities in the areas of emergency treatment, diagnosis and care of critically ill patients. Nurse practitioners with advanced preparation in specialized areas of clinical practice are increasing in numbers. It is fortunate for patients that nurses are gaining more clinical expertise since nurses spend more time with patients than physicians do.

As nursing activities become more sophisticated, so must nursing resources. We have attempted to provide a textbook of medical-surgical nursing that meets the requirements of current nursing practice. Basically the text has a psychophysiologic approach. The book is divided into three major sections. Section One considers unifying concepts basic to nursing practice, e.g., stress, adaptation, homeostasis, theories of disease causation, and the experience of illness. In Section Two psychophysiologic imbalances are discussed. Included in this section are discussions of: psychophysiologic responses to anxiety; cellular disturbances; the body's response to injury and infection; immunity, auto-immunity and hypersensitivity; fluid and electrolyte imbalances; physiologic shock; and the body's response to bed rest and immobilization. Section Three focuses on the clinical care of patients experiencing specific disorders of the various body systems and structures. Also included in Section Three are discussions of patients experiencing surgery, pain or disturbances of cellular function.

Throughout the text we have emphasized the psychosocial impact of illness, diagnostic techniques, symptomatology (with related anatomy and physiology) and specific methods of clinical care. Clinical care is heavily stressed and we have attempted to explain logically the reasons for clinical actions and observations. Patient teaching and rehabilitative processes are also accentuated. Numerous advanced nursing activities are discussed in detail, such as the care of critically ill patients requiring extensive surgery, cardiopulmonary resuscitation, intravenous therapy, respiratory therapy, closed chest drainage and tracheal intubation. Increasingly the importance of preventive care is being recognized, and throughout the text, preventive care is given appropriate coverage.

An attempt has been made to present the material in a manner that makes the learning process a dynamic experience. Learning techniques are interspersed throughout the units; periodically the reader is asked to pause in her reading to perform various activities or reflect in a directed manner on points emphasized. Some special aids to learning utilized in the book include: unit study guides; extensive bibliographies; comprehensive indexing; and frequent cross-referencing between units. Points of particular importance are summarized and highlighted with arrows, or they are boxed to facilitate review. When appropriate, overviews of anatomy and physiology are placed at the beginnings of units along with a summary of typical disorders that may affect the structures being considered.

Conscientious attempts have been made to bring out a book containing up-to-date information. However, the reader is advised to use this text in conjunction with recent professional journals to keep her level of nursing orientation truly current.

We will welcome and carefully review comments and suggestions which readers care to send concerning this text.

Although this text provides many basic guiding principles for adult patient care, each patient's care must be individualized depending upon his condition, his physician's philosophy and organizational policies. Basic guiding principles of care are, however, applicable in whatever setting a patient is located, e.g., home, clinic, hospital.

We are indebted to many people for their help and support in the preparation of this book. Special thanks are owed to John Dusseau, Robert E. Wright, Helen L. Dietz and Vern Tupper, all of the W. B. Saunders Company, for their long-sustained enthusiasm for and support of this project. We also gratefully acknowledge helpful consultations with the following nursing specialists: Barbara J. Fellows, Helon E. Hewitt, Joleen Klocke Heath and Virginia A. Mack. The librarians at the University of Washington Health Sciences Library have consistently been of valuable assistance in solving research problems associated with manuscript preparation. Mina Benjamin has been especially helpful in this way. With gratitude we acknowledge the contributions made to the text by Jo Ann Albers, Judith Atwood, Marie Cowan, Shirley Harlow, Rosemary Pittman and Joyce Zerwekh. We are appreciative of the accommodating manner with which Vy Creager assisted with typing. Finally, many thanks to our families, friends and colleagues for their continued encouragement of and interest in our writing.

Seattle, Washington

Joan Luckmann
Karen Sorensen

Contents

Section Two

Psychophysiologic Imbalances

Unit IV

Unit V

Section Three

Specific Problems in Medical-Surgical Nursing Practice

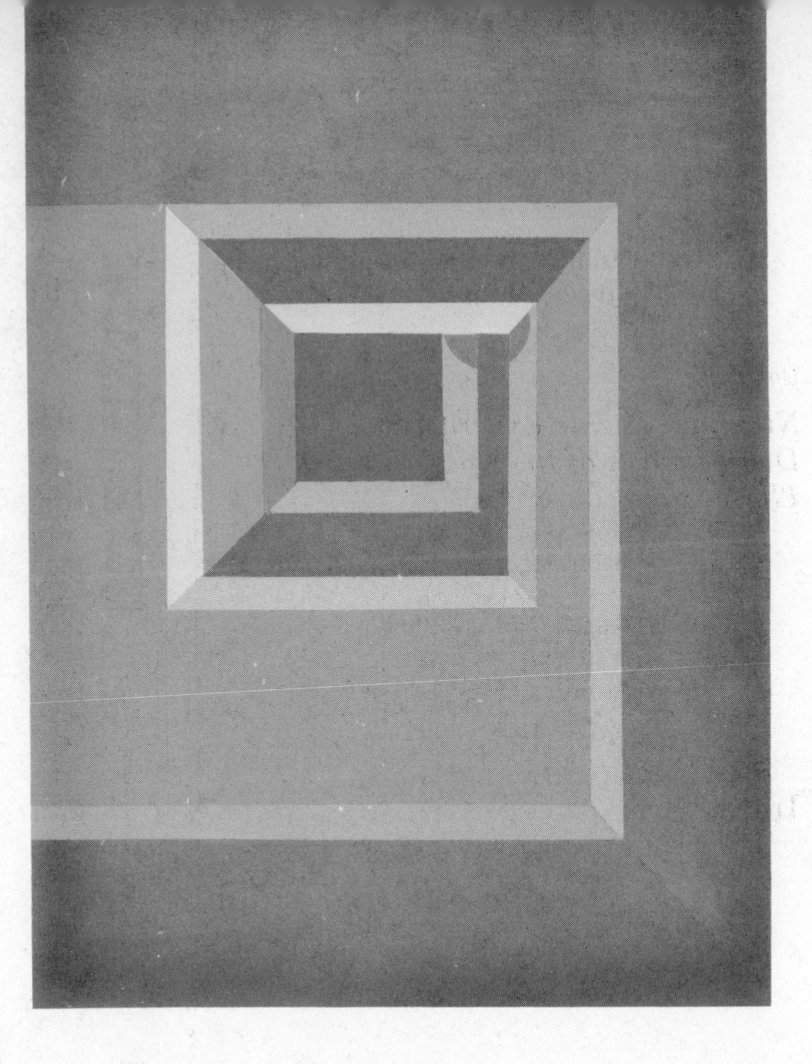

SECTION ONE

Unifying Concepts Basic to Nursing Practice

> STRESS, ADAPTATION, AND HOMEOSTASIS

> THEORIES OF DISEASE CAUSATION

> UNDERSTANDING THE EXPERIENCE OF ILLNESS

Whenever a large number of facts accumulates concerning any branch of knowledge, the human mind feels the need for some unifying concept with which to correlate them. Such integration is not only artistically satisfying, by bringing harmony into what appeared to be discord, it is also practically useful. It helps one to see a large field from a single point of view. When surveyed from a great elevation, some details in the landscape become hazy, or even invisible; yet it is only from there that we can see the field as a whole, in order to ascertain where more detailed exploration of the ground would be most helpful for its further development.

Hans Selye[47]

UNIT I

Stress, Adaptation, and Homeostasis

Introduction and Study Guide

Human beings adapting to various life stresses—both internal and environmental—are the central focus of every type of nursing. Medical-surgical nursing is concerned especially with disease processes and the care of sick patients.

The hospital is a world in itself, populated by people with special problems. Because patients *are* people, one finds in the hospital environment numerous personality types, cultural varieties, and endless human problems similar to those found in the larger world outside. But because patients are people *undergoing stress,* the hospital environment is one in which certain elements are exaggerated more than they are in the community at large. The hospital environment is intense, filled with strange odors, frightening sounds, and sudden tragedy; it is a place in which the extremes of infancy and old age, birth and death, anesthetized sleep and chronic pain come together.

Yet despite the range of human variability that exists in any hospital ward, there are certain *unifying concepts* that a nurse can use to bring a sense of order into her work with patients, and that can make her nursing care both comprehensive and meaningful. The purpose of this unit is to present those unifying concepts that will enable the nurse to view her patients as human beings, who—like herself—struggle daily to adapt to life's problems and to maintain balance in the face of stress. Unit I is divided into the following three sections:

> Chapter 1—Patients and Nurses Are People
> Chapter 2—Man Adapts to Stress
> Chapter 3—Man Struggles to Maintain a State of Balance

In Chapter 1 we consider man's general characteristics and needs, since in order to understand a patient's needs we must first be knowledgeable about people in general. In Chapters 2 and 3 we develop, in detail, those universal human problems of adaptation to stress and the maintenance of homeostatic balance; these are problems central to nursing and to patient care. The nurse who understands how people adequately adapt to stress, and how they normally maintain homeostatic balance, will have a basis for understanding *faulty* adaptation and the *breakdown of homeostasis* that occurs in illness.

Some of the terms and concepts discussed in this unit may be unfamiliar to you. Therefore, we suggest that you use the following *Study Guide* to make your reading more meaningful:

1. As you study this unit, strive to learn the general meaning of the following terms:

   cell; internal milieu; external environment; stress; adaptation—physiologic, psychologic, sociocultural, technologic; homeostatic mechanisms; negative feedback; positive feedback; thermostat-like regulators; servomechanisms; deviation; overshoot; oscillations—stable, unstable, damped, runaway.

2. As you read this unit, attempt to answer the following general questions:

   a. What biologic characteristics do all living organisms share?
   b. What common characteristics, experiences, problems, and needs do all human beings share?
   c. What are the stresses that act upon humans everywhere?
   d. How do people adapt to stress? What are the four levels of adaptation? What are the characteristics of adaptation?
   e. What are the results of homeostasis? Also, what are the basic characteristics of homeostatic mechanisms? What is the difference between positive and negative feedback?
   f. What happens when an error is signaled in a homeostatic system? What happens to a human organism when its attempts to maintain balance fail?
   g. In what ways can the concept of homeostasis be applied to the nursing care of patients?

Before beginning our discussion, two important points need to be made. First of all, much of the subject matter presented in this unit is controversial and lies in the area of theory and speculation. Although a great deal has been written about man and his adaptive abilities, we actually *know* very little about ourselves. The precise ways in which we function and adapt—physically, mentally, and emotionally—are only obscurely understood. Thus, theories about human nature are subject to correction and change as man better comprehends the mystery of himself.

Second, although unifying concepts such as those of adaptation and homeostasis are helpful in integrating seemingly unrelated data, it would be a gross oversimplification to imply that knowledge of ourselves can ever be reduced to any one common denominator. Unifying concepts have value for nurses mainly because they serve as reference points from which we can gain a perspective on the complexities of our own behavior and that of our patients.

CHAPTER 1

Patients and Nurses Are People

PATIENTS AND NURSES SHARE HUMAN BONDS

To be a successful nurse, you must be able to understand and apply scientific principles, to practice nursing care with technical skill, and to clearly communicate with a variety of patients in an empathetic, warm, and honest manner. Knowledge and technical skill often are more easily acquired by nurses and doctors than is the art of meaningful interaction with other people. Communicating with patients is especially difficult when the differences between yourself and your patients become exaggerated and the basic similarities that all individuals have in common are overlooked.

The purpose of this chapter is to discuss those human bonds that you, as a person, share with all other people—and thus with patients. Despite individual differences in age, appearance, personality, and social background, nurses and patients have in common many basic characteristics, problems, fears, and needs, and they face many of the same stresses. This commonality gives nurses and patients a meeting ground and it provides some basis, however slim, for communication and mutual understanding.

In a ward situation, knowledge of human bonds enables nurses to give compassionate care to persons of different cultures, races, religions, and ethnic backgrounds. As an example of the variety of personalities and the multitude of individual problems that nurses face daily, consider the following situation.

Today you have been assigned to care for four women occupying a four-bed ward. Both the head nurse and your instructor have briefed you concerning these patients, and now you are entering the room to survey the situation.

In one bed lies Mrs. Kowalski, an obese, jaundiced, Polish woman of about 55 years of age. Mrs. Kowalski has terminal cancer that has metastasized, or spread, throughout her body. Before becoming so very ill, she had been an obstetrical nurse in this very hospital. Consequently, she knows many doctors and nurses from different wards who come almost daily to visit and comfort her. One reason for their devotion is that she had herself assisted with the delivery of some of their children. You look carefully at her, now that she is sleeping, and you note that she breathes deeply and slowly. She has recently had the injection of morphine sulfate that she must receive frequently to subdue her constant pain. The head nurse has told you that Mrs. Kowalski is very bitter about her illness. She feels resentful toward all whom she has served—her children, her grandchildren, her patients. She views her life as one of sacrifice for others, which forced her to give up her own pleasures and happiness. Now she feels that her attitude toward life was a mistake and that she should have devoted more time to her own pleasure. Mrs. Kowalski has wanted to travel, to see the states, to see Europe, to see the world—and now she knows that she will never go.

In bed two lies Mary Murphy, a pleasant Irish woman. She smiles happily at you. She is young, 35, and today she has learned that she does not have what she so feared she had—cancer of the breast. She is wide awake and wanting to go home to her husband, who is an engineer, and her three children. She smiles at you, the uncertainty and apprehension gone that must have weighed upon her yesterday.

Mrs. Arethra Jones, an obese black woman, gazes pleasantly at you from bed three. She has suffered for many years from diabetes mellitus (a problem of faulty sugar metabolism), complicated by severe arteriosclerosis, a condition known to the laity as "hardening of the arteries." Mrs. Jones is the mother of 10 children, all of whom are devoted to her and who visit her almost daily, bringing, whenever possible, their own spouses and children. Mrs. Jones has worked much of her life in hospitals as a nursing assistant. Consequently she sympathizes with the nurses almost as much as they sympathize with her. Although she has been a diabetic for many years, she has never really accepted the limitations imposed by her condition in regard to diet and activities. Now, as a result of some severe indiscretions in diet, she is in the hospital, worried every minute about her finances, about her younger children, about her home.

Finally, you turn your attention to Miss Claire Hopkins, an aging spinster, propped up on pillows. She looks tired and faintly apprehensive, and she seems to breathe with difficulty. Miss Hopkins has severe congestive heart failure; in other words, her heart is failing to pump her blood adequately through her lungs and throughout her body. You give Miss Hopkins some oxygen, and when she feels better, she begins to talk to you. You find that she can't recall what she ate yesterday, or what she did, but she can remember the world of her youth with brilliant acuity. In her younger days Miss Hopkins was a secretary. In the evenings, she tells you, she attended night classes in many different fields—anthropology, history, art, civics. This kept her life from being too lonely. But, as she grew older and her vision failed, she found that she could no longer read as she once had. Thus, she tended to remain alone in her room for long periods, going over and over in her mind the fascinating things she had learned in school. This is how she passes time, even here in the hospital. In talking to her, you find that Miss Hopkins has the memory changes seen with age. You note that she is strangely distant and preoccupied, as if the world in which she lives has no link or connection with yours. You wonder about this woman, her life, her knowledge, her loneliness, her increasing isolation.

Now, with initial rounds made, you walk out the door and down the hall to the nurses' desk. You realize that within a few minutes you must pull together a plan of care that will give to each patient the emotional support, the instruction and guidance, and the physical care that she uniquely needs—a plan that will help each patient to obtain, if not optimum health, then at least a diminution of her suffering.

You consider the many problems that face you. You wonder how you should respond to Mrs. Kowalski's feelings about her disease, to her disappointment in her life. How should you interpret her pain—is it a completely physical phenomenon or does it have a mental component? What are her feelings about death? Does she think a great deal about it and is she afraid? Equally important, how can you, an inexperienced nurse, be empathic with this patient when you yourself have never known the pain of cancer, the fear of impending death, or the despair of a life ending before its time.

What about Mrs. Murphy? She has just experienced a severe psychologic trauma—the fear of possible breast cancer. Will you be able to understand the shock that she is just now recovering from? And then, there's Mrs. Jones. . . .

How can you approach her with instructions concerning a disease that she has lived with for so many years? Except for her hospital experience, what do you have in common with this patient when she is black and you are perhaps white or Oriental; when she has 10 children and you are perhaps not even married? When you consider Miss Hopkins, you feel an even greater gap between you as two people—a gap in age, a gap in life experience. You, who are probably young, healthy, and active, must work and communicate effectively with a woman who is aging, physically very ill, and emotionally isolated. What can you do with these problems?

Given this situation, there are three possible approaches that you can take: First, you can plan to care for these patients on a purely mechanical, technical level, ignoring all the intricate, painful, and delicate human problems that arise. That is, you make sure that Mrs. Kowalski receives her injections for pain, that Mrs. Jones is given instruction booklets concerning diabetes, that Mrs. Murphy is discharged properly, and that Miss Hopkins is given oxygen when necessary, as well as any medications that have been ordered. At the same time, you close your eyes and ears and ignore, as much as possible, Mrs. Kowalski's fears and bitterness, Mrs. Murphy's need for further instruction and reassurance regarding breast cancer, Mrs. Jones's basic misconceptions about her diabetes, and Miss Hopkins' pathetic attempts to establish contact with another person. As a result, you will "do your job" without either taxing yourself intellectually or investing yourself emotionally. A comfortable illusion of patient care will be created without any really thorough care ever being given. Unfortunately, this form of mechanized nursing practice is not uncommon.

Second, you can approach this group of patients in a helter-skelter fashion, recognizing that patient problems do indeed exist, but being unable to organize and understand the mass of signs, symptoms, clues, and responses that these problems create. Unlike the mechanically oriented nurse, you do not ignore the differences between patients, nor the many subtle details inherent in every human situation. Instead, you tend to think mainly in terms of differences and details without ever relating these details to each other or to any larger frame of reference. With this approach, you may feel that Mrs. Kowalski's bitterness over her illness, Mrs. Murphy's fear of cancer, Mrs. Jones's rejection of her illness, and Miss Hopkins' rejection of the real world are responses totally isolated from one another. Furthermore, you fail to see any interlinking threads between these four people and their problems, and yourself and your problems. Naturally, you come to feel frustrated and overwhelmed. To plan care with this attitude is like attempting to write a play without a plot, to create characters who act and react without basic human motivations. The end result, for both plan and play, is an unintelligible jumble of action without any unity of purpose.

Finally, you can approach nursing care with an appreciation of the diversity of human life and personality, but without losing sight of the basic similarities that unite all people, patients, and nurses. These similarities, consequently, make planning care easier. You recognize that Mrs. Kowalski, Mrs. Murphy, Mrs. Jones, Miss Hopkins and yourself are first of all people; consequently you all share certain basic human experiences. Furthermore, you all share the same basic human needs, some of which are satisfied and some of which are not. All of you are being acted upon by stresses arising either from within the environment or from within yourselves. Each of you is attempting to adapt as best you can to these stresses in the hope of reaching some sort of balance or equilibrium, both psychologically and physiologically. However, you tend to *differ* from one another in that some of you are meeting the challenges and stresses inherent in life more successfully than the others. And some of you have more stresses at this period in your individual lives than others.

In conclusion, if we view this ward with its four patients as containing a sample of the hospital population, and the hospital as containing a sample of persons drawn from the general population, then it is obvious that we must begin our study of patients by studying people. It has been pointed out by Martin and Prange that "nursing needs a better conceptualization of . . . the human phenomena with which it deals."[34] They continue by citing Galdston, who said about medicine:

> Medicine is founded on, pursues, and cultivates the knowledge and understanding of man as a living creature whose being is framed by a world of many and varied realities. Medicine is not only a body of knowledge and skills which aims at benefiting man, but also an understanding of the nature of the universe, and of man's position in it.[19]

In sum, nursing and medicine are concerned with total man, not a part of man. We strive for a holistic view of man, and begin by thinking of the broad science of man. It is people we care for, not facts or theories or principles. With this concept in mind, we shall now turn to a general discussion of man, both as a biologic being and as a thinking, feeling person, living in a complex social environment.

MAN AS A BIOLOGIC AND SOCIAL BEING

Man as a Living Organism

Western man, with characteristic egotism, likes to consider himself as being unique and totally different from the "lower" life forms surrounding him. The humiliating truth is that we have *much* in common with any cat, dog, fish, snail, gutter rat, or even the tiny amoeba. We share, with these and with all other living organisms, the struggle for life—for a continued existence in a changing environment. All of us, then, from the complex organism called man to one-celled amoebae, share the following biologic properties:

1. All living material, in whatever form, is chemically composed of carbon, hydrogen, oxygen, nitrogen, sulfur, phosphorus, calcium, iron, potassium, and magnesium. Sodium and chlorine, as well as smaller amounts of manganese, copper, and iodine, are typically present also. These chemicals interact together within the *protoplasm*, a viscous colloidal substance which constitutes the physical basis of living organisms.
2. With rare exceptions, *the protoplasm of living organisms is organized into cells.* We define a *cell* as a unit of life. A dynamic, highly organized structure, the cell is actively involved in the processes of growth and reproduction. Even those few organisms that appear to be noncellular (e.g., the virus) still contain the same basic substances found in ordinary cells. Thus, despite the great variety of living things that surround us (plant, animal, man), all life can be reduced eventually to the same vital components. Furthermore, all life today can be traced back to certain ancient and primitive cells that must have evolved at least two billion years ago.
3. In all living organisms, *respiration* is vital to the formation, maintenance, and eventual breakdown of the cells that form them.
4. *All organisms have an internal environment as distinguished from the exterior world or environment surrounding them.* This "internal milieu" is created by an encapsulating membrane which serves to protect the organism from the atmosphere external to it. The maintenance of the internal milieu is absolutely essential for life. Some of its major functions are to (a) help the organism adjust to changes in the external environment; (b) reduce the intrusion of noxious substances from the outside that could disturb the function of the organism; and (c) create a continuously open system for the exchange of vital substances between the internal and external environments. It is obvious that any breakdown or disruption of this internal milieu could be fatal to the organism.
5. All living things seem to pass through a *definite life cycle.* The processes of birth, growth and development, maturation and reproduction, decline and death surround us everywhere in nature. In man, as in other organisms, the regulation of these processes is primarily determined by genes, which are the units of heredity.
6. As implied above, all living things have the ability to *reproduce* themselves, resulting in the continuation of their species.
7. All organisms, if they are to survive and reproduce, must have *the capacity to adapt themselves internally to changes in the external environment.* This ability enables the organism to escape harm, to minimize injury, and to restore internal balance once this balance is lost. Hans Selye, an authority on stress, has written that "adaptability is probably the most distinctive characteristic of life."[47] Indeed, Selye goes so far as to equate adaptability with life and the loss of adaptability with death.

Thus, we and our patients share with all other living organisms a similar chemical structure. We and all other living things depend for life upon respiration, the maintenance of an internal milieu, the ability to grow and reproduce, and, finally, the ability to adapt to changing environmental conditions. Man's health can be upset if any of these vital functions are disturbed.

If these are the properties that man shares with other organisms, what then are the properties that set humans apart from other organisms and that humans share with each other?

Man as a Social Being

Basically, people everywhere are alike. On the other hand, we realize from personal experience that there is nothing quite so variable and seemingly unpredictable as individual human actions and reactions. This conflict between the variability of individual human beings and the universality of human nature has fascinated scholars for centuries. Over the years, scientists, artists, philosophers, and physicians have attempted to solve and resolve the basic contradictions inherent in man's personality.

In a profession such as nursing, we see these contradictions daily. Almost all our patients experience pain—but some cry, some react with bitterness, some are stoical. Almost all patients experience fear and apprehension—but some hide it behind a smile, some bury it in resignation, some express it in anger. What makes for this sameness in experience and yet these differences in reaction? Anthropologist Clyde Kluckhohn[28] attempted to summarize the essence of this enigma with elegant simplicity when he wrote that:

Every man is in certain respects
(a) like all other men
(b) like some other men
(c) like no other man.

Let's break this statement down and examine it for a moment as it applies to nursing. We will begin with the last statement.

Every man is in certain respects like no other man.

While we readily recognize our own individuality, we often find it difficult to realize the uniqueness of others. We tend to want to "group" others in our minds; at the same time we want others to recognize our special qualities and *not* group us. It is a fact, however, that every patient we care for *is* an individual; there is no other patient and no other person in the world exactly like him.

Our patients vary from each other for two main reasons: (1) they have inherited particular characteristics from their parents or earlier ancestors, and (2) they each come from a different environmental background (social, physical, psychologic, and economic). Each of our patients has grown up under different circumstances and has experienced dissimilar stresses, traumas, and triumphs. These experiences have been critical in shaping their unique personalities. Also, the distinct manner in which they view themselves and their relationship to the world around them contributes to their individuality. Past experience plays a significant role in determining how a patient will face a diagnosis and accept a regimen of treatment. Consequently it is possible for many patients to suffer from exactly the same disease, and yet for each to react so differently to the diagnosis that many divergent approaches are required in giving care.

For example, let us consider an actual situation involving two male patients, both of whom were very ill with coronary heart disease. One patient was a postman: he was a timid, small, fearful person who never took chances and avoided changes in his life as much as possible. The other patient was an attractive airline pilot, accustomed to a life of travel, glamor, and danger. His whole self-image revolved around seeing himself as *the* man of action. Both patients were faced with the real possibility of sudden death from a heart attack. To prevent another attack, it was imperative that they rest, change their diet, take prescribed medications, and, in general, follow prescribed treatment. The shy postman, terrified of dying, accepted without question the many restrictions placed upon him. The pilot, on the other hand, refused to drastically change his life or his diet. He rejected the thought that he should modify his activities. For this man, the possibility of dying was easier to accept than even a temporary dependence on other people.

Both these patients, interestingly enough, had the same doctor. This physician wisely realized that the classic rules of treatment expressed in textbooks must often be modified when applied to real people. Whereas a routine treatment program could be followed with the postman, it could not be with the pilot. The doctor accepted this fact and did not force the pilot into a way of life that would have destroyed him psychologically. Instead, he compromised with the patient's need for independence by allowing him as much freedom as possible, and by placing as few restrictions on him as necessary. As a result, the pilot did relax and rest, and eventually left the hospital, as did the postman. If the doctor had failed to consider individual differences and had rigidly adhered to "routine confinement," this patient's anxiety and anger over his restrictions might have precipitated a fatal heart attack or he might have become despondent and committed suicide.

This illustration indicates that while two patients may face the same problem, the same solution may not be applicable. Consequently, the skilled practitioner is not rigid in approaching patient care. What the book says about treatment should be weighed along with what the patient says about himself. Good care results only when both factors are carefully evaluated. Patients know themselves better than we know them, although they may sometimes be incapable of making sound judgments about what is in their best interest.

Every man is in certain respects like some other men.

Nursing care is complicated by the fact that we must consider our patients not only as individuals, but also as members of various groups. The ward situation developed earlier in this chapter provides us with a good example of the various group affiliations that patients are likely to have. For example,

Mrs. Kowalski and Mrs. Murphy are Polish and Irish, respectively. They belong to distinct ethnic groups, which may in turn affect their attitudes about diet, disease, hospitalization, and other matters. In this same room we have one black patient and three white patients. Although these patients share many things in common, there are certain cultural differences that must be considered in planning care.

Furthermore, not only do we have differing ethnic, racial, and economic groups present in this ward, but there are also different age and occupational groups. An elderly woman like Miss Hopkins cannot be approached in the same manner as a young woman of 35 like Mrs. Murphy. Consequently, we need to be well informed as to the general characteristics of the aged as compared to the characteristics of the mature adult. Two of the women, Mrs. Kowalski and Mrs. Jones, have worked in hospitals and that gives them a common bond with each other and with you, the nurse. It is possible that because of their experience, they will have to be approached somewhat differently from the person who has never worked in a hospital setting. Perhaps the two who have worked in a hospital are more anxious about being patients than the other two; perhaps this is not the situation at all. It must be considered and evaluated. Three of the women, Mrs. Kowalski, Mrs. Jones, and Mrs. Murphy, share the common bond of parenthood. Together they can discuss the trials and tribulations of child rearing, no matter how divergent their social and economic situations. All the women in this ward belong to the group, patient, as compared to the group of nurses, doctors, and technicians who surround them as staff members. The bond that patients feel toward each other is often extremely strong, especially among those with chronic illnesses.

Finally, we find that the group, patient, breaks down into groups of individuals with similar diseases. In fact, there are several groups of patients with similar conditions who have organized themselves on a national level. One such organization is Alcoholics Anonymous. Many other such groups exist, and these will be discussed at appropriate times throughout the text.

As a nurse, the more knowledge you have about different groupings of people—age, racial, ethnic, occupational, and religious—the more comprehensive and intelligent your care will be.

Every man is in certain respects like all other men.

Patients and nurses have their individual differences and their group differences. But, basically, we all belong to the same species and, consequently, we all have similar biologic characteristics. We all experience certain universal problems and share certain universal needs. It is this universality of need and experience that gives us a common stage upon which to act and interact with our patients. It is this mutuality, the sense of being part of humanity, that allows us to be empathic and to understand, to some degree at least, another human being.

What then is true of all people in terms of (1) basic needs and (2) universal experiences? What is the application to nursing?

Man's Basic Needs

Man has many needs, some of which are more vital than others. Physiologists, biologists, and psychologists have worked out many ways of grouping needs and the following scheme represents one such classification. According to Maslow,[35] there is a hierarchy of motivated needs, ranging from the most basic to the most sophisticated. In his scheme, there are the following six levels:

1. Survival needs: food, air, water, temperature, elimination, rest, pain avoidance.
2. Stimulation needs: sex, activity, exploration, manipulation, novelty.
3. Safety and security needs: safety, security, protection.
4. Love needs: love, belonging, closeness.
5. Esteem needs: esteem, self-esteem.
6. Self actualization: the process of making maximum use of one's abilities.

When we consider the area of human needs in relationship to patients, it is obvious that: (1) patients, as people, have the same basic needs as the nurse; (2) the patient cannot satisfy many of his needs while under care because of physical or

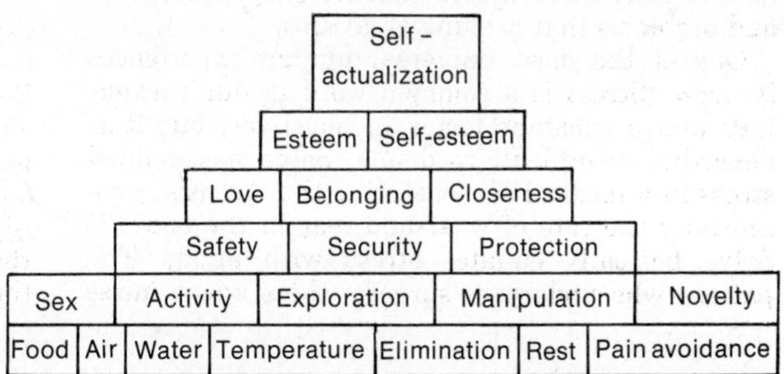

FIGURE 1–1. Maslow's hierarchy of needs, as adapted by Kalish. (From Kalish, R. A.: *The Psychology of Human Behavior.* Belmont, Calif., Wadsworth Publishing Co., 1966.)

mental incapacity or illness; and (3) it is the nurse's task to help the patient to gratify his needs realistically within the confines of his illness and hospitalization, preserving as much independence for him as possible and desirable, and permitting his dependence on her as necessary.

Some needs require constant gratification, whereas the attainment of other needs can be postponed. For example, we cannot live for long without air, but sexual activity can be postponed indefinitely. However, it must be recognized that, although the gratification of needs can be postponed or modified for varying lengths of time, *the needs are still present.*

Sensitivity to patients and intelligent nursing care depend upon a recognition of the entire gamut of human needs. Certainly we cannot ignore the patient's survival and protection needs. If he is cyanotic, he may need oxygen; if he is in pain, he may need medication or a position change; if he is unconscious or delirious, he needs the protection of side-rails on his bed.

On the other hand, the needs for love, stimulation, and esteem, though not so obvious, are equally important. For example, reconsider the case of the airline pilot with severe heart disease. His need for self-esteem, which involved the preservation of his masculine, daring self-image, was actually as great a need, if not greater, than his survival needs. Furthermore, patients on bed rest are known to deteriorate (mentally and physically) if their needs for mental stimulation and physical movement are not met. Children even under the most aseptic hospital conditions have failed to grow and have even died because of lack of affection and love.

In sum, patients, like ourselves, want to do more than just exist and survive. Too frequently in nursing care only the survival needs are considered. Patients want to live as completely as possible; they desire and need a certain amount of novelty, love, and esteem in their lives. They should not be denied self-actualization.

The Universal Experience of Stress

Because of the universality of human needs, it follows that there are certain human experiences and problems that are universal also.

One of the most universal human experiences is *stress.* Stress is a common word in our vocabulary and a constant factor in our lives, but it is nevertheless difficult to define. Selye has defined stress in a medical sense, stating that "stress is essentially the rate of wear and tear in the body."[47] Selye basically equates stress with aging. The patient who undergoes surgery, the student nurse who takes a difficult examination—both of these people are undergoing stress and both will change and age slightly as a result.

Another somewhat broader way of defining stress is "any influence, whether it arises from the internal environment or from the external environment, which interferes with the satisfaction of basic needs or which disturbs or threatens to disturb the stable equilibrium."[17] Stress, then, is anything that: (1) threatens or attempts to injure or destroy us; (2) keeps us from satisfying our basic needs; (3) interferes with our growth, development, and productivity; and (4) threatens to or actually does throw us out of balance, either physically or psychologically.

There are three *general* sources of stress:[47] First, stress can result from a *pathologic* change in the body as the result of disease or injury. Second, stress can be the outcome of *normal living* when no injury or illness has occurred. For example, daily commuting, entertaining, attending classes—all can be considered mildly stressful yet normal activities of modern life. Third, stress can be the outcome of planned activities or even therapies, and can be *curative.* For instance, competitive sports, though stressful, help us to work off certain emotions; electroshock therapy, a very stressful procedure, has proved helpful in working with the mentally ill.

Important *specific* sources of stress are:

> attacks by bacteria, viruses, and parasites
> trauma (injury, burns, assaults)
> inadequate food, warmth, protection
> disruptive social and family relationships
> conflicting social and cultural expectations
> basic needs that must be denied because of social pressure (e.g., forbidden sexual desires)
> imagined threats of injury (sources of stress do not have to be based in reality)
> changes in the internal physiology (e.g., puberty, menstruation, pregnancy, menopause)

Anthropologists in their study of man and stress have found that all people:[8, 28, 41]

> experience deprivation, frustration, and stress when needs are not satisfied
> tend to avoid stresses, such as injury, temperature extremes, and pain
> react in similar ways to extreme stress
> tend to adapt to stress and to satisfy basic needs by deliberately modifying the environment (e.g., inventing clothing, housing, medicines)
> tend to seek a state of equilibrium in the face of environmental and internal stresses

You and I share with all humans the universal experience of stress—a fact that should help us to feel a certain empathy with any patient in our care. Because patients are particularly vulnerable to stress, knowledge of the following processes is particularly important in nursing: (1) the nature of *human adaptation* to stress, and (2) the problem of reaching and maintaining *homeostatic balance* in the face of stress. We shall consider these areas in the following chapters.

CHAPTER 2

Man Adapts to Stress

Adaptation is a universal characteristic of life and, thus, serves as a unifying concept for understanding human behavior. Biologists and behavioral scientists have shown that whenever a person encounters stress, from whatever source, he attempts to adapt to it. If adaptation is successful, the individual's balance is not disturbed, or is restored. If adaptation is faulty, the individual becomes ill, and then as a sick person he must adapt to his illness. Thus, the concept of adaptation is of vital concern to nurses and physicians who daily cope with the adaptive changes that illness has forced upon patients.

THE MEANING OF ADAPTATION

The word "adapt" comes from the Latin *adaptare,* meaning to adjust. Thus, originally, adaptation simply meant adjustment. However, since the process of adaptation is characteristic of all living things, adaptation has been a subject for intensive study in many disciplines, ranging from plant biology to psychiatry. The result is that the word "adaptation" can be considered from the standpoints of both biology and human behavior. In its most comprehensive sense, the concept of adaptation includes the whole range of protective adjustments from the simplest motor action to the most complex interaction between individuals or entire nations. It involves organisms that are as simple as the one-celled amoeba and those as complicated as man.

In sum, adaptation is found at all levels of life; it is probably the one characteristic that separates living organisms from inanimate objects. At the human level adaptation is more complicated than among less complex organisms. It involves more than a simple biologic process. Man does not just react to his environment as an insect would; instead, he *responds* to his environment with its multiple stresses. With body, intellect, and emotion, man attempts to meet the challenges of life actively and aggressively.

LEVELS OF ADAPTATION

We may consider human adaptation as functioning at the following four levels: (1) the physiologic or biologic, (2) the psychologic, (3) the sociocultural, and (4) the technologic. For purposes of convenience, we shall examine these levels separately. However, it is essential to remember that, in terms of human experience, these levels are fully interrelated.

The Physiologic Level

Adaptation in the biologic sense is defined by Webster's New World Dictionary as a "change in structure, function, or form that produces better adjustment of an animal or plant to its environment." Physiologic or biologic adaptation involves compensatory changes that occur within the body in response to either (1) increased or altered demands being made upon the body, or (2) stresses (either internal or environmental) that are impinging upon the body and threatening to destroy its physiologic balance.

For example, consider the increased demands made upon the body by the popular form of exercise known as jogging. Jogging consists of running and walking alternately, at a slow to moderate pace, over varying distances. Many of the people undertaking this form of exertion have led sedentary lives before beginning a jogging program. Consequently, they experience a considerable degree of physical stress during their first exercise sessions. They may feel exhausted; they may experience muscular soreness and aching; their hearts may beat quite rapidly in an effort to circulate a sufficient blood supply to their muscles; their respirations may accelerate as a result of the additional amounts of oxygen needed. However, if these persons follow the recommended jogging schedule, increasing their efforts a little every day, they may eventually be able to jog quite a distance, at a moderate rate, without undue strain. Their muscles, hearts, and lungs will have gradually increased in strength and functional efficiency in order to best *adapt* to the additional demands placed upon them.

Man's ability to adjust to extreme changes in temperature and to climatic variations provides another example of physiologic adaptation. For instance, if a person is suddenly exposed to extreme cold, he tends to shiver, to stamp his feet, to wave his arms, and to move around generally. This muscular activity helps to increase his body's heat production, so that his body temperature remains normal despite the cold environment. On the other hand, individuals who live in cold climates for lengthy periods maintain the increased heat production necessary for survival by developing a higher rate of metabolism. Further, not only is heat production generally increased, but heat loss from the body is prevented by the development of protective mechanisms. For instance, sweating is reduced, the blood vessels that supply the skin tend to constrict more, and an insulating layer of subcutaneous fat develops as a result of an increased food intake. Because of these physiologic adaptations, and aided by such technologic adaptations as specially designed clothing, heating, and housing, explorers have been able to survive for considerable periods in extremely frigid environments in which they would normally perish. In contrast, the Eskimo, with a relatively simple technology, has developed genetic adaptations as a result of centuries of life in a frozen habitat. Consequently, these people have a short, thick body build with a heavy layer of subcutaneous fat. These physical attributes are most advantageous for life in cold climates.

The body's reaction to invading microorganisms serves as a further illustration of physiologic adaptation to stress. Man resists attacks by viruses and bacteria by developing an immunity to them. Briefly, immunity may be either inherited or acquired.* If inherited, an individual is born with a constitution *naturally* resistant to certain organisms. If acquired, the individual develops immunity as the result of either having a particular infectious disease and surviving it, or being inoculated against that disease. His body, in this situation, *adapts* to the presence of disease through forming antibodies in his blood that protect him. He thus develops immunity for specific diseases.

As a final example, in the field of sensory physiology, adaptation is viewed as a decrease in the intensity of a sensation resulting from "steady state stimulation" or continuous responses.[25] The olfactory sense provides a good example of sensory adaptation. We all know that when we come into contact with a noxious odor, we are immediately offended. However, if we remain in contact with this odor (steady state stimulation) and the odor remains constant, we become accustomed to it rather quickly; thus, there is a decrement in the intensity of sensation until we are oblivious of its existence. In other words, we adapt.

The Psychologic Level

Psychologic adaptation involves adjustment to stress through the use of learning, perception, and conscious and unconscious processes, including the various psychologic defense mechanisms.† This mode of adaptation is based primarily on complex neurochemical processes, many of which remain obscure and are as yet unexplained. It also involves our genetic endowment as well as the many associations, both pleasant and unpleasant, which arise from our past experiences.

As an illustration of psychologic adaptation, consider the intellectual and emotional adjustments that an average student must make within his various classes if he is to succeed, or indeed remain in college. Let us observe a hypothetic student named John who is pursuing a general academic course. A fairly intelligent, likable boy, John comes from high school to college with an above-average academic record.

At 8 o'clock in the morning John has a class in biology. The teacher, a woman, is very strict, demanding, and exacting in her approach to students. She expects immediate and precise recall of facts from the textbook and she does not encourage students to engage in free discussion of theory or areas of controversy. If John is to adjust satisfactorily to this class, he must always come with his lessons prepared and he must memorize verbatim the data in his text. If he wishes to argue a point, he must do it diplomatically.

At 10 o'clock John attends his history class. The professor, in this instance, is lenient, prefers to talk about everything but history, and gives very simple examinations. For this class, John does little preparation. Instead, he uses the time from this subject to prepare for biology. He does not let the fact that he is learning very little about history concern him particularly.

At 2 in the afternoon John has a class in American literature—a subject that he likes. Although the teacher spends almost the entire quarter discussing a few authors, his examinations make it clear that he demands a comprehensive knowledge of the entire scope of American literature. John realizes that success in this course involves independent study of material never alluded to in class. Students who are unable to grasp this fact eventually fail in the class.

In each of his classes John has had to make emotional and intellectual adjustments. When he changes classes, he is obliged to change his frame of reference to fit the subject being taught. When he changes teachers, he is obliged, to some degree, to change his attitude, his behavior, and his mode of approach. By so doing, John adapts to his role as a student; by functioning satisfactorily within that role, he remains in school. John has made a successful adaptation to the stresses in his life. He is using appropriate, healthy adaptive mechanisms that will ultimately help him to attain his goals.

While adaptation is always *useful* at the time it occurs, it does not always result in what is best for the *total* individual: *unhealthy adaptation* also occurs. In an attempt to respond to stress, an individual may adapt in a manner that may function temporarily to relieve his discomfort, but that ultimately may not be in his best interest.

For example, a man who unconsciously wishes to be dependent on other people may develop an incapacitating illness. This allows him to be dependent without experiencing guilt feelings over his dependency. He does not feel guilty because

*For a full discussion of immunity, see pages 165 to 191.

†This is discussed more completely on pages 113 to 116, Unit IV.

he accepts the idea that sick people can be dependent. This is not, of course, the situation with all illnesses. It does serve, however, as an example of adaptation that ultimately proves harmful to the individual, but that meets his immediate need to reduce the stress that his dependent feelings create.

Moreover, some psychiatrists believe that certain neurotic behavior has protective value. For instance, suppose that an obese individual cannot control his eating and feels driven to eat all the time ("compulsive" overeating). This is neurotic behavior, assuming there is no physiologic imbalance. The resulting obesity may protect the individual from becoming involved in threatening sexual relationships. If this person diets and loses weight, he will consequently become more sexually attractive. Then he will have to either come to terms with the problems of sexuality or develop a new protective neurosis. As long as he remains obese he is protected by his neurotic overeating. Even though he may say he wishes he were not so heavy, his neurotic need for protection is greater than his drive to be more attractive physically.

This person's adaptation is protective to him and should not be tampered with by unskilled persons. It may be that even though his adaptation appears unsuccessful, it is the most successful adaptation that he can make. Obese individuals have been known to commit suicide when losing weight because they could not adapt to the new problems created. For them, obesity was a successful, life-sustaining adaptation.

The student is cautioned not to generalize from this example or apply it to all obese people. Neurotic problems vary from individual to individual and are identified only through skilled exploration. This example is presented merely to illustrate neurotic adapatation.

Protection of the psyche from overwhelming trauma is seen not only in the neurotic, but in the extreme behavior of the psychotic as well. For instance, total withdrawal from the world serves to isolate the psychotic from an unbearable life experience; hallucinations may help him to recognize and control a threatening and chaotic existence. Thus, he is adapting to life in the only way he can at the time.

In summary, when we adapt psychologically to stress, we are attempting to protect ourselves so that we can continue to survive in life. Individuals adapt to stress in the best way they can at the time. Adaptive behavior may not always appear appropriate; however, it is always purposeful.

The Sociocultural Level

Adaptation at this level includes the various patterns of behavior by which people adjust to the society and the culture that surrounds them. More explicitly, sociocultural adaptation involves, first of all, the adjustment of an individual's actions and conduct to the norms, conventions, beliefs, and pressures of various groups. The family, professional societies, labor unions, social clubs, and sororities are but a few examples of the wide assortment of groups that demand our involvement and commitment. Second, adaptation at this level means adjustment of our behavior to the "total . . . ideas and institutions and conventionalized activities"[41] that define a culture. Examples of cultural groups include racial groups, geographic groups (e.g., American, European), and certain religious groups.

As an illustration of sociocultural adaptation at the *group* level, consider your own experience as a student preparing for the profession of nursing. When you first entered your school of nursing, you were probably exposed, almost immediately, to a new set of ethics that you had to accept, to a new vocabulary that you had to learn, and to certain standards of performance that you had to achieve. All these demands perhaps seemed overwhelming at first. Furthermore, your first experiences with patients may have been overshadowed by a sense of uncertainty, nervousness, and even fear. But gradually, over a period of months, you began to speak the medical language fluently, you came to believe in the values that you were taught, and you developed the confidence to function fairly efficiently in the nurse-patient relationship.

You may safely assume that the longer you remain in nursing, the more natural it will seem to you to be a nurse. This is because you, as an individual, will have adapted to the nursing profession. You will have become a bona fide member of the group. You may eventually become so well adapted to nursing that you will find it difficult to relate to other professional and social groups. This sense of exclusiveness is a common characteristic of professional societies, and one of the dangers of social adaptation. If this occurs, you will have adapted so exclusively to one group that you have lost your ability to adapt to others.

Adaptation at the *cultural level* can be exemplified in several ways. For instance, a cowboy who leaves the wilds of Wyoming to take up residence in Los Angeles must make many sweeping adjustments. He must adapt himself to urban sprawl, smog, roaring freeways, glaring lights, constant noise, numerous people, and the general turmoil of city life. He must adjust to crowding, competitive attitudes, emotional stresses, varying ideas and conventions, as well as to the multiple value systems found in a megalopolis.

The cowboy may at first feel awed and shocked by city life. He may even become emotionally disturbed by the changes in his own life style which this new situation demands. However, if he remains in the city long enough he may gradually develop the appropriate attitudes, habits, and behaviors. As a result, he will come to feel as at home in the heavily populated Los Angeles environment as he once did in the open country of Wyoming.

The process of cultural adaptation is also illustrated by the anthropologist who goes into the field to work with a group of primitive people, or by the

Peace Corps worker who volunteers to serve in an underdeveloped country. Both anthropologists and Peace Corps workers often tell of the "cultural shock" that they experienced when they first came into contact with the customs and activities of the people with whom they were working. Gradually, however, the sense of shock subsided as they became acclimated to the situation. Indeed, these workers sometimes become so well adapted to the foreign culture that the eventual reentry into the confines of their own culture proves difficult. Nurses may experience "cultural shock" as their nursing practice brings them into contact with various cultural groups.

In short, when we adapt to a group or to a culture, we modify and, in some instances, radically change our attitudes and behavior so that they merge with the norms, values, and institutions of the group or culture we are involved with. Of course, in order to adapt socially, we must also adapt psychologically, and in some instances, physiologically. For example, when the cowboy moved from Wyoming to Los Angeles, he was obliged to adapt psychologically to the emotional stresses inherent in city living, and physiologically to the air pollution characteristic of industrial areas.

The Technologic Level

Technologic adaptations are those scientific and industrial arts and innovations that man himself has created through the use of his cultural heritage. These adaptations have built for man an artificial world in place of the primitive pre-industrial world in which he once lived. Technology, an outgrowth of culture, has allowed us to modify and change our surrounding environment and to control many of the stresses that are part of that environment. Unfortunately, modern technology has also created certain new stresses to which man must adapt—for example, water, air, and noise pollution. On the whole, however, advances in science enable men to live longer with less discomfort than was ever before possible. Although we, as human animals, are still ruled by general biologic laws, we are more and more in control of our own destiny through industrial, scientific, and medical innovations.

Modern medicine, in particular, has evolved at a tremendous rate over the last decades. Because of medical science, man is adapting with greater success to the stresses of disease and injury, birth, and death than would have been believed possible in past centuries. For example, today medical technology eases population stresses through the use of contraceptives; emotional stresses through the use of tranquilizing drugs; the problems of infectious disease through the use of inoculations and sanitation; the dangers of childbirth through the development of better obstetric techniques; and the once fatal problems of heart and kidney failure through the use of transplants.

As a result of our technology, then, we are gaining a certain control over the universal problems of disease, pain, and death. The successes of medical science, however, have not been obtained without a price. Serious dilemmas (philosophic, ethical, and legal) have developed as a result of our technologic adaptations. These dilemmas are complex and far-reaching in their implications. These medical problems often have an effect on nursing practice, and they will be discussed as appropriate throughout the text.

CHARACTERISTICS OF ADAPTATION

All adaptive mechanisms (whether physiologic, psychologic, cultural, or technologic) tend to have certain common characteristics. These characteristics can be summarized as follows:

1. *All adaptive mechanisms are attempts to maintain within the individual optimum physical and chemical conditions.* Thus, through the process of adaptation, those physiologic processes necessary to life can be carried on to best effect. The process of maintaining a fairly steady internal environment for the individual is called *homeostasis.* The concept of homeostasis is so important that it will be explained at length in the following chapter.

2. *Individuals always retain their own identity despite the use of adaptive mechanisms.* Thus, we are able to adapt to changing conditions without losing those characteristics of appearance and behavior that particularly distinguish us. For example, we, as individuals, may undergo tremendous stresses during certain periods of our lives. We may be forced to adapt to painful trauma and to upsetting changes. As a result, we may wrinkle, develop gray hair, and age visibly. Nevertheless, we are still recognizable as human beings in general, and as ourselves in particular. We still retain the gross appearance and general behavior patterns that have characterized us throughout our lives. In sum, we exhibit a certain stability in the midst of change.

3. *Adaptation is a dynamic and active process.* Individuals do not passively submit to environmental or internal stresses; for example, such *internal* stimuli as hunger and thirst result in our *actively* seeking release from these tensions through such actions as seeking food and water. When *external* stresses threaten us, we may run from them, or block them from our consciousness (for example, by fainting), or actively struggle against them. Moreover, to further protect ourselves from danger, we may intensify the action of those sensory receptors that are necessary for our survival. For instance, in a life-threatening situation, our hearing tends to become more acute and our vision sharper than it "normally" is. Vision sharpens because the pupil of the eye dilates when we are under extreme stress. Involved in all these protective adaptive actions are the sympathetic and parasympathetic nervous systems as well as cer-

tain circulatory, endocrine, and sensory mechanisms.

4. *When individuals adapt to change or to stress, they tend to adapt as total organisms.* In other words, adaptation does not occur exclusively at any one level of human experience. Rather, it tends to embrace all levels—the physiologic, the psychologic, the sociocultural, and perhaps even the technologic. When you became a nursing student, you had to adapt physiologically to the greater work load, to the long hours of study, and to the muscular stresses required for lifting and moving patients. Psychologically you had to adapt on an intellectual level to the new and different subject matter, and emotionally to the responsibilities and problems inherent in patient care. At the sociocultural level you had to adjust to the ethics and norms of the nursing profession and of hospital culture. Technologically it was necessary to familiarize yourself with equipment new to you.

5. *Adaptation, as a process, has its definite limitations.* Although adaptive mechanisms and behavior exploit the available potentialities of the individual, they must also operate within the limitations of that individual's hereditary make-up, physiologic constitution, intelligence, and emotional stability. As one scientist has written, "a cornered amoeba cannot escape by flying."[17] Likewise, a man cannot flap his arms and fly or remain submerged in water indefinitely. He must adapt within the confines of his nature or through technologic innovations.

6. *Adaptive responses are much more limited in number and scope at the physiologic level than they are at the social and psychologic levels.* For instance, our blood sugar, the oxygen content of our blood, and our internal temperature can fluctuate only within certain narrow limits and still be consistent with life. On the other hand, there are many possible adaptive solutions available to us in situations involving emotional or social crises. However, even in these circumstances the number of possible solutions is finite.

7. *Adaptation can be viewed in relationship to time.* The individual who has sufficient time can adapt more readily to stress than can the individual who must adapt quickly. For example, the body is able to adapt remarkably well to a *gradual* blood loss. Individuals with hemorrhoids, slowly bleeding peptic ulcers, or unsuspected gastrointestinal tract cancer may lose up to one-half of their total red blood cell volume *without* experiencing the usual symptoms of anemia. This is because the blood loss is occurring over a prolonged period of time. Under these conditions, the bone marrow is able to increase the production of erythrocytes sufficiently to compensate for the blood loss.

In contrast, the body tends to adapt much less readily to a *sudden,* rapid blood loss. Consequently, persons suffering from sudden hemorrhage due to any number of causes *do* tend to develop anemia, with such symptoms as asthenia (weakness), fatigue, and pallor. If the blood loss has been considerable (1000 ml. or more), it may take two months or longer for the body to compensate adequately. Moreover, patients with sudden rapid bleeding may develop signs of shock such as rapid pulse, lowered blood pressure, and restlessness. These signs develop in response to the sudden drop in circulating fluid volume that occurs with hemorrhage. If the body is unable to compensate quickly enough and appropriate medical measures are not taken swiftly, the shock may become irreversible and death may result. *Time* is, thus, an important aspect of adaptation.

8. *Adaptability varies from individual to individual.* Flexible individuals who are readily responsive to change, and who employ a wide range of compensatory mechanisms, are more adaptable than those persons lacking these qualities. Consequently they are more likely to survive stress and change than are rigid individuals.

Although open to many philosophical interpretations, Franz Kafka's story, "The Hunger Artist" can be used to illustrate this principle as it applies to an individual life. "The Hunger Artist" centers around a man who practiced, for a livelihood, the highly specialized art of fasting. Living in a time when public fasting was popular, the Hunger Artist was very successful. He fasted while perched atop a pole or in other extreme situations. He was applauded and honored by people everywhere for his performances. Times changed, however, and people lost all interest in the art of fasting. The Hunger Artist, unfortunately, was unable to change with the times. Not only was he too old, but more importantly, he was too fanatically devoted to fasting to learn another profession. Fasting was the only thing he knew how to do well, and the only way of life he enjoyed. Finally, with no economic means left and deserted by everyone, the Hunger Artist joined a circus where he continued to pursue his art. There, in a cage, virtually unknown and almost completely neglected by the public he had once thrilled, the artist continued to fast day after day until finally he died in total obscurity. To sum up, the Hunger Artist had become extremely specialized and rigid in his response to the environment in which he lived. Consequently when that environment unexpectedly changed, he did not have the flexibility to change with it. As a result he could not adapt and he did not survive.

For the Hunger Artist, the ultimate price of an inability to adapt to change was death. For other individuals, the price of inadequate adaptation may be less drastic. Nevertheless, it may involve such serious problems as the development of mental illness, physical disease, or both.

Physical illness is not always the *result* of failure to adapt. Sometimes physical illnesses may *cause* problems in adaptation. Patients with an incapacitating disease such as a severe heart problem may be called upon suddenly to change their occupation and life style. Like the Hunger Artist, these changes may be demanded of them at a time in their life when they are most set in their ways and least able to change. Unless these patients are given reassurance and guidance in planning the future, they may not be able to adapt to the new way in which they must live to survive.

9. *Adaptation is a process that may make us, at the same time, less sensitive to some stimuli and more sensitive to other stimuli.* For example, when we attend a matinee on a sunny afternoon, entering a darkened theater from the outside, we are at first unable to see at all. Gradually, however, our eyes adapt to the dark and we are able to see fairly well. But while our eyes are becoming adjusted to the dark, they are becoming, at the same time, more sensitive to bright light. Consequently, by the time the show is over, we find that we can see very well inside the darkened theater, but when we go outside we are again temporarily blinded, this time by the light. In sum, exposure to darkness makes us more sensitive to light and vice versa.

10. Hans Selye suggests that "*an essential feature of adaptation is the delimitation of stress to the smallest area capable of meeting the requirements of the situation.*"[47] As an example of the principle of delimitation, Selye discusses the inflammatory process.

Inflammation, according to Selye, is a "local resistance to injury," characterized by heat, pain, redness, and swelling.*[47] This injury may result from the invasion of viruses or bacteria. It may also be caused by irritants and allergens. Inflammation serves the purpose of barricading off infected or irritated areas of tissue from those areas that are healthy. This localization of infection allows white blood cells to deal more effectively with dangerous invading organisms. Localization also prevents a serious infection from spreading throughout the body by way of the blood vessels to cause septicemia (generalized blood poisoning). In sum, then, the inflammatory process is an adaptive mechanism that *limits* a stress to the area capable of dealing with it. This localization of stress spares the individual from widespread trauma.

11. *Adaptive responses may be adequate to meet stress or change and to reestablish homeostatic balance. However, adaptive mechanisms may also be inadequate, excessive, or inappropriate.*

To illustrate, inflammation can, in some instances, serve *adequately* as an adaptive function. By means of connective tissue barriers, inflammation can prevent dangerous organisms from spreading throughout the body. If the inflammatory response to infection is *inadequate,* however, the body may be overwhelmed by the invading organisms. On the other hand, an inflammatory process can be maladaptive because it is *excessive.* If, for example, the irritant to our tissues is *not* a dangerous microbe but a harmless pollen, then inflammation acts as an excessive and *inappropriate* adaptive mechanism. Inflammation, in this case, is not aiding the individual; instead it is creating unnecessary pathologic changes that do not serve any protective purpose.

12. *Even though adaptation helps individuals to adjust to stress and to maintain or establish homeostatic balance, adaptive mechanisms may, in themselves, be stressful.* For instance, inflammation is an adaptive mechanism that can prevent the spread of highly infectious organisms throughout the body. However, the inflammatory process is, in itself, stressful for the individual because it causes certain physiologic changes that result in the symptoms of heat, swelling, redness, and pain. These symptoms are uncomfortable and, therefore, are stressful. In striving to achieve homeostatic balance, the individual may sometimes develop imbalances. These imbalances, in turn, will require the use of further compensatory adaptive mechanisms.

*For a detailed discussion of the inflammatory process, see Unit V, Chapter 22.

CHAPTER 3

Man Struggles to Maintain a State of Balance

A frequently observed truism might be stated thus: There is nothing so constant as change. Consequently there is nothing so vital to the preservation of life as the ability (1) to adapt satisfactorily to change, and (2) to maintain internal stability in the face of a variable and stressful environment. This constancy of change coupled with the necessity for stability has forced living creatures, over eons of time, to develop certain techniques for *automatically* maintaining balance despite constant threats to their equilibrium. Those self-regulatory techniques that preserve an organism's ability to adapt to stresses and yet to maintain its inner balance are called *homeostatic mechanisms.* A vital class of adaptations, homeostatic mechanisms operate at all levels of life, regulating biologic functioning and counteracting change and imbalance.

HISTORICAL PERSPECTIVES

Though the scientific study of homeostatic regulation is comparatively new, the concept of the need for physiologic balance has existed for centuries. Hippocrates, the father of medicine, conceived of health as the result of a balance or harmony between individuals and their environment. The French physiologist, Claude Bernard, around the middle of the nineteenth century, wrote of the *"milieu interne"* (internal milieu). He believed that life and health depended upon the constancy and stability of the circulating fluids of the body. In 1939 Cannon created the term *homeostasis* from the Greek words *homoios,* meaning "like," and *stasis* meaning "standing." In his classic text, *The Wisdom of the Body,* Cannon wrote:

> The constant conditions which are maintained in the body might be termed *equilibria.* That word, however, has come to have fairly exact meaning as applied to relatively simple physio-chemical states, in closed systems, where known forces are balanced. The coordinated physiological processes which maintain most of the steady states in the organism are so complex and so peculiar to living things—involving as they may, the brain and nerves, the heart, lungs, kidneys and spleen, all working cooperatively—that I have suggested a special designation for these states, *homeostasis.* The word does not imply something set and immobile, a stagnation. It means a condition—a condition which may vary, but which is relatively constant.[6]

Cannon conceived of homeostasis as a type of *dynamic* equilibrium as opposed to a static condition. His use of the term "homeostasis" applied mainly to the self-regulation of such internal physiologic processes as:

Body temperature	Electrolyte balance
Blood pressure	Muscle tone
Blood sugar concentration	Blood oxygen level
Water balance	Blood carbon dioxide level

Today, homeostasis has far wider applications. In addition to physiologic processes, the concept of homeostasis may be used to explain perceptual and cognitive processes; activities leading to the satisfaction of basic needs; instinctive reactions; and even intellectual and creative behavior.

Moreover, homeostatic principles have been applied to such diversified fields as genetics; growth; human, plant, and animal ecology; psychiatry; and engineering. In industry the basic concept of homeostasis has been used in the creation of such self-regulating devices as automatic airplane pilots, missile guidance systems, computers, and servomechanisms* for industrial automation. Although it is true that human technology has been able to produce very sophisticated self-regulating devices, these man-made mechanisms cannot begin to rival the biologic systems in complexity or in precision.

Thus, the concept of homeostasis has, in itself, adapted to changing environmental demands. Once thought of as simply the regulation of steady states in mammals, the term has now been expanded to include "any self-regulating system aiding survival."

BASIC CHARACTERISTICS OF HOMEOSTATIC MECHANISMS†

All homeostatic devices tend to be characterized by certain distinctive traits:

---

*This term is discussed on page 20.

†For information concerning the characteristics of homeostasis, the authors have relied especially on the work of Thomas Overmire.[39]

> *A. Homeostatic devices are compensatory in nature.*

In other words, homeostatic devices help to counterbalance any variation from those conditions that are most normal and optimal for the individual. Adjustments in the pH of the blood, the glucose level of the blood, body fluid and electrolyte levels, and body temperature, and the compensatory growth of tissues and proliferation of cells all provide examples of homeostatic *compensatory mechanisms.* Let us briefly discuss two of these examples: temperature regulation and compensatory growth.

1. *Temperature regulation.* As discussed earlier, a stable body temperature is vital for organisms that live in constantly changing climatic environments. For instance, normally our body temperature registers at 98.6° F. If we walk outside from a warm house into icy weather, our body temperature continues to remain at 98.6° F. instead of dropping to the low temperature reading registered outdoors. This remarkable stability of our body temperature is the result of certain *compensatory mechanisms:* specifically, vasoconstriction of our peripheral arteries and arterioles; pilomotor action resulting in "goose flesh"; increased muscular activity; and shivering.

Conversely, if we walk from an air-conditioned house out into a desert-like climate, our body temperature does not rise in response to this hot environment. Instead our body temperature again tends to remain fairly steady at 98.6° F. This stability is the result of the action of certain other *compensatory mechanisms:* namely, an increased circulation of blood to the peripheral blood vessels; an increase in sweating which leads to cooling; and an increase in thirst and water intake which prevents dehydration. As a result of these mechanisms for stabilizing temperature, we are able to adapt to changing climates while still retaining our internal equilibrium.

2. *Compensatory growth.*[20] The proliferation of cells and the enlargement or hypertrophy of organs and tissues provide further illustrations of the compensatory nature of homeostasis. For example, red blood cell levels rise in response to increased demands for oxygen; muscles hypertrophy or enlarge when additional demands are made upon them by exercise or stress; and the spleen and lymphatic organs increase in size when the body is invaded by infectious organisms. Moreover, when an organ such as a kidney is severely damaged or removed, the remaining kidney increases in size so that it is able to do the work of two organs instead of one. Finally, if the heart, for any reason, should begin to fail as a circulatory pump, the left ventricle of the heart enlarges or hypertrophies in order to pump out more blood into the arteries, thus *compensating* for the breakdown in circulatory function.

In summary, homeostatic mechanisms preserve the integrity of the body by counterbalancing stress and compensating for change.

> *B. Homeostatic mechanisms are self-regulatory.*

In other words, homeostatic devices *automatically* attempt to correct any deviation from what is characteristically normal function for the individual. It is fortunate for us as human beings that this is so. As Cannon expressed it:

> Without homeostatic devices we should be in constant danger of disaster, unless we were always on the alert to correct voluntarily what normally is corrected automatically. With homeostatic devices, however, that keep essential bodily processes steady, we as individuals are free from such slavery—free to enter into agreeable relations with our fellows, free to enjoy beautiful things, to explore and understand the wonders of the world about us, to develop new ideas and interests, and to work and play, untrammeled by anxieties concerning our bodily affairs.[6]

Homeostasis, then, provides us with the opportunity for a creative life rather than a bare existence

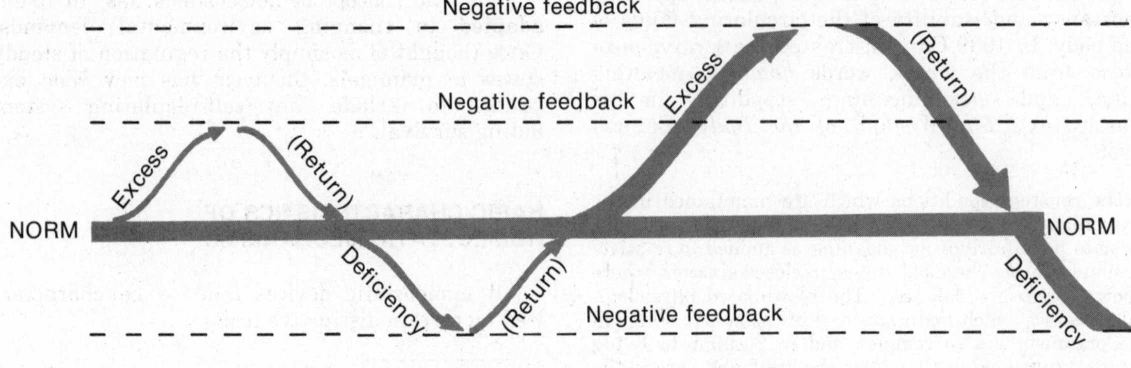

FIGURE 3–1. Negative feedback redirects toward the norm. It can be seen that negative feedback *negates* a deviation from normal which is *either* in *excess* of the norm or toward a *deficiency* from the norm. Negative feedback *always* directs the system *back to the norm.* The deviations from the norm may be slight or of a greater degree, as the size and length of the arrows indicate.

continually centered around the problems of *consciously* adapting to changes, both large and small.

Of course, it is only the healthy individual who enjoys the privilege of a body that is essentially self-regulating. When severe illness strikes, physiologic homeostatic mechanisms tend to break down and to lose their automaticity. It is at this point that doctors, nurses, and other medical personnel attempt to regulate those functions that are normally self-adjusting, by means of such technologic devices as intravenous fluids, hypothermia, and so forth.

C. Homeostatic systems tend to be negative feedback systems.

The main objective of a homeostatic mechanism is to minimize the difference between how a system *should* behave ideally and how it *is* behaving in reality. *Feedback* is the mechanism that enables the system to sense to what degree it is deviating from the set norm and to make the necessary adjustments to correct the deviation.

There are two major types of feedback: *negative* feedback, and *positive* feedback. *Almost all biologic systems are controlled by negative feedback rather than by positive feedback.* This is because a *negative* feedback system always leads the organism *back* to a state that is optimum for it. In other words, it *negates* and attempts to correct any radical change from the norm, either toward excess or toward a deficiency. This point is explained diagrammatically in Figure 3–1.

Positive feedback systems, on the other hand, tend to lead the organism consistently *away* from that state which is normal for it. The original error, rather than being corrected, is repeated again and again, thus compounding the problem. Consequently death or disaster results unless, at some point, the positive feedback is corrected or controlled by negative feedback. The essential difference between the two systems is shown diagrammatically in Figure 3–2.

HOW NEGATIVE FEEDBACK OPERATES

As stated earlier, negative feedback controls almost all biologic systems. To comprehend how a

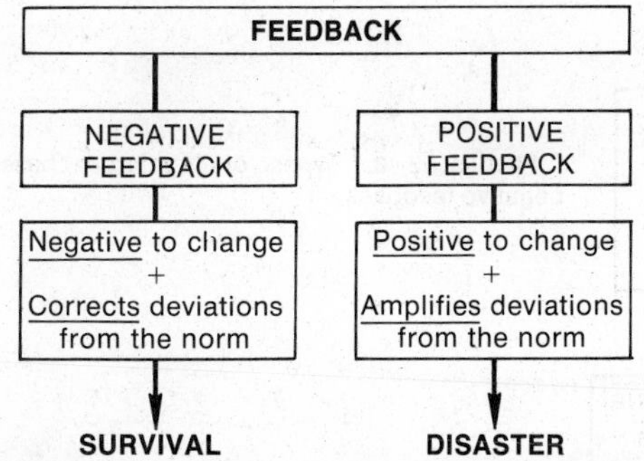

FIGURE 3–2. Comparison of negative and positive feedback mechanisms.

system of negative feedback operates within the body, it is helpful to first use a mechanical or electrical *model* for purposes of explanation. (Models are frequently used to explain biologic phenomena.) A model in this sense can be defined as a replica of a relationship or group of events, built to clarify a complex phenomenon, and expressed in a mathematical form or by means of mechanical or electrical apparatus.

Although models can be helpful, they can also be misleading, because mechanical models tend to *greatly oversimplify* the biologic activities and processes that they represent. Models serve only to provide us with a way of explaining complex phenomena; *they do not duplicate the physiologic phenomena* themselves. The ideas expressed by feedback mechanisms thus provide us with a way of thinking about the control of physiologic mechanisms, but they do not actually present distinct physiologic processes.

There are two major types of negative feedback mechanisms. One type is a *thermostat-like* mechanism, while a second type is a *continually fluctuating* mechanism. We shall first consider the thermostat-like regulator.

Thermostat-like Mechanisms

Thermostat-like regulators are distinguished by two features: First of all, these mechanisms operate by correcting deviations from a definite *predetermined goal* or "setting." Second, thermostat-like regulators operate intermittently rather than continuously, turning off and on as needed to correct errors. Thus, the system is triggered, whenever an error is signaled, toward that activity which will return it into the range of function normal for it.

There are many examples of thermostat-like regulators. One obvious example is the thermostat that controls the heating within our homes. Let us say that you have set the thermostat at 72° F., but the temperature of the house itself registers only 65° F. A small deviation from the goal is allowable, but if the deviation becomes too great, the system will be triggered into action. Once the heat turns on, the temperature in your house may increase to as much as 74 or 75° F.; i.e., the deviation will now be in *excess* of the goal. The error of overheating will be detected readily by comparing the actual temperature of the house and the thermostat setting. The furnace will then shut off until the house again becomes too cool. If the system is working properly, the house will remain at approximately the same temperature indefinitely despite weather conditions outside.

A second example of "stat" regulation is the *temperature control system within the body.* In this case the thermostat that controls temperature stability is located within the hypothalamus, a vital structure found at the base of the brain.

Operating by means of negative feedback, the thermostat control within the hypothalamus keeps our body temperature fairly steady at 98.6° F. despite environmental conditions. When a temperature elevation does occur, with resulting signs of fever, or when the temperature is subnormal, it is believed that the *goal* or *reference level* has been changed in some way. For instance, as we might accidentally set the thermostat within our homes incorrectly, the reference level within our hypothalamus may become altered by disease or accident. As a result, there is a corresponding alteration in body temperature.

A third illustration of "stat" control is the *regulation of food intake.* Physiologists now believe that there is an "appestat" (or appetite regulating center), which is also located in the hypothalamus. This structure contains two groups of cells with different functions. One group of cells constitutes the "feeding center," which causes us to want to eat. The other group of cells makes up the "satiety center," which signals us to stop eating when we have consumed sufficient food. Appetite regulation has been compared by physiologists with typical negative feedback systems. They theorize that such factors as blood sugar, hormones, changes in fat reserve levels, and psychologic factors possibly provide the signals that activate the feedback system. Variables such as body structure, state of health, psychologic make-up, and activity determine the *goal.* Appetite acts as a type of *error signal* that "turns on" when the individual has not consumed sufficient food to meet his needs. The *response* is that the individual continues to eat until he becomes satiated. His appetite then "shuts off," until the sensor is again activated. *Obesity* is sometimes explained by using this concept of homeostatic feedback. Physiologists now postulate that if any component of the feedback system is not working properly, appetite does not "shut off" and the person, as a result, overeats; eventually, obesity develops.

The *control of blood sugar levels* provides a final illustration of thermostat-like regulation. The *normal limits* for blood glucose are from 80 to 100 mg./100 ml. If we eat a substantial breakfast, our blood sugar will rise very rapidly until it passes the upper limits of normal. At this point there is, of course, a discrepancy between the *normal* blood sugar range and the *actual* glucose reading which registered following breakfast. As a result, an error is signaled, and the *excess* glucose is removed from the blood and stored in the liver as glycogen. As the day proceeds, however, we may, as a result of activity and metabolic demands, use up a large percentage of our circulating blood sugar. Consequently the level of glucose may drop below 80 mg./100 ml. This, in turn, results in an *error signal,* and the glycogen that has been stored is reconverted to sugar. This reconversion, in turn, raises the blood glucose level till it is again within a safe and normal range.

Continually Fluctuating Mechanisms

A *second* type of negative feedback control system is the *continually fluctuating mechanism (or servomechanism).* This system differs from the "stat" type regulator in two ways: First, the *goal* or reference point is *continually fluctuating,* and second, the *system is in continuous motion* rather than shutting off and on (see Fig. 3–3).

The control of hormonal levels within the body provides an illustration of this type of feedback. For example, let us consider the interrelationship between the adenohypophysis (anterior lobe of the pituitary gland) and the adrenal glands. The adenohypophysis secretes a hormone called "adrenocorticotropic hormone" or ACTH. When the ACTH level rises in the blood, the adrenal glands are stimulated to release hormones called glucocorticoids (G-C). However, when the blood level of

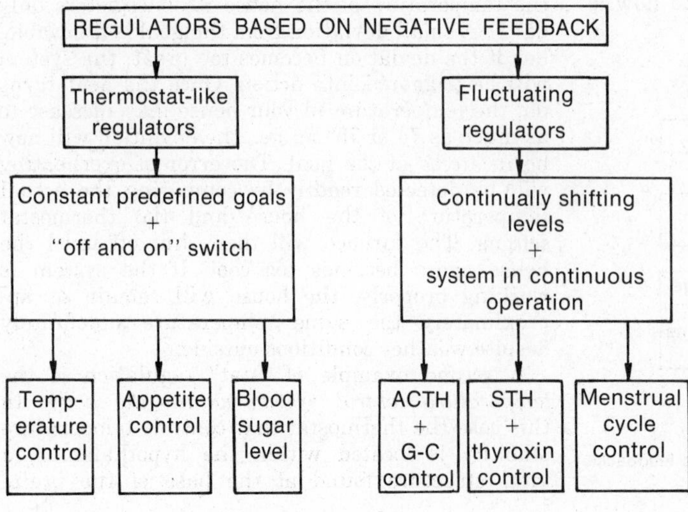

FIGURE 3–3. Types of regulators based on negative feedback.

G-C rises too high, the adenohypophysis is signaled by means of negative feedback to *inhibit* its release of ACTH. As a result, the blood level of ACTH drops and, consequently, so does the blood level of G-C. Eventually, the level of G-C drops so low that again the adenohypophysis is stimulated to release ACTH which, in turn, raises the level of G-C, and so forth. This process is illustrated in Figure 3–4.

Similar examples of feedback controls that involve endocrine balance are found in the relationship between the adenohypophysis and the thyroid gland, as well as in the complex hormonal control involved in the menstrual cycle. Both of these feedback mechanisms will be discussed in detail in appropriate sections of the text.

D. The regulation of a single physiologic process may require the operation of multiple homeostatic negative feedback systems.

In the examples given thus far, homeostatic regulation for a particular variable (temperature, appetite, etc.) has apparently been controlled by *one* negative feedback system. It is important, however, to realize that some variables (for example, blood pressure) may be under the control of *several* different feedback systems, which must *all* function so that they complement each other.

E. Some degree of deviation *or* error *exists in all homeostatic systems.*

The concept of homeostatic balance essentially represents an ideal. Actually in every self-regulating system there is *always* some degree of deviation from what is optimum or normal for that system. As Overmire states, "Homeostatic regulators can never be expected to function perfectly, since control is achieved only through adjustment of error."[39]

When an error is signaled in a homeostatic system, several problems may result, including the following:

1. A considerable *time lag* may be present between the moment the error is discovered and the moment corrective action is started.
2. As a result of this lag, the system may attempt to *overcompensate* for the error and what is called an *overshoot* will take place.[41]
3. This overshoot, in itself, is an error. Consequently a new time lag and another overshoot in the *opposite** direction will then result.
4. These overshoots in opposite directions create fluctuations or *oscillations* or *hunting* as the system attempts to correct itself and return to normal.
5. If the oscillations or overshoots *increase in size,* then a condition of *unstable oscillations* develops. This is a problem, and these unstable oscillations may result in disaster for the system. Another term for disaster, in this case, is *runaway.*
6. If, on the other hand, the oscillations are

*Note the difference between overshoots and positive feedback. Positive feedback, as we said earlier, goes continually *out* from the norm. Overshoots move back and forth around the norm.

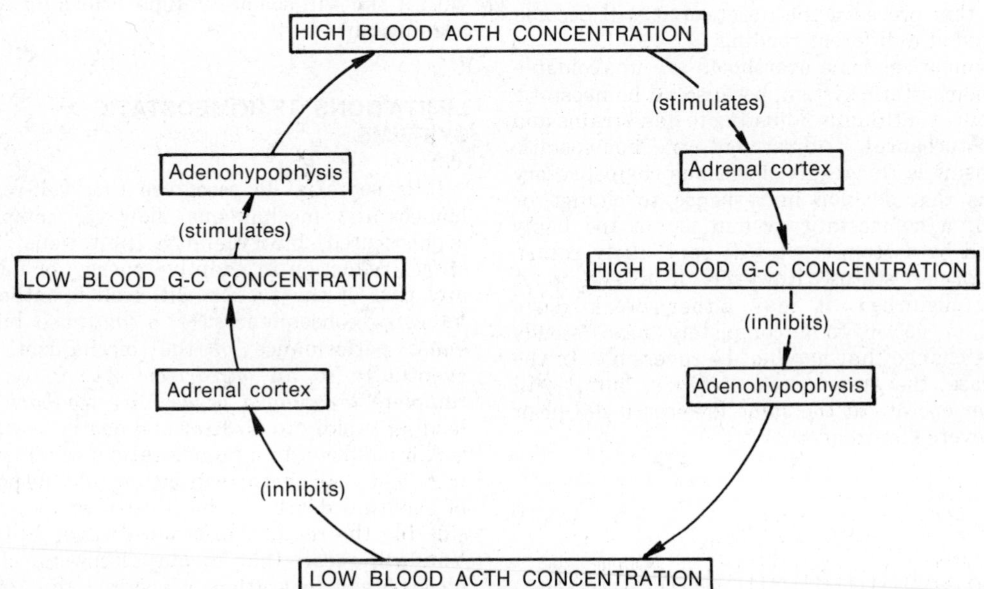

FIGURE 3–4. Control of ACTH secretion by the adenohypophysis—a feedback mechanism and also a homeostatic mechanism. High blood concentration of ACTH (adrenocorticotropic hormone) stimulates G-C (glucocorticoids) secretion, whereas resulting high blood G-C concentration inhibits ACTH secretion.

damped or they *decrease in size,* then the system can return to normal function (see Fig. 3–5).

Within the human body, homeostatic systems are *always* oscillating to some degree. However, these oscillations normally occur within *very narrow limits.* If the oscillations become too great, the continued existence of the individual is severely threatened.

As an example of oscillations in a negative feedback system, consider the control of arterial blood pressure. If, for some reason, arterial blood pressure begins to fall, an error is signaled. In response to this signal, and as a result of various physiologic mechanisms, the blood pressure will begin to rise. The problem is that the effect of the mechanism activated by the error signal to raise the blood pressure will persist not only until the pressure increases to the point considered normal but beyond that point, until the blood pressure is too high and another error is signaled. A new set of responses to this "too-high" error signal then acts to lower the blood pressure, but again the effect of the activity will persist beyond the "normal" point, the blood pressure will become too low, and still another error will be signaled.

Under these conditions, the blood pressure continues to *oscillate* or *overshoot* between high and low extremes. If the oscillations become too wild and unstable, the system may be driven to disaster. Fortunately, however, oscillations within the human body are readily *damped;* i.e., they decrease in size as a result of various compensatory physiologic reactions. Consequently, unstable blood pressure oscillations will most likely be damped. This means that either the blood pressure will return to that reading that preceded the upset, or it will become readjusted at a different reading.

To summarize, some overshoots are unavoidable in any homeostatic system, because all homeostatic systems are continually adjusting to new strains and new disturbances. Adjustment of homeostatic mechanisms is the result of various compensatory reactions that develop in response to change or stress. If a homeostatic system is not too badly disturbed by a stressor, it will very likely return to its former status. However, if a system is severely disturbed, it may either break down entirely or go on to a completely new "steady state," a change that may not be reversible. In the latter case, the system *will* stabilize, but it will no longer operate at the same level as it did prior to the severe disturbance.

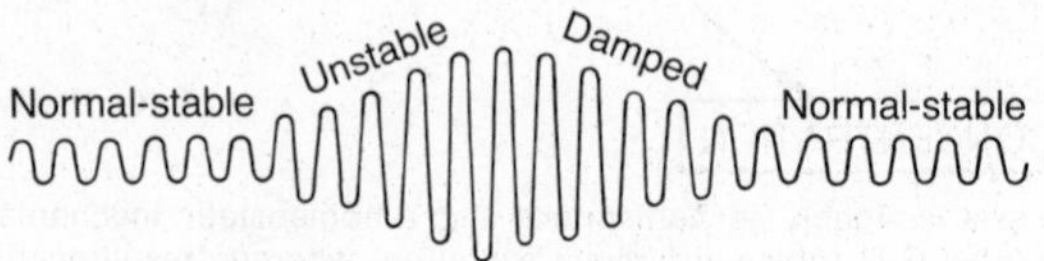

FIGURE 3–5. Types of oscillations.

THE PROBLEM OF POSITIVE FEEDBACK

Positive feedback is defined as "a situation in which an *increase* in response, when fed back to the control mechanism, causes a still *further increase* in response."[23] In other words, there is a continuous *reinforcing of the original error,* resulting in a *runaway* of the system. When this happens, negative feedback mechanisms break down; positive feedback causes an uncontrolled, constantly increasing deviation from the norm; and a vicious circle results, leading to disaster and death for the individual (see Fig. 3–6).

As an example of the dangers of positive feedback, consider the patient suffering from a sudden severe hemorrhage. First of all, as a result of blood loss, this person will experience a severe drop in his arterial blood pressure. The drop in pressure will then diminish the flow of blood to his heart muscle, and as a result his heart beat will be greatly weakened. This weakness, in turn, will lead to even less blood being pumped to the arterial system. Consequently the blood pressure will drop still lower, and even less blood will be returned to the heart. As a result, the heart beat will be further weakened, and so on. This vicious circle, unless stopped, will be repeated again and again until finally the patient dies. If, on the other hand, the patient receives medical and nursing care before his blood loss becomes too great, his body's negative feedback mechanisms will continue to operate. As a result, compensatory mechanisms involving blood pressure, the arterial system, and the heart beat will overbalance the positive feedback. A vicious circle will not occur, and the patient will live instead of die.

This example illustrates how valuable a knowledge of feedback can be to the nurse. Although the theory of homeostasis is initially somewhat complex, once the student familiarizes herself with it she will see daily implications for its use in nursing care.

LIMITATIONS OF HOMEOSTATIC SYSTEMS

It is essential to recognize that self-regulating homeostatic mechanisms, however complex and sophisticated, have definite limitations. Extreme stress, reduction in adaptive energy, or damage to any part of the system will lead to either of the following consequences: (1) a *continued* but *inadequate* performance of the mechanism, leading eventually to an *overdriven system,* or (2) the complete *breakdown of negative feedback* control, leading rapidly to disaster and death.

A breakdown in a homeostatic mechanism which may lead to an overdriven system and the possibility of eventual death can be illustrated by again considering the regulation of blood sugar in the body. You will recall that in our discussion of normal blood sugar regulation, we stated that our blood sugar must remain within certain clearly defined limits. We also stated that if the blood sugar exceeds these limits, glucose is then converted to glycogen and stored in the liver to be reconverted to glucose as needed. However, the smooth operation of this homeostatic mechanism depends upon a pancreatic hormone called *insulin*.

When an insulin *deficiency* exists, two things happen. First, sugar is not oxidized and utilized properly, and second, excess glucose cannot be converted to glycogen. These pathologic changes result in the individual's excreting large amounts of excess sugar in his urine. The abnormal excretion of sugar, in turn, leads to such compensatory mechanisms as a "craving for sweets," an increased urinary output, thirst, and so forth. This patient (who has developed the condition of *diabetes mellitus*) can survive for a while by means of these inadequate compensatory reactions. However, if his condition is not eventually diagnosed and treated with a proper diet and with insulin, his system will become overdriven. As a result of prolonged overworking of his system, he will suffer irreparable damage to his body organs, and without treatment he will eventually die.

The second limitation of homeostatic systems (more rapid breakdown of negative feedback control) is exemplified by the hemorrhaging patient described earlier, who continues to lose blood rapidly. At first, this patient's peripheral blood vessels will constrict, his blood pressure will oscillate for a while, and his heart, though weak, will beat very rapidly in order to compensate for the blood loss. Eventually, however, if this patient continues to bleed, negative feedback will totally break down. The patient's blood pressure will fall precipitously; his heart beat will become very weak, and then will stop entirely; his respirations will cease; and he will expire. The final evidence, then, that homeostatic mechanisms have limitations, and can fail, is death.

HOMEOSTASIS AS A UNIFYING CONCEPT

The concept of homeostasis has added a new and vital dimension to our comprehension of life processes. Knowledge of homeostatic mechanisms has contributed greatly to the study of (1) physiology; (2) health and disease; and (3) the general dynamics of living.

The field of physiology has benefited from the concept of homeostasis in at least three ways. First of all, the idea of homeostasis has brought a *sense of order and of unity* into the study of physiologic processes. Bodily changes and adjustments that formerly had seemed to conflict with each other can now be better understood as adaptive manifestations of homeostasis and as functions related to the *total* needs of the individual. Second, the concept of homeostasis has demonstrated the *interdependence of the body's systems*. For example, the circulatory, endocrine, and nervous systems are no longer conceived of as isolated units, operating independently of each other. Instead, they are now considered as part of a functioning whole, working

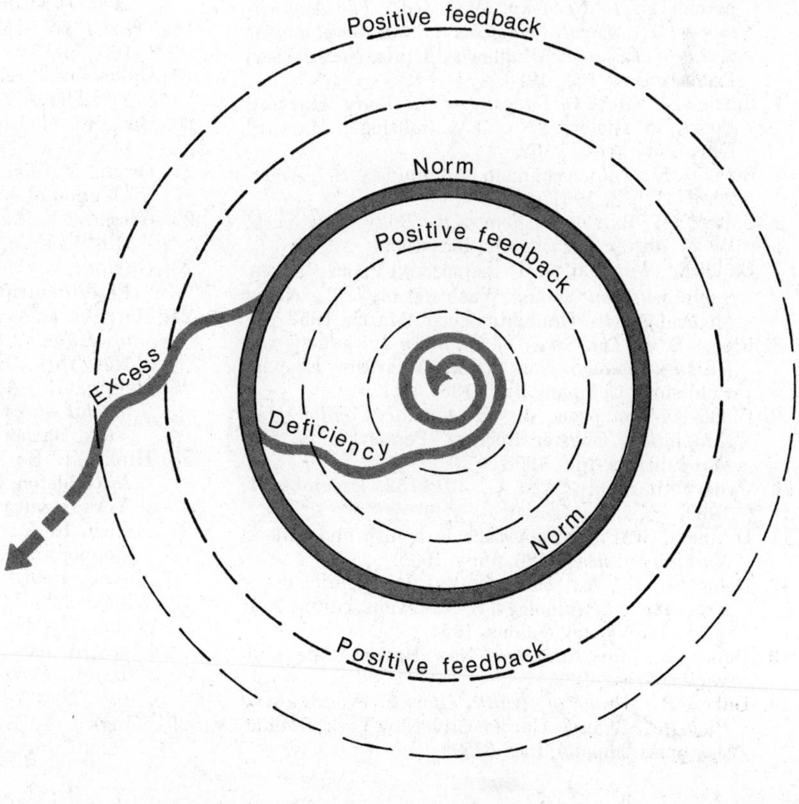

Positive feedback
Norm
Positive feedback
Excess
Deficiency
Norm
Positive feedback

FIGURE 3–6. Positive feedback constantly leads away from the norm. It can be seen that positive feedback *increases* a deviation from normal, which is *either* in *excess* of the norm or toward a *deficiency* from the norm. The result may be a *runaway* of the system leading to exhaustion and death.

together to enable the individual to survive emergencies and everyday stresses. Third, homeostasis has enabled us to see physiology as a *dynamic process* of continuous self-regulation and self-adjustment. Consequently we can better understand the many fluctuations and oscillations that occur constantly within the body. In the light of these factors, it is not surprising that many scientists conceive of homeostasis as the single most important concept in physiology.

Further, our appreciation of *health* and *disease* has been greatly expanded by the concept of homeostasis. A knowledge of basic homeostatic mechanisms has enabled persons in the allied medical fields to meet their responsibilities in a more logical and intelligent way. A brief summary of principles, based on the concept of homeostasis, that have implications for patient care follows:

> The body adapts to stress and defends itself against radical changes by means of self-regulating homeostatic systems.

> Self-regulating systems can break down as a result of extreme stress, a reduction in energy, or damage to a part of the system.

> Self-regulating systems that break down to any degree may elicit responses that are inadequate, inappropriate, unstable, or maladaptive.

> Homeostatic systems can destroy themselves through the continuous repetition of error, thereby leading to a vicious circle.

> Medical and nursing intervention, *if appropriate and timely,* can aid the body in returning to homeostatic balance—either to approximately the same level of balance or to a new "steady state" which may be irreversible but still functional.

Finally, we can see that all of life involves successful and unsuccessful attempts at developing and maintaining equilibrium. The process of living, then, on any level, from the cellular to the community, from the moment of birth to the hour of death, can be better appreciated when approached from the standpoint of homeostatic balance.

References for Unit I

1. Anthony, C. P.: *Textbook of Anatomy and Physiology.* 7th ed. St. Louis, The C. V. Mosby Company, 1967.

1a. Aspy, V. H.: Are patients people? *Nursing Times,* 68: 690, June 1, 1972.

2. Barrett, A. M.: *People Under Pressure.* New York, Twayne Publishers, Inc., 1960.

3. Bevan, W.: The concept of adaptation in modern psychology. *In* Goodsky, M. A. (ed.): *The Application of Biological Principles to the Development of Physical Systems.* Englewood Cliffs, New Jersey, Prentice-Hall, Inc., 1963.

4. Burnett, F. M.: *The Integrity of the Body.* Harvard Books in Biology, No. 3, Cambridge, Harvard University Press, 1962.

5. Burnett, M.: The mechanism of immunity. *Sci. Amer.* 204(No. 1):58, 1961.

6. Cannon, W. B.: *The Wisdom of the Body.* New York, W. W. Norton & Company, Inc., 1939.

7. Caudill, W.: Cultural perspectives on stress. *Symposium on Stress.* Washington, D.C., Army Medical Service Graduate School, March, 1953.

8. Clegg, E. J.: *The Study of Man: An Introduction to Human Biology.* New York, American Elsevier Publishing Company, Inc., 1968.

9. Cloudsley-Thompson, J. L.: *Animal Conflict and Adaptation.* Chester Springs, Pennsylvania, Dufour Editions, Inc., 1965.

10. Cybernetic man. *J.A.M.A.,* 210:1752, December 1, 1969.

11. D'Amelio, R. F.: An approach to health and illness. *Nursing Science,* 3:186, June, 1965.

12. Dempsey, E. W.: Homeostasis. *In Handbook of Experimental Psychology,* S. S. Stevens, editor. New York, John Wiley & Sons, 1951.

13. Dubos, R.: *Man Adapting.* New Haven, Yale University Press, 1965.

14. Dubos, R.: *Mirage of Health: Utopias, Progress and Biological Change.* Garden City, New York, Doubleday and Company, Inc., 1959.

15. Edholm, O. C., and Bacharach, A. L. (eds.): *The Physiology of Human Survival.* New York, Academic Press, Inc., 1965.

16. Engel, G. L.: A unified concept of health and disease. *Perspectives in Biology and Medicine* 3:459, Spring, 1960.

17. Engel, G. L.: Homeostasis, Behavioral Adjustment, and the Concept of Health and Disease, *In* Grinker, R. S. (ed.): *Mid-Century Psychiatry.* Springfield, Illinois, Charles C Thomas, 1953.

18. Fogel, S.: Total self and adaptation. *J. Soc. Psychosomatic Dentistry & Medicine,* 15:107, July, 1968.

18a. Fox, F. W.: Nature, nurture, and stress. *Lancet,* 2: 183, July 22, 1972.

19. Galdston, I. (ed.): *Beyond the Germ Theory.* New York, Health Education Council, 1954.

20. Goss, R. J.: *Adaptive Growth.* London, Logos Press, Ltd.; New York, Academic Press, 1965.

21. Grant, V.: *The Origin of Adaptations.* New York, Columbia University Press, 1963.

22. Gross, N. E.: *Living with Stress.* New York, McGraw-Hill Book Co., 1958.

23. Guyton, A. C.: *Textbook of Medical Physiology.* 4th Ed. Philadelphia, W. B. Saunders Company, 1971.

24. Harrison, G. A., et al.: *Human Biology: An Introduction to Human Evolution, Variation, and Growth.* New York, Oxford University Press, 1964.

25. Helson, H.: *Adaptation-Level Theory: An Experimental and Systemic Approach to Behavior.* New York, Harper & Row, 1964.

26. Hinkle, L. E.: Normal Stress in Normal Experience, *In* Galdston, I. (ed.): *Beyond the Germ Theory.* New York, Health Education Council, 1954.

27. Kalish, R. A.: *The Psychology of Human Behavior.* Belmont, California, Wadsworth Publishing Company, 1966.

28. Kluckhohn, C., and Murray, H.: Personality formation: The determinants. *In* Kluckhohn, C. and Murray, A. (eds.), with the collaboration of Schneider, D. M., *Personality in Nature, Society, and Culture.* New York, Alfred A. Knopf, 1959.

29. Langley, L. L.: *Homeostasis.* New York, Reinhold Publishing Corp., 1965.

30. Lantis, M.: Environmental stresses on human behavior—Summary and suggestions. *Arch. Environmental Health,* 17:578, October, 1968.
30a. Levine, S.: Stress and behavior: *Scientific American,* 224:26–31, January, 1971.
31. Libby, W. F.: Man's place in the physical world. *Health Physics,* 17:531, October, 1969.
32. Lissák, K.: *The Neuroendocrine Control of Adaptation.* New York, Pergamon Press, 1965.
33. McCulloch, W. S.: The stability of biological systems. *Brookhaven Symposia in Biology,* No. 10. Homeostatic Mechanisms, 1957.
33a. Man in his world. *Lancet,* 2:27, July, 1972.
34. Martin, H. W., and Prange, A. J.: Human adaptation—A conceptual approach to understanding patients. *Canadian Nurse,* 58:234, March, 1962.
35. Maslow, A. H.: *Motivation and Personality.* New York, Harper & Row, 1954.
36. Masuda, M.: Differing adaptive metabolic behaviors. *J. Psychosomatic Research,* 10:239, December, 1966.
37. Mathwig, G. M.: Living, open systems, reciprocal adaptation and the life process. *Nursing Research,* 18:523, November-December, 1969.
38. Murdock, G. P.: The common denominator of cultures. *In* Linton, R. (ed.): *The Science of Man in the World Crisis.* New York, Columbia University Press, 1945.
38a. Norris, C. M.: Delusions that trap nurses. *Nursing Outlook,* 21:18, January 17, 1973.
39. Overmire, T. G.: *Homeostatic Regulation.* American Institute of Biological Sciences, Biological Sciences Curriculum Study, Pamphlet 9, September, 1963.
40. Pantin, C. F.: Organism and environment. *Psychological Issues,* 6:113, 1969.
41. Rapoport, A.: Stochastic, mechanical, and teleological views of homeostasis. *Brookhaven Symposia in Biology.* No. 10. Homeostatic Mechanisms, 1957.
42. Redfield, R.: *The Primitive World and Its Transformations.* Ithaca, New York, Cornell University Press, 1953.
43. Richter, C. P.: Behavioral regulation of homeostasis. *Symposium on Stress,* 77, March, 1953.
44. Riggs, D. S.: Feedback: Fundamental relationship or frame of mind? *Advances in Enzyme Regulation,* 5:357, 1967.
45. Rock, I.: *The Nature of Perceptual Adaptation.* New York, Basic Books, Inc., 1966.
46. Romano, J.: *Adaptation.* Ithaca, New York, Cornell University Press, 1949.
46a. Roy, C.: Adaptation: A conceptual framework for nursing. *Nursing Outlook,* 18:42, March, 1970.
47. Selye, Hans: *The Stress of Life.* New York, McGraw-Hill Book Co., 1956.
48. Simpson, G. G., and Beck, W.: *Life: An Introduction to Biology.* 2nd Ed. New York, Harcourt, Brace and World, Inc., 1965.
49. Society for Experimental Biology: *Homeostasis and Feedback Mechanisms.* New York, published for the Company of Biologists on behalf of the Society for Experimental Biology by the Academic Press, 1964.
50. Spitz, R. A.: Aggression and adaptation. *J. Nervous & Mental Diseases,* 149:81, August, 1969.
51. Thompson, A. W.: Fight or flight response in clinical practice. *Med. Annals District of Columbia,* 38:496, September, 1968.
52. Torrey, H. B.: Adaptation as a process. *Scientific Monthly,* December, 1915.
53. Wallace, B., and Srb, A.: *Adaptation.* 2nd Ed. Englewood Cliffs, New Jersey, Prentice-Hall, Inc., 1964.
54. Wender, P. H.: Vicious and virtuous circles: The role of deviation amplifying feedback in the origin and perpetuation of behavior. *Psychiatry,* 31:309, November, 1968.

[Diseases] crucify the soul of man, attenuate our bodies, dry them, wither them, shrivel them up like old apples, make them so many anatomies.

Robert Burton

UNIT II

Theories of Disease Causation

Introduction and Study Guide

Disease is a predictable aspect of human life; it touches all of us in one form or another. Thus, disease and health concern us both personally and professionally. Diseases, injuries, and homeostatic imbalances—those painful adaptive failures that "crucify the soul of man"—are present everywhere in the world. Moreover, their number is staggering, their definitions variable, their causations multiple and complex, their symptoms numerous and sometimes apparently unrelated, their treatments subject to constant change and revision, and their prevention often questionable or unknown. It is no wonder that for the beginning student of nursing, the study of individual diseases—their causes, symptoms, and treatments—is almost overwhelming.

We shall try to simplify the task by first discussing disease causation in general terms and by broadly considering typical human responses to stress. Whereas the bulk of the text is concerned with *individual* diseases, the purpose of this unit is to explore the broad *overall* concepts of health and disease, thereby laying a basic framework for the study of individual maladies.

At this point we must caution you that even general information concerning health and disease is in a constant state of change and growth. Much of what was believed to have been true yesterday has been discredited today. What seems to be true today may be virtually meaningless tomorrow. Thus, it is best to approach the study of disease causation and theory with an open mind and in an inquiring and critical spirit.

As a brief overview, our objective in this unit is to explore with you the following important topics:

> the significance of disease for the individual
> changing concepts of health and disease
> traditional and modern theories of disease causation
> factors that cause disease
> human responses to disease
> nursing and a holistic approach to disease

Because this unit covers a large and complex subject area, it contains many terms, theories, and concepts that may be new to you. The following guides may help you to gain the most from your reading. Upon finishing this unit, you should be aware of the meaning of the following key terms: health, disease, stress; general adaptation syndrome (GAS), local adaptation syndrome (LAS); anti-inflammatory corticoids, pro-inflammatory corticoids; conditioning factors; socio-inheritance; stressors; "necessary and sufficient cause"; physiologic deprivation; psychologic stress; total life situation; sick role; ecology; iatrogenic disease; autonomic nervous system function; deficient response; excessive response; inappropriate response; anticipatory response.

You should be able to discuss, generally, the following theories of disease:

1. Theory of the body machine
2. Pathologic anatomic theories
3. Mind-body dichotomy
4. Germ theory
5. Cellular theory
6. Molecular theory
7. Multicausal theories
8. Bernard's theory of the disturbed internal milieu
9. Cannon's theory of homeostatic imbalance
10. Selye's theory of stress
11. (a) Harold Wolff's theory of inappropriate organ responses
    (b) Theory of rapid cultural change and disease causation
12. Stewart Wolf's theory of "disease as a way of life"
13. Theory of the brain's role in regulating, causing, and preventing disease (theories of Harold Wolff and Stewart Wolf)
14. Cybernetic theory of disease

You should be able to discuss generally the following concepts:

1. The changing definition of illness
2. The continuum of health and disease
3. Disease as a failure of adaptation
4. The false dichotomies of mind and body, mental and physical disease
5. The antiquity of disease
6. Man's life expectancy
7. Shifting geographic disease patterns
8. Characteristics of modern theories of disease
10. The diseases of adaptation
11. Stressors and five general ways in which they affect individuals
12. The seven major factors in the causation of disease
13. The body's response to physical injury
14. How the body protects itself against injury and its effects
15. The effect of psychologic stimuli upon the autonomic nervous system
16. Pleasurable emotion and physiologic changes
17. Maladaptive responses to stress
18. The development of multidimensional nursing care
19. Nursing and medicine as social sciences

Let us now turn to our discussion of health and disease and their significance and implications for man.

CHAPTER 4

The Concepts of Health and Disease

For most individual human beings the relative presence or absence of disease within themselves has always been a matter of tremendous importance. A person's abilities to work, to be productive, to love and to play are all related to how he feels and functions, both mentally and physically. Illness often also affects, in an adverse way, those with whom the ill person lives or works.

Furthermore, because some diseases may spread from one person to another, disease and health are important to the whole social order of man. Consequently, a variety of social institutions have focused attention and concern on these areas. Laws have been passed to control disease; philosophy and religion have attempted to explain disease and death; literature and art have endeavored to depict human suffering, as well as its powerful consequences; medical science has sought to diagnose and to treat disease and to alleviate suffering.

Because of the universal nature of disease, and its far-reaching personal and social consequences, thoughtful individuals have always asked questions about disease. Some of the most important questions are: What is disease and *why* does disease exist? What effect does disease have upon the individual and upon the society in which he lives? To what extent do the pressures exerted by society upon an individual cause disease? What can be done to alleviate disease, or at least to minimize its consequences? Will there come a time when all people are free from pain and disease—free to live a truly healthy and productive life?

A basic purpose of this unit is to explore these questions, all of which are central to the medical and nursing professions. Again, as in the preceding unit, much of the information imparted is of a theoretic and speculative nature. Man is only beginning to learn about himself as a total entity—a physical, intellectual, emotional, social being—struggling to adapt to a challenging environment. We are only beginning to study the broad concepts of health and disease in a manner that is holistic and yet precise.

HEALTH AND DISEASE: EVOLVING AND EXPANDING CONCEPTS

Health and disease are not static conditions. Rather, they are vital concepts that are variable in their meaning, and that are subject to the same continuous processes of evaluation and change as is man himself. In recent years, largely because of expanded medical and nursing research, our view of health and disease has changed in at least four major ways. These changes include the following:

1. Broader and more inclusive definitions and viewpoints of health and disease.
2. Awareness of changes in disease patterns and distribution.
3. Changes in our concepts of disease causation.
4. Changes in our approach to the treatment of disease.

We shall now pursue the first three points. The subject of treatment will be considered later in the text.

Changing Definitions and Viewpoints

The allied medical fields have only recently developed comprehensive definitions for health and disease. In the not so distant past, disease was often defined as "an absence of health," and health was defined as "an absence of disease"—definitions that obviously led nowhere. Some authorities saw disease and health as states of physical discomfort or well-being; unfortunately, such rigid, narrow viewpoints totally disregarded the emotional and social pressures that affect us all.

Today, experts define health and disease in terms that are at once broader and more precise. For instance, Romano defines health in the following way:

> *"Health, in a positive sense, consists in the capacity of the organism to maintain a balance in which it may be reasonably free of undue pain, discomfort, disability, or limitation of action."*[17]

Engel, in defining disease, states:

> *"Disease corresponds to failures or disturbances in the growth, development, functions, and adjustments of the organism as a whole or of any of its systems."*[17]

Thus, Engel implies that disease is not something that a person *has* and that is imposed upon him from the outside world; rather it is a failure of the *total* individual to grow, function, and adapt successfully to life's stresses.

Although it is difficult to define health and disease precisely, it is even more difficult to apply the concepts of health and disease to *people*. For example, consider the following individuals; which of them are sick and which are well?

> An American business executive has experienced two relatively severe heart attacks, yet continues to function satisfactorily on the job.

> A young housewife suffers every month from nervousness and instability due to premenstrual tension.

> A middle-aged hardworking engineer suffers from an aortic aneurysm but does not know it. This condition is often symptomless but is nevertheless life-threatening.

> A ballet dancer, though physically strong and lithe, tends when taxed by work to lose her sense of reality to the point of hallucinating.

> A college student occasionally escapes the realities and painful aspects of his life by using marijuana, a practice approved by his peer group.

> A lower class slum-dweller and his large family of thirteen all suffer from infected teeth, a condition that he and other members of the lower class accept as "normal."

> A young boy of Tristan da Cunha, an island in the South Atlantic, is a powerful swimmer and mountain climber even though he suffers from worm infestations, a condition he ignores because it is so common on his island.

> A Los Angeles salesman suffers from congested lungs and weeping eyes on smoggy days, a condition to which he has become accustomed.

Who is sick and who is well? Or are all these people sick to some degree and healthy to some degree? How does each of these individuals define sickness and health? Do their definitions differ markedly from doctors' or nurses' definitions?

It is almost certain that each of these people will view disease and health in a manner unique to himself and his group. Thus, they may define disease in terms of whether or not they can continue to work, produce, or study; whether signs and symptoms are present or absent; whether a state of discomfort is short or prolonged; whether a problem is physical, mental, or social. Their definitions of health and disease will vary according to their peer groups, their cultural setting, their geographic location, and their social class.

As you can see from the above, both medical and nonmedical people view health and disease in broad terms. Indeed, doctors' and laymen's views of health and disease have expanded over the past decades in the following ways:

1. We view health and disease as *relative* concepts and not as separate absolutes. All living things are diseased to some extent, they progressively undergo aging, and eventually die. Thus, it is important to consider health and disease as a *continuum,* or graduated scale, with excellent health at one extreme, while death is at the other. To illustrate, the individuals just described each occupy a certain position on this disease-health continuum, somewhere in between the two extremes. Moreover, their positions vary from year to year, day to day, hour to hour, depending upon their life situation. For example, the housewife with premenstrual tension will experience symptoms only at a certain time of the month; the ballerina hallucinates only when severely overtaxed physically. These women, then, are to some degree continually shifting up and down the continuum in response to various internal and environmental stresses.

2. We realize today that each person has his *own* unique definitions of health and disease. These personal definitions are based upon the individual's own life experience, which includes his cultural and social background and geographic setting. Thus, a man from Los Angeles might regard a worm infestation as a sign of illness, but will ignore the potentially dangerous physical discomforts stemming from a smoggy and polluted environment; on the other hand, a native of Tristan da Cunha would probably acknowledge himself as ill on a smoggy day in Los Angeles, but is able to ignore his worm infestation since it is common to his culture.

3. Disease, today, is defined not just as a morbid pathologic process within the body, but rather as a *failure of adaptation to the internal or external environment—a homeostatic imbalance that ultimately affects the total individual.*[29] For example, the housewife with premenstrual tension may become so irritable with her husband and children every month that her marriage and consequently her life becomes severely disrupted.

4. Finally, disease is now defined as including both the mental and physical aspects of illness; physical and mental diseases cannot be rigidly placed into separate categories. Thus, as Harold Wolff states, "It is unprofitable to establish a separate category of illness to be defined as psychosomatic or to separate sharply—as regards genesis—psychiatric, medical, and surgical diseases."[61]

To sum up, health and disease are now viewed as two sides of the same coin, a coin that is set in motion by unseen forces and that spins so rapidly that it is difficult to clearly distinguish one side of the coin from the other. As Romano states:

> Health and disease are not static entities, but are phases of life, dependent at any time on the balance maintained by devices, genetically and experimentally determined, intent on fulfilling needs and adapting to and mastering stresses as they may arise from within the organism or from without.[17, 18]

Shifting Patterns

Disease has always existed; in an infinite variety of ways it has manifested itself throughout man's history, from ancient times down to the present. However, the types of diseases most prevalent and the geographic distribution of certain diseases have been shifting over the centuries. For example, severe infectious diseases causing widespread epidemics and plagues were prevalent before the advent of the twentieth century. Since the twentieth century the mortality rate from infectious disease has been lowered drastically, and factors favoring its spread have been brought increasingly under control. In sum, the patterns and manifestations of various maladies have been significantly altered by modern advances in the medical sciences.

Similarly, during this century there have evolved distinctive differences in geographic disease patterns between the underdeveloped, overpopulated countries and the technologically developed countries of the Western world. For example, in such nations as India, tremendous overcrowding, poverty, and malnutrition are common. Consequently, in that nation in 1964, only one individual out of three at birth could expect to live as long as 50 years. Compare this to the life expectancy at birth in the United States, which in 1964 was 72 years. Twenty per cent of the children of India die from malnutrition, infection, and worm infestations before they are five! In the United States, 97 per cent of infants can expect to live to adulthood.[14]

From these statistics you can infer that the United States, by means of technologic advances, has partially eradicated such problems as starvation, severe overcrowding, and infection. Through the development and use of public health measures (e.g., chlorination of water, vaccines, and antibiotics), through the enforcing of pure food and drug laws, and by means of health education, the people in this country have been spared many of the infectious and depleting conditions common to non-Western countries. Life in America has been substantially enriched and improved, at least for the more affluent classes.

Further, modern medicine enables people today to live a considerably longer life than did their forefathers. For example, only 10 per cent of the prehistoric Neanderthal men lived past the age of 40, and only approximately one-half of the Neanderthal population lived past 20. The Greek citizens of the classic era lived only slightly longer than did their more primitive predecessors, while an average Egyptian of 2000 years ago lived only 22 years. A man born in the Middle Ages, as a result of some improvement in life style, could expect to live to be around 35. However, it was not until the nineteenth century, in the United States and England, that life expectancy increased to any appreciable degree. In 1900, as a result of both improvements in sanitation and in the control of some infectious diseases, a male at birth could expect to live to the age of 47.3 years. Today, because of our more sophisticated medical knowledge and practices, an American has a life expectancy of over 70 years—a tremendous increase in length of life as compared with the past.[63] Thus, not only have disease patterns varied widely over man's history, but his life span has increased greatly as a result of advances in medicine and public health.

On the other hand, however, technology and the "civilized" life of the cities have given birth to a whole new pattern of diseases—diseases that strike more slowly and more insidiously than infectious diseases, but that are just as deadly. Hence, whereas the people of underdeveloped countries are plagued by malaria, tuberculosis, diarrhea, gastroenteritis, and colitis, Americans suffer mainly from heart disease, cancer, vascular disease, diseases of the central nervous system, generalized arteriosclerosis, diabetes, and from the results of accidents. Americans may live longer lives than their less wealthy and sophisticated neighbors, but they suffer no less.

CHANGES IN THEORIES OF CAUSATION OF DISEASE

What factors ultimately cause disease? This question remains one of the great mysteries facing man—a mystery demanding solution.

Like all things mysterious, the question of disease causation has given rise to many theories over the centuries, some of which are still, in part, acceptable today. As a student of nursing, it is useful for you to have some idea of the changes in these theories. The changes in viewpoint have powerfully affected the philosophy of the medical and nursing fields—and consequently the goals of patient care. Let us first study the transition from the traditional theories of disease causation to the more modern theories of illness. Then, in the light of these transitional changes, let us examine more closely the current view of disease.

Transition from a Traditional View of Disease Causation to a Modern View

To study a mysterious object and to understand its many facets, it is usually necessary to take that object apart and examine its separate components. This is precisely what scientists and doctors, in the past, have done to human beings. In their effort to comprehend man, they have taken him apart, torn him away from his natural environment, divorced his mind from his body, fragmented even his physical being—dissecting system from system, organ from organ, and tissue from tissue. In the final analysis, science has reduced man to a molecular, even atomic level, so that he is no longer a whole and living being but rather a mechanized, dehumanized abstraction. Moreover, scientists in the past not only have split man into particles, but they have neglected to reunite him. Thus, until recently, man has been left in a sadly disjointed state, being appreciated as a group of parts rather than as a total entity.

It is not surprising, then, that traditional theories of human disease causation also tended toward a fragmentation of man, concentrating upon a single dimension of a patient's self, but never upon his whole being. Many of these traditional and limited theories of disease continue to influence modern medicine and nursing, creating a fragmentation in our patient care. Let us now briefly examine some of these older concepts that continue to influence us and the newer theories that are replacing them.

1. One early theory of disease causation viewed the *human body as a machine, and disease as the result of a defective part.* This old way of considering disease is sometimes termed the *pathologic-anatomic concept.*[29] The basis for the theory originated with Descartes, a seventeenth century French philosopher who envisioned man as a well functioning "body machine." Doctors, searching for ways to cope with disease processes, believed they saw in Descartes' mechanistic theories a solution to the problem of sickness. They reasoned that if disease was caused by a malfunctioning of the machine or by a defective part, then the cure for disease was simply to repair or remove the defective part or parts. Thus, the rationale for surgery as treatment is actually based upon Descartes' ideas, as are many other medical procedures.

Today newer theories have expanded upon this limited concept. For example, we now consider disease as *a failure in the growth, development, or adjustment of the organism as a whole rather than a part.* Moreover, we currently recognize the interrelationships which exist between the mind and the body as well as the total person and his environment. In sum, we see disease as more than a physiologic, pathologic process; instead we view it as a process that is intimately linked with the individual's total life experience.

2. A second traditional theory of disease is that *the disease process tends to be localized, affecting a single organ or system.*[60] This view of sickness, like the concept of the "body machine," is based upon the pathologic-anatomic concept of disease. It, too, tends to oversimplify highly complex phenomena. Advocates of this view stressed the importance of one individual organ or system in the study of disease because they noted that generally a single organ appeared pathologically altered. The effects that one diseased organ have upon the total body went undetected.

Today we recognize that *the body organs and the body systems are not separate entities but are closely interrelated* by means of the nervous, circulatory, and endocrine systems. Increasingly we realize that although disease may indeed affect one particular organ or system, the manifestations and consequences of that disease affect the entire body as well as the psyche of the individual. It is unfortunate that in spite of our present advanced medical knowledge, remnants of the outmoded "organ-centered" way of thinking still remain.

3. A third way of viewing disease in the past has centered around *the mind-body dichotomy.* Advocates of this obsolete point of view saw the mind and body as separate from each other; consequently they believed that no relationship existed between the intellectual-emotional component of man and bodily disease.

This dualistic theory, like the body machine theory, has dominated medical thinking since the days of Descartes. For centuries it has prevented nurses and physicians from developing a holistic view of disease. Only recently has science begun to conceive of man as a *total unit with body and mind integrated.* We realize today that every system of the body is capable of responding to psychologic pressures. The modern nurse recognizes that (1) certain diseases coincide with periods of emotional or mental stress in a patient's life, and (2) "purely" physical problems and disabilities such as a broken leg or arm can result in serious mental disturbance.

4. A fourth traditional view of disease causation is that *illness is the result of a single etiologic agent or cause.* Single-factor theories of disease causation have been popular in medicine because, like the preceding outdated concepts, these theories have tended to simplify the problems of diagnosis, treatment, and prevention. Doctors reasoned that if there was a single cause for disease, and that cause could be discovered and controlled, then disease could be eradicated.[17]

Medical history abounds with examples of single-factor theories. For instance, the body's chemistry was once regarded as the key to health and disease. Old medical writings emphasized that a proper balance of the four "humors" of the body—phlegm, blood, black bile, and yellow bile—guaranteed good physical health. Even a person's temperament was supposedly affected by the humors. For example, a phlegmatic man (a man with too much phlegm) was lazy; a sanguine person (from the Latin *sanguis* "blood") was hearty and sensual; too much black bile made a person melancholy, whereas too much yellow bile made him violent.

With the advent of Pasteur's *germ theory,* modern medicine was born. But even this theory, heralded by many scientists as the last word in disease causation, fell short. At first, physicians were hopeful that by simply identifying and killing dangerous microorganisms, disease could be eradicated forever. But we realize today that such a simple solution is not possible. Infectious diseases continue to exist despite the fact that many pathogenic organisms have been identified, vaccines and antibiotics have been developed, and public health and sanitation measures have been improved. Moreover, the germ theory, while partially solving the problem of infectious disease, is not applicable to the widespread pattern of noninfectious chronic disease which so drastically affects modern civilization.

Despite the failure of the germ theory to

explain all disease, doctors have continued to search for the one single causative agent behind many illnesses. Indeed, the tradition of the single-factor theory still flourishes to some extent in modern medicine. According to Engel, the "concept of the biochemical defect" provides one example of a contemporary single-factor theory.[17] The supporters of this concept hypothesize that defective enzymes or impaired biochemical systems cause disease. This viewpoint, to some degree, neglects emotional and environmental factors in disease causation, and instead stresses chemical and molecular factors.

Even in the field of psychiatry, single-factor theories are prevalent. For example, certain psychiatrists try to explain mental disease solely in terms of the person's early childhood. Other psychiatrists have concentrated upon thwarting of the sexual drive as the major problem in mental disease. More recently, some have theorized that biochemical changes are the cause of mental disturbance.

In sum, a wide variety of single-factor theories of disease have evolved over time. Although these theories help to explain certain aspects of disease, no single-factor theory has been shown to answer the *whole* question of disease causation. Even individual diseases do not seem to have a single cause or a single remedy. This discovery is slowly having an impact on modern medicine. As Selye points out:

> The principal endeavor of medicine in general is beginning to change. It is no longer the search for specific pathogens and for specific remedies with which to eradicate them. We always used to accept as a self-evident fact that each well-characterized disease must have its own specific cause. This tenet is self-evident no longer. It becomes increasingly more manifest that an agent does or does not produce disease, depending upon a variety of conditions.[48]

Only a *multicausal theory* of sickness, then, which takes into account all possible factors and predisposing conditions, can complete the puzzle of disease causation from which so many pieces are still missing.

5. A fifth traditional belief is that *the agents that cause disease are always external to man;* they are never a part of him. Since primitive times, man has tried to externalize and project away from himself those things that he considers evil or "bad." As Engel has said:

> The mechanism of projecting to the outside what is felt or experienced as uncomfortable, painful, or dangerous is universal in every human being and is characteristic of one phase of the psychological development of every child. So too is the idea that what is felt as bad or painful inside got there from the outside.[17]

Men consider disease to be painful, evil, and dangerous. It is not surprising, then, that people have thought of disease as an "invader" which enters a person's body from the outside world. This notion of disease is very old, dating back to primitive man, who viewed the world as a magical place filled with devils, charms, and spells.

In modern society, we too often view sickness as something apart from ourselves. Examples of this attitude are common in our everyday speech. We say we are "invaded" by microbes, "contaminated" by infectious material, we "breathe in" pollen and allergens, we "ingest" foods that sicken us, we "catch" colds, are "driven" by our primitive instincts, and we are corrupted by our vices. When we visit a physician, we want him to "rid us" of our disease with medicines and treatment. We want the surgeon to "cut out" the organ that has become diseased or the cells that have become cancerous. When mentally disturbed, we visit a psychiatrist who lets us "talk out" our feelings and objectify our fears. In sum, man, both primitive and modern, has tried to externalize disease by reducing it to a "bad thing" that has its own independent existence apart from the sufferer.

This objective way of thinking about disease is psychologically comforting to both patient and doctor. If we can project the cause of a disease outside ourselves, we can then put it under a microscope, study it, fight it, and cure it. However, this point of view can dangerously simplify the approach to nursing care. Nurses will feel no need to understand patients if they believe that what has caused disease is an external factor rather than an internal problem. Such nurses will believe their task ends with the giving of medications and the performance of procedures.

Conversely, the belief that disease is caused by some factor that is an intimate part of ourselves is psychologically disquieting. For then the enemy that causes us so much sickness, pain, and discomfort is no longer external to us—it is within us and *a part of us.* With such a view, the cause of illness cannot be exorcised like a devil or exterminated like a microbe. It becomes necessary for doctors and nurses to study *the patient himself* as well as the disease if they want to effect a cure.

Modern medical theorists are taking as much cognizance of the "enemy within" as they are of those disease-producing factors that exist in the external world. Consequently many broad questions are being asked today. Why, for example, when three people are exposed to the tuberculosis bacillus, does only one of the three develop tuberculosis? And why, since all of us are exposed to many different infectious microorganisms, does this one person develop tuberculosis and not some other infectious disease? Is it something in the person that predisposes him to tuberculosis or is it something in the *environment?* Or is it the result of some peculiar interrelationship between the two?

Such questions must be answered. However, the external-factor theory alone does not offer the solution. In recent years, science has been looking more carefully at man himself and at the way in which he *responds internally* to external stressors and invaders. Medicine has shifted its emphasis from the study of environmental factors to the study of man's internal milieu and his adaptive processes. As Stewart Wolf points out:

> Newer concepts of disease hold that illness and incapacity arise from efforts on the part of the body to deal with adverse forces in the environment more frequently than they do from the direct effect or intrinsic nature of the adverse stimulus itself. In a sense, disease is a reaction to rather than an effect of noxious forces.[60]

Thus, for the final answer to disease causation we must look to the individual man himself as well as to the external world surrounding him.

Comparison of Traditional and Modern Theories of Disease Causation

Traditional theories of disease causation are usually anatomically oriented and they tend to support etiologic concepts of illness that are rigid, narrow, and mechanistic.

Modern theories of disease differ from traditional theories in at least four ways: (1) Modern theories are based upon the *total man* rather than upon bodily processes. (2) They are more *unified* and less fragmented. The interrelationships between the various organs, between mind and body, and between the total man and his environment are increasingly being recognized. (3) Current theories consider man's unique *response* to disease as well as the disease itself. (4) Finally, the etiology of disease tends to be multicausal in scope rather than unicausal.

In this chapter we have discussed, in a general way, changes in theories of disease causation over the past centuries. We have commented on the transition from a traditional to a modern viewpoint of illness. Let us now briefly discuss selected outstanding modern theories of disease causation—theories that have virtually revolutionized the whole concept of illness and why it develops.

CHAPTER 5

Modern Unified Theories of Disease

A unified theory of disease has been the dream of scientists since the beginning of medical history. A perfectly unified disease theory appears impossible because of the tremendous variety of diseases and the endless number of factors in their causation. Nevertheless, certain physicians and other scientists have attempted to establish modern theories of disease causation that are broad enough to encompass a large percentage of the diseases as well as a majority of the causative factors. Scientists such as Bernard, Cannon, Selye, Harold Wolff, and Stewart Wolf, in particular, are responsible for the development of unified concepts of disease with which you should be familiar.

As a student of nursing, you may wonder why it is necessary to have a detailed theoretic knowledge of disease causation. Such knowledge is necessary because theory is not something that remains restricted to a book or laboratory; theories are eventually applied to patients. *You* are a vital link between a hypothesis formed in the mind of a scientist and the actual practical benefits which that hypothesis provides for sick individuals. In other words, you are the person who will help to put the theory into practice. Thus, you can never know too much about disease or why it occurs. Your whole professional life will revolve around questions of causation and treatment. Only by understanding what scientists presently believe to be true about disease can you hope to contribute to patient care. Let us now briefly summarize the important hypotheses that modern scientists have formulated.

THE THEORIES OF BERNARD AND CANNON

Claude Bernard, nineteenth century French physiologist, laid the foundation for the modern concept of disease causation with his experiments and hypotheses. His contributions to medicine and nursing are multiple. First of all, Bernard had a unique view of man, whom he described as "a piece of constancy moving in a world of variables."[19] He saw man not as a being set apart from his environment, but rather as an integral part of the environment.

Second, as mentioned previously, it was Bernard who first described the *internal milieu*, or the internal environment of the body. He hypothesized correctly that if an organism was to live, it must have the capacity to maintain its internal milieu in a relative state of constancy. As a result of his experiments, Bernard was able to describe some of the mechanisms that regulate the balance of our internal body fluids.

Third, Bernard saw illness in a new and enlightening way. He argued that sickness was the result of (1) imbalances in the internal environment of the body, and (2) breaks in the vital communication that must exist between the internal milieu and the external environment. As a fourth contribution, Bernard described disease not only as a disturbance of homeostatic balance, but as an *adaptive attempt* to restore balance. He taught that these adaptive attempts at balance were appropriate in kind, but were incorrect in magnitude. For example, an individual with pneumonia suffers from a lack of oxygen. In response to this deficit, the bone marrow produces more red blood cells, these being the oxygen-carrying cells of the body. These excess erythrocytes, however, thicken the blood, making it much more difficult for the heart to pump it through the lungs. Congestive heart failure may then result from the body's response, which, while appropriate to the situation, is excessive for the good of the total organism.

Today we carry Bernard's theory of adaptive responses a step further. We now believe that the body's adaptive reactions not only may be excessive but may also be *inappropriate* to the situation. We will elaborate more on this modern concept when we discuss the theories of Hans Selye and Harold Wolff.

The first physician to expand radically upon Bernard's hypotheses was Walter Cannon, who taught physiology at Harvard in the early part of this century. As we stated earlier, the term "homeostasis" was coined by Cannon, who was especially interested in the body's *self-regulating processes.* In particular, Cannon explored the "fight or flight" reaction of the body to emergency situations, and the nervous and adrenal apparatus involved in these reactions. On the whole, this American physiologist was mainly concerned with "the *wisdom* of the body" rather than with the body's mistakes and blunders; that is, he was more interested in health than in disease. Consequently, it was not until Hans Selye formulated his theory of stress that Bernard's contributions were fully applied to the problem of disease causation.

SELYE'S GENERAL THEORY OF STRESS

Hans Selye's contribution to the study of disease causation rests upon his hypotheses concerning stress* and the stress syndrome. Selye's interest in formulating a general theory of stress began many years ago when he was a medical student. At that time Selye noted that most diseases are characterized by only a *few* specific signs, and that almost all maladies share *many signs and symptoms in common*—for example, weight loss, fatigue, malaise, aches and pains, and gastrointestinal upsets. In other words, he observed that almost all patients, regardless of diagnosis, share the same pathologic changes. Selye subsequently called this phenomenon the "syndrome of just being sick." Later, after years of experimentation, Selye renamed it the *stress syndrome* or *general adaptation syndrome* (GAS). Furthermore, he suggested that certain hormones, called *adaptive hormones,* are released during stress, and that these hormones help to create the common symptoms seen in all patients.

From his observations, Selye finally concluded that *stress plays a role in every disease process* regardless of causation. Selye defines stress, for purposes of scientific investigation, as *"the state manifested by a specific syndrome which consists of all the non-specifically induced changes within a biological system."*[49]

According to Selye, the GAS appears whenever an organism is subjected to long-continued stress. Some of the manifestations of the GAS may include: the stimulation of the adrenal glands, with a release of hormones; the development of gastrointestinal ulcers; and the shrinkage of lymphatic tissues. The stressors that may bring about the GAS are nonspecific in nature and may be any of such common events as trauma, infection, burns, severe colds, emotional upsets, or others.

In addition to the body's general systemic response to stress, Selye proposes that the body can also adapt to local stressors. He has called this process of local response, which takes place within a single organ or specific section of the body, the *local adaptation syndrome,* or LAS. An example of an LAS is inflammation, a process which we shall discuss in Unit V.

Selye has suggested that both the GAS and the LAS develop in three distinct stages: (1) an alarm reaction, (2) the stage of resistance, and (3) the stage of exhaustion.[47] Let us look briefly at these three stages in terms of a generalized body reaction.

1. The Alarm Reaction. Essentially this stage is a "call to arms" of the body's defenses against any nonspecific stressor, e.g., cold, heat, x-rays, and so forth. The individual homeostatic mechanisms described by Cannon (regulation of body temperature, blood calcium, and fluids and electrolytes) are mobilized and coordinated to meet the aggressor that has challenged the body's resources. The noxious effects of the stressor are generalized to the whole body, because no one organ system is, at that point, able to cope with them.

Selye divided the alarm reaction into two phases: the shock phase and the countershock phase. During the *shock* phase, the autonomic nervous system becomes very active; moreover, large amounts of epinephrine and cortisone are released into the blood stream. Typical signs of shock appear (see Chapter 26, Unit V). The shock period may last from a few minutes to around 24 hours. If the person lives and the damage from the stressor has not been too great, the *countershock* phase follows, during which most of the changes produced during the shock period are reversed. This phase then merges into the next stage—that of resistance.

2. The Stage of Resistance. This is really the stage of adaptation. During this time the body uses its most appropriate channels to combat the stressor. It attempts to limit the noxious effects of the stressor to the smallest area of the body capable of dealing with them.

3. The Stage of Exhaustion. During the final phase of the GAS, the adaptation that the body has developed can no longer be maintained. The appropriate channels that have attempted to control the stressors become exhausted and break down as a result of wear and tear. Consequently the stress effects, which have been contained in the smallest area possible during the stage of resistance, again spread to the entire body. The manifestations that occurred during the alarm stage appear once more. This phase, depending upon the toxicity of the stressor, may terminate in total collapse and death. In other cases the exhaustion may be temporary; after a rest the individual may return to normal. With advancing age, however, it becomes increasingly difficult for the organism to recover and return to its former function. Thus life, according to Selye, is really a protracted GAS which develops as a result of the stresses of living and which inevitably ends in exhaustion and death.

Coordinating and Regulating Factors

What coordinates and regulates the GAS and LAS? Selye writes that many organs and systems contribute to the regulation of these stress syndromes; most important are the brain, the central and autonomic nervous systems, and the pituitary and adrenal glands. The adrenal and pituitary glands are particularly crucial to adaptation, for they release hormones that specifically combat stress and that inhibit or stimulate the body's defense mechanisms as necessary. Selye calls the hormones produced by the adrenal and pituitary

*Stress is discussed briefly in Unit I, on p. 10.

glands *adaptive hormones*. The group of adaptive hormones that *inhibit* excessively defensive activities on the part of the body have been termed *anti-inflammatory corticoids* or *glucocorticoids*. The release of glucocorticoids into the blood stream is stimulated by the pituitary hormone ACTH. An example of an anti-inflammatory corticoid is cortisone, one of the hormones secreted by the adrenal cortex. The other group of adaptive hormones *stimulate* the body's defenses. These secretions are known as *pro-inflammatory corticoids*, or *mineralocorticoids*. An example of a pro-inflammatory corticoid is aldosterone, also secreted by the adrenal cortex.

The body's ability to resist stress and adapt to noxious forces depends upon a proper balance of these essential chemical substances. In turn, the effect of these adaptive hormones upon the body's resistance to stress depends upon certain *conditioning factors*, i.e., circumstances that influence the course of the GAS without being a part of it. The most important conditioning factors are diet, climate, heredity, past experience, and past exposure to stressors. Such conditioning factors are responsible for the varying individual ways in which different persons react to the same degree of stress.

Diseases of Adaptation. What specifically is the relationship of the GAS to disease? First of all, as we have said, Selye theorizes that the GAS is an integral part of all pathologic processes, no matter what their cause; i.e., adaptation to stress on the part of the body plays a role in *every* disease. Second, Selye states that *faulty adaptation*, in itself, can cause disease. Selye has named these "derailments" of the adaptive syndrome the *diseases of adaptation*. These maladies are not due to any specific pathogen, but instead they are the direct result of a faulty response to a stressor. Usually adaptation to stressors involves a balanced blend of defense and submission on the part of the body. When the body overdefends itself and there is a surplus of pro-inflammatory hormones, such diseases as arthritis, allergy, and asthma develop. When the body does not defend itself sufficiently, as a result of the release or injection of too much anti-inflammatory hormone, then the individual may succumb to overwhelming infection. Further, sometimes adaptation can be faulty or inappropriate and result in such conditions as stomach ulcers, a disorder we shall discuss briefly below in connection with the theories of Harold Wolff.

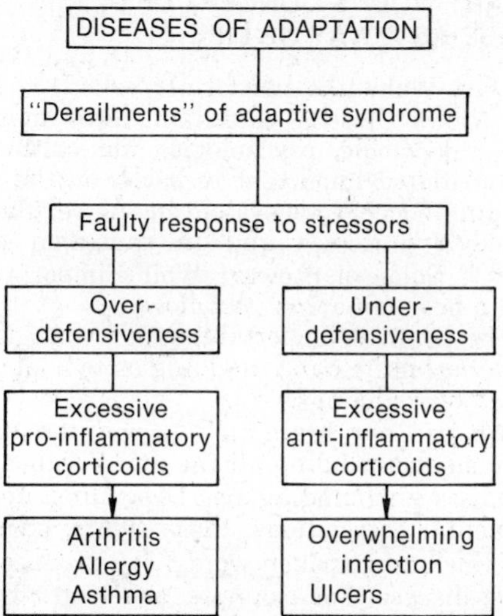

FIGURE 5–1. Selye's scheme of the major diseases of adaptation and the pathophysiologic factors that precipitate them.

HAROLD WOLFF'S THEORY OF STRESS, DISEASE, AND ORGAN MALADAPTATION[61, 62, 63]

Both Selye and Harold Wolff, a New York psychiatrist, have been interested in how people respond to stress, and how these responses, in themselves, can subsequently lead to a breakdown in homeostasis. Selye, however, was mainly concerned with *physiologic* processes and the responses of the body to such *acute* stressors as hemorrhage, burns, trauma, and shock. Wolff, on the other hand, was more interested in the responses of individuals, both *physiologically and psychologically*, to such *chronic* stressors as a frustrating job situation or an unhappy home life. Wolff believed that a person's "total life situation," with its sorrows, joys, successes, and frustrations, could profoundly affect his susceptibility to disease. Wolff's research in this area helped to lay the foundation for some modern theories of psychosomatic medicine.*

Like Selye, Wolff based much of his thinking on the concepts developed by Claude Bernard. As you will recall, Bernard believed that disease was often the result of adaptive attempts on the part of the body to restore homeostasis—attempts that were appropriate in kind but incorrect in magnitude. Wolff recognized, through his more sophisticated research methods, that adaptive responses are not only incorrect in magnitude but are also frequently blundering and *inappropriate* to the situation. He theorized that inappropriate attempts at adaptation occur in man for several reasons. First, a human being has a *highly developed nervous system and cerebral cortex*. Consequently man can symbolize, recall the past, and project himself into the future. Therefore, threats of possible danger and *symbols* of danger are just as important in human disease causation as are noxious microbial, chemical, and mechanical forces. Second, man is essentially a *tribal creature*. That is, he depends upon other people for many of his satisfactions in life. Stresses may be created by his need to work and to associate successfully with other persons, many of whom differ radically from himself. Often he responds in-

*Psychosomatic medicine is discussed on pp. 120 to 124.

appropriately to other individuals because his perception of certain human relationships is unrealistic and distorted; this distortion results, again, from the human ability to symbolize and to consider both past and future.

Distorted perception of a situation involving human relations can eventually lead to illness. For example, consider the following situation.

> A husband comes home from a long day's work; he is exhausted and still preoccupied with the day's business. His wife is also exhausted from coping all day with the demands of their children. Nevertheless, she has cooked a nice meal and cleaned the house. When the husband walks in the door, he looks disturbed; moreover, he fails to comment upon the clean house or upon his wife's efforts to cook. The wife interprets the husband's preoccupation with business and his lack of interest in the house as a lack of interest in *her*. (Her mother always said this would happen!) She does not kiss him, and now he believes that she is angry at him over an incident of the day before. Neither individual speaks to the other and the hostility builds between them. No one enjoys dinner, the children are cross, the parents are upset, and everyone eventually goes to bed with "a sour stomach" and a headache. If this situation occurs night after night, the headaches and upset stomachs become habitual. Eventually, as a result, a serious illness may develop in some member of the family.

To summarize, in this family's case essentially four things have happened: First, there was a distorted evaluation by two people of each other's behavior; second, this distortion resulted in blocked communication and guarded hostility; third, these negative reactions, in turn, led to further inappropriate responses on the part of husband and wife; finally, out of the frustration, disappointment, and anger came *physiologic symptoms* which further added to their misery.

Wolff's research indicates that certain individuals caught in this kind of vicious circle consistently respond to a frustrating situation through a *particular* body organ or system, perhaps the stomach, back, colon, or nasal membrane. The organ involved varies from person to person and seems to follow a built-in pattern specific for the individual. Mucous membranes (whether of the nose, stomach, rectum, bladder, or vagina) seem to be particularly susceptible to stress, probably because these tissues comprise one of the body's main lines of defense against stressful invaders from without the body. Mucous membranes can exhibit a variety of stress reactions: for instance, engorgement, edema, hemorrhage, ischemia, increased friability, faulty absorption, ulceration, inflammation, and altered reactions to chemical substances. Such pathologic changes occur frequently in response to traumatic personal situations. If these changes are habitual and are combined with other noxious, chemical, or physical stressors, such responses can eventually lead to irreversible tissue damage.

Selye points out that every organ responds in its *own particular way* to stress. For example, the liver may develop an abscess in response to stress, but it will never develop an ulcer no matter how great a stressor it is exposed to. Wolff carried the point further and proved that organs not only respond to stress in their own particular way, but they, like people, may also respond *inappropriately* to stressful situations; that is, organ functions such as digestion and elimination, which ordinarily benefit man under the proper conditions, may be activated inappropriately in response to a stimulus or need which these functions *are not equipped to satisfy or control*. Such troublesome patterns of organ response cannot help an individual to achieve his goals or to control his environment; instead, if prolonged, they may lead to serious illness. For example, when something irritates the colon (e.g., castor oil), diarrhea tends to develop and, as a result, the noxious substance is expelled. Such a response is appropriate and expected. It is inappropriate, however, to develop diarrhea as a result of unsatisfactory interpersonal relationships (e.g., forced association with a hated person). No matter how severe the diarrhea, it is not possible to get rid of the hated person in this way.

Let us now summarize Wolff's theory. Essentially he taught that (1) the development of illness was related to the total life pattern of an individual; (2) we, as individuals with highly developed nervous systems, are capable of symbolizing and reacting to these symbols. Consequently we may react inappropriately to situations, especially those involving interpersonal relationships. (3) Organs themselves can react *inappropriately* in a stressful situation, activating functions that cannot vanquish the stressor; and (4) such inappropriate organ responses, if prolonged, can result in disability, disease, and death.

STEWART WOLF'S CONCEPT OF DISEASE AS A WAY OF LIFE

Stewart Wolf, like his former colleague Harold Wolff, views disease causation from many aspects—physiologic, psychologic, and cultural. He has contributed important research on the role of the brain and nervous system in the regulation of the body's processes and in causation of disease.[59, 60] Some of Stewart Wolf's important find ings can be summarized as follows:

1. The brain is important both in maintaining our *internal* milieu and in aiding us to adapt to our *external* surroundings.

2. We use our brain to *interpret* the external environment, including all the many sights, odors, and noises surrounding us. Depending upon our past mental associations, these sights, odors, and noises (including spoken words) can produce symptoms of disease. For example, a person who fears pregnancy can become nauseated at the mere mention of pregnancy. Eating something with a disgusting taste or smelling a noxious odor can also

create nausea. This phenomenon is related to the activity of the brain and nervous system and the *meaning* that it gives certain experiences.

According to Wolf, man's ability to respond to symbols actually determines whether he will remain healthy or become diseased. Because man's responses to stresses of a symbolic nature involve his goals, aspirations, and values, these responses actually constitute his "way of life." Thus, if a person's responses are essentially and consistently negative and maladaptive in nature, *disease becomes a way of life* for that individual.

3. While neural processes can *cause* disease manifestations to appear, the power of the brain also can *relieve* the symptoms of disease and mitigate injury. For example, consider the *placebo effect*—an old and well known phenomenon in medicine. This occurs when, in certain cases, patients in severe pain are given injections of sterile water or normal saline ("the placebo"), which they believe to be morphine sulfate or some other narcotic. The placebo may produce definite pain relief. Moreover, placebo administration, whether pill, injection, or procedure, has at times been followed by "substantial and measurable changes in bodily mechanisms."[60] According to Wolf, a placebo works not because of any pharmacologic properties but because of the way in which the *brain interprets the therapeutic effort,* and the significance and meaning to the patient of the *total situation* surrounding that effort, e.g., the hospital environment and the attitudes of doctors and nurses.

Studies with *hypnosis* provide yet another example of the brain's ability to mitigate tissue damage. In an impressive experiment by Chapman and associates, subjects were exposed to thermal stimuli in precise quantities which were sufficient to produce burns. These stimuli were applied to both of their forearms. In the control group, no hypnotic suggestion was given and the right and left forearms of each subject developed virtually identical burns as a result of the stimulus. In the experimental group, however, the subjects were first placed under hypnosis and, while hypnotized, were told that the left arm would be impervious to the stimulus, but the right arm would be particularly vulnerable. Then the thermal stimulus was applied. In 30 out of 40 trials, the left arm of the subjects showed only a small burned area while the right arm incurred a substantial area of tissue damage. In these cases, mental suggestion and neural integrative action actually determined, in part, the response of the body tissues to an external stressor.[60]

4. In addition to the fact that the brain can create and mitigate the development of disease, the brain itself can be damaged by faulty interaction between an individual and his environment. This faulty interaction, in turn, leads to further maladaptation. Brain damage as a result of environmental stress has been particularly noted in prisoners of war. Such damage has been irreversible in some instances.

For example, a group of 100 Norwegian war veterans of World War II, who had been interned in concentration camps for three years, were examined 12 years after liberation. These men (all of whom had experienced humiliation, deprivation, isolation, beatings, floggings, and threats of execution at the hands of their captors) were found to suffer from a "more or less gross loss of brain substance."[61] In reviewing the life histories of these abused men following their release from prison and from the service, it was found that the men could not readjust to civilian life and that they complained of fatigue, irritability, mood swings, sleeplessness, memory loss, lack of initiative, and headache. Thus, for these men, the highly traumatic situation of internment had led to brain damage that resulted in a poor adjustment to civilian life.

5. If the cerebral hemispheres are destroyed, removed, or damaged, the signs and symptoms of systemic disease are greatly changed. For example, a cat without its cerebral cortex, but with brain stem and hypothalamus intact, will not respond with fever to the injection of pyogenic substances. Thus, the brain affects not only the development of disease but the manifestations of disease.

In sum, Wolf sees the brain as an integral part of the total organism or individual. In turn, he envisions the total individual as an integral part of the total environment. This environment includes all of the sights, sounds, and symbols, both pleasing and noxious, which surround each person, and which each individual interprets and makes meaningful through the use of his brain. Disease, then, cannot be separated from the total person, from his way of life, or from his interpretation of what life *means* to him. For this reason, Wolf believes that such terms as "psychogenic" disease, "functional" disease, and "organic" disease are inaccurate and misleading. All disease affects the function of some organ or system, and no disease in man can be completely divorced from the influence of the nervous system, the higher mental centers, and the meaning that these bodily components give to the stimuli and stresses that are a part of life.

THE CYBERNETIC CONCEPT OF DISEASE

The cybernetic theory of disease is based upon the concept of *feedback,* a principle discussed in Unit I. In review, feedback is defined as the mechanism that enables a self-regulating system to sense the degree to which it is deviating from the set norm and to make the adjustments necessary to correct the detected deviation.

Feedback is involved everywhere in the disease process. As Masturzo states in *Cybernetic Medicine,* "Wherever one views pathophysiology at any level of organization, disturbance of self-regulation emerges as one unmistakable mechanism of disease in every system of the body."[35] Thus, fever, injury, edema, heart failure, parkinsonism, cancer, and even death can be viewed as disturbed homeostasis—as "misfired self-regulation." As you will recall from Unit I, unstable oscillations and unmonitored positive feedback are the two most deadly problems resulting from disturbances in homeostatic balance.

The cybernetic theory is derived from Bernard's principle of the disturbed internal milieu and from Cannon's concept of upset homeostasis. The cybernetic theory plays an important role in *all* the modern theories of disease which we have been discussing. Let us now quickly review each theory. As you read them, identify how feedback is a part of the theory.

> *Selye* writes of the body's attempts to restore homeostatic balance by means of adaptive hormones. He explored the problems engendered by too little hormone, too much hormone, or an inappropriate release of hormones in response to stressors.

> *Harold Wolff* hypothesized that individuals attempt to adapt to or to correct situations that are experienced by them as deviant or abnormal. In their attempt to adapt, organ functions are often used inappropriately and to the detriment of the individual.

> *Stewart Wolf* concentrates on the action of the brain and the nervous system in upsetting the body's balance and in mitigating imbalances. As Wolf points out, health and disease may be determined by an interplay between too little and too much adaptive reaction "brought into play by feedback from the internal and external milieu."

CHAPTER 6

Stress and Disease: Major Causative Factors

As we indicated in the previous chapter, multiple factors are involved in disease causation. The nurse needs a precise knowledge of these factors to carry out her role of mitigating and preventing illness. In order to more fully appreciate the complexity of disease causation and, hence, the difficulty of controlling it, it is again necessary to look at man and his environment from many different aspects—the physical, the chemical, the biologic, the psychocultural, and the ecologic.

GENERAL CONSIDERATIONS

Before considering specific factors in disease causation, let us first briefly discuss *stressors*. We shall define stressors as agents or factors that challenge the adaptive capacities of an individual, thereby placing a strain upon that person which may result in stress and disease. Five general characteristics of stressors are of special importance here.

1. Stressors affect different people in different ways.

These differences in reaction depend upon the following factors:

a. *The stressor itself,* how suddenly it appears, how long it lasts, and how forceful it is. A very stressful situation that is short-lived is often better tolerated by an individual than a less stressful situation that tends to be chronic. This is because chronic stress demands continuous adaptive efforts. Eventually, because of constant wear and tear of a chronic nature, the individual actually changes, physically and psychologically, becoming more vulnerable to other stressors. If the stress has been both chronic and severe, the individual may be permanently and adversely altered.

b. The reaction to a stressor depends also upon the *limitations and potentialities of the individual* for dealing with stress. These factors are dependent upon the person's genetic constitution as well as his past history of adapting to stressful situations. For example, a person with diabetes mellitus, a hereditary disease of metabolism, is far less able to resist infection than one who does not have diabetes. Thus, the effect of a stressor is always *relative* and never absolute; it is relative to the individual undergoing stress, and in particular to his adaptive capabilities.

c. Certain stresses have more *meaning* and *importance* in the lives of some individuals than in the lives of others. This variation depends upon the person's family background and environment, and upon the values which he has developed as a result. For example, failure in school may not be stressful for a child from a lower socioeconomic group, since it actually releases him to go out and work. For a child of professional parents, however, failure in school can lead to mental illness, depression, even suicide.

2. Whenever a person encounters stress, from whatever source, he attempts to adapt to it.

If adaptation is successful, the individual's balance will not be disturbed or will be restored. Indeed, many people gain confidence in themselves, achieve goals, and develop new potentials as a result of a stressful encounter which they have successfully met and adapted to. Others are not successful in their adaptation to stressors. If adaptation is consistently faulty, these people will become ill.

3. Any one stressor is, in itself, a source of new stresses.

People often find themselves caught in a chain of events stemming from one original upset. For example, a patient with a communicable disease is undergoing stress because he is ill. He is usually placed in an isolation unit, which constitutes another stress. Consequently, he may become upset with the staff and they, in turn, with him. As a result, a third stress is created. These stresses, put together, may slow down his recovery. He is hospitalized longer, his finances are affected adversely, his job is threatened, his family is upset, and so one stress leads to another. Unfortunately the patient must adapt himself to many diverse stresses at a time when he lacks the resources to do so.

4. No one stressor or etiologic factor can, by itself, cause a disease.

As Engel points out, when a person is ill, one factor involved in his illness may be of greater importance than any other factor. This factor may be highly specific to the causation of his disease; indeed, it may be absolutely necessary for the development of the disease. However, *no one factor is both necessary and sufficient* for the development of a particular malady.[17]

For example, consider the nurse who develops staphylococcal boils as a result of working with a patient with a staphylococcus wound infection. For this nurse to become infected, it is of course necessary for her to be exposed to staphylococci. The staphylococcus, then, is a *necessary* agent in this case of contamination. However, the exposure to the staphylococcus, alone, is *not* an adequate reason for the development of an infection. Nurses are exposed daily to this organism, yet they do not become infected. Some other factors, one or more of which must be present for infection to occur, are: lowered resistance to disease, fatigue, emotional stress, poor handwashing technique, and poor dressing technique using contaminated tape, scissors, and other hospital equipment. In sum, it takes *both* exposure to the staphylococcus *and* some of these other factors to provide necessary and sufficient cause for the development of a staphylococcic infection.

In the instance of chronic diseases, such as cancer and heart disease, it is even more difficult to find the contributing causes necessary for their development. Exactly which etiologic factor must be present, and in what particular combination, for any one chronic disease to evolve remains a mystery.

> *5. Stress, of whatever nature, if too prolonged and too severe, can eventually overwhelm any person, no matter how well he has developed his adaptive capabilities.*

Research on the effect of combat duty and concentration camp experiences on the individual soldier has more than proved the eventual overwhelming effect of constant stress. Harold Wolff, for example, writes concerning the effects of battle:

> . . . it may be inferred that everyone has his breaking point, that there are stresses that no man can withstand. Conflict in excess of an individual's current integrative capacity may be a precipitating factor in such a "break." Conversely, whatever reduces integrative capacity may increase the possibility of an individual being overwhelmed by frustrations and conflicts, hitherto managed successfully. Loss of sleep, exhaustion, pain, very loud noises, starvation, malnutrition, infection, sepsis and intoxication, by decreasing integrative capacity, make conflict relatively excessive. Likewise, acts that terrorize, humiliate, destroy self-esteem and create a conviction of being isolated, abandoned or unwanted may reduce integrative effectiveness.[63]

Let us now summarize these general statements concerning stressful factors and their effects. First, people react in different ways to stressors, depending upon the stressor itself, the limitations and potentialities of the individual, and the special meaning that the stressor has for that individual. Second, persons always attempt to adapt to stress. Third, these attempts at adaptation inevitably lead to new stresses. Fourth, no single stress, by itself, is both necessary and sufficient to cause disease. Finally, there are stresses that are either so severe or so prolonged that they can eventually overwhelm the adaptive capabilities of the best-adjusted individual. Let us now turn to a discussion of specific stress-producing factors.

TYPES OF STRESSFUL FACTORS THAT CAUSE DISEASE

Selye has listed, in a general way, those stressors that can elicit an alarm reaction and subsequent adaptive activities on the part of the organism. This list of alarming stimuli that may result in disease is as follows:

ALARMING STIMULI (STRESSORS)[47]

Trauma	Deep anesthesia
Surgical interference with vital organs	Temporary blood vessel occlusion
Fractures	Reduced oxygen tension
Crushing of tissue	Burns
Infectious diseases	Drugs
Bacterial toxins	Hormones
Hemorrhage	Natural and synthetic folliculoids (estrogens)
Exposure to cold and heat	
Obstetric shock	Diet
Gravity shock	Fasting
Nervous stimuli	Overfeeding
Spinal transection	Vitamin deficiencies
Emotional stimuli	X-rays or radium rays
Rage, fear	Solar rays

For a more detailed discussion, stressful stimuli or factors can be broken down into the following groups: (1) hereditary or genetic factors, (2) physical and chemical factors, (3) microorganisms and parasites, (4) psychologic factors, (5) cultural factors, (6) ecologic factors, and (7) stressful factors resulting specifically from life in a technologic society. Let us now briefly consider each group and its relationship to disease.

1. Genetic Factors. These factors, according to Engel, underlie "the individual chemical characteristics of the cells of each person and as such contribute to the basic chemical structure underlying the capacity for growth and development of every cell and system."[17] Genes, then, influence the biochemical structure of the entire body. They consequently have a powerful effect on our appearance, longevity, and intelligence, as well as on our vulnerability to stresses and our susceptibility to disease.

The relationship between genetic inheritance and disease is increasingly becoming an area for scientific investigation. We know that defective or abnormal biochemical systems can be transmitted through the genes. Such defective systems or "inborn errors of metabolism" give rise to structural and developmental defects in the unfortunate individual who inherits them. Sometimes these defects appear in the newborn child and adversely affect his existence throughout his entire life. In other cases, inherited defects become evident only under certain conditions. For example, sickle cell anemia is a hereditary disease seen predominantly in blacks. Clinical manifestations of the disease do not appear unless the afflicted individual is exposed to a lowered oxygen tension. Thus, many blacks who were soldiers and airmen in World War II did not realize that they had sickle cell anemia until they flew at high altitudes in nonpressurized planes; only then did symptoms of this hereditary malady appear. In other types of hereditary disease, symptoms of the disorder may not appear or become troublesome unless precipitated by such factors as diet, climate, or emotional stress.

Whereas genetic factors influence our state of health and susceptibility to disease, environmental factors may influence the *extent* to which our heredity controls us. For example, individuals may lengthen or shorten their life span according to their mode of living. The person who is inclined to obesity, and consequently to other maladies such as hypertension, can choose to diet and exercise or he can choose to overeat and to underdo. Maladaptive and detrimental traits of character can be overcome by learning new behavior patterns.

In other words, we are all born with a certain inherited potential for self-realization or self-destruction. What we do with this potential depends upon ourselves and upon the environment in which we live. Therefore, even diseases that are inherited need not inevitably maim, disable, or kill. As a result of modern medicine and better education of the lay public, many of these inborn maladies are being identified and controlled.

2. Physical and Chemical Agents. According to Engel,[17] factors that are capable of injuring us because of their physical or chemical properties essentially fall into the following groups:

a. Dangerous substances or forces that impinge upon our bodies from the *external environment.* Examples of such factors are: mechanical forces, poisons, heat, cold, radiation, electricity, high or low atmospheric pressure, industrial poisons, and drugs. The extent to which these substances or forces can injure us depends, in turn, upon three additional factors. First, the individual's tolerance and ability to adapt to certain stressors. For example, tall, thin persons are less able to adapt to an extremely cold climate than are persons with a short, heavy body build. Individuals with light, sensitive skin can be severely burned by exposure to sun rays that would only tan a dark-skinned individual. Second, *social and psychologic factors* may be significant. For example, a person's work may bring him into contact with dangerous chemical substances or heavy machinery. The impulsive or accident-prone individual may be far more susceptible to mechanical injuries than is a cautious person. Third, the *virulence of the factor itself* is of critical importance. For instance, some highly concentrated chemical substances are capable of killing a person on contact. Likewise, a severe enough electric shock can quickly prove fatal to the unfortunate victim.

b. Substances or forces, *within our bodies,* that injure by being excessive or by being in contact with organs that are particularly sensitive to them. Excessive insulin production resulting in insulin shock, excessive cholesterol storage in the arteries leading to arteriosclerosis, and the action of refluxed gastric juices on the esophagus, resulting in ulcerations, are all examples of how our own internal secretions and products can injure us.

c. Physical or chemical substances *required* by the body which are *insufficient in amount or un-*

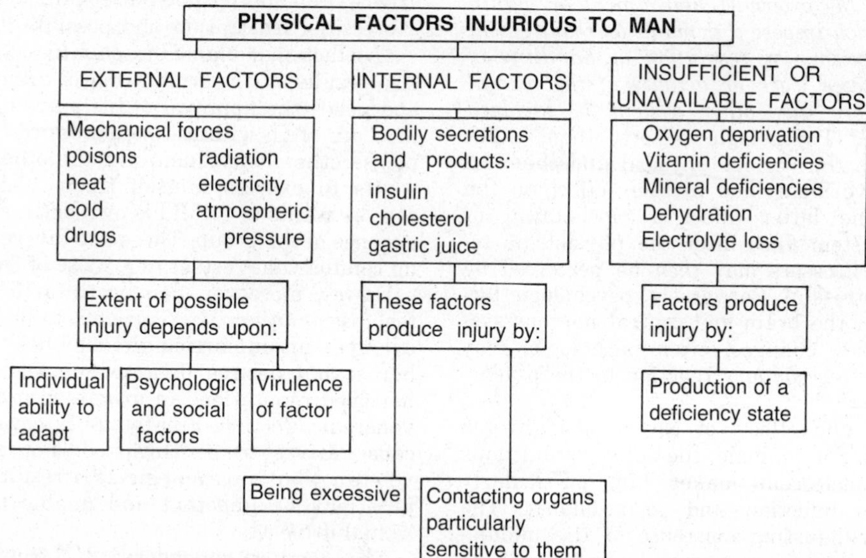

FIGURE 6-1. The three major types of physical stressors that can produce disease in man.

available. Lack of such vital substances can result in physiologic deprivation and injury. Examples of deprivation are many; the individual who has oxygen hunger, the person who does not receive proper vitamins and nutrients, the man who is severely dehydrated, and the patient with an electrolyte loss through vomiting or diarrhea are all suffering from the consequences of deprivation.

3. *Microorganisms and Parasites.* The extent to which microorganisms and parasites are capable of producing disease in another living organism depends upon their source, their ability to enter the body of the host and establish themselves in a tissue, organ, cell, or body fluid, their potency and virulence, and their number (especially in the case of parasites).

Microorganisms, then, vary in their ability to infect a host. For instance, some microorganisms are capable of infecting almost anyone exposed to them for the first time. Measles and smallpox viruses, prior to the development of vaccines, caused large-scale epidemics affecting thousands of people. Other microorganisms affect only a selected few persons out of a population; still others harmlessly occupy the tissues of the host, becoming destructive only when the individual's resistance is lowered. Such factors as fatigue, poor diet, and psychologic stress, or the presence of another disease condition such as diabetes mellitus or leukemia, is capable of lowering a person's defenses, thereby making him extremely susceptible to infection. To sum up, the characteristics of the microorganism, or parasite, the adaptive ability of the host, and those environmental stresses currently affecting the host all influence the causation of infectious or parasitic disease.

4. *Psychologic Factors.* Engel states that *"psychological stress refers to all processes, whether originating in the external environment or within the person, which impose a demand or requirement upon the organism, the resolution or handling of which necessitates work or activity of the mental apparatus before any other system is involved or activated."*[17] Psychologic factors, then, differ markedly from the various physical and chemical agents we have mentioned in their effect on the individual. The latter affect a biochemical or physiologic system *first;* after the physiologic reaction, these stressors may *then* be perceived by the mind as stressful. Conversely, psychologic factors *first* affect the brain and central nervous system; physiologic changes, often pathologic, may then follow as a *secondary* reaction to the psychologic trauma.

The causes and effects of psychologic stresses vary with age. For example, the active tumultuous life of the adolescent makes him particularly vulnerable to infection and to accidents. The competitive, exhausting existence of the middle-class adult makes him susceptible to such problems as stress ulcers, hypertension, heart disease, and alcoholism. The elderly person, his life lonely and his hopes diminished, often lapses into an inactive existence accompanied by various degenerative disorders. In sum, the coming of puberty with its physiologic changes, the adult years of responsibility, the advent of the climacteric and menopause, the years of retirement and aging, and the slow decline thereafter—all present unique psychologic stresses to which the individual must adapt.

What specific factors lead to the development of psychologic stress at any age? What is the possibility of disease resulting from such stresses?

Three major factors, as Engel points out,[17] are responsible for the development of psychologic stress. First of all, we are psychologically traumatized if we *lose* or fear losing something which we value or love, and which is especially important to us and to our self-concept. Persons, ideals, hopes, valued possessions, a prized job, the body image, social role, home, and country all represent objects of worth for different individuals. The loss of any one of these may result in a variety of psychologic experiences ranging from depression, grief, and mourning to feelings of anger and frustration.

Second, *injury and pain, or threats of the same,* almost always give rise to psychologic stress. One reason for this is that pain and injury are closely linked with loss and fear of loss. For example, if a person is injured in an accident, losing a leg, he will most definitely suffer from a sense of loss of body function and body image. Conversely, the loss of a loved person or object may compel certain individuals to attempt suicide. In general, however, persons respond to injury and loss by attempting to protect themselves and by making the most appropriate adaptations possible.

Frustration of drives is the third factor that gives rise to psychologic stress. Drives are frustrated for a number of reasons. During childhood, we learn that certain drives must be controlled, for example, the sexual drive. The need to control drives, however, often conflicts with the need to express our drives; if no appropriate outlet can be found for this expression, frustration and possibly illness result.

The fact that *man is essentially a tribal animal* also results in the frustration of drives. He wants and needs the approval of his peers. Consequently men are often willing to suppress certain drives to please other individuals. On the other hand, man wants to express himself freely and to be himself; he wants to fulfill his own desires, often at the expense of the group. These two divergent needs set up conflict that results in a sense of frustration.

Drives, moreover, can be thwarted because we feel *loss or injury* if we attempt to fulfill them. For example, an unmarried girl may hesitate to satisfy her sexual desires because she fears the loss of her good reputation, an unwanted pregnancy, or a venereal infection. Finally, an *injury* can, in itself, cause drives to be thwarted. For instance, the veteran who is paraplegic as a result of a war injury may be impotent and unable to satisfy his sexual drive.

The conflict engendered by frustrated drives

demands some resolution. As Engel points out, stress arises because the individual, on the one hand, feels compelled to satisfy his inner needs and yet, on the other hand, he can find no satisfactory or safe outlet for these drives. As a result, the drive goes unfulfilled, the conflict is unresolved, psychologic stress builds up, physiologic processes break down, and, finally, physical and mental diseases develop.

Although loss of a loved object, fear of injury, and drive frustration can all lead to psychologic stress, the *total life situation* of a person also has a most profound effect upon that individual's mental and physical well-being. In his study of various groups of workers, Hinkle[23] found that the healthiest individuals were also the happiest in their personal lives. They tended to be people who found satisfaction in their marriages, homes, and jobs. Conversely, unhappy, dissatisfied persons, who disliked their jobs and home lives, tended to be the sickest. These subjects expressed little hope for their futures and generally felt that they could never escape from the intolerable situations in which they lived or worked.

To summarize, the extent to which psychologic stress can result in an increased susceptibility to disease depends upon the following: (1) the person's age group; (2) the magnitude of the losses, injuries, and frustrations he must endure and his ability to adapt to these stresses; and (3) the types of life and work situations in which he is involved. People who lead generally satisfying lives and who feel fulfilled in terms of job, marriage, and general aspirations suffer from fewer illnesses than those persons who feel consistently frustrated in their present existence and are without hope for the future.

5. Cultural Factors. In large part, our particular way of viewing life and the world surrounding us originates in our cultural heritage. Cultural attitudes, beliefs, and traditions are all deeply ingrained in each of us. These factors can affect all aspects of our personality and life, including our attitudes toward health and disease.

Cultures vary widely in their traditions. It is not surprising, then, that cultural attitudes toward disease and injury vary throughout the world, and that a disease or injury that is considered serious in one culture may be looked on as trivial in another.

Conflicting cultural values are prevalent in the United States and in Europe; in certain instances, these conflicts lead to illness. For example, in the United States the individual is encouraged from earliest childhood to be competitive, to earn good grades, to accomplish goals, and to achieve high pay and an elevated status. The very human need to be dependent on other people is discouraged. Thus, a conflict is created between the American cultural values of assertiveness and independence, and the need to be loved and cared for. According to Parsons, one way in which an American can honorably resolve this conflict without losing face is to become legitimately ill.[39b] Thus, in our culture, the "sick role" has become an accepted defense against conflict. The person who is sick, and who "*tries* to get well," can have his needs for dependency met without seriously jeopardizing his place in American society.

Rapidly changing cultural values also can create a major source of anxiety. Old and traditional cultures appear to be less productive of stress and disease than are newer, more radical societies. Values in traditional societies change little, and there are sanctioned ways for resolving anxieties and conflict. On the other hand, in societies where the "old ways" of life are breaking down and the "new ways" have not yet been fully established, stress and disease tend to become more prevalent. Indeed, disease can become "a way of life" in a society, like our own, which is rapidly changing, where nothing is defined and nothing is sacred, where everyone is potentially mobile, and where there is open choice and constant conflict.

6. Ecologic Factors. Ecology can be defined as

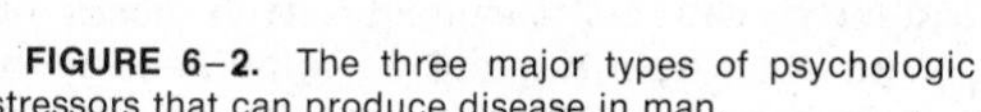
FIGURE 6-2. The three major types of psychologic stressors that can produce disease in man.

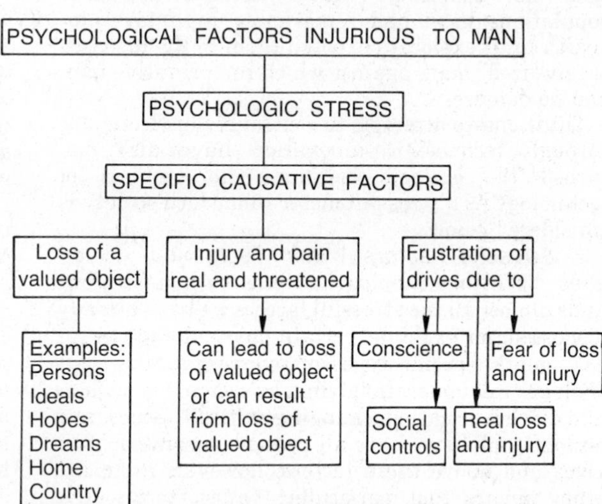

the branch of biology dealing with the mutual relations between organisms and their environment.[12] *Human ecology,* a science that particularly interests us in nursing, is "concerned with the reciprocal relations between man and his environment."[12]

In essence, human ecology implies a certain mutuality and balance between man and man, and man and nature. When man is in a state of ecologic balance, he is healthy; conversely, when a man is out of balance with his environment and with other men, and is no longer able to make successful adaptations, he is ill.

Ecologic balance is most easily maintained in environments that are stable and fairly settled, so that stresses and the need for change are at a minimum. However, when people must exist under environmental conditions that are upset, unsettled, or highly complex, ecologic balance tends to break down and morbidity and mortality rates rise.

War, for example, tends to upset the ecologic balance of both man and nature. War and disease are closely linked; over the centuries epidemics and plagues have followed battles, killing large numbers of the remaining populace. Even today, warfare and disease are inseparable. The large numbers of displaced persons, often poorly clothed and crowded together; the incapacitation of public health facilities with resultant pollution and general lack of sanitation; the defoliation of forest lands, the problems of food production and food supply; the cultural and psychologic deprivation; and the lack of medical care can all seriously upset the ecologic balance of a wartorn country. Such imbalances increase the vulnerability of a population to serious epidemics.[1]

Second, large-scale migrations and explorations also upset the ecologic balance. Whenever two different peoples come together, each group is exposed to new diseases for which they have developed no immunity. Many isolated primitive populations have had remarkably high levels of health until explorers exposed them to the diseases of "civilized" man, against which the primitive men had no defense.

Third, man's attempts to control his environment through technologic innovation have also disturbed the ecologic balance. The problem of technology as a stressful factor in modern society is considered below.

7. Stressful Factors Within Technologic Societies. Within technologic societies such as ours, one finds almost all the stressful factors we have already discussed; for example, certain physical and chemical agents, specific types of microorganisms, psychologic dilemmas involving loss of loved objects and drive frustration, changing cultural values, and ecologic imbalances are all present to some degree. Over and above these factors, however, there are other agents that particularly affect technologic societies and that are mainly responsible for the prevalence of chronic degenerative diseases within Western culture. Many of these underlying factors have been created, unwittingly, by man himself in his desire to control his environment, his health, his life, and his civilization.

More specifically, the major stressful factors within technologic societies are (1) products of our industrial technology, (2) products of our medical technology, and (3) the result of social conditions. Additional agents result from an interplay between social and technologic factors. Let us briefly discuss each of these areas.

First, some of the *industrial technologic* factors that contribute to the development of disease are:

> Pollution of air and water with gases, wastes, and poisons—for example, the dangerous by-products of factories, automobile exhausts, and cigarette smoking.
> Overuse of lethal insecticides and weed-killers, contaminating our water and food.
> Use of dangerous radioactive materials by science and industry.

Second, experts in *medical technology,* while alleviating many disease factors, have at the same time created new and perplexing problems by (1) developing numerous dangerous and powerful drugs and other forms of therapy, and (2) lengthening the human life span. The sheer number of drugs and medicinal preparations available to the public today is staggering. Ninety per cent of the drugs prescribed by the modern doctor did not exist 20 years ago. Many of these medications, while seemingly safe, have not been subjected to the long test of time. Consequently they may have some unexpected and frightening consequences. For example, when thalidomide (a sedative developed in Europe) was given to expectant mothers, the drug influenced the growth of the unborn child, producing severe deformities.

Even those drugs that have been in use for a long time often have dangerous side effects. Allergies to penicillin can be fatal. Chloromycetin, a broad-spectrum antibiotic, has frequently produced aplastic anemia—a potentially deadly disease in which the bone marrow ceases to produce blood cells. Moreover, certain antibiotics and sulfa drugs can destroy the natural flora of the intestinal tract or the vagina, thereby upsetting the ecologic balance of the body. Cortisone, the "miracle drug" that reduces the agony of inflammatory conditions, also leaves patients open to the menace of "silent" infections that develop without noticeable symptoms. Even aspirin, if taken in too large doses or too frequently, can be poisonous. High doses of phenacetin (a drug frequently combined with aspirin) may cause damage to kidney tissue. Tranquilizers, sleeping pills, weight reduction pills, contraceptive pills, along with thousands of other prescribed drugs, have their dangers. It is no wonder that, according to public health officials, 1.3 million Americans every year are incapacitated for at least one day—sometimes requiring medical aid—because of the side effects and untoward effects of drugs.[14]

Although drugs are the commonest offenders in terms of untoward effects, other medical therapies are not exempt from being potentially dangerous. Let us look at a few examples. Patients can develop serum hepatitis from a blood transfusion; intravenous fluids can overload the circulation, resulting in a filling of the lungs with fluid; irradiation can precipitate leukemia; prescribed bed rest can result in such complications as kidney stones, blood clots, and decubitus ulcers. Disease caused by the physician in his effort to treat the patient is called *iatrogenic disease.*

Modern medicine, moreover, has created certain problems by *extending the average person's life span* in Western society to around 70 years. A long life has always been the dream of man, but the increased longevity in technologic societies is unfortunately associated with a high incidence of chronic and degenerative diseases. At least 19 million Americans suffer from the chronic disorders of heart trouble, arthritis, and diabetes—all conditions that tend to appear in their most dangerous forms *after* the age of 50. Doctors speculate that these degenerative conditions seem to be related, in some way, to the longevity of the sufferer as well as to his way of life.

The *urban* way of life and the *social conditions* under which we live constitute the *third* agent responsible for disease-producing stresses in Western culture. People involved in technologic societies tend to live in cities where they are subjected to certain social stresses. Crowding, vehicular traffic, conflicting life styles, crushing loneliness, racial upheavals, student uprisings, as well as the breakdown of traditional values, eventually take their toll in disease of body and mind. The alienated workman, the disillusioned teacher, the angry slum dweller, the lonely old person aware of his obsolescence, the neurotic, the alcoholic, and the drug addict are common to our technologic society. These alienated products of urban life may be our friends and our patients; indeed, they may even be ourselves. As Eric and Mary Josephson express it in *Man Alone:*

> The alienated man is every man, and no man, drifting in a world that has little meaning for him and over which he exercises no power; a stranger to himself and to others. . . .[25]

Although our whole society is affected by social stresses, certain groups *within* the society seem to be affected more than others. People of the lower and working classes, as well as certain minority groups, suffer from a higher incidence of disease than do members of the middle and upper classes. In the United States, infections, chronic disease, mental disease, dental caries, cancer, and tuberculosis all occur more commonly among the poor. The higher incidences of these conditions among the lower class seem to be related to social isolation, malnutrition, ignorance, poor housing, and a generally low standard of living.[24]

Many of the agents that underlie chronic diseases are the result of an *interplay* among several different factors within our society. One example of such interplay is *obesity*—an important predisposing condition in hypertension and heart disease. The problem of obesity is related to overeating and lack of exercise, both of which are the result of technologic developments and/or emotional and social maladjustment. Technologically, modern farming and marketing methods have made many rich and potentially fattening foods easily available; also, the use of the automobile and various labor-saving devices has reduced physical exertion to a minimum for the average American. From a social viewpoint, our society, as we related earlier, is one in which many people are lonely, nervous, and under emotional stress. Often such people tend to chronically overeat, and eventually become obese. Thus, food, made readily available by modern technology, becomes a fattening and dangerous solace for those who live sedentary lives under stressful social conditions.

To summarize, while the urban way of life has reduced some health problems, it has obviously produced new problems that are equally serious. On the one hand, we live in a society in which technology gives us a long life, sanitation, pure food and drugs, and comparative freedom from infectious disease; on the other hand, this same society burdens us with choking pollution, iatrogenic disease, the pain of chronic maladies, and the evils of human alienation, mental illness, and prolonged old age.

CHAPTER 7

The Individual's Response to Stress-Producing Factors

As we have seen, many stressful agents can precipitate disease. However, it is our *individual reaction* to these stressors that ultimately determines the *extent* to which a potentially dangerous stressor can cause a breakdown of tissues, organs, or mental apparatus. Consider now the area of human response from the following three standpoints: (1) the body's response to physical injury, (2) the body's response to psychologic stimuli, and (3) attempts at adaptation that produce disease.

THE BODY'S RESPONSE TO PHYSICAL INJURY

Providing a degree of protection against bodily injury is one of the major functions of our skin, bones, gastrointestinal tract, blood, liver, and nervous system. For example, the *skin* is the first line of defense against invasion by microorganisms; moreover, its pigmentation protects man against the adverse effects of certain types of radiation. The *bones* protect man's vital organs; the *gastrointestinal tract* neutralizes certain poisons by means of mucous secretions; the *blood* contains antibacterial and antiviral substances; the *liver* detoxifies poisons and dangerous drugs; and, finally, the *nervous system* provides man with protective reflexes and instincts as well as with the reasoning and intelligence necessary to fight or to flee from stressful and dangerous situations.

Should the protective functions of these structures fail, and the individual subsequently develop a disease or injury, the body continues to respond in a protective manner, this time against the effects of injury and disease.

The body exhibits only a few types of reactions to physical injury. Selye has pointed out that the major reactions elicited by injury are *inflammation, sclerosis, increased capillary permeability, hormonal responses,* and certain *fluid* and *electrolyte shifts,* which will be discussed later in the text. In cases of infection, *antibodies* are usually built up as a defense against the troublesome organisms. When there has been a long-continued exposure to infectious disease, an *immune* reaction may develop as yet another type of bodily defense. Of course, the *nervous system and brain* continue to defend us against the effects of injury by promoting helpful adaptations and through the use of intelligence, knowledge, and will.

Inflammation is the most typical response by the

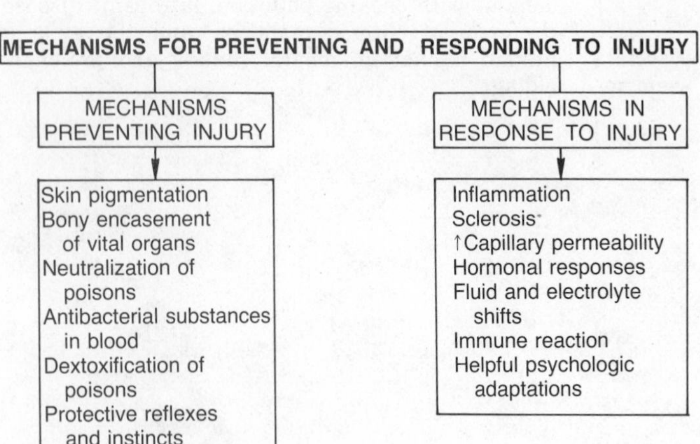

FIGURE 7-1. Major body mechanisms that prevent injury and defend man against injury once it occurs.

body to tissue injury from whatever cause. Because inflammation tends to remain localized, it is the outstanding example of the body's ability to respond to stress on a *limited basis,* or, according to Selye's stress theory, by means of the local adaptation syndrome (LAS). When stresses become overwhelming, the body *responds as a whole,* with the release of pituitary and adrenal hormones, an increase in blood sugar, and changes in blood pressure and temperature. In terms of Selye's theory, these responses are manifestations of the alarm reaction or first stage of the GAS, in which the entire body mobilizes for action.

In sum, body tissues and organs have only a limited number of defensive responses against a destructive stressor or against the effects of injury and disease. Responses may develop either at a local site undergoing stress, or they may involve the entire organism in an "all-out" encounter against the stressful invader.

RESPONSES OF THE BODY TO PSYCHOLOGIC STIMULI

The body is remarkably sensitive to even slight psychologic stimuli, responding in observable ways to almost every perceptible variation in the environment. Some impressive studies have been published concerning the effects of psychologic stimuli upon autonomic nervous system functions, i.e., those functions that are controlled by the sympathetic and parasympathetic nervous systems. Let us now summarize briefly some of these findings.

The Circulatory System. Slight changes in the environment are capable of affecting the heart rate, arteriole size, muscle tone of veins, and circulating blood volume. For example, listening to a faint whisper or hearing a door open can produce noticeable changes in arterial pressure, and driving an automobile in moderate traffic can cause alarming elevations of blood pressure. Thus, fairly minor and routine stimuli can result in noticeable physiologic responses.[52]

Although emotions do not have to be intense to produce an autonomic nervous system response, the type of emotional response is related to the type of circulatory change evoked. For example, when we feel angry, hostile, and anxious, the arterioles in the skin and kidneys and throughout the body constrict. This constriction of vessels, in turn, makes the heart beat faster, alters heart rhythm, and causes the arterial blood pressure to rise. On the other hand, when we feel fearful, depressed, or in despair, the opposite reactions occur: heart rate slows and blood pressure falls. If life seems truly bleak or shocking, we may attempt to escape it entirely by fainting.

Observable *local* changes also result from disturbances in the circulation due to emotional stimuli. Who has not observed the flush of anger, the pallor of fear, or the blush of embarrassment? All these color changes of the skin are under autonomic nervous system control, and thus are accompanied by alterations in blood pressure.

The Alimentary Tract. The digestive system, like the circulatory system, responds differently to different sets of emotional stimuli. For example, when one feels angry and hostile, the gastric mucosa reddens and the secretions and movements of the stomach increase in volume and magnitude. Moreover, the colon flushes and may become continuously spastic. Conversely, such feelings as sorrow, disappointment, and fear cause the mucosa of stomach and colon to pale and the movements of these organs to slow or cease. Anorexia, nausea, and vomiting may result. Even the salivary glands are affected by emotion. We all know that the mouth becomes very dry when we are afraid and that it literally "waters" when we are anticipating something pleasant, for example, a good meal. Thus, the body does not lie; through its response to psychologic stimuli it gives us a good indication of how we truly feel about a situation.

Other Systems. The *bladder,* like the circulatory and alimentary systems, also responds in predictable ways to opposing sets of emotions. For example, the person who feels resentful, frustrated, or upset tends to have an increase in bladder contraction and a resultant sense of urgency. Conversely, a sense of dejection or depression causes the bladder wall to relax and urine is retained. Fear can cause incontinence of urine in both children and adults.

The *pupil of the eye* is affected by emotion. It tends to become smaller when we are sleepy or uninterested in our environment and, conversely, to enlarge when we are stimulated, afraid, or in a state of rage; hence, the descriptive expression "wide-eyed with fear." The *bronchial muscle,* the *sweat glands,* and the *temperature-regulating mechanisms* are also subject to changes due to psychologic stress. We all know that breathing alters with excitement, sweating can result from fear or passion, and we can feel cold or hot depending upon the immediate events in our lives.

Variations and Inconsistencies in Responses

It is important to note that these autonomic responses to stimuli are typical responses; in other words, people generally react in these particular ways to certain stressors. However, two different people can react to similar psychologic stresses in directly opposite ways. For example, one man caught in a stressful situation might prepare physiologically for a fight; another person of different temperament and upbringing might faint when under comparable emotional pressure. Indeed, the *same* person may respond to similar predicaments in different ways at different times, depending upon his perception of the stressor and his defensive resources at the moment. In sum, the decision as to whether we should "stand and fight" or "faint and flee" depends upon our personality, our background, our level of vitality at the moment, the circumstances immediately surrounding us, and the way in which our brain perceives and interprets the situation.

Just as the uncomfortable emotions of grief, depression, anger, hostility, and fear all produce body responses, *pleasurable emotions* such as joy, love, and happiness can also lead to physical changes. For example, some people weep "tears of joy" or "scream with joy" when they feel a sense of extreme relief or happy emotion; individuals passionately in love experience changes in heart rate and rhythm, breathing, and muscle tone; a person who feels satisfied after a meal with pleasant companions tends to relax and even to sleep.

Unpleasant bodily responses may also arise on joyful occasions. These undesirable somatic changes appear to be related to one of two factors: First, joy may be mingled with a sense of fear or anxiety; indeed, an individual may *believe* that he feels happy in a certain situation when in reality he feels *both* happy and anxious—the anxiety leading to many upsetting symptoms. For example, a young person on his wedding day may express feelings of happiness and joy. However, he may also be experiencing various doubts, fears for the future, anxieties concerning parenthood, and so forth. It is these essentially unpleasant emotions, then, rather than the sense of joy or happiness, that give rise to the unpleasant bodily sensations.

Second, unpleasant bodily changes in response to joy may also occur in individuals who are physically too weak or ill to adapt to any intense emotion, even great happiness. Upon occasion such people have literally died in a transport of joy. For example, prisoners of Nazi Germany who were beaten, starved, and weakened by their stressful life were known to die during the excitement of being liberated. As one writer observed during just such a liberation:

> All these prisoners lit up with ineffable joy and hope when they saw the white Red Cross busses turn into the concrete square and grasped that they were to leave in them. For many, it was too much altogether, they hadn't the strength to grapple with so fantastic, so marvelous a prospect—they collapsed and died—literally—of joy.[54]

In summary, then, our bodies respond to emotional stimuli with certain definite physiologic changes which may be perceived by the individual as either pleasant or unpleasant. The autonomic nervous system, in particular, plays a vital role in the body's response to stressors through the regulation of heart action, blood pressure, pulse, sensory changes, digestive tract function, bladder function, and temperature regulation. The degree of functional change in these tissues and organs depends upon the *type* of stressor impinging upon the person and also upon its magnitude and force.

MALADAPTIVE RESPONSES PRODUCTIVE OF DISEASE AND DISORDER

Although many of our attempts to adapt to life's stresses prove satisfactory, some efforts tend to "backfire," causing injury and disease; still other attempts at adaptation fail because they are either inadequate or too chaotic to cope successfully with a stressful situation. Such maladaptive responses lie at the base of many illnesses.

Four major responses to stress that can be extremely costly to the individual in terms of health are the following: (1) the distorted anticipatory response; (2) the excessive response; (3) the deficient response; and (4) the inappropriate response.

1. The Distorted Anticipatory Response. Human reactions in anticipation of certain events can be helpful and protective if they are correct and appropriate. For example, as we pointed out earlier, saliva and gastric juices tend to flow in anticipation of a meal, or epinephrine is released and the pupil of the eye enlarges in anticipation of danger. These are appropriate adaptive responses. However, the anticipatory response can be overused, misused, and badly distorted. For instance, when a person thinks intensively about something unpleasant that *might* happen to him, his body reacts physiologically *as if* that unpleasant thing were actually taking place.

According to Stewart Wolf, faulty reactions "in anticipation" give rise to a group of diseases that he calls the "as if" disorders.[59] One example of an "as if" disorder is the gastric ulcer. Evidently individuals with gastric ulcers consistently behave physiologically "as if" they were going to kill and eat individuals with whom they are in conflict; i.e., their stomachs prepare for a meal whenever they are faced with a hated opponent. Wolf hypothesizes that such a reaction was appropriate under prehistoric conditions, since primitive man probably *did* want to kill and eat a dangerous opponent. Today, of course, cannibalism is inappropriate, and such behavior on the part of the stomach will not enable an individual to successfully handle a traumatic interpersonal relationship. The inappropriate digestive secretions will instead, over a period of time, lead to the development of gastric ulcers that will further aggravate the individual's life adjustment. Examples of other possible "as if" disorders are heart disease, diabetes mellitus, and hypertension.

2. The Excessive Response. Excessive responses are those "apparent attempts at adaptation which either destroy by sheer excess or that, in correcting one defect, involve the organism in other complications caused directly by this same homeostatic effort."[41] Examples of such reactions abound in medical literature. Anaphylactic shock resulting from an overdose of a drug to which one is sensitive; fibrosis and the overgrowth of scar tissue; and the collagen disease, arthritis, are all disorders resulting from excessive attempts by the body to adapt to stress. In the area of mental disorder, excessive response is evident in persons with manic behavior and in individuals who are obsessive, overly compulsive, hyperactive, or hypersensitive to small stimuli.

3. The Deficient Response.[41] Feebleness, inadequacy, and failure characterize the deficient response to stressors. In essence, the deficient reaction is representative of man's weakness of mind and body and his vulnerability to the endless stresses of life.

There are numerous examples of inadequate responses in human pathology. For instance, secondary infections represent a failure of tissue response; congenital malformation represents a failure of prenatal development. Nutritional deficiency, starvation, paralysis, atrophy, ischemia, necrosis, hypofunction, endocrine failure, impotence, and senility are all common examples of the body's inadequacy and failure to adapt because of deficient responses. The deficient response is characteristic of even the most vigorous people; everyone has his Achilles' heel—his area of special vulnerability. For instance, such problems as poor eyesight, poor digestion, and inadequate coordination are common.

4. The Inappropriate Response. In terms of human physiology and psychology, this type of response can be defined as "an ill-timed, inopportune, misguided, inappropriate, blundering reaction of whatever kind."[41] This is the type of reaction that tends to worsen an already stressful situation. One example of an inappropriate response is the body's tendency, when in heart failure, to absorb large amounts of salt and water—a response which only aggravates matters by overloading an already weakened heart with fluid.

SUMMARY

Let us now generally summarize the topic of human response to stress-producing factors. First of all, the body's organs and structures not only serve to protect us against injury, but they also serve to protect us once injury develops. The body responds to physical injury by means of inflammation, increased capillary permeability, sclerosis, fluid and electrolyte shifts, the production of antibodies, and the development of the immune reaction against infection. Body reactions to stressors—physical, chemical, or bacterial—may be local or generalized.

Second, the body also responds physiologically to psychologic stimuli. Changes in heart action, rate, and rhythm, changes in digestive and urinary tract function, and changes in muscle tone and body temperature all represent physical responses to both negative and positive emotional states. Many of these responses are mediated by the autonomic nervous system.

Third, distorted attempts to adapt to stress can lead to serious consequences for the health of the individual. Responses that are distorted, excessive, deficient, or inappropriate are all maladaptations that can result in injury, disease, and death.

THE MULTIDIMENSIONAL APPROACH TO HEALING

We have emphasized throughout this unit the multidimensional aspects of disease. We have pointed out that disease is not only the product of those noxious forces that impinge upon man from the external world, but that disease also results from man's personal responses to the various stressors external to him. We have attempted to discuss disease and man's reaction to it from the standpoint of multiple disciplines, namely, physiology, biology, medical science, anthropology, psychology, and human ecology.

If disease is the result of multiple factors, both in man and in the environment, it follows, then, that the healing and the treatment of disease by nurses and physicians must also take place on multidimensional levels. Healing in one dimension, whether physical, psychologic or social, is limited healing; it results in what Paul Tillich calls "unhealthy health."[57] This phenomenon of "unhealthy health" occurs if and when "healing under one dimension is successful but does not take into consideration the other dimensions in which health is lacking or even imperiled by the particular healing."

For example, a woman with breast cancer may undergo successful surgery; i.e., her cancerous breast will be removed without complication and she will leave the hospital "cured." This is one-dimensional healing unless the doctor and nurse caring for this woman recognize that the *psychologic trauma* created by the fear of cancer as well as the body mutilation resulting from the surgery must also be treated: anxiety cannot be cut out with a scalpel; fear and grief over loss cannot be excised as one would remove a tumor. Furthermore, the nurse and physician must also carefully consider the woman's *social adjustment* following her breast removal. What will she wear when she goes home? How will she look in a bathing suit or in an evening gown? Will her husband still love her or will he reject her and view her as mutilated? These are questions that the patient will have that are not answered by surgery; surgery can only eradicate the physical problem; it can only work successfully within the physiologic dimension. For a more complete cure to take place, the woman's social adjustment and psychologic problems must be evaluated and treated as well as her physical disease. This will result in more complete healing for the patient, since treatment and nursing care will include all dimensions of her problem.

Nursing, then, must be comprehensive in its scope and in its goals. The educated nurse must be able to understand man's basic needs, and the multiple forces that impinge upon him, as well as the many adaptive and maladaptive techniques that he uses in meeting stress.

Moreover, the modern nurse and doctor must recognize that curing disease and injury is not enough. Today we need to think in terms of man's *total life situation* and the *meaning* that that situation holds for him. We must consider man's adjustment to his environment and to society, as well as the effect of that adjustment or maladjustment on disease causation, cure, and eradication. This is why modern nursing and medicine are not only biologic sciences; they are also *social sciences*. The aims and goals of nursing today center around not just physiologic man or psycho-cultural man, but *total* man—the total patient.

References for Unit II

1. Alland, A.: War and disease: An anthropological perspective. *Bulletin of the Atomic Scientists,* June, 1968. Reprinted from *Natural History,* December, 1967.
2. Bajusz, E.: *Physiology and Pathology of Adaptation Mechanisms, Neural, Neuroendocrine, Humoral.* New York, Pergamon Press, 1968.
3. Beland, I.: *Clinical Nursing: Pathophysiological and Psychosocial Approaches.* New York, The Macmillan Company, 1965.

3a. Birley, J. L.: Stress and disease. *Journal of Psychosomatic Research,* 16:235, August, 1972.

4. Black, M., and Wagner, B.: *Dynamic Pathology: Structural and Functional Mechanisms of Disease.* St. Louis, The C. V. Mosby Company, 1964.

4a. Brock, J. F.: Nature, nurture and stress in health and disease. *Lancet,* 1:701, April 1, 1972.

5. Cameron, C. T.: Anticipated disease—A new concept. *Canadian Medical Association Journal,* 99:307, August 17, 1968.
6. Cammer, L.: The exhaustion of adaptive reserve and depression. *Diseases of the Nervous System.* 30(Suppl.):131, February, 1969.
7. Canter, A. et al.: The frequency of physical illness as a function of prior psychological vulnerability and contemporary stress. *Psychosomatic Medicine.* 28(No. 4, part 1):344, July-August, 1966.
8. Caudill, W.: Cultural perspectives on stress. *Symposium on Stress.* Washington, D.C., Army Medical Service Graduate School, March, 1953.
9. Clegg, E. J.: *The Study of Man: An Introduction to Human Biology.* New York, American Elsevier Publishing Company, Inc., 1968.
10. Clifford, M. C.: Health and the urban poor. *Nursing Outlook,* 17:62, December, 1969.
11. Cloudsley-Thompson, J. L.: *Animal Conflict and Adaptation.* Chester Springs, Pennsylvania, Dufour Editions, Inc., 1965.
12. D'Amelio, R. F.: An approach to health and illness. *Nursing Science,* 3:186, June, 1965.

12a. Diseases of civilization. London Medical Group Seventh Annual Conference. *Nursing Times,* 66: 251, February, 1970.

13. Dubos, R.: *Man Adapting.* New Haven, Yale University Press, 1965.
14. Dubos, R. and Pines, M.: *Health and Disease.* Life Science Library. New York, Time-Life Incorporated, 1965.
15. Dunbar, H.: *Emotions and Bodily Change.* 3rd ed. New York, Columbia University Press, 1946.
16. Edholm, O. C.: *The Physiology of Human Survival,* edited by O. G. Edholm and A. L. Bacharach. New York, Academic Press, Inc., 1965.
17. Engel, G. L.: A unified concept of health and disease. *Perspectives in Biology and Medicine.* 3:459, Spring, 1960.
18. Engel, G. L.: Homeostasis, behavioral adjustment and the concept of health and disease. *In* Grinker, R. L. (ed.): *Mid-Century Psychiatry.* Springfield, Illinois, Charles C Thomas, 1953.
19. Galdston, I. (ed.): *Beyond the Germ Theory; the Roles of Deprivation and Stress in Health and Disease.* New York, Health Education Council, 1954.
20. Harrison, C. A., et al.: *Human Biology: An Introduction to Human Evolution, Variation, and Growth.* New York, Oxford University Press, 1964.
21. Health in a changing world. *Medical Journal of Australia,* 1:37, January 10, 1970.
22. Hill, J. M., and Loeb, E.: The biologically defenseless patient. *Postgraduate Medicine,* 32:36, 1962.
23. Hinkle, L. E.: Normal stress in normal experience. *In* Galdston, J. (ed.): *Beyond the Germ Theory.* New York, Health Education Council, 1954.
24. Irelan, L. M.: *Low Income Life Styles.* Washington, D.C., U. S. Department of Health, Education, and Welfare, Welfare Administration, Publication No. 14, 1967.
25. Josephson, E., and Josephson, M.: *Man Alone: Alienation in Modern Society.* New York, Dell Publishing Company, 1962.
26. Kral, V. A., et al.: Long-term effects of a prolonged stress experience. *Canadian Psychiatric Association Journal,* 12:175, April, 1967.
27. Kruse, H. D.: The interplay of noxious agents, stress and deprivation in the etiology of disease. *In* Galdston, J. (ed.): *Beyond the Germ Theory.* New York, Health Education Council, 1954.
28. Kruse, H. D.: The ratios of health and disease—How the presence, excess, deficit, or absence of conditions evokes disease. *In* Galdston, J. (ed.): *Beyond the Germ Theory.* New York, Health Education Council, 1954.
29. Kuiper, F. C.: A few notes on the disease concept. *Psychiatria, Neurologia, Neurochirurgia,* 70:187, May-June, 1967.
30. Lazarus, R. S.: *Psychological Stress and the Coping Process.* New York; McGraw-Hill Book Company, Inc., 1966.

30a. Levine, M. E.: Holistic nursing. *Nursing Clinics of North America,* 6:253, June, 1971.

31. Levine, R.: Metabolic responses in chronic stress situations. *Symposium on Stress,* March, 1953, p. 46.
32. Lidz, T.: Chronic situations evoking psychological stress and the common signs of the resulting strain. *Symposium on Stress,* March, 1953, p. 116.
33. Lipowski, Z. J.: Psychosocial aspects of disease. *Annals of Internal Medicine,* 71:1197, December, 1969.
34. Martin, H. W., and Prange, A. J.: Human adaptation—A conceptual approach to understanding patients. *Canadian Nurse,* 58:234, March, 1962.

35. Masturzo, A.: *Cybernetic Medicine.* Springfield, Illinois, Charles C Thomas Company, 1965.
36. Masuda, M.: Differing adaptive metabolic behaviors. *Journal of Psychosomatic Research,* 10:239, December, 1966.
37. Meldman, M. J.: A general concept of disease. *Psychosomatics,* 6:383–90, November-December, 1965.
38. Mirsky, I. A.: Metabolic responses in acute stress situations. *Symposium on Stress.* Washington, D.C., Army Medical Service Graduate School, March, 1953.
39. Mumford, E.: Poverty and health. *Nursing Outlook,* 17:32, September, 1969.
39a. Niederland, W. G.: Introductory notes on the concept, definition and range of psychic trauma. *International Psychiatric Clinics,* 8:1, 1971.
39b. Parsons, T.: *The Social System.* Glencoe, Illinois, The Free Press, 1951.
40. Rahe, R., and Meyer, M., et al.: Social stress and illness onset. *Journal of Psychosomatic Research,* 8(No. 1):35, July, 1964.
40a. Reverby, S.: A perspective on the root causes of illness. *American Journal of Public Health,* 62: 1140, August, 1972.
41. Richards, D.: Homeostasis: Its dislocations and perturbations. *Perspectives in Biology and Medicine,* 3:238, Winter, 1960.
42. Richter, C. P.: Behavioral regulation of homeostasis. *Symposium on Stress,* March, 1953, p. 77.
43. Rubin, R. T., et al.: Life stress and illness patterns in the U.S. Navy. 3. Prior life change and illness onset in an attack carrier's crew. *Archives of Environmental Health* (Chicago), 19:753, November, 1969.
44. Sanford, N.: *Self and Society: Social Change and Individual Development.* New York, Atherton Press, 1966.
45. Schwaid, M. C.: A holistic understanding of health in the adult. *Nursing Science,* 3:194, June, 1965.
46. Selye, H.: Stress and the general adaptation syndrome. *British Medical Journal,* 1950, p. 1383.
47. Selye, H.: *The Physiology and Pathology of Exposure to Stress; A Treatise Based on the Concepts of the General Adaptation Syndrome and the Diseases of Adaptation.* Montreal, Acta, 1950.
48. Selye, H.: The physiopathology of stress. *Postgraduate Medicine,* 25:June, 1959.
49. Selye, H.: *The Stress of Life.* New York, McGraw-Hill Book Co., Inc., 1956.
50. Sigerist, H. E.: *Civilization and Disease.* Chicago, University of Chicago Press, 1943.
51. Sodeman, W. A., and Sodeman, W. A., Jr.: *Pathological Physiology: Mechanisms of Disease.* 4th ed. Philadelphia, W. B. Saunders Company, 1967.
52. Spalding, J. M. K.: The effects of psychological phenomena on autonomic function. *Journal of Psychological Phenomena on Autonomic Function,* September, 1965, p. 149.
53. *Statistical Abstract of the United States,* 1969. 90th Annual Edition. Prepared under the supervision of William Lerner, U. S. Department of Commerce, Bureau of the Census, 1969.
54. Stevenson, I.: Physical symptoms during pleasurable emotional states. *Psychosomatic Medicine,* 12:98, March-April, 1950.
55. Stewart, G. T.: Limitations of the germ theory of disease. *Dental Digest,* 74:475, November, 1968.
56. *Symposium on Medical Aspects of Stress in the Military Climate, Proceedings.* Washington, Walter Reed Army Institute of Research, Walter Reed Army Medical Center, 1965.
56a. Taylor, F. K.: A logical analysis of the medico-psychological concept of disease. *Psychological Medicine,* 1:356, November, 1971.
57. Tillich, P.: The meaning of health. *Perspectives in Biology and Medicine,* 5:92, Autumn, 1961.
58. Veith, I.: Historical reflections on the changing concepts of disease. *California Medicine,* 110:501, June, 1969.
58a. Weiss, J. M.: Psychological factors in stress and disease. *Scientific American,* 226:104, June, 1972.
58b. White, B. W.: Critical events in life histories. *Annals of the New York Academy of Sciences,* 193:248, August, 1972.
59. Wolf, S.: A new view of disease. *Journal of American Medical Association,* 84:129, April 13, 1963.
60. Wolf, S.: Disease as a way of life. *Perspectives in Biology and Medicine,* 4:288, Spring, 1961.
61. Wolff, H. G.: A concept of disease in man. *Psychosomatic Medicine,* 24:25, January-February, 1962.
62. Wolff, H. G.: Life situations, emotions, and bodily disease. *Symposium on Stress,* March, 1953, p. 132.
63. Wolff, H. G.: *Stress and Disease.* 2nd ed. Springfield, Illinois, Charles C Thomas, 1968.
63a. Wolfman, E. F., Jr.: Gastroduodenal stress ulcers. *California Medicine,* 116:62, January, 1972.
64. *World Almanac and Book of Facts.* 1970 edition. Luman H. Long, editor. New York, Newspaper Enterprise Association, Incorporated, 1970.

The startling strokes of fate bring mental conflict to man.

I Ching[172]

UNIT III

Understanding the Experience of Illness

Introduction and Study Guide

In illness, one's "normal" state of existence or life pattern is altered. The nature of this alteration is as varied as the individual lives of those who are ill. In order to help patients to adapt to illness and hospitalization the nurse must attempt to comprehend how the state of illness is experienced by each patient in her care. This unit will review some common experiences associated with illness and the existence of the ill. Obviously, because there are many possible interpretations of the meaning of illness, our discussion must be limited to those experiences that we believe are representative or "typical."

The unit will begin with a consideration of illness as a "normal" state of existence (we are not referring here to serious, critical, or terminal illness) and will review some typical experiences with minor illnesses such as we all have probably had. Because of the "shared nature" of illness it is possible for the nurse to reflect on her own experiences with illness and thus better understand how others who are ill may feel. Therefore, after we discuss some typical experiences with illness we shall examine some nursing implications and general conclusions concerning the state of illness which can be derived from our individual experiences and then abstractly applied to "the patient."

In Chapter 9 we shall discuss some of the reasons why people may not seek medical evaluation and care as readily as they perhaps should. The ways in which patients react to medical diagnoses are extremely variable; some typical reactions and the possible meanings to patients of such behavior are considered in Chapter 10. Although the entire unit might be considered a discussion of some of the worries that accompany illness, Chapter 11 will focus on these various concerns in greater detail. If one hopes to understand the existence of the ill it is necessary to examine the sick role in our society—the behavior that our society accepts and expects from the ill; this is taken up in Chapter 12.

Chapter 13 reviews some forms of disorganized behavior and disorganized thought processes that may occur with illness, e.g., confusion or disorientation, hallucinations, illusions, and delusional thinking. In Chapter 14 the concept of body image is reviewed briefly and disturbances of body image are discussed. Next, the care of patients who are terminally ill and in the process of dying is considered. The final chapter focuses on grief as a reaction to loss.

In order to obtain the most benefit from reading this unit, follow this *Study Guide:*

1. Devote some time to thinking carefully about your own experiences with illness. From these experiences, identify ways in which you can better understand how your patients may be feeling and how you can be of help to them.
2. In your own words discuss some of the reasons why people may not seek medical care as soon as they ideally should. Also, briefly discuss those persons who seek medical care more often than their physical condition warrants. In other words, what have you learned about hypochondriacs?
3. Identify and discuss some *general* factors that influence patients' reactions to diagnosis and the state of illness.
4. In giving patient care, attempt to identify how your patients each seem to be reacting *specifically* to diagnosis and the state of illness. Look for evidences of the specific reactions (e.g., shock, denial) discussed in Chapter 10.
5. In giving patient care, attempt to identify how illness has interfered with the usual patterns of gratification of the needs discussed in Chapter 11 (e.g., survival needs, stimulation needs). Then *plan* ways of helping to meet these needs for each patient in your care.
6. What is meant by a "role"? What four expectations do we tend to have of people we think of in the "sick role"? How can these expectations cause problems in patient care?
7. What is meant by confusion or disorientation? Can you give an example of your own of a hallucination, an illusion, and delusional thinking? As you meet confused or disoriented patients try to identify what is causing their confusion or disorientation. Review the medical histories and diagnoses of these patients and evaluate their environments. Incorporate in your nursing care of these individuals appropriate suggestions from Chapter 13.
8. State why knowledge of the concept of body image is important in nursing and how a nurse can help a patient to accept his changing body image.
9. Try to identify your feelings about death and caring for persons who are dying. What have your experiences with death been like? How do you think these experiences have influenced your present attitude? Review factors of importance in giving nursing care to patients who are terminally ill and in the process of dying.
10. What are the three phases of the process of grieving? Why should a nurse understand the grieving process?

CHAPTER 8

Illness: A "Normal" State of Existence

A certain amount of illness is normal in that it is an unavoidable aspect of life. Everyone has had a cold, the flu, measles, or a headache. What is it possible to learn from these experiences?

Let us begin our consideration of the existence of the ill by looking first at our own experiences with illness. In the process of doing this we shall identify some important "nursing insights," that is, insights that nurses should have into how patients feel and what they need when ill. When such insights about the behavior and feelings of patients are based on the recollections of a nurse's own experiences with illness, it is possible for her to give patient care based on "shared feelings" that both patient and nurse have experienced. Nausea, for example, is a common feeling with many illnesses; the nurse who has been nauseated can give more sensitive care to nauseated patients by thinking about her own experience with this symptom.

To begin with, try to recall your experiences with a recent illness—perhaps "the flu." Think specifically about the following three areas: (1) your mood during illness; (2) how medications affected you; and (3) your interests and sense of awareness when ill. Let us briefly discuss each of these topics and some appropriate nursing insights to be derived from them.

MOOD DURING ILLNESS

When you were ill, perhaps you felt something like this:

> Although my mood fluctuated I felt generally somewhat depressed and quite irritable. I had plans and obligations that I could not meet. It was an effort not to be cross and irritable with others who were trying to help me; somehow I felt as if they had let me down because they couldn't make me feel well. Everyone seemed to be full of energy and having a good time except me. Why me? Why did I have to get sick, and why just now? I was depressed and I resented everyone's trying to cheer me up. How did they know how I felt? On the other hand, I resented it if they seemed "long-faced" around me. I guess I didn't know what I wanted. Just when I thought I was feeling better I would get nauseated again or have a headache. It was discouraging. I felt I just wanted to be left alone, and yet, when I was left alone I felt neglected.

What nursing insights into patients' moods can we derive from the above recollections?

Nursing Insights

First of all, the nurse should *expect* that patients' moods and personalities will be affected by illness. Sick people simply do not act as they would if they felt well. Their moods may fluctuate, perhaps from an attempt at gaiety one moment to tears the next. Illness prevents people from doing what they want to do, and often even from being at home, where they want to be. Frustrated people are irritable, and irritable people often have rather rapid mood fluctuations.

In trying to evaluate a particular patient's moods, it is helpful if the nurse has some idea of what his pre-illness personality was like. If there is doubt about whether or not a patient's behavior is seriously "abnormal," that is, represents a gross deviation from his usual behavior, it is advisable to ask friends and family to describe his pre-illness personality.

People often feel *angry* because they have become ill, and they may project this anger onto persons caring for them; again, the nurse should expect that this might occur and not be surprised when it does. The nurse must guard against being so hypertensive that she takes personally patients' anger, tears, or general irritability. She should try to evaluate objectively whether she actually had a part in precipitating the reaction or whether it is attributable to other causes. The hypersensitive nurse who is upset by patients' expressions of mood or emotion adds to the frustrations of those in her care by making them feel badly for "upsetting the nurse."

Nursing requires an ability to be a sounding board for patients and to accept them during both pleasant and unpleasant moments. Although the nurse may feel a sense of discomfort in response to the *specific* manner in which a patient is acting, or his mood, she must be able to convey an attitude of *general* acceptance of the patient as a person. In other words, the attitude that she tries to convey to patients is: "I like you although this specific behavior of yours makes me uncomfortable." This acceptance of the person requires that the nurse demonstrate a genuine appreciation of the patient's frustrations rather than looking at his behavior alone and reacting to it without an understanding of what prompts it.

The hypersensitive nurse often conveys to patients the unfortunate impression that if they are "good" and don't upset her she will take care of them, but if they forget to say "thank you," or cry or are angry she will have hurt feelings and will leave them alone. This attitude places patients under a severe emotional strain.

Also, as we know, when patients must suppress their resentments, physiologic function is affected unfavorably. For fear of angering those persons they are dependent upon for care, patients may feel unable to unburden themselves of anxiety. This attempt to suppress emotion may express itself physiologically through such symptoms as: an increase in angina attacks; elevations of blood pressure in hypertensive patients; precipitation of asthmatic attacks; or an increase in inflammation, irritation, or ulceration in a diseased colon or stomach. A nurse's own mood may, therefore, actually increase the suffering of patients physically and psychologically and may delay their recovery!

We should add that although it is necessary to make allowances for patients' behavior and moods because they are ill, it is also necessary to evaluate such behavior, keeping in mind the fact that excessive and prolonged mood swings may indicate severe emotional difficulties requiring psychiatric aid. In addition, we do not mean to imply that the nurse should accept any behavior of an extreme nature. Obviously if a frustrated patient feels like pounding on the nurse, she cannot say, "Pound away, I understand." We are merely pointing out that a tolerant acceptance is essential, accompanied by an attempt to understand why the patient is acting as he is.

Realistically we expect mood fluctuations to occur even when we feel well; we feel more irritable one day than another. Sometimes we feel in harmony with everyone, and at other times everyone seems to misunderstand us. Patients cannot be unrealistically expected to behave "better" when they are sick than they would if they were well. A patient once said, "I am expected to be more pleasant than the staff and yet I'm the one who is sick!"

Second, because the hospitalized patient is under constant supervision 24 hours a day, his behavior may be subject to overevaluation. To appraise a patient's behavior realistically the nurse should remember that if her own behavior were under 24-hour surveillance, aspects of it might appear extreme. Whereas she can leave the presence of others if she feels upset, the patient has no place to go to be alone. Because of the lack of privacy, being hospitalized is like being in a fish bowl.

Finally, in appraising patients' mood fluctuations the nurse must be cognizant of the *physical* fatigue and discomfort that may be present. She must keep in mind how tired patients become from: (1) lack of sleep; (2) constant interruptions; (3) physical immobilization, e.g., traction, confinement to bed, and casts; (4) pain; (5) vomiting; and all sorts of other discomforts. Fatigue makes us all irritable.

The hallmark of a truly professional nurse is not her ability to take care of patients whom she personally likes and whose pleasant moods make *her* feel good. The professional person has the ability to care for, and about, those patients (often called "difficult") whom she may find personally upsetting. Such a nurse does not expect everyone to be of a similar disposition or even that a given individual will be consistently pleasant, nor does she expect other people to consistently attune their mood to hers. The nurse must be adaptable to patients' moods. She must sense when levity might be enjoyed and when it is out of place; when patients need to be alone as well as when her presence can be helpful. The professional nurse views mood fluctuations as a normal occurrence in the existence of the ill. She attempts to evaluate and understand the moods and behavior of patients in terms of her knowledge of the behavioral sciences and her own life experience.

In summary, moods and behavior generally should be expected to vary in illness from what they are in health. With illness, many signs of irritation may be noted. Such expressions of anxiety need to be evaluated in the light of both the psychologic and physiologic stresses to which patients are subjected.

EFFECTS OF MEDICATIONS DURING ILLNESS

Now, recall again your own experiences with "the flu." This time evaluate how medications affected you and made you feel. Does this sound familiar?

> I didn't take many medications. Really the medicines were a problem in some ways. I had a headache, but anything I took for that upset my stomach. I vomited a lot and had diarrhea. I was given some liquid medication to stop the diarrhea. but it coated my mouth and the taste nauseated me. I had some pills which were to help to prevent nausea, but at first when I took them I vomited them back. Later, when they did stay down I felt so terribly drowsy from them that it was an effort to be awake and I felt unpleasantly groggy. The medicine certainly did affect how I felt; sometimes it made me feel better, but at times it also made me feel worse. On the whole I felt weak, shaky, and very tired. I had been awake a lot at night because I was sick. One night the doctor gave me something to help me to sleep. It really hit me. When I got up to go to the bathroom I felt dizzy and unreal. I almost stumbled and fell.

Let us abstract some nursing implications from these experiences and see how we might better understand patients in terms of their experiences with medications.

A major factor in understanding the existence of the ill is understanding how medications affect the patient. We are not referring here to the specific physiologic actions or major functions of medication; these will be discussed in reference to specific illnesses later in the text. We refer here mainly to the psychologic effects of medications—i.e., alterations of alertness, mood, and behavior—and to the way in which the medication makes the patient feel physically—i.e., dizzy, drowsy, nauseated. These effects are often overlooked and may frequently be significant factors in accidents and misunderstandings that are disruptive to recovery.

For example, let us say that a drug causes a patient to feel mentally "groggy" and somewhat out of touch with his environment. If the nurse is unaware that the patient feels as he does, and moreover that medication is the cause of these feelings, she might make some of the following misinterpretations: (1) She might not realize that the patient requires safety precautions in his care and he might fall, choke, roll over on his I.V., be burned, or otherwise be injured or interfere with his treatment. (2) She might interpret his vague disinterest in his surroundings, and in her, as rudeness or unfriendliness on his part; that is, she may incorrectly infer that he is alert but is deliberately choosing to be uncommunicative. (3) She may think this patient is depressed because he sleeps a great deal or is unusually quiet. (4) She may believe that his physical condition is becoming more serious and that he is becoming unresponsive. All these are serious misinterpretations.

Almost all medications have effects that may be unpleasant for the patient; therefore, he may become discouraged with his treatment and wonder if it's all worth it. Because the doctor has ordered the medication and because the nurse gives it to him, the patient may feel resentful toward those caring for him and feel that they are adding to his misery rather than diminishing it. This is particularly true if the doctor and nurse appear disinterested in how the medication makes him feel. Supportive concern and recognition of the patient's feelings can do much to help him to accept his prescribed medication.

There are times, of course, when the side effects or untoward actions of medications warrant discontinuation of the treatment. In such a situation, the nurse's notes and observations are often helpful in deciding whether or not this is advisable.

Finally, medications may precipitate extreme behavioral changes in patients who are debilitated, very weak, or aged. For example, it is not at all uncommon for a sedative to produce gross confusion and disorientation in aged patients.

Because of the factors just discussed, behavioral evaluations, and evaluations of how the patient feels generally, must always be made carefully in full consideration of the medications the patient is receiving and the possible effects they might have. In attempting to understand the effects of medications upon patients it is useful to bear in mind the following important principle of pharmacology:

> *No drug introduces a new function into an organism; rather it inhibits, accentuates, or otherwise modifies a function that already exists.*

Application of this principle to patient care means that:

> *Medications will not make patients behave or feel totally different than they ever have before; instead, certain behavior, feelings, and so forth, will be exaggerated, diminished, or otherwise modified.*

INTERESTS AND AWARENESS DURING ILLNESS

As a final recollection on your part try to remember what your interests and awareness were like during your own experience with illness. Again let us imagine that the following description is by a "typical" person with "the flu."

> I noticed that it was difficult to be very interested in other people, or in what they were doing or talking about. I was mainly interested in *me* and how I felt from one moment to the next. It was like I was constantly taking my own pulse; i.e., "Do I feel like turning over? do I feel like going to the bathroom again? do I feel better or worse?" I was certainly more aware of my body than I usually am. Certain parts of my body seemed magnified in my mind, as if they were blown up out of all proportion and occupied all of my attention. When I felt sick to my stomach I felt as if I were all one stomach and it was all I could think about; when my head ached I felt as if I were all head. I also noticed that I was acutely aware of sensations, such as odor, movement, light, and sound. I simply felt too nauseated to move. Sudden movements on the part of others irritated me; noises and light seemed magnified in my senses and intensified my headache and irritability. Finally, I noticed that my awareness of time was altered. I dozed a lot, and since I was sick day and night for a couple of days, the light and darkness seemed all foggy and blended together. Somehow it was worse to be sick at night; I felt more alone. When I was sickest, and sleeping a lot, the time seemed to pass quite rapidly and all blur together. However, as I recovered and had a little energy, the time dragged and I felt discouraged that I didn't get well faster.

Once again, with this as an example of "typical" experience while ill, let us see what can be drawn from this example and applied to understanding patients generally.

Nursing Insights

As our example indicates, the ill person is primarily interested in and concerned about himself. This is to be expected for several reasons, the first of which is the fact that illness may threaten survival. When survival is threatened, all a person's adaptive skills are mustered and self-interest becomes paramount; the animal-like reaction of "every beast for himself" comes to the fore.

A second reason for self-interest in the ill is simply the fact that when we are in psychologic or physical pain it *is* most difficult to think of others. Thus, at such times, one becomes "inner-directed" to the self rather than "outer-directed" to others. When we are suffering, our energies are directed toward obtaining relief.

Because the ill person is inner-directed, most conversations with him (and this is most certainly the case with the acutely or critically ill) center on the patient himself. This is as it should be. A patient should not feel pressured to talk about the state of the world, the nurse's life and interests, or other topics. Likewise, he should not feel pressured to talk about himself, but should be encouraged to do so if he wishes. In sum, the patient who talks about himself and his condition is not egocentric, rude, or selfish; he is attempting to adapt to illness. The nurse will find that what a patient says helps her to understand him better; it also helps him to more effectively tolerate his situation.

A third reason for patients' self-interest is the fact that areas of bodily concern tend to be magnified during illness and thus are difficult to put out of mind. We all know that a tiny foreign particle in the eye seems much larger than it actually is, and removing that particle becomes our major concern. We are immobilized in terms of other tasks or interests until our discomfort is relieved. This mental magnification of physical problems is probably adaptive in nature, helping us survive; however, it is often helpful to the patient if the nurse helps to keep his problems in a somewhat "normal" perspective rather than adding to the magnification of them.

For example, if a patient has an abdominal incision he may feel aware only of that incision (it is magnified in his mind and dominates his attention) and thus he may say, "I'm afraid to move because that operation might break open." Although the nurse gives recognition to how he feels and does not belittle him for feeling as he does, she helps the patient to put the incision in perspective with the rest of his body and his total health. "I think I know how you feel, but your operation area is secure. It is important that you move about so that you will recover more rapidly. It hurts at first, but the pain will lessen and your abdomen will actually become stronger than if you just lie still. I want you to try to think about your legs and your lungs as well as your abdomen. By moving your legs around in bed you help your blood circulation, and by coughing and deep breathing you help to keep your lungs free from infection." Having broadened the patient's perspective, from his incision to his total body, the nurse then proceeds to teach him exactly what he can do to help himself.

A fourth reason why self-interest is so predominant in the ill is that their senses are often heightened, again as a protective means of adaptation. As the nurse proceeeds with her work she should constantly be striving to reduce unpleasant odors, disturbing noises, harsh lights, and sudden, jerky movements on her part. All these factors can be most irritating to patients in their state of heightened sensitivity. The nurse who smells of cigarette smoke, strong perfume, bad breath, or body odor often cannot be tolerated at the bedside and is as unwelcome there as the plague. She should have little cause to wonder why she is an ineffective nurse.

Smooth, confident movements, accompanied by explanations of what is going on and what the patient can do to help, are learned skills of immeasurable value in nursing practice. Sudden, rough, and jarring movements make the patient tense and frightened and are a cruel insult to his integrity. Of course, such movements may also be physically painful.

Finally, in addition to being heightened, senses may be distorted during illness. This is true of the sense of time. With illness, time may take on new meaning. It may seem more precious than ever or it may be cursed; it may seem to fly by, with the patient virtually unconscious of its passage, or, for the patient locked in agonizing suffering, it may seem motionless. A distorted sense of time can produce confusion and disorientation. These problems will be discussed in the next unit.

SUMMARY

We have noted the following major insights into patients' interests and awareness during illness:

> The ill person is primarily concerned about himself, because illness may threaten survival.

> When in pain it is difficult to be "other-directed."

> Areas of bodily concern tend to be magnified during illness.

> Senses are often heightened during illness.

> Senses may be distorted during illness.

CHAPTER 9

Recognizing the Need for Medical Attention

The realization that one needs medical care is generally a gradual process rather than a sudden revelation. Often it is extremely difficult for people to seek out and submit to medical evaluation. By the time the patient reaches the doctor's office, clinic, or hospital he may have experienced a great deal of anxiety about his condition. Weeks, months, and even years may pass between the beginning of an illness and the time when some patients finally come for an evaluation of their ailments; sometimes they arrive in an ambulance and sometimes their arrival is too late for help to be given.

REASONS WHY PEOPLE MAY NOT SEEK MEDICAL HELP

What are some of the reasons why seeking medical assistance can be so psychologically difficult? First of all, there is a *realistic financial concern* in many situations. Many people feel that they simply cannot afford to be sick and have to lose time from work or caring for a family, pay doctor and hospital bills, buy medications, and so forth. And so they postpone seeking help in the vain hope that their condition will improve. Also, there is the fact that sometimes it is *difficult to estimate the seriousness of the condition.* Often it takes time to determine whether or not an illness is a lasting condition, which requires professional treatment, or whether the illness will be brief and fleeting in nature. A period of time may pass while the person observes and evaluates his symptoms to decide whether they are getting better or worse.

Some people experience *doubt as to whether or not the symptoms are "real"* or "just something I imagine." It is rather common today to hear patients preface a discussion of their ailments with statements such as, "Maybe I'm neurotic, but . . . "; or "Maybe it's all in my head; however . . ."; or "I guess I'm just an old hypochondriac; nevertheless. . . ." Such statements reflect the fact that many people in our society today have a little bit of knowledge about anxiety, hypochondriasis, neuroticism, psychosomatics, and so forth, and, on the basis of their incomplete knowledge, become fearful that their symptoms might be "imaginary." Such people are reluctant to seek medical evaluation because of worry that the doctor may find nothing wrong with them and they will feel embarrassed for taking up his time. Such "neurotic" fears on the part of partially informed persons are not uncommon and have unfortunately kept some people from seeking treatment for physical conditions (e.g., heart conditions, diabetes, malignancies) until their condition passes beyond the treatable phase and death or disability ensues. Other people may spend long periods of time suffering from disorders that could easily be alleviated in a short time.

An individual's *conception of illness* is another factor that may cause delay in seeking medical aid. One study[180] has demonstrated, for example, that middle-class Americans generally believe that to be "ill" means that one has an ailment of recent origin that interferes with one's usual activities. Persons who view illness in this manner are oriented more toward acute infectious diseases with obvious symptoms (these diseases are decreasing) than they are toward chronic illnesses (which are becoming more common). In the early stages of chronic illness, symptoms may persist over a period of time without necessarily becoming worse or interfering with usual activities. Persons with the early stages of chronic illnesses may not think of themselves as ill and may delay seeking early diagnosis and treatment. Obviously, judgment as to whether one views himself as ill has a bearing on whether he will seek medical help.

There are additional reasons why people may not go to doctors even though they feel that something is wrong with them. At times people will neglect finding out what their problem is because they *"fear the worst."* They appear to feel that by ignoring the trouble, it will resolve itself; they live in the hope of wishing away their illness. Many people live in this state of fearful uncertainty. They will dread the worst rather than seek their doctor's opinion. Sometimes the illness does prove to be serious and the physician's diagnosis coincides with the patient's fears; i.e., he does need surgery, or has cancer, tuberculosis, or the heart problem he feared. Reluctance to learn of such problems is naturally understandable. However, more often than not the diagnosis will be of a less severe problem than that imagined. With any treatable condition, the sooner treatment can begin, the better it is for the patient's well-being. It should also be recognized that medicine and nursing can provide palliative and comfort measures for those with incurable illnesses.

The nurse may serve in her community as a bridge between patients and doctors. Because of her place in the health professions, the nurse who recognizes how difficult it is for many people to seek medical care will be in a unique position to help patients. Often people feel more comfortable in talking with a nurse than with a doctor. At home and in her community the nurse may frequently be approached by people asking her if *she* thinks they ought to go to the doctor. In effect they are asking her to make their decisions for them; also, however, they are asking for her support. Many people find it easier to go to the doctor or phone him if they can say, "A nurse I talked with thought I should come in." The nurse, of course, cannot diagnose and treat; however, she can provide real service by helping people to reach someone who can evaluate their symptoms. Often, after talking about his condition, his fears and his concerns with the nurse, the patient is relaxed enough that he feels comfortable in proceeding to the clinic or doctor.

Let us next examine some attitudes toward a patient or his condition that might be detrimental to him once he has reached the doctor and nurse, attitudes that might make him feel uncomfortable about having come in. (1) *Scolding* the patient for not coming in sooner is obviously embarrassing to him and might make him reluctant to return the next time for fear of further reprimands. (2) Any sign of irritation *minimizing* the patient's concerns, so that he is made to seem "silly" for being worried and coming in for care, is rude and belittling. Implying that he "pampers" himself and "gives in" to illness too readily or that he is overly concerned with his health will make it much more difficult for him to seek care again. Examples of statements that minimize the patient's concerns are: "You mean this is all that's bothering you?"; "Couldn't this have waited a day or so?"; or (in an irritated tone) "Everything has been checked out, nothing is wrong, you worry too much." (3) On the other hand, an attitude that *overalarms* the patient about his symptoms may frighten him away from further medical care by making him decide, "It's worse than I thought. There's no telling what will have to be done to me. Maybe it's too late anyway." (4) Finally, an attitude that is *too casual* and *joking* about a patient's condition may make him feel that his condition is not being taken seriously enough.

The psychologic discomfort of having to submit to a *physical examination* and a discussion of one's *intimate life history* are also factors that keep some patients from seeking medical evaluation. For many the physical contact necessary during a physical examination is sexually threatening or otherwise disturbing and emotionally charged. People dislike being poked, probed, peered into, and exposed, and often have feelings of helplessness, fear, and resentment toward the examiner. Submitting to diagnostic procedures also may be dreaded because of fear of pain, exposure, and the unknown. The nurse can be of direct assistance to patients and help to relieve or minimize fears and anxiety in all these areas.

Too often physicals, histories, and diagnostic examinations are conducted in a manner embarrassing and dehumanizing for patients, as in assembly-line fashion they are unhappily put through the mill of medical science: they are asked to talk and then are thoughtlessly interrupted; they are excluded from conversation and "talked around and about" even though they are often lying in the middle of the group and the conversation is about them; they are vacantly stared at, or gazed through, as if they were lifeless; they are crudely and needlessly exposed; they are whisked out of their room without explanation; they are bluntly asked tactless questions and subjected to rude comment, often in front of a group, as their private life and distresses are made public. When people are expected to surrender all claims to human sensitivity, as in the above instances, it is no wonder that many delay "medical assistance and care" as long as possible. Needless to say, none of these examples constitutes acceptable medical or nursing practice. If we really want to understand why patients are reluctant to seek medical aid and accept nursing care, we must look honestly and with sensitivity at existing practices.

Some patients avoid seeking medical care because of the *previous unfortunate experiences* which they, or others whom they know, have had with doctors, medicine, and surgery. Sometimes the criticisms leveled against the medical profession, nurses, and hospitals are justified; at other times they appear not to be. The important point, in terms of this discussion, is the feeling that one cannot trust those persons needed to give care. And, on the basis of this, even when feeling ill, people may not seek necessary medical care. Persons who feel that doctors and nurses have been rude, callous, incompetent, and indifferent to them will naturally be reluctant to seek out what they view as "more of the same." Winning back the confidence of such injured persons is a difficult task, but it is not an impossible one. Patients who feel they cannot trust us are frightened, and justly so, for they often place their life in our hands.

In such a situation, it is most important to let the person talk about what happened in the past and to remain nonjudgmental yet supportive. The listener should not rush to the immediate defense of the doctor, nurse, or hospital being criticized, with statements such as: "I'm sure they were just doing what had to be done and what was right . . . after all, the doctor or nurse knows best," or "It was probably hospital policy to do it that way." Reacting in this manner will cause the patient to feel that it is useless to talk further because the listener appears to have already made up her mind that no matter what the situation may be, the staff is always right.

Instead of leaping to judgmental statements, such as those above, it is often most helpful to begin by attempting to find out all the information the person has about the situation, and thus to generally encourage discussion of the incident, rather than implying that you are certain that the "medical people" were right and you don't want to discuss it further. Often broad, supportive statements are helpful, such as, "So much about illness is frightening, isn't it?" or "It's upsetting to hear about an incident like your friend's experience." It is possible to encourage the person to think more critically about what he heard, saw, or experienced by saying something like, "It is difficult to understand such occurrences. What do you think was actually happening?"

After the person has been allowed to talk about the incident that frightened him, it is helpful to proceed to talk about his own current situation. For example, if he has just learned that he is going to need surgery, and he has told you about the frightening things that happened to his friend who had surgery, you can say something like, "I guess you must be wondering what will happen to you now after hearing about your friend's experience." Then it is possible to begin to talk about how his experience and condition may differ from his friend's, and to identify some of his specific fears and concerns.

In sum, some of the reasons why people may not seek medical attention as readily as they should are:

> realistic financial concern

> difficulty in realizing the seriousness of the condition

> doubt concerning whether or not the symptoms are real

> confused concepts of illness

> fear of the worst

> discomfort of physical examinations and history-taking

> previous unfortunate experiences

Let us now look briefly at the other side of the coin and consider those patients who seek medical attention more often than their condition warrants.

PERSONS WHO SEEK MEDICAL CARE MORE OFTEN THAN NECESSARY

Patients of this nature are often referred to rather loosely as "hypochondriacs." Let us consider the concept of "hypochondriasis" briefly. The term is frequently heard in lay discussions; as far as professional usage goes, the term is actually a generic, *descriptive* one rather than a distinct nosologic entity. It is still found in some literature, however, and generally refers to persons who have a tendency to show somatic "overconcern" and who have physical symptoms with no basis in demonstrable organic changes. Thus, the concept is somewhat synonymous with psychogenic functional disorders.*

Without using the term "hypochondriasis" we would say that some individuals show a very high level of concern and preoccupation with their body functions. Such persons may seek out medical attention far more often than their physical condition warrants. Although these patients are a source of irritation to some medical personnel, two factors must be kept in mind: (1) At least they do seek out medical evaluation, and it is important that they do, for these patients can develop serious physical ailments as readily as anyone else; therefore they should *not* be discouraged from asking for care. (2) These patients *are* ill and *are* in need of care, for their bodily concern signifies a high level of anxiety and, in fact, they do not feel well.

*Psychogenic functional disorders are discussed in Unit IV.

CHAPTER 10

Reactions to the Confirmation of Illness

Illness lays bare the character of what may be called the patient's "security system." By this is meant the adequacy of the patient's behavior patterns in relationship to the demands of his environment. A weak security system is made even weaker by illness or disability, a strong security system is made even stronger. That is to say, illness is a crisis in the life of the individual, and any crisis serves to test and to display the strength of the person's resources for dealing with his world.

Reinhardt and Meadows[154]

In the previous chapter we have reviewed some of the difficulties that a patient may experience during the transitional period when he comes to realize that he is ill. In this chapter we shall continue ahead to that interval of time when the patient actually learns what his diagnosis is and thus faces the fact of a confirmed illness.

What are some typical reactions to illness and diagnosis? What are some of the general factors that contribute to how a patient thinks about his illness and reacts to it? These questions are the concern of this chapter.

GENERAL FACTORS INFLUENCING REACTIONS TO DIAGNOSIS AND ILLNESS

We could say, generally, that four factors combine to determine how a patient reacts to his diagnosis or illness: (1) the nature of the illness; (2) the nature of the patient; (3) the attitudes of others toward the illness; and (4) the patient's own attitudes toward the illness. Let us consider each of these factors in turn.

1. The Nature of the Illness. Illnesses have become departmentalized and differentiated within hospitals by the formation of special wards, and they have been segregated by professional persons into areas of specialization or interest, but illnesses cannot be categorized in terms of patient response to them. Each response is unique; the same illness holds different meanings for different individuals. The unique meaning of a given illness for a patient will, in part, determine his reaction to that illness. The disease or illness that one person dreads is not particularly frightening to someone else; conditions that may seem minor in nature to a professional person may be of major concern to a patient—in fact, may panic him. The type of illness that an individual has is thus of great personal importance to him. The prognosis, severity, and expected length of illness are additional factors of great concern to an ill person.

2. The Nature of the Patient. Individual responses to illness are largely determined by the characteristic responses to anxiety that every individual has developed during his life. Each person's pattern of using mental defense mechanisms* actually becomes his characteristic *personality pattern*. An individual will therefore respond to the anxieties of illness as he has responded to other anxiety-provoking situations, in accordance with his basic personality traits. One individual may calmly accept his fate and treatment, whereas another with the same diagnosis may become disorganized in behavior, depressed, argumentative, and resistive to medical care. We shall discuss some examples of specific defensive behavior later in the chapter.

In addition to his unique pattern of mental defense, an individual's *ideas about himself,* i.e., his self-concept, and his *personal philosophy of life* will also determine in part his reaction to his diagnosis and illness. A part of this general feeling about oneself and one's life is a feeling of motivation toward either health or sickness. These are subtle kinds of feelings that most of us are not even conscious of. Nonetheless, such feelings become apparent when life histories are subjected to careful evaluation. For example, we all know some people who tend to be ill more or less continually and others who are almost always well. For some people illness is more a life pattern than health is; it is actually a more manageable way of life for them than a healthy state. We do not mean to imply that all people who are ill at any given time are motivated to illness. We are referring instead to life styles, or long-range patterns. This motivation toward health or illness is a crucial factor in the reaction to illness, and in the patient's recovery pattern.

Other factors that influence individual reactions to illness are: age, social class, general state of personal happiness, financial position, and num-

*The mental defense mechanisms are discussed in Unit IV.

ber of past illnesses. Some brief examples of the influence of such factors follow: (a) *Age:* older people may be able to accept an illness with a poor prognosis more calmly than a younger person. (b) *Social class:* certain diseases tend to be accepted more readily in one social class than in another; e.g., venereal disease may be more accepted among lower class persons than those of middle class. (c) *General state of personal happiness:* persons who are happy and feel loved may find illness and hospitalization difficult to bear because it means separation from home and loved ones; on the other hand, lonely, unhappy people may feel that they receive more attention, and are the object of more concern, when ill than when they are well. (d) *Financial position:* for those of low to middle income, with no health insurance, an illness may rapidly plunge them into overwhelming debt, while well-to-do persons do not have this concern. (e) *Number of past illnesses:* One's first experience with major illness may seem almost unreal, because it brings the realization of one's vulnerability to illness.

3. The Attitudes of Others Toward a Patient's Illness are readily communicated to him, and will, in turn, influence his own reaction to his illness. For example, some illnesses are more socially "acceptable" than others and these are less anxiety-provoking for the patient. If the patient's illness is of an "unacceptable" nature, e.g., venereal diseases, he may feel rejected, "dirty," and victimized. Some illnesses are threatening to other people. Communicable diseases like tuberculosis and leprosy provoke fear in many people as a threat to their own health; they may, therefore, shun a patient with these illnesses. Conditions that are mutilating and disfiguring, e.g., burns, accidents, skin conditions, open ulcers, gangrene, may evoke strong reactions of disgust, fear, and revulsion in others. The same is true of conditions with offensive odors which may cause others to choke, gag, tear, and generally appear nauseated. Obviously such reactions are apparent to the conscious patient and decidedly mar his self-image and influence his reaction to his illness.

4. The Patient's Own Attitudes Toward the Illness. Illness is a major disruption to normal living for the patient and also is disturbing to his self-image. His self-concept may undergo rapid and extreme alterations as a result of the physical and mental effects of the illness, and its effects upon others in his life. If he is to live a life that is at all satisfactory during his illness, and afterwards, the patient must adapt psychologically; he must regain the psychologic equilibrium that his illness has disrupted.

The patient is called upon to adjust his needs to the demands that his illness imposes. He will attain psychologic equilibrium during illness (if he can) in exactly the same ways he has at other times in his life: through the trial and error process of learning. Those caring for him must give him the time to learn and must be patient with him as he undergoes the trials and errors of adaptation.

It has been observed[127] that everywhere in life, whenever disruption of functions takes place, spontaneous synthesis and regeneration occur. This is true of both mind and body. Just as the body immediately begins to try to protect itself and heal when it suffers an insult, so the mind begins to strive for adaptation when illness strikes. For successful recovery to take place, *both* physical and mental adaptive mechanisms must function successfully and have sufficient time to do so. Some individuals recover physically from a critical illness or injury but are unable to regain a healthy level of psychologic adaptation; others adjust to the reality of their infirmity with amazing psychologic tenacity and grace, but die.

Some of the early attempts that a person makes at psychologic adaptation to his illness, or to the knowledge of his diagnosis, may be impulsive and irrational in nature. He may be attempting to solve this problem by defensive patterns that have worked for him in the past but are inappropriate in this new situation. Indeed, some of the early or most immediate behavioral responses to an illness may not seem to be at all in a person's best interest, since his behavior may actually alienate him from those upon whom he depends for help and care. Also, under the stress of illness a patient may be unable to think rationally or to make sound decisions. However, whether these early attempts at adaptation appear "ideal" or not, the initial reactions to his illness are probably the most protective patterns of behavior upon which the patient can draw at the time.

SPECIFIC REACTIONS TO DIAGNOSIS AND THE STATE OF ILLNESS

In order for you to more readily comprehend the situations about to be discussed, pause to imagine that you have had some backaches over a period of time which have been growing steadily worse. You have had some diagnostic tests and are now hearing the results of these from your doctor. He tells you that there is no doubt about it, *you* have cancer of the spine! Before reading further, stop to think about this situation. It happens to people daily. What influence would this have on your life, right now? How does it make you feel? What might your response or reply to the doctor be? What is *your* reaction to the diagnosis?

Anxiety. The predominant early response to diagnosis and illness is a feeling of anxiety*—physical and mental. Why does this response occur? Probably the fundamental basis for feeling anxious at such times is that "any disease is a failure, more or less complete, of the organism. Complete failure, of course, is death. From the start, therefore, illness is allied with anxiety, and it tends to arouse all the anxiety-laden feelings of the patient."[154] Anxious feelings, then, are actually feelings of concern for one's life and well-being.

*Anxiety is discussed in detail in Unit IV.

The specific causes of anxiety are variable from person to person and are probably associated with the fact that the situation in which the person finds himself provokes into action many unconscious thoughts and feelings that have been repressed and inhibited up to that time. Fantasies, fears, dreams, and bits of repressed reality are all uncomfortably stirred up as awareness of an illness penetrates the mind. Anxiety, as we know, is capable of increasing physiologic and psychologic pain. We also know that high levels of anxiety can affect the course of treatment adversely. It is becoming increasingly clear, for example, that patients who are extremely anxious prior to surgery are poorer surgical risks and tend to have a stormier postoperative course than patients who are relatively at ease preoperatively.

Shock

> The internal and external communications needed for the integration of functions temporarily stop at the impact of catastrophe. The cerebral cortical awareness and the diencephalic adaptive controls no longer apply. We see this process of sudden disintegration most graphically in shock-phenomena.[127]

Many people experience a period of shock when they first learn of their diagnosis, particularly if it is serious in nature. They feel immobilized; things seem unreal and dream-like. Even their own behavior may seem unreal to them, as if they were watching a motion picture of themselves and time has slowed down. Often shock makes people incapable of thinking clearly or acting rationally. For a period of time their behavior may make no sense to themselves or to others; they may act automatically and like robots. For example, a patient when told that she has cancer may vacantly reply, "Yes—well, I'd better go and get the grocery shopping done." Indeed she may then walk out of the doctor's office, do the grocery shopping, and not even recall for a period of time what she has been told. She retreats for a time into the protective insulation of a dream-like state. When the period of shock begins to end, however, and an awareness of reality returns, she may collapse and sob or suddenly become extremely depressed, perhaps even suicidal. Individuals in a state of shock need protective care and understanding and must be helped especially as the shock lessens.

Denial. The person in shock is denying his illness. Denial of illness, however, often continues long after the initial shock has passed. "I'm really not sick." "How could *I* possibly have cancer? I don't believe it!" These are examples of verbal denial. The reasons why it is necessary for an individual to deny his illness are many. Whatever the reasons, the nurse should bear in mind that the denying patient is not being stubborn. What may appear to be obstinate behavior is generally a frightened attempt, on the patient's part, to fend off overwhelming threats. Denial is protective, and one must proceed with care in deciding how to approach this protective shield. Forcing the patient to lay down his armor too soon and "face facts" may mean making him vulnerable to a painful reality which he may be unable to endure.

The adaptive value of denial can be seen in the daily practice of nursing where it is not uncommon to meet patients who deny their illness for a period of time and then, upon finally accepting it, rapidly die. The process of denial appears to have been life-sustaining for such persons. Instances have been cited in which patients have committed suicide when they have finally come to "accept" their diagnosis. Is it wrong for such people to *live* in the dream that they are healthy? Some patients die denying that they are ill, and this has probably been felt to be therapeutically best for the patient. Their denial is left uninterrupted. Other patients are slowly helped to accept the reality of their illness and to adapt to it even though it may be fatal. The physician should determine how a patient's denial should be treated.

As we have seen, denial must be handled gently, for it is often a safety valve that prevents the emergence of sheer panic and terror. When you see a patient denying his condition you may think that he is merely pretending that he doesn't believe what he knows is true. The denying patient is not trying to fool anyone. In true denial the patient honestly believes that he does not have the problem that he is denying. He feels convinced that others are wrong, and will search desperately for evidence to support his belief. This quest for supportive evidence may lead such a patient to distort what he sees or hears, and therefore he may misquote you or his doctor. If this occurs, try to understand that his goal is not to make life difficult for anyone, but rather to make life bearable for himself.

Like any other behavior, denial occurs in various degrees. *Forgetting* is a mild form of denial; forgetting to take one's medication, forgetting to keep a doctor's appointment, or forgetting to stay on a prescribed diet are all mild forms of denial of illness. It is mentally convenient to "forget" what it is uncomfortable to remember. In situations of more extreme denial we find that, in a pathetic struggle to prove that they are well, some people will push themselves into states of overexertion or make hopeless pilgrimages from one consultation room to another. They are trying to reassure themselves that they are not ill and do not have the disease that has been diagnosed. The danger of such actions is, of course, that it will prove fatal to the patient.

As we have said, at times a patient may be allowed to continue to deny his actual diagnosis; when little hope or treatment can be offered, nothing would be gained in bringing him to an acknowledgment of his fate. The nurse must respect such a decision and reinforce it. As for those patients who die because their denial causes them to overexert or avoid treatment, who can judge their actions? Certainly the nurse cannot. For some people serious illness may mean invalidism, weakness, dependency—all unacceptable ways of life for them. Each patient's life is his own and how he chooses to live or die is his choice. Although the nurse must make every attempt to help a patient to accept treatment that will help him, she cannot force treatment on him or make decisions that are not hers to make.

Denial is very much a part of life. We all try to deny much of the unhappiness, suffering, and apparent waste of life that we know exists throughout the world. You, as a nurse, will find much that you may want to deny. However, nursing actions must be based on reality. Giving up denial means facing truths that are often difficult to accept. In nursing it means facing life as it is and then trying to do what can be done to make some of life's harsh realities more bearable.

Suspicion. Some people react to their diagnosis with suspicion. These feelings are closely related to those of denial, but the patient who is suspicious has not *completely* closed his mind to the possibility that his diagnosis may be true. He tries, however, to find many possible reasons for doubting the diagnosis. Suspicious statements will sound like these: "I'm fine—that doctor is just out to make some money." "The family just wants to put me in the hospital and be done with me." "The laboratory made a mistake; that report must be about someone else." "You are all lying to me, but I know what you're up to." You will find that some patients will be suspicious of their diagnosis if it *is* serious in nature, whereas others will be suspicious if their diagnosis does *not* prove to be serious. Therefore, one patient may say, "I don't believe you; it's not as serious as you make out," and another will say, "I don't believe you, this can't be all that's wrong with me. I know you're keeping something from me."

As we have said, adjustment and adaptation take time. If a person's life pattern has been one founded on suspicion, that is, "Everyone tries to take advantage of me," his initial reaction to the anxiety of illness and diagnosis will undoubtedly be one of suspicion. Some doubt is reasonable, but suspicion can grow out of proportion, so that the person becomes suspicious about everything. "My bill is going to be padded." "I don't believe that that medicine is for what you say it is." "Everyone is talking about me." "I know they're going to do more in surgery than they said they would." Such extreme suspicion is a serious, reportable condition.

Patients who are suspicious are not just complaining; they are frightened and feel that they must be on their guard or they will be hurt and taken advantage of. The suspicious person lacks trust in others, and the person who lacks trust asks a lot of questions. This may prove to be irritating; however, patience is necessary since trust is not easily or rapidly built.

Questioning. "Why me? Why did I have to get this? Why do I have to suffer?" People who are ill often scan their lives trying to find the answers to such questions and believing that there must be a reason for or a purpose to their illness. While some can find no answers to explain their misfortune of being ill, others find a variety of explanations such as: illness is a punishment for sin; illness results from neglect of one's health; or illness is predestined and is in one's best interest. Still other patients may view their illness scientifically in biologic or psychologic terms. Another answer to the question "Why me?" is simply that illness is a part of life, something we are susceptible to and which occurs purely as a random phenomenon of nature.

Regardless of the answers, there are many questions about illness that evoke anxious feelings. For example, why does one person have a cancer confirmed at surgery while another's condition proves to be benign? Why does one person recover while another dies? Why does one person escape from a serious accident unscathed while another is mutilated?

Insignificance and Loneliness. Illness makes one feel insignificant, like a grain of sand on a beach. It also causes one to feel alone in facing his problems. Illness brings with it the realization that we all pass through life in separate orbits. We cannot move out of ours and into that of another person if we find our journey is frightening or is soon to end. Patients often feel trapped in their illness. "I can see what is happening to me. I know what will happen to me. But I can't alter it and neither can anyone else."

Regression and Dependency. Regression is a common reaction to illness; it is a natural reaction, when not extreme, since it facilitates recovery by allowing the patient to be more dependent than usual. By allowing himself to rest and be cared for the patient can restore his strength and can progress to health.

It has been pointed out by Meerloo[127] that regression often acts as a defensive device against stress. Under stress all organisms tend to assume a less differentiated, more primitive way of life. On the microscopic level, multicellular organisms may become unicellular at times of stress or danger. In the body, "A temporary regression takes place when an injury occurs; more primitive cells, the fibroblasts, take over for regeneration and repair as if they temporarily returned to a state of omnipotent capacity."[127] Meerloo further points out that a different management of energy takes place with regression; the regressive principle leads the organism by means of the path of least resistance to a phase of greater inertia but regained stability. Regression thus helps in the process of attaining greater stability and better adaptation both physiologically and psychologically. It is a kind of "strategic retreat of the organism in order to mobilize new forces of resistance and regeneration."[127]

Therefore in illness it should be expected that patients will regress to levels of behavior that are not as mature as those which they assume when well. They need to be allowed sufficient and appropriate regression and dependence upon others in order to recover. In a state of regression the patient may think of the nurse as a sort of "mother figure"; he hopes for the ideal "mother" who will care for him lovingly, gently, and with concern. These are important qualities for any nurse.

Shame and Guilt. When patients believe that their illness is a punishment for sin or wrongdoing (either imagined or real), they may react with feelings of shame or guilt. Also, certain diseases may make an individual feel disgraced or ashamed, depending upon his family and cultural background. Some people feel that they shame their family by having certain "unacceptable" conditions (e.g., mental disorders, epilepsy, venereal disease, tuberculosis) and they feel responsible for having brought on the condition. Feelings of shame and guilt related to illness are damaging to the self-concept. In some conditions, such as alcoholism, the patient may be viewed by others as weak-willed, or he may think of himself in those terms.

Rejection. Illness may precipitate feelings of being rejected. Although some of these feelings of rejection may be imagined, often they are partially based on reality, since illness does actually cause one to be removed from his usual life patterns and state of health. Those illnesses that are socially unacceptable or socially threatening to others, e.g., communicable disease, cause the patient to be rejected and isolated even more. Prolonged illnesses create many feelings of rejection in the patient's personal life, as friends and loved ones may begin to take the illness for granted and proceed with their own lives. Because illness does cause the patient to be shut out from many activities of life, it is especially important to him to have warm relationships with those caring for him.

At times patients may imagine that they are rejected because of illness when this is really not the case. In such situations the patient may be using his illness as an excuse for not receiving the attention of others instead of looking objectively at his pre-illness behavior.

Fear. The fears that accompany the realization that one has a dreaded disease are many. Most of this unit is a discussion of such concerns and the ways in which people react to them. Here we shall present a brief list of some specific fears that often accompany illness:

> fear of a strange place, i.e., the hospital, nursing home, and so forth.
> fear of equipment—"Will it hurt me? What if it doesn't run right?"
> fear of pain, loss of body parts, or mutilation
> fear of being "experimented" on
> fear of having to suffer as punishment for past misbehavior
> fear of being abused, neglected, having one's feelings hurt, or in other ways being treated impersonally
> fear of being left alone or isolated from loved ones
> fear of loss of function or loss of self-control
> fear of death
> fear of burdening others

Many of these fears begin in childhood and accompany us, in various forms, throughout our lives. They are the subject of our fantasy and discussion, and, as we observe manifestations of these fears in others, they gradually become part of our own feelings. Much of this mental activity is repressed until illness, with its accompanying anxiety, reaches the tap roots of our minds and the fears resurface and magnify.

Often it is true that what is imagined and anticipated is more frightening than the actual experience; nevertheless, the dread is there. The fearful person may be hostile to others; he is on the defensive and trying to protect himself. He is ready to fight, but often he can't identify what he should strike out at. Anxiety and hostility are often interrelated.

Attempting to guess what a patient's fears may be is not good practice; through guessing you may suggest fears that he hadn't thought of but that will now disturb him. For example, suppose you are talking with a patient who is about to go to surgery. He appears fearful and so you guess at what his fears are and say, "Perhaps you're worried that you'll choke while you're unconscious because you can't swallow. Don't worry. Someone will suction you out until you are awake." Probably the patient didn't have that in mind at all, but he will now! Let the patient tell you what he is fearful of. You may make general comments, however, such as, "It isn't unusual to be frightened at a time like this. In fact it's perfectly normal. If you would like to talk about how you feel, I might be of some help to you."

Withdrawal and Depression

> The actions of withdrawal by human beings are numberless: fantasy, autistic image-making, inferiority feelings, shyness, delusions, illusions, melancholia, anxieties, fears, self-incriminations, and so on. The individual thus turns to an internal drama, with isolating themes, wish-fulfilling thoughts and actions, and actors formed in the molds of unrestrained impulse.[154]

Withdrawal and depression commonly occur as reactions to diagnosis and illness. Like most of the other reactions discussed so far, we expect some of this behavior to accompany illness. Excessive or prolonged withdrawal or depression, however, is a cause for real concern, and signs or symptoms of these conditions should be reported.

Let us briefly consider some common experiences and expressions during depression. The depressed person typically appears sad or shows little expression. The forehead is furrowed, the mouth turned down. Personal hygiene may be neglected. Women may not put on make-up and comb their hair; men may not shave even though they are physically able.

Physically the body as a whole appears to be slowed down or not working properly. This general slowing down process affects bowel function (constipation), the menstrual cycle, and sexual interest. Food may seem tasteless, and the appetite is poor. The depressed person often loses weight and may suffer from a feeling of choking or tightness in the throat and a hollowness in the stomach. Sleep disturbances may occur, with insomnia and early morning wakening. When sleep does come, it is often broken or disturbed by bad dreams and nightmares, and the person awakens fatigued. Often such a patient awakens in the early morning hours filled with self-torturing thoughts or, in the presence of illness, to the reality of illness and suffering. In a desperate attempt to escape both his physical and mental anguish he may attempt to take his life.

With depression there are often evidences of sloth, weariness, exhaustion, persistent lassitude, inner tension, inertia, and a general lack of energy. However, in states of *agitated depression,* the patient may be hyperactive: pacing, moving about, picking rapidly at the bed clothing, and so on. Patients in states of agitated depression should be protected against suicidal attempts. Some additional typical signs of depression are sighing, wringing the hands, slow speech, and frequent weeping.

The severely depressed person longs for an escape from his life situation, which he feels is intolerable. He may, therefore, be preoccupied with thoughts of death and/or suicide. Often it is difficult for the depressed individual to concentrate, and he may have difficulty remembering. His affect centers primarily around feelings of despair, hopelessness, isolation, and desolation. The depressed person often withdraws from others. He may pull the shades, turn out the lights, pull the covers up around his head and shoulders, and not respond to the presence of others. He is suffering and in need of medical and/or psychiatric aid.

It is not uncommon for people under the stress of serious or terminal illnesses to express fears of "losing their mind" because they are unable to take their minds off themselves and their troubles. They may feel that they cannot endure their state. These troubled persons should not have their concerns minimized; they need opportunities to discuss how they feel and what they are worried about. Sometimes just talking about the pressures they are under is of help. Notation should be made of such a patient's distress, for he may benefit from skilled psychiatric evaluation and consultation. Some patients find relief in talking with their spiritual adviser or the hospital chaplain.

Paradoxical Reactions. At times patients respond to their diagnoses in ways that are paradoxical, that is, not at all what we might expect. For example, they may joke about their condition, even though it is extremely serious. Individuals with neurotic tendencies may appear relieved to learn that they are ill or that they require surgery. These are not expected reactions and may catch the nurse unaware of what is happening. Like all other reactions, these should be accepted as the individual's unique reaction to stress.

SUMMARY

In this chapter we have discussed some various ways in which people react to a diagnosis and the state of illness. We identified four general factors that influence these reactions. These were: (1) the nature of the illness; (2) the nature of the patient; (3) the attitudes of others toward a patient's illness; and (4) the patient's own attitudes toward his illness. The specific reactions to diagnosis and the state of illness that were discussed include: (1) anxiety, (2) shock, (3) denial, (4) suspicion, (5) questioning, (6) feelings of insignificance and loneliness, (7) regression and dependency, (8) shame and guilt, (9) rejection, (10) fear, (11) withdrawal and depression, and (12) paradoxical reactions.

CHAPTER 11

Worries Illness Brings

Illness is a time beset with worries; it interferes with one's usual pattern of need-gratification and this disruption produces worries. In this chapter we shall identify some "typical" worries of the ill by reviewing common groups of human needs and then considering some concerns that result when satisfaction of those needs is blocked by illness.

With illness, the relative importance of needs may fluctuate markedly from one hour to the next. For example, some needs, which were satisfied with ease and only passing attention in health, may increase in importance and demand considerable attention in illness. Much nursing expertise involves the skillful recognition of impaired need gratification, a recognition of the effect of this on the patient, and the identification and implementation of precise actions designed to remedy the thwarted satisfaction of needs. Realistically the nurse cannot meet *all* of a patient's needs, just as no one person can ever do this for another. However, it is important to realize that nursing is concerned with the total picture of a patient's needs and a consideration of all of them. Nursing care does not focus exclusively on physiologic survival needs.

Let us identify some examples of worries that are frequently expressed by patients as a result of the frustration of various need gratifications because of illness. Earlier in the text we mentioned briefly some basic human needs that were presented diagrammatically in the form of a hierarchy (see p. 9). At this point we shall review this hierarchy more carefully. It is obvious that basic needs, i.e., survival needs, must be reasonably satisfied before it is possible to satisfy those higher on the hierarchy.

SURVIVAL NEEDS IN ILLNESS

In health, survival needs may receive relatively little conscious attention and are usually not a source of concern, we eat, breathe, eliminate, get a drink of water, and go to bed without realizing that we are actually doing these things to stay alive. In illness, however, we become acutely conscious of the life-sustaining necessity for survival needs to be met and regulated. A bout of diarrhea, for example, makes one keenly aware that elimination requires regulation and, at such a time, the need for balanced or controlled elimination occupies one's attention. We fear exhaustion and depletion.

Survival needs are essentially physiologic or bodily needs, for example, food, air, water, appropriate temperature, elimination, rest, and pain avoidance. The survival needs are thus the needs of major concern in critical illness. In this respect sickness is comparable to the experiences of early childhood, which also focus on bodily processes. When ill, one's primary worries for a period of time may thus be bodily worries: for example, "Can I pass gas? Can I keep this food down? Will bowel movements hurt after surgery?" Much nursing time is occupied with attempts to help patients to meet their survival needs comfortably and safely and, therefore, to lessen their worries in this area.

Patients' bodily concerns may often center around worries about how much pain and suffering they will have to endure. Accompanying these worries are fears that they will not be able to bear their pain in a manner acceptable to themselves and others. Patients, especially men, often worry that they will "cry like a woman," or "act like a baby." These fears of loss of behavioral control are also part of the worries that many preoperative patients have: namely, that they will "talk" or "fight" as they come out of the anesthetic.

Impaired survival needs naturally bring worries about the future. Patients may be deeply concerned about the future well-being of their families and loved ones since the illness also affects them. Future debts resulting from the illness are often the source of patients' worries. Indeed, patients often are realistically concerned about whether or not they have a future, for when survival needs cannot be met, the patient knows he is in danger of dying. Worries about dying, or living in a crippled state, i.e., "just surviving . . . like a vegetable," are basic concerns that accompany illness.

Patients may respond to worries like these by displaying a concern for their bodily processes that is exaggerated or disproportionate to the seriousness of the illness. The nurse will often find patients who have a heightened concern for their pulses, breathing, bowel movements, and so on. Because these patients are unable to distinguish between what is important and what is not, in regard to their body functions, they try, almost frantically at times, to observe and question anything they notice about their condition. The nurse must help by ruling out unnecessary concerns, and she must understand that these actions are an expression of fear and anxiety.

STIMULATION NEEDS IN ILLNESS

Although survival needs may come dramatically to the fore with illness, it should not be forgotten that other needs are also present. The needs for sex, novelty, activity, manipulation, and exploration may be suppressed during critical illness, but these stimulation needs do not entirely disappear. Although illness and hospitalization may block the overt expression and satisfaction of some needs, for example, the need for sexual activity, evidence of the continued presence of such needs may appear in sublimated forms. Thus, a male patient may joke and otherwise sexually banter with the nurse, expressing his sexual need in ways that he views as socially acceptable.

When the stimulation needs are denied their normal expression because of illness, many worries may develop that are related to the individual's life situation. Patients whose marriages are based primarily on sexual experience may worry that their marriage partner will be sexually unsatisfied while they are ill and may even be unfaithful while they are hospitalized. Certainly operations that interfere with attractiveness or sexual function will cause concern for the patient. In addition, patients who are accustomed to an active sexual life may find prolonged illnesses that require rest, restriction of sexual activity, and confinement (e.g., tuberculosis) difficult to bear and they naturally become restless and "on edge."

When needs for novelty, activity, manipulation, and exploration are thwarted by illness, people may become depressed and even disoriented. Man is generally an active being. Inactivity spawns introspection and, for many, introspection is depressing. Patients worry about how long they will have to be inactive and whether or not they will be able to return to their pre-illness level of activity. Just as inactivity can cause the muscles to contract and atrophy, it also can cause mental activity to become restricted.

Frustration of the stimulation needs becomes manifest in a convalescing patient's boredom and his attempts to introduce something new into his environment. Perhaps he plays a trick on the nurse, or decorates "his space" in the ward by hanging up cards, ribbons, creepy-crawlies, and so on. Orthopedic wards, occupied by many patients passing time while bones slowly heal and muscles strengthen, are often scenes of pranks as well as creative activities. In these situations the nurse must tax her ingenuity to combat patients' boredom and to help patients take their minds off their aching, often confined, bodies. Occupational therapy is of great help in such situations.

SAFETY AND SECURITY NEEDS IN ILLNESS

In illness, typical day-to-day patterns that one has established for feeling safe and secure are interrupted. Accidents and illnesses, in themselves, bring the realization that one is not invulnerable to suffering and death; confidence is shaken as the daily assumption that one will always be alive and well is jolted. Such realizations make the ill person feel unsafe and insecure. He realizes that he truly lives his life alone. Even though he may have lived with loved ones, who protected him from many of life's unhappinesses, he now knows that these protectors cannot shield him from illness, accident, or death.

Nevertheless, the ill person continues to want protection, and he now looks to his doctors and nurses to protect him from life's adversities and uncertainties. The ill person may think of a nurse as his protector in much the same way that he thought of his mother in this role. Thus, he may try to ascribe superhuman powers to the nurse. For example, in his state of wishing for protection, he may expect that his nurse will be omniscient, that is "all-knowing," so that she can see his future, protect him from harm, or make the right decisions for him. Obviously a nurse does not have such superhuman powers. However, she can recognize when a patient is looking for strengths in those caring for him, and, realizing this, she can be as supportive and protective of him as possible.

When illness threatens safety and security needs, a patient often becomes worried about being *left alone.* As we have said, he finds himself alone in his state of illness, often in the hospital, while those persons he is normally with are away from him. He goes to surgery alone, they wait; he feels pain alone, they look on; he gasps for breath, they breathe easily but cannot breathe for him. Nurses can help patients to feel less lonely.

Illness also makes patients feel helpless, and they worry about what will happen to them in their helpless state. Will an accident occur in their treatment? In this era of mass communication almost everyone knows that medical and nursing accidents happen. Many people are coming to feel that hospitals are places of "hazards rather than havens." They are aware of infections and malpractice, and fear being the victims of carelessness. "Do these people taking care of me know what they're doing?" Every attempt must be made to help the patient to feel and to *be* safe and secure.

Patients fear being *abandoned by loved ones* during their illness. As we mentioned earlier, the attitudes of others are readily communicated to patients. Some families feel relieved to have the ill person "taken off their hands," and once they have him in the hospital may feel relieved of their burden. Such people often do not visit or even telephone to inquire about the patient. Older patients particularly worry that they will be rejected by their families and "dumped into a nursing home where no one cares."

At the other extreme, some patients worry that they will be sent home or taken home before they are ready to go. For example, they may fear that they will be denied the care they need because of the cost involved. Indeed, this may happen since, at times, the family may pressure the doctor to send the patient home because of the cost. Cost cannot be minimized, but it is unfortunate when it interferes with the necessity for care. Another concern in this area is that of running out of money or insurance, having to go on welfare, and being sent to a "welfare ward." Often "welfare wards" are equated in patients' minds with neglectful care.

LOVE NEEDS IN ILLNESS

Separation from one's usual companions and way of life means that needs for love, belonging, and closeness are severely threatened in the existence of the ill. We are not referring to romantic or physical love when we refer here to the need for love, but rather to those strong feelings of affection, concern, kindness, closeness, and understanding that one shares with those close to him. These are shared feelings that are essential for a feeling of well-being and, therefore, to be denied these feelings from others creates a most unhappy situation. When ill and away from those persons they care about, patients obviously worry: "Will loved ones change? Will they no longer want me? Am I an unattractive burden?"

Like the stimulation needs and the needs for safety and security, the needs for love and belonging are present in all patients. These needs are not vaporized by illness. In fact, they may be intensified by the uncertainty of illness and by illness itself. As we mentioned, the persons who provide gratification of needs may shift somewhat with illness: when he was well, the patient's needs were gratified by individuals in his private life; with illness he now looks to those in the medical professions for need gratification. We do not mean to imply that staff members can ever take the place of friends and relatives for the patient; nor do we mean to imply that loved ones cease to provide need gratification for the ill. However, staff members *are* needed to contribute to the ever-present needs for safety, security, love, and belonging that continue into a patient's hospital existence. In the hospital the staff may be with a patient more than loved ones are, and also, they are often with him during "crisis moments" in his life and illness when loved ones may be excluded from his presence, i.e., surgery, intensive care, isolation, and emergencies.

A patient is not truly "taken care of" unless the nurse helps him to feel safe, secure, loved, and like one who "belongs," rather than an outsider who is viewed as an intruder. Patients worry about being treated impersonally. A touch of the hand, a stroke on the brow, a look, a pat, the way a patient is handled, made comfortable, and helped can all contribute to making him feel close to those caring for him. In all these "loving gestures" the nurse must bear in mind that her actions should not be seductive in quality but rather a sincere expression of appropriate concern.

ESTEEM NEEDS IN ILLNESS

If a patient's needs for love, closeness, and belonging are relatively satisfied through the concern and interest of clinic or hospital staff members, then he has also been helped to meet another group of needs: the needs for esteem and self-esteem. Because he receives love, concern, and respect from others, and because he feels he "belongs" and "is one" with others, the patient's feelings of self-esteem are enhanced. He is important enough that others care about his feelings. He is not overlooked, or impersonally treated as if he is merely one person out of thousands whose weight will leave an indistinguishable imprint on the mattress he lies on; he does not feel forgotten before he has left. The person who has a sense of esteem by others feels that he is regarded by them as an individual of worth and value, and if he has a feeling of self-esteem he feels this way about himself.

Illness can markedly interfere with the gratification of esteem needs. The ill person often does not feel that he is of worth and value to others, or to himself, but instead he feels he is a "drag on life," a burden, and an unpleasant reminder of those aspects of life that people prefer not to think about. All these feelings create intense worries.

In our society our bodies are seldom viewed by strangers and we are not usually touched by them except perhaps in a handshake. With illness comes the realization that one's body will be viewed and handled by strangers, and feelings of esteem may be threatened by such experiences. Once again, realizing the prevalence of worries about being physically handled and visually inspected, we emphasize the following rule:

> *Minimize exposure of the patient by means of proper draping and make physical contact of a firm, but gentle, professional quality.*

Observance of this rule is a prime obligation of all medical personnel, since few experiences are more disheartening or humiliating to a patient than to be the subject of indifferent exposure and careless handling.

SELF-ACTUALIZATION NEEDS IN ILLNESS

Probably the most difficult group of needs for a patient to satisfy during illness are self-actualization needs. By these needs we refer to (1) expressing one's personality, and (2) developing one's abilities. Illness makes it difficult for a person to be the kind of person he *really* is rather than the person he thinks others want him to be. Because he is dependent upon others for care and does not wish to arouse their displeasure, the patient often feels forced to succumb and act like the person others want him to be. He feels helpless to stand up and be himself because to oppose those caring for him means risking being cut off from their care and attention. Many of his concerns thus center around trying to please all the staff members. Patients also find it difficult to meet self-actualization needs because of other patients who may exert pressure on them to act in one way or another.

Illness may also severely curtail the patient's making maximum use of his abilities by preventing him from using and developing his personal talents. In some accidents or illnesses a patient may be left in a state in which he can never again use abilities that he has developed: he may be blind, or paralyzed, without a limb, without a voice, or permanently weakened. A large part of our unique identity and personality consists of how we use our individual abilities and talents; therefore, such losses are hard to bear and cause great concern.

SUMMARY

We have reviewed some typical worries and concerns of the ill that result because illness interferes with normal need gratification. In order to identify those worries that are fairly representative of ill persons, we have reviewed common groups of human needs. The *specific* worries and concerns of any given patient will depend largely upon the way in which his specific needs are blocked or frustrated by his specific illness. Nursing involves attempting to identify and understand such personal concerns and to provide supplementary need gratifications when the normal avenues of satisfaction are impaired.

CHAPTER 12

The "Sick Role"

> There appears to be a consensus throughout the population in terms of the behavioral expectations relevant to the sick role. Differences in role expectations regarding different illness states, therefore, appear to be related not to differing conceptions of the appropriate manner of treating the sick person, but rather to differing conceptions of who is and who is not sick.[68]

This unit has focused on the existence of the ill. One manner of thinking about existence is to consider the life process in terms of roles. In this chapter we shall discuss the "sick role."

Briefly stated, a social role is a pattern of *expected behavior;* therefore, the sick role is the pattern of behavior that we expect from persons whom we view as "sick." We tend to mentally categorize people into various roles all the time, e.g., sexual roles, status roles. This process is usually one that takes place more or less unconsciously.

The nurse, therefore, constantly is mentally assigning patients to various roles; often she lacks an awareness of doing this. However, she should try to become aware of this process, because the roles that she assigns to people (i.e., the way she thinks of them) will affect her expectations of them and her actions and attitudes toward them.

As the quotation at the beginning of this chapter indicates, one problem that we often experience in relation to roles is that of deciding whether or not a given person should be placed in a particular role. Once we have mentally categorized him, in terms of a role, we know how to react toward him. Thus, with the sick person, our problem is not one of knowing how to react to him when he is sick, but rather the problem lies in deciding in the first place if he really should be considered sick.*

Roles are *learned.* Just as the nursing student learns the nursing role from the nurses with whom she associates, so all of us have learned the sick role from those around us in life. We have formed our expectations of sick people as we grew and observed how our family and friends reacted toward the ill or how they themselves behaved when ill. We have also learned how we should act when we are ill. Patients have all undergone experiences like this and each has a concept of how he believes he is expected to behave and what he expects of those caring for him. From the cultural norms surrounding us as we grew, we all learned what the rules of behavior, the rights, and the obligations of the ill are in our social group.

We all tend to feel more comfortable when we know what behavior is expected of us in any given situation. If we feel we are not behaving as others expect us to, or if they are not behaving as we expect them to, uneasiness results and misunderstandings occur. Patients feel uncomfortable when they are not sure what behavior is expected of them or if they do not feel like behaving as others expect them to. At times, conforming to one's expected role may be difficult, or the role itself may not be clear. In fact, it appears that it is only with severe or critical illnesses, when the prognosis is clearly serious or is uncertain, that role definition is clear-cut. In this situation the "sick role" is quite evident.

Although individuals may vary to some degree in their role concepts, depending upon their individual upbringing, it is possible to look generally at some roles. Let us do this now with the "sick role."

THE COMPONENTS OF THE "SICK ROLE"

For centuries people have had ideas about how the ill can be expected to behave, and, in turn, how to behave toward them. However, it was not until the early 1950's, with the published work of Talcott Parsons,[138] that the formalized concept of the "sick role" began to receive attention. Parsons made, at that time, four major statements about the behavioral expectations that are relative to the sick role. See if your ideas about sick people agreee with his observations:

First, Parsons pointed out that *sick persons are exempt from normal social role responsibilities.* This exemption varies in degree, depending upon the nature and severity of the illness. For example, sick persons are not expected to do their usual work or to carry out their duties of father, mother, husband, or wife, as the case may be. The physician is often called upon to act as a legitimatizing agent for this suspension of obligations, i.e., to say about the patient, "He is sick and must have a rest and go to the hospital for treatment." Once the patient is told this by an authority, his claim to exemptions from his usual duties is typically viewed as legitimate by himself and by others. He has been told that he is sick and can act sick.

*Some of the problems involved in deciding who is sick are discussed in Unit II.

There are objective tests and criteria for the determination of whether or not one is ill, how sick one is, and what the nature of the illness is. Parents may serve as legitimatizing agents for children. A child may ask his mother to legitimatize his illness. Thus, he goes to her, says he is sick and doesn't feel like going to school, and then he waits to hear from her whether or not she says he is sick. She may say, "I don't know whether you are sick or not. I'll take your temperature." Thus she looks for objective criteria to help in her validation. If she says he is sick, he is exempted from his usual duty to go to school.

Although illness and the sick role may enable the ill person to be excused from his usual social role, it also can place an obligation on him, since others may tell him how he should act. For instance, when he is sick others can tell him that he *ought* to rest, stay in bed, not eat, take medicine, stay home, take care of himself, and so on, depending upon his illness. A patient may not want to give up his usual responsibilities and assume these new obligations that are part of the sick role. Also, these obligations may prove a source of difficulty in the transition period from illness to health, for, as the patient recovers, he may no longer want to do what others believe he "ought" to do; e.g., he may want to be out of bed while others think he should still remain in bed.

Second, *it cannot be expected that the sick person could "pull himself together" and get well merely by an act of will or decision on his part.* Because he cannot "help it" that he is ill, he must be "taken care of." And because the illness itself is "not his fault," the sick role once again excuses the ill person from his usual responsibilities in life. Even though the ill person may have been partially responsible for the fact that he did become ill or injured, now that he *is* sick he is incapable of terminating his "condition"; the illness is beyond his control. The condition itself must either heal of its own accord or be acted upon. The patient is viewed as "entitled" to help, for he cannot, by his own will, make himself recover. Just as he cannot recover by using his own *will,* the sick person also cannot heal himself by his own *knowledge;* he is not competent to diagnose and treat himself. He does not know what needs to be done.

Third, *there is an obligation on the part of the sick person to "want to get well," for the state of being ill is defined as being an undesirable situation.* Illness is a strain that involves discomfort, disability, suffering, the possibility of death, and, of course its reality at times. In most instances it is to a patient's best self-interest to get well. There are problems, however, that can prevent sick people from wanting to get well. Because the sick role is composed, in part, of privileges and exemptions from responsibilities for the ill person, these factors may become sources of "secondary gain" toward which the patient often is unconsciously motivated. When this is the case, individuals may not be motivated to "get well" as strongly as they are to "stay ill or become ill." They wish to remain in the sick role and enjoy its priviliges.

The fourth and final observation that Parsons made concerning the sick role was that *there is an obligation to seek technically competent help, usually from a physician, and to cooperate with him in the process of trying to recover.* This obligation varies in proportion to the severity of the condition. The patient is thus expected to act as he is directed to, even though the directions often involve requiring him to suffer, or risk death, disability, and/or financial loss. He may be expected to cooperate even as life slowly leaves him and he eventually dies.

While the ill are expected to seek competent help, they are often in the difficult position of not really knowing who is a competent doctor (or nurse). Therefore, they often select such "helpers" in random ways, such as picking a name out of the phone book or going to their neighbor's doctor. Thus, without really *knowing* the competency of those caring for him and asking him to risk suffering or death, the patient is expected to cooperate fully in whatever he is asked to do. The patient is, therefore, often expected to assume "on faith" that those caring for him know what they are doing and that they have his best interests in mind at all times. This puts him in a most difficult position and creates problems of trust.

These are the major aspects of the sick role that Parsons identified. They are the patterns of behavior which we expect from persons whom we view as sick.

People who do not act in accordance with the role in which we have placed them are disturbing to us. For example, a patient who is obviously sick but refuses to cooperate is disturbing to us since we expect patients to cooperate. Likewise, persons in the sick role who do not seem to want to get well are disturbing to us; we expect them to want to get better and find their reluctance to do so difficult to understand.

CHAPTER 13

Disorganized Behavior and Thought Processes Accompanying Illness

Because of the physiologic and psychologic stresses and the social isolation that illness often imposes, various aberrations of behavior and disorganized thinking processes may accompany illness. When behavior becomes disorganized it is not directed toward achieving reality goals; the behavior does not correspond with what is culturally expected and what would be in accordance with reality. Disorganized thinking processes fail to keep the patient in contact with reality and fail to help him to function effectively. The nurse needs to be knowledgeable about various types of disorganized thoughts and behavior, the causes of such disorganization, and the appropriate methods of treatment. The study of psychiatric nursing is helpful in this area of patient care.

SOME GENERAL CAUSES OF DISORGANIZED THOUGHTS AND BEHAVIOR

Many different *psychologic stresses* may cause various forms of disorganized thought and behavior. Such stresses are not so clearly understood as are those stresses that are basically physiologic. It is increasingly recognized that *social and sensory deprivation* can precipitate disorganized behavior.

Some of the *physiologic* stresses that may cause disorganized behavior and thought processes during illness are: temperature elevations; nutritional, fluid-electrolyte, and acid-base imbalances; impaired renal function; lack of sleep; and cerebral hypoxia interfering with the metabolic processes of the brain's cerebral neurons.[64] Older persons may be particularly susceptible to this last-mentioned type of confusion; indeed, older persons have been described as "living on the edge of cerebral hypoxia."[139] Noxious agents can also produce reversible or irreversible damage to cerebral neurons and thereby cause disorganized behavior. Numerous diseases that attack nervous tissue can cause behavioral changes. Although the precise etiologic mechanisms are poorly understood, a distended bladder or fecal impaction may have noxious effects upon brain cells that precipitate temporary confusion or delirium. Acidosis and increased levels of carbon dioxide are common causes of confusion. Also, hypertension contributes to brain ischemia.[64]

INDICATIONS OF DISORGANIZED BEHAVIOR

Some manifestations of disorganized behavior and thinking are confusion or disorientation, hallucinations, illusions, and delusional thinking. Terms such as these often are not correctly applied or uniformly understood. For example, what one person means when she says a patient is "disoriented" may be very different from what another person thinks of as disoriented behavior. Thus, accurate terminology must be appropriately used in describing behavior and thought processes that are disorganized.

CONFUSION AND DISORIENTATION

The terms *"confusion"* and *"disorientation"* can be used interchangeably, and it is repetitious to use them both and say that a patient is "confused *and* disoriented." Confusion[78] generally refers to a state of disordered orientation; it represents a disturbance of consciousness in the sense that awareness of time, place, or person is unclear. Confusion may be due to organic or psychic causes. Disorientation,[78] likewise, refers to impairment in the understanding of temporal, spatial, or personal relationships. The confused or disoriented patient thus may not know who he is; what time of day or what day, month, or year it is; and/or where he is.

Confusion and disorientation are not the same as delirium; a delirious patient may appear confused or disoriented, but not all confused or disoriented patients are delirious. Also, a comatose or semicomatose patient should not be called confused or disoriented. Before a patient can be described accurately as confused or disoriented he must be awake enough so that he can be expected to be properly oriented to his environment.[117] The levels of consciousness known as delirium, semi-coma, and coma are discussed in Unit VIII.

Confusion and disorientation represent less severe alterations in brain function than do coma or delirium. With confusion and disorientation there is a loss of the higher nervous activity within the central nervous system which typically functions to enable one to maintain normal relationships within one's internal and external environments. Loeser observes that while the dysfunctions within the brain during confusion or disorientation are minor, the social dysfunction is devastating: "One doesn't need a very severe brain injury or a very severe alteration in the metabolism of the brain cells to result in what is functionally an essentially useless human being. If you don't know where you are or what to do, you are of little value to yourself or to the rest of the world, in spite of the fact that the amount of dysfunction within your central nervous system is minimal."[117]

With confusion or disorientation there is loss of ability to adapt and to respond to normal stimuli and to maintain the normal cyclic patterns of day and night. Thus, it is not uncommon to find that the confused patient may want to sleep during the daytime and then is hyperactive at night.

The confused or disoriented patient is not comatose; he can perceive what is happening in his environment. He can hear and see, and can speak and respond in some way to what is happening around him. However, if we compare what is viewed as "normal" behavior with that of the confused patient we find that what he says and does is not the appropriate or culturally expected behavior.

Evaluating the Confused or Disoriented Patient. Confusion and disorientation may be transitory states that come and go, and thus they may be difficult to evaluate. These states may last minutes, hours, months, or years. One cannot decide on the basis of one question or one observation whether a patient is confused or disoriented; a series of questions and observations (of both verbal and nonverbal behavior) are needed. In the process of evaluation you might observe if the patient can find his way back to his room and his bed; if he appears to recognize his doctor and you; and if he seems to understand why he is in the hospital. Does he seem to know what time of day it is and where he is? How aware of current events is he? Does he know who the President is? If he has just listened to the news, does he seem to remember what he heard? Does he remember whether his doctor visited today, what he had for breakfast, or when he last saw visitors in the hospital? Much of this information can be obtained, without directly questioning the patient, by listening closely to what he says, and by observing his behavior. At times, however, specific questions are necessary.

The following guidelines will help you in interviewing a patient to evaluate whether he is confused or disoriented. In general, do not ask questions to which the patient can simply reply "Yes" or "No." His correct answer to such questions can simply be a guess on his part or an attempt to cover up his confusion. For example, do not say, "Do you know where you are?" for the patient may say, "Yes," although he doesn't really know where he is. Instead ask, "Can you tell me the name of this hospital and what city it is in?"

Also, in attempting to determine whether or not the patient is oriented to time, person, and place, evaluate your interviewing of the patient in light of the following:[117]

> Is the patient being asked realistic questions? What is his level of intelligence? What have his experiences been? How long has he been hospitalized?

> Is the patient fully awake when he is talked to or is he groggy and only half-awake?

> Does he have the aids to orientation and expression that he requires? For example, is he exposed to radio, television, newspapers, calendars? Does he have a clock or watch? Does he have his glasses on? Are his dentures in so that he can speak clearly? Does he require a hearing aid? If so, is it turned on?

> Do you have the patient's attention when talking to him? (You may want to touch him before speaking to gain his attention.) Are you giving the patient your attention and really trying to communicate with him?

> Does he speak English or are you talking to him in a language he does not understand?

> Can he speak? Is he perhaps aphasic, i.e., capable of receiving stimuli for speech but unable to handle symbolic expression through language? (A patient may be aphasic and not be confused.) Has he had a laryngectomy? Is he deaf? Is he mute?

> Does the patient have memory difficulties? (The confused patient cannot appropriately function here and now. Someone with memory difficulties may not be confused; he may be able to function appropriately here and now but cannot remember.) It is important to know if the patient is aware of his intellectual deficit. A person with memory difficulties may say, "I don't know the date. I can't remember things." A confused patient may say, "It is 1926."

In describing the confused or disoriented patient, it is often best not to use the terms "confused" or "disoriented" since these terms may mean different things to different people. It is much clearer, and more accurate, if you state as simply as possible: (1) how the patient appeared; (2) what you did to stimulate him; and (3) what his response was. For example: "While Mr. Smith and I were walking down the hall, I asked him if he could tell me how he happened to come to the hospital. He replied: 'I don't know where I am. How long have I been here?'"

Some Causes of Confusion or Disorientation. Confusion and disorientation are common signs of both physical and mental illness. Some causes of confusion[117] are listed below:

Congenital causes: relatively rare.

Degenerative causes (in any age group): relentlessly progressive diseases which may involve confusion, e.g., Huntington's chorea.

Infections (viral, bacterial, fungal): confusion may result from fever or infection.

Neoplasms (in brain or metastatic to brain): some tumors occur without neurologic findings but with confusion, e.g., frontal lobe, slow-growing tumors.

Vascular lesions: the most common cause in geriatric patients, e.g., repeated small strokes slowly destroying brain cells; ruptured aneurysms; arteriovenous malformations.
Trauma: mechanical deformation of the brain.
Metabolic factors: most commonly found causes in hospitalized patients, resulting from diabetes, electrolyte imbalance (prolonged vomiting), hormonal disturbances, hypothyroidism, drugs (side effect of steroids and some drugs used to treat Parkinson's disease; side effect of narcotics and sedatives and psychedelics). Alcohol is *the* most common cause of confusion found in the general hospital.
Seizures: confusion may occur during or following seizures.
Psychiatric causes: these may be numerous.
Sensory deprivation

Effects of Sensory Deprivation. Studies in sensory deprivation have established that when people are deprived of sensory stimulation they may develop confusion, inaccurate perception, faulty reasoning, impaired memory, and even hallucinations. In spite of this fact, one frequently finds that confused patients are restrained and isolated from others by being placed in a room alone or by having curtains pulled around their cubicles. Confused patients' perceptual fields are actually further decreased by such "treatment" and they are placed in a situation that actually fosters the perpetuation of confusion. "When you take a confused patient, tie him down in bed, all fours splayed out, looking up at a white ceiling and leave him alone, you are just putting him through more sensory deprivation."[117]

Blindness and deafness are principal causes of sensory deprivation and, hence, confusion; the individual whose senses are impaired, e.g., because of cataracts and/or partial deafness, is more likely to become confused than a person with intact sensation.

It is not surprising to learn that darkness and loss of spatial image can precipitate or intensify a state of confusion. Studies in sensory deprivation (in which the subjects wore various kinds of goggles) demonstrated that fewer hallucinations occur with complete darkness (or with opaque head coverings) than if the visual field is generalized with translucent goggles that let in some light but that do not allow patterns to be seen. Also, when slight stimulation is allowed, e.g., a low sound or low ambient light, there is a greater amount of distortion and hallucinatory activity than in the total absence of stimulation. Presumably there must be some kind of stimulus before it can be distorted.[47]

Emphasis has also been placed on the importance of *meaningful* contact with the environment in minimizing sensory deprivation. Some investigators believe that it is the restriction of meaning that is mainly responsible for the effects of sensory deprivation, rather than the quantitative physical limitation of stimuli per se.[56] Thus, patients need to have meaningful contact with their environment and with persons in their environment.

Nursing Care of Confused or Disoriented Patients

Confusion (or disorientation) is completely disabling to a patient; he is dependent on others for care and protection. Let us now examine some ways in which nurses may help these patients. Three major goals to keep in mind in the care of confused patients are: (1) preventing or modifying disorganization; (2) supporting and protecting the patient during aberrant behavior; and (3) reorienting him to reality.[64] It is desirable to evaluate the patient's level of comprehension and his emotional state before attempting to orient him to reality, since a sedated, drugged, highly anxious patient will be susceptible to reorientation efforts only after his level of anxiety and his medications are reduced.[64]

It is helpful if the confused person can be assigned to the care of the same nurse for consecutive days. Everything is bewildering enough for such a patient without adding to it the presence of many different people. For the confused patient one assigned nurse fulfills the role of an "anchor person" by serving as a steady point of reference.[155] Authorities suggest that this "anchor nurse" should be generally good-natured and even-tempered, available and accessible, noncoercive, and patient. The nurse should consider her posture, voice, and gestures when with the patient and make sure that these are friendly rather than threatening. Her movements should be slow and deliberate rather than sudden and sporadic. In her activities the nurse should strive to include rather than exclude the patient. That is, she should tell the patient what she will be doing and talk with him as she proceeds rather than remaining silent and simply doing things *to* him. This point will be discussed further later.

With professional skill the nurse can alter, manipulate, and plan the environment in which the patients in her care exist. The nurse governs "environmental input and output" and combats sensory saturation as well as sensory deprivation. She can alter the patient's physical environment to some extent and she can markedly alter his interpersonal environment. The professional nurse sets a "tone" of emotional care and respect for the disturbed patient. Others will be encouraged to follow her example, since the nurse serves as a model of behavior for other staff members and for a patient's friends and relatives. If the nurse treats a confused patient in a depersonalized, hopeless manner and makes fun of his behavior, then other people will follow the example that she has set. If the nurse shows respect for the patient, others will also.

The confused patient may say or do things that are foreign to our experience; he makes us feel uncomfortable and may appear to be teasing or funny. He may remind us of people "acting silly" or of comedians. However, unlike the clown or comedian, the patient is not acting or performing for our benefit. He is with us to receive professional care, understanding, and protection during his confusion. The comedian feels uncomfortable if we do *not* laugh at him; the disoriented patient feels uncomfortable if we *do* laugh at him, and he will become louder the more deeply confused he becomes. Unlike the comedian who can choose how he will communicate, the confused patient has no conscious choice regarding his communication. Laughing at or making fun of such a person is cruel. Also, joking about the confused patient within the hearing of other patients makes the others uncomfortable because they sense your lack of compassion and feel that you lack understanding of them.

How can a nurse helpfully regulate a disoriented patient's physical environment? Studies in sensory deprivation help a great deal and their findings can be implemented. A room should have adequate light and the light should vary between day and day. Night lights should be left on in the patient's room. Shades should not remain down during the daytime. As mentioned earlier, the patient should have the normal aids to orientation available and in use: e.g., radio, television, newspapers, magazines, a calendar, an accurate clock or watch, glasses, dentures, and a hearing aid if required. To be used properly the radio must be clearly tuned in to programs in keeping with the patient's interests, if possible, and loud enough to be understood (too loud or too soft will be annoying); the television must be in focus as well as close enough to see and loud enough to hear; radio and television should not be left on hour after hour or the patient becomes fatigued and may attempt to mentally tune them out (perhaps lapsing more deeply into confusion); newspapers and magazines must be in good repair and current; a calendar must be where it can be viewed and large enough to be seen clearly, and turned to the correct day, week, or month; clocks and watches must be kept wound, accurately set and placed so the patient can easily see them; glasses must be clean and in use; hearing aids need to be properly placed, maintained with batteries, and turned on when in use.

Other manipulations of the physical environment that the nurse can carry out include rearranging furniture for the patient's benefit so he can see outside or into the halls; placing the call bell within reach; and arranging flowers, or some of the patient's familiar belongings. Familiar objects can help a confused patient to become oriented, and colorful robes, curtains, bedspreads, pictures, and wall paint are visually stimulating.

Further physical management includes moving the patient himself. Again, studies of sensory deprivation guide the nurses' action. People become confused when they do not move, do not touch themselves, and are not touched by others. (Consider here the detrimental effect of wrist restraints that restrict movement and do not allow the patient even to touch himself.) Enclosure in a confined space for a period of time can cause confusion. The nursing implications of these studies begin with the nurse's recognition that touching and movement are very important for orientation and include plans for the integration of these activities into nursing care.

Touch the patient when talking to him and when caring for him. Movement is helpful in maintaining orientation to body image: therefore, passive exercises, encouraging the patient to move, turning and positioning the patient, rolling the bed up or down for various periods, and getting the patient out of bed and out of his room as much as possible are essential nursing actions. It is important also to reduce noises, shadows, and drafts that might disturb the patient or that he might misinterpret. Again, these are areas within the control of the nurse.

Because the confused person cannot respond appropriately to his needs, he must be periodically taken to the toilet, given fluids to drink, be supervised during meals, and helped to rest. Without such care the forgetful person can become impacted, incontinent, dehydrated, malnourished, and excessively fatigued. Intake and output records should be kept for all confused patients.

Incontinence contributes to confused patients' regression, feelings of helplessness, and lowered self-esteem. Every effort must be made to retrain the incontinent patient to normal bowel and bladder elimination or at least to prevent incontinence. The disoriented patient is not unconscious; he is not insensitive to the manner in which he is regarded or treated. If he is allowed to remain incontinent the feeling communicated to him is one of hopelessness and degradation; his animal nature is allowed to take precedence over his human nature. If he is roughly washed and diapered after incontinence he will not be encouraged to regain bowel and bladder control; he will instead actually be trained to be incontinent.

Contrast this type of "care" with an atmosphere of: (1) Staff *recognition* that disorientation means a lack of appropriate response to time. (2) Staff *expectation* that the patient may be incontinent unless they assume for him a "time awareness" regarding his needs to void or defecate; the confused patient cannot plan ahead and therefore once he is aware of having to eliminate he may not have time to find the toilet or to get help. (3) Staff *awareness* that they must form a retraining plan and keep records on all shifts in an attempt to determine the patient's pattern of bowel and bladder function. (4) Staff *acceptance* of this area of need for care. (5) Staff *enthusiasm* that the patient *can* be trained or at least that they themselves can be trained to anticipate and respond to the patient's pattern of intake and output so that he will not be incontinent. What a difference in atmosphere for the patient; the difference between feeling that one is a chore and an animal, and the feeling that one is a person who is ill, in need of help, and is receiving it!

All the nursing actions that have been mentioned thus far can be carried out without staff members ever talking to the patient. His furniture can be rearranged, his radio turned on, his elimination care given—all without ever talking to him, or at most giving only a few commands. However, if such is the situation, the patient's care is inadequate. A major portion of the plan of care must be directed toward thoughtful, preplanned, verbal communication—talking that is directed toward meeting the patient's need for reorientation.

Confused patients are uncertain about what is real, and so nursing efforts must be directed toward helping to reestablish with them those elements of reality that we share with one another. Reality comprises a mental experience or inner life that is private to each individual as well as aspects of life that are shared in common with others. For example, when a nurse sits at a desk, the nurse and the desk are obvious to all—they are a part of the "shared reality" that is available to everyone's experience; however, the nurse's thoughts are a part of her own inner reality and are not shared or obvious to the onlooker unless the nurse verbalizes what she is thinking. It is the shared facts of daily reality that the nurse may focus on initially in attempting to reorient the confused patient and to make him more comfortable.

Some important shared, basic factors in everyone's orientation are agreements about time, persons, and places. As we have indicated, an individual is disoriented when he doesn't know what time it is; what day, month, or year it is; who he is; who others are; where he is; and the geography and location of surrounding areas. In our waking lives we have mutual agreements in these areas; this constitutes an important part of reality, the awareness of which keeps us oriented.

If the nurse's goal is to focus on the shared elements of reality (i.e., concerning time, place, and person) it is in these areas that she will plan her "verbal care" of the patient. How? Instead of talking about abstract things she will talk about the *real things* in the environment and the *facts* that she knows about the patient. For example, instead of feeding the patient in silence, the nurse who is trying to reorient the patient verbally will talk about what the foods are, what meal it is, the tray, the dishes, and so on. Instead of saying, "Have some of this," she will say, "Would you like some of these green beans?" In stressing shared time she will identify the meal being served. Instead of saying, "It's time to eat," she will say, "It is Tuesday morning. I have brought you some breakfast."

In a continuing attempt to reorient the confused patient the nurse directs her comments to reality. She will *repeatedly* identify herself to the patient (because he does not remember) and she will focus on what time it is, who the patient is, where he is, and why he is there. Speaking slowly, so that the patient will have time to think about what is being said and have time to ask questions, the nurse moves from topic to topic. If the patient misunderstands she will attempt to clarify briefly. She should not contribute to a patient's disorientation by agreeing with his misinterpretations and she should not upset him by arguing but rather, work to understand what the patient may mean. The patient should be corrected gently and the comments refocused. For example, if the patient says, "Aren't you sister Mary?" She may respond, "No, I am Miss Thomas, your nurse at General Hospital. Who is sister Mary?"

When you are going to speak to the patient, gain his attention, look into his eyes when you speak so he can watch your lips move, and speak clearly, slowly, and in an appropriate tone and volume of voice. Talk to the patient as an adult, not with "baby talk." You may find initially that it is difficult to talk to people if they make no reply to what you have said. Lack of response may make you feel that you want to stop talking, or it may embarrass you. Disoriented people are sometimes a threat to our own reality and thus cause us to feel like retreating from them for fear that we also may become confused. Resist such feelings and try to understand them. Other feelings that you may have with a disoriented patient are: concerns that he may say something embarrassing to you: a belief that he may stay quiet and tranquil if you don't disturb him by talking; and worries about what other people will think about your attempts to communicate with the patient. Analyze such feelings, remembering that the confused patient needs your communication with him. It takes real effort to try to communicate with confused people, but it is of prime importance in their care.

Because confused people lose their awareness of the cyclic movement of time, they should be helped to dress in the daytime rather than remaining constantly in sleeping attire, which they may associate with night. Since medications such as sedatives may intensify confusion, first use other nursing measures to help restless, confused patients to sleep. For example, a brief talk, a back rub, a cup of warm milk, a trip to the bathroom, washing the hands and face can all help to relax a patient sufficiently so that sleep is possible without medication. Sedation may be contraindicated in patients who have impaired renal or cerebral functions.

Combat social isolation by: stopping in the confused patient's room frequently; bringing the patient's chair (or bed) into the doorway of his room or out into the hall or by the nursing station (during the day, evening, or at night); taking the patient for frequent walks or wheelchair rides; and encouraging visiting by friends, relatives, volunteers, staff, or other patients.

The confused patient's coherence and thinking ability are dulled; he is bewildered, forgetful, and perceives inadequately. Also, he may be inattentive, have sleep disorders, hallucinate, become agitated, talk incoherently, wander about, or get lost.[139] Such a patient obviously needs protective care. The confused person is a frightened person. He often feels defenseless in his bewilderment and is afraid of being taken advantage of. He tries to protect himself when he feels threatened and at such times may refuse care and try to keep people away from him. Forcing this patient or restraining him will add to his fear and aggressiveness. Often the more fearful and upset the patient becomes, the more confused and defensive he becomes.

Restraint policy varies from one hospital and one physician to another; however, the trend is to forbid the use of restraint or to use it only according to definite procedures which ensure protection of the patient. If restraints are used they should be applied only after a decision is carefully made that the restraints are necessary for the *patient's well-being* and not for the convenience of the staff. Some general points to bear in mind concerning restraints are: (1) Let the patient know that he is not being punished; inform him that he is being restrained for his own well-being so that he will not fall or injure himself. (2) Never place restraints around a patient's neck; he may suffocate. (3) Apply restraints snugly so the patient cannot get out of them or become entangled in them; however, do not impede the circulation. (4) Body restraints are preferable to wrist and ankle restraints because they allow greater freedom of movement. (5) Change the restrained patient's position often. (6) Remove the restraints frequently to give skin care and to allow the patient to move. (7) Put padding under the restraints to protect the skin; and (8) carefully supervise the restrained patient. Remember that the restrained person is totally dependent on others for his safety and care. This is a frightening condition for the patient and a situation of responsibility for the nurse.

Both physical restraint and the use of drugs to restrain the patient can contribute to a patient's confusion by impairing reality testing and communication. Remove restraints as soon as possible.

HALLUCINATIONS, ILLUSIONS, AND DELUSIONAL THINKING

Hallucinations, illusions, and delusional thinking are instances of disordered behavior and thought disturbances. Let us briefly consider these problems.

Hallucinations. Hallucinations[78] are sensory impressions occurring in the *absence of external stimuli,* whether or not accompanied by insight into their unreal nature on the part of the subject. Any of the senses may be affected, and so hallucinating patients may believe that they see, hear, smell, feel, or taste objects or stimuli that are not actually present. The hallucinated stimuli (whether a vision, a sound, an odor, or a taste) have no source in the environment; instead they are sensations arising within the patient himself.

The presence of visual hallucinations suggests that a patient's problem may be an organic disease of the brain rather than functional mental illness. Visual hallucinations most typically occur in the deliria of acute infectious diseases or toxic psychoses and most often occur with acute, reversible organic brain disorders. A variety of drugs may also cause visual hallucinations; such drugs include not only exotic drugs, e.g., mescaline, but also prescribed medications, e.g., amphetamines and antiparkinsonism medication. Also, the withdrawal of some drugs, e.g., alcohol and barbiturates, can produce visual hallucinations.[34]

Some additional causes of visual hallucinations with an organic basis are listed below:[34]

- brain tumors and other space-occupying lesions
- the aura of an epileptic attack or migrainous headaches
- metabolic disorders, e.g., adrenal insufficiency, dehydration, hypoparathyroidism, pernicious or addisonian anemia, hypoglycemia, anorexia, and uremia
- trauma
- collagen diseases
- cerebrovascular accidents
- degenerative diseases, e.g., Pick's and Alzheimer's diseases

Visual hallucinations are associated with mental illness as well as organic problems. Generally visual hallucinations are associated with the acute psychoses and auditory hallucinations with the chronic psychoses. Visual hallucinations may also occur as a result of sensory deprivation.[56]

Illusions. Illusions[78] differ from hallucinations in that with an illusion *a real stimulus is present* but the person *misinterprets* the actual stimuli from the environment. For example, a shadow may be present on the wall, but the patient misinterprets the shadow and believes that he sees a person standing by the wall.

Delusional Thinking. "Delusional thinking"[78] refers to thoughts or beliefs that are false; that is, they are contrary to demonstrable fact. For example, a person may believe that he is being persecuted by the police when this is not true.

CHAPTER 14

Disturbances of Body Image

One of the fascinating paradoxes of the human condition is that the human body, which unites and identifies man as a biologic species, gives rise, in each of us, on a psychologic level, to a body image that is one of the subtly unique features of the individual personality.[137]

Every person carries in his mind an image of his own body; this organic picture is called "body image." Body image forms an integral part of an individual's conception of his personality, his worth, and his relations with other people.[137]

Illness, surgery, and accidents can distort the body image and may make necessary its reorganization. The nurse needs to be familiar with this concept so that she can help patients with the distress which they may suffer from body image distortion. Disturbances of body image are believed to underlie many clinical syndromes of bodily dysfunction.[29]

The concept of body image provides a way of thinking about one's body and how, through the body, one relates to the environment. This internal mental representation of one's body is elaborated out of all the interoceptive* stimuli that reach the cerebral cortex and all the experiences in which an individual perceives his body as a meaningful part of his subjective world.[29] Body image also helps with the localization on the body surface of incoming sensory impulses and makes possible the performance of motor activities through the constant relationship of the body to other objects.[100]

Objects that are attached to the body or participate in the body's movement are often viewed as part of the body image, e.g., a cane or wheelchair, or eyeglasses. The body image and the corresponding body boundaries function, in part, to help one maneuver in the external world. For example, knowledge of one's size or body boundaries is necessary in judging whether or not one can fit into a given space.

Paul Schilder[165] is an important contributor to our present knowledge of body image. According to him, body image is a *gestalt* or a unified pattern for organizing sensory input. Although body image has a physiologic basis, it is composed of physical, psychologic, and social experiences. Thus, body image not only includes an individual's personal and psychologic investment in his body and its parts, but also has a sociologic meaning for both the individual and society. Body image is, to Schilder, a tridimensional unity involving interpersonal, environmental, and temporal factors.

Interoceptive stimuli are those coming to the brain from the body's internal surface field; stimuli from the body's external surface field are referred to as *exteroceptive* stimuli. *Proprioceptive* stimuli arise within bodily tissues (primarily the muscles, tendons, and labyrinth) and provide information about the body's position and movement.

DEVELOPMENT OF BODY IMAGE

Even during embryonic and infantile states multiple sensory impressions begin to lay the foundation for the formation of body image. As an infant grows into a child, and on through the life of that individual, his body image continues to be susceptible to new information.

Infancy and childhood are periods of direct exploration of one's body surface and body orifices. An awareness of internal organs comes from sensations of discomfort. Usually internal organs are only vaguely incorporated into the body image except when pain or discomfort is referred to the surface. Early sensory experiences are extremely important in the development of body image; sensations that subserve optic, olfactory, auditory, thermal, and pain stimuli are believed to be of secondary importance to the kinesthetic* and tactile exploration of the body during the formation of body image.[100] Movement, play, pain, and interactions with others all contribute to body image formation.[42]

Body protuberances and body orifices are highly important in orienting one to his own body, as well as to the environment and the bodies of others. At these points communication among the body, other persons, and the environment is most direct and closest. Therefore, body protuberances and orifices have particular value and meaning in body image.[42, 165]

Over the years, with growth, the body image is continuously modified and the mental images of the body and body parts that are developed remain as memory traces within the nervous system. In addition to knowledge about his own body, the growing child perceives the bodies of others, com-

*"Kinesthesia" refers to the sense through which we perceive muscular motion, weight, position, and so forth.

pares himself to them, and identifies with them. He learns to have certain attitudes toward his body and body functions. Such attitudes and affects generally are related to the individual's sex and are acquired through the process of socialization. Parental attitudes will strongly influence what the child perceives as "good, clean, loved, and pleasing" about his body and body parts, and what he views as "bad, dirty, disliked, or repulsive."[100] During the developmental process a value is attached to the body as a whole. However, "the psychic investment in some parts of the body appears to be greater than in others, and this differential evaluation appears to be related to the meaning which these particular parts have in the life of the individual."[43]

DISTURBANCES OF BODY IMAGE

Body-image phenomena, as observed in the general clinic, may represent either a healthy psychophysiologic reaction or be evidence of psychological and emotional maladaptation.[100]

Acute disturbances of body image may occur following surgical or traumatic dismemberment when the basic body image persists in spite of the visible or apparent loss of a body part. Crowley[42] comments that the body image is constantly the same and yet constantly different, in the same way that the body itself remains the same and yet changes. However, alterations in one's body image may lag far behind physical changes that occur, particularly if the changes occur traumatically or if they are undesirable.

When an individual fails to reorganize his body image over a period of time following distortions or changes in his body, he has not made the appropriate psychologic adaptation. Such maladaptive states often occur in individuals for whom the integrity of the pre-illness or pre-accident body image was overvalued in maintaining self-esteem. For example, limb amputees generally adapt poorly to limb loss if the integrity of a limb symbolizes either masculinity or femininity to them.[100] Thus, the *meaning* of the bodily defect to the individual is highly important. Kolb notes, "Depending upon the individual, the loss may have any meaning such as heroic sacrifice or a deserved punishment, a realization of helplessness and vulnerability, a conviction of loathsomeness, a despicable mutilation to be hidden or accepted, or a rejection of the part with defiance toward society and social customs."[100]

In our society, physical disfigurement is generally viewed with disapproval, repulsion, and rejection. Deformity and disfigurement are therefore anxiety-provoking. "Despite evidence of social, vocational, and intellectual competency, the deformed are exposed to a kind of stereotyping which is socially disadvantageous. Pervasive as these attitudes are, there is a reality basis for the high concern manifested by patients with physical deformities."[100]

Because they emulate the generally rejecting attitudes of their families, peers, and society as a whole, most patients with body defects manifest unhealthy attitudes and behavior in relation to their bodies. Indications of such rejection of one's body image are:[100] reticence to meet others; reclusive tendencies; unwillingness to look into mirrors; unwillingness to discuss the deformity; and unwillingness to accept corrective surgery, corrective aids, vocational rehabilitation, or other devices that aid rehabilitation.

A distortion of one's customary body image is experienced as a distortion of the self. A disfigured person may fear separation from and rejection by significant persons upon whom he is dependent. As a part of separation anxiety, such a patient may feel hostile toward these others. Also, he may feel hostile toward surgeons and others involved in his care. Distortions of body image also modify the patient's unconscious mental life. Thus, he may repeatedly dream of the incident that caused his disfigurement and/or may have a wish-fulfilling dream life in which the lost part plays an active role.[100]

Because disturbances in body image are threatening and anxiety-provoking, denial is frequently used by these patients. For example, paraplegic patients may deny that their paralysis is permanent.[42] Depressive reactions also occur frequently following disfigurement.[100]

In some patients the threat or actuality of trauma associated with surgical procedures may remobilize repressed fantasies of personal mutilation. It is not unusual for patients who are to have limb amputations to be highly concerned about how the separated limb will be handled and disposed of. Sometimes frank psychotic reactions, related to distortions of body image, follow acute trauma or prolonged somatic disease.[100]

Bellak[15] observes that when a person is ill with heart disease or disease of some other organ, the patient develops a special image of the involved organ which could be called an "organ image." When this occurs the organ looms predominantly in the patient's thoughts, and his attitude toward the sick organ may change in such a way that the organ itself becomes *anthropomorphized* in his thinking; i.e., he thinks of the organ as something independent, needing special care. The patient's attitude toward his sick organ (and thus, toward himself) may become overprotective and oversolicitous.

Alterations in body image have been demonstrated[6] to occur as a result of long-term confinement to a wheelchair. Because a wheelchair is present between the body and the external world the body itself ceases to perform its normal function of contact with the environment; body image boundaries deteriorate because of disuse, and judgments about body boundaries become inaccurate. In this situation, body image boundaries no longer have the needed contact with the environment that provides the body with the feedback necessary for a continuing evaluation of its status and boundaries.

SITUATIONS CAUSING BODY IMAGE DISTURBANCES

Kolb observes that body image disturbances may be classified as consequent to the following categories of illnesses: "(1) disorders following neurologic diseases and affecting any part of the sensory or motor system connected with movement and posture, whether involving the peripheral or the central nervous system; (2) disorders occurring with changes in the body structure as an expression of acquired or induced toxic or metabolic disorder; (3) disorders consequent to progressive deformation, occurring either late or early in life and caused by other somatic diseases; (4) disorders after acute dismemberment; and (5) disorders of personality development, including the psychoses, psychoneuroses, and psychopathic states."[100]

Body image disturbances can also be classified according to whether the body image is:[42] (1) exaggerated, e.g., during pain and with hypochondriasis; (2) diminished, e.g., following cerebral vascular accidents; (3) distorted, e.g., with drug intoxication, migraine headaches, vertigo, and syncope; and (4) phantom, e.g., phantom pain, phantom limb, and following mastectomy. It should be mentioned that phantom sensations are not necessarily painful. While phantoms of amputated limbs are the most frequently encountered, phantoms may also occur following removal of other body protuberances, e.g., the nose, eyes, teeth, nipples, breasts, and penis.[100]

Following cerebral vascular accidents resulting in paralysis of limbs, the patient often feels as if the limb were not a part of himself or as if it were gone, even though it is still a part of his body. Following amputation the opposite occurs, and the patient generally feels as if the missing body part were still present; he experiences a persisting phantom of the body part.[42]

The importance of body image and its distortion in illness can be illustrated by considering facial or mouth pain. Because of its importance in our communication with others, the face may frequently be involved in difficulties that we have with self-concept and in communicating our needs to others. The face becomes almost synonymous with the self.[145] When pain of the face or mouth occurs, therefore, the particular emotional significance of these body areas must be considered in understanding the total problem. Face pain after traumatic alteration of the facial configuration—i.e., through accident or surgery—may persist markedly past the time it might be expected to on the basis of the organic pathology. Such pain is understandable if we realize that the patient interprets the damaged face as damaged "self."

The individual whose body image is distorted feels like a stranger to himself and to others. "I look different. Will I be loved and accepted? Have I become repulsive and ugly? How changed am I?" Anxieties of this type cannot be surgically corrected but can be relieved only by loving and accepting responses from significant persons in the individual's life.[145]

Body image and self-image are also of importance in understanding the problem of obesity. In some instances the obese individual's self-image may provide an important cornerstone for his emotional adjustment, so that weight loss, with its accompanying change in self-image, is anxiety-provoking and perhaps is emotionally detrimental. Mathis comments on this:

> It is not enough to recognize that psychogenic factors exist. It is necessary to understand that although overeating has a significant meaning to the patient, the resulting obesity also may serve an important function. It is quite irrational to tamper with the overeating unless one is also prepared to deal with the function of the excessive weight. It is quite similar to the symptoms of a neurotic illness in that their removal without attention to the basic cause may produce more discomfort than the original symptoms. This means that the physician may at times decide that weight reduction is not in his patient's best interest, or that it should be combined with psychiatric assistance.[121]

Body image is related to a variety of diverse phenomena, such as sexual behavior, level of aspiration, ability to tolerate stress, and style of life. Body image is also related to choice of "psychosomatic" symptoms. For example, research with Rorschach responses demonstrates that persons whose symptoms involve the body's exterior (e.g., rheumatoid arthritics) tend to perceive their body boundaries as being firm and as a defense against the environment, while patients with symptoms involving the body's interior (e.g., patients with peptic ulcers) are likely to perceive their body boundaries as being infinite, vulnerable, and easily penetrated.[55, 203]

Nonsurgical treatment procedures can cause changes in body image. For example, side effects of medications can cause changes in secondary sex characteristics or the development of facial changes such as moon face; or changes may occur in skin color as a result of radiation.[27]

HELPING THE PATIENT TO ACCEPT HIS CHANGING BODY IMAGE

To quote Crowley:

> In working with the patient who is suffering from a serious disturbance in body image, one's goals are to reduce anxiety to the point where [the] patient is able to view his situation comfortably and support him as he begins the task of reconstructing or changing his body image.[42]

Crowley summarizes the following points in the nursing care of patients who have disturbed body images:[42]

> Listen to the patient to identify areas of confusion and to become aware of how his behavior makes sense to him.

> Support areas of health and avoid confrontation in troubled areas, thereby lessening anxiety.

> Encourage movement since movement helps to build body image (by bringing the body into new relationships with itself, the environment, and other people).

> Encourage interaction with other people. Experiencing the reaction of others to one's body and one's reaction to theirs is important in altering body image. The patient must learn to re-relate to others with his changed body.

> Help the patient to become involved in caring for his body so that he can learn to love his body as it now exists. Through self-care, the patient increases those visual, tactile, and proprioceptive stimuli that help him to learn to know his body once again.

> Communicate, through your nursing care, your concern for and interest in the patient's body. Through your ability to care for and respect a patient's mutilated body, he can learn to reassess his feelings of revulsion and dislike.

Whenever possible, patients should be psychologically prepared preoperatively for surgical procedures that may severely change their body image. Examples of such operations are: hysterectomy, radical mastectomy, amputation of the extremities, thoracoplasty, radical excisions of the head, face and neck, and colostomy, ileostomy, and abdominal-perineal resection.

CHAPTER 15

Terminal Illness, the Process of Dying, and Grief

> To be aware of the separateness of self is to be aware of one's insignificance and helplessness, and this entails the knowledge that one will die . . . death remains. Eventually nothing avails against it, for it is not a misfortune but an inevitability.[200]

For some nurses the care of patients who are experiencing terminal illness and the process of dying is one of the most uncomfortable situations in their nursing practice. Patients in this ultimate situation are greatly in need of the compassionate understanding and skills that they believe nurses should possess. Unfortunately, in the care of a dying patient, many nurses feel that they do not meet their own expectations or those of the patient.

Frequently a patient's last home is a hospital ward and his last contact with the living is with a nurse. Often, too, a nurse is the first staff member to meet with friends and relatives of a deceased person. The nurse has the daily care of the terminal patient and the minute-by-minute moments with him and his family. Both patient and family look to her for empathy, comfort, and direction.

Nursing interaction with a dying patient and the physical care given through terminal illness do *not* need to be sources of discomfort for nurses. Attitudes are learned, and they are amenable to change through introspection and education. Like any other nursing service, the care of the dying can become a source of pride for the nurse who achieves skill in this area and who obtains a sense of satisfaction in helping a patient through perhaps the most anxiety-laden period of his life. The care of the dying is a learned skill that will mature with increments of thoughtful practice. One nurse expresses her satisfaction in the care of the terminally ill as follows:

> Many people have said to me, "How depressing it must be knowing that in spite of all your efforts they will not get better." I suppose that it would be if one measured achievement in that way, but I believe that there is an entirely different way to look at this work. Surely, to provide the support and care and attention that practically every human being will need in his turn, is worthy of all the skill and thought and experience that nursing can provide.[63]

The needs of the dying are many, complex, individualized, and often are debatable. Some issues often discussed are: whether or not a patient should be told that his illness appears fatal; whether or not a patient should die at home or in a hospital; and euthanasia. The philosophic issues involved in the care of the terminally ill cannot be pursued in this text, but they are issues to which every nurse should address herself.

ANXIETIES ABOUT DEATH

There are many factors in growing up in our society today that tend to make us uncomfortable in thinking about death and to make it difficult for us to be with the dying. If the nurse hopes to help others to accept death, she must: reach certain philosophic conclusions about death herself; recognize that cultural and religious beliefs vary concerning death; and understand that each individual's personal experiences with the dying and dead markedly affect his perspective of death. The more completely the nurse can understand and accept various individual perspectives about death, the less pressured she will feel to force her own viewpoint upon others.

For some persons the mental preparation for death is more difficult than the physical act of dying. Anxiety must be coped with, a meaning must be assigned to death, and unresolved conflicts are often revived. Although terminally ill patients should not be pressured to discuss impending death, they should feel free to do so if they wish.

It is natural for frightened people to employ mental defense mechanisms in an attempt to protect themselves from anxiety. As a nurse you need to recognize defensive behavior in dying patients and to accept such behavior without retaliation. Also, since defensive behavior on your part can contribute to unhappiness for patients in your care, it is important to strive to consciously recognize your own defenses concerning death and how they cause you to act toward others. For example, avoidance of the dying may be a defensive behavior on your part, for the dying are a reminder that we are each vulnerable to death. We emphasize that the recognition of one's defenses does not mean becoming void of feeling or "hardened" toward death.

In lecturing to students of nursing about the care of the dying, Dr. C. W. Wahl said:

> Our task is analogous to that of the harp player. The harp player develops a callus on the tip of each finger so that his fingers won't bleed when he plays the harp and plucks the strings. Yet, if he is a good harp player, through these calluses he preserves an amazing sensitivity. Those calluses do not prevent him from being a good harp player; they make him a good harp player. . . . Courage is not the absence of fear, it is the ability to function effectively in the presence of fear.[198]

Nurses cannot handle their anxieties about death by running from the dying, denying death, or trying to conceal it from themselves. They have *chosen* to accept a professional responsibility that *requires* them to look at feelings that they may have harbored for years. If nurses cannot become death-accepting, they will become patient-rejecting! Accepting death may require a long and difficult process of thought, experience, and consultation with others. However, nurses who have gone through this process feel that it is most worthwhile.

IMPENDING DEATH: CLINICAL CARE

The nurse cannot control the inevitability of death, but there is much that she can control in an attempt to make the final stages of life as satisfying as possible for the terminal patient.

Cautiously, and with sensitivity, try daily to discern what the patient is capable of: when he needs to be dependent and when it is best to encourage or allow independency. From experience you will come to recognize when a patient seems to be "giving up too soon" or when he seems overly distressed and depressed. Psychiatric consultations can be helpful at such times, as well as conferences with the patient's doctor and a reevaluation of the nursing care plan. Patients who are terminally ill should be independent for as long as possible and helped to pursue activities of interest; they will *need* to be dependent soon enough. Help to maintain the terminal patient's normal physical appearance, bodily functions, and activities as long as feasible. Tub baths, showers, exercises, being up and dressed, shampoos, shaves, and hair sets—all should be continued as long as desirable without unduly fatiguing the patient.

By focusing on the *present,* the nurse can help to make the terminal patient's life as natural as possible. Actually we all live only in the present; although we may recall the past or try to think ahead to the future, we really only *live* in each present moment. The terminal patient is no different in that respect.

We all want to be physically comfortable, and we are typically in more or less constant motion in an effort to attain comfort. We change our position, brush our teeth, take a bath, and so on, to attain physical comfort. Much can be done to help the terminal patient to stay physically comfortable when he can no longer help himself, if you try to anticipate what he needs.

McClain and Gragg observe that "Many of the unpleasant characteristics of death are due to the cessation of normal body functions. If the nurse understands the reasons for these changes, she will be more able to meet the needs of the patient."[122] A summary of some changes that may occur with approaching death and at death are presented below.

TABLE 15-1. CHANGES THAT OCCUR WITH APPROACHING DEATH AND AFTER DEATH

A. *Facial Appearance, and Sight, Speech, and Hearing: Facial muscles* relax; cheeks become flaccid, moving in and out with each breath. Facial structure changes so dentures cannot be worn. With dentures removed, mouth structure may collapse, lips pucker and sink in. Loss of muscle tone and anemia cause *facies hippocratica:* prominent cheeks and chin; pinched sharp nose; pale ashy skin; and sunken, glazed eyes. Sides of nose draw in with each inspiration. *Sight* gradually fails. Patient instinctively turns toward light; eyes remain half open and glazed. With death, pupil fixes and does not react to light. *Speech* becomes increasingly difficult, confused, or unintelligible, and finally impossible. *Hearing* is believed to be retained longest.

B. *Skin and Muscular-Skeletal System: Muscles* relax gradually, lose their irritability, and patient is increasingly less able to move. Lips first lose reflexes, sensation and ability to move. Following death, muscles become fixated. *Rigor mortis* occurs: stiffening of body, beginning a few hours following death, starting with jaw and progressing successively down body. Immediately following death body movement of muscles may occur. With death's approach, *skin* becomes pale, cool, covered with profuse perspiration, and extremities mottled, all owing to peripheral circulatory failure. Following death, body cools rapidly initially, then gradually reaches environmental temperature.

C. *Respiratory System:* Respirations become: irregular, Cheyne-Stokes; rapid and shallow, or very slow; stertorous. Oxygen lack due to circulatory failure is ultimate cause of death in respiratory failure. When respirations cease, endoenzymes speed process of tissue hydrolysis.

D. *Central Nervous System:* Mental status varies from mental clarity to coma. Reflexes are gradually lost. Restlessness may occur owing to need for oxygen and sensation of heat experienced although body surface is cooling. Consciousness is lost with death; reflexes are absent.

E. *Circulatory System:* Circulatory changes cause alterations in temperature, pulse, and respiration as circulatory system gradually fails. Rapid, irregular pulse precedes death. Radial pulse gradually fails; once it stops, apical heart rate may continue briefly. Usually heart beats a while following cessation of respirations. Following death, blood may settle, causing *postmortem hypostasis:* bruise-like red or blue discolorations.

F. *Gastrointestinal and Genitourinary Systems:* Hiccoughs, nausea, vomiting, and weight loss occur. Impaction, urine retention, distention, and bladder and bowel incontinence may be present. Decreasing peristalsis prevents stomach from emptying its contents into intestine; stomach, thus, distends with whatever is swallowed. Impaction may occur because of lack of energy needed to evacuate bowels. Incontinence is due to relaxation of anal and bladder sphincters.

Nursing Actions In the Care of the Terminally Ill

Facial Appearance and Sight, Speech, and Hearing. Remove *dentures* if they obstruct breathing, contribute to nausea, or do not fit properly. Lubricate the patient's lips. Close the patient's mouth if it is open following death; place a rolled towel under his chin to keep mouth closed. As *vision* fails, communicate more with speech and touch. Tell the patient what you are doing. Keep the room comfortably illuminated; prevent bright lights from shining in the patient's face. If the patient's eyes are open during terminal stage, protect them with normal saline pads or protective ophthalmic ointment. After death, close the patient's eyes by gently pushing down on his eyelids. Keep a flashlight and ophthalmoscope at bedside. As *speech* fails, anticipate needs that the patient cannot express; continue to talk to him although he cannot reply. Since *hearing* remains longer than it appears to, say only what is appropriate for the patient to hear when in his presence. Speak clearly, close to the patient.

Skin and Muscular-Skeletal System. Patients in terminal stages of illness may be markedly "wasted" physically and lack sufficient adipose tissue to cushion bony prominences. Careful, frequent *skin inspection* and *care* are essential over all bony prominences. Pad the bedpan for emaciated patients. Weakened patients who cannot turn themselves should be placed on alternating pressure mattresses. Pad bony prominences. Make every effort to prevent decubitus ulcers; they are physically and mentally distressing, contributing to a sense of despair about dying.

Patients greatly appreciate being comfortably *positioned and frequently turned.* Movements should be accomplished as smoothly and effortlessly as possible so that the patient's increasing dependency is not emphasized. A patient having terminal cancer should be turned by two persons, even though he may not weigh much. Painful metastasis to the bone is common, and therefore smooth, gentle handling is important. Proper positioning can greatly lessen pain; even though it may be initially painful for the patient to be moved, he may feel markedly better in a few minutes than he did before he was turned. It is essential to use ample pillows, pads, towels, trochanter rolls, and so forth, to position patients correctly.

Continue *range-of-motion* exercises as long as the doctor believes it is advisable. Although the patient may see little purpose in this, such exercises may prevent discomforts of inactivity, e.g., aching, contractures, and so on. Exercises are carried out with the goal of maintaining *present* comfort in this situation, rather than enabling future function.

Keep the patient with *diaphoresis* dry, also his gown and bed. Following death, place patient in good body alignment as much as possible.

Respiratory System. It is distressing to feel *short of breath.* Thus, the patient who is alert, apprehensive, restless, and short of breath may be given inhalation therapy to ease his discomfort. However, this would not be given to prolong the life of a comatose patient expected to die. Elevation of head and shoulders may make breathing easier. Keep room air as fresh as possible with comfortable circulation. Observe respirations.

In the final stages of life the patient may be unable to move his secretions by coughing, swallowing, and turning in bed. As a result, his respirations become noisy (stertorous), and periodic suctioning is required. Suction gently, as necessary, to keep the patient comfortable. Avoid letting the patient remain too long in one position because this encourages pooling of secretions; keep him positioned on his sides rather than flat on his back.

Morphine may be given in an attempt to slow rapid respirations and prevent regurgitation and coughing. When respirations are very shallow, a mirror held up to the patient's nose and mouth may indicate if he is breathing; the clouding of the mirror with moisture indicates that he continues to breathe. Ultimately, respirations cease.

Central Nervous System. Some patients are alert and mentally clear until the moment of death; others may be confused, delirious, or only partially conscious; still others are comatose and unresponsive to external stimuli. Continuously evaluate the patient's mental status; plan care accordingly. For example, protect the restless patient with side rails and provide supervision; continue to inform the patient who appears comatose of what you are doing.

If the patient is conscious, evaluate the necessity for blankets according to what he says is comfortable. Even though his skin may feel cool to you, the patient may feel quite warm. Excessive covers can increase restlessness. Avoid exposing the patient; see that he is covered at least with a sheet.

Circulatory System. Follow the progression of the patient's circulatory vital signs. Have stethoscope and sphygmomanometer at bedside. Check both apical and radial pulse; when radial pulse ceases, continue to listen to apical. Following death, elevate the patient's head and shoulders to prevent discoloration of the face due to *postmortem hypostasis.*

Gastrointestinal and Genitourinary System. Often the terminally ill are nauseated and perhaps vomiting. They may ultimately be unable to tolerate food or oral liquids and may be placed on intravenous therapy. Oral liquid should be given cautiously, checking the gag reflex if in doubt. This can be done as unobtrusively as possible while giving mouth care. The patient may drown from oral liquids if the gag reflex is absent and he cannot swallow. Terminal patients may be very thirsty because of diaphoresis. Many patients will be on I.V.'s only, to relieve thirst, at the time of terminal care. Carry out I.V. therapy as ordered and monitor it carefully. The restless patient may dislodge the I.V. needle, causing painful infiltration.

Give frequent oral hygiene. If the patient is conscious and able to handle secretions, mouthwash may be used. Glycerin and lemon juice swabs are useful for persons who are semiconscious or unconscious.

Terminal patients may require assistance with drinking and eating. It may be helpful to give liquids from a teaspoon with the patient turned slightly onto one side. One of the most common causes of death in chronic illness is starvation. Attractive food service with foods served at their proper temperatures, small amounts of alcoholic beverages, medications, and mouth care are all activities that can help to stimulate the appetite. Moreover, the patient should ideally receive food when it is best for him rather than when it is most convenient for the staff. Intake, output, and weight should be recorded and subjected to careful evaluation.

Change of position and medications may help to control nausea and vomiting. Antiemetics may be given 30 to 45 minutes before meals. Other activities that may help to reduce nausea are to keep 7-Up, ginger ale, crackers, and ice chips at the bedside and to order small but frequent servings of food. Avoid jarring the patient, as this can upset the nauseated patient to the point of provoking vomiting.

Elimination can cause severe distress for the weakened, terminally ill. Common problems are: constipation, impaction, urine retention, distention, and bladder and bowel incontinence. Analgesics may cause constipation. Palpate the bladder to detect urine retention; check for abdominal distention; observe for signs of impaction. Each of these problems should receive appropriate treatment; each should be *prevented* if possible. The incontinent patient requires frequent and thorough skin, perineal, and catheter care. Every effort should be made to reduce both the physical and mental distress that incontinence can cause.

General Care. Hospital routines may need modifications for the terminal patient, and the nurse should make every attempt to modify her care to maintain the patient's welfare rather than for purposes of nursing convenience. For example, the patient who is restless from pain and bed rest should not be awakened for early morning care; his days of pain and discomfort are long enough and he should be allowed to wait to be washed and have his linens changed when he awakens. Moreover, it might be that the patient sleeps poorly at night and is in need of sleep.

Because the terminally ill person may tire easily, the nurse may need to limit visitors and to space procedures to prevent undue fatigue. The patient should be kept physically clean, but a "total bath" may not be necessary, and may be too painful or fatiguing.

Dressings should be changed as frequently as necessary, and the atmosphere around the patient kept fresh, without draft, comfortably lit, and quiet. Even though every effort is made to keep the patient and the environment clean, there may be situations in which distressing odors are present and pleasant air sprays may be helpful. These should be used as discreetly as possible to lessen the patient's feeling that he is offensive.

All unnecessary or soiled equipment should be removed from the room. Perhaps the patient will enjoy having some familiar objects in his room, and these should be permitted as much as possible.

Rest periods should be planned and maintained. A sign posted on the door when a patient is resting may spare him unnecessary interruptions or noises, e.g.: "Mr. Johnson is resting from 1 to 2 this afternoon. Please do not disturb him." However, he should not feel ignored or forgotten. It is possible to greatly relieve a patient's apprehensions by letting him know that you are keeping in touch with him. Drop in and visit at times when the patient hasn't called you so he won't feel he must call each time he needs help. He may feel relieved to know that you are watching out for him in the event that he should be unable to call you.

In managing the pain, nausea, and other problems of the terminally ill, the nurse will have opportunity to ease patients' discomforts by skillfully administering medications so that they will be most effective. Her consultations with physicians regarding the effectiveness of medications will help to keep orders current with patients' changing needs.

Pain of increasing intractability and severity will be a source of great distress for some patients. Pain control should be as intensive as possible; that is to say, the nurse should employ all her nursing skills to control it, and not rely just on medications.

A question that has long concerned people is whether or not the act of dying is itself painful. An expert on pain, Dr. W. K. Livingston, has discussed this question in the following way:

> I am convinced that neither a dying man nor a person undergoing anesthesia feels any pain, though their groans and body movements, those physical manifestations which we so naturally associate with pain, may seem to support the contrary view.
>
> With these convictions I can tell the man who fears death will be painful that dying is merely the closing event in a sequential loss of function which accompanies brain depression. . . . A dying man may welcome death because it offers his exhausted body rest. Before all his senses fail, before he loses all power of speech and movement, before his heart stops beating, long before his nerves lose their capacity to transmit pain signals, the ability of the brain to translate these signals into pain perception has been lost. For pain is a product of consciousness in which the essential element is awareness.[116]

GRIEF: REACTION TO LOSS

The process of grieving is frequently observed in nursing: people who are facing death grieve because they must die and leave family, friends, and life; those who have died are grieved for by the living who miss them; and patients who have lost a part of themselves (i.e., an organ or a limb) grieve for their loss of body part or body image that was familiar to them and a part of their essential narcissism. Because the grieving individual is often cared for by nurses, the nurse must understand the grief process.

The process of grieving is essentially a reaction to loss. For example, the reactions of a child to the loss of its mother are similar to the sequence of mourning behavior in adults. Bowlby[21, 22] noted these similarities and observed the following behavioral phase: First, a vehement *protest* that may be expressed behaviorally in many different ways, such as: confusion, negation, efforts to recover the lost one, crying, rage, self-mutilation, and introjection. The next phase is that of *despair,* which is manifested by apathy, disorganization of behavior, loss of appetite, solitary rumination, and isolation. The final phase is one of gradual detachment from the lost one, followed by a reattachment to surrounding persons and substitutes for the lost one.

The nurse who can understand these various phases of behavior will be able to apply this model in an attempt to understand the loss reactions that patients express. The patient who has lost a limb, for example, may at first protest the loss, then despair because of the loss, and, finally, gradually detach himself from the lost limb and direct his interests to mastering the use of a substitute one. The understanding nurse will, thus, not express retaliatory anger to a patient who expresses anger in the early stages of recovery from an amputation. Likewise, she will have insight into his moments of despair in the recovery process. In both of these situations she will recall this basic rule:

> *Persons who have experienced loss must be allowed to grieve.*

Rumination of the loss is necessary in grieving, and much nursing care will center around listening to what the grieving person has to say. Often there is no need for the nurse to say anything. The grieving person may be repetitious in the contemplation of his loss. It must be remembered that the purpose of his communication is not to tell news but to express feelings that require repetition. Tears may aid the grieving individual and should not be suppressed. Rather than feeling embarrassed about crying, the person experiencing loss should be helped to feel that it is perfectly natural that he cry and, moreover, that he need not cry alone. If mentioning the loss makes the grieving person cry, the nurse should not feel guilt over bringing the subject up. As indicated, a catharsis is needed to help with gradual emotional detachment from the loss.

Many people, even those with religious belief in an afterlife, often do not want to be reminded that they must face the uncertain aspects of death and leave life as they know it. Death evokes feelings of grief not only in those who will be left behind in life, but also in the dying who must leave life as they know it. Death means separation; the living and the deceased will be parted, each losing the other.

The grieving person appreciates those who can accept his grief and stay with him. There is little need for words, and much feeling can be conveyed with a touch of the hand or sitting silently together.

In the case of the person with a terminal illness, he must be allowed to grieve in advance of his loss or in anticipation of it. Anticipatory guidance[30] is helpful in adjusting to the impact of loss. This guidance involves talking about an impending loss and the meaning of the loss to the person. Based on her work with over 200 dying patients, psychiatrist Dr. Elizabeth Kubler-Ross[103–105] presents the following insights concerning grief: The terminally ill patient must grieve in order to prepare himself to leave this world. This has been referred to as "preparatory depression," and is thus distinguished from "reactive depression" that people may experience as a result of loss of a body part. The patient who is grieving about the coming loss of his life should be allowed to express his sorrow without being told not to be sad. He is not helped by being told to "look at the sunny side of things," for this would mean that he should somehow not contemplate his impending death.

Persons who are not allowed to express grief, or who have their grieving process excessively suppressed with medications (e.g., tranquilizers or sedatives), can become severely depressed. However, the nurse should recall that any behavior that is excessive or prolonged may indicate severe mental turmoil that might benefit from psychiatric help. Excessive, prolonged grieving may be indicative of marked depression.

Authorities have noted that in our society, with its small-family system and close relationships with only a few persons, we are susceptible to feeling loss through death more deeply than people in societies that encourage relationships with large numbers of people. Because we are close to so few people, those who die seem psychologically irreplaceable and we have difficulty turning to others.

Our society does not teach us how to grieve. As a matter of fact, we often stifle the grieving process and are upset if people appear to be grieving or if they attempt to act out their grief; we expect composure and for grief to be internalized. People who cry often make us uncomfortable. Other cultures have established behavioral expectations for grieving persons. Thus, it is possible for them to act out their loss more comfortably because they know what to do and what is expected.

Nurses often experience feelings of bereavement at

the death of a patient, but are unable to express their grief. Conflict of this nature produces a tension between the social role of bereaved person and the role of nurse.[150]

CONCLUSION

It is not easy to care for the dying—to give them the nursing care and support that they should have and need. Patients who die do not make us feel good as nurses, as do those who recover and bolster our feelings of healing omnipotence. Other peoples' deaths influence us and we feel their loss. John Donne wrote, "Any man's death diminishes me because I am involved in Mankind." Such losses hurt. Nevertheless, it would not be possible to feel a loss if we had not experienced gains from those same individuals.

There comes a time to die. It is as natural to die as it is to be born and to breathe. The acts of life are all interrelated, and in many ways there is a natural progression toward death throughout life.

References for Unit III

1. A time to die: Further reflections. *Medical Journal,* 1:127, January 18, 1969.
2. A way of dying. *Atlantic Monthly,* 199:53, January, 1957.
3. Aldrich, C. K.: The dying patient's grief. *J.A.M.A.,* 184:109, May 4, 1963.
4. Annis, J. W.: The dying patient. *Psychosomatics,* 10: 289, September-October, 1969.
5. Apple, D. (ed.): *Sociological Studies of Health and Sickness.* New York, McGraw-Hill Book Company, 1960.
6. Arnhoff, F. N., and Mehl, M. C.: Body image deterioration in paraplegia. *Journal of Nervous and Mental Diseases,* 137:88, July, 1963.
7. Arteberry, J. K.: Distance and the dying patient. *In* Bergersen, B. S., et al. (eds.): *Current Concepts in Clinical Nursing.* Vol. I. St. Louis, The C. V. Mosby Company, 1967.
8. Baker, J., and Sorensen, K.: A patient's concern with death. *American Journal of Nursing,* 63:90, July, 1963.
9. Barckley, V.: What can I say to the cancer patient? *Nursing Outlook,* 6:317, June, 1958.
10. Barckley, V.: The crisis in cancer. *American Journal of Nursing,* 67:278, February, 1967.
11. Barnes, E.: *People in Hospital.* New York, St. Martin's Press, 1961.
12. Baumann, B.: Diversities in conceptions of health and physical fitness. *Journal of Health and Human Behavior,* 2:39, Spring, 1961.
13. Beecher, H. K.: Nonspecific forces surrounding disease and the treatment of disease. *J.A.M.A.,* 179:437, February 10, 1962.
14. Bell, R. R.: The impact of illness on family roles. *In* Folta, J., and Deck, E. (eds.): *A Sociological Framework for Patient Care.* New York, John Wiley & Sons, Inc., 1966.
15. Bellak, L. (ed.): *Psychology of Physical Illness.* New York, Grune & Stratton, Inc., 1952.
16. Bernard, J., and Thompson, L.: *Sociology: Nurses and Their Patients in a Modern Society.* 7th ed. St. Louis, The C. V. Mosby Company, 1966.
17. Biase, D. V., et al.: Anticipated responses to short-term sensory deprivation. *Psychological Reports,* 24:351, April, 1969.
18. Blewett, L. J.: To die at home. *American Journal of Nursing,* 70:2602, December, 1970.
19. Bloom, S. W.: *The Doctor and His Patient.* New York, Russell Sage Foundation, 1963.
20. Bowers, M., et al.: *Counseling the Dying.* New York, Thomas Nelson & Sons, 1964.
21. Bowlby, J.: Childhood mourning and its implications for psychiatry. *American Journal of Psychiatry,* 118:481, 1961.
22. Bowlby, J.: Process of mourning. *International Journal of Psychoanalysis,* 42:317, 1961.
23. Brawley, P., and Pos, R.: The informational underload (sensory deprivation) model in contemporary psychiatry. *Journal of Canadian Psychiatric Association,* 12:105, April, 1967.
24. Brooks, B. R.: Aggression. *American Journal of Nursing,* 67:2519, December, 1967.
25. Brown, E. L.: *Newer Dimensions of Patient Care. Part I. The Use of the Physical and Social Environment of the General Hospital for Therapeutic Purposes.* New York, Russell Sage Foundation, 1961.
26. Brown, E. L.: *Newer Dimensions of Patient Care. Part III. Patients as People.* New York, Russell Sage Foundation, 1964.
27. Brunner, L. S., et al.: *Medical Surgical Nursing.* 2nd. ed. Philadelphia, J. B. Lippincott Company, 1970.
28. Burnside, I. M.: Sensory stimulation: An adjunct to group work with the disabled aged. *Mental Hygiene,* 53:381, July, 1969.
29. Cantrell, W. A., and Frazier, S. H.: Psychiatry for the general practitioner. *In* Arieti, S. (ed.): *American Handbook of Psychiatry.* Vol. III. New York, Basic Books, Inc., 1966.
30. Caplan, G.: *Principles of Preventive Psychiatry.* New York, Basic Books, Inc., 1964.
31. Cardone, S. S., et al.: Psychophysical studies and body-image, IV. Disturbances in a hemiplegic sample. *Archives of General Psychiatry* (Chicago), 21:464, October, 1969.
32. Carner, D. C.: You can manage people better if you tell them more. *Modern Hospital,* 109:96, September, 1967.
33. Cartwright, A.: *Patients and Their Doctors.* New York, Atherton Press, 1967.
34. Charlton, M. H.: Visual hallucinations. *Psychiatric Quarterly,* 37:489, 1963.
35. Chodil, J., and Williams, B.: The concept of sensory deprivation. *Nursing Clinics of North America,* 5:453, September, 1970.
36. Christman, L.: Assisting the patient to learn the "patient role". *Journal of Nursing Education,* 6: 17, April, 1967.
37. Clever, C.: Do you dare risk involvement with patients? *R.N.,* 30:69, November, 1967.
38. Connolly, M. G.: What acceptance means to patients. *American Journal of Nursing,* 60:754, December, 1960.

39. Corbeil, M.: Nursing process for a patient with a body image disturbance. *Nursing Clinics of North America,* 6:155, March, 1971.
40. Coser, R. L.: *Life in the Ward.* East Lansing, Michigan, Michigan State University Press, 1962.
41. Craven, P. K.: A facade for fear. *A.N.A. Clin. Sessions,* 28, 1966.
42. Crowley, D.: Body Image. (Mimeographed.) Presented at the Institute, "The Unconscious Patient and the Disoriented Patient," sponsored by the University of Washington School of Nursing, April 14, 1966.
43. Crowley, D.: *Pain and Its Alleviation.* Los Angeles, School of Nursing, UCLA, 1962.
44. Davidson, R. P.: Let's talk about death, Part 2. To give care in terminal illness, *American Journal of Nursing,* 66:74, January, 1966.
45. Dorfman, W.: *Closing the Gap Between Medicine and Psychiatry.* Springfield, Illinois, Charles C Thomas, 1966.
46. Duff, R., and Hollingshead, A. B.: *Sickness and Society.* New York, Harper & Row, 1968.
47. Dunham, J.: Perception and sensory deprivation. (Mimeographed.) Presented at the Institute, "The Unconscious Patient and the Disoriented Patient," sponsored by the University of Washington School of Nursing, April 14, 1966.
48. Dunlap, H. E.: Family and the dying patient. *Geriatric Nursing,* 3:15, June, 1967.
49. Eisman, R.: Why did Joe die? *American Journal of Nursing,* 71:501, March, 1971.
50. Elliott, S.: The day the students came. *American Journal of Nursing,* 69:551, March, 1969.
51. Elmore, J. L., and Verwoerdt, A.: Psychological reactions to impending death. *Hospital Topics,* 45:35, November, 1967.
52. Engel, G. L.: Grief and grieving. *American Journal of Nursing,* 64:93, September, 1964.
53. Feifel, H. (ed.): *The Meaning of Death.* New York, McGraw-Hill Book Company, Inc., 1959.
54. Field, M.: *Patients Are People.* 3rd ed. New York, Columbia University Press, 1967.
55. Fisher, S., and Cleveland, S. E.: *Body Image and Personality.* Princeton, N. J., D. Van Nostrand Company, 1958.
56. Flynn, W. R.: Visual hallucinations in sensory deprivation. *Psychiatric Quarterly,* 36:55, 1962.
57. Folta, J., and Deck, E. (eds.): *A Sociological Framework for Patient Care.* New York, John Wiley & Sons, Inc., 1966.
58. Freeman, H., et al. (eds.): *Handbook of Medical Sociology.* Englewood Cliffs, New Jersey, Prentice-Hall, Inc., 1963.
59. Freeman, V. J.: Human aspects of health and illness: Beyond the germ theory. *Journal of Health and Human Behavior,* 1:8, 1960.
60. Friedson, E.: *Patients' Views of Medical Practice.* New York, Russell Sage Foundation, 1961.
61. Fulton, R. L. (ed.): *Death and Identity.* New York, John Wiley & Sons, Inc., 1965.
62. Fulton, R. L., and Langton, P. A.: Attitudes toward death: An emerging mental health problem. *Nursing Forum,* 3:105, 1964.
63. Garland, D.: The care of the dying. *Nursing Times,* 64:355, March 15, 1968.
64. Gerdes, L.: The confused or delirious patient. *American Journal of Nursing,* 68:1228, June, 1968.
65. Glaser, B., and Strauss, A. L.: The social loss of dying patients. *American Journal of Nursing,* 64: 119, June, 1964.
66. Glaser, B., and Strauss, A. L.: *Awareness of Dying.* Chicago, Aldine Publishing Company, 1965.
67. Glaser, B., and Strauss, A. L.: *Time for Dying.* Chicago, Aldine Publishing Company, 1968.
68. Gordon, G.: *Role Theory and Illness: A Sociological Perspective.* New Haven, Connecticut, College and University Press, 1966.
69. Gould, D.: Power and sickness. *New Statesman,* 74:13, July 7, 1967.
70. Green, E. P.: How can we help the dying? *Consultant,* 7:46, June, 1967.
71. Gunther, J.: *Death Be Not Proud.* New York, Pyramid Books, 1957.
72. Hall, B. L.: Human relations in the hospital setting. *Nursing Outlook,* 16:43, March, 1968.
73. Hamilton, J. W.: Masked depression: Progressive somatiziation as a response to object loss. *Psychiatric Quarterly,* 44:583, 1970.
74. Hayes, W., and Gazaway, R.: *Human Relations in Nursing.* 3rd ed. Philadelphia, W. B. Saunders Company, 1964.
75. Hearn, C. R.: Evaluating patient's nursing needs. *Nursing Times,* 68:65 (insert), April 27, 1972.
76. Hecht, A.: Questions relatives ask. *Geriatric Nursing,* 4:23, February, 1968.
77. Henry, W. D., and Mann, A. M.: Diagnosis and treatment of delirium. *Canadian Medical Association Journal,* 93:1156, November 27, 1965.
78. Hinsie, L., and Campbell, R. J.: *Psychiatric Dictionary.* New York, Oxford University Press, 1960.
79. Hinton, J.: *Dying.* Baltimore, Penguin Books, Inc., 1967.
80. Hinton, J. M.: The physical and mental distress of the dying. *Quarterly Journal of Medicine,* 32:1, 1963.
81. Hinton, J. M.: Facing death. *Journal of Psychosomatic Research,* 10:22, July, 1966.
82. Hirt, M., et al.: Attitudes to body products among normal subjects. *Journal of Abnormal Psychology,* 74:486, August, 1969.
83. Hobart, C. W.: The meaning of death. *Journal of Existential Psychiatry,* 4(No. 15):219, Winter, 1964.
84. Hoffman, E.: Don't give up on me! *American Journal of Nursing,* 71:60, January, 1971.
85. Howell, T. H.: Some physical causes of mental symptoms. *Gerontologia Clinica,* 1:132, 1959.
86. Ingles, T.: Death on a ward. *Nursing Outlook,* 12:28, January, 1964.
87. Jackson, J. K.: The role of the patient's family in illness. *Nursing Forum,* 1:119, Summer, 1962.
88. Johnson, D. E.: Powerlessness: A significant determinant in patient behavior? *Journal of Nursing Education,* 6:39, April, 1967.
89. Jung, C.: The soul and death. *In* Feifel, H. (ed.): *The Meaning of Death.* New York, McGraw-Hill Book Co., Inc., 1959.
90. Kastenbaum, R.: Viewpoint: Helping the patient prepare for death. *Geriatrics,* 22:80, February, 1967.
91. Kaufman, R. V.: Body-image changes in physically ill teen-agers. *Journal American Academy of Child Psychiatry,* 11:157, January, 1972.
92. Keeping patients alive. Who Decides? *US News,* 72: 44, May 22, 1972.
93. King, J. M.: Denial. *American Journal of Nursing,* 66:1010, May, 1966.

94. King, S.: *Perceptions of Illness and Medical Practice*. New York, Russell Sage Foundation, 1962.
95. Kneisl, C. R.: Dying patients and their families: How staff can give support. *Hospital Topics,* 45:37, November, 1967.
96. Kneisl, C. R.: Thoughtful care for the dying. *American Journal of Nursing,* 68:550, March, 1968.
97. Kneisl, C. R.: Body image. Its meaning to the self. *Journal of New York State Nurses Association,* 2:29, Spring, 1971.
98. Knicely, K. H.: The world of distorted perception. *American Journal of Nursing,* 67:998, May, 1967.
99. Knutson, A.: *The Individual, Society, and Health Behavior*. New York, Russell Sage Foundation, 1965.
100. Kolb, L. C.: Disturbances of the body-image. *In* Arieti, S. (ed.): *American Handbook of Psychiatry*. Vol. I. New York, Basic Books, Inc., 1959.
101. Kraegel, J. M., et al.: A system of patient care based on patient needs. *Nursing Outlook,* 20:257, April, 1972.
102. Kram, C., et al.: The dying patient. *Psychosomatics,* 10:293, September-October, 1969.
103. Kübler-Ross, E.: *On Death and Dying*. New York, The Macmillan Company, 1969.
104. Kübler-Ross, E.: Dying with dignity. *Canadian Nurse,* 67:31, October, 1971.
105. Kübler-Ross, E.: What is it like to be dying? *American Journal of Nursing,* 71:54, January, 1971.
106. Kutscher, A. (ed.): *Death and Bereavement*. Springfield, Illinois, Charles C Thomas, 1969.
107. Larson, V.: What hospitalization means to patients. *American Journal of Nursing,* 61:44, May, 1961.
108. LeShan, L.: The world of the patient in severe pain of long duration. *Journal of Chronic Diseases,* 17:119, 1964.
109. LeShan, L., and LeShan, E.: Psychotherapy and the patient with a limited life span. *Psychiatry,* 24:318, 1961.
110. Levine, D.: Anxiety about illness. *Journal of Health and Human Behavior,* 35:30, Spring, 1962.
111. Levitas, I. M.: Treating hospital patients like people. *Medical Economics,* 43:85, December 12, 1966.
112. Levy, R.: Immobilized patient and his psychological well-being. *Postgraduate Medicine,* 40:74, July, 1966.
113. Lewis, F.: *Patients, Doctors, and Families*. New York, Doubleday & Company, Inc., 1968.
114. Lewis, F. C.: Patients who want to be sick. *Today's Health,* 46:21, January, 1968.
115. Lewis, W. R.: A time to die. *Nursing Forum,* 4(No. 1): 7, 1965.
116. Livingston, W. K.: What is pain? *Scientific American Reprint,* March, 1953.
117. Loeser, J.: The disoriented patient: Causes and effects. (Mimeographed.) Presented at the Institute, "The Unconscious Patient and the Disoriented Patient," sponsored by the University of Washington School of Nursing, April 15, 1966.
118. Macgregor, F. C.: *Social Science in Nursing*. New York, Russell Sage Foundation, 1960.
119. Magill, K. A.: How one patient handled fear. *American Journal of Nursing,* 67:1248, June, 1967.
120. Martin, H. W., and Prange, A. J.: The stages of illness—Psychosocial approach. *Nursing Outlook,* 10:168, March, 1962.
121. Mathis, J. L.: Obesity—Sin or savior? *Psychosomatics,* 6:171, May-June, 1965.
122. McClain, M. E., and Gragg, S. H.: *Scientific Principles in Nursing*. 5th ed. Saint Louis, The C. V. Mosby Company, 1966.
123. McCown, P. P., and Wurm, E.: Orienting the disoriented. *American Journal of Nursing,* 65:118, April, 1965.
124. Mead, M.: The right to die. *Nursing Outlook,* 16:20, October, 1968.
125. Mechanic, D.: The concept of illness behavior. *Journal of Chronic Disease,* 15:189, February, 1962.
126. Mechanic, D., and Volkart, E. A.: Stress, illness behavior, and the sick role. *American Sociological Review,* 26:51, February, 1961.
127. Meerloo, J. A. M.: *Illness and Cure*. New York, Grune & Stratton, 1964.
128. Meinhart, N. T., and Aspinall, M. J.: Nursing interventions in hypovigilance. *American Journal of Nursing,* 69:994, May, 1969.
129. Moriarty, D. (ed.): *The Loss of Loved Ones*. Springfield, Illinois, Charles C Thomas, 1967.
130. Morris, M., and Rhodes, M.: Guidelines for the care of confused patients. *American Journal of Nursing,* 72:1630, September, 1972.
131. Mosey, A. C.: Treatment of pathological distortion of body image. *American Journal of Occupational Therapy,* 23:413, September-October, 1969.
132. Myers, R. S.: Whatever is bad by day is worse at night. *Modern Hospital,* 110:91, January, 1968.
133. Myers, T. I.: Sensory and perceptual deprivation. *In Symposium on Medical Aspects of Stress in the Military Climate*. Washington, D.C., Walter Reed Army Institute of Research, 1964.
134. Nelson, A.: The hospital and the dignity of man. *Queensland Nurses Journal,* 9:5, January, 1967.
135. Nobbs, K. L. G.: Confusion in the elderly. *Nursing Times,* 58:1190, September 21, 1962.
136. Noyes, R.: The act of death, the art of treatment. *Medical Insight,* 3:22, March, 1971.
137. Olson, E. V.: Immobility: Effects on psychosocial equilibrium. *American Journal of Nursing,* 67: 794, April, 1967.
138. Parsons, T.: *The Social System*. Glencoe, Illinois, The Free Press, 1951.
139. Patrick, M. L.: Care of the confused elderly patient. *American Journal of Nursing,* 67:2536, December, 1967.
140. Pattison, E. M.: The experience of dying. (Mimeographed.) Presented at the Institute, "Death: Children and Adults." Sponsored by the University of Washington, School of Nursing, May 12-13, 1966.
141. Pearson, L. (ed.): *Death and Dying*. Cleveland, Case Western Reserve University, 1969.
142. Perrine, G.: Needs met and unmet. *American Journal of Nursing,* 71:2128, November, 1971.
143. Peterson, D. I.: Developing the difficult patient. *American Journal of Nursing,* 67:522, March, 1967.
144. Philip, S., et al. (eds.): *Sensory Deprivation*. Cambridge, Harvard University Press, 1961.
145. Pilling, L. F.: Psychosomatic aspects of facial pain. *In* Alling, C., III, et al. (eds.): *Facial Pain*. Philadelphia, Lea & Febiger, 1968.
146. Powers, M. E., and Storlie, F.: The apprehensive patient. *American Journal of Nursing,* 67:58–63, January, 1967.

147. Prange, A. J., Jr., and Martin, H. W.: Aids to understanding patients. *American Journal of Nursing,* 62:98, July, 1962.
148. Quint, J. C.: Obstacles to helping the dying. *American Journal of Nursing,* 66:1568, July, 1966.
149. Quint, J. C.: The dying patient: A difficult nursing problem. *Nursing Clinics of North America,* 2: 763, December, 1967.
150. Quint, J. C.: *The Nurse and the Dying Patient.* New York, The Macmillan Company, 1967.
151. Quint, J. C.: The threat of death: Some consequences for patients and nurses. *Nursing Forum,* 8:286, 1969.
152. Quint, J. C., et al.: Improving nursing care of the dying. *Nursing Forum,* 6(No. 4):368, 1967.
153. Reid, F. W., Jr.: Prolongation of life or prolonging the act of dying? *J.A.M.A.,* 202:180, October 9, 1967.
154. Reinhardt, J. M., and Meadows, P.: *Society and the Nursing Profession.* Philadelphia, W. B. Saunders Company, 1953.
155. Reusch, J.: Psychotherapy for the well and psychotherapy for the ill. *Psychotherapy and Psychosomatics,* 13:68, 1965.
156. Ritvo, M. M.: Who are "good" and "bad" patients? *The Modern Hospital,* 100:79, June, 1963.
157. Robinson, A. M.: Loss and grief. *Journal of Practical Nursing,* 21:18, May, 1971.
158. Rubenstein, V. M.: Symposium on the difficult patient. *Nursing Clinics of North America,* 2:691, December, 1967.
159. Rubin, R.: Body image and self-esteem. *Nursing Outlook,* 16:20, June, 1968.
160. Rudd, T.: Use and abuse of sedatives. *Gerontologia Clinica,* 1:148, 1959.
161. Sanders, R. A.: Improvement in time orientation in hospitalized geriatric patients. *Journal of American Geriatric Society,* 13:1013, December, 1965.
162. Sauer, J. E., Jr.: Preadmission orientation: Effect on patient manageability. *Hospital Topics,* 46:79, March, 1968.
163. Saunders, C.: The last stages of life. *American Journal of Nursing,* 65:70, March, 1965.
164. Savoie, Sister M. R.: The person before the disease. Journal of Nursing Education, 6:11, August, 1967.
165. Schilder, P.: *The Image and Appearance of the Human Body.* New York, International Universities Press, 1950.
166. Schlesinger, B.: *Higher Cerebral Functions and Their Clinical Disorders.* New York, Grune & Stratton, 1961.
167. Schoen, E. A.: Clinical problem: The demanding, complaining patient. *Nursing Clinics of North America,* 2:715, December, 1967.
168. Schultz, D. P.: *Sensory Restriction: Effects on Behavior.* New York, Academic Press, Inc., 1965.
169. Sharp, D.: Lessons from a dying patient. *American Journal of Nursing,* 68:1517, July, 1968.
170. Sigerist, H. E.: The special position of the sick. *In* Roemer, M. (ed.): *Henry E. Sigerist on the Sociology of Medicine.* New York, M. D. Publications, 1960.
171. Simpson, K.: Moment of death. *Nursing Times,* 63:1604, 1967.
172. Siu, R. G. H.: *The Man of Many Qualities: A Legacy of the I Ching.* Cambridge, The MIT Press, 1968.
173. Smith, D. W.: Patienthood and its threat to privacy. *American Journal of Nursing,* 69:509, March, 1969.
174. Sorensen, K. M., and Amis, D. B.: Understanding the world of the chronically ill. *American Journal of Nursing,* 67:811, April, 1967.
175. Sorensen, K., and Baker, J.: Curriculum implications for student-patient verbal interaction about death. *In* Pesznecker, B. L., and Hewitt, H. E. (eds.): *Psychiatric Content in the Nursing Curriculum.* Seattle, University of Washington Press, 1963.
176. Spiegel, A. D., and Demone, H. W., Jr.: Questions of hospital patients—Unasked and unanswered. *Postgraduate Medicine,* 43:215, February, 1968.
177. Steiger, W., and Hansen, A. V., Jr.: *Patients Who Trouble You.* Boston, Little, Brown and Company, 1964.
178. Sudnow, D.: *Passing On.* Englewood Cliffs, New Jersey, Prentice-Hall, Inc., 1967.
179. Susser, M., and Watson, W.: *Sociology in Medicine.* New York, Oxford University Press, 1963.
180. Sweetser, D. A.: How laymen define illness. *Journal of Health and Human Behavior,* 1:219, 1960.
181. Tagliacozzo, D. L.: The nurse from the patient's point of view. *In* Skipper, J. K., and Leonard, R. C. (eds.): *Social Interaction and Patient Care.* Philadelphia, J. B. Lippincott Company, 1965.
182. Tarnower, W.: The needs of the hospitalized patient. *Nursing Outlook,* 13:28, July, 1965.
183. Taylor, D. A., et al.: Personality factors related to response to social isolation and confinement. *Journal of Consulting and Clinical Psychology* (Washington), 33:411, August, 1969.
184. Thaler, O.: Grief and depression. *Nursing Forum,* 5(No. 2):8, 1966.
185. The care of dying older persons. *Geriatrics,* 22:91, September, 1967.
186. Thomas, M. D.: Anger in nurse-patient interactions. *Nursing Clinics of North America,* 2:737, December, 1967.
187. Toynbee, A., et al.: *Man's Concern with Death.* London, Hodder and Stroughton, 1968.
188. Ullman, M.: Disorders of body image after stroke. *American Journal of Nursing,* 64:89, October, 1964.
189. Ujhely, G. B.: Grief and depression: Implications for preventative and therapeutic nursing care. *Nursing Forum,* 5:23, 1966.
190. Ujhely, G. B.: What is realistic emotional support? *American Journal of Nursing,* 68:758, April, 1968.
191. Van den Berg, J. H.: *The Psychology of the Sickbed.* Pittsburgh, Duquesne University Press, 1966.
192. Vanden Bergh, R. L.: Let's talk about death. Part I. To overcome inhibiting emotions. *American Journal of Nursing,* 66:71, January, 1966.
193. Van Kaam, A.: The nurse in the patient's world. *American Journal of Nursing,* 59:1708, December, 1969.
194. Velazquez, J. M.: Alienation. *American Journal of Nursing,* 69:301, February, 1969.
195. Verwoerdt, A.: *Communication with the Fatally Ill.* Springfield, Illinois, Charles C Thomas, 1966.
196. Verwoerdt, A., and Wilson, R.: Communication with fatally ill patients—Tacit or explicit? *American Journal of Nursing,* 67:2307, November, 1967.
197. Wagner, N.: The loss reaction. (Mimeographed.) Presented at the Institute, "Death, Children and Adults," sponsored by the University of Washington School of Nursing, May 12, 1966.

198. Wahl, C. W.: Death. Mimeographed copy of lecture to students of nursing, University of California at Los Angeles, 1957.
199. Watson, J.: Death—A necessary concern for nurses. *Nursing Outlook,* 16:47, February, 1968.
200. Weelis, A.: *The Quest for Identity.* New York, W. W. Norton and Company, Inc., 1958.
201. Williams, B. P.: The problems and life-style of severely burned man. *In* Bergersen, B. S., et al. (eds.): *Current Concepts in Clinical Nursing.* Vol. II. St. Louis, The C. V. Mosby Company, 1969.
202. Williams, G. W.: Illness and personality. *American Journal of Nursing,* 63:85, June, 1963.
203. Williams, R. L., and Krasnoff, A. G.: Body-image and physiological patterns in patients with peptic ulcer and rheumatoid arthritis. *Psychosomatic Medicine,* 26:701, 1964.
204. Wolff, K.: Confused geriatric patient. *Journal of American Geriatric Society,* 12:266, March, 1964.
205. Wygant, W. E., Jr.: Dying, but not alone. *American Journal of Nursing,* 67:574, March, 1967.
206. Zimny, G. H.: Body image and physiological responses. *Journal of Psychosomatic Research,* 9:185, October, 1965.
207. Zubek, J. P. (ed.): *Sensory Deprivation: Fifteen Years of Research.* New York, Appleton-Century-Crofts, Inc., 1969.
208. Zubek, J. P., et al.: Relative effects of prolonged social isolation and confinement: Behavioral and EEG changes. *Journal of Abnormal Psychology,* 74:625, October, 1969.

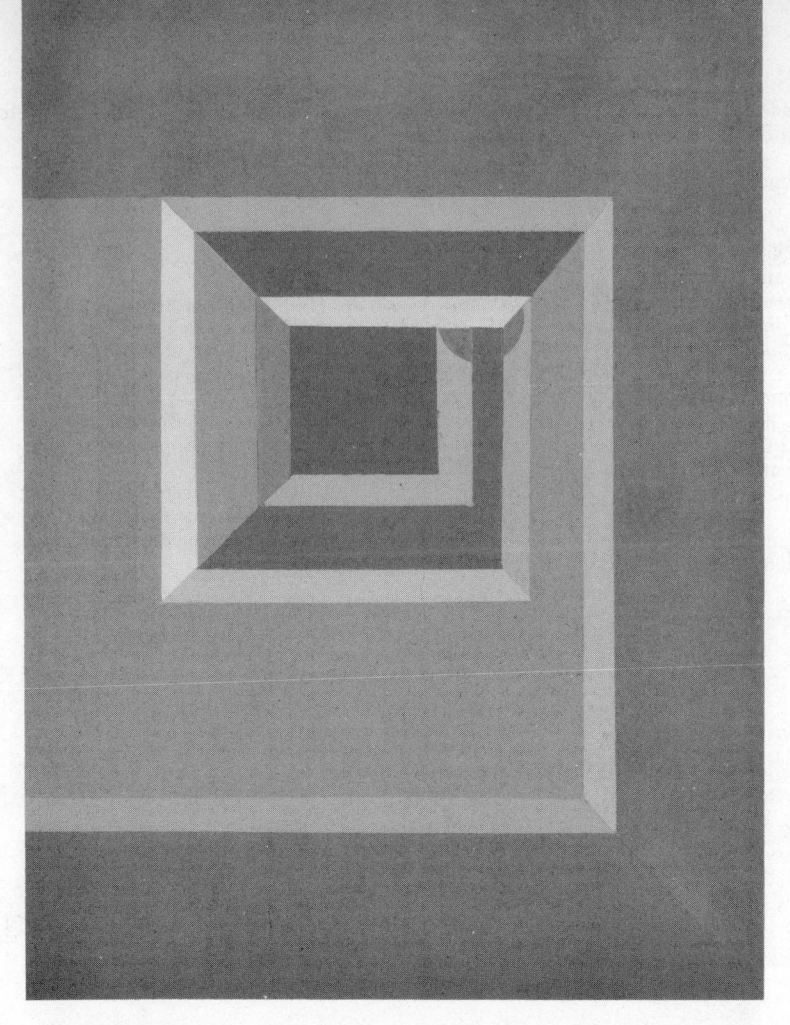

SECTION TWO

Psychophysiologic Imbalances

It is a natural law that the organism which is not sufficiently adaptable and tolerant must inevitably perish. For a failure to adapt, either in the individual or in the race, means a failure to evolve and this, in a competitive universe, is suicidal.[19]

UNIT IV

Disturbances in Homeostasis: Psychologic Imbalances

Introduction and Study Guide

Adaptation, as a general topic, was discussed at length in Unit I: psychologic adaptation was mentioned briefly as a part of general adaptation. We learned that psychologic adaptation involves adjustment to stress through the use of learning, perception, and conscious and unconscious processes, including the various psychologic defense mechanisms.

In this unit we shall pursue in greater detail some of the complexities of human psychologic adaptation and some consequences of failure to adapt. Adaptive failure takes its toll physically and psychologically, often resulting in illness. Because of the illness produced, adaptive failure, with its accompanying state of disturbed homeostasis, is of concern to the nurse.

Specifically, this unit will begin with an overview of psychologic homeostasis. Following this, the "normal" self and the self in illness will be discussed. Next, theories will be presented pertaining to anxiety, mental defense mechanisms (or mental adaptive mechanisms), and mind-body interaction. The latter part of the unit will focus on the ways in which theories of mind-body interaction contribute to "somatopsychic" and "psychosomatic" illnesses. The treatment of psychosomatic disorders also will be discussed briefly.

Perhaps you are wondering why some of these topics are included in a medical-surgical nursing textbook. Why, for example, is mind-body interaction discussed? As you will recall from Unit II, an understanding of illness and the ill person is based upon the knowledge that the mind does not exist separately from the body, and vice versa. This point has intentionally been emphasized repeatedly because if the nurse hopes to understand man's "behavior in illness," it is imperative that she realize that:

> *Every ill person is experiencing* both *physiologic and psychologic imbalances. Physiologic imbalance creates an emotional disequilibrium, and emotional imbalance causes physiologic disturbances.*

Moreover, the nurse must have an understanding of the *normal* self and its defenses as a basis for understanding the psychologic imbalances and disturbances that *illness* causes.

We wish to emphasize in this introduction that while we use such terms as "mental," "psyche," "emotional," and "psychologic," or "physical," "soma," "somatic," and "physiologic," it is not actually possible to dichotomize (separate) man into such entities. These terms have filtered down from the time in history when it was incorrectly believed that a separation did exist between mind and body. We continue to find evidence of this ancient idea of mind-body separation expressed daily in materials we read and statements we hear, such as, "I like medical-surgical nursing because I don't like to work with patients who have mental problems." A statement such as this indicates a belief that it is possible to classify patients as *either* physically sick *or* emotionally sick. As we have just indicated, this is simply not true; illness is not an "either-or" matter that involves either physical or mental problems.

The student of nursing will see the far-reaching effects of disturbed psychologic homeostasis as soon as she enters her clinical work. It has been estimated that out of *all* the patients seen in medical practice today, one third have psychosomatic disorders and another one third have somatic (physical) disorders that are complicated by psychiatric problems. Clearly, the nurse who is practicing "medical-surgical" nursing will not be caring for patients who have purely physical problems; she will have in her care many persons with significant psychologic disorders.

The reader should find the following study guide of help in reading the unit and in summarizing major ideas once the unit has been studied.

1. The following is a list of terms that may be new to you as you read the unit:

soma, somatic, dichotomize, affect, subjective, autonomy, introspect, alienation, defense mechanisms, rationalization, projection, regression, suppression, identification, compensation, denial, reaction formation, sublimation, displacement, Cartesian dualism, somatopsychic, psychogenic, psychosomatic, functional, psychophysiologic, and epidemiology

2. When you have completed the unit you should be able generally to discuss the following in your own words:

a. The concepts of mental balance and mental imbalance
b. The continuum of behavior
c. Components of the healthy self
d. Why it is difficult to gain self-understanding
e. Ways of meeting the needs of the normal self in illness
f. How self-understanding on the nurse's part can help her in giving patient care
g. Psychologic adaptation
h. The nature of emotions
i. Anxiety as a motivating force
j. What produces anxiety
k. Physiologic, psychologic, and behavioral responses to anxiety
l. Functions and general characteristics of defense mechanisms
m. Nursing implications of defense mechanisms
n. Mind-body interaction and its relevance to nursing
o. Evidences of mind-body interaction
p. Theories of mind-body interaction
q. How language contributes to our concepts of "mind" and "body"
r. Psychogenic etiology
s. Difference between somatopsychic and psychosomatic illnesses
t. Difference between psychophysiologic and functional illnesses
u. General theories of psychophysiologic etiology
v. The adaptive or maladaptive nature of psychophysiologic symptoms
w. General prevalence of psychosomatic disorders
x. Major concepts of treatment and nursing care for patients with psychosomatic disorders

CHAPTER 16

The Self in Health and Illness

PSYCHOLOGIC HOMEOSTASIS

If people are to adjust to the stressful conditions involved in everyday living, psychologic adaptation must take place. If individuals are to live in a state of health, their psychologic processes must operate within a framework of relative balance. Here we shall discuss, in a general manner, the process of psychologic homeostasis that has been previously referred to in Unit I. Since psychologic adaptation ultimately is based upon complicated neuroanatomic and neurophysiologic processes, it is understandable that some neurologic disorders will disrupt psychologic processes. (See Unit VIII.)

Mental health can be equated with mental balance; *mental illness* can be equated with mental imbalance of such a nature that the individual is unable to cope successfully with the stresses that are a part of his "normal" life. You will recall that stress is a highly individualized, personal matter; what is stressful for one person may not prove stressful for another.

The concepts of mental balance and imbalance are not fixed and separate entities, but rather exist in fluctuating relationships with each other. This is essentially the same kind of relationship as that involved in the concepts of health and disease, which have been discussed earlier in the text. Emotional balance is comparable to a fluid or moving phenomenon; like an ocean tide, or a wave, our feelings are in a state of constant motion. They vacillate and vary and their directions may change, yet they ultimately intermingle to become a part of the whole. Some feelings crest at one time and some at another; motion, fluctuation, and oscillation are the normal states of emotions—they change with time and circumstance.

We need a series of prolonged observations of an individual's behavior to gain some idea about his overall emotional balance. Therefore, rather than observing one fixed incident in a person's life it is necessary to get a general "life-feeling" about him over a period of time before we can begin to understand his relative state of emotional equilibrium. Only by doing this can we determine the significance of any imbalances observed; i.e., is the behavior observed relatively unusual for that person, or is it fairly typical of his life pattern? An individual's relative psychologic strengths and weaknesses can become apparent with prolonged observation in the same way that his physical strengths and weaknesses will present themselves.

Summarizing, it is not possible to state a single criterion for emotional balance. Rather, emotional balance (or imbalance) is usually discussed with reference to the interaction of various kinds of behavior or feelings and the complex manner in which they go to make up each individual's unique emotional life. Let us next consider how these *separate* emotional components can be viewed.

Any given individual behavior, mood, feeling, or attitude (e.g., aggression, depression, elation, joy) can be thought of as existing on a continuum; that is to say, various behaviors or feelings may range from being virtually absent in a given individual at a given time to being present to an excessive degree.

Minor states of psychologic disequilibrium are experienced by everyone and pose no threat to the healthy "self." However, when such states of disequilibrium are extreme or prolonged, even the most basically mentally and physically healthy individual may have difficulty in reestablishing an equilibrium. Physical illness can also contribute to various degrees of psychologic disequilibrium. When psychologic homeostatic failures occur, maladaptive behavior and/or psychosomatic illness are two possible results.

Before the nurse can understand psychologic imbalances and their effects, she must first come to know the general components of the healthy, balanced individual—or self. This general knowledge will serve several important functions for the nurse: (1) she will more completely understand man's "healthy" existence in a broad sense; (2) she can more readily identify how illness imposes mental strains on a patient, and she can thereby attempt to help him to experience as normal an existence as possible within the limitations of his illness; and finally (3) it will enable her to attain self-understanding in order to use her own "self" therapeutically in patient care.

THE HEALTHY SELF

> It is easier to sail many thousand miles through cold and storm and cannibals . . . than it is to explore the private sea, the Atlantic and Pacific Ocean of one's being alone.
>
> Henry David Thoreau—*Walden*

It is only through subjective reflection that we can explore what we mean by the "self." We have no conceptual definition of the self to begin with because no definition has been universally accepted. Descriptions of what the self is like invite disagreement, for we each tend to describe "the" self in terms of how we think about "our" self. It is possible, however, to pull together some generalizations about the healthy, normal self.

1. *The healthy, adjusted self is not entirely free from emotional conflicts or symptoms of illness.* A certain amount of illness, imbalance, or conflict is a natural aspect of life. The healthy self is able to live with and resolve conflicts rather than be overwhelmed or immobilized by them. Stress and conflict will produce some mental disequilibrium, even in the healthy self, and therefore some of the symptoms of mental illness may appear.

2. *Ample energy and a drive toward self-actualization characterize the healthy self.* It takes energy to resolve conflicts. The well adjusted individual is able to cope with his life's problems without depleting his supply of energy. He thus has ample energy to be productive in life and to enjoy the pleasures that are available to him. This means that it is possible for him to achieve a fairly high level of self-actualization, personally and with others.

a. *Some of the values and goals of life that people seek vary from culture to culture.* In addition, variation is found among personal goals and values. These are determined in part by an individual's personal constitutional endowment and also by his life experience. In spite of this diversification of cultural and personal goals, people everywhere strive toward self-actualization as fully as their cultural and personal situations permit. They strive to fulfill their potentials, to grow and to achieve as much as they can. None of this is possible without encountering conflict. The healthy individual attempts to learn from his conflicts so that he may achieve a higher level of self-actualization.

b. *Individuals vary in their ability to become aware of deeper levels of the self and to gain insight or self-awareness.* Although many people recognize the *need* for self-awareness, too few work to attain it.

> Avoiding responsibility and decision through avoiding inner resources and powers, we evade the challenge to be what we are or can be. We are truly adrift, like a ship in irons.[79]

Even for those who do work to attain it, complete self-awareness is impossible.

c. *The self is simultaneously composed of sameness and change.* We remain the same person, recognizable to ourselves and to others, even though we change and grow physically and psychologically.

> I was a moment ago; I am part of the past. Yet it is I who now am, who then was. Though I passed with time, I did persist.[147]

It is through this quality of persistence that we are able to remain ourselves while undergoing change. The fact that we remain the same and yet change in a nebulous manner makes it difficult to track the elusive self, much less to understand it.

3. *The healthy self has a sense of personal integration or of a coherent wholeness.* As individuals we must come to know ourselves, to develop a feeling and sense about the person we are. This involves reaching a consciousness of ourselves, our values, and our life directions. It further means forming our own values, thoughts, and opinions by choice from the complex variety of ideas and ways of life that surround us. In order to do this, life's contradictions and inconsistencies must be considered.

All this introspection about oneself, one's behavior, and the values of the outer world (that outside of the self) is carried out in an attempt to achieve some inner sense of order and meaning for life. We cannot live with too great a sense of disorder. We need to feel related to our world and to have a relatedness within ourselves. We must feel that we are not impulsive and erratic, lacking direction in our lives and buffeted by fate. It is important to feel able to predict, to some extent, what the world is like—to know it and to understand it. We must have a similar sense about ourselves and our self-concepts. If one hopes to know the world and himself, he must be prepared to look realistically and as objectively as possible at what he finds. This process is not easy, as Kierkegaard has demonstrated:

> To venture causes anxiety, but not to venture is to lose one's self. . . . And to venture in the highest sense is precisely to become conscious of one's self.

4. *The healthy self strives to maintain some autonomy and therefore it is not necessarily of a socially conformist nature.* Although we want to know what others are like, and wish to conform and be like them to some extent, the healthy individual also wants to maintain his own individuality. The strong self strives toward the idea of maintaining a sense of its own uniqueness or authentic being. However, by nature we are also social beings, and so, in addition to wanting autonomy, the self also seeks involvement with the world and with others.

5. *Owing to the unique consciousness of man, the self is capable of introspection and is aware of time.*

> What presumably began as some barely living jelly much like the protoplasm which still fills the cells of our bodies is now Man the Maker and Man the Thinker. Because something we call Mind has emerged from that merely mechanical ability to react, which is the most primitive characteristic of life, Man has taken control of his own destiny, to at least some limited extent, instead of leaving it

> in the hands of whatever mysterious power first created life. He can send capsules . . . far out into the measureless space which surrounds the globe to which he was once confined. What is much more remarkable and perhaps more fateful is that he can also wonder and speculate about his origins, his destiny and the meaning of his existence.
>
> Joseph Wood Krutch
> (Introduction to Eiseley[29])

Man has developed a unique consciousness. Loren Eiseley[29] writes that man evolved into something the world had never seen before—a "dream animal." Unlike the rest of the animal world, man escaped the eternal present into a knowledge of past and future.

Thus, it is possible for men to think of their lives in ways that animals cannot: imagining tomorrow, remembering yesterday, and dreaming about how things might be. This consciousness favors men above other animals, but it also carries with it burdens and responsibilities. Just as a man can imagine future good times and dream his future dreams, he can also imagine terror, suffering, and death. Through his unique consciousness, a man can become morbidly preoccupied with the past or the future to the point of becoming mentally ill. Or he can become so introspective that he shuts out the rest of the world.

The self is not "found," it is achieved through introspection. Many people speak of finding themselves as if, quite by accident, they had stumbled upon something lost. The self is ever-present, although it may be present behind a variety of masks; it is ever-evolving, ever-becoming; it is evanescent and appears as reflections of its parts. What it represents, at any given time, is the life achievement of the individual. We do not lose our old self, we outgrow it and achieve something more.

It is through the baffling ability for introspection that a man can know his consciousness. Man, unlike other animals, can perceive himself in the act of perceiving. That is, we can see ourselves seeing ourselves. We can question ourselves and what our existence is all about.

The healthy self uses introspection for growth and better self-understanding, striving for maximum achievement. Man's introspection generally serves to guide him in the direction best for him. Because he can transcend time, he can learn from the past and, to some extent, plan for the future. Thus, he can use the present creatively in a conscious, constructive effort for self-actualization.

Man is in the unique position of being aware of time's passage and also of living in knowledge of his fate. However, the healthy individual is able to use this knowledge constructively. Through developing a consciousness of the present, and by realizing that the present is all that he has, he can strive to make his time more meaningful. It is not the quantity of time that is important, but rather the quality of it. In discussing "Man, Transcender of Time," Rollo May states:

> It is by no means as easy as it may look to live in the immediate present. For it requires a high degree of awareness of one's self as an experiencing "I." . . . But the more awareness one has—that is, the more he experiences himself as the acting, directing agent in what he is doing—the more alive he will be and the more responsive to the present moment. Like self-awareness itself, this experiencing of the quality of the present can be cultivated.[88]

6. *The self is composed of a public self and a private self.* Karl Marx among others has called our attention to the division of man into a "public" and "private" person. We all know that our public self is often not quite the same as our real or private self since we may feign or disguise our real self in public. We also know that as individuals we are isolated from others in the sense that we can never become another person and no one can become us. We can present a part of ourselves to the world or to others, but we cannot give our self-perception to others.

The newborn baby is not aware of himself as existing separately from his environment or from others. It is as we grow that we learn of the distances between ourselves and the world around us.

> As man becomes aware of himself as apart from his environment and as separate from his fellow men, the original oneness of life with its matrix is lost.[149]

Because of the existence of a public and private self we have a consciousness of ourselves as separate from other people, i.e., a feeling of otherness. A part of this feeling is the realization that we exist alone. This separateness of the self makes one feel helpless and insignificant. We are not referring here to an absence of any religious unification, but rather to the fact that we are all our separate selves.

The healthy self is able to accept the division between the public and private self and the alienation from others. For the healthy self, the public self and the private self are fairly similar. Also, the sense of alienation and isolation from others is balanced by those life experiences that can be shared with others. These shared experiences become bonds that unite men in their experience, e.g., in the areas of religion, culture, family, groups, and roles. Thus, even though we are isolated and see things from our own viewpoint, we can communicate with others. However, if we hope to communicate as accurately as possible and to establish bonds we must carefully explore our private self. As Eiseley wrote: "Men see differently. I can best report from my own wilderness. The important thing is that each man possess such a wilderness and that he consider what marvels are to be observed there."[29]

7. *Even though individual "selves" are isolated from one another, it is possible to form bonds with others.* Communication and self-knowledge are the tools with which we subjectively work to leave the isolation of our own experience and form bonds with others. In doing this we attempt to look at our

own experience and to relate it to the experience of others, and then we turn the question around and look at the experience of others and try to relate it to our own. How are the experiences similar? How do they differ? Why do they differ? We constantly work to sharpen our awareness of our self and of others and to reduce our prejudices and biases. We try to sharpen the blunt tool of subjectivity. We look at the limitations of the tool and we consider its assets.

An ability to communicate with others is essential to the life of a healthy self. Communication is a bond with others; it is our means of feeling less like separate planets pursuing our individual orbits, and more like a united galaxy. The great philosopher Karl Jaspers repeatedly emphasized the necessity of communication. He wrote: "The thesis of my philosophizing is this: The individual cannot become human by himself. Self-being is only real in communication with another self-being. Alone, I sink into gloomy isolation—only in community with others can I be revealed in the act of mutual discovery."[72]

8. *The self is largely determined by and recognized from the values that it assumes.** Ultimately the search for oneself is the responsibility of oneself. Others cannot do this for us because we are isolated from them and live in a state of alienation. The self that we choose to be results to a large extent from our choice of values. In discussing values, Wheelis has discussed how alone we are in making our choices: "[The alienated person] is thrown back on his own resources, becomes himself the referent of meaning and value."[149] Wheelis continues to point out that in the end we decide for ourselves the values we will live by; they are a matter of choice. From all the possible variety of values that we might embrace, we select those by which we *will* live. We choose some values that we believe are "better than" others. Our values may or may not conform to those that predominantly surround us. Perhaps our values are valid and perhaps they are not; at times values transcend the evidence of proof for them at hand.

Our identity is ultimately founded upon the values that we assume, because our values determine our goals and our goals define our identity. Often our values change through life. Our values are *not* what we say, but rather are what we do, because "values cannot function as values unless they are held as such. A value which is forgotten or ignored is, empirically, not a value."[149]

9. *The concept of oneself is founded upon perceptions of oneself; at times we perceive ourselves differently from the way others perceive us.* As early as the 1700's, David Hume was aware of the fact that we see ourselves in terms of perceptions. When he wrote on "Personal Identity" he stated:

> For my part, when I enter most intimately into what I call *myself,* I always stumble on some particular perception or other, of heat or cold, light or shade, love or hatred, pain or pleasure. I never can catch *myself* at any time without a perception, and never can observe anything but the perception.[59]

We perceive ourselves, or think of ourselves, in many different ways. In part, we think of ourselves in terms of our feelings, abilities, and actions. Our perceptions evoke feelings about ourselves, and *our feelings about ourselves are usually intense.* This fact is easily verified from one's own experience. We know how easily our feelings may be hurt or how insecure we may feel if our self-image is threatened. We know self-disappointment as well as dreams of fulfillment. Surprisingly enough, however, we usually know very little about what we actually *are* like! *One's feelings about oneself (or one's self-concept) may correspond with the truth or reality or they may not.* In addition, *our behavior nearly always appears more consistent to us than it does to others who observe it.* We all tend to see what we want to see.

We may not be as we think we are. This fact of self-deception often goes unrecognized. When it is discovered, we may find that we are in truth a part of what we had denied that we were. This realization means that, unknown to us, we possess attributes that we have despised or disliked in others. We may also have qualities that we admire in others but do not realize that we also possess. If some of my ideas about myself are inaccurate, it may mean such diverse things as these: I may describe myself as friendly, while others say I am hard to get to know; or I may think I don't do well in some activity, whereas others may think I excel.

Self-knowledge will help one to obtain a more realistic view of himself over a period of time. It will enable one to better understand how he presents himself to others and to see those incongruities that may exist between how he appears to others and how he appears to himself. Such insight is essential, for regardless of the accuracy of one's self-concept, it greatly influences how others react to us and how we behave toward others.

Let us now look at some of the reasons why it is difficult to perceive oneself accurately or to gain self-understanding. *First* of all, the process is difficult because self-understanding involves attempting to understand our own unconscious psychologic defenses* and unconscious motivations. Thus, our vision is often distorted. *Second,* we may

*Certain philosophers believe that man does not determine what his own self will become, but rather that his self is determined for him by his heredity and environment. Today self-determination and free choice of values in life are being increasingly accepted by philosophers and psychologists.

*These defenses are briefly discussed on pp. 113 to 116.

find it too psychologically painful to *believe* facts about ourselves which do not support our own "good" self-image. If we are incapable of looking at aspects of ourselves that displease us, then we cannot hope to look honestly at ourselves. *Third,* because the process of self-understanding is psychologically painful and uncomfortable, we often prefer focusing our attention on the behavior of *others.* This is a hazard inherent in nursing and in other occupations that require some "understanding" of others. We must realize that *self*-understanding precedes the ability to begin to understand others. Because we never completely understand ourselves or others, the process becomes one continuous attempt at self-knowledge while engaged in trying to understand others.

A *fourth* factor that makes self-knowledge difficult to achieve is that some people may lack the intelligence, and thus the knowledge, that is necessary to penetrate the complex self with its hidden and disguised motivations and experiences. Language skills, vocabulary, memory, and foresightedness are closely related to intelligence and vary from person to person. In part, then, the self we can become is determined by our vocabulary and verbal ability because thinking requires the use of concepts, and our concepts are most often verbal. Therefore, the more concepts an individual can build and consider (in terms of his vocabulary), the better able he is to think. Individuals also vary in their ability to think in abstractions, e.g., mathematics and philosophy. Consequently they have difficulty in thinking about the self, or the mind, because the self is an abstraction.

Self-knowledge will help one to obtain a more realistic view of himself and to achieve a balance of *self-acceptance* and *self-rejection.* This means that the individual is able to maintain a kind of psychologic homeostasis or equilibrium about his self-concept. An individual who *completely* accepts himself "as is," cannot reach his full potential, for he does not grow. On the other hand, a person who is overly harsh or rejecting of himself suffers a crippling imbalance. It is the ability to change, evolve, and be flexible, then, that facilitates growth through self-knowledge. Flexibility thus makes healthy psychologic adaptation possible.

Because we are not bound to a static existence, change is possible and is our human privilege. As life progresses, change occurs. Some changes are beyond man's control (e.g., physical aging); other changes can be made voluntarily (e.g., behavior). Fortunately, awareness of oneself can lead to growth or productive change in behavior and insights. An individual is, thus, not bound to always act as he acts today.

10. *Each self is individual and unique from all others.* Although this fact increases the difficulties of knowing one another (because we cannot predict what individuals are like in advance of knowing them), it does make life the interesting experience that it is.

How can we best describe *why* each individual is unique? We can think of every organism and each part of every organism as consisting of the interaction of at least three factors: time, heredity, and environment. Each of these factors is indispensable for life. Time is the life span in which to grow and develop. This growth and development is guided by the blueprint of heredity which controls the selection and use of materials, and by the environment. Each individual or organism embodies a unique combination of these factors.[122]

We can read about man for just so long. And then, if we really want to strive to understand people, we must meet the people themselves. The nurse is in a unique position to do this. She meets people most often during periods of crisis or intense experience in their lives. These are times when pretense is reduced to a minimum and the true self appears more clearly. Such times call for wisdom.

THE SELF IN ILLNESS

How does all this information about the self relate to nursing? We shall now see.

1. *Healthy, adjusted individuals are not entirely free from emotional conflicts or symptoms of illness.* This statement can orient the nurse to the fact that conflict and illness are often "normal" life experiences. Since the nurse will often care for patients who are *not* healthy and adjusted, it will be helpful if she can view imbalances in their proper perspective. She needs to recognize those imbalances that are temporary, and view them as temporary, and she also must recognize those imbalances that are permanent and accept the fact that they cannot be reversed. In *both* situations, a nurse must look for and develop the strengths that her patients have as well as recognize and prevent a deepening of weaknesses. A nurse's concept of health, adjustment, and balance is as important as her concept of illness, maladjustment, and imbalance.

The nurse must also strive for an awareness of her own emotional conflicts so that she does not project these upon persons in her care and upon her co-workers.

2. *Ample energy and a drive toward self-actualization characterize the healthy self.* A lack of energy is a general characteristic of physical and mental illness. The *body* is often weak and fatigued when combating physical stresses and illness; the *mind* is likewise weary, and people lack energy when they are experiencing mental stress and anxiety. When one is ill, however, the drive toward self-actualization is not necessarily absent. The nurse's responsibility then becomes one of helping ill individuals to continue to fulfill their potentials, and to grow and achieve as much as they can within the limitations imposed by their illness. People can grow and learn *from* periods of stress and *within* such periods. They do not usually become emotionally and psycho-

logically immobilized and cease being themselves merely because they are ill.

The nurse also can learn from periods of stress that she herself experiences, and she can strive to become aware of the many possibilities for self-actualization in her personal and professional life.

3. *A sense of personal integration or a coherent wholeness about oneself is essential for healthy functioning.* An individual who is ill needs a sense of order and personal integration as much as a healthy individual. The nurse can help to keep order in the patient's universe by preparing him as best she can for what will be happening to him. She can do this in small ways, for it is mainly in small ways that we all order our lives. For example, she can tell the newly admitted patient what the general routine of the hospital is. The nurse can tell a patient *what* she will be doing for him when she is assigned to care for him and *when* she will do these things. She can allow the patient to order some of his time by making some decisions *with* him about when they should do something. For example, would he like his bath early this morning or later? When would be the best time to take him to a telephone so he can phone home?

People who are ill may become confused or disoriented so that they lose the important sense of personal integration. When this occurs the nurse can help to reorient the patient by telling him where he is, what time it is, what day it is, who she is, and so forth.

4. *The healthy self strives to maintain some autonomy, and therefore mentally healthy individuals are not necessarily social conformists.* Even when ill and hospitalized, the individual needs to maintain a sense of his own uniqueness and autonomy. Many of the daily "problems" that nurses encounter center around this fact. Individuals do not like to conform to enforced ways of behaving (and neither do nurses). Autonomy expresses itself in thousands of different preferences. These preferences come to the nurse as innumerable requests—requests that express the wish to be treated differently from the "rest of the group." Basically such requests are for recognition of individuality. No one wants to be thought of as a part of a nameless, faceless group in which individuals cease to exist. No one wants to be thought of as a "gallbladder" or "room 214." Patients fear that they may be thought of in this kind of depersonalized manner.

The requests directed to the nurse, then, are serious; they are important to the self-concept of the patient even though they may seem minute and unimportant to the point of being "picky." The bids for autonomy may sound like this: "This meat is overcooked. I like mine rare." "I don't want a spread on my bed." "I don't care if it isn't visiting hours, I'm expecting company." "I want to wear my own pajamas." "I don't like ice water, I want a cup of warm water." "My roommate wants the window up, but I want it down." "I want a scrambled egg, not a boiled one." "I simply *cannot* use a bedpan." And so, the nurse must mediate between the necessity for some conformity as a part of group living and the equally important necessity for some autonomy.

5. *Owing to the unique consciousness of man, the self is capable of introspection and is aware of time.* Let us first look at his introspective nature. Illness is often a time of great uncertainty and, thus, a time of deep introspection. Because man is (as Eiseley says) a "dream animal," because he is capable of introspection and of projecting his thoughts forward and backward in time, he will dream, muse, rejoice, fret, and worry in the presence of the nurse. Often a patient needs, and wants, to think out loud and to talk with those around him. This is perfectly natural. What is unnatural for the patient is that those around him, at this time of crisis or concern for him, are not his familiar friends and family. He must talk with strangers about concerns that are often deeply personal.

Through introspection a man comes to know his inner feelings. Through his communications *we* can come to know his feelings and concerns. Consequently nursing requires skills in communication. It is necessary that a nurse help people to feel comfortable with her. This requires sensitivity to *both* verbal and nonverbal communication—the nurse's own as well as that of others. Furthermore, a nurse must be able to talk with people from extremely divergent backgrounds. The ability to speak simply and slowly will greatly enhance clarity of communication. The nurse should attempt to speak to patients without using complicated terms and the jargon of her profession.

Let us now turn to a consideration of the relation of the self to time. It is not time in and of itself that is important, but the *quality* and *meaning* of time for the patient and the nurse. Because we can determine to a large extent what the quality of our time will be, the nurse can create a *quality* in the time she spends with patients. A conscious awareness of this ability can greatly influence the quality of nursing time spent with all patients.

It does not matter whether a nurse will be with a patient for one minute or eight hours, she will determine the quality of her relations with the patient (e.g., her pleasantness) and thus will determine the quality of that time. No one but the nurse herself determines how much she will consciously *give* to the time she spends with a patient. She can grudgingly merely "put in time," or she can spend time with the patient helpfully and creatively.

Let us look at another aspect of time. The present is all that any of us has. Although the past and future are important to us, we live only in the present. Occasionally people (both patients and nurses) view illness and hospitalization as a time *away* from life—that is, as if the patient's life were suspended in time and would begin again when he is well or out of the hospital. This negation of the present needs to be guarded against, for it is the present that is truly meaningful.

The nurse can help the patient to be a constructive agent of his time. One of the commonest examples of negation of the present is seen in the attitude that nurses often convey in their care of terminal patients. Because his future life appears brief, the nurse often overlooks the importance of the present for the patient. These patients need more than others perhaps the comfort, warmth, and security that any of us want. They still want the *quality of their present life to be meaningful*. The dying are still living, only the dead are dead. And the dying live in the present time, as they have always lived, and as we all live.

6. *The self is composed of a public self and a private self.* Both patient and nurse have public and private selves. We often "fool" with our own and are "fooled" by others' public selves. Occasionally we are brought to the realization that we really didn't know someone at all in terms of his private self; all we saw was the public self. Let us see how "Richard Cory" was known:

> Whenever Richard Cory went down town,
> We people on the pavement looked at him:
> He was a gentleman from sole to crown,
> Clean favored, and imperially slim.
> And he was always quietly arrayed,
> And he was always human when he talked;
> But still he fluttered pulses when he said,
> "Good morning," and he glittered when he walked.
>
> And he was rich—yes, richer than a king,
> And admirably schooled in every grace:
> In fine, we thought that he was everything
> To make us wish that we were in his place.
>
> So we worked and waited for the light
> And went without the meat, and cursed the
> bread;
> And Richard Cory, one calm summer night
> Went home and put a bullet through his head.
>
> E. A. Robinson[115]

Just as you may not appear to others as you think you appear, so your patients may not appear to you as they think they do. A patient may think he appears calm when, in fact, he looks very apprehensive. Or a patient may think he doesn't seem irritable, when he actually is very short-tempered. He may think you know that he feels faint as he stands by the bed, when you really can't tell this, and so on. A doctor may think he appears calm, when he actually looks very pressured and acts tense. You may think you don't appear hurried to your patient, but you make him feel rushed.

The nurse must strive to see both her public self and her private self. She will also need to try to distinguish between the public and private selves of her patients. Just as she understands that her own public behavior does not always express her private feelings, so she must understand the same thing concerning the behavior of patients. As she must become skilled in verbal communication, so she must develop sensitivity and awareness to nonverbal communication so that she can see glimpses of the veiled private self behind the public mask.

The private self is isolated and alienated from other selves. Understanding these feelings that *all men* have, the nurse can empathize with those who are feeling lonely, isolated, and alienated in their illness. Illness, misfortune, and suffering make people realize strongly how separate from other people they really are. *They* are in pain, *they* face death, *they* are frightened, but the world goes on. And no one can assume the pain, death, or fear of others. The nurse, however, can reduce the feelings of isolation by her skilled, comforting presence and by her willingness to allow the patient to talk with her about his life situation. She can work to alleviate pain and to reduce fears. She can strive to reduce the differences between the public and private self.

7. *Even though individual "selves" are isolated from one another, it is possible to form bonds with others.* Although our interpretation of the feelings and behavior of others is largely subjective, we can manage to find common bonds with other people. We all must work within the limitations of subjectivity. Thus, when a patient says, "I'm miserable and full of pain," or "The doctor told me this morning I have cancer," the nurse cannot factually say, "I know how you feel." The nurse can, however, draw on her own experience. She can look for common bonds of experience with which she can attempt to understand the feelings of other persons as she talks with them, observes them, and attempts to be "with" them. To use a phrase of Loomis, we hope the nurse and patient can, in the purest sense, "resonate together."

> To "resonate" with another human being is to know that when you speak you are heard by him. The echoes that reverberate to you in his voice are rich with the sounds of your own concern. Similarly, your own voice, echoing back to him, has been affected by what you have heard him say and what you felt that he believed.[79]

The nurse who is capable of this level of communication is a nurse who is a *student of man*. She understands his isolation from others and his bonds with them. She studies human experience as carefully as she studies anatomy and physiology. Such a nurse is an "idea person" as well as a "fact person." It has been pointed out that

> nursing needs a better conceptualization of its own functions and the human phenomena with which it deals. This path to better ways and techniques will be opened by ideas, not by discrete, poorly related principles to be slavishly followed as techniques.[84]

If we deal with separate facts we fail to see the relationships between them; if we think only of separate people we fail to recognize that there are bonds that unite them. A factual approach to nursing is oriented toward objects as instruments for health (e.g., medications, hypodermics, dressings) rather than people. On the other hand, the nurse who works with "ideas" recognizes that consciousness, subjectivity, and communication are instruments for health and that she *herself* is an instrument that can be therapeutically applied . . . or denied.

8. *The self is largely determined by and recognized from the values that it assumes.* A nurse's value system will greatly influence her nursing practice. It may not influence how she talks about her nursing practice, but it will be directly reflected in the actual practice itself. A nurse may say that she values and respects individual differences, but the manner in which she treats individuals with differences will ultimately show what her values really are. As we have said previously, values are not values unless they are held as such and are the basis for action.

A nurse must be able to tolerate ideas and values that are foreign to her. Eiseley has said, "On the world island we are all castaways so that what is seen by one may often be obscure to another."[29] It is the task of the nurse to try to understand the obscure; it is her privilege to come to know differing visions of life on this "world island."

9. *The concept of oneself is founded upon perceptions of himself; however, at times we perceive ourselves differently from the way others perceive us.* How fragile one's self-concept is! How easily it is influenced or damaged! Every time a nurse speaks of a patient, she is speaking of a self. Her challenge becomes one of seeing how honestly, how accurately, and how fairly she can refer to that self. In attempting to describe a patient, she must invest as much effort in that description as she would in her own self-description. If others see us differently from our own self-perception, and we see them differently from theirs, we must evaluate ourselves and others cautiously.

How do others describe you? Do they do it partially in terms of themselves and their needs? In part they do, and you too describe others partially in terms of yourself. The beginning, then, is self-knowledge. Your feelings and perceptions about yourself will serve as your "antenna," your baseline for understanding others.

10. *Each self is individual and unique from all others.* Realizing this, the nurse can *expect* and enjoy the differences in patients whom she meets. She will not personally like all those she meets, but she can find that one of nursing's most rewarding aspects is the fact that she will meet so many different people. An appreciation of individuality and a conscious effort to allow it to flourish as much as possible can contribute greatly to patient care.

CHAPTER 17

Anxiety . . . The Motivating Emotion

EMOTIONS

In order to understand the concept of anxiety it is necessary first to examine some basic facts about emotions. Emotions are feelings that prompt a person to observable action or to internal mental and physiologic changes. They are thus crucial in the adaptive process. Physiologic changes take place within the body when emotional states occur, and it is known that specific patterns of physiologic change are related to specific emotions.

Some physiologic activities that undergo changes as a result of emotional states are: (1) brain waves, (2) the electrical resistance of the skin surface, (3) heart rate, (4) muscular tension, and (5) breathing rate. All emotions may be said to exist on three levels: (1) a neuroendocrine level; (2) a motor-visceral level; and (3) a level of conscious awareness.

Emotions motivate behavior. The resultant behavior may be impulsive and maladaptive, or it may be appropriate and adaptive. Emotional development is influenced by both the maturation process and learning. Emotions can be aroused by projecting oneself ahead in time (anticipating the future) or by recalling the past.

In the mature adult a wide range of emotional behavior is possible. One familiar emotional state is *anxiety*. Since the concept of anxiety is essential for understanding psychic life, let us turn our attention to it at this time.

THE NATURE OF ANXIETY

Anxiety may be considered to be essentially a human experience, since it is associated with the capacity for delayed reaction, choice of action, self-reflection of motivation, and projection of the self into the future. Thus, anxiety can be present only in man, who has evolved a form of self-reflective consciousness.

We are said to be living in the "age of anxiety." Anxious feelings are familiar to us; however, these feelings are not unique to our period in history. Anxiety has always been a part of human existence because it is the result of frustrations and conflicts that occur with life. Of the variety of unpleasant emotions that are the end product of conflict and frustration, anxiety is the most outstanding.

Anxiety can be described as apprehension, dread, foreboding, or uneasiness that is related to an *unidentifiable* source of anticipated danger. "Anxiety" and "fear" are not the same, because with fear the source of danger is recognized and can be identified. Generally when we feel anxious we are aware of feeling uncomfortable; indeed, at times we may experience intense discomfort. Such feelings are usually an admixture of both physical and mental states: (1) we are aware of a feeling of nervousness or mental uneasiness, and (2) we also experience a variety of physiologic states that are disturbing. The results of such unpleasant feelings are a variety of manifestations of anxiety, for example, a quavering voice. Uncomfortable as we may be when anxious, we generally cannot identify exactly what it is that causes us to feel as we do. It is precisely because we cannot readily recognize its source that anxiety can become so disturbing. Usually we are unable to tolerate anxious feelings for a sustained period of time. As further discussion will demonstrate, we attempt to terminate anxiety in many different ways.

Even though anxiety may be uncomfortable to experience, it is, nevertheless, an essential life ingredient. Anxiety can be thought of as being helpful or harmful, depending on the following: (1) its degree of intensity, (2) its appropriateness, and (3) its duration.

An appropriate degree of anxiety serves a useful integrative purpose. Unless we are mildly anxious as students, for example, we tend to lack appropriate motivation to study and learn. Excessive anxiety, on the other hand, may have a disintegrative effect because it can immobilize an individual or lead to panic states in which appropriate goal-directed behavior is not possible. However, when anxiety is absent, in apathy for example, goal-directed behavior is also impossible. In nursing, one is often faced with the critical issue of how best to manage an apathetic patient. It is not uncommon to witness the death of patients who lack the will to live and thus become apathetic and die, even though their presenting illness need not have been fatal. Such events are further testimony to the fact that we cannot separate the mental and physical states—the one pervades the other and they are mutually interactive.

In addition to the degree of anxiety present, we must consider its appropriateness and duration. It is appropriate and expected that individuals experience anxiety in certain situations and not in others. Also, the expected duration of anxiety will vary with the situation itself and with the individual's perception of it. Ultimately, of course, we find that the same situation may prove to be anxiety-provoking for one person but not for another. Such matters of individual perception vary greatly, depending upon an individual's learning and degree of maturation.

As Figure 17–1 indicates, perception contributes greatly to the production of anxiety. As the photograph demonstrates, the emotional state of anxiety makes its appearance during infancy. Usually the first behavioral signs of anxiety appear at about seven or eight months of age. Did the picture on the left make you feel "anxious" when you first noticed it? Can you identify why it made you feel "anxious"?

Anxiety forces change. It is the piston-like driving force in the dynamics of all human adjustment. The important factor is the *direction* of the change, for anxiety can produce both constructive and destructive change. An individual can grow through the changes that anxiety forces or he can be destroyed by them. Sustained anxiety clearly can produce mental and physical illness if the individual's adaptive pattern is unhealthy for him. Anxiety is our life partner; either we can strive to recognize its presence and use it constructively, or we can succumb to it.

WHAT CAUSES ANXIETY?

A countless variety of situations involving frustration, conflict, and stress cause anxiety and are familiar to us all. We all have incentives or are motivated toward certain goals in life for a variety of reasons. However, life experience shows us that we do not always reach the goals we seek. Obstacles to goal satisfaction may be either external or internal. When our goal-directed behavior is thwarted or interfered with, we experience frustration. Frustration produces feelings of anxiety within us; these feelings are also produced by conflicting motives that force us to make choices.

Whether or not an event is perceived as anxiety-producing is an individual matter. Generally we may say that situations of frustration, conflict, or stress that threaten the physical or mental security of an individual produce anxiety. Certainly the major anxiety-producing conditions that the nurse will encounter are illness and death. Threats to physical existence can be recognized more easily than threats to one's mental self-concept. It is possible to see clearly an uncontrolled infection producing bodily changes that are life-threatening, but it is more difficult to identify the threats to the patient's mental self-image that such an illness produces.

Illness is both physically and mentally taxing. The skilled nurse recognizes that illness produces anxious feelings in patients; she also tries to be sensitive to the individual anxieties that patients experience when illness interferes with their unique self-expectations and needs.

ANXIETY IS COMMUNICATED

Both verbally and nonverbally we receive messages that tell us when other people are anxious. An individual's voice may shake or break; his words may convey anxiety; his manner of speaking may change from his usual pattern to one

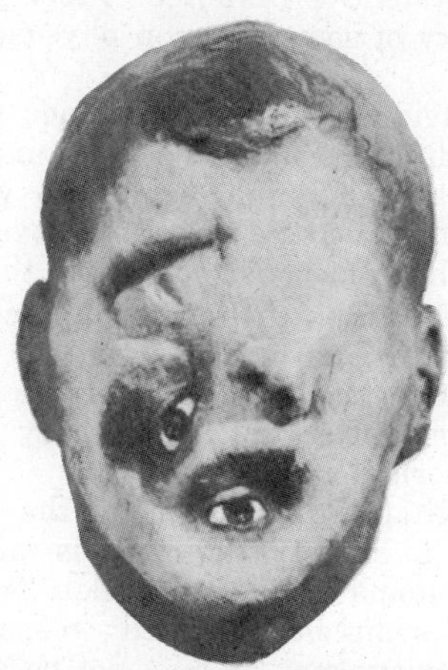

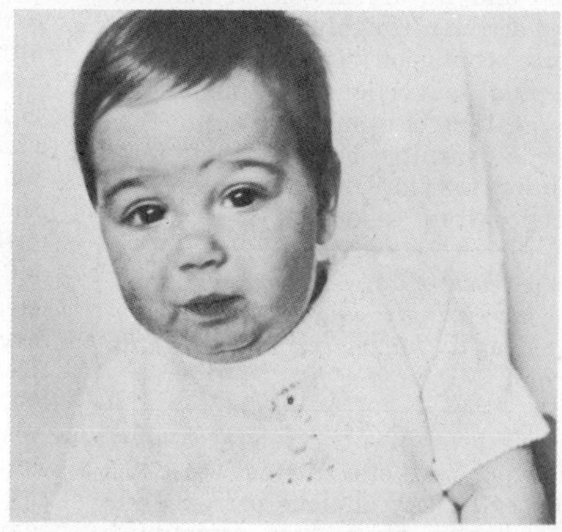

FIGURE 17–1. Perceptual distortion and anxiety. Violation of perceptual expectancies makes the baby of about eight months express anxiety when he sees the distorted mask at left. At an earlier period, before he learned what the human face is supposed to look like, he might have smiled at the mask. (From Kagan, J., and Havemann, E.: *Psychology: An Introduction.* New York, Harcourt Brace and World, 1968.)

more rapid or slow; the pitch of his voice may change. A tense posture, nervous movements, "wide-eyed" appearance, and perspiration are a few nonverbal clues to anxiety. Anxious feelings can be communicated from one person to another. One anxious patient in a ward can make other patients anxious; the anxious nurse communicates her anxiety to patients and co-workers.

LEVELS OF ANXIETY

It is important that the nurse understand the ways in which anxiety is believed to affect such important processes as learning, perception, awareness, and thinking. Because the nurse daily works with anxious people, she can help to meet their needs better if she can understand what their mental experiences are like. As always, she can learn best from her own experience.

Mild anxiety is an asset to successful adaptation in life. When we are mildly anxious we are alerted in such a manner that we can "take in" more than usual and thus our perception becomes keener, and we are in a state that is conducive to learning. A mild state of anxiety may thus help a nurse to function effectively; it may also help a patient to learn or to understand what the nurse or doctor may be attempting to tell him.

As the level of anxiety increases, however, we lose our ability to function effectively over a period of time. When anxiety mounts we become less able to consider a situation in its entirety; our perceptual field is reduced so that we perceive only part of a situation. In situations of extreme anxiety (panic) we may find that we "blow up" one area of concern out of all proportion and are unable to comprehend the total situation. Panic also may produce a state of mind in which our attention is greatly scattered and we are unable to maintain any goal-directed activity. Heightened anxiety thus tends to produce confusion and becomes maladaptive. Perceptual distortions of time, space, people, and the meaning of events also occur. Such distortions impede learning because they interfere with our ability to relate one item to another, to recall, or to concentrate generally.

> *As a patient's level of anxiety increases he will become increasingly unable to understand clearly what is happening to him and what is expected of him.*

Thus, if a patient's level of anxiety is excessively high, it will interfere with effective patient teaching. Because the extremely anxious person easily misunderstands what is said to him, communication with him should be clear and directions brief. Nonverbal motions may aid in clarifying communication at such times. The anxious person needs an opportunity to discuss his feelings with a calm person.

RESPONSES TO ANXIETY

Anxiety produces physiologic (somatic) responses and psychologic responses simultaneously; our awareness of these responses varies.

PHYSIOLOGIC RESPONSES

In response to anxiety the body alerts itself in preparation to "fight or flee." When we are anxious we can feel our heart beat faster (tachycardia) or "flutter" (palpitate); we may breathe rapidly (hyperventilate) or experience difficulty in breathing (embarrassed respirations); perhaps we yawn a lot or feel chest pain. Some other physiologic effects of anxiety that we may consciously experience are anorexia, nausea, vomiting, abdominal cramps, or diarrhea. We may feel flushed or perspire excessively. Some individuals experience an urgency to urinate or may need to urinate more frequently. Anxiety can produce dysmenorrhea and frigidity in women; men may experience impotence. The musculoskeletal response may be manifested as aching muscles or joints and complaints of arthralgia or arthritis. Backache, headache, or wryneck also may be attributable to anxiety. These are all physiologic results of anxiety that we may consciously be aware of and thus *feel.*

Other changes in body function occur that are *not* within our conscious awareness. For example, in order to force more blood into the muscles, the blood pressure is maintained or elevated. Moreover, blood is made available to the muscles by means of its temporary removal from the gastrointestinal tract. Also, the liver releases sugar, the adrenals produce epinephrine, and peristaltic activity is reduced. The pupils dilate so that we can "see more" and thus be ready to respond to emergencies. In general, the cardiovascular system is stimulated and the gastrointestinal system is inhibited. Table 17–1 presents a summary of some common physiologic effects of anxiety.

As individuals each of us tends to experience anxiety differently: one person may experience mainly gastrointestinal symptoms while another may most commonly notice cardiovascular symptoms. If the anxiety is short-lived, that is, successfully dealt with, these psychic and physiologic effects do no harm. However, it can be seen clearly that sustained or chronic anxiety will eventually take its toll of the body by keeping it in an abnormal state.

Although these are some of the typical major responses to anxiety, the nurse is cautioned not to assume automatically that anxiety is the sole basis for these symptoms or bodily responses. For example, anxiety may or may not be a contributing factor in the etiology of headache. Only a precise diagnostic work-up can demonstrate the specific etiology of such symptoms in a given patient.

TABLE 17–1. COMMON PHYSIOLOGIC EFFECTS OF ANXIETY

Effects Which May Be Consciously Felt	Effects Which Cannot Be Consciously Felt
Heart beats faster or flutters	Blood pressure rises
Difficult or rapid breathing	Blood temporarily removed from gastrointestinal tract and made available to muscles
Frequent yawning; dry mouth	Liver releases sugar
Chest pain	Adrenals produce epinephrine
Anorexia, nausea, vomiting, abdominal cramps, diarrhea, gas pains, "butterflies"	Peristaltic activity is reduced
Flushing, excessive perspiration, "cold sweats," shifts in body temperature	Pupils dilate
Urgency to urinate, frequent urination	
Dysmenorrhea, frigidity	
Impotence	
Aching muscles and joints	
Arthralgia, arthritis	
Backache, headache, wryneck	

Furthermore, if anxiety should prove to be a significant factor, the nurse must remember that the symptom is out of the patient's conscious control. The pain experienced from headache caused by anxiety may be as intense as that of a headache resulting from brain tumor.

The physiologic responses to anxiety that we have been discussing may exist in varying degrees or levels, depending upon the intensity of the anxiety. The greater the anxiety, the more extreme the physiologic response tends to be. These physiologic responses to anxiety are of obvious interest to the nurse as she studies the body in health as well as in conditions in which physiologic changes are disease-producing.

PSYCHOLOGIC AND BEHAVIORAL RESPONSES TO ANXIETY

Anxiety tends to motivate us to behaviors and attitudes that we hope will reduce the anxiety and the resultant discomfort that it produces. As individuals we each tend to develop our own patterns of reacting to the frustrations, conflicts, and anxious feelings that are a part of life. Much of our personality actually consists of our individual manner of dealing with anxiety.

Mental Defense Mechanisms

There are many different ways of classifying reactions to anxiety. Although our individual responses are all unique to some extent, there are broad common patterns of reacting that have been identified and named "defense mechanisms" or "adaptive mental mechanisms." These are mental processes and behavior that serve the important function of protecting our self-esteem by defending us against excessive anxiety.

Adequate self-esteem and self-respect are necessary for healthy function. We all use certain types

TABLE 17–2. COMPARISON BETWEEN GENERAL ADAPTATION SYNDROME AND PSYCHOLOGIC ADAPTATION PROCESS

Stage	General Adaptation Syndrome (Hans Selye)	Psychologic Adaptation Process
Stage 1	An initial alarm reaction alerting certain organs of the body (i.e., sympathetic nervous system arousal)	Frustrating situations produce heightened state of arousal manifested as (1) aggression (fight), (2) flight (withdrawal from the situation), or (3) diffuse anxiety
Stage 2	Stage of resistance: physiologic functions are at abnormal levels for prolonged periods in an attempt to defend the body against stress	To diminish anxiety there is an attempt to distort some aspect of thinking by means of defense mechanisms
Stage 3	Stage of exhaustion	If defense mechanisms fail or are overused, psychologic resources are exhausted

of behavior, especially in stressful situations, in attempts to maintain and improve our self-concept. All of us more or less regularly encounter anxiety-producing situations through which we feel our "self" threatened. Defense mechanisms comprise those habits that we have developed for defending our self-regard amd at times enhancing it. The self is protected, by means of defense mechanisms, not only from the threats that may present themselves in our external environment (i.e., from other people and from situations in which we find ourselves) but also from the dangers that arise from within ourselves (i.e., from our own impulses or affects).

Defense mechanisms have several general characteristics: First, they defend the self and protect it from injury by bolstering self-esteem or through self-enhancement. Second, defense mechanisms are not used deliberately, but rather they are unconscious, or at least partly so. Defense mechanisms also tend to have in common the quality of self-deception; that is, they operate by (1) masking or disguising our true motives, or (2) denying the existence within ourselves of impulses, actions, or memories that might be anxiety-provoking to us. Adaptive mental mechanisms thus protect us from anxiety by distorting (1) perception, (2) memory, (3) action, (4) motivation, and (5) thinking, or by completely blocking out some psychologic process.

Defense mechanisms are essential for healthy adaptation. A number of similarities have been observed between Selye's concept of the general adaptation syndrome (describing physiologic reactions to stressors) and our psychologic reactions to stressful situations. (See Table 18–2.)

Like anxiety, defense mechanisms can contribute in a positive sense to an individual's developing life or they can, through overuse or their failure

TABLE 17–3. DEFENSE MECHANISMS AND THEIR USAGE

Defense Mechanism	Description	Examples in Nursing Care
Rationalization	Assigning logical reasons or plausible excuses for what we have done impulsively or for motives that we do not wish to acknowledge; serves to maintain self-respect and prevents feelings of guilt	A patient is extremely rude and demanding; he thinks to himself that it is all right for him to behave this way because he is sick; he thus excuses his behavior
Projection	Attributing to others exaggerated amounts of undesirable qualities which we have but do not wish to recognize in ourselves	The patient above may not recognize his rude, demanding behavior; instead he thinks the nurse is behaving in this way—thus projecting his feelings onto her; actually her behavior is misinterpreted by him, as she has not been rude or demanding
Repression	Involuntarily forgetting about unacceptable ideas, impulses, or events; serves to protect us from being constantly aware of anxiety-producing situations	A patient had a sudden strong urge to defecate and was incontinent before the nurse could help her onto the bedpan; the patient was extremely embarrassed by the situation; a month later she had totally forgotten about the incident and did not remember it again
Suppression	Consciously putting unacceptable ideas, impulses, or events out of mind; the material can readily be recalled	A patient has been told by her physician that she needs to undergo surgery; this thought is upsetting to her; she leaves the doctor's office and says to herself, "I won't think about it now; I'll do some shopping instead"
Regression	Returning to an earlier level of emotional adjustment; an unconscious process	A patient is usually quite self-sufficient when he is feeling well; however, with his illness he becomes somewhat more dependent than his physical condition necessitates; thus, he returns to an earlier level of dependency
Identification	Unconsciously adopting the personality characteristics of another individual whom the subject admires—the opposite of projection; not consciously trying to be like someone else	Two patients with multiple sclerosis share a room in the hospital for several weeks; one admires the other very much and over a period of time her attitude toward her illness becomes similar to that of the friend she admires A nurse's professional, kind attitude with patients is unconsciously adopted by other members of the staff who admire her

when needed, lead to a disruptive, unhappy life pattern.

Defense mechanisms usually are studied in detail in courses in psychology and psychiatry. We include here a brief outline of some common defense mechanisms to facilitate the transfer of psychologic theory into patient care in a medical-surgical setting. (See Table 17–3.)

We can understand more clearly the fears and concerns of patients if we can identify when they use adaptive mechanisms and what their behavioral adaptive patterns are. Let us briefly summarize some major points concerning defense mechanisms and look at some nursing implications:

> Defensive behavior often evokes, in others, feelings of retaliation or retreat. The nurse who reacts to anxious patients in this manner (because she does not recognize their anxiety and understand it) may intensify a patient's anxiety rather than reduce it. Furthermore, the nurse should examine her own defensive behavior and recognize that such behavior, on her part, can create problems for her with patients and co-workers.

> While it is possible to describe defense mechanisms and resultant behavior, we often cannot identify or understand the specific needs that make the person rely on the mechanisms he is using. Therefore, the nurse should not tamper with a patient's system of defenses; rather, she should recognize the behavior as being defensive in nature and as serving the function of protecting the individual from anxiety. While a patient's behavior may seem maladaptive to her (because of the defenses used), it may be that the patient's defenses are serving adaptive purposes for him at the time. Without them his anxiety might be overwhelming.

> Defense mechanisms are not "abnormal" or "bad." They are used daily by everyone as a means of adaptation to life. They are helpful and necessary because they reduce anxiety and help us to retain emotional equilibrium. However, psychopathology or psychologic maladaptation can occur when (1) certain defense mechanisms are overused, and the individual becomes overly dependent on their usage; or (2) they fail to protect the individual as they once did. A nurse needs extensive education and experience before she can identify when the use of defense mechanisms is pathologic in degree. Patient behavior that she feels is questionable should be discussed with the attending physician.

> Defensive behavior, like all behavior, may be thought of as existing on a continuum or in various degrees. The

TABLE 17–3. DEFENSE MECHANISMS AND THEIR USAGE (*CONTINUED*)

Defense Mechanism	Description	Examples in Nursing Care
Compensation	A conscious or unconscious attempt to overcome real or imagined inferiorities	A patient paralyzed from the waist down works hard to develop the muscles in his trunk and arms to compensate for his inability to use his legs
Denial	Unconsciously refusing to acknowledge to oneself a known fact that is uncomfortable to accept; not consciously lying to oneself	A patient is proved to have cancer and is told the diagnosis by his physician; the patient does not consciously admit to himself that he has cancer; he denies the diagnosis
Reaction Formation	A forbidden motive or behavior is denied, and the individual develops behavior displaying the opposite motive	A patient is fearful of surgery but instead of appearing fearful he acts unconcerned and nonchalant about it; he jokes about surgery and says, "There's nothing to it. I don't know why some guys are such babies about going"
Sublimation	The "socialization of energy" by diverting unacceptable impulses into socially accepted behavior	A patient is angry because he was hit by a car, injured and is hospitalized for several weeks; he is missing work and his wife is home taking care of their three young children by herself; he directs his "angry energy" into pounding designs into leather and selling the purses, wallets, etc.; he sends home the small amount of money he makes and thus has a sense of contributing to his home and family
Displacement	Emotion or behavior is redirected from the original object or person to a more acceptable substitute object	A patient hopes to go home but is told by his doctor that he probably cannot be discharged for some time; the patient is angry at what the doctor says but doesn't want to appear angry at the doctor; the rest of the day he is short-tempered with the nurses; he thus displaces his anger from the doctor to the nurses

classification of behavior into defense mechanisms is an arbitrary procedure and it would be unfortunate if it resulted in the stereotyping or labeling of individuals. There are no clear borderlines between various types of defensive behavior. Often when an individual reacts to a stressful situation, his behavior is a combination of several mechanisms.

> Defense mechanisms normally function to help to conserve emotional energy. Healthy living should be a process of expedient use of energy—both physical and mental. An individual whose self-esteem is chronically low or who lacks self-respect (consciously or unconsciously) may utilize so much energy through overuse of defense mechanisms (in an attempt at self-justification) that he has little energy available for use in constructive self-realization. This may be the situation with a person experiencing an illness. Illness produces frustrations, conflicts, and anxiety. In trying to ward off anxiety and retain a satisfactory self-concept, a patient may overuse certain mechanisms, thus taxing his mental energy and flexibility. Also, he may find that certain mechanisms that helped him to adapt when he was well fail him in illness. Recognizing that illness and hospitalization are stressful experiences, the nurse should *expect* that patients may react to their situation with some exaggerated use of their defense patterns and with mental fatigue and irritability.

> When we say that a certain type of behavior serves as a defense mechanism we are speaking theoretically. Behavior that is classified as functioning as a defense mechanism in one situation may not be used as a defense mechanism in another situation. Whether or not the behavior is used defensively depends upon the individual's motivation and whether the behavior has distorted his sense of reality.

CHAPTER 18

The Mind-Body (Psyche-Soma) Problem

> Our present day Psyche-Soma Complex affects not only our scientific thinking and our research but also our diagnostic systems, our etiological thinking and our therapy. But, even more than that, it also influences our cultural and social functioning.[109]

We have seen thus far that men react to anxiety physiologically and psychologically, that is, with both body and mind. Now perhaps we should ask those difficult questions that have been pondered for centuries: "What is mind?" "What is body?" "Are they separate or related?" "Are they indivisible?" "Do mind and body really exist separately or do they exist only as words?" "Does one control the other; are they dualistic or part of a monistic system?" The questions become increasingly complex and are currently being answered in a variety of ways; the answers powerfully influence one's view of illness. Ultimately the answers lead to the acceptance or rejection of theories of psychosomatic medicine or the psychogenic etiology of any physical illness.

Let us proceed to look historically at the mind-body dichotomy and to a consideration of some evidence for mind-body interaction. We shall then discuss briefly some theoretical problems of the mind-body dilemma.

HISTORICAL BACKGROUND

Despite the fact that the mind-body relationship has a direct bearing on illness, and thus on nursing and medicine, the issue has received little formal attention, and personal views of the problem are rarely made explicit. An understanding of the mind-body problem is of importance in viewing disturbed homeostasis and the resultant illness as it affects the total individual. Far from being an "academic issue," the mind-body problem is of immediate concern to nurses and physicians because of the high incidence of psychosomatic disorders.

Let us look more closely at the term "psychosomatic." This term expresses the "mind-body" relationship in medical language: "psycho" refers to the "psychologic" and "somatic" refers to the "physical." Thus, in a very general way, the term "psychosomatic disease" refers to the belief that the mind and body are both involved in the illness. From this general viewpoint, psychosomatic disease is no new discovery, since Hippocrates was familiar with it. The belief that both mind and body are factors in illness was lost, however, for a period of time in history. Let us look more closely at how this came about.

It appears that in primitive society there was no division between physical and mental disease. Trephine holes found in ancient skulls indicate that an attempt was made to treat disease by enabling the physical departure from the body of evil spirits believed to have caused the illness. A holistic approach to disease in man, recognizing the importance of the interrelationship of mind and body, was present throughout the Babylonian-Assyrian, Greek, and Roman civilizations, and also during the Dark Ages. The nature of the mind-body interrelationship was, however, in keeping with the cultural and religious beliefs of those times. For example, during the Dark Ages, the psyche came to be viewed as a mystical and irrational force.

Subsequent to this, during the Renaissance the "mind" was claimed as the proper concern of religion and philosophy, and the "body" became the property of medicine. It was at this time that the belief that mind and body are interrelated was lost; it is the influence of the thinking prevalent during this period of history that we are still trying to overcome in medicine and nursing today.

Throughout the text we have made brief statements concerning the interrelationship of mind and body. Such remarks are necessary because current thinking still possesses remnants of the outdated mind-body model of Cartesian dualism previously alluded to in Unit II. This model resulted from one man's attempt to solve the "mind-body problem." René Descartes conceived of this dichotomous model in the 17th century, stating, in essence, that a clean-cut dualism of soul (mind) and body existed: the soul was thought of as conscious and the body as inanimate. For Descartes, mind and body were two distinct entities that were each subject to different laws of operation and principles of causality. And so, for centuries, men lived as divided beings and did not think of themselves as the beautiful complex of mind and body that they are.

Descartes' model made a tremendous impact on Western thought concerning the nature of man. However, a great deal has transpired since the 17th century, and with the emergence of more precise scientific thought, the model of Cartesian dualism has been unable to withstand the test of time. When Freud postulated the unconscious element of man's mental life, the model of the Cartesian dualism was destroyed. Descartes had not conceived of the unconscious and, therefore, it was not considered in his model.

The work of Freud thus led to a reversal of the Cartesian trend by increasing our awareness of the importance of emotions in producing mental and physical imbalances. Reluctantly and skeptically men began to think of themselves as whole beings again. The task of "reuniting" the divided man has been difficult and is by no means completed.

"PROOFS" OF MIND-BODY INTERACTION

Our personal experience tells us that our mind and body are unitary in nature; that is, we experience them together. We experience our "self" as a combination of physical and mental phenomena. Sometimes we may be more aware of our body (i.e., with pain) and at other times our mind (i.e., in solving an abstract mathematical problem), but we cannot experience one without the other. We cannot experience pain without consciousness, and we cannot experience mental states without the anatomic and physiologic functioning of a brain.

The concept of the interaction of mind and body can be established more clearly in our thinking by considering the effects of anxiety that were previously discussed. If you are not convinced that mind and body interact, evaluate how you feel "physically" the next time you are "mentally" anxious. You will find it most difficult (indeed impossible) to separate your feelings into "physical" and "mental" categories. By gaining insight into one's own experiences and feelings when anxious, it is possible to more readily understand the psychophysiologic illnesses that will be discussed in the next chapter.

Let us briefly consider some additional general evidence of mind-body interaction:

1. *Apathy*[134] of prisoners of war has been known to lead to death even though there was no evidence of physical illness and food was available. This occurred in prisoners with no evidence of psychotic reaction. Wild, healthy animals have also been known to die in confinement.

2. The *tickle*[95] serves as another example. Have you noticed that you cannot tickle yourself? The response depends on more than mere touch; certain mental interactions are necessary to make a touch a tickle. As Darwin observed, someone other than the tickled must do the tickling. This may seem like an obscure "proof" of mind-body interaction; however, deaths from tickling have actually been recorded in a number of instances.

3. *Voodoo* provides additional evidence of the monistic nature of mind-body. While the actual practice assumes many forms, in essence voodoo, or hexing, represents a "magical" suggestion that can produce illness and death. Voodoo could be said to demonstrate mind-body interaction when an individual is aware of being hexed and then develops physical problems. It has been suggested that the voodoo deaths of folklore were psychologically provoked through the development of psychosomatic disease.[86] Belief in such magical suggestion is not limited to the past; "rootwork"[137] appears to be a North American derivative of voodoo that is still in practice. Many questions remain unanswered concerning voodoo. One major question is: Does the individual become ill from the curse, or might he have become ill anyway as a result of other causes?

4. *Hypnosis* has provided some interesting connections between mind and body. One study demonstrated that it was apparently possible to produce ecchymotic (bruise-like) lesions in specific locations on the subject's body with hypnotic suggestion.[3]

The situations presented above demonstrate that the so-called borders between our conscious, unconscious, and physical selves are not rigid. Interactions occur that are not clearly understood at this time, but it is nevertheless clear that mind and body are not separate entities.

THEORIES OF THE MIND-BODY PROBLEM

Over the centuries a wide variety of theories have been constructed in an attempt to answer the ancient mind-body question. Today, new theories continue to try to resolve the riddle. Unfortunately considerable confusion still exists, and much of the research deals with the problem in a very inconsistent manner.

Two major groups of theories that should be discussed briefly are the theories of *interactionism* and of *independence* of mind and body. *Interactionist* theories maintain that the mind and body do somehow interact; there have been a variety of ideas about just where and how this interaction takes place. Hippocrates was the first interactionist. Although he derived the psychic from the somatic he nevertheless recognized, with his typical astuteness, that emotions in turn have physical effects. Theories of *independence* are simply those that maintain that mind and body exist completely separately and that they do not interact.

Today, most people tend to believe that, in ways which are not yet understood, mind and body interact. Theories of independence rarely are openly supported by anyone; however, such theories continue to permeate many persons' attitudes toward illness, as the following quotation demonstrates:

> Typically, the doctor and his patient oscillate between two mind-body theories—namely, interactionism and independence. If the ordinary physician is specifically asked to state his position, he will usually give an interactionist answer, such as "The body influences the mind and the mind influences the body." He may also include references to "psychosomatic versus somatopsychic." In less guarded moments he is likely to reveal a belief in mind-body independence, with a remark like "There is nothing physically wrong with you, it's all mental." Probably no one who has had experience with the contemporary medical scene could fail to recognize both of these as statements he has heard many times.[44]

This tendency to have such a vacillating viewpoint presents definite problems in medicine and nursing. Therefore, the nurse should consciously recognize her own viewpoint. If she considers the psychologic element as *the* basic cause of illness, then the physical aspect becomes neglected in her patient care or assumes secondary importance. The

opposite is also true. If illness is viewed by her as basically "physical," then psychologic factors may be overlooked. Such omissions may be crucial to the welfare of patients.

When thinking about the psychologic factors in an illness, physical factors should not be excluded . . . and vice versa.

Because the mind-body problem has proved to be a conceptual barrier posing problems in medical thinking, unifying concepts are needed rather than concepts that break a man apart and name the divisions. We need cohesive models that enable us to view mind and body as one indivisible monistic event; that is, to view man as a reality, one unitary whole, within his environment.

CHAPTER 19

Mind-Body Interaction in Illness: Psychosomatic and Somatopsychic Illness

Although it is generally recognized that emotional factors do contribute to physical disease, and vice versa, the exact mechanisms of the interaction of mind and body are not clearly understood. Indeed, discussions of these mechanisms are often heated and controversial. Both "psychosomatic illnesses" and "somatopsychic illnesses" involve mental and physical disturbances. They are similar in this respect, but they do differ significantly, as you will see in the following discussion.

BASIC CONCEPTS OF SOMATOPSYCHIC AND PSYCHOSOMATIC ILLNESSES

Generally speaking, it can be said that with somatopsychic illnesses physical diseases are influencing mental activity, and with psychosomatic illnesses extreme or prolonged emotional states are influencing body functioning. Let us examine these concepts more closely.

SOMATOPSYCHIC ILLNESS

In *somatopsychic illnesses* the *physical* problems or physical maladaptations *precede* and contribute to the emotional, behavioral problems or maladaptations. Organic disease is primary (that is, "first") and it causes or is associated with personality deviations and their related emotional and psychologic disturbances. Somatopsychic disorders thus include systemic disorders in which central nervous system symptoms, particularly behavioral change, are prominent. In such disorders the emotional complaints have a systemic, organic basis. Examples of such somatopsychic illnesses (in which the patient's behavior may be markedly influenced by his physical condition) are: inborn errors of metabolism, intrinsic or extrinsic intoxications, nutritional deficiencies, and disorders of the endocrine glands.

Consider another example of somatopsychic illness that will illustrate, in a slightly different manner from the preceding examples, how a physical disorder might affect a person mentally. When a patient realizes that he has cancer he may feel depressed; a realization of his physical state produces the depression. Here we see an obvious relationship between the organic disease (the cancer) and the emotional disturbance; also, notice that the organic disease precedes the emotional disturbance.

PSYCHOSOMATIC ILLNESS

In *psychosomatic illness* the *emotional* problems or maladaptations are believed to *precede* physical disorders in such a manner that the physical maladaptive process is said to be "psychogenic" in origin. By psychogenic we mean that the illness results from prolonged emotional or psychologic stress.

A broad view of psychosomatic etiology would be that emotional factors have a role in producing or aggravating many physical disorders. The exact mechanism of psychosomatic interaction is unknown at present. To use a familiar simile, psychosomatic illnesses are comparable to an iceberg: the symptoms and disorders that are observable are similar to the visible part of the iceberg; the multiple unobservable factors of stress represent the much larger mass of ice below the surface of the sea (Fig. 19–1).

To summarize: (1) *somatopsychic illnesses* are caused by nonpsychogenic factors and result in physical diseases that precede and contribute to psychologic problems; (2) *psychosomatic illnesses* are referred to as psychogenic in origin and, thus, psychologic maladaptions precede physical disorders.

Psychosomatic illnesses may be divided into two groups, both psychogenic in origin: (1) *functional*

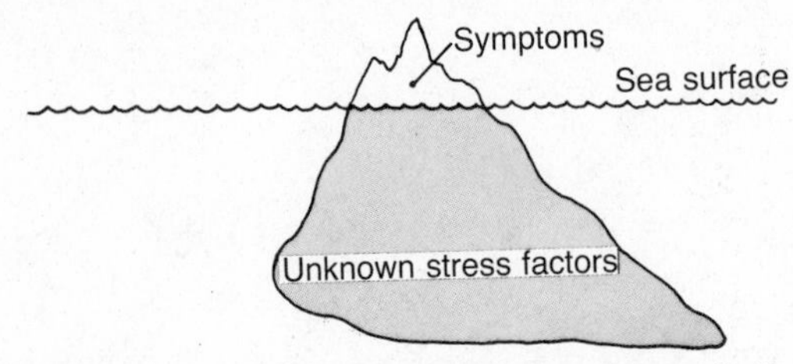

FIGURE 19–1. The iceberg simile of psychosomatic illness. Observable symptoms represent only a small part of the total disorder.

illnesses and (2) *psychophysiologic illnesses*. The presence or absence of bodily structural changes (that is, tissue changes or organic damage) constitutes a major difference between functional and psychophysiologic disease. Whereas functional problems result in no organic pathologic changes, psychophysiologic disorders do show pathologic changes. Figure 19–2 illustrates schematically the etiology of somatopsychic, psychosomatic, functional, and psychophysiologic illnesses.

Functional Illness

Illnesses are termed *functional* when organic pathologic changes cannot be demonstrated as providing a basis for the patient's symptoms. It has been estimated that one third of the patients who consult physicians are ill but have no definite bodily disease to account for their illness. Nurses thus meet many patients with functional disorders. Such patients are reacting to stress in the sense that they experience physical symptoms (pains, flutterings, and so forth), but structural tissue change has not taken place. Functional disorders are psychogenic disorders which involve no structural changes in tissue, but which produce problems in the *function* of the area involved.

Authorities emphasize that the diagnosis of functional illness must be established not simply by the exclusion of organic disease, but by its own characteristics as well. When there is no physical basis for a patient's symptoms, an attempt should be made to understand the symptoms in terms of their *meaning* from the standpoint of behavior. This may involve psychiatric investigation, since functional problems may have a symbolic meaning to the patient.

Disorders that can be classified in some instances as functional are: irritable bowel syndrome, hyperventilation, constipation, enteritis, some headaches, anorexia nervosa, disorders of menstruation, sexual disorders (i.e., impotence, frigidity), and psychogenic pain.

Psychophysiologic Illness

In *psychophysiologic* disorders pathologic changes actually do occur in the structure of tissue composing the organ affected. The symptoms experienced by the patient are believed by many to be the result of prolonged repression of emotion, which disturbs normal physiologic balance. Eventually this prolonged malfunctioning produces actual structural changes in visceral organs. The patient's defense against anxiety is said to be on a physiologic level, with his affect (mood) being expressed through the body viscera. Thus, psycho-

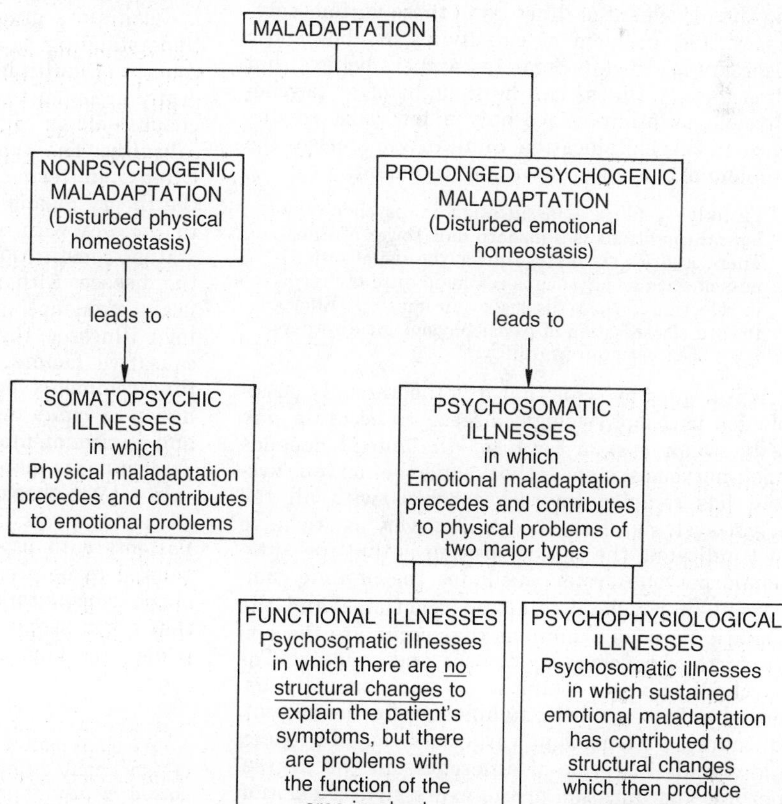
MALADAPTATION
NONPSYCHOGENIC MALADAPTATION (Disturbed physical homeostasis)
PROLONGED PSYCHOGENIC MALADAPTATION (Disturbed emotional homeostasis)
leads to
leads to
SOMATOPSYCHIC ILLNESSES in which Physical maladaptation precedes and contributes to emotional problems
PSYCHOSOMATIC ILLNESSES in which Emotional maladaptation precedes and contributes to physical problems of two major types
FUNCTIONAL ILLNESSES Psychosomatic illnesses in which there are no structural changes to explain the patient's symptoms, but there are problems with the function of the area involved
PSYCHOPHYSIOLOGICAL ILLNESSES Psychosomatic illnesses in which sustained emotional maladaptation has contributed to structural changes which then produce symptoms

FIGURE 19–2. The etiology of somatopsychic, psychosomatic, functional, and psychophysiologic illness.

logic factors are believed to play an important part in the formation or aggravation of the anatomicopathologic or physiopathologic changes that occur.

Authorities[63] believe that the affect most commonly implicated in psychophysiologic disorders is chronic anxiety; specific affective reactions, such as rage or depression, are less common. The *autonomic nervous system* is believed to be involved in producing the organic component of psychophysiologic reactions. The gastrointestinal, respiratory, cardiovascular, endocrine, and genitourinary systems are innervated by the autonomic nervous system and are thus locations of illness commonly classified as psychophysiologic. The skin also is often involved. Thus, some disorders that are commonly felt to be of psychophysiologic origin include: ulcerative colitis, duodenal ulcer, obesity, some headaches, many skin disorders, bronchial asthma, some endocrine disorders, essential hypertension, coronary heart disease, and accident proneness. During recent years research has also indicated that emotional factors may be significant in the etiology of pulmonary tuberculosis and cancer of various types.

In discussing functional, psychophysiologic, and somatopsychic illnesses we have attempted to list "typical" illnesses. It should be recognized, however, that wide varieties of opinion exist concerning the placement of illnesses in these various categories. The problem of classifying psychosomatic disorders is difficult. Some researchers believe that almost every illness can be thought of as psychophysiologic; others place only a few selected diseases in this classification. Shulkin summarizes the problem of classification in his statement:

> Frankly speaking, classification in psychophysiological conditions is a modern day Tower of Babel. There is a joyous disregard for the usual orderliness of science; physicians commonly use lay terms in referring to these disease syndromes. . . . Efforts toward classification of psychophysiologic disorders have been very unrewarding.[130]

It is argued by some that it is theoretically possible for psychophysiologic disease to occur in *any* body organ system because "the mind" depends upon nervous system activity, and the nervous system has complex interrelationships with all the organ systems of the body. However, as we have just indicated, the classic position is that the autonomic nervous system mediates the organic component of psychophysiologic reactions, and the somatic nervous symptoms that occur are the end products of psychologic stresses and conflicts. The psychophysiologic symptom is not generally believed to have symbolic significance for the patient. Of course, a tremendous variation is noted between individuals in terms of differences in the degree, nature, and duration of the expression of emotion through disturbances in various body organs.

Theories of Psychophysiologic Etiology. Systems of classification of disease often derive from theories of etiology. Let us now focus our discussion specifically on *psychophysiologic* disorders and consider some etiologic theories.*

In the early days of "psychosomatics" each specialized profession (i.e., psychology, psychoanalysis, neurology) had its own school of thought about the problem and there was little communication between the disciplines—each group held fiercely to its own point of view, believing its theory could not be improved by knowledge from other fields. At this time, rapprochement appears to be taking place between the various disciplines currently studying psychophysiologic conditions, and knowledge from epidemiology, biochemistry, physiology, psychiatry, psychology, neurology, pathology, and so on, is being "pooled" with greater frequency. Out of this interdisciplinary approach, eclectic theories are increasingly beginning to emerge.

Today much of the volatile theorizing and many of the sweeping generalizations, which characterized psychosomatic discussions in their infancy, are being slowly replaced by a more careful, scientifically delineated, experimental approach. However, much remains unclear, and a great deal of work must be done. At present the theories of psychophysiologic illness are still comparable to winds blowing in all directions at once, and while such winds continue to blow, it is impossible to identify what the true causes of psychophysiologic problems may be. Because of the wide variety of etiologic theories of psychophysiologic illness, it is difficult to group them in an all-inclusive, meaningful manner. However, certain points are rather commonly agreed upon.

Certainly a great boost toward interdisciplinary understanding came with the introduction of the concept of multiple causes of disease, and it is generally accepted today that the basic model of psychophysiologic disease is the *theory of multicausality*. The concept was discussed in Unit II. Briefly, in terms of psychophysiologic disorders, the theory means that psychic factors are believed to *interact* with somatic factors (i.e., nutritional status, constitution, organ pathology) to produce the disease. Although psychic factors have a significant influence on the etiology of psychophysiologic illnesses, they are not considered as the *only* causative factors. Psychophysiologic illnesses are thus commonly believed to result from the interaction of *many* determinants—organ, psychologic, and environmental. Let us examine some of these determinants more carefully.

In all the theories of psychophysiologic etiology, *anxiety* or *stress* is believed to be an initial factor. Patients with psychophysiologic illnesses are considered to be *organically vulnerable* to the physiologic concomitants of emotional arousal in a way that other people are not. In other words, psychic factors in themselves are not the only causative

*We shall omit a theoretical discussion of the etiology of functional disorders, since these are primarily discussed in psychiatric terminology, which is too involved to present in a medical-surgical textbook.

determinant of such disorders, since many people who experience anxiety do not develop somatic illness. A specific interaction of psychic factors with somatic factors, such as nutritional status, constitution, and organ vulnerability, is necessary to produce the disease state.

Although this basic theoretic model is generally accepted, debate exists concerning the interpretation of the model clinically and theoretically. For example, there are several theories about the issue of "symptom choice";* that is, why a person develops certain symptoms or pathology rather than developing other symptoms. Why is it that a particular organ is affected by emotional stress more than other organs in a given individual? In other words, why does one person react to stress with stomach trouble while another becomes hypertensive? There are three general approaches to answering the question of symptom choice in psychophysiologic illnesses: (1) that *specific* psychologic stresses produce *specific* symptoms; (2) that stress *in general* (rather than specific stresses) produces symptoms; and (3) that a wide range of stimuli may evoke a pattern of emotional arousal that consists of specific, consistent physiologic responses which are *characteristic of that individual* (i.e., the symptoms depend upon the individual's typical response pattern rather than the nature of the stimulus).

It can be seen that numerous psychophysiologic theories exist, and the reader is cautioned to remember that, at present, many questions about illnesses of this nature remain unanswered. The nurse's attitude toward psychophysiologic conditions will be reflected to the thousands of patients with these illnesses for whom she may care. Therefore, generalizations, misinterpretations, or reliance on outdated theories on her part could create unhappiness for many. Speculative theories carry with them both dangers and promises!

The nurse needs, of course, to keep informed of changes in theories that pertain to her area of practice. She cannot wait for clarity to emerge in the field of psychosomatic medicine before she begins to care for those persons who suffer from psychosomatic illnesses. These patients are with her each day; she cannot ignore the basic problems experienced by many patients in her care, but must provide knowledgeable care. The nurse must constantly explore the uncharted territory of mind-body interaction, keeping company with physicians, scientists, and philosophers. We all look forward to the time when order and definitive answers will emerge from the present admixture of psychosomatic theories, and suffering can be more effectively reduced or prevented. In the interval, we share the hope and professional concern of Michael Polanyi, philosopher of science, that it might be possible "to establish a better foundation than we now possess for holding the beliefs by which we live and must live, though unable adequately to justify them today."[106]

Psychophysiologic Symptoms: Maladaptive or Adaptive? Are the psychophysiologic symptoms that a patient develops maladaptive or adaptive for him? Do they tend to destroy him or do they instead help him to adapt to life? These questions will be discussed from both points of view.

Let us first briefly consider how these symptoms might be *adaptive*. It has been stated that while psychophysiologic symptoms have pathologic aspects (i.e., they produce structural changes in the body), they may serve a positive and constructive function in the patient's adjustment to the conflicts and anxieties of life.[104, 117] By permitting a protective integration of the patient's personality, the symptoms may protect him from a total mental breakdown. The physical symptom thus represents a more easily tolerated pain than the pain of anxiety. Psychophysiologic symptoms might in this sense be considered as a means of adjustment and could be helpful to the patient. For example, in his discussion of social class and illness, Jurgen Ruesch[118] states that for the lower middle class the only possible solution for unsolved psychologic conflicts lies in physical symptoms. Thus, it could be postulated that physical symptoms are actually serving a protective or restitutive function for this highly repressed group of people.

Other authorities, writing on the adaptive function of psychophysiologic symptoms, maintain that the homeostasis of the total organism (person) may be achieved at the expense of the integrity of one part of the organism.[49] Thus, one part saves the whole. This viewpoint is illustrated by the fact that it is a common clinical phenomenon for a patient with psychophysiologic symptoms to become emotionally disturbed, even psychotic, when the somatic aspects of his illness are resolved.

If symptoms can be viewed as adaptive, the nurse can consider the patient as a whole person whose behavior and symptom formation is not just a random event but is actually a meaningful search for identity and stability in a difficult world. On the other hand, psychophysiologic illnesses can also be considered from a *maladaptive* perspective. Thus, while it is possible to think of psychophysiologic symptoms as defensive physical adapatations to maintain psychologic homeostasis, it is debatable whether or not such symptoms can actually be considered helpful.[136] It is possible to have psychophysiologic problems that are so severe that they interfere with the afflicted person's ability to even live. Certainly it is doubtful whether somatic symptoms of this magnitude are protecting the patient.

Some investigators maintain that psychophysiologic symptoms do *not* diminish anxiety or tension and thus do *not* serve as psychologic defense mechanisms. Instead, they maintain that the symptoms appear when the psychologic defenses *fail* to reduce anxiety. The symptoms, thus, actually represent the physiologic concomitants of anxiety.

Finally, still other experts believe that it may be a matter of (1) the severity of a symptom (its degree

*See also Unit II, p. 36.

of usage by the patient) or (2) how the symptom fits into the patient's total life situation that determines whether psychophysiologic symptoms are adaptive or maladaptive for a given individual.

Incidence of Psychosomatic Conditions. It is erroneous to assume that everyone who develops an illness that might be classified as psychosomatic actually has a psychosomatic disorder. Headaches, for example, can result from brain tumor rather than mental stress, and likewise, back pain may be attributable to a herniated disk instead of anxiety. Evidence of disturbed psychologic adaptation must *precede* the ailment for an accurate psychosomatic diagnosis to be made; bodily symptoms alone do not constitute a psychosomatic diagnosis.

Although it is difficult to obtain accurate statistics on psychosomatic problems, illnesses of this nature clearly appear to be great in number and responsible for much suffering and death. It has been estimated that close to *one million* persons die annually from disorders that are primarily emotional in origin! Naturally much greater numbers of persons living are assumed to be afflicted with such disorders. As we mentioned in the introduction to this chapter:

> *It has been estimated that one third of all patients seen in medical practice today have psychosomatic disorders and that another third have somatic problems complicated by psychiatric problems.*[123]

An understanding of psychosomatic conditions is obviously of great importance in medical and nursing practice. These illnesses must be prevented when possible and recognized and treated when they do occur.

CHAPTER 20

Treatment of Psychosomatic Disorders

Inclusion of an illness in the psychosomatic group implies that, in a high percentage of cases, emotional conflict in one form or another has contributed to the causation of the disorder. Because psychosomatic illnesses involve psychologic factors, their ideal treatment involves attention to both physical and psychologic maladaptations. Recall that psychosomatic conditions may be divided into two groups: (1) functional illnesses, and (2) psychophysiologic illnesses.

A professional attempt to identify and understand the stress that the patient is subject to is an integral part of successful therapy. Unless the individual can be assisted to adapt successfully to his life stresses, his psychosomatic condition will undoubtedly recur despite medical therapy, or his illness may merely shift from one symptom to another. Successful treatment of psychosomatic conditions is extremely complex because, at present (1) there is no one answer to the question of etiology; (2) it is not agreed which illnesses should be considered psychosomatic; and, furthermore, (3) it is not known what specifically constitutes treatment of psychosomatic disorders.

FUNCTIONAL DISORDERS AND THEIR TREATMENT

You will recall that with functional disorders the problem is primarily one of psychologic imbalance expressed in physical symptoms. Also, no structural change is present to account for the symptoms. These patients are ill although they have no organic pathology. They are definitely in a state of maladaptation believed to be precipitated by stress, which creates an imbalance in psychologic homeostasis. Because of their discomfort, persons with functional disorders seek medical help, unaware that their illness does not have an organic basis. These patients will often be met by nurses in doctors' offices, as well as in hospitals where the patient may be undergoing a diagnostic work-up.

Authorities recommend that if the physician is satisfied that the patient has no organic disease (in other words, after careful and thorough work-up), he should stop the examinations and *discuss* with the patient the fact that no organic disease is present. The patient is then in need of psychiatric aid, either from his physician or a psychiatrist. It is not enough to rule out physical disease and send the patient home; he must be referred for more specific therapy.

In the course of psychiatric aid, the patient is helped to understand how the mind influences the body in terms of simple illustrations, e.g., blushing. Gradually the patient will be helped to discuss his life and the problems that he may be having. This is best accomplished indirectly rather than asking outright, "Are you worried about anything?" The therapist needs to come to know the patient as a human being, his ability to adjust to stresses in life, the degree of anxiety in his make-up, and the nature and seriousness of his conflicts. A genuine understanding of these factors involves far more than merely making a cursory examination of the patient's life and discovering "a problem." Discovering a problem does not mean that the present illness can be explained in terms of that problem. The psychiatric treatment of patients with functional illnesses is complex and specialized. Untrained persons should not attempt to discuss the patient's condition with him except to indicate that they realize he is uncomfortable. The illness may, in some way, be psychologically protective for the individual, and the patient's adaptive mechanisms must be treated with respect, knowledge, and sensitivity.

PSYCHOPHYSIOLOGIC DISORDERS AND THEIR TREATMENT

Let us quickly review what we might consider to be the "typical" development and progression of psychophysiologic disorders. As we have demonstrated earlier, bodily changes (e.g., increased heart rate) are concomitant with anxiety. When the body's stress mechanisms function at a heightened level for a prolonged period of time, the eventual result may be overreaction and organ damage or malfunction. Prolonged psychophysiologic reactions can produce chronic disease and death, although, in many instances, remission or recovery is possible. Schematically we can portray the possible progressions of psychophysiologic disease as shown in Figure 20–1.

An understanding of etiology is basic to successful treatment. In attempting to understand the causation of a psychophysiologic illness, it is helpful to speculate about the following three questions posed by Halliday:[50] (1) Why did this patient become ill in the manner he did? (2) What kind of person is he, that he should behave in this way? (3) Why did he become ill when he did? These questions lead us to speculate about: (1) the *physiologic* mechanism of the patient's illness, or what has happened physically; (2) the *individual,* in terms of what kind of person he is and what his physical and psychologic predispositions tend to be; and (3) his *environment* from the perspective of what he has met with generally—food, social and psychologic problems, irritants. When these three fields can be related to one another, we may say that the illness is explained.

What is the *treatment* of psychophysiologic disorders? When a patient with a psychophysiologic condition has organic pathologic changes, it is not sufficient to evaluate and care for only the physical problem. Purely physical treatment could only produce a temporary removal of symptoms since the individual's emotional capacity to cope with the same or new adverse situations may be unaltered or even worsened by his experience.[66] Ideally, in addition to physical care, the patient should receive the psychologic help that will enable him to deal with emotional difficulties. If patients with psychophysiologic disturbances are not provided with *both* physical and psychologic care, they may remain vulnerable to emotional conflict even though their physical problem appears to be corrected. Such vulnerability may mean recurrent attacks of their original psychophysiologic illness, or "syndrome shift" may occur, with the consecutive replacement of one syndrome by another and the production of a progression of various psychophysiologic illnesses, each differing from its precursor. It should be recognized, however, that many patients recover from psychophysiologic disorders without either recurrence or syndrome shift.

In establishing a diagnosis, a complete physical examination should be carried out.[123] Often this, in itself, is therapeutically valuable when proper reassurance is given the patient. The examination should include radiology, electrocardiography, and laboratory work. In addition, both a clinical history and a personal history of personality development should be taken. From these findings the physician searches for clues to a psychophysiologic diagnosis and for evidence to support the diagnosis.

At present, psychophysiologic treatment may be carried out by a medical physician or a psychiatrist, or by cooperation of a psychiatrist, clinical psychologist, or psychoanalyst with a medical physician. We shall not discuss the *medical treatment* in this section of the text; rather, the treatments are discussed later in the book in relation to specific conditions. Let us look briefly, however, at the approach of psychotherapy.

Vagueness shrouds many statements in the literature about the *psychiatric treatment* of psychophysiologic disorders. Little is published on the *specific* psychiatric treatment of these illnesses, and thus the field of therapy is permeated with generalizations. This lack of direction, in part, reflects a lack of specific etiologic knowledge. In spite of the problems, some guidelines for the psychotherapy of psychophysiologic disorders do exist.

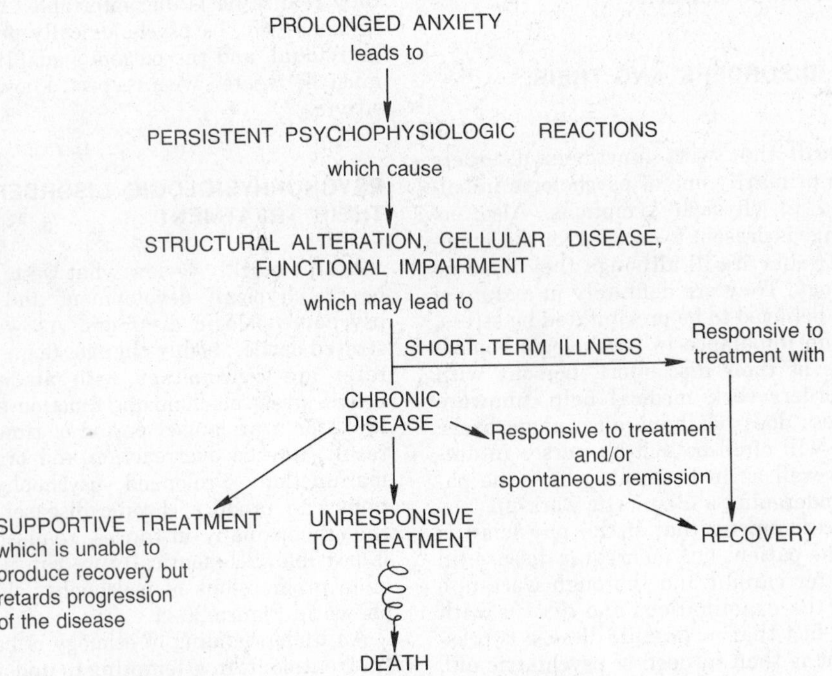

FIGURE 20–1. Possible progression of psychophysiologic disease.

For example, it is generally accepted by psychiatric experts that psychiatric therapy must be carefully managed so that it does not produce an emotional state that could aggravate the patient's psychophysiologic condition. The broad goal of psychiatric care is to reduce the patient's anxiety. To achieve this goal, much of the care during acute illness consists of support, reinforcement of defenses, reassurance, and gratification of dependency needs when appropriate. Tranquilizers may also be prescribed. Unfortunately psychotherapy has not proved to be as helpful in treating psychophysiologic disorders as it was originally hoped it would be.

One final consideration that we shall mention briefly is the use of "environmental prescriptions," which are guides for therapeutically manipulating a patient's environment. For example, the doctor may recommend a change in the patient's basic family environment or job setting. Such manipulations could obviously alter the patient's life markedly, and so they must be made only after an extensive evaluation.

NURSING IMPLICATIONS

The nurse will encounter patients with functional and psychophysiologic disorders in the doctor's office, clinics, on home visits, and in hospitals as they undergo medical evaluation and treatment. These patients pose complex diagnostic and management problems for the physician. The nursing care of such patients *must* involve both physical and mental care. Physical care varies with the area of involvement and is discussed later in the text with the appropriate illness. The emotional nursing care that such patients require is not complicated but it does require thought. Patients with psychosomatic conditions generally require a "giving" attitude on the part of those supplying care: an attitude of caring, support, understanding, warmth, and comfort. The major goal of emotional care is to reduce anxiety. This may involve allowing the patient to be dependent and reinforcing his mental defense pattern. Allowing a patient to be dependent does *not* mean keeping him dependent, fostering dependency, or allowing him to be so dependent that his physical condition is in jeopardy, e.g., allowing the patient to develop pneumonia from not coughing or moving about in bed.

Generally patients with psychosomatic problems are extremely sensitive to the attitudes that others have toward them. Feelings of rejection may readily intensify these patients' basic anxieties. It is of vital importance that nurses understand that patients suffering from psychophysiologic and functional disorders are *not* "pretending" to be ill; they are *not* malingering; they *are* suffering. The nurse's responsibility is to convey to the patient the feeling that she knows he is uncomfortable and that she will try to provide comfort for him. Tragically these patients are often not conscious of the emotional problems or stresses that may be perpetuating their illnesses. Even when the emotional problem is believed to have been identified, the relationship between the emotional situation and the pathophysiology involved may not be clearly understood —as testified by the variety of etiologic theories that currently exist.

Generally persons suffering from psychosomatic disorders genuinely desire relief from their illness and from the life problems involved in their illness. They desire to adapt to life without illness. Unfortunately *some* patients with illnesses of this nature have unmet needs (for love, dependency, attention, and so forth) that cause them *unconsciously* to remain physically ill so that these needs may be partially met. In essence, they are unable to adapt their needs to "wellness."

The nurse is in an important position to carry out environmental manipulation for the psychosomatic patient within the hospital. Since a major goal of care during the acute phase of psychosomatic illness is to reduce anxiety, the nurse should endeavor to provide a restful environment. The nurse is also in a key position to make professional observations concerning the patient's physical condition and his behavior. She should attempt to understand his personality so that she might anticipate what situations would be anxiety provoking to him. The nurse can also observe how the patient expresses his anxiety and allow him to do so when feasible.

Finally, the nurse should be familiar with any psychopharmacologic agents that the patient receives. Patients with psychosomatic disorders may be anxious and also have an underlying depression. If this is so, *both* an antidepressant and tranquilizer are often necessary, since it is known that (1) tranquilizers or sedatives (if given alone) may reduce anxiety but may fail to relieve the depression (in fact, may actually augment the depression); and (2) while antidepressant drugs alone may relieve depression, they have less effect on the tension state.[123] Increasingly we are becoming aware of the need for careful supervision of administration of these drugs, because of their potent nature and possible serious side effects. The nurse's observations of the patient's response to such medications will be most helpful to the physician as he attempts to find which psychopharmacologic agent and which dosage will be most helpful for the patient.

CONCLUSION

It is hoped that this unit has helped the reader to realize that concepts of mind-body interaction are in a state of tumult. However, such tumult should not be viewed with disdain, for some theories, although admittedly fragmentary at present, hold great promise for a future understanding of total man.

The area of mind-body interaction in the production of disease is of great importance to nursing. Increasingly it is recognized that we cannot think of the ill person as being only physically ill; concomitant mental reactions must also be considered. Concepts of psychophysiologic and psychosomatic disease are gaining an established place in medicine. These fields are far more complicated than they were once believed to be. Psychosomatic medicine is a field quite new to the sciences. As such it currently suffers from problems of definitions, classifications, and interpretations. Even the experts are confused. However, such confusion is part of any new scientific approach. We should be reminded that in the science of chemistry it took over a century of research before a clear definition of an element was formulated.

Realizing that the content of this unit has been based upon theoretic discussion more than fact, the nurse is cautioned to avoid narrow interpretations of "psychosomatic" problems in her practice. She is encouraged to view illness as a process of homeostatic disturbances composed of delicate psychophysiologic imbalances, and to keep an inquiring mind concerning the etiology of such imbalances. She can best serve her patients by assuming that their illnesses and problems have a multicausal basis.

References for Unit IV

1. Aasterud, M.: Defenses against anxiety in the nurse-patient relationship. *Nursing Forum,* 1:35, Summer, 1962.
2. Abrams, W. B.: Somatopsychic conditions: Classification and clinical orientation. *In* Nodine, J. H., and Moyers, J. H. (eds.): *Psychosomatic Medicine.* Philadelphia, Lea & Febiger, 1962.
3. Agle, D., Ratnoff, O., and Wasman, M.: Studies in autoerythrocyte sensitization. *Psychosomatic Medicine,* 29:491, September-October, 1967.
4. Alexander, F.: *Psychosomatic Medicine: Its Principles and Applications.* New York, W. W. Norton Company, Inc., 1950.
5. Basowitz, H.: *Anxiety and Stress: An Interdisciplinary Study of a Life Situation.* New York, Blakiston Division, McGraw-Hill Book Co., Inc., 1955.
6. Bertalanffy, L. V.: The mind-body problem: A new view, *Psychosomatic Medicine,* 26:29, January-February, 1964.
7. Bogardus, E. S., and Brethorst, A. B.: *Sociology Applied to Nursing.* 3rd ed. Philadelphia, W. B. Saunders Company, 1952.
8. Bojar, S.: The psychotherapeutic function of the general hospital nurse. *Nursing Outlook,* 6:151, March, 1958.
9. Boulette, T. R.: Anxiety and the nurse, *P.N.,* 17:28, August, 1967.
10. Braden, W.: *The Private Sea.* Chicago, Quadrangle Books, 1967.
11. Brady, J. V.: Experimental studies of psychophysiological responses to stressful conditions. *In Symposium on Medical Aspects of Stress in the Military Climate.* Washington, D.C., Walter Reed Army Institute of Research, 1964.
12. Brill, N. Q.: The importance of understanding yourself. *In* Mereness, D. (ed.): *Psychiatric Nursing.* Vol. I, Dubuque, Iowa, William C. Brown Company, 1966.
13. Buchan, D. J.: Mind-body relationships in gastrointestinal disease. *Canadian Nurse,* 67:35, March, 1971.
14. Burkhardt, M.: Response to anxiety. *American Journal of Nursing,* 69:2153, October, 1969.
15. Cattell, R. B.: The nature and measurement of anxiety. *Scientific American,* 96, March, 1963.
16. Chalke, F. C. R.: Effect of psychotherapy for psychosomatic disorders. *Psychosomatics,* 6:125, May-June, 1965.
17. Cleghorn, R. A.: Psychosomatic principles. *Canadian Medical Association Journal,* 92:441, 1965.
18. Cleland, V. S.: Effects of stress on thinking. *American Journal of Nursing,* 67:108, January, 1967.
19. Cloudsley, T., and Leonard, J.: *Animal Conflict and Adaptation.* Chester Springs, Pennsylvania, Dufour Editions, 1965.
20. Cooper, B.: The epidemiological approach to psychosomatic medicine. *Journal of Psychosomatic Research,* 8:9–15, July, 1964.
21. Dorfman, W.: *Closing the Gap Between Medicine and Psychiatry.* Springfield, Illinois, Charles C Thomas, 1966.
22. Dorpat, T. L.: Phantom sensation of internal organs. *Comprehensive Psychiatry,* 12:27, January, 1971.
23. Drage, E. M.: Recall of panic episodes. *American Journal of Nursing,* 68:1254, June, 1968.
24. Dubos, R.: *Man Adapting.* New Haven, Yale University Press, 1965.
25. Dumas, R. G.: Utilization of a concept of stress as a basis for nursing practice. *A.N.A. Clinical Sessions,* 193, 1966.
26. Dunbar, F.: *Mind and Body: Psychosomatic Medicine.* New York, Random House, 1947.
27. Durand, M.: The nurse and the anxious patient. Paper presented at the Institute "Anxiety, Depression and Suicide," sponsored by University of Washington School of Nursing, February 10, 1966.
28. Eaton, J. W., et al.: Resistance to psychiatry in a general hospital. *Mental Hospital,* 16:156, 1965.
29. Eiseley, L.: *The Immense Journey.* New York, Time-Life, Incorporated, Time Reading Program, 1962.
30. Engle, G. L.: A unified concept of health and disease. *Perspectives in Biology and Medicine,* 3: 459, Summer, 1960.
31. Engel, G. L.: *Psychological Development in Health and Disease.* Philadelphia, W. B. Saunders Company, 1962.
32. Ewalt, J. R.: Somatic manifestations of depression. *Hospital Medicine,* 2:60, October, 1966.
33. Farnsworth, D. L.: Mental health is a point of view. *American Journal of Nursing,* 60:688, May, 1960.
34. Fischer, H. K., et al.: Psychosomatic medicine. *Progress in Neurology and Psychiatry,* 25:409, 1970.
35. Folta, J., and Deck, E. (eds.): *A Sociological Framework for Patient Care.* New York, John Wiley & Sons, Inc., 1966.
36. Francis, G. M.: How do I feel about myself? *American Journal of Nursing,* 67:1244, June, 1967.
37. Freedman, A. M., and Kaplan, H. I. (eds.): *Comprehensive Textbook of Psychiatry.* Baltimore, The Williams & Wilkins Company, 1967.

38. Freeman, V. J.: Human aspects of health and illness: Beyond the germ theory. *Journal of Health and Human Behavior,* 1:8, 1960.
39. Fromm-Reichmann, F.: Psychiatric aspects of anxiety. *In* Stein, M., Vidich, A. J., and White, D. M. (eds.): *Identity and Anxiety.* Glencoe, Illinois, The Free Press, 1960.
40. Funkenstein, D. H.: The physiology of fear and anger. *Scientific American Reprint,* May, 1955.
41. Galdston, I. (ed.): *Beyond the Germ Theory.* A New York Academy of Medicine Book, 1954.
42. Gilbert, M. M.: Reactive depression as a model of psychosomatic disease. *Psychosomatics,* 11:426, September-October, 1970.
43. Glasrud, C. A. (ed.): *The Age of Anxiety.* Boston, Houghton-Mifflin Company, 1960.
44. Graham, D. T.: Health, disease, and the mind-body problem: Linguistic parallelism. *Psychosomatic Medicine,* 29:52, January-February, 1967.
45. Graham, D. T.: Psychophysiology and medicine. *Psychophysiology,* 8:121, March, 1971.
46. Greenfield, A. D. M.: The effects of emotion on the peripheral circulation. *Journal of Psychosomatic Research,* 9:155, September, 1965.
47. Gregg, D.: Anxiety, a factor in nursing care. *American Journal of Nursing,* 52:1363, November, 1952.
48. Gregg, D.: Reassurance. *American Journal of Nursing,* 55:171, February, 1955.
49. Grinker, R. R., and Robbins, F. P.: *Psychosomatic Casebook.* New York, Blakiston Division, McGraw-Hill Book Co., Inc., 1954.
50. Halliday, J. L.: Concept of a psychosomatic affection. *Lancet,* 2:692, 1943.
51. Hamilton, M.: *Psychosomatics.* New York, John Wiley & Sons, Inc., 1955.
52. Hammer, L. Z. (ed.): *Value and Man.* New York, McGraw-Hill Book Company, 1966.
53. Harms, E.: *Origins of Modern Psychiatry.* Springfield, Ill., Charles C Thomas, 1967.
54. Hayes, W., and Gazaway, R.: *Human Relations in Nursing.* 3rd ed. Philadelphia, W. B. Saunders Company, 1964.
55. Hinkle, L. E., Jr.: Human ecology and psychosomatic medicine. *Psychosomatic Medicine,* 29:391, July-August, 1967.
56. Hinkle, L. E., Jr.: Normal stress in normal experience. *In* Galdston, I. (ed.): *Beyond the Germ Theory.* A New York Academy of Medicine Book, 1954.
57. Hofling, C. F., Leininger, M. M., and Bregg, E.: *Basic Psychiatric Concepts in Nursing.* 2nd ed. Philadelphia, J. B. Lippincott Company, 1967.
58. Hughes, J. M.: Anxiety. *Nursing Mirror,* 132:17, March 12, 1971.
59. Hume, D.: Personal identity. *In* Hammer, L. Z. (ed.): *Value and Man.* New York, McGraw-Hill Book Company, 1966.
60. Kalkman, M. E.: Recognizing emotional problems. *American Journal of Nursing,* 68:536, March, 1968.
61. Kaplan, H. I.: History of psychosomatic medicine. *In* Freedman, A. M., and Kaplan, H. I. (eds.): *Comprehensive Textbook of Psychiatry.* Baltimore, The Williams & Wilkins Company, 1967.
62. Kemp, C. G.: Communication in the helping relationship. *Occupational Health Nursing,* 20:14, April, 1972.
63. Kessel, N., and Munro, A.: Epidemiological studies in psychosomatic medicine. *Journal of Psychosomatic Research,* 8:67, July, 1964.
64. Klerman, G. L.: Stress and adjustment reactions: Classification and clinical orientation. *In* Nodine, J. H., and Moyer, J. H.: *Psychosomatic Medicine.* Philadelphia, Lea & Febiger, 1962.
65. King, J. M.: Denial. *American Journal of Nursing,* 66:1010, May, 1966.
66. Kissen, D. M.: Physical disease and emotional factors—An approach to prevention. *Nursing Mirror,* 126:29, April 19, 1968.
67. Knapp, P. H.: The psychosomatic field. *Psychosomatic Medicine,* 32:425, July-August, 1970.
68. Kral, V. A., Pazder, L. H., and Wigdor, B. T.: Long-term effects of a prolonged stress experience. *Canadian Psychiatric Association Journal,* 12: 175, April, 1967.
69. Le Shan, L.: Psychological states as factors in the development of malignant disease: A critical review. *Journal of the National Cancer Institute,* 22:1, 1959.
70. Lee, E. N., and Mandelbaum, M. (eds.): *Phenomenology and Existentialism.* Baltimore, The Johns Hopkins Press, 1967.
71. Leigh, D.: The contributions of psychoanalysis and psychiatry to psychosomatic medicine. *Psychotherapy and Psychosomatics,* 15:153, 1967.
72. Levi, A. W.: Existentialism and the alienation of man. *In* Lee, E., and Mandelbaum, M. (eds.): *Phenomenology and Existentialism.* Baltimore, The Johns Hopkins Press, 1967.
73. Levine, M. E.: Holistic nursing. *Nursing Clinics of North America,* 6:253, June, 1971.
74. Lewis, J. A.: Reflections on self. *American Journal of Nursing,* 60:828, June, 1960.
75. Lief, H. I.: Anxiety reaction. *In* Freedman, A. M., and Kaplan, H. I. (eds.): *Comprehensive Textbook of Psychiatry.* Baltimore, The Williams & Wilkins Company, 1967.
76. Lief, H. I., et al.: *The Psychological Basis of Medical Practice.* New York, Paul B. Hoeber, 1963.
77. Lipowski, Z. J.: Review of consultation psychiatry and psychosomatic medicine: I. General principles. *Psychosomatic Medicine,* 29:153, March-April, 1967; and Review of consultation psychiatry and psychosomatic medicine: II. Clinical aspects. *Psychosomatic Medicine,* 29:201, 1967.
78. Lipowski, Z. J.: New perspectives in psychosomatic medicine. *Canadian Psychiatric Association Journal,* 15:515, December, 1970.
79. Loomis, E. A., Jr.: *The Self in Pilgrimage.* New York, Harper & Brothers, 1960.
80. Loudon, J. B.: Private stress and public ritual. *Journal of Psychosomatic Research,* 10:101–108, July, 1966.
81. Lucia, S. P.: The psyche of man and his illness. *Medical Times,* 99:140, August, 1971.
82. Lyons, Sister M. L.: The creative use of self in human relations. *AORN,* 5:47, February, 1967.
83. Macgregor, F. C.: *Social Science in Nursing.* New York, Russell Sage Foundation, 1960.
84. Martin, H. W., and Prange, A. J.: Human adaptation: A conceptual approach to understanding patients. *The Canadian Nurse,* 58:234, March, 1962.
85. Masserman, J. H.: Science, human values and psychiatry. *Psychotherapy,* 15:179, 1967.
86. Mathis, J. L.: A sophisticated version of voodoo death: Report of a case. *Psychosomatic Medicine,* 26:104, March-April, 1964.
87. May, R.: Centrality of the problems of anxiety in our day. *In* Stein, M., Vidich, A. J., and White, D. J. (eds.): *Identity and Anxiety.* Glencoe, Illinois, The Free Press of Glencoe, 1960.

88. May, R.: *Man's Search for Himself.* New York, W. W. Norton and Company, Inc., 1953.
89. Meldman, M. Jay: A general concept of disease. *Psychosomatics,* 6:383, November-December, 1965.
90. Meldman, M. J.: A model for resolving the mind-body problem. *Psychosomatics,* 6:150, May-June, 1965.
91. Meldman, M. J.: Hyperattentionism and hypoattentionism. *American Journal of Psychiatry,* 120: 805, 1964.
92. Meldman, M. J.: A nosology of the attentional diseases. *American Journal of Psychiatry,* 121:377, 1964.
93. Menninger, K., Mayman, M., and Pruyser, P.: *The Vital Balance: The Life Process in Mental Health and Illness.* New York, The Viking Press, 1963.
94. Menninger, W. C.: Are you mentally mature? *Life and Health,* 82:12, July, 1967.
95. Mintz, T.: Tickle—The itch that moves: A psychophysiological hypothesis. *Psychosomatic Medicine,* 29:606, November-December, 1967.
96. Mordkoff, A. M.: The relationship between psychological and physiological response to stress. *Psychosomatic Medicine,* 26:135, March-April, 1964.
97. Mowchenko, G.: Care of patients with GI diseases that have a psychological component. *Canadian Nurse,* 38:40, March, 1971.
98. Neyland, M. P.: Anxiety. *American Journal of Nursing,* 62:110, May, 1962.
99. Nodine, J. H., and Moyer, J. H. (eds.): *Psychosomatic Medicine.* Philadelphia, Lea & Febiger, 1962.
100. Norton, W. A.: Mind, body, and language. *Canadian Psychiatric Association Journal,* 12:93, April, 1967.
101. Nussbaum, K.: Somatic complaints and homeostasis in psychiatric patients. *Psychiatric Quarterly,* 34: 311, 1960.
102. Oskendorf, M.: Emotional responses of patients to physical illness. *ANA Clinical Sessions,* 145, 1966.
103. Parley, K.: How to balance your tensions. *American Journal of Nursing,* 67:2099, October, 1967.
104. Parsons, T.: Illness and the role of the physician: A sociological perspective. *In* Kluckhohn, C., and Murray, H. (eds.): *Personality in Nature, Society, and Culture.* New York, Alfred A. Knopf, 1959.
105. Peplau, H.: A working definition of anxiety. *In* Burd, S. F., and Marshall, M. (eds.): *Some Clinical Approaches to Psychiatric Nursing.* New York, The Macmillan Company, 1963.
106. Polanyi, M.: The body-mind relation. *In* Rogers, C., and Caulson, W. (eds.): *Man and the Science of Man.* Columbus, Ohio, Charles E. Merrill Publishing Company, 1968.
107. Polonia, P.: Body-mind problems from an empirical point of view. *British Journal of Psychiatry,* 118: 7, January, 1971.
108. Pollock, T.: Yes, you can work under pressure: Stress, properly harnessed, can bring out your best. *Hospital Management,* 103:32, June, 1967.
109. Pos, R.: The psyche-soma complex: An exercise in symbolic logic. *Canadian Psychiatric Association Journal,* 12:125, April, 1967.
110. Powers, M. E., and Storlie, F.: The apprehensive patient. *American Journal of Nursing,* 67:58, January, 1967.
111. Rahe, R. H., McKean, J. D. Jr., and Arthur, R. J.: A longitudinal study of life-change and illness patterns. *Journal Psychosomatic Research,* 10:355, May, 1967.
112. Rahe, R. H., et al.: Social stress and illness onset. *Journal of Psychosomatic Research,* 8:35, July, 1964.
113. Rahe, R. H., et al.: Prediction of near-future health change from subjects preceding life changes. *Journal of Psychosomatic Research,* 14:401, December, 1970.
114. Ramsey, I. T. (ed.): *Biology and Personality.* New York, Barnes and Noble, Inc., 1965.
115. Robinson, E. A.: Richard Cory. *In* Saunders, G., and Nelson, J. (eds.): *Chief Modern Poets of England and America.* 3rd ed. New York, The Macmillan Company, 1943.
116. Rogers, C. R., and Coulson, W. R. (eds.): *Man and the Science of Man.* Columbus, Ohio, Charles E. Merrill Publishing Company, 1968.
117. Rubin, J.: Positive functions of psychosomatic symptoms. *Medical Times,* 93:769, July, 1965.
118. Ruesch, J.: Social technique, social status, and social change in illness. *In* Kluckholn, C., and Murray, H. (eds.): *Personality in Nature, Society, and Culture.* New York, Alfred A. Knopf, 1959.
119. Ruesch, J., et al.: *Psychiatric Care.* New York, Grune & Stratton, Inc., 1964.
120. Russell, C., and Russell, W. M. S.: Raw materials for a definition of mind. *In* Scher, J. (ed.): *Theories of Mind.* New York, The Free Press, 1962.
121. Sanisbury, P.: Psychosomatic disorders and neurosis in out-patients attending a general hospital. *Journal of Psychosomatic Research,* 4:261, 1960.
122. Sartain, A., et al.: *Psychology: Understanding Human Behavior.* 2nd ed. New York, McGraw-Hill Book Company, Inc., 1962.
123. Schecter, N.: Management of emotional illnesses in general practice. *Psychosomatics,* 6:132, May-June, 1965.
124. Schottstaedt, W. W.: *Psychophysiologic Approach in Medical Practice.* Chicago, Year Book Medical Publishers, 1960.
125. Schwab, J. J., et al.: Problems in psychosomatic diagnosis: I. A controlled study of medical inpatients. *Psychosomatics,* 6:369, 1964; II. Severity of medical illness and psychiatric consultations. *Psychosomatics,* 6:69, 1965; III. Physical examinations, laboratory procedures, and psychiatric consultations. *Psychosomatics,* 6:147, 1965; IV. A challenge to all physicians. *Psychosomatics,* 6:198, 1965.
126. Schwab, J. J.: Enlarging our view of psychosomatic medicine. *Psychosomatics,* 12:16, January-February, 1971.
127. Selye, H.: *The Stress of Life.* New York, McGraw-Hill Book Company, Inc., 1956.
128. Selye, H.: The stress syndrome. *American Journal of Nursing,* 65:97, 1965.
129. Sheafer, D. W.: The symptom complex of anxiety: Its interplay with fear. *Medical Insight,* 3:16, April, 1971.
130. Shulkin, M. W.: Classification of psychophysiologic conditions. *In* Nodine, J. H., and Moyer, J. H. (eds.): *Psychosomatic Medicine.* Philadelphia, Lea & Febiger, 1962.
131. Smerdon, A. C.: The development of tension. *Occupational Health,* 19:15, January-February, 1967.
132. Stevens, L. F.: Understanding ourselves. *American Journal of Nursing,* 57:1022, August, 1957.
133. Stine, J. J.: Anxiety—A factor in somatic symptoms. *American Journal of Psychiatry,* 127:1099, February, 1971.
134. Strassman, H. D., Thalder, M. B., and Schein, E. H.: A prisoner of war syndrome: Apathy as a reaction

to severe stress. *American Journal of Psychiatry,* 112:998, 1956.
135. Sullivan, H. S.: The meaning of anxiety in psychiatry and in life. *Psychiatry,* 11:1, February, 1948.
136. Teitelbaum, H. A.: *Psychosomatic Neurology.* New York, Grune & Stratton, Inc., 1964.
137. Tinling, D. C.: Voodoo, root work, and medicine. *Psychosomatic Medicine,* 29:483, September-October, 1967.
138. Torrance, E. P.: *Constructive Behavior: Stress Personality and Mental Health.* Belmont, California, Wadsworth Publishing Company, Inc., 1965.
139. Vanderpool, J. P., et al.: Empathy: Towards a psychophysiological definition. *Diseases of the Nervous System,* 31:464, July, 1970.
140. Wahl, C. W. (ed.): *New Dimensions in Psychosomatic Medicine.* Boston, Little, Brown and Company, 1964.
141. Walike, B. C.: Personality factors. *American Journal of Nursing,* 67:1427, July, 1967.
142. Walker, L. O.: Every patient is unique. *Nursing Outlook,* 16:39, September, 1968.
143. Walton, H. J., and McPherson, F. M.: Clinicians as observers of psychological events. *Journal of Psychosomatic Research,* 8:319, December, 1964.
144. Watts, A. W.: *Psychotherapy East and West.* New York, Ballantine Books, Inc., 1961.
145. Webster, T. G.: Learning processes in physician education: Integrating psyche and soma. *Psychiatry in Medicine,* 2:67, January, 1971.
146. Weiss, E., and English, S. O.: *Psychosomatic Medicine.* Philadelphia, W. B. Saunders Company, 1957.
147. Weiss, P.: *Reality.* Carbondale, Illinois, Southern Illinois University Press, 1967.
148. Wenger, M. A., Bagchi, B. K., and Anand, B. K.: Voluntary heart and pulse control by yoga methods. *International Journal of Parapsychology,* 5:30, Winter, 1963.
149. Wheelis, A.: *The Quest for Identity.* New York, W. W. Norton and Company, Inc., 1958.
150. Wilson, M., and Meyer, E.: The doctors' vs. the nurses' view of emotional disturbances. *Canadian Psychiatric Association Journal,* 10:212, 1965.
151. Wittkower, E. D.: Twenty years of North American psychosomatic medicine. (Presidential Address.) *Psychosomatic Medicine,* 22:308, 1960.
152. Wittkower, E. D., and Lipowski, Z. J.: Recent developments in psychosomatic medicine. *Psychosomatic Medicine,* 28:722, September-October, 1966.
153. Wittkower, E. D.: Some selected psychosomatic problems of current interest. *Psychosomatics,* 12:21, January-February, 1971.
154. Wolff, H. G.: *Stress and Disease.* Springfield, Illinois, Charles C Thomas, 1953.

UNIT V

The Body's Response to Disturbances in Homeostasis

A wide variety of physiologic imbalances can occur that can disturb bodily homeostasis. Some of these imbalances are listed below:

1. Cellular disturbances
2. Inflammation
3. Drug intoxication*
4. Fluid and electrolyte imbalance
5. Acid-base imbalance
6. Anoxia and asphyxia*
7. Tissue repair and regeneration (the body's response to injury and infection)
8. Physiologic shock
9. Infection*
10. Immunity and hypersensitivity
11. Auto-immunity
12. Nutritional imbalance*
13. Genetic defects*
14. Disturbances in blood flow*
15. Hemorrhage*
16. Extremes in temperature,* and burns*
17. Ionizing radiation*
18. The body's response to bed rest and immobility

The starred items are discussed in other units of the text. This unit will focus on the following major areas of discussion, all of which are basic to nursing care.

> the cell and cellular disturbances
> responses to injury (inflammation and repair)
> the immune system (immunity, hypersensitivity, and auto-immune disorders)
> fluid and electrolyte and acid-base imbalances
> shock
> the body's response to bed rest and immobility

CHAPTER 21

The Cell and Cellular Disturbances

> Whatever its form, however it behaves, the cell is the basic unit of all living matter. In the cell, nature has enclosed in a microscopic package all the parts and processes necessary to the survival of life in an ever-changing world.
>
> John Pfeiffer, *The Cell*[9]

INTRODUCTION AND STUDY GUIDE

Cells are the basic units or building blocks that compose the bodies of all living organisms. Within the adult human body there are approximately 60,000 billion cells—each of them energetically multiplying, reacting to stimuli, producing enzymes, and carrying out many precise and highly specialized functions. Dynamic, frantically active, and yet orderly in its workings, the healthy cell exists as a miniature chemistry laboratory, powerhouse, factory, and duplicating machine—perfectly reproducing itself over and over again. Of course, when aging, illness, and injury strike the cell, as they inevitably will, pathologic changes develop which alter both cellular structure and function. As a consequence, the cell's ability to work and produce becomes curtailed and reduced, to the detriment of the total organism.

In this chapter, we shall discuss briefly the structure and function of the normal healthy cell as well as some of the major pathologic problems that affect, damage, and destroy cells. To aid you in your study of the cell, we refer you to the following guide:

1. Upon completion of this chapter, you should be aware of the definitions of the following key terms:

cytoplasm, nucleus, nucleoli, chromosomes, chromatin, nucleic acid, DNA, RNA, organelles, mitochondria, ribosomes, endoplasmic reticulum, lysosome, phagocytosis, pinocytosis, degeneration, infiltration, necrosis, cell death.

2. You should be able to discuss generally the following subjects:

a. The general functions of cells.
b. The major specialized cell groups.
c. The causes of cellular damage.
d. The major types of degenerations.
e. The major types of disturbances in cell growth.
f. The major types of cellular necrosis.

THE LIVING CELL: A STRUCTURAL AND PHYSIOLOGICAL UNIT

CELLULAR COMPOSITION

Cells are composed of protoplasm, a heavy, thick colloidal material that actively exhibits the basic properties of all living matter, namely, growth, movement, reproduction, secretion, irritability, ingestion, and assimilation.

A highly complex substance, protoplasm is composed of many different chemical materials, the most important being briefly listed and discussed below.

Water. Seventy to 85 per cent of protoplasm is water, which acts both as a universal solvent for cellular chemicals and as a fluid medium in which chemical reactions can take place.

Protein. Ten to 25 per cent of protoplasm is comprised of protein, which, in turn, is made up of atoms of hydrogen, oxygen, nitrogen, and carbon. *Structural* proteins make up the surrounding membranes of the cell as well as the membranes of many of the tiny structures that exist within the cell. *Enzymes* (which are a type of protein) are also found within the cell. These extremely important protein substances have the power to catalyze chemical reactions. thereby accelerating the speed of vital cellular activities.

Electrolytes. You will recall from chemistry that an electrolyte is a substance or compound composed of atoms which, when placed in solution, break up into separate, charged particles called ions. The most important intracellular electrolytes are potassium, magnesium, phosphate, sulfate, and bicarbonate. The role of these cellular electrolytes will be discussed in detail in Chapters 24 and 25.

Lipids. These fatty or fat-like substances, which are generally insoluble in water, make up approximately 2 or 3 per cent of the protoplasm. One of the most important cellular lipids is cholesterol.

Carbohydrates. Only 1 per cent of the protoplasm is composed of carbohydrate, which is stored within the cell as *glycogen.* The cell uses carbohydrate not as a building material like protein, but rather as a nutrient.

THE MAJOR COMPONENTS OF THE CELL: THEIR STRUCTURE AND FUNCTION

The cell is composed of three major parts: (1) the cell membrane, (2) the nucleus, and (3) the cytoplasm (Fig. 21–1). The cytoplasm, in turn, holds within its jelly-like substance several tiny, vitally important structures called organelles ("little organs"). Because each of these cellular structures performs highly specialized functions vital to the metabolism of both the individual cell and the total organism, we shall briefly consider them individually.

The Cell Membrane. This porous, thin, elastic membrane is composed mainly of protein and lipid substances. Only 100 angstrom units* thick, the cell membrane firmly encircles and encloses the cytoplasm, protecting it from the dangers of the external environment. The cellular membrane is a highly selective structure which allows only certain substances to enter and leave the internal environment of the cell through its minute pores. The cell itself works to maintain this controlled inward and outward flow of substances both actively and passively. Actively, it expends its energy to transport electrolytes and other materials across the membrane in either direction; passively, it allows certain substances to seep through the membranes in accordance with the laws of filtration, diffusion, and osmosis.* Potassium tends to be held within the cell, while most sodium ions and plasma are actively excluded from the cell. Water and food pass freely through the cell's semipermeable membrane, while waste products flow, unhindered, outward into the external environment. In sum, the cell membrane, although structurally flimsy, acts as a highly selective and effective casing that surrounds the cellular contents; thus, it is a major line of protection against intrusion into the cell by disruptive forces.

*One angstrom unit equals 1 ten-millionth of a millimeter.

*Fluid movement is discussed on pp. 198–199, and active transport is described on p. 199.

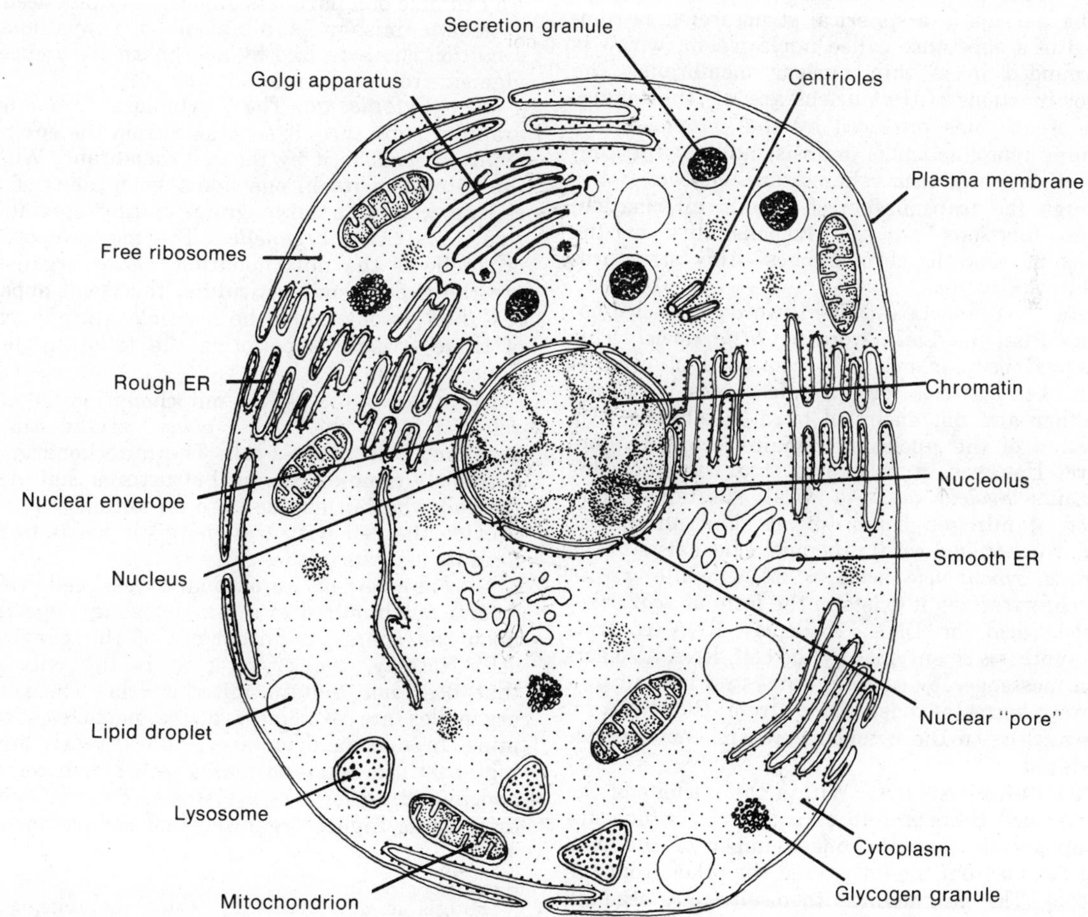

FIGURE 21–1. Diagram of a generalized animal cell. Although shown here as a round cell, animal cells may have many shapes. Note that ribosomes occur freely in the cytoplasm as well as attached to the endoplasmic reticulum. (Clark, M. E.: *Contemporary Biology.*)

It is fortunate indeed that the vital cell membrane can regenerate itself should it tear or rupture. Exactly how the cell membrane is repaired remains unknown. However, authorities do recognize that cellular membrane repair will not occur, following rupture, if there are an abnormally low number of calcium ions within the body fluid; calcium evidently helps to promote the health of the cell membrane, as well as the safety of the cytoplasm and the tiny nucleus that it envelops.

The Nucleus. The nucleus has been called the "heart" of the cell because it is so vital to cellular life. Indeed, it was once believed that no cell, with the exception of the mature red blood cell, could live without its nucleus. (An erythrocyte loses its nucleus just before it leaves the bone marrow for its maiden voyage into the general circulation.) However, we now recognize, through experiments involving microdissection of cells, that certain unicellular organisms can live even though their nuclei have been removed. Despite these few exceptions, the nucleus is, nevertheless, of monumental importance to the existence of almost all cells.

The nucleus is a spherical structure; it is composed of a substance called nucleoplasm, which is surrounded by a thin nuclear membrane. The major functions of the nucleus are: (1) the regulation of enzymes produced by the cytoplasm, (2) cellular reproduction or mitosis, and (3) the control of an organism's hereditary characteristics through the transmission of genetic information. These functions are the responsibility of the nucleolus, and the chromosomes—tiny structures within the nucleus.

THE NUCLEOLUS. The word "nucleolus" comes from the Latin word for *little kernel.* This spherical body is evidently composed of rows of bead-like particles or granules, loosely bound together and not encircled by a membrane. The function of the nucleolus remains somewhat obscure. However, it is known that the nucleolus contains *nucleic acid*—a vital substance composed of nitrogen bases, sugars, and phosphoric acid. Nucleic acid within the nucleolus exists in the form of *ribonucleic* acid, or RNA, while within the chromosomes it exists in the form of *deoxyribonucleic* acid, or DNA. Evidently RNA controls the synthesis of enzymes by the cell. RNA also acts as a messenger by carrying vital information concerning enzyme construction from the DNA of the nucleus to the cytoplasm where enzymes are produced.

THE CHROMOSOMES. Within the nucleus of the human cell there are 46 chromosomes, which are grouped into 23 pairs, one member of the pair originating from the father and the other from the mother. The chromosomes themselves are studded with from 50,000 to 100,000 genes. The genes carry hereditary information concerning both the species and the individual characteristics of an organism and transmit this information from generation to generation.

The genes are composed of chromatin, a substance which, when viewed under the microscope, seems to be coarse granules arranged in a fine network. These chromatin granules constitute the deoxyribonucleic acid, or DNA, of the cell. DNA contains within its structure, in a "double helix," the genetic code for that cell. Thus, when a cell divides by mitosis, the chromosomes first make doubles of themselves. The replicas migrate to opposite sides of the cell, and when the cell splits and divides, each daughter cell is identical in every way to the parent cell.* DNA, then, acts as the one single key to the once mysterious door of heredity. Finally, as we implied earlier, DNA also exerts control over RNA and the latter's function in enzyme production.

In such a complex operation as the transmission of heredity, it is not surprising that mistakes are made in the process of duplicating cells. Genes can be lost or they can change in ways that are unfavorable to the welfare of the organism. Such a change is called a *mutation.* Lost genes and abnormal genes can lead to inborn errors of metabolism and resultant diseases, as well as to organisms that are physically abnormal in appearance. Examples of diseases caused by an inborn error of metabolism are phenylketonuria (PKU) and sickle-cell anemia. An example of a harmless abnormality produced by a genetic mishap is albinism—a nonpathologic condition characterized by an abnormal absence of pigment from the skin, hair, and eyes.

The Cytoplasm. The cytoplasm, a fine, granular substance, is separated from the environment external to it by the cell membrane. Within the cytoplasm itself, one finds the nucleus of the cell as well as a large group of tiny specialized structures called *organelles.* The most important organelle is the mitochondrion. Other organelles are the endoplasmic reticulum, the Golgi apparatus, the lysosomes, and the centrioles. Briefly, each of these structures performs the following functions:

MITOCHONDRION. The mitochondrion is often referred to as the "power-house" of the cell, or as a tiny cell-within-a-cell. The mitochondria are extremely complex chemical structures that are to the cell what an engine is to an automobile; they provide the cell with the energy it needs to perform its many activities (Fig. 21–2).

The number of mitochondria per cell varies from a few hundred to a few thousand, depending upon the energy requirements of the particular cell. Notably, the erythrocyte is the only cell that does not contain mitochondria. These tiny organelles are extremely active particles, swimming through the cytoplasm and constantly breaking apart into bits and pieces which then reunite, end to end, to form new systems. Thus mitochondria, while highly organized and compartmental-

*Mitosis is the process by which the cells of the body multiply. It is a continuous process that involves four complex phases: the prophase, the metaphase, the anaphase, and the telophase.

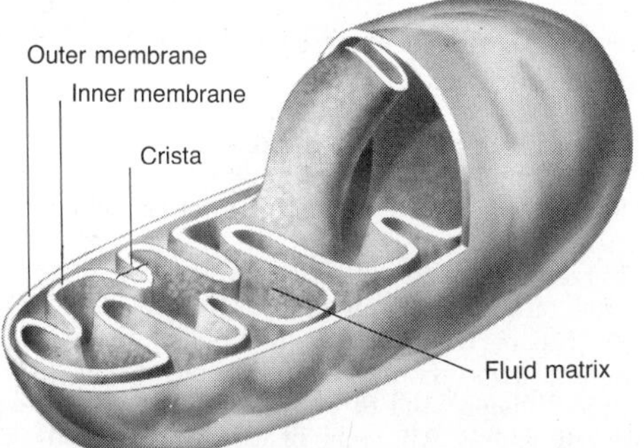

FIGURE 21–2. Structure of mitochondrion is basically that of a fluid filled vessel with an involuted wall. The wall consists of a double membrane, with infoldings of the inner one forming cristae. (Clark, M. E.: *Contemporary Biology.*)

ized, are not static structures but are instead very dynamic.

The major function of the mitochondria is the oxidation of foodstuffs and the changing of energy released by oxidation into adenosine triphosphate (ATP), a substance which supplies the energy needed by the cell in its daily work and which is necessary for protein synthesis.

ENDOPLASMIC RETICULUM. The endoplasmic reticulum (ER) is composed of a fine network of tiny hollow tunnels that branch like miniature arteries throughout the inside of the cell. The ER, along with its other functions, evidently operates somewhat like a railroad, transporting materials throughout the cell as needed.

Studding some of the ER tunnels, like so many unpolished gems, are the *ribosomes*—tiny spherical granular particles with a diameter of slightly less than one-millionth of an inch (Fig. 21–3). The ribosomes, some of which float free in the cytoplasm, are like the "factory hands" of the cell; they synthesize protein substances and align amino acids. The protein substances manufactured by the ribosomes are next transported as tiny protein granules into the ER tunnels and then on to the Golgi complex, the next station in the protein manufacturing assembly line.

GOLGI APPARATUS. The Golgi apparatus is a group of miniature sacs filled with protein, which evidently "package" proteins for distribution throughout the cell. The total workings of this organelle still remain a mystery.

LYSOSOMES. The lysosome, a vesicle surrounded by membranes, constitutes the cell's organ of digestion. Lysosomes contain powerful digestive enzymes that are capable of breaking down large molecules of fat, protein, and nucleic acid into smaller molecules so that they can be oxidized for energy by the mitochondria. By means of its membranes, the lysosome keeps its potentially dangerous digestive enzymes separate from the rest of the cell. Sometimes, however, when the intracellular contents become more acid in nature (e.g., as the result of a severe injury), the lysosome membranes rupture and the outpouring enzymes then destroy the cell as well as the bacteria—if any—that have created the lethal cellular disturbance.

While they obviously can be dangerous to the cell, lysosomes more often act as physiologic defense mechanisms. Authorities now believe that the polymorphonuclear white cells have the power to digest engulfed bacteria because they contain lysosomes within their cytoplasm. Lysosomes also perform the function of removing injured cells or cell parts from damaged tissues so

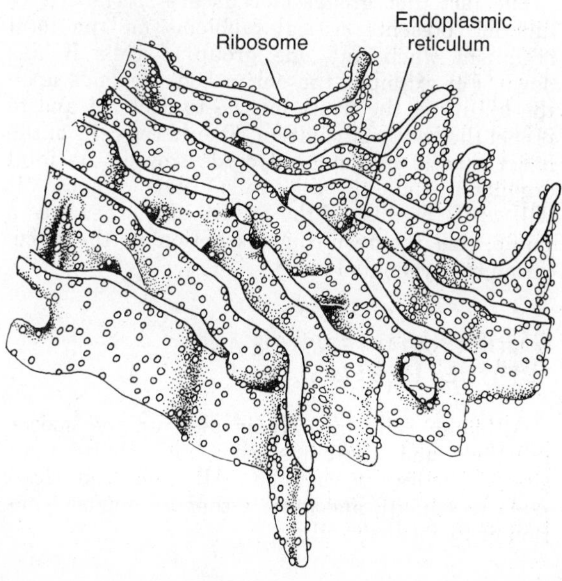

FIGURE 21–3. A joint operation. The ribosomes shown dotting the endoplasmic reticulum are thought to be made at the surface of or inside the nucleus and then sent out to produce their protein in the cytoplasm. Their teamwork with the ER is especially apparent in cells that make protein to be shipped out, but in many cells that do not export their products, the ribosomes float freely in the cytoplasm. (Modified from Pfeiffer, J.: *The Cell.* Life Science Library. New York, Time, Inc., 1964.)

that new cells can replace the old ones in the process of repair.

CENTRIOLE. The centriole is a tiny body that plays a role in cell division and reproduction.

In review, the cell is composed of many highly complex, minute structures that work together in a coordinated teamlike manner.

SPECIAL CELL UNITS

Somatic cells, while tiny compact worlds within themselves, nevertheless do not exist in isolation; instead, cells bond together, according to their special functions, and thereby form definite units or structures called *tissues*. In turn, tissues unite to form individual *organs*. The four major specialized types of cells of the body that we find united into larger tissue units are as follows:

> *Epithelial cells* are arranged in sheets and serve to cover the outside of the body; these cells also act as an absorptive covering, lining the inside of the body's cavities and tubular structures.

> *Nerve cells* form the highly specialized, irritable, and conductive nerve tissue. Injured or destroyed nerve cells cannot be replaced.

>*Muscle cells,* by means of shortening and extending themselves, do the physical work of the body. Contractility is the major characteristic of muscle cells.

> *Connective tissue cells* bind together and support other cells and tissues; they include blood cells and skeletal cells. *Blood cells* carry oxygen to the tissues, and carry carbon dioxide and wastes from the tissues. Also, they defend the body against microorganisms. *Skeletal cells* build the body's bony scaffolding.

The fact that groups of cells are *specialized* in function presents critical problems for the total organism when any one group of cells breaks down. For example, the entire body depends upon the ability of the heart muscle to contract and to propel the body's circulation. Should the cells of the heart muscle be damaged or destroyed, the total organism and all the cells that compose it will suffer because of the failure of the heart as a pump, and the resulting disruption in the circulation of oxygenated blood.

MAJOR CHARACTERISTICS AND ACTIVITIES OF CELLS

Although cells have their own unique special functions and attributes, they also share many characteristics in common. All cells reproduce, react to stimuli, and move either by ameboid motion or by means of cilia.

As you can see from the previous discussion, cells perform many activities. The most important activities are:

> Synthesis of large protein molecules.

> Production of energy for cellular work.

> Maintenance of a homeostatic environment within the cell.

> Ingestion and assimilation by the cell of materials from the outside environment by means of active and passive transport, pinocytosis, and phagocytosis.*

> Reproduction within unicellular organisms (by means of simple division) and in higher organisms (by means of mitotic division). All cells of the human body divide and reproduce with the exception of the cells of the brain, spinal cord, glomerulus of the kidney, and striated and cardiac muscles. These cells, which cannot be replaced, are called *permanent* cells. As you will see later, the process of mitosis contains implications for the problem of cancer.

In essence, the body cells, like the body itself, must eat, drink, digest, and assimilate substances, protect themeselves by reacting to stimuli, reproduce, build products, and expend energy. Also, like the total organism which they comprise, cells age, become sick and injured, lose their ability to function and to expend energy, die, and finally decay.

AGING AND INJURY OF THE CELL

THE AGING CELL

Like the human beings they compose, cells age, wither, and die. In a young healthy person, cells are constantly and rapidly multiplying and dividing and they function efficiently. As a person ages, however, his cells tend to multiply more sluggishly and to perform their tasks with less perfection. Thus, as time passes and the individual grows old, he usually suffers from a deficiency of cells, and he must also rely upon cells that no longer function quite so effectively.

What happens to our cells as they age? Many different untoward changes occur; for example, with aging, cells shrink in size, protein synthesis slows, the Golgi complexes begin to break apart, and the mitochondria may fragment into pieces. Ultimately the aged cell dies and disappears—its nucleus disintegrating and its cytoplasm liquefying.

Different types of cells have different life spans. For example, those epithelial cells lining the intestinal tract live only about a day and a half; red blood cells can live for 120 days; and at the opposite extreme are nerve cells, which have a potential life expectancy of 100 years.

Pinocytosis is the engulfment and ingestion of *liquid* droplets by the cell, whereas *phagocytosis* is the engulfment and ingestion of such large particles of matter as bacteria and other cells. Pinocytosis is derived from the Greek word that means *to drink,* while phagocytosis is taken from the Greek word meaning *to eat.*

THE INJURED CELL

To ascertain whether a cell is healthy or sick, alive or dead, is often a difficult task for the pathologist. Dead cells do not immediately show distinct necrotic changes. Often injured cells do not demonstrate any external evidence of disease or injury until the injury is far advanced. In other cases, the enzymes that the cell produces are poisoned, while the cell itself appears to be functioning satisfactorily. In addition, when injuries to the cell have been slight, cellular functions and structure remain essentially unchanged. Thus, despite the building of elaborate apparatuses for cellular study, the actual signs of sickness, and even of cellular death, may at times remain cloudy and obscure.

The Causes of Cell Injury

The extent to which any stressor can injure or kill cells depends upon the following three essential factors: (1) the *intensity* of the impact of the stressor upon the cell, (2) the *length of time* during which the cell has been under attack by the stressor, and (3) the *type* of cell under stress. Some cells are more vulnerable to injury or are more susceptible to certain stressors than other cells.

The major stressors that can injure cells seriously are: ischemia due to infarction or cessation of the blood flow, physical agents, chemical agents, microbial agents, and genetic disorders. These five categories were considered in Unit II under the general causes of disease (pp. 42 to 44).

Ischemia. Ischemia injures and kills cells by depriving them of the oxygen they need in order to perform their metabolic functions. Ischemia is usually caused by blood clots of sufficient size to occlude a vessel, thereby depriving the cells and tissues served by that blood vessel of oxygen. Ischemia can also result from peripheral vascular disorders in which the arteries become so narrowed and tortuous that they can no longer perform their function of transporting oxygenated blood to tissues.

Physical Agents. Physical agents such as heat, cold, trauma, radiation, and electrical shock can also damage cells.

Heat, if extreme, damages cells by literally "cooking them," thereby coagulating the protein within their cytoplasm. Even mild heat can result in permanent cellular damage if it is applied over a prolonged period of time to persons with peripheral vascular disorders. Irreversible damage occurs in these cases because heat increases the metabolic needs of cells and tissues—a dangerous situation when the circulation of oxygen to the cells is deficient and when the waste products from the increased cellular metabolism cannot be washed away.

Cold injures cells by constricting the blood vessels, thereby decreasing the circulation of blood and oxygen to tissue cells. Freezing temperatures, which result in frostbite, permanently injure involved vessels. Also, cold temperatures can cause blood clots to form by slowing the circulation. Thrombus formation, in turn, will occlude arteries, resulting in ischemia of those cells that are supplied with blood by the arteries. Cellular death and necrosis will be the final, unfortunate consequence.

TRAUMA. Trauma injures cells by ripping their membranes to pieces and by displacing the organelles of the cell.

RADIATION. Radiation can cause mutations, damage enzyme systems, and interrupt the process of cell division and multiplication. The fact that radiation can stop cell mitosis makes radiation therapy of importance in the treatment of cancer—a disease involving pathologic cell growth. While all cells can die as a result of radiation, certain cells are more susceptible than others. Germ cells, bone marrow cells, and lymphocytes are highly sensitive to radiation, while the cells of the cartilage, muscle, brain, kidney, liver, thyroid, pancreas, pituitary gland, adrenal gland, and parathyroid gland are relatively insensitive. Persons who are likely candidates for cellular damage from radiation are those who work with radioactive materials and nuclear fission reactors.

ELECTRICAL SHOCK. If severe, electrical shock can cause inflammatory reactions in nerve cells and nerve fibers, which will later be followed by degenerative changes. Damage to the brain may be permanent or temporary. The cells of other vital organs of the body are, of course, also damaged by a jolt of electricity. When voltages are high, the heart muscle may quiver or fibrillate rather than contract, and a usually fatal condition called *ventricular fibrillation* may result. Voltages too low to cause ventricular fibrillation can impair the action of the muscles of the respiratory system, and the jolted individual may die of anoxia.

Chemicals. Chemical agents harm cells by destroying or injuring their delicate structures and by disrupting their production of enzymes. The capacity of any chemical to produce cell injury depends upon the strength and toxicity of the chemical, and upon the susceptibility of the cell to the chemical. Thus salt water, which is normally considered harmless, can, in high concentrations, cause cells to shrivel and die. A small amount of cyanide kills cells because of its extreme toxicity. Carbon tetrachloride is notorious for its affinity to liver cells, while mercury is particularly dangerous to kidney cells. Certain drugs such as LSD and thalidomide are believed to cause genetic changes. The major portals of entry for chemicals toxic to cells are the lungs, the skin and mucous membranes, and the gastrointestinal tract.

Microorganisms. Microorganisms such as bacteria injure cells mainly by means of the *toxins* they produce, either endotoxins or exotoxins.* Other organisms, like certain of the viruses, produce no toxins, but live as obligatory parasites on the energy of living cells. Viruses are like cells in that they can multiply and can produce their own proteins. However, viruses do not, by themselves, have the *energy* for these dynamic activities. Thus, viruses penetrate cells, take over their enzyme systems, and then proceed to drain the doomed cell of its vitality and energy.

Genetic Disturbances. Genetic disorders can cause cellular damage through the development of mutant cells or through familial hereditary disorders which are passed on via the genes from generation to generation.

Major Types of Cell Disorders

There are several types of cell disorders. The major forms are degenerations and infiltrations and disorders of cell growth, including cancerous growth, atrophy and hypertrophy.

*An endotoxin is a toxic substance produced within a microorganism and is released when the cell in which it was produced is destroyed. An exotoxin is excreted by a microorganism into a surrounding medium.

Degenerations and Infiltrations. Pathologists can generally identify injured cells by means of observable changes within their cytoplasm and nucleus. Some of the commonest pathologic changes are the result of the processes of either degeneration or infiltration. Sometimes both conditions occur together, as is the case in fatty change and glycogen degeneration. These two major cellular disturbances are generally the result of nonfatal injuries, and their unhealthy effects upon the cell can usually be erased in time. Nevertheless, the tell-tale signs of degeneration or infiltration within the cells give the pathologist a basic clue that all is not well within the total organism. Such adverse cellular changes, according to Boyd,[1] truly represent the "fingerprints of disease."

The term *degeneration* implies that the cellular structures are in a state of deterioration or impairment and, as a result, cellular function and work are disrupted. On the other hand, *infiltration* means that a substance that is *external* to the cell filters into the cell, permeating it and damaging its ability to function. For example, when large amounts of fat globules are deposited within the cell as the result of a metabolic systemic illness, the process is called "fatty infiltration."

While infiltration and degeneration can be distinguished in terms of the process involved, they both represent disorders of the cell's basic biochemistry, resulting from such variable stressors as genetic disorders, metabolic disease, anoxia, and so forth.

The major types of degenerations and infiltrations are: cloudy swelling, fatty change, and glyco-

TABLE 21-1. DEGENERATIONS AND INFILTRATIONS: A SUMMARY OF IMPORTANT CONSIDERATIONS

Name of Degeneration or Infiltration	Conditions in Which Found	Pathologic Changes Within The Cell	Prognosis
1. Cloudy swelling	Infectious disease, fever, poisoning, anoxia, malnutrition, kidney, liver, heart, and glandular disorders	1. Protein substances become cloudy 2. Cells tend to swell owing to an increase in intracellular water 3. Protein metabolism is disturbed	Changes are rarely permanent
2. Fatty change	Starvation, malnutrition, cirrhosis of the liver, infectious hepatitis, poisoning with arsenic, bismuth, gold, or silver, liver intoxication due to chloroform or carbon tetrachloride	1. Excess fat accumulates within the cytoplasm following either disruption of enzyme systems within the cell, leading to faulty fat metabolism by the mitochondria, or infiltration of fat into the cell as a result of starvation or metabolic disease 2. Organs mainly affected by fatty change are the liver, kidney, and myocardium of the heart	This condition is usually reversible; however, it does indicate serious cell injury that may terminate in cellular death
3. Glycogen infiltration and degeneration	Diabetes mellitus	1. Abnormal accumulation of glycogen within the cells, especially of the kidney and heart 2. Usually there is no disruption of cellular function	Prognosis is good, as most changes are reversible

gen infiltration and degeneration. The major pathologic changes, the causes, and the prognosis for each of the above processes are included in Table 21-1.

Disturbances of Cell Growth. Some major disturbances of cellular growth involve the problems of atrophy, hypertrophy, and cancer.* We shall briefly define these terms as they specifically apply to cellular and tissue pathology.

Atrophy is defined as the wasting of a tissue or organ and a *decrease* in its size *following* both maturity and a normal development. This wasting condition is due to either a decrease in the *number* of cells composing the tissue or a decrease in the actual *size* of the cells themselves. Atrophy may follow disuse of an organ, disorders of a tissue due to disease, circulatory deficiencies, compression of a tissue or part, and nerve damage. Atrophy, although found in connection with many disorders, can also be a *normal* physiologic process that occurs as the individual ages and passes through the various stages of his life. Thus, the thymus gland atrophies when the child matures, and the ovaries atrophy as the mature woman passes into the menopause.

Hypertrophy is an increase in the size of an organ or tissue. This increased bulk is *not* the result of the appearance of additional cells; instead it is the result of an *increase in size* of the cells which already comprise the organ. Hypertrophy may represent the response of an organ to a greater load of work. For example, when the heart is subjected to great strain, the left ventricle of the heart enlarges or hypertrophies in order to handle the additional stress. A second example of hypertrophy is the increase in size of the biceps muscle in individuals engaged in hard physical labor.

Hypertrophy may occur in any tissue or organ; however, it most commonly affects the heart, kidney, endocrine glands, and skeletal muscles, and the smooth muscles of the intestinal tract.

Cancer is a disease in which cellular growth is disturbed and chaotic, and in which normal cellular function becomes modified and physiologically maladaptive. Of cancer cells, the responsible agents for this dread disease, Boyd states, "Cancer cells are the anarchists of the body, for they know no law, pay no regard for the commonweal, serve no useful function, and cause disharmony and death in their surroundings."[1] Cancer cells, moreover, are capable of migrating to different parts of the body, thereby causing the spread, or metastasis, of malignant tumors or neoplasms, which further disrupt and destroy the body's life-sustaining functions.

The causes of cancer as well as the measures that will cure and prevent this disorder are still mysteries that are being slowly and relentlessly unraveled by determined scientists. The unit on the nursing care of patients with cancer will discuss, in detail, some of the important theories of cancer causation. Also, it will describe the medical and nursing care involved in the current major treatments for cancer—namely, radiation therapy, surgery, and chemotherapy.

*The cancer cell is discussed in detail in Unit VII.

CELL DEATH AND CELLULAR NECROSIS

It is important *not* to use the terms "cell death" and "cell necrosis" interchangeably. *Cell death* occurs when the vital functions of the cell cease; *cell necrosis* follows cell death and includes morphologic changes that eventually result in the lysis and dissolving of the cell. Thus, cells evidently die long before signs of their death become apparent under the pathologist's microscope. Because of this fact, it is as difficult to accurately distinguish between an injured cell and a dead one as it is to differentiate between a normal cell and an injured cell. Thus, it may be difficult for a pathologist to determine the extent of damage caused by a disease process; sometimes only the signs of cellular necrosis can confirm the pathologist's suspicion of cellular death.

Cell Death

Cells die as a result of chemical poisons, bacterial toxins, anoxia due to thrombosis and infarctions, and powerful physical agents such as irradiation. As cells die, their vital functions may cease gradually, one by one. This dissociated cessation of functions makes it impossible for the pathologist to state the exact moment of cellular death.

Following the death of the cell, the process of cell necrosis begins, the nucleus breaks up, and the cytoplasm becomes liquefied. Finally, the dead cell loses its identity as a separate entity and the process of autolysis is complete.

Cell Necrosis

The process of cell necrosis *follows* the death of the cell. Enzymes within the cell as well as those exterior to it cause the necrotic breakdown. The morphologic changes involved in cell necrosis depend upon which type of necrosis the cell has undergone. The four major *types* of cellular necrosis are: coagulation necrosis, liquefaction necrosis, caseous necrosis, and gangrenous necrosis.

Coagulation Necrosis. This generally results from *anoxia* of the cell, which, in turn, may be caused by a loss of blood supply to the cell. An outstanding characteristic of coagulation necrosis is that a shadowy outline of the cell remains distinct for days or weeks following the death of the cell and the escape of its vital inner contents. This cell, then, can be compared to a rag doll which has lost all its stuffings or to an archeological ruin from which all detail has been erased by time.

Liquefaction Necrosis. This is a rapid and *total* destruction of the entire cell, including the cell's membrane. This type of necrosis most commonly affects the cells of the brain, as well as those cells that have been invaded by pus-forming bacteria.

Caseous Necrosis. This is generally associated with cellular destruction resulting from tuberculosis. Characteristically the dead cell affected by caseous changes develops the appearance of soft cheese. This form of necrosis is very distinctive and can be readily identified in the laboratory.

Gangrenous Necrosis. This necrosis results from ischemia of the cell, coupled with an infection by saprophytes, bacteria which can live only in ischemic tissues. The problem of gangrenous destruction will be discussed in appropriate areas throughout the text.

References

1. Boyd, W.: *An Introduction to the Study of Disease.* Philadelphia, Lea & Febiger, 1962.
2. Brachet, J.: The living cell. *Scientific American* 205:50, September, 1961.
3. Bresnick, E., and Schwartz, A.: *Functional Dynamics of the Cell.* New York, Academic Press, Inc., 1968.
4. Guyton, A. C.: *Textbook of Medical Physiology.* 4th ed. Philadelphia, W. B. Saunders Company, 1971.
5. Fox, C. F.: The structure of cell membranes. *Scientific American*, 226:31, February, 1972.
6. Hayashi, T.: How cells move. *Scientific American,* 205:62, September, 1961.
7. Holter, H.: How things get into cells. *Scientific American,* 205:167, September, 1961.
8. Kathari, M. L.: Genesis of cancer (a temporal approach). *Journal of Postgraduate Medicine* 14: 49–69, April, 1968.
9. Pfeiffer, J.: *The Cell.* Life Science Library. New York, Time, Incorporated, 1964.
10. Simard, P.: The nucleus: Action of chemical and physical agents. *International Review of Cytology* 28:169–211, 1970.
11. Sodeman, W. A., and Sodeman, W. A., Jr.: *Pathologic Physiology.* 5th ed. Philadelphia, W. B. Saunders Company, 1974.
12. Stent, G. S.: Cellular communication. *Scientific American,* 226:14, September, 1972.
13. Wallach, D. F.: The organization of cell membranes. *International Archives of Allergy* 36(Suppl.):672–701, 1969.
14. Wessells, N. K.: How living cells change shape. *Scientific American,* 225:76, October, 1971.

CHAPTER 22

Protective Responses to Injury

INTRODUCTION AND STUDY GUIDE

Stress and response to stress, healthy or faulty adaptation, as individual responses are the pivotal points of any discussion of health and disease. These factors determine whether a given disturbance will result in an individual's continuing life or his death.

To some extent, we have already considered these areas in earlier units. First of all, in both Units II and III we discussed many of the multiple stressful factors that continuously impinge upon man. You will remember that the most important physiologic stressors challenging man's adaptive resources are: (1) physical stressors such as heat, cold, radiation, and trauma, (2) chemical irritants such as strong acids, alkalis, and poisons, as well as certain substances which man manufactures within his own body, and (3) bacterial agents and microorganisms.

Second, we pointed out that if man is to survive, he must respond to these stressors with all the protective and adaptive mechanisms at his disposal. The major defensive systems, providing a high degree of protection against physical injury, are the intact skin, the mucous membranes, the bones, the blood, the gastrointestinal tract, the reticuloendothelial system, the endocrine system and the nervous system.

Third, we emphasized that despite the hundreds of stressors that can assault us, and despite the complexity of our protective systems, the human animal actually has a very limited repertoire of *physiologic reactions* specifically designed to counter physical stress. You will recall that those major reactions are inflammation, sclerosis, increased capillary permeability, hormonal responses, the immune response (the production of antibodies in reaction to antigens), and fluid and electrolyte shifts. Finally, we stated that *inflammation* is the most typical example of the body's ability to respond to tissue injury or bacterial invasion.

In this section of Unit V we shall explore in more detail the various means by which the body defends itself against attack and injury. The following areas will be discussed:

1. The body's defensive cells:
   > The cells of the reticuloendothelial system
   > The leukocytes
2. The body's major defensive organs:
   > Lymph nodes
   > Bone marrow
   > Spleen
   > Liver
3. The body's major physiologic responses to injury:
   > Inflammation
   > Repair

In discussing these areas we shall review the work of the reticulum cell, the white blood cell, and the macrophage; the purpose of capillary permeability; and the role of humoral and hormonal defenses in resisting infection. In the later chapters of this unit, we shall look at the immune reaction and at those fluid and electrolyte shifts that occur as a reaction to stress.

To help you to develop a better comprehension of this subject matter, we suggest that you make use of the following study guide:

Upon completion of this chapter, you should be aware of the meaning of the following key terms:

reticuloendothelial system, reticulum cell, tissue histiocyte, polymorphonuclear leukocyte, lymphocytes, monocytes, macrophages, phagocytosis, chemotaxis, chemical mediator, histamine, leukocytosis, leukopenia, leukocytosis-promoting factor, agranulocytosis, opsonins, antitoxins, inflammatory lymph, fibroblast, abscess, cellulitis, ulcer, fistula, boil, carbuncle, resolution, repair, parenchymal tissue, connective tissue, permanent cells, fibroblasts, granulation tissue, scar tissue, primary union, secondary union.

You should also be able to discuss generally the following topics:

1. The role of the reticuloendothelial system and leukocytes in protecting the body against invasion by dangerous aliens.
2. Distinguishing differences between the morphology and physiologic functions of the different leukocytes.
3. The roles of the liver, spleen, lymph nodes, and bone marrow in body defense.
4. The causes of inflammation.
5. The major components of the inflammatory response.
6. The overall characteristics of the inflammatory response to injury—the different defenses at work.
7. The different types or classes of inflammatory response.
8. Major factors affecting the outcome of inflammation.
9. Types of tissue repair.

10. The rate of wound healing in different types of tissues.
11. Factors that distinguish primary union from secondary union.
12. The formation of scar tissue.
13. Abnormalities that can result from a secondary union and from the formation of excessive scar tissue.
14. Treatment of the contaminated wound and other wound complications.
15. Factors that govern the success of the repair process.
16. The goals of medical and nursing care.

THE DEFENSIVE CELLS OF THE BODY

THE CELLS OF THE RETICULOENDOTHELIAL SYSTEM

While the typical inflammatory response can be likened to a fast-moving, hard-fought battle, the role of the reticuloendothelial system against injury is comparable to that of a vigilant national guard in a country that is currently peaceful, yet under constant threat of annihilation. Like silent sentries on guard, the cells of the reticuloendothelial system are located strategically throughout the body, awaiting possible action should disruption or invasion by foreign material occur. Some cells are stationary, seizing and killing potential invaders before they can enter the circulatory system, which is the body's mainstream. Other cells, such as the tissue histiocyte, are usually stationary, but can also quickly become mobile as the need arises, changing into powerful, motile, bacteria-ingesting macrophages. The cells of the reticuloendothelial system are not only capable of capturing and annihilating intruders, but they can also form immune bodies that serve to safeguard the body against future generations of the invaders.

Where is this remarkable protective system located? Of what is it composed? How does it operate?

The reticuloendothelial system is not localized to any one part of the body but instead is widely dispersed throughout many body organs. Its cells line blood vessels and lymph channels; they are found in the spleen, liver, lymph nodes, and bone marrow.

The major cells of the reticuloendothelial system are the *reticulum cells.* These cells perform two vital functions: first, they are the precursors of the body's erythrocytes and granulocytes; and second, they perform the essential task of phagocytosis (*see later*). In addition, reticulum cells that are located within the bone marrow operate as efficient "fine filters," removing from the blood such tiny particles as protein toxin.

Reticulum cells are remarkable for their ability to differentiate into many different types of cells and are truly the chameleons of the body. For instance, reticulum cells can change themselves into the following varied forms: hemocytoblasts, which later become red blood cells; myeloblasts, which eventually evolve into leukocytes; lymphocytes, which are a form of leukocyte; plasma cells, which play an important role in immune body formation; and tissue histiocytes.

The *tissue histiocyte* is so useful in the body's defense that it deserves special mention. This versatile cell is found scattered widely throughout the body's tissues, its function being to ingest debris and foreign bodies. Being both fixed and motile, tissue histiocytes are capable of swelling up, leaving their stationary posts, and traveling to the site of inflammatory action, where they then phagocytize invaders. When tissue histiocytes behave in this manner, they are called *macrophages*. Tissue histiocytes can also change into fibroblasts, cells that are capable of laying down collagen or connective tissue fibers. Thus, fibroblasts are formed when inflamed tissue needs to be walled off from healthy tissue by means of a collagen barrier, and when tissue damage needs to be repaired.

In sum, the cells of the reticuloendothelial system are both stationary and wandering. They are highly efficient in their efforts to corner and devour invaders and all manner of foreign materials. Moreover, they are efficient in the production of antibodies.

THE LEUKOCYTES

Like the cells of the reticuloendothelial system, the leukocytes or white blood cells (W.B.C.s) also play a vital role in the defense of the body against invaders and in the inflammatory reaction to injury.

The Classification and Function of White Blood Cells

The leukocytes comprise another motile unit of the body's defense system. One of the outstanding characteristics of leukocytes is their ability to go almost *immediately* to the scene of injury and to deal with harmful invaders in an on-the-spot death struggle.

These remarkable protective cells are divided into the following two major groups: (1) the *polymorphonuclear leukocytes,* which include neutrophils, eosinophils, and basophils; and (2) the *mononuclear leukocytes,* which include lymphocytes and monocytes. The relative numbers of the different white blood cells (average differential count for adults) are shown in Table 22–1.

Polymorphonuclear Leukocytes ("Polys"). The poly group is composed of three subgroups of cells: the neutrophil, the eosinophil, and the basophil. While each group has its own distinctive qualities, all these groups share several characteristics in common.

First of all, as the name implies, *poly*morphonuclear leukocytes have a *many-shaped* (poly) *nucleus.* A second important characteristic of the

TABLE 22-1. THE AVERAGE DIFFERENTIAL WHITE COUNT FOR ADULTS

Cell	Number of Cells per Every 100 White Cells
Neutrophils	62.0
Eosinophils	2.3
Basophils	0.4 to 1.0
Lymphocytes	30.0
Monocytes	5.3

poly group is their *granular* appearance when viewed under a microscope. Third, all polys are formed in the *bone marrow* and consequently they are sometimes referred to as *myelogenous cells* [*myelo,* bone marrow]. Finally, polys (neutrophils in particular) function to give the body *rapid* protection against any outside invaders. Thus, the polys are like the "marine corps" of the body or like "shock troops," because they arrive early at the scene of battle and bear the major brunt of the physiologic warfare. In a serious infection, polys may only live one or two hours before dying in the fray. Normally this group of leukocytes remains alive about 14 hours; at times, however, polys have been known to live for several days before disintegrating.

While all polys have similar origins and functions, each group has its own specialized tasks in the mechanism of defense.

THE NEUTROPHIL. These polys are the most important of the white cells and also the most numerous, comprising 50 to 70 per cent of all circulating leukocytes. Neutrophils are small, motile, highly phagocytic cells, for which reason they are sometimes called microphages (i.e., they are small ("micro") cells that are capable of ingesting bacteria and foreign matter).

Neutrophils play a vital role in the body's local inflammatory reaction because they are both the first and most numerous type of cell at any area of disease or tissue injury. Also, neutrophils play an important role as "scavengers," by cleaning up the debris that accumulates as a result of the inflammatory "battle." Even in death, neutrophils serve a useful purpose. By releasing a proteolytic enzyme, the dead and disintegrating neutrophil digests not only surrounding bacteria and dead cells but also *itself,* thus cleansing "the inflammatory battlefield" of even its own lifeless remains.

While inflammation is the major condition causing a neutrophilia (an increase in neutrophils), *any factor* that leads to the destruction of cells and tissue can give rise to an increase in the neutrophil count. Consequently, cancer, extreme fatigue, acute hemorrhage, a myocardial infarction with resultant necrosis of the heart muscle, poisons, surgery, and injections of foreign protein into the body all result in a degree of neutrophilia. In the case of a myocardial infarction (a form of "heart attack"), neutrophilia constitutes an important diagnostic sign.

Neutrophils, over and above their task in abating local tissue injury, may also play a part in the overall *systemic* reaction to the tissue destruction. Some authorities postulate that neutrophils possibly release a substance that produces *fever*—an important general symptom of inflammation and infection.

EOSINOPHILS. The eosinophil differs markedly in several ways from its sister cell the neutrophil. We have briefly contrasted the characteristics and functions of the two cells in Table 22-2.

Eosinophils are apparently a very important cell group in *parasitic* and *allergic* conditions, in which they may increase to form over 50 per cent of the total differential count. Their role in these conditions is quite obscure. Eosinophils apparently enter the circulation whenever foreign proteins are injected into the blood; they are also found in substantial numbers at the sites of antigen-antibody reactions. Moreover, some authors postulate that eosinophils evidently have the capacity to detoxify those harmful protein substances released by parasites. This theory helps to explain the increase of eosinophils in parasitic reactions.

Eosinophils appear to be under the control of the *adrenocortical hormones.* Selye and other scientists have found that eosinophils tend to disappear from the circulation whenever there

TABLE 22-2. CHARACTERISTICS OF NEUTROPHILS AND EOSINOPHILS

Neutrophils	Eosinophils
1. When stained and viewed under the microscope, granules in them appear as *gray.*	1. When stained and viewed under the microscope, granules in them appear *bright, pinkish red*
2. Comprise 50 to 70% of leukocytes	2. Comprise 1 to 2 per cent of leukocytes
3. Motile, fast-moving	3. Motile, but sluggish
4. The *first* cells to arrive at the site of inflammation	4. One of the *last* cells to arrive at the inflammatory site—often coming after healing has started
5. Excellent, effective phagocytes	5. Very weak phagocytes

is an excessive release of the cortical hormones as a result of stress, or when patients are receiving cortisone injections.

BASOPHILS. When stained and viewed under a microscope, basophils can be distinguished by the appearance of blue-black granules in their cytoplasm. This group of polys represents the smallest proportion of the white blood cells, comprising no more than 1 per cent of the total differential. This means that out of 1000 leukocytes, approximately 4 are basophils.

What are the functions of this white blood cell minority group? First of all, basophils, like eosinophils, increase in number during the healing phase of inflammation. Second, basophils evidently play an important role in proper blood circulation by releasing *heparin,* a powerful anticoagulant. It is theorized that the basophil's ability to liberate heparin causes a decrease in cell clumping and other aspects of blood coagulation that occur during the inflammatory process. Also, basophils apparently help to maintain proper circulation by eliminating from the blood those excess fat particles that accumulate following the ingestion of a high-fat meal.

Mononuclear Leukocytes. In contrast to the polys, mononuclear leukocytes do not have granules in their cytoplasm—a fact that has earned them the name of *nongranular* or agranular leukocytes. Also, mononuclear leukocytes are not produced in the bone marrow as polys are, but instead stem from *lymphatic tissue* such as that found in the lymph nodes and spleen.

This second major group of leukocytes is composed of the subgroups lymphocytes and monocytes.

LYMPHOCYTES. A much smaller blood cell than a poly, the lymphocyte is formed mainly in the lymph nodes and, to some extent, in the small lymphoid follicles of the tonsils, intestines, and bone marrow. In the event of an infectious or toxic condition, these lymphogenous tissues tend to hypertrophy greatly. Who has not, at some point in her life, experienced swollen painful nodes in the armpits, groin, or throat as a result of some infection or toxic condition?

Lymphocytes are fairly numerous cells, forming 25 to 33 per cent of the differential. When no infection exists within the body, there are approximately 2100 lymphocytes per cubic millimeter. However, with certain infections—for example, whooping cough—the lymphocyte count can go as high as 100,000 per cu. mm., although such a high count is generally quite rare!

Like the eosinophils, lymphocytes are under the control of the *adrenocortical hormones.* This statement holds important implications for the nurse. When working with patients on *steroid therapy,* remember these points:

1. When a patient is receiving steroid therapy, he will experience a decrease in the number of lymphocytes being produced as well as a shrinking of his lymphoidal tissues.
2. These events leave the patient receiving adrenocortical hormones dangerously susceptible to infection.

The lymphocyte is important to the body's well-being. Its outstanding function is the *release of antibodies*—a vital task that we shall discuss under the immune reaction. As a possible second function, lymphocytes are thought to aid in the *neutralization of the toxic byproducts of bacterial activity.* These byproducts are usually produced as a result of the conflict between bacteria and polys. Thus, it is appropriate that (unlike the polys) lymphocytes tend to appear and function *late* in the inflammatory process, when the hottest part of the battle is over. Indeed, an increase in the lymphocyte count is considered to be an indication of *chronic inflammation.* Consequently, an elevated lymphocyte count is often discovered in such long-term conditions as syphilis, tuberculosis, and infectious mononucleosis.

A final group of functions are based upon the great versatility of lymphocytes. Like the tissue histiocyte, to which they are closely related, lymphocytes are able to *transform themselves* into different types of cells, thereby serving varying and divergent purposes. Thus, when inflammation is present, a lymphocyte can leave the circulation, swell up, and become a powerful bacteria-ingesting macrophage. With the subsidence of inflammation, the lymphocyte can next transform itself into a tissue histiocyte and then into a fibroblast. In this final form, lymphocytes are able to lay down collagen fibers and aid in the task of tissue repair.

The life span of these highly useful white cells is usually only a few hours. However, radioactive studies have shown that when tissue needs are minimal, lymphocytes can live 100 to 200 days.

MONOCYTES. These cells form 4 to 6 per cent of the white blood cell differential count. Their numbers rise mainly in such conditions as tuberculosis and malaria. Like the lymphocyte, monocytes are formed in lymphoid tissue. Their potential life span and ultimate fate still remain a mystery.

Monocytes are closely related to the phagocytic macrophages of the reticuloendothelial system. Along with the reticuloendothelial cells, the monocyte forms the *second line of defense* against bacterial invasion by following close "on the heels" of the polys—the first line of defense. Thus, the monocytes arrive at the scene of battle after the initial encounter.

Once at the inflammatory site, the monocytes can act as extremely powerful macrophages, ingesting much larger particles than can the neutrophil, as well as at least five times as many particles in one ingestion. Tougher and less vulnerable than the neutrophils, or microphages, the monocyte is able to survive its fellow polys and live on into the late stages of the acute inflammation as well as into the chronic stages. Thus, like lymphocytes, increased numbers of monocytes are typically observed in *chronic inflammatory conditions.*

Monocytes also play an important part in the "clean up" procedures that follow any inflammatory battle. Active hungry scavengers, monocytes are capable of ingesting dead bacteria, wornout polys, and large amounts of protein debris, thereby clearing and preparing the field for the process of repair and healing.

White Blood Cell Count (Total W.B.C.)

The normal range for the total W.B.C. in adults is 6000 to 9000 per cu.mm. In infections the total W.B.C. in adults can increase to 30,000 per cu.mm. When such a radical increase in the circulating white cells occurs, the condition is called *leukocytosis*. Pneumonia, myocardial infarctions, malignant disease, and infections can all lead to high leukocyte counts. Conversely, the total W.B.C. can become abnormally low. A marked decrease in the leukocyte count is called *leukopenia*. For obscure reasons, a leukopenia sometimes develops in typhoid fever and occasionally in tuberculosis. Leukopenia may also result from a decreased production of white blood cells owing to extreme debilitation or severe deficits of vitamins, folic acid, and amino acids—those materials that are used extensively by the body in the formation of leukocytes. Finally, since the bone marrow produces a major portion of the body's leukocytes, any damage to the bone marrow can result in the suppression of white blood cell formation and in an extremely dangerous, often fatal, form of leukopenia called agranulocytosis. (See Unit XII.)

PLASMA CELLS

The small, round, irregularly shaped plasma cells are probably derived from either lymphocytes or reticulum cells. They exist predominantly in the connective tissue of the walls of the intestinal tract, as well as in the lymph nodes, spleen, and bone marrow. Large numbers of plasma cells are found when inflammatory reactions become chronic. As with the lymphocyte and monocyte, plasma cells are increased in syphilitic conditions.

The actual role and function of plasma cells is somewhat obscure. However, it is generally believed that they are a primary source of antibody production.

In summary, the major defensive cells of the body are the cells of the reticuloendothelial system, the leukocytes, and the plasma cells. Major facts about each cell type are summarized in Table 22–3.

BODY ORGANS INVOLVED IN DEFENSE: THE STRUCTURES OF THE RETICULOENDOTHELIAL SYSTEM

The major organs involved directly in body defense and in the production of protective cells are the *lymph nodes,* the *spleen,* the *liver,* and the *bone marrow*. These structures serve as efficient factories for the production and maturation of reticulum cells and leukocytes; moreover, they work as blood purifiers, filtering out the soot, foreign bodies, microorganisms and defective or malignant cells that threaten to harm or destroy the body. These organs, then, are vitally responsible for the *prevention* of *infection* and *disease*. Because of their important services, the body is often spared the pain and trauma of an inflammatory reaction, as well as the threat of annihilation by the many dangerous forces that continuously assault it.

THE LYMPH NODES

All foreign matter and all microbial, bacterial, and viral invaders must pass through the lymphatic system on their way to the general circulation. Strategically located along the course of the lymphatics are clusters of small structures called lymph nodes, or lymph glands. Some of these oval structures are as small as the head of a pin; others are as large as a lima bean. Rarely solitary, most lymph nodes are found in discrete groups. The major groups of lymph nodes and their locations are as follows:

1. *Submental* and *submaxillary nodes,* in the mouth.
2. *Superficial cervical glands,* in the neck.
3. *Superficial cubital nodes,* which can be found just above the bend of the elbow.
4. *Axillary nodes,* which are located under the arm and in the upper chest regions; 20 to 30 large nodes comprise this important group.
5. *Inguinal nodes,* within the groin.

Small lymphoid follicles are also found in the tonsils, intestinal tract, and bone marrow. The anatomic locations of the most important lymph nodes are illustrated in Figure 22–1.

Lymph nodes serve three important functions: First of all, they contain "passageways" or sinus channels for the transport of the important watery substance called *lymph*. Second, these same passageways, in addition to their role as transport systems, also function as vital defensive systems. Lined heavily with reticulum cells, the lymph sinuses are able to filter out and devour dangerous foreign materials. Finally, the lymph node serves as "parent and nursery" for the birth and growth of lymphocytes and monocytes. Thus, if you were to examine tissue from a lymph node, you would find it densely packed with lymphocytes.

Under normal conditions the lymph nodes serve as efficient filters. Unfortunately, however, the body is sometimes invaded by hordes of virulent microorganisms. When this happens, the nodes may be so overworked and overtaxed that they themselves succumb to infection. An infection of a lymph node is called *lymphadenitis* and is characterized by the signs and symptoms of inflammation that we shall discuss shortly.

TABLE 22-3. THE BODY'S DEFENSIVE CELLS: A SUMMARY OF FACTS

Cell Type	Number in Health and Disease	Place of Origin	Distinguishing Characteristics	Function
A. Reticulum cell	Large numbers line blood vessels and lymph nodes; also found in spleen, liver, lymph nodes, and bone marrow	Reticuloendothelial system	1. Both stationary and motile 2. Capable of differentiating into different cells as the need arises, e.g., into a tissue histiocyte and then into a fibroblast 3. Can become macrophages	1. Phagocytosis 2. Helpful in process of repair 3. Body's second line of defense against invasion
B. Leukocyte	1. In health, 6000-9000/cu. mm. 2. Increase up to 30,000/cu.mm.in infection			Motile unit of the body's defensive system
1. Polymorphonuclear leukocytes		Formed in bone marrow (myelogenous cells)	1. Many-shaped nucleus 2. Granular appearance under microscope	Give body rapid protection against outside invaders
a. Neutrophies (microphages)	1. In health, 50 to 70% of all circulating white cells 2. High counts in *acute* inflammation and whenever there is tissue damage (myocardial infarction)		1. Small 2. Motile 3. Highly phagocytic 4. Gray granules under a microscope	1. First cell type to arrive at inflammatory site (first line of defense) 2. Phagocytosis 3. Act as scavengers, cleaning inflammatory site 4. Possibly cause fever
b. Eosinophils	1. In health, 1 to 2% of circulating white cells 2. High counts in parasitic infestations and allergic conditions and during healing phase of inflammation		1. Granules stain red under microscope 2. Motile but sluggish 3. Phagocytic 4. Under control of adrenocortical hormones	1. Weak phagocytes 2. Can possibly detoxify foreign protein substances
c. Basophils	1. In health, 1% of circulating cells 2. Increase during healing phase of inflammation		Blue-black granules under a microscope	Release of heparin, which possibly causes a decrease in cell clumping during the inflammatory process
2. Mononuclear leukocytes		Produced in lymphatic tissue such as the lymph nodes and spleen	Nongranular appearance under the microscope	Important defensive cells in chronic inflammation
a. Lymphocytes	1. In health, 25 to 33% of all circulating white cells 2. Increase to great numbers in certain infections 3. Increase late in inflammatory process and in *chronic* inflammation	Formed mainly in lymph nodes and lymphoid follicles	1. Much smaller cell than the poly 2. Under the control of the adrenocortical hormones 3. Capable of differentiating into different types of cells	1. Release of antibodies 2. Phagocytosis 3. Helpful in tissue repair
b. Monocytes	1. In health, 4 to 6% of total circulating white cells 2. Numbers increase in tuberculosis and malaria and in chronic inflammatory conditions	Formed in lymphoid tissue	1. Large "tough" cells 2. Capacity to ingest large numbers of bacteria at one time	1. Along with reticulum cell, forms second line of defense against bacterial invasion 2. Phagocytosis 3. Act as scavengers, cleaning inflammatory site
c. Plasma cells	1. Normally found in large numbers in the walls of the intestinal tract, lymph nodes, spleen, and bone marrow 2. Increase in chronic inflammation	Probably derived from either lymphocytes or reticulum cells	1. Small 2. Round 3. Irregularly shaped	1. Role obscure 2. Possibly active in antibody formation

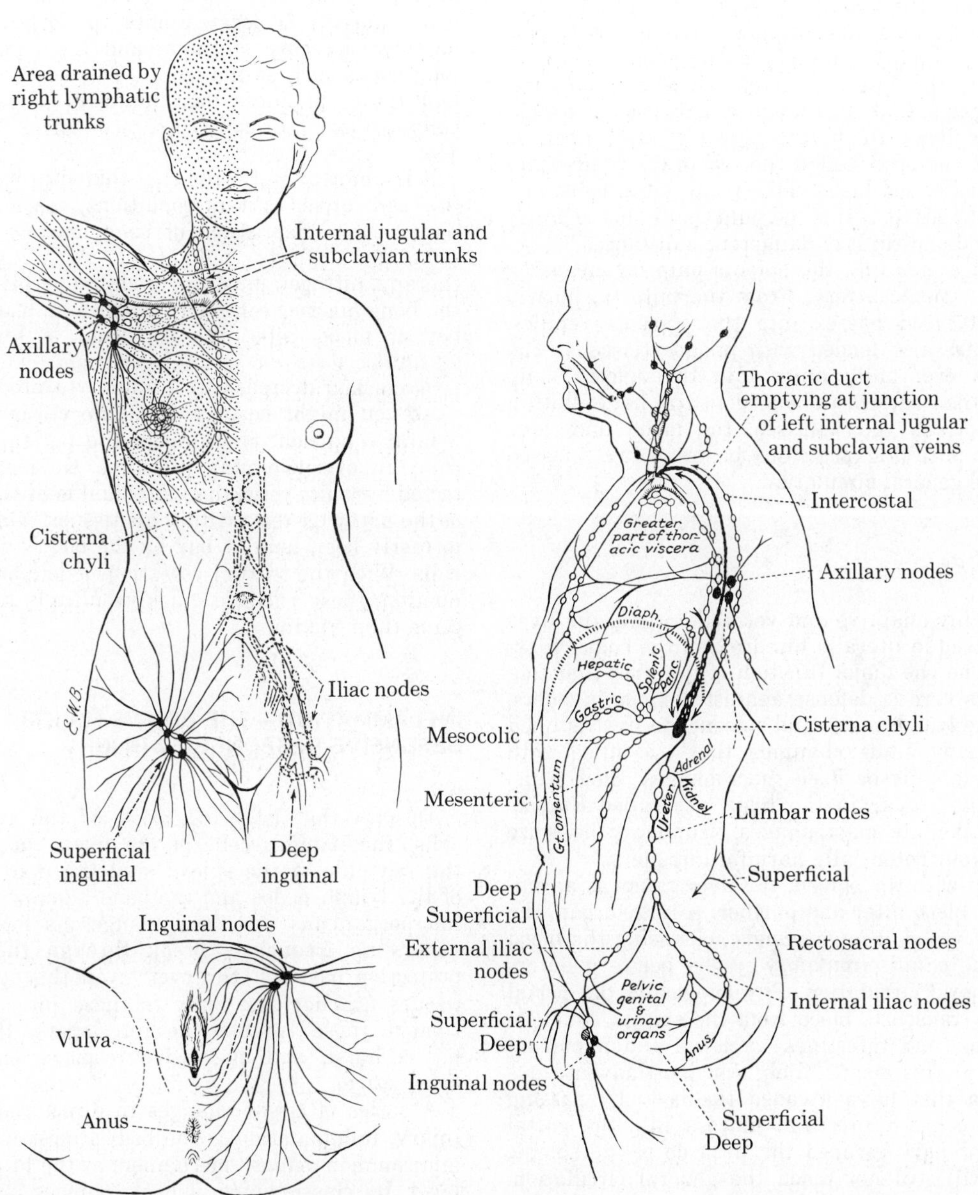

FIGURE 22–1. Diagram of superficial lymphatic vessels and lymph nodes. Shading indicates area drained by right lymphatic trunks. (From *Dorland's Illustrated Medical Dictionary*. 25th ed. 1974.)

*THE SPLEEN**

This highly vascular bean-shaped, gland-like organ lies beneath the diaphragm, and behind and to the left of the stomach. While the spleen serves many functions, its unique anatomic structure makes it highly valuable as a defensive organ. Basically the spleen is composed of a fibrous tissue capsule that surrounds a network or framework of fibers. In the interstices of these fibers is found a material called the *red pulp,* a substance composed of red blood cells, white blood cells, and macrophages. It is this red pulp that helps to purify the blood and rid it of dangerous substances.

Blood comes into the splenic pulp for cleansing via the splenic artery. From the pulp the nearly purified blood passes into the spleen's venules, which are also loaded with phagocytic cells. The venules eventually unite into the splenic vein, which then carries the blood to the liver. Within the liver, as you will see, the blood undergoes further purifying processes before being released into the general circulation.

THE LIVER

A highly adaptive and versatile organ, the liver is involved in literally hundreds of the body's functions. The one major function of the liver that concerns us here is defense against noxious invaders. Like the lymph nodes and spleen, the liver is lined with many sinus channels that are filled with reticulum cells or fixed macrophages. Such cells, when they occur in the liver, are called *Kupffer cells.* Like all macrophages, Kupffer cells seize and devour potentially harmful intruders.

Along with the spleen, the liver ranks as an important blood filter and purifier. A large organ, the liver serves as a mighty sieve, cleansing the blood from the *portal circulatory system* before it enters the general circulation. Physiologically the portal system transports blood from the spleen, stomach, pancreas, and intestines—a large and important territory. This means, then, that most adventurous bacteria that have invaded the body by passing from the gastrointestinal mucosa into the portal blood, or have escaped the hazards of the splenic pulp, will still not reach the general circulation. Instead, they will meet swift death in a Kupffer cell.

In reviewing these few facts about the liver as a protective organ, one can readily see the effect of liver disease upon the body's defense against microorganisms. Indeed, these points explain why individuals with cirrhosis of the liver—a condition involving destruction and scarring of the liver tissue—are so vulnerable to overwhelming infection.

*The spleen and its functions will be discussed in greater detail in the Units on Diseases of the Circulatory and Lymphatic systems.

THE BONE MARROW

The lymphatic tissues and the myeloid tissues (or red bone marrow) are the *hemopoietic* (also called hematopoietic) tissues of the body; i.e., they produce blood cells. In the adult human the red bone marrow is located only in certain bones, namely, the ribs, sternum, and the ends of the long bones such as the femur. This scattered myeloid tissue produces vast numbers of reticulum cells, remarkable cells discussed earlier on page 144.

It is unfortunately true that this vital bone marrow can, under certain conditions, cease to function. Such a depression of bone marrow activity sometimes affects individuals receiving x-ray therapy, nitrogen mustard, or chloromycetin. When the bone marrow refuses to produce its usual number of blood cells, the condition is known as *agranulocytosis* or *granulocytopenia;* i.e., there is a marked decrease in granulocyte production.*

As you might suspect, agranulocytosis is often a fatal condition, resulting in the patient's death from an overwhelming infection. No longer protected by white cells, the individual is at the mercy of the many bacteria within his tissues, which have formerly been held at bay by the body's defensive cells. With the virtual cessation of leukocyte production, these bacteria quickly multiply and overcome their victim.

INFLAMMATION—THE BODY'S MAJOR DEFENSIVE RESPONSE TO INJURY

Despite the defensive work of the reticulum cells, the Kupffer cells of the liver, the cells in the red pulp of the spleen, and the macrophages of the lymph nodes and the bone marrow, various microorganisms and other dangerous foreign invaders *do* frequently break through the body's protective barriers. However, even then the body tissues are not easy prey to these intruders. To combat these troublesome interlopers, the body has a harsh and aggressive response called *inflammation.*

A series of tissue changes in direct reaction to injury, inflammation is the body's most important and common defense mechanism at the local tissue level. Its classic signs of heat, redness, pain, and swelling accompany numerous disease states—both mild and severe—even though these conditions arise from vastly different etiologic origins. Thus it is the rare individual who has not suffered from the symptoms of inflammation at some point in his life.

*Agranulocytosis is discussed more fully in the Unit on Blood, p. 779.

Indeed, many of the patients in your care will be ill with an inflammatory condition. The common suffix "itis" means inflammation. Stomatitis, appendicitis, cellulitis, gastritis, nephritis, vaginitis, and colitis are all inflammatory conditions.

Since the subject of inflammation is so relevant to the everyday clinical situation, it is necessary to explore it more fully.

DEFINITION, EFFECT, AND CAUSATION

Inflammation can be defined as an immediate, aggressive response by the body to the injury or potential destruction of its cells and tissues. Inflammation is an essentially *local* tissue response as opposed to a more total-body, systemic response. You will recall that Selye has equated inflammation with the LAS or Local Adaptation Syndrome. (See Unit II, p. 36.) The specific *effect* of the inflammatory adaptive syndrome is to destroy or dilute the injurious agent as well as to prevent the spread of injury. Thus, inflammation acts adaptively to delimit the area of stress by walling off the injured site with barricades of fibrous tissue.

The *causes* of inflammation are many. We have already listed most of them in earlier discussions. In brief review, major etiologic factors resulting in inflammation are: physical injury such as trauma, burns, and frostbite; chemical irritants; bacterial irritants; and exudates formed within the body. It is important to remember that causative factors in inflammation may be either intrinsic or extrinsic.

AN OVERVIEW OF THE INFLAMMATORY RESPONSE AND ITS COMPONENTS

Inflammation can be compared to a melodrama played at the physiologic level since it involves all the elements of melodrama, including potential harm to the central character, a death struggle between opposing forces, and a sense of suspense or uncertainty as to the outcome of the battle.

Although the subject of inflammation is complex, it can be reduced to a few general principles:

> Inflammation always involves some type of *tissue injury*.

> The inflammatory *events* that follow tissue injury are almost always exactly the same, although they may differ in severity and outcome.

> The *components* involved in the inflammatory drama are always the same, as are their general roles and responses.

Thus, like a play replayed a million times on a million different stages, inflammation follows exactly the same script and has exactly the same characters and roles, regardless of the circumstances in which it is enacted.

The major *components* involved in inflammation are: (1) the blood vessels, (2) the blood itself, (3) the inflammatory exudate, (4) the defensive cells, including microphages and macrophages, (5) antibodies, and (6) the surrounding connective tissue. The major *responses* that characterize inflammation and that involve the above components include: (1) the vascular response, (2) the formation of the inflammatory exudate, (3) the defensive cell response, (4) the fibrin response, (5) the humoral response, and (6) the hormonal response.

The Vascular Response

When the tissues of an individual are injured, his blood vessels respond in the following manner:

1. The blood vessels *momentarily constrict* and then quickly *dilate*. These changes in the diameter of the blood vessels are believed to be due to the release of vasoactive substances at the site of injury. The first blood vessels to dilate are the arterioles, followed by the venules and, finally, the capillaries.

2. As a result of the vasodilatation of the blood vessels, more blood is quickly brought to the injured part. The *hyperemia* produced, in turn, results in the redness and heat so characteristic of inflamed tissues.

3. Not only do the blood vessels dilate during an inflammatory reaction, but the capillaries become highly *permeable* as well. The increased capillary permeability, in turn, leads to the passage of water, colloids, ions, and the body's defensive cells into the area of injury.* This fluid is usually called the *inflammatory exudate*.

What exactly causes this increased capillary permeability is still a matter for researchers to ponder. Thus far, scientists believe that when cells are damaged they manufacture and discharge certain substances that compel the capillaries to dilate. These substances are called *chemical mediators*. An important chemical mediator is histamine, a substance that evidently *initiates* the vascular response. However, since it is unable to sustain the increase in capillary permeability for any prolonged length of time, histamine is called a short-acting chemical mediator.

Physiologists are now searching for chemical mediators that play a role in delayed and sustained vascular reactions such as those that follow injury from ultraviolet rays and radiation. Bradykinin is believed to act in this way.

4. The blood flow, which has been rapid during the initial phase of inflammation, slows and may even stagnate. This *stasis of the blood* is the result of the packing of red cells in the capillaries; blood clots because of the heavy concentration of red blood cells and the pressure of the inflammatory exudate.

*The terms "ion" and "colloid" are defined and discussed on p. 196.

The Formation of the Inflammatory Exudate

The inflammatory exudate, as we just stated, is generally composed of water, colloids, ions, and defensive cells. This lymph-like substance collects readily at any site of tissue injury. In mild injuries the inflammatory exudate is mainly composed of serum; in more acute inflammations, however, the exudate contains fibrin and even red blood cells, which gives the exudate a hemorrhagic appearance.

Three factors are responsible for the formation of the exudate: one is the hyperemia that occurs after injury; a second is the increased capillary permeability; and a final cause is the increased filtration pressure created by hyperemia as the increased blood volume presses against the vessel wall. This increased pressure forces some of the blood and some of the cells out into the tissue spaces.

The inflammatory exudate has certain functions once it reaches the area of injury: (1) to dilute the toxins released by bacteria; (2) to bring to the site certain nutrients necessary for tissue repair, and (3) to carry the protective cells that will phagocytize and destroy bacteria.

While the inflammatory exudate is very useful to the body, it can and often does create serious problems for the injured person. First of all, the additional fluid in the area of injury causes swelling, and the swelling causes pain and sometimes immobility. This *swelling or edema,* which is often severe, can constitute a serious problem for the person whose injured arm or leg is in a cast that does not provide room to accommodate the swollen tissues. For these individuals the swelling and compression may result in a closing off of arterial flow to the damaged part as well as a restriction of venous return. Such symptoms as coldness, blueness, and swelling of the extremity may occur, along with sensations of pain, tingling, and numbness. Elevation of the injured and swollen part usually helps to increase venous return and to relieve the edema. At times a hole may have to be cut out of the cast, or the cast may have to be split and then taped together to allow for the swelling.

A second group of patients for whom inflammatory edema constitutes a dangerous problem are those with *head injuries.* When the tissues of the brain swell, the hard bony cranium cannot enlarge to make room for its increased contents. As a result, the patient develops an *increased intracranial pressure,* a neurologic complex of signs discussed later in the text.*

*For a discussion of the signs of intracranial pressure, see the neurologic unit, pp. 430 to 431.

The Defensive Cell Response

The inflammatory exudate that leaks into inflamed tissues as a result of increased capillary permeability is loaded with white blood cells and with macrophages of the reticuloendothelial system. This response by the body-protecting cells is highly complex and still somewhat of a mystery. The major components of the response are: (1) pavementing of leukocytes, (2) the migration of protective cells, (3) phagocytosis by the protective cells, and (4) leukocytosis—a systemic reaction.

Pavementing of Leukocytes. As stated under the *vascular response,* the blood flow tends to be rapid during the first part of the inflammatory response; then the circulation slows and even stagnates. With the slowing of the blood flow, the leukocytes (mainly neutrophils) leave the center of the blood stream in order to line the walls of the capillaries. When neutrophils stick to the vessel walls in this manner, the result is called *margination* or *pavementing* of leukocytes.

The Migration of Protective Cells. From this position, lining the vessel walls, the white cells begin their process of *migration* to the site of injury. Squeezing through the vessel walls by a process known as diapedesis, and slithering through the tissue spaces by means of ameboid motion, the vast army of phagocytic cells begins its journey to the site of invasion.

Even when a person is in a state of health, white blood cells are always migrating to the tissues in small numbers. Injury simply *speeds* this process of migration and greatly increases the number of defensive cells that are "on the move." A very important defense mechanism in injury, this migration of defensive cells serves three purposes: (1) to destroy injurious agents, (2) to neutralize the toxins produced by these agents, and (3) to remove the inflammatory debris of dead cells and dead bacteria. Migration begins within a few minutes after injury.

As we pointed out earlier, all the different types of defensive cells *do not* migrate to the site of injury at the same time. Instead, migration is quite *selective,* with some cells (like the neutrophils and macrophages of the reticuloendothelial system) coming early, while other cells (like the monocyte, lymphocyte, and plasma cell) arrive later.

What is the force that attracts these cells, drawing them like a magnet to the site of injury? One theory, questioned by some authorities, is that of *chemotaxis.* This hypothesis simply states that when certain chemicals are released by the tissues, defensive cells are either drawn *toward* the source of the chemical (positive chemotaxis) or they are propelled *away* from the source of the chemical (negative chemotaxis). The chemicals that evidently are responsible for chemotaxis in the inflammatory reaction are bacterial toxins, as well as the *polysaccharides* that are released by the injured tissues.

Phagocytosis

One of the most important tasks of the body's defensive cells is phagocytosis, the engulfing and ingestion of harmful foreign substances. The material ingested may be bacteria, parasites, dead cells, or foreign matter such as soot. The phagocyte digests its prey by means of the proteolytic enzymes that it produces. White cells also release bactericidal agents, such as lysozyme, which kill the bacteria before the bacteria can kill the white cell.

It is its own gluttony, however, rather than the foreign objects, that finally destroys the phagocyte. As the defensive cell ingests bacteria and other foreign particles, breakdown products accumulate within its cytoplasm. These breakdown products are harmful to the phagocyte and, by accumulating, they eventually bring its life to an end.

Leukocytosis—The Systemic Reaction

As we stated earlier, most infectious and inflammatory conditions are characterized by a marked increase in circulating white blood cells, called leukocytosis. The count may climb from between 6000 and 10,000 per cu. mm. up to 30,000 per cu. mm.

One explanation for this intensification of leukocyte production and release is that the inflammatory exudate contains a substance which is a *leukocytosis-promoting factor* (LPF). It is possible that this globulin factor promotes a hyperplasia of bone marrow tissue which, in turn, increases white blood cell production and release.

A second theory explaining leukocytosis is that the disintegrated white blood cells at the site of inflammation release a substance that promotes leukocytosis. Some physiologists believe that this substance is actually a form of the LPF.

In any event, leukocytosis is a cardinal sign, always present when inflammation occurs, and usually subsiding with the disappearance of the inflammatory reaction.

The Fibrin Barrier

Like the migration of leukocytes and macrophages, the formation of a fibrin barrier or net is a vital physiologic defense mechanism against the further spread of infection and inflammation. Exactly how this fibrin barrier works is still a mystery. Does it form a wall surrounding the inflamed area and encircling the bacteria, thereby trapping these undesirable aliens and making them available to the action of the phagocytes? Does it form a heavy net that catches dangerous intruders as a net catches fish? Or is it a bewildering maze in which the bacteria, on their way to new tissue territories, become endlessly lost and thus more vulnerable than ever to the hungry macrophages? No one knows for certain which answer is correct. We do know, however, that without the fibrin barrier, a simple local infection can easily spread to become a dangerous, even fatal, systemic malady.

How is this valuable fibrinous material formed? First of all, you will recall that both tissue histiocytes and lymphocytes are capable of transforming themselves into fibroblasts, thereby helping to form the fibrin mesh. Second, in the process of inflammation, fibrinogen escapes from the blood. Fibrinogen, an important blood component involved in the clotting mechanism, is then converted to fibrin.

The fibrin barrier, like all physiologic defenses, creates certain problems for the body, the most significant of which is the formation of *adhesions*. When such fibrous bonds or adhesions form between adjacent loops of bowel, they are an important cause of intestinal obstruction. Adhesions can also cause respiratory problems when they form between the pleura covering the lungs and the lining of the chest wall.

The Humoral Defense

While defensive cells phagocytize bacteria, and the fibrin mesh checks the spread of bacteria, the *humoral defense* fights and *neutralizes bacterial toxins*. This defense mechanism depends upon the antitoxins and antibodies that are contained within the inflammatory serum. These powerful substances are involved in the important antibody-antigen reaction, to be discussed in more detail in Chapter 23.

The Hormonal Response

You will recall from Unit II that Selye designated inflammation as the prime example of the Local Adaptation Syndrome or LAS. The LAS, like the GAS, is dependent upon the action of the brain and central nervous system and upon the hormones of the adrenal and pituitary glands. According to Selye, some hormones, such as cortisone, are *anti-inflammatory*, suppressing the formation of eosinophils and lymphocytes and causing the shrinkage of lymphoid tissue. As a consequence, these hormones *limit* the spread of the inflammatory reaction. Other hormones, such as *aldosterone*, are *pro-inflammatory* corticoids that stimulate the body's defensive activities and thereby promote and support the inflammatory reaction.[10]

In sum, there are many factors at the body's disposal for defensive purposes. Each factor has its own particular role to play, yet each factor must work in coordination with several other factors if the defense is to be successful.

SIGNS AND SYMPTOMS OF INFLAMMATION

The major local and systemic manifestations of inflammation and their causation are listed on the following page.

Pathophysiologic Basis	Signs and Symptoms
Local Reaction	
Blood vessels dilate and blood is brought rapidly to injured area; hyperemia results	Heat (calor) and redness (rubor) around the area of injury
Exudation of inflammatory lymph produces local edema around injured area	Swelling (tumor)
Nerve endings in the area of inflammation are painfully stimulated by both the pressure of the inflammatory lymph and the chemicals that are released by the damaged cells	Pain (dolor)
Pain and discomfort resulting from nerve ending involvement cause the patient to hold the injured part as immobile as possible; muscle spasms around the area of injury help to splint motion	Loss of function and the involuntary cessation of movement
Systemic Reactions	
Neutrophils may release enzymes that are fever-producing; in infections, bacteria release toxins that are absorbed into the circulation and then act upon the hypothalamus to produce fever	Fever accompanied by increased pulse and respiration rates; adults may experience chills; children may suffer from convulsions
Increased numbers of WBC are released from the bone marrow and lymph nodes into the blood; this is possibly the result of the leukocytosis-promoting factors (LPF)	Leukocytosis
A chilly sensation commonly precedes fever; it also is accompanied by a lowered skin temperature, which is caused, in turn, by marked vasoconstriction; the chill and shivering cause an increase in body metabolism and heat production; it is speculated that there may be a shivering center in the hypothalamus	Chills and "gooseflesh"
A thermoreceptive center in the hypothalamus is probably responsible for diaphoresis; this symptom usually accompanies fever and usually heralds the beginning of a fall in body temperature	Sweating
The exact cause for a decrease in appetite in inflammatory and infectious conditions is not known; environmental problems such as nauseating odors and sights and psychologic problems such as worry and depression probably contribute to the development of this problem	Anorexia
Fever, anorexia, and nausea predispose to a loss of weight	Weight loss
The exact cause for the achy, exhausted feeling accompanying inflammation and infection is not known	General malaise, "aches and pains," "feeling terrible"
Muscle groups are sometimes directly invaded by organisms; also, the inactivity of muscles that generally accompanies inflammation may lead to atrophy of the muscle and further weakening	Generalized weakness and an inability to sustain normal activity
High fever, sweating, and dehydration contribute to a sense of lethargy and depression; however, other factors of emotional origin are undoubtedly at work	Depression and a loss of enthusiasm
Some authorities believe that the general systemic symptoms that occur in inflammation are the result of the general adaptation syndrome (GAS); Selye states that persons suffering from such symptoms are involved in the "syndrome of just being sick"[10]	"The syndrome of just being sick"

WAYS OF CLASSIFYING INFLAMMATORY REACTIONS

While all inflammatory reactions share to some degree the same general and local manifestations, inflammatory reactions also *differ* from one another in a number of important ways. We find that there are four major ways of classifying inflammatory reactions, each type of reaction being distinguished by certain characteristics. Major criteria used in classifying inflammatory reactions are as follows:

1. Causation
2. Duration
   a. Acute
   b. Chronic
3. Type of exudate produced
   a. Serous
   b. Fibrinous
   c. Catarrhal
   d. Purulent
   e. Hemorrhagic
4. Location (the specific site and type of tissue involved in the process)
   a. Abscesses (fistulas, boils, carbuncles)
   b. Cellulitis
   c. Ulcers

CAUSATION

As stated earlier, inflammation can be caused by any agent that is capable of injuring or killing tissues and cells.

DURATION

Inflammatory reactions are classified as *acute* or *chronic,* mainly in terms of the length of time they have been in existence. However, chronic and acute inflammatory reactions also have many other distinctive and differentiating characteristics. In Table 22–4 we have outlined some of the most distinctive features of each.

One important type of chronic inflammation is *granulomatous chronic inflammation.* This inflammatory reaction develops in the following conditions: tuberculosis, syphilis, leprosy, brucellosis, and fungus infections. Characterized by a tumor-like proliferation of cells at the site of injury, granulomatous inflammations may eventually be replaced by large amounts of scar tissue.

It is important to remember that these classifications of inflammation, while useful, are nevertheless quite arbitrary. Acute inflammation can subside and become chronic, while chronic inflammations may develop as a low grade reaction to toxicity and never become an acute response.

EXUDATE

The major types of exudate produced in the course of inflammatory reactions are the following: serous, fibrinous, catarrhal, purulent, and hemorrhagic. These major forms of exudation are briefly compared and contrasted in Table 22–5.

The type of exudate produced in an inflammatory reaction often serves as an excellent guide to diagnosis. The physician may therefore request that the laboratory take a smear of the exudate from an inflamed area, especially if he suspects the presence of bacteria. The smear of material obtained is then used for a bacterial culture. From the culture it is possible to identify the type of organism present, as well as the antibiotics to which it is sensitive and susceptible.

TABLE 22–4. DISTINGUISHING CHARACTERISTICS OF ACUTE AND CHRONIC INFLAMMATORY REACTIONS

Distinguishing Characteristics	Acute Inflammatory Reactions	Chronic Inflammatory Reactions
Duration	Generally last from a few days to a few weeks; if inflammation lasts more than a few weeks, it is termed chronic	Generally persist over many weeks and may last for several months
Important anatomic changes	Vascular congestion; exudation of inflammatory lymph and defensive cells	Proliferative cell multiplication; proliferation mainly fibroblastic, which leads to scarring
Dominant cell at the site of injury	Polymorphonuclear leukocytes, with neutrophils arriving first	Mononuclear cells, especially lymphocytes and plasma cells
Symptoms	Redness, heat, pain, swelling, and all the general systemic signs	Symptoms may not be severe; because of proliferation of fibroblasts, scarring, deformities, and adhesions may develop, with *permanent* tissue damage

LOCATION AND POSITION

Inflammatory reactions are also classified according to their *location* within the body and according to the particular *organ* which they affect. Thus, the term "myocarditis" signifies inflammation of the heart muscle; "appendicitis," an inflammation of the appendix; "nephritis," an inflammation of the kidney nephron; and so forth.

A final way to group inflammatory conditions is according to the *position* that an inflamed area occupies within the particular tissue involved. There are three distinct types of inflammatory reactions that are based upon this classification and need clarification: abscesses, cellulitis, and ulcers.

Abscesses

An abscess is defined as a "localized collection of pus caused by suppuration in a tissue, organ, or confined space." Abscesses are usually formed as the result of tissue invasion by pyogenic bacteria. As you will recall, the pus produced is a mixture of necrotic tissue debris as well as dead and living bacteria and polys. Abscesses are also characterized by parenchymal and stromal cell destruction which, in turn, leads to scar tissue and to the production of permanent deformities.

Boils and carbuncles are common examples of the inflammatory abscess. A *boil* is an abscess of the root of a hair follicle; it results from bacterial infection. Staphylococci are the pyogenic organisms most frequently involved in the etiology of a boil. A *carbuncle* is a group of boils adjacent to one another. Because this type of abscess extends into the subcutaneous tissue, carbuncles are much more serious than boils. Suppuration is deeper and more extensive, healing is slower, and scarring may be quite extensive.

Abscesses may terminate in a variety of ways. First, some abscesses may extend from the involved organ or tissue to the surface of the body, where the accumulated pus is released. Abscesses frequently extend to the surface by means of either a sinus or a fistula. A *sinus* is a tract that drains pus to the outside from an abscess that is fairly deep within the tissues. A *fistula* is an abnormal tract that may form between two hollow organs or between a hollow organ and the skin. Examples

TABLE 22–5. A SUMMARY OF THE VARIOUS TYPES OF INFLAMMATORY EXUDATES

Type	Characteristics	Derivation	Typical Conditions in Which Exudate Appears
Serous	A watery, low protein fluid that is generally produced in large amounts	From blood serum and from the cells lining the peritoneal, pleural, and pericardial cavities and joint spaces	Skin blisters Pericarditis Pulmonary tuberculosis with effusion
Fibrinous	Exudate filled with large amounts of fibrinogen, which results in the precipitation of fibrin	If capillaries are damaged, the increase in their permeability leads to the escape of the large fibrinogen molecule into the inflammatory exudate	Occurs in severe acute inflammations Pneumococcal pneumonia
Catarrhal	Mucinous secretion	Released from tissues that are mucus-producing (nasopharynx, lungs, intestinal tract, uterus)	Common cold Smog may cause watering of eyes and nose
Purulent or suppurative	Characterized by the presence of *pus,* which is a thick fluid composed of partly liquefied necrotic tissue debris plus large numbers of dead and living bacteria and polys	Pus is mainly produced by such pus-producing (pyogenic) bacteria as staphylococci, pneumococci, meningococci, gonococci and certain streptococci; certain chemicals such as silver nitrate may also cause suppurative inflammations	Acute appendicitis Gonorrhea Abscesses Boils and carbuncles
Hemorrhagic	Red blood cells escape into the exudate; patients suffer from tiny hemorrhages into their skin and tissues (petechiae); the skin may be covered with small red areas; in severe cases, the patient's coloring may be very dusky	Results from damage to capillaries and blood vessels due to severe infection	Fulminating infection Subacute bacterial endocarditis The "black smallpox"

of fistulas are the channels that form between the rectum and vagina or between the interior of the bowel and the skin surface. Second, abscesses may burst *within* the body, releasing pus into a body cavity and thereby creating serious complications for the patient. For example, an appendix may rupture from an inflammatory process; as a result, the contents of the inflamed appendix flow into the peritoneal cavity, causing peritonitis. Third, small abscesses may be terminated by the process called *resolution,* in which the pus and debris of inflammation are simply digested by the macrophages rather than draining out or bursting forth from the area of tissue damage. Finally, as stated earlier, abscesses tend almost always to result in some permanent damage to the involved cell and in the formation of scar tissue.

Since abscesses are quite common in clinical practice and can be very dangerous, a few words of caution are in order. In working with patients with abscesses, remember these points:

1. *Never squeeze a pimple or boil forcefully, as this may cause the infection to extend.*
2. *Instruct persons with boils around the nose and within the nostrils to seek medical aid, as neglect can produce such serious complications as sinus thrombosis, meningitis, and septicemia.*
3. *The use of careful technique in the changing and discarding of dressings from patients with abscesses will prevent the transmission of infection to yourself or to other patients. Be sure to wear gloves or to use forceps when removing contaminated dressings.*

Cellulitis

Any inflammatory process that is poorly defined and diffuse and has a marked tendency to spread through solid tissues is called cellulitis. This type of inflammation usually involves the skin and subcutaneous tissues, although it may also extend to deeper tissues, as occurs in pelvic cellulitis. Any pathogen that can invade the body's tissue can cause cellulitis, although the *hemolytic streptococcus* is the most common and virulent cause.

Ulcers

An ulcer is a superficial defect of the surface of an organ or tissue that is caused by the sloughing of necrotic tissues destroyed by the inflammatory process. Ulcers are commonly found in the mucosa of the stomach, mouth, and intestines. For example, the gastric or stomach ulcer is frequently encountered in modern man. Persons with poor circulation as a result of peripheral vascular disease may develop multiple stasis ulcers on their legs. A third common site for ulcer formation is the cervix of the uterus. Each of these types of ulcer formation will be considered in appropriate sections of the text.

THE OUTCOME OF THE INFLAMMATORY PROCESS

THE RESULTS OF INFLAMMATION

An inflammatory process can eventually terminate in several ways—some adaptive and some maladaptive. Let us explore some of these possible outcomes.

First, as we stated earlier, mild inflammatory reactions are often *resolved* and heal quickly with no complications. Second, inflammation may be *inadequate* as a response to stressors. In this case the inflammatory defenses at work may be unable to contain dangerous infectious and foreign intruders within a limited area of the body. Thus, microorganisms and other foreign proteins are able to escape and to enter the general circulation and cause a serious *bacteremia.* If the bacteria begin to increase their numbers within the blood stream, a fatal *septicemia* may ensue. Third, the development of inflammation may result in an *overreaction* on the part of the body to a stressor. The etiologies of such diseases as arthritis and polyarteritis nodosa are possibly linked to an overly virulent and extensive inflammatory reaction. Finally, as stated previously, inflammation can result in a number of pathologic changes. Peritonitis, fistulas, ulcers, boils, adhesions, and permanent scars are some of the developments that can arise from the inflammatory process and cause serious and lasting problems for the patient.

FACTORS THAT AFFECT THE OUTCOME OF THE INFLAMMATORY PROCESS

The eventual outcome of inflammation rests upon (1) the nature of the stressor, and (2) the patient's ability to respond adaptively to that stressor. You will recall from Unit II that if the stressor is very powerful or if the patient's resistance is poor, the patient may be overcome and the stressor may emerge the victor over a weakened or dead host. Conversely, if the stressor is weak or the patient has strong resistance, the stressor will be weakened or eliminated, and the patient will continue to live and hopefully will regain his strength.

The Nature of the Stressor

Several factors may tip the scales in favor of victory for the stressor.

Number or Amount. The number of invading organisms or the amount of stressor (e.g., the dose of radiation that a patient receives). Generally speaking, the *greater* the amount of the stressor, the more likelihood that the stressor will create serious or possibly fatal illness in the patient.

Virulence. The virulence or *strength* of the invader. Even a brief exposure to strong radiation can give rise to serious burns. Infection by a few powerful (highly virulent) pyogenic organisms, such as the streptococci, can be more threatening than a similar invasion by a greater number of less virulent organisms.

The Spreading Factor. The ability of certain organisms to *spread* through tissues and to *dissolve fibrin barriers* enables those organisms to undermine the adequacy of the inflammatory process. The streptococcus and the staphylococcus, in particular, have this ability. Both these microorganisms are able to produce an enzyme called *hyaluronidase,* sometimes called the "spreading factor." Hyaluronidase, along with other factors, helps to increase the permeability of tissues and the consequent spread of organisms from diseased tissue to healthy tissue.

Resistance to Phagocytosis. The ability of certain organisms to resist phagocytosis increases their ability to live and to multiply. It is believed that some bacteria are enclosed in a polysaccharide capsule that protects them from the ever-present polys and macrophages. Thus, these organisms are able to go on living, thereby endangering the life and health of the host.

The Nature of the Patient and His Response to Stress

The presence of certain factors within a given patient modifies that patient's response to microorganisms and to other stressors. For example, consider the following case histories of two infected patients with inflammatory responses—one who lived and one who died. See if you can select those influences that made the crucial difference between recovery and death.

The Case of the Businessman's Son. One winter, Carl Young, the 19 year old son of a well-to-do business man, developed a case of the Asian flu, complicated by a severely inflamed throat. Carl, who had rarely been ill in his life, felt sick enough to go to bed. Carl's mother called their family physician, who told her to bring Carl into his office that very afternoon. After examining Carl and taking a smear for a throat culture, the physician ordered cough medicines, antihistamines, a mild pain medication, and an antibiotic. Carl went home to bed. His mother cooked him meat broths and gave him juices to drink. Within a few days Carl was feeling much better, and by the end of a week he felt well enough to return to his college classes.

The Case of the Retired Gardener. Philip Oldster, 68, lived in one room of a run-down rooming house. He was barely existing on his meager savings, money that he had carefully put away during his many years as a gardener. During his prime, Mr. Oldster had been a good gardener and had made a reasonable living. However, when he grew older the bachelor had to give up his livelihood because of the development of severe diabetes and a gradual worsening of his arthritic condition. As a result of such problems, this once active man had to radically change his life style, being forced to live on his savings and sometimes on welfare. Unable to afford the apartment he had lived in, Mr. Oldster moved to the least expensive room he could find. He found he could not afford fresh fruits, meats, and vegetables. Exhausted, crippled, and with only a hot plate for cooking, he was unable to prepare good meals. Increasingly he ate only bread, cereal, eggs, and macaroni or spaghetti. Besides, as he used to admit to himself, if he did cook, who would he eat with anyway?

As you might suspect, Mr. Oldster had few social contacts with the exception of his landlady, whom he saw briefly almost daily. One week, the landlady missed seeing Mr. Oldster for several days and decided to check on her tenant. She found him ill and feverish, almost delirious, and he was taken by ambulance to the county hospital. The young intern at the hospital decided that Mr. Oldster probably had Asian flu and had developed pneumonia. Despite the efforts of doctors and nurses, antibiotics, and IV's, Mr. Oldster died within 24 hours of admission to the hospital. Mr. Oldster's landlady was the only person who had to be notified of his death.

As you review these two histories, you can see several obvious reasons why one patient overcame infection while the other succumbed. Briefly, the major factors creating this difference are the following:

>*Age:* The younger the patient the more likely he is to adapt successfully to stressors that create inflammation.

>*Nutrition:* Patients who have received adequate protein and vitamin C tend to be less predisposed to tissue damage and are better candidates for healing and repair.

>*Economic standing:* Persons with adequate incomes tend to survive illness far better than the poor. Patients like Carl Young can afford *immediate* medical care from experienced physicians. On the other hand, patients like Mr. Oldster often will not seek care because of its expense or because they have no one to transport them to a doctor. Only when critically ill are they taken to a public hospital, where they are frequently treated by young and inexperienced interns.

> *Social setting:* Persons who live in comfortable surroundings and who have a family that cares about them survive illness better than those who live alone in an unpleasant environment, as did Mr. Oldster.

> *The Tissue Affected:* Some tissues are more vulnerable to infectious disease than are other tissues. As you will recall, Mr. Oldster's *lungs* were affected by his infection. Lung tissue is loose tissue filled with large spaces that allow infectious processes to spread rapidly despite inflammatory defenses. Infections also disseminate rapidly in peritoneal, pericardial, pleural, and joint spaces.

> *The Presence of Other Diseases:* Individuals having chronic diseases, such as arthritis, tend to succumb more

easily to infections since their resistance is lowered from years of illness.

> *The Presence of Diabetes.* The diabetic is less able to resist infection than the nondiabetic. This is because diabetics tend to have a poor vascular response to even slight invasions of microorganisms. Also, the diabetic's elevated blood sugar creates a good medium for the growth and multiplication of bacteria.

Other important factors affecting a host's responses to infections (which were not mentioned in our case histories) are:

> *The Presence of Arteriosclerosis.* Persons with vascular diseases have great difficulty in resisting infections, especially of the lower extremities. Often patients with sclerosed blood vessels, and a resultant inadequate blood supply, develop severe leg ulcers that do not heal.

> *Immunity.* Individuals are more highly resistive to certain infections if they have either a natural or an acquired immunity to the organism causing the infection. Immunity will be discussed in the next chapter of this unit.

> *Ionizing Radiation (X-radiation).* Exposure to ionizing radiation causes a lowered resistance to infection as well as impaired imflammatory defenses. This is because x-radiation causes the death of many of the body's cells, including the valuable lymphocyte. Moreover, x-radiation suppresses antibody formation. These facts were pitifully demonstrated at Hiroshima and Nagasaki, where many survivors of the atomic bomb died from overwhelming infection a few days following the bombing and their exposure to excessive radiation.

> *Cortical hormones.* As stated earlier, patients who either are receiving cortisone medicinally or are producing too much cortisone in their body have an increased susceptibility to infection. The exact reasons for this increased susceptibility will be considered under The Endocrine System (Unit XIX).

All the factors we have listed are important not only to the patient's ability to *resist* disease, but also to his body's ability to repair damaged tissue. Obviously both resistance and repair must take place for recovery to occur. Let us now consider the processes of repair and healing.

REPAIR AND HEALING

Repair is defined as the "replacement of dead or damaged cells by new healthy cells derived either from the parenchymal or connective tissue stromal elements of the injured tissue."[3] You will recall from physiology that the *parenchymal tissues* are the important, predominant, and functional tissues of an organ or gland, while the "connective tissue stromal elements" make up the framework or scaffold that serves to support and contain the parenchymal tissues.

A highly complex process, repair can ultimately produce different results in different cases, depending upon the type of tissue involved, the extent of tissue injury, and the general condition of the patient. For some patients, repair may lead to almost perfect healing of a wound, with minimal or no scarring; such excellent repair results from the healing of tissues that contain parenchymal elements. In other cases, in which healing is by connective tissue elements, the patient may be left with deforming, disabling, and permanent scars.

To better grasp the process of repair, it is helpful to explore the following six areas: types of repair, types of tissues and their regenerative capacity, types of repair by connective tissue—primary and secondary unions—complications of the repair process, factors that affect the repair process, and the treatment of wounds and injuries.

TYPES OF REPAIR

Injured tissues may be repaired by the process of *regeneration,* or they may be repaired by the formation of *scar tissue.* Regeneration occurs when injured cells and tissues are replaced by new cells and tissues that are identical or quite similar in nature and function to the damaged cells. Regeneration can follow both minor and serious tissue injuries. The ability of injured tissues to regenerate depends mainly upon two factors: the ability of the cells of the injured tissues to multiply, and the ability of the newly formed cells to coalesce into units that can function physiologically. For proper function, newly formed units must be equipped with a normal blood, lymph, and nerve supply.

A second type of repair is by means of scar tissue formation. Collagenous scars may form in the healing of tendons, fascia, connective tissue, and collagenous structures. Also, nonfunctioning fibrous scars may patch tissues that cannot be regenerated; for example, damaged heart muscle, brain; and some nerve tissue cannot regenerate and, therefore, these vital structures can heal only by scar tissue formation.

TYPES OF TISSUES AND THEIR REGENERATIVE CAPACITY

We have already indicated that different types of tissues have different capacities for healing. In sum, certain tissues can be almost perfectly reconstructed; other tissues are replaced by tissues that are similar in type; and, finally, certain tissues are incapable of any type of regeneration, and so injuries to these tissues are patched by a nonfunctional fibrous scar.

Tissues that Heal by Regeneration of Identical Tissue

Upon injury, the following tissues are able to heal with perfect regeneration of the injured parts:

Epithelial Tissues. Squamous surfaces of the skin, interior of the mouth, vagina, and cervix; the lining of the salivary glands, pancreas, and biliary tract; the vascular epithelium, the cellular layer of the cornea, the tubular epithelium of the kidney; the epithelium of the digestive and respiratory tracts. For the perfect reconstruction of epithelial tissue, the underlying structures that provide support for the epithelium must be intact.

Splenic and Lymphoidal Tissues. Periodic injury of these tissues results in scarring.

Hemopoietic Tissues. The bone marrow tissues.

Parenchymal Tissues of the Glands. The parenchymal elements of the liver, salivary glands, sebaceous glands, pancreas, and endocrine glands are all highly capable of regeneration. However, repair of the parenchymal tissues of glands cannot take place if the underlying framework of the gland is in poor condition or if the gland has been *completely destroyed.* For example, if the sweat glands or the sebaceous glands of a patient have been completely destroyed by a severe burn, these particular glandular structures will never regenerate.

Tissues that Are Replaced and Successfully "Mimicked" by Collagenous Scar Tissue

Tendons, fascia, connective tissue, and collagenous tissues heal by means of fibroblastic activity. The result of such healing is a tissue that closely resembles the original structure.

Tissues that Are Replaced by Nonfunctioning Scar Tissue

Unfortunately some of the most vital tissues of the body, if injured, cannot be replaced by either identical or similar cells and tissues. The tissues of the brain; the neurons of the central nervous system; the renal glomeruli; and striated, cardiac, and smooth tissue must last throughout a person's lifetime. All the above are highly specialized tissues with functions of a precise nature that cannot be simulated by other tissues. Moreover, these structures are composed of cells (sometimes called permanent cells) that are unable to undergo mitotic division except in utero. Consequently when these cells are severely injured or destroyed, the tissues that the cells have built are replaced by fibrous scars that do not contribute to the physiologic functioning of the organism.

For example, when an individual suffers a myocardial infarction or "heart attack," a part of the heart muscle dies. Cell death, in this disorder, is the result of an inadequate blood and oxygen supply to the involved tissue cells. As the necrotic area heals, a nonfunctioning fibrous scar replaces the specialized heart muscle tissue. As a result, the individual who has suffered and recovered from a myocardial infarction now has a heart that is damaged in its efficiency as a circulatory pump. If this same patient should have several more small infarctions his heart may become so scarred with fibrous tissue and so reduced in its efficiency as a pump that it will seriously fail in the performance of its functions. Consequently the patient who has suffered from multiple infarctions faces the possibility of dying in congestive heart failure.

TYPES OF REPAIR BY CONNECTIVE TISSUE: PRIMARY AND SECONDARY UNIONS

In most injuries both parenchymal and stromal cells are damaged or destroyed. Consequently healing *normally* involves not only the regeneration of parenchymal cells, but also the proliferation of fibroblasts and the resultant building of connective tissue. A repair by connective tissue also occurs whenever an injury has been very large or extensive; the fibrous scar tissue covers the large central area of the defect, and parenchymal regeneration occurs around the edges of the injured site. Finally, as you will recall, fibrous scar tissue is used in the repair of highly specialized tissue composed of permanent cells (e.g., the heart muscle).

Connective tissue repair can be beneficial to the patient in several ways: (1) it fills in defects after extensive injury; (2) it repairs areas damaged by thrombosis and infarction; (3) it gives added strength to blood vessels damaged by aneurysms;* and (4) it helps to form barricades between damaged, inflamed, and infected tissues and healthy tissues.

On the other hand, connective tissue repair can be as damaging as it is helpful. Crippling scars, obstructed blood vessels and nerve pathways, and permanent disfigurement are some of the complications of healing by fibrous tissue growth.

There are two major types of repair by connective tissue: The first is called *primary healing or union.* Primary union, such as the repair of a clean surgical incision by connective tissue elements, is often referred to as healing by *primary* or *first intention.* The second type of connective tissue repair is called *secondary union.* When this refers to the repair of contaminated surgical wounds, a secondary union is called healing by *secondary intention.*

As a brief comparison of the major characteristics of repair by first intention and by second intention, we quote from Cameron[3]:

> In essence, union by second intention differs from union by first intention in the following respects:
> 1. Loss of a greater amount of tissue.
> 2. Production of necrotic debris and inflammatory exudate requiring removal.
> 3. Formation of larger amounts of granulation tissue to fill the defect.
> 4. Slower replacement of the destroyed elements.
> 5. Production of larger amounts of scar.

COMPLICATIONS OF THE REPAIR PROCESS

Like all body responses to injury, the process of repair can sometimes end in new injury and in

*An aneurysm is an outpouching of the wall of a blood-vessel due to weakness of the vessel wall (see Chap. 64).

further disease for the patient. For example, repair as a response to infection and inflammation can be frustrated by the appearance of a new stressor, for example, a fresh invasion by bacteria or dangerous foreign substances; it can be inadequate, leading to poor healing of a wound with the formation of unstable and weak scars; finally, repair can be excessive, resulting in large amounts of ugly nonfunctional scar tissue that eventually strangles blood vessels and nerve pathways in its fibrous grip. Because such complications can obviously lead to serious, often irreversible problems for patients, let us briefly explore some of the most important types of pathologic healing.

Contaminated Surgical Wounds. Sometimes a clean wound that has been closed and properly sutured becomes infected. An infection of this type is often the result of cross-contamination from other patients or of poor handwashing or dressing technique on the part of the attending doctors or nurses. Such a wound will fill with pus and will need to be cleansed of foreign debris and necrotic tissue before healing by second intention is possible. Sometimes the surgeon will elect to close the wound and resuture it. Following this procedure, which is called *secondary closure,* the wound will then heal by *third intention.*

Unstable Scars. When an injury is quite large, the edges of the open wound may not be able to meet and mend properly. As a result, the new young vascular tissue that has been "granulating in" to fill the defect remains exposed. Eventually its blood supply diminishes, and the granulation tissue stops growing and slowly changes into an avascular unstable scar. Covered by a thin and delicate sheet of epithelial cells, this poorly nourished scar tissue is vulnerable to both ulceration and further injury. If, over several decades, ulceration occurs again and again, the unfortunate patient with an unstable scar may eventually develop a squamous carcinoma called *Marjolin's ulcer* at the site of ulceration. To prevent the formation of an unstable scar and its complications, the surgeon may employ a split skin graft or a pedicle graft to close the open wound and to cover the unprotected granulation tissue.

Excessive Granulation Tissue. When granulation tissue is unusually abundant and also swollen and edematous, it is called "proud flesh." Such an abnormal growth of granulation tissue can upset the process of repair by hindering the growth of epithelium over the wound.

Keloids. These huge, ugly, tumor-like overgrowths of scar tissue occur mainly among people with highly pigmented skins, particularly blacks. Keloids can be excised; however, they have an infamous capacity for recurring following surgical removal.

Hypertrophied Scars. Because they are red, large, raised, and hard, hypertrophied scars have an unpleasant appearance. Moreover, they produce an uncomfortable itching. Hypertrophied scars sometimes develop following inaccurate wound closure. The ugly appearance of these scars can be minimized to some extent by surgical revision.

Contractures. Contraction of scar tissue leading to disability and severe deformity occurs mainly when severe injuries are located on the face or over a joint and are healing by secondary union. Early surgical closure of open injuries by skin grafts can help to prevent contractures. However, in some cases the skin grafts themselves develop contractures unless splints and physical therapy are ordered by the physician.

Interference with Organ Function. Scar tissue, when excessive, can definitely interfere with an organ's physiologic functioning. Function can be impaired or destroyed when the scar tissue is abundant enough to close off and reduce the organ's vital blood supply and to choke its nerve pathways.

FACTORS THAT AFFECT THE REPAIR PROCESS

There are several important factors that affect the outcome of the healing process—some beneficially and some injuriously.

Favorable factors involving the patient and his physiological conditions are as follows:

> Youth.

> An adequate blood supply to the affected area, bringing oxygen and nutritive elements and removing the waste and debris from the inflammatory process.

> Good general health and stamina.

> Adequate nutritional intake, especially of protein and vitamin C, both of which favor healing.

Favorable factors involving the site of injury:

> Minimal or moderate tissue destruction rather than extensive destruction.

>An intact underlying framework upon which new tissues can be reconstructed.

> The presence of tissues that are capable of regeneration.

> The absence of infection with its accompanying exudate of pus and necrotic debris.

> Immobilization and rest of the injured part.

Adverse factors involving the patient and his physiologic condition:

> Old age.

> Easy fatigability and poor physical condition.

> An inadequate blood supply to the affected area due to severe peripheral vascular disease, varicose veins, excessive scarring from earlier injuries, edema around the injured area and/or venous stasis.

> The presence of diabetes mellitus, a condition that favors the development of severe infections.

> An excess of adrenocortical steroids within the body due to disease of either the pituitary gland or adrenal gland or due to chemotherapy with steroids. Excess steroids in the blood seem to depress the inflammatory reparative process.

> Protein and ascorbic acid deficiencies.

Adverse factors involving the site of injury:

> Total destruction of a complete physiologic unit (for example, a kidney nephron or a sweat gland). Once destroyed, individual physiologic and anatomic units cannot be regenerated.

> Destruction of the underlying framework upon which new tissues can be reconstructed. Such destruction leads, unfortunately, to extensive growth of scar tissue.

> The absence of tissues that can be regenerated.

> The presence of infection, with its accompanying pus and tissue debris.

> Excessive motion of injured parts and tissues.

> The use of large numbers of sutures in repairing an injury. Sutures, when used to close a wound, tend to act as foreign bodies.

>Paralysis of the limb in which the injured tissue is located.

> Hematomas, seromas, and severe trauma around the site of the wound.

THE TREATMENT OF WOUNDS AND INJURIES

By employing knowledgeable clinical care, doctors and nurses can greatly aid the work of nature in the inflammatory-reparative process.

Ten major principles of wound care that we can employ in our work with patients and that will aid the reparative process are the following:

Immobilize and Rest the Injured Tissues. Rest ensures better utilization of oxygen and nutrients by the body's injured tissues, whereas activity increases the metabolic needs of tissues. Also, activity creates additional waste products at the site of injury and irritates already inflamed tissues. Moreover, activity tends to foster the harmful migration of microorganisms from injured tissues into healthy ones by breaking down the fibrin barriers —major defenses against the spread of infection. To immobilize and rest injured tissues, we place broken legs in casts and injured arms in slings, we shade and bandage damaged eyes, and we place the patient with a damaged heart muscle on total bed rest.

Convert the Contaminated Wound into a Clean Wound Before Surgical Closure. As we said earlier, injured tissues that are filled with pus and necrotic debris cannot heal properly. Such wounds must be cleansed of foreign materials; also stagnant clotted blood must be removed because blood clots can become filled with bacteria. Some methods used for cleansing wounds are:

> *Irrigation* of the wound with sterile solutions of saline or hydrogen peroxide to wash out tissue debris and to reduce the number of bacteria.

> Surgical *debridement* of the wound, that is, excising by scalpel dead tissue and tissues in which foreign materials are embedded.

>Incision and drainage in order to remove from the wound *abnormal collections* of exudate, which act adversely to retard healing, to promote bacterial growth, and to cause pressure on organs nearby the injured area. Penrose drains of soft rubber are frequently used to drain out abnormal fluid collections. When a great deal of fluid is present within the injured area, the drain may be attached to low suction.

>*Homeostasis.* The surgeon always endeavors to control bleeding into the wounded area; also, he is careful to remove old, clotted, and possibly contaminated blood from the site of injury. The nurse has the responsibility to watch for signs of bleeding on a patient's dressing or cast, and to report the appearance of blood drainage or frank blood to the physician.

Protect the Wound from Further Injury and Infection. The meticulous use of sterile technique in dressing and in irrigating wounds is of the greatest importance in preventing infection. A second factor in preventing wound contamination is to isolate patients with clean wounds from those with contaminated wounds. Finally, in order to prevent further injury, physicians and nurses usually strive to manipulate injured tissues as little as possible. Excessive manipulations and the performance of unnecessary procedures can destroy new granulation tissue as well as break down fibrin barriers, thereby promoting the spread of bacteria.

Administer Antibiotics. To prevent and control infection, physicians often order penicillin or sulfonamides or one of the broad spectrum antibiotics.

Administer Steroids. In a few carefully selected cases, steroids may be given to reduce the virulence of the inflammatory reaction to injury, and to limit the spread of inflammation from injured tissues to healthy tissues. For example, cortisone may be given to reduce the severity of a serious eye inflammation.

Preserve the Blood Supply to the Injured Tissues. It is important to check bandages, casts, and splints for excessive tightness around an injured limb. If poorly applied, or in the presence of excessive tissue swelling, a splint can act as a tourniquet, completely shutting off the blood supply to the involved extremity. Tight surgical dressings that encircle an extremity can also act as constricting bands that reduce the tissue's arterial and venous circulation.

The application of warmth to an injured area *increases* the circulation to damaged tissues. Heat causes the blood vessels and capillaries to dilate; as a result, increased numbers of leukocytes and larger amounts of antitoxin are brought to the site of injury.

Elevate the Injured Part. Elevation of injured extremities helps to increase the venous return of blood to the heart; it also contributes to maintenance of proper wound drainage.

Promote Adequate Nutrition. An adequate intake of protein, calories and vitamin C tends to speed and to facilitate the reparative process.

Relieve Pain. Patients who have suffered injury or who have recently undergone surgery will naturally suffer some pain. Pain must be relieved in injured and postoperative patients, since discomfort can cause the additional problems of restlessness, insomnia, and anxiety—all factors that can act adversely on the healing process. For detailed information on various methods for the relief of pain, see Chapter 44, pp. 566–579.

Give Psychological Support. Patients whose bodies are undergoing the process of repair are often emotionally upset. If the patient has broken a limb, he may have to lie for long periods of time in a cast, losing valuable weeks away from work or school and family. An individual who has developed a severe inflammation of the eye may face the possibility of permanently impaired vision. The person who has suffered severe injuries in an accident will probably fear scarring, deformity, and life-long disability. A man who has had a heart attack worries about suffering another attack and about the possibility of dying. These are just a few of the worries that patients may have; it is not surprising that many injured persons suffer also from fear, depression, and despair, and look to their doctors and nurses for support.

How do you alleviate the anxiety of such individuals? A few helpful actions that you can employ are: (1) listen to your patient's concerns and do not minimize his worries. (2) Answer a patient's questions concerning his injury as honestly as possible. Consult with the physician as to what he has told the patient concerning the prognosis for his condition so that your comments do not conflict with the doctor's. (3) Convey the patient's questions to the doctor so that he can discuss these concerns with his patient at the first opportunity. A patient may be afraid to talk with his doctor, feeling the doctor is too busy to be interested in his questions. It is the nurse's responsibility to strengthen communication patterns between the patient and doctor. (4) Watch your patient carefully for signs of severe depression. A patient who suddenly finds himself scarred and crippled for life may think of suicide as an alternative to facing the difficulties of readjustment and the problems of rehabilitation. Such a patient should be brought quickly to the attention of the attending physician. Tranquilizers, antidepressants, and psychotherapy may be ordered for these troubled individuals. (5) Recognize that a patient who is convalescing from serious injuries or surgery may be very hostile or angry at times. Furthermore, his anger may be directed against you—an innocent bystander! Try to accept such a patient's hostility as gracefully as possible; recognize that his outbursts are probably temporary, and that they will pass as he slowly regains his grip on himself and his sense of hope for the future.

References

1. Auld, M. E., et al.: Wound healing. *Nursing '72* 2:36, October, 1972.
2. Beland, I. L.: *Clinical Nursing: Pathophysiological and Psychosocial Approaches.* 2nd ed. New York, The Macmillan Company, 1970.
3. Cameron, R.: Inflammation and repair. *In* Robbins, S. L.: *Pathology.* Philadelphia, W. B. Saunders Company, 1967.
4. Ganong, W. F.: *Review of Medical Physiology.* Los Altos, California, Lange Medical Publishers, 1967.
5. Guyton, A. C.: *Textbook of Medical Physiology.* 4th ed. Philadelphia, W. B. Saunders Company, 1971.
6. Liechty, R. D., and Soper, R. T.: *Synopsis of Surgery.* St. Louis, The C. V. Mosby Company, 1968.
7. Meyers, M. B.: Sutures and wound healing. *American Journal of Nursing* 71:725, September, 1971.
8. Pathology of injury. *Lancet* 2:911, October 28, 1972.
9. Roberts, D.: Wound healing: A scientific review. *Applied Therapeutics* 12:10–14, April, 1970.
10. Selye, H.: *The Stress of Life.* New York, McGraw-Hill Book Co., Inc., 1956.
11. Thomas, L., et al. (eds.): *International Symposium on Injury, Inflammation and Immunity.* Baltimore, The Williams & Wilkins Company, 1964.
12. Watts, G. T.: Closure of wounds. *British Medical Journal* 1:501–502, February, 1970.
13. Zweifach, B. W., et al. (eds.): *The Inflammatory Process.* New York, Academic Press, Inc., 1965.

CHAPTER 23

The Mechanism of Immunity—Normal and Pathologic Responses

The capacity to develop immunity, and thus to neutralize alien and often malevolent intruders, is one of the most important homeostatic mechanisms for survival in a sometimes hostile world. Vital as this immune response is to life, derangements can produce severe, even fatal disease.[47]

INTRODUCTION AND STUDY GUIDE

Since the earliest times, both men and animals have been plagued by unseen enemies—parasites, bacteria, viruses—which have continuously sought to enter and ravage the inner world of their bodies. Against these minute and dangerous living organisms, animals and men have had to develop some means of defense if they were to live and reproduce their own kind. Thus, over eons of time, there has evolved the homeostatic mechanism called *immunity*—a mysterious and complex process that protects men and animals against attacks by such tiny alien invaders as bacteria and viruses.

The subject of immunity raises many questions, some of which are only partially answerable at this time. Questions concerning immunity that are of particular concern in nursing are as follows:

1. What exactly is immunity and how and why did it evolve in the individual and in the species?
2. What are the major components of the immune response?
3. What theories are available to explain the development of immunity and the production of antibodies?
4. What are the major types of immunity?
5. What happens to the body when the immune response becomes pathologic?
6. In what ways can man suppress the immune response when it is either pathologic or disruptive to the success of such therapeutic measures as organ and tissue transplantation?

In order to answer these questions, the material in this chapter will focus upon the following three areas:

> Immunity as a normal adaptive mechanism.

> Pathologic conditions associated with the immune response.

> Immunologic aspects of transplant rejection.

Because the subject of immunity is difficult, challenging, and filled with many technical terms and confusing theories, we urge you to make use of the following study guide:

Upon completion of this chapter, you should be able to define generally the terms listed below. (To more easily learn the "vocabulary of immunity," write each of the following words [as it appears in the text] on a 3 × 5 card along with its definition. Review your cards frequently as you study this unit.) Important terms are as follows:

acquired immunity, active immunity, agammaglobulinemia, agglutination, allergen, allergy, allograft, allograft reaction, anaphylaxis, antibody, antigen, antilymphocyte serum (ALS), Arthus reaction, atopic allergies, autoallergen, autograft, autoimmune diseases, blocking antibodies, cellular immunity, clone, collagen diseases, complement, desensitization, eosinophilia, gamma globulin, hapten, hay fever, histamine, histocompatibility antigens (HL-A), humoral immunity, hypersensitivity, hypogammaglobulinemia, hyposensitization, immune response, immunity, immunologic tolerance, immunologically competent cells (I.C.C.), immunopathy, immunosuppressive techniques, incomplete antibodies, isotransplant, lymphocytes, lysis, lysozyme, neutralization, opsonization, passive immunity, plasma cell myeloma, precipitation, precipitin allergies, properdin, reagins, self-antigen, "self-markers," serum sickness, skin-sensitizing antibodies, species immunity, "take," thymus-dependent system, toxoids, tuberculin reaction, urticaria, vaccine, xenograft.

You should also be able to discuss, in general terms, the following concepts and theories:

1. "Self" tolerance or immunologic tolerance.
2. The "self-marker" hypothesis.
3. The six major types of immunity and their interrelationships.
4. The roles of plasma cells and lymphocytes in promoting the immune response.
5. The role of the thymus gland in the origin of the immune system.
6. The "instructive theory."

7. The "clonal selective" theory.
8. The difference between an immune response and an allergic response.
9. Allergens and antibodies involved in allergic responses.
10. The etiology, diagnosis, and treatment of allergic conditions.
11. Etiologic theories of autoimmunity.
12. The physiologic basis for transplant rejection.
13. Types of transplants.
14. Suppression and prevention of graft rejection.

Describe the etiology, symptoms, and clinical care for the following immunopathies:
1. Hypogammaglobulinemia.
2. Plasma cell myeloma.
3. Anaphylaxis.
4. Serum sickness.
5. Hay fever.
6. Urticaria.
7. Allergic asthma.
8. Autoimmune disease.

State the uses and side effects of the following medications:
1. Antihistamines (in particular, diphenhydramine hydrochloride).
2. Epinephrine.
3. Corticosteroids.
4. Levarterenol bitartrate.
5. Metaraminol bitartrate.
6. Tuberculin.
7. Cytotoxic drugs.
8. Antilymphocyte serum.

IMMUNITY AS A NORMAL ADAPTIVE RESPONSE

DEFINITION

Immunity is comprehensively defined by Mackay and Burnet as follows:

> (1) In the broadest terms, immunity is the essential function by which vertebrate organisms maintain their functional integrity insofar as this is threatened by the entry or appearance of foreign chemical substances in the body. More commonly, immunity is used to cover either (2) the whole complex of processes concerned with protection against pathogenic or potentially pathogenic microorganisms, or (3) the acquired and specific resistance to reinfection that follows infection by a pathogenic agent, and other phenomena of the same general quality, such as the development of antitoxin in response to toxoid.[35]

Immunity, then, is a homeostatic characteristic of vertebrate animals that ensures their survival; a complex group of biologic processes that protects the body against foreign invaders; and a process that builds up resistance in an organism, sometimes thereby preventing that organism from being infected *twice* by the same foreign protein matter. The general effects of immunity are (1) to neutralize and to destroy alien organisms and (2) to build up resistance to further attacks by alien proteins.

THE IMMUNE RESPONSE

Whenever the body recognizes the presence of an invading organism or a protein material that it cannot identify as a part of itself, the body normally protects itself by developing an *immune response*. In the *healthy* immune system, an immune response involves "the development of protective proteins" in response to an invasion of the body by foreign and dangerous protein substances. The *protective* proteins are called *antibodies* and the *foreign* proteins are called *antigens*. In an immune system damaged by *pathologic* changes, an immune response may occur in response to certain of the body's *own* proteins—these proteins being called *self-antigens* or autoantigens. Those pathologic conditions in which the body directs the immune response against itself are called *autoimmune* diseases and will be discussed in more detail later.

> *In sum, for an immune response to take place, two antagonists are required—an antibody and an antigen (either a foreign antigen or a self-antigen).*

Antigens

Antigens are chemical substances that are nearly always *protein* in nature, and are viewed by the body as an attacking force. Thus, we find that the structures of antigenic microorganisms such as bacteria and viruses are protein, as are almost all the toxins that they manufacture and release. Microorganisms and their toxins are termed *antigenic* because they stimulate the production of antibodies against themselves.

Antigens are capable of two highly sophisticated functions, both of which may result in the eventual destruction of the antigens by antibodies. One role of antigens is to *initiate* an *immune response*, i.e., antigens stimulate the development of antibodies against themselves. The second role of antigenic substances is to *react specifically with those antibodies* that have developed against them—a process that we shall discuss shortly.

Antibodies

Antibodies, sometimes called immune bodies or immunoglobulins, are protective substances composed of protein that can be detected in the blood. In simple terms, an antibody has been defined by Burnet as "a modified soluble protein with properties that make it stick to the type of molecule or microorganisms against which it was developed."[8]

Essentially, antibodies are globulins, a *globulin*

being a simple protein that is insoluble in pure water but is soluble in dilute salt solutions. Antibodies within the blood serum are found almost entirely within the *gamma globulin* fraction of the serum, gamma globulin being an important type of blood protein.

The major burden of antibody *production* rests upon the *plasma cells,* which are believed to synthesize all the body's circulating gamma globulin. However, minute amounts of antibodies are also produced by lymphocytes.

The major *function* of antibodies is to defend the body from foreign antigenic substances. By destroying invading microorganisms, antibodies also protect the body against the effects of those noxious toxins released by the antigens.

Antibodies perform their complex tasks of defending the body by reacting with antigens in several different ways. Some of the most important types of antigen-antibody reactions are:

> *Agglutination:* Antibodies disarm bacteria and render them harmless by causing them to clump together.

> *Opsonization:* Antibodies coat bacteria and make them more appetizing to the phagocytes.

> *Lysis:* Antibodies cause invading bacteria to dissolve or liquefy. In order to liquefy bacteria, a protein substance called *complement* must be in combination with the antibody. Evidently complement causes the membrane of the microorganism to rupture; this rupture, in turn, causes the inner substance of the bacteria to seep out into the body fluid. Once complement unites with the antigen and antibody, it becomes *fixed* or bound, which means that it cannot then combine with any other anti-antigen-antibody pair.

> *Neutralization:* Antibodies combine with toxic antigens and disarm the antigens by neutralizing their toxic components. Following the antigen-antibody reaction, the combined antigen-antibody pair are phagocytized by reticuloendothelial cells.

> *Precipitation:* Antibodies react with antigens in a fluid medium, causing an aggregation reaction which is visible, i.e., antigens and antibodies cluster together into a visible mass.

As a result of these adaptive antigen-antibody reactions, homeostatic balance is maintained in the face of hostile invasive forces.

"SELF"-TOLERANCE (IMMUNOLOGIC TOLERANCE)

If the purpose of the immune response is to recognize and then to destroy alien invaders, then how does the body *distinguish* alien invaders from substances that are part of the body itself? How does the defensive mechanism of the body know what to attack (foreign protein) and what to tolerate (body protein)? If such distinctions are not clearly made, the body could possibly mistake *all* proteins for foreign proteins, thereby injuring and even destroying itself. How can such a catastrophe be avoided?

Burnet has precisely formulated this problem of distinguishing between "self" and "not-self" in a theory that is sometimes called the *"self-marker hypothesis."*[8] He points out, first of all, that the cells of the body that are involved in the inflammatory response (i.e., reticuloendothelial cells and lymphocytes) not only rid the body of *foreign* protein and bacteria, but also rid the body of its *own* old and discarded cells. When the reticuloendothelial cells and lymphocytes destroy and phagocytize old, worn-out cells, it is very important that this process *not* elicit an immune response. According to Burnet, the body's own proteins have a particular molecular configuration that is marked "self"; these cells are sometimes called "self-markers." Moreover, the reticuloendothelial scavenger cells contain among themselves certain cells called "recognition units," which have evidently learned to "recognize" the self-markers. These recognition units can be compared to a home guard that recognizes the uniform of a friendly soldier as opposed to a dangerous alien. As a result of this recognition process, antibodies are produced *only* against substances that are marked not-self and are *not* produced against the self.

In sum, immunity depends upon the body's ability to recognize differences in the chemical structure of substances. As it comes to recognize what is self as compared to what is not-self, the body develops tolerance to itself. This form of tolerance is called *self-tolerance* or *immunologic tolerance.**

The concept of self as distinguished from not-self contains important implications for the fields of medicine and nursing; specifically, it helps to cast light upon the obscure subject of autoimmune disease, as well as upon the problem of transplant rejection. Briefly, in autoimmune disease, homeostatic mechanisms *fail to distinguish* between self and not-self, thereby leading the body to mistake its *own* protein for foreign protein, and consequently to form antibodies against itself. As a result of such physiologic confusion, there is destruction of self-components.

On the other hand, in transplant surgery it is the *successful recognition* by the body of foreign tissues as opposed to the self that results in transplant rejection. Thus, foreign tissues that are sutured to the body's tissues hold for a time only, and then are soon rejected by the body's immune system because they are not-self. It is indeed ironic that a homeostatic mechanism such as the immune reaction can ultimately work against man's efforts to treat his maladies and handicaps.

TYPES OF IMMUNITY

There are several specific types of immunity that you will be reading about in the clinical literature. Immunity has been traditionally classified as either

*A current theory explaining the development of immunologic tolerance during fetal life is discussed on pp. 171–172.

natural or acquired, active or passive, humoral or cellular.

Natural and Acquired Immunity

Natural immunity is defined as a natural resistance against infection that an individual inherits genetically and with which he is born, certain antibodies being naturally present within his body. For instance, an individual may have a high natural resistance throughout his life to colds and flu, whereas another person becomes ill with colds every winter. However, a person's natural resistance to infectious diseases can be greatly enhanced or reduced by such factors as diet, environment, body metabolism, state of mental health, and the virulence of the invading microorganism.

While individuals may inherit a natural resistance to certain organisms, natural immunity may also characterize a race or species. Indeed, the best example of natural immunity is *species immunity*. Because of species immunity, one species of animal will be highly resistant to an invading organism, whereas another species may be extremely vulnerable to that *same* organism. To illustrate, many bacteria have little effect on the human body, i.e., the human organism is highly resistant to them. Thus, man is totally resistant to distemper, a disease that kills 25 to 75 per cent of all dogs that contract it. On the other hand, human beings are susceptible to certain diseases that other animals resist. For example, while gonorrhea and typhoid fever have plagued man for centuries, these diseases are not found among other species. Also, while innumerable human beings have died from tuberculosis, the rat is highly resistant to this dangerous and deadly infection.

Substances that play important roles in natural immunity are the following: (1) gamma globulins, which act to destroy bacteria; (2) lysozyme, which acts to dissolve bacteria; (3) basic polypeptides, which inactivate certain types of gram-positive bacteria; and (4) the properdin system.[22]

Properdin is a serum protein of high molecular weight that is particularly valuable to the process of natural immunity. We speak of the properdin system because properdin acts only in conjunction with complement and magnesium. This system plays a part in bacterial destruction, the neutralization of viruses, and the hemolysis of red blood cells. Animals such as rats, which have a high titer of properdin, are highly resistant to infections, whereas guinea pigs, which have a low titer of properdin, are highly susceptible to infections.

The opposite of natural or innate immunity is *acquired immunity*. In acquired immunity, the individual is not born with an inherited resistance to a particular organism; instead he *develops* immunity against an organism either by *actively* producing his own antibodies (active immunity) or by *passively* receiving antibodies that have been manufactured within the bodies of other people or animals (passive immunity).

Acquired immunity may either develop *naturally* within an individual's body, or develop *artificially* as a result of a vaccination or inoculation. When acquired immunity develops *naturally,* it results from a disease process within the body. This form of immunity is produced during the *initial* attack by the causative bacteria or viruses and is probably one reason that the sick individual recovers.

To acquire immunity naturally, the patient depends, then, upon an innate ability to develop immune bodies against particular viruses or bacteria. Thus, when the individual's body is invaded by a specific organism for the first time, he may suffer a serious reaction. However, antibodies are built up against the initial invasion of this organism. A "memory" of the antigens produced by the organism is passed on to successive generations of body cells. As a result, when the body is attacked a second time by the same antigen, the reaction will be very slight or possibly no reaction will take place at all. Thus, the individual has *acquired* an immunity to an organism against which he had no natural immunity. This type of immunity, once developed, persists for years or even for the lifetime of the individual. For example, both smallpox and syphilis confer lifelong immunity upon their victims. However, as every cold sufferer knows, colds and many types of flu confer no immunity at all.

In some unfortunate cases, individuals can develop an acquired immunity against a particular organism, even though they still harbor the organism within their bodies. This organism, then, while harmless to its carrier, can be transmitted to other individuals and can infect them. The classic example of this situation is the *typhoid carrier*. In the case of a typhoid carrier, antibodies against typhoid are present in his blood, although typhoid bacilli continue to live in his gallbladder and intestinal tract. Thus, the individual, while protected by his own antibodies, remains highly infective to other susceptible individuals.

When acquired immunity develops *artificially,* as a result of vaccination or inoculation, it may be acquired either passively or actively.

Passive and Active Immunity

Passive immunity is a type of acquired immunity in which the individual receives or is given antibodies that have been manufactured in the bodies of other individuals or animals. For example, an unborn child may receive antibodies from his mother through the placental circulation. Or individuals may receive injections of serum containing antibodies that have been *actively* developed in the bodies of other people or animals. In both instances the individual who is passively receiving antibodies is being given specific gamma globulins that will be reactive against specific antigens. In neither case have the body cells of the individual actively undergone the changes that take place in the production of active immunity; instead the individual passively *accepts immunity.*

The major advantage of passive immunity is that it is *immediate* in its reaction, rescuing the patient almost at once from the adverse effects of an invading antigen. The patient is protected, even though he has not had time to form his own antibodies against the attacking antigen. The major disadvantage of passive immunity is that it is *temporary,* usually lasting for only a few weeks or months. How long passive immunity will last depends upon the source of the antibody, and also upon how well the antibody-producing mechanism of the individual works. Antibodies transmitted from a mother to her child in utero seem to last the longest of any type of passive immunity. Antibodies acquired in this fashion may circulate in the newborn child's blood for as long as six months. The fact that a newborn child receives antibodies from the mother is advantageous, because newborn children are unable to efficiently synthesize antibodies. Passive immunity that has been received from another adult tends to last from a few weeks to a few months. Gamma globulins are destroyed most rapidly when passive immunity has been transferred from an animal source to an adult; this type of immunity lasts from 10 days to two weeks.

In addition to the temporary nature of passive immunity, a second disadvantage is that an injection of immune serum can cause the patient to develop an allergic reaction called *serum sickness.* The symptoms of serum sickness and its treatment will be discussed later in this chapter.

In *active immunity,* as opposed to passive immunity, the individual does *not* receive immune bodies from other individuals or organisms; instead he manufactures antibodies himself against specific antigens. Moreover, the individual has the capacity to *continue* to manufacture these immune bodies even after the antigen has been vanquished.

Active immunity can be acquired either as the result of a *disease process* as discussed earlier, or from an inoculation with a suspension of either (1) killed bacteria, (2) attenuated living bacteria, or (3) the denatured toxins produced by bacteria. Substances used for an inoculation that are composed of killed or attenuated bacteria are called *vaccines,* whereas substances that are made from the denatured toxins of viruses and bacteria are called *toxoids.*

Let us first discuss the vaccines. As stated

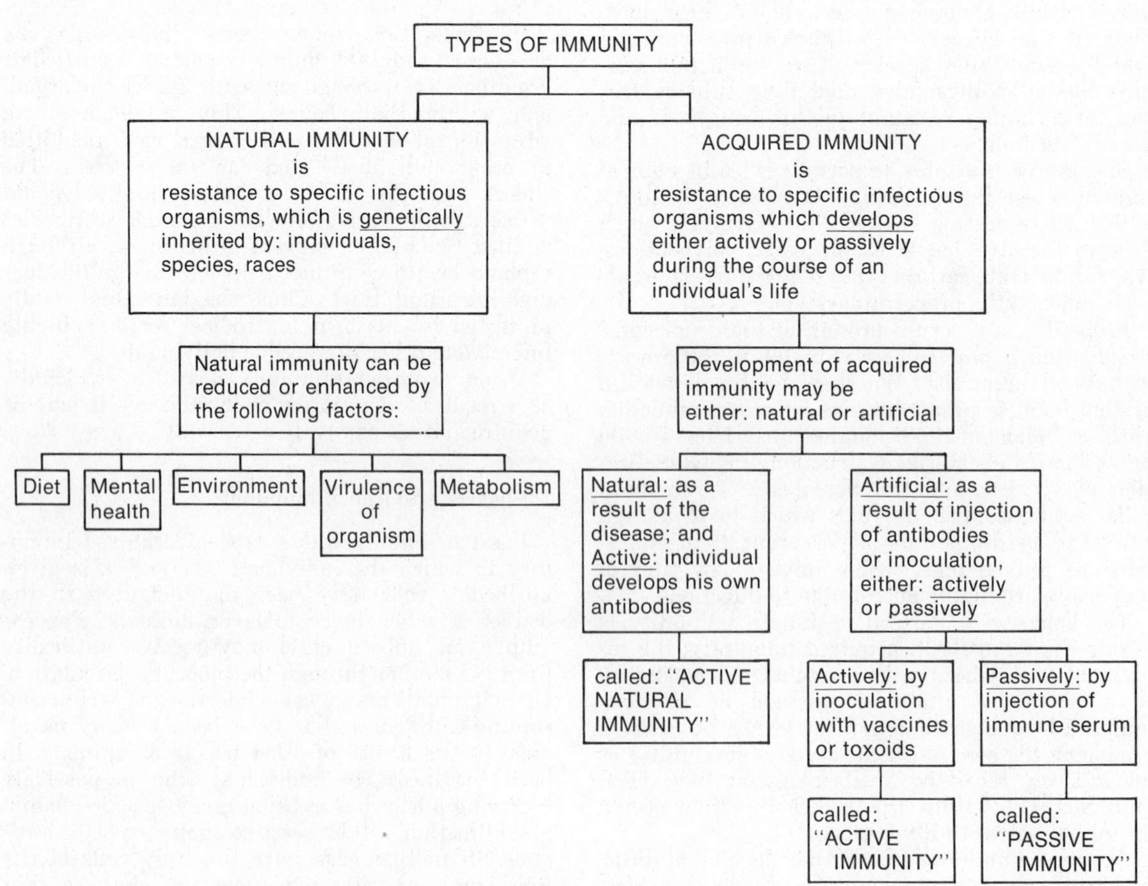

FIGURE 23–1. A comparison between natural and acquired immunity.

previously, vaccines may contain live viruses or bacteria that have been attenuated. For live virus vaccines to function successfully, they must be quite similar to the pathogenic virus, and yet they must be nonvirulent. To render a virus pathogenically harmless, it is passed from one animal to another over and over again, until at last the virus produces a mutant that is relatively harmless. Some examples of live virus vaccine preparations are: (1) the Sabin vaccine for polio, which is given orally; (2) the BCG (the Bacille Calmette-Guérin) vaccine against tuberculosis, which has been attenuated by years of artificial culturing; and (3) live virus vaccines, which have been developed against yellow fever and rabies.

More commonly, vaccines are composed either of killed microorganisms or of the dead products of virulent viruses or bacteria. Two examples of killed cultures are the typhoid vaccine and the Salk vaccine for polio. In the Salk method, killed viruses are injected into the skin, as opposed to the oral Sabin method.

How does the body respond to vaccination with a dead virus?[22] The *initial* reaction to the dead virus vaccine is slow, for it takes approximately seven days for antibodies to begin to appear in the blood. These antibodies rapidly increase their concentrations, reaching a top level of concentration at around the tenth to fourteenth day following vaccination. After the fourteenth day antibody concentration within the blood begins to drop. A few weeks following the initial vaccination, only traces of the antibodies produced remain in the circulation. However, if a patient is given a *second* injection of this same killed virus vaccine following cessation of the primary response, the antigens, this time, will stimulate antibody production within a few days as opposed to a week. Also, the antibodies produced will continue to circulate throughout the body for many months rather than for just a few weeks.

A third method for artificially conferring active immunity is by means of injecting a *toxoid.* Toxoids are bacterial toxins that have been chemically changed and denatured in such a way that they can no longer be harmful to the body. However, since the toxoids remain antigenic, they can act favorably to confer immunity upon the individual into whom they are injected. Two examples of toxoids are the tetanus toxoid and the diphtheria toxoid.

For a diagrammatic conparison of passive and active immunities, see Figure 23-2.

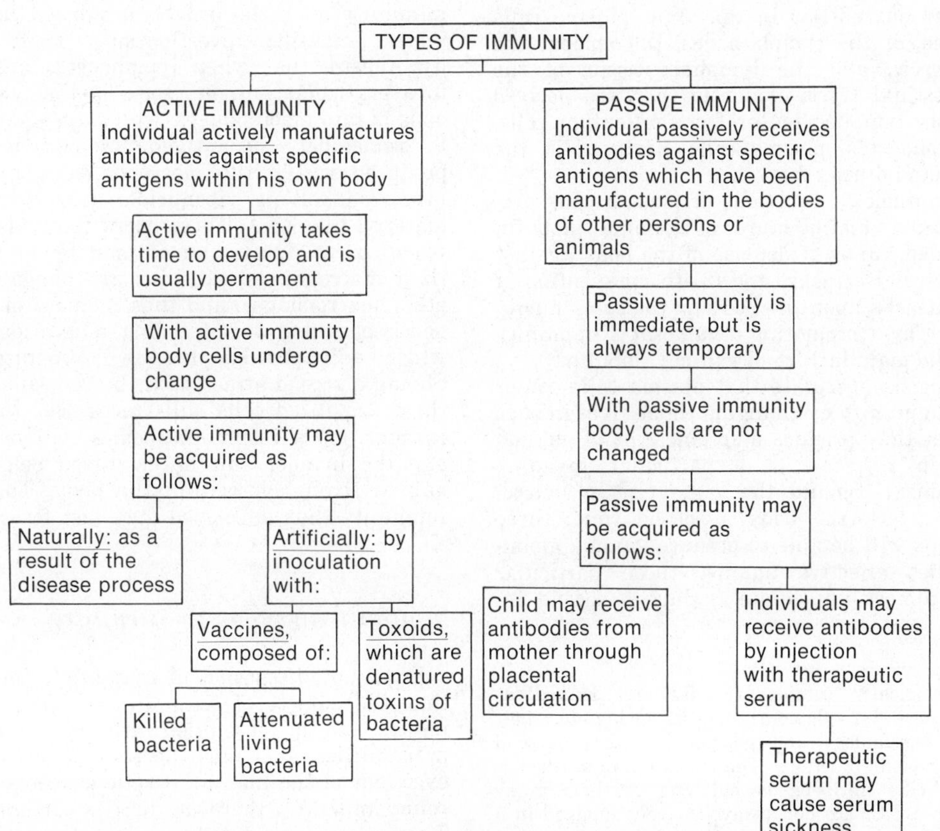

FIGURE 23-2. A comparison of active and passive immunity.

Humoral and Cellular Immunity

In the past, those who studied immunology were sharply divided into two schools of thought: one school was the humoral school of immunity, and the other was the cellular school. Advocates of the humoral school believed that immunity resulted from antibodies present in the body's *serum* rather than in the body's cells. Advocates of the cellular school stressed the notion that immunity relied solely upon *cells,* such as the small lymphocyte, for its transmission. Today these two schools of thought have merged. Modern immunologists now believe that *both* cells and factors in the serum must be present and normal if the immune process is to function successfully. Thus, both humoral and cellular immunity are important components in the body's complex system of defense.

Humoral immunity has been more thoroughly explored by immunologists than has cellular immunity. The antibodies that take part in humoral immunity are *gamma globulins.* Production of circulating gamma globulins and, consequently, of humoral immunity, is the responsibility of the *plasma cell.*

Plasma cells, like the small lymphocytes responsible for cellular immunity, are classified as *immunologically competent cells* (I.C.C.).* As we pointed out earlier in this unit, plasma cells are formed in the lymph nodes, the spleen, the bone marrow, and the lymphoid tissue of the gastrointestinal tract; evidently they are derived either from lymphocytes or from reticulum cells. Like lymphocytes, plasma cells originate in the thymus gland during fetal life.

The immunologic functions of plasma cells are: (1) the *rapid* manufacture of gamma globulin when needed, (2) swift defense of the body against *initial* bacterial attacks, and (3) the prevention of *repeated* attacks upon the body by the *same* microorganism by promoting *humoral* immunity through the manufacture of gamma globulin.

Physiologists speculate that plasma cells confer humoral immunity by changing themselves in such a way that they produce a *specific type* of gamma globulin in response to a particular invading microorganism. Should the same type of microorganism attack the body a second time, these altered cells will be able to produce gamma globulin supplies effective against these particular microbes almost immediately; thus, a second invasion by the microorganisms will be aborted. It is because of the role of plasma cells that we rarely contract the same infectious disease twice. Humoral immunity remains active over a period of from three months to three years.

In contrast to humoral immunity, *cellular immunity* depends upon the presence of *intracellular* antibodies that *remain* with the cells. Thus, those antibodies associated with cellular immunity do *not* circulate in the body fluids as do gamma globulins.

Also, cellular immunity is *slow* acting in comparison with the rapid action of humoral immunity. On the other hand, cellular immunity may last a lifetime in contrast to the rather limited protective span of humoral immunity.

Cellular immunity is established and transmitted by the *small lymphocyte,* an immunologically competent cell that is equal in importance to the plasma cell. Lymphocytes were discussed in some detail in the section on inflammation. You will recall that they originate in the thymus gland during fetal life and arise from the tissues of the lymph nodes, spleen, and bone marrow during adult life. The immunologic functions of lymphocytes are: (1) the promotion of graft rejection and delayed hypersensitivity reactions (sometimes called *cell mediated reactions*), (2) the release of antibodies against antigens during *initial antigenic attacks,* and (3) the prevention of second and third attacks upon the body by the *same* microorganisms by promoting *cellular* immunity within the cell.

Exactly how lymphocytes act to confer cellular immunity upon the body is a subject that is still under scientific investigation. Some theorists hypothesize that when lymphocytes are exposed to a particular antigen, some of the lymphocytes expand into macrophages, which are somehow able to "remember" the antigen.[2] Memory is probably produced within the macrophage by a chemical process involving ribonucleic acid (RNA), or a material like RNA. These particular cells are thus *sensitized* to a particular antigen. When the sensitized macrophages die, they are phagocytized by other macrophages, and thus memory of the antigen is passed on to succeeding generations of cells, which will possibly act as "recognizer cells." Should a second attack occur by the same antigen, these sensitized cells will "recognize" the specific invader. As a result, antibodies will be released and the invader will be destroyed before it can gain a stronghold within the body. The cellular immunity thus developed may last for a lifetime.

CURRENT THEORIES OF IMMUNITY

From our discussion of immunity, you can see that the subject of immunity is often vague in nature, and that it is filled with many possibilities, probabilities, and some theoretic guesswork. However, out of the many theoretic concepts that surround immunity, there are three important theories. These theories not only explain how the normal immune system develops, but they also form the

*Immunologically competent cells are defined as specialized cellular elements which, owing to their particular morphology and physiology, are concerned with immunologic functions. The formation of antibodies against specific antigens is but one of their many roles. While I.C.C. are not always actively engaged in a direct response to an antigen, they are fully competent to do so should the need arise.

basis for understanding the pathology of the immune system as well as the process of transplant rejections.

The first theory, which is widely accepted, explains the role of the thymus gland in the origin of immunologically competent cells, (i.e., plasma cells and lymphocytes). The other two theories explain how antibody production originates and how antibodies form against specific antigens. These theories are called the "instructive theory" and the "clonal selective" theory.

The Role of the Thymus Gland in Immunity

Ancient philosophers considered the thymus gland to be the "seat of the soul," but modern immunologists regard the thymus as the "cornerstone of immunology."[31, 47] The thymus gland is important in immunology because, as recent investigations have proved, the thymus acts as the site of origin for most of the antibody-forming cells that comprise the body's immune system.

Located in the mediastinal cavity, the thymus gland is composed of lymphoid tissue and is situated in front of and above the heart. The cells that comprise this gland are called thymic cells or thymocytes. These cells form rapidly during fetal and early postnatal life. While the thymus gland grows rapidly during the first two years of life, it atrophies during puberty.

Experiments have shown that there are two distinct cell systems that originate in the thymus gland.[36] One system is called the *thymus dependent system,* while the other group of cells is called the *thymus independent system.* Cells belonging to the thymus dependent system differentiate in the thymus gland and eventually develop into *small lymphocytes.* As the lymphocytes mature, they escape from the thymus gland and seed themselves throughout the peripheral lymphoid system, becoming embedded in the lymph nodes and spleen. Once the lymphocytes are mature, they begin to circulate throughout the blood and lymphatic systems, causing the cell-mediated immune responses of graft rejection and delayed hypersensitivity that we mentioned earlier.[34]

Cells belonging to the thymus independent system evolve from the same stem cell (i.e., a cell that gives rise to a specific type of cell), as those belonging to the thymus dependent system. However, thymus independent cells grow and mature in a different chemical environment than do thymus dependent cells. Eventually thymus independent cells come to lodge in the peripheral lymphoidal tissues where they finally are converted to reticulum cells and then possibly into *plasma cells.* Thymus independent cells are thus responsible for humoral immunity and for the secretion of immunoglobins, substances that serve to protect us against bacteria.

In sum, the thymus gland is the birthplace of both lymphocytes and plasma cells and, consequently, of cellular and humoral immunity. As you will see, this role of the thymus gland plays a vital part in the "clonal selective" theory to be discussed shortly, and in the explanation of self-tolerance and autoimmune disease.

Other investigations have demonstrated that the thymus gland, as the cradle of immunity, is vitally important to mammals during the early months of their lives. Immunologists experimenting on the thymus gland of adult and newborn mice have drawn certain conclusions that have implications for the health of mankind.[40] They have found that the thymus gland of an *adult* mouse can be removed with little change, whereas thymectomy in a *newborn* mouse produces the following profound effects upon the animal and upon its immune system: First of all, the animal may die, and at autopsy there may be little lymphoid tissue found; second, these animals fail to reject grafts, and, finally, the thymectomized mice cannot respond to new antigens with proper antibody formation. However, if thymic cells are transfused into thymectomized mice, lymphoid tissues grow again. Such experiments establish that the thymus gland is vital to the development of the immune system and possibly to its restoration following damage or destruction. Moreover, these investigations may have implications for the future of transplant surgery and for the overcoming of the graft rejection mechanism.

Pathology of the thymus gland has been linked with certain clinical problems in immunology in man. For example, tumors in the thymus gland have been found in autoimmune conditions. Also, atrophy of the thymus gland has been definitely associated with hypogammaglobulinemia, which is an abnormally low level of gamma globulin in the blood.[40]

Theories of Antibody Formation

How antibodies are actually formed within the body is a question for which there is as yet no definitive answer. It is clear that immunologically competent cells underlie *all* immune reactions, whether they be humoral or cellular in nature. However, scientists are still searching for the exact process by which these cells manufacture antibodies; this process may have profound implications for those pathologic conditions that are linked with the immune system.

Two major theories of antibody formation have evolved over recent years. They are the "instructive theory" and the "clonal selective" theory. The instructive theory is the older and more classic view. According to this hypothesis, the building up of antibodies against specific antigens is a *continuous* process and occurs throughout a person's life. In contrast, the newer clonal selective theory holds that antibody patterns are established *before birth.* Both theories are accepted in part by many immunologists, and each theory has made its own significant contributions to the field of immunology. Let us now consider the major points of each theory.

The "instructive theory" is based upon the following assumptions:[35]

1. When a foreign antigen enters the body, it makes contact with an immunologically competent cell—probably a plasma cell or lymphocyte. This is a purely random operation, as the antigen can establish contact with *any* immunologically competent cell, and that cell will be able to manufacture antibodies against the antigen. (This point is in direct contrast to the clonal selective theory, in which immunologically competent cells are able to produce only a single type of antibody against a specific antigen.)
2. The antigen, having randomly contacted the immunologically competent cell, is used by that cell as a mold in which to cast its own RNA.
3. The cell's RNA is then remolded and acts as a mold or template for the mass production of identical cells, which will then produce the antibodies that will specifically react against that particular antigen.
4. Thus the antigen (a) acts as a pattern and "dictates" to the immunologically competent cells or "instructs" them to manufacture specific gamma globulin molecules which are precisely tailored to neutralize or inactivate that antigen, and (b) the antigen apparently causes these "instructed" cells to proliferate and to produce large numbers of the necessary antibodies.

In sum, this theory holds that the antigen enters the body as a foreign and unknown substance, and then it imprints its own particular molecular configuration upon antibody-producing cells. These cells then proceed to produce the proper antibodies that will fit that antigen, as a key fits a lock.

Let us now turn to the clonal selective theory of antibody formation. Immunologists use the term "clone" to denote cells that are able to transmit "immunologic memory" to their descendents concerning specific antigens. How these cells develop this capacity to produce antibodies against foreign antigens can be summarized as follows:[35]

1. According to the clonal selective theory, antibody patterns are established around the time of birth or during early embryonic life, rather than following birth, as in the "instructive" theory.
2. In early life, thymic cells (the basis for immunologically competent cells) mutate frequently until a group of at least ten thousand different cells is created. This vast group of cells can *potentially* produce *all possible types of antibodies*—even antibodies against the body's own proteins.
3. During fetal life, body proteins contact these immature immunologic cells. If a cell has the *same* pattern as the *body antigen*, which makes it able to produce antibodies against that antigen, the immature immunologic cell will be destroyed and phagocytized by phagocytes that are circulating within the gland. Gradually, during fetal life, all the body's proteins pass through the thymus gland, and over a period of time, all cells that might potentially react against the body's own proteins are destroyed. The cells left cannot react any more against the "self," but only against those foreign materials that are "stamped" "*not*-self." As a result, the only cells remaining at birth are those cells that respond to *foreign* antigens; all cells that might respond to the body's own constituents will have been phagocytized; thus, *self-tolerance* or *immunologic tolerance* is established.
4. Those immunologic cells that have survived mature as the fetus matures. Then, as we stated earlier, the cells leave the thymus gland and seed themselves throughout the lymphoid tissue:
5. Each of the cells remaining at birth is able to produce only a *single* type of antibody against a *specific antigen*. (Note that this point is in contrast to the "instructive" theory, in which the antigen randomly "contacts" *any* immunologic cell, and that cell, after "instruction" by the antigen, can make antibodies against the antigen.)
6. After birth, should a foreign antigen gain access to the body, that antigen will then travel to the reticuloendothelial system, where it will find a mature immunologic cell with a *predetermined* ability to manufacture specific antibodies against it.
7. The antigen thus "selects" a reticulum cell and activates that cell. The reticulum cell changes into a plasma cell and produces antibodies. The plasma cell then divides and continues to divide for months and even for years. Thus, antibody formation persists and immunity becomes fairly lasting.

The clonal selective theory has not been conclusively proved. However, it explains more satisfactorily than the instructive theory how immunologic tolerance and self-recognition develop in the fetus. This theory also serves as an excellent basis for explaining the development of autoimmune diseases.

PATHOLOGIC CONDITIONS ASSOCIATED WITH THE IMMUNE RESPONSE

Normally the immune response is a homeostatic measure that protects the body from invasion by foreign, antigenic substances. However, the immune response can become pathologic. When immune responses are either deficient, excessive, inappropriate, or abnormal, the pathologic condition that results is called an *immunopathy*. There are four major types of immunopathies, which can be briefly summarized as follows:[48]

1. *Hypo- or agammaglobulinemia*. A failure of response or an inadequate response owing to an inability to synthesize and to maintain a normal level of gamma globulins.
2. *Plasma cell myeloma* (multiple myeloma). An excessive response involving neoplasia* of the immune system that leads to the manufacture of abnormal globulins and an excessive proliferation of plasma cells.
3. *Hypersensitivity or allergy*. An inappropriate and abnormal response to antigens originating outside the body. The allergic state results in such maladies as anaphylaxis, asthma, hay fever, and allergies—food, drug, and plant—and serum sickness.

*Neoplasia is the development of new and abnormal tissues, or neoplasms, which serve no useful purpose in the body.

4. *Autoimmune disease.* An abnormal response in which a person's *own* antibodies and immunologically competent cells react against the cells and tissues of his own body, resulting in symptoms and functional changes. In essence, autoimmune disease proves to be a sensitivity to one's own self and a loss of self-tolerance. Some important autoimmune diseases are Hashimoto's disease, polyarteritis nodosa, disseminated lupus erythematosus, scleroderma, and rheumatoid arthritis.

We shall now briefly discuss each of these important immunopathies. For more detailed information on these conditions, see appropriate sections of the text.

HYPO- OR AGAMMAGLOBULINEMIA—AN INADEQUATE RESPONSE

As we have seen, gamma globulins defend the body against the invasion of foreign antigens such as microorganisms and toxins; gamma globulins are produced by plasma cells in response to these antigens. As long as this mechanism works satisfactorily, the body remains relatively secure against attack by dangerous foreign antigenic substances. However, as with all protective mechanisms, the mechanism of gamma globulin synthesis can fail, or be so inadequate that it is unable to meet the defensive needs of the body. When this happens, the resulting condition is called either hypogammaglobulinemia or agammaglobulinemia. The term *hypo*gammaglobulinemia is more accurate, as gamma globulins are never totally absent from the body's circulation.[66]

There are two major types of hypogammaglobulinemia, congenital and acquired. Individuals with the *congenital* form usually suffer from an atrophy of lymphoid tissue, and they die during childhood from trivial infections. This condition usually appears when the infant is from one to three months old; at this point the antibodies that the mother has passed to her child through the placental circulation have been used up, and the child has lost this valuable form of passive acquired immunity. If congenital hypogammaglobulinemia is present, the child will be unable to synthesize the gamma globulin that will enable it to build an active form of immunity for self-protection.

The *acquired* form of hypogammaglobulinemia develops in adult life, usually in the wake of a serious illness. Adults with this condition suffer severely as a result of minor infections because they lack the antibodies necessary to fight microorganisms. However, persons with hypogammaglobulinemia are still capable of *cellular* immunity, as they usually have a normal number of lymphocytes. You will recall that the lymphocyte is the major element in the development of cellular immunity. Thus, patients with hypogammaglobulinemia experience delayed hypersensitivity reactions* and they reject transplants.

*Delayed hypersensitivity is discussed on p. 181.

The exact cause of hypogammaglobulinemia is not known. However, physicians believe that there may be a *hereditary* basis for this disorder, even in the acquired form.[48] It has been observed that acquired hypogammaglobulinemia often appears in conjunction with such neoplastic disorders as multiple myeloma, lymphoma, and lymphatic leukemia—all conditions that affect the body's reticuloendothelial system. Evidently cancer cells are capable of destroying the sites of gamma globulin production and of replacing lymphoid tissue with cancer cells that are physiologically nonfunctional. Acquired hypogammaglobulinemia also appears secondary to maladies that involve severe protein losses, for example, liver disease, nephrosis, and malnutrition. It is not clear precisely what role a protein deficit plays in the development of acquired hypogammaglobulinemia. Hypogammaglobulinemia is diagnosed on the basis of gamma globulin levels within the blood and by examination of the bone marrow and lymph node biopsy. Treatment of this condition involves the following measures:

1. Patients generally receive regular *monthly intramuscular injections of human gamma globulin,* which of course increases their resistance to infectious diseases.
2. Patients are taught to *increase their resistance* to infectious diseases by proper diet, adequate rest, appropriate clothing, and by avoiding persons with such minor infections as colds and influenza. It is important to remember that an infection that would be minor to the "normal" person could easily prove fatal to an individual with hypogammaglobulinemia.
3. Although *antibiotics* are rarely given prophylactically, for these persons they are immediately given in large doses in the event of infection.
4. In a few selected cases, surgeons have *transplanted lymph nodes* from one identical twin, who does not suffer from hypogammaglobulinemia, to his afflicted brother or sister. Unless transplants of lymph nodes are done between identical twins, the transplant will be rejected. You will recall that patients with hypogammaglobulinemia can reject transplants because these persons have cellular immunity even though they do not have humoral immunity and circulating gamma globulins. Patients receiving transplants who have *normal* gamma globulin production are given corticosteroids to suppress the rejection response. However, to give a patient with hypogammaglobulinemia corticosteroids would defeat the entire purpose of the transplant, because corticosteroids *lower* resistance to infectious diseases. For this reason, the patient with hypogammaglobulinemia who receives corticosteroids to suppress transplant rejection would continue to be highly vulnerable to infectious diseases *despite* his transplanted lymph nodes.[66]
5. In patients with the acquired form of hypogammaglobulinemia, physicians strive to *treat the primary cause* of the condition, for example, nephrosis or leukemia.

When nursing patients with hypogammaglobulinemia, it is your responsibility to guard these patients against dangerous infections. Some guidelines in caring for these individuals are the following:

1. Isolate patients with hypogammaglobulinemia from all other patients with infectious diseases or with contaminated wounds.
2. Observe good handwashing techniques when you work with these individuals.
3. Use careful sterile technique in catheterizations and in dressing changes.
4. Shield these patients from drafts or from becoming overly warm, as colds may result.
5. Do not take care of patients with this diagnosis if you are suffering from a cold, flu, or even a minor infection.
6. Report promptly to the physician any temperature elevation or any sign of infection or illness, so that the doctor may immediately institute antibiotic treatment.

PLASMA CELL MYELOMA (MULTIPLE MYELOMA)—AN EXCESSIVE RESPONSE

As the derivation of the name implies, plasma cell myeloma (*myelos,* marrow, and *oma,* tumor) is a tumor or neoplasm of the bone marrow. The bone marrow is a tissue that is composed of vast numbers of plasma cells. Since plasma cells manufacture gamma globulins, this disease is generally characterized by (1) production of excessive amounts of gamma globulin (hyperglobulinemia) or (2) synthesis of an abnormal and apparently useless type of gamma globulin that fails to properly perform its function of defending the body against foreign organisms.[66] Plasma cell myeloma is further distinguished by the appearance of large amounts of protein in the urine, by abnormal serum proteins, and, unfortunately, by the spread of the neoplasm from the zone of origin to other bones—thus the term "*multiple* myeloma."

This condition is rapidly fatal, killing its victims within six to 12 months. If possible, amputation of the affected bone is the treatment of choice; also, therapeutic agents such as chlorambucil have been given with some success. For further information on this condition, consult Unit XII.

HYPERSENSITIVITY AND ALLERGY—ABNORMAL REACTIONS OF THE IMMUNE SYSTEM

Whereas the immune response is a protective adaptive response designed to guard the body against the invasion of dangerous, toxic substances, the allergic response is an *oversensitive* and often harmful response on the part of the body against foreign substances that may actually be *harmless,* e.g., plant pollens. In other words, in the immune response the body's protective cells *correctly* recognize dangerous intruders, fight them, and often destroy them. Conversely, in an allergic response, the body's protective cells "*overestimate*" the danger from a harmless intruder, start a battle and, in the end, produce needless damage to the body's tissues. As Hans Selye points out: "Whether to fight or not to fight depends upon circumstances. . . . Yet all biologic groups from the microscopic to the geographic are singularly shortsighted when it comes to this alternative."[54] The body, then, like a man or a nation, can make a mistake in sizing up its foes. In the case of a nation, a small and foolish incident can lead to a deadly war. Similarly, in the case of the body, a pollen can lead to severe dyspnea and a tiny bee sting can end in death.

Definitions

The word "allergy" (from *allos,* other, and *ergon,* energy) signifies that the activity of an individual or the energy of the body has in some way been altered.[5]

To the general public, an allergy is an idiosyncrasy that usually develops in response to a pollen, food, dust, plant, or animal hair. Such allergies are widespread in our population. Indeed, they account for many of the constant complaints that we hear around us, such as "Keep the cat away from me. I can't stand cat hair—it makes me sneeze," "Don't give me any strawberries! I break out all over," or "My mother-in-law had a dose of penicillin and nearly died."

Although the term "allergy" is widely used by the public, the word *hypersensitivity* is sometimes used by language purists to designate only those allergic conditions in which a definite immunologic mechanism has been active. Nevertheless, most immunologists *do* use the terms allergy and hypersensitivity interchangeably.

Hypersensitivity is simply an abnormal or unusual reaction to an agent (usually a foreign agent, and commonly a protein) that does not normally produce symptoms in most persons. Thus, only certain people are allergic to pollens, while only certain *other* people are allergic to strawberries. For this reason, allergies are known as "idiosyncratic" disorders.

Types of Allergens

An *allergen* can be defined as any substance with the capacity to create a hypersensitive state or an allergy within the body. Although allergens are highly variable in their chemical makeup, most are protein in nature. However, there are a few nonprotein allergens. For example, some nonprotein drugs and some plant oils have the capacity to cause allergic contact dermatitis.

Major types of allergens can be categorized as inhalants, ingestants, contactants, injectants, and infectants. *Inhalants* include plant pollens and dusts. They may create such problems as seasonal hay fever, seasonal asthma, and allergic rhinitis. Tissues that are particularly vulnerable to inhalants are the conjunctival mucosa, nasal mucosa, and bronchial mucosa. *Ingestants* include foods and drugs. Allergies to ingestants may manifest themselves as allergic rhinitis, asthma, diarrhea, colitis, abdominal pain, dermatitis, urticaria, and migraine headaches. The major organs and tissues affected by ingestants are, therefore, the nasal mucosa, the bronchial mucosa, the gastrointestinal mucosa, the skin, and the brain. *Contactants* include soaps and plants and mainly affect the skin, resulting in such problems as contact dermatitis. *Injectants* include such preparations as foreign sera and drugs; these substances can affect any tissue in the body, causing drug allergy and serum sickness. Finally, *infectants* or *bacteria* can also infect any tissue in the body and can lead to bacterial allergy.

A final and mysterious group of allergens are termed *autoallergens*. Autoallergens are altered and modified tissue allergens that have become so changed by physical, chemical, or infective agents that they can cause a hypersensitive reaction or an allergic reaction within the individual. These allergens, then, develop *within* the body rather than entering the body as a foreign substance from the outside environment. Autoallergens evidently play an important role in the cause of autoimmune disease.

Antibodies Characteristic of Allergic Reactions

The major types of antibodies that are involved in allergic reactions are precipitin antibodies, reagins, and incomplete antibodies that are located within the cells. *Precipitin antibodies* are mature antibodies that are important both in antigen-antibody reactions and in allergic responses. They also play important roles in the more immediate types of hypersensitive reactions such as anaphylaxis and serum sickness. *Reagins* are antibodies that are particularly characteristic of allergic conditions. These antibodies produce no observable immunologic reactions within a test tube; the action of reagins can be demonstrated only in living tissues. A characteristic of reagins is that they become fixed to tissue cells. Sometimes also termed "*skin-sensitizing antibodies*," reagins occur most commonly in hay fever, asthma, and atopic dermatitis.[64] Finally, *incomplete antibodies*, which are still located within the cells, are associated mainly with such modes of delayed hypersensitivity as tuberculin allergy and allergic contact dermatitis.

General Etiologic Factors

The precise factors causing allergy are not known; however, *heredity, congenital factors,* and *contact* between an individual and an allergen are known to play important roles in the development of allergic reactions.

First of all, heredity has been linked with the etiology of allergy because some allergies definitely appear to run in families. Also, allergies appear to affect one tenth of the population more frequently and more severely than other individuals within the population. Moreover, heredity evidently not only determines that a particular individual will be allergic, but also determines the type of allergy that person will experience, as well as the precise allergens to which he will be susceptible. The exact manner in which heredity influences the development of allergic manifestations in a patient is still not clearly understood.

Congenital factors can influence an individual's susceptibility to allergens, because allergens can definitely be passed to the fetus via the placental circulation. Such an allergic sensitivity is *not* the result of hereditary transmission but is acquired, the fetus being actively sensitized during prenatal life. For example, if a mother, during pregnancy, eats large amounts of a high protein food, the child may become overly sensitized to that particular protein while it is still within its mother's uterus. After birth, when the child comes into contact with that protein food, he may then manifest certain clinical signs of allergy.

A final important etiologic factor in allergy is *contact* between the patient and a particular offending allergen. Although heredity plays a role in predisposing an individual to the development of a particular allergy, heredity alone *cannot* cause a person to become allergic. Contact with an allergen is *essential* to the development of any allergy. On the other hand, in certain allergies such as atopic dermatitis, seasonal hay fever, and allergic asthma, contact with the allergen is not sufficient in itself to produce the allergy, because heredity is a major factor. For example, although thousands of people within our population are exposed to certain seasonal pollens every year, only a limited number of persons, with a certain hereditary predisposition toward allergic reactions, develop seasonal hay fever.

There are certain *precipitating or modifying factors* that also influence the development of allergies. The most important of these are psychic stress, infection, endocrine disturbances and, in some instances, pregnancy. Such factors can upset the homeostatic balance between an individual with a hereditary predisposition toward the development of allergy and his allergenic surroundings. For example, some women when pregnant experience severe bronchial asthma attacks for the first time in their lives. Following pregnancy, the same women may have no further attacks. Similarly, certain individuals, when under great nervous stress, will break out in hives. Even the suggestion of an allergic condition can sometimes precipitate the development of an allergic attack. For example, a typist of our acquaintance developed a serious attack of hives while typing a paper on the subject! Thus, the mental state of an individual and his physiologic status *both* profoundly influence whether an individual with a hereditary predisposition toward allergy will actually develop the allergy.

Specific Etiologic Factors

The manifestations of any allergy will depend upon a number of specific factors in addition to the general factors just discussed. The most important are:

1. *The nature of the allergen.* What *type* of allergen is involved? Is it a pollen, dust, food, drug, or microorganism?
2. *The concentration of the allergen.* For example, did the patient receive a large dose of a drug to which he is allergic (i.e., penicillin), or did he receive a small dose? Did an individual with a food allergy eat a large portion of the food he is allergic to or only a bite of it? (Incidentally, chocolate and strawberries are common allergic foods.) Naturally the concentration or amount of the allergen taken in or ingested will make a great difference in the severity of the symptoms.
3. *The type of antibody involved in the reaction.* Is the antibody involved a precipitin, a reagin, or is it an immature antibody that is still located in the cells? As you recall, each type of antibody is important in a particular type of allergic condition.
4. *The type of organ or tissue that is affected by the allergen.* Almost any tissue in the body can be affected. Particularly vulnerable are the brain, skin, gastrointestinal tract, and the mucosa of the conjunctiva, the nose, and the bronchials. The organ affected will greatly influence the type of symptoms produced. Thus, an allergy affecting the gastrointestinal tract will produce diarrhea, nausea, and vomiting; a skin allergy may erupt into eczema and urticaria; and when the brain is affected, the patient may suffer a migraine headache.
5. *The toxic substances released as a result of the allergen-antibody reaction.* The major substances released through an allergic reaction are histamine, or histamine-like materials, acetylcholine, adenosine, bradykinin, heparin, and serotonin and, evidently, a proteolytic enzyme.[22]

Since the substances listed above circulate freely through the body fluids, they can cause symptoms not only at the site of the allergen-antibody reaction, but also at sites far removed from the initial area of contact.

Histamine and histamine-like substances play an important part in allergic reactions, being responsible in large part for many of the symptoms. The most important effects of histamine are upon the circulatory system and upon the bronchial tubes.

Histamine affects the *vascular system* by causing peripheral vascular dilatation which, in turn, leads to peripheral pooling of blood and a decrease in the output of the heart. As a result of the decreased coronary output, capillary pressure becomes great, causing fluid to leak from the vascular system into the tissues, thereby creating *edema* (i.e., excess fluid within the tissues).

Histamine produces a constriction of the smooth muscle of the bronchioles. The bronchiolar effects of histamine are very important in bronchial asthma, as you will see when you study the nursing care of patients with respiratory disease. In sum, many allergic symptoms, such as respiratory wheezing and edema, can be directly traced to the release of histamine during the allergen-antibody reaction.

Major Categories and Types of Allergic Reactions

Allergists usually divide the broad category of hypersensitivity or allergy into two subcategories: immediate hypersensitivity, and delayed hypersensitivity. In *immediate* hypersensitivity, the antibodies that cause the allergic reaction are *humoral* antibodies that circulate in the plasma of the afflicted animal or person. Because of the great importance of humoral antibodies in immediate hypersensitivity, some authorities recommend that immediate hypersensitivity be called *"humoral antibody hypersensitivity."*[11] In contrast, in *delayed* hypersensitivity, circulating humoral antibodies play no role. Instead, those antibodies that cause a delayed hypersensitivity reaction are associated with *lymphoid cells* rather than plasma cells; consequently some authorities recommend that delayed hypersensitivity be called *"cellular hypersensitivity."*[11]

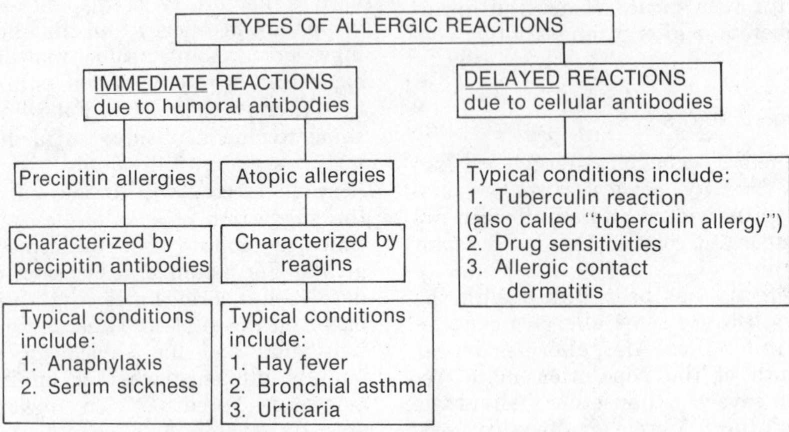

FIGURE 23–3. Major types of allergic reactions.

The two categories of immediate hypersensitivity and delayed hypersensitivity can be broken down further into several distinct subgroups of allergic conditions. Immediate hypersensitivity reactions can be divided into precipitin allergies and atopic allergies. *Precipitin* allergies are characterized by the presence of precipitin antibodies and include anaphylaxis, serum sickness, and the Arthus reaction, which is a local anaphylactic reaction. *Atopic* allergies are characterized by the presence of reagins, or skin-sensitizing antibodies, and include hay fever, urticaria, and bronchial asthma. These immediate hypersensitive states are generally characterized by an increased capillary permeability, edema, and, in some cases, by constriction of the arterioles. The *tuberculin reaction* is the best known subcategory of *delayed* hypersensitivity. Other types of delayed hypersensitivity reactions are allergic contact dermatitis and some drug sensitivities. For a diagrammatic summary of the major types of allergic reactions, see Figure 23–3.

Immediate Hypersensitivity: Precipitin Allergies. As stated previously, the most important precipitin allergies are anaphylaxis and serum sickness. Let us briefly look at these entities individually, and examine their relationship to each other.

ANAPHYLAXIS. Anaphylaxis is one of the most dramatic and also one of the most feared of the allergic reactions. Its development depends upon the presence of *circulating precipitating gamma globulin antibodies.* For this reason, anaphylaxis will not affect individuals suffering from hypogammaglobulinemia, although these people may develop *delayed* hypersensitivity reactions.[11]

Anaphylaxis can occur in any species of animal—man, dog, and guinea pig, to name but a few. Fortunately it is relatively rare in man, but anaphylaxis does occur in humans as a result of injections of vaccines, drugs, and sera. For example, penicillin and antidiphtheritic serum can cause anaphylactic reactions in susceptible individuals. Another important cause of anaphylaxis among human beings is bee or wasp stings. Indeed, individuals have been known to die as a result of a bee sting, being overwhelmed by the violent reaction.

The major characteristics of anaphylaxis are as follows:

1. Anaphylactic shock is *sudden* in its development, and its highly dramatic symptoms last for only a brief period of time.
2. Anaphylaxis is an *acquired* type of allergy and does not seem to depend upon hereditary factors.
3. The sera of individuals who have suffered from an anaphylactic attack contain circulating humoral antibodies. These antibodies can be *demonstrated in the laboratory.*
4. It is possible to induce anaphylactic shock artificially in laboratory animals, and to accidentally produce it in man by giving him a *second dose* or injection of an antigen against which he has been previously sensitized.

The *symptoms* of anaphylaxis are similar to those that occur after an injection of histamine. Thus, patients with anaphylactic shock suffer from spasms of their smooth muscles, urticaria, profound respiratory distress, asphyxia, and circulatory collapse. As a result of circulatory collapse, the patient's blood tends to pool in his vascular system and edema occurs; his heart decreases its output of blood, which creates signs of shock and fainting. Thus, an alternative term for anaphylaxis is *"anaphylactic shock."* Other symptoms are incontinence, fever, dilated pupils, a loss of consciousness, and convulsions. In extreme cases, death may result in from five to 10 minutes after the onset of the attack. Sometimes, following partial recovery from the attack, patients develop neurologic complications. Such complications, fortunately, are rare.

Anaphylactic shock occurs in human beings under the following conditions:

1. *The administration of* any drug, vaccine, *or* sera *given* parenterally, *provided the patient has been previously sensitized to these drugs, or to substances chemically similar to the drugs.*
2. *The administration of therapeutic sera, following a sensitizing dose of sera given 10 days earlier.*
3. *The administration of* oral *penicillin, provided the patient has been previously sensitized to penicillin.*

The necessary precautions that you should take in administering drugs parenterally or penicillin orally will be discussed shortly.

How is anaphylactic shock treated? First, anaphylaxis constitutes an *emergency.* There is no time to waste, as the patient may expire within minutes! This is an outline of the major therapies employed in anaphylactic shock.

1. Drug therapy to halt the deadly symptoms of anaphylaxis.
   a. Antihistamines to halt the action of histamine upon the blood vessels and bronchioles of the patient.
   b. Epinephrine solution to counteract the action of histamine.
   c. Corticosteroids such as hydrocortisone sodium succinate USP (Solu-Cortef) to aid in recovery following the initial attack.
2. Oxygen therapy to counteract asphyxia.
3. Maintenance of an airway.
4. Correction of shock.
   a. Trendelenburg position to counteract shock.*
   b. Levarterenol bitartrate USP (Levophed, norepinephrine) 0.2 per cent solution by intravenous drip to elevate blood pressure.*
   c. Metaraminol bitartrate USP (Aramine) by intravenous drip to elevate blood pressure.*

*The use of the Trendelenburg position and the administration of vasoconstrictors such as Levophed or Aramine are not accepted by all physicians. These controversial treatments are discussed further on pp. 282–286 in the chapter on shock.

Drug therapy. The major drugs used in anaphylactic shock are antihistamines, epinephrine, and the corticosteroids. These drugs should be on hand whenever parenteral medication is being given or whenever penicillin is being administered either orally or intramuscularly. Let us very briefly consider each of these drugs, as they are very important not only in anaphylactic shock, but in other allergies as well.

The antihistamines. You will recall from our previous discussion that histamine is released in antibody-antigen reactions. Moreover, it is histamine that causes the major vascular and bronchial symptoms seen in anaphylaxis. Consequently the administration of an *anti*histamine drug should help to abate the symptoms to a certain degree. Antihistamines cannot block the release of histamines, but they act to block the action of histamine upon blood vessels and bronchioles, thereby alleviating the symptoms caused by this action.

The antihistamine drug most commonly used in anaphylaxis is

> diphenhydramine hydrochloride (Benadryl) aqueous, 5-20 mg. I.V.

Benadryl has the following side effects: sedation, lowered concentration, headache, flushing, blurred vision, dizziness, lethargy, dermatitis, bronchial asthma, anorexia, nausea, vomiting, diarrhea, poor coordination, and paresthesias. In extreme cases, patients may develop insomnia, tremors, palpitation, and even convulsions—all symptoms of excitement.[20] When caring for patients on large doses of Benadryl I.V., remember:

1. *Make certain the side rails are up on patient's bed, as Benadryl produces sedation.*
2. *Watch for transitory irritation at injection site.*
3. *Do not allow patient to ambulate without supervision, or to operate an automobile until the effects of the drug have worn off.*

Epinephrine. An excellent preparation for emergency purposes, epinephrine is a hormone secreted by the medulla and is a sympathomimetic drug. Because its actions on the body are directly opposite to those of histamine, epinephrine acts to counteract the actions of histamine. Consequently it can halt anaphylactic symptoms and reverse those pathologic changes that have already taken place. Epinephrine acts to: stimulate the myocardium, increase cardiac output, increase blood pressure, and relax the smooth muscles of the respiratory tract (thereby relieving the asphyxia and the sense of suffocation associated with anaphylactic shock).

Epinephrine is a highly toxic drug, causing such symptoms as nervousness, tremor, palpitation, anxiety, headache, sweating, hypertension, dyspnea, tachycardia, ventricular fibrillation, pulmonary edema, and cerebral vascular accidents. When giving epinephrine, it is important to watch for signs of *hypotension,* one of the most important secondary effects of the drug. Since hypotension in an anaphylactic patient will only serve to increase his already shocked state, the blood pressure of a patient on epinephrine must be monitored continuously. The standard dose of epinephrine in the treatment of anaphylactic shock is as follows:

> Epinephrine solution, 1 ml. of 1:1000 solution (1 mg.) I.M. immediately, to be repeated in 5 to 10 minutes and as needed.[6]

If the patient fails to respond immediately to epinephrine given I.M., the physician may then order the following:

> Epinephrine solution 1:1000, 0.1–0.4 ml. diluted in 10 ml. of saline given *very slowly* I.V.[6]

As you prepare the epinephrine solution for administration to the patient, be careful not to use a bottle in which the solution has turned brown or has precipitated.

Corticosteroids. Corticosteroids are commonly given in allergic conditions for their anti-inflammatory action. In the treatment of anaphylactic shock, steroids probably act too slowly to be valuable in the initial attack of anaphylaxis, although they may be helpful once the emergency is over.[4] The steroids of choice to be used in anaphylaxis are the following:

> Hydrocortisone sodium succinate (Solu-Cortef), 100–250 mg.

or

> Prednisolone hemisuccinate (Metacortelone), 50–100 mg. in water or saline, given by intravenous infusion over a period of 30 seconds following the administration of epinephrine. Both these medications are used in prolonged reactions.

Although cortisone helps to reduce the inflammatory symptoms arising from allergies, it also has profound side effects: water retention, sodium retention and edema, hypertension, hyperglycemia, loss of potassium, negative nitrogen balance, hirsutism, acne, peptic ulcer, and lowered resistance to infectious agents.

Oxygen therapy. Since patients with anaphylaxis suffer from bronchial constriction and asphyxia, their need for oxygen is great. Blue recommends that 40 per cent oxygen be given rather than 100 per cent oxygen,[4] as the latter tends to actually depress the respiratory center. While some authorities recommend positive pressure oxygen therapy, another believes that positive pressure breathing is highly dangerous for the patient suffering from vascular collapse due to anaphylactic shock.[4, 6]

Maintenance of an open airway. Because asphyxia is present, cyanosis is a not uncommon symptom of anaphylactic shock.

> *Be prepared to administer mouth-to-mouth resuscitation should the patient become cyanotic.*

Remember, intermittent positive pressure breathing by means of mechanical respiration is risky in the patient suffering from severe vascular collapse.

Prevention and correction of shock. Severe shock in anaphylaxis may be prevented by: (1) the use of the shock or Trendelenburg position, (2) constant monitoring of blood pressure and pulse, and (3) the use of vasopressor drugs. Important vasopressors are:

- Levarterenol bitartrate (norepinephrine, Levophed) USP 0.2 per cent, 4 ml. per one thousand ml. of 5 per cent dextrose solution (or dextrose in saline solution) by intravenous drip.
- Metaraminol bitartrate (Aramine), a cardiotonic drug as well as a vasopressor, 0.5 to 5.0 mg. I.V. or 15 to 100 mg. by slow infusion in 250 to 500 ml. of 5 per cent dextrose solution I.V.

Both Levophed and Aramine are extremely dangerous drugs. Both are capable of causing sloughing of the tissues around the needle site as well as a severe elevation in blood pressure. In caring for patients on these vasopressor drugs, remember the following:*

> 1. *Check the injection site every few minutes for signs of infiltration of the medication. Remember that infiltration of Levophed or Aramine can cause tissue sloughing and gangrene!*
> 2. *Continually monitor the blood pressure and pulse of patients on these drugs. Adjust the rate of flow to maintain a constant blood pressure at the level ordered by the doctor.*
> 3. *Never leave a patient on Aramine or Levophen unattended. During your absence from the bedside, the I.V. drip may begin to accelerate or the needle may slip out of the vein, causing this necrotizing solution to infiltrate into the patient's tissues.*

Obviously it is far better to *prevent* the development of anaphylactic shock than to be forced to treat it. There are several precautionary measures that physicians and nurses can take to prevent anaphylactic shock. First of all, physicians should use *caution* in the prescription of potentially dangerous drugs, especially if the patient under their care has a history of such allergies as hay fever or bronchial asthma. Second, it is the doctor's and nurse's responsibility to ask the patient if he has suffered from allergic attacks in the past whenever *any* drug is to be administered parenterally, or penicillin is to be given *either* orally or parenterally. Some important questions that you might specifically ask your patient *prior* to the administration of these drug preparations are:

1. Has the patient ever been troubled by hay fever, asthma, dermatitis, or any other type of allergy?
2. Has the patient ever had an injection of the drug that you are now going to administer?
3. Has the patient ever experienced an allergic reaction to the particular drug that you are preparing to give him?
4. Has the patient who is to receive therapeutic sera containing gamma globulin had an earlier injection of sera within the last 10 days? (You will recall that anaphylactic shock may follow a second injection of therapeutic serum provided the person had been sensitized to the serum 10 days earlier.)

Carefully evaluate the patient's answers to these questions, and be prepared to take the following actions:

> Remember:
> 1. *If the patient does have a definite history of allergy, check with the physician* before *you give the drug to make sure that the doctor is aware of this fact.*
> 2. *If the patient has had a prior allergic reaction to the particular drug that you are now going to give him,* do not *give the drug either orally or parenterally! Report your findings immediately to the physician.*
> 3. *If you are preparing to give the patient a therapeutic serum, and he has had an injection of this same serum 10 days earlier,* do not *give the serum and report your findings to the physician. The doctor will undoubtedly wish to first test the patient for hypersensitivity to the serum by administering a small amount of the medication by intracutaneous injection.*
> 4. *If the patient has a history of allergy to any drug, mark this information* clearly *on the patient's chart, on the Kardex, and at the patient's bedside. Remember that a sick individual may not always be able to inform nurses and other personnel of his vulnerable allergic state.*

There is a third major preventive measure against anaphylactic shock. When you are preparing to give any drug parenterally or to administer penicillin either orally or parenterally, be certain that *emergency drugs are readily available.* As one authority states:

> No potentially anaphylactic parenteral medication should be given without an emergency tray ready at hand containing the following items: (1) injectable aqueous epi-

*Levophed and Aramine are discussed under Shock, and in the care of the patient with myocardial infarction.

nephrine 1:1000, (2) appropriate syringes and needles, (3) tourniquet or sphygmomanometer cuff, (4) oxygen supply, (5) tracheotomy set, (6) intubation and laryngoscopic equipment, (7) scalpels and forceps, (8) intravenous antihistamine solution, (9) polyethylene intravenous tubing, (10) intravenous drip equipment, (11) intravenous steroid solution ampules, and (12) cardiac stimulants.[4]

As a fourth precaution, some physicians recommend giving the patient a dose of an antihistaminic drug such as Benadryl prior to the parenteral administration of a medication to which the patient may be allergic, especially penicillin. Also, physicians may occasionally order that a small amount of cortisone be given prior to the administration of potentially dangerous drugs. However, the use of cortisone in this instance is controversial.

As a final preventive measure, if a patient is definitely allergic to a drug that he *must* receive, physicians will then attempt to *hyposensitize* or *desensitize* the patient against the allergic effects of the drug. Hyposensitization procedures will be discussed shortly.

Since anaphylactic shock may develop from *bee* or *insect stings* as well as from drugs, let us briefly consider some precautionary measures that persons susceptible to such stings should be taught to observe. Hypersensitive persons must avoid: (1) wearing perfume and bright colors, as these attract insects; (2) excessive exposure of their skin, especially around the neck; (3) sitting or lying down on the grass in areas where there are many bushes, hedges, flowers, and trees; and (4) going barefoot. Moreover, persons susceptible to insect stings should carry emergency insect bite kits and know how to use them.[4] One authority recommends that the doctor or nurse should teach hypersensitive persons to administer epinephrine to themselves.[13] At least, epinephrine should be carried by the individual along with a card stating that he is allergic to insect stings and should have *immediate* care if stung. Finally, victims of insect stings should be skin tested and then desensitized against the particular species of insect to which they are allergic.

SERUM SICKNESS. In contrast to anaphylactic shock, *serum sickness* is a generally nonfatal, self-limiting ailment that occurs within one to three weeks following exposure to an antigenic drug substance. On the other hand, serum sickness is similar to anaphylactic shock in that it can occur after the administration of *any* drug and after the administration of any foreign serum, such as the tetanus or diphtheria antitoxins.

Since serum sickness does not develop immediately, you may wonder why it is classified, along with anaphylactic shock, as an "immediate" hypersensitivity. Serum sickness is classified as an immediate rather than as a delayed reaction because it is attributable to the presence of *humoral antibodies* and not to the presence of cellular antibodies. It is because of this confusion in terminology that one authority suggests that we classify serum sickness as a "humoral antibody allergy of delayed appearance."[11]

Let us briefly consider the *pathogenesis* of serum sickness since it is the commonest of the precipitin allergies. The usual course of events that ultimately lead to serum sickness is as follows: (1) A patient is injected with a particular serum or he is given a particular drug against which he has no immune bodies. (Note how serum sickness differs from anaphylaxis in that the individual has *not* been previously sensitized to the drug or serum.) (2) Within 10 days antibodies have formed against the foreign antigen, which still continues to be present in the blood. (3) An extensive, overall allergic reaction takes place.

The *treatment* of serum sickness depends upon the severity of the reaction. The drugs generally used in mild reactions are antihistamines and aspirin. In more severe types of serum sickness reactions, not only antihistamines are given, but epinephrine and cortisone as well. Very severe forms of serum sickness should be treated in the same manner as anaphylactic shock.

Serum sickness can be prevented by the same precautions that prevent anaphylactic shock. In review, to prevent either of these reactions, remember the following rules:

1. *Know your patient's past history of allergy.*
2. *Know specifically what drugs your patient has been allergic to in the past.*
3. *Immediately report any unusual findings concerning the patient's allergic history to the doctor.*
4. *If the patient has a history of allergy, mark this information clearly on his chart, his Kardex, and at his bedside.*

Immediate Hypersensitivity: Atopic Allergies. The word "atopic" originally meant an atypical or strange disease. In contrast to precipitin allergies, atopic allergies are apparently linked with heredity. Thus, we find that atopic hypersensitivities to allergens appear in approximately 10 per cent of the population, and that the afflicted individuals typically have a family history of atopic allergies.

The *antibodies* involved in atopic conditions are called reagins or skin-sensitizing antibodies. As we said earlier, an outstanding characteristic of reagins is that they cannot be detected in a test tube, but only in living tissue.

Pathologically atopic hypersensitive reactions tend to affect the *skin* and *mucous membranes* in particular. The major *types* of atopic allergy are hay fever, eczema, urticaria, allergic purpura, allergic migraine, and allergic asthma.

HAY FEVER. Hay fever is a seasonal allergy that is caused by contact with such allergens as tree pollens, grasses, or plants, e.g., ragweed. The major problem in hay fever is edema and congestion of the mucous membranes of the nose as a result of the release of histamine. Major signs and symptoms of hay fever are: inflammation of the conjunctivae and tearing, bouts of violent sneezing, and discharge of watery substance from the nose. Hay fever can be treated by first skin testing the patient to see to what particular substances he is allergic, and then slowly hyposensitizing him against the particular allergen. The drugs of choice in the treatment of hay fever are *antihistamines,* which help to counteract the effects of histamines upon the blood vessels and thereby help to prevent the symptoms of hay fever.

URTICARIA. Urticaria comes from the Latin *urtica,* nettle. This atopic allergy, which is sometimes called "the hives," is the result of contact between a person with a hereditary predisposition and such allergens as plants, foods, pollens, certain drugs, and insect venom. Externally urticaria is distinguished by the appearance of large welts or wheals, and internally by small areas of edema that appear throughout the internal organs. The signs of urticaria are probably due to the dilatation of arterioles and to the leakage of fluid out of the capillaries into the tissue spaces. Treatment involves avoidance of the allergen, and drug therapy with antihistaminic drugs. For certain patients the doctor may order epinephrine or ephedrine subcutaneously. Cortisone is sometimes used in more severe cases of hives.

ALLERGIC ASTHMA. Allergic asthma, also known as bronchial asthma, is a common condition, affecting individuals with a hereditary predisposition to the development of allergy. In this type of asthma, the bronchial walls are hypersensitive to foreign substances such as egg whites, plant pollens, vegetable dust, and face powders. In addition, there can be sensitivity to certain bacteria that normally dwell within the respiratory tract. Thus, the individual may be hypersensitive to both intrinsic and extrinsic agents. Upon exposure to these antigenic agents, individuals prone to bronchial asthma suffer from constriction of bronchial passages and edema of the mucous membranes of the bronchi. Bronchial constriction and edema are the basis of such symptoms as dyspnea (especially upon exertion), severe wheezing, and a sense of suffocation.

In the treatment of bronchial asthma, antihistamines are of little value. For mild and moderate attacks, *epinephrine* is the drug of choice. The usual dosage is:

> Epinephrine injection (1:1000) 0.2 to 0.5 ml. subcutaneously. Repeat every 1 to 2 hours in moderate attacks.

Epinephrine may also be used in spray form. Other drugs that are used in the treatment of this condition are aminophylline, ephedrine, and ACTH. As in other atopic allergies, it is important for the patient to avoid, as much as possible, the specific allergen that is causing his problem.

Bronchial asthma is an important and common disease entity that will be discussed further in the unit on respiratory disorders.

Delayed Hypersensitivity (Hypersensitivity: Bacterial, Tuberculin, Infection, or Cellular). Delayed hypersensitivity is best exemplified by the *tuberculin reaction,* which will be considered further under the discussion of the *Care of the Tuberculosis Patient.*

The tuberculin test is used to detect the presence of tuberculosis infection in man, and it is based upon a positive reaction to an injection of tuberculin. Tuberculin is a sterile preparation of a bacterial protein obtained from a culture medium. Tuberculin is either injected intradermally as in the Mantoux test, rubbed onto the skin as in the von Pirquet test, or applied to the skin on a piece of gauze as in the Vollmer patch test. If the individual being tested does not have tuberculosis, there will be no reaction to these tests. However, if the patient is or has been infected by the tubercle bacillus, a local inflammatory reaction will occur on his skin within 48 to 96 hours. The fact that an individual with tuberculosis reacts in a positive manner to the tuberculin test indicates that his cells have become sensitized to the tubercle bacillus.

Other types of delayed reaction allergies are (1) *contact sensitivities,* which result from contact with such allergens as poison ivy; (2) *drug sensitivities* due to the administration of sulfonamides, penicillin, and other antibiotics;* and (3) *infection allergies* due to contact with certain bacteria, viruses, spirochetes, and parasites.[11, 22] In all these conditions, humoral antibodies within the plasma are unimportant and have no effect; the hypersensitive reaction takes place on the surface of, or within, cells that have previously been sensitized by contact with an allergen.

Diagnosis of Allergic Conditions

To discover whether a person has an allergy and, if so, exactly what allergen is creating the problem, it is necessary for the doctor, nurse, and patient all to act as detectives. Together they will need to explore the patient's past history, his present health status, his home environment, his social habits, and the conditions under which he generally works. To diagnose the presence of an allergy as well as the causative allergen involved, the following three avenues of investigation must be carefully pursued: (1) a complete history, including a medical history, family history, and a social history; (2) a complete physical examination, including certain laboratory procedures; and (3) allergy tests, which may include skin tests, mucous membrane tests, and elimination diets.

The Complete History. The complete history will include a past medical history, a family history, and a social history. We have listed some pertinent questions that should be answered concerning the patient's past and present life, and his state of health.

---

*Penicillin, one of the most common causes of anaphylactic shock, also can act as an etiologic factor in delayed allergic reactions.

I. *Past History of Allergic Problems*
1. Has the patient experienced an allergic reaction to such typical allergens as pollens, plants, certain foods, cat or dog hair, cleansing fluids, soaps, or face powders?
2. Has the patient noted any seasonal bouts of sneezing, wheezing, tearing, asthmatic attacks, or sensitivity to particular foods? Are the attacks seasonal, semiyearly, or yearly?
3. Has the patient been particularly prone to colds and flus over the years?
4. If the patient is presently experiencing allergic symptoms, has he experienced these same symptoms in the past?
5. Where was the patient living and what type of occupation was he in when he first experienced the symptoms of allergy?
6. What has been the course of the allergy since the first attack?

If the patient is a woman, you will want to ask her the following:

7. Did the patient develop her allergy during pregnancy? Do the symptoms of allergy appear during *every* pregnancy? Do the symptoms of allergy disappear following the child's birth?
8. Does the patient notice a change in her symptoms when she is menstruating?
9. Did the allergy first develop during the patient's menopause?

II. *Family History of Allergic Problems*
1. Does the patient have any relatives who have similar symptoms as a result of contact with particular allergens?
2. Have any relatives of the patient had to be treated for allergic conditions?
3. Specifically, what types of allergic conditions have family members suffered?

III. *Social and Environmental History*
1. In what type of physical environment does the patient live? Does he live in the country where he would contact various animal danders, or does he live in a factory area where various soots and pollutants might be in the air? Does he live in a heavily forested area where the air, during certain seasons, is heavy with pollens, or does he live in a very windy location where dusts and pollens are constantly circulating around him? Is his home located on a tree-lined street or are there trees surrounding his home—trees that might carry a pollen to which the patient is allergic?
2. Does the patient have a pet cat, dog, or horse, and are there many animals in his neighborhood?
3. What types of fabrics are used in the patient's home? Does the patient have cotton or wool blankets on his bed? Of what material are the curtains made? What types of rugs are on the floors?
4. What type of heating does the patient have in his home? Does he have air conditioning, or are the windows left open in the summer?
5. What types of foods do the patient and his family enjoy? What are some typical menus in his household? Does the patient eat a great deal of chocolate, eggs, shellfish, strawberries, or wheat products—all foods that can act on certain patients as allergens? If the patient does ingest these types of foods, has he noticed any reaction after eating them?
6. What types of drugs does the patient take? If he takes any particular drug continually, has he ever had a reaction to that drug? Has he ever experienced an allergic reaction to *any* drug?
7. Does the patient notice the appearance of allergic symptoms when he is overly tired or when he is under emotional tension or strain?

The answers to these questions can provide valuable clues as to whether a patient is experiencing an allergy and what the allergen involved might be. In no other condition is it of greater importance to take a thorough history and to investigate as many aspects of the patient's immediate and past environment as possible.

The Physical Examination. Following history taking, the patient will next be given a complete physical examination, with special attention being paid to the site of his symptoms. For example, if the patient has hay fever, the doctor will want to examine the mucous membranes of the nose very carefully. If the patient has hives, naturally the doctor will want to examine the skin. When a patient experiences dyspnea and asthma, the doctor may wish to order an electrocardiogram to rule out the possibility that the attacks of dyspnea are due to a heart condition. Finally, the doctor may also want to check the patient's sinuses, tonsils, and teeth to learn if these organs are acting as foci for infection.[64]

Laboratory work is an important part of the physical examination of the allergic patient. Be prepared for the doctor to order a urine specimen, blood serology, and a complete blood count. In addition, a differential white count will probably be ordered to detect eosinophilia (an increase in eosinophils), a condition that occurs in allergic reactions. In some cases the patient's nasal secretions and sputum may be examined for the presence of eosinophils.

Tests for Allergies. Major types of allergy tests are: skin tests, mucosal tests, and food diaries and elimination diets.

SKIN TESTS. If the patient's history and physical examination point to the possibility of an allergic condition, the doctor will then probably order skin tests in order to confirm that possibility. Skin tests are generally done in a series: for example, the first allergen to be used in testing might be made up from pollens, the second allergen from weeds, the third from dusts, the fourth from horse dander, and so forth.

The major types of skin tests are the scratch test, the intracutaneous test, and the patch or contact test. The *scratch* and *intracutaneous tests* depend upon the use of a control site and a test site. A small amount of allergen is placed on or into the test site, while only the diluent is used on the control site. After a predetermined time period, both sites are compared and the test is read as either positive or negative.

To administer a *scratch* test, the doctor or nurse first makes a small superficial test scratch approximately an eighth of an inch long on the patient's forearm or on the inner aspect of his arm, and a *control scratch* on the other arm. Next, the allergen is applied to the test scratch in either liquid, paste, or powdered form. When the allergen is in powdered form, a diluent is first placed on the test site and then the powdered allergen. Diluent only is placed on the control scratch. In approximately 10 to 30 minutes, the test scratch and the control scratch are compared. If the patient has had a reaction to the allergen, both a wheal and a zone of redness will appear around the test site. If the patient has had no reaction to the allergen being tested, both the control and the test sites will appear the same.

With the *intracutaneous test,* the allergen is diluted and then injected into and not through the epidermis. The equipment you will need to gather for an intracutaneous (or intradermal) test is as follows:[64]

> Sterile liquid allergen 0.02 ml.
> A tuberculin syringe
> A small needle, 26 gauge, one fourth of an inch long.

The intracutaneous test is similar to the scratch test in that there are a test site and a control site. To administer the test, the allergen is injected into the epidermis of the test site and only diluent is injected into the epidermis of the control site. Following approximately a 10-minute wait, both the control site and the test site are checked for a reaction. As with the scratch test, a positive reaction generally involves the appearance of a wheal and an area of redness that surrounds the test site.

A *patch test* is primarily used to test for allergens causing contact dermatitis. To perform a patch test, a little of the allergen is simply applied directly against the skin and then the allergen is covered with an airtight patch. After 48 to 72 hours the skin that has been in contact with the allergen may be examined for signs of redness, swelling, or the appearance of wheals. This test is particularly useful in testing for allergies to soap, cleansing agents, and hair dyes.

MUCOUS MEMBRANE TESTS. Two important mucous membrane tests are the ophthalmic or eye test, and the nasal or sniff test. To administer the *eye test,* the physician may choose to use either a liquid extract or a dry powder of the suspected allergen. In performing the test, the physician simply places a drop or two of the liquid or a few grains of the powder into the conjunctival sac of one eye, which is designated as the test eye. No preparations are placed in the opposite eye—the control eye. After five to 10 minutes, the two eyes are compared. If the eye test is positive, the patient may experience tearing as well as itching of the conjunctiva. When reactions are positive, it is important to remove the allergen from the conjunctival sac. Removal can be facilitated by flushing out the conjunctival sac with normal saline. Following removal of the allergen, one or two drops of aqueous epinephrine (1:1000) are then instilled into the conjunctival sac.[64]

In the *nasal* or *sniff test* one nostril serves as a test site, while the other nostril serves as a control. The patient sniffs the allergen (which is either in the form of a spray or dry powder) into one nostril, while holding the other nostril closed. If the patient has a positive reaction to the allergen, he will sneeze, cough, experience nasal congestion, and have a watery discharge from the nostril. The major limitation of this test is that it causes considerable discomfort by inducing troublesome nasal symptoms.

FOOD DIARIES AND ELIMINATION DIETS. Patients who appear to be suffering from a food allergy may be asked to keep a food diary in order to ascertain the particular food or foods to which they are allergic. In this method of testing, the patient first of all keeps a daily written record for a week or more of all the foods that he eats. Then the physician will ask the patient to remove one item of food at a time from his diet for a designated period. For example, the patient may be asked to remove all wheat products from his diet for a period of one week. If the patient continues to have allergic symptoms, he may then remove all milk products from his diet for a similar period. If the symptoms still persist, he may next remove chocolate preparations from his diet, and so on, until at last the specific allergen causing the problem is found. Sometimes elimination programs similar to that used with food are used to eliminate cosmetics and clothing believed to act as allergens. Such a program can be quite exhausting and sometimes disappointing to the patient. Therefore, it will be up to you as a nurse to encourage the patient to continue in the search for the allergen that is creating his symptoms. Often you will be the person designated to explain to the patient the process of an elimination diet, and perhaps even to set up a specific program for him.

In sum, the process of searching for a causative allergen in an allergic condition is an exhaustive, meticulous, and precise procedure. The time involved in diagnosing the allergen responsible for an allergy may run into weeks or even months. Once the allergen itself has been found, then the long process of treatment must begin.

General Principles of Treatment in Allergic Conditions

Although the treatment of individual allergies will be presented in appropriate sections of the text, we shall outline here some broad general principles of treatment that are used in many allergic conditions. Major methods of therapy are as follows:

Avoidance of Specific Allergens. Despite the fact that a specific allergen may cause a patient to suffer a multitude of miserable symptoms, the avoidance of that allergen may, nevertheless, cause considerable upheaval in the patient's life. Although avoiding the allergen may relieve symptoms, such avoidance may also mean that the patient may have to change his place of residence, change his job, or give up certain personal enjoyments in his life (for example, pets). Some of the most common means by which persons avoid specific allergens are as follows:

> The individual may move away from his neighborhood or, in extreme cases, may even move from one part of the country to another part (i.e., he may move from a wet area of the country like Seattle where pollens abound, to a hot dry section of the country such as Arizona).

> The person may be forced to change his occupation. For example, if the patient sells fabrics and is allergic to certain types of materials or to the lint that comes off the material, he may have to go into another type of sales.

> A change in eating habits is a common solution to allergic conditions. Such well-liked foods as shellfish, chocolate, and cakes and cookies made from wheat products may have to be totally eliminated from the diet.

> People may be forced to give up pets, such as a favorite cat or dog. Persons allergic to animal dander, despite their love for animals, may never be able to have a pet in their homes.

> The use of another soap or cleansing agent is oftentimes a simple solution to an attack of dermatitis-type allergy. Sometimes it is necessary to experiment to find a soap that does not create symptoms.

> Individuals with allergies to certain drugs will naturally have to avoid these drugs. If, on the other hand, it is essential that the drug be taken, it will be necessary to desensitize the person to that medication.

> Certain changes may have to be made within the allergic person's home environment. Damp dusting may have to be done daily, pillows filled with feathers may have to be changed to those made of sponge rubber; cotton blankets may have to be used instead of wool; favorite drapes and rugs may have to be removed.

> The avoidance of colds, flu, and infections is very important in the prevention of allergy. Thus, persons troubled with allergies must take special care to avoid infectious individuals, as well as to dress warmly in cold, damp weather.

> Since emotional upsets and extreme fatigue are important precipitating factors in allergy, patients must try to avoid the occurrence of such problems as much as possible. Adequate rest and a calm outlook on life's problems are helpful in decreasing the number and severity of attacks. When an individual is extremely disturbed mentally, the physician may decide on referral to a psychotherapist for treatment.

Drug Therapy. Patients generally require some drug therapy when suffering from allergic attacks. Drugs that provide systematic relief from allergic attacks are the following:

antihistamines	bronchodilators
epinephrine	sedatives
ACTH	tranquilizers
cortisone	

Antihistamines play a vital role in the treatment of all allergies, but especially in the treatment of anaphylactic shock, serum sickness, hay fever, and urticaria. Antihistaminic drugs commonly employed in the treatment of allergy are:[6]

> Chlorpheniramine (Chlor-Trimeton, Teldrin) 4 mg. q.i.d.*

> Tripelennamine (Pyribenzamine); 25 mg. q.i.d.*

> Promethazine (Phenergan), 12.5–25 mg. b.i.d.*

> Doxylamine (Decapryn), 12.5–25 mg. b.i.d.

> Methapyrilene (Semikon, Histadyl, Thenylene), 25–50 mg. q.i.d.

> Thonzylamine (Anahist, Neohetramine), 50–100 mg. q.i.d.

> Triprolidine (Actifed), 2.5 mg. b.i.d.

A number of side effects can be caused by the use of antihistamines; the major side effect is sedation or drowsiness. Other side effects are weakness, dizziness, gastrointestinal upsets, a dry mouth, and blurred vision. When large doses are given, excitement and insomnia may sometimes develop.

Hyposensitization (Desensitization, Hyperimmunization). A fairly successful, but very time-consuming, method for treating allergy is hyposensitization. Particularly effective in the treatment of hay fever, hyposensitization therapy is carried out in the following manner: The individual is first skin tested to determine the particular allergen (e.g., pollens, horse dander, household dust) to which he is allergic. Then the patient is given frequent injections of this antigen in very small amounts; as his treatment continues, he gradually receives progressively larger doses. In the early stages of treatment a mild allergic reaction is usually experienced. With continued treatment, however, the reactions become weaker until finally the allergen causes no reaction. Hyposensitization therapy is especially effective in patients subject to hay fever.

Hyposensitization dosages are usually given either daily, weekly, or monthly, depending upon the type of allergen that is affecting the patient as well as upon his particular allergic condition. For example, a patient with hay fever may receive a pollen extract by injection at four- to seven-day intervals. When the hyposensitization program is carried out by the oral method, the patient will probably take a daily dose of the allergen. As his condition improves, increasingly long periods of time will pass between hyposensitization treatments, until finally treatment is discontinued.[64]

Why exactly does hyposensitization work? Evidently the more an individual is exposed to the allergen to which he is allergic, the more he is able to develop what are called *blocking antibodies.*[22] Although no one knows exactly how blocking antibodies control allergic symptoms, physiologists postulate that blocking antibodies evidently slip in between an allergen and a reagin-containing cell. In this way, blocking antibodies prevent the allergen from contacting the reagin to produce an allergic response. Such blocking antibodies are always found in the blood of the hay-fever patient following hyposensitization treatment.

There are two major types of hyposensitization programs: specific hyposensitization, and nonspecific hyposensitization. The patient receiving *specific* hyposensitization treatment is given extracts of the specific allergen to which he is allergic. In other words, he is given daily, weekly, or monthly injections of particular dusts, pollens, molds, or danders. He receives these specific allergens until his allergic symptoms—usually those of hay fever—are relieved or cured. Patients receiving *nonspecific* hyposensitization treatment are given extracts of agents *other than the allergen* that is caus-

*Preparations for parenteral use are available.

ing their condition. This method of treatment is generally used when the physician has been unable to ascertain the specific allergen causing the allergy, or when the patient has not responded in a satisfactory manner to specific hyposensitization.

The most commonly employed nonspecific agents are *bacterial vaccines.*[64] These bacterial vaccines are prepared by swabbing the affected patient's nasal passage and bronchi and then using the collected secretions to grow a culture of the bacteria obtained. This form of hyposensitization is sometimes used in the treatment of asthma. *Histamine* is another substance that is used in nonspecific hyposensitization. Given subcutaneously in small dosages, at intervals from twice a day to once every two to four weeks, histamine injections help to alleviate symptoms and to improve the patient's tolerance to certain allergens. Histamine injections given in this manner have been particularly effective in urticaria and migraine, and in allergies affecting the skin and nasal mucosa.

As you can see, the treatment of allergy is frequently time-consuming, expensive, and exasperating. To be successfully treated, the patient may be forced to undergo many weeks of skin testing, and perhaps weeks or months of hyposensitization therapy. To obtain relief from symptoms, the patient may be required to take expensive or even dangerous drugs such as ACTH or cortisone. Finally, the treatment of allergy may require radical changes in the patient's life, such as moving, giving up pets, or changing jobs.

It is no wonder that individuals affected by allergies may become discouraged, despondent, and angry. As you care for allergic patients, it is important to be aware of their feelings and to try to understand how they experience their allergies. Your encouragement and continued interest in these people and in their condition can do much to help allergic patients to remain within a program of therapy.

AUTOIMMUNE DISEASE—AN ABNORMAL RESPONSE OF THE IMMUNE SYSTEM

In the past immunologists believed that the body reacted with an immune response only against proteins of foreign origin. Physiologists took it for granted that the body would always recognize its *own* proteins and would never make the frightening error of responding to its own materials by the formation of antibodies. The repellency of the very notion that the body might react against its own "self" is expressed clearly in Paul Ehrlich's descriptive term "horror autotoxicus."

Today we realize that it is possible for certain of our own body proteins to be regarded as not-self by the body, and consequently to be reacted against by the body's immunologic system. When such an unfortunate failure to distinguish self from non-self occurs, the pathologic condition is called an *autoimmune disorder.* The general nature of autoimmune disease is described clearly by Mackay and Burnet in the following statement:

> In autoimmune disease we are concerned with a group of conditions which result essentially from some breakdown in the processes by which the body insures that immune responses are directed only against foreign material. Immunity is normally concerned, not only with the inactivation and rejection of microorganisms and other foreign substances, but at least as importantly in recognizing that they are foreign. The essence of autoimmune disease is probably the failure at some point of this power of differentiating between the body's own material (self) and foreign material (not-self).[35]

Theories of Autoimmune Disease

In viewing the evolutionary background of human beings, it is generally true that those factors that are maladaptive have been eliminated, while factors which have adaptive value have been retained. If this is the case, why do autoimmune reactions still exist when they are so maladaptive in nature?

According to Crowle, there are two possible answers to this question:[11] Evolution is a continuous process, and man is forever adapting; in other words, a perfect man does not exist. Moreover, only those factors that are highly threatening to the survival of the organism are eliminated; moderately harmful factors tend to be eliminated slowly. Furthermore, in those cases in which a negative (harmful) factor is associated with a positive factor, which helps man to survive, the negative agent is eliminated at an even slower rate. Evidently the autoimmune response, which is maladaptive, is also associated with the body's *adaptive* ability to suppress the growth of abnormal tumor cells. Thus, the autoimmune process, while pathologic, has continued to survive in man. In sum, Crowle states that autoimmunity, seen in this light, can be considered "as an unfortunate side effect of a still imperfect protective immunological mechanism, as can also be said, for example, of anaphylaxis and immediate-type hypersensitivity."[11]

There is a second major reason for the existence of autoimmune disease. The immune system in man is very complex and, like any complex apparatus, is capable of making mistakes and therefore of reacting against itself, instead of against foreign proteins. How such mistakes are made is still somewhat obscure, although they are currently the subject of ardent research. Because you will be giving nursing care to many individuals who suffer from autoimmune conditions, we shall consider the major theories of why autoimmunity develops.

Currently, the major etiologic theories that are used to explain the development of autoimmune diseases are:

1. The "forbidden clone" theory.
2. The combining of a hapten with a body protein.
3. The release of inaccessible antigens.
4. Tissue injury.
5. Excessive delayed cellular immune reactions.
6. Genetic factors.

The *"fordidden clone" theory* is one of the most popular theories for explaining the cause of autoimmune disease. To understand the forbidden clone theory, it is helpful to first briefly review the clonal selective theory that we discussed earlier. Advocates of the forbidden clone theory state that *despite* the adaptive activities that take place during fetal life, a forbidden clone of cells *does* somehow emerge, reacts with the body's own proteins, and causes an autoimmune reaction. A clone of cells that is reactive against the self may emerge owing to either a mutation of an immunologically competent cell [I.C.C.], or activation of a forbidden clone of cells by injury, disease, or some change in the body's metabolism.

A second possible cause of autoimmune disease is the entrance of a hapten into the body. A *hapten* (from the Greek *to fasten*) is a normally nonantigenic substance that has the capacity to combine with a body protein. Evidently once a hapten combines with a body protein, the body protein can be modified in such a way that it will act as a foreign antigen. Important haptens that are believed to elicit autoimmune reactions are drugs, industrial chemicals, constituents in dust, and breakdown products from horse dander.[22] It is important to remember that the items just listed are not, in themselves, antigenic to the body. It is only when a particular drug or chemical, for example, an antibiotic, combines with a body protein, and only slightly modifies it, that the drug or chemical can cause the body to react immunologically.

A third possible cause of autoimmune disease is the *release of inaccessible antigens*. Inaccessible antigens are antigenic substances that normally do *not* circulate throughout the person's system, but instead remain enclosed within cells or tissues such as the thyroid gland, the lens of the eye, the adrenal glands, or the testes. Even during fetal life, these inaccessible antigens remain locked outside the circulation—inaccessible to the clones of immature immunological cells developing within the thymus gland. You will recall that, during fetal life, clones of cells that are active *against* the body's own protein are destroyed. Thus, when inaccessible antigens are released into the circulation, as a result of illness or accident, these antigens then activate clones of cells that were *not* destroyed during fetal life, since these cells had no opportunity to contact the once secluded antigens. The activation of these clones leads to cell multiplication and antibody formation. The antibodies formed then react with the once-inaccessible antigens that the body now interprets as not-self, and an immune response develops.[35]

A fourth condition that might create an autoimmune response is *tissue injury*.[47] Authorities believe that it is possible for such injuries as myocardial infarction and skin burns to alter certain of the body's tissues to such a degree that the body no longer is able to recognize certain body proteins as self. As a result of such changes, an autoimmune condition can be precipitated.

Finally, some authorities think that the symptoms and lesions of autoimmune disease result from an excessive *delayed cellular immune reaction* involving lymphoid cells.[24] Others believe that some *underlying agent* is causing damage to cells and tissues, and that it is the damaged cells themselves that act as antigens and promote the immune reaction. Almost all authorities seem to agree that autoimmune disease has a *genetic* or hereditary basis.[47] Thus, it may be that certain people have a definite predisposition to the emergence of forbidden clones. To date, however, we have no certain answer as to why some individuals are affected by autoimmune diseases and why others escape them entirely.

It is presently impossible to list with confidence those conditions that are actually autoimmune in nature. Many idiopathic conditions are listed as autoimmune, possibly for want of a better classification. Also, as Robbins points out, it has become somewhat "fashionable" in medical circles to state that a disease is of autoimmune origin. We can only, with great caution, make a list of probable and possible autoimmune conditions. Robbins has broken these conditions down as follows:[47]

Probable autoimmune diseases

1. Hashimoto's disease
2. Systemic lupus erythematosus
3. Autoimmune hemolytic anemia
4. Idiopathic thrombocytopenic purpura
5. Rheumatoid arthritis
6. Postviral encephalomyelitis
7. Lupoid chronic hepatitis
8. Autoimmune adrenalitis
9. Autoimmune orchitis
10. Autoimmune uveitis

Possible autoimmune diseases

1. Polyarteritis nodosa
2. Scleroderma
3. Dermatomyositis
4. Glomerulonephritis
5. Rheumatic fever
6. Wegener's granulomatosis
7. Multiple sclerosis
8. Demyelinating diseases of the brain

Sometimes you will find that the terms "diffuse collagen disease" and "connective tissue disease" are used in referring to the following conditions: systemic lupus erythematosus, polyarteritis nodosa, rheumatic fever, rheumatoid arthritis, and scleroderma. These disorders are called collagen diseases because they are generally characterized by changes in collagenous connective tissue—a type of tissue that is widely scattered throughout the body. The term "collagen disease," therefore, refers to the site of involvement, while the term "autoimmune disease" refers to the cause of the condition. Because collagen is located throughout the body's tissues, the signs and symptoms of the so-called diffuse collagen diseases tend to be referable to almost every organ and tissue of the body. Also, all the collagen disorders are characterized by an inflammatory response with the exception of scleroderma. Systemic lupus erythematosus, scleroderma, and polyarteritis nodosa are ultimately fatal.

General Treatment of Autoimmune Conditions

We shall be discussing the treatment of patients with specific autoimmune diseases as appropriate throughout this textbook. While treatment does vary for each condition, we can make a few general statements concerning the care of persons afflicted by any type of autoimmune disease.

The essential dilemma that physicians face as they attempt to treat autoimmune conditions is the following: how can they suppress the formation of antibodies that will react against self-constituents without also, at the same time, decreasing the body's defenses against microorganisms and other foreign intruders? Also, how can the physician destroy forbidden clones without also eliminating normal and useful cells? Unfortunately it is not yet possible to differentiate forbidden cells from normal cells or to eliminate harmful antigen-antibody reactions without also suppressing those reactions that are useful. Thus, the treatment of autoimmune conditions is always potentially dangerous. In attempting to eliminate the body's antigenic reaction against itself, we cannot help but upset those homeostatic mechanisms of immunity that serve to protect against foreign invaders.

The most commonly used general measures in autoimmune disease are: (1) the administration of corticosteroids, (2) the use of ionizing radiation, and (3) the administration of salicylates. The *corticosteroids* are highly beneficial in the treatment of autoimmune diseases because they produce anti-inflammatory effects, promote lymphocytolysis, suppress antibody production, and weaken or inhibit the effects of antigen-antibody interaction.[35] On the other hand, corticosteroids are dangerous in that they lower the patient's resistance to new infections. Moreover, since the corticosteroids suppress inflammatory reactions, the patient taking corticosteroids, who is also concomitantly suffering from an infection, may be without those symptoms (redness, heat, fever, pain, swelling) that would call attention to his malady.

Ionizing radiation, the second major form of treatment in autoimmune disease, helps to modify the immune response. This form of treatment is also used to prevent the rejection of transplants. The patient is treated by means of x-ray and radioactive isotopes, methods of therapy that will be discussed later in Chapter 35.

Finally, the *salicylates* have been used for years by physicians in their attempts to relieve the symptoms of rheumatic fever and rheumatoid arthritis. While aspirin is helpful in the relief of symptoms, it is not curative.

In sum, there is as yet no cure for autoimmune disease, nor is there any way to prevent it from developing. As immunologists focus more sharply upon the possible causes of autoimmune diseases, there may emerge in the near future some definitive curative help for those unfortunate people afflicted by these diffuse and deadly conditions.

IMMUNOLOGIC ASPECTS OF TRANSPLANT REJECTION

The successful transplantation of organs and tissues as a means of preserving life, correcting deformities, and repairing organic damage has been an age-old dream of physicians. In recent years, as a result of scientific advances in both surgery and physiology, that dream seems to be coming true. As a result of new discoveries in the field of immunology, complex types of transplant surgery have become more common, and these techniques are today a subject of intense interest and concern for professional personnel and laymen alike. Indeed, transplants have been highly newsworthy since December, 1967, when the first heart transplant was performed in Capetown, South Africa.

The major problem in transplanting organs and tissues from one body to another has not been the technical difficulties of surgery; rather the difficulty is that the body, because of the homeostatic mechanism of immunity, tends to immediately reject anything which is not-self. Thus, when an attempt is made to transplant an organ, such as the kidney or heart, from one person to another, the transplantation surgery is successful for only a brief time. Then, with deadly efficiency, rejection ultimately begins, and the transplanted tissue shrivels and dies.

Let us now focus our attention briefly on the actual *mechanism* of transplant rejection; which *types* of transplants are most likely to be quickly rejected; *therapeutic measures* that can be taken to suppress the transplant rejection reaction; and the future of transplant surgery.

THE VOCABULARY OF TRANSPLANTATION SURGERY

As you read about transplantation surgery, you will discover a number of terms that may be new to you. The most important terms that you need to know are:

> *Autograft* (autogenous transplant). This term is derived from "auto," which means self. An autograft is tissue that is transplanted from one part of a person's body to another part of his body; for example, a skin graft with a pedicle flap. This type of transplant, made of the patient's own tissues, is usually successful.

> *Allograft* (homotransplant or homograft) is a transplant that is made between *nonidentical* members of the same species; for example, a heart transplant between two nonrelated people. These transplants are usually unsuccessful unless potent immunosuppressive measures are taken. However, there are pronounced differences in the extent and type of allograft rejection that follows transplantation. As you will see, corneal transplants as well as bone and blood vessel grafts are much less adversely affected than are heart and kidney transplants.

> *Isotransplant* is a tissue exchange between *identical* twins. Isotransplants have a greater history of success than do allografts.

> *Xenografts* (heterografts) are tissues that are transplanted between species; for example, from a dog to a cat, or from a rat to a mouse. Xenografts are rapidly re-

jected because vascular anastomoses are almost never established.

The vocabulary of transplantation surgery involves not only types of grafts but also the possible outcome of the surgery. A few words that you may read or hear include:

> *"Take"* is a successful transplantation in which the wound heals and the transplant functions effectively.

> *Allograft reaction* is the customary type of transplant rejection, in which the allograft transplant is initially accepted and then rejected by the body and ultimately destroyed.

> *White graft reaction* is a rapid form of transplant rejection that occurs between species. For example, a skin graft that is transplanted between species is always white and bloodless in appearance. It soon dies, shrivels, and is then discarded, as a scale.

MECHANISM OF ALLOGRAFT REJECTION

Although a cause for considerable consternation among surgeons and physicians, allograft rejection is actually a normal homeostatic function of the body. Because an allograft is clearly not-self, allograft rejection is expected in a healthy organism. As stated earlier, the body's adverse reactions to transplants are evidently mediated by the lymphoid system and are a form of *cellular immunity* rather than humoral immunity.

Exactly what sequence of events occurs in graft rejection no one knows. However, there are a number of theories concerning the rejection process. Also the actual pathologic changes that occur in allograft rejection have been documented many times. According to one authority,[14] allograft rejection occurs in two stages. The first stage he refers to as the *afferent arc*. During this period the body, in some way, recognizes the foreign material as not-self. Unless recognition occurs, there will be no response and consequently no rejection. The precise process of "recognition" is not known; what is known is that when the blood circulates through the transplant, the lymphocytes within the blood stream, in some way, come to "recognize" the transplanted tissue as foreign.

Whereas the afferent arc of the rejection process involves recognition of foreign material on the part of the host, the *efferent arc* (or second stage of the rejection process) involves a definite *defensive reaction* by the body's immune system against the alien tissue or organ. As a result of the recognition of foreign material by the lymphocytes, *antibodies* are formed against the graft. These antibodies then circulate through the graft and, as a result, an antigen-antibody reaction takes place along with the production of an inflammatory reaction. During the inflammatory process, venules within the graft are the first blood vessels to be damaged, followed by the capillaries, and, finally, the small and then the large arteries. Because of injury and damage to the blood vessels, *ischemia* (a local anemia caused by the obstruction of circulation) develops, and cell damage and necrosis soon ensue. Thus, the graft is destroyed. This whole dramatic rejection process takes approximately 10 days. Should the host receive a *second* transplant from the *same* donor, his "sensitized" lymphocytes will produce antibodies very quickly against the tissues of the donor, and the second transplant will be rejected even more rapidly than the first—within four to five days as opposed to 10 days. This accelerated rejection response to the second transplant from the same donor is known as a *second set reaction*.[28]

As stated earlier, the extent of the allograft rejection process as well as the damage produced depends upon the *type* of tissue that is being transplanted between two unrelated members of the same species. For instance, *corneal transplants* are highly successful and are rarely rejected. There are two reasons that corneal transplants take so well. First of all, the cornea is poorly vascularized. Because of a lack of vascular connection between host and donor, the recognition or afferent arc of the rejection process is nullified, since without *recognition* of foreignness there can be no reaction. Second, the cornea contains few cells, and therefore little antigen can be released by the transplanted tissues.[26] Thus, corneal transplants tend to survive the body's usually relentless immunologic mechanism.

In contrast to a corneal transplant, a kidney transplant between an unrelated donor and host typifies the allograft rejection process with all its swift deadliness. For the first few days following the kidney transplant, the kidney is able to put out urine and it tends to function satisfactorily. However, when the rejection process begins, urine output diminishes dramatically, and the renal tissue becomes tender, swollen, and dusky in appearance. Within approximately 10 days the transplanted kidney will cease to be viable unless potent immunosuppressive techniques are employed.

With bone, fascia, and blood vessel grafts, the tissues do not survive the rejection process, *but* the transplant is nevertheless successful. In these types of grafts, the dead cells of the transplanted tissue simply serve as a "scaffolding" over which the patient's own tissues will eventually grow by means of a process called "creeping substitution."

While rejection rarely occurs in corneal transplants, and generally does not affect the success of bone, fascia, and blood vessel grafts, allograft rejection is the major problem surgeons face when performing any other type of transplant procedure. How is the rejection process slowed down or halted? Is there any way in which it can be prevented altogether?

Overcoming Transplant Rejection

To date there is no one method that is completely successful in overcoming the allograft rejection process. However, surgeons and immunologists are currently conducting extensive research to discover a method that will make the problem of organ and transplant rejection a concern of the past. Some of the major techniques that surgeons employ for suppressing and preventing rejection are briefly discussed below:

Immunosuppressive Techniques. These do not prevent transplant rejection from occurring; they simply suppress rejection once the process has started. All the following immunosuppressive agents are used to decrease the amount of lymphoid tissue in the body and to lower the number of circulating lymphocytes.

Corticosteroids suppress the destructive inflammatory reaction that occurs at the site of the transplant. Unfortunately the corticosteroids affect *all cells* rather than just lymphoid cells; moreover, they are capable of suppressing all immune responses and not just the rejection response. As a result of these widespread effects, corticosteroids produce extremely dangerous side effects, a susceptibility to infection being the most important. Thus, when corticosteroids are used for immunosuppressive purposes, physicians and nurses must use *flawless* sterile techniques during the surgical procedure and following it; also, they must carefully observe the patient for signs of such postoperative infectious complications as pneumonia. Despite the many dangers involved in the use of corticosteroids, they are still the therapeutic mainstay of renal and heart transplants.[41]

Cytotoxic drugs also serve to reduce the potency of the immune response by destroying or suppressing lymphoid tissue. Examples of useful cytotoxic drugs are: Imuran, 6-mercaptopurine, bromouracil, and the folic acid antagonists.[46] Unfortunately, these drugs, like the corticosteroids, cause many dangerous side effects.

Total body irradiation was once a popular procedure for suppressing transplant rejection but is rarely used today.[43] While total body irradiation suppresses transplant rejection by interfering with antibody synthesis, the procedure is extremely dangerous in that it stimulates the release of adrenocortical hormones, alters organ metabolism, and creates imbalances within the internal milieu.[14]

Antilymphocyte serum [ALS], and its derivative, antilymphocyte or antilymphoblast globulin [ALG], are important and fairly new immunosuppressive agents.[58] Once used only in animal transplants, ALS is now being prepared commercially on a large scale. While the exact mode of action is not clear, ALS apparently destroys lymphocytes, depletes the body's lymphoid tissues, and decreases antibody production. The major advantage of ALS over other immunosuppressive agents is that it affects *only* those lymphocytes that are involved in graft rejection, while lymphocytes that protect the body against bacterial invasion are spared.[26]

The Prevention of Transplant Rejection. This will, hopefully, be possible in the near future. Currently immunologists are working on a predominantly experimental basis with the following procedures:

Alteration of the graft itself by treating it with irradiation, chemicals, and freezing; this has been unsuccessful to date.

Splenectomy and thymectomy, operations for the removal of reticuloendothelial tissues, are theoretically feasible procedures for preventing graft rejection. You will recall that when the thymus gland is removed from a baby mouse, the mouse loses its ability to reject transplants. Unfortunately, however, in the adult human, a thymectomy has little effect upon immunologic response. However, immunologists are hopeful that in the future thymectomy may prove valuable for man when it is performed in conjunction with ALS administration.[41]

Tissue typing techniques are currently used with success prior to transplant surgery as a preventive measure against allograft rejection. The purpose of tissue typing is to match graft donors and graft recipients as closely as possible in order to reduce the severity of the rejection response. Thus, tissue typing is much like blood typing; in both instances an attempt is made to match donor and recipient and thereby minimize adverse reactions. The antigens that cause graft rejection are called *histocompatibility antigens* (HL-A). It is the hope of immunologists that some day great numbers of individuals will be grouped, not only by blood type, but in terms of their histocompatibility antigens. Such a procedure would greatly aid surgeons in their selection of a donor organ or donor tissues that would not be rejected by the body of the host.[14]

Induction of tolerance to a donor graft is a future possibility in transplant surgery. Histocompatibility antigens, prepared in such a way that they are no longer immunogenic, may someday be administered in minute dosages to a potential host. By this process of hyposensitization, the potential host will develop *tolerance* for the foreign antigens of the donor. When the transplant surgery is finally performed, the host's immunologic system will not react against the transplant, and there will be no rejection response.

THE FUTURE OF TRANSPLANTS

According to one authority, the most promising advances, that will make transplant surgery a safe procedure in the future, are:[14]

- Advances in tissue typing
  - Technical advances
  - Immunogenetics
- Advances in immunosuppression
  - The further development of ALS
  - Newer and safer drugs
- New methods for diagnosing rejection early in the process
- The elimination of complications that arise late in the process
- A better conception of the rejection process
- The storage of organs

However, once the transplant procedure becomes relatively easy and safe technically, there are still many ethical problems that must be considered in its use. Is the replacement of old and damaged organs in an elderly person a humane procedure? What are the ethical considerations in the use of donors? If vital organs are removed from a dying donor, how can the moment of death be precisely determined, so that removal of the organ will not cause the donor's death, and yet the removed tissues will be viable enough to become functional within the recipient's body? How will the widespread use of transplants ultimately affect the human species in terms of adaptation and evolution? These questions are among the major ethical dilemmas that physicians and nurses must face and solve.

References

1. Asperheim, M. K., and Eisenhauer, L. A.: *The Pharmacologic Basis of Patient Care.* 2nd ed. Philadelphia, W. B. Saunders Company, 1973.
2. Background: Immunology. *Nursing Times,* September 13, 1968, p. 1244.
3. Background: Organ transplants. *Nursing Times,* February 23, 1968, p. 260.
4. Blue, J. A.: Anaphylaxis and serum sickness. *In* Conn, H. F. (ed.): *Current Therapy 1969.* Philadelphia, W. B. Saunders Company, 1969.
5. Boyd, W.: *An Introduction to the Study of Disease.* Philadelphia, Lea & Febiger, 1952.
6. Brainerd, H., et al.: *Current Diagnosis and Treatment.* Los Altos, California, Lange Medical Publishers, 1959.
7. Burnet, Sir F. M.: Autoimmune disease. *In* Sodeman, W. A., and Sodeman, W. A., Jr. (eds.): *Pathological Physiology: Mechanisms of Disease.* 4th edition. Philadelphia, W. B. Saunders Company, 1967.
8. Burnet, Sir F. M.: How antibodies are made. *Scientific American,* November, 1954.
9. Collagen may be used for artificial organs. *J.A.M.A.* 200:22, May 3, 1967.
10. Craven, R. F.: Anaphylactic shock. *American Journal of Nursing* 72:718, April, 1972.
11. Crowle, A. J.: *Delayed Hypersensitivity in Health and Disease.* Springfield, Ill., Charles C Thomas, 1962.
12. Dave, V. K.: Contact dermatitis. *Nursing Times* 67:504, April 29, 1971.
13. Delayed reaction to bee sting: Risky. *J.A.M.A.* 208:254, April 14, 1969.
14. Feldman, J.: Graft rejection. *Archives of Internal Medicine* 123:713, June, 1969.
15. Flavell, S. G.: Asthma, *Nursing Mirror* 134:19, May 26, 1972.
16. Francis, B. J.: Current concepts in immunization. *American Journal of Nursing* 73:646, April, 1973.
17. French, R.: *Nurse's Guide to Diagnostic Procedures.* 3rd ed. New York, McGraw-Hill Book Company, 1971.
18. Gravis, G.: Allergies: A guide to practical diagnostic observations. *Journal of the New York State Nurses Teachers Association* 3:27, Winter, 1972.
19. Gonzalez, L. L.: New organs for old: Transplantation and its problems. *Clinical Anesthesia* 8:377, 1972.
20. Govoni, L. E., et al.: *Drugs and Nursing Implications.* New York, Appleton-Century-Crofts, Inc., 1965.
21. Good, R., et al.: Studies on transplantation biology. *In* Thomas, L., Urh, J., and Grant, L. (eds.): *International Symposium on Injury, Inflammation and Immunity.* Baltimore, The Williams & Wilkins Company, 1964.
22. Guyton, A. C.: *Textbook of Medical Physiology.* Philadelphia, W. B. Saunders Company, 1966.
23. Harvard, C. W. H.: Function of the thymus. *Nursing Mirror* 134:29, June 9, 1972.
24. Hong, R.: The physiology of immunity. *Minnesota Medicine,* September, 1969, pp. 1377–1380.
25. Humphrey, J. H.: The suppression of immune responses by nonspecific agents. *In* Samter, M., and Alexander, H. L. (eds.): *Immunological Diseases.* Boston, Little, Brown and Company, 1965.
26. Illingworth, Sir C.: Organ transplantation. *Nursing Times,* May 31, 1968, p. 743.
27. Immunology—What the future holds. *Nursing Mirror* 133:35, August 20, 1971.
28. Jones, C.: Transplantation and immunity. *Surgery, Gynecology and Obstetrics,* June, 1965, p. 1317.
29. Keefer, C., et al.: *The Merck Manual.* Rahway, New Jersey, Merck and Company, Inc., 1966.
30. Lessof, M. H.: The current status of transplantation immunology. *Scientific Basis of Medicine. Annual Reviews, 1972.* New York, Humanities Press, Inc., 1972, p. 16.
31. Levin, J., and Snyder, C.: The thymus gland and immunity. *The American Surgeon* 33:317, May, 1969.
32. Lockey, S. D., Sr.: Sensitizing properties of food additives and other commercial products. *Annals of Allergy* 30:638, November, 1972.
33. Lymphocyte changes in immune reaction measured by new test. *J.A.M.A.* 210:236, October 13, 1969.
34. Lymphoid "policeman" safeguarding organism. *J.A.M.A.* 207:853–856, February 3, 1969.
35. Mackay, I., and Burnet, F. M.: *Autoimmune Diseases: Pathogenesis, Chemistry and Therapy.* Springfield, Ill., Charles C Thomas, 1963.
36. Manipulating the new immunology. (Medical News.) *J.A.M.A.* 207:852, February 3, 1969.
37. McFarland, W.: Lymphocytes: Past, present and future. Immunology in Clinical Medicine—6. *Postgraduate Medicine* August, 1967, p. 92.
38. Medawar, P.: Immunosuppressive agents with special reference to antilymphocyte serum. *Proceedings of the Royal Society of London* 174:155, November, 1969.
39. Miller, J. F. A. P.: Biology of the immune (allergic) response. *In* Gell, P. C. H., and Coombs, R. R. A. (eds.): *Clinical Aspects of Immunology.* Philadelphia, F. A. Davis Company, 1968.
40. Miller, J. F. A. P.: The thymus and the development of immunologic responsiveness. *Science* 44:1544, June 26, 1964.
41. Nelson, P. S.: Immunological aspects of organ and tissue transplantation. *The Medical Journal of Australia,* October 12, 1968, p. 607.
42. Notkins, A. L., et al.: How the immune response to a virus can cause disease. *Scientific American* 228:22, February, 1973.
43. Organ transplants. *Nursing Times,* May 31, 1968, p. 724.

44. Owen, E. R.: Preventing the rejection response to transplanted organs. *The Medical Journal of Australia,* February 15, 1969, p. 354.
45. Patel, R., et al.: Serotyping for homotransplantation. *J.A.M.A.* 207:1319, February 17, 1969.
46. Roantree, R. J.: The uses of gamma globulin in prophylaxis and treatment. *Medical Clinics of North America* 49:1745, 1965.
47. Robbins, S. S.: *Pathology.* 3rd ed. Philadelphia, W. B. Saunders Company, 1967.
48. Roberts, A. C.: Modern materials, their contribution and use in the human body. *Nursing Mirror,* December 29, 1967, p. 1.
49. Rodman, M. S.: Drugs for allergic disorders: Anaphylaxis, asthma. Part 1. *R.N.* 34:63, June, 1971.
50. Rowlands, D. T., and Bassen, E. H.: Immunological mechanisms of allograft rejection. *Archives of Internal Medicine* 123:491, May, 1969.
51. Rowley, D. A., et al.: The immune response suppressed by specific antibody. *Immunology* 16:544, 1969.
52. Salaman, J. R.: Problems of transplantation. *Clinica Chemica Acta* 22:115–122, 1968.
53. Schechter, D. C.: Transplantation glossary. *New York State Journal of Medicine* 72:3013, December 15, 1972.
54. Selye, H.: *The Stress of Life.* New York, McGraw-Hill Book Company, 1956.
55. Shafer, K. N., et al.: *Medical-Surgical Nursing.* 5th ed. St. Louis, The C. V. Mosby Company, 1971.
56. Sherman, W. B.: Allergy. *In* Sodeman, W. A., and Sodeman, W. A., Jr. (eds.): *Pathological Physiology: Mechanisms of Disease.* Philadelphia, W. B. Saunders Company, 1967.
57. Silverstein, A. M.: Ontogeny of the immune response. *Science* 144:1423, June 19, 1964.
58. Simmons, R. S., et al.: Immunosuppressive assay of antilymphoblast globulin in man: Effect of dose, histocompatibility, and serologic response to house gamma globulin. *Surgery* 68:62, July 1970.
59. Sinclair, N. R., and Elliott, E. V.: Neonatal thymectomy and the decrease in antigen sensitivity of the primary response and immunological "memory" systems. *Immunology* 15:325, 1968.
60. Stinson, E. B., and Schroeder, J. S.: Cardiac transplantation in man. I. Early rejection. *J.A.M.A.* 207:2233, March 24, 1969.
61. Surgeons review and debate transplants to date. *American Journal of Nursing* 68:2318, November, 1968.
62. Taylor, H. E.: The clinical application of antilymphocyte globulin. *Medical Clinics of North America* 56:419, March, 1972.
63. Tests confirm immunity role of lymphocytes. *J.A.M.A.* 210:2344, December 29, 1969.
64. Tuft, L.: Allergy. *In* Tice, I. F. (ed.): *Practice of Medicine.* Vol. I. New York, Hoeber Medical Division, Harper & Row, 1968.
65. What's behind the puzzle of immunity? *Bulletin of the National Tuberculosis Association* 54:5, February, 1968.
66. Wilkinson, R.: Gamma globulins in health and disease. *Nursing Times* May 31, 1968, p. 725.
67. Williams, G.: Transplantation. *Nursing Times,* June, 1969, p. 711.
68. Williams, G. M.: What's new in surgery. Transplantation. *Surgery, Gynecology and Obstetrics* 136:212, February, 1973.
69. Williams, G., et al.: Antibodies and human transplant rejection. *Annals of Surgery* 170:603–616, October, 1969.
70. Winkelstein, A., et al.: Immunosuppressive therapy. *American Journal of the Medical Sciences* 265:92, May 25, 1973.
71. Zukoski, C. F.: Transplantation. *Surgery, Gynecology and Obstetrics* 134:280, February, 1972.

CHAPTER 24

Fluid and Electrolyte Balance

There are many ways of looking at man. Poets, psychologists, and politicians have their ways. Physicians, at times, must consider him a complex biochemical system, reacting to a myriad of influences and, in turn, trying to maintain a state of balance known by the happy term "homeostasis." Nowhere is this better seen than in that field of science known as fluid and electrolyte metabolism.[54]

INTRODUCTION AND STUDY GUIDE

Fluid and electrolyte balance, like man himself, can be considered from many different aspects. From the viewpoint of a chemist, the term connotes a highly complex and technical field of study, often seemingly remote from man. To the physician, fluid and electrolyte metabolism is the study of chemical reactions in man; to him, the term symbolizes an ever-broadening field of research—a field with vast therapeutic applications. To the nurse, the subject implies an exacting, sometimes burdensome, always vital part of the care of the whole patient. For her, the science of fluids and electrolytes involves the careful measurement of the patient's bodily intake and output of fluid, as well as the intelligent observation of a myriad of symptoms; it means alertness to the many subtle yet significant changes in the patient's psychologic affect and physiologic functioning. Finally, to the patient, fluid and electrolyte balance may mean a relative state of well-being, while severe imbalance may spell discomfort, mounting distress, coma, and even death.

The study of fluid and electrolyte balance and imbalance, then, has numerous practical and vital implications for nurses and their patients. Nurses are continually involved with problems of balance and imbalance as they perform such procedures as:

- Measuring a patient's food and fluid intake and measuring output from urine, stool, and vomitus, as well as gastric, intestinal, and bile drainage.
- Weighing patients daily.
- Starting intravenous infusions and adding electrolyte solutions and medications to intravenous infusions.
- Checking the flow rate of intravenously administered fluids.
- Irrigating nasal gastric suction tubes.
- Recording fluid balance at the end of each eight-hour shift and each 24-hour period.
- Reporting to the physician any deviation from normal fluid intake and output or any symptoms that might indicate a fluid or electrolyte imbalance.

These cardinal responsibilities, many of which may sound uninteresting, if not actually unpleasant, constitute some of the most significant services that patients require from their nurses. Although few patients actually die of fluid and electrolyte imbalance, imbalances can influence the possible outcome of a disease process. That is why fluid and electrolyte therapy is always a part of the total therapeutic plan for patients. The fact that doctors base many therapeutic decisions upon what is recorded by nurses, in terms of fluid intake, output, and the patient's weight, makes it imperative that nurses understand the importance of these measurements.

To provide the basic principles of fluid and electrolyte physiology and pathology, this chapter will discuss the following major concepts:

- Body water—its composition, volume, distribution, functions, and homeostatic regulation.
- Electrolytes and plasma proteins—their distribution, functions, and measurement.
- Water and electrolyte exchange between the fluid compartments.
- Homeostatic mechanisms that regulate water and electrolyte balance.

Because the topics just listed are complex and require a precise grasp of technical material on the reader's part, we offer the following guides to help you gain the most from your reading:

1. *Before* you begin to study the material in this chapter, *review* the following chemical terms and concepts:

   atom, element, molecule, compound, electrical charge, electrolytes, ions, ionization, cations, anions, the law of electrical neutrality, solutions, and pH

2. As you study the chapter, familiarize yourself with the following terms:

   semipermeable membrane, plasma protein, osmolarity, nephron, Bowman's capsule, ADH, aldosterone

Upon completion of this chapter, you should be able to generally discuss the following concepts:

a. The percentage of water in the adult human body.
b. Water distribution throughout the body's fluid compartments.
c. The composition of the body fluids in each of these fluid compartments.
d. Semipermeable membranes and control of body water distribution.
e. The role of proteins in plasma and in cell protoplasm.

f. The role of the kidney nephron in maintaining fluid and electrolyte balance.
g. The important hormones involved in the maintenance of fluid and electrolyte balance.

BODY WATER

Like a fish torn from the sea, a human being deprived of water cannot live for long. Without fluid, a man's skin dries and cracks, his temperature soars to burning heights, his mind deteriorates, his cells shrivel and, finally, he lies as withered and dead as an ancient Egyptian mummy. What, then, is this all-important substance so absolutely vital to life? What is its chemical makeup, and what are its functions? Where is water distributed in the body? How can water be lost from the body and, more vitally important, how can it be replaced? These are some of the important questions upon which our discussion will center.

BODY FLUID AND BODY WATER

Our cells depend upon an aqueous medium much as the bodies of our marine ancestors depended upon the sea for sustenance and for continued life. Like sea water, body fluid is not "pure," but contains both water and various "salts" which, technically, are termed *"electrolytes."* Electrolytes are substances that dissociate into ions or electrically charged particles when placed in water. In this chapter, then, the term *body fluid* refers to *both* water and electrolytes, while the term *body water* refers to water alone.

Body fluid is in a state of balance when its water and electrolyte components are present in the proper proportions, when losses of body water and electrolytes are replaced, and when excesses are eliminated.

TOTAL BODY WATER (TBW)

Water is the major constituent of the body; 60 to 70 per cent of the weight of the body is composed of water, while 30 to 40 per cent of the body is composed of solids. It is important to realize, however, that these figures apply to the "ideal man," and that there are tremendous variations between individual men, between men and women, and between adults and children.

First, adults vary significantly in the amount of water their bodies contain. This variance is due mainly to the amount of body fat present, since fat is essentially water free. Consequently a thin individual will have more fluid per pound of weight than a fat individual.

Second, a woman's body contains a smaller percentage of fluid in relationship to her total weight than does a man's. This is because a woman's body is composed of a larger amount of fat. It is estimated that the normal female body contains 50 to 54 per cent water, and 46 to 50 per cent solids.

Looking, finally, at the percentage of fluid present in the bodies of infants and children, one is struck by the difference in body composition between youngsters and adults. The figures in Table 24–1 compare the proportion of body water per pound of body weight at different ages.

Note that the percentage of water *decreases* with age. Also, note that there are no differences in the percentage of body water between the male and female until late adolescence or early adulthood, when the female body increases in the proportion of fat, and, at the same time, decreases in the proportion of water.

Important implications for the paramedical professions rest upon these facts. First, fluid balance is of greater importance in the *infant* than in the adult because so much of a baby's body is composed of water. The slightest imbalance in children immediately becomes evident. *The younger the child, the more serious is any decrease in the vital body fluids.*

Second, the *aged* need special nursing care because of their slowly diminishing body fluids; e.g., their *skin,* frequently dry and scaly, does not need to be bathed as frequently as does the skin of a young person. The use of soothing skin lotions is far more satisfactory in the care of the elderly than the use of drying alcohol. Also, it is important to realize that the *geriatric patient may easily become dehydrated because his percentage of body water is already somewhat depleted.* Indeed, a certain degree of dehydration appears to be always present in the very old, as typically evidenced by their lack of muscle tone, dry hair, and wrinkles.

WATER DISTRIBUTION

Water and electrolytes (i.e., body fluid) are distributed between two fluid compartments: the

TABLE 24–1. BODY WATER AT VARIOUS AGES AS PER CENT OF BODY WEIGHT

	Newborn	**6 mo.**	**2 yr.**	**16 yr.**	**20–39 yr.**		**40–59 yr.**	
					M	F	M	F
Total body water [TBW]	77	72	60	60	60	50	55	47

intracellular fluid compartment (ICF) and the *extracellular fluid compartment* (ECF). Seventy per cent of total body water is normally within the cells or in the ICF compartment, while 30 per cent of total body water is located outside the cells in the ECF compartment. Twenty-four per cent of the water in the ECF compartment occupies the tissue spaces (*interstitial* water), while 6 per cent appears in the vascular space as plasma (Fig. 24–1). The fluids contained within the intracellular and extracellular compartments are not static but *move freely* between the cells, the plasma, and the tissue spaces.

Despite the interchange between compartments, each type of fluid has its own particular functions.

> The *intracellular fluid* provides the cell with the internal aqueous medium necessary for its chemical functions.

> The *extracellular fluid* serves as the body's transportation system, carrying water, electrolytes, nutrients, and oxygen to the cells and removing the waste products of cellular metabolism.

Extracellular fluid is composed of: (1) interstitial fluid, (2) plasma, (3) transcellular fluids.

> *Interstitial fluid* lies outside both the vascular space and the cells; it provides the cells with the external medium necessary for cellular metabolism.

> *Plasma,* which contains colloids or plasma protein, is the liquid part of the blood; along with red blood cells, it maintains vascular volume.*

> *Transcellular fluids* are the body's secretions and excretions, e.g., saliva, gastrointestinal juices, cerebral spinal fluid, and urine.

THE FUNCTIONS OF WATER

The largest component of all living matter is water. The functions of water are as follows:

> Provides an aqueous medium for cellular metabolism.

> Transports materials to and from cells.

*In discussing fluid and electrolyte metabolism, we are concerned only with the *plasma* component of the vascular compartment, since red blood cells do *not* move out of the vascular compartment, and do not flow from one compartment to another.

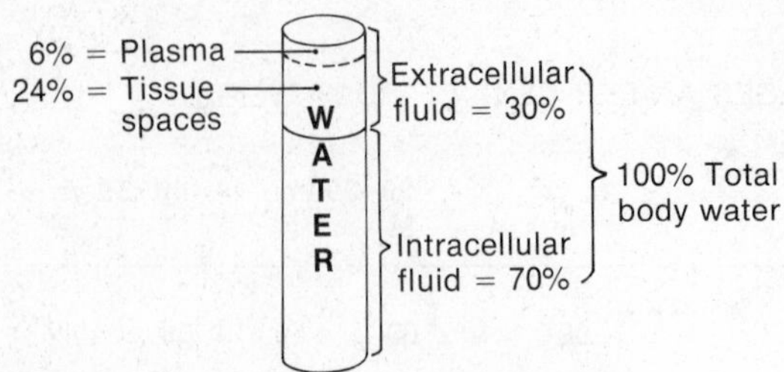

FIGURE 24–1. Total body water distribution in the adult.

> Acts as a solvent in which are dissolved the many solutes available for cell function.

> Regulates body temperature.

> Maintains the physical and chemical constancy of the intracellular and extracellular fluids.

> Maintains the vascular (blood) volume.

> Aids in the digestion of food through hydrolysis, which is the breakdown of molecules through the addition of water.

> Provides a medium for the excretion of waste from the body.

WATER BALANCE*

Body water *balance* is dependent upon a balance between water intake and output, i.e., gains in body water must equal losses in body water. Thus, water *imbalance* exists when water intake and output are unequal and gains in body water exceed losses, or losses exceed gains. In water imbalance individuals can become subject either to water overload or to dehydration. If overload becomes too great, a man will actually drown in his own fluids. If intake is not great enough or is entirely lacking, man becomes dehydrated.

In Table 24–2 a typical 24-hour water balance record provides an example of *normal* intake and output, which would keep the body of an adult in normal water balance.

Note that our greatest single source of water *intake* is from water or liquids ingested as beverages, while our second greatest source is the "hidden" water in foods. Indeed, it may surprise you that lean meats contain 75 per cent water, while fruits and vegetables contain an even greater percentage. However, if the intake of "hidden" water in foods and the water of oxidation are combined, these two sources of water *exceed* the oral intake.

Thus, to assess water balance, it is important to keep an accurate record of the intake of both solid *foods and liquids.*

Turning next to *output,* note that the largest proportion of water is eliminated from the kidneys, moderate amounts of water are eliminated from the skin and lungs (insensible or evaporate water loss), and only small amounts of water are normally eliminated from the gastrointestinal tract. The elimination and conservation of water are homeostatically controlled by the kidney, the gastrointestinal tract, various hormonal substances, and the brain (pp. 201–210). Because of the importance of the renal system in regulating output, it is possible to estimate the state of water balance by comparing the 24-hour intake volume with the 24-hour urine output volume, realizing that urinary output represents slightly over half the total water output.

Insensible water loss from the lungs and skin is not the same as visible sweating, or diaphoresis, which is an observable water loss. Insensible loss

*In discussing water balance, the authors have drawn extensively from personal communication with Joleen K. Heath as well as from her article. "A Conceptual Basis for Assessing Body Water Status."[37]

includes the 750 to 1000 ml. of water eliminated in the vapor of our breath and in the moisture that constantly forms on our skin, even though we may not be aware of it. These insensible losses are greatly increased when body metabolism is accelerated as in fevers, when respirations are significantly increased as in pneumonia, and when individuals live in hot climates. Consequently these insensible losses must be carefully estimated by the doctor when attempting to correct water imbalances. Nurses can help with the assessment of insensible losses by carefully noting and recording the patient's rate and depth of respiration and the presence of diaphoresis.

In summary, when a state of water balance exists, water intake, in the form of ingested food, fluid, and oxidation, equals the water output through the kidneys, bowel, skin, and lungs. Accurate interpretation of intake and output must take into consideration *all* sources of water gains and losses.

MINIMUM WATER REQUIREMENTS FOR SURVIVAL

In reviewing the chart of typical water balance for 24 hours you will see that an "average" person should take in approximately *2600 ml. of fluid per day* to meet the body's water requirements. If this is the case, how much water does an individual need for *survival?*

Over the years scientists have tried to establish the minimum food and water requirements for man. It is recognized that men and women can survive for remarkably long periods (up to 45 days) without food. This survival is possible because the body is able to convert its stored protein and fat supplies into needed energy when food is not available. However, there is no evidence that it is possible to survive without water for even half this period. The maximum amount of water produced by oxidation of fat stores would barely equal the amount of water lost by insensible sweating. Consequently, man *must* obtain his water supply through sources outside his own body.

While a minimum of 2000 ml. of fluid per day is required for *normal* balance, 1500 ml. per day is the basal* requirement for a 24-hour period. This basal water requirement applies *only* if the individual concerned is healthy, relatively inactive, and living in a temperate climate. Under these conditions an individual could live for a period of time, but he would not be in optimal balance. On the other hand, persons who live in a hot climate, who have high fevers with continued excessive perspiration, or who have a rapid respiratory rate may require up to *5000 ml. of water per day*. When these basal requirements are not met, *dehydration* is the inevitable result.

How long can a person live without *any* water? Adults can live up to 10 days and children up to five days, provided weather conditions are favorable. In the hot, drying desert, however, death may come within a few hours. With the loss of 1 per cent of body water, a man caught in the desert feels thirsty. When he loses 5 to 8 per cent of his body water, he feels weary, his pulse rate rises, his temperature soars (because he can no longer sweat), and his mental processes deteriorate. With the loss of 11 to 15 per cent of water, he develops delirium, deafness, and kidney failure. In the final stages of dehydration (more than 20 per cent), "his skin cracks, a blood-sweat oozes from his body, his eyes weep tears of blood, he becomes a 'senseless automaton,' digging desperately in the sand, and he passes beyond any possible revival by water."[87]

*Basal requirements are those absolute minimums that will sustain cellular activity if the individual is totally at rest.

TABLE 24–2. BODY WATER BALANCE IN THE ADULT OVER A 24-HOUR PERIOD

Intake	ml.	Output	ml.	
Oral fluids	1200	Urine from kidneys	1500	
"Hidden" water from foods	1100	Water vapor from lungs	400	insensible water loss
Metabolic sources	300	Sweat from the skin	600	
(Water of oxidation): Protein = 40 ml./100 Gm. Fat = 100 ml./100 Gm. CHO = 100 ml./100 Gm.		Feces from the bowel	100	
	2,600		2600	

Death from dehydration can occur anywhere, especially among children, and among the aged whose water intake is neglected. Children, because of their precise kidney function and greater metabolic rate, are particularly vulnerable. It is not uncommon in hospitals to see young, severely dehydrated children with sunken eyes and high fevers brought into the hospital too late to be saved. Like the man stranded in the desert, the small child with rapid fluid loss and lack of fluid replacement, can, within hours, pass "beyond any possible revival by water."

ELECTROLYTES AND PLASMA PROTEINS

A man cannot live long without water, nor can he hope to exist in a state of equilibrium or homeostasis without a proper balance of electrolytes and plasma protein substances, or colloids. Thus, it is important for nurses and doctors to consider carefully the role of electrolytes and colloids in the body's physiology: namely, their chemical nature, functions, measurement, balance, and concentration within the body's fluid compartments.

*THE CHEMICAL NATURE OF ELECTROLYTES**

An electrolyte is defined as a substance or compound composed of atoms, which, when placed in a solvent such as water, break up into separate charged particles called *ions*. Positively charged ions are called *cations,* and those negatively charged are called *anions*. Important cations in terms of body fluid metabolism are sodium (Na^+), potassium (K^+), calcium (Ca^{++}), and magnesium (Mg^{++}), while important anions are chloride (Cl^-), bicarbonate (HCO_3^-), phosphate (HPO_4^{--}), and sulfate (SO_4^{--}).

As a simple example of how ionization works, let us consider sodium chloride (NaCl). If we place NaCl into solution, it will dissociate or ionize into the positive cation Na^+ and the negative anion Cl^- ($NaCl \rightarrow Na^+ + Cl^-$). We can prove that sodium carries a positive charge and chloride a negative charge by placing sodium chloride in a wet electrical cell and then passing an electric current through the solution; as a result of this we find that Na^+ (a cation) travels to the *negative* pole or *cathode,* and Cl^- (an anion) travels to the *positive* pole or *anode*.

*We assume that the reader has taken at least one course in basic chemistry, and consequently is familiar with the terminology used in describing chemical elements and processes, as well as with some of the important chemical reactions that occur in the human body.

Body water contains cations and anions. Moreover, in the body fluids each cation is *always balanced chemically* by an anion. In essence, the body's electrolytes are governed by Faraday's *Law of Electrical Neutrality,* which states:

> *The sum of the number of negative electric charges must equal the sum of the number of positive electric charges in a solution.*

Thus, if the cations in our body fluids increase, the anions must increase; and if the cations decrease, the anions must also decrease. In this way the electrolyte balance is maintained.

Not all substances dissociate in solution. Substances which *do not ionize* and which, consequently, do not carry an electrical charge are called *nonelectrolytes.* An example of a nonelectrolyte is glucose, which remains a nondissociated, electrically neutral molecule in body water. Most organic compounds are nonelectrolytes.

THE CHEMICAL NATURE OF PLASMA PROTEINS

Protein plays a significant role in fluid and electrolyte metabolism. It is found both in cells and in plasma. Protein within the protoplasm of the cells is called *proteinate* (an anion), while protein in plasma is in colloid form. Colloids are macromolecules that are usually unable to pass through an animal membrane because of their size, and consequently these plasma proteins tend to remain within the blood vessels rather than diffusing out into the tissues. Some authorities believe that plasma proteins tend to behave like anions, having a negative charge and being balanced electrically by cations. The most important plasma proteins are *albumin, globulin,* and *fibrinogen.* These colloidal substances are synthesized in the liver.

THE PHYSIOLOGIC FUNCTIONS OF ELECTROLYTES AND PLASMA PROTEINS

Electrolytes and plasma proteins perform important physiologic functions within the body. The major functions of electrolytes are: (1) the promotion of neuromuscular irritability; (2) the maintenance of body fluid osmolarity; (3) the regulation of H^+ balance; and (4) the distribution of body fluids between the fluid compartments.

Plasma proteins, like electrolytes, play an important role in body water distribution. Basically, plasma proteins hold water within the blood vessels, thereby preventing the leakage of excess water into the tissues and the subsequent development of edema.

MEASURING FLUIDS AND ELECTROLYTES

In nursing care of patients with fluid and electrolyte imbalances, the correct measurement of the fluids and electrolytes used in parenteral therapy is of great importance. Even small errors in measurement while preparing intravenous infusions can result in serious fluid and electrolyte imbalances.

The most important measurements used in working with fluids and electrolytes are the following:

1. The *liter* [L.] and the *milliliter* (ml.) (or cubic *centimeter* [cc.]). The liter and milliliter are measures of *volume*. IV solutions are always measured in liters and milliliters. For example, the doctor may order one liter (or 1000 ml.) of normal saline for a patient with a fluid imbalance. (For all practical purposes the milliliter and cubic centimeter are equivalent, and fluid measurements are often expressed in cubic centimeters [cc.]).

2. The *gram* [Gm.] and the *milligram* [*mg*.]. These are units of *weight;* one gram equals 1000 mg. We can express serum electrolytes and plasma proteins in terms of *grams per cent* or *milligrams per cent*. This measurement simply tells us the number of grams or milligrams of an electrolyte or colloid in 100 ml. of fluid. For example, the normal plasma protein content of blood is 6 Gm. per cent. In other words, there are 6 Gm. (or 6000 mg.) of protein in every 100 ml. of plasma.

3. The *milliequivalent* [mEq.]. The electrolyte content within a water compartment can be most accurately expressed in terms of *milliequivalents per liter* (mEq./L.). The milliequivalent is the *measure of the chemical activity or chemical combining power of an ion*. In other words, the milliequivalent is a measure of the power of a cation to combine with an anion, thus forming a molecule.

Although two different chemicals may have equal weights, one chemical may have a greater chemical combining power or greater number of charges than does the other chemical. This is why ions are measured in terms of *milliequivalents* rather than milligrams (i.e., in terms of *chemical combining power* rather than weight).

Metheny and Snively have suggested the following analogy to clarify the concept of the milliequivalent:[55] In our civilization we use the word *horsepower* to designate physical power. For example, an old jalopy may have "30 horsepower," meaning it has the same amount of driving force as if 30 horses were pulling it. A powerful racing car, on the other hand, may have over 600 horsepower. The *weight* of the jalopy and the *weight* of the modern sports car have *nothing* to do with the *power* of these respective cars. Indeed, the slow jalopy will undoubtedly be far heavier than the speedy convertible. Thus, the difference in physical activity and performance between these two automobiles is best measured in terms of *mechanical* power rather than weight!

With electrolytes the unit of chemical power is the milliequivalent; one milliequivalent is *equivalent to the activity of 1 mg. of hydrogen.* One milligram of hydrogen, then, constitutes a "chemical horsepower," because 1 mg. of hydrogen exerts *1 mEq. of chemical activity.* By weight, 23 mg. of sodium, 39 mg. of potassium, 20 mg. of calcium, and 4140 mg. of proteinate each exert the same chemical power as 1 mg. of hydrogen.

In sum, 1 mEq. of *any* electrolyte is chemically equivalent to 1 mg. of hydrogen; therefore, 1 mEq. of any electrolyte is chemically equivalent to 1 mEq. of any other electrolyte, even though the *weights* of these two electrolytes may differ significantly. Moreover, the number of milliequivalents of cations in the body fluids must always balance the number of milliequivalents of anions for chemical neutrality to exist (Fig. 24–2). Chemical neutrality of the body fluids is essential for the maintenance of normal neuromuscular excitability.

NORMAL ELECTROLYTE AND PLASMA PROTEIN BALANCE

We normally obtain essential electrolytes and plasma proteins by ingesting a diet that is adequate in nutrients. A minimum daily intake of 2400 to 2600 ml. of water, 4.5 Gm. of sodium, 3 Gm. of potassium, and 0.05 Gm. of protein per kg. of body weight is required for healthy balance. Our normal output of water and electrolytes tends to roughly equal the intake.

It is important to remember that electrolytes are dissolved in the water that we lose through urination, defecation, or sweating. Thus, whenever water is replaced, electrolytes must also be replaced, and vice versa, to maintain water and electrolyte balance.

ELECTROLYTE CONCENTRATIONS IN THE BODY'S FLUID COMPARTMENTS

Water and electrolytes are distributed throughout the body's fluid compartments—the extracellular fluids compartment (made up of plasma, tissue fluid, and transcellular fluids) and the intracellular

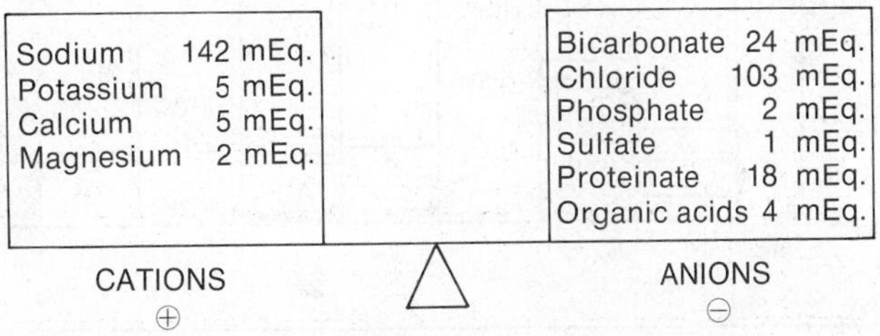

FIGURE 24–2. When their weights are written in milliequivalents, the cations and anions of extracellular fluid approximately balance each other. (Modified from Metheny and Snively.)

CATIONS ⊕	
Sodium	142 mEq.
Potassium	5 mEq.
Calcium	5 mEq.
Magnesium	2 mEq.

ANIONS ⊖	
Bicarbonate	24 mEq.
Chloride	103 mEq.
Phosphate	2 mEq.
Sulfate	1 mEq.
Proteinate	18 mEq.
Organic acids	4 mEq.

fluid compartment. Extracellular fluids and intracellular fluids contain the *same* electrolytes but in different amounts. The electrolytes contained in the *intracellular* fluid are potassium, magnesium, phosphate, and proteinate, and traces of sodium and chloride. *Potassium* is the major cation of the ICF and *phosphate* is the major anion. The electrolytes contained in the *extracellular* fluid are sodium, chloride, bicarbonate, and traces of potassium, magnesium, protein, and phosphate. *Sodium* is the major cation of the ECF and *chloride* is the major anion. In Figure 24–3 the relative proportions of electrolytes are shown for both the intracellular and extracellular compartments.

Samples of *plasma* are used by laboratories to measure electrolytes in the *extracellular* fluid compartment. This is because the plasma component of the ECF compartment has almost the *same electrolyte composition* as does the interstitial component, except that plasma contains the plasma proteins (colloids.) Normal approximate laboratory findings for electrolytes and plasma proteins within the plasma are:

Sodium	140 mEq./L.
Potassium	5 mEq./L.
Chloride	103 mEq./L.
Bicarbonate	24 mEq./L.
Colloids	6 Gm. per cent (6 Gm./100 ml.)

While electrolyte concentration of the ECF is measurable, scientists are not as yet able to analyze the concentration of electrolytes in the intracellular fluid.

The *transcellular* fluids (e.g., urine, bile, saliva) each have their distinct electrolyte composition which tends, in health, to remain fairly stable. When illness strikes, the transcellular fluids may become depleted through vomiting, diarrhea, excessive perspiration, and so forth. When such depletion occurs, electrolytes are lost along with water. Both water and electrolytes, then, must be replaced for balance to be restored.

FLUID AND ELECTROLYTE MOVEMENT

A knowledge of fluid and electrolyte transport throughout the body and its regulation is basic to an understanding of such pathophysiologic con-

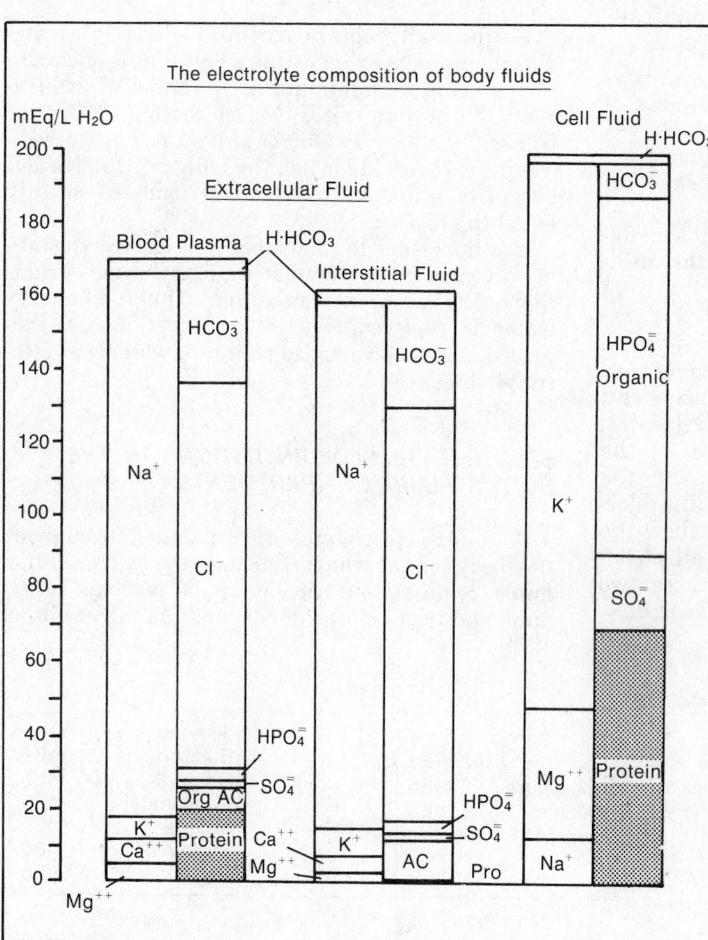

FIGURE 24–3. A comparison of the electrolyte composition of the extracellular and intracellular fluid compartments. (Modified, by permission, from Gamble, J. L., *Chemical Anatomy, Physiology and Pathology of Extracellular Fluid.* Cambridge, Harvard University Press, Massachusetts, 1947.)

cepts as edema, dehydration, circulatory overload, and water intoxication as well as numerous other fluid and electrolyte imbalances. To understand fluid and electrolyte movement within the fluid compartments of the body, one must carefully consider the following two processes: (1) the transport of fluid and electrolytes between the intracellular fluid and extracellular fluid compartments; and (2) the transport of fluids between the interstitial fluid compartment and the vascular compartment.

FLUID AND ELECTROLYTE TRANSPORT BETWEEN THE INTRACELLULAR AND EXTRACELLULAR FLUID COMPARTMENTS

The flow of fluids and electrolytes between the ICF and ECF compartments depends upon: the *osmolarity* of the fluid compartments and the phenomenon of *active transport.*

Osmolarity

Osmolarity[67] is defined as the total number of dissolved particles (solute) within a solution, or as the number of dissolved particles per liter. When two solutions of different osmolarities (i.e., solutions that contain differing concentrations of dissolved particles per liter) are separated by a membrane permeable to water, the *distribution* of water *shifts* so that the osmolarities of the two solutions equalize. Thus, the solution with the greatest osmolarity (i.e., the greatest concentration of dissolved particles per liter) *gains* water while the solution with the lowest osmolarity (i.e., the lowest concentration of dissolved particles per liter) *loses* water. Because water goes where the greatest number of electrolyte particles are, the two solutions will develop *equal* osmolarities (i.e., an equal number of particles per liter) as a result of the fluid shift. In the body, osmolarity controls water distribution between the ICF and ECF compartments. Water is normally distributed between the compartments so that the osmolarities remain essentially the same in the various fluid compartments.

The dissolved particles within the body fluids are primarily electrolytes and colloids—potassium, phosphate, and proteinate within the ICF compartment, and sodium, chloride, and plasma proteins within the ECF compartment. Should the ICF develop a greater osmolarity (more electrolytes per liter) than the ECF, water will shift from the ECF into the ICF and the cells will consequently *swell.* Conversely, should the ECF develop a greater osmolarity than the ICF, water will shift from the cells into the ECF compartment, and the cells will *shrivel.* Thus, osmolar changes affect cell volume.

While osmolarity controls water distribution, osmolarity itself is principally regulated by water *intake* and *output.* Water intake is controlled by thirst, while water loss is controlled by the antidiuretic hormone (ADH), the kidney nephron, and the gastrointestinal tract.

How is osmolarity measured? Laboratories use the *serum sodium level* as a measure of the osmolarity of the plasma. Because both the ICF and

ECF compartments have the *same* osmolarity, the serum sodium level, is an *indirect* measure of the osmolarity of the intracellular fluid compartment. The normal serum sodium level is 140 mEq./L. When sodium (the principal cation of the ECF) is elevated above normal limits, the osmolarity of the plasma, and consequently of the body, is increased. When the serum sodium level is depressed below normal limits, osmolarity is decreased.[67]

The patient with an elevated serum Na^+ level due to water depletion is suffering from a hyperosmolar imbalance; i.e., he has a decrease in water *relative* to Na^+ (hyperosmolarity). Thus, the concentration of electrolytes within his fluid compartments is too great to maintain balance. Conversely, when the patient has a lowered serum Na^+ and/or an increase in body water due to water retention or overload, the patient has a *hypo-osmolar* imbalance; i.e., he has an *increase* in water *relative* to sodium (hypo-osmolarity), and his electrolytes are diluted.* The concepts of hyperosmolarity and hypo-osmolarity are diagrammatically represented in Figure 24–4.

Active Transport

While osmolarity controls *water* movement and distribution, active transport applies to the work required to *transport ions* across a cellular membrane against chemical or electrical gradients.

The physiology of active transport remains obscure. However, authorities hypothesize that cells are able to transport sodium and other positively charged osmotic particles across cell boundaries and into the extracellular fluid where they balance the cell's anion, proteinate; the mechanism of this transport is called a "cation pump" or "sodium pump." If Na^+ were *not* "pumped" from the cells, intracellular protein could not stay in balance with

*Hyperosmolar and hypo-osmolar imbalances are discussed in detail in Chapter 25.

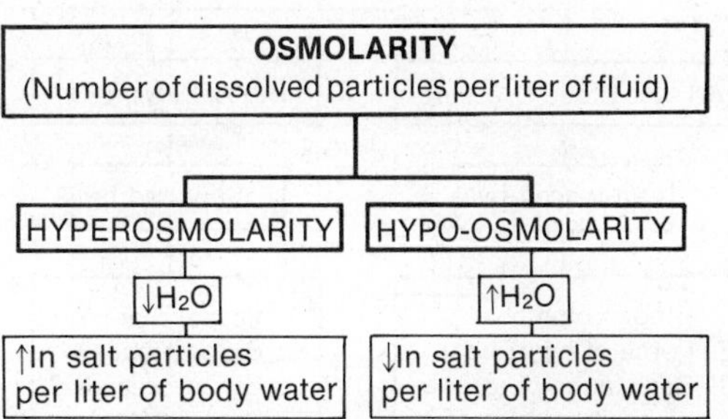

FIGURE 24–4. The concept of osmolarity as applied to water depletion and water excess in humans.

extracellular Na^+; consequently, water would be pulled into the cells, the cells would swell, and extracellular water would diminish. Thus, active transport insures normal cell volume.

FLUID TRANSPORT BETWEEN THE VASCULAR COMPARTMENT AND THE INTERSTITIAL FLUID COMPARTMENT

To grasp how fluid exchange occurs between the vascular (blood) and the interstitial (tissue) fluid compartments, it is necessary to consider briefly the following factors: plasma proteins, capillary permeability, plasma osmolarity, blood hydrostatic pressure, filtration pressure, colloid osmotic pressure, and the role of the lymphatic system.

The *plasma proteins,* as we stated earlier, are negatively charged particles found mainly in the blood or intravascular compartment. The normal level of plasma proteins in the blood is 6 to 8 Gm. per cent. *Albumin* makes up the largest fraction of plasma proteins.

Because they are large particles, the plasma proteins are generally unable to pass through the walls of the capillaries, although a small amount of protein does escape. Thus, while the capillary walls are *freely permeable* to water and to certain electrolytes, they are *not freely permeable* to protein; therefore, the concentration of plasma proteins within the blood vessels is high. Thus, plasma normally has a 0.5 per cent *greater* osmolarity than interstitial fluid; i.e., it has a 0.5 per cent greater capacity to attract and to hold water than interstitial fluid. Any reduction in plasma osmolarity results in swollen tissues (edema) and loss of blood volume.

The three major factors involved in the maintenance of blood volume, and the consequent avoidance of edema, are blood hydrostatic pressure, colloid osmotic pressure, and filtration pressure.

Blood hydrostatic pressure (B.H.P.) is the pressure of the blood cells and plasma within the capillaries. Blood hydrostatic pressure is dependent upon the level of the arterial blood pressure, the rate of blood flow through the capillaries, and the venous pressure. As you will recall from physiology, each of these factors is, in turn, influenced by other factors. Some of the major influences are diagrammed in Figure 24–5. The normal blood hydrostatic pressure within the arterioles is 32 mm. Hg, and within the veins it is 12 mm. Hg.

The next major factor in the transport of fluids between the vascular and interstitial compartment is the *colloid osmotic pressure* (also called "oncotic pressure," O.P.), or that pressure exerted by the plasma proteins. The colloid osmotic pressure is important in the transportation of fluid from the vascular system to the interstitial compartment and back again. The plasma proteins work somewhat like a sponge, holding water within the vessels and sucking back that water which escapes from the vessels. Normally the colloid osmotic pressure within the capillary is around 22 mm. Hg.

Finally, the *filtration pressure* (F.P.) is the pressure of the blood in the blood vessels minus the colloid osmotic pressure (F.P. = B.H.P. − O.P.). The filtration pressure in the arteriole is +10 and is a positive pressure $\left\{32\ \frac{\text{B.H.P.}}{\text{mm.Hg}} - 22\ \frac{\text{O.P.}}{\text{mg.Hg}} \rightarrow \frac{\text{F.P.}}{+10}\right\}$. In the venule, the filtration pressure is −10 and is a negative pressure $\left\{12\ \frac{\text{B.H.P.}}{\text{mm.Hg}} - 22\ \frac{\text{O.P.}}{\text{mm.Hg}} = \frac{\text{F.P.}}{-10}\right\}$. In terms of body functioning these figures imply that at the arteriolar end of the capillary, the blood hydrostatic pressure, or pressure of blood within the capillaries, is *greater* than the colloid osmotic pressure. Fluid is thus *forced out of the capillaries* into the tissues. At the venular end of the capillary, however, the blood hydrostatic pressure is *less* than the colloid osmotic pressure, and the water is *sucked back* into the vessels. Thus,

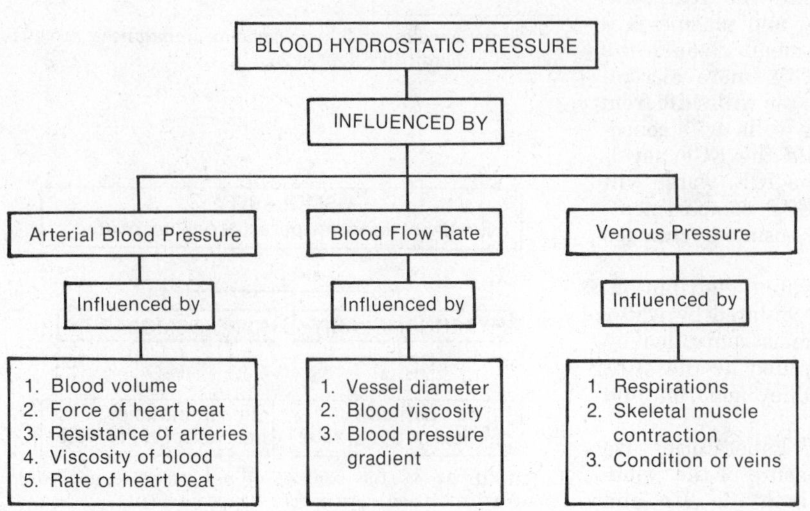

FIGURE 24–5. The major factors influencing blood hydrostatic pressure.

the filtration occurs at the arteriolar end of the vessel and reabsorption at the venular end of the capillary (Fig. 24–6). When the blood hydrostatic pressure gets too high, thereby increasing the filtration pressure, the protein sponge is subjected to a pressure over and above that which it can exert; thus, water goes into the tissues (edema). When the blood hydrostatic pressure drops to a certain level, the protein sponge is then able to soak up the lost water, bringing it back into the blood stream.

A final factor influencing fluid transport between the plasma and interstitial fluid is the *lymphatic system*. One function of this system is to return to the capillaries excess fluid as well as the small amount of protein that escapes from the plasma into the interstitial fluid.

Having considered the major factors that control the *return* of fluid to the vascular system, let us next discuss the major problems that can influence the *loss of water* from the plasma.

Rise in Blood Hydrostatic Pressure. This raises the filtration pressure, causing fluid to be squeezed out into the tissues more readily. The resulting edema or swelling of tissues results from fluid being forced into the interstitial spaces. A rise in the blood hydrostatic pressure occurs in hypertensive individuals and in those who receive an overload of intravenous fluids.

Drop in Colloid Osmotic Pressure. This reduces the rate of reabsorption of the fluid that was squeezed out at the arteriolar end of the capillary. As a result, fluid will accumulate in the tissues, with resulting edema.

A decrease in the colloid osmotic pressure is usually the result of protein loss. *Hypoproteinemia* (low plasma proteins) usually occurs in malnutrition, infection, hemorrhage, profuse serous drainage, in severe burn cases, in instances of renal, cardiac, and hepatic damage, and after lengthy operations. Patients afflicted with these conditions are usually edematous and perhaps *dehydrated* as well. Although patients with edema appear to have "too much water," they often actually suffer from the problem of water depletion. This is because their water is not being circulated properly; thus, water is not readily available for the body to meet its various needs.

Obstruction in the Lymphatic System. This can lead to fluid retention within the tissues, because fluid is blocked in its attempt to return to the circulation. For example, *lymphedema* can occur after a radical mastectomy for breast cancer, which involves removal of the lymphatics of the axilla. It can also result from tropical parasitic infections.

MAJOR HOMEOSTATIC MECHANISMS CONTROLLING FLUID AND ELECTROLYTE BALANCE

Water and electrolyte balance and their distribution throughout the body are homeostatically regulated by the endocrine system, the gastrointestinal system, the renal and cardiovascular system, the nervous system, and the respiratory system. These systems exercise control over water and electrolyte intake and excretion. Moreover, these systems are the *only* controls over body water and electrolyte exchange. For this reason, even minor breakdowns in the function of any one of these systems can lead to water and electrolyte imbalances.

THE ENDOCRINE SYSTEM AS A HOMEOSTATIC REGULATOR

The major hormones regulating fluid and electrolyte metabolism are the antidiuretic hormone (ADH) aldosterone, thyroid hormones, parathyroid hormone (PTH), and diuretic hormone (DH) (or diuretic principle).

Antidiuretic Hormone (ADH)

As the name implies, ADH prevents the body, under certain conditions, from losing fluid. It is

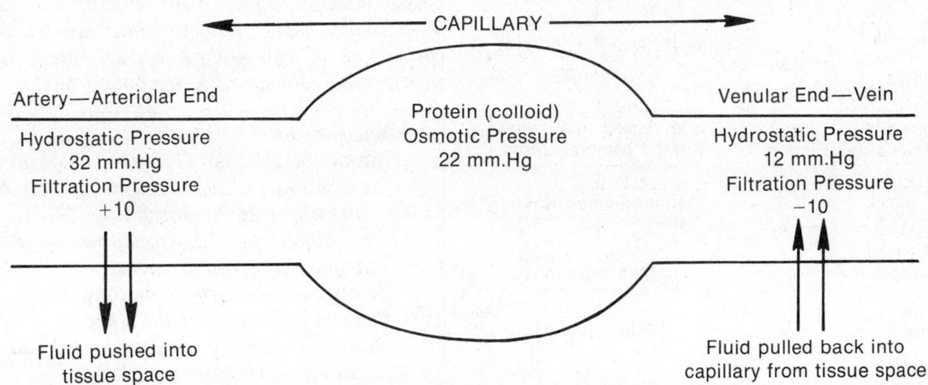

FIGURE 24–6. Pressure differences within the capillary function to push and pull fluid; fluid is pushed out of the capillary into the tissue spaces at the arteriolar end and is pulled back into the capillary from the tissue spaces at the venular end. (Modified from Dutcher and Fielo.)

"anti" or opposed to fluid loss. Some major facts concerning ADH are boxed below:

> ADH
> Major functions: *(1) water conservation by promoting water reabsorption by the kidney; (2) control of the osmotic pressure of the extracellular fluid (ECF).*
> Formed: *by neurosecretory cells of the hypothalamus.*
> Stimulus: *increased osmolarity of the ECF.*
> Released: *from the posterior lobes of the pituitary gland.*
> Site of action: *distal renal tubules and collecting duct of the kidney.**

The release of ADH is stimulated by an *increase* in the osmolarity (hyperosmolarity) of the extracellular fluid, which stimulates the osmoreceptors located in the hypothalamus.† Stimulation of the osmoreceptors, in turn, stimulates the release of ADH from storage in the posterior pituitary gland. In sum, an *increase* in the osmolarity of the ECF results in an *increased secretion* of ADH and a *decreased* urinary output. Conversely, a *decrease* in the osmolarity of the ECF leads to a *decreased secretion* of ADH and an *increased* urinary output. For a diagrammatic illustration of the effect of osmolarity on ADH release, see Figure 24–7.

There are at least nine circumstances that can *stimulate* ADH production and release with resultant water conservation: water loss that causes an increase in ECF osmolarity, reduced circulatory blood volume, morphine sulfate injections, pain, barbiturates, anesthetics, emotional stress, surgical trauma, and accidental trauma.

It is particularly important for nurses and doctors to recognize the interrelationship between surgical or accidental trauma and the release of ADH. The actions of ADH on the body and the physiologic reactions of the body to surgical or accidental trauma are similar. It appears that surgical procedures activate the patient's hypothalamic centers with the resultant stimulation of both the anterior and posterior lobes. Consequently, both ADH and ACTH are released in large amounts following injury. (You will recall from Unit II that ACTH is one of the hormones involved in stress reactions.) This means that following surgery or accident, *urine volume is reduced regardless of intake!* Remember, then, the following important rule:

> *Administer fluids* cautiously *during early postoperative and post-trauma periods while ADH is being released. "Forcing" fluids can result in overhydration and drowning.*

Factors suppressing ADH formation are: (1) hypo-osmolarity of the ECF or an increased water load, (2) increased blood volume, (3) cold, (4) acute alcohol ingestion, (5) CO_2 inhalations, and (6) diuretics. These conditions, then, cause an *increased urinary output.*

Diabetes insipidus* is an endocrine disease caused by a lack of ADH production. This condition is characterized by extreme thirst, high fluid intake, and the resultant daily voiding of large amounts of very dilute urine. Before the advent of hormonal therapy, patients with this malady were known, in extreme circumstances, to drink their own urine, so great was their misery from thirst and dehydration! For a diagrammatic summary of factors stimulating and inhibiting ADH release, see Figure 24–8.

Aldosterone

The second hormonal regulator of fluid and electrolyte metabolism is aldosterone. Whereas ADH is the body's great conserver of water, aldosterone is the body's great conserver of sodium (Na^+). Because sodium holds fluid within the body (more specifically ECF), aldosterone, like ADH, is also a conserver of the body's water. Some major facts concerning aldosterone are boxed below:

> Aldosterone
> Major functions: *(1) conservation of Na^+ excretion in such conditions as Na^+ depletion and hemorrhage; (2) regulation of blood and extracellular fluid volume.*
> Formed: *in adrenal cortex.*
> Stimulus: *Sodium depletion.*
> Released: *from adrenal cortex.*
> Site of action: *kidney nephron, sweat glands, and salivary glands.*

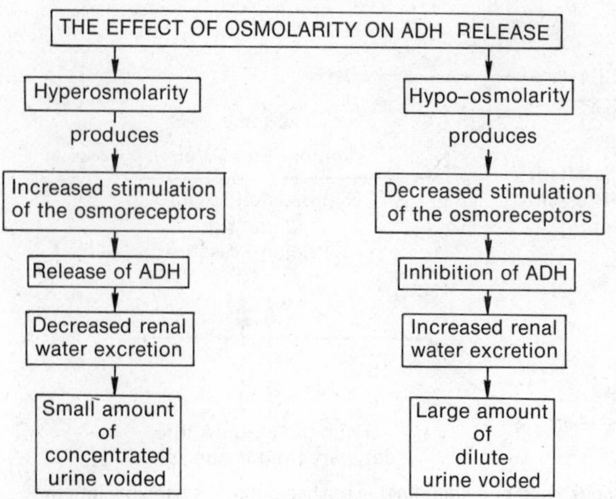

FIGURE 24–7. The effect of osmolarity on ADH release and inhibition.

*The role of the kidney in regulating fluid and electrolyte metabolism is discussed on pp. 204–207.

†Osmoreceptors are cells sensitive to slight osmotic changes in the blood bathing them.

†Diabetes insipidus is discussed in detail in Unit XIX.

There are at least six major factors that control the secretion of aldosterone.

Sodium Depletion. Sodium depletion appears to be the *greatest single stimulus* to aldosterone secretion. Sodium depletion occurs among people who are deprived of a sufficient NaCl intake, who sweat excessively, or who live in hot climates. These individuals suffer from a decrease in ECF and plasma volume, with a resultant reduced blood flow to vital organs such as the kidney. With the release of aldosterone, sodium is conserved and body fluid is retained.

Changes in the ECF Volume. These affect the *rate* of aldosterone secretion. An increase in the ECF volume causes a *decrease* in aldosterone secretion and an *increase* in renal sodium excretion. Thus, *dehydration* leads to an increase in aldosterone secretion.

Changes in Blood Volume. These are of great importance in influencing aldosterone excretion. An acute *loss* of blood as a result of *hemorrhage* is a major stimulus for aldosterone release, renal tubular reabsorption of sodium, and resultant water retention, which acts to keep the Na^+ in an isotonic solution.

Changes in the Electrolyte Composition of the Plasma. These changes also control aldosterone secretion. Increased sodium excretion, decreased potassium excretion, and/or increased potassium intake all result in increased aldosterone secretion.

Constriction of Two Major Arteries. Constriction of the carotid and the renal arteries stimulates an increased secretion of aldosterone.

Large Doses of ACTH. These also cause an increase in aldosterone secretion. This effect, however, is short lived in man.

Other factors that stimulate aldosterone secretion are nervous tension and anxiety, pregnancy, major surgery, and trauma. Also, an increased aldosterone within the circulating blood may be caused by *hepatic disease* or failure, because the liver is almost completely responsible for the removal of excess aldosterone from the body. Thus, individuals with liver disease tend to suffer from edema because of excessive sodium and water retention.

In addition to the two homeostatic regulating hormones just discussed, three other hormones—the thyroid hormone, the parathyroid hormone, and the diuretic hormone—should also be considered.

Thyroid, Parathyroid and Diuretic Hormones

The thyroid and diuretic hormones are both important for normal diuresis. The release of *thyroid hormone* increases renal blood flow, glomerular filtration rate, and urinary output. The second hormone that increases diuresis is the *diuretic hormone* (DH). DH is secreted by the anterior lobe of the pituitary gland and directly increases urinary output. Little is presently known about DH.

The parathyroid hormone, known as parathormone (PTH), is linked with the homeostatic regulation of calcium and phosphate ion concentration in body fluids. PTH acts mainly on the kidneys, bones, and gastrointestinal tract. Insufficient PTH can cause severe imbalances of calcium and phosphorus. The functions of calcium and phosphorus, the imbalances involving these two ions, and the specific role of PTH will be discussed further in the next chapter.

In sum, hormones that prevent an excessive loss of water from the body are ADH and aldosterone. ADH conserves body water and controls the ECF volume by promoting renal tubular reabsorption of water. Aldosterone conserves the body fluids by promoting reabsorption of sodium ions by the kidney, resulting in water retention.

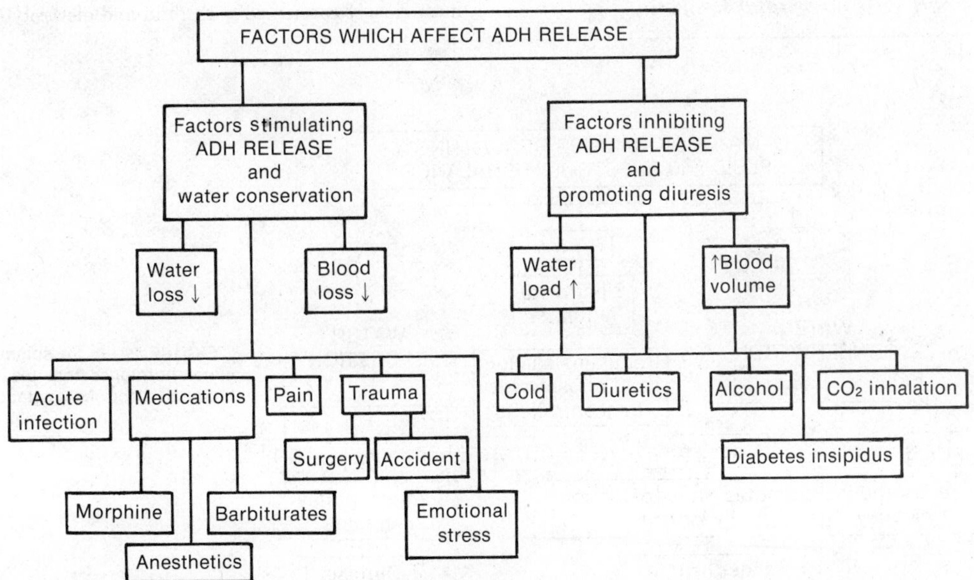

FIGURE 24-8. Factors that stimulate and inhibit the release of ADH.

In contrast, the two major hormones promoting diuresis and water loss are the thyroid and diuretic hormones. Parathormone acts mainly to establish proper calcium and phosphorus metabolism (Fig. 24–9).

THE GASTROINTESTINAL TRACT AS A HOMEOSTATIC REGULATOR

Another equally important mechanism for maintaining fluid balance is the gastrointestinal tract. Under normal conditions the gastrointestinal system is the sole route of intake for fluids and electrolytes. Thus, the major role of the gastrointestinal tract is the replenishment, by absorption, of the fluids and electrolytes lost from the body through the skin, respiratory tract, and kidney. The intestinal tract absorbs the fluids from dietary intake, as well as approximately 7 to 9 L. of glandular and gastrointestinal tract secretions. However, out of this enormous amount of fluid, only 100 ml. of water are lost from the bowel daily; the rest is reabsorbed.

Moreover, fluids and electrolytes within the intestinal tract are subject to rapid transport across the intestinal mucosa in both directions. Authorities estimate that every 90 minutes a volume of fluid equal to the volume of the body's blood plasma (i.e., 3000 ml. in a 70-kg. man) passes through the intestinal mucosa.[70] With such a rapid turnover of fluid, it is no wonder that the smallest upset in gastrointestinal tract function precipitates fluid and electrolyte imbalance.

> *The fluid imbalances and depletions most commonly encountered in clinical practice are gastrointestinal in origin.*

THE RENAL SYSTEM AS A HOMEOSTATIC REGULATOR

The kidney, the most complex organ of the body with the possible exception of the brain, is the *chief regulator of homeostasis and of the body's internal environment.* It carries the major responsibility for the regulation of water as well as of sodium and hydrogen ions. To understand the work of the kidney in maintaining fluid and electrolyte metabolism, we must review the anatomic structure of the kidney and those physiologic functions of the kidney specifically concerned with water and electrolytes.

Anatomic Structure of the Kidney*

The *nephron* is the kidney's functional unit, serving to clear the blood of waste materials, form urine, and regulate both the fluid and electrolyte and the acid-base (H^+) balance of the body. Within each human kidney there are approximately 1,000,000 nephrons. Each nephron is composed of a glomerulus, Bowman's capsule, proximal convoluted tubule, the loop of Henle, the distal convoluted tubule, the collecting tubule, an afferent and efferent vessel, as well as a capillary network. Each nephron is in communication with other nephrons by means of linking tubules.

The work of the nephron in the formation of urine is as follows: Blood, under high pressure, flows into the kidney from the renal artery—an artery that is derived directly from the abdominal aorta. Upon reaching the kidney, the blood is channeled into a cluster of tiny capillaries called a *glomerulus,* a word from the Latin meaning "little ball." Each glomerulus, in turn, is partly encapsulated within a double endothelial capsule called

*The anatomy of the kidney will be discussed in greater detail in Unit XI. In this chapter, we are mainly concerned with the kidney nephron, which is the structure most closely connected with fluid and electrolyte balance.

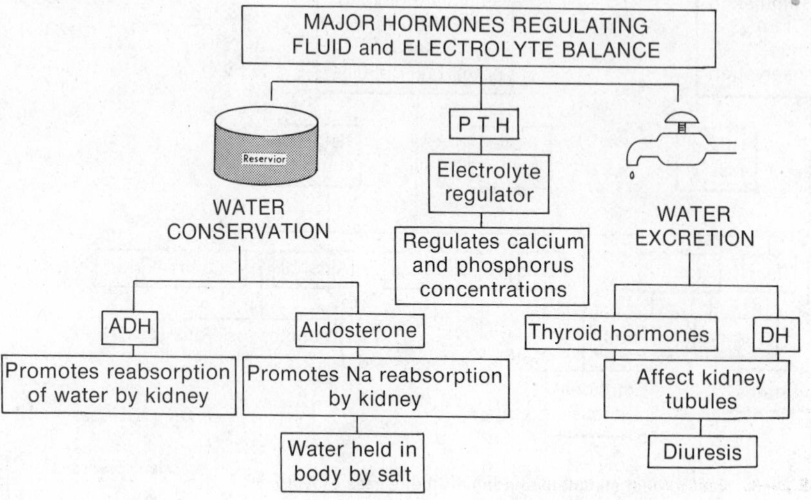

FIGURE 24–9. A summary of the major hormones that play a role in fluid and electrolyte metabolism.

Bowman's capsule. Because of the extremely high pressure of the blood within the capillaries encapsulated by Bowman's capsule, an act of filtration occurs and the Bowman's capsule extracts from the glomerulus a dilute, protein-free filtrate that is similar in composition to plasma. Plasma proteins and cells are left behind in the blood stream because the capillary walls and the walls of Bowman's capsule are semipermeable membranes through which only certain substances can pass. Many useful substances as well as waste products, however, do pass through the membrane walls into the filtrate. The Bowman's capsule forms this plasma-like ultrafiltrate at the average rate of 125–130 ml./minute.

From the Bowman's capsule the filtrate flows into the all-important renal tubules. Within the *proximal convoluted tubule* reabsorption of 85 per cent of the water, some sodium chloride and other electrolytes, as well as glucose, creatine, amino acids, vitamin C, and lactate, takes place. This process is called *obligatory* reabsorption, i.e., this is reabsorption that takes place *without regard* for the body's need for fluids and electrolytes. Within the *loop of Henle* further reabsorption of water occurs. Finally, within the *distal convoluted tubule, facultative reabsorption* of water takes place, a reabsorption of water governed by the body's *requirements* for fluids. Facultative reabsorption is controlled by ADH. This process is diagrammatically illustrated in Figure 24–11.

By the time the filtrate is ready to enter the *collecting tube,* where the process of urine formation will be finally completed, 98 per cent of the glomerular filtrate will have been reabsorbed! This means that out of every 125 ml. of fluid that pass through the glomerulus every minute, approximately 123 ml. of fluid will be returned to the blood stream, and only 2 ml. of filtrate will be finally transformed to urine. This 2 ml., then, will be carried to the renal pelvis to be excreted from the body. Because of their abilities, the kidneys are called the master chemists of the body. Any renal upset or disease, consequently, wreaks havoc on the body's fluid and electrolyte balance by destroying kidney function.

Physiologic Functions of the Kidney in Health and Disease

The major functions of the kidney are briefly listed in the box below:

The Kidney

1. *Selects and rejects materials according to the body's needs.*
2. *Removes wastes from the body.*
3. *Controls H^+ balance.*
4. *Regulates the composition of the blood and ECF.*
5. *Maintains volume and concentration of urine.*
6. *Regulates sodium.*

Kidney Selectivity. As you recall from our discussion of the structure of the nephron, most of the water, electrolytes, and other substances that pass through the glomerulus are normally returned to the blood stream. The selectivity of the nephron is markedly altered, however, in the very young, the very old, and in patients suffering from burns, shock, cardiovascular-renal disease, and various forms of stress. In these conditions, water tends to be retained and, consequently, the plasma and ECF volumes are maintained at the expense of the body's tonicity. In other words, under these particular circumstances, fluid is retained *in excess* of sodium. This retention of fluid leads to a *hypotonic* overexpansion of the ECF that is more persistent and more difficult to treat than is the problem of dehydration. Thus, an alteration of nephron selectivity can lead to a state of overhydration or hypo-osmolarity (water in excess of solute particles).

Removal of Wastes. The kidneys remove the waste products of metabolism, nitrogenous products, drugs, toxins, and other foreign substances that have been absorbed by the digestive tract.

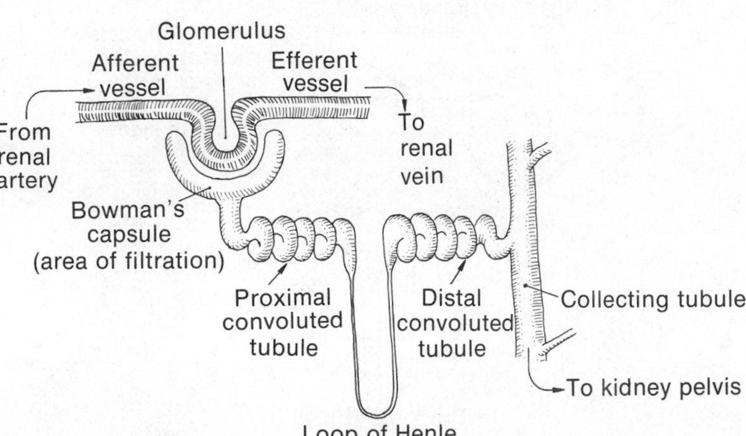

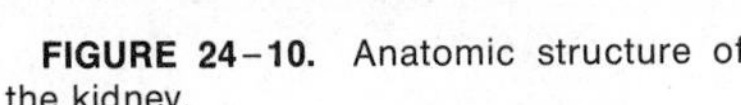
FIGURE 24–10. Anatomic structure of the kidney.

This function will be considered in detail in the unit on kidney disease.

H^+ Balance. One vital role of the kidney is to maintain the blood at the slightly alkaline pH of 7.35 to 7.45. The kidney is able to control the alkalinity of the blood by controlling the *rate* at which H^+ is excreted from the body. We shall discuss pH, and the control of H^+ balance in greater detail in Chapter 25.

Blood Composition. The kidney nephron, by means of its selective filtration process and its reabsorptive abilities, directly affects the composition of the blood and the ECF. By altering the osmolarity (number of particles per liter) of the ECF, the kidney indirectly affects the osmolarity of the ICF. For example, if the kidney becomes seriously damaged, blood composition may be radically changed because wastes and toxins, as well as excess acids, are not being excreted. This alteration in blood composition will eventually affect the water and electrolyte composition of the entire body—within the vascular system, within the tissues, and within the cells.

Maintenance of Volume and Concentration of Urine. Both the urine volume and the concentration of electrolytes within the urine vary widely from person to person as well as from day to day in the same person. For example, under extreme circumstances, urine volume output could vary from 200 ml. per day to 14 liters per day.

Electrolyte concentrations in the urine are equally variable. Sodium, chloride, potassium, calcium, and phosphorus may appear in small or large amounts, depending upon the body's needs at the time. Thus, there are not set norms for the concentration of electrolytes within the urine—there are just minimum, optimum, and maximum values.

While volume and concentration of urine are variable, this variability is, with health, in keeping with the body's requirements at the time. The volume and concentration of urine varies: if we ingest more fluids and electrolytes than the body needs, *excretion* results; and if we ingest fewer fluids and electrolytes than the body needs, *conservation* results.

This means that if a healthy person ingests a large amount of fluid, he will excrete a large volume of dilute urine. Conversely, if he ingests a small amount of fluid, he will excrete a small volume of concentrated urine. If he has a decreased intake of *both* water and sodium chloride or an increased loss of these substances, only the minimum volume of urine necessary for eliminating the nitrogenous wastes accumulated from the day's metabolic activities will be excreted. This volume is approximately 500 ml. As you can readily see, the capacity of the kidney to alter the concentration and volume of urine to be excreted is highly adaptive for man; without such a capacity we could not survive.

The ability of the kidney to concentrate urine is a good test both of kidney function and of the state of the body's fluid balance. The normal kidney is able to concentrate urine up to a specific gravity of 1.030.* When a person has healthy kidneys we can determine his fluid balance by measuring the specific gravity of his urine; a *low* weight indicates fluid excess, while a *high* weight indicates a fluid deficit.

*Specific gravity is the ratio of the weight of a substance to the weight of an equal volume of water. As a basis of comparison, laboratories use water as a constant against which to measure solutions such as urine. Distilled water has a specific gravity of 1.000 Gm/ml.; i.e., 1 ml. of water weighs 1 Gm. The normal range for the specific gravity of urine is from 1.010 to 1.030. In the case of urine and certain other solutions, the term "specific gravity" is also used to indicate the concentration of that solution.

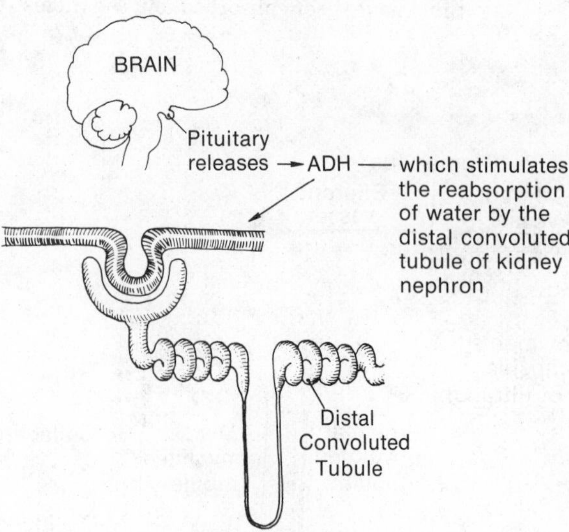

FIGURE 24–11. Action of the kidney.

The test for the specific gravity of urine has important implications for the surgical patient. It is necessary to know the concentrating powers of a patient's kidneys *before* surgery in order to maintain his fluid balance *following* surgery. The preoperative patient with *normal* kidneys will be able to concentrate urine to a specific gravity of 1.030. This means that he will be able to excrete in a 24-hour period 35 gm. of solutes in a liquid medium of 500 ml. This amount of solute waste is normal for a 24-hour period. If the preoperative patient has *impaired* kidneys, he may be able to concentrate urine to only 1.010; thus, he will require 1450 ml. of water to excrete the same 35 gm. of solutes in 24 hours. Following surgery, the patient with damaged kidneys will have an even larger load of solute wastes owing to the trauma he has undergone. As a result, it may take an even greater amount of urine to excrete his solutes!

You will recall that ADH normally conserves water in the body following trauma or surgery. In the patient with renal disease this mechanism will not be operative, and consequently he may lose much more fluid than he should at this critical time.

In addition to renal disease, any serious illness tends to impair the function of the nephron. Thus, in diseases unrelated to the kidney, the patient may also be subject to dehydration because of the kidney's inability to concentrate the urine.

To summarize, the kidneys alter the volume and concentration of urine in keeping with the body's requirements. When the ability to concentrate urine is lost, as a result of kidney or other disease, there is danger of developing dehydration.

Sodium Regulation. You will recall that sodium determines both the volume and the osmolarity of the ECF; the kidney, which controls the delicate balance of sodium within the body, is precise in its capacity to conserve sodium. Over a three- to four-day period, *intake of sodium almost exactly equals output.* Moreover, out of the 24,000 mEq. of Na^+ filtered by the glomeruli daily, 99.5 per cent is reabsorbed in order to keep the body in a steady state.

What controls the kidney in its regulation of sodium? Two factors seem important: First of all, aldosterone fosters sodium reabsorption; second, changes in body posture seem to be associated with changes in urine flow and sodium excretion. For example, when an individual first stands up after lying down, urine flow and sodium excretion are decreased. Conversely, if he has been standing up and then goes to bed, both urine flow and sodium excretion increase. These changes in posture have definite implications for patients on bed rest.* Individuals lying down may initially have a better urinary output than those standing for prolonged periods. Diuresis is thus temporarily facilitated by bed rest.

For purposes of simplification, we have discussed the kidney in isolation from the other organs of the body. Actually, the kidney is vitally linked with every other organ, particularly the hormonal and nervous systems. Moreover, the kidney forms a vital link in the cardiovascular-renal system. Consequently, hormonal diseases (especially those involving ADH and aldosterone), nervous system disorders, and cardiovascular disorders all affect kidney function and consequently fluid and electrolyte balance. Congestive heart failure, hypertension, diabetes insipidus, and disorders of the adrenal cortex are a few of the numerous diseases that can impair the work of the kidney nephron.

*For a further discussion of bed rest, see Chapter 27.

THE NERVOUS SYSTEM AS A HOMEOSTATIC REGULATOR

While the kidney is characterized as the "master chemist" of the body, the brain and nervous system can be characterized as the "master switchboard," regulating the kidney as well as the rest of the body. The overall function of the brain as a homeostatic regulator is to centrally control water and sodium intake and excretion. The brain accomplishes its role by means of the following:

The brain:

1. *Manufactures* ADH.
2. *Contains regulatory mechanisms for correcting changes in the* volume *of body water.*
3. *Contains regulatory mechanisms for correcting changes in the* osmolarity *of body water.*

Hormonal Production

The antidiuretic hormone, ADH, is secreted by the cells of the hypothalamus, a portion of the brain. ADH is stored in the posterior pituitary. See previous discussion, page 201.

Regulation of Body Water Volume

The midbrain contains a *volumetric monitoring system* that responds to variations in extracellular fluid volume. This system evidently receives information about fluid volume from various receptors located in the walls of the great veins, the arteries, and the atria. From the volumetric monitoring system, information concerning blood volume is relayed to those control systems that govern ADH release, thirst, and the release of aldosterone.

How are these mechanisms stimulated and inhibited? You will recall that receptors in the hypothalamus are responsible for stimulating the release of *ADH* from storage in the posterior pituitary gland. The *thirst center* is also located in the hypothalamus and may be turned off and on by changes in body fluid osmolarity. In addition, messages are somehow carried from the volumetric regulating center to the adrenal cortex for either the release or inhibition of aldosterone—the body's conserver of sodium, and, consequently, of water.

To illustrate how body water volume is regulated, consider the following examples of volume increase and decrease. When body water volume increases (*hypervolemia*), ADH release is inhibited and aldosterone is not secreted. As a result, the individual urinates a large amount of fluid. Because he is not thirsty, he does not drink to replace the water he is excreting, and his body fluid regains its normal volume. Conversely, when body water volume decreases significantly (*hypovolemia*), ADH is released. The thirst center is stimulated and the individual drinks; also, his urine becomes less in amount and is more concentrated. Moreover, because of aldosterone release, sodium is conserved and water is held in the body; thus, water balance is again achieved (Fig. 24–12).

Regulation of Body Water Osmolarity

While the *midbrain* apparently contains the volume receptors, the *hypothalamus* is believed to be the locus of activity for the regulation of body osmolarity. First, the hypothalamus manufactures ADH and contains osmoreceptors that signal the posterior pituitary gland to release or to retain ADH as needed. Osmoreceptors in the hypothalamus are believed to shrink when the osmolarity of the ECF increases and to swell when the osmolarity of the ECF decreases. Consequently, an increased osmolarity of the ECF (which causes the osmoreceptors to shrink) allows ADH to be released. Conversely, in patients in whom osmolarity of the ECF is decreased, the osmoreceptors swell and ADH is not secreted.

Second, the *thirst center* is very sensitive to the osmolarity of the body fluids. Basically, thirst results from (1) low water intake, (2) excessive water loss, (3) excessive Na^+ intake, and (4) excessive intravenous infusion of hypertonic solutions.* These circumstances result in cellular dehydration, reduced blood volume (hypovolemia), and hyperosmolarity of the ECF. These changes in osmolarity stimulate the thirst center, and nerve impulses are conveyed to the higher brain centers which then create "the drive to drink"—a drive that is controlled, to some degree, by cultural norms.

On the other hand, thirst is *inhibited* by (1) a large water intake, (2) water retention within the body, (3) a low Na^+ intake, and (4) excessive infusions of isotonic or hypotonic solutions.* These circumstances result in cellular overhydration, an increased blood volume (hypervolemia), and decreased osmolarity of the ECF, which, in turn, results in a diminished drive to drink.

A patient's complaint of thirst is of practical importance because thirst is the major symptom that people are *consciously* aware of in fluid imbalance and dehydration. However, the presence or absence of thirst, in clinical situations, is *not al-*

*An *isotonic solution* is one which has the *same* osmolarity as another solution, i.e., normal saline that contains 0.9 per cent NaCl is isotonic with plasma. A *hypotonic solution* is one that has a *lower* osmolarity than another solution to which it is compared. For example, distilled water is hypotonic to plasma. A *hypertonic solution* is one that has a *greater* osmolarity than another solution to which it is compared. For example, a solution of NaCl 5 per cent would be hypertonic to plasma.

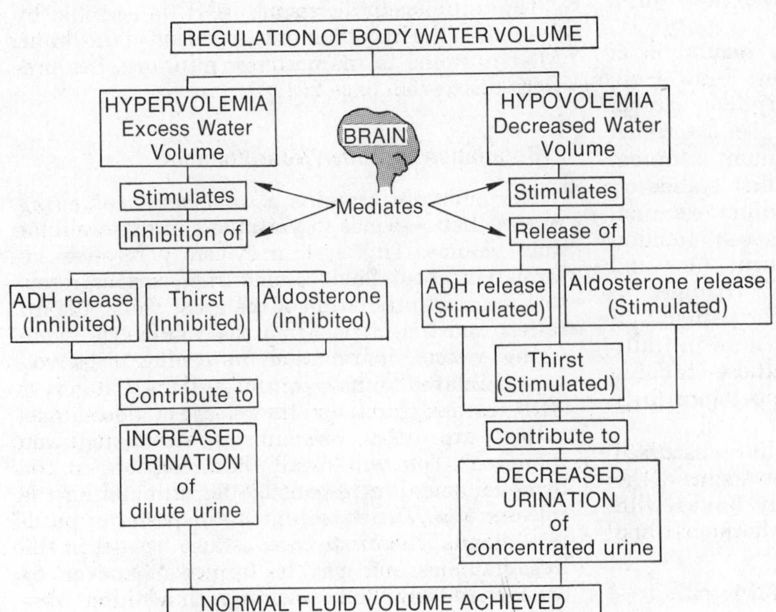

FIGURE 24–12. The regulation of body water volume depends upon ADH, thirst, and aldosterone. The release or inhibition of these mechanisms is mediated by the brain.

ways a true indicator of the state of fluid balance, for the following reasons:

1. *Edematous* individuals may be thirsty, although they appear to be overloaded with fluid. Their thirst develops because the blood volume of the edematous patient may actually be quite low as a result of the seepage of a large amount of plasma into tissue spaces, thereby causing a type of dehydration. Sufficient fluid is not available in the blood stream to effectively circulate to tissues and cells.

2. A *dehydrated* person may not be thirsty. For example, comatose or confused elderly patients may be severely dehydrated, and yet have no drive to drink.

3. A person with *hypo-osmolarity* of the ECF will not experience thirst even though the water volume of his body is lowered. In conditions in which the individual has lost more electrolytes than water, the drive to drink will be inhibited even though a state of dehydration exists.

4. An individual may be *either* dehydrated or in a state of fluid overload because his responses to the thirst drive are influenced more by the customs of his culture than by his actual fluid requirements. For example, in American culture it is customary to drink socially and at meals; we consider it impolite not to offer a guest a beverage. Consequently, at times, the drinking habits of Americans may be more influenced by social custom than by the physiologic need for fluid.

At this point, let us briefly review the mechanisms discussed. The overall function of the brain in the control of homeostatic mechanisms is to ensure the proper intake and excretion of sodium and water. As we have pointed out, the brain performs this function by means of hormonal production and secretion, and by the regulation of both body fluid volume and osmolarity. The role of the brain and nervous system in water and sodium control is briefly summarized in the outline that follows.

CENTRAL REGULATION OF WATER AND SODIUM HOMEOSTASIS BY THE BRAIN AND NERVOUS SYSTEM*

I. **Intake of Water**
   - A. *Regulated by midbrain volume receptors.*
     1. Increased volume of ECF leads to a decrease in ADH and inhibits thirst.
     2. Decreased fluid volume leads to an increase in ADH and stimulates thirst.
     3. Adrenal cortex stimulated to release or inhibit aldosterone. If fluid volume low, aldosterone released; if fluid volume high, aldosterone inhibited.
   - B. *Regulated by "thirst" osmoreceptors in the hypothalamus.*
     1. Hyperosmolarity of ECF is stimulus to thirst.
     2. Hypo-osmolarity inhibits thirst.

II. **Intake of Sodium**
   Probably regulated by a midbrain volume receptor, which signals adrenal cortex to release aldosterone.
   - A. "Salt hunger" (a desire for salty foods) stimulated by a negative sodium balance.
   - B. "Salt hunger" inhibited by a positive sodium balance.

III. **Excretion of Water**
   - A. *Midbrain volume receptors.*
     1. Stimulate water *excretion* when fluid volume is *high* (ADH inhibited).
     2. Stimulate water *retention* when fluid volume is *low* (ADH released).
   - B. *Osmoreceptors in hypothalamus.*
     1. ADH released in hyperosmolarity.
     2. ADH inhibited in hypo-osmolarity.
   - C. *Midbrain and renal volume receptors.*
     1. Stimulate *aldosterone* secretion if fluid volume low, retaining Na^+ and H_2O.
     2. Inhibit aldosterone secretion when fluid volume is high; thus, Na^+ retention is decreased and water is excreted.

IV. **Excretion of Sodium**
   Regulated by midbrain and renal volume receptors.
   - A. Na^+ depletion stimulates aldosterone secretion and sodium conservation.
   - B. Overloading with Na^+ inhibits aldosterone rerelease.

Two illustrations of how the brain normally responds to changes in fluid volume and osmolarity follow: First, consider what happens to a man who is vigorously exercising and consequently is losing a great deal of water and some Na^+ in his sweat. This man loses a certain amount of his blood volume, which can be demonstrated by a definite loss in weight. The receptors in his vascular system consequently respond to the loss of blood volume and relay the message to the midbrain.

From the volumetric center in the midbrain, messages are conveyed to the hypothalamus, which then stimulates the release of ADH from the posterior pituitary gland. Because the plasma is more concentrated than normal, fluid is pulled from the interstitial and intracellular compartments into the vascular system. Also, the hyperosmolarity of the ECF stimulates osmoreceptors in the hypothalamus, which further contribute to ADH release. With the secretion of ADH, the desire to urinate is diminished, and the urine produced appears somewhat concentrated. Thirst and "salt hunger" increase. Thirst is in response to changes in body fluid volume and osmolarity, which are conveyed to the thirst center, while "salt hunger" is apparently linked to stimulation of the volume receptors in the midbrain. As a result of the release of aldosterone, any Na^+ that this individual ingests will be retained, and Na^+ retention, in turn, holds fluid within his body. Thus, at the end of his tasks, this man, weary from exercise and possibly pleased with his weight loss, will probably be found resting, having a large cold drink, eating

*Adapted from Logothetis, J.: Postgraduate Medicine 40:408, October, 1966.

potato chips, and rapidly regaining both his fluid and weight losses!

Conversely, what happens to the individual who has a fluid overload, perhaps resulting from a big night out with the boys and too much to drink? Just the opposite changes occur in the overhydrated man as those present in the individual just described; in situations of fluid overload there are increased blood and ECF volumes. Volume receptors respond accordingly, and ADH and aldosterone are not secreted. However, DH is secreted, thirst and "salt hunger" are inhibited, and diuresis results. The overhydrated man, then, who has healthy nervous, renal, and hormonal systems will urinate a large amount of dilute urine. As a result, his blood and ECF volumes are again restored to normal.

References

The references for this chapter will be found at the end of Chapter 25.

CHAPTER 25

Fluid and Electrolyte Imbalance

INTRODUCTION AND STUDY GUIDE

We have discussed in the preceding chapter general concepts of fluid and electrolyte balance. In this chapter these general concepts are applied both to patients suffering from specific imbalances and to groups of patients who are particularly *prone* to imbalances, e.g., patients who are burned, vomiting, or undergoing surgical treatment. Guidance is given in the process of assessing patients with suspected imbalances as well as in caring for them once an imbalance is diagnosed. Throughout the chapter prevention of imbalances will be emphasized, for preventive care is always one of a nurse's most essential tasks. The major topics which are included in this chapter are:

> General concepts of fluid and electrolyte imbalance.
> Specific fluid and electrolyte imbalances.
> General principles of diagnosis, management, and treatment of various imbalances.
> The care of patients particularly susceptible to imbalances.

The reader may find the following chapter guide helpful:

1. Before beginning to study this chapter, be certain you understand the following concepts discussed in Chapter 24.

a. *Water.* Its functions; how it is gained and lost normally and abnormally by the body; requirements for daily living.
b. *Electrolytes.* Their functions; the maintenance of balance; electrolyte concentrations in the body's fluid compartments.
c. *Osmolarity.*
d. Colloid osmotic pressure.
e. Homeostatic mechanisms controlling fluids and electrolytes.

2. As you study this chapter familiarize yourself with the following terms:

volume deficit, volume excess, dehydration, water intoxication, circulatory overload, ascites, hypernatremia, hyponatremia, pH, buffer, steady state regulator, chloride shift, pO_2, pCO_2, acidosis, alkalosis, primary and compensatory H^+ imbalances, carbon dioxide narcosis, hyperkalemia, hypokalemia, tetany, Trousseau's phenomenon, Chvostek's sign, hypercalcemic crisis, delirium tremens, hypoproteinemia, central venous pressure, negative nitrogen balance, paralytic ileus, anasarca, and edema: pitting, dependent, refractory.

3. Endeavor to become acquainted with the following medications and solutions:

colloidal solutions, noncolloidal solutions, amino acid preparations, fat emulsions, alcohol preparations, electrolyte solutions, diuretics (mercurial and thiazide), potassium chloride, potassium triplex, potassium citrate, IV calcium salts, calcium gluconate, adrenocortical medications, THAM, 0.9 per cent ammonium chloride.

4. Upon completion of this chapter, you should be able to apply this knowledge to patients in your care. Thus, in the clinical situation:

a. Identify those patients assigned to you who are likely candidates for developing an imbalance.
b. *Prevent* imbalances from developing in your patients.
c. Look for the early signs of imbalance and report them accurately.
d. Assess patients' needs in terms of fluids and diet.
e. Participate knowledgeably in the treatment of fluid and electrolyte upsets, being fully aware of the medical problems that medical treatment can create.

GENERAL CONCEPTS OF FLUID AND ELECTROLYTE IMBALANCE

THE MAJOR TYPES OF IMBALANCES

Fluid and electrolyte imbalances can be categorized into three types of conditions, caused by: (1) a *deficit* or an *excess* of any one of the substances of which the body is composed, (2) a nutritional deficiency, and (3) a shift in the position of the extracellular fluid (ECF). Disorders that can be caused by a *deficit or excess of essential body substances* are:

> Water-sodium imbalances.
> Hydrogen ion imbalances.
> Potassium imbalances.
> Calcium imbalances.
> Magnesium imbalances.

Disorders caused by *nutritional deficiencies* are:

> Protein deficiency (hypoproteinemia).
> Caloric deficiency.

The two important *fluid shifts* are:

> Plasma shifts to the interstitial space.
> Interstitial fluid shifts into the plasma.

A given patient may have one imbalance or a combination of imbalances. For example, water and sodium deficit, potassium deficit and acidosis (hydrogen ion excess) may all occur together in a patient suffering from severe diarrhea.

PATIENTS MOST LIKELY TO DEVELOP IMBALANCES

Almost *every* patient, regardless of diagnosis, who is sick enough to be in the hospital has some problem with his water and electrolyte balance. This is because illness, by its very nature, upsets the body's delicate homeostatic mechanisms, thereby making imbalances inevitable. Certain patients, because of their particular illnesses, are especially vulnerable to fluid and electrolyte upsets. Persons suffering from the following conditions or undergoing the following therapies need special vigilance on the part of the nurse:

Conditions Contributing to Imbalances	Therapies Contributing to Imbalances
Ulcerative colitis	Surgery
Kidney disease	Diuretic therapy
Burns	Low sodium diets
Congestive heart failure	Hormonal therapy
Cirrhosis of the liver	Intravenous therapy
Severe diabetes	
Hormonal disorders	

These and all other patients whose conditions are serious or critical warrant a careful intake and output record, as well as continuous observation for symptoms of imbalance.

MAJOR FACTORS CAUSING IMBALANCES

Deviations of fluid and electrolyte balance from normal are caused by alterations in the *volume of water* in one or all of the body's fluid compartments, and alterations in the *concentrations of electrolytes* within the fluid media (osmolarity). The major causes for such deviations are listed below:

A. Fluids and electrolytes may be *deficient.*
   1. Intake may be below the minimum requirements of the body.
   2. Excretion or loss of fluid and electrolytes may be increased.
   3. Important substances or chemicals may be undergoing destruction within the body.

B. Fluids and electrolytes may be in *excess* of the body's needs.
   1. Intake may be greater in amount than a healthy body can excrete.
   2. Excretion may be impossible because of kidney or liver disease.
   3. Excessive amounts of electrolytes may *accumulate* in the body of the patient suffering from an extensive death of tissue, e.g., from burns or other severe injury.

C. Water and electrolytes may undergo *fixation* within the body. For example, in *ascites,* fluid collects within the abdomen; in *edema,* fluid accumulates within the tissue spaces. In both these conditions, fluids are lost from the body's vital circulation. As a result, the patient with either ascites or edema, or both conditions, actually suffers from a *water deficit,* even though he appears to be "water-logged."

D. The body may *increase its use* of fluids and electrolytes in the presence of high fever and infection.

E. Upsets in *homeostatic balance* or the breakdown of homeostatic-regulating mechanisms such as the kidney nephron may result in severe imbalance.

PHYSIOLOGIC CHANGES DUE TO IMBALANCES

> *Fluid and electrolyte imbalances, once they develop, tend to affect* every *system of the body.*

Calcium imbalance affects the bones, kidneys, and gastrointestinal tract; potassium imbalance affects the heart and muscles as well as the nervous system; and sodium imbalance affects blood volume and blood pressure as well as the nervous system. A water imbalance affects the entire body, including the eyeballs, the body tissues, and the brain. In sum, while the various imbalances do have specific causes, the *physiologic effects* of the imbalances tend to be somewhat nonspecific and to involve the total organism.

WATER-SODIUM BALANCE AND IMBALANCE

Because body fluids contain *both* water and sodium, and because variations in the water component affect the sodium component and vice versa, water and sodium balances and imbalances must be considered *together* and in *relationship* to each other.* Before describing disturbed relationships between water and sodium, normal water and sodium balance should be understood. Body water was discussed at length in Chapter 24.

SODIUM (Na^+) METABOLISM

The outline opposite summarizes basic facts concerning Na^+ balance.

*Sodium, potassium, calcium, hydrogen, and so forth, exist in the body in ionized form. Consequently, when we discuss sodium in this chapter, we are referring to the sodium ion (Na^+).

The following *general* statements can be made about sodium imbalance from the essential facts listed. First, deficiencies or excesses of body sodium result in the following problems:

> Blood volume changes:
Na^+ deficit ⟶ blood volume deficit (hypovolemia)
Na^+ excess ⟶ blood volume excess (hypervolemia)
> Blood pressure changes:
Na^+ deficit ⟶ hypotension
Na^+ excess ⟶ hypertension
> Upsets in body fluid osmolarity:
Na^+ deficit ⟶ decreased osmolarity
Na^+ excess ⟶ increased osmolarity
> Hormonal changes:
Na^+ deficit ⟶ increased aldosterone secretion
Na^+ excess ⟶ decreased aldosterone secretion
> Disturbances in brain cell function:
Na^+ deficit ⟶ swollen brain cells
Na^+ excess ⟶ shrunken brain cells
(due to changes in osmolarity)*
> Disturbances in muscle contractility*
> Changes in neuromuscular irritability*
> H^+ disturbances*

Second, hormonal imbalances, impaired Na^+ intake, or excessive losses of Na^+ in urine, sweat, feces, or gastric, pancreatic, and intestinal tract secretions all predispose the individual to sodium imbalance (either a deficiency or excess) which, in turn, leads to osmolar and volume imbalances.

*These pathologic changes occur in varying degrees in both Na^+ deficit and Na^+ excess.

TYPES OF WATER-SODIUM IMBALANCES

Water-sodium imbalances can be broken into the following subgroups:

1. Osmolar imbalances
   a. *Hyperosmolar* imbalances in which there is a decrease in H_2O relative to Na^+ or an increase in Na^+ relative to water. These disturbances lead to the *shrinking* of cells.
   b. *Hypo-osmolar* imbalances in which there is an increase in water relative to Na^+ or a decrease in Na^+ relative to H_2O. These disturbances cause *swollen* cells.
2. *Volume imbalances* (sodium, isotonic imbalances) in which water and Na^+ vary *together.* Cellular disturbances do not develop.

These major imbalances and their subgroups are diagrammatically represented in Figure 25-1.

OSMOLAR IMBALANCES

Osmolar imbalances basically involve disturbances in *osmolarity,* and consequently *water distribution,* throughout the body's fluid compartments. We stated earlier that osmolarity is the total number of dissolved particles per liter. Also, we said that osmolarity affects body water distribution, because water shifts from solutions of lesser osmolarity to solutions of greater osmolarity. When fluid shifts occur because of differences in the osmolarities of the fluid compartments, cellular and extracellular fluid volumes are altered accordingly.

Body Sodium (Na^+)—A Summary of Basic Facts

I. The body of a "normal" male of 70 kg. (154 lb.) contains 2700 to 3000 mEq. of Na^+.
II. Sodium is found in all fluid compartments.
   A. ECF contains 140 mEq./L. of Na^+. Na^+ is the dominant ion of the ECF compartment.
   B. ICF contains 10 mEq./L. of Na^+.
   C. Gastric mucus, bile, intestinal juices, and pancreatic juice all contain substantial amounts of Na^+.
III. Na^+ performs the following vital functions:
   A. Regulates fluid *volume* within the fluid compartments.
      1. Thereby regulates the *size* of the fluid compartments.
      2. Principally regulates the size of the *ECF compartment* where Na^+ is the dominant ion.
   B. Maintains blood volume and regulates the size of the vascular space.
   C. Controls body water distribution by maintaining an *osmotic* equilibrium between the ECF and the ICF.
   D. Increases cell membrane permeability.
   E. Acts as a buffer base (discussed under H^+ balance).
   F. Aids in the conduction of nerve impulses.
   G. Helps to control muscle contractility, especially heart muscle.
   H. Assists in the maintenance of neuromuscular irritability.
IV. Na^+ requirements for life:
   A. Normally, man needs 4.5 Gm. of Na^+ per day.
   B. These needs are usually met by a normal diet and by adding salt to food.
   C. Na^+ excretion in sweat, urine, and feces approximates intake.
V. The homeostatic regulation of sodium:
   A. Aldosterone, a mineralocorticoid, controls the excretion and retention of sodium. Aldosterone is probably controlled, in turn, by a midbrain volume receptor. (See Chapter 24.)
   B. The GI tract controls Na^+ excretion in the presence of Na^+ depletion.
   C. The corticosteroids promote Na^+ reabsorption by the kidney tubules.

You will recall that the osmolarity of the body fluids can be altered by altering either the amount of body water within the fluid compartments or the amount of Na^+ and other particles dissolved in the body water. Thus, in osmolar imbalances, water may be lost or gained *relative to* Na^+, or Na^+ may be lost or gained *relative* to H_2O.

Osmolar imbalances are diagnosed by means of the *serum* Na^+, which is elevated in hyperosmolarity and lower in hypo-osmolarity. The outstanding symptoms in osmolar disturbances are manifestations of *cerebral dysfunction,* e.g., confusion, agitation, depression, and coma. These symptoms develop in response to the *shrinking* of cells during hyperosmolar disturbances and the *swelling* of cells in the presence of hypo-osmolar disturbances. Treatment in osmolar imbalances generally involves *giving fluids* to correct hyperosmolar disturbances and *restricting fluids* during hypo-osmolar disturbances.

Hyperosmolar Imbalances

Etiology. Hyperosmolar imbalances result from either a water deficit or an extracellular Na^+ overload. In water deficit the numbers of Na^+ (sodium ions) are normal, but they are dissolved in too little water. In Na^+ excess there are too many sodium ions per liter of water. Both water deficit and Na^+ excess cause hyperosmolarity, shrinking of cells, and dehydration. Major causes of H_2O deficit and Na^+ excess are outlined below:

Etiologic Factors in Hyperosmolarity Due to Either Water Deficit or Sodium Excess

I. Water deficit
   A. Decreased water intake due to:
      1. Difficulty in swallowing.
      2. Impaired thirst (cerebral injury).
      3. Coma or semicoma.
      4. Unavailability of water.
      5. Extreme debility.
   B. Increased water output due to:
      1. Watery diarrhea.
      2. Diabetes insipidus.*
      3. Diabetic acidosis.*
      4. Tracheobronchitis. (This illness causes very rapid breathing, which, in turn, leads to a substantial water loss in the breath vapor.)
      5. Profuse diaphoresis.

II. Extracellular sodium excess
   A. Excessive infusions of hypertonic solutions
   B. The administration of a heavy solute load as medical therapy
      1. Excessive IV glucose administration.
      2. Excessive tube feedings of protein.
      3. Frequent feedings of milk and cream without adequate water replacement. (These heavy loads of solute materials cause an *obligatory loss of water* by the kidney, which, in turn, leads to *dehydration plus sodium excess.)*

Bases of Symptoms. The symptoms of hyperosmolar imbalances are primarily symptoms of *dehydration* since water is *decreased* relative to Na^+. In dehydration resulting from decreased water intake, excessive water output, or a heavy solute load, the ECF becomes *hypertonic* (the ECF has a greater osmolarity than the ICF) owing to the lack of water. As a result of hypertonicity, water leaves the cells and passes into the extracellular fluid. While the ECF is temporarily restored to proper tonicity, the cells become dehydrated and shrunken. As dehydration progresses, water becomes reduced in *all* compartments and the symptoms listed at the bottom of page 215.

In reviewing the patient's laboratory work, remember that the *serum* level of sodium may be normal in spite of an increase in total body sodium. This is because the excess sodium is in the tissues rather than in the plasma.

Clinical Care. The goals of care for the patient with a *hyperosmolar imbalance* are:

1. Fluid replacement.
2. Prevent complications of dehydration:
   a. Shock.
   b. Renal failure.
   c. Fever.

*Diabetes insipidus was discussed in Chapter 24. Both diabetes insipidus and diabetic acidosis (a complication of diabetes mellitus) will be considered in detail in the chapter on endocrine disorders.

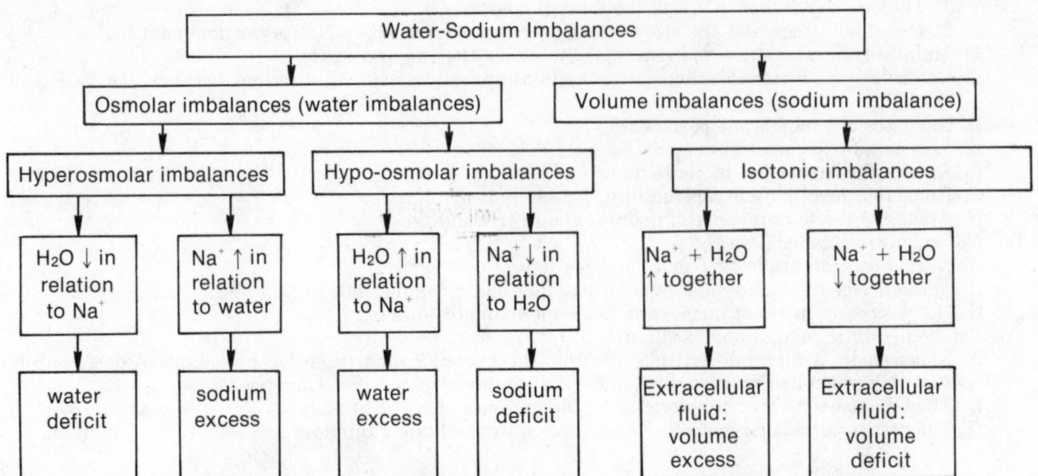

FIGURE 25–1. Diagrammatic summary of water-sodium imbalances.

3. Prevent complications of therapy:
   a. High blood sugar.
   b. Circulatory overload.
   c. Sodium overload.

FLUID REPLACEMENT.* Dehydration due to water deficit or solute overload is treated with fluids. If dehydration is mild, oral fluids may suffice; if dehydration is severe, intravenous infusions of 5 per cent glucose in water are usually recommended. If hyperosmolarity is due to excessive infusions of hypertonic solutions, intravenous therapy with saline solutions is discontinued.

The amount of fluid given to each patient depends upon (1) the degree of dehydration, (2) whether the patient is also losing water through vomiting or diarrhea, (3) the patient's size and weight, and (4) the presence of fever (a high fever requires more water for purposes of vaporization).

The nurse's role in treating patients with a hyperosmolar imbalance is as follows:

> Check weight upon admission and as ordered.

> Keep an accurate record of I and O (See pp. 246–247.)

> Check the temperature upon admission and every 2 to 4 hours.

> Carefully check IV infusions for proper flow rate. Guard against infiltration and infection. (See pp. 254–257.)

> Give adequate fluids (by route ordered) to patients who are comatose or paralyzed, or who are taking tube feedings. Also, carefully evaluate fluid needs of patients with excessive water losses due to watery diarrhea, rapid breathing, or metabolic disease.

> Evaluate fluid needs by checking (1) urinary output and concentration for signs of either oliguria or polyuria, (2) body weight for either a sudden gain or loss, (3) blood pressure for sudden fluctuations that might indicate fluid retention or dehydration. Be aware of laboratory findings such as an elevated serum sodium or elevated hemoglobin as indicative of hyperosmolarity.

> Instruct ulcer patients who are receiving half-and-half hourly to drink at least eight to 10 glasses of water daily.

When fluid replacement is adequate, and if other disease conditions are not present, urinary output improves, body temperature drops to normal, blood pressure stabilizes, serum Na^+ returns to normal, and the patient regains his weight losses.

PREVENT THE COMPLICATIONS OF DEHYDRATION. To prevent severe shock, renal failure, and fever from developing in dehydrated patients, the nurse needs to take the following actions:

Shock. Check the vital signs at least every two hours (pulse, blood pressure, respiration). Report a drop of blood pressure below normal for the patient, and any rise in pulse rate.

Renal failure. Check the urinary output at least every two hours if the patient is severely dehydrated. The patient will probably need an indwelling catheter.

*Fluid replacement is discussed in detail later in this chapter.

Symptoms	*Bases of Symptoms*
Increased blood viscosity; lowered blood pressure; lowered venous pressure	H_2O is reduced in all fluid compartments
Thirst	Increase in osmolarity in all fluid compartments stimulates "thirst" osmoreceptors in the hypothalamus
Poor skin turgor (especially over forehead and upper chest); skin that is pinched over these sites remains in the pinched position for several seconds	Loss of normal elasticity of skin
Dryness of skin and mucous membranes; tongue dry and furrowed	Cells of the skin and mucous membranes "dry out"
Skin cool and pale	Peripheral vascular constriction to compensate for hypotensive state due to hypovolemia
"Doughy" skin in severe cases	Na^+ excess of ECF causes fluid to be held in tissue spaces
Eyeballs soft and sunken; dark circles under eyes	Water tension in eyeballs decreases
Mild cases result in 2 per cent loss of total body weight; *moderate to severe* cases result in 6 per cent loss of total body weight; *very severe* cases result in 7 to 14 per cent loss of total body weight	Water losses are not being replenished through proper intake
Elevated temperature	Regulation of body temperature is disturbed by water lack (normal temperature control requires 800 ml. of H_2O intake over every 24 hour period)
Apprehension and restlessness; coma in severe cases	Cellular dehydration in brain due to shift of water from cells to extracellular fluid compartment
Concentrated urine and a high specific gravity above 1.030	ADH released in response to increased osmolarity of body fluids
Renal shutdown in severe dehydration	Decreased plasma volume results in decreased blood flow to kidney; oliguria and anuria
Laboratory findings: Elevated hemoglobin	Blood viscosity increases as water decreases
Elevated serum Na^+ above 150 mEq.	Osmolarity of plasma increases.

> *Report a urinary output of* less than *25 ml. per hour or 500 ml. in a 24-hr. period.*

Fever. Report any elevation of temperature over 100° F. If the temperature is over 101° F. orally, begin cooling measures. In the severely dehydrated patient, check the temperature at least every two hours.

PREVENT THE COMPLICATIONS OF THERAPY. Watch for indications of a *high blood sugar* when giving IV glucose in water: thirst, fatigue, large urinary output, and sugar in the urine. Prolonged intravenous feeding with sugar solutions may overtax the islet tissue of the pancreas. This, in turn, may lead to a lowered production of insulin.

Watch also for signs of *circulatory overload* when a patient is receiving IV therapy. This condition is discussed later.

Hypo-osmolar Imbalances

Etiology. Hypo-osmolar imbalances result from either water excess or Na^+ deficit. In water excess the number of Na^+ ions is normal, but they are diluted in *too much water.* In Na^+ deficit, the amount of water in the body may be normal, but there are *too few* Na^+ *ions* per liter of water. Both H_2O excess and Na^+ deficit are characterized by *swollen cells.* Major causes of H_2O excess and Na^+ deficit (both of which result in hypo-osmolarity) are outlined below:

Etiologic Factors in Hypo-osmolarity Due to Either Water Excess or Sodium Deficit

I. Water excess (water intoxication) may be due to:
  A. Excessive fluid intake.
    1. Schizophrenics may drink excessively while hallucinating.
    2. Alcoholics may develop water intoxication on a drinking bout.
  B. Inability to excrete water excesses due to:
    1. Kidney disease.
    2. Brain injury due to trauma.
  C. Iatrogenic problems.
    1. Forcing fluids (IV or oral) on patients with increased ADH secretion.
      a. Following surgery or trauma.
      b. Following injections of morphine sulfate.
      c. Following anesthesia.
    2. Excessive infusions of 5 per cent dextrose in water.
    3. Excessive tap water enemas.
      a. Tap water is hypotonic and is absorbed by the bowel.
      b. As a result, body water is diluted and osmolarity is lowered.

II. Sodium deficit (hyponatremia) may be due to:
  A. Poor NaCl intake.
  B. Iatrogenic problems.
    1. Diuretics.
    2. Low salt diet.
    3. Replacement of H_2O and Na^+ losses with *water only:*
      a. Allowing patients to drink large amounts of plain water when perspiring and losing Na^+.
      b. Irrigating nasal gastric tubes with *plain water* (this causes Na^+ to be literally washed out and suctioned from the stomach).
      c. Giving a patient who is vomiting ice chips made of *plain water;* again, Na^+ is washed out of the stomach with no replacement.
      d. Excessive IV solution of dextrose in water instead of isotonic solutions.

Bases of Symptoms. In hypo-osmolar imbalances, the cells swell with H_2O and neuromuscular symptoms predominate. Common symptoms of hypo-osmolar imbalances are listed at the bottom of the page along with their causative factors:

Clinical Care. To treat hypo-osmolar disturbances, it is necessary to *restrict water intake* by mouth and intravenously. When cerebral edema is severe and when renal failure is not a problem, hypertonic saline will be given IV.

To *prevent* the needless development of water excess, remember these rules:

> Do not give excessive tap water enemas.

> Do not overload renal, neurologic, and postoperative patients with intravenous fluids.

> Do not force fluids on patients with increased ADH secretion. Keep careful track of intake and output to prevent excessive intake.

> Do not replace losses of both sodium and water with plain water alone! Replacements should be made with isotonic IV solutions and/or oral liquids containing both electrolytes *and* water, e.g., isotonic ice chips, bouillon, fruit juices.

> Do not irrigate a nasogastric tube with plain water. Instead use *normal saline* for irrigations.

> Do not indiscriminately overload patients with glucose and water, either intravenously, by tube feedings, or orally.

When hyponatremia is present, and the patient must be treated with hypertonic solutions, remember:

> *1. Observe for signs of* Na^+ *excess (hypernatremia, hyperosmolarity).*
> *2. Observe for signs of circulatory overload (extracellular volume excess).*

Symptoms	*Bases of Symptoms*
Absence of thirst (in contrast to the thirst present during hyperosmolar imbalances)	Decrease in osmolarity in all fluid compartments decreases stimulus to "thirst" osmoreceptors in the hypothalamus
Polyuria if kidneys are healthy, oliguria if kidneys are diseased; oliguria further contributes to H_2O excess	Release of ADH inhibited
Twitching; hyperirritability; mental disturbances; disorientation; convulsions; coma	Cells swell with fluid, which gives rise to cerebral edema
Nausea; vomiting; weakness; muscle twitch	Serum Na^+ level depressed
Serum Na^+ level depressed below 120 mEq./L.	Laboratory changes

In isotonic or volume imbalances (also classified as sodium imbalances), Na^+ and H_2O increase or decrease *together* in roughly the same proportions as found in the extracellular fluid, rather than *disproportionately* as in osmolar imbalances. Consequently, when Na^+ is retained, H_2O is also retained, and the extracellular volume is excessive. Conversely, when Na^+ is lost, proportionate amounts of H_2O are also lost, and the extracellular volume is depleted.

Volume (isotonic) imbalances, then, are characterized by fluctuations of the ECF volume. When ECF volume *increases,* circulatory overload and edema result. When ECF volume *decreases,* dehydration and circulatory collapse result. Since osmolarity throughout the body fluid compartments remains unchanged, the cells neither shrink nor swell; consequently, there are *no* cerebral symptoms in isotonic imbalances as there are in osmolar imbalances.

Changes in extracellular fluid volume are detected by means of the physical examination, history, hematocrit, serum protein levels, and urine chloride. Clinical care involves the administration of isotonic fluid in volume depletion and the restriction of fluid in volume excess.

Extracellular Volume Depletion

Etiology. Extracellular volume depletion results from losses of both Na^+ *and* water. The majority of ECF losses are from the gastrointestinal tract and skin. Conditions which can result in large and unusual losses of Na^+ and H_2O are: hemorrhage, diarrhea, vomiting, kidney disease, excessive sweating, burns, draining fistulas and abscesses, fever, decreased production of aldosterone, and internal sequestration of fluids—peritonitis, edema fluid under burns, and so forth.

How long does it take for the body fluids to become depleted through abnormal losses? It is imperative to realize that *individuals vary markedly in the rapidity with which water depletion occurs.* Generally, however, it is recognized that losses from *frequent* diarrhea and vomiting can deplete the *extracellular* fluid within a *few hours,* leading to fatal shock. On the other hand, *gradual* losses of intestinal secretions may not deplete the body's store of extracellular fluid for *several days.* Even when a marked reduction in extracellular fluids occurs *gradually,* the body's *cellular* fluids are eventually drained to replenish the extracellular fluid losses. Once the cellular fluid has been depleted, it will take three or four days for replenished extracellular fluid to make up this vital deficit; these exchanges take time. Often the body will be unable to meet the problem of fluid depletion through its own resources, especially if the depletion involves cellular fluid. Consequently the patient will require outside assistance in the form of intravenous fluids if life is to be sustained.

Bases of Symptoms. The symptoms of extracellular volume deficit are mainly *symptoms of dehydration and circulatory collapse.* Common symptoms and their causation are listed at the bottom of the page.

Clinical Care. Extracellular volume depletion is usually treated by *intravenous infusions of isotonic solutions.* Adults with an extracellular volume deficit of 3 to 6 liters usually receive 1 to 3 liters of isotonic solutions *in addition* to those fluids needed to maintain water-sodium balance. As symptoms subside, additional water can be given in smaller amounts.

Extracellular Volume Excess

This condition is sometimes called *circulatory overload.* Both water and Na^+ are significantly *increased* in roughly the same proportions. Extracellular volume excess occurs in the following groups of patients:

Symptoms	*Bases of Symptoms*
Weakness; nausea; vomiting; poor skin turgor; shrunken tongue; sticky mucous membranes; weight loss	H_2O and Na^+ are deficient in the extracellular fluid compartment, resulting in dehydration
Decrease in fullness of the neck veins when patient lies flat*	Venous pressure is decreased due to loss of plasma volume
A postural systolic blood pressure fall in excess of 10 mm. Hg*	Blood volume is inadequate
Oliguria and anuria (in severe cases)	Decreased plasma volume, resulting in decreased blood flow to kidney
Shock	Circulatory system may collapse as a result of inadequate blood volume
No thirst usually	Osmolarity of the cells is not disturbed
Laboratory findings: Elevated hemotocrit and protein concentration	Plasma volume is reduced
Urine chloride excretion below 50 mEq./L.	Decreased urine chloride is a first sign of Na^+ lack
Normal serum Na^+ concentration	Na^+ and H_2O are lost proportionately

*How to correctly "read" neck vein fullness is discussed in the unit on the Heart, Unit X.
*Postural changes in blood pressure can be detected by taking the patient's blood pressure first in the supine position, and then in the seated position.

> Patients who have received IV *saline* in excessive amounts, too rapidly, or at night when they are sleeping and renal function is normally slowed.
> Patients with *cardiac failure, chronic kidney failure, liver disease,* or *cerebral damage.*
> Patients who receive *cortisone injections* often suffer from sodium and water retention as a side effect.

The major *pathologic effect* of a volume excess is an overloading of all fluid compartments with water *and* saline. The main signs and symptoms of *too much body fluid* are: weight gain; pitting edema (see p. 258); pulmonary edema (a condition caused by excessive serous fluid in the alveolar spaces and characterized by dyspnea, cough, sweating, and frothy or pinkish sputum); puffy eyelids; and ascites (an accumulation of fluid in the abdomen). Note that the patient does *not* develop cerebral signs as during water excess. This is because, with extracellular volume excess, there is no change in the tonicity of the body fluids, or in the osmolarity of the cells, including the brain cells.

The treatment for volume excess includes the administration of *diuretics* and the *restriction of sodium.* Procedures useful in the correction of this condition include weighing the patient daily, strict monitoring of IV infusions, and the recording and evaluation of intake and output.

To *prevent* a volume excess from developing, remember these rules:

1. *Do not, on your own impulse, increase the rate of drip of an IV infusion simply because the IV is behind schedule. Instead, consult the patient's doctor concerning the possibility of a new IV schedule.*
2. *Attempt to plan your patient's IV schedule with the doctor so that the majority of the fluid is given during the day. Do not overload the "resting kidney" by running IV infusions too rapidly during the night.*

HYDROGEN ION (H^+) BALANCE*

Hydrogen ion (H^+) balance is vital to human life and health. Some essential factors concerning the hydrogen ion—its normal concentration within the body fluids, functions, production, measurement, excretion, via the kidneys and lungs, and homeostatic regulation—are outlined below:

*Traditionally, hydrogen ion balance and imbalance have been referred to as "acid-base" balance and imbalance. Today, authorities are finding the use of the term *acid-base* confusing, and instead they are concentrating more on the central role of the H^+ in acid-base relationships within the body fluids. Consequently this discussion will focus on H^+ homeostasis rather than upon acid-base balance.

Hydrogen Ion (H^+) Balance—A Summary of Basic Facts

I. H^+ is normally present in body fluids in a concentration of 0.00004 mEq. per liter.
   A. H^+ exists in far lower concentrations within the body fluids than do other ions, e.g., Cl^- and K^+.
   B. Fluctuations of H^+ are tolerated better by the body than fluctuations of other ions.
II. H^+ is found in both the cellular and extracellular fluids. Physiologists hypothesize that cellular fluid has a higher H^+ concentration than extracellular fluid.
III. H^+ plays a vital role in the regulation of the following biochemical and metabolic activities:
   A. Must be present for proper cellular function.
   B. Is necessary for the efficient function of enzyme systems.
   C. Is essential for the binding of oxygen by hemoglobin.
   D. Acts as a powerful chemical agitator within the body fluids.
IV. H^+ concentration determines the relative *acidity* or *alkalinity* of a solution.
   A. The greater the number of H^+ present, the more *acid* the solution.
   B. The smaller the number of H^+ present, the more *alkaline* the solution.
V. The acidity and alkalinity of a solution (i.e., H^+ concentration within a solution) is measured in terms of pH.
   A. pH is chemical shorthand for the *negative* logarithm of the hydrogen ion (H^+) concentration.
   B. Neutral pH is a H^+ concentration of 0.0000001 Gram per liter or 10^{-7} Gram per liter or a pH of 7.
   C. The total pH scale extends from 0 to 14, with 7 being neutral.
   D. The *higher* the pH the *lower* the H^+ concentration of a solution and vice versa.
      1. A solution with a pH less than 7 is *acid.*
      2. A solution with a pH greater than 7 is *alkaline.*
VI. The pH's of some of the body fluids are as follows:
   A. The *blood* pH is 7.40.
      1. When the pH of the blood drops *below* 7.40, the individual has *acidosis.*
      2. When the pH of the blood rises *above* 7.40, the individual has *alkalosis.*
      3. The range of blood pH compatible with life is from 6.8 to 7.8.
   B. *Intracellular* fluid pH probably ranges between 6.9 and 7.2. The pH of cells has, to date, been measured only by indirect methods.
   C. pH for important transcellular fluids:
      1. Urine pH is approximately 6.0.
      2. Central spinal fluid pH is from 7.36 to 7.44.
      3. Pure gastric juice pH is from 1.0 to 2.0.
      4. Intestinal juice pH is from 6.5 to 7.6.
      5. Bile from gallbladder pH is from 5.0 to 6.0.
      6. Liver bile pH is 7.4.
      7. Pancreatic juice pH is from 7.6 to 8.2.

(Outline continued on the opposite page.)

Because the homeostatic mechanisms regulating H^+ concentration are extremely complex, we shall explore these in greater detail.

Homeostatic Regulation of Hydrogen

Dilution of H^+ Excess. H^+ can become heavily concentrated in a single tissue or area of the body. For example, if you exercise your arm excessively, H^+ builds up in the arm muscles. When such a build up occurs, the excess H^+ are quickly whisked away by the rapidly moving circulation so that they can be distributed more evenly throughout the body fluids. Dilution is a rapid-acting mechanism sometimes termed the *first line of defense* against a shift in pH.

Buffers and Buffer Systems. In its broadest sense, a buffer is a type of "shield" which, by intervening between two machines, chemicals, and so forth, prevents dangerous or explosive interaction. For example, we speak of "buffer zones" between warring nations.

Within the body fluids, buffers are mixtures of acidic and alkaline substances that act to protect the body against dangerous fluctuations of H^+ concentration when excess acids or alkali are added to the body fluids. Buffers protect by "soaking up" excess hydrogen or hydroxyl ions (OH^-).* This sponge-like action of the buffer removes the additional acidic or alkaline ions from the circulation. As a result, these ions are unable to affect, to any great degree, the pH of the solution.

For example, note the equation below. If a strong acid† like HCl is added to a buffered solution, the result is a weaker acid and a salt.

HCl		$NaHCO_3$		H_2CO_3		NaCl
Hydrochloric acid (strong acid)	+	Sodium bicarbonate (strong buffer base)	→	Carbonic acid (weak acid)	+	Sodium chloride (salt)

*Hydroxyl ions (OH^-) are *released* when a base dissociates in water.

†Strong acids and bases ionize readily in an aqueous solution, whereas weak acids and bases do not.

Hydrogen Ion (H^+) Balance—A Summary of Basic Facts (Continued)

VII. H^+ circulates throughout the body fluids in the following two forms:
 A. *Volatile* H^+ of carbonic acid.
  1. Volatile H^+ are found mainly in the form of CO_2 and water.
  2. Volatile H^+ must be constantly excreted in gaseous form from the lungs.
 B. *Nonvolatile* H^+ (or metabolic H^+).
  1. Nonvolatile H^+ are produced as the result of various metabolic processes within the body.
   a. Some H^+ are produced in the form of organic acids, e.g., uric acid.
   b. Other H^+ are found in the form of sulfuric and phosphoric acids.
  2. Normally a person ingesting a balanced diet will produce 50 to 100 mEq. of nonvolatile H^+ daily.
  3. Nonvolatile H^+ are eliminated by the kidney.

VIII. The body obtains H^+ in the following ways:
 A. The largest number of H^+ arise from the body's many complex metabolic processes.
  1. The metabolic process that produces *volatile H^+* is the complete metabolism of fat and carbohydrate to CO_2 and H_2O, which yields nearly 14,000 mEq. of carbonic acid daily.
  2. Some of the metabolic processes that yield *nonvolatile* H^+ are:
   a. The incomplete breakdown of carbohydrates and fats to form lactic acid, pyruvic acid, acetoacetic acid, and citric acid.
   b. The oxidation of nucleoproteins and phosphoproteins.
   c. The oxidation of sulfur-containing amino acids to yield sulfuric acid residues.
 B. Excess H^+ can be produced as a consequence of *disease.*
  1. Excess H^+ may be released in cases of trauma and burns as a result of tissue damage and protein breakdown.
  2. H^+ retention and excess occur in renal failure.
 C. Additional loads of H^+ may be ingested by means of *medications* that contain ammonium or mineral salts.
 D. A small amount of H^+ is ingested in the normal diet.

IX. H^+ are excreted from the body as follows:
 A. The *lungs* eliminate the volatile H^+ of carbonic acid as CO_2 and H_2O.
 B. The *kidneys* excrete nonvolatile H^+ in the following three forms:
  1. A very small amount of *free H^+* is excreted in the urine. These ions determine the urine pH, which ranges from 4.0 to 8.0.
  2. Sixty per cent of nonvolatile H^+ is excreted as ammonium ions [NH_4^+].
  3. Forty per cent of nonvolatile H^+ is excreted in the form of weak acids.

X. H^+ concentration within the body fluids is homeostatically regulated by means of the following mechanisms:
 A. Dilution of H^+ excess by the extracellular fluid.
 B. Buffering by the following buffer systems:
  1. The H_2CO_3-$NaHCO_3$ buffer system.
  2. Protein buffer system.
  3. Phosphate buffer system.
 C. Respiratory control of volatile H^+.
 D. Renal control of nonvolatile H^+.

As you can see, the additional hydrogen ions released by the strongly ionized hydrochloric acid are used in forming weak carbonic acid. Because carbonic acid ionizes only slightly in solution, the H^+ donated by the HCl remain "tied up" within the newly formed H_2CO_3 and the pH change of the solution is slight.

The same general role of the chemical acidic buffer is illustrated in the equation below. If a *strong* base, such as sodium hydroxide, is added to a buffered solution, the result is the production of a weaker base and water:

NaOH Sodium hydroxide (strong base)	+	H_2CO_3 Carbonic acid (acidic buffer)	→	$NaHCO_3$ Sodium bicarbonate (weak base)	+	H_2O Water

In this instance, the additional hydroxyl ions are used in forming a large amount of weak sodium bicarbonate. Again, as a result of buffering, the pH of the solution remains stable despite the addition of a strong base.

Within the body fluids, H_2CO_3 and $NaHCO_3$ operate *together* as a *buffer system,* protecting the body from overwhelming amounts of acid or alkali. A buffer system is composed of a weak acid which coexists together with its salt. For example, in the H_2CO_3–$NaHCO_3$ buffer system, the weak acid is H_2CO_3, which ionizes slightly to H^+ and HCO_3^-. The salt of the acid is $NaHCO_3$, which ionizes freely to Na^+ and HCO_3^-. Together, this weak acid and its salt "patrol" the extracellular fluids, "seizing" excess hydrogen or hydroxyl ions wherever they find them.

Buffer systems circulate throughout the body's fluid systems: within the plasma, within the cells, and throughout the extracellular fluid. Three major buffer systems operate to control these vital fluids: (1) the *carbonic acid-bicarbonate system* (which we just mentioned); (2) the *protein buffer system*; and (3) the *phosphate buffer system*:

THE H_2CO_3–$NaHCO_3$ BUFFER SYSTEM. The H_2CO_3–$NaHCO_3$ buffer system is the most important system of the ECF, but is the least important buffer operating inside the cell. This system buffers up to 90 per cent of the H^+ of the extracellular fluid. It is closely regulated by the lungs and kidneys, the lungs excreting H_2CO_3 and the kidneys excreting $NaHCO_3$.

The most important thing to remember about the H_2CO_3–$NaHCO_3$ system is that it is *not* the *absolute* amounts of each component of the system that regulates H^+ concentration; rather, it is the *ratio* of H_2CO_3 to $NaHCO_3$ that controls H^+ equilibrium. For example, the normal ECF concentration of H_2CO_3 is 1.37 mEq./L. while the concentration of $NaHCO_3$ is approximately 27 mEq./L. The concentrations of these two chemical components represent a 1:20 ratio – 20 parts of $NaHCO_3$ to every 1 part of H_2CO_3. Remember:

The 1:20 ratio of H_2CO_3 to $NaHCO_3$ is crucial to H^+ balance. When ratio is disturbed, balance is upset.

This means, then, that the pH of the body fluids will remain within normal limits even if absolute amounts of each chemical vary. The ratio could conceivably be 2:40 or 0.05/0.10 and still be considered normal. Of course, there are several factors that can disturb the H_2CO_3:$NaHCO_3$ ratio. These upsetting factors will be considered in detail under H^+ imbalances.

PHOSPHATE BUFFER SYSTEM. The phosphate buffer system is almost identical in its actions to the bicarbonate system. The major components of the system are NaH_2PO_4 and Na_2HPO_4. The phosphate buffer is abundant within the cell; thus, it plays a more important role within the cell than within the ECF.

PROTEIN BUFFER SYSTEM. The protein buffer is the most plentiful and most powerful buffer in the body. It is active in the ECF, the plasma, and especially in the cell. Within the cell, it is the hemoglobin of the erythrocyte (a protein substance) that provides nearly three fourths of the chemical buffering power of the body's fluids. Proteins are powerful buffers because they are highly versatile, performing either as acid or base, as the occasion demands.

The efficiency of all the buffer systems working together is truly remarkable. Out of every one million hydrogen ions added to the body fluids, all but five are successfully and rapidly buffered! However, buffer systems have their limitations in handling the body's acids and bases. Hydrogen ions that the body fails to control become the responsibility of the body's most powerful steady state regulators – the lungs and the kidneys.

Respiratory Control of H^+ Balance. The respiratory system (including its neurologic centers in the medulla) controls the H_2CO_3 part of the H_2CO_3–$NaHCO_3$ buffer system. This control is exercised by means of feedback mechanisms operating between the respiratory center in the medulla of the brain and the lung. Healthy lungs are rapid regulators, partially correcting H^+ irregularities within one to three minutes following their development.

To comprehend the role of the lung as a homeostatic regulator of the H^+, we shall explore the following areas:

1. Respiratory gases.
2. CO_2 transport to and elimination from the lungs.
3. Chemical feedback control of CO_2 elimination.
4. Limitations of the lungs as H^+ regulators.

THE RESPIRATORY GASES. The gases that are most important in human physiology are carbon dioxide and oxygen. The amounts of these gases in the body fluids are usually measured in terms of their *partial pressures.*

The *partial pressure of a gas* is defined as "the pressure which any one gas exerts, whether it is alone or mixed with other gases." The pressure which any one gas exerts will determine that gas's chemical and physiologic activities.

The partial pressure of *carbon dioxide* (pCO_2) is usually referred to as carbon dioxide pressure or carbon dioxide tension. Likewise, the partial pressure of *oxygen* (pO_2) is called oxygen pressure or oxygen tension. In the normal resting adult (breathing quietly) the pCO_2 of the alveolar air and venous blood is 40 mm. Hg, while the pCO_2 of the *arterial* blood is 35 to 38 mm. Hg. The pO_2 of *arterial blood* is 95 to 100 mm. Hg, while that of *venous blood* is between 35 and 40 mm. Hg. When the pCO_2 becomes elevated due either to CO_2 retention or to an overly great CO_2 production, the condition is called *hypercapnia*. When the pCO_2 becomes abnormally low due to excessive "blowing off" of CO_2, the condition is called *hypocapnia*. Finally, a decrease of pO_2 is called *hypoxia*.

THE TRANSPORT OF CO_2 AND ITS ELIMINATION FROM THE LUNGS. Carbon dioxide is produced constantly in large amounts as a byproduct of both the body's metabolic activities and the oxidation of carbon in foods. Because CO_2 is a potentially deadly acidic substance, it *must* be eliminated via the lungs. But how does CO_2 reach the lungs for elimination and what happens to CO_2 while en route?

The major steps in the formation and transport of CO_2 to the lungs are: (1) CO_2 is formed by various intracellular and metabolic processes; (2) CO_2 is then released into the interstitial fluids from which it passes into the plasma, with some CO_2 passing into the erythrocytes; and (3) from the plasma, CO_2 goes to the lungs where it is released into the air. However, CO_2, during the transport period, goes through a number of important processes, these occurring within the plasma and red blood cells.

Three things can happen to CO_2 when it enters the *plasma* from the interstitial fluid:[17]

I. A part of CO_2 remains *dissolved* in the blood where it can be measured in terms of the pCO_2.
   A. Dissolved CO_2 reacts with water to form H_2CO_3 (carbonic acid):

$$CO_2 + H_2O \longrightarrow H_2CO_3$$

   B. When the arterial blood becomes venous, the increase in CO_2 causes H_2CO_3 to ionize into H^+ and bicarbonate (HCO_3^-):

$$H_2CO_3 \longrightarrow H^+ + HCO_3^-$$

   C. The hydrogen ions, which are added to the circulation, are buffered by plasma buffers.
   D. As a result, little change in H^+ concentration occurs.

II. A part of CO_2 joins with the proteins of the blood to form *carbamino compounds.*

III. A large proportion of CO_2 passes into the erythrocytes.

Within the erythrocytes, CO_2 again undergoes three distinct processes:

I. Some CO_2 simply remains *dissolved* within the red blood cells.

II. A substantial amount of CO_2 combines with hemoglobin to form *carbamino compounds.*

III. The largest part of the CO_2 combines with water to form H_2CO_3.
   A. H_2CO_3 then ionizes to yield H^+ and HCO_3^-.
   B. The hydrogen ions are buffered by hemoglobin, while the majority of bicarbonate ions pass into plasma in exchange for Cl^-. This exchange of ions is called the *chloride shift* and serves three purposes:
      1. The exchange of negatively charged ions preserves the electrical neutrality of the cells and plasma.
      2. The passage of HCO_3^- into the plasma helps to maintain the 1:20 ratio of H_2CO_3 to $NaHCO_3$.
      3. The transfer of HCO_3^- into the plasma allows large amounts of CO_2 to be carried to the lungs in the form of bicarbonate ions. Thus, the pH of the blood is only slightly disturbed by the additional CO_2.

Following these complex processes, CO_2, mainly in the form of HCO_3^- and carbamino compounds, finally reaches the lungs via the venous blood at a partial pressure of 46 mm. Hg. Since the pCO_2 within the alveolar spaces of the lung is 40 mm. Hg, CO_2 diffuses fairly readily from the venous blood into the alveolar air. While CO_2 is being released into the alveolar spaces for expiration, a "reverse chloride shift" takes place within the body fluids. In this process, all the reactions involved in CO_2 transport reverse themselves:

1. Cl^- returns into the plasma in exchange for HCO_3^-.
2. H_2CO_3 diffuses back into the cells where it ionizes into CO_2 and water.
3. The CO_2 thus formed quickly diffuses into the plasma.
4. From the plasma, the CO_2 passes into the alveolar air where it joins the CO_2 from the venous blood.
5. The CO_2 thus accumulated from these two sources is finally excreted from the alveoli into the atmosphere.

The entire physiologic process of CO_2 transport that we have just described normally takes only a few minutes from the production of CO_2 at the cellular level to the time of final release of CO_2 from the lungs.

FEEDBACK MECHANISMS IN THE REGULATION OF CO_2 EXCRETION. The H^+ concentration of the blood and the amount of CO_2 build-up within the body fluids both have a direct effect upon respiration, the respiratory center (including the respiratory neurons in the medulla), and the 1:20 ratio of H_2CO_3 to $NaHCO_3$.

The three major factors that affect the respiratory center in the medulla are the pH of the blood, the pCO_2 and the pO_2. As shown in Table 25–1, increases or decreases of these factors result in significant alterations in pulmonary ventilation.

The roles of the blood pH and plasma pCO_2 and the roles of the respiratory center in the brain and the lungs are well integrated in the overall tasks of controlling H^+ concentration and the ratio of H_2CO_3 to $NaHCO_3$. For example, note what happens within the body when either side of the ratio of acid to base is disturbed.

First, consider the body's response to a build-up of CO_2, possibly resulting from exercise. When CO_2 within the body fluid increases the pH of the blood drops below 7.4, the acid side of the H_2CO_3;$NaHCO_3$ ratio increases, and the pCO_2 increases. As a result, the individual responds by breathing more rapidly than usual (hyperventilates) and the extra CO_2 is thereby excreted from the lungs. Because the air expired is moist, CO_2 is actually eliminated as

H_2CO_3, thus lowering the concentration of H^+ within the body fluids.

On the other hand, when the bicarbonate side of the 1:20 ratio increases or the acid side decreases the pH of the blood rises above 7.4, the base side of the H_2CO_3:$NaHCO_3$ ratio decreases, and the pCO_2 is lowered. As a result, the person affected breathes more slowly than usual (hypoventilates) and CO_2 is held back and not released from the lungs. CO_2 then unites with H_2O, and more H_2CO_3 is formed which *then* increases the H^+ concentration of the body fluids.

These events, which occur following CO_2 build-up and excretion, are summarized in Figure 25–2.

Note that the negative feedback control system governing H_2CO_3 concentration and the elimination of CO_2 is of the *servomechanism* type as opposed to "stat" type regulation. (See Unit I.) The levels of CO_2 and H_2CO_3 are continuously shifting, thereby requiring constant monitoring. If this system is disturbed for even very brief periods of time, H^+ balance is seriously upset.

THE LIMITATIONS OF THE LUNGS AS STEADY STATE REGULATORS. The lungs are vital regulators of H^+ balance because they have an enormous surface area from which CO_2 can be readily diffused; they can bring about rapid changes in H^+ concentration when necessary. However, the lungs have definite limitations in this role. First of all, the lungs can excrete, retain, or inactivate only the H^+ of H_2CO_3. Handling those excess hydrogen ions that arise from other sources is the burden of the kidney. Second, the lungs can help to compensate only *temporarily* for changes in H^+ concentration. If the problem in H^+ balance lies *outside* the respiratory system, responsibility for regulation again falls to the kidney.

The respiratory tract can only *partially* correct deviations in pH from normal. For example, if the pH of the blood should fall from the normal of 7.4 to 7.0, the lungs will be able to restore the pH to around 7.2 or 7.3 within a minute or so. However, they cannot restore the pH of the blood to 7.4.

Renal Control of H^+ Concentration

The *kidneys* regulate the $NaHCO_3$ part of the H_2CO_3–$NaHCO_3$ buffer system. As indicated earlier, the kidney eliminates *nonvolatile* H^+, whereas the lung eliminates *volatile* H^+. Also, unlike the lung, the kidney works slowly, taking up to half a day to correct an imbalance. However, the renal system is powerful and efficient, neutralizing *almost completely* any excess acid or base that is disturbing the delicate balance of the body fluids. To compensate for H^+ imbalances, the kidney alters the *rate* of excretion of various electrolytes such as H^+, Na^+, and K^+, thereby correcting the concentrations of H^+ and other electrolytes within the body fluids.

Four major processes are involved in the kidney's regulation of H^+ homeostasis:

1. H^+ secretion by the proximal and distal tubules.
2. Exchange of H^+ for Na^+ in the tubular urine.
3. Excretion of H^+ as ammonia.
4. Suppression of H^+ and Na^+ exchange.

Secretion of H^+. When CO_2 joins with water, hydrogen ions are released along with bicarbonate ions.

$$3\,(CO_2 + H_2O) \longrightarrow 3\,H^+ + 3\,HCO_3^-$$

The hydrogen ions thus formed are secreted by the epithelial cells of the proximal tubules, distal tubules, and collecting ducts of the kidneys into the urine for excretion.

The exact mechanism that controls H^+ secretion is unknown. However, scientists agree that H^+ secretion is regulated mainly by the *concentration of CO_2 in the ECF*. Thus, the greater the concentration of CO_2 in the ECF, the faster hydrogen ions are secreted; conversely, the lower the concentration of CO_2 in the ECF, the fewer the hydrogen ions secreted.

Hydrogen Ion–Sodium Ion Exchange. As H^+ are secreted from the tubular cells into the tubular urine, they are *exchanged* for sodium ions and then excreted. The *sodium ions* within the tubular urine are usually in partnership with an anion—either HCO_3^- or HPO_4^{--}. When H^+ ions are secreted into

TABLE 25–1. THE EFFECT OF pH, pCO_2 AND pO_2 UPON RESPIRATION

Factor	Effect of Increase on Respiration	Effect of Decrease on Respiration
pCO_2 (has most profound effect on respiration): normal = 40 mm. Hg	Respiration is stimulated; pCO_2 of 50 mm. Hg causes pulmonary ventilation to triple	Respiration is inhibited; pCO_2 of 30 mm. Hg causes pulmonary ventilation to decrease to one fourth of normal
pH of blood (has the second most serious effect on respiration): normal = 7.40	If above 7.41, respiration is inhibited; if above 7.50, pulmonary ventilation is reduced by one half	If below 7.41, respiration is stimulated; if below 7.20, pulmonary ventilation quadruples
pO_2 (has least effect on respiration): normal = 98 to 100 mm. Hg	Increase has very little effect on respiration	Respiration is stimulated and CO_2 is blown off

the urine, the Na^+ ions are "forcibly grabbed" from the urine filtrate and from their partner anions by the kidney cells and returned to the plasma. Within the plasma, the "captured" sodium ions are quickly reunited with HCO_3^- to again form the compound $NaHCO_3$. Thus, as a result of the $H^+ = Na^+$ exchange, $NaHCO_3$ is regenerated and the $H_2CO_3:NaHCO_3$ ratio is held steady.

And what happens to the secreted hydrogen ions? Their fate ultimately depends upon which anion Na^+ is linked with while in the tubular urine. For example, if the anion is HCO_3^-, as is frequently the case, the following reaction will take place:

HCO_3^-		H^+		CO_2		H_2O
Bicarbonate ion—released from its partnership with Na^+	+	Secreted hydrogen ions	→	Carbon dioxide which diffuses into cell	+	Water excreted as urine

The *rate* of $H^+ = Na^+$ exchange and HCO_3^- reabsorption is influenced by several factors. Chloride deficiency, an increased pCO_2, and an increased aldosterone secretion (which causes Na^+ retention) all *stimulate* the exchange process. Conversely, a decrease in the pCO_2 and a decrease in aldosterone secretion both *inhibit* $H^+ = Na^+$ exchange.

A final influence on the exchange mechanism is the *pH of the urine.* If the pH of the urine reaches between 4.0 and 4.5, H^+ secretion stops. This, in turn, halts the $H^+ = Na^+$ exchange. At this critical point, the body must rely upon the *ammonia mechanism* for continued H^+ secretion.

Ammonia Mechanism. Upon the breakdown of certain amino acids, ammonia (NH_3) is formed within the distal tubule cells of the kidney. When the NH_3 formed diffuses from the cells into the urine, it reacts with some of the free H^+ present in the urine to form ammonium molecules (NH_4^+). The NH_4^+ molecules then join with anions such as chloride or sulfate ions, and together they (NH_4^+ + anion) are excreted in the urine. The overall effect of this mechanism is to *increase* the bicarbonate side of the $H_2CO_3:NaHCO_3$ ratio by eliminating excess H^+.

Also, as stated earlier, the ammonia mechanism controls H^+ secretion when the urine pH rises too high. In this case, the mechanism operates by "soaking up" the free H^+ in the urine, thus *lowering* the urinary pH. As a result, the renal tubule cells are soon able to operate again in their job of secreting H^+ into the urine for $H^+ = Na^+$ exchange.

Suppression of $H^+ = Na^+$ Exchange and NH_3 Secretion. The purpose of this mechanism is to *increase the excretion of $NaHCO_3$ in the urine.* Suppression of the $H^+ = Na^+$ exchange and NH_3 secretion occurs in response to either increases in plasma $NaHCO_3$ or decreases in plasma H_2CO_3.

In sum, the kidney (like the lungs) has several ways of coping efficiently with the acid-alkali load, being able to remove substantial amounts of acids or alkali daily. As long as the kidneys and lungs remain healthy, and the acid-alkali loads are not too great, pulmonary and renal systems serve as a powerful line of defense against H^+ imbalance.

HYDROGEN ION (H^+) IMBALANCES

The maintenance of H^+ balance depends upon the healthy function of the kidneys, lungs, and brain. These remarkable organs can normally adjust swiftly and efficiently to fluctuations of H^+ concentration. However, when subjected to unusually heavy loads of acid or alkali, or in the presence of renal, respiratory, or brain disease, the body's ability to cope with H^+ regulation fails and imbalances result. The imbalances created are of two major types: *acidosis* or *alkalosis.*

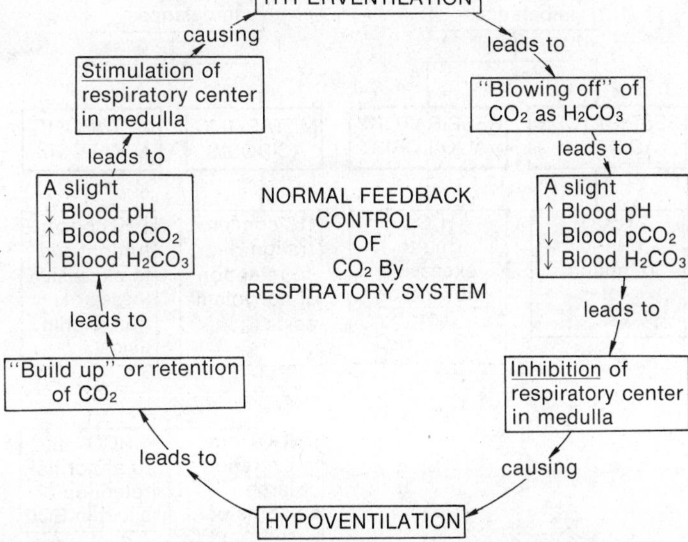

FIGURE 25-2. Feedback control of H+ concentration and the elimination of CO_2.

Definitions

> Acidosis *is a condition in which the H^+ concentration is elevated above normal, or the alkali reserve of the body is reduced below normal.*
> Alkalosis *is a condition in which the H^+ concentration of the body fluid is decreased below normal or the body base is increased above normal.*

If the basic failure rests with the *pulmonary* system, the condition is called *respiratory acidosis or alkalosis.* In *respiratory acidosis,* H^+ are being retained within the body fluids as excess H_2CO_3; in *respiratory alkalosis,* H^+ are being excreted too rapidly from the body in the form of CO_2 and water vapor.

When the basic failure is *renal* in nature, the imbalance is called *metabolic acidosis* or *alkalosis.* In *metabolic acidosis* excessive nonvolatile or metabolic H^+ are being retained within the body fluids, or HCO_3^- is being lost in abnormally large amounts from the kidneys. Conversely, in *metabolic alkalosis* there is either an abnormal loss of nonvolatile H^+ from the body or an abnormal gain in HCO_3^- by the ECF. These various conditions are represented graphically in Figure 25–3.

There are several different names for the four major imbalances, that you may find in use on patients' charts. The most representative are listed in Table 25–2.

TABLE 25–2. TERMS COMMONLY APPLIED TO THE FOUR MAJOR IMBALANCES

Imbalance	Names in Common Usage
Metabolic acidosis	Nonrespiratory acidosis Primary base bicarbonate deficiency
Metabolic alkalosis	Nonrespiratory alkalosis Primary base bicarbonate excess
Respiratory acidosis	Primary CO_2 excess Carbon dioxide retention Hypercapnea
Respiratory alkalosis	Primary CO_2 deficiency

Besides classifying imbalances on a physiologic basis, they may also be grouped as *primary* imbalances, *secondary* or *compensatory* imbalances and *mixed* imbalances. A *primary* imbalance is one arising *directly* from an acid or base overload or from disease of the lungs or kidneys. A *secondary* or *compensatory* imbalance is one that arises in *response to the primary disturbance* in H^+ equilibrium. Finally, imbalances can be *mixed,* i.e., a patient can conceivably have two primary imbalances, one metabolic and one respiratory. In *mixed*

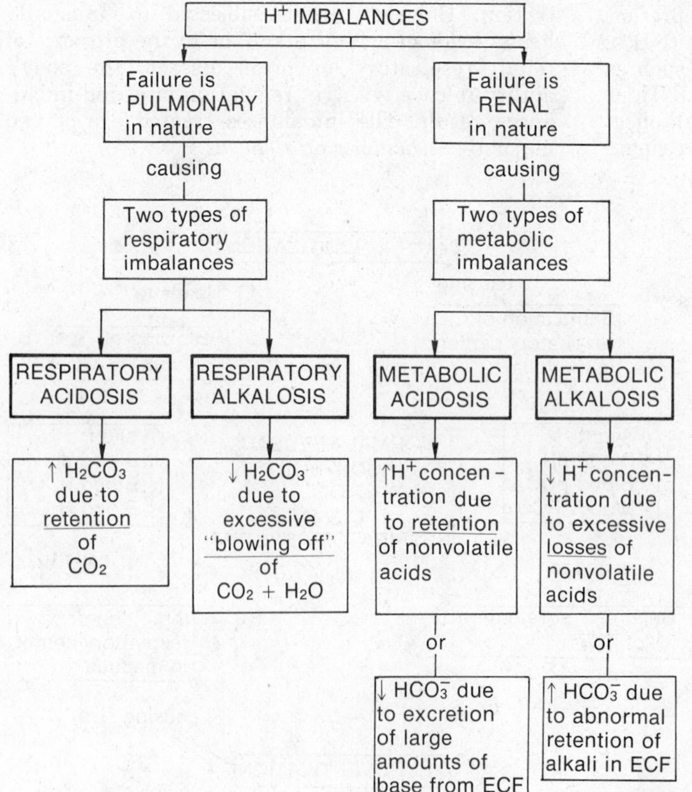

FIGURE 25–3. Classification of the four major H^+ imbalances.

conditions, neither imbalance is compensating for the other; instead, both imbalances are the result of two distinct disease processes or their complications. For example, a patient could have a primary respiratory acidosis resulting from lung disease and a primary metabolic alkalosis as the result of a gastric disorder causing excessive vomiting of HCl.

The Effect of H^+ Imbalance

H^+ imbalances produce many critical pathologic disturbances within the body. You will find it much easier to learn the signs and symptoms of the different imbalances if you thoroughly acquaint yourself with the following points:

1. *In H^+ imbalance all the major signs and symptoms are the result of* disturbances of the central nervous system *(CNS).*
2. *In* acidosis *(either respiratory or metabolic) the major problem is* depression *of the* CNS. *Decrease in mental capacity, delirium, coma, and death may result.*
3. *In* alkalosis *the major problem is* overexcitability *of the CNS. Extreme nervousness, overexcitability, and tetany result. In susceptible persons (e.g., epileptics)* convulsions *may develop. Death may follow* tetany of the respiratory tract.

The number of symptoms seen in an imbalance and their severity depend largely upon the *length of time* the patient has suffered the imbalance, the *magnitude* of the H^+ or HCO_3^- deviation, and the efficiency of the kidneys and lungs in compensating for the imbalance. For example, a patient may die as a result of a rapidly developing, severe imbalance that overwhelms the body's compensatory mechanisms. Conversely, a patient suffering from a mild imbalance over a long period of time may experience few or no symptoms because of the development of compensatory mechanisms. Indeed, symptoms will appear in patients *only* when the kidneys and lungs have failed to compensate, either partially or completely.

Compensatory Mechanisms Resulting From H^+ Imbalance

What are the major lines of defense against H^+ imbalances?

The first *line of defense against H^+ imbalances is the dilution of H^+ in the ECF and* buffering.

As stated earlier, the major buffer systems of the body are the H_2CO_3–$NaHCO_3$ system, the protein buffer system, and the phosphate buffer system.

The second *line of defense against H^+ imbalances is the* respiratory system.

If the patient has a lowered pH, the lungs compensate for the acidosis by increasing respirations. Conversely, if the blood pH is elevated, the lungs compensate for the presence of alkalosis by decreasing the rate of respiration.

The third *line of defense against H^+ imbalances is the* renal system.

Diseased kidneys are ineffective in excreting nonvolatile acids. To compensate for the kidney's failure, the *lungs* attempt to lower the body's total acid content by increasing the rate of CO_2 excretion. By eliminating some of the body's volatile acid, the lungs, in the absence of proper renal function, help to raise the pH of the blood toward normal. If the lungs become diseased, the kidneys compensate for increased acid retention by excreting nonvolatile acids more rapidly, thereby lowering the body's total acid content.

The Diagnosis of H^+ Imbalance

Disturbances of H^+ balance are difficult to diagnose for at least three reasons: First of all, H^+ imbalances rarely appear spontaneously; they are almost always the result of *primary underlying conditions* such as diabetes mellitus or emphysema, which may be diagnosed before the H^+ imbalance can be treated effectively. Second, the symptoms of the primary imbalance are often *masked* by the symptoms of a *compensatory imbalance.* For example, a patient who is hyperventilating may have a respiratory alkalosis resulting from hysteria. Hyperventilation, in this case, is a *symptom* of respiratory alkalosis. On the other hand, a rapidly breathing patient might have a metabolic acidosis. Hyperventilation in this latter case represents a *compensatory* reaction to the build up of H_2CO_3 within the body. A third difficulty in diagnosis is that definite signs and symptoms of imbalance may be minimal or absent for long periods of time, during which compensatory mechanisms are functioning adequately.

Because of these problems in diagnosis, doctors must rely heavily upon the following laboratory tests when working with patients suffering from H^+ disorders:

> *Blood pH.* Determines whether a H^+ imbalance exists. Although the test confirms the presence of either an acidosis or alkalosis, it *does not* tell whether the imbalance is respiratory or metabolic. The *normal* blood pH reading is 7.40. An *elevated* pH indicates alkalosis; a *lowered* pH indicates acidosis.

> *pCO_2 determination.* Measures the amount of *carbon dioxide dissolved in the plasma.* Normally carbon dioxide pressure is 35 to 50 mm. Hg. The pCO_2 is *elevated* when the acid part of the H_2CO_3:$NaHCO_3$ ratio is increased and *acidosis* is present. The pCO_2 is *lowered* when the acid part of the H_2CO_3:$NaHCO_3$ ratio is decreased and *alkalosis* is present.

> *CO_2 combining power.* Measures the alkali reserve of the body, i.e., the amount of HCO_3^- present. The *normal*

value is between 52 to 58 vol. of CO_2 per ml. serum (22–30 mEq./L.). *An elevated* CO_2 combining power indicates *alkalosis,* whereas a depressed CO_2 combining power indicates *acidosis.* This test is currently being replaced in many hospitals by the determination of *plasma total CO_2 content.*

> *Plasma total CO_2 content.* Measures amount of the body's HCO_3; it indicates to what degree bicarbonate has increased or decreased. *Normal* plasma CO_2 content is between 20 and 30 mEq. per L. An *elevation* of plasma CO_2 content indicates an elevation of the bicarbonate ions and alkalosis; a *depression* of plasma CO_2 content indicates a depletion of the bicarbonate ions and acidosis.

In sum, the laboratory findings for *acidosis* are: lowered pH, increased pCO_2, depressed CO_2 combining power, and a depression of plasma CO_2 content. Conversely, laboratory findings for *alkalosis* are: elevated pH, decreased pCO_2, elevated CO_2 combining power, and an elevation of plasma CO_2 content.

To diagnose *respiratory* imbalance, the doctor will generally order the pH, pCO_2, and plasma total CO_2 content. To diagnose *metabolic* disorders, the plasma total CO_2 content determination is generally considered sufficient.

Basic Clinical Care in H^+ Imbalances

However complex the various imbalances are, four basic rules of care apply to all of them:

1. Treat, and if possible remove, the primary disease or disorder that is creating the imbalance.
2. Through supportive medical and nursing care, aid the renal and respiratory systems in their struggle to compensate for imbalance.
3. Carefully observe and record rate and depth of respiration and abnormal behavior.
4. Medicate with drugs that will neutralize excess acid or base, as the condition warrants.

In acidosis, acids are most commonly neutralized by such drugs as: *sodium bicarbonate, sodium lactate,* and *sodium gluconate.* The neutralization of excess base may be achieved by administering *ammonium chloride,* either orally or intravenously.

Now let us consider the specific imbalances.

Metabolic Acidosis

Etiology. The basic defects that can cause metabolic acidosis are: (1) an abnormal loss of $NaHCO_3$, which decreases both the base side of the H_2CO_3:$NaHCO_3$ ratio and the pH of the body fluids; and (2) a heavy production of nonvolatile acids, which overloads the kidneys and exceeds renal capacity for the secretion of excess acid. Major causative factors resulting in these defects are:

OVERPRODUCTION OF METABOLICALLY PRODUCED ACIDS. In conditions such as diabetes mellitus, hyperthyroidism, starvation, severe infections with fever, and prolonged fasting or vomiting, proteins and fats are burned for energy instead of carbohydrates. The result is an accumulation of ketone bodies, which create an acidosis.

Some studies state that *anesthesia* can also cause acidosis in certain individuals. Because anesthesia is a stress that increases the body's metabolism markedly, additional proteins and fats are burned, causing the production of increased acid.

EXCESSIVE INGESTION OF METABOLIC ACIDS. Patients on ketogenic and high fat, low carbohydrate diets can develop acidosis. Also, the oral ingestion of such organic acids as salicylic acid or boric acid will result in the formation of excess H^+. Finally, excessive ingestion of such medications as ammonium chloride, ferrous sulfate, and paraldehyde (a drug commonly used in treating acute alcoholism) all promote the development of H^+ overload.

INADEQUATE RENAL FUNCTION. In renal disease the kidney loses its ability to compensate adequately for acid overloads. Thus, H^+ are not excreted at a normal rate, nor is $NaHCO_3$ sufficiently conserved.

ABNORMAL LOSSES OF ALKALI. Severe diarrhea and the loss of pancreatic, biliary, and lower bowel secretions result in acidosis. In these cases, HCO_3^- is being lost in large amounts from the body which, in effect, is the same thing as adding acid to the body. *Prolonged vomiting* of *deep* gastrointestinal contents also causes acidosis owing to loss of base. In contrast, acute vomiting of *stomach contents* results in *alkalosis* owing to the loss of HCl.

SEVERE TISSUE ANOXIA. Patients who suffer from severe tissue anoxia resulting from pulmonary disorders, hepatic disease, or serious anemia produce excessive amounts of lactic acid. The circulation of large amounts of lactic acid in the blood can result in a critical metabolic acidosis termed *lactic acidosis.* The onset of lactic acidosis is usually sudden, and the prognosis is almost always poor, since this condition is highly resistive to treatment.

Compensatory Mechanisms. The body fights metabolic acidosis in the following ways:

RESPIRATORY DEFENSE

Kussmaul respirations (air hunger)

1. Breathing increases in rate and depth.
2. Excess H_2CO_3 is "blown off."
3. *Result:* H^+ concentration of ECF is lowered.

RENAL DEFENSE

1. $Na^+ = H^+$ exchange is increased, which reresults in the excretion of H^+ in the urine.
2. Rate of the ammonia mechanism is increased.
3. *Result*
   a. An acid urine is produced.
   b. Large numbers of H^+ ions are excreted as NH_4.
   c. There is a greater return of HCO_3^- to the ECF where it joins with Na^+ to form $NaHCO_3$.
   d. The base side of the H_2CO_3:$NaHCO_3$ ratio is increased.

If the acidosis is compensated, H^+ levels in the ECF will decrease and the plasma bicarbonate level will rise. A possible *complication* resulting from the compensatory mechanisms just discussed is the development of secondary or compensatory metabolic alkalosis.

Bases of Symptoms. The symptoms seen in metabolic acidosis are the result of both the primary imbalance and the compensatory reaction of the body. At the bottom of this page, major symptoms are listed along with their causative factors.

Clinical Care. The major goals of clinical care for patients with metabolic acidosis are:

1. The restoration of proper blood volume and osmolarity.
2. The correction of HCO_3 deficit.
3. Correction of K^+ excess.

THE RESTORATION OF PROPER BLOOD VOLUME AND OSMOLARITY. Patients with acidosis are often seriously dehydrated from vomiting, diarrhea, and so forth. Consequently the doctor will need to have a precise record of the patient's weight fluctuations as well as a record of his intake and output. A Foley catheter will be ordered, and in severe cases, hourly urine measurements may be necessary to observe for fluid depletion. Also, sodium chloride or Ringer's lactate are usually administered intravenously to compensate for fluid losses.

THE CORRECTION OF THE HCO_3 DEFICIT. $NaHCO_3$, or molar Na lactate, is often added to the IV solution to correct the $NaHCO_3$ deficiency and to neutralize the excess acid. In severe acidosis patients may receive IV administration of 1/6 molar sodium lactate – a potent solution.

CORRECTION OF K^+ EXCESS. Patients with metabolic acidosis who have severe tissue damage frequently develop hyperkalemia. Because a serious K^+ excess can result in toxic heart symptoms or even cardiac arrest, every effort must be made to reduce K^+ in the plasma. (See later discussion.)

The general treatment listed above can expose the patient to new dangers. One common complication of therapy in metabolic acidosis is *rebound respiratory alkalosis.* This imbalance commonly occurs following $NaHCO_3$ replacement. The symptoms of respiratory alkalosis are discussed on p. 232. A second complication of therapy is tetany due to *hypocalcemia.* This imbalance occurs upon *correction* of the metabolic acidosis for the following reasons:

When the body fluids are *acid,* calcium is available in ionized form; this is the most effective form for maintaining normal muscle contractility and the proper transmission of nerve impulses. However, when the body fluids become *alkaline, less* calcium is ionized and, consequently, the body's Ca^{++} is *not* very effective in preventing neuromuscular irritability.

Patients with metabolic acidosis have predominantly acid body fluids, thus, calcium exists in a highly ionized form. If the patient is suffering from a Ca^{++} deficit, symptoms will *not* appear because his Ca^{++} is being utilized. Once the acidosis is corrected, however, the patient's body fluids will become more alkaline. As a result, less Ca^{++} will exist in ionized form, and *neuromuscular irritability* and *tetany* may develop. The treatment of choice, should this complication appear, is the intravenous administration of calcium gluconate. (See p. 237 for precautions in the administration of this drug.)

Nursing Implications. When caring for patients with *metabolic acidosis,* watch for the following symptoms: (1) increased rate and depth of breathing; delirium; coma; and (2) neuromuscular signs of K^+ excess, such as weakness, flaccid paralysis, and cardiac arrest. Following therapy, observe for: hypoventilation due to respiratory alkalosis, and tetany due to Ca^{++} deficit. Take safety precautions when working with patients in metabolic acidosis. Do not leave a delirious patient unattended. Always make certain that the siderails are up if you must leave the bedside. Remember that disorientation and weakness may cause the acidotic patient to fall from his bed and injure himself seriously, thereby complicating his condition further.

Metabolic Alkalosis

Etiology. The basic problems characterizing metabolic alkalosis are: (1) an abnormal rise in the base bicarbonate of the plasma which increases the alkali side of the H_2CO_3:$NaHCO_3$ ratio; and/or (2) a decrease in the H^+ concentration of the plasma, with a resultant rise in blood pH. Important causes of metabolic alkalosis (or base bicarbonate excess) are described on page 228.

SYMPTOMS OF METABOLIC ACIDOSIS

Symptoms	*Bases of Symptoms*
Apathy; disorientation; delirium; weakness; stupor; coma	Central nervous system depression resulting from the accumulation of acids and loss of HCO_3^-
Kussmaul respirations	Compensatory reaction by the lung
Laboratory findings: Blood pH below 7.35; plasma HCO_3^- below 25 mEq./L.	Accumulation of metabolic acids in the plasma or loss of base from the plasma
Acid urine with pH below 6.0	Compensatory reaction by the kidney; H^+ secretion and $Na^+ - H^+$ exchange increased
Severe arrhythmias; cardiac arrest	Serum K^+ excess is a common complication of metabolic acidosis, especially if the patient has suffered from severe tissue damage (intracellular K^+ shifts into the plasma to create hyperkalemia)

EXCESSIVE LOSS OF H^+ FROM THE BODY. Patients who are particularly susceptible to H^+ depletion are: (1) those who are vomiting stomach contents (not deep gastrointestinal contents as in metabolic acidosis), and (2) those on gastric suction who are losing electrolytes and who are *not* receiving adequate electrolyte replacement. In both of these situations patients are *losing large amounts of HCl,* which leads to the following problems:

> The loss of excessive H^+ from the body in emesis or drainage.
> The loss of Cl^-, which leaves Na^+ unattached and free to unite with HCO_3 to form $NaHCO_3$.
> The conservation of the anion HCO_3^-, which serves to replace the lost anion Cl^-, and thus preserve the electrical neutrality of the body.

As a result of these chemical changes, H^+ is lost and excesses of $NaHCO_3$ are produced; consequently, the 1:20 ratio of buffer acid to buffer base is upset in favor of buffer base. To make matters worse, if the body has been subjected to severe trauma or stress, Na^+ is retained in unusually large amounts because of an increased secretion of aldosterone. The increased Na^+ in the body fluids combines readily with HCO_3^- to form a heavy alkaline load. Thus, the patient who has suffered from an accident or burns and who is on gastric suction must be carefully observed for the signs of alkalosis.

EXCESSIVE INGESTION OF ALKALI. Patients with peptic ulcers or "acid stomach" often take ordinary baking soda or milk of magnesia, thinking that self-medication with alkaline substances will relieve their symptoms.* Actually baking soda, indiscriminately used, often causes an "acid rebound" as a result of the release of CO_2. This reaction causes increased acidity, which makes the patient uncomfortable; thus, he ingests more baking soda and a vicious circle begins which finally ends in metabolic alkalosis. Ulcer patients who are *both* vomiting and ingesting alkali medications are particularly vulnerable to this imbalance, as they are losing H^+ in the emesis at the same time that they are ingesting HCO_3^-.

Compensatory Mechanisms. Major ways in which the body tries to compensate for metabolic alkalosis are as follows:

THE BUFFER DEFENSE. As HCO_3^- increases in the ECF, it reacts with acid buffer salts. This results in a decrease in bicarbonate and an increase in the carbonic acid partner of the H_2CO_3:$NaHCO_3$ ratio.

RESPIRATORY DEFENSE. Hypoventilation is the major defense; this conserves CO_2, which increases the pCO_2 and H^+ concentration of the ECF. Two complications can result from hypoventilation: (1) secondary respiratory acidosis owing to retention of CO_2; and (2) decreased O_2 intake and resultant hypoxia from the shallow, slow respirations.

RENAL DEFENSE. H^+ is conserved and large amounts of K^+ and Na^+ are excreted with the excess of HCO_3. This can produce a dangerous K^+ deficit. Ammonia production slows and H^+ is conserved. This results in an alkaline urine rather than the normal slightly acid urine.

Note how the compensatory mechanisms used by the body to fight metabolic alkalosis are almost exactly the opposite of those used to ward off metabolic acidosis. In acidosis the person hyperventilates and excretes an acid urine. In alkalosis the person hypoventilates and excretes an alkaline urine. In both any malfunctioning of buffers, kidney, or lungs results in an imbalance that is uncompensated and dangerous.

Bases of Symptoms. The signs and symptoms of metabolic alkalosis appear in the lungs, neuromuscular system, kidneys, and heart. As in metabolic acidosis, symptoms are the result of both the primary imbalance and compensatory mechanisms. Major symptoms and their causative factors are: listed at the bottom of the page.

Clinical Care. To correct the metabolic alkalosis and alleviate the symptoms, the following therapeutic steps are necessary:

TREATING THE PRIMARY CONDITION. The major causative factors in alkalosis are loss of acid, overingestion of alkali, and loss of electrolytes, especially Cl^- and K^+.

First, patients who are losing acid because of vomiting or gastric suction will need appropriate replacement fluids. Second, to prevent electrolyte

* For a more complete discussion of the relationship of the milk-alkali syndrome and metabolic alkalosis to peptic ulcer, see the discussion of gastrointestinal tract disorders, Unit XV.

SYMPTOMS OF METABOLIC ALKALOSIS

Symptoms	*Bases of Symptoms*
Belligerence; irritability; disorientation; lethargy; tetany; convlusions	Overexcitability of the central nervous system due to the accumulation of bicarbonate and loss of H^+
Shallow, slow respirations· decreased thoracic movements; cyanosis and periods of apnea	Compensatory mechanism by the lungs
Irregular pulse; muscle twitch; paralytic ileus, cardiac arrest	Abnormal losses of K^+ from the ECF in exchange for H^+
Laboratory findings:	
Plasma pH 7.45; plasma bicarbonate above 29 mEq./L.	Increase in HCO_3^- side of H_2CO_3:$NaHCO_3$ ratio
Urine pH above 7.0 (alkaline)	Compensatory reaction by the kidney

losses, irrigate the patient's gastric tube with isotonic solution rather than with plain water, and always give the patient isotonic fluids to drink when fluids are ordered. Third, ulcer and other patients must be instructed *not to medicate themselves* by taking large amounts of baking soda at home.

Warn ulcer patients who are taking *prescribed* alkaline substances at home to stop the medication and call their physician should they develop a distaste for milk, dryness of mouth, anorexia, weakness, and lethargy. These are signs of the milk-alkali syndrome.

CORRECTION OF ALKALOSIS. The alkalosis is usually treated by giving Ringer's solution, which contains 10 mEg./L. of chloride. This solution not only corrects the alkalosis, but alleviates the chloride deficit as well. In severe cases the doctor may order 0.9 per cent ammonium chloride (NH_4Cl) intravenously. This drug causes the release of HCl, thus restoring both the normal H^+ concentration of the ECF and normal Cl^- levels. Ammonium chloride 0.9 per cent is an *extremely dangerous* medication. When administering this drug intravenously, remember these points:

1. *Give 0.9 per cent ammonium chloride (NH_4Cl) at a rate of 1 liter in 4 hours or 2-3 ml./minute.*
2. *A faster rate of administration may result in* hemolysis of the red blood cells.
3. *NH_4Cl is contraindicated in hepatic and renal patients.*
4. *Excessive administration of NH_4Cl may cause a rebound metabolic acidosis.*

The use of 0.9 per cent NH_4Cl intravenously is a somewhat controversial subject. Some physicians think that the drug is worthwhile despite its dangers, while others believe that its toxic effects negate its value as a corrective drug in alkalosis.

CORRECTION OF H_2O, Na^+, Cl^-, AND K^+ DEFICITS. Sodium, H_2O, and Cl^- deficits are usually corrected by administering normal saline. To correct K^+ deficits, KCl is given IV; cathartics may be withheld and thiazide-type diuretics discontinued.

The correction of K^+ deficits is particularly important in the treatment of alkalosis. K^+ deficits that have developed prior to or during the course of metabolic alkalosis must be replaced before H^+ balance can be restored for the following reasons:

1. When body fluids become too alkaline, the kidneys fight to preserve H^+ by *substituting* K^+ for H^+ in the H^+–Na^+ exchange. Thus, large amounts of K^+ are excreted in the urine. The result is *extracellular K^+ loss.*

2. If these extracellular losses of K^+ are not corrected, K^+ is then pulled from the cells to replace the extracellular losses. This results in *intracellular K^+ loss.*

3. In response to decreasing amounts of intracellular cation K^+, the cations Na^+ and H^+ enter the cell in order to balance the losses and thus preserve the electrical neutrality of the body fluids. The result is an *intracellular acidosis* and an *extracellular alkalosis.*

The metabolic alkalosis that has contributed to the development of a K^+ deficit in the first place is now complicated further by the problems listed below:

> When a K^+ deficit occurs, the kidneys (for unknown reasons) are unable to excrete HCO_3^-.

> When K^+ losses are severe, the kidney "frantically" tries to preserve K^+ are the expense of H^+, which it excretes. The loss of H^+ then, coupled with the retention of HCO_3^-, worsens the alkalosis that is already present. To correct the alkalosis, K^+ *deficits* must be immediately replaced. Moreover, to sustain the body's K^+ at a normal level, the alkalosis must be corrected.

The patient's response to therapy can be followed on the basis of a daily electrolyte analysis, weight, and hemoglobin readings. Generally it takes 12 to 24 hours to correct the NaCl and water deficits, around 42 hours to correct the K^+ deficit, and between 48 and 72 hours to fully reverse the alkalosis.

Respiratory Acidosis

Etiology. As the name signifies, respiratory acidosis is an imbalance in which abnormalities of respiration cause an increase in the H^+ concentration of the body fluids. You will recall that the problem in *metabolic acidosis* is an excessive loss of sodium bicarbonate coupled with overproduction and retention of nonvolatile acids. In *respiratory acidosis,* the causative defect is the *excessive retention of CO_2*, resulting in: (1) the combining of retained CO_2 with H_2O to form excess H_2CO_3; (2) a decrease in the ratio of $NaHCO_3$ to H_2CO_3; (3) an increase in the pCO_2 and H^+ concentration of the body fluids; and (4) a lowering of the blood pH. If respiratory acidosis is severe, the amount of H_2CO_3 in the body fluids may be twice the normal amount.

The factors creating this situation include: First, respiratory acidosis can be voluntarily caused by *breath holding.* However, it is more commonly the result of *respiratory diseases* that halt or hinder the gaseous exchanges normally occurring between the blood and alveolar air. Major physiologic disorders resulting in the reduction of CO_2 and O_2 exchange in the alveoli are:

> Damage to the respiratory center in the medulla.

> A decrease in the surface area of the lung which, in turn, reduces the diffusion of gases.

> Obstruction of the passageways of the respiratory tract. There are many diseases and injuries that can produce the changes just listed. The major conditions are: emphysema, bronchiectasis, pneumothorax, hemothorax, bronchial asthma, drug intoxication (resulting in respiratory depression), use of O_2 tents (cause excessive inhaling of CO_2), bronchial pneumonia, poliomyelitis, pulmonary fibrosis, acute alcoholism, burns of the respiratory tract, congestive heart failure, and poor gaseous exchange during surgery.*

*The development of respiratory acidosis during surgery is discussed in Unit VI.

Compensatory Mechanisms. The major ways in which the body attempts to compensate for respiratory acidosis are as follows:

DEFENSE BY THE BUFFER SYSTEM. The body increases the *rate of the chloride shift* and a larger than normal number of chloride ions pass into the red blood cells from the plasma in exchange for HCO_3^-, which passes into the blood. The result is that excess H_2CO_3 is neutralized, and the increased proportion of H_2CO_3 to $NaHCO_3$ is corrected and the normal 1:20 ratio is restored.

RESPIRATORY DEFENSE. Hyperventilation (increase in the rate and depth of breathing) is the main defense occurring in response to the increased pCO_2 and lowered pH of the plasma. The result is that large amounts of CO_2 and H_2O (H_2CO_3) are "blown off," pCO_2 drops toward normal, and the pH rises.

RENAL DEFENSE. The kidneys labor to lower the concentration of H^+ in the body fluids by: (1) increasing the rate of $H^+ - Na^+$ exchange (this results in H^+ excretion and reabsorption of Na^+, which joins with HCO_3^- to form $NaHCO_3$); and (2) increased formation of ammonia, which results in an increased H^+ excretion. The total result of renal defense is that excess H^+ ions are excreted in an acid urine, and the base portion of the H_2CO_3:$NaHCO_3$ ratio is increased. Compensation by the kidney is complete; however, it takes about half a day for a plasma pH to return to normal.

The individual with pulmonary disease must rely heavily upon the renal compensatory mechanisms for the control of respiratory acidosis. However, in severe cases, the kidney with its slow but steady regulation of blood pH may not be able to act quickly enough to compensate for the acidosis. Thus, the pH may drop to dangerously low levels before compensation finally takes place.

Bases of Symptoms: The major symptoms of respiratory acidosis are cardiopulmonary. Often the only sign of imbalance is *dyspnea upon exertion.* However, other serious symptoms may occur. These are listed below along with their causative bases.

When a patient has chronic lung disease (e.g., emphysema), he may develop a severe complication called *CO_2 narcosis.* This condition is the result of the following chain of pathologic events:

(1) The diseased lung cannot excrete CO_2 in large amounts; (2) CO_2 accumulates within the blood; (3) the pCO_2 rises and the pH falls; (4) the respiratory center in the medulla is overwhelmed by the rising CO_2 concentration of the body fluids; (5) the respiratory center loses its sensitivity to the elevated CO_2 concentrations and fails to respond (the medulla responds only to slight changes in blood pH; CO_2 concentrations of over 9 per cent cause depression of the respiratory center); (6) the patient, instead of breathing rapidly in order to "blow off" CO_2 now hypoventilates; (7) CO_2 builds up in the body fluids and chronically remains elevated; (8) the constant elevation of CO_2 levels in the body fluids leads to the condition of CO_2 narcosis.

Symptoms of CO_2 narcosis are the result of huge accumulations of CO_2 within the blood. They involve the sensorium, the respiratory center, the heart, and the neuromuscular system. The major symptoms are:

Sensorium: drowsiness, irritability, depression, hallucinations, coma.
Respiratory system: poor ventilation, shallow respirations.
Heart: tachycardia, arrhythmias.
Neuromuscular: paralysis of extremities, tremors of face, convulsions.

> Remember:
> *CO_2 narcosis can be precipitated by giving excessive oxygen therapy to patients with poor ventilation (e.g., postoperative patients and patients with emphysema).*

These people, because their respiratory centers are no longer responding adequately to plasma CO_2 concentrations, depend upon *anoxia* as their major respiratory stimulus. Therefore, when too high a concentration of O_2 is given to patients with emphysema or to postoperative patients, they lose their *one* reason for breathing, namely, the *need to correct O_2 lack.* As a result, the patient may cease to breathe altogether and will die! Thus, there is need to use caution and judgment when administering O_2 to dyspneic patients.

Clinical Care. As stated earlier, in respiratory acidosis the major problem is poor ventilation and the consequent accumulation of elevated CO_2 levels within the blood. Therefore, the major goal of therapy is to correct or at least to *control the respiratory disease,* thereby improving ventilation. Other goals

SYMPTOMS OF RESPIRATORY ACIDOSIS

Symptoms	*Bases of Symptoms*
Hyperventilation at rest; wheezing; tachycardia; cyanosis; mental disorientation	Inadequate pulmonary ventilation and hindrance of the normal O_2–CO_2 exchange between the blood and alveolar air
Laboratory Findings:	
Plasma pH below 7.35; plasma bicarbonate 29 mEq./L.; acid urine with pH below 6.0	Renal compensation
In decompensated cases: shallow respirations; rapid respirations; severe dyspnea; suprasternal retraction	Lung disease exists and the kidney is unable to act rapidly enough to control the pH

of therapy are to *neutralize the excessive acid,* and *correct H_2O, K^+, and Cl^- imbalances* if they exist.

IMPROVEMENT OF RESPIRATORY FUNCTION.* Some of the typical treatments often ordered to improve respiratory efficiency are: antibiotics to curb respiratory infections; postural drainage; bronchodilators and detergents; inhalation therapy with nebulization; breathing exercises that increase the efficiency of respiration; mechanical respirators; and oxygen administered with extreme caution.

CORRECTION OF THE ACIDOSIS. Important drugs and solutions used in treating respiratory acidosis are:

> THAM given intravenously at 300 ml. per hour. This organic buffer compound is used in very severe cases of respiratory acidosis. THAM reduces the CO_2 concentration of the ECF and increases both the HCO_3^- concentration and the pH of the blood. While THAM is a useful drug in acute cases, it is dangerous in that it depresses respiration and can result in apnea. Consequently, THAM should not be given to patients with *chronic* respiratory acidosis because of the danger of CO_2 narcosis.

> Ringer's lactate solution IV is given in severe cases of respiratory acidosis.

> Sodium bicarbonate 5 Gm. orally every 30 minutes or 0.25 Gm./kg. of body weight, IV.

> One sixth molar solution of sodium lactate, 20 mg./kg. of body weight, IV until the urine has an alkaline reaction.

These drugs and solutions need to be administered with caution. As you will recall, the intravenous administration of sodium bicarbonate to patients with acidosis may result in *tetany* once the acidosis is corrected and the body fluids become more alkaline. Thus, as in metabolic acidosis, *calcium gluconate* should be on hand in the event of this complication. Some doctors may order a prophylactic dose of 10 ml. of 10 per cent calcium gluconate to be given intravenously *before* sodium bicarbonate administration, thereby alleviating the possibility of tetany.

Occasionally, in addition to the above drugs and solutions, patients may be placed on *gastric suction* to remove excess HCl, thereby raising the pH of the body fluids.

THE CORRECTION OF WATER AND ELECTROLYTE IMBALANCES. To correct dehydration, the doctor may order the intravenous administration of hypotonic solutions containing carbohydrates and electrolytes. If K^+ levels are elevated, appropriate measures will be taken to correct the hyperkalemia.

As with all the imbalances discussed, treatment unfortunately can create new complications. In respiratory acidosis, three iatrogenic conditions may occur as a result of therapy: (1) *tetany,* which results from the administration of $NaHCO_3$ and the consequent correction of the lowered pH of the blood; (2) *CO_2 narcosis,* which results from the administration of large quantities of O_2 to patients with longstanding chronic CO_2 retention; and (3) *rebound respiratory alkalosis,* which results from too rapid compensation of respiratory acidosis, overzealous use of mechanical respirators, and the excessively rapid administration of $NaHCO_3$.

*Methods of treating respiratory problems are discussed in detail in Unit XIV.

Respiratory Alkalosis

Etiology. The major problem that characterizes respiratory alkalosis is the *excessive secretion of CO_2* resulting from hyperventilation. This loss of CO_2 results in (1) a decrease in the H^+ concentration of the body fluid, (2) a decrease in the pCO_2, (3) an increase in the ratio of $NaHCO_3$ to H_2CO_3, and (4) a rise in the blood pH.

These disturbances are almost always the result of hyperventilation, and overstimulation of the respiratory center in the brain. *Hyperventilation* with resultant respiratory acidosis most frequently develops as a result of the following conditions:

> Hysteria and anxiety reactions.

> The aftermath of severe exercise.

> Anoxia at high altitudes, which leads to increased respirations and an increased loss of CO_2.

> Poorly adjusted respirations, which cause patients to hyperventilate.

Overstimulation of the respiratory center in the brain can result from:

> Fever.

> C.N.S. diseases (e.g., meningitis and encephalitis).

> Intracranial surgery.

> Aspirin poisoning.

Both respiratory alkalosis and acidosis are imbalances that can be caused voluntarily. For example, acidosis can be caused by purposely holding one's breath, and alkalosis can be caused by voluntary hyperventilation. However, while respiratory acidosis is caused by definite physiologic disorders that interfere with pulmonary ventilation, respiratory alkalosis is more often the result of psychologic and environmental factors and diseases that are not necessarily respiratory in nature.

Compensatory Mechanisms. The body strives to correct respiratory alkalosis as follows:

DEFENSE BY THE BUFFER SYSTEM. The body increases its production of organic acids, and the acids react with excess bicarbonate ions. The result is that excessive base is neutralized, and there is restoration of the normal 1:20 ratio of H_2CO_3 to $NaHCO_3$.

RESPIRATORY DEFENSE. Respirations decrease or even cease until CO_2 levels rise to a high enough level to again stimulate respiration. The result is that the decrease in plasma H_2CO_3 is compensated and a H^+ excess results, and the excess H^+ is then excreted by the kidneys as necessary.

RENAL COMPENSATION. The kidney halts the reabsorption of HCO_3^- and hastens its excretion; it also diminishes the production of NH_4. The result is that H^+ is retained in the body until the normal 1:20 ratio of H_2CO_3 to $NaHCO_3$ is restored.

Thus, the body compensates for respiratory alkalosis by decreasing respiration and producing an alkaline urine.

Bases of Symptoms. The most outstanding characteristic of respiratory alkalosis is *increased neuromuscular irritability*. Therefore, patients with this imbalance develop hyperreflexia, a positive Chvostek's sign, and muscular twitch. Also, generalized convulsions sometimes occur. Characteristic laboratory findings are: urine alkaline with pH above 7.0, and plasma pH above 7.45. Sometimes K^+ depletion may occur if the attack of respiratory alkalosis is prolonged over several days. Hypokalemia, in this case, can be controlled by administering 1 mEq. of K^+/kg. of body weight per day.

Clinical Care. In treating respiratory alkalosis, the first step is to eliminate the cause of the hyperventilation. Psychotherapy may be required for the hysterical or highly anxious patient. Some doctors have hysterical patients rebreathe their own CO_2 from a paper bag, thus increasing the H^+ concentration of their blood. Other doctors order whiffs of 5 per cent CO_2—a therapy that sometimes "backfires" by increasing instead of decreasing hyperventilation. Patients suffering from neurologic disorders or from aspirin poisoning require, first and foremost, treatment of the primary condition. Respirators used for ventilation should be checked hourly and adjusted as needed for optimal but not excessive ventilation.

POTASSIUM BALANCE

Essential facts concerning potassium [K^+] balance are summarized at the bottom of this page.

In reviewing the outline below, it is apparent that *anything that reduces the integrity of the cell will produce a K^+ imbalance.* For example, trauma, burns, and starvation are all factors that impair cellular metabolism, thereby creating potassium upsets. When potassium imbalances *do* occur, symptoms involving *cardiac, cellular,* and *neuromuscular function* develop. *Kidney function* is also disturbed since the kidney is the major organ of potassium excretion. We shall now explore the specific problems of potassium deficit and excess.

POTASSIUM IMBALANCES

Potassium Deficit (Hypokalemia)

This is a common imbalance and one that is potentially deadly in its pathologic effects.

Etiology. The major causes of potassium deficit are summarized on the opposite page.

Bases of Symptoms. A potassium deficit of the ECF (hypokalemia) basically affects *cellular metabolism* which, in turn, affects the functions of the neuromuscular system, and cardiovascular system, gastrointestinal tract, respiratory tract, and kidney. H^+ balance is also upset. These disturbances are listed at the bottom of page 233 along with the specific symptoms they produce.

Body Potassium (K^+)—A Summary of Basic Facts

I. The body of a normal 70-kg. (154-lb.) male contains approximately 3500 mEq. of K^+.
II. K^+ is found in all fluid compartments.
   A. It is the dominant ion of cellular fluid (which contains approximately 2950 mEq. of the body's K^+).
   B. The extracellular fluid contains only about 4 mEq./L. of K^+.
   C. The normal serum K^+ concentration ranges from 3.8 to 4.5 mEq. per L.
III. K^+ performs the following valuable functions:
   A. Regulates the intracellular osmolarity.
   B. Promotes cellular growth.
   C. Helps to promote the conduction of nerve impulses.
   D. Helps to promote proper skeletal muscle function.
   E. Helps to promote proper heart muscle activity.
IV. K^+ ingestion and excretion.
   A. Normally a person requires 40 mEq. of K^+ per day.
   B. Eighty to 90 per cent of ingested K^+ is excreted in the urine while 10 to 20 per cent is excreted in the stools.
V. The conservation of cellular K^+.
   A. The amount of K^+ in the cell depends upon the following factors:
      1. The integrity or general health of the cell.
      2. The sodium pump, which maintains a high K^+ cellular content by actively excluding Na^+.
      3. The ability of the cell to store some surplus K^+.
      4. The ability of the kidney to conserve K^+ to some degree when the cells become depleted.
   B. K^+ moves *into* the cells when glucose is being metabolized by the body.
   C. K^+ moves *out* of the cells under these conditions:
      1. During strenuous exercise.
      2. When cellular metabolism is impaired.
      3. When the cell dies.
   D. When K^+ *is lost* from the cell, the following happens:
      1. Other ions shift into the cell in order to maintain cellular tonicity, e.g., Na^+ and H^+ ions shift into the cell from the ECF to replace lost K^+.
      2. The cell, due to the H^+, then becomes more acid while the ECF becomes more alkaline.

Causes of Potassium Deficit

I. Inadequate intake of K^+ due to:
  A. Poor dietary habits.
  B. Nausea.
  C. Poor appetite.
  D. Acute alcoholism.
  E. Extreme dieting.
  F. Parenteral fluids that are low in K^+ and high in Na^+. The kidneys and cells are apparently unable to conserve K^+ when the body is deprived of a K^+ intake at the same time that it is receiving a large Na^+ load. For obscure reasons, the body tends to conserve Na^+ at the expense of K^+.

II. Increased utilization of K^+ during the healing phase of burns and as a complication of diabetic acidosis.

III. Excessive loss of K^+ due to:
  A. Therapeutic agents.
    1. Thiazide-type diuretics (e.g., Esidrix, Enduron, Naqua) retard reabsorption of K^+.
    2. Adrenal steroid therapy, causing Na^+ retention and increased K^+ excretion.
    3. Excessive infusions of IV solutions (especially saline) without adequate K^+ replacement.
    4. Excessive enemas and laxatives lead to loss of K^+-rich mucous lining the colon.
    5. Gastric and intestinal suction.
    6. Operations in which large amounts of K^+ are lost in the drainage from the surgical site, e.g., colostomies, ileostomies, large or small bowel resections.
  B. Conditions of the gastrointestinal tract.
    1. Vomiting, because K^+ is lost with the regurgitated mucus and gastric juices.
    2. Ulcerative colitis and diarrhea.
    3. Fistulas of the small or large intestine.
  C. Metabolic disorders.
    1. The stress syndrome:
      a. Occurs in response to fear, severe psychologic upsets, burns, extensive surgery, untreated diabetes, and tissue cell damage.
      b. Affects adrenal and pituitary action.
      c. Mobilizes K^+ from tissue cells and excretes it in large amounts.
    2. Conditions causing an increased corticosteroid production, e.g., Cushing's syndrome.
  D. Trauma, e.g., severe burns and crushing injuries.
  E. Renal disorders: K^+ deficit usually results from a defect of tubular reabsorption.

Symptoms of Potassium Deficit

Symptoms	*Bases of Symptoms*
Anorexia; weakness; lethargy; irritability; mental confusion; flabby muscles (like half-filled hot water bottles); a rounded body contour; flaccid paralysis; shallow respirations	Reduction of neuromuscular irritability
Arrhythmias; congestive heart failure; heart block; cardiac arrest	Necrosis and fibrosis of heart muscle
Hypotension (possibly part of the shock syndrome that results from surgery)	Vascular weakness
Decreased intestinal motility; abdominal distention; paralytic ileus	Weakness of smooth muscles of gastrointestinal tract
Reduced concentrating power	Structural changes in the kidney
H^+ and Na^+ enter the cell to replace K^+; cell becomes acidic	H^+ disturbances

The diagnosis of a potassium deficit is usually made on the basis of the above signs and symptoms and the patient's history. An EKG tracing, while often ordered, gives only a vague idea of the seriousness of the K^+ deficiency. Laboratory findings show only the amount of *extracellular* K^+ available, giving *no* measurement of cellular K^+ content. Cellular K^+ replaces extracellular K^+ when it becomes depleted. Thus, while a patient may actually be suffering from a serious *intracellular* K^+ deficit, it is possible that his *extracellular* K^+ may be within normal limits. Nevertheless, the serum K^+ level is the major diagnostic test for K^+ deficit.

Clinical Care. The goal of care in a potassium deficiency is to supply sufficient K^+ to make up for the deficit. The major methods of treatment are as follows:

ORAL REPLACEMENT OF POTASSIUM. Physicians generally agree that it is less dangerous to use the oral route in replacing K^+ than the more rapid-acting intravenous route. The most natural way to correct a K^+ deficit is through the use of a *high potassium diet.* Some dietary sources of K^+ are listed in Table 25–3.

A second important method of K^+ replacement is with *oral medications.* Some of the most common medications are the following:

1. Potassium chloride (KCl) 5-10 Gm. per day (enteric-coated pill). Potassium chloride, despite its tendency to cause gastric irritation, has been widely used for years; however, the safety of KCl in the correction of K^+ deficit has come into serious question. In recent studies small groups of patients have developed stenosis and ulcers of the small intestine following the ingestion of this drug. As a consequence, some doctors believe that a chloride-free K^+ salt (such as potassium triplex or potassium citrate) should be given in place of potassium chloride.

2. Potassium triplex, 5 ml. (15 mEq. K^+) orally, 3 times daily. Potassium triplex, a liquid medication, contains equal amounts of potassium acetate, potassium bicarbonate, and potassium citrate. Because this drug has an unpleasant taste, it is best administered in juice.

3. Potassium citrate, 1 or 2 Gm. orally, daily in divided doses.

4. Potassium gluconate (Kaon), 30 ml. (40 mEq.) orally, daily.

In dispensing oral medications containing potassium, implement the following rules to ensure greater safety:

1. *Dispense oral medications containing K^+ with caution since potassium excess can result from excessive dosages.*
2. *Watch carefully for oliguria in patients receiving K^+ supplements (an important sign of toxicity).*
3. *Question the administration of K^+ to patients with renal disease, because K^+ may be retained if renal output is poor.*
4. *Question the administration of K^+ to patients with dehydration and resultant oliguria.*

TABLE 25–3. IMPORTANT DIETARY SOURCES OF K^+*

	Potassium-Milli-equivalents
Fruits	
Apricots, raw, 2-3 medium	7.06
Banana, 1 medium	16.12
Dates, dried, 3-4	5.78
Figs, raw, fresh, 2 large	4.86
canned in syrup, 3 figs, 2 tbsp. syrup	2.68
dried, 7 small	19.96
Oranges, 1 medium 3″	9.21
Peaches, dried, 1/2 cup, uncooked	28.16
Prunes, dried, raw, 5 large	7.68
Raisins, dried, seedless, 2 tbsp.	3.68
Juices	
Tomato, 1/2 cup, canned	7.29
Orange, 1/2 cup, fresh	5.68
Miscellaneous	
Brazil nuts, shelled, 4 medium	2.56
shelled, 1/3 cup	17.15
Instant coffee, 2 Gm., dry in 240 ml. water	6.14

*Adapted from Snively, W. D., and Westerman, R. L.: Minnesota Medicine 48:713, June, 1965.

Because of the dangers involved in potassium replacement, K^+ is usually given only to those patients who have been deprived of, or have been losing, potassium for at least three days. Potassium salts are administered with extreme caution to postoperative patients. Medications containing K^+ are not given until urinary function is firmly reestablished.

INTRAVENOUS ADMINISTRATION. K^+ is administered by means of commercially prepared electrolyte IV solutions containing K^+, or by ampules of liquid potassium salts that are added to liters of such IV fluids as 5 or 10 per cent glucose in water. Generally, 40 mEq. of K^+ is administered daily. Since potassium is potentially highly toxic, the nurse needs to observe carefully the following general rules pertaining to its administration:

> Do *not* give K^+ salts in concentrated form directly into the vein: *Cardiac arrest can result!* K^+ salts are always administered diluted in solutions when given by IV drip.

> Dilute each small ampule containing potassium salts in at least one liter of solution prior to starting the infusion. If by accident the IV should drip too rapidly, the dilution of the potassium in a large amount of solution will help to prevent a deadly toxic reaction.

> Carefully watch the *rate* of drip of solutions containing potassium. Give no more than 20 mEq. of potassium per hour to an adult patient. For example, if the infusion contains 40 mEq. of potassium in 1000 ml. of solution, drip the solution no faster than 8 ml./min. A *faster rate of infusion can lead to cardiac arrest.*

> When solutions containing fairly high levels of K^+ (40 mEq./L.) are administered the patient may develop severe pain along the vein being used for the infusion. This

discomfort can be controlled by slowing the rate of drip. Also, the doctor may order either 5 mg. heparin, 5 to 10 ml. of 2 per cent procaine, or 1 mg. of prednisone to be added to each liter of fluid to relieve the pain.

> Do not give IV potassium solutions *unless renal flow is adequate.* If administering 40 mEq. of potassium salts in 1 liter of fluid, urine flow should be at least 1 ml. per minute.

> It may be necessary to monitor IV potassium administration with an EKG; K^+ toxicity with impending cardiac arrest is clearly heralded by changes in the T-waves. (See Unit X.)

It usually requires several days for the correction of a potassium deficit, especially in the presence of large intracellular losses.

Preventive Measures. Because many dangers are involved in potassium replacement, it is obviously essential to prevent K^+ deficits from developing. Some specific ways of preventing the development of K^+ deficits are:

> Know the following facts about your patient: What medications has he been taking? Diuretics? Cortisone? Has he been vomiting? If so, what is the amount and color of the vomitus? Does he have diarrhea? How many stools per day? What kinds of foods does he select? Are they adequate in K^+ content? What is the amount of his urinary output?

> Carefully observe patients undergoing emotional and/or physical stress, as well as postoperative patients, for signs of potassium deficiency.

> Chart and report to the doctor any findings that might suggest a K^+ deficit.

> Always irrigate nasal gastric tubes and intestinal drainage tubes with normal saline to prevent washing out valuable K^+ ions.

> Watch carefully for signs of digitalis toxicity in patients receiving *both* digitalis and thiazide type diuretics—both of which lower cellular K^+. Digitalis acts with greater potency on the heart in a thiazide-induced hypokalemia.

> Remember:
> 1. *Digitalis toxicity can occur in a patient receiving both digitalis and thiazide diuretics* even *if the patient is receiving a non-toxic dosage of digitalis.*
> 2. *Signs of digitalis toxicity are: nausea, vomiting, anorexia, and arrhythmias, preceding the heart block.*

> If a patient has a K^+ deficit and must receive replacement therapy, watch carefully for the symptoms of K^+ excess and toxicity.

Potassium Excess (Hyperkalemia)

Etiology. The major causes of potassium excess are:

RETENTION OF K^+ WITHIN THE BODY. Patients who are particularly affected are those in renal failure, postoperative patients with a poor renal output, and those with adrenocortical insufficiency.

EXCESSIVE RELEASE OF K^+ FROM THE CELLS. Patients suffering from serious burns, crushing injuries, or infection all face the problem of potassium toxicity, especially if renal function is poor.

INTRAVENOUS INFUSIONS CONTAINING K^+. These should not be given in excessive amounts or administered too rapidly in an attempt to treat K^+ deficits.

Bases of Symptoms. The major systems affected by K^+ excess are the cardiac, renal, and neuromuscular as shown at the bottom of the page.

Clinical Care. The goal of care for patients having K^+ excess is to reduce the serum K^+ immediately.

> Remember: *A seriously elevated serum potassium constitutes a* medical emergency. *Cardiac arrest may be imminent.*

To accomplish a rapid reduction of serum K^+ levels, the factors which cause potassium excesses are promptly eliminated as follows:

REDUCTION OF RETENTION OF K^+ WITHIN THE BODY. K^+ is reduced by promoting a greater urinary output. In event of renal shutdown, the *artificial kidney* may be used or, in some cases, *peritoneal dialysis* may be instituted. (See Unit XI.)

Another way to remove excess K^+ from the body is through the use of *ion exchange resins,* such as Kayexalate, which act to remove K^+ from the intestinal tract. They are administered either by enema or by mouth. Resins work by exchanging their Na^+ ions for serum K^+ ions as they pass along the bowel, thus the name "ion exchange."

MINIMIZATION OF EXCESSIVE RELEASE OF POTASSIUM. K^+ is minimized by controlling the breakdown of tissue. Tissue breakdown is prevented by

Symptoms of Potassium Excess

Symptoms	*Bases of Symptoms*
Slight hyperkalemia is manifested by intestinal colic and diarrhea; *severe* hyperkalemia creates symptoms of weakness, flaccid paralysis, paralysis of muscles of phonation	Neuromuscular irritability is *increased* in slight hyperkalemia and *reduced* in severe hyperkalemia (as in K^+ deficit)
Cardiac arrest is usually preceded by a bradycardia	Cardiac toxicity produces impaired conduction of heart impulses
Oliguria; anuria	Renal shutdown develops as a complication of burns, shock, or dehydration
Serum K^+ in excess of 5 mEq./L.	Changes in laboratory findings

controlling infection and ensuring intake of *adequate calories and carbohydrates.* Such actions serve to spare protein and, consequently, to eliminate the wasting of tissue.

ELIMINATION OF EXCESSIVE K^+ INTAKE. Excessive K^+ intake is eliminated by stopping *all* sources of potassium—oral and parenteral.

The fate of the patient with potassium excess depends ultimately upon the speed of diagnosis and the promptness with which the corrective measures are carried out.

CALCIUM BALANCE

The outline at the bottom of the page summarizes some important facts about calcium.

What are the implications for imbalance that can be drawn from Figure 25–4? First, the maintenance of a normal serum calcium depends upon proper intake of calcium, the availability of vitamin D, the level of blood phosphorus, and the proper functioning of the parathyroid glands. Consequently any factor that significantly alters Ca^{++} intake, the mobilization of Ca^{++} by vitamin D, the blood level of phosphorus, or the functioning of the parathyroid gland can create an imbalance. Second, in specific imbalances—either excesses or deficiencies—we can expect symptoms involving the *neuromuscular system,* the *heart,* and the *bones*—all systems with which the Ca^{++} ion is vitally involved. The *kidneys* are also affected, particularly in excesses, because it is the kidney that excretes calcium.

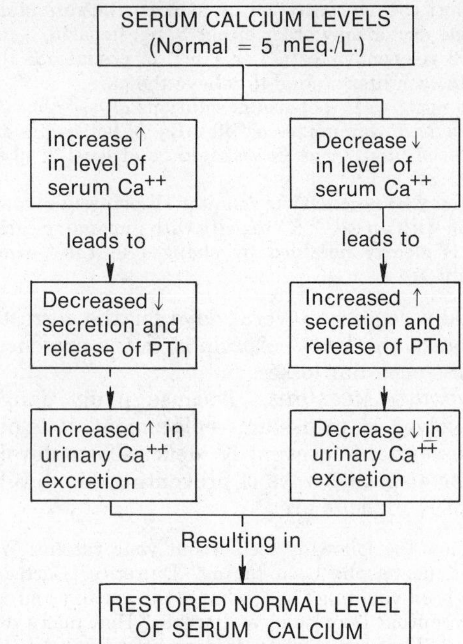

FIGURE 25–4. The effect of the serum calcium level upon the excretion of parathormone (PTH).

Body Calcium (Ca^{++})—A Summary of Basic Facts

I. Normal serum Ca^{++} is approximately 5 mEq./L.
II. Distribution of Ca^{++}:
  A. Nearly 99 per cent in the bones.
  B. Fraction of Ca^{++} in the blood plasma.
III. Ca^{++} performs the following functions:
  A. Decreases neuromuscular irritability.
  B. Decreases capillary permeability.
  C. Promotes normal muscle contractility.
  D. Promotes transmission of nerve impulses.
  E. Essential for blood clotting.
  F. Essential for building of bones and teeth.
IV. Ca^{++} requirements:
  A. Adult requires 0.8 Gm. Ca^{++} daily.
  B. Children and infants require 0.7 to 1.4 Gm. daily.
  C. Pregnant and lactating women require 1.3 to 1.5 Gm. per day.
V. Ca^{++} intake, absorption, and excretion:
  A. Food intake:
    1. Three fourths of Ca^{++} requirement is supplied by milk and milk products.
    2. One fourth of Ca^{++} is supplied by vegetables and fruit.
  B. Absorption of Ca^{++}:
    1. Depends in part upon the presence of vitamin D.
    2. Controlled by the parathyroid glands.
  C. Ca^{++} is excreted in the urine.
VI. Relationship between calcium and phosphorus:
  A. Inverse relationship exists for obscure reasons:
    1. When calcium is elevated, blood level of phosphorus is low.
    2. When blood level of calcium is low, phosphorus level is elevated.
VII. The regulation of Ca^{++}:
  A. Depends upon parathormone [PTH], a parathyroid hormone.
  B. Release of PTH depends upon the level of serum calcium. (The effect of fluctuation in the serum Ca^{++} upon PTH is diagrammed in Figure 25–4.

Calcium Deficit (Hypocalcemia)

Etiology. A calcium deficit can occur in one or more of the following instances:

> An excessive loss of Ca^{++} from the body. This problem often arises in acute pancreatitis.
> Following a *thyroidectomy* in which one or more of the parathyroid glands are accidentally removed.
> During *pregnancy* and *lactation* when Ca^{++} requirements are higher.
> When there is a lack of *vitamin D* in the diet.
> Following the *correction of acidosis.*
> Following the excessive administration of *citrated blood*—a product capable of inactivating calcium.

Calcium deficiencies are also seen in hypoparathyroidism, rickets, osteomalacia, and chronic renal disease.

Bases of Symptoms. When there is a severe hypocalcemia, a condition called *tetany* develops. Tetany is characterized by the symptoms listed at the bottom of the page.

Both Trousseau's sign and Chvostek's sign are important diagnostic tests for tetany. To test for *Trousseau's sign,* a blood pressure manometer is inflated on the patient's arm (creating enough pressure to stop the circulation) for from one to five minutes. If, as a result, contractions of the fingers and hands (carpal spasms) develop, tetany is present. To test for *Chvostek's sign,* tap the patient's face just below the temple where the facial nerve emerges. If, as a result, there is a momentary contraction of the lip, nose, or side of the face, Chvostek's sign is positive. A positive finding indicates *hyperirritability of the facial nerve*—an important sign of tetany.

Clinical Care. Calcium deficiency is corrected by oral, intramuscular, or intravenous administration of calcium salts. When hypocalcemia is mild and is *not* accompanied by tetany, the following drugs are given orally.

1. Calcium lactate, 5 Gm. orally, 3 times daily.
2. Calcium chloride, 1 Gm, Q.I.D. Calcium chloride can be given intraveneously as well as orally; however, it should not be given intramuscularly, as it is irritating to tissues.
3. Calcium gluconate, 4 to 15 Gm. orally, daily. This drug may also be given IV and IM. Give medication containing calcium one half hour before meals and/or at bedtime for best absorption. Often the doctor will order large doses of vitamin D (50,000 to 400,000 U.S.P. units) to be given in conjunction with the calcium.

In patients in whom tetany is anticipated or actually present, prompt treatment with IV medication is necessary. One drug commonly used is:

4. 10 per cent calcium gluconate solution, IV. Calcium gluconate should be administered slowly. If the symptoms of tetany are not relieved, 10 ml. can be given. In patients with severe hypocalcemia, 80 ml. of 10 per cent calcium gluconate may have to be added to each liter of 5 per cent glucose in water that the patient receives until the signs of tetany disappear.

The following rules are guidelines for working with intravenous infusions containing calcium:

1. *Guard against the infiltration of IV solutions containing calcium. Tissue sloughs will result.*
2. *Do not add calcium to solutions containing carbonate or phosphate.* Dangerous precipitations *will form.*
3. *Question giving IV calcium therapy to pations receiving digitalis. Calcium ions have an action similar to that of digitalis; consequently, if calcium salts are given at the same time,* digitalis toxicity *can result.*
4. *Watch for signs of hypercalcemia. Intravenous calcium therapy can result in* cardiac arrest.

If tetany is present in the patient or if the development of tetany is anticipated, remember that *convulsions* may result.

Calcium Excess (Hypercalcemia)

While calcium deficit tends to affect mainly the neuromuscular system, calcium excess produces

SYMPTOMS OF CALCIUM DEFICIT

Symptoms	*Bases of Symptoms*
Painful tonic muscle spasms; facial spasms ("tetany facies"); grimacing; tingling of fingers; fatigue; laryngospasm; Trousseau's sign; positive Chvostek's sign; convulsions	Increased neuromuscular irritability producing hyperreaction of motor and sensory nerves to stimuli
Tingling and numbness of fingers	Vascular spasms
Definitive EKG tracing; palpitations; arrhythmias	Increased irritability of the heart muscle
Serum Ca^{++} decreased below 4.5 mEq./L.; serum phosphorus elevated; Sulkowitch test of urine shows no precipitation*	Laboratory changes

*For the Sulkowitch test, a 24-hr urine sample is collected and tested for Ca^{++}ions.

diffuse symptoms affecting many of the body's systems.

Etiology. The major factor that can create a Ca^{++} excess is an overactivity of the parathyroid glands (hyperparathyroidism). Other factors are:

> Excessive mobilization and absorption of Ca^{++}.
> Decreased renal excretion of Ca^{++}.
> Tumors of the parathyroid glands.
> Excessive intake of vitamin D.

The problem of calcium excess is most commonly linked with hyperparathyroidism; however, it is also seen in various bone diseases, malignant metastases to bone, and hyperthyroidism. Patients with ulcers who consume large amounts of milk daily, as well as various alkaline medications, frequently develop hypercalcemia as a part of the milk-alkali syndrome.

Bases of Symptoms. When there is a calcium excess in the body, blood calcium levels become abnormally high while serum phosphorus levels become abnormally low. These abnormal blood levels, in turn, give rise to many diversified symptoms. Note, in the list below, that the pathologic changes produced by calcium excess are chiefly related to the *gastrointestinal* tract, the *kidneys,* the *neuromuscular* system, and the *skeletal* tissues.

Because of these many and varied symptoms, it is often difficult for physicians to diagnose Ca^{++} excess and to differentiate it from other medical problems. The only reliable way to diagnose Ca^{++} excess is by means of laboratory studies of Ca^{++} and P^{+}. Since such studies are not always ordered, patients may be ill for months and even years with an undiagnosed calcium excess. Moreover, a few patients may develop the critical problem of hypercalcemic crisis before treatment is instituted. *Hypercalcemic crisis* is heralded by: severe nausea and vomiting dehydration, mental confusion, coma, and renal failure. This condition constitutes a *medical emergency* and demands immediate care.

Clinical Care. Traditionally, patients with calcium excess have been treated with steroids, parenteral isotonic saline, and a limited calcium intake. In recent studies physicians with small groups of patients have tried the following newer methods of therapy for calcium excess:

> Isotonic disodium phosphate and/or monopotassium phosphate given orally or intravenously.
> Isotonic sodium sulfate in water, 2 liters, IV.

These potent medications can result in hypocalcemia (tetany) as well as minor disturbances of serum K^{+}, Mg^{++}, and Na^{+}.

Emergency treatment for hypercalcemic crises does not, of course, take the place of needed medical, surgical, and nursing care for the correction of underlying causative factors.

MAGNESIUM (Mg^{++}) BALANCE

Physicians have only recently explored the importance of a proper intake of Mg^{++} in the daily diet as well as the clinical problems of Mg^{++} deficit. The difficulty of measuring the level of Mg^{++} within the body fluids is perhaps responsible for the small amount of clinical knowledge available regarding this ion. However, some important facts are available concerning normal Mg^{++} metabolism. These are summarized on the opposite page.

Because Mg^{++} is essential for neuromuscular integration and for providing a sedative effect upon the body, disturbances in Mg^{++} balance produce disturbances in *neuromuscular function. Deficits* of Mg^{++} produce central nervous system irritability, convulsions, and extreme behavioral changes (e.g., wild combative actions); Mg^{++} *excess* can produce paralysis, hypotension, and sedation of the neuromuscular system.

MAGNESIUM IMBALANCES

Magnesium Deficiency

Etiology. The major cause of a Mg^{++} deficiency is a low intake of Mg^{++} over a long period without adequate Mg^{++} replacement coupled with prolonged

Symptoms of Calcium Excess

Symptoms	*Bases of Symptoms*
Bone pain; osteoporosis; osteomalacia (softening of bone); pathologic fractures	Decalcification of bones (calcium drains from the bones into the blood)
Flank pain; kidney infection; kidney stones; kidney loses its ability to concentrate urine; renal failure, which may result in death	Hypercalciuria due to increased Ca^{++} deposits in the renal pelvis and parenchyma
Diarrhea; faintness; constipation; atony of intestinal tract; peptic ulcer (in 8 per cent of patients); anorexia; nausea; vomiting	Gastrointestinal disorders due to an increase of Ca^{++} ions in sympathetic ganglia; this impedes transmission of afferent stimuli
Extreme lethargy; exhaustion; mental confusion; loss of interest in surroundings; irritability	Behavioral changes due to neurologic malfunctioning
Plasma calcium levels above 5.8 mEq./L.; definitive EKG tracing; serum phosphorus decreased; Sulkowitch test of urine shows increased Ca^{++} precipation	Laboratory changes

and abnormal losses of magnesium from the gastrointestinal tract or kidney. These problems are most commonly seen in *surgical* patients.

Other groups of patients particularly prone to Mg^{++} deficiency are persons with the following conditions or during the following phases: chronic and severe malnutrition, chronic alcoholism accompanied by delirium tremens*, chronic nephritis, the diuretic phase of renal failure, prolonged severe diarrhea, prolonged IV therapy without Mg^{++} replacement, intestinal malabsorption, and hypoparathyroidism.

Since Mg^{++} is abundant in many of the foods that we normally eat, Mg^{++} deficiency is rarely the result of inadequate diet. When Mg^{++} deficit does occur due to nutritional problems, it tends to develop over a prolonged period of time; the dietary inadequacies are extreme; and the effects of the deficit tend to be cumulative.

Bases of Symptoms. As we stated earlier, Mg^{++} deficiency is particularly characterized by *increased neuromuscular and central nervous system irritability.* Below are listed the major pathologic effects of Mg^{++} deficit and the corresponding symptoms.

*Delirium tremens [DT's] is an acute toxic psychosis common among chronic alcoholics. It is characterized by confusion, combative behavior, and terrifying hallucinations.

Body Magnesium (Mg^{++})—A Summary of Basic Facts

I. A "normal adult male body" contains approximately 25 Gm. of Mg^{++}.
II. Distribution of Mg^{++}:
  A. Seventy per cent of Mg^{++} is combined with Ca^{++} and P^{+} in the bones.
  B. Thirty per cent of Mg^{++} is in the soft tissues and body fluids.
  C. Predominantly an intracellular ion with a concentration of 28 mEq./L.
  D. Extracellular concentration of Mg^{++} approximately 1.5-2.5 mEq./L.
    1. Blood serum level 1.4-2.5 mg/100 ml.
    2. Mg^{++} within vascular system mainly within blood cells and not within the serum.
III. Mg^{++} performs the following functions:
  A. Essential for integrity of neuromuscular system.
  B. Has sedative effect upon the body which is opposed by Ca^{++}.
  C. Activates many enzymes essential for proper carbohydrate metabolism.
  D. Promotes regulation of blood phosphorus level.
IV. Mg^{++} ingestion, absorption, and excretion:
  A. Food intake:
    1. Adults normally require 200 to 300 mg. of Mg^{++} per day.
    2. Mg^{++} is abundant in food; it is a vital constituent of chlorophyll.
    3. Nuts, soybeans, cocoa, seafood, whole grains, dried beans, and peas are excellent sources of Mg^{++}.
    4. With the intake of a *normal* diet, it is virtually impossible to develop a Mg^{++} deficiency.
  B. Absorption of Mg^{++}:
    1. Forty-five per cent of ingested Mg^{++} is absorbed while the remainder is excreted in the feces.
    2. Factors inhibiting Mg^{++} *absorption* are the presence of excess fat, phosphates, Ca^{++}, and alkalosis.
    3. Increased absorption of Mg^{++} by the intestinal tract is stimulated by parathyroid hormone (PTH).
  C. Mg^{++} excretion:
    1. Fifty-five per cent of Mg^{++} is excreted in the feces.
    2. Renal excretion of Mg^{++} is low, because kidney tends to conserve Mg^{++}.

SYMPTOMS OF MAGNESIUM DEFICIENCY

Symptoms	*Bases of Symptoms*
Frank tetany; hyperactive reflexes; positive Chvostek's sign; facial twitching; jerking; convulsions; plucking at bed sheets	Neuromuscular irritability is increased
Psychotic behavior; hallucinations; delusions; wild combative behavior; extreme confusion	Central nervous system is greatly stimulated
Symptoms appear when Mg^{++} levels are at 1.5 mEq./L.; *severe* symptoms appear when Mg^{++} levels are at 1.25 mEq./L.	Laboratory changes

Magnesium deficit is not always easy to diagnose on the basis of symptoms alone because the tetany produced by Mg^{++} deficit is almost indistinguishable from that produced by Ca^{++} deficit; however, laboratory tests will show a decreased serum magnesium and a normal serum Ca^{++}. Also, the symptoms of Mg^{++} deficit greatly resemble those of water excess; convulsions and mental disturbances occur in both conditions. It is necessary to rely heavily upon laboratory tests as well as upon the patient's history for an accurate differential diagnosis.

Clinical Care. The goals of care in Mg^{++} deficit are:

1. To replace the Mg^{++} deficiency.
2. To replace continuing Mg^{++} losses.
3. To quickly control symptoms.

For rapid results, Mg^{++} replacement is usually parenteral, either intravenously or intramuscularly. Common dosages of magnesium sulfate are:

1. $MgSO_4$ 10 Gm. dissolved in 1000 ml. of 5 per cent G/W given IV over a 1½- to 2-hour period.

2. $MgSO_4$ 8 Gm. IM daily, in 4 divided doses. After the first 48 hours, 4 Gm. daily in 4 divided doses. This injection should be given deep in the muscle. Certain precautions should be observed when administering magnesium sulfate, especially by the intravenous route:

> Remember:
> 1. *Give IV infusions containing magnesium sulfate* slowly. *Too rapid a drip rate will cause the patient to suffer from an uncomfortable feeling of heat.*
> 2. *Question giving IV magnesium to any patient with poor renal function. Magnesium excess may result from urine retention.*
> 3. *Stop the IV* at once *if the following signs of Mg^{++} excess develop:*
>   a. *Weak or absent deep reflexes.*
>   b. *Sharp decrease in systolic pressure.*
>   c. *Elevated T waves (as in K^+ excess) on ECG.*
>   d. *Skeletal muscle paralysis.*
>   e. *Extreme sedation and coma. The patient may progress to a* cardiac arrest *if these symptoms develop.*
> 4. *Have injectable* calcium gluconate *available. Calcium antagonizes the sedative action of magnesium and will help to reverse the above symptoms.*

The prevention of Mg^{++} deficiency is a major goal of patient care today. Preventive medical care involves the following practices:

> Patients who are NPO and who are on prolonged IV therapy should receive daily Mg^{++} supplements (10 to 20 mEq. of magnesium sulfate are generally ordered to be added to the parenteral fluids).

> Patients with a suspected Mg^{++} deficit owing to gastrointestinal tract losses usually receive 64 to 128 mEq. of magnesium IM over a 24- to 72-hour period.

When giving Mg^{++} supplements, be alert to the possible development of a Mg^{++} *excess.*

Magnesium Excess

This imbalance may be caused by the following conditions:

> Renal insufficiency causing Mg^{++} retention.
> Overdoses of Mg^{++} during replacement therapy.
> Severe dehydration resulting in oliguria and retention of Mg^{++}.
> Repeated enemas with magnesium sulfate (epsom salt), a potent saline cathartic.
> Use of antacids containing Mg^{++} by patients with renal failure (e.g., Gelusil, magnesium oxide, and hydrated magnesium aluminate).

The main physiologic alterations in Mg^{++} excess, as in K^+ excess, are *oversedation of the neuromuscular system* and a *pronounced reduction in neuromuscular irritability.* Major symptoms are:

> A warm sensation throughout the body.
> Paralysis similar to that seen with curare-like drugs.
> Hypotension.
> Sedation.
> Respiratory embarrassment.
> Cardiac arrhythmias progressing to arrest.

Clinical Care. The goals of care for patients with a Mg^{++} excess are: (1) to treat underlying causative conditions or circumstances that are creating a Mg^{++} excess; and (2) to offset the toxicity and life-threatening symptoms of Mg^{++} excess.

TREATMENT OF UNDERLYING CONDITIONS. Patients suffering from renal failure are treated with peritoneal dialysis or with the artificial kidney, whereas dehydrated patients are given fluids. These measures increase urinary output and, consequently, Mg^{++} excretion. Moreover, any medications or compounds containing Mg^{++} (enemas, antacids, IV solutions) are withheld from patients with suspected or confirmed Mg^{++} imbalances or with renal failure.

TREATMENT OF Mg^{++} TOXICITY. Patients with symptoms of Mg^{++} excess are given 10 per cent calcium gluconate immediately. This medication antagonizes the sedative action of Mg^{++}, reversing the symptoms of toxicity.

FLUID SHIFTS

Fluid shifts are basically position changes of the extracellular fluid and electrolytes. There are two main types of fluid shifts: (1) plasma to interstitial fluid shift, and (2) interstitial space to plasma fluid shift.

Little is known today about the dynamics of fluid shifts or their purpose in the body's reaction to trauma and disease. As Metheny and Snively state, "These mysterious tides of disease represent a curious response to unseen, unfathomed forces set in motion by certain illnesses and injuries."[55] Despite their elusive nature, the shifts create very real and dramatic changes within the traumatized human body.

On the opposite page, the two major fluid shifts are compared and contrasted with each other in terms of characteristics, cause, symptoms, and clinical care.

Nursing Implications

Fluid shifts are potentially dangerous mechanisms: a plasma to interstitial fluid shift can result in *shock;* an interstitial fluid to plasma shift can lead to *pulmonary edema* – both critical, life-threatening complications.

In caring for patients particularly subject to the development of fluid shifts, you need to consider the following points in mapping out a plan of care. First, be aware of *which type* of fluid shift your patient may develop as well as its major signs and symptoms.

Second, be aware of specific ways to protect patients from developing further complications as a result of fluid shifts. With patients suffering from a *plasma to interstitial fluid shift,* the *major goals of preventive care are:* (1) to prevent irreversible shock; (2) to prevent tissue breakdown and decubitus ulcer formation; and (3) to prevent iatrogenic complications of therapy.

> Remember:
> 1. *A patient who has* just recently *suffered a serious burn, trauma, or obstruction will develop a* plasma to interstitial fluid shift. *The main signs will be those of* circulatory collapse.
> 2. *A patient who has suffered a burn or crushing injury three to five days earlier will develop an* interstitial fluid to plasma shift. *The main signs will be those of* circulatory overload.

Fluid Shifts—A Comparison of Characteristics, Causative Factors, Symptoms, and Clinical Care

Plasma to Interstitial Fluid Shift

I. Characteristics:
   A. Following severe trauma or injury, fluid, sodium salts, and bicarbonate shift from the injured areas into noninjured areas
   B. Fluid also shifts from the plasma into the peritoneum and into the pleura
II. Causative factors:
   A. Massive crushing injuries
   B. Burns (shift occurs on the 1st or 2nd day following injury)
   C. Following perforation of a peptic ulcer
   D. Intestinal obstruction
   E. Lymphatic obstruction
   F. Venous thrombosis
   G. Obstruction of major vessel
III. Bases of symptoms:
   A. Mechanism causing shift is obscure, but it is possibly of neurogenic origin
   B. The shift results in:
      1. Loss of fluid from the blood which leads to shock
      2. Edema of noninjured areas
      3. Dehydration of the injured area
IV. Common symptoms:
   A. Signs of *shock:*
      1. Pallor
      2. Hypotension
      3. Tachycardia
      4. Weak to absent pulse
      5. Cold extremities
      6. Oliguria
      7. Unconsciousness
      8. *No* weight loss as fluid is not lost from the body
   B. Laboratory Findings due to the loss of fluid from the blood:
      1. Hemoglobin elevated
      2. Red blood cell count elevated
V. Clinical care:
   A. The specific factors causing the shift are treated (e.g., burns, injury, obstruction)
   B. Fluids and electrolytes lost from the plasma are *judiciously* replaced
   Pulmonary edema and circulatory overload can result when the interstitial fluid to plasma shift occurs on the 3rd to 5th post-trauma day

Interstitial Fluid to Plasma Shift

I. Characteristics:
   A. Fluid and electrolytes shift from the interstitial spaces into the vascular system, usually following a plasma to interstitial fluid shift
II. Causative factors:
   A. Remobilization of edema fluid following burn or severe injury (occurs on 3rd to 5th day)
   B. Compensation following internal or external hemorrhage
   C. Excessive infusions of hypertonic solutions:
      1. Serum albumin
      2. Plasma
      3. Dextran
III. Bases of symptoms:
   A. Mechanism causing shift following burns and injury is obscure
   B. Excessive infusions of hypertonic solutions increase the osmolarity of the blood, consequently drawing fluid from the interstitial spaces
IV. Common symptoms:
   A. Following loss of whole blood signs are similar to shock:
      1. Weakness
      2. Pallor
      3. Tachycardia
      4. Hypotension
   B. Following shift of fluid resulting from administration of hypertonic solution or from burns:
      1. Bounding pulse
      2. Pulmonary edema
      3. Hypertension
      3. Cardiac enlargement
      5. Engorgement of peripheral veins
   These signs result from an overloading of the vascular system
   C. Laboratory findings due to shift of fluid into plasma:
      1. Hemoglobin decreased
V. Clinical care:
   A. Generally excess fluid is excreted naturally, if the patient has normal heart and kidney function
   B. In the presence of heart or renal disease, rotating tourniquets may be ordered to counteract pulmonary edema. (See pp. 641–642.)
   C. Following hemorrhage, a blood transfusion may be ordered

*Prevent Irreversible Shock.** The shock that typifies a plasma to interstitial fluid shift is due to the sudden fluid loss from the vascular system. Such a fluid loss from the blood stream into the tissues can be just as serious and deadly as a hemorrhagic loss of fluid from the body. Vital signs, urinary output, and the patient's sensorium are all profoundly affected. Consequently, in your plan of care for patients with this condition, you will:

> Check blood pressure every one to two hours for hypotention. (Be sure that you have a baseline blood pressure with which to compare subsequent blood pressures.)

> Check pulse every one to two hours for tachycardia or for a pulse over 100 beats per minute. Check the *quality* of pulse. Is it thready? and weak? These are signs of shock!

> Check the patient's state of consciousness. Does he seem confused? Is his alertness to the environment decreasing?

> Check urinary output hourly; oliguria and renal failure are important signs of circulatory collapse.

> Check the patient's skin color as well as the "feel" of his skin. A cold moist skin and an ashen pallor may be indicative of shock.

> Watch for oxygen hunger, i.e., does your patient seem to be gasping for air?

Be certain to chart your findings carefully. Of course, report to the physician significant changes or observations concerning symptoms. Careful, frequent observations are essential during the critical periods of shock.

Prevent Tissue Breakdown. Remember that in a plasma to interstitial fluid shift, the injured area becomes *dehydrated* while the noninjured area becomes *edematous.* Because edematous tissue is very fragile, it is prone to breakdown and to decubitus ulcer formation. Thus, noninjured areas of the body in a plasma to interstitial fluid shift must be carefully observed for *beginning* signs of breakdown. Frequently check the patient's skin for small areas of skin redness and tenderness; especially observe the skin overlying the sacrum, hips, and other bony prominences. Turn and move the patient every hour on a *specific turning schedule.* (See p. 298.) Position properly with pillows.

Prevent Iatrogenic Complications of Therapy. Patients suffering from a plasma to interstitial fluid shift are usually treated with IV fluids. Remember that fluid overload may result when the inevitable interstitial to plasma fluid shift occurs on the third to fifth day post trauma. Do not speed up the rate of IV fluid administration. Observe for signs of pulmonary edema.

Second, to prevent interstitial fluid to plasma shift, *remember:* never overload a patient with fluid who has just suffered a burn or trauma, and never overload *any* patient with hypertonic saline solution.

*For a further discussion of shock, see Chapter 26.

NUTRITIONAL DEFICIENCIES*

No discussion of fluid and electrolyte imbalance would be complete without considering caloric and protein deficits, those important nutritional deficiencies that have spelled misery for mankind over the centuries and that continue to plague people even in this modern age. Persons in underdeveloped countries still face starvation; vast numbers of people in the United States do not eat correctly because of ignorance concerning proper diet; patients in hospitals and at home often do not receive adequate nutrition, and their need for additional proteins, vitamins, and calories go unrecognized and untreated. Thus, even in a technological society, the nutritional problems are ever-present.

Despite many gaps in our knowledge, we are becoming increasingly aware of the role of nutrition and diet in the promotion of health and in the causation of disease. Today, we recognize that the health of an individual may, to a large extent, depend upon what he eats, how much he eats, and how well he digests, absorbs, and utilizes his food.

While all aspects of nutrition are pertinent to the study of health and disease, the following problems in nutrition are particularly relevant to the area of fluid and electrolyte balance.

Caloric Metabolism

When we eat, our bodies convert the ingested foodstuffs into energy. Energy, the force of life sustaining activity, is measured in terms of *heat equivalents* or calories. The outline on the opposite page summarizes a few essential facts about calories.

Caloric Deficit

Major causes of caloric deficit serious enough to create symptoms are:

Decrease in Caloric Intake. Decreased intake is found in persons suffering from starvation and those undergoing strenuous therapeutic reducing diets. A lowered caloric intake also develops with nausea and vomiting, e.g., in patients with gastrointestinal disorders.

Abnormally Increased Utilization of Calories. This problem arises in persons with a higher than normal metabolic rate, e.g., hyperthyroidism, cancer, and infection. For every degree of fever as measured on the centigrade scale, the BMR rises 7 per cent. Thus, patients with elevated temperatures require a greater caloric intake. Hypertension, anemia, burns, and dyspnea can also cause an increase in the BMR and in caloric needs.

Faulty Absorption and Utilization of Food. Even if food intake is normal, the person who cannot properly absorb or metabolize his food actually suffers from a form of starvation. For example, an individual with diabetes mellitus cannot properly metabolize carbohydrates. Consequently, he burns protein and fat in place of carbohydrates to meet his energy needs. As a result, the severe diabetic develops metabolic acidosis.

*Owing to problems of space, no attempt has been made to present nutritional disorders in detail in this textbook.

The major physiologic result of any caloric deficit is a *protein deficit,* because in the absence of adequate calories, body tissues are burned to supply needed energy for metabolic processes.

The most important *symptoms* of a caloric deficit are: mental depression, shortness of breath (SOB), loss of muscle tone and mass, increased acetone in the urine, weakness, fatigue, weight loss, and malaise.

The prevention of caloric deficits, and consequently of protein deficits, is of importance in the treatment of any patient, but especially those who are burned, have had surgery, or are bedridden. Individuals who are unconscious or NPO must have replacement fluids carefully calculated in terms of calories. How physicians estimate caloric needs for patients on parenteral therapy will be discussed on p. 255.

Protein Metabolism

The word protein is derived from the Greek word *proteios* meaning "primary" or "holding first place." Indeed, protein does hold first place in the animal body because it is the essential life-giving, life-sustaining substance comprising living cells and tissues. Major facts concerning protein that are pertinent to patient care are summarized on the following page.

Within this outline of normal protein metabolism, certain points demand reemphasis because they contain vital implications for patient care.

First, note that essential proteins cannot be made within the body, and that protein substances form the bulk of muscle and tissue and are being *constantly used* by the body's cells, tissues, and fluids to maintain themselves. This means that a person must eat a certain amount of essential protein substance every day or a deficiency develops. If an individual is *ill,* his appetite decreases, he may be nauseated, or vomiting, and, as a result, will probably not ingest sufficient protein for his body's needs. Without adequate diet or parenteral replacement, a state of *hypoproteinemia* and *negative nitrogen balance* develops, further jeopardizing his health. Protein replacements and protein-sparing nutrients* must always be considered when working with the anorexic or nauseated patient.

*Protein-sparing nutrients are foods high in carbohydrates or fat content. These foods are used by the body for energy in place of protein; thus, the term, "protein sparing."

The Calorie—A Brief Summary of Basic Facts

I. The calorie (Latin, *calor,* heat) is a measure of heat.
   A. In nutritional terms, the calorie measures the energy value that a definite proportion of food will yield upon oxidation within the body or upon being burned within a laboratory.
   B. The large calorie or kilocalorie is the unit of measurement used in dietetic laboratories and studies. The kilocalorie is equal to the amount of heat needed to raise 1 kg. of H_2O 1° C.
II. Calories are drawn from the following three major groups of nutrients.
   A. Proteins:
      1. One gram of protein is equivalent to 4 calories. This is termed the "fuel factor" or average caloric value of protein.
      2. Proteins supply approximately 15 per cent of the average daily caloric intake.
   B. Fats:
      1. One gram of fat is equivalent to 9 calories.
      2. Fats supply 40 per cent of the average daily caloric intake.
   C. Carbohydrates:
      1. One gram of carbohydrate is equivalent to 4 calories.
      2. Carbohydrates supply approximately 45 per cent of the average dietary intake.
III. The caloric needs of the healthy individual vary with the following factors:
   A. Basal metabolic rate (BMR):
      1. Defined as the amount of energy that a physically, mentally, and emotionally relaxed person must expend in order to maintain the basic physical processes of life.
      2. Metabolic rates are determined by measuring the number of calories produced during a certain time period, e.g., over 24 hours.
      3. The BMR is higher in men than in women; it is increased during periods of growth, during pregnancy and lactation, and during emotional upsets.
      4. The BMR is lower in elderly persons, and in conditions of starvation and malnutrition.
   B. Surface area of the body:
      1. Surface area is a measurement that takes both height and weight into account. It can be computed from specially designed tables.
      2. A large person has a greater surface area, greater metabolic rate, and greater need for calories than a smaller individual.
   C. Activity:
      1. Sedentary activity requires fewer calories than physical activity.
      2. Mental activity, however difficult and demanding, requires very few calories.
   D. Age:
      1. A younger person has a greater metabolic rate and higher caloric needs than does an older person.

Protein—A Brief Summary of Pertinent Facts

I. Protein is an *organic* substance composed of carbon, hydrogen, oxygen, and nitrogen.
II. When proteins are digested, they break down into *amino acids,* the basic structural units of proteins.
III. Amino acids are classified as either *essential* or *nonessential.*
   A. Essential amino acids:
      1. Are absolutely necessary for body growth and cellular life.
      2. Must be *obtained in food* as they are not produced in the body.
   B. Nonessential amino acids:
      1. Are not absolutely necessary for body health and growth.
      2. Can be manufactured within the body.
IV. Proteins are classified as either *complete* or *incomplete* according to the type of amino acids they contain.
   A. Proteins that contain all the essential amino acids are *complete proteins,* e.g., those found in meats and dairy foods.
   B. Proteins missing one or more of the essential amino acids are *incomplete proteins,* e.g., those in grains and vegetables.
V. The *functions* of protein:
   A. The most basic and vital constituent of living cells.
   B. Comprises bulk of muscle, visceral, and epithelial tissue.
   C. Important constituent of plasma and hemoglobin.
   D. Essential for body growth.
   E. Essential for maintenance and repair of tissue.
VI. Dietary requirement of protein:
   A. Quantity:
      1. One gram of protein daily per kg. of body weight is recommended for people in the United States.*
   B. Quality:
      1. *Complete* proteins, containing all the essential amino acids, should be a part of the health diet.†
VII. Phases of protein metabolism:
   A. Anabolism:
      1. Following absorption, amino acids are incorporated into the body tissue protein (tissue protein synthesis).
      2. In this process, complex substances are built up from simpler substances and *energy is used.*
   B. Catabolism:
      1. Complete protein substances are broken down into simpler substances, oxidized, and excreted; energy is released.
VIII. The concept of *nitrogen balance*:
   A. Nitrogen is present in protein substances and in nonprotein substances such as urea, uric acid, ammonia, and creatinine.
   B. Nitrogen from all the above sources (both protein nitrogen and nonprotein nitrogen) comprises the *total nitrogen balance.*
   C. Negative nitrogen balance exists when the *output* of nitrogen exceeds *intake.*
   D. Positive nitrogen balance exists when *intake* of nitrogen-containing substances exceeds the *output.*

---

*Protein, 0.85 Gm. daily per kg. of body weight, is recommended by the World Health Organization (WHO). People in underdeveloped countries, however, are surviving on far less protein than this.

†The Food and Agriculture Organization, a division of WHO, has ranked eggs and milk as the most complete protein foods; i.e., egg and milk contain the largest amount of those amino acids that are absolutely necessary for health.

Second, note that protein is absolutely necessary for the *building of tissues.* Following injury, surgery, or a severe burn, the body desperately needs protein to rebuild those tissues that have been traumatized. Unfortunately patients may be unconscious, unable to eat, or anorexic at the time they are in need of additional protein. The prevention of hypoproteinemia is, thus, a matter of vital clinical concern during the critical periods of many patients' lives. Let us explore this important topic further.

Hypoproteinemia

The main causes of a protein deficit are as follows:

1. Inadequate intake of protein.
2. Severe loss of protein, e.g., hemorrhage, burns, draining ulcers, ascites.
3. Increased utilization of protein for the rebuilding of tissues, e.g., following burns or trauma.
4. Increased catabolism, e.g., fever, elevated BMR, infection, malignancy.

The major physiologic result of hypoproteinemia is a breakdown of the body tissue protein for use to meet the body's needs. Some outstanding symptoms are: weight loss, fatigue, anemia, hemoglobin decreases, anorexia, loss of muscle mass and tone, and plasma albumin level decreases below 6 Gm./100 ml. In addition, surgical patients with protein deficiencies also suffer from *retarded healing* of incisions and may also develop a condition called *nutritional edema,* a complication resulting from a lowered colloid osmotic pressure owing to inadequate serum proteins. You will recall that lowered colloid osmotic pressure results in a loss of fluid from the vascular system into the tissues, which then become edematous.

How can protein deficits be *prevented or at least corrected,* especially in patients who are burned, critically ill, or undergoing surgery? Physicians may order the following measures in an attempt to return the patient to a positive nitrogen balance:

> A regular diet that is appetizing to the patient and that is high in carbohydrates is a vital protein sparer. Why is a regular diet ordered and not a high protein diet? The answer is that diets high in protein also have a high satiety value; consequently, patients may fail to eat a large enough portion of their food. Moreover, patients on high protein diets often excrete large amounts of protein in their urine (azoturia), thus defeating the beneficial effects of the diet.

> *Protein hydrolysates,* either parenterally or by tube feeding.

You, as the nurse, can help to prevent protein deficiencies by carefully evaluating patients' daily dietary intakes:

> Make patient rounds during mealtimes whenever possible and note the following: Does the patient seem pleased with his diet? Are there any foods that he dislikes? Is he eating a balanced diet rather than just the dessert or just the soup? Does the patient have his dentures in? Does the texture of the food seem correct for him? Can he feed himself or does he require assistance? Is he too proud to ask for help?

> Check on the timing of your patients' meals. Some people will find six small meals a day much more satisfying than the traditional three large meals per day.

> If the patient is dissatisfied with his diet, or if more satisfactory timing of meals seems desirable, request the dietitian to consult with the patient or with you, as appropriate.

> Make certain that before discharge both patient and family understand the diet and the need for adequate protein.

Adequate protein should cause weight to stabilize, muscle tone and mass to improve, and wounds to heal without painful time-consuming, expensive complications.

GENERAL PRINCIPLES OF ASSESSMENT, MANAGEMENT, AND TREATMENT OF FLUID AND ELECTROLYTE IMBALANCES

In this section we shall draw upon our knowledge of specific imbalances to consider some general principles for observing, assessing, and treating *any* patient believed to have an imbalance. Our discussion will explore the following basic steps that nurses and physicians observe in caring for patients with imbalances.

Step 1: Assess patients in terms of fluid and electrolyte balance.

Step 2: Arrive at a medical and nursing diagnosis.

Step 3: Develop a plan of care for patients with imbalances.

Step 4: Manage fluid and electrolyte therapy.

These topics will be discussed in terms of *both* medical and nursing actions, for physicians and nurses today must function as a coordinated team to ensure successful diagnosis and treatment.

ASSESSING THE PATIENT

In assessing a patient for possible imbalances, both doctor and nurse explore many different avenues of inquiry. They must learn about the patient's usual living patterns and past complaints, his present signs and symptoms, and his actual physical status (through diagnostic and laboratory studies). Such information is then used by the physician to diagnose the patient's particular imbalance, and by the nurse to diagnose the needs of the patient resulting from that imbalance. Let us now consider the roles of both doctor and nurse in patient assessment and diagnosis.

In evaluating a patient for possible imbalances, the physician generally considers the patient in terms of the following questions:

1. Have there been abnormalities in the volume of ECF? increase? decrease?
2. Have there been abnormalities in the electrolyte composition of the ECF? Are the serum concentrations of Na^+, K^+, Ca^{++} Mg^{++}, and sodium bicarbonate normal, excessive, or deficient?
3. Have there been abnormalities in the position of the ECF? fluid shifts?
4. Does the patient show evidence of nutritional deficiency?

To answer these questions, the doctor takes a detailed history, does a thorough physical examination, carefully evaluates the patient's fluid balance record, and orders various laboratory studies. The nurse usually assists the physician as he examines the patient. She also contributes her observations and findings to those made by the doctor and other paramedical people. Moreover, she makes sure laboratory tests ordered by the doctor are carried out; explains these tests to the patient; withholds fluids, food, and medications as necessary; and reports unusual laboratory findings to the physician.

The Clinical History

The physician asks the patient for facts about his past health:

> Has the patient recently gained or lost weight?

> Has the patient been taking any drugs, e.g., cathartics, diuretics, digitalis, thiazide type drugs, or cortisone?

> Has he been on any restricted or unusual diets, e.g., a low calorie or low sodium diet?

> Is there any disease condition present that might upset the body's balance, e.g., endocrine or metabolic disease?

> Has the patient received any therapeutic fluids intravenously or by tube feeding?

> Does the patient seem to have a satisfactory intake and output balance record?

> Does the patient suffer from incontinence, excessive diaphoresis, vomiting, or wound drainage? These three factors could cause intake and output (fluid balance) records to be inaccurate.

As doctor and nurse talk with the patient, they should note his sensorium, affect, and level of energy. Does the patient seem confused, belligerent, lethargic, or unusually fatigued? These signs can be important diagnostic observations related to imbalance.

Physical Examination

Following the taking of the clinical history, the physician usually examines the patient, aided by the nurse, for clinical symptoms of imbalance. Symptoms may be minimal or prominent; also symptoms of one imbalance may mimic those of another imbalance. To offset such confusion, any patient examination, whether a formal physical examination or a daily nursing evaluation, must be systematic and thorough.

You will want to search for symptoms of deviations from normal fluid and electrolyte balance by evaluating the following factors: blood pressure, pulse, respirations, temperature, odor of the skin, moistness or dryness of the skin, skin turgor, appetite for food, thirst (presence or absence), weight, behavioral changes, changes in urinary volume and concentration, sensation (e.g., tingling or numbness), condition of the mucous membranes, breath odor, intraocular pressure, heart action, neuromuscular function (include deep tendon reflexes), gastrointestinal function, circulatory changes, and orthopedic status.

These factors, as mentioned earlier, vary distinctively with the different imbalances.

Fluid Balance Record

The fluid balance record is a record maintained for a given patient showing his fluid intake (oral, parenteral, and by feeding tube) and his fluid output (urine, stool, gastric suction, wound drainage, and vomiting). When accurately recorded, the fluid balance record is a valuable aid in diagnosing imbalances and in calculating fluid replacement needs. Unfortunately fluid intake and output are not always precisely measured, nor are the findings always accurately recorded.

One study has shown that a significant proportion of the patient's daily fluid intake is his oral medications. Indeed, daily fluid intake with medicines was found to range from approximately 249 to 472 ml. This study further demonstrated that in some patients water intake with medicines actually *exceeded* by 30 per cent the daily intake order for the patient. Failure to measure and record water given to patients on medicine rounds can result in a serious fluid overload.[38]

Other errors in recording intake and output include the following (1) Bottles of intravenous solutions may actually contain 1100 ml. of fluid rather than the usual 1000 ml. (2) Bottles of blood or intravenous solution may contain 600 ml. of solution rather than 500 ml. (3) Small sips of water or mouth rinsing, when repeated throughout the day, can actually total 1000 ml. per 24 hours.[54] One can see that it is possible for a patient's intake record to be in error by as much as 2000 ml.! Such a lack of accuracy can result in serious consequences for patients with kidney disease, burns, severe diarrhea, and so forth.

Other common sources of error, in evaluating and recording intake and output, involve the following:[55]

> Poor communication among staff members about which patients are on fluid balance.

> Failure to communicate with patients and visitors recording intake and output.

> Guessing at intake and output measurements rather than actually measuring fluids.

> Failure to record fluid taken in as ice chips (a 200-ml. glass of ice chips equals approximately 100 ml. of water).

> Failure to record intake of solid foods (recall that solid foods also contain water).

> Failure to indicate loss of water by perspiration (i.e., whether patient is perspiring excessively, moderately, or mildly).

> Failure to estimate fluid loss from incontinence of stool or urine, or from wound exudate.

> Failure to measure fluid used as irrigating solutions (e.g., for bladder or wounds).

> Failure to accurately weigh a patient at the same time every day on the same scale and in clothing of the same approximate weight (remember: daily weights are one of the best indicators of fluid gain or loss).

Any of the above errors may result in incorrect diagnosis and treatment of imbalances.

Although a recording of intake and output is not ordered for every patient, *every* patient does require evaluation of his state of fluid balance. In caring for patients not on intake and output measurement, oversights can be avoided by asking yourself the following questions:

> Is the patient drinking at least 1500 ml. of fluid per day?
> Is he voiding at least once every eight-hour shift?
> Is his skin dry and loose?
> Is a fever present?
> Is he perspiring excessively?
> Is his urine concentrated?

If the answers to these questions produce doubts about the patient's state of hydration, the situation should be discussed with the doctor, and accurate measurement of intake and output started.

Diagnostic Tests

Although the nurse and physician can make a general estimate of the patient's problem from his history and physical examination, laboratory tests are regularly used to confirm or establish a diagnosis or to distinguish one imbalance from another. Standard diagnostic tests include:

> *Complete blood count* (CBC).
> *Hemoglobin estimates.* Hemoglobin (Hgb) is generally higher than normal in dehydration and lower than normal in overhydration. Normal Hgb for men is 14.5-16.5 Gm./100 ml. blood and for women is 13.0-15.5 Gm./100 ml.
> *Urinalysis.* This includes a description of the odor of the urine, amount of sedimentation, pH, specific gravity, and tests for protein and glucose.
> *Electrolyte concentration.* Analysis of electrolyte concentrations generally includes the serum concentrations of Na^+, K^+, Ca^{++}, Mg^{++}, H^+ (pH), and protein. In Table 25–4 dangerously high and low levels of these electrolytes in plasma are recorded.

Blood Urea Nitrogen (BUN). Normal range is from 8 to 28 mg. per 100 ml. blood; BUN tends to be elevated during water and Na^+ depletion and when kidney function is poor.

Plasma Proteins. As stated earlier, the normal amount of plasma proteins in blood is approximately 6 Gm. per cent. When the amount of plasma protein is below normal, retention of fluids occurs owing to the blood's decreased colloidal osmotic pressure.

Electrocardiogram (EKG). This is especially important in diagnosing K^+, Mg^{++}, and Ca^{++} imbalances; when these imbalances are severe, an EKG can give warning of impending cardiac arrest.

After the physician receives the results from these tests, he can more precisely make his final diagnosis. Of course, you as the nurse can also make use of diagnostic test results in periodically evaluating a patient's progress and in planning daily care.

Making the Diagnosis

The following examples illustrate how appropriate information concerning patients is gathered and fit together to diagnose and treat fluid and electrolyte imbalances.

Clinical Case No. 1. Mr. M., an elderly man, is admitted during a severe flu epidemic. He tells you that for two days he has been: too nauseated to eat or drink; has had severe vomiting and diarrhea; and has been sweating a great deal. His admission record indicates a 10-pound weight loss, a temperature of 102° F., and blood pressure of 118/92—a low reading for a man his age. Mr. M. physically appears dehydrated: his mouth appears dry; his tongue has deep furrows running longitudinally; his eyes seem sunken; his skin turgor is very poor; he seems tired and lethargic. Laboratory studies report an elevated hemoglobin and an elevated BUN. Also, the specific gravity of his urine is high, indicating a concentrated urine.

When put together the pieces of this puzzle indicate *volume deficit.* With this knowledge, you can surmise that daily weights, intake and output, and IV replacement fluids will all be a part of the care of this patient.

Clinical Case No. 2. Mr. R. has been admitted on numerous occasions highly intoxicated. When he is admitted today, Mr. R. is semistuporous; however, as the day progresses, he becomes increasingly belligerent and confused and appears to have various visual and auditory hallucinations. In addi-

TABLE 25–4. DANGEROUS HIGH AND LOW LEVELS OF SOLUTES IN PLASMA*

	Too High		Too Low	
	Mild to Moderate Symptoms	*Severe Symptoms*	*Mild to Moderate Symptoms*	*Severe Symptoms*
Sodium (mEq./L.)	155-170	>170	120-130	< 120
Potassium (mEq./L.)	7-9	>9	2.2-3.0	< 2.2
Calcium (mEq./L.)	6-7	>7	3-4	< 3
Magnesium (mEq./L.)	>5	>10(?)	1 and below(?)	< 1(?)
Hydrogen ion, as pH	7.5-7.6	>7.6	7.0-7.5	< 7.0
Glucose (Mg. %)	1000 or above(?)	–	40-60	< 40
Protein (Gm. %)	–	–	3.4-5	< 3

*From Keitel, H. G.: *Consultant* 3:42-47, February, 1963.

tion, his face is twitching and he plucks almost incessantly at the bedclothes. When the doctor inquires about the laboratory work you inform him that the patient's serum Mg^{++} levels are at 1.25 mEq./L., a common finding in cases of delirium tremens.

When the pieces of this puzzle are put together, Mr. R. is diagnosed as a chronic alcoholic in delirium tremens with a Mg^{++} deficiency. You can surmise that intravenous replacements of Mg^{++} will be ordered, and you can thus review the relevant nursing care before starting the medication.

We have greatly oversimplified the case of Mr. R. Actually, as a severe alcoholic he is probably suffering not only from a Mg^{++} deficiency, but also from water, protein, and vitamin deficits.

Having considered how to assess a patient in terms of imbalance, we shall now proceed to discuss the goal of all diagnoses, laboratory work, and systematic assessment, namely, clinical care.

COMPOSING A PLAN OF CARE

The Emergency Patient

Severely dehydrated persons, burned patients, hemorrhaging patients, and accident victims will die in a state of fluid and electrolyte imbalance if they do not receive adequate and prompt treatment. Some important lifesaving measures are as follows:[43]

> Treat *shock* immediately. Keep a constant check on the vital signs and on the patient's state of consciousness.

> Prepare for the doctor to order an electrolyte analysis followed by IV replacement therapy for any serious electrolyte deficits.

> For a patient with severe extracellular fluid deficit and oliguria, prepare for the doctor to order IV fluid replacement. A Foley catheter will probably be indicated. It will be necessary to measure urinary output on the critical patient hourly.

Patients with severe life-threatening imbalances will need constant *planned* nursing observations and care until the vital signs stabilize and urinary output is adequate, i.e., at least 25 ml. per hour.

The Seriously Ill Patient with an Imbalance

Any seriously ill person is a potential candidate for fluid and electrolyte imbalances. Consequently, in your plan of care for any seriously ill person, whether suffering from acute or chronic illness, be certain to include the following tasks that are summarized from preceding material:

> Evaluate daily the patient's food intake compared with his nutritional needs. For example, a postoperative patient needs protein to rebuild tissues and to encourage wound healing. Does this patient order and eat foods high in protein? A patient with diarrhea loses large amounts of K^+. Does he eat foods high in K^+, e.g., bananas and orange juice?

> Daily *evaluate* the patient's intake and output record. Is intake adequate in relationship to output and vice versa? An accurate record of intake and output is not useful unless it is reviewed to identify and correct significant discrepancies or deviations from normal.

> Evaluate the patient's need for fluids, electrolytes, and foods, considering the presence of: fever, severe dyspnea, nausea, vomiting, anorexia, and draining wounds. Do not forget that severe emotional stress can also seriously affect the fluid and electrolyte balance.

> Daily examine the patient in relationship to the multiple factors listed under the physical examination. Remember that new fluid and electrolyte imbalances may develop at any time during the course of an illness. You, as the nurse, often are in a position to make the *first* observations of an imbalance that is in the early stages of development.

A GUIDE TO FLUID REPLACEMENT

Major goals of fluid replacement are:

1. Correct preexisting deficits of water and electrolytes, and restore, as quickly as possible, the *vascular fluid volume,* thus reducing shock and dehydration.
2. Meet the patient's maintenance (or life-sustaining) needs for fluids, electrolytes, and calories.
3. Replace *dynamic* or *concurrent losses* of fluid and electrolytes from suctioning, vomiting, diarrhea, and so forth.

In ordering fluids, the doctor considers: (1) the *patient* and his clinical record, (2) the *route* of fluid administration, (3) the *type* of solution to be given, and (4) the *rate* of administration.

Some general guides for ordering fluid replacements based on the *patient's clinical status* are:

> The patient's appearance, complaints, daily weight, and vital signs.

> Daily intake and output requirements.

> The laboratory reports.

The major *routes* for fluid replacement are oral, rectal, and parenteral.

Oral Route

Replacement of fluids and electrolytes by mouth is generally considered to be the safest method. Oral replacement should be used when the patient is not vomiting and does not have dysphagia, and when the situation is *not* an emergency. During emergencies, fluids are generally administered parenterally for rapid absorption.

Patients receiving oral fluid replacements are usually given *prescribed* amounts of water, milk, fresh fruit juice, and beef extracts. These fluids supply needed calories, proteins, sodium, and potassium, as well as serving to replace any fluid volume deficit.

Because oral fluid replacement is considered safe, doctor's orders and nurses' records concerning oral fluid replacement are not always as precise as they should be. As a result, the patient may not receive the proper type or amount of fluid necessary to meet his needs. In caring for patients receiving oral liquids:

> Remember:
> 1. *Question vague orders concerning fluid replacement (e.g., "fluids ad lib" and "force fluids").*
> 2. *Know the* exact *amount and type of fluid a patient should receive for replacement purposes.*

For patients unable to drink fluids, the doctor may order tube feedings as an oral fluid replacement procedure. (See Unit VIII for discussion of tube feeding.)

Rectal Fluid Replacement

Proctoclysis, or rectal fluid replacement, is not a very reliable method for replacing an electrolyte deficit so it is infrequently used today. Since only water, sodium, and chloride are absorbed by the large intestine, proctoclysis cannot be relied upon to meet a patient's caloric needs and, consequently, is not used for maintenance purposes. Nevertheless, you may occasionally receive an order to give a rectal feeding. For greater success with this procedure, be sure to observe the following points:

> Check the patient for diarrhea; you cannot give a proctoclysis if diarrhea is present.

> An enema is routinely ordered one to two hours prior to giving a rectal feeding.

> A No. 18 to 22 French catheter is generally used for the feeding.

> Make certain that the solution is warmed prior to administration.

> Drip the solution into the patient at a rate of 10 to 60 drops per minute; if given too rapidly the patient will expel the fluid.

> Do not give more than 2000 ml. of fluid in 24 hours.

Parenteral Administration

The parenteral route is the most controlled and expedient method of fluid administration, because the solutions go directly into the body's fluid compartments. It is also the most dangerous method of fluid administration, giving rise to potential complications which often rival in severity the imbalance being treated. Nevertheless, parenteral fluid replacements frequently are absolutely necessary; therefore, you must be fully acquainted with the subject in order to handle the procedure safely and effectively.

Because parenteral solutions are fast acting and potentially dangerous, specific questions need to be answered concerning their use:

1. Under what circumstances are parenteral fluids administered?
2. What major principles serve as guides in parenteral fluid administration?
3. What routes can be used for parenteral fluid replacement? What are the advantages and disadvantages of each method?
4. What are the major types of solutions that can be ordered?
5. Upon what bases does the physician estimate a patient's parenteral fluid requirements? Why does he order particular fluids for particular patients?
6. How does the physician translate his plan of parenteral therapy into a nurse's fluid order? What should the order include? What are the nurse's responsibilities in carrying out a fluid order?

In the discussion below, we shall briefly explore the answers to these questions.

Why Parenteral Fluids Are Ordered. Parenteral fluid replacements are generally ordered under the following circumstances:

> The patient is NPO or is physically incapable of taking oral liquids.

> The patient requires *rapid* fluid and electrolyte replacements.

> The patient requires a medication that will be destroyed by the gastric juices if it is administered orally.

> The patient requires a medication that, if given orally, can not be absorbed by the gastrointestinal tract.

Guiding Principles in Parenteral Fluid Administration. Some important considerations when giving parenteral fluids to patients are as follows:

> *Adequacy of renal function* is the single most important factor to consider in parenteral fluid administration.

> Remember, during parenteral fluid administration:
> *If a patient suffers from any form of renal disease, careful observations of flow rate, meticulous recording of intake and output, and prevention of circulatory overload and pulmonary edema are vitally important!*

> Whenever possible fluids and electrolytes should be given by the *oral route* in preference to the parenteral route.

> Daily measurement of *weight* is a helpful guide in evaluating a patient's hydration. Sudden weight shifts are highly significant. Any sudden variation in a patient's weight in excess of 5 per cent is usually the result of body water loss or retention.

> When a seriously ill patient is receiving parenteral fluids, the insertion of a *Foley catheter* along with measurements of the *hourly urine volume* provides a useful indication of hydration.

> Whenever possible, administer parenteral fluids during the day when renal function is at its best.

> When a patient must receive IV parenteral fluids for a period of days or even weeks, do all you can to: keep the patient comfortable, prevent infiltration of fluid into the tissues, prevent infection at the site of administration, and to preserve the patient's veins. These topics are considered below.

Major Routes for Parenteral Fluid Therapy and Their Dangers. The two major routes used for administering parenteral fluids are the subcutaneous route (hypodermoclysis) and the intravenous route.

SUBCUTANEOUS ROUTE: HYPODERMOCLYSIS. Like proctoclysis, hypodermoclysis is infrequently used. Subcutaneous fluids, when employed, are mainly given to obese patients, young children, and aged patients with badly sclerosed veins. In such patients hypodermoclysis is advantageous because it is easier to start and maintain than an intravenous infusion.

Commonly used sites for subcutaneous infusions are the lateral and anterior aspects of the thigh, the abdomen, the lateral chest, the buttocks, and beneath the breasts.

Few fluids are suitable for hypodermoclysis administration since they must closely resemble the plasma in tonicity and electrolyte content. In Table 25–5 we have listed some solutions that are either suitable or unsuitable for subcutaneous infusion.

Solutions that *do not* contain electrolytes may cause hypotension and possibly shock. These complications develop because nonelectrolyte solutions, when given subcutaneously, tend to pull electrolytes from the plasma and adjacent tissues into the area around the clysis. The result is a dangerous decrease in plasma volume. On the other hand, hypertonic solutions tend to pull water from the plasma into the subcutaneous spaces because of their high osmotic pressure; this also results in plasma volume reduction. Alcohol, amino acids, and fat emulsion are irritating to tissues, while gastric replacement solutions differ considerably from the normal pH of the body. *Always question* the subcutaneous administration of any of these solutions.

In adults receiving hypodermoclysis, solutions are generally allowed to drip at a rate of 30 to 40 drops per minute, depending upon how well the solution is being absorbed by the tissues. When absorption is somewhat slow, the enzyme *hyaluronidase* [Wydase] may be given to facilitate dispersion and absorption of the solution. Wydase is usually injected either into the tissues surrounding the clysis site or into the clysis tubing. When using Wydase watch for signs of *allergic reaction* at the injection site as well as a *generalized fluid overload* due to rapid absorption of the clysis fluid.

While a hypodermoclysis is easy to start and does supply needed fluids, it can be a dangerous procedure. Problems at the site of administration that are linked with this method of fluid administration include: infection, with abscess formation; tissue sloughing due to poor absorption; and extreme discomfort, especially if the solution is allowed to run too rapidly.

INTRAVENOUS ROUTE. Parenteral fluids are most commonly administered intravenously. This is often a lifesaving procedure in hemorrhage or shock because the fluids enter the vascular system directly, thereby immediately increasing the plasma volume. Also, IV fluids can be given to patients over long periods of time if necessary. Fluids given by this route can be calculated daily to supply needed calories, carbohydrates, proteins, vitamins, and electrolytes.

TABLE 25–5. A COMPARISON OF SAFE AND CONTRAINDICATED SOLUTIONS IN HYPODERMOCLYSIS

Safe Solutions	Contraindicated Solutions
1. Isotonic saline 0.9%	1. Electrolyte-free solutions
2. Half-isotonic saline (0.45%) with 21% dextrose	2. Hypertonic solutions
3. Ringer's solution	3. Alcohol
4. Lactated Ringer's solution	4. Amino acids
5. Darrow's solution	5. Fat emulsions
	6. Gastric replacement solution

Remember, during hypodermoclysis:

1. *Observe for redness and irritation around the injection site when Wydase is used.*
2. *Observe for signs of infection. Always use sterile technique when starting a clysis. When the clysis is discontinued, cover the injection site with a sterile dressing.*
3. *Observe for swelling around the injection site.*
4. *Watch for signs of circulatory overload.*

Choice of site for IV infusions depends upon the length of time IV therapy will be required, and whether the physician has ordered a simple venipuncture or a venisection (cutdown). The simple venipuncture is the procedure of choice for patients on short-term therapy, while the cutdown is used for those patients who must remain on IV therapy for an extended period of time. For short-term therapy, veins in the antecubital space and on the dorsum of the hand are used. For long-term therapy, a leg vein that is free of varicosities may be selected. Other suitable veins are the accessory cephalic or median antebrachial on the flat surface of the forearm, the saphenous vein at the ankle and the femoral vein in the thigh. For a cutdown procedure the physician often selects the saphenous vein at the ankle, because this site is more comfortable and allows the patient greater movement—important considerations in long-term therapy.

While IV therapy may indeed be lifesaving, it clearly involves multiple dangers. Major complications of IV therapy are:

> *Infiltration* of IV solutions into the tissue spaces, possibly resulting in a hematoma. Infiltration of certain medications (Levofed, Aramine, calcium gluconate) can cause dangerous tissue sloughs.

> *Thrombophlebitis* owing to trauma of the vein.

> A *pyogenic reaction due to contaminated fluids or* equipment.

> *Speed shock,* a severe systemic reaction to IV fluids containing drugs that are administered too rapidly.

> *Air embolism,* which results from a failure to clear the tubing of air before administering fluid.

> *Circulatory overload.*

Symptoms of these complications as well as nursing actions are summarized on the opposite page.

*Major Types of Parenteral Solutions.** Many different types of parenteral fluids are available today. Each of the important groups of parenteral fluids is briefly considered on page 252.

*For a more thorough discussion of parenteral fluids, it is helpful to consult the pamphlets on water and electrolyte balance published by the major drug houses. Both Abbott and Baxter Laboratories have published informative brochures on the different solutions they manufacture.

The Complications of IV Therapy—Symptoms and Relevant Nursing Actions

Complication	*Symptoms*	*Nursing Actions*
I. Infiltration of IV solution	A. Infusion rate slows or stops completely B. Swelling, hardness, and pain around the needle site C. A feeling of coldness around the injection site D. When the bottle is lowered below the level of the needle, blood fails to return into the tubing E. Signs of tissue necrosis	1. Immediately stop the infusion 2. Apply warm towels to the swollen area 3. If necessary, restart the infusion at another site
II. Thrombophlebitis	A. Pain along the vein B. Area of redness and swelling around the affected vein C. Generalized symptoms such as fatigue, fever, rapid pulse, malaise	1. Stop infusion 2. If necessary, restart the infusion at another site 3. Apply warm moist compresses 4. Do *not* massage or rub the affected limb 5. To prevent thrombophlebitis, 1 mg. of hydrocortisone is sometimes added to each liter of fluid
III. Pyogenic reaction	A. Symptoms generally appear 30 min. after the infusion is started B. Temperature elevation and chills C. Headache D. Nausea and vomiting E. Circulatory collapse, if severe	1. Immediately stop infusion 2. Check vital signs 3. Notify doctor 4. Save IV solution so that it can be examined for pathogens 5. Do *not* give any solution that is cloudy
IV. Speed shock	A. Pounding headache B. Fainting C. Rapid pulse D. Apprehension E. Chills F. Back pain G. Dyspnea Symptoms are variable and will depend upon the drug being used.	1. Stop or slow infusion, depending upon the severity of the symptoms 2. Notify physician
V. Air embolism	The main problem is sudden vascular collapse due to occlusion of vessel by embolism; as a result, tissues which are normally supplied with blood by the involved vessel will not receive adequate oxygen. Signs are: cyanosis, low blood pressure, tachycardia, rise in venous pressure, unconsciousness	1. Check vital signs 2. Give oxygen 3. To prevent this complication: a. Make certain that air is out of the tubing before injecting needle into the vein b. Do *not* elevate the arm or leg receiving the infusion above the heart; a negative pressure will be created in the vein and air will be drawn into the vein should there be any leaks in the IV apparatus c. Do not allow the IV to "run dry"; there should be a little fluid left in the tubing when you disconnect the infusion
VI. Circulatory overload	This problem was discussed on pp. 217–218.	

Major Types of Parenteral Solutions

I. Carbohydrate solutions:
  A. Purposes and advantages:
    1. Provide needed calories and nutrition.
    2. Provide fluid replacement.
    3. Increase the glycogen content of the liver.
    4. Are an effective cardiac stimulant.
    5. Provide water for the body's numerous needs from oxidation.
    6. Act as a protein sparer.
    7. Prevent starvation ketosis.
  B. Limitations:
    1. Dextrose solutions do not replace electrolyte losses.
    2. Dextrose solutions are of no value in shock.
  C. Major types of solutions available:
    1. 2.5, 5, 10, and 15 per cent dextrose in water.
    2. 5 and 10 per cent dextrose in saline.
    3. Invert sugar solutions in water or saline. Invert sugar is composed of equal parts of glucose and fructose.
    4. 50 per cent glucose:
      a. This solution is sometimes given to individuals who need calories but are unable to cope with large amounts of fluid, e.g., patients with severe cardiac or kidney problems.
      b. Such a concentrated solution should be given *very slowly.*
  D. Untoward effects:
    1. Concentrated carbohydrate solutions (over 5 per cent dextrose in water or saline) may irritate the veins and cause thrombophlebitis.
    2. A high blood sugar may result. (See p. 216.)

II. Electrolyte solutions containing sodium:
  A. Purposes:
    1. Treatment of dehydration.
    2. Satisfy daily salt requirements.
    3. Correct low salt syndromes.
    4. Treatment of shock.
    5. Treatment of H^+ imbalances.
  B. Limitations: Will not correct multiple electrolyte imbalances.
  C. Major types of solutions available:
    1. Physiologic solution of sodium chloride (normal saline or N.S.).
    2. Hypotonic saline (0.45 Gm. NaCl/L.).
    3. Hypertonic saline in strengths of 3 and 5 per cent.
    4. One-sixth molar sodium lactate is used to treat acidosis.
  D. Complications:
    1. Circulatory overload.
    2. Sodium overload.

III. Special purpose electrolyte solutions:
  A. Examples of solutions available are:
    1. Potassium solutions. (For discussion of IV K^+ see pp. 234–235.)
    2. Ringer's solution:
      a. A normal saline solution to which K^+ and Ca^{++} have been added in place of some of the Na^+.
      b. Used in hypohydration and electrolyte losses due to vomiting, diarrhea, and gastric suction.
    3. Lactated Ringer's solution:
      a. Similar to plasma.
      b. Supplies lactate ions.
    4. Multiple electrolyte solutions, for example, Butler's and Darrow's solutions.
    5. Gastric replacement solution: replaces losses due to vomiting or gastric suction.

IV. Protein hydrolysates (also called amino acid solutions):
  A. Purposes:
    1. Supply proteins for tissue repair.
    2. Correct negative nitrogen balance states.
  B. Contraindications:
    1. Should not be given to patients with severe renal disease.
    2. Give with caution to patients with *liver* disease or with history of *allergy.*
  C. Types of solutions available:
    1. Amigen
    2. Aminosol
    3. Stuart amino acids
  D. Untoward effects:
    1. Allergic reactions.
    2. Fever.
    3. Nausea and vomiting (may result if solution given too rapidly).
    4. Headache.
    5. Thrombophlebitis at the injection site.
  E. Special precautions for greater safety in administration:

(Outline continued on the opposite page.)

Remember, *in administering* protein hydrolysates:

1. Do not *keep a solution in the refrigerator once it has been opened. Use at once or discard!*
2. Do not *use solutions that are cloudy or contain precipitate matter.*
3. Do not *add other mixtures to amino acid solutions.*
4. *Give* slowly. *The usual dose of amino acid is 100 to 200 Gms per 24 hours.*

V. Fat emulsions:
  A. Purposes and advantages:
    1. Provide excellent source of calories.
    2. Can be used for severe nutritional disorders coupled with a poor oral intake.
    3. Beneficial for long-term unconscious and semiconscious patient.
    4. Sometimes administered to patients with malignancies, burns, severe renal disorders, ulcerative colitis, or with nonfunctional gastrointestinal tracts.
    5. Sometimes given to preoperative and postoperative patients.
  B. Types of solutions available:
    1. Lipomul. Contains cottonseed oil; provides 800 calories in 500 ml.
    2. Intralipid. Contains soybean oil.
  C. Possible contraindications:
    1. The "perfectly safe" fat emulsion does not yet exist.
      a. Fat emulsions *should always be used with caution.*
      b. Patients with liver diseases, coagulation problems, and acidosis should be meticulously observed for side effects.
  D. Adverse side effects (especially to Lipomul):
    1. Early reaction:
      a. Apparently due to introduction of colloids into the blood stream.
      b. Characterized by a shock-like syndrome, severe back pain, cyanosis, urticara.
    2. Later reaction:
      a. Occurs around the third week following the infusion.
      b. Characterized by anemia, blood clotting, and hemorrhage.
  E. Special precautions to observe:

Remember, *in administering* fat emulsions:

1. *Give slowly according to the following schedule:*
   First 5 minutes – 10 gtts./min.
   Next 25 minutes – 40 gtts./min.
   Then – 60 gtts./min.
2. *Use sets developed for Lipomul infusion.*
3. Do not *mix Lipomul with other medicines or liquids.*

VI. Solutions containing alcohol:
  A. Indications and advantages:
    1. Gives the patient needed calories while sparing the patient's body fats, proteins, and carbohydrates.
    2. Has a sedative effect.
    3. Gives an increased sense of well-being.
    4. May act as an analgesic.
  B. Examples of solutions available:
    1. 5 per cent alcohol, 5 per cent dextrose in water.
    2. 5 per cent alcohol, 5 per cent dextrose in saline.
    3. 10 per cent alcohol, 10 per cent glucose in water.
    4. Trinidex, 5 per cent alcohol, 5 per cent dextrose with vitamins in water.
  C. Contraindications: Patients with epilepsy, liver, or kidney disease or in shock should not receive alcohol solutions.
  D. Dosage and rate:
    1. 200 to 300 ml. of a 5 per cent solution per hour provides sedation without intoxication.
    2. On the average, patients are given one to two liters of alcohol solutions in 24 hours.
  E. Side effects:
    1. Cerebral depression.
    2. Loss of alertness.
    3. Restlessness and coma (in an overdose).
  F. Special precautions:
    1. Watch carefully for signs of infiltration, tissue slough can result.
    2. Observe for signs of phlebitis around the injection site.

VII. Colloidal solutions*:
  A. Indications:
    1. Expansion of a depleted plasma volume.
    2. Support of the plasma osmotic pressure. Additional protein materials are supplied by colloidal solution which, in turn, holds fluid within the vessels.
    3. Prevention of shock and circulatory collapse.
  B. Examples of solutions available:
    1. Whole blood.
    2. Plasma.
    3. Human serum albumin.
    4. Plasma expanders (dextran and gelatin).

*The giving of blood and plasma will be discussed more fully in the unit on blood, Unit XII.

The preceding outline does not list all the IV solutions available.

Out of the great number of available solutions, how does the doctor know which solution to choose for his patient? How does he evaluate his patient's replacement needs? What observations must the nurse make to help the doctor in this assessment?

Evaluating the Patient's Parenteral fluid and Electrolyte Needs. As stated earlier, a patient's fluid requirements fall roughly into three broad groups: (1) fluids to meet *basal requirements* or maintenance needs; (2) fluids to keep pace with *dynamic* or *continuing* losses; and (3) fluids to replace any old or *prior* losses. In the outline below, we have presented some of the major areas generally considered in assessing a patient's fluid needs and in developing a plan of care.

Once the physician has assessed the patient's fluid and electrolyte needs, he then transforms his evaluation into a nurse's fluid order. Let us now consider what this order should contain and the nurse's responsibilities in regard to carrying it out.

Orders for Parenteral Fluids. Physicians' orders involving fluid and electrolytes should be as precise and as exact as prescriptions for dangerous or potentially lethal medications. Unfortunately physicians, like nurses and other professional people, are sometimes careless or hurried and, as a result, neglect to write clear and complete orders. A safe order for

---

*Assessing the Patient's Parenteral Fluid Needs**

I. Basal requirements:

To assess a patient's basal requirements, physicians and nurses must evaluate the patient's needs for water, electrolytes, carbohydrates, and vitamins.

A. Water requirements:

Patients require approximately 1500 to 2500 ml. of water per day if they are not sweating excessively, high fever is not present, and renal function is normal. In writing individualized parenteral fluid orders, physicians usually consider the following:

1. The basal metabolic rate is considered in terms of:
   a. The patient's age, sex, activity, thyroid function, and diagnosis.
   b. Conditions that increase the patient's metabolic rate (i.e., fever, hot weather) or decrease metabolic rate (i.e., cardiac failure, renal shock).
2. Water losses from the following sources:
   a. Urine.
   b. Perspiration (sensible and insensible).
   c. Feces.
   d. Respiratory tract. Water losses vary with state of cardiovascular-renal function.
3. The intake and output record in terms of balance and the adequacy of both intake and output.
4. Daily weight:
   a. An important aid in calculating those water losses that cannot be readily measured (i.e., from sweating or incontinence).
   b. The *ideal* weight should be used in calculating water requirements for patients who are obese or edematous.
5. Body surface area. Calculated from tables based on height and weight measurements.
6. Solute loads. Postoperative patients and patients with metabolic disorders need more water intake to excrete wastes, toxins, and excess sugar.
7. Central venous pressure (CVP):
   a. The pressure of blood within the right atrium is the central venous pressure. It can be measured in the peripheral veins of the arms or in the femoral vein.
   b. Normal venous pressures in the antecubical vein is 6 to 10 cm. of H_2O.
   c. The CVP procedure provides a most accurate guide in body fluid replacement because it is a good index of the body's circulating blood volume.†
   d. An elevated CVP indicates an overloading of the circulatory system.
   e. An abnormally low CVP indicates an inadequate circulatory volume.
   f. CVP is normally performed on oliguric patients receiving parenteral fluids to prevent fluid overload.

B. Basic electrolyte requirements:

1. In general, patients have the following daily electrolyte requirements:
   Na^+ 60 – 1000 mEq./day
   K^+ 40 – 75 mEq./day
   Cl^- 80 110 mEq./day
   NaCl 3.5 – 6.0 Gm./day (average 4.5 Gm.)
2. In evaluating electrolyte needs, physicians use the clinical history, the physical examination, and laboratory findings.
3. Following surgery, physicians generally use caution in prescribing NaCl solutions. This is especially true if patients are old, debilitated, or have renal or cardiac dysfunction.
4. Precautions are always used when prescribing K^+ solutions or additives.

(Outline continued on the opposite page.)

*In discussing the assessment of parenteral need, the authors have relied heavily upon Reese, L.: *Applied Therapeutics* 7:719, September, 1965.

†The procedure for CVP is discussed in the unit on the circulatory system, Unit X.

parenteral infusions should include the following items:

1. The *specific solution* or solutions the patient is to receive; if more than one bottle of solution is to be given, the bottles should be numbered consecutively.

2. The *additive solutions,* if any, should be written out, as well as the number of milliliters or milliequivalents to be given. The doctor should specify whether the solution is to be added to the bottle or placed into the tubing.

3. A rough *time schedule* should be included if more than one IV is ordered.

4. If a single IV is ordered, either the time for its *completion* or the drip rate per minute should be specified.

5. A *maximum drip rate* should be ordered in case the IV or IV's get behind schedule.

The following is an example of an *acceptable* order for parenteral fluids:

Date
8/17 #6 IV 1000 ml. 5% dextrose/water add to bottle KCl 20 mEq.
Start at 8 A.M. and run to 4 P.M.
#7 IV 1000 ml. 5% dextrose/saline
Start at 4 P.M. and run to midnight
Then discontinue IV's
Run IV's #6 and #7 no faster than 150 gtts. per minute even if behind schedule.

An example of a *questionable* order that you should not accept without further clarification from the doctor is:

Date
8/17 #6 IV 1000 ml. 5% dextrose/water add KCl 20 mEq.
#7 IV 1000 ml. 5% dextrose/saline
Discontinue IV's following this infusion.

This order leaves far too much to the discretion of the nurse. A schedule, maximum drip rate, and in-

Assessing the Patient's Parenteral Fluid Needs (Continued)

C. Basic carbohydrate requirements:
   1. A 70-kg. patient requires approximately 1800 calories per day for nourishment, to prevent starvation ketosis, and to spare protein.
   2. The physician usually orders the carbohydrates to be given in the form of 5 or 10 per cent glucose in water or saline.
   3. Glucose solution *alone* cannot supply a patient's total caloric needs over a sustained period of time.
      a. One liter of 5 per cent glucose in water supplies only 50 Gm. of glucose or 200 calories.
      b. Generally, patients receive 2500 ml. of glucose in water or saline per day. This amounts to only 500 *calories per day*—not sufficient to meet the 1800 calories required by a patient over a 24-hr. period.
      c. For long-term patients, physicians may order in addition to glucose solution, the following calorie-supplying preparations: protein hydrolysates, emulsified fat preparations, solutions containing alcohol, or tube feedings.
      d. For those patients requiring parenteral nutrition for only a few days, physicians are concerned mainly with *fluid* replacement rather than caloric requirements.

D. Basic vitamin requirements:
   1. Vitamin supplements are usually ordered for the patients:
      a. Who are NPO and receiving parenteral therapy for more than three days.
      b. Who are severely malnourished, e.g., alcoholics.
      c. With acute illnesses or infections.
      d. Who are recovering from surgery.
      e. Who are burned.
   2. Vitamins commonly used in parenteral fluid administration are vitamin C and members of the vitamin B complex group.

II. Replacing dynamic losses
   A. These represent losses over and above basal losses of fluids and electrolytes.
   B. The main causes of dynamic losses are:
      1. Vomiting.
      2. Diarrhea.
      3. Gastric or intestinal suction.
      4. Wound drainage.
      5. Fluid shifts between compartments as seen in patients with burns and trauma.
   C. Special purpose electrolyte solutions are often ordered for replacing continuing gastrointestinal tract losses.

III. Replacing prior losses
   A. Prior deficits represent those deficiences or imbalances of fluids and electrolytes that the patient had *prior* to current treatment.
   B. The major types of prior deficits are:
      1. Water depletion.
      2. Electrolyte deficits or imbalances.
      3. Red blood cell mass deficit.
      4. Deficiency of plasma proteins.
   C. To treat these problems, the physician may order:
      1. Glucose and water solutions.
      2. General or special purpose electrolyte solutions.
      3. Whole blood to replace red cell mass.
      4. Salt-poor human albumin to replace plasma proteins.

structions concerning additive medicines are all missing. With this order, it would be possible to either overload the patient with fluid, or to fail to hydrate him rapidly enough. Such serious errors can be avoided by clarifying with the physician any sketchy instruction concerning parenteral fluid infusions.

The most precise way to keep an IV infusion *on schedule* is to calculate the number of drops (gtts.) per minute the IV must run in order to finish within a certain time period. For instance, in the example above, the physician has ordered IV #6 (1000 ml. 5% D/W) to start at 8 A.M. and be completed by 4 P.M.; i.e., 1000 ml. of fluid are to be administered in an 8-hour period. To find the number of drops per minute the IV must run, follow these steps:

1. Consult the directions on the IV apparatus as to the number of drops that are necessary to administer one ml. of fluid to the patient (different commercial sets vary in this respect). For example, the Baxter Laboratory's regular sets deliver 1 ml. in 10 gtts; the Abbott sets deliver 1 ml. in 13 to 15 gtts. Let us say, for purposes of our example, that we are using a *Baxter Laboratory set.*
2. Calculate the number of drops per minute necessary to administer IV #6 to the patient within the time allotment of 8 hours.* Use the following formula:

$$\text{Drops/min.} = \frac{\text{Total volume infused} \times \text{drop/ml.}}{\text{Total time of infusion in minutes}}$$

3. Total volume infused = 1000
   Drops/ml. = 10 in a Baxter set
   Total time in minutes = 8 × 60 = 480
4. $\text{gtts./min.} = \frac{1000 \text{ ml.} \times 10}{480} = $ approximately 20 gtts./min.
5. Thus, to infuse 1000 ml. 5% D/W in 8 hours, you would need to run IV #6 at around 20 gtts./minute.

A second way to keep an IV on schedule is to place a long strip of adhesive tape on the side of the IV bottle next to the ml. calibrations. The tape is then marked to show the amount of solution that the patient should receive every hour in order to complete the IV on time. For example, if the patient is to receive 1000 ml. in 8 hours, you know that he will have to receive 125 ml. every hour. If the IV starts at 8 A.M., the tape is then marked to show that by 9 A.M. 125 ml. should have been infused, and 875 should be left in the bottle; by 10 A.M. 250 ml. should have been infused, with 750 ml. left, and so forth. This simple and practical method of IV scheduling is illustrated in Figure 25–5.

There are several factors that can either increase or decrease the rate of drip from the desired setting.

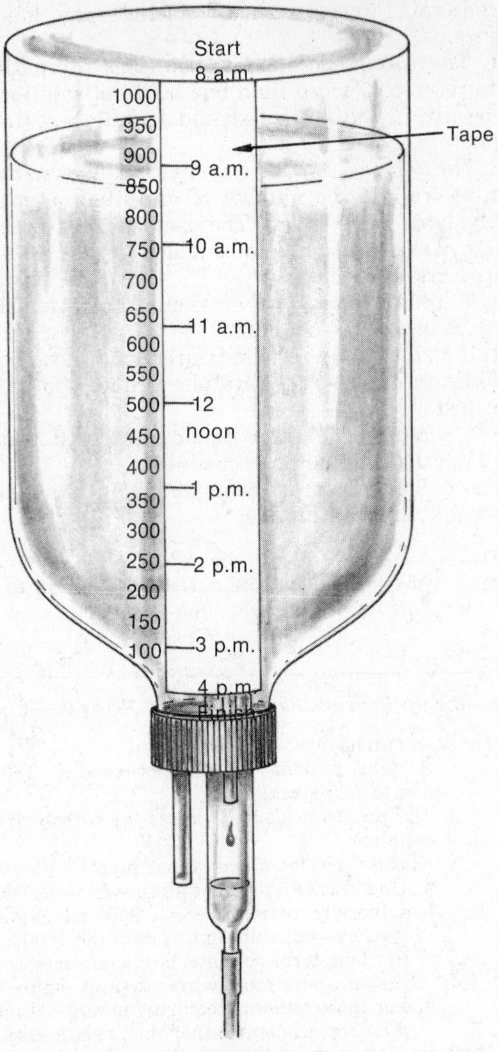

*Slide rule IV drop calculators are available through some of the commercial drug houses such as Abbott Laboratories, Cutter Laboratories, and Baxter Laboratories.

FIGURE 25–5. Tape attached to I.V. bottle to assist with keeping intravenous infusions on schedule.

Consequently, you should check the IV drip rate at least every 15 minutes once the setting has been made. Some of the most important of these disturbing factors include the following: (1) The needle's position in the vein may change due to the patient's position or movements. (2) The distance between the site of administration (i.e., the vein in which the needle is inserted) and the height of the bottle may be altered. For example, the IV *bottle* may be *raised* or *lowered* in relationship to the site of injection. The higher the bottle is raised, the faster the flow, and vice versa. Also, the patient's *bed* may be *lowered* or *raised*; if the bed is lowered and the IV pole is not adjusted, the IV will tend to drip more rapidly; conversely, the IV will drip more slowly if the bed is elevated. (3) The needle can become obstructed by a tiny clot, that will, in turn, slow the rate of drip. (4) Kinks in the tubing as well as the pressure of the bedclothes on the tubing can obstruct the flow.

In addition to checking the IV drip rate, other observations will need to be made. As stated earlier, many complications can arise as a result of IV parenteral fluid therapy. You will want to review frequently all untoward effects of IV infusion in order to prevent them effectively.

PATIENTS ESPECIALLY SUSCEPTIBLE TO FLUID AND ELECTROLYTE IMBALANCES

Fluid and electrolyte imbalances, like death and taxes, affect everyone at certain points in their existence. Of course, some individuals, because of their particular ailments, are more vulnerable to imbalances than other persons are. Ill persons particularly prone to fluid and electrolyte upsets and who require careful evaluation and observation are: (1) patients with diarrhea, (2) patients who are vomiting, (3) patients with edema, (4) postoperative patients, and (5) patients with burns. In the short discussion that follows we shall briefly list the imbalances most common to each of these patients and then pose a few questions concerning the prevention and care involved. These questions should aid you in reviewing some of the essential points considered in this chapter and Chapter 24.

THE PATIENT WITH DIARRHEA

Diarrhea is a commonly encountered clinical problem, occurring both in the hospital and at home. Some common causes of diarrhea are intestinal infections, toxic poisoning, drugs, fecal impactions, carcinoma, ulcerative colitis, pancreatic insufficiency, and certain neurologic diseases such as tabes dorsalis and diabetic neuropathy.

Diarrhea causes four major fluid and electrolyte imbalances.[3] They are:

> Dehydration (volume deficit).
> Na^+ deficit.
> K^+ deficit.
> Acidosis (this problem develops in response to decreased kidney function and Na^+ loss).

As you can see, diarrhea causes decreases in both blood volume and electrolytes. The major homeostatic mechanisms that occur in response to diarrhea are the fluid shift mechanism, the aldosterone mechanism, and the ADH mechanism (Figure 25–6).

A few important questions for review of the problems of diarrhea are:

1. What precisely stimulates aldosterone release in diarrhea? What stimulates ADH release? What other circumstances, besides diarrhea, cause the release of these hormones?
2. Does a patient with diarrhea suffer from hyperosmolarity or hypo-osmolarity or does he have an "isotonic" type of imbalance? Will he be thirsty? Why or why not?
3. When a patient suffers from frequent and profuse diarrhea, how long does it take to deplete the ECF? What important complications develop as a result of fluid depletion?
4. Which will constitute the more serious electrolyte imbalance resulting from diarrhea—a K^+ deficit or a Na^+ deficit? Why? How is the Na^+ deficit treated? What precautions must you observe in administering K^+ supplements intravenously or orally?
5. What are the three major complications that patients develop as a result of dehydration? How are these complications treated? What secondary problems may result from treatment?
6. In severe dehydration, you should check the urinary output every two hours. What findings will you report?

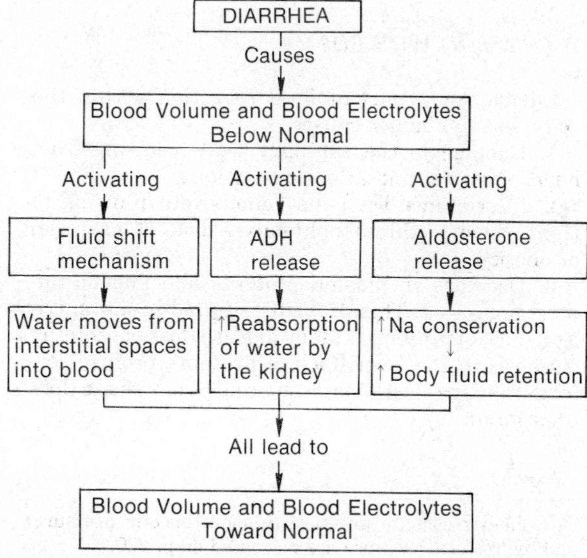

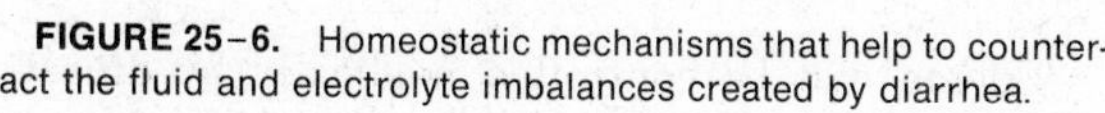
FIGURE 25–6. Homeostatic mechanisms that help to counteract the fluid and electrolyte imbalances created by diarrhea.

THE PATIENT WITH LOSSES FROM VOMITING OR SUCTION

The patient who is vomiting and the patient receiving gastric suction may suffer from large losses of fluid and electrolytes. For example, in 24 hours a patient may lose up to 2500 ml. of gastric fluid plus an additional loss of 1500 ml. of saliva. Water, H^+, Na^+, K^+, Cl^-, and small amounts of Mg^{++} are all present in gastric juice; consequently, deficits of these ions cause the different types of imbalances that result from vomiting.

Vomiting and gastric suction cause:

> Fluid volume deficit.
> Na^+ deficit.
> K^+ deficit.
> Metabolic alkalosis (H^+ and Cl^- are lost in vomiting. HCO_3^-, a base, is retained to compensate for the Cl^- loss.)
> Mg^{++} deficit.
> Ketosis of starvation.

These imbalances can be prevented or at least minimized by the nursing care discussed earlier.

As a review of relevant nursing implications, see if you can answer the following questions:

1. What nursing actions can help to prevent the development of Na^+ deficit ("depletion hyponatremia") in the patient who is vomiting and the patient on gastric suction? What are the most common signs of this imbalance?
2. Patients suffering from either vomiting or diarrhea require careful recording of their intake and output. Can you list 10 ways in which nursing staffs may fail to keep an accurate record? How would you correct these problems?
3. What types of IV solutions do you think will be ordered for the patient who is vomiting?
4. Should you use saline or distilled water when irrigating a patient's Levin tube? Give a reason for your choice.

THE PATIENT WITH EDEMA

Edema, an abnormal fluid retention within the body, has five major causes:

1. Damage to the capillary wall resulting from burns, trauma, and allergic reactions.
2. Interference with the venous return owing to tight garters, thrombophlebitis, lack of exercise, or obesity.
3. Decrease in plasma proteins and plasma oncotic pressure.* This problem is found in malnutrition (lack of protein), kidney disease (loss of protein), cirrhosis of the liver (lack of protein), profuse serious drainage (loss of protein), and hemorrhage (loss of protein).
4. Rise in blood hydrostatic pressure, which causes fluid to be squeezed into the tissues. This problem is due to circulatory overload and occurs in the following conditions: heart failure (due to salt and water retention), kidney failure (due to salt and water retention), and excessive infusions of hypertonic saline.
5. Obstruction of the lymphatic system, which may follow a radical mastectomy.

Symptoms that commonly accompany edema are weight gain, high blood pressure, and dyspnea.

The principal types of edema that can be identified in clinical practice are: pitting, dependent, and refractory. The major factors that distinguish one form of edema from another are listed below:

Pitting Edema. To test for pitting edema, press the edematous area of the patient, usually the ankles or sacrum, with your finger. If the indentation from your finger remains in the patient's flesh for a period of time, pitting edema is present.

Dependent Edema. This type of edema is related to gravity and to the patient's position. The excess water flows to the most dependent portion of the patient's body. In observing for dependent edema:

1. Check the sacral area and buttocks of patients on *bed rest.* Because the patient is in a prone position, the tissues of the buttocks and sacrum are most likely to become receptacles for excess fluid.
2. Check the ankles and buttocks of patients who have been *sitting* for extended periods of time. Edematous fluid will tend to flow to these dependent parts.

Refractory Edema. Edema that persists despite diuretic therapy and salt-restricted diets is said to be "refractory." Patients with this type of edema will also tend to have persistent weight gain and perhaps hypertension.

While edema may be described as pitting, dependent, or refractory, it can also be classified in relation to *where* it develops within the body. Some technical words that are used to describe edema in terms of location are listed below:

1. Anasarca – severe *generalized* edema.
2. Ascites – an excessive accumulation of fluid within the peritoneal cavity.
3. Pulmonary edema – excess fluid within the lung tissue.
4. Subcutaneous edema – excessive fluid in the subcutaneous tissues. This condition is common in heart failure.
5. Hydrothorax – effusions of fluid into the pleural cavity.
6. Hydropericardium – effusions of fluid into the pericardial cavity.

Edema can be controlled medically by diuretic therapy, the prescription of salt-poor diets, and occasionally by the parenteral administration of salt-poor proteins. Water may also be moderately restricted.*

*Colloidal osmotic pressure (plasma oncotic pressure) and hydrostatic pressure are discussed on p. 200.

*The medical and nursing care of edematous patients is discussed more thoroughly in the units on heart and kidney disease, Units X and XI.

There are several points to remember when you give nursing care to patients with edema. Major considerations are boxed below.

1. *Carefully regulate the IV fluids that you administer to patients with edema, especially those having pulmonary edema.*
2. *Observe carefully and frequently for decubitus ulcer formation, since edematous tissue is fragile and prone to breakdown. Patients with edema require frequent position changes. If possible, procure an alternating pressure mattress.*
3. *Edematous patients are usually malnourished. Unless contraindicated, encourage these patients to eat substantial amounts of protein.*
4. *Observe edematous patients for thirst. You will recall that edema fluid is trapped in the tissues and, thus, is not available for the body's needs. Patients with edema may therefore actually suffer from dehydration.*

As with any condition, patients being treated for edema are subject to iatrogenic complications. The most important iatrogenic problems are: (1) low salt syndrome resulting from the low sodium diet, and (2) hypokalemia, or K^+ deficit, resulting from the administration of diuretics.

We have listed a few important questions in relationship to edema. Answers to these questions may be found in earlier reading. (See Chapter 24 of this unit.)

1. What are plasma proteins? What are their normal levels in the serum? Which plasma protein is the most abundant when no pathology is present.
2. What does it mean when we say that the plasma has a 0.5 per cent greater osmolarity than the interstitial fluid? What happens when there is a reduction, however small, in colloidal osmotic pressure?
3. What is the blood hydrostatic pressure? What factors determine blood hydrostatic pressure? What pathologic conditions can create an excessive blood hydrostatic pressure and what will be the result of the excess?
4. Why are patients who are edematous sometimes advised to "eat beefsteak"? What other dietary changes may the doctor recommend?
5. What are the symptoms of low salt syndrome? What are the major symptoms of K^+ deficit? How can K^+ deficit be prevented in patients on diuretic therapy?

THE SURGICAL PATIENT

During the preoperative period, the major imbalance facing surgical patients is *dehydration* due to losses of ECF. These losses are usually the result of vomiting, diarrhea, gastrointestinal tract drainage, and intestinal obstructions (in which fluid is trapped in the obstructed loops of bowel). Because of such problems, patients often are treated with vigorous IV therapy *before* surgery can be performed.

During the first 24 to 48 hours of the postoperative period, you can expect certain characteristic shifts in the patient's fluids and electrolytes. These adjustments seem to be related to the alarm reaction of the GAS as described by Selye. During the early *postoperative period* the following adjustments occur:

> ADH is released.
> Urine volume is *decreased* regardless of intake, and water is retained.
> Aldosterone secretion is increased (especially following major surgery).
> Na^+ is retained.
> K^+ excretion is increased.

If the patient vomits or is on *gastric* suction following surgery, he may develop the imbalances discussed on p. 258, whereas if he has intestinal drainage or suction, he will probably present a clinical picture similar to that described on p. 257. Postoperative patients who are NPO, nauseated, or anorexic also face the crucial problems of caloric, protein, and vitamin deficiencies unless these nutrients are replaced.

In sum, the most typical complications following major surgery are:

1. Water overload (due to ↑ ADH).
2. Volume excess (due to ↑ Na^+).
3. Abdominal distention } (due to K^+ deficit)
4. Paralytic ileus } (due to K^+ deficit)
5. Shallow respirations
6. Hemorrhage and shock.
7. Acute renal insufficiency.
8. Signs of tetany (occasionally Ca^+ fall to a dangerous level).
9. Arrhythmias (due to ↓ K^+ and ↓ Ca^{++}).
. Respiratory acidosis (generally due to poor ventilation during and following surgery).

Some review questions centered around the care of the surgical patient are:

1. Why is it important to know the concentrating powers of a patient's kidneys before surgery? What is the concentrating power of a normal kidney? What problems does the postoperative patient face who has damaged kidneys and impaired concentrating power?
2. Does a decreased urinary output in postoperative patients indicate dehydration? Is it typically permissible to force fluids on postoperative patients?
3. The postoperative patient is often on scheduled IV's for a few days following surgery. In planning the patient's IV's with the doctor, what factors should be considered?
4. K^+ deficits are common in the postoperative period. Are K^+ supplements often added to a patient's IV's immediately postoperatively? Why or why not?
5. What types of surgical operations are most likely to lead to a K^+ deficit?
6. What three circumstances occurring together postoperatively, will definitely lead to a K^+ imbalance?
7. Do laboratory reports on K^+ levels tell the whole story about a patient's state of K^+ balance? Why or why not?
8. What is a safe rate of drip when administering

K^+ intravenously? What will happen to the patient if you allow the IV to drip too quickly?

9. Patients undergoing what type of surgical operations are particularly likely to develop a Ca^{++} deficit? What are the signs of tetany and what are the underlying pathologic changes?

10. Both K^+ and Ca^{++} must be administered with caution to patients receiving digitalis. Why is this so?

11. In the surgical patient, what is the major cause of a Mg^{++} deficit? What are the major pathologic disturbances? Why must clinicians rely so heavily on laboratory tests in diagnosing Mg^{++} deficit? What precautions are important to observe in administering Mg^{++} intravenously?

THE BURN PATIENT

Individuals suffering from serious burns are prime candidates for multiple severe imbalances.

Important imbalances that may develop as a result of burns are:

> Water deficit.
> Sodium deficit.
> K^+ excess during first 48 hours (due to cellular trauma).
> K^+ deficit after first 48 hours (due to shifts of K^+ from ECF into cells).
> Metabolic acidosis.
> Plasma to interstitial fluid shift (during first 48 hours).
> Interstitial fluid to plasma shift (following first 48 hours).
> Ca^{++} deficit.
> Negative nitrogen balance (during convalescent period).

Immediate recognition and care of the above imbalances and fluid and electrolyte shifting mechanisms is essential in attempts to save the life of the severely burned individual. Some questions that may help the reader to review and correlate these multiple imbalances follow:

1. What signs and symptoms of imbalance do burn patients have during the *first* 48-hour period post trauma? How do these early signs and symptoms compare with those that develop during the second 48-hour period post trauma and thereafter? What major physiologic reactions create these differences in symptomatology?

2. What is the best method for replacing K^+? What foods would you recommend for K^+ replacement? What oral medications are given?

3. What are the goals of treatment and nursing care for the two types of fluid shifts resulting from burns?

4. What is meant by the term "negative nitrogen balance?" How can such a problem be minimized?

References for Chapters 24 and 25

1. Abbey, J. C.: Nursing observations of fluid imbalance. *Nursing Clinics of North America* 3:77, March, 1968.
2. Affara, F. A.: Blood gases. Part 2. *Nursing Times* 69: 80, January 18, 1973.
3. Anthony, P.: Fluid imbalances—Formidable foes to survival. *American Journal of Nursing* 63:75, December, 1963.
4. Asperheim, M. K., and Eisenhauer, L. A.: *The Pharmacologic Basis of Patient Care.* 2nd ed. Philadelphia, W. B. Saunders Company, 1973.
5. Ayres, S. M., et al.: Pulmonary physiology at the bedside: Oxygen and carbon dioxide abnormalities. *Cardiovascular Nursing* 9:1, January/February, 1973.
6. Bartler, F.: Hyper- and hypo-osmolarity syndromes. *American Journal of Cardiology* 12:650, November, 1963.
7. Beland, I., et al.: *Clinical Nursing.* 2nd ed. New York, The Macmillan Company, 1970.
8. Best, C., and Taylor, N.: *The Physiological Basis of Medical Practice.* 8th ed. Baltimore, The Williams & Wilkins Company, 1966.
9. Betson, C.: Blood gases. *American Journal of Nursing* 68:1010, May, 1968.
10. Birch, C. A.: Aldosterone. Part III. *Nursing Times* 61: 502, April 9, 1965.
11. Borow, M.: The use of central venous pressure as an accurate guide for body fluid replacement. *Surgery, Gynecology and Obstetrics* 120:545, March, 1965.
12. Brainerd, H., et al.: *Current Diagnosis and Treatment.* Los Altos, California, Lange Medical Publishers, 1969.
13. Burgess, R. E.: Fluids and electrolytes. *American Journal of Nursing* 69:90, October, 1965.
14. Cerebral extracellular fluids in respiratory control. *Nursing Mirror,* February 9, 1968, p. 25.
15. Chapman, W. H., et al.: *Urinary System Syllabus.* Seattle, Washington, University of Washington Medical School, 1969.
16. Clack, B.: Intravenous infusions—Uses and contraindications. *Nursing Times* 63:1068, August 11, 1967.
17. Davenport, H. W.: *The ABC of Acid-Base Chemistry: The Elements of Physiological Blood-gas Chemistry for Medical Students and Physicians.* 5th ed. Chicago, University of Chicago Press, 1969.
18. Davenport, R.: Tube feeding for long term patients. *American Journal of Nursing* 64:121, January, 1964.
19. DeVeber, G. A.: Fluid and electrolyte problems in the postoperative period. *Nursing Clinics of North America* 1:275, June, 1966.
20. Dudrick, S. J., and Rhodes, J. E.: Total intravenous feeding. *Scientific American* 226:73, May 1972.
21. Dutcher, I., and Fielo, S.: *Water and Electrolytes: Implications for Nursing Practice.* New York, The Macmillan Company, 1967.
22. Dutcher, I. E., and Hardenburg, H. C.: Water and electrolyte imbalances. *In* Meltzer, L. E., Abdellah,

F. G., and Kitchell, J. R. (eds.): *Concepts and Practices of Intensive Care for Nurse Specialists.* Philadelphia, The Charles Press, Inc., 1969.

23. Fenton, M.: What to do about thirst. *American Journal of Nursing* 69:1014, May, 1969.
24. Fielo, S.: Teaching fluid and electrolyte balance. *Nursing Outlook,* March, 1965, pp. 43–44.
25. Fisch, C.: Relation of electrolyte disturbances to cardiac arrhythmias. *Circulation* 47:488, February, 1973.
26. Frisell, W. R.: *Acid-Base Chemistry in Medicine.* New York, The Macmillan Company, 1968.
27. Ganong, W. F.: *Review of Medical Physiology.* Los Altos, California, Lange Medical Publications, 1967.
28. Gantt, C. L.: Water and electrolyte disorders associated with renal vascular lesions. *Postgraduate Medicine* 40:344, September, 1966.
29. Gillies, J. C.: Fundamentals of surgery. 3: Fluid balance. *Nursing Times* 62:1493, November 11, 1966.
30. Grollman, A.: Diuretics. *American Journal of Nursing* 65:84, January, 1965.
31. Gumnit, R. J.: Fluids and electrolytes in the comatose patient. *Geriatrics* 21:131, August, 1966.
32. Gump, F. E., and Kinney, J. M.: Caloric and fluid losses through the burn wound. *Surgical Clinics of North America* 50:1235, December, 1970.
33. Gutman, R., and Burnell, J.: Paraldehyde acidosis. *American Journal of Medicine* 42:435, 1967.
34. Guyton, A. C.: *Textbook of Medical Physiology.* 4th ed. Philadelphia, W. B. Saunders Company, 1971.
35. Hallberg, D., et al.: Fat emulsion for complete intravenous nutrition. *Postgraduate Medicine* 42:A-149, November 19, 1967.
36. Harrington, J. T., and Lehmann, J., Jr.: The metabolic production and disposal of acid and alkali. *Medical Clinics of North America* 54:1543, November, 1970.
37. Heath, J. K.: A conceptual basis for assessing body water status. *Nursing Clinics of North America* 6:189, March, 1971.
38. Holmes, J. H.: Fluid intake with medication. *Archives of Internal Medicine* 116:813, November, 1965.
39. Johnson, G., Jr., et al.: Management of fluids and electrolytes in surgical patients. *Review of Surgery* (Philadelphia) 27:87–94, March-April, 1970.
40. Kassirer, J., and Schwartz, B.: Correction of metabolic alkalosis in man without repair of potassium deficiency. *American Journal of Medicine* 40:19, 1966.
41. Katsikas, J. L., and Goldsmith, C.: Disorders of potassium metabolism. *Medical Clinics of North America* 55:503, March, 1971.
42. Kee, J. L.: Fluid imbalance in elderly patients. *Nursing '73* 3:49, 1973.
43. Keitel, H. G.: A primer for understanding and recognizing fluid and electrolyte imbalances. *Consultant* 3:42–47, February, 1963.
44. Kerpal-Fronius, E.: Iatrogenic damage in fluid replacement therapy. *Triangle* 6:217, July, 1964.
45. Krieger, H.: Guides to electrolyte balance in the postoperative patient. *Hospital Medicine* 3:62, August, 1967.
46. Lapides, J.: Clinical signs of dehydration and extracellular fluid loss. *J.A.M.A.* 191:413, February 1, 1965.
47. Leonhardt, K. O.: Electrolyte, acid-base and water metabolism: An introduction for the anesthetist. *Journal of the American Association of Nurse Anesthetics* 35:429, December, 1967.
48. Liebenberg, J., et al.: Fluid therapy during surgery. *British Medical Journal* 4:494, November 22, 1969.

48a. Liechty, R. D., and Soper, R. T.: *Synopsis of Surgery.* 2nd ed. St. Louis, The C. V. Mosby Company. 1972.

49. Logothetis, J.: Neurological effects of water and sodium disturbances. 1. General mechanisms: Hypernatremic syndromes. *Postgraduate Medicine* 40:408, October, 1966.
50. Logothetis, J.: Neurologic effects of water and sodium disorders. 2. Hyponatremic syndromes and changes in blood volume. *Postgraduate Medicine* 40:621, November, 1966.
51. Luppi, A. P.: Homeostatic problems in general surgery. *California Medicine* 102:412, June, 1965.
52. MacConnachie, H. F.: An old-fashioned approach to acid-base balance. *American Journal of Medicine* 49:504, October, 1970.
53. Mason, E. E., and Liechty, R. D.: Fluids and electrolytes—Parenteral fluid orders. *In* Liechty, R. D., and Soper, R. T.: *Synopsis of Surgery.* St. Louis, The C. V. Mosby Company, 1968.
54. Medical Staff, Lilly Research Laboratories: Clinical application of fluid and electrolyte balance. *Physicians' Bulletin* 26:2, February, 1961.
55. Metheny, H. M., and Snively, W. D.: *Nurses' Handbook of Fluid Balance.* Philadelphia, J. B. Lippincott Co., 1967.
56. Moravec, D. F.: A review for nurses: The intravenous route of administration. *Hospital Management* 106:78–79, July, 1968.
57. Moravec, D. F.: A review of pharmacy for nurses: The nature of parenteral administration. *Hospital Management* 105:72, March, 1968.
58. Notter, D., et al.: *General Medicine.* Seattle, Washington, University of Washington School of Medicine, 1970.
59. Nuttall, F. Q.: Serum electrolytes and their relation to acid-base balance. *Archives of Internal Medicine* (Chicago), 116:670–680, November, 1965.
60. Pearson, J. B.: Water and electrolyte balance. *Nursing Times* 63:415, March 31, 1967.
61. Potassium imbalance. Programmed instruction, *American Journal of Nursing* 67:343, February, 1967.
62. Reed, G. M., and Sheppard, V. F.: *Regulation of Fluid and Electrolyte Balance: A Programmed Instruction in Physiology for Nurses.* Philadelphia, W. B. Saunders Company, 1971.
63. Reese, L.: Fluid and electrolyte therapy in the adult. *Applied Therapeutics* 7:719, September, 1965.
64. Rothe, C. F.: Fluid dynamics. *In* Selkurt, E. (ed.): *Physiology.* 2nd ed. Boston, Little, Brown and Company, 1966.
65. Rubini, M. E., and Chojnacki, R. E.: Principles of parenteral therapy. *American Journal of Clinical Nutrition* 25:96, January, 1972.
66. Schneider, W. J., and Boyce, B. A.: Complications of diuretic therapy. *American Journal of Nursing* 68:1903, September, 1967.
67. Scribner, B. H. (ed.): *University of Washington Teaching Syllabus for the Course on Fluid and Electrolyte Balance.* 7th ed. Seattle, University of Washington School of Medicine, 1969.
68. Seizures and hypoparathyroidism. *J.A.M.A.* 201:123, August 28, 1967.
69. Shaw, D. H.: Potassium and water distribution in depression. *British Journal of Psychiatry* 112:269, March, 1966.

70. Shields, R.: Surgical aspects of the absorption of water and electrolytes by the intestine. *Monographs in the Surgical Sciences* 1:119, June, 1964.
71. Snively, W. D.: Toward a better understanding of body fluid disturbances. *Nursing Forum* 3:60, 1964.
72. Snively, W. D., and Westerman, R. L.: The clinician views potassium deficit. *Minnesota Medicine* 48: 713, June, 1965.
73. Stevenson, J. A. F.: Current concepts of the regulation of water and salt exchange. *Applied Therapeutics* 7:713, September, 1965.
74. Strydon, N. B., and Holdsworth, L. D.: The water requirements of humans. *Journal of Occupational Medicine* 7:581, November, 1965.
75. Swartz, C. D.: Post-operative fluid and electrolyte management in the elderly. *Geriatrics* 22:231, March, 1967.
76. Tranquada, R., et al.: Lactic acidosis. *Archives of Internal Medicine* 117:192, February, 1966.
78. Vanderwerf, C. A.: *Acids, Bases, and the Chemistry of the Covalent Bond.* New York, Reinhold Publishing Corporation, 1964.
79. Verne, D.: Water and electrolyte balance: A review. *Journal of Oral Surgery* 23:609, November, 1965.
80. Waddy, F. F.: Intravenous injections and infusions. *Nursing Times,* October 13, 1967, p. 1361.
81. Weisberg, H. F.: Parenteral fluid therapy in adults. *In* Conn, H. F. (ed.): *Current Therapy 1969*. Philadelphia, W. B. Saunders Company, 1969.
82. Westerman, R., and Snively, W.: Potassium deficit: Clinical aspects. *General Practitioner* 33:85, June, 1966.
83. Williams, F. H.: Potassium overdose. A potential hazard of non-rigid parenteral fluid containers. *British Medical Journal* 1:714, March, 1973.
84. Williams, J. T., and Moravec, D. F.: Intravenous therapy: Intravenous additives. Part 12. *Hospital Management* 102:57, December, 1966.
85. Williams, S. R.: *Nutrition and Diet Therapy.* St. Louis, The C. V. Mosby Company, 1969.
86. Winters, R. W.: Terminology of acid-base disorders. *Annals of Internal Medicine* 63:873–884, November, 1965.
87. Wolf, A. V.: Thirst. *Scientific American* 194:70, 1956.

CHAPTER 26

Physiologic Shock

Active research interest in shock dates back to the early years of this century. Awareness of the clinical problem existed much before this. The history of this long effort to determine the true nature of the syndrome provides eloquent testimony to its inherent complexity. For at this moment, the critical shock mechanism still remains an elusive entity.[32]

INTRODUCTION AND STUDY GUIDE

"Is the patient going into shock? Is he already in shock?" A nurse often asks herself these critical questions as she gives patient care.

> *In its most basic sense, shock is a generalized state of inadequate circulation.*

The patient in shock, or threatening to go into shock, is seriously ill; the nurse must act rapidly and precisely to protect him from the complications and possible fatal outcome of his condition.

It is thought that 100,000 deaths and an unknown number of permanent injuries occur annually in the United States from shock. As recently as 1967 it was estimated that 9 to 10 per cent of persons who go into shock fail to recover.[53] Therefore, the nurse must promptly recognize and treat symptoms of *early* circulatory failure before severe shock ensues.

Let us emphasize to the reader that most of the research conducted on shock mechanisms and treatment is based upon hemorrhagic or traumatic shock. This chapter thus focuses on these forms of shock. Much less information is available regarding shock associated with myocardial infarction than other categories of shock, largely because of the absence of any satisfactory laboratory animal models. Therefore, myocardial shock is often excluded from general discussions of shock, and is only briefly discussed in this chapter.

Because of the basically lethal nature of shock, research on shock is usually performed with laboratory animals rather than human subjects. This poses problems in determining which aspects of the experimental data are valid for application to the treatment of shock in man. Nevertheless, it is believed that the basic hemodynamic disturbances caused by prolonged shock, whatever the cause, are similar in the dog (used experimentally), in man, or in any other of the mammalian species. Apparently the differences among various members of the species lie in the susceptibility of differing tissues to the basic hemodynamic disturbances shared by them all.[46]

We shall discuss four different types of shock: (1) hematogenic, (2) cardiogenic, (3) neurogenic, and (4) vasogenic. Because shock varies in form it is technically more accurate to refer to specific types of shock, or "patterns of shock,"[6] instead of making broad, general references to "shock." Nonetheless, shock is often discussed in a broad sense in medical literature and in clinical situations. In these instances, *"shock" in general terms refers to a state of generalized inadequate circulation which causes decreased perfusion of the body tissues with blood and produces a wide range of systemic effects.*

Shock may arise from many different etiologies since it can be an untoward effect of numerous disease conditions. Moreover, shock usually is a complex phenomenon to treat because its initiating factors are often multiple, e.g., physical injury plus blood loss plus infection. In addition, each patient's general physical status and medical background are unique, and the physiologic responses of different individuals to similar noxious events are never the same.[19]

In studying the clinical syndrome commonly called "shock," you, as a nurse, will be concerned with three major factors: (1) patients' responses to the particular insults leading to shock (e.g., traumatic hemorrhage); (2) their responses to the shock episode itself; and (3) the nature of those responses that determine whether recovery will be possible.

In reading this chapter, the following study guide should be helpful:

> Identify major groups of shock and state examples of each group.

> In your own words state the major physiologic problems that contribute to irreversible shock.

> Recall the compensatory body mechanisms that operate to combat shock and how these "defenses" can both help and harm the individual in shock.

> Review the major changes that occur during shock in: the microcirculation; the blood; the reticuloendothelial system; the liver, intestines, kidneys, and lungs. Also, review fluid shifts that occur during shock, and the metabolic problems that develop owing to inadequate tissue perfusion.

> Familiarize yourself with the various signs and symptoms of shock.

> In what position should the patient in shock be placed? What are the advantages and disadvantages of vasopressor drugs and of vasodilator drugs in treating

shock? Why might adrenocorticoids and antibiotics be administered to a patient in shock? What treatment may be necessary to provide cardiac support, renal support, and respiratory support? Why is fluid replacement so highly important in the treatment of shock? What are some of the factors evaluated in deciding whether fluid replacement is adequate? Why is fluid replacement frequently in excess of the estimated fluid loss?

CIRCULATION: A BRIEF REVIEW

Several major components or divisions make up the circulatory system: namely, the heart, the large blood vessels, and the microcirculation.* Each of these major subdivisions is, in a sense, designed for and concerned with separate and distinct intrinsic activities. Therefore, each of these subdivisions encompasses a separate area of homeostasis.[31] However, *the circulation is a closed system,† and all parts of the circulation are interdependent, so that an alteration in one part will have an effect on the other parts.*[71]

The operational activities of the heart and large blood vessels are regulated by the vasomotor center of the brain, the autonomic nervous pathways, and the monitoring devices (baroreceptors and chemoreceptors)** located in the walls of the heart, and the large vessels. Regulation of the microcirculation, however, is a different matter.

Once the blood flow passes "the arteriolar floodgates"[31] and enters the tissues proper by way of the microcirculation, it is regulated by a completely new set of devices that are primarily of a chemical nature. The microcirculation is governed locally by those substances that are "liberated into the local tissue environment by the metabolic activities of its literally millions of cells."[31] Such local regulation gives the body a sensitive, discriminating mechanism by means of which the blood flow can be adjusted according to the needs of the tissues from one moment to another.

For adequate circulation of blood the following three basic factors must function effectively together: (1) *vascular tone,* or resistance of the blood vessels; (2) *blood volume,* or the total amount of blood in the body; and (3) *cardiac pump,* or the pumping action of the heart.

When the body is in a state of health the volume of the blood, the size of the vascular bed (as determined by vasoconstriction and vasodilation), and the cardiac muscle pump action are all operating in balance with one another. This balanced situation is referred to as a state of "dynamic equilibrium"; that is, all parts of the body are receiving the amount of blood that they need to sustain circulatory health.[6]

As long as two of the basic components are able to maintain satisfactory compensatory action, adequate circulation of the blood can be maintained even though the third component may not be functioning normally. Thus, if one function fails, other parts of the system will put compensatory mechanisms into effect: e.g., vascular tone may increase (thereby causing vasoconstriction and reduced vascular capacity), cardiac pump action may increase, or blood volume may increase. However, when compensatory mechanisms fail or when more than one of the three components malfunction, circulatory failure results, throwing the individual into a state of shock.

DEFINITIONS AND BASIC PATHOLOGY OF SHOCK

> From the earliest recognition of shock as an entity, attempts to define it have been almost as difficult as attempts to determine its mechanisms.[25]

Much confusion exists concerning the definition and classification of shock. The word "shock" is commonly used to refer to a *group* of signs and symptoms that could be caused by a *variety* of disorders, such as hemorrhage, infarction, or coronary thrombosis. One general definition of shock is presented herewith:

> Shock *is an abnormal physiologic state in which there is a disproportion between the circulating blood volume and the size of the vascular bed, resulting in circulatory failure and anoxia.*[6]

In most cases of shock the decreased perfusion of the microcirculation is caused by a fall in the cardiac output. A variety of factors may be responsible for this fall in cardiac output: (1) the myocardium itself may fail, as in coronary thrombosis; (2) the heart chambers may not fill adequately, as in cardiac tamponade; or (3) there may be a decrease in the amount of blood returned to the heart by way of the great veins. Decreased venous return to the heart may be due to: (a) an increase in the volume capacity of the veins themselves (that is, vasodilation), as in septic shock which is secondary to severe infection; or (b) an actual deficit of available blood, as in shock due to hemorrhage or wounds.[71]

Various situations obviously can occur within the body that disrupt adequate vascular tone, adequate blood volume, and/or cardiac pump action. The events of these vicious circles are shown diagrammatically in Figure 26–1. Failure of both the respiratory and circulatory systems contributes to progressive circulatory failure. Circulatory

---

*Terms used interchangeably with "microcirculation" are "peripheral circulation," "capillary circulation," and "terminal vascular bed."[32]

†Blood does not actually come into direct contact with the cells, other than those lining the blood vessels, except in the sinusoids of the liver and in the spleen.[71]

***Baroreceptors* are sensory nerve terminals that are stimulated by changes in pressure. *Chemoreceptors* are receptors or sense organs that are excited by chemical substances.

failure produces ischemia of the tissues. This may result in death if the ischemia is so severe or prolonged that the cells are unable to continue with the metabolic activities (e.g., nutrition, elimination of wastes) that are necessary to sustain life.

CLASSIFICATIONS OF SHOCK

Although shock can be classified in several different ways, one concise classification is that proposed by Blalock in 1934 and modified by Bordicks:[6]

1. *Hematogenic shock* (decreased blood volume)
   A. Hemorrhagic shock (loss of whole blood)
   B. Burn shock (loss of plasma fluids and electrolytes)
   C. Diabetic shock, acidosis (loss of fluids and electrolytes from all three body compartments)
2. *Cardiogenic shock* (failure of the heart to pump adequately)
   A. Left myocardial infarction
3. *Neurogenic shock* and *vasogenic shock* (an increased size in the vascular bed)
   A. Neurogenic shock
      1. Spinal anesthesia shock
      2. Insulin shock
   B. Vasogenic shock
      1. Anaphylactic shock
      2. Toxic shock

As you will observe, this classification is based upon the three previously discussed predominant physiologic mechanisms that support adequate circulation: blood volume, cardiac pump action, and vascular tone.

In *hematogenic shock* the primary cause is a marked *decreased volume of blood,* so that the metabolic needs of the body cannot be met. Any condition that can cause a marked reduction in the blood volume can cause hematogenic shock; some prime examples are:

> *Hemorrhagic shock,* which is a loss of whole blood. Shock will develop fully in a previously healthy person when he has lost about one third of his normal blood volume. The loss of smaller amounts of blood may result in shock in persons less able to compensate rapidly.

> *Burn shock,* also referred to as "electrolyte shock" or "plasma loss shock," is primarily caused by the rapid shift of plasma fluid from the vascular compartment, across heat-damaged capillaries, and into the interstitial compartments and/or the burned area's surface. Also, with burn shock there is a loss of plasma, fluid, and electrolytes from all three body compartments—plasma from the vascular compartment, sodium from the vascular and interstitial compartments (ECF), and potassium from the intracellular compartment.

Regardless of the cause of large losses of plasma the result is always decreased blood volume and a greatly increased viscosity of the blood, which also adds to the slowness of blood flow.

Burn or electrolyte shock can also be produced in other conditions, e.g., *fistulas* and *diarrhea.* Other disorders in which the loss of plasma may be profuse are: severe venous obstruction, nephrotic syndrome, intestinal obstruction, starvation (nutritional hypovolemia), and severe trauma.

> *Diabetic shock* (acidosis, coma) consists of metabolic acidosis and severe dehydration of all three body compartments—intracellular, interstitial, and vascular. Without insulin replacement, death may result. Once the insulin-glucose-water-electrolyte balance is restored, those metabolic deficiencies that result from insulin insufficiency (dehydration and reduced cellular utilization of glucose for energy) will be corrected.

Cardiogenic shock (also called "cardiac shock") results from *failure of the cardiac muscle pump.* When the heart muscle can no longer perform adequately (i.e., heart failure) it can no longer pump blood in sufficient amounts to all parts of the body. As with all forms of shock, cardiogenic shock results ultimately in deficiencies in cellular supplies and the removal of wastes.

Left myocardial failure is the most common cause of cardiogenic shock. For example, if there is an occlusion of a left coronary artery, then an adequate supply of blood cannot reach areas of the left myocardium (*left myocardial infarction*). As a result of tissue hypoxia and lack of nutrients, the left heart muscle becomes increasingly weak and unable to contract forcefully. Blood dams up in the left atrium and left ventricle of the heart and in the pulmonary venous circuit. Pulmonary congestion, pulmonary hypoxia, and marked dyspnea occur.

Neurogenic shock and *vasogenic shock* are types of shock that result from inadequate vascular tone. Both these forms of shock are caused by an *increase in the size of the vascular bed due to massive vasodilatation.* In both patterns of shock the blood volume remains "normal"; therefore, a disproportion occurs because the normal amount of blood cannot adequately fill the increased size of the capillary area.

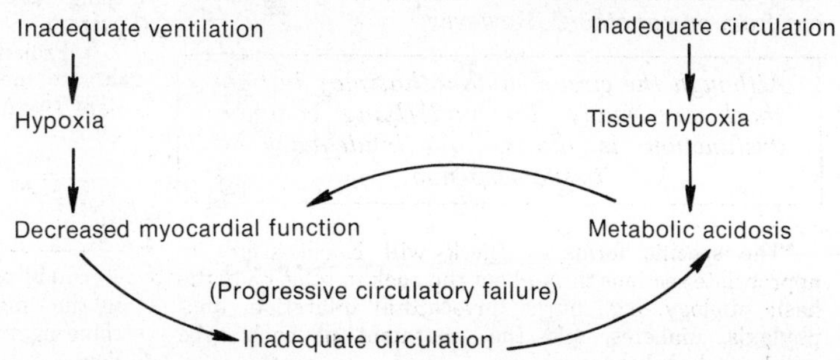

FIGURE 26–1. Progressive circulatory failure in shock. (From Vandermeer, B. L.: *Journal of the American Association of Anesthetists.* April 1965.)

Following this extensive vasodilatation there are decreased blood pressure, decreased return of venous blood to the heart, and decreased cardiac output. The end result of these developments is, as in other forms of shock, tissue anoxia and, ultimately, cell destruction.

Although vasodilatation occurs in both neurogenic and vasogenic shock, the mechanisms that cause the vasodilation differ: Neurogenic shock results from a diminished vasomotor tone, hence, a diminished vasoconstrictor tone that produces vasodilatation throughout the body.

Vasogenic shock results from loss of vasomotor activity caused by toxic substances acting directly on the blood vessels, producing vasodilatation.

Neurogenic shock is caused by dilation of the blood vessels secondary to nervous factors. Among the possible causes are: brain damage, deep general anesthesia, spinal anesthesia, and fainting.

Vasogenic shock is caused by dilation of the blood vessels brought about by humoral (vasoactive) substances. Two examples of vasogenic shock are *anaphylactic shock* and *toxic shock* (also known as bacterial shock, septic shock, bacteremic shock, endotoxic shock, or exotoxic shock).

Insulin shock can be classified as either cardiogenic or neurogenic shock. You will recall that diabetic shock is caused by hyperglycemia, which results from too little insulin (hypoinsulinism) in the body. In insulin shock we find hypoglycemia resulting from too much insulin (hyperinsulinism) in the body. Both the heart and central nervous system are adversely affected by hyperinsulinism. The metabolism of glucose provides essentially all the energy for the central nervous system. Among other problems caused by hyperinsulinism, the vasomotor nerves lose their ability to maintain the tonus of the blood vessels, and vasodilatation with hypotension results.

We have just reviewed some broad basic patterns of shock (hematogenic, cardiogenic, neurogenic, and vasogenic), each of which has a different primary etiology. Of course, some cases of shock are due to combinations of problems and do not fit into a single category. It is becoming increasingly clear that the *initial clinical course and the initial treatment of the various primary events causing shock* (e.g., hemorrhage, infection, coronary thrombosis, immune reaction) *are quite different from one another.** However:

> *Although the circumstances that may initiate shock are many, the underlying common dysfunction is always an inadequacy of tissue perfusion.*

*The specific forms of shock will be discussed in appropriate sections throughout the book in relation to the basic etiology, e.g., burns, myocardial infarction, anaphylaxis, diabetes, and the treatment of each type will be included there.

STAGES OF SHOCK

Shock is a dynamic condition in which a patient's status is constantly changing; its progression can be divided into stages for easier discussion:[25]

Initial Stage. The cardiac output is insufficient to supply the normal nutritional needs of the body's tissues, but it is not low enough to cause serious symptoms.

Compensatory Stage. The cardiac output is reduced further, but because of compensatory vasoconstriction, the blood pressure tends to remain within a normal range. Blood flow to the skin and kidneys decreases, while blood flow to the central nervous system and the myocardium tends to be maintained. A decrease occurs in the blood reservoirs.

Progressive Stage. The unfavorable changes become more and more apparent: falling blood pressure, increasing vasoconstriction, increased heart rate, oliguria. The compensatory mechanisms are unable to cope with the reduced cardiac output and, therefore, the status quo is not maintained. During this stage, the shock becomes progressively more severe, even though the initial cause of the shock is not itself becoming more severe. In other words, intrinsic factors in the person, aside from the original cause of the shock, are causing his condition to deteriorate.

Irreversible Stage. In the final stage of shock no type of therapy can save the patient's life. There is myocardial depression and a loss of arteriolar tonus, and infused blood tends to remain in the dilated capillary bed.

A variety of physiologic events occur in shock that set up various feedback patterns that can lead to progression of shock (Fig. 26–2).

PHYSIOLOGIC EFFECTS OF SHOCK

The reduced blood flow through the tissues during the shock syndrome, by its very nature, impinges on almost every facet of homeostasis.[93]

Some of the physiologic mechanisms believed to be responsible for the development of irreversible shock leading to death are:

> Cardiac failure and "shock lung."

> Failure of the microcirculation and pooling of blood.

> Sludged blood† combined with resulting intravascular aggregation, agglutination, and thrombosis.

> The release of toxic products and/or bacteria from the liver, muscle, and/or intestine.

> Metabolic derangements; loss of the liver's detoxifying abilities; depression of the reticuloendothelial system.

> Prolonged vasoconstriction, causing visceral damage due to mechanical limitation of blood flow and attendant stagnant anoxia; tissue necrosis and cellular death.

†Sludging of the blood refers to a situation occurring in the smaller blood vessels in which the red cells become aggregated into masses, thereby slowing the blood flow.

NEUROENDOCRINE AND OTHER TYPES OF DEFENSES DURING SHOCK[6]

The neuroendocrine responses during shock are bodily defensive reactions that occur during the stage of resistance of the general adaptation syndrome (GAS) discussed in Unit II. Remember that the length of the stage of resistance varies from one individual to another and is determined by the individual body's ability to compensate for its deficiencies. Therefore, one patient may be able to combat shock for a longer period of time than another. For example, a previously healthy person will have a longer stage of resistance against shock than a previously debilitated person.

Keep in mind that:

> *The main purposes of the body's defenses in shock are to: (1) establish a depot of readily available energy, and (2) to maintain a state of circulatory balance so that the vital organs will have the blood needed for life.*

Some basic features of the neuroendocrine responses to shock follow:

> The body is prepared for "fight or flight" and, economically, *supports vital body functions.*

> Under the control of the sympathetic nervous system, the adrenal medulla releases two hormones (norepinephrine and epinephrine) that produce effects similar to those caused by direct sympathetic stimulation (e.g., *vasoconstriction* and *increased heart rate*).

> The anterior pituitary secretes ACTH, which stimulates the adrenal cortex to produce mineralocorticoids (which act generally to *control fluid and electrolyte balance*), and glucocorticoids (which mainly *affect energy and tissue resistance*). The antidiuretic hormone (ADH) is secreted by the posterior pituitary.

Generally the hormonal response to stress results in the rapid provision of fuel for the body's various tissues, organs, and systems. These fuels (e.g., amino acids, fatty acids, glucose, sodium, and water) are produced by breaking food down into sugars, fatty acids, and amino acids that are converted into energy by a chemical process, resulting in the formation of adenosine triphosphate (ATP), the main source of energy produced and used inside the body's cells.

The glucocorticoids, particularly hydrocortisone, *mobilize energy stores.* During the initial period of shock the small stores of available carbohydrate are rapidly depleted and it becomes necessary to mobilize protein and fat stores to meet the body's energy requirements. Protein catabolism and negative nitrogen balance occur as a part of the metabolic response, as a result of gluconeogenesis (resulting from glucocorticoid action) and starvation.

The *sympathetic nervous system* and the hormones of the *adrenal medulla* initially help to maintain the arterial blood pressure. The adrenal medulla secretes epinephrine in copious amounts in response to stress; this substance accelerates the heart rate. This *increased heart rate* works together initially with *increased peripheral vascular resistance* (caused by vasoconstriction resulting from stimulation by the sympathetic nervous system) to maintain the body's blood pressure.

The veins are a reservoir for blood and, thus, the initial constriction of the veins in shock remedies

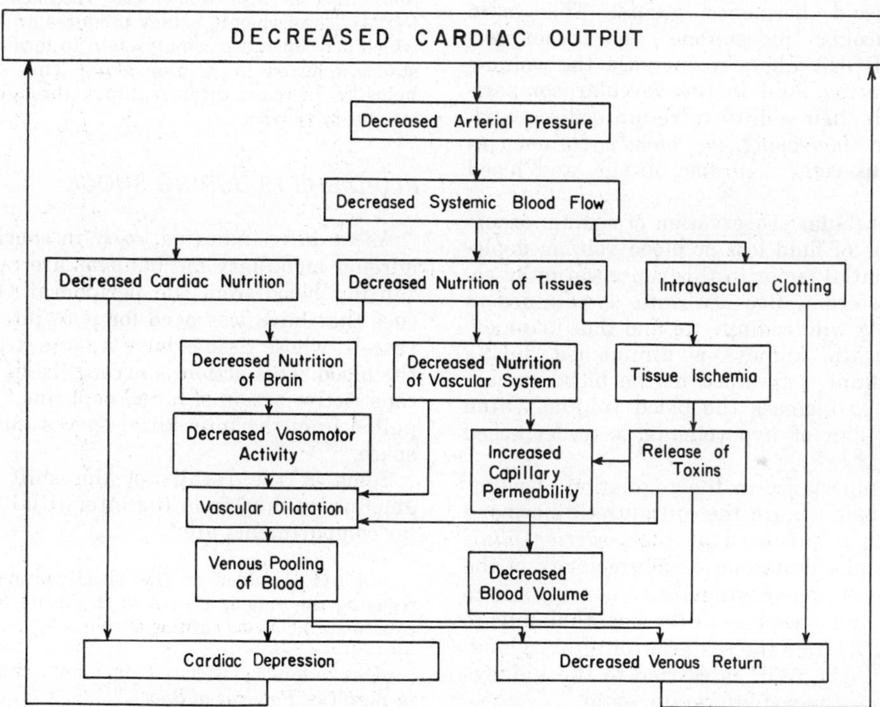

FIGURE 26–2. Different types of feedback that can lead to progression of shock. (From Guyton, A. C.: *Textbook of Medical Physiology*, 4th ed. 1971.)

the slack in the circulating blood volume by squeezing blood into the circulation from the venous reservoir. The resultant *increased venous return* to the heart may be as great as two-and-a-half-fold. Consequently the heart has more blood to pump back out into the circulation since it can pump only the amount of blood that it receives from the venous circuit.

With the development of shock, the blood pressure generally tends to drop, owing to an inadequate circulating volume of blood and decreased cardiac output. As a result of the decline in blood pressure, a reflex *compensatory vasoconstriction* occurs that is initially helpful but dangerous if prolonged. Vasoconstriction does provide some protection for such "high priority" organs as the brain and the heart. Also, the increased heart rate, increased peripheral resistance, and the addition of blood volume from reservoirs all help initially to maintain the blood pressure in shock.

The *vasoconstrictive activity that is triggered by the sympathico-adrenal system is harmful if it is sustained,* for it further decreases the microcirculation through most tissues and organs of the body. "While it is of immediate survival value, this reaction cannot continue for longer than a few minutes because of the resulting metabolic derangement."[71] It can be seen that if the shock state is prolonged, serious problems ensue, and reactions that are initially helpful, such as vasoconstriction, may actually become life-threatening.

Increased production of the adrenocortical and mineralocorticoid hormones occurs. The main mineralocorticoids, aldosterone and desoxycorticosterone (DOCA), help to increase the volume of the circulating fluid in the vascular compartment through their ability to retain sodium and, hence, water. *Increasing the blood's volume* increases venous return, cardiac output, and blood pressure.

The renal tubular conservation of sodium occurs with any type of fluid loss or blood volume depletion. An essential factor in this conservation of sodium is aldosterone. Because water is retained in the body along with sodium, we find that urine excretion from the kidneys is diminished during shock. This fluid is retained in the blood stream in an effort to increase the blood volume. Often the earliest sign of hypovolemia is a decreased urine volume.

Of major importance in the regulation of water and sodium balance are the antidiuretic hormone (ADH), which is produced by the *posterior pituitary gland,* and aldosterone. The osmolarity of the blood increases in dehydration states, causing stimulation of the osmoreceptors in the hypothalamus to release the ADH from the posterior pituitary gland. Via the blood, the ADH is carried to the kidneys where it causes the body to retain water.

Other Compensatory Mechanisms

In addition to the responses of the sympathetic nervous system and the adrenal glands to shock, many other compensatory factors operate initially in shock in an attempt to maintain the blood volume. Some of these mechanisms and their actions in hemorrhagic shock are outlined below:*

Red Bone Marrow. Stimulated by the hypoxic effects produced by a decreased blood volume, the red bone marrow produces and *releases additional red blood cells into the circulation.* An increased oxygen-carrying power is made available with the increased number of red cells. Because the red cell formation takes place at an abnormally rapid speed, immature red cells are passed into the blood stream. Immature red cells have less oxygen-carrying power than mature red cells, however, for the hemoglobin content of red blood cells increases with the cells' maturity.

Liver and Spleen. *Extra red cells* are squeezed into the circulation by the liver and spleen.

Interstitial Compartment. *Fluid passes from the interstitial compartment into the vascular compartment.* (See later.)

Carbon Dioxide. Increased carbon dioxide *dilates the arterioles located in active tissues and constricts those in nonactive tissues.* Because the heart is the most active tissue at this time, excessive CO_2 is produced in the myocardium. This directly dilates the coronary arteries leading to the myocardium and thereby allows this tissue to receive more arterial blood (with its oxygen and nutrients). CO_2 is also a powerful stimulant of the vasoconstrictor center in the sympathetic nervous system. With vasoconstriction of nonactive tissues, the blood is shunted to the more active tissues which have a greater immediate need of it.

Kidneys. A renal pressor substance (RPS) is released by the kidneys into the blood stream as a result of renal arteriolar vasoconstriction, regulated by sympatho-adrenal medullary mechanisms. RPS increases the tone of arterioles and thus *aids in arteriolar constriction.* RPS is also known as vasoexcitor mechanism (VEM). The ischemic kidney produces an enzyme, renin, which acts upon a plasma protein to form a pressor substance referred to as *angiotonin.* This substance also helps to increase cardiac output through its vasoconstrictor properties.

FLUID SHIFTS DURING SHOCK

As we have indicated, *early* in shock, sympatho-adrenal medullary mechanisms are responsible for shifting blood from the peripheral vessels of tissues that have less need for it to internal visceral vessels, whose tissues have a more urgent need for the blood. This action is accomplished by the vasoconstrictive action of norepinephrine.[6] Also, fluid is pulled from the interstitial spaces into the venous space.

Some of the results of the shift of excessive amounts of fluid from the interstitial to the vascular compartments are:[6]

> Fluid is added to the blood volume, thereby increasing the venous return to the heart which, in turn, causes an increased cardiac output.

---

*This summary is based upon information presented in Bordicks: *Patterns of Shock.*[6]

> Although the fluid from the interstitial compartment expands the volume of blood, it also causes a hemodilution of the blood.

> Also, the interstitial compartment becomes markedly depleted of fluid, producing tissue dehydration.

> Laboratory findings at the time of this hemodilution and tissue dehydration are: decreased red blood cells, decreased hematocrit, decreased plasma proteins, hyperglycemia, acidosis, hypochloremia, elevated blood urea nitrogen, increased polymorphonuclear leukocytes.

> The patient experiences the signs and symptoms of dehydration, e.g., thirst, dry and cracked lips, and dry mucous membranes.

During the *later* stages of shock a serious problem is that if vasoconstriction is prolonged, it increases the pressure in the capillaries and thus forces fluid to be lost from the vascular compartment into the interstitial compartment.[56] One phenomenon consistently associated with the later stages of hemorrhagic shock is the presumed loss of extracellular fluid into the wall and the lumen of the bowel. This causes liquid, bloody stools.[67]

CARDIAC FUNCTION DURING SHOCK

Basically there are two causes of decreased cardiac output: cardiac depression, and decreased venous return. Any circulatory change that initially decreases the cardiac output can lead to progressive shock, e.g., hemorrhage, anaphylaxis, septicemia, dehydration. Also, a variety of disorders can cause the heart to fail as a pump, e.g., myocardial infarction, heart rate arrhythmias, cardiac tamponade, or a massive pulmonary embolism that obstructs blood flow from the right ventricle.

The heart appears to deteriorate severely as shock progresses; this deterioration is one of the major causes of death. Once the heart has deteriorated beyond a certain level, irreversible shock occurs and the patient's life cannot be saved. Cardiac deterioration may not be detected until almost terminal conditions have developed, because cardiac depression is frequently masked by the tremendous cardiac reserve of the normal individual. Because of this reserve, the heart can deteriorate to less than one third, or sometimes less than one fifth, of its normal pumping strength without any measurable evidence of cardiac failure.

THE MICROCIRCULATION DURING SHOCK

Shock does not develop because the circulation is impaired in one specific organ but, rather, the common denominator in the problem is the fact that the microcirculation in *all* organs is decompensated.[21]

The portion of the cardiovascular system between the arteriole and the venule is termed the *microcirculation*.[2] It is this portion of the cardiovascular system that comes into intimate contact with the cellular elements of the body, for the microcirculation is the end point of the transport system of the blood vessels. It is through the vessels of the microcirculation that tissue environment is maintained, since it brings nutrition to the tissues and removes waste products.

The microcirculation is the largest organic unit of the body, encompassing some 60,000 miles of vascular channels and containing well over 90 per cent of all the blood vessels in the body. Because of its very size, the microcirculation can disrupt the functioning of the entire body; if these small vessels are unable to operate properly, in even a relatively small area, serious problems may develop.[21, 31]

Capillaries are so widely distributed that no cell is more than 25 to 50 μ away from a capillary. However, in spite of the fact that the microcirculation has an enormous *potential* capacity, normally the capillaries are relatively ischemic, containing only some 6 to 7 per cent of the body's volume of blood. As a general rule, the flow of blood through the capillary bed is influenced by the particular needs at any given time of the cells that are located by (juxtaposed to) the vessel.[21, 31] The capillaries open in rotation upon demand of the cells adjacent to them. For example, when they become anoxic, the mast cells secrete histamine to cause the capillary sphincters to open.[27, 30]

While the body's larger blood vessels are regulated by the autonomic nervous system, this is not true of the microcirculation. Arteriole and capillary sphincters are separate mechanisms that are governed by different controls. The muscle located in the microcirculation is highly sensitive and is capable of producing behavior that is precise and well coordinated and that governs the various pathways of blood flow through the capillary bed.

Microcirculatory insufficiency is the final common sequence of events caused by the basic etiologic mechanisms that precipitate shock; peripheral vascular failure or microcirculatory failure is, therefore, a phenomenon common to all the etiologic factors in various forms of shock.[16] Microcirculatory failure (i.e., peripheral vascular failure) consists physiologically of two sets of factors: microvessel dysfunction, and dysfunction of the tissues that lie closest to these vessels. These two components are functionally inseparable and act in an interdependent manner.

Regardless of the initiating circumstances, or the level of impact, an identical sequence of events occurs within the microcirculation.[31] These events are shown diagrammatically in Figure 26–3.

One of the most striking characteristics of the microcirculation is its autonomy as a functional entity. The microcirculation's patterns of behavior, in both normal and abnormal environmental situations, are notably independent of those vasomotor influences that affect the major divisions of the circulatory system lying next to it (i.e., the systemic circulation). It is noteworthy that the systemic circulatory bed and the microcirculatory bed do not appear to have developed sensing devices; thus, events taking place within one bed do not effectively modulate or influence the events in the other. As we shall next see: *the relative autonomy of the microcirculation and the lack of modulation between the systemic circulation and the microcirculation are critical factors in determining the ultimate course of events in shock.*[31]

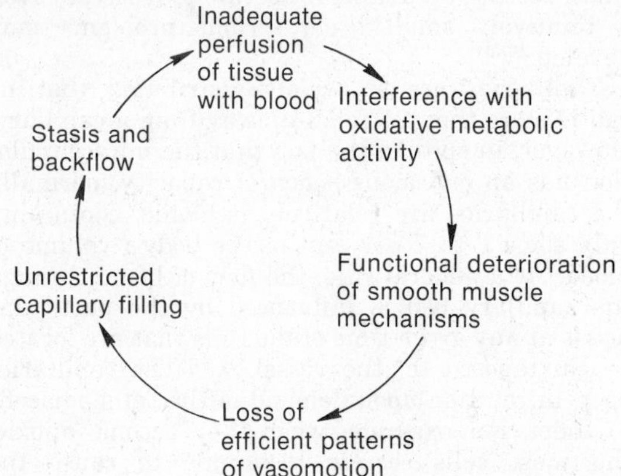

FIGURE 26–3. Microcirculatory hemodynamic events in shock.

> With the *onset* of shock, during the compensatory phase, the systemic circulation and the microcirculation work together. Both undergo an overall readjustment in which their activities are *coordinated* and are operating to preserve the entire system. The heart and the large vessels accomplish their part in this coordinated effort by *cardioacceleration* (increased heart rate) and *vasoconstriction;* the microcirculation acts by altering its patterns of vasomotion to pass the blood through the microcirculation as rapidly as possible so that it can be returned more efficiently to the venous reservoir.

> As the state of shock *progresses,* however, the compensatory phase cannot be maintained, and the blood flow becomes inadequate to meet the tissues' minimal needs. The systemic circulation and the microcirculation begin to function in *opposite directions,* opposing one another in an *uncoordinated* manner. The systemic circulation sustains its initial compensatory readjustment (vasoconstriction) while the microbed does not and, thus, the response of the circulation as a whole is no longer coordinated. Specifically, the microcirculation dilates and reverses its adjustment from that of an effort to curtail blood flow toward actually trying to secure more of the limited supply of available blood for itself. The blood supply is thereby progressively sequestered in the capillary beds, i.e., the blood is said to "pool" in the microcirculation. Because the cells demand greater perfusion time, many or most of the capillaries remain open at any one time, thus increasing the vascular space.[21, 27, 30, 31]

> "An increase in the vascular capacity, a decrease in the blood volume, or decreased heart action will reduce the mean circulatory pressure.* In turn, the pressure gradient for the venous return of blood is decreased, which results in a venous 'pooling' of blood, a decreased venous return to the heart, and decreased cardiac output."[6]

In the absence of modulating feedback mechanisms, the process described becomes progressively more severe, resulting in total circulatory disruption. Once the vascular space is enlarged, as a result of vasodilatation of the microcirculation, even a normal blood volume is insufficient to fill all these small vessels and also leave enough remaining volume to fill the veins. A low central venous pressure and inadequate venous return to the right heart result, with a further decrease in cardiac output.[27, 30]

BLOOD FACTORS DURING SHOCK[44]

Relationships have been established between the degree of hemorrhagic shock and derangements in various blood factors. (See Table 26–1.) For example, the degree of shock is more than slight when a third of the blood volume is lost; a severe degree of shock exists when one half of the blood volume has been lost. The loss of hemoglobin also parallels the degree of shock; however, the percentage of hemoglobin loss is typically greater than the volume loss.[21]

Some of the more important alterations in blood composition during shock are changes in hemostatic (blood coagulation) and immunologic mechanisms, in the content of various vasoactive substances, and in the levels of certain hormones.

Coagulation. During shock some anoxia of tissues results from the slow movement of blood in the capillaries, and anaerobic metabolism (see later) begins, causing an increase in the production of lactic acid. The slow-moving, acid blood is *hypercoagulable.* The blood, however, will not actually coagulate unless some clot-initiating factor is present. Such factors include bacterial toxins and thromboplastin of red blood cells liberated by hemolysis. Hemolysis accompanies trauma, especially trauma which causes massive crushing. When any of these factors is present, along with the stagnant acid blood of shock, widespread (disseminated) clotting occurs in the vessels. This, in turn, causes a clotting defect resulting in possible capillary oozing if a wound is present, and the occlusion of many capillaries with clots which completely halt tissue perfusion.[27, 30]

Later on, the activation of endogenous fibrinolysin accompanies the widespread coagulation, and clots tend to lyse and wash away. However, if the clots have been in place long enough to cause much focal tissue necrosis, failure of vital organs may occur.[27, 30] Once this is initiated, collapse of the microcirculation becomes progressively unremittent so that correction of the initiating causes can no longer halt or reverse the outcome, i.e., the patient moves into progressive and then irreversible shock and dies.

Vasoactive Materials. Both the *polypeptides* (e.g., bradykinin, angiotensin II, and vasoexcita-

*Mean blood pressure = $\frac{\text{systolic + diastolic}}{2}$

tory material*) and the *amines* (e.g., histamine, serotonin, and ferritin) undergo changes in various types of shock and thereby cause changes in vasoconstriction and vasodilatation, which are discussed later.

Hormones. During shock the endocrine glands secrete increased quantities of hormones, notably catecholamines, vasopressin, and adrenocortical hormones. Increased blood catecholamine levels are found in several types of shock, e.g., hemorrhagic, toxic, traumatic, and anaphylactic forms.[44] (See previous discussion.)

Immunologic Factors. All forms of shock produce a severe depression of the reticuloendothelial system (RES) and of antibacterial defense mechanisms. Alterations occur in the immunologic factors circulating in the blood stream.

The disturbances in the blood proper are partially due to tissue hypoxia as well as to an impairment of the monitoring activities of the RES. Indeed, the stasis, sludging, tendency to venular thrombosis, impaired capillary permeability, and subnormal vascular reactivity that occur during shock can all be traced back to dysfunction of the RES. The capacity of the RES to remove bacteria and the constantly formed endotoxins from the blood stream is greatly reduced during shock.[93]

The impaired ability of the RES to ward off toxic agents is critical, since the reduced blood flow through the intestines during shock impairs the vitality of intestinal tissue so extensively that bacterial products from the intestine gain access to the blood stream. To further compound the problem, the individual in a state of shock is more susceptible than normal to bacterial products, particularly bacterial endotoxins,[93] since interference with the RES leads to a reduced capacity to withstand stress.

INADEQUATE TISSUE PERFUSION DURING SHOCK

In any type of shock, regardless of etiology, the fundamental problem is inadequate tissue perfusion *owing to a marked reduction of blood flow through the tissues.*

Any tissue that is deprived of an adequate blood supply will suffer progressive damage and will ultimately be destroyed. Some tissues may be so damaged that their ultimate recovery is not possible and, consequently, death results if the tissue involved performs a vital function. Since various tissues have differing oxygen requirements, some organs will be irreversibly damaged before other tissues have reached this stage of destruction.

In shock, inadequate tissue perfusion does not occur uniformly in all tissues. This failure, for example, does not appear to develop to any recognizable extent in musculoskeletal areas; on the other hand, the liver and small intestine suffer marked damage. Microcirculatory failure appears to have a predilection for the abdominal visceral tissues; however, even there the changes are not uniform. For example, the *spleen* and *adrenals* demonstrate considerable changes, which are typical of vascular insufficiency; however, they *do not* develop serious cellular metabolic derangements during the lethal stages of the syndrome.[31]

Liver and Intestine Function During Shock[46, 66]

Shock states are believed to cause important changes in the functions of the liver and the intestines. Because some aspects of these changes are interrelated, the liver and intestines will be discussed together.

During shock both the liver and the intestines suffer from impaired circulation and both are believed to be possible sources of toxic materials.

> The splanchnic area blood vessels are those most strongly constricted by reflex sympathetic nervous system activity and by vasopressor agents. Thus, splanchnic circulation is highly susceptible to the deleterious effects of prolonged vasoconstriction during the development of shock.

> The liver has an important role in the metabolism of carbohydrate, protein, and fat and, also, is a major detoxifying organ. Under normal circumstances the liver is believed to protectively trap and dispose of toxic materials (released from the bowel contents) that are the products of the action of bacterial enzymes. During

*Vasoexcitatory material (VEM) is also known as renal pressor substance (RPS).

TABLE 26–1. DATA INDICATING RELATIONSHIP BETWEEN DEGREES OF SHOCK AND DERANGEMENT IN BLOOD FACTORS

Degree of Shock	Blood Loss Volume (% of normal)	Hemoglobin (% of normal)	Hematocrit (% cells)	Plasma Protein (Gm. %)
None	14.4 + 3.9	20.0 + 5.2	42.5 + 1.7	6.6 + 0.1
Slight	20.7 + 4.3	29.7 + 4.1	38.4 + 1.5	6.4 + 0.1
Moderate	34.3 + 3.5	46.1 + 3.4	34.6 + 1.0	6.2 + 0.1
Severe	45.9 + 4.7	54.4 + 4.3	31.5 + 1.5	6.0 + 0.1

Data summarized from Beecher, H. K.: *Resuscitation and Anesthesia for Wounded Men.* Springfield, Illinois. Charles C Thomas, 1949, by Gladish, J. T., Winnie, A. P., and Collins, V. J.: *Postgraduate Medicine,* July, 1967, p. 44.

shock the anoxic liver develops metabolic deficiencies and probably an impaired ability to detoxify.

> With shock, enhanced bacterial invasion of the liver from the intestine appears to occur.[66] In addition, the anoxic liver may itself release vasotoxic substances. The depressed protective action of the reticuloendothelial system (previously discussed) also allows the release of bacterial endotoxins (*Escherichia coli, Brucella melitensis*), which appear to destroy the integrity of the microcirculation.

> The liver plays a key role in the splanchnic circulation. With shock, pooling of blood occurs in the splanchnic area. Pooling of blood in the liver and portal bed may be caused by the plugging of large numbers of small hepatic vessels, sinusoids, and intrahepatic radicles of the portal vein and hepatic artery with masses of agglutinated blood. The persistence of an extreme state of resistance to portal blood flow may lead to stagnation of the blood in the portal system. This presumably results in blood backing up into the vessels of the intestines, adding to mucosal congestion and pooling of blood that is present in the intestinal capillaries.

Intestinal changes seem to play a significant role in irreversible hemorrhagic and bacteremic shock. It should be emphasized that ischemic changes within the intestine are not believed to be responsible for the death of all patients suffering from prolonged hemorrhagic or bacteremic shock; gastrointestinal changes are now believed to have a more vital role in the progression of shock than was previously thought. In the human the submucosa of the bowel is the layer that "suffers first the ravages of ischemia."[46] As the period of congestion and subsequent stagnant anoxia becomes prolonged, there are actual tissue necrosis and loss of integrity of the mucosa of the bowel. Bacteria are believed to contribute to irreversible shock by escaping into the systemic circulation as a result of destruction of the intestinal mucosal barrier.

The arterioles and venules of the intestine are evidently highly susceptible to the extensive vasoconstriction that occurs during shock. The massive amounts of tissue destruction that result from vasoconstriction and tissue anoxia are sufficient to produce death even in the absence of bacteria. Drugs that decrease peripheral vascular tone (e.g., vasodilators) are productive of more normal blood flows to organs and thereby preserve visceral integrity and improve survival rates. Of course, the circulating blood volume that has already been lost must be restored prior to the administration of such drugs. (This point will be discussed further in the section on treatment.)

Kidney Function During Shock

The rate of urine production reflects visceral blood flow and body fluid balance. Thus, urinary output indicates the status of the circulation through the vital organs; a good urine output indicates adequate circulation, even if the arterial blood pressure is lower than normal.[6] During shock the urine output is measured and compared with normal urine production. One ml. (or cc.) of urine per minute, or 60 ml. per hour, is the normal excretion of urine from the kidney. The patient who becomes acutely hypovolemic cannot maintain an hourly output of 40 to 60 ml. of urine.[21] A decreased urine output (*oliguria*) typically occurs in shock. In many instances during shock the urine output may stop completely (*anuria*); when this occurs, the patient is said to be in "renal shutdown."

Glomerular filtration within the kidney depends upon the pressure at which the blood is circulated through the glomerular capillaries. As a general rule, the average capillary pressure of blood is much higher in the glomeruli than it is in the other capillaries. Interestingly enough, under usual circumstances the kidney is able to maintain this heightened capillary pressure in the glomeruli in spite of changes in the systemic blood pressure. It is not clear exactly how this is accomplished; however, it is known that the afferent arterioles supplying the glomeruli dilate as the blood pressure falls and constrict as it rises. However, there are limits beyond which this adaptive mechanism can no longer protect the kidney against the hazards of a falling systemic blood pressure. Thus, shock produces oliguria and anuria.

We should remember that the reduction of urinary volume in itself is not of significance; the importance lies in the fact that the oligemia is due to inadequacy of the *general circulation* which, in turn, causes poor renal perfusion.[6] Thus, oligemia reflects inadequate circulation to the kidneys and to the body as a whole.[86] Obviously a patient in such a state is threatened with the progressive deterioration of his general circulatory function unless adequate treatment is provided immediately.

During shock, when there is a steady decline of blood volume and blood pressure, the glomerular filtrate is progressively reduced. Because it cannot be excreted by the kidneys, sodium, along with the water, leaves the body through the sweat glands. (In uremia, the frost which forms on the skin is actually sodium chloride.)[6] The damaged kidney loses its crucial ability to regulate electrolyte and acid-base balance.

Inadequate perfusion of the renal capillaries with blood is believed to be the cause of *early* renal failure in shock. The afferent and efferent arterioles constrict, and blood is shunted away from the glomeruli. *Later*, if shock persists, actual renal shutdown is caused by focal tubular necrosis.

We have indicated previously that the kidney may suffer from renal ischemia during shock because the microcirculatory failure has a predilection for the abdominal visceral tissues. Because the kidney has a high rate of metabolism, it is highly susceptible to injury of the tubule cells when the blood supply is deficient. Vasoconstriction in the kidney may unfortunately continue for a long time after the blood pressure has been restored to normal levels. When injury to the kidney is extensive and renal failure ensues, tubular necrosis occurs. The kidney can repair this condition, so that normal function will return in 10 to 14 days if the patient can be given appropriate therapy during this time and is not overloaded with fluids.

Oliguria does not contraindicate the administration of large volumes of fluid in treating shock. In fact, the restoration of renal capillary perfusion along with that of other vital capillaries restores urine volume production as long as tubular necrosis is not already present. Indeed, fluid administration may prevent renal tubular necrosis.[30]

Lung Function During Shock

Pulmonary lesions are seen in humans dying of shock. Such lesions are produced, in part, by thrombi in the pulmonary microcirculation. They have been observed in hemorrhagic and toxic shock and shock resulting from thrombosis.[30]

While respiratory insufficiency may precede shock in some patients, it may appear in others following the correction of the basic problem causing the shock. In fact, some persons may survive the shock period but die subsequently from respiratory failure, even though they had no pulmonary disease before they developed shock. The respiratory lesion produced is called "shock lung," or acute pulmonary failure. As indicated, the lesion may progress to death even though blood pressure, lactic acid, urine output, and other conditions are restored to normal. Shock lung is characterized by: pulmonary congestion, hemorrhage, atelectasis, edema, capillary thrombi, and the decrease or disappearance of pulmonary surfactant.* Increasing pressure is often needed to assist respiratory exchange. The PO_2 falls progressively and death occurs.[30]

In addition to direct structural and functional changes during shock, pulmonary function may also be impaired as a result of pulmonary edema developing secondary to heart failure.

METABOLIC CHANGES DURING SHOCK

As we have previously emphasized, shock produces prolonged circulatory insufficiency, which leads to variable and inadequate perfusion of certain organs and tissues, particularly at the microcirculation level. Such circulatory deprivation results in tissue hypoxia; many of the biochemical effects of shock are largely due to this. In addition, a variety of metabolites accumulate because of diminished venous blood flow and diminished lymphatic flow (except from areas that are traumatized directly, where lymph flow is usually increased). Widespread "toxic" effects may be produced owing to the escape of certain intracellular metabolites, which results in profound metabolic changes. The accumulated metabolites may affect local tissue circulation and metabolism as well as the circulation and metabolism of other areas to which they are eventually transported.[43]

Anoxia; Hypoxia

Tissue anoxia (or most usually "hypoxia," a deficiency of oxygen) occurs in all types of shock as a result of decreased circulation of blood to the body tissues. Cells are dependent upon an adequate circulation if they are to function properly, because it is by means of circulation that the cells: (1) receive their nutrients, electrolytes, and oxygen; and (2) have waste products removed.

Anoxia and hypoxia can both be tolerated for a short period of time. However, as the time lengthens, the chances of recovery diminish because oxygen lack appears to be a stimulus for the development of irreversible shock. If the available oxygen in the body is sufficient to meet the need, irreversible shock should not occur. Conversely, the greater the disparity between oxygen need and available oxygen, the more rapidly irreversible shock will develop.

In view of these facts, those factors that increase the body's need for oxygen would be detrimental to the person in shock (e.g., increased metabolic rate, high temperature, physical activity); beneficial factors would be those that decrease the need for oxygen (e.g., hypothermia or low metabolic rate). Factors that increase the available oxygen (e.g., increased cardiac output or vasodilators with the arterial pressure remaining constant) would be helpful.

The flow of blood through the microcirculation of organs and tissues is so diminished in shock that there is *inadequate or no delivery of the oxygen and substrates* that are necessary for living cells to maintain normal metabolism and energy production.

Oxygen and substrates are essential to life because they make possible a series of complex chemical transformations that result in the synthesis of adenosine triphosphate (ATP), which is the ultimate source of energy for life processes.[71]

Anaerobic Metabolism; Metabolic Acidosis

When oxygen is not present, ATP is produced through a different set of reactions referred to as *anaerobic metabolism* or "fermentation." Production of ATP in this manner is a useful emergency measure; however, it is inefficient compared with the normal process of aerobic (oxidative) metabolism. Anaerobic metabolism produces anaerobic metabolites such as lactic acid (which causes intracellular acidity with consequent cellular damage) and substrates of the adenylic acid system (which depress the heart).[14]

Because lactic acid is nonvolatile, it accumulates in the tissue fluids, causing them to become increasingly acid and ultimately producing a *metabolic acidosis*. During metabolic acidosis we find that blood pH, pCO_2 and bicarbonate fall, while a rise occurs in pyruvate, lactate, phosphate, and sulfate. *Respiratory alkalosis* or *respiratory acidosis* (induced by pulmonary ventilatory or diffusion changes) may be superimposed on the metabolic

**Surfactant* is a lipoprotein that reduces surface tension within the alveoli. Surface tension rises in the alveoli and atelectasis results when surfactant is reduced or destroyed, e.g., with shock, trauma, or anoxia.

acidosis. This situation will become progressively worse the longer the living cells are deprived of necessary blood.[43]

Unless the circulation is restored, the acidotic reaction, resulting from metabolic acidosis, will ultimately kill the cells.[71] The build-up of lactic acid causes such a severe, local acidosis that cellular enzymes become inactivated and, as a result, the cells soon die.[27, 30]

Intracellular or Lysosomal Enzymes[36]

It now appears that lysosomal enzymes not only are released in dead cells that are undergoing autolysis, but also are released just prior to cell death as a result of cellular anoxia or some other form of injury; e.g., these enzymes may be liberated as a result of trauma and endotoxins. Research on shock suggests that disruption of lysosomes and the release of their contained enzymes in free, active form occurs in the liver during shock, and that this is one mechanism of cell destruction that results from prolonged shock.

Lysosomal enzymes become most active in an acid pH range. Thus, as long as physiologic acid-base balance is maintained within the body, these enzymes are repressed within normal cells. However, in hypoxic tissues during shock states, the accompanying metabolic acidosis accelerates the solubilization and activation of these enzymes.

Activation of lysosomal hydrolases within the cells, and their release into the circulation, markedly exacerbates the tissue injury that is produced in shock. The release of active lysosomal proteases and other enzymes from damaged tissue into the blood stream, and their action on extracellular as well as intracellular structures, probably contributes to the progression of injury from cell to cell.

The presence of hepatic lysosomal active enzymes in the blood stream, along with blocking of the reticuloendothelial system, is a potential factor in the lethal outcome of shock. As previously indicated, blockade of the reticuloendothelial system drastically reduces its capacity to clear bacteria from the blood stream.

SIGNS AND SYMPTOMS OF SHOCK

The classic signs and symptoms of shock following hemorrhage (hematogenic shock) and wounds are given below. The signs and symptoms of shock due to other causes are basically similar to those listed, although they may differ in specific details.

COMMON INDICATIONS OF HEMATOGENIC SHOCK

Cold, moist skin (some types of shock cause skin to be dry and/or warm)
Ashen pallor (some types of shock cause cyanosis or rubor)
Dryness of mucous membranes
Decreased body temperature
Low systolic and diastolic blood pressure (hypotension is usual, but normotension or hypertension occurs with some types of shock)
Slow capillary filling; collapse of superficial veins of extremities
Oliguria; anuria
Pilomotor and sudomotor activity
Thirst
Cold
Restlessness, nervousness, apprehension, irritability, drowsiness, stupor
Weakness
Rapid, shallow respirations; air hunger
Rapid, weak ("thready") pulse
Nausea, vomiting
Metabolic acidosis
Patient steadily progresses toward a so-called irreversible phase

RESPIRATORY RATE IN SHOCK

Rapid, shallow respirations typically result from decreased tissue perfusion.[8] The respiratory rate increases as the oxygen-carrying power of the blood decreases. Also, the respiratory rate is increased because the accumulation of excessive amounts of carbon dioxide (due to metabolic acidosis) serves as a stimulus to the respiratory center.[6]

PULSE RATE IN SHOCK

As a general rule, the pulse rate *increases* in shock as a result of increased sympathetic stimulation. The body's compensatory mechanisms further accelerate the pulse rate by increasing the number of contractions of the heart per minute. This occurs in an attempt to maintain adequate circulation of the blood when the circulating volume of blood is not adequate. This sequence of events is particularly true in shock states caused by fluid loss or acute myocardial infarction.[8]

In addition to being more rapid, the pulse is typically weak and thready. At the onset of shock the pulse rate is not so directly related to the severity of the pathology as is the blood pressure. This is because, in the early stage of shock, worry, excitement, and fear may influence the heart rate out of proportion to the underlying conditions. However, when emotional factors are no longer significant, serial observations of the pulse rate over a period of time may be highly useful in evaluating the patient's condition and the direction of the shock state. Simeone[71] notes that elderly patients (with and without various degrees of heart block) are an exception to this. These patients may show little change in their heart rates in spite of the presence of conditions that cause circulatory failure (e.g., hemorrhage).

The pulse rate may become extremely slow in the terminal stages of irreversible shock. If the radial pulse is irregular, you should simultaneously check the apical pulse. The difference between the count of the apical pulse and the count of the radial pulse is known as the *pulse deficit.* Ideally two persons should determine the pulse deficit together; one person listens with a stethoscope to the heart sounds at the heart's apex while the other person feels the radial pulse. If the radial pulse cannot be felt, you may find that the pulse is detectable in the facial, temporal, carotid or femoral areas.

BLOOD PRESSURE IN SHOCK

> *The blood pressure is inversely related to the heart rate, so that a decreased blood pressure is accompanied by an increased heart rate.*[6]

The systolic blood pressure indicates the integrity of the cardiac mechanism, the arteries and the arterioles,[21] while the diastolic blood pressure indicates the resistance of blood vessels.

The amount of peripheral resistance (or vasoconstriction) is indicated by the level of the diastolic blood pressure. For example, an increasing diastolic pressure indicates increasing resistance of the peripheral blood vessels; conversely, a declining diastolic pressure is indicative of decreasing peripheral resistance. When the diastolic pressure falls significantly, we know that vasoconstriction is being lost as a compensatory mechanism. When vasoconstriction is replaced by marked vasodilatation there is no resistance to blood flow and, thus, blood pressure cannot be maintained.[6]

It is usual for the blood pressure to begin to fall when the total blood volume is decreased by about 15 to 20 per cent of normal; however, it is not unusual for some persons to lose as much as 25 per cent of their total blood volume without showing signs of shock.[6]

Typically, through the progressive stages of shock the systolic and diastolic arterial pressures drop, the systolic pressure usually dropping more than the diastolic. The pulse pressure* also falls, since pulse pressure is equal to the difference between the systolic and diastolic pressures. Actually *evaluation of the pulse pressure is more significant than evaluation of blood pressure,* since it tends to parallel the cardiac stroke volume.[56]

It should be remembered that the significance of the blood pressure in an individual patient depends to some extent upon his *usual* blood pressure. While some persons normally have a systolic blood pressure of about 100 mm. Hg, others may have high blood pressure, with a usual systolic pressure of 210 mm. Hg. Obviously a blood pressure of 100 mm. Hg would mean two vastly different things for these two groups of persons. A blood pressure of 100 mm. Hg or less is significant for persons whose systolic pressure usually ranges from 110 to 140 mm. Hg. In order to maintain the coronary circulation, it is necessary to have a minimal systolic pressure of from 60 to 70 mm. Hg. In interpreting blood pressure readings it is always helpful to know what the individual's usual blood pressure has been. Also, remember that when the patient is in a supine position, a decline in blood pressure may be a late finding. Brand and Thal present the following words of caution concerning the clinical interpretation of hypotension:

> It is important to realize that hypotension, by itself, is not shock, and that unless other clinical manifestations are present, a low systolic pressure should not be construed as shock. In many instances a systolic pressure of only 70 to 80 mm. of mercury may be of sufficient magnitude to permit adequate tissue perfusion in vasodilated patients.[8]

While the auscultatory blood pressure and pulse pressure are *usually* reduced in shock, some patients with all the peripheral manifestations of shock, may have normal intra-arterial pressure despite markedly reduced or absent cuff pressure and upper extremity pulses. Such a discrepancy between intra-arterial and cuff pressures in patients in shock can have important clinical implications.

> *Failure to recognize that low cuff pressure does not necessarily indicate arterial hypotension can lead to dangerous errors in therapy.*

For example, should vasopressor medications be administered (as they might be because of a false impression of hypotension), they could produce hypertension and acute heart failure. Valuable information about the level of arterial pressure in vasoconstricted patients can be gained by evaluation of the strength of femoral pulsations. However, direct measurement of the arterial pressure may be the only accurate way to assess the status of the patient in some situations.[10] This will be discussed again later on.

There are additional problems that need to be considered in evaluating blood pressure during shock. The following facts make blood pressure per se (and particularly the systolic pressure) an unreliable criterion for determining the presence and severity of shock:

> In the early stages of shock blood pressure changes are generally unreliable because the arterial pressure may actually be normal or even high even though the factors that are initiating the shock are present. In fact, blood volume deficits of a liter or more may occur even though arterial and venous pressures are normal or elevated.[46]

> When severe vasoconstriction is present the blood pressure may be normal even though the circulation is actually highly inadequate. Also, conversely, the blood flow may not be inadequate even though the blood pressure is decreased, e.g., owing to mechanisms such as vasodilatation.

> An unobtainable blood pressure generally indi-

*Pulse pressure is often less than 20 mm. of mercury.

cates a very low pulse pressure and cardiac output; it does not necessarily indicate a low blood pressure.[56]

As indicated, while shock is usually associated with systemic hypotension, there are situations in which it may be associated with normal or even high blood pressures in spite of serious injury or blood loss. Such cases are referred to as "compensated shock," because vigorous sympathicoadrenal activity is "compensating" for the oligemia by precariously sustaining the blood pressure through neuroendocrine defenses. In such situations relatively small additional blood losses, anesthesia, or even a change in the patient's position can lead to "decompensation and catastrophe."[71]

Hardaway and his associates clinically classify hypotensive, and normotensive or hypertensive shock as follows:[30]

- I. Hypotensive shock
  1. Cold skin (arterioles constricted, low central venous pressure, low cardiac output)
     - a. Low blood volume (responds well to transfusion)
       - (1) Hemorrhage
       - (2) Fluid loss (burns, massive wounds, infection, dehydration, etc.)
     - b. Normal blood volume (poor response to transfusion)
       - (1) Septic shock
  2. Warm skin (arterioles dilated, not real shock as capillaries are often well perfused. Increased cardiac output)
     - a. Arsenic poisoning
     - b. Spinal shock
     - c. Shock due to any anesthesia
     - d. Shock due to vasodilators
  3. Heart failure (arterioles constricted, decreased cardiac output, high central venous pressure)
- II. Normotensive or hypertensive shock (arterioles constricted, decreased cardiac output, low vena cava pressure)
  1. Compensated shock
  2. Epinephrine shock
  3. "Overcompensation" shock
  4. Pheochromocytoma

SKIN APPEARANCE IN SHOCK

As you can see from the preceding outline, the status of the skin during shock varies, depending on the etiologic basis of the shock state. Thus, you will notice clinically a striking contrast between the pallor and collapsed veins of a patient suffering from shock due to hemorrhage and/or trauma, and the cyanosis and venous distention of a patient in shock caused by pulmonary embolus or heart failure.[71]

Generally during shock decreased tissue perfusion causes the skin to feel *"cool and clammy"* and to appear *pale*. Since blood provides warmth and color to the skin, a decreased blood volume and vasoconstriction of the blood vessels in the skin (as in hemorrhage) cause the blood supply to the skin to be deficient, and pallor results.[6, 8, 71] Coolness and a clammy feel to a patient's skin during shock result from constriction of the peripheral blood vessels caused by increased activity of the sympathetic nervous system (an early sign of shock).[8] Clamminess is also suggestive of an acute deficit of vascular fluid (e.g., blood and plasma) and an extensive sodium and chloride deficit.

Diaphoresis occurs in the late, severe stages of hemorrhagic shock because aldosterone secretion is decreased. As a result, sodium can no longer be retained in the body; in turn, water cannot be retained either and it leaves the body via the sweat glands.[6]

"Clammy" skin is especially common in shock associated with overwhelming infection, with nervous reaction, or in wound shock following medication with opiates.[71] Prior to the administration of opiates in wound shock the skin is often *cold and dry*. Also, it should be noted that in some cases of infection and hypotension the characteristic signs are *warm dry skin with rubor* (redness) and *plethora* (florid complexion) of the face.

As we have indicated, *cyanosis** may also be present during some forms of shock. Cyanosis typically occurs with pulmonary embolus or heart failure. Also, late in hemorrhagic shock the blood within the vessels is insufficient in both quantity and quality to give the skin a normal hue; the low volume of arterial blood has a proportionately low volume of hemoglobin and, thus, a decreased oxygen content. Cyanosis that appears late in hemorrhagic shock is usually caused by the presence of excessive amounts of deoxygenated blood in the skin capillaries. Also, blood flow in these vessels is very sluggish.[6] In the old and the very young the fingernail beds and the lips will often become cyanotic before the rest of the body begins to appear blue.

One means of evaluating peripheral circulation is to observe the effects of circulation in the nail beds. This is done by pushing down with the thumb nail on one of the patient's fingernails and then releasing the pressure and observing the return of color to the nail bed. Normally a compressed nail bed fills within a fraction of a second after the pressure is released. Capillary filling, after compression of the skin and particularly the nail bed, is slow in shock and may take several seconds. Another means of evaluating peripheral circulation is to apply digital pressure to a peripheral vein (i.e., to "stroke" the vein) and see if it collapses. Venous collapse with digital pressure indicates that very little blood is within the vein.

LEVEL OF CONSCIOUSNESS IN SHOCK

Early in shock hyperactivity of the sympathetic nervous system, with increased secretion of

*Cyanosis is discussed further in Unit X.

epinephrine, usually causes the patient to feel anxious, nervous, and irritable, and to have an anxious, worried expression.[8, 71]

Those signs and symptoms that are associated with a lack of blood supply to the brain are determined by the *suddenness* with which the shock develops and the *severity* of the insult. If the onset of the shock is sudden and the degree of shock is severe, the body may not have time to initiate its compensatory mechanisms of adjustment and, consequently, the brain is deprived of its blood supply, and fainting and unconsciousness result. The patient in a horizontal position may feel dizzy and faint if he assumes an upright position. If shock develops more gradually, over a period of several hours, some of the early signs may be apathy, lethargy, and confusion. On the other hand, the patient may be restless and unusually alert. Thus, changes in the degree of alertness in either direction are of importance in evaluating shock.

With shock, the amount of blood flowing to the brain may become insufficient to maintain normal mental functioning and a normal level of consciousness. When the supply of blood is limited, a decreased supply of oxygen and glucose to the brain results. The primary source of energy for the nerve cells is the oxidation of glucose. The brain cells are highly sensitive to a shortage of oxygen. Because the functioning brain cell depends on carbohydrate metabolism, and because the metabolic process depends on oxygen, the metabolism within the brain is decreased in the presence of an oxygen shortage. The systolic blood pressure is an important factor in maintaining cerebral blood flow since at least 40 mm. Hg of pressure is required to deliver blood to the brain. Usually a decrease in the systolic pressure is accompanied by a decrease in the flow of blood to the brain.[6] However, the vessels of the brain, like those of the heart, are not constricted by the vasoconstrictor center and, thus, blood from the peripheral vessels can be shifted to the brain as an emergency compensatory measure.

The level of consciousness decreases as the circulation to the brain tissues becomes increasingly impaired, and the patient may then become confused, agitated, and restless. In severe and late shock, apathy may ensue. Drowsiness and stupor are more likely to occur in shock related to severe infection than in shock caused by trauma and hemorrhage. A comatose condition may ultimately be reached terminally. Because coma is unusual, except terminally, the possibility of intracranial damage must be ruled out when it does occur.[8, 71]

KIDNEY FUNCTION IN SHOCK

The urine output is one of the most sensitive indices in shock. A decreased urine volume often is the earliest sign of hypovolemia, and may occur even while the arterial blood pressure and pulse remain stable.

An indwelling urinary catheter, which allows measurement of urine produced, is useful in determining the status of the patient and the effectiveness of therapy.[21] Because an indwelling catheter predisposes the patient to the danger of ascending urinary tract infection, *extreme* caution and careful technique must be used to prevent this from happening. *Remember, the patient in shock has a lowered resistance to infections!*

Urine flow should be kept above 50 ml. per hour. If the hourly output of urine diminishes significantly, treatment must be instituted to prevent renal shutdown. It is recommended that a urine output of less than 30 cc. per hour be reported at once; urine flow less than 20 ml. per hour can cause renal tubular necrosis, which results from inadequate renal circulation. Actually, the nurse should strive to recognize impending renal failure prior to the appearance of oliguria. Some of the changes that indicate nonoliguric renal failure are: (1) reduced specific gravity and osmolarity of the urine, (2) reduced urine creatinine clearance, (3) a rise in sodium urine concentration relative to the amount in the serum, and (4) a progressive rise in the blood's urea nitrogen, creatinine, and potassium.

METABOLIC ACIDOSIS IN SHOCK

In shock the metabolic products of cellular metabolism accumulate and produce a state of acidosis as a result of the stasis of blood and inadequate circulation. Although the body tries to compensate for this acidosis by using its many buffer systems, these compensatory mechanisms may fail. Such failure allows a dangerous state of overt acidosis to develop.[8] For a discussion of acidosis and its signs and symptoms, see the preceding chapter.

BODY TEMPERATURE IN SHOCK

In severe shock the thermoregulatory mechanism is disturbed, causing the body temperature to fall. While the body metabolism normally produces heat, in severe shock metabolism is extremely low.[6]

SUMMARY

In summary, some major manifestations of decreased tissue perfusion are: cold and "clammy" skin; anxiety progressing to a declining level of consciousness, oliguria or anuria, hypotension, increased pulse rate, rapid and shallow respirations, and metabolic acidosis. In addition to the above, some other findings are: peripheral cyanosis, collapsed peripheral veins, elevated or reduced body temperatures, and (in cardiogenic shock) distended neck veins. These signs vary according to the etiology of the shock and are thus not present in all patients.[8]

In Table 26–2 the clinical signs and symptoms of various degrees of shock are listed, both for conditions involving blood volume loss and those in which there is no blood loss.

As you realize, it is difficult to know when shock actually exists and when therapy should begin. Because of this difficulty it has been established that in clinical shock, as a general rule, treatment should be instituted whenever at least two of the following conditions prevail: (1) systolic blood pressure of 80 mm. Hg or less; (2) pulse pressure of 20 mm. Hg or less; and (3) pulse rate of 100 or more.[21]

CLINICAL CARE OF THE PATIENT EXPERIENCING SHOCK

> The primary aim of the treatment of shock is to increase tissue perfusion. Unless this is accomplished early after onset, subsequent therapeutic measures are of no avail and death can be anticipated.[9]

The patient lies in a state of shock. In addition to a urinary catheter, he has catheters placed in the radial artery, the right atrium of the heart, and the pulmonary artery. He is being attended by senior physicians and nurses, who will remain with him until he is out of danger. The patient's bed is custommade, so that it is a little narrower and higher than the usual hospital bed. This makes it suitable for use as an operating table for minor surgeries, such as tracheotomy or cutdown procedures. The head and foot of the bed easily lift off so that tracheal intubation and other therapeutic maneuvers can be readily performed. Special holders for transducers, etc., are also present on the bed. A portable image intensifier can be used (i.e., to place a pulmonary artery catheter) at the bedside because the mattress and springs are made of a plastic material, so that x-rays can penetrate the bed. The patient's radial artery pressure, central venous pressure, pulmonary artery pressure, electrocardiogram, and rectal and skin temperature are continuously monitored on a multichannel recorder and screen. A device regulates body temperature by warming or cooling the patient. Cardiac output is measured by the cardiac green dye method, and a computer calculates the curve. To help in monitoring fluid intake, output, and retention, the bed sits on a metabolic scale that is accurate to the nearest gram.

Adjoining the patient's room is a nursing station that serves as a supply center (i.e., for drugs, intravenous solutions, emergency resuscitation equipment, respirator, tracheotomy, and cutdown trays) and a data recording and processing center. A laboratory is only a few steps from the bed. It is equipped for a wide variety of blood coagulation tests, including factor assays. A diagram of the clotting process is drawn by a thromboelastograph. From the same blood sample the red blood cell mass and plasma volume are measured (with a Hemolitre). Other equipment is available for the performance of an average of more than 300 laboratory determinations per patient per day. The following is a list of some of the indices that can be determined:

1. Hemodynamic measurements
   a. Arterial blood pressure (radial artery)
   b. Central venous pressure
   c. Pulmonary artery pressure
   d. Cardiac index
   e. Peripheral resistance
   f. Mean transit time
   g. Central blood volume
2. Hematologic measurements
   a. Hemoglobin and hematocrit
   b. Red blood cell mass (determined with sodium chromate ^{51}Cr)
   c. Plasma volume (determined with iodinated ^{131}I serum albumin)
   d. White blood cell count
   e. Platelet count
   f. Fibrinogen concentration
   g. Prothrombin time
   h. Partial thromboplastin time
   i. Thromboelastograph clotting time
   j. Assays of proteolytic enzyme activity
   k. Individual clotting factor assays (I, II, IV, V, VII, VIII, IX, X, XI, XII)
3. Metabolic measurements
   a. Frequent precise weighing
   b. Serum and urine electrolyte concentration
   c. Lactate and pyruvate concentration
   d. Blood urea nitrogen, creatinine, and liver function studies
   e. Catecholamine assay
   f. Oxygen consumption study
   g. Core and skin temperature
4. Respiratory system studies
   a. Blood pH
   b. Blood gas studies (arterial and venous oxygen and carbon dioxide pressure)
   c. Minute volume
5. Others
   a. X-ray studies as indicated
   b. Electrocardiographic monitoring

The situation that we have just described approaches being an ideal treatment and research clinic for shock.[30] Probably the area in which you will work will not have all the features mentioned; however, you will undoubtedly be involved with many of these aspects of care. Regardless of where you are practicing you will undoubtedly care for patients in shock, for shock is a common condition.

> Shock can occur in any hospital area—medical, surgical, orthopedic, obstetric, operating and recovery rooms, psychiatry, dermatology, metabolic, etc. Shock can occur in any home, on any street, in any doctor's or dentist's office. In a word, shock can occur anywhere. Sometimes shock occurs when it could and should have been prevented.[6]

Caring for a patient in shock is one of the most complex, demanding and critically important areas of nursing practice. Frank observes that, "Early in-

TABLE 26-2. CORRELATION OF CLINICAL SIGNS AND SYMPTOMS OF SHOCK WITH BLOOD VOLUME LOSS*

A. LOSS OF BLOOD VOLUME—TRAUMA AND HEMORRHAGE

Degree of Shock	Blood Pressure	Skin			Thirst	Mental Status	Blood Loss (% of normal volume)	Blood Loss (cc., approx. quantity)
		Temperature	*Color*	*Response to Pressure Blanching*				
None	126/75	Normal	Normal	Normal	Normal	Clear, distressed	14.4	750
Slight	109/66	Cool	Pale	Definite slowing	Normal	Clear, distressed	20.7	1000
Moderate	95/58	Cool	Pale	Definite slowing	Marked	Clear, some apathy	34.3	1750
Marked	49/25	Cold	Ashen to cyanotic	Very sluggish	Severe	Apathetic to comatose; little distress except thirst	45.9	2250

B. NO BLOOD LOSS—MEDICAL CONDITIONS: INFECTIONS, PERICARDITIS, MESENTERIC THROMBOSIS, ETC.

Degree of Shock	Blood Pressure	Skin		Respirations	Pulse	Mental Status	Average Blood Lactic Acid (mEq. per L.)
		Extremities	*Cyanosis*				
Minimal	Slight fall	Pale and cool	Lips, extremities or both	Normal	Thready and rapid	Restless and apprehensive	5
Moderate	80/60 to 60/40	Cold and clammy	Lips, extremities or both	Rapid and shallow	Thready and rapid	Apprehensive and confused	6
Marked	60/40 to 40/20	Cold and clammy	Lips, extremities or both	Often Cheyne-Stokes or sighing	Thready and rapid	Confused to stuporous	11
Extremely marked	20/1 to 20/0	Cold and clammy	Lips, extremities or both	Often Cheyne-Stokes or sighing	Rapid, slow or unobtainable	Stuporous to comatose	17

*Breed, E. S.: The diagnosis and management of shock. *Medical Clinics of North America* 41:669–683, May, 1957.

tensive and meticulous management is much more likely to succeed than last-ditch heroics."[19] When a patient is in shock, or close to it, constant attendance is required, with a senior, well informed physician close at hand. Physician and nurse must observe physiologic changes as they occur and at that time make the therapeutic adjustments that are required. Shock is an emergency that often necessitates team action on the part of many: nurse, physician, laboratory technician, pharmacist, and inhalation therapist—each has a vital role. Each person must know his or her job and perform it skillfully and rapidly, anticipating what the next action might be.

At the bedside, immediate laboratory evaluations are essential in treating shock. Blood chemistries, blood gases, pH, and electrolytes need to be determined frequently and reported promptly so that therapy can be adjusted to the patient's rapidly changing physiologic status.

For the treatment of shock to be successful, it must be based upon: (1) a recognition of the various pathophysiologic changes that are associated with *specific* shock conditions, and (2) an understanding of the *general* problem of inadequate tissue perfusion that is common to all shock states.[8, 71] Since the methods for treating inadequate tissue perfusion vary according to the specific etiology, an *accurate differential diagnosis,* which will establish the specific etiology of the shock state, is the *first* step in treatment. The differential diagnosis is usually readily made unless the patient is in an advanced state of shock, in which several specific forms of shock may exist concomitantly. Some forms of shock that are usually easily recognized are: hemorrhagic shock due to extensive bleeding, burn shock caused by extensive burns, and cardiogenic shock typified by severe chest pains and ECG readings indicative of acute myocardial infarction. Probably the least obvious diagnosis is that of toxic (i.e., septic) shock. Identification of toxic shock requires "astute clinical suspicion which is later confirmed by laboratory identification of the bacterial agent."[8]

OVERVIEW OF MODES OF TREATMENT

The treatment of shock, in a general sense, has changed markedly during the past few years.

> Lower his head, keep him warm, and use vasopressor drugs to elevate his blood pressure were once traditional practices in the care of the patient in shock. Now, as a result of new knowledge, all of these measures are being seriously questioned, and principal emphasis is being placed on maintenance of adequate capillary blood flow throughout the body tissues and organs.[71]

As with many areas of clinical care, clear-cut and final answers concerning the treatment of shock cannot be presented. Accordingly, the concepts of treatment outlined in this chapter will surely change over a period of time with the acquisition of new knowledge.

As we have indicated, clinical care varies according to the specific etiology of the type of shock being treated. For example, the patient in hemorrhagic shock primarily requires blood replacement; the treatment of traumatic and burn shock mainly involves the replacement of electrolytes and plasma fluids; and diabetic shock indicates insulin administration in addition to the proper replacement of fluids and electrolytes.[6]

The treatment of all forms of shock must be directed toward improving and maintaining tissue perfusion rather than merely elevating the blood pressure, for it is apparent that pressure is one of the lesser factors involved in maintaining adequate blood flow to the tissues served by the microcirculation.[21]

Of central importance in the current treatment of shock is the establishment and maintenance of an adequate blood volume. However, in addition to supplying an adequate circulating volume of blood, other adjuncts are necessary to facilitate the distribution of this blood to the body and to enhance the perfusion and oxygenation of the tissues with the circulating blood.

In the treatment of shock *all* the basic pathophysiologic changes associated with the development of shock must be corrected. For example, some of the problems that must often be treated are: the *vascular* problem of vasoconstriction, with its resultant diminished tissue perfusion; the *intravascular* problem of coagulation and sludging of cells; and the *extravascular* problem of extravasation of fluid into the extravascular space.

Characteristically impairment of tissue function is correctable at an early stage, but may lead to death if treatment is inadequate or if the condition goes untreated. It is generally held that in the later stages of shock the condition becomes "irreversible," leading inexorably to death in spite of treatment. Before it may be concluded that shock has become irreversible the following possible causes for failure of therapy must be excluded:[71]

> Inadequate restoration of circulating blood volume.

> Failure to recognize occult bleeding (into the abdominal or thoracic cavity or into the extremities).

> Failure to recognize interference with cardiopulmonary function (cardiac tamponade, pulmonary embolism, fat embolism, coronary thrombosis, tension pneumothorax, massive atelectasis).

> Failure to recognize overwhelming infection.

Let us hasten to point out that clinical treatment for "irreversible" shock is never abandoned while the patient remains alive.[43]

> The term "irreversible shock" has no meaning in the clinic and can only be justified after the fight has been lost.[19]

ASSESSMENT OF THE PATIENT IN SHOCK

A variety of different measurements are used to determine the patient's status and the effectiveness of treatment in shock states. In addition to actual *measurements* (e.g., blood volume, central venous pressure, and so forth), it is important that repeated *observations* be made, on a planned basis, of the clinical signs characteristic of shock (e.g., sympathetic nervous system activity causing increased pulse, pallor, cool skin, perspiration).

Monitoring of Urine Flow

A bladder catheter is a simple means of monitoring the patient in shock. By enabling the continuous measurement of urine flow, the bladder catheter provides important information about the peripheral blood flow and the function of the kidneys. Since the amounts of urine that are excreted during shock are often very small, it is important to have an accurate, calibrated urine collector. In some settings, the indwelling Foley catheter may be attached to a urinometer collector or to a more complex electric urinometer.[19]

Because changes in urine volume are highly important as an index of the success or failure of therapy, it is recommended that the nurse check the urine output every few minutes and measure it at least every half hour.[8]

In some forms of shock, such as toxic shock, renal shutdown is common and may produce a rapidly increasing state of metabolic acidosis.

Monitoring of Blood Volume *

The blood volume in shock is a fluctuating value of key importance in determining fluid replacement therapy. It is particularly important in hypovolemic shock to know the actual blood volume. Isotope techniques can usually provide this measurement rapidly and easily.[8, 19]

Some physicians believe that many patients who are suffering profound or irreversible shock are undertransfused because their blood volumes are believed to be normal. Some believe that a central venous pressure (CVP) measurement gives more information than a determination of blood volume. Others believe that the Volematron technique for determining blood volume is easy to perform at frequent intervals and is accurate and highly helpful.[30, 46]

Recently a chlorpromazine test (CPZ test) has been reported for determining blood volume. Normovolemic patients do not become hypotensive following the intravenous injection of a small dose of chlorpromazine (0.1 to 0.2 mg. per kg. of body weight). A 25 per cent or greater drop in the systolic blood pressure following the administration of 0.2 mg. of chlorpromazine indicates a significant degree of hypovolemia. This test can be clinically useful, as follows: When a patient's vital signs begin to stabilize following transfusion for hemorrhagic shock, the question of whether he needs additional blood may be resolved by performing an adrenergic block with a small dose of chlorpromazine. The replacement is probably adequate if the drop in the systolic blood pressure is less than 25 per cent; if the test shows a deficiency in blood volume, it may be repeated following the administration of additional colloid.[21]

The hematocrit is not a reliable index for measuring the blood volume during shock. The hematocrit can be misleading, for if it is checked before the passage of fluid occurs from the interstitial space into the blood stream, it would appear normal or near normal in spite of a reduction of blood volume, owing to the hemoconcentration caused by the compensatory actions of the red bone marrow, spleen, liver, and venous reservoirs. On the other hand, the hematocrit would show a decline if measured after this fluid shift, since the passage of interstitial fluid into the blood stream causes hemodilution.[6, 19]

*Blood volume is discussed further in the unit pertaining to the heart, Unit X.

Measurement of the Degree of Blood Lactic Acidosis

The extent of the acid-base derangement accompanying shock can be estimated by measuring the pH, pCO_2, and the standard bicarbonate levels of the blood. A low pH and a low standard bicarbonate indicate metabolic acidosis.[8] *Other laboratory tests* that may be performed include blood hemoglobin, hematocrit, red cell count, serum electrolyte, pO_2, and blood lactate and pyruvate.

Monitoring of Pulmonary Artery Pressure (PAP)

Because it is a direct measurement within the lesser circulation, the pulmonary artery pressure (PAP) is often a more sensitive index of adequate fluid volume replacement and impending right heart failure than the central venous pressure measurement (CVP). At present a determination of pulmonary artery pressure is not recommended for routine clinical use; however, it has provided useful information on a research basis.[30]

Measurement of Cardiac Output

While the measurement of cardiac output is a useful technique in assessing the clinical course of cardiogenic shock, the procedure is in its experimental stages and there are no simple techniques for performing these determinations.[8] Cardiac output is discussed further in the unit on the heart.

Continuous Monitoring of Systemic Arterial Blood Pressure

A helpful record of the pressure at each heart beat (systolic blood pressure) can be obtained by attaching a brachial artery needle (Rochester or Cournand type) to a strain gauge and to a direct writing instrument.[19] Brand and Thal[8] report a simple, effective method for monitoring the arterial blood pressure as follows:*

Materials Required

1. An intravenous pole
2. Adhesive tape, 65–70″ in length, 1½″ wide
3. Extension tubing (Bardic # 1750), 30″ long with a capacity of 5.8 cc. (4 tubes)
4. Three-way stopcock
5. An arterial catheter
6. Venesection tray
7. An empty sterile bottle
8. A 500-cc. flask (containing saline with heparin) along with intravenous tubing for flush purposes (flush solution)

Procedure (See Fig. 26–4)

1. Extend the intravenous pole to its maximum height.

*This method was devised by Robert F. Wilson, M.D., Assistant Professor of Surgery, Wayne State University, College of Medicine. (From Brand, L., and Thal, A. P.: Shock. *In* Meltzer, L. E., Abdellah, F. G., and Kitchell, J. R. (eds.): *Concepts and Practices of Intensive Care for Nurse Specialists.* Philadelphia, Charles Press Publishers, Inc., 1969.)

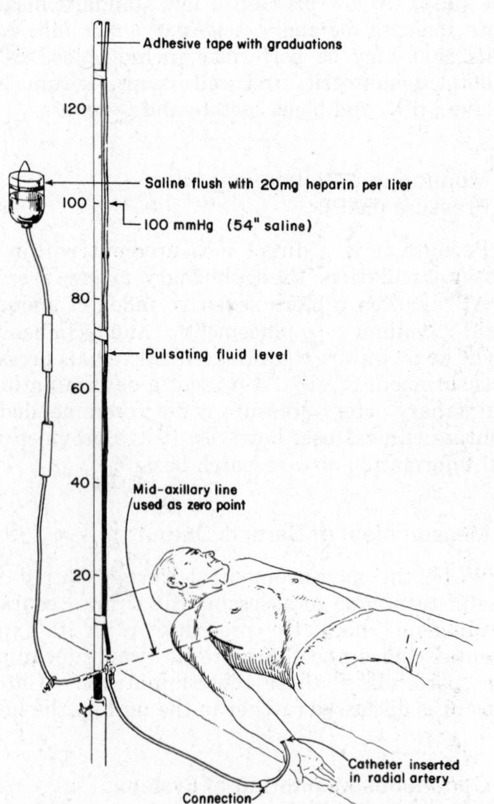

FIGURE 26–4. Direct measurement of arterial blood pressure. (From Brand and Thal: *In* Meltzer, Abdellah and Kitchell: *Concepts and Practices of Intensive Care for Nurse Specialists.* Philadelphia, The Charles Press. 1969.)

2. The adhesive tape is marked at successive intervals of 5.4″. The bottom line is labeled as zero and each successive interval as 10, 20, 30, etc. Since each 5.4″ represents 10 mm. Hg, a reading scale for pressure measurement is available.
3. Secure the calibrated adhesive tape to the length of the intravenous pole with the zero point at the level of the patient's midaxillary line.
4. Connect three extension tubes together and fasten adjoining tubing to the intravenous pole so that one end extends over the top and into an empty sterile bottle and the other end (the male tip) extends free below the zero point for subsequent attachment.
5. The free end of the extension tube and the end of the intravenous tubing from the flush bottle are connected to two of the arms of a 3-way stopcock.
6. The fourth extension tube is attached to the third arm of the stopcock.
7. The entire system is filled with flush solution (the sterile bottle at the top of the tubing will catch the overflow when filling and washing out the tubing).
8. The fourth extension tube (Step 6) is then connected to an arterial catheter that has been placed in the radial artery.
9. The stopcock is turned so that the fluid in the extension tube on the intravenous pole is in continuity with the arterial system.
10. The level of fluid in the long extension tube represents the *mean* arterial blood pressure.
11. When the system is functioning correctly, the fluid level in the extension tube should fluctuate with each heart beat. If this does not occur, the arterial line is partially occluded and flushing is required.

Monitoring of Central Venous Pressure

The central venous pressure (CVP) is a measurement of great importance in the treatment of shock. CVP determination measures adequacy of vascular volume and the pumping action of the heart. By monitoring the CVP the physician can follow an index of right ventricular function at the bedside. This cardiovascular response to fluid load is believed to be the single most important measurement that can be made in hypovolemic shock. The CVP is also useful in the assessment of the venous return in other forms of shock. By monitoring the CVP it is often possible to discern whether circulatory failure is due to congestive heart failure or hemorrhage.[8, 21] For a more complete discussion of the CVP see Unit X, Chapter 48.

Estimation of Fluid Loss

Since adequate fluid replacement is of central importance in the treatment of shock, it is vitally important for fluid loss to be estimated as accurately as possible. The estimation of fluid loss has been previously discussed in detail in Chapter 25.

Red blood count, blood hemoglobin, hematocrit, blood pH, blood gases, central venous pressure, blood volume, and urine output are determined as frequently as necessary to evaluate the results of therapy in the treatment of shock.

POSITIONING

The patient in shock is generally positioned so that the lower extremities are elevated to an angle of 45 degrees; the knees are straight, the trunk is horizontal or very slightly inclined, so that the thorax is lower than the pelvis; and the neck is comfortably positioned, with the head on a level with the chest or slightly higher[71] (Fig. 26–5). The advantage of this position is that it promotes increased venous return from the lower extremities without affecting blood flow through the brain. Elevation of the legs mobilizes the blood pooled in the lower extremities and, by the force of gravity, this additional circulating blood increases venous return to the heart, thereby improving the cardiac output. While this position is of temporary value in moderate oligemia, it is without value in severe oligemia because the extremities would have very little blood in them.[71, 78]

Until quite recently the Trendelenburg position was recommended in the treatment of shock. The patient was placed in a head-down position with his feet at least 30 cm. higher than his head, in the belief that this position would effectively increase cardiac output by facilitating venous return from the lower extremities and would also improve circulation to the brain. However, the Trendelenburg position is now known to: *impair* cardiac output, *decrease* the effectiveness of respiration and, at times, actually *decrease* the circulation to the brain. The reasons follow:

> Trendelenburg position does not facilitate the flow of venous blood from the brain to the right atrium, or the flow of oxygenated blood from the pulmonary blood stream to the left atrium.[6]

> If too steep, the Trendelenburg position causes the abdominal organs to push against the diaphragm, thereby decreasing the area for pulmonary expansion and decreasing the respiratory pump's effectiveness.[6]

> Trendelenburg position may initiate aortic and carotid sinus reflexes, causing constriction of the blood vessels supplying the brain and, thus, decrease in blood flow to the brain.[3]

TEMPERATURE

Until recently it was standard procedure to apply external heat to the patient in shock. Now it is realized that:

> *Heat, in any form, should not be applied to the patient in shock.*

Heat application causes the peripheral blood vessels to dilate and draws blood back from the vital organs into the vessels of the skin, thus interfering with the body's initial compensatory mechanism of peripheral vasconstriction. Also, heat increases the body's metabolism, thus increasing the need for oxygen and substrates and thereby putting an added strain on the heart.[6, 71] However, the patient should be kept comfortably warm, and every care should be taken that he does not become chilled.

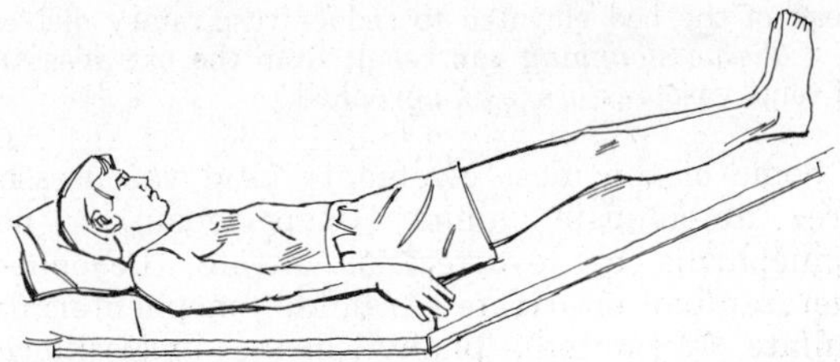

FIGURE 26–5. Recommended position for the treatment of shock. Legs should be elevated with the knees kept straight and the head should be on a level with, or slightly higher than, the chest. (Modified from Simeone: *American Journal of Nursing*, June, 1966.)

Elevated body temperatures should be returned to nearly normal if the elevation is serious in degree; however, hypothermia for the treatment of shock is generally not advisable, since it increases the blood's viscosity and slows the flow of blood through the microcirculation. Also, hypothermia slows the heart, increases the possibility of ventricular fibrillation, and inhibits the body's reparative processes.

VASOCONSTRICTION AND VASODILATION[56]

For some time a dichotomy of opinion has existed in the treatment of shock concerning the use of *vasopressors,* to *increase* peripheral resistance and systemic blood pressure, and the use of *vasodilators,* to *decrease* peripheral resistance and blood flow. Generally the cardiovascular effects of these two procedures are diametrically opposite. While pressor drugs, e.g., adrenergic drugs (sympathomimetic amines), have been used to elevate the systemic blood pressure, physicians now realize that excessive vasoconstriction may impede, rather than enhance, tissue perfusion.

> Mounting laboratory and clinical evidence suggests that pressor drugs are not an unmixed blessing in shock. Their ability to produce an increase in systemic arterial pressure, largely as a result of increased peripheral resistance, offers . . . a sense of security that is often false because the response is unsustained and diverts attention from the lethal mechanisms that are in progress.[19]

As previously indicated, vasoconstriction in various vascular beds (the major effect of pressor drugs) is now accepted as a central feature of the shock syndrome. Interestingly, all the classic signs of shock are also signs of increased sympathetic nervous system activity and/or vasoconstriction: pallor; cold, sweating extremities; oliguria; collapsed veins; and slow capillary filling. Physicians and nurses frequently observe, while at the bedside, that *factors that promote vasoconstriction* (e.g., pain, fear, hypoxia) *tend to accentuate the development of shock.* Studies also demonstrate that the infusion of relatively small amounts of epinephrine or norepinephrine causes vasoconstriction, which hastens circulatory failure in shock due to hemorrhage.

On the other hand, controlled experiments prove that certain *agents that induce vasodilatation, or inhibit vasoconstriction, significantly increase the survival rate or survival time in shock.* Included in this group of helpful agents are adrenergic blocking agents, ganglionic blocking agents, and direct-acting peripheral vasodilators.

Adrenergic blockade will *prevent* the following harmful effects of prolonged vasoconstriction in shock:

> Prolonged vasoconstriction increases the pressure in capillaries and thereby promotes a loss of fluid from the vascular to the interstitial compartment.

> Prolonged vasoconstriction can alter the local distribution of blood flow, especially in the splanchnic area, so that a considerably increased proportion of blood passes through channels from which an exchange of metabolites with tissue cells does not readily occur. Cellular nutrition is thus impaired and waste products accumulate.

Not only will adrenergic blockade prevent the above changes in circulation, it may helpfully induce changes in the opposite direction. As various workers have commented, in the treatment of shock it is easy to lapse into the treatment of the patient's blood pressure per se, rather than focusing therapy on promoting the perfusion of tissues with blood.

In sum, while vasopressor drugs were once believed to be of great value in treating shock, many modern practitioners and researchers believe that the basic treatment for many forms of shock is to dilate the peripheral blood vessels (and spare visceral organs from the devastating effects of prolonged vasoconstriction) instead of contributing to the vasoconstriction already present in shock. At present the value of vasodilators is being carefully considered. However, investigators are optimistic about this form of treatment and believe that it should be included in the armamentarium of shock therapies.

Present Role of Vasopressor Drugs

Although pressor therapy is being critically evaluated at present, it is also cited as having some *favorable effects.* For example, *increased blood flow to the brain and heart* is believed by many to be a desirable outcome of pressor therapy. Such increased blood flow may be particularly beneficial in elderly patients who cannot tolerate prolonged severe hypotension because they have arteriosclerotic narrowing of the coronary or cerebral arteries. The reduced perfusion of tissues with blood, when arterial pressures are below 60 to 70 mm. Hg, may result in myocardial infarction or a cerebral vascular accident.[19]

> *Perfusion of vital organs is impossible if the systolic blood pressure is below 50 mg. of Hg.*

The physician may prescribe a vasopressor agent for brief use if the degree of vasoconstriction in shock is not sufficient to maintain blood flow to vital organs such as the brain and heart. Pressor drugs may also be used to *correct hypotension that is secondary to paralysis of vasoconstrictor nerves,* e.g., in spinal anesthesia. Although vasopressor drugs may be used in the treatment of neurogenic shock, they are usually not used in treating traumatic and hemorrhagic shock. Whether vasopressor drugs should be used in treating cardiogenic shock is at present an unresolved dilemma.[21, 54, 71]

Usually the goal of vasopressor therapy is to achieve and maintain a mean blood pressure of 70 to 80 mm. of Hg, thus maintaining a blood pressure level that is sufficient to insure perfusion of tissues, rather than to attain normal blood pressures. Generally attempts to increase the blood pressure beyond the recommended level are inadvisable, since these drugs increase the oxygen demand of the heart and may thereby cause death-producing arrhythmias.[8]

Pressor therapy is used for as short a time as possible, for while drugs that cause vasoconstriction may initially be helpful in supplying improved circulation to the heart and brain, prolonged use of these drugs may cause irreversible damage in the tissues of the kidney, liver, lungs, and gastrointestinal tract.[21] Some of the *major adverse effects* of pressor therapy are:[8, 19, 54]

> Pressor drugs *potentiate the action of endotoxin* (or vice versa).

> These drugs appear to *cause a further reduction of the blood flow* to the kidneys and *to the entire splanchnic area.*

> An excessive and/or sudden rise in the arterial blood pressure, which vasopressors could cause, may precipitate *heart failure.*

> *Overloading of the vascular system* can occur, because pressor drugs must be diluted in rather large volumes of fluid before they are administered. The use of an infusion pump, which enables the controlled delivery of minute amounts of the undiluted drug, is one solution to this problem.

> *Ventricular arrhythmias* may develop during the administration of pressor drugs. ECG monitoring should be used and the physician notified at once if frequent premature ventricular contractions* are observed.

> *Pulmonary edema or left ventricular decompensation* can occur. Vasopressors cause a rise in blood pressure as a result of peripheral vessel constriction. This promotes a possibly dangerous overloading of the pulmonary circulation because blood is diverted to the central circulation from peripheral areas. When such problems appear, the IV flow should be slowed to a minimum, the physician should be notified at once, and the head of the bed elevated to reduce respiratory distress.

> *Tissue sloughing* can result from the extravasation of some vasopressors, e.g., Levophed.

Some of the most commonly used vasopressors are: angiotensin amide (Hypertensin); 1-norepinephrine or levarterenol bitrate (Levophed); metaraminol bitartrate (Aramine); mephentermine sulfate (Wyamine); phenylephrine hydrochloride (Neo-Synephrine); and isoproterenol (Isuprel).

*See Unit X for additional information about heart beats.

While Aramine and Wyamine can be administered either intravenously or intramuscularly, Levophed (probably the most frequently used vasopressor) can be given only intravenously. Levophed should be injected into large and central veins after it has been previously diluted in an intravenous dextrose solution. The intravenous drip should be stopped at once if tissue infiltration occurs.[54]

When any vasopressor is administered the arterial blood pressure should be carefully monitored to watch for undesirable elevations in blood pressure. Flow of the intravenous solution is carefully adjusted to establish and maintain the desired blood pressure.

Remember as you administer these drugs (and other intravenous infusions) that when a patient who is receiving intravenous infusions changes his position, the rate of flow of the solution may be altered, causing an undesirable change in the amount of medication being delivered.

Present Role of Vasodilator Drugs

When vasoconstriction is severe and persists despite the infusion of what should be adequate fluid replacement, vasodilators may be helpful. Vasodilators are used on the premise that the peripheral blood vessels are fully constricted during shock owing to the large output of norepinephrine (which occurs as a compensatory action on the part of the body) and that *if this vasoconstriction were inhibited* a beneficial redistribution of blood would occur. The blood trapped peripherally would thus become available for enhancing tissue perfusion and the vascular volume should be increased.

Peripheral vasoconstriction decreases capillary blood flow and is deleterious in many hypotensive states; conversely, vasodilatation, *after adequate volume addition,* may improve capillary flow, tissue perfusion, and cellular metabolism and thus increase survival rates.[30]

When shock is caused by hypovolemia, rapid and adequate fluid replacement must be achieved when vasodilators are used.[8] Vasodilators are dangerous because they will result in a fall in the arterial blood pressure *if* they are given while circulating blood volume is deficient and the body is depending upon vasoconstriction for arterial pressure. However, if the vascular space is full and the cardiac venous return is adequate, then vasodilatation should result in the opening of arterioles in the lungs and elsewhere, letting the blood through and increasing the cardiac output and capillary perfusion. When a vasodilator is administered *after* adequate filling of the expanded vascular space, the resultant vasodilatation should not cause a systemic blood pressure drop. Indeed, at times a vasodilator may produce a dramatic and sustained rise in the systemic arterial pressure.[30]

Blood pressure and central venous pressure should be continuously monitored when vasodilator drugs are being used. Usually a mean blood pressure of 70 is considered acceptable; however, if abrupt severe hypotension should occur, administration of the drug is generally stopped and fluid administration increased.

The CVP will drop substantially if there is a marked decrease in peripheral resistance. The blood volume needs to be expanded as the vascular space enlarges, and CVP measurements are used to gauge the amount of fluid needed to fill the enlarging vascular space. The rate of fluid replacement is adjusted to maintain the desired CVP. If the CVP continues to fall in spite of fluid replacement the situation is *critical,* for this means that the rate and volume of fluid replacement are insufficient to meet the physiologic needs of the patient.

It is important to realize that with vasodilators the tissue perfusion may be improved even though the arterial blood pressure may be lower than normal. Patients receiving vasodilators should be kept in a flat position in bed; elevation of the head could produce a dangerous orthostatic hypotension.[8]

Because of the presence of sclerotic vessels, older patients may not be able to tolerate the hypotension that may accompany treatment of shock with vasodilator drugs. When this is the situation, a cardiogenic drug may be given in combination with the vasodilator to increase the cardiac output and thus help to maintain or raise the blood pressure.

Antiadrenergic drugs appear to have prophylactic value in several types of shock. However, such drugs are potentially dangerous in that they can precipitate lethal complications.[30] Some investigators[19] are evaluating splanchnic autonomic blockade accomplished by the introduction of long-acting local anesthetic agents (lidocaine and others) into the retroperitoneal space via paravertebral needle or catheter. This procedure is done in an effort to limit the site of antiadrenergic action to the area of greatest apparent need (the splanchnic area) and thus minimize or avoid the hypotensive effect of total body adrenergic blockade.

Some examples of drugs used to produce vasodilatation and reduce peripheral resistance are: phentolamine (Regitine), phenoxybenzamine (Dibenzyline), chlorpromazine (Thorazine), and hydrocortisone.

Phenoxybenzamine (Dibenzyline) is one of the more powerful antiadrenergic drugs. This medication reduces peripheral resistance by blocking the alpha adrenergic receptors in the walls of the blood vessels so that the blood vessels do not respond to the norepinephrine that is produced during shock. Dibenzyline also reduces the small vessels' responses to histamine and serotonin. The heart's effectiveness is increased when this vasodilator is given because it does not change the cardiac catecholamines, e.g., epinephrine and norepinephrine.

Interest has developed in the use of phenoxybenzamine as a pretreatment for surgical procedures (e.g., open-heart surgery) that are often associated with a postoperative shock-like pattern as a result of poor perfusion of vital tissues during surgery.[46]

As we have indicated, Dibenzyline is likely to cause a further fall in blood pressure if it is given in the presence of hypovolemia, because the adrenergic blockade that it produces will increase the size of the vascular space. However, this can be remedied by giving the medication as a slow drip at the same time that plasma or blood is being given to fill up the increasing vascular space. It is important to remember that the volume of plasma needed to treat shock in such a situation is far in excess of measured losses. In other words, the best clinical results are not obtained by merely replacing estimated plasma losses. If adequate fluid replacement is not given and the Dibenzyline is administered by itself, death will rapidly follow because the blood pressure will drop to disastrously low levels, resulting in respiratory arrest. Dibenzyline may be administered in a dose of 1 mg. per kg. of body weight given intravenously over a one- to two-hour period, combined with plasma and blood administration.[46]

Chlorpromazine also antagonizes vasoconstriction during shock. Small doses of chlorpromazine (0.1 to 0.2 mg. per kg. of body weight) have been found to adequately produce the desired alpha adrenergic blockade without the excessive sedation produced by higher doses. As with phenoxybenzamine, chlorpromazine should not be given unless suitable fluid can be administered to fill the expanded space in the vascular compartment that results from adrenergic blockade.[21]

ADRENOCORTICOIDS

The early use of adrenocortical hormones in the treatment of shock was based on pioneer demonstrations that, under stress, the adrenocortical function increases. However, as yet the precise mechanisms that underlie the action of these hormones remain unidentified.[62]

Today many investigators recommend the administration of large doses of adrenocorticoids in the treatment of shock. However, while glucocorticoids (e.g., cortisone, hydrocortisone)* have an established place in the treatment of some types of shock, the therapeutic indications for use of the mineralocorticoids (e.g., aldosterone and desoxycorticosterone) have *not* been satisfactorily established.[62]

*Examples of synthetic glucocorticoids are prednisone, prednisolone, methylprednisolone, triamcinolone, and dexamethasone.

Experimental evidence indicates that adrenocorticoids may exert both cardiotonic (e.g., increased cardiac output) as well as vascular effects. Glucocorticoids may counteract the reduced cardiac output and the accompanying increased total resistance to blood flow that are the two basic hemodynamic inadequacies of shock. Thus, corticosteroids may be administered in the treatment of shock on the basis that they increase blood flow and decrease blood resistance, thereby augmenting the beneficial effects of vasopressor agents.[77] When given large doses of glucocorticoids, patients in shock may maintain a more adequate blood pressure level owing to improved systemic blood flow. Inactive pools of venous blood evidently cause reduced cardiac output in toxic shock; adrenocorticoids seem to contribute toward mobilizing such pools.[62]

The *antitoxic effect* of the adrenocorticoids is another reason for their use in the treatment of shock.[62] In addition, it is known that steroids *stabilize the lysosomal membrane* and prevent the intracellular release of enzymes. Also, they *increase blood volume* by increasing sodium retention.

When steroid therapy is used in managing shock it is agreed that the dosages should be in pharmacologic quantities rather than merely in the range of replacement therapy. At least 3000 mg. of hydrocortisone per day is recommended by some.[8] Some typical dosage schedules of corticoids in treating shock follow.[62]

> Intravenous doses of 500 mg. hydrocortisone (Solu-Cortef), and 100 mg. prednisolone or methyl-prednisolone (Hydeltrasol, Solu-Medrol), or 20 mg. dexamethasone (Decadron) may be used every 4 to 6 hours for a period usually not exceeding 3 to 5 days.

> The initial injection is twice the amount listed above, i.e., 1 gm. of cortisol, 200 mg. of prednisolone, or 40 mg. of dexamethasone.

> Some physicians prefer direct, slow, intravenous injection to a more prolonged infusion by intravenous drip.

> A gradual reduction of dosage is not necessary for corticoid treatment of such short duration; it may be stopped abruptly.

> Doses of corticoids smaller than those listed above may prove inadequate in treating shock.

Adrenocortical hormones provide *specific* treatment for those rare instances of shock that are due to adrenal insufficiency, e.g., addisonian crisis.

Some *general* situations in which adrenocortical therapy might prove helpful include: (1) the treatment of cases of protracted hypotension associated with severe allergic (hypersensitivity) reactions, and (2) counteracting the detrimental effects of gram-negative endotoxins. Steroids improve the survival rate of patients in shock from gram-negative bacterial infection of the blood stream. In such circumstances the drug must be given in very high doses.

In spite of advances in treatment, the mortality rate in gram-negative shock remains at about 50 per cent.

Considerable interest is being expressed in the role of corticoids in combination with vasopressor agents in treating shock. Some believe that the efficiency of the hormones appears to be much greater if they are given in combination with various pressor agents.[44]

The conventional clinical practice of administering corticosteroids only as a final and desperate measure after vasopressor therapy has failed is not recommended.[62] When used, corticosteroids should be administered early in the course of shock, rather than as a last resort after other medications have proved unsuccessful.[8]

Several theoretical dangers to the patient may accompany steroid therapy in the high dosage ranges used in treating shock: acute gastrointestinal bleeding; the aggravation of diabetes; and inhibition of the antibody response, thereby making possible uncontrollable infection. Since patients receiving high doses of steroids are susceptible to infection, they should be protected in every way from potential sources of infection. The prevention of pneumonia, wound infection, and bacteremia should be kept in mind. Also, excretions (e.g., vomitus, urine, feces) from patients receiving large steroid doses should be examined for blood, since steroids can induce internal bleeding.[8]

ANTIBIOTICS

When shock is due to an infection, antibiotic therapy is highly important and must be instituted immediately. When bacteremic shock is suspected, a blood specimen, for culture and sensitivity, is taken at once and then antibiotics are started even though the infecting organism has not been identified. At the same time that the blood sample is drawn, samples of urine, sputum, and any fluid from draining wounds, sinuses, and so forth, should be taken for culture. Since toxic shock is often caused by gram-negative enteric bacteria, a combination of ampicillin, polymixin, and cephalothin may be used until the findings of the cultures and sensitivities are available.[8]

CARDIAC SUPPORT

Medications that will improve myocardial contraction are basic in treating those forms of shock that cause a decreased cardiac output, e.g., hypovolemic shock and cardiogenic shock. (See also Unit X.) Various medications may be employed to improve cardiac efficiency:

> *Digitalis* is frequently used if there is evidence of cardiac failure.[30] By strengthening and slowing the heart beat, digitalis gives support to a weakened heart and may reduce the rate of heart beats to a more normal level. *Ouabain* and *deslanoside (Cedilanid D)* are examples of rapidly acting digitalis preparations that may be given intravenously early in the course of shock. These medications are not given to patients who are already digitalized. In addition to being given to treat patients with pre-existing or present evidence of cardiac failure, digitalis is indicated for patients with increased central venous pressure, digitalis-responsive arrhythmias, and, controversially, in myocardial infarction. Digitalis is without value in treating shock due to other causes.

> *Isoproterenol* (Isuprel) is more effective than digitalis in strengthening the force of myocardial contraction and thus improving cardiac output.

> *Quinidine* and *procainamide* may be given to treat arrhythmias that tend to reduce cardiac efficiency. These medications, however, do reduce myocardial contractility.

> Atropine may be used for bradycardias, which predispose to cardiogenic shock.

For a further discussion of medications used to improve cardiac efficiency see the unit on the heart. The precautions necessary in using such medications should be observed as detailed in that unit.

Continuous cardiac monitoring is desirable, particularly if beta-mimetic adrenergic drugs are being administered. The use of vasopressor drugs in treating myocardial infarction is controversial. Phlebotomy may be employed to treat cardiac failure.

RENAL SUPPORT

Impaired kidney function and acute renal tubular necrosis may result from shock, as we have discussed earlier. Thus, oliguria is often a concomitant of shock. Simeone comments:

> In the early phase of the shock immediately subsequent to severe burns, trauma, and hemorrhage, the subnormal urinary output can be corrected by restoring the circulating blood volume to normal and by providing the normal daily requirements of water and electrolytes. However, in other forms of shock (septic shock, in particular), late in severe burns, and in oligemic shock which has progressed into the late phase, restoration of normal circulating blood volume and composition may not correct the oliguria or anuria. Indeed, the cardiovascular failure may no longer exist, while the oliguria progresses to a lethal anuria.[71]

In an attempt to prevent acute renal damage the urine output is monitored with an indwelling catheter and osmotic diuretics, e.g., urea and mannitol, may be given.[8] The correction of metabolic acidosis and the utilization of other measures to increase blood volume and improve cardiac output will also benefit the kidney as well as other tissues. If tubular necrosis is present, artificial dialysis may be needed until the regeneration of functioning renal tubular epithelium can take place.[71]

Mannitol is the reduced form of the 6-carbon sugar mannose; it is filtered in the urine and is neither reabsorbed nor metabolized. Mannitol acts as an osmotic diuretic and, thus, helps to rid the body of hemolyzed cells and other wastes that accumulate in the renal tubules. By restoring to active circulation the fluid that was lost (due to the block of the microcirculation), mannitol helps to alleviate the microcirculatory block in shock. Large amounts of hemoglobin or myoglobin may be in the circulation during shock. At the glomerular level these substances are filtered, and if the urinary flow is inadequate (because of the pronounced water reabsorption that occurs during shock) these substances will precipitate in the tubule. By maintaining an adequate output of urine, mannitol helps to prevent tubular damage.[21]

Furosemide (Lasix) has also been recommended for similar use (instead of mannitol) in patients with oliguria or in whom oliguria is anticipated.

RESPIRATORY SUPPORT

The patient in shock must be checked immediately to be certain that the airway is open and functioning. If necessary, ensure ventilation by mouth-to-mouth breathing. Circulatory improvement depends on adequate respiratory function, for the arterial blood must be oxygenated by the lung and carbon dioxide must be exchanged into the atmosphere in order to help to correct the metabolic acidosis that develops with shock. By increasing the rate of pulmonary ventilation (by spontaneous or mechanical hyperventilation) it is possible to correct *minor* degrees of metabolic acidosis. The "blowing off" of carbon dioxide into the expired air results in a return of the blood pH to normal.[71]

The pCO_2 is measured to determine whether the metabolic acidosis is being effectively combated by hyperventilation: a low pCO_2 along with low pH and bicarbonate levels (metabolic acidosis) indicates that hyperventilation is compensating; a rising pCO_2 in the presence of a persistently low pH indicates that respiratory assistance will be needed because hyperventilation is failing. As hyperventilation fails, the patient's rate and depth of respiration decline and cyanosis appears. In this situation the accumulated carbon dioxide can be removed only with a respirator to assist ventilation; oxygen administration is valueless.[8]

In treating the earliest stages of respiratory failure due to metabolic acidosis, a pressure-controlled respirator that is triggered by the patient's demand (e.g., Bird respirator) may be adequate. However, if there is obvious respiratory failure and pCO_2 levels are quite high, a volume displacement, piston-type respirator is indicated, such as the Engstrom, Morch, or Emerson. Brand and Thal observe that those powerful respirators can convert respiratory acidosis to respiratory alkalosis in 10 to 30 minutes.[8]

Some of the causes of respiratory failure in shock are:[19]

> Respiratory overload due to fever, infection and/or metabolic acidosis.

> Cerebral arterial insufficiency which obtunds the gag and cough reflexes as well as the respiratory center's sensitivity.

> Stupor, coma, or aspiration of gastric contents, causing airway obstruction.

> Physical exhaustion from long, severe illness existing before the onset of shock or resulting from the shock episode itself. The patient in shock works hard to move air in and out of his lungs since he is dyspneic.

To relax the exhausted patient in severe or prolonged shock, and to correct respiratory failure, treatment often needs to include tracheal intubation or tracheostomy. An endotracheal tube may be used or a cuffed tracheostomy tube may be inserted following tracheostomy. The ventilatory dead space is reduced by a tracheostomy, and more thorough tracheobronchial hygiene can be performed. Intubation or tracheostomy may be followed promptly by an increase in blood pressure.[30, 71]

In all cases of shock, regardless of cause, the patient must receive supplemental oxygen to protect him against hypoxemia. Oxygen concentrations above 30 per cent appear adequate to protect against hypoxemia.[21] The prolonged administration of 100 per cent oxygen is contraindicated because of the danger of inducing oxygen toxicity.[71] Usually the lowest concentration of oxygen that will maintain a pO_2 of 60 mm. of Hg or higher is prescribed, since high oxygen concentrations are known to be damaging to the lung.

In treating shock oxygen may be indicated to correct hypoxia caused by disorders such as pneumonia and cardiac failure.

FLUID REPLACEMENT

> The most important treatment of noncardiac shock is fluid volume administration given, if necessary, to the point of an elevated central venous or pulmonary artery pressure. Adequate volume is more important than the type of fluid administered. Blood is given only up to a normal red cell mass.[30]

Most forms of shock (excluding that associated with myocardial infarction) involve a decreased effective circulating blood volume, owing to the external or internal loss of whole blood, plasma, and/or relatively protein-free plasma water. Recognizing this fact, the mainstay of shock therapy has been established as the expansion of the circulating blood volume by the intravenous administration of blood or other appropriate fluids.[56]

Various fluids are given to correct specific problems, such as electrolyte or protein deficiencies or other defects of the blood, including acidosis and hyponatremia. However, in treating shock, the *immediate* results of therapy seem to depend less on the type of fluid used for fluid replacement than upon the *amount* of fluid administered. Generally enough fluid is given so that the normal blood volume is exceeded. In part, this "extra" fluid is required because of the expanded vascular space caused by the dilation of the microcirculation. Therapy must be monitored to prevent circulatory overload. Hypervolemia can be lethal.

In replacing fluids, enough volume must be added to fill the capillaries and run through into the veins. Such fluid replacement maintains the central venous pressure and provides an adequate venous return to the heart, which, in turn, promotes additional cardiac output.[30] In addition, adequate fluid replacement will decrease the blood catecholamine level and thus produce a physiologic vasodilatation that promotes capillary flow. This adequate flow of fluids in the capillaries, in turn, perfuses tissues and prevents sludging and coagulation within the vessels.[30]

As we have indicated earlier, a phase of *hypercoagulability* occurs in several forms of shock, producing intravascular thrombosis. Indeed, such clotting of the blood within the capillaries may begin quite early in the hypotensive period. It has been observed in experimentally produced ventricular fibrillation that minute clots appear in the circulating blood and pulmonary capillaries if resuscitation is delayed beyond five minutes. In traumatic shock thrombi occur in the region of the crushed tissue, and in hemorrhagic shock thrombi appear in the vascular beds of the lungs, liver, intestines, kidneys, and other tissues.[44]

An important aspect in preventing irreversible shock is, thus, treatment that prevents hypercoagulability in the blood or that promotes the lysis of thrombi that have already formed. Heparin has been observed to prolong survival time or to reduce the mortality rate in toxic shock, acute circulatory arrest, and hemorrhagic shock, as well as in those forms of shock resulting from the administration of incompatible blood or amniotic fluid. In hemorrhagic shock the dissolution of clots by fibrinolysin therapy may at times avert irreversibility even though intravascular coagulation has occurred.[44]

Patients in shock may have multiple clotting defects involving deficiencies of several clotting factors. Fibrinogen often is high, indicating that an increase in the manufacturing of this element has exceeded the increase in its utilization. Other factors are typically decreased and may become extremely low, resulting in a tendency to hemorrhage and serious capillary bleeding. Platelet defects are also common in shock. The *rapid* administration of fresh whole blood or fresh frozen plasma may quickly and effectively treat the coagulation and platelet defects.[30]

Whole Blood Replacement*

If hemorrhage is the primary cause of shock, the rapid administration of large volumes of whole blood may be necessary. The blood will act as a hypothermic agent unless it is warmed to body temperature. This can be hazardous in the presence of shock, because slowing of cardiac action, with decreased cardiac output or ventricular fibrillation, may result if body temperatures fall below 32°C.[8]

When treating shock resulting from hemorrhage, plasma is usually given as an initial emergency treatment to sustain blood pressure. The acute anemia, resulting from the hemorrhage, must then be corrected by replacement with whole blood to prevent hypoxemia. The physician determines the amount of blood to be given by evaluating the patient's clinical response and hematocrit. Blood volume studies are also evaluated when they are available.

In fluid replacement a normal red blood cell mass should be maintained; however, fluids that are given in excess of normal volume should be fluids other than blood to allow for their easy removal from the circulation once shock is over. If the normal red blood cell mass is exceeded, it is difficult for the body to get rid of the excess when the vascular volume contracts back to normal after adequate perfusion of the tissues is achieved. Also, since there are dangers involved in blood transfusions, blood should not be used as long as another fluid can satisfactorily maintain an adequate oxygen-carrying capacity and sufficiently increase blood volume. Saline or other fluids can be as effective as blood in increasing blood volume. While colloid (e.g., dextran or normal serum albumin) remains in the vascular system longer than electrolytes, the immediate effect is the same.[30]

*For additional information on the administration of whole blood see Unit XII.

Plasma Expanders

Fluids that contain molecules large enough to be retained in the blood vessels are necessary in the treatment of shock in which plasma loss is excessive, e.g., burns, acute pancreatitis, and peritonitis. Plasma, electrolyte solutions containing albumin, or dextran of high or low molecular weight may be administered. Concentrated albumin may be used to increase the colloidal osmotic pressure; thus, fluid escape from the vascular system due to protein depletion can be controlled.[8]

Dextran is frequently used in fluid replacement therapy in shock. Both regular (also called "high-molecular weight" or "clinical") and low-molecular weight (LMW) dextran have been recommended for use as plasma expanders that will rapidly expand the plasma volume.[8] Human blood plasma carries the risk of transmitting viral hepatitis; therefore, pharmaceutical plasma expanders are generally recommended.[71] LMW dextran (Rheomacrodex) appears to be less effective as a volume expander than regular dextran or another colloidal agent known as hydroxy-ethyl starch,[8] and LMW dextran is now used mainly to reduce the blood's viscosity and reduce red cell aggregation.

Colloidal solutions may be administered in the treatment of oligemic shock if properly matched whole blood is unavailable or cannot be obtained rapidly. While normal saline solutions, which are readily available, can be used in emergencies to begin the correction of oligemia, colloidal solutions are recommended, since they remain in the circulation longer than crystalloids.[71]

In treating oligemic shock,[78] a plasma volume expander, e.g., dextran, or human serum albumin, may be given until properly cross-matched whole blood is available. Before the dextran is administered a blood sample should be taken for blood grouping and cross matching.

High molecular weight dextran is most often used in amounts not exceeding 1 liter in the adult, or one third the expected volume of blood to be replaced.[71] While high molecular dextran tends to remain in the blood more readily than LMW dextran, excessive amounts can interfere with blood-clotting mechanisms and promote erythrocyte aggregation. This, of course, adds to the problems of slow-moving blood.

Balanced Electrolyte Solutions

During oligemic shock the loss of circulating blood volume is associated with a redistribution of extravascular fluid. Thus, a sizable amount* of fluid leaves the extravascular, extracellular space *in addition* to the fluid lost from the circulating volume as a result of hemorrhage. In fluid replacement therapy, therefore, *both* the deficit of whole blood lost from the circulation and the additional fluid lost from the extravascular space must be replaced in the form of lactated Ringer's solution or other balanced saline solutions.[71] When the loss of free water has been great (as in burns) 5 per cent dextrose in water may be given, since fluid replacement with dextrose solution is preferable to salt solutions in order to avoid electrolyte overloading.[8]

When severe metabolic acidosis is present, a buffer often needs to be added to the circulating blood, e.g., tris-(hydroxymethyl)aminomethane (THAM), or sodium bicarbonate.[71] (THAM is a complex organic agent.) It should be remembered that solutions containing sodium are frequently contraindicated in cardiac disorders. Sometimes large quantities of normal saline may be administered in treating shock.

Electrolyte solutions such as Ringer's lactate or saline buffered with bicarbonate help expand extracellular volume, reduce viscosity and prevent sludging.[8] When lactate levels are abnormally high and lactate is not being metabolized properly, it is undesirable to administer lactate and it is believed to be better to treat acidosis with sodium bicarbonate. However, lactated Ringer's solution has recently been advocated for the initial treatment of shock because it contains the electrolyte content that the kidney requires to maintain an adequate level of renal function.[78] This solution is frequently given by intravenous infusion for rapid expansion of the vascular volume.[8]

Specific abnormalities of electrolyte and acid-base balance are corrected as they are identified. Therapy is gauged by serial arterial pH determinations. (See Chapter 25.)

Care of the Patient Receiving Fluid Replacement for Shock

In a majority of cases of shock, fluid replacement is the only treatment required. In some instances up to 8 to 12 liters of fluid may be administered in only a few hours. As mentioned earlier, the volume of fluid given generally exceeds estimates of blood or fluid loss or volume deficit.[30]

Often it is difficult to evaluate whether the fluid replacement is adequate. Internal losses of circulating fluid volume, including whole blood, into areas of trauma, infection, and so forth, are most difficult to estimate and, if a vasoconstrictor drug has been administered or if vasoconstriction has persisted for a considerable length of time, an additional considerable loss of circulating volume may have occurred as a result of the vasoconstriction.[56] The volume of fluid administered may be pushed until either (1) systemic blood pressure, urine volume, and lactate levels return to a relatively normal level; or (2) central venous or pulmonary artery pressures, or both, become elevated.[30]

Central venous pressure (CVP) measurement is one of the first steps in the treatment of shock since it is an important means of estimating fluid loss. The infusion of blood or other fluids is usually continued only as long as the CVP is low, below 10 cm.; when the CVP is higher than normal (e.g., 10 or 12 cm.) benefit cannot be expected from the continued infusion of fluids or blood. A phlebotomy may be performed if the CVP becomes elevated to 15 cm. or more. When the CVP is low and the patient's lungs are clear, with no signs of cardiac asthma or left ventricular failure, fluids are administered to improve the return of blood to the heart. However, there are patients who have a normal or low CVP in spite of faulty left ventricular function; these patients readily develop pulmonary edema or cardiac asthma. Thus, a low or normal CVP does not always mean that fluid administration is advisable.[71]

The administration of fluids should be stopped prior to extremely high elevations of *pulmonary artery pressure* if an adequate systemic response has been achieved. An adequate volume of fluid causes an adequate venous return to the right heart with the result that the output of the right heart will be increased. If there is continued pulmonary obstruction due to coagulation in the microcirculation and vasoconstriction, then pulmonary artery hypertension may result; this would be reflected in the pulmonary artery pressure. In the presence of right heart failure this increase in pressure may back up through the right heart, causing an abnormal elevation in the central venous pressure. Vasodilators may be helpful in opening this partially blocked pulmonary microcirculation.[30]

While *red blood cell mass measurements* are reasonably accurate in shock, the same is not true of *plasma volume measurements*. Accurate measurements of plasma volume are not possible in shock since by the time the iodinated ^{131}I serum albumin has properly mixed in the slowly circulating blood, significant amounts have already leaked out of the vascular tree.[30]

The measurement of blood volume by *dilution techniques* does not appear to solve the problem of estimating fluid loss because of technical difficulties and also because there are no standards available for estimating the circulating volume that is optimal for a given individual subjected to a particular type, severity, and duration of stress.

*This extravascular loss can amount to some 4 liters in moderately severe shock.

The administration of *phenoxybenzamine* provides a simple and reliable test for measurement of the adequacy of prior blood and other fluid volume therapy and allows for the more rapid administration of larger amounts of intravenous fluids in patients with myocardial adequacy. Any considerable fall in blood pressure during the administration of phenoxybenzamine suggests an inadequate circulating blood volume, since in well ventilated, normovolemic, supine humans, adrenergic blockade will produce little or no fall in the systolic blood pressure and only a limited decrease in the diastolic pressure. The blood pressure may start to fall rapidly in *hypovolemic* patients when as little as 10 per cent of the usual dose of phenoxybenzamine has been infused.[56]

GENERAL CARE

As a nurse you should be alert for early signs of shock, since treatment must be started as soon as possible to prevent irreversible shock.

Some general points to keep in mind in caring for patients in shock are:

> Assemble all equipment and supplies (suction, emergency drugs, and so forth) and have them in working order.

> Prevent the complications that the patient can develop from enforced immobilization.

> Continuous monitoring and observation of the patient is imperative, since changes in cardiovascular and respiratory functions can occur rapidly, and treatment must be adjusted accordingly.

> Help the patient to feel at rest physically and emotionally to reduce his physical needs for oxygen and nutrients.

> Strive to reduce the patient's fears and anxieties about what is happening to him and about the equipment being used.

> Keep the room temperature somewhat cool (65 to 68° F.) to reduce the patient's metabolic rate.

> Provide adequate pain relief, since pain intensifies shock. However, do not give unnecessary narcotics and sedatives. Remember that restlessness may be due to a lack of oxygen to the brain rather than pain. Since impaired circulation can cause the delayed absorption of drugs, hypodermic injection is not advisable. For example, if morphine is given subcutaneously to the patient in shock it may not be absorbed and repeated doses will accumulate. Then when adequate circulation is restored, morphine poisoning can occur, for excessive amounts of the drug are then absorbed. Analgesics or narcotics should be given intravenously to patients in shock, the usual dose being one half to two thirds the customary hypodermic dosage.[8]

Bordicks[6] states that there are two prime roles that the nurse must fulfill in caring for all patients in any pattern of shock. These important functions are: (1) The nurse must *expedite therapeutic orders* that will help the body to *obtain homeostatic balance,* without the need for compensatory mechanisms. (2) The nurse must also *understand* the compensatory mechanisms that are operative at the time and *support* them.

References

1. Ayres, S. M., and Gianelli, S.: *Care of the Critically Ill.* New York, Appleton-Century-Crofts, Inc., 1967.
2. Baez, S. and Orkin, L. R.: Microcirculatory effects of anesthesia in shock. *In* Hershey, S. G. (ed.): *Shock. International Anesthesiology Clinics.* Vol. 2. No. 2. Boston, Little, Brown and Company, 1964.
3. Beland, I. L., et. al.: *Clinical Nursing.* 2nd ed. New York, The Macmillan Company, 1970.
4. Birch, C. A.: *Emergencies in Medical Practice.* 8th ed. Baltimore, The Williams & Wilkins Company, 1967.
5. Booth, B. H., et al.: Anaphylaxis: A consideration in the differential diagnosis of shock. *Journal of Allergy* 42:364, December, 1968.
6. Bordicks, K. J.: *Patterns of Shock: Implications for Nursing Care.* New York, The Macmillan Company, 1965.
7. Bradley, E. C.: Blood volumes measured in patients during shock states. *Journal of Trauma* 9:145, February, 1969.
8. Brand, L., and Thal, A. P.: Shock. *In* Meltzer, L. E., Abdellah, F. G., and Kitchell, J. R. (eds.): *Concepts and Practices of Intensive Care for Nurse Specialists.* Philadelphia, Charles Press Publishers, Inc., 1969.
9. Chandler, J. G.: The physiology and treatment of shock. *RN* 34:42, June, 1971.
10. Cohn, J. N.: Blood pressure measurement in shock. *J.A.M.A.* 199:972, March 27, 1967.
11. Cohn, J. N.: Treatment of shock following myocardial infarction. *California Medicine* 111:66, July, 1969.
12. Cook, G. C.: Hepatic changes associated with shock. *International Anesthesiology Clinics* 7:883, Winter, 1969.
13. Corday, E., et al.: Pressor agents in cardiogenic shock. *American Journal Cardiology* 23:900, June, 1969.
14. Crowell, J. W., and Guyton, A. C.: Cardiac deterioration in shock: II. The irreversible stage. *In* Hershey, S. G. (ed.): *Shock. International Anesthesiology Clinics.* Vol. 2. No. 2. Boston, Little, Brown and Company, 1964.
15. Doty, D. B.: The practical value of the central venous catheter for monitoring the patient in shock. *Journal of Trauma* 9:148, February, 1969.
16. Eastridge, C. E., et al.: Shock: The hemodynamic diagnosis and treatment. *Southern Medical Journal* 62:665, June, 1969.
17. Fowler, A. W.: Treatment of shock. *British Medical Journal* 4:494, November 21, 1970.
18. Fox, C. L., and Lasker, S. E.: Fluid therapy in surgical emergencies. *Surgical Clinics of North America* 35:335, 1955.
19. Frank, E. D.: Septic shock. *In* Hershey, S. G. (ed.): *Shock. International Anesthesiology Clinics.* Vol. 2. No. 2. Boston, Little, Brown and Company, 1964.

20. Frieden, E.: The enzyme-substrate complex. *Scientific American.* 201:125, August, 1959.
21. Gladish, J. T., Winnie, A. P., and Collins, V. J.: Shock: Recognition and modern management. *Postgraduate Medicine* 42:41, July, 1967.
22. Gil-Rodriguez, J. A.: Emergency extracorporeal circulation. *International Anesthesiology Clinics* 7:921, Winter, 1969.
23. Goldfarb, D.: Mechanical circulatory assist techniques in the treatment of cardiogenic shock. *Journal of Surgical Research* 9:493, August, 1969.
24. Greenbaum, R.: The blood and transfusion fluids in shock. *International Anesthesiology Clinics* 7:775, Winter, 1969.
25. Guyton, A. C., and Crowell, J. W.: Cardiac deterioration in shock: I. Its progressive nature. *In* Hershey, S. G. (ed.): *Shock. International Anesthesiology Clinics.* Vol. 2. No. 2. Boston, Little, Brown and Company. 1964.
26. Hanquet, M., et al.: Changes in catecholamine levels during shock in man. *Canadian Anaesthetists' Society Journal* 17:201, May, 1970.
27. Hardaway, R. M.: *Syndromes of Disseminated Intravascular Coagulation: With Special Reference to Shock and Hemorrhage.* Springfield, Illinois, Charles C Thomas, 1966.
28. Hardaway, R. M.: Current aspects of shock management. *Current Practice in Orthopedic Surgery* 4: 185, 1969.
29. Hardaway, R. M.: Treatment of shock. *Southwest Medicine* 52:26, February, 1971.
30. Hardaway, R. M., et al.: Intensive study and treatment of shock in man. *J.A.M.A.* 199:779, March 13, 1967.
31. Hershey, S. G.: Dynamics of peripheral vascular collapse in shock. *In* Hershey, S. G. (ed.): *Shock. International Anesthesiology Clinics.* Vol. 2. No. 2. Boston, Little, Brown and Company, 1964.
32. Hershey, S. G., (ed.): *Shock. International Anesthesiology Clinics.* Vol. 2. No. 2. Boston, Little, Brown and Company, 1964.
33. Hewer, C. L.: The physiology and complications of the Trendelenburg position. *Canadian Medical Association Journal* 74:295, 1956.
34. Hill, D. W.: Computers in the management of shock. *International Anesthesiology Clinics* 7:1035, Winter, 1969.
35. Hinshaw, L. B.: Role of the veins in shock. *Journal of Oklahoma State Medical Association* 63:106, March, 1970.
36. Janoff, A.: Alterations in lysosomes (intracellular enzymes) during shock: Effects of preconditioning (tolerance) and protective drugs. *In* Hershey, S. G. (ed.): *Shock. International Anesthesiology Clinics.* Vol. 2. No. 2. Boston, Little, Brown and Company, 1964.
37. Kamada, R. O., et al.: The phenomenon of respiratory failure in shock: The genesis of "shock lung." *American Heart Journal* 83:1, January, 1972.
38. Kelman, G. R.: Cardiac output in shock. *International Anesthesiology Clinics* 7:739, Winter, 1969.
39. Kovaric, J. J., et al.: The use of fresh blood to correct coagulation defects associated with trauma and shock. *Military Medicine* 133:534, July, 1968.
40. Kurihara, M., and Moody, F. G.: The complications of general surgery. *In* Meltzer, L. E., Abdellah, F. G., and Kitchell, J. R. (eds.): *Concepts and Practices of Intensive Care for Nurse Specialists.* Philadelphia, Charles Press Publishers, Inc., 1969.
41. Learning about shock. *Nursing Mirror* 133:27, October 8, 1971.
42. Ledingham, I. M.: Hyperbaric oxygen in shock. *International Anesthesiology Clinics* 7:819, Winter, 1969.
43. Levenson, S. M., Nagler, A. L., and Einheber, A.: Some metabolic consequences of shock. *In* Hershey, S. G. (ed.): *Shock. International Anesthesiology Clinics.* Vol. 2. No. 2. Boston, Little, Brown and Company, 1964.
44. Levy, M. N., and Blattberg, B.: Blood factors in shock. *In* Hershey, S. G. (ed.): *Shock. International Anesthesiology Clinics.* Vol. 2. No. 2. Boston, Little, Brown and Company, 1964.
45. Lewin, I., et al.: Pulmonary failure associated with clinical shock states. *Journal of Trauma* 11:22, January, 1971.
46. Lillehei, R. C., et al.: The nature of experimental irreversible shock with its clinical application. *In* Hershey, S. G. (ed.): *Shock. International Anesthesiology Clinics.* Vol. 2. No. 2. Boston, Little, Brown and Company, 1964.
47. Litton, A.: Microvascular effects of vasoactive agents in shock. *British Journal of Surgery* 55:751, October, 1968.
48. MacBryde, C. M. (ed.): *Signs and Symptoms.* 4th ed. Philadelphia, J. B. Lippincott Company, 1964.
49. MacLean, L. D., et al.: The patient in shock. I. *Canadian Medical Association Journal* 105:78, July 10, 1971; II. 182, July 24, 1971.
50. Mazzia, V. D. B., and Rapaport, F. T.: Management of traumatic shock. *In* Hershey, S. G. (ed.): *Shock. International Anesthesiology Clinics.* Vol. 2. No. 2. Boston, Little, Brown and Company, 1964.
51. McLaughlin, J. S., et al.: Cardiovascular dynamics in human shock. *American Surgeon* 35:166, March, 1969.
52. McLaughlin, J. S., et al.: Pulmonary function in shock in humans. *British Journal of Surgery* 56:696, September, 1969.
53. Medical news, *J.A.M.A.* September 4, 1967.
54. Meltzer, L. E., Pinneo, R., and Kitchell, J. R.: Acute myocardial infarction. *In* Meltzer, L. E., Abdellah, F. G., and Kitchell, J. R. (eds.): *Concepts and Practices of Intensive Care for Nurse Specialists.* Philadelphia, Charles Press Publishers, Inc., 1969.
55. Moyer, J. H., et al.: Cardiogenic shock. I. *Pennsylvania Medicine* 71:53, December, 1968.
56. Nickerson, M.: Vasoconstriction and vasodilatation in shock. *In* Hershey, S. G. (ed.): *Shock. International Anesthesiology Clinics.* Vol. 2. No. 2. Boston, Little, Brown and Company, 1964.
57. Nickerson, M.: Vascular adjustments during the development of shock. *Canadian Medical Association Journal* 103:853, October 17, 1970.
58. Perlroth, M. G., et al.: Cardiogenic shock: A review. *Clinical Pharmacology and Therapeutics* 10:449, July-August, 1969.
59. Prys-Roberts, C.: Lung function in shock. *International Anesthesiology Clinics* 7:759, Winter, 1969.
60. Rosen, S. M.: Renal failure during and after shock. *International Anesthesiology Clinics* 7:861, Winter, 1969.
61. Rutherford, R. B.: Current concepts in the use of whole blood in the management of hemorrhagic shock. *Maryland Medical Journal* 17:65, September, 1968.

62. Sambhi, M. P., et al.: Adrenocorticoids in the management of shock. *In* Hershey, S. G. (ed.): *Shock. International Anesthesiology Clinics.* Vol. 2. No. 2. Boston, Little, Brown and Company, 1964.
63. Schloerb, P. R.: Shock and metabolism. *Surgery, Gynecology and Obstetrics* 128:315, February, 1969.
64. Schumer, W., et al.: The role of corticoids in the management of shock. *Surgical Clinics of North America* 49:147, February, 1969.
65. Schumer, W.: Evolution of the modern therapy of shock: Science vs. empiricism. *Surgical Clinics of North America* 51:3, February, 1971.
66. Selkurt, E. E.: Role of liver and toxic factors in shock. *In* Hershey, S. G. (ed.): *Shock. International Anesthesiology Clinics.* Vol. 2. No. 2. Boston, Little, Brown and Company, 1964.
67. Shires, G. T., Carrico, C. J., and Coln, D.: The role of the extracellular fluid in shock. *In* Hershey, S. G. (ed.): *Shock. International Anesthesiology Clinics.* Vol. 2. No. 2. Boston, Little, Brown and Company, 1964.
67a. Shires, G. T., et al.: *Shock.* Philadelphia, W. B. Saunders Company, 1973.
68. Shock lung. *California Medicine* 112:43, February, 1970.
69. Shoemaker, W. C.: Sequential hemodynamic patterns in various causes of shock. *Surgery, Gynecology and Obstetrics* 132:411, March, 1971.
70. Shoemaker, W. C., et al.: The dilemma of vasopressor and vasodilators in the therapy of shock. *Surgery, Gynecology and Obstetrics* 132:51, January, 1971.
71. Simeone, F. A.: The nature and treatment of shock. *American Journal of Nursing* 66:1289, 1966.
72. Sladen, A.: Pathogenesis of the shock lung. *Texas Medicine* 67:67, June, 1971.
73. Sonnenschein, H.: Treatment of shock. *J.A.M.A.* 217: 697, August 2, 1971.
74. Sun, R. L.: Trendelenburg position in hypovolemic shock. *American Journal of Nursing* 71:1758, September, 1971.
75. Symposium on current concepts and management of shock. *Journal of the Maine Medical Association* 59:191, October, 1968.
76. Trauma at first sight. *Emergency Medicine* 131:3, October, 1971.
77. Udhoji, V. N., Weil, M. H. and Sambhi, M. P.: Pressor amines and angiotensin in the treatment of shock. *In* Hershey, S. G. (ed.): *Shock. International Anesthesiology Clinics.* Vol. 2. No. 2. Boston, Little, Brown and Company, 1964.
78. Vandermeer, B. L.: Shock, blood pressure, and anesthesia. *Journal of American Association of Nurse Anesthetists,* April, 1965.
79. Vasopressors and other drugs used in shock. *British Medical Journal* 3:756, September 26, 1970.
80. Vitek, V., et al.: Blood lactate in the prognosis of various forms of shock. *Annals of Surgery* 173:308, February, 1971.
81. Watt, D. A., et al.: Treating shock. *British Medical Journal* 1:507, February 22, 1969.
82. Weil, M. H.: Progress in the bedside management of shock. *Journal of Trauma* 9:154, February, 1969.
83. Weil, M. H., and Shubin, H.: *Diagnosis and Treatment of Shock.* Baltimore, The Williams & Wilkins Company, 1967.
84. Weil, M. H., and Whigham, H.: Head-down (Trendelenburg) position for treatment of irreversible hemorrhagic shock. *Annals of Surgery* 162:905, November, 1965.
85. What CVP can and cannot tell you about patients in shock. *Patient Care* 5:102, March 15, 1971.
86. Wilson, J. N.: The management of acute circulatory failure. *Surgical Clinics of North America* 43:469, 1963.
87. Wilson, R. F., et al.: Factors affecting prognosis in clinical shock. *Annals of Surgery* 169:93, January, 1969.
88. Wilson, R. F., et al.: Central venous pressure and blood volume determinations in clinical shock. *Surgery, Gynecology and Obstetrics* 132:631, April, 1971.
89. Wilson, R. F., et al.: Hemodynamic changes, treatment, and prognosis in clinical shock. *Archives of Surgery* 102:21, January, 1971.
90. Zimmerman, B.: Postoperative management of fluid volumes and electrolytes. *Current Problems in Surgery.* Chicago, Year Book Medical Publishers, Inc., 1965.
91. Zipes, D. P.: The management of shock. *North Carolina Medical Journal* 29:420, October, 1968.
92. Zweifach, B. W.: Etiology of the shock syndrome. *The Heart Bulletin* 14:26, March-April, 1965.
93. Zweifach, B. W.: Relation of the reticulo-endothelial system to natural and acquired resistance in shock. *In* Hershey, S. G. (ed.): *Shock. International Anesthesiology Clinics.* Vol. 2. No. 2. Boston, Little, Brown and Company, 1964.

CHAPTER 27

The Body's Response to Bed Rest and Immobility

It is always assumed that the first thing in any illness is to get the patient to bed . . . yet we should think twice before ordering our patients to bed and realize that beneath the comfort of the blanket there lurks a host of formidable dangers.[1]

INTRODUCTION AND STUDY GUIDE

The patient who lies in bed day after day with little reason to move, little appetite to eat, and little capacity for hope is a vulnerable person. While he lies "resting" and inert, such a patient (especially if he is aged and weak) is susceptible to many dangerous conditions, e.g., thrombosis, decubitus ulcers, pneumonia, renal calculi, osteoporosis, contractures, footdrop, and mental disturbances.

The benefits of rest for such an individual are obviously negated if he develops any one of these immobilization disabilities—disabilities which can usually be prevented by foresight and by careful planning on the part of the nursing and medical staffs. For example, consider the following description of Mr. R. Jones, an elderly bedridden man of 71, whose condition has deteriorated as a result of oversights and misconceptions on the part of the hospital staff.

Mr. Jones lies in his bed on the top floor of the city hospital, which is the geriatric division. On this floor patients sometimes wait for months to be transferred to a rest home where they will live out what remains of their lives.

The ward has 16 beds crowded closely together; two overworked aides care for the patients as best they can. The entire geriatric floor consists of four wards like Mr. Jones' and is supervised by one R.N. who rarely has time to leave her desk because of excessive paperwork; as a result of inadequate supervision, there is little organized planning of patient care.

Mr. Jones has been on this ward for two weeks following a massive stroke which left him paralyzed and unable to turn himself. He spends the greatest portion of his time in bed with the side rails up. He is turned twice during the night, once during the afternoon and again in the evening. In the morning, following breakfast, Mr. Jones, along with other patients, is lifted from bed and placed into a wheelchair by his bed where he remains until two in the afternoon. Sitting for hours in his wheelchair, Mr. Jones usually slumps and sleeps. The aides believe that getting Mr. Jones up and into a chair every day will prevent the development of pressure sores. Thus, today, the aides were shocked to discover the beginning of a decubitus ulcer on Mr. Jones' sacrum—an ulcer which was actually produced by sitting for long hours, immobile, in a wheelchair.

Decubitus ulcers are not Mr. Jones' only problem. He is dehydrated, malnourished, and severely constipated. His joints are getting stiffer daily, and he is developing a noticeable footdrop.

Mr. Jones' mental state has also deteriorated. Although he was once a jovial and talkative person, this patient has gradually withdrawn into himself. To whom, after all, can he talk? The patient on the right side of his bed lies silent and coiled into the fetal position; the patient on his left seems incoherent, muttering to himself all day long; the patient across the ward is dying; the aides are impersonal; the nurses and doctors are busy and seldom in his room; and his relatives come only rarely as he upsets them by crying throughout their visit.

Mr. Jones will soon be transferred to a nursing home where his condition may continue to deteriorate. Even if he should be cared for by an interested and motivated nursing staff in the nursing home, Mr. Jones' present immobilization disabilities would be extremely difficult and expensive to correct. The tragedy is that Mr. Jones' disabilities could generally have been *prevented.* Intelligent, conscientious care on the part of the nursing staff could have made the last period of Mr. Jones' life comfortable, active, and meaningful.

It is the purpose of this chapter to discuss the patient on bed rest, the helpful and hazardous effects of bed rest and immobility upon the patient, and the major nursing actions that help to prevent the complications of bed rest from developing. Our discussion will briefly cover the following areas:

> The problem of defining bed rest
> The beneficial and untoward effects of bed rest
> The responses of the body to bed rest and immobilization.

More specifically, we shall review the responses of the skin, the musculoskeletal system, the cardiovascular system, the respiratory system, the renal system, the gastrointestinal tract, the metabolic system, and the psyche to prolonged "rest."

As an aid to your study of this chapter, we urge you to make use of the following brief study guide.

Upon completion of this chapter, you should be able to do the following:

1. Define generally the following terms: bed rest;

immobilization disability; decubitus ulcer; shearing force; disuse atrophy; contracture; disuse osteoporosis; orthostatic hypotension; venous thrombosis; embolism; Valsalva maneuver; urinary stasis, and renal calculi.

2. Discuss generally the following:
   a. The major benefits of bed rest.
   b. The pathologic effects of bed rest upon every major system of the body.
   c. Which groups of patients are most prone to the development of the complications of bed rest.
3. Perform the following nursing actions when caring for patients:
   a. Identify among patients assigned to you those who are most susceptible to the complications of bed rest.
   b. Assess patients on bed rest in order to prevent the possible complications of immobilization.
   c. Draw up a specific plan of care for patients on bed rest and put the plan into action.

THE PROBLEM OF DEFINING BED REST

In general terms, "bed rest" is an activity status which specifies that the patient be put to bed for the purpose of "rest." Bed rest is either specifically prescribed for a patient by his physician, or it is simply assigned to a patient by the staff on the basis of that patient's inability to walk, move, and perform activities for himself. In clinical practice you will find that the status of bed rest is actually a hazy concept and that few doctors and staff members define bed rest in precisely the same way.

For example, when a doctor prescribes bed rest for a patient, he may *assume* that the staff will allow the patient to perform certain simple activities such as using a bedside commode, washing his face and hands, and feeding himself. To his dismay, the physician may discover that his patient has been almost totally immobilized by the hospital staff, because the head nurse views bed rest as meaning complete confinement for the patient, with no self-care activities allowed on his part. As a result of such confusion in defining bed rest, the physician may become angry, the staff may be upset, and the patient may actually develop potentially fatal complications owing to his total immobilization. This type of confusing and dangerous situation is all too common in hospital settings. Thus, it is important that *all* members of a hospital staff, from the doctor to the aide, agree upon a definition of bed rest, upon the amount of activity a patient on bed rest is to be allowed, and upon the exact means by which the complications of bed rest are to be prevented.

THE BENEFICIAL AND UNTOWARD EFFECTS OF BED REST

BENEFICIAL EFFECTS

While the emphasis in this chapter is upon the complications and the development of disabilities consequent to bed rest, we wish to emphasize that there are many benefits to be derived from bed rest. Some of its beneficial aspects and some important indications for its use are as follows:

> To *relieve pain* due to coronary ischemia, surgical procedures, trauma, fractures, and wounds. Rest, by decreasing movement, prevents excessive irritation of injured tissues, and it reduces the oxygen demands of such vital organs as the heart muscle, thereby easing discomfort.

> To *promote healing and repair* of injured tissues by reducing the metabolic need of tissues and by preserving the fibrin barriers that prevent the migration of microorganisms from sick tissues into healthy tissues.

> To *relieve ankle edema and venous congestion* by placing the patient in bed and elevating his legs.

> To *give support* to the weak, exhausted, perhaps febrile patient who, because of illness, is simply unable to remain standing and active, e.g., patients debilitated by carcinoma or by severely incapacitating neurologic diseases.

To be of any benefit to a patient, bed rest must, of course, *be restful*—physiologically and psychologically. This vital requirement, which sounds so simple to achieve, is commonly overlooked by nurses and doctors alike. How often we order a patient who is beset with worry, harassed by pain, and panicked from fear "to rest." Such a patient may be in bed quietly enough, but his mind may be churning and his emotions in a state of flux; in other cases, the patient may become bored, depressed, and withdrawn. If the patient is to truly benefit from rest, his pain must be eased, his concerns and fears must be allowed open discussion, and his interests in life and in his surroundings must be kept alive.

UNTOWARD EFFECTS

Even when properly prescribed, defined, and carried out, bed rest like any treatment has its hazards as well as its benefits. The complications of bed rest are sometimes called *dependent disabilities* or *immobilization disabilities.* Such complications constitute the *iatrogenic* consequences of rest in bed. The bulk of the information in this chapter pertains to these disabilities and their prevention.

Briefly, immobilization disabilities affect every system and major organ in the body, i.e., the skin, muscles, bones, heart, brain, kidneys, and lungs. The most important immobilization disabilities and their consequences according to physiologic systems are summarized on the following page.

These disabilities mainly affect patients who are elderly, malnourished, critically ill, paraplegic, and/or comatose. Prevention of the complications of bed rest is one of the major goals in nursing today.

RESPONSES OF THE BODY TO BED REST AND IMMOBILITY

Each system responds in its own way to prolonged bed rest and immobility. In this chapter we shall briefly investigate the major responses of each system to bed rest, the major complications of bed rest, and the planned prevention of disabilities.

THE EFFECTS OF PROLONGED BED REST UPON THE SKIN

The continuous hard pressure of a bed mattress or chair seat against the skin eventually results in the production of a pressure sore or *decubitus ulcer*. First of all, the skin layers are gradually worn away from rubbing against the sheet or chair; second, the compressed skin and tissue eventually become necrotic because of ischemia produced by the pressure. A decubitus ulcer is therefore defined as "an area of the skin in which pressure has destroyed the surface tissue with progressive destruction of the underlying tissue."[2]

The major sites of the body that are most prone to the development of pressure sores are: the back

IMMOBILIZATION DISABILITIES AND THEIR CONSEQUENCES

Organ System	Mobilization Disability	Consequence
Skin	Decubitus ulcers	Osteomyelitis
Musculoskeletal system	Muscle weakness, backache, muscle atrophy, joint stiffness	Contractures, deformities
	Disuse osteoporosis	Pathologic fractures* renal calculi,* deformities, osteoarthropathy*
Cardiovascular system	Increased work load of the heart, increased use of the Valsalva maneuver	Tachycardia,* cardiac arrest
	Orthostatic hypotension, thrombus formation	Pulmonary embolism*
Respiratory system	Decreased chest expansion, stasis of secretions, CO_2 narcosis,* respiratory acidosis*	Hypostatic bronchopneumonia*
Renal system	Difficult micturition, urinary stasis, renal calculi	
Gastrointestinal system	Anorexia,* negative nitrogen balance, constipation*	Fecal impaction, bowel obstruction
Metabolic system	Decreased production of adrenocortical hormones, increased protein breakdown	
Psyche	Depression, boredom, increased introspection	Insomnia

*Starred items will be discussed in greater detail in appropriate sections of the text.

of the head, the spines of the scapula, the heels, the palms of the hands, the iliac crests, and the lower sacrum. These locations are particularly vulnerable to pressure because: (1) the skin lies over sharp, prominent bones; (2) these tissues are not adapted, as are our feet, to the bearing of a large amount of weight; and (3) the patient's weight, when lying supine, is borne *specifically* by these 10 small sites rather than by the total posterior of the body. No wonder these areas are the ones that we must inspect carefully, *at least daily,* when caring for the bedridden patient.

Groups of patients who are particularly susceptible to the development of pressure sores are the following:

> Patients whose general condition is *rapidly deteriorating.* Such patients may have: sudden loss of appetite, dehydration, development of urinary or fecal incontinence or both, increasing confusion, a sudden elevation in temperature, the onset of diarrhea or constipation, and/or new complaints of pain. When any of these signs appear suddenly in a bedridden patient not previously bothered by them, that patient must be carefully observed for the development of pressure sores.

> *Newly admitted patients* whose condition prior to admission has so deteriorated that it is necessary for them to come to the hospital and be placed on bed rest. One investigator discovered from a study of 250 elderly patients admitted to the hospital that of the 59 patients who developed ulcerations, 70 per cent did so within the first two weeks after admission and 34 per cent did so within the first week.[28]

> *Elderly* bedridden patients who make few spontaneous bodily movements.

> *Obese* patients whose extra weight creates additional pressure over weight-bearing areas.

> Very *thin* emaciated patients whose skin lies in a thin layer over the body's bony prominences.

> *Sedated* patients who are taking large doses of tranquilizers or sleeping pills and who consequently are not moving readily.

> *Paralyzed* patients who have suffered spinal cord injuries (e.g., paraplegics and quadriplegics).

> *Neurologic* patients with diseases of the central nervous system such as disseminated sclerosis and Parkinson's disease and patients in coma due to cerebral vascular accidents, trauma, and so forth.

> *Edematous* patients, especially those with edema of the sacrum and buttocks.

> *Malnourished* patients with protein and vitamin deficiencies.

There are several physiologic factors that contribute to the development of pressure sores. They are: (1) severe elevations in the capillary pressure; (2) prolonged pressure on a body tissue; (3) decreases in the number of spontaneous bodily movements, and (4) an increase in the shearing force.

Landis, who studied the capillary pressure in ischemic areas, was one of the first investigators to attempt to explain the etiology of decubitus ulcers. In his studies he found that the blood pressure in capillaries normally ranges from 16 to 33 mm. Hg. He theorized that *prolonged tissue ischemia* causes extremely *high elevations of the capillary pressure,* resulting in death of cells in the ischemic area and in ulceration. Landis found that a person sitting on a wooden chair without padding would have, over his ischial tuberosities, a capillary pressure of up to 300 mm. of mercury! However, when he experi-

mented with an alternating pressure pad, Landis discovered that pressure in all body positions was reduced toward more normal limits.[34]

In similar studies Rudd emphasized the factor of *time* in the development of pressure sores. From his investigations, Rudd concluded that *less pressure over a prolonged period* of time contributes more to the possible formation of pressure sores than more pressure over a short period of time. Thus, patients who are acutely or chronically ill, heavily sedated, or unconscious are all in grave danger of developing pressure sores because they cannot readily move themselves, and therefore tend to lie in one position for long periods.[34]

Any decrease in the number of spontaneous bodily movements that a patient makes during the night will result in an increase in decubitus ulcer formation. Investigators discovered that: (1) normal people made as many as 400 spontaneous movements of some kind during an eight-hour night, (2) elderly patients who made 25 to 225 movements during the night did not develop pressure sores, and (3) patients with a nightly average of less than 25 movements *all* developed tissue damage.[28]

Another important etiologic factor contributing to the formation of decubitus ulcers is a "pushing" pressure described in clinical literature as the *shearing force.* This force is in play when the head of a patient's bed is raised or when a patient is allowed to assume a slumped sitting position. Because a *pushing* force is being exerted on the tissues, tissues tend to tear, producing deep and serious pressure sores. Ulcers created by the shearing force most often develop upon the sacrum and heels (Fig. 27–1).

There are four major stages in the progression of a deep penetrating pressure sore: (1) *irritation* of the skin with a resultant redness, (2) *edema* and swelling due to the leakage of fluid from dilated damaged blood vessels, (3) *tissue necrosis* with the

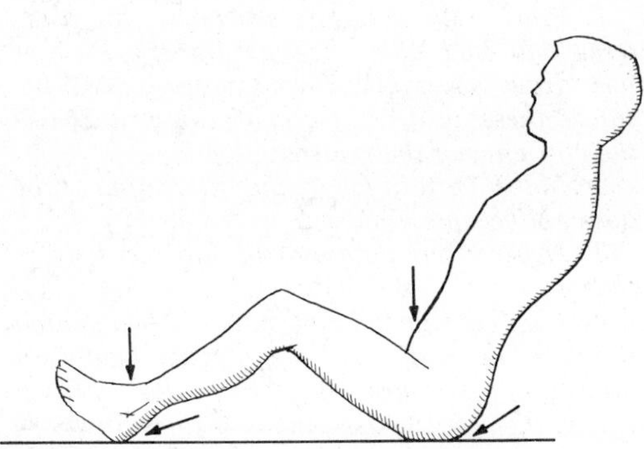

FIGURE 27–1. The shearing force exerts a downward and forward pressure. (After Norton, *Nursing Times,* March 27, 1964.)

result that the reddened area turns bluish and then black (the dead skin, at this point, separates from the necrotic tissue; this exposed area of necrosis is called the slough), and (4) *healing by second intention,* which can easily break down again. During this stage, granulation takes place, and the area finally becomes fibrotic and scarred. The scar tissue which develops is not so strong as normal tissue, and, with pressure, the area can easily become ulcerated once more.

Prevention of Decubitus

This unfortunate sequence of pathologic events leading to the development of severe ulcerations can be prevented by means of intelligent observation, planning, and patient care on the part of the nursing staff. Indeed, it is far easier to prevent the development of decubitus than to treat it. Some of the most important preventive measures, all of which should be used, are the following:

> The identification of patients who are particularly prone to the development of decubitus ulcers, e.g., patients with a deteriorating general condition, emaciated patients, and so forth.

> *Daily examination* of decubitus-prone patients for redness, discoloration, or a blistering of their back, buttocks, or heels.

> The immediate institution of a *preventive regimen* for any patient who is liable to develop pressure sores or whose condition is rapidly deteriorating.

Such a preventive regime should include the following:

> The use of an *alternating-pressure pad or mattress.* This is a pneumatic mattress, electrically operated, with air strips that cyclically inflate and deflate alternately, at three- to five-minute intervals. As a result of this device, no one area of the body is exposed to pressure for more than a few minutes at a time. In many hospitals, nurses can use this mattress without a doctor's order.

In caring for patients on an alternating-pressure mattress, remember the following points:

1. *Place* only *a bottom sheet over the mattress and tuck this sheet in lightly. Do not use draw sheets or incontinence pads, because these added layers of linen decrease the efficiency of the mattress.*
2. *Make certain that the air input tube does not become kinked.*
3. *Never insert a pin into the mattress for any reason.*
4. *Place a sign on the patient's bed which informs the staff that the patient is on an alternating-pressure mattress, and which warns them not to use pins or added linens.*
5. *Inspect the mattress at least twice daily to make certain that it is working properly.*

If an alternating-pressure mattress develops any defect, however small, it *must* be replaced at once as it will no longer provide the patient with maximum protection.

> *Turn patient* a minimum of once every two hours from the prone to the supine to the side-lying positions. Sometimes a *Foster* or *Stryker* frame is used to facilitate the turning of paralyzed patients. It is important to post a precise turning schedule both on the patient's bed and in the Kardex. The times for turning and the positions in which the patient should be placed need to be clearly noted.

While a strict turning schedule is of real value, Bliss and McLaren warn us not to rely *exclusively* upon turning the patient to prevent pressure sores. It is recommended that, in addition to turning, the patient be placed upon an alternating pressure mattress. If an alternating pressure mattress is not available, the patient should be placed and turned upon layers of pillows for the best results.[4]

> Keep the decubitus-prone patient *in bed* and care for him in as *flat a position* as possible. By means of these measures you will reduce the problem of shearing force and the deep and dangerous ulcerations that it can produce. If it is necessary for the patient to be rolled up in bed due to severe dyspnea, heart disease, or pulmonary edema, be sure to support the soles of the patient's feet with an added *footboard,* thereby counteracting the shearing force to some extent.

> Use a *bed cradle* to keep the weight of the bed blankets off the patient's feet. This device, along with the use of an alternating-pressure mattress, helps to prevent the development of heel sores, and it keeps the patient more comfortable.

> *Bed socks or boots* made of foam rubber help to reduce friction between the patient's heels and the bed sheets and thus reduce the incidence of heel sores.

> *Avoid* the use of *doughnuts* and *rubber rings* since these devices compress the area of skin beneath them, decreasing blood supply around points of pressure. As a result, doughnuts and rubber rings can actually cause large decubiti to form around the very area that they are designed to protect, thus enlarging the ulcer.

> *Avoid* the use of *rubbing alcohol* for back rubs; alcohol dries the patient's skin and makes it more prone to breakdown.

> *Avoid* the overuse of *sedatives* and *tranquilizers,* as these drugs tend to reduce the patient's desire to move and turn.

> Provide the patient with adequate *fluids* and with a *nutritious diet* that is high in protein and vitamin C—nutrients that encourage tissue build-up and repair.

> Keep the patient's *skin clean, dry, and well lubricated.* However, as Bliss and McLaren point out from their investigations:[3]

Skin care alone, *including the use of pHisoHex, silicone preparations, and zinc oxide, will* not *prevent the development of pressure sores.*

Bliss and McLaren discovered that placing a patient on a sheepskin to aerate his skin (a commonly used preventive device) is also not particularly helpful in the decubitus-prone patient.[4]

> *Teach* patients and their relatives the value of frequent turning and movement. Also, alert patients can be taught to examine their own skin on a daily basis for the slightest signs of pressure. Finally, the patient confined to a wheelchair can be taught to lift his buttocks off the seat of the wheelchair by pressing down with his hands on the arms of the chair. This maneuver, if done at least twice an hour, reduces the shearing force. Paraplegics, in particular, benefit from learning to perform this technique.

Treatment of Decubitus

Despite the conscientious use of the preventive measures just listed, certain patients, because of their extremely debilitated condition, *do* develop pressure sores. Also, you may be assigned patients who have pressure sores that they developed before admission to the hospital. When a pressure sore is present, what are some of the treatment measures that you can take?

Because decubitus ulcers are extremely difficult to treat, numerous methods of treatment have evolved over time. Some of these treatments (e.g., flotation therapy) are based on strictly scientific principles, while others, such as the pouring of granulated sugar into the wound, are derived from folk medicine. Below are listed some of the major methods of treatment, both new and old, that are being employed in hospitals today.

Special Mattresses. Special mattresses such as the alternating-pressure mattress and special *turning devices* such as the Foster and Stryker frames are used not only as preventive measures against the development of decubiti, but are employed in treatment as well.

Flotation Therapy. Flotation therapy is a sophisticated form of therapy in which the patient is placed upon a plastic tarpaulin which, in turn, floats upon water.[37] Flotation therapy is based upon Archimedes' principle that when a body is partially submerged in water, it gives up its weight. Thus, when a patient with a decubitus ulcer is allowed to float upon water, his body displaces some of the liquid which fills the "water bed." As a result, the patient's body becomes lighter and the pressure exerted against the patient's skin by the "water mattress" is far less than that which would be exerted by an ordinary mattress. This form of therapy is highly successful with paralyzed patients and with burn victims. In these cases, the "water bed" definitely seems to promote healing of the ulcer. Another advantage of flotation therapy is that the routine constant turning and positioning normally required by paralyzed patients is not necessary and can be virtually discontinued; as a result, these individuals receive more rest.

Unfortunately not all patients can tolerate weightlessness. Individuals with serious emotional problems sometimes experience hallucinations and nightmares; others become emotionally isolated and withdrawn. Also, because flotation therapy reduces the need for turning, some patients on "water beds" have developed contractures and other immobilization disabilities. To prevent these iatrogenic problems, nurses must put patients on flotation therapy through range-of-motion exercises at least two or three times a day. Also, the nursing staff must constantly observe for the signs of thrombus formation, renal calculi, anorexia, and constipation.

Air-fluidized Bed. The air-fluidized bed is another new and sophisticated method for preventing decubitus ulcers.[20] The patient who lies upon this special device floats upon a loose polyester filter sheet placed over a bed filled with fine sterile glass beads. Air, which is delivered by a blower, continuously flows upward through the beads (Fig. 27–2). As a result of the constant airflow, the patient's body is supported and his weight is evenly distributed. This form of therapy has proved to be of special value in the care of paraplegics with ulcerations of the chest wall, sacrum, and the ischial tuberosities. With this treatment, hallucinations and other mental disturbances have not been reported to date.

Local Therapeutic Measures. Numerous different types of local therapeutic measures (i.e., therapies that are applied directly to the ulcerated area) are used, despite the fact that many of these therapies are without a known scientific basis. Some of the more common local treatment measures are listed below. All these "therapies" are applied directly to the pressure sore.

granulated sugar
Elase ointment
A and D ointment
salt solutions
desloughing agents (e.g., Euresol)
exposure to the air
exposure to ultraviolet light
mixtures of tincture of benzoin and mineral oil
sheepskins
yeast

Anabolic Steroids. Anabolic steroids are sometimes given to promote the retention of nitrogen. The rationale for this use is to counteract the state of negative nitrogen balance which seems to characterize most patients with decubiti.

Surgical Intervention. Surgical intervention is sometimes used when the decubitus ulcer is healing very slowly, thereby leaving the patient open to infection and increasing disability, owing to loss of serum and protein from the draining sore. In surgery, the ulcer is usually debrided and then closed. In some cases, skin must be grafted over the ulcerated site.

The doctor may choose any one of the treatment measures just listed. However, no matter which treatment is instituted, it is important that the nurse carry out the following:

> Institute immediately a program containing the vital preventive measures discussed earlier (i.e., patient teach-

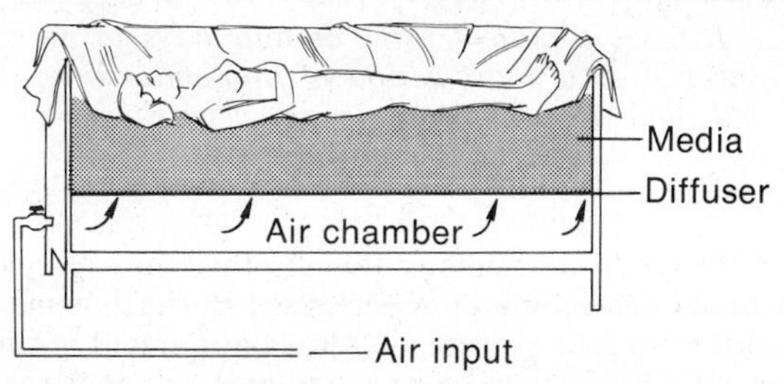

FIGURE 27–2. Air-fluidized bed.

ing, ordering of nutritious diet, placing the patient on a special mattress, and so forth).

> Give the patient firm psychologic support. Remember that this patient faces the additional trauma of seeing and smelling a draining, foul sore that is actually eroding *his* body. Also, the sick individual who develops a pressure sore will now be confined for a longer period because of his new affliction.

> Prevent the ulcerated area from becoming infected. Infection will retard healing of the ulcer and may eventually result in *osteomyelitis*—a condition characterized by inflammation of the bone marrow. Patients with a pressure sore in the early stages should have the ulcerated site cultured for the presence of *staphylococcus aureus*. Antibiotic therapy will need to be started immediately if organisms are present in the drainage.

THE EFFECTS OF PROLONGED BED REST UPON THE MUSCULOSKELETAL SYSTEM

While relief from the stress of activity is helpful in certain orthopedic conditions, immobilization of the body's bones, muscles, and joints can result in severe and permanent disabilities. Major musculoskeletal problems created by bed rest are: (1) weakness; (2) backache; (3) muscle or disease atrophy, joint stiffness, and contractures; and (4) disuse osteoporosis.

Weakness. Any person who has been confined to bed for even three or four days feels weak and wobbly when he first gets up. This weakness upon ambulation is attributable both to the underlying illness and to the weakening of antigravity muscles, i.e., those muscles that support the body while standing, walking, and balancing movements. To prevent excessive weakness, patients should be ambulated as soon as it can be tolerated. Also, patients who have been bedridden will feel more comfortable and less apprehensive if they are ambulated gradually, first being "dangled," then guided to a chair placed near the bed, and then walked to the bathroom or day room where they can remain for a longer period of time each day. By means of a planned program of ambulation, bedridden patients will slowly regain confidence concerning their ability to walk and to balance themselves. The longer a patient has remained in bed, the longer it will take him to regain his strength, balance, and coordination. Remember:

> *It takes a patient three or four days to recover from a short period of immobilization, but four to six weeks to recover from six weeks of immobilization.*[8]

Backache. Patients confined to bed for a period of time often complain of backache. Backaches may result from poor posture, awkward alignment of the patient's body when in bed, and/or a soft mattress that gives poor support to the patient's back. To combat backache, the following measures are helpful: (1) scheduled position changes, (2) a firm mattress and/or bedboards placed under the mattress, (3) frequent back rubs, (4) a daily exercise program, and (5) physiotherapy.

Muscle Atrophy, Joint Stiffness, and Contractures. For the body's muscles and joints to remain healthy and mobile, they must be subjected to a certain amount of daily stress and strain and they must be put through a normal range of movements. Without daily strain and movement, muscles quickly weaken, atrophy, and shorten, and joints become stiff and immobile. Indeed, when muscles are not sufficiently exercised and joints are allowed to remain immobilized in one position for a prolonged time, *contractures* result that can doom the patient to permanent crippling deformities that resist all attempts at treatment!

A *contracture* is defined as a permanent contraction of a muscle in which the muscle is fixed, shortened, and resists stretching. Contractures can result from: (1) lack of exercise, (2) muscle spasticity, (3) prolonged joint immobilization, (4) pain that prevents movement, and (5) edema and swelling which can splint an area and thereby limit muscular activity. Three of the most common deformities that result from prolonged bed rest are footdrop, wrist drop, and external rotation of the hip.

Contractures are an extremely difficult disability to treat once they form; indeed, the treatment of a contracture involves extensive physiotherapy and may even require surgery. Thus, as with all immobilization disabilities, it is best to *prevent* contractures from developing in the first place. Some important preventive measures are the following:

> Frequent scheduled position changes.

> Range-of-motion exercises in which each joint is put through as complete a range of motion as possible without producing pain. Each range-of-motion exercise should be done five times during each of three periods scheduled throughout the day.

> Isometric exercises during which the patient, at first, need not move his joints but can simply contract his various limb and trunk muscles. Later the patient may exercise against resistance by pushing against a weight or sandbag.

> Shoulders, in particular, must be put through a full range of motion several times daily.

> *Elderly patients who are receiving intravenous infusions, and whose arms are immobilized for even an hour a day, may develop a "frozen shoulder" if their arms are not exercised.*[16]

> The use of bedboards and a firm mattress ensures better alignment of the patient's body.

> A padded footboard placed *firmly* against the patient's feet helps to prevent footdrop.

> A trapeze over the patient's bed will encourage him to move and turn himself and to perform self-care activities.

> Handrolls help to maintain the patient's hand in a position of function.

> A soft foam-rubber sponge for the patient to squeeze

helps to prevent finger flexion contractures, particularly at the metacarpophalangeal joint.

> A trochanter roll (made by folding a bathtowel or bath blanket into thirds lengthwise and then in half) can be tucked under the patient's thigh and hip and then rolled firmly under itself to prevent external rotation of the hip.

> Avoidance of the use of the knee-gatch bed position helps to prevent hip and knee flexion contractures.

*Disuse Osteoporosis.** This painful, crippling condition is the most frequently seen metabolic bone disease in the United States. The word "osteoporosis" means *porosity of bone*. The increased bone porosity is caused by a substantial loss of bone calcium, phosphorus, and matrix. These losses result from an increase in the rate of bone destruction, which *exceeds* the rate of bone production.

While osteoporosis can be caused by several different factors, *disuse* osteoporosis develops because the musculoskeletal system is immobilized and is not being used. This condition is very common among paraplegics and severe arthritics, and it affects *all* immobilized patients on bed rest. Because some degree of osteoporosis always occurs in the immobilized patient, Browse states that osteoporosis is actually a *physiologic* reaction to bed rest rather than a pathologic one.[8]

While disuse osteoporosis inevitably affects the bedridden, one must nevertheless make every effort to prevent the occurrence of a severe degree of osteoporosis, along with its attendant complications, namely:

> Renal calculi due to the draining of calcium from the patient's bones.

> Pathologic fractures due to the bone's lack of structural firmness.

> Deformities due to the bone's soft sponginess.

> Osteoarthropathy due to the deposit of calcium in the joints.

To prevent disuse osteoporosis, authorities recommend that patients be allowed to stand and to bear weight as soon as possible. The paralyzed patient can obtain the effect of weight bearing by being placed for a period each day on a tilt table or oscillating bed, either of which is raised and locked into a standing position. Patients who can ambulate to some extent can learn to stand or walk between parallel bars. All patients need to exercise and to contract their muscles daily, particularly against resistance. While a nutritious diet is essential, increasing calcium intake definitely does *not* prevent osteoporosis; indeed, additional calcium in the diet simply adds to the large load of minerals that the patient is already excreting.

THE EFFECTS OF PROLONGED BED REST UPON THE HEART AND VASCULAR SYSTEM

There are four major effects that prolonged bed rest has upon the heart: (1) an increased load of work upon the heart, (2) the development of orthostatic hypotension, (3) an increased use of the Valsalva maneuver, and (4) an increased incidence of thrombus formation and pulmonary embolism.

*Osteoporosis will be discussed in greater detail in Unit XVII.

Work Load of the Heart

Bed rest may rest a person's muscles and bones, but it definitely does *not* rest his heart. Indeed, when one lies down there is a 25–30 per cent increase in cardiac output, a 40 per cent increase in the stroke volume (amount of blood that the heart puts out at each beat), and a 30 per cent increase in the total work of the heart.[8] According to one study by Deitrick et al., four normal, healthy subjects, at the end of a six-week period of immobilization, had an average increase in their heart rates of 3.8 beats per minute.[13] This progressively increasing heart beat indicates that prolonged immobilization produces a decline in cardiovascular function.

Another investigator reports that in the supine position, the heart works 30 per cent harder than in a sitting position.[12, 31] Thus, a patient whose heart needs rest should actually be nursed in a sitting position rather than supine for the best results.

Despite the fact that bed rest does cause the heart to work harder, there is no evidence that bed rest harms the heart. Indeed, with prescribed rest, large hearts do become smaller, since the general stresses and muscular strains to which ambulatory patients are subjected are reduced. Rest in an armchair is an alternative that protects the patient both from the stresses of active ambulation and from the increased cardiac output stimulated by rest in bed.

The Valsalva Maneuver

When a person uses his arm and upper trunk muscles to move in bed or when he strains to defecate, he performs the Valsalva maneuver. In other words, the individual fixes his thorax and holds his breath, which is consequently forced up against his closed glottis. As a result, the patient's intrathoracic pressure increases, his pulse increases, blood flow to the heart slows, and venous pressure rises. When the patient finishes moving or straining, he lets his breath out, which, in turn, causes his intrathoracic pressure to decrease and his pulse to decrease. As a result bradycardia develops. In the vulnerable heart, angina and even sudden death due to decreased coronary blood flow may ensue.

Patients on bed rest have been shown to perform the Valsalva maneuver 10 to 20 times per hour. Because of the danger of cardiac arrest, coronary patients on bed rest must be taught not to strain while defecating. It is preferable that these individuals use a bedside commode for defecation rather than a bedpan, because the commode allows the patient to assume a normal sitting position, which reduces the need to strain. Of course, every effort must be made to prevent constipation in the heart patient. (See later discussion.)

Orthostatic Hypotension

As we stated earlier, all patients when they first get up after a period of bed rest feel weak, wobbly, and dizzy. The dizziness and faintness are due, in part, to muscular weakness; however, faintness also results from hypotension or a low blood pressure which is caused, not by cardiac disease, but by a failure of arteriolar vasoconstriction upon assuming an erect position.

The exact etiology of orthostatic hypotension is still somewhat obscure. Evidently when a patient is in bed for a prolonged period of time, the parts of his circulatory system that respond to changes in posture (i.e., going from the supine to the erect position or vice versa) deteriorate in their ability to function. Thus, upon rising after a prolonged period in bed, the splanchnic and muscle arterioles do not constrict but dilate; blood pools in the abdominal viscera and muscles, and the patient faints. Exactly why vasoconstriction fails is not known. Browse hypothesizes that, since the nervous system is intact, the problem of orthostatic hypotension must result from a *local* failure of the blood vessels. He believes that the patient's vessels have become habituated to the bed rest state, in which they generally remain somewhat dilated. Consequently, when the patient suddenly stands up, these "habituated" vessels are unable to constrict appropriately in response to nervous stimuli, and the blood pressure drops.[8] Other authorities suggest that because muscle tone generally decreases during bed rest, there is a decrease in the efficiency of those muscles that press against the veins, thereby aiding venous return to the heart. When this factor, known as the "vasopressor mechanism" is diminished, venous blood pools in the lower parts of the body rather than being propelled through the heart and out into the arterial circulation.[31]

The problem of orthostatic hypotension cannot be completely prevented. Some suggestions for lessening the severity of the problem are:

> Try to have the patient ambulate as soon as permissible.

> Get the patient up very gradually. At first only raise the head of the bed and let the patient become accustomed to that position. Slowly increase his period of ambulation each day.

> Place pressure bandages on the patient's legs. This will aid venous return to the heart and augment the vasopressor mechanism.

Thrombus Formation and Pulmonary Embolism*

Deep vein thrombosis (i.e., the formation of a blood clot within the deep veins) is unfortunately a common complication of bed rest that seems to be related to the *length of time* the patient is in bed. However, bed rest is not an absolute necessity for the development of thrombi, for blood clots sometimes form in the veins of normal, healthy individuals. In either case, the major danger from thrombus formation is *pulmonary embolism,* in which the clot breaks loose from the vein wall and is carried to the lungs where it blocks off the blood supply to a portion of the lung tissue. If the embolus is a small one, damage may be minimal; if damage is extensive, the patient may die.

Authorities generally agree that there are three factors which contribute to the formation of thrombi and potential emboli.[8, 31]

An Increase in Blood Coagulability. In general medical patients on bed rest there apparently are no changes in the blood due to immobility other than an increase in plasma volume which, in turn, decreases the viscosity of the blood. However, in post-trauma cases (following either surgery or an accident) there tends to be an increase in blood viscosity, platelet count, platelet stickiness, and prothrombin time—all of which increase blood coagulability. Also, if the bedfast patient is dehydrated, his blood will be more viscous and thus more prone to clot formation. While these changes may not actually cause thrombi to form, they possibly *accelerate* their formation.

Venous Stasis. A slowing of the flow of blood in the veins can result from a lack of muscular contraction in the legs. Evidently venous stasis alone will not cause thrombosis. However, venous stasis *in addition* to another factor, such as hypercoagulability or damage to the intima of the vein, can cause thrombosis.

Damage to the Intima of the Vein Wall. When the intima or inner coat of a vessel is damaged, platelets quickly cover the defect and intimal cells grow over the platelets, thereby restoring the vessel wall. Generally the process of healing terminates at this point; however, in some cases, the plaque of platelets continues to grow and a thrombus develops.

How do vein walls become damaged during bed rest? Several factors are known to promote damage. One is the use of the *lateral recumbent position,* especially following anesthesia or when the patient is heavily sedated. In this position the tibia of the lower leg is compressed by the calf of the upper leg; moreover, the femoral vein of the upper leg is squeezed and possibly damaged as it presses against the lower leg. To correct this uncomfortable, potentially dangerous position, the upper leg should be lifted off the lower leg and placed so that its total length and weight rest upon a pillow (Fig. 27–3). A second factor promoting intimal

---

*For a detailed discussion of thrombus formation and pulmonary embolism, see Unit XIII.

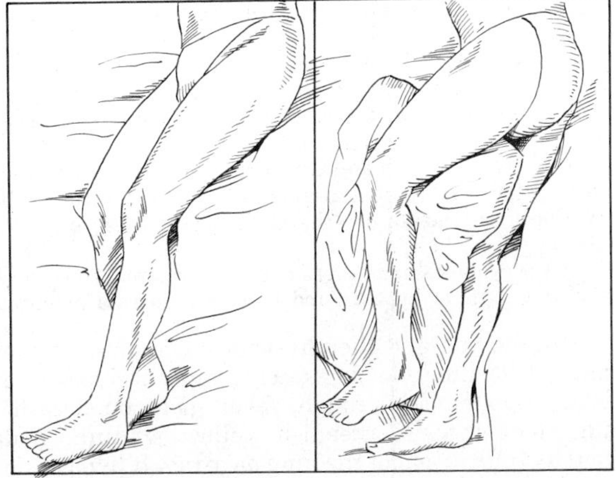

FIGURE 27-3. *A,* The lateral recumbent position as an etiologic factor in venous thrombosis. *B,* Correct positioning will prevent thrombosis. (After Browse, *The Physiology and Pathology of Bedrest.* Springfield, Ill., Charles C Thomas, 1965.)

damage is the use of the Fowler position, in which the knees are flexed over a bent-knee gatch. Third, the placing of pillows directly under the patient's knees may lead to blood clot formation.

Prevention of Thrombus and Embolism. Because of the danger of pulmonary embolism, it is naturally most important to prevent thrombus formation. Some important preventive measures are:

> Encourage patient to move his legs throughout the day.

> Set up a definite program of complete range-of-motion exercises three times daily.

> Encourage the ingestion of fluids to decrease the viscosity of the blood.

> Use pressure bandages to augment venous return to the heart.

> Never rub the patient's legs, as you can dislodge a clot that may have formed, thereby releasing an embolus into the circulation.

> Avoid the use of the knee gatch, pillows beneath the knees, and the lateral recumbent position.

THE EFFECT OF PROLONGED BED REST UPON THE RESPIRATORY SYSTEM

Prolonged bed rest apparently has little direct effect upon pulmonary function, once the patient's lungs have made certain adjustments to the supine position. However, respiratory problems secondary to immobilization may develop. For example, the general muscle weakness that results from bed rest may cause respiratory difficulties, since greater effort is required to breathe while lying down.

Under certain conditions, prolonged bed rest can result in respiratory problems that can lead to such grave complications as bronchopneumonia and carbon dioxide narcosis. These are brought on by: (1) decreased chest expansion and decreased chest movements, (2) stasis of secretions and pooling of mucus, and (3) CO_2 narcosis and respiratory acidosis.

Decreased Chest Expansion and Decreased Chest Movements

The prolonged pressure of a bed mattress against a patient's chest will tend to decrease the expansion of his chest cage. Decreased chest expansion and weakness of the muscles of respiration cause a decrease in ventilation. This, in turn, results in a decrease in the oxygenation of the blood and an inadequate expiration of CO_2. Factors that contribute to a limited chest expansion and that must be controlled or avoided are: heavy sedation and narcotics, which depress the respiratory center in the medulla; and tight abdominal or chest binders, and abdominal distention due to ascites, feces, or flatus, which interfere with the normal descent of the diaphragm. To encourage maximum chest expansion, the patient on bed rest must periodically breathe deeply. A program of specific deep breathing exercises will be discussed later under preoperative care, pp. 318–319.

Stasis and Pooling of Secretions

When secretions and mucus begin to pool in the bronchi and lungs of the bedridden patient, the patient becomes highly susceptible to the development of *hypostatic bronchopneumonia.** Major factors leading to the stasis and pooling of secretions and thus to bronchopneumonia are:

The patient's *underlying weakness,* which results in reduced bodily movements and a decrease in the efficiency of the cough reflex. This weakness is usually due both to the disease condition requiring bed rest (e.g., cancer, heart disease, recent surgery, burns, accident trauma) as well as to prolonged immobilization itself.

While a normal healthy person will move around in bed and will cough up any secretions that pool in his bronchi during the night, a sick, weakened individual may not have the strength to do so. Thus, the bedridden are prone to pooling of mucus, bacterial invasion, and atelectasis (collapse of a portion of lung) as a result of the obstruction of bronchi. If the patient on bed rest is also taking *narcotics or sedatives,* his muscle strength is further weakened and his chest expansion further decreased.

The supine position causes *disturbance of the normal distribution of mucus around the bronchi.* Normally mucus is spread out rather evenly around the bronchial tubules. However, in the supine position, mucus tends to pool on the dependent sides of the bronchi while the upper surfaces may become very dry. Both the pooling of mucus and the drying of the upper bronchial walls interferes with adequate functioning of the cilia (whose job

*Bronchopneumonia is discussed in greater detail in Unit XIV.

it is to sweep excess mucus up and out of the bronchi). As a result, there is an even greater pooling of mucus and an increased possibility of infection and obstruction.

The mucus that pools during bed rest may be *abnormal in consistency.* Sometimes the mucus is watery and so copious in amount that it cannot be expectorated by the weakened patient. Other patients, e.g., those who are dehydrated or on anticholinegic drugs, may have heavy, thick mucus which they cannot cough up and which tends to obstruct the bronchi. Such mucus is sometimes referred to as being "ropey" or "stringy" in character. If the secretions are very thick or copious, suctioning of the patient may be necessary.

When caring for a patient who seems too weak to cough up his secretions or to turn himself, make certain that you help him to move, cough, and deep-breathe at scheduled times. As you observe the patient's respiratory rate, carefully note his breathing patterns. Ask yourself these questions as you evaluate his pulmonary function:

> Are the patient's respirations shallow rather than full and deep? If so, the patient's chest expansion may be seriously restricted by one of the factors that we just discussed.

> Does he have to labor to get his breath? Labored breathing may indicate hypoxia and clogged respiratory passages due to mucus secretions.

> Do his respirations sound moist or wet? If so, the patient may be developing a hypostatic bronchopneumonia.

> Is the patient trying to cough up mucus? Is the mucus thick or thin in consistency, white or greenish yellow in color, copious or sparse in amount? Ropey thick mucus might indicate that the patient is dehydrated and needs fluids. Thin, copious mucus indicates that the patient may need suctioning if he is very weak. Greenish yellow mucus is one diagnostic sign of hypostatic bronchopneumonia.

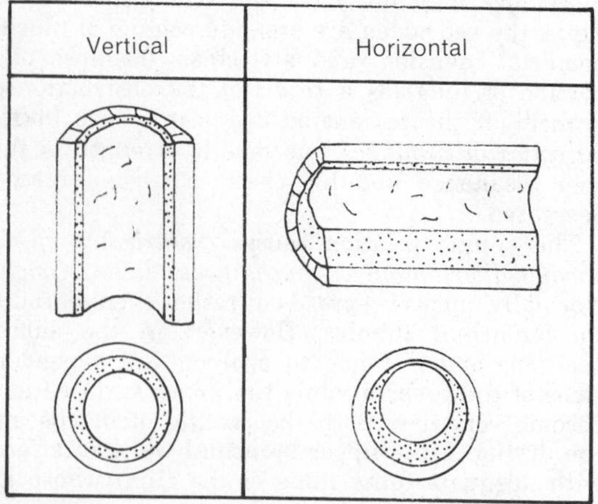

FIGURE 27–4. Gravity's effect upon mucous distribution within a bronchial tube. (After Browse, *The Physiology and Pathology of Bedrest.* Springfield, Ill., Charles C Thomas, 1965.)

> Is the pulse rapid? A rapid pulse is one of the *first* indications of oxygen lack.

> Is the patient's temperature elevated? If so, the patient may be developing bronchitis or bronchopneumonia.

> Does the patient seem irritable, confused, or disoriented? If so, the patient may need oxygen.

> Is the patient using his neck muscles to breathe rather than his abdominal muscles? The use of the axillary neck muscles to breathe is a *late* sign of severe respiratory disability.

> Are cyanosis and severe dyspnea present? These are the *late* signs of hypoxia and must be reported at once.

Finally, you and the physician must observe the patient for the following *specific* signs of hypostatic bronchopneumonia: cough, fever, pain on breathing, leukocytosis, greenish yellow sputum, and patchy infiltration of the lung on x-ray. If hypostatic pneumonia is present, antibiotics and vigorous coughing are the treatment measures of choice.

Carbon Dioxide Narcosis and Respiratory Acidosis

When a patient's respiratory movements decrease and his cough reflex diminishes, the oxygen-carbon dioxide exchange in his lungs is severely affected. As a result, CO_2 accumulates in his blood; at the same time the oxygen tension of the blood decreases and tissue hypoxia develops.

At first, the increase in plasma CO_2 stimulates the respiratory center in the medulla with the result that respirations increase. At the same time the lowered oxygen tension of the blood stimulates the aortic and carotid bodies, which also stimulate the respirations. These compensatory changes, however, are only *temporary.* As you will recall from Chapter 25, the medulla soon refuses to respond to the rising CO_2 blood level. Carbon dioxide continues to build up in the blood, and CO_2 narcosis develops. At the same time, the responses of the carotid and aortic bodies are weakened, and the oxygen levels of the blood continue to drop. Without prompt treatment, such patients can rapidly progress to states of respiratory acidosis, respiratory and cardiac failure, coma, and death. For a more detailed description of respiratory acidosis and CO_2 narcosis, their symptoms and treatment, refer back to Chapter 25.

THE EFFECT OF PROLONGED BED REST UPON METABOLISM

Prolonged bed rest has the following effects upon metabolism:[8]

> The basal metabolic rate (BMR) tends to fall slightly; however, it returns to normal within three weeks following the patient's return to ambulatory status.

> Muscle mass decreases; however, the patient's total body weight tends to remain stable.

> A state of negative nitrogen balance develops within four days following the patient's immobilization. By the tenth day of bed rest, the state of negative nitrogen balance reaches its peak; then gradually the patient returns to a normal state of balance.

> There is a decreased production of adrenocortical hormones—"stress hormones."

To counteract these changes in metabolic function, make certain that the patient receives a diet that is adequate in protein. Also, to reduce the problem of muscle atrophy, encourage active and/or passive exercises and movement.

THE EFFECT OF PROLONGED BED REST UPON THE GASTROINTESTINAL TRACT

Immobility has little effect upon the functional activities of the gastrointestinal tract. Thus, both digestive and bowel function remain relatively unchanged during bed rest; however, as the energy requirements of the patient's cells are lessened, appetite may decrease. Also bowel habits may change as a result of shifts in the patient's routine and environment.

Adverse Effects upon Ingestion

Anorexia may develop due to the patient's underlying malady as well as from the general weakness, worry, and boredom accompanying immobility. *Hypoproteinemia* is a common problem in the bedridden patient. Lowered blood protein levels are due to anorexia; to some disease conditions, e.g., cancer and tuberculosis; and to the increased catabolic activity that immobilization causes.

To *prevent* patients on bed rest from becoming seriously malnourished, the following suggestions may prove useful: (1) help the patient to select foods that have high nutritional value; (2) encourage the patient to eat foods that are high in protein, e.g., cheese, milk, meat, fish, and eggs; (3) serve small, frequent feedings; (4) ask the dietitian to visit the patient to determine his food preferences and dislikes; (5) chart carefully exactly how much the patient eats and which foods he leaves on his tray; and (6) notify the physician if the patient has a poor appetite and is refusing his meals.

Adverse Effects upon Elimination

Constipation is a frequent complication for patients on bed rest. Many factors can contribute to its development. First of all, patients who are sick enough to be on bed rest experience changes in their diet, changes in their daily schedule and routine, and a decrease in their general level of activity—all of which can lead to a change in bowel habits. Second, patients often feel embarrassed to use a bedpan and they find bedpans uncomfortable; consequently, patients frequently suppress their desire to defecate. Many patients on bed rest who have the desire to defecate find that they simply cannot do so in this unnatural position. Finally, the general muscle weakness that characterizes the immobilized patient also extends to those muscles that are involved in the act of defecation, e.g., the abdominal muscles, the diaphragm, and the levator ani. Particularly in the elderly, muscle weakness and poor sphincter tone often contribute to problems with constipation.

In sum, the immobilized patient, his diet and routine changed, and his natural desire to defecate inhibited by embarrassment, discomfort, and muscle weakness, gradually neglects his body's urgings. In time, owing to habitual neglect, the patient loses even his *desire* to defecate. As a result, his rectum becomes chronically distended and the patient becomes severely constipated. Malaise, headache, dizziness, loss of appetite, and abdominal distention often accompany constipation.

Fecal impactions will develop if the patient's severe constipation is not treated conscientiously. A fecal impaction is a hardened or putty-like stool that remains in the rectum or colon; it must often be removed manually or even surgically. Impactions can be diagnosed by (1) the presence of a distended abdomen; (2) in some cases watery diarrhea (which passes around the impacted stool); and (3) the identification of a hard mass in the rectum or colon upon digital examination or sigmoidoscopy. Without proper intervention, a fecal impaction can lead to a mechanical bowel obstruction.

It is of prime importance to prevent fecal impactions from developing in immobilized patients with heart disease, in those who have suffered a cerebral vascular accident, and in postoperative patients who have undergone eye surgery. When patients with these particular conditions develop a fecal impaction, they often try to expel the hardened stool by excessive straining. Straining, in turn, may lead to such complications as cardiac arrest, additional cardiovascular accidents, and serious damage to the operated eye.

Careful observation is very important in the *prevention* of constipation and the development of fecal impactions. Note the frequency, color, consistency, amount, and shape of the patient's stools. The absence of stools for over three or four days, frequent stools (three or more per day), hard dry stools, watery stools, blood-tinged stools, and thin ribbon-like stools (indicating a possible bowel obstruction) should be charted and reported to the doctor.

If you suspect the development of a fecal impaction, digitally examine the patient's rectum for the presence of a hard mass and examine his abdomen for distention.

In addition to careful observation and reporting, constipation can be prevented by placing the immobilized patient upon a regimen that encourages good bowel habits. If possible, get the patient up to the bathroom or to the bedside commode each day at the same time. For best results, identify the time of day during which the patient normally has a bowel movement. Encourage the patient to drink ample fluids, to eat fruits and vegetables, and to drink a glass of prune juice whenever his bowels fail to move for a few days; discourage him from becoming dependent upon laxatives and enemas. Also, help the immobilized patient to exercise his abdominal muscles daily since this will help him to strengthen those muscles used in defecation.

The *treatment* of constipation and fecal impactions will probably require the use of stool softeners, mineral oil, enemas, and digital removal of the stool. For more complete instructions concerning the treatment of constipation, see Unit XV.

THE EFFECT OF PROLONGED BED REST UPON RENAL FUNCTION

Prolonged bed rest has relatively little direct effect upon the work of the kidney nephron; however, when a patient is *first* immobilized, his renal functioning is almost immediately affected by the supine position in the following ways: (1) renal blood flow greatly increases, in turn increasing the cardiac output; and (2) blood volume increases by 10 to 15 per cent owing to both a slight increase in capillary filtration and a large increase in the volume of tissue fluid being reabsorbed into the plasma. This increase in blood volume creates a temporary increase in urinary excretion.[8]

After the patient has adjusted to the state of bed rest (this usually takes around three weeks) the immediate increase in blood volume described above is followed by, first, a slow decrease in blood volume and then a slow increase.[8, 13]

Although immobility has no ill effects upon the functioning of the kidney nephron itself, the patient on prolonged bed rest may experience the following adverse effects upon his urinary excretory functions: difficulty in urinating, urinary stasis, and the formation of renal calculi.

Difficulty in Urination

To urinate normally it is necessary to have integrated action of the internal uretheral sphincter, the external uretheral sphincter, and the detrusor muscle of the bladder wall.* When the bladder fills with urine its walls are stretched and the individual experiences a sensation of bladder fullness or pressure. Urination can occur by voluntarily relaxing the perineal muscles and the external sphincter. Relaxation of the external sphincter, in turn, initiates the micturition reflex (an autonomic nervous system reflex) in which the detrusor muscle contracts. Upon contraction of the bladder wall, intrabladder pressure increases, the internal sphincter relaxes, and urine flows out through the urethra.

When patients are immobilized, they continue to experience normal sensations of bladder fullness. However, despite their desire to void, most bed patients experience difficulty in actually passing their urine. Common causes for difficult micturition are as follows:

- Hypertrophy of the prostate gland is a common cause of difficult micturition among elderly males. The enlarged prostate acts as a mechanical obstruction to urine flow, and it frequently causes such acute urinary retention that catheterization is required.
- Embarrassment may inhibit a patient from asking for the bedpan or urinal.
- The use of a bedpan or urinal, while in bed, makes the act of urination both uncomfortable and awkward. In the supine position it is difficult to relax the perineal muscles or to consciously bear down, as one normally does, to raise the intrabladder pressure. When these voluntary actions are not carried out, detrusor muscle contraction cannot be initiated.

When patients have difficulty in urination, because of any of the above causes, their bladders tend to become overly distended. Bladder distention results in an excessive stretching of the detrusor muscle, which, over a period of time, results in a decrease in the sensation of bladder fullness. The patient, consequently, has little desire to void even though he needs to do so. As pressure from urine in the bladder builds up, the patient may experience an overflow incontinence. Catheterization may be necessary to gradually relieve bladder distention. Without catheterization back pressure from the bladder distention may become so great that it actually damages the kidney nephron. However, the catheterization procedure itself is always hazardous because it can lead to serious urinary tract infections. Because of the dangers inherent in catheterization, emphasis should be placed on preventing bladder distention.

To *prevent bladder distention* due to difficulty with micturition, the nurse must first make careful observations. She needs to note and chart: (1) how frequently the patient voids, (2) the amount of urine that the patient passes with each voiding, (3) urinary incontinence, (4) any pain or difficulty that the patient experiences while voiding, and (5) the presence of bladder distention. If the patient has not voided for over eight hours despite adequate fluid intake or if he "dribbles" urine continuously and if his bladder is distended, you will need to try various appropriate measures to help the patient void. Some of the fundamental methods are: (1) allowing the male patient to stand beside his bed to void and the female patient to sit on a bedside commode, (2) running water, the sound of which may help the patient to relax his perineal muscles, (3) pouring warm water over the perineum itself, and (4) placing gentle manual pressure on the lower abdomen. If these methods fail, you should request an order for catheterization. When catheterization is necessary, it must be performed with strict aseptic technique to prevent infection.

Urinary Stasis and Renal Calculi

When human beings stand in their normal erect position, the force of gravity enables urine to flow

*For a more complete discussion of the micturition reflex, see p. 715.

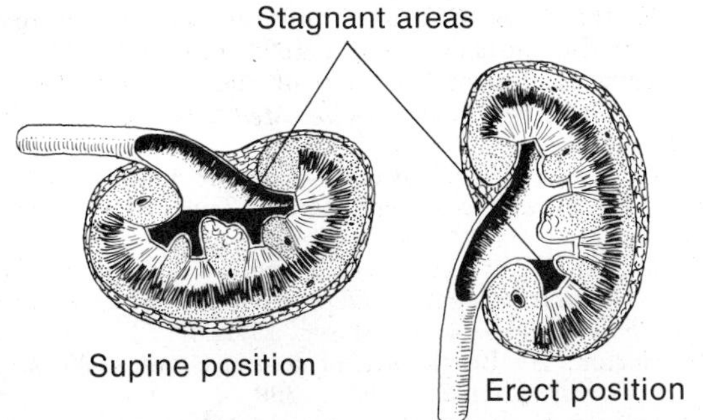

FIGURE 27-5. The effect of gravity upon renal flow out of the renal pelvis. (After Olson and Schroeder: *American Journal of Nursing,* April, 1967.)

freely from the renal pelvis and out through the ureter. However, when they are lying supine, gravity no longer aids the flow of urine and it tends to collect and to *stagnate* in the renal pelvis (Fig. 27–5).

As the urine stagnates, various tiny particles and crystals in the urine also remain in the stagnant pools of the renal pelvis where they may form the nuclei of renal calculi.

Renal calculi, sometimes called "kidney stones" or "recumbency stones," occur in 15 to 30 per cent of all immobilized patients. Most commonly, calculi develop after at least 14 to 21 days following the initial immobilization; they may develop sooner in patients with diseases characterized by elevated urine calcium concentration.[8]

Major factors contributing to the formation of renal stones in patients on bed rest are:*

> Urinary stasis.
> A slightly alkaline urine (which is common in patients on bed rest).
> Urinary tract infection.
> Elevated calcium concentrations in the urine. The amount of urine calcium can triple after only two weeks in bed. This increase is due to the draining of calcium from the bones as a result of disuse osteoporosis.
> Elevated phosphorus owing to disuse osteoporosis.
> A decrease in the *ratio* of citric acid to calcium in the urine. Citric acid normally acts to keep calcium in solution.

When the above factors are present, the patient in the supine position develops renal stones within his bladder and renal pelvis. These stones, which are composed mainly of calcium salts, can cause bleeding (hematuria), severe pain (renal colic), backache, nausea, and vomiting.

To *prevent* renal calculi, it is important to (1) combat urinary stasis by ambulating the patient as soon as permissible and by scheduling passive and active exercises; (2) keep the urine diluted by forcing fluids; (3) in some cases, lower the urinary pH by means of an acid-ash diet that includes cereals, poultry, meat, and fish; and (4) eliminate possible urinary infection by avoiding catheterization unless absolutely necessary.

*The etiology of urinary calculi is discussed more fully on p. 727.

THE EFFECT OF PROLONGED BED REST UPON THE MENTAL STATE

Persons on prolonged bed rest often feel lethargic, lonely, and depressed. Removed from their usual routine of work and play, bedfast patients may also suffer from acute anxiety and insomnia as they worry about their homes, families, jobs, and finances. Moreover, immobilized patients with neurotic or psychotic tendencies may tend to become emotionally disturbed. Some may act in hostile, belligerent ways; others may become severely withdrawn; still others may become disoriented, losing all track of time and place.

To help patients adjust emotionally to bed rest, consider the following suggestions:

> If possible, place the immobilized patient in a room with patients who are oriented and interested in their surroundings. Contact with such individuals may help the bedridden patient to feel less isolated and less out of touch with the world.
> Attempt to bring the outside world to the patient by having a bedside telephone and radio and a television with remote controls.
> Allow the patient, as much as possible, to help in the planning of his own care. This will help the patient feel that he is an active participant in his own program of care and rehabilitation.
> Identify patients with exaggerated or inappropriate emotional responses and report your observations to the physician so that a psychiatric consultation can be arranged if necessary.
> Allow patients on bed rest to openly discuss with you their anxieties and worries. Such discussion, while momentarily taxing, may serve to ease the patient's mind enough so that he can truly rest—both physically and mentally.

References for Unit V

1. Asher, R. A. J.: The dangers of going to bed. *British Medical Journal,* October 13, 1947, p. 967.
2. Bardsley, C., et al.: Pressure sores: A regimen for preventing and treating them. *American Journal of Nursing* 64:82, May, 1964.
3. Bliss, M. R., and McLaren, R.: Preventing pressure sores in geriatric patients. *Nursing Mirror* 123:379, January 27, 1967.
4. Bliss, M. R., and McLaren, R.: Preventing pressure sores in geriatric patients. *Nursing Mirror* 123:405, February 3, 1967.
5. Bliss, M. R., and McLaren, R.: Preventing pressure

sores in geriatric patients. *Nursing Mirror* 123:434, February 10, 1967.
6. Bliss, M. R., et al.: Preventing pressure sores in hospital: Controlled trial of a large-celled ripple mattress. *British Medical Journal* 1:394, February 18, 1967.
7. Brower, P., and Hicks, D.: Maintaining muscle function in patients on bed rest. *American Journal of Nursing* 72:1250, July, 1972.
8. Browse, N. L.: *The Physiology and Pathology of Bedrest.* Springfield, Illinois, Charles C Thomas, 1965.
9. Bruce, R.: Don't let the patient be nursed to death. *Nursing Mirror,* November 3, 1967, p. 124.
10. Carnevali, D., and Brueckner, S.: Immobilization—reassessment of a concept. *American Journal of Nursing* 70:1502, July, 1970.
11. Clay, E.: Operation bedsore, Part I. *Nursing Times,* March 22, 1968; Part 2, March 29, 1968.
12. Coe, S. W.: Cardiac work and the chair treatment of acute coronary thrombosis. *Annals of Internal Medicine* 40:42, January, 1954.
13. Deitrick, J. E., et al.: Effects of immobilization upon various metabolic and physiologic functions of normal men. *American Journal of Medicine* 4:3, January, 1948.
14. Dowling, A. S.: Pressure sores—their course, prevention and treatment. *Maryland State Medical Journal* 19:131, June, 1970.
15. Edberg, E. L.: Prevention and treatment of pressure sores. *Physical Therapy* 53:246, March, 1973.
16. Fisk, G. D.: Isometric and isotonic exercise for geriatric patients. *Geriatrics,* January, 1967, p. 175.
17. Gilstone, A.: Bedsore of the ear. *Lancet* 2:1313, December, 1972.
18. Goldstrom, D. K.: Cardiac rest: Bed or chair? *American Journal of Nursing* 72:1812, October, 1972.
19. Gosnell, D. J.: An assessment tool to identify pressure sores. *Nursing Research* 22:55, Jan-Feb, 1973.
20. Harvin, J. S., and Hargest, T. S.: The air-fluidized bed: A new concept in the treatment of decubitus ulcers. *Nursing Clinics of North America* 5:181, March, 1970.
21. Holley, L.: The physical therapist—Who, what and how. *American Journal of Nursing* 70:1521, July, 1970.
22. Johnson, M. L.: Problems involved in the prevention of pressure sores. *Nursing Mirror* 135:37, July, 1972.
23. Isler, C.: Decubitus: Old truths and some new ideas. *RN* 35:42, July, 1972.
24. Kottke, F. S.: Effects of limitation of activity upon the human body. *J.A.M.A.* 196:830, June 6, 1966.
25. Levy, R.: Immobilized patient and his psychological well-being. *Postgraduate Medicine* 40:74, July, 1966.
26. Lowthian, P. T.: Bedsores—Current methods of prevention and treatment. *Nursing Times* 67:501, April, 1971.
27. Mutter, D., et al.: Isometric exercise and the cardiovascular system. *Modern Concepts of Cardiovascular Disease* 41:11, March, 1972.
28. Norton, D.: Breakdown of pressure areas. *Nursing Times,* March 27, 1964, p. 399.
29. Olivari, H., et al.: The surgical treatment of bedsores in paraplegics. *Plastic and Reconstructive Surgery* 50:477, November, 1972.
30. Olson, E. V., and Edmonds, R. E.: The hazards of immobility: Effects on motor function. *American Journal of Nursing* 67:788, April, 1967.
31. Olson, E. V., and Johnson, B. J.: The hazards of immobility: Effects on cardiovascular function. *American Journal of Nursing* 67:781, April, 1967.
32. Olson, E. V., and McCarthy, J.: The hazards of immobility: Effects on gastrointestinal function. *American Journal of Nursing* 67:785, April, 1967.
33. Olson, E. V., and Schroeder, L. M.: The hazards of immobility: Effects on urinary function. *American Journal of Nursing* 67:780, April, 1967.
34. Olson, E. V., and Thompson, L. F.: The hazards of immobility: Effects on respiratory function. *American Journal of Nursing* 67:783, April, 1967.
35. Olson, E. V., and Wade, M.: The hazards of immobility: Effects on metabolic equilibrium. *American Journal of Nursing* 67:793, April, 1967.
36. Olson, E. V., et al.: The hazards of immobility: Effects on psychosocial equilibrium. *American Journal of Nursing* 67:779, April, 1967.
37. Pfaudler, M.: Flotation, displacement, and decubitus ulcers. *American Journal of Nursing* 68:2351, November, 1968.
38. Pressure sores: Successful trial of a new treatment. *Nursing Times,* April 21, 1967, p. 513.
39. Spencer, W. A., et al.: Physiologic concepts of immobilization. *Archives of Physical Medicine and Rehabilitation* 46:89, January, 1965.
40. Taylor, J. C.: Decubitus ulcers. *Nursing Science,* August, 1964, p. 293.
41. Thornhill, H. L., and Williams, M. L.: Experience with the water mattress in a large city hospital. *American Journal of Nursing* 68:2356, November, 1968.
42. Torelli, M.: Topical hyperbaric oxygen for decubitus ulcers. *American Journal of Nursing 73*:494, March, 1973.
43. Wallace, C. M.: To bed or not to bed? *Nursing Mirror* 128:26, March 28, 1969.

SECTION THREE

Specific Problems in Medical-Surgical Nursing Practice

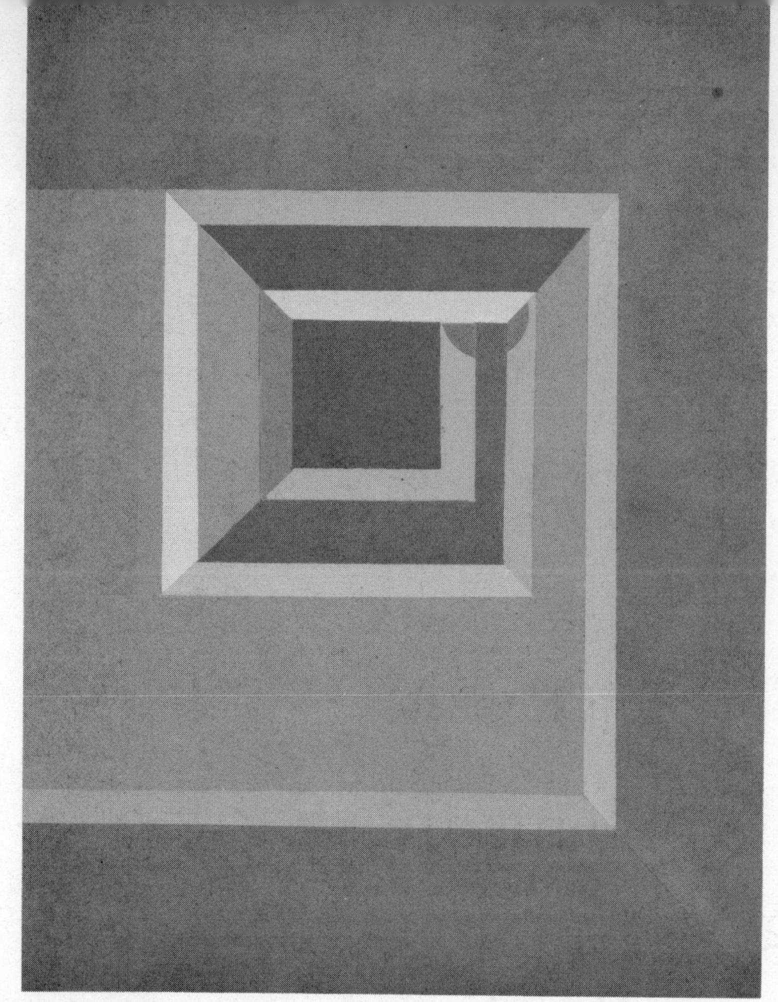

surgical risk
operative permit
general anesthesia total unconciousness & affects entire organism
regional " no uncon.; loss of painful sensation in 1 region
laryngospasm mucosa goes into spasm due to irritation by anesthetic or allergic Rx to anesth. - produces obstruction which can be prevented by endo. tube
bronchospasm chronic bronchitis asthma, emphesyma, gastric juices - wheezing
hypothermia
purposeful hypotension
airway
"fistula-forming" tubes - T-tubes - tubes into organ to outside
wound dehiscence opening of wound edges
evisceration protrusion of loops of bowel through the incision
acute gastric dilatation
paralytic ileus
acute parotitis

We operate every day and an operation is but an incident in our day's work. For the patient, it is his whole life and he must and will walk through the valley of the shadow of death alone. He certainly cannot pay us a greater compliment than by putting his life into our hands and nothing but the very heart- and backbreaking best must be given back in return.[43]

UNIT VI

Nursing Patients Experiencing Surgery

Unit Introduction and Study Guide

The nursing of patients who are experiencing surgery is an exacting, difficult, demanding task. Yet for many nurses surgical nursing is a most challenging and gratifying specialty. The modern surgical nurse works with a wide variety of interesting patients; owing to advances in anesthesia and in surgical techniques, she frequently has the pleasure of seeing her patients recover quickly from their operations and return home to a productive life.

Basically, you perform your duties as a surgical nurse during the following three periods:

> The *preoperative period,* during which you admit the patient to the surgical floor and prepare him physically, emotionally, and legally for his operation. The emphasis, during this period, is upon the correction of physiologic and psychologic problems that might increase surgical risk, and upon instructing the patient in exercises that will benefit him during the postoperative period.

> The *operative period,* during which you transfer the patient to the operating room where he is anesthetized and undergoes the scheduled surgical procedure. The emphasis, during the surgery itself, is upon asepsis, hemostasis, and the safe induction of anesthesia.

> The *postoperative period,* during which you observe and assist the patient as he recovers from the anesthesia and from the stress of surgery itself. The emphasis, during this period, is upon the maintenance of proper respiratory and circulatory function, the alleviation of pain and discomfort, and the prevention of postoperative complications.

To aid you in your study of this material, we offer the following guides:

1. As you study this unit, familiarize yourself with the following terms:

   surgical risk, operative permit, general anesthesia, regional anesthesia, laryngospasm, bronchospasm, hypothermia, purposeful hypotension, airway, "fistula-forming" tubes, wound dehiscence, evisceration, acute gastric dilatation, paralytic ileus, acute parotitis.

2. Upon completion of this unit, you should be able generally to discuss the following concepts:

a. The four major types of conditions that generally require surgical intervention.

b. The usual classification of surgical procedures.

c. The estimation of surgical risk and your role in assisting the surgeon as he gathers information concerning the patient.

d. The typical preparation of a patient for surgery from the time he enters the hospital until the time he is transported to the operating room.

e. The major differences between general and regional anesthesia.

f. The complications of anesthesia—their treatment and prevention.

g. Typical care of the patient in the recovery room.

h. The goals of surgical care and their achievement.

i. The major symptoms that herald the development of postoperative complications.

j. The major postoperative complications—their prevention and treatment.

CHAPTER 28

The Patient Undergoing Surgery: General Considerations

Today surgery takes place in a thoroughly equipped, aseptic environment. The surgeon is aided in his task by recent advances in medical technology and by knowledge of man's physiologic responses to stress. The anesthesiologist's responsibilities have been lightened in recent years by the development of safe yet potent anesthetic agents. The modern nurse can effectively care for surgical patients within the specialized environment of a well equipped recovery room.

However, despite such advances, for the *patient himself,* the decision to undergo surgery stands as a moment of crisis in his life. Surgery represents a personal crisis because any operation, however minor, always carries some risk; moreover, surgery inevitably involves a certain amount of expense, discomfort, pain, and emotional stress for the patient as well as a disruption of his usual life pattern.

What conditions force a patient to undergo the risk of surgical procedure? What are the major types of surgeries and what are some of the general effects upon the patient? How do surgeons estimate the amount of risk that a patient will face as he lies anesthetized upon the operating table? What is the role of the nurse in reducing surgical risks and in making the operation and its aftermath successful?

BASIC TYPES OF CONDITIONS REQUIRING SURGERY

Despite the large number of individual conditions that are treated by surgeons, there are four basic pathologic processes that are the cause of almost all surgical problems.[38]

The four pathologic processes responsible for most surgical conditions are:

1. Obstruction *2. Perforation*
3. Erosion *4. Tumors*

Obstruction or blockage mainly affects arteries (e.g., the coronary or cerebral arteries), tubes (e.g., the bronchial and eustachian tubes), and ducts (e.g., the cystic duct). For example, when the coronary arteries are blocked, a myocardial infarction results, whereas a blockage of cerebral arteries produces a cerebral vascular accident ("stroke"). Atelectasis or lung collapse results from an obstructed bronchial tube, whereas a middle ear infection can be caused by an obstructed eustachian tube. When a "stone" blocks the cystic duct, cholecystitis or inflammation of the gallbladder results.

Obstructions of passageways within the body are dangerous because they block the flow of such vital substances as blood, air, cerebral spinal fluid, urine, and bile.

Perforation is the rupture of an organ, artery, or bleb. Examples of perforation are: perforated duodenal ulcer, ruptured bladder, and cerebral hemorrhage due to the rupture of a major cerebral artery. Perforation is a dangerous event that usually calls for emergency surgery.

Erosion is the wearing away or eating away of the surface of a tissue as a result of continuous physical irritation, infection, ulceration, or inflammation. The process of erosion may wear away blood vessel walls, resulting in bleeding. Cancerous tumors, bladder stones, duodenal ulcers, and tuberculosis can all lead to the erosion of blood vessels and resultant bleeding.

Tumors are abnormal growths of tissue that form masses serving no physiologic function within the body, and that may be malignant. Tumors often grow very large in size before they are detected. Also, since tumors often may not initially produce symptoms, a patient may neglect his condition and fail to seek prompt medical advice. At times such neglect may be fatal. One of the commonest methods of treating tumors is by surgical excision of the mass.

MAJOR CATEGORIES OF SURGICAL PROCEDURES

Surgical procedures are classified according to their: (1) purpose, (2) degree of risk to the patient, and (3) urgency.

Types of surgeries classified to *purpose* are: diagnostic, exploratory, curative, (including ablative, reconstructive, and constructive) and palliative.

Diagnostic surgery enables the surgeon to make or to verify a suspected diagnosis. A common type of diagnostic surgery is the *biopsy,* in which the surgeon excises a small amount of tissue and sends it to the pathology laboratory for microscopic examination, which will establish a diagnosis. For instance, surgeons commonly take a biopsy of breast tissue if they suspect the presence of breast cancer. If the specimen of tissue is found to contain cancer cells, the surgeon then proceeds to excise the tumor and often removes the entire breast and surrounding lymph nodes.

Exploratory surgery enables the surgeon to estimate the extent of disease and, at times, to make or confirm a diagnosis. A common example is an exploratory laparotomy, during which the surgeon makes an opening in the abdomen, explores the abdominal area and organs for signs of cancer, bleeding, and so forth, hopefully diagnoses the patient's condition, and determines the need for more extensive surgery.

Curative surgery (ablative, reconstructive, and constructive) is performed to remove or to repair damaged, diseased, or congenitally malformed organs or tissues. *Ablative* surgery involves the removal of diseased organs (e.g., nephrectomy, or the removal of a kindey; *reconstructive* surgery is the partial or complete restoration of a damaged organ or tissue to its normal appearance and function (e.g., plastic surgery of the facial structures following a severe burn); *constructive* surgery is the repair of a congenitally defective organ to improve its function and appearance (e.g., plastic surgery of a congenitally deformed nose); and *palliative* surgery relieves symptoms, although it does not cure the disease causing the symptoms. For example, nerves supplying a diseased organ may be cut to reduce or to alleviate severe pain; infected necrotic tissues may be removed to reduce pain and for esthetic purposes; an intestinal bypass operation is sometimes performed to relieve symptoms of intestinal obstruction caused from an inoperable bowel cancer.

Types of surgeries classified according to *magnitude* and *degree of risk* for the patient are: major surgery and minor surgery.

Major surgery involves high risk for the patient because he may be on the operating table for a prolonged period of time; a large amount of blood may be lost; vital organs will be handled and may be removed; and postoperative complications may develop. Examples of major surgery are open-heart surgery, nephrectomies, and abdominal-perineal resections.

Minor surgery, on the other hand, is generally not prolonged, engenders few serious complications, and involves little patient risk. An example of minor surgery is a skin biopsy.

Operative procedures may also be classified according to *urgency.* Principal categories are emergency surgery, imperative or urgent surgery, planned required surgery, elective surgery, and optional surgery.

Emergency surgery must be performed *immediately* in order to: (1) save the life of the patient; (2) save the function of an organ or limb; (3) remove a damaged organ or limb as necessary; or (4) stop hemorrhage. Examples of clinical situations requiring emergency surgery are: severe trauma resulting from an automobile accident, severe and extensive burns, a perforated ulcer, and gunshot or stab wounds.

Imperative or urgent surgery must be performed as soon as possible, preferably within 24 hours. Examples of conditions that must be surgically corrected within 24 to 48 hours are: kidney stones, severe bleeding hemorrhoids, and cancerous tumors that are beginning to erode major blood vessels or obstruct a bronchus.

Planned required surgery is *necessary* for the patient's well-being but is *not* urgent. This required surgery may be scheduled weeks or months ahead of the proposed operation. Examples of conditions that require correction by planned surgical procedures are tonsillitis and eye cataracts.

Elective surgery is surgery which should be performed for the patient's well-being but which is not absolutely necessary. Examples of conditions requiring elective surgery are: hemorrhoids that are not bleeding, simple hernias, and scars correctable by plastic surgery.

Optional surgery is surgery that the patient requests, generally for esthetic or psychologic reasons, e.g., a face lift.

THE EFFECT OF SURGERY UPON THE PATIENT

A surgical procedure, whether major or minor, emergency or optional, *always* affects the patient, both physically and emotionally. Although each type of operation creates its own specific problems, some *general* effects of surgery upon the patient are listed and discussed below.

Effects of Surgery

1. *The stress response is elicited.*
2. *The defense against infection is lowered.*
3. *The vascular system is disrupted.*
4. *Organ functions are disturbed.*
5. *The body image may be disturbed.*
6. *Life styles may change.*

Stress Response Is Elicited

As a result of surgery, patients experience an activation of the stress response triggered by an increased production of epinephrine by the adrenal glands. The release of epinephrine produces the following physiologic effects: (1) an increased heart rate, (2) a more forceful heart beat (which causes greater amounts of oxygenated blood to be forced into the arteries), and (3) peripheral vascular constriction. Moreoever, the increased circulation of epinephrine causes the release of other vital hormones that play a role in the patient's response to stress.

The success of the stress response in maintaining homeostatic balance is determined, to a large degree, by the age and physical condition of the patient as well as by the duration of the stress. In the aged or debilitated person, the ability to withstand stress and to tolerate surgery and anesthesia is often markedly reduced. One reason that the aged and debilitated respond poorly to stress is that their adrenal glands are often atrophied and reduced in size.[27] As a result, less epinephrine is released and the stimulation of ACTH and corticoid production is decreased.

Specific disorders that decrease the body's adaptive mechanisms and that should be treated prior to surgery are: liver disease, shock, hemorrhage, dehydration, electrolyte imbalance, acidosis, alkalosis, hypoproteinemia, vitamin deficiency, anemia, adrenal insufficiency, alcoholism, pulmonary disorders, heart ailments, vascular insufficiency, renal insufficiency, obesity, hyperthyroidism, diabetes mellitus, and emotional instability.

In any person, young or old, healthy or sick, prolonged stress eventually depletes the "stress hormones" as well as the substances composing them.

The need for a powerful stress response can be minimized by careful, thoughtful medical preparation and nursing care. The well prepared, calm preoperative patient and the comfortable postoperative patient rely far less on the stress response for survival than do frightened, uncomfortable patients who are left alone in pain and uncertainty.

Defense Against Infection Is Lowered

When the surgeon's scalpel incises the patient's skin, the first line of defense against bacterial invasion is destroyed. Despite sterile equipment and meticulous technique on the part of all members of the surgical team, infection remains as an ever-present potential danger for the surgical patient.

Vascular System Is Disrupted

As the surgeon incises more deeply into the patient's tissue, blood vessels are severed and must immediately be clamped. However, despite the quick response of surgeons in clamping these bleeding vessels (known as "bleeders"), some blood loss always occurs during surgery. At times, hemorrhage and shock may develop during the course of the operation or postoperatively.

Organ Functions Are Disturbed

During surgery, organs are manipulated, causing the organ function to be temporarily disrupted during the postoperative period. Also, some operative procedures involve the removal of organ tissues or total organs. As a result of more radical surgeries, the physiologic functioning of the entire body may be seriously affected. For example, a patient with cancer of the stomach may require a total gastrectomy, and removal of the stomach may cause great difficulty in maintaining adequate nutrition. As a result, the patient may develop anemia, become weak and apathetic, and spend the rest of his life as a semi-invalid.

Body Image May Be Disturbed

Disturbances of body image may occur as the result of (1) amputations of a limb or breast, (2) mutilating operations, e.g., radical neck surgery, and (3) operations during which organs of symbolic or emotional importance are removed. For example, the removal of a woman's uterus is not visibly apparent. However, the woman who has lost her uterus may *feel* that she is irreversibly changed and is no longer a "complete woman."

Life Styles May Change

Certain types of operations may force a patient to radically alter his whole way of life, at least during a postoperative period of learning and retraining. For example, the amputee has to learn to use an artificial limb; this takes time and effort on his part. Job retraining may also be needed, as well as modification of recreational activities.

In sum, surgery solves certain problems only to create others. To face surgery requires courage on the patient's part as well as the ability to adapt to stress. One role of the surgeon and the nurse is to prepare the patient for the stresses and problems that he will inevitably meet. The preparation of the preoperative patient for his operation is discussed in Chapter 29.

THE ESTIMATION OF SURGICAL RISK

The degree of surgical risk is based upon four factors: (1) the physical and mental condition of the patient; (2) the extent of the disease; (3) the magnitude of the required operation; and (4) the resources and preparation of the surgeon, nurses, and hospital.[36]

ASSESSING THE PATIENT'S PHYSICAL AND MENTAL CONDITION

The degree of surgical risk is affected profoundly by the following factors: (1) the patient's age, (2) his state of nutritional balance, (3) his state of fluid and electrolyte balance, (4) his general health, (5) the types of drugs that he takes regularly, and (6) his mental health. Let us briefly examine each of these factors.

Age

Children and young and middle-aged adults generally tolerate surgery fairly well, while the premature baby and the aged tolerate surgery poorly. Operating on older persons is risky for the following reasons:

> The aged are highly sensitive to stress, to anesthetics, and to certain drugs that are used pre- and postoperatively, e.g., scopolamine, morphine sulfate, and barbiturates.

> The elderly are often dehydrated and malnourished, making them prone to shock and retarded tissue healing. Senescent patients frequently are victims of degenerative diseases (e.g., congestive heart failure and arteriosclerosis) as well as chronic respiratory diseases (e.g., emphysema). Moreover, many elderly male patients have prostatic hypertrophy, which can lead to postoperative urinary and renal problems.

One authority states that the most common problem seen in the aged preoperatively is a lower than normal *total blood volume.*[59] Patients with a lowered blood volume prior to surgery are unable to tolerate even a small amount of bleeding, and go rapidly into shock. Thus, many old persons require blood transfusion *before* their operation in order to decrease risk.

In general, operative risk for older patients is lower in those operations that are brief in duration, elective, cause little blood loss, and statistically incur a low percentage of postoperative complications. On the other hand, lengthy surgery, emergency surgery, hemorrhage, and a high percentage of postoperative complications all increase risk.

Nutritional Status

Major preoperative nutritional problems are: (1) debilitation and malnourishment due to protein, iron, and vitamin deficiencies, and (2) obesity.

Nutritional deficiencies mainly affect the aged, the chronically ill, persons with cancer, and patients with gastrointestinal conditions that cause severe diarrhea and/or vomiting, e.g., ulcerative colitis and pyloric stenosis.

To treat preoperative patients who are malnourished, encourage a high intake of carbohydrate (needed for energy); protein (needed for wound healing); vitamins (also needed for healing); and vitamin K (necessary for proper blood coagulation). Although patients should be encouraged to gain weight if they are abnormally thin, a substantial weight gain is *not* absolutely essential for the success of the surgery.

Obesity must be corrected by weight loss prior to an operation that is not of an emergency nature. The severely obese patient faces an increase in surgical risk for every pound he is overweight. As some authorities point out, an additional 25 miles of blood vessels are needed to supply 30 lb. of excess fat! In turn, these miles of additional vessels place a tremendous strain upon the patient's heart. Thus, the obese individual with his overburdened body and laboring heart often cannot withstand the additional stress of surgery.

Other reasons why surgical risk is increased in the obese are:

> Obese persons frequently suffer from hypertension, congestive heart failure, and metabolic problems such as diabetes mellitus—all of which may complicate their operative and postoperative course.

> Fatty tissue is difficult for the surgeon to approximate and to suture, especially in abdominal operations. Thus, the obese patient is prone to wound dehiscence.

> Fatty tissue is liable to postoperative infection.

Treatment of the obese patient prior to surgery requires a strict reducing diet and evaluation and care of conditions such as hypotension and diabetes mellitus.

Fluid and Electrolyte Balance

Dehydration and hypovolemia predispose the patient to complications both during surgery and postoperatively. Dehydration, as stated in Unit V, may result from prolonged vomiting, diarrhea, and bleeding, coupled with inadequate fluid intake. To correct dehydration, fluids are usually administered intravenously or by hypodermoclysis during the preoperative period.

Electrolyte imbalances, like water imbalances, also increase operative risk. It is particularly important to correct K^+, Mg^{++}, and Ca^{++} deficiencies and H^+ imbalances prior to surgery by means of proper diet, IV infusions, and so forth. (See Unit V.)

General Health

The presence of any *infectious* process or any serious *physiologic malfunctioning* increases the operative risk. Thus the surgeon, aided by the nurse and laboratory personnel, examines the surgical candidate for the presence of infection and to determine the adequacy of: cardiovascular function, pulmonary function, genitourinary function, metabolic function, neurologic function, and hematologic factors.

Infection. *Any* infection, even a minor cold on the day of surgery, can affect the course of surgery adversely. Thus, physicians and nurses must be alert to the presence of such symptoms as sneezing, coughing, a sore throat, an elevated temperature, and the appearance of skin lesions, boils, or rashes. An elevated white count should also be reported to the surgeon. Any of the preceding findings may result in the cancellation or postponement of surgery.

Cardiovascular Function. The presence of

minor or well controlled heart ailments generally has little effect upon operative risk. Heart conditions that *do* increase risk are angina pectoris, a recent myocardial infarction (within the previous six months), malignant hypertension, and severe uncompensated congestive heart failure. In the elderly, risk is also increased by hypovolemia and anemia. Also, the presence of peripheral vascular disease can result in impaired tissue healing if the operation involves the extremities.

Patients suspected of having cardiovascular disease should be carefully observed for an elevated blood pressure, rapid, irregular pulse, edema, cold, blue extremities, weakness, and fatigue. Typical *laboratory* and *diagnostic studies* of cardiovascular function ordered preoperatively are: electrocardiogram, central venous pressure, red blood count, hematocrit, hemoglobin, and serum Na^+.

Preoperative *treatment* of patients with cardiovascular disease includes rest, a low sodium or low cholesterol diet, heart medications such as digitalis, and the judicious administration of fluids.

Pulmonary Function. Crippling pulmonary conditions, such as emphysema and bronchiectasis, increase operative risk because they impair the patient's ability to exchange CO_2 and O_2. These conditions also predispose the patient to severe pulmonary infections.

In determining the presence of hazardous pulmonary malfunction, observe patients for: shortness of breath, wheezing, clubbed fingers, chest pain, and coughing with the expectoration of copious and/or purulent mucus. Question the patient carefully concerning smoking habits; also obtain a history of his respiratory allergies and infections. The doctor will order a chest x-ray for diagnostic purposes.

Patients with severe respiratory disease are usually treated preoperatively with aerosol treatments, postural drainage, antibiotics, and restricted smoking. To prevent postoperative respiratory complications, these individuals need preoperative instruction in the deep breathing and coughing exercises that they will practice following surgery (see p. 318).

Genitourinary Function. The surgical patient needs adequate renal function to eliminate protein wastes from his body and to preserve fluid and electrolyte balance. Genitourinary conditions that increase operative risk are advanced renal insufficiency, acute nephritis, and prostatic hypertrophy. As stated earlier, in the elderly male patient, prostatic hypertrophy obstructs the normal flow of urine and predisposes the patient to urinary infection.

To assess genitourinary function, observe the preoperative patient carefully for the serious symptoms of frequent urination, dysuria, and anuria. Also, check the appearance of the patient's urine; if it is cloudy or bloody rather than clear amber in color, renal disease may be present. Of course, report any abnormal findings to the surgeon.

The most commonly ordered preoperative tests of renal function are:

URINALYSIS. Urinalysis is performed on either a clear voided specimen or a catheterized specimen to check the urine for: red or white blood cells (may indicate an infection or tumor), casts (may indicate renal disease), protein (may indicate renal disease), sugar (usually indicates diabetes), and specific gravity (if low, i.e., under 1.010, the kidney is evidently unable to concentrate urine; if elevated, i.e., over 1.025, the patient is dehydrated).

BLOOD UREA NITROGEN (BUN) OR NON-PROTEIN NITROGEN (NPN). These laboratory studies test the ability of the kidney to excrete urea and protein wastes. If the findings are seriously abnormal, the patient is a poor surgical risk since he may develop postoperative renal failure.* To decrease risk, serious kidney diseases and urinary infections must be treated with appropriate measures *prior* to surgery.

Metabolic and Liver Function. Untreated *diabetes mellitus* greatly magnifies surgical risk as it predisposes the patient to infection and to poor tissue healing. As you will see in Unit XIX, diabetes is diagnosed by means of urine and blood tests and is generally treated by proper diet, proper exercise, and insulin injections.

Liver disease, such as Laennec's cirrhosis, also increases risk because an impaired liver is unable to detoxify dangerous drugs, to produce and excrete bile, and to metabolize carbohydrates, fats, and amino acids. Patients with a history of alcoholism and with signs of jaundice and ascites require a careful examination for liver disease prior to surgery. Since these persons are usually malnourished and debilitated, the doctor will generally order a high caloric diet, IV solutions, and vitamins as a part of their preoperative regimen.

Neurologic Factors. Serious neurologic conditions, such as uncontrolled epilepsy or severe Parkinson's disease, increase surgical risk. Important neurologic findings in preoperative patients are: severe headaches, frequent dizziness, lightheadedness, ringing in the ears, unsteady gait, unequal pupils, and a history of convulsions.

Hematologic Factors. Most surgical procedures result in some blood loss, even in persons whose blood coagulates normally. Thus, patients with missing or abnormal coagulation factors face the complications of severe bleeding, hemorrhage, and shock coincident with surgery. Findings of importance that point to abnormal hematologic factors are:[5]

> A history of bleeding tendencies.

> Symptoms such as easy bruising, excessive bleeding following dental extractions and shaving, severe nosebleeds.

> The presence of hepatic or renal disease.

> Prior use of anticoagulants.

---

*For more information concerning tests of renal function, see Unit XI.

- Abnormal bleeding time, prothrombin time, or platelet counts (discussed in Unit XII).

Patients with the above findings are given blood transfusions prior to surgery to correct blood volume deficits or anemia. Additional blood is always on hand for patients with coagulation problems in event of hemorrhage during surgery or during the postoperative period.

Use of Drugs

Many preoperative patients take prescribed or nonprescription drugs that can increase operative risk by: (1) increasing coagulation time, and (2) interacting unfavorably with the anesthetic. Drugs that may result in complications for the surgical patient are:

- Anticoagulants: can cause hemorrhage during surgery.
- Antibiotics: can combine unfavorably with the anesthetic agent, thereby causing untoward effects.
- Tranquilizers: increase hypotension and, thus, can cause shock.
- Thiazide diuretics: can create potassium imbalances.

Mental Outlook

The patient who greatly fears his impending operation, the anesthetic, and postoperative pain and discomforts significantly increases his surgical risk. Fears of surgery are not always in proportion to the seriousness of the surgery; therefore, the fact that a contemplated operation is minor in nature does *not* mean that a patient will be free from fear. Indeed, apprehensive patients undergoing a minor orthopedic operation or tonsillectomy have been known to die in surgery from a cardiac arrest, possibly triggered by their extreme anxiety.

A patient who feels and states that he is doomed to die in surgery or who is greatly afraid of surgery needs opportunities to talk of his fears with concerned staff members. Do not give false reassurance to such a patient or dismiss his fears. An extreme fear of surgery is a dangerous problem; it must be taken seriously by the staff responsible for the patient's operative course. The attending physician should be alerted to such fears when they are detected in preoperative patients.

Maladjusted patients with a past history of severe depression, paranoia, and other mental illnesses may also adapt poorly to the stress of surgery. Sometimes mentally disturbed persons, who are generally able to function at home and at work despite their emotional problems, develop full blown psychoses or neuroses postoperatively.

THE EXTENT OF THE DISEASE

Although surgical risk clearly rests upon the physical and mental condition of the patient, the degree of risk also depends upon the *disease* being treated, more specifically the *nature* of the disease, the *site* of the disease, and the *length of time* the patient has been ill with the disease.

Nature of the Disease

Is the disease *benign* or *malignant*? This is one of the gravest questions a surgeon must answer, for malignancy greatly increases risk at the same time that it often makes surgery the treatment of choice for removal of the cancerous cells. When the surgeon must partially or totally remove an organ because of cancer or another disease, the extent of risk depends upon the *importance of function* of the excised organ. For example, removal of the gallbladder is not so serious as removal of the stomach.

Location of the Disease

Operative risk depends upon the location of the disease and of the organ or organs requiring surgery. Surgical risk decreases in descending order in the following sites: heart, thorax, esophagus, brain, rectum, colon, stomach, lung.[36]

Duration of the Disease

The longer a patient has had a disease, the greater the surgical risk involved in correcting the disorder. Risk increases with chronicity because chronic diseases such as cancer tend to severely debilitate the patient, thereby lowering his resistance to stress and infection.

EXTENT OF THE SURGICAL PROCEDURE

Operative risk increases proportionately to the magnitude of the operation. Thus, the risk involved in minor surgery, e.g., a D and C (dilatation and curettage), is far less than in extensive major surgery such as colon resection. In major surgery, factors such as blood loss, tissue and organ trauma, and prolonged operating time all increase risk.

CALIBER OF THE PROFESSIONAL STAFF

Risk decreases for the surgical patient when the hospital staff is competent and well trained and when the hospital is well equipped and fully staffed. Even very sick patients with prolonged illnesses who are facing lengthy operations have a greater chance of survival among interested, highly knowledgeable physicians and nurses working efficiently in a fully equipped setting.

CHAPTER 29

Preparing the Patient for Surgery

In this chapter we shall discuss preparing patients for operations that are either required or elective and that have been scheduled by the surgeon a few days or weeks prior to the patient's hospital admission date. In the case of emergency surgery and certain urgent procedures, some of the preparation that we discuss in this chapter cannot be carried out fully owing to lack of time. However, it is the responsibility of the nurse and of the surgeon to prepare every patient *as fully as possible*, despite intervening circumstances, in order to decrease operative risk and to insure the patient's postoperative safety.

Generally, the specific preparation of a patient for a planned operation takes place during three time periods: (1) upon admission and during the day or days prior to the operation, (2) the night before surgery, and (3) on the morning or day of surgery.

PREPARING THE PATIENT PRIOR TO THE OPERATION

The preoperative patient may be admitted to the surgical floor the day before or several days prior to his surgery, depending upon the extent of preoperative treatment required. For example, alcoholic patients or cachectic patients suffering from cancer may be admitted a week or more before their scheduled operation in order to correct nutritional and fluid-electrolyte deficiencies.

When you admit a preoperative patient, your first duties will be to: (1) introduce yourself to the patient; (2) obtain his blood pressure, pulse, respiration, and temperature; (3) weigh the patient; (4) order laboratory tests as needed; and (5) briefly interview the patient in order to obtain essential information as well as to help him to feel secure and to enable him to ask questions that he may have. Questions that you will ask are:

> Has the patient had any serious illnesses or previous operations?

> What drugs is the patient currently taking and what drugs has he taken recently?

> Does the patient have any allergies or dietary restrictions?

> Is the patient experiencing any symptoms or discomforts at this time?

> Does the patient have any questions about the coming operation or what is going to be expected of him?

Following the preliminary admission procedure (including interview and charting), you will next consider in some detail the following aspects of preoperative care: psychologic, legal, physiologic, and instructional and preventive.

PSYCHOLOGIC ASPECTS

As we emphasized in the first chapter of this unit, all patients are somewhat fearful of surgery—some more so than others. The *extent* to which people are afraid of surgery depends upon their basic personalities, habitual reactions to stress over the years, general state of mental health, and the preconceptions that they have concerning surgery and anesthesia.

Typical fears harbored by preoperative patients center around postoperative pain, the discovery of cancer, the loss of organs that have special meaning for them, the hazard of death, anesthesia hazards, vulnerability while unconscious, saying "bad things" while under the anesthetic, the possibility of disfigurement and disability, and the problem of being separated from loved ones and former activities.

As you will recall from Unit III, patients react in many ways to fear. When facing an operation, patients may express their fears through a variety of behavior, e.g., by becoming silent and withdrawn, hopeless and helpless, childish, belligerent, evasive, tearful, or clinging. Almost all patients, regardless of diagnosis, regress to some degree when hospitalized and feel helpless when first admitted into the hospital environment.

What can you do to help the preoperative patient adjust to the hospital and overcome his fear of surgery? A few suggestions that you might try with the apprehensive preoperative patient are:

> Give the patient a booklet containing information about hospital routines, visiting hours, mealtimes, the location of the chapel, and so forth.

> Explain to the patient what to expect in the operating room and recovery room without introducing new fears or worries. If the doctor plans to transfer the patient to the intensive care unit following surgery, answer his questions concerning intensive care.

> Allow the *patient* to ask questions concerning his operation and the postoperative period; tell him only as much as he wishes to know. However, if the patient

is very withdrawn or aggressive, tactfully inquire into his fears and encourage him to express his concerns.

> Patients undergoing major procedures such as a mastectomy, laryngectomy, or colostomy may profit from being introduced to former patients who have successfully recovered from these operations. For example, you may wish to contact the local laryngectomy or colostomy club and arrange for a club member to visit the patient.

> Occupational therapy can be arranged for patients who are facing an extended preoperative period. Games, handicrafts, and television all serve to distract the patient and ease his fear and loneliness.

Handling a patient's fears in these ways can smooth his operative course. Studies show that the calm, emotionally prepared preoperative patient is better able to withstand the induction of anesthesia; he also experiences less postoperative vomiting and fewer postoperative complications.

LEGAL ASPECTS

Any patient undergoing a surgical procedure, however minor, *must* sign an operative permit. The operative permit guards the *patient* against submitting to operations that he does not know about or does not want; it also protects the *hospital staff* and the *surgeon* from legal action in which the patient or his family claim that an operation was performed without the patient's permission or knowledge.

> *Signed permission is needed for each procedure, however minor, if the surgeon plans to enter a body cavity.*

The patient should have a full explanation of the operation *before* he signs the permit; pictures and diagrams may be necessary. Moreover, the patient must be told about possible complications and disfigurements that may result from the surgery; he needs to know if any organs or parts of his body may be removed. In sum, the patient needs an honest and fair statement of what he faces both in surgery and following his operation.

Adults sign their own operative permits unless they are unconscious or mentally incompetent; in these instances a relative or guardian will sign the form. Children under 18 must be signed for by an adult, preferably a relative. If the child's family cannot be present to sign the permit, permission can be obtained from a parent by telephone, wire, or letter. When the minor's relatives cannot be located at all, the surgeon may sign the permit himself depending on the laws in his state, or he may need to obtain a court order to operate.

Once the permit has been signed, it becomes a permanent part of the chart. Make certain that the operative permit accompanies the patient's chart to the operating room.

PHYSIOLOGIC ASPECTS

As we emphasized in Chapter 28, the patient should be in as optimum a state of health as possible if surgical risk is to be kept to a minimum. Thus, the patient's past medical history will need to be explored carefully as well as any current medical problems. Prior to the date of surgery, the staff must make every effort to (1) correct dietary deficiencies if they exist; (2) reduce the obese patient's weight; (3) correct fluid and electrolyte imbalances; (4) restore an inadequate blood volume with blood transfusions; (5) treat any specific ailments, e.g., diabetes, heart disease, renal insufficiency; (6) halt or cure any infectious process; and (7) treat the alcoholic patient with intravenous infusions, vitamins, and proper fluids.

INSTRUCTIONAL AND PREVENTIVE ASPECTS

Patients need to be carefully instructed preoperatively concerning the proper way to cough, deep breathe, turn, and move their extremities during the postoperative period. Such instruction, given in sufficient detail and at the correct time, greatly reduces operative and postoperative complications.

The best *time* to instruct patients concerning their role in preventive techniques is relatively close to the time of the surgery, e.g., the afternoon or evening prior to their operation. If instruction is given several days in advance, the patient may forget the instructions; on the other hand, if the patient is taught preventive measures an hour or so before surgery, he may be too apprehensive to listen or too heavily sedated to comprehend.

Preoperative instruction must, first of all, include the practice of proper deep breathing and coughing maneuvers. These exercises are particularly valuable for patients over 50 years old, as well as for any patient experiencing shortness of breath, severe coughing, large amounts of mucus, and other respiratory problems.

The correct form of *breathing* for postoperative patients is *diaphragmatic-abdominal* breathing. You can instruct the patient in this technique as follows:[32]

> Ask the patient to lie on his back and flex his knees. (If it is impossible for the patient to lie flat on his back, he may be on his side.)

> Have the patient place his hand upon his mid-abdomen.

> Tell the patient to inhale through his nose until his upper abdomen balloons outward.

> Next have the patient exhale through his mouth by contracting his abdominal muscles and squeezing the air out.

> Inform the patient that he will need to breathe in this manner five to 10 times every hour during the postoperative period.

Coughing exercises can be given next. Tell the patient to inspire and expire several times. Then have him expire forcefully, and tell him to make an explosive sound as he lets the air out through his mouth. These breathing and coughing exercises will help to expand collapsed lungs and prevent postoperative pneumonia and atelectasis.

Finally, the patient will need to practice *turning* from side to side, using the siderails to help him in his movements. Turning will help to prevent respiratory problems. Finally, ask the patient to flex his hips, knees, and ankle joints and to move his foot in a circle. These last exercises will help to prevent circulatory problems such as thrombophlebitis and postoperative "gas pains" or flatus.

PREPARING THE PATIENT ON THE EVE OF SURGERY

Major considerations on the evening before surgery are: (1) preparing the patient's skin, (2) preparing his gastrointestinal tract, (3) preparing for anesthesia, and (4) promoting rest and sleep.

PREPARING THE PATIENT'S SKIN

The object of a thorough bath and a skin "prep" of the operative area is to reduce to a minimum the bacteria on the patient's skin. Such preparation reduces the number of bacteria that will be carried into the deeper tissues from the skin when the surgeon makes the incision with a sterile scalpel.

"Prep" procedures are done by different staff members in different hospitals. Some institutions have a prep orderly or prep nurse who does all the skin preparation of preoperative patients. In other hospitals, the nurse in charge of the preoperative patient does the prep for patients assigned to her the evening prior to their surgeries.

The actual prep procedure also differs according to specific hospital's policy. In most institutions an antiseptic soap is used to gently scrub the skin. This type of soap may be applied to the operative site repeatedly several days before surgery; it may also be left on the skin for five to 10 minutes following application. These soaps are valuable in that their repeated use leads to a substantial reduction in the number of bacteria on the skin.

Some surgeons recommend preparing the skin with benzalkonium chloride solution (Zephiran Chloride). When using Zephiran Chloride, remember not to soap the skin prior to use, as soap causes Zephiran to precipitate and thereby reduces its effectiveness.

No matter which cleansing agents or what prep procedure you use, you will find the following principles useful:

> The areas of the prep should always be wider and longer than the area of the proposed incision, because the surgeon may unexpectedly need to make a larger incision.

> Use a strong light, well focused, and a sterile safety razor with a new blade.

> Shave *against* the grain of the hair shaft to insure a clean, close shave.

> While doing the prep, check the skin for nicks, irritations, and cuts; all these are potential sites for infection. Chart the presence of these.

In some hospitals a *depilatory* cream is used instead of the customary "shave." Depilatory cream is a chemical compound that is applied to the surgical site, left on for 10 minutes, and then removed along with the hair. Some transient rashes occasionally result from the use of depilatory cream.

PREPARING THE GASTROINTESTINAL TRACT

The patient's gastrointestinal tract needs special preparation on the evening before surgery to: (1) reduce the possibility of vomiting and aspiration during anesthesia, and (2) prevent contamination from fecal material during intestinal tract or bowel surgery.

Preparation of the gastrointestinal tract involves: food and fluid restriction, the administration of enemas, and sometimes the insertion of a gastric or intestinal tube.

The *restriction of foods and oral fluids* is essential to prevent vomiting during surgery, the aspiration of any vomitus, and the resultant development of aspiration pneumonia. Because solid food must be withheld seven to 10 hours before the operation, most patients receive nothing by mouth (NPO) after midnight; however, water can usually be given up to four hours before surgery, depending upon the hospital policy. When surgery is not scheduled until late afternoon, the patient may eat a light breakfast in the morning.

When a patient is NPO, the staff usually (1) tells the patient he is not to eat or drink and why; (2) removes food and water from the patient's bedside stand; (3) places a "NPO" sign on the door and on the bed; (4) marks the patient's Kardex "NPO," (5) informs the diet kitchen that the patient is awaiting surgery, and (6) informs the oncoming staff that the patient is to receive nothing by mouth. Patients who are extremely debilitated or malnourished may receive intravenous infusions of glucose, amino acids, or plasma up to the moment of surgery.

Enemas are not routinely ordered preoperatively in most hospitals because enemas are upsetting both psychologically and physiologically. However, two or three enemas are generally given the evening prior to operations on the *intestinal tract* or *colon* in order to prevent contamination of the peritoneal cavity from the spillage of fecal matter during surgery. In some cases the surgeon may order laxatives and enemas to be given over two to three days before the patient undergoes colonic surgery.

Tubes for gastric or intestinal suction are sometimes inserted the evening before or the morning of surgery in order to remove gastric or intestinal contents. This procedure is usually performed on patients about to undergo major abdominal surgery or intestinal tract surgery.*

PREPARING FOR ANESTHESIA

The anesthesiologist usually visits the preoperative patient the evening before his surgery. During his visit, he generally examines the patient for evidence of pulmonary problems or upper respiratory infections, and he investigates the patient's smoking habits. Usually he discusses with the patient the type of anesthetic he plans to use, the sensations the patient will experience as he undergoes anesthesia, and any fears the patient has concerning anesthesia.

At times patients are reluctant to disclose their anxieties to the anesthesiologist but may feel comfortable in talking about them with the nurse. The nurse can then tell the anesthesiologist what the patient's anxieties appear to be, and ask him to explore these areas further. As we have emphasized, a calm confident patient undergoes the induction of anesthesia more smoothly than the nervous frightened individual.

PROMOTING REST AND SLEEP

The preoperative patient will rest more completely on the night before surgery if he is physically comfortable, mentally at ease, and adequately sedated. He will sleep better in a freshly made bed and in a well ventilated room. In preparing the patient for rest, give him a soothing backrub, and perhaps a glass of warm milk or weak tea, if fluids are not contraindicated. Talk with the patient as you care for him, and allow him to speak openly about any last moment doubts or fears that he may have concerning his surgery. Try to express a positive attitude toward the surgery.

On the night before surgery, the surgeon will undoubtedly leave an order for a sleeping medication. Two commonly used sleep medications are:

>Pentobarbital sodium (Nembutal Sodium) 50–100 mg. orally.

> Secobarbital sodium (Seconal Sodium) 50–100 mg. orally.

*The insertion of gastric and intestinal tubes is discussed in Unit XV on gastrointestinal tract disease.

Encourage patients (especially apprehensive persons) to take their h.s. medications so that they will have a good night's sleep to start the operative day.

PREPARING THE PATIENT ON THE DAY OF SURGERY

EARLY MORNING CARE

On the morning of surgery, the nurse usually awakens the patient about an hour before he is scheduled to receive his preoperative medications. During that time period, the nurse performs the following general tasks:

> Records the patient's *blood pressure* upon awakening so that the anesthesiologist and recovery room personnel will have a baseline blood pressure reading against which to compare later readings.

> Records the patient's *temperature, pulse,* and *respiration.*

Report to the surgeon any elevation of temperature, because surgery may need to be cancelled due to infection.

> Checks to make certain that the skin prep has been completed in a thorough manner.

> Asks the patient to void and then measures and records the amount of urine.

> Gives the patient *oral hygiene* and removes any dentures or removable bridge work. (Be certain to store these valuable items according to hospital procedure.)

> Removes and stores the patient's *jewelry.* Usually patients are allowed to wear their wedding rings, which are either tied on or taped on.

> Dresses the patient in a clean gown and perhaps leggings. Covers the patient's head. If the patient has very long hair, braids the hair into two braids.

> *Removes colored nail polish,* because the operating room personnel frequently check the patient's nail beds for cyanosis.

> *Questions the patient* to make certain that he has neither eaten for the last 10 hours nor drunk fluids during the preceding four hours.

> *Carries out any special orders* for the administration of enemas, insertion of a Levin tube, or the starting of an intravenous infusion.

> *Checks the patient's identification band* for accuracy and to make certain that it is secure.

Following these procedures, the patient is finally given his *preoperative medications* (see below).

To prevent errors or omissions in the performance of these many preoperation tasks, most hospitals supply nurses with a checklist somewhat like that shown below. As each task is completed, it is checked off.

Preoperative Check List

Patient's Name
Jane Doe

Room Number
206

Date
Jan. 1, 1974

✓ 1 Vital signs (record below):
BP 120/80; Pulse 80; Respiration 20; Temperature 98.6°.
✓ 2 Skin prep completed.
✓ 3 Operative permit signed.
✓ 4 Voided. Time: 6:30 A.M. Amount 200 ml.
✓ 5 Valuables removed and stored.
✓ 6 Rings taped.
✓ 7 Nail polish removed.
✓ 8 Dentures removed and stored.
✓ 9 NPO for last 10 hours (or for length of time designated by hospital policy).
___ 10 Enemas given. Results: None ordered.
✓ 11 Other procedures: Levin tube inserted and clamped.
✓ 12 Identification band present.
✓ 13 Contact lenses removed.
✓ 14 Preoperative medications:

Medications ordered and *times given:*
6:45 A.M. Nembutal 100 mg. IM
7:15 A.M. Demerol 100 mg. IM
Atropine sulfate 0.4 mg. IM

THE PREOPERATIVE MEDICATIONS

Preoperative medications are given to allay anxiety, decrease the flow of pharyngeal secretions, reduce the amount of anesthesia to be given, and create amnesia for the events that precede surgery. The four major types of preoperative medications are: sedatives, tranquilizers, analgesics, and vagolytic and drying agents.

Sedatives are given to decrease the patient's anxiety, to lower his blood pressure and pulse, and to reduce the amount of general anesthetic to be given in surgery. Examples of preoperative sedatives are:

> Pentobarbital sodium (Nembutal Sodium) 100 mg. IM 90 minutes before surgery.
> Secobarbital sodium (Seconal Sodium) 100 mg. IM 90 minutes before surgery.

An overdose of any sedative can lead to respiratory depression.

Tranquilizers are useful drugs for lowering a patient's anxiety level. Examples of tranquilizers that are given preoperatively are:

> Thorazine 12.5 to 25 mg. IM 1 to 2 hours before surgery.
> Phenergan 12.5 to 25 mg. IM 1 to 2 hours before surgery.

Tranquilizers can cause a dangerous hypotension both during and after surgery. Nevertheless, one geriatrics specialist recommends using tranquilizers as a premedication for elderly patients in place of opiates. He points out that while tranquilizers cause hypotension, opiates can lead to severe respiratory depression in older patients—a potentially more dangerous situation.

Analgesics are given preoperatively to relax the patient and to decrease anxiety; they are not necessarily given to relieve pain. Typical preoperative analgesic agents are:

> Morphine sulfate 8 to 15 mg. SQ 1 hour preoperatively.
> Demerol 50 to 100 mg. IM 1 hour preoperatively.

Narcotic analgesics such as these are dangerous drugs because of their tendency to cause vomiting and respiratory depression. Thus, some surgeons do not use analgesics preoperatively unless the patient is in pain; instead, they order barbiturates and tranquilizers to relax the patient.

Vagolytic and drying agents are given for the following reasons: (1) to reduce the amount of *tracheobronchial secretions,* which can clog the pulmonary tree and result in pneumonia and atelectasis; and (2) to *interrupt vagal nerve impulses,* which act to slow the heart. Tracheobronchial secretions increase during surgery because the mucus-secreting cells of the pharynx, larynx, and tracheobronchial tree are irritated by the anesthesia, whereas vagal impulses are stimulated by procedures such as intubation during surgery.

Typical vagolytic and drying agents are:

> Atropine sulfate 0.3 to 0.6 mg. IM given about 45 minutes before surgery.

Atropine sulfate, an anticholinergic drug, is given to inhibit parasympathetic stimulation when parasympathetic anesthetic agents such as halothane and cyclopropane are used. Without the vagal block produced by atropine, the parasympathetic stimulation caused by the above anesthetic agents can result in cardiac arrest. Also, atropine sulfate reduces tracheobronchial secretions and dries the mucous membranes. An overdose of atropine sulfate can cause severe tachycardia.

> Scopolamine (Hyoscine) 0.3 to 0.6 mg. SQ 45 minutes before surgery.

Along with drying the mucous membranes, scopolamine causes sedation, amnesia, and euphoria. Unfortunately scopolamine can cause confusion, restlessness, and even hallucinations, especially in the elderly. Elderly patients should be given a smaller than usual dose. Overdoses of scopolamine can result in severe respiratory depression, which may have to be treated by means of prolonged artificial respiration.

When you administer preoperative medications, be certain to give the correct drug in the correct dosage by the correct method at precisely the time ordered. If preoperative medications are administered too early or too late, the induction of anesthesia may be more difficult. Before giving the medication, note whether the blood pressure has been taken and recorded. If the blood pressure has not been taken, obtain a reading *before* giving the medication.

After administering the preoperative medication, put the bed siderails up, lower the shades, turn off bright lights, and tell the patient not to try to get up. Once the patient has slipped into a peaceful, drowsy state, speak to him only when necessary and then briefly and quietly.

Sometimes preoperative medications are not given according to a prepared schedule, but instead are administered "on call" just before the patient goes to surgery. Medications are usually given in this manner when the surgery schedule is tentative or is irregular. Some surgeons question whether preoperative medications given "on call" are of any value. Certainly it is a practice to be avoided whenever possible.

TRANSPORTING THE PATIENT TO SURGERY

When the surgical personnel call for the patient to be transported to surgery, you as a floor nurse must carry out a number of tasks. First you must check the patient's chart for the following:

✓ 1 The operative permit is present and signed.
✓ 2 Blood and urine studies have been completed and are on the chart.
✓ 3 Vital signs are recorded.
✓ 4 The disposition of valuables and dentures is recorded.
✓ 5 Preoperative medications are charted, including dosage, time given, and patient's reaction.
✓ 6 Any significant observations of the patient have been noted.

Next, the sedated patient should be gently moved to a stretcher, covered with blankets to protect him from drafts, and secured with a restraining belt. His chart will accompany him to the operating room. The person responsible for wheeling the patient to surgery should be cautioned not to "swing" the cart roughly or walk too rapidly, as this type of movement can cause nausea and dizziness.

After the patient has left the floor, you will need to prepare the patient's room for his return, especially if the hospital does not have a recovery room. Setting up the patient's room for postoperative care includes:

> Arranging furniture so the stretcher can easily be brought to the bedside.
> Making a surgical bed.
> Setting out an emesis basin in event of vomiting.
> Bringing in additional equipment such as blood pressure equipment, IV standards, and a suction machine.
> Checking all equipment to make certain it is in working condition.

THE PATIENT'S FAMILY

During surgery the patient's relatives usually wait in a waiting room or in the hospital lobby. If the patient's family must leave the hospital for any reason, ask them for a phone number where they can be reached; also give them the phone number of the hospital and the extension of the surgical floor.

It is always considerate to spend some time talking with the patient's family about what they may see when they visit their relative in the recovery room or intensive care unit or when he returns to his room. They should be prepared for the sight of tubes, intravenous infusions, oxygen, and so forth.

In talking with the family, it is best to keep the conversation centered rather generally upon postoperative care and the recovery room rather than commenting specifically about the patient's operation and its possible outcome. You cannot know the exact outcome of an operation any more than can the family or even the surgeon. You can only encourage the family to maintain a positive outlook while they wait to speak to the surgeon following the operation. Inform the family when you receive word that the surgery is completed, and make certain that the doctor receives word in surgery that the family is waiting to see him.

CHAPTER 30

The Patient in Surgery

ADMITTING THE PATIENT TO SURGERY

When the preoperative patient leaves the surgical floor and is wheeled to the operating room he is transferred to the care of the surgical team, a group of highly trained individuals who must work together as a coordinated team for the welfare and safety of the patient.

THE SURGICAL TEAM

The surgical team is composed of the surgeon, his assistants, the anesthesiologist, the scrub nurse, and the circulating nurse (Fig. 30–1).

The *surgeon* heads the surgical team and carries, along with the anesthesiologist, the major responsibility for the patient's life and welfare. It is the surgeon who must make the major decisions as to the course of the surgery, e.g., whether to remove an organ, amputate a limb, or make radical or extensive repairs. The surgeon must be constantly alert to the changing physiologic needs of the patient as the patient strives to adjust to the stress of surgery.

The *assistants* to the surgeon are other surgeons or surgical residents who plan to make surgery their career. These doctors expose the operative site by retracting tissues away from the site and by sponging and suctioning blood and serum obscuring the surgeon's vision of the site.

The *anesthesiologist* anesthetizes the patient in order to alleviate pain and induce relaxation. In addition to this major task, the anesthesiologist must: maintain the patient's airway; ensure the patient an adequate O_2–CO_2 exchange; infuse blood, fluids, and drugs as necessary; monitor the patient's circulation and respiration; and alert the surgeon immediately in the event of complications. The anesthesiologist carries a heavy responsibility, for it is his role to maintain the pa-

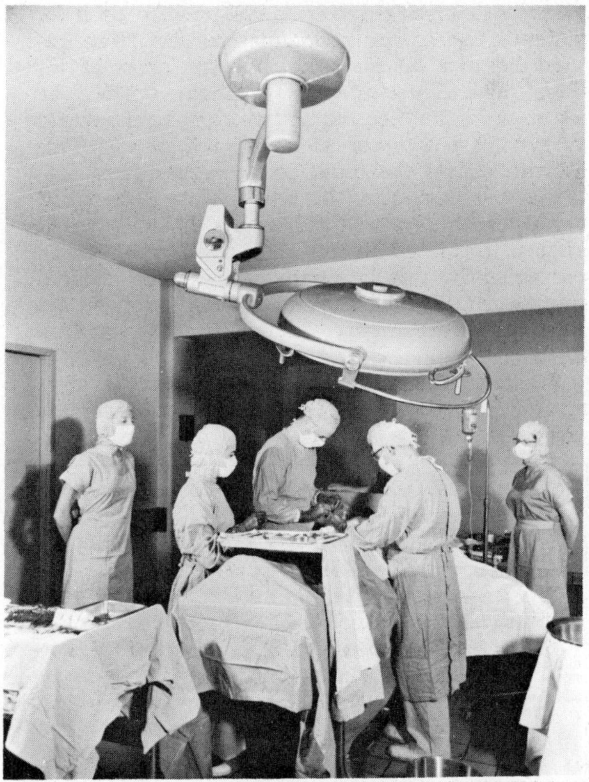

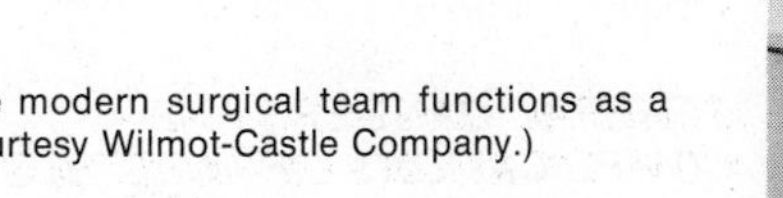

FIGURE 30–1. The modern surgical team functions as a coordinated unit. (Courtesy Wilmot-Castle Company.)

tient safely in a state that lies somewhere between deep sleep and death.

The *scrub nurse* stands beside the surgeon throughout the operation and supplies him with instruments, sutures, sterile towels, sponges, and so forth. She is called a "scrub" nurse because she scrubs her arms and hands before donning her sterile gown and gloves and handling sterile equipment. The surgeon and surgical assistants also scrub; the anesthesiologist does not.

The circulating nurse does not "scrub in" or wear sterile gowns or gloves. She is the manager of the operating room—a taxing job indeed! The circulating nurse must make certain that all equipment is working properly before the surgery, must prepare and autoclave instruments for the surgery, alert team members of any breaks in sterile technique, label specimens, and contact the x-ray and pathology departments at the surgeon's request. Her job is to keep the operating room running smoothly and safely as she "circulates" around the operating suite bringing needed supplies and drugs to the table and taking away unneeded items or specimens.

POSITIONING THE SURGICAL PATIENT

The position of the patient upon the operating table will vary with the surgery. For example, the *dorsal recumbent position* is customarily used for patients undergoing abdominal surgery. The patient lies flat on his back with his arms at his sides. The *Trendelenburg* position, with head lower than the feet, is the position of choice for surgery of the lower abdomen and pelvis. This position causes the intestines to be displaced into the upper abdomen. In the *lithotomy* position, the patient's legs and thighs are flexed to right angles, exposing the perineal and rectal areas; consequently this position is used for vaginal repairs and D and C's. Various other positions are used for neurosurgery, kidney surgery, and so forth.

Whatever the patient's position upon the operating table, there are certain rules of safety to observe:

> *When positioning a patient on the operating table,* remember:
>
> 1. *Strap the patient to the table with straps that are* well padded.
> 2. *Do not strap the patient so tightly that circulation is impaired.*
> 3. *Do not allow the patient's arms or legs to dangle over the sides of the table.*
> 4. *Pad all bony prominences (e.g., the elbow, ankle, knee) to prevent nerve and tissue damage.*

Remember that the patient will remain immobile in one position for a long period of time, in some cases for hours! Even with careful positioning, most patients are stiff and sore postoperatively if they must spend a prolonged period on the operating table.

Following positioning, the patient is next prepped by the circulating nurse, draped by the scrub nurse, and anesthetized by the anesthesiologist.

Because all surgical patients regardless of diagnosis and type of surgery undergo anesthesia, we shall discuss in some detail the purpose of anesthesia, the types of anesthesia, and the dangers and complications of anesthesia.

ANESTHESIA

The anesthetized state is easy but dangerous to induce. In man's more primitive past, a blow on the head or a heavy draft of liquor sufficed; today we have many new and sophisticated means. However, despite improvements, anesthesia remains difficult to control and regulate precisely. As one authority observes:

> It [the anesthetized state] must be considered as a comatose state produced by severe drug poisoning during which the patient is subjected to trauma, hemorrhage, starvation, and other abnormal conditions.[20]

If the anesthetized state is so filled with dangers, what then are its benefits and what, more precisely, are its complications?

THE BENEFITS OF ANESTHESIA

Anesthetics are given primarily to completely eradicate the pain of surgery during the operative period. They are also given to relieve fear and anxiety and to relax tissues. Because of new and sophisticated types and methods of anesthesia, even severely ill heart and kidney patients can be now operated upon and be expected to survive the operation.

GENERAL DANGERS AND COMPLICATIONS OF ANESTHESIA

The major complications of anesthesia affect the circulatory and respiratory systems, although all physiologic functions are somewhat disturbed or suppressed by anesthesia. Specifically, the major dangers of anesthesia are:[20]

Cardiac Arrest. Certain anesthetics result in the retention of carbon dioxide which, in turn, leads to anoxia, CO_2 narcosis, respiratory acidosis, and cardiac arrest.*

*CO_2 narcosis and respiratory acidosis were discussed in Unit V, Chapter 25.

Respiratory Depression. Respiratory complications due to anesthesia usually result from one of the following problems:

1. *Excess mucus* may be produced as a result of irritation of the respiratory passages by the anesthetic agent. The excess mucus, in turn, causes airway obstruction, anoxia, and respiratory failure.
2. *Central nervous system depression* due to the use of depressant drugs may lead to hypoxia, anoxia, and respiratory failure.
3. Peripheral *neuromuscular conduction* may be disturbed owing to the use of muscle relaxants such as curare. Drugs such as curare and anectine interrupt the transmission of nervous impulses from nerves to muscles. When the respiratory muscles are affected, respiratory depression results.

Bronchospasm and Laryngospasm. Bronchial and laryngeal mucosa may go into severe spasm, producing a deadly airway obstruction. Both bronchospasm and laryngospasm can result from the irritating effects of anesthetics on the bronchial or laryngeal mucosa or from an allergic reaction to the anesthetic. These complications can be prevented by the insertion of an endotracheal tube (see Unit XXII).

Diminished Circulation. The circulation may be impaired and diminished, mainly because of the following three problems:

1. The *venous system may fail* in its job of returning blood to the heart to be pumped out to the arterial system. Evidently certain anesthetic agents interfere with autonomic nervous system control of the vein walls; the walls become dilated, and blood, which should be returning to the heart, pools within the relaxed veins. Thus, circulation to the heart and tissues decreases.
2. The *contractility of cardiac muscle* may diminish owing to anesthetic agents, and this, in turn, decreases cardiac output.
3. Blood, which is already diminished in amount, may be *poorly distributed* throughout the body, so that it fails to reach vital organs such as the kidney, liver, and heart in sufficient amounts. Anesthesia can upset the delicate mechanisms that control blood distribution and guarantee an adequate circulation to vital organs.

Hypotension and Shock. Preoperative medications, powerful anesthetics, and blood loss can all lead to surgical shock during the operation. In addition, the use of anesthetics lowers the body's adaptive responses to shock, thereby compounding the problem.

Loss of Protective Responses to Pain. When a person is properly anesthetized, he cannot feel pain and thus he fails to respond normally to pain. Because this defensive reaction is lost, patients may be accidentally injured during surgery. For example, they may be burned from a cauterizing instrument, may suffer circulatory impairment from being too tightly strapped to the operating table, and may undergo nerve trauma or paralysis as a result of improper or careless positioning during the operation.

Vomiting and Aspiration. Vomiting and aspiration of vomitus into the respiratory tract sometimes occurs during the second or excitement stage of anesthesia induction (see p. 000) as a result of reflex stimulation of the patient's vomiting center. Also, patients admitted for emergency surgery may have a full stomach and will vomit and aspirate unless an endotracheal tube is inserted prior to the induction of anesthesia.

While the respiratory and circulatory systems are most vulnerable to complications from anesthesia, all systems of the body are disturbed. Gastrointestinal motility and renal function decrease and may fail entirely; metabolic activities are slowed and become disturbed; and often dangerous neurologic changes occur. For example, elderly persons may suffer from a cerebral vascular accident (CVA) due to the spasmotic effects of certain anesthetic agents upon the sclerotic, partially occluded arteries that are commonly found in geriatric patients. In other cases, anoxia due to airway obstruction may lead to convulsions.

The complications listed above are most likely to occur during the *induction* of the anesthesia. At this critical time, overdoses of the gas or drug can result in severe respiratory and circulatory problems.

TYPES OF ANESTHESIA

There are two major classifications of anesthesia: general and regional. *General* anesthesia produces total unconsciousness and affects the entire organism. *Regional* anesthesia, on the other hand, produces a loss of painful sensation in one region of the body only and does not result in unconsciousness. Table 30-1 compares the purpose, method of administration, advantages and disadvantages of these two major types of anesthesia.

Types of General Anesthesia

As is pointed out in Table 30-1, anesthesia can generally be administered via three methods: (1) by inhalation, (2) intravenously, and (3) rectally.

Inhalation Anesthesia. This type of anesthesia is administered by giving the patient gases or liquids in volatilized form which he inhales through a mask or endotracheal tube directly into his lungs. Inhalation anesthesia is the standard anesthesia used in most major surgeries involving the upper abdomen, head, neck, and thorax. The *advantages* of inhalation anesthesia are the prevention of pain, the relaxation of tissues, and the alleviation of anxiety through producing a state of total unconsciousness. The major *disadvantages* of this type of anesthesia are circulatory and respiratory depression. Also, certain of the gases and liquids used in inhalation anesthesia are highly *flammable* and *explosive* when they are mixed with air or oxygen, e.g., cyclopropane, ether, and ethylene.

When flammable and explosive anesthetic agents are being used, observe the following rules:

> Remember:
> 1. *Do not wear slips or uniforms of nylon or rayon and do not use wool blankets; these materials can set off a static spark.*
> 2. *Do not allow smoking in the vicinity of the operating room.*
> 3. *Do not allow the use of electrocautery.*
> 4. *Do not touch the patient in the vicinity of his breathing mask as it may cause an electric spark.*
> 5. *Do not allow the patient to smoke for 12 hours postoperatively or his visitors to smoke for six hours postoperatively.*

The major methods for administering inhalation anesthesia are: the open drop method, by mask, and by endotracheal tube. When the *open drop* method is used, the anesthetic liquid is dropped directly onto the layers of gauze or onto an absorbent face mask that is held over the patient's mouth and nose. When a *mask* is used, the gases generally flow into the mask via a tube from a supply tank where the gases are held under pressure. Finally, when an *endotracheal tube* is employed, the gases flow from a supply tank directly into the patient's tracheobronchial tree.

The induction of inhalation anesthesia takes place in four distinct stages: Stage I—the beginning of induction; State II—loss of consciousness; Stage III—surgical anesthesia and relaxation; and Stage IV—the danger stage. These stages and appropriate nursing actions are described in Table 30–2.

There are many different liquids and gases used in inhalation anesthesia. Two of the most commonly used *volatile liquid* anesthetics are ethyl ether and halothane (Fluothane); two com-

TABLE 30–1. TYPES OF ANESTHESIA COMPARED

General Anesthesia	Regional Anesthesia
1. *Purpose:* To cause total loss of sensation and complete loss of consciousness by blocking the "awareness centers" within the brain.	1. *Purpose:* To reduce all painful sensation in one region of the body without inducing unconsciousness. Produced by blocking sensory impulses to the brain.
2. *Methods* employed: a. Inhalation of gases or vaporous liquids. b. Intravenous infusion of anesthetic agent. c. Rectal induction of agent.	2. *Methods* employed: a. Topical anesthesia. b. Local block. c. Nerve block. d. Spinal anesthesia. e. Saddle block. f. Epidural block. g. Caudal block.
3. *Advantages:* a. *Flexibility:* General anesthesia can be used and modified for any type of surgery, and for any patient despite his age or physical condition. b. *Adequate time factor:* Can be employed during lengthy procedures with maximum comfort for the patient. c. *Better monitoring:* When caring for an extremely anxious patient, the anesthesiologist is often able to better control respiratory and circulatory functions when the patient is unconscious rather than awake and fearful.	3. *Advantages:* a. *Better airway control.* The patient who is awake is better able to maintain his own airway and to control mucous secretions and vomitus should vomiting occur. b. *Fewer respiratory complications:* Because patient is awake, he is able to cough and breathe normally, which prevents a dangerous pooling of mucus in the bronchi.
4. *Disadvantages:* a. *Respiratory and circulatory depression:* Most anesthesia deaths result from such depressions of function. b. *Explosion hazards:* Explosions occur infrequently with the use of inhalation anesthesia.	4. *Disadvantages:* a. Anxiety and fear are not allayed. Patient continues to see and hear throughout operation. b. *Lack of flexibility:* Difficult to use with small children, elderly senile persons, and uncooperative persons. c. *Short time period:* Generally cannot be used for lengthy operations. d. Drugs employed can cause systemic depression. e. *"False security":* It is incorrectly believed that regional anesthesia will not cause respiratory or circulatory problems.

monly used *gas* anesthetics are nitrous oxide and cyclopropane. These specific agents—their advantages and disadvantages—are presented diagrammatically in Table 30–3.

Other important anesthetic gases and liquids are:

> *Vinyl ether (Vinethene):* An explosive anesthetic agent used mainly in brief operations in which both rapid induction and rapid recovery are required.
> *Trichloroethylene* (Trilene): A noninflammable, rapid-acting anesthetic commonly employed in obstetrics.
> *Ether:* An explosive anesthetic producing deep and prolonged anesthesia. Ether rarely produces cardiovascular complications and, consequently, is sometimes used for high risk patients.

Intravenous Anesthesia. When general anesthesia is administered intravenously the patient experiences a simple, pleasant, and extremely *rapid* induction; unconsciousness generally occurs only 30 seconds following the initial IV administration of the anesthetic agent. Intravenous anesthesia is sometimes given to relax a patient *prior* to the administration of the more powerful (*and* more harmful) inhalation anesthetic agents. However, intravenous anesthesia is sufficiently potent to be used alone in such minor procedures as dental extractions and pelvic examinations.

The major *advantages* of IV anesthesia are: (1) rapid pleasant induction; (2) absence of explosive hazards; and (3) a low incidence of postoperative nausea and vomiting. Major *dangers* are: (1) *laryngospasm* and *bronchospasm,* owing to excitement of laryngeal reflexes by the drug, (2) *hypotension,* owing to depression of the vasomotor center in the brain, and (3) *respiratory arrest,* owing to drug overdosage, which may also result in cardiac arrest. Be prepared for the above complications of intravenous anesthesia by having on hand: oxygen; an endotracheal tube; emergency drugs to stimulate the heart and respirations; and vasopressor drugs to counteract hypotension and shock should they occur.

> *Thiopental sodium* (Pentothal Sodium) is the most commonly used intravenous anesthetic.
> Pentobarbital sodium (Nembutal Sodium) and secobarbital sodium (Seconal Sodium) are two other drugs that are sometimes employed.

TABLE 30–2. FOUR STAGES OF ANESTHESIA*

	From	To	Patient Status	Nurse Should
STAGE I	Beginning administration of gas or drug	Loss of consciousness	May appear inebriated, drowsy, dizzy	Close OR doors; keep room quiet; stand by patient to assist, if necessary
STAGE II	Loss of consciousness	Relaxation	May appear excited; may breathe irregularly; may move arms and legs or body; patient very susceptible to external stimuli (noise, being touched suddenly)	Be ready to restrain patient if needed; remain at patient's side, quiet and alert; assist anesthesiologist, if needed
STAGE III	(Surgical anesthesia stage) relaxation	Loss of reflexes; depression of vital functions	Regular respiration, contracted pupils, eyelid reflexes disappear, jaw relaxed; auditory sensation lost during this stage	Begin prep only when anesthesiologist indicates Stage III has been reached and patient is under good control
STAGE IV	(Danger stage) vital functions too depressed	Respiratory failure; possible cardiac arrest	Not breathing; little or no heartbeat or pulse	If arrest occurs, react immediately to assist in establishing airway; provide cardiac arrest tray, drugs, syringes, long needles; assist surgeon with closed or open cardiac massage

*Nursing Care of the Patient in the O.R. Ethicon Division, Inc., Somerville, N. J.

Rectal Anesthesia. This form of general anesthesia is given via a rectal tube and is sometimes used for very minor procedures such as a pelvic examination. Rectal anesthesia does not produce complete unconsciousness and, therefore, it must always be supplemented by other types of anesthesia for more extensive procedures. The *advantages* of rectal anesthesia are: (1) fairly rapid induction (usually within 5 minutes); (2) reduction of preoperative anxiety; and (3) ease of administration. Rectal anesthesia can be given in the patient's room following a cleansing enema. *Disadvantages* and complications of rectal anesthesia are: (1) respiratory rate and depth are decreased; (2) mild hypotension is produced; and (3) central hepatic necrosis can result from the use of tribromoethanol (Avertin).

Two typical rectal anesthetic agents are:

> *Avertin;* this drug can cause respiratory depression, hypotension, and liver damage.

Avertin should not be administered to patients with known liver or kidney disease or to very elderly persons.

> *Thiopenthal Sodium;* this drug may cause respiratory depression and hypotension.

Whenever Avertin or thiopenthal is being administered to a patient on the ward, remember the following rules:

1. Watch for respiratory depression and have respiratory stimulants and oxygen on hand.
2. Check the patient's blood pressure every 10 to 15 minutes and report serious deviations from normal.
3. Do not leave the patient unattended.

Types of Regional Anesthesia

As shown in Table 30–1, regional anesthesia is used to anesthetize one region of the body only. When regional anesthesia is being administered, the anesthetic agent is deposited either upon the surface to be anesthetized or upon a particular nerve or nerve pathway that lies between the area to be incised and operated upon and receptors of painful stimuli located within the central nervous system. This procedure, then, blocks the transmission of painful stimuli to the brain.

Types of regional anesthesia are: (1) topical anesthesia; (2) local block; (3) field block; (4) nerve block; (5) spinal anesthesia; (6) saddle block; (7) epidural block; and (8) caudal anesthesia.

The major differences between these various types of regional anesthesia are the *rate* at which the anesthetic agent diffuses from the site of application or injection, and the *size* of the re-

TABLE 30–3. SOME AGENTS USED TO PRODUCE ANESTHESIA BY INHALATION; THEIR ADVANTAGES AND DISADVANTAGES

Volatile Liquid Anesthetics		Gas Anesthetics	
Ethyl Ether	*Halothane*	*Nitrous Oxide*	*Cyclopropane*
		Advantages	
1. Safe 2. Relatively nontoxic 3. Good relaxant	1. Nonexplosive 2. Rapid induction and rapid recovery 3. Highly potent 4. Nonirritating to respiratory and GI tracts	1. Noninflammable 2. Nonexplosive 3. Relatively nontoxic 4. Rapid induction and rapid recovery 5. Of special value in dental extractions and obstetrics	1. Potent 2. Relatively nontoxic 3. Rapid, pleasant induction and recovery 4. Of special value in major surgery of chest and abdomen
		Disadvantages	
1. Irritates eyes, skin, kidneys 2. Causes postoperative nausea and vomiting 3. Causes increased secretions in respiratory tract	1. Complications of hypotension and cardiac arrest occur *rapidly*	1. Can cause hallucinations and dreams 2. Weak anesthetic 3. Must be used in conjunction with another anesthetic or a barbiturate for adequate anesthesia	1. Highly flammable 2. Highly explosive 3. Powerful respiratory depressant 4. Can cause cardiac arrest and laryngospasm 5. No analgesic effect 6. Patient is restless and noisy
		Caution	
1. Avoid in presence of severe respiratory disease	1. Have cardiac resuscitation equipment on hand and working		1. Have available cardiac resuscitation equipment 2. Observe explosion precautions

gion that is anesthetized. Topical and local anesthesia block only peripheral nerves around the area of the incision; field anesthesia blocks the area *around* the incision; spinal anesthesia, saddle block, epidural blocks, and caudal anesthesia all block areas that are even further removed from the operative site.[2]

Topical Anesthesia. When an anesthetizing drug is sprayed or dropped onto an area to be desensitized, topical anesthesia is achieved. This short-acting form of anesthesia can block peripheral nerve endings in the skin as well as those in the mucous membranes of the vagina, rectum, nasopharynx, and mouth. Topical anesthesia is employed in minor procedures, e.g., rectal examinations when painful hemorrhoids are present, or to desensitize the bronchi prior to a bronchoscopic examination. *Advantages* of topical anesthesia are: (1) speed of action, and (2) general nontoxicity. *Disadvantages* are that the patient's tissues are not relaxed nor is his anxiety reduced. An unusual complication of topical anesthesia is an anaphylactic reaction resulting from prior sensitization to the drug. One drug commonly used for topical anesthesia is:

> *Cocaine* in a 4 to 10 per cent solution. This drug is for topical use *only,* and is mainly used to anesthetize the eye and the mucous membranes of the nose, mouth, and urethra. Cocaine is a highly poisonous drug if it enters the circulatory system. If accidentally injected, cocaine may cause severe excitement followed by shock, respiratory failure, and cardiac arrest. Oxygen and artificial respiration will be required to save the patient's life in event of such a severe reaction.

Other drugs used for topical anesthesia are butacaine, Pontocaine, and lidocaine (Xylocaine).

Local Block. In contrast to topical or surface application of an anesthetic agent, local anesthesia is dependent upon the *injection* of an anesthetic agent such as procaine by needle and syringe into the skin and subcutaneous tissues of the area to be incised. As a result of local anesthesia, only the peripheral nerves around the area of the incision are blocked. Local blocks are used in short minor operations and prior to the administration of spinal anesthesia.

When a local anesthetic is administered, it is important that the doctor not allow the needle to slip into one of the patient's veins. If a local anesthetic agent is accidentally given intravenously, dangerous *anaphylactic shock* may result. For this reason, the doctor should always withdraw the plunger of the syringe before injection to make certain that the needle is not in a vein.

Field Block. In a field block, the area *surrounding* the incision is injected and infiltrated with local anesthetics; this is in contrast to local anesthesia, in which only the area of the incision is injected. Thus, a field block actually "walls in" the area around the incision, and thereby prevents the transmission of sensory impulses to the brain from that area. The same precautions must be taken in performing field blocks as in local blocks.

Nerve Block. A nerve block acts to block nerves or individual plexuses of nerves that are further removed from the operative site than those nerves that are anesthetized by a field block.

Nerve blocks may be employed to anesthetize: an entire finger (digital nerve block), the entire upper arm (axillary block), or the chest or abdominal wall (intercostal nerve block). Nerves most commonly blocked are the brachial, intercostal, radial, and femoral. Drugs generally used for nerve blocks are procaine and lidocaine. Once the drug has been injected, the area is generally anesthetized within several minutes; this effect will last longer than that produced with local or topical anesthesia.

Nerve blocks, like local blocks, can produce severe allergic responses if the drug is accidentally injected into a blood vessel. A second rare complication is *ischemic necrosis* of an extremity (particularly a digit).

Ischemia develops because the nerve blockage encircles the extremity and, as a result, circulatory function is reduced. During the postoperative period, carefully check the warmth and color of the extremity anesthetized with a nerve block. Notify the surgeon if the extremity appears pale and is cold.

Spinal Anesthesia. The spinal block is a commonly used method of producing anesthesia. Spinal anesthesia can be employed for almost any type of major procedure that is performed below the level of the diaphragm; e.g., hysterectomy, appendectomy.

Spinal anesthesia is administered by the anesthesiologist in the following steps as outlined:

STEP 1. POSITIONING. The patient is placed on his side in a flexed position. He is held by the nurse and is cautioned not to move. As you can see in Figure 30–2, the patient's neck is sharply flexed, his upper arm is placed across his chest and his lower arm is placed at right angles to his body.

STEP 2. LUMBAR PUNCTURE AND SPINAL TAP. A lumbar puncture is performed in the lower back between the levels of the second or third lumbar vertebrae (L_2L_3) and the fifth lumbar and first sacral vertebrae (L_5S_1). There is no danger of piercing the spinal cord during this procedure as the spinal cord stops at L_2.

1. The anesthesiologist, wearing sterile gloves, first preps the patient's skin in the vicinity of the puncture with a skin antiseptic such as tincture of Zephiran and then drapes the patient with a sterile towel.

2. Next the doctor draws an imaginary line between the patient's iliac crests in order to approximate the exact site for the puncture.

3. The area over the site of the puncture is then infiltrated with procaine, thereby producing a local block.

4. Once the area is anesthetized, the doctor inserts a spinal needle at the proper level and he

then observes the spinal fluid, which should be clear in color and flowing freely.

STEP 3. INJECTION OF THE ANESTHETIC AGENT

1. If the spinal fluid appears bloody or is obstructed in its flow, the anesthetic medication is not injected through the spinal needle.

2. If the spinal fluid is clear and flows freely, a local anesthetic agent is injected through the spinal needle into the subarachnoid space (i.e., between the pia mater and the arachnoid membrane). Thus, the anesthetic agent passes into the spinal fluid.

3. Almost any local anesthetic agent can be used for spinal anesthesia. The most common drugs are:

> *Procaine hydrochloride* (Novocain)—the shortest acting of the spinal anesthetics.
> *Dibucaine hydrochloride* (Nupercaine)—the longest acting agent.
> *Tetracaine hydrochloride* (Pontocaine)—most widely used agent for safe, long-acting anesthesia.

Sometimes epinephrine is added to the local anesthetic agent in order to give a more prolonged anesthetic effect, e.g., Pontocaine mixed with epinephrine provides adequate anesthesia for up to three to four hours. Epinephrine causes local blood vessels to constrict; this prevents rapid absorption of the anesthetic agent.

4. If the anesthesiologist wishes to prolong the spinal anesthesia for an even greater length of time, he may give the patient a *"continuous spinal."* To administer continuous spinal anesthesia, the anesthesiologist inserts a semirigid catheter into the subarachnoid space and then injects the anesthetic agent intermittently as necessary. The catheter remains in place throughout the operation.

STEP 4. POSITIONING THE PATIENT FOLLOWING THE ADMINISTRATION OF SPINAL ANESTHESIA

1. Place the patient on his back following the injection of the anesthetic agent, and on his side if he is receiving a continuous spinal.

2. For a high level of anesthesia, lower the patient's head and shoulders to degree ordered by the anesthesiologist.

3. After 10 to 20 minutes the anesthesia level is set and the patient may be placed in any position desired without disturbing the anesthesia level.

Within a few minutes following induction of spinal anesthesia, the patient experiences a loss of sensation and a paralysis of his toes, then feet, then legs, and finally his abdomen. Spinal anesthesia causes the nerve roots and spinal cord to be blocked in the transmission of impulses just as local anesthesia causes peripheral nerve fibers to be blocked. As one anesthesiologist emphasizes:

> The physiologic effect of spinal anesthesia is due to its neuroblockage. Vasodilatation (and hypotension if it occurs) results from autonomic block, anesthesia from sensory block, and muscle paralysis from motor block. Respiratory effects are due to motor blockage.[10]

Autonomic nerve fibers are the first fibers to be blocked by spinal anesthesia and the last to recover. Following autonomic blockage, temperature, touch, pain, motor pressure, and proprioception fibers are blocked, in that order.

Spinal anesthesia offers many advantages for patients undergoing surgical procedures involving the lower half of their bodies. Major benefits of spinal anesthesia are:[10]

1. Ease of administration.
2. Expensive equipment and drugs not necessary.
3. Relative safety of method.
4. Excellent muscle relaxation provided.
5. Does not cause fetal depression, and thus can be used for cesarean sections.
6. Does not cloud patient's consciousness or alertness. However, anxious patients can be given a small dose of barbiturate, which will enable them to rest and even to sleep throughout their operation.
7. Can be used for patients with a full stomach since the patient will be awake to maintain his own airway in event of vomiting.

Complications of spinal anesthesia are listed in Table 30–4, along with their causes, prevention, and treatment.

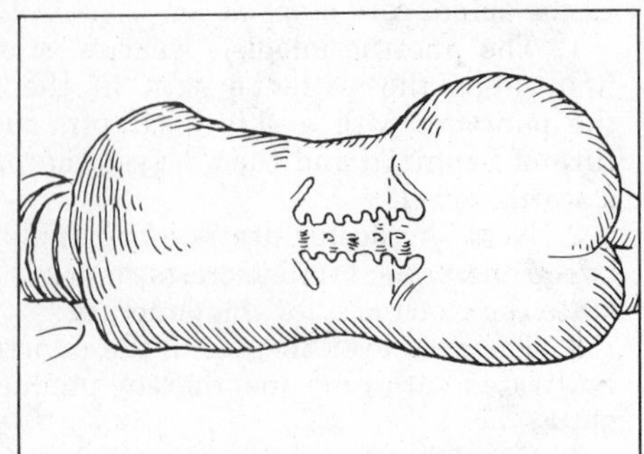

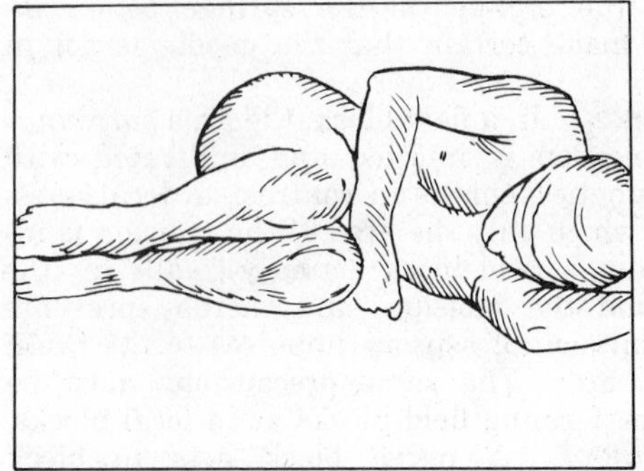

FIGURE 30–2. The proper position for the administration of spinal anesthesia.

When caring for a patient who has undergone spinal anesthesia, remember that he is a potential candidate for serious respiratory or cardiovascular problems. Check the patient's blood pressure and his rate and depth of breathing every 10 to 15 minutes during the recovery period. If the blood pressure begins to fall rapidly and breathing becomes difficult, notify the surgeon or anesthesiologist at once so that treatment measures can be started promptly.

As the anesthesia wears off, observe the patient carefully. To make sure he has an adequate return of motion to his extremities, ask him if he can move his toes. However, as one anesthesiologist warns, the patient who can wiggle his toes has *not* necessarily recovered completely from the "spinal." A patient's ability to move his toes simply means that the motor blockade is wearing off, although autonomic blockade is still *present.* Patients who are still experiencing autonomic blockade are prone to *hypotension* despite their

TABLE 30–4. COMPLICATIONS AND DISCOMFORTS OF SPINAL ANESTHESIA

Complications and Discomforts	Causes	Clinical Care	Prevention
Hypotension	Paralysis of vasomotor nerves; usually occurs shortly after induction of anesthesia	Administer: 1. Oxygen by inhalation 2. Blood or plasma IV 3. Stimulant drugs, e.g., ephedrine or methoxamine (Vasoxyl) IV 4. Trendelenburg position if level of anesthesia is fixed, 10 to 20 minutes after induction	Administer ephedrine or methoxamine preoperatively
Nausea, vomiting, and pain during surgery	Occurs mainly during abdominal surgery, due to traction placed on various structures within abdomen		Give weak solution of thiopenthal IV at same time that spinal anesthesia is induced
Headache (can be extremely painful and may last days or weeks)	Cerebral spinal fluid (which cushions the brain) is lost through dural hole; Leakage of fluid and loss of cushioning effect increased by: 1. Use of a large spinal needle 2. Poor hydration 3. Hypersensitivity of the patient	To treat: 1. Apply tight abdominal binder 2. Administer fluids 3. Administer analgesics 4. Administer caffeine sodium benzoate (medication used for migraine headache) 5. Inject saline into subarachnoid space as last resort	To prevent: 1. Use of very small spinal needle reduces incidence of spinal headache to 0.9 per cent 2. Administer IV and oral fluids before and after induction of spinal anesthesia 3. Keep patient flat and quiet
Respiratory paralysis	Occurs if drug reaches upper thoracic and cervical cord in large amounts or in heavy concentrations	Give artificial respiration by anesthesia machine, hand-held resuscitator, or mouth-to-mouth breathing	Avoid use of Trendelenburg position before level of spinal anesthesia set, i.e., 10 to 20 minutes following induction
Neurologic complications (e.g., paraplegia, severe muscle weakness in legs)	Paralysis postoperatively may be due to 1. Use of unsterile needles, syringes, and anesthetic medications 2. Preexisting diseases of the central nervous system (e.g., multiple sclerosis and spinal cord tumors), which cause paralysis rather than the spinal anesthesia itself	See neurologic section, Unit VIII, for treatment of paraplegia	To prevent: 1. Use of strict sterile technique 2. Use of heat-sterilized drugs 3. Use of sterile disposable needles 4. Careful preoperative neurologic examination to ascertain the presence of neurologic disease

ability to move their toes and extremities.[10] Therefore, patients who have undergone spinal anesthesia and who are discharged from the recovery room to the surgical floor still require careful monitoring of their blood pressure. Watch these patients carefully for sudden drops in blood pressure and for other signs of shock.

Saddle Block. This form of anesthesia, commonly used in obstetrics, is sometimes referred to as a "low spinal" because: (1) it is induced in a similar way to spinal anesthesia except that the anesthetic drug is injected into the dural sac at the 3rd and 4th lumbar space, and (2) it mainly produces anesthesia of the perineal area, thus the term, "saddle block." Its physiologic effects are generally like those of spinal anesthesia.

Caudal Block. Like the saddle block, caudal anesthesia is used in obstetrics. The caudal block is somewhat more extensive in its effects than is the saddle block, producing anesthesia from the umbilicus to the toes.

SPECIALIZED METHODS OF PRODUCING ANESTHESIA

Specialized anesthesia techniques are used for certain types of operations; e.g., open heart surgery. These techniques may be used alone to provide anesthesia, or they may be used to supplement other types of anesthesia.

Muscle Relaxants

Muscle relaxants are given mainly to supplement other more powerful general anesthetic agents. When given in combination with muscle relaxants, potent general anesthetic drugs can be administered in a smaller dose. This ensures greater patient safety.

Muscle relaxants produce their physiologic effects by blocking the transmission of nervous impulses to the muscle fibers. This blockade produces temporary paralysis of all voluntary muscles, including the muscles that control respiration. One dangerous complication produced by muscle relaxants is severe *respiratory depression.*

The two major drugs that act as muscle relaxants are:

> *Curare,* which is capable of producing muscle relaxation in from one to three minutes. Muscles are blocked by curare in the following order: eyelids, eyeballs, face, neck, throat, trunk and, finally, the muscles of the extremities. Within one to two hours the effects of curare wear off and the muscles become activated again, but in the reverse order: i.e., muscles of the extremities, trunk, throat, and so forth. The most dangerous untoward effect of curare is respiratory depression.

> *Anectine* is a more rapid-acting muscle relaxant than curare; its action takes place in from 60 to 90 seconds. In addition, Anectine is rapidly eliminated, usually within three to five minutes! Consequently, Anectine is often administered many times during an operative procedure as needed for muscle relaxation. Like curare, Anectine can cause respiratory depression.

Hypothermia

A highly specialized method of anesthesia, hypothermia is the deliberate reduction of the patient's body temperature to between 28 and 30° C. or 82 and 86° F. The purpose of hypothermia is to reduce the rate of tissue metabolism and consequently, the rate of O_2 uptake by the body's cells and tissues. *Situations* in which hypothermia is employed are: heart surgery, brain surgery, surgery on large vessels supplying major organs (e.g., renal and carotid arteries and the aorta), and the treatment of severely injured persons with an impaired blood supply to their vital organs.

Methods and *apparatus* for producing hypothermia are: ice water immersion, molding of partially filled ice bags over the patient's extremities, and extracorporal cooling devices which cool the blood outside of the body and then reinfuse the cooled blood back into the patient.

Major complications of hypothermia are respiratory depression and cardiac arrest.

Following surgery the body of the patient who has received hypothermia is generally allowed to rewarm slowly at its own rate.

Purposeful Hypotension

Anesthesiologists use this unusual technique in operations in which a reduction of bleeding at the operative site is particularly advantageous, e.g., brain surgery, radical neck surgery, and radical pelvic surgery. Purposeful hypotension is produced by either administering drugs that paralyze the patient's autonomic nervous system, or inducing a deep level of general anesthesia. One general anesthetic agent commonly employed in purposeful hypotension is halothane.

As the surgeon places his last suture and the operation ends, the patient enters the third and final phase of his operative odyssey—the postoperative period. It is during this last period that the nurse's observations and actions must be particularly skillful if the patient is to recover safely from the anesthesia and the operation itself.

CHAPTER 31

General Care of the Patient Following Surgery

IMMEDIATE CARE OF THE PATIENT RECOVERING FROM ANESTHESIA

TRANSPORTING THE PATIENT FROM THE OPERATING ROOM

Following the completion of the operation, the operating room staff generally dress the patient in a clean gown and move him to a stretcher. In moving the patient from the operating table to the stretcher, the operating room personnel strive to avoid the following three problems:

> *Exposure,* which predisposes the patient to respiratory infections and shock.

> *Rough handling,* which may place a strain upon the patient's sutures.

> *Hurried movements and rapid changes in position,* which predispose the patient to hypotension. In particular, the patient should be moved gradually from the lithotomy to the horizontal position and from the prone to the supine position.

Always have adequate help when moving or transferring a postoperative patient. Never try to move an unconscious person by yourself or with just one other person.

When the patient is on the stretcher, he should be covered with blankets and secured with safety belts or restraints over the knees and elbows. The side rails of the stretcher should be up to ensure patient safety in case the patient begins to awaken from anesthesia during his trip from the operating room. The anesthesiologist and sometimes the surgeon accompany the patient to the recovery room.

The Recovery Room

Within the specialized confines of the recovery room the patient, under constant nursing supervision, recovers from the anesthesia (Fig. 31–1).

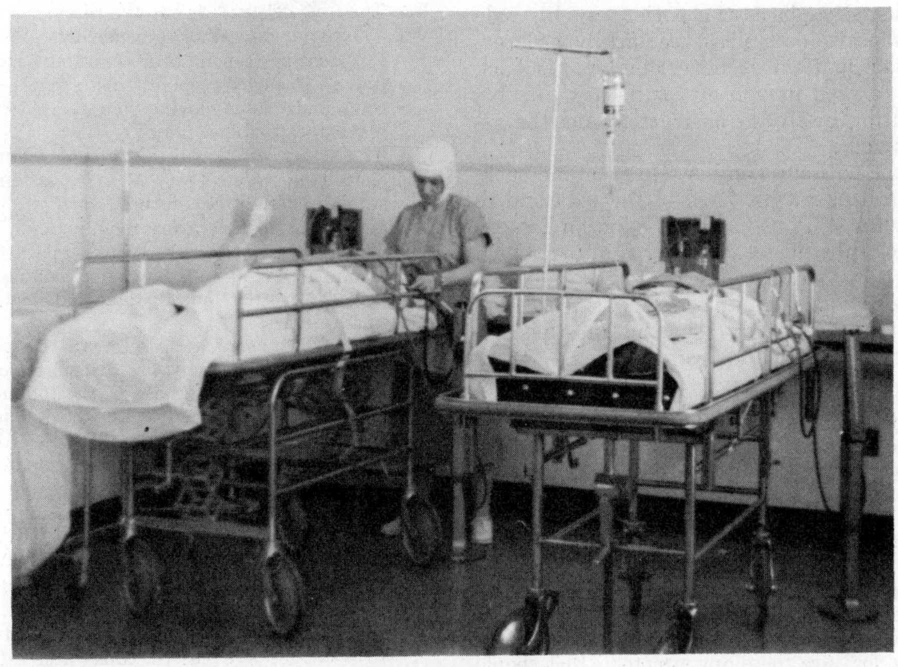

FIGURE 31–1. A typical scene in a modern recovery room. (From Le Maitre, G., and Finnegan, J.: *The Patient in Surgery. A Guide for Nurses.* 2nd ed., 1970.)

Once his vital signs have stabilized and he responds to simple commands, the patient is then transferred to the surgical floor where he will complete his convalescent period. In certain cases, recovery room patients may be transferred to the Intensive Care Unit (ICU) for continued specialized care with constant nursing supervision. Patients who are transferred to the ICU usually are patients who (1) are a poor risk; (2) have undergone major vascular surgery (e.g., resection of an aortic aneurysm), transplant or endocrine surgery (e.g., surgery of the adrenal gland); or (3) have suffered from cardiac arrest or respiratory insufficiency during or following surgery.[33]

Admission of the Patient to the Recovery Room. In the morning the recovery room nurse (a specially trained person) usually receives a list of the patients who are scheduled that day. Before the arrival of each patient from surgery, the nurse generally checks each individual patient cubicle for the following equipment: a sphygmomanometer and stethoscope, IV equipment, suction apparatus, tongue depressors, an airway, an emesis basin, mouth wipes, and monitoring devices. Other supplies which should be close at hand and ready for use if needed are: emergency drugs, narcotics, tracheostomy set, airway, oxygen, cutdown tray, universal donor blood, plasma expanders, endotracheal tube, catheterization sets, defibrillator, Bennett or Bird respirator, and gastric suction apparatus.

Once the patient arrives from surgery, he is either moved from the stretcher to a bed, or he is left on the stretcher while in the recovery room. The nurse usually places the patient on his side in the Sims position. Unless specifically ordered, an unconscious patient is never left on his back because his relaxed tongue may fall back into his throat, resulting in airway obstruction and the aspiration of mucus.

Whether the patient is on his side or on his back, it is essential to turn his head to the side and to extend his chin (Fig. 31–2). This position lessens the danger of aspiration of mucus or vomitus, which would cause airway obstruction.

Once the postoperative patient is safely positioned, the nurse generally asks the anesthesiologist or surgeon about the following factors:

> What is the patient's general condition?
> What type of operation was performed?
> What type of anesthesia has the patient received?
> Did the patient suffer from any problems or complications during surgery that will affect his course postoperatively?
> What pathologic disorders were encountered during surgery? Was cancer discovered? If so, has the family been informed? Will the patient be told that cancer is present?
> Are there any particular symptoms or complications to observe for? Are there any symptoms that should be reported immediately?
> Are there any orders that must be carried out immediately?

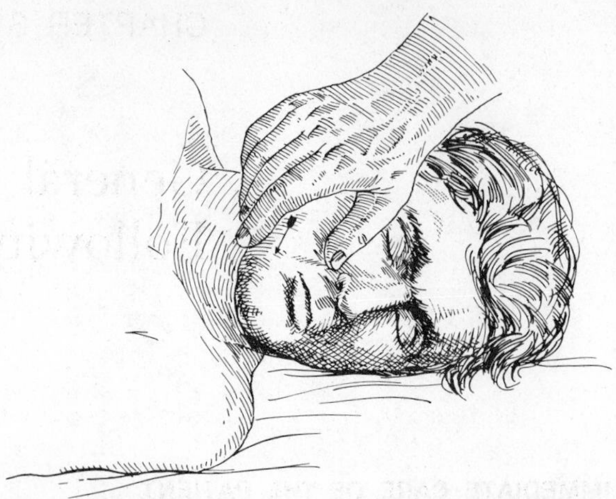

FIGURE 31–2. Position of hand to hold the jaw forward after inhalation of anesthesia. Note that the fingers are placed behind the angle of the jaw, and the direction of the arrow shows the direction of pressure being exerted on the jaw. As the jaw is pushed forward the tongue is brought forward so as to keep an open airway. This is important, especially after operation under general anesthesia in children, for instance, in tonsillectomy.

With the doctor, the recovery room nurse next reviews the patient's chart in terms of the anesthesia record; drugs, IV's and blood received during surgery; and the length of time the patient was in surgery. Later, the nurse reads the patient's history.

Typical Observations and Orders

After positioning the patient and talking to the doctor, the following routine observations are made and the findings are recorded:

> The *time* of admission to the recovery room.
> The patient's *level of responsiveness* upon admission; e.g., does he respond at all to stimuli such as light or touch? Does he respond to his name or to simple commands? Is he moving voluntarily or making audible or intelligible sounds?
> The *temperature* and *vital signs*. The vital signs should be taken every 15 minutes until they are stable and the temperature every two to four hours, depending upon recovery room policy.
> *Skin color and dryness.* A dusky, pale, cold, wet skin is one important sign of shock and should be reported. Also note the lips and nail beds for paleness and cyanosis.
> The presence of an *airway* in the patient's oropharynx. An airway is a hollow rubber or plastic tube that passes over the base of the tongue and acts to keep the tongue from falling back and obstructing the natural airway (Fig. 31–3). The patient normally pushes the airway out by himself as he regains consciousness.
> The absence of *reflexes*, e.g., the gag reflex.
> The condition of the *dressing*, e.g., dry or soiled. If soiled, note the color, type, and amount of drainage (e.g., "Is the spot of drainage the size of a quarter?").
> The presence of *drainage tubes*, e.g., a T-tube or gastric tube.* Is the T-tube unclamped and attached to a bottle? Are gastric tubes and intestinal tubes hooked up to suction as ordered? Make sure the

*Gastric tubes and T-tubes are discussed in Unit XV.

tubes are not kinked and that the patient is not lying on them and thus obstructing drainage.

> *The IV infusion.* Note the type of IV solutions that are running. Also check the *amount* of IV solution left in the bottle, the *rate* of drip, if the solution has infiltrated, and orders for other IV solutions to follow. Check to see if any medications have been added to the IV or if any are ordered to be added.
> The presence of a *blood* transfusion. Note if a blood transfusion is running or if one is ordered. Check the rate of drip. Watch carefully for signs of a reaction, as discussed in Unit XII.
> The quality and rate of the *respirations.* If the patient has dyspnea, check to see if oxygen is ordered. Make certain that mechanical breathing aids are close at hand and in working order.
> The presence of a bladder *catheter.* If the catheter is inserted into the bladder, make certain that it is unclamped, is hooked to a drainage bag or bottle, and is freely draining. Note any abnormalities in the appearance of the urine.
> *Any unusual symptoms.* Constantly observe for marked elevations in temperature, signs of shock, hemorrhage, or a blocked airway, and signs of circulatory overload from excess IV fluids.

Typical orders for a patient in recovery room are:

1. NPO, except for isotonic ice chips.
2. Vital signs q. 15 minutes until stable, then q. ½ hour for next 2 hours.
3. Oropharyngeal suctioning prn.
4. Complete IV solution that is currently running, then discontinue IV.
5. Phenergan 12.5 mg. IM prn for nausea and vomiting once vital signs have stabilized.
6. Demerol 75 mg. IM q. 3 to 4 hr. prn for pain.
7. I and O.
8. Have patient cough, turn, move legs, and deep breathe every 2 hours.
9. Hematocrit and electrolyte studies in the morning.
10. Catheterize if patient does not void in 10 hours.
11. Reinforce dressings prn.

In addition to routine orders, the surgeon will also write special orders that apply only to specific types of operations, e.g., neurosurgery, eye surgery, or which apply to an individual patient's problem (e.g., diabetes).

GOALS OF CARE THROUGHOUT THE POSTOPERATIVE PERIOD

From the moment the patient is admitted to the recovery room to the time when he has recovered from his operation, there are certain definitive goals that act as guides throughout the postoperative course. These goals are outlined in the box below.

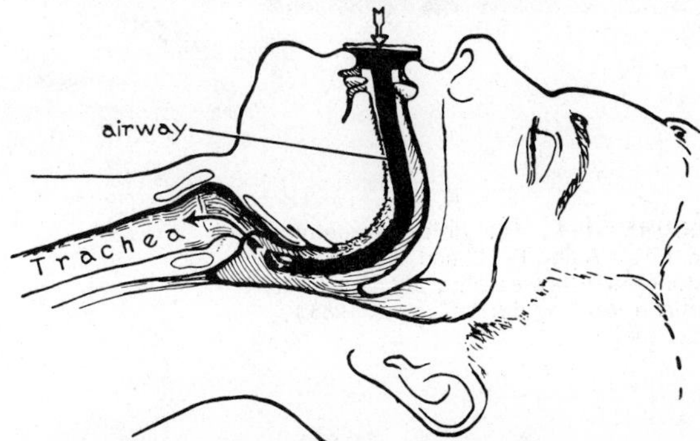

FIGURE 31–3. An airway functions by preventing the tongue from falling back to obstruct the patient's airway. (From Sutton, A. L.: *Bedside Nursing Techniques in Medicine and Surgery.* 1969.)

Goals of Care for Postoperative Patients
Goal 1: Promote cardiovascular function and tissue perfusion.
Goal 2: Promote respiratory function by maintaining open airway.
Goal 3: Promote nutrition and elimination.
Goal 4: Promote fluid and electrolyte balance.
Goal 5: Promote renal function.
Goal 6: Promote rest and comfort.
Goal 7: Promote wound healing.
Goal 8: Promote early movement and ambulation.
Goal 9: Prevent postoperative complications.

GOAL 1: PROMOTION OF CARDIOVASCULAR FUNCTION AND TISSUE PERFUSION

A satisfactory cardiac output is the basis for good tissue perfusion. Measures of cardiac output and consequently of tissue perfusion are:

A. Arterial blood pressure
  1. *Normal* findings: Whether or not a blood pressure reading is low depends upon the baseline blood pressures taken *before* surgery.
  2. *Abnormal* readings that are reportable:
    a. Fall in systolic pressure of more than 20 mm. Hg.
    b. Systolic blood pressure below 80 mm. Hg.
    c. Blood pressure that is continually dropping by 5 to 10 mm. Hg over several readings.
  3. Causes of postoperative low blood pressures:
    a. Muscle relaxants.
    b. Spinal anesthesia.
    c. Overdosage of premedication.
    d. Changes in the patient's position.
    e. Blood loss.
    f. Poor lung ventilation.
    g. Peripheral pooling of blood.

B. *Pulse*
  1. *Normal* finding: The pulse is usually slightly rapid immediately following surgery.
  2. *Abnormal* findings that are reportable:
    a. Bradycardia
      (1) Pulse below 60 beats per minute.
      (2) Can be caused by anesthetic agents.
      (3) Generally of little consequence if the patient has no other symptoms.
    b. Tachycardia
      (1) Pulse above 110 beats per minute.
      (2) Causes:
        (a) Excess blood loss.
        (b) Cardiac arrhythmias.
        (c) High fever.
        (d) Atelectasis.
        (e) Pneumonia.
        (f) Anxiety.
        (g) Nitrous oxide anesthesia.
        (h) Oxygen lack.

c. Irregular pulse.
(1) May be a regular irregularity, an irregular irregularity or a skipped beat.
(2) Sometimes caused by cyclopropane.

C. *Respiration*
1. *Normal* finding: Respirations usually slow and deep when patient is anesthetized.
2. *Abnormal* findings: In certain cases, abnormal respirations represent a cardiovascular problem rather than a pulmonary problem.
3. Abnormal findings that signify a cardiovascular problem and that are reportable:
a. Rapid difficult respirations may indicate anoxia, shock, and oxygen lack.
b. Shallow, quiet, slow respirations may indicate depression of the respiratory tract.
c. Shallow difficult respirations in which the patient uses his neck and diaphragmatic muscles may indicate paralysis of the intercostal muscles from anesthesia. Artificial respiration is indicated!

GOAL 2: PROMOTION OF RESPIRATORY FUNCTION

Normal respiratory function depends upon the maintenance of an open clear airway during and following surgery.

A. Causes of a *closed* airway:
1. Obstruction due to:
a. Mucus collection in the throat.
b. Aspiration of mucus or vomitus.
c. Loss of the swallowing reflex.
d. Loss of control of the muscles of the jaw and tongue. As a result, the tongue slips back against the pharynx and blocks the airway.
2. Laryngospasm due to:
a. Intubation.
b. Irritating effects of anesthetics.
3. Bronchospasm due to:
a. Prior respiratory diseases, e.g., chronic bronchitis, emphysema, asthma.
b. Inhalation of gastric juices during surgery.

B. Signs of poor respiratory function:
1. Restlessness (an early sign).
2. Fast, thready pulse (an early sign).
3. Confusion.
4. Air hunger (i.e., rapid, shallow breathing).
5. Nausea.
6. Apprehension.
7. Cyanosis (a late sign).
8. Snoring (appears when tongue causes airway blockage).
9. Respiratory stridor (seen in larygospasm).
10. Wheezing (may appear in bronchospasm).

C. Results of untreated hypoventilation and respiratory obstruction are:
1. Atelectasis.
2. Pneumonia.

D. Emergency care of respiratory complications:[32]
1. *Oral airway* insertion prevents tongue from occluding airway.
2. *Endotracheal intubation* provides clear airway. Endotracheal tube can be attached to a mechanical respirator.

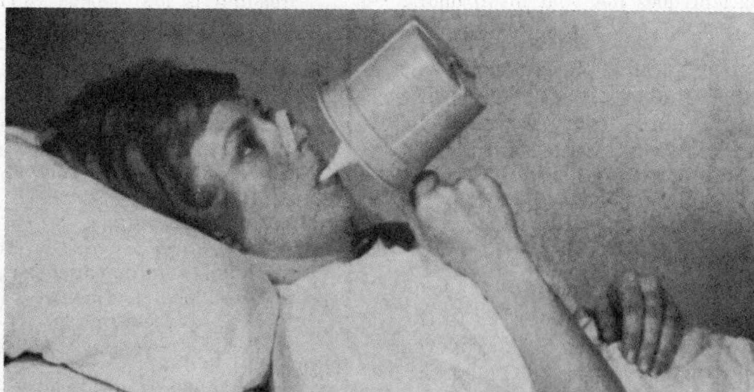

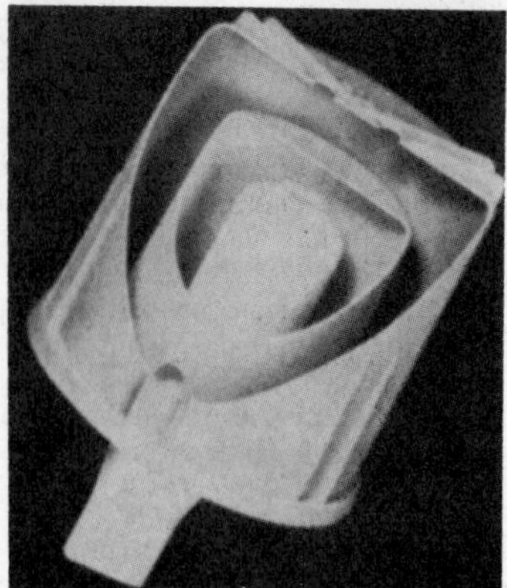

FIGURE 31–4. The Adler rebreathing tube. (From Adler, R. H., and Brodie, S. L.: Postoperative rebreathing aid. *American Journal of Nursing 68*:1287, June, 1968.)

3. *Oxygen* administration by means of a mask catheter or endotracheal tube.
4. Intermittent positive pressure breathing (IPPB)* to give continuous ventilation to patients with airway obstruction.
5. *Drugs* commonly used in respiratory emergencies are:
   a. Antibiotics.
   b. Bronchodilators (e.g., aminophylline).
   c. Expectorants (e.g., potassium iodide and ammonium chloride).
   d. Liquefying agents (e.g., Alevaire, Mucomyst).
   e. Respiratory stimulants (e.g., Coramine, caffeine sodium benzoate).
6. Tracheostomy* is indicated for patients with complete or prolonged partial airway occlusion and for patients who cannot tolerate endotracheal intubation.

E. Methods of promoting adequate respiratory function.
   1. Methods useful in early postoperative period:
      a. Whenever possible, position patient on side so that tongue does not fall back into throat and occlude airway.
      b. Suction mouth and pharynx gently to remove mucus.
      c. Leave airway in place until patient pushes it out of his mouth himself.
      d. Use of a mechanical respirator, such as Bird or Emerson, beneficially controls rate and depth of respirations; also prescribed mixtures of air and oxygen can be forced into respiratory system.
      e. Use of rebreathing device forces patient to breathe his own exhaled air with its increased CO_2 content, e.g., the Adler rebreathing tube that is pictured in Figure 31–4.
   2. Methods useful throughout postoperative period.
      a. Encourage the patient to breathe deeply every two hours in the manner described on p. 318.
      b. Encourage the patient to cough every two hours.
         (1) Splint the patient's incision so that coughing will be less painful and less likely to cause the incision to rupture.
         (2) Have patient cover his mouth, and turn your face away from him so that you avoid breathing in the spray from his mouth.
         (3) Check the color and consistency of mucus he expectorates. If a respiratory infection is present, the mucus may be thick, greenish, and foul smelling.

GOAL 3: THE PROMOTION OF NUTRITION AND ELIMINATION

Following surgery, the patient typically first receives parenteral fluids, next liquids, then solid foods and, finally, a full diet.

A. Parenteral fluids given during the immediate recovery period include:
   1. Intravenous fluids.
   2. Amino acids.
   3. Blood.

B. Liquids, administered when vomiting stops, include:
   1. Broth.
   2. Tea with lemon and sugar.
   3. Fruit juices.
   4. Jello.
   5. Soups.

*IPPB and tracheostomies will be discussed further in Units XIV and XXII.

C. Early solid foods include:
   1. Toast.
   2. Light cornstarch puddings.
   3. Easily digested meats and vegetables.

D. A full diet is started as soon as possible to promote vitamin and mineral balance and proper nitrogen balance.

E. The patient generally has a bowel movement by the second or third postoperative day. If the patient's bowels do not move, the surgeon generally orders an enema.

GOAL 4: PROMOTION OF FLUID AND ELECTROLYTE BALANCE

Following surgery, promotion of proper fluid and electrolyte intake and electrolyte output is crucial. Imbalances postoperatively can lead to retention of metabolic wastes, neurologic and cardiac problems, and problems of over- or underhydration.

A. The goals of postoperative fluid and electrolyte therapy are twofold:
   1. To give sufficient fluids to maintain extracellular fluid volume and blood volume. Proper fluid volume ensures:
      a. Adequate blood pressure.
      b. Adequate cardiac output.
      c. Adequate urinary flow.
   2. To prevent fluid overload with resultant congestive heart failure and pulmonary edema.

B. Normal fluid and electrolyte adjustment during the first three to four days following surgery:
   1. Renal retention of H_2O and Na^+.
   2. Expansion of ECF in excess of Na^+ and Cl^-.
   3. Transient decrease in ECF Na^+ and Cl^-.
   4. Increase in K^+ excretion.
   5. Decrease in hematocrit as a result of the expansion of ECF.

C. Normal fluid and electrolyte adjustments during the fifth through seventh day following surgery:
   1. Diuresis.
   2. Return of ECF volume to normal.
   3. Serum Na^+ returns to normal.
   4. Reduction of K^+ concentration in urine.

D. *Abnormal* fluid and electrolyte changes as a result of surgery are presented in Unit V, Chapter 25.

E. Principal causes of postoperative *dehydration* and *electrolyte deficits:*
   1. Failure to replace deficits existing prior to surgery.
   2. Inadequate replacement of *normal* postoperative losses.
   3. Excessive postoperative losses as a result of sweating, hyperventilation, wound drainage, gastrointestinal tract drainage, diarrhea, and vomiting.

F. Principal causes of *fluid overload* are:
   1. Excessive administration of fluids.
   2. Inadequate renal function.

G. Principal causes of *respiratory acidosis* (a common postoperative H^+ imbalance):
   1. *Anesthesia* can cause an excessive intake of CO_2 and a reduction in respiratory rate.
   2. *Narcotics* (especially in the elderly) reduce respiratory efficiency.

3. *Postoperative pain* and *bulky uncomfortable dressings* make most patients reluctant to cough and deep breathe.
4. *Abdominal distention* (a common postoperative problem) crowds diaphragm and makes deep breathing difficult.
5. *Surgery with high incision* involving the diaphragm reduces ventilation, e.g., hiatus hernia repair and gallbladder surgery.
6. *Postoperative complications,* e.g., *atelectasis, pneumonia,* and *bronchitis,* cause respiratory obstruction and poor ventilation.

H. Nurses can help to prevent postoperative fluid and electrolyte imbalances:
1. Record I and O accurately.
2. Report abnormal laboratory findings to surgeon immediately.
3. Administer intravenous infusions on time and at the proper rate.
4. Obtain an order for an antiemetic (e.g., Phenergan) for patients with severe, prolonged vomiting.
5. Irrigate gastric suction tubes properly (see Unit V, Chapter 25).
6. Instruct patient to cough and to deep breathe to prevent respiratory acidosis.

GOAL 5: PROMOTION OF RENAL FUNCTION

A. Normally patient should void within eight to 10 hours following surgery, particularly following abdominal and gynecologic surgeries.

B. Causes of an inability to void postoperatively:
1. Effects of the anesthesia.
2. Pain.
3. Fear and tension.
4. Unfamiliar surroundings.
5. Clogged catheter.

C. Signs of bladder distention are:
1. A fullness above the symphysis pubis that can be palpated.
2. Voiding 1 to 2 oz. of urine every 15 to 20 minutes (retention with overflow), or a complete inability to void.

D. Bladder distention may be relieved:
1. Induce patient to void by means described in Unit V, Chapter 27.
2. Obtain order for catheterization only as last resort.

E. Keep an accurate record of intake and output on all postoperative patients for at least 24 hours following surgery.

GOAL 6: PROMOTION OF COMFORT, REST, AND FREEDOM FROM PAIN

Rest is essential if patient is to recuperate successfully. To rest properly patient must be as free as possible from the following problems:

A. Pain.
1. Factors related to high incidence and intensity of postoperative pain:
   a. *Type of anesthesia* used.
      (1) Cyclopropane and nitrous oxide are soluble agents that are eliminated rapidly from body; consequently, patients are restless and in pain early in postoperative period with use of these agents.
      (2) Soluble anesthetics, e.g., diethyl ether, cause central nervous system depression; their anesthetizing effects continue for hours following surgery.
   b. High level of anxiety.
   c. Extensive surgical procedures.
   d. Lengthy procedures.
   e. Poor state of mental health.
2. Postoperative pain that occurs within the *first 24 hours* following surgery is usually relieved by the administration of *narcotics.*
   a. Drugs commonly used:
      (1) Morphine.
      (2) Demerol.
      (3) Levo-Dromoran.
      (4) Pantopon.
      (5) Nalline.
      (6) Codeine.

   While narcotic agents are routinely given for pain during the first 24 hours postoperative, do not overmedicate the patient! Narcotic overdosages can cause severe complications.
   b. Complications of postoperative drug therapy:
      (1) Lung complications (due to depression of the cough reflex).
      (2) Increased nausea and vomiting.
   c. *Before* administering narcotic agents:
      (1) Check blood pressure: if low, give only small doses of narcotics.
      (2) Check for presence of painful *pressure points* if patient has cast or splint;* if present, notify surgeon. Surgeon will split or cut window in cast; when pressure is relieved, narcotics are unnecessary.
      (3) Check for *distended bladder;* if present, obtain order for catheterization if patient is unable to void.
      (4) Check for *abdominal distention* and *flatulence.* Obtain order for a rectal tube or Harris flush if the patient is suffering from gas pains, a common postoperative complaint.
      (5) Try pain-relieving techniques, e.g., back rub, position change before giving analgesics; narcotics may be unnecessary.
   d. As convalescence progresses, administer pain medication in decreasing dosages and strengths.
      (1) Narcotics are usually administered by injection every 3 to 4 hours prn during the first 24 hours postoperatively.
      (2) After the first 24 to 48 hours, the surgeon usually writes new orders for pain medication which include:
         (a) A less potent agent (e.g., codeine in place of Demerol).
         (b) A smaller dosage.
         (c) Oral administration of the agent rather than parenteral administration.
      (3) The nurse should discourage an overreliance by the convalescent patient upon narcotics.
         (a) Change patient's position and rub his back in order to relieve pain.
         (b) Give the patient adequate reassurance concerning his operation; relieve pain-producing anxiety.
         (c) Notify the surgeon if the patient asks for narcotics at frequent intervals several days after the operation. The patient may be developing a postoperative complication, or an overreliance upon narcotics.

*See Unit XVII.

B. *Restlessness.*
1. Factors that cause restlessness:
   a. Pain.
   b. Bladder distention.
   c. Abdominal distention.
   d. Fear.
   e. Anxiety.
   f. Oxygen lack.
   g. Wet, tight dressings.
   h. Hemorrhage.
2. To relieve restlessness:
   a. Obtain order for pain medication or barbiturate.
   b. With physician, evaluate whether patient needs oxygen.
   c. Change patient's position and massage his back.
3. If the patient is agitated and restless, pad the side rails. Watch that the patient does not pull out his drainage tubes or IV infusion and that he does not tamper with his dressing or injure himself in other ways.

C. Nausea and Vomiting.
1. From 30 to 40 per cent of all surgical patients vomit.
2. Incidence of postoperative vomiting is related to:[39]
   a. *Sex:* Female patients vomit more than male patients.
   b. *Type of surgery:* Vomiting is more common following gynecologic surgery.
   c. *Age:* Male patients under 30 vomit more than male patients over 30.
   d. Type and level of *anesthesia:* Higher incidence of vomiting is associated with:
      (1) Use of cyclopropane and ether.
      (2) Deep levels of anesthesia.
      (3) Anesthesia given by mask.
   e. *Premedication used:* Vomiting more common when Demerol is administered instead of morphine.
3. To relieve postoperative nausea and vomiting:
   a. Administer antiemetic drugs, e.g., the phenothiazides.
   b. Administer small doses of sedatives, e.g., the barbiturates.
4. Antiemetic agents have dangerous side effects:
   a. Hypotension.
   b. Prolong effects of anesthesia.
   c. Bone marrow suppression (in some cases).
5. To *prevent* postoperative vomiting:
   a. Prepare patient mentally and physically during preoperative period for stress of surgery.
   b. For patients undergoing surgery with high incidence of postoperative vomiting (e.g., eye surgery, and surgery of the vestibular region), surgeon may order:[12]
      (1) The administration of an antiemetic drug:
         (a) 30 to 40 minutes before the end of surgery.
         (b) As soon as the patient arrives in the recovery room.

GOAL 7: PROMOTION OF WOUND HEALING

Maintenance of *strict asepsis* during surgery and during the postoperative period is the most important single factor in promotion of wound healing. Contamination and infection disrupt process of wound repair.

A. Ways in which healing is promoted and infection prevented are:
1. Covering the wound with a *sterile* dressing.
   a. Dressings may or may not be ordered depending on surgeon's policy. Dressings are usually ordered for:
      (1) Wounds draining heavily.
      (2) Wounds that can be contaminated by urine or feces.
      (3) Wounds requiring immobilization.
      (4) Wounds bleeding or oozing.
   b. Use strict aseptic technique when applying dressings.
2. Insertion of *drains* (e.g., Penrose drain) into wounds filled with harmful collections of fluid.
   a. Fluid collections are harmful:
      (1) Fluid places pressure upon surrounding organs.
      (2) Collections of bile, urine, pus, and pancreatic juice cause tissue irritation and necrosis.
      (3) Collections of stagnant fluids act as bacterial culture media.
   b. When large amount of fluid drainage is present, drainage tube is often attached to tubing and to low suction.
   c. When suction is applied to a draining wound, make certain that the drainage tubing is not kinked or twisted, because the flow of drainage will be curtailed.
3. Insertion of a hollow tube into an internal organ in order to carry drainage from organ to outside of body.
   a. These tubes are sometimes called "fistula-forming" tubes; they make a hollow connection between internal organ and outside of body.
   b. Examples of fistula-forming tubes are T-tubes, gastrostomy tubes, cecostomy tubes, and cystostomy tubes.
   c. Within 7 to 10 days, these tubes are usually surrounded and walled off by fibrous tissue.

> *Handle "fistula-forming" tubes with care! Should you or the patient accidentally remove the tube before the fibrin wall forms, the drainage will leak into the peritoneal cavity, often with fatal results.*[16] *Remember also that infection can travel from outside the body, up the tube, and into the body.*

B. Nursing observations
1. Check dressing when you first arrive to assume patient's care.
2. Check dressing every two hours thereafter for drainage, and so forth.

GOAL 8: PROMOTION OF EARLY MOVEMENT AND AMBULATION

In Chapter 27 we emphasized that patients who are immobilized for long periods of time develop weakness, respiratory diseases such as pneumonia and atelectasis, circulatory problems such as thrombophlebitis, osteoporosis, urinary retention, bladder stones, and a negative nitrogen balance. These problems apply to the surgical patient as well as to the medical patient.

A. To prevent the complications of immobilization following surgery:
   1. Encourage patient to move, turn, cough, deep breathe, and flex ankles and legs upon awakening from anesthesia, and to perform these activities repeatedly throughout his postoperative course.
   2. With surgeon's permission, allow patient to stand to void within a few hours after surgery.
   3. Allow postoperative patients to bathe themselves and to assume their own personal care as soon as possible.
   4. Encourage patients to begin to ambulate within a day or two after surgery, upon surgeon's order.

GOAL 9: PREVENTION OF POSTOPERATIVE COMPLICATIONS

Observe the patient constantly for the following postoperative complications:

Shock.
Hemorrhage.
Pneumonia.
Atelectasis.
Gastric dilatation.
Paralytic ileus.
Renal failure.
Acute parotitis.
Wound infection.
Wound dehiscence.
Urinary infections.
Thrombophlebitis.
Hiccoughs.
Decubitus ulcers.
Emotional disturbances.

CONVALESCENCE AND DISCHARGE

The length of time that a patient needs to recuperate from his operation depends upon (1) the patient's physical and mental condition prior to surgery; (2) the magnitude of the operation; and (3) whether postoperative complications develop.

To prepare the patient and his family for the patient's discharge from the hospital is an important nursing duty. Patients who have undergone minor surgery (e.g., a D and C) require little instruction upon discharge. In such cases you will probably make an appointment for the patient to return to the hospital clinic or doctor's office for a final postoperative examination. On the other hand, patients who have undergone extensive surgery (e.g., colostomy, laryngectomy, radical mastectomy) require careful instruction before discharge. Such instruction should begin prior to the day of discharge and may include information about diet, elimination, exercises that they should perform, activities that must be limited, and possible complications of which they must be aware. Special instructions for specific operations are discussed in appropriate sections throughout the textbook.

CHAPTER 32

Preventing and Treating Postoperative Complications

The surgical patient not only faces the risk of undergoing an operation, he also faces the possibility that dangerous complications may develop during the postoperative period.

> *No matter how seemingly minor an operation is, the danger of postoperative complications is* always *present.*

Patients have hemorrhaged to death following a tonsillectomy and have gone into severe shock following a simple hernia repair.

The prevention of the development of postoperative complications should be one of your primary goals in caring for surgical patients. The prevention of postoperative complications enables the patient to convalesce swiftly, saving him time, expense, worry, and pain, perhaps even saving his life. Once postoperative problems develop, they are difficult to treat. Often one complication leads to other complications, greatly prolonging the patient's hospitalization. For example, the patient who develops pneumonia following surgery will be placed on bed rest. Immobilization in bed can lead to further problems such as thrombophlebitis, osteoporosis, and the formation of renal stones. With pneumonia, the patient's appetite frequently fails and he may develop a negative nitrogen balance which, in turn, affects the rate of wound healing. The patient, if very ill with postoperative pneumonia, will experience fever and diaphoresis, which can result in fluid and electrolyte imbalances. Intravenous fluids will probably be ordered, and the patient then suffers additional discomforts and is immobilized even more strictly. Finally, these many problems cause mental anguish for the patient and his family.

OBSERVING FOR POSTOPERATIVE COMPLICATIONS

To prevent postoperative complications, you must *know* the significant symptoms that herald the onset of a complication and be able to *recognize* quickly these symptoms once they develop. What are some important symptoms that you must be able to recognize? One authority states:

> *Fever is the commonest evidence of postoperative complications. Cardiovascular collapse, although less common, is more dramatic and emergent. Together these two signs forecast at least 90 per cent of postoperative complications.*[37]

Because recognition of these two signs will enable you to recognize the majority of postoperative complications, we shall briefly discuss their significance during the postoperative phase.

FEVER

You should expect the average postoperative patient to have a slight elevation of temperature during the first day or so following surgery. However, a marked elevation of temperature (above 100° F.) or a *persistent* fever needs to be investigated.

A sustained temperature elevation following surgery usually signals the onset of one of the following problems: (1) pulmonary complications; (2) wound infection or dehiscence; (3) urinary infections; or (4) thrombophlebitis. To remember these four complications seen in connection with fever, Liechty offers the following helpful advice:

> These causes of fever occur so frequently that they should be committed to memory as the 4 W's: "wind, wound, water, and walk." When fever occurs, these common sources should be systematically and repeatedly evaluated.[37]

Pulmonary Complications

Pulmonary problems generally develop within the *first* 48 hours after surgery. Postoperative respiratory complications may be caused by one or several of the following factors:

>Colds, flu, and sore throats that were not brought under control during the preoperative period.

> Exposure to respiratory infections following surgery.

> Use of anesthetics, endotracheal tubes, and oxygen—all of which irritate the tracheobronchial tree and cause increased mucous secretions.

> Aspiration of vomitus.

> Prolonged immobilization of patients upon the operating table during lengthy operations.

> Inability of the anesthetized patient to cough, expectorate mucus, and maintain his own airway.
> Depressing effects of many narcotics upon the coughing reflex.
> Collapse of the lung during surgery and inadequate reexpansion of lung tissue following surgery.
> Severe postoperative pain, which makes the patient reluctant to turn, cough, and deep breathe.
> Surgery with a high abdominal or chest incision that causes the patient to neglect deep breathing exercises because of pain.
> Extreme debilitation and old age, which lower the patient's resistance to pulmonary infections.
> Prolonged postoperative immobilization, which leads to decreased chest expansion, the pooling of mucus in the bronchi, and hypostatic pneumonia.

The most common lung problems seen postoperatively are atelectasis (collapse of a lung or lobe of a lung), pneumonitis, bronchitis, pneumonias (bronchial, lobar, and hypostatic) and pleurisy.*

As emphasized earlier, these conditions can be *prevented* by careful preoperative instruction concerning moving, coughing, and breathing exercises and by vigilant and repeated postoperative coaching on a planned basis (e.g., every two hours) in all these areas. The maintenance of an open airway, adequate hydration (which thins mucous secretions), and early ambulation are also of vital importance in the maintenance of respiratory function.

Should respiratory complications develop, the patient may need to undergo uncomfortable procedures, e.g., bronchoscopy (to remove mucous plugs) and postural drainage (to move secretions in the lung). Also, he may be placed on a course of antibiotic therapy. If his respiratory problems are severe, the patient will need oxygen and he may even require the use of a mechanical respirator in order to breathe.

Wound Infection

Wound infections generally occur around the fifth postoperative day, although the initial inflammatory process is often evident within 36 to 48 hours after surgery. Important factors which predispose the patient to wound infections are:

> *Obesity.* Fatty tissues do not heal readily and are difficult for the surgeon to approximate and suture.
> *Debilitation.* Persons debilitated by cancer, malnutrition, ulcerative colitis, and so forth, have a lowered resistance to *all* infection.
> *Old age.* Elderly individuals with arteriosclerosis and poor circulation have lowered defenses against infection.
> *Lengthy, complicated operations.* Complex operations place an increased stress upon the patient, which lowers his resistance.
> *Therapy with steroids, irradiation, and anticancer drugs.* These drugs and treatments can reduce the body's leukocyte count drastically.
> *The presence of other diseases,* in particular hypogammaglobulinemia, diabetes mellitus, obstructive jaundice, ulcerative colitis, uremia, leukemia, aplastic anemia, and malignant neoplasms greatly lowers the patient's resistance to wound infection.

Wound infections can also result from poor technique in the operating room, and from careless dressing techniques postoperatively.

Studies show that the general *attitude* of a hospital staff toward infection control is an important factor in the prevention or promotion of infection. For example, some surgeons and nurses have a false confidence about infection control, fostered by the availability of multiple antibiotics. The attitude of, "Oh, well, if a wound infection develops, we can always clear it up with antibiotics" remains prevalent. Also, staff personnel are sometimes careless in their aseptic technique because they fail to recognize the importance of asepsis; as a result, pick-up forceps, dressing trays, bandage scissors, and adhesive tape may often be grossly contaminated. Some people almost seem to think that "bugs just aren't there if you can't see them." Thus, *education* of hospital staff members in various positions (e.g., nurse, aide, orderly, maid) about the principles of asepsis is one important way to prevent wound infections.

The *organism* most commonly responsible for wound infections is *Staphylococcus aureus,* a gram-positive, nonmotile organism. Staphylococci produce *pyogenic* infections; their presence in a wound is usually diagnosed by laboratory examination of a specimen of wound drainage. This organism can be transmitted to the surgical patient from contaminated dressing cart equipment, and from staff members and patients who are carriers harboring the organism in their noses and throats. Failure to *isolate* patients with infections from patients with clean wounds is another common factor in the transmission of "Staph" infections.

Other organisms responsible for wound infections are *Escherichia coli, Proteus vulgaris, Aerobacter aerogenes,* and *Pseudomonas aeruginosa.*

Major symptoms of wound infection are redness, tenderness, and heat in the area of the wound or incision, coupled with the appearance of wound drainage.

Check obese patients carefully for signs of wound infection; surplus fatty tissue often obscures the presence of infection.

To *treat* wound infections, the surgeon generally irrigates and cleanses the wound with sterile normal saline solution, inserts a drain into the incision, cultures the infected drainage, and, on the basis of the findings of the culture, orders appropriate antibiotic therapy.

*These pulmonary conditions are discussed in Unit XIV.

Wound Dehiscence and Evisceration

Wound dehiscence is an opening of the wound edges, whereas wound evisceration is characterized by the protrusion of loops of bowel through the incision. Malnourished, chronically ill, and obese patients are those most prone to wound dehiscence. Related causative factors are:

> The presence of wound infections.
> Faulty closure of the wound in surgery.
> Severe stretching of the abdominal wall as a result of coughing and retching.

Although wound dehiscence and evisceration can occur at anytime, they generally occur on the 6th to 7th postoperative day. At this time, the patient's suture line is weaker than it was on the first three days after surgery. Therefore, you will want to encourage patients to cough vigorously during the first few days following surgery, while the suture line is strongest.

Make every effort to prevent the patient from developing pulmonary complications that will force him to cough vigorously on the 5th, 6th, and 7th days postoperatively, when the suture line is weaker and the wound can possibly rupture.

Any wound can rupture. However *midline abdominal incisions* are most prone to dehiscence and evisceration.

Typical *symptoms* of wound dehiscence are often dramatic. When an abdominal wound ruptures suddenly and evisceration occurs, coils of intestine protrude from the incision. When the wound edges part slowly, a gush of pinkish serous drainage is usually the major symptom.

In any postoperative patient, the sudden escape of a profuse, pink serous drainage from the wound is an ominous sign and must be investigated quickly.

To *treat* wound dehiscence, the surgeon generally orders the patient back to surgery where he resutures the wound.

The nurse's role in event of wound dehiscence is:

> Remain calm.
> Ring the emergency bell, put on the call light, or phone the hospital operator and have her notify the nurse's station on your floor to send help immediately.
> Have another nurse notify the surgeon of the emergency while you remain with the patient.
> Cover any protruding coils of intestine with sterile towels or dressings moistened with normal saline.
> Moisten the sterile towels and dressing frequently with sterile normal saline.
> Check the patient's vital signs because he may go into shock.
> Reassure the patient that the doctor is on his way. Wound dehiscence is a frightening experience!
> Set up IV equipment and have a nasal gastric tube and gastric suction equipment on hand.
> Notify surgery that the patient will be returning to the operating room.

Wound dehiscence can often be *prevented* by the proper application of a scultetus binder. However, some surgeons object to use of scultetus binders on the grounds that a binder tends to weaken the patient's muscles. Other preventative measures are the correction of nutritional deficiencies and of obesity prior to surgery.

Urinary Infections*

The most common cause of urinary infection postoperatively is catheterization. Typical symptoms of urinary infection generally occur between the 5th and 8th postoperative day. Symptoms include dysuria, frequency, and fever. To *treat* urinary infections, the surgeon will ask you to send a specimen of urine to the laboratory for culture and sensitivity. In other words, he wants to find out what organism is causing the infection (culture) and to what antibiotic the organism is sensitive (sensitivity). The doctor will then order appropriate antibiotics based upon the laboratory findings.

To prevent bladder infections, *avoid catheterization* if at all possible. Try to help the patient to void by means of the various techniques discussed in Chapter 27.

Thrombophlebitis†

Postoperative thrombophlebitis generally occurs seven to 14 days following surgery. Thrombophlebitis is sometimes caused by injury to the vein wall from the use of tight leg straps and leg holders during gynecologic surgery. Also, stasis and an increased blood coagulability (etiologic factors in thrombophlebitis) may develop postoperatively because of dehydration and an inadequate circulation resulting from hemorrhage. Obesity, prolonged immobilization, and senility are also associated with this complication.

Thrombophlebitis can be *prevented* by the use of leg exercises postoperatively, early ambulation, and wrapping the patient's legs in ace bandages while he is in bed and prior to the first time he ambulates. *Treatment* includes rest and the administration of anticoagulant drugs.

The greatest danger with thrombophlebitis is that the clot will break loose from the vein wall in the leg and will travel as an embolism to the patient's lungs, heart, or brain.

*Urinary stasis and infection are discussed in Unit V, Chapter 27, and in Unit XI.

†Thrombophlebitis is discussed in Unit V, Chapter 27, and in Unit XIII.

CARDIOVASCULAR COLLAPSE (Shock)

The commonest causes of postoperative shock are:

> Bleeding and hemorrhage (hypovolemic shock).
> Sepsis (septic shock).
> Cardiac arrest and myocardial infarction (cardiogenic shock).
> Drug sensitivity (anaphylactic shock).
> Transfusion reactions.
> Pulmonary embolism.
> Adrenal failure.

With the exception of septic shock, these specific forms of shock are discussed in appropriate sections of the text. Because sepsis is one of the most important causes of postoperative shock (indeed, some authorities state that it is the *most* common cause), we shall briefly discuss this complication.

The causes of *septic shock* are twofold. As one authority states:

> Septic shock has at least two distinctly different mechanisms for producing shock: (1) extensive cellulitis or diffuse infections of body cavities (peritonitis) cause sequestration of large amounts of plasma-like fluid into the injured tissue to produce hypovolemia, and (2) toxins produced by the infecting organisms exert profound effects upon circulation.[51]

Shock produced by gram-negative organisms is more profound that that produced by gram-positive organisms. Characteristics of shock produced by gram-negative organisms are: profound vasoconstriction, toxemia, acidosis, tissue anoxia, oliguria, heart failure, and hypotension. Gram-positive organisms, on the other hand, produce vasodilatation; acidosis and anoxia do *not* occur.

Septic shock is treated by administering massive doses of antibiotics IV, fluids, and corticosteroids.

OTHER POSTOPERATIVE COMPLICATIONS

Other important postoperative complications are: gastric dilatation, paralytic ileus, renal failure, acute parotitis, hiccoughs, decubitus ulcers, and emotional disturbances. The causes, symptoms, and clinical care of these postoperative problems are outlined below.

Acute Gastric Dilatation

This is an uncommon complication that is usually relieved within 48 hours by gastric intubation. However, death from shock may occur within a few hours.

Etiology

1. Exact etiology unknown.
2. Several liters of air and dark-colored, foul-smelling material collect in the stomach.

Symptoms

1. Overflow type vomiting.
   a. No retching present.
   b. Nausea may not be present.
   c. Vomitus tends to pour from the mouth.

Clinical Care

1. Immediate gastric intubation and suction.
2. Replacement of fluids and electrolytes.

Adynamic or Paralytic Ileus

X-rays reveal a dilated bowel, with gas distributed throughout the digestive tract.

Etiology

1. May be a reaction to anesthesia, trauma, or abdominal operations.
2. Electrolyte imbalance.
3. Wound infection.
4. Metabolic diseases.

Symptoms

1. Peristaltic activity of the gastrointestinal tract stops temporarily.
2. Bowel sounds are absent.
3. Neither gas nor feces are passed by rectum.

Clinical Care

1. Nasogastric suction.
2. IV fluid administration.
3. The Miller-Abbott intestinal tube is sometimes used.
4. A rectal tube is used to relieve flatus.

Renal Failure

This is a rare postoperative complication, but carries a high mortality rate. It is discussed in more detail in Unit XI.

Etiology

1. Prolonged preoperative or postoperative hypotension.
2. Postoperative septicemia.
3. Preexisting renal disease that was not corrected prior to surgery.

Symptoms

1. Oliguria or anuria despite adequate fluid intake.
2. Low urinary specific gravity.
3. Increased urinary sodium output.

Clinical Care

1. Early peritoneal or renal dialysis.
2. Strict fluid restriction.
3. Protective isolation to prevent infection.

Hiccoughs

Hiccoughs are usually no more than an uncomfortable nuisance that disappears after a short period. However, they may persist for weeks and, in this case, indicate a serious underlying condition. They are most likely to develop following abdominal surgery.

Etiology

1. Irritation of the phrenic nerve due to:
   a. A distended abdomen.
   b. Abscesses close to the diaphragm.
   c. Gastric dilatation.
   d. Peritonitis.
2. Anxiety.
3. Acidosis.
4. Surgical procedure performed close to the diaphragm.

Symptoms

1. Intermittent spasms of the diaphragm produce a typical sound; i.e., "hic."
2. Hiccoughs can result in:
   a. Exhaustion.
   b. Vomiting.
   c. Fluid and electrolyte imbalances.
   d. Malnutrition.
   e. Wound dehiscence.

Clinical Care

1. Rebreathing own air from a paper bag.
2. Whiffs of carbon dioxide.
3. Gastric lavage or suction.
4. Sedatives.
5. Tranquilizers.
6. In extreme cases:
   a. Phrenic nerve block.
   b. Phrenic nerve crush.

Acute Parotitis ("Surgical Mumps")

This is a rare complication of surgery. It should be given prompt attention because a secondary staphylococcal infection may develop.

Etiology

1. Poor oral hygiene following surgery.
2. Extreme debilitation.

Symptoms

Inflammation of the parotid gland which produces:

a. Pain.
b. Swelling.
c. Redness.

Clinical Care

1. X-ray therapy during the early stages.
2. Surgical incision and drainage.
3. Antibiotics.
4. Prevent by:
   a. Frequent oral hygiene.
   b. Giving fluids when allowed.
   c. Giving the patient pieces of hard candy to suck.

Decubitus Ulcers

These were discussed in detail in Chapter 27.

Etiology

1. Immobility.
2. Extreme debilitation.
3. Prolonged pressure over bony areas.
4. Preexisting arteriosclerosis.

Symptoms

Necrosis and ulceration of tissues overlying bony prominences.

Clinical Care

1. To *prevent:*
   a. Frequent movement.
   b. Early ambulation.
   c. Cleanliness.
2. For treatment, see Chapter 27.

Emotional Disturbances

Etiology

1. Grief over loss of a body organ or part.
2. Disturbances of body image.
3. Prior emotional problems.
4. Exhaustion and extreme debilitation, which lower resistance to stress.

Symptoms

1. Insomnia.
2. Restlessness.
3. Hopelessness.
4. Agitation.
5. Delusions.
6. Suicidal thoughts.

Clinical Care

1. Report these symptoms to the surgeon.
2. Give reassurance and emotional support.
3. In extreme cases use precautions against suicide:
   a. Do not leave knives or razors with the patient.
   b. Observe continuously.
   c. Make certain that patient swallows sleeping medications and does not hoard them.
   d. Do not allow near unprotected windows, especially if high, or by fire escapes.

References for Unit VI

1. Adler, R. H., and Brodie, S. L.: Postoperative rebreathing aid. *American Journal of Nursing* 68: 1287, June, 1968.
2. Brenkenridge, F., and Bruno, P.: Nursing care of the anesthetized patient. *American Journal of Nursing* 62:26, July, 1962.
3. Browse, N. L.: *The Physiology and Pathology of Bedrest.* Springfield, Illinois, Charles C Thomas, 1965.
4. Brunner, L., et al.: *Textbook of Medical-Surgical Nursing.* 2nd ed. Philadelphia, J. B. Lippincott Company, 1970.
5. Buckwalter, J. A.: Blood coagulation and transfusion. *In* Liechty, R. D., and Soper, R. T. (eds.): *Synopsis of Surgery.* St. Louis, The C. V. Mosby Company, 1968.
6. Buckwalter, J. A., and Smith, I. M.: Surgical infections. *In* Liechty, R. D., and Soper, R. T. (eds.): *Synopsis of Surgery.* St. Louis, The C. V. Mosby Company, 1968.

7. Bukutis, A.: Anesthetic reactions. *Nursing, 72* 2:16, September, 1972.
8. Burgess, M. G.: A nursing care plan for the postoperative patient in the recovery room and the intensive care unit. *Nursing Clinics of North America* 3:499, September, 1968.
9. Che-Lu, T.: The fine points of acupuncture. *AORN Journal* 17:59, January, 1973.
10. Clark, R. B.: The case for spinal anesthesia. *American Journal of Nursing* 67:294, February, 1967.
11. Cullinon, J.: Anesthesia by acupuncture. *Nursing Times* 68:1019, August 17, 1972.
12. Downs, S.: The control of vomiting. Part I. *Nursing Mirror,* January 12, 1968, p. 349; Part 2. January 19, 1968, p. 388.
13. Dumas, R., and Leonard, R. C.: The effect of nursing on the incidence of postoperative vomiting. *Nursing Research* 12:12, Winter, 1963.
14. Eisler, J., et al.: Relationship between need for social approval and postoperative recovery and welfare. *Nursing Research* 21:520, November-December, 1972.
15. Fischer, R. P., et al.: Postoperative renal failure. *Journal-Lancet* 88:42, February, 1968.
16. Furnas, D. W., and Liechty, R. D.: Wounds, wound healing, and drains. *In* Liechty, R. D., and Soper, R. T. (eds.): *Synopsis of Surgery*. St. Louis, The C. V. Mosby Company, 1968.
17. Giese, H. A., Jr.: Comparison of three agents used in surgical scrubs. *Ohio State Medical Journal* 68:855, September, 1972.
18. Gilston, A.: Recent advances in anaesthesia. *Nursing Mirror* 129:29, May 23, 1969.
19. Goegli, E. H., et al.: Can preoperative learning be improved? *AORN Journal* 16:43, November, 1972.
20. Hamilton, W. K.: Anesthesia. *In* Liechty, R. D., and Soper, R. T. (eds.): *Synopsis of Surgery*. St. Louis, The C. V. Mosby Company, 1968.
21. Heironimus, T. W.: Postoperative respiratory problems of the surgical patient. *Nursing Clinics of North America* 3:495, September, 1968.
22. Hellewell, J.: The nurse's role in anesthesia. Preoperative preparation. Part 1. *Nursing Times* 68:400, April 6, 1972.
23. Hellewell, J.: Postoperative care. Part 2. *Nursing Times* 68:443, April, 1972.
24. Hellewell, J.: Respiratory failure. Part 3. *Nursing Times* 68:467, April 20, 1972.
25. Hellewell, J.: Cardiac arrest and resuscitation. Part 4. *Nursing Times* 68:512, April 27, 1972.
26. Howat, D. D. C.: Drugs and anaesthesia. *Nursing Mirror* 128:31, April 18, 1969.
27. Inglis, J. M.: Premedication in the geriatric patient. *Geriatrics,* September, 1967, p. 115.
28. James, D. G.: The operative umbrella. Part II. *Nursing Times* 66:624, May 14, 1970.
29. Johnston, D. F.: *Essentials of Communicable Disease*. St. Louis, The C. V. Mosby Company, 1968.
30. Johnson, J. E., et al.: Psychosocial factors in the welfare of surgical patients. *Nursing Research*. 19:18, January-February, 1970.
31. Kanof, N. M.: Who needs hexachlorophene? Hospitals and some people. *J.A.M.A.* 222:409, April, 1972.
32. Kurihara, M., and Moody, F. G.: The complications of general surgery. *In* Meltzer, L. E., et al. (eds.): *Concepts and Practices of Intensive Care for Nurse Specialists*. Philadelphia, The Charles Press Publishers, Inc., 1969.
33. Lawson, L. J.: Intensive care of the surgical patient. *Postgraduate Medicine* 43:263, April, 1967.
34. Le Maitre, G., and Finnegan, J.: *The Patient in Surgery. A Guide for Nurses*. 2nd ed. Philadelphia, W. B. Saunders Company, 1970.
35. Levine, E. C., and Fielder, J. P.: Fears, facts, and fantasies about pre- and postoperative care. *Nursing Outlook* 18:26, February, 1970.
36. Liechty, R. D.: Preoperative care. *In* Liechty, R. D., and Soper, R. T. (eds.): *Synopsis of Surgery*. St. Louis, The C. V. Mosby Company, 1968.
37. Liechty, R. D.: Postoperative care. *In* Liechty, R. D., and Soper, R. T. (eds.): *Synopsis of Surgery*. St. Louis, The C. V. Mosby Company, 1968.
38. Liechty, R. D., and Soper, R. T. (eds.): *Synopsis of Surgery*. St. Louis, The C. V. Mosby Company, 1968.
39. McCarthy, R.: Vomiting. *Nursing Forum* 3:49, 1964.
40. MacIntosh, O. C.: Defining hospital infections. *Postgraduate Medicine,* November, 1967, A-119.
41. Marrow, N.: The care of the anaesthetised patient. *Nursing Times* 65:133, August 21, 1969.
42. Minckley, B. B.: Physiologic hazards of position changes in the anesthetized patient. *American Journal of Nursing* 69:2606, December, 1969.
43. Moynihan, B. G. A.: *Abdominal Operations*. Philadelphia, W. B. Saunders Company, 1905.
44. Newman, B.: The hex on hexachlorophene. *Medical Times* 101:33, February, 1973.
45. Olson, E. V., and Schroeder, L. M.: The hazards of immobility: Effects on urinary function. *American Journal of Nursing* 67:780, April, 1967.
46. Pleitz, J. A.: Psychological complications of the surgical patient. *AORN Journal* 16:137, August, 1972.
47. Reece, E. L.: Drugs that complicate anesthesia. *Journal of the American Association of Nurse Anesthetists* 38:227, June, 1970.
48. Rutherford, A. M.: Inhalation therapy in the recovery room. *Nursing Clinics of North America* 3:497, September, 1968.
49. Seymour, C. A.: Anaesthetics for the student nurse. *Nursing Times,* July 2, 1970, p. 844.
50. Smith, W. O.: Magnesium deficiency in the surgical patient. *The American Journal of Cardiology,* November, 1963, p. 667.
51. Soper, R. T.: Shock. *In* Liechty, R. D., and Soper, R. T. (eds.): *Synopsis of Surgery*. St. Louis, The C. V. Mosby Company, 1968.
52. Streeter, S., et al.: Hospital infection—A necessary risk? *American Journal of Nursing* 67:526, March, 1967.
53. Sutton, A. L.: *Bedside Nursing Techniques in Medicine and Surgery*. Philadelphia, W. B. Saunders Company, 1969.
54. Swartz, C. D.: Postoperative fluid and electrolyte management in the elderly. *Geriatrics* 22:231, 1967.
55. Vain, E. H.: Obesity in surgery. *AORN Journal* 16:85, September, 1972.
56. Veber, G. A.: Fluid and electrolyte problems in the postoperative period. *Nursing Clinics of North America* 1:275, June, 1966.
57. Waddy, F. F.: Post-operative care. *Nursing Times,* April 21, 1967, p. 510.
58. Weiler, Sister M. C.: Postoperative patients evaluate preoperative instruction. *American Journal of Nursing* 68:1465, July, 1968.
59. Ziffren, S. E.: Geriatric surgery. *In* Liechty, R. D., and Soper, R. T. (eds.): *Synopsis of Surgery*. St. Louis, The C. V. Mosby Company, 1968.

Knowledge is a powerful weapon against cancer.[1]

UNIT VII

Nursing Patients Experiencing Neoplastic Disorders

Unit Introduction and Study Guide

One purpose of this unit is to inform the student about the nature of cancer and to present relevant facts and theories concerning its prevalence, etiology, pathogenesis, diagnosis, and treatment.

A second purpose is to examine the fear of cancer that is so prevalent in our society. Fear can prevent a patient with a suspicious lump from seeking medical advice; fear can make a physician feel too uncomfortable to speak frankly with a patient who has cancer; fear can cause a nurse to view cancer nursing as a depressing and hopeless field of work, and to either resent or avoid the cancer patient. In this unit, we attempt to examine the roots of this fear both in United States society and in ourselves.

A third and final purpose of the unit is to present the challenge of cancer nursing. For too many years the care of patients with cancer has been depreciated and devalued. Fortunately, today, nurses are becoming more aware of the rewarding aspects of cancer nursing. Indeed, the modern nurse plays a vital role in both the prevention and treatment of malignant tumors. Among her many responsibilities are: (1) educating the public concerning the danger signs of cancer and the need for a yearly physical examination; (2) gathering data for cancer research projects; (3) administering dangerous chemotherapeutic drugs; (4) promoting the physical and psychologic well-being of the patient following radical surgery; (5) safeguarding the patient, herself, and others during the administration of radiotherapy; and (6) giving physical care and empathetic support to the patient with terminal cancer. It is no wonder that Barckley states:

> If we fail to perceive the excitement and challenge in cancer nursing, we miss the opportunity, given to so few, to learn the difference our own care can make in enhancing the comfort and the survival of such patients.[6]

In the following study guide, we have prepared questions and listed some basic terms and theories that will help you meet the objectives listed above:

1. Before you begin your reading ask yourself the following questions: What does the word "cancer" mean to me? What

have I already read and heard about cancer? What would I do if I discovered a suspicious lump or developed a symptom suggestive of cancer? How would I react if my doctor told me I had cancer, and that it was far advanced? How do I feel about radical surgery as a treatment for cancer? What have I read or heard about radiation therapy?

2. As you read the unit, familiarize yourself with the following terms:
cancer cure, neoplasia, benign neoplasm, malignant neoplasm, carcinoma in situ, anaplastic cells, differentiation, metastasis, cachexia, carcinoma, sarcoma, carcinogen, oncogene, precancerous lesion, Papanicolaou test, exfoliative cytology, biopsy, sentinel metastasis, intra-arterial infusion, intra-arterial perfusion, radiation, isotope, radioisotope, half-life, alpha particles, beta particles, gamma rays, sealed radioisotopes, unsealed radioisotopes, tracers, curie, roentgen, rad, scintillation counter, scintillation scanner, radiosensitivity, radioresistance, external radiotherapy, x-ray therapy, teletherapy, internal radiotherapy, interstitial therapy, intracavitary therapy, distance, time, shielding, external hazard, internal hazard.

3. Familiarize yourself with the following theories and concepts concerning cancer: multistage theory, progression, multifactoral theory, viral theory, oncogene theory, biologic determinism, immune theory, spontaneous regression.

4. Following your reading, attempt to answer the following questions:

a. What is the difference between a benign and a malignant neoplasm?

b. What are the seven warning signs of cancer?

c. What are the seven safeguards against cancer?

d. What is the purpose and value of the Papanicolaou test?

e. What is the purpose of a biopsy?

f. What are the manifestations of cancer?

g. What are the four major types of surgery performed in the management of cancer?

h. What are the major classes of agents used in cancer chemotherapy?

i. What are the toxic effects of cancer chemotherapy? How can these effects be prevented or treated?

j. What are the two *regional* methods of drug administration?

k. What is the procedure for an "organ scan"?

l. What precautions must the nurse observe during external radiotherapy?

m. What precautions must the nurse observe during internal radiotherapy? with sealed sources? with unsealed sources?

n. What are the toxic effects of radiotherapy?

o. What problems does the patient with terminal cancer face? How can you alleviate or lessen the severity of these problems?

CHAPTER 33

Introductory Concepts in Cancer Nursing

When Dr. Oliver Wendell Holmes discovered that the author Nathaniel Hawthorne had cancer, he is said to have remarked, "The shark's tooth is upon him."[2]

Cancer, "the shark's tooth" that unrelentingly strikes and kills its victims, is characterized by the disorderly, uncontrolled multiplication and growth of abnormal cells and by the spread of these cells into normal tissues throughout the body. The dissemination of cancer cells into healthy tissues eventually leads to widespread tissue destruction and to the death of the host unless medical therapy is instituted.

The word *cancer* is derived from the Latin word meaning "crab." No one knows why this term is used to designate malignant disease. There is no evidence that the ancient Greeks or Romans connected the advent of malignancy with the influence of the crab, one of the constellations of the zodiac. Perhaps the word "cancer" is simply descriptive of the crablike extension of malignant cells into healthy tissue and the deadly "hold" or crablike grip that the disease has upon its victims.[4]

The victims of cancer are not only human beings, but animals and plants as well. Indeed, malignancy in animals has given scientists an opportunity to study the growth and development of cancer cells in vivo—study that has implications for the development of cancer in humans.

Within the United States and throughout the world, cancer has been and continues to be a tremendous social and economic problem. Today, cancer ranks second as a cause of death in this country, preceded only by the cardiovascular disorders. Cancer develops and grows in one out of every four persons and strikes two out of every three families. When cancer strikes, it kills unless there is rapid medical intervention. Statisticians estimate that approximately 3 to 5 million persons will die of cancer during the 1970's, while 6.5 million persons will develop cancer and 10 million people will be under medical supervision for the disease.

Moreover, cancer is costly in dollars as well as lives. Over 12 billion dollars a year are spent on the care of patients with cancer and on cancer research. And still the precise interplay of those factors that probably cause cancer remains unknown.

BASIC CHARACTERISTICS OF CANCER CELLS: AN OVERVIEW

What is a cancer cell? How does it differ from a normal cell and what are the factors that cause cancer cells to develop? (See also Chapter 34.)

You will recall from Chapter 21 that the cell is the basic unit or building block of structure for all forms of plant and animal life, and that within the human body there are approximately 60,000 billion cells. Each of these cells carries out precise and highly specialized functions that are harmoniously interlocked with the activities and functions of other cells; as a result of coordinated cellular activities, the body grows and performs as an integrated whole.

Unfortunately a normal cell can undergo changes that transform it into a cancer cell, which has different characteristics from other cells in the same tissue. The cancer cell, like the normal cell, can exactly and endlessly reproduce itself. However, unlike normal cells, cancer cells serve no useful purpose, and they grow in a disorderly and unrestricted fashion.

Exactly what causes this transformation from normal cell to malignant cell is not known; however, there is evidence that viruses, certain physical and chemical agents, and radiant energy may, in some way, cause the change.

Cancer, then, generally begins as a "localized" disease; it is initiated by the transformation of a single normal cell or cells into an abnormal cell or cells. As the malignant cells reproduce, a visible tumorous growth is produced. The tumor may remain localized for a time in its place of origin (in situ). Later, the cancer cells may begin to invade surrounding tissues and structures (invasive cancer). Still later, the malignant cells may leave their site of origin and spread or metastasize via blood vessels and lymph nodes to other tissues. This deadly form of cancer is called *metastatic* cancer. Once cancer has reached the metastatic stage, it is extremely difficult to treat or cure.

STATISTICAL CONSIDERATIONS

CANCER INCIDENCE AND MORTALITY RATES WITHIN THE UNITED STATES

According to the 1973 *Cancer Facts and Figures,* 1,025,000 Americans were being treated for cancer in 1973, and 665,000 more persons were predicted to develop cancer during the year and be diagnosed for the first time. Statisticians predict that more than 53 million persons living in the United States today will develop cancer.

The incidence of reported cases of cancer has been steadily increasing since 1900. There are at least five reasons for this apparent rise in incidence. First of all, *diagnostic methods* are far more precise today than in the past. Thus, many more persons are now being diagnosed who would have died from "unknown causes" years ago. Second, the gathering, analysis, and publication of *statistics* concerning cancer has become more sophisticated over the years. In the past many persons with cancer were undoubtedly overlooked in the gathering of information and were not included in the yearly reports on cancer morbidity and mortality. Third, the *classification* of cancer disorders has grown to include Hodgkin's disease and leukemia. In 1973 alone, 19,000 persons were diagnosed with leukemia and 4,800 persons with Hodgkin's disease. Fourth, the *entire population* of the United States has increased substantially since the turn of the century. Finally, due to advances in medical science, people are *living longer* today than even a few decades ago. Because older persons are more vulnerable to cancer than young persons, the incidence of cancer is higher now than when more people died at an early age. In sum, the apparent rise in the incidence of cancer is somewhat misleading; it may simply reflect more precise diagnostic and statistical methods as well as alterations in age span of the population.

Like the incidence rate, the mortality rate for cancer is also rising. In 1900 cancer ranked seventh as a cause of death in the United States; today it ranks second, preceded only by cardiovascular disorders. Thus, today one person dies of cancer for every five persons who die from all other causes, including accidents.

While the overall incidence and mortality rates for cancer are on the increase, the incidence of the *various types* of cancer varies. Below we have briefly summarized the relative incidence of the principal types of cancer.

Breast cancer is the leading cause of cancer deaths in American women. Of every 100 women, 7 will some day suffer from breast cancer.

Lung cancer is the leading cause of cancer death in American men. Among both sexes (but particularly in males) the incidence of lung cancer is rising rapidly. The rate of deaths of American males from lung cancer is 18 times higher today than 40 years ago. Researchers believe that the risk of developing lung cancer is definitely increased by habitual heavy cigarette smoking.

Colon-rectal cancer has a higher incidence in the United States than any other form of cancer with the exception of skin cancer. Both sexes are equally susceptible to this form of malignancy.

The death rate from *uterine cancer* is fortunately decreasing; indeed, the rate is down one third from what it was 35 years ago. This decline in deaths from uterine cancer probably reflects more precise diagnostic and treatment methods as well as the widespread schooling of women concerning the necessity for a "pap" smear.

Skin cancer has the highest incidence of all forms of cancer; fortunately, however, skin malignancy is also the most preventable form of cancer and has the highest cure rate.

Oral cancer and *cancer of the prostate* also affect considerable numbers of persons in the United States and elsewhere. Prostatic cancer predominantly affects men over 60.

CURE RATES

A patient who is cured of cancer is defined as an individual who "is without evidence of disease for at least five years after diagnosis and treatment."[12] Of course, there are many exceptions to this definition. For example, some patients may be cured after two years, while other patients may suffer for 10 years before they are free of cancer. However, the medical consensus is that it takes approximately five years for the average patient with cancer to be cured of his disease.

Although cancer incidence and mortality rates are increasing, cancer cure rates are fortunately accelerating even more rapidly. Early in this century, most patients who developed cancer died. By the late 1930's less than one person out of five was cured; by the late 1940's one patient out of every four with cancer was cured. Today the cure rate has risen to a ratio of one cancer cure to every three deaths—a significant saving of human life.

However, if more individuals sought early diagnosis and treatment for suspicious symptoms, many more lives could be saved. The American Cancer Association points out:

> Of every six persons who get cancer today, two will be saved and four will die. Numbers 1 and 2 will be saved. Number 3 will die but might have been saved had proper treatment been received in time. Numbers 4, 5, 6 will die of cancers which cannot yet be controlled; only the results of research can save these patients. This means that about half of those who get cancer could and should be saved—by early diagnosis and prompt treatment. Thus the immediate goal of cancer control in this country is the annual saving of 333,000 lives, or half of those who develop cancer each year.[12]

THE IMPACT OF CANCER UPON THE PATIENT, THE NURSE, AND THE COMMUNITY

When cancer strikes, it affects a number of different people. Naturally it most intimately injures the patient and his immediate family. Also, a diagnosis of cancer may cause adverse reactions in the nurses, doctors, and other personnel who must care for the patient. Finally, cancer disrupts the community as a whole in a variety of ways.

CANCER, THE PATIENT AND THE FAMILY

Different people react in different ways to a suspicious lesion or symptom, to a confirmed diagnosis of cancer, and to the daily progression of the disease. Reactions generally depend upon the patient's age, maturity, family relations, economic situation, emotional stability, and knowledge of cancer causation and cure. For example, consider the following case histories.

Miss Jones, an attractive 32 year old woman, noted a lump in her breast one morning when she was showering. Every day thereafter she would examine her breast with the hope that the lump had disappeared. Miss Jones, who was a high school science teacher, knew that she should immediately make an appointment to see her doctor; however, she always found excuses for not doing so. Having an attractive body was important to Miss Jones; she realized that if the lump was cancerous, she might be permanently disfigured by the loss of a breast. Finally, she convinced herself that the lump was probably harmless. By the time Miss Jones did seek medical aid the tumor had grown to a considerable size. Upon biopsy, the growth was found to be malignant, and Miss Jones was forced to undergo a mastectomy.

When Mr. Carl learned from his doctor that he had cancer of the rectum, he became extremely depressed. The news that he would have to undergo a bowel resection and the creation of a permanent colostomy upset him terribly; he doubted that he could live through the surgery. Between the time of his diagnosis and the day of surgery, Mr. Carl's whole personality and outlook on life changed. A usually gregarious, cheerful person, he became silent and withdrawn. He had little to say to family and friends; and his fear of death grew, he sought only his priest. Even following relatively successful surgery, Mr. Carl remained depressed and despondent for months. He felt disgusted by the sight of his colostomy, and believed that it made him offensive to friends and family.

Mrs. Gray, a young mother of one child, had deeply wished for a second child to complete her family. Her husband also wanted another child. When Mrs. Gray's doctor discovered that she had cervical cancer and would require a hysterectomy, Mrs. Gray became quite anxious about the effect of the surgery upon her marriage; nevertheless, she agreed to undergo the operation. Following surgery Mrs. Gray began to develop severe anxieties concerning herself and her role as wife and mother. She increasingly deprecated her value as a person. Frequently she made statements such as "I'm only half a woman now"; "I'm no good to my husband, he won't love me any more"; "I can't have children like other women." As her distress increased, Mrs. Gray even contemplated suicide. Alarmed, her husband and doctor insisted that she seek psychiatric help. Eventually, with the aid of her doctors and husband, Mrs. Gray was able to accept herself and the realities of her situation.

Mrs. Heath, 42, a housewife with a large family, had had a radical mastectomy for breast cancer. Three years later she discovered a lump in her groin. However, she did not inform her husband or doctor of the growth. Instead she sent away for some herbal medications for cancer that were advertised in a magazine. She hoped that the medicine would make the lump "go away." Mrs. Heath did not feel that she could stand the pain of another radical procedure. She chose instead to seek "painless" but totally unreliable, unorthodox methods of "treatment" in the hope of a miraculous cure.

Note that each of the individuals described above responded to the diagnosis of cancer and the need for extensive surgery with *fear*. However, the fear experienced by these patients took different forms. Miss Jones feared destruction of her feminine appearance and her body image; Mr. Carl feared the loss of life and later of his friends and family; Mrs. Gray feared the loss of her ideal feminine role as mother and wife; whereas Mrs. Heath feared the pain, misery, and discomfort involved in radical surgery. Moreover, not only did each cancer patient fear something different, but each person's response to fear varied. Thus, Miss Jones denied the possibility of a cancerous lump in her breast; Mr. Carl retreated from life and loved ones; Mrs. Gray became agitated and suicidal; and Mrs. Heath turned to quackery and resorted to "magical" thinking. Some patients meekly resign themselves to their fate, whereas others commit suicide in the belief that their life is no longer worth living.

Of course, not all patients respond so negatively to a diagnosis of cancer. Some persons, as the result of a strong religious belief or a stoic philosophy of life, are able to accept their condition with equanimity and courage despite underlying fears.

The patient's *family* is also profoundly affected when a member is diagnosed as having cancer. The advent of cancer within a family can mean the loss of a spouse, the loss of a parent, or the loss of a child. Furthermore, the family suffers economically as well as emotionally when a member develops cancer. Diagnostic tests, hospitalization, radiation therapy, chemotherapy, and surgery are all very expensive. Paying for needed medical services may keep a family in debt for years. Also, if the husband or wife dies of cancer, the family loses the earning power of that individual. If the mother of young children dies, the father will need to either hire domestic help to take her place or send the children away to live with relatives. Thus, the advent of cancer may severely disrupt family life and even destroy it.

Like the patient himself, the patient's family may react to a diagnosis of cancer in several ways. Some family members feel guilty, believing that they are somehow responsible for the patient's illness. Others feel depressed and despondent over the possible death of someone they love. Still others may feel resentful and hostile; the financial burden plus the emotional burden of caring for a sick relative may be too heavy for some persons to bear. Some family members may beg the patient's doctor to do everything possible to save the patient's life; others may ask the physician to "let the patient be," to let him die in peace.

CANCER AND THE NURSE

Nurses and doctors, despite their scientific training, are as vulnerable to the fear of cancer as are other persons. Let us briefly examine the roots of this fear and the effect that fear has upon the nurse's ability to care for persons with cancer.

First of all, doctors and nurses know, perhaps better than anyone else, that cancer brings disfigurement, pain, tissue destruction, and death to its unfortunate victims. Thus, cancer is firmly linked, even in the minds of nurses, with an image of despair, destruction, and decay. Moreover, cancer has not been romanticized and ennobled in the minds of laymen and professionals as have other diseases. As one author explains:

> Many of us continue to think of heart disease as a badge of honor, signifying the wearer has an important job where stress has made its inroads, or that he has been an exceptionally hard worker. All forms can be discussed anywhere with melancholy pride. But this is not true of cancer. If heart disease is equated with the strains of command, and tuberculosis with poverty, cancer still has an image of mystery tinged with doom.[6]

Thus, doctors and nurses, because of their own anxiety concerning the destructiveness and ignominy of cancer, may find themselves avoiding the care of cancer patients in favor of caring for patients with other less frightening diseases.

Another reason that nurses and doctors may fear cancer is because our knowledge of cancer causation and cure is still so incomplete. Professional persons in the allied medical fields realize that they are as prone to the development of cancer as is the layman. This frightening realization, whether conscious or unconscious, can cause some nurses and physicians to avoid caring for patients with cancer.

Our lack of scientific knowledge concerning cancer has yet another adverse effect upon the nurse. Because of current inadequacies in cancer diagnosis and therapy, nurses who work with cancer patients see their patients die more often than patients with other diseases. Thus, the care of cancer patients is often a source of frustration and a sense of failure for the nurse.

And yet the patient with cancer needs, above all, a sympathetic and empathetic nurse, a person who is interested in him, who wants to care for him, and *who does not fear him* because of his disease. In other words, the cancer patient needs a nurse who has faced and overcome her own fear of cancer to the extent that she can consistently give empathetic care. To give such care to the terminal patient, the nurse must believe that the patient's life holds *meaning for him* despite the fact that it is ending.

Second, biochemists, physiologists, physicians, nurses, and others are endeavoring to alleviate cancer by means of painstaking research into its causes and cure. The major goal of cancer research is to find answers to the following basic questions:

> What factor or factors cause a normal cell or cells to become cancerous? What predisposing events promote the development of cancer?
>
> What part do viruses play in the causation of cancer? What is the role of immunity in preventing cancer?
>
> What methods can be used to identify cancer-prone individuals? What methods will enable doctors to diagnose cancer early in the course of the disease?
>
> What drugs can be developed that will stop the unrelenting division and multiplication of cancer cells?
>
> What improvements can be made in cancer surgery and irradiation?

We may learn the answers to these questions soon. Scientists are hopeful that they will find the cure for cancer during the 1970's. George Tadaro of the National Cancer Institute states hopefully, "We may well be the last generation of mankind to carry the burden of cancer on our shoulders."[2]

CANCER AND THE COMMUNITY

Cancer not only adversely affects individuals; it also produces devastating effects upon the community at large. Cancer exacts a heavy toll from the community in terms of both dollars and man-hours of labor.

The community also loses the abilities, skills, and working hours of the cancer victim, who is often in the prime of his life and at the peak of his efficiency. The President's Commission on Heart Disease, Cancer, and Stroke stated that cancer among persons under 65 costs the nation "72,000 man-years of productivity among the labor force, 44,000 man-years among those keeping house, and 52,000 man-years among those unable to work."[12] Cancer, more than any other disease, causes women to lose working years from their lives, and among men, cancer ranks third as a cause of loss of working years, preceded only by accidents and heart disease.

What has the nation and the community at large done to control and alleviate this costly and demoralizing disease? First of all, both professional and lay members of society have formed and organized cancer agencies and organizations that are devoted to education, research, prevention, early diagnosis, and services for persons suffering from cancer. The two major organizations devoted to cancer control are as follows:

American Cancer Society, Incorporated (ACS) is a national voluntary agency through which approximately 2.25 million persons are involved in the fight against cancer. The ACS has its main office in New York City and 58 Chartered Divisions and 3100 Units scattered over the 50 states. The society is involved in public and professional education and in the formation of research programs and the training of research personnel. Units of the ACS also work with cancer patients and their families.

The *National Cancer Institute* within the National Institutes of Health was created in 1937 in order to develop extensive cancer research programs.

CHAPTER 34

Neoplastic Disease: Tumor Growth and Theories of Causation

The word "cancer" is synonymous with the term malignant neoplasm. The word *neoplasm* is derived from the Greek *neo* which means "new" and *plasia,* "growth." Thus the term, literally defined, means the growth of new tissues. Defined medically, a neoplasm is an *abnormal* new growth of tissue which serves no purpose and which can be highly damaging to the host.

A neoplasm may be either benign or malignant. A *benign* neoplasm is an abnormal growth of tissue that is relatively harmless and does not spread to and infiltrate other tissues. On the other hand, a *malignant* neoplasm is an abnormal growth that is always harmful to the body and that may spread or metastasize to other tissues far removed from the site of origin.

The term neoplasm is often, somewhat incorrectly, equated with the term *tumor*. Strictly defined, a tumor is simply an abnormal swelling or enlargement, and is one of the four signs of inflammation—redness, heat, pain, swelling (or *tumor*). Whereas the proliferation of neoplastic cells results in a tumor, tumorous swellings can also develop as a result of either inflammatory changes or abnormal accumulations of fluid or blood within a limited area of tissue, e.g., a hematoma or blood tumor. The terms tumor and neoplasm, then, are not truly synonymous.

STRUCTURE AND GROWTH OF NEOPLASTIC CELLS

Neoplastic cells differ from normal cells in terms of appearance, patterns of growth, and physiologic function. In *appearance,* neoplastic cells are usually larger than are normal cells and they have a bigger nucleus; also neoplastic cells tend to differ substantially from *each other* in terms of size and shape while normal cells are more homogeneous.

The *extent* to which neoplastic cells are abnormal in appearance depends upon whether the tumor they form is benign or malignant. In *benign* tumors neoplastic cells tend to closely resemble healthy cells. On the other hand, *malignant* tumors are characterized by cells that may bear almost no resemblance to those cells that normally compose the afflicted tissue. Neoplastic cells that are strikingly deviant from normal cells are called *anaplastic cells*. Anaplastic cells tend to be primitive and embryonic in type, and they characteristically grow into disorganized, irregular cellular nests or sheets. The presence of anaplastic cells in a tumor is the "best criterion of malignancy."[41]

In terms of *growth,* neoplastic cells seem to proliferate in response to abnormal stimuli (physical, chemical, hormonal, and viral agents). Furthermore, the rules of growth that normally govern healthy cellular reproduction seem unable to halt or restrict the proliferation of neoplastic cells. Why neoplastic cells continue to reproduce themselves endlessly and abnormally is an important question.

In reference to *function*, malignant cells, unlike normal cells, serve no purpose. The end result of neoplastic cellular growth is an abnormal tissue mass which does not function in any useful way and consequently cannot contribute to the well-being of the host.

In sum, neoplastic cells are the anarchists of the body. They are primitive in appearance, and they divide and multiply endlessly without regard for the normal physiologic rules of growth that dominate normal cells. Moreover, neoplastic cells exist as parasites, occupying space and drawing nutrition and sustenance from the host's body while contributing nothing in return.

FORMATION OF NEOPLASMS

Neoplastic cells mass together to form neoplastic tissue growths or tumors. Each neoplastic tumor is composed of two parts: (1) the *parenchyma* of the tumor, which is the major part, and which is composed of parenchymal tumor cells, and (2) the *stroma,* which is composed of connective tissue and blood vessels and which supports and provides structure for the parenchymal tumor cells.[41] The blood vessels of the stroma feed and nourish the tumor, especially when it first forms and begins to grow.

The tissue of a neoplastic tumor may closely resemble the normal tissue of the structure on which it grows or it may look completely different. The extent to which the tissue cells of the parenchyma of the tumor resemble normal cells is termed *differentiation.* A tumor is *well differentiated* if its cells appear to be almost normal; benign tumors are almost always well differentiated. Conversely, a tumor is *poorly differentiated* if it is composed largely of primitive, anaplastic cells. Malignant tumors, which are composed mainly of anaplastic cells and which bear little resemblance to normal tissue masses, are said to be *dedifferentiated.* The degree of differentiation of tumor cells is sometimes calculated on a graded scale ranging from I to IV. Grade I implies that the tumor cells closely resemble normal cells, while Grade IV implies that the tumor cells deviate widely from normal.

How do neoplasms develop? Slowly or rapidly? According to the *multistage theory* of tumor evolution, malignant neoplasms grow and develop slowly and pass through two or more different stages during their period of maturation. Also, this theory supports the view that cancerous tumors *gradually* acquire their characteristics over a period of time rather than all at once; this phenomenon by which malignancies attain their characteristics slowly is called *progression.*[41]

CHARACTERISTICS OF BENIGN AND MALIGNANT NEOPLASMS

As we have already implied, neoplastic tumors are classified as either benign neoplasms or malignant neoplasms.

> *Deciding whether a tumor is benign or malignant is probably the most important decision a physician must make when treating a patient with a tumorous growth.*

Let us first consider the *benign tumor.* The word *benign* comes from the Latin *bene* meaning "good" and *genus* which means "sort." Thus a benign tumor is a "good sort of tumor," or at least it is a tumor of limited growth that will not radically harm or kill the host. But the benign tumor, however harmless, does *occupy space.* Consequently, if a benign neoplasm is located in a strategic position, it can cause the obstruction of tubes and the compression of vital tissues. As a rule, however, if a tumor is benign, the patient will generally have a good prognosis because the tumor can be readily excised.

Malignant tumors, on the other hand, represent a serious threat to the life and well-being of the host. The word *malignant* comes from the Latin word *malus* which means "bad." Thus a malignant tumor is a "bad sort of tumor" that, in contrast to the benign tumor, brings pain and death to the host. Malignant neoplasms are dangerous not only because they occupy space but because they grow in a radical and disorganized fashion. Also, they release their cancerous cells for dissemination throughout the body. Moreover, they sap and drain the metabolic and nutritional resources of the host, leaving the patient weak, anemic, and subject to fatal infections. Thus, the individual with a malignant neoplasm often has a poor prognosis. Malignant neoplasms, because of their invasive and metastatic nature, cannot be readily excised or cured, as can the benign tumor. Table 34–1 compares the characteristics of these two major types of neoplasms.

METASTASIS

Because *metastasis* is the most dangerous and life-threatening aspect of neoplastic disease, we are going to discuss this phenomenon in more detail. Some important questions and answers concerning the causes and effects of metastasis are considered below.

Q. What is the exact meaning of the term *metastasis?*
A. The word metastasis is derived from the Greek word *meta* meaning "beyond" and *stasis* meaning "standing." Metastasis means the capacity of cancer cells (or in some cases bacteria) to move from one body tissue or organ to another body tissue or organ. *Metastases,* then, are secondary tumor growths that result from the migration and spread of malignant tumor cells from the *primary* site or original area of neoplastic activity. The capacity of a neoplastic tumor to metastasize to other sites is a major characteristic of malignancy, and it definitely distinguishes malignant from benign growths.
Q. What tissues and organs of the body are most frequently invaded by metastasizing cancer cells?
A. The lymph nodes, liver, lungs, bones, and brain are the most common sites for metastasis. Also tissues that have been previously injured are highly susceptible to metastasis. Statistics concerning preferred sites for metastasis are as follows:[36]

> *Lymph node* involvement occurs in approximately 50 per cent of terminal cancer patients.

> *Liver metastases* develop in 36 per cent of patients.

> *Lung metastases* occur in 30 per cent of patients.

> *Bone* involvement occurs in approximately 15 to 20 per cent of terminal patients. The bones most commonly involved (in descending order) are the vertebrae, ribs, skull, femur, pelvis, humerus, and sternum.

> The *brain* develops metastatic growths in approximately 5 per cent of terminal patients, especially those with primary cancer of the breast, lung, and kidney.

> *Sites of metastasis* can also metastasize to other organs, further complicating the patient's condition.

Q. Do all malignant tumors metastasize?
A. No, even though all tumors that metastasize are malignant, not all malignant tumors metasta-

size. Some *types* of malignant tumors metastasize more readily than others, and some patients are apparently more susceptible to metastatic growths than are other individuals.

Q. What factors are believed to cause malignant tumors to metastasize?

A. Knowledge is incomplete concerning the factors responsible for metastasis. However, the factors listed below are believed to play an important role in the spread of cancer cells:

> Malignant cells have a *lower cohesiveness* than normal cells, which enables them to break away easily from their parent tumor and travel to new locations.

> Cancer cells have the ability to *survive* for a period of time *independent* of other cells; thus, malignant cells are able to stay alive long enough to be transported as separate entities via blood or lymph from one site to another.

> Malignant cells are *invasive,* a quality that facilitates their passage through various defensive barriers (e.g., fibrous tissue barricades), into normal tissues.

Q. What steps are involved in the formation of a metastasis?

A. Robbins points out that there are three steps involved in the formation of a secondary growth. They are:[41]

Step 1: Separation of the malignant tumor cells from their parent tumor; these liberated cells now begin a period of travel through the body,

TABLE 34-1. A COMPARISON OF THE CHARACTERISTICS OF BENIGN AND MALIGNANT NEOPLASMS

Characteristic	Benign Neoplasm	Malignant Neoplasm
Speed of growth	Grows slowly usually continues to grow throughout life unless surgically removed; may have periods of remission during which growth stops for a time	Grows usually rapidly, tends to grow relentlessly throughout life; rarely, neoplasm may *regress spontaneously*
Mode of growth	Grows by enlarging and expanding; always remains localized; never infiltrates surrounding tissues	Grows by infiltrating surrounding tissues; may remain localized (in situ) but usually spreads out to infiltrate other tissues
Presence of capsule	Almost always contained and confined within a fibrous capsule; capsule does not prevent expansion of neoplasm but does prevent growth by infiltration; capsule advantageous because it and enclosed tumor cells can be easily removed surgically	Never contained and confined within a capsule; absence of capsule allows neoplastic cells to invade surrounding tissues; absence of capsule makes surgical removal of tumor more difficult
Characteristics of cells composing tumor	Usually well differentiated; mitotic figures absent or scanty; cells appear adult; anaplastic cells absent; cells function poorly in comparison with normal cells from which they arise; if neoplasm arises in glandular tissue, cells may be capable of secreting hormones	Usually poorly differentiated; large numbers of normal and abnormal mitotic figures present; cells tend to be anaplastic, i.e., young, embryonic type cells; cells too abnormal to perform any physiologic functions; occasionally a malignant tumor arising in glandular tissue may secrete hormones
Recurrence	Recurrence extremely unusual when surgically removed	Recurrence common following surgery because of spread of tumor cells into surrounding tissues
Metastasis or spread of tumor from original site to other organs of body	Metastases never occur	Metastases very common; most dangerous and deadly aspect of neoplastic disease (see discussion below)
Effect of neoplasm on tissues and body as a whole	Not harmful to host unless neoplasm located in area where it causes compression of tissues or obstruction of vital organs; does not produce *cachexia* (weight loss, debilitation, anemia, weakness, wasting); neoplasm located in glandular tissue may secrete the hormone normally produced, resulting in *excess* of hormone in blood	Always harmful to the host; will result in death unless removed surgically or destroyed by radiation or chemotherapy; causes disfigurement of the body, disrupted organ functions, and nutritional imbalances; may result in ulcerations, sepsis, perforations, hemorrhage, and tissue slough; almost always produces cachexia, which leaves patient prone to pneumonia, anemia, etc.; infrequently malignant tumors secrete hormones, causing a hormonal imbalance; usually cells too poorly differentiated to produce normal body secretions
Prognosis	Very good; tumor generally removed surgically	Depends upon speed with which cancer diagnosed; poor prognosis indicated if cells are poorly differentiated and evidence exists of metastatic spread; good prognosis indicated if cells still resemble normal and there is no evidence of metastasis

during which time they are dependent upon their own resources for survival.

Step 2: Spread of the tumor cells from the primary site to the secondary site via one of the following three pathways:

> The *lymphatic channels:* These vessels constitute the most common route for widespread dissemination of cancer cells. For example, there are numerous lymph channels around the breast and particularly in the axilla. Thus, in patients with breast cancer, some cancer cells may spread through the lymph channels into the lymph nodes where they form metastatic growths. Other cancer cells may travel from the lymph channels around the breast to distant sites all over the body.

> The *blood vessels* (including both veins and arteries): these channels typically carry cancer cells from the primary tumor to the lungs, liver, and bones.

> *Transplantation* or the *direct transport* of tumor cells from one site to another site: this phenomenon can occur accidentally during surgery; malignant cells are carried via instruments or gloves. Also, malignant cells can slough off from diseased organs within the peritoneal cavity and drop down onto an ovary or onto the mesentery.

Step 3. Establishment and *growth* of the tumor cell at the secondary site: For the metastasizing cells to develop, the environment of the new site must be suitable to the growth of the cancer cells. Exactly why certain metastasizing cells grow well in one site but not in another remains unknown.

Q. How long does it take for a metastatic growth to be detectable?

A. A new neoplastic growth cannot be detected until it contains around 500 cells and is approximately 1 cm. in size. The length of time needed to produce a nodule 1 cm. in diameter depends upon the particular reproductive cycle of the malignant cells composing the growth. If the cells reproduce rapidly, the metastatic growth may obtain a size of 1 cm. within months; if the cells proliferate slowly, it may be many years before the metastatic growth is large enough for detection.

Q. What is the effect of metastasis upon the patient?

A. The growth of a secondary tumor puts severe additional stress upon the host, whose strength has already been sapped by the primary growth. Thus, the patient with metastases becomes rapidly cachexic. Cancer with metastasis generally terminates in the patient's death.

CLASSIFICATION OF BENIGN AND MALIGNANT NEOPLASMS

Neoplasms are classified not only in terms of whether they are benign or malignant; they are also grouped according to the tissue from which they arise (Table 34–2).

As you study Table 34–2, note that almost all names for tumors end in the suffix "oma" meaning "tumor." In turn, the suffix "oma" is usually attached to a term for the parent tissue of the tumors; thus adenoma comes from the Greek *aden,* "gland" plus "oma." When more than one parent tissue enters into the formation of a neoplasm, the names of the tumors are even more descriptive. For example, an adenomyoma is a benign neoplasm that contains both glandular and muscle cells; a leiomyofibroma is a fibroid tumor of the uterus that contains both smooth muscle and fibrous connective tissue.

Benign tumors of *epithelial origin* are not so easily classified and named as are tumors arising from mesenchymal origin, i.e., fibrous tissue, bone, muscle, blood vessels, lymphatics, and nerves; this is because epithelial tissues are of many different varieties. For this reason, benign tumors of epithelial origin are classified according to either their microscopic appearance (e.g., an adenoma is a tumor with glandular elements) or their gross structure; e.g., a polyp (from the Greek *polys* many + *pous* foot) is a benign tumor of epithelial origin with a pedicle or stem that attaches the growth to a mucous membrane.

Three of the most common benign tumors listed in Table 34–2 are the fibroma, lipoma, and leiomyoma.

The *fibroma* may grow anywhere in the body, but it very frequently makes its home in the uterus. Fibromas are generally small, but occasionally they grow to great size. These encapsulated, relatively harmless tumors do not cause symptoms unless, due to location, they place pressure on a bone or nerve. Fibromas are easily removed surgically.

The *lipoma,* which is a very common benign tumor, arises in adipose tissue. Lipomas rarely cause symptoms; however, they are poorly encapsulated and they may put pressure on surrounding tissues as they expand.

The *leiomyoma,* a benign neoplasm of smooth muscle origin, is the most common benign tumor in women. Leiomyomas may develop anywhere in the body, but they most commonly grow in the uterus. Rarely (in approximately 1 per cent of cases), these tumors become malignant.

Let us next consider the classification of malignant tumors. A malignant tumor that arises from *epithelial* tissue is called a *carcinoma,* whereas a malignant neoplasm that arises from *mesenchymal* origins (i.e., blood vessels, lymphatics, nerve tissue) is called a *sarcoma* (Greek *sarc* means flesh).

Three representative examples of malignant neoplasms are carcinoma in situ, fibrosarcoma, and bronchogenic carcinoma.

Carcinoma in situ is a neoplasm of epithelial tissue that remains *confined* to the site of origin. In situ carcinoma typically affects the uterus, developing in the squamous epithelium along the surface of the cervix. This form of cancer usually remains localized and thus can be removed surgically. However, it is well to remember that in situ carcinoma can become invasive, eroding into surrounding tissues.

The malignant fibrosarcomas are similar to

benign fibromas. Fibrosarcomas tend to grow in the same sites and may originate as benign fibromas, later becoming malignant. These bulky, well differentiated tumor masses are usually responsive to surgery. Fortunately, fibrosarcomas rarely metastasize.

Bronchogenic carcinoma is the cause of 90 per cent of all cases of lung cancer. Bronchogenic carcinoma usually develops in the lower trachea and lower bronchi. Surgical excision of the tumor is the treatment of choice. However, this type of cancer readily gives rise to metastases, and if this occurs, surgical treatment can be only palliative.

PATHOGENESIS AND ETIOLOGY OF CANCER

The pathogenesis of cancer is the mechanism by which etiologic agents transform normal cells into tumor cells. Although scientists have learned a great deal about the etiologic agents responsible for cancer (viruses, chemicals, radiation), the *exact* mechanism by which these agents transform healthy cells into neoplastic cells still remains obscure.

One premise that most scientists accept today is that cancer develops as a result of some irre-

TABLE 34–2. CLASSIFICATION OF NEOPLASMS*

Tissue of Origin	Benign	Malignant
Connective tissues		Sarcoma
Embryonic fibrous tissue	Myxoma	Myxosarcoma
Fibrous tissue	Fibroma	Fibrosarcoma
Adipose tissue	Lipoma	Liposarcoma
Cartilage	Chondroma	Chondrosarcoma
Bone	Osteoma	Osteogenic sarcoma
Epithelium		Carcinoma
Skin and mucous membrane	Papilloma	Squamous cell carcinoma
Glands	Polyp	Basal cell carcinoma
		Transitional cell carcinoma
	Adenoma	Adenocarcinoma
	Cystadenoma	
Pigmented cells (melanoblasts)	Nevus	Malignant melanoma
Endothelium		Endothelioma
Blood vessels	Hemangioma	Hemangioendothelioma
		Hemangiosarcoma
Lymph vessels	Lymphangioma	Lymphangiosarcoma
		Lymphangioendothelioma
Bone marrow		Multiple myeloma
		Ewing's sarcoma
		Leukemia
Lymphoid tissue		Malignant lymphoma
		Lymphosarcoma
		Reticulum cell sarcoma
		Lymphatic leukemia
Muscle tissue		
Smooth muscle	Leiomyoma	Leiomyosarcoma
Striated muscle	Rhabdomyoma	Rhabdomyosarcoma
Nerve tissue		
Nerve fibers and sheaths	Neuroma	Neurogenic sarcoma
	Neurinoma	
	(Neurilemoma)	
	Neurofibroma	(Neurofibrosarcoma)
Ganglion cells	Ganglioneuroma	Neuroblastoma
Glia cells	Glioma	Glioblastoma
		Spongioblastoma
Meninges	Meningioma	Malignant meningioma
Gonads	Dermoid cyst	Embryonal carcinoma
		Embryonal sarcoma
		Teratocarcinoma

*Adapted from Bouchard, R.: *Nursing Care of the Cancer Patient.* 2nd ed. St. Louis. The C. V. Mosby Co., 1972.

versible cellular alteration at the molecular level that is caused by the action of one or more etiologic agents and that results in uncontrolled cellular reproduction and growth. These irreversible changes evidently develop within the cell's nucleus. Deoxyribonucleic acid (DNA), a basic constituent of the nucleus, is in some way altered so that its structure becomes abnormal. As a result, the cell changes into a cancerous cell. When this defective cell divides, the daughter cells are modeled upon the defective molecular code contained within the DNA of the mother cell. Over time, the defective daughter cells divide and multiply, and the malignancy develops and grows.

Theories attempting to explain this cellular alteration are constantly being formulated and proposed. One theoretical agent that has been suggested is the oncogene. This is a growth-promoting agent supposedly present in all cells, but normally active only early in life during the growth period. It is suggested that in some manner this agent may become reactivated later in life and may cause unwanted cell proliferation. Further, it may enter other cells and distort the code contained in the DNA of the normal cells.[2]

It is still not known whether the cellular derangements that result in cancer are caused by a single agent or by multiple agents acting together. Laboratory experiments tend to support the *multifactoral theory of pathogenesis,* which holds that cancer develops in response to the combined action of several etiologic factors.

There are approximately 150 different types of cancer found in humans, and there are probably at least 500 different agents that can act as causative factors. In addition to etiologic agents, there are also *predisposing factors,* such as age, sex, and occupation, that can influence the *host's susceptibility* to various etiologic agents.

ETIOLOGIC FACTORS

Causative agents that are chiefly responsible for the development of cancer in man and animals can be categorized as follows:

> Viruses.
> Chemical agents.
> Physical agents.
> Hormones.

Such agents are often referred to as *carcinogens;* i.e., these agents can cause malignant changes in normal cells provided the cells are exposed to the agent over a sufficient period of time.

Carcinogens are everywhere in our environment, but not all persons are equally susceptible to the same carcinogens; for example, smokers have a higher incidence of lung cancer than nonsmokers, but not all smokers develop cancer; radiologists have a higher incidence of leukemia than do physicians in other fields, but not all radiologists develop leukemia. Exactly what causes different individuals to respond differently to the same carcinogen is not yet known.

Viruses

The study of viruses as carcinogens is one of the most promising areas in cancer research today. In spite of earlier doubts as to the validity of the theory of viral causation, there is now abundant proof that viruses cause cancer in animals. Viruses have been identified and photographed within cancerous lesions. Also scientists have injected filtrates taken from virus-infected cancerous tissue into healthy animals, and these animals have later developed cancer. Since scientists cannot experiment on human beings as they do on laboratory animals, it is difficult to obtain evidence that viruses cause human cancer. However, indirect evidence is accumulating that strongly supports the theory that certain forms of human cancer are caused by viruses.

How do viruses change normal cells into cancer cells? The complete answer to this question is still not known. Some hypotheses are as follows: Viruses may upset the cell's metabolic processes or block metabolic pathways in such a way that *virus* particles are reproduced in place of the normal healthy cell. This process is called *replication;* it involves destruction of the cell by the virus. Viruses may promote adverse changes in the cell's genetic code, along the lines described previously. As a result, cells are reproduced on the basis of faulty information concerning their structure and functions. This process is called *transference;* the cells are not destroyed but they are altered so that their characteristics differ from normal cells.[47]

Chemical Agents

Some of the most common chemical carcinogens are: chromium, cobalt, tar, soot, asphalt, the nitrogen mustards, certain plastics, aniline dyes, the hydrocarbons in cigarette smoke, air pollutants from industry, crude paraffin oil, fuel oils, nickel, asbestos, and arsenicals. Most of these cause cancer only after close and prolonged contact, and those affected are usually workers in industries where these chemicals are employed or occur as byproducts.

The most highly publicized chemical carcinogens are air pollutants and the hydrocarbons in cigarette smoke. These two carcinogenic agents will be considered in the discussion of lung cancer (Unit XIV).

Physical Agents

The major physical agents believed to be associated with the causation of cancer are as follows:

Ionizing radiation, whether from x-rays or radioactive isotopes. Persons who work with radiant energy face the threat of developing leukemia. For example, as stated earlier, radiologists suffer a substantially higher rate of death from leukemia than do doctors in other fields. Also, there has been a substantial increase in the incidence of leukemia among victims of atomic fission and fallout (for example, the Hiroshima and Nagasaki survivors).

Sunlight and ultraviolet radiation may cause skin cancer in persons whose skins are exposed to strong sunlight over a substantial period of time. The degree to which persons expose themselves to sunlight depends, to some extent, on their *location*. For example, skin cancer is more prominent among sunbathing Californians than it is among persons who live in cloudier northern areas; also, it is more common among rural inhabitants than among urban dwellers. Further, skin coloring affects the degree to which the sun can damage the skin. For example, dark-skinned persons (blacks, Puerto Ricans) are less likely to develop skin cancer upon exposure to the sun than are fair-skinned Nordic populations. Evidently the greater pigmentation of the dark person's skin protects him from the carcinogenic effects of strong sunlight.

Physical trauma such as mechanical blows to the body or chronic irritations may possibly cause cancer. Whether a *single physical blow* can cause cancer is a controversial question. It is true that neoplasms are sometimes discovered at the site of an injury following an accident or beating. However, one can argue that the neoplasm was located at that site already and that the physical blow or accident simply called attention to its presence.

While a single blow is a questionable carcinogen, there is more likelihood that *repeated minor trauma* associated with *infection* may give rise to malignancy. For example, pipe smoking is linked with cancer of the lip; a jagged tooth may be a causative factor in cancer of the tongue; women who have borne many children may develop cancer of the cervix.

Hormones

There is much to learn about the role of hormones in the causation of cancer. In animal experiments scientists have demonstrated that a relationship exists between hormonal secretion and action and tumor development and growth. Exactly what the relationship is remains obscure. Do hormones actually cause normal cells to change into cancer cells? Or do hormones simply lower the host's resistance to other carcinogens? Do hormones act only to promote the growth of tumors caused by other factors? The answers to these questions lie in the future.

PREDISPOSING FACTORS

What factors cause some individuals to be more sensitive to the carcinogens than other individuals?

Age

Cancer strikes and kills persons of all ages—children, youths, adults, and the aged. However, as we stated earlier, older persons develop cancer more readily than do younger individuals. For example, more than one half of the persons who died from cancer in 1971 were over 65. Older persons may be susceptible to cancer simply because they have been exposed to carcinogens over a longer period of time than younger persons.

Sex

Women are more susceptible to *certain types* of cancer than men and vice versa. For instance, females are more susceptible to breast cancer and cancer of the intestines, whereas males are more susceptible to cancer of the lung and stomach. However, since 1949 more men have died from cancer of *all types* than women. For example, in 1971, 183,000 men died of cancer in comparison to 152,000 deaths among women. The increased incidence of cancer deaths among males is apparently related to the higher incidence of lung cancer. With the current increase in women smokers, statistical differences between men and women may eventually even out.

Urban Versus Rural Residence

Cancer is more common among urban dwellers than among inhabitants of rural communities. The greater susceptibility of urbanites to cancer is probably related to their greater exposure to air pollutants.

Geographic Distribution

The susceptibility of individuals to different types of cancer varies on a national basis. For example, the incidence of cancer of the stomach is higher in Japan than it is in the United States, while cancer of the breast is rare in Japan but has a high incidence in the United States. Breast cancer is also common in Europe. These differences in susceptibility to different forms of cancer probably result from environmental factors (e.g., national diet, ethnic customs, types of pollutants found in environment) rather than from genetic differences between races and nationalities.

Occupation

Persons in some occupations are more susceptible to cancer because of their greater contact with certain carcinogens; e.g., workers in chemical factories suffer from a heavy exposure to chemical carcinogens; persons who handle radioisotopes are exposed to heavy doses of radiant energy.

Familial Susceptibility

The tendency of inbred strains of mice to develop cancer of one particular site has been definitely demonstrated in the laboratory. However, there is no conclusive evidence that heredity plays a vital role in the development of human cancers. Nonetheless, a hereditary predisposition toward malignancy of a particular organ or site is sometimes apparent in the family histories of patients with cancer.

Cancerous and Precancerous Lesions

The presence of malignancy in one tissue appears to increase the patient's susceptibility to the development of cancer in other tissues. Also *precancerous* lesions and some benign tumors are dangerous because they may later undergo transformation into cancerous lesions and tumors. Some common precancerous lesions are pigmented moles, burn scars, senile keratosis (brown scaly patches on the epidermis), leukoplakia (whitish areas in the mouth), and benign adenomas or polyps of the colon or stomach. All these lesions need to be carefully and periodically observed for malignant changes.

THE PATIENT'S PROGNOSIS: CANCER GROWTH VERSUS HOST RESPONSE

There are two major factors influencing prognosis in cancer: the rate of tumor growth and spread, and the host's physiologic reaction.

Cancers vary in their growth rates. Some may develop and grow slowly, not causing symptoms or death for many years; other cancers may grow, spread, and kill with terrifying speed. Also, patients differ in their responses to cancer. Some patients with cancer may succumb rapidly, whereas others may continue to live and work for many years despite their condition. What creates these differences in tumor growth and patient response?

First, let us consider *tumor growth.* Some authorities hypothesize that the malignant tumor's growth and metastatic potentials are genetically predetermined from the very beginning of the tumor's development; this is the theory of *biologic determinism.* According to this hypothesis, tumors that evolve slowly will retain the characteristic of a slow growth pattern throughout their development. On the other hand, tumors that display rapid growth and invasiveness from their inception will continue to grow and spread rapidly. Patients with slow-growing, noninvasive tumors naturally have a better prognosis; they can look forward to a longer life span, and they also have a higher cure rate, than do patients with rapid-growing, invasive tumors. In sum, then, the theory implies that the patient's prognosis and his duration of survival are predetermined during the genesis of his malignant disease.

However, both the growth and metastatic potential of the tumor are also influenced by the individual patient's *reaction* to his cancer. Some individuals are more vulnerable to the development and spread of cancer than are others. The host's (patient's) degree of vulnerability may depend, to a large extent, upon heredity and the efficiency of his immunologic defenses.

Heredity possibly plays a role in (1) the initial response of the host to a carcinogen, (2) the competency of the host's defense mechanism against cancer (i.e., histiocyte response, inflammatory response, fibrin production), and (3) the manner in which the body metabolizes or disposes of carcinogenic agents.

The role of *immunity* in preventing and controlling the growth and spread of cancer cells is an area of great interest for cancer researchers. As you recall from Chapter 23, the immune system protects the body against the invasion of foreign substances (including viruses) by the production and release of antibodies that act to destroy the foreign antigens. If the immune system can protect the body against viruses that produce infections, it may also be able to guard the body against the viruses that possibly cause cancer.

Supporting evidence for this theory has been obtained from the postoperative experiences of heart and kidney transplant patients. Because the immune response causes rejection of newly transplanted organs, patients undergoing transplants are given large doses of immunosuppressive drugs such as cortisone. It would appear that the risk of developing cancer is greater among persons who have undergone transplantation surgery than among the population as a whole.

Also, evidence that the immune system plays a role in cancer control is accumulating in the laboratory. Researchers now know that human tumors release antigens that stimulate the patient's immune system to produce antibodies; these antibodies, in turn, act to destroy the cancerous cells. However, in some cases the tumor is not destroyed. Why is this so?

Experiments on mice have indicated that malignant tumor cells are capable of releasing "blocking agents" or "antibodies" that interfere with the action of the host's own antibodies, thereby preventing tumor destruction. However, other experiments demonstrate that the immune systems of mice can thwart the action of "blocking antibodies" by releasing *"deblocking antibodies."* These deblocking agents upset the action of the blocking agents which, in turn, allows the host's antibodies to act against the tumor cells.[25, 26]

Thus, failure of the immune system to suppress a cancerous growth may be related to either an excess of circulating blocking antibodies or a deficiency of deblocking antibodies. Research on blocking and deblocking antibodies is still in a highly experimental state. Nevertheless, cancer researchers are hopeful that new forms of immunotherapy will eventually evolve from these findings.

The *spontaneous regression* of tumors is another phenomenon that may be controlled by the immune system. Spontaneous regressions of cancers occur in about one in every 100,000 cases. Exactly how the immune response brings about this miraculous change, or if it plays any role in spontaneous regression at all, is still a provocative and unanswered question.

CHAPTER 35

Treating and Caring for Patients with Cancer

CANCER CONTROL AND PREVENTION

Programs of cancer control center around three major objectives: the prevention of cancer by means of research and public education, the elimination or control of factors and agents predisposing patients to cancer, and diagnosis of cancer during its earliest stages when curative treatment is still possible.

The first step toward the control of cancer is *education* of both professional persons and laymen concerning the warning signs of cancer and the detection and prevention of cancer. The American Cancer Society (ACS) is constantly circulating information in order to school the public in these vital areas. Table 35–1 lists the seven warning signs of cancer and the seven protective measures against cancer emphasized by the ACS.

A second step toward cancer prevention is *increased government controls* of potential carcinogens. For example, cigarette packages must now carry a warning concerning the danger of smoking; strong drives to control air and water pollution are occurring all over the country; also government specifications have been developed that protect factory workers, x-ray technicians, and others against undue exposure to ionizing radiation.

Third, the ACS and other organizations are endeavoring to *change habits and customs* that are known to predispose Americans to cancer. For example, persons are urged, via short television presentations, to "kick the habit," i.e., to stop smoking; sunbathers are cautioned about the danger of overexposure to strong sunlight; pediatricians are strongly urging circumcision of newborn males because uncircumsized males have a higher incidence of penile cancer.

DIAGNOSING CANCER

Although prevention is the ideal method of cancer control, the second best method involves early diagnosis of malignant diseases and the removal of precancerous lesions. Nurses and physicians must emphasize to their patients and to the general public the importance of discovering and eradicating cancerous lesions *early, before* they begin to metastasize from the primary site. Nurses can help in this educational process by emphasizing the need for an annual physical examination, by stressing the importance of a yearly Papanicolaou test for women and by teaching women the technique for the monthly breast self-examination. (See Unit XVIII.)

TABLE 35–1. SEVEN WARNING SIGNS OF CANCER AND SEVEN SAFEGUARDS AGAINST CANCER (AMERICAN CANCER SOCIETY)

Cancer's Seven Warning Signs	Seven Safeguards Against Cancer
1. Change in bowel or bladder habits	1. *Breast:* Regular monthly self-examination of breasts for lumps, nodules, or changes in contour
2. A sore that does not heal	2. *Colon-Rectum:* Annual proctoscopic examination in persons over 40
3. Unusual bleeding or discharge	3. *Lung:* Control and preferably elimination of the cigarette smoking habit; annual chest x-ray
4. Thickening or lumps in breast or elsewhere	4. *Oral:* Annual examinations of the mouth and teeth
5. Indigestion or difficulty in swallowing	5. *Skin:* Avoidance of undue exposure to sunlight
6. Obvious change in wart or mole	6. *Uterus:* Annual Papanicolaou smear for all female adults
7. Nagging cough or hoarseness	7. *Basic:* Yearly complete physical examination for all adult men and women; annual urinalysis and blood work

MANIFESTATIONS OF CANCER

When a malignant growth is in its early stages, it often fails to produce symptoms. Thus, tragically, many patients fail to seek early medical care because they are asymptomatic. By the time manifestations appear and the patient is examined, the malignant growth may have reached such an advanced stage that hope of cure is greatly diminished. It is precisely because malignancies tend to lie dormant for years that cancer detection techniques such as the "Pap" smear and sigmoidoscopy should be a routine part of the yearly physical examination.

What finally causes the manifestations of malignancy to become apparent? What are the major symptoms of cancer?

Manifestations generally appear once the neoplasm has grown to a sufficiently large size to cause one or several of the following problems:

> Pressure upon surrounding organs.
> Distortion of surrounding tissues.
> Obstruction of lumens of tubes.
> Interference with the blood supply of surrounding tissues.
> Interference with organ function.
> Disturbance of body metabolism.
> Parasitic use of the body's nutritional supplies.
> Mobilization of the body's defensive responses, resulting in inflammatory changes.

Major manifestations of cancer, their accompanying symptoms, and their causation are outlined below.

Anemia

Etiology

1. Bleeding from ulcerated lesions or erosion of a blood vessel.
2. Infection.
3. Bone metastases (when present) prevent bone marrow from replacing worn-out or damaged erythrocytes.
4. Chemotherapy and radiation therapy can cause bone marrow depression.

Symptoms

1. Tachycardia.
2. Palpitations.
3. Dyspnea.
4. Dizziness.
5. Easy fatigability.
6. Weakness.

Infection of Surface of Tumor

The most common site for the development of infected ulcerated cancer lesions is the breast. This results from necrosis and death of the tissues covering the neoplasm.

Symptoms

1. Fever.
2. Leukocytosis.
3. Elevated sedimentation rate.
4. Anorexia.
5. Malaise.

Serous Effusions

Serous effusions often accompany breast, lung, and ovarian cancers. They frequently result from the metastasis of tumor cells.

Symptoms

PLEURAL EFFUSIONS

1. Dyspnea.
2. Decreased breath sounds.
3. Cough.

PERITONEAL EFFUSIONS

1. Ascites.
2. Anorexia.

Pain

Pain is one of the late developments of cancer, but its appearance depends on the organ system involved. It is most likely to occur when there is obstruction or destruction of a vital organ, pressure on sensitive tissues or bone, or involvement of nerves. Bone cancer is particularly painful because the rigidity of the bone allows for little or no expansion as the tumor cells proliferate.

Etiology

1. Tumor infiltration and swelling of tissues that are enclosed in membrane that is richly supplied with sensory nerves.
2. Obstruction of a hollow viscus.
3. Nerve compression by a tumor mass or by direct infiltration of the tumor into the nerves.
4. Obstruction of blood vessels by pressure of tumor mass or by infiltration into the vessel by tumor cells.
5. Reaction of tissues surrounding tumor, leading to inflammation, infection, and necrosis.

Symptoms

1. Tachycardia and rapid pulse if pain is superficial in nature.
2. Bradycardia if pain is severe and deep.
3. Rapid, shallow respiratory rate if pain is severe.
4. Nausea and vomiting.
5. Hypoxia may accompany severe pain.
6. Irritability and insomnia.

Syndrome of Cancer Cachexia

Cachexia weakens the patient and predisposes him to other problems, such as pneumonia.

Etiology

1. Origin obscure.
2. In some cases, ulceration and infection predispose patient to a "wasting" syndrome.
3. Possibly toxic products released by the tumor promote wasting.

Symptoms

1. Weight loss.
2. Muscular weakness.
3. Anorexia.
4. Severe depression.
5. Pain.
6. Acidosis.
7. Toxemia.

Malignant disease that remains untreated or that is in a far-advanced metastatic stage when diagnosed is fatal. Death results from the widespread biochemical and metabolic disturbances caused by the growth and spread of the malignancy. More specifically, death typically follows the development of one of the following complications:

> Metastasis to the brain.
> Uremia resulting from obstruction of a ureter.
> Severe hemorrhage.
> Intestinal obstruction.
> Obstruction of a bronchus.

THE CANCER DETECTION EXAMINATION

The physician employs both general and special techniques in a complete cancer detection examination. General techniques include obtaining the patient's familial and environmental histories, performing a thorough physical examination and ordering and evaluating laboratory examinations of the patient's blood and urine. The more specialized techniques used for purposes of cancer detection are the following:

Cytologic Examination or Papanicolaou Test ("Pap" Smear)

This valuable diagnostic test was developed by George N. Papanicolaou in 1943. The original purpose of this test was to discover cancer of the cervix during the early noninvasive asymptomatic stage. Today, the test is also used to detect early cancers of the digestive, respiratory, and renal tracts, and occasionally of the breast. Also the Pap smear is currently employed to evaluate the patient's response to chemotherapy and radiation therapy, as well as to detect malignant disease when it recurs postoperatively.

Materials used for Pap smears include: (1) cervical scrapings, (2) bronchial secretions and washings obtained by bronchoscopy, (3) urine sediment, (4) coughed up sputum, (5) aspirated gastric secretions, and (6) mammary gland discharge fluid.

The method for obtaining a Pap smear is fairly simple. First of all, the doctor either scrapes cells from a tissue (e.g., the cervix) or obtains cells by aspirating fluid or sediment from an organ (e.g., the stomach or bronchi). Next, the doctor fixes the smear by immersing it in a chemical solution of equal parts of ether and 95 per cent ethyl alcohol. Finally, the fixed slide is allowed to dry and then is sent to a cytotechnologist or pathologist for staining and evaluation.

The laboratory technique used to analyze the Pap smear is called *exfoliative cytology,* which means the examination of desquamated or sloughed-off cells. Under the microscope the cells may have either a normal or an anaplastic appearance. The appearance of the cells is graded on the following five-point scale:

Class I—Normal.
Class II—Probably normal.
Class III—Doubtful (may be malignant).
Class IV—Probably malignant.
Class V—Malignant.

The doctor will repeat the Pap smear if the desquamated cells being examined are classified as "doubtful" (Class III). If the cells are "probably malignant" (Class IV), the physician will perform a biopsy in order to further evaluate the patient's condition.

Biopsy

A biopsy is the surgical excision of a small piece of tissue for microscopic examination; this is the method most commonly used to either rule out or confirm a diagnosis of malignancy.

The patient is usually scheduled for minor surgery. If the site for biopsy is easily accessible (e.g., cervix, breast), the patient is appropriately draped, a local anesthetic is administered, and a piece of the suspicious tissue is removed by the surgeon. Additional procedures (e.g., bronchoscopy, cystoscopy, and sigmoidoscopy) are necessary if the tumor is internal.

There are two types of biopsy procedures; the type used depends upon the *size* of the tumor. If the suspicious tumor is *small,* the entire tumor is excised for examination; this is called a *total* or *excision* type biopsy. If the tumor is *large,* only a part of the neoplasm is excised; this is called a *subtotal* or *incisional* type biopsy. There is some question as to the safety of the subtotal biopsy. Some surgeons believe that this procedure opens vascular channels and releases tumor cells that may then metastasize to other sites during the time when the excised tissue is being examined. However, there are no studies to date that definitely confirm this fear.

Following the excision, the material obtained by the biopsy goes to the pathologist, who generally uses one of two methods for examining the specimen: the frozen (rapid) section or the permanent paraffin section. To prepare a *frozen* section, the pathologist first freezes the tissue; next he dices the tissue into thin sections; finally, he examines the tissue slices. The main advantage of the frozen section is the *speed* with which the section can be prepared and the diagnosis made—only minutes are required. In contrast, the slower more classic method of embedding the tissue in paraffin takes about 24 hours; however, the paraffin section provides the pathologist with clearer detail than does the frozen section.

Needle Biopsy. In this method of biopsy, tissue is aspirated from a suspicious nodule or mass rather than excised. Needle or aspiration biopsy is used mainly to obtain tissue samples from the liver, kidney, spleen, and lung.

X-ray Examinations

X-ray techniques are particularly useful in the diagnosis of obstructive tumors of the gastrointestinal, respiratory, and renal tracts. They are also valuable in the identification of bone malignancies. In addition, radiographic procedures are helpful in pinpointing the location of brain tumors and the degree to which the tumors are compressing surrounding tissues.

Sometimes the suspicious lesion that brings the patient to his doctor for a cancer detection examination is not the primary lesion, but a *metastatic* or secondary lesion. A metastatic lesion that becomes evident *before* the primary lesion appears is called a *sentinel metastasis.*[40] Of first priority in the examination of patients with sentinel metastases is a thorough search for the hidden primary site so that treatment can be started at once.

PSYCHOLOGIC ASPECTS OF CANCER DIAGNOSIS

In Chapter 33 we discussed the psychologic impact of cancer upon the patient and his family, as well as the great fear of cancer that touches all of us. Because cancer is so dreaded, we can assume that the patient who visits his physician with a suspicious lump or symptom fears the results of his examination. If the patient does indeed have cancer, a major question is raised: *Should the patient be told the truth about his condition or should he be left in ignorance?*

There is no one correct answer to this question; all we know with certainty is that patients differ greatly in their response to a diagnosis of cancer. Some patients might be crushed by the knowledge that they have cancer and give up the struggle for life; others might deny the brutal fact; still others might seek a swift end in suicide. On the other hand, there are patients who must feel in control of their destinies and who therefore must know the truth however frightening; to withhold information from these patients tends only to increase their suspicions and worsen their mental outlook. In essence, then, the decision to tell or not tell the patient about his diagnosis depends upon the physician's subjective evaluation of both the patient's personality and psychologic resources for withstanding stress; the decision is also influenced by the opinions, feelings, and wishes of the patient's family. It is the nurse's role to support whatever decision the physician and patient's family finally make, and to give the patient only that information that all have agreed is pertinent and helpful.

THE TREATMENT OF PATIENTS WITH CANCER

The major objective of cancer therapy is to completely remove or destroy the malignant neoplasm as early in the course of the disease as possible. If cure is not feasible, important alternate goals are to prevent further metastases, relieve symptoms, and preserve the patient's life for as long as possible.

Three major methods for treating patients with cancer are: surgery, chemotherapy, and radiation therapy. A fourth form of therapy that is still in the experimental stages is immunotherapy.

SURGICAL THERAPY

There are four major types of surgery performed in the management of cancer.

Diagnostic Surgery

The purpose of diagnostic surgery is to either confirm or rule out a possible diagnosis of malignancy. The biopsy, which we have just discussed, is the procedure of choice.

Radical Surgery

Radical surgery is the most widely employed method of cancer therapy. The aim of *radical* surgery is to remove all the tumor without disturbing the structure or function of the host too extensively.[36] This form of therapy is particularly useful in the treatment of those cancers of the skin, colon, rectum, breast, cervix, prostate, and stomach that are still in the early stages of development. Once cancer becomes invasive and metastatic, surgery is no longer curative.

One commonly employed radical procedure is the en bloc resection. The purpose of this procedure is to excise both the original growth and the lymph channels that drain the area around the tumor. The term "en bloc" means that both the tumor and the lymph nodes are removed together; thus, the surgeon avoids slicing across lymphatic pathways. The en bloc method is employed in radical mastectomy for breast cancer and radical neck resection for cancers of the head and neck.

Unfortunately radical surgery, if it is to be curative, often involves the sacrifice of an organ, the disruption of organ functions, or permanent disfigurement. For example, the surgeon may be forced to amputate a limb, remove the patient's breast or colon, remove a portion of the jaw, and so forth. Such extensive surgical measures, however necessary, are almost always extremely difficult for patients to accept psychologically. Immediately following radical surgery, patients may suffer from strong feelings of anxiety, dependency, and depression. Upon discharge, patients may develop hypochondriasis, feelings of paranoia, and obsessive-compulsive habits.

Prophylactic Surgery

You will recall that precancerous lesions (e.g., warts, polyps, senile keratosis), if left untreated, sometimes evolve into cancer later in the patient's life. The purpose of prophylactic surgery is to remove precancerous lesions while they are still harmless and nonmalignant.

Palliative Surgery

The fundamental aims of palliative surgery are: (1) to retard the growth of the tumor, and (2) to relieve the distressing manifestations of cancer when a cure is no longer possible. Let us briefly consider these two aspects of treatment.

First, the *growth* of malignant tumors, in some cases, depends upon the secretion of certain hormones into the circulation, e.g., estrogens and testosterone. To slow the growth of a neoplasm, the surgeon may remove those glands (ovaries, testes, adrenal glands, pituitary gland) that secrete hormones known to stimulate the growth of cancers in certain parts of the body. For example, a bilateral oophorectomy in a premenopausal female may abate the progress of breast cancer; a hypophysectomy or bilateral adrenalectomy may further retard tumor growth in women with recurrent breast cancer following oophorectomy; removal of the testes may retard the growth of prostatic malignancies.

Second, certain *distressing manifestations* of cancer can be relieved by palliative surgery, e.g., ulcerations, obstructions of the gastrointestinal tract, and severe or intractable pain. *Ulcerations* are removed by excision of the necrotic tissues and by antibiotic therapy. The relief of *obstructions* depends upon the site of involvement; e.g., obstruction of the gastrointestinal tract can be relieved by a gastrointestinal bypass; obstruction of the colon can be relieved by a colostomy. *Severe pain* can be relieved by the blocking of nerves with neurolytic agents or by the surgical interruption of sensory nerve pathways; when pain is *intractable,* a cordotomy may be necessary.

Following denervation procedures, remember that the denervated tissues are no longer sensitive to painful stimuli and that the patient will therefore need protection against heat and pressure. These patients require special nursing care, e.g., positioning on an alternating pressure mattress, frequent position changes. (See Unit VIII for further discussion.)

Preoperative and postoperative care for patients undergoing these four types of surgery (diagnostic, radical, prophylactic, and palliative) is essentially the same as it is for any other type of surgery. For discussions of specific operations (radical neck resection, mastectomy, bowel resection) and the care involved, see the appropriate unit.

CHEMOTHERAPY

Objectives and Uses

The goal of cancer chemotherapy is to destroy all the malignant tumor cells without causing excessive destruction of the patient's healthy cells and disruption of the patient's normal cellular processes. How do drugs destroy cells? Evidently certain drugs are capable of interrupting cellular production of nucleic acids, which, in turn, interfere with cellular growth, development, and replication.

Unfortunately there is to date no anticancer drug capable of completely destroying a neoplasm. However, chemotherapy is helpful in those cases in which cure by surgery or radiation is not feasible; e.g., patients with diffuse cancers that are too widespread to be either surgically excised or pinpointed for destruction by radiation. Drug therapy is also helpful in the palliation of solid tumors of the prostate, kidney, breast, ovary, uterus, lung, large intestines, and adrenal cortex, and it is useful in the treatment of leukemia and lymphomas.

Classification of Drugs Used in Cancer Chemotherapy

There are relatively few drugs that have proved useful in cancer chemotherapy. Over the last decade approximately 300,000 drugs have been tested, but only about 200 of this group have been found to be capable of destroying tumor cells, and fewer than 20 are now in clinical use. However, there are currently a number of anticancer agents under investigation that may eventually be used in patient care.

Agents being used today in cancer chemotherapy are classified into the following categories:

Steroid Compounds. These function by creating a hormonal imbalance within the body which acts to suppress tumor growth.

Estrogens are mainly used to treat carcinoma of the breast and carcinoma of the prostate; *androgens* are used to treat carcinoma of the breast; *adrenocortical hormones* are administered in the care of leukemias, lymphomas, and multiple myeloma.

Radioactive Isotopes. Radioactive isotopes are used to selectively destroy malignant cells, thereby eradicating tumor growth. (See later discussion of radiation therapy.)

Included in this category are compounds containing radioactive iodine (^{131}I), radioactive phosphorus (^{32}P) and radioactive gold (^{198}Au).

Alkylating Agents. Cell poisons act by damaging DNA within the cell nucleus, which, in turn, disrupts cell growth and division. They also produce *radiomimetic* results, i.e., the effect of these agents on cells is similar to the effects of radiation therapy. They are used in Hodgkin's disease,

TABLE 35-2. DRUGS FOR TREATING CANCER*†

Classes and Names of Drugs	Clinical Use(s)
Antimetabolites	
Cytarabine (Cytosar)	Acute granulocytic and lymphocytic leukemias
5-Fluorouracil (Fluorouracil) Floxuridine (FUDR)	Carcinomas of breast, uterus, GI tract, and other organs
Mercaptopurine (Purinethol)	Acute leukemia, chronic granulocytic leukemia
Methotrexate (formerly Amethopterin)	Acute leukemia, choriocarcinoma, lymphosarcomas of head, neck, and pelvis
Thioguanine	Acute leukemia, chronic granulocytic leukemia
Alkylating agents	
Busulfan (Myleran)	Chronic granulocytic leukemia
Carmustine (BCNU)‡	Acute lymphoblastic leukemia, glioblastoma, carcinomas of lungs and pancreas
Chlorambucil (Leukeran)	Chronic lymphocytic leukemia, malignant lymphoma, Hodgkin's disease
Cyclophosphamide (Cytoxan)	Acute lymphoblastic leukemia, lymphoma, Hodgkin's disease, multiple myeloma
Mechlorethamine (Mustargen; nitrogen mustard)	Hodgkin's disease, lymphoma, control of effusions
Melphalan (Alkeran)	Multiple myeloma
Thiotepa (triethylenethiophosphoramide)	Carcinomas of breast, ovary, and lungs; malignant lymphoma, control of effusions
Triethylenemelamine (TEM)	Chronic lymphocytic and myelocytic leukemias, malignant lymphoma
Natural Anticancer Agents (Antibiotics and Alkaloids)	
Dactinomycin (Cosmogen; actinomycin D)	Wilms' tumor, choriocarcinoma, testicular tumor
Daunorubicin (Daunomycin)	Acute lymphocytic leukemia, neuroblastoma
Mithramycin (Mithracin)	Testicular tumor
Vinblastine (Velban)	Hodgkin's disease and other lymphomas, reticuloendothelial malignancies
Vincristine (Oncovin)	Acute lymphoblastic leukemia, choriocarcinoma, malignant lymphoma
Antitumor Steroid Hormones	
Adrenocorticosteroids	
Prednisolone sodium hemisuccinate (Meticortelone et al.) Prednisone (Deltasone, Meticorten, et al.)	All used in acute lymphoblastic leukemia and other malignant hematologic diseases, lymphoma, multiple myeloma
Androgens	
Fluoxymesterone (Halotestin et al.) Testolactone (Teslac) Testosterone cypionate (Depo-Testosterone) Testosterone enanthate (Delatestryl) Testosterone propionate (Perandren et al.)	All used in breast cancer
Estrogens	
Diethylstilbestrol (Stilbestrol et al.) Ethinyl estradiol (Estinyl et al.)	All used in prostatic carcinoma and in metastatic mammary cancer in postmenopausal women
Progestins	
Hydroxyprogesterone caproate (Delalutin) Medroxyprogesterone acetate (Provera) Megestrol (Megace)	All used in metastatic endometrial carcinoma
Miscellaneous Anticancer Chemicals	
Hydroxyurea (Hydrea)	Chronic myelocytic leukemia,melanoma
L-Asparaginase‡	Acute leukemia, lymphoma
Mitotane (Lysodren)	Carcinoma of the adrenal cortex
Procarbazine (Matulane)	Hodgkin's disease and other lymphomas

*From Rodman, M. J.: Copyright, 1972, by Medical Economics Company. Reprinted with permission from *RN*, Vol. 35, No. 2, February, 1972.

†Each entry on this list gives the generic or commonly accepted name of the drug, followed in parentheses by its trade name(s) and/or synonym.

‡On clinical trial.

chronic leukemia, lymphosarcoma, and multiple myeloma, and also used palliatively for inoperable cancers. Included in this category are the nitrogen mustards, ethylenamines, and sulfuric acid esters. Principal drugs are mechlorethamine, busulfan, chlorambucil, cyclophosphamide, triethylenemelamine (TEM), and melphalan.

Antimetabolites. Antimetabolites promote injury of both normal and cancer cells by interrupting the manufacture of certain metabolites that are needed for the normal functioning of cells. They also imitate certain essential components of nucleic acid and compete with these components for sustenance. Thus, these agents retard cell reproduction and consequently tumor growth. Representative antimetabolites include methotrexate, 6-mercaptopurine, and 5-fluorouracil.

Miscellaneous Drugs. This group of drugs includes: antibiotics—dactinomycin (actinomycin D, Cosmegen), and alkaloids—vinblastine (Velban), vincristine (Oncovin). Numerous other drugs have been used on a tentative basis for cancer chemotherapy, and still other new agents are constantly being introduced on an experimental basis.

In Table 35–2 specific agents used in cancer chemotherapy are listed in conjunction with information concerning clinical uses.

See Table 35–3 for a list of the neoplastic diseases that are responsive to chemotherapy and the types of drugs administered in each case.

Drug Administration

When neoplastic disease is widely disseminated, antineoplastic agents are administered via the systemic route (oral, IM, IV). When malignant tumors are still localized, drugs are administered via localized or regional methods. Neoplasms treated regionally may include tumors of the head and neck, advanced pelvic tumors, metastatic tumors of the liver, and various types of tumors of the extremities.

There are two *regional* methods of drug administration: intra-arterial infusion, and intra-arterial perfusion. Both these methods enable the physician to administer large doses of potent antineoplastic drugs directly into the blood vessels supplying the tumor without introducing a toxic drug into the general circulation.

In *intra-arterial infusion* an antimetabolite is injected into an artery supplying the tumor, usually the brachial, axillary, carotid, or femoral artery. At the same time a metabolite, a substance that counteracts the effects of the antimetabolite, is injected intramuscularly in order to protect the remainder of the body from cell injury. The citrovorum factor, a bacterial derivative, is usually used for this purpose. Figure 35–1 shows the procedure. The artery is cannulated and a high dose of antimetabolite is continuously pumped to the tumor site by a hydraulic pump. The drug is usually given at a rate of 1.0 to 1.5 liters every 24 hours, and the treatment may be continued for five or six days or longer.

In *regional intra-arterial perfusion* the region of the body to be perfused is isolated from the general circulation and connected to a source of extracorporeal circulation. Large doses of the antineoplastic agent can then be directed to the tumor without entering the general circulation and damaging major organ systems. Figure 35–2 shows the circuit employed in the treatment of a melanoma of the knee area. The isolated circuit is maintained for a half hour to an hour, after which a fluid not containing the drug is run directly into the extracorporeal circuit to dilute the drug and remove it from the tumor site. Because of the complex nature of this procedure, it is difficult and dangerous and is performed only in centers where skilled personnel and appropriate equipment are available.

Both regional techniques may produce the toxic effects of the drugs used (see later) in spite of precautions.

Toxic Effects of Antineoplastic Drugs

> *All antineoplastic drugs are potentially dangerous agents; their use results in a 2 to 4 per cent mortality rate. Patients receiving antineoplastic drugs must be vigilantly observed for signs of toxicity.*

Even following discontinuation of the drug, patients require careful observation, because *maximum toxicity tends to develop five to seven days following cessation of chemotherapy.*

Why are these therapeutic agents so toxic? Antineoplastic drugs are dangerous because they are capable of damaging and destroying not only malignant cells but certain normal cells as well. *Normal* cells that are vulnerable to the antineoplastic drugs are those that are characterized (as are cancer cells) by rapid cell division and proliferation. Such cells are principally located in the blood-forming organs (e.g., the bone marrow), the lining of the gastrointestinal tract, and the hair follicles. Thus, the three major forms of drug toxicity are bone marrow depression, alopecia, and gastrointestinal tract disorders.

Bone Marrow Depression. This is the most severe and dangerous complication of cancer chemotherapy; it can be caused by almost any one of the antineoplastic drugs. When the bone marrow becomes depressed, it is unable to produce thrombocytes (platelets), leukocytes (white blood cells), and erythrocytes (red blood cells); thrombocytopenia, leukopenia, and anemia result. Symptoms accompanying each of these blood dyscrasias are:

- *Thrombocytopenia:* petechiae, ecchymosis, epistaxis.
- *Leukopenia:* easy susceptibility to infection.
- *Anemia:* weakness, easy fatigability, pallor.

To continuously evaluate the effect of antineoplastic drugs upon the bone marrow, the physi-

TABLE 35–3. DRUG TREATMENT OF SOLID MALIGNANT TUMORS*†

Specific Solid Malignant Tumor	Primary Drugs Employed	Specific Solid Malignant Tumor	Primary Drugs Employed
Choriocarcinoma	Methotrexate and dactinomycin (Cosmegen) in combination	Testicular cancer	Chlorambucil (Leukeran) Methotrexate and dactinomycin (Cosmegen) in combination Mithramycin (Mithracin)
Uterine cervix	Alkylating agents, antimetabolites, experimental methylmitomycin (porfiromycin)	Ovarian cancer	Cyclophosphamide (Cytoxan) and other systemic alkylating agents
Uterine endometrium	Hydroxyprogesterone caproate (Delalutin) Medroxyprogesterone acetate (Depo-Provera) Megestrol acetate (Megace)	Control of abdominal effusions	Local instillation of Gold ^{198}Au (Aurcoloid 198, Aureotope) Mechlorethamine (Mustargen) Thiotepa
Mammary carcinoma in *Pre*menopausal women (following ovariectomy)	Testolactone (Teslac) Testosterone cypionate (Depo-Testosterone) Testosterone enanthate (Delatestryl) Testosterone propionate (Perandren)	Adrenocortical cancer Gastrointestinal cancer (colorectal and gastric)	Mitotane (Lysodren) 5-Fluorouracil (5-FU)
*Post*menopausal women (and for control of pleural effusions)	Estrogens, androgens, and mechlorethamine (Mustargen) Thiotepa Quinacrine (Atabrine)	Liver cancer Malignant melanoma	Floxuridine (FUDR) given intra-arterially Hydroxyurea (Hydrea) Melphalan (Alkeran)
Prostatic carcinoma	Chlorotrianisene (Tace) Diethylstilbestrol (Stilbestrol)	Wilms' tumor	Dactinomycin (Cosmegen) combined with surgery and irradiation
		Neuroblastoma and Ewing's sarcoma	Cyclophosphamide (Cytoxan) Vincristine (Oncovin)

*From Rodman, M. J., Copyright, 1972, by Medical Economics Company. Reprinted with permission from *RN*, Vol. 35, No. 3, March, 1972.

†In the column at right, the generic name of each drug is given first, followed in parentheses by its trade name(s) or synonym.

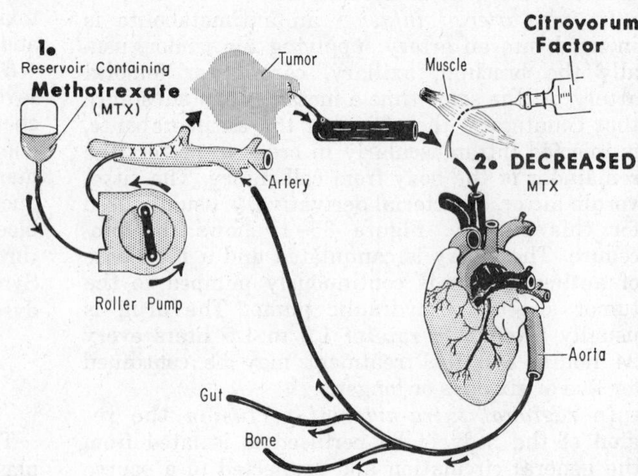

FIGURE 35–1. Regional intra-arterial infusion. (From Lawton, R. L., and Liechty, R. D.: Malignant Neoplasms. *In* Liechty, R. D., and Soper, R. T. (eds.): *Synopsis of Surgery.* St. Louis, The C. V. Mosby Company, 2nd ed. 1972.)

cian generally orders a daily complete blood count and platelet examination during their use.

Alopecia. The development of alopecia, while not a dangerous side effect of cancer chemotherapy, is nevertheless a traumatic experience for the patient, especially for the female patient. In our society there is much emphasis upon beautiful hair as a prerequisite for femininity. The woman who is losing her hair may fear that she is also losing her desirability as a woman. This feeling of loss adds more weight to the sense of despair that already burdens most patients with cancer. Indeed, the psychologic stress imposed by balding may cause some individuals to withdraw almost completely from social contacts; their state of depression and despondency may be overwhelming. You will need to talk to these patients about the temporary nature of their condition. Emphasize that their baldness is simply a side effect of the anticancer drug that they are taking and that, once the drug is discontinued, their hair will grow out again. In the meanwhile, the patient's morale can be greatly bolstered by the purchase of an attractive wig or some bright scarves. Male patients may also feel in better spirits if you encourage them to wear a hair piece or colorful cap.

Gastrointestinal Tract Disorders. The four gastrointestinal tract disorders that can result from cancer chemotherapy are:

SLOUGHING OF THE COLONIC MUCOSA. This is the most severe form of drug toxicity; it is associated with bleeding and infection.

NAUSEA AND VOMITING. When prolonged, nausea and vomiting result in dehydration. Also, vomiting causes a loss of H^+ and Cl^- which, in turn, leads to hypochloremic alkalosis. For care of the vomiting patient with fluid and electrolyte imbalances, see Chapter 25.

DIARRHEA. Prolonged diarrhea also causes fluid and electrolyte imbalances. When uncontrolled, diarrhea results in dehydration, hypokalemia (loss of K^+), hyponatremia (loss of Na^+), hypochloremia (loss of Cl^-), and acidosis (loss of $HCO^3)^-$.

STOMATITIS. This condition is characterized by inflammation of the oral mucosa. Early symptoms are dry mouth and burning of the lips; sometimes both painful ulcerations and secondary infections of the oral mucosa develop. It becomes difficult for the patient to chew his food or to eat or drink substances that have a high acid content. Stress to the patient that he should avoid eating hot spicy foods, drinking alcoholic beverages, and smoking cigarettes, since these activities will further irritate his mouth. Examine the patient's mouth frequently for signs of infection or ulceration, and administer meticulous oral care on a scheduled basis several times a day. For a more complete discussion of stomatitis, see Unit XV.

RADIOTHERAPY

The goal of radiotherapy is to destroy the malignant tumor without unduly harming surrounding tissues. "The fundamental concept underlying irradiation treatment of tumors is that tumor cells are more susceptible to the effects of irradiation than are normal cells."[36] Thus, it is possible to destroy malignant cells while inflicting only temporary injury upon neighboring cells that are normal.

Radiation has many specific medical uses. It can be employed as a *diagnostic tool* to locate malignant tissue as well as to measure blood volume, blood circulation time, red blood cell turnover, glandular activity, and the rate of formation of red blood cells. Radiation can be used

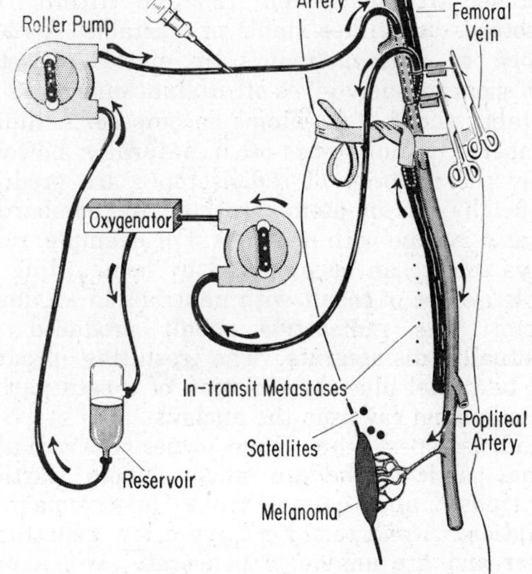

FIGURE 35-2. Regional intra-arterial perfusion. (From Lawton, R. L., and Liechty, R. D.: Malignant Neoplasms. *In* Liechty, R. L., and Soper, R. T. (eds.): *Synopsis of Surgery.* St. Louis, The C. V. Mosby Company, 1972.)

therapeutically to *destroy tumor growths;* it can be prescribed alone or in combination with either surgery or cancer chemotherapy. Radiotherapy is administered by means of roentgen therapy, large radioisotope sources ("bombs"), and local or internal applications of radium or radioisotopes.

In addition, radiation is useful as a *palliative measure.* For example, in patients in whom a malignancy is far advanced, radiation of the tumor can relieve the patient's pain for sustained periods of time, ranging from months to years. One condition in which radiation is frequently used to relieve pain is metastatic cancer of the breast to the bone. Finally, radiation is a vital area for *medical research;* many experimental radioisotope compounds are being tested currently with the hope that some of them will lead to a cancer cure.

Basic Concepts Underlying Radiodiagnosis and Radiotherapy

Let us briefly review some of the definitions and concepts basic to the study of radiation and radioisotopes.

Radiation is the emission of waves or particles of radiant energy. Examples of radiation are radio waves, infrared red waves, ultraviolet light, x-rays, alpha particles, beta particles, and gamma rays. A substance that is *radioactive* has the property of spontaneously emitting some form of radiant energy, e.g., a radioisotope.

You will recall that an isotope is a chemical element having the same atomic number as another (i.e., the same number of nuclear protons), but having a different atomic mass (i.e., a different number of nuclear neutrons). The chemical properties of the two forms are the same. For example, the element hydrogen has three isotopes: common hydrogen (H), deuterium (H^2) and tritium (H^3).

Isotopes are either stable or unstable. A *radioisotope* or *radionuclide* is an unstable isotope that spontaneously gives off radiant energy as the unstable nuclei of its atoms decompose. A limited number of radioisotopes occur naturally; however, today the majority of radioisotopes are produced artificially in an atomic reactor by bombarding a stable isotope with neutrons. For example, radioactive cobalt can be produced by bombarding the stable isotope of cobalt with neutrons in an atomic reactor. The radioactive cobalt produced will eventually disintegrate. The resulting products will be nickel plus the emission of a beta particle and a gamma ray from the nucleus.

Radioisotopes emit three types of radiation: alpha particles (helium nuclei), beta particles (electrons), and gamma rays (electromagnetic radiation). *Alpha particles* have a low penetrating power and are unable to penetrate even a piece of paper; *beta particles* have a moderate penetrating power but are unable to penetrate a piece of wood; *gamma rays* have an intense penetrating power; however, they cannot penetrate a thick piece of concrete (Fig. 35–3). Beta particles and gamma rays are used in cancer detection and therapy.

The *half-life* of a radioisotope is the time it takes for one half of the atoms composing the radioisotope to decay (i.e., the time required for the radioisotope to lose one half its original energy). Some radioisotopes have a half-life of a few days, whereas others have a half-life of many years. For example, iodine-131 has a half-life of about eight days, cobalt-60 has a half-life of five years, and radium-226 has a half-life of 1620 years.

The length of the half-life is an important consideration in the choice of radioisotopes for medical use. Radioisotopes with short half-lives can be used in an *unsealed* form; for example, iodine-131 is usually administered by mouth; gold-198, which has a half-life of 2.7 days, is administered by injection. These radioisotopes expend their energy rapidly and are excreted readily by the body. On the other hand, radioisotopes with longer half-lives must be administered to the patient *sealed* in some type of metal container so that they can be removed upon discontinuation of radiotherapy. For example, radium, with a long half-life of 1620 years, is administered encased in metal seeds or needles that can be removed when the course of therapy is completed.

Radiation is *measured* in several ways. The activity of a radioactive substance or its rate of disintegration is measured by the *curie.* One curie (Ci) is equivalent to the amount of any radioisotope that undergoes 3.7×10^{10} disintegrations per second (i.e., a curie measures the number of atoms in a particular radioisotope that disintegrate in one second).[3, 19] One millicurie (mCi) equals one thousandth of a curie; one microcurie (μCi.) equals one millionth of a curie. The *roentgen* is the international unit of measurement of x-rays and gamma rays. The *milliroentgen* (mr.) is one thousandth of a roentgen. The *rad* is the measure of radiation dosage used for diagnosis and therapy. Dosages of radiation used to destroy malignant growths are measured in hundreds or thousands of rads, whereas tracer doses of radioisotopes used for diagnostic purposes are measured in millirads.

Radiation cannot be detected by ordinary methods; i.e., we cannot see, hear, smell, taste, touch, or feel radiation. Consequently sensitive

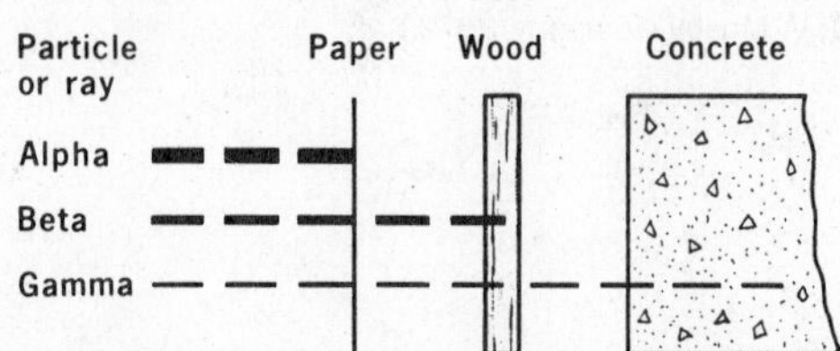

FIGURE 35–3. Relative penetration of alpha, beta, and gamma radiation. (From Phelan, E. W.: Radioisotopes in Medicine Booklet. *In Understanding the Atom Series.* U.S. Atomic Energy Commission, Division of Technical Information, 1966, p. 8.)

instruments have been designed to detect and measure radioactivity; these instruments measure and record the physical, chemical, and electrical effects of radioactive substances upon materials. Examples of measuring instruments that are used in medicine are Geiger-Muller counters, scintillation counters, specimen counters, scanners, gamma cameras, and whole body counters (see below).

Radiation, even in small doses, is somewhat injurious to all cells. However, it exerts its most destructive effects upon cells that are in rapid mitosis. Because cancer cells are characterized by rapid cellular division, they are more vulnerable to the destructive aspects of radiation; thus, the rationale for radiotherapy in the treatment of cancer. Unfortunately radiation in high doses can permanently damage even normal cells or the body as a whole. Also, when the gonads or sex glands are irradiated, genetic mutations can result.

The Role of Radioisotopes in Diagnosis. When diagnostically employed, radioisotopes are used as *tracers*. A tracer is a material that can be administered to the patient, either orally or by injection, and then identified, located, and traced by sensitive apparatus as the radioactive material circulates through the body and concentrates in particular organs and tissues.

The *scintillation counter* is the most popular instrument used to measure radioactivity for diagnostic purposes. A photoelectric cell within the counter is able to detect radiant energy; flashes of light occur whenever particles or rays of radiant energy strike certain phosphors, such as sodium iodide crystals, that are located within the apparatus. Each light flash represents a radioactive signal, and the intensity of the flash measures the intensity of the signal. The light flashes

are converted within a photomultiplier tube into electrical impulses, amplified, and then recorded on sensitized paper by a synchronously moving pen. This type of recording is similar to the recording of electrical impulses within the heart (electrocardiogram) or electrical impulses within the brain (electroencephalogram).

The *scintillation scanner* is a device for locating and pinpointing malignant growths by measuring the uptake of a radioisotope. An important part of this apparatus is the *probe,* a container that houses the phosphor crystals and photomultiplier tube. To examine the patient, the scintillation scanner is passed back and forth over the area of the body that is being studied. If the liver is being examined, the probe will be passed back and forth over the right hypochondrium and epigastrium (Fig. 35-5).

Brain scan may be done by a *scintillation camera* that produces many images in rapid sequence, showing the transit of an isotope through cerebral vessels (Fig. 35-4).

Radioisotopes are useful in the diagnosis of cancer and other entities for several reasons. First, radioisotopes can be administered in extremely small doses; e.g., one billionth of a gram of a radioisotope can be measured for administration as a tracer dose. With such small doses, the body absorbs a minimal amount of radiation, and consequently the cells suffer no damage. Thus, radioisotopes can be employed diagnostically without the danger of cellular destruction.

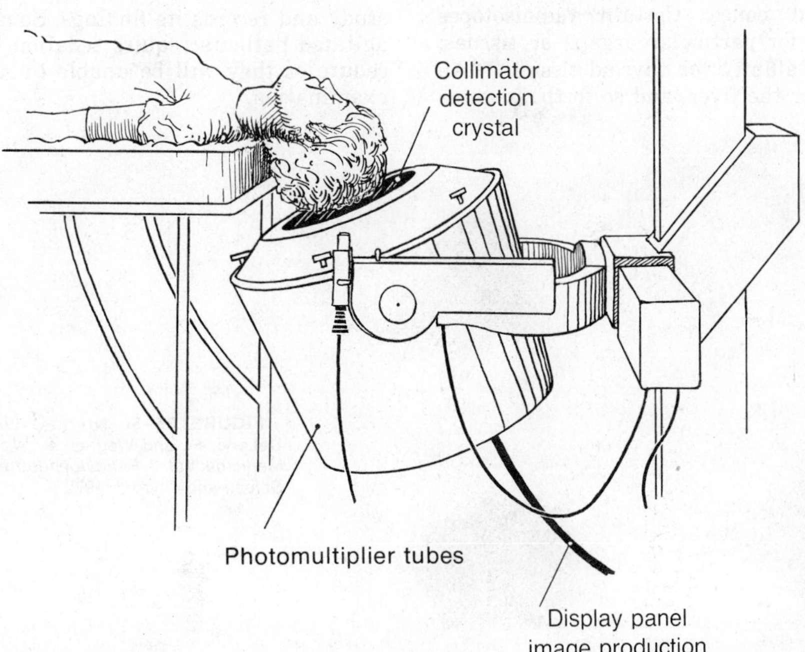

FIGURE 35-4. Scintillation camera. (From James, A. E., Jr., and Squire, L. F.: *Exercises in Diagnostic Radiology. Nuclear Radiology,* 1973.)

Second, radioisotopes can be used to study the functions of specific organs and tissues. A classic example of this type of study is the ^{131}I uptake test that is used to evaluate thyroid function. If the presence of thyroid disease is suspected, the patient receives a tracer dose of radioactive iodine (^{131}I). The radioactive iodine will circulate to the thyroid gland and there be converted into thyroxine in precisely the same manner as regular (nonradioactive) iodine. In other words, the body cannot distinguish between radioactive or "tagged" atoms of iodine and regular iodine; it processes both types of atoms in exactly the same way. However, tagged atoms of iodine and other substances (iron, gold, sodium, phosphorus) differ from regular atoms in one important respect: the doctor can trace, locate, and measure the tagged atoms by means of scintillation counters or scanners. Consequently, by tracing and measuring the number of tagged atoms of iodine that pass into the thyroid and the number that are secreted, the doctor can determine whether the thyroid gland is diseased. For instance, the normal thyroid picks up 30 per cent of the tracer dose of iodine and excretes 60 per cent in the urine. However, if the patient has hyperthyroidism, the thyroid will take up 70 per cent of the tracer dose and excrete 10 per cent in the urine.

Radioisotopes are also employed to measure blood volume, blood circulation rate, red blood cell turnover, cardiac output, and lung blood flow, using the same types of procedures.

Finally, radioisotopes are used to locate tumors and lesions within the brain, kidneys, liver, lungs, pericardium, and bones. Certain radioisotopes have an affinity for particular organs or tissues; e.g., ^{131}I has an affinity for thyroid tissue, ^{198}Au has an affinity for the liver, and so forth. In some cases, if the organ harbors a malignant tumor, the tagged atoms will tend to *concentrate* in the area of tumor growth; consequently a scan of the organ will reveal a high uptake of the radioisotope at the site of the tumor. For example, ^{131}I is used to locate cancerous tissues that have metastasized from the thyroid gland to other parts of the body (Fig. 35–6). An area in which the concentration of a radioisotope is unusually high is called a "hot spot." In other cases, the tagged atoms tend to concentrate *less* densely in the diseased portion of the organ than in the normal portion. For example, examine the lung scan shown in Figure 35–7. Note that the tumor growth that has involved the right upper lobe has failed to concentrate the radioisotope, and it appears as a blank area or "cold spot" on the scan.

For the patient, undergoing an organ scan is a simple and completely painless procedure. There are three steps involved.

STEP 1: ADMINISTRATION OF THE RADIOISOTOPE. The patient is given a tracer dose of the appropriate radioisotope either orally (in an "atomic cocktail") or by injection.

STEP 2: WAITING PERIOD. Before the scanning procedure can be performed, the radioisotope must be assimilated by the organ under study. The length of time required for assimilation varies; for example, it takes one hour for radioactive gold to be assimilated by the liver; therefore, the patient must wait for one hour following an IV injection of ^{198}Au for his liver scan. For a brain scan, the patient must wait one and one half hours following an injection of radioactive mercury, and 18 to 48 hours following an injection of RIHSA (radio-iodinated human serum albumin).

STEP 3: THE SCANNING PROCEDURE. The patient is simply asked to lie still and breathe normally while the scintillation scanner measures the radioactive atoms concentrated in the organ under study and records its findings. Sometimes restless, agitated patients require sedation before this procedure or they will be unable to relax during the examination.

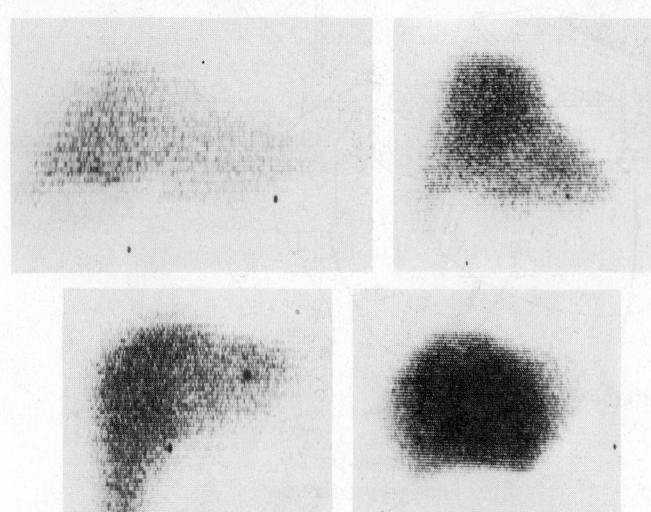

FIGURE 35–5. Normal liver scan. (From DeLand, F., and Wagner, H. W.: *Atlas of Nuclear Medicine, Vol. 3, Reticuloendothelial System, Liver, Spleen and Thyroid,* 1972.)

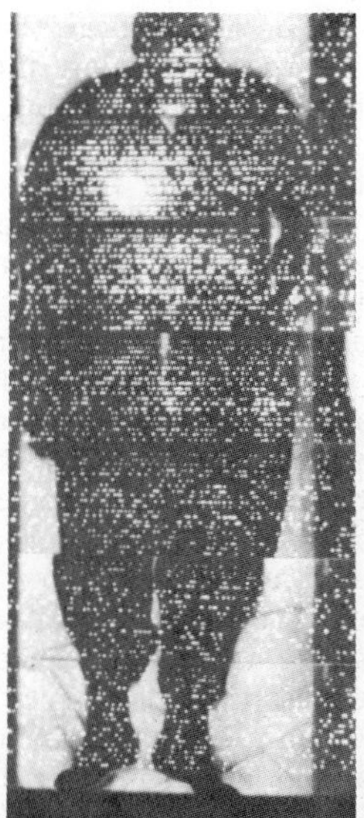

FIGURE 35-6. ^{131}I is used to locate tumors which have metastasized from the thyroid gland. (From Phelan, E. W.: Radioisotopes in Medicine Booklet. *In Understanding the Atom Series.* U.S. Atomic Energy Commission, Division of Technical Information, 1966.)

The Role of Radiation in Therapy. As we stated earlier, radiation is used therapeutically to destroy malignant cells and also as a palliative measure to relieve pain in cases of far-advanced malignant disease. Radiotherapy may be used alone or in combination with surgery or cancer chemotherapy.

In what types of tumors is radiotherapy successful? First of all, for successful radiotherapy the tumor must be radiosensitive rather than radioresistant. A tumor that is *radiosensitive* is composed of cells that can be destroyed by radiation, whereas a tumor that is *radioresistant* is composed of cells that resist the destructive effects of radiant energy. Cells that are most radiosensitive are: (1) rapidly dividing; (2) poorly differentiated, embryonic, and immature; and (3) characterized by increased metabolic activity.

Second, tumors must be located in areas where they can be treated with fairly large doses of radiation without causing serious injury to neighboring tissues. Consequently, radiosensitive tumors that are located deep within the body cannot be safely irradiated because large doses of radiation would have to first pass through normal tissues before reaching the tumor; as a result, healthy tissue as well as malignant tissue would be destroyed. On the other hand, tumors that are located on the skin or mucous membranes are most successfully treated by radiotherapy because they can be directly subjected to large doses of radiation without great harm to adjacent structures.

More specifically, radiotherapy produces the most favorable results in medulloblastoma (tumors of the cerebellum), lymphomas, metastatic breast cancer, and tumors of the skin, lip, mouth, tongue, uterine cervix, urinary bladder, larynx, tonsils, nasopharynx, and sinuses. Radiation is least successful in the treatment of malignant melanoma, metastatic lung cancer, fibrosarcoma, myosarcoma, osteogenic sarcomas, and tumors of the stomach, pancreas, liver, and prostate.

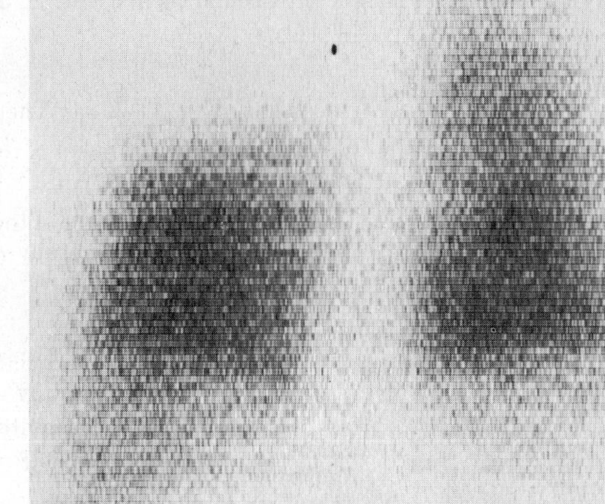

FIGURE 35-7. Scan showing presence of tumor in right lung. (From DeLand, F., and Wagner, H. W.: *Atlas of Nuclear Medicine. Vol. 2, Lung and Heart,* 1970.)

Administering Radiotherapy

Radiotherapy can be administered in a variety of ways. Note in Figure 35–8 that there are two major types of radiotherapy: external radiotherapy, and internal radiotherapy. *External* radiotherapy is administered either by x-ray machines or by radioisotopic sources. Common forms of x-ray therapy are:

> Low voltage roentgentherapy (100 to 125 kv.), which is used primarily in the treatment of skin cancer.

> High voltage roentgentherapy (200 to 250 kv.), which is used to treat deep-seated cancers.

> Supervoltage roentgentherapy (voltages of more than 800 kv.), which is the equivalent of cobalt-60 or cesium-137 teletherapy.

Patients differ in their responses to x-ray therapy. Consequently the dose of radiation delivered during each treatment and the number of treatments prescribed depend upon the radiologist's evaluation of the patient's individual case. Sometimes the patient must receive more treatments than were originally planned; in other cases x-ray therapy has to be discontinued because of pronounced side effects.

Radioisotopes. Radioisotopes are used as an *external source* of radiation, either in the form of "*bombs,*" which are employed in teletherapy, or in the form of *external molds,* which can be topically applied to the surface of the skin or eye.

Teletherapy. Teletherapy (*tele*—"distance") utilizes extremely high intensity sources of cobalt-60 or, sometimes, cesium-137. The cobalt-60 is enclosed and shielded within a protective casing called a "cobalt bomb." The bomb is located either a short distance above the area of the body being irradiated or it is attached to a movable carrier that revolves completely around the patient. When a revolving device is used, the patient must be positioned so that the high intensity beams strike the malignant growth throughout the entire rotation of the radiation source (Fig. 35–9). During this treatment the patient receives only gamma rays, because the beta particles are screened out by a filter located between the cobalt-60 and the area being irradiated.

The major advantage of teletherapy is that it can be used to irradiate and destroy deep internal cancers without seriously damaging the overlying skin. Consequently teletherapy can be successfully employed in the treatment of deep-seated malignancies of the brain, head, neck, esophagus, lung, and bladder without fear of incurring severe skin reactions. A second advantage of teletherapy is that it causes fewer cases of radiation sickness than does x-ray therapy.

Radioisotopes can also be incorporated into *external molds* and applied topically to the skin and the eye. For example, cobalt-60 can be encased within a protective mold or container and then applied to carcinomas of the ears, lips, scalp, mouth, larynx, and penis. Radioactive tantalum (^{182}Ta) can be enclosed in a flexible wire that is then bent to fit to various anatomic structures. For example, in cases of retinoblastoma (a malignancy of the retina), a wire containing ^{182}Ta can be molded into a circle and then placed directly over the tumor.

Internal Radiotherapy. This involves placement of specially prepared radioisotopes directly into the tumor itself or into the systemic circulation. The three major types of internal radiotherapy are as follows:

INTERSTITIAL THERAPY. In this method, the radioisotope of choice (e.g., cobalt-60, iodine-125, tantalum-182, cesium-137, iridium-192, gold-198, radon-222, or yttrium-90) is packed into either needles, beads, seeds, ribbons, or catheters and then implanted directly into the malignant tumor. For example, implantations of cobalt-60, encased in gold or silver needles, are used to treat cancer of the cervix or other sites. In some cases the needles are bent so that they correspond to the

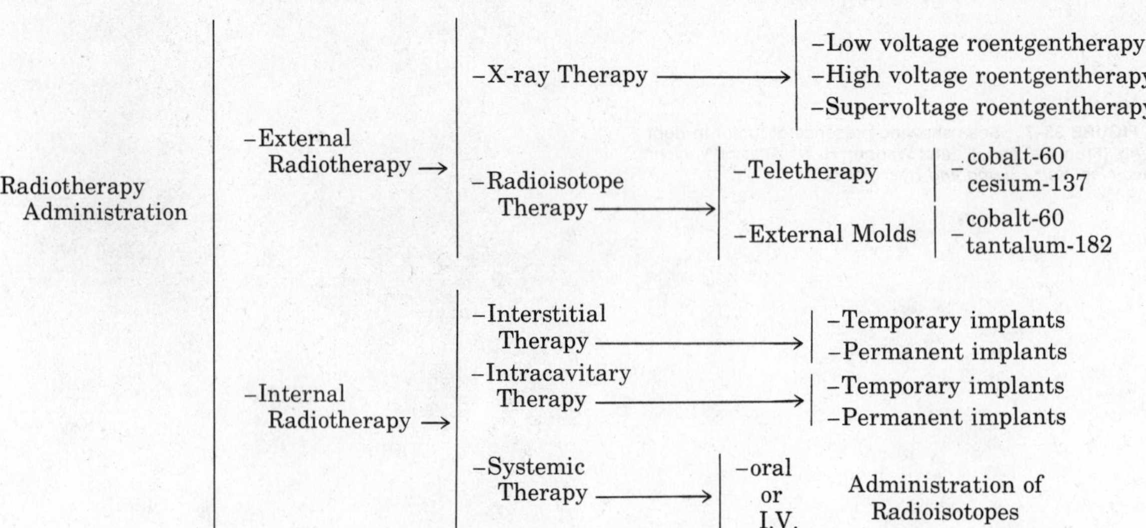

FIGURE 35–8. Forms of radiotherapy.

shape of the tumor. In other cases the needles are spaced along a plastic ribbon that can easily be molded to the structure of the organ being irradiated. Also, implantations of ceramic beads containing yttrium-90 are sometimes used to destroy the pituitary gland, thereby slowing down tumor growth in other parts of the body.

Because accurate placement of the radioactive needles or beads is absolutely necessary, radioisotopes are implanted surgically. Implants may be left in the tumor either temporarily or permanently.

INTRACAVITARY ISOTOPE THERAPY. The two types of malignant disease that are most amenable to intracavitary therapy are cancer of the uterus and cancer of the bladder. The radioisotopes used in intracavitary therapy can be encapsulated into needles that are inserted into the uterine tumor; placed in plastic tubes that are sutured into the cancerous tissues; or poured, in liquid form, into balloons that are positioned inside the bladder. Implants may be removable or permanent. Radium, cobalt-60, iridium-192, and tantalum-182 are used for removable implants, whereas radon-222, gold-198, and iridium-192 are used for permanent implants.

SYSTEMIC THERAPY. Radioisotopes are sometimes administered intravenously. For example, sodium phosphate (^{32}P) is used in the treatment of polycythemia vera and myelogenous leukemia.

Dangers of Radiation Therapy

While radiation can be beneficial in that it destroys malignant cells, it is also extremely dangerous because it damages and destroys *normal* cells at the same time. The extent to which

cells and tissues can be damaged by radiation depends upon the following four factors:

Intensity of Prescribed Dose. The patient who receives one large dose of radiation is more likely to develop tissue damage than the patient who receives multiple small doses over several treatment sessions.

Degree of Exposure. Irradiation of a large portion of the body produces more tissue damage than irradiation of a small area.

Radiosensitivity of the Cells. As we stated earlier, cells that are dividing rapidly and that are poorly differentiated are more vulnerable to radiation than are highly differentiated cells that are not dividing.

Individual Differences. Apparently some persons are inherently more susceptible to irradiation than are other individuals.

Important toxic effects resulting from radiotherapy are as follows:

Radiation Sickness. In its early stages, this systemic reaction is characterized by nausea, vomiting, and malaise; later the patient may develop purpura, petechiae, diarrhea, and inflammation of the mouth or throat. In its most severe form, this condition can be fatal.

Treatment of the patient includes: (1) bed rest; (2) small frequent feedings of a high caloric, high protein diet; (3) adequate fluid intake; and (4) the

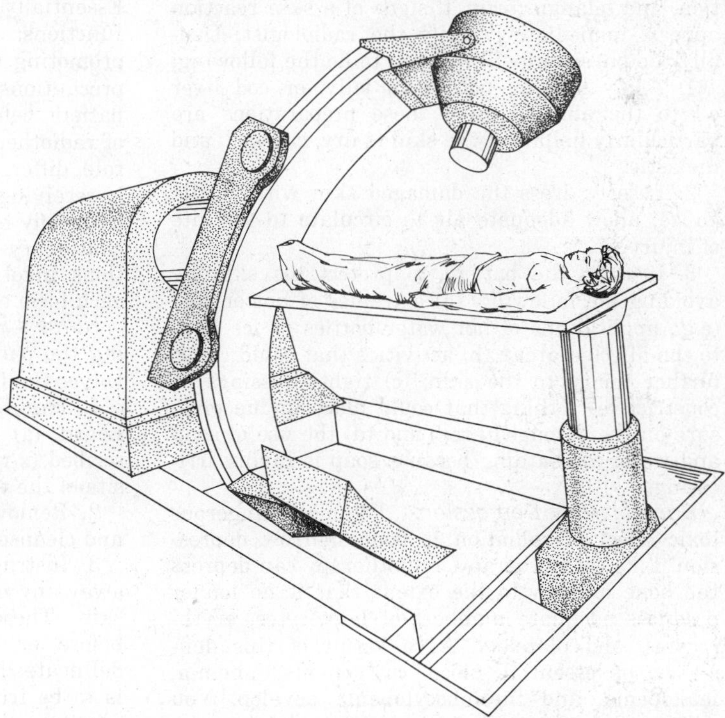

FIGURE 35–9. Teletherapy administered from a movable source. (From Phelan, E. W.: Radioisotopes in Medicine Booklet. *In Understanding the Atom Series.* U.S. Atomic Energy Commission, Division of Technical Information, 1966, p. 42.)

administration of vitamin B_{12}, sedatives, antihistamines, and antiemetics. It is important to maintain accurate records of the patient's intake and output. If the patient continues to vomit, he will require intravenous infusions of glucose in physiologic solutions of sodium chloride in order to maintain adequate nutrition and hydration.

Skin Reaction. When any part of the body is irradiated, the skin, because it is the body's outer protective covering, is also irradiated; consequently, skin reactions resulting from radiotherapy are extremely common. Once damage occurs, the skin tends to heal slowly and scar easily. Healing is retarded because radiation primarily damages those rapidly proliferating cells that are needed for tissue repair. Erythema, desquamation, and abnormal pigmentation of the skin may develop during or soon after radiation therapy. More serious problems such as atrophy or shrinking of the epidermal layer, telangiectasis (dilatation of capillaries due to vessel damage), depigmentation of the skin, and subcutaneous fibrosis sometimes occur months or years following discontinuation of radiotherapy. The most severe late manifestations of skin damage are skin cancer and necrotic and ulcerative lesions of the skin; fortunately these conditions develop only occasionally.

When caring for patients receiving radiotherapy, examine the skin frequently for redness, desquamation, and telangiectasis. If signs of a skin reaction appear, immediately notify the radiologist. Usually the physician will ask you to do the following:

1. Apply lanolin, petroleum jelly, or cod liver oil to the affected area; these preparations are particularly helpful if the skin is dry, cracked, and inelastic.

2. Loosely dress the damaged skin with sterile gauze; allow adequate air to circulate to the site of injury.

3. Instruct the patient to protect his skin by avoiding the following: (a) extremes of hot or cold (e.g., applications of hot water bottles or ice bags to the affected area); (b) activities that could cause further injury to the skin; (c) tight dressings or constrictive clothing that could place undue pressure on the damaged area; and (d) the use of soap and water for bathing because soap is highly irritating.

Bone Marrow Depression. The most dangerous toxic effect of radiation is bone marrow depression. Like chemotherapy, radiotherapy can depress the bone marrow to the extent that it no longer produces adequate numbers of leukocytes, erythrocytes, and platelets. As a result of this deficiency of essential blood components, anemia, leukopenia, and thrombocytopenia develop. You will recall that patients with these blood dyscrasias suffer from weakness, easy susceptibility to infection, and bleeding tendencies.

Because bone marrow depression is so dangerous, it is important to be aware of the patient's complete blood count and hemoglobin levels both *before* and during radiotherapy. By ordering weekly hematologic examinations, the physician and nurse can observe the effects of radiation on the blood cell and platelet production. If erythrocyte, leukocyte, and thrombocyte levels begin to fall dramatically, the radiologist may be forced to discontinue radiotherapy altogether. In other patients, the doctor may continue radiotherapy but, at the same time, treat the manifestations of bone marrow depression. For example, if severe anemia develops, the doctor will order blood transfusions to raise the patient's erythrocyte level. Also, prophylactic antibiotics will be administered to offset the patient's susceptibility to infection.

Increased Susceptibility to Cancer in Irradiated Areas. Cancer sometimes develops at the site of irradiation 20 or more years following the administration of radiotherapy; sites that are particularly vulnerable to this long-term effect of radiotherapy are the skin, lungs, and bones.

Birth Defects Due to Irradiation. If a pregnant woman's reproductive organs are exposed to radiation during the second to sixth weeks of gestation, the offspring may be born with congenital defects.

Other Toxic Effects. Leukemia, radiation cataracts due to excessive irradiation of the eye, and lung fibrosis due to excessive irradiation of the thorax may also develop.

Nurse's Role in Radiotherapy

The nurse plays a key role in radiotherapy. Essentially she performs the following three functions: preparing the patient for therapy, promoting radiation safety by observing radiation precautions; and psychologically supporting the patient before and throughout the administration of radiotherapy. These three aspects of the nurse's role differ, depending upon whether the patient is receiving external or internal radiotherapy. Let us briefly examine the preparatory measures, precautionary measures, and psychologic considerations involved in caring for patients undergoing each form of radiotherapy.

Nurse's Role in External Radiotherapy. *Preparing* the patient for external radiation typically involves the following steps:

1. Familiarize yourself with the patient's chart. Learn: (a) the type of external radiotherapy prescribed (x-ray therapy or teletherapy), and (b) the site of the tumor undergoing irradiation.

2. Remove dressings or bandages from the site and cleanse the skin.

3. Instruct the patient not to remove or wash away any marks that the radiologist makes on his skin. These marks, made in indelible ink just before or during the patient's first treatment, delineate the exact area of the patient's body that is to be irradiated; they are usually not removed until the patient's course of radiotherapy is completed.

4. Accompany the patient to the radiology de-

partment and remain there until treatment is completed.

During the radiotherapy procedure itself, what precautions are necessary? In what ways can you protect yourself from exposure to x-rays or gamma radiation while the patient is undergoing treatment? In essence, protecting oneself against exposure to excessive radiation (from either external or internal sources) depends upon three basic factors: distance, time, and shielding. Let us briefly examine these three precautionary measures.

DISTANCE. The greater distance you maintain from a source of x-rays or gamma rays, the less you will be exposed to radiation. To compute the amount of radiation that a person receives at varying distances from a radiating source, employ the inverse square law. According to this law, by simply doubling your distance from a source of x-ray or gamma radiation, you can reduce your exposure by one fourth. For example, if you stand four feet away from a source of radiation, you will be exposed to approximately one fourth the intensity of radiation received at two feet; two feet from the source, the intensity of radiation will be one fourth of that received at a distance of one foot, and so forth.

In sum, to protect yourself from x-rays or gamma rays, do not work any closer to the source of radiation than is absolutely necessary.

TIME. The *less time* you spend close to a radiating source, the less you will be exposed to radiation. For example, if you remain near a source of radiation for five minutes instead of 10 minutes, you will reduce your exposure by one half.

SHIELDING: The best protection for a doctor, nurse, or technician who must work close to a source of radiation over a period of time is *shielding,* or the use of appropriate materials to halt and absorb rays of radiant energy. The type of shielding used depends upon the type of rays emitted by the source of radiation. Lead shields are needed to halt x-rays and gamma rays; consequently, persons working in the radiology department wear leaded gloves and aprons. Also, radioisotopes emitting gamma rays must be kept in leaded containers. Glass, lucite, and aluminum shields are used to screen beta rays. No shield is needed for alpha particles, because these are incapable of penetrating even a piece of paper.

Remember:

1. *Maintain distance: Do not remain in the room while a patient is undergoing x-ray therapy or teletherapy unless absolutely necessary.*
2. *Limit time exposure: If requested to hold a baby or confused person during therapy, ask to be rotated with other personnel during subsequent treatments.*
3. *Use proper shielding: If you must hold a patient during therapy, always wear a leaded apron and gloves.*

It is important to talk to the patient about the external radiotherapy procedure, and to discuss the reasons for the safety precautions listed above. Proper psychologic preparation and adequate explanations can help the patient to accept therapy with a minimum of anxiety and fear. Questions that patients often ask about external radiotherapy and some appropriate answers are listed here.

Q. Is radiotherapy painful?
A. Radiotherapy is absolutely painless; you will not experience any sensation during treatment.
Q. What will I be asked to do during my treatment?
A. You will simply be asked to lie very still on a special table while the treatment is being given. If you find it difficult to remain in one position for long, we will support you with pillows or sandbags.
Q. Will I be left alone during treatment?
A. Yes, as a safety precaution, you will remain alone in the treatment room while the x-ray or teletherapy units are in operation. Although the radiation coming from the treatment apparatus is benefiting you, scattered radiation within the room can harm personnel who are exposed to it.
Q. What if I should become sick during my treatment and need a nurse? What should I do?
A. Although you will be alone in the room, you will be able to talk at any time to the x-ray technician via an intercom system. Also, the technician will be right outside your room and will be observing you constantly through a window. Should you need help, the technician or nurse will shield herself with a leaded apron and leaded gloves and then enter the room to assist you.
Q. Will I be radioactive after my treatment? Will I have to be isolated in a room away from everyone?
A. Fortunately, safety precautions are necessary only during that time you are actually undergoing radiotherapy. Once your treatment is completed, you will be transported from the radiology department to your own room, and all safety precautions and isolation policies will be discontinued.

Nurse's Role in Internal Radiotherapy. Preparation of the patient for internal radiotherapy differs, depending upon whether the radioisotope is to be implanted or administered systemically. If the radioisotope (sealed in needles, beads, or wires) is to be implanted into either a tissue or organ cavity, the patient is prepared for surgery. No special preparation is required when the radioisotope is unsealed and is to be administered either systemically (orally or intravenously) or injected directly into a body cavity.

Following administration or implantation of a radioisotope, the patient requires special care. Unlike the person undergoing external radiotherapy, the patient who receives internal radiotherapy must be isolated once the radioisotope is within his body. Isolation is necessary because the patient is *himself* a source of radioactivity as long as the implanted or injected radioisotope remains within his body and continues to emanate rays of radiant energy. Key points that will help you to care for the patient receiving internal radiotherapy with either sealed or unsealed radioisotopes are as follows:

1. Familiarize yourself with the patient's chart, learn: (a) what radioisotope is being used; (b) the type of source (i.e., is the radioisotope sealed in an applicator, seeds, beads, needles, or in unsealed form); (c) the mode of administration (interstitial implantation, intracavitary insertion or implantation, or systemic administration); (d) the date when treatment started; (e) the site of implantation (if a sealed source); and (f) the number of days during which the patient must be isolated.

2. Familiarize yourself with the *radioisotope* being used; learn: (a) its half-life; (b) the type of radiation emitted (gamma rays or beta particles); and (c) if an unsealed source, the manner in which it is metabolized and excreted.

3. Familiarize yourself with the *hospital's policy* concerning radiation safety. Study the radiation instruction sheet that should be in the patient's chart. Learn where you can contact the radiation officer should radioactive contamination occur.*

4. *Isolate* the patient receiving internal radiotherapy. The patient should be assigned a private room that has a phone, an intercom system linked to the nurse's desk, and an observation window through which the patient can be observed by the staff. Instruct visitors not to enter the room but to stand outside the observation window or at the door. Wear a gown and gloves when caring for the patient, and discard these items into special hampers and containers before leaving the room.

5. *Identify* the patient receiving internal radiotherapy. Note the necessity for radiation precautions on the patient's chart and Kardex; place a sign that displays the radioactive symbol on the patient's door (Fig. 35–10).

6. Maintain *distance* from the patient; stand within three feet of the patient only long enough to give basic care.

7. Recognize the *time* factor: give necessary care as rapidly as possible.

8. *Protect youself.* Wear an exposure meter (film badge) on your pocket if you are working daily near radioactive sources. If the badge indicates that you are receiving more than the maximum permissible dose (MPD) advocated by the National Committee for Radiation Safety (NCRS), make certain that you are temporarily relieved from the care of patients undergoing radiotherapy.

*Radiation officers are persons who have been specially trained and licensed by the U.S. Atomic Energy Commission to work with radioactive sources.

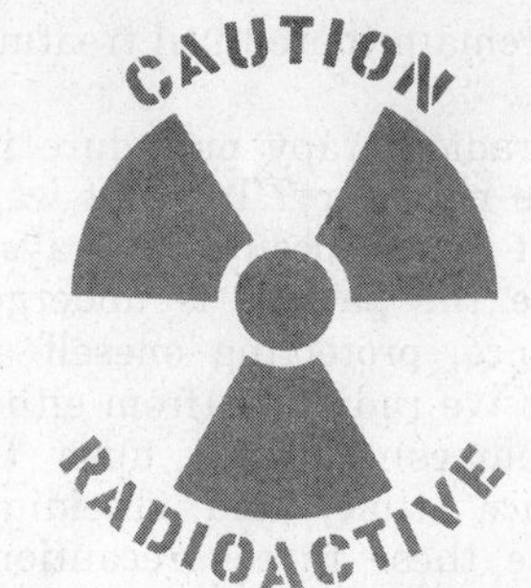

FIGURE 35–10. Radiation symbol.

9. Give *psychologic support* to the patient and his family during this trying period of physical and social isolation. Explain to the patient and his relatives the rationale for radiation precautions. Emphasize that isolation is a temporary measure and that it will be discontinued as soon as the radioisotope is either excreted (if an unsealed source) or removed (if a sealed source). The patient's sense of loneliness can be somewhat abated by listening to the radio, watching television, and talking with family and friends on the telephone.

10. Immediately notify the *radiation officer* should a radioactive source be spilled, dropped on the floor, lost, or accidentally discarded; if there is any question of radioactive contamination, the room will need to be monitored with special apparatus designed to detect the presence of radioactivity.

The general points of care and the precautions listed above apply to *all* forms of internal radiotherapy as well as to both sealed and unsealed sources of radioactivity. However, because sealed and unsealed sources differ from each other in certain respects, each type requires the employment of *additional* precautionary measures for safe use.

Sealed sources of internal radiation differ from unsealed sources in that the radioisotope is completely enclosed by a nonradioactive material. Thus, the radioisotope cannot circulate through the patient's body nor can it contaminate the patient's urine, sweat, blood, or vomitus. Consequently, you can dispose of the patient's body discharges and excretions without exposing yourself to radiation.

Contamination from sealed sources can result from the following *external* forms of exposure: (1) direct (external) contact with the sealed radioisotope, i.e., touching a sealed source with bare hands; and (2) lengthy exposure to the gamma rays that emanate from the tumor site where the radioisotope is implanted.

To prevent external hazards arising from contact with sealed sources of radioactivity, remember the following rules:

1. Limit your time *with the patient in order to decrease exposure to gamma rays.*

2. Maintain distance *from the source; e.g., if the sealed source is implanted in the pitui-*

tary gland, as often as possible stand at the foot of the bed rather than at the head of the bed.

3. Use shielding. *If a sealed source is dislodged and falls into the bed or onto the floor, pick it up with long-handled forceps and place it into a leaded container.* Never touch a radioactive source with your bare hands!

4. Before discarding used dressings, always check the dressing thoroughly for sealed sources that may have become dislodged. Transfer a dislodged source with forceps from the dressing to a leaded container. Report the incident to the radiologist and radiation officer.

Unsealed sources used for internal radiotherapy are given by intravenous injection, by mouth, or by instillation directly into a body cavity. Unlike sealed sources, unsealed radioisotopes are not encased in nonradioactive protective containers. Consequently, unsealed sources can result in two types of contamination hazards: (1) an *external* hazard due to the emission of gamma rays or beta rays from the patient's body; and (2) an *internal* hazard due to radioactive contamination of one or all of the patient's body fluids and products, e.g., feces, urine, sweat, vomitus, cavity drainage. Thus, when you care for patients receiving unsealed internal radiation, remember these rules:

1. Maintain distance *and observe the* time *factor in order to avoid (external) exposure to the rays of radiant energy emanating from the patient.*

2. Avoid contact with and properly dispose of all contaminated body discharges.

The three principal radioisotopes used for unsealed internal radiotherapy are iodine-131, phosphorus-32 and gold-198. No special precautions are required when the patient receives tiny tracer doses of these substances; however, strict precautionary measures are needed when the patient is receiving therapeutic dosages. Below are summarized the precautions that you should observe when caring for patients receiving unsealed radiotherapy with ^{131}I, ^{32}P, or ^{198}Au.

Iodine-131 (^{131}I). Half-life of this radioisotope is eight days. The patient's body will emit gamma rays. The medication is administered orally and the major source of radioactive contamination will be the urine, with lesser hazard from sputum, vomitus, sweat, feces, and blood.

PRECAUTIONARY MEASURES

1. Observe principles of distance, time, and shielding.
2. Mark bedpans for patient's use only.
3. Pour urine into leaded container and transfer to radiology department for safe disposal.
4. Wear gloves when touching bedpans, bedclothes or patient's linens.
5. Wash patient's dishes within the room and then monitor them for radioactivity or use paper plates.

6. Following removal of isolation precautions, thoroughly scrub and air the room until monitoring equipment indicates that the environment is safe.

Phosphorus-32 (^{32}P). ^{32}P may be administered orally, intravenously, and by intracavitary insertion. Its half-life is 14 days, and the patient's body poses no hazard as the beta rays emitted are not considered dangerous. Vomitus, wound seepage, and feces should be handled with special care.

PRECAUTIONARY MEASURES

1. Remove dressings with long-handled forceps.
2. Place used dressing in leaded container; carry to radiology department for disposal.
3. Wash hands carefully with soap and water following patient care.

Gold-198 (^{198}Au). Gamma rays may be emitted by the body of the patient who has had ^{198}Au inserted into a body cavity. Half-life of the isotope is 2.7 days. Wound seepage and cavity drainage will require special care.

PRECAUTIONARY MEASURES

1. Observe principles of distance, time, and shielding.
2. Remove dressings with long-handled forceps, place in leaded containers, and transport to proper area for disposal.

NURSING CARE OF PATIENTS WITH TERMINAL CANCER

The patient who is dying of cancer suffers from any of a variety of physical and emotional problems: e.g., complications of bed rest, severe depression, social isolation, anorexia, dehydration, nausea, vomiting, incontinence, decubitus, bone metastases, severe unrelenting pain, and fear of death. To prevent, alleviate, or at least lessen the severity of these problems, include the following nursing actions in your plan of care.

Encourage Physical Activity

In Chapter 27 we pointed out that immobility can lead to many complications, e.g., decubitus, contractures, renal stones, depression, and so forth. To prevent these complications, allow the patient to remain ambulatory as long as possible; plan scheduled periods of activity and rest. Should he become bedridden, obtain an alternating pressure mattress to prevent decubitus formation. In your daily plan of care also include schedules for turning the patient, performing passive exercises, inspecting the skin (particularly the buttocks, hipbones, shoulders, and ears), administering skin care, and helping the patient to cough and deep breathe. For a more detailed discussion of essential nursing care for immobilized patients, see Chapter 27.

Encourage Intellectual and Social Activity

The patient with terminal cancer almost always feels depressed, isolated, and lonely. Activities that may help to occupy his or her mind and to lessen the depression are painting, knitting, embroidery, sewing, reading, and watching television. To lessen social isolation, encourage the patient who is still ambulatory to visit with other patients in the day room and, when possible, to eat his meals with fellow patients in the hospital cafeteria if the hospital has one for patients. Once the patient becomes bedridden, he may enjoy frequent visits with his family, friends, and priest or minister. The extremely despondent patient who has lost all hope and sense of meaning in life may benefit from visits from members of one of the special cancer clubs (e.g., the colostomy clubs, ileostomy clubs). Talking to other people who have experienced cancer and who are still living and active may encourage the patient to continue his struggle to remain alive, alert, and active for as long as possible.

Promote Adequate Nutrition and Hydration

Encourage the patient to eat a diet that is adequate in protein and carbohydrates and to drink at least eight glasses of fluid a day. Order small frequent servings of food for the patient with anorexia. Take time to feed the patient who is weak and to give him sips of water or juices throughout the day. As you care for the patient, observe for the signs of cachexia: wasting, weakness, weight loss. Keep a careful record of the patient's daily weight; also record his intake and output. Note if the patient suffers from: (1) an inadequate fluid intake, (2) a poor renal output, (3) vomiting, (4) diarrhea, or (5) wound or cavity drainage. Watch for signs of dehydration, malnutrition, vitamin deficiency, or electrolyte imbalance (Chapter 25). If a fluid and electrolyte imbalance develops, or if the patient becomes comatose and unable to eat, intravenous feedings are ordered and fluid and electrolyte replacements administered.

Control Incontinence

Patients with terminal cancer often suffer from urinary and fecal incontinence. To promote the patient's comfort and prevent skin excoriation and decubitus: (1) obtain an order for an indwelling catheter; (2) bathe the patient's genital and rectal areas frequently; (3) protect the mattress with a plastic cover; and (4) diaper the patient if absolutely necessary.

Control Odors

Far-advanced cancer causes tissue necrosis and sloughing, which, in turn, results in a foul odor. To minimize odors: (1) bathe the patient frequently, (2) change soiled dressings promptly, (3) ventilate the room adequately, and (4) use deodorants, e.g., electric deodorizers, spray deodorants, powdered charcoal in the dressing, Airwick, and so forth.

Protect Patients with Bone Tumors or Metastases from Pain and Injury

Patients with primary or metastatic bone cancer characteristically suffer severe pain; also, because of the fragility of the involved bone, these patients are often victims of pathologic fractures. To prevent pain and accidental fractures: (1) place the patient on a firm mattress; (2) support the patient's back, head, and neck with small pillows; (3) obtain adequate help when turning the patient; (4) use a turning sheet so that the patient can be turned and moved "in one piece"; and (5) place side rails on the bed to prevent falls.

Relieve Pain

Patients in the final stages of cancer often suffer severe unrelenting pain, which can be relieved by: (1) analgesics, sedatives, and narcotics; (2) radiation therapy; (3) hypnosis; (4) nerve blocks; or (5) various palliative operative procedures.

Analgesics, Sedatives, and Narcotics. When treating the pain with cancer, one should first administer nonaddicting non-narcotic analgesics, and proceed to the use of narcotics only when pain becomes extremely severe. Non-narcotic analgesics, such as the salicylates or the coal tar analgesics, are frequently of great benefit in controlling cancer pain. Therefore, these nonaddictive medications should be exploited to maximal use until more powerful medication becomes necessary. If pain increases as the disease advances, 30 to 60 mg. of codeine may be given orally every 4 to 6 hours along with such non-narcotic analgesics as 600 mg. of aspirin, and 65 to 130 mg. of Darvon. Surprisingly enough, patients with fairly advanced metastatic cancers may sometimes obtain adequate relief with aspirin.

When pain does become severe enough that narcotic administration is required, the following two therapeutic guidelines should be considered:

1. When life expectancy is believed to be less than three months, continued narcotic administration is the management of choice; however, if life expectancy is greater than three months, some method other than narcotic administration becomes advisable.

2. When narcotics are given for a prolonged period of time, the problem of addiction can be deferred as long as possible by: (a) limiting the use of any one narcotic to a three-week period and then changing to a different drug; and (b) rotating the narcotics sooner than three weeks if the patient is making repeated demands for increased dosage.

Wang suggests that the following additional

principles of chemotherapy be followed in controlling pain in terminal cancer patients:[48]

1. Use long-acting narcotics rather than short-acting ones.

2. Administer medications orally as long as possible. This will eliminate the immediate satisfying response and avoid the shorter duration of analgesic activity by the parenteral route.

3. Administer narcotics on a p.r.n. basis to avoid unnecessary doses.

4. If sedatives or tranquilizers are used to allay anxiety and fear, smaller doses of the narcotic analgesic may be effective. Individualize dosage to provide adequate but not excessive sedation.

5. Chart degree of pain observed and frequency of drug administration.

6. Narcotic dosages should be increased only when indicated and only after the preceding points have been considered.

7. Whenever possible narcotic dosages should be reduced.

In sum, narcotics must be administered cautiously to patients with malignant conditions. As Bonica observes:

> While the proper use of [narcotics] . . . can be considered of great value and a true blessing to patients with cancer pain, the simplicity of their administration and their inexpensiveness—desirable qualities of any drug—frequently favors their misuse. It should be remembered that narcotics, while effective in making pain more bearable for the patient, never really abolish it.[8]

Radiation Therapy. Radiation therapy is also widely used in managing pains caused by various *malignant* conditions. For example, in the treatment of bone metastases involving weight-bearing bones, radiation therapy spaced over a period of weeks usually gives excellent pain relief. Although the patient may complain of more pain during treatment, there is usually a dramatic relief of pain immediately following completion of the series of treatments. A single treatment may effectively control pain originating from lesions that are not in weight-bearing bones and do not produce pressure.

Some other malignant conditions in which excellent pain relief may sometimes be obtained by radiation therapy are: carcinoma of the pancreas; carcinoma of the urinary bladder; carcinoma of the prostate; and metastases to the eye. In addition, radiation therapy can produce a dramatic relief of pain and a decrease in symptoms caused by metastases from adenocarcinoma of the colon involving the sacral plexus or invasion of retroperitoneal structures. Radioactive colloidal gold may be helpful in controlling pleural effusion or ascitic fluid resulting from malignant disease.

Hypnosis. The therapeutic use of hypnosis can also provide substantial relief in the terminal stages of malignant disease.

> Patients with malignant disease are frequently better candidates for successful pain relief through hypnosis than patients with other painful states. This may relate to their desperate need for pain relief or to the fact that denial of pain is compatible with the wish to deny the existence of the disease.[35]

While hypnosis is helpful in treating persons with terminal malignant disease, it should be realized that in most cases neither pain nor the need for some medication will be abolished completely. It may be, however, that with hypnosis as an adjunct to other therapies, a patient's pain can be controlled with a non-narcotic analgesic or a small infrequent dose of a narcotic. If this is possible, then a great service is accomplished for the patient, since he will be spared the potential discomforts of addiction, toxicity, and side effects from high, frequent doses of narcotics.

Nerve Block. The block of sensory nerves is particularly useful in managing cancer pain. While they have some limitations, sensory nerve blocks have more to offer than narcotic analgesics and may therefore be utilized as a complement to these drugs, as may neurosurgery. When they are effectively carried out, nerve blocks are not accompanied by some of the problems inherent in narcotic therapy, such as depression of respiration, circulation, gastrointestinal function, and other visceral disturbances. Neurolytic substances may be injected when neurosurgical procedures are not feasible and when the patient's life expectancy is no longer than two months.

Operative Procedures. Intractable pain can sometimes be relieved by such operative procedures as rhizotomy, gastrointestinal by-pass operations, bilateral adrenalectomy, hypophysectomy.

For a further discussion of pain, see Unit IX.

Psychologic Support. Give psychologic support. It is never easy to talk to a dying patient, or to listen to a patient's feelings concerning his coming death. As one patient with cancer poignantly writes:

> We embarrass our friends, for Emily Post has provided no rules for conversation with the dying. We know our friends guard their tongues, and they force us to watch our words even more. Mentioning that we won't be here next year, or even perhaps next month, is not in good taste. We have to talk about "when the children are grown," or "when the house gets too big for just the two of us," because the sensibility of our friends to death will not allow them to face what we face each minute: the fact of our dying.[44]

To give empathetic care to a patient dying of cancer, it helps to put yourself in the place of the patient. Imagine what it would mean to have your lifetime cut in half; to lose your spouse, children, and friends; to renounce forever your dreams and hopes; to face the final extinguishing of your personality. Allow yourself to feel some of the fear and despair that your patient is feeling. Accept the patient's expressions of anger, guilt, and bitterness, but focus, whenever possible, upon the areas of the patient's life that are still meaningful. In essence, help the patient to live what remains of his life as well and as fully as possible.

References for Unit VII

1. *A Cancer Source Book for Nurses*. New York, American Cancer Society, Inc., 1963.
2. Anderson, A. H., Jr.: Cancer: Blunting the shark's tooth. *Nature Science Annual,* 1972 Edition. New York, Time-Life Books, 1972.
3. Andrews, J. T., and Pope, R. A.: Radio-isotopes in medicine. *Nursing Mirror,* February 16, 1968, p. 23.
4. Asimov, I.: *Words of Science and the History Behind Them*. New York, The New American Library, Incorporated, 1959.
5. Baker, C. G.: Assessments of new methods of cancer therapy. *Postgraduate Medicine* 48:119, November, 1970.
6. Barckley, V.: The crisis in cancer. *American Journal of Nursing* 67:278, February, 1967.
7. Bodey, C. P.: Supportive care of the cancer patient. *Postgraduate Medicine* 48:203, November, 1970.
8. Bonica, J. J.: *Clinical Applications of Diagnostic and Therapeutic Nerve Blocks*. Springfield, Illinois, Charles C Thomas, 1959.
9. Bonica, J. J.: Management of intractable pain. *In* Way, E. L. (ed.): *New Concepts in Pain and Its Clinical Management*. Philadelphia, F. A. Davis Company, 1957.
10. Bouchard, R., and Owens, N. F.: *Nursing Care of the Cancer Patient*. 2nd Ed. St. Louis, The C. V. Mosby Company, 1972.
11. Brauer, P. H.: Should the patient be told the truth? *Nursing Outlook* 8: 1960.
12. *'73 Cancer Facts and Figures*. New York, American Cancer Society, Inc., 1973.
13. Chesney, D. N.: Scintiscanning: A new light on diagnosis. *Nursing Times,* August 18, 1967.
14. Cole, W. H. (ed.): *Chemotherapy of Cancer*. Philadelphia, Lea & Febiger, 1970.
15. Craytor, J. K.: Talking with patients who have cancer. *American Journal of Nursing* 69:744, April, 1969.
16. Cullinan, J.: Radioisotopes in medical diagnosis and investigation. *Nursing Times,* March, 1968, p. 287.
17. Fox, J. E.: Reflections on cancer nursing. *American Journal of Nursing* 66: June, 1966.
18. Francis, G. M.: Cancer: The emotional component. *American Journal of Nursing* 69:1677, August, 1969.
19. French, R. M.: *Nurse's Guide to Diagnostic Procedures*. 3rd Ed. New York, McGraw-Hill Book Company, Inc., 1971.
20. Grivelle, M. G.: An intra-arterial perfusion for the treatment of a parotid tumour. *Nursing Times,* February 16, 1968.
21. Gross, L.: Transmission of cancer in man. *Cancer* 28: 784, September, 1971.
22. Gunn, W. G., et al.: Palliation of pain in cancer patients. *G.P.* 40:125, September, 1969.
23. Hall, T. C.: Philosophy and pain control in cancer patients. *Postgraduate Medicine* 48:223, November, 1970.
24. Healey, J. E.: Beyond definitive treatment: A new emphasis in cancer care. *Postgraduate Medicine* 48:214, November, 1970.
25. Hellström, K. E., and Hellström, I.: Some aspects of the immune defense against cancer. I, In vitro studies on animal tumors. *Cancer* 28:1268, November, 1971.
26. Hellström, K. E., and Hellström, I.: Some aspects of the immune defense against cancer. II, In vitro studies on human tumors. *Cancer* 28:1269, November, 1971.
27. Hanschke, V. K.: *Primer on Radiation Therapy*. New York, New York Memorial Center, 1966.
28. Hodes, P. J.: Advances in diagnostic radiology. *Postgraduate Medicine* 48:79, November, 1970.
29. Huck, P.: Coping with cancer. *Nursing Mirror,* April 5, 1968, p. 28.
30. Huggins, C. B.: Adrenalectomy as palliative treatment. *J.A.M.A.* 200:165, June 12, 1967.
31. James, A. E., and Wagner, H. N.: Role of nuclear medicine in cancer. *Postgraduate Medicine* 48:88, November, 1970.
32. Karnofsky, D. A.: Cancer chemotherapeutic agents. *Cancer* 18:72, 1968.
33. Klagsburn, S. C.: Communications in the treatment of cancer. *American Journal of Nursing* 71:944, May, 1971.
34. Knudson, A. G.: Genetics and cancer. *Postgraduate Medicine* 48:70, November, 1970.
35. Lauer, J. W.: Hypnosis in the relief of pain. *Medical Clinics of North America* 52:217, January, 1968.
36. Lawton, R. L., and Liechty, R. D.: Malignant neoplasms. *In* Liechty, R. D., and Soper, R. T.: *Synopsis of Surgery*. 2nd ed. St. Louis, The C. V. Mosby Company, 1972.
37. LeShan, L.: The world of the patient in severe pain of long duration. *Journal of Chronic Diseases* 17: 119, 1964.
38. Phelan, E. W.: Radioisotopes in medicine. Booklet in *Understanding the Atom* Series. Washington, D.C., U. S. Atomic Energy Commission, Division of Technical Information, 1966.
39. Pilowsky, I., et al.: Pain and its management in malignant disease. *Psychosomatic Medicine* 31:400, September-October, 1969.
40. Pories, W. J., and Morton, J. H.: Solitary and selected multiple metastases: Diagnosis and management. *Postgraduate Medicine* 48:107, November, 1970.
41. Robbins, S. L.: *Pathology*. 4th ed. Philadelphia, W. B. Saunders Company, 1974.
42. Rummerfield, R. S., and Rummerfield, M. V.: What you should know about radiation hazards. *American Journal of Nursing* 70:780, April, 1970.
43. Santos, G. W.: Immunologic concepts and their potential role in cancer therapy. *Postgraduate Medicine* 48:194, November, 1970.
44. Shepardson, J.: A team approach to the patient with cancer. *American Journal of Nursing* 72:488, March, 1972.
45. Talley, R. W.: Chemotherapy of solid tumors. *Postgraduate Medicine* 48:182, November, 1970.
46. Turnbull, F.: Pain and suffering in cancer. *Canadian Nurse* 67:28, August, 1971.
47. Viruses as a Cause of Cancer: A Report on Research. New York, American Cancer Society, Inc., 1969.
48. Wang, R. I. H.: Control of pain. *American Journal of the Medical Sciences* 246:590, November, 1963.

UNIT VIII

Nursing Patients Experiencing Disturbances of Neurologic Function

INTRODUCTION AND OVERVIEW

The nervous system is the body's most highly organized system. The nervous system is highly valued, having both structural (i.e., anatomic) and functional (i.e., physiologic) preference among body systems. This unit will discuss why the nervous system is of such vital importance to human life and what the major consequences are from neural* disorders. The onset of neurologic disorders may be sudden, e.g., traumatic severence of the spinal cord or rupture of a cerebral aneurysm, or insidious, e.g., Parkinson's disease or multiple sclerosis. We are able to discuss in detail only the most common neurologic disorders and their clinical management. Some less common disorders are briefly mentioned to give a more complete picture of neurologic problems. Of necessity our discussion of neurosurgical procedures is brief.

Neurologic nursing is an intriguing area of practice which is both highly demanding and highly rewarding for the nurse practitioner. The nurse's understanding of neurologic and neurosurgical problems is based upon a discernment of the interrelated aspects of neurologic functioning. Such an understanding requires a sound basic knowledge of the anatomy and physiology of the nervous system. With such knowledge you, as a nurse, can *logically* understand how a specific neurologic disorder causes the resulting symptoms that the patient assigned to your care experiences—the symptoms which you will try to alleviate and with which you will help the patient to cope. The nurse's ability to make precise clinical observations of neurologic symptoms is also highly important and often ultimately helps to establish an accurate diagnosis that correctly localizes the area of disturbance.

Neurologic disorders are often frightening for patients to experience. They may interfere with an individual's means of keeping in touch with his environment, e.g., by blinding him or numbing him; they may rob a person of the vital need to move, e.g., through paralysis; or they may prevent communication, e.g., through loss of the ability to speak or to understand the spoken or written word. Diagnostic tests pertaining to neurologic disorders are also frequently frightening, and dis-

*Neural is frequently used as the adjective for nerve or central nervous system (CNS).

turbances of the brain are viewed by many patients as occurrences shrouded with mystery. Also, surgery on the brain or spinal cord is often a terrifying experience for the patient. Certainly such procedures have hazardous potential postoperative sequelae and therefore require skilled management. The patient with a neurologic problem is often forced into situations in which he is dependent upon others to help him; indeed, in some instances such a patient may be totally dependent—unconscious and relying on a respirator for his next breath.

Neurologic nursing requires an abundance of patience on the nurse's part. For example, the movements of patients with neurologic disturbances are frequently extremely slow and inaccurate. However, it is advisable to remember that the patience required of *you*, the nurse, is nominal when compared with the infinite patience required by the victim of neurologic disease. The patient must adjust to the changes in himself that have been imposed by his illness* and also work to relearn those skills and abilities that most adults take for granted. For example, the patient may be incontinent and have to relearn bowel and bladder control, or he may have to relearn how to feed and dress himself or how to talk, write, and walk. The frustrations are many, and a nurse's encouragement and enthusiasm are needed many times each day.

At the same time that the nurse assists the neurologic patient with tasks that he cannot perform for himself, she constantly works to find ways to rehabilitate the patient so he may eventually regain functions that are presently lost. *Rehabilitative care is an integral part of nursing care in both acute and chronic neurologic disturbances.* Through her imagination and creativity the nurse can inspire the patient to become a part of the rehabilitation process. Without the patient's efforts and determination, rehabilitative procedures eventually are doomed to failure.

> *Preserving and restoring function are ever-present goals for nurse and patient, even though ultimate complete restoration of function may be impossible.*

Muscle tone, range of motion, and proper positioning need to be constantly maintained in a paralyzed limb in hopes that the patient may be able to again use that limb at a later date. Nothing is more tragic than for a patient to survive the initial insult of a "stroke" (cerebrovascular accident), for example, only to face living with a withered, contractured arm or leg which is useless to him because it was not properly cared for while he was helpless. Possibly such neglect occurred because a staff member falsely believed that any return of function was "hopeless."

Recent advances in the control of neurologic disorders are impressive. New medications, improved surgical techniques,

*See discussion of *body-image*, p. 82.

and advances in knowledge of neuroanatomy and neurophysiology are today bringing relief and hope to many patients who were once actually hopeless. For example, the promising medication L-dopa has provided relief for many persons from the confining rigidity and stiffness associated with Parkinson's disease; improved neurosurgery has provided relief from many excruciating pain syndromes once considered to be "intractable" pain problems; and today recent research indicates that even the problem of neural regeneration in man should no longer be viewed as insolvable.[179]

> *The functional interrelationship between mind and body expresses itself constantly in neurologic patients.*

Neurologic nursing is truly psychophysiologic nursing, for in the nervous system more than any other system of the body psyche and soma are one. Because mental experience is housed in the brain, it is natural that disorders of the brain often cause disturbed mental experiences. Thus, patients with various neurologic disorders may experience personality or behavioral changes as a result of their illnesses; some patients with neurologic problems may hallucinate or experience illusions as a result of organic brain changes. Total nursing care of patients with neurologic conditions therefore requires implementation of a plan of care which meets both the physical and mental needs of individual patients.

Before proceeding to the study guide, let us briefly clarify that *neurology* is basically concerned with disorders of the nervous system in which *organic* disorders are apparent, whereas *psychiatry* is fundamentally concerned with *functional* disorders lacking a demonstrable physical basis. Of course such distinctions are obviously not clear-cut in practice since much is unknown about the physical basis of the psyche, and also since it is sometimes impossible to demonstrate physical disorders of the nervous system even though it is known that something is organically wrong.

STUDY GUIDE

The following guides will help you as you study this unit.

1. Chapter 36 outlines basic anatomy and physiology of the nervous system. You can understand neurologic disorders only if you understand how these disorders affect the *normal* structure (anatomy) and function (physiology) of the nervous system. Do not skim over the outline in Chapter 36, but rather read it slowly, pausing to ask yourself if you are really familiar with the points included. Review those you are not familiar with *before* proceeding to read Chapter 37. Do the following as part of your review.

> Name the main functions of the nervous system and identify and discuss the three divisions of the nervous system.

> Describe the autonomic nervous system. What are the two main parts of the autonomic nervous system and how do they function?

> Describe a neuron, how it functions, and its basic parts.

> Locate and name the brain's main parts and the major functions of each area. State the functions of the cerebrospinal fluid.

> Locate and describe the spinal cord and its major functions.

> Review the names and functions of the cranial nerves. Describe a plexus. Locate and name the three major plexuses of the spinal nerves.

> Name the covering of the brain and spinal cord and its layers. What are the functions of the layers?

2. Chapter 37 discusses how the nervous system is clinically examined and assessed. Some aspects of the neurologic examination are performed by the nurse as she gives "routine" care to selected patients; for example, the nurse often tests certain reflexes and sensations. Study carefully those aspects of the neurologic examination that you will perform (they are identified throughout the Unit). Chaper 37 also contains discussions of diagnostic tests and procedures commonly used in evaluating the status of a patient's nervous system. The nurse prepares patients for these tests (physically and emotionally), assists with the performance of some of these tests, e.g., the lumbar puncture, and gives care to the patient following the tests. The care given following some neurologic diagnostic tests, e.g., pneumoencephalogram and myelogram, is perhaps of greater importance than the care given following many of the tests which investigate the functioning of some of the other body systems. The nurse knowledgeably assesses the patient's condition following the various neurologic tests and procedures and alerts the physician when symptoms of impending danger appear. Study with special attention the section of Chapter 37 that discusses neurologic diagnostic tests and procedures.

3. Chapter 38 discusses some common clinical problems that occur as a result of altered neuroanatomy or neurophysiology. Such clinical problems include: altered states of consciousness, increased intracranial pressure, abnormal body temperature elevations, seizures and convulsions, neurogenic shock, respiratory failure, infection, problems related to spinal disorders, hemiplegia, language disorders, and emotional and behavioral changes. The clinical care discussed in Chapter 38 is of central importance not only in the nursing care of patients with primarily neurologic disorders but also in caring for patients with numerous other primary disorders. For example, patients may be unconscious for numerous reasons. Because the care discussed in Chapter 38 is of importance in many of your responsibilities as a nurse, you will want to be thoroughly familiar with its content. We have emphasized in Chapter 38 the *reasons why* the various aspects of clinical care are of importance. Focus on those reasons in your studying so you will know why you perform certain actions and will not simply perform them automatically.

4. Chapter 39 discusses specific neurologic disorders. Limited space requires that we discuss only the more common disorders and makes it necessary for even those discussions to be brief. Of the conditions discussed in Chapter 39, some occur with greater frequency than others and should therefore receive greater consideration in your studies, e.g., meningitis, intracranial tumors, transient cerebral attacks, intracranial

aneurysms and primary (spontaneous) subarachnoid hemorrhage, cerebrovascular accidents (CVA's), parkinsonism, myasthenia gravis, multiple sclerosis, epilepsy, vascular headaches (e.g., migraine), muscle contraction headaches, head injury, spinal injury, sciatic nerve injury, and trigeminal neuralgia. The discussions of clinical care are generally brief in this chapter; only points that specifically and commonly apply to a given condition are discussed, since common clinical problems were discussed in detail in Chapter 38. Refer back to Chapter 38 as necessary.

5. The discussions of head injuries and spinal injuries presented in Chapter 39 form a basis for discussion in Chapter 40 of clinical care of patients undergoing neurosurgery; therefore, you may need to refer back to these discussions as you study Chapter 40. You may also need to refer back to Chapter 38, e.g., for discussions of increased intracranial pressure, paralysis, and so forth.

In conclusion, if you study this unit carefully and in the manner just outlined you will obtain a firm foundation of knowledge upon which to base your nursing actions. The study of neurologic disorders is *complex,* because the nervous system affects all the other systems of the body. However, the study of the nervous system is *difficult* only if it is approached illogically or haphazardly. As you can see, the chapters of this unit are placed so they logically build upon one another. Appropriate medications are discussed throughout the unit; however, you should consult a textbook of pharmacology for detail.

OVERVIEW OF BASIC TYPES OF NEUROLOGIC DISORDERS

Neurologic disorders are complex because of the anatomic variability of the nervous system. Moreover, almost all diseases use the nervous system to express themselves. For example, while such symptoms as pain, weakness, sensory loss, disturbed thinking, and impaired mood or alertness may be symptoms of *primary* disease of the nervous system, even more often they are of a *secondary* nature, reflecting disease in some other bodily organ or system. Also, such symptoms are most frequently expressions of man's faulty adjustments to his environment. Possible *psychophysiologic* bases for symptoms must be carefully evaluated since the nervous system expresses psychologic and somatic symptoms in response to both real and symbolic threat or injury.

There are many different ways to classify neurologic disorders. We have chosen to follow the classification in the table, which lists typical examples of neurologic disorders. In Chapter 39 we shall discuss the various disorders listed in the table on page 390.

As indicated previously, the nervous system may become involved in a wide variety of diseases that are not neurologic diseases per se, i.e., not primary neurologic diseases. For example, pernicious anemia can cause subacute combined degeneration of the spinal cord (which selectively affects the long tracts of the posterior, lateral, or anterolateral areas of the cord), and diabetes may cause neuritis (involvement of the peripheral nerves) or central nervous system symptoms. Such secondary causes of neurologic disorders are discussed in appropriate sections elsewhere in the text.

TYPICAL EXAMPLES OF NEUROLOGIC DISORDERS

Causative Factor	Examples of Disorders
Infection	Acute (Sydenham's) chorea; brain abscess; infections of meninges; subdural and epidural infections, e.g., empyema and abscess; virus infections, e.g., acute anterior poliomyelitis and herpes zoster; rickettsial infections, e.g., spotted fever and typhus fever; syphilis; infections from other microorganisms
Tumors	Intracranial tumors, e.g., tumors of meninges, cranial nerves, supportive tissue, ductless glands, congenital tumors, granulomas; spinal tumors; tumors of peripheral nerves
Vascular lesions	Vascular lesions of brain, e.g., cerebral infarction (embolism and thrombus), cerebral hemorrhage, hypertensive encephalopathy, subarachnoid hemorrhage, intracranial aneurysms; vascular lesions of spinal cord
Developmental defects	Developmental defects of brain, e.g., congenital hydrocephalus; developmental defects of spinal cord, e.g., spina bifida
Heredofamilial and degenerative diseases	Presenile dementia (Pick's disease, Alzheimer's disease); cerebral palsy; chronic (Huntington's) chorea; Parkinson's syndrome; spasmodic torticollis; amyotrophic lateral sclerosis (ALS); syringomyelia and syringobulbia; progressive muscular dystrophy; myasthenia gravis
Demyelinating disease	Multiple sclerosis
Paroxysmal disorders	Epilepsy (convulsive disorders); syncope (fainting); Meniere's syndrome; migraine, and other forms of headache
Nutritional disorders	Deficiencies of vitamins, trace minerals, and amino acids
Trauma, e.g., puncture, blows, fracture, crush, chemicals, ionizing radiation, electrical injuries, decompression sickness	Injuries to head (craniocerebral trauma); injuries to spinal cord or its roots; injuries to cranial and peripheral nerves

CHAPTER 36

Basic Anatomy and Physiology of the Nervous System

Although various aspects of the anatomy and physiology of the nervous system will be referred to throughout this unit in greater detail, the following outline of basic facts is presented to help you to orient yourself to the nervous system as a whole. Refer as necessary to a good textbook of anatomy and physiology.

I. Nervous System
   A. *Functions.* Controls and coordinates all parts of the body (each structure of the body communicates directly with the brain); receives stimuli from body's interior and external environments through sensory systems (i.e., organs of special sense), and largely determines body's responses to these impulse-messages; contains man's higher functions, e.g., memory, reasoning.
   B. *Divisions* (Fig. 36–1)
      1. CENTRAL NERVOUS SYSTEM (CNS). Brain and spinal cord. Cranial cavity (containing brain) and spinal canal (containing spinal cord) form body's *dorsal cavities;* these cavities join, forming a continuous space.
      2. PERIPHERAL NERVOUS SYSTEM. Cranial and spinal nerves. Cranial nerves carry impulses to and from brain; spinal nerves carry impulses to and from spinal cord.
      3. AUTONOMIC NERVOUS SYSTEM. Functional classification of a certain group of peripheral nerves, some cranial and some spinal, governing functions that usually occur automatically.
         a. Regulates action of glands and involuntary smooth muscles located in walls of tubes, hollow organs and heart.
         b. Divisions (Fig. 36–2)
            (1) *Sympathetic nervous system.* Origin in thoracolumbar area; accelerates some body processes.
            (2) *Parasympathetic nervous system.* Some originate in cranial, others in spinal (sacral) regions; balances action of sympathetic system.

II. Brain (encephalon) (Fig. 36–3)
   A. *Major Fissures (Sulci).* Longitudinal fissure, central fissure, lateral fissure.
   B. *Ventricles.* Four irregularly shaped spaces; filled with cerebrospinal fluid (CSF), which cushions shock.
   C. *Main Parts.* Cerebrum (two hemispheres); brain stem (interbrain or diencephalon, including thalamus and hypothalamus); midbrain; pons (medulla oblongata); cerebellum.
      1. CEREBRUM. Two cerebral hemispheres, right and left, covered by cerebral cortex (outer nerve tissue)—highest functions of brain performed here. Cerebral cortex receives and analyzes all impulses; stores knowledge of impulses received; controls voluntary movements (i.e., movements subject to conscious deliberation), thought, association, discrimination, and judgment; memory allows much knowledge to be produced again for reuse.
         a. *Cerebral cortex* of each hemisphere is divided into four major lobes (named from overlying cranial bones).
            (1) *Frontal lobe.* Is subdivided into (a) the precentral gyrus, (b) the cortical area in front of the precentral gyrus, and (c) the prefrontal "lobe," which is the most important anterior expansion. The precentral gyrus is called the "motor cortex" because it has a motor function. The left side of the brain controls the right side of the body; right side of brain controls left side of body. Upper portion of motor center controls lower parts of body. Area in front of precentral gyrus is also associated with motor activities and is called "premotor area." Broca's speech area, which has a

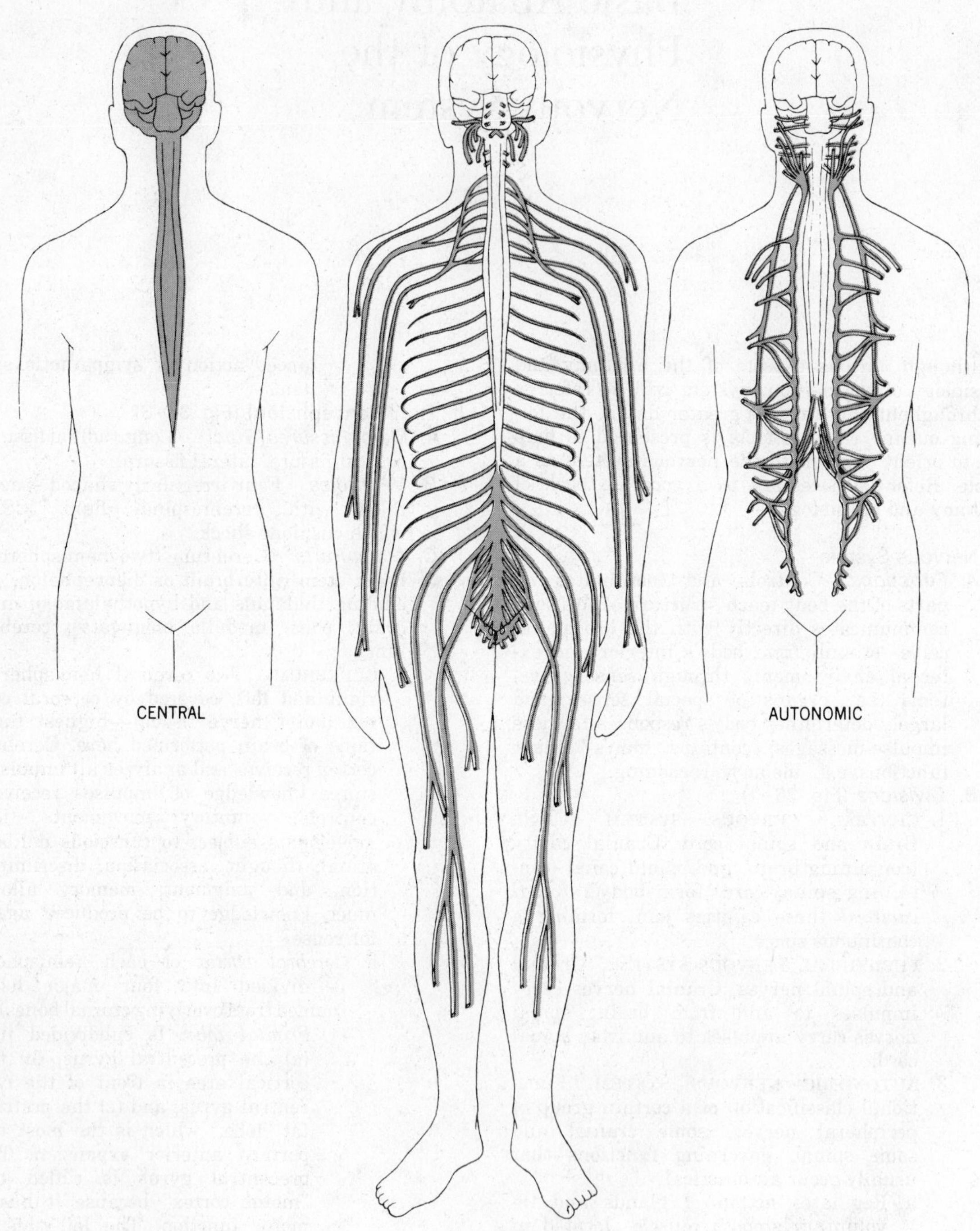

FIGURE 36–1. Divisions of the nervous system. (From Schifferes, J. J.: *Essentials of Healthier Living.* 4th ed. New York, John Wiley & Sons, Inc., 1972.)

role in motor aspects of vocalization, lies in premotor area. Prefrontal lobe is important in subtle expressions, e.g., concern with social attitudes, anxiety, placidity, drive.

(2) *Parietal lobe.* Contains sensory area for interpretation of pain, touch, temperature, pressure, and so forth; also functions in determination of size, shape, and distance. The postcentral gyrus, in parietal lobe, is also called the "general sensory cortex" and is the primary receptive area for the general senses.

(3) *Temporal lobe.* Contains auditory center.

(4) *Occipital lobe.* Contains visual area.

Two additional lobes are sometimes referred to: (5) central lobe (insula); and (6) limbic lobe.

b. *Speech centers.* Closely connected with learning, are located in cerebral hemispheres (Fig. 36–4).

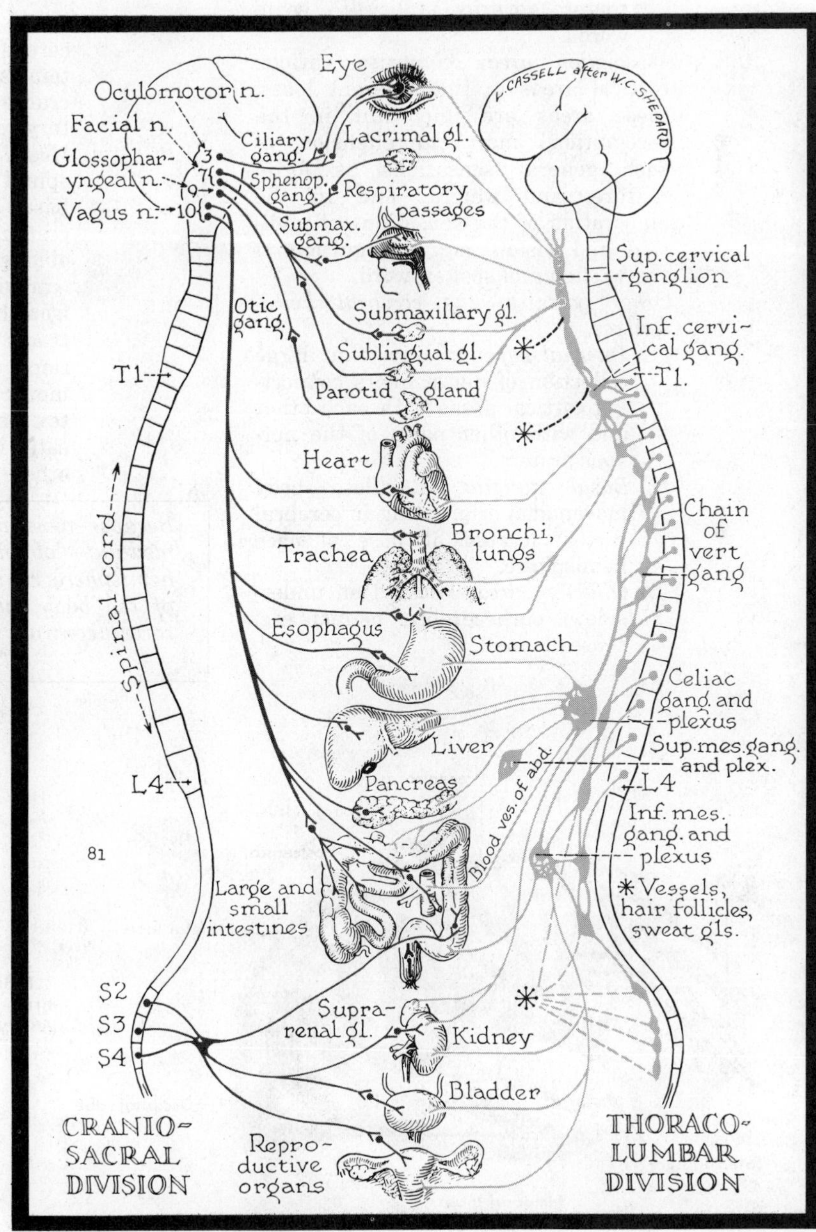

FIGURE 36–2. Diagram of the autonomic nervous system. (From King, B. G., and Showers, M J.: *Human Anatomy and Physiology,* 6th ed. 1969.)

(1) *Auditory speech center.* Located in temporal lobe near auditory center; makes possible the understanding of words.
(2) *Visual speech center.* Located in occipital lobe near visual center; governs ability to read with understanding.
(3) *Motor speech center.* Located in frontal lobe in front of lowest part of motor cortex; controls muscles of speech.
(4) *Written speech center.* Located in frontal lobe above motor speech center; governs ability to write words.

c. *Association areas* comprise various cortical areas in the different lobes; these areas are important in the recognition and comprehension of such general sensations as form, texture, and weight, and in the elaboration of the sensations of audition and vision, e.g., recognition of the written and spoken word.

d. *Other parts of the cerebral hemispheres.*
(1) *Internal capsule.* Important large collection of nerve fibers connecting cortical areas with each other and with other parts of the nervous system.
(2) *Basal ganglia.* Regulate body movements originating in cerebral cortex; located at base of each hemisphere.
(3) *Olfactory area.* Located on underside of each cerebral hemisphere; sense of smell.

2. BRAIN STEM. Includes the deeper parts of the brain not visible when viewing the intact brain, and a series of smaller parts extending toward spinal cord.

a. *Diencephalon* (interbrain) including thalamus and hypothalamus.
(1) *Thalamus.* Relays impulses and monitors sensory stimuli (e.g., suppresses or magnifies them).
(2) *Hypothalamus.* Controls some emotions (e.g., pleasure, fear), water balance, sleep, appetite, body temperature, and both divisions of autonomic nervous system.

b. *Midbrain.* Conducts impulses between "lower centers" (i.e., pons, medulla oblongata, cerebellum) and "higher centers" (i.e., cerebrum) of brain. Also relays some eye and ear reflexes.

c. *Pons.* Bridges or connects many structures, e.g., midbrain and medulla, cerebellum and rest of nervous system; also connects with four pairs of cranial nerves; controls some respiratory reflex (involuntary) actions.

d. *Medulla oblongata.* Joins brain and spinal cord through large opening in base of skull. Last four pairs of cranial nerves connect with medulla oblongata. Contains nerve fibers (carrying messages up to and down from brain) grouped together forming tracts (bundles) according to function. In medulla oblongata most motor fibers coming from motor cortex in cerebral hemispheres decussate, i.e., cross from one side to the other.

Because most motor fibers decussate in the medulla oblongata, the right cerebral hemisphere controls muscles in the left side of the body, and the upper portion of the cortex controls muscles in the lower parts of the body.

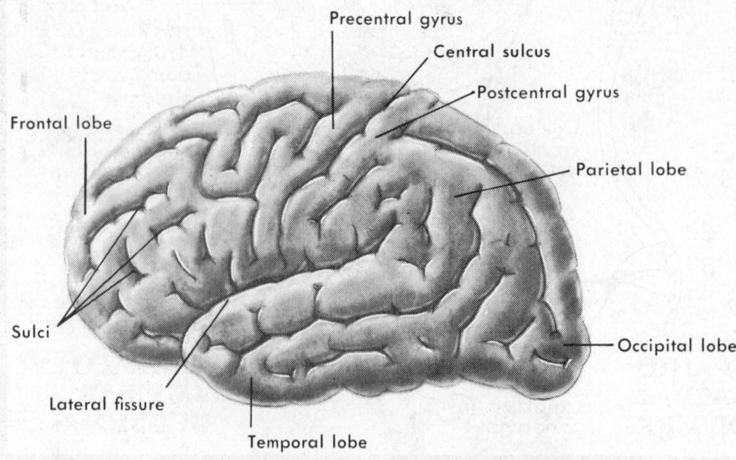

FIGURE 36–3. The external surface of the brain. (From Dienhart, C. M.: *Basic Human Anatomy and Physiology* 2nd ed. 1973.)

Important reflex center; some neurons end in medulla oblongata and impulses are relayed to other neurons. Contains various *centers* or *nuclei* (collections of cell-bodies, i.e., gray matter); location of vital centers:

(1) *Cardiac center.* Slows heartbeat.

(2) *Respiratory center.* Controls respiratory muscles.

(3) *Vasomotor center.* Affects blood pressure by acting on blood vessel wall muscles.

3. CEREBELLUM. "Little brain" aids in coordination of voluntary muscles, balance, maintenance of muscle tone. Is attached much like a large seashell to lower portions of the brain (i.e., the brain stem).

III. Spinal Cord

A. Structure. H-shaped gray matter (nerve cell bodies), surrounded by white matter (thousands of nerve fibers); all inside spinal canal.

B. Function

1. SENSORY (AFFERENT) PATHWAY. From afferent nerves through ascending tracts up to brain.
2. MOTOR (EFFERENT) PATHWAY. From brain through descending tracts down to nerves supplying muscles, glands.
3. REFLEX PATHWAY. Forms reflex arc in spinal cord. Rather than being relayed to and from brain for action, spinal reflexes (e.g., knee jerk) take place at cord level; *sensory* neuron relays impulses from receptors to *central neurons* (located entirely within cord); central neurons, in turn, send impulses to motor neuron leading to glands or muscle (Fig. 36–5). Sensory neurons begin in a receptor and lead to cord, having their cell-bodies located in *dorsal root ganglia* outside the cord; motor neurons have cell bodies located in *anterior* (ventral) *horns* of spinal cord and emerge from cord in bundles, forming *ventral roots.*

IV. Meninges

A. Function. Connective tissue covering and completely enclosing brain and spinal cord, providing protection and, in part, carrying blood supply.

B. Structure (3 layers)

1. DURA MATER. "Hard matter" or outermost membrane, thickest, toughest. Covers brain and lines skull interior; these two layers of dura mater are separated in places, forming spaces (i.e., *cranial venous sinuses*) filled with blood flowing out of brain. In the spine the space between walls of the vertebral canal and the outer surface of dura mater is *epidural* or *extradural space* (contains blood vessels, adipose, and areolar connective tissue). The inner dura mater in the brain's medial aspect is tautly extended between the occipital lobe of the cerebrum and the cerebellum. This structure, which helps to support the occipital lobe, is called the *tentorium.*
2. ARACHNOID MEMBRANE. "Spider-web-like," loosely attached to pia mater by web-like fibers. Subarachnoid space for fluid occurs between arachnoid and pia mater in brain. Also, cranial portion of arachnoid sends tiny finger-like projections (*arachnoid villi*) through dura mater's inner layer, into cranial venous sinuses, aiding in return of cerebrospinal fluid to blood stream.
3. PIA MATER. "Gentle mother", or innermost layer of meninges. Unlike other two layers, pia mater is attached to nerve tissue of brain and spinal cord and follows dips and curves of brain and cord surface. Delicate membrane containing blood vessels. Brain's larger blood vessels lie in subarachnoid space; branches from these pass through pia mater into brain substance providing large amount of brain's blood supply. Also nourishes spinal cord cells.

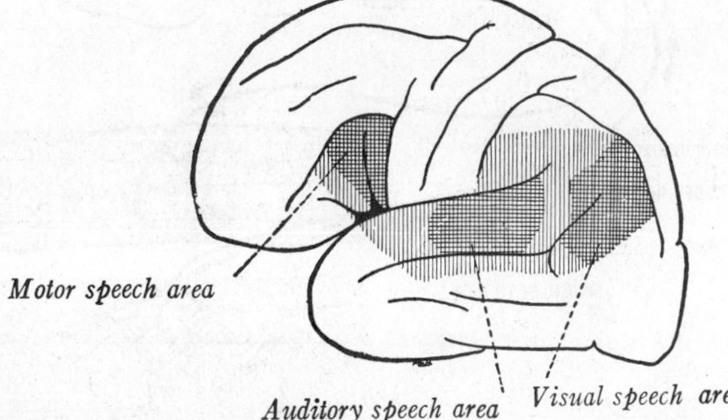

FIGURE 36–4. The three principal speech areas. (From Ranson, S. W., and Clark, S. L.: *Anatomy of the Nervous System.* 10th ed. 1959.)

V. Nerves. Basic units of nerve tissue are individual *nerve cells* (neurons) made up of: *cell body; nerve fibers (axons, dentrites).* Dendrites conduct impulses to cell body; axons conduct impulses away from cell body. *Nerves* are bundles of individual nerve fibers, bound together with connective tissue, which carry impulses and are located outside CNS.

A. *Afferent (Sensory) Nerves.* Carry impulses *to* CNS; connected with *sensory receptors* or *end-organs,* i.e., nerve endings which receive stimuli from environment. Two kinds of receptors: those generally located throughout body responsive to general sensations (e.g., pain, temperature, touch); those responsive to special sensations (e.g., taste, sound, vision) carried by cranial nerves. Afferent dendrites usually are single, very long, and do not have tree-form appearance typical of other dendrites.

B. *Efferent (Motor) Nerves.* Carry impulses *from* CNS out to muscles, glands.

C. *Mixed Nerves.* Composed of mixture of afferent and efferent fibers.

D. *Peripheral Nerves*

1. CRANIAL NERVES (12 pair)

a. *General functions.* To conduct special sense impulses (e.g., smell, visual, hearing); general sense impulses (e.g., pain, pressure, touch, vibration, temperature, and deep muscle sense); voluntary muscle control or somatic muscle impulses; involunatry control or visceral effector messages to glands and involuntary muscles.

b. *Names and functions. I. olfactory* (smell); *II. optic* (vision); *III. oculomotor* (contraction of most eye muscles); *IV. trochlear* (supplies one eyeball muscle); *V. trigeminal* (great sensory nerve of head and face; general sense impulses; motor to chewing muscles); *VI. abducens* (supplies one eyeball muscle); *VII. facial* (largely motor, muscles of facial expression; sensory for taste; secretory to lacrimal, submaxillary, sublingual glands); *VIII. acoustic* (hearing); *IX. glossopharyngeal* (general sense impulses from tongue, pharynx, i.e., throat; taste; secretory to parotid; motor for swallowing muscles in pharynx); *X. vagus* (longest cranial nerve; secretory to glands producing digestive and other secretions; supplies most abdominal and thoracic organs); *XI. accessory* (motor to two neck muscles); *XII. hypoglossal* (motor to tongue muscles).

2. SPINAL NERVES (31 pair). Eight cervical; 12 thoracic; 5 lumbar, 5 sacral, and 1 coccygeal (Fig. 36–6).

a. *Structure.* Each nerve attached to spinal cord by two roots forming nearly continuous rows along the cord; dorsal root; ventral root.

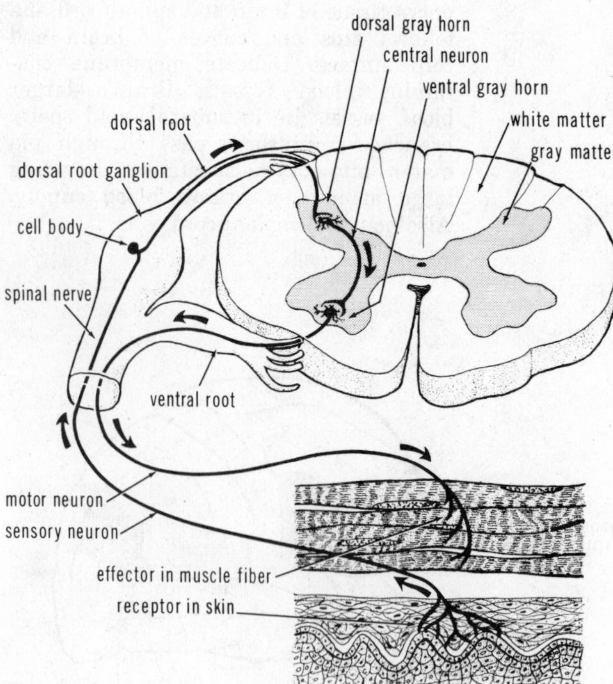

FIGURE 36–5. Spinal reflex arc. (From Memmler, R. L., and Rada, R. B.: *The Human Body in Health and Disease.* 3rd ed. Philadelphia, J. B. Lippincott Company, 1970.)

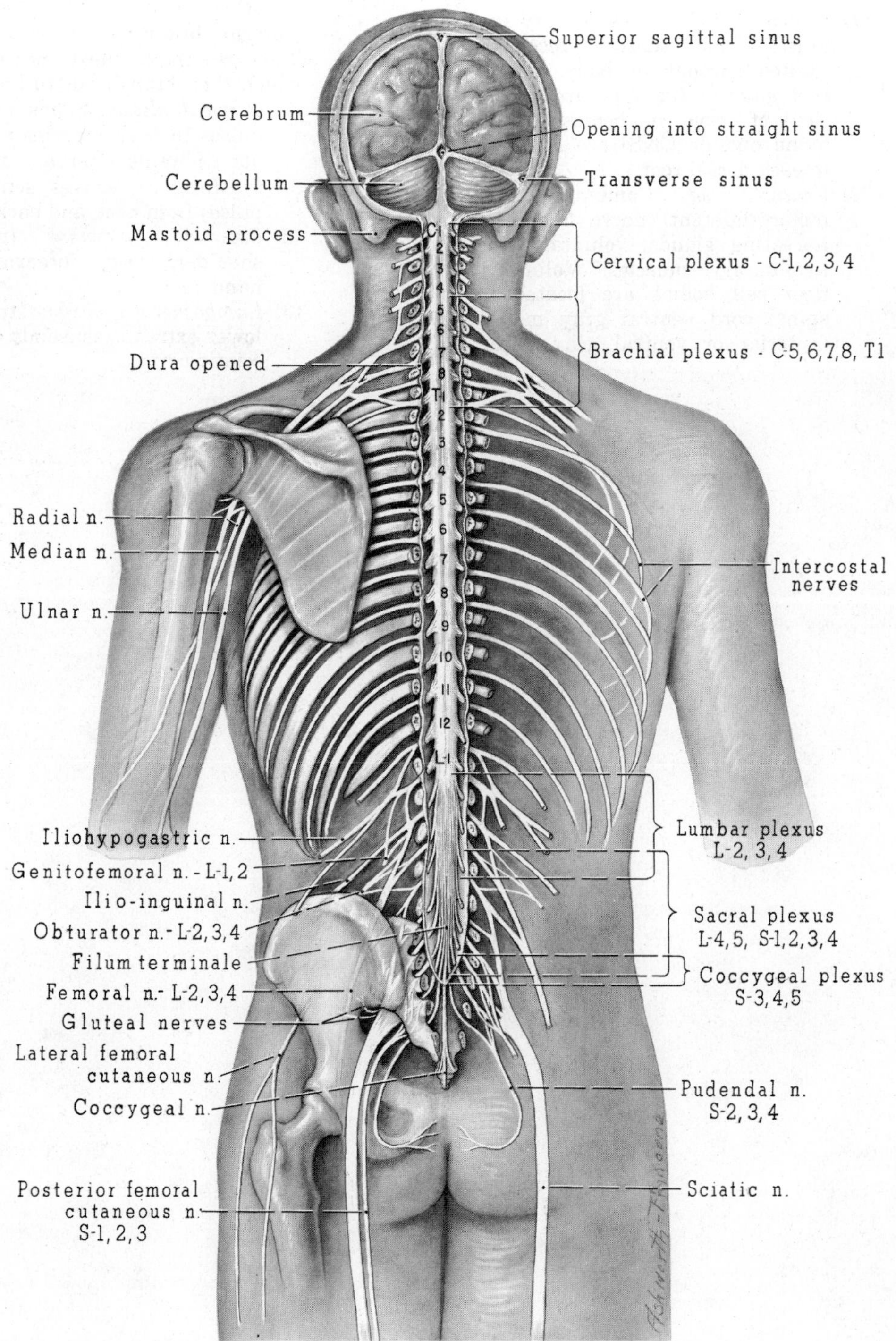

FIGURE 36–6. Spinal cord and nerves emerging from it. (From Jacob, S. W., and Francone, C. A.: *Structure and Function in Man.* 3rd ed. 1974.)

(1) *Dorsal root.* Receives sensory impulses from sensory receptors located throughout body. *Dorsal root ganglia* (ganglia are collections of nerve cell bodies usually found outside CNS) are attached to each dorsal root.
(2) *Ventral root.* Combination of motor (efferent) nerve fibers innervating glands, voluntary and involuntary muscles. Voluntary fiber cell bodies are located in spinal cord ventral gray matter (anterior or ventral gray horn); involuntary fiber cell bodies are located in spinal cord lateral gray horns.

b. *Spinal nerve plexuses.* A short distance from spinal cord each spinal nerve branches into small posterior divisions and large anterior divisions. Anterior branches interweave, forming three major plexuses (networks) which then branch out to body parts.
(1) *Cervical plexus.* Sends motor impulses to neck muscles and sends out phrenic nerve, activating diaphragm; receives sensory impulses from neck and back of head.
(2) *Brachial plexus.* Innervates shoulder, arm, forearm, wrist, hand.
(3) *Lumbosacral plexus.* Innervates lower extremities; sends out large sciatic nerve.

CHAPTER 37

Examination of the Nervous System and Assessment of the Neurologic Patient

The neurologic examination begins with a careful history and thorough physical examination. To these processes are added a variety of special diagnostic tests and procedures which supplement and add precision to clinical neurologic diagnosis. While some of these special tests are painless to the patient and simple to perform, others are complex and cause pain and discomfort. Since some neurologic diagnostic procedures are actually potentially life-threatening, the nursing and medical staff in attendance must be prepared to promptly correct possible complications. Observations of the patient's condition, made and recorded by members of the nursing staff, can be an additional source of helpful information during the diagnostic process as well as during the later therapeutic process.

Remember that preparation for any diagnostic examination or test involves both physical and psychologic preparation of the patient in addition to assembling necessary equipment for the doctor's convenient use. The supportive care the nurse gives to a patient undergoing diagnostic and evaluative procedures is extremely important. She can be of great benefit and enhance this patient's well-being by not only allowing him to discuss his concerns, but also by giving appropriate patient education and by instilling confidence in him concerning the abilities of persons caring for him.

In addition to scheduling diagnostic tests, preparing the patient, and assisting the physician as indicated, the nurse has the important responsibility of caring for the patient following completion of the various diagnostic procedures. Such care basically centers around: (1) keeping the patient comfortable; (2) observing for the onset of complications resulting from the procedure and reporting these; (3) helping the patient's friends and family during this stressful time; and (4) protecting the patient from injury or complications during his recovery from the diagnostic procedures. Protecting the patient involves such activities as observing for specific potential complications following diagnostic tests (discussed with the various tests) and keeping all staff members informed of specific orders following the tests. For example, if a patient's bed is to be kept flat following a procedure, the patient should be informed of the order and a sign indicating the order should be placed on the patient's bed where it can be clearly seen by all persons coming into the room. Keeping the patient and all persons coming to the patient's bedside informed of necessary restrictions is a highly important aspect of nursing practice. Failure to conscientiously perform this responsibility can not only delay a patient's recovery and cause him discomfort, but at times may be life-threatening. Additional precautions, e.g., siderails, assistance in walking, and so forth, should be used as indicated for the patient's safety.

The nurse can provide further assistance during neurologic examinations by screening and protectively draping the patient, encouraging relaxation, and providing a darkened, quiet, and comfortably warm setting.

THE NEUROLOGIC EXAMINATION

The principal object of the neurologic examination is to determine and to localize disorders of the nervous system by recognizing disturbances in function and determining the degree to which these symptoms depart from normal.

Prior to a complete neurologic examination a general physical examination is performed, and general medical, family and social histories are obtained. Then the neurologic history is taken, and neurologic physical examination is carried out. The routine neurologic examination includes a systematic examination of the *cranial nerves,* the *sensory system,* the *motor system* (including tests for coordination and reflexes), as well as observations of autonomic function. The patient's *psychologic state* is also evaluated.

Because the history and examination are observations rather than a diagnosis, the examiner attempts to avoid diagnostic terms, e.g., "aphasia," in recording his findings. Instead he describes clearly what his observations are. This procedure should also be followed by the nurse in reporting her observations.

EQUIPMENT

Equipment which may be used during the neurologic examination includes:

> Flashlight
> Tongue depressors
> Cotton applicators
> Pins (to test for pain perception)
> Soft brush, e.g., camel's hair (to test for touch perception)
> Snellen chart or Jaeger test chart (to test for visual acuity)
> Compass (for two-point discrimination)
> Tuning fork (to test vibratory sense and hearing)
> Stethoscope
> Ophthalmoscope (to examine fundi of eyes)
> Otoscope (to examine ears)
> Reflex (percussion) hammer
> Tape measure (to measure various lengths and circumferences, e.g., infant's head, extremities)
> Clean medicine droppers

In addition to the above equipment it is helpful to have on the neurologic examination tray some stoppered bottles containing various substances to test the patient's sense of taste and smell, and his perception of temperature (e.g., bottles filled with hot and cold water).

The completed examination tray should also have small pieces of assorted materials to test texture perception (e.g., silk cloth, terry cloth, sandpaper) and a jar of various common articles to test the patient's ability to identify form and to test speech (e.g., items such as a screw, safety pin, button, key, and matches). A printed page should be available to test the patient's ability to read.

HISTORIES

Significant factors in the *family history,* pertaining to neurologic evaluation, include the incidence of symptoms similar to those of the patient, as well as the occurrence in family members of muscular and neurologic diseases.

The *neurologic history,* taken from the patient concerning his present illness, focuses on his symptoms and their onset, and on data needed to clarify diseases which primarily attack the nervous system or which produce obvious neurologic symptoms.

The following symptoms are especially important in the neurologic history and are carefully evaluated:[232a] changes in consciousness; headache; dizziness; pain, numbness, and dysesthesia, i.e., impairment of any sense (especially the sense of touch), or a painful, persistent sensation induced by gentle touching of the skin; disturbances of vision; disturbances of smell and taste; convulsions ("fits"); vomiting; motor weakness; bladder difficulty; difficulty in gait (i.e., how the patient walks) and station (i.e., how the patient stands); disturbances of speech and expression; disturbances of sleep; and autonomic and trophic disturbances.*

INITIAL OBSERVATIONS

The examiner begins his neurologic evaluation the moment he first sees the patient. Naturally, observations are most complete if the patient is ambulatory and fully conscious. Initial observations include the patient's *general appearance,* e.g., personal appearance (neatness, and so forth); mannerisms, e.g., quick and energetic or slow moving and sluggish; and *obvious disturbances,* e.g., in speech, articulation, coordination, and movement. Notation is also made of *obvious physical defects,* e.g., amputations, and the patient's *level of consciousness.* An interview with a witness, friend, or relative is essential when the patient is comatose or psychotic, and in the presence of diffuse organic brain disease with dementia, severe personality disorders, or such toxic metabolic processes as delerium tremens. Under these conditions the nurse should ask persons accompanying the patient to the hospital to remain until the doctor can talk with them.

PSYCHOLOGIC EVALUATION

During the neurologic examination the physician attempts to actively involve the patient *intellectually* and *emotionally* as well as physically. The interview with the patient during the examination can reveal disorders of psychologic function related to disturbances of higher cortical function, e.g., memory defects. The patient's *personality* and *mood* are also noted. The preceding factors are also important for the nurse to evaluate in her contacts with the patient; she should record her observations.

EVALUATION OF THE CRANIUM AND NECK

The patient's cranium and neck are examined during the neurologic examination. The size and shape of the head are noted, and the scalp and skull are inspected and palpated to detect any scars, deformities, or tenderness. This is especially important in examining patients with a history of *trauma.* Auscultation over the skull, mastoid areas, orbits, and carotid and subclavian arteries is important when *vascular tumors* or *anomalies* are suspected. *Bruits* (i.e., abnormal sounds or murmurs heard in auscultation) may be heard over the skull, and at times may be transmitted down to the neck's upper carotid level. Tenderness and spasm of the neck muscles can also be important findings.

*Changes in tissues which occur secondary to loss of muscular tone in the blood vessels or faulty innervation of the blood vessels feeding these tissues.

EVALUATION OF THE CRANIAL NERVES

The cranial nerves are evaluated during the neurologic examination as follows:

Olfactory (I). The blindfolded patient is asked to sniff and identify various nonirritating, easily recognizable odors.

Optic (II). Each eye is separately examined. The *fundi* are examined with an ophthalmoscope in a darkened room; the eye's retina, retinal arteries and veins, and optic nerve head are examined. Congestion of retinal veins and swelling or congestion of optic nerve head, i.e., choked disc or papilledema, is a manifestation of *increased intracranial pressure. Visual acuity* is grossly tested by having the patient read something, count fingers, and so forth. Also, the Snellen chart or Jaeger type test chart may be used. *Visual fields* are evaluated. Loss of vision in one-half of a field of vision is called *hemianopia.* (For a detailed discussion of examination of the eye see Unit XXI).

Oculomotor (III), Trochlear (IV), and Abducens (VI). Nerves III, IV and VI are tested together. These three nerves innervate the upper eyelid, supply the extrinsic ocular muscles, and provide parasympathetic innervation to the pupils. Therefore, examination of these nerves involves observation for *ptosis* (i.e., drooping of the upper eye lid from paralysis of the third nerve), testing of the pupil's size, convergence, and reaction, and the eye's movements (i.e., extraocular muscle movements).

Trigeminal (V). The fifth cranial nerve has a motor and a sensory division. The *motor division* is tested by asking the patient to clamp his jaw, open his mouth against resistance, widely open his mouth, move his jaw from side to side, and make chewing movements. The *sensory division* is tested by evaluating areas of sensation from the vertex (i.e., top of the head) to the chin. Sensitivity to pain (e.g., pinprick), touch (e.g., wisp of cotton or soft brush), and temperature (e.g., hot and cold bottles of water) is tested, as well as the corneal reflex. (Corneal reflex is discussed on p. 403). The oral and nasal cavities are also tested for sensory changes.

Facial (VII). Trismus, tremor and involuntary chewing movements may appear. The face is observed for symmetry and the ability to contract facial muscles. The patient is asked to smile, frown, elevate his forehead and eyebrows, tightly close his eyes and resist attempts to open them, whistle, show his teeth, and blow out his cheeks. The sense of taste is tested with various sweet, salty, acidic (sour), or bitter substances.

Acoustic (VIII). The eighth cranial nerve has two divisions: The *cochlear nerve* is tested for *auditory acuity* by having the patient listen to the whispered voice, the tick of a watch, and a tuning fork at various distances from the ear. Testing of bone and air conduction is carried out with a tuning fork. Additionally, an audiometer may be used for a precise evaluation of auditory acuity. The *vestibular nerve* is concerned with reflexes that maintain equilibrium in space by coordinating muscles of the eye, neck, trunk, and extremities. Various tests may be employed to evaluate vestibular function, e.g., cold caloric test, rotation, and galvanic. (For detailed discussion of evaluation of hearing and equilibrium see Unit XXI).

Glossopharyngeal (IX) and Vagus (X). Because of the overlapping innervation of the pharynx, the ninth and tenth cranial nerves are examined together. The patient is asked to open his mouth widely and say, "Ah." While he does this the palate's elevation, position, and movement are checked. The gag reflex is checked, and also the patient's ability to swallow some water. The posterior third of the tongue is tested for taste, as with the seventh cranial nerve. The patient is asked to cough and to speak to test the vagus nerve; involvement of this nerve results in an ineffectual cough and a weak, hoarse voice.

Spinal accessory (XI). This nerve innervates the upper portion of the trapezius and sternocleidomastoid muscles. In testing, the patient is asked to elevate his shoulder tips up toward his ears (with and without resistance), and to turn his head to one side and resist the attempts of the examiner to pull the chin back toward midline.

Hypoglossal (XII). The twelfth cranial nerve provides the tongue with motor innervation. The patient is asked to open his mouth widely, stick out his tongue, rapidly move his tongue from side to side and in and out. Also, the strength of the tongue is tested by having the patient push his tongue against the inside of his cheek and resist pressure applied to the area externally by the physician.

EVALUATION OF THE SENSORY SYSTEM

The complete sensory examination can be performed only on the conscious patient because the patient must be able to focus his attention on the stimuli and cooperate with the examiner. The stuporous patient may be tested for the presence of responses to painful stimuli (e.g., reflex withdrawal of limbs, wincing, grimacing), but it would be impossible to perform other aspects of the sensory examination. In performing the complete examination sensation is tested with the *patient's eyes closed.*

We have already discussed some aspects of the sensory examination; you will recall that we mentioned evaluation of vision, hearing, smell and taste, as well as touch, pain, and temperature.

Various disturbances of sensation may occur. For example, *dysesthesias* are well-localized sensations that are irritative to the patient, such as sensations of warmth, coldness, itching, tickling, crawling, prickling, and tingling. *Paresthesias* are distorted sensory stimuli; for example, light touch may be experienced as a burning or painful sensation. Absence of the sense of touch is called *anesthesia,* while reduced sense of touch is *hypesthesia* and an overly sensitive sense of touch is *hyperesthesia.* An area of reduced sensation of pain is termed *hypalgesic;* increased is *hyperalgesic,* and absence of pain is *analgesic.* Other disturbances of sensation are discussed throughout the unit.

Routinely during the sensory examination tests are carried out for touch, pressure, movement, position (proprioception), vibration, and pain. When there is a loss of the sense of pain, tests for temperature awareness are performed. In the sensory examination *stereognosis* (i.e., the form and configuration of felt objects or three-dimensional discrimination) is also tested. The loss of this sense is called "astereognosis."

EVALUATION OF THE MOTOR SYSTEM

During the neurologic examination the motor system is examined in terms of: *general appearance,* e.g., notation is made of contractures, abnormally large muscle masses, or evidence of muscle wasting; *muscular tonus; coordination; muscular movement; station; gait; posture;* and *muscular strength. Grip* is commonly tested by asking the patient to strongly grip the examiner's hand or index finger, which the examiner then tries to withdraw. *Abnormal movements* and *muscular spasms* are also noted. *"Motor signs,"* that is, indications of motor damage, include *restlessness, tremor,* and *involuntary movements.*

Impaired Coordination

A defect in the performance of coordinated, skilled muscular acts is called *apraxia.* Tests for coordination are usually divided into tests for equilibratory and nonequilibratory coordination. *Equilibratory coordination* involves coordination of the body as an entire unit, especially in maintaining upright posture. Such activities involve cerebellar, proprioceptive, and vestibular antigravity mechanisms. *Ataxia* refers to a disturbance in equilibratory coordination. A positive *Romberg's sign* means that ataxia is present, causing a tendency to sway and fall when the patient *closes his eyes* and stands with his feet close together. The tests of nonequilibratory coordination involve *successive movements,* e.g., tapping the fingers rapidly up and down, as well as such tests as the *finger-to-nose test* (in which the patient is told to extend his arm, pointing the index finger, and then swing his arm in an arc to touch the tip of his nose).

Abnormal Movements

Abnormal involuntary movements that may be observed during the neurologic examination include: choreatic movements, athetoid movements, dystonic movements, choreoathetosis, tremors, and muscular fasciculations.

Choreatic movements asymetrically involve first one muscle group and then another in jerky, quick, involuntary movements. *Athetoid movements* are writhing, twisting movements that are slower and more continuous than choreatic movements. Both choreatic and athetoid movements typically disappear during sleep. *Dystonic movements* are athetoid-like movements, involving large segments of muscle; the muscle tonus characteristic of dystonic movements varies between hypotonia (particularly at rest) and hypertonia (during movement). *Choreoathetosis* is a combination of athetoid and choreatic movements.

Various types of *tremor* appear with disorders of the nervous system. Tremors are movements in which the opposing muscle groups involuntarily contract, producing alternating or rhythmic movements of groups of joints or a single joint. The rate (slow, rapid) and amplitude (fine, coarse) of tremors varies. The rate and amplitude of tremors can be altered by rest or action. Some tremors (*rest tremors*) diminish or entirely disappear with action, whereas other tremors (*action* or *intention tremors*) appear with the initiation of certain actions. Tremors are also described in terms of being *constant* or *inconstant,* and *regular* or *irregular.*

Muscular fasciculations are fine twitching movements of small segments of resting skeletal muscles. These movements occur first in one part of the muscle and then in another and do not cause joint movements.

Muscular Spasms

Four types of muscular spasms are discussed here: clonic or myoclonic, tonic or tetanic, occupational, and tics.

Spasms that appear as a sudden jerk or series of rapid jerks of a muscle group, single muscle, or part of a muscle are called *clonic* or *myoclonic spasms.* Continuous muscular contractions, brief or prolonged, are called *tonic* or *tetanic spasms.* Writer's cramp is an example of an *occupational spasm* in which spasms occur in muscles used in performing various habitual acts. Muscle spasms repeatedly occurring in the same muscle group are called *tics.* Tics are also sometimes described as "nervous twitches" or "habit spasms."

Associated Movements

Associated movements are muscular motor patterns and contractions which *involuntarily* accompany various voluntary movements, thereby adding to the balance and gracefulness of such voluntary movements, giving them skill. (For example, normally one extends the wrist in making a fist.) Associated movements are considered to be extrapyramidal motor patterns. Various disorders of the nervous system can modify normal associated movements, e.g., by increasing or reducing them.

Abnormal Gaits and Postures

Neurologic disorders may seriously interfere with a patient's posture and the way he walks. Gait disturbances can best be observed as the patient walks naturally in a straight line. Some of the most easily recognizable gait and posture disturbances seen in neurologic conditions are discussed in Chapter 39.

EVALUATION OF REFLEX ACTIVITY

Evaluation of a patient's reflexes is part of the diagnostic neurologic examination of a patient as well as an important procedure in the ongoing clinical assessment of a patient with an established neurologic disorder. Evaluation of reflex responses can provide information about the nature, location, and progression of neurologic disorders.

A wide variety of reflexes may be evaluated clinically. Four major groups of reflexes are discussed below, along with examples of each group and explanations of how various reflexes are clinically elicited.

1. *Superficial or cutaneous reflexes* are produced by cutaneous or mucous membrane stimulation. The stimulus is produced by stroking a sensory zone. Examples of superficial reflexes are: the *abdominal reflex,* in which scratching of the skin of a quadrant of the abdomen normally results in contraction of the abdominal muscles of that quadrant; and the *plantar* or *sole reflex,* in which scratching of the plantar surface of the foot (i.e., the outer sole of the foot), from the heel toward the toes, normally contracts or flexes the toes and sometimes the foot.

Other superficial reflexes are: the *corneal reflex,* in which gentle stroking of cornea with a wisp of cotton causes reflex blinking (to test the left eye have the patient look up and to the right—vice versa for the right eye—and bring the stimulus in from the side in such a manner that the patient cannot see your hand, then very gently touch the outer edge of the cornea); and the *pharyngeal reflex* or *"gag" reflex,* in which gentle stimulation of the back of the throat and the pharynx with a tongue blade produces gagging.

In testing various superficial reflexes the examiner may use such implements as a wisp of cotton, an applicator stick, a double tongue blade, or a pin.

2. *Deep or tendon reflexes* are of greater diagnostic value than are superficial or cutaneous reflexes. Deep or tendon reflexes result from stimulation of deep structures, i.e., stimulation of muscle tendons. Such reflexes are called *muscle stretch* or *mystatic reflexes* since the reflex contraction of a muscle results from stimulation by rapid stretching of the muscle. This is clinically achieved by sharply striking the muscle's tendon of insertion with a sudden, brief blow.

Tendons usually examined are the Achilles, patellar, biceps, and triceps. Tapping the Achilles tendon normally produces an *ankle jerk,* resulting in plantar flexion of the foot; tapping the quadriceps femoris tendon just below the patella normally produces a *knee jerk, quadriceps jerk* or *patellar reflex,* resulting in extension of the leg; tapping the biceps brachii tendon normally produces a *biceps jerk,* resulting in flexion of the forearm; and tapping the triceps brachii tendon at the elbow normally produces a *triceps jerk,* resulting in extension of the forearm.

3. *Special reflexes* involve structures other than the skeletal muscles. For example, reflex mechanisms normally help to maintain respiration and keep blood pressure within normal limits. Reflex salivation may follow a taste of food. Flashing a light in an eye normally causes the diameter of the pupils of both eyes to lessen, thereby limiting the amount of light that can enter; this is known as the *light reflex* or *pupillary reflex.* (See also p. 423.)

4. *Pathologic* or *abnormal reflexes* are exaggerations of normal reflexes, or they are reflexes which do not normally occur. The presence of such reflexes can indicate neurologic disorders, frequently of the spinal cord or higher centers. The *jaw reflex* (in which the jaw contracts and closes the mouth as a result of a downward blow on the lower jaw, when the mouth is relaxed and hangs passively partially open) occurs only rarely in healthy individuals, but is noticeably present in sclerosis of the spinal cord's lateral columns. The jaw reflex is also called the *mandibular reflex* or the "jaw jerk."

The *palm-chin reflex* is another pathologic reflex produced by vigorous, rapid irritation with a blunt instrument of the mound on the palm at the thumb's base, causing the muscles of the chin to be pulled up on the same side.

"Clonus" refers to rapidly alternating flexions and extension at the joint, resulting from the continuous rhythmic contractions of a muscle subjected to stretch. This is unlike the normal stretch reflex, which typically produces one reflex action; with clonus, the action continues.

Babinski reflex occurs when the sole of the foot is scratched with a blunt point, causing dorsiflexion of the big toe and frequently fanning of the other toes, instead of normal plantar flexion (Fig. 37–1). This is accompanied by dorsiflexion of the foot at the ankle and flexion at the knee and hip. The Babinski reflex is probably the most important single pathologic sign in neurology.

In eliciting the Babinski reflex the stimulus is started at the midpoint of the heel and is carried upward and laterally along the sole's outer border until the ball of the foot is reached; there the stimulus is directed across the ball of the foot toward the medial side. Or the stimulus may be started at the midlateral sole and carried down toward the heel.[232]

Generally, exaggerated deep reflexes are accompanied by diminished or absent superficial reflexes, or by such pathologic reflexes as the Babinski toe sign.[111]

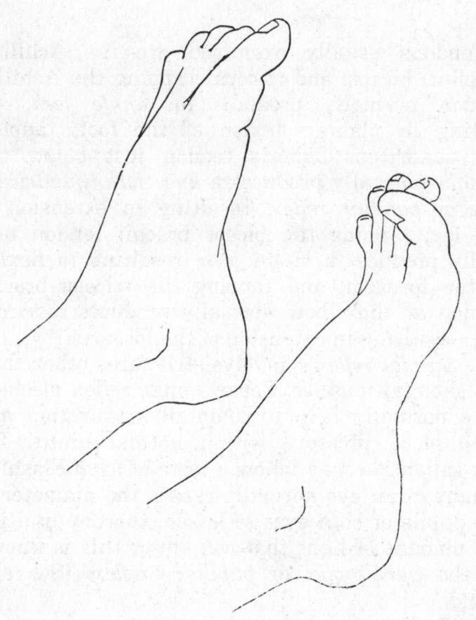

FIGURE 37–1. Normal plantar flexion compared with pathologic or Babinski response. (From Gardner, E.: *Fundamentals of Neurology*. 5th ed. 1968.)

EVALUATION OF THE AUTONOMIC NERVOUS SYSTEM

Many diseases that are not primarily of the nervous system have symptoms related to impaired autonomic function, e.g., postural hypotension, Raynaud's disease. Unit XIX discusses autonomic disorders related to the endocrine organs e.g., symptoms of overaction of the sympathetic system are outstanding in hyperthyroidism. In this unit we shall focus on disorders in which neurologic components are of major significance, e.g., causalgia, syringomyelia, and peripheral neuropathy.

Some general symptoms of autonomic dysfunction include: alterations in patterns of perspiration; faulty body temperature regulation (i.e., hypothermia and hyperthermia); abnormal pulse rate and pilomotor responses; as well as trophic, vasomotor, and pupillary changes. Autonomic dysfunctions in organic disease are often localized in a certain area of the body.

In examining for autonomic disturbances the physician also inquires about *polyuria, abnormal motility of* the *gastrointestinal tract,* and possibly *urinary* or *fecal incontinence.* He examines the abdomen for evidence of *bowel* and *urinary bladder distention. Changes in thirst, energy, potency, libido, weight,* and *appetite* may also be significant.

The patient's skin, mucous membranes, hair, and nails are examined for obvious *trophic changes.* Trophic changes occur in various diseases and cause the loss of innervation incorporating the autonomic nerve supply. Trophic disturbances may be manifested by changes in the affected area's temperature, sweating, and color, e.g., pallor, cyanosis, and erythema. Paralyzed limbs may be cooler to touch than other areas of the patient's body. Also, with trophic changes the nails may become curved, brittle, broken, and thickened; the skin may be painlessly ulcerated, thickened, atrophied, pigmented, oily, scaly and rough, or tight, shiny and dry. The hair may become oily, brittle, and dry, or loss of hair or abnormal hair growth may occur. Painless ulceration may be present on the fingers, toes, or other regions.

An additional trophic change, which nurses constantly combat, is decubitus ulceration, which tends to occur in denervated regions of the skin, beginning at areas subjected to prolonged pressure. (The prevention and clinical care of decubitus ulcers has been discussed in Unit V.) *Palpitation,* i.e., unduly rapid action of the heart which is felt by the patient, may also indicate autonomic dysfunction.

DIAGNOSTIC TESTS AND PROCEDURES

SKULL X-RAY

When the doctor orders "routine" skull x-rays, the radiologist takes films in the following projections: lateral, half axial, axial, and posteroanterior. Additional specialized views may also be ordered and/or tomograms may be taken. Tomograms are selected horizontal or vertical layered exposures taken at measured depths. When tomograms are sequentially reviewed it is possible to obtain some idea of the two-dimensional shape of a defect, e.g., an abscess.

BRAIN SCAN

Brain scanning is an innocuous procedure. Following intravenous injection of a radioactive substance the patient is taken to the radioisotope laboratory and a scan is done with a sensing device, e.g., a Geiger-Müller counter. The scanning takes only a few minutes, and the patient is returned to the ward. This procedure is used on all patients who are suspected of having a brain tumor. Other lesions that may be detected with a brain scan include brain abscesses, hematomas, and arteriovenous malformations. A brain scan helps to determine whether more intensive studies are needed; it is also possible to evaluate the effects of surgery, radiotherapy, or chemotherapy.

Brain scans are done in the anteroposterior (AP) and lateral positions. The basis for the procedure is that radioactive elements emit rays (beta, gamma, or x-ray) that can be measured electronically. These tracer substances tend to concentrate more readily in pathologic regions than they do in normal tissues; thus, areas of abnormal brain tissue are evident when a diagnostic brain scan is performed (Fig. 37–2). Readings are made at various times according to the wishes of the physician. For example, readings may be made immediately following injection, and then additional scannings may be performed two hours following the injection and at subsequent intervals of 24, 48, and 72 hours.

LUMBAR PUNCTURE ("SPINAL TAP"; SPINAL PUNCTURE)

A lumbar puncture refers to puncture of the lumbar region of the spine in such a manner that the needle enters the lumbar subarachnoid space of the spinal canal and cerebrospinal fluid (CSF) can be withdrawn. This is a procedure with which the nurse frequently assists the physician.

Lumbar puncture is one of the most common diagnostic tests performed on neurologic patients. It is the only accurate procedure for establishing intracranial pressure when the pressure is believed to be elevated. LP is often carried out immediately if meningitis and other infections of the CNS (viral and spirochetal as well as bacterial) or subarachnoid hemorrhage are suggested.

Because LP is uncomfortable for the patient and is not without hazards (e.g., leakage of CSF,

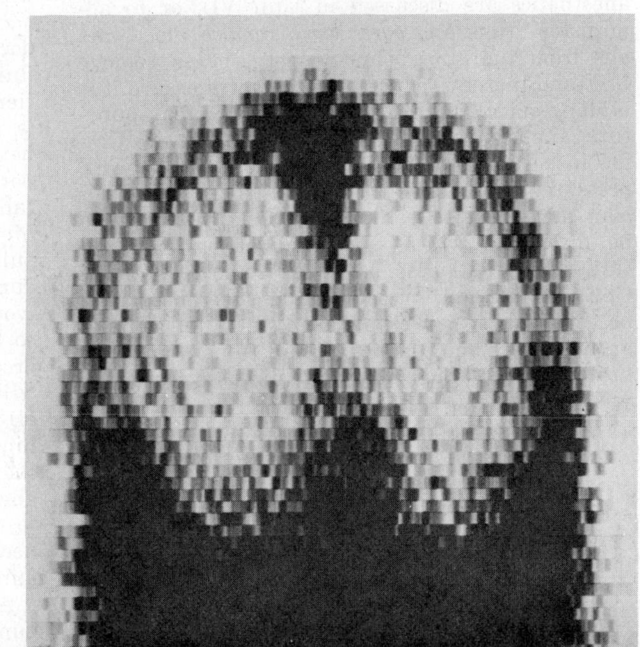

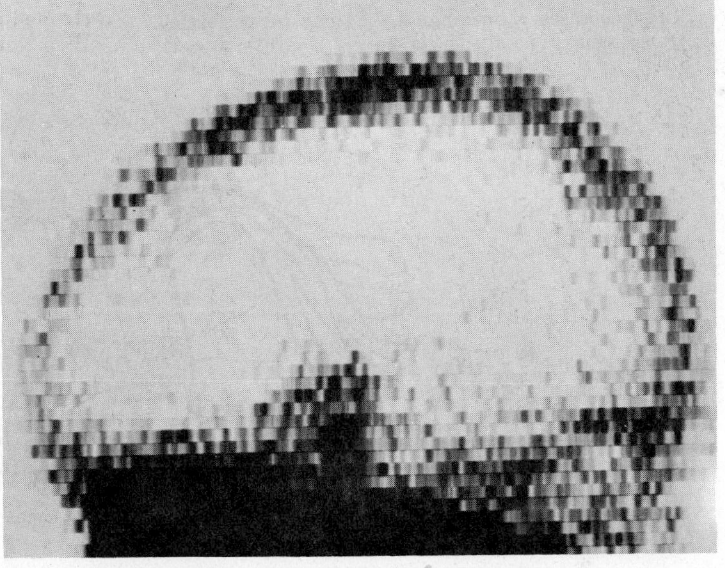

FIGURE 37–2. Scan of brain showing pituitary tumor. *A*, Anterior view indicates area of abnormal activity at base, almost in midline; *B*, lesion is in region in lateral view of pituitary fossa. (DeLand, F., and Wagner, H. W.: *Atlas of Nuclear Medicine.* Vol. I. Brain. 1969.)

infection, damage to intervertebral discs, respiratory failure, postpuncture headache), the necessity for the procedure is carefully evaluated before it is carried out.

Let us emphasize the need for *strict aseptic technique* in the performance of lumbar puncture (and in all procedures in which the CNS is directly penetrated); the introduction of an infectious agent could produce a serious, perhaps fatal, infection.

Lumbar puncture may be performed for a variety of therapeutic as well as diagnostic purposes. *Therapeutically* lumbar puncture may be performed *to administer* spinal anesthesia (spinal anesthetics are discussed in Unit VI), or to administer drugs and sera; or *to remove* blood and pus from the subarachnoid space, or to remove CSF and thereby reduce intracranial pressure if it is dangerously high. *Diagnostically* lumbar puncture enables the removal of a sample of CSF for inspection and the measurement of the CSF pressure. At the time that this is done, the physician may elect to perform "spinal dynamics" (to be discussed) which could indicate a block in CSF circulation. Also, following removal of some CSF, air, oxygen, or radiopaque substances may be injected and x-rays taken (e.g., encephalograms) which may help to locate tumors or other brain disorders. Such x-rays are discussed later.

> *Lumbar puncture is* contraindicated *if there is evidence of greatly increased intracranial pressure (e.g., papilledema),* if an intracranial tumor is suspected, and in the presence of an infection at the site of the puncture.*

The presence of a space-occupying lesion within the cranium, e.g., tumor, may greatly increase the CSF pressure, producing papilledema. In such conditions, LP is contraindicated because the rapid reduction in pressure caused by removal of CSF can cause herniation of the brain structures into the foramen magnum. This, in turn, puts pressure on the vital centers in the medulla, e.g., the respiratory center, and could cause sudden death.

> *Should displacement of the brain cause sudden collapse, the emergency treatment consists of artificial respiration and maintenance of a patent airway. Removal of CSF from the lateral ventricles may also be indicated.*

For our purposes in the following discussion assume that the lumbar puncture is being performed to obtain a CSF specimen and to measure the CSF pressure.

Prior to the procedure tell the patient that the doctor is going to take a small sample of spinal fluid from the lower spine. Even though the patient appears confused or stuporous, tell him what is going to happen to him and what to expect next as the procedure is being performed. If the patient is capable of understanding a more detailed explanation, prior to the procedure instruct him that: (1) he will lie on his side with his legs pulled up close to his chin; (2) he should not move during the procedure but should lie still (you may need to help to hold a restless patient so he cannot move during the procedure); (3) the procedure may be slightly painful, but mostly he will have a feeling of pressure from the needle; (4) he may have brief, flitting pains in his legs or hips if the needle touches nerves that run to these areas; (5) the doctor will give a little local anesthetic (usually 1 per cent procaine) in the area to help to reduce the feeling caused by the needle; and (6) the procedure takes only a few minutes to perform.

Although a headache may follow a lumbar puncture, it is best not to discuss this possibility with the patient, since the power of suggestion is strong in an untoward reaction of this nature.

If a signed permit is necessary for lumbar

*In some cases of meningitis, LP may be performed in the presence of papilledema.

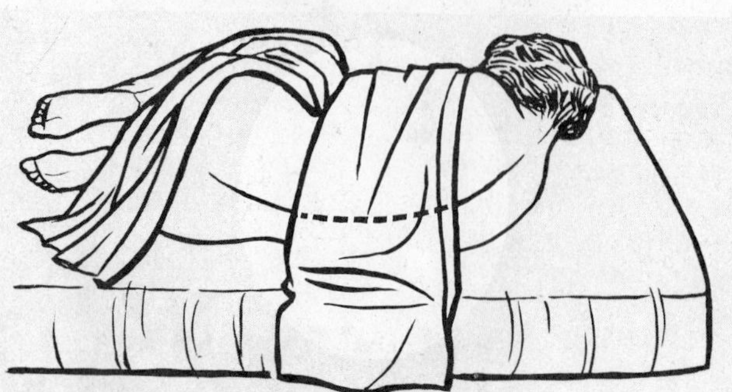

FIGURE 37–3. Lateral position for lumbar puncture.

puncture (it is in some hospitals), have one signed prior to the procedure. Next assemble the equipment for the doctor, clear a clean working area beside the treatment table or at the bedside, and have the area well lighted. Usually hospitals have a preassembled sterile spinal tray which contains most of the equipment the doctor needs, e.g., the needles, syringes, manometer, test tubes, and sponges. You may need to obtain a local anesthetic, sterile gloves, and a band aid to be placed over the puncture area following the procedure. Also you may need a laboratory slip and a marking pencil to number the specimens.

Prior to the procedure, have the patient empty his bowels and bladder. During the procedure the nurse encourages the patient to breathe normally and to relax as much as possible.

The lateral recumbent position of the patient for a spinal tap is shown in Figure 37–3. As you can see, the patient is placed on his side with his back close to the edge of the bed; this makes his back readily accessible to the physician. The patient's knees are drawn up, curving his back, thereby separating his vertebrae and increasing the space between them so the needle can be introduced more readily. A small pillow is placed under the patient's head to keep his spine on a horizontal plane; a large pillow may be placed between the patient's knees.

The nurse usually stands in front of the patient and places one hand behind the patient's knees and the other on his shoulder, thereby reminding him to keep the desired position. Also, the nurse helps to keep the patient's "up" shoulder from falling forward to prevent rotation of his spine. During the procedure the patient should be reassured as needed and should be reminded not to make sudden movements.

The physician wears sterile gloves when performing a spinal tap. He may prepare the skin of the patient's back over the site to be punctured, or he may have you do the skin preparation. A sterile drape may or may not be used, depending upon the preference of the doctor. All equipment, including a spinal manometer for measuring the CSF pressure, is sterile.

The spinal puncture is generally performed between the third and fourth lumbar vertebrae (Fig. 37–4). Since the spinal cord ends at the lower border of the first lumbar vertebra or the upper border of the second lumbar vertebra, puncture between the third and fourth lumbar vertebrae minimizes danger of injuring the spinal cord. The puncture in the adult is about level with the top of the hip bones, i.e., the iliac crests.

With a small needle, syringe, and a local anesthetic agent the doctor anesthetizes the area. Next he introduces the large spinal needle. The needle has a stylus which the doctor removes upon entering the spinal canal. Next the doctor attaches a stopcock and the manometer to measure the initial CSF pressure before removing any fluid.

In measuring the CSF pressure the doctor watches to see how high the fluid rises within the manometer's column. He may say the pressure reading out loud so you can help him to

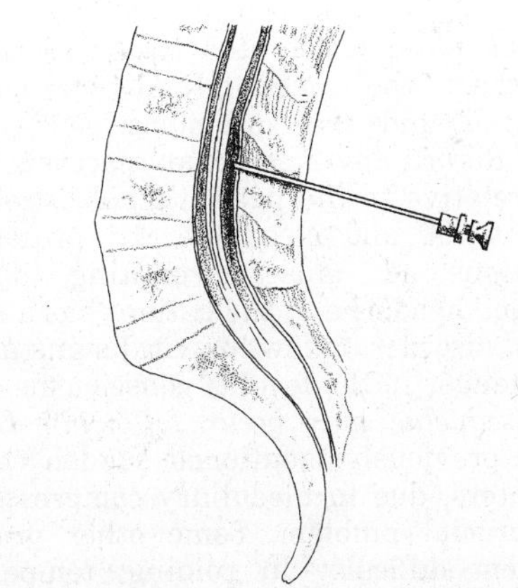

FIGURE 37-4. Position and angle of needle for lumbar puncture; it is in 4th lumbar interspace below level of spinal cord.

remember the figure. The doctor may ask you to steady the manometer or to help him to hold it straight. If you are not wearing sterile gloves, hold only the very top of the manometer with your fingers to steady it.

The first stabilized CSF pressure reading that the doctor makes is called the *"initial pressure."*

Normal initial CSF pressure (with patient in horizontal position) is 6 to 13 mm. Hg or 80 to 180 mm. of H_2O. Pressures over 200 mm. of H_2O are considered abnormal.

Normally the CSF oscillates in the manometer, readily responding to coughing, straining, and changes in the patient's breathing.

In collecting specimens of CSF the doctor allows the fluid to drip into a series of small, sterile test tubes. The tubes are numbered in the sequence of their collection, e.g., No. 1, No. 2, and No. 3; the doctor may hand the tubes to you to number. Two to three ml. of fluid is collected in each tube; a total of 8 to 10 ml. may be removed. As you take the tubes from the doctor be careful not to contaminate his gloves or the sterile field. Also, since CSF may contain highly virulent organisms, e.g., those causing meningitis, be extremely careful that you do not contaminate yourself. Wash thoroughly after handling the specimen tube; keep your hands off your uniform and away from your face until you can wash.

Specimens of CSF should be taken *directly* to the clinical laboratory so they can be examined as quickly as possible. If allowed to stand, changes take place in the fluid which alter the findings.

Following the LP chart that the procedure was performed, the time, the attending doctor's name, and how the patient tolerated the procedure. In addition, chart the amount and character of fluid removed and the specimens sent to the laboratory. Record any significant reactions to the procedure relative to the patient's pulse, coloring, and respirations, and also note the presence of such reactions as nausea, vomiting, dysuria, retention, and headache. If the patient has a known intracranial disorder, follow his vital signs and observe for changes in the level of consciousness.

Various sequelae may occur following LP. Of course, the previously mentioned sudden collapse of vital centers, due to medullary compression, is the most crucial problem. Some other problems are: transient difficulty in voiding; temperature elevation preceded by meningeal irritation; local pain, edema, or hematoma resulting from trauma at the puncture site; and pain radiating to the thigh caused by nerve root irritation. An additional common problem following LP is headache (to be discussed next). It is estimated that one out of four patients suffers from some kind of sequelae following LP.[37]

Postpuncture Headache ("Spinal-puncture Headache"; "Spinal Headache")

Postlumbar-puncture headache is typically bifrontal and suboccipital, appears a few hours to several days following the procedure, and is characteristically relieved when the patient is lying down but resumes upon his sitting up. Postpuncture headache is worsened by a sudden jolt of the head and by jugular compression. Usually the headache is of a throbbing nature. Although such headaches frequently disappear within 24 hours, they may last for several days. The precise etiology of postpuncture headaches is unknown.

It has been found that postpuncture headaches do not occur more often in patients who are ambulatory following the procedure than in those who are conservatively treated with bed rest. Nonetheless, while most physicians believe it unnecessary to keep the patient in bed following LP, others try various measures to prevent postpuncture headache. Some doctors order recumbency in bed for various lengths of time, e.g., 12 to 24 hours following LP. If the patient is to remain flat, immediately place a sign on his bed to inform all staff members and visitors of this order; remember, of course, to also inform the patient.

Once a postpuncture headache begins, various *treatments* may be ordered. Commonly the patient is placed on bed rest in a quiet darkened room, an ice cap is applied to the head, and analgesic medications are administered as ordered. Forcing fluids may also help to reestablish the CSF level.

Queckenstedt Test (Spinal Dynamics; CSF Pressure Readings; Manometric Tests)

This procedure is carried out when the physician suspects compression of the spinal cord, e.g., due to the presence of a spinal tumor, or following dislocation or fracture of vertebrae. These disorders may produce partial or complete blockage of CSF circulation in the spinal subarachnoid space. The physician looks for indications of such obstruction by noting the manner in which CSF pressure readings vary following timed compression of the jugular veins on each side of the neck. (Consult a textbook of neurologic nursing for details concerning this test.) Performance of the Queckenstedt test is contraindicated in the presence of intracranial disease, particularly in the presence of indications of hemorrhage or increased intracranial pressure.

CISTERNAL PUNCTURE

Cisternal puncture is puncture of the cisterna magna (the space between the cerebellum and the medulla) by the introduction of a short-beveled needle below the occipital bone and between the first cervical lamina and the rim of the foramen magnum. The CSF system may be tapped in this manner for a variety of reasons, e.g., to drain CSF or to obtain a CSF specimen in the presence of a subarachnoid block, or if lumbar puncture is contraindicated; to perform encephalography or inject air or dye for myelography. Cisternal puncture may be performed, instead of a lumbar tap, on ambulatory patients, because it is generally accompanied by minimal risks and side effects.

Usually postpuncture headache does not follow cisternal puncture; however, immediately following the procedure the patient should be observed for apnea, cyanosis, and dyspnea. These complications are rare, however, and typically the patient is able to assume his prepuncture activities soon after the cisternal puncture is completed.

Preparation of the patient for cisternal puncture includes explanation of the procedure to the patient and signing by him of a permit. The nape of the patient's neck may be ordered shaved up to the external occipital protuberance in the midline. Because this puncture is closer to the brain than a lumbar puncture, patients are frequently fearful. The patient's cooperation is important. Along with offering appropriate reassurance, the nurse instructs the patient to not move during the procedure.

The patient is positioned at the edge of the treatment table, or his bed, on his side. A sandbag is slipped under the patient's head to keep his cervical spine and head on a straight line with his thoracic spine; his head is flexed forward and held firmly in position by the nurse. Following skin preparation, as for lumbar puncture, a local anesthetic may or may not be injected. Then the

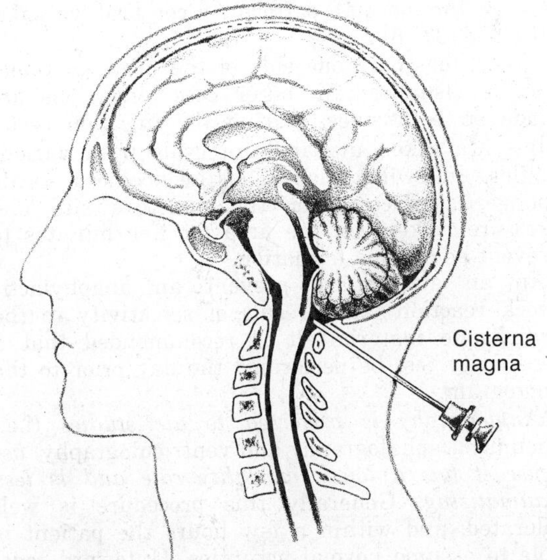

FIGURE 37–5. Position of needle for cisternal puncture. Note short bevel and length of needle.

cisternal needle with stylet in place is inserted to a depth of about 5 cm. (Fig. 37–5).

LABORATORY EXAMINATION OF CEREBROSPINAL FLUID

A few helpful "rules of thumb" concerning cerebrospinal fluid (CSF) laboratory findings are as follows:

> *Blood,* i.e., many RBC, in the CSF indicates hemorrhage somewhere in the CNS, e.g., torn or ruptured blood vessels from injury, or ruptured aneurysm.

> *Increased cells* may indicate infection somewhere in the CNS. For example, polymorphonuclear leukocytes may be increased as a result of pyogenic infection; increased lymphocytes may occur with viral infections and tuberculosis. If extremely large numbers of cells are present, the CSF may actually appear cloudy.

> *Lowered blood sugar* often results from bacterial infections of the CNS.

> *Lowered chloride level* also often results from bacterial infections of the CNS.

> *Increased protein level* usually occurs in the presence of a brain tumor or degenerative diseases.

CEREBRAL ANGIOGRAPHY, PNEUMO-ENCEPHALOGRAPHY, VENTRICULOGRAPHY AND VENTRICULAR PUNCTURE

General Remarks

Cerebral angiography, pneumoencephalography, and ventriculography are all contrast studies used in neuroradiology. Briefly, these procedures are as follows: (1) *cerebral angiography* is visualization of the brain's vascular system by injection of a contrast dye into the circulating blood; (2) *pneumoencephalography* is visualization of the brain's ventricles and subarachnoid spaces, i.e., the CSF spaces in and around the brain, by withdrawal of CSF and the injection of air or oxygen into the spinal subarachnoid space through a LP; and (3) *ventriculography* is the visualization of the brain's ventricles by removal of CSF and injection of air or oxygen directly into the ventricles through burr holes in the skull.

Before proceeding to discuss these procedures individually, let us summarize some facts which apply to all three of these diagnostic tests:

> A signed permit, i.e., permission slip, is required.

> Prior to these procedures vital signs are taken and recorded to establish a baseline of information. Additionally, the size and reaction of the pupils, facial symmetry, level of consciousness, and the motion and strength of the extremities, e.g., hand grip, should be ascertained and the observations charted for similar control purposes. These same points are evaluated periodically by the nurse following the procedure.

> The procedure is discussed with the patient as his condition indicates. The physician discusses any risks involved with the patient's next of kin and the patient.

> A general anesthetic may or may not be given for these procedures. (For discussion of the care of patients following general anesthesia see Unit VI.)

> For some of these procedures the patient is prepared as for surgery, e.g., food and fluids are withheld for six hours, sedatives and analgesics are administered, and so forth. (See Unit VI.) Indeed, surgery sometimes does immediately follow the diagnostic procedure.

> An emergency tracheotomy set and emergency drugs should be available, e.g., an ampule of epinephrine (adrenaline), because these diagnostic tests may produce respiratory distress and shock.

Orders specific to each procedure are carried out as ordered before the procedure. In addition to the discussions in this text concerning cerebral angiography, pneumoencephalography, and ventriculography, consult your hospital procedure book and a textbook of neurology for further information concerning these specific procedures and the nursing responsibilities associated with them. Of course, you should also consult the doctor's order sheet for specific orders for each individual patient.

Cerebral angiography, pneumoencephalography, and ventriculography are all potentially hazardous procedures. The contrast dyes used in angiography may be irritating to the vessels and, also, since the dye is a foreign substance, some patients may experience allergic reactions and possibly go into anaphylactic shock as a result of sensitivity to the dye. Likewise, the gases (air or oxygen) injected during a pneumoencephalogram and a ventriculogram are foreign substances and can cause irritative cellular reactions. An increase in intracranial pressure may occur as a response to irritation from the injected gas.

An additional hazard with pneumoencephalogram is that the rapid withdrawal of a large amount of CSF from below the tentorium can cause downward dislocation of the medulla into the foramen magum. The disastrous result of such dislocation may be severely depressed respirations, leading to death. Pneumoencephalogram is not performed if evidence of increased intracranial pressure is present.

Cerebral Angiography (Arteriography)

Angiography has become increasingly important among neurologic diagnostic procedures. In this procedure intracranial and extracranial blood vessels are visualized by injecting a radiopaque compound into an artery in the neck or arm and then x-raying the head as the material circulates through the cerebral vessels. By visualizing the cerebral veins and arteries it is possible to localize lesions which are of sufficient size to distort grossly the normal pattern of cerebral vascular flow (Fig. 37–6).

Sometimes only one side of the brain's circulation is visualized; in other cases injections are made on both sides. During the injection serial films are taken at rapid intervals from various angles. Following removal of the needle a sterile sponge is placed over the puncture site and pressure is kept on the area for five minutes to prevent hematoma formation.

In an attempt to prevent an anaphylactic shock reaction (as a result of sensitivity to the radiopaque material) it is recommended that a sensitivity test be performed the day prior to the angiogram.

Angiography is preferred to air studies (i.e., pneumoencephalography and ventriculography) *because it has a lower mortality rate and is less traumatizing.* Generally this procedure is well tolerated, and within a few hours the patient is able to assume normal activities. Untoward reactions rarely occur, but when they do they usually take place during the procedure or immediately following it. Most often they result from vasospasm or local hemorrhage. However, both local untoward reactions and those central in origin may occur. Centrally, changes in the level of

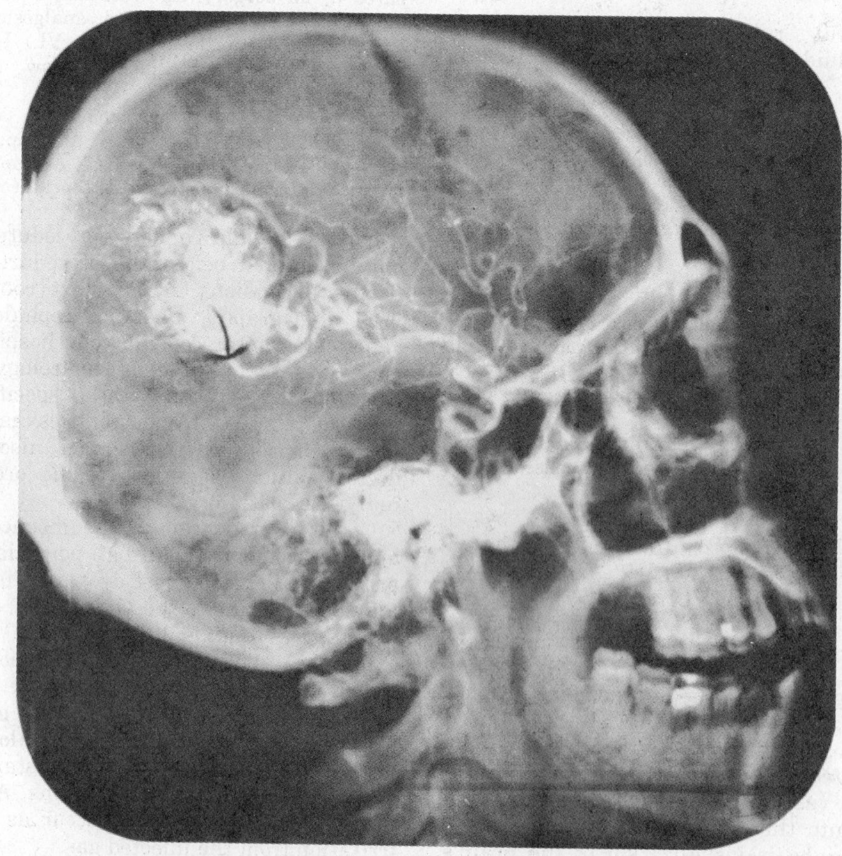

FIGURE 37–6. Arteriovenous malformation of parieto-occipital region as demonstrated by angiography. (Courtesy Dr. Juan Taveras.) (From Merritt, H. H.: *A Textbook of Neurology.* 4th ed. Philadelphia, Lea & Febiger, 1967.)

consciousness, aphasia, hemiplegia, or hemiparesis may occur; locally, a hematoma may develop at the site of the puncture. If such a hematoma is large it can necessitate immediate tracheostomy, because it compresses the trachea and esophagus, producing difficulty in breathing and swallowing. If an anaphylactic reaction occurs, the procedure should immediately be terminated and vigorous treatment initiated. (See Unit V.) Such untoward side symptoms as general prostration, convulsive seizures, or an increase in focal symptoms occurs in less than 10 per cent of patients; these symptoms are usually transient in nature.

Following angiography the patient is positioned comfortably in bed. In addition to taking vital signs the nurse may apply an ice collar to the patient's neck to relieve local discomfort and to reduce superficial swelling. Usually the site of injection is somewhat tender, painful, and slightly swollen. Periodically the patient's neck is observed for increasing swelling, which indicates possible formation of a hematoma. If a patient experiences difficulty in breathing or swallowing, the doctor is promptly notified. Decreased hand grip and facial weakness, on the side opposite the injection, are also significant and are reported.

Observe the patient for a delayed reaction to the dye. Nausea, vomiting, numbness or weakness of the extremities, speech disturbances, profuse sweating, and alterations in level of consciousness may indicate such a delayed reaction. If the patient has headache he is medicated as ordered and kept quiet. After nausea has subsided, encourage the patient to take fluids in spite of pain on swallowing.

Pneumoencephalography (Encephalography; Air Encephalography)

When a LP or cisternal puncture is performed, air or oxygen may be introduced into the subarachnoid space. The air rises to outline the ventricular system and intracranial space, i.e., meningeal spaces, so that these areas can be visualized by x-ray. The resultant x-ray is called a "pneumoencephalogram"; the procedure itself is sometimes briefly referred to as a "pneumo."

Pneumoencephalography may be performed either for diagnostic purposes or therapeutically (to relieve intractable headache). If a space-occupying lesion is identified in the pneumoencephalogram, immediate surgery is required because the pressure alterations within the brain following the introduction of air will increase cerebral edema and the possibility of acute respiratory failure and death. The contraindications for pneumoencephalography are the same as those for LP.

Vital signs are followed carefully during the procedure and following it. During the pneumoencephalogram pulse, respiratory rate, and blood pressure are elevated. During the procedure the patient sits in a special chair with casters. For the first hour following the procedure vital signs are taken every 15 minutes, then every half hour, then every hour until stabilized and, finally, they are taken every four hours. Patients are generally kept flat in bed without a pillow for 12 hours following pneumoencephalography. During this period the patient is observed carefully for signs of increased intracranial pressure and other signs of possible untoward reactions such as convulsions, shock, prolonged headache, respiratory difficulty, sustained vomiting, chills, or fever.

Because the injected air is light, it tends to pocket in the uppermost ventricle. The ventricle has no method for absorption; thus, in order to hasten the passage of the air from the ventricles into the CSF circulation the patient is turned from side to side (while flat) at least every two hours. Also, fluids are usually forced (to 3000 ml.) and are taken through a straw once nausea subsides. Sometimes it is necessary to force fluids containing salt, e.g., vegetable juices. Rolling over is painful for the first day, but encourage the patient to do this and help him to turn over smoothly without jarring himself. If the patient does not roll from side to side his recovery from the procedure will be delayed.

It is not unusual for patients to have *severe headaches* during pneumoencephalography and for 12 to 36 hours following this procedure. Medications are administered as indicated and as ordered for the relief of headache. Caffeine sodium benzoate, 0.5 Gm., I.M., may be ordered p.r.n. for the relief of intractable headache or for stimulation. Other medications which may be given to relieve headache include Darvon (dextropropoxyphene hydrochloride), Demerol (meperidine hydrochloride), codeine and acetylsalicylic acid. An ice cap may also help to relieve headache. Once the intracranial air is absorbed and is replaced with CSF, the headache subsides; generally this takes 24 to 36 hours. In addition to headache, some *nausea* and *vomiting* frequently occur. Special attention is necessary to prevent aspiration of vomitus. Parenteral fluids may be required for the first 24 hours. Also, the air in the patient's ventricles may cause him to temporarily hear "noises" in his head. Although aggravating, this symptom gradually disappears once the gas is absorbed.

Closely supervise the patient for the first day or two following the procedure and see that he is kept flat and is assisted as necessary, e.g., in eating and in turning. Once the order is given to begin elevating the patient's head, the head of the bed is generally elevated *slowly* and progressively a little bit every few hours. If nausea and headache increase when the patient is up, they are generally relieved by having the patient lie flat again.

Pneumoencephalography is a hazardous procedure which is not undertaken lightly. Therefore, patients must be closely observed and protected from possible life-threatening sequelae. Because it is safer and less traumatic, angiography has almost replaced pneumoencephalography.

Ventriculography and Ventricular Puncture

A ventricular puncture is insertion of a special short-beveled ventricular needle directly into the lateral ventricle. In adults it is necessary to make small scalp incisions and drill small burr holes in the skull cap through which the needle may be inserted (Fig. 37–7). This drilling is not necessary in infants; the needle with stylet is pushed through the infant's scalp and anterior fontanel.

A *ventriculogram* is a radiogram of the brain's ventricles filled with air or oxygen. The air or oxygen is introduced into the ventricles through a needle thrust through the brain into the ventricles. Sometimes a catheter is inserted in place of the needle after the ventricle has been tapped. The catheter is left in place until the x-ray films have been taken and read. The CSF is replaced with air, which is introduced directly into the lateral ventricles.

Some of the reasons *ventricular punctures* are carried out are: (1) to inject air or oxygen directly into the ventricles in the performance of a ventriculogram when pneumoencephalography is contraindicated; (2) to establish a route for ventricular drainage; and (3) when lumbar or cisternal punctures are contraindicated.

Ventriculograms may be used to study the patency of the ventricular system, to localize brain tumors, or to detect such cerebral anomalies as atrophy and porencephaly. Ventriculography may be performed under local, intravenous, or general anesthesia. The procedure is usually performed in the operating room with the patient sitting in a special chair. It is generally necessary to shave a part of the head. If a craniotomy is to immediately follow the ventriculography, appropriate preoperative preparation of the patient must be carried out. (See Unit VI.)

Following the procedure a sterile dressing is applied, covering the tissues and the skin sutured over the burr holes. Prevention of infection in the areas of the burr holes is imperative, since the route of infection leads directly into

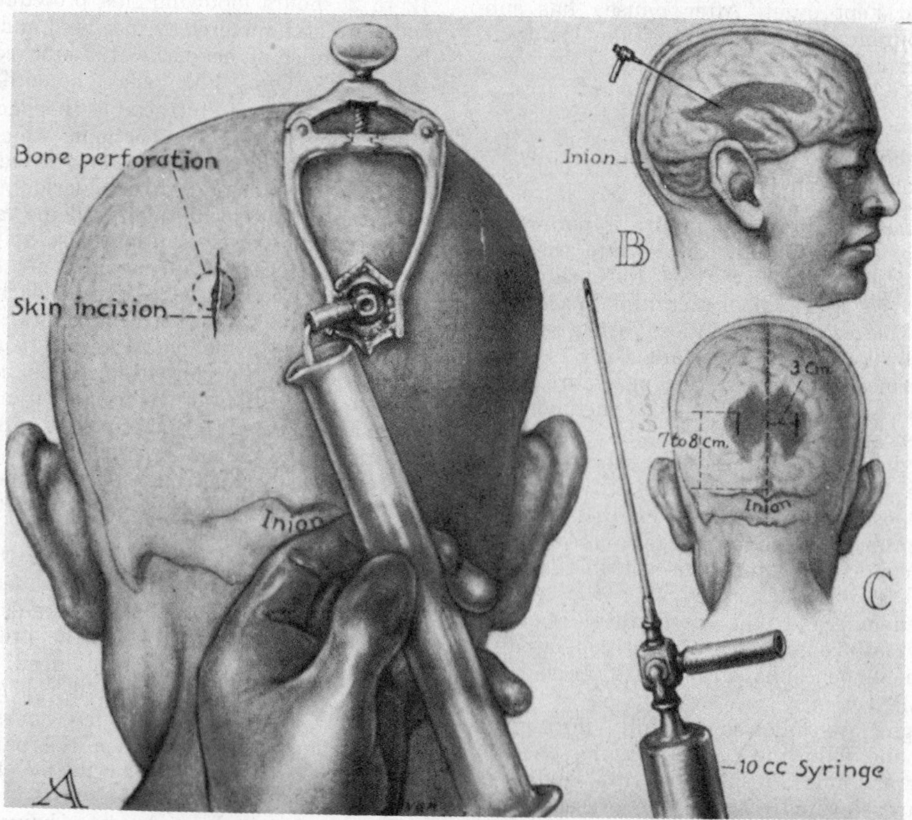

FIGURE 37–7. Ventriculography. *A*, Location of incisions and burr holes with a needle in the ventricle. *B* and *C* show further details. (From Sachs, E.: *Diagnosis and Treatment of Brain Tumors and Care of the Neurosurgical Patient.* 2nd ed. St. Louis, The C. V. Mosby Co., 1949.)

the brain. Periodically the dressing is observed for signs of infection, bleeding, or drainage.

Generally the head of the bed is elevated 10 to 15 degrees following the procedure, and the patient's position is changed every two hours. Vital signs are taken immediately following the procedure and then at half-hour or hourly intervals, depending upon the x-ray findings and the patient's condition. Significant changes in the patient's condition are reported at once to the appropriate person. Some of the serious complications that may occur following ventriculography are: shock, respiratory collapse, hemorrhage, and increasing intracranial pressure. A lumbar puncture x-ray may be kept at the patient's bedside so the doctor can immediately perform a spinal tap if the CSF pressure suddenly increases.

Analgesics and stimulants may be ordered and an ice bag to relieve headache. Fluids and food are given as tolerated. The head of the bed is elevated as tolerated on the day following the procedure.

MYELOGRAPHY

Myelography is x-ray examination of the spinal cord and vertebral canal following injection of positive or negative contrast media into the lumbar (Fig. 37–8) or cisternal subarachnoid space. The spinal subarachnoid space which surrounds the spinal cord is visualized. Recently the examination has been extended to also include examination of the posterior fossa of the skull. Myelography is a particularly valuable diagnostic procedure when the spinal cord is believed to be compressed, e.g., from spinal cord tumor, and in the detection of herniation or rupture of an intervertebral disc. *Discography* may be performed as a diagnostic procedure in a suspected rupture of an intervertebral disc. This is radiographic visualization of the disc by injection of an absorbable contrast medium directly into the disc. Prior to either procedure a permit is obtained from the patient following explanation of the process.

Air is a "negative" contrast medium, whereas various radiopaque oil dyes, e.g., Pantopaque and Lipiodol are positive contrast media. Air studies may be preferred since some available dyes may be irritating if left in the subarachnoid space, causing inflammation of the arachnoid membrane. Often, when oils are used the physician attempts to remove the oil following completion of the x-rays by drawing the oil back through the needle itself. Irritation of nerve roots from such manipulation is often painful.

For *positive contrast* studies a lumbar puncture is performed, spinal dynamics are determined, and a radiopaque oil with a high iodine content is injected into the subarachnoid space. Following injection of the oil the patient is screened under fluoroscopy by the radiologist and then turned onto his abdomen and tilted on the x-ray table. During the tilting process (to facilitate flow of the dye into the subarachnoid space) the patient is held secure on the table by foot and shoulder supports. If the LP has been performed *above* the level of suspected compression, the patient is tilted so the oil flows downward; if the LP has been performed *below* the suspected level of compression the patient is tilted so the oil flows toward the head. The oil will not be able to flow beyond an area of compression.

Following positive contrast myelography the patient is observed for indications of meningeal irritation from the dye. If the dye has been completely removed, the patient is usually kept flat in bed for several hours before he is allowed to resume his usual activities. However, if the dye has not been completely removed following *positive* contrast myelography, the patient's head should be kept *elevated* above the

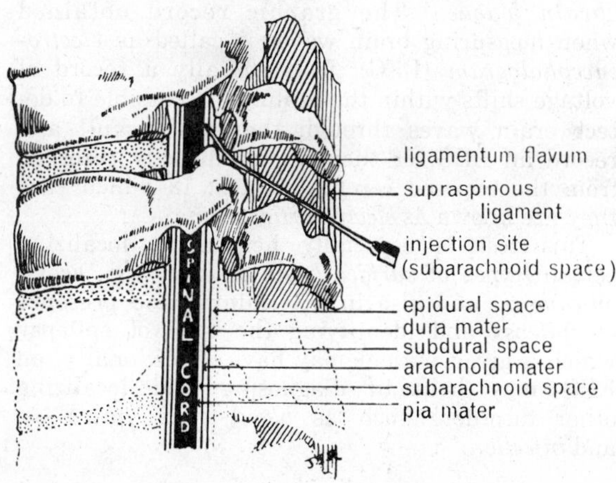

FIGURE 37–8. Diagram of section of spinal column showing site for injection of contrast medium for myelography. (From Fairburn, B.: Neurosurgery today. Spinal cord surgery. *Nursing Times.* Feb. 24, 1967.)

level of his spine. If this is not done the dye will gravitate from the spinal region to the brain, possibly causing irritative cerebral meningitis.

For *negative contrast* (air myelography) studies, the cisterna magna is tapped with the patient in a lateral recumbent position and with the head of the table tilted down 20 degrees. Spinal fluid is removed and is replaced with air. Tomograms are then taken which outline the spinal cord. Following negative contrast myelography the patient's head is kept *lower* than his trunk for 48 hours to prevent the trapped air from entering the intracranial subarachnoid space. The patient's head can then usually be elevated since, by this time, most of the air should be absorbed.

ELECTROENCEPHALOGRAPHY AND ELECTROMYOGRAPHY

Electrical changes in the body can be diagnostically evaluated by means of the *electrocardiogram* (a measurement of the activity of the heart's muscle), the *electromyogram* (a measurement of the activity of peripheral muscles), and the *electroencephalogram* (a measurement of the brain's electrical activity). The electrocardiogram is discussed in Unit X.

Electroencephalography

The brain's neurophysiologic activity produces spontaneous variations in electrical potentials that can be recorded with electrodes placed on the surface of the scalp. The patient's hair is *not* cut or shaved off for this procedure. The electrodes may be attached to the scalp with colloidion or they may be small pins stuck into the scalp. Since the scalp has few nerve endings, the placement of the pin-like electrodes is not particularly painful.

The oscillations or rhythmic electrical discharges produced by the brain's electrical activity are called "*brain waves.*" The graphic record obtained when measuring brain waves is called an *electroencephalogram* (EEG); it is actually a record of voltage shifts within the brain. It is possible to detect brain waves through the intact skull and record an EEG, or they can be directly recorded from the exposed cerebral cortex, in which case they are known as *electrocorticograms.*

This test is especially helpful in localizing certain types of *surface brain lesions* (e.g., scars) or *tumors*, and also in determining the presence of *epilepsy* and identifying the type of epilepsy which a given patient may have. Additionally, an EEG may help in diagnosing and localizing other disorders such as *blood clots, abscesses,* and *infection.*

Electroencephalograms can be taken in the office or laboratory or at the patient's bedside with lightweight, compact, wheeled instruments. Once a record of brain wave activity is obtained, specialists interpret the record according to the brain wave's characteristics, frequency, and amplitude.

If the physician believes the risk of precipitating seizures will not be too great, he may order that anticonvulsant medications should not be given during the 48-hour period before the EEG is taken. Sedatives are also generally withheld unless a sleep record is desired. Also, because fasting can affect the brain wave pattern, the patient should not be fasting prior to the test, unless specifically ordered. On the day of the test the patient should take no stimulants or depressants of any kind (e.g., coffee, tea, Coca-Cola, alcoholic beverages) since these would alter the EEG.

The EEG is obtained with the subject resting in a darkened room or with his eyes closed. Movements, interruptions, and external distractions of every kind should be minimal. When possible the test is performed with the patient in a sitting position.

Electrodes are placed in standard locations on the subject's scalp on both sides of the head, and the various wire leads from these standard locations are hooked up to the recording machine. Some patients fear they could be electrocuted or receive an electric shock during the procedure; such fears should be allayed with the reassurance that the machine is not sending electricity into the patient but is simply recording the electrical activity present in the patient's brain. During the recording of the brain waves the patient merely rests and relaxes. Abnormal EEGs are shown in Figure 37–9.

During the test the patient is asked to hyperventilate (30 to 40 respirations per minute as deeply as possible for three minutes). Hyperventilation accentuates any abnormalities that may appear on the record. The patient may also be asked to perform some simple kind of mental activity.

Electromyography (EMG)

As previously indicated, electromyography (EMG)[12, 73, 102, 148] is a diagnostic procedure that measures and records electrical currents, i.e., muscle action potentials or muscle nerve impulses, induced by muscular action. EMG is helpful in diagnosing neuromuscular diseases because this procedure enables the physician to detect and to characterize small changes within the patient's neuromyal system. The instrument used is the electromyograph.

EMG is particularly useful in evaluating patients with symptoms of abnormal sensation or weakness. EMG can *determine the presence of disease* of the motor unit (i.e., a single motor neuron, its axons, and all the muscle fibers innervated by its branches) and *localize the site.*

Thus, EMG helps in the differentiation of any one kind of lower motor-neuron disease or any one myopathy from others in the same disease category. Also, EMG provides useful indications of the *source, extent, and prognosis* of the disorder. Frequently the processes of peripheral nerve degeneration and regeneration can be monitored electromyographically before clinical changes appear. In some cases, identification can be made of the *time at which* lower motor neuron *damage occurred.*

In the diagnostic electromyography either surface electrodes (applied to the surface of the skin) or needle electrodes (inserted into the muscle) may be used.

MUSCLE BIOPSY

Muscle biopsy is of value in diagnosing neuropathies and myopathies. An electromyogram is helpful in locating those areas of muscle that are most abnormal. It is important that the areas that have actually been traumatized by the needle electrodes be avoided when tissue is taken for biopsy.

NERVE CONDUCTION STUDIES

Nerve conduction studies enable measurement of the excitability and conduction velocity of the motor and sensory fibers of peripheral nerves in the limbs. A stimulating electrode and a recording electrode are placed over different areas along the path of the nerve being studied. Then an electrical impulse is applied to the stimulating electrode and a measurement is made on an oscilloscope of the time it takes for the impulse to reach the recording electrode. This time interval is called the *"latency period."* By combining the latency period with the distance between the electrodes, conduction velocities are calculated. Conduction velocities are expressed in meters per second. It is important that both motor and sensory conduction velocities be obtained from the uninjured extremity as

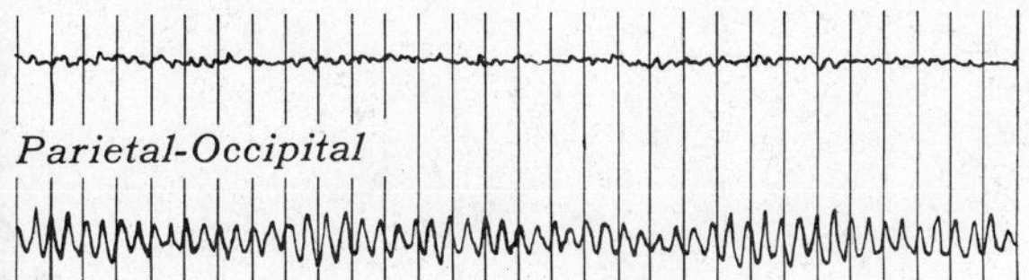

NORMAL ADULT
10/sec. activity in occipital area

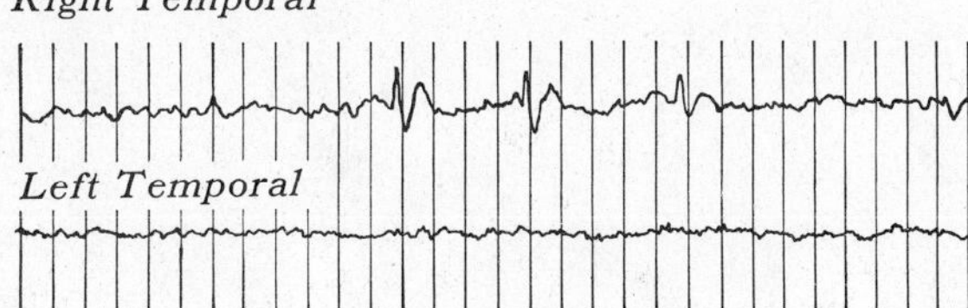

TEMPORAL LOBE EPILEPSY
Right temporal spike focus

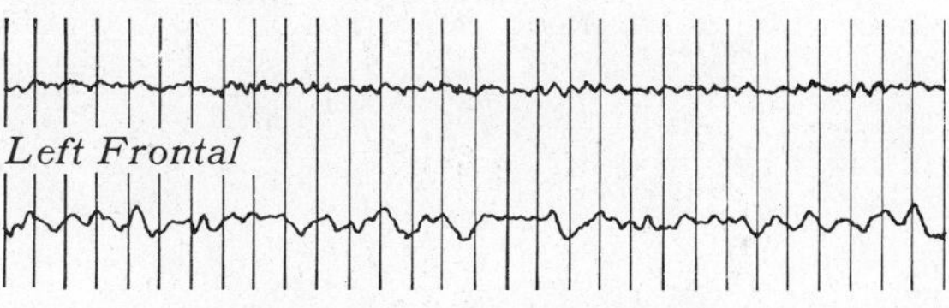

PETIT MAL SEIZURE
Synchronous 3/sec. spikes & waves

BRAIN TUMOR
Left frontal slow wave focus

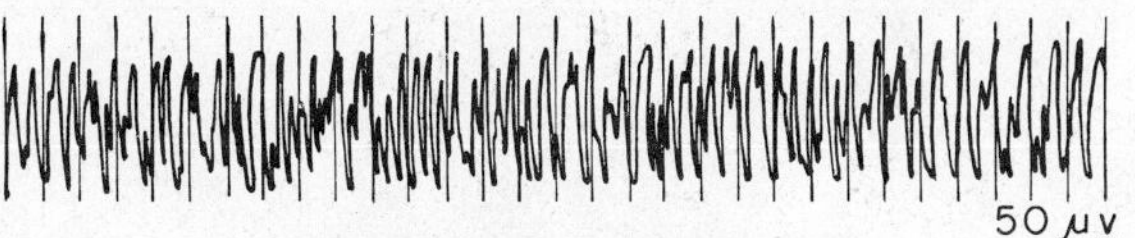

GRAND MAL SEIZURE
High voltage spikes, generalized

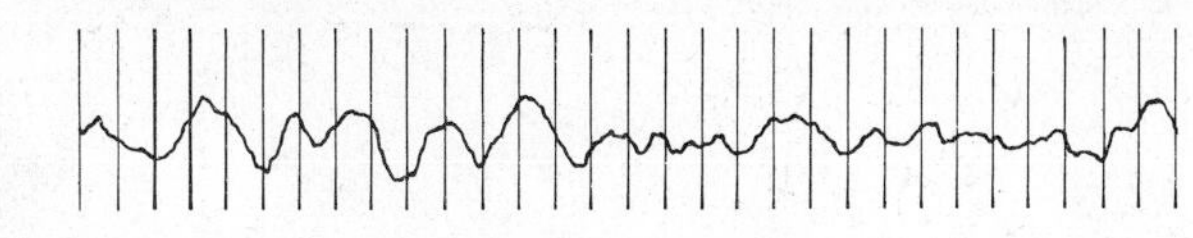

ENCEPHALITIS
Diffuse slowing

FIGURE 37–9. Examples of normal and abnormal EEG's. (From Lyght, C. E., et al. (eds.): *The Merck Manual,* Rahway, N.J., Merck Sharp and Dohme, 1966.)

well as from the injured extremity in evaluating peripheral nerve injuries.

SPECIAL TESTS OF BIOLOGIC TISSUES[232]

Chromosome analysis is used to help to diagnose certain abnormal neurologic conditions and to provide the basis for genetic counseling in families manifesting evidence of congenital neurologic malformations. Chromosomes can be prepared for microscopic examination from the tissue culture of cells obtained from peripheral blood, bone marrow, or skin.

Mental retardation and/or *convulsive seizures* may result from neurologic dysfunction associated with inborn *errors of metabolism.* The diagnosis of disorders of carbohydrate and lipid metabolism may necessitate measurement of the concentration of a specific enzyme in blood cells or tissue obtained by biopsy of the brain, muscle, liver, or peripheral nerve. Usually disorders of protein metabolism are indicated by increased amounts of particular amino acids in the urine or blood.

ECHOENCEPHALOGRAPHY

Echoencephalography is a diagnostic technique that utilizes sound. In 1956 it was first demonstrated that by passing a beam of pulsed ultrasound through the head in the temporoparietal region, and recording the returning echoes, it was possible to measure the position of structures in the cerebral midline and to determine whether these had been displaced to one or the other side of the midline by deforming intracranial disease. The midline structures, especially the lateral walls of the third ventricle but also some other structures, send back echoes that can be used to determine the presence or absence of displacement of these structures.

CHAPTER 38

Clinical Problems Resulting from Altered Neurologic Structure and Function

The nervous system functions basically to transmit information in the body; therefore, when disorders occur within the nervous system a patient may experience various clinical problems which are manifestations of bodily "communication problems." For example, disorders of the nervous system may cause the patient to experience distorted mental activities (e.g., hallucinations, memory difficulties, or perceptual distortions) or perhaps to lose entirely some mental activities (e.g., coma may occur). Disorders of the nervous system may also result in the distortion or loss of regulation of body movements, e.g., reflexes may be exaggerated or paralysis may develop. Additionally, autonomic and trophic activities may be altered by disorders of the nervous system, e.g., muscle atrophy may occur or changes may develop in the temperature or sweating pattern of an affected area.

Numerous clinical problems, such as the above examples, can result from altered neurologic structure and function. In this chapter we shall focus on some of the more common clinical problems associated with neurologic disorders.

ALTERED STATES OF CONSCIOUSNESS

INTRODUCTION AND DEFINITIONS

Total consciousness implies various *subjective processes* which can be thought of as an awareness of surroundings. However, because it is often difficult or impossible to properly evaluate these subjective factors in patients with reduced levels of consciousness, clinically we often observe a patient's objective *responses* to various stimuli, e.g., *auditory-visual, tactile-painful.* Other nonintellectual responses that are assessed include: (1) *motor activity* (e.g., in deep coma there may be flaccidity, hyperkinesia, or little or no spontaneous activity); (2) *reflexes* (e.g., in deep coma the pupillary, corneal, and plantar reflexes are absent); and (3) *autonomic* or *"vegetative" activities* (e.g., vital signs vary in various levels of consciousness, depending upon the causative factor).

LEVELS OF CONSCIOUSNESS AND CONFUSIONAL STATES

Consciousness actually occurs on a continuum. Attempts have been made to identify various phases of this continuum for purposes of discussion; these "landmarks" are referred to as "levels" or "planes" of consciousness. One way of thinking of consciousness is as a "graded form of awareness" ranging from simple perceptual discriminations (e.g., "hot", "cold") to highly complex mental activities such as mathematical abstraction and philosophic thinking. Daily we each normally experience fluctuations in our state of consciousness, ranging from highly alert periods productive of complex mental activity to periods of sleep.

Depressed Levels of Consciousness

It is often said that a patient moves through various depressed levels of consciousness as he either progressively loses or regains consciousness. The various sequential levels of depressed consciousness can be categorized thus:

Level 1: Consciousness. The person is alert, awake, and responsive to stimuli.

Level 2: Lethargy, Somnolence, Drowsiness, or Obtundation. There are blunted alertness and dulled behavior in which parts of the content of consciousness are lost, excessive drowsiness, or falling asleep under inappropriate conditions. The patient responds appropriately and usually briskly to painful stimuli.

Level 3: Stupor. Physical and mental activities are minimal and the person is inaccessible to many stimuli. Verbal stimuli, e.g., commands, usually elicit poor or inadequate responses. The person is incapable of sustained attention. He may react to strong stimuli (e.g., bright light, loud noises) or noxious stimuli (e.g., pressure over supraorbital notch or pinprick) by reflex withdrawal, grimacing, or making unintelligible sounds. Usually reflexes and sphincter action are not changed. Restless motor activity may occur.

Level 4: Light Coma, Semicoma. The person does not respond to ordinary stimuli but may respond to painful stimuli, e.g., pinprick or pressure over sternum. Reflex reactions may be preserved, but plantar reflexes are often extensor in nature.

Level 5: Deep Coma. There is profound insensibility; limbs are flaccid and motionless; muscle, tendon, and plantar reflexes are usually absent. No reaction to painful stimuli, except for occasional fragmentary, abnormal motor responses, e.g., decerebrate posturing. Incontinence is usually present. Pupils may be constricted or dilated and are unresponsive to light; corneal and pharyngeal reflexes are minimal or absent. Vital regulatory mechanisms (e.g., thermal, respiratory) in brain may be disturbed. Periodic or depressed respirations are common. As long as the vital centers are intact, the patient remains alive.

Confused States

The levels of depressed consciousness described above are phenomena somewhat different from the so-called confusional states, that is, *confusion or disorientation* and *delirium.*

Confusion or Disorientation. This involves mildly disturbed consciousness, with impaired perception, poor memory, poor capacity to think clearly, and defective attention. Disorientation in time and place, along with some irrelevancy of thought processes, is often an early indication of confusion.

Refer back to Unit III for discussion concerning some causes of confusion or disorientation and the nursing care of confused or disoriented patients.

Hallucinations, Illusions, and Delusional Thinking. These are also discussed in Unit III.

Delirium. This occurs in infections causing high body temperature, and in toxic conditions, e.g., alcoholic delirium, also called delirium tremens. Confusion occurs in delirium along with increased psychomotor and autonomic activity. *Content* of consciousness is basically disturbed rather than *degree* of consciousness. The patient responds to questions but does so in an extraneous manner. Talkativeness, overalertness, and insomnia occur. Clouding of consciousness and perceptual disorders are present, with illusions, hallucinations, restlessness, and tremulousness of the lips and fingers. A low seizure threshold is present. With *delirium tremens* ("D.T.'s") the patient characteristically has visual and tactile hallucinations in which he sees and feels animals and creeping creatures crawling over his skin.

Confusion and disorientation are not the same as delirium. The delirious patient may be confused or disoriented; however, not all confused or disoriented patients are delirious.

While the comatose person is *hypo*active, the delirious person's behavior is at the opposite extreme—he is *hyper*active. Activity of the nervous system is greatly slowed down during coma and, conversely, it overfunctions during delirium.

Delirium frequently develops suddenly and may disappear with equal rapidity. Usually the symptoms are most prominent at night. Delirium basically results from interference with metabolic processes of the brain's neurons. The physician primarily directs his efforts to treating the disorder causing the delirium, e.g., infection, fever, drug toxicity. The nurse carries out prescribed treatments, attempts to minimize the confusion or disorientation, and protects the patient. Some of the nurse's efforts are also directed at reducing fever in the hyperthermic patient.

The following points are important in caring for the delirious patient:

> *Keep in mind that the patient cannot control his behavior.* His behavior is unpredictable, irrational, and impulsive.

> *Protect the patient from injury.* Accidents happen easily. Keep siderails up, keep the patient closely supervised, and use restraints only as a last resort (and then with a doctor's order if that is the hospital policy). The patient may feel less restless if he can sit up in bed. Keep objects away from the patient which could be used for self-injury. Reassure the patient frequently and keep your manner calm and nonaggressive. Speak quietly, slowly, and repetitively to help to orient the patient, e.g., "You are in the hospital. I am your nurse." Give simple, brief explanations of your actions.

> *Supervise eating and drinking.* Usually the delirious patient cannot "calm down" enough to pause to eat or drink by himself. Feed him and give him fluids. Sometimes extra fluids and between-meal feedings are indicated.

> *Reduce sensory stimuli to a minimum to prevent increasing confusion and hyperactivity.* The patient's environment should be kept quiet and softly lighted (keep light on at night). Conversation at the bedside should be minimal and appropriate.

Although the most dramatic examples of altered states of consciousness most commonly come to mind, e.g., deep coma following head injury, the nurse should remember also some of the more subtly altered states of consciousness present in patients under her supervision. For example, when a patient is given a tranquilizer or sedative, an organic disorder of brain function which alters that patient's state of consciousness is being imposed on him.

CAUSES OF ALTERED STATES OF CONSCIOUSNESS

Careful inquiry into the circumstances under which a patient lost consciousness, plus his medical history, often produces information of diagnostic value.

For purposes of discussion the causes of unconsciousness can be divided into those resulting from brain disorders, metabolic disorders, and functional or psychiatric disorders as shown in the diagram on the opposite page.

Local brain disorders are suggested by neurologic findings, either cranial nerve abnormalities or unilateral long tract signs. Coma due to local brain disorders most often results from supratentorial mass lesions and/or brain edema, causing unconsciousness from downward pressure on the brain.

Cranial Lesions

Supratentorial lesions (i.e., lesions located above the tentorium, which divides the cerebrum from the cerebellum), which commonly produce stupor and coma include: cerebral hemorrhage, large cerebral infarction, subdural hematoma (trauma), epidural hematoma, brain tumor, meningitis, and brain abscess (rare).[189]

Supratentorial mass lesions usually interfere with consciousness by compressing the diencephalon as they shift and squeeze the contents of the supratentorial compartment. As the lesion enlarges it demands more room for expansion. Eventually the expanding lesion may cause the diencephalon to be displaced downward, through the tentorial notch, i.e., *transtentorial herniation*. This herniation results because the bones of the base of the skull and the fibrous tentorium resist movement of the cranial contents, except in a direction toward the tentorial opening (Fig. 38–1).

The presence of stupor or coma in patients with supratentorial lesions is serious because it indicates compression or distortion of the deeply located upper brainstem and also that downward herniation of the forebrain is about to occur through the tentorial notch. Tentorial herniation generally impacts the midbrain and usually results in permanent brain damage or death. Indications of possible herniation, therefore, must be recognized and reported before an advanced stage is reached. With sufficient warning, osmotic decompressing agents or surgical treatment may be instituted and the possibilities of death or serious neurologic injury averted.

Symptoms of impending transtentorial herniation include: (1) gradually deeper levels of unconsciousness; (2) sighing, yawning, periodic respirations; (3) pupillary changes (e.g., the pupils may shrink yet retain reflexes to light, or one or both pupils may dilate widely and become unreactive to light); (4) outward deviation of one eye; and (5) bilaterally stiff, rigid, or spastic extremities.

Subtentorial (or infratentorial) lesions cause stupor or coma if they compress or destroy the brainstem's centrally located activating systems anywhere above the midpons. Stupor or coma also results if expanding lesions of the posterior fossa compress the midbrain upward. Subtentorial lesions may obstruct cerebrospinal fluid flow, leading to herniation of the cerebellum into the tentorial notch. Usually subtentorial lesions produce early localized brainstem signs, e.g., cranial nerve paralysis, nystagmus, ophthalmoplegia. Subtentorial lesions include: pontine or cerebellar hemorrhage, brainstem infarctions, basilar artery aneurysms, brainstem and cerebellar tumors, trauma, and (rarely) cerebellar abscess.

Metabolic Depression of the Brain

Metabolic depression of the brain may result from primary or secondary causes. *Primary causes* are conditions in which there is intrinsic failure of the metabolism of neurons or glial cells; these frequently cause dementia, but usually do not cause coma until their terminal phase. *Secondary causes* are extracerebral conditions that produce

COMMON CAUSES OF UNCONSCIOUSNESS

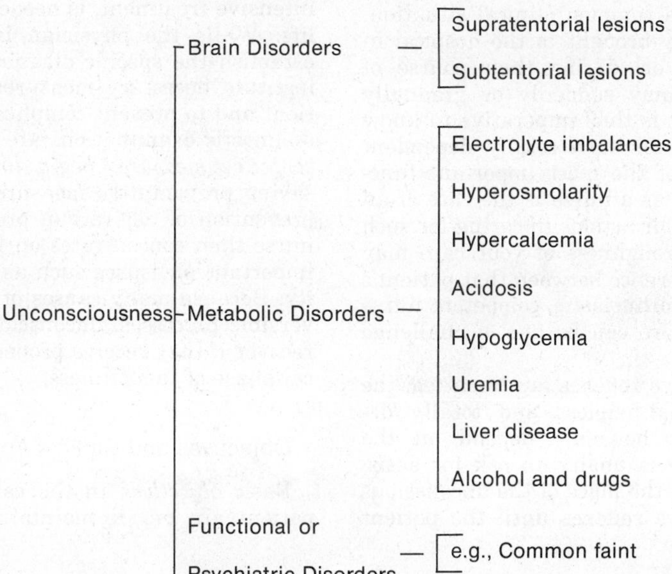

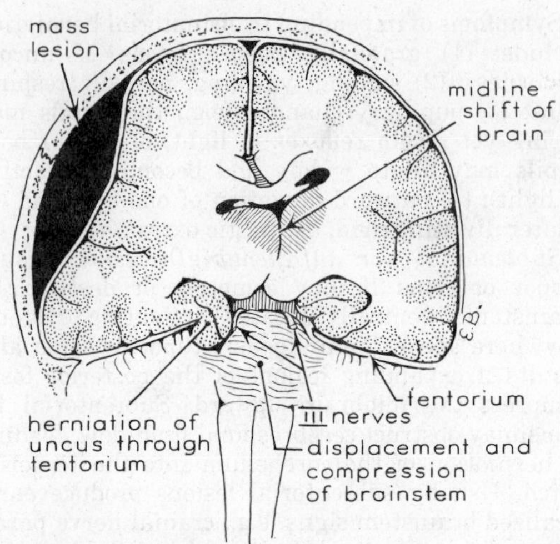

FIGURE 38–1. Mechanism of uncal herniation. (From Young, J. F.: Recognition, significance, and recording of the signs of increased intracranial pressure. *Nursing Clinics of North America 4* (No. 2):225, June, 1969.)

disruption of brain metabolism by either: (1) the effects of ingested or endogenous toxins, e.g., depressant drugs or products of uremia; or (2) interfering with the brain's supply of necessary substances, e.g., oxygen, glucose, or thiamine. It is not clear whether most metabolic agents cause depressed consciousness mainly by affecting the cerebral cortex or the brainstem's reticular formation.

CLINICAL CARE OF THE UNCONSCIOUS PATIENT

Unconsciousness is a common clinical situation. Patients are frequently brought to the hospital in an unconscious state or, during their course of hospitalization, they may suddenly or gradually become unconscious. It is thus imperative to know how to care properly for such totally dependent persons. Indeed, one of the most important functions you will perform as a nurse is the care of an unconscious person. Your actions in caring for such a patient and the thoroughness of your care may actually mean the difference between that patient's life or death. For the enthusiastic, competent nurse this area of clinical care can be one of challenge and reward.

Because his protective reflexes are impaired, the unconscious patient is helpless and totally dependent upon others; he must depend on the nurse even though he is unable to ask for assistance. The nurse takes the place of the unconscious patient's lost protective reflexes until the patient once again regains them or until he dies. By recalling what some of the protective reflexes are, the nurse can identify some of her functions in the care of the comatose patient. For example, because he does not have normal spontaneous movements, the patient needs protection from skin breakdown due to prolonged pressure on bony prominences, and he needs protection from the pooling of secretions in his lungs. Likewise, because he cannot swallow or cough, the unconscious patient needs protection from choking and needs to have his fluid and electrolyte balance maintained in ways not dependent upon his ability to swallow. Because he cannot blink, the unconscious patient needs his eyes protected if they are open, and since he cannot maintain his own body hygiene, this must be attended to by others. Also, since he is unaware of his environment (and thus of external stimuli) he needs protection from the environment and help in adjusting to environmental changes. Because of his lack of awareness of his body position in space, the patient needs to be positioned correctly so that his limbs will not be injured from the weight of his body on them or from being left in awkward positions for long periods of time. Because he cannot move about and keep his joints lubricated and mobile, the dependent patient needs to have his limbs exercised passively.

For a complete discussion of the problems and potential complications associated with prolonged bed rest and the clinical care of the patient immobilized for prolonged periods of time, see Unit V. Here we shall discuss specific clinical care related to the fact that a patient is unconscious.

We have demonstrated that coma may result from numerous causes. Our emphasis in this section is on therapeutic measures that are common to the care of all unconscious patients regardless of the etiology of the coma. Special care required by the specific causes of the state of unconsciousness is discussed in other appropriate sections of the text. Care of the postoperative patient who is unconscious from anesthesia is discussed in Unit VI.

Unconsciousness is frequently a *medical emergency* because often specific therapy, requiring intensive treatment, is needed to save the patient's life. While the physician is busy attempting to establish the specific diagnosis, nursing personnel institute necessary measures to maintain the patient and to prevent complications during the time diagnostic examinations are being performed. *Preventative measures begin immediately.* Once lifesaving preventative measures are completed, e.g., prevention of aspiration, prevention of shock, the nurse then concentrates on less urgent but highly important measures such as prevention of deformity. Because many causes of coma are actually reversible processes, unconscious patients may often recover if they receive proper care during the critical phase of their illness.

Objectives and Clinical Approach

Basic *objectives* in the care of the unconscious patient are to: (1) maintain and support normal body activities and functions; (2) prevent the development of complications that may prevent the patient's recovery or that could cause him residual problems once he regains consciousness; (3) treat the trauma or disorder that produced the unconsciousness; and (4) treat the unconscious state itself.

Life-saving measures may be necessary in treating the unconscious patient before a specific etiologic diagnosis can be established. Once immediate life-saving treatment is given, the physician pauses to carefully evaluate the cause of coma; additional actions, without such specific knowledge, are potentially dangerous.

The general initial clinical approach to the unconscious patient is usually as follows:

> *First, prevent additional injury to the brain and other vital organs. Ensure open airway!*

> *Quickly check vital signs* (rate and depth of respirations, pulse rate, heart sounds, blood pressure); observe color of skin, lips, and fingernails; look for evidence of incontinence and for secretions from the mouth, nose, or ears; observe for tremulousness, muscular jerking, convulsive movements, and posture.

> *Immediately treat shock, correct pulmonary obstruction and other causes of anoxia, maintain blood pressure, meet oxygen and metabolic needs.* Check airway carefully and be certain patient is breathing deeply enough to oxygenate his lungs and to eliminate CO_2. Next check heart and blood pressure more carefully and look for evidence of possible sources of bleeding. Be certain that cardiac output and blood volume are sufficient to supply brain's and kidney's metabolic requirements.

> *Start an intravenous infusion* (with a large bore needle) on all patients in coma. When starting I.V., obtain blood samples for typing and cross matching.

> *Evaluate depth of consciousness* by observing responses to stimuli and *determine presence of localizing neurologic symptoms* pointing to focal intracranial disease.

> *Examine pupil sizes and reactivity to light for indications of increased intracranial pressure* or other indications of the cause of the coma.

> *Examine deep and superficial reflexes* (e.g., determine if they are overactive, underactive, absent, unequal on the body's two sides, or unaltered). Examination of the reflexes is particularly valuable in the comatose patient because they give objective indications of the patient's condition in a manner not requiring the patient's conscious participation. Check corneal reflex.

> *Examine for response to painful stimuli.* Other aspects of the sensory examination are not possible or are unreliable in patients with reduced consciousness.

> *Examine for evidence of trauma.* Remember that trauma may be the *result* of some causes of coma rather than the *initial cause* itself of the coma, e.g., a bitten tongue may result from a convulsion. Examine pupils and optic fundi for signs of increasing intracranial pressure; examine ears for ruptured tympanic membranes.

> *Obtain blood sample* for sugar determination. Glucose, 50 per cent, 50 ml. I.V., may be administered when symptoms indicate a metabolic disease (other than *hyper*glycemia) or if the cause of coma is not clear. This prompt intravenous administration of *glucose* prevents further cerebral damage during the time laboratory tests are being performed if the cause of coma is hypoglycemic encephalopathy. Even if the coma is later proved to have some other cause, the I.V. sugar does no harm.[189]

> *Thiamine,* 50 to 100 mg., is also injected if possible alcoholic (Wernicke's) encephalopathy exists.

Nursing Observation and Reporting

The unconscious patient cannot be properly cared for unless his entire body is inspected periodically. Thus, *nursing care of the unconscious patient includes carefully making frequent, objective observations, followed by evaluation of the observations and detailed, accurate recording and reporting.* Physicians rely heavily upon nurses to observe, assess, and record an unconscious patient's neurologic status and to report significant changes.

A set of *serial observations* is valuable for comparison when a change occurs or a new sign appears. Even though the findings may seem unremarkable for long periods of time, a record or pattern is being established as a baseline for future observations. *Level of consciousness, pupillary responses, and vital signs are evaluated together.* The symptoms probably most indicative of increasing cerebral dysfunction are a lowering level of consciousness and a change in pupillary equality and reactivity. A fixed, dilated pupil indicates increasing intracranial pressure. If pressure is not reduced, herniation of the uncus may result within 15 to 60 minutes. Level of consciousness and pupil reactivity and equality are evaluated every 15 minutes for the first few hours of unconsciousness. If the patient's condition permits, the time interval may then be lengthened.

As the nurse examines the body of the unconscious patient she notes any lacerations, bruises, or ulcerations, as well as the color, texture, and temperature of the skin. She also looks for possible fractures, dislocations, and contractures. If the patient has been injured and has received first aid at the site of the accident, his extremities are checked to be certain no tourniquets have been applied and left tightened. If dressings are present, inspect them frequently for bloody drainage, or if on the head, for indications of possible leakage of CSF.

As she observes and evaluates the unconscious patient the nurse asks herself many questions. Some of these are:

> Are the circulation and respiration effective? Is his pulse slowing while his BP is widening? (If so report at once, for this indicates possible increasing intracranial pressure.) Does the patient appear to be going into shock?

> Is his airway patent? Is the color normal in his nail beds and mucous membranes?

> Are his pupillary responses normal and are corneal responses present? Are the pupils of equal size? Are abnormal eye movements or position present?

> Are some normal reflexes absent? Are some abnormal reflexes present?

> In what position are the patient's head, limbs, and trunk? Does he change these positions? Is his neck rigid or stiff? Are there other indications of meningeal irritation? Are there changes in muscle tone? Is paralysis evident? Is the patient making voluntary movements?

> Are convulsions present? (Give a detailed report of the onset and progression of any convulsions—focal or generalized.)

> Is the patient incontinent? Is his abdomen distended?

> Are there indications of fluid or electrolyte imbalances?

> Is periocular or facial edema present following head injury or cranial surgery?

> Does the patient respond to noxious stimuli? Is he resistive to care? Is spontaneous behavior present? What is his level of consciousness?

Maintaining Circulation and Respiration

Partial airway obstruction is the commonest source of harm to patients with depressed consciousness. *Support the unconscious patient's circulation; establish and maintain the airway, and prevent aspiration of secretions and vomitus.* When a person is found unconscious *loosen all tight clothing,* particularly around the neck, and *clear his airway immediately!*

Partial airway obstruction typically manifests itself through noisy respirations and/or obvious efforts in breathing. *Remember: a noisy airway is an obstructed airway.* Measures must be taken to protect the patient against partial airway obstruction even though obstruction is not obvious. The simplest measure is keeping the patient properly positioned. The *lateral* or *semiprone* position facilitates drainage of respiratory secretions and prevents the tongue from falling backward and obstructing the airway. In positioning the patient to facilitate easy respiration do not acutely flex the patient's neck by placing a large pillow under his head; such flexion could compress the airway. *Frequently* check the patient's position. Be certain that comatose patients are kept in the lateral position if they are transported to other areas of the hospital.

However:

> *CAUTION: Do not change the position of a recently injured patient until you have reasonable assurance that his cervical spine has not been injured.*

Until the patient can be positioned on his side it may be necessary to manually hold his jaw forward (to keep the tongue forward) and to use an oral airway.

> Never allow an unconscious patient to remain unattended on his back *because his tongue may fall back, occluding his airway; also, secretions pool in the pharynx.* Aspiration is a serious threat to the unconscious patient *because it may cause blockage of the airway, leading to respiratory failure or other pulmonary complications, e.g., infection.*

Why is the airway especially important in this group of patients? The reason is that patients with depressed consciousness often have brain disorders which have already caused some increase in intracranial pressure and *airway obstruction (however subtle) increases* an abnormal *intracranial pressure* or may itself cause such pressure.

Inadequate respiratory exchange may cause: (1) CO_2 retention, which causes diffuse cerebral edema and increases intracranial pressure, or (2) decreased arterial O_2 level, resulting in lack of oxygen to brain tissue. Obviously the balance of O_2 and CO_2 in the blood stream must be carefully maintained at proper levels if respiration is to be adequate. *Respiratory failure* will occur if the patient has insufficient lung ventilation and inadequate gas exchange (as revealed by arterial blood gas measurements). To prevent respiratory failure in such a situation, *O_2 therapy, positive pressure assisted breathing techniques,* or *artificial ventilation with a respirator* is indicated. (See Unit XIV.)

When observing the status of a patient's airway also observe his *rate and rhythm of respiration. Cyclic* or *slowed* respirations may indicate increased intracranial pressure. These findings should be reported at once, so that proper treatment can be instituted. Respirations are discussed in Unit XIV.

If the unconscious patient is not breathing or is in cardiac arrest, *heart-lung resuscitation* is immediately instituted to reestablish satisfactory cardiac and pulmonary function. (See Unit X.) This is imperative to provide emergency oxygenation to the brain. Remember that CNS tissue cannot be deprived of its blood supply for very long before irreversible damage and death occur.

An *oropharyngeal airway* may be used for a short period of time. Then, if necessary, a *cuffed endotracheal tube* is inserted to: (1) allow long-term positive-pressure ventilation; (2) allow removal of tracheobronchial secretions; and (3) seal off the digestive tract and prevent aspiration. Many semiconscious or unconscious patients have food in their stomachs. The cuffed endotracheal tube prevents aspiration of vomitus because the inflated cuff prevents regurgitation into the tracheobronchial tree. (See Unit XIV.) The tube is kept in place until the patient is sufficiently awake so that secretions or vomitus will not be aspirated or until the decision is made to insert a *cuffed tracheostomy tube.* Often an open route for suction of the trachea in a comatose patient is lifesaving. Significant respiratory changes or hypoxia should be reported at once. *Suction equipment should constantly be available at the bedside of the comatose patient, ready for instant usage.*

Because the comatose patient lacks pharyngeal reflexes and is unable to swallow, the accumulation of secretions in the pharynx creates the potential danger of aspiration. *Suctioning* of the posterior pharynx and upper trachea should be performed as indicated. (See Unit XIV.)

In addition to suctioning, *frequent turning* and *postural drainage* (see Unit XIV) are employed to facilitate proper drainage of secretions and thus to prevent atelectasis and hypostatic pneumonia. The prone position may be ordered periodically to give additional gravity drainage by exploiting the natural anatomy of the tracheobronchial system (which slopes posteriorly at about 17 degrees). In some instances the foot of the bed may be ordered elevated to facilitate postural drainage.

> *Never place an unconscious patient in Trendelenburg position without an order; this position increases intracranial pressure.*

Blood Pressure, Pulse, and Temperature Patterns

It is difficult to evaluate *initial* pulse or BP observations if a patient's vital signs are not known *prior* to the present incident. However, these initial readings establish a baseline. *Serial* recorded observations of blood pressure and pulse are necessary because serial changes in vital signs are of critical importance. For example, a widening pulse pressure (i.e., the systolic blood pressure widens while the diastolic remains the same or falls) may indicate increasing intracranial pressure. A low pulse rate and/or a high blood pressure also may signal high intracranial pressure. Vital signs are usually measured every 15 to 30 minutes until they appear stable.

The unconscious patient's temperature is initially measured *rectally* every two hours unless there is indication of rising temperature. Then it must be taken more frequently. Temperature elevation may indicate the development of such complications as hyperthermia, urinary tract infection, pneumonia, dehydration, or wound infection. Hypothermia occurs in some patients. Indications of the possible onset of any complications are reported promptly. (Hypothermia and hyperthermia are discussed later.) *Oral temperatures are never taken on unconscious patients.*

State of Consciousness

> *Level of consciousness is the most important single indication of a patient's cerebral function.*

Changes in a patient's level of consciousness can occur quite rapidly. Patterns of change are observed by means of frequent checking. Whenever a change occurs, check the patient again in 5 to 15 minutes. The condition of consciousness is best described in simple terms rather than through terms such as "coma," "stupor," or "unconsciousness," which are frequently as misleading as they are helpful. For example, chart such observations as: "Alert, awake, oriented to time, place and person"; or, "Restless, acts drowsy or lethargic." Other statements might include such observations as: "Incontinent. Correctly carries out verbal commands. Responds to painful stimuli in purposeful manner, e.g., pushes away examiner's hand when pinched"; "Responds to painful stimuli in nonpurposeful manner, e.g., grimacing or decerebrate posturing"; "No response to painful stimuli, no gag reflex, no cough reflex, no corneal reflex." Specific, objective descriptions of a patient's responses (or lack of them) provide a good basis for subsequently identifying changes in his level of response.

In describing a patient's state of consciousness it is important to *describe the apparent level of consciousness* in addition to the *approximate duration of that level* of consciousness, e.g., momentary or transitory, or prolonged for several minutes, hours, or days.

In estimating a patient's level of responsiveness keep in mind the following important points: (1) before beginning the examination *arouse the patient* to his maximal capacity for response (brisk massage of the area around the lips and mouth helps to arouse the patient); (2) during testing *respect the patient's dignity and well-being* (when employing painful stimuli be particularly careful not to cause unnecessary injury, and explain this testing process to the patient's family or friends who may be present). *Strong* painful stimuli should be applied judiciously and only by the physician. The nurse may use milder stimuli, e.g., a pinch, pulling a hair, or the application of something cold.

Remember that a patient needs reorientation as he regains consciousness.

Pupil Size and Reactions to Light

> *Changes in pupil equality and reactivity are primary indications of increasing cerebral dysfunction.*

Examine both pupils to see if they are of equal size and if they react to light by constricting. Also, determine the absolute size of both pupils, i.e., large or small. Pupils may be abnormally small or abnormally large. *An alarming finding is unequal pupil size in which one pupil is abnormally large and does not react to light.* If this change occurs the physician should be notified at once. An abnormally small pupil may be important but is less significant.

When examining a patient's pupils keep in mind the following: (1) examination should be carried out in a darkened room; (2) observe *both* pupils simultaneously because you cannot be certain the pupils are equal unless you view them simultaneously (you may need help to do this correctly as it is difficult to hold both the patient's eyes open when using a flashlight); (3) remember some patients normally have unequal pupils; (4) make certain the patient does not have an Argyll Robertson pupil* or an artificial eye (this mistake has occurred and the pupil in the prosthesis was reported as "fixed"†); and (5) remember you are examining the size of the *pupil* (which depends on how much the iris is open), not the size of the eye in general, e.g., "wide-open," "closed."

When charting pupil size make a labeled drawing of the relative size of both pupils. A small ruler that is graduated in millimeters is useful in measuring pupil size.

Remember the pupils are examined for reactivity by observing the constriction of the pupil when a light is shone into each eye from the side. Observe whether the pupil reacts to light briskly or sluggishly.

Body Tone

In assessing body tone (particularly that of the extremities) make comparisons, e.g., compare right side with left side, upper with lower. Observe for such factors as weakness, rigidity, and flaccidity. Tonic states may be observed in the trunk, e.g., the entire trunk may be extended. Increasing spasticity may indicate increasing cerebral involvement.

Reflexes

The nurse may be asked to check the *Babinski reflex*. Two other important reflexes that the nurse checks are the *corneal reflex* and the *gag reflex*. (See Chapter 37.) Absence of the corneal reflex usually indicates pressure on the trigeminal (fifth cranial) nerve. When this reflex is absent the nurse gives appropriate eye care. Absence of the gag reflex means danger of aspiration and requires special nursing measures, e.g., positioning, suctioning.

Body Movements

Are voluntary or spontaneous movements present? If so, what are they? Stand and watch the patient. A semiconscious patient may be moving his arms but not his legs; this may be the first indication of a previously undetected spinal cord lesion. Perhaps the patient moves his arm and leg on one side of his body, but not on the other; this may indicate a hemiplegia.

Observe the extremities of the patient for the presence of rhythmic, spontaneous movements indicative of a convulsive *seizure*. *Early* recognition of limited, confined rhythmic movements (e.g., of a finger, toe, calf muscle, or facial muscle) is important. When such mild rhythmic twitching is observed in a patient who is not receiving anticonvulsant medication, the physician should be notified. Anticonvulsant therapy may then be started. This could prevent a major convulsive seizure which could possibly seriously aggravate intracranial disorders.

The onset of *restlessness* in a previously quiet patient may be the first indication that compression is occurring from a space-occupying intracranial lesion, e.g., increased intracranial pressure developing due to a slowly forming subdural hematoma. Restlessness may also indicate other problems, e.g., cerebral anoxia, hypoxia, partially obstructed airway, hemorrhage, distended bladder, fracture, tight dressing. Restlessness may favorably indicate that the patient is regaining consciousness.

General Hygiene; Room Environment

The unconscious patient should be *bathed,* have his *hair combed,* and *receive skin and nail care* the same as any other patient receiving total care. Patients often tend to scratch themselves as the depth of their consciousness lessens; thus, their nails should be trimmed and filed. Patients who are comatose for long periods of time may be lifted occasionally into a bathtub half filled with warm water. For unconscious patients (or any patient with long-term debilitating disorders) application of superfatted solutions, e.g., castile, baby oil, cold cream, may be substituted for a bath every fourth or fifth day. This prevents loss of cutaneous oils and the subsequent development of skin irritations or dryness. When unconsciousness persists for long periods of time, the physician usually allows a *shampoo* every ten days to two weeks. Environmental temperature is determined according to the patient's condition, e.g., if he is hyperthermic he may be covered with only a sheet or loin cloth.

Safety and Preventive Measures

Side rails should be kept up at all times when the comatose patient is not receiving direct care or is unattended. Observe seizure precautions for persons with seizure histories and for those patients who could possibly have a seizure for the first time.

When moving or turning the unconscious patient give adequate support to his limbs and head. An unsupported limb may dislocate if allowed to fall unsupported. Also, when turning the unconscious patient always turn him toward you or toward another person so he will not roll off the bed. In addition, protect the unconscious patient from external sources of heat, e.g., hot water bottles, heating pads, radiators, exposed light bulbs, and heat lamps.

Remove and safely store an unconscious patient's dentures and dental bridges; they could cause airway obstruction or could be swallowed or broken. Also, examine the patient for contact lenses and remove and store them if they are present.

**Argyll Robertson pupil* (or "stiff" pupil) is one which is contracted and which responds to accommodation effort but not to light. It is often seen in neurosyphilis.

†A *fixed pupil* does not react either to light or on convergence, or in accommodation.

Protect the patient from injuring himself during convulsions or periods of hyperexcitability. Such protection may be provided by physical measures, e.g., padded side rails and keeping the patient's nails short and clean, or by chemical measures; e.g., paraldehyde, 5 ml., or sodium phenobarbital, 30 to 60 mg. (½ to 1 grain) may be prescribed when seizures occur or during periods of excitability or overactivity. Caution must be observed that the unconscious patient is not overly sedated because *excessive sedation depresses vital functions and increases the hazards of immobilization.*

Avoid restraining the patient unless absolutely necessary. Remember the restrained patient is likely to become increasingly confused and combative.

Unconscious patients ideally *should not be left unattended.* However, some patients (whose conditions are not critical) can be left for periods of 15 to 30 minutes. Because emergencies can develop rapidly in the unconscious patient, routine *emergency equipment* is kept readily available, e.g., tracheotomy tray, airways, suction, oxygen, respirators, I.V. standard, cutdown tray, I.V. solutions, and emergency medications.

The use of *prophylactic antibiotics* is *not* recommended in the long-term management of unconscious patients because of the danger of superinfection from resistant organisms. When infections occur they are treated vigorously with an appropriate course of a suitable antibiotic.

The judicious use of *elastic stockings* may forstall thrombophlebitis (a frequent complication of bed rest). These should be removed several times each day.

Positioning and Exercises

By keeping the unconscious patient properly positioned at all times and by periodically moving him about and passively exercising his extremities, the nurse can prevent the development of numerous complications.

Remember that devitalized, i.e., denervated, tissue in a paralyzed area easily breaks down, forming decubitus ulcers. *The prevention of decubitus ulcer formation is thus highly important in unconscious and paralyzed patients.* Because the patient may remain absolutely still in any position in which you place him, make certain that the position will be a safe one for him. An alternating air pressure mattress should be used for all unconscious patients, in conjunction with turning and passive exercises, to prevent tissue ischemia, which predisposes to decubitus ulcer formation. Patients with neurologic disorders are also particularly prone to the development of *deformities and contractures* since the nervous system controls muscle action.

A hand roll may be used to maintain the hand in a position of function. If the patient's thumb tends to fall forward so that it does not grip the roll, gauze may be placed over the thumb and then loosely taped to the hand roll to keep the thumb in a position of function. Of course, such supportive bandages must be removed to properly exercise the hand, wrist, and fingers. The hand roll prevents *flexion contractures of the fingers.* "Cock-up" arm splints may be employed to prevent *wrist drop* (Fig. 38–2).

Foot drop is a deformity which is all too often overlooked. The traditional footboard is not effective for the unconscious patient because of the necessity of keeping the patient in a lateral position. Posterior splints and passive exercises are thus used to prevent foot drop in these patients. Special skin care and frequent observations are required to prevent the formation of decubitus ulcers on the heels of patients in posterior splints. Prevention of *hip and knee flexion contractures* is a critical element in positioning the lower extremities.

Shoulder tightness, which could result in *"frozen shoulder"* can be prevented not only by passive exercises, but also by alternate positioning of the shoulder joint from the abducted to the extended position.

Eye Care

Normally the cornea functions as an anatomic shield which protects vision. However, this natural shield is injured if the eyes remain open for long periods of time; i.e., the cornea dries, becomes irritated, and may develop ulcers. Corneal reflexes may be absent, and excessive dryness of the cornea may occur in unconscious patients. The eye will be vulnerable to damage, even from the fine dust particles normally present in the air. *Protective eye care may include frequent inspections with a flashlight, shielding an open or partially open eye, simple eye irrigations, and instilling protective eye drops.* Damage to the eye, corneal ulcerations, keratitis, or drying of the cornea can result in blindness if proper eye care is not given.

A covered tray should be kept set up at the patient's bedside for eye care, and the appropriate care should be given *at least* every four hours as a *scheduled* treatment. Be certain to wash your hands before and after carrying out eye care.

The eye may be *irrigated* with normal saline solution. Then the eyelids are dried with cotton and one or two drops of mineral oil or methyl cellulose (0.5 to 1 per cent solution) are instilled to protect the eye and to prevent drying of the cornea.

A protective *eye shield* should be applied if the corneal reflex is absent and if the eyes are open and/or appear irritated. This prevents the cornea from being scratched or otherwise irritated. Or it may be desirable to close the eyelids of the unconscious patient with a small *"Butterfly" collodion dressing* or *adhesive strip,* but unless properly applied, such butterfly dressings may irritate the eye rather than protect it. When patients are unconscious for long periods of time their eyelids may be sutured closed, i.e., *temporary tarsorrhaphy.*

Nose and Ear Care

Nasal passages may become occluded in the unconscious patient because he is unable to sniff, blow, or normally clean his nose. To clear the nasal passages of mucus and crust formations, first gently swab the nose with an applicator moistened with water or normal saline; next, use one lightly lubricated with mineral oil. A steam vaporizer in the room may relieve the excessive dryness of the mucous membranes of the nose and mouth which commonly accompanies mouth breathing in the unconscious patient. Of course, caution must be exercised to prevent burning the patient with steam.

Never clean or suction the nasal passages or ears of patients who have had brain surgery or suffered a head injury without a specific doctor's order. If *bleeding* is noted from the patient's ears or nose, or if *cerebrospinal fluid* (looking like a watery dis-

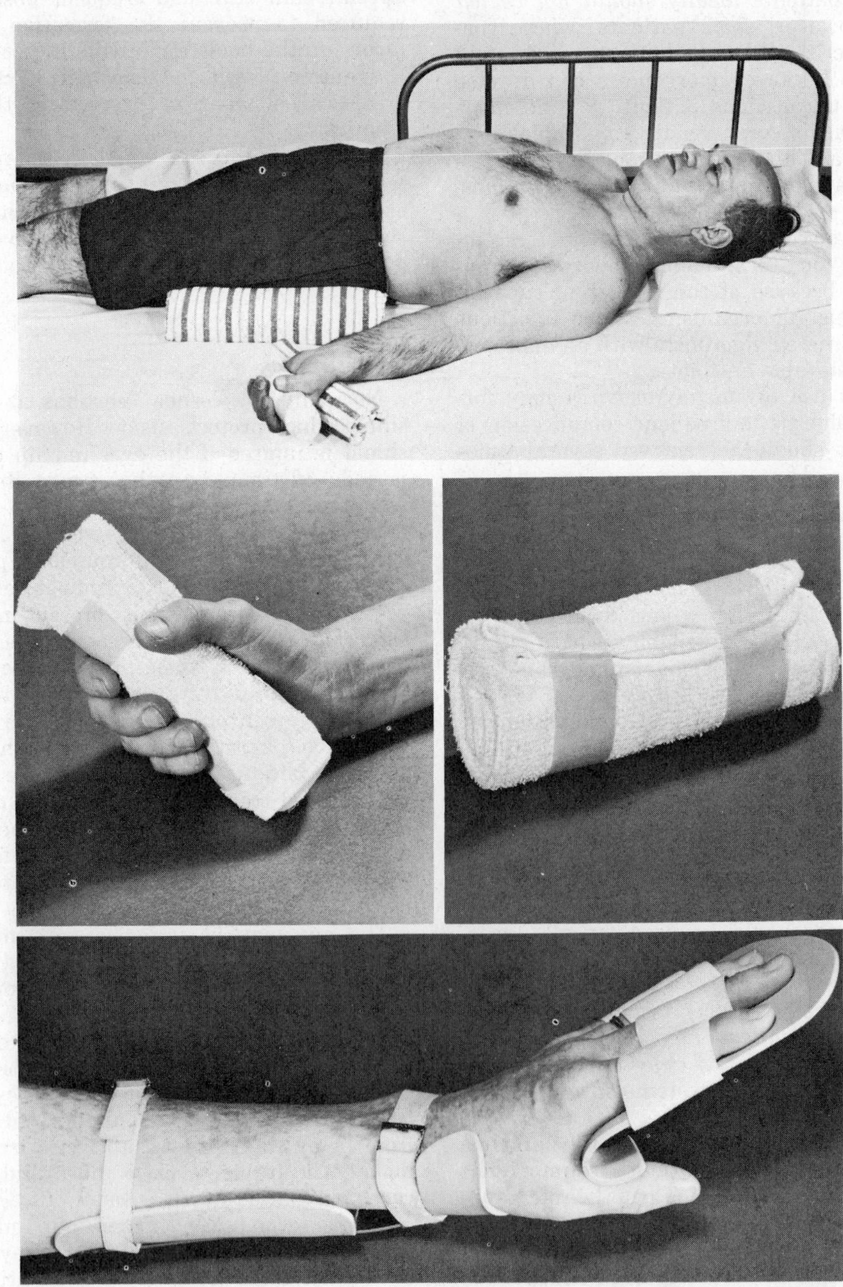

FIGURE 38-2. Wrist and hand positioning. (From Krusen, F. H., Kottke, F. J., and Ellwood, P. M., Jr.: *Handbook of Physical Medicine and Rehabilitation*, 2nd ed. 1971.)

charge) appears to be draining from these areas, *notify the physician at once!*

Mouth Care

Mouth care is conscientiously given *every two hours* (as a *scheduled* treatment) to: (1) provide oral hygiene; (2) prevent excessive drying of the oral mucous membranes; and (3) prevent other complications such as parotitis, sordes, herpes simplex, aspiration, and respiratory tract infection. *Aspiration and respiratory tract infections are common causes of death in unconscious patients.*

A mouth care tray is kept assembled and covered at the bedside. Mouth care is performed gently but thoroughly. To perform mouth care place the unconscious patient well over on his side to prevent possible aspiration. The affected side should be uppermost in patients with facial paralysis. Have the bottom sheet protectively covered and place a towel under the patient's chin and over his shoulder. Place the emesis basin beside the mouth. Prop the mouth open by placing a padded tongue blade or soft roll between the patient's jaws. Do not put your fingers in the unconscious patient's mouth when giving mouth care. If the prop slips out you could be bitten accidentally.

The unconscious patient's teeth are carefully brushed with a small toothbrush at least twice daily. The mouth's mucous membranes, tongue, and gums are cleansed with glycerin and lemon juice swabs or Cook's mouth ointment. The mouth is then rinsed out with Gly-Oxide, an oral lavage solution. Gauze wrapped around a tongue depressor or around a toothbrush (and saturated with Gly-Oxide or covered with Cook's mouth ointment) may be useful in carrying out some aspects of mouth care. *During mouth care of the unconscious patient excess secretions should be removed with suction.* It is easiest if two persons perform mouth care together; one person does the cleansing while the other suctions as necessary.

Particular care should be given to the area around the uvula in patients breathing with their mouths open for long periods of time. Crusts may form in this area which may break off and be aspirated.

Use a flashlight and tongue depressor to inspect the patient's mouth daily. Keep the patient's lips coated with a soothing lubricant to prevent the formation of encrustations, drying, and cracking. Remember to have good light when giving mouth care and wash your hands prior to the procedure and upon its completion.

The mouth care described above for unconscious patients is also indicated for all patients who are seriously ill, are febrile, have facial or bulbar palsy or trigeminal neuralgia, or have had cranial surgery.

Maintaining Nutrition and Fluid Balance

Because he cannot swallow normally and would thus aspirate, the unconscious patient is not given food or liquids by mouth. Therefore, his nutritional and fluid-electrolyte needs are met in other ways, e.g., through nasogastric tube feedings, hypodermoclysis, or intravenous infusion.

Fluid balance is generally maintained by intravenous infusion (or occasionally hypodermoclysis) for the initial 24 to 48-hour period of unconsciousness and then, if coma continues, nasogastric tube feedings are started. These may be started earlier if the patient's veins are poor or to facilitate frequent position change.

Tube Feedings. Tube feedings are the most desirable method of providing prolonged nourishment for the unconscious patient because, while protein and carbohydrates can be administered parenterally, fats are not routinely administered intravenously. Paralytic ileus occurs fairly often in unconscious persons, and a nasogastric tube assists with gastric decompression.

Tube feedings may be used not only for the unconscious patient, but also for patients with such disorders as: paralysis of throat musculature; senility with loss of desire to eat; cancer of the lip, tongue, pharynx, esophagus, or stomach; fistula of the gastrointestinal tract; chronic brain syndrome; or multiple sclerosis.

When tube feedings (i.e., gavage, from the French word for "crammings") are ordered, a nasogastric tube is inserted through the nostril into the stomach, and small amounts of liquids and blenderized foods are periodically administered through a funnel or Asepto syringe attached to the tube.

Commercially prepared tube feeding formulas are available which provide the daily required nutrients, including vitamins and minerals. These solutions are usually low in bulk and high in protein and calories. (The high protein content helps to prevent decubitus ulcer formation.) If a commercial formula is not used, the feeding may be prepared in the diet kitchen. It is noteworthy that gastrointestinal complications (e.g., diarrhea) can be reduced by substituting a blenderized well-balanced soft diet for the traditional tube feeding mixtures or commercial preparations.

The insertion of a nasogastric tube is *contraindicated* in patients with nasal disease, bilateral nasal obstruction, and recent gastric surgery (there is danger of pushing the tube through the incision). Also, once the tube is inserted, various *complications and problems* in maintaining the tube may ensue. Among these are: (1) trauma to the stomach mucosa if the distal end of the tube hardens, as happens after a period of time; (2) vomiting and aspiration if the stomach is overfilled; (3) plugging of the tube; (4) misplacement of the tube into the trachea or lungs, thereby causing aspiration of anything passed through the tube; (5) development of ulcerations and crustations in the nares; and (6) tracheoesophageal fistula; the latter breakdown of the anterior esophageal wall results from prolonged contact between the nasogastric tube and the tracheostomy tube (if present). Tracheoesophageal fistula requires immediate treatment and becomes apparent when gastric contents appear in tracheal excretions.

Some important facts to remember in caring for patients who require tube feedings are:

> *Prior to the feeding place the patient in Fowler's position,* straighten his body trunk so it is not flexed sharply, and elevate the head of the bed 45 degrees.

> *Check position of tube* (to be certain it is in the stomach and *not* in the tracheobronchial tree) *prior to administering the feeding* by: (1) placing end of tube in glass of water and looking for bubbles, which would indicate tube is in lung or trachea; (2) aspirating a small amount of gastric secretions back into a 20-cc. syringe; and (3) administering 30 to 50 ml. of water before administering the formula. This water clears the tube of mucus and, also, if the water is aspirated it is less dangerous than other liquids (e.g., milk formula or fruit juice), which would be a cause of lung infection and irritation).

> While the physician orders the daily amount and type of gastric feedings for a patient, the nurse will usually *determine the frequency and amount of each individual feeding.* Only about 100 to 200 ml. of liquid or the feeding mixture is usually administered at one time. Never give more than 300 ml. at one time if you do not know the patient's tolerance, i.e., 50 ml. of water prior to feeding, 200 ml. of feeding, and 50 ml. of water to wash the tube out following feeding to prevent blockage. A regimen of 150 to 200 ml. of clear fluid, saline solution, or dextrose and water (depending upon caloric requirements) can be alternated with fruit juices, salty broths, and high-protein liquids. *Before each feeding the gastric contents should be aspirated,* and if more than 50 ml. is returned, it is recommended that the aspirate be reintroduced through the tube and that the scheduled feeding be omitted. To help to maintain electrolyte balance, *gastric contents which are aspirated should be replaced.*

> Generally adults tolerate feedings of 200 ml. every two to three hours. However, the total amount of each feeding varies with the individual patient's stomach capacity, tolerance, age, nutritional needs, and so forth. Some adults are tube fed three times each day. *Overfilling of the stomach is hazardous, because it may precipitate vomiting or regurgitation. Suction immediately if this occurs.* It may be necessary to force the patient's jaws open to insert the suction tube if the patient is choking. To try to prevent regurgitation give smaller, more frequent feedings, and have the patient rest undisturbed for a short period of time following the feeding. *Reposition patient on his side following feeding. Do not allow the funnel to become empty during the feeding* because this allows air to enter the stomach.

> Tablet medications should be crushed and completely dissolved in 15 to 30 ml. of water before they are administered through the tube. After instilling the medication always administer water through the tube to be certain all the medication reaches the stomach.

> *Give frequent mouth care and observe for irritation of the nostril* through which the tube passes.

> *Observe the restless or confused patient to be certain he does not pull out the tube.* Aspiration may result if the tube is pulled out during a feeding session or any time it is unclamped. During feeding sessions, cloth wristlets or wristlet restraints may be needed.

> *Measure and record all intake.* Be sure to include amounts of liquids taken in with medications and those taken in when the tube is rinsed out before and after feedings. Observe carefully for symptoms of dehydration, alkalosis, and acidosis.

> *Before removing the tube, clamp it to prevent aspiration.* Also *clamp the tube after each feeding* if it is left in place.

Aspiration pneumonia is always a hazard for the tube-fed patient. If the patient's head is elevated to a 45 degree angle while he is fed, this hazard is reduced because, if the tube is displaced, there is less possibility of food entering the trachea. A patient should not be fed in the supine position unless it is impossible to position him otherwise. The Trendelenburg position and any motion conducive to nausea should be avoided for two to three hours following a large feeding.

Mechanical pumps are available to provide the unconscious patient who has a nasogastric tube with a slow, steady delivery of formula or other liquids. These pumps may be adjusted to deliver from 40 to 200 ml. of liquid per hour. However, it has been noted that diarrhea frequently results from continuous drip.

Nasogastric tubes are traumatizing since they are a foreign object in the gastrointestinal tract. Often bright blood or small amounts of old blood may be aspirated with gastric contents while the tube is in place. Obviously, trauma should be minimized in every possible way.[48]

Try to position the tube so it is not pulled to one side or the other of the nares, causing excessive pressure which could lead to ulceration of that area. Change the tube as ordered. Some physicians believe that polyvinyl tubes are less irritating than the formerly used rubber tubing and can be left in place several weeks at a time; others say that the tube should be changed every five days. When changing the tube, alternate nares to reduce irritation of mucous membranes. Lubricate the nares frequently to prevent crust formation, and give frequent mouth care. Observe for lesions of the nose, mouth, tongue, and gums. Also, watch for signs of tracheoesophageal fistula in patients with tracheostomy tubes.

Other problems encountered with tube feeding are the growth of bacteria in the excellent nutrient media of food particles in the tube, and the precipitation of protein material within the tube with subsequent clogging. These problems are reduced by *always* rinsing the tube out with water following each feeding, and by avoiding formulas that tend to occlude the lumens of small tubes, e.g., formulas containing egg.

Maintaining Fluid and Electrolyte Balance. Important aspects in maintaining fluid balance in the unconscious patient are: accurate intake and output records; weighing the patient daily; and awareness of the significance of such symptoms as excessive sweating, diarrhea, or vomiting.

Before the physician can plan fluid and electrolyte therapy[91] for a comatose patient he must determine if the coma itself is related to a disturbance in the patient's fluid or electrolyte state, or if the patient has a normal electrolyte state that must be maintained during the period of coma. In order to detect electrolyte imbalances various tests are made, e.g., blood sugar, blood urea nitrogen or creatinine, serum sodium, potassium, and chloride, and carbon dioxide. Dehydration and water intoxication (true hyponatremia) are two common causes of electrolyte imbalance associated with coma.

Remember, I.V. solutions and blood transfusions must run slowly in patients with intracranial conditions. They may increase intracranial pressure if given too rapidly (60 drops per minute is average rate of flow). Although some physicians attempt to avoid *cerebral edema* by withholding fluids following head trauma or other neurologic problems, this method is generally viewed as an ineffective maneuver. As a rule, such patients should receive a normal amount of fluid and electrolyte solution. When necessary, cerebral edema can be controlled by high doses of potent steroids or, for brief periods of a few hours, by rapidly infusing urea or mannitol.

Returning to Oral Feedings

> Never *give an unconscious patient food, fluids, or medications by mouth.*

When the patient begins to respond to verbal stimuli and has a gag reflex, his ability to suck and swallow water is tested. In some settings the physician does this test; in others, the nurse. Prior to the test the patient is placed well over onto his side and suction is started, to be used if needed. Water is used in testing the ability to swallow to reduce the dangers in case of aspiration. The patient may be given water to suck through a straw, or on a wet swab.

Once it is established that the patient can safely swallow, small oral feedings may be started. Nasal feedings are terminated when the patient is able to take sufficient nutrition orally. Initially, for patients who cannot suck through a straw or drink from a glass due to facial paralysis, fluids may be placed into the unaffected side of the patient's mouth with an Asepto syringe with about two inches of rubber tubing on the end (to protect the patient from the glass tip, which could accidentally be broken).

During his first attempts to eat by himself again, the patient needs the nurse's quiet reassurance and her calm advice and reminders, e.g., to eat slowly, to swallow, and so forth. The patient should not be hurried or feel rushed. Gradually he progresses to a soft diet. Positioning is important as the patient begins to eat and swallow. Food and fluids should be taken into the unaffected side of the mouth if the patient has residual facial paralysis. This makes chewing easier and reduces drooling. In bed the patient with residual facial paralysis should be positioned with his affected side up before he is fed.

Maintaining Elimination

Frequently both urinary and fecal incontinence occur in the unconscious patient. For esthetic reasons, as well as to prevent decubitus ulcer formation, the incontinent patient's skin is kept clean and dry. Incontinence is always recorded, and the amount excreted estimated as accurately as possible. It is important to record what time incontinence occurred so some idea of the patient's pattern of elimination can be established. This can be helpful in retraining the patient as he recovers or in preventing incontinence by placing him on the bedpan at about that time. Even while the patient remains unconscious the urinal may be placed or the patient put on the bedpan at times when his "pattern" shows he may eliminate.

Urinary incontinence may be contained by the use of an indwelling catheter (Foley) or an external drainage apparatus. Occasionally a form of tidal drainage may be employed to maintain bladder capacity and muscle tone and to try to prevent bladder infection. The physician decides whether a catheter should be inserted. Because catheters are possible sources of infection and are "foreign bodies," they should be removed as soon as possible and bladder training started. Careful observations and cystometrogram studies determine when the catheter can be removed. Bladder retraining is often possible by encouraging the patient to maintain a regulated fluid intake and to develop a pattern of habitually emptying the bladder. If a vaginal discharge or odor is noted, the physician may order cleansing douches. Unconscious female patients also need hygienic menstrual care.

The abdomen of the unconscious patient should frequently be checked for indications of bladder or bowel distention. A full bladder may be an overlooked cause of incontinence; i.e., dribbling may indicate retention with overflow. (See Unit XI.) Also, constipation and fecal impaction may occur; small, frequent liquid stools may indicate impaction. (See Unit XV.)

The unconscious patient requires a program of *bowel care* planned to control bowel movements and keep them on a fairly normal schedule and to prevent involuntary stools and fecal impaction or constipation.

Bowel problems can usually be avoided or eliminated by: mild cathartics; regular daily fluid intake of 3000 ml.; 1 to 3 oz. of prune juice each A.M.; rectal suppositories; and *regular* toileting.

As soon as the patient is able, a program of bowel training should be instituted. Cathartics and lavages are discontinued as soon as possible to prevent the patient from becoming overly dependent on them. Maintenance of a *regular* schedule is important in establishing a bowel control program. Thus, bowel care, e.g., cathartics (if used), suppositories, digital removal, are administered at approximately the *same time* each day. Unit XV of this text discusses specific problems with elimination, and Unit XI discusses catheters.

The Family of the Unconscious Patient

Unconsciousness is upsetting for a family to witness. They cannot communicate with the patient; they fear for irreversible brain damage; they may worry that his condition will remain the same for a long period of time; or they may be anxious about possible death. The expense of highly specialized, long-term care is an additional concern. Family members and friends receive comfort from seeing the unconscious patient kept clean, comfortable, and attractive in appearance and also from seeing (and being in) his well-kept room. Remember that although the patient appears unable to hear, he may actually hear everything that is said near him. Discuss this fact with the family and remember yourself to keep your conversation appropriate in the presence of the patient.

INCREASED INTRACRANIAL PRESSURE

In discussing altered states of consciousness, we of necessity mentioned increased intracranial pressure, which is commonly associated with factors that may cause altered states of consciousness. In this section we shall summarize some earlier statements regarding increased intracranial pressure and also enlarge our discussion of this common clinical problem.

There is no room for expansion within the adult cranial cavity; therefore, there can be no increase in the bulk of any element within the cranial cavity except at the expense of some other element or structure. Increased intracranial pressure occurs with increased intracranial bulk, regardless of the cause of the increased bulk. Excessive, prolonged, increased intracranial pressure ultimately produces anoxia of the brain cells and cellular death, resulting in permanent brain damage or death of the patient.

The nurse needs to be familiar with the causative mechanisms and the symptoms of this condition. Of course, one goal of clinical care with neurologic patients is to *prevent* increased intracranial pressure; however, when it does occur it must be *recognized early* so that prompt treatment can be started. Often the nurse is the person who remains with the patient to watch for symptoms of increasing intracranial pressure.

CAUSES AND MECHANISMS

Increases in the amount of CNS tissue, in the size of cerebral blood vessels, or in the amount of cerebrospinal fluid (CSF) may each increase pressure in the cerebral compartment. Common causes of increased intracranial pressure are lesions of the brain, including edema, hemorrhage, tumor, infection, abscess, or injury.

Cerebral edema, a condition associated with many CNS disorders, may be interstitial (14 to 35 per cent of the brain's weight is made up of interstitial fluid) or intracellular. Intracellular cerebral edema resolves very slowly; thus, the symptoms of increased intracranial pressure may be slow in disappearing even though the increased pressure has been relieved. Brain edema may occur postoperatively or may result from injury or any condition in which there is arteriolar spasm which reduces the volume of blood circulating in the capillaries and greatly increases capillary permeability, e.g., acute nephritis or malignant hypertension.

Following a head injury, or occasionally following intracranial surgery, *intracranial bleeding* may occur. This blood (a high protein fluid) attracts and holds water, thus adding to the problem of compression and accumulation of bulk within the skull's rigid confines. And, as indicated, *added bulk within the skull, from any source, results in potentially dangerous increased intracranial pressure.*

The symptoms produced by increased intracranial pressure result from distortion of tissues secondary to the increased pressure as well as direct pressure on cerebral contents. Because the skull prevents outward expansion of the brain, the pressure is transmitted downward so that with increasing pressure a portion of the temporal lobe eventually herniates. We have previously discussed tentorial herniation (p. 419).

SYMPTOMS

Early recognition of the symptoms of increased intracranial pressure and *prompt treatment* are necessary to ensure the patient's recovery. The symptoms may occur gradually, e.g., over a period of days or weeks, or with dramatic suddenness, e.g., within minutes or a few hours. Cerebral hemorrhage, for example, may cause the rapid development of intracranial pressure; a supratentorial tumor, on the other hand, may have a gradual onset.

Generalized symptoms result because the increased pressure is exerted throughout the brain, producing widespread dysfunction of the nervous system. Generalized symptoms are superimposed on *focal symptoms* produced by the primary lesion. Of course, with increasing intracranial pressure the cerebrospinal fluid pressure readings will be found to be elevated.

Restlessness and Decreased Levels of Consciousness

Increasing restlessness, irritability, confusion, disorientation, delirium, or subtle decreases in levels of consciousness are the earliest symptoms of increasing intracranial pressure and transtentorial herniation. With increasing pressure the patient's level of consciousness declines. Deepening of coma is a serious sign.

Headache

Generally, headache associated with increasing intracranial pressure is constant and of increasing intensity. It may be accompanied by failing vision. Usually it is aggravated by straining (coughing, straining at stool) or movement and is somewhat relieved by elevating the head and lying quietly in bed. Since lowering the head increases pressure, *a patient with increased intracranial pressure should never be placed in Trendelenburg position without a specific physician's order.* Vomiting may or may not accompany the headache.

Vomiting

When it occurs, vomiting is recurrent and may be projectile in nature. It may or may not be accompanied by nausea, and may not be related to eating.

Eye Changes

Various eye changes occur as the third cranial (oculomotor) nerve is compressed by the herniating temporal lobe or is stretched by the descending brainstem. *Slow or "sluggish" pupillary reactions* to light indicate impaired function of the third cranial nerve. *Unequal pupil size,* i.e., one pupil is normal in size while the other is much smaller, indicates irritation of the third cranial nerve to the abnormal side.

Pupils may be *unilaterally dilated and fixed* initially with increased intracranial pressure, and then as the patient's condition worsens they may become *bilaterally dilated and fixed* (a terminal sign). A fixed, dilated pupil must be reported immediately!

Because the dura which covers the CNS extends to ensheath the optic nerve, increased intracranial pressure is transmitted through the CSF to the head of the optic nerve. This causes: (1) an *increase in the normal blind spot* (i.e., the area on the retina where the optic nerve leaves the eye), because it lacks visual receptors; (2) *decreased visual acuity;* and (3) *papilledema,* i.e., edema of the optic nerve head, or "choked disc." Double vision or progressive failure of vision may result from papilledema.

Vital Signs

Changes in vital signs indicative of increased or increasing intracranial pressure are *slowly falling pulse and respiration,* accompanied by a *rise in blood pressure.* This pattern should be reported at once. If untreated, lengthening periods of apnea and cyclic respirations follow, and eventually respirations cease entirely. REMEMBER: the comatose patient cannot clear his airway, and airway obstruction increases intracranial pressure.

With increasing intracranial pressure, compression may cause a *terminal rise in temperature* due to failure of the thermoregulatory mechanism. (See hyperthermia, p. 433.) Otherwise, body temperature measurements do not give useful information concerning the increasing intracranial pressure. Frequent temperature recordings may be made using an electric or battery-operated thermometer with a rectal lead.

Neurologic Symptoms

Worsening of focal neurologic symptoms or the appearance of new neurologic symptoms may indicate an increase in intracranial pressure. *Aphasia* may appear, indicating worsening of the basic disorder. *Hemiparesis* or *hemiplegia* may occur on the side opposite the lesion in a patient with increasing intracranial pressure.

Increasing motor weakness may be detected by noting weakness of grasp. A *positive Babinski reflex* may occur, as well as *decorticate* or *decerebrate posturing.* With *decorticate posturing* both arms are abducted and in rigid flexion, the hands are rotated internally, and the fingers are flexed. With *decerebrate posturing* all extremities are in rigid extension, with the arms abducted, back arched, and toes pointed inward. *Seizures* may occur, particularly with transtentorial herniation. Irritation of cortical and subcortical areas may cause generalized or focal seizures.

Tense bulging decompression or elevation of the bone flap may occur in patients following cranial surgery. This symptom of increased intracranial pressure is an important one following craniotomy. During the surgery all or part of the temporal bone is removed in front of the ear on the side of the surgery to allow for some expansion of the cranium when postoperative edema occurs. Without contaminating the incision, the nurse may occasionally palpate this area gently. The amount of tension in the skin flap over this area indicates roughly the amount of intracranial pressure; e.g., if the area is tense and bulging, then this region is being used to help to decompress the raised intracranial pressure.

TREATMENT

The ideal treatment of increased intracranial pressure is to remove the basic cause of the pressure increase, e.g., drain a hematoma, treat an infection, or remove a tumor. When surgical removal of the cause is impossible, attempts are made to temporarily reduce the pressure by such measures as: (1) the use of medications that promote osmotic diuresis in an attempt to reduce cerebral edema; or (2) mechanical decompression by the removal of some cerebrospinal fluid or surgically providing space for brain expansion. Measures like these may allow the patient's condition to stabilize sufficiently for surgery at a later date.

In the *conservative treatment* of the patient with increased intracranial pressure the patient is positioned with his *head elevated* to increase venous drainage from the brain. In addition, a *dehydrat-*

ing regimen may be instituted. Such therapy may include:

> *Hypertonic solutions intravenously.* Substances relatively impermeable to the blood-brain barrier, e.g., urea or sucrose, may be used to reduce brain swelling. The intravenous injection of such substances in hypertonic solution causes the rapid movement of water from the ventricles into the blood. This produces a temporary brain volume reduction. Examples of hypertonic solutions are: 250 ml. of 25 per cent glucose; 50 ml. of 50 per cent glucose; urea (Urevert) or mannitol; and concentrated proteins (serum albumin and plasma).

> *Steroids* have been effective in reducing the incidence and severity of postoperative cerebral edema. Corticosteroids may be given following the administration of a hypertonic solution to sustain the therapeutic effect; hypertonic solutions *rapidly* reduce pressure, whereas the corticosteroids are *slow* in action. Among the most commonly used of these medications are dexamethasone (Decadron) and methylprednisolone (Solu-Medrol).

> *Restricted (limited) fluid intake:* 800 to 1200 ml. each 24 hours. This procedure is not so common as it formerly was.

> *Dehydrating, diuretic medications:* Caffeine sodium benzoate, I.M., theobromine or other diuretic drugs, or magnesium sulfate, I.M., may be used. The latter may also be given orally or rectally.

Mechanical decompression may be accomplished by removing CSF to decrease pressure or by removing a piece of skull to provide room for the brain to expand. In the latter procedure positioning the patient on the operative side is contraindicated postoperatively.

When intracranial pressure is increasing at a rapid rate, CSF is generally removed via ventricular puncture to decrease the pressure. This route is preferred in such situations because of the danger of cerebral herniation, which can occur with lumbar puncture in the presence of increased intracranial pressure.

In some cases *continuous ventricular drainage* may be instituted. This may be achieved by the continuous withdrawal of ventricular fluid through a special device which automatically maintains intracranial pressure at any specified level.

NURSING CARE

As we have emphasized, the *early* detection of increasing intracranial pressure is of vital importance, since the process is frequently reversible. The frequency with which nursing observations are made is determined by the patient's condition, the rapidity with which his intracranial pressure appears to be rising, and the appearance of new, significant symptoms. It is important to begin treatment, when possible, *before* such serious symptoms as pupillary fixation, spastic hemiplegia, and cyclic respirations develop.

The nurse explains to both patient and family that the frequent testing she performs is done routinely and does not indicate that the patient's condition is worsening. A brief explanation of the reasons for the tests helps to reassure the patient and to engage his cooperation for the multiple necessary interruptions at this time.

Summarized below are some important nursing activities concerning the care of patients with possible or actual increased intracranial pressure.

> *Observe the patient closely and regularly; frequently check vital signs and evaluate findings for symptoms of increasing intracranial pressure.* Check patient's *level of consciousness* and report any significant changes in level of responsiveness. *Check pupils* for changes in absolute pupil size, pupil equality, and reactivity to light. Vital sign changes occur somewhat later than changes in level of consciousness and pupillary changes. Thus, the nurse should promptly report the earlier changes (in levels of consciousness and pupils) to the physician without waiting for vital sign changes to develop. Record *temperature* frequently. Institute appropriate measures to reduce *temperature elevations.* (See hyperthermia, p. 433.)

> *Prevent hypoxia* by keeping the patient's airway clear. As mentioned earlier, hypoxia may cause brain swelling, which further accentuates elevation of intracranial pressure.

> *Maintain elevation of head.* Unless contraindicated the patient is kept sitting up, out of bed. If bed rest is indicated, his head should be elevated above the level of his heart at a 30 to 40 degree angle (without acutely flexing the neck). This upright position improves drainage from the brain, reduces venous congestion, may reduce headache and may prevent a further increase in intracranial pressure.

> *Administer fluids as ordered.* In an attempt to decrease interstitial fluid (and thus reduce or prevent cerebral edema), the fluid intake of patients with increased intracranial pressure may be limited to cover only obligatory losses. Fluid intake should be spaced over a 24-hour period so the patient does not receive a large amount at any one time. Patients receiving steroids or intravenous urea or mannitol may have their fluid intake maintained up to 2500 ml.; special attention is given to maintain fluid-electrolyte balance. (See Unit V.)

> *Run intravenous solutions and blood transfusions* slowly and keep the rate of delivery even, e.g., 60 drops per minute. If given too rapidly, the added circulatory volume may further elevate the intracranial pressure.

> *Accurately measure and record intake and output.* Because osmotic diuresis stimulates a large urinary output, patients receiving diuretics such as intravenous urea or mannitol should have their output measured frequently and accurately so the physician can maintain fluid-electrolyte balance. Periodically check to be certain the patient's bladder is not distended, and observe for retention of urine even though the patient may be incontinent or urinating frequently. Bladder distention may cause restlessness, which can be incorrectly viewed as a symptom of increasing intracranial pressure.

> *Reduce straining by the patient,* e.g., by instituting nursing measures to reduce vomiting and excessive coughing, by keeping the patient calm without restraint, and by giving appropriate bowel care to prevent constipation. Straining increases intrathoracic and intra-abdominal pressures, and these, in turn, increase intracranial pressure. *Enemas may be contraindicated* in patients with increased intracranial pressure; however, stool softeners and mild laxatives may be administered. If suctioning is necessary, it is performed gently to try to minimize the coughing which results from nasotracheal suctioning. Straining at restraints also increases intra-

cranial pressure; thus, *restraints should not be used* without specific orders. In an attempt to keep the patient calm, be calm yourself. *Instruct the conscious patient regarding necessary restrictions;* e.g., caution him not to strain. Some patients will require total care. *Supervise the patient during strenuous activities,* e.g., while on bedpan, while vomiting, and evaluate his condition a few minutes after these activities for indications of serious increase in intracranial pressure.

> *Administer medications as indicated for pain relief.* For example, administer acetylsalicylic acid compounds and caffeine as ordered to reduce headache. *Opiates are contraindicated* because they decrease the rate and efficiency of respirations. Reduced respirations increase intracranial pressure. *Sedatives* are usually not given to a patient with increased intracranial pressure because they tend to depress the level of consciousness and obscure the symptoms of increasing pressure. Pain is evaluated carefully before it is treated, and significant new developments are reported, e.g., sudden sharp head pain or the occurrence of headache in a patient who was previously free of pain for some time.

> *Administer other medications as indicated.* As discussed earlier, cerebral edema may be treated with high doses of corticosteroids or with hypertonic solutions.

> *Familiarize yourself thoroughly with the differences between the symptoms of rising intracranial pressure and those of cardiovascular shock.* For example, with cardiovascular shock there is no pupillary change, the blood pressure falls, the pulse rate rises, the skin is usually pale, cold, clammy and moist, and loss of motor power results from low blood pressure, but there is no paralysis. (Shock is discussed in Unit V.)

> *Observe posture and presence of spontaneous movements and test motor strength.* Compare the right extremities with the left. Simultaneously test the grasp of each hand for strength of grasp, ability to release, and equality. If the patient does not respond to commands, evaluate extremity movements in response to painful stimuli.*

Figure 38–3 illustrates a form used at Toronto General Hospital for recording observations on neurosurgical patients in order to detect changes indicative of increasing intracranial pressure. The top sample (Fig. 38–3*A*) shows appropriate designations to be used, while the bottom sample (Fig. 38–3*B*) presents an example of the completed record for one patient over a three-hour period. The abbreviations used for recording pupillary findings are: (RB) "reacting briskly," the normal reaction; (R) "reacting," the constriction is both less and slower than in the opposite eye; (RS) "reacting slowly," the response is markedly slower; and (F) "fixed," the pupil fails to constrict when the retina is stimulated with light. Observe that the relative sizes of the pupils are schematically drawn by the observer. Concurrent with slowing down in reflex constriction, the pupil begins to increase in size; it is widely dilated when "fixed."[273]

ABNORMAL BODY TEMPERATURE ALTERATIONS

The normal range of oral temperature in a resting person is from 36.5 to 37.5°C. (97.7 to 99.5°F.). Body heat must be regulated within a relatively small range in order for various physiologic processes to operate successfully. CNS function is impaired when body temperature varies 4°C. (9°F.) either above or below the normal range, and convulsions frequently occur when body temperature exceeds 41°C. (105.8°F.). Thermal death results from irreversible changes that occur if body temperature rises above 44 to 45°C. Unassisted survival is generally impossible if body temperature exceeds 8°C. above normal or drops to 10°C. below normal. The body protects itself more vigorously against overheating than against excessive cooling.

HYPERTHERMIA

Hyperthermia (hyperpyrexia) is a body *temperature elevation* to 41°C. (106°F.) or above. During hyperthermia body metabolism continues to produce heat; however, very little heat is dissipated from the body. Because the patient does not perspire and because his superficial blood vessels fail to dilate, his fever continues to rise. Typically the hyperthermic patient's skin appears pale and is perhaps mottled instead of red. While his trunk feels hot and dry, his limbs may feel cold. A shaking chill or quivering of the arms and legs may occur.

At temperatures above 41°C. (106°F.) the rate of cellular metabolism is so greatly increased that physiologic regulation can no longer overcome the rapid rate at which heat is produced. Because the patient's own cooling mechanisms are inadequate, death will occur unless intensive treatment is instituted immediately.

For each centigrade degree of rise in body temperature the body tissues' oxygen requirements increase by approximately 13 per cent (or 7 per cent for each Fahrenheit degree). Brain tissue is highly susceptible to hypoxia. To prevent brain tissue damage from the hypoxia which occurs with hyperthermia, prompt therapy is needed to reduce the body temperature to safe levels.

Causes of Hyperthermia

Hyperthermia may result from various causes, e.g., from infection, from malfunction of the body's thermoregulatory center, or from prolonged exposure of an individual to excessively high environmental temperatures.

The body's thermoregulatory center may malfunction, producing hyperthermia, in the following instances: (1) as a result of cerebral edema; (2) following cerebrovascular accidents; (3) following intracranial surgery; (4) following head injury; or (5) as a result of brain tumors or other lesions.

As stated, hyperthermia also occurs as a result of excessive exposure to high environmental temperatures. This condition, called *"heatstroke"* or *"sunstroke,"* develops because the body cannot dissipate heat faster than it is being received ex-

TORONTO GENERAL HOSPITAL

NEUROSURGICAL

CRANIO-CEREBRAL NURSING RECORD

1 – 6 – 69

27457 Jan. 6-69 1 2 C B

DUE 32

MR. JOHN

222 GREEN RD., TORONTO, ONT.

DR. J.T.

DAY Monday DATE Jan. 6 19 69

ABBREVIATIONS: RB - REACTING BRISKLY, R - REACTING, RS - REACTING SLOWLY, F - FIXED

HOUR	LEVEL OF CONSCIOUSNESS	B.P.	PULSE	PUPILS RIGHT	PUPILS LEFT	MOVEMENT & STRENGTH OF ARMS AND LEGS RIGHT (R)	LEFT (L)	TEMP.	RESP.	OTHER SYMPTOMS & OBSERVATIONS
	ALERT – Describe	Record	Record	Record		**Compare** right with left		Record	Record	**For example**
	e.g. – orientation	each	rate	– size		**Record** – equal or unequal		each	rate	Abnormality of pulse,
	– ability to obey commands	Reading		– reaction		**Hand grasps** – strong, weak, absent		Reading		respiration, voiding, stools
	DROWSY – Describe			to light		**Arms and legs**				Fluid leak: site, appearance,
	e.g. – orientation					Movement – describe				amount
	– ability to obey			RB ●	● RS	e.g. – spontaneous				Intravenous or blood: Reading
	commands			R ●	● R	– to command				and amount absorbed
	STUPOROUS – Describe			RS ●	● RS	– to pain – light,				Drugs – only those ordered
	e.g. response			RS ●	● RB	moderate or deep.				for a specific symptom
	– to questioning			RB ●	● RS					Special tests – e.g. arteriogram
Times	– to light pain			F ●	● F					Headache
as	– Ability to obey commands			F •	• F					Vomiting
Order-	**SEMI-COMATOSE**									Unusual behaviour
ed	Responds only to pain –									Speech disturbances
	light, moderate or deep.									Difficulty swallowing
	COMATOSE									Seizure: Describe
	No response to deep pain									Eyes: Ptosis, ocular deviation
	Any other observations									

TORONTO GENERAL HOSPITAL

NEUROSURGICAL

CRANIO-CEREBRAL NURSING RECORD

1 – 6 – 69

27457 Jan. 6-69 1 2 C B

DUE 32

MR. JOHN

222 GREEN RD., TORONTO, ONT.

DR. J.T.

DAY Monday DATE Jan. 6 19 69

ABBREVIATIONS: RB - REACTING BRISKLY, R - REACTING, RS - REACTING SLOWLY, F - FIXED

HOUR	LEVEL OF CONSCIOUSNESS	B.P.	PULSE	PUPILS RIGHT	PUPILS LEFT	MOVEMENT & STRENGTH OF ARMS AND LEGS RIGHT (R)	LEFT (L)	TEMP.	RESP.	OTHER SYMPTOMS & OBSERVATIONS
1330	Drowsy – rouses easily.	110/70	74	RB ●	● RB	Moves arms & legs spontaneously.		100	22	Haematoma – R.
	Orientated to name only.					Grasps firm and equal.				temporal – Seen by Dr. B.
	Obeys simple commands.									
1400	No change	115/70	74	RB ●	● RB	No change		100	22	Emesis 100 c.c.
										Brownish fluid.
1445	Stuporous – responds only to	115/80	70	R ●	● RB	Moves arms & legs to light pain.		100	22	Echogram done.
	light pain.					L. slower than R.				
1540	Semi-comatose – Responds to	130/80	68	RS ●	● RB	Moves arms & legs to moderate pain.		100	24	Twitching – L. side of mouth.
	moderate pain.					L. slower and weaker than R.				Seen by Dr. B.
				TOTAL FLUID INTAKE 60 c.c. – sips of water						
				TOTAL FLUID OUTPUT Emesis 100 c.c.						*J. Jones*
				Voided 350 c.c.						
1615										500 c.c. Mannitol 20%
										I.V. started.
1630	Semi-comatose – Responds only	136/80	70	RS ●	● R	R. moves to	L. slight mov't.	101	18	Seen by Dr. B. & Dr. T.
	to deep pain.					deep pain				
1645	Semi-comatose – Responds to	160/86	56	RS ●	● R	R. moves slowly	L. slight mov't. –	101	16	
	repeated deep pain.					to deep pain.	weak.			Seen by Dr. T.
				Taken to Surgery						

(*See opposite page for legend.*)

ternally. Hence, environmental heat gain occurs and the body's temperature increases. Additionally, another source of heat is produced within the body because this increased tissue temperature increases cellular metabolism. For example, at 42°C. (107.6°F.) cellular metabolism is increased to a rate 50 per cent higher than that of tissues at normal temperatures.

Early symptoms of heatstroke include visual disturbances, headache, nausea, and vomiting. Additional symptoms include: rapid respirations, rapid bounding pulse, weakness and muscle flaccidity. As the condition progresses the patient becomes delirious and eventually lapses into coma. The thermoregulatory center appears to fail when body temperature exceeds 41°C. (106°F.). At this time, in addition to the presence of a high temperature, the patient typically collapses and there is a noticeable *absence* of sweating. Sweating normally is a protective mechanism which cools the overly heated body; however, in this instance sweating fails to occur (even though desperately needed) because of CNS damage. Without proper therapy, death results within a few hours. (*Note:* Heatstroke differs from *heat cramps* or *heat exhaustion* [heat prostration], in which a marked body temperature rise does not occur.)

Clinical Care of the Febrile or Hyperthermic Patient

Clinical care focuses on reducing the elevated body temperature. Temperature reduction may be accomplished in a variety of ways.

When a patient's temperature is moderately elevated, e.g., 38.4°C. (101°F.), the room temperature should be maintained at 70°F. and blankets and excess clothing removed from the patient. The patient may be covered only by a sheet or occasionally both sheet and gown are removed and only a breast covering and loin cloth are used. Various methods of cooling (discussed on p. 436) may be prescribed by the physician if the patient's temperature continues to rise.

Unless contraindicated, fluid intake is increased to 3000 ml. every 24 hours. In the presence of increased intracranial pressure, the fluid intake may not be increased.

Antipyretics may or may not be ordered. Antipyretic drugs appear to act on hypothalamic centers and obtain their effects through normal physiologic processes, e.g., by reducing the thermoregulatory center's sensitivity and producing diaphoresis. These drugs are of little or no value in treating hyperthermias resulting from hypoxia, heat stroke, or injured thermoregulatory centers, e.g., from CVA, cerebral tumor, or following head injuries or brain surgery. Antipyretic drugs are most useful in treating fever caused by the effects of pyrogens on the thermoregulatory centers.

Symptomatic systemic treatment is indicated when hyperthermia has an obvious cause, e.g., phlebitis, cystitis, wound infection, meningitis, or pneumonia.

General comfort measures are important in the care of any patient with an elevated body temperature. For example, the patient should be kept dry and clean (this is especially important if he is perspiring heavily) and he should be given frequent skin, mouth, and nose care.

Rectal temperatures are taken frequently on hyperthermic patients, so that appropriate artificial cooling measures can be planned by the physician. The patient with a mild to moderate temperature elevation has his temperature checked every four hours. A patient with a temperature elevation over 40°C. (104°F.) has his temperature checked every hour until it levels off at a lower, safer level.

Induced hypothermia (discussed below) may be necessary to protect the patient from the hazards of excessively high body temperatures.

HYPOTHERMIA

The body may be cooled either *locally* (e.g., by packing a limb in crushed ice) or *generally* (e.g., by immersing the body in a tub of ice water or placing an electrically controlled cooling blanket over the body). These are methods of deliberately inducing hypothermia. The body can also become hypothermic *accidentally,* e.g., from prolonged exposure to an excessively cold environment. This discussion focuses on general hypothermia which is induced for therapeutic purposes.

By definition, *"induced hypothermia"* is the controlled reduction of body temperature to a level considerably below normal (e.g., 32° to 26° C. or 89.6° to 78.8°F.) and the maintenance of the temperature at that level. Given proper care it is possible for an individual to survive induced hypothermia that reduces body temperature to below 24°C. In practice generally, however, body

FIGURE 38-3. *A,* Form for recording results of craniocerebral testing by the nurse, showing appropriate designations to be used. *B,* Completed craniocerebral record for one patient for three hours. (From Young, J. F.: Signs of increased intracranial pressure. *Nursing Clinics of North America. 4*(No. 2):225, June, 1969.)

temperature is not allowed to reach such a low level. The level of hypothermia desired for a given patient varies, depending upon the reasons for employing the procedure. The physician determines the level of hypothermia to be maintained and the length of time the patient will be maintained at that subnormal temperature. Hypothermia may be described as mild, moderate or deep, depending upon the level of temperature maintained.

Uses of Hypothermia

Hypothermia may be employed for either medical or surgical purposes.

Surgically hypothermia is used to: facilitate selected procedures by reducing blood flow; lower the operative risk in severely debilitated "poor risk" patients; relieve intractable pain (e.g., in terminal cancer); and reduce the amount of anesthesia necessary during surgery. Surgical procedures for which hypothermia may be utilized include: amputations, cardiac surgery, vascular surgery, and lengthy brain operations. By reducing cerebral blood flow, hypothermia is useful in intracranial operations for aneurysms and highly vascular tumors.

During some surgery hypothermia may be used in conjunction with general anesthesia to decrease metabolism and thereby reduce oxygen requirements. The use of hypothermia influences the amount of anesthetic needed and the speed with which the anesthetic agent is eliminated from the body. (Surgery is discussed generally in Unit VI.)

Medically hypothermia may be employed to: decrease circulation time; reduce intracranial pressure; control cerebral edema; reduce oxygen requirements by decreasing metabolic activity; decrease circulation time; and treat or prevent extreme temperature elevations. Hypothermia may be used in the treatment of shock, cardiac arrest, and gastrointestinal hemorrhage.

Responses to General Hypothermia

Among the physiologic changes which take place as body temperature is lowered are the following:

> *Rate of metabolism decreases.* Body metabolism is reduced by almost 50 per cent when body temperature is reduced to 30°C. (86°F.), and is reduced to 25 per cent of normal if temperature reaches 20°C. (68°F.). Death may then occur suddenly.

> *Endocrine, liver, and kidney functions decrease* as the rate of metabolism decreases.

> *Heart's pacemaker is affected.* The critical level below which arrhythmia occurs (due to altered myocardial irritability) varies with the anesthetic agent used and the patient's age and condition.

> *Circulation slows.* The volume of circulating blood is reduced as plasma pools in peripheral capillary beds. Slowing occurs as the heart's neuromuscular tissue is affected by the reduced temperature.

> *Oxygen consumption is reduced.*

> *Pulse, respiration, and blood pressure fall.*

> *Venous and cerebral spinal fluid pressures decrease.*

> *Cerebral function is reduced.* Cerebral blood flow is reduced about 6 per cent for every degree the centigrade temperature is reduced below normal; brain bulk is reduced.

While observing and caring for the patient as his level of body temperature is reduced, the nurse keeps in mind the expected responses to hypothermia so she can quickly identify responses indicative of the development of possible complications. Typical responses to reduced body temperature occur in the following sequence: (1) rate of metabolism decreases and heart rate and respiratory rate are reduced at 35.5°C. (96°F.); (2) impairment of higher mental processes occurs, and the patient responds to verbal commands but has difficulty performing complicated acts at 33.3°C. (92°F.); (3) patient becomes stuporous and has reduced responses to external stimulation at 32.2°C. (90°F.); (4) unconsciousness ensues, although heart action is not disturbed at 30°C. (86°F.); also, at this temperature the body's temperature regulation is almost completely lost, and the patient becomes poikilothermic (i.e., his body temperature varies with the environmental temperature) and rewarming will not occur without external heat; and (5) at 27.8°C. (82°F.) the heart rate, blood pressure, and respiratory rate continue to fall and ventricular fibrillation may occur. At this final level the patient is comatose; pupillary reaction to light and corneal and gag reflexes are absent.

Methods of Inducing General Hypothermia

Some methods used to reduce body temperature include:

> *Chemical hypothermia.* A combination of drugs known as a *"lytic cocktail"* may be given to suppress the brain's heat regulatory center, reduce temperature to a subnormal level, sedate the patient, and prevent shivering. The medications most commonly used in such combinations are chlorpromazine hydrochloride (Thorazine) and meperidine hydrochloride (Demerol) or promethazine hydrochloride (Phenergan). Body temperature may be reduced about 4° by this method.

> *Ventricular cooling.* An indwelling catheter is inserted into a cerebral ventricle and a hypothermic physiologic solution is instilled.

> *Internal surface cooling.* Various body surfaces may be cooled internally. For example, the nurse may give ice water enemas or the surgeon may pour cold saline solutions into the abdominal or thoracic cavities. Gastrointestinal bleeding may be treated by circulating ice water in a balloon inflated in the stomach. The latter procedure is called "intragastric cooling."

> *Extracorporeal cooling.* Blood stream cooling is accomplished by removing blood from a large vessel, cooling it, and returning it to the body's circulation. Extracorporeal cooling is performed with special ap-

paratus, a heart-lung machine. The blood is cooled as it passes through coils within the machine. During the procedure heparin is given to prevent blood clotting. Extracorporeal cooling rapidly produces hypothermia and is mainly used during cardiac and vascular surgery. At the termination of surgery the blood may be rewarmed by changing the machine's settings. (Heart surgery is discussed in Unit X.)

> *External surface cooling.* The body's external surface may be cooled by methods such as: immersion in ice water; covering with electrically refrigerating (hypothermia) blankets; exposure to cool air (e.g., from an electric fan); or application of cracked ice or ice bags.

Because the nurse is most often involved in methods of external surface cooling, let us discuss these procedures further and the general clinical care given a hypothermic patient.

Surface cooling which is performed in a patient's room is typically used to prevent cerebral edema and to reduce dangerously high temperatures. Surface cooling may also be used in surgery.

Surface cooling may reduce body temperature to as low as 25°C. (77°F.). However, surface cooling to such a low temperature is used only in surgery. More commonly body temperature is reduced by only a few degrees. For example, typically in treating a high temperature elevation the body temperature is reduced and maintained at 35 or 36°C. (96 to 98°F.). Body temperature is lowered to about 31 to 35°C. (87.8 to 95°F.) in the prevention of cerebral edema. As a general rule, surface hypothermia is maintained above 27.8°C. (82°F.) to prevent irreversible complications, e.g., irreversible ventricular fibrillation.

When surface cooling is used, treatment is directed at not only cooling the body, but also at *preventing shivering,* e.g., by the intravenous administration of such medications as chlorpromazine and sodium phenobarbital. Shivering during the cooling procedure must be prevented, since it increases metabolic activity, produces heat, markedly increases oxygen usage, increases circulation, may produce hypoglycemia (by using up muscle and liver glycogen), and may cause hyperventilation and respiratory alkalosis. Also, it takes a longer time to reduce body temperature in a shivering patient.

As previously indicated, temperature reduction can be accomplished by various methods of surface cooling. An *electric fan* may be placed at the patient's bedside and directed toward the patient to cool his body by evaporation. A loin cloth may be placed over the patient and a *bath towel or sheet saturated with cold water* placed over his trunk. The towel is periodically resaturated and an electric fan is directed toward the towel. Also, *ice caps* may be placed at the patient's groins and axillas.

Iced alcohol sponges may be ordered if body temperature reaches 103°F. or above. These sponges reduce body temperature by increasing body surface evaporation of heat. Iced alcohol sponges are contraindicated in very young and very old patients and in the presence of convulsions, chills, systemic shock, and severe cachexia or debility.

Occasionally, in emergency situations, a hyperthermic patient may be placed in a *tub of ice water* to halt a rapidly rising fever. However, *tepid sponges* are tolerated better than such cold baths. Also, because they are less likely to cause shivering, tepid sponges are often more effective. Solutions used for tepid sponges include water, alcohol, or a mixture of both.

A cold sponge bath or tub bath causes heat loss by conduction and evaporation, i.e., some of the body's heat is transferred from the skin surface into the bathing solution and other body heat is lost as the heat of vaporization. With a tepid sponge, heat loss occurs by evaporative cooling. Because cooling results from continuous evaporization of moisture into the air, an electric fan is frequently used to keep the air in motion over cooling sponges.

Sponge friction massage may be employed if the patient's skin is cold during a temperature elevation. After the patient is packed in ice for 15 minutes his skin is rubbed with a towel. By improving cutaneous vasodilation this procedure draws more warm blood to the body's surface where it can be cooled and the heat dissipated.

Remember, if a cooling sponge bath is not properly administered or is of too brief a duration, the procedure may only stimulate shivering, and thereby cause the adverse effect of increasing heat production rather than contributing to heat loss.

If cooling sponges fail to reduce body temperature, the physician may order an *oxygen tent* (used for its air conditioning effects) and *cool to ice-cold lavages or enemas.* A persistent fever may require that the patient be packed in ice, put in a tub of cold water, or placed on a *hypothermic mattress.*

Most hospitals have hypothermic mattresses, i.e., a refrigerating machine and cooling blankets made of rubber or vinyl. A cooled solution of alcohol and water is circulated through coils in the blanket (Fig. 38–4). (*Note:* To rewarm the patient the machine is reset and the solution is warmed.) Several different hypothermic units are on the market. The hypothermic blanket causes heat loss by conduction and convection, i.e., heat is transferred from the body surface to the cooling blanket. Use of a hypothermic unit is the procedure of choice for treating hyperthermia related to hypothalamic damage. For details of the operation of hypothermic units consult manufacturers' information booklets.

Hypothermic mattresses are the simplest, most efficient and most precise method of inducing general hypothermia. By the setting of a gauge at the desired level of coolness, the fluid flowing through the coils is maintained at the desired temperature.

Clinical Care Associated with Hypothermia

Skilled nursing care is necessary with induced hypothermia.

The following activities are typically of importance *prior to* prolonged hypothermia (i.e., hypothermia to be maintained possibly for several days): (1) bathe the patient, inspect his skin for discolorations or lesions, and apply a thin coating of lanolin, oil, or cream to the entire body; (2) administer a cleansing enema; (3) insert a retention urinary catheter (to evaluate renal function and renal output); (4) start an intravenous infusion or assist with an intravenous cutdown (to maintain fluid-electrolyte balance); (5) administer preinduction medications such as meperidine hydrochloride (Demerol), chlorpromazine (Thorazine), or promethazine hydrochloride (Phenergan) to depress the heat-regulating center of the brain, prevent shivering, and help the conscious patient to relax during the cooling procedure; (6) make baseline observations and recordings of the patient's vital signs, level of consciousness, and responsiveness; and (7) assemble emergency equipment and medications, e.g., vasopressors, cardiac stimulants, respiratory stimulants, respirators, and tracheostomy tray. Intravenous infusions must be started prior to the procedure, since the peripheral veins collapse in the hypothermic state.

Prior to any hypothermic procedure briefly explain the procedure to the conscious patient and reassure him that he will be constantly attended and will not be excessively uncomfortable. Give appropriate explanations and reassurance to family members.

During prolonged hypothermic therapy the following activities are of importance:

> *Take, record, and evaluate vital signs frequently.* During hypothermic therapy an electric thermometer (with a probe inserted into the patient's rectum) is commonly used to check the patient's temperature. By this device the body temperature is continually monitored when attached to a recording device. The most accu-

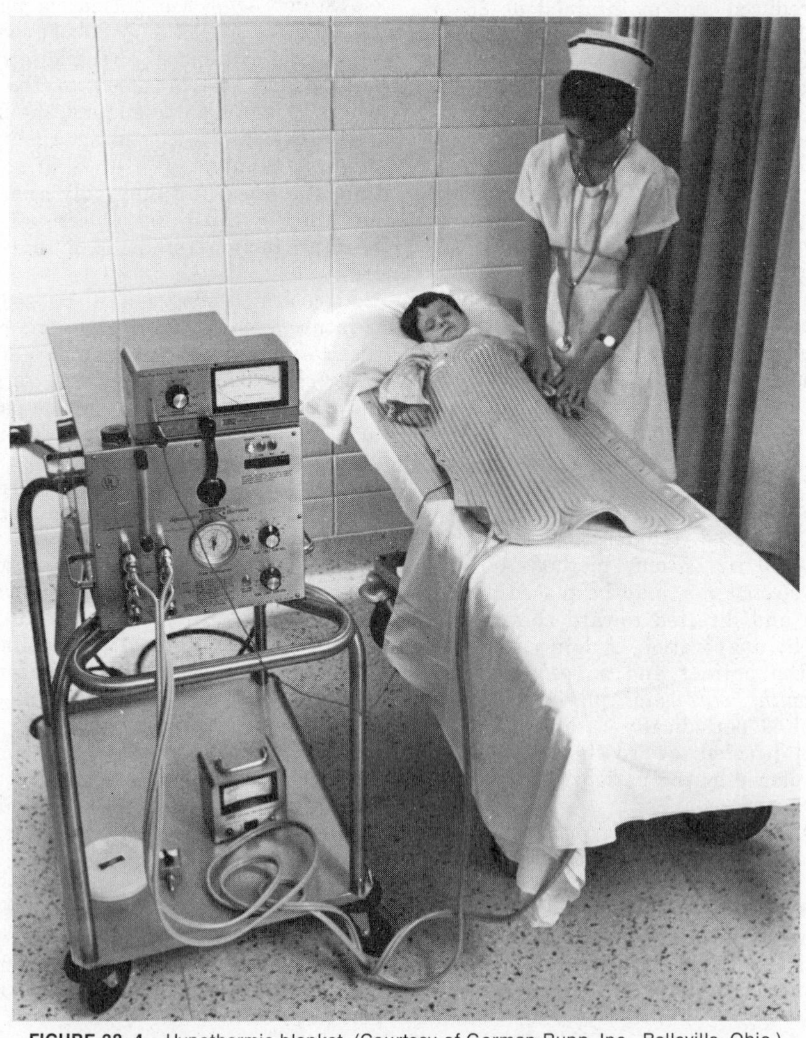

FIGURE 38–4. Hypothermic blanket. (Courtesy of Gorman-Rupp, Inc., Belleville, Ohio.)

rate indication of body temperature may be obtained if the rectal temperature probe is inserted at least three inches and is angled anteriorly. An electric thermometer (thermisto probe) may also be placed in the patient's esophagus (e.g., in the anesthetized patient). The goal of therapy is to maintain the desired level of hypothermia. Because a downward drift of one or two degrees typically occurs after the cooling procedure is terminated, it is customary to stop the procedure, or to reduce it, when the patient's body temperature is within one or two degrees of the desired temperature. An electrocardiograph and electroencephalograph may be used during hypothermia to detect cardiac arrhythmias and cerebral anoxia. It is expected that vital signs will gradually be reduced as body temperature is being lowered. *Report immediately* undesired levels of body temperature, shivering, marked changes in cardiac rate, irregular cardiac rhythms, or other fluctuations or abnormalities in vital signs. If the temperature is undesirably low, cardiac arrest may occur.

> *Administer medications as ordered to prevent shivering.* Shivering typically occurs when body temperature reaches 30°C. (86°F.).

> *Make certain the patient is attended constantly.* If you cannot remain with him yourself, see that he is cared for by a competent person.

> *Maintain a patent airway,* e.g., by suctioning and correct positioning. Because the gag reflex may be absent, the patient must be protected from aspiration. If indicated, use a respirator to support ventilation.

> *Protect the patient's eyes* in the absence of the corneal reflex and when protective eye secretions are reduced. (See Unit XXI.)

> *Prevent complications of immobility.* (See Unit V, Chap. 27). For example, turn the patient at least every two hours, correctly position him, carry out range-of-motion exercises passively. Turn the patient frequently if cooling blankets are used. Sometimes patients undergoing hypothermia are placed on CircOlectric beds so they can be turned more easily.

> *Periodically fill and reposition ice bags* if they are being used.

> *Observe the patient's skin* every one or two hours for indications of pressure, discoloration, edema, or frostbite (e.g., immovable firm areas of skin caused by fat necrosis or crystallization of tissue).

> *Give frequent oral hygiene* and *remove crusts from the nares.* (See discussions on pp. 426 to 427).

> *Measure and evaluate urinary output periodically.* It is expected that urinary output will decrease when the temperature is lowered to 32°C. (89°F.). Urine specimens for analysis may be collected frequently.

> *Provide intake as ordered,* e.g., intravenously and/or via nasogastric tube. Oral intake is not permitted because hypothermia may depress or remove the gag reflex. (Other reflexes are also altered.)

Clinical care *during and immediately after rewarming* of the patient continues to be intensive. The physician decides when to terminate hypothermia and rewarm the patient to a normal level of body temperature. Rewarming may be accomplished by: (1) changing the setting on a warming-cooling blanket so that warm liquid is circulated through the blanket; (2) removing the cooling blanket, ice bags, and so forth, covering the patient with regular blankets, and allowing him to rewarm by exposure to a warmer natural environment; (3) diathermy; or (4) partially immersing the patient in warm or tepid water.

During the rewarming procedure, be careful not to burn the patient or to expose him to excessively warm temperatures. Attend the patient constantly and evaluate his vital signs. Report immediately any abnormalities. Usually the rewarming procedures are terminated (e.g., extra blankets are removed or the warming blanket is turned off) once the patient's temperature reaches a level that is 1 to 2 degrees below normal. The procedure is terminated at this time because some upward temperature drift usually occurs. Consciousness is usually regained when body temperature reaches around 32°C. (89°F.).

Following hypothermia the patient's temperature is closely observed for several days, e.g., every 3 or 4 hours. Excessive temperature elevations may occur, because the temperature-regulating mechanism is often unstable for a while. Also, because cardiac irregularity and fibrillations can occur after rewarming, the patient's pulse is checked frequently for one or two days.

With assistance the patient gradually regains independence, e.g., begins to take oral nourishment, has urinary catheter removed, and increases activities as his general condition permits.

SEIZURES AND CONVULSIONS

Seizures may be manifestations of numerous diverse disorders. Here we focus on the clinical care of any patient experiencing a seizure from any cause. Seizures are sudden episodes of varying severity precipitated by abnormal, excessive neuronal discharges within the brain. In its broadest sense, the term "epilepsy" is synonymous with "seizure." A seizure is a phenomenon, not a disease. We shall not go into a detailed discussion here of the causes of seizures. Let us simply say, for purposes of this discussion, that seizures may be symptomatic of any condition that interferes with neuronal metabolism or that injures neurons. Actually at least 50 various conditions are *known* to induce seizures. However, *the causes of most seizures remain unknown.*

In common usage the term "seizure" is often used synonymously with "convulsion." Such usage is inaccurate, however, since "convulsion" correctly refers only to the muscular contractions that may be one component of a seizure. Technically a *convulsion* is a violent involuntary contraction or series of contractions of the voluntary muscles. The nurse should familiarize herself with the following *types of convulsions:*

> *Clonic convulsion.* Alternating contraction and relaxation of opposing muscle groups, producing a jerky, convulsive movement.

> *Tonic convulsion.* The persistent contraction of a muscle or set of muscles, not atrophic or due to muscular shrinkage.

> *Tetanic convulsion.* Any form of spasm characteristic of tetanus; a tonic convulsion without loss of consciousness.

> *Epileptiform convulsion.* Any convulsion with loss of consciousness.
> *Local convulsion.* Any minor spasm affecting only one muscle or only one part or member of the body.
> *Hysterical convulsion.* Any spasmodic movement accompanying a hysterical disorder.
> *Central, essential, or spontaneous convulsion.* Any convulsion due to a lesion of the CNS rather than one resulting from excitement from an external source.

Occasionally lay persons refer to a seizure or convulsion as a "fit" or "attack."

CLINICAL CARE DURING SEIZURES AND CONVULSIONS

Seizures range in intensity from imperceptible impulse changes within the brain to highly dramatic episodes in which a person suddenly falls unconscious and begins to thrash about, salivates heavily, and becomes cyanotic. (Various types of seizures are discussed in Chapter 39.)

Seizures and convulsions are frequently frightening for the nurse to witness a first time. It is helpful, however, if focus is kept on the patient's needs to be protected and observed during the seizure so effective therapy can be planned, rather than on your own feelings at the moment. You may find it helpful to remember that you are merely observing *exaggerations* of normal actions during seizures, e.g., exaggerated movements, exaggerated salivation, and so forth. These observable behavioral exaggerations result from exaggerated neuronal impulses.

To protect the patient during seizures and convulsions:

> Stay with and help the patient. Send someone else for additional help.
> Protect patient from injury to himself, particularly respiratory aspiration and obstruction. Screen the patient, remain calm, give reassurance.
> Administer anticonvulsant medications as ordered. Observe for side effects. (See p. 510.)
> Lower siderails during seizure so patient will not injure himself by banging them, and stay with patient. Between seizures keep siderails up and padded. If advisable, pad head of bed also.
> Accompany patients who have frequent seizures if they are up walking or up to go to the bathroom. If left unattended they could suddenly have a seizure and fall.
> If an ambulatory patient has a grand mal seizure preceded by an aura (p. 508), he may have enough time to lie down and place a folded handkerchief between his teeth before the seizure starts. If the patient is in a wheelchair when a severe seizure begins, immediately slide him gently onto the floor. If patient is standing and you have hold of him when seizure begins, lower him gently to the floor (away from furniture and other hard objects). If standing by patient's bed, lower him onto it. However, *do not attempt to lift the patient during a seizure.* To do so may injure him. Instead of moving the patient during a seizure, move away from him things against which he could bang and injure himself.

> *Maintain patent airway and adequate ventilation.* Loosen tight clothing, e.g., belt, collar; insert plastic airway if possible; turn patient onto his side (lateral position facilitates drainage), or turn his head to the side and point his chin downward (so saliva and mucus will run out of the mouth and not be aspirated, and so tongue will drop forward away from airway). During convulsions the patient is unable to swallow. This increases the possibility of aspiration because vomitus and increased secretions are frequently present. *The usual causes of death in convulsing patients are aspiration and asphyxia. Pharyngeal and, if necessary, endotracheal suctioning are used as indicated.* To maintain adequate ventilation *oxygen may be administered* to assist in the control of hypoxia.
> If possible, i.e., if the patient's jaw is relaxed, *insert plastic airway, hard rubber wedge, or padded tongue blade* between back teeth to protect tongue and mouth (from biting) and to maintain airway (tongue may fall back, obstructing airway). If patient is making chewing motions, try to place a soft object between his teeth during the relaxing phase of the chewing cycle. *Keep padded tongue blade and plastic airway readily available at bedside of any patient with known or suspected seizure disorder.*
> *Do not attempt to forcibly open convulsing patient's mouth if his jaws are clenched, and do not attempt to push an airway or tongue blade forcibly between the patient's front teeth.* To do so may break or loosen teeth or injure lips. *Never put your fingers into the patient's mouth;* he may accidentally bite you during the seizure.
> *Place pad* (folded blanket, jacket, towel, bathrobe) *under patient's head,* so he won't bang his head on the floor, siderails, and so forth. Provide protection without possibility of suffocation.
> *Do not attempt to restrain the patient's movements during convulsions.* Restraint may increase the movements and could cause fracture if extreme spasticity is present. Lightly hold the patient's hands to prevent him from banging them. The patient having a psychomotor seizure, in which he wanders around, should not be forcibly restrained (unless he is in danger of injury) since this may increase the severity of the seizures.

Observation of Patient During Seizures and Convulsions

Observe and record the following:

> Preconvulsive signs; presence or absence of an aura. Position of head, body, and extremities prior to onset and following onset of seizure.
> Initial activity. First thing patient does, e.g., emits a cry. How did he attract your attention? Did he fall at beginning of seizure?
> Progression and type of muscular activity, e.g., tonic, clonic, localized (focal), generalized. Turn back covers, if patient is in bed, so you can observe the patient completely during the seizure. What parts of the body are involved? Where did movements begin and to where did they progress? Did the movements change in character? Note nature of any automatisms in psychomotor seizure. Note presence of diaphoresis or clenching or grinding of the teeth.
> Presence of any deviation of tongue or eyeballs in the head, e.g., deviated up, down, to side. Did pupils change in size, become unequal, react to light during and after the seizure?
> Patient's level of consciousness prior to, during, and following the seizure. Was consciousness lost? Was he confused or sleepy during or following the seizure? Following the seizure did the patient have a memory for the event? Did he have a headache?

> Note presence of: incontinence (urinary or fecal or both); thick salivation and mucus; vomiting (type); bleeding (from bitten tongue).
> Describe respiratory character, e.g., apnea, stertor, and respiratory rate. Describe skin color of face and lips.
> Presence of apparent injury as a result of falling or other activity during the seizure.
> Presence of muscular weakness, pain, discomfort, paralysis, or aphasia following seizure. Before or after the seizure did patient notice any disturbances in coordination, impaired speech or thought processes, changes in vision or hearing, changes in motor power, paresthesias, or other symptoms?
> Following seizure, record vital signs. Are any sudden changes present?
> Finally, be certain to record the length of the entire seizure, length of period of unconsciousness, length of time of clonic phase or tonic phase. In patients having multiple seizures, record the frequency and number of seizures.

Your observations may help the physician to: (1) identify which area of the brain is involved; (2) determine if the seizure resulted from idiopathic epilepsy or is a symptomatic disorder; (3) plan appropriate medical or surgical treatment; and (4) plan appropriate patient teaching and counseling.

Once convulsive movements have stopped, the patient should be moved to a quiet place, turned on his side, and allowed to regain consciousness naturally. Suction as necessary during this time. A period of quiet rest is advisable. The patient may feel drowsy or have a headache following the seizure. Reassure the patient and reorient him if necessary.

In planning care for the seizure-prone patient, plan individualized care that does not impose unnecessary limitations on the patient's activities. It is best, of course, for the patient to be ambulatory if possible. The patient having frequent seizures may not be allowed to wear dentures until seizure control is achieved, since the dentures could become broken or aspirated during a seizure. *Always take rectal temperatures on patients prone to seizures.* If a seizure occurred while patient had an oral thermometer in his mouth, serious injury could result. The patient who may have seizures is best placed in areas on the hospital ward where he can be observed easily.

NEUROGENIC SHOCK

Shock[21] is discussed generally in Unit V, Chap. 26. You will recall from that section that shock results from a disproportion between the circulating blood volume and the size of the vascular bed. During health an adequate blood supply is maintained to all the body's tissues because a dynamic equilibrium is maintained between the blood volume, the heart pump mechanism, and the size of the vascular bed.

With neurogenic shock the volume of blood in the body is normal, but the *vascular bed is greatly increased in size.* This increased vascular capacity means that the normal blood volume is incapable of adequately filling the blood vessels. This disproportion reduces the mean circulatory pressure. The pressure gradient for the return of venous blood is, in turn, decreased, resulting in: (1) venous "pooling" of blood; (2) decreased venous return to the heart; and (3) decreased cardiac output. Following this, generalized tissue anoxia occurs along with other signs and symptoms of oxygen deficiency. Cyanosis, however, rarely occurs in neurogenic shock.

Neurogenic shock may occur from brain injury, deep general anesthesia, fainting, and spinal anesthesia (common cause). It is important that the nurse be able to differentiate neurogenic shock (due to peripheral vasodilatation) from hemorrhagic shock (due to reduced blood volume). Failure to make this differentiation could cause the nurse to make the possibly fatal mistake of increasing the rate of flow in a blood transfusion being received by a patient in neurogenic shock, because she incorrectly thought the cause of the shock was decreased blood volume. Such an overloading of circulating blood volume would place a burden on the patient's heart once his vasomotor tone has been restored or stimulated, e.g., with levarterenol drugs. If this added burden to the heart occurred in a patient with any cardiac weakness, congestive heart failure and pulmonary edema could develop, and the patient would literally drown in his own blood.

The *treatment* of neurogenic shock centers around *administration of a vasopressor,* i.e., vasoconstrictor, intramuscularly or parenterally in solution. Such a drug is discontinued once the effects of the spinal anesthetic have worn off, so that the patient's vasomotor nerves once again receive sympathetic stimulation. Once the immediate danger of shock has passed the vasopressor therapy is stopped to prevent pulmonary and renal problems. Severe *ischemic nephrosis,* causing oliguria or anuria as a result of intense, prolonged renal vasoconstriction, can be caused by the indiscriminate administration of vasopressors. For several days following vasopressor treatment of neurogenic shock the patient's urine volume is measured hourly. An indication of the development of ischemic nephrosis is the presence of a *sharp decline in renal output,* in the absence of symptoms of shock. When this happens the doctor usually limits fluid intake and potassium.

RESPIRATORY FAILURE FROM NEUROLOGIC DISORDERS

Neurologic disorders frequently cause respiratory failure by: (1) depressing or destroying the cells in the lower brainstem that integrate respiration; (2) damaging the spinal motor pathways for breathing, their nerves, or respiratory muscular structures; or (3) producing paralysis or sensory loss that results in airway obstruction. Providing appropriate respiratory assistance is therefore an important aspect of the clinical care of many patients with neurologic disorders. (Respiratory failure is discussed in detail in Unit XIV.)

INFECTION COMPLICATING NEUROLOGIC DISORDERS

Neurologic disorders mainly predispose to possible infections as a result of the depressed levels of consciousness, immobility, and paralysis that they may cause. Some of the major potential infections that may occur are respiratory infections (e.g., pneumonia), skin infections (e.g., decubitus ulcers), and infections of the genitourinary tract.

The use of antimicrobials is generally reserved for the specific, vigorous treatment of bacteriologically identified infections *after* the infection has appeared and findings from a culture or smear have been reported. However, chemoprophylaxis does reduce the incidence of pneumonia during convalescence from short episodes of coma, e.g., those resulting from drug poisoning. The use of chemoprophylaxis in such circumstances is the exception rather than the general practice with unconscious or immobilized patients.

PROBLEMS RELATED TO SPINAL DISORDERS

This section focuses on a variety of problems that result from impaired functioning or altered structure of the spinal cord. Although the discussion focuses mainly on the more extreme degrees of clinical problems, the reader is encouraged to remember that spinal disorders may also cause similar problems of lesser degrees.

Clinical care varies with the level and extent of damage to the spinal cord and the appropriate treatment. Refer as necessary to other areas of the text; e.g., the unconscious patient is discussed on p. 420; the patient with bulbar involvement on p. 463; and spinal surgery is discussed on p. 536. Also see discussions of injuries affecting the spinal cord in Chapter 39.

CAUSES AND SIGNIFICANCE OF SPINAL DISORDERS

Injury, disease, or surgery of the spinal cord may cause striking impairments because of the important functions carried out by the cord, and also because these functions are carried out within such a small, compact and complex structure.

Diagnosis of Cord Damage

Damage to the spinal cord may be diagnosed from a history, physical and neurologic examinations, x-rays of the spine, myelograms, and lumbar puncture. Typically cord injury manifests itself by loss of sensation and/or inability to move an extremity. Pain may also occur. Since only a few diseases of the spinal cord can be treated effectively, an early differential diagnosis is important whenever a spinal deficit is discovered.

Cord compression causes a lesion of the cord at a particular level, marked by motor, reflex, or sensory levels above which findings are normal and below which they are abnormal.

LEVEL AND EXTENT OF CORD DAMAGE

The symptoms related to cord damage vary, depending upon the level, severity, and extent of the damage.

Level of Injury

Damage to the spinal cord may cause paralysis of the body parts innervated by nerves leaving the cord below the level of the spinal disorder. The resultant symptoms thus vary with the level of damage. Figure 38–5 illustrates quadriplegia, paraplegia, and hemiplegia. Some typical results of injuries at various cord levels are summarized below:

> *Cervical injury* may cause *quadriplegia,* i.e., paralysis of all four extremities and the trunk. Respiratory failure may occur as a result of paralysis of the diaphragm and intercostal muscles. Initially the patient experiences paralysis of bowel and bladder function, is unable to void, and has fecal incontinence. Also, initially perspiration may not occur in paralyzed regions below the level of the cord injury; this may at first cause a temperature elevation. Later on, excessive perspiration may occur in the unaffected regions.

> *Thoracic injury* may cause *paraplegia,* i.e., paralysis of both lower extremities and more or less of the trunk. Bowel and bladder functions are typically paralyzed initially. A flaccid paralysis is usually followed by a spastic paralysis.

> *Lumbar injury* may cause paralysis of the lower extremities, which remain flaccid. Paralysis of bowel and bladder also occurs.

Because they are protected by the rib cage, the thoracic vertebrae are seldom injured. The 5th and 6th cervical vertebrae and the 1st and 5th lumbar vertebrae are the most common levels of injury. Fractures in the cervical region commonly result from acute hyperflexion of the neck crushing the body of one or more cervical vertebrae.

Extent of Injury

The spinal cord may be completely severed or only partially destroyed. As one would expect, *partial destruction* of the cord causes symptoms that are less severe than those resulting from complete transection or from hemisection (or bisection) of the cord. Symptoms from partial cord destruction are nonetheless still serious problems, e.g., decreased awareness of pain and temperature, weakness, paresthesias, increased deep reflexes, and disturbed urinary sphincter control.

During the early stages of cord injury it may be impossible to determine if the cord has actually been transected or is merely traumatized and edematous.

Hemisection (or bisection) of the spinal cord refers to a lesion that cuts or affects one-half of the cord. Resultant symptoms depend on the area sectioned.

Complete transection of the spinal cord produces serious problems, such as loss of all sensation, spastic paralysis, impaired sexual functioning, loss of urinary and rectal sphincter control, and vasomotor instability of the body beginning a little higher than the level of the lesion. Isolated cord reflexes remain that are cut off from any inhibiting control from the CNS above the level of transection; such reflexes are often problematic rather than helpful to the patient.

When the spinal cord is transected by accident or disease it is, in effect, separated from the brain. In essence the patient then has two central nervous systems: (1) the brain and a certain length of spinal cord above the transection; and (2) the rest of the spinal cord. However, there is no neural connection between these two systems. When transection of the cord is functionally complete, afferent impulses cannot ascend from below the level of the lesion to the brain, and efferent impulses cannot descend to body areas innervated below the break in the cord's continuity.

As indicated, lesions at the level of the thoracic cord or above affect the patient's respirations; the danger of possible pneumonia is then greatly increased because of weak chest movements which do not adequately expand lung tissue and move lung secretions.

Nontraumatic transection of the cord may occur, but more commonly cord transection results from trauma.

PARAPLEGIA AND QUADRIPLEGIA

Paraplegia

Paraplegia is a condition resulting from injury to the spinal cord at the thoracic or lumbar level (due to accident or disease) which causes paralysis of the lower limbs, depending upon the level of injury to the spine.

Some *causes* of paraplegia are: hemorrhage, embolus or thrombus caused by direct injury to the spine; infection; spinal tumor; developmental defects or disease, e.g., spina bifida, cerebral palsy; poliomyelitis; multiple sclerosis; and syphilis. Paraplegia most frequently follows trauma, e.g., automobile accidents, falls, gunshot or shrapnel wounds, diving, or football injuries.

The *onset* of paraplegia may be either gradual or sudden, depending upon the cause. Usually with injury to the cord the onset is sudden. There may be either total or partial damage to the spinal cord at the site of the lesion, resulting in complete or partial paralysis of the lower extremities. *Once completely severed, the spinal cord will not grow together again.* Some spinal cord injuries are not complete, and in time there may be some return of function. If the paralysis is due to injury and there

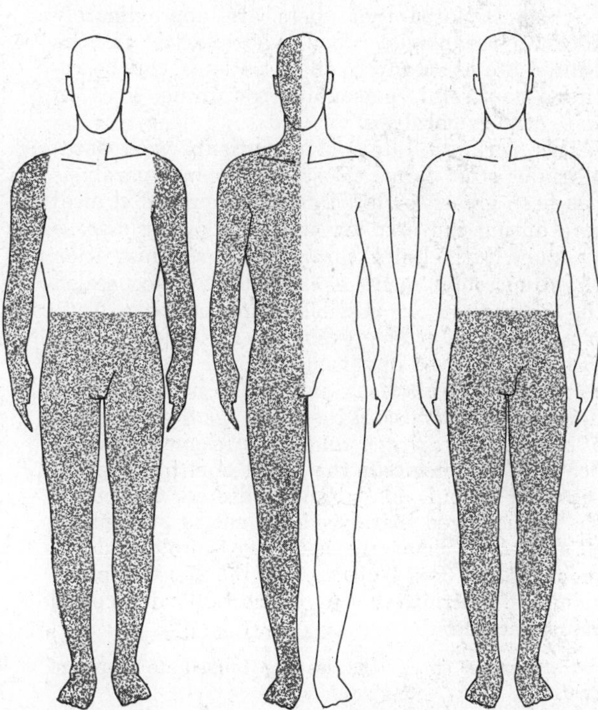

FIGURE 38–5. Areas of paralysis. Left, quadriplegia; center, hemiplegia; right, paraplegia. (From Culver, V. M.: *Modern Bedside Nursing.* 8th ed. 1974.)

is no evidence of bone damage or fracture, there may be a spinal cord contusion. If such is the case, there is a better chance of total return of function.

If the cause of the paralysis cannot be found and corrected within 24 hours after the sudden onset of the paraplegia, there is little chance that correction after that period will be effective in completely restoring the spinal cord's function.

The extent of the total recovery of function cannot be determined definitely for 18 to 24 months. However, a person with a spinal cord injury who is to regain some muscle function generally begins to do so within a few months following insult to the cord.

Quadriplegia

Quadriplegia is the same as paraplegia except that the level of injury to the spinal cord is cervical and thus the upper extremities are affected as well as the lower extremities. Quadriplegia (also called "tetraplegia") is, therefore, loss of motion and sensation in both the arms and the legs.

Home care of the quadriplegic requires the coordinated efforts of many persons. It is possible only as a result of comprehensive planning and in the presence of strong family relationships. Twenty-four-hour care may be necessary for the patient who is paralyzed below the neck, particularly if he has a tracheotomy.

Care in Paraplegia and Quadriplegia

It is estimated that there are approximately 100,000 paraplegics and quadriplegics in the United States. Many of these patients can be restored to useful, personally rewarding lives in spite of their paralysis.

The mortality rate among patients with paraplegia or other forms of extensive spinal paralysis has been greatly reduced due to improved clinical care during the first few weeks following disease or injury. Such clinical care employs administration of antimicrobial agents as indicated and focuses on the prevention of possible complications. Antibiotics now delay or prevent the early deaths that formerly occurred in paraplegics and quadriplegics as a result of infections. In spite of such progress, however, *infections still constitute the highest cause of death to paraplegics and quadriplegics.* Usually death in paraplegics is the result of either urinary sepsis or trophic ulcers and bedsores. Of course, the immobilized, paralyzed patient is susceptible to all the problems associated with prolonged immobilization. (See Unit V, Chapter 27.) Complications and reactions that may occur following spinal injury include:

> Systemic shock (the leading immediate cause of death).
> Paralysis.
> Spinal shock.
> Flaccidity.
> Hyperreflexia; spinal automatisms.
> Muscle spasms, spasticity, rigidity.
> Pains, e.g., joint and muscle, visceral, pains at level of injury.
> Urinary tract infections, e.g., pyelonephritis, renal calculi (kidney stones).
> Pneumonia; respiratory failure.
> Poor circulation.
> Decubitus ulcers (pressure sores).
> Impotence.
> Burns and other injuries (resulting from loss of sensation).
> Tendon contractures, e.g., foot drop, wrist drop.
> Ankylosis of joints.
> Malnutrition.
> General debility.
> Paralytic ileus, bowel impaction, fecal incontinence.
> Urinary incontinence.
> Changes in body image, grief, depression.
> Sensory deprivation.

Most of the above problems are discussed in detail in following sections. Systemic shock is discussed in Unit V, Chapter 26.

Goals of rehabilitation must be established early. The goal for paraplegics is *at least* brace and crutch locomotion, since eventually, almost without exception, every paraplegic can become independent with the use of braces and crutches. The goal for quadriplegics is *at least* wheelchair locomotion (with as much additional activity and movement as the individual's injury and his self-determination allow).

Once broad goals are established, then daily, weekly, and monthly objectives can be determined. Because no two patients have exactly the same problems, goals for rehabilitation as well as the techniques of rehabilitation vary from one individual to another.[71]

Numerous *operations* and *mechanical devices* have been developed to compensate for paralyzed muscles. As indicated, mobility can often be restored with braces, crutches or wheelchairs. By means of bracing or surgical procedures it is frequently possible to reconstruct the important pinch between thumb and forefinger, which may have been lost as a result of paralysis. This enables the patient to again perform such activities as feeding and shaving himself. *Tendon transfers* may be performed in the hands and forearms of patients following spinal injury. Following muscle reeducation, these tendon transfers may be highly effective.

Automatic lifts make it possible for anyone to transfer a paralyzed patient from his bed into a chair. Such lift devices need to be readily available to persons caring for paralyzed patients. Be certain you are thoroughly acquainted with how the lift operates before using it to transport a patient. Also, always use proper body mechanics in moving paralyzed patients.

Physiotherapy and occupational therapy are highly valuable in the treatment of the immobilized or paralyzed patient, having both physical and psychologic value. Occupational therapy is started once convalescence begins. Paralyzed patients are encouraged early to be as active and independent as they safely can be. Only *necessary* restrictions are imposed to prevent fostering unnecessary dependence. During convalescence the patient is kept out of bed as much as possible and is dressed in his own clothing.

The paralyzed patient needs to be taught the meaning of his symptoms, how they can be relieved, and how he can help himself. The patient must also be taught to recognize symptoms that could indicate progression of his disorder, or the development of complications, e.g., infection, pressure areas, contractures, impaction.

The nurse is frequently the person who gives instructions to those who will be assisting the paralyzed patient with his care at home. The thoroughness of her teaching can make for a more harmonious, less taxing relationship between the patient and those he is with at home. Friends and family are the source of the patient's greatest long-term support and encouragement. Therefore, the instruction of these persons is an important responsibility in helping the patient to adjust to his paralysis.

A great deal of advance preparation is needed before the paraplegic or quadriplegic patient can return home. It may be necessary for new housing to be acquired to meet the patient's new needs, or remodeling of the present home may be needed.

After the patient leaves the hospital or rehabilitation center it is important that he continue to receive continued medical evaluation and periodic supervisory visits from a visiting nurse.

*FIRST AID FOLLOWING SPINAL INJURY**

A patient with suspected spinal injury must be handled with *extreme* care! If there is even the slightest possibility that the spine has been injured, the patient should be treated as if there were a known injury. *Death or permanent disability results more frequently from improper transportation of a patient with a fracture of the spine, sometimes unrecognized, than from any other injury.* Therefore, do not lift or move an injured person or his head until he has told you where he has pain and until he has shown you that he can wiggle his fingers and toes. If the patient complains of back pain, his back may be broken. This pain may radiate to his abdomen and chest or down to his legs. If a patient has neck pain he may have broken his neck. If he cannot wiggle his toes or move his legs, his back is broken; if he cannot move his fingers, his neck is broken. Such symptoms of spinal injury must be carefully searched for.

Spinal injuries may easily be overlooked in the unconscious patient. The unconscious patient should be handled in such a manner that a spinal injury would not be aggravated or worsened if it is present. If a fracture of the spine might be present and the patient is unconscious, he should be handled as though his neck is broken.

Spinal injuries should be suspected following falls, blows to the head from a heavy object, automobile accidents, football injuries, or diving accidents.

Fractures of the spine may exist without cord injury. However, if such fractures are improperly handled and the spine is twisted or bent, cord injury may occur. For example, if the patient with a broken back is carried in such a manner that his body is bent, e.g., in a soft canvas stretcher or in a blanket, or if the head of a patient with a fractured cervical spine is lifted or propped up, the spinal cord may be ground between parts of the broken spine. Any useful remnant of the cord that may have escaped injury initially may thus be destroyed.

> *Patients with spinal injuries should be moved on a firm board or door rather than on a sagging stretcher which flexes the spine.*

Do not allow bystanders to hastily move the patient, flexing his spine. *Never* allow the patient with an injured spine to sit up. The patient should not be moved until a firm, flat support is prepared beside the patient and until a sufficient number of helpers (at least four persons) are present and are instructed how to gently lift the patient and hold him in proper alignment with firm traction on the head and neck to prevent any motion of the head. Only then is the patient moved with extreme caution. When moving a patient with a cervical fracture on or off a stretcher, manual traction *must* be applied. The door or board should extend at least 4 inches beyond the top of the victim's head.

Following admission to the hospital the physician evaluates the level and extent of the injury by performing a physical examination and diagnostic tests and x-rays as indicated. Every attempt is made to prevent unnecessary movement of the patient, e.g., x-rays are taken with the patient on the litter rather than moving him to the x-ray table. If symptoms of cord compression are present, then decompressive surgery may be performed to prevent additional squeezing of the cord by relieving the pressure of the vertebral bones on the cord.

IMMOBILIZATION AND POSITIONING FOLLOWING SPINAL INJURY AND SURGERY

Following spinal injury a patient may be immobilized due to resultant paralysis, or he may be immobilized because his doctor has ordered him not to move (to prevent additional injury and to allow injured tissues time to heal). Patients may be immobilized for varying lengths of time following spinal surgery. Some patients who have spinal

*For details concerning the movement and transportation of a patient following spinal injury, consult a textbook of first aid or neurologic nursing.

injuries are unconscious as a result of other injuries. The immobilized patient may require complete care.

To prevent unnecessary movements the patient with damage to the spinal cord or spine is not moved into a bed upon admission until the doctor has decided what type of immobilization he wants for the patient and which type of bed or frame the patient is to be placed on, whether a fracture bed, i.e., a regular bed with a fracture board under the mattress, a CircOlectric bed, or a Foster or Stryker frame (to be discussed).

Because *proper alignment and support of the spine are highly important aspects of the treatment of spinal disorders,* the physician carefully selects how he wishes to accomplish these measures. Traction may be employed, or the physician may order the bed to be hyperextended or kept flat. The selection as to the type of bed or frame needed varies with the physician's preference, the type and level of injury, the equipment available, and the size of the patient. Every attempt is made in the clinical care of patients with spinal disorders to prevent sagging of the bed and motion or poor alignment of the spine. The length of the period of immobilization following acute injuries of the spinal cord varies with the level of the injury and the prescribed treatment; in some cases immobilization may last for months.

Explanations are given to the conscious patient of necessary restrictions of motion as well as movements that he can safely make and should make, e.g., deep breathing and coughing (if allowed). The patient's cooperation in his treatment may thus be obtained and he may attain peace of mind in some respects and be less fearful.

Fracture Bed

A "fracture bed" can be made from a regular hospital bed by placing sponge rubber mattresses and an alternating air pressure mattress over a fracture board. In some instances a firm horsehair mattress may be used instead of a foam mattress. Mattresses with springs are not used. Plastic sheeting is placed over the sponge rubber mattress. Only one sheet is placed over the alternating air mattress if it is used.

If the patient is to be placed in a position on the fracture bed which hyperextends his spine, the bed is made up so the patient's head will be at the foot of the bed. A hinged fracture board is placed under the mattress in this instance, and the knee gatch is elevated to provide hyperextension. A footboard is placed on all fracture beds.

Stryker and Foster Frames

Advantages of the Stryker or Foster frame over a regular hospital bed in treating spinal injuries are that continuous cervical traction can be maintained if necessary, and the patient can easily be turned manually to face-up or face-down positions. It is important that these frames be adjusted to the measurements of a given patient; such adjustments add to the patient's comfort and prevent the development of deformities. As with the patient in a regular hospital bed, the patient on a frame must be kept in proper body alignment to prevent deformities and contractures. For example, arm rest wings on the frame should be at the level of the shoulder so that strain is not placed on the shoulder girdle. Footboards, hand rolls, aluminum or plastic wrist splints, and posterior splints are employed as indicated.

The *Stryker frame* has two metal frames (an anterior frame and a posterior frame) with taut canvas covers and a thin protective padding over each frame. These frames are supported on a movable cart which has a pivot apparatus at each end. By securing one frame over the patient while he lies on the other it is possible for one person to easily change the position of the patient from his back to his abdomen, and vice versa. Thus, for turning purposes the patient is briefly "sandwiched" between the frames. Once the patient is safely turned the uppermost frame is removed. During the turning process the patient is prevented from falling or sliding by placing straps around both frames. If the patient can, he is instructed to fold his arms around the anterior frame as he is turned. If he cannot use his arms they are safely strapped in to prevent injury. A small canvas strip across the middle of the posterior frame, i.e., the one the patient is on when lying on his back, is removable for use of the bedpan. The anterior frame has a space for the patient's face so that when he lies on his abdomen he can rest, read, or eat, without turning his head to the side. Arm rests may be fastened to the sides of the anterior frame if desired.

The conscious patient must be prepared for use of the Stryker frame so he will not be afraid of falling while being turned and so he can understand the purposes and advantages of such a device. Always tell the patient which direction you will turn him and tell him when you are ready to turn him. Give such explanations even to the patient who has an altered state of consciousness; he may be able to hear you.

The Stryker frame may be used for treating fractures and injuries of the spinal column and following spinal surgery, e.g., following spinal fusion. It may also be used generally to facilitate care of any chronically ill, disabled patient. The frame greatly facilitates care. The Stryker frame cannot be used when hyperextension is necessary without the use of Crutchfield tongs. Figure 38–6 illustrates the Stryker frame.

The *Foster frame* is similar to the Stryker frame except that it is more stable, takes up more space, and is heavier. Also, the Foster frame has a hyperextension regulating bar which enables placement of the patient in a position of hyperextension or flexion if this is indicated. Remember not to use this regulating bar as a handle when you are turning the patient in the frame; to do so could cause an undesirable alteration of the patient's position away from the degree of hyperextension or flexion ordered by the physician. Uses of the Foster frame are similar to those of the Stryker frame.

CircOlectric Bed

The CircOlectric bed may be placed in various horizontal and vertical positions and also in sitting positions if the patient's condition allows. Levers are provided for head and knee gatches. As indicated by its name the bed is electrically operated. A pushbutton on an electrical switch is depressed to move the patient to "face" and "back" positions.

Equipment is available to set up cervical, pelvic, and Buck's traction on this bed. A transfer sling, siderails, and additional special equipment are also available for use on the CircOlectric bed. When changing the patient's position from prone to supine (or vice versa) the change of position is accomplished by vertically turning the patient in a circle as he lies between anterior and posterior frames (Figs. 38–7 and 38–8). The position of the bed can be stopped and maintained at any specific level during the turning process. Thus, the CircOlectric bed can be used in helping the patient to gradually assume an upright standing position by using it like a tilt table. (See also Figure 38–12.)

For details concerning the actual manipulation and set-ups for Stryker and Foster frames or the CircOlectric bed, consult procedure books and the manufacturers' product information. Of course, you should be thoroughly familiar with how this equipment operates and what it feels like to have it used on you before you use it on a patient.

Moving the Patient with a Spinal Injury

When moving the patient with a spinal injury from the stretcher onto his bed or frame, a team of three to five persons is necessary. Usually the physician supervises moving the patient and directs the team members. If a physician is not available a nurse acts as leader and gives directions, e.g., "At the count of three everyone lift together." (Before moving the patient, an inexperienced team should practice moving one of the team members from a stretcher to a bed.) Proper alignment of the patient's body is necessary while he is being moved. Everyone must keep in line and lift together so the patient's spine is not twisted or bent. If necessary the physician applies manual hyperextension to the patient's spine while the patient is being moved into his bed.

A patient arriving on a board or stretcher can be laid directly onto a Stryker or Foster frame while still strapped to the board. He is then transferred onto the frame by having the other section

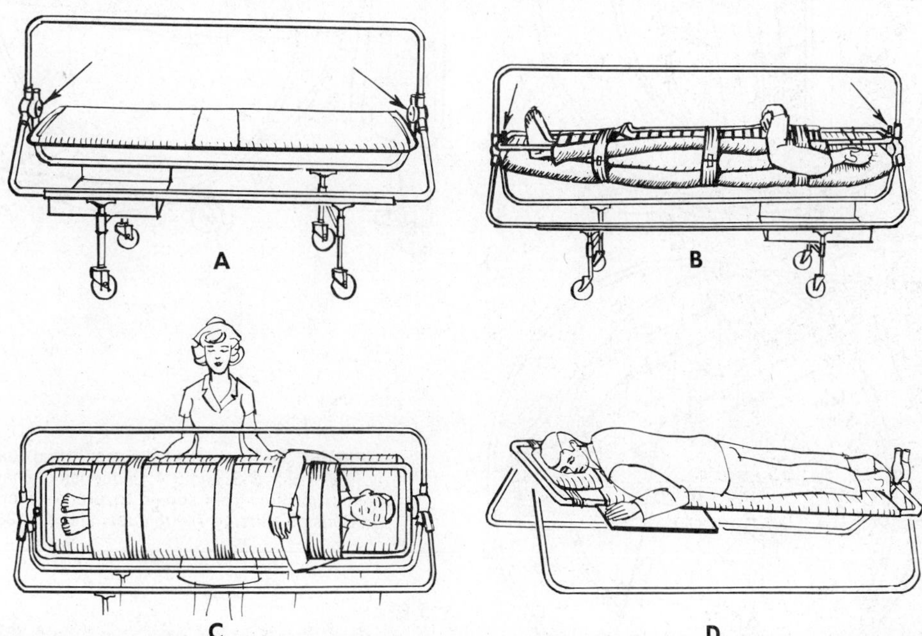

FIGURE 38–6. *A*, Stryker frame, unoccupied. *B*, Patient positioned for turning between anterior and posterior frames (note protective straps). *C*, Patient being turned by one nurse. *D*, Patient prone on anterior frame with arm rest fastened to side of frame. (From Sutton, A.: *Bedside Nursing Techniques, 2nd ed. 1969.)*

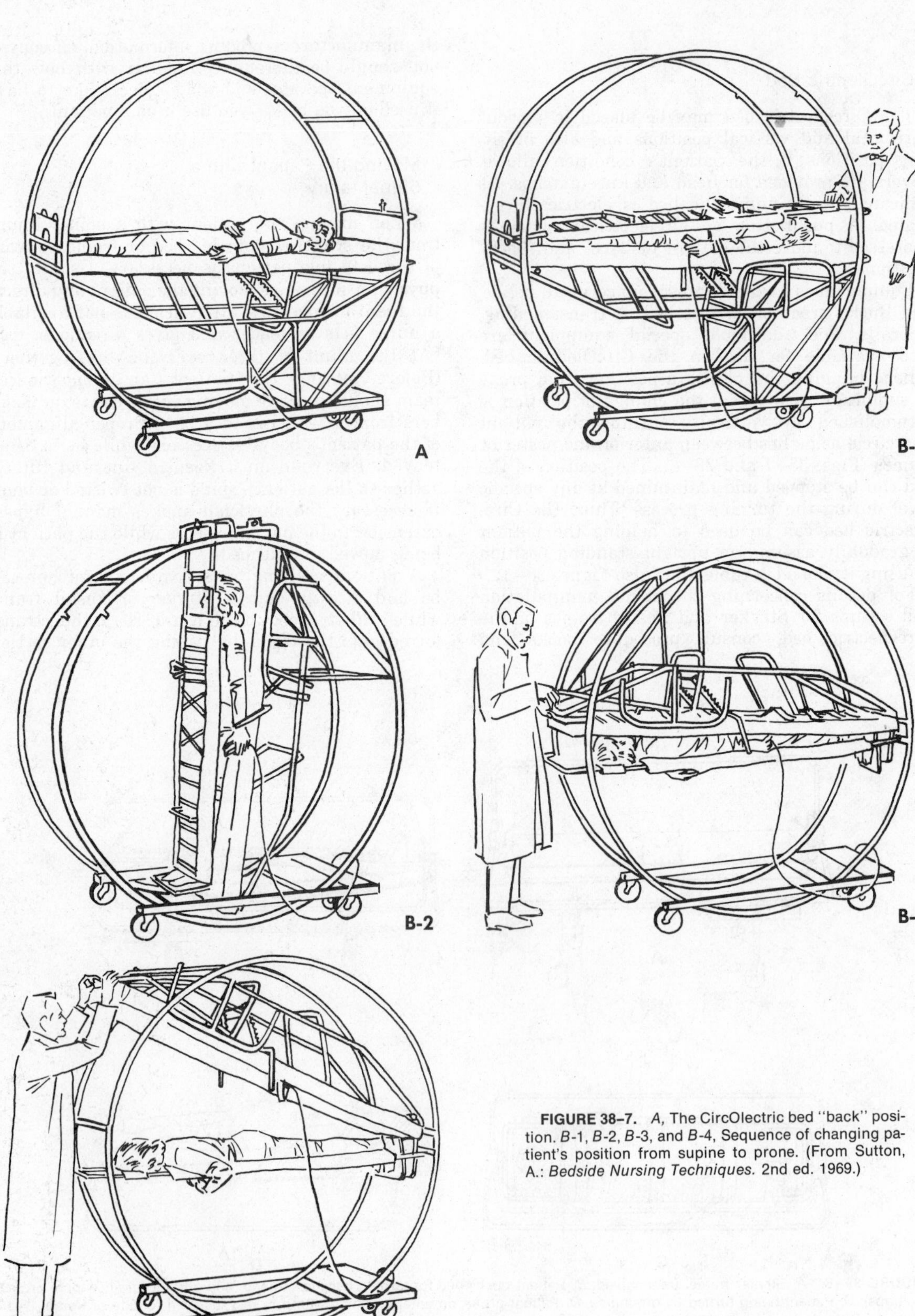

FIGURE 38–7. *A,* The CircOlectric bed "back" position. *B*-1, *B*-2, *B*-3, and *B*-4, Sequence of changing patient's position from supine to prone. (From Sutton, A.: *Bedside Nursing Techniques.* 2nd ed. 1969.)

of the frame brought down and being turned onto that section.

Everything is made ready before the patient with a spinal injury is moved into his bed or frame. Place a *lifting or turning sheet* on the bed or frame of any patient with a spinal disorder. Be certain the sheet is placed so it extends from above the patient's head to below his buttocks for cervical injuries, or from above the level of the shoulders to below the buttocks for thoracic or lumbar injuries. With this sheet the patient can be turned or lifted with a minimum of spinal motion if turning is allowed. Have the bed gatched as necessary if it is to be in a position of hyperextension or have traction ready if that is to be used.

Hyperextension

To reduce pressure on the spinal cord the patient with a spinal fracture may be placed in a position of hyperextension. This position may be maintained by: (1) gatching a fracture bed with the patient placed with his head at the usual foot of the bed; or (2) application of head or neck traction.

> *Patients in hyperextension should not have their positions changed or their traction released without specific orders from the physician.*

Since injuries at the *cervical level* often result from crushing of the cord by acute hyperflexion of the neck, the treatment involves extending the

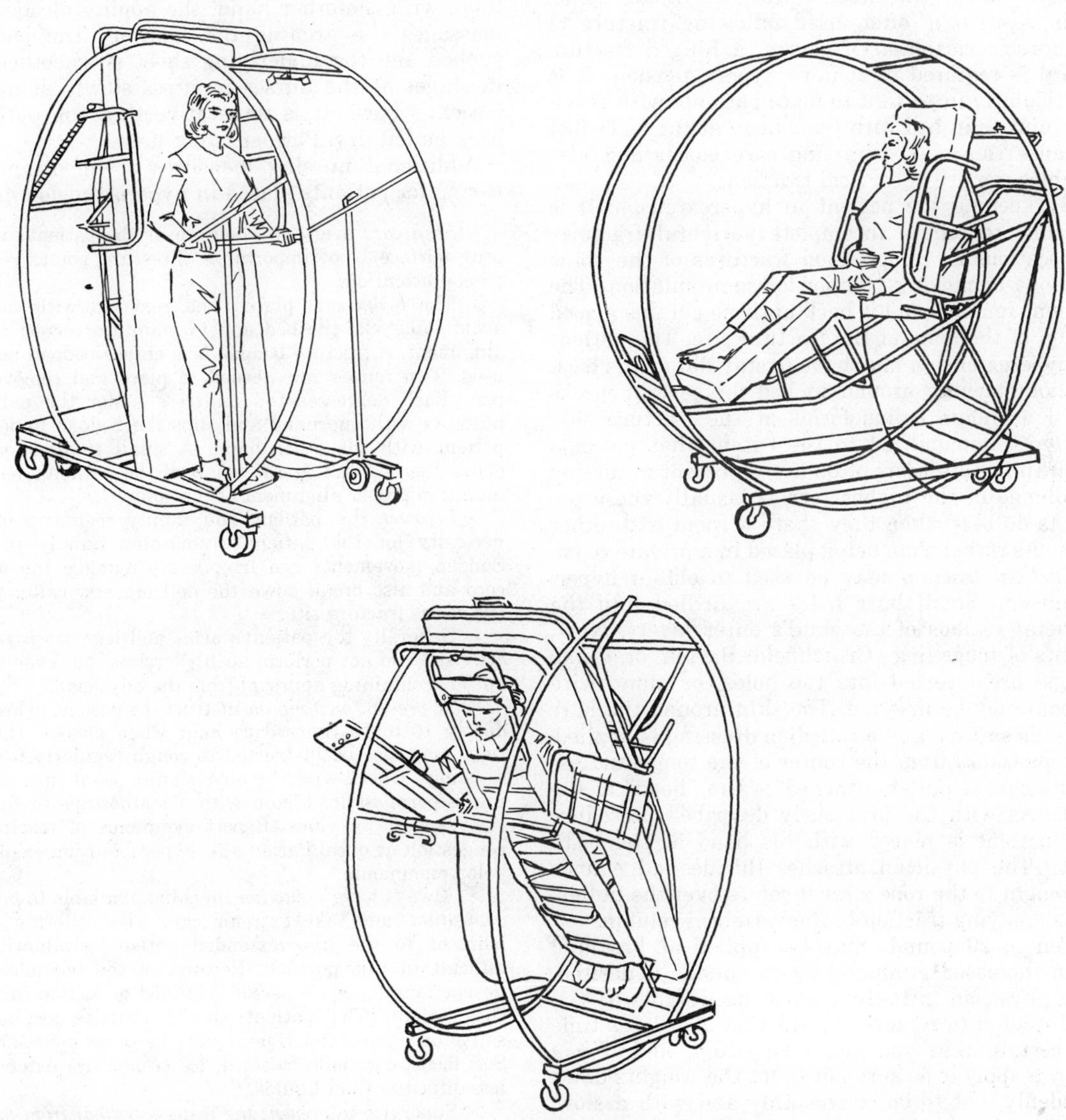

FIGURE 38–8. Other positions possible with CircOlectric bed. (From Sutton, A.: *Bedside Nursing Techniques*, 2nd ed. 1969.)

neck and holding the head back in a position of extension to relieve pressure on the cord. As mentioned earlier, such hyperextension is necessary even in the first aid treatment of these patients; to prevent or minimize cord damage the fracture is reduced early and head or neck traction is employed. Fractures at a *lower level* than cervical injuries may be treated by hyperextension on a Bradford frame, Foster frame, or gatched fracture bed.

When *gatching a fracture bed* the patient is placed so his head is at the usual foot of the bed, as indicated. The "knee" gatch is thus located under the patient's back rather than under his knees. The patient may then be placed so that the high point of the angle of the gatch is located directly under the area of fracture in his spine. This position is often used following fracture of a thoracic vertebra. Of course, a hinged fracture board is required to achieve hyperextension. It is particularly important to place patients with cervical injuries in bed with their head at the bed's foot because this makes nursing care easier and also enables the use of cervical traction.

By keeping the patient in hyperextension it is possible to reduce incomplete vertebral fracture-dislocations or compression fractures of the spine without employing traction or manipulation. The patient remains on his back until he obtains a good union of the bone at the fracture site. The patient in hyperextension may have to stay flat on his back without moving around in bed for several weeks until adequate callus forms at the fracture site. Patients immobilized to the extent that patients with spinal disorders often are represent a nursing challenge of the highest order. Usually these patients do best when they share a room with other patients rather than being placed in a private room.

Skeletal traction may be used to obtain hyperextension. Small burr holes are drilled into the parietal regions of the skull's outer layers. Next, points of tongs (e.g., Crutchfield, Barton, or Vinke tongs) are inserted into the holes, or piano wire (Hoen) may be inserted. The skin around the burr holes is sutured and a collodion dressing is applied. A rope comes from the center of the tongs and extends over a pulley attached to the "head" of the bed. (As with the previously described procedure the patient is placed with his head at the bed's foot.) The physician attaches the desired pounds of weight to the rope after it comes over the pulley, thus applying traction to the vertebral column.

Ten to 20 pounds may be applied at first and then increased gradually to 30 pounds if desired. The physician initially applies the weights. If you are ordered to remove the traction at a later time be certain that you do so smoothly, and if you then reapply it be sure not to let the weights down suddenly, but to do so smoothly and with a slow, steady motion.

Care is taken to prevent infection at the site at which the tongs enter the patient's skull. These areas are inspected daily and any signs of infection are reported. Sterile dressings may be placed over these areas. Also, pressure areas must be watched for, particularly on the shoulders, sacrum, heels, and back of the head.

Skeletal traction may be maintained 4 to 6 weeks. Turning the patient who has tongs in place is discussed below. When allowed the patient should be turned onto his side for feeding to reduce the danger of possible choking and aspiration. Skeletal traction on the head is illustrated in Figure 38–9.

As with any form of traction, the nurse makes certain that the patient being hyperextended with skeletal traction is receiving full benefit from his treatment. (See Unit XVII.)

If the patient is hyperextended on his back (or is otherwise immobilized on his back) and not allowed to turn, *two* nurses are needed to adequately administer *back care* every two hours. Working on opposite sides of the bed, each nurse depresses the mattress on her side by the patient's back and then, with the other hand, she applies alcohol and massages the area to the midline. The back is rubbed and the underlying sheet is smoothed out in stages as the nurses progress slowly along the patient's back. It is imperative that the patient's back be left dry. Powder is not used.

Additional nursing measures of importance in caring for patients placed in hyperextension are:

> *Skin care* every two hours over the patient's entire body surface is of importance. Pressure points require special attention.

> The *bedpan* is placed and removed with care to avoid soilage of the bed and to maintain correct spinal alignment. A fracture bedpan or a child's bedpan may be used. Two nurses are needed to place and remove the pan. Each depresses the mattress under the patient's buttocks with one hand and slips the bedpan under the patient with the other hand. A small towel is placed above the bed pan at the small of the patient's back to maintain proper alignment of the spine.

> *Instruct* the patient and family members of the necessity for the patient's remaining quietly in bed. Sudden movements can irreparably damage the spinal cord and also break down the delicate new callus forming at the fracture site.

> Generally the patient's arms and legs are *passively exercised.* Do not perform such exercises, however, without first obtaining approval from the physician.

> To *prevent pneumonia* instruct the patient to breathe deeply 10 to 15 times each hour when awake. The patient may also be instructed to cough regularly to clear his lungs. Check with the physician to see if such coughing is permissible. Listen with a stethoscope to the patient's chest for rales. Report symptoms of respiratory congestion at once. Patients in hyperextension easily develop pneumonia.

> Always have a *suction* machine available to *prevent aspiration,* and take extreme care when offering nourishment to the hyperextended patient; swallowing is difficult in this position. Because of the possible need for suctioning, only a person qualified to suction can feed the patient. The patient should practice swallowing saliva or water a few times before he takes nourishment. Soft foods, e.g., jello, custard, ice cream, are eaten with less difficulty than liquids.

> Supervise to *prevent the restless patient from falling* out of bed or moving about excessively in bed. The

hyperextended patient frequently feels more secure when sleeping if he has "reminders" not to move, e.g., sandbags placed on both sides of his body or a draw sheet placed across his abdomen and tucked in under both sides of the mattress.

Seeing the patient in traction is frequently frightening for family members, and it helps if the nurse discusses this treatment briefly with family members before they visit the patient the first time. Traction achieved with tongs is particularly distressful. Explain that the tongs are not actually going through the patient's skull but are merely in the bony outer layer. Although hyperextension appears extremely uncomfortable to the onlooker, patients often adjust to it very nicely and find it gives them welcome relief from pain.

Turning

Once a patient is allowed to turn onto his sides following spinal injury or spinal surgery he is turned in a *log rolling* manner. In other words, he keeps his body rigid, with his arms folded across his chest, and is then rolled over and turned as a whole, as if he were a solid log. A turning sheet is kept under the patient and one nurse stands on either side of the bed. The patient's head pillow is removed prior to the turn and is replaced after the turn is completed. Prior to the turn a pillow may be placed between the patient's legs to prevent his upper leg from falling over and dropping down during the turn—a movement that could jar the spine. If it is necessary to support the patient's head and neck during the move, a third nurse is used for this purpose.

After the head pillow is removed, and the patient has folded his arms over his chest, he is lifted to the side of the bed while resting on his back in preparation for the turn. This lift is accomplished by the nurses on either side of the bed rolling the turn sheet up close to the patient's body and then lifting together and shifting the patient to one side of the bed. The leg pillow mentioned above is then placed and the patient is log rolled toward the opposite side of the bed. For example, if the patient were being rolled onto his right side the nurse on the patient's left side pulls the turn sheet upward; this motion rolls the patient over. The other nurse supports the patient at his shoulders and hips, as he rolls toward her, so he does not roll too far over, e.g., onto his abdomen (Fig. 38–10).

Following the turn, the turn sheet is drawn taut and smooth and is anchored on either side under the mattress. The patient is left comfortable and in good alignment, with his head pillow replaced and his upper leg flexed on top of the leg pillow (to relieve strain on his spine and to help to maintain his position). The patient's hips are pulled back slightly so he can stay comfortably on his side with his spine straight.

With the physician's order, a patient with *skeletal tongs* (who is not on a Stryker frame) *may be*

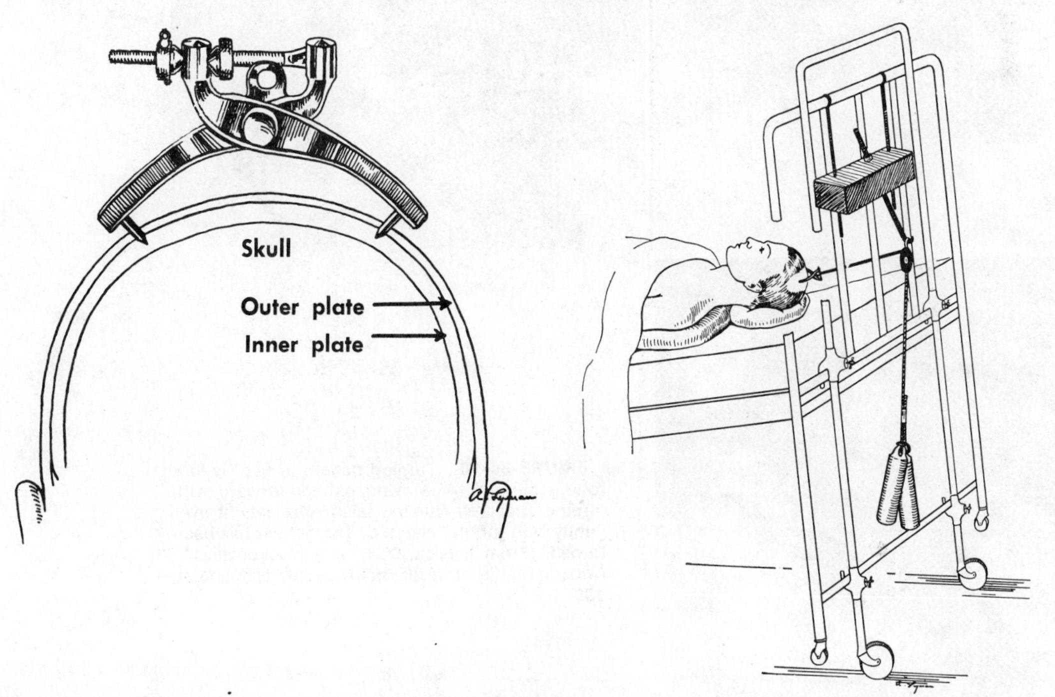

FIGURE 38–9. Crutchfield tongs. (From Larson, C. B., and Gould, M.: *Orthopedic Nursing.* 7th ed. St. Louis, The C. V. Mosby Co., 1970.)

turned in bed. This is accomplished as follows: (1) a pillow is placed between the patient's legs (to keep the upper leg from dropping and jarring the patient's spine and head as he is turned); (2) a pillow is placed longitudinally on the patient's chest and his upper arm is rested on it (to prevent the shoulder from dropping and twisting the patient's neck as he is turned); (3) a team of three persons *plans* together to turn the patient by rolling him like a log while being certain that his head is kept at all times in a direct line with the cervical spine's axis (without being flexed either forward or laterally) and making certain his shoulders turn with his neck and head; (4) one person supports the patient's head and directs the other two team members during the turning; (5) the second team member supports and rolls the patient's shoulders while the third person supports and rolls the patient's hips and legs; (6) during the turning process the patient is positioned so that his head and cervical spine are in a direct line with the traction's pulley; and (7) a small pillow is slipped under the patient's head while the patient's head is still manually supported in the lateral position by the team captain (this support maintains cervical alignment).

When turning a patient with a cervical fracture, e.g., in tongs, observe him closely for indications of respiratory difficulties.

CAUTION: Do not exert heavy traction on the shoulder girdle when moving or turning paralyzed patients or those with depressed levels of consciousness; injuries could be caused to the brachial plexus.

IMPAIRED CARDIORESPIRATORY AND VASCULAR FUNCTIONS

Respiratory failure may result from cervical injuries or bulbar involvement, and immediate respiratory assistance may be necessary.

Equipment should be available to accomplish

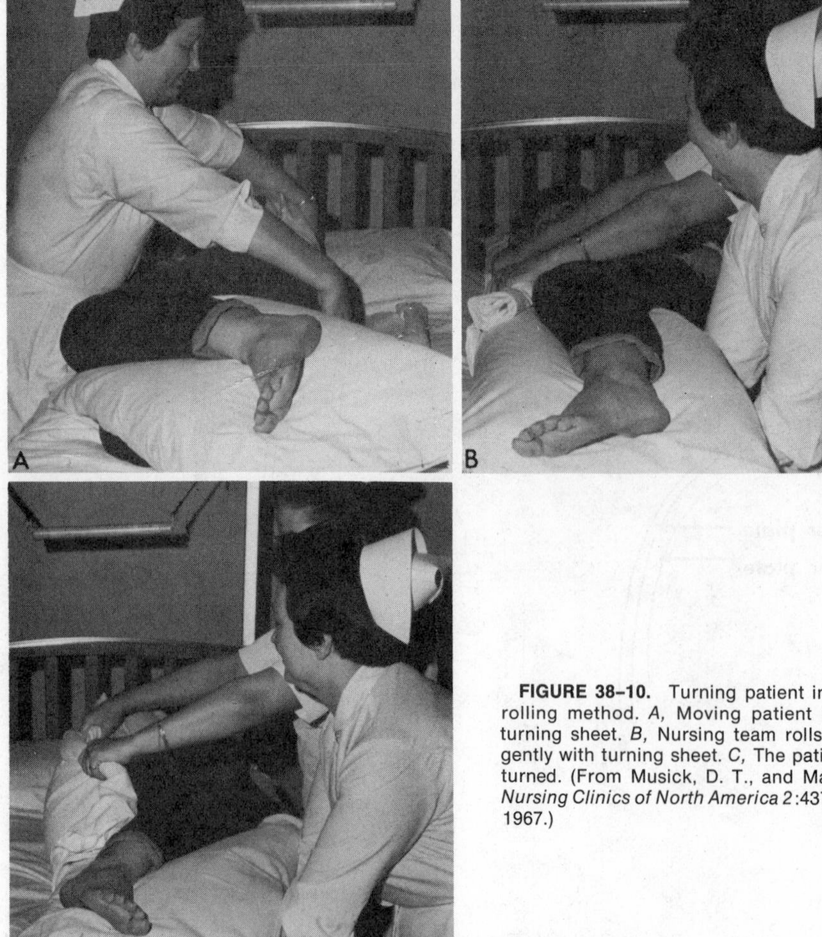

FIGURE 38–10. Turning patient in bed by log-rolling method. *A*, Moving patient forward with turning sheet. *B*, Nursing team rolls patient over gently with turning sheet. *C*, The patient has been turned. (From Musick, D. T., and MacKenzie, M.: *Nursing Clinics of North America* 2:437, September, 1967.)

suctioning, perform tracheostomy, and mechanically assist respiration. Mechanical respiratory assistance is required when a definite loss or impairment of respiratory muscle function occurs. A chest respirator or rocking bed may be necessary. Respiratory failure resulting from neurologic disorders is discussed in Unit XIV. Careful preventative care, e.g., coughing and deep breathing, is established to *prevent pulmonary infection.*

Because of *venostasis* in the lower limbs, the incidence of *pulmonary embolus* is increased in paraplegics confined to bed. Passive exercises and elastic supports on the legs may help to reduce the incidence of this complication.

Periodic hypertension may accompany filling of the bladder or rectum following spinal injury. Following cervical injuries the intercostal muscles are paralyzed, leaving only *diaphragmatic respiration.* Patients with this condition rapidly develop dyspnea when they exert themselves. Thus, they have a low tolerance and have only limited use of such fatiguing devices as braces and hand-powered wheelchairs.

SPINAL SHOCK (DIASCHISIS, "SHOCK REACTION")

Following injury the spinal cord at first does not show any activity; this period of inactivity is called the period of "spinal shock." Spinal shock is the immediate, complete loss of motor, reflex, sensory, and autonomic activity below the level of a spinal lesion. Although spinal shock typically occurs with complete, sudden transverse sections of the spinal cord and with acute cerebrovascular accident (CVA), some degree of spinal shock also occurs with incomplete cord transection.

Initially the urinary bladder is paralyzed and atonic; however, after parasympathetic activity returns, automatic bowel and bladder control may be obtained. Gradually autonomic activities return. Initially during spinal shock reflexes are absent, but then hyperreflexia develops (during which even light cutaneous stimulation evokes reflex movements). Also, a flaccid paralysis is initially present, which may become a spastic paralysis as spinal shock subsides.

SPINAL AUTOMATISMS

Following transection of the spinal cord the lower part of the cord eventually works automatically on its own; the brain can no longer influence those reflex movements that are "built into" the spinal cord. Spinal reflex activities which *automatically occur* following severence of the cord are called *"spinal automatisms,"* e.g., the flexor withdrawal reflex, and the reflex emptying of the urinary bladder and bowel.

Spinal automatisms are primitive spinal mechanisms normally kept inactive by higher centers. However, when these normal inhibitions of the higher centers are destroyed by severe spinal cord disease or decerebrate states at the midbrain level, the spinal automatisms are "released." (*Decerebration* refers to interruption or sectioning of the nervous system below the level of the cerebral hemispheres. Do not mix the terms *decerebration* and *decortication* in your thinking. Decortication refers to destruction of the cerebral cortex.)

When the spinal cord is severed the blood pressure and temperature in the part of the body supplied by the isolated spinal cord fall markedly and respond poorly to reflex stimuli. Other functions may occur reflexly, e.g., control of the urinary bladder, but lack integration with other visceral activities. Visceral activities may be initiated by stimuli which are normally ineffective, e.g., scratching of the skin may cause vasodilatation, sweating, and perhaps emptying of the bladder.[72]

The "release" of spinal automatisms causes the patient to respond to stimuli in ways which can be puzzling to both the patient and the nurse unless they understand the origin of such responses. For example, stimulation of the limbs (perhaps by flexion of the toes while drying the patient's foot during the bed bath) causes the flexor reflexes to predominate, and *mass flexion* of the upper and lower extremities occurs. Mass flexion reactions also may be accompanied by massive contractions of the abdominal wall, evacuation of the urinary bladder and bowels, and such autonomic responses as sweating, flushing, and pilomotor reactions below the level of the lesion.

Lesions of the nervous system may produce defective urinary bladder function often referred to as *"cord bladder."* For example, stimulation of the skin of the lower abdomen or thighs may cause reflex micturition, i.e., reflex emptying of the urinary bladder. This form of cord bladder is called an *"automatic bladder."*

It is important for the nurse to realize that stimulation of the skin of the lower abdomen or thighs may also cause, in the male, *reflex ejaculation* of seminal fluid and *priapism,* i.e., persistent abnormal erection of the penis, generally without sexual desire. Obviously in giving nursing care unnecessary stimulation of those areas that elicit such reflex spinal automatisms should be avoided. When such reactions do occur, the nurse's unembarrassed, accepting response to the situation will help to relieve the patient's anxiety. An explanation of the cause of some of these spinal patterns of movement may help the uninformed patient to understand why his body is reacting as it does.

SPASTICITY; MUSCLE SPASMS

Spasticity may result from various causes, e.g., cerebrovascular accidents, spinal cord injuries, and cerebral palsy. Spasticity may develop two weeks to several months following injury to the spinal cord. This spasticity may be relieved by physical exercise, hydrotherapy, Hubbard or whirlpool baths (Fig. 38–11), exercises under water, standing, or such medications as Paraflex, Robaxin, carisoprodol, Tolserol, or Prostigmin.

Spastic movements may be initiated by such emotions as apprehension, crying, anger, or laughing, or from cutaneous stimulation, e.g., tickling, stroking, or pinching. While spastic movements may be annoying to the patient, he may also learn to recognize events which trigger such movements and then use some of these triggering activities to assist him with various activities such as emptying his bladder.

Following traumatic complete transverse lesion of the spinal cord, painful intense *spasms of the muscles* of the lower extremities occur. (Such spasms may also occur with other severe neurologic disorders.) The paralyzed patient must tactfully be told that the occurrence of muscle spasms does not mean that voluntary movement is returning, but rather that these spasms occur involuntarily. Muscle spasms vary, according to the patient's posture, from mild muscular twitchings to vigorous mass reflex states. Because violent involuntary muscle spasms can actually throw the paralyzed patient off his bed or frame, it is important to protect him from such falls by keeping bed siderails up and by always having restraining straps comfortably secured over the patient's body when he is lying on a frame or is being transported on a stretcher. Muscle spasms are typically aggravated by cold weather, sitting for prolonged periods of time, and emotionally upsetting events.

Reflex spasms may become intolerable and may be triggered by extrinsic or visceral stimuli, e.g., a distended bladder.

A certain amount of muscle spasm may actually help the paraplegic to support his trunk or to position an extremity. However, painful or recurrent spasms that forcibly flex or adduct the lower limbs prevent rehabilitation by interfering with sitting and ambulation. These flexor spasms are reflex responses. Thus, to try to prevent their occurrence it is necessary to remove sources of noxious stimulation that could trigger the reflex spasms, e.g., treat bladder infections and decubitus ulcers if present.

Medications employed in treating muscle spasms include: methocarbamol, meprobamate,

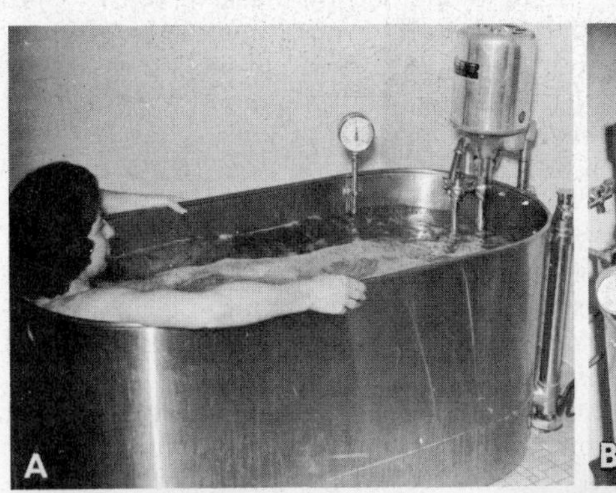

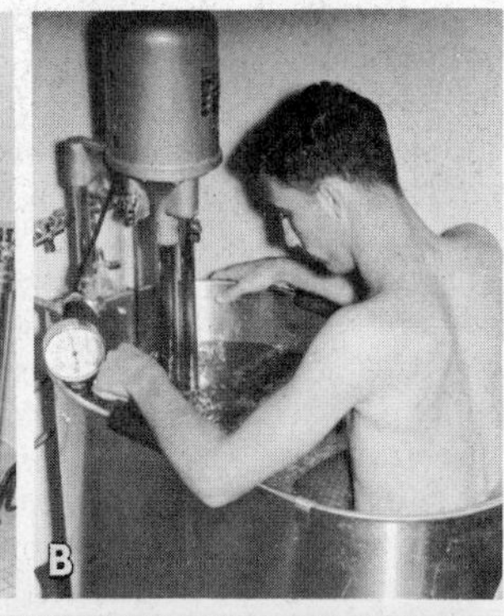

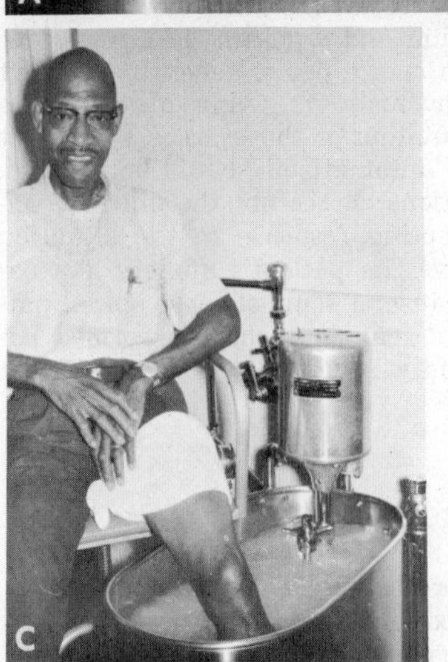

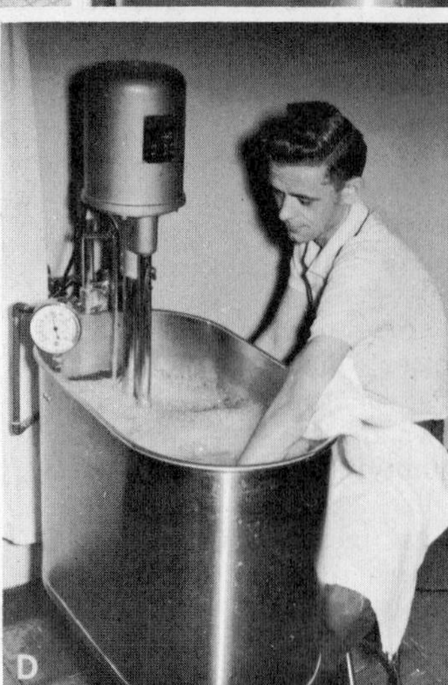

FIGURE 38–11. Whirlpool bath therapy. (From Krusen, F. H., Kottke, F. J., and Ellwood, P. M., Jr.: *Handbook of Physical Medicine and Rehabilitation.* 2nd ed. 1971.)

and chlordiazepoxide hydrochloride. Side effects of such medications include drowsiness and muscle weakness. Muscle spasms may also be treated with such physical therapy practices as stretching exercises and warm tub baths. Exercises under water and Hubbard baths may not only relieve muscle spasm, but may also relieve pain, improve muscle tone, and stimulate circulation.

When painful, severe muscle spasms or spasticity cannot be controlled by conservative measures, e.g., with specific pharmacologic agents or physical therapy, it may be necessary to employ more drastic measures. Possible *surgical procedures* include: excision of the distal end of the spinal cord; anterior rhizotomy; chordotomy; frontal myelotomy; nerve resection; peripheral neurotomy; tendon resection; tendon transplantation; cordectomy; surgical section of the sciatic, obturator, or lumbosacral nerve roots; and division of muscles and tendons. Recently attempts have been made to correct spastic deformities with *neuroelectric stimulation.*

RIGIDITY

Rigidity is a state of increased resistance to passive stretch. Various disorders cause rigidity. The basic problem with rigidity is a difficulty in initiating movement; in spontaneous actions rigidity is characterized by a paucity of associated movements (e.g., as with Parkinson's disease). A variety of physical therapy measures may be employed to treat rigidity, e.g., passive and active exercise, warm baths.

PAIN

Often patients with spinal injuries have pain present at the level of the injury which radiates along the spinal nerves originating in that area. For example, chest pain may occur following a thoracic injury, while leg pain may follow an injury at the lumbar level. Analgesics, (acetylsalicylic acid, narcotics) may be prescribed and should be given as indicated for pain relief. However, remember:

> *Narcotics are* not *administered in the presence of high cervical injuries because they tend to add to respiratory depression.*

Patients with thoracic level injuries often tend to splint their chests and to breathe shallowly to avoid pain. Of course, these actions set the stage for the development of respiratory complications. To prevent this, narcotics may be given for pain control and then deep breathing and coughing (unless contraindicated) are encouraged to areate the lungs and to move secretions in the respiratory passages. Thoracic pain may also be relieved by paravertebral nerve blocks.

Usually pain occurs later than muscular spasms. Some paraplegic and quadriplegic patients have both pain and muscle spasms. Pain most frequently occurs in the lower extremities.

Pain associated with spasticity may be treated with such drugs as opiates, sedatives, antispasmodics, anticonvulsants, or ataractics. When medical pain relief cannot be obtained, neurosurgery may be considered, e.g., neurectomy, chordotomy. (Pain is discussed further in Unit IX.)

TENDON CONTRACTURES; ANKYLOSIS OF JOINTS; MUSCLE SHORTENING

Other complications of paralyzed limbs are muscle shortening, tendon contractures, and ankylosis of joints. These problems are caused from improper positioning of the patient in bed or chair and by lack of joint movements. Measures that can prevent such complications are: position changes; proper positioning of joints at all times; use of footboard in supine position; draping bedding over frames to keep pressure of pull of bed linens off feet; maintenance of 15 degree flexion of knee joints in supine position; conditioning exercises (active and passive); and other physiotherapeutic measures *performed regularly.*

Passive exercises prevent contractures as well as future painful reflex dystrophies of the hand and shoulder. Passive exercises may be started 48 to 72 hours after spinal injury if ordered. Passive exercises should be performed as early as prescribed by the physician; check with him to determine when exercises may be started. When the patient's condition permits, *active exercises, massage,* and *electrical stimulation* may also be prescribed. If the patient has fractured his spine, resulting in paraplegia, exercises to develop his upper extremities, shoulders, chest and back are started once x-ray examination shows that a callus has adequately formed at the fracture site.

Standing for at least a few minutes each day prevents contractures that could otherwise develop in the hips from long periods of sitting. The patient may stand supported in a walker or he may learn to stand supported between two stable chairs or on crutches.

MUSCLE WEAKNESS; FATIGUE

Wrist drop and foot drop *will* develop following paralysis of the extremities unless proper preventative measures are carefully taken. These problems and contractures may take months to overcome once they develop and may prevent some patients from ever walking, even with crutches and braces.

> *Provide continual support for paretic or paralyzed extremities.*

To counteract the force of gravity on weakened

muscles and thereby prevent foot drop keep the patient's feet firmly supported in dorsiflexion at right angles to his hips. A paralyzed upper extremity is supported in a sling when the patient is out of bed and with cock-up splints while he is in bed. Usually the hand end of the splint is given a two-inch elevation to support the wrist, and the fingers are maintained in a position of function. Posterior molded casts may be used instead of splints to support a paralyzed wrist while the patient is in bed. For some patients pillows and a hand roll suffice.

Rehabilitative programs often require strength and endurance on the part of the patient. To prepare him for ambulation the unaffected parts of the patient's body are strengthened, and a diet is usually provided that is high in protein, vitamins, and calories. Suitable exercises are started early in preparation for ambulation, and the patient's tolerance for activity is gradually increased. Care must be taken not to *fatigue* the patient. Periods of planned rest and recreation are important.

Weight Bearing; Assuming an Upright Position

Following cord injury weight bearing is started as early as possible to stimulate osteoblastic activity and thus decrease the demineralization of bone or osteoporosis that develops with prolonged immobilization. (See Unit V, Chap. 27.)

If a CircOlectric bed to *gradually* assist the patient to a standing position is not available, standing boards or tilt tables can be used (Fig. 38–12).

Wheelchairs

Many patients are mobilized by modern, folding *wheelchairs.* Wheelchair selection needs to be tailored to meet the needs of the individual patient because the wheelchair is the most important orthopedic appliance for persons whose normal means of locomotion is either completely abolished or impaired due to limb paralysis or physical loss of limbs.

Let us emphasize that:

> Prolonged, unrelieved *periods of sitting in a wheelchair are hazardous since they may lead to various complications, e.g., flexion contractures, decubitus ulcers, bone atrophy, loss of calcium from bones, pathologic fractures, and renal calculi.*

When sitting up, e.g., in wheelchair, the paralyzed patient needs to periodically shift his weight and lift his weight (by pushing with his arms) to relieve the constant pressure on his buttocks. Failure to perform these pushups, either through neglect or forgetfulness, results in skin breakdown. Electronic devices are available that ring a bell when it is time for a pushup.[66]

Braces; Corsets; Orthopedic Shoes

A back brace or corset is often prescribed and custom fitted to a patient following ruptured lumbar intervertebral disks or other spinal injuries. (See also Unit XVII). The appliance, e.g., a *Taylor back brace* or splint (Fig. 38–13) or a heavy muslin corset with stays, may initially be prescribed to be worn for periods of time while the patient is in bed and turning. Later it may be worn only when the patient plans to get up. The patient is turned to one side, the brace or corset is then placed up

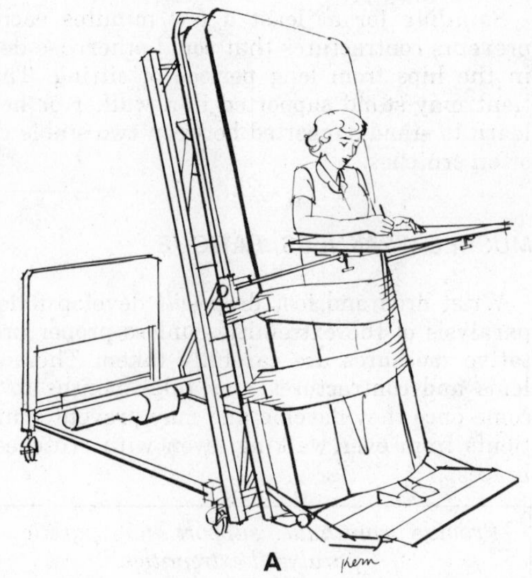

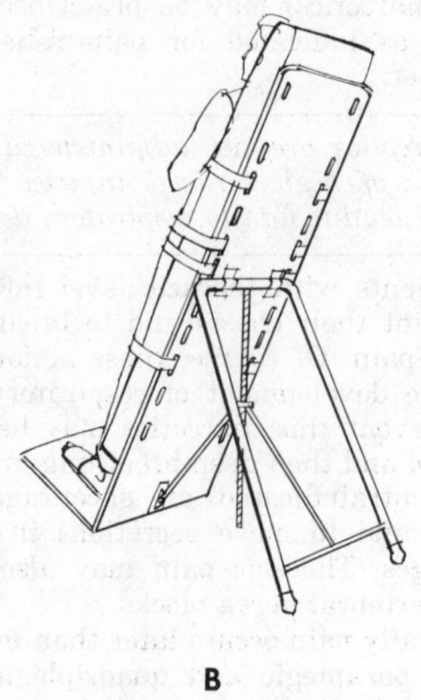

FIGURE 38–12. *A*, Example of a tilting hospital bed. *B*, Example of a tiltboard (also called tilt-table). (From Sutton, A.: *Bedside Nursing Techniques*, 2nd ed. 1969.)

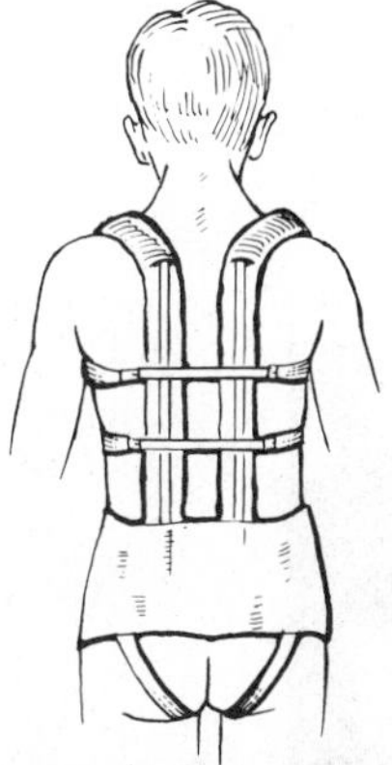

FIGURE 38-13. Taylor splint. (From *Dorland's Illustrated Medical Dictionary.* 25th ed. 1974.)

against his back, and he is then rolled back into the appliance. Finally, the brace or corset is secured with straps while the patient lies on his back in bed. It is desirable for a thin knitted undershirt to be worn next to the skin under a brace, to protect the skin and also to keep the brace clean. The brace or corset is applied *before* the patient is helped out of bed. As improvement occurs, and with teaching, some patients learn to apply their own braces and corsets while in bed. Other patients continue to need help even after discharge.

A *neck brace* (fitted so the patient's chin rests on a cup and the neck is kept hyperextended), a *Thomas collar* (which extends up under the chin and prevents flexion of the neck) or a *Chandler felt collar splint* may be necessary following fracture of a cervical vertebra or rupture of a cervical disk. Such appliances may be worn following "whiplash" injuries resulting from automobile accidents (Fig. 38-14).

The patient wearing a brace must learn to be careful not to fall or otherwise lose his balance because of his brace. The weight of a brace may be surprisingly heavy at first to a patient who is weak from lying in bed and from being ill. Neck braces tend to limit vision, since the patient cannot look down at his feet.

Shoes should be worn, rather than slippers, by all patients who have had spinal injuries, and indeed by any patient learning how to walk again after any injury or prolonged illness. Preferably the shoes should tie (so firm support is possible) and they should have a low heel. Of course slick soles and slick heels are hazardous. Orthopedic shoes may be advisable. Wearing shoes also helps to prevent foot drop when the patient lies down.

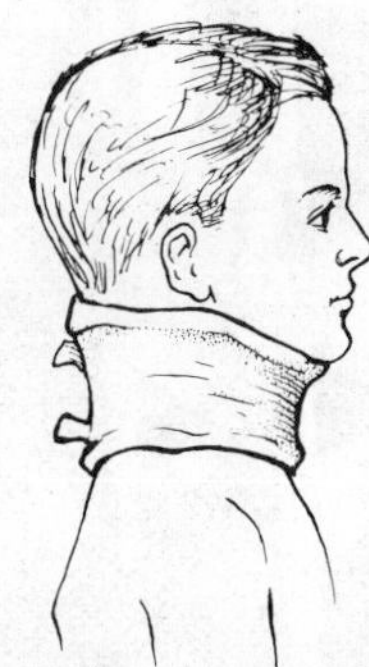

FIGURE 38-14. Chandler felt collar splint. (From *Dorland's Illustrated Medical Dictionary.* 25th ed. 1974.)

Transfers

The paraplegic patient must learn a variety of transfers to become self-sufficient. A few of these are pictured in Figures 38-15, 38-16 and 38-17. Before he can transfer, he first learns to sit up.

IMPAIRED CIRCULATION; DECUBITUS ULCERS; ABSENCE OF SENSATIONS

> Decubitus ulcers *(pressure sores) are a dread complication of paralysis since* circulation is poor *in denervated tissue because of lack of muscle activity.*

Because of loss of sensation in an anesthetic area, pain and pressure which normally prompt a change in position are not felt. Sometimes merely the weight of bedding can cause the tips of the toes to break down. Skin breakdown may also occur when plaster casts are applied over anesthetic areas. Decubitus ulcers have been known to develop within a period of six hours. This complication can be prevented, however, by the administration of careful nursing care and by teaching the patient self-help measures. The prevention and care of decubitus ulcers is discussed in Unit V, Chapter 27.

Like renal calculi, decubitus ulcers can be partially prevented if the patient stands in braces in an upright position. Range-of-motion exercise and gentle total body massage improve the paralyzed patient's circulation. Elastic stockings may improve circulation in the lower extremities.

The paralyzed patient is taught to frequently and regularly inspect his skin for signs of pressure or irritation which could progress to ulcer formation. A mirror may be used as necessary for this inspection. Persons caring for the patient also maintain a constant vigilance for the appearance of red spots or other indications that the patient's skin is being rubbed or chafed. *The paralyzed patient's entire body is inspected daily for skin breakdown.*

The paralyzed patient's skin is kept clean and dry; special attention is given to the perineal area. When the patient is confined to bed, skin care is given every two hours, immediately after the patient is turned. Let us reemphasize that the paralyzed patient must be turned every two hours—

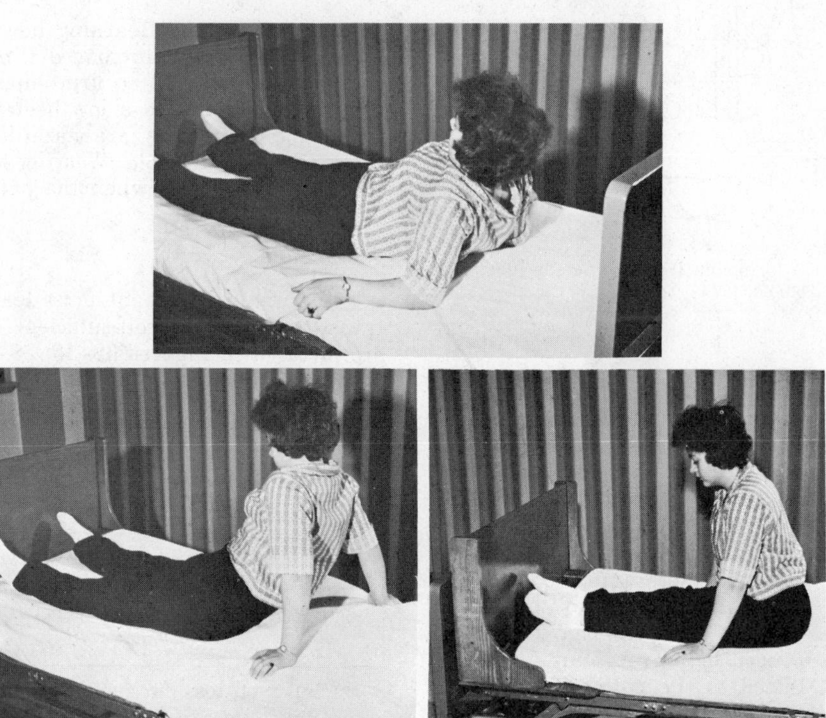

FIGURE 38–15. Paraplegic patient coming to sitting position. (From Krusen, F. H., Kottke, F. J., and Ellwood, P. M., Jr.: *Handbook of Physical Medicine and Rehabilitation,* 2nd ed. 1971.)

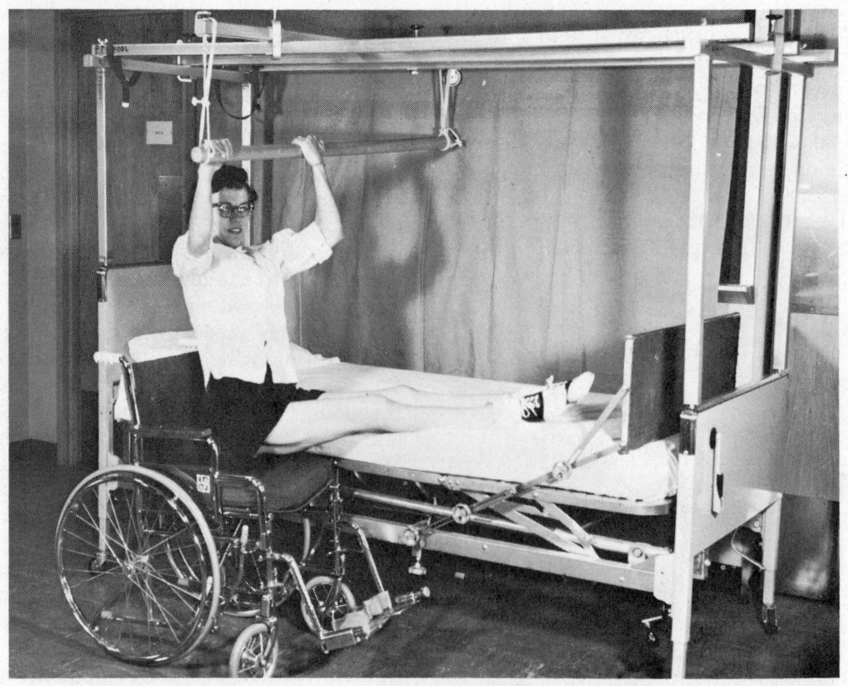

FIGURE 38–16. Paraplegic patient transfering from bed to wheelchair using a 4-foot trapeze bar. (From Krusen, F. H., Kottke, F. J., and Ellwood, P. M., Jr.: *Handbook of Physical Medicine and Rehabilitation,* 2nd ed. 1971.)

day and night—to compensate for the loss of spontaneous movements.

> *Do not apply external heat if there has been a loss of sensation. Be careful that bath water is not excessively warm.*

Sensory loss poses serious problems for the paralyzed patient because he cannot feel the pain or pressure that signals tissue damage. The paralyzed patient (or any patient with impaired sensation) should thus avoid wearing tight, restrictive clothing and improperly fitting shoes or braces. Because of impaired sensation the patient cannot feel areas of injury to his skin in the affected areas; therefore, he must gear himself to *preventative thinking,* which will enable him to avoid potential sources of danger. He must avoid close proximity to sources of heat(e.g., heaters, radiators, fireplaces) and avoid the use of heating pads or hot water bottles. Burns can pose serious problems because of impaired circulation.

Foot care and nail care on paralyzed limbs need to be regularly and carefully performed to prevent nails from rubbing or cutting the skin and from becoming ingrown. Foot infections must be prevented, e.g., the patient is instructed to not cut at corns or calluses. (Foot care is discussed further in Units XIII and XIX.)

It is advisable to give injections of medications *above* the level of the patient's cord lesion when-

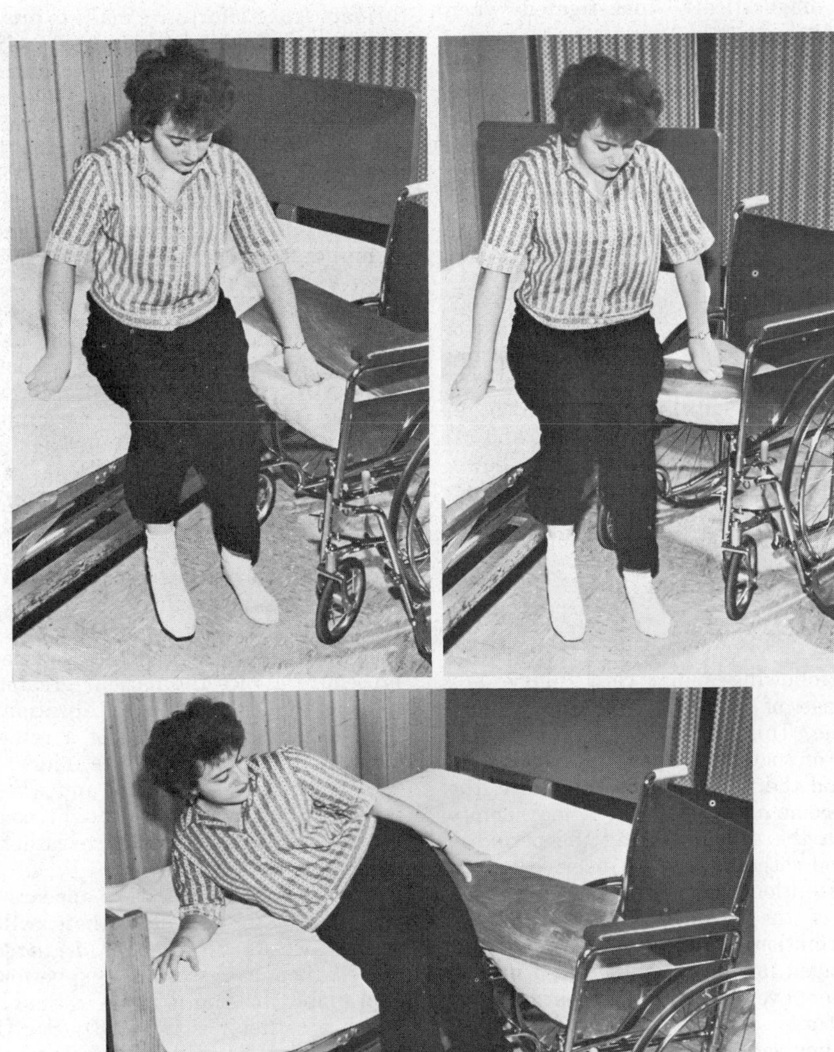

FIGURE 38-17. Paraplegic bed to wheelchair lateral transfer using a sliding board. (From Krusen, F. H., Kottke, F. J., and Ellwood, P. M., Jr.: *Handbook of Physical Medicine and Rehabilitation,* 2nd ed. 1971.)

ever possible. Adequate absorption of injectable medications is not likely to occur in denervated areas of the body which have impaired capillary and precapillary circulation.

BOWEL AND URINARY BLADDER FUNCTION

Disorders of both the brain and the spinal cord can alter *urinary bladder function.* Patients with CNS disorders therefore need to be observed for incontinence, retention, urgency, dribbling, frequency, enuresis, precipitate micturition, and other indications of faulty bladder control. Such observations should be recorded. Possible bladder infections are diagnostically investigated when symptoms appear.

Central nervous system disorders may also *impair* the *bowel's* sphincter control. Therefore, observe and report constipation, diarrhea, and tenesmus, i.e., ineffectual, painful straining at stool. (For detailed discussion of significant observations and nursing care of patients with intestinal disorders, see Unit XV.)

In planning care of the paralyzed patient's urinary bladder and bowels, the nurse keeps several objectives in mind. Among these are: (1) prevention of urinary tract infection; (2) preservation of normal bladder and bowel capacity and normal muscle tone in these areas; (3) preservation of a normal, routine pattern of elimination which requires a minimum of artificial assistance; and (4) teaching the patient to regain bladder and bowel control (by means of governing reflex functioning) when this is possible, and when this is not possible teaching him self-help measures to maintain regularity and to prevent complications.

Urinary Bladder Function

Immediately following spinal cord injury, i.e., during the phase of spinal shock, the urinary bladder is *atonic.* This period of atony may last several weeks or months. Upon recovery from spinal shock, and the return of the reflex arc, the bladder may become *automatic;* i.e., it may empty reflexively as in the infant. During the period of atony a retention catheter may be inserted to prevent bladder distention and to prevent bed soilage. *Overdistention* of the bladder causes stretching and fissure formation which can predispose to *infection.* Prolonged use of a catheter also predisposes to infection even though every attempt is made to prevent it.

Remember, when sensory pathways are affected, the patient may be unable to feel the discomfort of bladder distention. The nurse periodically checks the patient for distention; maintains an accurate record of intake and output; maintains aseptic technique when giving care related to indwelling catheters (because of the possibility of urinary tract infections); and observes for symptoms of bladder infection.

Renal calculi, pyelonephritis, and hydronephrosis are major causes of death in paraplegics and cause considerable disability in patients with less extensive paralysis.

The above renal complications begin as a result of incomplete emptying of the bladder, which initially necessitates catheterization; catheterization is then followed by secondary infection and vesicoureteral reflux.

Bladder or *kidney infections* are difficult for the patient to experience, in addition to being a serious threat to the paralyzed patient's life. Thus, everything possible must be done to prevent the possible occurrence of these complications. (See Units V and XI.)

Along with preventing infections of the genitourinary tract, efforts are made to prevent the formation of *renal calculi* (kidney stones). The prevention of calculi formation is partially dependent on having the patient drink substantial amounts of water. While for some patients this increases the problems of keeping dry, it is nonetheless a necessary measure. It is recommended that adequate fluid balance be maintained with a minimal output of 2000 ml. every 24 hours; this generally requires a minimal 24-hour fluid intake of 4000 ml. (See Unit V, Chap. 27.)

The prevention of calculi and renal infections is also dependent on having the patient stand on his feet in his braces for about an hour a day. Some sources recommend that x-rays (a flat plate of the abdomen) be taken monthly in an attempt to identify the presence of calculi early in their formation in paralyzed persons. Periodic turning and other position changes are also important in preventing stasis of urine within the kidney pelvis and resultant infection.

Generally it has been established that paraplegic patients are most effectively rehabilitated by initially using a *retention catheter* attached to a suitable drainage bag or "up" bottle (see Unit XI); this procedure allows the patient greater mobility and reduces the length of hospitalization. Few patients need to continue the use of a retention catheter. Depending on the site of the injury, many patients who are highly motivated, and whose intelligence is not impaired, can be taught complete bladder control without the use of a catheter if they are otherwise in good health.

If urinary tract infection appears likely, or if it appears that an internal catheter will be needed for several weeks, *suprapubic drainage* may be required, i.e., a cystostomy is performed (a small suprapubic incision is made in the bladder through which a catheter is inserted). (See Unit XI.) However, this decision is carefully made since it is more difficult for patients to recover bladder function at a later date following suprapubic drainage.

The retention catheter may be removed early and *incontinent* males can be connected to bedside drainage with a condom tube. However, a catheter is generally necessary for a longer time with incontinent females. Catheterization is necessary for both males and females when *urinary retention* occurs. A Foley catheter is usually needed for chronic retention. Single catheterizations may take care of episodic retentions or those unlikely to recur, e.g., acute poliomyelitis or multiple sclerosis.

Once the catheter is removed it may still be necessary to catheterize the patient periodically to measure residual urine. Vesicouretheral reflux can damage the kidneys if the residuum of urine is too large. It is thus highly important to determine if the patient is adequately emptying his bladder.

Attempts at *bladder training* are started once the bladder begins to empty reflexively following spinal injury. The goal is to establish an automatic bladder trained to empty at regular intervals. The *automatic voiding* reflex may be weaker than the normal voiding reflex; however, the reflex may be increased in various ways, e.g., from stimulation below the level of the lesion in the spinal cord, by exerting gentle pressure over the bladder, or by stroking the lower abdomen or inner aspects of the thighs. The patient may be taught various exercises for conditioning the voiding reflex if he is capable of performing them. *Spontaneous automatic voiding is established in many patients by maintaining a fluid intake of 3000 to 5000 ml. daily, then intermittently clamping the catheter, and finally making regularly scheduled attempts to void without the catheter.* The patient is instructed so that he can participate in the program. Important points are: (1) establishment of a *regular routine;* (2) a carefully scheduled program of fluid intake so the bladder will empty at a convenient time; and (3) recording of fluid intake and voiding times by the patient.

When bladder retraining is first started the patient may attempt to void hourly. Once this is achieved, the interval is lengthened gradually. The schedule is maintained for 24 hours. Patient and staff should realize that it may take weeks or months for successful retraining to occur. Unrealistic expectations discourage the patient.

Until a schedule is finally achieved (and sometimes even afterwards), a continual dribbling of urine occurs. The patient who is on a voiding schedule may use some form of *external drainage apparatus* or a padded *penile incontinence clamp* which mechanically compresses the uretheral wall and prevents dribbling. Because penile clamps can cause circulatory obstruction and are generally uncomfortable, they are usually worn for only brief periods of time and are alternated with an external form of drainage collection. The penile clamp must be released at least every two hours and repositioned to ensure adequate circulation to the penis. The paralyzed patient who lacks penile sensation must be certain to release the clamp as instructed, since he cannot feel the discomfort that impaired circulation causes, signaling tissue damage.

External drainage for the male can be provided in various ways; e.g., a urinal may be placed in the bed, or a male leg urinal may be attached with a soft rubber shield that fits snugly over the penis. Various types of male urinals are available. Female urinals of various types are also available but may be less satisfactory. The female may do better with an incontinent panty of some type or sanitary perineal pads under plastic or rubber-lined panties. With any incontinent patient, every effort is made to prevent odor and skin irritation. External appliances must be kept clean and aired daily; thus, more than one appliance per patient is necessary.

Broad spectrum antibiotics allow control of bladder infections associated with indwelling catheters, so that today the development of "automatic" bladder function with a *tidal drainage apparatus* is not so important as it formerly was. Thus, tidal drainage is rarely used currently in treatment of paraplegic or quadriplegic patients.

Paralyzed individuals should have periodic evaluations by a urologist because they are susceptible to renal damage from various sources. (See also Unit XI.)

Bowel Function

Fecal incontinence occurs during the acute phase of spinal shock. Also, *hypomotility* of the bowel may be a problem resulting from immobility. However, it is estimated that bowel training is possible in more than 80 per cent of paraplegic and quadriplegic patients. Specifically, nursing care is directed at: (1) prevention of constipation, distention and impaction; (2) early detection and treatment of these conditions if they do occur; and (3) reestablishment of habitual, controlled bowel movements by conditioned reflex activity. (See also section on bowel and urinary bladder control, p. 429, and Unit V, Chap. 27.)

Paralytic ileus commonly occurs for a few days following spinal injury or acute poliomyelitis. (See Unit XV.) Oral feedings are eliminated until bowel activity returns. A nasogastric tube may be used to decompress the intestinal tract if abdominal distention occurs.

During the *acute phase* of the patient's illness he may be given an enema or colon lavage* every three to four days, or more often if necessary. However, attempts are made to prevent dependency upon such procedures for evacuation. Suppositories are tried before resorting to enemas or lavages. If a colon lavage is indicated, a cathartic may be given the night before as ordered. One-half hour prior to the lavage, Pitressin or Prostigmin may be administered to increase the effectiveness of the lavage by stimulating peristalsis.

When giving an enema or lavage to the paraplegic or quadriplegic it must be remembered that

*Colon lavage is the filling of the lower bowel with a solution under low pressure and then emptying it by utilizing the flow caused by gravity with siphonage.

the patient cannot retain the solution. Protectively cover your uniform and drape the patient's bed.

CAUTION: *Because the paralyzed person's intestine distends easily, enemas should be given carefully, taking care to not administer excessive amounts of fluid.*

Bowel retraining is accomplished (as with bladder retraining) by (1) keeping a careful record of the patient's individual pattern of intake and elimination, and then (2) by establishing routine patterns of bowel elimination through the use of suppositories and other means of stimulating evacuation until (3) reflex evacuation at desirable times is possible. An adequate fluid intake is important. Also, to achieve desirable bowel control the patient must adhere strictly to a diet that is individually planned to avoid tendencies toward diarrhea or constipation. Normal bulky foods should be in the diet; however, excessive high-residue food may cause loose stools. The patient must develop muscle tone and drink 3000 to 4000 ml. of fluids daily.

Training the patient to have habitual, controlled bowel movements (by conditioned reflex activity) is started as soon as the patient is able to sit up in a chair. The patient must be able to sit on the toilet (or a commode if necessary) since the bedpan impedes normal bowel evacuation. Privacy, a sitting position, and the patient's active participation are important if successful bowel movements are to be achieved.

Attaining continence once more may determine a patient's vocational future and may make a difference in his ability to continue family and social relationships which are meaningful to him. In addition, bowel and bladder training may give a patient the self-confidence and psychologic boost necessary to withstand the other problems created by his paralysis.

REPRODUCTIVE AND SEXUAL FUNCTIONS

Following injury to the spinal cord the paralyzed female is usually still capable of procreation; however, the paralyzed male is usually unable to procreate. Disturbances in the male's sexual functions vary according to the level of the lesion; while ejaculation is usually not possible following complete cord transection, reflex erection can usually be achieved. Complete rehabilitation includes counseling from a neurologist concerning reproductive and sexual activities.

PSYCHOLOGIC ADJUSTMENTS TO PARALYSIS

Adjustment to paralysis is frequently extremely difficult both physically and psychologically. The sudden paralysis of a previously healthy, active individual poses many profound psychologic problems for both patient and family. While hemiplegia (see p. 464), following a cerebrovascular accident, occurs most often in older persons, paraplegia and quadriplegia most often occur in adolescents or young adults.

Paralysis from vertebral trauma usually occurs suddenly, whereas that from disease of the spinal cord, e.g., multiple sclerosis, develops gradually. Often it takes time for the patient to realize fully the extent of his disability and the effects this disability will have on his life style. Naturally, acceptance of such problems as hemiplegia, paraplegia, and quadriplegia is psychologically very difficult, and the patient may employ various psychologic defense mechanisms. (See Units III and IV.) For example, patients experiencing loss of function, e.g., from paralysis, frequently react with initial bitterness and hostility. Mood swings may occur rapidly.

The nurse tries to evaluate carefully the reasons for a given patient's behavior, e.g., hostility, depression, withdrawal. By employing all her skills and her knowledge related to the patient's problems, the nurse tries to help him to achieve a healthy adjustment (rather than mere passive acceptance) to his new physical status.

Paralysis causes complex changes in a person's self-image and body image. Immobilization may also contribute to sensory deprivation and its associated results, e.g., hallucinations. Grieving feelings and behavior are common and must be normally expressed and accepted before they can be resolved. (See Unit III.) Appropriate attempts are made to increase sensory input to minimize sensory deprivation. For example, the patient's environment is kept pleasantly stimulating.

Paralyzed persons do best initially in an environment in which they are with others who face and must overcome similar problems. The patient should be dressed in his own clothing as soon as possible and encouraged to be out of bed and out of his room. Social activities are planned to reduce feelings of social isolation and to help the patient to regain self-confidence.

A sense of security is important to everyone. It is particularly important for the newly paralyzed person to feel secure as he begins to adjust to the necessary aspects of dependency which accompany his condition. Your frequent drop-by visits can give him a feeling of security. Also, he should always have available a means of summoning help. The paralyzed person needs to learn that it is safe for him to be alone for periods of time. Gradually he learns to trust his own abilities and resourcefulness and then to relinquish his reliance on others as much as possible.

To avoid unnecessary frustrations the nurse works to keep the patient's environment comfortable and pleasant in appearance; she keeps items conveniently placed, e.g., telephone, call bell, television controls; she is sensitive to the fact that it is difficult to have to ask for help repeatedly.

While a great change has occurred in the past half century regarding the rehabilitative prognosis of paraplegics and quadriplegics, the wise nurse is realistic as well as optimistic in her viewpoint and tries to understand the tremendous changes in life style that the patient is experiencing. Although some paraplegics happily progress to achieve complete rehabilitation, most have lives that are "burdensome, frustrating, and physiologically complex."[248] Indeed, so great are the trials faced by most paraplegics that suicide is the second most frequent cause of death.[248] At times a severe mental depression may appear as the patient realizes that his paralysis and the need to be partially (or perhaps almost completely) dependent are permanent. Depth of depression must be carefully evaluated and psychiatric help given as indicated.

NUTRITION

It is best to not feed patients with neurologic disorders until they have been examined to be certain that their condition has not impaired the mechanics of swallowing and that their stomachs are not distended.

The paralyzed patient or the immobilized patient often must be fed by others for a period of time. With special devices the paralyzed patient can often learn eventually to feed himself. As discussed, patients in hyperextension may have difficulty swallowing. Take care in feeding such a patient or giving him liquids. Always have suction apparatus ready to use if the patient chokes.

Numerous problems can lead to nutritional difficulties in paralyzed patients, e.g., inactivity, anorexia, decubitus ulcers, paralytic ileus. Osteoporosis causes excessive calcium loss; the alkalinization of urine by citrus fruits can contribute to the occurrence of urinary sepsis and the formation of renal calculi; and decubitus ulcers contribute to hypoproteinemia. A protein loss over a period of time can lower tissue resistance and lower resistance to infection, in addition to causing weight loss and malnutrition.

It is essential that the paraplegic or quadriplegic patient's diet have an average daily protein intake of 150 to 300 grams and that it is also high in vitamins and calories. Since B vitamins occur in high protein foods, a deficiency of these vitamins generally accompanies an inadequate intake of protein. A high protein, high caloric diet helps to heal injured tissue and to prevent decubitus ulcer formation. At first 2000 to 3500 calories may be given daily. However, in order to avoid obesity, this may need to be lowered later on. Obesity greatly complicates the problems of a paralyzed person and increases the possibilities of complications. To minimize the possibility of urinary calculi formation, the calcium intake is kept below 0.5 gram daily during the first few months.

BULBAR INVOLVEMENT

Various neurologic diseases involve the lower brainstem, producing difficulties in respiration, talking, swallowing, and coughing, e.g., tetanus, myasthenia gravis, bulbar poliomyelitis.

Bulbar involvement in such conditions manifests itself by the following *symptoms:* pooling of food and saliva in pharynx and increased accumulation of secretions in the oropharynx; inability or difficulty in swallowing (dysphagia); hypoxia; hoarseness; and perhaps laryngeal stridor. Accumulations of food or secretions cause airway obstruction; pulmonary aspiration, and asphyxia. Mortality is high during the early stages of bulbar involvement.

In caring for patients with bulbar involvement the nurse is alert for early evidence of hypoxia, e.g., anxiety, restlessness, apprehension, sleeplessness, increasing respiratory effort, and increasing pulse rate. The onset of hypoxia may be only subtly indicated (e.g., small, apparently insignificant requests by the patient) and thus its early detection requires the nurse's careful observation.

Indications of hypoxia in a patient with bulbar involvement require investigation by the nurse for possible causes of the airway obstruction. Frequently a tracheotomy is performed on patients with bulbar involvement, and mechanical ventilatory help may be necessary. (See Unit XIV.) Increasing respiratory paralysis, air hunger, loss of respiratory function and difficulty in communicating require careful management and are frightening for the conscious patient.

The nursing care of patients with bulbar involvement is similar to that previously described (for the care of patients with altered states of consciousness) with regard to observation of vital signs, deformity prevention, and maintenance of airway and fluid balance.

The nurse may test the patient's ability to swallow before she offers him food or fluids. This is done by first placing the patient well over onto his side. Next the nurse takes a teaspoon of water in one hand and a suction catheter in the other. If the patient is unable to swallow the water, it is suctioned back.

A bulbar diet, which eliminates milk products and many sticky carbohydrate foods, is ordered in small, frequent feedings, when dysphagia is present. A calorie count may be needed to be certain of adequate caloric intake. Usually a bulbar diet is tolerated better than a puréed or full liquid diet. A small glass or cup is desirable in administering liquids because the patient may have increased difficulty sucking and swallowing if a straw is used. With progressive dysphagia it may be necessary to maintain nutrition with tube feedings or a gastrostomy.

The extent of bulbar paralysis and the return of muscle function vary. The patient who retains some bulbar paralysis is particularly handicapped. Such a person may need to continuously wear a tracheostomy tube (which must be periodically removed and cleansed, see Unit XXII), and often must have expensive suction equipment in his home (and a person qualified to use it). Eating, drinking, and common colds are all potentially hazardous.

HEMIPLEGIA

Hemiplegia is unilateral paralysis of one-half of the body. A complete hemiplegia thus involves one-half of the face and tongue, the arm and the leg of the same side. Aphasia may be present. The muscles of the thorax and abdomen are usually not paralyzed because they receive innervation from both cerebral hemispheres. Hemiplegia *typically* results from a cerebral vascular accident (CVA, also called "stroke" or "apoplexy") involving one hemisphere of the brain, but it may also be caused by other cerebral disorders. The specific causes of CVA and its immediate treatment are discussed more completely in Chapter 39.

The *clinical assessment* of the hemiplegic patient includes evaluation of motor function and reflex activity, and evaluation of defects of cerebral function, e.g., perception, cognition, comprehension, communication, memory, and orientation. The patient's mental attitudes, personality pattern, and awareness of his disability are also evaluated, and his potential for recovery is estimated. It is of course necessary for the nurse to realize in which areas the patient's defects occur so she can plan and give appropriate care. Many problems associated with paralysis have been discussed in the preceding section on spinal disorders. The hemiplegic patient may have many of the problems that patients have as a result of impaired spinal cord functioning, e.g., spasticity, muscle spasms, rigidity, pain, tendon contractures, ankylosis of joints, muscle shortening, muscle weakness, fatigue, paralysis, impaired circulation, decubitus ulcers, absence of sensations, and psychologic adjustments to paralysis. Additionally the hemiplegic patient (who is typically an older person) may have impaired bowel and urinary bladder functions.

As with paraplegics and quadriplegics, the rehabilitation program for patients with complicated hemiplegia is most effective when it involves a comprehensive approach supported by a variety of trained paramedical personnel. A highly optimistic morale and a high level of motivation are important for successful rehabilitation. Staff members set this tone on a ward.

ORIGIN OF HEMIPLEGIA

The paralysis of hemiplegia results from destruction in the *motor area of the cortex* or the fibers in the *pyramidal tract.* A disorder, e.g., hemorrhage or clot, in the brain's right side causes a left-sided hemiplegia, and vice versa. This is because there is a crossover of nerves in the pyramidal tract as they course down from the brain to the spinal cord. *Other cortical areas* may be affected also, producing additional localizing symptoms, e.g., hemianesthesia, hemianopia, apraxia, agnosia, aphasia.

UNCOMPLICATED HEMIPLEGIA; COMPLICATED HEMIPLEGIA

Hemiplegia may be referred to as "uncomplicated" or "complicated." *Uncomplicated hemiplegia* is relatively uncommon. In this condition the patient is unable initially to move his affected arm or leg, but has no other disorder of cerebral function and no active disease elsewhere in his body. The prognosis is good.

Complicated forms of hemiplegia include bilateral hemiplegia, hemiplegia accompanied by cranial nerve abnormalities, or hemiplegia accompanied by other disorders such as hemianesthesia and hemianopia. The prognosis in hemiplegia is influenced by the presence of such neurologic complications and is also greatly influenced by the presence of additional related or unrelated diseases, e.g., cardiac, respiratory, or renal insufficiency.

RETURN OF FUNCTION

The degree of hemiplegic paralysis is usually greater, i.e., more complete, early in the illness than it will be later on. This is because edema and pressure from other sources may be impairing nerve function in some areas only temporarily. False hopes are never raised, but the patient is given realistic encouragement, and every attempt is made to prevent the development of complications that will add to the patient's confinement or impede or prevent optimum recovery. *The return of functional use of an involved upper extremity is not so frequent as the return of functional use of the affected leg.*

EXAMINATION OF THE COMATOSE HEMIPLEGIC

In a comatose patient hemiplegia may be identified by *flaccidity of the limbs* occurring on the paralyzed side; this occurs during the stage of spinal shock. The unsupported paralyzed leg of the hemiplegic patient typically lies with the foot everted; the leg must be supported to keep a position of normal alignment and function. You will also notice in a hemiplegic patient that if both eyelids are lifted together, then suddenly released, the *eyelid* on the affected side may *not close completely.* Or if it does close, it usually closes more slowly than the lid on the unaffected side. Indications of *lower facial weakness* are also frequently apparent in the comatose hemiplegic patient. For example, you may observe ballooning of the cheek on the paralyzed side during expiration; weakness of the muscles of elevation around the mouth; and asymmetry or drooping of the mouth on the affected side. These lower facial weaknesses are clearly apparent from observation of the patient's facial response to painful stimuli, e.g., pressure over the supraorbital notch; his facial grimacing in response to the pain is asymmetrical.[232]

REHABILITATION POTENTIAL; REHABILITATION GOALS

After the nurse has helped the hemiplegic patient to survive the acute phase of his illness and has prevented the formation of complications and deformities, she then assumes the challenge of helping to continue to rehabilitate the patient to a life that holds meaning for him. This challenge requires patience, ingenuity, and knowledge of the rehabilitative process. *Successful rehabilitation is not achieved without detailed planning.* Numerous modifications may be necessary in the patient's home and in his daily living activities. All members of the rehabilitation team work together to help the patient to relearn lost abilities and to learn new abilities. For the aphasic hemiplegic the special skills of a speech therapist are needed in addition to those of other specialists.

Among the *goals of a rehabilitation program* for the hemiplegic are: (1) prevention of complications during the acute phase; (2) correction of any deformities that have developed; (3) retraining of the patient to achieve maximum independence, e.g., to walk, to use the affected upper extremity to the maximum, to perform self-care activities, to be employable (if of employable age); and (4) helping the patient to adapt successfully psychologically and socially. *Remember: rehabilitation begins with admission!*

The patient is made to realize early in his illness that he is expected to do certain things for himself and that the activity prescribed by his doctor is good for him. Encouragement is frequently needed to get the patient to use the paretic limb to its maximum potential; there is a tendency to do everything with the unaffected limb.

As soon as he can sit up in bed the patient is encouraged to perform all the *self-care activities* he can by using his unaffected hand, e.g., brush teeth, feed himself, comb hair, shave, and bathe. This strengthens the unaffected side in addition to encouraging independence. The nurse assists as necessary but does not needlessly "rush in." Various *hemiplegic transfers* are illustrated in Figure 38–18.

The complete rehabilitative care of the patient with hemiplegia is beyond the scope of this book. Many helpful sources are available, however. With the doctor's approval the nurse may obtain a copy of the pamphlet *Strike Back at Stroke* for use by the patient and his family. *Strike Back at Stroke* is a well-illustrated brochure published by the Public Health Service (Publication No. 596) and may be obtained from the Superintendent of Documents, U.S. Government Printing Office, Washington, D.C. 20402. Write for a copy for your professional use.

POSITIONING AND EXERCISING THE HEMIPLEGIC

Proper positioning, exercising, and turning of the hemiplegic patient can prevent many deformities and complications from developing at a later date.

Frequently the hemiplegic prefers to lie on his involved side and may not want to turn over onto his unaffected side. However, lying on either side too long may cause skin breakdown over the external malleoli and greater trochanters. The sacral and heel areas are particularly vulnerable to breakdown if the patient lies on his back too long.

> *The hemiplegic patient is turned mainly onto his unaffected side.* He may be positioned briefly on his affected side (taking care that body weight is not causing harm to paralyzed extremities) or he may lie for short periods of time on his back. He should not be allowed to sit upright in bed for extended periods of time because this position may contribute to *hip flexion deformity.* The flat position is best. When he is on his side, the upper thigh should not be flexed acutely. The patient's *position should be changed every two hours.*

> When the patient is turned prone (as he should be for 15 to 30 minutes several times daily), hyperextension of the hip joints may be obtained by placing a small pillow under the pelvis from the umbilicus down to the thighs' upper third.

> *A pillow should not be placed under the affected knee* because this encourages a flexion deformity and impedes circulation. However, if there is a tendency to develop *hyperextension of the knee,* a folded towel may be placed under the knee for short periods of time while the patient is on his back.

> Place a *footboard* to prevent (1) *foot drop and heel cord shortening* and (2) plantar flexion caused by the weight of bed linens. The best preventatives of foot drop are avoidance of pressure, frequent passive range-of-motion (ROM) exercises, and early sitting up with the feet flat on the floor.

> A *padded posterior splint* may be applied to the affected leg at night to maintain correct positioning and prevent *flexion of the leg.*

> A *trochanter roll,* extending from the crest of the ilium to mid-thigh, prevents *external rotation at the hip* by wedging under the projection of the greater trochanter and preventing the femur from rolling.

> *Support the affected leg* when turning and positioning the hemiplegic patient. If the flaccid leg falls forward and downward when the patient is turned onto his unaffected side, a *complete dislocation of the hip joint* may occur as the head of the femur slips out of its socket. A pillow placed between the patient's legs provides adequate support.

The return of motor impulses, following CVA, usually begins sometime within the period of two to 14 days. When these impulses begin to return, the affected part (which was initially flaccid) becomes spastic as the muscles tighten. With spasticity the problem of contractures occurs. However, even before spasticity sets in, passive exercises are started to prevent contractures and "frozen" joints.

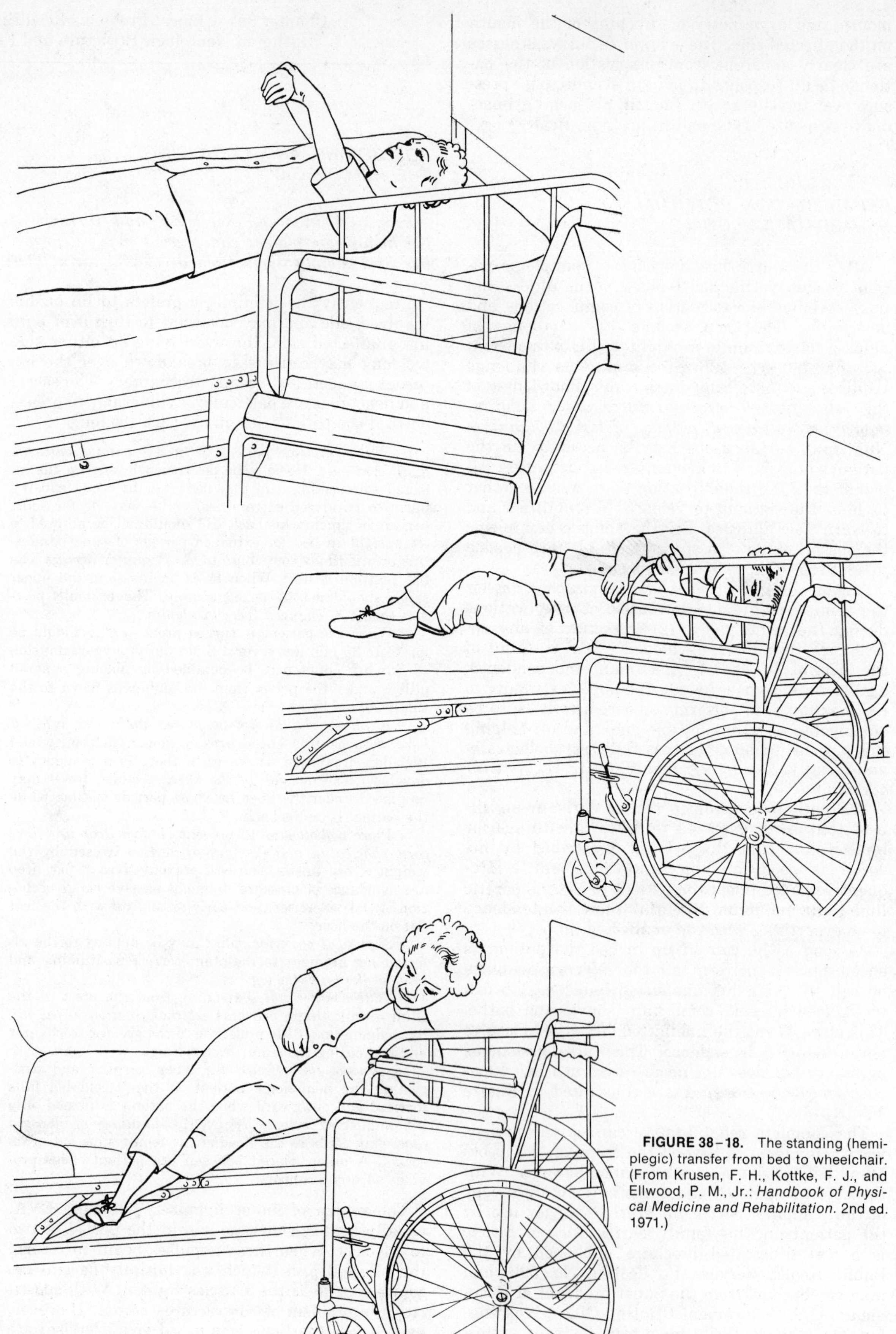

FIGURE 38–18. The standing (hemiplegic) transfer from bed to wheelchair. (From Krusen, F. H., Kottke, F. J., and Ellwood, P. M., Jr.: *Handbook of Physical Medicine and Rehabilitation.* 2nd ed. 1971.)

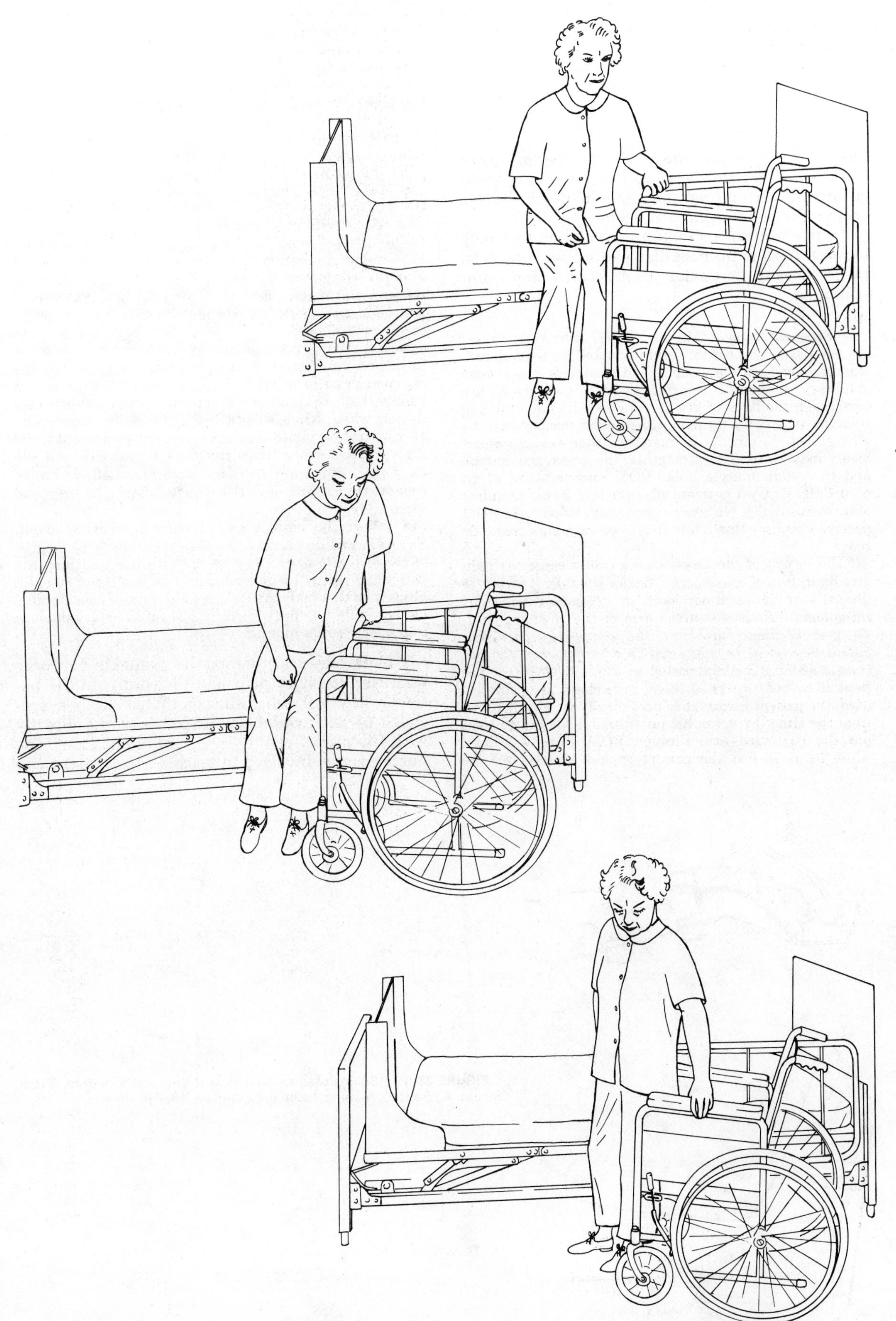

Passive exercises are more difficult to perform once the affected muscles begin to tighten, and in exercising the extremities they should not be forced beyond the point of initiating pain.

Passive exercises stimulate circulation and help to reestablish neuromuscular pathways in addition to preventing muscular contractures and joint stiffening.

> Frequent *range-of-motion (ROM) passive exercises* are employed to prevent joint immobility, tendon contractures, and muscle atrophy and weakness. Once some voluntary movement returns, assisted movements are performed; the force of gravity can be eliminated during such movements by utilizing *sling-suspensions*. When the strength of movements is increased, then *resisted movements* may be used to strengthen the weakened muscle and to restore muscle bulk. ROM exercises are given q.i.d. daily for CVA patients after the first 24 hours unless otherwise ordered. No order is necessary to perform ROM passive exercises this often; it is good nursing care to do so.

> The *weight of the immobile arm* may cause (1) pain and limitation of movement ("frozen shoulder") owing to fibrositis of the shoulder joint, or (2) *subluxation,* i.e., incomplete dislocation, of the arm at the shoulder joint. To prevent these problems the *completely paralyzed flaccid arm must be supported in a sling when the patient is walking,* and supported on a pillow when the patient is in bed or seated in an arm chair. If a sling is used, the patient is taught to periodically remove his arm from the sling (by using his unaffected arm) and to then put the paralyzed arm through ROM exercises. Even while he is in bed the patient should exercise his affected arm by grasping it at the wrist with his unaffected hand and raising the affected arm over his head.

While in bed, *adduction of the affected shoulder* is prevented by placing a pillow in the axilla, between the upper arm and chest wall, to keep the arm in abduction at an angle of about 60 degrees. The arm is slightly flexed in a neutral position. The forearm is placed on another pillow in a "modified Statue of Liberty" position, with the elbow above the shoulder and the wrist above the elbow. This position stretches tight the shoulder's internal rotators. *Elevation of the arm* also helps to prevent *edema* with resultant *fibrosis*.

The *affected hand* is placed in a *position of function,* i.e., slight supination with the fingers slightly flexed and the thumb in the position of opposition. A *hand roll* or *splint* may be used to prevent *flexion of the fingers* and *adduction of the thumb,* and frequent passive *ROM exercises* are used. If the wrist and fingers are quite spastic a splint may be required to prevent the tendency to flexion contracture. Some physicians believe that the common practice of giving a patient a ball of yarn or a rubber ball to squeeze is harmful since it promotes flexion when extension is what is desirable. Figure 38–19 illustrates splints that may be used to prevent *wrist drop* and *foot drop*. Teach the patient to *stretch and rub the fingers of his affected hand* with his unaffected hand several times each day. Each finger should be exercised separately.

> Assist the patient as necessary in moving about. *Siderails* and an *overhead trapeze* or a *rope from the foot of the bed with a hand grasp bar* attached will help the patient in sitting up and turning if he is allowed to exert himself in this manner. He can help himself considerably by using his unaffected arm and leg if he is taught how to properly assist himself.

When a physical therapist is available he works with the doctor to plan and to coordinate the patient's physical rehabilitation. When such a specialist is not available, the doctor works directly with the nurse, patient, and family members. The nurse may be involved in teaching the patient and

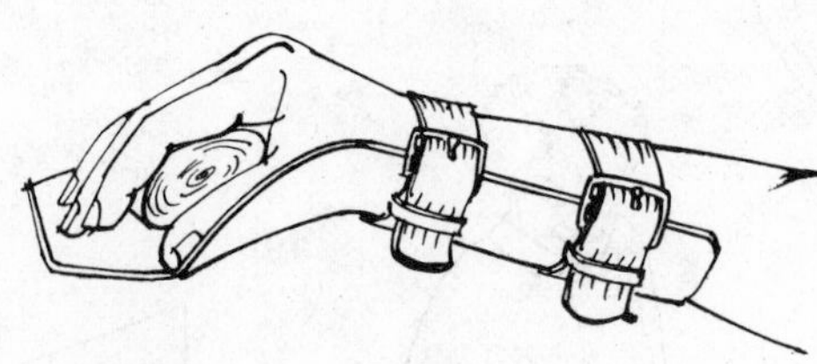

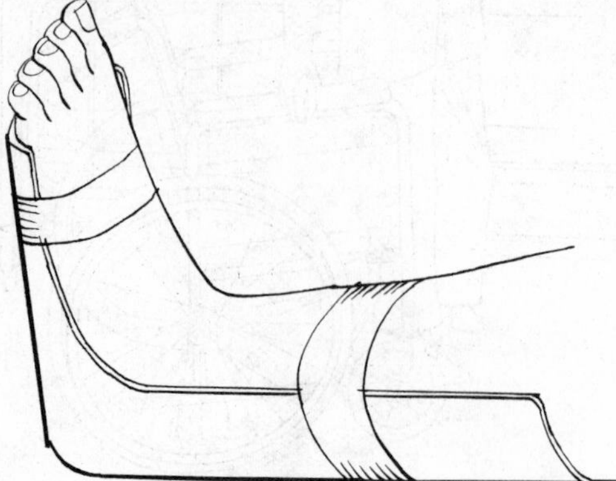

FIGURE 38–19. Splints used to prevent wrist drop and foot drop. (From Sutton, A.: *Bedside Nursing Techniques,* 2nd ed. 1969.)

his family activities that the patient should perform or have performed for him. A written schedule of exercises is best. It should be emphasized that *regularity and frequency are important in exercise performance.* Short regular periods of exercise cause less fatigue to the patient and maintain better range of motion and muscle tone than do infrequent, longer periods of exercise.

EXERCISES IN BED

The performance of exercises while the patient is still in bed not only helps to prepare the patient for later activities, e.g., walking, but also instills hope and a feeling in the patient that he will improve. The hemiplegic patient can learn to move his affected leg, when he is moving and exercising, by sliding his unaffected leg under the affected one and then moving his functioning leg. Also, while in bed the hemiplegic patient can prepare for ambulation by carrying out quadriceps muscle setting and gluteal setting exercises. Instruct the patient as follows:

> *Gluteal setting.* "Pinch" or contract the buttocks together and count to five; then relax and count to five. Repeat.

> *Quadriceps setting.* Contract the quadriceps muscle, on the anterior portion of the thigh, while raising the heel and attempting to push the popliteal space against the mattress. While holding the muscle contracture count to five, then relax and count to five. Repeat. Perform on each extremity if possible.

Quadriceps setting exercises are started once consciousness is regained. During the day they should be repeated every hour, beginning with five repetitions and increasing gradually to 20 repetitions each time. The quadriceps muscle is the most important muscle in giving the knee joint stability when walking.

SITTING UP

The patient is helped out of bed as soon as the doctor permits. It should be remembered, however, that *the sense of balance is severely affected when half the body is paralyzed.* Thus, the patient is given adequate preparation before he sits up and adequate help so he feels secure.

The patient's head is *slowly* raised in bed, and he is given time to become accustomed to having his head elevated after lying flat. Often the hemiplegic tends to lean toward his paralyzed side and to lose his balance when he first tries to sit up. To correct this he is taught to lean toward his uninvolved side. Initially his paralyzed side is supported by the nurse. The patient must also be taught to balance his head. When the patient first sits up, his back and head are supported. Gradually he learns to sit by himself and with the head of his bed elevated. Then he learns to sit on the edge of the bed, with his feet on a firm surface. The patient can help to maintain his balance by extending his affected arm and placing his hand flat on the bed beside him. Be patient and encouraging as the patient relearns how to balance himself.

Eventually the patient learns to raise his paralyzed leg with his unaffected leg and to then swing both legs laterally over the side of the bed onto the floor. The hemiplegic patient can get up most easily if his paralyzed side is *away* from the side of the bed from which he gets up.

WHEELCHAIR

The hemiplegic patient is taught how to safely transfer from his bed into a chair, onto a commode, or into a wheelchair. He can propel a wheelchair with his unaffected arm and leg. One-arm drive wheelchairs are available for patients with unilateral paralysis. Once he is in a wheelchair, the patient's level of independence increases greatly.

STANDING AND WALKING

In preparation for walking the patient is helped out of bed and into a standing position as soon as possible. This helps him to maintain a sense of balance and prevents disuse atrophy.

In spite of weakness in the affected limb, the hemiplegic often develops extensor reflex, i.e., reflex patterns of extension, which enable him to stand. A tilt table may be used if the patient has difficulty in achieving standing balance.

Using a wheelchair is helpful, but walking is best for the patient, and so he continues to work and to relearn this basic skill. As soon as the quadriceps muscle on the unaffected side has regained its normal strength, practice in standing begins. The patient may be seated at the foot of his bed and instructed to rise, using the muscle power of his unaffected leg while steadying himself with his good hand. He may have a tendency to swing round toward the affected side. The patient gradually learns to take an increasing amount of weight on his weaker side. Most hemiplegic patients can be taught to walk. The patient is frequently reminded to keep the weight of his body forward over his feet.[132]

It is important that the patient practice and learn to walk correctly. If he develops incorrect habits they may be extremely difficult to overcome later. The nurse supervises the patient until he is capable of walking alone without fear of falling. Heel-toe walking with a reciprocal gait pattern is the goal of ambulation. The patient who has been properly trained to walk should not show circumduction, scraping of the toes, or any other disabilities said to be commonly characteristic of the hemiplegic gait.

BRACING

Usually the decision regarding the need for *leg bracing* is deferred until after training for standing and ambulation has started. This is because the hemiplegic frequently does not need any leg bracing for ambulation. If a brace is necessary, the most commonly used *short leg brace* for a hemiplegic patient is the double-bar 90 degree ankle stop with a posterior metal calf band (Fig. 38–20). An orthopedic type oxford shoe, properly fitted to the patient, is used as a basis and support for the brace.

Any patient with a brace must be taught to properly apply and remove the brace, give proper skin care, observe for skin breakdown, and properly care for the brace itself.

SAFETY

Siderails are kept up while the "new" hemiplegic is in bed because he has a poor sense of balance and can easily roll out of bed. As the patient's condition improves he may use the siderails to pull himself up or to help to turn himself. Once the patient is able to get out of bed unassisted, full siderails may prevent him from being as ambulatory as he should be. At this stage the patient may find half siderails useful. The patient who has *impaired sensation* must take care not to injure himself and should inspect his body frequently for signs of skin lesions. *Visual disturbances* may also increase the hazards to a hemiplegic's safety.

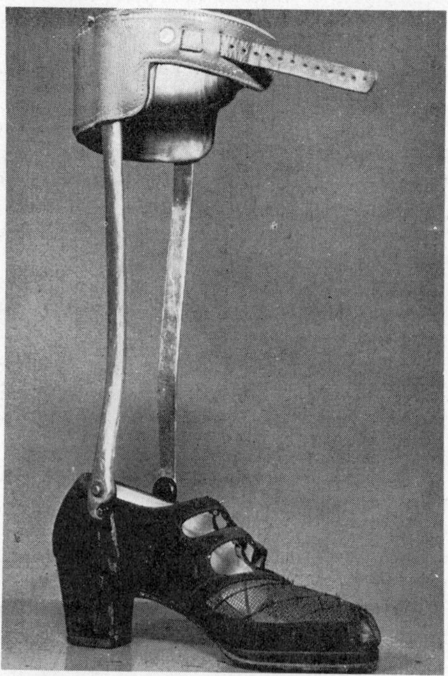

FIGURE 38–20. Short leg brace. (From Krusen, F. H., Kottke, F. J., and Ellwood, P. M., Jr.: *Handbook of Physical Medicine and Rehabilitation*, 1971.)

Hemiplegic patients are more likely to *fall* than other persons. To prevent a fall the patient must be taught to stand and walk slowly, rest adequately between intervals of walking, have adequate light, and watch carefully where he is going.

FEEDING THE HEMIPLEGIC

Feeding the patient who has partial paralysis of his tongue, mouth, and throat must be done carefully to prevent choking and aspiration. The patient is often fearful of choking and is frustrated by the difficulty he encounters in eating. The person feeding the patient must appear unhurried and encourage the patient to persist in his attempts to swallow. The patient does best if turned onto his back or unaffected side to eat. If he has difficulty in swallowing he cannot be on his back because of the increased danger of aspiration. Place the food into the *unparalyzed side of the mouth.* By lying on his unaffected side the patient will not have the problem of the food or liquids spilling out of the paralyzed side of his mouth, and he can swallow more easily. It is often best to begin the feeding by letting the patient take some water. This tests his swallowing ability and lets him practice swallowing. Then food is given in small bites. Foods that can easily cause choking are best eliminated from the diet, e.g., stringy meats, unboned fish, semicooked vegetables.

The patient's nutritional status is carefully evaluated to ensure adequate nutrition. His intake is recorded, and supplemental feedings are given as indicated. If the patient is incapable of swallowing, tube feedings may be given.

It is desirable for the hemiplegic to learn to feed himself and thus regain independence. Numerous devices are available to help him to do so, but he must be patiently helped and encouraged (Fig. 38–21).

Food may need to be cut into bite size pieces, but the patient should be helped to feed himself; this improves appetite and the patient's self-image. The patient may need to be protected from spillage while eating, and if he spills should be given a clean gown or shirt. Bed linens soiled during a meal should also be changed promptly. Following the meal the patient's face and hands are washed and he is given oral hygiene; food tends to accumulate in the paralyzed side of the mouth, and this area is given special attention to make sure it is cleansed thoroughly.

HEMIPLEGIC DEFORMITIES AND OTHER COMPLICATIONS

Needless to say, all the previously described activities are more difficult (sometimes impossible) for the hemiplegic patient to perform if he has been allowed to develop deformities and if other complications are present.

The flexor muscles *are the body muscles that will cause hemiplegic deformities and contractures following CVA unless the patient is properly positioned and exercised.*

When control of voluntary muscles is destroyed, the strong flexor muscles exert control over the extensors. This natural tendency can cause serious deformities. For example, in the patient with hemiplegia the affected arm tends to adduct, since the adductor muscles are stronger than the abductors, and to rotate internally. The elbow, wrist, and fingers tend to flex on the affected arm. The affected leg tends to rotate externally at the hip joint, flex at the knee, and plantar flex and supinate at the ankle joint (Fig. 38–22).

The two most common complications associated with hemiplegia are: (1) a frozen shoulder; and (2) a shortened heel cord, with plantar flexion of the foot. Both these complications are preventable *if proper care is given during the acute phase of paralysis.*

INCONTINENCE

Incontinence of urine in the hemiplegic patient is not the result of brain damage following CVA unless there is extensive encephalomalacia. Research has demonstrated that there is no physiologic reason for the patient with CVA to be incontinent. Rather, much of the incontinence that occurs in this group of patients, or other hemiplegic patients, results from inattention, memory lapses, emotional factors, use as attention-getting mechanism, and inability to make needs known.[226] The patient is thus often dependent on the nurse to anticipate his elimination needs, make provisions for them, and train him to a program of bowel and bladder rehabilitation.

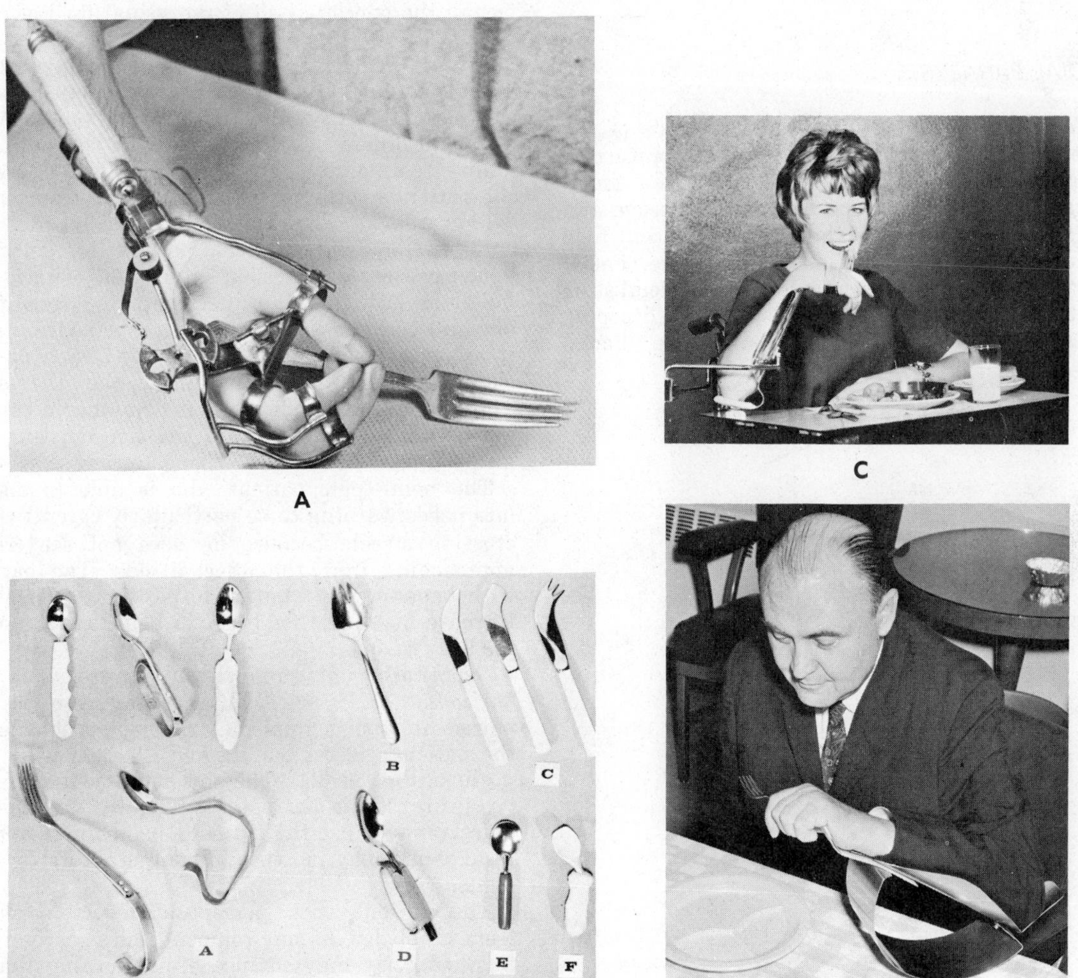

FIGURE 38–21. Devices that paralyzed patients can use to feed themselves. (From Krusen, F. H., Kottke, F. J., and Ellwood, P. M., Jr.: *Handbook of Physical Medicine and Rehabilitation*, 1971.)

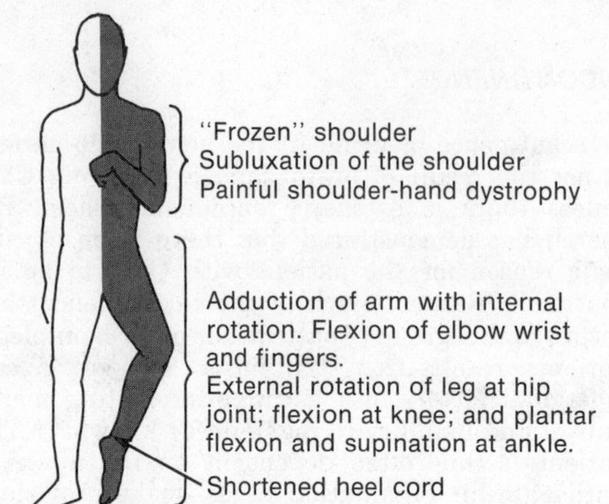

FIGURE 38–22. Hemiplegic deformities to be prevented. Note that the elbow is bent, the wrist is flexed and the fingers are curled into palmar flexion; the knee is bent and the heel cord shortened.

FACIAL PARALYSIS

Facial paralysis of the lower two-thirds of the face may occur with hemiplegia; usually, return of function occurs. However, until it does a *facial sling* (Fig. 38–23) may be used, and massage and electrical stimulation of the facial nerve will help to retain the tonus of the facial musculature. (Facial paralysis may also follow craniotomy.) A facial sling on the affected side gives support to the drooping mouth and lessens excessive drooling. Facial paralysis is generally on the same side as the hemiplegia. When facial paralysis is present it may be helpful at first to give liquids through a rubber tipped Asepto syringe. Special care must be taken in feeding the patient, as discussed earlier.

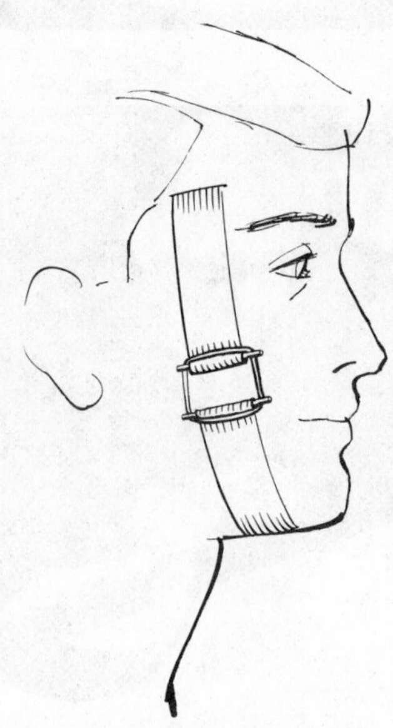

FIGURE 38–23. Facial sling; used with facial paralysis. (From Sutton, A.: *Bedside Nursing Techniques,* 2nd ed. 1969.)

EMOTIONAL LABILITY

Emotional lability, i.e., "emotional incontinence," may follow a CVA. This condition is characterized by a tendency to burst into tears or burst out laughing (less commonly) without any provocation. While the patient appears highly distressed, he is not really experiencing unhappiness. This condition differs from an affective depressed state. Family members often need help to understand this condition.

VISUAL DISORDERS

Lesions in the parietal and temporal lobes may interrupt visual fibers of the optic tract (en route to the occipital cortex) and produce visual defects. A lesion on one side of the brain produces a defect in the opposite half of the visual field of each eye.

Visual deficiency problems commonly occur in association with hemiplegia and may prevent the patient from seeing recognizable cues. Also, visual disorders may interfere with the patient's ability to relearn motor skills and may increase the patient's susceptibility to accidents and physical hazards.

Homonymous hemianopia refers to defective vision or the loss of vision in one-half of *each* visual field such that the affected patient sees only one-half of what a person with normal vision sees in any position. The patient may see clearly on one side of the midline but nothing on the other side. The patient with homonymous hemianopia cannot see past the midline toward the side opposite the lesion unless he turns his head toward that side.

The hemiplegic patient who is able to ambulate needs warning to be particularly careful when crossing streets because he does not see traffic approaching from the affected side. The patient with hemianopia is taught to position his head to increase his visual field and to help to reestablish his body image.

Depth perception and *visual perception in the horizontal and vertical planes* may also be impaired in the hemiplegic, causing problems in the patient's motor performance, both in gait and posture (Fig. 38–24). The patient may or may not be aware of his perceptual difficulty. Perceptual defects may cause the patient's behavior to appear bizarre and may increase his vulnerability to accidents.

The patient with perceptual defects benefits from simplicity. An environment that is excessively busy or noisy may confuse him. Clothing that is simply designed and easy to put on, directions that are simply given in a brief, concise manner, and food trays that are set with a minimum number of

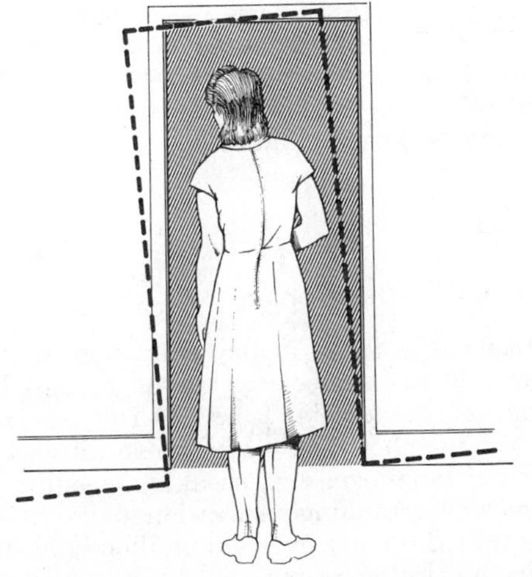

FIGURE 38–24. Perceptual disturbance in hemiplegia. (From Krusen, F. H., Kottke, F. J., and Ellwood, P. M., Jr.: *Handbook of Physical Medicine and Rehabilitation*, 2nd ed. 1971.)

utensils, dishes, and foods are easiest for the patient to cope with, because decision making and complexity are thereby reduced.

For more complete discussions of how to help the patient who has visual deficits, consult M. M. Burt's article "Perceptual Deficits in Hemiplegia,"[35] and R. Piggott and F. Brickett's article "Visual Neglect."[188]

HEMIANESTHESIA; PARESTHESIA; LOSS OF MUSCLE-JOINT SENSE

The *hemianesthesia* that may accompany hemiplegia is generally incomplete. It may be unnoticed by the patient, or he may experience *paresthesia* on the affected side. Some patients experience unpleasant sensations of numbness or heaviness. Occasionally the hemiplegic suffers with persistent, boring pain, i.e., thalamic pain. An additional problem that may accompany hemianesthesia (or may occur alone) is a *disturbance of proprioception* and *postural sense* with *loss of muscle-joint sense.* This disability may interfere seriously with the patient's ability to ambulate, because of lack of balance control and inappropriate movements. A patient with this impairment must learn to walk with his eyes on his feet. The risk of falling is high because of the tendency to misplace the feet when walking.

AGNOSIA

Loss of muscle-joint sensation may be accompanied by *agnosia;* i.e., the interpretation of visual, tactile, or other sensory information in the brain is disturbed. With agnosia *a loss occurs of the ability to recognize objects.* Whether the patient has visual, auditory or tactile agnosia, he demonstrates an impairment in the transmission of sensory signals to the conceptual level. *Agnosia* does *not* refer to deafness, blindness, or loss of touch.[99]

As indicated, agnosias of various kinds may occur. For example, loss of muscle-joint sensation may be accompanied by *delusional beliefs about the position of a limb in space or its existence or ownership.* In such conditions the patient may not feel that his arm is actually a part of his own body; he may not be aware of the position of his arm; or he may deny that a limb is paralyzed when it obviously is.

Another type of agnosia affects only one-half of external space, and objects on one side are correctly interpreted while those on the other side are ignored, e.g., the patient may be able to tell time only if it is between 12 and 6 o'clock and not if it is between 7 and 12 o'clock. A patient with this condition, of *neglecting the left half of space,* generally has left hemiplegia and may tend to avert his head and eyes to the right.

Naturally the nurse needs to be aware of these conditions and plan accordingly. She helps the patient so he does not overlook important left-sided objects or events, if that is the affected side; e.g., she sees that he eats the food on the left side of his plate and she helps him to groom the left side of his head and body. Additionally, the patient is protected from being injured by objects close to or approaching on his left side.

When the patient neglects his affected side the nurse can either arrange the patient's environment so that important items are on the involved side, or she can train the patient to take care of his affected side, e.g., by instructing the patient to turn his head and frequently look at his affected side, and to follow simple cue cards that list the steps of such procedures as dressing.[35]

A patient with *visual agnosia* sees objects but does not recognize them or attach meaning to them. He may become disoriented because he cannot recognize environmental cues; he may fail to recognize familiar faces or symbols. The patient with visual agnosia is frequently seen picking up objects, curiously examining them, and then replacing them—still puzzled about their function. The patient may need assistance with eating or dressing and other activities of daily living because he does not know what to do with such objects as silverware, clothing, or toilet articles. This condition leaves the patient highly vulnerable to injury, because he fails to recognize the symbols man has learned to associate with danger, e.g., a skull and cross-bones signifying poison, a red stop light. *Extensive visual agnosia* can result in such extreme behavioral effects that the patient is frequently diagnosed as having diffuse dementia. In such a patient an accurate diagnosis is difficult to establish.[64]

"Word blindness" and "word deafness" are specific localized forms of visual or auditory agnosia, which are mentioned in the section on aphasia.

APRAXIA

Brain damage may also cause *apraxia;* i.e., the patient is *able to move the affected part* (it is *not* paralyzed or uncoordinated), *but* he *cannot use the part for specific purposeful actions,* e.g., walking, speaking, or dressing.[107] While the apraxic patient can conceive or conceptualize the content of the message he wishes to send to his muscles (e.g., "stand"), he is unable to reconstruct those motor patterns or schema that are necessary to convey the impulse message. Thus, accurate "instructions" do not reach the limb from the brain concerning specific movements.[128]

Numerous variations of apraxia occur, ranging from relatively simple to highly complex disorders. Apraxia may occur in any or all modalities, and may vary from one modality to another; e.g., a patient may have less difficulty writing than speaking, or vice versa.

Generally in hemiplegic patients apraxic and agnosic states occur along with other manifestations of brain damage and have a poor prognosis for functional recovery. And so, for some patients, problem compounds upon problem, and while such patients are often known as hemiplegic patients, "the paralysis of the affected side is almost the least of their difficulties."[107] The disorders of cortical function, which we have been discussing, make rehabilitation highly difficult unless spontaneous recovery of the affected cortical functions returns. Aphasia is another disorder of cortical function, which is discussed in the following section.

LANGUAGE DISORDERS

Many neurologic patients may have language disorders of various kinds that may be related to their neurologic disorders. The nurse assists with the identification and evaluation of these language disorders as well as with language rehabilitation.

Many hospitals today have available a *speech doctor* and/or speech therapist. The nurse may work with a patient who has a language disorder under the direction of these speech specialists, or with a physician. In some areas speech therapy consultation can be arranged by contacting the nearest appropriate voluntary or governmental service agency.

The nurse can help patients with speech disorders in a variety of ways, depending on the specific problem. When a patient is not speaking loudly enough, the nurse can advise him to take a deeper breath; this will enable him to use more energy when speaking. If the quality of a patient's speech is too nasal, the nurse can help him correct this by having the patient open his mouth wider while speaking; this allows more sounds to come through the mouth instead of being diverted through the nose. A patient who speaks too rapidly can be reminded to slow his speech pattern down and to practice pacing himself.

APHASIA

Definition of the Problem

Aphasia is a defect in the utilization and interpretation of the symbols of language caused by a disorder of the cerebral cortex. The defect is a symptom complex that may involve all aspects of the use of language, e.g., speaking, reading, writing and understanding spoken language. It is estimated that there are over one million aphasic persons in the United States.

Types of Aphasias and Speech Patterns

An aphasia may be of a *sensory* nature (receptive aphasia), which affects the comprehension of speech, or it may be of a *motor* nature (expressive aphasia or executive aphasia), which affects the production of speech.

Sensory aphasias involve loss of the ability to comprehend written (or printed) or spoken words. For example, with *auditory* or *acoustic aphasia* ("word deafness") the patient has difficulty understanding what is said to him. He is not deaf; he hears sounds but they fail to make sense to him because he cannot understand the symbolic communication associated with the sounds. *Visual aphasia* ("word blindness") is similar, except that the patient cannot read words even though he can see them. He has lost the ability to understand the symbolic content of the printed or written figures.

Motor aphasias encompass any of the varieties of aphasia in which the power of expression by writing, making signs, or speaking is lost. For example, with motor aphasia a patient may find that even though he can recall words, he has lost the ability to combine speech sounds into words and syllables.

Pure motor or pure sensory aphasias rarely occur. Thus, the most common aphasias are of a *mixed* nature (expressive-receptive aphasia) in which both expressive and receptive elements are affected. Also, most aphasias are partial rather than complete. *Global aphasia* (total aphasia) is of such a degree that neither expressive nor receptive language abilities are retained.

Causes

The pathology of aphasia depends more on the lesion's location than its histologic abnormality, since numerous variable pathologic lesions can cause aphasia. However, *the most common cause of aphasia is vascular disease of the brain. The middle cerebral artery is the most common site of involvement in CVA.* All lobes but the occipital are supplied by branches of the middle cerebral artery. *Cerebral edema* may cause a temporary aphasia (e.g., following trauma or surgery) which resolves when the edema is reduced.

Aphasia may result when circulation to the patient's speech center is cut off. *The condition is most common when hemiplegia involves a patient's dominant side and his brain lesion involves the posterior aspect of the inferior frontal gyrus.* The speech center for a right-handed person is located in his left cerebral hemisphere, while the speech center for a left-handed person lies on the right side of his brain. Thus, a right-handed person with a right-sided hemiplegia may have aphasia, since his speech center is in the affected left hemisphere.

Severity of Aphasic Involvement

The severity of aphasic involvement varies with the area and the extent of cerebral damage. Severe brain damage may deprive the patient of any meaningful relationship with his environment.

Communication involves the dual process of both sending and receiving language as mentioned. While either dimension can be equally affected, the more common pattern, following initial recovery, is for the expressive defect to be greater than the receptive.

Occasionally the residual brain function is not adequate for the aphasic to relearn the complicated processes of communication. However, it is frequently possible to train the dormant speech centers in the brain's unaffected hemisphere to supplement or replace the functions of the areas damaged in the affected hemisphere. Many aphasics do well with speech therapy or show a tendency to spontaneous recovery. Because it cannot be assumed that spontaneous recovery will occur, speech therapy should ideally be started early. However, some benefit from speech therapy may be derived even two or more years following the origin of the speech disorder.

Clinical Care

The nurse can frequently continue and reinforce lessons that the speech therapist has initiated. In the absence of a therapist, the nurse may conduct language rehabilitation sessions with the physician's approval. During such sessions the nurse takes care to not fatigue the patient and to remember that the patient may have a short attention span.

The following ideas are useful as the nurse administers care to the aphasic patient:

> When a patient cannot understand the spoken word, repeat simple directions until they are understood, e.g., "Drink this juice." Also use nonverbal techniques of communication.

> When a patient cannot identify objects by name, give him practice in receiving word images. For example, point to an object and clearly enunciate its name, e.g., "hand," "glass."

> When a patient cannot express himself verbally, give him practice in repeating words after you. Begin with simple words and then progress, e.g., "Yes," "No," "Here is breakfast."

> When working with the aphasic patient, practice expanded speech (a slower rate) and self-pacing (permitting the individual time to respond).

> Help the patient's family, friends, other patients, and staff members to communicate with the aphasic patient. The nurse acts as a model by showing others how she communicates with the patient. Her attitude is one of calmness, patience, and helpfulness. She explains how damaging it can be to the patient's self-image if others act embarrassed or amused by his attempts to communicate.

> Listen and watch carefully when the aphasic patient attempts to communicate and try especially hard to understand him. This reduces the patient's frustration.

> Anticipate the aphasic patient's needs so he will feel less helpless because of his communication handicap.

> Gradually shift topics of conversation when talking to the patient who has receptive difficulty. It may be necessary to tell the patient that you are going to change the topic.

> Sometimes it is helpful, when talking to an aphasic patient who has receptive difficulty, to be within six feet or less of the patient and to face him directly.

> If the patient has *word deafness,* give him simple directions. Repeat directions until they are understood.

> If the patient has *naming aphasia,* help him to practice naming objects frequently used. This gives practice in recalling word images.

> If the patient has *motor aphasia,* have him practice trying to repeat words and sounds after you.

Initial care involves trying to put the aphasic patient at ease and to reduce the feeling of panic which he may have when he first realizes that he cannot communicate as he formerly could. It is important for the nurse to speak slowly and clearly to the patient and offer him calm reassurance that she understands his problem and will help him.

The nurse shows the patient his call bell and lets him practice using it. She tells the patient that she will watch him carefully and he can signal his needs with sign language. It is important to talk to the patient without exerting pressure on him to respond verbally. When the patient appears ready the nurse may introduce picture or word cards or picture books to temporarily facilitate communication.

Aphasic patients often express their emotional state by irritability and periods of "moodiness." Often these frustrated people are anxious, bewildered, and depressed. Emotional lability may be an additional result of cerebral damage. Such behavior is accepted matter of factly but kindly and without embarrassment. Every attempt is made to reduce the patient's frustrations and to teach him to communicate effectively once again. The nurse can supplement her knowledge of aphasia and its management by obtaining literature from a speech pathologist, from the library, and from appropriate associations, e.g., the American Heart Association and the Institute of Physical Medicine and Rehabilitation.

DYSARTHRIA

Dysarthria (anarthria) is a difficulty in speaking which *results from imperfect articulation*. It is important to differentiate between dysarthric and aphasic speech. With dysarthria the patient understands and comprehends language, but he has difficulty pronouncing words and may slur them, enunciating poorly. No disturbance occurs with grammar or in the construction of a phrase or sentence. The dysarthric patient can understand verbal speech, can read, and can write (unless his writing hand is paralyzed, absent, or injured).

Dysarthria may result from a weakness or paralysis of the muscles of the lips, tongue, and larynx or a loss of sensation. Patients with dysarthria often have difficulty chewing and swallowing food because of lack of muscle control, in addition to speaking problems.

Generally the *evaluation* of dysarthria includes: examination of the peripheral speech mechanism, tests for specific speech skills, otolaryngologic consultation, and assessment of the patient's functional ability based on the clarity of his speech in conversation. *Speech therapy* is of benefit to many dysarthric patients.

CHAPTER 39

Specific Neurologic Disorders

This chapter focuses on specific neurologic disorders. Because the major areas of clinical care of neurologic patients have been discussed in Chapter 38 only details of care which are highly specific to a given disorder are presented in this chapter. Refer back to appropriate areas of Chapter 38 as necessary.

INFECTIONS AFFECTING THE NERVOUS SYSTEM

Practically all the pathogenic microorganisms may invade the parenchyma, coverings, and blood vessels of the nervous system. Frequently, in order to clarify discussion, the various infectious syndromes are divided according to the main area of involvement, e.g., infections of the meninges, subdural and epidural infections, and so forth. There are two terms of importance to clarify in discussing infectious processes involving the nervous system: (1) *meningitis,* inflammation of the meninges, and (2) *encephalitis,* inflammation of the brain.

GENERAL CARE IN INFECTIONS

The treatment and clinical care of patients with infections that affect the nervous system consist basically of: (1) administering antibiotics as ordered that are specific for the causative organism; (2) treating increased intracranial pressure and/or hyperthermia if they occur; (3) protecting the delirious patient (see Unit III); (4) providing symptomatic care, e.g., keeping the patient's linens dry if he perspires excessively, keeping the room quiet and darkened if the patient has a headache or is photophobic, offering oral hygiene if emesis occurs, handling the patient gently and unhurriedly if he is nauseated or has unusual sensitivity of his skin and muscles, placing a cool cloth over the patient's forehead and eyes if he so wishes; (5) maintaining fluid-electrolyte balance; (6) enforcing isolation as necessary; (7) preventing complications of bed rest; and (8) making frequent observations of the patient, because rapid worsening of his condition may occur. Observations include looking for symptoms of meningeal irritation, increased intracranial pressure, changes in level of consciousness, and hyperthermia. The nurse makes detailed notes concerning how the patient appears and how he says he feels.

BRAIN ABSCESS

A brain abscess is the presence of encapsulated or free pus in the brain's substance following an acute purulent infection. Abscesses vary in size from an area of purulent necrosis involving the major part of one hemisphere of the brain, down to lesions of microscopic size.

The commonest infecting organisms are the pneumococci, *Staphylococcus aureus, Streptococcus viridans,* and *Streptococcus hemolyticus,* although infection may be caused by any of the common pyogenic bacteria. By the time surgery is performed the abscess is frequently sterile.

Brain abscesses may arise from: direct extension from infections within the cranial cavity (mastoid, nasal sinuses, osteomyelitis of the skull); infections secondary to fractures of the skull; or metastases from infection elsewhere in the body (heart, lungs, tonsils, upper respiratory tract).

Brain abscesses today are relatively rare, constituting less than 2 per cent of patients coming to intracranial surgery. The *symptoms* of brain abscess are basically similar to those of any expanding brain lesion. Headache, nausea, vomiting, and convulsions (focal or generalized) commonly occur as a result of edema of adjacent brain tissue and increased intracranial pressure, which develops rapidly. The *treatment* of brain abscesses is surgical *evacuation* of the pus combined with pre- and postoperative administration of *antibiotics. Untreated brain abscesses are usually fatal.*

Because recurrent convulsive seizures may develop or continue following brain abscess, prophylactic treatment with phenobarbital or diphenylhydantoin sodium is generally administered to all patients who have been treated for an abscess in the cerebral hemispheres. Such prophylactic therapy continues for at least a year.

INFECTIONS OF THE MENINGES

Meningitis proper, or leptomeningitis, is subdivided into two groups according to the severity of the inflammatory reaction; this, in turn, is partially related to the nature of the infecting organism. The two groups are: (1) acute purulent meningitis, and (2) subacute purulent meningitis.

Acute Purulent Meningitis

The most frequent causative organisms of acute purulent meningitis are the meningococcus, pneumococcus, streptococcus and influenza bacillus, although almost any pathogenic bacteria may cause this disorder. Viral meningitis also may occur.

Pathogenic microorganisms obtain access to the meninges and ventriculosubarachnoid space in a variety of ways. For example, they may accidentally be introduced at the time that a lumbar puncture is performed, or they may enter the subarachnoid space through a compound skull fracture or fractures through the mastoid or nasal sinuses. Organisms may also invade the meninges by the direct extension of an infected area in the skull, spine, or parenchyma of the nervous system. Similarly, pathogenic microorganisms may metastasize from infections of the viscera (e.g., heart, lung), or they may migrate to the ventriculosubarachnoid space through the blood stream.

Diagnosis and therapy of acute purulent meningitis depend upon isolating and identifying the specific microorganism and determining the source of the infection. Antibiotics have been highly beneficial in reducing the mortality rate of all forms of meningitis in recent decades. Complications and sequelae of meningeal infection rarely occur with modern treatment, and those complications caused by involvement of other parts of the body by meningococci or other intercurrent infections are more easily controlled than in the past.

The onset of meningitis is typically manifested by headache, prostration, nausea and vomiting, back pain, stiff neck, and chills and fever. Although the patient is usually irritable at the onset of the illness, as the infection progresses the sensorium often becomes clouded, and stupor or coma may develop. Generally the patient with meningitis appears acutely ill and confused, stuporous, or semicomatose. Focal neurologic signs rarely occur; however, convulsive seizures are often an early symptom.

Usually with meningitis there is rigidity of the neck (nuchal rigidity) with positive Kernig and Brudzinski signs.

> *Brudzinski's sign.* The patient's chest is held down as the head is rapidly elevated from the bed. In meningeal irritation such passive flexion of the neck produces flexion of both thighs at the hips, as well as flexure movements of the ankle and knee.

> *Kernig's sign.* The patient is recumbent and his thigh is flexed to a right angle, i.e., toward his abdomen, keeping the knee flexed at a 90 degree angle to the thigh. Extension of the leg upward then causes spasm of the hamstring muscles, resistance to additional extension of the leg at the knee, and pain.

Subacute Meningitis

Usually subacute meningitis is caused by infection with tubercle bacilli or mycotic organisms. Subacute meningitis typically differs from acute purulent meningitis in the following ways: the degree of inflammatory reaction is less severe; the onset of symptoms is less acute; the course of the illness is more prolonged; and relapses are apt to occur (particularly with mycotic infection).

VIRUS INFECTIONS

In spite of the fact that multiple viruses exist, *virus infections are not a common cause of disease of the nervous system of man.* Some of the diseases whose etiology is unknown at present may eventually prove to be caused by viruses.

Among the viral diseases that may affect the nervous system, probably the most common are herpes zoster, poliomyelitis, and various forms of encephalitis and myelitis in which the brain and/or spinal cord are attacked as part of a systemic viral infection. Rabies, potentially the most dangerous viral infection of the nervous system, is rarely seen. Only poliomyelitis and herpes zoster will be discussed in any detail here.

While immunization procedures are available for rabies, poliomyelitis and some of the encephalitides, they are not available against most of the viral encephalitides. *At present, mass immunization has proved to be practical only for acute anterior poliomyelitis.* The greatest hope for the control of other viral diseases is believed to lie in the identification and elimination of the vectors responsible for their transmission. *No adequate treatment exists for the majority of the CNS viral infections.*

Acute Anterior Poliomyelitis (Infantile Paralysis)

The development of an effective vaccine has caused acute anterior poliomyelitis, formerly the most common form of CNS viral infection, to greatly decrease in incidence. Today paralytic poliomyelitis ("polio") is virtually a clinical rarity in the United States, and also worldwide except in isolated areas where the population has not received vaccination. Acute anterior poliomyelitis is a generalized disease characterized by the destruction of the motor cells (particularly the anterior horn cells in the spinal cord and the brain stem, especially the medulla) and the appearance of a flaccid paralysis of those muscles innervated by the affected neurons. This disease is caused by a virus that is almost entirely neurotropic and spreads from the gastrointestinal tract to the nervous system.

Cases of poliomyelitis are divided into two groups, depending upon whether paralysis is present. Paralytic cases are subdivided into spinal forms and bulbar forms. In the spinal form paralysis is restricted to the spinal segments. Such paralysis is flaccid in nature, usually is asymmetrical, and is scattered in distribution, although it tends to be more severe in one extremity (most frequently the legs are involved). Involvement of the diaphragm and intercostal muscles or damage to the medulla oblongata's respiratory centers may produce respiratory paralysis. Occasionally a transient bladder paralysis may occur. In the *bulbar form of paralytic acute anterior poliomyelitis* there is involvement of the muscles supplied by the cranial nerves, because the bulbar nuclei are involved. These muscles may be affected alone or in combination with spinal musculature. The disorder is commonly unilateral. Respiratory paralysis results from lesions in the reticular formation.

Patients with paralysis of the respiratory muscles require prompt, intensive care. At the first indication of respiratory embarrassment, the patient should immediately be placed in a respirator and given frequent reassurance that his breathing will be supported. Such treatment, *before* serious respiratory paralysis develops, greatly increases chances of recovery. Some physicians routinely perform a tracheotomy on all patients receiving respirator care; tracheotomy is always indicated in the presence of spasm of the laryngeal muscles or when mucus occludes the air passages.

As mentioned earlier, in recent years immunization with either killed virus (Salk) intramuscularly, or the live attenuated virus (Sabin) by mouth has caused a remarkable reduction in the number of cases of paralytic acute anterior poliomyelitis. It is recommended that a series of three or four immunizing doses of either vaccine be administered to all persons between the ages of one and 45 years; the second dose is given a month to six weeks after the first, and the third dose seven to nine months after the second. In subsequent years booster inoculations can be given. Obviously such prophylactic measures are highly advisable.

For a more complete discussion of poliomyelitis consult a textbook of neurologic nursing or communicable disease.

HERPES ZOSTER ("SHINGLES")

Herpes zoster is an acute viral infection of nerve structure caused by a neurotropic variety of the chickenpox virus (the varicella-zoster virus). The disease involves inflammation of the cerebral ganglia and ganglia of the posterior nerve roots. In herpes zoster a nodular or vesicular eruption of the skin (herpes) occurs in conjunction with acute segmental neuralgia (zoster). The zoster or neuralgia occurs first, and is followed in three to four days by the development of the skin lesions in the same area. During the acute stage of the illness a meningitis with fever, stiff neck, malaise, and headache may occur, preceding or accompanying the selective nerve root involvement.

Typically herpes zoster is characterized by a grouping of painful nodules or vesicles that are arranged along the course of a nerve or group of nerves, usually on only one side of the body. The intercostal nerves (branches of the thoracic spinal nerves in the area of the waist) are most commonly affected. Another relatively common site is the first branch of the fifth cranial nerve, causing pain in the eyeball and surrounding tissues (ophthalmic herpes zoster). Herpes zoster occurs more commonly in older patients.

Cross-immunization studies have demonstrated that exposure to herpes zoster may cause chickenpox, and vice versa. Recurrence is uncommon. Generally a lasting immunity follows an attack.

The acute, painful stage of herpes zoster generally lasts 10 to 21 days before it gradually subsides and the pain disappears. There is no medication available to specifically treat herpes zoster, as is true of nearly all other virus infections. *Nursing care centers around prevention of infection of the skin lesions and keeping the patient as comfortable and pain-free as possible.* Wet dressings may be applied to acute and extensive inflammatory lesions. Some physicians order calamine lotion or other shake lotions that are cooling, drying, and antipruritic. Apply such lotions liberally and cover them with a protective layer of cotton batting to protect the lesions from trauma. Some sources recommend that unbroken lesions be painted with tincture of benzoin or collodion. During the acute phase of the illness, bed rest and symptomatic care are given as indicated. Nonaddicting analgesics may be ordered for pain relief. If bacterial infection of the rash develops, local or systemic treatment with antimicrobial medications is indicated. Some physicians administer high doses of adrenal steroids during the acute phase. If trigeminal herpes involves the cornea, local antimicrobials and adrenocorticosteroids are instilled into the eye. Barbiturates or bromides may help to control the tension and nervousness that may be associated with the neuralgia.

The patient with *uncomplicated* herpes zoster makes an uneventful recovery as the lesions dry and disappear along with the pain. A scar may remain, and the area may remain painful for about two weeks. With *complicated* herpes zoster the patient may develop a postherpetic neuralgia that causes pain of varying severity and intractability. This develops because the sensory ganglia located on the posterior nerve roots are affected.

Postherpetic neuralgia may be difficult to treat and may in fact cause intractable pain. Intercostal nerve blocks may be performed. The involved area may be infiltrated with Kenalog suspension and lidocaine. Sometimes a small dose of radiotherapy may help. Deep x-ray may be given to the posterior ganglia.

NEUROSYPHILIS

Syphilis is discussed generally in Unit XX. In this unit we shall discuss only some major types of syphilis affecting the nervous system, i.e., neurosyphilis. Neurosyphilis does not develop in all patients with syphilis. However, all patients who do develop neurosyphilis will have passed through a stage of asymptomatic syphilitic meningitis that is recognizable upon examination of the CSF; i.e., white cells are increased, with or without a protein increase, and a positive serologic reaction is present. Thus, every patient with known syphilis should be followed with appropriate spinal fluid examinations, whether or not he has been treated for the primary infection.[207]

The incidence of neurosyphilis is decreasing, probably because penicillin is generally effective in treating early syphilis. Neurosyphilis does not develop in patients who have received adequate penicillin therapy in the primary or secondary stage. The causative organism, *Treponema pallidum,* invades the CNS within the first few weeks or months of the original infection; however, clinical evidence of this involvement usually does not appear for many years. As a rule, the only indication of CNS involvement in the first few years following the primary infection is an abnormality of the CSF.

Asymptomatic neurosyphilis is treated with penicillin. Penicillin therapy readily reverses the CSF changes and usually eliminates the dangerous possibility of the later development of paretic or tabetic neurosyphilis. Generally 15 to 20 million units of penicillin are given intramuscularly in a period of 14 to 21 days and, if necessary, repeated after six months. If the patient is sensitive to penicillin, aureomycin, erythromycin, or terramycin may be substituted.[161]

Meningeal and vascular neurosyphilis may occur any time following the primary infection and may appear during the course of paretic or tabetic neurosyphilis. Generally, however, meningeal involvement appears within the first two years following the initial infection and frequently the symptoms occur at the time of the secondary rash. [161] The cerebral meninges may be involved either diffusely or focally. When the meningitis is focal, there is granuloma formation (gumma). A gumma is a circumscribed mass of granulation tissue. When they occur, gummata typically grow from the pia mater, compressing and invading the brain's parenchyma. Although the symptoms of diffuse syphilitic meningitis readily respond to treatment with penicillin, intracranial gummata are not responsive to such therapy and must be surgically removed. Following such surgery, antisyphilitic chemotherapy, i.e., penicillin, is administered.

Cerebral vascular neurosyphilis (producing endarteritis with thrombosis and encephalomalacia) clinically produces various focal neurologic symptoms, e.g., aphasia and hemiplegia. Usually about seven years pass between the primary infection and the appearance of symptoms.

The two main forms of late neurosyphilis, also called *parenchymatous neurosyphilis,* are tabes dorsalis and dementia paralytica (also called general paresis of the insane, syphilitic meningoencephalitis, and paretic neurosyphilis). Both these conditions occur many years after the primary syphilitic infection.

Tabes dorsalis is also called progressive locomotor ataxia because ambulation difficulties predominate. Although *rare* at present, formerly this condition developed in approximately 9 per cent of all persons with syphilis. Typically the first symptoms appear 10 to 25 years following the primary infection. Pathologically, degenerative changes occur in the posterior funiculi of the spinal cord and in the brainstem. Clinically, tabes dorsalis is easily diagnosed by the following findings: lightning pains (usually in the legs); dysuria; ataxia; peculiar slapping gait; Argyll Robertson pupils;* absent deep reflexes and loss of proprioceptive sensibility; and zones of hyperesthesia and hypalgesia. A principal group of symptoms are *arthropathies* (commonly called *Charcot joints*) characterized by enlargement of the joint, hypermotility, and deformity resulting from dislocations, deposition of new bone, fractures and erosions. Charcot joints are also common in syringomyelia. The joints may become quite large; however, the bone destruction also allows remarkable mobility. An impressive finding is the absence of pain upon squeezing or manipulation of the joint. Arthropathies may occur in any joint.[232]

Dementia paralytica was formerly one of the most common causes of admission to mental hospitals; admissions from this disorder have greatly decreased in recent years. Dementia paralytica is actually a chronic spirochetal meningoencephalitis that produces such a disruption in the function of the cerebral cortex that a general dissolution of mental and physical capacities results. Clinically the symptoms of both the major and minor psychoses occur; dementia paralytica may simulate any type of mental disturbance with either a functional or organic basis.

*Argyll Robertson pupils may be seen in disorders other than neurosyphilis, e.g., multiple sclerosis, epidemic encephalitis, diabetes mellitus, midbrain and pineal tumors, and chronic alcoholism.

TUMORS OF THE NERVOUS SYSTEM

Various tumors affect the nervous system; some originate within the nervous system (i.e., primary tumors) and others (secondary tumors) are implanted there as a result of metastases from different regions of the body. The large majority are primary tumors. Some tumors are malignant, whereas others are benign. Our discussion focuses mainly on intracranial tumors and spinal tumors. Tumors of the peripheral nerves are mentioned only briefly.

INTRACRANIAL TUMORS

Overview

All intracranial tumors, whether benign or malignant, are potentially fatal unless they are treated, since there is no room for excess tissue within the skull. Death from untreated brain tumors results either from (1) primary brain damage, i.e., the local destructive, irritative, or compression effect of the tumor; (2) progressively increasing intracranial pressure, which most brain tumors produce.

Probably more than half of brain tumors are malignant, infiltrate the brain substance, and are thus not amenable to complete surgical removal. In this group fatal recurrence often occurs within two years.

The *clinical course* of patients with intracranial tumors is closely related to the type of tumor. *Generally the symptoms of intracranial tumors are of slow onset and they typically progress until the patient dies if he is not treated.* Although remissions are relatively infrequent, they occasionally occur, even with a highly malignant tumor.[161]

It is helpful to realize that there are two basically different categories of tumors of the brain: (1) those intracranial tumors that are *inside the brain substance,* e.g., tumors of the supportive tissue (gliomas) and tumors of the blood vessels; and (2) those intracranial tumors that are *outside the brain substance,* e.g., tumors of the meninges (such as meningiomas), tumors of the cranial nerves (such as acoustic neuromas), and tumors of the pituitary region. Metastatic tumors may occur either inside or outside the brain substance, or in both areas.[207] *Primary brain tumors occur more frequently within the brain than outside it, and practically all primary tumors within the brain are gliomas.*

Intracranial tumors occur predominantly in early adult life or in middle age; however, all types of intracranial tumors may present their initial symptoms at any age.

Localized (Local) Symptoms of Intracranial Tumors

The localized symptoms of intracranial tumors are those caused by localized destruction, irritation, or compression by the tumor of that part of the brain in or near which it lies. These symptoms vary, depending upon the specific area of the brain affected. Such symptoms may include: paresthesia, anesthesia, muscular weakness, olfactory hallucinations, language disturbances, staggering gait, changes in hearing, and visual disturbances, e.g., diplopia, hemianopia.

Generalized Symptoms of Intracranial Tumors

Generalized symptoms of intracranial tumors are caused by such factors as distortion of various areas of the brain, cerebral edema, and increased intracranial pressure. Choked disks, headache, and nausea and vomiting are the classic triad of symptoms that are commonly considered to be characteristic of brain tumors. (You will recognize these as symptoms of increased intracranial pressure.) However, experts state that the appearance of these symptoms is highly variable during the course of the growth of brain tumors, and in some cases these symptoms do not appear at all. Therefore, no constellation of symptoms is pathognomonic of intracranial tumors.

In addition to choked disks, headache, and nausea and vomiting, other common generalized symptoms of intracranial tumors include mental symptoms (e.g., personality changes, lethargy) and seizures. Frequently seizures are the first symptom of an intracranial tumor. When headaches occur they tend to be: (1) generalized; (2) most intense in the frontal or occipital areas; (3) of increasing frequency and duration; (4) intensified by straining; and (5) irregular in their occurrence. Intracranial tumors may also cause diplopia or blurred vision.

Diagnosis of Intracranial Tumors

A physical examination and history that reveal the above symptoms of intracranial tumor are helpful in diagnosis. Additionally, special tests and laboratory evaluations may include: skull x-rays, examination of CSF, electroencephalography, echoencephalography, radioactive brain scanning, angiography, and ventriculography or pneumoencephalography. Details of these procedures were previously discussed in Chapter 37. In addition to skull x-rays, the patient's chest is also x-rayed to exclude primary cancer of the lung.

Examination of the CSF is frequently helpful in establishing the diagnosis of brain tumor. An increased pressure and an increased protein content are abnormalities of the CSF that characterize brain tumor. *The performance of a lumbar puncture is hazardous if a high degree of choked disk is present.*

Electroencephalography is especially helpful in localizing tumors near the surface of the cerebral hemispheres. *Echoencephalography* is a safe procedure, and experts recommend that it be performed on all patients believed to have brain tumors. On the other hand, although *ventriculography* and *encephalography* are helpful in diagnosing brain tumors and determining the general location of almost all brain tumors, both these procedures are accompanied by a definite risk in patients with intracranial tumors.

Angiography is highly valuable in diagnosing and localizing brain tumors. The tumors are localized by noting the displacement of arteries and veins and by finding abnormal vascular patterns on the angiogram. Often the type of the tumor can be determined by the nature of its vasculature. Like angiography, *radioactive scanning* is highly valuable in localizing brain tumors (by means of their differential uptake of gamma-emitting labeled carriers).

Usually the process of assessment to establish the diagnosis is carried out over a period of several days. However, in urgent cases it can be performed within a few hours.

Tumors of the Cranial Nerves

The cranial nerves may be compressed or invaded by benign or malignant tumors, or they may be the primary site of tumors. Here we shall consider the latter. While any of the cranial nerves may be the site of origin of a tumor, those most commonly affected are the optic nerve (by glioma), the eighth cranial (acoustic) nerve (by neurofibroma), and the fifth cranial nerve (by neurofibroma). Of these, the eighth cranial is most commonly affected.

Neurofibromas of the eighth cranial, i.e., *acoustic nerve,* are acoustic neuroma, acoustic neurinoma, cerebellopontine angle tumor, or perineural fibroblastoma of the eighth nerve. These tumors constitute 5 to 10 per cent of all intracranial tumors. Typically the onset of symptoms is between the ages of 30 and 60. Acoustic neuromas grow slowly, and usually the symptoms are present several months or years prior to diagnosis. Tinnitus is an early symptom, followed by a degree of deafness. Other symptoms that occur frequently are: (1) sensation of giddiness or unsteadiness of gait; (2) facial paralysis (as a result of seventh nerve involvement); and (3) loss of the corneal reflex (as a result of trigeminal involvement). If untreated, death is almost inevitable. Surgical removal is the treatment for acoustic neuromas, since they do not respond to radiation therapy. Frequently by the time the patient comes to surgery the tumor is quite large and removal is difficult. Thus, this benign tumor that occurs outside the brain substance still has a relatively high mortality rate.

Blood Vessel Tumors and Malformations

Numerous malformations of blood vessels are sometimes included in the literature under tumors; there are a number of different classifications of these vascular anomalies and malformations. Generally there are two main groups: (1) *angiomas,* which are malformations composed of blood vessels of adult structure; and (2) *angioblastomas* (also called hemangioblastomas), which are tumors comprised of embryonic vascular channels and blood vessel-forming cells. The latter are the only true tumors of blood vessels in the brain. These tumors are cystic lesions (often red and hemorrhagic) that are quite rare and generally occur in early middle life in the area of the cerebellum. The diagnosis of a tumor of the cerebellum is established by ventriculography. Complete surgical cure is possible in patients with a single tumor.

Granulomas

Granulomas are tumors or neoplasms composed of granulation tissue. Granuloma formation may occur in the nervous system following infections with syphilis, the larvae of various intestinal parasites, fungi, sarcoidosis, and tuberculosis. *Tuberculomas* of the brain are always secondary to tuberculosis elsewhere in the body; however, the tuberculosis need not necessarily be active. (See Unit XIV.) The symptoms of tuberculomas are similar to those of other brain tumors. Tuberculomas are amenable to surgery when proper chemotherapy is administered to prevent spread of the tuberculosis.

Metastatic Brain Tumors

Metastatic brain tumors are generally a manifestation of generalized metastases. (See also Unit VII.) Almost all carcinomas or sarcomas located elsewhere in the body may metastasize to the brain or its coverings; however, in approximately 40 to 60 per cent of patients *the most common primary sites of intracranial metastatic tumors are the lung (bronchus) or breast.* For this reason, as mentioned earlier, a chest x-ray is routinely taken on all patients who are suspected of having an intracranial tumor. Carcinomas of the prostate and cervix uteri may involve the brain's dura or the skull, but they rarely involve the brain substance itself. While metastatic tumors of the brain may develop at any age, they typically parallel the age incidence of malignant tumors in general, thus occurring most often between ages of 40 and 70.

Usually metastatic tumors are characterized by a rapid onset and progression of symptoms; death usually occurs within a few months of appearance of the first symptoms. Typically dozens of metastatic nodules are found in the brain at autopsy. However, in approximately 25 per cent of patients a solitary nodule occurs. When a single metastasis does occur it can be removed, if it is in a suitable area of the brain, and the patient experiences temporary relief of symptoms and may gain several useful months of life. However, generally the metastases are multiple, as mentioned, and operation is rarely advisable. An exploratory craniotomy may be performed when there is reasonable doubt as to whether the lesion is truly metastatic. X-ray therapy may be given to retard the growth of intracranial metastases. Also, recently corticosteroids have been found to be valuable in obtaining symptom relief and increasing life span, although they are not curative.

Treatment of Intracranial Tumors

Some comments concerning the treatment of intracranial tumors have already been made. *Early treatment is important. Intracranial tumors are treated by surgical removal of the tumor when possible.* If indicated, this is followed by radiation therapy (Fig. 39–1). In those patients in whom the tumor cannot be completely removed, the period of remaining useful life may be lengthened if the partial removal is followed by radiation therapy. *Usually cure of the following types of tumors can be obtained by surgical removal:* lipomas, acoustic neuromas, meningiomas, cystic astrocytomas of the cerebellum, colloid cysts of the third ventricle, angiomatous malformations, and some of the granulomas and congenital tumors. Chemotherapy of malignant gliomas is being tried experimentally. Some drugs that have been administered in association with radiation therapy and surgery in the treatment of malignant gliomas include: nitrogen mustard, vincristine sulfate, mithramycin and methotrexate. These drugs have been therapeutically effective in some patients.

When surgical consultation is not readily available, *temporary measures may be necessary to reduce increased intracranial pressure.* Intracranial surgery is discussed in Chapter 40.

Clinical care varies with the location of the tumor and the patient's symptoms. In Chapter 38 we have discussed the care of patients who are unconscious, or have seizures, increased intracranial pressure, and other symptoms found in patients with brain tumors. Care of the patient receiving radiation treatment has been covered in Unit VII.

The nurse's observations are important with regard to all the preceding areas. Specifically, when caring for a patient with a brain tumor (or suspected brain tumor) you routinely observe for indications of increasing intracranial pressure, symptoms of impaired motor function, significant alterations in vital signs or pupils, evidence of hyperthermia, seizures, pain, and vomiting. With reference to pain, note the location, duration, and severity of headache and the position that the patient assumes to obtain maximum comfort during the headache. Caution the conscious patient not to strain (e.g., while vomiting or using the bedpan), because this increases intracranial pressure and can result in respiratory failure. Note whether the vomiting is related to meals, whether it is projectile, and if it is accompanied by nausea (often abbreviated "N & V").

As you might expect, patients who suspect or know they have a brain tumor are often frightened and require kindness, patience, and understanding from the nurse. They often have questions about brain surgery. Find out from the doctor if a patient's tumor is malignant and what he has discussed, concerning the diagnosis, with the patient and relatives. Relatives also need the support of the nurse.

SPINAL TUMORS

Spinal tumors most frequently occur in young or middle-aged adults and most often involve the thoracic region. The symptoms of spinal tumors vary widely, depending upon the level of cord involvement. For example, tumors at the cord's caudal end may produce bowel and urinary bladder symptoms, whereas cervical lesions may produce such symptoms as paralysis of the diaphragm and spastic tetraplegia.

The histology of the various types of primary and secondary spinal tumors is generally exactly the same as that of intracranial tumors.

Most tumors affecting the spinal cord are attached to the meninges or spinal nerve roots, whereas brain tumors most often occur within the brain itself. Tumors of any kind within the substance of the spinal cord are relatively rare, representing only slightly more than 10 per cent of all spinal tumors. Metastatic tumors are quite common in the epidural space (because of involvement of the contiguous vertebrae), but they are exceedingly rare in the substance of the cord itself. Carcinoma far more frequently metastasizes to the vertebrae than it does to the bones of the skull.

Spinal tumors occur only about one-fourth as often as intracranial tumors.

Metastatic tumors in the vertebral column may cause pressure on the cord and may extend directly into the cord. Usually the symptoms worsen steadily as the tumor enlarges. Such metastatic tumors may actually destroy the vertebral column which surrounds and supports the cord. Primary cord tumors also occur but are rarer than metastatic tumors.

Classification of Spinal Tumors

Spinal tumors are often classified by location in reference to the dura, i.e., extradural and dural; and in the intradural group with reference to the cord, i.e., intramedullary or extramedullary.[207] Tumors within the spinal canal originate either

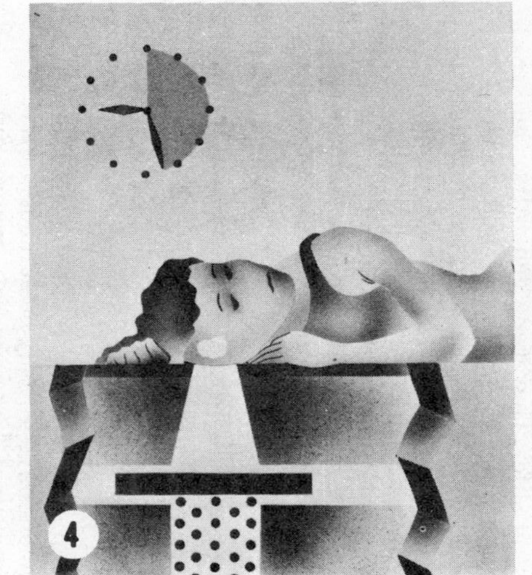

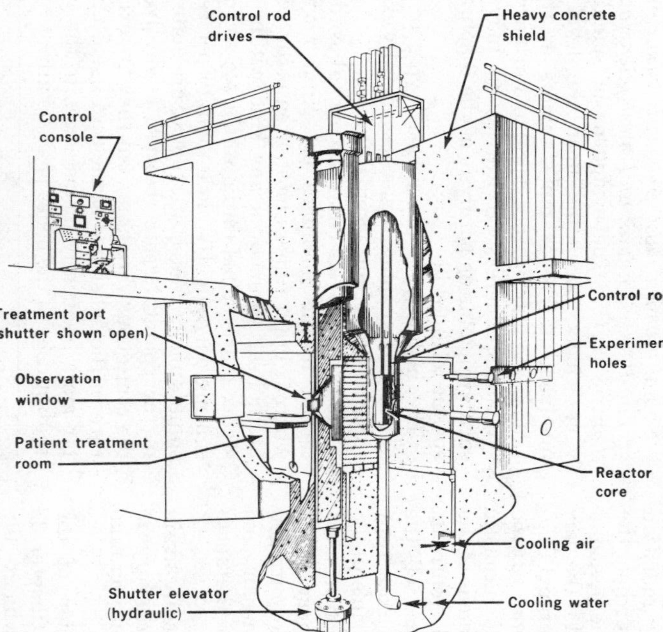

Neutron capture treatment of a brain tumor, using the Brookhaven National Laboratory research reactor (center). (1) A lead shutter shields the patient from reactor neutrons. (2) A compound containing the stable element boron is injected into the bloodstream; the tumor absorbs most of the boron. (3) After 8 minutes, when the tumor is saturated, the shutter is removed and neutrons bombard the brain, splitting boron atoms so that fragments destroy tumor tissue. (4) Twenty minutes later the shutter is closed and the treatment ends.

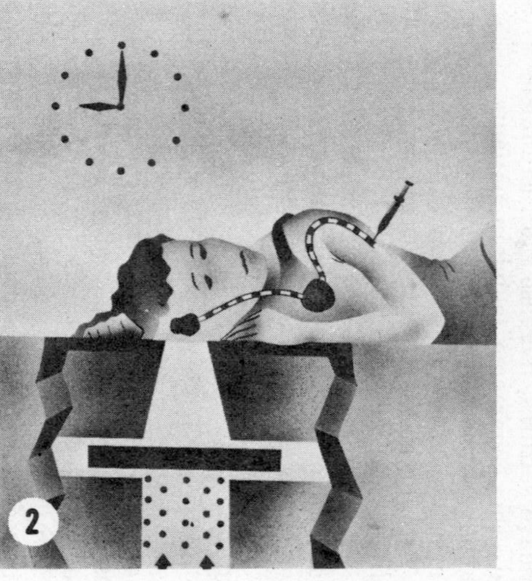

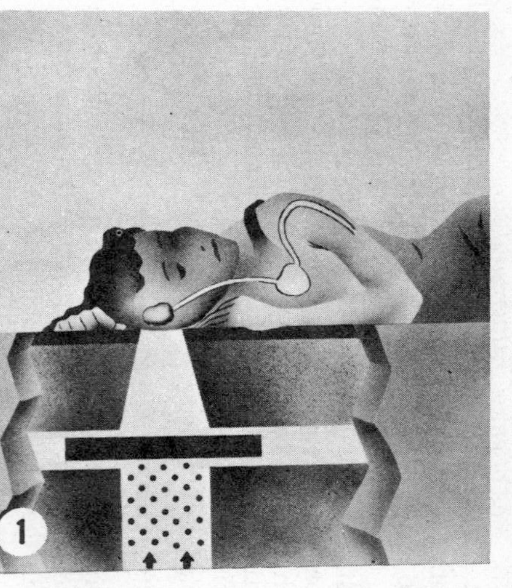

FIGURE 39–1. Neutron capture treatment of a brain tumor. (From Phelan, E. W.: *Radioisotopes in Medicine.* United States Atomic Energy Commission, Division of Technical Information, 1966.)

from the surrounding tissues, i.e., extramedullary, or from the cord's substance, i.e., intramedullary.[9] Approximately 50 per cent of spinal neoplasms are extradural, 40 per cent extramedullary, and 10 per cent intramedullary. Neurofibromas and meningiomas are the two commonest tumors affecting the spinal cord. Both are benign, operable, and may not produce permanent damage if removed early enough.

Symptoms of Spinal Cord Compression

Cord compression is the common pathologic feature of all tumors within the spinal canal, since there is little room for expansion in the canal. Compression of the spinal cord interrupts the function of nerve fibers in the cord's peripheral portions. *Early symptoms of cord compression* include:

> Spastic weakness of muscles below the level of the lesion.
> Impaired cutaneous and proprioceptive sensation below the level of the lesion.
> Impaired control of urinary bladder and rectum (to less extent).
> Increased reflexes, with extensor plantar responses and loss of appropriate abdominal skin reflexes.

A wide variation occurs in the distribution and severity of motor weakness and sensory loss, depending in part on whether the tumor affects the anterior, lateral, or posterior portion of the cord.

Diagnosis of Spinal Tumors

Complete general medical and neurologic examinations are given to the patient suspected of having spinal tumor. Additionally, x-rays are taken of the spine, spinal puncture is performed, and the spinal subarachnoid space is visualized with Pantopaque or air (myelography).

Treatment of Spinal Tumors

The treatment of spinal tumors is more frequently effective than that of brain tumors. The treatment of spinal tumors is by radiation (see Unit VII) or surgery (spinal surgery is discussed in Chapter 40).

The treatment of extramedullary tumors is surgical removal. Benign *extramedullary* tumors have an excellent prognosis as long as the cord has not been severely damaged by compression. Typically, benign tumors of the spinal cord grow slowly and may progressively produce symptoms over a period of years.

Cord compression resulting from *extradural* neoplasms may be relieved by surgical laminectomy, radiation, chemotherapy, or combinations of these. Radiation, either alone or in combination with chemotherapy, produces particularly good results in treating myelomas or metastatic lymphomas.

Intramedullary tumors usually cannot be completely removed surgically. Some gliomas respond to radiation therapy to some degree, but usually only symptomatic improvement occurs and the prognosis is very poor. Sometimes spinal cord gliomas are extremely slow growing.

PERIPHERAL NERVE TUMORS

While solitary tumors (generally neurofibromas) may develop on any of the peripheral nerves, most often multiple tumors occur and are part of the syndrome of *neurofibromatosis* (*von Recklinghausen's disease*). The symptoms that result from tumors of the peripheral nerves are similar to those caused by other peripheral lesions.

VASCULAR LESIONS OF THE NERVOUS SYSTEM

VASCULAR LESIONS OF THE BRAIN

Cerebrovascular diseases are diseases of the brain's blood vessels. As elsewhere in the body, hypertension and arteriosclerosis are the major underlying causes of cerebrovascular diseases.[207]

Cerebrovascular lesions are the commonest cause of brain disturbances.[161] In the United States vascular lesions in the CNS rank third as a major cause of death, exceeded only by heart disease and cancer. In addition to being a major cause of death, cerebrovascular diseases also leave millions of persons handicapped. The incidence of cerebrovascular diseases is particularly high in persons over age 65. Because of the population's increasing longevity, the magnitude of this problem will increase. While a growing number of these patients are older persons who are incurable by any prospective means, many such patients benefit from preventative measures, precrisis recognition, and effective postcrisis treatment. In elderly patients, specific surgical measures for the treatment of cerebral disturbances are rarely applicable.

Cerebral Circulation

In order to understand CNS vascular conditions the nurse must familiarize herself with knowledge of cerebral circulation: that is, knowledge of the nervous structures to which major vessels run, and from which arise the principal symptoms of a CVA. Also, in order to understand the pathology of cerebrovascular diseases and, thus, the effects they produce, it is essential to understand a few facts about the physiology of cerebral circulation. *The most important fact to bear in mind is that the brain has a tremendous oxygen requirement.*

The carotid and vertebral-basilar systems provide the brain's blood supply. Blood supply to the brain may be altered (slowly or rapidly) by such local disorders as thrombi, emboli, hemorrhage, or vascular spasms, or by such generalized disorders as ineffective heart-lung actions.

Extensive interruption of the brain's circulation causes *cerebral anoxia,* i.e., inadequate oxygenation of the brain's tissues resulting from deprivation of blood supply to the total brain. The effects of such anoxia are reversible in the adult for up to four to six minutes. The effects may vary under individual circumstances but irreversible changes always occur when cerebral anoxia lasts more than 10 minutes. Anoxia may be caused by various disorders, a principal one being cardiac arrest.

Cerebral anoxia results from interference with the brain's total blood supply; *cerebral infarction* refers to deprivation of blood supply to a localized area of the brain. Cerebral infarction may result from disorders such as a thrombus or embolus occluding a vessel, or from spasms of a vessel which interfere with cerebral circulation. The extent of the infarction depends upon such factors as the location and size of the occluded vessel and the adequacy of collateral circulation to the area supplied by the occluded vessel.

Atherosclerotic disease frequently affects the arteries leading to the brain. Common sites of plaque formation in these arteries are shown in Figure 39–2. Thrombi may form on atherosclerotic plaques, or blood may clot in an area of stenosis where the blood stream is slowed or where eddying occurs. Thrombi can break loose from a blood vessel wall and become emboli carried in the blood stream. Thrombi and emboli are discussed further in the following section.

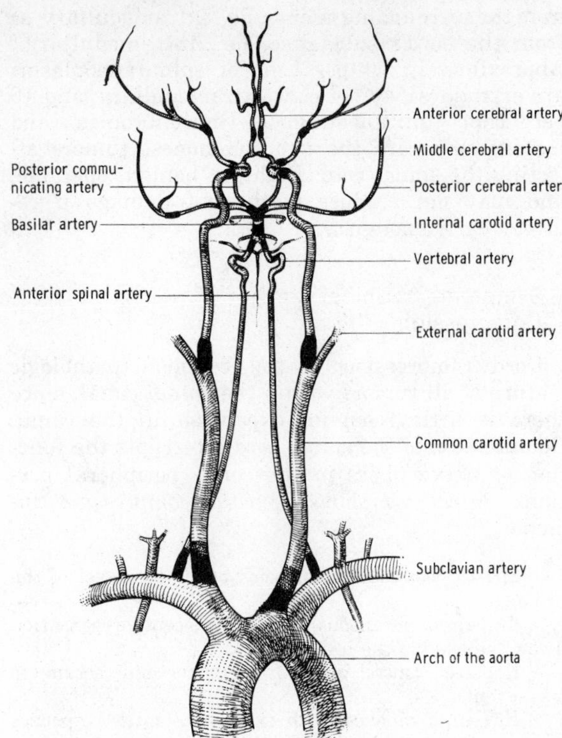

FIGURE 39–2. Common sites of extracranial atheroma formation. (From McDowell, F. H.: *In* Beeson, P. B., and McDermott, W. (eds.): *Cecil-Loeb Textbook of Medicine.* 13th ed., 1971.)

Cerebrovascular Accidents (CVA's, Strokes, Apoplexy)

A *cerebrovascular accident (CVA)* is a condition caused by any *acute* vascular lesion of the brain. Over 500,000 Americans suffer a CVA each year. It is estimated that eight out of 10 patients who have a stroke survive the initial phase. Skilled medical and surgical care, emphasizing prevention of complications and planned early rehabilitation, make it possible for 30 to 60 per cent of patients who survive a CVA to return to productive work. Nevertheless, more than 200,000 persons die in the United States annually from cerebrovascular diseases. Over half these deaths result from cerebral hemorrhage.

The consequences of severe, sudden derangements in the nervous system's blood supply, e.g., from thrombus, embolus, or hemorrhage, are familiar to almost all lay persons as "stroke" or "apoplexy" (from the Greek, meaning to "strike down.") In Greek times it was believed that persons suffering strokes (and grand mal seizures) were struck down by some external force, such as an act by one of the gods.

CVA's may produce an almost unlimited variety of neurologic symptoms, and the onsets of CVA's are highly variable. At times the onset is relatively mild, and the patient may merely experience transient symptoms, e.g., slight disturbances of speech. Consciousness may or may not be altered, and symptoms may last for only a few seconds or minutes or may persist indefinitely. The more severe CVA's may have a violent onset in which the patient falls to the floor and then lies inert, comatose, breathing stertorously or cyclically, face flushed, cheek puffing out on the paralyzed side with each expiration, and arm and leg flaccid on that side. Seizures (usually generalized but at times focal) may also occur.

Numerous methods for investigating the causes of CVA and improved means of diagnosing and preventing this disorder are being researched. Arteriography, isotope brain scanning, and ophthalmodynamometry, to measure the pressure in the retinal artery, are used in diagnosis. Anticoagulation has been used for some time to prevent repetition of arterial occlusion by thrombi and emboli. More recently attempts have been made to dissolve an already existing clot by using thrombolysins.

Research is underway to try to predict fairly exactly when a likely candidate for a stroke (or heart attack) will actually suffer the attack. By identifying various risk factors it is possible to identify persons who are particularly prone to developing ischemic thrombotic cerebrovascular disease (and ischemic heart disease). One possibility is that by studying the liquidity of the blood of such persons it might be feasible to recognize the early indications of beginning coagulation. The patient might then be treated with anticoagulant drugs to bring about a return to normal liquidity before thrombosis can occur.

Etiology of Cerebrovascular Accidents. As stated earlier, a common cause of stroke is a narrowing or complete closing of one of the blood vessels supplying the brain, i.e., occlusive vascular disease. Several events that impair brain function can occur in the cerebral circulation. These include thrombosis (blood clot formation), embolism (blocking of a vessel by a blood clot floating in the blood stream), hemorrhage (bleeding), compression (pressure), and spasm (tightening and closing down of the walls of an artery due to vasoconstriction).

SPASM. Arterial spasm reduces blood flow to the area of the brain supplied by the constricted vessel. Spasm of short duration does not necessarily cause permanent brain damage.

COMPRESSION. Compression of cerebral vessels may result from a tumor, a large blood clot, swollen brain tissue, or other disorders. While compression or arterial spasm can cause infarction of the brain, *the three most common causes of CVA's are thrombosis, embolism, and hemorrhage.*

THROMBOSIS. *Thrombosis is the commonest cause of CVA.* Thrombosis results from occlusion of a vessel, most often due to atherosclerosis. Occlusion may also be secondary to an inflammatory reaction in vessel walls.

The vessel affected by thrombosis may be intracerebral; however, *the main site of obstruction usually is not within the brain but is in the extracerebral vessels.* Formerly it was thought that most cases of cerebral infarction resulted from thrombosis within the three main cerebral arteries (or their branches) intracerebrally or intracranially. However, the importance of the vessels in the neck and their points of origin from the aorta in the etiology of CVA is now established. The presence or absence of symptoms in patients with occlusive lesions in the neck depends on the adequacy of the collateral circulation.

Thrombosis produces an *ischemia* of the brain tissue that is supplied by the affected vessel, and edema and congestion in the surrounding areas. The area of *edema* may cause greater dysfunction than that caused by the infarct itself. The edema subsides after a few hours in some patients, although it may take several days in others. As the edema subsides the patient begins to show improvement and may regain some functions that were impaired by the edema.[161]

A stroke caused by thrombus formation tends to develop while the patient is asleep or within an hour after arising. This differs from a stroke caused by hemorrhage, which most often occurs during active waking hours. (Strokes resulting from embolism occur at any time without an apparent time pattern.) Cerebral thrombosis may also occur during vascular collapse in myocardial infarctions and following surgery.

The *symptoms* of thrombosis are highly variable, depending on the site of the vessel occluded and the size of the area affected in the brain. The symptoms of thrombosis may take several days to develop.[25] This clinical picture is exceedingly different from a stroke caused by cerebral hemorrhage (in which symptoms occur within minutes, or hours at the longest) and that caused by cerebral embolism (in which the symptoms follow even more rapidly). Symptoms appear more slowly with a thrombus than with an embolus because a thrombus more gradually produces ischemia.

EMBOLISM. The incidence of cerebral embolism occurs most often after age 40. "Cerebral embolism" refers to the occlusion of a cerebral vessel by such substances as a fragment of clotted blood, tumor, fat, bacteria, or air. Typically, cerebral embolism is associated with heart diseases in which fragments of clotted blood or bacterial vegetations are released from the heart's walls or valves and then lodge in the cerebral arterial system.

Occlusion of cerebral vessels by an embolus causes necrosis and edema similar to that following thrombosis, unless the embolus contains bacteria. If it is septic, and the infection extends beyond the walls of the vessel, an abscess forms or encephalitis develops. If the infection remains contained within the occluded vessel, an aneurysmal dilation of the vessel, called a *mycotic aneurysm,* may develop. This is dangerous because cerebral hemorrhage may occur later if the aneurysm ruptures.

As indicated earlier, the onset of cerebral embolism typically occurs rapidly. Symptoms may develop, without warning, within from 10 to 30 seconds. The embolus most often lodges in the middle cerebral artery. The extent of damage is often less severe and the recovery more rapid following embolism than following thrombosis or cerebral hemorrhage.

INTRACEREBRAL HEMORRHAGE. Let us first clarify that hemorrhage may occur outside the dura mater (extradural hemorrhage, p. 516), beneath the dura mater (subdural hemorrhage, p. 515), in the subarachnoid space (subarachnoid hemorrhage, p. 496), or within the brain substance (cerebral or intracerebral hemorrhage). In this section we are concerned only with the last-named hemorrhage.

Intracerebral hemorrhage results from rupture of a cerebral vessel. Cerebral hemorrhage is most common after age 50. These hemorrhages usually cause the most extensive residual functional deficits and the slowest recoveries of the various types of CVA's. Large hemorrhages usually come from arteries, whereas small extravasations may come from the veins and capillaries. As with the previously discussed conditions, the effects of intracerebral hemorrhages vary, depending on the site of the hemorrhage and its extent.

The *rupture of arteriosclerotic vessels, in the presence of hypertension, is the cause of most hemorrhages into the brain.*[207] Most intracerebral hemorrhages are very large; therefore, it is not surprising that *hypertensive hemorrhage into the brain is the most common cause of death in the group of cerebrovascular diseases.*[207] While infarcts from thrombosis occur more commonly, they do not cause death unless they are massive. Although recovery is possible following hypertensive hemorrhage, it is more unlikely. (Intracerebral hemorrhage following head injury is discussed on page 516).

Onset, Symptoms and Clinical Course of CVA's. The nurse caring for a patient with CVA needs an understanding of the etiology of stroke and must be able to recognize its precipitating as well as its progressive symptoms.[87] Often the patient with cerebral vascular disease first comes to the attention of nurses and physicians following the sudden, frequently dramatic, onset of coma or focal neurologic symptoms, e.g., hemiplegia, aphasia. CVA's most often occur suddenly, the symptoms reaching maximal intensity within a few minutes or few hours at most. *Premonitory symptoms* seldom occur. However, when they do occur these "warning" symptoms may include mental confusion, drowsiness, dizziness, and headache. Occasionally with thrombosis or a spasm of a vessel, focal premonitory symptoms may occur. For example, a transient loss of speech, hemiplegia, or paresthesias of half of the body may precede the onset of a severe paralysis by a few hours or days.

Typical symptoms associated with a CVA include: *generalized symptoms* such as headache, vomiting, convulsions, coma, nuchal rigidity, fever, hypertension, abnormalities of the heart, sclerosis of peripheral and retinal vessels, confusion, disorientation, memory impairment and other mental changes; and *focal neurologic symptoms* related to the site of the hemorrhage or infarct, e.g., paralysis, sensory loss, language disorders, and reflex changes.

Usually the *general symptoms* are most intense immediately after the onset of the CVA; however, sometimes there is a gradual increase in the depth of the coma. The *focal symptoms* also are typically most severe immediately following onset. However, occasionally following intracerebral hemorrhage the focal neurologic symptoms may increase in severity or extent for a few hours as the hemorrhage continues to enlarge in size. Progression of focal neurologic symptoms may sometimes occur following cerebral thrombosis or embolism.

The focal symptoms that result from cerebral hemorrhage vary, depending on the site of the hemorrhage. However, *complete hemiplegia* (with or without a hemianopia or hemianesthesia) *commonly occurs, since the basal ganglia and adjacent internal capsule are affected in more than two-thirds of these patients.* It is in this region that the motor nerves to the body are gathered together into a relatively small space before they pass down into the spinal cord. Thus, the hemorrhage destroys or compresses those nerves, and the motor impulses are cut off from the muscles. As a result, the side of the body, e.g., face, arm, leg, that is supplied by the side of the brain affected by the hemorrhage is paralyzed, i.e., becomes hemiplegic.[25]

> *Because the motor nerves from one side of the brain cross to the opposite side before passing down the cord, hemorrhage on the brain's right side causes left-sided hemiplegia, and vice versa.*

Additionally, it is significant that the speech center in right-handed persons is on the brain's left side, i.e., in the dominant hemisphere; thus, hemorrhage into the left side often produces aphasia as well as right-sided hemiplegia. The symptoms of cerebral hemorrhage vary with the areas of the hemisphere involved.

The focal symptoms produced by thrombosis or cerebral embolism within the arterial system supplying the brain are highly characteristic of the area of involvement. Thus, these symptoms are extremely helpful in establishing a precise diagnosis, and the nurse's observations of these symptoms are important.

The *thalamic syndrome* is frequently observed following a CVA that involves the region of the thalamus. Typically this syndrome is manifested by a burning or aching dysesthesia which involves an entire half of the body. Discomfort is most intense in the extremities, especially the hand. This pain usually begins first several weeks following the CVA. Thalamic pain is intensified by emotional disturbances. Increased emotional lability, with unmotivated crying or laughing, is often associated with the thalamic syndrome.[63]

Extensive cerebral lesions (resulting from hemorrhage more often than from thrombosis) often produce *conjugate deviation of the eyes,* or *head and eyes,* toward the side of the lesion. The comment is often heard that the patient's eyes "look toward his lesion." Usually when such deviation is present the patient also has only limited movements of the head and eyes toward the opposite direction. As the patient's condition improves generally, these symptoms tend to resolve.

Pupillary abnormalities vary in type and frequency following CVA; however, frequently inequalities of pupil size occur. Typically the larger pupil is on the side opposite the cerebral lesion.

Changes in the patient's reflexes and plantar responses and other symptoms of focal brain damage, e.g., hemiplegia, aphasia, hemianopia, are related to the lesion's site.

CVA's, with the exception of rupture of a large aneurysm, are not the cause of sudden death. When sudden death does occur it is usually due to heart failure. However, if the intracerebral hemorrhage ruptures into the ventricles in the course of a day or two, this complication is fatal. Symptoms of increased intracranial pressure may develop.[207]

In fatal cases of CVA's of all types the duration

of life varies from a few hours to several months following the original attack. Death may occur within three to 12 hours, but it usually is delayed for a period of one to 14 days.

Almost always in patients with any type of *fatal CVA* there is a rise of temperature, pulse rate, and respiratory rate several hours or days before death. These symptoms result from impairment of vital centers. Increase in depth of coma or lapse into coma also occurs. These symptoms indicate a collapse of the vasomotor and heat-regulating centers. Common *contributory causes of death* in patients with intracerebral hemorrhage, primary subarachnoid hemorrhage, or cerebral thrombosis are bronchopneumonia, lobar pneumonia, cardiac failure, uremia, and pulmonary infarction.

Diagnosis of CVA's. Diagnostic methods that may be employed in the evaluation of CVA's typically include: skull x-ray, blood work (particularly WBC, nonprotein nitrogen, blood sugar), urinalysis (obtained by catheterization only if necessary), and examination of CSF. Sometimes other procedures may be necessary, such as an electroencephalogram (EEG), echoencephalogram, radioactive brain scan, pneumoencephalogram, ventriculogram, or cerebral angiography. Some physicians routinely perform angiograms, whereas others do not. Of course, physical and neurologic examinations are done.

When a patient has a suspected CVA the physician must reach three important diagnostic conclusions: *First,* he must diagnose if the patient actually has a CVA, or if the patient has another disorder instead. *Second,* once he has determined that a CVA has occurred, the physician diagnoses the basic cause. *Third,* the physician determines if the patient is suffering from more than one disorder. It is important for the specific cause of a CVA to be identified, because treatment is directed at the cause and also because the prognosis varies with the cause.

Possible intracerebral hemorrhage must be ruled out before anticoagulant therapy is administered. The administration of an anticoagulant in the presence of hemorrhage would gravely worsen the hemorrhage by preventing clotting.

Clinical Care During Acute Stage of CVA. The treatment of CVA is generally divided, for purposes of discussion, into care during the acute phase and care during the stage of recovery or convalescence. In the acute stage, or the period immediately following onset of the CVA, the clinical care is directed mainly at saving the patient's life. During the convalescent stage residual defects are treated. Here we focus on the acute stage. See the section on hemiplegia (Chap. 38) for further discussion of the rehabilitative aspects of care. Refer also to other parts of Chapter 38 as appropriate.

FIRST AID FOR THE STROKE VICTIM. When a stroke occurs, the first consideration is to *maintain the patient's airway.* Loosen tight clothing to facilitate respirations and circulation to the head. If the patient is unconscious turn him onto his affected side (detected by the ballooning of the cheek with expiration) to prevent aspiration of saliva. Care of the unconscious patient, including airway maintenance, is discussed in Chapter 38. If the patient is conscious, he may assume a position of comfort. Elevate the patient's head slightly to minimize cerebral edema or to relieve increased intracranial pressure or headache. Start oxygen inhalation if the patient is cyanotic or appears to have difficulty breathing. Keep the patient warm. Offer reassurance to the conscious patient. Send for medical help at once and keep the patient quiet.

GENERAL CARE. Shortly after the patient is first admitted to the hospital his head is carefully examined for indications of external injury, and presence or absence of stiffness of the neck is noted. His temperature, pulse, respirations, and blood pressure are checked, as well as his optic disks and the size and reactions of his pupils. The odor of the patient's breath is noted, and he is examined for paralysis (particularly hemiplegia) and other focal neurologic symptoms. Examination of the comatose hemiplegic is discussed in Chapter 38.

Skilled nursing care is essential during this acute period while the patient is on complete bed rest. The patient is handled carefully to avoid injury; if he is unconscious or has increased intracranial pressure, appropriate care is given as discussed in Chapter 38. Let us summarize some essential points concerning general care of the patient following CVA:

> *Maintain patent, adequate airway and oxygenation.* An artificial airway is usually inserted if stertorous respirations occur. At times, tracheostomy is indicated. Frequent suctioning may be necessary. It may be advisable to administer oxygen.

> *Make frequent observations and take vital signs.* Observe for symptoms of hyperthermia, shock, increasing intracranial pressure, seizures, and worsening of level of consciousness. Specifically, make frequent observations and recordings concerning: pupillary reactions, posture, motor abilities (presence or absence of voluntary or involuntary movements, grip), loss of sensation or heightened sensation, pain, bulbar symptoms, respiratory symptoms, level of consciousness, stiffness or flaccidity of neck, vital signs, skin color, skin temperature, skin moistness or dryness, input and output, vomiting, incontinence, abdominal distention, and bladder distention.

> *Observe for recurrent CVA's.* Remember that stroke may be preceded by headache, flushing of the face, vertigo, subjective feeling that something is about to happen, sudden loss of consciousness, or convulsions. Pulse may be rapid and bounding, blood pressure elevated, respirations labored and stertorous.

> *Ensure adequate fluid-electrolyte balance.* For a few days fluids may be restricted in an attempt to reduce intracranial pressure. (See Unit V, Chapters 24 and 25.) Intravenous feedings are typically given for the first several days. Then if the patient continues comatose or has impaired swallowing (dysphagia), tube feedings may be given. Maintain proper nutrition.

> *Maintain proper positioning and alignment; turn and reposition frequently; maintain muscle tone.* (See

discussions in Chapter 38.) *Prevent complications of bed rest,* e.g., pneumonia, urinary stasis, contractures, decubitus ulcers, and so forth. (See Unit V, Chap. 27.) Experts make the following recommendations pertinent

> *Do not leave the patient on his affected side for more than 20 minutes four times each day. As soon as the patient responds to commands, encourage deep breathing and coughing each time the patient is turned. Start range-of-motion exercises for all extremities on day of admission.*

> *Maintain adequate elimination.* A urinary catheter may be inserted initially when the patient is unconscious or stuporous. Later, bladder and bowel training is started. However, some physicians[130] do not think a catheter should be inserted routinely merely to keep the bed dry, since a catheter makes retraining more difficult and is a primary cause of severe urinary tract infection. Some patients regain bladder control within three to five days. Thus, rather than catheterize for incontinence alone, catheterization is avoided unless it is necessary for other reasons. If a patient is not catheterized, the urinal or bedpan is offered every two hours, *day and night,* for the first 48 to 72 hours. If a catheter is inserted, a completely closed, sterile set-up is necessary and fluids are forced, to 3000 ml. per day unless contraindicated. Following removal of the catheter watch for *urinary retention.* Bladder and bowel retraining have been discussed in Chapter 38. The patient should be reassured that his bowel and bladder control will probably improve daily.

> *Prevent constipation and impactions,* as discussed in Chapter 38 and Unit V, Chapter 27. It is important that the CVA patient *not strain at bowel movements,* because this increases intracranial and vascular pressures, which, in turn, encourages hemorrhage, rupture of aneurysms, and so forth. Be prepared for *fecal incontinence* during the early stages. Give frequent skin care to the incontinent patient to prevent skin breakdown.

TABLE 39–1. DIAGNOSIS OF CEREBROVASCULAR DISORDERS

	Intracerebral Hemorrhage	**Cerebral Thrombosis**	**Cerebral Embolism**	**Subarachnoid Hemorrhage**	**Vascular Malformation and Intracranial Bleeding**
Onset	Generally during activity. Severe headache (if patient is able to report findings).	Prodromal episode of dizziness, aphasia,etc,often with improvement between attacks. Unrelated to activity.	Onset usually within seconds or minutes. No headache. Usually no prodrome. Unrelated to activity.	Sudden onset of severe headache unrelated to activity.	Sudden "stroke" in young patient. No headache. Unrelated to activity.
Course	Rapid hemiplegia and other phenomena over minutes to one hour.	Gradual progression over minutes to hours. Rapid improvement at times.	Rapid improvement may occur.	Variable; apt to be at worst in initial few days after onset.	Most critical period is usually in early stages.
History and related disorders	Suspect diagnosis especially if other hemorrhagic manifestations are present and in acute leukemia, aplastic anemia, thrombopenic purpura, and cirrhosis of the liver.	Evidence of arteriosclerosis, especially coronary, peripheral vessels, aorta. Associated disorders: diabetes mellitus, xanthomatosis.	Evidence of recent emboli: (1) other organs (spleen, kidneys, lungs), extremities, intestines; (2) several regions of brain in different cerebrovascular areas.	History of recurrent stiff neck, headaches, subarachnoid bleeding.	History of repeated subarachnoid hemorrhages, epilepsy.
Sensorium	Rapid progression to coma.	Relative preservation of consciousness.	Relative preservation of consciousness.	Relatively brief disturbance of consciousness.	Relatively brief disturbance of consciousness.
Neurologic examination	Focal neurologic signs or special arterial syndromes; nuchal rigidity.	Focal neurologic signs or special arterial syndromes.	Focal neurologic signs or special arterial syndromes.	Focal neurologic signs frequently absent; nuchal rigidity, positive Kernig and Brudzinski signs.	Focal neurologic signs; cranial bruit.

(*Table continues on opposite page*)

> *Measure and record intake and output.* (See Unit V, Chaps. 24 and 25.)

> *Include family members in your plan of care.* Let them help when possible, if they desire to do so, and help them to understand the patient's condition.

> *Provide a restful, quiet atmosphere* in the patient's room and provide *planned periods of rest.* Attempts are not made to awaken the comatose patient except for necessary care, e.g., bedpan, neurologic testing, and so forth.

> *Administer respiratory and circulatory stimulants* to comatose patients as ordered.

> *Administer other medications as ordered,* e.g., antibiotics, medications to control blood pressure and anticoagulants. Use sedatives and tranquilizers cautiously. Avoid opiates because they tend to depress respiratory centers and may obscure important observations.

> *Assist with diagnostic procedures and prepare the patient for surgery if surgery is ordered.*

> *Observe for visual and perceptual defects* and plan care accordingly.

> *Protect the patient's eye on the affected side* if necessary. Irrigate with physiologic saline and instill Tearisol drops in affected eye t.i.d. Cover with patch as necessary.

> *Give mouth care at least every three to four hours day and night,* giving special attention to the paralyzed side of the tongue and mouth.

> *Prevent intellectual regression and disorientation. Reorient the patient regaining consciousness, the confused, and the aphasic patient.* Establish communication with the aphasic patient.

Cerebrovascular diseases contribute to numerous *behavioral* as well as neurologic and physiologic deviations. Some of the associated behavioral changes that may follow CVA are confusion, loss of memory, language disorders, and emotional lability. Behavioral changes may also accompany the problems of paralysis, and there may be changes in body image, sensation, vision and perception. (See appropriate sections in Chapter 38.) Cerebral edema may contribute to a patient's confusion for a while.

Empathetic understanding is necessary as the pa-

TABLE 39–1. DIAGNOSIS OF CEREBROVASCULAR DISORDERS *(Continued)*

	Intracerebral Hemorrhage	Cerebral Thrombosis	Cerebral Embolism	Subarachnoid Hemorrhage	Vascular Malformation and Intracranial Bleeding
Special findings	Hypertensive retinopathy, cardiac hypertrophy, and other evidences of hypertensive cerebrovascular disease may be present.	Evidence of arteriosclerotic cardiovascular disease frequently present.	Cardiac arrhythmias or infarction (source of emboli usually in the heart).	Subhyaloid (preretinal) hemorrhages.	Subhyaloid (preretinal) hemorrhages and retinal angioma.
Blood pressure	Arterial hypertension.	Arterial hypertension frequent.	Normotensive.	Arterial hypertension frequent.	Normotensive.
CSF	Grossly bloody.	Clear.	Clear.	Grossly bloody.	Grossly bloody.
Skull x-ray	Shift of pineal to opposite side.	Calcification of internal carotid artery siphon visible; shift of pineal to opposite side may occur.	Pineal apt to show little if any displacement.	Partial calcification of walls of aneurysm sometimes noted.	Characteristic calcifications in skull x-rays may be present.
Cerebral angiography	Hemorrhagic area seen as avascular zone surrounded by stretched and displaced arteries and veins.	Arterial obstruction or narrowing of circle of Willis (internal carotid, etc).	Arterial obstruction of circle of Willis branches (internal carotid, etc).	Typical aneurysmal pattern in circle of Willis arteries (internal carotid, middle cerebral, anterior cerebral, etc).	Characteristic pattern showing cerebral arteriovenous malformation.
Brain scan	May show increased uptake in affected cerebral area. Most marked in 2–3 weeks, with diminution or clearing thereafter.			Apt to be normal.	Increased uptake may be seen in area of arteriovenous malformation.
Echoencephalography	May show shift of midline toward opposite side in those patients with a cerebral lesion acting as a mass.				

*Reproduced with permission from Chusid, J. G., and McDonald, J. J.: *Correlative Neuroanatomy and Functional Neurology.* 15th ed. Los Altos, Calif., Lange Medical Publications, 1973.

tient regains consciousness following CVA. Imagine what it would be like to regain consciousness following a stroke and find that your right arm and leg are paralyzed and that you cannot talk to anyone about your situation. Perhaps you cannot even understand what is said to you. This is the plight of the hemiplegic, aphasic patient.

The length of time that a patient must remain on bed rest following a CVA varies, depending on the preference of the physician and the cause of the CVA. Some physicians believe patients should be mobilized early, whereas others prefer a rather prolonged course of bed rest. One fairly standard practice is to begin mobilization and active rehabilitation as soon as consciousness is regained if the cause of hemiplegia is from a cerebral thrombosis. If a cerebral hemorrhage has caused the CVA, the patient cannot begin active mobilization until the bleeding appears to have stopped entirely; this may take weeks or months.

Some hospitals now have intensive care units (ICU) for neurologic patients. This is an area where the patient with a stroke may be given intensive treatment during the acute phase of his illness.[130] It is important to help the patient and his family to realize that such an area is not just for treatment, but also is designed to help the patient to avoid becoming more ill. The ICU may have such equipment as: oxygen and suction apparatus, endotracheal tubes, respirators, cardiac monitors with heart-rate meters and alarm systems, cardiac defibrillator, cardiac internal-external pacemaker, hypothermia equipment, alternating air pressure mattresses, emergency drug carts, and intravenous equipment. Figure 39–3 shows a patient receiving intensive care after a stroke.

The nurse caring for a CVA patient realizes that *cardiovascular considerations* are important during the patient's acute care for the following reasons:[130]

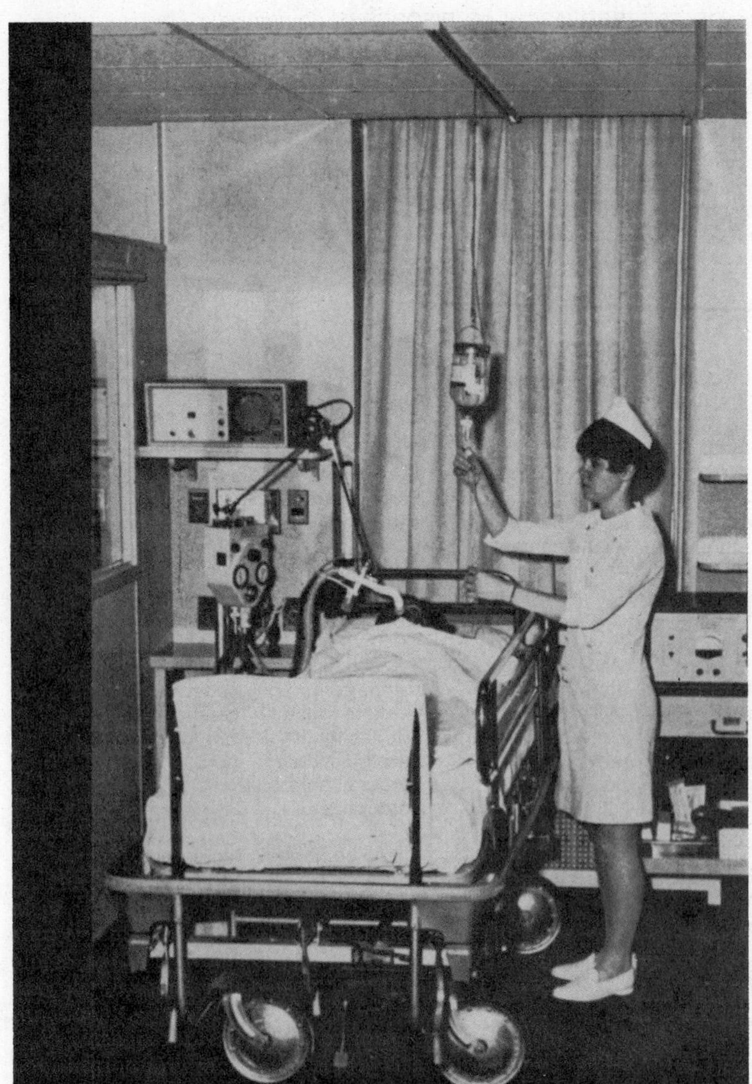

FIGURE 39–3. Patient receiving intensive care after stroke. (From Large, H., et al.: In the first stroke intensive care unit. *American Journal of Nursing* 69:76, January, 1969.)

> Stroke patients have a relatively high incidence of *arteriosclerosis*.
> Stroke may be a complication of *heart disease.*
> Hemorrhagic strokes are generally associated with longstanding *hypertensive cardiovascular disease.*
> *Arrhythmias* may develop from pressure being exerted on those brainstem centers of importance in heart regulation.
> *Pulmonary emboli* are a relatively common complication in immobilized patients.

Thus, if the CVA patient is receiving intensive care, the nurse needs to be able to recognize common arrhythmias on cardiac monitors; participate in emergency treatment of arrhythmias both by drugs and D.C. countershock; and know when it is appropriate to administer oxygen and when it is not.[130] (Cardiac disorders are discussed in Unit X.)

SPECIFIC TREATMENT. Once a specific diagnosis is established the physician institutes appropriate treatment based on the specific etiology. First we shall discuss treatment of a patient with a cerebral infarction resulting from thrombosis and embolism, followed by consideration of appropriate treatment of a patient with a CVA caused by hemorrhage (Table 39–2).

1. *Treatment of cerebral infarct (thrombosis, embolus).* The management of a recent cerebral infarct centers basically around attempts to: (a) increase perfusion of cerebral tissues with newly oxygenated blood; (b) support marginal tissue around the infarct; (c) stimulate restitution of function in those neurons in which the damage is reversible; and (d) prevent further clot formation and additional cerebral impairment. Recently additional attempts have been made to dissolve or surgically remove existing clots, and to surgically reconstruct partially occluded arteries.

Treatment of cerebral infarct may be directed at:

> *Maintaining cerebral blood flow.* Bed rest, with the head lower than the heart, helps to maintain cerebral blood flow.
> *Reducing the brain's metabolic requirements. Hypothermia* has been advocated for this purpose, but as yet is of questionable value.
> *Maintaining blood pressure and reducing any factors that acutely reduce cardiac output.* Maintenance of circulation, prevention of shock.
> *Correcting any conditions that may have precipitated the infarct,* e.g., treatment of myocardial infarction.
> *Reducing pooling of blood in the lower extremities* by applying elastic stockings.
> *Avoiding sudden postural changes.*
> *Improving cerebral circulation,* e.g., by a *block of the stellate ganglion* and administration of *vasodilators.*
> *Preventing further clot formation. Anticoagulants,* e.g., Dicumarol and heparin, may be administered.

Many strokes progress in a fluctuating or stepwise pattern. Such progressing strokes, due to an enlarging cerebral thrombus with downstream propagation and embolization, are often called *strokes-in-evolution* or *strokes-in-progress.* These stroke patients may benefit from *immediate* anticoagulant therapy. It is thus important for physician and nurse to: (a) identify *early* those strokes due to thrombo-occlusive disease which develop gradually over several hours or days in a fluctuating or stepwise progression; (b) rapidly establish a diagnosis of thrombosis (and rule out intracranial hemorrhage); and (c) immediately institute appropriate anticoagulant therapy.[251]

Agreement has not been reached concerning how long anticoagulant therapy should be continued. However, the *appearance of signs of bleeding anywhere in the body* (e.g., gums, urine) *indicates that treatment should be stopped immediately and vitamin K administered.* The nurse should thus watch for signs of bleeding when patients are on anticoagulant therapy. (Anticoagulant therapy is discussed further in Unit X.)

Recently attempts have been made to *dissolve a fresh clot* by immediately administering plasminogen activators, plasmin, and proteolytic enzymes. The value of this therapy is yet to be evaluated.

Also attempts have been made to *surgically* reestablish circulation to the brain by: (a) removing clots from thrombosed carotid or vertebral arteries, or (b) reconstructing arteries that are partially or completely occluded. The latter form of surgery appears useful in treating carotid or basilar insufficiency. It is debatable whether a fresh clot can be removed from a major vessel in time to prevent necrosis in the region of infarction. Intracranial surgery is discussed in Chapter 40.

A long-term treatment goal is the prevention or alleviation of atherosclerosis and hypertension, e.g., by low fat diet, weight reduction, prophylactic surgery, and reduction of hypercholesterolemia.

2. *Treatment of intracerebral hemorrhage.* Goals of therapy are to: (a) preserve life; (b) minimize resultant disability; and (c) prevent recurrence. The clinical care specifically centers on:

> *Control of hyperthermia.* Often mass intracerebral hemorrhages are accompanied by a rapid increase in temperature. A refrigerator blanket or ice packs may be indicated.
> *Control of convulsive seizures.* In cases complicated by seizures diphenylhydantoin (Dilantin) may be given I.M. every 4 hours. Intravenous amobarbital (Amytal) and other intravenous sedatives should be avoided.
> *Prevention or alleviation of hypertension.* When blood pressure is *elevated* it must be gradually returned to nearly normal levels. If blood pressure is lowered rapidly, a hypotension-induced cerebral ischemic infarct may be precipitated. (Hypertension is discussed in Unit X.) Controlled diet may be necessary for weight reduction in the obese patient.

Five important symptoms that may foreshadow cerebral hemorrhage in the hypertensive patient are: *(1) severe occipital (back of head) or nuchal (nape of neck) headaches; (2) vertigo (dizziness) or syncope (fainting); (3) motor or sensory disturbances (e.g., tingling, paresthesias, transient paralysis); (4) nosebleeds; and (5) retinal hemorrhages. Report such symptoms so that prophylactic measures can be employed to try to prevent CVA.*

> *Symptomatic treatment of severe headache, stiff neck, restlessness, and delirium.* Delirium can last for as long as two weeks. (The clinical management of delirium is discussed in Unit III.) *Relief of headache.* An acetylsalicylic acid compound (Empirin) with codeine by mouth, or codeine hypodermically may be given. At times codeine sulfate orally or parenterally may be necessary as often as every two hours to relieve headache. Frequently this also relieves restlessness. Avoid other narcotics for analgesia since they depress respiration. *Control of restlessness.* At times it is necessary to administer chlorpromazine (Thorazine) intramuscularly every three to four hours as indicated. Make certain the patient is not restless for preventable reasons, e.g., a full bladder.

TABLE 39–2. THERAPY IN CEREBRAL VASCULAR DISEASE (FROM REPORT OF THE CEREBRAL VASCULAR STUDY GROUP OF THE NATIONAL INSTITUTE OF NEUROLOGICAL DISEASE AND BLINDNESS)*

Aim	Methods
1. AIMS WHICH MIGHT BE INCLUDED IN A TREATMENT PROGRAM	
a. Infarction	
(1) Atherothrombosis	
(*a*) Restore circulation when stroke has occurred	position, CO_2 inhalation, vasodilation, etc. fibrinolysin thromboendarterectomy
(*b*) Prevention of a thrombotic stroke of which there has been prodromal ischemia (*c*) Arrest progression of thrombosis-in-evolution	improved early diagnosis position anticoagulant fibrinolysin surgical endarterectomy
(*d*) Prevention or alleviation of atherosclerosis	low-fat diet reduce hypercholesterolemia; estrogens weight reduction prophylactic surgery
(*d*) Prevention or alleviation of hypertension	
(2) Embolism	
(*a*) Restore circulation when stroke has occurred	as above (1) (*a*) embolectomy
(*b*) Prevent occurrence or recurrence of embolism	anticoagulant corrective cardiac surgery prevent coronary heart disease
b. Hemorrhage	
(1) Intracerebral hemorrhage	
(*a*) Surgical evacuation of hemorrhage	
(*b*) Prevention or alleviation of hypertension	
(2) Ruptured saccular aneurysm	
(*a*) Surgical evacuation of intracerebral hemorrhage	
(*b*) Prevention of recurrence of bleeding	surgical obliteration of sac ligation of vessel on which aneurysm lies application of plastic, *etc.*

To the above methods of management must be added (*a*) General medical management of the patient in the acute phase and (*b*) Rehabilitation of the patient physically, psychologically and socially.

*From Merritt, H. H.: *A Textbook of Neurology.* 4th ed. Philadelphia, Lea & Febiger, 1967.

> *Prevention of straining,* e.g., straining at stool, excessive coughing, vomiting, or lifting. Constipation must be avoided and mild laxatives, stool softeners, or colon lavages may be given (particularly when codeine is required for pain relief). Prevent aspiration, choking, excessive coughing, and vomiting by withholding oral fluids and food for 24 to 48 hours, followed by clear liquids for another 24 to 48 hours, and then a soft diet.

> *Provision for rest and quiet.* During the acute phase following intracerebral hemorrhage the patient is typically kept in bed for as long as the presence of stiff neck, headache, and prostration require. Since rebleeding usually does not occur when rupture is due to hypertensive vascular disease or A-V anomaly, the patient may be up as soon as he feels well enough. Some physicians believe that following intracranial hemorrhage moderate sedation, hypotensive drugs and bed rest should be continued for 10 to 14 days, or longer if indicated.

> *Reduction of increased intracranial pressure.* This may be achieved by the rectal administration of 25 per cent solution of magnesium sulfate, or by lumbar puncture. The patient must not be excessively dehydrated, and only enough fluid is removed to relieve severe headache. If a lumbar puncture is carried out, the physician does *not* perform the Queckenstedt test. The value of LP in patients with intracerebral hemorrhage is uncertain, and at times the procedure may be hazardous; e.g., it may cause serious uncal or cerebellar herniation. On the other hand, if a large amount of blood has accumulated in the subarachnoid space, an LP may help to relieve increased intracranial pressure.

> *Operative removal of blood clot.* Whether or not to operate on the patient who has had an intracerebral hemorrhage, and when to operate, are widely debated topics. In carefully selected patients this surgery may be lifesaving and may reduce the neurologic consequences of the CVA. Many patients are not suitable candidates for surgery because of their poor general condition.

Some physicians recommend that arteriograms not be performed until it appears that the patient will survive the initial hemorrhage (seven to 10 days). At that time it can be determined if surgical intervention is possible. Surgery is not contemplated when angiography shows that severe vascular spasm is still present. There is no known method of stopping a hemorrhaging vessel without surgery.

3. *Summary.* To *summarize the basic treatment of all CVA's* during the acute phase, remember that the treatment of CVA hinges on a specific diagnosis of the cause of the stroke. Once this is established, proper treatment is provided which is directed at the specific cause of the CVA. Basically treatment may include:

> *Anticoagulants* for strokes resulting from infarction (thrombus, embolus); these are given to slow the blood's coagulation time with the goal of preventing clot formation. Anticoagulants are given only if hemorrhage has been ruled out.

> *Medications* may also be given to reduce dangerously high *blood pressure,* or to elevate alarmingly low blood pressure.

> *Surgery* may be employed in selected cases to control some hemorrhages, to remove clots, or to sew a graft into an artery before it can rupture. CVA's may result from a plugged artery in the neck, which can be surgically corrected.

Transient Cerebral Ischemic Attacks ("Little Strokes")

Transient ischemic attacks (TIA's) are *brief, reversible* episodes of neurologic dysfunction caused by a temporary focal cerebral ischemia. TIA's are also called "intermittent cerebrovascular insufficiency." The basic abnormality common to all patients with TIA's is a *transient* decrease in delivery of blood to a focal area of the cerebrum or brainstem. Numerous factors can cause this ischemia.

Occlusive disease of the extracranial cerebral vessels is the most common cause of TIA's, as with cerebral vascular accidents, although there are many other causes. The most frequent site of this occlusion is the origin of the internal carotid artery; however, lesions may also occur at the origin of the common carotid or vertebral arteries. The symptoms vary, depending upon which area of the brain is ischemic. Examples of the types of symptoms produced by TIA's are: visual, auditory, or vestibular disturbances; various motor and sensory disturbances; headache; slowing of mental processes; or convulsions.

Generally TIA's last only minutes (often two to 10 minutes) to an hour. Occasionally they may last only a few seconds or as long as 24 hours. While the attacks are frequently recurrent, some patients have only one or two TIA's. TIA's may occur for as long as two years prior to cerebral infarction, or clusters of TIA's may first appear only a few hours or days before cerebral infarction occurs. Between attacks a patient's neurologic examination is generally entirely normal.

Three important investigations in the *diagnosis* of TIA's involving the internal carotid artery are: (1) stethoscopic examination for bruits; (2) ophthalmodynamometry, i.e., indirect measurement of pressure in the retinal artery; and (3) angiographic studies of intracranial and extracranial blood vessels.

Vascular surgery or anticoagulation may prevent fatal attacks in some patients who have TIA's. At the present time *surgical treatment* is available only for obstructive lesions within the extracranial vessels. The procedure most commonly performed is *endarterectomy,* i.e., surgical removal of the thickened areas of the innermost lining of the affected artery. Surgery is most successfully performed before a stenotic artery has become completely occluded. Those patients who are unable to have surgery may benefit from prolonged *anticoagulant therapy* in an attempt to: (1) reduce the incidence of emboli; (2) prevent thrombus formation; and (3) alter blood coagulation factors or reduce blood sludging. Not all persons are candidates for anticoagulant therapy. Patients are selected cautiously for this therapy to prevent hemorrhagic complications.

Intracranial Aneurysms and Primary (Spontaneous) Subarachnoid Hemorrhage

Statistics indicate that approximately 10 per cent of all cerebrovascular lesions result from ruptured aneurysms occurring in one of the vessels in the subarachnoid space. *This serious condition is the cause of death in over 50 per cent of all fatal cerebrovascular lesions in patients below age 45.* The symptoms resulting from aneurysms in the subarachnoid space can occur at any age, but most commonly occur between the ages of 35 and 65. Thus, this condition typically affects a younger population than most CVA's.

Hemorrhage into the subarachnoid space may occur spontaneously in patients with blood dyscrasias, intracranial tumors, vascular anomalies (angiomas), intracerebral hemorrhage, or infections of the nervous system. *The most common cause of subarachnoid hemorrhage is trauma to the head which ruptures meningeal vessels;* this form of subarachnoid hemorrhage is discussed later. Spontaneous hemorrhage in the subarachnoid space may also occur following *rupture of an aneurysm in the subarachnoid space.* This type of hemorrhage is considered here.

Congenital saccular aneurysms are the most common type of aneurysm of the brain's blood vessels. These aneurysms, which result from a congenital weakness of the vessel, *are the most frequent cause of primary uncomplicated subarachnoid hemorrhage.* Although any of the intracranial vessels may be the site of an aneurysm, they most often occur on the internal carotid or middle cerebral artery.

The *symptoms* of intracranial aneurysms are usually of two kinds: those due to *compression* of the brain tissue or cranial nerves, and those resulting from *leakage* from or rupture of the aneurysm. The symptoms resulting from compression are less common. When they do occur the most common focal symptoms are caused by the partial or complete paralysis of the muscles supplied by the third or sixth cranial nerves. Visual defects or convulsions may also be present, and cranial bruits may be heard over the affected side. Some patients experience headaches. However, let us emphasize that *in most cases the aneurysm is "silent" and produces no symptoms until it begins to bleed.*

In over 90 per cent of patients with intracranial aneurysms the *onset of symptoms occurs suddenly,* due to leakage or rupture from a "silent" aneurysm. When this happens, the *patient experiences sudden severe headache* followed by mental cloudiness or confusion. Almost always stiffness of the neck and Kernig's sign occur within a few hours of the onset; pain may also occur in the lower back and legs. Prognosis is poor if loss of consciousness occurs at the onset. About one-third of patients develop paralysis or aphasia immediately or a few hours after the onset. Cranial nerve palsies may also develop.

Following small hemorrhages the vital signs may be normal. However, they are more likely to be altered for a few days, with moderate temperature elevation (100 to 102°F.) and slightly increased pulse and respiratory rates. In over half the patients the blood pressure is elevated. Intracranial pressure is usually increased and the CSF is bloody. The CSF white count and protein count are increased in proportion to the amount of blood in the fluid. Usually the diagnosis of intracranial aneurysm as the cause of primary subarachnoid hemorrhage can be definitely established by cerebral angiography.

The *clinical course* is variable for patients who survive the attack. Sometimes the aneurysm continues to leak slowly and then after a few days ruptures severely, causing death. At other times the aneurysm may seal off and then suddenly rupture later. It is unusual for rupture to occur after six months. In patients who recover, the bleeding stops and improvement takes place gradually.

Treatment may include the following:

> *Quiet, undisturbed bed rest, flat in bed,* and *avoidance of straining.*

> Administration of *analgesics to relieve headache.*

> *Lumbar puncture,* to establish diagnosis, and *angiography,* if surgery is contemplated.

> *Surgery* is indicated when there is evidence of a large intracortical clot. In addition to evacuating the clot the surgical treatment may include: ligation of the common or internal carotid artery in the neck, clipping or ligating the neck of the aneurysm, or wrapping it with muscle or other substances. Sometimes the aneurysm is "trapped," with clips placed on either side of it.

Debate exists as to whether the patient with an aneurysm should be treated conservatively (quiet bed rest for a number of weeks) or surgically, as discussed. The choice of surgery as opposed to medical treatment is governed by such factors as the location and size of the aneurysm, the patient's clinical status, and the surgeon's skill and experience. Many neurosurgeons believe that operation is essential because of the high mortality rate with conservative treatment and because of possible recurrence of the hemorrhage.

VASCULAR LESIONS OF THE SPINAL CORD

Vascular lesions that occur in the spinal cord are similar to those occurring in the brain in that they are caused by rupture, thrombosis, or embolism of the blood vessels supplying the spinal cord. Trauma is usually the cause of *hemorrhage* into the spinal cord or its covering. *Embolism* of the spinal vessels rarely occurs except in caisson disease, i.e., decompression sickness. Unlike the cerebral blood vessels, arteriosclerosis of the spinal vessels is not a common cause of *thrombosis.* Thrombosis of the spinal vessels most often is secondary to an inflammatory reaction in the meninges, or else it results from compression of the vessels by tumors, granulomas, and abscesses in the epidural space.

Myelomalacia

Myelomalacia, or *softening of the spinal cord,* develops as the result of vascular *occlusion.* Myelomalacia is a serious condition which has a poor prognosis because there is usually little or no return of function to the involved areas. The diagnosis is presumed whenever there is the *sudden* appearance of symptoms of a transverse myelitis.

The *symptoms* of myelomalacia vary, depending upon the level of the thrombosis. For example, a cervical level occlusion produces *sudden* quadriplegia. Occlusion at the thoracic level produces similar symptoms except that the arms are not affected. Involvement at the level of the lumbar spine results in paraplegia, disturbed bladder and bowel function, and impaired pain and temperature sensation. (See Chapter 38.)

The *treatment* of myelomalacia is two-pronged: one aspect is concerned with the symptomatic care of the problems resulting from the cord lesion, e.g., the paralysis, loss of sensation; the other is directed at treatment of the disease that caused the vascular lesion in the first place. Treatment of the cause of the condition does not produce any significant degree of improvement in symptoms resulting from the myelomalacia. This is because, as we have emphasized before, it is impossible to restore nervous tissue that has been destroyed.

Hematomyelia

Hematomyelia refers to *hemorrhage into the substance of the spinal cord.* This condition almost always follows trauma. The symptoms vary, depending upon the size of the hemorrhage. Typically, symptoms develop *suddenly,* immediately after a spinal injury.

Diagnostically the physician must identify whether the cause of the sudden symptoms (following trauma) is hematomyelia or a fracture and dislocation of the vertebrae. If a fracture dislocation is discovered immediate surgery is indicated to relieve cord compression. A fracture dislocation is identified by seeing the area of involvement on x-ray and by the presence of complete subarachnoid block when a lumbar puncture is performed. Because hematomyelia has a better prognosis for spontaneous return of function than does myelomalacia, rehabilitative care is highly important.

VASCULAR LESIONS OF THE CEREBRAL VEINS AND SINUSES

Lesions do not often occur in the small *cerebral veins;* however, they may be affected by extension of an infectious or thrombotic process in the large dural sinuses. Focal neurologic symptoms are produced when occlusion of the cortical and subcortical veins does occur. The large *dural sinuses* may become thrombosed if they are infected or if there is infection in the epidural or subdural spaces. In adults the dural sinuses may be occluded by trauma, tumor masses, or such conditions as the formation of clots in polycythemia. The dural sinuses that are most often thrombosed are the lateral, cavernous, and superior sagittal.

The *superior sagittal sinus* is less commonly affected by an infective thrombosis than either the lateral or cavernous sinus. Thrombosis of the *lateral sinus* is generally secondary to otitis media and mastoiditis; however, this condition rarely occurs today due to effective antibiotic chemotherapy of these conditions.

Cavernous sinus thrombosis typically occurs secondary to suppurative processes in the orbit, nasal sinuses, or upper half of the face. The infective process commonly first involves one sinus and then rapidly spreads to the opposite side. Symptoms of a septic thrombosis occur suddenly. The patient is acutely ill, has a septic kind of febrile reaction, and experiences pain in the eye. Visual acuity may or may not be affected, and pupillary reactions may or may not be preserved. The pupils may be small or dilated; the corneae are cloudy and corneal ulcers may develop. Although fatal until recently, this condition may now be treated with antibiotics, and possibly anticoagulants.

DEVELOPMENTAL DEFECTS OF THE NERVOUS SYSTEM

Congenital defects of the nervous system range from minor defects which are practically unnoticeable (such as a slight decrease in intelligence due to abnormal development) to striking, sometimes fatal, gross abnormalities, such as: absence of the head *(acrania);* absence of the brain *(anencephalus);* extremely small brain *(microcephalus);* and excessive enlargement of ventricular cavities of the brain *(hydrocephalus).*

The central nervous system begins to develop early in intrauterine life and continues to develop both functionally and structurally for several years. Various defects of the brain or spinal cord may be present at birth. Such developmental defects include the *absence of a part or the whole of various structures* of the brain and *failure in the development of or closure of the cranial or spinal bones,* with or without accompanying damage to the brain or spinal cord.

HYDROCEPHALUS

Hydrocephalus refers to an abnormal accumulation of cerebrospinal fluid in the cranial vault. This condition most frequently occurs in infants. Since the bones of the skull are not fused together in the infant, the pressure of the accumulating fluid forces the head to actually enlarge, sometimes tremendously, and the forehead to become prominent (Fig. 39-4). Adults have no cranial enlargement with hydrocephalus because the cranium is fixed in size and cannot give. In both infants and adults, the mounting pressure caused by excess fluid with-

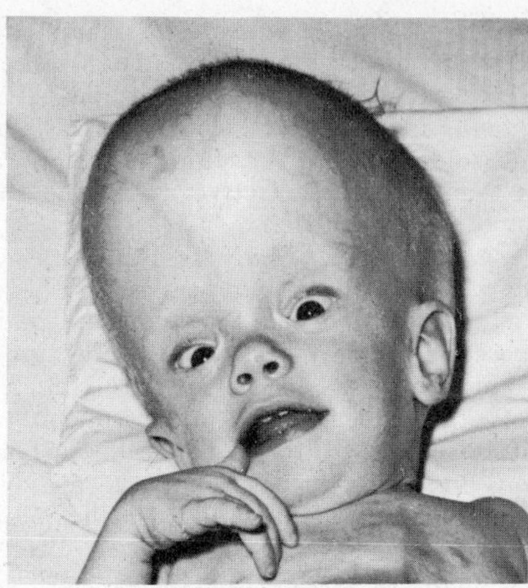

FIGURE 39-4. Hydrocephalus. (From Marlow, D. R.: *Textbook of Pediatric Nursing.* 4th ed. 1973.)

in the skull squeezes the brain tissue against the skull, causing tissue atrophy and tissue death, convulsions, and mental weakness.

Hydrocephalus present at birth is called *congenital, primary,* or *chronic hydrocephalus. Secondary* or *acute hydrocephalus* may result from meningitis (e.g., tubercular meningitis), obstruction of the brain's venous outflow, or spread of the inflammation of otitis media from the ear to the cranial cavity.

Various surgical procedures have been developed to treat hydrocephalus by implanting artificial drains in the brain and creating new paths of circulation for the cerebrospinal fluid. For example, silicone tubes or tubes of various other compositions may be placed from the brain ventricle, behind the ear, and down the neck under the skin. Finally, the tube is spliced into the jugular vein where the fluid can drain into the circulating blood.

SPINA BIFIDA

Spina bifida is a term used to cover a wide range of closure defects which generally occur in the lower lumbar region. A minor defect may occur only in the bony vertebral arches; however, in a more severe defect, the meninges or the meninges along with the spinal cord are displaced backward, although the defect remains covered with skin.

A *meningocele* (protruding sac of meninges) or a *meningomyelocele* (protruding sac containing meninges, spinal cord, and roots) may occur with spina bifida as elements in the spinal canal balloon out through the defect. In the latter unfortunate condition, the infant is generally paralyzed in both motor and sensory spheres below the level of the deformity. Neural control of bladder and bowel function is also typically absent. Additionally, the protruding sac, containing CSF, is often dangerously fragile and infection is possible, producing fatal meningitis. Developmental defects are discussed more completely in pediatrics textbooks.

HEREDOFAMILIAL AND DEGENERATIVE DISEASES OF THE NERVOUS SYSTEM

Numerous conditions that affect the central nervous system have unknown causes. Most of those to be discussed in this section fall into this category.

Research may some day demonstrate that some disorders that are currently of unknown etiology result from damage caused by exogenous or endogenous toxins or genetically conditioned metabolic defects. Recently there has been increasing interest in the possibility that some chronic diseases of the nervous system (e.g., amyotrophic lateral sclerosis, multiple sclerosis) could be caused by slow and latent viruses. Currently there is no proof that any neurologic disease of man is caused by such organisms, but research is underway which could prove differently.

EXTRAPYRAMIDAL DISORDERS

Various disorders that involve the basal ganglia are referred to as extrapyramidal disorders. These conditions are characterized by abnormal involuntary movements (dyskinesias), disturbances in bodily posture, and changes in muscle tone. We shall consider two extrapyramidal disorders in this section: Huntington's chorea, and parkinsonian syndrome.

Huntington's Chorea

Huntington's chorea is also called hereditary chorea, adult chorea, and chronic progressive chorea. Huntington's chorea is a hereditary disease of the basal ganglia and cerebral cortex that typically appears in adult life (ages 35 to 50). It is characterized by choreiform (rapid, jerky) movements and mental deterioration.

Although this disorder is relatively rare, its incidence may be high in areas where affected families have lived for several generations. The condition may be transmitted by either sex, and both sexes are equally affected. About 50 per cent of offspring inherit the disorder.

No effective treatment exists for Huntington's chorea. This fact plus the hereditary nature of the disease should make it inadvisable for any member of an afflicted family to produce children; genetic counseling is imperative. Huntington's chorea relentlessly progresses, producing total incapacity and ultimately death (generally 15 years after onset).

Parkinsonism (Parkinson's Disease)

Parkinsonism, formerly called Parkinson's disease, is now viewed as a clinical syndrome rather than as one specific disease. Therefore, the term "parkinsonism" has come into frequent usage. There are several forms of parkinsonism. The original, which Dr. James Parkinson first wrote about in 1817, is now called "idiopathic parkinsonism," (also known as shaking palsy, or paralysis agitans). Parkinsonism may be classified etiologically as follows:[177]

> *Idiopathic* (most common).
> *Postencephalitic* (declining numbers).
> *Atherosclerotic* (parkinsonism with other signs produced by atherosclerosis of the CNS).
> *Drug induced* (especially by certain tranquilizers).
> *Toxic,* due to *carbon monoxide poisoning* (rare); *chronic manganese poisoning* (rare); or *chronic mercury poisoning* (rare).
> *Midbrain compression* (not uncommon).
> *Traumatic* (rare).

Whatever the specific classification, parkinsonism is generally considered as an extrapyramidal disorder affecting the basal ganglia. The disorder results from interruption of the balance-coordinating extrapyramidal tracts, whose main cell stations are located in the brain's basal ganglia.

Etiology. As we have shown, the clinical syndrome of parkinsonism may result from or occur in association with numerous factors. In the majority of cases the cause is unknown, i.e., the disease is *idiopathic. This type of illness is one of the most common nonvascular causes of neurologic disability. Postencephalitic* parkinsonism formerly occurred as a sequel in a large percentage of persons who suffered from epidemic encephalitis, but now is rarely seen. There is no evidence that *atherosclerosis* actually causes a true parkinsonism syndrome; however, when the CNS is affected by atherosclerosis some manifestations of parkinsonism may occur.[177] As indicated in our classification, conditions resembling parkinsonism may result from poisoning with carbon monoxide, mercury, or manganese. These are rare conditions, as are parkinsonism resulting from trauma to the head and following CVA.

It is well known that symptoms typical of parkinsonism may develop in patients who are given large doses of tranquilizers for an extended period; following withdrawal of the offending medication these symptoms disappear. The *piperazine group* of drugs, e.g., trifluoperazine (Stelazine), is the most likely to produce parkinsonism. Drugs of the *chlorpromazine group,* e.g., Largactil, will produce similar symptoms if given in large doses. Less than half the patients on tranquilizers develop symptoms of parkinsonism. Sometimes parkinsonian effects occur as a result of *midbrain compression.* For example, parkinsonism can occur postoperatively from brainstem compression as a result of postoperative edema. In sum, while the majority of patients with parkinsonian symptoms probably have some form of degeneration involving the basal ganglia and substantia nigra, similar disorders of motor function can result from other pathologic processes.

It is not unusual to find multiple cases of idiopathic parkinsonism in a family, but more frequently the condition occurs sporadically and is not considered to be a familial disorder.

Course and Symptoms. Parkinsonism is slowly progressive. The course is often rapid for the first few years and then levels off. The advance of symptoms most often extends over several decades. The first symptoms most often appear in the sixth decade, and slightly less often in the fifth.

Early in the illness the patient may notice a slight *slowing up* of the ability to perform usual activities. A general feeling of *stiffness* may be noticed, along with *mild diffuse muscular pains.*

Tremor is a common early symptom of parkinsonism. It usually occurs in one of the upper limbs. Tremor is commonly accompanied by *"pill-rolling" movements* of the thumb against the fingers. Typically the tremor is an alternating tremor (i.e., it consists of alternating movements of opposing muscles) and it varies in intensity and distribution. Usually tremor is reduced or abolished by voluntary movement; however, some patients have an intention tremor (i.e., voluntary movement worsens the tremor). In such a case, the tremor may be the main cause of disability; however, more often the main cause of disability is *akinesia* (i.e., absence or poverty of movements) or *dyskinesia* (i.e., impaired voluntary activity resulting in fragmentary or incomplete movements).

Dyskinesia, another frequent early symptom, often begins by affecting one arm, or only the fingers and thumb. Complicated movements are slow and difficult to perform. Muscular power usually becomes affected when the disease is well advanced. Failure to swing the affected arm while walking, i.e., *loss of automatic associated movements,* is one of the earliest symptoms of parkinsonism. *Poverty and slowness of movements* may occur in all the normal activities of daily living, e.g., dressing, eating. *Impaired handwriting* is another early symptom. Rigidity of the arms results in *jerky, "cogwheel" motions.*

The effects of parkinsonism on the legs appear as *various disorders of locomotion.* In the early stages there may be a slight stiffness of one leg in walking, and the corresponding arm may be held flexed at the elbow and abducted at the shoulder. Also, the patient may catch or drag one foot. Later, when both sides of the body are involved, a typical *shuffling gait with little steps* appears. Some patients begin to take quicker and quicker steps *(propulsive gait);* occasionally this occurs in the backward direction *(retropulsion).* The patient with a propulsive gait is in danger of falling and at times has difficulty stopping unless he can grasp something or have someone slow him down by holding his arm. Some patients have difficulty starting locomotion, and then break into a propulsive gait, whereas others merely walk with a slow, shuffling gait without swinging their arms. In advanced cases the *posture* becomes affected so that the patient stands with his head flexed, shoulders stooped, and spine arched forward.

Often a *characteristic facial appearance* occurs with parkinsonism and the face appears stiff, mask-like, and staring (Fig. 39–5). Sometimes *oculogyric crises* occur, and the patient's eyes are fixed upward, upward and to one side, or downward. These crises may last for several hours. *Blepharospasm* producing almost total closure of the eyelid is a symptom in some patients.

Typically the *speech* of a patient with parkinsonism is low pitched, monotonous, slow, lacks modulation, and is poorly articulated (dysarthric). Frequently *saliva flows involuntarily from the mouth* because it is not directed to the back of the mouth and swallowed. Various *autonomic effects* accompany parkinsonism, e.g., lacrimation, constipation, incontinence, and decreased sexual capacity. Excessive perspiration and undue sensitivity to heat also commonly occur.

Parkinsonism does not usually affect the *intellectual faculties*. However, because the emotional strain of living with such a condition is great, *mood disturbances* often occur. Usually the symptoms of parkinsonism are greatly intensified during periods of emotional tension.

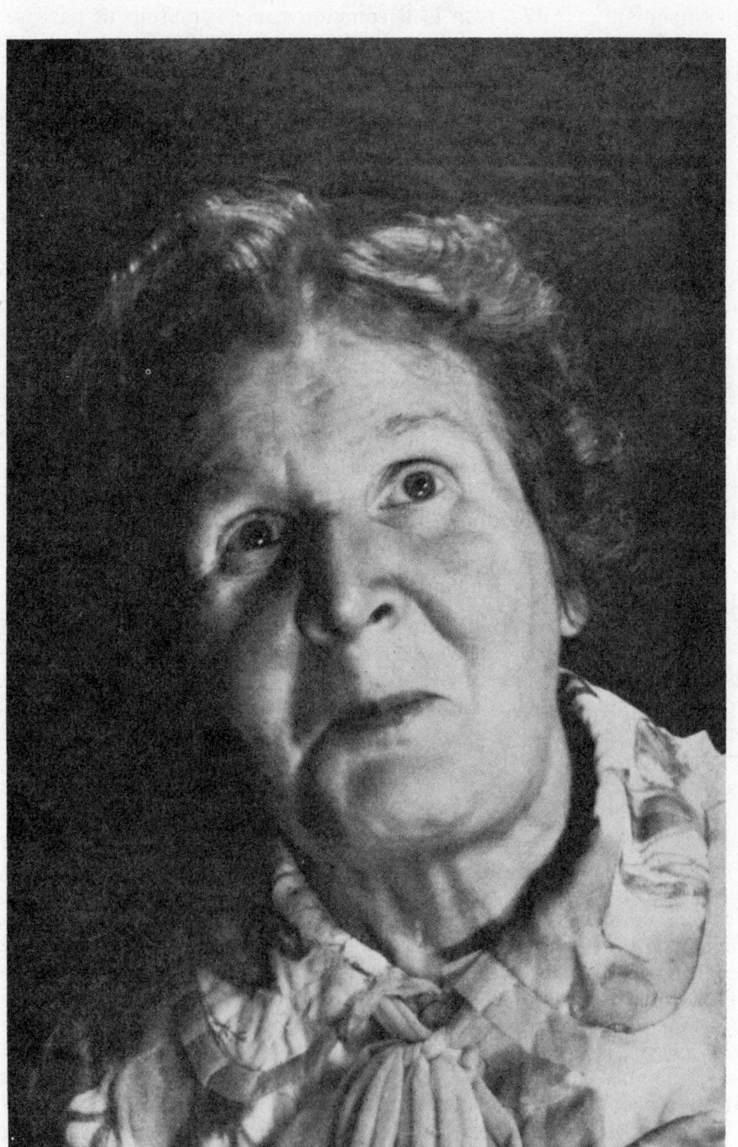

FIGURE 39–5. Typical "mask-like" expression occurring with parkinsonism. (From Oliver, L.: *PARKINSON'S DISEASE.* Courtesy of Charles C Thomas, Springfield, Ill., 1967.)

Many symptoms of parkinsonism vary in degree, are seldom proportional to each other, and are highly individualized.

Clinical Care. In well advanced cases of parkinsonism the *diagnosis* is easily made by finding the characteristic manifestations of the disorder. Generally the results of laboratory examinations are within normal limits.

It has been said that *parkinsonism is the U.S.A.'s third most crippling illness.* Thus, the nurse needs to be thoroughly acquainted with the clinical care indicated for this condition. *Treatment* may include such measures as: medications, surgery, physical therapy, psychologic support and education (for both patient and family), rehabilitative efforts, and efforts to maintain a general state of good health.

> *Physical therapy* helps to combat the muscular rigidity that accompanies the illness and helps to prevent contractures.

> The patient must be taught to pay attention to his *posture* and prevent postural deformities from occurring. Observe carefully for the tendency of the head and neck to become flexed. *Prevention* is imperative. Postural exercises are important to keep the head and neck erect. During periods of rest the patient should lie on a firm bed without a pillow (to prevent the spine from being flexed forward); periodically the patient should lie prone.

> *Gait training* is also important because of the tendency for the gait to become shuffling and propulsive.

> All measures that *improve general health* are encouraged, e.g., fresh air, moderate exercise, adequate periods of rest, and a good diet. The progress of the illness may be slowed by such measures. The patient with parkinsonism often has *difficulty maintaining weight* because of problems with eating and side effects from medications. The patient should be weighed periodically. Supplementary feedings may help to keep up the patient's caloric intake. Electrical food warming trays keep the patient's food hot and yet allow him time to rest while eating.

> The patient with *excessive tremor* may find he can partially control the tremor of his hands and arms if he sits in an arm chair and grips the arms of the chair.

> A *moderate consumption of alcohol* is frequently beneficial in parkinsonism; it reduces tremor and also has a *tranquilizing effect.* Various medications may be prescribed to help the patient to rest well at night.

> If the patient's *voice* is extremely weak he may benefit from using a small electric voice amplifier, such as is used following laryngectomy. (See Unit XIV.)

> *Constipation* often poses problems for the patient with parkinsonism because of side effects of medications, lack of exercise, lack of saliva in the gastrointestinal tract (lost through drooling), and weakness of the muscles necessary for adequate defecation. If swallowing is impaired the patient may not be taking an adequate fluid intake. Factors that may help to reduce constipation are discussed elsewhere.

> The patient with far advanced disease may have extreme *difficulty in swallowing* and is in danger of choking while eating or drinking. Have suction available and do not rush the patient as he eats. Aspiration pneumonia is a serious, sometimes fatal, occurrence.

> *Lassitude* is frequently present with parkinsonism and the patient may therefore want to accept more help than is necessary or is good for him.

A cheerful mental outlook is to be encouraged, and it is helpful if the patient can live in a pleasant emotional climate. As his condition progresses he will need increasing help, which should be given as unobtrusively as possible. Patient and family need to realize that parkinsonism does not impair sight or hearing, nor does it shorten life. Education about the illness should be given to both patient and family. It should be emphasized that the condition does *not* cause eventual paralysis and is painful only if the patient neglects to perform his proper exercises and movements faithfully (or if this is neglected by others).

While considerable advances have been made in the surgical treatment of parkinsonism recently, medical treatment is still the backbone of therapy. Certain factors are of importance in the *drug therapy of parkinsonism:*

> All antiparkinsonism medications are given after meals to obtain an even effect, to prevent gastric irritation, and to minimize dryness of the mouth during meals.

> Great individual variation exists in the responses to antiparkinsonian medications. Dosages are individualized. Usually small doses are given at first and then increased to the maximum point of tolerance. Combinations of drugs are more effective than single medications. A variety of medications that can be used in various combinations are available.

> Long-term chemotherapy is necessary and can give symptomatic improvement.

> Sudden withdrawal of medications is inadvisable, since it may precipitate a parkinsonian crisis. This may happen if a patient is admitted to a hospital and his medications are taken from him. If treatment is temporarily interrupted for any reason, the medications should be given in small doses once treatment is resumed. Tolerance is lost rapidly and is regained slowly. Old medications are gradually withdrawn when a new medication is being introduced.

> In all parkinsonian conditions the rigidity is favorably affected by medications, whereas tremor is not often diminished.

Recently *synthetic medications with an atropine-like action* have been developed and have almost entirely replaced the formerly used belladonna alkaloids. The synthetic compounds have less severe toxic side effects and are longer acting. *Most medications used today are anticholinergic, antispasmodic, and antihistaminic. The anticholinergic effect is the most important factor in the treatment of parkinsonism.*

The *synthetic compounds* commonly used today include: benzhexol or trihexyphenidyl (Artane), biperiden (Akineton), phenglutarimide hydrochloride (Aturbane), benztropine methanesulphonate (Cogentin), diethazine hydrochloride (Diparcol), orphenadrine hydrochloride (Disipal), procyclidine hydrochloride (Kemadrin), ethopropazine hydrochloride (Lysivane), cycrimine hydrochloride (Pagitane), methixine hydrochloride (Tremonil), chlorophenoxamine (Phenoxene), and ethopropazine (Parsidol). These compounds may be used in conjunction with antihistaminic drugs or cerebral stimulants to combat the lethargy that occurs with parkinsonism or that is induced by other therapies.

Other medications that are occasionally used for parkinsonism include: imipramine hydrochloride (Tofranil), an antidepressant that improves the dyskinesia of parkinsonism; trimeprazine tartrate (Vallergine), a hypnotic and antihistaminic that can alleviate the muscular pain which sometimes occurs in parkinsonism; methylpentynol carbamate (Oblivon C), a night-time sedative useful for restless patients; amyl nitrite, inhalation of which provides temporary relief of tremor; mephenesin (Myanesin), used in treating parkinsonian rigidity since it causes a transitory relaxation of voluntary muscle; and Benzedrine, a cerebral stimulant given to counteract the drowsiness produced by some medications used in treating parkinsonism and also used for oculogyric crises. Analgesics, e.g., aspirin, are useful in relieving cramplike pain. Phenobarbital often relieves insomnia.

Two *promising new medications* in the treatment of parkinsonism are levodopa (L-Dopa) and amantadine hydrochloride (Symmetrel). Levodopa has been referred to as the most important contribution to the medical therapy of a neurologic disorder in the past 50 years. This significant new medication is administered orally and is basically a form of replacement therapy in which the patient is given increasing doses of the medication to the point of control of symptoms and tolerance. For further discussion of levodopa see articles by Fangman[61] and Robinson.[207] The results of Symmetrel treatment resemble those for levodopa although they are not so dramatic. Symmetrel and levodopa do not appear to be antagonistic. In fact, combination of the two may well be synergistic, requiring lesser amounts of L-Dopa.[217]

Occasionally patients with parkinsonism experience what is called a *"parkinsonian crisis"* as a result of psychologic trauma or the sudden withdrawal of antiparkinsonism medications. In the crisis a sudden severe exacerbation of tremor, rigidity, and dyskinesia occurs, accompanied by acute anxiety, sweating, tachycardia, and hyperpnea. Sometimes there is also an oculogyric crisis.

A parkinsonian crisis calls for immediate treatment. The patient is placed in a quiet room with subdued light. An intramuscular or intravenous injection of sodium phenobarbital, 180 mg., may be given, or in moderately severe cases sodium amylbarbital, 180 mg., may be given orally. Antiparkinsonism medications are also given.

Numerous operations have been devised in an attempt to relieve the symptoms of parkinsonism. Over a period of time many of these procedures have been replaced by newer techniques with fewer side effects. Currently attention is being focused on procedures for destruction of the inner segment of the globus pallidus, the ansa lenticularis, and the ventrolateral nucleus of the thalamus. Destruction in these areas can be produced by stereotaxis employing alcohol, freezing (cryosurgery), electric cautery, ultrasound, or other means. Carefully placed lesions in these areas can reduce the severity of rigidity and tremor with little or no evidence of weakness. Such operations have proved highly beneficial in carefully selected patients. However, usually not more than one patient out of ten will meet the criteria and thus possibly benefit significantly from thalamotomy. Stereotactic surgery is discussed further in Chapter 40.

AMYOTROPHIC LATERAL SCLEROSIS

Amyotrophic lateral sclerosis (ALS) is a chronic progressive disease of unknown etiology that affects the spinal cord. ALS is characterized by atrophy and fibrillation of the somatic musculature as a result of degeneration of the motor cells in the spinal cord and medulla oblongata. This degenerative disease is relatively common. Over 80 per cent of the affected persons manifest the first symptoms of the illness between the ages of 50 and 70; however, onset may occur at any age. It is generally believed that inheritance is not a significant factor; however, a number of families have been reported in which one or more members of several generations have been afflicted with ALS.

Amyotrophic lateral sclerosis is a lower motor neuron disease. Both flaccid bulbar and spastic bulbar paralysis occur. However, in the late stages of the illness only true bulbar, flaccid paralysis is present. Usually muscular weakness is the initial symptom; it most often occurs in the distal portion of the extremities. Occasionally dysarthria or dysphagia are initial symptoms. Both weakness and atrophy of the muscles occur along with muscular fibrillations and fasciculations. Other possible symptoms are aching pains and paresthesias in the extremities and mental symptoms in the form of affective outbursts, e.g., explosive uncontrollable outbursts of laughing, crying, or a mixture of both.

Weakness of the muscles of the palate, pharynx, and tongue are initial symptoms in approximately one fourth of patients. This poses difficult problems for the patient, e.g., deglutition is impaired, solid foods are swallowed with difficulty, and fluids are regurgitated through the nose. In the last stages of the illness complete aphagia may occur, necessitating tube feedings. Also in the late stages of ALS, urinary frequency, urgency, difficulty in initiating the stream, or incontinence may occur. Terminally, muscular weakness and atrophy are generalized and often there is quadriplegia and bulbar paralysis.

No treatment is available to alter the course of ALS. The patient's condition progressively worsens without remission. Death most often occurs about three years after the initial symptoms.

SYRINGOMYELIA AND SYRINGOBULBIA

Syringomyelia is a disease of the spinal cord and medulla of unknown origin, characterized by muscular weakness and wasting, various sensory defects, symptoms of injury to the cord's long tracts, and trophic disturbances. Symptoms result from the presence of abnormal cavities filled with yellow liquid in the substance of the spinal cord, especially the cervical cord. Scar tissue surrounds the cysts. *Syringobulbia* refers specifically to the presence of these cavities in the medulla oblongata. Such cavities may occur only in the medulla (without involving the spinal cord), but they more frequently occur in combination with cervical syringomyelia. Typical symptoms of syringobulbia are atrophy and fibrillation of the tongue, loss of pain and temperature sense in one or both sides of the face, nystagmus, respiratory stridor or dysphonia.

Syringomyelia is believed to be a developmental anomaly since it is fairly often associated with other developmental defects. Symptoms may begin at any age but most often occur at ages 30 to 40. Symptom onset is insidious. With cervical syringomyelia the early symptoms often include: atrophy, weakness, and fibrillations of the small muscles of the hands; loss of pain sense in the fingers or forearm; weakness and atrophy of the muscles of the shoulder girdle; Horner's syndrome; nystagmus; and vasomotor and trophic disturbances of the upper extremities. Although there is segmental loss or impairment of the sensibility for pain and temperature there is preservation of sensibility for light touch. Segments of sensory loss may be separated by zones of normal sensibility. Spasticity, ataxia, or paralysis of the lower extremities may occur as well as disturbed bladder control.

Cranial nerve involvement may introduce additional problems, e.g., impairment of pain and temperature sense in the face, loss of the corneal reflex (necessitating protection of the eye, dysphagia, dysarthria, laryngeal stridor (which may necessitate tracheotomy to enable normal respiration), nystagmus, and atrophy and fibrillation of the tongue muscles.

Kyphosis (i.e., abnormally increased convexity in curvature of the thoracic spine when viewed from the side, referred to as "humpback" by lay persons) and scoliosis (i.e., a noticeable lateral deviation in the normally straight vertical line of the spine) often occur in syringomyelia, along with club foot. Charcot joints occur more frequently with syringomyelia than with tabes dorsalis.

The *course* of syringomyelia is a progressive one; however, it may remain stationary for many years. Some patients live 40 years after onset. In others the disease is rapidly progressive, causing incapacitation (from paralysis or sensory defects) or death within a few years.

No effective treatment exists for syringomyelia or syringobulbia. X-ray treatment has been recommended to the affected areas of the cord, but has not been successful in preventing further damage. Surgical drainage of the cystic cavity after laminectomy (see Chapter 40) may be beneficial, especially when a complete subarachnoid block exists. In such cases incising and evacuating the contents of the cavity may relieve pressure on the cord. Symptomatic treatment is given to Charcot joints, sores, felons, and so forth. The patient is instructed to be particularly careful of analgesic areas of his body to prevent injury, e.g., chafing of the skin, ulceration, burns.

PROGRESSIVE MUSCULAR DYSTROPHY

Progressive muscular dystrophy is a common *inherited disease* characterized by weakness and degeneration of the affected muscles. The pattern of muscular involvement tends to follow a characteristic distribution in members of the affected family. In most cases the major pathologic findings are confined to the muscles, while the peripheral and central nervous systems remain normal. It is not precisely known why the degenerative changes occur in the muscles; however, it is known that various disturbances occur in the enzyme systems concerned with muscle metabolism.

The major symptoms result from muscle weakness, mostly limited to the muscles of the trunk and extremities, with the girdle musculature affected more severely than the distal parts of the extremities. Occasionally pseudohypertrophy occurs in almost all the muscles. An advanced degree of lumbar lordosis, (i.e., an abnormally increased concavity in the curvature of the lumbar spine as viewed from the side) results from weakness of the trunk muscles and is characteristic of the posture occurring with progressive muscular dystrophy. The gait is characteristically a steppage, waddling gait resulting from weakness of the pelvic muscles. Pain seldom occurs, and there are no sensory symptoms.

Wide variation occurs in the *course* of progressive muscular dystrophy. When the onset of symptoms occurs after age 20, the prognosis is improved. The usual pattern is for the affected muscles to weaken gradually. Atrophy slowly progresses to the unaffected muscles. It is not uncommon for a patient to have had the condition for 40 to 50 years and still be able to walk; however, some patients are confined to a bed or wheelchair after five to 15 years. Braces make walking possible for some patients. The small muscles of the hands and feet are the last to be affected. Death may result from involvement of the bulbar, respiratory, and cardiac musculature or from intercurrent infection.

As muscle weakness progresses, patients with muscular dystrophy benefit from the use of various self-help devices. Individualized exercise programs are also of importance. There is *no effective treatment* that will stop the progression of muscular dystrophy; therefore, *prevention is important* by means of effective genetic counseling.

MYASTHENIA GRAVIS

Myasthenia gravis is a relatively common disease, characterized by weakness and rapid exhaustion of striated muscles following exertion. The basic problem appears to be a defect in the transmission of a nerve impulse at the myoneural junction. It is not known what causes this serious problem in impulse transmission; however, recent studies indicate that myasthenia gravis is possibly an autoimmune disease. While the familial incidence of myasthenia gravis is higher than chance, there is currently little other evidence to indicate that the disease is inherited. It occurs slightly more often in women. Onset of symptoms is most commonly between ages 20 to 40; however, it may occur at any age.

Usually *symptom* onset is insidious. The outstanding characteristic of the disease is the relationship of muscular weakness to muscular activity. The power of contraction rapidly diminishes after a few repeated activities of the muscles involved; then with rest the muscles rapidly regain their power of contraction. Not all muscles recover in this fashion, however, and certain muscles have a continually reduced function. The muscles affected by residual weakness vary somewhat in location and degree of weakness. However, the extraocular muscles are affected at some time during the course of myasthenia in almost all patients. Involvement of the ocular muscles is the most common initial symptom.

Weakness of facial and levator palpebrae muscles produces the expressionless appearance of the myasthenia patient, characterized by: droopy eyelids, smoothed features, full lips with underlip slightly everted, and a tendency for the mouth to hang open. The patient often seems to be snarling when he tries to smile. Other ocular palsies may occur, with diplopia and nystagmus. Variability in ocular symptoms from day to day is characteristic.

With progression of the disease other muscles become involved. Involvement of the muscles of deglutition results in choking spells and nasal regurgitation. Involvement of the muscles of speech causes a nasal voice; aphonia may develop with severe involvement. When the muscles of mastication are affected the jaw sags. The flexors of the neck are frequently involved, so that the patient may constantly hold his hand under his chin to support his head. The extremities are often involved. The upper are usually affected before the lower and the proximal muscles before the distal ones. Early in the disease the patient may thus notice difficulty in brushing his teeth, shaving, and combing his hair.

Clinical Care. Some of the major problems of the patient with myasthenia and some nursing measures that can be taken include:

> *Difficulty taking nourishment.* Involvement of the muscles of chewing and swallowing makes eating a difficult and slow process. Sometimes weakness of the palate and pharyngeal muscles causes regurgitation of fluid through the nose. Suction apparatus must be readily available. Tube feedings and I.V feedings may become necessary.

> *Dyspnea and impaired ability to cough and swallow.* Involvement of the muscles of respiration may cause weakness of cough, attacks of dyspnea following exertion, and finally, dyspnea occurs even at rest. The patient has difficulty clearing the respiratory tract of mucus and fluids. If the patient is unable to swallow saliva, a tracheotomy is performed. Respiratory distress necessitates artificial respiration. Preferably, use of a respirator should be preceded by tracheotomy.

> *Weakness.* Weakness is greatest following exertion and at the end of the day. The patient's activities must be carefully planned to avoid excessive fatigue. As mentioned, with rest there is typically improvement in muscle strength. When the muscles of mastication and swallowing are involved, the patient may be able to eat the first part of his meal without difficulty, but with each successive bite the chewing and swallowing become progressively more difficult. It is thus important that the meal not be rushed, and it is helpful if food is served on a warming tray. Smaller but more frequent feedings may be helpful. Sometimes a patient's muscles become weak even without exercise. Occasionally a patient's neck muscles may be so weakened that he is unable to lift his head from the pillow. Care of the bedfast patient is discussed in Unit V, Chap. 27. In a severe attack the patient may be completely paralyzed and the muscles of respiration, which may have been uninvolved previously, may be affected.

The *course* of myasthenia gravis may be characterized by *remissions* and *exacerbations.* Symptoms may fluctuate in severity from day to day, and spontaneous remissions may develop which last for many years. Some patients experience a gradual extension of the involved areas which progresses to a relatively steady state of weakness, remaining unchanged for many years except for moderate changes in severity. Others experience rapid progression of involvement, leading to death within a few months.

Generally myasthenia gravis can be easily *diagnosed* by finding the characteristic relationship of activity to the involved muscles, the location of the involved muscles, and the fluctuating course of the illness. Additionally, dramatic improvement in muscular strength typically occurs following the injection of neostigmine or edrophonium chloride (in a previously untreated case), and this phenomenon is used for diagnostic testing and for the regulation of drug dosage. Further investigation for diagnostic purposes may include: (1) electrical stimulation, which demonstrates fatiguability of the affected muscles (Jolly reaction); and (2) electromyography, which demonstrates a similar but less dramatic diminution of the action potentials of the muscles.

The *treatment* of patients with myasthenia gravis basically relies on administration of *short-acting anticholinesterase compounds* e.g., neostigmine (Prostigmin), pyridostigmine (Mestinon), and ambenonium (Mytelase).

The optimal drug regimen for a patient with myasthenia is the smallest dose that will produce the greatest strength. Excessive dosage may cause generalized weakness as a result of anticholinesterase intoxication (*"cholinergic crisis"*). This state is often accompanied by parasympathomimetic side effects and a variable degree of muscular "tightness" and fasciculations. Dysphagia and respiratory weakness may result from overdose and may be so severe that they necessitate endotracheal intubation and artificial respiration.

Many patients receiving anticholinesterase compounds develop excessive salivation, sweating, nausea, diarrhea, abdominal cramps, and occasional vomiting. To prevent or alleviate such visceral disturbances, tincture of belladonna or atropine sulfate may be prescribed with the anticholinesterase agent. For some patients ephedrine or potassium chloride may produce a slight increase in strength when administered as adjuvants to anticholinesterase medication. Corticotropin or cortisone is sometimes recommended for a patient with severe myasthenia who is responding poorly to the usual treatment; however, several fatalities have followed their use and they are not currently recommended as a routine form of treatment. The administration of curare, quinine, quinidine, morphine, neomycin, and large doses of barbiturates may be dangerous for the patient with myasthenia gravis. *No type of sedative should be given to any myasthenic who is having breathing or swallowing difficulties.*

Treatment with the anticholinesterase compounds (with or without adjuvant therapy) is continued indefinitely. Often the patient is allowed to regulate his own drug dosage according to need.

Sometimes a *"myasthenic crisis"* occurs in which there is exacerbation of the disease accompanied by a diminished response to and increased requirement for anticholinesterase medication. The patient may become refractory to neostigmine regardless of the size of the dose. The patient is placed on complete bed rest and, if he can swallow, small amounts of neostigmine are administered orally. Dysphagia and respiratory distress may develop and are usually managed by intramuscular neostigmine and supplementary atropine and suction to diminish and remove secretions. If acute paralysis of the respiratory muscles develops, the patient is placed in an artificial respirator and is given neostigmine I.M. or I.V. if necessary. Tracheotomy may be performed.

In some cases it is difficult to determine whether a patient's increased weakness is caused from an overdosage of anticholinesterase medication ("cholinergic crisis") or from exacerbation and progression of the myasthenic involvement and the need for more medication ("myasthenic crisis"). A small dose of edrophonium chloride (Tensilon) (2.0 mg.) may be given I.V. to help in making a differential diagnosis. If myasthenic crisis is present the patient's condition may show a transient increase in strength, whereas if cholinergic crisis is present the weakness will become severe following the injection.

Thymectomy, i.e., removal of the thymus gland, is sometimes employed in treating myasthenia gravis. It is still not possible to conclusively evaluate the effects of this procedure.

It is important that the patient with myasthenia gravis realize the nature of his illness and the objectives of treatment, i.e., that the anticholinesterase compounds are administered for the amelioration of weakness, and that they do not produce a "cure." It is also important for the patient to make every effort to maintain his general health and to avoid respiratory infections (which could progress to a fatal pneumonia or result in strangulation because of inability to cough productively). Vocational rehabilitation may be necessary. Also changes may be necessary in the patient's pattern of activities and the arrangement of his home to prevent excessive expenditure of energy. During acute periods of the illness a suction machine, respirator, and tracheostomy tray should be available. As indicated the patient may require total care, including tube feedings or intravenous feedings. The extremely weak patient is totally dependent on others. An eye patch may help to eliminate diplopia and "lid-crutches" may help ptosis. The dysphagic patient requires a diet that can be swallowed easily, e.g., minced food.

The patient should wear a bracelet or necklace identifying him as a myasthenic, and should be given the address of the Myasthenia Gravis Foundation.*

DEMYELINATING DISEASES OF THE NERVOUS SYSTEM

The myelin of the nervous system may be affected by numerous disorders. For example, demyelination or myelin breakdown may be a *secondary* aspect of infections, deficiency states, intoxications, or degenerations affecting the nervous system. There are numerous other conditions in which the myelin is *primarily* affected. *The most common of these primary demyelinating diseases is multiple sclerosis.* The causes of most demyelinating disorders remain unknown. Currently evidence indicates that an allergic basis might be present for most of the primary demyelinating disorders, with genetic and geographic factors influencing susceptibility.

MULTIPLE SCLEROSIS

Multiple sclerosis (MS) is a chronic, slowly progressive disease of the CNS, characterized pathologically by the presence of numerous dissemi-

*Myasthenia Gravis Foundation, Inc., New York Academy of Medicine Bldg., 2 East 103rd St., New York, N.Y. 10029. Informative literature is available from this agency.

nated areas of demyelination and clinically by numerous, varied neurologic symptoms that have a tendency toward alternating *remission and exacerbation.*

This remitting and relapsing disease primarily affects the white matter of the CNS and is *one of the most frequent nonvascular causes of neurologic disability.* MS has been reported from all parts of the world. The incidence is much higher in the cold and temperate climates than in the tropics and subtropics. In the U.S.A. the incidence is estimated to be five to seven times lower in the southern states than in the northern states.

It is not clear whether genetic factors are important in MS. The incidence is about equal in the sexes. MS is predominantly a disease affecting young adults. The onset of symptoms typically occurs between the ages of 20 and 40. Although numerous factors have been cited as possible causes of MS, the definite cause remains unknown.

Because the lesions of multiple sclerosis are diffusely scattered throughout all parts of the brain and spinal cord, *the symptoms of multiple sclerosis are highly variable.* Hallmarks of MS are: (1) the chronic and relapsing nature of the illness punctuated by remissions and exacerbations (although as many as 30 per cent of affected patients steadily worsen from the onset); and (2) the multiplicity of the symptoms and their tendency to vary in nature and severity with the passage of time.

Weakness of the extremities is the most common symptom of the illness. There may also be generalized weakness which is out of proportion to the demonstrable muscular weakness. Usually weakness begins or is most noticeable in the lower extremities. When both lower extremities are involved, urinary disturbances (e.g., urgency, frequency) often appear. The extent of impairment ranges from minor weakness to total paralysis. Spasticity, hyperreflexia, and pathologic reflexes are often present.

Multiple sclerosis has no classic form; however, most patients who have had the illness for many years display the triad of symptoms originally described by Charcot (known as *"Charcot's triad"*): (1) nystagmus; (2) intention tremor; and (3) scanning speech, i.e., slow enunciation with a tendency to hesitate at the beginning of a word or syllable. Loss of coordination frequently causes the MS patient to be ataxic and clumsy, and to walk with a combination spastic-ataxic gait. An impairment of pain and temperature sense occurs fairly often in one-half of the trunk and in the corresponding lower extremity. A patient with this involvement requires special attention to prevent injury to these areas of anesthesia. A common early finding in MS is deficiency of touch sensation of one hand. Complete blindness rarely occurs; however, considerable permanent visual loss is common.

Some of the milder *mental changes* that commonly appear with MS are: euphoria, apathy, poor judgment, and poor attention. While transient psychotic episodes can occur, severe mental deterioration generally does not appear until the terminal stages of the illness (then it occurs in about one-fourth of the patients involved). It is not unusual to find mild emotional disturbances in the early course of the illness. Such disturbances make diagnosis difficult; it is not uncommon for patients early in the course of MS to be viewed as neurotic because of their varied, temporary symptoms and emotional instability.

Terminally, paresis or complete paralysis of the lower extremities is almost always present. The use of the arms may be severely limited as a result of ataxia or cerebellar involvement.

As mentioned, the *clinical course* of MS is highly variable and is punctuated by periods of remissions and exacerbations. It appears that partial healing may occur in the areas of degeneration and that this accounts for the transitory character of many of the early symptoms. Over a period of years increasing neurologic deficits occur as a result of an increasing number of disseminated lesions and lesion enlargements. Remissions usually last for several months to two years, but the length of the remissions is highly variable.

Generally the course of the illness extends over a period of 10 to 20 or more years.

When death does occur it is most often from some intercurrent disease or infection, e.g., respiratory or urinary infection. This usually happens after the disease has progressed to the extent that the patient is completely incapacitated.

Exacerbations may be precipitated by such factors as: fatigue, chilling, malnutrition, emotional disturbances, acute febrile illnesses, and exposure to cold, damp weather.

There is no specific diagnostic test for multiple sclerosis. The *diagnosis* is based on the presence of multiple symptoms of CNS involvement and a history of remissions and exacerbations of the symptoms. The only significant findings in the laboratory examination are those in the cerebrospinal fluid. In about two-thirds of patients the gamma globulin content is elevated. Also there may be an abnormal colloidal gold curve which is accompanied by a negative serologic test for syphilis. Electroencephalographic findings are mildly abnormal in about two-thirds of patients. A definite diagnosis can seldom be made at the time of the first attack.

There is no specific *therapy* for multiple sclerosis, although numerous types of therapy have been advocated over the years. Currently the corticosteroids are being extensively used. It appears that the administration of cortisone and corticotropin produces some temporary beneficial effects but does not appreciably alter the ultimate course of the disease. The use of anticoagulants, e.g., heparin and bishydroxycoumarin, is experimental and can cause serious hemorrhage. Various vitamin preparations may be administered for their psychotherapeutic and tonic effects.

Because of the relatively low incidence of multiple sclerosis in warm climates, it is sometimes recommended that patients with MS move to such a climate if possible.

Since no specific therapy exists, the care of the patient with multiple sclerosis is basically a matter of symptomatic general care which varies with the patient's current needs. In general, the following are advocated: a *regular* daily program of activity, rest, and relaxation; avoidance of overwork and fatigue; moderate exercise and physiotherapy; warm baths; psychotherapy; a calm, relaxed environment which does not demand that the patient respond rapidly (either physically or emotionally); a well-balanced diet with ample high vitamin foods and fluids; fresh air and sunshine; and avoidance of overheating and chilling. As with all patients who have neurologic disabilities, the patient with multiple sclerosis is encouraged to remain active as long as possible, and every attempt is made to prevent invalidism. The patient benefits from the cultivation of hobbies and activities that can replace activities that are no longer possible. Social activities are encouraged, and the patient's normal social contacts should continue. Vocational retraining may be indicated.

The patient's family and friends need to be helped to understand the patient's condition and such manifestations of his illness as emotional lability, slowness of speech, and slowness in ability to respond. The patient's major disabilities are spasticity, disturbances of coordination, and disturbances of bowel and bladder function. (See Chapter 38.)

If some muscles are permanently affected it is frequently possible to train other muscles to assume the lost action. Self-help devices are useful to the patient with multiple sclerosis, enabling him to remain independent longer. The patient's environment at home may require installation of ramps, handrails, and so forth. The patient may require the care discussed in the sections pertaining to hemiplegia or paraplegia in Chapter 38. Also refer to Chapter 27 of Unit V for a discussion of the care of the patient confined to bed. Unnecessary catheterization is avoided (as with all patients) because of the possible serious consequences. Visual disturbances may pose special problems for the patient by further curtailing his activities. Safety measures are of prime importance because of the patient's multiple impairments. Some physicians recommend bed rest during periods of acute exacerbation. Others believe the patient should remain active but avoid fatigue.

The National Multiple Sclerosis Society has local organizations in many larger cities. The home office is at 257 Park Avenue South, New York, N.Y. 10010. This voluntary organization acts as an information center for patients and the general public and conducts a research and educational program regarding multiple sclerosis. Local units provide patients with direct services.

PAROXYSMAL DISORDERS OF THE NERVOUS SYSTEM

EPILEPSY (CONVULSIVE DISORDERS)

The millions of epileptics in the United States have a nervous system disorder which is becoming increasingly better understood and treated. Today epilepsy is viewed as a condition that is often reversible or can at least be controlled as well as diabetes if the affected individual seeks medical care. Unfortunately in spite of this encouraging progress many epileptics still do not seek medical help and try to conceal their disability.

Definition

"Epilepsy" is derived from the Greek word *epilepsia,* meaning to "take hold of" or "seize." In early times epilepsy was viewed as being of divine origin and was called "the sacred disease" because it was believed that the epileptic was seized by the gods. This ancient explanation has been replaced with the current concept that *epilepsies are paroxysmal disorders of the nervous system that result in recurrent attacks of loss of consciousness or other types of seizures in which convulsive movements or other motor activity, sensory phenomena, or behavioral abnormalities may occur.*

It is more appropriate to refer to "the epilepsies" rather than merely "epilepsy," since many types of *recurrent* seizures occur. These seizures result from paroxysmal excessive neuronal discharges in different parts of the brain. It is not known exactly what prompts the brain tissue to discharge abnormally. However, it is speculated that an abnormal concentration of acetylcholine makes the cells more reactive to stimuli in the affected areas.[161] The acute disturbance in cerebral function that produces a seizure can usually be demonstrated on EEG. More males are afflicted with epilepsy than females. Seizures occur in all races and all climates.

"Symptomatic" and "Idiopathic" Epilepsy

Convulsive seizures can be divided into two broad groups: (1) *symptomatic or secondary epilepsy,* in which the probable cause of the seizures has been determined; and (2) *idiopathic or primary epilepsy,* in which study of the patient has failed to reveal a definite cause for the seizures. In approximately 75 per cent of adults with seizures no obvious cause of the attacks can be found.

There is a great deal of dispute concerning the role of inheritance in the occurrence of *idiopathic* convulsive seizures. It is thought by some that the disorder is not directly inherited, but rather that a predisposition to seizures or a lowered seizure threshold may be inherited, and that consequently a disturbed chemical balance can precipitate a seizure in such a susceptible person. The theory of a genetic basis for these convulsive seizures is not completely accepted, however, and has possibly been overemphasized.

Usually, idiopathic seizures have their onset

early in life (although they may start at any age); the vast majority of seizures begin prior to age 25, generally from the third to the fifteenth year of life.

The causes of *symptomatic* epilepsy, i.e., due to organic factors, are multiple. Among these are: hyperpyrexia, CNS infections, cerebral hypoxia, toxic agents or poisons, metabolic intoxications and disturbances, convulsive agents, parasitic infections, cerebral trauma, brain defects, expanding brain lesions, anaphylaxis, and degenerative brain disease.

In many of the above conditions convulsive seizures may appear as only a transient symptom which does not recur following treatment of the basic disorder. However, recurrent seizures may persist for years or indefinitely if a permanent lesion or scar remains in the CNS.

It is important to remember that convulsive seizures may be caused in "normal" persons by electrical stimulation or by administration of convulsion-causing drugs. Also, occasionally simulated convulsive attacks occur in hysterical or other psychoneurotic patients; usually persons having such simulated attacks do not injure themselves during the attack or as a result of falling from the seizure. Such attacks are not a type of "true" epilepsy.

Types of Seizures

It is difficult to categorize precisely the numerous manifestations of seizures; however, certain types of epileptic seizures can be distinguished. The most common of these are grand mal, petit mal, and psychomotor. The majority of epileptics have only one type of seizure; some have two or more types.

Grand Mal Seizures. Grand mal seizures are also called "major convulsions." Approximately 90 per cent of epileptics are subject to these seizures. Grand mal seizures may be subdivided into two groups: focal or jacksonian, and typical grand mal seizures.

FOCAL OR JACKSONIAN SEIZURES. These are precipitated by organic lesions in the motor or sensory cortex, which often makes it possible to identify the area of the brain involved. Close observation of this type of seizure is thus important in order to identify precisely the area in which the focal cerebral lesion is located. In focal jacksonian motor seizures the seizure begins with convulsive twitchings in one part of the body, e.g., the distal part of one extremity, and then the involuntary movements spread or "march" (jacksonian march) centrally to affect other areas of the body. *Sensory* focal seizures may also occur, in which the patient experiences transient abnormal sensations (e.g., numbness, tingling) in specific areas of the body. If the seizure spreads to involve the entire body, i.e., becomes "generalized," the patient loses consciousness and displays the manifestations of a typical grand mal seizure.

TYPICAL GRAND MAL (TONIC-CLONIC) SEIZURES. There are many varieties of grand mal seizures; however, the typical sequence is:

> *Prodromal phase.* Some grand mal seizures are preceded by a prodromal phase in which a vague change occurs in emotional reactivity or affective responses, e.g., increasing depression or anxiety. This phase may last minutes or even hours.

> *Aura.* More often an "aura" occurs at the onset of the seizure. An aura is generally a brief sensory experience directly related to the point of origin of the seizure, e.g., a feeling of weakness, dizziness, strange sensations in an arm or leg, numbness, or an unpleasant odor. Usually the aura precedes the other manifestations of the seizure by only a few seconds. Occasionally the aura may give the patient enough time to lie down, or may not even be followed by a complete seizure.

> *"Epileptic cry."* The cry, which precedes loss of consciousness and falling, is caused by a thoracic and abdominal spasm which expels air through the narrowed spastic glottis.

> *Convulsions.* During the *tonic phase* the muscles are held in rigid tonic contraction, i.e., tonic extensor rigidity of the trunk and extremities occurs, the respirations may be suspended, and the face becomes cyanotic. The jaws are fixed and the hands clenched. The eyes are opened widely; the pupils dilate and become fixed. Usually this phase lasts only a few seconds. With the onset of the *clonic phase* respirations are jerky and become stertorous. During this phase jerky movements occur (which may last a minute or more) and saliva is blown from the mouth and creates a froth at the lips. Urinary or fecal incontinence may occur, and the lips and inside of the cheeks may be bitten.

Following the clonic phase the convulsion gradually subsides, excessive motor activity ceases, respirations become more normal, and the patient slowly returns to consciousness.

A *postictal state* often follows a grand mal seizure and is characterized by the presence of headache, general fatigue, confusion, and sometimes specific residual neurologic symptoms, e.g., hemiparesis or monoparesis (called *Todd's paralysis*). This postictal paralysis may last from a few minutes up to several hours. During this time automatic behavior may also occur.

Following a grand mal seizure the patient usually falls deeply asleep for several hours. When he awakens he often has a headache, a sense of depression, and complete amnesia for the seizure episode except for some memories of the prodromal phase or the aura. He may feel nauseated and have stiff, sore muscles. Following a very severe grand mal seizure a period of mental confusion may be present for several days. Because the patient does not protect himself when he loses consciousness and falls, he may be injured. It is thus important to examine the patient for indications of bruises, lacerations, or fractures following a seizure.

Grand mal seizures vary in their intensity and frequency, e.g., from many times daily to once or twice yearly. Generally the attacks may occur at any time of day or night.

Petit Mal Seizures. These seizures occur mostly in children (commonly between the ages of three and 10) and seldom have an onset after age 20.

They characteristically are a form of idiopathic epilepsy; however, they may also follow birth injuries or acute febrile childhood illnesses. Petit mal seizures are, as their name implies, "little" seizures or minor seizures. These seizures occur with great frequency in a given patient, unlike the grand mal seizures. While some patients may have a few attacks daily or every few days, others may have several hundred each day. Generally attacks do not occur during active exercise. Usually, but not always, the seizures diminish or perhaps disappear entirely after puberty. Grand mal or psychomotor seizures may develop at any time in a patient who initially had only petit mal seizures.

Petit mal seizures are characterized by a brief lapse or loss of consciousness during which the patient suddenly stops whatever activity he may be performing and stares blankly. He may blink rapidly, slightly deviate his eyes and head, or briefly make minor movements of his lips and hands. The patient seldom falls; however, he may stagger a few steps, droop his head, or lose urinary bladder control. Upon termination of the attack the patient is immediately alert and continues with his previous activities. Some seizures last merely one or two seconds, others may persist from 15 to 90 seconds. Because of the frequency of such petit mal seizures an affected child may have difficulty with his schoolwork.

Myoclonic seizures, i.e., sudden involuntary contractions of a single muscle or small groups of muscles of the trunk and extremities, may occur during petit mal seizures, but they are equally frequent during grand mal seizures. *Akinetic seizures,* characterized by a sudden loss of muscle tone in all the muscles of the body which causes the patient to fall to the ground, can occur in association with petit mal seizures or grand mal seizures. A brief lapse of consciousness may occur, but typically the patient is on his feet again so quickly that he may not be aware that a loss of consciousness actually occurred.

Psychomotor Attacks. Psychomotor attacks are generally associated with brain damage, frequently involving the temporal lobe. These attacks may thus develop at any age following brain damage. Psychomotor attacks are usually characterized by a brief lapse of consciousness, during which the patient does not fall to the ground or lose consciousness. Superficially psychomotor attacks are somewhat similar to petit mal seizures *except* that: (1) the duration of the attack is longer, usually lasting from 30 seconds to two minutes; (2) the range of muscular movements is greater; (3) clouding of consciousness is deeper, the patient being completely amnesic during the attack, and clouding of consciousness may continue for a brief period of time following the attack; and (4) EEG abnormalities differ from those during a petit mal seizure.[161] Rarely, periods of mental cloudiness, fugue states, or periods of amnesia may last several hours or days. During the attack automatic activity occurs that often follows a repeatable pattern and may include inappropriate or asocial behavior.

Status Epilepticus. Status epilepticus (abbreviated "status") refers to successively recurring grand mal seizures, between which the patient does not regain consciousness. Unless the seizures can be terminated, death occurs. Many epileptics have one or more episodes of status epilepticus.

Precipitating Factors

Most seizures occur without obvious precipitating factors. However, in some patients the seizure activity may be related to some specific stimulus. Among these stimuli are: sudden loud noises, music, flickering light, prolonged reading, coughing, drugs, and sleep. It is not clear whether emotional stimuli can precipitate an attack.

Status epilepticus may be precipitated by the sudden withdrawal of anticonvulsant medication, e.g., 1 to 4 days following discontinuance of phenobarbital, or 7 to 21 days after discontinuance of Dilantin sodium.

Diagnosis

It is difficult to determine whether a patient has idiopathic epilepsy or seizures resulting from an identifiable (and possibly treatable) cause. Epileptic seizures also must be differentiated from hysterical episodes. To accomplish this the patient is asked for a complete history and undergoes general medical and neurologic examinations, skull x-rays, cerebrospinal fluid examination, determination of the nonprotein nitrogen and calcium content of the blood, and electroencephalogram. Additional evaluation measures may include cerebral angiography, echoencephalography, pneumoencephalography, and assigned nursing observations.

The nurse's observations are highly important during a patient's seizures, since the nurse is more likely to observe the seizures than the physician. Seizures should be described in minute detail, including the sequence of the appearance of the phenomena which occur.

The EEG helps to establish the diagnosis of epilepsy and determine specific types of seizures. However, a normal EEG does not always exclude a diagnosis of epilepsy; likewise, the finding of minor abnormalities does not always confirm the diagnosis. During a seizure the EEG abnormalities involve all portions of the cortex. Between seizures patients with epilepsy may show short bursts of abnormal EEG activity and other EEG abnormalities.

Treatment

For purposes of discussion the treatment of epilepsy can be divided into four areas: (1) elimination of factors that may cause or precipitate seizures; (2) physical and mental hygiene; (3) medical treatment; and (4) surgical treatment.

Elimination of Causative Factors. When definite factors or disorders are known to be the underlying cause of symptomatic epilepsy every attempt is made to correct these disorders with specific medical or surgical therapy.

Physical and Mental Hygiene. It is important that the patient with epilepsy live as normal a life as possible and not be made to feel excessively "different" from others. Both patient and family members must learn to accept the patient's condition and not exaggerate it or make the patient into an invalid through overprotection. While certain dangerous activities should be avoided by the patient or should be engaged in only with special safeguards, e.g., swimming or horseback riding, there are still a wide variety of activities that can be enjoyed. The driving of motor vehicles will depend on local laws and the patient's medical control. Family members should be taught how to care for the patient during a seizure. The epileptic should always carry identification which states that he has epilepsy and lists the name of his physician.

It is important that the patient establish and adhere to a *regular* pattern of adequate diet, fluid intake, and sleep, and moderate recreation and exercise. Alcoholic beverages are contraindicated. Some patients seem to have fewer seizures if they are mildly dehydrated, possibly because this reduces potential cerebral edema.

Persons with epilepsy often have a poor *self-image,* feelings of inferiority, self-consciousness, and other emotional problems that can be overcome through education and the support and understanding of persons who care about them. Social attitudes concerning epilepsy have changed a great deal in recent years, but more education of the public will be necessary before this illness will lose the mystery and fear with which so many lay persons continue to view it. Only when social attitudes are changed, and informed legislation is enacted, will the epileptic be able to lead a realistic life. Various organizations exist that are trying to accomplish these goals and assist the epileptic with the problems he has because of his illness, e.g., the National Epilepsy League, Inc., with headquarters at 130 North Wells St., Chicago, Ill., 60606, and the National Association to Control Epilepsy Inc., with headquarters at 22 East 67th St., New York, N.Y., 10021. The adult epileptic may benefit from vocational rehabilitation. Selected patients may also benefit from psychotherapy.

Medical Therapy. The successful treatment of epilepsy rests ultimately on preventing the occurrence of seizures.[161] The most effective method of controlling seizures is the use of anticonvulsive drugs, of which there are many. The *ketogenic diet,* a high-fat diet which produces a mild ketosis or acidosis, was formerly used extensively in the treatment of petit mal seizures in children. However, since medical therapy is now effective in most patients with such seizures, the diet is rarely used. Table 39–3 lists four of the most commonly used anticonvulsant drugs, with usual dosages and effects. Some other anticonvulsants used to treat epilepsy are the following:

TABLE 39–3. COMMON ANTICONVULSANTS

Drug	Dosage	Side Effects	Toxicity
Diphenylhydantoin (Dilantin)	Average:0.3 gram q.d. Range: 0.06–0.6 gram q.d. Children: 0.15–3 grams Therapeutic level: 10–25 mcg./ml. serum	Ataxia, drowsiness, gum hyperplasia, hypertrichosis, nystagmus	Rash, serum sickness, pseudolymphoma, Stevens-Johnson syndrome, lupus erythematosus, macrocytic anemia, rare hepatic or marrow toxicity; cerebellar degeneration; peripheral neuropathy; possibly teratogenic in high dosage.
Phenobarbital	Average: 0.12 gram q.d. Range: 0.03–0.24 gram q.d. Children: 0.045–0.1 gram Therapeutic level: 15–30 mcg./ml. serum	Drowsiness, ataxia, nystagmus	Rare; rash; possibly teratogenic in high dosage.
Primidone (Mysoline)	Average: 1 gram q.d. Range: 0.5–2.0 gram q.d. Children: 0.25 gram	Drowsiness, nausea, ataxia, nystagmus (tachyphylaxis usual)	Rash, adenopathy, lupus erythematosus, macrocytic anemia, arthritis, edema.
Ethosuximide (Zarontin)	Average: 1 gram q.d. Range: 0.5–2.0 gram q.d. Children: 0.75–1.0 gram	Nausea, abdominal pain, drowsiness, personality change, headache	Rash, nephropathy, marrow depression.

*Modified from Van den Noort in Conn, H. F.: *Current Therapy 1973.*

Hydantoins (used primarily in grand mal and psychomotor attacks): Peganone, Mesantoin, Phenantoin
Succinamides (used in petit mal seizures): Celontin, Milontin
Oxazolidines (used in petit mal): paramethadione (Paradione), trimethadione (Tridione)
Barbiturates: mephobarbital (Mebaral)

Other drugs such as tranquilizers (Valium) or the carbonic anhydrase inhibitor acetazolamide (Diamox) are occasionally used in various types of epileptic seizures.

No one anticonvulsant medication will achieve complete seizure control in all patients. Chemotherapy for epilepsy thus involves various programs of drugs, which are carefully selected for each individual. This process may require weeks of trial and error and adjustment. During this period the patient, the family (and frequently the nurse) must observe carefully any seizure activity and side effects from the medications. Also, the patient being treated for the first time should try to identify any factors that may precipitate a seizure, e.g., menstruation or other stresses. The decision as to which medications to administer to a given patient rests basically on correctly identifying the nature of the attack. Some patients respond better to two or more medications.

Anticonvulsant medications must be built up in dosage during observation to see that they do not produce untoward toxic side effects. The patient must realize that he should *take his medicine regularly* and that he should neither increase nor decrease his dosage without consulting his doctor. The physician will decide if and when a patient who has remained seizure-free for a prolonged period of time can stop taking his medication. Frequent and rapid shifting or replacements of drugs are undesirable. Generally, when drug changes are being made, the old drug is continued for several days while the full dosage of the new drug is gradually established.

While specific anticonvulsant drugs are not available for each type of seizure, one major therapeutic division is noteworthy:[85] petit mal seizures respond best to either succinamide or oxazolidines (methadiones), but these drugs are not effective in the treatment of major generalized (grand mal) or focal cerebral seizures. Likewise, while the hydantoins are useful in grand mal and other seizures, they are not effective in petit mal. Patients with generalized grand mal and focal motor seizures are best treated with Dilantin (diphenylhydantoin) and phenobarbital, frequently in combination.

The treatment of status epilepticus is a medical emergency and, as with any emergency, first an open airway and adequate pulmonary ventilation are established. The patient is constantly observed and protected from exhaustion and self-injury, e.g., by padded siderails. Pulmonary edema occasionally occurs as a complication. The patient may remain comatose and have repetitive seizures for 12 to 24 hours or longer.

An intravenous infusion is started and kept open. Attempts are made to terminate status seizure activity by intravenous injection of sodium phenobarbital (5 mg./kg.) dissolved in distilled water and a single dose of Dilantin (5 mg./kg.). The sodium phenobarbital may be repeated at 20- to 30-minute intervals as necessary. If the patient does not respond to the preceding therapy, then 4 to 6 ml. of paraldehyde may be given in 100 ml. of isotonic saline solution as an I.V. drip until the seizures are controlled.

The use of other barbiturates, e.g., Amytal (sodium amobarbital) or Seconal (sodium secobarbital), is discouraged in treating status not only because these are less effective anticonvulsants, but also because they are more dangerous owing to their greater respiratory depressive effect. Recently Valium (diazepam) has been used in doses of 5 to 15 mg. I.V. over a period of a few minutes, and it has been reported to have excellent results.

In some cases if seizure activity cannot be terminated, the patient may be anesthetized with one of the volatile anesthetics, e.g., chloroform or ether. In some refractory cases anesthetic doses of sodium pentobarbital (intravenously or rectally) may be necessary; in others, hypothermia may be helpful. Oxygen and cardiac stimulants may be required and should be available, as should a suction machine. To prevent aspiration of mucus the patient's head may be lowered and he may be turned on his side. The room should be quiet and darkened.

Because status epilepticus is a condition especially difficult for a patient's friends and family to witness, they should be given special consideration and assisted in every way possible.[42] Even after the seizures are controlled, the patient may continue to be unconscious for several days. *The development of recurrent seizures is an immediately reportable condition.*

Surgical Treatment. As mentioned earlier, some convulsive seizures are caused by lesions of the brain which can be surgically removed, e.g., operable brain tumors, cysts, or abscesses. In addition to removing such expanding lesions, it may be possible in carefully selected patients to remove cortical scars. Surgical treatment of this nature, which removes a focus of abnormal discharge, is usually performed only on patients with focal attacks who have not responded to anticonvulsant therapy. Following surgery the patient must generally continue to take anticonvulsant medication. (See Neurosurgery, Chapter 40.)

SYNCOPE (FAINTING)

Syncope (fainting) is a transient loss of consciousness, for a few seconds up to one or two minutes, resulting from cerebral ischemia. Typically syncope occurs when the person is standing; he experiences prodromal symptoms for a few seconds or a minute or two before losing consciousness. Common prodromal symptoms are dizziness, sweating, epigastric discomfort and lightheadedness. While unconscious the patient is pale or ashen in color, perspires heavily, feels cold to the touch, and has a weak pulse and dilated pupils. Upon recovering consciousness the patient is usually immediately mentally alert but may feel weak.

Most frequently syncope results from a sudden decrease in the brain's circulation. The most common type of attack is *vasovagal syncope*. In this condition, which usually occurs in normal adults, there is a sudden loss of resistance in the peripheral blood vessels. Because the blood pools in the dilated peripheral vessels, the circulation to the brain becomes inadequate, producing cerebral ischemia. This common cause of fainting is often associated with gastrointestinal disturbances, anxiety, tension states, and so forth, which are precipitated by emotional or environmental stresses. At the immediate onset of symptoms the patient should lie down or sit down with his head between his knees.

The second most common cause of syncope is *orthostatic hypotension*. Cerebral ischemia occurs when a patient whose cardiovascular reflexes are impaired assumes an erect posture and he experiences an excessive drop in blood pressure. Numerous disorders can cause orthostatic hypotension, but it most often occurs with various organic conditions of the central or peripheral nervous system, e.g., parkinsonism, after sympathectomy, or with diabetic neuritis. Persons affected by orthostatic hypotension are taught to exercise their extremities while lying down before they sit up, then to exercise them again while sitting on the edge of the bed, and finally rise *slowly*. This gradual change from a recumbent posture to an erect posture often prevents syncope. Some patients require an abdominal support and leg bandages.

MENIERE'S DISEASE

Meniere's disease is a disorder of unknown etiology affecting the inner ear. It is characterized by recurrent episodes of severe vertigo, accompanied by progressive deafness and tinnitus in the affected ear. A feeling of fullness or pressure may be present in the involved ear. Meniere's disease most typically occurs in men 50 to 60 years of age. The condition is relatively common.

During acute attacks the patient experiences severe vertigo, spinning of surrounding objects, nausea and vomiting, profuse perspiration, and headache. Nystagmus may be present, and at times a brief loss of consciousness may occur. The onset of an attack is usually sudden and sometimes so violent that the patient falls to the ground. Hearing loss and tinnitus occur during the attack and persist between attacks. Hearing loss is apt to be progressive and is unilateral in 90 per cent of patients. Most often the hearing loss is of a nerve type rather than a conduction type.

Meniere's disease is a chronic disease with symptoms that are recurrent over the years. While temporary or complete remission of the attacks of vertigo may occur (either spontaneously or following treatment), the tinnitus and hearing loss are usually permanent. Some attacks are only of a few minutes' duration, whereas others may last several hours. The attacks occur irregularly.

Diagnostically, caloric or Bárány tests of labyrinthine function may or may not show altered function. Audiometry shows decreased speech discrimination and may identify a nerve type hearing loss.

Attempts have been made to relieve the acute attacks of vertigo by both medical and surgical treatments. The *medical treatment* may include such measures as:

> *Dietary alterations.* The patient may be placed on restricted fluid intake and a salt free or low sodium diet (to decrease fluid retention). Patients with a hypoglycemic tendency may be given a diet that is low in carbohydrates, moderate in fats and high in protein. Between-meal and bedtime feedings may be given to maintain blood sugar level. In some patients attacks appear to be triggered by food allergies. Allergy tests may identify hypersensitivities to any of the common food allergens. In the presence of an allergy the food is avoided.

> *Medications.* Medications that may be used between attacks include: histamine subcutaneously (in desensitizing doses); antivertiginous medications such as dimenhydrinate (Dramamine), nicotinyl alcohol-trimethobenzamide hydrochloride (Tigacol), meclizine-nicotinic acid (Antivert), nicotinic acid, eriodictyon glycoside, or diphenylhydantoin. Medications are changed if relief is not rapid. Oral medications are prescribed until the patient obtains relief. If a patient is having a *"cluster" of attacks* histamine may be given intravenously (daily for 4 to 6 consecutive days); generally the complete I.V. injection takes 90 to 180 minutes. During *severe acute attacks* diphenhydramine (Benadryl) or dimenhydrinate is given parenterally. Also, an attack may be terminated in 15 to 20 minutes with a fairly high dose of atropine sulfate subcutaneously. The patient should seek such medical help upon the first indication of an attack. Some patients can be taught to self-administer the atropine.

Some physicians prescribe diuretics, e.g., potassium chloride, acetazolamide (Diamox), chlorothiazide (Diuril), in the medical treatment of Meniere's disease. Mild sedation and tranquilizers may be used to help to calm the patient. Emotional support and reassurance are important. Patients may be advised to discontinue smoking to avoid vasospasm and vasoconstriction.

> *Surgery.* About 10 per cent of all patients with Meniere's disease require surgery. Among the surgical procedures which may be used are: (1) *surgical destructive labyrinthectomy;* (2) *ultrasonic or cryosurgical labyrinthectomy;* and (3) *section of eighth cranial nerve.* Some of these procedures may cause loss of hearing. Relief from vertigo may not occur for several weeks in some cases.

The nurse caring for a patient hospitalized with Meniere's disease must try to understand how frustrating, incapacitating, and uncomfortable acute attacks of this disease are for the patient. The patient is handled gently and is allowed to do as much of his own care as possible, and at his own pace, to minimize possible vertigo, nausea and vomiting. Because the patient can fall during a severe attack of vertigo, his environment is kept safe (e.g., bed siderails up) and he is assisted when out of bed. The patient is instructed as to any limitations concerning his activities, and a call bell is kept close at hand at all times. He is encouraged to notify the nurse at the first indication of an attack so that medications can be given. If surgery is performed, the nurse explains and carries out the physician's instructions regarding pre- and postoperative care. The patient may be hospitalized seven to eight days following labyrinthectomy. Dietary instruction is given as indicated.

HEADACHE (CEPHALALGIA)

Headache, man's most common pain, may occur either in the absence of organic disease or as a manifestation of serious disease. It is estimated that *some form of headache affects 90 per cent of the population.* While most headaches are transient and of only moderate or slight severity, a few are chronic, intense, and frequently recurrent over a period of months or years. Headache is *a symptom of an underlying disorder,* rather than a disease in itself. It is thus important that the cause of this symptom be identified in any given patient so that treatment can be directed at the underlying cause.

Some of the more important disorders that commonly give rise to headache include: intracranial tumors and infections; acute systemic infections; head injuries; cerebral arteriosclerosis; cerebral hypoxia; severe hypertension; and chronic or acute diseases of eye, ear, nose, or throat.

Vascular Headaches

"More than 90 per cent of all headaches result from painful dilation and distention of cranial arteries or sustained contraction of skeletal muscle around the face, scalp and neck; these headaches occur in a life setting that engenders frustration, resentment, anxiety, emotional tension and fatigue."[190] Vascular headaches are basically caused by the dilation and distention of one or more of the extracranial and, probably, intracranial (i.e., dural) branches of the external carotid artery; edema of the adjacent tissues also occurs. *The most familiar vascular headache syndrome is the migraine.*

Migraine. Migraine headaches are paroxysmal disorders characterized by periodic, recurrent attacks of headache in an individual who is in good health in the intervals between headaches. Migraine is said to be more common among women and to have a typical onset during the second and third decades of life. The pathogenesis includes both physical and psychologic factors. All writers stress the hereditary and familial character of this disorder. Remission commonly occurs after the menopause in women or in late middle life in men. It is estimated that migraine occurs in 5 to 10 per cent of the population. The headaches may recur several times weekly or only several times a year.

The migraine headache may be preceded by an *aura or prodromal phase* in which the patient may feel depressed, irritable, restless, and perhaps anorectic. During this period the patient may also experience various other symptoms, e.g., visual disturbances (flashes of lights, diplopia, transitory impaired vision), paresthesias, vertigo, or transient hemiparesis. The prodromal symptoms may last only a few minutes or several hours.

The *headache itself* is believed to result from dilatation of the vessels of the head which lie outside of the brain substance, i.e., dural arteries or arteries of the scalp. The head pain may be generalized or unilateral. The pain may be localized to the front, back, or side of the head. The temple is the most common location. The prodromal symptoms and the head pain rarely recur in the same location in every attack. The pain varies in intensity from mild discomfort to a prostrating, throbbing pain that forces the patient to seek seclusion and take to bed in a darkened room. During this period the patient is acutely ill. Migraine attacks most commonly last for six to 18 hours. Various somatic manifestations may accompany severe attacks: photophobia, nausea, vomiting, vertigo, tremor, diarrhea, and excessive sweating or chilliness. During the attack the arteries on the head may be prominent and the amplitude of their pulsations increased. Swelling, redness, and excessive tearing of the eyes and swelling of the nasal mucosa (with or without epistaxis) may also occur along with the headache. Initially the pain is throbbing but later it becomes a steady ache. The pain of migraine can be reduced by applying pressure on the common carotid and the affected superficial artery. It is typically reduced or eliminated by such vasoconstrictor drugs as ergotamine tartrate, if taken early enough.

Cluster headaches (histamine headaches; Horton's syndrome) are a variant form of migraine formerly believed to be caused by a sensitivity to histamine. Patients with this condition have headaches that tend to occur in clusters, i.e., numerous attacks occur in a period of a few days, weeks, or occasionally months, and then there is a remission with no symptoms for months or years; following the remission the headaches again recur in clusters. Men are affected more frequently than women with this agonizing head pain, and the attacks usually begin between the ages of 30 and 60.

The individual attacks begin suddenly and may last only a few minutes or as long as two hours (seldom more). During the attack the patient experiences intense throbbing pain arising high in the nostril and localized to one side of the forehead; the pain typically spreads from the nostril to involve the region behind the homolateral eye, and sometimes the forehead. During the attack, on the side of the pain the nose and eye water and the skin reddens. These individual attacks of headache tend to occur from once to several times daily. Without any apparent reason, the cluster of attacks subsides as suddenly as it began.

The *treatment of migraine* involves both preventative aspects and the treatment of an acute attack. Patients may benefit from psychotherapy, which helps to give them a basic understanding of their tensions and assistance in resolving major life conflicts.

Methysergide (Sansert) (2 mg. three or four times daily orally) may help to prevent migraine headache; it will not stop a migraine attack in progress, however. This medication also has prophylactic value in the treatment of cluster headaches. Additional prophylactic measures may include relaxation and improved sleep obtained through the judicious administration of analgesics, tranquilizers, and hypnotic drugs, e.g., salicylates, meprobamate, and barbiturates.

Treatment during an acute attack of migraine varies with the intensity of the attack. *Mild attacks* may be treated with common analgesics e.g., aspirin, with or without the addition of caffeine citrate or codeine. *Severe vascular headaches* require the administration of ergot derivatives to restore the painfully dilated vessels to a nonpainful constricted state and restore the pain threshold to normal. These medications provide relief only if taken *before* the headache has lasted two hours, i.e., before the vessels become rigid from edema of their walls. Ergotamine tartrate (Gynergen) or dihydroergotamine should therefore be given as soon after the onset of symptoms as possible.

During an acute attack of migraine the patient benefits from rest in a quiet darkened room. Some patients find some additional relief from damp compresses.

Muscle Contraction Headaches (Tension Headaches)

Muscle contraction headaches result from long-sustained contraction of skeletal muscles around the scalp, face, neck, and upper back. Vasodilatation of the associated cranial arteries also may contribute to the irritability of the involved muscles and the head pain. The long-sustained contraction causes the muscles to become tender and, as a result, the patient further restricts their motion. This prolonged muscle contraction is the primary source of many headaches that are associated with states of excessive emotional tension. Sustained muscle contraction may also cause headaches secondary to painful stimuli from other cranial structures, e.g., brain tumor, the distended arteries of vascular headache, inflammation in the eye, ear, nose, paranasal spaces, or teeth.

Muscle contraction headaches cause a steady, nonpulsatile ache (unilateral or bilateral) in any region of the head. The headaches may last unrelieved for weeks, months, or years. The pain may be localized or change frequently in location and intensity. Sometimes these headaches are fleeting but recurrent. The headache may be spontaneously accompanied by dizziness, tinnitus, or lacrimation, or these symptoms may be elicited by pressing on the tender muscles. Palpation may demonstrate contracted muscles with localized painful areas or nodules. The patient may experience pain if he combs his hair or wears a hat, and exposure to cold may precipitate or aggravate a headache.

Muscle contraction headaches are *treated* when possible by removing the primary source of stimulation, e.g., treating disease of the teeth or nose when this is present. Persons with prolonged or frequently recurrent muscle contraction headaches of psychologic origin are treated with psychotherapy (as discussed under migraine) to remove or to reduce the basic cause of the headaches. The symptomatic treatment of the headaches themselves includes: aspirin, phenobarbital, massage, manipulation and manual stretching of the affected muscles, local heat, warm baths, and bed rest.

Head Pain and the Eyes, Ears, Teeth, and Paranasal Structures

Eyes. Headaches may result from errors of refraction, glaucoma (with increased intraocular pressure), inflammation, and disturbances of ocular muscle equilibrium.

Ears. Primary ear disease which produces headache is relatively rare, but when it does occur the process is usually inflammatory or destructive.

Teeth. Painful stimuli in a tooth produce local toothache, which may be accompanied by a secondary headache resulting from prolonged muscle contraction.

Paranasal Structures. The openings to the sinuses are more highly sensitive to pain than the sinuses' walls, and thus the pain associated with sinus infection is most likely due to irritation and inflammation of these openings. The pain of the *sinus headache* is typically reduced or eliminated by the intranasal application of vasoconstrictor agents or topical anesthetics, particularly around the openings to the sinuses.

Diagnosis of Headache

To determine the cause of recurrent or chronic headaches the physician takes a detailed history, thoroughly studies the patient both physically and psychologically, and routinely performs such tests as: skull x-rays, EEG, CSF examination, echoencephalography, and radioactive scanning. Occasionally pneumoencephalography or angiography may be performed when it is believed that an intracranial lesion may be causing the headaches. The history includes questioning the patient concerning: (1) localization and paths of pain radiation; (2) character of the headache; (3) intensity of pain; (4) incidence, mode of onset, duration, and frequency of headache; (5) mode of cessation of headache; (6) localized tenderness; and (7) associated phenomena.

The *nurse's observations* of a patient's headaches can help to establish the diagnosis and should thus be detailed and precise.

Headaches are commonly "self-treated" with drug store medications available without prescription. The nurse should encourage persons with persistent or repetitive headaches to seek medical evaluation. Excessive use of coal-tar analgesics or any habit-forming drug for relief of pain is to be discouraged.

TRAUMA AFFECTING THE NERVOUS SYSTEM

The nervous system can be traumatized in numerous ways, e.g., through various types of physical injuries, and by the effects of agents such as chemicals, electrical currents, and radiation. The primary focus of this discussion is on accidental injuries resulting in forceful puncture, blows, fractures, or crushing injuries.

INJURIES TO THE HEAD (CRANIOCEREBRAL TRAUMA)

Traumatic brain injury is the most common cause of death between the ages of one and 35.[186] While it is not known exactly how many persons sustain head injury in all types of accidents, it is known that in vehicular accidents 70 per cent of the injuries involve the head.[197]

Although the physician or nurse has no way of preventing the *primary* brain trauma caused by the original accident (e.g., contusions and hemorrhages), prompt treatment may minimize the development of *secondary* lesions resulting from circulatory impairment and cerebral edema.[183] Vigorous treatment of hypoxia and acid-base disturbances (which almost always occur in comatose patients) may prove be the most effective means of reducing head injury mortality in the years ahead.[129]

Many patients suffer primary, irreversible brain injury at the time of the original accident which ultimately causes death. Brainstem hemorrhage is the most common cause of death from such injuries. *Severe cerebral swelling,* i.e. cerebral edema, commonly follows brain injury and is probably the most common cause of death in those patients who survive the initial injury and who do not develop intracranial mass lesions. Some patients survive the initial trauma of head injury only to later develop *expanding hematomas,* e.g., epidural and subdural hemorrhages, which may be fatal unless promptly diagnosed and treated.

Types and Effects of Head Injuries

Head injuries are frequently classified on the basis of the nature of the injury to the *skull* rather than the actual brain injury. Three common groups of craniocerebral trauma are: (1) closed head injuries; (2) depressed skull fracture; and (3) compound skull fracture.

> *Closed head injuries* (also called *nonpenetrating*). With these injuries there is no skull injury, or only a linear skull fracture with no displacement of bone fragments. Closed head injuries can be subdivided according to the severity of injury to the underlying cerebral substance: (1) *simple concussion,* which occurs when there is a physiologic impairment of neuronal function but there is no visible structural (anatomic) damage to the brain; and (2) *destruction of brain tissue* related to *edema, contusion* (bruising of the cortex resulting from percussion of the brain against a bony prominence), *laceration,* and *hemorrhage* (to be discussed further.)

> *Depressed skull fracture.* With a simple depressed skull fracture the pericranium is intact, but a fragment of fractured bone is depressed inward; this compresses or injures the underlying brain.

>*Compound skull fracture.* A fracture of this nature tears the pericranial tissues, causing direct communication between the lacerated scalp and the cerebral substance through the depressed or comminuted fragments of bone and lacerated dura.

The above classifications are mainly of importance in deciding whether surgical treatment is necessary; *the patient's prognosis for life and recovery of function depends more on the actual brain injury rather than on the skull injury per se.*[161] In terms of the patient's clinical appearance it may not be possible to tell whether his brain has been concussed, contused, or lacerated.

Subdural Hemorrhage

A subdural hematoma is a collection of blood between the dura and arachnoid in the subdural space. Blood which escapes into the subdural space is not absorbed but rather is organized or encapsulated by the dura. As the blood organizes into a clot the blood cells within the clot's membrane lyse, forming a fluid of high osmotic character. Water from the surrounding subarachnoid space is drawn into the clot, producing a gradually increasing intracranial mass. Large clots may produce such high intracranial pressure that cerebral herniation occurs and death may result.

Generally subdural hematomas are divided into acute, subacute, and chronic types. *Acute subdural hematomas* result from laceration of the brain, with a tear in the arachnoid allowing blood (from the small pial veins bridging the subdural space) and CSF to collect in the subdural space. Occasionally acute subdural hematomas may also result from a ruptured saccular aneurysm or intracerebral hemorrhage if there has been tearing of the arachnoid over the source of the hemorrhage. Usually acute subdural hematomas develop within the first few days following injury. The increase in intracranial pressure generally develops slowly since the blood forming the subdural hematoma is usually of venous origin. *Acute subdural hematomas are a serious complication requiring prompt treatment since they compress and distort an already damaged and edematous brain.*

The patient developing an acute subdural hematoma may remain unconscious following the injury, or his state of consciousness may be variable (depending partially upon the extent of injury). If the patient is conscious, headache is usually present. The patient may then become irritable, confused, and lapse again into coma or show fluctuating levels of consciousness. Symptoms of increasing intracranial pressure occur. A lumbar puncture is contraindicated since it may precipitate foraminal herniation. However if CSF is obtained it may be bloody or xanthochromic, have increased protein, and show elevated pressure. Usually patients who develop acute subdural hematoma have underlying brain damage and severe brain swelling.

Most patients with acute subdural hematoma are operated on within three days following injury. Surgical treatment consists of evacuation of the hematoma, removal of macerated brain, and vigorous treatment of the brain swelling at the time of surgery with hypertonic solutions and periods of hyperventilation.

Usually the prognosis is poor, mainly because of the primary brain damage. Of course, every attempt is made to identify the presence of a subdural hematoma early, before herniation can occur. The nurse must therefore be alert to the development of typical symptoms of increasing intracranial pressure as she cares for the patient who has sustained craniocerebral trauma. Occasionally symptoms of acute subdural hematoma may develop within a few hours following injury.

Surgery for *subacute subdural hematoma* is usually performed between three days and three weeks after injury. *Chronic subdural hematoma* may not come to treatment for many weeks or months following injury. With subacute and chronic subdural hematomas there is a latent interval during which the patient appears to be recovering from the initial injury or seems completely recovered, and then days, weeks, or months later he develops gradually progressive neurologic symptoms. Although similar, the symptoms and associated brain damage are much less severe in subacute or chronic subdural hematoma than in the acute form. The symptoms are similar to those of any increasing intracranial mass, e.g., headache and slowly deteriorating level of consciousness.

Although nonsurgical treatment appears to be successful in some cases of chronic subdural hematoma (e.g., by osmotherapy using 20 per cent mannitol),[238] the most commonly employed form of treatment is surgical removal of the hematoma.

The most useful procedures in *diagnosing* subdural hematomas are trephination, carotid or retrograde brachial angiogram, and radioisotopic brain scanning.

Extradural or Epidural Hemorrhage

Extradural hemorrhage most frequently results from a tear in the wall of the middle meningeal artery. As a result, blood hemorrhages into the extradural space, separating the dura from the skull. Usually extradural hematomas form on the side of the injury. Extradural hemorrhage is uncommon compared to cerebral contusion and subdural hematoma. Unless the mass is evacuated surgically, tentorial herniation eventually occurs, resulting in death.

Extradural hemorrhage manifests itself in the following ways: Consciousness may or may not be lost at the time of the initial head injury, and the initial injury may or may not be severe. If consciousness is lost, the patient may regain consciousness and have a "lucid interval" of several hours' duration before the symptoms of the extradural hemorrhage begin to appear, or he may not regain consciousness. Usually symptoms of extradural hematoma appear within a few hours after the accident. These symptoms include indications of brain compression, coma, and hemiplegia.

Extradural hemorrhage is the most serious complication following head injury. In untreated cases the mortality rate is nearly 100 per cent, and in treated cases it is over 50 per cent (due partially to delay in establishing diagnosis and in part to the severity of concomitant brain damage).[161] While there may be no clinical symptoms of this complication immediately following the initial trauma, once the hematoma grows to a critical level in several hours, deterioration progresses rapidly, and the patient may die if he has been sent home with inadequate observation. For this reason patients are usually hospitalized for a period of time, even following relatively minor head injuries. In spite of their rarity, extradural hemorrhages are important because they are potentially fatal, and also because prompt, proper treatment can be followed by successful recovery if the patient has not suffered other injuries.

Diagnosis of extradural hematomas may include: typical history and symptom progression, x-ray evidence of fracture through one of the meningeal arteries or large sinuses, diagnostic exploratory trephine openings, and angiography. *Rapid diagnosis and prompt treatment are essential,* and the nurse's observations and notification of the physician of significant changes in the patient's condition are imperative. *Treatment* of extradural hematomas is temporal craniectomy or craniotomy. Operative results depend heavily upon the extent of associated brain damage or other injuries.

Other Results of Head Injury

Intracerebral Hemorrhage. Multiple, scattered, small hematomas may accompany head injury; they may occur in the area of the contused or lacerated brain or at some distance from the original injury. Occasionally a single, large subcortical hematoma may form which can be evacuated surgically if diagnosed in time. The symptoms of such a hematoma are indistinguishable from those of extradural or subdural hemorrhages; the diagnostic processes are also similar. Generally, increased intracranial pressure and focal neurologic symptoms (e.g., hemiplegia) develop a few hours or a few days following the injury. Operative results are often poor because of damage to brain tissue caused by the hemorrhage.

Cerebral Thrombosis. Cerebral thrombosis may follow distortion of the brain by an extradural or subdural hematoma, or injury to artery walls. Cerebral thrombosis was discussed earlier.

Arteriovenous Aneurysms. Common causes of arteriovenous aneurysms are trauma which lacerates the internal carotid artery (as it passes through the cavernous sinus) such as by penetrating missiles or fracture of the sphenoid bone. Immediately after the accident the patient may notice a bruit, synchronous with the pulse. Other symptoms may include exophthalmos, distended orbital and periorbital veins, and paralysis of cranial nerves. These symptoms result from increased tension in the cavernous sinus due to the accumulation of arterial blood. It may be necessary to surgically ligate the internal carotid artery in the neck and intracranially ligate the internal carotid and ophthalmic arteries.

Mental Disturbances. A variety of mental disturbances may occur as sequelae of head injuries, e.g., confusion, inability to concentrate, emotional disturbances, changes of personality, transient psychotic episodes, mental deterioration, post-traumatic personality disorders, and amnesia. The severity of the mental disturbance is variable as well as the duration of the problem. Following head injury it is important to determine the degree and duration of any change in consciousness. *Traumatic amnesia* is divided into: (1) *retrograde amnesia,* loss of memory of events preceding the injury, and (2) *anterograde amnesia,* amnesia for events following the injury.

It has long been recognized that following head injury a patient may experience what is collectively called a "*post-traumatic syndrome.*" Such a syndrome may include the following symptoms: headache, poor concentration (especially in reading), dizziness, and unsteadiness related to sudden head movements, irritability, sensitivity to noise, insomnia, restlessness, hyperhidrosis, depression, personality changes, nervousness, impaired memory, anxiety, alcohol intolerance, and easy fatiguability. While as many as half of the number of head-injured patients may experience these symptoms in mild form for a short time, the symptoms are not referred to as "post-traumatic" or "postconcussional syndrome" unless they persist for weeks or perhaps years and incapacitate the patient for work.

Traumatic Delirium, Automatic Behavior. Once a patient begins to regain consciousness following head injury, after a period of perhaps several days of unconsciousness, it is not unusual for him initially to be noisy and generally disturbed and confused. Such a patient is often experiencing *traumatic delirium* resulting from cerebral irritation.

This is a temporary phase during which the patient must be protected, reassured, humored, and cared for as with other delirious states. (See Chapter 38 and Unit III.) Because the patient may remain in this partially confused state even after he can clearly speak and cooperate in some respects, the nurse may incorrectly believe that the patient is being wilfully uncooperative. After this phase comes a period of time in which the patient appears to have fully regained his mental faculties. He may be up and about, recognize his visitors, cooperate, and so forth, yet his memory of these activities is impaired. During this phase of recovery the patient is in a state of *automatic behavior* during which he has no memory of day-to-day events and yet is able to carry on his activities in a seemingly normal manner.

Convulsive Seizures. Post-traumatic epilepsy occurs following head injury in about 10 per cent of all patients who sustain head injury. The incidence is as high as 50 per cent when there has been penetration of the dura and laceration of the underlying cortex with formation of a cerebromeningeal scar.

Occasionally post-traumatic convulsive seizures may occur immediately following the injury or within the first few days postinjury. When this is the case, the seizures are believed to be related to acute brain damage or to the presence of hematomas, abscesses, or meningitis. Such seizures rarely persist for long and have a good prognosis. The more typical picture of post-traumatic seizures is for seizures to begin six to 18 months following the initial injury. Post-traumatic seizures are more often generalized than focal. In some cases the seizures may spontaneously cease or decrease in frequency.

Following head injury attempts of various kinds may be made to try to prevent the development of post-traumatic epilepsy. These *prophylactic measures* may include:

> Elevating depressed skull fractures.

> Thoroughly debriding compound skull fractures and suturing the dura to decrease the amount of scar formation (and thus the likelihood of seizures).

> Administering anticonvulsant medications prophylactically for one to two years (1) to patients who have sustained a severe head injury, and (2) to those patients who have a persistent focus of abnormal activity in their EEG.

GENERAL CLINICAL CARE FOLLOWING HEAD INJURY

Two major goals in the care of the head-injured patient are: (1) prompt recognition and treatment of hypoxia and acid-base disturbances that can contribute to cerebral edema; and (2) prompt recognition and treatment of increasing intracranial pressure resulting from such factors as cerebral edema and/or expanding hematoma. (Review carefully Unit V, Chaps. 24 and 25; Unit XIV; and Chapter 38 of this unit.)

Among the most significant recent advances in the care of patients with head injuries are: (1) increasing knowledge of how to properly care for an unconscious patient; and (2) recognition of the contribution of respiratory insufficiency to secondary brain swelling and neuronal dysfunction. We have previously discussed care of the unconscious patient. Let us reemphasize here that of primary importance in the care of an unconscious person is the *maintenance of a clear airway and effective respirations.* Inadequate respiratory function causes cerebral hypoxia and contributes to cerebral edema in ways previously mentioned.

Few patients die immediately from head injury; however, many die within the first few minutes from associated difficulties with respiration or shock. Early death may result from damage to the brainstem. Because severe mechanical trauma to the brain is associated with a high rate of morbidity and mortality, vigorous treatment must be started immediately if the patient's prognosis is to be improved. Initial care is directed at saving the patient's life, preventing the development of secondary brain injury as much as possible, and preventing further injury to the entire body.

Overview. Summarized below are important aspects in the general clinical care of head-injured patients. Details are presented in following sections.

> First, establish an airway and adequate respiratory exchange.
> Prevent aspiration.
> Check for the presence of shock; insure regular heart rate and adequate blood pressure.
> Search for evidence of spinal injuries.
> Observe for scalp and skull injuries.
> Prevent infection.
> Observe for cerebrospinal fluid leakage.
> Prevent the patient from unnecessary straining.
> Maintain normothermia.
> Establish baseline observations of the patient's neurologic status and vital signs; make frequent repeated observations.
> Observe for symptoms of increasing intracranial pressure.
> Observe for nuchal rigidity.
> Maintain fluid-electrolyte, acid-base balances and nutrition; record and evaluate intake and output.
> Control restlessness and pain; reorient the patient as he regains consciousness.
> Observe for seizures and be prepared to care for the patient during seizures.
> Position the patient as indicated and/or ordered.
> Prevent stress ulcers.
> Ensure rest; prevent complications of bed rest and of unconsciousness.
> Obtain history of how the injury occurred and how it affected the patient, e.g., did the patient lose consciousness?
> Observe for the various sequelae that can follow head injury.

Airway Establishment; Maintenance of Respirations. In caring for head-injured patients who are unconscious, first establish an airway and adequate respiratory exchange. With sufficient help, and while supporting the spine and keeping it in proper alignment, *logroll the patient onto his side* to prevent aspiration. Place a support under the patient's head to keep his cervical spine straight (Fig. 39–6). A *tracheostomy* may be performed or a *cuffed endotracheal tube* inserted to make a watertight seal. *Blood gases* are studied to determine adequacy of respiratory exchange. *Assisted ventilation* may be necessary to make sure the patient is adequately exchanging air. Carefully evaluate the patient's respiratory status. Prevention of respiratory complications in the comatose patient have been discussed in Chapter 38. (Respiratory care is discussed in Unit XIV.)

Cerebral anoxia from inadequate respiratory exchange is a leading cause of death in head-injured patients. In the brain-injured patient intracranial pressure is highly sensitive to changes in the blood's O_2 and CO_2 content and pH. Therefore, relatively mild degrees of hypoxia or hypercapnia cause great increases in intracranial pressure and can rapidly result in the patient's death. Hyperventilation, hypoventilation, and impaired cellular respiration can rapidly add to the development of secondary brain injury, e.g., circulatory dysfunction and cerebral edema. The mechanisms by which such respiratory changes cause brain damage in head injury are clearly summarized by Parsons.[183]

Aspiration Prevention. In addition to use of the side-lying position, aspiration may be prevented in the unconscious head-injured patient by other treatment measures, e.g., suctioning, nasogastric tube, tracheostomy. Aspiration can occur from inhalation of vomitus, blood, secretions, and so forth. Head-injured patients often vomit; some have been drinking alcoholic beverages prior to their accidents. Hemorrhage may result from nasopharyngeal injuries. Additionally, highly anxious patients may swallow large amounts of air following an accident. The air may then acutely dilate the stomach and produce emesis. The stomach may also be acutely dilated by ileus following severe injuries. A *nasogastric tube* may be passed to prevent emesis and aspiration of the stomach's contents. Treatment of severe nasopharyngeal bleeding may involve *emergency tracheostomy* and *suctioning* of the bronchi. The hemorrhaging head-injured patient is more likely to die from respiratory obstruction than from blood loss.[91]

Initially it is safer to suction the head-injured patient through the mouth rather than the nose *because of the close proximity of the cerebrum and nasopharynx; nasal suctioning could further damage these areas.*

Cardiovascular Complications. Check for the presence of shock; insure the presence of a regular heart rate and adequate blood pressure. Keep the patient quiet and comfortably warm. Frequently evaluate pulse and blood pressure. *If the patient appears to be in hypovolemic shock elevate his extremities; do not put him in the head-down position,* i.e., Trendelenburg position. If the brain is damaged, the head-low position increases intracranial pressure, produces cerebral venous stasis, and produces respiratory embarrassment (by causing pressure of the abdominal contents against the diaphragm). Elevation of the extremities does not contribute to cerebral edema; it favorably increases return of blood to the heart. (Shock is discussed in Unit V, Chap. 26.) Some head-injured patients experience *cardiac arrest* and other cardiovascular complications. (See Unit X.)

Spinal Injuries. The patient is carefully examined for spinal injuries. Do not allow the newly injured patient to move about even though he is conscious. Assume that all patients who are unconscious from head injuries have a spinal fracture until proved otherwise. Use extreme care in moving the patient. Unless contraindicated, turn the patient by the logrolling method every two hours to reduce pulmonary complications and other complications of bed rest. *Head injury is quite often associated with spinal cord damage.*

Skull and Scalp Injuries. Cover *open head wounds* with the cleanest material available at the scene of the accident. Apply pressure to bleeding scalp wounds only if there does not appear to be an underlying depressed or compound skull fracture. Do not attempt to remove foreign objects, or any objects causing penetrating injuries, from the wound. In the emergency room uncomplicated scalp wounds (which do not lie over depressed or compound skull fractures) are anesthetized locally, cleansed, and sutured.

Simple skull depressions are *electively* treated in surgery by elevation of the depressed bone fragment and repair of the dura if it is lacerated. All bone fragments are removed. *Compound depressed skull fractures* are *immediately* treated surgically; the scalp, skull, and devitalized brain are debrided and the wound cleansed thoroughly. Unless all foreign material is removed, a brain abscess develops. Debridement of a penetrating wound or depressed skull fracture frequently leaves a cranial defect that is cosmetically unsightly. Fortunately, *cranioplasty* can be performed to correct this defect. Cranioplasty has been simplified and cosmetic

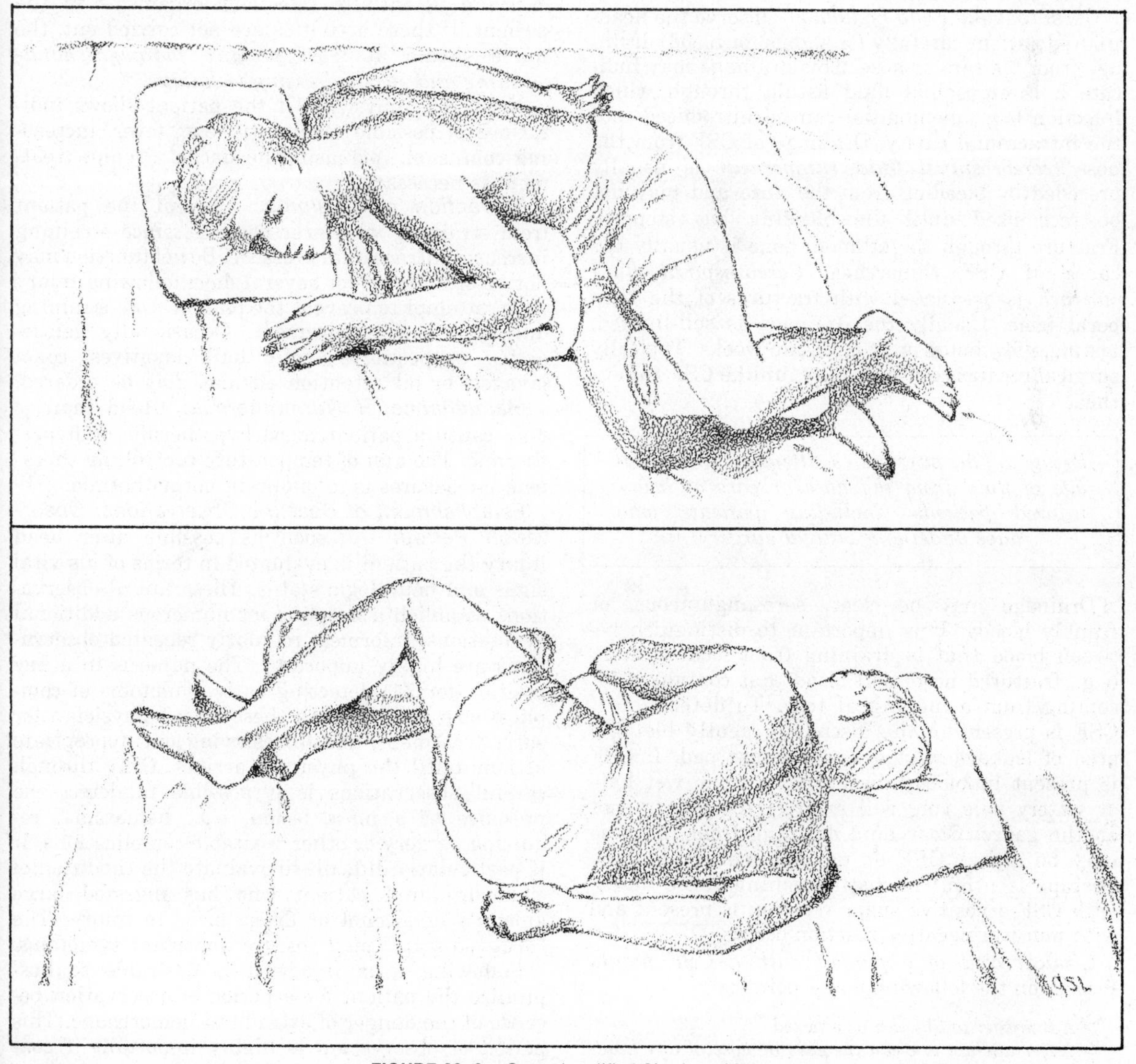

FIGURE 39–6. Coma (modified Sims) position.

results improved by the current use of various synthetic materials, e.g., acrylic plastic, tantalum, and stainless steel.

Infection Prevention. The risks of infection are more serious in a head wound than elsewhere in the body. In the emergency room antibiotics and prophylatic drugs for tetanus are administered if scalp lacerations or open fractures are present. Do not make vigorous efforts to clean up the patient during the acute period following head injury; rest is important. Use meticulous aseptic technique for all dressing changes and other sterile procedures. Early surgical treatment of compound skull fractures establishes a basis for infection-free healing. Possible infections that may occur following head injury include: extradural infections, osteomyelitis of the skull, external wound infections, brain abscesses, and meningitis.

Cerebrospinal Fluid Fistulas. Observe the head-injured patient carefully for serous (or blood) drainage from his ears or nose. This drainage may indicate a cerebrospinal fluid fistula through which infection (e.g., meningitis) can be introduced into the intracranial cavity. Drainage of CSF from the nose *(cerebrospinal fluid rhinorrhea)* is usually preceded by bleeding from the nose and may not be recognized until the bleeding has stopped. Fracture through the ethmoid bone is usually the cause of CSF rhinorrhea. *Cerebrospinal fluid otorrhea* is associated with fractures of the temporal bone. Usually the drainage is self-limited, lasting a few hours or at most two weeks. Typically surgical repair is not necessary, unlike CSF rhinorrhea.

> *Bring to the physician's attention any seepage of fluid from the nose or ears of head-injured patients (including patients who have undergone cranial surgery).*

Drainage may be clear, serosanguineous, or frankly bloody. It is important to distinguish between blood that is draining from local trauma (e.g., fractured nose) and blood that contains CSF coming from a meningeal tear. To determine if CSF is present in the discharge, gently blot the area of leakage with a *sterile* gauze pad. If CSF is present in bloody discharge, a clear wet halo or watery pale ring will encircle the bloody spot on the gauze. Clear fluid draining from the nose may be either CSF or normal watery mucus. Testape is useful in distinguishing these fluids; with CSF a positive sugar reaction is present and with mucus a negative reaction occurs.[175]

Clinical care of a patient with a CSF fistula focuses on the following major points:

> *Administer antibiotics* as ordered.

> *Never attempt to clean the ears or nose of any head-injured patient until the doctor gives his approval to do so.* If a CSF fistula is present, cleaning may introduce infection.

> *Never use nasal suction,* for to do so could cause serious additional brain damage or possibly introduce infection.

> *Instruct the patient not to cough, sneeze, or blow his nose.* These activities increase the likelihood of meningitis developing and may also allow air to enter the cranial cavity (forming a *pneumocele* which may further increase intracranial pressure).

> *Gently place loose, sterile cotton* in the *outer* opening of the ear or nose for absorbency or place a loosely slung external bandage, e.g., sterile pad, over the *external* ear to absorb the discharge. Do not pack cotton or gauze in place so that it obstructs the fluid's free flow.

> *Replace dressings as soon as they become moist* to prevent germs from passing through the moisture of the cotton and subsequently traveling to the brain.

> *Note color, consistency, and approximate amount of drainage.*

> *Instruct the patient to remain on bed rest.*

Some sources recommend that the patient with a CSF fistula be placed in *protective isolation* and that personnel wear masks and gowns to prevent carrying potentially infectious organisms to the patient. If these activities are not carried out, the nurse should at least *practice thorough handwashing and sterile dressing technique.*

Notify the physician if the patient shows indications of possible meningitis, e.g., fever, increasing confusion, increasing headache. Prompt treatment is necessary.

Prevention of Straining. Prevent the patient from straining whenever possible, since straining increases intracranial pressure. Bowel function may not be stimulated for several days following injury in an attempt to prevent the patient from straining during a bowel movement. Occasionally gentle-acting suppositories, mild bulk laxatives, colon lavages, or oil retention enemas may be ordered.

Maintenance of Normothermia. Head injuries may cause a patient to be hypothermic or hyperthermic. The aim of temperature-controlling therapeutic measures is to maintain normothermia.

Establishment of Baseline Observations: Observation Period. As soon as possible after head injury the patient is evaluated in terms of his vital signs and neurologic status. These initial observations establish a baseline for numerous additional evaluations. Informed, regularly repeated observations are highly important. The nurse is in a key position for: (1) detecting early symptoms of complications; (2) reporting these to the physician for early treatment; and (3) carrying out appropriate actions until the physician arrives. Only through careful observations is it possible to detect the presence of a mass lesion, e.g., hematoma, requiring surgery or other treatable complications. It is particularly difficult to evaluate the condition of a head-injured patient who has ingested large amounts of alcohol or drugs prior to injury. The "drugged state" may obscure important symptoms.

Following head injury it is desirable to hospitalize the patient for a period of observation because of the danger of extradural hemorrhage. This period of observation is highly important if consciousness was lost at the time of the accident (or later). The minimal period of observation is six hours, and the ideal period of observation is 48 hours for all patients who have been unconscious following head injury, even though the period of unconsciousness was only minutes or seconds long. If the patient remains at home, instructions must be given to the family: to awaken the patient hourly; how to examine him and what to look for; and what to do in the event of seizures or other symptoms of complications. The importance of these repeated examinations following head injury are emphasized both to the conscious patient and to his family.

In the hospital the frequency of vital sign measurements varies with the patient's condition, but usually these measurements are taken every 15 minutes until they are stable within safe limits. Often it is necessary to awaken a head-injured patient hourly during the first 24 to 48 hours following injury to evaluate his vital signs and neurologic status. The various parameters evaluated may include: level of consciousness and responsiveness; pupillary diameters and responses to light; pulse; blood pressure; respiratory rate; temperature (rectal); motor strength; speech; vision; reaction to auditory and painful stimuli; response to command; spontaneous activity; and general responsiveness to stimulation. During the observation period sedatives and narcotics are contraindicated except when specifically ordered; they are sometimes ordered if the patient is highly restless and an intracranial hematoma has been ruled out by surgery or angiography. (Evaluation of vital signs in the unconscious patient and in a patient with intracranial pressure is found in Chapter 38; shock is discussed in Unit V, Chap. 26.)

Decreasing level of consciousness is the single most important criterion of increasing intracranial pressure, e.g., from an expanding hematoma or cerebral edema. However, the patient may show worsening of any or all of the following parameters during observation: (1) responsiveness; (2) focal motor ability; (3) pupillary reactions and size; and/or (4) vital signs.

Be sure to inform the physician immediately of symptoms and signs such as: deepening levels of consciousness, restlessness, bradycardia, sudden temperature alterations, increasing blood pressure, sudden drop in blood pressure, cyanosis, or worsening of focal symptoms.

Nuchal Rigidity. Nuchal rigidity, i.e., involuntary stiffness of neck muscles, may indicate cervical spine injuries, meningeal irritation, or subarachnoid bleeding following head injury. In the presence of nuchal rigidity immobilize the patient's head until cervical spine injuries are ruled out.

Fluid-Electrolyte, Acid-Base Maintenance; Nutrition. Maintain fluid-electrolyte and acid-base balances and nutrition; record and evaluate intake and output. In the severely head-injured patient continuous intravenous infusion is maintained and fluid-electrolyte and acid-base balances are carefully managed. (See Unit V, Chaps. 24 and 25, and Chapter 38 for sections of related importance). Periodically laboratory evaluation may be made of such factors as blood electrolytes, blood urea nitrogen, blood gases, and pH.

A properly balanced fluid intake is gradually given to the patient as ordered. *Intravenous feedings* may be continued for several days. *Tube feedings* cannot be given until adequate peristalsis returns (usually about 48 hours after the accident) and cannot be used if marked abdominal distention or gastric retention develops following feedings. *Oral feedings* are avoided if they could precipitate vomiting, since vomiting increases intracranial pressure and can also result in aspiration.

As discussed previously, some physicians restrict both oral and parenteral fluids in some head-injured patients in an attempt to prevent excessive intracranial pressure. Intravenous fluids are typically administered at a minimal flow rate because of the possible danger of cerebral edema.

A retention catheter (or condom drainage apparatus for male patients) may be used to provide a means for accurately measuring urinary output and to avoid incontinence and restlessness. *Initially check urinary output regularly* to ascertain the adequacy of the circulatory system in the semiconscious or unconscious head-injured patient. Occasionally severe brain injury is associated with impaired renal function of unknown etiology. In spite of treatment the patient may die from renal failure.[195]

Restlessness; Pain; Disorientation. Evaluate and control restlessness and pain; reorient the patient as he regains consciousness.

Pain in the head-injured patient is best relieved by carefully administering codeine or other ordered mild analgesics. Occasionally if a major bone is fractured and the patient does not have symptoms of increased intracranial pressure, an opiate may be ordered to be given *with caution* so that pain is relieved without excessively depressing the patient.

Narcotics are generally contraindicated following head injury. Narcotics are not given if increased intracranial pressure is present.

Evaluate *restlessness* in an attempt to identify its cause. Restlessness in a head-injured patient may result from: (1) brain injury; (2) returning consciousness; or (3) other causes, e.g., increasing intracranial pressure, pain, full bladder, respiratory insufficiency, uncomfortable position, tight dressing. Try to correct manageable situations that may be causing the patient's restlessness, e.g., change his position. If the patient remains restless, inform the physician.

Sometimes the physician tries to relieve the patient's restlessness by prescribing *hypotensive drugs* (to reduce intracranial pressure) or by performing a *lumbar puncture* (to remove a small amount of CSF). At other times the physician prescribes *light sedation* with small initial doses of short-acting, mild medications. *Excessive sedation must be avoided in head-injured patients.* It is better to let the patient be a little noisy and a little restless rather than oversedating him. Restraints are generally undesirable since they may increase the patient's agitation and thereby increase his intracranial pressure. Protect the restless patient from injury. (See Chapter 38 and also Unit III).

As the patient gradually regains consciousness he needs to be *reoriented,* e.g., tell him generally what has happened to him, where he is, and that he is being taken care of.

Seizures. Be prepared to care for the head-injured patient if he develops seizures. Observe the patient closely for indications of seizure activity. Seizures may worsen a head-injured patient's condition; therefore, every attempt is made to prevent them, e.g., anticonvulsants may be prescribed prophylactically. Anticonvulsants are always ordered once a seizure does occur. If appropriate orders have not been left by the physician, be certain to inform him of any indications of threatening seizures.

Positioning. Position the head-injured patient as indicated and/or ordered. The patient frequently is placed in semi-Fowler's position unless he is comatose, in shock, or has spinal injuries. (Positioning appropriate in treating these complications has been previously discussed).

Stress Ulcers. Frequently stress ulcers occur (in the stomach and duodenum) following head injury, probably caused by postinjury autonomic imbalances. Atropine (which inhibits vagal impulses) may be prescribed prophylactically. Also, once peristalsis returns, nasogastric tube feedings with antacids may be ordered.

Rest; Complications of Inactivity. Rest is important following head injuries and therefore the patient is aroused only as often as absolutely necessary. However, it is of equal importance that the patient be kept active enough to prevent the complications associated with inactivity (Chapters 27 and 38). The conscious head-injured patient may become very tired because he may be awakened hourly for testing for the first 24 to 48 postinjury hours. Keep the patient's environment quiet. Plan clinical care to ensure rest periods.

History. A history of how a patient was injured can be helpful to the physician. Therefore when accident witnesses accompany a newly injured patient to the hospital, ask them to wait to talk with the doctor.

Observation for Sequelae. Following head injury the patient is closely observed (for as long as necessary) to detect possible disorders which may have been caused by his injury, e.g., mental changes, headache, dizziness. Possible results of head injury have been discussed.

INJURIES TO THE SPINAL CORD OR ITS ROOTS

Spinal cord injuries may occur from numerous causes, e.g., penetrating or crushing wounds, spinal fractures, spinal dislocations, compressing spinal tumors, or ruptured disks. Symptoms that develop from trauma to the spine may result from injury to the substance of the spinal cord or injury to the nerve roots. Injury to the bony spine is in itself not of practical importance except when the injury affects the spinal cord or its roots. Damage to the spinal cord may result from: (1) simple concussion which does not directly traumatize the cord; (2) penetrating missiles or fracture dislocations which compress, contuse, or lacerate the cord substance; (3) hemorrhage into the cord's substance, i.e., hematomyelia, and (4) compression of the cord's vascular supply.[161] As discussed previously, the symptoms that result from cord injury vary, depending on the seriousness of the injury and the level of the injury. The care of patients with spinal cord injuries has been covered earlier.

Ruptured Intervertebral Disk

In 98 per cent of instances ruptured, prolapsed, or herniated intervertebral disks occur at the 4th and 5th intervertebral spaces in the lumbar spine. Less frequently herniation of a disk occurs in the cervical region. Herniation of lumbar intervertebral disks is the most common cause of pain of sciatic distribution. The intervertebral disks (particularly between the 4th and 5th lumbar vertebrae and between the 5th lumbar and sacrum) are subject to tremendous forces and degenerative changes. When the surrounding ligaments are also injured and weakened, disk material (the nucleus pulposus) begins to extrude through the ligaments and compress the spinal cord and/or displace spinal nerve roots (Fig. 39–7). Ruptured disks cause an estimated 10 per cent of the backaches that prompt patients to seek the help of a physician. When the herniation occurs rapidly the patient experiences "acute low back syndrome"; if it occurs gradually the resulting persisting pressure causes "chronic low back" pain. Often younger patients report a history of a flexion injury, e.g., injury caused by heavy lifting from a stooped position during which they "feel something give way" in their backs. In older patients with degenerative changes, even trivial trauma, e.g., sneezing, or a misstep, may cause disk herniation.

Common *symptoms* of *lumbar* disk herniation include: low back pain radiating down the posterior thigh; muscle spasm; aggravation of pain by straining, e.g., coughing, defecation, bending, lifting, and straight leg raising; depression of deep tendon reflexes; and hypesthesia in the distribution of the affected nerve roots. Myelography may be normal or may show narrowing of one of the lower disk spaces. Rupture of a small laterally placed *cervical* disk typically causes stiff neck, shoulder pain radiating down the arm into the hand, and paresthesias and sensory disturbances in the hand. Electromyography or electrical testing of the peripheral nerves is valuable in localizing the site of ruptured disk. (See Chapter 37.)

Conservative methods of treating disk herniation are tried initially unless there are symptoms of cord compression, e.g., severe motor loss or loss of bladder function. In the presence of cord compression, immediate decompressive surgery is indicated, e.g., laminectomy. Acute *lumbar* disk herniation is treated with complete bed rest, often without toilet privileges. The patient may be allowed to assume the position of greatest comfort or he may be placed in traction to increase the distance between adjacent vertebrae or to relieve spasm of the thigh and back muscles, e.g., pelvic traction or simple Buck's extension (4 to 10 pounds). The mattress should be firm. A bed board may be placed under the mattress. Additionally the patient may be treated with local heat, massage, adhesive strapping, or a well-fitted, properly padded pelvic support or brace, or by muscle relaxants and analgesics. It should be remembered that prolonged heat increases congestion and is thus undesirable. Morphine may be indicated for severe pain, but the nurse must not forget the

potential dangers of addiction with prolonged usage. Once the acute pain subsides the patient is started on appropriate exercises.

While on bed rest the patient is encouraged to systematically change his position in bed (when not in traction). The patient with back pain may be most comfortable with the backrest elevated 20 to 30 degrees and his knees slightly flexed. Other positions that may be comfortable include: (1) supine, with pillows under the legs or (2) on either side, with a thin pillow between the knees. Physicians who prescribe the semisitting position (which encourages forward flexion of the lumbar spine and thus reduces strain on the back) do not permit the patient to lie in the prone position at any time since this causes hyperextension of the spine. Also, the patient should not use an overbed trapeze. In

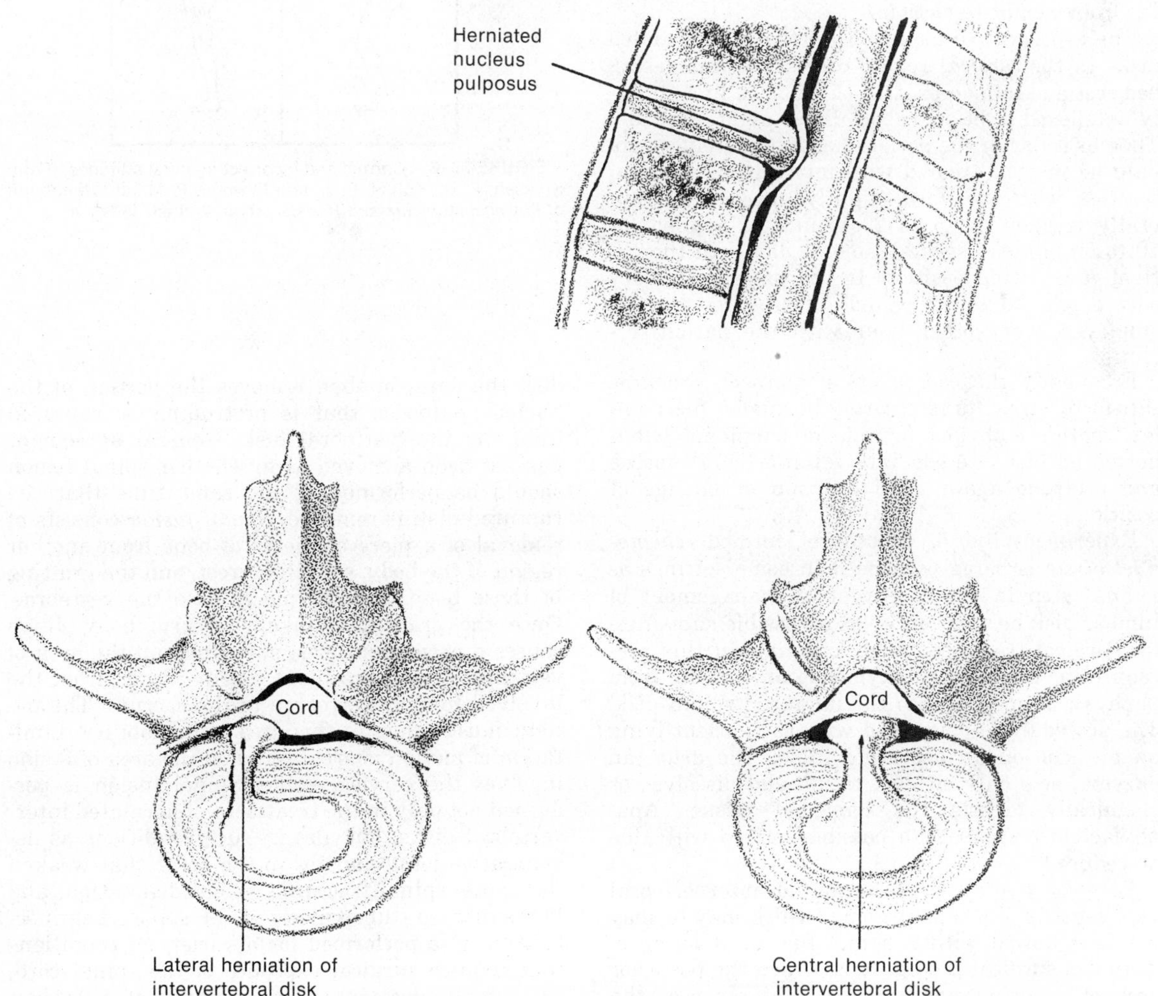

FIGURE 39–7. Forms of vertebral herniation.

bed the patient is turned in a logrolling manner and is given a fracture bedpan or child's bedpan. In placing the bedpan the patient is rolled onto his side (be sure to have a turning sheet on the bed), the bedpan and a small pillow or roll are placed to ensure adequate support to the lumbar region, and the patient is then rolled back onto the pan. *Proper alignment while the patient is in bed is of utmost importance in the treatment of patients with back disorders.*

When the patient is allowed out of bed he usually wears a back brace or a corset at first. Since restricted back motion progressively weakens the musculature and causes further degeneration of spinal structures, back supports generally should not be used after symptoms have been relieved. Postural training and teaching the patient how to stoop and lift correctly are important. Teach the patient to concentrate on lifting and not to lift until he has thought about *how* he intends to lift the object. The obese patient with back pain benefits from weight reduction.

The conservative approach in treating herniated disks in the *cervical* region consists of analgesics, bed rest and immobilization of the neck in a slightly anteflexed position, especially at night, e.g., in a Thomas collar. If the patient has moderately severe pain he may be treated with intermittent cervical traction with the head slightly anteflexed. Generally traction of 15 to 20 pounds is applied for 20 to 60 minutes several times a day with the patient in a sitting position. In the presence of very severe pain, 8 to 12 pounds of traction may be employed every other hour with the patient reclining.

Frequently the conservative approach produces satisfactory results in treating herniated disk, unless there are obvious neurologic symptoms. Often herniated disks recede into intervertebral spaces and protrude again upon exertion or change of position.

Experimentally a procedure termed *chemonucleolysis* is being performed in some settings as a final step in the conservative management of lumbar disk herniations or as a possible substitute for surgical treatment of disk injury. In this procedure a new drug, chymopapain (made from papaya), is injected into the damaged spinal disk. The procedure is performed with the patient lying on his side on an operating table. The drug, an enzyme, acts only on disk tissue and dissolves or chemically digests the damaged tissue. Anaphylactoid response is a possible hazard with this procedure.[146]

Surgical treatment of herniated intervertebral disk consists of a laminectomy, which may or may not be followed with a spinal fusion. A *laminectomy* is a surgical procedure in which the posterior arch of a vertebra is removed. This exposes the spinal cord. In treating a herniated intervertebral

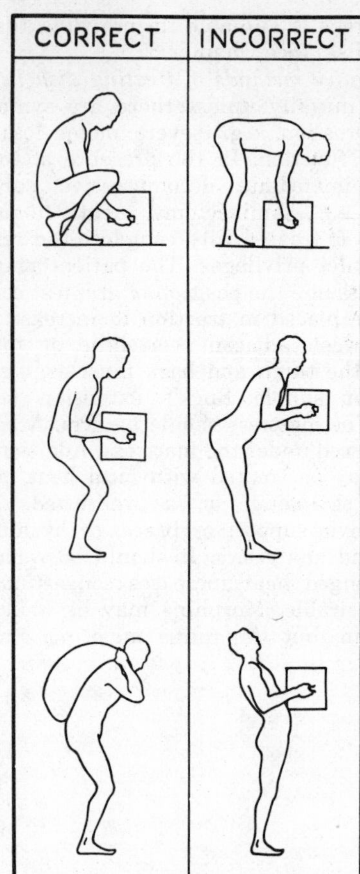

FIGURE 39–8. Correct and incorrect postural attitudes. (From Krussen, F. H., Kottke, F. J., and Ellwood, P. M., Jr.: *Handbook of Physical Medicine and Rehabilitation.* 2nd ed. 1971.)

disk the surgeon then removes the portion of the nucleus pulposus that is protruding or ruptured from the intervertebral disk. General agreement has not been achieved as to whether spinal fusion should be performed at the same time that the ruptured disk is removed. *Spinal fusion* consists of removal of a piece or pieces of bone from another region of the body, e.g., iliac crest, and the grafting of these bone chips or pieces onto the vertebrae. Once the graft has "taken," a firm bony union causes a permanent area of stiffness in the area of vertebrae that were fused together, e.g., from the involved lumbar vertebrae to the sacrum. The patient must adjust to this area of immobility. Limitation of motion is greatest when the area of fusion involves the cervical spine. Spinal fusion is performed not only in the treatment of herniated intervertebral disks, but also in such conditions as degenerative joint changes in the spine that weaken the spine, spinal fractures, spinal dislocation, and Pott's disease (tuberculosis of the spine). Laminectomy is also performed for a variety of conditions that require surgical exposure of the spinal cord, e.g., spinal decompression, removal of a broken bone fragment, removal of a spinal blood clot, or tumor. Nursing care following spinal surgery is discussed in Chapter 40.

INJURIES TO PERIPHERAL NERVES

Only some of the most common injuries of the peripheral nerves are considered here. The peripheral nerves can be injured in numerous ways, e.g., fractures of the bones and stretching of the nerves, constriction by fascial bands, pressure, trauma associated with perforating wounds, or the injection of drugs. The nerves most commonly subjected to external pressure are the radial, common peroneal, ulnar, and long thoracic nerves. The median nerve is most often affected by constriction by fascial bands; the axillary nerve is commonly affected in an allergic reaction to injections of serum; and the sciatic is commonly injured by the direct injection of medications. Of course, any of the peripheral nerves can be injured by bone fractures or perforating wounds.[161]

When a peripheral nerve is traumatically severed the ends should be anastomosed surgically to enable healing. When nerves are only slightly damaged, mild edema occurs at the site of the injury; this may cause temporary symptoms which recede in a period of only a few days or possibly weeks. The nearer the site of injury occurs to the central nervous system, in a completely severed peripheral nerve, the poorer the chance of regeneration occurring.

Median Nerve Compression at the Wrist (Carpal Tunnel Syndrome)

Carpal tunnel syndrome may develop spontaneously without a known cause or may occur as a result of disease or injury. A common known cause is trauma to the wrist involving the distal end of the radius and the carpal bones.

When the symptoms are mild and of short duration, or if the patient is opposed to surgery, the wrist may be immobilized on a splint, or temporary relief may be obtained by the injection of hydrocortisone acetate suspension into the carpal tunnel. Surgery is indicated when the symptoms are severe and of long duration, when muscle atrophy occurs, or when the sensory loss in the fingers and hand is progressive. Standard surgical treatment for carpal tunnel syndrome is decompression of the medial nerve by section of the transverse carpal ligament[63] (Fig. 39–9).

The counterpart of the carpal tunnel syndrome in the lower extremity is the *"tarsal tunnel syndrome,"* in which the posterior tibial nerve is trapped beneath the flexor retinaculum and deep fascia along the medial border of the foot.

Ulnar Nerve Compression at the Elbow

Lying within a bony groove at the elbow the ulnar nerve is susceptible to compression either from direct trauma to the elbow (hitting the "crazy" bone) or from changes within the groove that cause the nerve to be gradually squeezed. Repeated mild trauma (e.g., habitual leaning on the elbows upon a hard surface) can also injure the ulnar nerve. Resultant sensory changes occur in the ulnar aspect of the hand and wrist. The usual treatment for ulnar nerve compression at the elbow is transplantation of the ulnar nerve.[63]

Sciatic Nerve Injury

The sciatic nerve is the longest nerve in the body. *The common peroneal nerve (a terminal branch of the sciatic) is more often subject to trauma than any other nerve in the body.* Because of its peculiar course and distribution the sciatic nerve is more exposed to internal and external trauma and inflammation than any other nerve. Nurses are aware that sciatic nerve injury can result from faulty injection technique.

Sciatica refers to severe pain in the lower extremity that occurs along the course of the sciatic nerve and its branches. There are numerous causes of sciatica, but in about 90 per cent of patients the causes are rupture of an intervertebral disk and osteoarthritis of the lumbosacral spine producing mechanical pressure on the nerve or its spinal roots. Typically the pain of sciatica begins in the buttocks and extends down the back of the thigh and leg to the ankle. Usually sciatic pain is constant. Any movement of the lower extremity that stretches the nerve causes pain and involuntary resistance. Straight leg raising on the affected side is limited, and complete extension of the leg is not possible when the thigh is flexed on the abdomen *(Lasègue's sign)*. The treatment of sciatica is based upon treating the underlying cause when possible. (See also discussions of ruptured intervertebral disk and arthritis.)

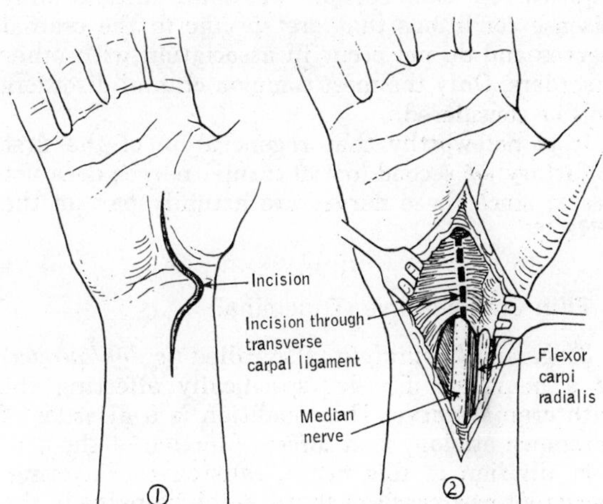

FIGURE 39–9. Technique of section of transverse carpal ligament. (From Finneson, B. E.: *Diagnosis and Management of Pain Syndromes.* 2nd ed. 1969.)

DISEASES OF THE CRANIAL AND PERIPHERAL NERVES

The cranial and peripheral nerves may be damaged by: tumors, infections, trauma, vascular and metabolic disturbances, and toxic agents. *Neuritis* refers to nerve damage from any cause. *Mononeuritis* refers to injury to a single nerve as a result of localized injury; *polyneuritis* refers to diffuse damage to many nerves as a result of toxic agents and metabolic disturbances.

The symptoms that develop following nerve damage are related to the type of nerve injured and the extent of damage. When *motor* nerves are damaged, the resultant symptoms may include: flaccid paralysis, muscle wasting, and loss of reflex in the muscle innervated by the injured nerve. When *sensory* nerves are damaged, loss of sensation occurs in the area of anatomic distribution of the nerve. When *mixed* nerves or sensory nerves are affected, vasomotor disorders and trophic disturbances typically result; these disorders may follow either partial or complete interruption of the nerve. Following partial injury or incomplete division of a nerve the patient may experience stabbing pains, dysesthesias, e.g., pins and needles sensations, and occasionally the burning pains of causalgia.

CRANIAL NERVES

The cranial nerves can be affected in numerous ways in association with various disorders of the nervous system as we have seen. For example, they may be secondarily affected from compression resulting from increased intracranial pressure or they may be directly injured as a result of head injuries. In this section we shall discuss only disease conditions that are specific to the cranial nerves and do not occur in association with other disorders. Only the most common cranial disorders will be considered.

It is noteworthy that regeneration of the first (olfactory) or second (optic) cranial nerves does not occur, since these nerves are actually part of the CNS.[161]

Fifth Cranial Nerve (Trigeminal)

Trigeminal neuralgia (also called *tic douloureux*) is a neuralgic disorder specifically affecting the fifth cranial nerve. This condition is a disorder of unknown etiology that affects function of the *sensory* division of this nerve, causing excruciating, recurrent paroxysms of sharp, stabbing pains in the distribution of one or more of the nerve's three branches. The trigeminal nerve is one of the largest of the cranial nerves and consists of the following divisions: I, ophthalmic; II, maxillary; and III, mandibular (Fig. 39–10).

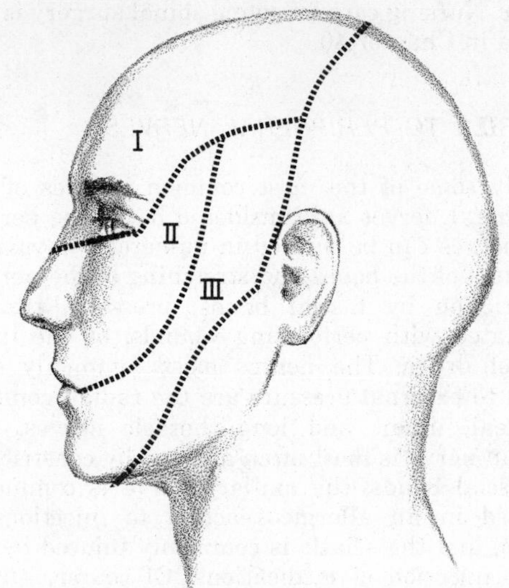

FIGURE 39–10. Trigeminal nerve distribution.

Trigeminal neuralgia is possibly the most agonizing benign condition, and has been known to prompt severe depression and suicide. This neuralgia is called tic douloureux because patients often wince repeatedly at the severity of the pain. The attack of pain typically begins suddenly, e.g., like a tooth fracturing. The pain is limited strictly to one or more branches of the fifth cranial nerve and does not spread beyond the nerve's distribution of innervation. The second and third divisions of the nerve are most commonly involved with the pain.

Trigeminal neuralgia attacks are characterized by the presence of sensitive *trigger zones,* the stimulation of which sets off one of the paroxysms of pain. These trigger areas are often small areas on the patient's upper or lower lips, gums, side of the nose, or cheek. A zone may be triggered into producing pain if it is stimulated, e.g., by cold wind, shaving, washing, chewing, swallowing, or talking. The fearful patient may try to prevent the paroxysms of pain by going without nourishment, oral hygiene, or shaving for days, or by trying to keep his face immobile while talking. Pain may interfere with the patient's sleep. In an attempt to avoid drafts, the patient may keep his face and head covered. Often the patient is fearful of being approached by other persons who might inadvertently trigger an attack.

Trigeminal neuralgia is the *most frequent of all primary neuralgias.* It affects more women than men and most often appears in middle or late life.

Numerous *medical and surgical treatments* have been tried for trigeminal neuralgia. Analgesic medications usually will not relieve the severe pain, except for morphine (and *narcotics are contraindicated* because of possible addiction with prolonged, frequent use). Recently, however, advances have been made in the non-narcotic treatment of this disorder. A suspension of mephenesin carbamate (a low-toxicity non-narcotic) effectively controls pain in some patients and may provide sufficient relief to eliminate the need for surgery. The administration of mephenesin should be followed by juice or milk since these liquids may reduce the gastrointestinal discomfort that the medication occasionally causes. Some patients with trigeminal neuralgia respond to pentazocine (Talwin). This powerful non-narcotic analgesic may be administered parenterally every four hours. The inhalation of drops of trichlorethylene on cotton produces variable degrees of pain relief.

Diphenylhydantoin (Dilantin) will abort an acute attack of trigeminal neuralgia if injected intravenously. The daily administration of this anticonvulsant may prevent recurrent attacks in some persons. Recently carbamazepine (Tegretol), another anticonvulsant, has been found to be more effective than Dilantin and to have fewer side effects. Tegretol may be given alone or in combination with Dilantin.

When medical management fails, the patient with tic douloureux is referred for *surgical treatment.* The trigeminal system may be treated surgically in a variety of ways intracranially or peripherally. *Peripheral measures* may include alcohol injection or avulsion of the supraorbital nerve, infraorbital nerve, or mandibular division. *Intracranially* the sensory root of the trigeminal nerve can be divided, providing permanent relief from the attacks.

Total severance of the sensory root of the trigeminal nerve produces *permanent* aftereffects. Permanent anesthesia of the innervated area results and the patient may also experience various disturbing sensations, e.g., numbness, stiffness, and occasionally burning. Often an alcohol injection is performed before the nerve is sectioned so the patient can *temporarily* experience the aftereffects before deciding upon the surgery. Whenever possible, *partial sectioning* of the nerve is carried out to spare the division or divisions of the nerve not affected. For example, since severance of the first section of the nerve results in corneal anesthesia, this section is not cut unless it is affected with the pain. Recently microsurgery has improved the precision with which the fibers can be selectively cut. For example, while eliminating the sensations of pain and temperature it is possible to preserve the corneal reflex and the sensation of touch.

Points of importance in the *nursing care* of patients with tic douloureux are summarized below:

> Observe and record *characteristics of the attack,* including precipitating factors, description of the pain. (Pain is discussed in Unit IX.)

> Note *ways in which* the patient tries to *protect himself* from precipitating attacks, e.g., avoids drafts and remains in his room, avoids chewing and shaving.

> *Individualize diet and fluids,* e.g., frequent, small feedings of semiliquid foods served at room temperature may be preferred. Avoid very hot or cold nourishments and fluids.

> *Encourage maximum activity and self-help.* Older patients especially should be encouraged to remain active. Often the patient prefers to care for himself, since he knows how to avoid trigger areas which others might accidentally stimulate.

> *Avoid triggering attacks.* Protect the patient from drafts. Avoid jarring the patient or his bed. Do not force him to perform activities that may trigger pain. If it is necessary to insert a nasogastric tube for feeding, be certain to insert it in the nostril on the unaffected side of the face.

> *Administer medications* as ordered; record apparent effects.

> *Postoperatively,* know which branches of the nerve have been sectioned and provide appropriate protection and patient teaching. For example, if the first (ophthalmic) branch is severed completely, the corneal reflex on that side will be absent and the patient should receive appropriate *protective eye care* and instructions about how to care for his eye. (See Unit XXI.) If the second and third branches of the nerve are cut the patient must: (1) avoid hot beverages and foods that could burn oral mucous membranes; (2) avoid biting oral mucous membranes while chewing; and (3) routinely visit his dentist semiannually since pain will not be felt in the areas innervated by the second and third branches of the nerve. Eating may be initially difficult if the nerve's lower branches are cut; the patient should be told to take food in on the mouth's unaffected side. Because food may accumulate in the mouth and not be felt on the affected side, frequent oral hygiene is necessary. The male patient must be especially careful not to cut himself while shaving. Often herpes simplex (cold sores) develop following section of the fifth cranial nerve, due to injury to the gasserian ganglion, or hyperthermia or dehydration. Such lesions are best treated with frequent applications of Campho-Phenique. These lesions usually heal in a week.

> *Offer emotional support* both preoperatively (because the patient suffers from the painful attacks and the fear of repeated attacks) and postoperatively (when the patient must adjust to the aftereffects of the surgery).

Seventh Cranial Nerve (Facial)

Our discussion here is concerned with the motor aspects of the facial nerve. The facial nerve is the main motor nerve of the muscles of the face. *Paralysis of the facial nerve occurs more commonly than paralysis of any other nerve, cranial or somatic.*

Facial paralysis may be central or peripheral in origin. A *central facial palsy* is an upper motor neuron paralysis or paresis. Sometimes central facial palsy produces dissociation of motor function such that the patient cannot voluntarily show his teeth on the paralyzed side of his face, but he can show his teeth with emotional stimulation which causes him to smile or laugh. This phenomenon is called "voluntary-emotional dissociation."[232]

The most common type of *peripheral facial paralysis* is called *Bell's palsy.* This is paralysis of the muscles of expression of one side of the face, when no evidence can be found of any pathologic cause.

With Bell's palsy there is typically: (1) an upward movement of the eyeball on the affected side upon closing the eye, i.e., "Bell's phenomenon"; (2) drooping of the mouth on the affected side; (3)

flattening of the nasolabial fold; (4) widening of the palpebral fissure on the affected side; and (5) a slight lag on the affected side upon closing the eyes. Note in Figure 39–11 the weakness of the face on the affected side.

Bell's palsy affects males and females about equally. While all age groups (from ages two to 85 years) have been affected, the most common age range is between ages 20 and 40. There is no known cure for Bell's palsy. Various palliative measures may be employed, including:[261] (1) analgesics if discomfort is present due to herpetic involvement; (2) cortisone drugs for the first few days (to possibly decrease nerve tissue swelling); (3) physiotherapy, e.g., moist heat, gentle massage, stimulation of the facial nerve with faradic current; (4) support of sagging facial muscles with strips of adhesive or with a facial sling; and (5) protection of the cornea, e.g., with artificial tear solution, sunglasses, eyepatch at night, periodic gentle manual closure of the eye. The patient with Bell's palsy needs to be reassured that he has not had a stroke and that his chances of complete recovery in a few week's time are good. Eating may be difficult.

The patient can participate in his recovery by performing passive exercises which improve muscle tone and position. When active exercise of the facial muscles becomes possible, grimacing exercises are to be performed in front of a mirror (three times each day for five minutes each).[261]

More than 80 per cent of patients with Bell's palsy recover within a few weeks, without residual symptoms. When permanent complete facial paralysis results, surgery may be performed. Anastomosis of the peripheral end of the facial nerve with the spinal accessory or the hypoglossal nerve allows closure of the eye during sleep and restores tone to the facial musculature.

Eighth Cranial Nerve (Acoustic)

Each eighth cranial nerve has two divisions: the auditory (cochlear), and the vestibular portions (the nerve to the semicircular canal system). Symptoms of involvement of the cochlear branch include loss of hearing and tinnitus; those of involvement of the vestibular portion include vertigo, disturbance of equilibrium, and impaired ocular movements. Tinnitus and loss of hearing are considered in Unit XXI.

Functional disturbances of the labyrinth may occur either as recurrent attacks, i.e., Meniere's syndrome, or as an isolated event, i.e., acute labyrinthitis.

The cause of *acute labyrinthitis* is unknown. While the condition may follow a head cold, it may also occur without antecedent infection of the nasopharynx. Typical symptoms include: severe sudden vertigo, nausea, sudden disturbance of equilibrium, and sudden nystagmus. During the attack the patient prefers to lie in a darkened room; lies quietly in bed without turning his head; is photophobic; has a headache; has an ataxic gait; and may refuse food. No specific treatment exists. To relieve the vertigo the patient may be given dimenhydrinate (100 mg. once to several times daily) or perphenazine (4 mg. t.i.d.). Because of the patient's severe vertigo he should be assisted when walking, and siderails are kept up on the bed. If the patient prefers, his room is kept darkened. Feedings are individualized in the presence of nausea and vomiting. Generally after a period of several days or weeks the nystagmus disappears and the vertigo diminishes.

POLYNEUROPATHIES

Polyneuritis or "multiple peripheral neuritis" refers to the clinical syndrome produced by *widespread involvement* of the peripheral nerves, with resultant sensory loss and reflex impairment. Generally a polyneuritis is related to either a toxic or metabolic condition. Examples of some polyneuropathies are: alcohol-vitamin deficiency polyneuritis; arsenic or lead polyneuritis; polyneuritis associated with deficiency states; diabetic polyneuritis; polyneuritis associated with carcinoma and other malignant neoplasms; diphtheric polyneuritis; and the Guillain-Barré syndrome.

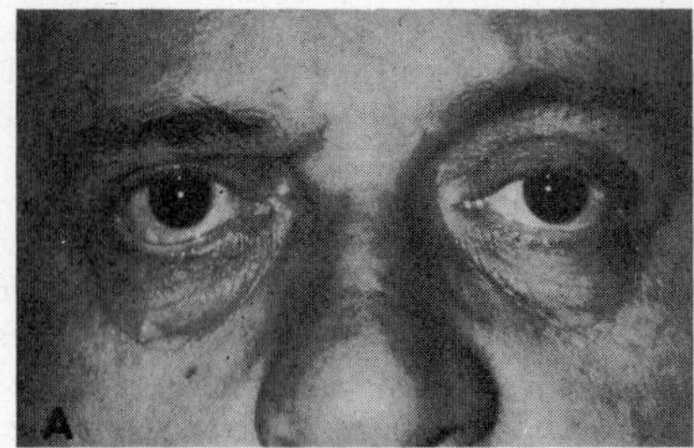

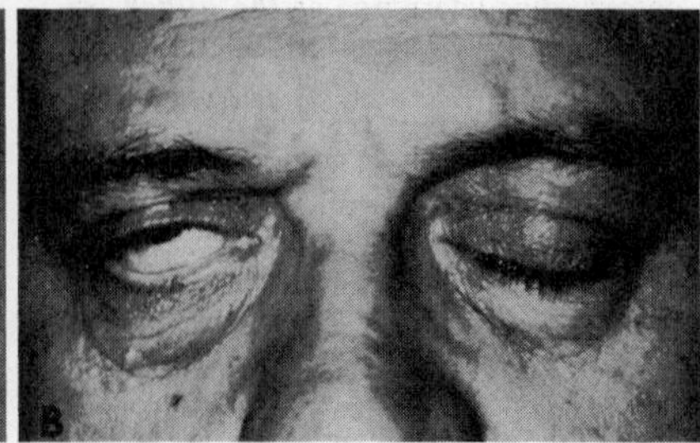

FIGURE 39–11. Bell's palsy of the right side. *A*, Eyes open in primary position. Note ptosis of left lid. *B*, Attempted lid closure. Note weakness of right orbicularis and upward rotation of right eye, or Bell's phenomenon. (Courtesy of Dr. David J. McIntyre.) (From Delp, M. H., and Manning, R. T.: *Major's Physical Diagnosis.* 7th ed. 1968.)

Guillain-Barré Syndrome

Guillain-Barré syndrome is an acute infectious neuronitis, of unknown etiology, characterized by widespread peripheral nerve and cranial nerve involvement. It may occur at any age, but is most frequent between the ages of 30 and 50. Both sexes are equally affected. A mild upper respiratory infection or, less often, gastroenteritis usually precedes development of the syndrome. The symptoms of the infection usually last for only a few days, and the neuritic symptoms appear anywhere from four to 21 days after the symptoms of the infection subside. The initial neurological symptom is usually weakness of the lower extremities; after 24 to 72 hours the weakness extends to the upper extremities and facial muscles. Sometimes paresthesias in the extremities precede the weakness. Usually the paralysis reaches its maximum within a few days of the onset. Cranial nerve paralysis frequently occurs and may cause facial paresis and difficulty in swallowing, talking, and mastication.

Generally the motor weakness in the muscles of the trunk and extremities is quite severe and may result in a flaccid quadriplegia and weakness of the muscles of respiration. About one-fourth of the patients require a mechanical respirator. Respiratory failure may occur anywhere from two to 21 days after onset of symptoms. In some cases severe impairment of cutaneous sensibility may occur, but generally sensory changes are minor. In severe cases rapid pulse, low grade fever, and moderate hypertension may occur. Most patients experience muscle tenderness or sensitivity of the nerves to pressure. The most common laboratory finding is an increased CSF protein content.

If death occurs, it most commonly results from respiratory failure or intercurrent infection. The mortality rate is reported as varying between 15 and 60 per cent. The rate of recovery in patients who survive is variable and is related to the degree of involvement. Usually recovery is slow and is not complete for many months. With marked quadriplegia full recovery may take up to 18 months. The disease does not recur and is not transmissible from one person to another.

There is no specific treatment for Guillain-Barré syndrome. It is vital that the patient be observed carefully for symptoms of respiratory paralysis and that an artificial respirator be promptly used when indicated. Administration of corticosteroids has given good results.

CHAPTER 40

Neurosurgery

Various modern surgical techniques have greatly reduced the risks of intracranial surgery. For example, *improved anesthetic procedures* relax the brain, making the patient easier to handle. Medications such as *urea* and *mannitol* may be given to reduce intracranial tension by dehydrating cerebral tissues; this makes possible easier retraction of brain tissue during surgery. *Hypotensive drugs* may be administered to lower the blood pressure when bleeding is especially likely to cause difficulties. *Hypothermia* is not used so frequently now as formerly; however, it may still be used for surgery on aneurysms or arteriovenous malformations.

Today, *stereotaxic instruments* permit precise local stimulation or destruction of areas of the brain. Such instruments essentially are metal frames in which the patient's head can be clamped in a standard position, and on which a needle holder can be moved in three planes along graduated scales. The needle tip can be guided accurately to reach calculated areas within the brain. Cannulas can also be stereotactically inserted into the brain. Through the cannulas refrigerants may be introduced (e.g., liquid nitrogen) which freeze surrounding nervous tissue, thereby causing either permanent or reversible changes. This procedure is a form of *cryosurgery*. Similar results may be obtained by stereotactically focusing a beam of *ultrasound* vibrations. Ultrasound beams can be applied through the intact skull (or vertebrae).

Microsurgical techniques are now applied to neurosurgery (Fig. 40–1). These techniques have enabled breakthroughs in neurosurgery such as improving classic techniques and making possible new approaches to the cranial structures, e.g., transsphenoidal, translabyrinthine. Microsurgical techniques are also used in some spinal surgery.

Improved clinical care of unconscious patients and head-injured patients is an additional and important factor in making surgery on the nervous system more effective.

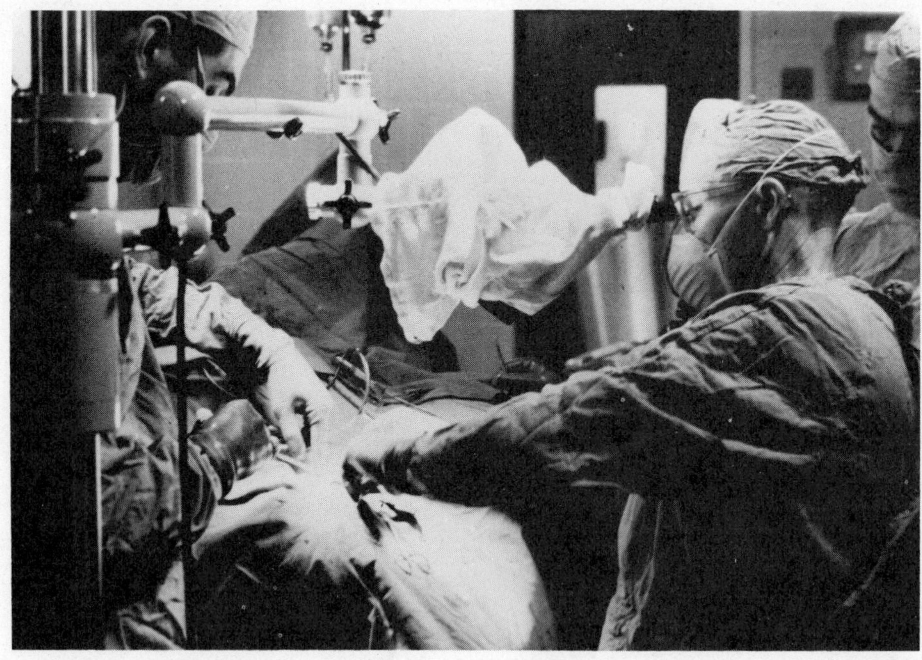

FIGURE 40–1. Operating microscope in use for nerve suture. (From Rowe, S. N.: Surgical treatment of nerve lesions. *In* Vinken, P. J., and Bruyn, G. W. (eds.): *Handbook of Clinical Neurosurgery.* Vol. 8. New York, American Elsevier Publsihing Co., Inc., 1970.)

INTRACRANIAL SURGERY

A craniotomy is an opening into the skull. Such openings may be made in several ways; for example: (1) "attached cranial section," in which the bone flap remains attached and hinged to muscles and other structures; (2) "detached cranial section," in which a section of cranium is detached from its attachments and temporarily removed for surgical exposure of the cranial contents; (3) "trephination," in which a circular piece or "button" of cranium is removed by a trephine; and (4) "craniectomy," in which a portion of cranium is removed and not replaced, e.g., for decompression.

As with many other surgical procedures, neurosurgical procedures are often described in terms of the operative approach taken, e.g., subtemporal, suboccipital, transmastoidal, transorbital, anterior, posterior. Craniotomies may be described in relation to the tentorium, e.g., supratentorial, infratentorial.

PREOPERATIVE CARE

Generally the preoperative preparation of a patient for intracranial surgery differs very little from that necessary for general surgery, particularly when the operation is not performed as an emergency measure, and the patient's general condition is good.[151] However, there are a few factors of importance which should be emphasized concerning preoperative preparation for intracranial surgery. (See also Unit VI on general surgery.)

> Preoperative bowel care is given cautiously and *only as ordered.* The patient is instructed not to strain at defecation since this aggravates increased intracranial pressure. A *small* enema or colon lavage is given cautiously and large enemas are never given. Sometimes enemas are not ordered because of the possibility of dangerously increasing intracranial pressure by fluid absorption or straining.

> Withhold food and fluids as ordered. Some patients may already be on restricted fluids because of cerebral edema.

> Explain preoperative procedures even though the patient may be stuporous or even appear unconscious; he may be able to hear.

> See that operative permission has been obtained from the patient (if capable) or a close relative. Often it is the physician's responsibility to obtain such permission after explaining the proposed surgery to the patient and family.

> Administer preoperative medications as ordered. Any order for narcotics, except codeine, is carefully checked by the nurse because of the danger of further depressing cerebral function. Generally morphine is not given to patients with cerebral lesions because of the danger of respiratory depression. Atropine may be ordered alone. A barbiturate may be ordered to reduce the patient's apprehension, if his condition permits.

> Follow instructions regarding scalp preparation. A shampoo may be ordered. At the time of the shampoo the patient's scalp is examined carefully. The nurse must be careful that her fingernails are short and clean so she does not scratch the patient's scalp while giving the shampoo. Report any unusual scalp conditions, e.g., dermatitis, infections. The patient's head may not be shaved over the operative area until he has been anesthetized in the operating room. Usually only a small area of the head is shaved, and care is taken to attempt to preserve hair on the patient's head in such a manner that it can be drawn over the scar after convalescence. Reassure the patient that his (or her) hair will grow back in the area shaved. Some hospitals request that the patient's cut hair be saved; some patient's wish to have pieces of their long hair made into hairpieces. Today the availability of commercial wigs and other hairpieces reduces the depersonalizing effects that patients often experience when their hair is cut for cranial surgery. Generally the scalp is prepared immediately prior to surgery so that if the scalp is accidentally lacerated during the shaving the wound will not have time to become infected. If preparation of the patient's head is done on the ward, a clean towel is pinned around the patient's head following the preparation.

> If there are no contraindications to activity, the patient should be gotten out of bed and walked around before the preoperative medication is given. This stimulates circulation.

> Have the patient void. Check the paralyzed patient for distention of the urinary bladder; retention of urine can occur.

> The patient with elevated intracranial pressure may be on a dehydrating regimen preoperatively. If so, follow orders concerning dehydration measures.

> Inspire confidence in the patient concerning his surgeon and members of the staff. Set an example through your own skillful, understanding care. Provide a relaxed, restful atmosphere in which the patient feels comfortable in expressing his concerns. Direct your help and attention not only to the patient but also to his family members and friends.

> Evaluate and note such factors as the patient's: temperature (rectal), pulse, respirations, blood pressure, level of consciousness, orientation (e.g., concerning person, place, time), awareness of what is happening and ability to follow instructions, mental status generally and mood, pupil size, pupil equality and reaction to light, limb movements, strength in extremities (e.g., grip), skin color and palpable skin temperature (e.g., cool, warm). Note also any paresis or paralysis, limitations or exaggerations of movements, sensory abnormalities, indications of skin pressure, burns, irritations, abrasions, bruises, hematomas, or edema. Finally, note any other abnormal observations, e.g., symptoms of dehydration, chest congestion, seizures, aphasia, visual or auditory disorders. (Report immediately any symptoms of increasing intracranial pressure or respiratory congestion.) The preceding observations provide a basis for comparison with postoperative findings and it is thus possible to determine if the patient's condition is worsened, improved, or unchanged in these various parameters as a result of surgical intervention.

POSTOPERATIVE CARE

Usually following cranial surgery the patient is kept in the intensive care unit until his condition is stabilized and he can safely be returned to the ward for general care. Care of the unconscious patient and care of the head-injured patient have been discussed previously (Chapter 38). Following intracranial surgery the patient has, in effect, a head "injury." Thus, the principles of care for head-injured patients apply to care of the patient following cranial surgery. Here we summarize some points of outstanding importance regarding postoperative care of patients who have had cranial surgery:

> Prevent aspiration and ensure adequate respiratory ventilation; promptly treat respiratory obstruction or respiratory failure.

> Appropriately position and turn the patient; enforce necessary restrictions of activity and position, and encourage allowed activities.

> Attempt to prevent postoperative complications.

> Frequently observe and evaluate the patient, watching closely for indications of developing complications, e.g., cerebral edema, bleeding, CSF leakage.

> Promptly report indications of developing complications and take necessary emergency actions.

> Observe for, evaluate cause of, and provide adequate protective care when restlessness occurs.

> Observe for and relieve periocular edema.

> Observe for, report, and administer appropriate care for such postoperative residual disorders as paralysis, muscle weakness, corneal anesthesia or other sensory losses, difficulty in swallowing, visual or language disorders, and/or personality disorders.

> Observe for indications of seizure activity; when possible prevent convulsions; administer appropriate care in the presence of convulsions or status epilepticus.

> Frequently inspect dressings and reinforce as necessary. Report abnormally tight dressings, abnormal bleeding, or CSF leakage. Maintain sterile technique to prevent wound infection and possible meningitis.

> Administer medications as ordered, bearing in mind the special precautions of importance following intracranial surgery.

> Take appropriate action to relieve headache.

> Prevent straining by the patient, e.g., at restraints, during bowel movements, during coughing.

> Provide a quiet, restful environment.

There are several important "DO NOT'S" which should be remembered when caring for patients following intracranial surgery:

> *Do not* suction the patient's nose without a written order.

> *Do not* lower the patient's head or place him in Trendelenburg (head-low) position without a written order.

> *Do not* place the patient on his operated side if a large tumor was removed or if bone was removed and not replaced following supratentorial surgery.

> *Do not* flex the patient's neck or allow him on his back following infratentorial surgery.

> *Do not* allow the unconscious or obtunded patient to lie on his back.

> *Do not* restrain the restless patient unless all other measures fail to control his restlessness or to protect him. If restraints seem necessary, never apply them without a written order; try applying protective mittens before using wrist restraints.

> *Do not* take the patient's temperature orally.

> *Do not* heavily sedate the patient.

> *Do not* administer narcotics unless you have double checked an order to do so.

> *Do not* administer intravenous solutions rapidly.

> *Do not* administer fluids orally until they are ordered, and then do so only after the patient's gag and swallowing reflexes have been tested.

> *Do not* administer cathartics, enemas, and so forth, or attempt to remove impactions unless ordered.

Following surgery the patient may have an IV running into his arm, an indwelling catheter in his urinary bladder, a Levin tube in his gastrointestinal tract, a nasal oxygen catheter in one nostril, and a tracheostomy tube in his throat. Possibly he may have his breathing assisted by a respirator and his body temperature controlled with a hypothermic blanket. Additionally the patient may have a catheter placed in one of the cerebral ventricles; this is attached to a drainage system and collection bottle (kept at the same level as the ventricle). Obviously the care of such a patient is complex and requires skill. Even such maneuvers as turning and positioning a patient who is attached to and probed by so much equipment is difficult. In some settings the patient's temperature, respirations, pulse, and intracranial pressure are monitored continuously and his cerebral blood flow is measured. Currently these are not routine practices. However, it is not unusual to have investigations by EEG, ECG, radiography or ultrasound performed at the bedside. The nursing staff must be prepared for such emergencies as cardiac or respiratory arrest and have appropriate equipment and drugs readily available to treat such complications if they occur.

In spite of the long duration of many intracranial operations, surgical shock is not a common aftereffect. However, these operations are associated with special hazards of their own, which can be prevented only by keen observation. The recognition of these hazards forms the basis of postoperative care following intracranial surgery.[151]

Observation and Evaluation

In caring for a patient following intracranial surgery the nurse makes frequent, careful neurologic observations, measurements of vital signs, and evaluations of her findings. Periodically she evaluates the various parameters she evaluated preoperatively. If the patient is stuporous or unconscious the nurse tests for reaction to stimuli, e.g., insertion of the rectal thermometer, mildly painful stimuli, and the patient's reflex status. These findings are compared with those recorded preoperatively. The frequency with which the various observations are made varies with the patient's condition and the doctor's preferences and may range from every five minutes to every two hours during the first few hours following surgery.

It is important to realize when making observations on a patient who has been operated on for removal of a brain tumor that preoperatively a dye, e.g., fluorescein sodium, may have been injected intravenously to help to localize the tumor at the time of surgery. Given one hour preoperatively, the dye causes the patient's skin and sclera (i.e., whites of the eyes) to appear jaundiced for several days postoperatively.

In evaluating the findings of her observations the nurse watches especially for indications of such *complications* or results of intracranial surgery as: shock; increased intracranial pressure; seizures and convulsions; CSF leakage (e.g., otorrhea, rhinorrhea, saturation of the dressing with CSF); hemorrhage; worsening of focal symptoms; lowering of level of consciousness; impaired motor function, e.g., paresis, paralysis (monoplegia, hemiplegia); facial weakness or facial paralysis; respiratory complications; abnormal body temperatures, e.g., hypothermia, hyperthermia; meningitis or wound infection; bowel and/or urinary bladder complications; impaired functioning of the vagus and glossopharyngeal nerves, e.g., difficulty in swallowing, loss of gag reflex; corneal anesthesia or other alterations in sensation or reflex actions; pain; headache; periocular edema (puffing or swelling of the eyelids); ecchymosis; visual or speech disturbances; changes in personality or behavior; herpes simplex; sordes; parotitis; all the complications of bed rest, e.g., thrombophlebitis, decubitus ulcers; and fluid-electrolyte imbalances, e.g., dehydration.

Airway Care

Prevention of the hazard of respiratory obstruction requires special attention following intracranial surgery since the lesion itself or the operative interference may cause paralysis of swallowing muscles and the risk of inhalation of vomitus and secretions.[151] The unconscious patient with a lesion in his brain tends to have excessive secretions in his respiratory tract and inadequate expulsion of such secretions by coughing. The patient must be carefully positioned on his side with his head low or at least flat unless his condition requires elevation of the head. In any event the lateral position is maintained to help to keep the tongue from falling back and obstructing the oral pharynx.

Nasal oxygen may allow adequate respiratory exchange. The nurse never inserts a nasal catheter following brain surgery without a written order stating it is safe to do so; in some cases the area of surgery may be injured (the same is true for nasal suctioning). Vigorous coughing is dangerous following intracranial surgery because it increases intracranial pressure. Thus, suctioning is carefully performed and the conscious patient is instructed to deep breathe periodically to clear his lungs, but not to cough strenuously. When tracheobronchial secretions are profuse, and neither oral suctioning nor medications provide adequate relief, a tracheostomy is quickly performed. Even mild hypoxia increases swelling of the brain; thus, every attempt is made to prevent this disorder.

Position, Turning, Activity

Sometimes following intracranial procedures bone flaps are left out postoperatively to allow expansion of inoperable tumors and/or to reduce pressure from postoperative edema. The bone may be saved and later replaced, or cranioplasty may be performed at a later date in surviving patients. If bone is removed and not replaced, the patient is nursed on the nonaffected side.

There are some general guidelines to follow in positioning patients following intracranial surgical procedures:

> *Following infratentorial surgery* keep the patient positioned *flat* on *either side* with his *head properly aligned* with his spinal column, e.g., a small pillow may be necessary under the head. Keep the patient off his back for the first 24 to 48 hours; after this period of time the physician may order the head of the bed gradually elevated over a period of several days.

> *Following supratentorial surgery* the patient is *not allowed* to lie *on the operated side if a large tumor has been removed* since the force of gravity could cause displacement of brain structures. Usually following supratentorial surgery the patient is positioned on his side with his *head elevated 45 degrees* (unless in shock). The upright position is maintained in an attempt to: (1) reduce cerebral edema; (2) minimize the possibility of hemorrhage; and (3) improve CSF circulation.

Following intracranial surgery *do not lower the patient's head* without written permission from the neurosurgeon since the head-low position increases the brain's blood supply and may precipitate venous bleeding. The patient in shock may be ordered to be placed flat with his extremities elevated. The Trendelenburg position is contraindicated because it increases intracranial pressure by increasing the brain's blood supply and may therefore start a hemorrhage.

As with any patient in bed, frequent *turning* (at least every two hours) is important for the postoperative patient following intracranial surgery to prevent the complications of immobility. For the first 48 postoperative hours the patient is turned cautiously with the help of several persons. The patient who has had infratentorial surgery should be *positioned* and turned in such a manner that his head is kept properly aligned with his body at all times. In turning the patient one nurse supports the patient's head, preventing twisting of the neck; the patient is positioned in such a manner (on his side) that his nose is in line with his breastbone.

Instruct the postoperative patient concerning any limitations of activity and position. Tell him how you will help him to move, and so forth. Place a sign on the head of the bed clearly stating any restrictions regarding his position. Discuss these limitations with family members if they visit.

Usually the patient who has had intracranial surgery is kept quiet (except for necessary interruptions) and is given total care for the first 48 hours after surgery. In some hospitals this care is given in an intensive care unit. If in bed on the ward, the patient is usually positioned with his head at the foot of the bed to facilitate observation, support, and positioning of the head. A turning sheet is placed on the postoperative bed; put the sheet on the bed so that it will extend well above the patient's head.

On the third postoperative day, if complications are not present, the patient is often allowed to assume some self-care. Occasionally the patient may be allowed up in a bedside chair on the day of surgery if the nature of his surgery and his condition permits. Typically, following infratentorial surgery patients may not be allowed up until the 10th postoperative day, and following supratentorial surgery the patient is allowed up in a chair on the third to fifth postoperative day.

Intracranial Pressure, Cerebral Edema, Intracranial Bleeding

Varying degrees of cerebral edema occur following intracranial surgery, and occasionally bleeding may also occur. Both these factors may cause increased intracranial pressure. If this is not rapidly relieved the brain's vital centers become arrested and death ensues. The nurse observes for symptoms of increasing intracranial pressure and attempts to control postoperative edema by following the physician's orders. Orders may concern positioning, use of hypothermia, administration of hypertonic urea, mannitol, or adrenocorticosteroids or cortisone-like compounds, e.g., dexamethasone and methylprednisolone, which diminish the entry of water into the traumatized brain. Additional measures used to combat cerebral edema may include: dehydration measures which limit fluid intake (watch output record carefully); ventricular tapping when the ventricles are large; and perhaps continuous catheter drainage attached to a sterile reservoir maintained at a level which roughly equals normal CSF pressure.

When continuous ventricular drainage is employed to drain off excess spinal fluid, the nurse takes care to: (1) prevent traction on the tubing, which could displace the catheter in the ventricle; (2) prevent kinks in the tubing, which could obstruct free flow of CSF; (3) keep the patient's head and drainage receptacle at proper heights to maintain approximately normal CSF pressure; (4) keep the tubing and collecting bottle sterile to prevent introduction of pathogens into the brain; and (5) notify the physician if the drainage appears to stop so he can evaluate the problem. Generally the doctor removes the catheter after 24 to 48 hours.

Dressing

Frequently observe the dressing. Report at once indications of hemorrhage, excessive CSF leakage, and tightness of the dressing. Clear or yellow drainage may indicate loss of CSF.

Reinforce dressings as necessary with *sterile* dressings to prevent the absorption of pathogens through the dressing to the wound by capillary action. Meningitis can result from wound infection following cranial surgery. Sometimes a *drain* is left in place for 24 to 48 hours; if so, reinforce the dressing as necessary and cover the reinforcement with a sterile towel. Change the towel every half hour and hold the towel in place with tape. Observe a restless patient carefully to be sure he does not disturb his dressing or contaminate the wound, e.g., by stretching.

The frequency with which the physician removes and changes dressings varies. Fluid may be noticed to collect under the scalp, and the physician may aspirate it when he changes the dressing.

Generally supratentorial incisions are made behind the hairline somewhere on the anterior two-thirds of the head; infratentorial incisions are made just above the nape of the neck. Following supratentorial surgery the patient may have a firm dressing of crinoline and starch which covers the head like a bathing cap. Following infratentorial surgery the patient usually has a firm dressing which encircles the head and also gives firm support to the neck in such a manner that it prevents flexion of the neck.

After the dressings have been removed, following suture removal, it may be noticed that the scalp has become encrusted and may have some dried blood on it. Hydrogen peroxide is used to remove the dried blood. The crusts may be softened and then removed by: (1) oiling the scalp with olive oil or mineral oil or coating it with yellow petrolatum jelly; (2) covering the oiled or greased scalp overnight with a soft towel; and (3) gently washing the area the next morning with soap and water. When cleansing the scalp rub lightly; do *not* rub over the operated area, and make the rubbing motions *toward* the suture line (do not pull or rub the scalp in such a manner that you place stress on the suture line). After the dressings are removed the nurse inspects the wound at least twice daily looking for bulging (indicative of increasing intracranial pressure or fluid accumulation) or signs of injury to the wound.

After the wound is healing the patient may wear a protective stockinette cap or scarf over his or her head. The patient is warned not to scratch his head and to take care not to bump his head. This is particularly important if a portion of the brain is unprotected because bone was removed at the time of surgery and not replaced.

Hyperthermia, Hypothermia

Surgery in the region of the hypothalamus may disturb the nerve cells responsible for temperature control. As a result, the patient's body temperature may either drop or increase until death. If temperature disturbances seem to be developing, the patient's temperature is taken every 15 minutes to assess the problem and permit institution of proper treatment.

Hyperthermia may result not only from damage to the heat controlling mechanisms of the hypothalamus and brainstem, but also from excessive dehydration, thrombophlebitis, or local or general infection. Hyperpyrexia may last for 48 hours postoperatively owing to the presence of blood in the cranium.

Convulsive Seizures

Patients with intracranial lesions and particularly head-injured patients, including the head injury caused by intracranial surgery, may develop epilepsy. These persons may have only a single seizure, or they may have many and even progress into the serious condition of status epilepticus. Because convulsive seizures increase cerebral edema or bleeding in the postoperative patient, the physician frequently attempts to prevent their initial occurrence by prophylactically administering such medications as diphenylhydantoin or phenobarbital.

Restlessness

Restlessness, ranging from moderate restlessness to wild thrashing about, is generally most acute the second or third postoperative day when the patient's general condition has improved enough for him to move about, but mental confusion may still persist. Evaluation of restlessness and care of the restless patient have been previously discussed. Following cranial surgery restless may last for several days. The administration of barbiturates may make the patient even less manageable. Paraldehyde is possibly the most satisfactory sedative. Tranquilizers, e.g., chlorpromazine, may be ordered.

Headache

Severe headache may occur for 24 to 48 hours postoperatively. The patient may be given an ice bag to the head p.r.n. Do not jar the patient's bed or move him suddenly. Keep his environment quiet, calm, and dimly lit. Administer appropriate medications as indicated for pain relief. Remember: barbiturates and narcotics are generally contraindicated because of possible medullary (and hence respiratory) depression and masking of symptoms of increasing intracranial pressure. Medications that may be ordered include: aspirin, caffeine citrate, codeine, or Demerol (given in conjunction with a tranquilizer).

Bowel, Urinary Bladder

Periodically check the patient for distention of the bowel and urinary bladder. Often the postoperative patient can go as long as 12 hours following intracranial surgery without voiding if he is dehydrated. The incontinent patient may or may not be catheterized, depending upon the doctor's wishes. Because metabolic disorders of CNS origin can cause a decrease in urinary output, the nurse reports significant decreases to the physician. An intake and output record is kept on all patients.

Never administer a cathartic, colon lavage, or enema following intracranial surgery without permission in writing from the doctor. Straining at stool may dangerously increase intracranial pressure. Some physicians ask the patient not to try to have a bowel movement for several days. Sometimes a cathartic is given on the third postoperative day and a small, low enema on the fourth day. Tell the patient not to strain at expelling the enema. Report impactions to the physician for removal. The patient who was able to have adequate preoperative bowel preparation benefits from this during the postoperative period. However, in some instances it is not possible to cleanse the colon prior to surgery.

Fluids, Food

Many physicians today believe it is unnecessary to restrict fluids postoperatively in an attempt to offset cerebral edema. However, some physicians still limit fluid intake to 1500 ml. for several days. Do not administer intravenous fluids rapidly following intracranial surgery; this could cause a dangerous increase in intracranial pressure or pulmonary edema.

Following supratentorial surgery, in contrast to abdominal operations, there is no contraindication to giving fluids orally and food by mouth as soon as the patient is alert and can swallow. In such cases fluids may be ordered orally on the day of surgery. If vomiting is present, e.g., from increased intracranial pressure, oral intake may be temporarily discontinued since the strain of vomiting could cause intracranial bleeding. *Following infratentorial surgery* the patient may be kept NPO for 24 hours because of impaired swallowing and gag reflexes. After 24 hours the physician may test these reflexes and, if they appear to be functioning, water may be given (with suctioning equipment at hand), followed later by other fluids. Withhold all oral feedings if any symptoms of difficulty in swallowing appear. Tube feedings may be necessary if there is paralysis of the muscles that govern swallowing. When necessary, tube feedings are usually started 48 hours postoperatively. The physician inserts the tube if there is a possibility that tube insertion may endanger the patient.

Once patients are alert, able to swallow, and have oral feedings ordered, they are usually fed for the first 48 hours to insure adequate intake and prevent unnecessary motion.

Metabolic Disturbances

Following intracranial surgery metabolic disturbances of various types may occur as a result of surgical trauma. These disturbances may potentially lead to coma. They must rapidly be identified and the imbalance corrected.[239]

Ecchymosis, Periocular Edema

Following surgery, ecchymosis and edema, e.g., periocular edema, may distort the patient's features. The family should be told generally how the patient appears before they are allowed to see him for the first time postoperatively. Additionally, if any noticeable defects have been detected postoperatively, e.g., facial paralysis, aphasia, the family should be prepared for these.

Relieve periocular edema by applying a light coating of petrolatum around the patient's eyes and on the eyelids, and then periodically applying light cold compresses (of crushed ice in Pliofilm taped over the affected eye).

Complications of Bed Rest

Following intracranial surgery the nurse works to prevent all the complications of bed rest (as discussed in Unit V, Chap. 27) as long as the patient is immobilized. Check with the physician concerning when to begin passive exercises and whether you can ask the patient to cough routinely.

Emotional Support

Provide emotional support to the patient and family members during the postoperative period. This support and understanding are particularly important if postoperative defects occur, e.g., paralysis, skull defects, if complications develop, or if the surgery appears unsuccessful. If a defect remains in the skull owing to removal of bone, the physician should discuss with the patient plans for cranioplasty (to protect the area and improve appearance) before the patient sees his defect.

Convalescence

During convalescence the patient may have to adapt to various residual disorders. Some are of a temporary nature, e.g., double vision, whereas others may be permanent, e.g., paralysis, aphasia. The patient's concern about double vision may be relieved by alternately covering one eye each day with an opaque eye shield. The management of other defects and complications has been discussed previously in this unit. Eventually plans may be carried out for restyling the patient's hair and, if desired, obtaining a wig or hairpiece.

SPINAL SURGERY

Laminectomy and spinal fusion have been discussed previously, in the section on herniated vertebral disk (Chapter 39). Here we shall discuss the pre- and postoperative care of patients undergoing these operations. Generally, postoperative restrictions are fewer following laminectomy than following spinal fusion.

In caring for spinal fusion patients it is important to know whether anterior fusion or posterior fusion was done. Anterior fusion is performed by reaching the lumbar spine through the abdomen, or by removal of midline disks and bony spurs in the cervical spine through an anterior approach to the spinal canal in such a manner that the vertebral bodies are exposed through the anterior aspect of the neck. Posterior fusion is performed by reaching the spine directly through an incision in the patient's back, e.g., back of the neck or back of the lumbar spine. Postoperative positions vary, depending upon whether the fusion was anterior or posterior. It is helpful to remember that the goal of care is to prevent strain or flexion at the surgical site.

Since posterior lumbar fusions are the most common type of spinal fusion, our discussion focuses mainly on the care of patients who have undergone that procedure.

PREOPERATIVE CARE

The patient is prepared for spinal surgery as ordered. (The routine preparation of a patient for surgery has been discussed in Unit VI.) Summarized below are a few important points which pertain specifically to preoperative preparation for spinal surgery.

> Teach the patient how he will be turned postoperatively in the logrolling manner and teach him how to do muscle conditioning exercises which may be ordered postoperatively. If the patient's condition permits, have him practice turning and practice the exercises with your help and guidance. Familiarize the patient with the Stryker frame or any other special equipment that will be used postoperatively. Tell the patient that he will be turned frequently after surgery as his doctor orders and that turning in the correct manner will not be harmful to him but will actually benefit him. Instruct the patient about necessary postoperative limitations of activity, and measures he can take to help himself, e.g., periodic deep breathing. Instruct him not to reach for anything after surgery which could cause a strain (e.g., telephone, water, urinal) but rather to ask for these items to be handed to him for a few days. Tell him his call bell will be close at hand. Teach the patient how he will roll onto the bedpan rather than lift his hips; have him practice this with your help.

> Discuss the surgery with the patient and try to identify his fears. Many patients dread spinal surgery because they fear possible paralysis postoperatively; if the patient does not mention this fear do not suggest it to him and thus possibly add new worries. Allay anxieties whenever possible and encourage patient and family to express their concerns.

POSTOPERATIVE CARE

Following spinal surgery, postoperative care is directed at preventing complications, preventing further spinal injury, and providing an opportunity for the wound (and graft if present) to heal. It is of critical importance to *be certain the patient's spine is in a position of correct alignment at all times and that his bed is flat.* Postoperative orders vary with the surgery performed and the physician's preferences. Some physicians allow greater activity than others. Check postoperative orders carefully concerning the amount of activity the patient may have and positions he may assume.

Postoperative Transfer

When transferring the patient to his bed postoperatively, at least four people should assist. They gently and smoothly transfer the patient while keeping his spine supported and properly aligned. The stuporous or unconscious patient is never positioned on his back.

Positioning

Keep the patient's bed flat. Sometimes the head of the entire bed is elevated on 6-inch blocks, but the bed itself is not flexed. The mattress is firm, and a bedboard is usually placed under the mattress. Place a sign on the bed stating the bed is to be kept flat, and inform the patient and the relatives of this important restriction.

When the patient is positioned on his *back,* the back muscles may be relaxed somewhat if pillows are placed under the *entire length* of the patient's legs. This may also reduce the possibility of thrombophlebitis occurring in the femoral vessels.[131] Take care, however, that you *do not* flex the patient's knees by placing a folded pillow under the popliteal space; this is a hazardous practice.

When positioning the patient on his *side* following spinal surgery prevent strain on the back muscles by: (1) keeping the spine straight; (2) pulling the hips slightly back so the patient is balanced; (3) flexing the upper leg and placing a pillow between the legs; and (4) placing a pillow to support the upper arm, thus preventing the upper shoulder from sagging.

Place the *call bell* conveniently so the patient will not strain in reaching for it or in reaching for objects he needs but cannot grasp. Once the patient is allowed to reach for things, see that the objects he needs are conveniently placed.

Support the patient's back and legs while he is on the *bedpan* so that all sections of his body are on the same plane. Use a fracture bedpan or a small child's bedpan. *Stimulate circulation* in the patient's back, head, and neck following spinal surgery. Give frequent back rubs that include the scalp, neck, and thighs. When permitted it is desirable to reestablish circulation in the dependent areas of the back and thighs by having the patient lie prone periodically.[131] Explaining the importance of the prone position helps the patient to tolerate it better.

Turning

Be sure the patient's bed has a turning sheet placed on it postoperatively. When turning the patient to his side, logroll him. Avoid twisting the patient's spine or twisting him at his hips. Eventually the patient is able to turn himself while keeping his spine rigid.

To maintain the best spinal alignment, some doctors order the patient to be turned only from back to abdomen, or vice versa, and to avoid the side-lying position. Some physicians order the patient to remain supine for several days following spinal fusion, without being turned. Others order the patient to remain prone for several days (allowing turning only for voiding.)[131] Still other surgeons have other turning schedules. Check turning orders carefully for a given patient. Turning a patient following spinal surgery is facilitated by the use of such equipment as the Stryker frame, CircOlectric bed, or Foster bed.

Have extra help in turning the patient the first few times. If a fusion was performed, be certain the leg from which the graft was taken is well supported during the turn as well as afterward. During the first turning sessions the patient will be apprehensive. If he is not turned smoothly, with confidence, and with a minimum amount of discomfort, his anxiety will increase and he will be fearful of future turning sessions. It is equally important to keep up vigilance and continue to practice *careful turning* with adequate help even after several weeks have passed and the patient is able to help in the turning process. Particular care is needed during the fourth and fifth postoperative weeks. Spinal bone grafts are delicate and heal slowly. Gentleness, proper handling, and avoidance of twisting, bending, and sagging are needed at all times to encourage sound healing.

Observation and Evaluation

Postoperatively following surgery on the *cervical spine* observe the patient carefully for indications of respiratory paralysis resulting from cord edema. A respirator should be readily available. During postoperative care prevent flexion of the neck.

Every two to four hours during the first 48 postoperative hours evaluate the patient's motor abilities and sensation in his extremities. Progressive *worsening* of motor and sensory functions is indicative of spinal cord edema or hemorrhage compressing the cord; promptly report indications of cord damage or cord compression. If sensory losses are present, take precautions to prevent injury, e.g., from heat. Chart indications of any postoperative *improvement* that the patient may note compared with how he felt preoperatively, e.g., "the tingling I had in my leg is gone."

Dressing

Skin incisions for laminectomies and posterior spinal fusions are about 4 inches long and are made directly over the spinous processes. Observe the wound or dressing for indications of hemorrhage or

CSF leakage; if present, notify the surgeon. Reinforce the dressing as necessary with sterile compresses. If the dressing becomes contaminated, e.g., with urine from the bedpan, it must be changed. Some physicians wish to do the first dressing change themselves. As with any wound, observe the surgical wound for indications of infection. When spinal fusion has been performed be certain to also inspect the dressing at the site from which the bone graft was taken.

Pain, Muscle Spasms

Spinal cord edema may cause pain for some time postoperatively. Spasms may occur in the back and thigh muscles as a result of irritation of nerves during surgery. The area from which bone was taken for a spinal fusion may also be quite painful for several days. Provide pain relief as ordered and as indicated and take appropriate nursing actions to prevent or minimize pain. (See Unit IX.) Keeping the operated leg and the spine correctly and comfortably positioned helps to reduce pain and muscle spasms.

Complications of Bed Rest

Prevent the complications that can develop from prolonged immobility. (See Unit V, Chap. 27.) Don't forget to place a footboard on the patient's bed and to correctly position the patient against it.

Food, Fluids

Usually fluids are encouraged as soon as nausea subsides, and diet is increased as tolerated following spinal surgery.

Urinary Bladder, Bowels

Check the patient every two to four hours postoperatively for bladder or bowel distention. Bladder and bowel dysfunction may occur for several days postoperatively. Force fluids as ordered, encourage a regular time for bowel movements and bowel care, provide roughage in the diet (when allowed), and administer medications and enemas as ordered, e.g., mild bulk laxative, Dulcolax suppository. Inactivity often causes problems with bowel elimination. Instruct the patient not to strain at bowel movements; straining increases pain and also increases CSF pressure.

Activity

Supervise physical therapy as ordered. Check with the physician concerning active and passive exercises; some are contraindicated because of the strain they place on the back, e.g., straight leg raising while lying flat in bed. Supervise new activities as they are ordered. Provide appropriate teaching, e.g., concerning exercises, lifting, limitations of activity (avoid straight leg raising, avoid bending at the waist). Teach the patient how to move correctly, how to dress himself, how to get up off the bed, how to hold his spine straight, and how to prevent reinjury to his spine.

When he is allowed to be up in a chair instruct the patient to select a straight, firm chair and to keep his feet flat on the floor—not up on a footstool and not with legs crossed. When getting the patient up for the first time (whether on the day of surgery or after several weeks of bed rest) *have ample help,* and observe the patient closely for indications of dizziness, weakness, or fainting. Postural hypotension may pose a problem since the patient cannot have the head of his bed elevated gradually because of the danger of flexing the spine. If the patient should collapse and faint when getting up, the consequences could be disastrous if adequate help is not available to prevent him from falling and reinjuring his spine. If the patient collapses, the team helping him must be prepared to continue to support him and return him to bed while maintaining proper spinal alignment.

Have the patient wear stockings and firm walking shoes when ambulating, not slippers. Slippers do not provide adequate support, and the patient may fall if they are of a soft or slick material or if they fit poorly and slip off. If the soles of the patient's shoes are slick, apply strips of adhesive tape across them to improve traction.

When the patient sits in a chair have him keep his back straight when sitting down and standing up. Be certain to hold the chair, and perhaps to have it placed against a wall to prevent the chair from slipping away as the patient sits down or gets up.

Teach the patient that when he wants to pick something up from the floor he should squat down, with his back held straight and his knees and hips sharply flexed. Demonstrate this to him. Caution the patient to take special care not to suddenly stretch, twist, flex or jar his back, e.g., in stepping off a curb, turning his ankle on a rock, stepping into a hole, stubbing his toe. The patient must learn to walk carefully and to keep close watch of the terrain over which he is walking. Stair climbing, weight lifting (greater than 5 lbs.), and automobile driving may be prohibited for a while to prevent strain on the back.

Braces, Body Casts

Following spinal surgery the patient may wear a body cast, brace, or corset. Initially back braces or corsets may be worn at all times while the patient is in and out of bed; eventually the patient is allowed to be up for short periods without them. (Braces are discussed further in Unit XVII.)

Sometimes body casts are applied following spinal fusion. Such casts are usually worn six to eight weeks. After cast removal the patient is fitted with a back brace, which is worn for an additional three to six months. Activities allowed for patients in body casts vary. Some patients are allowed up in the cast, whereas others are confined to bed. (Cast care is discussed in Unit XVII.)

Patients who must be inactive for long periods following spinal surgery often become bored and restless during their convalescence. It is a challenge to the nurse's imagination to keep them occupied in an interesting manner. Occupational therapy, radio, television, reading material, and the company of others helps the time to pass. Such patients do best in a ward setting where they can visit with other patients and where they can be distracted by the various activities of ward living.

References for Unit VIII

1. Agranowitz, A., and McKeown, M. R.: *Aphasia Handbook for Adults and Children.* Springfield, Ill., Charles C Thomas, 1964.
2. Aldes, H. J.: Rehabilitation of multiple sclerosis patients. *Journal of Rehabilitation* 33:10, March-April, 1967.
3. Alvarez, W. C.: *Little Strokes.* Philadelphia, J. B. Lippincott Company, 1966.
4. Asso, D., et al.: Psychological aspects of stereotactic treatment of parkinsonism. *British Journal of Psychiatry* 115:541, May, 1969.
5. Ausman, J. I.: New developments in anticonvulsant therapy. *Postgraduate Medicine* 48:122, December, 1970.
6. Bakay, L.: Neurosurgery. *In* Nardi, G. L., and Zuidema, G. D. (eds.): *Surgery.* 2nd ed. Boston, Little, Brown and Company, 1965, pp. 755–789.
7. Ballantine, H. T., and Prieto, A.: Early recognition and management of neurosurgical emergencies. *Surgical Clinics of North America* 46:527, June, 1966.
8. Barton, J.: To help a hemiplegic, you have to know how it feels to be one. *Modern Nursing Home* 24:37, April, 1970.
9. Beeson, P. B., and McDermott, W. (eds.): *Cecil-Loeb Textbook of Medicine.* 13th ed. Philadelphia, W. B. Saunders Company, 1971.
10. Beland, I. L.: *Clinical Nursing: Pathophysiological and Psychosocial Approaches.* 2nd ed. New York, The Macmillan Company, 1970.
11. Bell, D. S.: Dangers of treatment of status epilepticus with diazepam. *British Medical Journal* 1:159, January 18, 1969.
12. Bender, L. F.: Diagnostic electromyography. *J.A.M.A.* 199:137, March 6, 1967.
13. Bergersen, B. S., and Krug, E. E.: *Pharmacology in Nursing.* 12th ed. St. Louis, The C. V. Mosby Company, 1973.
14. Bergstrom, N. I.: Ice application to induce voiding. *American Journal of Nursing* 69:283, February, 1969.
15. Bickerstaff, E. R.: *Neurology for Nurses.* London, The English Universities Press, 1965.
16. Biddle, A. S.: The unconscious patient and nursing observations essential to his good medical care. (Mimeographed.) Presented at the Institute, "The Unconscious Patient and the Disoriented Patient," sponsored by the University of Washington School of Nursing, April 14, 1966.
17. Bishop, G., in a personal letter to Beecher, H. K.: *Pharmacological Review* 9:59, 1957.
18. Boegli, E. H., and Steele, M. S.: Scoliosis. *American Journal of Nursing* 68:2399, November, 1968.
19. Boone, D. R., and Landes, B. A.: Left-right discrimination in hemiplegic patients. *Archives of Physical Medicine* 49:533, September, 1968.
20. Boone, E. T., and Self, L. H.: Nursing care of the paraplegic using an experimental electronic spinal neuroprosthesis to activate voiding. *Journal of Neurosurgical Nursing* 4:61, July, 1972.
21. Bordicks, K. J.: *Patterns of Shock: Implications for Nursing Care.* New York, The Macmillan Company, 1965.
22. Boshes, L. D.: Management of Parkinson's disease. *In Parkinson's Disease Symposium, 1965.* Chicago, United Parkinson Foundation, 1966.
23. Bouchard, J.: *Radiation Therapy of Tumors and Diseases of the Nervous System.* Philadelphia, Lea & Febiger, 1966.
24. Boyarsky, S., (ed.): *The Neurogenic Bladder.* Baltimore, The Williams & Wilkins Company, 1967.
25. Boyd, W.: *Introduction to the Study of Disease.* 6th ed. Philadelphia, Lea & Febiger, 1971.
26. Braaf, M. M., and Rosner, S.: More recent concepts on treatment of headache. *Headache* 5:28, July, 1965.
27. Brainerd, H., Margen, S., and Chatton, M. J.: *Current Diagnosis and Treatment.* Los Altos, Calif., Lange Medical Publications, 1969.
28. Branson, H. K.: The epileptic: How you can help. *RN* 35:48, June, 1972.
29. Branson, H. K.: The epileptic and the nurse. *Hospital Management* 100:144, October, 1965.
30. Brooks, H. L.: The golden rule for the unconscious patient. *Nursing Forum* 4:12, March, 1965.
31. Brown, J. R., and Opitz, J. L.: Treatment of neuropathies. *In* Vinken, P. J., and Bruyn, G. W. (eds.): *Handbook of Clinical Neurology.* Vol. 8. New York, American Elsevier Publishing Co., Inc., 1970.
32. Brunette, J. R.: Visual field disturbance associated with hemiplegia. *Canadian Journal of Ophthalmology* 2:16, January, 1967.
33. Brunner, L. S., et al.: *Textbook of Medical-Surgical Nursing.* 2nd ed. Philadelphia, J. B. Lippincott Company, 1970.
34. Burrell, Z. L., Jr., and Burrell, L. O.: *Intensive Nursing Care.* St. Louis, The C. V. Mosby Company, 1964.
35. Burt, M. M.: Perceptual deficits in hemiplegia. *American Journal of Nursing* 70:1026, May, 1970.
36. Butts, C. L., and Canney, V. E.: The Unresponsive Patient. *American Journal of Nursing* 67:1886, September, 1968.
37. Carini, E., and Owens, G.: *Neurological and Neurosurgical Nursing.* 5th ed. St. Louis, The C. V. Mosby Company, 1970.

37a. Carroll, B.: Fingers to toes. *American Journal of Nursing* 71:550, March, 1971.
38. Caveness, W. F., and Walker, A. E.: *Head Injury* (Conference Proceedings). Philadelphia, J. B. Lippincott Company, 1966.
39. Chaffee, E. C., and Greisheimer, E. M.: *Basic Anatomy and Physiology.* 2nd ed. Philadelphia, J. B. Lippincott Company, 1969.
40. Chusid, J. G., and McDonald, J. J.: *Correlative Neuroanatomy of Functional Neurology.* 13th ed. Los Altos, California, Lange Medical Publications, 1967.
41. Clark, K., and Grossman, R. G.: Injuries to the central nervous system. *In* Shires, G. T. (ed.): *Care of the Trauma Patient.* New York, McGraw-Hill Book Co., 1966.
42. Clipper, M.: Nursing care of patients in a neurologic intensive care unit. *Nursing Clinics of North America* 4:211, June, 1969.
43. Conant, R. G., et al.: Stroke morbidity, mortality and rehabilitative potential. *Journal of Chronic Diseases* 18:397, April, 1965.
44. Conn, H. F. (ed.): *Current Therapy.* Philadelphia, W. B. Saunders Company, 1974.
45. Cooper, I. S.: Cryogenic neurosurgery. *The American Academy of General Practice* 39:96, February, 1969.
46. Culp, P.: Nursing care of the patient with a spinal cord injury. *Nursing Clinics of North America* 2:447, September, 1967.
47. Cunningham, M. E.: Intensive nursing care of the neurological patient. *Hospital Management* 108: 79, September, 1969.
48. Davenport, R. R.: Tube feeding for long-term patients. *American Journal of Nursing* 64:121, January, 1964.
49. DeBakey, M. E., et al.: Surgical treatment of cerebrovascular disease. *Postgraduate Medicine* 42: 218, September, 1967.
50. De Jong, R. N.: *The Neurologic Examination.* 3rd ed. New York, Harper & Row, 1967.
51. Devney, A. M., and Kingsbury, B. A.: Hypothermia: In fact and fantasy. *American Journal of Nursing* 72:1414, August, 1972.
52. Drury, J. H.: Handbook of range-of-motion exercises. *Nursing '72* 2:19, April, 1972.
53. Duffy, G. P.: Lumbar puncture in presence of raised intracranial pressure. *British Medical Journal* 1:407, February 15, 1969.
54. Eckstein, H. B., and Macnab, G. H.: Myelomeningocele and hydrocephalus. *Lancet* 1:842, April 16, 1966.
55. Elizabeth, S. R.: Sensory stimulation techniques. *American Journal of Nursing* 66:281, February, 1966.
56. Elliott, H. C.: *Textbook of Neuroanatomy.* 2nd ed. Philadelphia, J. B. Lippincott Company, 1969.
57. Elson, R.: *Practical Management of Spinal Injuries for Nurses.* Baltimore, The Williams & Wilkins Company, 1966.
58. Epstein, L. J., and Simon, A.: Organic brain syndrome in the elderly. *Geriatrics* 22:145, February, 1967.
59. Espir, M. E., and Millac, P.: Treatment of paroxysmal disorders in multiple sclerosis with carbamazepine (Tegretol). *Journal of Neurology, Neurosurgery and Psychiatry* 33:528, August, 1970.
60. Fairburn, B.: Neurosurgery Today, Part 1. *Nursing Times* 63:75, January 20, 1967; Brain tumours, Part 2, 63:108; Head injuries, Part 3, 63:143; Subarachnoid haemorrhage, Part 4, 63:177; Parkinson's disease, Part 5, 63:207; Spinal cord surgery, Part 6, 63:249, February 24, 1967.
61. Fangman, A., and O'Malley, W. E.: L-Dopa and the patient with Parkinson's disease. *American Journal of Nursing* 69:1455, July, 1969.
62. Felstein, I.: Yesterday, today and tomorrow: Parkinsonism. *Nursing Mirror* 126:19, June 21, 1968.
63. Finneson, B. E.: *Diagnosis and Management of Pain Syndromes.* 2nd ed. Philadelphia, W. B. Saunders Company, 1969.
64. Foley, J. M.: Agnosia. *In* Beeson, P. B., and McDermott, W. (eds.): *Cecil-Loeb Textbook of Medicine.* 12th ed. Philadelphia, W. B. Saunders Company, 1967.
65. Fordyce, W. E., and Jones, R. H.: Efficacy of oral and pantomine instructions for hemiplegic patients. *Archives of Physical Medicine* 47:676, October, 1966.
66. Fordyce, W. E., and Simons, B. C.: Automated training system for wheelchair pushups. *Public Health Reports* 83:527, June, 1968.
67. Fox, J. L.: Recent advances in neurological surgery. *RN* 35:OR/ER 1, May, 1972.
68. French, R. M.: *Nurse's Guide to Diagnostic Procedures.* 3rd ed. New York, McGraw-Hill Book Company, 1971.
69. Friedman, A. P.: How to prevent tension headache. *Consultant* 7:16, January, 1967.
70. Frost, A.: *Handbook for Paraplegics and Quadriplegics.* Chicago, National Paraplegia Foundation, 1964.
71. Gage, E. L.: Diagnosis of brain tumors in middle age. *Geriatrics* 22:150, October, 1967.
72. Gardner, E.: *Fundamentals of Neurology.* 5th ed. Philadelphia, W. B. Saunders Company, 1968.
73. Gardner, M. A. M.: Responsiveness as a measure of consciousness. *American Journal of Nursing* 68: 1034, May, 1968.
74. Garland, H.: Medical aspects of head injury. *Nursing Mirror* 118:i, April 17, 1964.
75. Garland, H.: Neurological problems. Special investigations. Part 1. *Nursing Times* 64:39, January 12, 1968; Part 2, 64:89, January 19, 1968.
76. Gatz, A. J.: *Manter's Essentials of Clinical Neuroanatomy and Neurophysiology.* 4th ed. Philadelphia, F. A. Davis Company, 1970.
77. Gaul, A. L., et al.: Hyperbaric oxygen therapy. *American Journal of Nursing* 72:892, May, 1972.
78. Gerdes, L.: The confused or delirious patient. *American Journal of Nursing* 68:1228, June, 1968.
79. Gersten, J. W., Jung, A., and Brooks, C.: Perceptual deficits in patients with left and right hemiparesis. *American Journal of Physical Medicine* 51:79, April, 1972.
80. Geschwind, N. N.: Language and the brain. *Scientific American* 226:76, April, 1972.
81. Gibbs, G. E.: Perineal care of the incapacitated patient. *American Journal of Nursing* 69:124, January, 1969.
82. Gilbert, M. M.: Etiology and treatment of post concussion syndrome. *Headache* 7–8:57, July, 1968.
83. Gilland, O.: How to take the headache out of spinal taps. *Headache* 8:154, January, 1969.
84. Gilson, A. J.: Brain scanning: Localization of nonneoplastic intracranial lesions. *In* Croll, M. N., and Brady, L. W. (eds.): *Recent Advances in Nuclear Medicine.* New York, Appleton-Century-Crofts, Inc., 1966.
85. Glaser, G. H.: The epilepsies. *In* Beeson, P. B., and McDermott, W. (eds.): *Cecil-Loeb Textbook of Medicine.* 13th ed. Philadelphia, W. B. Saunders Company, 1971.

86. Goda, S.: Communicating with the aphasic or dysarthric patient. *American Journal of Nursing* 63:80, July, 1963.
87. Goode, M. A.: The patient with a cerebral vascular accident. *Nursing Outlook* 14:60, March, 1966.
88. Green, J. R. (ed.): Seminar on the Management of Head Injuries. *Arizona Medicine* 25:123, February, 1968.
89. Greenhouse, A. H.: Modern concepts in cerebral vascular disease. *The American Academy of General Practice* 35:99, May, 1967.
90. Gumnit, R. J.: Fluids and electrolytes in the comatose patient. *Geriatrics* 21:131, August, 1966.
91. Gumnit, R. J.: The medical management of closed head injuries. *Geriatrics* 22:112, December, 1967.
92. Guyton, A. C.: *Textbook of Medical Physiology*. 4th ed. Philadelphia, W. B. Saunders Company, 1971.
93. Haber, M. E.: Parkinson's disease: Challenge to the health professions. *Nursing Clinics of North America* 4:263, June, 1969.
94. Halper, A. S., et al.: Communication problems of the stroke patient. *Nursing Homes* 16:16, October, 1967.
95. Hamby, W. B.: Remarks concerning intracranial aneurysmal surgery. *In* Ojemann, R. G., et al. (eds.): *Clinical Neurosurgery*. Baltimore, The Williams & Wilkins Company, 1970.
96. Hickey, M. C.: Hypothermia. *American Journal of Nursing* 65:116, January, 1965.
97. Hirsch, C. J., and Caulfield, P. A., Jr.: The acute brain syndrome: Early recognition and management. *General Practitioner* 35:87, January, 1967.
98. Hoffman, W. W., and Ryan, R. L.: A controlled study of L-Dopa in Parkinson's disease. *California Medicine* 112:9, February, 1970.
99. Holmes, G.: Some clinical aspects of pain. *In* Ogilvie, W., and Thomson, W. (eds.): *Pain and Its Problems*. London, Eyre and Spottiswoode, Ltd., 1950.
100. Hooper, R.: *Neurosurgical Nursing*. Springfield, Ill., Charles C Thomas, 1964.
101. Horwitz, N. H., and Rizzoli, H. V.: *Postoperative Complications in Neurosurgical Practice: Recognition, Prevention, and Management*. Baltimore, The Williams & Wilkins Company, 1967.
102. Howard, F. M., Jr.: The electromyogram and conduction velocity studies in peripheral nerve trauma. *In* Ojemann, R. G., et al. (eds.): *Clinical Neurosurgery*. Baltimore, The Williams & Wilkins Company, 1970.
103. Hrobsky, A.: The patient on a CircOlectric bed. *American Journal of Nursing* 71:2352, December, 1971.
104. Hughes, M. T.: Neurology; A sub-specialty. *Journal of Neurosurgical Nursing* 4:83, July, 1972.
105. Hunkele, E., and Lazier, R.: A patient with fractured cervical vertebrae. *American Journal of Nursing* 65:82, September, 1965.
106. Hyman, M. D.: The stigma of stroke. Its effects on performance during and after rehabilitation. *Geriatrics* 26:132, May, 1971.
107. Isaacs, B.: *An Introduction to Geriatrics*. Baltimore, The Williams & Wilkins Company, 1965.
108. Iverson, S. M.: Helping a quadriplegic patient to adjust. *American Journal of Nursing* 64:128A, January, 1964.
109. Jackson, F. E.: The pathophysiology of head injuries. *Clinical Symposia* 18:77, July-December, 1966.
110. Jackson, F. E.: Treatment of head injuries. *Clinical Symposia* 19:4, January-March, 1967.
111. Jacob, S. W., and Francone, C. A.: *Structure and Function in Man*. 3rd ed. Philadelphia, W. B. Saunders Company, 1974.
112. Jacobansky, A. M.: Stroke. *American Journal of Nursing* 72:1260, July, 1972.
113. Jacobs, E. M., and Denault, P. M.: *Neurology for Nurses*. Springfield, Ill., Charles C Thomas, 1964.
114. Jennett, W. B.: Mental symptoms after head injury. *Nursing Times* 63:1226, September 15, 1967.
115. Jennett, W. B.: Symptomatic epilepsy. *Nursing Mirror* 124:602, September 29, 1967.
116. Jennings, C. R.: The stroke patient—His rehabilitation. *American Journal of Nursing* 67:118, January, 1967.
117. Kaplan, G.: The psychogenic etiology of headache post lumbar puncture. *Psychosomatic Medicine* 29:376, July-August, 1967.
118. Karvounis, P. C., Chiu, J., and Sabin, H.: The use of prefabricated polyethylene plate for cranioplasty. *The Journal of Trauma* 10:249, March, 1970.
119. Kast, E. C.: A limited discussion of the treatment of Parkinson's disease. *Diseases of the Nervous System* 28:684, October, 1967.
120. Kaufmann, G. E., and Clark, W. K.: Transmission of increased intracranial pressure across the tentorium in man. *Surgical Forum* 20:437, 1969.
121. Kaufmann, G. E., and Clark, W. K.: Emergency frontal twist drill ventriculostomy. *Journal of Neurosurgery* 33:226, August, 1970.
122. Kempe, L. G.: *Operative Neurosurgery*. 2 vols. New York, Springer-Verlag, 1970.
123. Kennedy, R. H. (ed.): *Emergency Care*. Philadelphia, W. B. Saunders Company, 1966.
124. King, R. B.: The value of mephenesin carbamate in the control of pain in patients with tic douloureux. *Journal of Neurosurgery* 25:153, 1966.
125. Kirgis, H. D., et al.: Strokes and their treatment. *Geriatrics* 23:144, February, 1968.
126. Knapp, M. E.: Practical physical medicine and rehabilitation: Spinal cord injury, Part 1. *Postgraduate Medicine* 42:A–95, August, 1967; Part 2, 42: 111, September, 1967.
127. Krenzel, J. R., and Rohrer, L. M.: *Paraplegic and Quadriplegic Individuals*. (Handbook for Nurses.) Chicago, The National Paraplegia Foundation, 1966.
128. Krusen, F. H., Kottke, F. J., and Ellwood, P. M., Jr. (eds.): *Handbook of Physical Medicine and Rehabilitation*. 2nd ed. Philadelphia, W. B. Saunders Company, 1971.
129. Langfitt, T. W.: Head injuries in adults. *In* Conn, H. F. (ed.): *Current Therapy*. Philadelphia, W. B. Saunders Company, 1969.
130. Large, H., et al.: In the first stroke intensive care unit. *American Journal of Nursing* 69:76, January, 1969.
131. Larson, C. B., and Gould, M.: *Orthopedic Nursing*. 7th ed. St. Louis, The C. V. Mosby Company, 1970.
132. Levenson, C.: Rehabilitation of the stroke hemiplegic patient. *In* Krusen, F. H., Kottke, F. J., and Ellwood, P. M., Jr. (eds.): *Handbook of Physical Medicine and Rehabilitation*. Philadelphia, W. B. Saunders Company, 1965.
133. Levine, M. E.: *Introduction to Clinical Nursing*. Philadelphia, F. A. Davis Company, 1969.
134. Levy, R.: Immobilized patient and his psychological well-being. *Postgraduate Medicine* 40:74, July, 1966.

135. Lewin, W.: *The Management of Head Injuries.* Baltimore, The Williams & Wilkins Company, 1967.
136. Livingston, S.: *Drug Therapy for Epilepsy.* Springfield, Ill., Charles C Thomas, 1966.
137. Locke, S.: The neurological aspects of coma. *Surgical Clinics of North America* 48:251, April, 1968.
138. Locksley, H. B.: Hemorrhagic strokes. *Medical Clinics of North America* 52:1193, September, 1968.
139. Long, J.: Carotid thromboendarterectomy. *American Journal of Nursing* 9:1969, September, 1966.
140. Luessenhop, A.: Care of the unconscious patient. *Nursing Forum* 4(No. 3):6, 1965.
141. Luessenhop, A.: Nursing care: A critical factor in unconscious patients' survival. *Hospital Topics* 43:1244, July, 1965.
142. Lundy, J. S.: Short methods of treatment for spinal-puncture headache. *Headache* 7–8:85, July, 1967.
143. Luria, A. R.: *Human Brain and Psychological Processes.* New York, Harper & Row, 1966.
144. Luria, A. R.: The functional organization of the brain. *Scientific American* 222:66, March, 1970.
145. Lyght, C. E., et al. (eds.): *The Merck Manual.* 11th ed. West Point, Pa., Merck, Sharp & Dohme, 1966.
146. Macnab, I., et al.: Chemonucleolysis. *Canadian Journal of Surgery* 14:280, 1971.
147. Mancall, E. L., and Hirschhorn, A. M.: Dynamic factors in the pathogenesis of cerebrovascular disease. *Geriatrics* 22:168, March, 1967.
148. Marinacci, A. A.: Clinical electromyography: A review. *Bulletin of the Los Angeles Neurological Societies* 35:181, October, 1970.
149. Marshall, A. M.: Neurosurgical nursing with relation to rehabilitation. *Rehabilitation Literature* 11:342, November, 1967.
150. Marshall, J.: *The Management of Cerebrovascular Disease.* Boston, Little, Brown and Company, 1965.
151. Marshall, J., and Mair, J.: *Neurological Nursing.* 2nd ed. Oxford, Blackwell Scientific Publications, 1967.
152. Martin, M. A.: Nursing care in cervical cord injury. *American Journal of Nursing* 63:60, March, 1963.
153. Martin, M. A.: Care of a patient with cerebral aneurysm. *American Journal of Nursing* 65:90, April, 1965.
154. McAlpine, D., Lumsden, C. E., and Acheson, E. D.: *Multiple Sclerosis: A Reappraisal.* 2nd ed. Baltimore, The Williams & Wilkins Company, 1965.
155. McDowell, F. H.: Cerebrovascular diseases. *In* Beeson, P. B., and McDermott, W. (eds.): *Cecil-Loeb Textbook of Medicine.* 13th ed. Philadelphia, W. B. Saunders Company, 1971.
156. McDowell, F. H. (ed.): Symposium on Levodopa in Parkinson's Disease. Held at Roche Research Tower, Hoffmann-La Roche Inc., Nutley, New Jersey, June 17, 1971. *Neurology* 22 (part 2): 1–102, 1972.
158. McHenry, L. C., and Jaffe, M. E.: Cerebrovascular disease, Part I: Diagnosis. *The American Academy of General Practice* 37:88, March, 1968; Part II: Management, 37:98, April, 1968.
159. McKenzie, S.: Stereotaxic radiofrequency coagulation: A treatment for trigeminal neuralgia. *Journal of Neurosurgical Nursing* 4:75, July, 1972.
160. Memmler, R. L., and Rada, R. B.: *The Human Body in Health and Disease.* 3rd ed. Philadelphia, J. B. Lippincott Company, 1970.
161. Merritt, H. H.: *A Textbook of Neurology.* 4th ed. Philadelphia, Lea & Febiger, 1967.
162. Miller, B., and Coyle, N. R.: Guillain-Barré syndrome: Nursing care. *American Journal of Nursing* 66:2224, October, 1966.
163. Miller, B. E.: Assisting aphasic patients with speech rehabilitation. *American Journal of Nursing* 69: 983, May, 1969.
164. Millichap, J. G.: *Febrile Convulsions.* New York, The Macmillan Company, 1968.
165. Millikan, C. H., Siekert, R. B., and Whisnant, J. P. (eds.): *Cerebral Vascular Diseases.* New York, Grune & Stratton, Inc., 1966.
166. Mindham, R. H. S.: Psychiatric symptoms in parkinsonism. *Journal of Neurology, Neurosurgery and Psychiatry* 33:188, April, 1970.
167. Moidel, H. C., et al.: *Nursing Care of the Patient with Medical-Surgical Disorders.* New York, McGraw-Hill Book Company, 1971.
168. Morrison, S. T., and Arnold, C. R.: *Landon and Sider's Communicable Diseases.* 9th ed. Philadelphia, F. A. Davis Company, 1969.
169. Mueller, A. D.: Psychological factors in rehabilitation of paraplegic patients. *Archives of Physical Medicine* 43:151, April, 1962.
170. Murphy, J. J., and Schoenberg, H. W.: Principles of management of the neurogenic bladder. *Hospital Medicine* 3:88, March, 1967.
171. Musick, D. T., and MacKenzie, M.: Nursing care of the patient with a laminectomy. *Nursing Clinics of North America* 2:437, September, 1967.
172. Nathan, P.: *The Nervous System.* Philadelphia, J. B. Lippincott Company, 1969.
173. Nishioka, H.: Neurosurgery. *In* Liechty, R., and Soper, R. T. (eds.): *Synopsis of Surgery.* St. Louis, The C. V. Mosby Co., 1968.
174. Noback, C. R.: *The Human Nervous System.* New York, McGraw-Hill Book Company, 1967.
175. Nulsen, F. E., and Gardner, M. A. M.: Head injuries. *In* Meltzer, L. E., Abdellah, F. G., and Kitchell, J. R. (eds.): *Concepts and Practices of Intensive Care for Nurse Specialists.* Philadelphia, The Charles Press Publishers, Inc., 1969.
176. Ojemann, R. G., et al. (eds.): *Clinical Neurosurgery.* Proceedings of the Congress of Neurosurgical Surgeons, Boston, Mass., 1969. Baltimore, The Williams & Wilkins Company, 1970.
177. Oliver, L.: *Parkinson's Disease.* Springfield, Ill., Charles C Thomas, 1967.
178. Olson, E. V.: The hazards of immobility: Effects on psychosocial equilibrium. *American Journal of Nursing* 67:794, April, 1967.
179. Ommaya, A. K.: Nervous system injury and the whole body. *The Journal of Trauma* 10:981, No. 11, 1970.
180. Overs, R. P., and Belknap, E. L.: Educating stroke patient's families. *Journal of Chronic Diseases* 20:45, 1967.
181. Parent, A. D., Meyer, G. A., and Tindall, G. T.: Blood chemistry changes in head-injured patients. *Journal of Neurosurgical Nursing* 4:9, July, 1972.
182. Parkinson, J.: *An Essay on the Shaking Palsy.* London, Sherwood, Neely & Jones, 1817.
183. Parsons, L. C.: Respiratory changes in head injury. *American Journal of Nursing* 71:2187, November, 1971.
184. Parsons, M.: Intracranial venous thrombosis. *Post-*

graduate Medical Journal 43:409, June, 1967.

185. Patrick, M. L.: Care of the confused elderly patient. *American Journal of Nursing* 67:2536, December, 1967.
186. Patterson, R. H., Jr.: Injuries of head and spine. *In* Beeson, P. B., and McDermott, W. (eds.): *Cecil-Loeb Textbook of Medicine.* 13th ed. Philadelphia, W. B. Saunders Company, 1971.
187. Pharmacologic and clinical experiences with levodopa: A symposium. (Held at Georgetown University School of Medicine, Washington, D.C., January 14, 1970.) *Neurology* 20(Part 2):1–65, December, 1970.
188. Pigott, R., and Brickett, F.: Visual neglect. *American Journal of Nursing* 66:101, January, 1966.
189. Plum, F.: The pathogenesis of stupor and coma. *In* Beeson, P. B., and McDermott, W. (eds.): *Cecil-Loeb Textbook of Medicine.* 13th edition. Philadelphia, W. B. Saunders Company, 1971.
190. Plum, F.: Headache. *In* Beeson, P. B., and McDermott, W. (eds.): *Cecil-Loeb Textbook of Medicine.* 13th ed. Philadelphia, W. B. Saunders Company, 1971.
191. Plum, F.: Axioms on coma. *Hospital Medicine* 4:20, May, 1968.
192. Plum, F.: Physiology and diagnosis of coma. *Bulletin Mason Clinic* 23:53, June, 1969.
193. Plum, F., and Posner, J. B.: *Diagnosis of Stupor and Coma.* Philadelphia, F. A. Davis Company, 1966.
194. Plummer, E. M.: The MS patient. *American Journal of Nursing* 68:2161, October, 1968.
195. Potter, J. M.: Head injuries today. *Postgraduate Medical Journal* 43:574, September, 1967.
196. Quesenbury, J. H.: Nursing action—not reaction—for a stroke patient's rehabilitation. *In* Bergersen, B. S. et al. (eds.): *Current Concepts in Clinical Nursing.* Vol. 2. St. Louis, The C. V. Mosby Company, 1969, p. 86.
197. Quesenbury, J. H., and Lembright, P.: Observations and care for patients with head injuries. *Nursing Clinics of North America* 4:237, June, 1969.
198. Ramey, I. G.: The stroke patient is interesting. *Nursing Forum* 6:273, Summer, 1967.
199. Ransohoff, J., and Sadik, A. R.: Spinal cord injury: Current status and some recent advances. *Journal of Neurosurgical Nursing* 4:49, July, 1972.
200. Raskind, R.: Lumbar disc herniation: An occasional emergency. *Consultant* 12:45, March, 1972.
201. Rees, J. E., et al.: Regional cerebral blood-flow in transient ischaemic attacks. *Lancet* 2:1210, December 12, 1970.
202. Reeves, E. W.: The aphasic patient. *Nursing Outlook* 11:522, July, 1963.
203. Regan, P. A.: A patient-centered approach to neurologic nursing. *Nursing Clinics of North America* 4:201, June, 1969.
204. Regina, S. E.: Sensory stimulation techniques. *American Journal of Nursing* 66:281, February, 1966.
205. Rhoads, J. E., et al.: *Surgery: Principles and Practice.* Philadelphia, J. B. Lippincott Company, 1970.
206. Rob, C. G., and De Weese, J.: Surgical treatment of transient strokes. *Postgraduate Medicine* 42:19, July, 1967.
207. Robbins, S. L.: *Pathology.* 3rd ed. Philadelphia, W. B. Saunders Company, 1967.

207a. Robinson, M. B.: Levodopa and parkinsonism. *American Journal of Nursing 74*:656, April, 1974.

208. Ross, G. S.: Trigeminal pain. *Journal-Lancet* 88:47, February, 1968.
209. Rovit, R. L.: Surgical treatment of epilepsy. *Postgraduate Medicine* 41:355, April, 1967.
210. Rowe, S. N.: Surgical treatment of nerve lesions. *In* Vinken, P. J., and Bruyn, G. W. (eds.): *Handbook of Clinical Neurology.* Vol. 8. New York, American Elsevier Publishing Co., Inc., 1970.
211. Sacks, E., Jr.: Translabyrinthine microsurgery for acoustic neuromas. *Journal of Neurosurgery* 22: 399, April, 1965.
212. Samra, K., et al.: Relief of intention tremor by thalamic surgery. *Journal of Neurology, Neurosurgery and Psychiatry* 33:7, February, 1970.
213. Sarkisov, S. A.: *The Structure and Functions of the Brain.* Bloomington, Indiana University Press, 1966.
214. Sawtell, R. R., and Martin, G. M.: Perceptual problems of the hemiplegic patient. *Journal-Lancet* 87:193, June, 1967.
215. Saxon, J.: Techniques for bowel and bladder training. *American Journal of Nursing* 62:69, September, 1962.

217\. Schoenberg, B. S.: Strokes in women of childbearing age: A population study. *Neurology* 20:181, February, 1970.

217\. Schwab, R. S., et al.: Amantadine in the treatment of Parkinson's disease. *J.A.M.A.* 208:1168, May 19, 1969.

218. Schwartz, M. L., and Dennerll, R. D.: The employable epileptic: Fact, fiction, and contradiction. *Journal of Rehabilitation* 33:36, January-February, 1967.
219. Schwartz, W. S., et al.: Management of transient cerebral ischemic attacks. *California Medicine* 107:471, December, 1967.
220. Scott, D. F., and Dodd, B.: *Neurological and Neurosurgical Nursing.* Elmsford, New York, Pergamon Press, 1966.
221. Shapiro, W. R., and McDowell, F.: Spontaneous subarachnoid hemorrhage. *Hospital Medicine* 3: 19, October, 1967.
222. Shaw, D. A.: Parkinson's disease. *Nursing Times* 63: 1740, December 29, 1967.
223. Shafer, K. L., et al.: *Medical-Surgical Nursing.* 4th ed. St. Louis, The C. V. Mosby Company, 1967.
224. Shenkin, H. A., and Haft, H.: Forminotomy in the surgical treatment of herniated lumbar disks. *Surgery* 60:274, 1966.
225. Siekert, R. E.: Symposium on neurologic disorders. *Medical Clinics of North America* 52, July, 1968.
226. Sister Regina Elizabeth: The scientific rationale of bowel and bladder training. *Arizona Medicine* January, 1966, p. 13.
227. Smith, G. W.: Care of the patient with a stroke. New York, Springer-Verlag, 1967.
228. Smith, S. W.: Subdural hematoma in adults. *Postgraduate Medicine* 42:A–59, August, 1967.
229. Sodeman, W. A., and Sodeman, W. A., Jr.: *Pathological Physiology: Mechanisms of Disease.* 5th ed. Philadelphia, W. B. Saunders Company, 1974.
230. Spector, M. (ed.): *Dizziness and Vertigo: Diagnosis and Treatment.* New York, Grune & Stratton, Inc., 1967.
231. Spencer, W. A., et al.: Physiologic concepts of immobilization. *Archives of Physical Medicine* 46: 89–100, January, 1965.

232. Steegman, A. T.: *Examination of the Nervous System.* 3rd ed. Chicago, Year Book Medical Publishers, Inc., 1970.
233. Stern, W. E.: Tumors of the brain. *California Medicine* 102:40, January, 1965.
234. Stevens, V. C.: Clinical hypothermia: Some nursing concepts. *Journal of Neurosurgical Nursing* 4:33, July, 1972.
235. Strang, R. R.: The etiology of Parkinson's disease. *Diseases of the Nervous System* 31:381, June, 1970.
236. Suggs, K. M.: Coping and adaptive behavior in the stroke syndrome. *Nursing Forum* 10(No. 1): 100, 1971.
237. Sutton, A. L.: *Bedside Nursing Techniques in Medicine and Surgery.* 2nd ed. Philadelphia, W. B. Saunders Company, 1969.
238. Suzuki, J., and Takaku, A.: Nonsurgical treatment of chronic subdural hematoma. *Journal of Neurosurgery* 33:548, November, 1970.
239. Sweet, W. H.: Surgery of the nervous system. *In* Moyer, et al. (eds.): *Surgery: Principles and Practice.* 3rd ed. Philadelphia, J. B. Lippincott Company, 1965.
240. Sweet, W. H.: Trigeminal neuralgias. *In* Alling, C., III, et al. (eds.): *Facial Pain.* Philadelphia, Lea & Febiger, 1968.
241. Symposium on levodopa. *J.A.M.A.* 218:1903, December 27, 1971.
241a. Take a look at the unconscious patient. *Emergency Medicine* 4:143, April, 1972.
242. Talbot, H. S.: Adjunctive care of spinal cord injuries. *Surgical Clinics of North America* 48:737, August, 1968.
243. Taren, J. A., and Martin, M. A.: Cerebral aneurysm and care of the patient with a cerebral aneurysm. *American Journal of Nursing* 65:90, April, 1965.
244. Tasker, R. R.: Increased intracranial pressure. *Canadian Nurse* 61:207, March, 1965.
245. Taylor, D. C.: Treatment of epilepsy. *In* Crammer, J. L. (ed.): *Practical Treatment in Psychiatry.* Oxford, Blackwell Scientific Publications, 1969.
246. Tolley, J. A., III: Carotid artery occlusive disease. *California Medicine* 107:254, September, 1967.
247. Toole, J. F., and Whisnant, J. P. (eds.): *Cerebral Vascular Diseases.* New York, Grune & Stratton, Inc., 1968.
248. Travis, G.: *Chronic Disease and Disability.* Berkeley, University of California Press, 1961.
249. Trigiano, L. L.: Independence is possible in quadriplegia. *American Journal of Nursing* 70:2610, December, 1971.
250. Tweed, G. G., Coyle, N. R., and Miller, B.: Guillain-Barré syndrome. *American Journal of Nursing* 66: 2222, October, 1966.
251. Udall, J. A.: Anticoagulant therapy for progressing strokes. *Postgraduate Medicine* 42:212, September, 1967.
252. Ullman, M.: Disorders of body image after stroke. *American Journal of Nursing* 64:89, October, 1964.
253. U.S. Public Health Service, Chronic Diseases Program: *Strike Back at Stroke.* Publication No. 596. Washington, D.C., U.S. Government Printing Office, 1962.
254. VanderArk, G. D., et al.: Repair of cerebrospinal fluid fistulas using a tissue adhesive. *Journal of Neurosurgery* 33:151, August, 1970.
255. Vinken, P. J., and Bruyn, G. W. (eds.): *Handbook of Clinical Neurology.* Vol. 8. New York, American Elsevier Publishing Co., Inc., 1970.
256. Walsh, J. J.: *Understanding Paraplegia.* Philadelphia, J. B. Lippincott Company, 1964.
257. Walsh, T. J., and Smith, J. L.: Tegretol—A new treatment for tic douloureux. *Headache* 7–8:62, July, 1968.
258. Wells, R. W.: Huntington's chorea: Seeing beyond the disease. *American Journal of Nursing* 72: 954, May, 1972.
259. White, D. N.: The six "laws" of echoencephalography. *Neurology* 20:435, May, 1970.
260. Whitehouse, F. A.: Stoke—Some psychological problems and causes. *American Journal of Nursing* 63:81, October, 1963.
261. Whiteman, M.: Bell's palsy. *American Journal of Nursing* 71:2139, November, 1971.
262. Wilcoxson, H. L.: Cerebrovascular accident: The role of the public health nurse. *Nursing Clinics of North America* 1:63, March, 1966.
263. Wilentz, J. S.: *The Senses of Man.* New York, Thomas Y. Crowell Company, 1968.
264. Wilson, J. C., Jr.: Low back pain and sciatica. *J.A.M.A.* 200:129, May 22, 1967.
265. Wilson, S. A. K.: *Neurology.* 2nd ed. Vol. 2., A. N. Bruce, ed. Baltimore, The Williams & Wilkins Company, 1955.
266. Wise, C. S., et al.: Rehabilitation of the stroke patient. *Postgraduate Medicine* 42:262, October, 1967.
267. Wolff, H. G.: *Headache and Other Head Pain.* 2nd ed. New York, Oxford University Press, 1963.
268. Woodburne, L. S.: *The Neural Basis of Behavior.* Columbus, Ohio, Charles E. Merrill Publishing Company, 1967.
269. Wylie, C. M.: Hospital care for patient with strokes in the acute stage. *J.A.M.A.* 193:791, September 16, 1965.
270. Yahr, M. D., and Duvoisin, R. C.: Drug therapy in parkinsonism. *New England Journal of Medicine* 287:20, July 6, 1972.
271. Yahr, M., et al.: *Parkinson's Disease, Present Status and Research Trends.* U.S. Public Health Service Publication No. 1491. Washington, D.C., Government Printing Office, 1966.
272. Yaryura-Tobias, J. A., et al.: Action of L-dopa in drug induced extrapyramidalism. *Diseases of the Nervous System* 31:60, January, 1970.
273. Young, J. F.: Recognition, significance, and recording of the signs of increased intracranial pressure. *Nursing Clinics of North America* 4:223, June, 1969.
274. Young, J., and Reid, M.: Neurosurgical nursing care in the surgical management of intracranial aneurysms. *Journal of Neurosurgical Nursing* 4:21, July, 1972.
275. Zohn, D. A., et al.: Bell's palsy: Management based on prognosis. *The American Academy of General Practice* 36:99, October, 1967.
276. Zubek, J. P. (ed.): *Sensory Deprivation.* New York, Appleton-Century-Crofts, Inc., 1969.
277. Zulch, K. J.: *Brain Tumors: Their Biology and Pathology.* 2nd ed. Translated by A. B. Rothballer and J. Olszewski. New York, Springer-Verlag, 1965.

UNIT IX

Nursing Patients Experiencing Pain

INTRODUCTION AND STUDY GUIDE

A nurse needs to have a thorough understanding of the pain phenomenon. You will recall and use "pain theory" many times during your professional life, for much of a nurse's time is spent in attempts to understand, evaluate, and reduce the pains that patients suffer. Pain is one of the most important symptoms which you will encounter, not only because of its frequency, but principally because of the distress and suffering that are a part of it.

You may find the following study guide helpful:

1. Reiterate in your own words what some fallacies are about pain and why pain is so difficult to describe and define. Also, keep in mind one definition of pain.

2. Recall some reasons why the pain experience is a complex mind-body experience. Also, state in your own words what you know about the various ways that pain is described.

3. As you will see, there are many types of pain. Distinguish the different types in your mind. In your own words, tell what you know about the function of pain, acute pain, chronic pain, and the evaluation of pain.

4. In your own words state how nerve blocks, radiology, hypnosis, physical therapies, and pain clinics contribute to comprehensive pain therapy.

5. Nurses frequently give medications for purposes of pain relief. Concentrate when studying Chapter 44 on how you can most effectively, and safely, utilize medications to relieve pain. Remember the basic rule for nurses in giving medications is to *be familiar* with a medication *prior* to administering it. Use this chapter as a clinical guide in planning the pharmacologic aspects of care of patients having pain. Refer as needed to pharmacologic texts.

6. You should become thoroughly familiar with the content of Chapter 45 and apply the content of this chapter to your patient care. Use this chapter as a reference in giving patient care and in evaluating and planning care of the patient having pain. Remember also the hazards that the absence of pain creates.

CHAPTER 41

The Phenomenon of Pain

Bodily pain was regarded for hundreds of years as a means of obtaining religious grace, or as a punishment considered to be God-given and "good for the soul." This acceptance and affirmation of physical pain underlay all Oriental as well as Western religions. Because of this attitude toward pain, for a long period of time, efforts to control or abolish it were inhibited.[75]

It has been only recently that medicine has been able to bring multiple treatment methods to focus on the goal of pain control. A variety of approaches are found in the pain therapy of today, e.g., chemotherapy, hypnotism, nerve blocks, open and closed stereotaxic surgery and other surgical approaches, behavior modification techniques, and psychiatric therapies. *Scientifically* pain is currently subjected to the scrutiny of many disciplines. *Philosophically* the problem of pain continues to pose enduring questions such as, "Why must man suffer and be subjected to pain?"

Although major advances have been made within the past few decades in both understanding and alleviating pain, much remains to be learned and many fallacies about pain still exist. The nurse must be able to discriminate between fact and fallacy in this important area of her practice.

FACTS AND FALLACIES ABOUT PAIN

Listed below are some misconceptions about pain as well as a few statements that are generally accepted as accurate—or as facts:

Fallacy	*Fact*
All persons who are critically ill or gravely injured experience intense pain.	Persons who are critically ill, e.g., have terminal cancer, or are gravely injured, do *not* inevitably experience pain. While some persons do have pain at such a time, others may not.
The greater the pain, the greater the amount of tissue damage.	Intensity of pain is *not* directly proportional to the severity or extent of tissue damage.
Pain is symptomatic of *incurable* illnesses, e.g., "If I have pain, it's probably 'too late' for a doctor to help me."	Pain is an important symptom which often indicates that treatment is necessary. Many painful conditions *are* treatable, indeed curable!

THE UNIQUE NATURE OF PAIN

Although much *is* predictable about the pain response, there are aspects of it that remain incomprehensible. In a way, attempting to understand and describe pain is like trying to talk about the wind—*only its effects can be observed.* Thus, with pain we see the grimace, the clenched fist; *the phenomenon itself cannot be seen,* is difficult to describe, and is often hard to recall precisely. "The symptom which most frequently warns the patient of the presence of a pathological condition, and which most often causes him to seek medical advice, is at the same time that about which he remembers least."[113]

Following are some statements about the complex, unique experience of pain:

> Pain is mediated by receptors that are chemosensitive.*

> Pain is difficult to evaluate because it is an entirely subjective phenomenon. Also, it is especially difficult to differentiate psychologic from organic factors. Both "organic pain" and "psychogenic pain" are called "pain" and are experienced in the same way even though there are differences in how they develop.

> Whereas slight wounds may be quite painful, it is also possible to have extensive wounds that are painless. Under certain stressful conditions, even severe wounds may not be painful.

> Pain does not indicate the seriousness or the amount of tissue damage, but rather it is generally indicative of the *rate* of tissue damage. Pain, thus, indicates that tissue damage is in progress.

> Pain patterns (e.g., intensity, duration, rhythmicity) vary, depending upon the etiology or the organ system involved.

> Individuals vary in their ability to withstand the same pain. The same stimulus may produce varying results in various persons and even in the same person if conditions are altered. The female is generally conceded to be able to withstand pain better than the male.

> Pain intensity has a definite ceiling or maximum. Studies with heat demonstrate that even though the rate of pain-stimulation and tissue damage continues to increase, there is a point at which pain intensity fails to increase.

> The word "pain" is often inaccurately used to refer to feelings (both physical and mental) that are actually not painful. For example, feelings of "pressure" may be confused with feelings of "pain."

> There are distinguishable qualities of pain (e.g., burn, prick, sharp, dull) and distinguishable intensities (e.g., minor, slight, excruciating).

---

*Chemosensitive means sensitive to changes that occur in chemical composition.

> Interpretations of the pain sensation vary: It is debatable whether pain is always an "uncomfortable" experience. Some believe that pain is not an unpleasant sensation to persons with masochistic tendencies or to persons who have had leukotomy (prefrontal lobotomy).

> Pain that originates from bodily disorders is believed to differ from pain that is experimentally produced. Also, pain that is self-inflicted is believed to be experienced differently from pain that has its source outside of oneself.[96]

> Pain may be present in the absence of demonstrable bodily disease, injury or noxious stimulation, e.g., "phantom limb pain."

DEFINITIONS OF PAIN

An accurate definition of the term "pain" is difficult to arrive at. One dictionary defines pain as "a feeling of distress, suffering or agony, caused by stimulation of specialized nerve endings." Pain cannot be satisfactorily defined in other than subjective terms.[98] W. K. Livingston, a pioneer in the study of pain, writes: "I am unwilling to call anything pain unless it is perceived as such."[85] Thus, if a person has what appears to be a "painful" injury but experiences no pain himself, the injury cannot accurately be called painful.

It has been said simply that, "Pain is what the subject says hurts."[98] *Pain is ultimately defined by every individual introspectively in terms of his own experience and the "meaning" that pain holds for him.*

PAIN AS A PROTECTIVE MECHANISM

Pain is an important warning of danger to man; however, it is not essential for biologic adjustment, since persons who have pain pathways surgically or pathologically interrupted, and those persons born without the ability to experience pain, can adjust themselves to their environment.[141] Nevertheless, the loss or absence of the ability to feel and respond to pain predisposes an individual to repeated bodily injury.[63]

Let us examine more closely the function of pain and how some of man's defenses against injury are related to one another.[85]

> The *withdrawal reflex* is the simplest and the most familiar defense, e.g., pulling away from something hot. These reflexes are violent and irrepressible when the threat is great. The muscular reflexes act as a *first* line of defense against injury and often effectively help us to break contact with an offending stimulus by causing us to pull away from it. In order to reduce the length of contact with the stimulus to a minimum—and thus to reduce or prevent tissue damage to the body—the withdrawal reflex occurs with fantastic speed. The impulses race over the shortest possible route from the injury site to the spinal cord and back again to the musculature in the area of injury.

> *Visceral reflexes* involving the glands of internal secretion act as a *second* line of defense against bodily injury. By preparing us for "fight or flight" such reflexes can give us the almost superhuman agility and strength needed in a crisis to save us from real danger.

> *Voluntary responses* to a situation (those responses that we willfully or consciously decide to perform) are a *third* line of defense. Once a noxious stimulus is translated by the brain into perceived pain, the individual, having felt pain, can locate its source and decide, on the basis of his past experience, what he should do.

These three lines of defense are intimately related, and all are activated by the same noxious stimuli. Because reflex responses occur much faster than voluntary ones, they give better protection against injury. However, reflexes are always stereotyped and may be totally inappropriate to a situation, but they occur whether or not they will serve any useful purpose. Thus, if injury or pain is sustained or repeated, these reflexes may actually waste and deplete bodily resources to the extent that new stresses or infection cannot be withstood. Livingston points out: "As a matter of fact, actual tissue injury need not be present to cause this exhaustion. Fear can do exactly the same thing. Often the threat of pain does a person more harm than the injuries that taught him to fear it."[85]

In sum, while pain is protective in some situations, it is useless in others. For example, pain serves a useful function when abdominal tenderness shields an inflamed gallbladder; however, the pain associated with a phantom limb apparently has no protective value.

THE "COMPONENTS" OF PAIN

The entire pain experience is complex in nature, involving an interplay of perception, physiology, feeling states or emotions, and other reactions. Thus, pain is evidently linked to a group of complex experiences rather than to a single sensation produced by a specific stimulus.

> *Pain is a complex "mind-body" experience involving the total person rather than only the mind or only the body. Indeed, the mental and physical experiences of pain are inseparable.*

Therefore, although we shall discuss pain in terms of its *"component parts"* (e.g., perception, reaction), the reader is asked to bear in mind that this is done only for purposes of discussion and has no basis in actual experience.

The sensation of pain may be said to have three component parts: (1) *reception* of the pain stimulus by the pain receptors (free nerve endings in the skin and certain other tissues) and *conduction* of the pain impulses by nerves; (2) *perception* of pain in the higher centers of the brain (e.g., thalamus and cerebral cortex, [Fig. 41–1]); and (3) *reactions* to pain, which are physical, emotional, and psychologic in nature.[92]

The *perception* of pain is a neurophysiologic

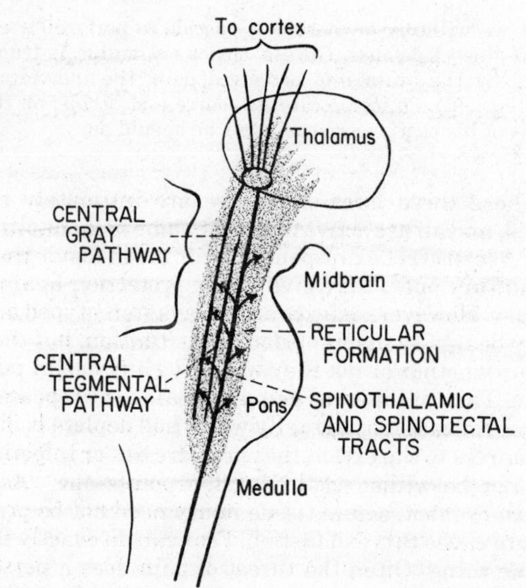

FIGURE 41-1. Transmission of pain signals into the hindbrain, thalamus, and cortex through multiple diffuse pathways. (From Guyton, A. C.: *Textbook of Medical Physiology.* 4th ed., 1971.)

process that can be modified by drugs and psychic factors. Moreover, it can even be completely prevented by interrupting the nerve pathways by surgical or chemical procedures (e.g., surgery or nerve blocks).

The *reaction* to pain is a complex physiopsychologic process involving the cognitive functions (e.g., awareness, reasoning). Reactions to pain are highly individualistic and may vary for a given individual from one time to another in his life. Reactions may be *anticipatory*, occurring prior to the pain-producing stimulus and in expectation of it, or they may occur *after* pain perception as a response to it.

Physiologic and emotional reactions contribute to every individual's unique perception of his pain; many factors influence this perception.* For example, it was observed that some soldiers severely wounded in battle during World War II said that they felt no pain and wanted no pain-relieving drugs. Because they had lived through battle, and believed that being wounded meant that they would be sent home, they experienced no pain, but rather felt relief.[9] Therefore, these men did not perceive their wounds as terrible, painful experiences, but rather as a means of relief and escape from an intolerable situation.[9] Other examples are known of soldiers failing to perceive pain from their wounds because they were under the influence of rage or of the exaltation of battle.[29]

On the other hand, it has been observed[7] that victims of automobile or industrial accidents (whose ages and types of wounds were similar to those of wounded soldiers) overwhelmingly sought relief by medication from what they experienced as excruciating pain. These wounds, to accident victims, *meant* a sudden deterioration from an existing acceptable situation into an impossible one, the consequences of which would be loss of income, unexpected expenses, and mutilation.

Some factors that influence the perception and meaning of pain and the reactions to pain are: (1) attitude toward pain; (2) past experience with pain; (3) value judgment, e.g., pain is "good" or "bad"; (4) mood; (5) emotional status, e.g., stable or unstable; (6) will and self-control; (7) state of the nervous system and the various cerebral processes, e.g., fatigue, disease; (8) situational and environmental components; (9) social, cultural, and economic elements; and (10) the presence or absence of anxiety.

Mental faculties play a definite part in reactions to pain. It has been observed,[113] for example, that: (1) patients with *severe, chronic painful conditions* gradually become free of pain with a decrease in mental capabilities, e.g., with senility; (2) patients with *moderate mental deficiency,* e.g., due to retardation, may react abnormally strongly to painful stimuli because they lack the intelligence to reason out beforehand the extent of the discomfort that will be produced by the noxious stimuli. In addition, *personality defects,* as well as level of intelligence, are evidently factors in the pain reaction. "Those persons who display an abnormal mental reaction to pain will frequently display corresponding mental instability on other occasions."[113] Emotionally unstable individuals seem extraordinarily prone to develop pain.[108]

THE PAIN THRESHOLD

The pain threshold is the smallest perceivable pain, i.e., "the lowest perceptible intensity of pain."[141] Various factors may alter the pain threshold. For example, inflammation or injury of tissues near the nerve endings which subserve pain may *lower* the threshold for pain. This means that stimuli which ordinarily are nonpain-producing (i.e., "nonnoxious") may induce pain; also, stimuli which previously produced mild pain may now produce a more intense pain. Such situations are referred to as *hyperalgesia,* meaning a state of excessive sensitiveness to pain.

Wolff and Wolf[141] report that all persons having healthy body structures have approximately the same *capacity* for perceiving pain, that is, the threshold for the perception of pain is approximately the same in all normal subjects. However, the threshold for *reaction* to pain, unlike that for perception, varies between wide limits for given individuals and for the same person under differing circumstances.

The intensity of two pains which exist separately but at the same time is no greater than that of the more intense of the two. It has long been observed that the existence of one pain may actually raise the

*Students desiring to read further about the psychologic and interpersonal functions of pain are referred to Engel[45] and Szasz.[131] For a discussion of the symbolic and communicative aspects of pain read Szasz.[131]

threshold for perception of another; thus, the person in intense pain may bite his lip or squeeze his fingernails into the palms of his hand and, by creating this "counter pain," lessen the intensity of the original pain.

THE LOCALIZATION OF PAIN

The cerebral cortex functions to localize the sensation of pain. The accuracy with which this occurs varies with (1) the abundance or sparseness of sense organs present in various bodily regions, and (2) the frequency with which the entire sensory circuit is utilized. Physiologically, resistance at the synapses is reduced in a pathway that is frequently used. Thus, the more often that a sensory circuit is used to transmit a sensation, the more readily that sensation will be transmitted. Because the lips, hands, and tongue are diffusely impregnated with sensory nerve endings and are frequently employed to identify objects, these areas undergo a rapid surface localization of painful stimuli that is highly precise and accurate.

It is possible to compare the nerve endings of the tongue, eyes, and hands with fire alarm boxes in a building. Both the nerve endings and the fire alarm boxes help in the process of localizing disturbances. Nerve endings will identify an area of pain (on the tongue, for example) just as the fire alarm boxes will pinpoint the location of a fire in a building. Moreover, if the signal relay system, e.g., from the alarm box to the fire station (or from the nerve ending to the brain), is frequently subjected to drills or usage, then each part of the system, or each member of the team, knows what functions need to be performed and operates smoothly and rapidly, thus reducing resistance in the transmission of the signal.

In contrast to the areas of the tongue, lips, and hands, visceral pain is usually poorly localized because of: (1) the relative paucity of nerve endings, and (2) the relative lack of use of this sensory pathway. Therefore, there is a relative absence of cortical training in the brain in the process of identifying the area affected. However, those deeper structures that are subject to more frequent stimulation by contacts giving rise to sensory impulses may have more clearly localized pain sensations; for example, muscles and periosteum of bones near the body surface.

Pain-producing stimuli almost invariably excite other forms of sensation: a pinprick, thus, usually evokes sensations of touch or pressure and of penetration of the skin; a bruise produces feelings of pressure; and a burn is accompanied by a sensation of heat. These sensations, which are evoked at the same time as pain, probably also provide a basis for localizing and discriminating painful experiences.[62]

CHAPTER 42

Types of Pains

> We all know from our own experience that there is not just pain, but pains, many different kinds of pain with a wide range of varying sensory qualities. . . . Pain, moreover, is rarely experienced in isolation, but is commonly associated with other sensations such as touch, pressure, heat and cold, and also with elements, which though we may not consciously isolate them, are concerned with its location.[24]

It is important for a nurse to realize that there are many different types of pain, so that she can more knowledgeably participate in the specific treatment and nursing care of patients in pain. Familiarization with types of pains will enhance the nurse's skills in observing patients with pain and in accurately reporting her observations and planning patient care.

There are various ways of discussing types of pains. For example, pain may be referred to in terms of:

> *Time of occurrence,* e.g., "postoperative"* pain.
> *Duration or length of time* experienced, e.g., "chronic pain" or "acute pain," and *"intensity of pain,"* e.g., "severe pain," "mild pain."
> *Force or agent causing pain to occur,* e.g., "spontaneous pain," "self-inflicted pain," or "other-inflicted pain."
> *Mode of transmission,* e.g., "projected or referred pain."
> *Ease of transmission,* e.g., "facilitated pain" or "inhibited pain."
> *Location or source,* e.g., "pain from the gallbladder" or "superficial, deep or central pains."
> *Symptoms or manner in which pain is experienced,* e.g., "sharp pain," "burning pain."
> *Causation,* e.g., "organic pain," "pretended pain," "psychogenic pain," "psychophysiologic pain."

This chapter will discuss further: (1) chronic and acute pain; (2) projected or referred pains; (3) superficial, deep, and central pains; (4) pretended, psychogenic, and psychophysiologic pains; and (5) facilitated and inhibited pains.

CHRONIC PAIN AND ACUTE PAIN

In general, *acute pain* is temporary, has immediate onset, and eventually subsides after successful treatment, or often without treatment. Examples of acute pain are the pains of traumatic injury, ordinary headache, and renal colic. Acute pain may be useful in that it causes the sufferer to attempt to determine its cause and to seek relief from suffering, e.g., to notice that his finger is on a hot stove and to pull it away.[4]

In contrast to acute pain, *chronic pain* is continual, may begin gradually, persists or recurs for an indefinite period of time and is refractory to treatment.[135] Examples of chronic pains are those caused by trigeminal neuralgia, severe rheumatoid arthritis, and advanced cancer. Prolonged pain has deleterious effects on vital organs such as the heart and kidney. Moreover, chronic pain is often frustrating to experience, because it does not provoke defensive reflexes and gives the patient no clue as to how he might lessen it.[81]

The mental reaction to pain depends on the duration of the pain and, to a far lesser extent, its intensity.[113] Pain that is constant, continuous, and moderate is much more difficult to bear than that which is paroxysmal and intense. A patient who has a continuous sensation of pain (e.g., in anesthesia dolorosa*) will become increasingly engrossed by his illness, fearful, tense, depressed, and may appear somewhat mentally withdrawn, whereas a patient with an acute attack of intense pain (e.g., in trigeminal neuralgia) may come to terms with his periods of pain. Although he may have an agonized appearance at the time of an attack, he appears normal between attacks.

Pains caused by cancer vary in their intensity, but they rarely, if ever, reach the *severity* of some of the other pains that humans suffer, for example, those of tic douloureux or of renal colic. Thus, rather than the intensity of such pains, it is their *chronic and prolonged natures* which at times make them exhausting and virtually unbearable.[46] Let us emphasize again that not all persons with cancer experience pain. However, when pain is present and is intractable, it drags the patient on a downhill course manifested by emotional deterioration, insomnia, anorexia, weight loss, and loss of strength.

Extremely intense pain is unlikely to be felt over a long period, because pain of high intensity usually means that the nerve endings themselves are being destroyed. Once nerve endings are destroyed, pain is likely to cease or at least diminish in intensity. However, an important exception occurs with causalgia, when the nerve trunk itself is damaged and intense pain is experienced over long periods.[87]

Pains caused by *organic* diseases are seldom constant in nature, but rather they vary because the or-

---

*See Unit VI for a discussion of postoperative pain.

*_Anesthesia dolorosa_ is a condition occurring in paralysis or in some spinal cord diseases in which there is tactile anesthesia with severe pain in the part.

ganic etiologic factors usually fluctuate from time to time, and also because nerve centers periodically tire. Often, although not always, a patient's pain is diagnosed as *psychoneurotic* in origin if the patient says that he has the same pain constantly.[87]

Intractable, chronic pain states, producing *prolonged* and *intense* bombardment of the central nervous system, create a destructive effect on the sufferer. These pain states "may too often—and not unexpectedly—terminate in a self-dissolution of life."[63] This mental state is typified in the final entry that was made in the *Journal* of Alice James (sister to Henry James) two days prior to her death:

> I am being ground slowly on the grim grindstone of physical pain, and on two nights I had almost asked for K's lethal dose; but one steps hesitantly along such unaccustomed ways, and endures from second to second.

PROJECTED OR REFERRED PAINS

Projected or referred pain is that felt in an area *different* from the place where the pain impulses originated; the pain is, thus, "referred" from its original source to another area of the body. A disturbance of the pain pathways produces a sensation of pain in a region supplied by peripheral nerve branches. For example, an acoustic neuroma may produce trigeminal neuralgia. Projected or referred pains will be briefly mentioned again in the following section.

SUPERFICIAL PAIN, DEEP PAIN, AND CENTRAL PAIN

Superficial (cutaneous) *pain* is sometimes called "direct pain" because the pain accurately localizes where the point of disturbance is. Two types of superficial pain have been described: (1) that with an abrupt onset and pricking quality, and (2) pain of slower onset with a burning quality. Superficial pain occurs in the skin or the second sensitive layer, that is, the deep fascia of the limbs and trunk and any subcutaneous ligament or tendon.

Pain arising from structures deeper than the surface structures is termed *deep pain*. Three varieties of deep pain may occur: (1) true visceral (splanchnic) and deep somatic pain, which is felt at the point of noxious stimulation and may or may not be associated with referred pain; (2) referred pain, which is pain experienced at a site other than the area of stimulus; and (3) pain from secondary skeletal muscle contraction. *Central pain* is pain for which no peripheral cause exists at the time the pain is perceived by the subject.

Deep pain can further be compared with, and distinguished from, superficial pain as shown in the table on the following page.

Superficial pain is relatively uncomplicated since it is directly perceived and can readily be localized. Let us turn our attention now to the more complicated phenomena of deep pains and central pain.

DEEP PAIN SYNDROMES

It is impossible to consider all the various deep pain syndromes at this point. Many of them will be mentioned in appropriate sections of the text; however, we shall make some summarizing comments here.

Visceral Pain

A viscus (plural, viscera) is any of the large interior body organs occupying one of the body's cavities, such as the cranial, thoracic, abdominal, or pelvic cavity. The word "splanchnic" pertains to the viscera; thus, visceral pain may also be called splanchnic pain. Usually the term "viscera" refers to the ab-

TABLE 42–1. THREE MAJOR GROUPS OF PAIN SYNDROMES

Superficial Pain	Deep Pain	Central Pain
1. Abrupt onset—pricking quality 2. Slower onset—burning quality	1. True visceral and deep somatic pain a. True visceral (splanchnic)—from diseased body organ b. Deep somatic—segmental distribution, from lesion of vertebra, muscle, or other neuromuscular origin 2. Referred pain—projected from viscus or other deep structure to surface of body 3. Secondary skeletal muscle contraction—pain from spread of excitation within spinal cord	1. Causalgia—from injury to peripheral nerve 2. Phantom limb pain—after amputation 3. Central pain—from lesions within CNS that affect pain pathways

dominal viscera. Some typical visceral pains that will be discussed more completely in appropriate sections of the text are the pains of: acute appendicitis; cholecystitis; inflammations of the biliary-pancreatic tract; gastroduodenal disease; cardiovascular disease; pleurisy; and renal and ureteral colic.

While some bodily areas are highly sensitive to pain, others are not. For example, gross insults can be given to the body's viscera without exciting pain, such as clamping the stomach (so long as the mesentery is not pulled upon), or pinching or pricking the heart.[99] Holmes[62] observes that it is not surprising that most of the viscera are insensitive to those stimuli that will excite pain in somatic structures (such as cutting, burning, or pressure) since the viscera are not normally exposed to such trauma. Therefore, they cannot be expected to be endowed with a nervous apparatus to respond to them. However, while these stimuli do not produce pain in most of the viscera, other stimuli, such as violent or abnormal contractions of hollow viscera (like the ureters and alimentary tract), may cause severe pain.

Pain in the alimentary tract is a common medical occurrence and appears to emanate mainly from the muscular and serous coats. Such pains are believed to occur when the abdominal mucosa is inflamed, ulcerated, or otherwise abnormal, or when the visceral muscles contract strongly or pass into spasm. Thus, although the wall of the intestine itself may be insensitive to cutting, burning, or crushing, it does produce pain under other conditions.

The parietal peritoneum, the mesentery, and many blood vessels are sensitive to injuries such as cutting, stretching and handling. Moreover, the mucosal linings of the urethra, bladder, ureters, and kidney pelvis are sensitive to pain.[141]

Abdominal pain may also be caused by the perforation of bodily organs with the resultant drainage of various amounts of their contents into the peritoneal cavity. Table 42–2 indicates the irritating properties of abnormal intraperitoneal fluid extravasation, listed in order from the most irritating to the least irritating.

In the *chest* the parietal pleura is found to be richly supplied with pain endings through the intercostal nerves, and on the diaphragmatic surface, by the phrenic nerve as well. The visceral pleura in the chest, however, is insensitive to pain. Elsewhere and throughout their serous surfaces both the visceral and parietal pericardia are insensitive to pain, with the exception that the lower portion of the fibrous pericardium appears to be supplied with pain fibers from the phrenic nerve.[141]

At this point let us look more closely at *pains due to inflammation, vascular pains, and pains of muscular origin.* Some important points about these types of pains are summarized below:[1, 141]

Pains due to Inflammation. Inflammation induces a hyperalgesic state in the affected tissue; in-

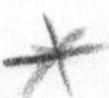

Superficial Pain	*Deep Pain*
Associated symptoms may be hyperalgesia, paresthesia, analgesia, tickling, or itching. Also associated with brisk movements, a quick pulse, and a sense of invigoration.	*Associated symptoms* due to autonomic responses include: pallor, sweating, nausea, vomiting, and, at times, bradycardia, fall in blood pressure, syncope, faintness, and perhaps even death in shock. Also associated with quiescence and sometimes local muscular rigidity of the abdominal wall.
Nausea never occurs.	*Nausea* ("sickening pain") is found only when deep structures are involved, e.g., in renal and intestinal colic, gallstones, and angina.
Quality of pain is a sharp, bright sensation felt superficially.	*Quality* of pain is primarily dull, aching. May be described as boring, crushing, throbbing, or cramping, or, if less intense, as a soreness or hurting.
Duration is typically shorter than deep pain.	*Duration* is often fairly long.
Localization tends to be more precise than with deep pain. Pain is often experienced as a point, surface, or line.	*Localization* is often diffuse and inaccurate; seems to originate in a fairly broad area. Pain frequently is felt as if it were of three dimensions and occupied space.
Hyperalgesia of a primary nature may occur with superficial pain. The hyperalgesia occurs at the site of the original noxious stimulation.	*Hyperalgesia* secondary in nature may exist with deep pain, occurring at a distance from the original noxious stimulus. Thus, in referred pain, a superficial hyperalgesia may be associated with deep pain.
	Muscle contraction and tenderness occur often.
	Segmental spread of pain is frequently noted. Pain may not remain confined to the original spinal segment, but false localization may spread into one or more neighboring spinal cord and skin segments.

flammation is one of the commonest pathologic conditions that influences pain sensitivity.

Vascular Pains. The precise vascular pain mechanism is not understood, but it is believed to originate from some pathologic condition of the vessels or perivascular tissues. Also considered of importance is the participation of some pain-producing chemical substances.

The blood vessels are frequently involved with the mediation of pain. Blood vessels are believed to be associated with pain induced by cold. Also, distortion of cranial vessels by pulling, displacement, or distention is the source of a large proportion of headaches including: migraine; headaches associated with arterial hypertension; headaches of brain tumor; and headaches associated with variations in the hydrodynamics of the cerebrospinal fluid.

Pains of Muscular and Bony Origin. The primary cause of muscle pain is believed to be not muscle tension itself, but rather the compression or constriction of blood vessels within the muscle. The sustained clenching of muscles or their continued overwork may produce muscular pain.

> Ligaments, joint capsules, fascia, tendons, and muscle all vary in the density of their innervation; the periosteum is the most sensitive.

> Spontaneous pain may be induced by spasms, rupture, ischemia, inflammation, or other disturbances of the ligaments, tendons, muscles, and periosteum of bones and joints.

> While chemical irritants injected into muscles may give rise to considerable pain, the usual ways in which muscular pains occur are in association with stretching, ischemia, or forceful or sustained contractile activity. In both the latter cases the nerve endings are believed to be stimulated by an excessive concentration of potassium.

> When muscle pain causes a sustained reflex contraction of the muscle, a vicious circle of pain may occur; the contraction successively increases muscular pain and the pain gradually radiates into adjacent areas.

> A large proportion of headaches, especially those accompanied by stiffness or tenderness in the neck and occipital region, originate from sustained contraction of underlying head muscles.

> Muscular ischemia induces pain in the extremities in intermittent claudication and occlusive vascular disease and is the basis of the pain of coronary occlusion.

Referred Pain

Whereas deep pain may arise from disease of the viscera or from a lesion of a deep somatic structure

(such as one of the vertebrae, a muscle, or an interspinous ligament), both visceral and somatic pain may be, and in fact usually are, referred to a segment of the skin.[99] The referral of pain to a segment of the skin is clearly illustrated in herpes zoster, in which inflammation of the ganglion of a particular posterior nerve root (lying beside the spinal column) causes lesions and sensations to appear on the surface of the body on the segment of skin that is innervated by the affected nerve.

Referred pain is curious because in some instances it may be intense, whereas there may be little or no pain *in situ*, i.e., at the point of noxious stimulation. In other situations, the *in situ* pain may predominate. Referred pain may occur with or without hyperalgesia, and in the presence or absence of pain or tenderness due to secondary muscle spasm.

Referred pains are often baffling and call for a careful differential diagnosis. For example, spinal cord tumors may cause pain that mimics the pain of gallbladder disease because of irritation of nerves which supply the abdomen's right upper quadrant. Diabetics may have a right lower quadrant pain suggestive of appendicitis when disease of the appendix is actually not present.[99] Figure 42–1 illustrates some patterns of referred pain.

Identification of the segment of the spinal cord that is involved in transmitting the pain is diagnostically helpful. Pain arising from a deep structure, whether a viscus or a deep somatic structure, will have a referred segmental distribution, or pattern of pain, that is determined according to the segment of the spinal cord that is supplying the structure.

Central Pain Syndromes. Causalgias, phantom limb pains, and central pains are sometimes spoken of collectively as "central pain syndromes," even though their etiologies differ. The etiologies for these pain syndromes can basically be distinguished in the table on the following page.

Causalgia is sometimes listed separately from central pain, but the fact remains that *causalgia, phantom limb pain,* and *central pain* are all related because all three are *autonomic reflex pain syndromes*. Thus, despite having widely differing etiologies, these disorders have a striking similarity of underlying pathophysiologic mechanisms and clinical features.

TABLE 42–2. ABNORMAL INTRAPERITONEAL FLUID ACCUMULATIONS (IN THE ORDER OF THEIR PAINFULLY IRRITATING QUALITIES)*

1. Pancreatic enzyme fluid
2. Gastric or duodenal fluid
3. Fecal fluid
   a. Colon
   b. Appendiceal
   c. Small bowel
4. Bile
5. Urine
6. Blood
7. Lymph

*Dorsey, J. M.; *Medical Clinics of North America* 52:103, January, 1968.

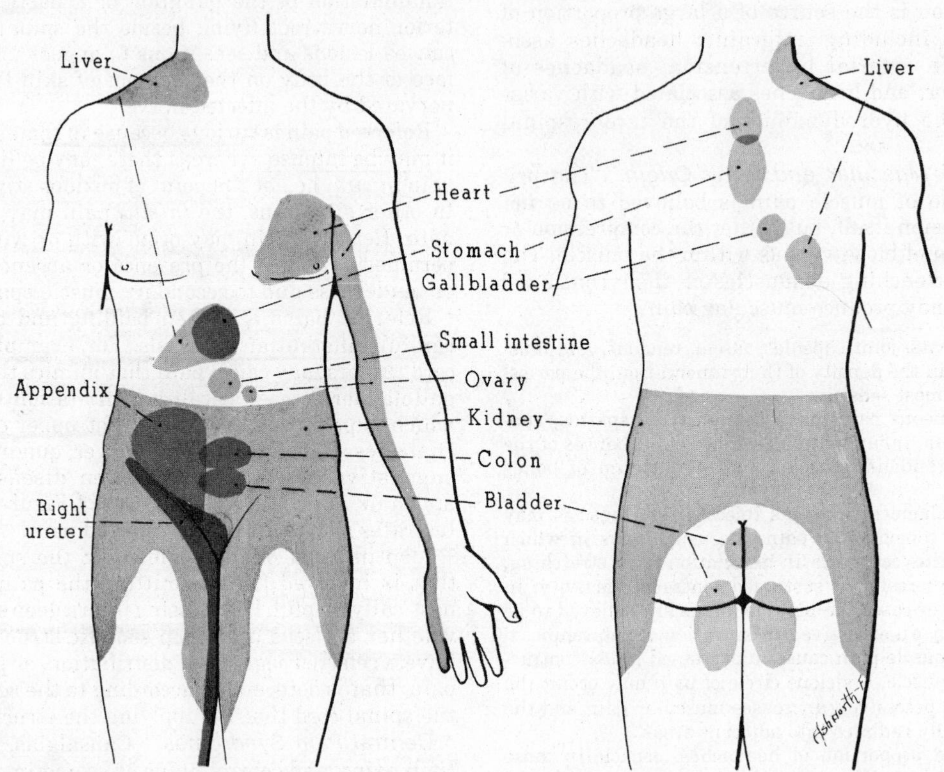

FIGURE 42–1. Areas of referred pain, anterior and posterior views. (Jacob and Francone: *Structure and Function in Man*, 3rd Ed. 1974.)

THE ETIOLOGY OF CENTRAL PAIN SYNDROMES

Type of Pain	*Usual Etiology*
Causalgia	High-velocity, penetrating wounds damaging peripheral nerves, usually the brachial plexus and median and sciatic nerves; the wounds typically injure but do not completely divide the nerves
Phantom limb pain	Following amputation
Central pain	Lesions within the central nervous system that directly affect pain pathways

Central pain syndromes have been clinically observed to have the following factors in common:

> All patients with central pain complain of pain that is present in the absence of peripheral stimulation or of an obvious pathologic process to account for the pain.[105]

> Peripheral stimulation will usually increase the pain in those areas in which the pain is localized.[105]

> All types of stimuli cause pain, including those that do not evoke pain when they are applied to normal areas in the same patient.[105]

> Although the change in cutaneous sensibility may occur in a variety of ways, the main common denominator is that there is damage to the afferent* pathways. Loss of function is always present.[105]

> There is frequently total loss of sensory communication from the part to which the pain is referred. Thus, sensations appear to arise in a part in which central afferent connections have been severed. When viewed in this manner causalgia and central pain are somewhat "phantom-like," even though they differ from true phantom limb pain in which there are actually feelings in an absent part of the body.[96]

Syndromes with the above features are called central pain syndromes because the damage is central to the peripheral receptors. Lesions of the peripheral somatic afferent nerves are included within this definition. "These conditions may be found with traumatic lesions of peripheral nerves such as causalgia, lesions of the spinal cord, vascular lesions of the brainstem, the thalamus syndrome, certain subcortical or even cortical lesions."[105] Another example is postherpetic neuralgia (see later).

Let us now proceed to examine some of the specific types of pain that we have just been referring to, namely, causalgia, phantom limb pain, and some examples of central pain (i.e., postherpetic neuralgia, and spinal cord lesions, brainstem lesions, thalamic lesions, and lesions of the cerebral cortex with central pain). Treatments for these painful conditions will also be discussed.

Causalgia. The term "causalgia" and its classic description resulted from observations of Union soldiers who sustained injuries to peripheral nerves during the Civil War. The pain syndrome of causalgia follows injury to a peripheral nerve and is characterized by burning pain that is often severe, persistent, diffuse, spontaneous, and aggravated by motion, touch, or emotional stimuli. Generally the pain is associated with dystrophic† and vasomotor changes and may cause emotional disturbances and changes if it is prolonged. The brachial plexus and the median and sciatic nerves are involved most frequently. While peripheral nerve damage is the usual cause, other conditions may rarely precipitate the problem, for example: sprains, bruises, fractures, amputations, and arterial and venous occlusions.

Since virtually any stimulus may set off paroxysms of excruciating pain (e.g., stimuli such as drafts of air, eating, temperature changes, contact with clothing), the person with prolonged causalgia pain may develop "into a nervous recluse who adopts such elaborate precautions to prevent paroxysms of pain that they may seem absurd. Apathy associated with a haggard and woebegone expression reflecting constant, severe suffering is the typical picture of this disease. . . . The symptoms may increase in intensity and area of involvement, the intractable pain leading eventually to drug addiction, invalidism, and even suicide."[46] In an attempt to prevent pain, the patient may maintain the affected joints rigidly, and in an effort to obtain partial relief he may keep the part wrapped in a moist cloth.

Neuralgia differs from causalgia in that the pain of neuralgia is typically throbbing or tingling, whereas that of causalgia is burning. Also, the pain of neuralgia is less severe and is generally restricted to the field of the affected nerve.

Phantom Limb Pain. Various sensations may be felt by patients in their phantom limbs (amputated extremity). These paresthesias (abnormal sensations) may commonly be: feelings of itching in the palm of the missing hand or sole of the foot; pressure sensations, tingling feelings, or the sensation described as "pins and needles." A throbbing, burning sensation of the hand or foot is the most persistent and common pain. "Another common pain is appreciated as a cramped and twisted abnormal posturing of the limb, which is maintained immovably rigid in spite of the desire of the patient to change position. This latter type of pain does not occur when the patient has the illusion of being able to move the phantom voluntarily. The fist may be clenched tightly with the nails tearing into the palm."[46] Patients with amputated legs or feet may feel their missing toes are tightly curled and cramped. Phantom pains may be of a stabbing, boring, or vise-like nature.

Although most phantom paresthesias are tolerable to those persons with them, there are some phantom pains that are intensely intolerable. Pain quality varies widely, but exacerbations may be precipitated by fatigue, excitement, sickness, weather changes, emotional stress, and other stimuli. A painless phantom limb may gradually become painful, but the more typical occurrence is for those phantoms that pose severe problems to be painful immediately postamputation. It is now clearly established that phantom limb pain affects only those who are born with a limb and lose it. Even so, only a small proportion of persons with a phantom limb have significant pain in it.[96]

Stump pain often is associated with phantom limb pain but is not necessarily related to it. Although patients usually experience some stump discomfort along with their phantom pain, some persons have phantom pain but have no stump problems.

Central Pain. This refers to that pain that is pri-

**Afferent* nerves transmit impulses from the periphery toward the central nervous system, i.e., sensory nerves; *efferent* nerves transmit impulses from the central nervous system toward the periphery.

†Reflex sympathetic dystrophy is a disorder of the sympathetic nervous system that may follow injury to the nerves or blood vessels, fracture, or sprain. It is characterized by rubor or pallor, sweating, edema, pain, or skin atrophy.

marily produced by lesions *within* the central nervous system which *directly* affect the pain pathways. Pain that is secondarily or indirectly related to central lesions (e.g., headache from increased intracranial pressure due to brain tumor) is *not* central pain.

Lesions producing central pain may involve the spinothalamic tract at any level from the spinal cord to the thalamus as well as the thalamocortical radiations from the thalamus to the cerebral cortex. Central pain is typically spontaneous; variable in severity, although usually constantly present; and subject to spontaneous aggravation, although its intensity may also be increased by such specific stimuli as sudden temperature changes, anxiety, and emotional stress. Overreaction to stimuli may occur, so that normally nonpainful stimuli may be experienced as painful. Also, there may be an unusually prolonged time lag between the initiation of a painful stimulus and the feeling of pain; moreover, the feeling of pain may then long outlast the stimulus. Frequently signs of autonomic dysfunction, such as increased perspiration, cyanosis, and lowered skin temperature, may accompany the pain. While many patients with central pain find it difficult to describe the quality of their sensations, others refer to their pains as boring, cold, burning, aching, or gnawing.

The *mechanism* by which central pain occurs is not precisely known, but it is speculated that "irritation" at the lesion site and/or "reduction of central inhibition" are factors important in central pain production. Also, since psychologic stress obviously aggravates central pain, doctors believe that regardless of what the specific pain mechanism is, pain production is somehow connected (in the highest integrative levels of the brain) to those neurologic circuits relating to emotions.

One type of central pain that presents some interesting histologic changes in nerve structure is *postherpetic neuralgia.* Following the extremely painful acute vesicular eruption of herpes zoster, and after these vesicles have subsided and disappeared, some patients will have a persistent, severe, intractable pain within the area of the original skin eruption, or postherpetic neuralgia. This pain syndrome is one of the most annoying and tormenting, with the unrelenting pain causing sleepless nights and virtually unbearable days. Patients may be willing to undergo any treatment in hopes of relief. However, the results of therapy are often poor, and frequently the postherpetic pain is intractable to all forms of treatment.[46]

The cause of the persistent pain which is present in postherpetic neuralgia is not fully understood. However, scarring and degenerative changes involving the spinal cord, ganglia, nerve trunks, and skin may be important factors in this pain problem.

> *Spinal cord lesions,* which may produce central pain, may arise from syringomyelia, trauma to the spinal cord, and spinal cord tumors.

> *Brainstem lesions* may produce central pain that has a crossed pain pattern such that the face is involved on the side of the lesion (i.e., "ipsilateral" facial pain) while the trunk and limbs are affected on the side opposite the lesion (because of the fact that spinothalamic fibers are involved which cross to innervate the opposite side of the body). Only a small proportion of brainstem lesions produce pain; these lesions are typically those involving the medulla and pons (which contain the descending sensory nucleus of the trigeminal nerve) rather than those in the mesencephalon (which has no sensory nuclei).

> *Thalamic lesions* are the most common cause of central pain and typically produce symptoms that affect the side of the body opposite the lesion. Vascular lesions of the thalamus, which involve the lateral nucleus of the thalamus, are the most common thalamic source of central pain, although tumor, trauma, or inflammation of this area may also produce spontaneous pain. When thalamic infarct or thrombosis occurs, the pains usually do not occur for several weeks. These pains may range from paresthesia to agonizing, boring, burning pains which are often associated with a sensation that the hand or foot is being twisted. Such thalamic pains following thalamic infarct (cerebrovascular accident or stroke) may involve an entire half of the body. The pain, following the stroke by several weeks, is generally most intense in the extremities, especially the hand. Thalamic pain may be intensified by emotional disturbances and increased emotional lability; i.e., unmotivated crying or laughter is often associated with this syndrome.[46]

The syndrome produced by thalamic lesions is referred to as the *thalamic syndrome,* and typically consists of the following signs and symptoms (all of which appear on the side opposite the lesion): (1) transient hemiparesis or hemiplegia; (2) loss of deep sensation and impairment of superficial sensation; (3) tremor, ataxia, and choreoathetoid movements; and (4) spontaneous, excruciating pains, hyperalgesia, and excessive reaction to stimulation of involved bodily areas. Hyperpathic pain may be present in the entire contralateral half of the head and body, or smaller contiguous areas may be affected.

The nurse caring for patients with thalamic syndrome will want to bear in mind that these patients will overrespond to stimuli, such as pinprick, stroking, and deep pressure on the involved area of the skin. Also, bright light, sudden noises, temperature changes (cold especially), fatigue, debilitation, and apprehension will all intensify the pain. In addition, these patients may laugh or cry without apparent motivation, since extreme emotional lability is a part of their illness.

Cerebral cortex lesions, such as brain tumors and other mass lesions, as well as cortical ischemic lesions resulting from cerebrovascular occlusive disease, may involve the cerebral cortex and not the thalamus. These may produce central pain in the contralateral side of the body. A careful neurologic examination must be carried out before treating a patient for "thalamic pain," so that a possible surgical lesion is not overlooked.

PRETENDED PAIN, PSYCHOGENIC PAIN, AND PSYCHOPHYSIOLOGIC PAIN

Pretended Pain

Pretended pain is neither psychogenic nor physiologic (organic) in origin, for pain is actually present in both these situations, whereas it is *not present* in persons who pretend to be in pain.

What are some reasons why people might pretend to have pain when pain is actually absent? Rasmussen[113] identifies three reasons why people might continue to act as if they were in pain, although they really are not: (1) they use pain as a means of concentrating interest and sympathy upon themselves; (2) they may escape the demands and boredom of everyday life (e.g., "I can't do the dishes, I have a headache"); and (3) pain may be pretended in an attempt to obtain some economic gain in the form of damages (i.e., compensation neurosis). In addition to these reasons, pain may also be simulated for purposes of (4) obtaining narcotics. In each of these four situations the individual is pretending to have pain in an attempt to control how others will act toward him. For example, "You should help me by giving me medicine (money) (doing my work) because I'm in pain."

PSYCHOGENIC PAIN*

Psychogenic pain can be defined as follows:[96] pain (1) that is independent of peripheral stimulation or of damage to the nervous system and due to emotional factors, or (2) in which any peripheral change, such as muscle tension, is a consequence of emotional factors.

> *An estimated 50 per cent of pain symptoms seen in general medicine are psychogenic in nature.*[73]

Wang[135] offers some additional criteria for determining whether pain is psychogenic in origin. He states that pain is psychogenic when no anatomic or physiologic explanation can be detected, when narcotics do not provide relief, when much relief is obtained with sedatives and placebos, and when it is possible to alleviate the pain by distracting the patient's attention.

PSYCHOPHYSIOLOGIC PAIN

Psychophysiologic pain is pain produced as a result of a chronic and exaggerated state of the normal physiologic expression of emotion, e.g., rage, fear. These long-continued visceral changes, resulting from repressed feelings, may eventually produce structural changes. While psychophysiologic leg pains, back pains, and abdominal pains are not uncommon, the most common pain of this nature is tension headache resulting from muscle spasms secondary to anxiety.

FACILITATED AND INHIBITED PAINS

Sensitivity to pain varies widely.

> There are some patients with pain whose symptoms are difficult, if not impossible, to relieve, even by surgery that interrupts all known nervous pathways connecting the site of injury or disease with the cerebral cortex. At the other extreme are persons without any detectable development or other lesion of their nervous systems who do not experience pain as a result of any form of injury or disease.[138]

*See also Chapter 43.

One explanation of such wide divergencies of response to pain is that in some instances the perception of pain may be "facilitated," whereas, at the other extreme, the perception is "inhibited."

Facilitated pain means that various phenomena have taken place that facilitate or "make it easier" for pain to occur. For example, after repeated stimulation, the sense-perceptive areas of the brain may become hypersensitive and, thus, easily triggered. Habitual pain pathways can be thought of schematically as being overused and worn smooth, so that less resistance to the emergence of pain takes place. Resistance at the synapses is reduced in such frequently used pathways. Slight structural changes at or near the original local site of pain production may thus cause stimuli to be transmitted and perceived with greater rapidity and sensitivity.

Because of overused pain pathways, a person who has long suffered with chronic cholecystitis may have typical gallbladder pain even *after* the removal of that organ. Also, the cortical threshold may be lowered generally as well as locally, e.g., a marked general hyperalgesia may be experienced with pneumonia. Another example of "supersensitive" pain pathways (which facilitate the transmission of stimuli producing pain) are those of the individual with chronic rheumatism who can predict weather changes by means of exacerbations of his pain.

Inhibited pain responses are those which "make it harder" for pain to be experienced. We have seen that *emotional attitudes* toward pain can greatly alter perception of the stimulus, and thus the learning process can influence perception. Through training and will power some persons can inhibit and control their responses to pain.

We have indicated that during periods of excitement or hysteria, an injury may not be felt as painful. Also, chronic *schizophrenics* have been observed to show no painful response to severe physical disease which might be expected to produce pain. Moreover, persons who are *severely subnormal mentally* have been known to harm themselves without apparent discomfort.[96]

In addition to these situations there are several other types of indifference to pain that are of importance.[96] A lack of pain perception or *"nonpain"* may be *clinically produced,* e.g., by surgically severing nerves for purposes of pain control, or may occur by *accident,* e.g., traumatic injury to the spinal cord.* Other persons may have been born with an abnormally weak mental reaction to pain. Some of

*For a further discussion see the unit on neurology, Unit VIII.

these congenital cases are probably attributable to a developmental defect, most likely central in origin.

Rarely one encounters a patient who has an apparently normal sensibility of pain, but an absence of mental reaction to it; this is referred to as *pain asymbolia*.[113] Asymbolia refers to loss of the ability to understand symbolic things. Thus, with pain asymbolia the patient loses the ability to understand the symbolism of pain. A person with such an affliction might wince upon noxious stimulation, but not withdraw from the pain-producing stimulus nor respond to other threats of damage. Since the threats are not symbolically thought of as damaging or harmful, the individual does not respond even though he appears to feel pain. This condition has been related to cerebral lesions.

CHAPTER 43

Evaluation of Pain and Patients Experiencing Pain

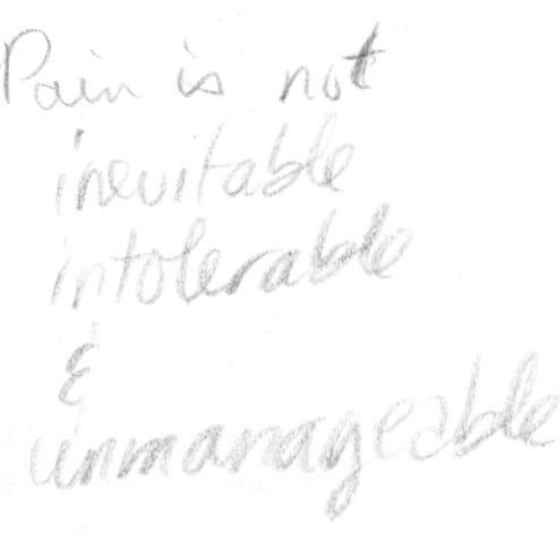

> The evaluation of pain so that it can be treated adequately is made difficult by its being an entirely subjective phenomenon. It is especially difficult to differentiate organic from psychic factors. The problem is further complicated because in most, if not all, patients, both factors contribute to the final expression of the pain. Furthermore, the proportion of contributions by the somatic and psychic spheres changes constantly.[46]

The evaluation of pain and of patients experiencing pain is an activity that nurses perform frequently. As we have demonstrated, pain is difficult to assess because it is a highly personalized, subjective experience which is manifested uniquely in each patient and which stems from diverse etiologies.

THE NURSE; THE PATIENT

Important areas in the evaluation of a patient experiencing pain are: (1) the nurse's evaluation of the patient's personality; and (2) her impression of herself as she is reflected in the patient's response to her.[37]

Does one ever become accustomed to witnessing pain in others? It is hoped that a nurse never becomes "hardened" to the presence of pain. But, certainly, she must build a constructive attitude toward pain if she is to encounter and help to alleviate suffering.

To form such a constructive attitude, a nurse must clarify her own feelings about suffering. For example, she will not be able to help a patient to find meaning in his pain-filled life if she does not truly believe that his life is meaningful; she cannot hope to clarify the "nightmare" of pain for a patient if she is not willing to look at the nightmare herself; and she cannot help a patient to break out of his shell of isolation if she, because of her anxiety, encloses herself in a shell. The nurse must come to the realization that pain, though subjective, is also a very real and universal experience, and that to understand it, and hopefully to alleviate it, is one of her greatest challenges.

Before planning specific care, evaluate how you feel about a patient having pain—your attitude toward him as a person and toward pain and suffering generally. If you possess the attitude that *pain is not inevitable, intolerable, and unmanageable*, you will be in a position to be helpful to patients who are afraid that they will have pain, as well as to those who currently have it. *Thoughtful, intelligent nursing care can prevent, reduce, make bearable, and control pain.* An optimistic, informed attitude toward pain control can bring to the fore each patient's strengths in responding to pain and help each to achieve a more realistic view of his situation.[11]

Because a patient's pain has special meanings *to him,* he may expect that those caring for him will, intuitively, understand his individual view of his situation and will respond appropriately. If your view of a patient's pain fails to coincide with *his* view of it, problems ensue.

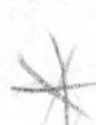

Evaluate how you think the patient having pain perceives you. For example, does he act toward you as if you are there to help him, or as if you are there to inflict further pain and add to his misery? Does he seem to feel that you believe what he is telling you about his pain and will act to help him, or as if he feels you doubt what he says and will dismiss it without seeking relief for him? Does he view you as interested and concerned, or bored and unimpressed with his situation?

Further discussion of ways in which a nurse can help the patient having pain, by means of her interaction with him, is presented further on. The individual personalities of both patient and nurse are important determining factors in the specific process of interaction. The meanings that both nurse and patient assign to pain are also important and must be evaluated.

EVALUATING THE MEANINGS OF PAIN

> The alleviation of pain on a professional level does not take place in a social vacuum. It takes place in a social situation. The patient in pain reacts diffusely to painful experiences and to the efforts of those who are trying to help him. The efforts expended on his behalf, as well as the pain itself, have meaning for the patient. Existing potentialities for alleviating pain can only be fully exploited when the meaning to the patient is given careful consideration.[37]

SOCIOCULTURAL FACTORS

As we have previously demonstrated, the experience of pain cannot be explained in purely physiologic or biologic terms; cultural and social aspects of pain must also be considered. For example, as a result of cultural influences, manifest (i.e., observable) behavior in pain experiences will vary. Some patients will quietly accept intense pain, whereas others quake, wail, and show other obvious signs of distress at the thought of a small needle prick.

Zborowski[143] points out that cultural influences may affect attitudes concerning *pain expectancy* (i.e., the anticipation of pain viewed as unavoidable in certain situations) and *pain acceptance* (i.e., the willingness to experience pain). For example, while pain may be "expected" as a part of medical treatment, some patients will be less willing to "accept" the pain than others.

Pain expectancy influences the perception of pain. Thus, in a person who has a morbid fear of cancer, every pain he develops will be intensified because to him it suggests the onset of cancer, which the individual "expects" he will develop. Expectations of pain are often out of proportion to the actual situation. For example, not all persons with cancer experience pain; however, most people with cancer "expect" that they will have pain. Such expectations can cause people to misinterpret other discomforts, such as pressure, for pain. Postoperative pain represents another situation in which pain expectations are important. Not all postoperative patients have pain.

In addition to pain expectancy and pain acceptance, other factors that may culturally vary are *pain apprehension* and *pain anxiety*. Pain apprehension is related to the tendency to avoid pain. Pain anxiety refers to the state of anxiety that the pain experience provokes; it mainly focuses on the cause of pain, the meaning of pain, and its significance for the welfare of the individual. Several factors have been identified as contributing to the anxiety of the patient experiencing pain. Some of these are: the element of the unknown; the loneliness of pain, and the helplessness engendered by pain; and the threat to the self or body image.[11, 37, 81]

Past experiences with pain, and past observations of others in pain, markedly affect individual perceptions of pain-producing situations. Therefore, learning and experience *condition* one's reactions to pain and add to the meaning that pain has for each different individual.

> The pain that a child experiences is often conditioned by the fears, attitudes and afflictions of his parents. Indeed, parental influences may be decisive factors in determining the amount of pain their children will suffer from minor injuries throughout the rest of their lives.[85]

Zborowski[143] concludes that there are ethnic variations in attitudes toward pain. In each culture, parents' approval or disapproval of their children's responses to pain promotes in the children specific acceptable forms of behavior in reaction to pain. When the responses to pain of three ethnic groups were studied it was observed that: (1) the model "Italian" patient responded to pain by *complaints* of discomfort caused by the pain as such; (2) the model "Jewish" patient mainly worried about the extent to which the pain indicated a *threat* to himself; and (3) the model "Old American" tended to avoid complaining and provoking pity and *minimized* his pain.

The Old American group provides the dominant values and attitudes in the United States, and thus represents those attitudes toward pain which many patients, doctors, and nurses have in this country. In his survey, Zborowski observed that the Italian and Jewish subjects manifested suffering and admitted to pain more readily than the Old Americans. Thus, depending on their culture, some persons will readily say that they are in pain whereas others are hesitant to mention it.

Moreover, it has been noted that pain occurring in "culturally unacceptable" body areas, e.g., areas embarrassing to the patient like the rectum, anus, genitalia, or buttocks, appears to be underreported compared with pain in more "acceptable" areas.

In striving to accept cultural differences in response to pain, the nurse needs to realize that the responses to pain of persons of cultural groups that differ from her own are as valid as her own responses to pain would be. Obviously, one must be cautious in judging how severe another person's pain may be.

INDIVIDUAL FACTORS

In addition to those cultural factors that affect reactions to pain, the nurse evaluating pain also considers the variety of individual meanings that pain may hold for different patients. Pain is a concept with wide connotations and with multiple meanings which often are difficult to identify since they derive from peoples' individual experiences.

Because of its central importance, the nurse attempts to understand how pain is viewed by each patient and what meaning it may have for him. It is also important to identify the patient's level of *anxiety* in response to the meaning. As anxiety increases, so does suffering; anxiety increases a patient's estimation of the intensity of his pain and his emotional responses to it. Uncertainty or fear of the meaning or significance of pain also exaggerates responses.

Emotional states and the *observable behavior* related to them reflect, as a rule, the meaning or significance of the pain to the subject.[87] Thus, observations should include watching for signs of depression, anger, fear, excitement, weeping, and so forth. Because people in pain are suffering, they may be jumpy, cross, bitter, fearful, depressed, childlike, and so on. Acceptance of such behavior and an understanding of its origin will lessen the strain on the patient.[11]

In addition to observing the patient's behavior you can also obtain some idea of the meaning of pain to a patient by *listening* carefully to what he says. Perhaps he views his pain as deserved punishment; he may think that pain means he is getting worse. Many meanings are possible. Patients who have had severe pain may be fearful of going to sleep and of relaxing because they are afraid their pain will return or that the pain means that they may die because the condition is critical.[11] Once the nurse has evaluated the meaning of pain to a particular patient, she can plan her care and design it to meet his needs more accurately.

For example, if a patient perceives of himself as being trapped and helpless in his painful state, the nurse can alleviate some of these perceptions by planning with the patient what she and he can both do to reduce or prevent his pain. Together they can decide: how to best position the patient; how he can help to move himself; and how often to change his position. Also, they can determine activities that he can do by himself to prevent or to reduce his pain, e.g., slow deep breathing through open mouth when pain increases, or exercises in bed to maintain and strengthen muscle tone. By identifying together ways to reduce or to prevent pain, both patient and nurse will feel less helpless against pain.

Important pain-conditioning experiences take place during childhood. The nurse will see in patients the results of such experiences. "A child learns many of his responses from his family during his early, formative years. A mother, by belittling, or, conversely, by comforting and cajoling, may implant in her small son the basis of the reaction the nurse meets when the son, grown to manhood, recovers from anesthesia following a surgical operation."[69] Pain can cause some adults to *regress* to childlike behavior patterns since basic patterns of responding to pain were learned then. Patients' expectations of how they should be treated when they are in pain vary from individual to individual. A patient can be made more comfortable if the nurse responds to him in a manner that he feels is appropriate and helpful to him.

When the nurse cares for the patient who regresses, she may respond with sympathy to his needs but she must *never* treat such a patient with pity. LeShan[81] observes that pity is an extremely corrosive emotion. Pity for a person who is already unsure of his status and uncertain of the meaning of his life only confirms his uncertainty. Pity enforces regression because it carries with it a sense of condescension. It confirms the patient's feeling of childish helplessness and loss of dignity and status. Consequently, the nurse needs to strive to treat patients as equals and as adults who are worthy of her esteem and her respect. Only thus can a nurse halt regression and help patients to rebuild self-images equal to their former stature.

Finally, in evaluating the individual meaning of pain, recall that in some situations, pain actually *benefits* a patient psychologically. While this is not usually so, it may be the case in some psychogenic pain or secondary pain. Moreover, under some conditions, pain may be a welcome sign of improvement and, as such, may be associated with pleasurable emotion, e.g., pains such as those that occur upon the return of sensation or feeling to a previously analgetic paralyzed limb.[87]

PSYCHOGENIC FACTORS

Perhaps the most obscure meanings of pains are those attached to psychogenic pains. Psychogenic pains have highly individualized meanings that are generally imperceptible to observers. The dualistic "mind-body" assumption, which permeates much of our medical philosophy as well as our language, is a major cause of confusion in thinking about pain. "When pain is regarded as a psycho-physiological phenomenon it becomes easier to talk and write about, but more difficult to understand."[96]

We have said that pain is always accompanied by some psychologic or emotional meaning. And yet, because such meanings are difficult to identify and verbalize, patients will rarely discuss their painful feelings except in medical, somatic, or physical terms.

One physician writes, "No matter what the patient's problem, he often feels that he must speak to his doctor in medical terms. . . . The patient wants to be accepted and understood by his doctor; therefore, he talks of somatic pain rather than of painful emotional experiences. The doctor, on the other hand, because of his limited time and his own emotional needs, often would rather hear and discuss somatic pains than . . . complicated emotional pains."[110]

Psychogenic pain raises, in an acute form, the problem of communication. Many people find it difficult to believe that pain in the absence of discoverable organic disease is the same kind of sensation that is felt when organic disease is present.[24]

EVALUATING PAIN

THE NATURES OF PAIN

Numerous factors, joined together, contribute to the "natures" of various pains. Some general factors that influence the nature of pains are:[87]

> *The integrity of the patient's nervous system.* If the nervous system is impaired so that it cannot maintain normal functioning, then the patient's responses to pain-producing situations will be altered, e.g., a nerve lesion causing diminution in sensation reduces all reactive responses. If the nervous system is faulty, the patient cannot be expected to have typical reactions to pain or, at times, even to feel pain.

> *The patient's state of consciousness.* The meaning of pain depends upon the state of consciousness, since past and present experiences have symbolic meanings that influence perception of a sensation.

>*Previous experience, training, or conditioning.* Depending on the person and the previous pain experiences, the reactions may be either increased or decreased. For example, one individual suffering extremely severe pain may at first bear it stoically, but, with repetition of the experience, become so fearful of additional pain that anticipation of it alone causes vomiting, fainting, or other physical-emotional reactions. Another person, in a similar

situation, may develop fortitude or resignation in response to repetition of painful experiences and progressively show a decrease in psychologic reactions.

> *The patient's racial or ethnic background.* In general, Anglo-Saxon or Nordic individuals are relatively less sensitive or less reactive to pain, whereas Jews and Latins are more sensitive and more reactive.

>*The patient's age.* Sensitivity to pain varies with age since learned emotional attitudes alter greatly the perception of pain. Infants are less sensitive to pain than adults. Repeated studies demonstrate that in any one individual sensitivity is learned as an infant, it increases as the person grows to adulthood, and then gradually diminishes with advancing age. In fact, the intensity of pain in the elderly may be of such low quality that it may be *overlooked* or its significance discovered later than is desirable.

> *Fatigue, debility,* and *repeated painful procedures* can all reduce the ability to tolerate pain. Likewise, *worry, lack of sleep,* and *prolonged suffering* (e.g., nausea, vomiting, diarrhea) can reduce a patient's ability to tolerate pain and, thus, increase his magnification of it. The exhausted patient's powers of self-control and resistance may become so depleted that one more pain becomes unbearable. In such conditions, a hypodermic injection may precipitate extreme psychologic responses, and the patient may weep uncontrollably, cry out, or attempt to flee or withdraw. On the other hand, some patients become so weary that their attention is withdrawn from their injuries and they almost apathetically accept any painful experience directed at them.

Detailed information concerning the nature of any pain is essential for accurate diagnosis and treatment. For example, to make a diagnosis of organic pain, medical personnel must be able to document clear objective changes in the nature of the pain or to recognize the extent to which the pain conforms to a known syndrome. In evaluating the nature of a patient's pain the information discussed in the previous chapter concerning various types of pains must be considered.

In formulating a complete clinical picture of any pain it is helpful to evaluate the following factors about the nature of the pain.[87, 106, 113]

ASSESSMENT OF THE NATURE OF PAIN

1. *History* of the origin and occurrence of pain.
   a. When did it begin?
   b. Has it interfered with sleep, other vital functions, or the performance of duties?
   c. Is it a factor in litigation or could it be related to malingering?
2. *Localization* of the pain in the body.
   a. In what area or areas of the body is the pain felt? Do the areas of pain differ under differing circumstances?
   b. If several parts of the body are painful, do the pains occur simultaneously and are they dependent on one another?
   c. Is the pain unilateral or bilateral? If bilateral is it present in identical areas on the two sides of the body? (Pain such as thalamic pain can be localized to the whole of one side of the body.)
3. *Extension, radiation, and depth:* A description of the "size and shape" of the pain.
   a. Does it extend diffusely over a large area or can it be pinpointed? Is the area poorly or well defined?
   b. Does the pain originate in a definite area and then radiate to other areas? Both the point at which the pain starts and its radiation are important in diagnosis and treatment.
   c. Can the pain be described in terms of three dimensions, e.g., width, length, and depth? Generally, the patient is able only to determine whether the pain is localized to the skin or to deeper structures. Usually it is not possible for him to give a more exact description of depth localization.
4. *Duration:* How the pain occurs in time or its time-relations. Often separate paroxysms of pain are assembled in series. When a patient speaks of the "duration of an attack" he usually means the duration or length of such a series.
   a. How long does the pain last?
   b. Is it paroxysmal, intermittent, steady or continuous, rhythmic, throbbing or pulsating? These are some terms commonly used to describe the nature of pain.
5. *Onset or pattern:* Occurrence and character of the attack as a whole.
   a. What time did the pain begin? Is it seasonal? (For example, peptic ulcer pain tends to recur in the spring and fall, possibly due to changes in diet.)
   b. Do any events, activities, or persons precipitate the pain? Can times or patterns be identified when pain is anticipated to occur? Is a stimulus, precipitating factor, or trigger zone identifiable? Is pain associated with changes in position or weather?
   c. What factors alter the character of the pain, increase, reduce, or otherwise modify it?
   d. Does an attack begin gradually or acutely? Does the pain reach a "peak" and then rapidly diminish after reaching maximum? Does the pain have a "plateau" at which it remains at a constant intensity for a period of time? Between attacks is the patient without pain or other symptoms, or does he have mild pain, paresthesia, or other symptoms?
   e. Have changes occurred in the pain pattern or in the patient's life, e.g., weight loss, stress, working conditions, or way of life?
6. *Day pains.* Some pains usually occur during the day since they are made worse by mental or physical activities. Examples are: locomotor pains such as rheumatism, sciatica, and flat foot; eye pain; neurasthenic pain; gastrointestinal pain; and morning sinus pain caused by no chance for sinuses to drain at night.[87]
7. *Night pains.* Pains occurring at night, particularly if they awaken the patient, are typically characteristic of organic disease (as opposed to psychogenic pains). However, some psychogenic pains may occur at night if the patient has insomnia and if, freed from the distractions of the day, he becomes fearful and anxious. Colic and ulcer pains typically occur at night, since at night our bodies are largely governed by autonomic nerve control, and, therefore, it is the time of vagus and parasympathetic activity. Also, because relaxation of protective muscle contraction occurs at night, involuntary movements occur. Thus, the pains of joint disease (e.g., tuberculosis of the bone and rheumatic disorders) are mainly nocturnal.[87] The patient whom the nurse finds sleeping well or resting quietly is not likely to be having pain.[11]
8. *Character or quality* of the pain: Is it dull, sharp, shooting? Often the character of pain is dependent on both its localization and its duration. It is not unusual

for the character of a pain to alter during its course. The character of pain is often used in the classification of painful conditions, and particular types of pain are associated with special types of attack, e.g., paroxysms of pain occur in neuralgia, whereas dull, boring pains are associated with a constant course without attacks.[113]

MacBryde[87] lists the following conditions and bodily areas and the quality of the pain associated with each:

Aneurysmal erosion: boring, pounding
Bones: deep, aching, boring
Muscles: sore, aching
Colic: twisting, griping, clamping
Angina: compression, constriction, comes on with exertion, great weight, agonizing, impending death
Pleuritis: stabbing, knifelike, with each breath
Peptic ulcer: burning, sharp, associated with hunger
Tabes: lightning-like, shooting, stabbing
Neuritis: burning, stinging
Neuralgia: sharp, cutting, paroxysmal, intermittent
Causalgia: burning, peculiar stinging
Burns, blisters, superficial skin lesions: burning, smarting, stinging, hot

9. *Intensity* of the pain must be determined to delineate proper therapy; e.g., morphine would not be given for a *mild* headache. Because of variable, individual psychologic factors it is often difficult to determine the intensity of pain. Some idea of the intensity can be obtained by noting the patient's physical appearance and whether the pain interferes with his activities.
   a. Does the patient describe his pain as mild, moderate, intense, severe, or excruciating? Such terms indicate intensity.
   b. What is his physical appearance, e.g., grimacing, curled up in bed?
   c. Does the pain interfere with sleep, employment, eating, conversation, and so forth? Does the patient have to go to bed or stay in bed because of his pain?
10. *Cessation* of a pain is important to note.
   a. When did it stop?
   b. Did it stop suddenly or gradually?
   c. Was anything done to stop it or did it stop spontaneously?
11. *Associated symptoms* should be evaluated. For example: skin changes (e.g., glossy skin); sensory changes (e.g., numbness); vomiting; photophobia; fever; abnormal glandular secretions (e.g., excessive sweating); and fever.
12. *Presumptive etiologic factors.*[113] Most patients have a definite opinion about what is causing their pain, and their views about the etiology should always be noted. Hereditary conditions should also be considered.

The cause of a pain should always be sought since pain is a symptom, not a disease itself.

When a patient's pain stops suddenly, changes in character, or appears in a new or unexpected area, it should be noted and, if the change seems to be highly significant, reported to the physician. Also, a point to remember in the evaluation of a patient following injury (a car accident, for example) is that *pain may initially be absent following sudden trauma.* Thus, the patient will need ongoing reevaluation since pain may begin to appear some time after the accident, heralding the discovery of previously undetected injuries.

The nurse evaluating pain will want to recall that patients may have pain even though no adequate organic cause can be found. She should also keep in mind that patients with a primarily psychiatric disorder may have pain arising from some associated physical disease. For example, a patient with a psychiatric disorder may also have a peptic ulcer that causes him pain.

RECOGNIZING PSYCHOGENIC PAIN

Although many writers believe it is futile to attempt to tell the difference between physical and psychogenic pains,[96] doctors often need to make such a differential diagnosis. This is an important decision. For example, it may mean the difference between whether or not a patient should have surgical therapy. The doctor has a legitimate concern not to misdiagnose physical illness, and he also has a concern to recognize psychologic illness and to provide suitable treatment for it.[96] A nurse's careful observations may be helpful in evaluating whether a pain is believed to be psychogenic.

The following are some factors of importance in identifying psychogenic pain:

> Pain symptoms do not fit into any known anatomic pattern.[3]

> Pains recur at precise intervals or under conditions of emotional disturbance.[3]

> Pain symptoms are not relieved by ordinary analgesic measures.[3]

> Pain symptoms cannot be explained by the presence of demonstrable organic disease or structural abnormalities.[99]

> Evidence exists of psychiatric illness that is sufficient to account for the development of the pain symptoms.[96]

> Pain tends to be located centrally in the head and trunk, or where lateral, tends to occur on the left.[96]

> Pain occurs continuously from day to day, without disturbing sleep.[96]

> Pain arises at irregular times for no apparent reason and lasts for a few hours.[96]

When some of these factors begin to appear together, there is a strong presumption that the psychologic aspects of the pain problem are important. Grounds for a psychogenic diagnosis must always be found by means of psychiatric investigation. Painful conditions should never be considered as psychogenic merely because no explanation for the symptoms has been found.[113]

PHYSIOLOGIC BASES OF PAIN

Although innumerable conditions can give rise to pain, the actual factors leading to the excitation of pain fibers can be reduced to simple proportions. Some pathophysiologic processes that stimulate pain are:[3, 87]

> Direct irritation of nerve endings, e.g., by mechanical factors operating in exposed tissues.

- Chemical substances, e.g., those occurring in acute inflammations (globulin, bradykinin, histamine, serotonin).
- Certain pathologic processes, e.g., some forms of ulceration and new growth.
- Irritation of peripheral nerves or of nerve roots, e.g., from a foreign body, displaced bone, or from local pressure caused by a neoplasm or inflammatory products in a confined space.
- Muscle spasm, e.g., from myocardial ischemia, or cramps from Buerger's disease.
- Overstretching, e.g., from acutely distended viscus or the passage of a calculus through a narrow duct.

Although such classifications are not all inclusive (e.g., central pains do not fit into the above outline) and are oversimplifications, they are nevertheless useful guides for evaluating the more common causes of pain and thus make it easier to clearly identify the measures necessary to bring relief. Therefore, in evaluating a patient's pain the nurse should try to identify the cause of the pain anatomically and physiologically so that she can give the patient appropriate help.

COVERT AND OVERT SIGNS AND SYMPTOMS OF PAIN

It is possible to divide the *signs* and *symptoms* of pain into two groups:[37] (1) those that are essentially of sympathetic origin and (2) those primarily of parasympathetic origin. This division is presented in Table 43–1 along with other signs of pain.

Wolff and Wolf[141] observe that, characteristically, pain sets off protective reactions within the body which may include occlusion of nasal passages with or without lacrimation, cardiospasm, cardiac arrhythmias, disturbances of gastric and colonic function, and elevation of arterial pressure. As we indicated earlier, if such body changes are sustained, they may themselves lead to a significant impairment of function or perhaps to actual tissue damage. Shock and even death may be caused by severe pain.

A patient malingering or pretending to have pain cannot imitate the facial expression of true pain, e.g., the pallor, pinched features, knotted brow, clammy skin, and dilated pupils.[92]

Since some patients hesitate to say that they have pain, you will need to observe carefully for the physiologic signs of discomfort; on the other hand, it is equally important to observe the patient's reactions, since physiologic signs may not be helpful. For example, in severe abdominal pain there is often an increased pulse rate and a decreased blood pressure; however, during a bout of tic douloureux there may be no circulatory change, even though the intensity of the pain is probably unparalleled.[62]

THE PATIENT'S COMPLAINTS ABOUT PAIN

It is not always accurate to conclude that a patient who does not complain of pain is comfortable. He may have severe pain but may not say that he does. Nevertheless, complete descriptions of pain are an aid to accurate diagnosis and the effective treatment of pain syndromes. Because pain is subjective, the nurse's evaluation should include listening to what a patient says about how he feels as well as watching for observable signs and symptoms of pain.

TABLE 43–1. OBSERVABLE SIGNS AND SYMPTOMS OF PAIN

Sympathetic in Origin (Vital functions are stimulated)	**Parasympathetic in Origin (Vital functions are depressed)**
A basically sympathetic response occurs with pain of low to moderate intensity or superficial pain.	A basically parasympathetic response occurs with pain of severe intensity or deep pain.
Observable signs and symptoms are: pallor elevated blood pressure dilated pupils skeletal muscular tension increased respiratory rate increased heart rate	Observable signs and symptoms are: pallor decreased blood pressure decreased heart rate nausea and vomiting weakness and fainting prostration possible loss of consciousness
The body prepares to act by either overcoming or fleeing from an external threat as epinephrine output is increased.	The body tries to minimize the effects of an internal threat.
Bodily defenses are mobilized.	Bodily defenses may collapse.

Other Signs of Pain

Patient assumes a posture or position that will minimize his pain, i.e., draws up knees or lies rigidly.
Patient may moan or make other sounds indicating his discomfort and may blink rapidly.
Patient may cry and appear frightened or restless; or, may lie quietly, afraid to move, withdrawing from being touched.
Patient may grimace and clench jaw or fists; his face may have a drawn expression and muscles may twitch.
Patient may perspire profusely (have diaphoresis).
Patient may hold or protect the painful area with his hands; the physical attitude may thus indicate pain and its location, e.g., holding head, pressing on abdomen.

Communication about pain is often a problem. When we deal with patients, we encounter the double difficulty of first defining an experience and then of communicating it: "The patient must find a word to describe the pain, and we must then understand it. Communication implies translating the patient's experience into one of our own."[24] Often it is hard to be sure of what is happening; the patient may be trying to explain an experience we may not have had, e.g., referred pain, spontaneous pain, or phantom pain. Because of these factors it is helpful to:

> Have the patient who states he has pain point to the area of pain and describe it. Avoid leading questions that could result in the patient's giving misleading information[11] and avoid opening up new areas for worry or arousing false hopes.[37]

> In charting, use the patient's own words about his pain, e.g., "Patient states: 'I feel like I have a tight band around my head,' or, 'It feels pricking.'" Patients often have difficulty finding words to describe what a pain is like. Nevertheless, the words that they use should be charted.

> Help the patient to talk objectively about his pain, to describe it as accurately as possible, and to distinguish between pain and other unpleasant bodily feelings, e.g., pressure, soreness, itching.

> Clarify what a patient means when he says he is "uncomfortable"; do not assume that he means he is "in pain." Perhaps he feels nauseated, dizzy, and so forth.

Mettler[98] believes that it is not justifiable to neglect a patient's *own* estimation of his pain, since few people complain of pain who are not, in fact, miserable. Because of its subjective nature, the nurse must be guided by what a patient tells her; however, a patient's description of pain (for example, its severity) must not be accepted without evaluating many other factors, since he may consciously or unconsciously minimize or exaggerate his symptoms. Remember:

A patient's description of his pain is influenced by his perception of the pain and what the pain means to him.

CHAPTER 44

The Treatment of Pain

> It is rather astonishing to contemplate how successful we have become in relieving pain, without knowing what pain actually is or what we are really doing when we use drugs to relieve it. Pain relief remains an empirical art, where experience counts greatly.[78]

How to avoid or treat pain has been a concern of man through the ages. Even though impressive gains have been made during the past two decades in knowledge of pain mechanisms, and consequently in pain control, clinical practice is still frequently bedeviled with situations in which pain relief is far from ideal.[139]

As noted earlier, pain prompts patients to seek medical help more often than any other symptom. Usually the causes of such pain are medical or surgical disorders that can be relieved with medications or by a surgical procedure. Thus, most pains are "acute" in nature and are amenable to therapy, or they may simply be self-limiting and vanish with the passage of time. As we have previously indicated, however, some pains are chronic and intractable.

OVERVIEW OF PAIN THERAPY

> Despite the potential aid of modern medicine, it is surprising how patient morbidity is seemingly accepted. Too often the physician is unaware of the magnitude of the pain problem while the nurse and relatives, too well aware of the problem, are unaware of the potential alleviation that can be made available from sources other than drugs.[63]

The comprehensive management of patients having pain requires a multiphasic approach. This is particularly true of those pains that become severe and intractable. Several therapeutic measures may be necessary, each precisely selected for certain desired effects. All forms of pain therapy should be carried out with consideration for both the physical and mental aspects of the pain experience and in an attempt to avoid overtreatment.

> *"The most important principle in the management of pain is avoidance of overtreatment."*[46]

Since pain often functions as an indicator of disease, the presence of pain usually calls for an *investigation* of its *underlying cause* rather than merely the relief of the patient's suffering. For example, the patient suffering pain from an inflamed appendix needs an appendectomy rather than aspirin. Logically, whenever possible, the treatment of pain should center around the elimination of the underlying cause of the pain rather than palliative measures.

In approaching treatment the physician differentiates between pains that are primarily structural, primarily psychologic, and primarily physiologic in origin. Once a diagnosis is established and the mechanism of pain determined, treatment must be planned carefully based upon consideration of:[18] (1) the pain's cause, site, type, mechanism, intensity, and probable duration; (2) nature of disease causing the pain; (3) the patient's age, mental and physical status, life expectancy, and his obligations to his family and community; (4) methods of treatment that are practical and are locally available; and (5) the complications that could develop consequent to each method of treatment.

> *A goal of pain therapy is to dampen responses to pain or perception of pain without the loss of consciousness or other sensations.*[75]

This means that: *surgically* the goal of therapy in pain-relieving procedures is to free patients of their pains without causing unnecessary loss of function or of other sensations (e.g., without producing permanent numbness of an area as a result of interruption of cutaneous sensation); *medically* the relief of pain by chemotherapeutic means strives to relieve pain without creating other new problems for the patient (e.g., addiction, constipation, dizziness).

A wide variety of clinical measures can be employed in pain therapy. Some of these are:

> *Specific medical and surgical therapy* directed at the pain-producing problem, e.g., antibiotics can relieve the pain of infection by reducing the infection; inflamed or malfunctioning organs can be removed surgically.
> *General measures,* e.g., positioning, distraction.
> *Physical therapies,* e.g., rest, heat, cold, massage.
> *Radiology,* to relieve pain caused by pressure from neoplasms by shrinking the tumor in size.
> *Reduction of pain-producing anxiety,* e.g., hypnosis, psychotherapy, sedatives, ataractic drugs, placebos, prefrontal lobotomy.
> *Production of analgesia or anesthesia,* e.g., analgesic medications, nerve blocks, general anesthesia, neurosurgery.

"Pain clinics"[17, 18] exist in various parts of the country for the diagnosis and management of pain syndromes. Such clinics usually consist of: a neu-

rologist, neurosurgeon, internist, general surgeon, orthopedist, psychiatrist, radiologist, anesthesiologist, social worker, and nursing staff. These clinics can make a valuable contribution to the patient in pain because of their comprehensive approach to pain therapy.

In those painful conditions caused by medical disorders that are *self-limiting* and in those pain problems that can be solved by the specific surgical extirpation of an organ (e.g., appendectomy) or specific medications, pain problems can be solved relatively simply, and the management is clear-cut. However, in situations of *intractable* protracted pain the problem is difficult to comprehend and solve. Examples of such chronic pain syndromes are: (1) visceral pain; (2) neuralgia; (3) myofascial syndromes; (4) reflex sympathetic dystrophies; and (5) cancer. In those situations in which the cause of pain is not known or, if known, cannot be eliminated, then the pain itself must be treated, and the services of a pain clinic may be helpful.

SPECIFIC MEDICAL AND SURGICAL THERAPIES

Much of the therapy of pain is conducted by administering medications that will act on the particular end-organ that is the source of pain, e.g., the heart, the gallbladder. For example, medications such as amyl nitrite and nitroglycerine relieve the pain of angina pectoris by direct action on the heart—the "painful end-organ." Such medications act directly on the pain-producing organ itself rather than on the higher centers responsible for pain perception. Such medications are *not* analgesics; analgesics act peripherally and/or centrally to modify pain perception or reaction. For example, while atropine may relieve pains caused by smooth muscle spasm by relieving the muscle spasm, and while ergotamine constricts overdistended arteries in the brain, thereby relieving the pain of migraine headaches, neither of these medications can accurately be called an analgesic.[141]

Specific medications having direct effects upon specific pain-producing end-organs are discussed in appropriate sections of the text (e.g., for a discussion of medications affecting the heart see the unit on cardiovascular function, Unit X). Likewise, *specific surgical procedures* that eliminate pain by removing or correcting the specific pain-producing organ are discussed in appropriate sections of the text; e.g., appendectomy is discussed in the unit on gastrointestinal function (Unit XV) and fractures are discussed in the muscular-skeletal unit (Unit XVII).

GENERAL MEASURES

In pain therapy, general procedures are always employed in an attempt to interrupt the pain-producing mechanism before resorting to more radical procedures that could create iatrogenic problems, e.g., analgesic medications, surgical procedures, nerve blocks. For the nurse this means she should remember to:

> *Try general nursing care measures to relieve pain* before *resorting to analgesics.*

For example, you may find that a patient is in pain because of his position in bed; perhaps he has a cast on his leg and the leg has rolled off a pillow and is uncomfortably twisted. By correctly positioning the patient's leg, his pain may be relieved so that he requires no analgesic. Always evaluate a patient in pain to determine general measures of care that may help him, and employ these measures first. There are many general nursing measures that can be employed in caring for a patient having pain. These are discussed further in Chapter 45.

PHYSICAL THERAPIES

Various types of physical therapy may be employed in the treatment of pain, e.g., rest, passive and active exercise, massage, heat and cold. Balme[3] observes that such therapies may be of great value in the early stages of painful conditions; all are greatly appreciated by patients. In the past there was a tendency to overemphasize the more *passive* forms of *physiotherapy;* today the more active forms of physiotherapy are also recognized. For example, while some alleviation of the pain of a sprained ankle may be obtained by rest, *active exercise* rather than passive physiotherapy is the best means of removing inflammatory exudate, which is pain-producing.

Rest is not without its value, however. Indeed, rest, proper positioning, and posture "take pride of place"[3] in the physical treatment of many painful disorders. This is especially true in the period of time immediately following trauma, as well as during any period of acute inflammation. Complete, prolonged immobilization is dangerous, however, since among other problems, muscle atrophy can occur along with the formation of painful adhesions. (See Unit V.) When rest is therapeutically indicated, those muscles that are guarding inflamed or injured tissues should be supported in a fashion that insures complete relaxation. Only when complete relaxation is accomplished will physiologic rest be possible for the affected part.

The use of *heat and cold* will be discussed further in Chapter 45. We shall merely mention here that moist heat is typically prescribed for the relief of pains due to superficial swelling or inflammation; dry heat is generally used to relieve the discomfort of congestion in the deeper tissues. Both heat and cold may be applied either wet (e.g., soaks) or dry (e.g., diathermy, electric pad, heat lamp, ice bag or hot water bag).

Massage is another form of physical therapy. It is most useful in the early stage of inflammatory swellings and in treating the pain of various forms of myalgia as well as fibrositis. Massage used in combination with some form of heat is useful in advance of more active forms of remedial exercise.

Numerous *local applications,* such as nonadherent dressings, analgesic ointments, and analgesic liniments may be beneficial in treating the more superficial forms of pain. Such pains may be due to neuritis, ulceration, and inflammatory conditions.

RADIOLOGY[54]

Because of multiple possible complications, it is not generally advisable for radiation therapy to be used in the treatment of *benign* diseases if the condition can be managed by less drastic measures. Although there are a few indications for radiation treatment of benign conditions for the symptomatic relief of pain, these indications are becoming fewer in number each year. Radiation therapy is extensively employed, however, in treating pains due to *malignant* conditions. (See Unit VII.)

REDUCTION OF PAIN-PRODUCING ANXIETY

Since heightened *anxiety* is known to increase pain, a variety of therapeutic measures may be employed to relieve anxiety and thereby *dissociate* the pain from responses to it; that is, the pain is still perceived but suffering is abolished or reduced. For example, the patient may say that he is aware that pain is present, but he just does not care that he has it. Examples of therapies that can cause such an altered reaction are: leukotomy (prefrontal lobotomy), electroshock therapy, psychotherapy, and ataractic drugs. Religious or hysterical mental states may, likewise, cause such dissociation.[87]

Pain that is primarily *psychogenic* in nature generally is more difficult to treat than that which results from demonstrable physical pathology. Since psychogenic pain may result from an inability to cope with reality, and an unconscious escape from such an intolerable reality, the sufferer needs treatment by means of *psychotherapy* and *reeducation.* "Alleviation of the symptom without producing a fundamental change in the patient's idea of himself and his reality will accomplish very little. If the underlying mechanism is not discovered and if the patient does not develop insight into his problems, the symptomatic relief will be short-lived."[31] Actually psychotherapy can be a valuable adjunct to any type of pain therapy (for both organic and psychogenic pain), since even intense pain caused by physical pathology may be partially reduced by giving adequate, positive psychologic support to the patient.[31]

Hypnosis

In the eighteenth century Mesmer introduced hypnosis as a treatment in formal medical practice. Since then the use of hypnosis in medicine has been disputed by some physicians and praised by others. One of Mesmer's followers accidentally discovered the level of trance that became classically recognized as hypnosis, i.e., the somnambulistic state of deep trance or hypnotic sleep associated with amnesia. This state was utilized for surgical anesthesia; however, once safe chemical anesthetics became available hypnosis was virtually abandoned in operative procedures. Only in the past two decades has there been a reawakening of interest in the use of hypnosis in the operating suite as an adjunct to chemical anesthetics.

Hypnosis has multiple uses, one of the most rewarding of which is the reduction of pain. Hypnosis is a type of pain therapy that is based on the power of suggestion and the process of focusing attention. An individual's reactions to pain can be decidedly altered by hypnosis. Hypnosis may be used as an adjunct to other pain-relieving therapies and is useful in a number of types of pain problems, e.g., dentistry, surgery, childbirth, and malignant diseases. Although hypnosis should be utilized only by properly trained persons, any nurse can use the power of suggestion to relieve pain, e.g., "Here is some medicine that will help to stop your pain." The hypnotic trance has been divided into three stages: light, medium, and deep.[77] Most investigators believe that 20 per cent of the general population can attain the stage of deep trance.

Lauer[77] observes that the depth of trance seems not to be related to the degree of success achieved in pain therapy. A variety of procedures may be employed to relieve pain following induction of the trance state, e.g., suggestion to alter the character of pain or the patient's attitude toward it; body disorientations and dissociations; anesthesia and analgesia for superficial and deep sensation.

Hypnosis cannot change organic lesions that are producing pain, but it can be used to reduce discomfort in a wide range of medical and surgical conditions. For example, hypnosis either by itself or in conjunction with other therapeutic measures has proved useful in decreasing discomfort associated with: peptic ulcer, painful conversion reactions, cervical disk disease, causalgia, postherpetic neuralgia, and trigeminal neuralgia. Moreover, along with producing analgesia, hypnosis has been helpful in the treatment of burned patients by improving their fluid balance, nutritional status, cooperation with treatment, and the will to live.

Hypnosis is not without its hazards. The procedure itself is relatively simple and innocuous compared to the administration of many anesthetic and analgesic drugs. However, the operator must be skilled and informed and the patient carefully selected to assure that he will not suffer untoward effects from hypnosis.

Attempts to remove symptoms by means of hypnosis must be tempered with the realization that for some patients symptoms may satisfy certain needs and may perform an adaptive or defensive service. Also, posthypnotic suggestion must be used cautiously, even though it is a valuable reinforcing mechanism in the prolonged relief of pain.

In situations of chronic pain, posthypnotic suggestion may be used in combination with autohypnosis (self-hypnosis) to provide prolonged relief. It is possible for many hypnotic subjects to be successfully trained in deliberate spontaneous trance induction or autohypnosis. The subject must be cautioned to use this procedure appropriately.

Placebos

Placebos are "nonspecific medications," which is to say they are inactive substances intended to have no pharmacologic effects. Placebos may, at times, be ordered for pain relief. Their use demonstrates that the "psychologic action" of a "medication" is often of prime importance in producing analgesia. Beecher and many other workers have shown that over 30 per cent of patients display analgesic response to placebo therapy.[75]

Whereas some persons react to placebos, others do not. Some patients are almost consistent "placebo reactors" or "nonreactors"; others may respond at some times to placebo medications, and at other times they will not.

Examples of substances used as placebos are: sodium bicarbonate, vitamins, distilled water, lactose capsules, or physiologic saline solution. With placebos, it is the power of *suggestion* that acts in relieving pain, since the patient *believes* that he is receiving a pain-relieving medication that will help him. The expectations of patient, nurse, and physician thus become of importance in placebo therapy. Remember that suggestion is a powerful tool. Placebo therapy needs careful management and should be carried out only on order of a physician.

Placebos may be potent in producing both side effects and toxicity in many patients; they have been shown to actually cause changes in laboratory data, such as the sedimentation rate, carbon dioxide-combining power, and the white blood cell count.[46] Once again it is demonstrated that the psyche and soma cannot be separated.

The patient is generally not told that he is receiving a placebo, but rather that he is being given a medication "to ease the pain" or whatever the desired action is. Some persons feel that the doctor who prescribes placebo medication is following the course of least resistance. On the other hand, there are doctors who think that the use of a placebo is justified in the *evaluation* of pain. However, the abuse of placebo administration has caused some patients to be unduly suspicious of all medications.[31]

PRODUCTION OF ANALGESIA OR ANESTHESIA

Analgesia and Anesthesia[83, 111]

An *analgesic* is defined as a substance that "reduces or abolishes suffering from pain without producing unconsciousness."[111] Thus, in *analgesia* the sensation of pain and the associated psychic reactions are abolished or reduced without impairment of consciousness; the perception of pain is altered. By changing a patient's attitude and mood toward his pain, analgesics induce apathy to the pain and promote feelings of well-being and freedom from anxiety.[55] *Anesthesia* refers generally to a loss of feeling or a loss of sensation, particularly a loss of the sensation of pain. There are many different types of anesthetics; e.g., spinal anesthesia, general anesthesia, and local anesthesia.

Analgesia can be produced at any of the points in the pathway of pain. A procedure frequently used in minor surgery is the *local infiltration* of an *anesthetic agent* to produce loss of sensation; or, to produce a *local nerve block,* the sensory nerve trunk may be infiltrated. At certain critical points almost any spinal or cranial nerve can be blocked with local anesthetic agents or neurolytic agents. Temporary or reversible nerve blocks are produced by local anesthetics; *neurolytic agents,* like phenol and alcohol, produce prolonged effects since they are destructive of the nerve ("neuro" refers to "nerve"; "lysis" means "destruction").

Local anesthesia is also called "regional anesthesia." In this state a particular region of the body is rendered insensible to pain, although the patient's general state of consciousness or awareness is not otherwise affected. Local anesthetic agents, whether applied topically, by the intravenous route, or by regional nerve trunk blocks, act by blocking the nerve impulse between the peripheral structures and higher centers. Sensory nerve conductivity is interrupted from the area of the body to be anesthetized. Local anesthetics do not cause a loss of consciousness, but there is a specific loss of pain sensation.

The *injection of anesthetic agents into the spinal fluid* anesthetizes both dorsal and ventral nerve trunks, producing loss of both motor and sensory functions. Patients under *spinal anesthesia* may not complain of pain, and yet they retain tactile discrimination and motor function. Such a patient may say that he can "feel the doctor working" on him, but he does not complain of pain. He may be able to move his toes and retains some of his reflex mechanisms. This is because local anesthetics block the smaller nerve fibers before the larger ones.[64]

A *general anesthetic agent,* acting directly upon central function, will produce various degrees of depression of total response or the total depression of all sensation. General anesthetics render the patient unconscious and thereby relieve him of pain over his entire body. Obviously general anesthesia is practical only for the relief of pain that would be caused by surgical procedures or orthopedic procedures. Anesthetics are discussed in Unit VI.

The pain threshold can be raised or obliterated by local anesthetization; analgesics can also raise the pain threshold. Analgesics, like morphine and alcohol, tend to have a much greater effect upon the reaction to pain than they do upon the perception of pain. Thus, while the pain is actually felt at almost the same intensity, the patient loses reactions such as anxiety, which usually accompany his perception of pain.[87]

Generally it is assumed that the analgesics, like the general anesthetics, produce their effects by acting on the *central* nervous system. However, some analgesics block the nerve-endings or receptors for pain and, thus, act peripherally.[83] This point will be discussed again.

Nerve Blocks

Essentially, nerve blocks are injections of various substances (for example, local anesthetics) close to nerves, thereby "blocking" off the conductivity of those nerves. Nerve blocking techniques may be employed to produce a complete, *reversible* interruption of nervous pathways for four different purposes:[17] (1) to eliminate a local focus of noxious stimulation or nervous irritation; (2) to interrupt the perception of pain, either at the source of the pain or anywhere along the peripheral afferent neurons; (3) to interrupt reflex mechanisms that are maintaining an abnormal activity of blood vessels, glands, skeletal or smooth muscle; and (4) to eliminate such reflex responses by direct infiltration of the skeletal muscle and other involved structures. Some *irreversible* nerve blocking procędures are also possible, as we have stated.

Most nerve blocks are used for the purpose of providing *symptomatic relief of severe pain;* however, they may also be used for other purposes, e.g., diagnosis, prognosis, prophylaxis.[17] Blocks given for pain relief are called "analgesic blocks." The analgesia, which is generally produced by means of the injection of a local anesthetic agent, provides relief of pain and may also serve to make use of additional kinds of treatments which would otherwise be excessively painful. For example, manipulation of a painful joint would be possible following a nerve block. Sometimes, due to interruption of those reflexes that operate to cause sustained pain, analgesic blocks can produce a beneficial effect which is prolonged beyond the effective duration of the agent injected.

Analgesic blocks are useful in a variety of acute and chronic disorders and often serve to reduce the amounts of narcotic agents that might otherwise be needed to control pain. Injection of procaine in the muscle or skin of an area of referred pain may greatly modify pain from visceral or other deep noxious stimulation. However, the pain cannot be eliminated unless the primary afferent impulses are terminated or blocked at their source by surgical or chemical means.[87, 141]

It should be emphasized that, while nerve blocks may be extremely helpful, not all patients benefit from such procedures. Also, the chemical interruption of nervous pathways by nerve block techniques constitutes only one aspect of the management of any pain syndrome.

Because all drugs used for local anesthesia are vasodilators, it is possible to potentiate the action of local anesthetic agents through the *supplementary use of epinephrine,*[17, 100] which is a vasopressor or a vasoconstrictor. The addition of a vasoconstrictor to the local anesthetic makes it possible to decrease the blood flow and thus: (1) prolong the effect of anesthesia by causing a local vasoconstriction that will allow the anesthetic agent to stay in contact with the tissues for a longer time; and (2) retard the absorption of the anesthetic into the general circulation.

In addition to prolonging the effects of the anesthesia, the supplementary use of a vasopressor with the local analgesic prevents the anesthetic from reaching a toxic blood level. The toxicity of local analgesic drugs depends upon their concentration in the blood; this, in turn, depends upon the speed of absorption. By causing vasoconstriction, vasopressor drugs delay absorption of the local analgesic solution and thus prevent a suddenly high blood concentration. This gives the body more time to metabolize and detoxify the medication. Also, bleeding is reduced by the vasopressor.

Two local anesthetics used for nerve blocks with which the nurse should be particularly familiar are procaine and lidocaine.[46]

Procaine (Novocain). This, the most commonly used local anesthetic, produces an analgesia in three to 10 minutes which lasts usually less than one hour. Never more than 15 mg. per kg. of body weight in adults, or 5 mg. per kg. of body weight in children should be given. Procaine cannot produce effective surface analgesia of mucous membranes by topical application.

Lidocaine (Xylocaine). Lidocaine offers the following advantages over procaine: (1) prompter action; (2) equal effectiveness with one-half the concentration of procaine; (3) twice the duration of effect as procaine for the same concentrations; and (4) effective surface analgesia of mucous membranes by topical application.

Other local anesthetic agents sometimes used for nerve block include Pontocaine, Metycaine, Nupercaine, and Intracaine.

Examples of some *acute* painful situations which may be relieved with nerve blocks are:

> Herpes zoster.
> Some neuralgias.
> Thrombophlebitis.
> Musculoskeletal problems, e.g., acute, severe post-traumatic pain following ligamentous tears, herniated intervertebral disk, fractured vertebrae and fractured ribs.
> Visceral conditions e.g., coronary occlusion, mesen-

teric thrombosis, perforated peptic ulcer, pancreatitis, and severe renal or biliary colic.

It has been observed that even heavy doses of narcotics administered intravenously may be ineffective in combating such acute pains and may, in fact, increase smooth muscle spasm and thus further intensify the pain. Therapeutic nerve blocks, which can be maintained for days if necessary, provide relief from such intense pain as that resulting from sudden, acute circulatory insufficiency created by embolus, vasospasm, thrombus, or trauma.

Sensory nerve fibers are more readily affected by local anesthetics than are motor fibers. For example, if a mixed (motor and sensory) nerve were infiltrated, a complete anesthesia could be produced in the absence of any detectable motor weakness. In addition to pain fibers, local anesthetics will also affect the small thinly myelinated or unmyelinated fibers carrying sympathetic impulses.

Some of the major types of nerve blocks are: (1) local blocks (infiltration and topical application); (2) paravertebral and prevertebral sympathetic (autonomic) blocks; (3) somatic nerve blocks of spinal nerves; (4) extradural blocks (caudal and segmental spinal epidural block); (5) subarachnoid blocks; and (6) blocks of cranial nerves.

Various nerve blocking procedures may be useful in managing *chronic* pain. Indeed, nerve blocks can be more desirable than the prolonged administration of addictive analgesics. Such blocks may provide pain relief to patients who would have developed tolerance to the analgesic action of narcotics—such that even high doses of narcotics would not alleviate the pain. Bonica observes:

> The administration of narcotics to patients with chronic pain is a frustrating, short-lived type of kindness; such a sense of mistaken humanitarianism is inevitably productive of tolerance and other phases of addiction. It is really a great disservice to the patient because with continued use of the addictive analgesics tolerance to the analgesic action develops until eventually an impasse is reached in which the patient's daily narcotic requirements are high while the alleviation of pain is inadequate.[17]

Lest we give the impression that nerve blocks provide a simple solution to the complex problems of disease and pain, let us consider some of the problems, contraindications, and complications of these procedures.

Nerve blocks may often be *unsuccessful* due to *problems* such as: (1) difficulties in identifying the pain pathways or in locating the correct nerve for injection, and (2) the complexity of pain psychophysiopathology involving, as it does, the patient's subjective reactions, central nervous system, and peripheral structures. Some additional problems are caused by the fact that only small volumes of solution can be injected at one time.

Nerve blocks are *contraindicated* in patients who (1) are psychoneurotic or psychotic; (2) have an infection at the site of injection; and (3) are in shock or are debilitated, especially if extensive vasomotor paralysis will be produced or if large amounts of local anesthetic solution are required.

> *Because of potential complications, nerve blocks should be performed with resuscitative equipment and necessary drugs on hand to combat untoward reactions.*

Some medications that may be required are: vasopressors (e.g., ephedrine, phenylephrine, or methoxamine); fast-acting barbiturates (e.g., thiopental or thyamylal), and rapid-acting muscle relaxants (e.g., succinylcholine).

Some *complications* of nerve blocks are:[17] hypotension; hypertension; mild, moderate, or severe toxic reactions to local anesthetic drugs; idiosyncratic reactions; overdosage of epinephrine or other vasoconstrictors; allergic reactions; pneumothorax; psychogenic reactions; inadvertent subarachnoid (spinal) block; hematoma; postinjection neuropathy; respiratory dysfunction and paralysis; and cardiac arrest.

Topical Applications for Pain Relief. Topical applications of dilute solutions of local anesthetics may be applied locally in the form of pastes, sprays, or other preparations. This may be effective in reducing the severe pain of burns, abrasions, and necrosis of the mucous membranes and skin. However, if these conditions are extensive (e.g., extensive burns or pruritus), the intravenous administration of local anesthetics such as procaine or tetracaine may be preferable to the form of topical application.

Cocaine, a highly toxic agent, is sometimes used for topical anesthesia, but *never* for infiltration anesthesia. No more than 100 to 150 mg. of cocaine, in a 4 per cent concentration, should be applied at one time. Cocaine may also be used in an atomizer for topical spray in a 10 per cent solution.

Toxic reactions to overdosages of topical medications can easily occur, and therefore you should use dilute solutions of the drugs and take care not to exceed the recommended total dosage. The following fact should be kept in mind concerning topical application:

Remember:

> *Following the application of local anesthetic drugs to burned or abraded skin or mucous membranes, the absorption of the medication is almost as rapid as following intravenous administration!*

Ethyl chloride may be used as a spray in treating some myofascial pain problems and other disorders that are caused and maintained by trigger areas located in superficial tissue. Several points to bear in mind for the successful use of this spray are: (1) have the patient comfortable, prior to beginning, with the body area that is to be sprayed well supported so muscles are relaxed; (2) apply the spray from 12 to 24 inches above the skin at an angle to the skin; (3) maintain slow, even sweeping motions moving in one direction rather than back and forth; (4) begin the sweep of direction at trigger areas and move toward the reference zone; (5) shield the patient's face; (6) repeat in a few seconds and then wait a few seconds until the entire reference zone is sprayed; and (7) if aching develops, lengthen the interval between sweeps.[17]

Cranial Nerve Blocks. Those cranial nerves that can most easily be blocked are the 5th (trigeminal), 7th (facial), 9th (glossopharyngeal), 10th (vagus), 11th (spinal accessory), and 12th (hypoglossal). Cranial nerve blocks are useful in managing the pain of idiopathic neuralgias, mechanical neuropathy, neuritis, and neoplastic lesions of the head. Also, certain autonomic disturbances involving pathways associated with these cranial nerves may be partially managed by nerve blocks.

Space does not permit discussion of each of these blocks. Our presentation is limited to the *block of the trigeminal nerve* or its branches. This nerve becomes involved in many painful and autonomic disorders because it supplies sensory fibers to the entire face as well as two-thirds of the head. Because of this extensive area of innervation, some of the most frequently used nerve blocks are those of the trigeminal (gasserian) ganglion or one or more branches of the nerve. These blocks aid in the differential diagnosis of painful conditions, e.g., tic douloureux of the trigeminal and glossopharyngeal nerves, herpes zoster, migraine headaches, cancer, and atypical facial neuralgia. Moreover, they help to differentiate pain due to conditions in the face from those caused by intracranial disorders.

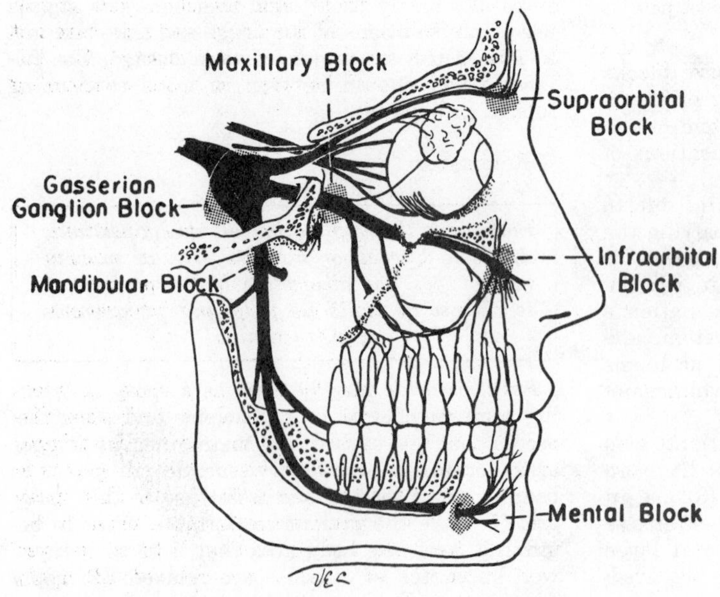

FIGURE 44–1. Diagram showing the anatomy and distribution of the trigeminal nerve and the optimal site of injecting it (stippled areas). (From Bonica, J. J.: *CLINICAL APPLICATION OF DIAGNOSTIC AND THERAPEUTIC NERVE BLOCKS.* 1959. Courtesy of Charles C Thomas, Publisher, Springfield, Illinois.)

Most of the trigeminal nerve is purely sensory; also, the major branches of the nerve are separated anatomically some distance from each other (Fig. 44–1). Because of the distribution of the trigeminal nerve, it is possible to interrupt one of its branches without involving the other major nervous pathways.

Following a nerve block procedure, in addition to observing for and reporting complications and untoward effects, the nurse should observe for and record the apparent amount, type, and duration of relief as well as the patient's complaints and the analgesics she administers for pain relief. Such observations may continue for several weeks and will help the physician to determine how effective the block was. It should be realized that when alcohol has been used for the block, the maximal effects do not occur for several days.

Administration of Medications for Pain Relief

> *The administration of medications is* not *the first action that should be taken to relieve pain.*

Kaufmann and Brown discuss the importance of knowledgeable nursing practice* in pain therapy below:

> Administering a medication, while a primary means of relieving pain, may or may not be the best means. Too often, by giving a shot or a pill, the nurse can practice "avoidism"—avoiding listening and understanding, avoiding nursing measures which might bring comfort in conjunction with or even instead of the medication. By so doing she may well withhold the support, assurance, and understanding which may relieve the patient of the necessity of having intense pain.

*Nursing care concerning the administration of medications for pain relief is discussed further in Chapter 45 of this unit.

A reverse aspect of this is the delay or withholding of a drug by the nurse, or by the patient himself. At times the nurse will put off giving a medication until the patient demonstrates marked discomfort. By the same token, the patient may fail to report pain until it becomes intense. He may do so to avoid being a nuisance, because he feels it is more courageous, because he is in one way or another opposed to taking medication, or for other reasons.[69]

The usual clinical practice for controlling pain is to give analgesic medications *along with* other supplementary medications or therapeutic measures, e.g., rest, proper position, and so forth. While analgesic medications, especially the narcotics, are the most frequently used type of therapy, they must be used *discretely* because of their undesirable side effects. Generally narcotics should not be utilized in treating pain unless other methods of treatment are not feasible or have failed.[18]

Although habituation, tolerance, and addiction are potential serious complications that can occur when potent analgesics are given, this does not mean that these medications should be withheld unnecessarily. In the presence of both short-term and long-term pain, narcotics can be highly useful if employed wisely. Habituation, tolerance, and addiction are not likely to occur in *short-term* pain therapy. Patients should not be made to suffer by unnecessarily withholding narcotics.

Medications used in pain therapy are many and they are administered in a variety of ways, e.g., by mouth, by topical application, by inhalation, or by injection. Medications may be injected by the usual subcutaneous, intramuscular, and intravenous routes. Also, in some instances, certain medications may be injected spinally, paravertebrally, or into selected nerves to produce nerve blocks, as discussed in the previous section. The latter types of injections are performed by physicians; although the nurse often assists with such procedures, she does not actually perform the injection.

Some of the types of medications used in alleviating, or at least reducing, pain are outlined in Table 44–1. *Systemic analgesic drugs* are the prevalent and most frequently used means of pain control.[135] *Analgesics include the most commonly prescribed drugs,*[111] *and therefore are the most widely used of all medications.*[55] This is not unexpected, since pain is usually the first symptom of injury and most diseases begin with or include pain as a symptom at some time during their course. It can readily be seen that:

> *Analgesics may well be the medications that you will administer* most frequently *in your nursing practice. Familiarize yourself with them.*

The "Ideal" Analgesic

Investigators and clinicians constantly speak of the elusive search for the ideal drug for this illness or that disorder. Unfortunately, as a rule, increased potency produces increased toxicity. Nevertheless, pharmacologists indefatigably strive to reach this goal.[75]

It can be seen that the task of the pharmacologist is difficult indeed: to prepare a medication that will have the desired effects while excluding the undesirable ones. Actually, pharmacologists have come a long way toward achieving the separation of clinical analgesia and dependence liability. With further research an even more successful separation of analgesic and physical-dependence properties may be hoped for. Some of the requirements of the ideal analgesic are that it would:[55, 75]

> Have rapid onset and long duration of action.

> Obliterate pain, diminish the anxiety associated with pain, and relax muscle spasms.

> Be effective for all patients regardless of age or disease.

> Be effective orally as well as parenterally.

> Be well tolerated and capable of prolonged use.

> Be free of side effects such as respiratory depression, constipation, nausea, vomiting, and circulatory depression.

> Exert a minimal degree of stupefaction and narcosis, i.e., be nontoxic.

> Have no tendency to allow the development of tolerance, addiction, or habituation.

> Act not only at the chemoreceptor level but also by blockage of the peripheral transmission system within the neuraxis.

> Be easily sterilized and possess a long shelf life.

> Be relatively inexpensive.

The ideal analgesic does not exist; instead, an overwhelming number of drugs are available for pain therapy.

Mechanisms of Analgesia. Analgesics do not all

TABLE 44–1. SOME TYPES OF MEDICATIONS USED FOR PAIN RELIEF*

Non-Narcotic Analgesic Agents
- I. Salicylates
- II. Para-aminophenols
- III. Pyrazolines
- IV. Other synthetic analgesics
- V. Skeletal muscle relaxant analgesics

Narcotic Analgesic Agents
- I. Opiates
  - A. Natural opiates
  - B. Synthetic opiates
- II. Nonopiate, addicting analgesics (Opioids)

Analgesic Adjuncts
- I. Barbiturates
  - A. Short-acting barbiturates
  - B. Intermediate-acting barbiturates
  - C. Long-acting barbiturates
- II. Amphetamines
- III. Opiate antagonists
- IV. Tranquilizers
  - A. Rauwolfia compounds
  - B. Phenothiazine derivatives

*Outline based on Kolodny, A. L., and McLoughlin, P. T.: *Comprehensive Approach to the Therapy of Pain.* Springfield, Ill., Charles C Thomas, 1966.

act in the same way. For example, acetylsalicylic acid, acetanilid, acetophenetidin, and aminopyrine act mainly on the *threshold for pain perception* and appear to have relatively little effect on the reaction to pain. On the other hand, opiates and alcohol owe their analgesic effects to their ability to control *reaction to pain* as well as to raise the pain perception threshold. The freedom from anxiety, relaxation, and apathy that follow the administration of morphine long outlast its effects on the threshold for pain perception.[141]

Recent evidence indicates that analgesics act *peripherally as well as centrally.* Peripheral action of analgesics is independent of any anti-inflammatory action that they may exert. Generally analgesics can be viewed as medications that modify the central reception of pain within the central nervous system, i.e., spinal cord and brain, by: "(1) blocking the facilitating reflexes and thereby elevating the pain threshold; (2) interrupting pathways for transmission of pain impulses in the brain, thereby modifying the central perception, interpretation, and reaction to the painful stimulus; and (3) modifying the central perception of pain and reducing psychogenic pain by depressing reflex activity."[55]

Types of Analgesics. For many years analgesics have been divided into two classes on the basis of their clinical effectiveness: (1) the "strong" narcotic analgesics; and (2) the "weak" non-narcotic, antipyretic analgesics.[83] Differences between the two classes clinically are based upon the nature of the pain condition for which each has been found to be effective rather than on analgesic potency. Generally the narcotic analgesics are administered for the relief of severe pains resulting from burns, fractures, coronary occlusion, renal colic, and so forth, whereas the non-narcotic analgesics are usually given for muscular aches, headaches, and pains of inflammatory origin.

STRONG NARCOTIC ANALGESICS. These consist of morphine itself, plus various morphine-like agents differing from morphine only in characteristics such as: rate of onset, duration of action, route of administration, adverse side effects, and chemical configuration. Drugs in this class induce drug dependence and tolerance. Since these drugs have structural similarities, it is relatively easy to classify them on the basis of chemical composition (Table 44–2).

The narcotic analgesic group includes morphine and a large number of morphine-mimetic drugs, e.g., the opiates (or morphine congeners) and the opioids (nonopiate addicting analgesics). Pharmacologic actions of the congeners of morphine are similar to those of the parent compound, morphine. Differences occur in: potency; effects on respiratory depression; histamine release; and, to a lesser degree, liability to tolerance and addiction. These drugs share the "ability to act in the place

TABLE 44–2. CHEMICAL BASES OF "STRONG" ANALGESICS*

Morphine	→	Codeine Heroin Pantopon
Semisynthetic compounds Numorphan	→	Paracodin Dilaudid Metapon
Synthetic compounds Meperidine	→	Demerol Nisentil Leritine Alvodine
Methadone	→	Dolophine Pipadone Palfium
Morphinan	→	Dromoran Phenazocine
Antagonists Nalorphine	→	Levallorphan Pentazocine Cyclazocine

*From Poswillo, D. E.: *In* Alling, C., III, et al. (eds.): *Facial Pain.* Philadelphia, Lea & Febiger, 1968, p. 65.

of morphine, not only in producing analgesia, but also in supporting physical dependence. . . . They are all, with the possible exception of codeine, potent systemic pain-relieving drugs, even though their potencies relative to one another may differ. . . . The adjective 'strong' applied to their analgesic potential should not be confused with 'potent.' "[111]

Morphine is probably the most useful drug in clinical practice, when given under appropriate circumstances and with the proper indications. Codeine is probably second only to morphine as a drug of choice for pain relief. Codeine has the advantage of being particularly useful in combination with nonaddicting analgesics.

Narcotic analgesics are *slowly absorbed* from several sources: the gastrointestinal tract, subcutaneous tissues, muscles, and intravenously. Even when analgesics are given intravenously, the full effect is not reached for at least 20 minutes. Although the narcotic effects last only about 4 to 6 hours, the *detoxification* of the drug is only about 90 per cent completed 36 hours after administration. Thus, both detoxification and absorption are slow processes. Detoxification occurs primarily in the liver by the process of conjugation; the kidneys excrete the main byproduct.

The morphine-mimetic drugs can cause many serious side effects, in addition to their potential for addiction.

> *The morphine-mimetic drugs affect* every *organ of the body!*

WEAK NON-NARCOTIC ANALGESICS. These are a diverse group of synthetic chemical agents. The pharmacologic properties of the weak analgesics overlap, but it is possible to classify them on the basis of their chemical structures into the six subgroups presented in Table 44–3.

Although described as "weak," the non-narcotic analgesics are actually highly effective in relieving pain in many situations; variables of dose and route of administration affect the potency of these medications. Non-narcotic analgesics are all readily absorbed from the gastric mucosa and rapidly hydrolyzed in the plasma, and the metabolites are excreted.[111]

Toxic reactions can be produced by all weak analgesics. Aminopyrine and phenylbutazone have adverse effects on blood-forming tissues. The phenacetin compounds have been demonstrated as toxic to the kidneys following prolonged administration. The salicylates probably are the most effective analgesics, having the least adverse reactions.[111]

"MIXED" OR COMBINED ANALGESICS. A combination of drugs acting by different mechanisms may exert a synergistic additive effect. By selective mixing the effects of individual drugs (e.g., analgesic, anti-inflammatory, antipyretic, muscle-relaxant, tranquilizing) may be combined. A wide variety of mixed compounds are available for clinical therapy, "utilizing the sum of the properties of the components."[111] Examples of some analgesic combinations are: *A.P.C. Compound* (containing aspirin, phenacetin, caffeine); *Darvon Compound* (aspirin, phenacetin, caffeine, propoxyphene); *Edrisal* (aspirin, phenacetin, amphetamine); *Empiral* (aspirin, phenacetin, phenobarbital); *Fiorinal* (aspirin, phenacetin, caffeine, isobutylallyl-barbituric acid); and *Phenaphen* (aspirin, phenacetin, hyoscyamine, and phenobarbital).

It is clearly established that the administration of mood-changing medications along with analgesics is helpful. The use of such potentiating adjuncts, e.g., barbiturates, tranquilizers, which not only affect the emotional input but also permit lower doses of narcotic agents, can significantly reduce suffering.[75]

TABLE 44–3. CHEMICAL BASES OF "WEAK" ANALGESICS*

Salicylates →	Aspirin Salamide Salophen
Anilines →	Phenacetin Antifebrin Tempra
Pyrazolines →	Phenazone Pyramidon Butazolidin Tanderil
Mefenamic acid →	Ponstan
Amphetamines →	Benzedrine Dexedrine Apamine Preludin
Muscle relaxants and tranquilizers →	Carisoprodol Chlorpromazine

*From Poswillo, D. E.: *In* Alling, C., III, et al. (eds.): *Facial Pain.* Philadelphia, Lea & Febiger, 1968, p. 62.

Complications and Misuse of Analgesics. The administration of narcotics and other analgesics may produce pain relief; however, *both short-term and long-term analgesic administration is fraught with problems.* While potential complications should not prevent the use of analgesic agents, these drugs must be used with caution and with an understanding of possible side effects and how these hazards might be reversed or avoided. Although the nature and incidence of complications associated with the administration of narcotic and similar drugs for pain relief will vary from patient to patient, it is possible to identify some common problems. Let us briefly examine some of the complications of analgesic therapy and how they might be reversed or avoided.

NAUSEA AND VOMITING. Narcotics may frequently precipitate nausea and vomiting. Indeed, it has been reported that in selected surgical patients the incidence of emesis associated with morphine may be as high as 46 per cent, and with meperidine as high as 36 per cent.[127]

PARESTHESIA. The subcutaneous or intramuscular injection of analgesic drugs is generally not irritating to the local tissues. However, if the drug is deposited in the region of a nerve, paresthesia and paresis may be precipitated along its course of distribution.[127] The nurse will, thus, want to be familiar with the "safe" sites for injections so that these distressing symptoms from nerve injury will be avoided.

ADDICTION. The problem of drug addiction has cast its shadow over pain therapy for centuries; a major problem in the chemotherapy of pain is the development by the patient of physical and psychologic dependence on the drugs used. This problem is of particular importance in persons who have pain with a considerable psychogenic overlay, since such persons are particularly prone to the development of drug dependency.[31]

With the development of drug dependency, the patient begins to rely or depend on the drug to remove him from reality or to change his reality. Such a patient, thus, asks increasingly frequently for the drug and steadily wants larger doses so that he can obtain the physical and psychologic feelings that the drug produces. The original need for the drug (i.e., to alleviate pain) thus becomes replaced by the acquired physical and psychologic dependence on it, so that the patient comes to feel that he *must* have the drug.

Closely observe patients receiving addicting drugs for signs of drug dependency.

When a patient has developed drug addiction and is then deprived of the drugs, he must be observed carefully for withdrawal symptoms such as anxiety, abdominal cramps, diarrhea, sweating, restlessness, and rhinorrhea.

CIRCULATORY DEPRESSION. Another complication of analgesic therapy that must be kept foremost in the nurse's mind is circulatory depression. Following the injection of certain narcotic drugs, hypotension may occur. At times this hypotension is of such a serious degree that cardiovascular collapse ensues. Although the exact etiologic mechanisms for these cardiovascular changes are not known, it appears that: (1) hypotension may be caused by a direct dilating action on peripheral vessels; and (2) a shock-like state may also be secondary to a release of histamine.[127]

> *Because of potential circulatory depression with hypotension, patients under the influence of narcotic drugs should* not *be allowed to walk and they should* not *be transported in a wheelchair. A stretcher should be used.*

RESPIRATORY DEPRESSION. Respiratory depression is a common complication of analgesic therapy. It is caused by the diminished sensitivity of the respiratory center to carbon dioxide. This problem is dose-related and accompanies the administration of all potent analgesic drugs, whether narcotics or narcotic antagonists. Stephen observes: "Each new potent analgesic is usually introduced with claims that it has a relative sparing effect on the respiratory center; however, up to now these claims have not withstood the test of careful investigation."[127] The problem of respiratory depression is particularly dangerous for elderly persons with respiratory impairment.

SHOCK*

> *Extreme caution must be observed in administering analgesic medications to a patient in shock.*

You will recall that with the syndrome of shock there is peripheral circulatory impairment. This means that intramuscular or subcutaneous injections of analgesics may be absorbed slowly, if at all, into the circulation with, consequently, little relief of pain. Because the patient continues to suffer, the nurse may be tempted to give repeated analgesic injections. Should she do so, the vital centers will be exposed to a relative overdose of narcotics when the shock is alleviated and the peripheral blood vessels are no longer constricted. When the vessels reexpand to normal size, the medication that has accumulated in the tissues will enter body circulation and be carried to the vital centers. To *prevent* this potential disaster and to give adequate pain relief to the patient in shock, it is recommended that intravenous injection of selected analgesics be given in doses just adequate to relieve pain.[127] (Note: Some preparations cannot be given safely by the intravenous route.)

Evaluation of the Patient for Pain Relief. Assume that you are at the bedside of a patient who needs a morphine-like analgesic to relieve moderate-to-severe pain. What factors about such a patient and his situation should be considered *before* a chemotherapeutic agent is given to relieve pain? Why, for example, isn't the patient in pain just routinely given an injection of morphine?

Evaluation of a patient prior to initiating analgesic chemotherapy is imperative so that the patient's pain relief will be obtained safely and will be adequate. Some factors to be evaluated are:[70] (1) the patient's body weight; (2) his individual pain experience; (3) his age, general state of health, general mental status, probable duration of his pain, and probable life expectancy; (4) his cardiac, respiratory, renal, and nervous system status; and (5) the presence or absence of cross tolerance.

BODY WEIGHT. The dose of morphine listed as the standard is 10 mg. per 70 kg. of body weight, although some patients require more and others less. Both the analgesic effect and the side effects of morphine, such as vomiting and respiratory depression, are dose-related. It has been demonstrated that the amount of analgesia produced with 15 mg. of morphine is only slightly greater than that with 10 mg.; however, the increase in side effects is proportionately greater than the increase in analgesia. This evidence further supports the use of 10 mg. of morphine as an average dose.

INDIVIDUAL PAIN EXPERIENCE. The great variation in the individual pain experience probably outweighs any effect of body size in pain and analgesia. The need for analgesic medications for the relief of postoperative pain clearly demonstrates the spectrum of individuality associated with "painfulness." Figure 44–2 represents a formulation put together from data from several sources, all pertaining to postoperative pain, expressed in terms of the drugs and doses required to relieve the pain. As you see, some patients have little pain, others have a great deal of pain. Some interesting groups of patients represented in the figure are: (1) those who have no pain postoperatively; (2) those who have pain that is relieved by a placebo; and (3) those who obtain no relief from narcotics at any dose, probably because they "interpret any relief short of complete analgesia as 'no pain relief.' "[70]

AGE, GENERAL STATE OF HEALTH, GENERAL MENTAL STATUS, PROBABLE DURATION OF PAIN, PROBABLE LIFE EXPECTANCY. By itself, *age* is not important in analgesic dosage. It is often said that "old people and young people are the most sensitive to the effects of narcotic and sedative drugs." Nonetheless, it has been established that no marked difference exists in the response of *healthy aged* persons to narcotics as compared to the response of younger patients when medications are given on a weight basis. However, de-

*For a more complete discussion of Shock, see Chapter 26.

bilitating illnesses are more common among older persons, and:

> *Patients with debilitating diseases, whether old or young, have a heightened sensitivity to the effects of narcotics.*

A patient's *general mental status*, the *probable duration of his pain*, and his *probable life expectancy* should also be considered in planning chemotherapy for pain. The mentally anxious individual may benefit from a tranquilizer in addition to an analgesic. The patient whose life expectancy is short may be given narcotics more readily than the individual with a chronic pain problem that will probably continue for a long period. If a patient will require prolonged therapy for relief of chronic pains, the side effects of analgesics (especially the addicting quality of morphine) must be considered.

CARDIAC, RESPIRATORY, RENAL, AND NERVOUS SYSTEM STATUS. Since many analgesic agents depress breathing or produce hypotension, an evaluation of the patient's cardiac, respiratory, renal, and nervous system status is of importance. The presence of increased intracranial pressure is cause for special concern.

> *Increased intracranial pressure.* Potent narcotic analgesics are contraindicated in patients with increased intracranial pressure because narcotics further increase cerebrospinal fluid pressure. This increase is secondary to carbon dioxide retention (increased arterial carbon dioxide tension), which always follows narcotic-induced respiratory depression.

A point of interest is that patients who are being artificially ventilated will not suffer from respiratory depression and carbon dioxide retention after receiving morphine, so they can receive narcotics in spite of an elevated cerebrospinal fluid pressure.

> *As a general rule, morphine is not given to patients who are suffering from* internal abdominal injuries, respiratory distress, *or* head injuries.

In all three of the above conditions morphine may cause vomiting, with serious effects. Suppression of the respiratory center in patients with respiratory distress may prove fatal: *morphine should not be given to patients with respirations of 12 per minute or less.* Concerning head injuries, we have just mentioned the danger of increasing the cerebrospinal fluid pressure. In addition, internal cerebral hemorrhage may also be present, causing depression of the respiratory center, which morphine would worsen. Moreover, the fact that morphine affects pupil size* could confuse clinical observations of pupil size, which are important with head injuries.†

CROSS TOLERANCE. The presence of cross tolerance can make effective chemotherapeutic pain relief difficult to achieve.

> *Cross tolerance.* The use of tranquilizers during the day, hypnotics at night, and alcohol in between has caused numerous persons in our fast-moving society to become tolerant to sedatives and narcotics. "For some persons it has brought death. A usual dose of hypnotics, which is large because of tolerance, after an extra large alcohol intake has led to asphyxia, either by simple respiratory obstruction or secondary to vomiting and aspiration."[70]

Tolerance develops to both the sedative and analgesic effects of narcotics, so that chronic users of tranquilizers, hypnotics, and alcohol become resistant to potent analgesics.

Before leaving the discussion of tolerance we should briefly discuss the patient with *liver disease.* Although pharmacologists classically teach that patients with liver or kidney disease should not receive medications that have to be excreted by these organs, clinical practice shows that there is no reason for withholding medications such as pentobarbital from a person with decreased liver function if the possibility of a longer effect is anticipated. The administration of drugs that are excreted through the liver or kidney to persons with

*Morphine acts as a miotic; that is, it constricts the pupil of the eye.

†Head injuries are discussed in the unit on Neurology.

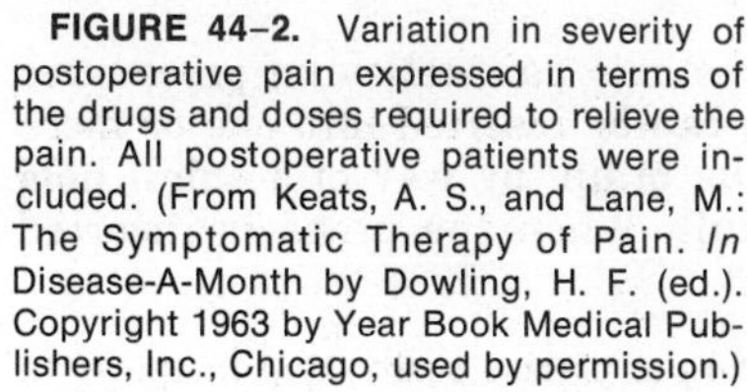

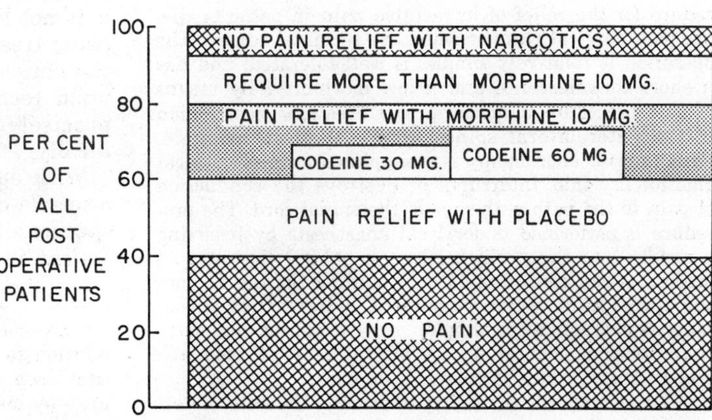

FIGURE 44–2. Variation in severity of postoperative pain expressed in terms of the drugs and doses required to relieve the pain. All postoperative patients were included. (From Keats, A. S., and Lane, M.: The Symptomatic Therapy of Pain. *In* Disease-A-Month by Dowling, H. F. (ed.). Copyright 1963 by Year Book Medical Publishers, Inc., Chicago, used by permission.)

liver or kidney disease will not greatly increase the intensity of the effect of the drug, but rather will prolong its action.[70]

NEUROSURGICAL PROCEDURES FOR PAIN RELIEF

When there is persistent, intractable pain of high intensity, neurosurgical procedures may be employed. Utilizing all the available knowledge of neuroanatomy and neurophysiology, the neurosurgeon attempts various procedures in an effort to effect relief from pain by interrupting parts of the paths in the nervous system that relay sensations to the brain from their point of origin. The goal of such surgery is to provide pain relief without causing the unnecessary loss of other sensations, for example, the loss of all feeling in an area.

Such operations may be performed peripherally or centrally on the spinal cord and brain itself. In addition, surgery on the autonomic nervous system, *sympathectomy,* may be performed alone, or in combination with other procedures for the pains of causalgia or vascular disease.

Summarized below are a few of the various neurosurgical procedures utilized in pain therapy:

> *Neurectomy* is the interruption of cranial or peripheral nerves by means of incision or injection. This procedure is employed when pain is localized to a small part of the body. When a cranial neurectomy is performed, a craniotomy is necessary.

> *Rhizotomy* is the interruption of the anterior or posterior nerve root area close to the spinal cord. Rhizotomy is performed when pain is more widely distributed than that occurring in a small area of the body. As many roots are divided as necessary to control the pain. A laminectomy is necessary for this procedure.

> *Chordotomy* is the surgical interruption of the pain-conducting pathways within the spinal cord. An incision a few millimeters in length is made in the anterolateral pathway opposite the side on which the pain is located. When pain is midline in nature, a bilateral chordotomy must be performed. A laminectomy is necessary for this operation.

> *Percutaneous cervical chordotomy* is a preferred procedure for the relief of intractable pain in patients who are poor surgical risks or who have terminal cancer. The operation is relatively simple, is well tolerated, and has a short convalescence and a low morbidity. By means of this procedure a nonsurgical stereotaxic destruction of the anterolateral spinothalamic tracts is possible. Percutaneous chordotomy is a simplified form of surgical chordotomy that interrupts or destroys the conduction of pain in the pain pathways of the spinal cord. The procedure is performed under local anesthesia by inserting a needle into the neck, below and behind the mastoid process. X-ray control is used in guiding the needle into the spinal cord. Some physicians believe that percutaneous chordotomy is simpler, more accurate, and safer than surgical chordotomy. A lateral cervical approach and an anterior approach have been used.

> *Tractotomy* is the surgical division of the anterolateral pathway in the brainstem. A craniotomy is necessary in order to accomplish this procedure.

> *Gyrectomy* involves the removal of the postcentral gyrus corresponding to the painful part. This is done to attempt to remove the registration of pain within the cortex of the brain. Therefore, this is a cerebral operation.

> *Frontal leukotomy (lobotomy)* causes the destruction of cerebral tissue in the frontal lobes of the brain.

Some neurosurgical procedures designed to alleviate pain are schematically illustrated in Figure 44–3.

It should be remembered that when *sensory* nerves are cut, the tissues which are no longer supplied with sensory innervation become highly susceptible to injury. With sensory innervation gone, feelings of pain, pressure, and temperature are no longer present, and injury can occur without the patient's even being aware that it has happened. Because the interruption of sensory nerve pathways deprives body tissues of these protective mechanisms, this procedure is usually not carried out unless other less radical treatment measures have failed.

Interruption of sensory nerves deprives tissues of protective reflexes, such as feelings of pain, pressure, and heat.

*STEREOTAXIC PAIN SURGERY**

In 1920 it was suggested that application of the techniques of stereotaxic surgery be used for the treatment of pain, by the section of deep fiber tracts in the brain. The first stereotaxic operations for pain were done around 1930, and the animal-perfected technique was then applied to man in the 1940's.

Stereotaxic brain surgery, aiming at the modification of cerebral function by the section of tracts and destruction of nuclei, may now be divided into two categories according to method of approach: (1) *open* stereotaxic surgery, using electrodes or other techniques, i.e., cryogenic surgery, radio frequency heating, implantation of radio isotopes, ultrasound; and (2) *closed,* bloodless stereotaxic *radiosurgery* with ionizing radiation, i.e., gamma rays, x-rays, protons, and other heavy particles.

Open stereotaxic techniques have been successfully developed for the treatment of intractable pain. Although the surgery is referred to as "open," it is not like conventional surgery where the area being treated is visually seen and manually felt by the surgeon. Stereotaxic operations are dependent upon technical apparatus, and the operation is precisely precalculated anatomically and technically.

With open stereotaxic pain-relieving procedures a needle or probe can be inserted into one or more specific sites in the brain, by way of a small hole drilled in the skull. When the probe is inserted

*"Stereotaxic" refers to precise positioning in space. In relation to surgery it connotes the location of operative sites deep within the body—frequently within the cranium—by instrumentation from outside the body.

the physician applies a heating current that results in coagulation of adjacent tissue; if a needle is inserted, a neurolytic agent is injected.

Many agents can be neurolytic, i.e., can destroy either nerve fibers themselves or their cells of origin. The effectiveness of injectable agents is variable and is influenced by such factors as the location of the injection and the concentration and volume of the neurolytic agent. Hot water, disinfectants (e.g., phenol), and alcohol are examples of injectable neurolytic agents. Other agents that can be neurolytic include high frequency sound, radiation, and dry ice.

Stereotaxic procedures can be accomplished with a high degree of accuracy and with little discomfort to the patient. By referring to right-angle coordinates, standard charts, and special x-rays, it is possible to selectively destroy tissue in preselected sites deep within the brain.

Both the size of the lesion and the position of the target are determined preoperatively. Although it is technically possible to place an accurate stereotaxic lesion anywhere in the depth of the brain with minimal risk, the surgery is not without problems, i.e., there is often a tendency for pain to recur in time, as with the more conventional pain surgery. However, it is also possible for such minute lesions to produce a permanent cure. The clinical result often cannot be judged for several months after the operation.

With *radiosurgery,* as well, the operative effect does not appear immediately, but rather after a latent period that varies with factors such as the dose of radiation. Some of the advantages of radiosurgery over the open method are: (1) there is no operative shock and practically no mortality risk; (2) the risks of infection and bleeding are eliminated; and (3) the patient can leave the hospital the day after the procedure. Since the lesion produced by radiosurgery continues to grow progressively for several months, care must be taken that the ultimate size of the lesion will not produce undesirable side effects.

For the patient suffering from longstanding pain, his pain becomes a force completely dominating his life. When such pain is removed, by surgical interruption of pain pathways, with resultant abolition of pain perception, the problem is not entirely solved. Because of the complicated nature of chronically painful conditions, such a patient frequently requires long-term psychotherapeutic and rehabilitative measures after surgery. Once surgical pain relief is obtained, function must be restored and new goals found. Occupational therapy and family training may be necessary.

TREATMENT OF CENTRAL PAIN SYNDROMES

Causalgia

Treatment for causalgia should be initiated promptly to prevent progressive incapacitation and suffering. The treatment of choice is interruption of the sympathetic chain that supplies the painful

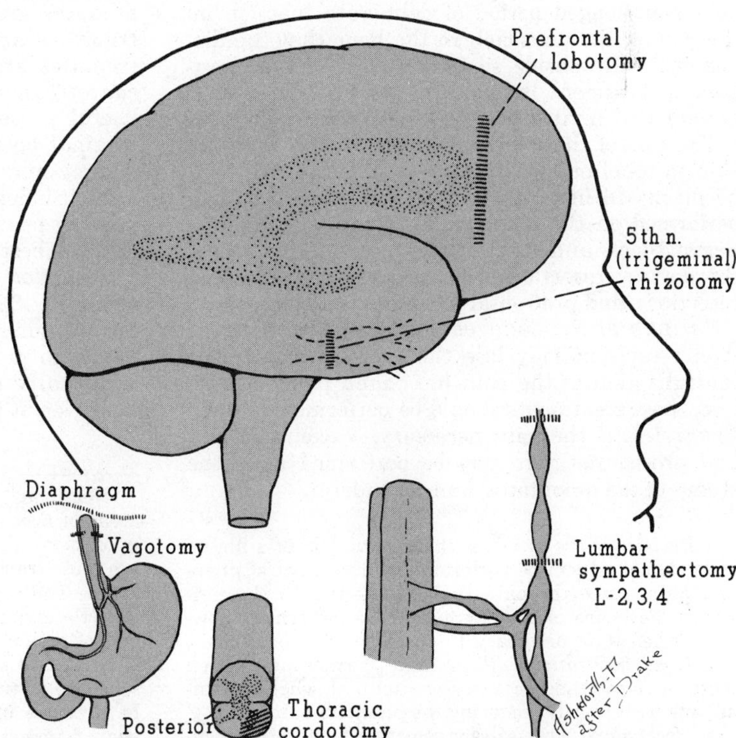

FIGURE 44-3. Surgery of pain. (From Jacob, S. W., and Francone, C. A.: *Structure and Function in Man.* 2nd ed., 1970.)

part. Sympathetic blocks with local anesthetics may be used both diagnostically and therapeutically. Successive blocks may produce effects of increasing duration such that the symptom may be mild and relatively undisturbing or may entirely vanish. However, a *sympathectomy* may be necessary if several blocks fail to provide satisfactory relief. A dorsal preganglionic sympathectomy is the procedure of choice for causalgias of the upper extremities; lumbar sympathectomy is the surgical approach for causalgias of the lower extremities. Once severe pain has been relieved, the patient should benefit from whirlpool baths, gentle massage, and active and passive movement.

Phantom Limb Pain

Treatment for phantom limb pain poses frustrating problems, since uniform success has never been obtained from any one type of treatment. It appears that with the passage of time there is a progressive "centralization" of the pain process. That is to say, a movement of the factors predominant in the production of pain occurs in a direction *away* from the peripheral site of the amputation and to a more central part of the nervous system. Thus, as the painful condition becomes long-term and chronic in nature, the cerebral cortex of the brain becomes predominantly involved in the projections of the phantom pain. "This progressive centralization of the pain process makes inadvisable a prolonged period of deliberate inaction on the part of the physician in the hope that the discomfort will subside spontaneously."[46] Also, postponing treatment is mentally discouraging to the patient and invites problems with drug addiction.

The role of the following procedures in relationship to relief or modification of phantom pain will be discussed briefly: local, peripheral procedures performed on the amputation stump, sympathetic nerve block and sympathectomy, anterolateral chordotomy, resection of the sensory cortex (cortical resection), and prefrontal lobotomy (leukotomy).

Peripheral Procedures. Procedures such as stump revision may lose their effectiveness once centralization of the pain has taken place. Therefore, these treatments should be performed as early as possible if they are necessary. Various peripheral procedures that may be performed upon the stump of the amputated limb include:

> *Revision of the stump,* with *reamputation* at a higher level should seldom be performed for the relief of phantom pain, since the pain typically recurs in the new stump. Revisions of the stump may be performed, however, when it is necessary to do so to fit a prosthesis.

> *Local infiltration with procaine* may be used when there is point tenderness in the stump or when a painful, adherent scar is producing the phantom pain.

> *Mechanical percussion* of sensitive amputation neuromas* may be employed when phantom limb pain is associated with a locally painful area in the stump. This unusual method of treatment is believed to produce progressive fibrosis of the nerve end and shrinkage of the neuroma as a result of the continued trauma.

The percussion is obtained by (1) striking the sensitive area of a *digital* stump vigorously and repeatedly against a solid object; (2) placing one end of a wooden peg which is about one inch in diameter over the sensitive area of a *lower extremity stump* and striking the other end with a wooden mallet for 10 to 20 minutes; or (3) using a mechanical vibrator for *either* a digital or lower extremity stump. While the percussion is initially performed several times per day, the duration and frequency of the percussion sessions are reduced with improvement.

> *Resection of a painful neuroma* may be attempted *one* time if repeated infiltrations with procaine and percussion fail to bring sustained relief and if the pain is localized and can consistently be relieved for short periods of time with procaine infiltration.

Sympathetic Nerve Block and Sympathectomy. These may relieve phantom limb pain when it is associated with vasomotor and sudomotor disturbances in the stump. An amputation stump that has such disturbances may be cold, cyanotic, hyperesthetic (excessively sensitive), painful, and covered with excessive perspiration during periods of discomfort. Exposure to cold and heightened emotional stress may increase the pain. Following a successful sympathetic ganglion nerve block, which denervates the sympathetic outflow to the stump, the affected area becomes warm, nontender, and dry. If the nerve block proves to be successful, it should be followed by a sympathectomy to insure more permanent results.

Anterolateral Chordotomy. This may be performed if the previously discussed procedures are unsuccessful or are not indicated, and if the patient is incapacitated by his painful phantom limb.

Chordotomy is technically easier to perform, and produces greater pain relief, when the lower extremities are involved than when the upper extremities are affected. *Percutaneous high cervical radiofrequency chordotomy* has proved to be a useful procedure that enlarges the scope of the original open surgical operation. Although chordotomy may relieve stump pain and local tenderness, it is less effective in relieving the pain in the missing phantom limb. Nonetheless, chordotomy is still the best available neurosurgical approach.

Resection of the Sensory Cortex (Cortical Resection). This should be an excellent procedure for relieving phantom pain, since this pain is believed to progressively migrate to the brain and eventually be projected by the cerebral cortex. However, it has been demonstrated that the major-

**Neuromas* are tumors growing from a nerve. These areas of new growth or tumors are predominantly made up of nerve cells and nerve fibers. *Amputation neuromas* are those traumatic neuromas that occur following amputation. The neuroma that often develops on the proximal end of a divided nerve consists of numerous naked fibers, and of others that do not have fully developed sheaths, embedded in a mass of new tissue. The neuroma is often sensitive to traction and pressure and, in addition, may be a source of pain referred to the phantom extremity apart from external excitation.[62]

ity of patients who have had cortical resection for phantom pain have had a recurrence of their symptoms. In addition, since the operation involves scar formation adjacent to the motor strip in the brain, epilepsy is a common complication. For these reasons, cortical resection is not a standard treatment for phantom pain.

Prefrontal Lobotomy (Leukotomy). This is a surgical procedure that poses many problems, although it may still be performed in managing phantom pain after careful consideration is given to its long-term effects. The primary problem is that when sufficient damage is done to the frontal lobes, so that pain appreciation is altered, then mental deterioration results. *Bilateral* destruction of the frontal lobes produces severe mental deterioration, although it does alter pain appreciation. On the other hand, unilateral frontal lobotomy does not produce prolonged pain relief.

Various psychologic theories have been proposed to account for phantom limb experiences and phantom limb pain. Psychiatrists have treated patients with phantom limb pain, and they report some successes and some failures from psychotherapy, hypnosis, narco-analysis, and electric shock. Clearly there is an interrelationship between attitude and the experience of pain, and although the exact psychophysiologic mechanism may be disputed, there is no doubt that there is such a mechanism.[96]

The psychologic significance of phantom limb pain and similar central pains is most often considered in relation to its *effects* rather than its *causes.* At times formal psychiatric treatment may help patients with various forms of neurogenic or central pain. In some cases an associated depressive illness may be treated with some benefit to the pain. However, more often the appropriate treatment measures involve the use of tranquilizers, local anesthesia, vibrators, and relatively minor surgical procedures.[96]

CHAPTER 45

Nursing Care of Patients Experiencing Pain

Divine is the work of subduing pain.
—*Hippocrates*

Caring appropriately for a patient experiencing pain calls for a high level of nursing acumen, sensitivity, and skill. One nursing leader summarizes this as follows:

> Nursing the patient in pain demands all the imagination, all the knowledge and skill and all the humanity the nurse has at her command. It is a mature kind of seasoned thoughtful nursing that the patient requires whether he knows it or not.[60]

If you observe a skilled nurse caring for patients having pain, you will see in practice what is described above. Watch the experienced nurse at work as she cares for numerous patients who are having a variety of pains; you will see that she has learned, in the hard school of clinical practice, to evaluate and respond to both the physical and emotional aspects of pain.[99] Versed in both the art and science of nursing she patiently appraises these patients' personalities, analyzes the physical and behavioral evidence that they present, and strives to constantly cultivate deeper insight into their characters and problems. Alert for changes, she constantly reevaluates her assessments and actions. All successful nurses are good psychologists in a sense, and all are multidisciplinary in their practice.

> *The clinical care of any patient experiencing pain, whether acute or chronic, must be based upon an understanding of: the* pain *being treated; the* individual *being treated; and the* mode *of* treatment.

The care of the patient who has pain is a complex activity requiring many skills on the nurse's part. In order to perform adequately, the nurse must have some knowledge of: the nature of pain and how it is experienced; the anatomy and physiology of pain; types of pain and the problems created when awareness of pain is absent; evaluation of pain; and medical, surgical, and nursing measures that can be taken to reduce or prevent suffering. Appropriate professional nursing intervention in caring for patients having pain obviously involves far more than merely giving a medication. Some additional factors involved in this clinical area are:[37]

> Concern with the physiologic, environmental, sociocultural and psycho-emotional components of pain.

> Awareness of both nurse's and patient's perceptions of pain, as well as reactions to pain.

> Consideration of the individual as a person as well as a member of a social unit, e.g., a family.

> Dedication to the prevention of pain as well as its alleviation.

As with other nursing activities, the clinical care of the patient in pain begins with the nurse's assessment or evaluation of the patient's condition. On the basis of her observations, the nurse next decides on the course of action that she believes is appropriate. In addition to trying to prevent or alleviate pain, the nurse relieves and comforts the patient by giving him hope and strength, even though it may be possible to achieve only limited goals in some situations.[37] The final step in the nurse's plan of care is to reevaluate her actions to determine the accuracy of her judgments and the effectiveness of her course of action. In actual practice these steps do not occur separately from one another but are part of an ongoing process.

THE NURSE: AN AGENT OF PAIN PRODUCTION AND PAIN RELIEF

The nurse acts as both an agent who produces pain and an agent who relieves patients' pains. She cares for many patients whose medical or surgical therapies are pain-producing; such pains are thus added to pains that may already be present from disease. Persons who are made to suffer, as patients must often be, frequently experience feelings of fear and anger directed at those who cause the suffering. This may be so even though the patient's best interests are being followed. It is naturally essential that you carry out pain-producing procedures as gently and skillfully as possible, and that you administer them while giving the patient emotional support and recognition of his discomfort.

Because the nurse can, within the sanctions of society and the realm of her responsibility, produce pain in others, she is in a position of power over patients and must be aware of the psychologic impact that this fact has upon them. The production of pain or discomfort in patients should never result from an intention to punish. The nurse must consciously evaluate her behavior so that a patient can in no way interpret what she is doing to him as punishment. Because medical, surgical, and nursing therapies may produce pain, the nurse will need to give constant support and encouragement to those in her care, so that they will not refuse treatments that are in their best interests. However, remember always that:

It is the right of a rational person to refuse treatment. Far too many patients refuse treatment because they have not received the mental preparation and support that would enable them to receive the care they need.

Broadly speaking, the nurse will work to prevent, alleviate, or remove the cause of pain and also strive to reduce the patient's perception of pain. Her clinical care will encompass three broad areas: (1) psychologic, (2) physical, and (3) pharmacologic or medical. The nurse's practice will involve all these areas in an integrated manner, although at one moment she may emphasize one aspect of care and then shift to concentrate on another as she works to prevent, palliate, and attenuate or remove pain.

GENERAL ASPECTS OF CARE

Earlier in this unit we reviewed details to be considered in evaluating the patient experiencing pain. As we emphasized, the nurse evaluates many factors: the patient's statements, his personality, her own personality and view of pain, the source of noxious stimulation, and the types of pains. She carefully surveys the patient to determine the extent of his suffering, realizing that there are wide variations in the physiologic manifestations of pain. She also knows that, due to the diversity of psychosocial responses and the various threats that pain poses, all patients do not manifestly express pain to the same extent.

Before you do anything to try to relieve a patient's pain, talk with him to find out more precisely what the problem is. Rather than assuming that you know how he feels, *find out from him* how he feels. For example, a patient who is only 12 hours postoperative may tell you he has pain; do not assume that he means pain in the area of the surgical procedure. He may have a headache, perhaps severe chest pain, or pain in the calf of his leg. Therefore:

Evaluate a patient's pain prior to taking any action to relieve it.

Also, evaluate whether he is actually in *pain* or whether he is uncomfortable. For example, a patient may say he is in pain when he actually has a feeling of pressure from flatus (gas).

On the basis of her evaluation, the nurse must decide whether the patient is having pain, and if it *is* present, whether it is of such intensity that it requires relief. Next she decides the appropriate method of providing relief and plans her care.

The following general statements about the clinical care of patients experiencing pain are important to consider as you begin to formulate a plan of nursing care:

> Pain is a *"cry for help"* that the able clinician will recognize and attempt to eliminate, whether the cause is physical or mental.[1]

> Pain should be respected and treated as pain, *regardless of its origin.* There is no subjective difference between psychogenic pain and organic pain. Psychogenic pain exists; it is not "imaginary."

> The *entire patient*—as a whole—should receive attention and care, rather than just the patient's pain symptom.[110, 120]

> *Specific therapy,* directed at the cause of the pain, must be used to treat pain whenever possible. For example, if a patient has pain caused by uric acid deposits in gout, it would not be sound therapy to give analgesics while neglecting to give specific therapy for gout.[120] Try to *identify the source* of discomfort or pain and then take *appropriate action* to reduce it, e.g., padding, positioning, turning, medication.

> *Ancillary problems,* which contribute to discomfort or aggravate pain, require treatment as well as the major pain problem. Examples of ancillary problems are: constipation, diarrhea, cough, anorexia, and frequent urination.[120]

> *Plan with the patient, listen to his suggestions, encourage his help,* and *let him know if something is going to be painful.* Plan with the patient what you will be doing for him so that he feels a part of his treatment rather than like an object that is constantly having something done to it. Listen to his suggestions about how something might be done, such as moving him. He knows what hurts; you don't. With the patient's help, you can identify situations, movements, and so forth, that cause pain, and those measures that bring the greatest relief. Always forewarn a patient if a procedure is expected to be painful. Help him to understand what to expect as well as what will be done to minimize the pain. Such information may make the pain more bearable.

> While *palliation* is not a substitute for treating the source of a pain, it may be: (1) employed as a relief-giving measure in situations in which the source of pain cannot be treated or removed; (2) used as a temporary measure until the source of the pain can be established; or (3) utilized as a supplement to other measures in the treatment process.[37]

Skill should be developed in administering *all* nursing procedures. A sympathetic approach and the careful use of preventive measures should help each patient to realize that he will not be hurt through clumsiness, thoughtlessness, or a hurried approach. Balme[3] points out that even so ordinary a procedure as the giving of hypodermic or intramuscular injections can be robbed of its terrors for the nervous patient if scrupulous attention is paid to details such as: the site of injection, the sharpness of the needle, the complete relaxation of the part to be injected, the use of a stabbing motion rather than a slow push, the avoidance of injecting a hypodermic injection into the skin, the realization that an intramuscular injection contains irritants to subcutaneous nerves and must therefore be deposited in the muscular layers, and avoidance of injecting too rapidly.

PSYCHOLOGIC ASPECTS OF CARE

Broadly speaking, there are three major areas of psychologic care to be considered in providing relief from pain; these are relieving anxiety, utilizing distraction and diversion, and combating anticipatory fears.

Relieving Anxiety

Excessive anxiety, which pain or the threat of pain often produces, must be reduced or attenuated, since it can lower a patient's pain reaction threshold and trigger systemic responses that make pain harder to combat. Generally, the more severe a patient's anxiety is, the greater will be his overreaction to pain stimulation. Thus, fear of pain and conditions that promote anxiety must be controlled.[13]

Just as anxiety can cause physical illness that may result in pain, so can pain produce anxiety. A few ways to diminish a patient's anxiety are to: let him talk; rub his back; stay with him for a while or at least do not appear rushed during the time you are with him; communicate your empathy; and help the patient to deal with situations that are stressful to him. Unless a patient can be helped to reduce excessive fears and anxieties, he is likely to become caught in the vicious circle depicted in Figure 45–1.

Much pain can be prevented by lessening a patient's fearful attitude toward pain. This can be accomplished in part by: (1) trying to determine the meaning that pain has for the patient, how fearful he is about experiencing pain, and what his reactions to pain are, e.g., physical tension, weeping, silent suffering; (2) helping the patient to describe accurately how he feels and to distinguish between pain and other sources of discomfort, e.g., between a feeling of pressure and one of pain; and (3) talking with the patient about his pain so that he realizes he can communicate with others about it rather than having to suffer alone.

Help the patient to gain some sense of control over the situation he is in.

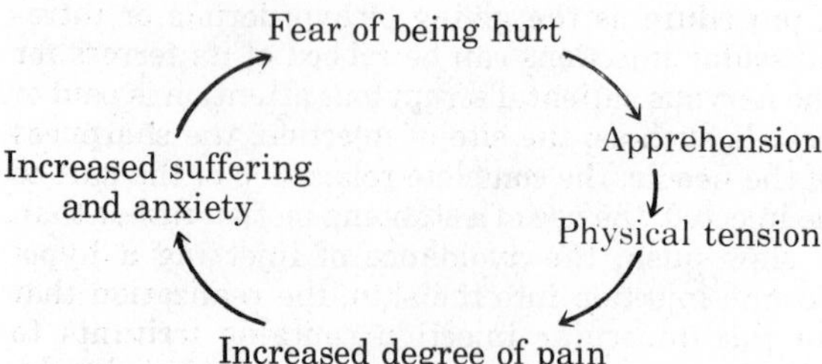

FIGURE 45–1. A vicious cycle of suffering which the nurse strives to break.

A patient's fearful attitude toward pain can also be reduced by helping him to realize that his pain will not necessarily get worse, become as severe as he might have anticipated, or remain as intense as it may be at the moment. Reassurance that everything possible will be done to prevent pain and to lessen pain when it does occur can be most comforting. Another way to reduce the patient's fear of pain is to let him know that he is *not completely helpless* as far as his pain is concerned; he can do a variety of things to help to prevent or lessen his pain, e.g., splint his incision when coughing. Also, he can tell the nurses how best to move him, or he can decide how to move himself in the least painful manner. A patient can also prevent some pain by not waiting until the pain is intense before requesting help for it.

Reassurance and hope increase tolerance for pain.

The nurse can give reassurance and hope and thereby help to keep a patient's morale high. It has, in fact, been observed that in the pain of cancer, the pain may depend more on a patient's morale than on his physical condition. "There can be no pain without involvement of the higher nervous centers and it is how these centers handle, absorb and integrate the pain that will determine its perception and the ability to resist it."[81]

Utilizing Distraction and Diversion

The conversion of a sensation into a painful experience is mainly an emotional reaction or a psychologic phenomenon. Reaction to pain, unlike perception of it, is a complex physiologic and psychologic response involving the highest cognitive mechanisms. In general, the intensity of suffering depends upon the extent to which pain is allowed to dominate the conscious mind.[13] "The use of drugs to alleviate suffering makes us all aware of the relationship between pain and the state of consciousness."[85] *Since pain perception is a conscious process, the nurse can reduce pain perception if she can reduce a patient's conscious awareness of his pain.*

Focusing a patient's attention on a painful procedure will increase his pain; conversely, distracting him may reduce his suffering.[87] There are times when it is necessary for a patient's well-being to focus his attention on his pain, e.g., telling a patient he will have pain associated with a procedure you are performing, such as an injection; and when making a thorough evaluation of the pain and of the helpfulness of measures that have been taken to reduce the pain. However, it is never advisable to excessively focus a patient's attention on what is being done to him or on the pain he is having. Skillful nursing is a combined effort to keep the patient informed and to turn his attention away from himself and his suffering.

Diversion must be carried out with sensitivity on the nurse's part. Attempts at distraction are not so successful in severe pain as in pain that is milder. Appropriate timing and a sincere manner are necessary, or the patient may feel that his pain is being minimized or that it is viewed as "all in his mind" and not real. Distraction maneuvers, therefore, call for skill, subtlety, and planning so that the patient's attention will be diverted to an area of interest and benefit to him. Individualized activities in occupational therapy or vocational rehabilitation may beneficially redirect a patient's concern and attention. Conversation, reading, and television watching are other types of distraction. "Small talk," however, is not a satisfactory diversion; rather it tends to increase the patient's tenseness and discomfort.[124] Likewise, excessive noise is tiring rather than being helpfully distracting. While one patient in pain may want his radio on, another may prefer as quiet an atmosphere as possible.

On the basis of one's individual nature and his past experiences with pain, as well as other life experiences that he has had, each person selects certain patterns of behavior in response to pain that may help to divert his attention from the pain. For example, pacing the floor may reduce one patient's pain, while another clenches his fist, holds his breath, or grasps a bed rail. Frustration ensues if these usual patterns of response are blocked, as they may be by a patient's physical, mental, or environmental circumstances. A patient confined to bed cannot pace the floor, for example, or a patient paralyzed from stroke cannot clench his fist. In situations such as this, the nurse will need to help the patient to identify new ways of coping with his painful situation;[37] he must learn new distractions.

Both *physical activities* and *mental activities* may serve as ways of attenuating or removing pain. In severe pain, *self-hypnosis* and *autosuggestion* may raise the pain threshold and may thus be a source of comfort to a patient. Also, it is possible to distract a patient from his pain by involving him actively with things he can do physically to help himself, e.g., "move your legs," "hold onto the siderail and roll onto your side," "breathe through your mouth."

Patients differ from one another concerning whether they want company if they are having pain. Some patients who are in pain feel most comfortable if they are left by themselves and not disturbed; others desire companionship at such a time and want the nurse to stop by frequently or to have a friend or relative at the bedside. Your sensitivity to such preferences will be appreciated by the patient.[37]

As distractions are reduced, a patient's attention may focus more completely on himself and his pain. Thus, pain often seems worse at night or in the early morning hours when the activities of the daytime are absent.[124]

Combating Anticipatory Fears

As stated earlier in this unit, pain is a combination of reception, perception, and reaction. *Reactions* may be *anticipatory,* occurring prior to the pain-producing stimulus and in expectation of it, or they may occur *after* the perception of pain and as a response to it.

The nurse is in an excellent position to help to combat fearful anticipatory reactions since she is often with a patient when he undergoes painful treatments and because she, herself, may be instrumental in producing some pain. An important nursing service is, thus, to help to prepare a patient to meet the pains that he will have by talking with him about the pain that he fears.[37] Talking about what the patient may expect to happen can help him to relax and to reduce muscle resistance that could be pain-producing; also, the nurse can help a patient to assume correct body alignment and positioning, which can help him to more comfortably tolerate a painful procedure.

It is helpful to patients if they can try to reason out beforehand the extent of discomfort that will be caused by a particular stimulus, e.g., a needle. Thus, it is beneficial to discuss procedures in advance so the patient will have some idea of what to expect. Prior to catheterization, for example, a patient may be told: "You will feel pressure as I insert the tube. It will probably not be painful although it may be uncomfortable."

Mental preparation of a patient preoperatively can help to allay fears of uncontrolled postoperative pain. One common fear about pain is that it will not be controlled or minimized. The preoperative suggestion that medications *will* help to alleviate much postoperative discomfort and that they *will* be given as needed can help a patient to benefit more from his postoperative medications.

As noted in Unit VI, the preoperative teaching of ways in which postoperative discomforts can be minimized or prevented is of great value. "In the fight to control pain, the valuable minutes before the pain commences—when the patient can give his full attention to learning how to cope with it—are indeed too precious not to be fully exploited. In any situation in which a patient could have been taught how to deal with his pain and has not been, a valuable opportunity has been wasted."[37]

The power of suggestion is a useful agent in combating fears of pain—an agent that can serve as the nurse's constant ally in her efforts to prevent or reduce pain. If a patient *believes* that a measure that is taken to reduce his pain *will indeed* reduce his pain, then the measure will often be successful.

It has long been recognized that the personality of a person (e.g., nurse) who is administering a treatment, and that person's verbal and nonverbal suggestions to a patient about the effectiveness of the treatment, play a powerful part in determining the ultimate therapeutic effect. Because this suggestive element is present in clinical care, it should be utilized whenever possible. Thus, a patient who is being given a medication to reduce his pain should enthusiastically and sincerely be told that the medication *will* help to relieve his pain and about when it should begin to be effective. At times a placebo may be ordered for pain relief; this, too, should be administered with an air of confidence that it *will* reduce pain. Of course, the patient is not told that he is receiving a placebo.

> *Gaining the patient's* trust *and* confidence *is of vital importance in pain therapy.*[120]

A *fear of future pain,* rather than present discomfort, may prompt some requests for medications; i.e., some patients will request analgesics on the basis of fear that pain will begin rather than the actual presence of pain. Evaluate whether the fear seems out of proportion to the patient's physical condition.[122] Try to prevent the use of analgesics *in anticipation* of pain rather than for relief of pain. Related to this is the fact that patients may occasionally want more medication than they need for pain relief because they *want to be "knocked out"* so that they can become oblivious to reality.[122] It is not in the long-term best interests of patients to give them more medication than they actually require. If drug usage is controlled, patients having long-term pain are less likely to reach a point at which they cannot obtain relief. Persons experiencing long-term pain need reassurance that their medications are being regulated carefully for their well-being and that every attempt will be made to keep them as comfortable as possible.

> All patients with chronically painful conditions live in dread, partly of the pain increasing in intensity, and partly of the knowledge that there is no effective therapy.[113]

In sum, everything possible should be done to give the patient the feeling that he will be protected from pain and spared pain in all possible ways. Gentleness, patience, and tolerance are essential qualities for the nurse to project when she is caring for the patient in pain. A lack of these will create fear and tension in the patient, causing increased pain and distress, and resistance in cooperation. The patient who is aware that the nurse is trying to do everything possible to avoid pain will be able to relax more readily and will have less pain than if he were tense and fearful.

PHYSICAL ASPECTS OF CARE

General supportive nursing care should be directed at minimizing or relieving any irritations that could lower the patient's pain tolerance. The patient should be kept warm, dry, and comfortable. Backrubs and exercise are also of importance.

In attempting to prevent pain and complications the nurse strives to *protect the patient from pain-producing situations* such as: local irritation or inflammation; muscle spasm or muscle strain; interference with local blood supply or venous and lymphatic drainage; and distention of hollow visceral organs. Specifically, the nurse evaluates each patient to see how she might prevent such painful complications as: infection, thrombophlebitis, decubitus, contractures, muscle strain, muscle spasm, pulmonary congestion, impaired circulation, bladder and bowel distention, and other painful conditions. Moreover, nursing care is planned to avoid further damage to traumatized tissue.[37]

All injured tissue should be handled gently! Lacerated tissue is more sensitive than intact skin and should not have anything dragged across it, e.g., bedcovers, or have adhesive substances, such as dressings, pulled off. Anything adhering to an open wound should be bathed with warm sterile water to soak it off, rather than being pulled off. Open wounds should never have irritating antiseptics, e.g., surgical spirit, tincture of iodine, applied to them. Protective dressings may prevent pain.

Painful dressing changes or pain-producing manipulations, such as bed change, can be planned to be carried out at a time when pain-relieving medications will be having their greatest effect on the patient.

To prevent pain or complications from *drainage tubes,* periodically check the tubes to be certain that they are not caught, stretched, or pulled; they are patent and not kinked, looped, or higher or lower than they should be in relationship to the patient's body plane; and they are in place.

Fatigue can lower tolerance to pain. All activities (including visits from family and friends) should be structured by the nurse so that the patient will not become overly tired. Planned periods of rest will greatly reduce discomfort and should, thus, follow periods of activity.

Immobilization may reduce pain caused by inflammatory lesions as well as pain caused by the interruption of blood supply to some local bodily area. In pain due to inflammation, immobilization reduces pain that would be caused by local pressure or mechanical friction. When pain is due to interruption of a local blood supply, immobilization acts therapeutically by: (1) reducing the oxygen requirements of the tissue that is deprived of its arterial blood supply, and (2) reducing the formation of metabolic wastes that would build up in the area as a result of circulation that is impaired and inadequate to carry wastes away.[27]

Elevation of a swollen part uses the force of gravity to reduce painful swelling. Edematous and casted limbs should be elevated, since increased tissue fluid can produce pain. Elevation facilitates the drainage of fluid by way of the lymph channels and also reduces the production of fluid in the area of inflammation. Also, a sitting position helps to alleviate the pains of cervical lymphadenitis, tonsillitis, and acute sinusitis.

A *position of semiflexion* reduces the pains of those painful joint disorders, e.g., arthritis, in which an increase in pressure within the joint cavity increases the severity of pain. When a joint is partly flexed, the capacity of the joint cavity is greatest, and thus the pressure of synovial fluid is at a minimum.

A *change of position* may help to relieve pain by relieving muscle spasm and reducing muscle strain. Frequent position changes and keeping the patient in good body alignment prevents painful muscle contractions. The patient should be told that his position is being changed to lessen pain. For some patients it is desirable to have a schedule of times posted for position changes as well as suggested positions for each time. The time of position change, the type of position the patient was placed in, and the patient's apparent comfort or discomfort in the position should be charted.

The patient in pain may avoid *movement,* since movement usually increases pain. Explain why certain movements are necessary, e.g., to prevent complications or to ultimately increase comfort. Demonstrate to the patient that future discomfort can be prevented by procedures carried on in the present. When movement is important following a painful procedure, such as following surgery, do patient teaching whenever possible in advance of the procedure so that the patient will expect to move and will know how to do so most comfortably.

The following points are helpful to recall when moving a patient:[11, 124]

> Tell the patient what you are going to do, why the move is necessary, and what he can do to help.

> Listen to the patient's suggestions about the move and do not hurry; give him time to think about the move.

> Let the patient move himself as much as possible since he knows what hurts and you don't. He can protect himself from unnecessary pain better than you can protect him.

> Consider and maintain body alignment and support in preparing for the move and in moving the patient. Utilize knowledge of correct anatomic position and normal range-of-motion of bodily parts. Remember that some painful parts may be fixed by muscular spasms or have range of movements restricted.

> Injured limbs should be held firmly but without being squeezed. Support extremities from underneath, cradling them on the flat of your hand and arm rather than grasping them from above in pinching fashion.

> Have the patient keep his spine stiff and move his body or body parts as a unit. Limbs should be moved as a whole, as support is given to the joints. Never allow a part of a limb to drag while other parts are being moved. While supporting the injured part and letting the patient help, accomplish the move slowly and steadily, stopping if the patient requests you to, and pausing if muscular resistance is incurred.

> If the patient needs help to move, make certain you have adequate help available. Before lifting or moving the patient appoint yourself or another person as leader and inform each helper and the patient what each person is to do, so that everyone will work together as a team. The leader should direct the activities out loud, e.g., "When I count to three we will all move smoothly together. You support Mrs. Jones' head and shoulders and I will lift her legs and buttocks. Mrs. Jones, you try to keep your spine stiff as we move you. Now. Ready? One, two, three." Always have several people help to move a patient with bone and joint problems (e.g., bone cancer) regardless of the patient's size, since these conditions are most painful.

Pillows, braces, casts, or splints may be necessary for the support of painful body parts during movement or for purposes of immobilization. "Splinting" may also be accomplished by manually supporting an area during movement. For example, painful incisions may be splinted with the hands, a folded towel, or a small pillow during periods of postoperative movements, coughing, sneezing, and so forth. Abdominal binders are also a splinting device that may be used postoperatively to give added support to the incisional area during periods of stress.

Following a move, *arrange pillows* so that they support and relax all muscles acting on an injured part and so that proper alignment is maintained. Also, combine gentle traction with the support of an injured limb.

The accumulation of toxic substances in muscles can be a cause of muscle pain. *Massage* can relieve such pain since it increases the flow of blood to the area. This, in turn, relieves hypoxemia and carries off some of the toxins that have accumulated. However, remember:

> Never *massage the calf of the leg! Since blood clots may form in that area, massage could break loose the clots and possibly cause a fatal embolism.*

Hot and cold applications,[27, 37] e.g., wet compresses or dry heat, are useful in relieving some pains by: (1) altering the rate and volume of regional blood flow; (2) decreasing pain sensitivity; and (3) relieving muscle spasm. Heat acts, generally, by producing a depressing action on the central nervous system; cold produces a local anesthetic effect. The specific actions of hot and cold applications are outlined below:

Hot Applications

Dilate local superficial blood vessels.
Increase blood flow (perhaps more than doubling the flow).
Increase capillary pressure, thus causing more transudation of fluid through capillary walls with increased lymph formation and accelerated lymph flow.
Reduce local inflammatory swellings, reduce tissue pressure, and reduce pain from pressure.
Reduce painful muscle spasm by causing muscle to relax.
Increase peristaltic movement in intestines if the abdominal wall is heated. (This is important in treating painful abdominal distention caused by paralytic ileus of the bowel.)

Cold Applications

Constrict local superficial blood vessels.
Decrease blood flow.
Produce temporary reduction of inflammatory swelling which, in turn, reduces pain.
Reduce pain sensitivity since marked chilling acts as a local anesthetic.
Decrease peristaltic movement in intestines if the abdominal wall is cooled. (This is important in the treatment of inflammatory disorders in the peritoneal cavity since intestinal immobilization slows down spread of infection.)

PHARMACOLOGIC ASPECTS OF CARE

Before a nurse is qualified to administer analgesic agents, she should possess knowledge of the nature of pain and the processes through which it is mediated.[55] Also, in order to effectively administer pain medications, the nurse will need to familiarize herself with expected patterns of pain. For example, the intensity of postoperative pain is related to the type of anesthetic used as well as to the patient and his operation.

> *The aim of giving pain medications should be to control the pain while preserving the patient's personality and maintaining his morale.*

These goals should be attained ideally without upsetting the patient's clarity of vision, his digestion, bowel function, or balance.[51]

Guidelines

As you administer analgesic medications you may find the following guidelines helpful to recall:

> Just as people vary in their responses to pain, they vary in their sensitivity to pain and to pain-relieving drugs.

> Individual patients may require different doses of an analgesic, and the same patient may also, at different times, have a variable requirement.[55]

> Pain relief should provide comfort without producing harm as a result of the medications administered.

> Use potent narcotics wisely by avoiding excessive or unnecessary administration. Avoid administering narcotics on a "routine" basis in the absence of actual need.

> Use non-narcotic drugs, rather than narcotics, if they will relieve symptoms.

> Know the basic actions, doses, routes of administration, side effects, and precautions for use of analgesic agents prior to their administration.

> Chart the apparent effectiveness of the analgesic and chart and report any apparent side effects, e.g., drug dependency, respiratory depression.

> Opiates should be used with extreme caution in patients with increased intracranial pressure, hepatic insufficiency, severe CNS depression, myxedema, acute alcoholism, delirium tremens, convulsive disorders, and Addison's disease.

> When patients are being treated with several medications simultaneously, patterns of drug interactions must be considered in selecting narcotic analgesics. For example, severe adverse reactions have been reported in patients receiving monoamine oxidase inhibitors who were given meperidine for pain. (Reactions of this nature have not been reported for morphine.) Similarly, chlorpromazine may intensify and prolong the respiratory depression produced by meperidine.

> Timing *is more important to successful pain chemotherapy than is drug or dose or interval.*[70]

Early, adequate relief is an important principle in pain therapy, because if pain can be treated effectively soon after its onset, it is relatively easier to control. The longer a patient suffers, the greater his apprehension becomes and, consequently, the more difficult it becomes to achieve pain relief with medications.[70]

It is *not* considered to be good practice to administer analgesic agents *routinely*. Too often one finds "routine" pre- and postoperative medication orders. As we have emphasized, reactivity to pain is highly variable from one individual to another. A "routine" approach to pain therapy ignores individual patient variability and can thereby result in either overuse or underuse of analgesics. This results in either: (1) a negation of the potential strength of the analgesic, with consequent inadequate pain relief, or (2) "snowing" the patient and increasing the incidence of undesirable side effects. Analgesic agents of appropriate strength need to be utilized for the varying degrees of pain that individual patients are experiencing. As the pain increases so must the potency of the drug; the opposite is also true. *Both the prescription and the administration of a drug should be tailored to meet each patient's individual needs.*

Only a very incomplete idea of the intensity of pain can be obtained from the *quantity* of drugs that patients may require. It has been observed that patients with pain that is constant and of moderate intensity have a far greater drug requirement than those with transient, intense pain.[113]

Working with the Physician

Physician and nurse must coordinate their efforts to provide pain relief.

In some situations analgesics are withheld until diagnosis of the patient's condition is established. Analgesics may be contraindicated for a period of time because they may mask or confuse the diagnosis. However, once the diagnosis is made, appropriate pain relief is in order.[55]

> *Because pain often is an important diagnostic aid (e.g., abdominal pain), it is frequently hazardous to administer analgesics before the cause of pain is reliably determined.*[141]

Generally analgesic medications are ordered on a *p.r.n. basis,* with specific directions concerning the drug, the dose, and the time interval between doses. However, the actual administration of the drug or its timing is left to the nurse's discretion. Sound nursing judgment is called for when pain-relieving medications and treatments are ordered p.r.n.

Physicians may leave more than one analgesic order for a patient, and it is up to the nurse to decide which medication to administer at the appropriate time. Moreover, at times more than one dosage may be ordered, so that the nurse must decide which she should administer. Such flexibility of orders permits the patient to receive medication that is appropriate to meet his variable needs. Thus, pain relief can be made adequate while avoiding overmedication or inadequate medication. A system of this nature is obviously advantageous; however, at the same time it requires that the nurse make informed decisions based on numerous facts about analgesics, such as their: benefits; side effects; indications; contraindications; duration and onset of action; typical doses; routes of administration; mixing properties with other medications; and the type of pain they most effectively relieve.

The effectiveness of medications given for the relief of pain should be *charted.* The nurse should check patients approximately one-half hour after they receive analgesics. The effects of the analgesic should be charted as well as the duration of pain relief. From such charting, doctors and other nurses will be able to discern which medications are most effective, and in what doses. Information about *which drugs* are effective and *how much* medicine is used can be helpful to the physician in diagnosing the etiology of a patient's pain. By knowing how much medicine is used the doctor can also form an opinion of the patient's general condition, especially with regard to his renal function. When a patient's drug requirement is high, it must be determined whether his pain is great enough to require such high doses of medications, or whether he is addicted to drugs.[113]

Working with the Patient

At times the nurse may *plan with the patient* when he may need medication; at other times the nurse will make such a decision on the basis of her own judgment. Obviously the administration of ordered medications for the relief of pain must be based on the nurse's anticipation of the patient's needs, as well as on her own observations of the signs and symptoms of pain.

As previously mentioned, it is well recognized that the efficiency of drug therapy is not solely dependent upon the nature of the drugs. Therefore, even though pain in severe physical disease has a physiologic basis, psychologic mechanisms greatly influence a patient's reaction.[16] Such *psychologic factors* need consideration in planning care. The nurse administering medications for purposes of pain relief should always make use of the augmentative effect on drug therapy that the *situation,* the *personality* and *attitude of the person administering the drug,* and the *patient's suggestibility* have on the results achieved.[37]

The very presence of the nurse should indicate to the patient her willingness to help. This is an important first step in pain therapy.[17] "Giving a medication" involves both the process of "giving" and "the medication" itself. The two are inseparable, but often the nurse's manner or attitude in giving medications does not receive sufficient attention. As we have previously indicated, the power of suggestion is strong and is a power that should be used in administering medications. Thus, when a medication is being given for pain relief, the patient might experience greater relief if he is told, "This medication will help to relieve your pain. I'll check back with you in a little while to see how you are feeling."

Prior to administering an analgesic, place the patient in a *comfortable position* and attend to other activities that will help the patient to relax generally, e.g., open the window and draw the curtain. Plan your care and the activities of others (e.g., other staff members, visitors) so that once the medication is given the patient will not be disturbed further.

Following administration of an analgesic allow the patient to rest so that the medication's helpful effects can provide maximum relief. With most narcotics dizziness and vomiting are observed more often in ambulatory patients than in those who are in bed. *Patients receiving narcotics should remain in bed, have siderails up, and be transported by stretcher.*

CHRONIC, INTRACTABLE PAIN[81]

General Considerations

As previously mentioned, there are some individuals whose pains become chronic and intractable in nature. When pain cannot be relieved by physical means, the nurse may find some of the following suggestions and insights helpful.

After working for 10 years with patients suffering chronic pain from neoplastic conditions, LeShan reached the following philosophic conclusions about chronic pain and the world of the patient in pain of long duration:[81]

> The patient in chronic, intractable pain lives during his waking moments in the cosmos of a nightmare. There are three basic similarities between the terror dream and the universe of the patient in chronic pain: (1) terrible things are being done to the person and worse are threatened; (2) others, or outside forces are in control and the will is helpless; and (3) there is no time limit set and one can, therefore, not predict when it will end.

> The above factors give rise to fearful feelings of helplessness and uncertainty, leading to a sense of futility. The patient's futility is made worse by the fact that his pain seems to serve no purpose in his life—it is meaningless and inexplicable.

> Meaningless and purposeless suffering is much harder for a person to accept and resist than pain that the subject can place in a coherent frame of reference.

> Chronic pain indicates only a state of existence; it does not warn or tell us what to do, in the way that acute pain does. It does not help us to act. Instead, it may be so severe that it disrupts potentially useful habits and activities.

> It is important to ourselves that we *respond* to strong stimuli, that we are connected to and react to our environment. However, this is difficult with chronic pain, since we are pushed toward suffering rather than reacting. Thus, we cannot act, we can only bear.

> When filled with pain, a patient is pulled to the immediate present, and goals for the future are lost. Pain forces personal existence to continue with little assistance from our usual orientations, defenses, safeguards, and associations.

We should not leave the chronically suffering individual alone and suspended in his pain-filled existence. Let us identify some actions that can be taken to lessen suffering through effective clinical care of the patient experiencing intractable pain.

One of the hardest basic tasks of a nurse is to help such a patient to formulate for himself suitable meanings for his pain that are not based on old guilts, fears, and anxieties. Each patient must be helped to find a meaning that makes sense to *him*, whether or not it makes sense to the nurse.[81] For example, if the patient is from a different cultural or social background than the nurse, the nurse must realize that this patient may have an entirely different set of values from her own. Instead of imposing her values on the patient, she should help the patient to reaffirm his own values and rediscover his own meaning in life.

Emphasis can helpfully be placed upon the patient's ability to find purpose and meaning in his life in spite of his difficult circumstances and his hopeless feelings about the future. The fact should be emphasized that no one, sick or well, knows the future. We, as human beings, can only hope that we shall live to have a future, but there is no guarantee. Such insecurity is a universal human condition, the reality of which must be accepted.[81] When a patient having chronic pain has lost interest in the present and has lost hope in the future, he needs the nurse's encouragement to turn his energies outward from the pain to other activities and to establish new goals. LeShan points out that the therapist must avoid being too gentle with the patient who needs such direction. High demands imply high respect, and consequently give strength to the patient.[81]

When the nurse helps her patient to set up new goals, she must remember that these goals are for a patient who is an individual; consequently, the goal must suit the individual patient's needs rather than the nurse's needs.[63]

A sense of loneliness is said to haunt sufferers of chronic pain, since the patient in pain cannot share his feelings of pain with others so that others may realize his suffering. He can only try to express his feelings in words or actions that frequently are not structured to fully communicate the depth of his pain or despair. In such a situation the nurse must make every attempt, even in minor ways, to let the patient know that she understands him, uncritically accepts him, and has an appreciation for what he is enduring.

The nurse who understands that she is not concerned with a sensation (pain) but rather with a human being experiencing a sensation will make a conscious effort to bring a sense of companionship to even the most lonely sufferer. "The nurse may decide that in a particular situation the most appropriate ministration is not a *doing* but a *being*. Just being there as a nonverbal comforter or a listener may help the patient to drain off psychic pressure which has translated itself into physical pain."[69]

We have indicated that the patient in chronic pain has been described as living in a nightmare—a terrible and timeless cosmos in which the patient feels helpless and alone. How can a patient who lives in such a waking state be helped? Hundreds of years ago Spinoza wrote, "Suffering ceases to be suffering as soon as we form a clear and precise picture of it." This statement implies that knowledge of precisely what is happening to cause suffering will help to abate the suffering. The patient must be helped to *reach conscious awareness* of the "nightmare" in which he lives, so that he can better understand it and accept it.[81] If the doctor and nurse could clarify for the patient why he has pain and why he is afraid of the pain, it might help to relieve much of the nightmare quality of the patient's existence.

Also, it may help some persons having chronic pain to realize that the experience of pain, though unique to each individual, is also a *universal* experience, touching all people at some time in their lives. Albert Schweitzer wrote eloquently of "a fellowship of pain" in which human beings all over the world are united by the desire to be free from pain.[81] The individual sufferer who realizes that he has a common bond and shares a common problem with all people who suffer pain, may, through his identification with mankind, lose some of his sense of hopeless isolation in a nightmare.

One final insight concerning chronic, intractable pain is this: Remember that for some individuals, *pain serves positive functions* as: (1) a form of communication, an attempt to say something that words alone cannot convey[81] and (2) a means of adaptation to the world.[44] Pain, thus, for some persons, fills an inner need and acts to maintain the psychodynamic structure of the person. LeShan observes that "our cultural orientation towards pain that it is evil and must be immediately relieved is so strong that, in spite of our knowledge of the cases when chronic pain has been relieved, to be followed immediately by emotional breakdown or suicide, we often ignore this problem."[81]

Long-Term Pain Chemotherapy

In treating patients having severe *chronic pain* of *nonmalignant* origin, narcotic analgesics must be given judiciously. The development of addiction could ultimately cause the patient greater distress than his momentary pain. Only during episodes of severe pain should one of the potentially less addicting narcotics (e.g., codeine) be used for a brief period along with large doses of non-narcotic analgesics.[135]

While addiction poses potential problems, the nurse must guard against withholding *necessary* medication for fear that addiction will occur. If a patient is in need of a narcotic, has it ordered, and shows no toxic effects, then the nurse should not indiscriminately prolong the interval between narcotics or withhold them. Signs of tolerance to narcotics should, of course, be observed for and reported, but it is ultimately the physician's decision whether the medication regimen should be changed. Patients in pain whose analgesics are indiscriminately withheld by the nurse will become fearful, panic-stricken, and angry. They will lose confidence in both the staff and the ability of their medications to lessen their pains. Moreover, their pain may increase to an intolerable intensity, taxing the limits of human suffering.

Narcotics should be avoided as a *primary* medication for controlling pain in *chronic* pain syndromes. When they are used, their usage should be intermittent, at most. Even when this is done, it is not unusual to note that the patient begins to request the narcotic with increasing frequency and at shorter intervals. The mildest drugs should be used first, with the doses spaced as far apart as possible and with the lowest effective dosage being used. In some situations the patient may be given a narcotic if the pain cannot be controlled on a given day. Generally, however, the morning and noontime medications should be non-narcotic. The dose of a narcotic ordered at night may be larger than that used at other times.[120]

Adequate therapy for pain, particularly when the pain is expected to continue for some time, brings with it the problems of increasing requirements, by the patient, of the narcotic medication prescribed, with ultimate tolerance, dependence, and addiction.[75]

One means of trying to avoid (or at least to prolong the occurrence of) the above problems is to utilize other agents, nonanalgesic in themselves, to potentiate the action of the analgesics by sedation and tranquilization of the patient. Therapy of this nature is an attempt to reduce the patient's discomfort to what might be considered a baseline, in order for treatment with minimal doses of narcotic agents to be as effective as possible.[75]

Pain tends to be worse when it occurs at night; it interferes with sleep and consequently makes a patient tense and exhausted during the day. The sedative hypnotic drugs are useful adjuncts to pain therapy. Sleeplessness is, in itself, a difficult clinical problem to manage, since habituation, tolerance, and mild addiction are potential problems. As a general rule, the nonbarbiturate hypnotics are useful since they are typically faster acting than barbiturates (usually act within 15 or 20 minutes) and they are short-acting, thereby causing relatively little feeling of "hangover."[120]

With prolonged pain chemotherapy the development of toxic manifestations may preclude the use of many excellent analgesics unless frequent, careful observations of the patient are made. Particularly in treating chronic pain, it is necessary that laboratory work and physical follow-up examinations be done periodically. When these details are attended to conscientiously, it is possible to prevent iatrogenic diseases that might be caused by prolonged analgesic usage. Some of the more common side effects to be anticipated are those affecting the hematologic, renal, hepatic, and dermatologic systems.[75] Thus, in situations of prolonged pain management the physician usually tries to prescribe the minimal dosage of medication that will control pain. An attempt is also made to use least potent drugs first, in order to save the more powerful drugs for later use and to prevent addiction.

ABSENCE OF PAIN

The destruction that can occur in the absence of pain demonstrates its value. Some cancers are painless until they become well entrenched and have spread to adjacent areas. A patient whose legs are without sensation owing to a spinal injury will not feel the pain of an overheated hot-water bottle, and severe burns may result.[124]

While the nurse is most frequently involved with caring for patients experiencing chronic and acute pains, she will also have patients in her care who *lack* the ability to experience pain. Such persons lack the sensory coordination that is necessary for the perception and interpretation of pain. A few persons are *born with* this deficit, but it occurs more commonly as a result of *injury,* e.g., traumatic severance of the spinal cord; *disease* process, e.g., tabes dorsalis; or *therapy,* e.g., neurolytic nerve block or surgical severance of sensory branches of nerves.

Persons lacking the protective mechanism of pain are handicapped in some ways and are less perfectly equipped to withstand the hazards of the environment. As a result, repeated traumatic incidents leading to severe tissue damage may be endured unconsciously when pain is absent, e.g., deep perforating ulcers of the feet may occur in tabes dorsalis.[92]

A prime goal of nursing therapy for patients who lack awareness of pain is to prevent injury and to teach the patient how he can prevent injury.

Without awareness of heat, pressure, and pain it is difficult to realize when tissue is injured. Thus, if tissue is in contact with injurious agents, is exposed to noxious agents for a dangerous length of time, or is exposed to them in dangerous amounts, unnoticed injury will result. Both patient and nurse must learn to think *ahead* to prevent injury by protecting and frequently inspecting affected areas for signs of injury that may already have occurred.

> Prevent burns from radiators, hot water, heating pads, electric elements, cigarettes.

> Prevent cuts, scrapes and bruises, e.g., from wheelchairs.

> Prevent pressure sores. Use alternating pressure mattress, sheepskin, cradle; keep bed free from wrinkles and crumbs.

> Teach patient to change his position, lift himself up, smooth his clothing and bed linens, and inspect his skin at least every two hours for redness or blanching. Perform these activities for patients who cannot help themselves.

References for Unit IX

1. Alling, C. C., III, et al. (eds.): *Facial Pain.* Philadelphia, Lea & Febiger, 1968.
2. Analgesics: The special challenge of chronic pain. *Patient Care* 6:135, March 15, 1972.

3. Balme, H.: Principles of treatment. *In* Ogilvie, W., and Thomson, W. (eds.): *Pain and Its Problems.* London, Eyre and Spottiswoode, 1950.
4. Bandler, R. J., Jr., et al.: Self-observation as a source of pain perception. *Journal of Personality and Social Psychology* (Washington) 9:205, July, 1968.
5. Batterman, R. C.: Pain relief with analgesic agents. *Disease-a-Month* 1:43, August, 1968.
6. Battista, A. F.: Subarachnoid cold saline wash for pain relief. *Archives of Surgery* 103:672, December, 1971.
7. Beecher, H. K.: Pain in men wounded in battle. *Bulletin U. S. Army Medical Department* 5:445, 1946.
8. Beecher, H. K.: Relationship of wound to pain experienced. *J.A.M.A.* 161:1609, 1956.
9. Beecher, H. K.: An inspection of our working hypotheses in the study of pain and other subjective responses in man. *In* Keele, C. A., and Smith, R. (eds.): *International Symposium on the Assessment of Pain in Man and Animals.* Edinburgh, E. and S. Livingstone, Ltd., 1962.
10. Beecher, H. K.: Anxiety and pain. *J.A.M.A.* 209: 1080, August 18, 1969.
11. Beland, I. L.: *Clinical Nursing: Pathophysiological and Psychosocial Approaches.* 2nd ed. New York, The Macmillan Company, 1970.
12. Bellville, J. W., et al.: Influence of age on pain relief from analgesics. A study of postoperative patients. *J.A.M.A.* 217:1835, September 27, 1971.
13. Blaylock, J.: The pathological and cultural influences on the reaction to pain: A review of the literature. *Nursing Forum* 7:263, 1968.
14. Bobey, M. J., et al.: Psychological factors affecting pain tolerance. *Journal of Psychosomatic Research* 14:371, December, 1970.
15. Boehm, G.: At last–A nonaddicting substitute for morphine. *Today's Health* 46:69, April, 1968.
16. Bond, M. R., and Pilowsky, I.: Subjective assessment of pain and its relationship to the administration of analgesics in patients with advanced cancer. *Journal of Psychosomatic Research* 10:203, September, 1966.
17. Bonica, J. J.: *Clinical Applications of Diagnostic and Therapeutic Nerve Blocks.* Springfield, Illinois, Charles C Thomas, 1959.
18. Bonica, J. J.: Management of intractable pain. *In* Way, E. L. (ed.): *New Concepts in Pain and Its Clinical Management.* Philadelphia, F. A. Davis Company, 1967.
19. Bonica, J. J.: Introduction. *In* Alling, C. C., III, et al. (eds.): *Facial Pain.* Philadelphia, Lea & Febiger, 1968.
20. Bonner, C. D., et al.: The team approach to hemiplegia. *Postgraduate Medicine* 40:708, December, 1966.
21. Boshes, B., and Arieff, A.: Clinical experience in the neurologic substance of pain. *Medical Clinics of North America* 52:111, January, 1968.
22. Botton, J. E.: Neurosurgical procedures for the management of intractable pain. *Clinical Orthopaedics and Related Research* 73:101, November–December, 1970.
23. Boucher, J. D.: Facial displays of fear, sadness, and pain. *Perceptual and Motor Skills* 28:239, February, 1969.
24. Brain, L.: Presidential address. *In* Keele, C. A., and Smith, R. (eds.): *International Symposium on the Assessment of Pain in Man and Animals.* Edinburgh, E. and S. Livingstone, Ltd., 1962.
25. Bronzo, A., Jr., et al.: Relationship of anxiety with pain threshold. *Journal of Psychology* 66:181, July, 1967.
26. Bruegel, M. A.: Relationship of preoperative anxiety to perception of postoperative pain. *Nursing Research* 20:26, January-February, 1970.
27. Brunner, L. S., et al.: *Textbook of Medical-Surgical Nursing.* 2nd ed. Philadelphia, J. B. Lippincott Company, 1970.
28. Buytendjik, F. J. J.: *Pain: Its Modes and Functions.* Chicago, University of Chicago Press, 1962.
29. Cahn, J., and Herold, M.: Pain and psychotropic drugs. *In* Soulairac, A., Cahn, J., and Charpentier, J. (eds.): *Pain.* New York, Academic Press, Inc., 1968.
30. Campbell, D.: The management of pain in the intensive care unit. *British Journal of Surgery* 57:721, October, 1970.
31. Carini, E., and Owens, G.: *Neurological and Neurosurgical Nursing.* 5th ed. St. Louis, The C. V. Mosby Company, 1970.
32. Carruyo, L., et al.: The effect of narcotics and narcotic-antagonists on the electrical activity of the brain: Its relationship with their pain-obtunding activity. *In* Soulairac, A., Cahn, J., and Charpentier, J. (eds.): *Pain.* New York, Academic Press, Inc., 1968.
33. Cashatt, B.: Pain: A patient's view. *American Journal of Nursing* 72:281, February, 1972.
34. Chaffee, E., and Greisheimer, E.: *Basic Physiology and Anatomy.* 2nd ed. Philadelphia, J. B. Lippincott Company, 1969.
35. Chambers, W. G., and Price, G. G.: Influence of nurse upon effects of analgesics administered. *Nursing Research* 16:228, Summer, 1967.
36. Copple, D.: What can a nurse do to relieve pain without résort to drugs? *Nursing Times* 68:584, May 11, 1972.
37. Crowley D. M.: *Pain and Its Alleviation.* Los Angeles, School of Nursing, UCLA, 1962.
38. de Grood, M. P.: Stereotaxic treatment of pain. *Journal of Neurology, Neurosurgery and Psychiatry* 34:106, February, 1971.
39. Derrick, W. S.: Subarachnoid alcohol block in the control of pain. *CA* 21:249, July-August, 1971.
40. Ditzler, J. W.: Epidural anesthesia in the management of pain. *Medical Clinics of North America* 52:209, January, 1968.
41. Dorsey, J. M.: Problems with pain in a general surgical practice. *Medical Clinics of North America* 52: 103, January, 1968.
42. DuGas, B. W.: *Kozier-DuGas Introduction to Patient Care.* 2nd ed. Philadelphia, W. B. Saunders Company, 1972.
43. Dundee, J. W.: Management of chronic pain. *Transactions of the Medical Society of London* 85:153, 1969.
44. Engel, G.: Psychogenic pain and the pain-prone patient. *American Journal of Medicine* 26:899, June, 1959.
45. Engel, G.: Psychogenic pain. *Journal of Occupational Medicine* 3:249, 1961.
46. Finneson, B.: *Diagnosis and Management of Pain Syndromes.* 2nd ed. Philadelphia, W. B. Saunders Company, 1969.
47. Fisher, A. L.: The psychiatric aspects of pain. *Headache* 7:63, July, 1967.
48. Fitzgerald, G.: When you feel pain. *Science Digest* 42:61, August, 1957.
49. Fordyce, W. E.: Operant conditioning as a treatment method in the management of selected chronic

pain problems. *Northwest Medicine* 69:580, August, 1970.
50. Frances, L. E.: Clinical applications, analgesics. *In* Alling, C. C., III, et al. (eds.): *Facial Pain.* Philadelphia, Lea & Febiger, 1968.
51. Garland, D.: The care of the dying. *Nursing Times* 64:355, March 15, 1968.
52. Gildea, J.: The relief of postoperative pain. *Medical Clinics of North America* 52:81, January, 1968.
53. Gillman, J.: Pain relief and other effects following barbotage. *Lancet* 1:746, April 1, 1972.
54. Griem, M. L.: The radiologist and the relief of pain. *Medical Clinics of North America* 52:203, January, 1968.
55. Grollman, A.: Use of drugs in relief of pain. *In* Finneson, B.: *Diagnosis and Management of Pain Syndromes.* 2nd ed. Philadelphia, W. B. Saunders Company, 1969.
56. Gunn, W. G., et al.: Palliation of pain in cancer patients. *GP* 40:125, September, 1969.
57. Guzman, F., and Lim, R. K. S.: The mechanism of action of the non-narcotic analgesics. *Medical Clinics of North America* 52:3, January, 1968.
58. Hackett, T. P.: Pain and prejudice. Why do we doubt that the patient is in pain? *Medical Times* 99:130, February, 1971.
59. Harris, A. B.: Critical evaluation and the neurosurgical treatment of pain. *Northwest Medicine* 69:576, August, 1970.
60. Hassenplug, L. W.: Introduction. *In* Crowley, D. M.: *Pain and Its Alleviation.* Los Angeles, School of Nursing, UCLA, 1962.
61. Hilgard, E. R.: Pain as a puzzle for psychology and physiology. *American Psychologist* 24:103, February, 1969.
62. Holmes, G.: Some clinical aspects of pain. *In* Ogilvie, W., and Thomson, W. (eds.): *Pain and Its Problems.* London, Eyre and Spottiswoode, 1950.
63. Hunter, J.: The mark of pain. *American Journal of Nursing* 61:96, October, 1961.
64. Inman, V. T.: Clinical pathologic consideration of pain mechanism. *In* Way, E. L. (ed.): *New Concepts in Pain and Its Clinical Management.* Philadelphia, F. A. Davis Company, 1967.
65. Jacob, S. W., and Francone, C. A.: *Structure and Function in Man.* 2nd ed. Philadelphia, W. B. Saunders Company, 1970.
66. Jaffee, J.: Narcotics in the treatment of pain. *Medical Clinics of North America* 52:33, January, 1968.
67. Kahn, J. P.,: How a psychiatrist looks at pain. *Medical Times* 98:127, December, 1970.
68. Kane, J., Jr., et al.: A case of congenital indifference to pain. *Diseases of the Nervous System* 29:409, June, 1968.
69. Kaufman, M. A., and Brown, D. E.: Pain wears many faces. *American Journal of Nursing* 61:48, January, 1961.
70. Keats, A. S.: Use of analgetics at the bedside. *In* Way, E. L. (ed.): *New Concepts in Pain and Its Clinical Management.* Philadelphia, F. A. Davis Company, 1967.
71. Keele, C. A., and Smith, R. (eds.): *International Symposium on the Assessment of Pain in Man and Animals. London, 1961.* Edinburgh, E. and S. Livingstone, 1962.
72. Kent, J. R.: Nursing care of the patient with a percutaneous cordotomy. *Journal of Neurosurgical Nursing* 1:53, October, 1969.
73. Klein, R. F., and Brown, W.: Pain descriptions in the medical setting. *Journal of Psychosomatic Research* 10:367, 1967.
74. Knighton, R. S., and Dumke, P. R. (eds.): *Pain: International Symposium on Pain.* Henry Ford Hospital. Boston, Little, Brown and Company, 1966.
75. Kolodny, A. L., and McLoughlin, P. T.: *Comprehensive Approach to the Therapy of Pain.* Springfield, Illinois, Charles C Thomas, 1966.
76. Lasagna, L.: Use of analgetics in clinical practice. *In* Way, E. L. (ed.): *New Concepts in Pain and Its Clinical Management.* Philadelphia, F. A. Davis Company, 1967.
77. Lauer, J. W.: Hypnosis in the relief of pain. *Medical Clinics of North America* 52:217, January, 1968.
78. Leake, C. D.: Introduction. *In* Way, E. L. (ed.): *New Concepts in Pain and Its Clinical Management.* Philadelphia, F. A. Davis Company, 1967.
79. Leffert, R. D.: Neurophysiology of pain. *Bulletin of the Hospital for Joint Diseases* 31:199, October, 1970.
80. Leksell, L.: Some principles and technical aspects of stereotaxic surgery. *In* Knighton, R. S., and Dumke, P. R. (eds.): *International Symposium on Pain.* Boston, Little, Brown and Company, 1966.
81. LeShan, L.: The world of the patient in severe pain of long duration. *Journal of Chronic Diseases* 17:119, 1964.
82. Lim, R. K. S.: Pharmacologic viewpoint of pain and analgesia. *In* Way, E. L. (ed.): *New Concepts in Pain and Its Clinical Management.* Philadelphia, F. A. Davis Company, 1967.
83. Lim, R. K. S.: Sites of action of narcotic and non-narcotic analgesics: Mechanism of pain and analgesia. *Headache* 7:103, October, 1967.
84. Lishman, W. A.: The psychology of pain. *Nursing Times* 66:1577, December, 1970.
85. Livingston, W. K.: What is pain? Reprinted from *Scientific American,* March, 1953. San Francisco, California, W. H. Freeman and Company, 1953.
86. Locke, S.: The neurological aspects of coma. *Surgical Clinics of North America* 48:251, April, 1968.
87. MacBryde, C. (ed.): *Signs and Symptoms: Applied Pathologic Physiology and Clinical Interpretation.* 4th ed. Philadelphia, J. B. Lippincott Company, 1964.
88. Markham, M. M.: The relief of pain. *Nursing Times* 66:1579, December 10, 1970.
89. McBride, M. D.: Pain and effective nursing practice. *ANA Clinical Sessions, 1966.* New York, Appleton-Century-Crofts, 1967, p. 75.
90. McBride, M. D.: The additive to the analgesic. *American Journal of Nursing* 69:974, May, 1969.
91. McCaffery, M.: *Nursing Management of the Patient with Pain.* Philadelphia, J. B. Lippincott Company, 1972.
92. McCaffery, M., and Moss, F.: Nursing intervention for bodily pain. *American Journal of Nursing* 67:1224, June, 1967.
93. Meares, A.: *Relief Without Drugs: The Self-Management of Tension, Anxiety, and Pain.* Garden City, New York, Doubleday, 1967.
94. Merskey, H.: Psychologic aspects of pain. *Postgraduate Medical Journal* 44:297, April, 1968.
95. Merskey, H.: Pain. *Nursing Times* 67:988, August 12, 1971.
96. Merskey, H., and Spear, F. G.: *Pain: Psychological and Psychiatric Aspects.* London, Baillière, Tindall and Cassell, 1967.
97. Merskey, H., et al.: The concept of pain. *Journal of Psychosomatic Research* 11:59, June, 1967.

98. Mettler, F. A.: Pain, I: What is it? *The Journal of the Medical Society of New Jersey* 61:10, January, 1964.
99. Moran, Lord: The meaning and measurement of pain. *In* Ogilvie, W., and Thomson, W. (eds.): *Pain and Its Problems*. London, Eyre and Spottiswoode, 1950.
100. Mörch, E. T.: Pain relief for office procedures. *Medical Clinics of North America* 52:173, January, 1968.
101. Moss, F. T.: The effect of a nursing intervention on pain relief. *ANA Regional Clinical Conferences*, 1967. New York, Appleton-Century-Crofts, 1968, p. 247.
102. Mullan, S.: Modern techniques in the management of pain. *Illinois Medical Journal* 133:598, May, 1968.
103. Murray, J. B.: The puzzle of pain. *Perceptual and Motor Skills* 28:887, June, 1969.
104. Murray, J. B.: Psychology of the pain experience. *Journal of Psychology* 78:193, July, 1971.
105. Noordenbos, W.: Physiological correlates of clinical pain syndromes. *In* Soulairac, A., Cahn, J., and Charpentier, J. (eds.): *Pain*. New York, Academic Press, Inc., 1968.
106. Ogilvie, W. H., and Thomson, W. A. R. (eds.): *Pain and Its Problems*. London, Eyre and Spottiswoode, 1950.
107. Parker, R. G.: Pain relief for the cancer patient through selective radiation therapy. *Northwest Medicine* 69:665, September, 1970.
108. Pennmann, J.: Pain as an old friend. *Lancet* 1:633, 1954.
109. Petrie, A.: *Individuality in Pain and Suffering*. Chicago, University of Chicago Press, 1967.
110. Pilling, L. F.: Psychosomatic aspects of facial pain. *In* Alling, C. C., III, et al. (eds.): *Facial Pain*. Philadelphia, Lea & Febiger, 1968.
111. Poswillo, D. E.: Pharmacodynamics of pain relief. *In* Alling, C. C., III, et al. (eds.): *Facial Pain*. Philadelphia, Lea & Febiger, 1968.
112. Raney, J. O.: Pain, emotion and a rationale for therapy. *Northwest Medicine* 69:659, September, 1970.
113. Rasmussen, P.: *Facial Pain*. Copenhagen, Ejnar Munksgaard, 1965.
114. Richardson, D. E.: Recent advances in the neurosurgical control of pain. *Southern Medical Journal* 60:1082, October 6, 1967.
115. Rickels, K.: *Non-Specific Factors in Drug Therapy*. Springfield, Illinois, Charles C Thomas, 1968.
116. Rodman, M. J.: Muscle relaxants: The drugs of many uses. *RN* 27:59, August, 1964.
117. Rodman, M. J.: Drugs for neuromuscular pain and spasm. *RN* 29:62, May, 1966.
118. Rodman, M. J.: Drugs for pain problems. *RN* 34:59, April, 1971.
119. Rose, A. S.: Anxiety and pain. *J.A.M.A.* 210:1103, November 10, 1969.
120. Sadove, M. S., and Albrecht, R.: Sedatives and tranquilizers in the treatment of pain. *Medical Clinics of North America* 52:47, January, 1968.
121. Schultz, N. V.: How children perceive pain. *Nursing Outlook* 19:670, October, 1971.
122. Sharp, D.: Lessons from a dying patient. *American Journal of Nursing* 68:1517, July, 1968.
123. Small, L. J.: Pain is partially what you make it. *Life and Health* 82:14, March, 1967.
124. Smith, D. W., Germain, C. P., and Gips, C.: *Care of the Adult Patient*. 3rd ed. Philadelphia, J. B. Lippincott Company, 1971.
125. Smith, L. A., et al.: *An Atlas of Pain Patterns: Sites and Behavior of Pain in Certain Common Diseases of the Upper Abdomen*. Springfield, Illinois, Charles C Thomas, 1961.
126. Soulairac, A., Cahn, J., and Charpentier, J. (eds.): *Pain*. Proceedings of the International Symposium on Pain. April 11–13, 1967. New York, Academic Press, Inc., 1968.
127. Stephen, C. R.: Complications of analgetic therapy. *In* Way, E. L. (ed.): *New Concepts in Pain and Its Clinical Management*. Philadelphia, F. A. Davis Company, 1967.
128. Sternbach, R. A.: *Pain: A Psychophysiological Analysis*. New York, Academic Press, Inc., 1968.
129. Swerdlow, M.: Four Years' Pain Clinic Experience. *Anaesthesia* 22:568, October, 1967.
130. Szasz, T. S.: The nature of pain. *Archives of Neurology and Psychiatry* (Chicago) 74:174, 1955.
131. Szasz, T. S.: *Pain and Pleasure: A Study of Bodily Feelings*. New York, Basic Books, 1957.
132. Szasz, T. S.: The psychology of persistent pain: a portrait of l'homme douloureux. *In* Soulairac, A., Cahn, J. and Charpentier, J. (eds.): *Pain*. New York, Academic Press, Inc., 1968.
133. Travelbee, J.: What's wrong with sympathy? *American Journal of Nursing* 64:70, 1964.
134. Turnbull, F.: Pain and suffering in cancer. *Canadian Nurse* 67:28, August, 1971.
135. Wang, R. I. H.: Control of pain. *The American Journal of the Medical Sciences* 246:112, November, 1963.
136. Way, E. L. (ed.): *New Concepts in Pain and Its Clinical Management*. Philadelphia, F. A. Davis Company, 1967.
137. Way, E. L.: Significant pharmacologic contributions in the development of analgetics. *In* Way, E. L. (ed.): *New Concepts in Pain and Its Clinical Management*. Philadelphia, F. A. Davis Company, 1967.
138. Weddell, G.: The relationship between pain sensibility and peripheral nerve fibers. *In* Knighton, R. and Dumke, P. (eds.): *Pain*. Boston, Little, Brown and Company, 1966.
139. White, J. C.: Foreword. *In* Knighton, R., and Dumke, P. (eds.): *Pain: International Symposium on Pain*. Henry Ford Hospital. Boston, Little, Brown and Company, 1966.
140. Wolf, S.: Placebos: Problems and pitfalls. *Clinical Pharmacology and Therapeutics* 3:254, 1962.
141. Wolff, H. G., and Wolf, S.: *Pain*. Springfield, Illinois, Charles C Thomas, 1958.
142. Woodforde, J. M., et al.: Pain and cancer. *Journal of Psychosomatic Research* 14:365, December, 1970.
143. Zborowski, M.: Cultural components in responses to pain. *Journal of Social Issues* 8:16, 1952.
144. Zborowski, M.: *People in Pain*. San Francisco, Jossey-Bass, Inc., 1969.

UNIT X

Nursing Patients Experiencing Disturbances of Cardiovascular Function and Blood Flow

Unit Introduction and Study Guide

The care of patients with heart disease is one of the most progressive areas in nursing today. The field of cardiology has advanced extremely rapidly in the last 15 years, and with each advance have come new responsibilities and challenges for nurses.

Today, nurse specialists who work in coronary care units (special areas of the hospital where critically ill heart patients are grouped together for comprehensive care) must have a knowledge of cardiology which is almost comparable to that of physicians. They must be able to swiftly identify life-threatening arrhythmias on an electrocardiogram and to perform emergency resuscitation measures, if necessary, without the aid of a doctor. The CCU nurse has truly become a significant and respected figure in the total field of health care.

Our goal in this unit is to give you a basic knowledge of heart disease—its cause and treatment—which will help you give comprehensive care (under supervision) to critically ill cardiac patients. Because cardiology is a vast and complex area of medical and nursing practice, this unit is both large and complex. In the study guide below we have listed only the most vital terms, diets, and drug groups that we feel are absolutely basic to a knowledge of cardiac nursing.

1. Chapter 46 of this unit is a basic review of material from anatomy and physiology which is pertinent to the discussions of heart disease which follow. Careful study of the normal cardiac structure and function presented will help you to understand the abnormalities of cardiac structure and function that we discuss throughout this unit.

2. As you study this unit familiarize yourself with the following terms: cardiac reserve, cardiac output, circulatory failure, thrombosis, embolism, infarction, arrhythmia, cardiogenic shock, anastomosis, coronary care unit (CCU), the Fick principle, fluoroscopy, angiocardiography, cardiac catheterization, electrocardiogram, leads, ballistocardiogram, phonocardiogram, cardiac compensation, cardiac decompensation, forward failure theory, backward failure theory, low-output failure, high-output failure, cardiac arrest, cardiopulmonary resuscitation, ectopic foci, precordial shock, defibrillation, cardioversion, pacemaker,

coronary heart disease (CHD), atherosclerosis, angina pectoris, myocardial infarction, hypertension (malignant and benign, primary and secondary), rheumatic fever, bacterial endocarditis, valvular stenosis and regurgitation, ball-in-cage valve prosthesis, pericarditis, cardiac tamponade, open heart surgery, hypothermia, extracorporeal circulation (ECC), heart-lung machine.

3. Familiarize yourself with these diets: low sodium and low cholesterol.

4. Carefully study the following drug groups, which are used to correct heart conditions: cardiac glycosides, cardiac depressants, diuretics, coronary dilators, antihypertensive agents, vasopressors, anticoagulants.

CHAPTER 46

The Cardiovascular System: An Overview of Normal Anatomy and Physiology

The human heart beats approximately 72 times per minute, forcing oxygen-carrying blood into the arterial system with every stroke. Moreover, this small, powerful pump contracts between 70 and 80 times *every* minute of *every* day throughout a person's lifetime, resting only 0.4 of a second between beats. Unlike other muscles of the body, the heart cannot stop and rest when tired and worn from work. Instead, it must keep pumping regularly, continuously, and with sufficient force for blood and oxygen to circulate properly to all parts of the vascular system and, thus, to all parts of the body.

The job of carrying oxygen and nutrients to cells, and metabolic wastes from cells for excretion, is a task that the heart and circulatory system must perform whether we are asleep or awake, active or sedentary. Therefore, not only must the heart labor constantly to meet the body's basal needs for oxygen and nutrients, it must also be able to *increase* its work output four or five times the normal if it is to sustain the body during periods of stress, e.g., hard exercise, great emotion, illness, and high fever. In sum, the heart, in addition to maintaining a steady normal workload, must also be able to quickly adjust and adapt to the various pressures of life.

One authority describes the enormity of the heart's tasks:

> The work done by the heart is out of all proportion to its size. Let us look at some figures. Even while we are asleep the heart pumps about two ounces of blood with each beat, a teacup with every three beats, nearly five quarts per minute, 75 gallons per hour. In other words, it pumps enough blood to fill an average gasoline tank almost four times every hour just to keep the machinery of the body idling. When the body is moderately active, the heart doubles this output. During strenuous muscular efforts, such as running to catch a train or playing a game of tennis, the cardiac output may go up to 14 barrels per hour. Over the 24 hours of an average day, involving not too vigorous work, it amounts to some 70 barrels, and in a lifetime of 70 years the heart pumps nearly 18 million barrels![171]

Although normally a remarkably precise, durable and efficient structure, the heart, like any machine, can unfortunately develop defects of structure and disturbances of function. What happens to the body when this mechanism, so necessary to life, begins to weaken and fail? What happens to the tissues and cells of the brain and other vital organs when oxygenated blood is no longer pumped to them in adequate amounts?

Before considering these questions, let us first review aspects of *normal* cardiovascular structure and function basic to the discussions of pathologic conditions in the following chapters. In the discussion below, the heart's major structures and the important mechanisms controlling the heart and circulation are presented. As you study this outline, ask yourself these questions:

1. In what ways can each of the cardiac structures and functions listed in the outline be adversely altered?
2. What physiologic disturbances can result from these alterations?
3. What effects do major pathologic alterations in the heart and circulatory system have upon the body as a whole? The answers to these questions are discussed in Chapter 47.

BASIC REVIEW OF THE NORMAL ANATOMY AND PHYSIOLOGY OF THE CARDIOVASCULAR SYSTEM

Function of the Cardiovascular System

The role of the *circulation* is to:

1. Continuously deliver oxygen, nutrients, hormones and antibodies to organs, tissues and cells throughout the body in response to varying tissue demands.
2. Remove end products of metabolism from tissues and cells.

The role of the *heart* is to:

1. Pump oxygenated blood into the arterial system, where it is carried to the capillaries supplying tissues.
2. Collect oxygen-poor blood from the venous system and pump it through the lungs to be reoxygenated.

The role of the *blood vessels* (arteries, capillaries, veins) is to carry blood to and from the body's tissues and cells.

Structure of the Heart

The heart is a cone-shaped, hollow, muscular organ, weighing 300 grams, located in the *medias-*

tinum, a space between the lungs within the thoracic cavity. Its base is directed toward the body's right side. Its apex is directed toward the left and rests upon the diaphragm.

The heart is a double pump having two sides. The *right* side receives *deoxygenated* blood from the body and pumps it to the lungs to be oxygenated; the *left* side receives oxygenated blood from the lungs and pumps it out through the aorta to all parts of the body (Fig. 46–1).

The *pericardium,* the loose fitting covering of the heart, is composed of:

1. *Fibrous pericardium,* a tough fibrous membrane attached to the great vessels.
2. *Serous pericardium,* composed of two layers: (a) outer parietal layer which lines fibrous pericardium, and (b) inner visceral layer, i.e., epicardium, which adheres closely to heart.
3. The *pericardial space*, between the visceral and parietal layers, filled with *pericardial fluid* (5 to 20 ml.). The fluid (a) lubricates the heart's surfaces as they slide over each other, and (b) alleviates friction between the heart's surfaces as the heart beats.

The *cardiac layers* are:

1. *Epicardium*—outer layer—same structure as visceral pericardium.
2. Myocardium—middle layer—composed of *striated* muscle fibers, interlaced together into bundles. This muscle causes the heart's contraction, which squeezes blood out of the heart into the arterial system.
3. Endocardium—innermost layer—composed of endothelial tissue and continuous with the blood vessels. It lines the heart's cavities and covers the heart valves.

The *cardiac chambers* are:

1. *Atria,* or *auricles*—the two upper "receiving" chambers: (a) The *right atrium* receives deoxygenated blood from all over body via the superior and inferior venae cavae, and pumps blood received into the right ventricle from whence it is pumped to the lungs. (b) The *left atrium* receives *oxygenated* blood from the lungs, and pumps oxygenated blood to the left ventricle, from which it is pumped out to the body. The *interatrial septum* separates the atria.
2. *Ventricles*—the two lower "distributing" chambers. The inner wall of the ventricles is characterized by: *trabeculae carneae,* interlacing bundles of muscle; *papillary muscles,* finger or nipple-shaped projections; and *chordae tendineae,* cord-like structures (composed of dense fibrous connective tissue) that are attached to the valve leaflets. (a) The *right* ventricle: receives blood from the

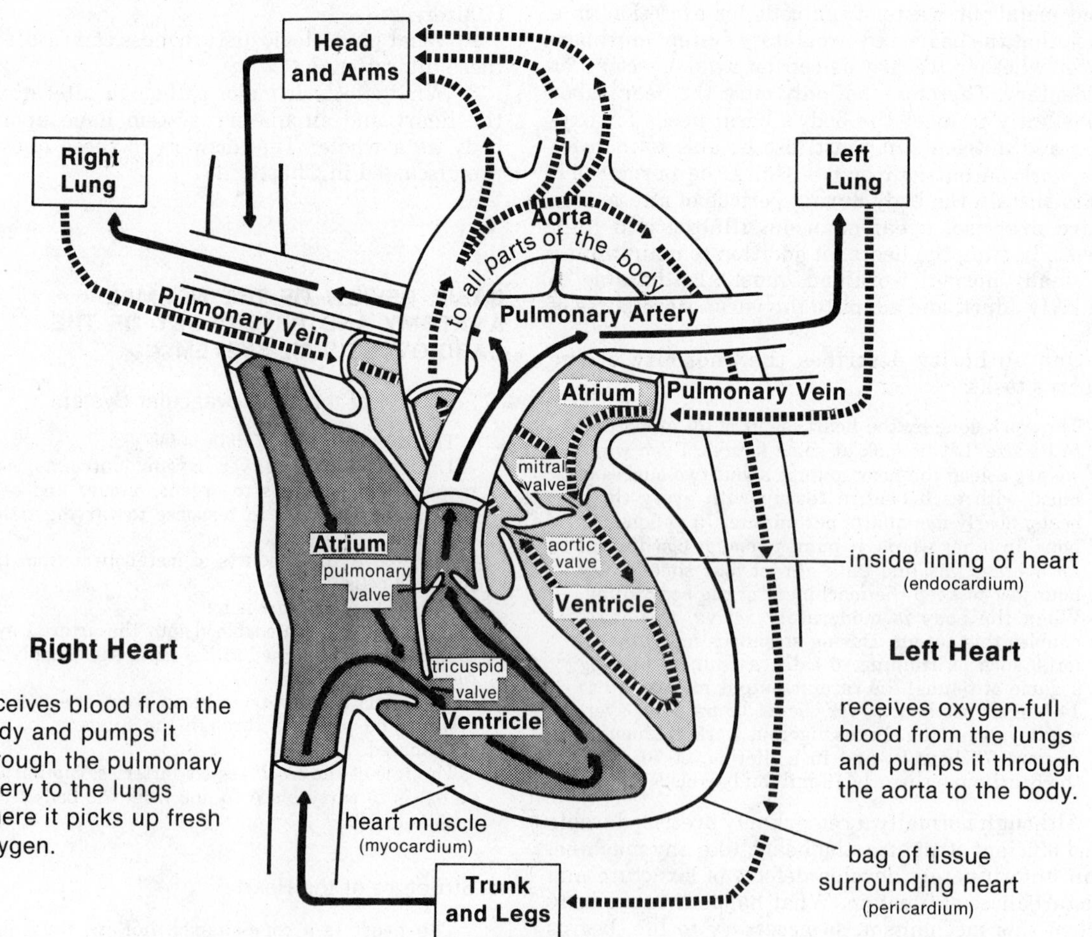

FIGURE 46–1. Schematic diagram of the heart. (Courtesy of American Heart Association.)

right atrium, and pumps out blood received to the lungs via the *pulmonary artery*. (b) The *left ventricle*—the heart's largest, most muscular chamber—receives *oxygenated* blood from the lungs via the left atrium, and pumps out blood received to all parts of the body; the *interventricular septum* separates the ventricles.

The *cardiac valves* are:

1. The *atrioventricular valves,* i.e., the tricuspid and bicuspid (mitral) valves, which guard openings between the atria and ventricles, forcing blood to flow forward from atria to ventricles, and preventing blood from flowing backward from ventricles to atria. The *tricuspid valve* guards the opening between right atrium and right ventricle. It is composed of three cusps (flaps) of endothelium, which close and unite to prevent backward flow of blood upon ventricular contraction. The *bicuspid valve* guards the opening between the left atrium and the left ventricle; it is composed of two cusps of endothelium.

2. The *semilunar valves* are half-moon-shaped flaps preventing blood from flowing back into the ventricles. The *pulmonary semilunar* valve lies between the pulmonary artery and the right ventricle; the *aortic semilunar* valve lies between the aorta and the left ventricle (Fig. 46–2).

Coronary Circulation

The *coronary arteries* (right and left) branch off the aortic arch, encircle the heart, and penetrate the myocardium. They supply the capillaries of the myocardium with blood (Fig. 46–3). Coronary blood flow *increases* with (1) increased activity (i.e., exercise); (2) increased heart rate; and (3) increased stimulation of the sympathetic nervous system.

The *coronary veins* return blood from the myocardium to the right atrium via the *coronary sinus.*

The *capillaries* of the heart muscle exchange oxygen and nutrients for waste products which are later excreted via the kidneys and lungs.

> *Myocardial capillaries are the heart's most essential structures; they* must *receive an adequate blood supply or heart failure will result.*

Pulmonary Circulation

The pulmonary circulation involves blood flow from heart to lungs and back to heart. Blood flows from the right ventricle, through the semilunar valve, to the pulmonary artery, to the lungs, to four pulmonary veins, and back to the left atrium.

Heart Rate

The normal heart rate is 60 to 90 beats per minute. *Sinus tachycardia* is a rate of over 100 beats per minute; it can follow exercise or emotional upset. *Sinus bradycardia* is a rate of less than 60 beats per minute.

Variations in heart beat are normally caused by:

1. *Exercise:* Increased activity causes increased need for oxygen and elimination of CO_2, which, in turn, causes increased heart rate.
2. *Size of individual:* Larger person has slower heart rate.
3. *Age:* Beat is fastest in fetus (120 to 160 beats per minute) and lowest in adults (65 to 80 beats per minute).
4. *Sex:* Women have a faster rate than men.
5. *Hormones:* Epinephrine and thyroxine cause increased rate.
6. *Temperature:* Fever causes increased heart rate; hypothermia causes decreased heart rate.
7. *Blood pressure:* Hypotension causes increased heart rate.

Regulation of Heart Rate and Rhythm*

Seven special properties of *cardiac muscle* are necessary for regulation of heart rate and rhythm:

1. *Rhythmicity:* Rhythm in both the formation and conduction of electrical impulses from atria to ventricles. The heart beats with a definite rhythm based on four phases: (a) stimulation, (b) transmission, (c) contraction, and (d) relaxation. Each contraction is accompanied by an electrical charge, thus forming the basis for electrocardiography.
2. *Irritability* (excitability): The ability of cardiac muscle cells to respond to stimuli. When irritable, heart muscle responds to stimuli with the strongest possible contraction (all-or-nothing law). Irritability is influenced by: (a) neural, hormonal, and nutritional balance; (b) adequacy of oxygen supply; (c) drug therapy; and (d) products of infection.
3. *Refractoriness:* This prevents heart muscle from responding to a new stimulus while the heart is still in a state of contraction due to an earlier stimulus, and thus helps to preserve heart rhythm. Irritability is lowest during refractory period. During the *absolute refractory period* the heart muscle

*Electrophysiology of the heart is discussed in more detail in Chapter 48.

VALVES

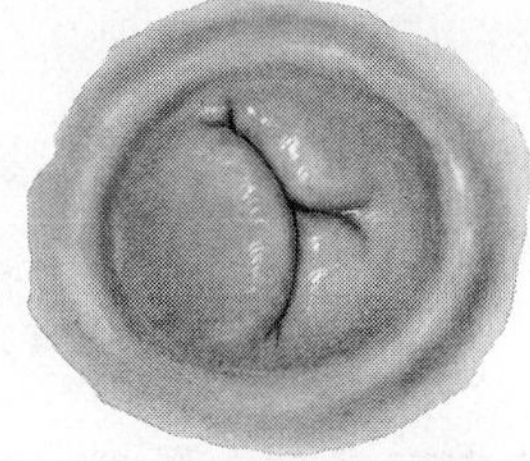
Tricuspid

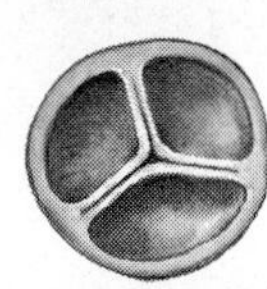
Aortic or Pulmonary

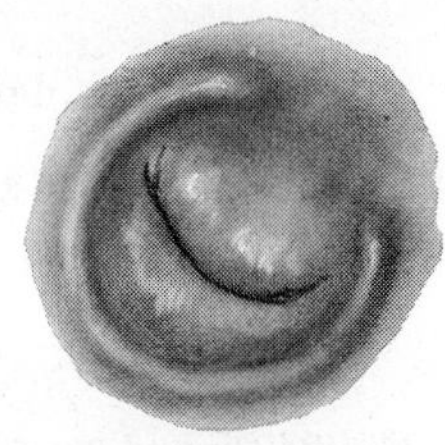
Mitral

FIGURE 46–2. Schematic "transparent" drawing of the heart showing the relations of the various heart valves. (From Jacob, S. W., and Francone, C. A.: *Structure and Function in Man.* 2nd ed., 1970.)

will not respond to *any* stimulus, however strong; during the *relative refractory period* the heart muscle slowly regains irritability.

4. *Conductivity:* Ability of heart muscle fibers to transmit electrical impulses.

5. *Contractility:* Shortening of heart muscle fibers in response to stimuli.

6. *Automaticity:* Ability of heart to beat spontaneously and repetitively without external neurohormonal control. The heart is capable of beating outside the body, given proper laboratory conditions. Automaticity is evidently linked to fluid and electrolyte balance rather than to nervous system control.

7. *Extensibility* (expansibility): Ability of heart muscle to *stretch* as the heart fills with blood between contractions. *Starling's "law of the heart"* states: the greater the stretch of cardiac muscle, the more forceful are the heart's contraction and beat. However, when muscle is *overstretched,* the force of contraction may *decrease* below normal level, causing circulatory failure.

The *cardiac conduction system* is composed of modified cardiac muscle cells characterized by the ability to conduct electrical impulses. The *purpose* of the conduction system is to enable atria and ventricles to contract at the *same rate,* rather than separately and at different rates. The *structures* of the conduction system are:

1. *Sinoatrial node* (S-A node) or *pacemaker,* located at junction of superior vena cava and right atrium. The S-A node initiates each heart beat. It elicits electrical impulses approximately 72 times per minute to cause atrial contractions. The S-A node is under the control of the sympathetic and parasympathetic nervous systems. Other areas of specialized tissue in atria, ventricles, and A-V node can take over the role of pacemaker if they elicit impulses at a faster rate than the S-A node.

2. *Atrioventricular node* (A-V node, or A-V junction), located in the lower aspect of the interatrial septum. The A-V node receives electrical impulses from the S-A node. Within the A-V node, the impulse is delayed 7/100 of a second while the atria finish contracting. The A-V node generates impulses when the S-A node fails to function. It generates only 40 to 50 impulses per minute, which is sufficient to sustain human life with reduced activity. Should the A-V node also fail, *lower pacemakers* take over the job of impulse formation; they maintain a very low heart rate.

3. The *bundle of His–Purkinje system* is continuous with the A-V node. The bundle of His (now often called the A-V bundle) is composed of special cardiac muscle fibers that originate in the A-V node; these fibers break into branches that extend down the interventricular septum where they are continuous with Purkinje fibers. The function of the bundle of His is to relay impulses from A-V node to ventricles. The function of the Purkinje fibers is to enable electrical impulses responsible for myocardial contraction to spread rapidly over all parts of the ventricles (Fig. 46–4).

Neurohormonal control of the heart rate and rhythm takes place as follows:

1. *Efferent* fibers transmit impulses from the cardiac center in the medulla oblongata to the heart. This enables the heart to adjust its rate to meet the body's changing needs. (a) *Sympathetic,*

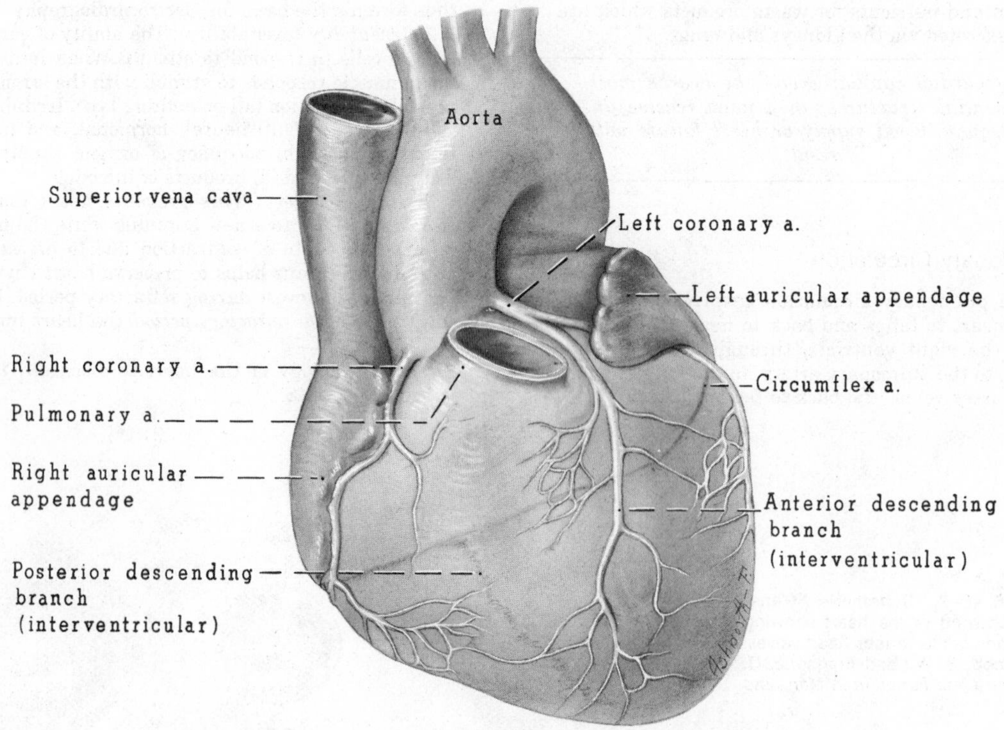

FIGURE 46–3. Coronary arteries which supply the heart. (From Jacob, S. W., and Francone, C. A.: *Structure and Function in Man.* 2nd ed., 1970.)

or accelerator, fibers *speed* heart rate and *strengthen* force of contraction. *Norepinephrine* is evidently released from the heart's sympathetic nerve endings when nerves are stimulated. It acts to increase heart rate, decrease the refractory period of the A-V node, increase cardiac workload, and impede coronary circulation by acting as a powerful vasoconstrictor. (b) *Parasympathetic,* or inhibitory, fibers travel in the two *vagus* nerves and act to *slow* heart rate, to *weaken* the force of contraction, and to *lengthen* the heart muscle's rest period. *Acetylcholine* is released by vagal nerve endings in the S-A node, A-V node, and bundle of His. It acts to decrease heart rate and increase the refractory period.

2. *Afferent* fibers conduct *pain* impulses only from the heart to the brain (e.g., when the myocardium's oxygen supply is decreased).

Cardiac Cycle

One cardiac cycle is equivalent to one complete heart beat; it lasts 0.8 second. It consists of two parts:

1. *Systole,* or contraction of both atria and then both ventricles; systole is initiated by release of an impulse from the S-A node.
2. *Diastole,* or relaxation of both atria and then both ventricles.

Heart Sounds

The *first* sound, "lubb," is of dull quality and low pitch; it signals:

1. Onset of ventricular systole.
2. Abrupt closure of atrioventricular valves; closure sets up vibrations in blood and heart walls; these vibrations are transmitted to the chest wall.

The *second* sound, "dubb," has a snapping quality; it signifies:

1. Onset of diastole.
2. Closure of semilunar valves, which causes vibrations in blood and heart walls.

Cardiac Output

Cardiac output is equivalent to *stroke volume* (i.e., amount of blood ejected with each beat) times *heart rate* (i.e., number of beats per minute).

Cardiac output = stroke volume × heart rate.

1. Stroke volume is approximately 70 ml. of blood ejected per heart beat.
2. Heart rate is normally 72 beats per minute.
3. Cardiac output is, thus, approximately 5040 ml. of blood per minute, i.e., 70 × 72. Cardiac output depends upon: (a) venous return; (b) cardiac rate; and (c) strength of contraction. Cardiac output can increase four to five times when the healthy body is subjected to strenuous exercise.

Cardiac Reserve

Cardiac reserve is the ability of the heart to adjust and to adapt to increased demands placed upon it from stresses such as: exercise, excitement, fever, cold, acceleration, deceleration, or disease states. Normally the heart is able to greatly increase its output of energy to meet demands made upon it.

Blood Pressure

This is defined as the pressure exerted by the blood against the walls of the vessels—i.e., arteries, veins, capillaries.

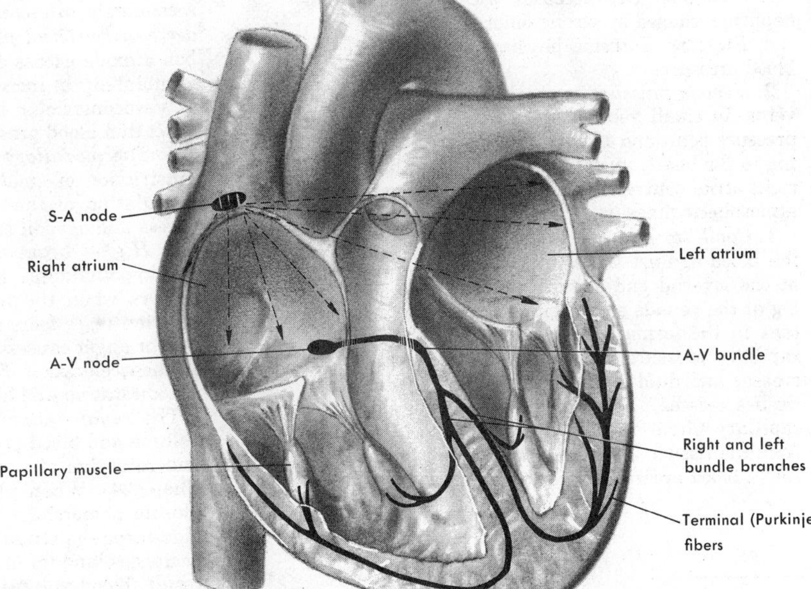

FIGURE 46–4. The Purkinje system. (From Dienhart, C. M.: *Basic Human Anatomy and Physiology.* 2nd ed. 1973.)

The *difference* in blood pressure in arteries, capillaries and veins, or *blood pressure gradient,* is the force that enables blood to flow throughout the body. The farther blood flows *from* the heart, the lower the pressure. Pressure is highest in arteries, drops significantly in capillaries, and is almost zero in great veins.

The three *types* of blood pressure are:

1. *Arterial* pressure: pressure of blood against arteries' walls. (a) *Systolic pressure* is *maximum* pressure of the blood exerted against the artery walls when the heart *contracts* and is working; it is normally 115 to 120 mm. Hg. (b) *Diastolic pressure* is the force of blood exerted against the artery walls when the heart is *relaxing;* it is normally 75 to 80 mm. Hg. (c) *Pulse pressure* is the *difference* between systolic and diastolic pressures; it is normally 40 mm. Hg.

Circulatory factors influencing arterial pressure include:

a. *Cardiac output:* Increased output increases arterial pressure; decreased output decreases arterial pressure.

b. *Peripheral resistance:* Narrowed arterioles increase blood pressure; dilated arterioles decrease blood pressure.

c. *Arterial elasticity:* Elastic vessels accommodate to changes in blood flow, whereas rigid sclerotic vessels cause increases in systolic and pulse pressures.

d. *Blood volume:* Decreased blood volume (e.g., due to hemorrhage) results in decreased pressure.

e. *Blood viscosity:* Increased blood viscosity, due to overabundance of RBC's or plasma proteins, results in *high* pressure; decreased viscosity from anemia or lack of RBC's results in *lower* pressure.

Other factors influencing arterial pressure are:

a. *Age:* BP is lowest in newborn babies and highest in adults.

b. *Weight:* BP increases with excess weight.

c. *Emotions:* BP increases with release of epinephrine, caused by strong emotion.

d. *Exercise:* Extreme physical activity increases blood pressure.

2. *Venous pressure* is the blood pressure in the veins. In small veins there are no pulsations; the pressure is around 12 mm. Hg. In large veins leading to the heart, pulsations are reflected back from right atrial contractions; blood pressure is around 0 atmospheric pressure.

3. *Capillary pressure* is the pressure exerted by the blood against the capillaries. It is 22 mm. Hg at the arterial end of the capillaries and 12 mm. Hg at the venous end. Capillary pressure is important in the formation of interstitial fluid.* When capillary pressure is *high,* capillary filtration increases and fluid shifts from vascular system into tissues (edema). When capillary pressure is *low,* capillary filtration decreases and fluid is drawn from the tissues into the circulatory system, which raises blood pressure.

*Capillary blood pressure and filtration were discussed in Unit V, Chapter 24.

Factors Regulating Circulation

The *nervous system* acts to regulate heart rate, degree of arteriolar constriction, and arterial blood pressure, in order to maintain homeostasis. Neural reflexes are controlled via the *vasomotor center* in the medulla oblongata. This comprises four centers controlling the heart and blood vessels:

1. *Vasoconstrictor* center, which *reduces* diameter of blood vessels.

2. *Vasodilator* center, which *increases* diameter of blood vessels.

3. *Cardioaccelerator* center, which *increases* heart rate.

4. *Cardioinhibitory* center, which decreases heart rate.

These four centers are stimulated or inhibited by:

1. *Pressoreceptors,* or baroreceptors—specialized nerve endings affected by changes in pressure of blood in arteries.

a. *Arterial* pressoreceptors are located in the walls of the aortic arch and the carotid sinuses. When arterial pressure *increases:* arterial pressoreceptors are stimulated and impulses are carried to the medulla oblongata, where vasodilator and cardioinhibitory centers are stimulated. As a result, heart rate and arterial pressure *decrease.* When arterial pressure *decreases,* arterial pressoreceptors receive inadequate stimulation and fewer impulses are carried to medulla oblongata. Thus, vasoconstrictor and cardioaccelerator centers are stimulated. As a result, heart rate and arterial pressure *increase.*

b. *Venous pressoreceptors* are located in terminal sections of the venae cavae and the right atrium. When blood pressure *increases* in venae cavae and the right atrium (e.g., from exercise), venous pressoreceptors and the cardioaccelerator center are stimulated. As a result, heart rate increases; blood is transferred rapidly into arterial system; and systemic blood pressure rises (*Bainbridge reflex*). When pressure of blood *decreases* in venae cavae and the right atrium, the reverse of the above occurs.

2. *Chemoreceptors:* receptors and organs located in the aortic arch and carotid bodies. Chemoreceptors are primarily sensitive to *oxygen* lack and secondarily to *increased blood carbon dioxide* and *decreased arterial pH.* When oxygen lack and carbon dioxide excess develop: (a) chemoreceptors are stimulated; (b) increased impulses are transmitted to vasoconstrictor center, and (c) arterioles constrict and blood pressure increases.

3. The *medullary ischemic reflex* produces vasoconstriction of small blood vessels in response to stimulation of the vasoconstrictor center by CO_2 excess and oxygen lack.

4. *Higher brain centers,* in the cerebral cortex and hypothalamus, transmit impulses to medullary centers when the individual experiences extreme emotion (e.g., fear, rage, embarrassment). Intense fear or anger causes vasoconstriction of arteries and cardioacceleration. Extreme embarrassment causes vasodilatation and blushing.

The *renal system* regulates circulation, blood volume and blood pressure by controlling excretion and retention of water in urine (see also Unit V, Chap. 24). When blood volume and BP *decrease* (due to hemorrhage, etc.): (a) release of ADH and aldosterone is stimulated; (b) glomerular filtration decreases; and (c) urine production decreases. As a result, blood volume and blood pressure rise. The opposite set of events occurs with an *increase* in blood volume and blood pressure.

CHAPTER 47

Abnormalities of Cardiac Structure and Function: An Overview

This chapter provides an overview of the following general concepts: (1) the causes of cardiovascular failure; (2) the effects of cardiovascular failure upon the body; and (3) methods by which cardiovascular failure can be reversed and its effects minimized.

THE CARDIOVASCULAR SYSTEM IN FAILURE

In the preceding chapter, we pointed out that it is the role of the cardiovascular system to deliver oxygen and nutrients to every cell and tissue of the body *without interruption,* and in amounts sufficient to meet the specific needs of each tissue and cell at any given moment. In order to meet the body's continuous metabolic demands, the cardiovascular system must fulfill the following requirements:

1. The heart must be able to adequately *pump blood* to all parts of the body. For effective pumping, the cardiac muscle and the cardiac conduction system must be in good working order.
2. The circulating *blood volume* must be sufficient to meet the body's needs.
3. *Peripheral vascular resistance* must be sufficient to maintain an adequate blood pressure.

When severe heart disease, hemorrhage, shock, or extreme hypotension, i.e., low blood pressure, develops, the heart and circulation will fail.

> Circulatory failure *is defined as the "inability of the circulation to maintain an adequate minute volume blood flow to supply the needs of the tissues."*[64]

Circulatory failure can be either acute or chronic. *Acute* circulatory failure develops rapidly with severe symptoms; it is best exemplified by the clinical pictures of shock, cardiac arrest, syncope, and sudden death.

Shock and *cardiac arrest* are discussed in detail elsewhere.* *Syncope* or fainting results from an intense, temporary cerebral ischemia. Causative factors include emotional shock, extreme fear, various arrhythmias (disturbances of heart rate and rhythm), flying at high altitudes, and standing for long periods in one position. Syncope is characterized by a severe drop in blood pressure and a sudden loss of consciousness. Generally the individual who faints revives quickly once he is placed in a horizontal position, e.g., on a bed or on the floor, with his head on a level with the rest of his body.

Sudden death occurs when the heart swiftly and without warning stops pumping. The resultant intense and irreversible cerebral anoxia brings life to a sudden end. Factors that may be responsible for the development of sudden death are: (1) severe hemorrhage into the brain or pericardial sac; (2) massive pulmonary embolism resulting in obstruction of blood flow to the brain; (3) ventricular fibrillation; and (4) sudden brain injury due to trauma, toxins, metabolic factors, or vascular occlusion. Other precipitating factors of sudden death are extreme fear or rage, heavy exercise in very hot or cold weather, straining while defecating, anesthesia, and withdrawal of fluid from the pleural or peritoneal cavities.

Chronic circulatory failure, on the other hand, develops gradually with more moderate symptoms; chronic failure is more specifically described by the term "*chronic congestive heart failure.*"

Failure of the heart and circulation adversely affects all organs throughout the body, causing them to function poorly. In particular, the brain, kidneys, and liver are vulnerable to circulatory failure; striking symptoms characteristically develop due to oxygen lack and the build-up of metabolic products in these organs.

CAUSATIVE FACTORS PRODUCING CARDIAC DYSFUNCTION

Table 47–1 lists factors associated with the development of cardiovascular diseases and their clinical manifestations. Although these factors are discussed throughout the unit, we shall briefly define them now and state their role in the causation of heart disease.

*Shock in general is discussed in Chapter 26, Unit V; cardiac arrest is discussed in this unit, Chapter 50.

DISTURBANCES OF BLOOD VOLUME

A normal *inflow* of blood from the venous system is a basic requirement for adequate cardiac function and output. The volume of blood entering the heart must be neither too small nor too great. Too *small* a blood volume entering the heart will cause a *decrease* in cardiac output and circulatory collapse; too *great* a volume of blood entering the heart will overwork the heart and will result in a circulatory overload.

Fluid Loss

A *decreased* blood volume results from fluid loss, which may have developed as a result of dehydration, hemorrhage, or shock. *Dehydration,* you recall, results from severe fluid losses as a result of vomiting, diarrhea, profuse diaphoresis, draining wounds, etc.* These fluid losses, in turn, rapidly deplete the extracellular fluid, leading to an inadequate cardiac output with consequent shock and circulatory collapse.

Hemorrhage is a second important factor that lowers blood volume, decreasing the inflow of blood to the heart. Hemorrhage is defined as the escape of blood from the vessel in which it is normally confined. Factors causing hemorrhage are: trauma that results in a vessel's rupture; *spontaneous* rupture of the vessel, e.g., a ruptured aortic aneurysm* or the rupture of a vessel in the brain of a hypertensive patient; *defects of the clotting mechanism* as a result of a deficiency of certain blood factors; and the effects of certain medications that interfere with the clotting mechanism, e.g., heparin, bishydroxycoumarin (Dicumarol).

Bleeding may be local or systemic. *Small* local hemorrhages are not dangerous unless they occur within the pericardial sac (where a blood collection can cause pericardial rupture) or in the brain.

On the other hand, *large systemic* hemorrhages are always dangerous because they adversely affect circulatory dynamics by drastically reducing blood volume, venous return to the heart, cardiac output, and the arterial blood pressure. To compensate for these dangerous changes, the cardiovascular system reflexively reacts in the following ways:

1. The *heart* beats more rapidly, i.e., tachycardia, in order to speed circulation to vital organs.
2. The *vessels* of the skin and abdominal viscera constrict. This increases arterial blood pressure and increases blood distribution to the vital organs, while reducing blood volume within the vessels of the skin and abdominal viscera.
3. The *liver* and *spleen* discharge additional red blood cells, which are stored for emergencies.
4. The *colloidal osmotic pressure,* i.e., oncotic pressure, within the capillaries increases owing to the decreased filtration pressure within the capillaries. Increased colloid osmotic pressure causes tissue fluid to be sucked back into the blood ves-

*Dehydration is discussed at length in Unit V, Chapter 25.

*An aortic aneurysm is an abnormal dilatation of a localized area of the aorta.

TABLE 47–1. FACTORS ASSOCIATED WITH THE DEVELOPMENT OF CARDIOVASCULAR DISORDERS

Causative Factors	Cardiovascular Disorders
Disturbances of blood volume	Shock; hemorrhage; fluid overload
Obstructions of blood flow	Thrombosis; embolism; infarction
Ischemia of heart muscle	Angina pectoris; myocardial infarction; coronary insufficiency
Cardiac infectious processes	Rheumatic heart disease; subacute bacterial endocarditis; syphilitic heart disease
Cardiac structural abnormalities	Congenital defects; acquired pathologic changes in structure of valves and heart walls
Hypertension	Arterial hypertension; pulmonary hypertension
Cardiac tumors	Primary; secondary
Trauma to heart	Penetrating cardiac lesion; nonpenetrating cardiac lesion
Alterations in cardiac rate, rhythm, and conduction	Disturbances of impulse formation; failures of conduction
Additional noncardiac factors	Prolonged fevers; anemia; hyperthyroidism; severe anxiety; polycythemia

sels, thereby increasing blood volume and the arterial blood pressure.*

5. The *kidneys* slow urine production, thereby conserving body fluid and blood volume.

When the above mechanisms fail to bring the hemorrhage under control and bleeding continues without medical treatment, irreversible shock soon develops, followed by death.

Shock, a third factor resulting in decreased blood volume and cardiac output, results not only from hemorrhage, but also from other events such as burns, severe blows to the body, severe allergic reactions (anaphylactic shock), terrifying or upsetting emotional experiences, and from heart failure or mechanical abnormalities that hinder cardiac function, i.e., cardiogenic shock.

Cardiogenic shock occurs when the heart fails as a pumping device and cardiac output is grossly inadequate to meet the body's needs. This form of shock results most frequently from damage to the heart muscle, severe arrhythmias, and compression of the heart as a result of cardiac tamponade. Cardiogenic shock is discussed further in Chapter 49 of this unit.

Fluid Overload

An abnormally *increased* blood volume results from a fluid overload. In Unit V, Chapter 25, we discussed the problem of extracellular volume excess. You will recall that patients who are most prone to a circulatory overload are those who have received excessive I.V. fluids; patients with heart, kidney, liver, or brain disease; and patients receiving cortisone injections. When administering fluids to patients with heart disease, remember this rule:

> *Be extremely careful not to overload a patient with heart disease with rapidly administered infusions of I.V. solutions. Acute pulmonary edema may result because the damaged heart muscle will be unable to pump out and circulate the excess fluid.*

OBSTRUCTIONS OF THE BLOOD FLOW

For adequate circulation to take place, not only must the blood volume be adequate, but the blood must also be able to reach the heart so that it can circulate properly through the lungs and heart chambers and out into the arterial system. Blood flow to the heart can be disturbed or obstructed by thrombi, emboli, areas of infarction, and constrictive pericarditis.

Thrombosis

A *thrombus*† (plural, thrombi) is a blood clot that has formed within a blood vessel or within the heart. Thrombus formation is dangerous because: (1) thrombi can occlude blood vessels, thereby obstructing blood flow to vital organs; and (2) thrombi can break free from their attachments to the vessel walls and travel in the blood stream to the heart, lungs, and brain, thus forming emboli.

Thrombi do not normally form within blood vessels because: (1) the healthy blood vessel has an inner wall lined with endothelial tissue which is so *smooth* that fibrin and platelets cannot adhere to form the genesis of a clot; and (2) blood flow through the vessels is generally so *rapid* that there is little chance that formed elements within the blood will settle out to form clots. Instead, these formed elements are swept swiftly and smoothly along the circulatory route.

Consequently, factors which lead to the formation of blood clots are those which (1) decrease the smoothness of the endothelial lining of the vessel walls and the heart valves; (2) decrease the rate of blood flow; and (3) increase blood coagulability and the viscosity of the blood. Table 47–2 lists these three major factors, along with the physiologic disturbances that cause them.

A thrombus is formed when intact and ruptured platelets adhere together on a vessel wall. This tiny

TABLE 47–2. CAUSATIVE FACTORS IN THROMBUS FORMATION

Major Factors	Contributing Factors
Damage to endothelial lining of blood vessels	Hardening or sclerosis of vessels due to aging; injury to arterial walls; neoplasms affecting arteries; damage to heart valves due to bacteria and the growth of vegetations
Decrease in rate of blood flow	Lack of muscular contraction in legs due to immobility and prolonged bedrest; spasm of arterial walls as in hypertension; narrowing of arterial walls as result of disease, e.g., atherosclerosis; increased viscosity of blood due to polycythemia or dehydration
Increase in blood coagulability	Increase in platelet count or platelet stickiness (often seen following surgery or trauma); use of vitamin K

*Fluid transport between compartments is discussed in Unit V, Chapter 24.

†Thrombus formation as a complication of bedrest is discussed in Unit V, Chapter 27.

mass of platelets, which projects slightly into the vessel lumen or out from the heart lining, is called a *plaque*. The platelets that compose the plaque cause the precipitation of fibrin and the accumulation of formed blood elements, which form a blood clot. This fibrinous mass, which started as a small plaque, is now called a *mural* thrombus, i.e., a thrombus attached to the wall of a vessel or the heart. Once formed, a thrombus may: (1) partially obstruct the lumen of a blood vessel; (2) completely obstruct the vessel's lumen (*occlusive* thrombus); (3) grow in size as a result of the addition of more platelets and formed blood elements (*progressive* or *propagating* thrombus); or (4) break free from the wall and travel in the blood stream (*embolus*).

Thrombosis may affect either the arterial or venous systems. Thrombi which occlude *arteries* usually result from extensive lesions of the arterial walls; because these thrombi obstruct the flow of blood to tissues, they may lead to ischemia or infarction of the dependent tissues.

Venous thrombosis is more common than arterial thrombosis since venous blood flow is slower than arterial, and also because the vein walls are thinner and more delicate than arterial walls and, thus, more susceptible to injury. Clots most commonly form within the veins of the legs and pelvis. The major danger in venous thrombosis is that the clot will break loose from the vein wall and embolize to the lungs.

Embolism

An *embolus* is a mass of undissolved matter in a blood or lymphatic vessel brought there by the blood or lymph flow. Emboli are composed of various types of materials: fat globules, bubbles of air, clumps of bacteria, tumor cells, foreign bodies (e.g., bullets), and clusters of parasites. The most common types of emboli, however, arise from preexisting thrombi in the veins and arteries which have become fragmented. In Table 47–3 we have listed the four most important types of emboli along with their causative factors and pathologic consequences.

Infarction

An *infarct* is a localized area of tissue, within an organ or part, which has become ischemic and necrotic due to the complete or total blockage of its blood supply. The formation of an infarct in the lung, usually as a result of a pulmonary embolus, is called a *pulmonary infarction*. The formation of an infarct in the myocardial tissue owing to blockage of the coronary arteries is called a *myocardial infarction*.

The commonest causes of infarction are thrombosis and embolism. Other causes are twisting of an internal organ or its parts so that the organ's blood

TABLE 47–3. TYPES OF EMBOLI: SOURCES AND POSSIBLE PATHOLOGIC CONSEQUENCES

Classification	Source of Emboli	Pathologic Consequences
Venous emboli	Fragmented thrombi within leg veins; most commonly deep calf muscles; fragmented thrombi within pelvic veins; thrombi on walls of heart's right side	May occlude a pulmonary vessel, coronary artery, or cerebral vessel; small emboli may cause small areas of infarction; large emboli may cause death
Arterial emboli	Mural intracardiac thrombi; vegetative masses on heart valves as result of bacterial endocarditis; atherosclerotic plaques; aortic aneurysms	Same as above
Fat emboli (minute globules of fat which are carried in the blood)	Fractures of the long bones; severe burns; soft tissue injuries; fatty changes in the liver; iatrogenic causes: orthopedic procedures: I.V. injections of oily radiographic media	Globules usually remain in lungs; globules may travel to the brain, kidneys, and liver, producing severe damage and death; globules may pass to the brain, causing unconsciousness and severe neurologic damage
Air or gas emboli (bubbles of air or gas within the circulation)	Chest injuries (air may enter a large vein during inspiration); pneumothorax procedure (large artery or vein may be ruptured by introduction of needle into chest)	Frothy masses may form which can occlude vessels, particularly in the lungs; large masses of gassy bubbles may become caught in right atria and ventricles and block pulmonary artery

supply is impaired, e.g., twisting of a testis or bowel loop; and compression of arteries and veins, thereby cutting off circulation to the tissues they supply.

The development of an infarction can be extremely dangerous, and infarctions are common causes of critical illnesses and deaths. Exactly how damaging an infarct will be depends upon its size and location.

Whether an organ will become infarcted as a result of thrombosis or embolism depends upon the *organ's blood supply*. Some organs, e.g., spleen and kidney, receive their blood supply from a *single* vessel called an "end artery." While the end artery has branches, it does not have any blood vessels *between* the branches, i.e., anastomoses.* Thus, if an end artery becomes obstructed, there are no "detour channels" or anastomoses to carry the blood to the organ's tissues by bypassing the obstruction. In such a situation infarction is almost inevitable.

In organs which have a *double* blood supply, one vessel can take over for the other in event of thrombosis or embolism. For example, the arms are supplied with blood from both the ulnar and radial arteries, while the legs receive blood from both the tibial and fibular arteries. Finally, organs such as the bones, muscles, uterus, thyroid gland, and skin are served by blood vessels with *many anastomoses;* consequently these organs do not often develop infarcts.

Unfortunately the coronary arteries that supply the myocardium contain very few anastomoses. However, numerous anastomoses exist between the heart's *small* vessels; these vascular connections can grow and provide the heart with sufficient collateral circulation if the artery occludes gradually over a period of time, or if the occlusion is only partial. But, if a *large* embolus *suddenly* blocks a coronary artery, infarction of the myocardium is inevitable because of the lack of anastomoses between the large arteries and the inability of the channels between the small vessels to swiftly provide collateral circulation under these circumstances.

ISCHEMIA OF THE HEART MUSCLE

As stated before, the heart muscle must receive adequate amounts of oxygenated blood and nutrients if it is to effectively pump blood throughout the cardiovascular system. *Should the coronary arteries, which supply the myocardium, become blocked, the heart muscle will suffer from oxygen deprivation* (i.e., *ischemia*). Insufficient blood supply to the myocardium results in such disorders as obliterative atherosclerotic heart disease, angina pectoris, coronary insufficiency, and myocardial infarction. These four serious disorders are grouped under the terms *coronary artery disease* (CAD) or ischemic heart disease and are discussed in detail in Chapter 51.

*An arterial anastomosis is a branch of an artery that is attached either to another artery or to itself at a more distant point. There are also arteriovenous anastomoses.

INFECTIOUS PROCESSES AFFECTING THE HEART

The structures of the heart, like any other body structures, are vulnerable to attacks by microorganisms and can be adversely altered by the resulting inflammatory and fibrous processes. The walls of the heart (epicardium, myocardium, and endocardium) can become dangerously infected and inflamed. As a result, valves may become narrowed, deformed and sclerosed, and their function may become seriously impaired.

The infectious processes which most commonly affect the heart are:

Rheumatic Fever. A systemic inflammatory disorder affecting the body's connective tissue, which may involve the endocardium, myocardium, and pericardium.

Rheumatic Heart Disease (RHD). A chronic cardiac condition which usually follows one or several episodes of rheumatic fever, and which is characterized by valvular deformity and dysfunction.

Bacterial Endocarditis (BE). A serious bacterial infection of the endocardium and valves that is caused by several types of organisms.

Myocarditis. Infection and inflammation of the myocardium resulting from many types of viral, bacterial, and parasitic disorders.

Pericarditis. Inflammation of the pericardium, which may follow rheumatic fever, penumococcal infections, and tuberculosis.

Syphilitic Heart Disease. A condition which may adversely affect the heart valves and aorta and which may not become evident until 10 to 20 years following the initial syphilic attack. (See Unit XX for a discussion of syphilis.)

Among the most serious complications arising from infectious processes within the heart are *damaged valves*. The valves may either develop *stenosis* (narrowing of the valves) or *insufficiency* (the valves are so eroded by infection that they cannot close properly). Both stenosis and insufficiency eventually lead to heart failure unless corrective measures are taken.

STRUCTURAL ABNORMALITIES DUE TO FACTORS OTHER THAN INFECTION

Structural abnormalities may be either congenital or acquired. *Congenital* heart disease results from faulty development of the heart's structures in utero. *Acquired* structural defects occur as a result of various disease processes that develop following birth.

Congenital malformations are of several types:*

1. The *valves* may be stenosed, deformed, or absent.

*For further information on congenital malformations, consult a textbook on Pediatrics.

2. The *arteries* (pulmonary and aortic) may be stenosed or malformed.

3. Abnormal *shunts* may be present. As their name implies, *left-to-right shunts* carry *oxygenated* blood from the left atrium or ventricle to the right atrium or ventricle; examples of conditions with left-to-right shunting are atrial septal defect and ventricular septal defect. These disorders *do not produce cyanosis* because the blood passes through the lungs before being shunted back to the heart's right side.

Right-to-left shunts carry venous, *nonoxygenated* blood from the right atrium or ventricle to the left atrium, left ventricle, or aorta. These conditions *produce cyanosis* since the pulmonary circulation is bypassed.

Acquired structural changes occur in the heart valves, the endocardium, myocardium, and pericardium. *Valvular* diseases are most commonly the result of infection or congenital abnormalities; they may also result from trauma. *Endocardial* disease may result from disseminated lupus erythematosus—an autoimmune disorder. Also, endocardial changes are sometimes seen in conjunction with rheumatoid arthritis.

The *myocardium* can be affected by diverse factors—tumors, metastases, toxins, chemicals, physical trauma (electric shock, radiation), immunologic responses, autoimmune diseases, and nutritional disorders. The conditions resulting from the effects of these factors on the heart are grouped into a single category called *cardiomyopathies*. Most cardiomyopathies are rare and of obscure etiology.

Pericardial disease usually occurs in conjunction with another disease that is affecting either the heart itself or surrounding structures, e.g., metastatic tumors.

HYPERTENSION—ARTERIAL AND PULMONARY

Hypertensive heart disease resulting from *arterial hypertension* is one of the most common forms of heart disease. (See also Chapter 52.) It is also a significant causative factor in death from heart failure. The major characteristic of hypertensive heart disease is hypertrophy of the left ventricle, which eventually leads to congestive heart failure. Left ventricular hypertrophy results from the heart's increased workload as it attempts to pump blood into resistive narrowed vessels.

There are two major types of arterial hypertension:

1. *Essential* hypertension: A common form of hypertension, which is of unknown origin.

2. *Secondary hypertension:* A less common form of the disease, which develops secondary to renal disorders, toxemia of pregnancy, endocrine disorders, and so forth.

Pulmonary hypertension (chronic cor pulmonale or heart-lung disease) is the analogue of hypertensive heart disease. In pulmonary hypertension, the pulmonary pressure is elevated rather than the arterial pressure. This condition most commonly results from chronic lung diseases such as emphysema; however, it may also be caused by thrombosis or emboli within the pulmonary circulation. Pulmonary hypertension leads to a thickening of the right ventricle. Because of the excessive workload placed upon the right ventricle, the right side of the heart eventually fails as a pump.

TUMORS AND TRAUMA

Primary tumors of the heart are exceedingly rare and are generally benign. On the other hand, *secondary* tumors, resulting from metastases, are not uncommon, and often develop from the spread of bronchogenic carcinomas arising in the mediastinal nodes.

Traumatic heart disease may occur as a result of: (1) *penetrating* wounds of the chest wall, e.g., bullets, needles; (2) nonpenetrating lesions, e.g., a blow to the chest; or (3) excessive physical strain or exertion.

DISTURBANCES OF RATE, RHYTHM, AND CONDUCTION

Disturbances of rate, rhythm, and conduction, i.e., arrhythmias, occur in both normal and diseased hearts. Arrhythmias develop when the muscle fibers of the heart are unable to properly elicit and transmit electrical impulses. Arrhythmias produce their effects on the body by altering circulatory dynamics. The arrhythmias will be discussed in Chapter 50.

NONCARDIAC FACTORS IN HEART DISEASE

The heart can be adversely affected by: disease processes in other parts of the body, nutritional factors, and emotional factors. Noncardiac problems damage the heart by[65] increasing the heart's workload, decreasing the heart's oxygen supply, disturbing the heart's metabolic processes, and interfering with the heart's nutrition.

Disease processes most likely to strain the heart and result in heart failure are systemic infections, fevers, autoimmune disorders, anemia, leukemia, hyperthyroidism, and electrolyte imbalances. Malnutrition can also produce heart disease, as exemplified by beriberi heart and cardiac disease associated with alcoholism. Finally, emotional stress and anxiety seems to produce transient adverse effects on cardiac rate, rhythm, output, and blood pressure.

CLASSIFICATION OF HEART DISEASE

From the preceding overview of some of the diverse factors that play a role in heart disease, you can see that there are several possible ways to classify the various heart maladies. For instance, heart diseases can be divided into two basic groups: *congenital heart disease,* and *acquired heart disease.* Another way to group heart diseases is according to the specific *structure* within the heart that is affected, e.g., valvular heart disease, diseases of the myocardium, pericardium, endocardium, and diseases of the coronary arteries. Or cardiac dysfunctions can be classified according to a *specific etiology,* e.g., ischemic heart disease, traumatic heart disease, and infectious processes within the heart.

Heart conditions may also be grouped according to which *side* of the heart they affect or whether they affect the *heart as a whole.* For example, conditions which affect the *right* side of the heart are right ventricular failure, chronic cor pulmonale, pulmonary hypertension, and congenital shunts. The *left* side of the heart is involved in left heart failure, mitral and aortic stenosis and regurgitation, myocardial infarction, and arterial hypertension. The heart as a *whole* is disturbed by the arrhythmias.

A particularly helpful way to classify a heart disease is according to the major type of *physiologic disturbance* responsible for its development.

Note that the different conditions listed in Figure 47–1 have one characteristic in common; they all eventually lead to a *reduction* in *cardiac reserve.* In other words, *the ability of the heart to meet the body's metabolic needs, under both basal conditions and stress, is impaired by all cardiovascular diseases.* Grades of reduction in cardiac reserve are discussed more fully in Chapter 49.

OVERVIEW OF THERAPY IN CARDIOVASCULAR DISEASE

BROAD GOALS OF CLINICAL CARE

The overall broad goals of clinical care for patients with cardiovascular ailments may be listed thus:

1. Prevention and early recognition of cardiovascular disease.

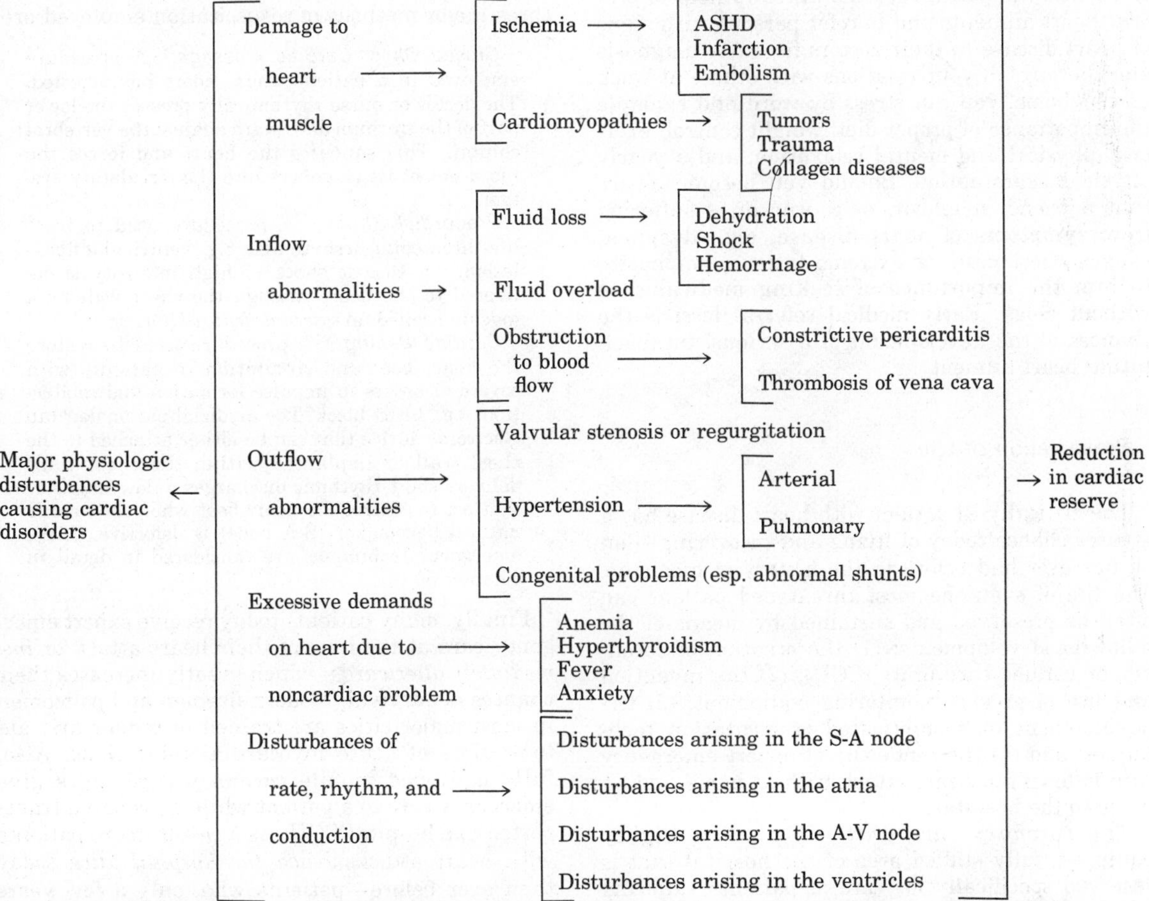

FIGURE 47–1. Classification of cardiac disorders according to the major type of physiologic disturbance.

2. Preservation of life in event of critical cardiovascular illness by means of: (a) coronary care units (CCU), (b) precise monitoring equipment, and (c) new resuscitation techniques.

3. Rehabilitation of patients with cardiovascular disease.

Prevention of Heart Disease

Heart disease is the leading cause of incapacitation and death in the United States and Europe today. The prevalence of cardiovascular ailments in these countries is possibly due to the fact that people are living longer and are more sedentary. Statistically, cardiovascular disease seems to most commonly affect obese, middle-aged persons who lead physically inactive lives. Also, some authorities believe that the high incidence of heart disease is linked to the constant emotional stress and anxiety under which many persons must function in their jobs and at home.

Because heart disease is so prevalent and because it can bring suffering and death in its wake, it is vitally important for the nurse to help to *prevent* heart ailments and to refer persons with signs of heart disease to their doctors for early diagnosis and therapy. In your relations with others at work and at home, you can stress by word and example the importance of proper diet, weight control, exercise, physical and mental relaxation, and a yearly physical examination. Should you become aware that a friend, neighbor, or co-worker is suffering from symptoms of heart disease, e.g., dyspnea, edema, chest pain, or extreme fatigue, emphasize to him the importance of seeking medical care without delay. Early medical referral lessens the chances of the development of a serious, incapacitating heart ailment.

Preservation of Life

The critically ill patient with heart disease has a greater chance today of living and recovering than he has ever had before in the history of medicine. The life of even the most threatened patient can often be preserved and sustained by means of the following developments: (1) the creation of coronary or cardiac care units (CCU); (2) the invention and use of precise monitoring equipment; (3) the development of sophisticated resuscitation techniques; and (4) the rendering of expert emergency care following a heart attack both at home and en route to the hospital.

The *coronary care unit* (CCU) is a highly equipped, fully staffed area of the hospital that is reserved specifically for care of patients suffering from acute myocardial infarction, dangerous arrhythmias, and severe heart failure. Within the CCU the patient critically ill with heart disease receives the constant care and supervision of skilled nurses who have received advanced education and experience in the field of cardiology. In most units the patient's pulse, blood pressure, venous pressure, and electrocardiogram readings are kept currently recorded for instant staff evaluation. In the event of any emergency, the necessary equipment, drugs, and personnel are on hand to immediately and skillfully treat the patient.

Monitoring equipment, which constantly records the patient's vital signs, venous pressure, and electrocardiogram tracings, is the second factor that helps to preserve patients' lives. The electrocardiogram monitor is basic to any coronary care unit. Pulse and blood pressure monitors are also commonly employed.

Such monitoring devices provide continuous data concerning the patient's condition. Today the majority of monitoring mechanisms contain an alarm system which sounds whenever an emergency situation arises or if the patient's vital signs deviate significantly from the norm. The use of these electronic devices allows nurses and doctors to care for several critical patients at once without worry that a patient will undergo dangerous alterations in his heart rate and rhythm without their knowledge.

Sophisticated *emergency techniques* constitute the third factor that has enabled physicians and nurses to save the lives of critically ill patients. The three major methods of resuscitation employed are:

> Closed Chest Cardiac Massage. A procedure employed in a patient whose heart has arrested. The doctor or nurse rhythmically presses the lower part of the sternum downward against the vertebral column. This squeezes the heart and forces the blood out of its chambers into the circulatory system.
>
> Precordial Shock. A procedure used to treat life-threatening arrhythmias, e.g., ventricular fibrillation. An electric shock of high intensity is delivered to the heart through the chest wall by a machine called an *external defibrillator*.
>
> Cardiac Pacing. A procedure used to restore the heart beat and circulation in patients with severe disorders in impulse formation and conduction, e.g., heart block. The artificial pacemaker (an electronic device that can be either attached to the chest wall or implanted within the chest wall) delivers short rhythmic discharges of low intensity that act to control the heart beat when the heart's natural pacemaker (S-A node) is defective. These emergency techniques are considered in detail in Chapter 50.

Finally, many patients today receive expert emergency care at the *time* of their heart attack or *immediately afterwards,* which greatly increases their chances of survival. Modern firemen and policemen in most major cities are trained to render first aid to victims of acute myocardial infarctions. Also, fully equipped mobile coronary care units give emergency care to a patient while he is being transported to a hospital CCU. As a result, more patients with heart attacks *reach the hospital alive* today than ever before—patients who, only a few years ago, would have died agonizing deaths either at home or on their way to the hospital.

REHABILITATION OF PATIENTS WITH CARDIOVASCULAR DISEASE

In the recent past persons with damaged hearts frequently believed that heart disease would incapacitate them, making them "cripples" for life. Such patients often became despondent, even suicidal, because they felt that the joys and responsibilities of an active life would no longer be theirs. Today one of the prime goals of doctors and nurses is to teach the patient with heart disease to live as fully and as actively as possible with minimal strain on his heart. Thus, following serious illness a patient usually is instructed to increase his activities gradually until he is able to resume his former duties and recreations.

It is true that some patients with heart disease must make rather drastic changes in their life style. For example, heart patients who have worked at hard labor or those whose jobs are extremely stressful may have to change occupations; the housewife with small children may have to hire help and rearrange her kitchen and house so that her workload is lighter; also, patients and their families may be forced to move from a two-story house to a one-story house to prevent overexertion from stair climbing.

However, the modern patient is not alone as he struggles to make these kinds of adjustments. The doctor, hospital nurse, public health nurse, industrial nurse, physical therapist, occupational therapist, social worker, and the patient's employer and family can all assist him as he reestablishes his life following serious illness. Moreover, patients who are compelled to make significant changes in their life style may obtain guidance from the Office of Vocational Rehabilitation and the American Heart Association.

CLINICAL GOALS AND TECHNIQUES

Specific therapeutic techniques and medications differ somewhat for each major cardiovascular problem. However, since the pathologic problems in all heart conditions tend to be somewhat similar, we can mention some important goals of care which generally apply to almost all dysfunctions of the cardiovascular system:

1. Improve cardiac output and increase cardiac reserve.
2. Correct arrhythmias and heart block.
3. Control sodium balance and edema.
4. Supply adequate fluid, nutrition, and oxygen to all tissues of the body.
5. Minimize the undesirable effects of therapy.

Drugs used in the treatment of cardiovascular disease will be discussed in later chapters of this unit. Here we shall simply mention the principal categories of drugs used to treat cardiovascular disorders.

1. Cardiac glycosides (e.g., digitalis).
2. Antiarrhythmic agents (e.g., procainamide, quinidine).
3. Diuretics (e.g., thiazides, mercurials).
4. Coronary dilators (e.g., nitroglycerin).
5. Antihypertensive agents (e.g., phentolamine, hydralazine, ganglionic blocking agents).

CHAPTER 48

Diagnosing and Assessing the Patient with Heart Disease

To diagnose heart disease the physician, assisted by the nurse, usually:

1. Inquires about the patient's *present* symptoms and complaints.
2. Determines the *etiology* of the heart ailment. He explores the patient's past history, habits, and working schedule; he also orders laboratory tests to verify the presence of infection, or any electrolyte abnormalities, abnormalities in the blood count, and so forth.
3. Determines, by physical examination and radiologic studies, what adverse *structural* changes have occurred within the heart, e.g., damaged valves.
4. Determines what *physiologic* problems and alterations have developed, e.g., a reduction in cardiac reserve.
5. Evaluates the extent of *cardiac reserve remaining*, and determines what *limitations* must be placed upon the patient so he may safely live within the limits of his heart's remaining functional capacity.

In this chapter we shall investigate: the typical medical history of the patient with heart disease, the classic symptoms of heart disease, the typical physical examination, diagnostic procedures, and nursing evaluation of the patient.

THE PATIENT'S MEDICAL HISTORY

Asking a patient relevant questions about himself and his present and past life patterns is just as important diagnostically as taking an ECG reading or listening to the heartbeat. As one authority states:

> It may be easier to listen at once with the stethoscope, but at the present time most cardiac diagnoses, and certainly the functional ability of the heart, are determined by what the patient tells us rather than by what the heart tells us.[155]

What exactly do we want to know about the patient with suspected heart disease? First of all, the doctor explores the patient's *past medical history*. This reveals what type of person the patient is, his general health record throughout his life, and etiologic factors that may have contributed to the development of his present cardiovascular symptoms. Answers to the following questions are generally obtained:

1. What important childhood diseases did the patient have? Was there evidence of rheumatic fever? Does the patient remember having symptoms of rheumatic fever—sore throat, "growing pains," nosebleeds, nervousness?
2. Did the patient ever have tuberculosis or pneumonia? These diseases are sometimes associated with constrictive pericarditis.
3. Does the patient recall having had such viral infections as mumps, chickenpox, and influenza? These childhood disorders sometimes contribute to the later development of cardiac dysfunction.
4. What drugs has the patient taken? digitalis? quinidine? diuretics? tranquilizers?
5. Has the patient ever experienced a direct blow or heavy pressure upon the chest?
6. Has the patient ever had thrombophlebitis or any other clotting disorder? You will recall that thrombophlebitis can precede pulmonary embolism.
7. Does the patient have a history of gout or diabetes? Metabolic disorders tend to be linked with the development of atherosclerosis.
8. Has the patient's weight remained fairly stable since the age of 20, or has he tended to gain weight steadily over the past years? Obesity and lack of exercise appear to be important factors in the development of hypertension and coronary artery disease.
9. Has the patient ever had a venereal disease, particularly syphilis?
10. Has the patient suffered from any severe emotional problems in the past? How does he generally react to upsetting experiences?
11. What are the patient's living habits, e.g., alcohol, coffee, and tea consumption; number of cigarettes smoked per day, amount of daily physical exercise, hours of sleep per night, frequency and length of vacations? Cigarette smoking, lack of physical exercise, and lack of rest as a result of stress and overwork are linked to the development of cardiovascular disease.

Second, the doctor may ask about the patient's *family history*. He may inquire if any member of the patient's family has had diabetes, tuberculosis, rheumatic fever, congenital heart disease, or if any relatives died prematurely as a result of hypertension or coronary disease.

The patient's *occupational* history, the third area of investigation, is of great importance in the diagnosis of heart disease. The doctor inquires into the physical and emotional demands of the patient's job, asking about what types of stresses the individual faces at work every day. The physician may also ask the patient about his transportation to and from his job, since modern commuting is a definite source of stress. For example, does the patient commute a long distance? Does he drive his own car? Does he drive during peak hours of traffic?

Finally, the patient's *marital* history is investigated. Domestic problems are possibly even more significant than occupational stress in the development of heart disease. Thus, the physician inquires into the number of marriages, divorces, and separations, the number and ages of the patient's children; adequacy of sexual relations; and the physical and mental health of the patient's marriage partner.

SYMPTOMS OF HEART DISEASE

> *The six cardinal symptoms diagnostic of heart disease are chest pain, dyspnea, fatigue, palpitations, syncope, and edema.*

Other important common symptoms are cyanosis, distended neck veins, murmurs, cough, and headache. When attempting to evaluate a patient's symptoms and their significance, answers are sought to the following questions:

1. How long (days, weeks, months, years) has the patient been experiencing the symptom?
2. How much does the symptom bother the patient?
3. Does any particular type of incident or episode trigger the symptom?

CHEST PAIN

Pain in the chest is a very common complaint, occurring in such cardiac diseases as angina pectoris, myocardial infarction, and pericarditis, and in such pulmonary diseases as pleurisy, pneumonia, and pulmonary embolism and infarction. Because chest pain can be caused by a number of different conditions, it is highly variable in its nature. To correctly evaluate chest pain and its causation, one must ask the patient about: (1) the *quality* of the pain (dull, sharp, crushing); (2) its *location;* (3) its *duration;* (4) points to which it *radiates* (arms, wrists, neck); and (5) *factors that precipitate, aggravate,* or *relieve* the pain (exertion, emotion, movement, and deep breathing). It is essential to obtain an accurate description of a patient's chest pain whenever it occurs, because the doctor uses this information to help to decide whether the patient has a cardiac or pulmonary condition.

DYSPNEA

Dyspnea is defined as *labored* or *difficult breathing.* Like chest pain, this common symptom affects patients with cardiac diseases and also those with respiratory ailments. Dyspnea can also trouble patients experiencing anxiety, depression, and a psychosomatic condition called "cardiac neurosis."

Although dyspnea can develop in any form of heart disease, it almost always occurs in conjunction with cardiac enlargements and other pathologic structural and physiologic changes within the cardiovascular system. This symptom is most severe and incapacitating when the patient's lungs are congested and edematous and his heart is in failure.

There are several types of dyspnea or breathing patterns that are abnormal or difficult; e.g., exertional dyspnea, orthopnea, paroxysmal nocturnal dyspnea, cardiac asthma, and Cheyne-Stokes respirations.

Exertional dyspnea, the most common form of cardiac dyspnea, occurs when the patient exercises moderately and disappears when he rests. Such noncardiac conditions as poor physical health, old age, obesity, anemia, and obstructions of the nasal passages may also lead to dyspnea with mild exercise.

Orthopnea is difficult breathing that occurs when the patient is resting flat in bed and is relieved when the patient assumes an upright or semivertical position. Usually placing two or three pillows under the patient's head relieves orthopnea. This symptom is always indicative of advanced heart disease and is far more serious than is exertional dyspnea.

Paroxysmal nocturnal dyspnea is a form of difficult breathing that occurs in terrifying attacks during the night, thus the term "paroxysmal" (sudden attacks which occur periodically), "nocturnal" (night), "dyspnea" (difficult breathing). One author vividly describes the attacks:

> The patient is aroused from his sleep gasping for air, and must sit up or stand to catch his breath. He may sweat profusely. Sometimes he throws open a window widely to relieve the oppressive sensation of suffocation. The chest tends to become fixed in the position of forced inspiration. Both inspiratory and expiratory wheezes, often simulating typical asthma, are heard. . . . Occasionally these attacks may occur several times a night, necessitating sleeping upright in a chair.[106]

These attacks occur at night because, normally, when we lie down to sleep, body fluids redistribute themselves and a state of *hypervolemia* develops. The diseased heart, however, is unable to adequately pump the extra fluid out into the circulatory system. Thus, the lungs become congested, and this, in turn, leads to difficulty in breathing.

Paroxysmal nocturnal dyspnea is most common in those cardiovascular conditions that overwork the left ventricle; e.g., hypertension and aortic stenosis or insufficiency. Factors that can lead to attacks of paroxysmal nocturnal dyspnea in heart patients are: coughing, nightmares, abdominal distention, full bladder, heavy evening meal, or frightening noises. These factors place an additional strain upon the heart, causing it to beat faster. Tachycardia in conjunction with the hypervolemia raises the blood pressure within the pulmonary circulation, thereby causing the development of congestion and even pulmonary edema.

Cardiac asthma is a term used to describe the *asthmatic wheezes* frequently heard in patients suffering from dyspnea in conjunction with pulmonary congestion and heart disease. The wheezes are caused by the following factors:

1. The lumens of the small bronchioles are reduced by the accumulation of edema fluids, which, in turn, increases resistance to airflow.
2. The walls of the bronchioles are thicker than normal because of the edema.
3. The small bronchioles are narrowed, and even collapsed, by the high intrathoracic pressure needed to overcome the obstruction to airflow within the bronchioles during expiration.*

The terms "cardiac asthma" and "paroxysmal nocturnal dyspnea" are sometimes used interchangeably, because cardiac asthma also occurs frequently at night when the patient is sleeping in a horizontal position.

Cheyne-Stokes respirations, or periodic breathing, is characterized by alternating periods of hyperpnea and apnea. In this form of dyspnea, the patient's breathing, at first shallow and slow, gradually becomes deeper and faster until it reaches a maximum point of depth. Next, the patient's breathing rate is slow and becomes more shallow until breathing stops all together, and a period of apnea lasting 10 to 20 seconds ensues. Following the apneic period, the breathing once again increases in depth and rate, and so on in a continuous cycle. This unusual breathing pattern characteristically appears in heart failure, certain neural disorders, and following large doses of sedatives (Fig. 48–1).

Evidently the basic cause of Cheyne-Stokes respirations is an alteration in the sensitivity of the respiratory center in the brain to changes in the blood gases, particularly carbon dioxide.

FATIGUE

Easy fatigability upon mild exertion, which is relieved by rest, is often the chief complaint of patients with heart disease. Fatigue due to heart ailments is a sign that the heart is unable to pump out sufficient blood and oxygen and to meet even a small increase in the metabolic demands of cells and tissues.

*See the discussion of asthma in Unit XIV for further information.

PALPITATIONS

The term palpitation is derived from the Latin word *palpitare,* meaning "to throb." Palpitation is a common symptom in patients with organic heart disease as well as those patients whose cardiac symptoms have a neurotic basis. The individual with palpitations from whatever cause typically complains of the unpleasant sensation of being conscious of his heart's action. Thus, the patient may state that he can feel his heart "beating rapidly" or "forcefully" or "irregularly," i.e., he is overly aware of the beating of his heart to the exclusion of other sensations.

The major causes of palpitations are:

1. Nonfatal arrhythmias, e.g., premature beats and atrial paroxysmal tachycardia.
2. Noncardiac organic problems, e.g., anemia, hyperthyroidism, debility, infection.
3. Nonpathologic factors, e.g., excessive exercise, excitement, large meals, alcohol, tobacco, excessive intake of coffee or tea.
4. Nervous and emotional disorders in which there is undue worry over heart action and excessive fear of heart disease; e.g., palpitation is the chief symptom of cardiac neurosis.

Persons with cardiac neurosis are often so conscious of their heart's action that they may say they feel palpitations even when their heart rate and rhythm are absolutely normal. On the other hand, persons with organic heart disease may become so habituated to disturbances in cardiac rate and rhythm that the palpitations can occur without the patient's being consciously aware of the symptom.

The two most common types of palpitations are sinus tachycardia and premature ventricular systoles. *Sinus tachycardia* is a rapid forceful beating of the heart that may begin suddenly or slowly and subsides gradually. We have all experienced sinus tachycardia as it commonly occurs whenever we exert ourselves or become unduly excited. *Premature ventricular systoles* give one the unpleasant sense that the heart is "skipping a beat" or "doing flip-flops." The existence of these and other types of palpitations can be diagnostically confirmed by electrocardiography.

SYNCOPE

Syncope or fainting, you recall, is the loss of consciousness as the result of a sudden decrease in blood flow to the brain. In patients with heart disease, syncope indicates that an adverse change in circulatory dynamics has suddenly and violently interfered with the individual's cardiac output and rhythm; e.g., there may have been the sudden development

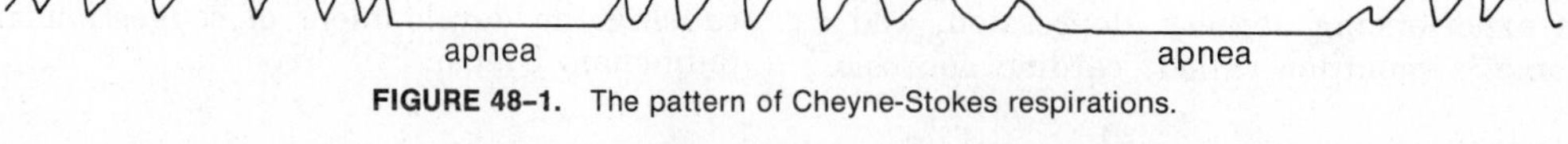

FIGURE 48–1. The pattern of Cheyne-Stokes respirations.

of heart block, cardiac arrest, or severe ventricular arrhythmias.

EDEMA*

Edema, a common symptom in many disorders, is defined as an "abnormal accumulation of extravascular, extracellular (interstitial) fluid that results from an abnormal expansion of extracellular fluid."[143] All edema fluid is drawn from the blood plasma and is similar in chemical composition to plasma. Edema may be localized to one specific organ or tissue, or it may be so severe that it affects the entire body (anasarca).

The major causes of edema in patients with heart disease and heart failure are: (1) obstruction of the blood flow *into* the heart, which leads to venous congestion; (2) obstruction of the blood flow *from* the heart, which results in pulmonary edema; (3) fluid overload, which leads to circulatory overload; (4) abnormal renal retention of water and electrolytes in response to hormonal and neural regulatory mechanisms; (5) increased renal, arterial and venous pressure; (6) increased capillary permeability; (7) decreased colloid osmotic pressure due to loss or destruction of plasma proteins; and (8) disturbances in those factors that regulate the formation and flow of lymph.

When caring for patients with heart disease, watch carefully for the following signs indicative of edema:

> *Sudden weight gain (from 10 to 20 pounds), which may* precede *the appearance of edema.*

> *Puffiness of ankles and hands in ambulatory patients.*

> *Swelling of tissues over the sacrum, buttocks, and posterior thighs in bedridden patients.*

OTHER SIGNS OR SYMPTOMS

Cyanosis

Cyanosis is a bluish discoloration of the skin that results from increased amounts of reduced hemoglobin within the blood. How *intense* the bluish skin hue is depends upon two factors: the *amount* of reduced hemoglobin present in the blood, and the extent to which one can *see the blood* within the superficial capillaries and venules of the skin. Visualization of blood within these vessels is dependent upon the patient's skin thickness and pigmentation. In certain areas of the body, cyanotic discoloration may be intense, and in other areas it may be obscured entirely.

When examining patients for the presence of cyanosis:

> *Observe color of ear lobes, lips, and fingernail beds.*

> *Observe color of mucous membranes and retina of the eye in dark-skinned persons.*

> *Observe patient in bright daylight if possible; fluorescent lighting distorts true color.*

Cyanosis may be either central or peripheral. *Central cyanosis* results from a low oxygen saturation of the arterial blood. Low arterial oxygen saturation may be caused by congenital right-to-left shunts (which cause the blood to bypass the lungs), or by pulmonary diseases, e.g., pneumonia. The central cyanosis appears on *warm* mucous membranes such as the conjunctiva and inside the lips and cheeks. The presence of central cyanosis is confirmed by testing the patient's arterial blood for the level of arterial oxygen saturation. In some extreme cases, arterial oxygen saturation may be as low as 75 per cent as compared to the normal 94 to 100 per cent.

Peripheral cyanosis differs from central cyanosis in that the arterial oxygen saturation is normal; however, the oxygen saturation within the peripheral vascular bed is poor. Extensive lack of oxygen saturation within the peripheral bed results from slowed circulation within the capillaries and venules. Thus, peripheral cyanosis develops in conditions such as heart failure and shock (in which circulation time is prolonged), and in polycythemia (in which the blood is thick and sluggish in its flow), as well as in certain peripheral vascular diseases. In contrast to central cyanosis, peripheral cyanosis appears only on *cool* parts of the body such as the nose, cheeks, and ears.

Hypoxemia

Hypoxemia, or insufficient oxygenation of the blood, is common in patients with cardiac disease and also those with lung disease.

When caring for patients with serious cardiac ailments, watch carefully for the following signs of hypoxemia:

> *An* increase *in* pulse rate; *the heart is trying to compensate for oxygen lack by pumping more blood more quickly.*

> *Signs of* cerebral anoxia; *e.g., irritability, restlessness, disorientation.*

> Asterixis *or* "liver flap"; *i.e., when the patient reaches for an object, his hands tend to flutter.*

> Cyanosis. *Cyanosis is a very* late *sign of oxygen lack. Do* not *wait for the appearance of cyanosis to notify the physician of suspected hypoxemia!*

Murmurs

The identification of a murmur, or abnormal heart sound, is one of the most important diagnostic indications of valvular heart disease. Normally blood

*Edema is discussed in detail in Chapters 24 and 25.

flows through the heart valves and blood vessels in a smooth, quiet fashion, and no audible sounds are produced. However, when there is turbulence within the blood stream, abnormal sounds develop and are called murmurs. Basically murmurs result from one of the following three factors: (1) high rate of blood flow through either a normal or abnormal valve; (2) blood flow into either a sclerosed or abnormal valve or into a dilated heart chamber or vessel; or (3) blood flow regurgitated backward through an incompetent valve or septal defect.

Murmurs are generally classified by means of the following factors:

> *Timing.* If a murmur occurs during systole, it is called a *systolic* murmur; if during diastole a *diastolic* murmur; if during both systole and diastole a *holosystolic* or *holodiastolic* murmur. Systolic murmurs, which occur when the valves are normally *open,* indicate obstruction to the blood flow, probably owing to a stenosed valve. Diastolic murmurs, which occur when the valves are normally *closed,* usually indicate regurgitation of blood as a result of incompetent valves.

> *Intensity.* Murmurs are graded on a scale that ranges from grade I (least intense or loud murmur) to grade VI (most intense murmur).

> *Location.* Designation of the place on the chest where the murmur is most clearly heard.

> *Quality.* Description of the sound, i.e., harsh, musical, blowing, rumbling.

> *Pitch.* Murmurs may be either high-pitched or low-pitched sounds.

> *Radiation.* Murmurs sometimes radiate to the neck, head, and extremities.

It is generally difficult for physicians to diagnose and interpret murmurs in the presence of severe heart disease.

Venous Engorgement of the Neck Veins

Distended neck veins are a common finding in congestive heart failure.

Engorgement of the cervical veins indicates a high central venous pressure. In the section on diagnostic tests we shall discuss how to estimate venous pressure by examination of the neck veins.

Other symptoms of cardiac disorders that you may observe while giving patient care include:

> *Cough.* Usually develops in patients suffering from heart failure and pulmonary edema.

> *Dizziness and headache.* Commonly observed symptoms in patients with hypertension and cerebral arteriosclerosis.

> *Visual disturbances.* An early sign of hypertension due to sclerosed vessels within the retina of the eye.

> *Abdominal pain.* Usually occurs in persons with liver engorgement resulting from heart failure.

> *Nosebleed.* Frequent nosebleeds in young persons may indicate rheumatic fever; in older persons, hypertensive heart disease.

THE PHYSICAL EXAMINATION OF THE HEART

The three main methods physicians use to examine the heart and its surrounding structures are percussion, palpation, auscultation.

PERCUSSION

When the cardiologist uses percussion to examine the heart, he lightly but sharply taps the area of the chest overlying the heart. The pitch of the resulting sounds aids in determining the *position* and *size* of the heart. By the use of percussion, the doctor can often diagnose cardiac enlargement or displacement—signs indicative of congestive heart failure. This diagnostic method is not ordinarily used to examine obese persons, athletic persons with very muscular chest walls, or patients with emphysema.

PALPATION OF THE PRECORDIUM

The precordium is that part of the anterior surface of the body that lies over the heart, the heart's great vessels, and the pulmonary structures that are located anterior to the heart. By palpating the precordium the physician is able to estimate *heart size;* also, he may be able to detect certain *abnormal vibrations* originating in the heart that are difficult to hear through a stethoscope.

AUSCULTATION

Auscultation, or listening to the patient's heart and chest with a stethoscope, is used to discover structural and functional abnormalities within the heart and lungs. Listening to the heart sounds is a particularly valuable diagnostic aid in thin individuals, because the sounds are far clearer than in obese persons. By careful auscultation with the stethoscope, the physician or specially trained nurse is able to:

1. Identify abnormal first or second heart sounds.
2. Note the appearance of abnormal heart sounds.
3. Analyze adventitious pulmonary sounds, e.g., rales and wheezes.
4. Note nonpathologic heart sounds.

The most important sounds to note are the first and second heart sounds. The *first* heart sound ("lubb"), which results from the closure of the mitral and tricuspid valves, indicates how well the left ventricle is contracting. If the sound is very loud, the left ventricle is probably contracting normally.

The second heart sound ("dubb"), which results from the closure of the aortic and pulmonic semilunar valves, gives information concerning the blood pressure within the vascular system—both arterial and pulmonary. Normally the second heart sound should be softer than the first sound. A very loud second heart sound may indicate either arterial or pulmonary hypertension.

Abnormal heart sounds can be differentiated from *normal* and *nonpathologic* sounds by means of auscultation. The normal heart sounds are usually of very brief duration, consisting only of a few vibrations, and are the result of a change in the velocity of the blood flow owing to closing of the valves. Examples of *nonpathologic* sounds are a "splitting" of the first sound, and an occasional added third heart sound. *Pathologic murmurs* are usually prolonged and have definite characteristics that are related to time, duration, intensity, location, and radiation.

Listening to the patient's *lungs* for abnormal sounds is an important method for diagnosing both heart and pulmonary abnormalities. *Moist rales,* which are fine crackling sounds like the crinkling of cellophane, are an important physical finding in patients with left ventricle failure. Rales may result from pulmonary infection, pulmonary edema, or aspiration of fluid; they generally indicate the presence of fluid within the patient's lungs.

Wheezes, a second type of abnormal chest sound, usually indicate narrowing of the bronchioles and the presence of bronchospasm. Wheezing is a common finding in acute pulmonary edema, asthma, and acute allergic reactions.

DIAGNOSTIC PROCEDURES

The four most common types of diagnostic procedures used to diagnose cardiovascular disease are: laboratory tests, measures of circulatory dynamics, x-ray techniques, and graphic procedures.

LABORATORY TESTS

The major types of laboratory tests that physicians commonly order for patients with suspected heart ailments are: (1) blood count, (2) blood sedimentation rate, (3) prothrombin time, (4) kidney function tests, (5) serum cholesterol, (6) blood smears and cultures, (7) blood serum protein, (8) serologic tests, (9) urinalysis, and (10) enzyme tests. Let us briefly explore the purpose of each of these tests, the normal values, and the meaning of abnormal findings.

*Blood Count.** A complete blood count is routinely ordered on all patients with suspected heart disease. The erythrocyte count is normally between 4 and 5.5 million/cu.mm. The erythrocyte count usually *decreases* in rheumatic fever and subacute bacterial endocarditis; it is usually *increased* in heart diseases in which inadequate oxygenation of tissues is a problem, e.g., right-to-left congenital shunts and heart conditions accompanied by pulmonary insufficiency.

The normal leukocyte count is from 5 to 10 thousand/cu.mm. The leukocyte count is *elevated* in infectious diseases of the heart (e.g., acute bacterial endocarditis), and following a myocardial infarction. The white count rises following a myocardial infarction because large numbers of white cells are necessary to dispose of the necrotic tissue resulting from the infarction.

Blood Sedimentation Rate. The blood sedimentation rate is a measure of the rapidity with which red blood cells settle out of the unclotted blood in one hour. The rate of settling is evidently influenced by changes in the levels of the blood proteins. The normal "sed" rate varies with the laboratory method used and with the sex of the patient. An approximately normal reading is between 6 and 20 mm. in one hour; the readings are generally higher for women than for men.

Examination of the blood sedimentation rate allows the physician to *roughly* follow the course of acute rheumatic fever, acute myocardial infarction, and infectious heart disease. However, the blood sedimentation rate is *not* a very accurate test, because it can be influenced by a number of physiologic factors other than disease. Although measuring the "sed" rate has been a helpful "old standby" in many hospitals, newer and more sophisticated tests are being developed which may eventually replace it.

Blood Coagulation Tests. As the name implies, blood coagulation tests examine the ability of a patient's blood to clot. Clotting is a complex physiologic phenomenon that is dependent upon the presence of blood clotting factors.

The *Lee-White coagulation time test* involves the examination of all the coagulation factors within the blood. The "normal" findings for this test vary with the laboratory method used. Daily coagulation times are ordered for patients who have suffered an acute myocardial infarction or who are receiving *heparin*—a potent anticoagulant that interferes with the clotting mechanism and helps to prevent further infarctions.

Prothrombin time determination, sometimes referred to as the "pro time," determines the activity of prothrombin, fibrinogen, and three other coagulation factors. This test is performed daily on the blood of patients receiving anticoagulant drugs that interfere with the synthesis of prothrombin in the liver, such as coumarin (Dicumarol) and warfarin sodium (Coumadin Sodium). The prothrombin time determination is also performed on patients suspected of having a tendency toward the formation of thrombi.

Blood Urea Nitrogen (BUN). The BUN is a test of renal function. *Urea* is an important nonprotein nitrogenous substance that is formed in the liver and found in the blood, lymph, and urine. Urea is the final end product of protein metabolism, and is the major nitrogenous factor within the urine. The BUN test measures the nitrogen faction of urea circulating in the blood.

The normal BUN is 8-28 mg./100 ml. of blood. BUN levels are elevated in kidney diseases and in heart ailments that adversely affect the renal circulation, e.g., congestive heart failure.

Serum Cholesterol. This laboratory test measures the level of cholesterol in the blood. Cholesterol is an alcohol released upon the breakdown of

*Leukocyte counts are discussed in Chapter 23; erythrocyte count is discussed in Chapter 61.

fats within the body. It is found in bile and blood and in the brain and spinal cord tissues. Cholesterol is most commonly ingested in egg yolk and in certain fats and oils.

The normal range for blood cholesterol is from 150 to 280 mg./100 ml. of blood. An increase in blood cholesterol is possibly associated with the development of atherosclerosis and coronary occlusion. We further consider the possible role of cholesterol in the etiology of coronary artery disease in Chapter 51.

For accurate results, patients should be *fasting* prior to the drawing of blood for the serum cholesterol test.

Serum Protein. You will recall from Chapter 24 that plasma proteins are large particles within the blood that exert a force called the *colloid osmotic pressure;* this pressure draws fluid from the interstitial fluid compartment into the vascular compartment or capillaries, thereby counterbalancing the force of hydrostatic blood pressure, which forces fluid out of the capillaries into the tissues. Thus, when the level of plasma proteins (especially serum albumin) drops below normal, the colloid osmotic pressure is diminished, and fluid escapes from the vascular compartment into the tissues. The result of diminished plasma proteins is *edema;* consequently the physician always checks the level of serum proteins in patients with edema.

The *normal* level of serum protein is 6-8 Gm./100 ml. of blood. A substantial decrease in the level of serum protein (below 5 Gm./100 ml.) results in edema. Hypoproteinemia (especially a reduction in serum albumin) is associated with longstanding cardiac failure as a result of malnutrition, decreased production of albumin by the liver in right-sided heart failure, and the loss of albumin in the urine and peritoneal effusions over a long period of time.

Blood Cultures. This form of laboratory study is ordered for patients with infectious diseases of the heart, e.g., bacterial endocarditis. The blood for the culture is obtained by venipuncture and is then inoculated into a culture medium. The bacterial colony that grows on the culture medium enables the doctor to identify the organism causing the infectious disease. Once the organism has been identified, the sensitivity of the organism to various antibiotics is tested to ascertain the proper course of therapy.

Serologic Tests. Because of the important role of syphilis in infections of the aorta and in the production of aortic aneurysms, the doctor frequently orders serologic examinations. Common serologic tests are flocculation tests, complement-fixation tests, and the *Treponema pallidum* immobilization (TPI) test.

Urinalysis. Heart disease (in particular, congestive heart failure) can result in damage to the kidneys. Thus, in congestive heart failure, casts are usually present in the urine, albuminuria is common, and the urine's specific gravity is high.

You will recall from Chapter 24 that the specific gravity of urine (or the concentration of urine) is between 1.010 and 1.025. Patients suffering from congestive heart failure typically have a dark, concentrated urine with a *high* specific gravity of between 1.020 and 1.030; sodium content of the urine is very low. The urine is concentrated in these individuals, because Na^+ and H_2O are being held in the tissues as edema fluid, cardiac output is reduced, and circulating blood volume is diminished. Diuresis and Na^+ restriction help to lower the specific gravity of the urine.

Albuminuria, as stated earlier, may also develop in patients suffering from congestive heart failure who have impaired renal function.

Enzyme Tests. Enzymes found within the heart muscle, which are released into the circulation whenever the myocardium is injured, are serum glutamic oxaloacetic transaminase (SGOT), creatine phosphokinase (CPK), and lactic dehydrogenase. Specific information concerning the normal serum levels of these enzymes and their role in the diagnosis of heart disease is summarized in Table 48–1.

MEASURES OF CIRCULATORY DYNAMICS

Four important diagnostic procedures that measure how effectively the blood is circulating through

TABLE 48–1. ENZYME TESTS: NORMAL LEVELS AND SIGNIFICANCE IN HEART DISEASE

Enzyme Test	Normal Level in Blood Serum	Tissues in Which Enzymes Normally Found	Significance of Elevated Blood Serum Levels
SGOT (serum glutamic oxaloacetic transaminase)	10-40 units (U)	Myocardial tissue, liver cells, muscle cells	Levels as high as 500 U indicate myocardial infarction; levels over 500 U indicate liver disease
CPK (creatine phosphokinase)	0-200 sigma units	Striated muscle, myocardium, liver and lung tissue in small amounts	Levels greatly elevated in myocardial infarction (MI); most useful in the early diagnosis of MI
LDH (lactic dehydrogenase)	165-300 units	Many body cells, including myocardial cells	Elevated levels following myocardial infarction and many other conditions; nonspecific for diagnosis of acute MI

the heart and vascular system are: circulation time determination, measures of cardiac output, blood pressure readings, and venous pressure measurements.

CIRCULATION TIME DETERMINATION

The circulation time is the length of time it takes for a special solution (either sodium dehydrocholate or calcium chloride) injected intravenously to circulate from the patient's arm to his tongue, where it can be tasted. Sometimes this test is called a "circ time." This test is employed mainly to establish a diagnosis of congestive heart failure or to follow the course of patients with this disease. The circulation time is *prolonged* in congestive heart failure because the patient's *blood volume* is *increased* (owing to fluid retention) and renal dysfunction, and because the *cardiac output* is reduced (owing to the heart's decreased pumping action).

The actual procedure for the circulation time determination is relatively simple. Here are the major steps:

1. Assemble equipment: a sterile syringe and needle, a tourniquet, antiseptic solution for the skin, an ampule of test solution, alcohol sponges, and a stopwatch.
2. Have the patient lie down and rest for at least 20 minutes prior to the test.
3. Help the patient to relax as completely as possible so that his body's metabolic needs are reduced; project a calm, reassuring attitude.
4. Explain the patient's role in the procedure. Tell the patient not to hold his breath when the doctor injects the test solution, because this will prolong the venous return to the heart. Explain to the patient that he will experience a bitter taste on his tongue shortly after the injection of the solution. Stress that he must tell the doctor as soon as he tastes the bitter substance.
5. The test may need to be repeated to double-check the results.

The normal systemic circulation time (from arm to tongue) is *15 seconds*. Circulation time is *prolonged* in congestive heart failure, polycythemia vera, and myxedema; it is *reduced* in hyperthyroidism, anemia, pregnancy, fever, congenital heart disease with right-to-left shunts, and after eating and exercise.

CARDIAC OUTPUT

You will recall from Chapter 46 that the cardiac output is the amount of blood pumped out of the left ventricle into the arterial system every minute; i.e., cardiac output is equal to the stroke volume (volume of blood pumped out with each beat) times the rate. Therefore, if the stroke volume of the left ventricle is between 50 and 90 ml., with an average of 70 ml., and the heart rate is 72 beats per minute, the normal cardiac output of the left ventricle is roughly between 4 and 7L. The cardiac output of the right ventricle is considered equal to that of the left; this is because the right ventricle, while it is not so muscular as the left ventricle, pumps against lighter resistance.

There are two major methods for measuring cardiac output: application of the Fick principle, and indicator dilution methods.

The *Fick principle* implies that the cardiac output per minute from the *right* ventricle (and consequently the *left* ventricle) can be determined by measuring the amount of blood that the right ventricle pumps into the lung capillaries within one minute. The amount of blood flowing through the capillaries of the lungs within 1 minute can be determined by: (1) measuring the amount of *oxygen* that the blood has absorbed within 1 minute, which is dependent upon the patient's basal metabolic rate, and (2) measuring the difference between the oxygen content of the oxygen-poor venous blood entering the lungs and the oxygen-rich arterial blood that flows from the lungs into the left side of the heart and the arterial system.

To estimate the cardiac output by applying the Fick principle, three laboratory measurements are needed:

1. A measure of the patient's oxygen consumption in milliliters per minute when the patient is resting; this measure is obtained by means of a basal metabolism machine.
2. A measure of the oxygen content of arterial blood, which is obtained by direct venipuncture of any artery.
3. A measure of the oxygen content of the mixed venous blood, which is customarily taken from the right ventricle or pulmonary artery during cardiac catheterization.

After obtaining the above measures, the physician next applies this formula to the data:[64]

$$\frac{O_2 \text{ absorption ml./min.}}{\begin{matrix}O_2 \text{ content of} \\ \text{arterial blood} \\ \text{in ml./L.}\end{matrix} - \begin{matrix}O_2 \text{ content of} \\ \text{mixed venous} \\ \text{blood in ml./L.}\end{matrix}} = \text{cardiac output in L./min.}$$

As an example of the application of this formula, consider the following measurements for a typical patient.[64] (1(O_2 absorption per minute = 200 ml.; (2) oxygen concentration of arterial blood = 190 ml./L.; (3) oxygen content of venous blood = 150 ml./L.

$$\frac{200 \text{ ml./min. (oxygen absorption)}}{\begin{matrix}190 \text{ ml./L.} \\ (\text{arterial } O_2)\end{matrix} - \begin{matrix}150 \text{ ml./L.} \\ (\text{venous } O_2)\end{matrix}} = \frac{200 \text{ ml./min.}}{40 \text{ ml./L.}} = 5 \text{ L. Blood}$$

This is equal to (1) the cardiac output of the right ventricle, and (2) the amount of blood that has passed through the lungs in 1 minutes. Because the outputs of both the right and left ventricles are approximately equal, 5 L. per minute is also the cardiac output of the left ventricle.

Indicator dilution methods provide a second means for obtaining a measure of cardiac output. In this procedure the patient receives a measured intravenous injection of dye (e.g., indocyanine green). Next, blood samples are drawn from an artery, and the concentration of dye within the blood is calculated by means of precise measuring devices. Then this reading, which shows the amount of time required for the blood to absorb the measured amount of dye, is amplified; it appears as a curve on graph paper. The size of the curve indicates how much blood the heart has pumped out into the arterial system in a given amount of time, i.e., the cardiac output. Blood samples for the dye dilution method can be obtained during cardiac catheterization.

The *normal* cardiac output for the calm, resting patient (who has been NPO for 12 hours) spans a range of from 4 to 7 L. per minute, with an average of 5.3. Table 48–2 lists the conditions that elevate and depress cardiac output.

ARTERIAL BLOOD PRESSURE

The most accurate blood pressure reading is obtained when the patient is truly resting. In other words; "the physical, metabolic, mental, and emotional stimuli that elevate blood pressure have been eliminated."[89] Naturally this is an ideal state for which we strive but rarely, if ever, achieve.

In earlier courses you have probably studied the basic equipment needed and the method for taking a blood pressure reading.* In this section we shall briefly emphasize those factors that decrease or increase the chances of error. Because the blood pressure is a common diagnostic and evaluative measurement and because it is primarily a nursing procedure, we cannot emphasize enough the importance of an accurate reading and the elimination of error. Blood pressure readings are *most accurate* when you adhere to the following basic rules:

1. Instruct the patient to neither eat, drink, nor exert himself for at least one half hour prior to his blood pressure reading. Try to have the patient in a quiet room that has a comfortable temperature. If he is ambulatory, allow him to remain comfortably seated for at least 5 minutes before taking the reading.
2. Place the seated patient's arm on a table in such a way that it is at *heart* level; likewise, position the bed patient's arm at heart level, supporting it comfortably. If the patient's arm is *not* at heart level, both systolic and diastolic readings may be in error by as much as 10 mm. Hg.
3. Make certain that the blood pressure cuff is the *correct width.* A cuff that is too *narrow* for the arm will give a falsely high reading; a cuff which is too *wide* will result in a falsely low reading. Generally, a cuff 12 to 14 cm. (about 6 in.) wide is suitable for the average adult.
4. Make certain that you apply the cuff snugly and evenly and that the bag is *completely deflated* prior to the first reading and between readings. Always center the cuff's bladder over the artery that you plan to occlude. Be sure that the stethoscope bell does not touch the tubes, cuff, or patient's clothing, as you may hear confusing extraneous sounds as a result.
5. Inflate the cuff as rapidly as possible (within 7 seconds or less) and deflate it at 2 to 3 mm. per heartbeat until you no longer hear Korotkoff's sounds.
6. When viewing the blood pressure gauges, remember these rules: (a) Observe the *aneroid* guage from directly in front of it and from no farther than 3 feet away. (b) Observe the *mercury* guage (which must be in a vertical position) with your eye at the level of the meniscus and from no farther than 3 feet away.
7. Take several blood pressure readings over a period of time; ask another nurse to take the patient's blood pressure so that you can compare readings.
8. When you record your findings: (a) Record the position of the patient during the reading. Blood pressure is usually higher in the standing position than in the lying position. Abbreviate lying (L) or standing (ST). (b) Record the arm used for the reading: right arm (RA) or left arm (LA). (c) Record the *muffling* of Korotkoff's sounds as the diastolic reading. Also record the point at which Korotkoff's sounds disappear; e.g., 142/80/78; 142/76/76.*

What is a "normal" blood pressure reading? Insurance companies often place the normal blood pressure reading at around 120/80. However, it is essential to remember that blood pressure readings

*When reviewing the blood pressure procedure, refresh your memory in regard to these terms: systolic blood pressure, diastolic blood pressure, Korotkoff's sounds, sphygmomanometer, blood pressure cuff, aneroid gauge, mercury gauge, auscultatory method, palpatory method.

*For years there has been a lively debate between the "muffled sound" school of authorities and the "last sound" school concerning which level provides the more accurate index of the diastolic pressure. In 1967 the American Heart Association settled the dispute by recommending that clinicians record *both* muffling of sounds and the disappearance of sounds as the diastolic pressure.[89]

TABLE 48–2. CONDITIONS THAT CAUSE A CHANGE IN CARDIAC OUTPUT

Conditions Decreasing Cardiac Output	Conditions Increasing Cardiac Output
1. Acute congestive heart failure	1. Hypoxia
2. Pericarditis with effusion	2. Hyperthyroidism
3. Old age	3. Excitement
4. Arterial hemorrhage	4. Exercise
5. Standing motionless, which decreases the venous return to the heart	5. Food intake
6. Myxedema	6. Oral and intravenous fluid intake
7. Atrial fibrillation	
8. Heart block	
9. Shock	
10. Valvular heart disease	

vary greatly among healthy individuals. For some persons a blood pressure of 120/80 would be abnormally high; for other persons it might be abnormally low. It is wise to consult the patient's former history or even the patient himself in regard to blood pressure readings taken in the past. What may appear to be an abnormal reading may actually be a normal reading for a particular individual.

Hypertension, a common problem, refers only to conditions in which the recorded pressure is *persistently* higher than normal.[115] Generally a blood pressure that is persistently above 160 systolic or 100 diastolic is considered hypertensive.

VENOUS PRESSURE

The central venous pressure (CVP) is a measurement of the pressure within the superior vena cava. CVP reflects the pressure under which the blood is returned to the superior vena cava or the right atrium.

The normal CVP usually is between 5 and 10 cm. H_2O. In situations in which the blood volume is *reduced* (e.g., hemorrhage or fluid loss from other causes), the *CVP is lower than usual;* thus, values below 5 cm. H_2O may indicate a decreasing circulating volume.

In situations in which the circulatory system is *overloaded* (e.g., due to excessive administration of fluids or congestive heart failure) the *CVP will be higher than normal.* Thus, values above 10 cm. H_2O indicate overloading of the right heart.

One may estimate venous pressure by: (1) examination of the neck veins or cervical veins; or (2) examination of veins on the dorsum of the hand; or (3) the venous pressure may be measured with a saline manometer.

Examination of the neck veins is an excellent means for estimating the venous pressure. One authority states:

> Examination of the cervical veins is the most reliable means of clinical estimation of venous pressure and actually often exceeds in accuracy the measurement of venous pressure with a saline manometer in inexpert hands.[58]

To estimate the cervical venous pressure, the physician or nurse should follow this procedure:

1. Have the patient lie on a bed or table and raise the head of the bed so the patient is sitting at a 30- or 45-degree angle. Use a table or bed that breaks at the patient's hipline; otherwise, the patient's neck will be flexed, making it impossible to properly examine the neck veins.
2. Remove clothing that compresses the neck or upper thorax.
3. Use a pocket flashlight or place a gooseneck lamp in a position so that small shadows are cast on the patient's neck, thereby making the veins more apparent (Fig. 48–2). Good lighting is important in this examination.
4. Locate the external jugular veins on each side of the neck and detect their pulsations.
5. Estimate the venous pressure by measuring the level to which the veins are distended up the neck toward the head *above* the level of the manubrium (i.e., the upper bone of the sternum, which articulates with the clavicle); also estimate how high the venous pulsations extend. In a healthy individual seated at a 45-degree angle, the venous pulses should not ascend any higher than 1 or 2 cm. above the manubrium. In a patient with a high venous pressure of 25 cm. or more (e.g., in severe congestive heart failure), the cervical veins may be distended from the level of the manubrium up to the angle of the jaw (Fig. 48–3).

It is possible to roughly estimate the venous pressure by *examining the veins on the back of the patient's hand* as he raises and lowers his arm. As the

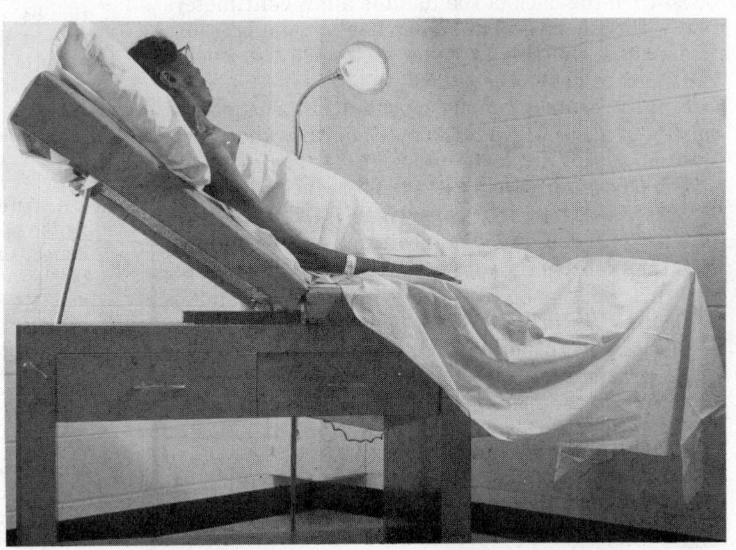

FIGURE 48–2. Cardiac patient in proper position for examination of cervical venous pulse. Note that the examining table breaks at the patient's hips so that the neck is not flexed. (From Fowler, N. O.: *Examination of the Heart.* Part 2: *Inspection and Palpation of Venous and Arterial Pulses.* Prepared for the Committee on Medical Education of the American Heart Association. New York, American Heart Association, 1970.)

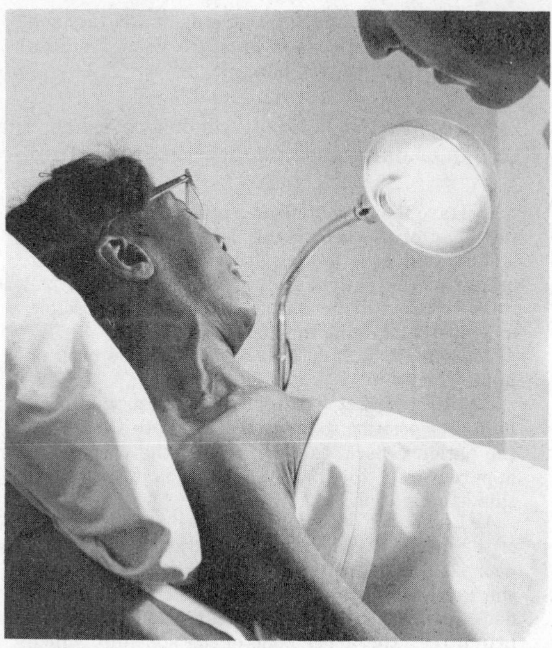

FIGURE 48–3. Close-up view of the patient, demonstrating greatly distended external jugular vein. The systemic venous pressure exceeded 30 cm H_2O. (From Fowler, N. O.: *Examination of the Heart. Part 2: Inspection and Palpation of Venous and Arterial Pulses.* Prepared for the Committee on Medical Education of the American Heart Association. New York, American Heart Association, 1970.)

patient raises his hand, observe for that point above the sternal notch at which the veins on the dorsum of his hand collapse. Normally collapse of the veins occurs when the back of the hand is a few centimeters above the sternal notch. When the venous pressure is elevated, the veins remain distended for several centimeters above the sternal notch.[4]

Finally, central venous pressure is measured by means of a *saline manometer.* Generally the procedure is carried out as follows:

The physician injects a needle, attached to a three-way stopcock and a 10 cc. syringe filled with 5 ml. of 3 per cent sodium citrate solution, into a vein; he will then release the tourniquet and withdraw a few milliliters of blood into the syringe so that it mixes with the citrate.

The physician next attaches a manometer to the stopcock and injects the mixture (blood mixed with citrate) into the manometer. The mixture flows into the veins and the level of fluid within the manometer drops. In a minute or so the level of fluid ceases to fall and fluctuate and then stabilizes. Note the level on the manometer at which the fluid stabilizes and chart it as the CVP.

Sometimes a critically ill patient requires *constant* monitoring of his CVP. In these instances the doctor may perform a cutdown or venous section and insert a polyethylene or polyvinyl catheter directly into the patient's right atrium or adjacent vena cava. The median basilic or cephalic vein is commonly used. If a cutdown is not practical, then the jugular or subclavian vein may be directly punctured, using a Teflon intracatheter for insertion. Teflon catheters with plastic styluses make the insertion an easy, simple procedure.

When the catheter is in place and the physician has removed the plastic stylus, a "flush bottle," which the nurse has ready is promptly started. A "flush bottle" is a 500-ml. bottle of 5 per cent dextrose in water, to which 10 mg. of heparin is frequently added to prevent clotting in the lumen of the catheter. The catheter can also serve as a source for intravenous fluids. To maintain patency, the flush bottle is regulated to drip slowly through use of the microdrip technique.

> *Remember that the fluid that the patient receives intravenously from the flush bottle could cause a circulatory overload unless it is carefully observed and adjusted to a slow rate of drip.*

A manometer is attached to the catheter. Kurihara and Moody offer the following information pertaining to establishing a baseline for the position of the monitor and measuring the pressure:

1. *Establishing a Baseline for Manometer Position.* The manometer is so positioned that the zero mark is at the level of the right atrium, using the left or right midchest (Fig. 48–4). The right atrium is located inferiorly to midsternum and halfway between the front to the back of the chest laterally. . . . If the patient has pulmonary emphysema, a lung disease or a barrel chest, use the lower third of the lateral chest in locating the right atrium. This then establishes the reference position prior to each subsequent CVP measurement and reading. . . .

If the patient cannot tolerate a flat supine position because of orthopnea with left-sided heart failure, he may sit at a 45-degree angle with the zero point of the manometer adjusted to the level of the right atrium in the sitting position. This then becomes the established reference position. Between measurements the patient may lie or sit in any position of comfort.

2. *Measurement of Pressure*

a. After the catheter has been properly positioned by the physician and the reference position is established, the nurse regulates the fluid from the flush bottle to run directly through the catheter into the vein ("solution arm" to "delivery arm" in diagram), in order to maintain the patency of the system.

b. By turning the stopcock from "solution arm" to "manometer arm," the manometer is then filled to a level of 20 to 25 cm.

c. The stopcock is then turned from the "manometer arm" position to "delivery arm" position for the actual pressure reading. With each respiration, the meniscus of the column of water in the "manometer arm" fluctuates. The reading is taken at the maximum level the meniscus reaches after it attains an average level in the column, indicating equal pressure in the manometer and the vena cava.

d. To keep the system open for subsequent readings, the stopcock is returned to its original position ("solution arm" to "delivery arm") and the flow is controlled by a microdrip method.

e. It is essential that the patient be relaxed at the time measurement is made, because straining, coughing, or any other activity that increases the intrathoracic pressure will cause spuriously high measurements. When CVP is measured while the patient is receiving mechanical respiratory assistance, the respirator must be temporarily disconnected to obtain a meaningful reading.[95]

Frequently check the connections between the catheter and the attachments to be certain that they are secure; if they are not secure, the danger of *air embolism is present.* If the original reference position was established with the patient in a flat position, this same flat position must be resumed again at the time of repeated pressure readings. False readings can result from even a slight elevation of the head of the bed.

X-RAY TECHNIQUES

X-ray techniques are one of the major tools for diagnosing various types of heart disease. Some of the major purposes of x-ray techniques in making an evaluation of cardiac structure and function are:

1. To provide information about: heart size and volume, the size of the individual chambers, the appearance of the vessels extending from the heart, and the presence and location of calcifications.
2. To reveal, by means of motion pictures (cineangiograms), any abnormal shunts or regurgitations within the heart.

The major types of x-ray techniques are fluoroscopy, angiocardiography, and cardiac catheterization.

Fluoroscopy

This simple, economical, and popular method of x-ray examination reveals the action of the heart at work. The patient stands in back of a fluorescent screen and in front of an x-ray tube. The examiner stands in front of the screen and is able to observe the continuous action of the heart.

This method of examination is used mainly to search for: (1) abnormal tumors, structures, and calcifications within the heart; (2) signs of lung congestion; and (3) signs of pleural or pericardial effusion.

Fluoroscopy is a safe procedure with one exception—it is possible to overexpose the patient and examiner to ionizing radiation during the examination.

Angiocardiography

This procedure involves the intravenous injection of a radiopaque solution or dye into the patient's veins, followed by a series of x-rays which reveal the course of the solution as it circulates through the patient's heart, lungs, and great vessels.

The purposes of angiocardiography are to:

1. Check the valves of the heart for competence.
2. Diagnose congenital septal defects.
3. Reveal calcifications or occlusions of the coronary arteries by means of selective coronary angiography.
4. Confirm diagnoses that cannot be confirmed by simpler means.
5. Study the structure and function of the heart in detail prior to cardiac surgery.

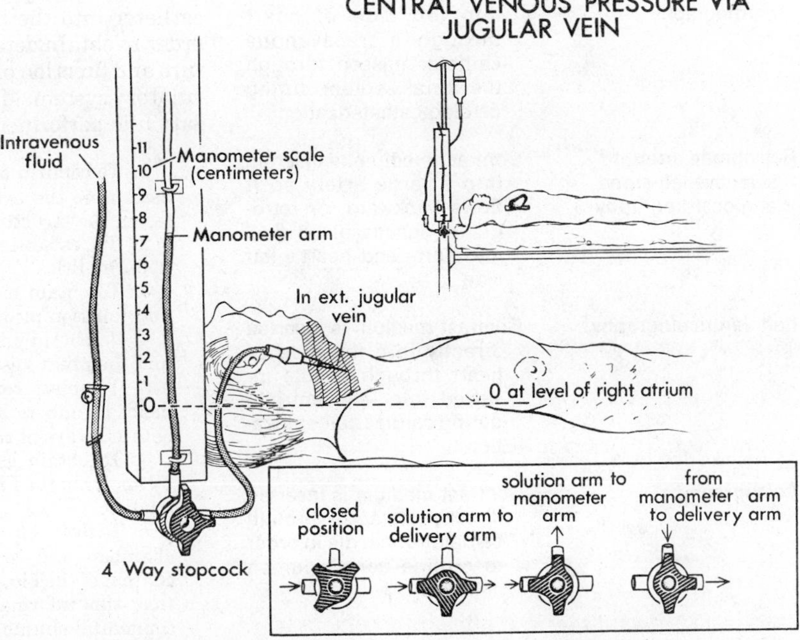

FIGURE 48-4. Central venous pressure obtained from the jugular vein. (From Kurihara, M., and Moody, F. G.: The complications of general surgery. *In* Meltzer, L. E., Abdellah, F. G., and Kitchell, J. R. (eds.): *Concepts and Practices of Intensive Care for Nurse Specialists.* Philadelphia, Charles Press Publishers, Inc., 1969.)

Angiocardiography is a complex and somewhat dangerous procedure, and thus is performed only when absolutely necessary. The major types of angiocardiography are listed and defined in Table 48–3. These procedures are usually performed in conjunction with cardiac catheterization.

The *contrast medium* used for angiocardiography is usually an organic iodine medium such as diatrizoate sodium (Hypaque Sodium), diatrizoate methylglucamine (Cardiografin), or sodium diprotrizoate and diatrizoate (Ditriokon). The physician calculates the dosage of contrast medium to be inserted into the patient's heart and vessels by determining the patient's weight in kilograms. Standard dosage for contrast media in angiography is 1 ml. per kg. of body weight.

TABLE 48–3. MAJOR TYPES OF ANGIOCARDIOGRAPHY

Angiocardiography Procedure	Method Employed
I.V. angiocardiography	Contrast medium is rapidly injected into a peripheral vein by means of a needle and syringe
Selective I.V. angiocardiography	Contrast medium is injected into the right heart chambers or pulmonary arteries by means of a catheter threaded up a vein and into the heart
Left-sided angiocardiography	Contrast medium is inserted into left side of heart through a transvenous catheter passed through the atrial septum during cardiac catheterization
Retrograde arterial selective left-sided angiocardiography	Contrast medium is inserted into a large artery so it flows backward, or retrograde, against blood flow into aorta and heart's left side
Left ventriculography	Contrast medium is inserted directly into left side of heart through needle inserted into left ventricle during cardiac catheterization
Aortography	Contrast medium is inserted directly into aorta through catheter or needle in order to outline aorta's lumen and branches

Preparation of the patient for the procedure is minimal. The nurse's duties prior to angiocardiography are:

1. Weigh patient and send weight record to x-ray department.
2. Withhold breakfast or lunch and fluids if patient is to receive any type of anesthetic agent.
3. Obtain order for mild sedative to be given one half hour before the procedure if patient appears anxious or fearful.
4. Question patient carefully concerning any allergies; report history of any allergic reactions to the physician *prior* to the procedure.

Patients sometimes react allergically to iodine-base contrast media. In some cases the doctor may wish to skin test the patient for a possible allergic reaction on the day prior to the angiocardiography. Be on guard for such allergic symptoms as flushing, nausea and vomiting, tingling and numbness, weakness, and urticaria. Fortunately, anaphylactic shock is rare. Nevertheless, oxygen, antihistamine drugs, and epinephrine should be on hand whenever angiocardiography is performed.

Other complications that occasionally develop are *tissue slough* due to leakage of the contrast medium into the area surrounding the vein, and *venous thrombosis*.

Although fatalities rarely occur during angiocardiography, deaths can result from the rapid injection of large doses of contrast medium directly into the coronary arteries or cerebral vessels; the large bolus of medium evidently acts as a type of thrombus.

Nursing care of the patient following angiocardiography usually consists of checking the area of the incision for tenderness, swelling, infection, or thrombosis. If the area is excessively sore, warm compresses usually ease the pain.

Cardiac Catheterization

This complex procedure involves the insertion of a catheter into the heart and surrounding vessels in order to obtain detailed information about the structure and function of the heart, the valves, and the circulatory system. More specifically, cardiac catheterization is performed for the following reasons:

1. To confirm a diagnosis of heart disease and to determine the extent to which the disease has affected the structure and function of the heart.
2. To establish the existence of congenital abnormalities.
3. To obtain a clear picture of cardiac structure and function prior to heart surgery.
4. To obtain pressures within the heart chambers and the great vessels.
5. To inject contrast medium directly into the heart chambers and adjoining vessels in order to obtain x-rays of the heart (i.e., angiocardiography).
6. To obtain estimates of cardiac output either by applying the Fick method or by indicator dilution studies.
7. To draw blood samples directly from the heart chambers and vessels in order to measure the O_2 content of the blood and the extent of oxygen saturation; this information indicates whether abnormal congenital shunts are present in the heart.

8. To enable the physician to perform specialized cardiac techniques, e.g., internal pacing of the heart.

Patients must be carefully prepared for this procedure, both physically and emotionally. Cardiac catheterization is as important and as potentially dangerous as surgery. Major steps in preparing the patient are:

1. Have the patient sign a *permit* for the procedure. Make certain that the doctor has explained the procedure—its purpose and its hazards—prior to the patient's signing the form.
2. Ask the patient whether he has ever suffered from allergies; the doctor may order a skin test with an iodine-containing solution on the day before the procedure.
3. Withhold solid foods for 8 hours and liquids for 3 hours prior to the procedure.
4. Drugs commonly ordered are: penicillin injection on the day of the procedure to prevent possible infection; atropine or scopolamine to decrease secretions when general anesthesia is employed; and Nembutal and morphine, which may be administered 30 minutes prior to the procedure to relax and sedate the patient.

To prepare the patient psychologically for this procedure, it is helpful to include the following questions and information in your preparatory discussion.

1. Let the patient relate to you what the doctor has told him about cardiac catheterization. Ask the patient if he has any questions about the procedure. (Remember that many patients find it extremely difficult to express themselves freely to their doctor.)
2. Note the patient's general attitude toward the procedure. Does he seem extremely nervous, anxious, or apprehensive? If so, encourage him to express his fears openly. If the patient continues to appear very anxious, report this to the doctor.
3. Tell the patient that he will experience little or no pain; however, he may feel fatigue because he will have to lie quietly for a period of 3 or more hours. Also, he may experience certain sensations; for example, he may at times have a fluttery sensation around his heart (this occurs if the catheter is being passed backward through an artery into the left side of the heart; his arm may feel like it is going to sleep; he may experience a flushed warm feeling (this happens when contrast medium is injected for the angiocardiogram).
4. Let the patient know whether he will be transported to the x-ray department or to the operating room. Right-sided cardiac catheterization is usually performed in the x-ray department, whereas left-sided catheterization may be done in an operating room.
5. Explain that he will lie on the x-ray or operating table and that electrocardiogram leads will be attached to one arm and to both legs, and that readings will be recorded constantly. Also inform him that the room will be darkened at some point during the procedure to take x-rays.

A *right*-sided cardiac catheterization is simpler and less dangerous than a left-sided procedure. For a right-sided cardiac catheterization, the physician first performs a cutdown on the antecubital vein and passes a sterile, radiopaque catheter 100 to 125 cm. long through the vein into the superior vena cava, then through the right atrium and ventricle into the pulmonary artery. The ECG is constantly monitored during the procedure, and x-rays are taken at some point during the proceedings. Pressures within the right atrium, ventricle, and pulmonary artery are measured and blood samples are drawn.

Left-sided cardiac catheterization allows the cardiologist to measure pressures and draw blood samples from the aorta and the left atrium and ventricle. Also, he can inject contrast medium into these areas and take x-rays. Catheterization of the left heart can be performed in a number of ways:

1. The catheter can be passed retrograde from the brachial or femoral artery into the left ventricle.
2. Following right heart catheterization, the atrial septum can be punctured with a special needle and the catheter passed from the right heart into the left heart.
3. The left atrium may be reached directly by inserting an 18-gauge, 6-inch needle with a stylet through the patient's back into his heart; following the puncture, the stylet is removed and the catheter is maneuvered into position within the left chambers of the heart and the aorta. This procedure, which may also be used to study the right heart, is called a *posterior percutaneous* or *transthoracic left atrial puncture*. Sometimes the doctor will elect to study both sides of the heart at once and will insert two needles into the heart—one into the right atrium and one into the left atrium.[156]
4. The left ventricle may be reached directly by puncture of the anterior chest with a special needle, followed by passage of a catheter into the left heart.

Once the catheter is successfully maneuvered into position, pressures, blood samples, and x-rays (angiocardiograms) are taken. *Pressure* readings are obtained from the vena cava, right atrium, pulmonary artery, left atrium, and left ventricle. Also, a pulmonary "wedge pressure" is obtained, which is a measure of pulmonary "capillary" pressure. Average pressures are listed in Table 48–4.

TABLE 48–4. AVERAGE PRESSURES WITHIN THE HEART CHAMBERS AND VESSELS*

	mm. Hg
Right atrium	
Mean	5
Right ventricle	
Systolic	25
Pulmonary artery	
Systolic	25
Mean	15
Left atrium or pulmonary artery wedged	10
Left ventricle	
Systolic	120
End-diastolic	10

*From Stanton, A.: Cardiac Catheterization. *Nursing Times*, June 28, 1968, p. 860.

Pressures are valuable diagnostic tools in two ways: elevated pressures are indicative of stenosed valves, and an elevated left ventricular end-diastolic pressure is one of the first signs of left ventricular failure.

Whenever the doctor suspects the existence of congenital shunts or septal defects, samples of blood are drawn from the various chambers and arteries to determine oxygen content and the percentage of oxygen saturation. The oxygen content of the blood in the different chambers shows whether the blood is circulating in the proper sequence through the heart. For example, the doctor can confirm the existence of a left-to-right shunt by noting that the oxygen content of the blood is abnormally high in the right side of the heart and pulmonary artery. Normal oxygen saturation values are listed in Table 48–5.

Remember that oxygen requirements of the tissues increase when an individual is excited or very restless; thus, the oxygen saturation values for patients who are frightened or restless may be quite inaccurate.

Care for patients following cardiac catheterization varies, depending upon the institution, but the following points are basic to good aftercare:

1. Allow the patient to rest for a full 24 hours following the procedure.
2. Check the patient's pulse every 10 to 15 minutes during the first hour and then every 30 minutes for the next 3 hours or until stabilized. Observe for arrhythmias and tachycardia and report these to the physician.
3. Check the patient's temperature every 6 hours, as it may become slightly elevated.
4. Observe for nausea and vomiting.
5. Check the site of the cutdown for signs of swelling, infection, bleeding, or thrombosis. If the arm is painful, obtain an order for warm, moist compresses.
6. Allow the anxious patient to discuss his experience with you if he wishes. Patients often recall the procedure vividly, particularly their sensations when the catheter was passed into the heart. "Talking out" feelings after a stressful experience often helps the patient to relax and to turn his mind to new experiences.

Complications are rare, but they can develop both during and following the cardiac catheterization procedure. During the catheterization, arrhythmias, including ventricular fibrillation, may develop as the catheter is passed into the ventricle; also *pneumothorax* and *hemopericardium* occasionally occur. Following the procedure there may be allergic reactions to the iodine-containing contrast medium (see Angiocardiography), thrombophlebitis of the vein used for the cutdown, or infection of the cutdown site.

TABLE 48–5. NORMAL OXYGEN SATURATION VALUES WITHIN THE CHAMBERS OF THE HEART AND GREAT VESSELS*

Site	Saturation	Site	Saturation
Inferior vena cava Superior vena cava Right atrium Right ventricle Main pulmonary artery	65-80%	Wedged pulmonary capillary Left atrium Left ventricle	95-98%

*From Stanton, A.: Cardiac Catheterization. *Nursing Times,* June 28, 1968, p. 860.

GRAPHIC TECHNIQUES

Graphic devices are used to record and graphically represent various aspects of cardiac function. Major graphic techniques are: (1) the electrocardiogram (ECG); (2) the phonocardiogram; and (3) the ballistocardiogram.

Electrocardiogram

An electrocardiogram or ECG is a graphic record of the *electrical impulses* that are generated by depolarization and repolarization of the myocardium. These impulses are conducted to the external surface of the body where they are detected by electrodes and measured by a galvanometer.

The ECG is employed mainly to diagnose coronary heart disease and such abnormal cardiac rhythms as atrial fibrillation. However, as one authority warns:

> It is important to realize that the electrocardiogram (ECG) does not depict the actual physical state of the heart or its function. An ECG may be normal in the presence of heart disease unless the pathologic process disturbs the electrical forces.[118]

At this point let us briefly review some general facts about the electrophysiology of the heart. You will recall from Chapter 46 that the S-A node (pacemaker of the heart) initiates each heart beat by discharging an electrical impulse. These electrical impulses, which are normally discharged in a rhythmic manner 60 to 100 times per minute, spread throughout the atria and then the ventricles. As a result, atrial contraction is followed by ventricular contraction, and blood is propelled with each beat from the atria into the ventricles and from the ventricles into the aorta.

You will remember that each heart beat is equivalent to one cardiac cycle. Each cardiac cycle consists of: (1) contraction or systole or *depolarization* of first the atria and then the ventricles, and (2) relaxation or diastole or *repolarization* of both atria and then both ventricles.

Through the action of the sodium pump, depolarization takes place as impulses move across cell membranes, and repolarization follows. Now let us apply this electrophysiologic process to cardiac muscle cells and to the myocardium as a whole. When the S-A node (pacemaker) elicits an electrical "spark" or impulse, that electrical spark stimulates the resting polarized myocardial cell. As a result, a wave of depolarization moves down the cell, causing the inside of the cell to become positively charged and the outside negatively charged. Soon a large group of myocardial cells are depolarized, which creates an electrical imbalance between the polarized section of the myocardium, which is *positive* in relationship to the depolarized section. The area of electrical imbalance produced is called an *electrical field*.

As the wave of depolarization spreads throughout the muscle cells of both atria and ventricles, first the atria and then the ventricles contract. When the depolarized cells become repolarized, the atria and then the ventricles relax. This process normally takes place with each beat of the heart—60 to 100 times per minute.

The recording of the electrical activity of the heart generally takes place as follows:

1. The body, and in particular the body fluid, is an excellent *conductor* of electrical current.
2. When the depolarization process sweeps in a wave across the cells of the myocardium, the electrical current generated is conducted to the *body's surface* where it is detected by special *electrodes* placed on the patient's limbs and chest.
3. The electrodes are attached to *two* points on the body and are then connected to the ECG machine in order to complete the electrical circuit. Each pair of attachments is called a *lead*. The most commonly used leads (I, II, and III) are depicted in Figure 48–5.
4. The ECG machine graphically records the *difference* in voltage between these two points during cardiac depolarization and repolarization. For example, it records voltage differences between the right and left arm for lead I; between the right arm and left leg for lead II, and so on. The ebb and flow of the electrical impulses produced during each cardiac cycle are amplified and recorded by the ECG machine as deflections or waves.

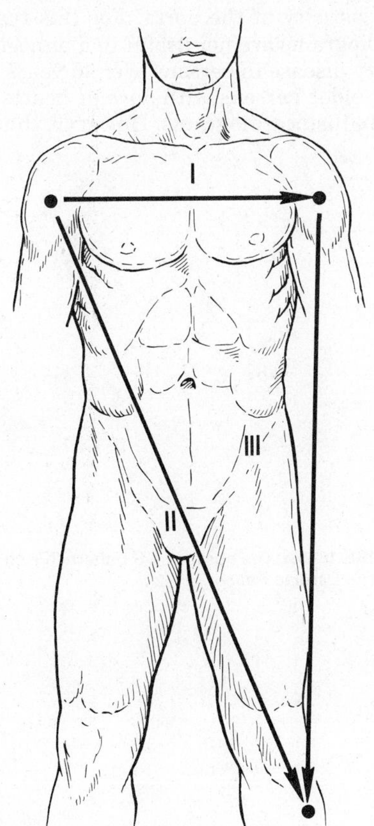

FIGURE 48–5. Points for obtaining ECG leads I, II, and III. (From Committee on Coronary Care Units and Cardiopulmonary Resuscitation: *Introduction to Arrhythmia Recognition*. California Heart Association, San Francisco, 1968.)

The waves of excitation recorded by the ECG machine onto graph paper are arbitrarily designated by the following letters: P, Q, R, S, T. The QRS letters are generally referred to as the "QRS complex." The typical ECG pattern formed by these waves is illustrated in Figure 48–6. As you study Figure 48–6 note the following:

> The P wave represents depolarization of the atria.
> The P-R interval represents the time it takes for the impulse to spread from the atria to the ventricles.
> The QRS complex indicates ventricular contraction.
> The T wave indicates repolarization of the ventricles.
> The S-T segment indicates that ventricular depolarization is completed and repolarization is about to begin.
> The U wave (not shown) is a small wave that sometimes follows the T wave; it is usually diagnostic of K^+ depletion.

An electrocardiogram tracing also shows the *voltage* of the waves and the *time duration* of both waves and intervals. As you can see in Figure 48–6, ECG graph paper is divided into horizontal lines and vertical lines, large squares and small squares. *Voltage* is represented by horizontal lines. Each small square is 1 mm. in height. Five small squares is equivalent to 5 mm. which, in turn, is equivalent to 0.5 mV. *Time* duration is measured by means of the vertical lines. Each *small* square signifies the passage of 0.04 second; and each *large* square, the passage of 0.20 second. Time durations for waves and intervals are as follows:

P wave—0.08 second
PR interval—less than 0.20 second;
average, 0.16 second
QRS complex—0.08 second
S-T segment—0.12 second
T wave—0.16 second

By studying the amplitude and time duration of the waves and intervals, doctors and nurses are able to diagnose disorders of both impulse formation and conduction.

When a cardiologist suspects that a serious arrhythmia is present, he usually orders a standard 12-lead ECG in order to comprehensively observe the electrical activity of the heart. The 12 leads are designated by Roman numerals and letters, e.g., I, II, III, V, aVR, aVL, aVF. These leads are classified as follows:

Standard limb leads (3 in number):

> Lead I: Measures the difference in electrical potential between the left arm and right arm.

> Lead II: Measures the difference in potential between the left leg and right arm.
> Lead III: Measures the difference in potential between the left leg and left arm. (Review Figure 48–5.)

Precordial leads (also known as V leads—6 in number):

> Electrodes placed at 6 different points on the chest wall overlying the heart.

Augmented unipolar limb leads (modified standard limb leads—3 in number):

>aVR: Checks electrical potential of right arm (*a* stands for augmented, *V* for unipolar, *R* for right arm).
> aVF: Checks electrical potential of left leg (*F* stands for left leg).

Augmented leads have wave deflections that are increased in amplitude by 50 per cent for easier reading.

Figure 48–7 is an example of a standard 12-lead ECG that is diagnostic of a right bundle branch block—a disorder of ventricular conduction discussed later. Generally a single lead ECG (employing lead II) is used for routine physical examinations, and for monitoring patients whose arrhythmias or cardiac disorders have already been diagnosed.

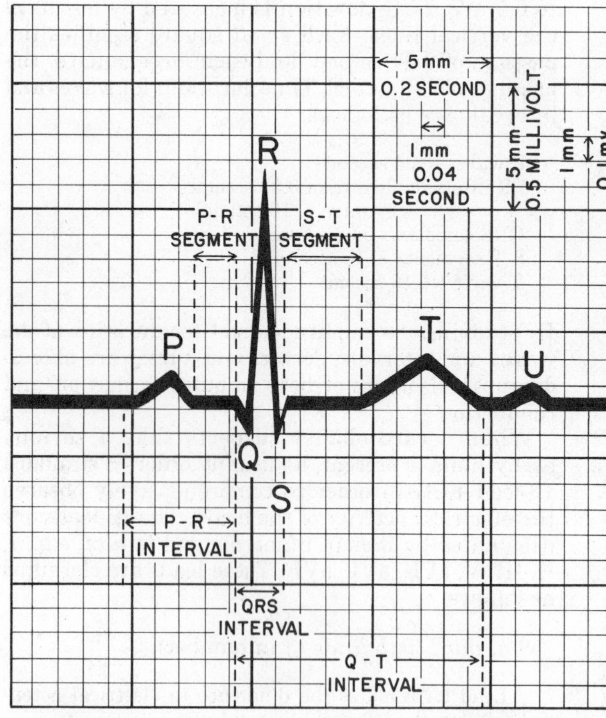

FIGURE 48–6. The normal ECG pattern. (From Sanderson, R. C.: *The Cardiac Patient.* 1972.)

When the physician orders an ECG for his patient, take a moment to reassure the patient that the procedure is absolutely safe and that he will *not* be electrocuted! Explain to the patient that an ECG simply records the electrical activity of his heart and that the procedure will help the physician to make a more accurate diagnosis if a cardiac problem is present.

Ballistocardiogram

A ballistocardiogram is a graphic recording of body movements that result from the force of the heart beat. This diagnostic method is used to: (1) measure cardiac output; (2) determine the strength of myocardial contraction; (3) measure the degree of elasticity of the aorta; and (4) diagnose the presence of coronary artery disease, mitral stenosis, and chronic constrictive pericarditis.

During this procedure the patient lies on a special table or board which is balanced and suspended by appropriately placed levers. The force of the patient's heart beat as his heart ejects blood causes his body to rapidly oscillate first backward away from the aorta and then forward. These tiny oscillations are converted by a transducer or pickup device into an electrical potential. The resulting waves are amplified and are recorded on graph paper by an ECG machine.

Abnormal ballistocardiograms appear characteristically in older individuals with hearts that are apparently normal, but who probably have some loss of elasticity of the aorta. For this reason, ballistocardiograms are not useful in diagnosing coronary artery disease in persons over 45 years old, since so many older persons with *normal* hearts have abnormal ballistocardiograms. However, this diagnostic tool can be used to predict the *possibility* of a second or third myocardial infarction in older persons. Abnormal ballistocardiograms occur following smoking or eating and in persons suffering from obesity, orthopedic problems, pulmonary disease, neural disorders, anemia, and fevers.

Ballistocardiography is a relatively simple procedure and it is a useful tool in research. However, some cardiologists feel that the information it gives is not completely accurate.

Phonocardiography

The technique of phonocardiography involves the electronic measurement, amplification, and recording of cardiac sounds onto special phonograph paper. For recording purposes a specially designed microphone is placed upon the patient's chest; this device picks up the low-frequency cardiac vibrations for amplification and recording.

This diagnostic procedure does not replace auscultation; indeed, certain murmurs can be identified more accurately by the use of a stethoscope in skilled hands than by this electronic device. However, some cardiologists find it helpful to keep a permanent record of their patient's heart sounds to review both before and following cardiac surgery.

NURSING ASSESSMENT OF THE CARDIAC PATIENT

It is generally the physician's task to thoroughly examine the newly admitted patient with heart disease and to diagnose his problem. However, no patient remains in the same state of health or disease as on the day of his admission; his condition naturally changes continuously. For this reason every seriously ill patient requires a *daily* assessment of his physiologic and emotional status and a daily critical evaluation of the success of treatment measures. This process of daily assessment is a primary task of the nurse.

As you care daily for the patient with heart disease, first of all *listen* to the patient. Does he have any new complaints, any new aches or pains, any new fears? Or has he ceased to make certain complaints that he formerly made daily? Has he ceased to complain because he is feeling better, or because he is becoming lethargic and despondent?

Second, observe the patient for *changes in his physiologic status*. Use these steps as a guide:

1. When you approach the patient's bed, first note his *position*. Is he lying flat or is he sitting up because of difficulty in breathing, i.e., orthopnea? Note his breathing. Does it appear difficult, wheezy, rapid, etc.? Is he coughing? Is the cough productive? Assess his general *coloring*. Is he flushed or feverish? Is he perspiring? Is there a bluish or cyanotic tinge to his skin? Is he perspiring? Take the patient's hand in yours and note the feel of his skin. A cold, clammy feeling hand could indicate poor circulation or shock; a hot dry feel to the skin might indicate dehydration or fever.
2. Talk with the patient. Note particularly complaints of *fatigue, dyspnea* (especially during the night), *headache, palpitations,* and *chest pain.* If the patient complains of *pain,* learn all you can about its location, radiation, quality, and intensity; also inquire about factors that precipitate and relieve

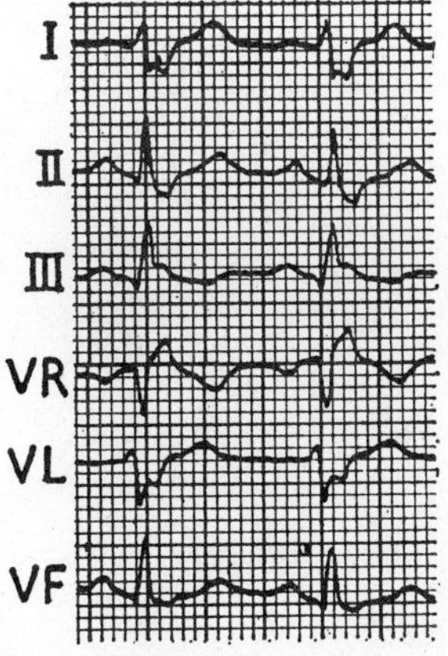

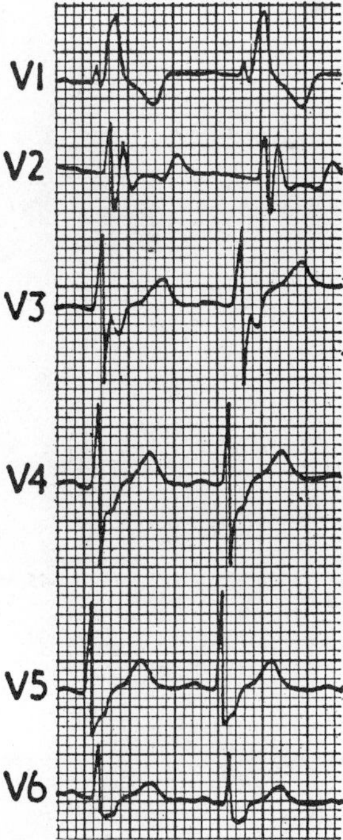

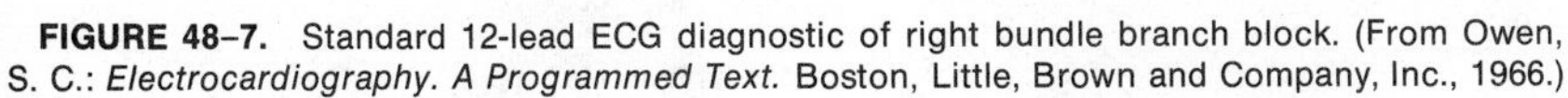
FIGURE 48–7. Standard 12-lead ECG diagnostic of right bundle branch block. (From Owen, S. C.: *Electrocardiography. A Programmed Text.* Boston, Little, Brown and Company, Inc., 1966.)

pain. As you converse with the patient, note his *affect*. If the patient acts confused, restless, or belligerent, he may need oxygen.

3. Check the patient's *pulse*, both at the apical and radial sites. Note the *rate*. Is the heart beating rapidly in order to compensate for a diminished cardiac output? Is it beating extremely slowly as a result of a blockage in the conduction system? Note the rhythm. Is the beat regular in its rhythm or is an arrhythmia present? Note the *amplitude* or strength of the pulse. Remember that the amplitude is partially determined by the force with which the heart ejects blood with each beat. A weak, fast pulse may signify shock and circulatory collapse.

4. Take the blood pressure on *both* arms. Always know the patient's normal *baseline* for blood pressure. Remember that a blood pressure reading that is considered abnormal for the population at large may not be abnormal for this patient.

5. Check the patient's *neck veins*. Look for engorgement of the external jugular vein; this is an important sign of congestive heart failure.

6. Listen to the patient's *chest* with a stethoscope. Listen for the presence of rales and wheezes.

7. Note the patient's *intake* and *output* record and his daily *weight*. If daily intake exceeds daily output and if the patient has suddenly gained weight, he is probably retaining fluid.

8. Examine the patient's *back, buttocks,* and *ankles* for signs of pitting edema.

If pitting edema, dyspnea, chest pain, and distended neck veins are present at the same time, the patient probably has heart failure.

9. Carefully evaluate the patient's *response to treatment*. Are symptoms lessening, remaining the same, or becoming worse? Does the patient feel that his treatment is not helping him, or is he optimistic about his program of care? Are any untoward symptoms developing as a *result* of treatment?

Your findings from your daily examination and assessment of the patient need to be carefully charted and discussed in conference with the physician and other staff members. Your observations, if carefully done, will give the physician valuable clues as to the course of the disease and the type of therapy that should be instituted.

CHAPTER 49

Chronic Congestive Heart Failure

Heart failure is the result of undue stress upon the heart; essentially it represents failure of the cardiac muscle to pump sufficient blood to meet the body's metabolic needs. As stated in Chapter 47, cardiac failure may be either acute or chronic. *Acute* heart and circulatory failure develop swiftly when the heart muscle suddenly, and often totally, fails in its function as a pump; the dramatic results of sudden failure are shock, cardiac arrest, syncope, and sudden death. On the other hand, heart failure that develops slowly and has milder symptoms manifests itself in a clinical syndrome called *chronic congestive heart failure* (CHF). This syndrome, which eventually affects 50 to 60 per cent of all patients with organic heart disease, is defined as "the clinical state resulting from inability of the heart to expel sufficient blood for the metabolic demands of the body."[20] Basically, CHF is identified by the following characteristics:

1. The development of *compensatory mechanisms* which enable the weakened heart to continue to function. The three major mechanisms are tachycardia (rapid heart beat), ventricular dilatation, and hypertrophy of the heart.
2. A *low cardiac output* that is inadequate to meet the metabolic needs of the body's tissues.
3. The accumulation of *abnormal amounts of blood* in the systemic or pulmonary circulations, or both, with resultant *congestion* of these systems.

CAUSATIVE FACTORS

The heart is doomed to gradual failure when one or more of the following conditions persists:*

1. The *inflow* of blood to the heart is greatly *reduced* because of hemorrhage, dehydration, and so forth.
2. The *inflow* of blood to the heart is greatly *increased* as a result of excessive I. V. fluids, Na^+ and water retention, and so on.
3. The *outflow* of blood from the heart is *obstructed* owing to damaged valves and narrowed arteries.
4. The *heart muscle* itself is *damaged* from either ischemia or inflammatory processes.
5. The *metabolic* needs of the body are increased as a result of fever, pregnancy, and so forth.

*See Figure 47–1.

Clinical entities that most commonly result in congestive heart failure and that develop as a result of the above factors are: arteriosclerotic heart disease, hypertensive cardiovascular disease, valvular heart disease, ischemic heart disease, rheumatic heart disease, constrictive pericarditis, the myocardiopathies, circulatory overload, pulmonary diseases, and such noncardiac entities as hyperthyroidism, obesity, pregnancy, anemia, fever, and infection.

> *Arteriosclerotic heart disease:* Arteriosclerosis, a condition characterized by a hardening and loss of elasticity in the walls of the arteries, increases the peripheral resistance against which the heart must pump. The resulting overwork forces the cardiac muscle to enlarge slowly. Sooner or later the muscle outgrows its blood supply and fails.

> *Hypertensive cardiovascular disease:* Hypertension, if sustained for a long period of time, causes irreversible degenerative changes within the arterial walls. These changes, in turn, result in a permanent narrowing of the arteries, which overtaxes the heart, causing it to enlarge and finally fail.

> *Valvular heart disease:* Narrowed or *stenosed* valves increase the work of the heart by forcing the heart to pump blood into the arterial system against considerable resistance. Dilated valves, which allow blood to regurgitate backward, also add to the work of the heart by increasing the amount of blood that it must try to pump forward with each stroke.

> *Ischemic heart disease:* The myocardium may not receive sufficient oxygen and nourishment as a result of either (1) narrowing of the coronary arteries owing to atherosclerotic changes or thrombosis, or (2) enlargement of the heart muscle fibers to the extent that they outgrow the blood supply.

> *Rheumatic heart disease:* Rheumatic fever usually damages the heart valves, causing them to become either narrowed or incompetent, which consequently puts strain on the heart.

> *Constrictive pericarditis:* As a result of infection, the pericardium may become inflamed and later scarred and constricted. When the heart becomes encased by the dense fibers of the scarred pericardium, the inflow of blood to the heart is obstructed; also, constriction may prevent the heart from expanding and filling with blood between contractions. The result of decreased cardiac expansibility is a low cardiac output and increased venous pressure.

> *Myocardiopathies:* This group of conditions can cause such extensive damage to the myocardium that it eventually fails.

> *Circulatory overload:* Too much fluid input to the heart, as a result of an overload of I.V. fluid, excessive

Na^+ retention, or renal shutdown, can overwhelm the heart's pumping capacity.

> *Pulmonary diseases:* Chronic emphysema, bronchiectasis, silicosis, and chronic tuberculosis all damage and constrict the arterioles of the lungs. Constriction of the pulmonary arterioles greatly augments the work of the *right* heart as it struggles to pump blood into the pulmonary circulation. As a result of these pulmonary diseases, the right ventricle enlarges and eventually fails, followed by failure of the left ventricle.

> *Hyperthyroidism, obesity, pregnancy, anemia, fever,* and *infection:* These conditions increase the demands of the tissues for oxygen as well as the amount of metabolic waste materials that must be eliminated. If any of the above problems continue for too long or are too severe, the heart eventually fails from overwork.

Factors that may *precipitate* CHF in *individuals with diseased hearts* are pregnancy and childbirth, severe tachycardia or bradycardia, severe overexertion and overwork, great mental strain, and a sudden elevation of the environmental temperature and humidity. These factors should be guarded against in individuals with known heart conditions.

CARDIAC RESERVE, COMPENSATION, AND DECOMPENSATION

The seriousness of a patient's cardiac disability is directly correlated with the extent to which his cardiac reserve is diminished. You will recall from Chapter 46 that cardiac reserve is the ability of the heart to adjust to increased demands placed upon it by exercise, excitement, fever, and so forth. When the heart loses its ability to adjust to various stresses by increasing its output, symptoms of heart disease develop.

> *The most typical first sign of reduced cardiac reserve is a* decreased tolerance to exercise.[19]

While cardiac reserve is most often lost gradually, it can also be lost *suddenly,* with resulting death.

In cases of gradual failure, how does the heart compensate for a loss in cardiac reserve? How does it augment its output in order to meet any increased demands placed upon it? The three major mechanisms by which the heart is sometimes able to increase its output are ventricular dilatation, ventricular hypertrophy, and tachycardia.

Ventricular dilatation refers to an increase in the *length* of the muscle fibers and is characterized by an increase in the *volume* of the heart chambers. With dilatation comes an increase in the systolic output because (according to Starling's law), a muscle when stretched contracts more forcefully. However, dilatation as a compensatory mechanism is limited. First, muscle fibers, if *stretched beyond a certain point,* cease to increase the contractile power of the heart. Second, a greatly dilated heart requires more oxygen to meet its metabolic needs. Thus, the dilated heart with a normal coronary blood flow can suffer from a serious lack of oxygen. Hypoxia of the heart muscle will, in turn, *decrease* the muscle's ability to contract.

Ventricular hypertrophy, on the other hand, refers to an increase in the *diameter* of the muscle fibers. It is characterized by a *thickening of the walls* of the chambers and a corresponding increase in the weight of the heart. Hypertrophy generally follows *persistent* dilatation, further increasing the contractile power of the muscle fibers.

However, hypertrophy, like dilatation, is limited as a compensatory mechanism. A hypertrophied heart does far greater work than a normal heart and, as a consequence, has greater demands for oxygen. Unfortunately, as the heart's muscle mass increases, the capillaries supplying the muscle fibers remain the same in number. Thus, in time, the hypertrophied heart, with its increased muscle mass, may simply *outgrow* its coronary blood supply and become hypoxic. Its contractile power then lessens.

Tachycardia, or an acceleration in heart rate, is the least effective compensatory mechanism. When the heart rate becomes too great, the ventricles are unable to fill adequately, with resultant hypotension and shock.

When these three mechanisms—tachycardia, dilatation, and hypertrophy—*succeed* in maintaining an adequate flow of blood to the tissues, *without symptoms* and in the presence of pathologic changes, the heart is in a state of *compensation. Cardiac decompensation* occurs when the heart, despite these mechanisms, is *unable* to cope with the work demands put upon it and must expend most of its reserve. At this point, symptoms develop upon activity, because the heart is unable to maintain adequate circulation.

FORMS OF CONGESTIVE HEART FAILURE

As we stated in Chapter 46, the heart is composed of two pumps—right and left—each of which bears its own stresses and has its own role in maintaining the circulation. For this reason, it is possible for one pump or side of the heart to fail independently of the other pump or side. For example, *left-sided* heart failure develops when the left pump of the heart fails, whereas *right-sided* heart failure occurs when the right pump fails. Generally, however, because the circulatory system is a closed circuit and because the work of the heart is dependent upon the smooth functioning of *both* pumps, left- and right-sided heart failure occur almost together—one closely following the other.

Left-sided heart failure practically always results from damage to the left ventricular myocardium. Clinical entities which most frequently cause left ventricular damage are: (1) hypertensive heart disease; (2) ischemic heart disease; and (3) aortic valvular disease resulting from rheumatic heart disease, syphilis, and congenital anomalies. In rare instances left-sided heart failure may begin in the left atria as a result of mitral stenosis.

Thus, in left-sided heart failure, the basic fault

lies in the heart muscle itself. The muscle may be diseased and unable to meet normal circulatory demands, or the heart muscle may be intrinsically normal but unable to meet increased circulatory needs. When failure first begins, the left ventricle fails to eject its full quota of blood. At this point the compensatory mechanisms of tachycardia, dilatation, and hypertrophy come into play. When these mechanisms fail, some residual blood remains in the dilated ventricle. This residuum, in turn, decreases the ventricle's capacity to receive blood from the left atrium. The left atrium, because it must now work harder to eject its blood, hypertrophies and dilates. As a result, it is unable to receive the full amount of incoming blood from the pulmonary veins. This leads to congestion of the *pulmonary system* and to symptoms that are *respiratory* in nature.

The *right* ventricle, because of the increased pressure in the pulmonary vascular system, must now dilate and hypertrophy in order to meet its increased workload. It eventually fails. Engorgement of the venous system then extends backward to produce congestion in the gastrointestinal tract, viscera, and kidneys, with *edema* as the main manifestation. This condition is referred to as *right heart failure.*

Right-sided heart failure almost always follows left-sided heart failure; it develops as a result of the stress placed upon the right ventricle as it attempts to pump blood against resistance into the patient's congested lungs. Occasionally, however, right-sided heart failure does develop *independently* of left-sided heart failure. Common causes are:

1. Infarction of the right ventricle.
2. Pulmonary diseases, e.g., chronic emphysema and chronic tuberculosis, which force the right ventricle to pump blood against damaged and obliterated arterioles within the lungs.
3. Constrictive pericarditis, which obstructs the inflow of blood to the heart from the venous system.
4. Tricuspid stenosis and congenital pulmonic stenosis (both of which are rare), causing undue exhaustion of the right ventricle.

Eventually the venous congestion created by right-sided heart failure causes the circulation of blood to slow, thereby lowering the output of the heart's left-side.

At this point we must emphasize that only in the *early* stages of cardiac failure do left- and right-sided heart failure occur independently of each other. In the later stages of CHF *both* sides of the heart fail to function and both pulmonary congestion and venous congestion are present.

Both right- and left-sided heart failure are sometimes referred to as *low output* failure because these two clinical entities are basically characterized by a reduction in cardiac output. *High output failure,* on the other hand, develops when the heart's output of blood is adequate or high but the metabolic demands of tissues are above normal. While low output failure results mainly from *primary* heart disease (i.e., the adverse alterations have developed within the heart itself), high output failure results from heart disease that develops secondary to other conditions. Hyperthyroidism, severe anemia, beriberi, arteriovenous fistula, and pregnancy often make such exorbitant demands upon the pumping action of the heart muscle that the heart, exhausted by its excessive efforts, finally fails.

THE MANIFESTATIONS OF CONGESTIVE HEART FAILURE

The symptoms of CHF result from a *decrease in cardiac output.* They involve congestion of either the pulmonary circulatory system, the venous system, or both. Almost all the manifestations of congestive heart failure affect tissues and organs that are located *away* from the heart, e.g., kidney, brain, liver, and extremities.

In the following discussion, we have divided the symptoms of CHF into symptoms of left-sided heart failure and symptoms of right-sided failure. Again we wish to emphasize that in advanced CHF, *both* sides of the heart fail and all the symptoms discussed below are present.

SYMPTOMS OF LEFT-SIDED HEART FAILURE

The following symptoms of left-sided heart failure develop as a result of congestion of the lungs with fluid owing to the back pressure of blood, and a decrease in cardiac output.

Dyspnea, Orthopnea, and Paroxysmal Nocturnal Dyspnea

These symptoms are caused by lung congestion and by the failure of the left side of the heart to maintain cardiac output. Dyspnea, you recall, means shortness of breath. It results from congestion of the patient's lungs owing to pulmonary engorgement. This congestion can eventually reduce the vital capacity to 1500 ml. or less.

The severity of dyspnea depends not only on the amount of pulmonary engorgement and resultant decrease in vital capacity, but also on the volume of air respired per minute. A patient with moderate pulmonary engorgement may not experience dyspnea at rest. However, when the same patient exercises, he may experience dyspnea because a greater volume of air is required.

Because dyspnea is a subjective complaint it cannot always be closely correlated with the extent of CHF. Thus, an apprehensive person with moderate, pathologic changes may be more aware of dyspnea than a phlegmatic person with advanced disease.

Orthopnea, you recall, is a more advanced stage of dyspnea in which the patient cannot lie flat in bed because recumbency increases his difficulty in breathing. Blood pools in the lower body while the patient is sitting up. When the patient lies flat, the blood returns from the lower part of the body via the venous system to the lungs and heart, which are already congested. The result is orthopnea or increased dyspnea in the recumbent position.

Paroxysmal nocturnal dyspnea is often one of the first signs of left ventricular failure. As stated in Chapter 48, this most frightening form of dyspnea awakens the patient from his sleep and forces him to get up from his bed and catch his breath.

Cheyne-Stokes Respirations

We stated earlier that Cheyne-Stokes respirations are a cyclical type of breathing in which periods of apnea are replaced by periods of rapid deep breathing and then by apnea, and so forth. The exact reason why Cheyne-Stokes respirations develop in CHF is not known. They may occur as a result of the prolonged circulation time between the pulmonary circulation and the central nervous system, which, in turn, affects the respiratory center. This symptom may also be related to the respiratory alkalosis* that so often develops in patients with congestive heart failure.

Pleural Effusion and Pulmonary Edema

These problems are the result of pulmonary congestion which is so severe that the distended capillaries leak fluid into the interstitial and alveolar spaces of the lungs.

Cough and Cardiac Asthma

Cough is a common symptom of left-sided heart failure. The cough is usually productive of large amounts of frothy, blood-tinged sputum. The patient coughs because a large amount of edema fluid is trapped within the pulmonary tree, irritating the delicate mucosa of the lungs. The expectoration of mucus is a result of severe pulmonary congestion and edema.

Wheezing or *cardiac asthma* is another sign of CHF; its exact etiology is as yet unknown.

Decreased Renal Function, Edema, and Weight Gain

Kidney function is adversely affected by the development of CHF, with the result that sodium and water are retained within the body. The probable sequence of events causing edema in left-sided heart failure is as follows: (1) Cardiac output is decreased because of heart failure; as a result, arterial pressure in the kidneys is diminished, reducing glomerular filtration and the output of sodium chloride and water. (2) Reduced effective circulating blood volume in some way triggers an increase in aldosterone secretion by the adrenal cortex; this then increases the rate of reabsorption of sodium by the renal tubules. (3) Because aldosterone causes sodium to be reabsorbed, the concentration of the extracellular fluid is increased. (4) The resulting increased osmotic pressure causes an increase in the release of antidiuretic hormone (ADH) from the neurosecretory cells of the hypothalamus, which results in the increased tubular reabsorption of water. The final result is edema.*

*Respiratory alkalosis is discussed in Chapter 25.

Cerebral Anoxia

A decrease in the amount of oxygen carrying blood to the patient's brain causes irritability, restlessness, and a shortened attention span. Cerebral anoxia develops because of the decrease in cardiac output characteristic of left-sided heart failure.

Fatigue and Muscular Weakness

The profound exhaustion that patients with congestive heart failure experience is due to a decrease in cardiac output and prolonged circulation time. Decreased cardiac output diminishes oxygen to the tissues and decreases the speed with which metabolic wastes are swept up into the circulation for excretion.

SYMPTOMS OF RIGHT-SIDED HEART FAILURE

When the right side of the heart fails, the symptoms produced center around edema and venous congestion within the organs.

Liver Enlargement and Abdominal Pain

As the liver becomes congested with venous blood, it enlarges. If this occurs rapidly, stretching of the capsule surrounding the liver causes severe discomfort. The patient may either complain of a constant aching in the right upper quadrant or of sharp pain.

In severe congestive heart failure, lobules of the liver may become so congested with venous blood that they become anoxic. Anoxia leads to necrosis of the lobules. In long standing CHF, these necrotic areas may become fibrotic and then sclerotic. As a result, the patient develops a condition called *cardiac cirrhosis,* manifested by ascites and jaundice—symptoms of liver damage.

*See Chapter 24 for a more detailed explanation of the role of hormones and the kidney in the development of edema.

Anorexia, Nausea, and Bloating

These symptoms develop secondary to venous congestion of the gastrointestinal tract. Anorexia and nausea may also result from digitalis toxicity—a common problem because digitalis is the drug of choice in treating congestive heart failure.

Dependent Edema

Among the early signs of right-sided heart failure are edema of the ankles and lower extremities. Evidently edema results from venous congestion of the kidneys, producing compensatory vasoconstriction that, in turn, decreases renal blood flow. As a result, sodium excretion is impaired and edema fluid is retained.

Coolness of the Extremities

Venous congestion throughout the body reduces peripheral blood flow. As a result, the extremities are cool and the nail beds are often cyanotic.

Anxiety and Fear

Every layman knows that the heart pumps blood through the body, and that without the vital work of the heart, life ends. For this reason, most individuals with a diagnosis of CHF feel anxious and depressed about their condition. As the course of the disease progresses and symptoms worsen, the fear of permanent disability and death may overwhelm even the most stoic patient. Patients express their fears in a number of ways; for example, they may have frequent nightmares, they may suffer from acute anxiety states or deep depressions, or they may withdraw completely from reality.

SYMPTOMS OF ADVANCED CONGESTIVE HEART FAILURE

Weight Loss and Cachexia

The individual with advanced congestive heart failure suffers from malnutrition of his tissues as a result of low cardiac output and venous congestion. Indeed, malnutrition may be as pronounced as it is in patients with advanced malignancies. However, because of the severe edema, patients with CHF look puffy and bloated and appear to be overweight. If diuresis is successful and edema is relieved, the patient's cachexic state becomes obvious.

Shock Syndrome

The typical clinical picture of shock usually appears during the terminal stages of CHF. Typical symptoms are: stupor, pallor, rapid thready pulse, cold sweats, restlessness, and profound hypotension. These symptoms develop because of a critical decrease in cardiac output due to almost total failure of the heart in its pumping action.

DIAGNOSING CONGESTIVE HEART FAILURE

Heart failure is generally diagnosed on the basis of the following:

> Presence of characteristic symptoms.
> Muffled heart sounds.
> Abnormal heart sounds.
> Rales at the bases of the lungs.
> X-ray showing hazy lung fields and prominent, distended pulmonary veins.
> Elevated venous pressure.
> Distended neck veins.
> Prolonged circulation time.
> Reduction in cardiac output.
> Presence of albuminuria.
> Elevated BUN.

Early recognition of these signs can forestall the development of advanced CHF and its complications.

GOALS OF CARE

The overall goal of care for patients suffering from CHF is to reduce or eliminate those causative factors that lead to symptoms and complications.

Individual goals of care to reduce or alleviate the causative factors responsible for CHF are as follows:

1. Enlist the cooperation of the patient and his family in pursuing a plan of care.
2. Diagnose and eliminate disease conditions and circumstances within the work and domestic environments that could contribute to the development of congestive heart failure.
3. Strengthen the heart and decrease its workload.
4. Reduce venous congestion in the lungs and body.
5. Supply oxygen and better nutrition to the heart muscle and to body tissues.
6. Decrease sodium and water retention.
7. Recognize, minimize, and alleviate the untoward effects of therapy: digitalis toxicity, thrombophlebitis, other complications of bed rest, low salt syndrome, and potassium deficiency resulting from mercurial diuretics.

The attainment of these goals depends upon the following therapeutic measures:

Therapy in CHF

1. *Physical and mental rest.*
2. *Digitalization.*
3. *Low caloric diet.*
4. *Reduction of H_2O and Na^+ retention by means of:*
   a. *Low Na^+ intake.*
   b. *Diuretics.*
   c. *Reduced fluid intake.*
   d. *Reduction of anxiety.*

5. *Oxygen therapy.*
6. *Mechanical removal of pleural and peritoneal effusions.*
7. *Education of the patient.*

REST

In Chapter 27, we pointed out the many advantages and disadvantages of bed rest. For patients suffering from CHF, bed rest is truly beneficial; some of its advantages for such patients are:

1. Reduction in heart's workload.
2. Promotion of diuresis.
3. Reduction in work of respiratory muscles (decreases dyspnea).
4. Reduction in tissues' demands for oxygen (lessens circulatory demands).
5. Decrease in venous return (lessens pulmonary congestion and dyspnea).
6. Lowered blood pressure (diminishes arterial resistance against which heart must pump).
7. Lowered heart rate (prolongs the recovery period of cardiac muscle, thereby resulting in a more efficient cardiac contraction).

Whether a physician will prescribe complete bed rest or a program of modified bed rest depends upon the seriousness of the patient's condition. As a guide to the amount of activity that is safe for a patient, the doctor may refer to the functional and therapeutic classifications of heart disease shown below and assign his patient to one of the classes within each classification.

FUNCTIONAL AND THERAPEUTIC CLASSIFICATION OF HEART DISEASE*

Functional Capacity (four classes)

Class I: No limitation of physical activity. Ordinary physical activity does not cause undue fatigue, palpitation, dyspnea, or anginal pain.

Class II: Slight limitation of physical activity. Comfortable at rest, but ordinary physical activity results in fatigue, palpitation, dyspnea, or anginal pain.

Class III: Marked limitation of physical activity. Comfortable at rest, but less than ordinary physical activity causes fatigue, palpitation, dyspnea, or anginal pain.

Class IV: Unable to carry on any physical activity without discomfort. Symptoms of cardiac insufficiency, or of the anginal syndrome, may be present even at rest. If any physical activity is undertaken, discomfort is increased.

Therapeutic Classification (five classes)

Class A: Physical activity need not be restricted.

Class B: Ordinary physical activity need not be restricted, but unusually severe or competitive efforts should be avoided.

Class C: Ordinary physical activity should be moderately restricted, and more strenuous efforts should be discontinued.

Class D: Ordinary physical activity should be markedly restricted.

Class E: Patient should be at complete rest, confined to bed or chair.

The length of time patients are confined to bed and restricted in their activities varies. Patients are generally confined to bed for a long enough period to regain cardiac reserve but not so long that disability and other complications of bed rest are promoted. Patients with *milder* cases of CHF may require only one to four weeks of bed rest, whereas those suffering from extremely *severe* heart failure may need to remain in bed for from 12 to 72 weeks. The optimum period of bed rest for patients with heart failure of varying degrees of severity is still under study.

The patient with heart disease who is confined to bed must *rest physically and mentally* if he is to benefit from his program of care. To help the patient rest, the physician may order a mild sedative or small doses of barbiturates and tranquilizers to overcome problems of restlessness and insomnia. The following nursing actions are also helpful in promoting the patient's rest:

1. Place the patient in a cool quiet room; do not locate him next to excessively noisy or talkative patients.
2. Keep the patient's toilet articles, books, radio, water, and so forth, close at hand so that he does not have to strain to reach them.
3. Allow the patient to use a bedside commode rather than a bedpan. Sitting on a bedpan is uncomfortable and it does not promote proper elimination.
4. Make the patient as comfortable as possible. Give backrubs, prop the pillows, change the patient's position as necessary.
5. Have a confident reassuring attitude when with the patient; endeavor to reduce his anxiety. Studies show that fear and anxiety can produce various transient cardiovascular responses; e.g., changes in heart rate, cardiac output, abnormalities in rhythm, change in blood pressure, peripheral resistance, blood viscosity, blood clotting time, and serum cholesterol level.

Whenever a patient is placed on a program of prolonged complete bed rest, you will naturally observe constantly for signs of thrombophlebitis, pulmonary embolism, hypostatic pneumonia, renal calculi, and mental depression. These problems and their prevention were discussed in Chapter 27.

The rate at which the patient is allowed to return to his normal activities depends upon the severity of his condition. The patient who has been on prolonged complete bed rest usually resumes his activities very gradually. At first he may be allowed to walk to the bathroom once a day; later he may be given full bathroom privileges and allowed to sit up for meals. As the patient becomes more independent and active, it is important to observe for weight gain, edema, dyspnea, and distended neck veins; the appearance of such symptoms is a

*These classifications were delineated by the Criteria Committee, New York Heart Association. From Brainerd, H.: *Current Diagnosis and Treatment,* Los Altos, California, Lange Medical Publications, 1969.

warning that a longer period of bed rest is necessary.

When the patient finally leaves the hospital and returns home, he will need to adjust his schedule so that he does not become overly exhausted. A nap in the afternoon, shorter working hours, early retirement at night, and frequent vacations may be necessary. As the patient's condition continues to improve, he may gradually undertake a program of mild exercise, e.g., walking short distances on level ground, playing a few holes of golf, and simple calisthenics. Such exercises, when performed sensibly, can strengthen the heart muscle and improve its performance.

DIGITALIZATION

The most important cardiac action of digitalis is a direct beneficial effect on myocardial contraction. Digitalis also increases the force of systolic contraction, the completeness of ventricular emptying, and the capacity of the heart for work. Digitalis preparations cause a sustained increase in the output of the failing heart.

Other effects of cardiac glycosides are reduction in the size of the dilated failing heart, depression of conduction through the bundle of His, reduced refractoriness and increased myocardial instability, a facilitation of vagal effect on the sinoatrial node, and diuretic action leading to salt and water elimination.

There are a number of different digitalis preparations, and all have approximately the same effect upon heart action. However, digitalis drugs differ significantly in their potency, speed of action, elimination from the body, and the extent of irritating action on the gastrointestinal tract. Table 49–1 lists commonly used digitalis preparations along with their distinguishing characteristics.

The *rate* of digitalization and the *method of administration* depend upon the severity of the patient's condition. Oral digitalis preparations are generally employed in less serious cases and are given in divided doses. The patient may receive the total digitalizing dose of an oral digitalis drug within 24 to 72 hours. In emergency situations when the patient is critically ill, the doctor generally orders deslanoside (Cedilanid-D) or digoxin intravenously for rapid digitalization. Intravenous and intramuscular preparations are generally employed only in acute situations in which the patient's life is threatened; otherwise, digitalis drugs are almost always administered orally.

When administering digitalis, one must constantly be on guard for signs of *digitalis toxicity* or intoxication. Patients most prone to digitalis toxicity are the elderly and persons with advanced heart disease, severe arrhythmias, or acute myocardial infarction. Also, individuals with cor pulmonale, hypothyroidism, hepatic disease, hypokalemia, or alkalosis readily develop signs of toxicity.

Major symptoms of digitalis toxicity are:

System	*Symptom*
Gastrointestinal tract	Anorexia, nausea, vomiting, diarrhea
Central nervous system	Headache, lethargy, restlessness, irritability, convulsions, delusions, hallucinations, aphasia, memory loss, coma, pain similar to trigeminal neuralgia
Eyes	"Colored" vision—usually yellow, sometimes blue; photophobia
Cardiovascular system	Arrhythmias, tachycardia or bradycardia with pulse rate *below 60,* heart block, cardiac failure

If any of the above signs are present, *do not* give the drug; report the symptoms at once to the physician. If digitalis toxicity is present the physician will probably order the following:[146]

1. Discontinue the drug.
2. Administer potassium salts intravenously to correct arrhythmias.

TABLE 49–1. TIME COURSE OF ACTION OF DIGITALIS PREPARATIONS*

	Onset of Action		Maximum Effect			
Glycoside	*I.V. or I.M.*	*Oral*	*I.V. or I.M.*	*Oral*	**Physiologic Half-time†**	**Total Duration of Action**
Ouabain	3–10 min.	——	30–120 min.	——	22 hr.	1–3 days
Deslanoside	10–30 min.	——	2–3 hr.	——	36 hr.	3–6 days
Digoxin	10–30 min.	1–2 hr.	2–3 hr.	3–6 hr.	33 hr.	3–6 days
Digitoxin	——	2–4 hr.	——	8–10 hr.	102–112 hr.	2–3 weeks
Digitalis leaf	——	2–4 hr.	——	8–10 hr.	——	2–3 weeks

*From Narliner, J. S., and Braunwald, E.: *In* Conn, H. F.: *Current Therapy,* 1973.

†Time required for disappearance of one-half of physiologic activity measured by changes in the ejection time index.

3. Administer *procainamide* (Pronestyl) intravenously to correct ventricular tachycardia if present.
4. Administer *propranolol (Inderal)* intravenously to control tachyarrhythmia if present.
5. Give EDTA (ethylenediaminetetraacetate) to block the action of digitalis.

Because of the danger of digitalis toxicity, the administration of digitalis is an important nursing action.

> When administering digitalis:
>
> 1. *Read the* labels *of all digitalis preparations with extreme care; these drugs have* similar names *(digitalis, digitoxin, digoxin) but* different strengths *and* dosages!
> 2. *Always take the patient's pulse for* one full minute *apically* before *administering a dose of digitalis.*
> 3. *Carefully note both the rate and rhythm of the pulse and chart them accurately.*
> 4. *If the heart beat is very rapid, below 60, or irregular, withhold the drug and notify the doctor.*
> 5. Observe *the patient carefully for all signs of digitalis toxicity; when severe symptoms are present, call the physician before giving the drug.*

DIET

Diet for the patient with CHF should be low calorie, bland low residue, divided into small feedings, and low in Na^+ content.

The *low caloric diet,* supplemented with vitamins, benefits the patient with heart failure in several ways: weight loss is promoted, thereby reducing the workload of the heart; cardiac output, pulse rate, and blood pressure are decreased and basal metabolic rate is lowered, reducing the demands of tissues for nourishment and oxygen.

A *bland low residue* diet is generally more palatable for patients with congestive heart failure. Raw fruits and vegetables are usually poorly tolerated because they cause gastric distention and heartburn. Also, patients should avoid foods belonging to the cabbage family, pastries, carbonated water, and fried foods because they tend to create flatulence and distention.

Small frequent feedings are preferable to three heavy meals a day. Large meals tend to create gastric distention, flatulence, and heartburn.

REDUCTION OF SODIUM AND WATER RETENTION

Methods employed to reduce edema are bed rest, digitalization, restriction of Na^+ in the diet, fluid restriction, diuretics, and reduction of anxiety.

Sodium-restricted Diets

Healthy adults on a regular diet generally ingest from 3 to 12 Gm. of Na^+ daily, depending upon their individual tastes. The most common source of Na^+ in the diet is table salt added to food, during preparation or at the table. Other less common sources of Na^+ are medications containing Na^+, baking soda, baking powder, and sodium-containing toothpastes. Foods and drinks that are particularly high in Na^+ are smoked meats and fish, canned soups and vegetables, beer, Pepsi-Cola, meat extracts, potato chips, olives, pickles, catsup, salad dressings, most candy bars, spaghetti, macaroni, breads, and crackers.

Patients who must restrict their Na^+ intake are usually placed on one of the diets described in Table 49–2. The strictness of the diet prescribed depends upon the severity of the patient's heart condition.

Low Na^+ diets can be made more palatable by adding salt substitutes to foods in place of table salt. Popular salt substitutes include Diasol, Adolph's salt substitute, Cosalt and Neocurtasal. Cooking with imagination and making food servings attractive can also help to make the low Na^+ diet more appetizing. Seasoning foods with onions, pepper, lemon and lime juice, vinegar, basil, bay leaves, chili powder, dill, mint, caraway seeds, paprika, garlic, mushrooms, taragon, and wine greatly improves the flavor of low Na^+ foods which might otherwise taste flat without added salt.

Sodium restriction is generally tolerated fairly well by most patients. However, patients sometimes develop *low salt syndrome.* Manifestations of Na^+ deficit include weakness, nausea, and vomiting. Generally, increasing the patient's Na^+ intake corrects this problem.

Diuretics

Because diuretics are powerful, potentially dangerous drugs, they are usually ordered only when digitalization and Na^+ restriction have failed to correct Na^+ and water retention. When diuretics are used, both physician and nurse should carefully observe the laboratory reports for abnormalities in electrolytes, pH, and the BUN. Both electrolyte balance and kidney function may be disturbed when diuretics are used for prolonged periods.

Diuretics may be grouped into those that are *rapid-acting* and are employed in *severe* CHF, and *maintenance* diuretics, which are used once the patient's condition has stabilized. *Rapid-acting* diuretics include the mercurials, furosemide (Lasix), and ethacrynic acid. These drugs are compared in Table 49–3.[140]

Maintenance diuretics include thiazide diuretics, triamterene (Dyrenium), chlorthalidone (Hygroton), and aldosterone antagonists (Aldactone A). These drugs are compared in Table 49–4.

All diuretics, when used in conjunction with a low Na^+ diet, may produce *dilutional hyponatremia* (water intoxication) unless the patient's water intake is curtailed. For the symptoms and treatment of dilutional hyponatremia, see Chapter 25.

TABLE 49–2. CLASSIFICATION OF LOW SODIUM DIETS

Diet	Amount Na^+ Allowed/Day	Indications	Food Substances and Beverages Allowed
Mild Na^+ restriction	2–3 Gm.	For patients with mild CHF	Do not add table salt; avoid obviously salty foods, e.g., salted nuts, potato chips, smoked meats, bouillon
Moderate Na^+ restriction	800–1200 mg.	For patients with serious CHF	Do not add salt to food at the table *or* during cooking; avoid salt-preserved foods and highly salted foods, condiments (e.g., catsup, soy sauce, chili sauce), cheese, peanut butter, canned vegetables and soups, frozen vegetables to which salt has been added, baking powder, prepared mixes, baking soda, and regular breads and rolls; use low Na^+ products
Strict low Na^+ diet	500 mg.	Patients with severe CHF	Observe all restrictions indicated for the moderate low Na^+ diet; avoid commercial salad dressings and mayonnaise, commercial candies, more than one pint skimmed milk a day (including milk used in coffee and on cereal), ice cream, ice milk, milk shakes, artichokes, beet greens, beets, carrots, celery, dandelion greens, mustard greens, spinach, Swiss chard, white turnips
Severe Na^+ restriction	250 mg.	Patients with very severe or intractable CHF	Observe all restrictions noted above; avoid regular milk (use low Na^+ milk only), more than 2 to 4 oz. meat daily and more than 3 eggs per week

TABLE 49–3. RAPID-ACTING DIURETICS

Drug	Usual Dose	Action Time	Indications	Hazards
Mercurials: Meralluride (Mercuhydrin); Mercaptomerin (Thiomerin)	1–2 ml. I.M.	Onset: 1–2 hr. Duration: 12–24 hr.	Acute edematous states	Frequent use causes hypochloremia with alkalosis, which produce refractoriness to the drug
Furosemide (Lasix)	50–100 mg. I.V. push 40–80 mg. P.O. 1–4 times daily 20 mg. I.M.	Onset: 5 min. Duration: 2–3 hr. Onset: 1 hr. Duration: 6–8 hr. Onset and results: 10–30 min.	Acute pulmonary edema Refractory edema	K^+ depletion, which may induce digitalis poisoning in patients taking digitalis; alkalosis; excessive diuresis, which can result in circulatory collapse
Ethacrynic acid (Edecrin)	0.5 mg./kg. I.V. push 50–100 mg. P.O. b.i.d.	Onset: 15 min. Duration: 6 hr. Onset: 30 min. Duration: 6 hr.	Acute pulmonary edema	Severe Na^+, K^+, and Cl^- depletion; nausea and diarrhea; agranulocytosis

Fluid Restriction

Generally fluid restriction is unnecessary, as Na^+ restriction and diuretics provide adequate diuresis. However, patients with severe refractory heart disease may need to restrict their fluid intake to less than 1000 ml. per day, and in extremely severe cases to 500 ml. per day.

Reduction of Anxiety

A reassuring attitude on the part of doctors and nurses is important in ensuring diuresis. A study by Barnes and Schottstaedt points out that a prolonged state of tension or depression can precipitate retention of sodium and water, whereas reassurance on the part of the physician or nurse can result in diuresis.[10]

Nursing Actions and Observations in Edema

The nurse has the following responsibilities in caring for patients who are being treated for severe edema:

1. Carefully record intake and output. Stress the importance of accurate records to all personnel caring for the patient.
2. Weigh the patient daily on the same scale, at the same time, and wearing the same amount of clothing.
3. Help the patient to rest as much as possible because recumbency favors diuresis in patients with heart failure.
4. Observe the patient for signs of dehydration from rapid diuresis. Observations of stability of blood pressure, fullness of the neck veins, hematocrit, urinary output, and skin turgor are helpful in determining the presence of dehydration.
5. Give the patient meticulous skin care, because edematous tissue is likely to break down. Check bony prominences at least daily. If possible, place the patient on an alternating pressure mattress, thereby lowering the possibility of decubitus development.

Criteria for evaluating the success of dietary and diuretic therapy in the patient with CHF are: a decrease in pitting edema, weight loss, good urinary output, absence of neck vein distention, decrease in pulmonary congestion as evidenced on x-ray, absence of rales and dyspnea, and a decrease in the circulation time and in the venous pressure.

OXYGEN THERAPY

Dyspnea is often greatly relieved by the administration of high concentrations of oxygen by means of nasal cannulas, tents, or masks. Oxygen therapy is particularly helpful in patients with CHF complicated by pulmonary disease or coronary thrombosis.

*PARACENTESIS AND THORACENTESIS**

Occasionally patients suffer from such severe peritoneal effusion that agonizing dyspnea and ab-

*Abdominal paracentesis is discussed in Unit XV; thoracentesis is discussed in Unit XIV.

TABLE 49–4. MAINTENANCE DIURETICS USED IN CHF

Drug	Usual Dosage	Hazards	Comments
Thiazide diuretics Chlorothiazide e.g. (Diuril)	250–1000 mg. P.O.	Hypokalemia, which may cause digitalis toxicity in digitalized patients; hyperglycemia; elevated serum uric acid, which may precipitate attacks of gout, and may precipitate occurrence of glaucoma	Modifications of Diuril (the parent thiazide) are: Hydrodiuril, Esidrix, and Naturetin; with small doses of thiazides, give patients orange juice to replace K^+ lost; with large doses of thiazides, doctor will order supplemental K^+
Triamterene (Dyrenium)	100 mg. q.d. or b.i.d. P.O.	K^+ retention with hyperkalemia; rarely causes hyperglycemia	Does not cause serious K^+ loss, as do other diuretics; moderately effective diuretic when used alone; very effective when combined with other diuretics
Chlorthalidone (Hygroton)	50–100 mg. q day *or* 100–200 mg. on alternate days P.O.	Side effects unusual; may cause attacks of gout by increasing uric acid levels	Long-acting drug; give once a day in morning with breakfast
Aldosterone antagonists spironolactone (Aldactone A)	25–50 mg. q.i.d. P.O.	May cause K^+ retention	Slow-acting diuretic; provides good diuresis when combined with thiazides

dominal distention result. Today, with modern diuretic drugs, excess peritoneal effusion is relatively rare. However, when excess fluid does accumulate within the peritoneal cavity, the physician can mechanically remove the fluid by means of abdominal paracentesis.

Excess fluid can also collect in the chest, causing severe dyspnea. Rarely, when diuretic drugs and Na^+ restriction fail to relieve pleural effusion, thoracentesis is indicated. However, repeated thoracenteses are dangerous, because they may cause Na^+ depletion, hypotension, and shock.

EDUCATION OF THE PATIENT AND HIS FAMILY

The treatment of CHF involves a long, often difficult period of adjustment for the patient and his family. Patterns of activity and patterns of eating and drinking must often change radically; furthermore, some changes must be accepted as necessarily being lifelong. Thus, without the patient's wholehearted cooperation, the treatment program may fail once the patient goes home from the hospital. Four reasons why patients fail to adhere to their prescribed treatment plan are:[163]

1. *Lack of knowledge concerning the disease process.* Patients who understand the mechanisms causing their heart to fail and the methods by which heart failure can be reversed are usually much more cooperative.
2. *Lack of motivation.* Some patients believe that their condition is hopeless and that there is little point in undergoing the rigors of a treatment program, particularly the Na^+ restricted diet. It is difficult to change such attitudes. However, the constant encouragement and reassurance of physician and nurse are helpful.
3. *Cultural and personal patterns.* Mexican and Italian patients, who are accustomed to spicy foods, may find it extremely difficult to eat a diet that differs so radically from the natural diet of their friends and family. Energetic persons whose self-image involves being active and outgoing may be unable to restrict their activity without becoming severely depressed. In such patients the nurse and physician may have to tolerate occasional lapses from the program and settle for less than total cooperation from the patient.
4. *Economic deprivation.* Some patients cannot afford expensive medications or special low Na^+ foods. Also, elderly, debilitated individuals may be unable to prepare special diets for themselves. These individuals will lapse from their treatment program unless they receive financial assistance.

COMPLICATIONS OF CONGESTIVE HEART FAILURE

The major complications of CHF are the complications of bed rest (Chapter 27), acute pulmonary edema, and refractory heart disease.

ACUTE PULMONARY EDEMA

Acute pulmonary edema is a medical emergency that usually results from left-sided heart failure. In patients with severe cardiac decompensation, the capillary pressure within the lungs may become so elevated that fluid pours from the circulating blood into the alveoli, bronchi, and bronchioles. The resulting pulmonary edema, if untreated, may cause death from suffocation. The patient literally drowns in his own fluids.

Symptoms of acute pulmonary edema are dramatic to view and terrifying for the patient. Typical manifestations include severe dyspnea, orthopnea, pallor, tachycardia, expectoration of large amounts of frothy, blood-tinged sputum, fear, wheezing, sweating, bubbling respiration, and cyanosis.

Treatment of acute pulmonary edema must be instituted immediately! Therapy includes the following steps:

1. *Positioning:* Place the patient in a semi-Fowler's position or in a chair in order to ease dyspnea.
2. *Sedation:* The physician generally orders morphine sulfate, 8 to 15 mg. subcutaneously, to alleviate anxiety, promote sleep, decrease pulmonary reflexes, and reduce venous return.
3. *Oxygen:* Administer oxygen in high concentrations by mask or by tent to relieve hypoxia and dyspnea and to lessen pulmonary capillary permeability. Always use a humidifier when giving oxygen; otherwise, bronchial secretions will thicken and dry. The administration of intermittent positive pressure breathing (IPPB) also helps to improve ventilation.
4. *Digitalization:* Rapid digitalization also promotes diuresis. Deslanoside intravenously is usually the drug of choice.
5. *Diuresis:* Rapid-acting diuretics usually help to promptly relieve fluid retention. The drug of choice in acute pulmonary edema is ethacrynic acid (Edecrin) 25 to 50 mg. I.V.
6. *Relief of bronchospasm:* Aminophylline, 500 mg. I.V. given slowly, helps to relieve severe bronchospasm and to increase cardiac output, renal flow, and urinary output of sodium and water. Aminophylline may also be administered in rectal suppositories containing 0.25 to 0.5 Gm.
7. *Reduction of blood volume:* Two methods for reducing blood volume are rotating tourniquets and venesection.

a. *Rotating tourniquets:* Soft rubber tourniquets or blood pressure cuffs are applied to three limbs with enough force to obstruct venous flow but not arterial flow, and are rotated every 15 minutes. Because approximately 700 ml. of blood are trapped in the patient's extremities, this procedure acts to retard venous return to the heart.

Rotating tourniquets is a potentially dangerous procedure. Basic rules to remember are given below:

Precautions when Rotating Tourniquets

1. *Occlude the vessels of each limb for* no more *than 45 minutes at a time.*
2. *Prepare a diagram of the procedure so that each member of the hospital team will*

know at what time to move the tourniquets and in which direction (Fig. 49–1).

3. Observe the patient's skin carefully throughout the procedure for signs of beginning irritation.

4. Remove tourniquets gradually, *or all the fluid trapped in the limbs will flood the heart at one time.*

Some hospitals use special electric automatic rotating tourniquet machines which have advantages over the manual application of tourniquets. First, timing of the inflation and deflation of the cuffs is precise, every 11¼ minutes. One cuff automatically deflates while the other cuffs automatically inflate. A complete rotation of the tourniquets takes place every 45 minutes.

Second, the correct amount of pressure is automatically applied to the blood vessels so that venous flow to the extremities is properly obstructed, but arterial flow is not. Finally, the automatic rotation of tourniquets frees the nursing staff to care for other patients.

b. *Venesection:* Removal of 300 to 700 ml. of blood can be performed when the rotation of tourniquets is unsuccessful in curtailing venous return to the heart. If circulatory collapse and shock have already developed, phlebotomy should not be performed as it will aggravate the shock state.

REFRACTORY HEART FAILURE

Heart failure is termed "refractory" or "intractable" when recommended diet, drugs, and treatments fail to alleviate symptoms and restore at least partial cardiac reserve; i.e., refractory heart disease is stubborn and difficult to manage.

To treat refractory heart disease, the physician usually reviews the patient's entire course and reassesses the medical treatment. Measures that the physician may then take include:

1. A prolonged period of complete bed rest in the hospital.
2. Severe Na^+ restriction, e.g., 250-mg. Na^+ diet.
3. Fluid restriction to 100 ml. per day.
4. Combined diuretic therapy using several different types of diuretics.

PROGNOSIS

The prognosis for patients with CHF depends upon: (1) the patient's age, (2) the degree of cardiac hypertrophy, (3) the amount of cardiac reserve, and (4) the presence of other heart or associated disorders. Patients generally survive five to eight years. The prognosis can generally be predicted by observing the patient's response to therapeutic measures. If the patient responds slowly or inadequately to prescribed medications, special diets, bed rest, and so forth, the prognosis is poor. Also, the patient's life and health are endangered if he develops any of the complications of bed rest, e.g., pneumonia, pulmonary embolism.

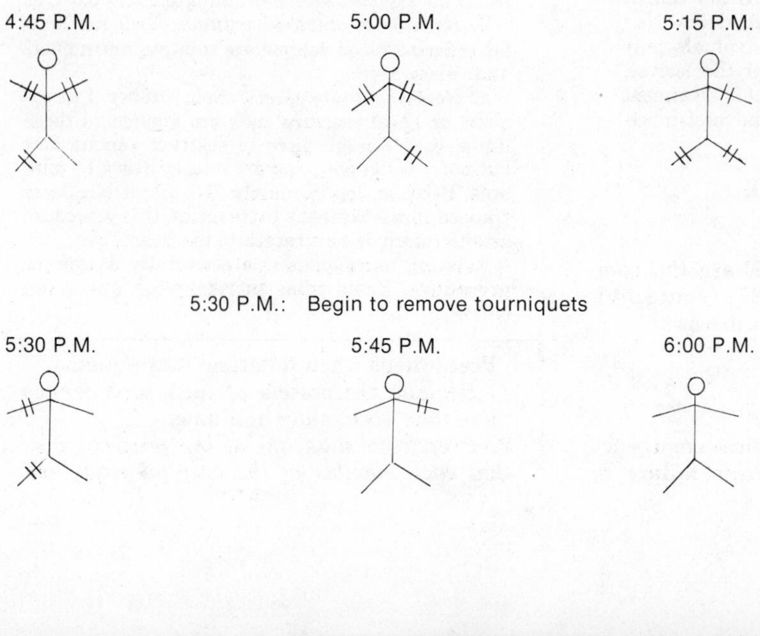

4:00 P.M.: Begin rotating tourniquets

4:00 P.M. 4:15 P.M. 4:30 P.M.

4:45 P.M. 5:00 P.M. 5:15 P.M.

5:30 P.M.: Begin to remove tourniquets

5:30 P.M. 5:45 P.M. 6:00 P.M.

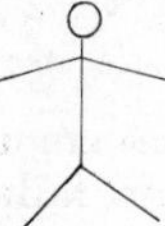

FIGURE 49–1. Rotating tourniquets: Diagram showing direction of rotation and time of rotation and removal.

CHAPTER 50

The Arrhythmias

Arrhythmias are disorders of the heart rate and rhythm that often lead to dramatic alterations in circulatory dynamics. For example, a *rapid* ventricular rate can precipitate angina pectoris, myocardial infarction, acute heart failure, pulmonary edema, syncope, and cerebral thrombosis. Conversely, abrupt *slowing* of the ventricular rate can cause heart block, fainting, and convulsions.

Arrhythmias affect both normal and diseased hearts. Persons with normal hearts may develop arrhythmias secondary to exercise, fever, hyperthyroidism, emotion, shock, and anemia. In other cases, arrhythmias arise as a direct result of coronary artery disease, rheumatic heart disease, and arteriosclerotic heart disease. Finally, many arrhythmias are caused by digitalis toxicity and electrolyte imbalances.

The most *frequently encountered* arrhythmias are sinus arrhythmia, sinus tachycardia, sinus bradycardia, atrial and ventricular premature beats, and paroxysmal atrial tachycardia. Six arrhythmias that can produce *critical alterations in circulatory dynamics* are: (1) ventricular fibrillation, (2) cardiac standstill, (3) ventricular tachycardia, (4) ventricular flutter, (5) sinus bradycardia, and (6) complete atrioventricular heart block.

> *The two potentially lethal arrhythmias are ventricular fibrillation and ventricular standstill; patients stricken by these arrhythmias must receive* immediate medical attention *or they will die within a few minutes or suffer irreversible brain damage.*

THE NORMAL AND ABNORMAL ECG

In Chapter 46 we discussed the normal electrophysiology of the heart. In Chapter 48 we considered the normal electrocardiogram which is, as you recall, a graphic tracing of the electrical activity of the heart as it completes each cardiac cycle. In this chapter we shall consider abnormalities in the electrocardiogram resulting from disturbances in the heart's electrophysiology. In Table 50–1 we briefly compare the significance of the waves and intervals of the *normal* ECG with the significance of *abnormal* waves and intervals.

TABLE 50–1. WAVES OF EXCITATION SEEN IN A TYPICAL ELECTROCARDIOGRAM

Wave	Meaning and Significance	Time Period	Abnormalities
P Wave	Signifies depolarization and contraction of the atria	0.08 sec.	Abnormal or absent P waves imply that another area of the heart muscle is acting as pacemaker in place of S-A node
P-R Interval	Section from beginning of P wave to beginning of QRS complex; signifies time it takes impulse to pass from atria to ventricles	Average time = 0.16 sec. Usually less than 0.20 sec.	*Prolonged P-R interval:* Impulse being conducted more slowly than normal through A-V node *Shortened P-R interval:* impulse being conducted over a shortened abnormal route from atria to ventricles
QRS Complex	Depolarization and contraction of ventricles (repolarization if atrial contraction is buried in the QRS complex)	0.08 sec.	Prolonged QRS complex signifies abnormal conduction or delay of conduction through the ventricles
S-T Segment	Period following completion of depolarization of ventricles and preceding repolarization of ventricles	0.12 sec.	*Elevation* or *depression* of S-T segment indicates ischemia of myocardium and infarction of the heart muscle
T Wave	Repolarization of ventricles following contraction	0.16 sec.	*Inverted* T wave: implies ischemia or infarction of heart muscle

Remember when studying arrhythmias that the shapes of the P waves and QRS complexes remain normal in appearance as long as the wave of depolarization travels the normal route from atria to ventricles; i.e., from the S-A node to the A-V node, to the bundle of His, and down the right and left bundle branches into the specialized network of the Purkinje system. The P wave and QRS complex become *aberrant* in appearance when abnormalities arise either in the pacemaker or S-A node, or along the pathway of impulse condition. As one authority points out, the key to the diagnosis of any arrhythmia is the presence and appearance of P waves or atrial activation and their relationship to QRS or ventricular complexes.[129]

DIAGNOSING AND ANALYZING ARRHYTHMIAS

Arrhythmias are diagnosed on the basis of the patient's medical history, the cardiovascular examination, and the ECG tracings. First of all, the patient may give a history of suddenly developing one or more of the following conditions: tachycardia, palpitations, anginal pain, extreme dyspnea, edema, and faintness.

Second, upon physical examination the doctor may discover the following evidence which points to the presence of a significant arrhythmia:

> A heart rate that is below 40 or above 140 beats/minute.
> An extremely irregular heart rhythm.
>A heart rate that does not increase with exercise or holding of the breath.
> A first heart sound which varies in intensity.
> The presence of the symptoms of congestive heart failure, shock, angina pectoris, syncope, or significant heart murmurs; these conditions may develop as a result of the effect of arrhythmias upon circulatory dynamics.

Finally, the physician will order a 12-lead electrocardiogram for the purpose of diagnosing the type of arrhythmia and the location of the cardiac disturbance. When examining an ECG tracing, one must carefully consider the following aspects:

Rate. The rate can be calculated by determining the distance between R waves (Fig. 50–1). Note: If there are two large squares between R waves, the rate is 150 beats per minute. Three large squares between R waves signifies a heart rate of 100 beats per minute, while four large squares is equivalent to 75 beats per minute. Remember that the heart rate per minute is equal to the number of squares between R waves divided into 300; for example, if there are two squares between R waves, 300 divided by 2 equals 150 beats per minute.

Regularity of Rhythm. The ventricular rhythm is regular if the R waves occur at *regular* intervals; the rhythm is *irregular* if the succession of R-R intervals fails to occur in a regular, normal time sequence. Some irregularities of rhythm occur regularly, whereas others occur spasmodically; the first group of arrhythmias are called *regular irregularities,* while the latter group are called *irregular irregularities.*

Appearance of the Waves or Deflections

P waves, when normal, are identical in contour and precede the QRS complexes. P waves remain *normal* in appearance in arrhythmias in which the S-A node continues to act as pacemaker, e.g., sinus tachycardia. P waves become *abnormal* in contour, inverted, or buried in the QRS complex in arrhythmias characterized by *ectopic foci* (*i.e.,* abnormal, out of place spots of irritable tissue located in either the atria, A-V node, or ventricles). Ectopic foci disturb heart rate and rhythm by initiating impulses at a faster rate than the S-A node, thereby taking over the role of pacemaker (e.g., atrial tachycardia).

The *QRS complexes* appear normal in arrhythmias in which the ventricles contract normally, e.g., all disturbances arising in the S-A node, atria, and A-V node. QRS complexes, on the other hand, appear grotesque and bizarre in ventricular arrhythmias. In disturbances arising in the A-V node, QRS complexes often *precede* P waves owing to the abnormal upward spread of impulses from the A-V node.

The *T waves* may be inverted following ventricular muscle damage resulting from myocardial infarction.

Length of the ECG Intervals. Prolonged intervals indicate disturbances in the rate of conduction of impulses from atria to ventricles. *Shortened* intervals may indicate an *abnormal route* of conduction of impulses from atria to ventricles.

CLASSIFICATION OF THE ARRHYTHMIAS

Arrhythmias may be classified in a number of ways, e.g., fast or slow, regular or irregular, atrial or ventricular, paroxysmal or constant, due to disturbances in impulse formation, or due to distur-

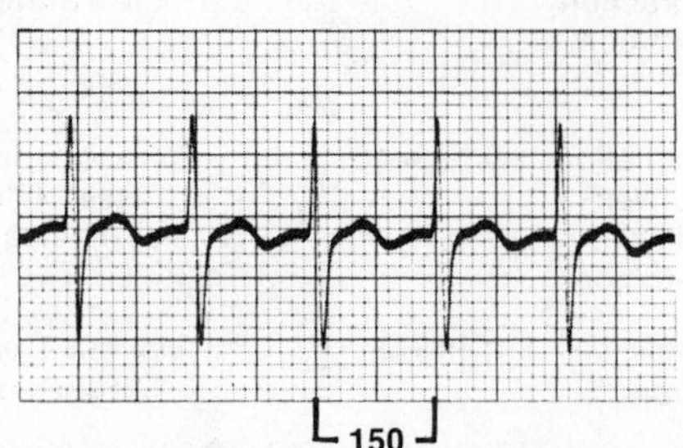

FIGURE 50–1. Calculating the rate of the heart beat. (From Phillips, R. E., and Feeney, M. K.: *The Cardiac Rhythms.* 1973.)

bances in conduction. In this discussion the arrhythmias are classified according to the part of the heart in which they originate, as follows:

- A. Disorders arising in the sino-atrial node
  1. Sinus tachycardia
  2. Sinus bradycardia
  3. Sinus arrhythmia
  4. Sinus arrest
- B. Disorders arising in the atria
  1. Premature atrial contractions (P.A.C.)
  2. Paroxysmal atrial tachycardia (P.A.T.)
  3. Paroxysmal atrial tachycardia with A-V block
  4. Atrial flutter
  5. Atrial fibrillation
- C. Disorders arising in the A-V node (or A-V junction)
  1. Disorders in which the A-V node takes over the role of pacemaker
     - a. Nodal (A-V junctional) rhythm
     - b. Premature nodal (junctional) contractions (P.N.C.)
     - c. Paroxysmal nodal (junctional) tachycardia (P.N.T.)
  2. Disorders of conduction through the A-V node
     - a. First degree heart block
     - b. Second degree heart block
     - c. Third degree heart block
- D. Disorders arising in the ventricles
  1. Disorders caused by ventricular irritability
     - a. Premature ventricular contractions (P.V.C.)
     - b. Ventricular tachycardia
     - c. Ventricular fibrillation
  2. Disorders of conduction
     - a. Right bundle branch block (R.B.B.B.)
     - b. Left bundle branch block (L.B.B.B.)

DISORDERS ARISING IN THE S-A NODE

You will recall from Chapter 46 that impulses normally originate in the S-A node or pacemaker, and that the S-A node is under the control of both the sympathetic and parasympathetic nervous systems. Also, remember that the heart rate speeds when the sympathetic nervous system is in control and slows when the parasympathetic nervous system is in control.

S-A node disturbances generally result from overactivity of either the sympathetic or parasympathetic nervous systems and rarely from disease of the S-A node itself. Factors that affect the sympathetic and parasympathetic nervous systems and interfere with the role of the pacemaker are: (1) excitement or emotion, (2) changes in the metabolic rate, (3) alterations in blood chemistry, (4) drug effects, (5) noncardiac diseases such as anemia and thyrotoxicosis, and (6) heart disease. As a result of any of these factors, the pacemaker may produce impulses too quickly (sinus tachycardia) or too slowly (sinus bradycardia); it may fail to initiate one or more beats (sinus arrest); or it may synchronize impulse formation with the individual's respiratory cycle (sinus arrhythmia).

In S-A node disturbances the heart *rate* varies between 60 and 160 beats per minute, the *rhythm* is regular with the exception of sinus arrest, and the ECG configuration remains unaffected. The P wave is normal because impulses are originating (as they should) in the S-A node; the QRS is normal because ventricular contraction is undisturbed.

In general, the sinus arrhythmias are of rather minor significance. However, prolongation of sinus tachycardia may place a strain on the heart muscle, and marked sinus bradycardia may lead to a severe decrease in cardiac output.

DISORDERS ARISING IN THE ATRIA

Atrial arrhythmias are caused by ectopic foci which develop in one of the atrial walls and which act to "take over" the role of the S-A node or pacemaker.

Atrial and nodal arrhythmias are sometimes called *supraventricular arrhythmias* because the abnormal foci for ectopic beats originate at a site above or within the A-V node. Ventricular arrhythmias, in contrast, are caused by abnormal foci within the ventricles.

How does an atrial ectopic focus affect heart rate and rhythm? First of all, such a focus may release an impulse *before* the S-A node is due to release its *normal* impulse; this premature impulse produces a *premature* atrial contraction (P.A.C.). Second, an atrial ectopic focus may become so irritable that it produces impulses *extremely rapidly,* thereby totally taking over the role of pacemaker. Such rapid rates of impulse formation occur in paroxysmal atrial tachycardia (160-240 beats/minute), atrial flutter (250-400 beats/minute), and atrial fibrillation (over 400 beats/minute). These extremely rapid atrial rates are dangerous because the heart muscle cannot contract efficiently, nor can it recover sufficiently between contractions. Ineffective myocardial contractions result in decreased coronary blood flow, which gives rise to anginal pain and congestive heart failure.

Atrial arrhythmias sometimes occur in conjunction with atrial-ventricular block. When atrial rates of impulse formation are very rapid (as in atrial tachycardia and flutter), the A-V node is unable to respond to each beat; it may respond only to every *other* beat (2:1 block), every *third* beat (3:1 block) or every *fourth* beat (4:1 block). In these arrhythmias with block, the ventricular rate is *always slower* than the atrial rate. Thus, the pulse (which reflects ventricular rate) may be normal in persons with atrial flutter or tachycardia even though the atrial rate is very rapid.

Characteristics of atrial arrhythmias are abnormally shaped P waves due to abnormal foci in the atria which initiate impulses rather than the S-A node, and normal QRS complexes because the ventricles are unaffected by the atrial disturbance.

Treatment of atrial arrhythmias centers on: (1) stimulation of the vagus nerve, which normally acts to slow the heart (digitalis and mechanical measures such as carotid sinus massage); (2) depression of myocardial irritability and contractility (quinidine and procainamide are drugs of

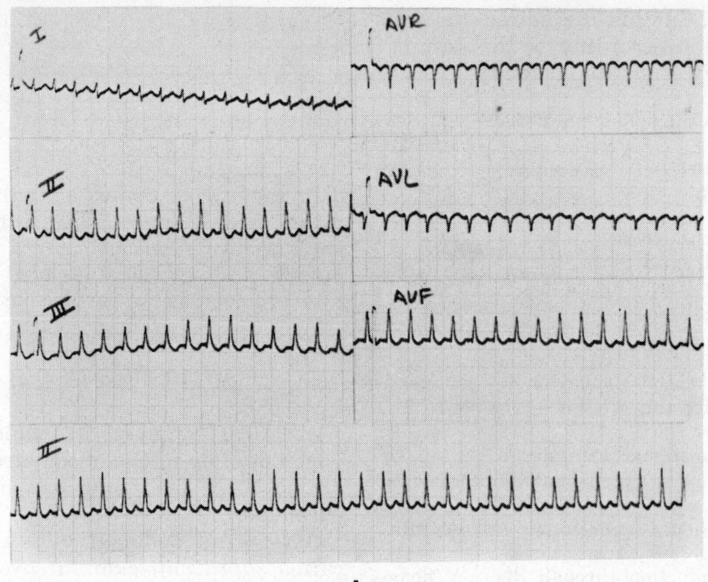

A

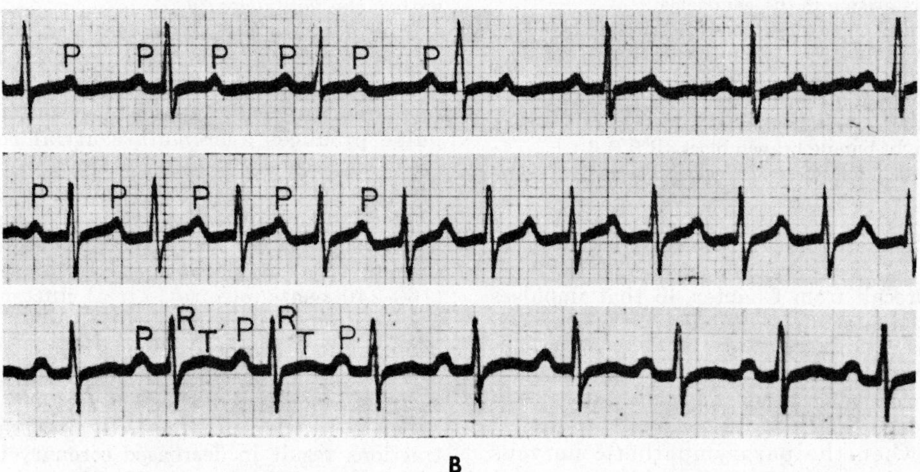

B

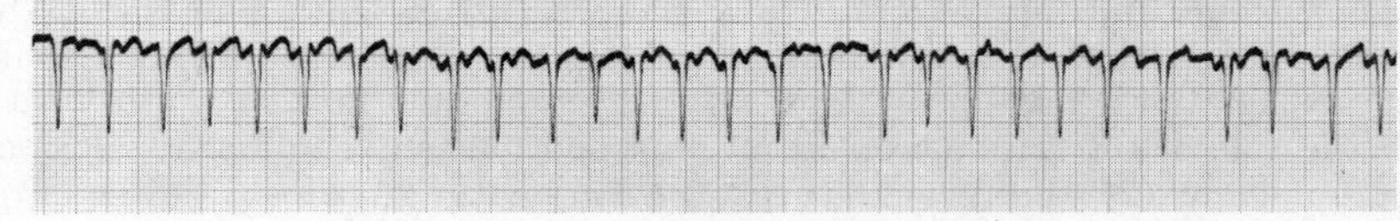

C

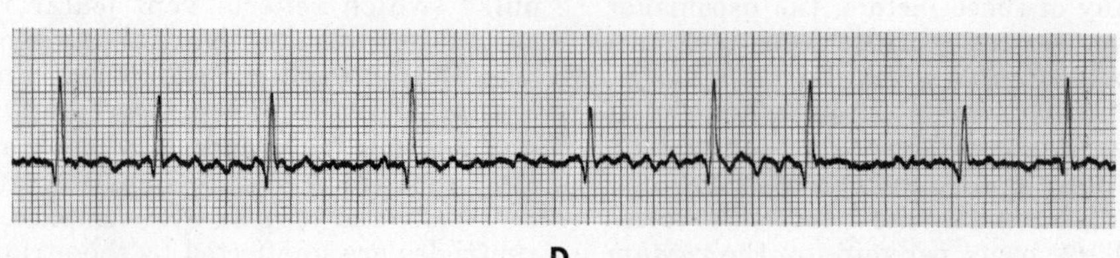

D

FIGURE 50–2. Atrial arrhythmias. *A,* Paroxysmal atrial tachycardia at a rate of 250 per minute. The P waves are superimposed on the T waves of the preceding beats. *B,* Paroxysmal atrial tachycardia with 2:1 A-V block. Atrial rate of 184 per minute and ventricular rate of 92 per minute. *C,* Atrial flutter with 2:1 block (lead V_1). The atrial flutter waves are regular at 375 per minute and some are "buried" in the QRS complexes. The ventricular response is somewhat irregular at 188 per minute. *D,* Atrial fibrillation with a moderate ventricular response (lead V_1). (*A, C,* and *D* from Sanderson, R. G.: *The Cardiac Patient,* 1972; *B* from Bellet, S.: *Essentials of Cardiac Arrhythmias,* 1972.)

choice); and (3) rapid conversion to normal rhythm (precordial shock) (see later in this chapter).

In Figure 50–2 ECG's of the chief atrial arrhythmias are shown.

*DISORDERS ARISING IN THE A-V NODE (OR A-V JUNCTION)**

Two major types of arrhythmias arise in the A-V node: (1) disturbances in which the pacemaker role of the S-A node is taken over by the A-V node; and (2) disturbances in which the A-V node blocks impulses journeying from the A-V node to the ventricles.

The *first* group of disturbances is characterized by the *upward* spread of impulses from the A-V node to the atria rather then the normal downward transmission of impulses from the S-A node to the A-V node. The abnormal upward direction of impulses is evident on the ECG; e.g., P waves are usually inverted and they may follow the QRS complex; the QRS complex is normal because the ventricles are contracting normally; and the P-R interval is shortened.

The major nodal arrhythmias are *nodal rhythm,* in which the A-V node acts as pacemaker, *nodal premature beats,* and *paroxysmal nodal tachycardia.*

The principal danger in untreated nodal arrhythmias is overwork of the heart and decreased output. Treatment of rapid nodal rhythms centers around drug therapy and precordial shock. Nodal rhythm is occasionally treated with an artificial pacemaker.

Heart Block

In the second group of nodal disturbances, impulses passing from the atria to the ventricles are *blocked* at the A-V node, so that the conduction of impulses from atria to ventricles slows or stops entirely.

Normally the impulse coming from the S-A node is delayed at the A-V node for less than 0.20 second before traveling on to the bundle of His. However, when the A-V node has been damaged by ischemia, rheumatic fever, or drug toxicity, impulses are delayed at the S-A node for abnormally long periods of time, depending upon the degree of heart block.

In *first degree heart block,* conduction in the A-V node is slowed, so that the P-R interval is longer than 0.20 second. This type of block is often associated with rheumatic fever or coronary artery disease, and may result from treatment with digitalis or quinidine. The rate and rhythm are normal and regular. The P wave is normal, but there is a prolonged P-R interval because of the prolonged A-V conduction time. Treatment may be required to increase the conduction rate; occasionally the use of a temporary pacemaker may be required.

In *second degree heart block,* every second, third, or fourth impulse from the atria is fully blocked; this creates a discrepancy between the atrial and ventricular rates, as mentioned in our discussion of atrial arrhythmias. This degree of block often occurs in arteriosclerotic heart disease, and also sometimes results from digitalis or quinidine therapy. It may proceed to third degree block.

There are two recognized subdivisions of second degree block: (1) The Wenckebach phenomenon, or Mobitz Type I block, is composed of recurrent cycles in which the P-R interval is progressively prolonged, until eventually no QRS complex follows the P wave. The cycle is then repeated (Fig. 50–3). (2) The Mobitz Type II block differs in that the P-R interval is constant in length. The P waves are normal and are followed by normal QRS complexes at regular intervals, until suddenly a ventricular beat is dropped (Fig. 50–4).

Third degree heart block, or complete A-V block, usually results from infections (i.e., rheumatic fever), fibrosis (scarring from myocardial infarction), digitalis toxicity, or congenital abnormalities. In third degree heart block, *all* impulses from the atria are blocked at the A-V node, and the atria and the ventricles become *completely dissociated;* i.e., the atria and the ventricles each have their own pacemaker and beat completely independently of each other (Fig. 50–5). When third degree heart block develops, there may be a pause before the pacemaker within the ventricles becomes active and begins to produce impulses. During this delay, cardiac output from the ventricles ceases and the patient faints or develops convulsions (Stokes-Adams syndrome). Once the ventricular pacemaker takes over, the ventricles begin to beat slowly (30 to 40 beats per minute) and the patient regains consciousness.

The greatest danger inherent in third degree heart block is ventricular *standstill* or *asystole* characterized by the Stokes-Adams attack. Ventricular standstill causes death within minutes unless an artificial pacemaker is employed at once (see later in this chapter).

A second danger in second and third degree heart block is *impaired cardiac output and circulatory function* owing to the slow ventricular rate that develops once the ventricular pacemaker takes over impulse production.

*Recent investigations have shown that previous conceptions of the atrioventricular node as an entity which possessed a high degree of automaticity, and hence could be regarded as a pacemaker, may be incorrect. Current terminology often refers to the A-V "node" as the A-V "junction," a term that embraces a somewhat larger area than was previously designated as the node. There is also some uncertainty as to the precise mechanisms by which the so-called nodal rhythms arise, and these arrhythmias are frequently referred to currently as "junctional arrhythmias." For the present we shall retain the more traditional nomenclature.

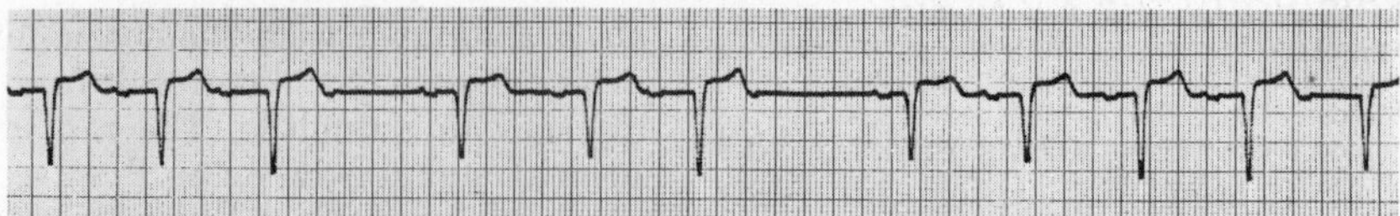

FIGURE 50–3. Second degree A-V block (Mobitz type I). The atrial rhythm is basically regular at a rate of 80 per minute, with some slight irregularity. After three beats with progressively lengthening P-R intervals, the fourth P wave is blocked, causing a pause. The cycle is then repeated—a 4:3 Wenckebach phenomenon. The pattern is not repeated in the third cycle. (From Sanderson, R. G.: *The Cardiac Patient*, 1972.)

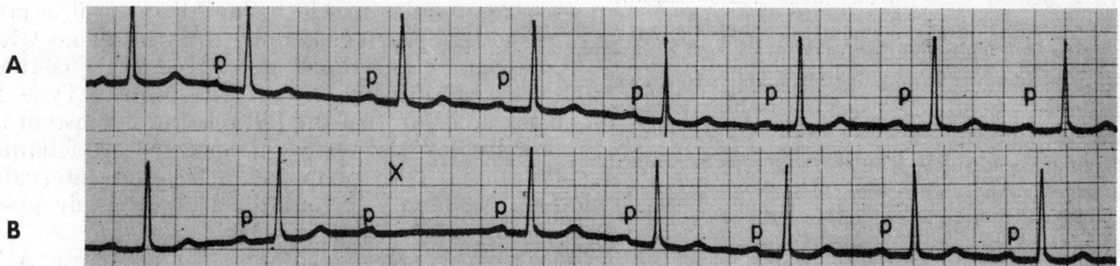

FIGURE 50–4. Second degree A-V block (Mobitz type II). *A* and *B* are a continuous record. There is a constant P-R interval prolongation at 0.28 second. Note the sudden appearance of a 2:1 A-V heart block in cycle X of strip *B*, followed by one slightly shorter P-R interval, and then a return to the cycles of P-R prolongation. (From Bellet, S.: *Essentials of Cardiac Arrhythmias*, 1972.)

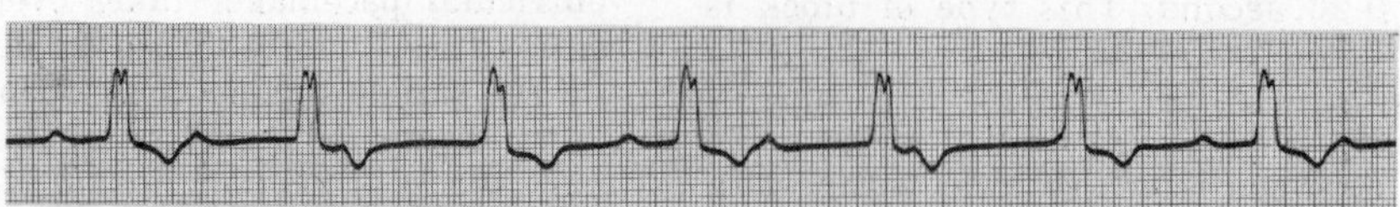

FIGURE 50–5. Complete A-V block. The atrial rate is 75 per minute. The completely unrelated ventricular rhythm has a rate of 44 per minute. (From Sanderson, R. G.: *The Cardiac Patient*, 1972.)

Heart block is generally treated with atropine or isoproterenol to speed the rate of impulse conduction. When heart block is severe, an artificial pacemaker is ordered for either temporary or permanent use.

DISORDERS ARISING IN THE VENTRICLES

Disorders of ventricular origin can be divided into the following two groups:

1. Arrhythmias that result from irritability of the ventricles.
2. Disturbances of impulse conduction through the ventricles as a result of injury of either the right or left bundle branches.

1. The first group of ventricular arrhythmias is characterized by ectopic impulses which result from myocardial irritability and which arise *below* the level of the A-V node. Irritability of the ventricles progresses on a scale from slight irritability (occasional premature ventricular contractions) to marked irritability (ventricular tachycardia) to extreme irritability (ventricular fibrillation).

Ventricular arrhythmias are generally more serious and life-threatening than are atrial or nodal arrhythmias. One reason for this difference is that ventricular arrhythmias are almost always associated with *intrinsic heart disease,* whereas atrial arrhythmias may develop in *normal* hearts that have been affected by emotion, fatigue, and so forth. Second, the ventricles are generally *protected* from the full impact of the atrial arrhythmias by the intervention of the A-V node. For example, in atrial flutter or tachycardia, the A-V node blocks one half to two thirds of the rapid, abnormal impulses fired from atrial ectopic foci. As a result, the abnormal impulses never reach the ventricles; thus, despite atrial disorders, the ventricles are able to contract at a normal rate and cardiac output is maintained. On the other hand, when the *ventricles* become highly irritable, cardiac output fails because the pumping of blood from the heart ultimately depends upon the smooth functioning of the ventricular muscles.

Premature ventricular contractions (PVC's) (also called ectopic beats and ventricular extrasystoles) are the most common of all arrhythmias. They are usually caused by irritable foci in the myocardium. An ectopic impulse forms before the next expected impulse from the S-A node and takes the place of the normal beat. Therefore, no P wave appears ahead of the QRS in the ECG. PVC's are innocuous when they are infrequent or isolated and require no treatment. They are dangerous when they are: (1) frequent (more than five per minute); (2) coupled with normal beats (*bigeminy*); (3) multifocal; or (4) when they follow a period of bradycardia.

Ventricular tachycardia occurs when an irritable ectopic focus in the ventricles takes over the role of pacemaker. There are rapidly occurring series of PVC's with no normal beats in between. In the ECG the P waves are often buried in the QRS, which has a wide, bizarre shape. The P-R interval is not measurable. The heart rate is 140–250/minute. Ventricular tachycardia is an *extremely dangerous* arrhythmia, producing a very low cardiac output which can lead to myocardial infarction and cerebral ischemia. At any time ventricular tachycardia can develop into ventricular fibrillation.

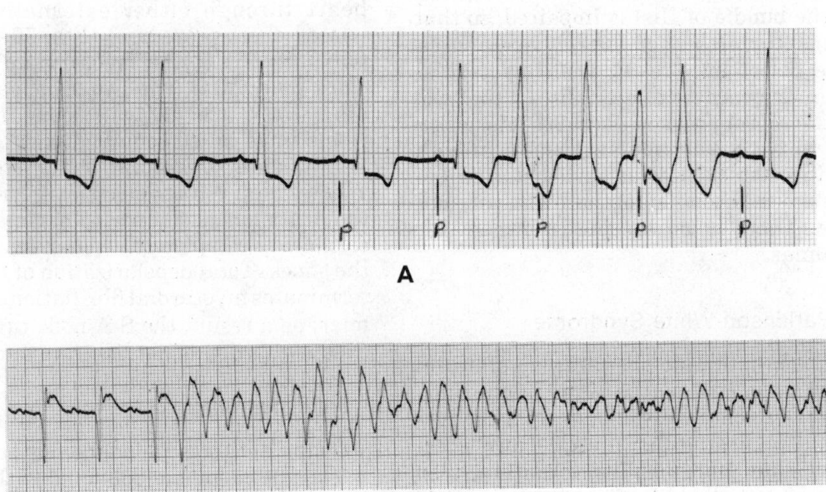

FIGURE 50–6. *A,* Ventricular tachycardia. After five normal sinus beats, four consecutive ectopic beats are present. The P waves are independent, continuing undisturbed at the basic sinus rate. A normal sinus beat then follows the brief run of ventricular tachycardia. *B,* Ventricular tachycardia and fibrillation following a PVC which occurs during the T wave of the preceding beat. (From Sanderson, R. G.: *The Cardiac Patient,* 1972.)

Ventricular tachycardia occurring at a rate of about 200 per minute is sometimes called *ventricular flutter*. Here the ECG shows continuous waves and the QRS cannot be distinguished from the S-T segment and the T wave.

Ventricular fibrillation is a *lethal* arrhythmia, and death results within minutes if treatment is not immediate. This is an advanced stage of ventricular tachycardia characterized by extremely rapid impulse formation and irregular impulse transmission. It usually results from severe myocardial damage, and may be the result of toxicity from quinidine, epinephrine, or digitalis. The heart rate is rapid and chaotic, and no rhythm of any kind can be discerned. The ECG has bizarre wave patterns and P waves and QRS complexes cannot be identified.

The treatment of the ventricular arrhythmia depends upon the degree of irritability of the myocardium. Infrequent premature ventricular contractions are usually not treated. Frequent P.V.C.'s are controlled with quinidine, lidocaine (Xylocaine), and procainamide (Pronestyl). *Ventricular tachycardia and fibrillation are emergencies that are swiftly treated with precordial shock and drug therapy* (procainamide, lidocaine, quinidine, vasopressor drugs). In ventricular fibrillation, procainamide sometimes is injected directly into the heart to produce cardiac arrest, and is followed by epinephrine or cardiac massage.

2. Disturbances of conduction through the ventricules (intraventricular block) result in either a right bundle branch block (R.B.B.B.) or a left bundle branch block (L.B.B.B.). Bundle branch block (B.B.B.) is generally considered to be a benign arrhythmia.

The arrhythmia derives its name from the fact that conduction in the right or left bundle branch (branches of the bundle of His) is impaired, so that the impulse must travel through the ventricular muscle itself. The defect may result from myocardial fibrosis or from an overdose of digitalis. Of the two, L.B.B.B. has the poorer prognosis because it is usually associated with left ventricular disease. In both types, the QRS complex is wide and distorted because of the abnormal conduction pathway through the ventricles. There is no specific treatment for these arrhythmias.

The Wolff-Parkinson-White Syndrome

This arrhythmia falls into the category of a preexcitation syndrome, that is, the sinus impulse bypasses, partially or completely, the normal conduction pathway. The ventricular muscle thus is activated earlier than normal. The condition, also called the "accelerated conduction syndrome," is often referred to as the W-P-W syndrome. The syndrome is quite common and is manifested by sudden attacks of supraventricular arrhythmias, especially atrial tachycardia. These are difficult to diagnose because the ECG resembles that of severe heart disease. It is thought that about 60 to 70 per cent of adults with this syndrome have normal hearts. However, if the tachycardia attacks are frequent, they may lead to myocardial fatigue and exhaustion. The attacks are treated by various drugs, chiefly digitalis, propranolol, quinidine, and procainamide.

GENERAL CLINICAL CARE IN THE ARRHYTHMIAS

The four major goals of care in the treatment of patients with arrhythmias are:

1. To convert an abnormal heart rhythm to a normal sinus rhythm.

2. To slow the ventricular rate when rapid.

3. To prevent further attacks of paroxysmal arrhythmias.

4. To decrease the degree of atrioventricular block if one exists.

Medical and nursing care generally revolves around the following therapeutic approaches: (1) drug therapy, (2) precordial shock (defibrillation and cardioversion), and (3) artificial cardiac pacing.

DRUG THERAPY

Important drugs commonly used in the treatment of patients with arrhythmias are: quinidine, procainamide (Pronestyl), lidocaine (Xylocaine), propranolol (Inderal), isoproterenol (Isuprel), atropine, and diphenylhydantoin (Dilantin). Facts concerning these drugs are summarized in Table 50–2.

PRECORDIAL SHOCK[97]

Precordial shock is a procedure used to halt life-threatening and dangerous arrhythmias; it is accomplished by delivering electric current to the heart through either externally placed paddles (closed chest procedure) (Fig. 50–7) or paddles applied directly to the myocardium in surgery (open chest procedure). The two principal forms of precordial shock are defibrillation and cardioversion (sometimes called countershock).

How does precordial shock stop arrhythmias? When a high voltage electrical current is delivered to the heart for a brief period of time, the entire myocardium is completely depolarized at the moment of the shock. Total depolarization of the cells generally terminates myocardial fibrillation and other arrhythmias; as a result, the S-A node can once again take over regulation of cardiac rate and rhythm.

Defibrillation[97]

Defibrillation is an emergency procedure in which an electric current is delivered to the heart to terminate a *life-threatening* arrhythmia, usually ventricular fibrillation. Specially trained physicians and nurses may be called upon to perform the procedure in case of emergency.

TABLE 50–2. DRUGS COMMONLY USED IN THE CARE OF PATIENTS WITH ARRHYTHMIAS

Drug	Action	Indications	Contraindications	Dosage and Route of Administration	Side Effects
Quinidine	Depresses myocardial excitability; slows conduction time in atria and ventricles, prolongs P-R and QRS intervals; prolongs refractory period; depresses myocardial contractility; reduces vagal tone.	Ventricular tachycardia; premature ventricular contractions; atrial flutter and fibrillation; ectopic beats (atrial or ventricular)	Sensitivity or allergy to drug; usually not given to persons with complete heart block, bundle branch block, thyrotoxicosis, acute rheumatic fever, or subacute bacterial endocarditis	Orally: 0.2 Gm. q.i.d., as maintenance dose I.M.: 0.4 Gm. I.V.: 0.3-0.8 Gm. quinidine gluconate given in emergency situations	Hypersensitivity: fever, rash, hypotension; neurologic effects: tinnitus, diplopia, confusion, headache, delirium; gastric effects: anorexia, nausea, vomiting, diarrhea; myocardial effects: heart block, nodal rhythm, ventricular arrhythmias; emboli when the heart is converting to normal rhythm
Procainamide (Pronestyl)	Depresses ectopic pacemakers; action on heart similar to quinidine	Premature ventricular contractions; ventricular tachycardia; ventricular fibrillation when defibrillator not available; atrial tachycardia	Severe heart damage and shock because of hypotensive effect; complete heart block; allergy	Orally: 0.25-1.0 Gm. q. 4-6 hr. I.M.: 1 Gm. ampule in 10 ml. dilutant I.V.: 1 Gm. ampule in 10 ml. dilutant given very slowly in emergency situations	Same as quinidine; severe hypotension with parenteral use
Lidocaine (Xylocaine)	Rapid-acting local or topical anesthetic agent; depresses myocardium; decreases excitability, conduction, and force of contraction; action similar to procainamide	Ventricular arrhythmias; sometimes used in open heart surgery as a direct topical anesthetic	Bradycardia; heart block; give with caution in liver disease, as drug is metabolized by liver	I.V. drip: 1 mg. per kg. body weight, given very slowly	Neurologic signs: dizziness, blurred vision, sweating, progressing to coma, hypotension, and convulsions; cardiac signs: large doses occasionally cause subendocardial ischemia
Propranolol (Inderal)	Beta adrenergic blocking agent; blocks the actions of the catecholamines upon the heart; decreases heart rate and ventricular volumes; decreases rates of S-A node and ectopic pacemaker sites; decreases A-V node conduction and ventricular irritability	Prolonged angina (see Chap. 51); premature ventricular contractions; atrial and ventricular tachycardias; tachycardia in Wolff-Parkinson-White syndrome; myocardial infarction.	Congestive heart failure and cardiogenic shock because patients in congestive heart failure or shock require catecholamine effects to stimulate force of myocardial contractions; A-V or bundle branch block; bronchospasm	Orally: 20-30 mg. t.i.d. or q.i.d. I.V.: 1 mg./q. 3 to 5 minutes (up to total dose of 5 to 10 mg.)	Bradycardia; hypotension; acute heart failure in persons with a damaged myocardium
Isoproterenol (Isuprel)	Increases heart rate, stroke volume, coronary blood flow; increases rate in A-V block by acting on sinus node and A-V node	Stokes-Adams syndrome; sinus bradycardia; sinus arrest; heart block	Use with caution in patients with hyperthyroidism, glaucoma, and limited cardiac reserve	I.C.: (directly in cardiac muscle) 0.2 mg. vial diluted in 19 ml. of normal saline I.V. push: 0.2 mg. diluted in 5-10 ml. normal saline Sublingual: 10-15 mg. q. 1-6 hr. Suppository: 5-15 mg. q. 1-6 hr.	Tachycardia; palpitations; weakness; sweating; nausea; angina; headache
Atropine	Vagolytic drug; abolishes vagal reflexes during cardiac arrest or hypoxia	Drug of choice in nodal rhythms; often used in surgery to control anesthesia-induced arrhythmias	Glaucoma; parotitis; tachycardia	I.V.: 1-2 mg. I.M.: 0.3-2.0 mg. Subcut: 0.6-0.8 mg.	Dry mouth with thirst; blurred vision from dilated pupils; disorientation; hallucinations; delirium; difficult voiding; decreased respirations
Diphenylhydantoin (Dilantin)	Suppresses myocardial irritability	Used when etiology of arrhythmia is obscure; e.g., failure of patient to take medications, metabolic imbalance, digitalis toxicity	Drug allergy; hepatic disease because drug is inactivated in liver	I.V.: 3.5-5.0 mg./kg. body weight, diluted in 5 ml. normal saline Orally: 200-400 mg. capsule daily	Transient hypotension due to peripheral vasodilatation; respiratory or cardiac arrest; shock

Preliminary Measures. When a patient is being monitored and the monitor alarm sounds, or when a threat to life is noted in some other manner, the patient's condition is evaluated immediately. The ECG reading is checked, and the leads are checked for loose connections. The patient's pulses are checked. If the emergency is confirmed, the code alarm is given over the hospital intercom system to summon the emergency team (e.g., "Dr. Blue, Code 99," or whatever). In the meantime, resuscitation measures are started by the first person on the scene. These include cardiac massage and mouth-to-mouth resuscitation (see below). During this time the defibrillator is being set up, turned on, and allowed to warm up. The machine is set at 400 watt-seconds unless the patient is in digitalis toxicity, in which case a lower setting is used. The synchronizer switch on the machine is turned to "off" (synchronization is not possible during ventricular fibrillation).

Preparation of Patient. Unless an I.V. is already running, one is started immediately. Sodium bicarbonate is given to combat acidosis, and lidocaine to prevent development of arrhythmias during or following shock. No anesthesia is used. Turn off the ECG machine, but leave the monitor turned on. Hyperventilate the patient with O_2 before and after the procedure. Remove oxygen from room during procedure.

Administration of Shock. The paddles are lubricated with electrode paste to prevent burning the skin. To save time, one paddle is usually placed over the *right sternal border*—the second intercostal space—and the other over the *apex of the heart.* The paddles can also be placed anteroposteriorly if convenient. All personnel, including the person administering the shock, *must stand back from the bed! Never touch bed or patient* when shock is being administered.

Evaluation of Procedure. Paddles are removed from chest at once by a qualified person and an ECG tracing is taken. A successful response is indicated by cessation of fibrillation, restoration of sinus rhythm, and normal contraction of heart muscle. A poor or dangerous response is indicated by failure of the arrhythmia to convert to normal rhythm or development of asystole.

Aftercare. A special steroid cream is applied to the skin where the electrodes had been applied. The patient is observed carefully, especially his pulse, state of consciousness, and patency of airway. Ventricular fibrillation can recur!

Cardioversion

This is an elective procedure in which electric current is delivered to the heart to terminate dangerous arrhythmias. The usual indications are tachycardias developing in patients who have had a myocardial infarction, e.g., atrial, nodal, or ventricular tachycardia. It is also used at times for atrial flutter or fibrillation. The procedure is performed *only* by specially trained physicians.

Preliminary Measures. ECG readings are taken to diagnose the type of arrhythmia present. The procedure is scheduled for a specified hour; it can be performed in the operating room or the CCU. No resuscitation measures are required.

Preparation of Patient. The patient is given a full explanation of the procedure. An I.V. is started before the procedure begins and is allowed to run for several hours after the procedure. Lidocaine is given to prevent development of arrhythmias, and potassium salts are given if the patient has hypokalemia.

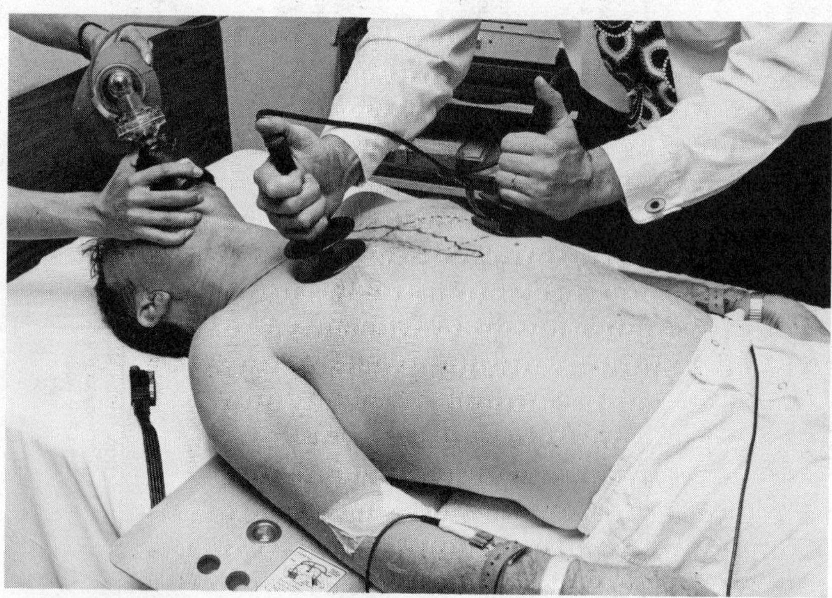

FIGURE 50–7. The emergency administration of precordial shock. (From Sanderson, R. G. (ed.): *The Cardiac Patient.* 1972.)

Quinidine is given several days prior to the procedure to prevent the development of arrhythmias. Anesthesia is used to reduce fear and pain; diazepam, sodium pentothal, and methohexital are commonly used.

Operation of the Machine and Administration of the Shock. The machine is set within a range of 50 to 400 watt-seconds. The synchronizer switch is turned to "on" in order to deliver the shock during the QRS complex. The paddles are lubricated with electrode paste. One paddle is placed on the patient's back, slightly medial to the tip of the left scapula, and the second is placed anteriorly over the base of the heart. The same precautions are observed during administration of the shock that were mentioned under defibrillation.

Evaluation of Procedure. Paddles are removed from the chest at once, and an immediate ECG tracing is done. In some cases ventricular fibrillation or tachycardia may occur. This indicates a poor response to the treatment; a successful response, of course, is indicated by the termination of the arrhythmia.

Aftercare. If the result is favorable, the patient remains in the recovery room or CCU until his condition stabilizes; he then returns to his room and may be discharged the following day.

As noted, cardioversion may not always restore normal heart rhythm in patients with severe arrhythmias. Disorders that may prevent the patient's heart from converting to normal rhythm following precordial shock are *hypoxia, acidosis,* and *drug toxicity.* The physician usually treats these disorders before he attempts precordial shock for the second time.

ARTIFICIAL CARDIAC PACEMAKERS

Definition and Uses

An artificial cardiac pacemaker is an electronic apparatus that is used to initiate the heart beat when the S-A node is seriously damaged and unable to act as pacemaker. The artificial pacemaker controls the heart beat by means of electrical stimulation of the ventricles. If the stimulating electrodes are placed *inside* the chest wall, the device is called an *internal* or *implantable* pacemaker. If the electrodes are placed *outside* of the chest wall, the device is called an *external* pacemaker.

Artificial pacemakers are used to stimulate the heart beat in the following conditions:[129]

1. Partial or complete A-V block with Stokes-Adams attacks that do not respond to medical therapy.
2. Complete heart block.
3. Acute myocardial infarction with partial or complete heart block.
4. Acute myocarditis with heart block.
5. Heart block following cardiac surgery.
6. Intermittent sinus arrest.
7. Sinus bradycardia with syncope.

Types of Pacemakers

There are two major types of pacemakers: *temporary* pacemakers and *permanent* pacemakers. These two categories can be further subdivided as follows: temporary pacemakers, for emergency and short-term pacing; and permanent pacemakers, for epicardial and endocardial pacing.

Temporary emergency pacing is used principally to correct asystole due to third degree heart block. Methods of artificially pacing the heart in emergency situations include the following:

1. *Direct application* of electrodes to the chest wall, which delivers a series of shocks ranging between 50 and 150 volts. This procedure, while often lifesaving, is painful for the patient; also it may cause burns of the chest.
2. *Percutaneous insertion* of electrodes through the chest wall directly into the myocardium.
3. *Insertion* of an insulated electrode wire *through a vein* in the arm to the right atrium, and then through the tricuspid valve into the right ventricle where it is wedged under the trabeculae; this method is called *emergency or temporary transvenous pacing.* The electrode positioned within the ventricle forms the negative pole of the circuit, while a wire loop sutured subcutaneously into the patient's arm forms the positive pole. Both these leads are connected to an external pacemaker, which stimulates the heart with a regular series of shocks ranging between 1 and 5 volts. This method of pacing is not painful as long as the amount of voltage is low. However, a higher number of volts causes muscle spasm and twitching in the area surrounding the subcutaneous loop.

Short-term pacing, the second form of temporary pacing, is useful in such disorders as myocardial infarction with temporary heart block, sinus arrest, and sinus bradycardia. The most popular method of short-term pacing is the insertion of a temporary transvenous pacing catheter as described above. This form of temporary pacing can be employed for several weeks if necessary. However, transvenous pacemakers should not be used for longer than one month, because the presence of the pacing catheter severely limits patient mobility, which can lead, in turn, to the complications of bed rest.

When weaning the patient from a temporary pacemaker upon which he has relied for several weeks, the nurse and physician must frequently evaluate the patient's cardiac rate and rhythm; also they must give the patient encouragement and emotional support.

To discontinue use of the pacemaker, the physician turns the *external* pacemaker off, but leaves the temporary transvenous pacing catheter in the right ventricle as a safety precaution. If heart block continues and the S-A node is still unable to initiate its own beats, the electronic pacemaker can quickly take over the role of the damaged node. It is important to tell a nervous patient that the artificial pacemaker will be activated immediately in event of any problem with his heart during this weaning period.

In contrast to temporary pacemakers, *permanent* pacemakers can be used for months to years. The most important indication for permanent pacing is persistent *chronic heart block with Adams-Stokes attacks.* Approximately one third of patients with chronic heart block and Adams-Stokes syndromes are successfully treated with drug therapy. However, a remaining two thirds of patients fail to respond adequately to drugs; this group must be treated with implantable permanent cardiac pacemakers.

There are two principal types of electrode placement for permanent pacing: endocardial and epicardial. The procedure for inserting an *endocardial,* or transvenous, pacemaker (the most common type) is similar to the insertion of a transvenous temporary pacemaker. Under fluoroscopic observation, a transvenous pacing catheter is passed through the *right external jugular vein* or through the *subclavian vein* beneath the clavicle (note that a superficial arm vein is *not* used as in temporary pacing) into the right atrium and then the right ventricle. This electrode within the right ventricle forms the negative pole of the circuit. The proximal end of the pacing wire or catheter forms the positive pole of the circuit and is attached to a battery-operated *pulse generator* (Fig. 50–8). The pulse generator is buried in a subcutaneous pocket, surgically placed beneath the clavicle or under the axilla; this completes the electrical circuit (Fig. 50–9). Note in Figure 50–9 that a small stab wound has been made in the "pocket," and that a drainage catheter is inserted and attached to low suction; the pocket is usually drained for 24 hours to prevent the accumulation of drainage and the possibility of infection.

The major early complication of endocardial pacing is *displacement of the endocardial leads* within the right ventricle. When endocardial leads become dislodged, the myocardium is only stimulated spasmodically and sometimes receives no stimulation at all. Generally the malpositioned electrode can be manipulated back into position without serious consequences.

A later complication of endocardial pacing is *breakage* of the *electrode wires* or *cracking* of the *wiring insulation.* The major sign of an insulation breakdown is the occurrence of missed beats in a radial pulse which is otherwise regular. Fortunately this malfunction is fairly uncommon today thanks to advanced research in pacemaker design.

Implantation of an *epicardial* pacemaker is a much more dangerous and complicated procedure than that described above. To institute epicardial pacing, the surgeon must perform a thoracotomy, expose the heart, and then sew electrodes onto the epicardium or heart's outer surface. Wires from these electrodes are then attached to a battery-operated pulse generator placed surgically in the anterior abdominal wall.

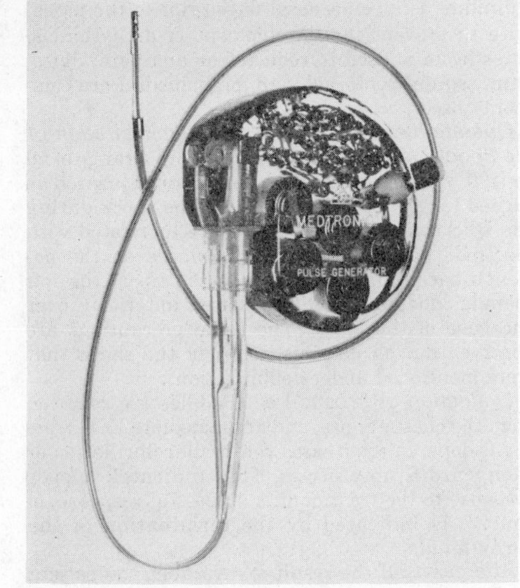

FIGURE 50–8. A permanent transvenous (endocardial) pacemaker. (Courtesy of Medtronic, Inc.)

The major early complications of epicardial pacing are the same as the complications arising from any type of thoracic surgery. Patients (who are generally in an older age group) may develop pulmonary infections, thrombophlebitis, decubitus, and all the other complications that accompany a prolonged immobilization period.

A *later* complication of epicardial pacing is the development of infected and inflamed areas around the electrodes which, in turn, necessitates increased power to stimulate the heart to contract. If infection is truly severe, epicardial pacing is discontinued in favor of endocardial pacing.

In sum, the major advantage of implanted pacemaker systems (endocardial and epicardial) is that

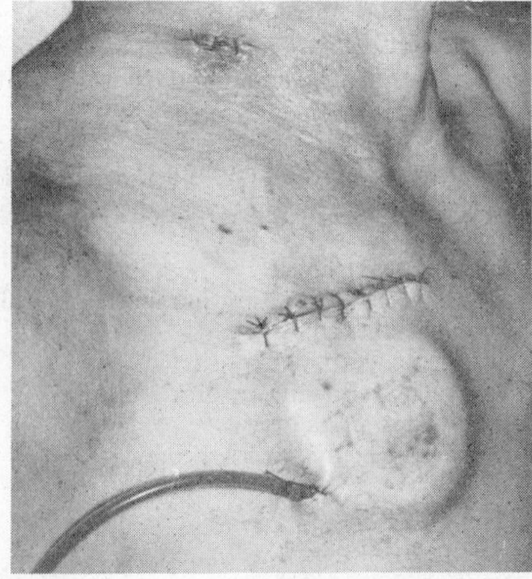

FIGURE 50–9. Pulse generator in subcutaneous pocket. (Courtesy of Medtronic, Inc.)

they are entirely subcutaneous. As a result, the patient is free to move, turn, bathe, ambulate and, in time, lead a normal life.

Methods of Pacing

The three major methods of cardiac pacing are: (1) fixed rate asynchronous pacing; (2) demand or standby pacing; and (3) atrial-triggered pacing.

The *fixed rate continuous asynchronous pacemaker* was the first pacing device to appear on the market. It is called a "fixed rate" pacemaker because it stimulates the ventricles to contract at a fixed or preset rate regardless of the body's metabolic requirements at the time. The term "continuous asynchronous" means that the pacemaker is not synchronized to the patient's ECG pattern; thus, it fires as set regardless of the ECG configuration.

The major advantage of the fixed rate pacemaker is its relative simplicity of operation. However, fixed rate pacemakers have three major disadvantages: First, the rate at which this pacemaker fires does not increase with the patient's metabolic needs. Second, some patients, following insertion of a fixed rate pacemaker, convert back to a normal rhythm; as a result, impulses released by the S-A node *compete* with impulses released by the artificial pacemaker. Fortunately, if the voltage is low, competition between the two pacemakers is not a serious problem ; an irregular pulse is generally the only sign. Finally, fixed-rate pacemakers can precipitate ventricular fibrillation if an artificial pacemaker impulse is released during the vulnerable period of ventricular repolarization following release of a normal impulse by the S-A node.

Demand pacemakers fire on demand, or when needed to stimulate ventricular contraction. Therefore, if the S-A node stimulates the appearance of a QRS wave, the demand pacemaker does not fire. On the other hand, when the S-A node is unable to trigger the apperance of a normal QRS, the demand pacemaker goes into action and stimulates ventricular action. Thus, the ECG readings of patients on demand pacemakers indicate the presence of an artificial pacemaker only when the natural QRS is not present.

Demand pacemakers are advantageous for patients who are frequently in normal sinus rhythm, but who nevertheless suffer periodically from attacks of severe bradycardia or syncope. In recent years, this type of pacing has supplanted the fixed rate type to a large degree.

Atrial-triggered synchronous pacemakers are more sophisticated devices than either fixed-rate or demand pacemakers. Essentially they operate as an electronic bundle of His; in other words, they detect the atrial P wave and then deliver a stimulus to the ventricles following a time delay identical to the P-R interval. Should atrial fibrillation develop, the atrial-triggered pacemaker is able to block every other impulse (2:1 A-V block), thereby ensuring that the ventricular rate does not rise above a predetermined safe level. Should atrial P waves fail to appear, the atrial-triggered pacemaker converts to a fixed-rate pacer.

The major disadvantage of these units is that they must be *surgically* implanted on the atrial surface in order to perceive the P wave. Because of the dangers of thoracic surgery, atrial-triggered pacemakers are infrequently used.

Technical Problems Associated with Cardiac Pacing

Technical problems that interfere with pacemaker operation are decreasing as scientists continue to perfect pacemaker design. Problems that still occur, however, include the following:

1. Dislodgement and migration of endocardial leads.
2. Wire breakage.
3. Cracking of insulation surrounding wires.
4. Infection of sites surrounding either pacing wires or pulse generator.
5. Interference with pacemaker function by TV channels transmitting at a frequency that distorts the pacemaker transmission. Laws are being enacted to assign frequencies to TV stations that will not disrupt pacemaker function.
6. Battery exhaustion occurring after 15 to 24 months. This unavoidable problem manifests itself by an initial tachycardia, followed by a bradycardia once the battery becomes sufficiently depleted. The implanted unit must be changed in the operating room.

Clinical Care of Patients with Artificial Pacemakers

The nurse has many responsibilities when caring for patients with pacemakers. In Table 50–3 the care of patients with temporary and with permanent pacemakers is outlined and compared.

The patient who is to be discharged with a pacemaker permanently implanted needs to receive several special cautions and instructions. Some of these are:

1. He should take his pulse once daily for one full minute and should note and report to the physician irregularities in rate and rhythm.
2. He should take frequent rest periods at home and at work.
3. He should be warned to avoid the use of electrocautery devices, ungrounded power tools, large electrical devices, and microwave ovens.
4. He should be warned not to come close to a running car, boat, or lawnmower engine.
5. The use of a safety razor rather than an electric razor should be encouraged.
6. Prolonged hiccoughs should be reported to the doctor; rarely, the catheter tip might perforate

TABLE 50–3. CLINICAL CARE OF PATIENTS WITH TEMPORARY AND PERMANENT PACEMAKERS

Therapeutic Measure	Temporary Pacemakers	Permanent Pacemakers
Activity	Immobilize extremity where transvenous catheter is inserted through a superficial vein; guard against *any* tension being placed on pacing catheter, in order to prevent displacement of catheter within ventricle	Moderately restrict patient's activities during first 24 hours following pacemaker insertion to observe pacemaker function under basal conditions; promote deep breathing, leg movements, and early ambulation following thoracotomy
Prevention of sepsis	Check temperature immediately following procedure and every 4 hours thereafter; report elevations of temperature at once; daily cleanse arm in which transvenous catheter is inserted, cover the area with an antibiotic ointment and sterile dressing; use sterile technique; oil the skin surrouding the catheter in the area outside the dressing where the wires of the external pacemaker may touch the skin; pad site under the catheter wires to prevent tissue injury	Same; antibiotics administered for 5 to 7 days following procedure; low suction to subcutaneous pouch following implantation of pulse generator in order to prevent accumulation of drainage
Postoperative care	Watch for signs of thrombophlebitis and infection at site of entry of transvenous catheter	Following thoracotomy: check vital signs q. ½ hour until stable; check chest tubes and suction; examine dressing for drainage; record I and O; give small amount of meperidine hydrochloride (Demerol) to relieve pain; ambulate day after surgery following endocardial implantation: regularly exercise arm on operated side to prevent frozen shoulder
Promote environmental safety	Check all equipment in patient's room for *proper grounding* when externally powered pacemaker is used; improperly grounded equipment may allow the escape of small amounts of electrical current which could reach the heart through the pacing catheter and cause ventricular fibrillation	Not applicable because entire pacemaker unit is subcutaneous.
Monitor heart rate and rhythm	In fixed rate pacemakers, pacemaker spike or artefact should precede each QRS complex on ECG; check for signs of competition between natural pacemaker and artificial pacemaker	Same; check for missed beats or tachycardia followed by bradycardia which may indicate battery failure; pulse generator x-rayed periodically to determine degree of battery depletion
Provide emotional support	Give full explanation of function and use of pacemaker; project a confident attitude when the patient is being weaned from the pacemaker	Encourage the patient throughout convalescent period following thoracotomy; explain that battery failure is not a problem if patient reports to his doctor or clinic for periodic checkups
Discharge home	Patients usually discharged once they have been completely weaned from temporary pacemaker and cardiovascular function has stabilized	Patients usually in hospital for two weeks following implantation of pacemaker; this time interval gives staff sufficient time to evaluate pacemaker function and wound healing. See text for special patient cautions and instructions.

the heart and migrate to the diaphragm, causing hiccoughs.

7. The patient should have a clinic appointment or see his private physician every three months.

CARDIAC ARREST AND CARDIOPULMONARY RESUSCITATION

Cardiopulmonary resuscitation (CPR) techniques are used to artificially maintain both circulation and ventilation in persons suffering from *cardiac arrest.* Cardiopulmonary resuscitation techniques involve: (1) external (closed chest) cardiac massage (manual heart compression), and (2) artificial ventilation by either mouth-to-mouth, mouth-to-nose, or mouth-to-airway techniques.

The term *cardiac arrest* is synonymous with the term *sudden death;* it means that the victim's heart beat, circulation of blood, and respirations have *suddenly* and *unexpectedly* stopped as a result of trauma, electrical shock, disturbed electrical activity within the heart, and so forth. Table 50–4 lists principal causes of cardiac arrest.

The terms *sudden* and *unexpected* are important in this definition because only the victims of *sudden* death are generally resuscitated. For example, a young healthy telephone repairman who suddenly receives a powerful jolt of electric current while working on telephone lines will undoubtedly suffer both cardiac and respiratory arrest; he is, thus, a candidate for immediate resuscitation measures. On the other hand, an elderly person who dies from cancer does *not* experience a cardiac arrest in the strictest sense of the term. When this patient's heart ceases beating, death comes as a *natural* event for which the patient and his family are prepared. Therefore, this patient is *not* a candidate for resuscitation measures; indeed, such measures would only prolong his suffering.

THE RESUSCITATOR AND HIS RESPONSIBILITIES

Cardiac arrest or sudden death can occur *anywhere*—in the home, on the street, in a general hospital ward, or in a highly specialized CCU. For that reason both professional persons and trained laymen are qualified to perform emergency cardiopulmonary resuscitation procedures. Within the hospital setting *nurses,* in particular, must be experts in resuscitation measures, because they are generally the first persons to discover a patient who has "arrested." It is typically nurses who must diagnose the problem, start cardiac massage, call for medical help, prepare emergency drugs, set up and sometimes even use the defibrillator. Because these tasks must be carried out *immediately,* every nurse needs accurate knowledge of resuscitation procedures of life-saving techniques.

Any person trained in resuscitation techniques has three major responsibilities that he must swiftly fulfill upon discovery of a victim of cardiac arrest.

TABLE 50–4. CAUSES OF CARDIAC ARREST

Causes Associated with Surgery*	Causes Not Associated with Surgery
Hypotension	Acute myocardial infarction
CO_2 retention	Electrical shock
Reactions to anesthesia	Sensitivity to insect bites
Depression from anesthesia	Anaphylactic reactions
Coronary occlusion	Suffocation, e.g., in plastic bag or abandoned refrigerator
Acute myocardial infarction	Airway obstruction, e.g., due to a foreign body
Inadequate ventilation of the lungs	Drug sensitivity
Anoxia due to airway obstruction	Digitalis poisoning
	Cardiac catheterization
	Drowning
	Carbon monoxide poisoning

*Approximately one cardiac arrest occurs in every 1200 operations.

> Responsibilities of the Resuscitator
>
> 1. Recognize *the* signs *of cardiac arrest.*
> 2. Protect *the patient's* brain *from* anoxia: *(a) immediately begin* external cardiac massage *in order to provide continuous artificial circulation to brain and vital organs; (b) rapidly begin* artificial ventilation *of the lungs.*
> 3. Summon help—*either doctor, resuscitation team, or ambulance.*

Signs of Cardiac Arrest

> *Signs of cardiac arrest are as follows:*
>
> *1. Abrupt and complete unconsciousness.*
> *2. Apnea or gasping respirations.*
> *3. Absence of heartbeat and femoral, radial, and carotid pulsations.*
> *4. Dilation of the pupils.*

The outstanding sign of cardiac arrest is the absence of a carotid pulse. In some cases, however, the carotid, femoral, and radial pulses may be present but very feeble. In these instances it is still necessary to begin resuscitation measures at once, because cardiac output is undoubtedly poor, and the patient's brain, kidneys, and liver will suffer from inadequate oxygenation without artificial ventilation.

If the resuscitator is unable to make a definite diagnosis of cardiac arrest based on the signs listed above, most authorities recommend that he begin resuscitation measures anyway, and leave the final decision to stop resuscitation for the physician when he arrives. There are, however, two groups of individuals who should *not* be resuscitated: they are patients in the last stages of an incurable illness and persons whose heart beat and respirations have been absent for more than six minutes.

Protection of the Brain from Anoxia

Once an individual suffers a cardiac arrest, he is considered *clinically* dead; i.e., his heart has stopped beating. The patient, however, is still *biologically* alive, i.e., his brain tissues and other organs still contain some oxygen and are therefore living. Indeed, the brain and other central nervous system tissues remain alive for a period of from four to six minutes, while other body tissues survive for even longer periods of time. Unfortunately, once this grace period of from four to six minutes following cardiac arrest passes, *biologic* death ensues and the patient's brain, now irreparably damaged, dies. Once biologic death occurs, resuscitation attempts are futile because the brain tissues are already severely damaged. Therefore, *remember:*

> *External cardiac massage and artificial ventilation* must *be started within* four to six minutes *following cardiac arrest or* irreversible brain damage *will develop as a result of oxygen deprivation and lack of circulation.*

Summon Help

It is extremely difficult for one person to carry out a successful cardiopulmonary resuscitation alone. It is almost mandatory that two persons assist the victim—one providing artificial ventilation, and the other providing cardiac compressions. Even when two persons are present, it is still absolutely essential to obtain expert medical help. The patient may need special drugs, countershock, intubation, and other emergency measures in order to reactivate his heart and respiratory system.

Within the hospital setting, special notification systems are generally used to quickly gather emergency resuscitation team members at the patient's bedside. Various codes are used; for example, "Alert—Room ___." "Doctor Blue—Room ___ stat." or "Code 99—Room ___ stat." Once the team arrives, each person performs the specific task for which he is especially trained.

STEPS IN THE TREATMENT OF CARDIAC ARREST

Treatment of victims of cardiac arrest can be divided into three stages: emergency care, specific medical therapy, and postresuscitation care.

Emergency Care

The major steps in emergency cardiopulmonary resuscitation are outlined and illustrated at right.

HEART-LUNG RESUSCITATION*

(For treatment of asphyxia or cardiac arrest.)

First Aid (Emergency Oxygenation of the Brain)

Must be instituted within 3 to 4 minutes for optimal effectiveness and to minimize permanent brain damage. Do not wait for confirmation of suspected cardiac arrest.

Step 1: Place patient in a supine position on a firm surface (not a bed). (A 4 × 6 foot sheet of plywood should be available at emergency care centers.)

Step 2: Tilt head backward and maintain in this hyperextended position. Keep mandible displaced forward by pulling strongly at the angle of the jaw. If victim is not breathing:

Step 3: Clear mouth and pharynx of mucus, blood, vomitus, or foreign material.

Step 4: Separate lips and teeth to open oral airway.

Step 5: If Steps 2 to 4 fail to open airway, forcibly blow air through mouth (keeping nose closed) or nose (keeping mouth closed) and inflate the lungs 3 to 5 times. Watch for chest movement. . . .

Step 6: Feel the carotid artery for pulsations.

a. If Carotid Pulsations Are Present: *Give lung inflation by mouth-to-mouth breathing (keeping patient's nostrils closed) or mouth-to-nose breathing (keep patient's mouth closed) 12 to 15 times per minute–allowing about 2 seconds for inspiration and 3 seconds for expiration–until spontaneous respirations return. Continue as long as the pulses remain palpable and previously dilated pupils remain constricted. Bag-mask techniques for lung inflation should be reserved for experts. If pulsations cease, follow directions as in 6b, below.*

b. If Carotid Pulsations Are Absent: *Alternate cardiac compression (closed chest cardiac massage) and pulmonary ventilation as in 6a, above. Place the heel of one hand on the sternum just above the xiphoid. With the heel of the other hand on top of it, apply firm vertical pressure sufficient to force the sternum about 2 inches downward (less in children) about once every second. For children use only one hand; for babies use only 2 fingers of one hand, compressing 80-100 times/minute.*

After 15 sternal compressions, alternate with 3 to 5 deep lung inflations. Repeat and continue this alternating procedure until it is possible to obtain additional assistance and more definitive care. If two operators are

*Modified from Safar, in Chatton, M. J., et al.: *Handbook of Medical Treatment.* 12th ed. Los Altos, Calif., Lange Medical Publications, 1970.

available, pause after every fifth compression while the partner gives mouth-to-mouth inflation. Check carotid pulse after 1 minute and every 5 minutes thereafter. Resuscitation must be continuous during transportation to the hospital.

As resuscitation efforts continue, the resuscitator must decide whether his attempts to reestablish the patient's circulation are effective. For resuscitation efforts to be judged *effective,* at least *one* of the following signs must be present.

Signs of Effective Resuscitation
1. Constriction of the pupils—key sign *that the brain is sufficiently oxygenated.*
2. Distinct carotid pulsations with each cardiac compression.
3. Blinking upon stimulation of the eyelid.
4. Breathing that begins spontaneously.
5. Movement and struggling.
6. Decreased cyanosis.

Unfortunately, resuscitation does not always succeed in reviving the patient. Factors responsible for *ineffective resuscitation* are listed in the next column:

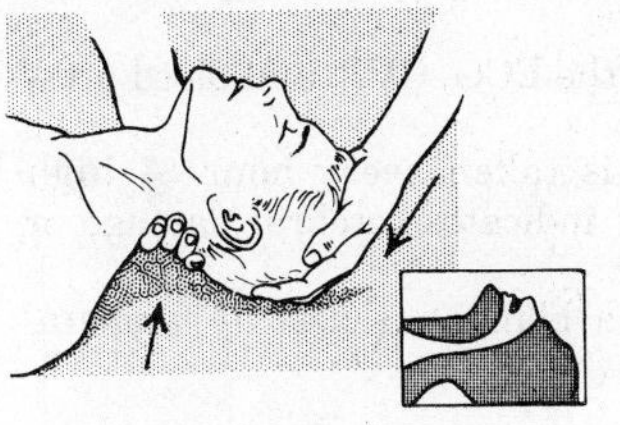

(1)
The operator takes his position at the patient's head.

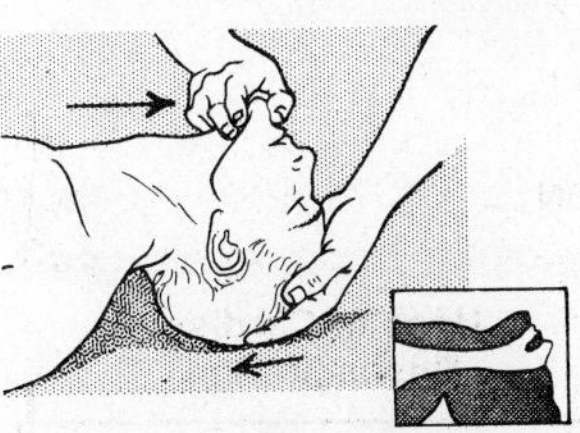

(2)
With the right thumb and index finger he displaces the mandible forward by pressing at its central portion, at the same time lifting the neck and tilting the head as far back as possible.

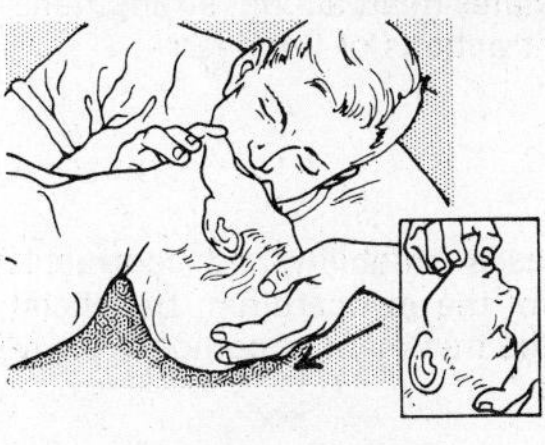

(3)
After taking a deep breath, the operator immediately seals his mouth around the mouth (or nose) of the victim and exhales until the chest of the victim rises.

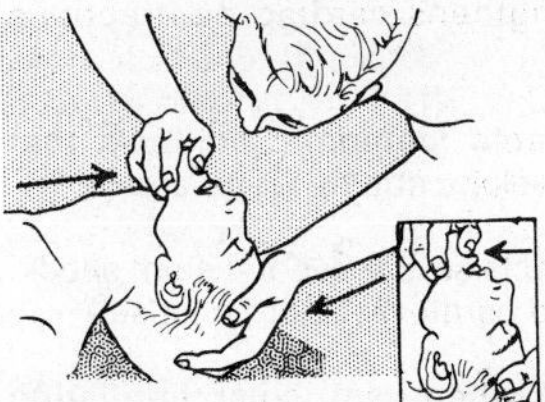

(4)
The victim's mouth is opened by downward and forward traction on the lower jaw or by pulling down the lower lip.

FIGURE 50–10. Technique of mouth-to-mouth resuscitation. (From Chatton, M. J., et al.: *Handbook of Medical Treatment.* 12th ed. Los Altos, Calif., Lange Medical Publishers, 1970.)

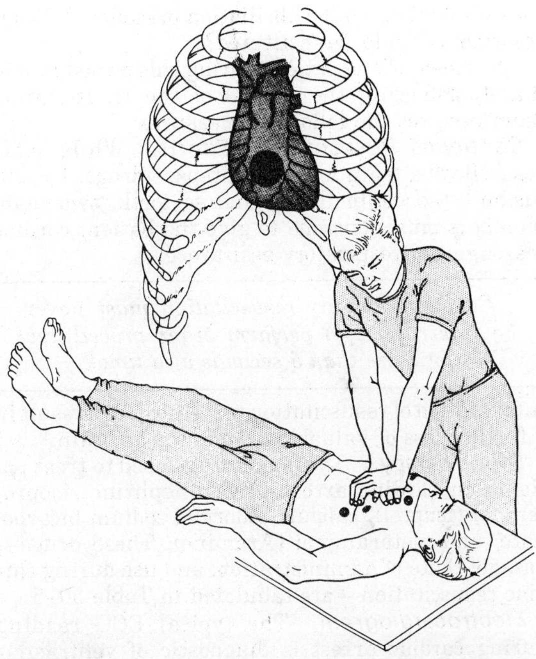

FIGURE 50–11. Technique of closed chest cardiac massage. Heavy circle in heart drawing shows area of application of force. Circles on supine figure show points of application of electrodes for defibrillation. (From Chatton, M. J., et al.: *Handbook of Medical Treatment.* 12th ed. Los Altos, Calif., Lange Medical Publishers, 1970.)

1. Incorrect resuscitative techniques.
2. Heart is drained of its blood by hemorrhage or cardiac tamponade.
3. Blood supply to the heart is obstructed by presence of a pulmonary embolus.
4. Severe chronic lung disease has destroyed lung's capacity to oxygenate blood.
5. Lungs are filled with vomitus as a result of aspiration during cardiac massage.

Ineffective resuscitation is characterized by continuous coma, absence of compression pulsations, and persistence of dilated pupils. Even though resuscitation appears to be ineffective, authorities recommend that the resuscitation effort continue for at least one hour following the initiation of resuscitation procedures.

Specific Medical Therapy

Definitive medical therapy commences once the patient has either been admitted to the emergency room or a special resuscitation team has arrived to take over the patient's care. At this time, three considerations become paramount:[36] (1) What is the underlying cause of the cardiac arrest and can it be corrected? (2) What type of arrest has occurred? Is asystole or ventricular fibrillation present? (3) What treatment should be instituted?

Treatment of the patient during this period immediately following the arrival of the resuscitation team involves the following measures:

Continued Resuscitation Efforts. While some resuscitation team members prepare drugs, I.V. infusions, the defibrillator, and so forth, two team members must continue to give the patient cardiac massage and respiratory assistance.

> *Cardiopulmonary resuscitation must* never *be interrupted to perform other procedures for more than 5 seconds at a time!*

Interruption of resuscitation procedures can result in a further loss of valuable oxygen to the brain.

Drug Therapy. The major drugs used to treat patients in cardiac arrest are epinephrine, isoproterenol (Isuprel), calcium chloride, sodium bicarbonate, and metaraminol (Aramine). These drugs—dosage, route of administration, and use during cardiac resuscitation—are tabulated in Table 50–5.

Electrocardiogram. The typical ECG reading during cardiac arrest is diagnostic of ventricular fibrillation; less commonly a reading will show asystole or a complete lack of wave configurations. However, an ECG may be normal in appearance although the heart is actually pumping very feebly with little cardiac output. Thus, ECG tracings cannot be used to rule out the possibility of cardiac arrest.

> *Remember that ECG tracings show only the electrical activity of the heart; they cannot serve as a guide to the heart's pumping efficiency.*

Precordial Shock. When the patient's heart is in ventricular fibrillation, the doctor uses either a direct current (D.C.) or alternating current (A.C.) defibrillator to shock the heart, thereby halting the chaotic bizarre movement of the ventricles. The defibrillator is not used when the heart is in complete asystole, as defibrillation has no effect on cardiac standstill.

Oxygen. The patient is given 100 per cent oxygen by means of an endotracheal tube in order to fully oxygenate his brain and other vital organs.

Nasal Gastric Intubation. The patient with a full stomach is intubated at once to prevent vomiting and aspiration of vomitus. Even patients with an empty stomach often require intubation, because gastric dilatation may result from mouth-to-mouth and mouth-to-nose resuscitation.

Postresuscitation Measures

Skilled aftercare of the patient who has suffered cardiac arrest is crucial to his survival. Typical orders and their rationale are given below:

1. If the patient is not already in the ICU or CCU he is admitted there because of his need for constant observation, monitoring equipment, defibrillators, and so forth.
2. Monitoring of the ECG, CVP, and blood pressure is instituted.
3. Temperature is taken every hour. A high temperature usually indicates cerebral damage or cerebral edema.
4. A hypothermia blanket is used if tempera-

TABLE 50–5. DRUGS USED IN CARDIAC RESUSCITATION

Drug	Dosage	Route of Administration	Uses in Cardiac Resuscitation
Epinephrine	0.5 mg. (in a solution prepared by diluting 1 mg. (1 ml.) of epinephrine in 9 ml. normal saline 0.5 mg. q. 5 min. as necessary	Administered directly into myocardium with 3½-inch 22-gauge needle I.V.	Stimulates heart action; strengthens contractions of the heart
Isoproterenol (Isuprel)	1-3 mg. in 250-500 ml. 5% dextrose in water	I.V. drip	Increases irritability and contractility of the myocardium; beneficial in the treatment of complete asystole
Calcium chloride 10%	5-10 ml.	I.V.	Strengthens cardiac contractions
Sodium bicarbonate	50 ml. (44.6 mEq. or 3.75 gm.) q. 5 min.	I.V.	Corrects metabolic acidosis that develops due to tissue anoxia
Metaraminol (Aramine)	200 mg. diluted in solution of 500 ml. 5% dextrose in water	I.V. drip	Corrects severe hypotension, shock, and cardiovascular collapse
Lidocaine (Xylocaine) 1% solution	50-150 mg.	I.V. push q. 15 min.	Used when ventricular fibrillation continues despite countershock measures

ture is over 101°. Hypothermia helps to lessen cerebral edema.

5. Blood gas and pH determinations are done to detect metabolic acidosis, which may have developed owing to poor tissue oxygenation during arrest.

6. Amobarbital sodium is given intravenously in case of convulsions, which may occur because of brain damage or acidosis. Dilantin is given if convulsions continue.

7. A chest X-ray is taken using portable equipment. Ribs often are accidentally fractured during cardiac massage.

8. Insert endotracheal tube if not already in place. This maintains an open airway for the unconscious patient who cannot clear his secretions by coughing. If patient is breathing satisfactorily, but remains unresponsive, leave tube in place for 48 hours. If he does not respond after 48 hours and if respirations are depressed, notify the physician and set up for a tracheostomy; have a volume respirator at the bedside.

9. Give oxygen continuously for 48 hours following resuscitation, by endotracheal tube, tent, or mask. This is required because respirations are depressed for some time after arrest.

10. Insert Foley catheter. Urine output is one measure of cardiovascular status. A very low urine output after cardiac arrest indicates cardiovascular collapse. Notify the physician if the urinary output is below 30 ml. per hour.

Complications

The patient may develop complications due to the cardiac arrest itself or as a result of the resuscitation measures used to save his life. Common complications are the following:

> *Pneumothorax* as a result of ribs fractured during cardiac massage.

> *Hemorrhage* from a ruptured liver or spleen due to faulty resuscitation techniques. Damage to liver and spleen can occur if the resuscitator applies pressure over the epigastrum rather than over the sternum.

> *Brain damage* as a result of cerebral hypoxia.

> *Seizures* due to either brain damage or metabolic acidosis.

CHAPTER 51

Coronary Heart Disease

For the heart muscle to contract properly, it must have an adequate blood supply. You will recall from Chapter 46 that the myocardium receives its blood supply from the coronary arteries. Should one or both of these arteries be blocked for any reason or should collateral circulation fail to develop, ischemia and infarction of the heart muscle are inevitable. The *major disorders* resulting from an insufficient blood supply to the myocardium are arteriosclerotic heart disease, angina pectoris, coronary insufficiency, and myocardial infarction; all these entities are grouped under the term *coronary heart disease* (CHD), also known as coronary artery disease and ischemic heart disease.

Blockage of blood to the myocardium may be partial and temporary (e.g., angina pectoris) or complete and protracted (e.g., myocardial infarction).

OVERVIEW OF CORONARY HEART DISEASE

INCIDENCE OF CHD

> *Coronary heart disease ranks* first *as a cause of death among persons in North America and Western Europe.*

Over half a million people die every year of CHD and its complications. Death rates due to CHD are influenced by the age, sex, and race of the patient and the social and economic environment in which he lives. Let us now briefly consider each of these points.

Age. Pathologic changes within the coronary arteries, which are severe enough to cause symptoms, appear predominantly in persons over 40. However, individuals in their 30's and even 20's have been known to suffer anginal attacks or myocardial infarction.

Sex. As a group, men are *four* times as likely to suffer from CHD as are women.[30] However, this marked difference in susceptibility to CHD between the sexes tends to even out among the older age groups. For example, men below the age of 40 are eight times as likely to be stricken with CHD as are young women; however, by the age of 70, just as many women are diagnosed with CHD as are men.

Race. White males die more frequently from CHD than do nonwhites.[30] On the other hand, the rate of deaths among white females is generally a little lower than among nonwhite females. However, among elderly women death rates tend to be about the same for both whites and nonwhites.

Environment. CHD is seven times more prevalent in North America, Australia, Europe, and New Zealand than in Japan, Africa, and South America.[30] Also, incidence is higher among urban populations than among those in rural areas.

CAUSATIVE AND PRECIPITATING FACTORS

The major cause of CHD is the development of *obliterative atherosclerotic* lesions within the coronary arteries, which act to narrow or obstruct these vital vessels.

> Atherosclerosis, *a disorder of lipid metabolism (characterized by deposits of fat-containing substances along the intima of blood vessels), is "the commonest underlying cause of cardiovascular disease and death."*[20]

In fact, 99 per cent of all cases are caused by narrowing of the coronary arteries due to atherosclerotic changes. Other rare causes of CHD are: (1) congenital abnormalities of the arteries; (2) luetic changes in the arteries due to earlier syphilitic infection; (3) vascular changes due to autoimmune disorders; and (4) coronary embolism.

Predisposing factors which apparently precipitate the onset of CHD are many and varied. The most significant factors are the following:[47]

1. *Personal factors*

   a. *Genetic predisposition:* Frequently members of the patient's family have suffered from CHD at an early age.

   b. Certain *personality traits:* Hard driving, competitive individuals who worry excessively about deadlines and who consistently overwork are *possibly* more prone to coronary disease.

   c. *Professional stresses:* Doctors and executives seem to be more readily stricken with CHD than persons with occupations imposing less responsibility.

2. *Disease patterns*

   a. *Hypertension:* Sustained BP of over 160/95 mm. Hg.

   b. *Obesity:* Weight 30 or more per cent above that considered standard for an individual of a certain height and build.

c. *Lipid abnormalities:* Serum cholesterol of over 200 mg. per 100 ml., or a fasting triglyceride of more than 250 mg. per 100 ml.

d. *Diabetes:* Fasting blood sugar of more than 120 mg. per 100 ml., or a routine blood sugar of 180 mg. per 100 ml.; evidence of sugar in the urine, decreased glucose tolerance.

e. *Gout:* Uric acid level elevated over 7.5 mg. per 100 ml.; past history of gout.

f. *ECG abnormalities:* e.g., left ventricular hypertrophy, intraventricular block, unexplained atrial fibrillation, myocardial infarction.

3. *Adverse environmental problems*

a. *Heavy cigarette smoking:* Evidently large amounts of nicotine absorbed into the blood stream may severely damage blood elements or the intima of arteries.

b. *Sedentary occupation and life style:* Lack of exercise tends to promote mental depression and obesity.

c. *Stressful situations:* Emotional problems tend to indirectly promote compensatory overeating and excessive drinking and smoking. Also, nervous tension elevates blood pressure. However, to what extent emotional stress may *directly* cause CHD is still not known, and all theories are highly speculative.

d. *High-caloric, high-fat diet:* Overeating and consuming fatty rich foods promotes obesity, lipid abnormalities, and diabetes.

PREVENTION AND GENERAL TREATMENT OF CHD

The prevention of CHD at this time rests on the recognition, control, and prevention of the high risk factors just listed. A typical prevention and treatment program includes the following factors:

Weight Reduction. This is achieved by means of a low-caloric diet. Instruct the patient to reduce *gradually*. Rapid weight loss can suddenly overload the blood with an excess of fatty substances which can, in turn, precipitate an anginal attack or a myocardial infarction.

Modified Low-cholesterol Diet. To reduce elevated serum lipid levels, patients generally restrict their intake of saturated fat, cholesterol, and simple sugars, and substitute *polyunsaturated* fats for saturated fat whenever possible. It is important to remember, however, that the role of diet in the pathogenosis of CHD is still a highly controversial subject.

Avoid Stress. Avoidance of situations that can precipitate anginal attacks is imperative; patients should avoid large heavy meals, intense emotional states, unusual strenuous exercise, and excessively hot or cold environments.

Correction of Preexisting Medical Problems. Treat problems that might contribute to the development of CHD (e.g., hypertension,, anemia, hyperthyroidism, aortic valvular disease).

Physical Examination. Yearly physical examinations and additional examinations are given as necessary; persons with recurrent indigestion, "heartburn," chest pain, and pain above the waistline that is associated with activity or emotional stress should see their physician.

Drug and Hormonal Therapy. *Anticoagulants* are used to treat and to prevent thrombosis. *Heparin* and *estrogens* have beneficial effects upon blood lipoproteins; however, these drugs have dangerous side effects. Heparin can cause bleeding, hematoma at the injection site, and dangerous allergic reactions. Estrogens can cause menorrhagia, breast soreness, and edema. *Nicotinic acid* given orally in large doses (3 to 6 Gm. daily in divided doses) substantially reduces serum cholesterol level. Side effects are gastrointestinal irritation, nausea, vomiting and diarrhea. *Thyroid* extract also lowers serum cholesterol but produces many undesirable side effects, e.g., nervousness, insomnia, palpitations.

Surgical Techniques. The goals of surgery in managing patients with CHD are to: relieve pain, reduce the heart's workload, and supply the heart muscle with sufficient blood to carry on its tasks. Today surgeons seek to control CHD principally by employing procedures that bring more blood to the heart. Four major methods are currently used: (1) *aortocoronary artery bypass* with an autograft of saphenous vein, which is the most common direct vascular reconstructive technique used today; (2) *thromboendartectomy,* during which the surgeon removes or cores out the obstructing material within the coronary blood vessels, thereby providing a larger lumen; (3) *resection* of the diseased portion of the coronary artery followed by anastomoses of the two normal ends; (4) *internal mammary artery implantation,* in which the surgeon implants an actively bleeding internal mammary artery into the left ventricular myocardium, thereby supplying the heart with blood from a source other than the coronary arteries; and (5) *cardiopericardiopexy,* in which the surgeon introduces sterile talcum powder into the pericardial sac, which results in an inflammatory process. The sterile pericarditis produced leads to the development of anastomotic intercoronary vessels and a better blood supply to the heart (this procedure is rarely performed anymore).

FORMS OF CHD

The major forms of CHD are: (1) arteriosclerotic heart disease (ASHD), also known as obliterative atherosclerotic heart disease; (2) angina pectoris; (3) coronary insufficiency; and (4) myocardial infarction (MI).

There is some disagreement among authorities concerning the classification of these disorders. Some authorities group angina pectoris, coronary insufficiency, and MI under ASHD. Others consider ASHD to be a specific type of CHD which differs in its manifestations from the other conditions listed. However, all authorities agree that there is much overlap between these disorders. Thus, some view ASHD, angina pectoris, coronary insufficiency, and MI as *stages* within a common, continuous disease process; this is the viewpoint which we assume in this unit.

ARTERIOSCLEROTIC HEART DISEASE (ASHD)

DEFINITION AND GENERAL DESCRIPTION

Arteriosclerotic heart disease (ASHD)* is a slowly progressive heart condition characterized by: (1) internal thickening and plaque formation within the coronary arteries due to the deposition of fatty substances along the intima; (2) resultant fibrosis, calcification, and narrowing of the coronary arteries; and (3) a slow constriction of the blood supply to the myocardium, which can finally give rise to symptoms of angina.

Atherosclerotic changes within the coronary vessels as well as within the aorta and cerebral vessels generally occur in the following three stages:

Stage 1: Fatty Streak Formation. Fatty streaks, which are thin, slightly elevated, smooth, yellow lines or dots, first appear during childhood. In some cases, these streaks regress completely.

Stage 2: Fibrous Plaque Formation. The development of fibrous plaques reflects both a low-grade inflammatory reaction and a healing response. When this stage is reached, there is likelihood of further progression of the disease.

Stage 3: Stage of Complication. This stage involves necrosis, calcification, and vascularization of the plaque, with or without hemorrhage into the plaque. Such changes predispose to thrombosis.

ASHD is the *most common clinical form of CHD.* Predisposing factors leading to ASHD are the same as those related to CHD.

THEORIES OF CAUSATION

Although it is a great killer and crippler of man, the exact cause of atherosclerosis is unfortunately unknown. More questions have been posed than answers given, and conflicting etiologic theories are constantly argued. The most pertinent questions troubling medical researchers are these:[64]

1. Is atherosclerosis an integral, uncontrollable part of the aging process? Or is atherosclerosis a pathologic condition resulting from disease-producing factors that are subject to human control?
2. Are the atherosclerotic changes within the major blood vessels the result of primary abnormalities of the vessels themselves? Or do the atherosclerotic changes in the vessel walls develop secondary to a primary metabolic abnormality that is present elsewhere in the body?

In an attempt to answer these questions several theories have evolved—the aging theory, the metabolic theory, the stress theory, the hormonal theory, and the multifactoral theory.

According to the *aging theory,* the development of atherosclerotic changes within the arteries is a normal part of aging, which affects *all* persons to a greater or lesser degree. Some authorities believe that atherosclerotic changes begin even in the very young, and that these changes almost universally affect persons over 20. Objections to the aging theory are based mainly on findings at autopsy; some elderly persons show no signs of atherosclerotic changes at autopsy, whereas young persons may show severe atherosclerotic changes.

Advocates of the *metabolic* theory state that atherosclerosis is the result of disturbances in *lipid metabolism*—in particular, cholesterol metabolism. Large numbers of research projects and studies have focused upon the role of cholesterol in the causation of atherosclerosis. Evidence for the metabolic theory is as follows:

1. Laboratory analysis of atherosclerotic lesions reveals the presence of large amounts of lipids, especially cholesterol esters and free cholesterol.
2. Numerous population studies conducted throughout the world show a correlation between *elevated serum cholesterol levels* and the development of CHD.[118]* For example, advocates of the metabolic theory point out that serum cholesterol levels are as high as 200 to 250 mg. per 100 ml. in the United States where the disease is common, whereas serum cholesterol levels are as low as 100 to 150 mg. per 100 ml. in Japan and Korea where the disease is uncommon.
3. Other comparative population studies reveal a correlation between a *high intake of animal fats* and the development of atherosclerosis. For example, deaths from CHD were statistically lower during World War II when fatty foods were scarce than during postwar years. With the postwar improvement in the economy, both the consumption of animal fat and the death rate from atherosclerosis rose. Another study comparing Japanese populations living in Japan, Hawaii, and Los Angeles revealed that CHD is relatively low among Japanese living in Japan, and moderately high among the Japanese in Hawaii; Japanese living in Los Angeles (Nisei) had rates comparable to those of the Caucasian population.

Other observers believe that the high incidence of atherosclerosis among persons in the United States, Denmark, and other highly technological countries is due to the economic and social *stresses* that are so abundant in Western civilization. Supporters of this theory point out that ASHD occurs far less frequently among more primitive peoples. However, advocates of the "stress theory" cannot explain precisely how life stresses cause athero-

*ASHD is one type of obliterative atherosclerosis. Obliterative atherosclerosis occurs not only in the heart, but also affects the aorta and the larger arteries of the brain. In this unit, obliterative atherosclerosis is discussed only in relation to heart disease.

*In reviewing these and other population studies, it is important to remember that the statistical data upon which the research is based are often inconclusive or unreliable.

sclerotic changes within the major arteries. One authority points out that anxiety and stress may well increase the needs of the heart for blood over and above the normal demands; however, it is unlikely that stress could cause hemorrhage into an atheroma or rupture of a plaque.[136]

Others point to *endocrine factors*—in particular, the *estrogens*—as a possible explanation for the onset and progress of atherosclerosis. The theory that sex hormones play an important role in the development of atherosclerosis rests upon the following evidence:

1. Atherosclerosis is prevalent among males, whereas females *prior* to the menopause are relatively immune to the process.
2. Young females (prior to the menopause) have a lower serum level of certain types of lipoprotein than do young males.
3. Serum levels of lipoprotein tend to equalize between the sexes during the years following the females' menopause; also, during the middle and late periods of life, atherosclerosis is equally prevalent among members of both sexes.

On the basis of these facts, some authorities conclude that the estrogenic hormones affect the release and distribution of plasma lipoproteins, which, in turn, influence the time of onset of atherosclerosis in each sex.

Finally, the *multifactoral theory* of atherosclerosis has many supporters. One authority states:

> It is more probable that atherosclerosis is a disease of multifactoral etiology in which inborn or genetic factors and environmental factors are concerned in varying degree in different persons.[64]

Genetic factors are particularly important in families with a history of diabetes or familial hypercholesterolemia. Outstanding environmental factors contributing to the development of atherosclerosis are diet, chain smoking, emotional stress, and a lack of physical exercise.

CLINICAL COURSE OF ATHEROSCLEROSIS

Atherosclerosis, by itself, does not necessarily produce symptoms. For symptoms to develop, there must be *critical deficit* in blood supply to the heart in proportion to the demands of the myocardium for oxygen and nutrients. When atherosclerosis progresses slowly, the collateral circulation that develops can generally meet the heart's demands under normal conditions. Thus, whether or not symptoms of ASHD develop depends upon the *total* blood supply to the myocardium (by way of coronary arteries *and* collateral circulation) and not just upon the condition of the coronary arteries alone.

Because the extent of collateral circulation varies from person to person, the development and progress of atherosclerosis follow one of the following courses:

1. *Unrecognized ASHD:* The individual suffers no symptoms during his life time; atherosclerotic changes are found at autopsy.
2. *Asymptomatic ASHD:* The arteries undergo extensive pathologic changes, but the patient remains symptom free as a result of establishment of good collateral circulation.
3. *Clinical ASHD:* Signs of heart disease are present. Cardiac manifestations of obliterative atherosclerosis include episodes of chest pain, myocardial infarction, congestive heart failure, heart block, gastrointestinal tract symptoms, and sudden death.

DIAGNOSIS

ASHD is diagnosed by the following methods:

1. A *history* of attacks of anginal pain.
2. *Coronary arteriography* helps to demonstrate the presence of calcification within the coronary arteries, and the degree to which the arteries are obstructed.
3. *ECG tracings* are examined for evidence of past myocardial infarction and the presence of T waves and Q waves.
4. *Laboratory tests* for total blood cholesterol. Hypercholesterolemia or a total blood cholesterol of more than 250 mg./100 ml. suggests the presence of atherosclerosis.

CLINICAL CARE

Clinical care of the patient with ASHD generally centers around prevention and treatment of the specific manifestations of the particular disease process, e.g., angina pectoris, MI, CHF. General treatment and prevention of ASHD is the same as that for CHD. The specific treatment for angina pectoris and MI is discussed in the next sections.

ANGINA PECTORIS

DEFINITION

Angina pectoris, which is also known as "cardiac pain of effort and emotion," is a clinical entity characterized by transient paroxysmal attacks of substernal or precordial pain that may radiate to the left shoulder and down the inner side of the left arm. (Other patterns of pain radiation also may occur with angina pectoris.)

The word "angina" is derived from a Greek word meaning "strangling," while the word "pectoris" refers to the breast or breast bone.

The pain of angina is precipitated by exertion, emotion, and exposure to cold, and is relieved by rest and the use of nitroglycerin tablets. *Unlike acute MI, the anginal pain is temporary, and myocardial tissues are not permanently damaged.*

CAUSATIVE FACTORS AND UNDERLYING PATHOLOGY

Angina pectoris is a temporary state of myocardial hypoxia, the exact cause of which is still obscure. However, each of the variables listed below can result in myocardial ischemia and anginal pain.[20]

1. *Decrease in myocardium's oxygen supply* (delivered by the coronary arteries)
   a. *Vessel factors:*
      (1) *Atherosclerosis,* narrowing the lumen of coronary vessels, is the most common cause of anginal attacks.
      (2) *Arterial spasm* and *reflexive narrowing* of coronary vessels, resulting from cold, emotional stress, and smoking.
      (3) *Coronary arteritis,* or inflammation of the coronary arteries, due to infections, autoimmune disease, and so forth.
   b. *Circulatory factors:*
      (1) *Hypotension* due to spinal anesthesia, potent antihypertensive drugs, blood loss, and so forth, resulting in decreased blood return to myocardium.
      (2) *Aortic stenosis* or *aortic insufficiency,* due to congenital anomalies or infectious processes, resulting in decreased filling pressure of the coronary arteries.
   c. *Blood factors:*
      (1) *Anemia* and *hypoxemia,* resulting in decreased oxygen flow to myocardium.
      (2) *Polycythemia,* causing increased blood viscosity, which slows blood flow through the coronary arteries.
2. *Increase in cardiac output*
   a. *Physiologic factors:* Exercise, emotion, digestion of a large meal.
   b. *Pathologic factors:* Anemia, hyperthyroidism.
3. *Increased myocardial need for oxygen*
   a. *Damaged* myocardium unable to properly utilize oxygen.
   b. *Hypertrophied* myocardium that has "outgrown" its normal blood supply and requires added supplies of oxygen.
   c. *Aortic stenosis* or *insufficiency* and *diastolic hypertension,* causing heart to work harder.
   d. *Thyrotoxicosis,* increasing oxygen consumption.
   e. Strong *emotion* and heavy *exertion,* increasing heart's and body's need for oxygen.

Atherosclerosis is by far the most common cause of angina pectoris. As you recall, if atherosclerosis develops gradually, collateral circulation is usually established. However, while collateral circulation can supply the heart muscle with *just* enough blood to meet normal circulatory requirements, it is generally unable to oxygenate the myocardium when the body is undergoing excessive stress, e.g., heavy exercise, running up a flight of stairs, walking against the wind, great emotional excitement, and after ingestion of a heavy meal. It is at these critical moments that the pain of angina strikes, generally forcing the individual to stop his activities and rest.

DIAGNOSIS

Angina pectoris is diagnosed on the basis of the following:

Patient's History

The key to the proper diagnosis of angina is a complete, detailed history of the patient's attacks, which the patient is encouraged to describe in his own words. Typically the patient describes his attacks as usually following exertion, emotion, or a heavy meal.

The *pain* of angina, the most important aspect of the history, usually has the following characteristics:

Sensation. Squeezing, burning, pressing, choking, aching, bursting. The patient often says the pain feels like "gas" or "heartburn" or "indigestion." Pain is never described as sharp or knifelike.

Location. In 80 to 90 per cent of patients the pain is experienced as retrosternal or slightly to the left of the sternum.

Radiation. Usually the pain radiates to the left shoulder and upper arm; it may then travel down the inner aspect of the left arm to the elbow, wrist, and fourth and fifth fingers. Less commonly, the pain may radiate to the right shoulder. The patient rarely experiences the pain as localized to any one single small area over the precordium.

Duration. Anginal attacks are usually of *short* duration, lasting less than three minutes. However, attacks precipitated by a heavy meal or extreme anger may last from 15 to 20 minutes.

Relief. Most anginal attacks quickly subside with the administration of nitroglycerin and with rest.

The typical "exertion—pain—rest—relief" symptom pattern is the major clue to the diagnosis of angina pectoris. Other symptoms accompanying the pain of angina are dyspnea, pallor, sweating, faintness, palpitations, dizziness, and digestive disturbances.

Physical Examination

Twenty-five to 40 per cent of patients with angina pectoris have no signs of cardiac pathology. Thus, the physical examination is rarely diagnostic.

ECG Findings and Angiocardiography

The electrocardiogram tracings are normal in 25 to 30 per cent of patients with angina pectoris. However, 70 per cent of patients with angina have ECG abnormalities following mild exercise.

Selective

X-rays of the coronary arteries may reveal atherosclerotic changes and evidence of CHD.

Nitroglycerin Test

The diagnosis of angina pectoris is fairly certain if glyceryl trinitrate (nitroglycerin), 0.4 mg. or 1/150 gr., invariably shortens an attack of anginal type pain or increases tolerance to exercise.

CLINICAL CARE

The care of patients with angina pectoris centers around two goals: relief of acute attacks, and prevention of further anginal attacks.

Relief of Acute Attacks

To relieve the severe pain of angina, the patient is instructed to do the following:

1. Stop all activity and sit down or lie down as soon as the attack begins, remaining quiet until the pain subsides. Patients must be warned against trying to "heroically" continue on with their normal activities in spite of the pain.

2. Take either glyceryl trinitrate (nitroglycerin) or amyl nitrite as soon as the pain begins.

Nitroglycerin has been the drug of choice against anginal attacks since 1867, and today is still the physician's major weapon against acute attacks. Administered sublingually, nitroglycerin acts to relieve the pain of angina within 1 or 2 minutes by producing dilatation of the coronary blood vessels. The usual dose is 0.3 mg. (1/200 gr.). If this dosage proves ineffective, the physician may then increase the dosage to 0.4 to 0.6 mg. (1/150 to 1/100 gr.) Side effects of nitroglycerin include headache, hypotension, dizziness, and flushing. Patients taking nitroglycerin need the following special instructions to receive full benefit from the drug:

a. Carry nitroglycerin tablets at all times. Family should know where the supply is kept at home.

b. Place one tablet under the tongue at the first indication of an attack and allow the tablet to dissolve completely. Retain saliva briefly before swallowing. If possible, lie down for a while after using the drug.

c. Always have "fresh" nitroglycerin tablets, as they lose their potency after six months. The patient will experience a burning sensation on his tongue and a full, throbbing sensation in his head if the tablets have full potency.

d. Repeat the drug dosage every 5 to 10 minutes until relief is obtained. The patient should know that the drug is not habit forming and that he cannot take an overdose.

e. Warn the patient that he will experience side effects such as headache and flushing. Tell him that the discomfort from side effects tends to lessen as tolerance develops.

Amyl nitrite is given in the form of pearls or ampules which are crushed or broken into handkerchief and inhaled. Dosage is usually 0.2 mg. Amyl nitrite is a potent drug that gives prompt relief from attacks. Side effects include flushing of the face, pounding pulse, dizziness, and headache. However, unlike nitroglycerin, this drug must not be taken repeatedly because it produces syncope.

3. A small amount of *whisky* or *brandy* (30 to 60 ml.) acts to promote the dilatation of blood vessels and general relaxation.

Prevention of Attacks

Measures that may be helpful in the prevention of attacks are outlined below:

Control of Precipitating Conditions and High Risk Factors

1. Anxious, nervous persons are often referred for psychiatric help. Also, they may be given mild, tranquilizing drugs.

2. Overweight patients are urged to reduce. All patients are encouraged to: eat small meals, avoid high-caloric and high-cholesterol diets, abstain from gas-forming foods, and rest for short periods following meals.

3. A regular program of daily exercise is planned for most patients in order to promote improved coronary circulation.

4. The patient who leads an active hectic life must learn to adjust his activities to a level below that which precipitates anginal attacks. Brief rest periods throughout the working day, an early bedtime, and longer vacations are "musts."

5. The physician tries to protect the patient from further anginal attacks by correcting any coexisting medical or cardiovascular problems, e.g., hyperthyroidism, hypertension, congestive heart failure. The doctor may prescribe digitalis and diuretics to lessen the workload of the heart.

Drug Therapy

1. *Nitroglycerin,* 0.4 to 0.6 mg. (1/150 to 1/100 gr.), may be used freely to prevent attacks. Patients must be taught to place a nitroglycerin tablet under their tongues *prior* to: exercising, eating a large meal, engaging in emotionally stressful situations, or having sexual intercourse.

2. *Long-acting nitrites* act to maintain *coronary artery vasodilatation,* thereby promoting a greater flow of blood and oxygen to heart muscle. Important long-acting nitrites are pentaerythritol tetranitrate (Peritrate), erythrityl tetranitrate (Cardilate), isosorbide dinitrate (Isordil) and trolnitrate phosphate (Metamine). Long-acting nitrites produce the same general side effects as nitroglycerin and amyl nitrate, i.e., severe headache, flushing of the skin, nausea and vomiting, hypotension, vertigo, and syncope. Recommended dosage, route of administration, onset and duration of action and general comments are listed in Table 51–1.

Although long-acting nitrites are helpful in preventing anginal attacks, they are disappointing in that many patients develop tolerance to them within a few weeks. Once tolerance has developed, patients must resort again to the use of nitroglycerin sublingually. Regularly and carefully question all patients receiving long-acting nitrites concerning the degree of relief that they are receiving from the drug. Remember that tolerance develops rapidly.

3. *Propranolol (Inderal),* a beta adrenergic blocking agent, is given orally in dosages of 10 to 30 mg. t.i.d. to decrease the number of anginal attacks and the consumption of nitroglycerin. Inderal acts by reducing the oxygen requirements of the myocardium. This, in turn, increases the exercise tolerance of patients with reduced coronary blood flow. However, because Inderal interferes with the pumping action of the heart, use extreme caution when administering this drug to persons with any degree of heart failure. Side effects of Inderal are usually transient and include nausea, vomiting, mental depression, and mild diarrhea.

4. *Sedatives, tranquilizers,* and *antidepressants* may lessen the frequency and severity of attacks. Commonly used tranquilizing drugs are phenobarbital, amobarbital, meprobamate, and diazepam. Drugs helpful against depression are methylphenidate and amitriptyline.

5. *Drugs* that *lower serum cholesterol* levels are sometimes ordered. Heparin, estrogen, and nicotinic acid were discussed earlier.

6. *Radioactive iodine* (^{131}I) is occasionally given to patients who have been refractory to treatment for three months, in order to decrease the activity of the thyroid gland. The resultant hypothyroidism produced by ^{131}I slows the patient's metabolism and lowers the workload of his heart. However, the side effects (induced hypothyroidism or myxedema) are so unpleasant that this method of treatment is employed only as a last resort.

Surgical Techniques. Surgical procedures, discussed earlier, are sometimes employed in angina pectoris to increase coronary blood flow. Some heart surgeons are using coronary angiography to more precisely locate lesions and points of narrowing within the coronary arteries preoperatively, which, in turn, enables them to perform more precise corrective surgery. Nevertheless, at present, surgical methods only ease the patient's symptoms; surgery as yet cannot halt the process of atherosclerosis, repair a hypertrophied or damaged myocardium, or prolong the patient's life better than chemotherapy.

In summary, there is to date no cure for the syndrome of angina pectoris. Nitroglycerin remains the drug of choice for alleviating the pain of angina and preventing further anginal attacks. Long-acting nitrites, propranolol, ^{131}I-induced hypothyroidism, and surgery are all useful methods for reducing anginal attacks, but they remain controversial. Selective coronary angiography may enable physicians to diagnose angina pectoris more accurately, thereby making treatment more precise.

PROGNOSIS

The prognosis for angina pectoris depends upon the underlying disorder, the amount of collateral circulation, and the patient's ability to control those personal and environmental factors that precipitate his attacks. The course of this disorder is generally prolonged. Attacks, which are typically interrupted by periods of remission, tend to become more severe and increasingly frequent. Patients usually survive from 5 to 10 years following the initial attack. One half of all sufferers from angina pectoris die suddenly; one third die following acute myocardial infarction.

TABLE 51–1. LONG-ACTING NITRITES

Drug	Dosage	Route of Administration	Action: *Onset*	Action: *Duration*	Comments
Pentaerythritol tetranitrate (Peritrate)	10 mg. t.i.d.	Oral	1 hr.	3–4 hr.	Tolerance develops rapidly if given regularly
Erythritol tetranitrate (Cardilate)	5–30 mg. t.i.d.	Oral or sublingual	5–10 min.	2–4 hr.	
Isosorbide dinitrate (Isordil)	5–30 mg. q.i.d. 5–10 mg. q.i.d.	Oral Sublingual	30 min. 2–3 min.	3–4 hr. 1½–4 hr.	Action may be hastened by chewing tablets
Trolnitrate phosphate (Metamine)	2–10 mg. q.i.d.	Oral	10 min.	Up to one week	Widely used as a prophylactic agent
Nitroglycerin ointment (Nitrol)	½ inch squeezed from tube, increasing to one inch	Applied to skin		3–4 hr.	May cause skin rash

ACUTE MYOCARDIAL INFARCTION (MI)

DEFINITION AND GENERAL DESCRIPTION

Acute myocardial infarction (MI), also known as coronary occlusion or just "a coronary," is a life-threatening condition characterized by the formation of localized *necrotic areas within the myocardium.* MI usually follows the sudden occlusion of a coronary artery and the abrupt cessation of blood and oxygen flow to the heart muscle.

Because heart muscle must function continuously, blockage of blood to the muscle and the development of necrotic areas within the myocardium represents a catastrophic blow to the body which may claim the patient's life. Indeed, even if the patient survives the initial attack, he is faced with a host of deadly complications, and with the dreaded but real possibility of suffering a second or third heart attack—attacks which may finally prove fatal.

Observation of a patient suffering from an acute MI leaves an unforgettable impression. The patient, sensing strongly that death is impending, is almost always frightened, in shock, and in extreme pain. Even if he lives, fear and the remembrance of the pain remain with the patient long after he recovers and begins the difficult struggle to reconstruct his life.

INCIDENCE AND PREDISPOSING FACTORS

Myocardial infarction is the leading cause of death in North America, Australia, Europe, and New Zealand. In the United States, 15 to 20 per cent of Caucasians die from "coronaries;" the figure is somewhat lower among blacks.

Predisposing factors for myocardial infarction are the same as for all forms of CHD.

ETIOLOGIC AND PATHOLOGIC FACTORS

The most common cause of myocardial infarction is complete or nearly complete occlusion of a coronary vessel by thrombus formation. Other less common causes are:

1. Hemorrhage of an atheromatous plaque, which initiates thrombosis or completes a partial thrombotic occlusion.
2. *Hypertrophy* of the heart muscle, causing the myocardium to outgrow its blood supply. Myocardial hypertrophy results from congestive heart failure and hypertension.
3. *Embolism* to a coronary artery.
4. *Gradual sclerotic occlusion* of a vessel without thrombosis.
5. Temporary *reduction in blood flow* to the coronary arteries resulting from postoperative or traumatic shock, gastrointestinal bleeding, severe dehydration, and hypotension from any cause.

> *When a coronary artery is suddenly blocked and blood and oxygen can no longer reach the heart muscle, the myocardial tissue supplied by that artery dies and becomes necrotic.*

Morphologic changes following an infarction include the following:[136]

1. First 12 hours. Heart tissue appears normal upon gross examination.
2. 18–24 hours. Infarcted area looks anemic and gray-brown in contrast to normal red-brown color of myocardium.
3. 2nd to 4th day. Necrotic area becomes sharply defined.
4. 4th to 10th day. Necrotic area very apparent. Central tissue soft and may contain areas of hemorrhage.
5. 10th day. Necrotic tissue beginning to be replaced by ingrowth of gray, fibrous, vascularized scar tissue.
6. 10th day to 6th week. Scar tissue continues to advance and replace necrotic tissue.

The most common site for myocardial infarction is the *anterior wall of the left ventricle* near the apex. Infarction of the anterior left ventricles results from thrombosis of the descending branch of the left coronary artery. The second most common site for a myocardial infarction is the *posterior wall of the left ventricle* near the base and behind the posterior cusp of the mitral valve. Infarction of the posterior left ventricle results from occlusion of the right coronary artery or circumflex branch of the left coronary artery.

The right ventricle and the atria are affected only 5 per cent of the time; the left ventricle is almost always affected because it carries a far heavier workload.

SYMPTOMS

The major symptoms of an MI vary, depending upon whether pain, shock, or pulmonary edema dominates the clinical picture. Typical symptoms and their causation are listed on the following page.

To understand more fully how an individual experiences pain and discomfort during an acute MI, pause to perform this brief experiment. Grasp firmly your lower left arm with your right hand. Tighten your grip to occlude circulation to your lower arm and hand and then pump your left hand. Continue this pumping action (while occluding the circulation) and you will feel an increasing sense of tension and painful discomfort. Magnify this feeling in your thoughts *many* times and imagine that it is occurring like a band around your chest and down your arm. These feelings are similar to those experienced during acute MI.

DIAGNOSIS

The diagnosis of acute myocardial infarction is based upon the following findings:

1. Typical *pain* of infarction—an intense crushing, substernal, anterior chest pain of longer duration than anginal pain and not relieved by nitroglycerin.
2. Development of profound *hypotension* and *shock.*
3. *Typical ECG findings* including abnormal Q waves and elevation of the S-T segment and T wave. Later, T waves become symmetrically inverted.
4. *Laboratory* findings include:* *leukocytosis* of 10 to 20 thousand cells/cu. mm. appearing on the second day following MI and disappearing in one week; *elevated sedimentation rate; elevated SGOT:* serum levels rise within 6 to 12 hours following infarction, reach a peak in 24 to 48 hours, and decrease to normal in 3 to 5 days; and *elevated LDH:* serum levels may remain elevated for from 5 to 7 days.

*Laboratory findings have been discussed in Chapter 48.

PROGNOSIS

Seventy to 80 per cent of patients survive the initial attack. Chances for patient survival are greatly diminished by the presence of the following:

> Old age.
> Evidence of other cardiovascular diseases, respiratory diseases, or uncontrolled diabetes mellitus.
> History of previous infarcts.
> Occlusion by a large thrombus.
> Sudden rapid occlusion.

The danger of death from myocardial infarction is greatest during the first two weeks, but is particularly severe during the first 24 to 48 hours.

Deaths generally result from the following complications:

> Severe arrhythmias—in particular, ventricular fibrillation (which causes 40 to 50 per cent of deaths following acute MI).
> Shock due to severe myocardial damage (9 per cent of deaths).
> Congestive heart failure (40 per cent of deaths).
> Rupture of the heart (5 to 10 per cent of deaths).
> Recurrent myocardial infarction (5 per cent of deaths).

Patients fortunate enough to avoid the development of complications following MI still require a period of from 6 to 12 weeks for complete recovery. Unfortunately, however, 50 per cent of those individuals who do completely recover from their first

Symptom	*Basis of Symptoms*
Pain: Crushing, severe, prolonged, unrelieved by rest or nitroglycerin, often radiating to one or both arms, the neck, and back.	Complete stoppage of blood supply to myocardium caused by thrombotic occlusion evidently causes accumulation of unoxidized metabolites within ischemic part of myocardium; this affects the nerve endings.
Shock: Systolic B.P. below 80 mm. Hg, gray facial color, lethargy, cold diaphoresis, peripheral cyanosis, tachycardia or bradycardia, weak pulse.	In some cases, shock caused primarily by the severe pain; in others, by a severe reduction in cardiac output and by inadequate tissue perfusion resulting in tissue hypoxia.
Oliguria: Urine flow of less than 20 ml./hr. as measured by indwelling Foley Catheter.	Inadequate urine flow indicates renal hypoxia owing to inadequate tissue perfusion resulting from shock.
Low-grade fever: Temperature rises within 24 hours and lasts 3 to 7 days; usually 100 to 103°F., accompanied by leukocytosis, elevated sedimentation rate, LDH, and SGOT.	Fever and elevated white counts result from destruction of myocardial tissue and the ensuing inflammatory process; fever drops when fibroblasts begin to replace leukocytes and scar tissue starts to form.
Apprehension, great fear of death, restlessness.	The severe pain of a heart attack is terrifying; also, most laymen are aware of the heart's importance and the significance of a heart attack; restlessness results from shock and pain.
"Indigestion," "gas pains around the heart," nausea and vomiting.	Patients may prefer to believe that their pain is caused by "gas" or "indigestion" rather than by heart disease; nausea and vomiting may result from severe pain or from vagovagal reflexes conducted from the area of damaged myocardium to the gastrointestinal tract.
Acute pulmonary edema: Sense of suffocation, dyspnea, orthopnea, gurgling; bubbling respirations.	In some cases, the left ventricle becomes severely crippled in pumping action owing to infarction; severe pulmonary congestion results, accompanied by low cardiac output and shock.

coronary will die within 5 years; 75 per cent will die within 10 years from massive infarctions.

CLINICAL CARE OF THE PATIENT WITH A MYOCARDIAL INFARCTION

The major *goals of care* for patients with acute MI are: (1) successful treatment of the acute attack and prompt alleviation of symptoms; (2) prevention of complications and further attacks; and (3) rehabilitation and education of the patient and his family.

Treatment of Acute Attack

The patient who is suffering from an acute MI must be treated immediately! The severe pain must be alleviated, the ensuing shock reversed, and restlessness and fear eased. Complete rest, sedation, narcotics, oxygen, I.V. fluids, continuous monitoring, observation, and additional care are essential if the patient is to survive the first crucial 48 hours following his attack.

Typical therapeutic measures ordered for the newly admitted patient with an MI are listed in Table 51–2 along with the rationale for each measure and the supportive nursing care.

TABLE 51–2. TYPICAL THERAPEUTIC ORDERS EMPLOYED IN THE TREATMENT OF MYOCARDIAL INFARCTION: RATIONALE AND SUPPORTIVE NURSING CARE

Typical Order	Rationale	Supportive Nursing Care
Admit to CCU stat	CCU ensures constant supervision, monitoring, expert nursing care, and immediate attention in event of emergency	Relieve anxiety; reassure patient and family about CCU; explain in simple terms use of monitor; explain that skilled nurses and physicians are in constant attendance
Semi-Fowler's position	Position is comfortable; lowers diaphragm, thereby increasing lung expansion and promoting better ventilation; decreases venous return to heart, which prevents excessive pooling of blood within pulmonary vessels	If possible, have bed prepared prior to admission; support patient's shoulders and head adequately; reposition patient frequently (do not allow him to slide down in bed); do not use gatch (flexed knees promotes thrombus formation)
Complete bed rest for 3–5 days	Bed rest decreases stress and strain on damaged heart	Place call light, water, bedside stand, within easy reach of patient; if necessary, feed and turn patient; omit baths until critical stage has passed; give care in a calm, quiet, efficient manner; limit visitors; promote emotional and mental relaxation; give reassurance; allow patient to discuss problems; watch for and prevent complications of bed rest
Bedside commode for bowel movements; allow patient (if male) to stand with help by bedside to void (critically ill patients have Foley catheter)	Using a bedpan or urinal in bed is fatiguing; also, elimination is almost always incomplete; constipation, impaction, and urinary retention can result	Place call light within easy reach; assist patient out of bed; lift critically ill patient to commode with help of other nurses or an orderly; warn patient *not* to strain at stool; carefully chart bowel movements and voidings
Colace, 50–200 mg. orally daily	Stool softness prevents obstipation and straining	Give colace (liquid) in fruit juice to mask bitter taste; if patient fails to have a bowel movement, notify doctor and obtain laxative order
Patient may feed and shave self (if mild attack)	Feeding and shaving self usually lessens emotional trauma and sense of helplessness; activity allowed depends upon severity of infarction, development of complications, presence of other illnesses, and patient's response to the activity	Arrange patient's tray or shaving equipment so that little exertion is required; watch patient carefully for signs of fatigue, and chart; consult doctor if patient appears to be overly tired from activities

(Table 51–2 continued on the following page.)

TABLE 51–2. TYPICAL THERAPEUTIC ORDERS EMPLOYED IN THE TREATMENT OF MYOCARDIAL INFARCTION: RATIONALE AND SUPPORTIVE NURSING CARE (*Continued*)

Typical Order	Rationale	Supportive Nursing Care
Clear liquid diet for 48 hours, then 1500 - calorie, soft, 2000-mg. Na^+ diet in 6 small feedings	Clear liquids reduce hazard of vomiting and aspiration should resuscitation be necessary; small, soft, low-calorie meals are easily digested; low Na^+ diet diminishes fluid retention, thereby decreasing work of the heart	Explain purpose of diet; serve food attractively; if diet unpalatable for patient, have dietitian consult with patient
Analgesia: Morphine sulfate, 8–15 mg. (1/8–1/4 gr.) subcut. for pain as needed Morphine sulfate, 10–15 mg. (1/6–1/4 gr.) slowly I.V. for severe pain; repeat in 15 minutes if pain not relieved (some physicians order Demerol or Dilaudid because each produces less vomiting)	Severe pain of infarction requires use of a powerful drug such as morphine to prevent development of severe shock	When patient complains of pain, evaluate situation immediately; carefully check BP, pulse, and respirations before and after giving drug (morphine causes hypoventilation and hypotension); *do not* give morphine if respirations less than 12 per minute; morphine and other narcotics may cause dizziness and fainting if patient stands; always put bedside rails up following injection of narcotics; encourage deep breathing to prevent pneumonia and atelectasis
Hypnotics: Phenobarbital, 1/4–1/2 grain t.i.d. orally; pentobarbital, 100 mg. orally H.S.	Rest of the total patient (heart, body, and mind) is absolutely essential following trauma of acute MI; sedatives and hypnotics reduce fear and restlessness	Observe patient for effect of drugs; if restlessness continues, consult with physician; provide patient with as restful an atmosphere as possible; schedule "quiet periods" during the day when patient will not be disturbed
Oxygen, 10 liters per minute (may be given by mask, nasal catheter, or cannula)	Arterial pO_2 decreases following MI; oxygen helps to relieve dyspnea, chest pain, shock, cyanosis, and pulmonary edema	Check oxygen cylinder frequently; make certain there is always O_2 in tank; have another tank on hand; check humidifier for H_2O level ("dry" oxygen can damage bronchial tubes); enforce safety precautions when O_2 being used, e.g., no smoking
BP, pulse, respiration q. 1–2 hrs. (vital signs may be continuously monitored by electronic means)	Vital signs give essential information; hypotension may foreshadow development of shock; rise in pulse rate may indicate shock; changes in pulse rhythm may precede life-threatening arrhythmia; very slow respirations may indicate morphine toxicity; gasping respirations (air hunger) may indicate oxygen lack; gurgling respirations indicate pulmonary edema	Explain to patient and family that frequent taking of vital signs is routine; report immediately BP above 170 or below 100, pulse above 110 or below 60, arrhythmias, respiration below 12 or above 24, and dyspnea and respiratory distress

(Table 51–2 continued on the opposite page.)

TABLE 51–2. TYPICAL THERAPEUTIC ORDERS EMPLOYED IN THE TREATMENT OF MYOCARDIAL INFARCTION: RATIONALE AND SUPPORTIVE NURSING CARE (*Continued*)

Typical Order	Rationale	Supportive Nursing Care
Temperature q. 4 hrs.	Patient usually develops fever 24–48 hrs. after MI	Report temperature over 101°F.; report fever that persists after 6 or 7 days (pulmonary infection or infarction may be developing); observe for signs of dehydration; use cooling measures as necessary
Twelve-lead ECG stat; continuous ECG monitoring, rhythm strip q. 2 hrs.; PVC count q. 2 hrs. for 48 hrs.	Twelve-lead ECG done soon after admission to evaluate cardiac status; rhythm strips used to observe changes in heart rhythm; frequent PVC's (3 per min.) indicate ventricular irritation and may precede ventricular fibrillation	Reassure patient; explain use of ECG monitor; explain that ECG alarm signifies that an electrode has come off patient's chest, *not* cardiac irregularity; explain that *static* on monitor indicates only muscular movement; have emergency drugs and defibrillator on hand in event of life-threatening arrhythmia
Measure and record central venous pressure (CVP) q. 1–2 hrs.; keep CVP catheter open with 5% D/W	An elevated CVP may indicate failure of right ventricle to handle venous return; low CVP usually indicates shock and circulatory failure	Report CVP above 12 or below 3 cm. H_2O
Intake and output	Fluid *intake* should be just adequate (around 2000 ml. daily); too much may result in CHF, too little may cause dehydration—especially with elevated temperature	Inform all personnel that patient on I & O; label bed, Kardex, etc.
Foley catheter to measure urine output and specific gravity q. 1–2 hrs. (this order for critically ill patient)	Oliguria indicates inadequate renal perfusion and shock; concentrated urine (high specific gravity) usually indicates dehydration	Report urine output below 30 ml. per hour and specific gravity of 1.020 or higher; maintain sterile technique when inserting and irrigating Foley catheter to prevent bladder infection
I.V. fluids: 5% dextrose in water by CVP catheter; keep open with 10–20 microdrops per minute	Vein should be kept open in case emergency I.V. drugs or a rapid phlebotomy is necessary	Watch I.V. infusions closely; if I.V. runs too rapidly, circulatory overload and pulmonary edema will result; maintain sterile technique in I.V. procedures
Special orders in event of complications include: antiarrhythmic agents, digitalis, diuretics, anticoagulants, K^+ medications, vasopressors or vasodilators	These orders discussed under Complications of MI.	

Prevention of Complications and Further Attacks

The possibility of death from complications always accompanies an acute MI. Thus, the prevention of life-threatening complications or at least their early recognition is one of the prime goals of clinical care. The major complications, their incidence, cause, prevention, and treatment are briefly outlined below.

*Arrhythmias.** Specifically, ventricular premature beats, ventricular tachycardia and fibrillation, atrial fibrillation, heart block.

SIGNIFICANCE. Forty to 50 per cent of deaths occur because of arrhythmias.

CAUSATION. Ectopic rhythms arise in or near borders of intensely ischemic and damaged myocardial tissues; damaged myocardium may also interfere with conduction system, causing dissociation of atria and ventricles (heart block).

SYMPTOMS. Typical rate, rhythm, and ECG findings for specific arrhythmias; heart block with Stokes-Adams syndrome characterized by syncope.

PREVENTION. PVC counts every 2 hours; report to physician if more than three PVC's per minute; prompt treatment of minor arrhythmias.

TREATMENT. *Frequent PVC's*—quinidine sulfate or lidocaine intravenously; *ventricular tachycardia*—quinidine, Pronestyl, lidocaine, Dilantin, precordial shock; *ventricular fibrillation*—immediate precordial shock; *atrial fibrillation*—digitalis, quinidine, precordial shock; *heart block*—isoproterenol, use of temporary pacemaker.

Shock†

SIGNIFICANCE. Shock is responsible for 9 per cent of the deaths from myocardial infarction; an estimated 80 per cent of patients who develop shock die from the complications.

CAUSATION. Severe pain, decreased myocardial contraction and diminished cardiac output; undetected arrhythmias.

SYMPTOMS. Systolic BP below 80 mm. Hg, diaphoresis, rapid pulse, restlessness, cold clammy skin, gray skin color.

PREVENTION. Rapid relief of pain and sufficient I.V. fluids to prevent circulatory collapse may help to prevent shock; rapid identification of arrhythmias is also important.

TREATMENT. Vasopressors such as levarterenol and aramine to raise blood pressure by increasing peripheral resistance; in other cases vasodilators such as phenoxybenzamine to promote better blood flow in the microcirculation; isotropic agents such as isoproterenol sometimes used to increase cardiac contractility and cardiac output, and to improve tissue perfusion; oxygen therapy; continuous CVP monitoring; antiarrhythmic agents.

Congestive Heart Failure

SIGNIFICANCE. Some authorities maintain that some degree of CHF and pulmonary edema is always present following acute MI.

CAUSATION. Left or right ventricular failure.

SYMPTOMS. CHF may be present at the onset of the infarction or it may develop weeks later following an arrhythmia or pulmonary embolism. Typical symptoms are dyspnea, orthopnea, weight gain, edema, enlarged tender liver, distended neck veins, basal rales.

PREVENTION. Low-sodium diet, restricted fluid intake, strict monitoring of I.V. fluids to prevent circulatory overload, bed rest.

TREATMENT. *CHF*—bed rest, digitalization, sodium-restricted diet, fluid restriction, diuretics; *pulmonary edema*—morphine, ethacrynic acid intravenously, phlebotomy of 300 to 500 ml. or rotating tourniquets; intermittent positive pressure breathing.

Rupture of the Heart

SIGNIFICANCE. A rare complication that usually develops one week to ten days following the infarction and is generally fatal.

CAUSATION. May result from a dissecting hematoma that completely lacerates a part of the infarcted area of the myocardium that is soft and necrotic. When the heart ruptures, blood collects in the pericardial sac (hemopericardium) and the heart is unable to dilate.

SYMPTOMS. Sudden death, although patient occasionally lives for a half hour or more.

PREVENTION. Hypertension, exertion, and straining at stool are factors that increase susceptibility to cardiac rupture. Preventive measures are complete rest during the first two weeks after the infarction, control of hypertension by medical means, stool softeners and laxatives to prevent constipation and impactions, and use of the bedside commode, which allows the patient to have a bowel movement more easily. *Caution the patient not to strain when having a bowel movement.*

TREATMENT. Pericardial aspiration, transfusions, possibly emergency surgery, immediate treatment of shock.

Pulmonary Embolism. This may be secondary to phlebitis of the leg or pelvic veins.

SIGNIFICANCE. Occurs in 10 to 20 per cent of patients at some point during either the acute attack or convalescent period.

CAUSATION. Prolonged bed rest, increased blood viscosity, increased blood coagulability, use of the gatch for flexing patient's knees.

SYMPTOMS. *Venous thrombosis*—pain and swelling of the affected leg, pain in the calf upon dorsiflexion of the foot, fever; *pulmonary embolism*—dyspnea, tachycardia, tachypnea, cough, pleuritic pain, pulmonary rales, cyanosis, fever, sometimes shock and cardiac arrest.

PREVENTION. Encourage patients to move legs and feet frequently; avoid placing pressure under patients' knees with pillows or bed gatch; apply Ace bandages or elastic stockings to legs; administer sufficient fluids to prevent dehydration and increased blood viscosity; anticoagulant therapy.*

TREATMENT. Sedation, I.V. therapy, oxygen,

---

*See Chapter 50 for a complete discussion of arrhythmias, antiarrhythmic drugs, resuscitation measures, and precordial shock.

†Shock is discussed in detail in Chapter 26.

*Anticoagulant therapy as a general preventive measure against thrombus formation and embolization following MI is highly controversial. In severe cases of myocardial infarction, however, most physicians do order intravenous administration of heparin upon the patient's admission, followed by an order for oral anticoagulants some days later. Anticoagulant therapy is discussed in detail in Unit XII.

heparin intravenously, oral anticoagulants, pulmonary artery embolectomy.

Recurrent Myocardial Infarction

SIGNIFICANCE. Occurs in about 5 per cent of patients during the period of recovery from the first acute attack.

CAUSATION. Possible overexertion, embolization, further thrombotic occlusion of a coronary artery by an atheroma.

SYMPTOMS. Same as for first acute MI.

PREVENTION. Bed rest, oxygen, sedation, anticoagulants.

TREATMENT. Same as for the original acute attack.

Shoulder-hand Syndrome

SIGNIFICANCE. A very rare disorder that is preventable.

CAUSATION. Prolonged immobilization of the patient's arms and shoulders.

SYMPTOMS. Affected shoulder becomes painful and tender; next, the hand becomes swollen, painful, and weak.

PREVENTION. Daily active or passive exercise of the arms and shoulders, physical therapy.

TREATMENT. Physical therapy.

Rehabilitation of Patient

A successful rehabilitation program begins the moment a patient with a "coronary" enters the CCU for emergency care and continues for months and even years following his discharge home from the hospital.

The overall goal of rehabilitation is to help the patient to live as full, vital, and productive a life as possible and yet remain within the limits of his heart's ability to respond to increases in activity and stress. In sum, the patient must avoid both invalidism and reckless overexertion.

Four important subgoals of rehabilitation are: (1) to develop a program of progressive physical activity; (2) to educate the patient and his family concerning cause, prevention, and treatment of CHD; (3) to help the patient to accept the limitations imposed by his illness; and (4) to aid the patient as he adjusts to changes in his occupational goals.

Program of Physical Activity. Patients who have suffered a heart attack usually remain on bed rest for only a few days, unless complications such as congestive heart failure or arrhythmias develop. The typical program of activity for patients recuperating from an acute MI is as follows:[160]

First week postinfarction (*immediate* phase):

1. Admission to the coronary care unit; room should be equipped with a calendar, clock, and window to help keep patient oriented.
2. Complete bed rest for first day or so with use of bedside commode for bowel movements.
3. Liquid diet for first 48 hours.
4. Shaving and feeding self, moving around in bed, and brushing teeth may be allowed once blood pressure and vital signs have stabilized; passive exercises should be started by coronary care nurse or physiotherapist.
5. As patient gains strength, he may sit for brief periods on side of bed and dangle his feet.
6. Ambulation to a bedside chair for 15 to 20 minutes three or four times per day often permissible after third day.

Second and *third weeks* postinfarction (*intermediate* phase):

1. After fifth day, discharge from CCU to intermediate or regular unit if no complications have developed. Monitoring of vital signs by wireless telemetry should be continued.
2. Self-care of majority of hygiene needs encouraged during second week; brief supervised walks in hall allowable if no signs of complications.
3. Patient must avoid fatigue. Dyspnea, chest pain, tachycardia, and a sense of exhaustion are warning signals that patient is attempting to do too much.

Fourth week through *third month* postinfarction (*long-term* phase):

1. If no complications arise, patient is discharged home after third week. Essential to counsel family against treating patient as an invalid.
2. Sexual intercourse may be allowed six to eight weeks after an MI. Caution patient not to eat or drink alcoholic beverages immediately prior to intercourse.
3. Smoking must be completely discontinued.
4. Frequent walks are permissible, but strenuous activities such as shoveling snow must be avoided.
5. Jogging may be undertaken during the eighth week provided the patient tests out satisfactorily using a treadmill or other graded exercise testing device.
6. Some patients may be able to return to work at the end of eight or nine weeks if they remain asymptomatic. Persons with professional or white-collar jobs may be able to work full time, but manual laborers may have to work part time or find more sedentary work.

Education of Patient and Family. Following an acute MI, the patient and his family must make many changes in their work patterns, life styles, diet, and so forth. Significant changes in life style are always easier to make if a person understands the basic reasons for change and the benefits he will ultimately obtain.

When teaching the patient about his condition, it is helpful to follow these steps:

1. Consult with the physician as to when the patient will be ready to learn about his condition; find out what information the doctor has already given the patient and family, and especially if there is any information that he wishes you to withhold.
2. Select the proper time to begin instruction; make certain that the patient is calm, comfortable, and rested, so that he will be receptive to learning.
3. Find out what the patient already knows or believes about CHD; correct any false notions or misconceptions.
4. Encourage the patient to ask questions about his condition. Give the patient paper and pencil and ask him to write down any questions that come to his mind throughout the day; later he can discuss these questions with your or the doctor.
5. Do not overload the patient with information; allow him to learn at his own pace. If the patient

appears bored, tired, or preoccupied, continue your discussion at a later time.

The family also needs help and instruction, especially when the patient is discharged home. In particular, family members will need to know: (1) exactly how much activity the patient can tolerate when he first goes home; (2) medications the patient will be taking and their side effects; (3) details of a special diet if one is ordered; and (4) signs of complications (such as CHF) that they should report to the physician.

Emotional Support for Patient and His Family. As indicated, suffering an acute MI is one of the most terrifying events that a person can experience. Because the pain and fear are so devastating, most patients react to their heart attacks in distinct and dramatic ways. There are several coping devices that patients use to adjust to the realities (or to *obscure* the realities) of their illness. Common ways by which patients cope with the fact they have had a "coronary" are: denial, euphoria, intellectualization, anger, hypochondriasis, regression, and depression. These coping devices have been discussed in Unit III.

Return to Occupation. Approximately two thirds of patients who have suffered a first myocardial infarction are able to return to their former occupations. However, certain occupations, such as driving public vehicles or working in heavy construction, are too hazardous. For example, the patient might have a second MI while driving a bus and endanger the lives of other persons as well as himself. In some cities, there are *cardiac work classification teams* composed of cardiologists, psychiatrists, social workers, and nurses who help patients who are bus drivers, heavy laborers, and so forth, to find more suitable work.

Self-employed and professional persons also need special guidance. The demands of the business and professional worlds are great, and competition is keen. The person with a heart condition who is a doctor, lawyer, or executive must learn to delegate duties to his associates and to make time for recreation and rest.

Housewives constitute another group of workers who need special counseling. They need to be instructed in how to simplify household chores and arrange working areas for maximum efficiency. In certain cases, housewives may need to employ a cleaning woman.

Finally, some patients are forced to retire completely from work. These persons may become depressed and bored unless they find interesting and useful ways to spend their time. Hobbies, television, movies, and card playing are all helpful diversions.

CHAPTER 52

Arterial Hypertensive Cardiovascular Disease

HYPERTENSION

DEFINITION AND SIGNIFICANCE

Although hypertension is a common cardiovascular ailment, there is no single definition of the term that is universally recognized. However, most definitions are similar to the following one accepted by the World Health Organization and many life insurance companies:

> *Hypertension is a persistent elevation of the systolic blood pressure above 140 mm. Hg and of the diastolic pressure above 90 mm. Hg.*

Many writers feel that the term "hypertension" does not necessarily denote a disease process, but is simply a physical finding that may or may not be medically significant.

Despite disagreement upon the exact definition of hypertension, authorities do agree that a sustained elevation of blood pressure is of clinical significance because of its effects upon the heart, the vascular system, the kidneys, and the eyes. These effects are important medically because they can lead to such conditions as *hypertensive heart disease,* with resultant heart failure, myocardial infarction, cerebral vascular accidents, and kidney failure; *arteriolar nephrosclerosis,* with eventual renal failure; and *retinal abnormalities* terminating in blindness.

CLASSIFICATION

The three general ways of classifying hypertensive cardiovascular disease are:

Systolic and Diastolic Hypertension

Systolic hypertension is apparently related to loss of elastic tissue and to arteriosclerotic changes occurring in the aorta and other large blood vessels with advancing years; the systolic blood pressure is also influenced by emotional stress.

Diastolic hypertension is a true disease phenomenon. It reflects the amount of pressure exerted on the arterial walls of the small arteries, exclusive of the pulse pressure (i.e., pressure caused by contraction of the left ventricle).

Intermittent and Continuous Hypertension

Intermittent hypertension occurs when the blood pressure is variable, fluctuating between normal and moderately elevated. Caused by alternating constriction and then relaxation of the blood vessels, intermittent hypertension may continue for months and even years.

Continuous hypertension develops when the arterioles throughout the body are seriously damaged.

Primary and Secondary Hypertension

Primary hypertension, also known as *essential* or *idiopathic hypertension, constitutes 90 per cent of all cases of hypertension.* Its etiology is unknown. Types of primary hypertension are:

1. *Benign* hypertension. Characterized by a gradual onset and prolonged course.
2. *Malignant* hypertension: Characterized by abrupt onset and a short dramatic course which is rapidly fatal unless treated.

Secondary hypertension develops as a result of other primary diseases of the cardiovascular system, renal system, adrenal glands, or neurologic system.

INCIDENCE AND PREDISPOSING FACTORS

Primary (essential) hypertension affects at least one person in every 10 in the United States or about 5 to 15 per cent of the adult population. Hypertensive heart disease, the result of a longstanding elevation of blood pressure, takes approximately 100,000 lives per year.

Hypertension most commonly develops in middle-aged and older persons, although it can strike youths and even infants. Females develop hypertension twice as frequently as males but are less dramatically affected by a sustained elevation of blood pressure. Blacks in the United States develop hypertension more readily than the white population; also, persons living in stressful urban environments and those frequently subjected to emotional trauma become hypertensive far more frequently than persons who live in rural or tropical environments and those living relaxed lives. Finally, studies show a link between obesity and hypertension and consistently demonstrate that a reduction in weight is usually accompanied by a reduction in blood pressure.

The malignant form of essential hypertension affects 1 to 5 per cent of those diagnosed as hypertensive. Males and blacks are particularly prone to this deadly form of the disease.

BENIGN PRIMARY (ESSENTIAL) HYPERTENSION

Theories of Causation

The causative factors resulting in the development of primary (essential) hypertension are unknown. However, several theories of causation are being investigated. Briefly, these theories are: (1) hypertension is caused by an excessive flow of vasoconstrictor nerve impulses from the vasomotor centers to the blood vessels; (2) hypertension results from kidney failure of unknown cause; (3) psychogenic factors such as continuous emotional disturbance can cause high blood pressure, (4) ischemia or irritated lesions of the brain cause hypertension; (5) hypertension is caused by a masked hormonal imbalance; (6) hypertension is a result of an inherited factor causing an increased thickness in the arterial walls; and (7) not one but many different factors are involved in the development of hypertension.

Pathophysiology

From a pathologist's viewpoint, essential hypertension is a disorder in which the arterioles offer abnormal resistance to blood flow; also, there is usually a concurrent elevation of systolic blood pressure attributable to changes in the aorta's distensibility.

Early in the course of essential hypertension there may be no obvious pathologic changes in the blood vessels and organs, and few or no symptoms occur other than intermittent elevations of the blood pressure. However, as time passes widespread pathologic changes take place in both the large and small blood vessels and in the vital organs supplied with blood and oxygen by these vessels, namely, the heart, kidneys, and brain.

The *large* vessels such as the aorta, coronary arteries, basilar artery to the brain, and peripheral vessels in the limbs become sclerosed and tortuous; also, their lumens narrow, resulting in decreased blood flow to the heart, brain, and lower extremities. As the damage continues, large vessels may become completely occluded or hemorrhage may occur.[122]

Small vessel damage is equally dangerous, causing additional adverse structural changes within the heart, kidney, and brain. The severely elevated diastolic blood pressure causes damage to the intima of the small vessels. Because of intimal damage, fibrin accumulates in the vessels, local edema develops, and intravascular clotting may occur. The final result of these adverse changes is a decreased blood supply to the tissues of the heart, brain, and kidneys and progressive functional insufficiency of these organs.[122]

As stated earlier, one of the results of a long-sustained elevation of diastolic pressure is hypertensive heart disease, which may terminate in kidney failure. In the development of hypertensive cardiovascular disease, one sees the following vicious circle of pathologic changes in which each new manifestation of the disease further complicates all other manifestations of the disease: (1) the heart is meeting increased peripheral resistance because of constricted arterials, but must continue to maintain normal cardiac output for the body to function without symptoms; (2) to accomplish this augmented work, the heart increases its *expenditure of energy* (this is accomplished by physiologic stretching of muscle fibers); (3) the stretching of muscle fibers leads to *hypertrophy* of the heart; (4) hypertrophy of the heart may lead to coronary insufficiency and *resultant myocardial infarction* because the enlarged heart muscle has outgrown its blood supply; (5) if the hypertrophied state of the heart is able to maintain proper cardiac output, a state of *compensation* exists and *left-sided cardiac failure* ensues; (6) as the diastolic pressure rises in the failing left ventricle and atrium, the congestion extends back to involve the entire pulmonary tree, leading to a state of *pulmonary congestion,* which, in turn, affects the *vessels of the kidney;* (7) the increased pressure of blood in the arteries coupled with the fact that arteriosclerosis weakens the blood vessels can cause blood vessels to rupture, producing *hemorrhage;* (8) when a blood vessel ruptures in the *kidney*, the latter becomes thrombosed. The area of the kidney supplied by the vessel becomes ischemic and dies, and this further aggravates the hypertension. Eventually, as this process occurs again and again, the kidney fails.

Death due to hypertensive cardiovascular disease results either from irreparable damage to the kidneys, brain, and myocardium as a result of small vessel damage, or from occlusion of a large vessel (e.g., acute MI) or hemorrhage from a large vessel (e.g., CVA).

Basis of Symptoms and Complications

As stated previously, the symptoms of prolonged, primary (essential) hypertension are due to pathologic changes in large and small vessels throughout the body. Typical symptoms and their causation are listed on page 679.

Like the symptoms, the *complications* of hypertension also affect the heart, brain, eyes, and kidneys. Thus, patients with longstanding primary (essential) hypertension may eventually suffer from congestive heart failure, acute myocardial infarction, cerebral vascular accidents, blindness, and uremia.

SECONDARY HYPERTENSION

Etiology

The causes of secondary hypertension are many, including:

1. Coarctation of the aorta.

2. Adrenal causes, e.g., pheochromocytoma, primary aldosteronism, Cushing's syndrome.
3. Renal disease, e.g., renovascular disease, parenchymal disease.

The etiology, pathogenesis, symptoms, and physical findings for these conditions are briefly outlined in Table 52–1. Hypertension can also be secondary to Na^+ retention during pregnancy, increased intracranial pressure from brain tumors and hematomas, and advanced collagen diseases.

Diagnostic Approaches

When the physician examines a hypertensive patient, he carefully evaluates the following four areas:

1. The *form* of hypertension, i.e., essential or secondary. To make a diagnosis of essential hypertension, the doctor first rules out all secondary causes of hypertension by means of the history, physical examination, and laboratory studies.
2. Whether a *curable* form of hypertension is present. Hypertension caused by coarctation of the aorta, adrenal dysfunction, primary aldosteronism, renovascular disease, or brain tumors is potentially curable.
3. The *severity* of the hypertension is evaluated on the basis of the degree of adverse changes within the arterioles supplying the retina, the presence of ECG abnormalities, the extent of cardiac enlargement, and the degree of renal failure.
4. The *rate of progression* of cardiovascular damage. Cardiovascular pathology is evident if the patient complains of anginal pain or suffers from the symptoms of CHF.

The *diagnosis* of hypertension is confirmed by: the patient's history, physical examination, and laboratory studies. When taking the patient's history, the physician or nurse asks the following questions:

1. At what age did the patient's blood pressure first become elevated?
2. Has anyone in the family suffered from high blood pressure?
3. Has the patient suffered at any point in his life from renal or cardiovascular disease?
4. Has the patient recently experienced dyspnea, fatigue, weakness, anginal type pain, swelling of the feet, or nocturia?
5. Has the patient suddenly lost weight (sign of pheocromocytoma) or suddenly gained weight (edema)?
6. Has the patient recently experienced severe headaches or drenching sweats (signs of pheochromocytoma)?

As the doctor or nurse talks with the patient, she notes if he has the hard driving personality usually associated with the hypertensive individual. She also notes the patient's appearance. Does the patient have the moon facies and peculiar distribution of fat characteristic of Cushing's syndrome? If a woman, is hirsutism present? Does the patient have a flushed appearance and anxious expression, as characteristic of pheochromocytoma?

Following history taking, the doctor next performs a physical examination which includes the following:

> *Blood pressure* readings taken on both arms in the supine and erect positions and on one leg. To obtain a truly reliable estimation of the patient's average blood pressure, readings should be taken every one to two hours over an eight-hour period for one to two days.

Symptoms	*Basis of Symptoms*
BP persistently elevated above 140/90.	Arterioles are constricted, causing abnormal resistance to blood flow.
Anginal pain.	Insufficient blood flow through coronary arteries to the myocardium.
*Intermittent claudication.**	Decrease in blood supply from peripheral vessels to the legs.
Retinal hemorrhages and exudates.	Damage to arterioles that supply the retina.
Severe *occipital headaches* associated with nausea and vomiting, drowsiness, giddiness, anxiety, and mental impairment.	Vessel damage within the brain.
Polyuria; nocturia; diminished ability of kidneys to concentrate urine; protein and RBC's in urine.	Arteriolar nephrosclerosis (hardening of arterioles within the kidney).
Dyspnea upon exertion.	Left-sided heart failure.
Edema of the extremities.	Right-sided heart failure.

*Intermittent claudication is a severe pain that develops in the patient's calf muscles when he walks and subsides when he rests; this is a symptom of peripheral vascular disease.

Remember: *A* single *blood pressure reading is almost always inaccurate.*

> Ophthalmoscopic examination for evidence of such vascular changes as arteriolar tortuosity, increased light reflex, narrowing, and irregularity of the arteries. Vascular damage within the retina has definitely occurred if hemorrhages, soft exudates, and papilledema are present.

> Examination of the *heart* and *aorta* by means of auscultation, ECG readings, and aortography; x-ray is also used to determine heart size.

> *Palpation of the arteries* in the neck, wrists, femoral areas, and feet for evidence of coarctation of the aorta.

> *Neurologic examination* for signs of cerebral thrombosis or hemorrhage. Signs of pathologic changes within the cerebrum range from a positive Babinski or Hoffman reflex to hemiplegia or paralysis of one side of the patient's body.*

Large numbers of *laboratory studies* are next ordered for the purpose of diagnosing the type of hypertension present. General screening tests include:

> Urinalysis and urine cultures to determine the presence of protein, RBC's, pus cells, and casts—all evidence of possible renal disease.

> Blood count and sedimentation rates.

> Serum sodium, potassium, chloride, and carbon dioxide.

More specific laboratory tests include:

> Test for *pheochromocytoma:*† Analysis of urinary catecholamine metabolites, histamine test, and cold pressor test.

> Tests for *primary aldosteronism:* Repeated electrolyte determinations of potassium, sodium, and carbon dioxide.

> Tests for *Cushing's syndrome:* Urine 17-ketosteroids, blood corticoids.

> Tests for *renal disease:* Intravenous pyelogram, urine cultures, radioisotope renogram, renal arteriography, intravenous urograms.

If the clinical work-up produces no evidence of coarctation of the aorta, adrenal disease, or primary renal disease, the doctor then diagnoses the condition as *essential hypertension.*

*Neurologic reflexes are discussed in Unit VIII.

†Tests for pheochromocytoma, primary aldosteronism, and Cushing's syndrome are discussed in Unit XVIII. Renal tests are discussed in Unit XI.

TABLE 52–1. SECONDARY HYPERTENSION

Cause	Etiology	Symptoms	Physical Findings
Coarctation of aorta	Constriction of portion of aorta causes elevated blood pressure proximal to obstruction	Absence of femoral pulses; decreased BP in legs as compared to arms; weight loss	X-ray shows notching of ribs; intercostal bruits on auscultation
Pheochromocytoma	Adrenal medullary tumor causes excess secretion of catecholamines	Half of all patients have sudden attacks of severe headache with palpitation; hypermetabolic state; excessive sweating; meat intolerance; flushed, anxious appearance	Elevated BMR; elevated fasting blood sugar; excess excretion of catecholamines in urine
Primary aldosteronism	Functioning adenoma of adrenal cortex	Moderate elevation of blood pressure; muscular weakness; polyurea; nocturia; polydipsia; tetany; paresthesias; headache	Dilute alkaline urine; persistently low serum K^+ levels
Cushing's syndrome	Excess glycocorticosteroids excreted from adrenal cortex; cause may be an adrenocortical adenoma (or carcinoma) or adrenocortical hyperplasia	Mild hypertension; moon facies; "buffalo" hump on back; edema; hirsutism	Excretion of large amounts of 17-hydroxycorticoids and 17-ketosteroids in urine
Vascular renal hypertension	Narrowing of renal artery due to atherosclerosis, fibrosis of wall of renal artery, or trauma to renal area	Hypertension; fluid retention with edema	Difference in length of kidneys; delayed appearance of dye from one kidney during intravenous pyelogram (IVP); decreased urine and Na^+ output
Parenchymal disease (acute and chronic glomerulonephritis)	Allergic response to infection in body (usually streptococcal), causing inflammatory changes in glomeruli	Hypertension; sodium and water retention; edema; oliguria; orthopnea; dyspnea; pulmonary edema; uremic odor	Cardiac enlargement; evidence of myocardial failure on ECG; elevated nonprotein nitrogen (NPN)

CLINICAL CARE OF THE PATIENT WITH HYPERTENSION

> The aim of treatment [of patients with hypertension] should be reduction of blood pressure to normal and its maintenance at normal levels in the hope that cardiovascular and renal damage, the late complications of prolonged hypertension, will be prevented.[13]

The following therapies are used to treat patients suffering from hypertension: general nonspecific therapeutic measures, drug therapy, surgical techniques, and specific therapies for hypertension of varying severity.

General Nonspecific Measures. General measures in the care of patients with essential hypertension include the following:

1. Weight reduction if the patient is obese.
2. Moderate salt-restricted diet.
3. Planned program of regular physical exercise.
4. Changes in job or domestic setting for patients who work or live under considerable stress.
5. Mild tranquilizing drugs for patients who are nervous and apprehensive.
6. Short period of psychotherapy for individuals with serious emotional problems.

General *nursing care* of the patient with hypertension includes:

1. Provision of a restful, quiet hospital atmosphere.
2. Explanation of all procedures and diagnostic studies. Remember that most patients with hypertension are nervous, high-strung, compulsive individuals who may find it difficult to relax while undergoing renal function tests, ECG readings, and so forth.
3. Listening to the patient's fears and worries and offering reassurance when appropriate.
4. Explanation of diet restrictions (caloric and sodium restrictions). Patients suffering from CHD in addition to hypertension should also be instructed to reduce their consumption of animal fats.
5. Careful and accurate recording of the patient's blood pressure in both the standing and lying positions two or three times a day.
6. Administration of potentially dangerous hypotensive drugs with close observation of the patient for side effects.

Drug Therapy. The most specific form of therapy today for the control of essential hypertension is chemotherapy. Important drugs used for the reduction of blood pressure are: reserpine (Serpasil), guanethidine (Ismelin), hydralazine (Apresoline), alpha methyldopa (Aldomet), pargyline (Eutonyl), pentolinium tartrate (Ansolysen), chlorisondamine chloride (Ecolid), mecamylamine hydrochloride (Inversine), trimethaphan (Arfonal), chlorothiazide (Diuril) and other thiazides, and spironolactone (Aldactone). The use of these drugs is summarized in Table 52–2.

Patients receiving antihypertensive drug therapy may develop acute hypotensive reactions, which are characterized by faintness, weakness, nausea and vomiting. Patients on drug therapy must be taught how to prevent acute hypotensive reactions as well as what to do should a reaction occur. When a patient with hypertension is soon to be discharged from the hospital, you will want to alert him and his family to these precautions.

If taking antihypertensive drugs:

1. Lie down immediately if faintness, weakness, nausea and vomiting occur; put feet higher than head; flex thigh muscles and wiggle toes. This position promotes cerebral blood flow and lessens pooling of blood in limbs. Muscular activity decreases pooling of blood in lower extremities.
2. Avoid hot baths, excessive amounts of alcohol, and immobility following exercise. Vasodilatation is promoted by heat, alcohol, and immobility after exercise, which may cause fainting when coupled with the effects of an antihypertensive drug.
3. Always rise *slowly* from a lying to a sitting position and from a sitting to a standing position. Slow motion allows the vascular system to adjust to positional changes.
4. Avoid standing motionless (e.g., at bus stops, in telephone booths, on subways, in supermarket lines, in the shower), especially within the first hour or two after receiving the medication. Standing causes vessels within the legs to relax, which allows blood to pool within the lower extremities; draining of blood from the brain and other vital organs can cause fainting.
5. Use caution when driving an automobile or when operating heavy or dangerous machinery, especially within two hours after taking the drug. A serious or fatal accident could occur if acute hypotension develops suddenly.
6. Avoid cheese, beer, or wine when taking a monomine oxidase inhibitor, (e.g., pargyline, Eutonyl). A severe reaction may occur, with the possibility of cerebral hemorrhage.
7. Avoid constipation; ask the doctor for a gentle laxative should bowels fail to move regularly. Exercise daily and take adequate fluids and roughage. Constipation may cause either an increased or irregular absorption of hypotensive drugs, which can result in critical hypotensive reactions.
8. Should hypotensive crises occur frequently, wrap legs firmly with Ace bandages when ambulating. Ace bandages help to promote venous return from the lower extremities and decrease pooling of blood within the legs.

Surgical Techniques. Surgical techniques for the control of primary hypertension have decreased greatly in popularity with the advent of potent antihypertensive agents. Surgery, however, is still employed in the correction of secondary forms of hypertension.

In *repair of coarctation of the aorta* the constriction is removed from the aorta and the upper and lower ends of the aorta are united, sometimes by means of a graft.

Adrenalectomy, or surgical excision of the adrenal tumor, is employed to correct pheochromocytoma, primary aldosteronism, and Cushing's syndrome.

Correction of renal artery stenosis may be done to

TABLE 52–2. DRUGS USED TO CONTROL HYPERTENSION

Drug	Classification	Action
Reserpine	Hypotensive	Depletes brain and peripheral tissues of norepinephrine; produces sedation; decreases peripheral vasoconstriction, heart rate, and standing blood pressure
Guanethidine (Ismelin)	Postganglionic blocking agent	Produces postganglionic sympathetic blockade, depletes tissue stores of norepinephrine
Hydralazine (Apresoline)	Hypotensive	Dialates peripheral blood vessels; increases cardiac output and renal blood flow
Alpha methyldopa (Aldomet)	Hypotensive	Biologic and hemodynamic effects uncertain; lowers supine and standing blood pressures; dilates peripheral arterioles; usually increases glomerular filtration and cardiac output
Pargyline (Eutonyl)	Monamine oxidase inhibitor	Prevents or reduces destruction of amines such as norepinephrine and serotonin; reduces peripheral resistance
Pentolinium tartrate (Ansolysen)	Ganglionic blocking agent	Blocks transmission of impulses through sympathetic ganglia, causing blood vessels to dilate; extremely potent
Chlorisondamine chloride (Ecolid)	Ganglionic blocking agent	More potent than Ansolysen
Mecamylamine hydrochloride (Inversine)	Ganglionic blocking agent	Same as Ansolysen
Trimethaphan (Arfonal)	Ganglionic blocking agent	Promotes pulmonary and peripheral vasodilation and emptying of the left ventricle
Chlorothiazide and other thiazides (Diuril)	Oral diuretic	Promotes excretion of Na^+, H_2O, and $K+$
Spironolactone (Aldactone)	Aldosterone inhibitor and diuretic	Inhibits Na^+-conserving effect of aldosterone; promotes renal Na^+ excretion without depleting $K+$

TABLE 52–2. DRUGS USED TO CONTROL HYPERTENSION (*Continued*)

Indications for Use	Dosage	Side Effects
Mild and moderately severe hypertension	0.25 mg. daily in single dose	Depression; nasal stuffiness; peptic ulceration; insomnia; Na^+ retention
Severe, moderately severe, renal, and essential hypertension	10-150 mg. daily in divided doses	Severe orthostatic hypotension; diarrhea; inability to ejaculate
Moderately severe hypertension	10-50 mg. q.i.d.	Tachycardia; angina pectoris; gastric irritation; palpitations; headache; arthritis; lupus erythematosus
Severe and moderately severe hypertension	500-3000 mg. daily in divided doses	Initial drowsiness; skin eruptions; dryness of mouth; fluid retention; fever; occasionally liver damage
Moderately severe hypertension; depressed patients with hypertension	50-75 mg. daily	Postural hypotension; severe hypertensive crises with possibility of cerebral hemorrhage if taken with beer, cheese, or wine; contraindicated in hypothyroidism, pheochromocytoma, advanced renal disease, and paranoid schizophrenia
Hypertensive crises and malignant hypertension	60-600 mg. orally daily in divided doses; 2.5-3.5 mg. as initial parenteral dose	Postural hypotension; diarrhea; muscle ache; inability to ejaculate
Same as Ansolysen	Initially 12-5 mg. daily orally; average dose 50-100 mg. b.i.d. orally	Same as Ansolysen
Same as Ansolysen	Average dose, 25 mg. daily orally in 3 portions	Same as Ansolysen; also mental confusion, tremors, psychiatric problems
Hypertensive crises, to lower blood pressure rapidly	One 5 mg. ampule diluted with 500 ml. of dextrose to start treatment	Excessive hypotension
May be effective alone or in combination with reserpine in the treatment of mild hypertension	0.5-1 Gm. daily in divided doses	Hypokalemia; hyperuricemia; hyperglycemia
Helps to combat hypokalemia produced by chlorothiazide	25 mg. b.i.d. or q.i.d.	Breast stimulation is rare side effect

alleviate hypertension caused by renal vascular disease.

Sympathectomy results in the blockage of stimuli from the sympathetic nerve fibers to the blood vessels innervated by the fibers. This surgery is performed only on those few patients who cannot tolerate chemotherapy or who will not take their drugs.

Before the advent of antihypertensive chemotherapy, sympathectomies were commonly done to correct hypertension. In many cases blood pressure was reduced, retinal abnormalities disappeared, headaches were eliminated, and life was prolonged. However, a sympathectomy can result in many discomforts and problems for the patient. Some of the untoward effects of this operation are severe postural hypotension lasting for months postoperatively, neuritis, loss of ejaculation in the male, and loss of perspiration in areas innervated by severed sympathetic fibers, with excessive perspiration in areas innervated by sympathetic fibers that are intact.

Specific Therapies for Hypertension of Varying Severity. There are six different phases of hypertensive disease: the prehypertensive, mild benign, moderately severe benign, severe benign, malignant, and acute emergency (acute hypertensive crisis).

Each of these phases has certain characteristics and requires a specific type of therapy; this information is briefly summarized in Table 52–3.

Rehabilitative and Educational Approaches

The nurse caring for the patient with hypertension usually has the responsibility for educating the patient in a program of lifelong blood pressure control as well as reinforcing the physician's instructions and explanations. As a general rule, physician and nurse must carefully tailor the rehabilitation program to the specific needs and personality of the patient. They must take into consideration the patient's habits, life style, and general outlook. Patients who are depressed or belligerent, who drink excessively, who are severely neurotic, or who have deteriorated mentally must be given special consideration in any teaching plan.

The most important point that the hypertensive individual and his family must understand is that *essential hypertension is a chronic condition* that cannot be cured but can be *controlled* by means of continuous chemotherapy, weight control, dietary restrictions, moderate exercise, sufficient rest and, if necessary, modifications in life style. As you and the doctor set up a teaching program for the patient about to be discharged home, make certain you include the following areas in your discussion:

TABLE 52–3. PHASES OF HYPERTENSION

Phase	Characteristics	Therapy
Prehypertensive	Blood pressure mildly elevated: systolic pressure below 200 mm. Hg, diastolic pressure below 100 mm. Hg; symptoms of anxiety may be present: headache, insomnia, irritability, forgetfulness	No specific therapy; occasionally tranquilizers or sleeping medication
Mild benign	Systolic pressure remains below 200 mm. Hg, diastolic pressure above 100 mm. Hg; vague symptoms of anxiety; headache, fatigue, palpitations	Weight reduction; Na^+-restricted diet; mild antihypertensive drugs; diuretics with K^+ replacements
Moderately severe benign	Systolic blood pressure above 200 mm. Hg, diastolic pressure above 110 mm. Hg; no evidence of vascular damage	Weight reduction; Na^+-restricted diet; more potent drugs: Aldomet, Apresoline, Eutonyl
Severe benign	Systolic blood pressure up to 250 mm. Hg or higher, diastolic blood pressure persistently above 120 mm. Hg; abnormal neurologic signs: severe occipital headaches, anginal pain	Postganglionic blocking agents, e.g., Ismelin; ganglionic blocking agents if postganglionic blocking agents fail to control BP, e.g., Ansolysen
Malignant	Sudden sharp elevation in blood pressure: diastolic pressure above 130 mm. Hg; papilledema; rapidly progressive renal failure with albuminuria, proteinuria, decreased specific gravity, increased blood urea nitrogen; severe epigastric pain; left ventricular failure; mortality 100% in 2 years if not treated	Most potent antihypertensive drugs available, e.g., Ismelin, administered concomitantly with thiazides and reserpine; hospitalize promptly
Acute	Greatly elevated diastolic blood pressure (above 140 mm. Hg); rapid development of following conditions: Hypertensive encephalopathy, severe headache, mental confusion, nausea, vomiting, convulsions, coma, papilledema, retinal hemorrhages; intracranial hemorrhage; acute congestive heart failure with pulmonary edema	Medical emergency requiring immediate treatment; diastolic blood pressure must be reduced rapidly; chemotherapy with reserpine I.M. or I.V., Aldomet I.V., ganglionic blocking agents subcut. or I.V., Arfonad I.V. diluted in dextrose; have patient in sitting position; monitor BP continuously while patient is receiving parenteral medications; when BP controlled, Ismelin or ganglionic blocking agents and reserpine may be given orally

Home Blood Pressure Recordings. The patient will need to learn how to wrap the blood pressure cuff, position his arm correctly, listen for systolic and diastolic sounds and record his pressure accurately. Except perhaps in the extremely anxious patient, taking his own blood pressure reading is often a great incentive for the patient to take his medications as prescribed and to control his weight and diet. The patient can see for himself that his blood pressure remains lower when he follows his treatment program and that it rises when he forgets to take his drugs, goes off his diet, or becomes unduly angry or excited.

Self-medication with Antihypertensive Drugs. As emphasized earlier, antihypertensive drugs have dangerous side effects. Patients who are going to administer their own drugs need to be given the following precautions:

> 1. *Never take a larger dose of drug than prescribed without consulting the doctor.*
> 2. *Always take the drug on time; do not skip doses.*
> 3. *Never suddenly discontinue a drug without the doctor's permission, because severe hypertension may develop.*
> 4. *Always report untoward effects to the physician.*

Also, patients need to be cautioned about *acute hypotensive reactions;* they need specific rules for preventing and treating hypotension should it occur.

Dietary Restrictions. The doctor will probably want the patient to see a dietitian before he is discharged. You or the dietitian can give the patient printed information listing low-calorie, low-sodium foods. Also, caution the patient to avoid eating large heavy meals, because the digestion of large amounts of food puts an unnecessary burden on his heart. He should also avoid drinking large amounts of fluid, because excess fluids increase the blood volume, which, in turn, increases blood pressure.

Exertion. Heavy, overly strenuous exercise is harmful for patients with hypertension; however, a planned, moderate exercise program is beneficial. Daily walks are an excellent means of exercise, although hills and stairsteps should be avoided. Gardening and golf are also enjoyable forms of exercise for many people.

Interpersonal Relations. The patient with hypertension recovers best in home and working environments that are relatively harmonious and peaceful. If the patient works under a supervisor who constantly harasses and pressures him, it may be necessary for the patient to find a more suitable employer. An upsetting domestic atmosphere may not be so easily changed. However, you and the physician can counsel the patient's spouse and older children concerning the importance of making the patient's home environment relaxed and pleasant. Once the patient's family understands the correlation between high blood pressure and emotional tension, they will hopefully ease the patient's home responsibilities and give him greater emotional support.

Hobbies. Encourage the patient to engage in hobbies that are stimulating and interesting but do not cause great anxiety or high emotion. Because people vary widely in their emotional responses to different activities, the selection of an appropriate hobby is a highly individual matter. For example, card playing for some persons is a pleasant social pastime, whereas for others it is competitive and nerve wracking. Likewise, sports viewing, political rallies, horse racing, and miniature golf each carry a different significance for different individuals. As you discuss various hobbies with the patient, try to evaluate his emotional response to the activity. Guide the patient as much as possible into hobbies that are engrossing but not stressful.

Prognosis

With the advent of effective antihypertensive chemotherapy, the outlook for patients suffering from hypertension is far brighter than it was in the past. Before antihypertensive drugs were brought on the market, 70 per cent of patients with hypertension died of heart failure, 15 per cent of cerebral hemorrhage, and 10 per cent of uremia. Today, most patients with hypertension die of complications of the basic atherosclerotic process, which affects the cerebral arteries, renal arteries, and coronary arteries, e.g., "stroke," renal failure, myocardial infarction. When hypertension arises as a secondary process, patients may die of the primary disease, e.g., polyarteritis, Cushing's disease, or nephritis.

Patients with malignant hypertension also have a far more favorable prognosis today than in former years. Before the advent of antihypertensive drugs, patients with malignant hypertension rarely lived for more than two years following the onset of the disease. Today, 50 to 60 per cent of patients are still living five years following diagnosis.

CHAPTER 53

Disorders that Affect Specific Structures of the Heart

You recall from Chapter 46 that the major structures of the heart are the pericardium, the myocardium, and the endocardium. Many different factors are capable of adversely affecting these vital structures, e.g., viruses, bacteria, toxins, tumors, trauma, and various systemic diseases. In some cases these factors affect only one structure of the heart; in other cases, all structures of the heart undergo pathophysiologic changes.

PANCARDITIS: RHEUMATIC FEVER AND HEART DISEASE

GENERAL CONSIDERATIONS

Rheumatic fever is an acute or chronic systemic inflammatory process characterized by attacks of fever, polyarthritis, and carditis; the latter may eventually result in permanent valvular damage.

While CHD and hypertension mainly affect individuals over 50, rheumatic fever is the most common cause of heart disease in persons under 50. No one knows the exact incidence of rheumatic fever because it is not reportable. However, authorities estimate that 2 to 3 per cent of persons who have suffered a beta-hemolytic streptococcal infection will develop rheumatic fever. Because most children and young people suffer at some time from a streptococcal infection, we can assume that the incidence of rheumatic fever is high. Fortunately, however, rheumatic fever is rapidly becoming less common as a result of prophylactic antibiotic therapy; for example, modern physicians immediately administer antibiotics to patients with streptococcal infections, thereby preventing the later development of rheumatic fever.

What are the major factors that *predispose* an individual to rheumatic fever and control *distribution* of the disease throughout the population?

First of all, *age* is a major consideration. Rheumatic fever primarily strikes children and teenagers. Children between the ages of five and 15 are particularly vulnerable; indeed, 90 per cent of first attacks of the disease affect this age group. Also, rheumatic fever is the principal cause of fatalities among youngsters between five and 19. However, while rheumatic fever mainly affects the young, it also attacks the aged, causing severe cardiac disability and death.

Second, rheumatic fever is influenced by *economic* factors; it strikes the slum dweller much more frequently than the suburbanite, the city dweller more frequently than the farmer. Evidently poor persons living in urban areas are more prone to rheumatic fever because of malnutrition, greater exposure to bacterial infections, and less money for medical care.

Finally, rheumatic fever may possibly have a *genetic* basis. Some authorities suggest that persons can inherit a Mendelian recessive trait for rheumatic fever. Other authorities, however, point out that rheumatic fever may appear "to run in families" only because all family members are exposed to the highly infectious group A streptococcus when one family member has an infection.

ETIOLOGY

The exact cause of rheumatic fever is unknown. A few authorities believe that viruses are the major etiologic agents, whereas others feel that rheumatic fever develops as a hypersensitivity reaction to certain allergens. However, most evidence points to the *poststreptococcal hypersensitization* theory. Facts supporting this hypothesis are as follows: Rheumatic fever almost always develops following upper respiratory tract infection by the *beta-hemolytic group A streptococcus*. The *time* interval between the development of the streptococcal upper respiratory infection and the advent of rheumatic fever is almost always around five weeks; this is the approximate amount of time needed for the patient to become sensitized to the organism and to undergo an immune reaction.* However, since only 2 to 3 per cent develop rheumatic fever following streptococcal infections, researchers hypothesize that these susceptible persons have a greater immunologic response to streptococci.

PATHOPHYSIOLOGY

Rheumatic fever is classified by most authorities as a hypersensitivity "collagen" disorder;† thus, it is

*See Chapter 23 for a discussion of the immune reaction.

†Collagen disorders (e.g., lupus erythematosus, polyarteritis nodosa) are discussed in Chapter 23.

characterized by an inflammatory process that affects connective tissue in organs throughout the body, i.e., the heart, joints, nervous system, respiratory system, and so forth.

While the effects of rheumatic fever upon the joints, tendons, skin, respiratory system, and serosal membranes are temporary and fairly benign, it often produces permanent damage of the heart. As one author states:

> The heart bears the brunt of the attack, suffers the most disabling injuries, and damage to it is the reason for the importance of rheumatic fever as a cause of disability and death.[136]

Rheumatic carditis, then, is the most important consequence of rheumatic fever; this condition develops in approximately three fourths of patients. Carditis generally appears during the first or second week following the development of rheumatic fever, and it involves one or all three layers of the heart (myocardium, endocardium, and pericardium). When all three layers are affected simultaneously, the condition is called *pancarditis.*

In Table 53–1 are summarized the pathophysiologic effects of rheumatic fever upon the myocardium, endocardium, and pericardium.

Rheumatic fever can lead to permanent heart damage if the endocardium and valves become involved in the inflammatory process. Damage is permanent because the valve leaflets encrusted with vegetations become shriveled and shortened, producing valvular dysfunction and poor cardiac activity. First, the damaged valve may become narrowed or *stenosed,* greatly increasing the heart's labors as it struggles to propel blood forward through its chambers and into the aorta. Second, the valve leaflets may become so shortened that they cannot close securely. As a result, blood *regurgitates* or leaks backward through the damaged valve into the chamber from which it was ejected. The final consequence of both valvular stenosis and regurgitation is heart failure owing to strain and overwork.

Noncardiac changes that result from the widespread inflammatory process are: (1) red, swollen, tender joints; (2) tissue edema; (3) large subcutaneous nodules under the skin; (4) thickened, red, granular synovial membranes; and (5) occasionally pneumonitis.

ONSET AND SYMPTOMS

As we stated earlier, rheumatic fever almost always follows a streptococcal infection. There are typically three phases in its onset.

Phase 1: The patient suffers from an acute streptococcal infection, e.g., scarlet fever, streptococcal sore throat, or streptococcal tonsillitis. During this period the patient experiences chills, fever, swollen lymph nodes, and sore throat.

Phase 2: Patient recovers from the acute infection and appears symptom-free. This latent period of sensitization lasts for from one to five weeks.

Phase 3: Symptoms of rheumatic fever develop and the patient is once again acutely ill.

While symptoms of the acute streptococcal infection result from the direct invasion of tissues by bacteria, the manifestations of rheumatic fever evidently result from a *hypersensitivity reaction* to those streptococci that invaded weeks earlier and were vanquished by the body's defense mechanisms. (See Chapter 22.) Thus, the symptoms result mainly from inflammation of connective tissues. The symptoms are many and varied. The most important manifestations of this diffuse inflammatory disease process are briefly summarized below:

> *Arthralgia* or joint pain is the most prominent mani-

TABLE 53–1. EFFECTS OF RHEUMATIC FEVER UPON THE MYOCARDIUM, ENDOCARDIUM, AND PERICARDIUM

Condition	Characteristic Lesion	Factors in Causation of Lesion	Significance of Pathophysiologic Involvement
Rheumatic myocarditis	Aschoff bodies, minute nodules, usually found in connective tissue around small arteries in myocardium	Formed by leukocytes that mass in inflamed tissues	Nodules may eventually become fibrotic; damage from fibrosis may eventually damage arteries in myocardium; myocarditis may cause a temporary loss in contractile power of the heart; permanent damage rarely results
Rheumatic endocarditis	Tiny *vegetations* resembling little beads form along line of closure of valve flaps	Probably result from inflammation, ulceration, and erosion of valve flaps	Inflammatory damage of valves results in *permanent* severe heart disease
Pericarditis	Nonspecific lesions	Result from a diffuse, nonspecific fibrinous or serofibrinous inflammatory reaction	May cause pericardial friction rub; usually no serious sequelae

festation of rheumatic fever. Joints affected are the ankles, knees, shoulders, elbows, and wrists. Arthralgia usually has a rapid onset and subsides after a period of several hours to several days. During this time young patients may complain of "growing pains."

> *Carditis* is the second most common manifestation of rheumatic fever; it is by far the most dangerous and destructive consequence of this disease (Table 53–1).

> *Fever* of 100.4°F. (38°C.) or higher temperature elevations alternate with periods when temperature is normal (relapsing fever).

> *Subcutaneous nodules* are small nodules that adhere loosely to the patient's tendon sheaths; they usually occur in children and are evident only during the first week or so following the onset of the disease.

> *Erythema marginatum* is a migratory rash that usually appears on warm areas of the body. The lesions are crescent shaped and have clear centers.

> *Abdominal pain* is a common symptom that varies in site and severity; the pain may be related to engorgement of the liver.

> *Sydenham's chorea* is a nervous disorder characterized by grimacing and constant jerky purposeless movements. It is common in children, especially young girls; characteristically, chorea does not appear until the late stages of the disease.

> *Malaise, asthenia, weight loss, and anorexia* probably develop as a result of fever, pain, and the general debilitation that is characteristically linked with any serious illness.

DIAGNOSTIC MEASURES

Laboratory Studies. There are no specific laboratory studies for diagnosing rheumatic fever. At best, laboratory findings only serve to confirm the presence of acute infection. Thus, one finds an elevated sedimentation rate and an elevated leukocyte count of from 15,000 to 30,000. One helpful, nonspecific laboratory finding that occurs in 85 to 90 per cent of patients with rheumatic fever is an elevation of *antistreptolysin serum titers;* a positive finding indicates that the patient's body has formed antibodies against one or more streptococcal antigens. Also, 50 per cent of patients with active rheumatic fever have a throat culture that is positive for *beta-hemolytic group A streptococci.*

ECG Findings. The presence of rheumatic carditis is best established by serial ECG tracings. A prolonged P-R interval, irregular rhythm, and signs of atrial fibrillation are the major evidence of myocardial damage.

Physical Examination. The final diagnosis of rheumatic fever rests upon the following physical findings: the presence of two or more of the following symptoms: carditis, Sydenham's chorea, subcutaneous nodules, erythema marginatum, and polyarthritis; evidence of a recent beta-hemolytic streptococcal infection; and prompt relief of fever and joint pain by salicylate administration.

Evidence of rheumatic *carditis* is based on typical ECG findings; presence of mitral or aortic diastolic murmurs; and signs of fibrous or pleuritic type pericarditis and/or CHF.

CLINICAL CARE

The major goals of care in the treatment of patients with rheumatic fever are:

1. To control and alleviate the infecting streptococci.
2. To protect the heart against the highly damaging effects of carditis.
3. To relieve joint pain, fever, and other symptoms.

Typical measures used in the care of patients with rheumatic fever are bed rest, proper diet, and chemotherapy with penicillin, salicylates, and steroids.

Bed Rest. A patient with rheumatic fever must rest for two reasons: to reduce strain on his heart, and to minimize metabolic needs during the acute, febrile stage of the disease.

When on bed rest the patient may be allowed by his doctor to perform certain self-care activities, e.g., turning himself, brushing his teeth, feeding himself, combing his hair. He may also enjoy nonstrenuous diversional activities such as watching television, reading, and listening to the radio. Short visits from relatives and friends are usually permitted, provided the visitors are free from colds, flus, and sore throats.

The patient must generally remain on bed rest for a period of several weeks or longer. He may not begin to ambulate or care for himself until the following criteria are met: his *temperature* remains normal without the use of salicylates; his *resting pulse* (in adults) remains under 100; his *ECG* tracings show no signs of myocardial damage; and his *sedimentation rate* returns to normal.

Once the patient is up and about, he must still be cautioned not to overdo. How long the patient's activities must be restricted depends upon whether carditis develops and the extent of permanent heart damage resulting from such carditis.

Restrictions may extend for many months; in severe cases of rheumatic carditis, patients may even be forced to undergo restrictions on a permanent basis; e.g., they may have to change occupations if their job is strenuous, move from a two-story house to a one-story house, and so forth. When significant changes in life style are necessary, patients can obtain guidance from the Crippled Children's Division of the Federal Children's Bureau and from the American Heart Association.

Diet Therapy. The patient with rheumatic fever needs a bland, high-protein, high-carbohydrate diet in order to maintain adequate nutrition in the face of fever and infection. The doctor may also order supplements of vitamins and minerals. Fluids should be forced to prevent dehydration due to fever. If the patient shows signs of severe carditis or CHF, a low-sodium diet is necessary; fluids may also be restricted.

Encourage the patient (who is often anorexic) to eat all his meals. You may have to feed him if his activity has been severely curtailed because of cardiac involvement.

Drug Therapy. The three major groups of drugs used to treat rheumatic fever are antibiotics, salicylates, and steroids. The antibiotics employed are *penicillin* and the *sulfonamides.* These drugs are given for 10 days following the onset of rheumatic fever in order to destroy any streptococci remaining alive in the upper respiratory tract. Following this 10-day period, prophylactic doses of these drugs are given to prevent fresh attacks of streptococcal infection.

The *salicylates* are given to control fever and to relieve joint pain. *Sodium salicylate* is the most commonly used drug in the salicylate group. The maximum adult dose of this drug is 1 to 2 Gm. (15 to 30 gr.) every 2 hours orally. For patients with heart failure, aspirin is ordered in place of sodium salicylate. Observe patients taking salicylates carefully for early signs of toxicity.

> *Early signs of salicylism include tinnitus, nausea, and vomiting.*

To reduce gastric irritation, salicylates are usually given with an antacid, or enteric-coated tablets are used.

Steroids are frequently given to patients with severe rheumatic fever to relieve symptoms. Fever, joint pain, and swelling are often dramatically reduced within 24 to 48 hours. However, steroid therapy probably neither prevents nor minimizes rheumatic carditis and its damaging aftereffects.

PROPHYLAXIS

First attacks of rheumatic fever are entirely preventable today, provided patients with streptococcal infections receive prompt antibiotic therapy. Also, patients who have recovered from an attack of rheumatic fever may prevent *subsequent* attacks by taking prophylactic doses of antibiotics and observing good health practices. Patients should be told that it is important that they avoid subsequent attacks of rheumatic fever, since repeated attacks may lead to serious heart disease, which can result in permanent cardiac disability and failure.

Penicillin is the prophylactic drug most frequently given, although the sulfonamides may be ordered if the patient is sensitive to penicillin. Two typical orders are penicillin, 200 to 250 thousand units orally before breakfast, or benzathine penicillin (Bicillin), 1 million units monthly. Additional doses of prophylactic penicillin must be taken before and after undergoing surgical procedures and dental extractions. Prophylactic drugs are usually given for a period of five years following the initial attack; after five years, recurrences are uncommon.

The patient must also take good care of teeth and gums and receive prompt dental care for cavities and gingivitis. Persons who have upper respiratory infections or who have had a streptococcal infection within the last three months should be avoided. Finally, the physician should be called immediately if any of the symptoms of streptococcic sore throat (pharyngitis) develop; it is extremely important that antibiotic therapy be received promptly for any infection.

The symptoms of streptococcic sore throat are an elevated temperature of 38.9° to 40° C. (102 to 104° F.), chills, sore throat, and enlarged painful lymph nodes. The patient must take excellent care of himself and guard against infections for the *rest of his life* if he is to avoid the possible development of heart disease.

PROGNOSIS AND COMPLICATIONS

Since the advent of antibiotic therapy, the prognosis for patients with rheumatic fever is generally good. Today, only 1 to 2 per cent of patients die during the initial attack; in these cases, death usually results from acute myocarditis. Most patients recover rapidly; laboratory and clinical signs generally completely subside within one to two months following therapy. However, some patients have residual heart damage, which may lead to either valvular stenosis or regurgitation. Should these patients have recurrent attacks of rheumatic fever, residual heart damage may eventually terminate in congestive heart failure. Fortunately, in some cases valvular disease can be successfully corrected by surgery before failure ensues.

Serious complications of rheumatic fever that may disable the patient or claim his life are: CHF (the major cause of death); infarctions of the brain or kidneys due to embolization of valvular vegetations or mural thrombi within the heart; bacterial endocarditis; and pulmonary congestion due to left-sided heart failure, which may result in deadly pulmonary infections.

DISEASES THAT AFFECT THE ENDOCARDIUM

You will recall from Chapter 46 that the endocardium is a layer of endothelial tissue that lines the heart's cavities and aids in the formation of the valves. Diseases that may affect the endocardium are bacterial endocarditis (acute and chronic), chronic valvular heart disease, and rheumatic endocarditis.

BACTERIAL ENDOCARDITIS

Definition and Characteristics

Bacterial endocarditis is a severe bacterial infection of the endocardium. It is characterized by the formation of friable vegetations on the heart valves, and by the metastatic spread of bacteria from the valves via the blood stream to organs and tissues all over the body. Bacterial endocarditis is usually fatal unless the patient receives antibiotic therapy.

There are two classic forms of bacterial endocarditis: acute bacterial endocarditis (ABE) and subacute bacterial endocarditis (SBE).

Acute bacterial endocarditis is a severe infection of fulminating onset characterized by high fever, heart murmurs, embolic phenomena, and splenomegaly. It is usually caused by highly pathogenic organisms capable of producing widespread damage, such as *Staphylococcus aureus,* pneumococci, beta-hemolytic streptococci, and gonococci. The infection follows a rapid course, and the endocardium may be severely damaged early in the disease. It is responsive to antibiotic therapy.

Subacute bacterial endocarditis is a smoldering infection manifested by a continuous fever, weight loss, fatigue, joint pains, and splenomegaly. The causative organisms are indigenous to the body and cause relatively little destruction; they include *Streptococcus viridans, S. faecalis,* and *Staph. aureus.* The onset is insidious and the course prolonged, but with adequate antibiotic therapy, there is little or no damage to the endocardium.

The incidence of bacterial endocarditis is much lower today than in the past because of the development of antibiotics. It is estimated that it currently represents approximately 1 per cent of all cardiac disorders. Persons between the ages of 20 and 40 are most susceptible to this disorder; however, bacterial endocarditis is currently striking older persons far more often than it did formerly.

Predisposing Factors

How do bacteria enter the body, overcome the body's natural barriers against invasion, and reach the heart valves? To quote Robbins:

> Two considerations are important in the production of these infections on the heart valves: (1) factors that predispose to the bacterial invasion of the heart valves and (2) portals of entrance of organisms into the blood.[136]

One factor that *predisposes* the patient's heart valves to bacterial invasion is *preexisting disease or injury* of the heart valves as a result of rheumatic, syphilitic, or arteriosclerotic heart disease or congenital anomalies. A second factor to consider is the *virulence* of the attacking bacteria. Bacteria of low virulence attack only damaged valves, but bacteria of high virulence can attack and destroy normal valves in patients with no preexisting heart disease.

Bacterial endocarditis usually follows *acute infection* of the tonsils, kidneys, gums, teeth, or lungs. However, bacteria can also enter the circulation following such simple maneuvers as vigorous brushing of the teeth or chewing hard foods or candies. It may also follow *heart surgery,* as a result of poor surgical technique or contamination. Finally, bacteria can be introduced into the body by contaminated needles and careless technique in the parenteral administration of drugs; for this reason, drug addicts are often victims of bacterial endocarditis.

Causative Organisms

In recent years, antibiotic therapy has brought about a substantial change in the organisms responsible for bacterial endocarditis. The incidence of infections caused by staphylococci has at least doubled in the last 30 years while frequency of infections due to *Streptococcus viridans* has been cut almost in half. The increased incidence of the staphylococci and *Streptococcus faecalis* as causative factors is evidently due to the development of antibiotic-resistant strains of these organisms. Other antibiotic-resistant organisms that are causing increased numbers of infections are fungi and gram-negative bacilli. On the other hand, pneumonococci, gonococci, and meningococci have been virtually eliminated as causative agents because these organisms are so highly sensitive to penicillin and other antibiotics.

Pathophysiology

As in rheumatic endocarditis, the lesion characteristic of bacterial endocarditis is a *friable vegetation* that forms on the valve leaflets. Such vegetations can severely damage not only the heart valves but other organs located throughout the body. The amount of damage caused depends on the type and virulence of organisms causing the infection; e.g., staphylococci are far more virulent organisms than is *Streptococcus viridans* and thus they cause larger vegetations more rapidly. Common complications resulting from the growth of vegetations on the valves are: perforation of the valve leaflets; extension of the bacteria to the aorta or to the pericardium; metastatic spread of the infecting organism from the valves through the blood stream, causing abscess formation within the myocardium, spleen, kidneys, and brain; and infarction of the spleen, brain, gastrointestinal tract, and other sites as a result of shedding of vegetations into the blood stream as *emboli.*

Symptoms and Complications

The signs of bacterial endocarditis can be categorized into three major groups:[164]

1. Those due to infection.
2. Those due to cardiac involvement.
3. Those due to emboli.

The signs of *infection* comprise the most outstanding manifestations of bacterial endocarditis. The most reliable sign of infection is *fever,* a manifestation of bacterial endocarditis present in all patients. Typically the fever is *remittent* in nature, with afebrile periods lasting from days to weeks. Other signs of infection are chills, night sweats, fatigue, anorexia, weight loss, "aches and pains," cough, and loss of libido.

Signs of *cardiac involvement* are usually related to the presence of either rheumatic heart disease or congenital heart disease. Typical manifestations include: tachycardia, splenomegaly, petechiae of the skin and mucous membranes, clubbing of the fingers and toes in longstanding cases of heart disease, pallor, joint swelling and pain, arthritis, and painful nodes of the finger and toe pads, which occasionally result from endothelial swelling.

The most important cardiac sign is a *cardiac murmur,* which varies in character from day to day. These variations represent the growth and fragmentation of the valvular vegetations.

Finally, *embolic phenomena* disrupt organ functions all over the body, causing widely divergent symptoms. When the left side of the heart is involved, vegetation fragments are swept into the arterial circulation, which carries them to the spleen, kidneys, gastrointestinal tract, brain, and extremities where they then create large and small areas of infarction. When the *right* heart is involved, emboli pass into the pulmonary circulation; these fragments may then clog the arterioles of the lungs, causing pulmonary infarction.

The *spleen* is the organ most commonly affected by emboli, followed next by the kidney. Signs of *splenic* infarction are tenderness and enlargement of the spleen, and pain in the upper abdomen. Key signs of *renal* involvement are flank pain and hematuria. When the arterioles of the *brain* are obstructed by emboli, the patient typically experiences sudden visual problems, an inability to speak, and paralysis of one side of the body. When emboli lodge in the arterioles of the *extremities,* gangrene of the toes or fingertips may result. Finally, *pulmonary* embolism is characterized by severe dyspnea, hemoptysis, cough, and pleuritic pain.

The symptoms of ABE and SBE were mentioned previously. Patients afflicted with ABE suffer higher fevers than those with SBE, severe chilling, and rapid weight loss. The vegetations produced on the valve leaflets are larger, and embolic phenomena are far more severe than in the subacute form of the disease. Patients with SBE appear to be chronically ill rather than acutely ill; they look thin and drawn, are tired, and are ashen in color.

The *complications* of bacterial endocarditis are many; the most dangerous are congestive heart failure, which often results directly from endocarditis; perforation or destruction of the aortic valve; infarction of the spleen, kidney, and so forth; embolism; anemia; and metastatic abscess formation.

Diagnosis

Correctly diagnosing bacterial endocarditis is a challenging task even for the most experienced physician. The reason the disease is so difficult to diagnose is because the majority of its symptoms are vague and nonspecific and could easily be attributed to several different infections and cardiac ailments. Even though embolic phenomena produce dramatic specific symptoms, the organs involved are generally far removed from the heart; consequently, many physicians fail to connect splenic or renal infarction with infectious heart disease.

The major method of diagnosis is examination of *blood cultures.* Typically, three to five blood specimens are drawn over a 36- to 48-hour period. In 85 to 90 per cent of patients blood cultures are positive by the third day. Other helpful but nonspecific laboratory findings in bacterial endocarditis are elevated sedimentation rate, anemia, leukocytosis, and microscopic hematuria, proteinuria, and casts.

Clinical Care

The five major aims of clinical care for patients with bacterial endocarditis are:

1. To identify the infectious organism.
2. To destroy the infectious organism, thereby halting the growth of vegetations on the heart valves.
3. To protect the heart from permanent damage and valvular destruction.
4. To prevent relapses and recurrent fevers.
5. To surgically correct reparable valvular deformities, congenital defects, and so forth.

These goals are met by means of general therapeutic measures, antibiotic therapy, and surgical techniques.

General Therapeutic Measures. Patients are generally hospitalized for from two to six weeks. Complete bed rest is generally not enforced unless fever or signs of heart damage are evident. Fever, when present, is relieved by means of rest, cooling measures, forced fluids, and the administration of aspirin. As in most infectious processes, the patient should be encouraged to eat a nutritious diet, to drink sufficient fluids, and to rest mentally and physically.

Antibiotic Therapy. The mainstay of treatment in bacterial endocarditis is the administration of antibiotics. Before the advent of antibiotics almost all persons afflicted with bacterial endocarditis died; patients still die when antibiotic therapy is not adequate.

The major principles of antibiotic therapy in the treatment of bacterial endocarditis are as follows:

> By means of blood cultures, the physician must discover to which antibiotic the infecting organism is *sensitive.*

> The antibiotic used must be *bactericidal* rather than bacteriostatic.

> The antibiotic must be ordered in *sufficiently large doses;* the serum level of the drug should be at least five to 10 times that needed to destroy the organism.

> Drug therapy needs to be continued for at least *four to six weeks* or the patient may suffer a severe relapse once the drug is discontinued.

> Antibiotics must be administered *exactly at the specified time intervals* or the blood levels of the antibiotic will fall, which, in turn, leads to the further multiplication and growth of organisms.

For most cases of bacterial endocarditis the ideal antibiotic is *penicillin;* this drug is particularly useful in the control of *Streptococcus viridans* infections. The dosage prescribed depends upon how sensitive the organism is to penicillin. Dosages range from 2.4 million units per day (for sensitive organisms) up to 100 million units per day (for penicillin-resistant organisms). In some cases streptomycin is given concurrently with penicillin. The combination of streptomycin and penicillin is particularly effective against *S. faecalis.*

Penicillin is almost always given *parenterally,*

either in divided doses I.M. or by a slow continuous I.V. drip. When given intravenously, the penicillin dosage is diluted in 1 to 2 liters of physiologic saline or glucose and administered to the patient over a 24-hour period. Because the patient will receive the I.V. drip over a long period of time (four weeks or longer), it is important to prevent complications from inactivity. Encourage the patient to turn, move, and deep breathe. If the needle is securely in the vein and the I.V. tubing is sufficiently long, movement should not disrupt the infusion. Once the patient begins to ambulate, obtain a movable I.V. stand so that the patient can push the stand and I.V. bottle ahead of him as he walks. Emphasize to patients that they should not remain immobile simply because they have an I.V. running.

Some patients are allergic to penicillin. In these cases the doctor may attempt to control the allergy with antihistamines and steroids. If severe allergies persist, the doctor then discontinues penicillin altogether and orders another antibiotic such as tetracycline, erythromycin, or chloromycetin. Unfortunately these drugs are not so effective as penicillin, and the patient will almost always suffer a relapse following therapy.

Criteria indicating control of the infection are the following:

> Fever, sweats, fatigue, tachycardia, and anorexia should gradually disappear within three to five days following the beginning of therapy.

> Weight gain and improvement in the blood picture should occur during the second week.

> Urinary function should steadily improve over the four- to six-week period of therapy.

Two major *complications* that can arise during the treatment period or soon afterward are embolic episodes and relapses. *Emboli* are fairly common during the first three months following the initial administration of antibiotics. Evidently emboli result from the shrinking and shedding of vegetations as the endocardium undergoes healing and repair. Fragmentation of vegetation with resultant embolism sometimes continues for as long as one to two years following the beginning of therapy.

Relapses usually occur within one to two weeks following cessation of therapy, although patients sometimes relapse months after treatment. Some reasons for relapses are ineffective antibiotic therapy, too short a period of treatment, drug reaction, embolism, metastatic abscess formation resulting from seeding of the blood with bacteria, thrombophlebitis, superinfection with other organisms, or the presence of an underlying disease such as rheumatic fever. Relapses are diagnosed on the basis of symptoms (a rise in fever, nodules, anorexia) and positive blood cultures. The physician generally treats the patient with a higher dosage of antibiotic given over a longer period of time or with a different antibiotic.

Surgical Techniques. Although surgery is sometimes a factor in causing bacterial endocarditis, it also plays a significant role in its cure. Some of the current uses of surgery in treating bacterial endocarditis and its sequelae are: removal of infected valves, drainage of abscesses in the heart and elsewhere, removal of congenital shunts, repair of injured valves and chordae tendineae, and splenectomy for splenic abscess or infarction.

Prognosis

Only 10 per cent of patients with bacterial endocarditis die of the primary disease; deaths are due to antibiotic-resistant infections or occur during relapse. Another 20 per cent die from complications: *cardiac failure* as a result of valvular damage or aortic insufficiency, *embolization* due to fragmentation of vegetations, or *renal insufficiency* caused by renal infarction. Of the 70 per cent of patients remaining, some will recover almost totally, whereas others may be burdened with a permanently damaged heart and possibly renal insufficiency.

Factors that determine the prognosis of bacterial endocarditis are: (1) the presence of preexisting heart damage; (2) the development of distorted valves and/or cardiac failure during the course of the disease; (3) the severity of embolic episodes; (4) the nature of the infecting organism (virulent or nonvirulent); (5) the duration of time between onset of the disease and therapy; (6) response of the organism to the antibiotic (antibiotic-sensitive or -resistant); (7) degree of kidney damage; and (8) the valve affected (aortic valve involvement is more serious than mitral valve involvement). The outlook is excellent for patients who are properly treated early in the course of the disease and who do not develop serious cardiac or renal lesions.

CHRONIC VALVULAR HEART DISEASE

The heart valves, when healthy, keep blood flowing through the heart and lungs in the proper direction. Diseased valves may *impede* the flow of blood from one chamber to the next (valvular *stenosis*) or they may allow blood to leak or regurgitate back into the chamber from which the blood is being propelled (valvular *insufficiency* or *regurgitation*). Either problem places great stress upon the heart. For a time the heart may be able to compensate for the additional strain by myocardial hypertrophy. However, if valvular damage worsens and the patient is not treated, CHF will eventually develop.

While any valve can be damaged, the mitral valve is the most commonly affected, followed in incidence by the aortic valve and the tricuspid valve. It is rare for the pulmonary valve to be involved. Below is listed the incidence of various forms of valvular disease.

Mitral valvular disease—50 to 60 per cent of all cases.

Combined mitral and aortic valvular disease—20 per cent.

Aortic valvular disease—10 per cent.

Pulmonic valvular disease—very rare.

The *diagnosis* of valvular heart disease is based upon: the patient's past history of heart disease (e.g., evidence of rheumatic fever or bacterial endocarditis); the presence of a significant murmur; and the detection of valvular lesions on x-ray, fluoroscopy, angiography, or ECG studies, or during cardiac catheterization.

Valvular heart disease is almost always treated *surgically*. The damaged valve may be repaired or it may be removed and a prosthetic valve sutured into its place.

One commonly used prosthetic valve is the *ball-in-cage* type, which is sewn into the valvular opening when the diseased valve is removed (Fig. 53–1). All parts of this metallic valve but the stainless steel ball within the cage are covered with woven Dacron mesh, a material upon which endothelial cells will grow rapidly. Advantages of this type of valve over the *homograft* valve (Fig. 53–2) are that it can be stored indefinitely until used, and it cannot be destroyed by the disease process that destroyed the patient's own natural valve.

Complications resulting from the insertion of ball-in-cage type valves are: (1) displacement of the valve owing to broken sutures; (2) loss of the ball or entire valve; (3) leakage within the artificial valve system, resulting in regurgitation; and (4) ventricular arrhythmias and trauma due to irritation of the ventricles by an improperly fitted metal cage. However, despite such problems, prosthetic valve replacements are enabling many patients with valvular heart disease to lead fuller and more productive lives.

Mitral Valvular Disease

As you recall from Chapter 46 the mitral or bicuspid valve lies between the *left* atrium and ventricle.

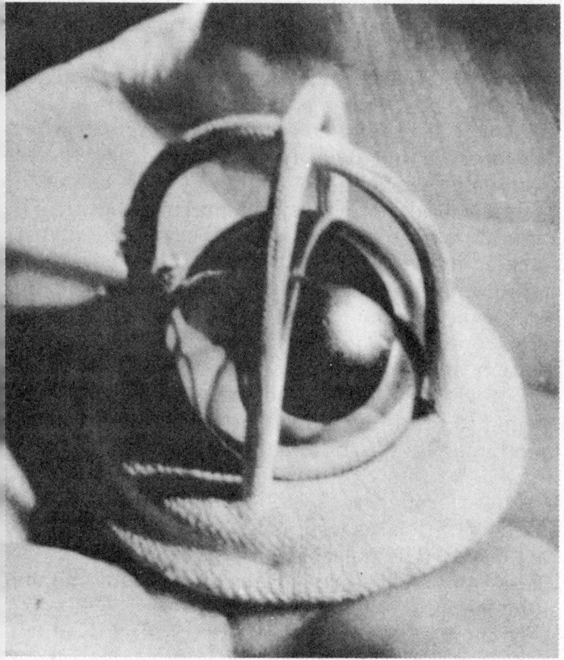

FIGURE 53–1. A prosthetic ball-in-cage type valve. (From Longmore, D.: *The Heart.* World University Library. New York, McGraw-Hill Book Company, 1971.)

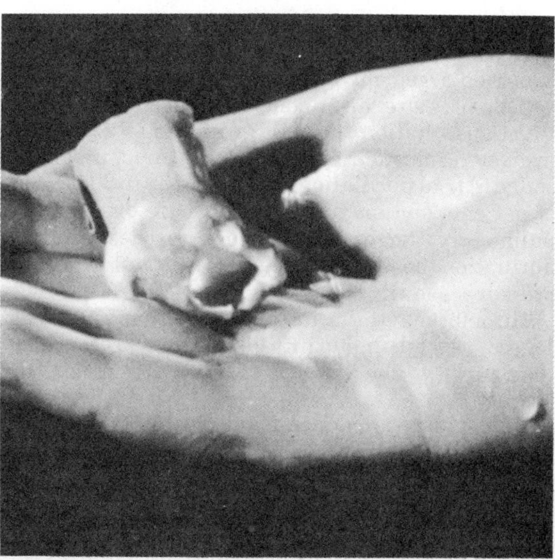

FIGURE 53–2. An aortic homograft valve reconstructed from its freeze-dried state by immersion in normal saline solution. (From Longmore, D.: *The Heart.* World University Library. New York, McGraw-Hill Book Company, 1971.)

It is the primary task of the mitral valve to promote blood flow *forward* from the left atrium to the left ventricle and to prevent the *backward* leakage of blood from the ventricle to the atrium. Lesions of the mitral valve tend either to obstruct the flow of blood from atrium to ventricle (stenosis) or to allow blood to leak back from ventricle to atrium (regurgitation). In either case, the left atrium is overworked. As a result, left atrial hypertrophy develops, followed by pulmonary congestion, overwork of the right ventricle, and right heart failure. Without treatment, patients with either mitral stenosis or regurgitation will die in CHF.

Mitral Stenosis. Mitral stenosis is the commonest lesion of the mitral valve. About three fourths of the patients are women under the age of 45. As acute rheumatic endocarditis heals, the valve leaflets retract, the chordae tendineae contract and shorten, and the mitral commissures fuse. As the valves become calcified and immobile the valvular orifice narrows, preventing normal passage of blood from left atrium to left ventricle. The left atrium hypertrophies to compensate for the strain of pushing blood through the narrowed orifice. The overload of blood trapped in the atrium causes pulmonary hypertension and congestion, the congestion, in turn, overworking the right ventricle and causing right ventricular failure. The inadequate filling of the left ventricle leads to reduced cardiac output and fatigue. In longstanding cases the left ventricle may shrink and even atrophy.

The symptoms of mitral stenosis may appear gradually or quite suddenly. The first symptom is usually excessive fatigue, but this may be accompanied by shortness of breath, cough, bronchitis, orthopnea, paroxysmal nocturnal dyspnea, cyanosis, and pulmonary edema. Failure of the right heart may cause enlargement of the liver, edema, increased venous pressure, and abdominal discomfort.

On auscultation there is a rumbling, low-pitched presystolic murmur and a snapping, loud, first heart sound. Atrial fibrillation develops in 50 to 80 per cent of patients and may precipitate acute dyspnea and pulmonary congestion. During episodes of atrial fibrillation the pulse is irregular and faint; the blood pressure is low.

Thrombi may form in the left atrium and be released as emboli during fibrillation. The emboli may travel to the kidneys, spleen, extremities, and brain.

Hemoptysis is common and results from long-standing pulmonary venous hypertension; it may be mild or severe.

Mitral stenosis may be diagnosed by angiography, cineangiography, catheterization of the left heart, ECG to determine signs of right ventricular hypertrophy, or ultrasound techniques to determine mobility of the mitral valve.

Treatment is surgical and consists of commissurotomy or prosthetic valve replacement. (See Chapter 54.)

Mitral Regurgitation. Mitral regurgitation is a less common phenomenon than mitral stenosis. The majority of patients are men. Although rheumatic fever is the principal cause, it may be a congenital anomaly or develop secondary to bacterial endocarditis or aortic valvular disease.

When the mitral valves atrophy, the left atrium dilates and hypertrophies to compensate for the increased load of blood leaking back from the left ventricle through the valve. This also causes pulmonary congestion and resulting right heart failure and its sequelae.

Many patients never develop cardiac symptoms, but most feel great fatigue, followed by dyspnea on exertion, and cough. The pulmonary symptoms are less severe than in mitral stenosis, but when the right heart is affected, the symptoms are the same.

On auscultation there is a blowing, high-pitched systolic murmur, and a third heart sound is present. Atrial fibrillation may occur, but does not precipitate acute pulmonary congestion.

The pulse is usually normal and adequate in volume, but will become irregular if fibrillation occurs. The blood pressure is normal or low.

Although emboli and hemoptysis do occur, their appearance is far less frequent than in mitral stenosis. Fatigue is quite pronounced because of the left ventricular failure.

Diagnosis is made by fluoroscopy and by injection of indicator dye into the left ventricle; prompt appearance of the dye in the left atrium gives a positive diagnosis.

Treatment is surgical and may be either valvuloplasty or valve replacement with a ball-in-cage prosthesis.

Aortic Valvular Disease

The aortic valve lies between the aorta and left ventricle. During systole it opens so that blood can flow from the ventricle into the aorta; during diastole it closes to prevent leakage of blood from the aorta back into the left ventricle.

Aortic valvular disease is far less common than is mitral valvular disease, although it often occurs in conjunction with mitral disease. Lesions of the aortic valve act to obstruct the flow of blood forward from the left ventricle into the aorta and systemic circulation (stenosis) or they allow blood to leak back from the aorta into the left ventricle (regurgitation or insufficiency). Both aortic stenosis and regurgitation overwork the left ventricle. Left ventricular hypertrophy develops as a compensatory measure and, in turn, is followed by atrial hypertrophy, pulmonary congestion, and right ventricular failure. Thus, aortic valvular disease, like mitral valvular disease, ends in CHF.

Atrial fibrillation and embolic phenomena are characteristic of mitral valvular disease, whereas angina pectoris and syncope result from aortic valvular disease.

Aortic Stenosis. Aortic stenosis accounts for one fourth of the patients suffering from chronic valvular disease; 80 per cent are male. It may be either congenital or acquired. Acquired disease may result from rheumatic endocarditis or, among the elderly, atherosclerosis.

In stenosis the aortic valve opening narrows, and the valve flaps fuse as a result of inflammation or growth of atherosclerotic plaques. The left ventricle hypertrophies without dilating to compensate for the stress of pumping blood through the narrowed opening. The cardiac output is low. The left atrium cannot empty normally, and pulmonary circulation becomes congested, placing the right ventricle under such stress that it will fail if treatment is not received.

Patients may remain asymptomatic until they are 30 or 40 years old. The first symptom is usually fatigue, followed by angina pectoris and dyspnea on exertion. The dyspnea is caused by the elevation of the left ventricular end-diastolic pressure, which also increases left atrial and capillary pressures. Late in the disease orthopnea, paroxysmal nocturnal dyspnea, and pulmonary edema may occur. The anginal pain probably develops because the hypertrophied left ventricle requires less blood as a result of the stenosis of the valve, causing a decreased cardiac output and a shortened diastole.

Syncope often occurs on exertion or change in position and may be caused by insufficient aortic output which produces inadequate flow of blood and oxygen to brain, by overactive carotid sinus reflex, by Adams-Stokes syndrome, or by transient arryhthmias.

A harsh, rough midsystolic murmur may be heard on auscultation, as well as a systolic thrill over the aortic area. The pulse is slow and small in volume. The systolic blood pressure is normal, but the diastolic is high.

Symptoms usually arise late in the disease and include extreme weakness, fatigue, debilitation, venous hypertension, edema, hepatomegaly, and ascites.

Diagnosis is made by left heart catheterization; aortic, coronary, and left ventricular angiograms, and ECG.

Surgery is the treatment of choice but is performed only when lesions are severe because of the high risk. Either valvulotomy or cusp or valve replacement by a prosthesis may be done.

Aortic Regurgitation. Aortic regurgitation occurs one half as frequently as aortic stenosis, and once again the majority of patients are male (75 per cent). It, too, may be congenital or acquired. Rheumatic endocarditis is the principal cause; syphilis may be an occasional etiologic factor.

The opening of the aortic valve widens, and valve flaps, deformed by infectious processes, fail to close properly during diastole, allowing blood to regurgitate from the aorta back into the left ventricle. The left ventricle dilates and hypertrophies to compensate for the greater load of blood. Unless treated, left ventricular failure will be followed by right heart failure.

The first symptom is usually sinus tachycardia or premature systoles, and is followed by dyspnea on exertion and angina pectoris. These symptoms may not appear until the patient is 30 or 40. The exertional dyspnea, as well as orthopnea and paroxysmal nocturnal dyspnea, develops as a result of pulmonary congestion. Late in the disease the patient may experience dyspnea at rest. Anginal pain develops for the same reasons as in aortic stenosis. Late in the disease the symptoms are similar to those experienced by patients with aortic stenosis.

On auscultation there is a soft, blowing aortic diastolic murmur and a forceful apical impulse. The systolic blood pressure is normal or slightly elevated, but the diastolic is low.

Diagnosis is made by angiocardiograms, ECG, and indicator dilution studies with opaque dye.

Treatment by surgery is undertaken only when disease is severe, and consists of the removal of the damaged leaflet and the suturing of the two normal cusps together to form a bicuspid valve, or replacement of the cusp or valve by a prosthesis.

Tricuspid Valvular Disease

The tricuspid valve guards the opening between the right atrium and right ventricle. Pure lesions of the tricuspid valve are relatively uncommon. Usually tricuspid stenosis or regurgitation develops in combination with other structural disorders of the heart.

Lesions of the tricuspid valve place great stress on the right side of the heart. As a result, these disorders inevitably produce *right heart failure.* Treatment involves correction of the valvular deformity and alleviation of the heart failure.

Tricuspid Stenosis. Tricuspid stenosis occurs predominantly in females. It is a relatively rare phenomenon and usually occurs in combination with mitral and/or aortic valvular disease. It may be congenital. It is most commonly a sequela of rheumatic fever.

The valve opening narrows and the valve flaps fuse as a result of endocardial inflammation. Blood is blocked on its return to the heart and lungs, with resulting venous engorgement and right heart failure. Failure of the right heart produces hepatomegaly, dependent edema, ascites, extreme fatigue, and cardiac cirrhosis. The resulting jaundice and cyanosis give the patient a slate-colored complexion.

Auscultation shows a rumbling diastolic murmur. There is a presystolic pulsation in the liver.

Chest x-rays show an enlarged right atrium. The diagnosis is confirmed by angiogram.

Treatment may be medical (low-sodium diet, diuretics, and digitalis) or surgical (valve repair or prosthetic replacement).

Tricuspid Regurgitation. Tricuspid regurgitation is relatively rare; it is found more frequently in children than in adults. It may be congenital, but more frequently follows rheumatic fever, bacterial endocarditis, or trauma.

As a result of inflammation the tricuspid valve widens and the valve flaps are unable to close securely. Blood leaks back into the right atrium as well as being pushed forward into the pulmonary circulation, causing venous engorgement and right heart failure.

Symptoms are the same as in tricuspid stenosis and the slate-colored complexion is sometimes seen.

A blowing holosystolic murmur is heard on auscultation. Atrial fibrillation is usually present.

An angiogram is diagnostic. Chest x-rays show an enlarged right atrium and ventricle.

Treatment is the same as for tricuspid stenosis.

Pulmonic Valvular Disease

Lesions of the pulmonic valve are extremely rare and will not be discussed.

DISEASES THAT AFFECT THE MYOCARDIUM: MYOCARDITIS

Acute myocarditis is an inflammatory condition of the myocardium. It develops either during or following diseases of viral, bacterial, rickettsial, spirochetal, fungal, or parasitic origin. Frequently acute myocarditis develops secondary to acute endocarditis or pericarditis.

The major cause of acute myocarditis is *rheumatic fever;* diphtheria, subacute bacterial endocarditis, trichomoniasis, and influenza are also associated with the development of this condition.

The symptoms are generally vague and nonspecific. In mild cases of myocarditis, symptoms are absent and diagnosis is made only on the basis of serial ECG readings, which typically reveal T wave abnormalities. In more severe cases the manifestations of myocarditis are generally obscured by the manifestations of the primary disorder, e.g., rheumatic fever, SBE, diphtheria. Thus, the patient may experience a variety of symptoms: fever, leukocytosis, fatigue, nausea and vomiting, anorexia, tachycardia, and chest pain. Shock and death may occur in young adults affected with severe myocarditis.

Myocarditis is diagnosed on the basis of ventricular enlargement and heart failure that develops suddenly and without apparent cause; i.e., there is no evidence of valvular heart disease or any other heart condition that can cause failure.

Patients with acute myocarditis are treated with digitalis and placed on complete bed rest until symptoms of infection and inflammation lessen and disappear. Overexertion and stress during the critical symptomatic period of myocarditis can result in sudden death.

DISEASES OF THE PERICARDIUM: ACUTE AND CHRONIC PERICARDITIS

Pericarditis is an inflammation of the visceral or parietal pericardium, or both, often resulting in compression of the heart, critical decrease in ventricular filling and empyting, and cardiac failure. This inflammatory process may develop either as a primary condition or secondary to a number of different diseases and circumstances, e.g., rheumatic fever, uremia, tuberculosis, collagen diseases, various infections (bacterial, viral, fungal), cancer, myocardial infarction, toxic overdose, and trauma.

Pericarditis is classified as either acute or chronic. Acute pericarditis, in turn, is classified as *dry* (fibrinous) or *exudative* (pericarditis with effusion). The exudate may be serous, purulent, or hemorrhagic. When fluid accumulates very rapidly or accumulations are large, *cardiac tamponade* develops and the heart is unable to expand and fill with blood; decreased filling, in turn, leads to drastically reduced cardiac output, shock, and death.

Chronic pericarditis is usually called *chronic constrictive* or *adhesive* pericarditis. A constrictive, sometimes calcified membrane around the heart prevents filling and emptying of the ventricles, eventually resulting in cardiac failure.

Acute Pericarditis

As stated previously, acute pericarditis is an acute inflammation of the pericardium that may be either dry or exudative.

Acute Fibrinous Pericarditis. This may result from virus infections, tuberculosis, bacteremia or septicemia of the pericardium, or spread from a contiguous organ. Delicate "violin string" adhesions form and may completely obliterate the pericardial sac, but they rarely spread to the thoracic wall, diaphragm, or lungs, and cardiac action is infrequently hampered.

On auscultation there is a to-and-fro friction rub over the precordium that is synchronous with the systole and diastole. The sound, which usually persists for seven to 10 days, may be soft and scratchy, loud and leathery, or low and grating.

Dyspnea is often present. There is chest pain that varies from mild to severe over the precordial or substernal area. It radiates to the shoulder and neck and down the left arm; it is aggravated by swallowing, coughing, and lying supine. The temperature may be elevated to 37.8 to 39.4° C. (100-103° F.), depending on the underlying infection. Fever also increases the pulse rate. Tachycardia is usually present. The patient is pale, anxious, and restless, and appears acutely ill.

Blood tests show a leukocytosis of 10,000 to 20,000. Chest x-ray will usually reveal cardiac dilatation. ST-T changes on the ECG are probably related to the myocarditis that so frequently accompanies pericarditis.

Treatment includes bed rest, analgesics (acetylsalicylic acid for mild pain, morphine sulfate for severe), and appropriate antibiotics.

Acute Pericarditis with Effusion. Acute pericarditis with effusion may follow acute fibrinous or acute purulent pericarditis or be caused by tuberculosis, malignant disease, myxedema, nephrosis, or advanced congestive heart failure.

Fluid accumulates within the pericardial sac, compressing the heart and reducing ventricular filling and arterial pressure. Cardiac action is severely hampered, leading to heart failure. Dyspnea and orthopnea are always present.

The friction rub heard in acute fibrinous pericarditis usually disappears when effusion develops but may occasionally be heard.

Pain may or may not be present; when present it may resemble that caused by acute fibrinous pericarditis or be dull, diffuse, and oppressive. The distended pericardium compresses the bronchi and lungs, causing a cough and making it necessary for the patient to sit up and lean forward to breathe.

The temperature may be elevated. The pulse is paradoxic; it fluctuates with respiration and is lowest at the end of each full inspiration. Neck veins are distended as a result of the reduced ventricular filling. The patient is acutely ill.

Leukocyte counts are elevated to 10,000 to 20,000. Pericardial fluid is aspirated for culture, for cytologic examination, and for determination of specific gravity and protein content. With large effusions the normal contours of the heart may not be discernible on chest x-ray. Fluoroscopy will reveal a decrease in the pulsations of the heart. Cardiac catheterization and angiocardiography are also useful diagnostic aids.

Bed rest, analgesics, and antibiotics are ordered. The physician may tap the pericardial sac, aspirating the collected fluid and instilling penicillin or streptomycin directly into the sac. Drainage may require incision of the chest wall.

Complications of Acute Pericarditis. The only important complication of acute fibrinous pericarditis is *pericardial effusion*. The major complication of pericarditis with effusion is *cardiac tamponade*.

Cardiac tamponade signifies an acute compression of the heart due to an accumulation of fluid within the pericardial sac. This critical condition develops when either the amount of fluid within the pericardial sac is very large or fluid has accumulated rapidly; e.g., sudden hemorrhage into the pericardial sac. Large or rapidly accumulating effusions raise the intrapericardial pressure to a point at which venous blood is unable to flow into the heart, which, in turn, decreases ventricular filling. As a result, venous pressure rises and cardiac output and arterial blood pressure fall. The heart attempts to compensate in this emergency by beating rapidly (tachycardia). However, tachycardia can sustain the patient's cardiac output for only a short period of time; without immediate treatment, the patient is doomed to die in shock.

The symptoms of cardiac tamponade are the same as the manifestations of shock, pericarditis with effusion, and venous congestion. In shock the patient experiences hypotension, tachycardia, cyanosis of lips and nails, restlessness, pallor, and diaphoresis. A paradoxic pulse, muffled heart sounds, and dyspnea result from the pericardial effusion. When the veins become congested those in the neck are distended, there is increased venous pressure, liver enlargement, ascites, and edema of the legs.

The patient with cardiac tamponade needs immediate treatment! The emergency treatment of choice is a pericardial paracentesis (i.e., aspiration of fluid from the pericardial sac). This relieves the pressure on the heart and thereby improves cardiac function. In many cases this procedure is lifesaving.

Chronic Constrictive Pericarditis

Chronic constrictive pericarditis is a chronic inflammatory condition in which the pericardium changes into a thick, fibrous, sometimes calcified band of unyielding tissue that encircles, encases, and compresses the heart, thereby preventing proper ventricular filling and emptying. The eventual result of this slow, unrelenting compression is cardiac failure.

Frequently a sequel to tuberculosis, chronic constrictive pericarditis is characterized by symptoms of right heart failure and inadequate cardiac output; e.g., fatigue on exertion, dyspnea, leg edema, ascites, low pulse pressure, distended neck veins, and prolonged circulation time. However, this condition is occasionally asymptomatic.

Chronic constrictive pericarditis is treated both medically and surgically. The patient is treated to relieve symptoms of congestive heart failure, with the doctor ordering digitalis, diuretics, and a low sodium diet. Surgical treatment involves excision of the damaged, constricting pericardium (i.e., pericardectomy). Surgery offers hope of cure to approximately 60 per cent of persons disabled by constrictive pericarditis.

CHAPTER 54

Care of Patients Undergoing Heart Surgery

In 1925 Sir Henry Soutlar of London performed the first heart surgery—a closed repair of a stenosed mitral valve. Since that time heart surgery has been revolutionized by the development of open heart techniques that allow the surgeon to directly visualize the heart while he explores, cuts, repairs, and sutures. Such optimal operating conditions have enabled modern surgeons to replace diseased valves with prosthetic valves, to repair severe congenital lesions, and to perform heart and heart-lung transplants.

TYPES OF HEART SURGERY

There are two major types of cardiac surgery: closed heart surgery, and open heart surgery. *Closed heart* surgery is performed without the benefit or hazards of *extracorporeal circulation* (ECC; cardiopulmonary bypass). ECC is a procedure in which a machine (the *pump oxygenator* or *heart-lung machine*) completely controls cardiopulmonary function, thereby enabling surgeons to operate for lengthy periods without the patient's becoming anoxic. Examples of closed heart procedures are (1) closed mitral commissurotomy to correct mitral stenosis (Chapter 53), (2) implantation of an internal mammary gland (Vineberg operation) to perfuse the heart with blood from a source other than the coronary arteries (Chapter 51), and (3) procedures that correct abnormal congenital shunts.

Conversely, *open heart procedures,* because of their lengthiness and complexity, must be performed with the aid of ECC. Examples of major open heart procedures are: total replacement of a diseased valve with a prosthetic valve (Chapter 53) and heart transplants.

HEART TRANSPLANTS

Since the 1960's heart transplants have been widely publicized and discussed throughout the world. The first successful human heart transplant was performed in Cape Town, South Africa, by the then obscure surgeon, Christiaan Barnard. By the end of 1970, 166 more heart transplants had been performed, but only 23 patients were living; i.e., the heart transplant procedure had had a discouraging 85 per cent mortality rate.[161]

The greatest single problem in performing heart transplants is not the surgical procedure itself, but the *rejection* process by which the patient's body rejects the donor's heart.* This process is poorly understood; however, physiologists do know that following implantation of the donor heart, plasma cells attack the donor cells and destroy them by upsetting their metabolic processes. Also, the patient forms antibodies against the foreign heart tissue, which leads to an antigen-antibody reaction. As a result, the heart's lining hemorrhages, the heart walls thicken, and the myocardium assumes a mottled appearance; finally, the new heart fails to function altogether and circulatory collapse ensues. As one surgeon sadly states:

> If only we could overcome rejection, the transplantation of the heart would become as routine as valve replacement now is (and that was rare enough only five years ago). Nothing is more encouraging than the *immediate* betterment that follows the replacement of a worn-out heart by one that is young and vigorous. Men and women who could not cross the room without the most crippling and undignified pain are younger and more sprightly almost from the moment they gain consciousness.... Few surgical procedures offer such a rapid and deep-reaching improvement.[103]

Unfortunately, until medical scientists overcome the rejection process, the gratifying results described above are only temporary; the majority of patients respond briefly and brilliantly only to die soon after surgery.

OPEN HEART SURGERY: BENEFITS AND PROBLEMS

As stated before, the greatest advantage of open heart surgery is that it allows the surgeon to directly visualize the heart while he operates. However, before open heart procedures could be developed, surgeons had to discover how to either: (1) slow or halt the patient's circulation for a period of time without causing brain anoxia (hypothermia), or (2) detour the blood that would normally enter the heart

*The process of allograft rejection is discussed in Chapter 23.

and lungs through an artificial heart-lung machine (ECC).

*Hypothermia** was the first technique to make open heart surgery possible. One purpose of hypothermia is to *decrease* the patient's *metabolic needs,* thereby automatically lowering the rate at which he uses oxygen. Another purpose is to provide the surgeon with a *bloodless field* in which to operate; the patient's reduced need for oxygen allows the surgeon to clamp off the venae cavae and azygos veins, thereby halting circulation through the heart for a period of time.

How long circulation can be stopped depends upon the *depth* of hypothermia. At normal body temperature the circulation can be stopped for only 2 to 3 minutes without tissue damage from anoxia. However at 28°C. (moderate hypothermia), circulation can be stopped for a period of 15 to 20 minutes—adequate time to complete certain simple procedures. At 10°C. (profound hypothermia) circulation can be halted for about 1 hour, during which time the blood is pumped through a heat exchanger; however, surgery must be completed within the hour or the patient may die unless rewarmed.

To induce hypothermia, the patient is anesthetized; next, his body is cooled in a hypothermia blanket that maintains his temperature at the desired level.†

The major danger of hypothermia is *ventricular fibrillation,* which occurs when the temperature drops to around 26°C. Other complications are cardiac arrest and cardiac failure.

Today, hypothermia is being almost universally replaced by total cardiopulmonary bypass (ECC). However, some surgeons continue to use moderate or profound hypothermia in combination with ECC.

*Hypothermia is discussed briefly in Chapter 28.

†Use of the hypothermia blanket is discussed in Unit VIII.

While hypothermia is suitable for surgery of short duration, only ECC can be used for extremely complex surgical procedures such as valve replacement or heart transplants. Thus, the heart-lung machine, more than any other apparatus, has made sophisticated open heart surgery possible.

The first pump-oxygenator was used with a human patient in 1951 in an unsuccessful attempt at ECC. Two years later the machine was used again in the successful repair of an atrial septal defect; the patient lived for 30 minutes while on cardiopulmonary bypass. Since 1955 improved versions of the machine have been built, and ECC is now routinely used throughout the world for open heart surgery.

The purposes of the heart-lung machine are four: (1) to divert the circulation from the heart and lungs which, in turn, provides the surgeon with a bloodless field in which to operate; (2) to perform all gas exchange functions for the body while the patient's heart and pulmonary systems are at rest (i.e., O_2-CO_2 exchange); (3) to filter, rewarm, or cool the blood; and (4) to circulate the oxygenated, filtered blood back into the patient's arterial system.

Briefly, the procedure for ECC is as follows: first the machine is primed (filled) with 3 or 4 liters of either heparinized blood or a blood substitute such as low molecular weight dextran (Rheomacrodex) or Ringer's lactate solution. When the patient's chest is opened the surgeon inserts two large bore cannulas through the right atrium into the superior and inferior venae cavae. The venous blood is next aspirated from the venae cavae by a vacuum pump into the heart-lung machine (Fig. 54–1). An oxy-

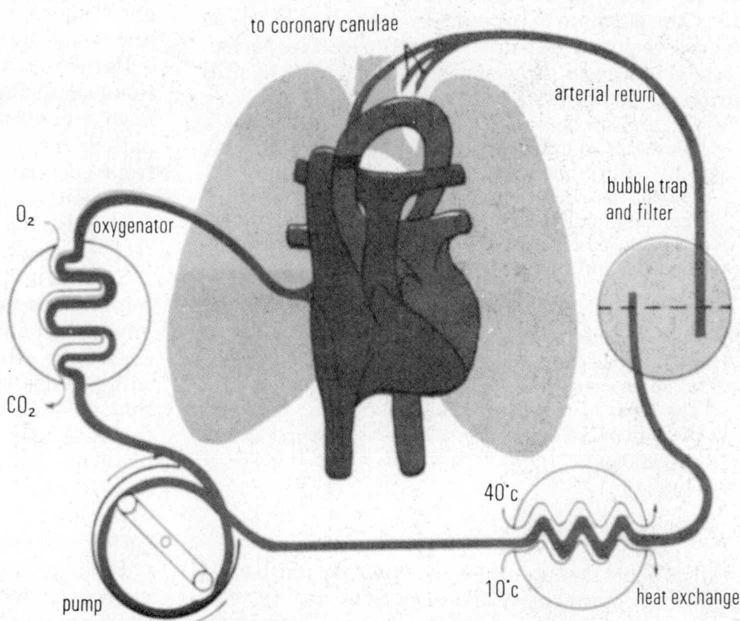

FIGURE 54–1. Schematic circuit of a heart-lung bypass. (From Longmore, D.: *The Heart,* World University Library, New York, McGraw-Hill Book Company, 1971.)

genator removes CO_2 from the blood and adds oxygen. The oxygenated blood is then pumped to a heat exchanger where it is rewarmed (or cooled if the surgeon desires hypothermia). Next the blood passes through a filter that removes air bubbles and other emboli. Finally, the blood is returned to the body via either the aorta or femoral artery.

Despite its beneficial effects, the use of the heart-lung machine is not without its dangers. For example, the pump can crush and destroy blood cells; also, sludging of cells sometimes occurs, leading to thrombus formation. Finally, air emboli can form as a result of excess oxygen absorption.

Other specific complications which are apparently related to ECC are: low cardiac output syndrome (shock), hemolysis and hemorrhage, lung damage, and kidney damage. These complications will be discussed under postoperative care.

PREOPERATIVE CARE

In Unit VI we discussed in detail the preparation of a patient for general surgery. All the information given in Unit VI is applicable to patients about to undergo heart surgery. However, because heart surgery is a particularly stressful experience, patients facing cardiac operations need special preparation and instruction in certain areas.

Patient's History

The patient you admit for heart surgery has probably suffered from cardiac and pulmonary symptoms for months or years. The extent of the patient's cardiac and pulmonary disability will naturally affect the outcome of his surgery as well as the type of care required during the postoperative period. Facts you need to know about the patient's physical status are as follows:

> The heart condition for which the patient is being surgically treated and its duration.

> The purpose of the surgery and the risk involved.

> Past cardiopulmonary illnesses that may predispose the patient to postoperative complications, e.g., bacterial endocarditis, pulmonary embolus, allergy, abnormal bleeding.

> The degree of cardiac impairment that the patient suffers; i.e., does he have symptoms or is he asymptomatic? Does the patient have symptoms when at rest or only when he exerts himself?

> The types of medications and therapeutic measures that the patient has received or is currently receiving, e.g., digitalis, quinidine, IPPB, oxygen.

Psychologic Preparation

All patients facing surgery, of whatever nature, are somewhat apprehensive. Those patients facing *heart* surgery often develop feelings of fear, depression, and despair that are overwhelming. Because fear can adversely affect the patient's *physiologic* response to surgery, it is important to allow the patient to ask questions and freely express his emotions about the coming operation. A preoperative program of instruction designed to reduce anxiety concerning heart surgery and the recovery period should include these four areas:

General Information. Information should be given concerning hospital rules and regulations; visiting hours in the ICU; the priest, rabbi, or minister who will be on duty and his visitation hours; and the house doctors and nursing supervisor whom the patient's family can contact for information on the day of his surgery and throughout the postoperative period

Most patients benefit from a tour of the recovery room and intensive care unit. It is helpful to introduce patients to the staff who will be caring for them. Familiarize the patient with the equipment that he will be seeing and using in the ICU, e.g., chest drainage tubes, oxygen apparatus, cardiac monitors, and I.V. setups.

Verbal Instruction. Instruct the patient concerning his heart condition, contemplated surgery, preoperative care and convalescence. However, before giving instruction in these areas, always ask the doctor what information he has already given the patient; also find out if the doctor wants any information withheld. Let the patient tell you in his own words what he understands to be wrong with his heart. Correct any misconceptions the patient may have about his disease and the corrective surgery he will undergo. Simple graphic charts and a model of the heart and its valves will help the patient to learn and to remember more easily.

Preparing for surgery is an area of concern for many patients. One study indicates that patients want to learn about the following aspects of preoperative care: diagnostic tests (electrocardiograms, electroencephalograms, and pulmonary function tests); blood replacement therapy; the surgical prep; and anesthesia (sleeping medications, anesthesiologist's visit on the eve of surgery, and state of consciousness immediately prior to the operation).[21]

Patients tend to ask the greatest number of questions about the *recovery room* and *ICU;* therefore, it is wise to discuss these two areas thoroughly. If the patient has not toured the facilities, he will benefit from a description of the areas. Patients feel far more confident once they learn that highly skilled nurses will care for them in a well-equipped, heavily staffed, special area of the hospital.

Second, prepare patients for what to expect as they regain consciousness in the recovery room. For example, tell the patient that he will awaken with a chest tube, which drains blood and air from his chest so his lungs can reexpand. Also inform the patient that he will be receiving oxygen via tent or mask, that an I.V. or blood transfusion will be running into his arm, and that he will be attached to a cardiac monitor. Emphasize that although the patient will experience pain, the pain will be relieved by medication and comfort measures.

Finally, explain to the patient that he will be awakened frequently in the ICU to receive vital nursing care. Give him examples of the types of scheduled activities for which he will be aroused; i.e., vital signs every 15 minutes; temperature every 2 hours; turning, coughing, deep breathing every hour; blood drawn for tests every morning, and so forth.

Patients also need information concerning discharge from the ICU and hospital. Areas of interest are the average length of stay in the ICU, the room to which the patient will return from the ICU, the average length of stay in the hospital, and the diet and activities permitted on return home. Be very general in your discussion of these points; remember that many unforeseen events can arise in surgery and in the ICU that can greatly alter the patient's postoperative course.

Demonstrations and Practice Sessions. Demonstrate deep breathing, range of motion, and coughing exercises, and use of the IPPB. Allow the patient to practice these activities under your supervision. Emphasize the vital importance of proper breathing, coughing, and movement.

Postoperative patients have expressed conflicting views about what they felt patients should be told beforehand concerning pain, hallucinations, and so forth. It is evident that patients differ significantly in the types of information they find helpful. Some wish to know everything and others nothing. Thus, the instruction of patients prior to heart surgery *must be highly individualized.*

Physiologic Preparation

It is important for patients to be in the best physical condition possible before undergoing the stresses of heart surgery. Thus, patients are generally admitted to the hospital a few days prior to the surgery for a thorough medical evaluation. During the preoperative period the goals of care are: (1) to conduct diagnostic and laboratory studies; (2) to correct any metabolic imbalances, infections, and arrhythmias; and (3) to establish baselines for vital signs, weight, ECG, and so forth—signs that can be used for comparison during the postoperative period.

Preoperative *laboratory tests* include urine, blood, electrolyte, and enzyme studies. Important *diagnostic studies* that give valuable information about cardiac status are the ECG, phonocardiogram, vectorcardiogram, chest x-rays, and cardiac catheterization.

Second, *existing imbalances* and *cardiac and pulmonary ailments* are corrected by means of rest, diet, and drugs. For example, CHF is treated with digitalis, low-sodium diet, rest, and diuretics; arrhythmias are corrected with quinidine or cardioversion; latent or residual infection is corrected by antibiotic therapy; K^+ imbalance is controlled by potassium triplex.

Finally, to establish *baselines* for postoperative comparisons, weigh preoperative patients daily and take their vital signs (including apical-radial pulse) every 4 hours.

Immediate Preoperative Care

The preparation of patients on the evening before and the day of heart surgery is essentially the same as the preparation of patients for chest surgery.* The patient's skin is prepped for a thoracotomy; if cardiopulmonary bypass is to be done, the inguinal area is also shaved. The nurse usually inserts a nasogastric tube and a Foley catheter on the morning of surgery.

POSTOPERATIVE CARE

General Observations and Orders

Following heart surgery the patient is admitted to the recovery room or intensive care unit. For the first 48 hours following his operation the patient needs constant professional observation and care, for it is during this period that the most serious complications arise.

Typical observations and orders for patients immediately following general surgery have been discussed in Unit VI. In addition to these general duties, you will also perform special tasks when caring for patients following heart surgery.

A summary of the early postoperative care is given herewith:

> Check blood pressure and pulse every 15 minutes for 12 hours; report systolic BP of below 80 or 90 mm. Hg, depending on the surgeon's order.

> Check all pulses (apical, radial, and pedal).

> Note level of consciousness; report to surgeon if patient does not awaken within 1 hour after surgery.

> Check pupils for size, equality, and reaction to light. Report to physician if pupils are unequal in size, are dilated, or fail to react to light.

> Connect central venous pressure catheter to a manometer at level of heart, monitor CVP continuously, and record findings every 15 minutes. Report CVP to surgeon if above 12 cm. H_2O or below 8 cm. H_2O.

> Elevate head of bed to semi-Fowler's position to facilitate chest drainage and lung reexpansion.

> Continuously monitor ECG. Note and report frequent premature contractions (atrial, nodal, or ventricular). These arrhythmias foreshadow more serious arrhythmias.

> Continuously administer oxygen to patient via tent or mask for first 24 hours following surgery, then discontinue oxygen if patient's condition has stabilized.

> Milk chest tubes hourly to dislodge clots; prevent kinking of tubing; record amount and color of drainage hourly.

> Measure urine volume hourly. Report to surgeon if urine output is below 20 ml. for 2 consecutive hours. Note color of urine and record specific gravity. Keep a cumulative hourly intake and output record.

> Begin deep breathing, coughing, IPPB, and range of motion exercises as soon as patient fully regains consciousness.

> Measure temperature hourly; report elevation of over 101°F.

*Review immediate preoperative care for patients undergoing general surgery, Unit VI.

> Administer I.V. infusions and blood transfusions per cutdown according to physician's orders.
> Schedule chest x-ray daily per doctor's order.
> Schedule daily electrolyte studies as ordered.

GOALS OF CARE FOR PATIENTS FOLLOWING CARDIAC SURGERY

Goal 1: Promote cardiovascular function, tissue perfusion, and stabilization of vital signs.
Goal 2: Promote respiratory function by promoting chest drainage and use of IPPB.
Goal 3: Promote fluid, electrolyte, and nutritional balance.
Goal 4: Promote renal function.
Goal 5: Promote rest, comfort, and relief from pain.
Goal 6: Promote neurologic function.
Goal 7: Promote psychologic adjustment to postoperative period.
Goal 8: Promote early movement and ambulation.
Goal 9: Prevent postoperative complications.

Goal 1: Promote Cardiovascular Function, Tissue Perfusion, and Stabilization of Vital Signs

The most reliable measures of cardiovascular function and tissue perfusion are the vital signs. Stabilization of vital signs following heart surgery usually indicates adequate cardiovascular function, whereas severe deviations indicate complications such as hemorrhage, shock, cardiac tamponade, or infection. The normal ranges for each vital sign following cardiac surgery and the meaning of deviations are as follows:

Arterial Blood Pressure

1. Maintain systolic BP between 20 mm. above and 20 mm. below normal baseline BP taken preoperatively. Following mitral and aortic commissurotomy, patients tolerate low systolic blood pressure of 90 or 80 mm. Hg without difficulty. Following surgery on coronary arteries, patients cannot tolerate systolic BP drop of more than 10 mm. Hg below preoperative baseline because myocardium will be inadequately perfused.
2. Causes of decreased blood pressure following heart surgery are pain, inadequate movement, cardiac tamponade, fear, low cardiac output syndrome, thrombosis blocking site of graft or anastomosis, metabolic acidosis, hemorrhage, overmedication with narcotics, arrhythmias, and hypovolemia.
3. Complications resulting from persistent hypotension are cerebral ischemia, renal shutdown, and myocardial infarction.

Pulses (Radial, Apical, Temporal, Posterior Tibial and Dorsalis Pedis)

1. Check *radial pulse* for rate, rhythm and volume. *Rapid* radial pulse may indicate arrhythmias, shock, fear, fever, hypoxia, CHF, or hemorrhage. *Slow* radial pulse may indicate heart block or severe anoxia.
2. Check *apical-radial pulse* for a difference in number of beats per minute. *Pulse deficit* may indicate atrial fibrillation—a frequent complication of mitral stenosis.
3. Check for presence of *pedal pulses* (over posterior tibial artery and dorsalis pedis artery). Absence of pedal pulses may indicate presence of peripheral emboli blocking blood vessel in extremity; report immediately to surgeon. If pulses are absent, check skin of lower extremities for coldness and cyanotic appearance.

Venous Pressure

1. Normal reading: 4 to 12 cm.
2. Normal range following heart surgery: 12 to 30 cm.; higher venous pressure promotes more efficient filling of heart and stronger ventricular contractions.
3. Causes of abnormally *elevated* CVP are hypervolemia, and ineffective myocardial contractions.
4. Abnormally *decreased* CVP results from hypovolemia.

Temperature

1. Normally the temperature rises 2 or 3 degrees above normal during the first or second day postoperatively and remains elevated for 3 to 4 days. Treat with aspirin (on doctor's orders) and minimal bed covering; for persistent elevations, icebags or a hypothermia blanket may be ordered.
2. Reportable abnormal findings are elevation to 102.2° F. (38.9° C.) or higher, or an elevation that persists for more than 4 or 5 days. Abnormal temperature elevation may be caused by infection, dehydration, hemolysis due to transfusion reaction, or atelectasis. The untoward effects of the elevated temperature are increased metabolic demands, which augment work of the heart, and dehydration and hypovolemia.

Abnormally low temperatures range from 34.4°C. (94°F.) to 36°C. (96.8°F.) and may be caused by shock or cardiac decompensation. The physician may order an electric blanket to increase temperature.

Electrocardiogram

1. Electrical activity of patient's heart is monitored continuously for at least 3 or 4 days following surgery.
2. Observe carefully for abnormal ECG tracings; heart block, ventricular tachycardia, and atrial fibrillation are common complications of open heart surgery.

Goal 2: Promote Respiratory Function and Sufficient Oxygenation by Promoting Chest Drainage and Use of Intermittent Positive Pressure Breathing Treatment (IPPB)

Adequate respiratory function depends upon the maintenance of a clear and open airway, removal of excess pulmonary secretions, proper aeration of lungs and oxygenation of blood, and the maintenance of chest tube patency and drainage. Observations of respiratory function and care of respiratory problems and complications include the following:

Observe and Promote Patency of Airway. See also Unit VI.

Observe Respirations

1. *Rate: Rapid* respirations may indicate airway obstruction, atelectasis, pain, fear, anoxia, excessive respiratory secretions, respiratory and metabolic acidosis, and acute gastric dilatation; *slow* respirations may indicate pain, extreme carbon dioxide retention, and overmedication with narcotics—particularly morphine sulfate.
2. *Depth:* Shallow respirations may be due to pain; give small dose of narcotic if vital signs are stable.
3. *Dyspnea:* Difficult breathing may be result of retained secretions in lungs, acidosis or hemorrhage; treat with oxygen set at 5 liters/min. per nasal cannula or at 10-12 liters/min. per oxygen tent.
4. *Cheyne-Stokes pattern:* May indicate onset of CHF.
5. *Grunting upon expiration:* Usually indicates airway obstruction; endotracheal intubation may be necessary.
6. *Wheezing:* Results from pulmonary edema, bronchospasm, or airway obstruction.

Observe and Control Pulmonary Secretions

1. Observe *amount:* Copious or scant.
2. Observe *color:* White or pale yellow secretions are normal; green and brown secretions may indicate pulmonary infection; large amounts of frothy secretions usually indicate pulmonary edema.
3. Observe for *accompanying signs* of retained secretions: apprehension, perspiration, rapid pulse, dyspnea, cyanosis, gurgling respirations.
4. Carefully avoid *complications* of retained secretions—atelectasis and cardiac failure.
5. Control *retained pulmonary secretions* by deep breathing exercises 5 to 7 times per hour, coughing, and turning every hour; endotracheal suction; IPPB with aerosol therapy (mucolytic agent used to help thin viscous secretions); open top tent with high humidity to help liquefy and loosen secretions; or bronchoscopy or tracheostomy if thick secretions obstructing airway cannot be removed.

Observe Skin. Observe patient's skin coloring for duskiness, mottling, or frank cyanosis; if duskiness appears, oxygen is usually given at 5 liters/min. per nasal cannula.

Chest Drainage. Check chest drainage from chest tubes.*

1. Chest tubes are indicated for pleural cavity; tubes drain fluid and air from the cavity, thereby allowing the lungs to reexpand following surgery. They are also used for drainage of the pericardial sac.
2. Measure and observe chest drainage by collecting drainage in a calibrated cylinder. Measure findings and record hourly. In *normal findings* the amount of drainage varies with the nature of the surgery and the patient's general condition. Up to 100 ml. of drainage may be lost during the first hour postoperatively as a result of reexpansion of the lungs, which forces drainage through chest tube. There will be approximately 500 ml. of drainage over first 24 hours, with an average of 20 to 30 ml. lost per hour. Large gushes of drainage are sometimes expelled when the patient turns or coughs. Drainage is usually dark red during the early postoperative period; it gradually becomes more serous as time passes.

Abnormal findings, which are reportable, include amounts of drainage in excess of 5 ml./kg. of body weight/hour; a sustained hemorrhage that lasts for more than 1 minute; and sudden cessation of chest drainage accompanied by increase in venous pressure, dyspnea, and oliguria, which may indicate intrathoracic bleeding with accumulation.

Blood is replaced by transfusion. The chest drainage is usually replaced milliliter for milliliter with intravenous blood. In some cases, blood transfusions continue until the CVP is normal.

Chest tubes are milked every hour to express clots, which could block drainage, and checked for kinks or bending. Chest wound infection is prevented by prophylactic administration of antibiotics. Portable chest x-rays are taken daily until lungs have reexpanded.

*Care of patient with chest tubes discussed in Unit XIV.

Goal 3: Promote Fluid, Electrolyte, and Nutritional Balance

Following heart surgery, the patient typically receives parenteral fluids, blood transfusions, water within 12 hours after surgery, clear liquids, solid foods, and then a full diet, which is usually low in sodium.

Parenteral Fluids

1. I.V. fluids are administered judiciously for the first 3 days postoperatively to avoid overload of the circulatory system, which can result in overwork of the heart.
2. Typically administer 500 to 700 ml. per square meter body surface per 24 hours (including oral intake).
3. Parenteral fluids most commonly used include Ringer's lactate solution and dextrose in water.
4. Sodium-containing fluids are rarely used, as they may lead to circulatory overload (hypervolemia) and heart failure.

Blood Transfusions. These are administered to replace blood lost in chest drainage.

Oral Liquids and Solids

1. Water is allowed 12 hours postoperatively if patient is fully responsive and not nauseated; clear liquids are allowed next, followed by solid foods.
2. Watch for signs of abdominal distention and paralytic ileus (see Unit VI); if either of these conditions develops, stop oral fluids at once and notify physician.

Electrolyte Balance

1. Daily electrolyte studies are ordered to determine blood levels of Na^+, K^+, Mg^{++}, and Cl^-; electrolytes are replaced parenterally if deficient.

2. Hematocrit, hemoglobin, prothrombin time, serum fibrinogen and euglobulin tests are ordered daily to determine extent of blood loss or hemorrhage.

3. Blood gas determinations of pCO_2 and pO_2 are ordered. (See Chapter 25.)

Nursing Duties

1. Careful measurement and recording of intake and output.

2. Daily weighing of patient to determine if he is holding fluids within his tissues or is losing excessive fluid rapidly; significant fluctuations in weight act as a guide to fluid replacement.

Goal 4: Promote Renal Function

To estimate the adequacy of the patient's renal function, carefully note and record volume, color, and specific gravity of urine; also check patient for signs of subrapubic distention.

Volume

1. Measure hourly for first 8 to 12 hours following surgery; patient almost always has a Foley catheter.

2. *Normal* findings: Output of 20 to 30 ml. per hour.

3. Reportable *abnormal* findings: Urine output less than 20 ml. for 2 consecutive hours.

4. Causes of oliguria or anuria are hypovolemia; hemolysis of erythrocytes during cardiopulmonary bypass, which causes sludging of blood in renal tubules; hypotension; and low output failure.

5. *Treatment* of oliguria involves increase in fluid intake if dehydration is present; correction of shock or low output failure; mannitol intravenously to increase renal blood flow, if indicated; and use of peritoneal dialysis or the artificial kidney in patients with renal shutdown.

Color. Urine color may be bloody as a result of hemolysis of erythrocytes during ECC.

Specific Gravity

1. Normal finding: 1.015 to 1.020.

2. Specific gravity may be *elevated* because of oliguria or presence of RBC's.

3. *Lowered* specific gravity results from overhydration and inability of kidney tubules to filter waste products.

Nursing Observations

1. Note intake and output.

2. Observe patient carefully for signs of bladder distention. (See Unit VI.)

Goal 5: Promote Rest, Comfort, and Relief from Pain

If the patient is to rest and sleep comfortably, pain must be relieved. Causes of pain and restlessness and their treatment are discussed in Unit VI. Some points specific to the relief of pain following heart surgery are outlined below:

Pain Medication

1. Administer Demerol hydrochloride 50-100 mg. every 3 to 4 hours for the first 24 to 48 hours postoperatively; administer judiciously, because large doses of narcotics suppress cough reflex.

2. Avoid overmedicating a patient who is still recovering from hypothermia; the body at this time is unable to metabolize the narcotic as quickly as normal, and the drug may accumulate in the patient's system.

3. Attempt to relieve patient's pain and restlessness with comfort measures prior to administering narcotic; e.g., change patient's position, splint incision during coughing, properly place pillows for support, give oxygen if anoxic, and so forth.

Splint Incision. Splint patient's incision firmly during his coughing and deep breathing exercises.

1. Use small pillow or hands to splint an anterior sternal splitting incision.

2. Use towel or hands to splint a lateral thoracic incision.

Goal 6: Promote Neurologic Function

Following heart surgery, you must carefully observe the patient's level of consciousness, pupil size and reaction, orientation, and ability to move extremities.

Level of Consciousness

1. Patient should awaken within 1 to 2 hours following surgery.

2. Failure to awaken may result from embolization of air, calcium, fat, or thrombotic particles to the brain.

3. *Slow* return of consciousness (over 2 to 4 days) may result from a diffuse neurologic deficit owing to poor cerebral capillary perfusion during ECC.

Eyes

1. Check pupils hourly during early postoperative period for size, equality in size, and reaction to light.

2. Pupils dilate when blood contains excess carbon dioxide.

Orientation

1. Disorientation and restlessness may indicate anoxia or embolization to the brain.

2. Mental confusion may also result from great fatigue or fear.

Ability to Move Limbs

1. Hemiplegia, inability to move an extremity, or extreme weakness of an extremity may indicate embolization to the motor area of the brain.

2. Check pedal pulses; absence of pulses may indicate presence of peripheral emboli blocking blood vessel to extremity.

Goal 7: Promote Psychologic Adjustment to the Postoperative Period

Following cardiac surgery, patients may become disoriented, delusional, and frankly psychotic; the majority of patients experience auditory or visual hallucinations. Also, severe depressions are not uncommon.

Causes of Confusion, Hallucinations, and Psychotic Behavior

1. Isolation within ICU.

2. Sensory deprivation.

3. Lack of rest and sleep over an extended period of time.

4. Fear and anxiety.

5. Depersonalization of the patient because of staff's preoccupation with monitors and machines.

6. Absence of normal day and night patterns (ICU's are active and well lighted 24 hours a day).

Causes of Postoperative Depression

1. Extreme fatigue and debility following surgery.

2. Prospect of future responsibilities that patient will face as he grows strong and well.

Prevention of Mental Confusion, Undue Fear, Anxiety, and Tension

1. Always address the patient by name and introduce yourself by name.

2. Have a calendar and clock beside the patient; orient him to the date and time of day.

3. Take an active interest in the patient; do not ignore *him* as you work with his monitor, IPPB apparatus, and so forth.

4. Position cardiac monitor so that it is out of the patient's view. Many patients are made unduly nervous by witnessing their own heart action.

5. Schedule the patient's day so that periods of nursing care alternate with periods of rest and relaxation.

6. Encourage patients to freely discuss their fears and anxieties.

7. Prepare patient's family for changes in patient's sensorium following surgery. Before the visiting hour, warn family members that patient is hallucinating or is severely depressed so that they are not unduly shocked.

Goal 8: Promote Early Movement and Ambulation

Prolonged periods of bed rest following heart surgery (or any surgery) may cause weakness, pooling of respiratory secretions, atelectasis, thrombophlebitis, osteoporosis, urinary retention, renal calculi, and a negative nitrogen balance. (See Chapter 27.) *Planned activity* is the most important single factor in preventing the complications of bed rest. The type and amount of activity that each patient is allowed will depend upon the type of surgery and the patient's general postoperative condition. Important considerations are as follows:

Position in Bed

1. Patient usually remains flat in bed until systolic blood pressure is over 100 mm. Hg; then patient may be placed in a semi-Fowler's position. Check BP again 5 minutes after patient assumes new position.

2. Patients recovering from coronary artery surgery should remain flat on their backs for 48 hours following surgery to prevent hypotension.

3. *Never elevate the patient's knees* because this position exerts pressure against the vessels of the lower extremities and may cause thrombosis.

Turning and Exercising

1. Following mitral, aortic, or congenital heart surgery patients are usually turned from side to side every 2 hours.

2. Following coronary artery surgery, patients may be turned from back to right side every 2 hours, once 48-hour period of rest flat in bed has passed.

3. Passive exercises and leg flexion every 2 hours to prevent thrombosis of lower extremities.

4. Active exercise of left shoulder is necessary to prevent "frozen shoulder," which results from lack of use of shoulder because of severe postoperative pain.

Typical Ambulation Schedule

1. On evening of operative day patient usually dangles for short period.

2. First day following surgery patient is generally allowed to sit in chair for a brief period of time.

3. Fifth to seventh day postoperatively patient begins to ambulate in room and down hallway.

4. By twelfth to fourteenth day patient is usually fully ambulatory.

5. Eight to 10 weeks is the normal length of time usually needed for patients to fully regain strength following surgery. Upon discharge home, the patient should gradually increase his activity until he can take moderate walks and climb stairs without undue fatigue. The patient usually returns to work between the second and third months following surgery.

Goal 9: Prevent Postoperative Complications

Observe the patient constantly for the following postoperative complications:*

1. Postoperative hemorrhage.
2. Shock due to hemorrhage, pain, or trauma.
3. Cardiac tamponade. (See Chapter 53.)
4. Renal insufficiency and renal shutdown due to shock, hemolysis, and afferent arteriolar vasoconstriction during ECC procedure.
5. Cardiac arrhythmias caused by K^+ imbalance, hypoxia, and acidosis. (See Chapter 50.)
6. Low cardiac output syndrome resulting from heart failure and metabolic acidosis.
7. Hypovolemia due to dehydration or severe bleeding.
8. Hypervolemia owing to fluid overload.
9. Electrolyte imbalances.
10. Respiratory insufficiency caused by inadequate exchange of respiratory gases during ECC.
11. Pneumothorax (inadequate lung expansion) resulting from blockage of chest tubes by kinks, blood clots, and so forth. (See Unit XIV.)
12. Wound infection, usually resulting from staphylococcal invasion.
13. Convulsions, hemiplegia, or limb weakness owing to embolization.
14. "Stress" ulcer resulting from reaction of body to prolonged physiologic stresses imposed by extensive surgery. (See Unit XV.)

*Postoperative complications are also discussed in Unit VI.

References for Unit X

1. Aagaard, G. N.: Treatment of hypertension. *American Journal of Nursing 73*:621, April, 1973.
2. Alexander, J. K., and Pettigrove, J. R.: Obesity and congestive heart failure. *Geriatrics 22*:101, July, 1967.
3. American College of Cardiology and Baptist Hospital, Nashville, Tennessee: *Advanced Cardiac Nursing*. Philadelphia, Charles Press Publishers, Inc., 1970.
4. Andreoli, K., et al.: *Comprehensive Cardiac Care: A Handbook for Nurses and Other Paramedical Personnel*. St. Louis, The C. V. Mosby Company, 1968.
5. Anthony, C. P.: *Textbook of Anatomy and Physiology*. 7th ed. St. Louis, The C. V. Mosby Company, 1967.
6. Baden, C. A.: Teaching the coronary patient and his family. *Nursing Clinics of North America 7*:563, September, 1972.
7. Bain, B.: Pacemakers and the people who need them. *American Journal of Nursing 71*:1582, August, 1971.
8. Bain, W. H., and Watt, J. K.: *Cardio-Vascular Surgery for Nurses and Students*. E. & S. Livingstone, Ltd., 1970.
9. Barbata, J. C., et al.: *A Textbook of Medical-Surgical Nursing*. New York, G. P. Putnam's Sons, 1964.
10. Barnes, R., and Schottstaedt, W. W.: The relation of emotional state to renal excretion of water and electrolytes in patients with congestive heart failure. *American Journal of Medicine 29*:227, August, 1960.
11. Barstow, R. E.: Diseases of the heart. *In* Moidel, H. C., et al. (eds.): *Nursing Care of the Patient with Medical-Surgical Disorders*. New York, McGraw-Hill Book Company, 1971.
12. Barstow, R. E.: Nursing care of patients with pacemakers. *Cardiovascular Nursing 8*:7, March-April, 1972.
13. Batson, H. M., et al.: Hypertension: Current trends in diagnosis and treatment. *Geriatrics 22*:134, November, 1967.
14. Beahrs, O. H., et al.: Goiter: The therapeutic choices. *Geriatrics 28*:80, July, 1973.
15. Beaty, H. N.: Bacterial endocarditis. *In* Conn, H. F. (ed.): *Current Therapy 1969*. Philadelphia, W. B. Saunders Company, 1969.
16. Beeson, P. B.: Bacterial endocarditis. *In* Beeson, P. B., and McDermott, W. (eds.): *Cecil-Loeb Textbook of Medicine*. 12th ed. Philadelphia, W. B. Saunders Company, 1967.
17. Bergersen, B. S., and Krug, E. E.: *Pharmacology in Nursing*. 11th ed. St. Louis, The C. V. Mosby Company, 1969.
18. Best, C. H., and Taylor, N. B. (eds.): *The Physiological Basis of Medical Practice*. 8th ed. Baltimore, The Williams & Wilkins Company, 1966.
19. Brachfeld, N., and La Due, J. S.: Congestive heart failure, coronary insufficiency and myocardial infarction. *In* Sodeman, W. A., and Sodeman, W. A., Jr. (eds.): *Pathologic Physiology: Mechanisms of Disease*. 4th ed. Philadelphia, W. B. Saunders Company, 1967.
20. Brainerd, H., et al.: *Current Diagnosis and Treatment*. Los Altos, California, Lange Medical Publications, 1969.
21. Brambilla, M. A.: A teaching plan for cardiac surgical patients. *Cardio-Vascular Nursing*, January-February, 1969.
22. Braunwald, E.: Chronic valvular heart disease. *In* Beeson, P. B., and McDermott, W. (eds.): *Cecil-Loeb Textbook of Medicine*. 12th ed. Philadelphia, W. B. Saunders Company, 1967.
23. Brener, E. R.: Surgery for coronary artery disease. *American Journal of Nursing 72*:469, March, 1972.
24. Brooks, S. M.: *Integrated Basic Science*. 2nd ed. St. Louis, The C. V. Mosby Company, 1966.
25. Browse, N. L.: *The Physiology and Pathology of Bed Rest*. Springfield, Ill., Charles C Thomas, 1965.
26. Buchholz, P. K.: Understanding the ECG. *R.N. 35*: 38, February, 1972.
27. Burke, G.: The treatment of angina pectoris. *Geriatrics 22*:168, May, 1967.
28. Burrell, Z. L., Jr., and Burrell, L. O.: *Intensive Nursing Care*. St. Louis, The C. V. Mosby Company, 1969.
29. Butler, H. H.: How to Read an ECG. (pictorial) Part 1. *R. N. 36*:35; (pictorial) Part 2. *36*:49, 1973.
30. *Cardiovascular Diseases in the U.S.: Facts and Figures*. New York, American Heart Association, 1965.
31. Carnes, G. D.: Understanding the cardiac patient's behavior. *American Journal of Nursing 71*:1187, June, 1971.
32. Carter, A. B.: Hypertension—Its causes and treatment. *Nursing Times 67*:531–33, May 6, 1971.
33. Cassem, N. H., et al.: Reactions of coronary patients to the CCU nurse. *American Journal of Nursing 70*:319, February, 1970.
34. Chaffee, E. C., and Greisheimer, E. M.: *Basic Anatomy and Physiology*. 2nd ed. Philadelphia, J. B. Lippincott Company, 1969.
35. *Chardack-Greatbatch Implantable Cardiac Pacemakers: Endocardiac and Myocardial Systems*. Technical Information Distributed by Corvek Medical Equipment Company, Portland, Oregon, for Medtronic, Inc.
36. Chatton, M. J., et al.: *Handbook of Medical Treatment*. 12th ed. Los Altos, Calif., Lange Medical Publications, 1970.
37. Clark, D. A., et al.: Cardiac transplantation in man. *American Journal of Medicine 54*:563, May, 1973.
38. Cogen, R.: Cardiac catherization: Preparing the adult. (Pictorial.) *American Journal of Nursing 73*:77, January, 1973.
39. Committee on Cardiopulmonary Resuscitation of the American Heart Association: *Emergency Resuscitation Team Manual: A Hospital Plan*. New York, American Heart Association, 1968.
40. Committee on Coronary Care Units and Cardiopulmonary Resuscitation: *Introduction to Arrhythmia Recognition*. California Heart Association, 1968.
41. Connar, R. G.: Cardiac arrest. *In* Conn, H. F. (ed.): *Current Therapy 1969*. Philadelphia, W. B. Saunders Company, 1969.
42. Coodley, E.: Anatomy of circulation: The failing heart. *Consultant 23*:106, July, 1972.
43. Coronary thrombosis. *Nursing Times 67*:744, June 17, 1971.
44. Correcting common errors in blood pressure measurement. (Programmed Instruction.) *American Journal of Nursing 65*:133, October, 1965.

45. Culbert, P., and Kos, B.: Teaching patients about pacemakers. *American Journal of Nursing 71*:523, March, 1971.
46. Davis, M. Z.: Socioemotional component of coronary care. *American Journal of Nursing 72*:1426, August, 1972.
47. Dawber, T. R., and Thomas, H. E.: Risk factors in coronary heart disease. *Cardio-Vascular Nursing 6*:29, January-February, 1970.
48. Dawson-Butterworth, K.: Heart-block and the nurse's role in treatment. *Nursing Mirror,* July 21, 1967, p. 372.
49. Delano, A., et al.: Monitoring the acutely ill cardiac patient. *Cardio-Vascular Nursing,* January-February, 1971.
50. Dembo, D. H.: Drugs for revival and survival. *Emergency Medicine 3*:27–30, June, 1971.
51. Drugs used in the care of the cardiac patient. *Nursing Clinics of North America 4*:645, December, 1969.
52. Dublin, L. I.: *Factbook on Man from Birth to Death.* 2nd ed. New York, The Macmillan Company, 1965.
53. Eich, R. H.: Tachycardia. *In* Conn, H. F. (ed.): *Current Therapy 1969.* Philadelphia, W. B. Saunders Company, 1969.
54. *Emergency Measures in Cardiopulmonary Resuscitation: Discussion Guide for Slide-Set.* Prepared by the Committee on Cardiopulmonary Resuscitation of the American Heart Association, 1969.
55. Escher, O. J. W.: Medical aspects of artificial pacing of the heart. *Cardiovascular Nursing 8*:1, January-February, 1972.
55a. Favaloro, R. G., et al.: Acute coronary insufficiency (impending myocardial infarction) and myocardial infarction: Surgical treatment by the saphenous vein graft technique. *The American Journal of Cardiology 28*:598, November, 1971.
56. Fisher, S.: Psychological factors and heart disease. *Circulation 27*:113, January, 1963.
57. Foster, S., and Andreoli, K. G.: Behavior following acute myocardial infarction. *American Journal of Nursing 70*:2344, November, 1970.
58. Fowler, N. O.: *Examination of the Heart: Part 2: Inspection and Palpation of Venous and Arterial Pulses.* Prepared for the Committee on Medical Education of the American Heart Association. New York, American Heart Association, 1970.
59. Fowler, N. O.: Sinus tachycardia—How to identify common causes. *Consultant 12*:47, March, 1972.
60. *Framington Heart Study: Detection of Factors Increasing Risk of Coronary Disease.* Bethesda, Maryland, The National Heart Institute, 1964.
61. Freis, E. D.: Office Evaluation of the Hypertensive Patient. Prepared for the Committee on Medical Education of the American Heart Association, 1969.
62. French, R. M.: *Nurse's Guide to Diagnostic Procedures.* 2nd ed. New York, Blakiston Division, McGraw-Hill Book Company, 1962.
63. Friedberg, C. K.: Coronary heart disease (ischemic heart disease). *In* Beeson, P. B., and McDermott, W. (eds.): *Cecil-Loeb Textbook of Medicine.* 12th ed. Philadelphia, W. B. Saunders Company, 1967.
64. Friedberg, C. K.: *Diseases of the Heart.* 3rd ed. Philadelphia, W. B. Saunders Company, 1966.
65. Friedberg, C. K.: Treatment of shock in acute myocardial infarction. *Postgraduate Medicine 42*:281, October, 1967.
66. Gazes, P. C.: Cardiac failure in adults—Signs and symptoms. *Postgraduate Medicine 49*:130, June, 1971.
67. Gazes, P. C.: Treatment of angina pectoris. *Postgraduate Medicine 50*:73, August, 1971.
68. Gilston, A.: Cardiac resuscitation: Some questions and answers. *Nursing Mirror,* June 2, 1967, p. VII.
69. Glassmon, E.: Direct current cardioversion. *American Heart Journal 82*:128, July, 1971.
70. Gold, R. G.: Cardiac dysrhythmias. I. *Nursing Times,* July 9, 1965.
71. Gold, R. G.: Cardiac dysrhythmias—Ventricular Dysrhythmias. *Nursing Times,* July 16, 1965.
72. Grollman, A.: How drugs work: Diuretics. *Consultant 12*:53, July, 1972.
73. Guyton, A. C.: Advanced Cardiac Pathophysiology for Nurses. *Proceedings: Advanced Coronary Care.* Nursing Course, October 12–16, 1970. Sponsored by the Washington/Alaska Regional Medical Program.
74. Hamilton, M.: Management of hypertension. *Nursing Mirror 132*:33, January 15, 1971.
75. Harris, A.: Cardiac pacing. *Nursing Mirror 130*:25, February 6, 1970.
76. Helfant, R. H.: Coronary arteriography. *American Family Physician 4*:75, November, 1971.
77. Hockberg, H. M.: Effects of electrical current on heart rhythm. *American Journal of Nursing 71*: 1390–94, July, 1971.
78. Hopkins, S. J.: Hypertension and cardiac failure. Part 1. *Nursing Times 68*:841, July 6, 1972.
79. Hull, E.: Cardiac output, hypertrophy and dilatation, valvular diseases, congenital defects; extracardiac factors. *In* Sodeman, W. A., and Sodeman, W. A., Jr. (eds.): *Pathologic Physiology: Mechanisms of Disease.* 4th ed. Philadelphia, W. B. Saunders Company, 1967.
80. Hussan, D. A.: Cardiac drugs today: Part I, Anticoagulants. *Nursing '73 3*:11, 1973.
81. Jacob, S. W., and Francone, C. A.: *Structure and Function in Man.* Philadelphia, W. B. Saunders Company, 1965.
82. Jarvis, D.: Open heart surgery: Patients' perceptions of care. *American Journal of Nursing 70*:2591, December, 1970.
83. Johnston, F. D.: The electrocardiogram. *In* Sodeman, W. A., and Sodeman, W. A., Jr. (eds.): *Pathologic Physiology: Mechanisms of Disease.* 4th ed. Philadelphia, W. B. Saunders Company, 1967.
84. Jokl, E.: Exercise and the heart. *Consultant 12*:46, July, 1972.
85. Jude, J. R., and Nagel, E. L.: Cardiopulmonary resuscitation 1970. *Modern Concepts of Cardiovascular Disease 34*:133, November, 1970.
86. Killip, T.: Arrhythmia, sudden death and coronary artery disease. *The American Journal of Cardiology 28*:614, November, 1971.
87. Kim, K., et al.: Problems in therapy for the hypertensive patient. *Geriatrics 28*:122, March, 1973.
88. King, J., et al.: Recent advances in therapy for refractory congestive heart failure. *Geriatrics 28*:94, March, 1973.
89. Kirkendall, W. M., et al.: *Recommendations for Human Blood Pressure Determinations by Sphygmomanometers.* Authorized by the Central Committee for Medical and Community Program of the American Heart Association on May 5, 1967. New York, American Heart Association, 1967.
90. Kirkendall, W. M.: What's with hypertension these days? *Consultant 11*:13, January, 1971.
91. Kleiger, R. E.: The patient with angina: Medical

management plus sympathetic continuous care. *Geriatrics 28*:74, March, 1973.
92. Koerner, S. K.: Oxygen in ischemic heart disease. *American Heart Journal 82*:269, August, 1971.
93. Kos, B. A., and Culbert, P. A.: Teaching the patient with a pacemaker. *Cardio-Vascular Nursing 6*:57, November-December, 1970.
94. Kratz, A. M., and Kratz, J. L.: Cardiac drugs today: Part II, Vasodilators. *Nursing '73 3*:33, 1973.
95. Kurihara, M., and Moody, F. G.: Complications of general surgery. *In* Meltzer, L. E., et al. (eds.): *Concepts and Practices of Intensive Care for Nurse Specialists.* Philadelphia, Charles Press Publishers, Inc., 1969.
96. Lamberton, M. M.: Cardiac catherization: Anticipatory nursing care. *American Journal of Nursing 71*:1718, September, 1971.
97. Lasry, J. E., and Glasser, M. L.: *Precordial Shock: Defibrillation–Cardioversion.* Prepared for the San Diego County Heart Association, May, 1970.
98. Lavin, M. A.: Bed exercises for acute cardiac patients. *American Journal of Nursing 73*:1226, July, 1973.
99. Lehmann, J.: Auscultation of heart sounds. *American Journal of Nursing 72*:1242, July, 1972.
100. Leonard, J. J., and Kroetz, F. W.: *Examination of the Heart: Part Four: Auscultation.* Prepared for the Committee on Medical Education of the American Heart Association. New York, American Heart Association, 1967.
101. Logue, B.: Angina Pectoris. *In* Conn, H. F. (ed.): *Current Therapy 1969.* Philadelphia, W. B. Saunders Company, 1969.
102. London, S. B., and London, R. E.: Critique of indirect diastolic end point—"muffling" vs. "last" sound. *Archives of Internal Medicine 119*:34, January, 1967.
103. Longmore, D.: *The Heart.* World University Library. New York, McGraw-Hill Book Company, 1971.
104. Luckey, E. H.: Diseases of the myocardium and mural endocardium. *In* Beeson, P. B., and McDermott, W. (eds.): *Cecil-Loeb Textbook of Medicine.* 12th ed. Philadelphia, W. B. Saunders Company, 1967.
105. Lukas, D. S., and Barr, D. P.: Cyanosis. *In* MacBryde, C. M. (ed.): *Signs and Symptoms: Applied Pathologic Physiology and Clinical Interpretation.* 4th ed. Philadelphia, J. B. Lippincott Company, 1964.
106. Lukas, P. S.: Dyspnea. *In* MacByrde, C. M. (ed.): *Signs and Symptoms: Applied Pathologic Physiology and Clinical Interpretation.* 4th ed. Philadelphia, J. B. Lippincott Company, 1964.
107. Magidson, O.: Refractory heart failure. *Geriatrics 22*:132, May, 1967.
108. Marriott, H. J. L.: Premature beats (extra-systoles). *In* Conn, H. F. (ed.): *Current Therapy 1969.* Philadelphia, W. B. Saunders Company, 1969.
109. Massie, E.: Palpitation and tachycardia. *In* MacBryde, C. M. (ed.): *Signs and Symptoms: Applied Pathologic Physiology and Clinical Interpretation.* 4th ed. Philadelphia, J. B. Lippincott Company, 1964.
110. Mayer, G. G., et al.: Arrhythmias and cardiac output. *American Journal of Nursing 72*:1597, September, 1972.
111. Mayer, J.: Low sodium diets. 2. Severe restriction. *Postgraduate Medicine 50*:49, July, 1971.

112. Mazzarella, J. A., and Burnham, P.: Pacemakers—Challenge to medicine and nursing. *Advanced Coronary Care Nursing Course Proceedings,* October 12–16, 1970, Seattle, Washington.
113. McIntyre, H. M.: The prevention of heart disease: A greater challenge. *Cardio-Vascular Nursing 7*: 77, September-October, 1971.
114. McIver, C.: Blood pressure: A consideration of terminology. *Canadian Medical Association Journal 91*:578, September 12, 1964.
115. Measurement of arterial blood pressure and the interpretation of blood pressure reading. (Programmed instruction.) *GP* July, 1964, p. 133.
116. Meehan, M.: EKG primer—A programmed instruction unit. *American Journal of Nursing 71*:2195, November, 1971.
117. Meltzer, L. E., et al.: *Concepts and Practices of Intensive Care for Nurse Sepcialists.* Philadelphia, Charles Press Publishers, Inc., 1969.
118. Meltzer, L. E., et al.: *Intensive Coronary Care.* Philadelphia, Charles Press Publishers, Inc., 1970.
119. Mendlowitz, M.: Hypertension. *In* Conn, H. F. (ed.): *Current Therapy 1969.* Philadelphia, W. B. Saunders Company, 1969.
120. Meserko, U.: Preoperative classes for cardiac patients. *American Journal of Nursing 73*:665, April, 1973.
121. Moidel, H. C.: Section I: Diseases of the heart. *In* Moidel, H. C., et al. (eds.): *Nursing Care of the Patient with Medical-Surgical Disorders.* New York, McGraw-Hill Book Company, 1971.
122. Notter, D., Giblett, E. R., and Finch, C. A.: *General Medicine.* Seattle, University of Washington Medical School, 1970.
123. Oshsner, J. L.: Surgery for myocardial revascularization. *Postgraduate Medicine 49*:127, April 20, 1971.
124. Owen, S. C.: *Electrocardiography: A Programmed Text.* Boston, Little, Brown and Company, 1966.
125. Page, I. H., and Dustan, H. P.: *Drug Treatment of Arterial Hypertension.* Booklet prepared by the American Heart Association, 1966.
126. Parmley, L. F.: Pericarditis. *In* Conn, H. F. (ed.): *Current Therapy 1969.* Philadelphia, W. B. Saunders Company, 1969.
127. Pearce, M., et al.: Management of heart arrest. *Nursing Mirror 133*:25–28, August 6, 1971.
128. Peart, W. S.: Arterial hypertension. *In* Beeson, P. B., and McDermott, J. W. (eds.): *Cecil-Loeb Textbook of Medicine,* 12th ed. Philadelphia, W. B. Saunders Company, 1967.
129. Perloff, D., and Sokolow, M.: Selected topics in cardiac arrhythmias. *Geriatrics 22*:190, September, 1967.
130. Pitorak, E. F., et al.: *Nurses' Guide to Cardiac Surgery and Nursing Care.* New York, Blakiston Division, McGraw-Hill Book Company, 1969.
131. Preston, T., et al.: Three therapeutic approaches in tachycardia. *Geriatrics 28*:110, March, 1973.
132. Putt, A. M.: A comparison of blood pressure readings by auscultation and palpation. *Nursing Research 15*:311, 1966.
133. Ramsey, M. A.: The failing heart. *Nursing '72 2*:18, October, 1972.
134. Redwood, D. R.: Heart block and cardiac pacemakers. *Nursing Times,* May 12, 1967, p. 614.
135. Reynolds, E. W.: Atrial fibrillation. *In* Conn, H. F. (ed.): *Current Therapy 1960.* Philadelphia, W. B. Saunders Company, 1969.
136. Robbins, S. L.: *Pathology.* Philadelphia, W. B. Saunders Company, 1967.
137. Roberts, G.: The coronary care unit. *Nursing Times 68*:181, November 16, 1972.
138. Roberts, J. T.: Dynamics and circulation of heart mus-

cle, cardiac reserve, heart pain, and cardiac cycle. *In* Sodeman, W. A., and Sodeman, W. A., Jr. (eds.): *Pathologic Physiology: Mechanisms of Disease.* 4th ed. Philadelphia, W. B. Saunders Company, 1967.

139. Rogoz, B.: Nursing care of the cardiac surgery patient. *Nursing Clinics of North America 4*:645, December, 1969.
140. San Diego County Health Association: *Cardiovascular Drugs.* Distributed by the California Heart Association, 1970.
141. Schlant, R. C.: Heart Block. *In* Conn, H. F. (ed.): *Current Therapy 1969.* Philadelphia, W. B. Saunders Company, 1969.
142. Schlant, R. C.: *Examination of the Heart: Part Three: Inspection and Palpitation of the Anterior Chest.* Prepared for Committee on Medical Education of the American Heart Association. New York, American Heart Association, 1970.
143. Schroeder, H. A.: Edema. *In* MacBryde, C. M. (ed.): *Signs and Symptoms:Applied Pathologic Physiology and Clinical Interpretation.* 4th ed. Philadelphia, J. B. Lippincott Company, 1964.
144. Seller, R. H., and Brest, A. N.: Heart failure in the elderly. *Geriatrics 22*:225, March, 1967.
145. Shafer, K. L., et al.: *Medical-Surgical Nursing.* 4th ed. St. Louis, The C. V. Mosby Company, 1967.
146. Shaver, S. A., and Leonard, J. J.: Congestive heart failure. *In* Conn, H. F. (ed.): *Current Therapy 1969.* Philadelphia, W. B. Saunders Company, 1969.
147. Shields, H. E.: Cardiac anatomy and physiology. *Nursing Clinics of North America 4*:563, December, 1969.
148. Short, F. A.: The normal 12-lead ECG and common variances including acute, resolving, and old infarcts: Digitalis effect, electrolyte imbalances and others. *Proceedings: Advanced Coronary Care Nursing Course,* October 12–16, 1970. Sponsored by the Washington/Alaska Regional Medical Program.
149. Slessor, G.: Auscultation of the chest—a clinical nursing skill. *Canadian Nurse 69*:40, April, 1973.
150. Smith, C. A.: Body image changes after myocardial infarction. *Nursing Clinics of North America* 7:663, December, 1972.
151. Smith, J. R., and Paine, R.: Thoracic pain. *In* Mac Bryde, C. M. (ed.): *Applied Pathologic Physiology and Clinical Interpretation.* 4th ed. Philadelphia, J. B. Lippincott Company, 1964.
152. Smith, S. E.: Drug therapy 1972: Drugs and the heart. Part 3. *Nursing Times 68*:317, March 16, 1972.
153. Sowton, E.: Cardiac pacemakers and pacing. *Modern Concepts of Cardiovascular Disease 36*:31, June, 1967.
154. Spencer, R. F.: Neurocirculatory asthenia. *In* Conn, H. F. (ed.): *Current Therapy 1969.* Philadelphia, W. B. Saunders Company, 1969.
155. Sprague, H. B.: *Examination of the Heart. Part One: History Taking.* Prepared for the Committee on Medical Education of the American Heart Association. New York, American Heart Association, 1967.
156. Stanton, A.: Cardiac catheterization. *Nursing Times,* June 28, 1968, p. 860.
157. Stead, E. A.: Pathologic physiology of heart failure. *In* Beeson, P. B., and McDermott, W. (eds.): *Cecil-Loeb Textbook of Medicine.* 12th ed. Philadelphia, W. B. Saunders Company, 1967.
158. Stead, E. A.: Treatment of congestive heart failure. *In* Beeson, P. B., and McDermott, W. (eds.): *Cecil-Loeb Textbook of Medicine.* 12th ed. Philadelphia, W. B. Saunders Company, 1967.
159. Sutton, A.: *Bedside Nursing Techniques in Medicine and Surgery.* 2nd ed. Philadelphia, W. B. Saunders Company, 1969.
160. Thomas, J.: Care and rehabilitation after myocardial infarction. *In* Conn, H. F. (ed.): *Current Therapy 1975.* Philadelphia, W. B. Saunders Company, 1975.
161. Thompson, T.: The year they changed hearts. *Life 71*: 56, September 17, 1971.
162. Tompsett, R., and Skripka, C.: Reappraising clinical features of bacterial endocarditis. *Postgraduate Medicine 42*:462, December, 1967.
163. Torrens, P. R., and Hanchett, E. S.: Public health nursing and the congestive heart failure patient. *Cardio-Vascular Nursing 3*:4, July–August, 1967.
164. Tumulty, P. A.: Management of bacterial endocarditis. *Geriatrics 22*:122, June, 1967.
165. Tweiski, A. J.: Psychological Considerations on the coronary care unit. *Cardio-Vascular Nursing,* 7:65, March–April, 1971.
166. Tyzenhouse, P. S.: Myocardial infarction: Its effect on the family. *American Journal of Nursing 73*:1012, June, 1973.
167. Warren, J. V.: Pericarditis. *In* Beeson, P. B., and McDermott, W., (eds.): *Cecil-Loeb Textbook of Medicine.* 12th ed. Philadelphia, W. B. Saunders Company, 1967.
168. Weiler, Sister M. C.: Postoperative patients evaluate preoperative instruction. *American Journal of Nursing 68*:1465, July, 1968.
169. Wessler, S., and Alexander, B.: *A Guide to Anticoagulant Therapy.* Prepared for the Committee on Medical Education of the American Heart Association. New York, American Heart Association, 1970.
170. What is a coronary thrombosis? *Nursing Times,* June 28, 1968.
171. Wiggers, C. J.: The heart. *Scientific American,* May, 1957.
172. Wild, J. B.: Emergency care of ventricular standstill. *Nursing Times 67*:734, June 17, 1971.
173. Williams, R. C., Jr.: Subacute bacterial endocarditis as an immune disease. *Hospital Practice 6*:111, June, 1971.
174. Williams, S.: *Nutrition and Diet Therapy.* St. Louis, The C. V Mosby Company, 1969.
175. Yokes, J.: The influence of bioengineering on the nurse and the cardiac patient. *In* Bergersen, B. S., et al. (eds.): *Current Concepts in Clinical Nursing.* St. Louis, The C. V. Mosby Company, 1967.
176. Yokes, J. A., and Reed, W. A.: Heart Surgery. *In* Meltzer, L. E., et al. (eds.): *Concepts and Practices of Intensive Care.* Philadelphia, The Charles Press Publishers, 1967.
177. Young, C. C., and Barger, Y. O.: *Introduction to Medical Science.* St. Louis, The C. V. Mosby Company, 1969.

UNIT XI

Nursing Patients Experiencing Dysfunction of the Kidney and Urinary Tract

Jo Ann Albers

Unit Introduction and Study Guide

The nursing of patients experiencing dysfunction of the kidneys and the urinary tract may encompass all aspects of nursing, from the care of patients with short-term, easily cured difficulties to long-term maintenance care or care of the dying. Kidney and urinary tract dysfunctions may affect males and females from birth to advanced age. Onset may be sudden, or slow and insidious.

Urology and nephrology are terms often used to distinguish disease entities. Urology refers to the study of disorders of the urinary tract, that is, ureters, bladder, and urethra, while nephrology refers to the study of disorders of the kidney itself. This is oftentimes an inadequate division, as disorders of the lower urinary tract soon affect the kidney and vice versa. These terms, urology and nephrology, are also used to designate specialties in medicine: the urologist is a surgeon concerned mostly with anatomic disorders, and the nephrologist is an internist concerned with physiologic disorders. This unit will not attempt to separate these two divisions.

As a nurse caring for patients experiencing dysfunction of the kidney and urinary tract you would be involved with patients in the following situations:

> Persons requiring a urinary catheter because of either incontinence or urinary retention.

> Persons with congenital defects of the kidney or lower urinary tract who may experience dysfunction for the first time at birth or in advanced age.

> Persons who suffer neoplasms, infections, and trauma, and experience damage to the kidney as well as other organs of the body.

> Persons whose kidney function may fail because of disease that is either primary, or secondary to some other malfunction of the body.

> Persons whose dysfunction of the urinary tract may involve fluid and electrolyte disturbances.

To aid in your study of this material, we offer the following guides:

1. Prior to studying this unit you should have a good grasp of the material on fluid and electrolyte balance and imbalance found in Unit V and particularly of the role of the kidney in maintaining balance.

2. As you study this unit familiarize yourself with the following terms: renal, urethra, ureter, micturition, nephron, tubules, glomerulus, parenchyma, renal pelvis, calyces, infundibula, blood urea nitrogen, creatinine, reflux, sphincter, strictures, incontinence, nocturia, hematuria, pyuria, voiding, fluid balance, catheter, urology, nephrology, catheterization, meatus, retention, specific gravity, creatinine clearance, urinalysis, concentration, pyelography, cystoscopy, urethrography, angiogram, retrograde, pyelonephritis, perinephric, ureteritis, cystitis, urethritis, nephritis, hydronephrosis, calculi, lithiasis, polycystic, glomerulonephritis, nephrotic, dialysis, diffusion, hemodialysis, peritoneal dialysis, dialysate, semipermeable membrane, hemograft, immunosuppressive, autoimmune, renal transplantation, cannula, arteriovenous shunt, and internal arteriovenous fistula.

3. Upon completion of this unit you should be able to discuss generally the following concepts:

a. General anatomy and physiology of the kidney and lower urinary tract.

b. Major anomalies of the kidney and urinary tract.

c. The nurse's role in assessing and maintaining adequate fluid and electrolyte intake and output.

d. The use of catheters in relieving retention.

e. Various diagnostic studies employed to detect kidney and urinary tract dysfunctions.

f. Major types of disorders causing dysfunction of the kidneys and lower urinary tract.

g. Typical nursing care of patients undergoing diagnosis or treatment of urinary tract dysfunction.

h. The signs, symptoms, and causes of renal failure.

i. The differences between acute and chronic renal failure.

j. The underlying principles of dialysis.

k. The major goals and outcomes of dialysis and renal hemografts in the care of persons experiencing renal failure.

CHAPTER 55

The Urinary System: Normal Anatomy and Structural Disorders

The kidney is a complex organ that is responsible for the formation of urine and largely controls its volume and concentration. Normally each individual has two kidneys. Urine leaves the kidneys by way of tubes called ureters and enters a muscular sack called the bladder. The bladder serves as a temporary reservoir for the urine until micturition, a reflex normally under voluntary control, sends the urine outside the body by way of a tube called the urethra.

THE KIDNEYS

ANATOMY-PHYSIOLOGY REVIEW

The kidneys lie one on each side of the spinal column and just below the diaphragm (Fig. 55–1). They are usually about 12 cm. long in the adult. The adrenal glands lie just above each kidney. The position of the liver causes the right kidney to be slightly lower than the left. The duodenum and ascending colon lie in front of the right kidney, while the spleen and descending colon lie in front of the left one. Each kidney is surrounded by fat and encapsulated in fibrous tissue.

Blood is supplied to the kidneys by way of the renal artery, which is a branch of the abdominal aorta. This artery subdivides into smaller arterioles that enter the nephrons, forming little tufts of capillaries called glomeruli. From the glomeruli the arterioles pass to the tubules. From the tubules the blood enters the venous system, leaving the kidney by way of the renal vein.

The kidney can be divided into two distinct areas: the parenchyma, and the pelvis. The parenchyma contains about one million nephrons, which are the functioning units of the kidney. (See Unit V for a description of the anatomy and physiology of the nephron.) The pelvis of the kidney is the start of the urine collecting system. It is made up of cup-like structures called calyces attached to funnel-like structures called infundibula. The pelvis normally holds only 3 to 5 ml. of urine. Peristaltic action transports the urine from the pelvis into the ureter.

The role of the kidney in maintaining adequate fluid and electrolyte balance is covered in Unit V.

In addition to regulating the volume and concentration of body fluid, the kidney removes waste products from the body. As protein is metabolized (broken down in the body) certain waste materials are formed. Some of these are urea, creatine, creatinine, and uric acid. Normally these are filtered out of the blood by the tubules of the kidney, but in malfunctioning states the kidney is unable to do this; consequently, abnormally high concentrations of these substances accumulate in the body. If this process is sudden, that is, if the malfunction of the kidney occurs quickly and these nitrogenous end products of protein metabolism accumulate rapidly, the body has little tolerance and the patient will become critically ill within about 48 hours of the occurrence. If the kidney slowly loses its ability to filter and eliminate the urea, creatinine, and other wastes, the body shows a surprising tolerance, and the patient can function quite effectively for a long time in spite of the abnormally high concentration of these substances in the blood. This situation will be discussed in greater detail in Chapter 57.

CONGENITAL ANOMALIES OF THE KIDNEY

The kidney may be unusually located, malformed, cystic, or absent. A single kidney is not uncommon and presents no difficulty if it functions properly. Absence of both kidneys does not permit life to continue. Newborn infants with congenital absence of kidneys usually have eyes set wide apart, low set ears and a small lower jaw.

Cystic disease will be discussed in Chapter 57.

When the kidney is located in an unusual place, for example, low in the body, it is called an ectopic kidney.

The kidney may be unusually large or small and may be shaped like a pancake or a horseshoe. The kidney may be duplicated on one side, usually within one capsule, with two separate drainage systems.

THE URETERS

ANATOMY-PHYSIOLOGY REVIEW

The ureters arise from the pelvis of their respective kidneys and provide a 25- to 30-cm. long passageway to the bladder. A ureter is about 5 mm. in inner diameter and narrows significantly at three different points: (1) where it joins the kidney, called the ureteropelvic junction; (2) where it joins the bladder, called the ureterovesical junction; and (3) where it crosses the bifurcation of iliac vessels and enters the bony pelvis.

Ureters in the female pass behind the uterus, whereas in the male the ureter enters the bladder in front of the seminal vesicles.

The ureters have a peristaltic action that propels urine toward the bladder and a sphincterlike action that prevents the flow of urine back up the ureters from the bladder. This backward flow of urine is called a *reflux*. Reflux of urine can be caused by any significant build-up of pressure in the urinary tract. Since the kidney pelvis holds only 5 ml. of urine, serious damage can be done to the kidney if any large reflux of urine occurs. Reflux can lead to inflammation of the kidney, or pyelonephritis.

CONGENITAL ANOMALIES

The ureteropelvic or the ureterovesicular junction can be congenitally obstructed. There may be more than one ureter draining a single kidney, or the ureter may enter the bladder from other than

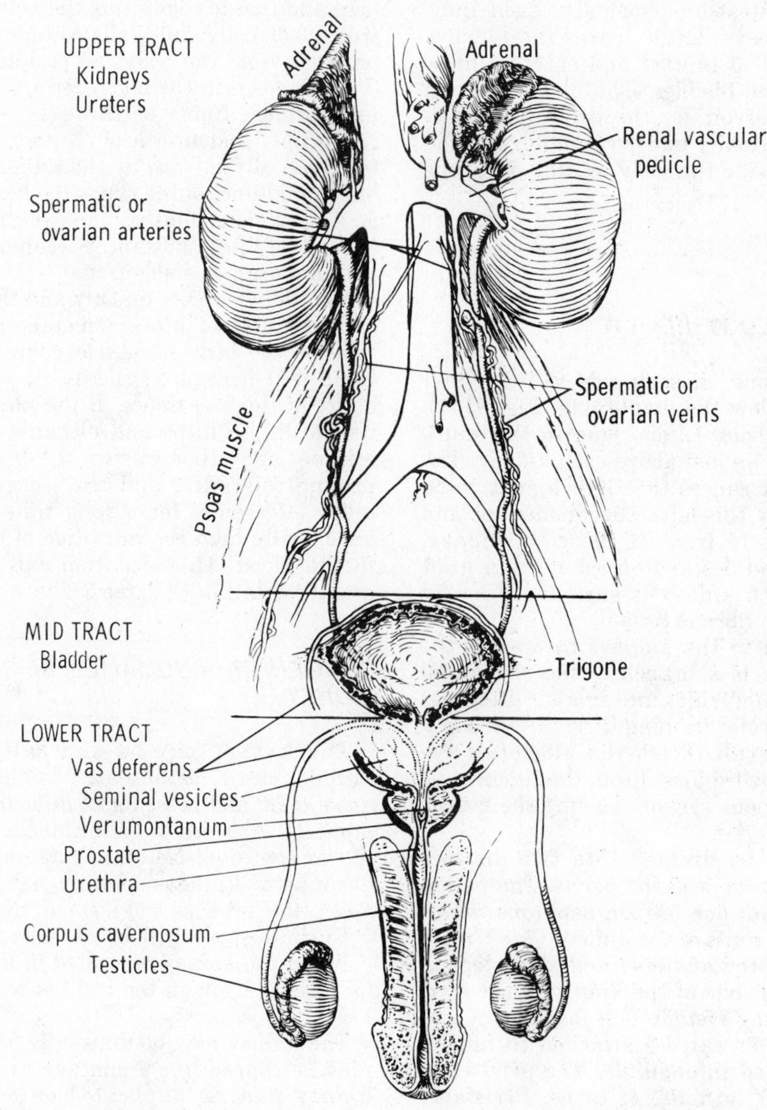

FIGURE 55-1. Anatomy of the male genitourinary tract. The upper and mid tracts have urologic function only. The lower tract has both genital and urinary functions. (From Smith, D. R.: *General Urology.* Los Altos, Calif., Lange Medical Publications, 1969.)

the usual place. At the corner of the bladder trigone the ureter may not enter the bladder but open instead into the urethra or vagina.

THE BLADDER

ANATOMY-PHYSIOLOGY REVIEW

The bladder is a muscular sac freely movable except at its base, where it is continuous with the urethra below. When empty it lies in folds, but as urine enters the bladder from the ureter in rhythmic spurts, the pressure within the bladder increases and the bladder muscle, called the detrusor muscle, relaxes, allowing the bladder wall to expand. When 300 to 500 ml. of urine is contained in the bladder, nerve endings in the detrusor muscle receive stimuli that are transmitted to reflex centers in the spinal cord. The internal sphincter located just above the point of insertion of the urethra into the bladder is opened, allowing urine to enter the urethra. The external sphincter then relaxes, allowing the expulsion of the bladder contents. The external sphincter is normally under voluntary control after about the age of 3 years; therefore, micturition can be delayed by contraction of this sphincter.

When the bladder becomes distended to 1000 ml. or more, bladder tone may be lost and tissue damage can occur.

CONGENITAL ANOMALIES

Tightening of the lumen of the bladder can be caused by a fibrous ring at the point of insertion of the urethra at the base of the bladder, commonly called the bladder neck.

A large-capacity bladder lacking in tone is called megalocystis. Both the bladder-neck contractures and megalocystis tend to occur more often in girls and cause recurrent urinary tract infections.

Exstrophy of the bladder is a condition resulting from a lack of closure of the symphysis pubis. There is no anterior abdominal wall, and the open bladder protrudes through to the surface. Since the bladder is not closed, urine leaks continuously, keeping the child wet and damaging the surrounding tissue. The bladder is usually removed and urine is drained by bringing the ureter through an opening in the skin or diverting its flow to the bowel. Plastic repair of the abdomen is necessary. All this requires many surgical procedures and frequent hospitalization. Children with this defect, and their families, require much skilled nursing care to help them to cope with this difficult situation.

Fistulas, or abnormal openings into the bowel or vagina, sometimes occur, as well as separated bladder compartments and diverticuli.

URETHRA

ANATOMY REVIEW

The female urethra is 3 to 5 cm. long and opens just above the vagina. The external opening is called the meatus. The external sphincter is located in the middle of the urethra. The urethra serves simply as a tube through which the urine flowing from the bladder makes its exit from the body.

The male urethra is about 20 cm. long, originating at the bladder and traversing the length of the penis. The urethral meatus, through which urine is discharged, is located at the tip of the glans penis.

CONGENITAL ANOMALIES

Hypospadias is a defect of the male urethra in which the meatus is located along the under surface of the penis or, occasionally, in the scrotum or perineum. This defect does not cause incontinence and can usually be surgically repaired, though several procedures may be required.

Epispadias is much less common and almost always accompanies exstrophy of the bladder. In this condition the dorsal urethra is not closed or is absent.

Urethral strictures and fistulas also occur.

CHAPTER 56

The Nurse's Role in Assessing and Maintaining Adequate Kidney and Urinary Tract Function

ASSESSING THE PATIENT

Assessment of the function of the patient's kidney and lower urinary tract is the first step in planning care for the patient with a urologic disorder. Only that part of assessment concerned with malfunction of the urinary tract will be discussed in this section.

Because of the key role of the kidney and urinary tract in maintaining adequate fluid and electrolyte balance, many patients with malfunction of this system will have imbalances. Assessment of such imbalances has been extensively discussed in Unit V. The patient's voiding patterns and observations of his urine are of prime importance in making an assessment and plan of care. Does he have a history of urinary tract problems? Does he have, or has he had in the past, any external drainage devices? How many times a day does he normally void? Is he required to get up during the night to void? Has he a feeling of urgency occurring frequently? Is the amount at each voiding scanty or copious? Does he experience difficulty in starting to void? Is there pain or a burning sensation? Is there any unusual color or odor to his urine?

A careful measurement should be taken of the blood pressure, as hypertension is often the cause, or the result, of kidney disease. The patient should be asked if he is currently taking a drug to control his blood pressure or a diuretic to eliminate fluid.

If the patient is receiving antihypertensive drugs, his blood pressure should be measured in a supine position and again when he has been standing for a few seconds. These drugs often cause postural hypotension, so that a normal or elevated blood pressure will drop to a very low level when the patient stands. (See also Unit X.)

The patient should be asked about any unusual tendency toward bruising or bleeding, since fragility of the capillaries accompanies early kidney failure.

Restlessness, insomnia, fatigue, and itching of the skin are frequent complaints of patients with renal disease.

The fluid balance record is a useful observation to determine adequacy of kidney function. In addition, the patient may have a need for a restricted fluid intake if he has been retaining excess fluid, or he may be on a forced fluid regimen to dilute his urine and increase urinary flow.

Weighing the patient each morning on the same scale, with the same amount of clothing, after voiding and before breakfast, will be a good guide to the adequacy of his fluid intake and output.

NURSING MEASURES IN RELIEVING URINARY INCONTINENCE OR RETENTION

PURPOSE OF INDWELLING CATHETERS

Catheters are inserted to drain urine from the urinary tract when there are obstructions to the flow of urine, when it is desirable to prevent urine from entering a particular part of the urinary tract, and also when a person is unable to void or to completely empty the tract. Catheters are also sometimes used to collect the urine when the patient is incontinent.

> *Urinary retention causes a reflux of urine back up the tract, leading to kidney damage.*
> *Urinary stasis leads to infection.*
> *Urinary retention causes pain.*

Catheters are inserted above the point of obstruction or the area that is to be kept free of urine.

URETHRAL CATHETERIZATION

Urethral catheters, to drain urine from the bladder, are the most commonly used catheters. Most often the nurse will be responsible for insertion of these catheters. It is important to remember that patients with urologic disorders may have obstructions or strictures that make the insertion of the catheter difficult. The nurse should seek help from the physician whenever she encounters difficulty in inserting a urethral catheter, because severe trauma and even puncture of the urethera and bladder can occur. Usually the physician will insert the catheter if it requires the use of a metal guide or other rigid device to guide it into place.

A catheter should be inserted gently, using strict aseptic technique. Even under optimal conditions a catheter can irritate the membrane lining of the urethra and can introduce or spread infection in the urinary tract.

There are several types of catheters that are used for urethral catheterization (Fig. 56–1). The size is graded in the French system and for adults the usual size range is 14 to 22 Fr. A curved-tipped catheter is frequently used for male catheterizations, while a straight-tipped catheter is used for the female. These catheters are made of soft rubber and have a solid round tip that has slits in the side for drainage. When a catheter is to be left in for continuous drainage of the bladder, an indwelling Foley catheter is used. This catheter has an inflatable balloon just below the tip which will, when inflated, prevent the catheter from slipping back down the urethra. Catheters must be sterile when inserted into the meatus.

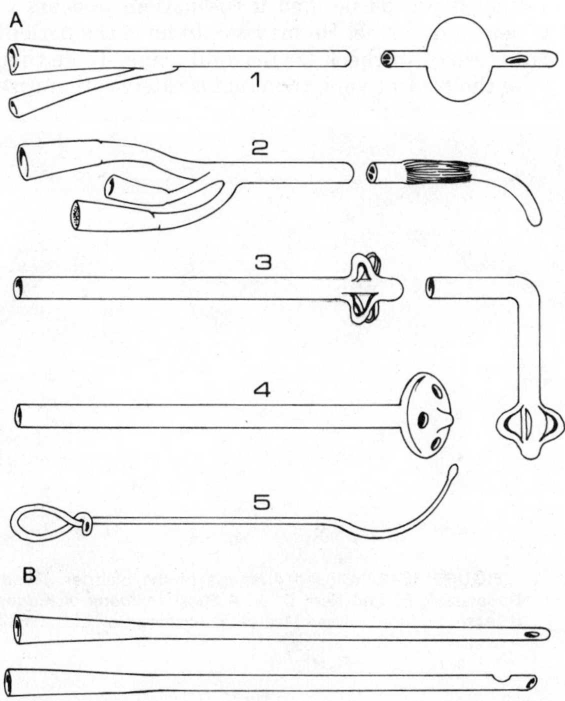

FIGURE 56–1. *A,* Self-retaining catheters. 1, The Foley catheter; 2, the three-way Foley catheter; 3, the Malecot catheter; 4, the Pezzer catheter. These catheters are able to maintain themselves in cavities. They come in various sizes and may be straight or angulated. Both types of Foley catheters are introduced into a cavity and the self-retaining balloon is inflated thereafter. The self-retaining protuberance at the tip of the Malecot and Pezzer must be elongated with a stylet (5) which is passed through the lumen before insertion. After insertion, the stylet is removed and the protuberance secures the catheter in place. *B,* Straight catheters. The straight catheter may have a single eye or many eyes; it may have a round tip or a whistle tip. These catheters are not self-retaining and must be secured with adhesive tape when being utilized as indwelling tubes. (From Whitehead, S.: *Nursing Care of the Adult Urology Patient.* New York, Appleton-Century-Crofts, Inc., 1970.)

Insertion of a Urethral Catheter

In addition to a sterile catheter you will need a sterile field on which to place it, sterile drape, sterile gloves, sponges, lubricant, and forceps. If specimens are to be collected, the appropriate containers should be at hand. A mild disinfectant solution and sponges for cleansing the area around the meatus are also necessary. It is important to have a good light to aid visualization of the meatus, especially in the female. If a self-retaining catheter is being inserted, a syringe of the appropriate size to inflate the balloon of the catheter must be available as well as tubing and a receptacle to connect the catheter for permanent drainage.

The procedure should be completely explained to the patient before beginning. Apprehension and tenseness may lead to a tightening of the sphincter, which will cause the insertion of the catheter to be painful and irritating. Providing privacy and appropriate draping will also help the patient to relax.

When catheterizing a woman have her lie on her back with her knees flexed, thighs apart. If this is a difficult position for the patient, good visualization of and access to the urethral orifice is possible with the patient on her side with her knees drawn to her chest and her shoulders bent forward.[17]

The male patient should be in the dorsal recumbent position for catheterization.

After the patient has been prepared for the procedure and the equipment is assembled and opened, sterile gloves are put on. The female labia should be well separated with one hand and kept separated until the catheter is passed. Using sterile forceps to hold disinfectant-soaked swabs, the meatus and surrounding area should be cleansed.

The foreskin of the penis, in the male, should be retracted and the meatus cleaned well. The catheter should be sterile, lubricated with a water-soluble lubricant and held in a sterile gloved hand as it is passed. The catheter should be inserted very gently into the meatus to avoid trauma.

The catheter should never be forced when resistance is encountered. Some resistance will be felt at the urethral sphincter, but waiting a moment for it to relax will usually permit the catheter to move in smoothly. The catheter should be inserted about 3 inches into the female and 8 to 10 inches into the male. If the catheter is to remain in the bladder it should be moved about an inch farther than the point where urine first began to flow. The balloon should be inflated at this point if this type of catheter is being used. No pain will be felt unless the balloon has not advanced completely into the bladder. If it is not, the balloon should be deflated, the catheter advanced and the balloon inflated again.

The catheter is then connected to a straight drainage system. Suction is never applied to drain a urethral catheter, but it should be placed so that urine may flow freely by gravity (Fig. 56–2).

The catheter should be anchored with tape to the thigh and brought out over the leg to connect to the drainage tubing. The collecting receptacle should always be kept below the level of the bladder to prevent a reflux of urine back up the tubing. The catheter may be irrigated to insure patency, but this should be done aseptically using sterile saline solution. Saline should return promptly through a patent catheter.

The area around the meatus should be inspected carefully to make certain it is clean and dry. It should be washed every few hours and all crusts and mucus removed to guard against infection, which is always a potential problem with indwelling catheters. Any swelling of the tissues around the meatus should be reported to the physician. This can be a very painful symptom, especially in the male. Sitz baths and local cleaning can help to reduce edema.

Following catheterization, ingestion of fluids should be encouraged, unless contraindicated, so that the urine will be diluted and increased in volume, thus helping to ensure patency of the catheter and preventing infection.

Catheters should never be pushed back up into the bladder if they should slip down for any reason. Always remove the catheter and insert another one, using aseptic technique.

The flow of urine from the catheter should be observed every 2 or 3 hours. If the urine is bloody, the catheter should be checked frequently to be certain it is not plugged with clots and to note the amount of blood loss.

Removal of the Catheter

Before removal of the catheter the procedure should be explained to the patient. He may have concerns about his ability to void without the catheter. If he was previously incontinent, he may be concerned that this will recur.

The balloon of the catheter must be deflated by withdrawing the contents with a syringe. The catheter is then gently but firmly pulled out.

The time and amount of each voiding should be recorded for 24 to 48 hours after removal of a catheter. Voidings of 100 ml. of urine or less frequently indicate incomplete emptying of the bladder. The doctor should be notified if the patient appears to be retaining urine. He may ask to have the patient catheterized to check for residual urine. To do this, have the patient void, then immediately catheterize

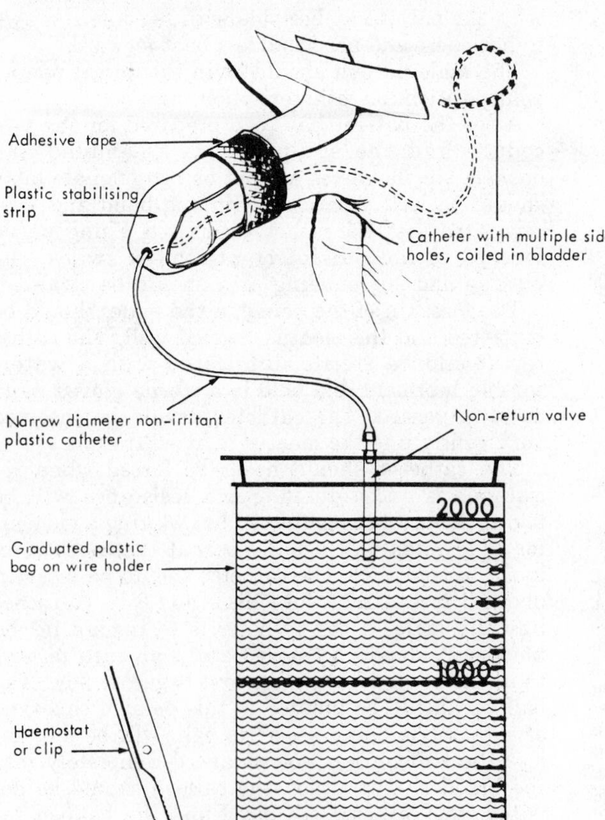

FIGURE 56–2. Closed drainage of the bladder. (From Douglas, A. P., and Kerr, D. S.: *A Short Textbook of Kidney Disease.* London, Pitman Medical Publishing Co., Ltd., 1968.)

him. If a volume greater than 50 ml. is obtained through the catheter, the patient is not adequately emptying his bladder.

Ureteral Catheters and Devices for Draining the Kidney Pelvis

Ureteral catheters are inserted into the ureters either for drainage of urine or for splinting. Sometimes the tip of the catheter is placed in the pelvis of the kidney. These tubes may be inserted during cystoscopy or during urologic surgery. The catheter may be inserted up through the urethra and bladder or may enter the kidney through abdominal or flank incisions.

It is of special importance to ensure that catheters draining above the bladder are kept patent. The kidney pelvis holds only 5 ml., so any reflux of urine can overfill the kidney, causing pressure damage to the tissues. A tubing stiff enough to prevent kinking should be used for drainage. The entire length of the tubing should be checked frequently to make sure it is patent.

The catheters are easily plugged with mucous shreds, blood clots, and chemical sediment. The doctor should be questioned before irrigating is done. If irrigation is carried out, aseptic technique must be used. A maximum of 5 ml. of irrigating solution should be allowed to flow in by gravity. If patency cannot be established, the doctor should be notified immediately.

OTHER NURSING MEASURES TO ASSIST THE PATIENT WITH URINARY RETENTION

When urinary retention is not the result of an obstruction, catheterization should be avoided until all other measures have been tried. Often hospitalized patients have difficulty voiding. This is especially true after surgery. Tenseness and anxiety can inhibit relaxation of the urinary sphincters. The patient may find he is unable to void into a bedpan or urinal while confined to bed, or he may be inhibited by the feeling of a lack of privacy. Placing the patient on a very cold bedpan can constrict the sphincter, making it difficult for her to initiate voiding.

Providing the patient with privacy, warming the bedpan before offering it to the patient, and placing the patient in a sitting position may all help to relieve the problem. Sometimes it is necessary to get the patient out of bed before he can void. Sometimes the stimulus of hearing water running, washing the hands in warm water, or pouring warm water over the perineal area will help the patient to initiate voiding. If the person is very tense and anxious, any measure that will help him to relax may help to relieve the retention.

Urinary retention should not be assumed to be present unless the patient has clearly taken in more fluid than he has lost, or he complains of discomfort from a full bladder, or bladder distention can be felt by examining the abdomen. That is, always be certain the patient is adequately hydrated when he is not voiding.

CARE OF THE PATIENT WITH URINARY INCONTINENCE

Because of the danger of infection with the continued use of indwelling catheters, they are not recommended as a solution to the problem of urinary incontinence. The person with urinary incontinence presents a serious nursing care problem.

One of the principal problems is the great embarrassment felt by patients who are aware they are incontinent. Lack of control of voiding is associated with an infantile state. In addition, our culture tends to view the act of elimination as a private matter and an impolite topic to be discussed in casual social situations. Loss of control of voiding may be viewed by some as a loss of control of one's environment and may lead to feelings of helplessness, hopelessness, and frustration.

Every effort should be made to maintain the patient's privacy and dignity. He should be consulted on all decisions concerning his care and permitted to do as many things for himself as possible in order to preserve his feelings of independence and autonomy. The nurse should discuss the problem of incontinence openly and matter of factly with the patient and allow him to express his feelings of concern. The patient will need much emotional support until a satisfactory solution has been reached.

Care of the patient's skin becomes a major problem when he is incontinent. Unless the patient is kept meticulously clean and dry, severe rashes and ulcerations of the skin will occur.

If the patient is not conscious or there is no hope that he will be able to void at specified intervals, then measures should be taken to keep urine off the skin. There are devices, sometimes called condom catheters or Texas catheters, that consist of a latex sheath that fits around the penis, with drainage tubing that can be connected to a drainage bag. These external catheters are sometimes difficult to keep in place and also may be a source of infection unless changed often and kept very clean. Bed pads treated with solutions that prevent the formation of ammonia in urine can be used under the patient. Women may be fitted with waterproof type pants with absorbent pads.

The patient's skin should be washed thoroughly with soap and water and dried well promptly after each voiding. All linen that has been soiled should be changed. Often the patient can be kept dry by simply offering the bedpan or urinal at frequent, regular intervals. Many elderly incontinent patients will remain dry if they are helped to a bedside commode.

Patients with spinal cord injuries and patients who have had a cerebrovascular accident frequently have lost neurologic control of the bladder; these patients can often be helped to control voiding by a program of bladder retraining. Assisting a patient with bladder retraining should not be undertaken by a nurse unless she has confidence that it can be successful. The patient must be motivated to regain control of voiding and must be made aware that it will require a period of time and a lot of patience. At first, the patient is asked to void every half hour or every hour day and night. When this program results in his being dry in between voidings, the interval is lengthened. Sometimes the patient can learn to hold urine up to 4 hours. Usually an external drainage device is used at night, after control is established, to avoid interrupting sleep.

Those assisting the patient should avoid all association with childhood toilet training. The patient should be helped to understand that accidents will occur. He will need much support and reassurance if success is to be achieved.

SPECIFIC DIAGNOSTIC STUDIES

EXAMINATION OF URINE

An analysis of the urine is such a useful guide to a person's general health that it is usually done as a routine test in most hospitals. The first voiding in the morning will usually contain the greatest concentration of abnormal constituents, so it is preferable for the specimen. The specimen should be obtained after cleaning the external genitalia and should be voided either directly into a clean specimen bottle or into a clean receptacle, from which it is poured directly into the specimen container. Seventy-five to 100 ml. of urine is required for the analysis.

Normal Urinalysis

Color	Clear yellow or straw
Acidity	pH 4.8–7.5
Protein	None
Glucose	0–trace
Red blood cells	0–3
White blood cells	0–4
Casts	Rare
Specific gravity	1.003–1.030

BACTERIOLOGIC STUDIES

A culture of the urine will be done when infection is suspected. The specimen may be voided or collected by catheterization. It must, in either case, be obtained under aseptic conditions, collected in a sterile receptacle, placed in a sterile specimen container, labeled with the patient's name, the date, the time collected, and whether it is a voided or catheterized specimen. The specimen should be either transported immediately to the laboratory to be set up on culture plates or refrigerated to avoid multiplication of bacteria and decomposition of the urine.

A voided specimen for culture may be collected from a male in the following manner:

1. Retract the foreskin.
2. Clean the penis and especially the meatus with a mild antiseptic.
3. Have the patient void a small amount (15 to 50 ml.) into the toilet or urinal.
4. Have the patient void about 10 ml. either directly into the sterile specimen receptacle or into a sterile pitcher. If a sterile pitcher is used, pour the urine immediately into the sterile specimen receptacle.
5. Cap the specimen, label appropriately, and transport to laboratory or refrigerate.

A voided specimen for culture may be collected from a female using the following procedure:

1. Cleanse the perineum with soap and water.
2. Using sterile gloves, separate the labia and cleanse the meatus with a mild antiseptic.
3. Keep the labia separated and have the patient void.
4. After the stream has started, place a sterile container to collect the specimen. Transfer the specimen to a sterile specimen receptacle.
5. Cap the specimen, label appropriately, and transport to the laboratory or refrigerate.

Urine specimens collected in this way are referred to as "mid-stream" or "clean catch" urines.

The patient may collect the sample herself if she is well instructed and physically able to do so. Explain the purpose of collecting the sample under aseptic conditions and have the patient repeat the procedure before allowing her to obtain the sample alone.

RENAL FUNCTION STUDIES

Blood Chemistry

(See Unit V for a discussion of electrolyte imbalances and diagnostic tests for abnormal levels of solutes in the plasma.)

With significant decreases in kidney function, the waste products of protein metabolism, normally removed from the body by the kidney and excreted via the urinary tract, may be found in abnormally high concentrations in the blood. The blood urea nitrogen (BUN) and serum creatinine are commonly measured to detect loss of kidney function. The BUN is normally 10 to 20 mg. per 100 ml. and the serum creatinine 0 to 1 mg. per liter. The specimen is obtained from the patient by venipuncture and the test is performed in the laboratory.

Measurements of blood levels of calcium, phosphorus, and uric acid are often done, especially when renal calculi are suspected.

Concentration and Dilution Studies

Loss of the ability of the kidney to dilute or concentrate urine is one indication of serious renal disease. With normal kidney function the number of dissolved particles in the urine (urine specific gravity) will increase with fluid restriction or loss; that is, the kidney will reabsorb more of the plasma fluid to compensate. Likewise, more fluid will be excreted in the urine, causing it to be more dilute (low specific gravity) when large amounts of fluids are ingested. With loss of renal function the specific gravity may remain low (1.008 to 1.012) regardless of the amount of fluid intake.

Concentration tests (e.g., Fishberg, Addis) involve some degree of purposeful dehydration of the patient for a given period of time. Specimens are then collected at specified times and the specific gravity of the specimens measured. If it remains low, this indicates an inability of the kidney to adequately concentrate the urine.

Dilution tests involve having the patient empty his bladder, then having him consume a large amount of fluid (up to 1200 ml. in half an hour). Urine specimens are then collected at specified intervals. With normal kidney function the fluid will all be excreted within 3 hours and will have a low specific gravity.

It is well for the nurse to ponder the discomfort one might feel if asked to restrict fluid intake completely for several hours and then to be asked to consume an unpleasant amount in half an hour. It is extremely important that the patient understand the diagnostic purpose of the procedure to avoid confusion in his mind. Often either he has been instructed previously to restrict his fluid intake, if he has been retaining too much fluid, or he has been asked to "force fluids" to increase his output.

Clearance Studies

The kidney's ability to remove or "clear" the plasma of a particular substance may be measured. Normally the kidney can remove urea from 60 to 80 ml. of plasma per minute. The *urea clearance test* involves having the patient fast for several hours. He voids, and the exact time of this voiding is recorded. The specimen is discarded. He drinks two or more glasses of water and in one hour he voids again. The exact time of this voiding is recorded and the entire specimen sent to the laboratory. A blood sample for measuring blood urea nitrogen is taken. The patient drinks more water. One hour from the last voiding he voids again. The entire specimen is sent to the laboratory carefully labeled with the exact time of voiding. The blood level and urine level of urea are compared. In patients with loss of kidney function the blood urea level will be elevated and the urea in the urine decreased.

Since the urea clearance test is dependent on a urine flow of 2 ml. per minute, it may not be a suitable test for some patients, especially those with a markedly decreased output.

The *creatinine clearance test* may be used and is actually a more accurate measure of the kidney's ability to filter the plasma. The patient voids, and at this time a 24-hour urine collection begins, starting and ending in the morning. At the end of the 24-hour period a fasting blood sample for a serum creatinine determination is obtained. An adult normally excretes 1.2 to 1.7 Gm. of creatinine in a 24-hour period.

Phenolsulfonphthalein (PSP) Test

PSP is a red dye that the kidney can completely excrete when functioning normally. It is injected intravenously, and urine samples are collected and sent to the laboratory. The dye is not visible in acid urine. In the laboratory the urine is alkalinized, turning it pink. Each specimen is compared with a standard color chart to determine the amount of dye excreted.

The patient should void and the specimen be discarded. It is extremely important that *exactly* 1 ml. (6 mg.) of dye is injected and the time recorded accurately. In exactly 15 minutes and exactly every 15 minutes for 1 hour the patient voids, and the individual samples, carefully labeled, are sent to the laboratory. Time intervals vary in different laboratories, but it is important to have the patient void at the exact specified intervals. Forcing fluids shortly before the test begins and during the test will help the patient to produce the samples on time.

If the patient's urine has a red color for any reason, such as bleeding or because of a drug he is taking, the PSP test will not be useful. Warn the patient that the dye may turn his urine red so he will not fear that he is bleeding.

Normally 25 per cent of the dye will be excreted within 1 hour.

RADIOLOGIC STUDIES OF THE KIDNEY

An x-ray of the kidney, ureters, and bladder is called a KUB. This simple x-ray will provide quite a bit of information, entails no risk to the patient, and may be performed without regard to the amount of kidney function remaining.

The outline of the kidneys and urinary tract can detect enlarged or contracted kidneys and help to diagnose hydronephrosis or the presence of some chronic disease process in the kidney. Being radiopaque, about 90 per cent of calculi will be visible on x-ray, thus aiding greatly in this diagnosis.

There are a number of studies that utilize radiopaque substances excreted by the kidney after injection intravenously or instillation through catheters directly into the kidney and urinary tract. Two commonly used substances are diatrizoate sodium (Hypaque) and meglumine diatrizoate (Renografin). These substances contain iodine and may cause severe allergic reactions in hypersensitive people. Skin testing is recommended prior to their use, but a negative reaction is no assurance that there will be no reaction. Any signs of allergic reaction, such as itching, hives, wheezing, or other respiratory distress, call for discontinuing the injection and treating the patient with antihistamines and providing emergency care for shock or respiratory difficulty.

Intravenous Pyelography (IVP)

This x-ray study involves the intravenous injection of a radiopaque substance followed by a series of films of the kidney and urinary tract. The films are taken at intervals of 2, 5, 10, and 15 minutes after the injection. If excretion is delayed, films should be taken continually at intervals for up to 4 hours or more. This x-ray provides a means of visualizing the kidney, showing the size, location, and shape, as well as the filling of the kidney pelvis and the ureters.

Preparation of the patient should include a clear explanation of the purpose of the procedure and how it is carried out. Food and fluids are withheld from midnight prior to the day of the examination. This relative dehydration allows the radiopaque substance to be more concentrated when it enters the kidney, thus providing clearer films. A larger dose of the radiopaque substance is usually necessary if this dehydration is contraindicated or if the patient's kidney function is too poor to concentrate the substance. An IVP should not be done on patients suspected of having multiple myeloma, because serious complications have been reported.

Most often castor oil or other cathartic is administered the night before the examination. This decreases gas and fecal matter in the bowel and provides clearer pictures of the urinary tract. Because the kidneys lie retroperitoneally, any barium remaining in the bowel following bowel studies must be removed prior to the IVP or the kidney may be obscured.

The nurse should be attentive to the fact that catharsis plus fasting from midnight can cause weakness, especially in a person already debilitated by age or illness. Patients should be instructed to call for assistance when they need to get up, and the staff should be alerted to the need to answer the call bell with special promptness.

When the patient is returned to his room, observation for reactions to the injection must be continued. Food, and especially fluids, should be given the patient as soon as possible to counteract his fast and dehydration.

Cystourethrography

Cystourethrography provides a visualization of urethral lesions, vesicoureteric reflux, and bladder neck or urethral obstructions. The radiopaque substance is instilled into the bladder through a urethral catheter. The patient may be asked to void while films are obtained.

Renal Angiograms

In this procedure a small catheter is placed in the femoral artery and passed into the aorta or renal artery. Radiopaque fluid is introduced via the catheter and serial films are taken. This study gives an excellent view of the renal arterial circulation and is especially useful in studying renovascular hypertension; it is also useful in the differential diagnosis of tumors and cysts.

Physical preparation of the patient is the same as for the IVP. Usually the patient is placed on bed rest for a few hours after the examination. The femoral area is observed for signs of bleeding, and pedal pulses are checked to detect any decreased circulation to the feet. A pressure dressing is usually applied to the femoral incision for a few hours.

Cystoscopy and Retrograde Pyelography

A cystoscope is a metal instrument constructed for insertion into the bladder by way of the urinary meatus. It consists of a sheath into which a telescope may be inserted for magnification. There is a light on the tip of the sheath to provide illumination, which allows the examiner an excellent view of the inside of the bladder.

The procedure is performed under either local or general anesthesia. If it is felt the patient will be unable to avoid sudden movements, which could cause injuries to the bladder or urethra, general anesthesia is indicated. Usually a sedative or narcotic is administered prior to the procedure.

Generally the patient fasts from midnight on the day of the procedure. Fluids are given in large amounts for several hours before the procedure, usually intravenously. This is necessary to ensure an adequate flow of urine for the collection of specimens and for retrograde pyelography if it is to be performed. Cleansing of the bowel as for an IVP is usually done.

The patient should be well instructed by the nurse in order to relieve any apprehension and thus avoid as much as possible the painful bladder spasms that can accompany the procedure. He should be told that he will be placed in a lithotomy position (legs in stirrups) and that this can be tiring and uncomfortable. He should be informed that deep breathing and general relaxation will decrease the discomfort of introducing the cystoscope. The desire to void will be pronounced as the cystoscope passes the neck of the bladder and also when the bladder capacity is measured by filling it with water.

Ureteral catheters may be placed into each ureter through the cystoscope. Specimens are then collected from each kidney.

A radiopaque substance may be instilled into the kidney through these catheters and x-ray films taken immediately. The patient will feel some discomfort as the injection is made, but pain should be felt only if the kidney pelvis is overdistended.

Cystoscopy is a very useful tool for both diagnosis and treatment. Its diagnostic uses include:

1. Direct inspection of the bladder, making it possible to see tumors, calculi, ulcers, or other defects.
2. Collection of urine directly from the kidney pelvis and from each kidney separately.
3. X-ray visualization through the retrograde pyelogram.

4. Measurement of bladder capacity and evidence of vesicoureteral reflux.
5. Biopsy of the bladder and urethra.

Treatment uses of the cystoscope include:

1. Resection of tumors.
2. Removal of stones and foreign bodies.
3. Dilatation of the ureters.
4. Emptying of the renal pelvis.
5. Implantation of radium seeds.

Care of the patient after cystoscopy should include bed rest for a short time. The patient should not stand immediately after removal of his legs from the stirrups, as this sudden circulatory change can cause dizziness and syncope.

Pink-tinged urine is quite common following cystoscopy, but any bright red bleeding or clots in the urine should be reported to the doctor. If dyes have been used in the procedure, the patient should be warned that his urine may have an unusual color. Pain in the back and a feeling of fullness and burning in the bladder may be experienced. Warm tub baths and mild analgesics are usually sufficient for relief. The patient should be encouraged to take large amounts of fluids after the procedure. This dilution of the urine will help to prevent further irritation to the tissues. Some chilling and a rise in temperature often occur following cystoscopy. If these symptoms do not subside readily as a result of providing extra warmth and offering frequent fluids, further investigation should be done. Cystoscopy may spread infection in the urinary tract and can cause a bacteremia. If the patient complains of abdominal pain following the procedure, the doctor should be notified, as accidental perforation of the bladder or ureters might be the cause.

Patients are often discharged within a couple of hours after cystoscopy. Written as well as verbal instructions should be given, as the patient may not be able to remember instructions given immediately after his having undergone this stressful procedure.

RENAL BIOPSY

Renal biopsy is a procedure in which a specially designed needle is inserted, piercing the skin and entering the kidney, to obtain a small sample of tissue for examination. The patient is in a prone or a sitting position. Local anesthetic is used.

An x-ray or a pyelogram is done just before the biopsy, so that markings can be made on the skin to guide the investigator in inserting the needle in the proper place.

Microscopic hematuria will occur whenever kidney tissue is obtained, but in about 5 per cent of patients there is visible blood in the urine. Perinephric hematoma occurs in about 1 per cent of patients who have a renal biopsy. Because of the danger of bleeding, platelet counts and bleeding and clotting times should be normal before a biopsy is performed. There is a 0.1 per cent mortality with biopsy even when done by experienced persons.

After biopsy the patient should be kept in bed for several hours. The nurse should observe the urine carefully and continue to observe every voiding until no blood is appearing. The patient should be encouraged to take large amounts of fluid to avoid clot formation and retention, which could obstruct urine flow.

A urine sample should be obtained for culture after the procedure, as perinephric infection is sometimes a complication of renal biopsy.

Renal biopsy has been most useful as a research tool to increase knowledge and understanding of many diseases. It is useful in determining the amount of kidney involvement in systemic diseases, such as lupus erythematosus, gout, polyarteritis nodosa, and amyloidosis, in which uremia is a major cause of death.

Before transplantation, renal biopsy is used to determine if the patient has active progressive disease that could recur in a newly transplanted kidney. It is also used to diagnose early rejection in a transplanted kidney.

Usually biopsy is not performed unless the knowledge gained would be likely to affect the treatment regimen for the patient.

CHAPTER 57

Specific Disorders of the Kidney and Lower Urinary Tract

PSYCHOLOGIC REACTIONS TO URINARY PROBLEMS

Because of the close anatomic relationship of the urinary and genital systems, patients, especially men, fear difficulties with their sexual functions when they have urologic disorders.

The patient's fears must be discussed openly and honestly with him so that he may use his available resources to cope with the real problems while false fears are allayed. The patient often feels inhibited in discussing his fears and finds it helpful for someone to inquire matter of factly if he has these specific concerns.

The social taboos our culture places on free discussion of urination sometimes causes the patient to avoid asking questions. Also, our cultural traits of keeping the genitalia hidden from view causes the examinations for urologic problems to be especially stressful to some people.

The act of urination is often performed in complete privacy, especially by women, so that being asked to void with others present may provoke anxiety and embarrassment.

The male patient may feel quite anxious and embarrassed when it is necessary for the female nurse to catheterize him or to inspect his genital area. If the nurse feels confident, is not embarrassed, and proceeds in a businesslike way, the patient is often able to relax. It is especially helpful to the patient if the nurse tells him exactly what she is going to do, what observations need to be made, and the reasons for them.

People are usually concerned that their kidney functions will be adversely affected by any urologic difficulty. Again, this concern should be discussed with the patient as honestly as possible.

GENERAL NURSING MEASURES TO SUPPORT THE PATIENT

Relief and control of pain is a major nursing measure in the care of patients with urologic disorders.

Pain is often quite severe and general discomfort almost always present. This aspect will be pointed out as we discuss the individual disorders. Many of the various diagnostic procedures commonly done also are most uncomfortable.

Medications as prescribed by the physician should be given as needed. Sitz baths or warm soaks may relieve the pain of urethritis. Forcing fluids to dilute the urine is often a most effective measure in the relief of pain.

Skin care is one important aspect of nursing these patients. Ammonia is formed from urea by bacterial action and causes the urine to take on an unpleasant odor. When urine remains on the skin it is highly irritating and becomes increasingly malodorous. Constant leaking of urine onto the skin causes a severe, painful rash and this, combined with the unpleasant odor, is a most distressing situation for the patient. Relief is aimed at preventing the leaking of urine as much as possible, protecting the skin with absorbent pads and protective creams such as zinc oxide, and meticulous cleaning of the skin.

Pruritus (itching) is often very severe, especially in the patient with uremia. There is no remedy that is effective in relieving the itching for all patients, but keeping the skin clean and dry is usually helpful. Various creams, lotions, astringents, and anesthetic ointments might be tried after consulting with the physician. A narcotic is sometimes required when the itching reaches intolerable levels.

Relief of thirst in patients on fluid restriction is a challenging nursing problem. Rinsing the mouth with water and sucking on ice can easily cause an excess of fluid to be ingested, so these measures should be used very sparingly and recorded each time. Sucking on hard candy, especially sour lemon drops, seems to help some patients. Offering the patient some distraction from his thirst sometimes makes it more bearable. Screening the patient from other patients who are being given fluids might be considered.

The patient should be told exactly what the doctor has recommended for his total liquid intake and why the restriction has been recommended. Careful planning should be done with the patient about when he wishes to receive his allotted fluid and what kind he prefers. Careful attention to meeting his requests may relieve some of his frustration over the situation.

Meticulous oral hygiene is necessary to preserve the health and comfort of the mouth and gums when liquid intake is severely limited.

Forcing fluids is frequently necessary for many patients with urologic disorders. Again, the patient needs to be told the total required, why it is important, and consulted about the type of liquid most palatable to him. When the daily oral fluid requirement is as high as 3000 ml. the patient should be drinking something at least hourly during his waking time.

SPECIFIC DISORDERS

INFECTIOUS PROCESSES

Pyelonephritis

Pyelonephritis is an inflammation of the kidney caused by a bacterial infection. There is overwhelming evidence to support the theory that most infections are caused by bacteria traveling up the urinary tract from the bladder through the ureter to the kidney. In many cases there are symptoms of cystitis (bladder inflammation) or ureteritis (ureteral inflammation) prior to the symptoms of pyelonephritis.

It is believed that reflux of urine from the bladder into the ureter caused by obstruction in the urinary tract commonly leads to pyelonephritis. In addition, obstruction causes stagnation of residual urine in the bladder, which allows the multiplication of bacteria and eventual invasion of surrounding tissue.

Pyelonephritis is much more common in females than in males. This is believed to be due to the shorter urethra in the female, which permits bacteria to reach the bladder more easily.

Catheterization and other instrumentation of the urinary tract is known to lead to bacteria in the urine in 4 per cent of those people who had normal bladders beforehand; in people with obstructions, the incidence increases to 30 per cent.

Acute pyelonephritis may cause minimal symptoms and may even be asymptomatic. Typically, though, the person complains of a need to void frequently, and the urine causes a burning sensation in the urethra. There may be severe flank pain, chills and fever, and weakness. The urine frequently has a foul smell and may be cloudy or bloody. The white blood count is usually elevated, and the urine contains many bacteria, pus cells, and red blood cells.

The urine will contain at least 100,000 organisms per milliliter when cultured. The urine sample for culture and sensitivity should be obtained before antibiotic therapy is begun.

Antibiotics will usually cause the urine to be sterile in 48 to 72 hours. The drugs are continued for at least two weeks after the first sterile urine is achieved. The urine should be recultured one week after the antibiotics are stopped, and periodically for a year after the infection. The greatest incidence of reinfection is at four months after treatment is discontinued. Infection will recur in about 35 per cent of patients.

Nursing care during the acute attack of pyelonephritis will be directed toward relief of the uncomfortable symptoms. Forcing fluids will offer the quickest relief for the burning on urination and will help to control the fever. The increased urine flow will also help to wash bacteria out of the urinary tract. Prompt and careful collection of specimens for culture of the urine will greatly aid the physician in determining the appropriate antibiotic.

When the acute infection has subsided, the patient should be instructed in the importance of continuing follow-up to prevent further infection, which can lead to chronic pyelonephritis and kidney failure. The patient should understand the importance of continuing the antibiotic even though he may feel fine. Some patients, particularly when there is a recurrence of infection, will be studied further with IVP or cystoscopy to determine the presence of a correctable obstruction.

Chronic pyelonephritis is caused by bacterial inflammation of the kidney that has left scarring, fibrosis, and tubular dilatation. The patient is usually hypertensive and shows signs of renal failure. At this stage of the disease there may be no bacteria in the urine on culture, but diagnosis is made by an IVP and renal biopsy.

If bacteria are found, the treatment is the same as for acute attacks. Hypertension must be controlled or it will further damage the kidney.

Nursing care of the patient in renal failure will be discussed in Chapter 58.

Perinephric Abscess

This is usually due to a staphylococcal infection that travels to the perinephric space by way of the blood stream from some other place in the body.

There is usually fever, pain, and tenderness in the flank and sometimes swelling. Antibiotics are given to eradicate the infection. Incision and drainage of the abscess may be required.

Ureteritis

Ureteritis is associated with pyelonephritis. Curing the kidney infection cures the ureteral inflammation, except when chronic infection causes the ureter to become fibrotic and strictures occur.

Cystitis

Cystitis is an inflammation of the bladder wall. It is much more common in females than in males. In the female it often occurs 36 to 72 hours after sexual intercourse. In the male it is usually associated with urinary retention caused by an obstruction from an enlarged, infected prostate gland.

The symptoms are usually localized to the urinary

tract; burning, frequency and urgency of urination, and some low back pain may occur.

Antibiotics and other chemotherapeutic agents are given to sterilize the urine. Hot sitz baths may relieve much of the discomfort. Unless there is some complicated underlying cause, cystitis should clear rapidly with this treatment. If it continues to recur, further diagnostic measures must be taken.

Urethritis

Urethritis is an inflammation of the urethra. It can occur as a sudden, acute infection and it may also be found in a chronic state. Its usual cause is bacterial but it can be chemical. Bubble bath has especially been noted to cause urethritis in small children, and some spermicidal jellies have produced it in women.

Symptoms, as in cystitis, include burning on urination, frequency, and nocturia. There may be pain in the urethra with movement. There is redness and irritation of the lining of the urethra; the lips of the meatus may be swollen. There is frequently a discharge in the male but not usually in the female.

Treatment includes removal of the cause of the urethritis and administering antibiotics if it is caused by an infection. Sitz baths, forcing fluids, and avoiding intercourse until symptoms subside usually result in a rapid clearing of symptoms.

Tuberculosis of the Kidney

Tuberculosis of the kidney occurs when tubercle bacilli are brought to the kidney by the blood stream from some other source in the body. Most often the body's natural defense mechanisms will prevent disease from occurring. Sometimes the organisms begin to grow slowly in the medulla of the kidney. It may take 15 to 20 years for significant kidney damage to occur. There are few, if any, symptoms until very late in the disease, at which time frequency of urination, burning, and other symptoms of cystitis may occur. Pus may be found in the urine.

Calcifications in the kidney seen on x-ray may suggest the diagnosis of tuberculosis. Cystoscopy will show the characteristic ulcers and lesions of tuberculosis. Growth of a culture of tubercle bacilli from the urine will confirm the diagnosis.

The primary treatment is the long-term administration of antituberculosis drugs. Surgery may be necessary to repair fibrotic or stenosed ureters.

The nurse should help the patient to understand the need for two or three years of continuous drug taking and the necessity for continuing follow-up even though he may feel well.

Tuberculosis is a disease that arouses a great deal of fear and a feeling of social isolation. The patient should be helped to understand the process and reassured that he is not necessarily contagious to others.

OBSTRUCTIVE DISORDERS

Hydronephrosis

Hydronephrosis is a dilatation of the pelvis of the kidney due to an obstruction in the urinary tract that prevents the normal flow of urine. Attacks may occur repeatedly with no permanent damage to the kidney. However, in severe obstructions nephrons are destroyed and will never completely recover. There is a great risk of pyelonephritis because of the urinary stasis and reflux.

Treatment should be aimed at preventing infection and permanently relieving the obstruction.

A heavy diuresis may occur just after an acute attack or just after a severe obstruction has been relieved. The nurse should be on the alert for this and consult the doctor about fluid and electrolyte replacement. Circulatory collapse can occur as a result of depletion of extracellular fluid.

STRICTURES AND CONTRACTURES

The *neck of the bladder* is a common site of contracture. It can be congenital but frequently follows chronic prostatitis in men or cystitis in women. Early symptoms include difficulty in starting to void and dribbling at the end of voiding.

Chronic retention leads to infection, hydronephrosis, and renal failure. Sometimes acute retention will occur, and this aids in the detection of the problem.

Treatment may be surgical, particularly if the cause is an enlarged prostate. Usually the patient is treated by sterilizing the urine with antibiotics and encouraging double voiding in an attempt to empty the bladder. The patient should be checked frequently for any symptoms of infection or hydronephrosis.

Urethral stricture often occurs as a result of the healing process when the urethra has been injured. Fibrous tissue is produced to fill in the injured area and this may lead to contractures.

Symptoms are much the same as in bladder neck obstruction, as are the complications.

Treatment consists of dilating the urethra with metal instruments, called sounds, of increasing size. If this is not effective, plastic repair may be necessary. Control of infection and prevention of retention are primary treatment goals, as in all urinary tract difficulties.

Ureteral strictures and *stenosis* are found at the ureteropelvic or ureterovesical junction. These are caused by reflux of urine when there is an obstruction lower in the urinary tract or by a hypertrophy of the smooth muscle ring at the ureterovesical junction.

Often symptoms are absent, and a kidney can be destroyed by hydronephrosis before the condition is detected. Occasionally patients may have pain akin to appendicitis or costovertebral angle pain. Some infection may be present, and if the hydronephrotic kidney is large enough it may be felt on physical examination.

Repair of the stricture and surgical correction of all areas of obstruction is the usual treatment.

Calculi (Nephrolithiasis)

Most calculi, or stones, are formed in the kidney, but they may also form in the bladder. Kidney stones may be very large and remain in the kidney, but most are passed down the ureter into the bladder, then voided. Small sandlike particles are called gravel, while the large branching stones are called staghorn calculi.

Most often stones are composed of a calcium salt. In some patients the cause is an excess excretion of calcium in the urine but others have a normal level of secretion. In these latter patients, the cause is generally an alkaline urine, which allows the calcium to come out of solution and crystallize. Some stones are composed of uric acid; urinary hyperacidity and gout are the usual causes of these. Cystine stones occur when cystinuria of over 25 mg. a day occurs. Most stones are radiopaque, but uric acid stones are not.

Sometimes stones are very small and are voided easily with no symptoms. When the stone is very large it can block the ureter, causing hydronephrosis and extreme damage to the kidney. When a large stone enters the ureter, renal colic occurs. This is a severe pain in the flank which radiates down the length of the urinary tract. The patient appears to be in acute distress, with sweating, pallor, and nausea and vomiting. If there is infection, high fever and pyuria may be present. Red blood cells are often seen in the urine. Frequency of urination is present throughout the attack, which lasts anywhere from a few minutes to several hours.

Nursing care during the acute attack of renal colic should be directed toward relief of pain and anxiety and control of fever and nausea. All urine voided should be strained to detect stones that are passed. When the stone passes, a marked relief from pain occurs, but soreness will persist for a while.

Sometimes it is necessary to remove the stone surgically or through cystoscopy. Occasionally multiple stones in the kidney require partial or total nephrectomy.

After the acute attack the nurse should arrange to instruct the patient on the particular diet prescribed to prevent further calculus formation. She should emphasize the importance of adequate fluid intake to dilute the urine and to maintain a large volume.

Cystic Disease

Polycystic disease of the kidneys is a hereditary disorder in which grapelike cysts replace some of the normal tissue of the kidney. It is usually bilateral and affects males and females equally. Symptoms usually appear around age 40, but sometimes do so as early as 20 or as late as 80.

Symptoms are varied. Pain frequently occurs and may be felt as a dull ache in the flank or as an acute renal colic. Hematuria is common, and infection occurs frequently. Hypertension with resulting cardiac enlargement and heart failure occurs in about 50 per cent of patients. Sometimes the kidneys are palpable on examination. The kidney can become so enlarged as to cause severe pressure on other organs. As the disease progresses, renal function deteriorates and ultimately uremia results.

There is no known way to arrest the progress of the obstructive cysts, so treatment is directed toward preservation of the kidney function. Surgical draining of the cysts has no effect on the progress of the disease. Prevention and control of infection and hypertension are essential. Principles of nursing care of the patient, once renal failure is evident, are the same regardless of the cause of the failure. These principles will be discussed in Chapter 58.

If the diagnosis of polycystic kidneys is made during childbearing years, genetic counseling should be offered to the patient because of the hereditary basis of the disorder.

Medullary sponge kidney is a cystic disorder that occurs late in life and does not appear to be hereditary. Infection, pain, and hematuria are common, as in polycystic disease, but renal function usually does not deteriorate unless infection is uncontrolled.

Neoplasms

Benign tumors of the kidney are rare. When large ones occur it is relatively impossible to distinguish them from malignant tumors by x-ray, so the kidney usually must be removed.

Tumors of the ureter, bladder, or urethra are not so common as those of the kidney. Symptoms of obstruction are most common, with difficulty in starting the urinary stream, decreased size and force of the stream, and dribbling at the end of voiding. Hematuria is common and sometimes causes colicky pain from the passage of clots or masses of cells. About four fifths of renal tumors are adenocarcinomas and two thirds of these occur in men.

Symptoms are often absent until very late in the disease. Gross hematuria without pain occurs in two thirds of the patients. Pain is usually a very late symptom, if it occurs. Sometimes the patient may notice a mass in the flank, or it may be discovered on routine physical examination. Many times symptoms do not appear until metastasis has occurred, with accompanying weight loss, weakness, and anemia.

Renal adenocarcinomas usually do not respond to x-ray therapy or chemotherapy; therefore, nephrectomy is the treatment of choice. See Unit VII for a discussion of the care of the patient with cancer.

TRAUMA TO THE KIDNEYS AND URINARY TRACT

Kidney Trauma

Serious injury to the kidney is relatively rare because of the protection afforded by the rib cage and the heavy muscles of the back. Traffic accidents and falls in which the person lands on his abdomen, flank, or back are the most common causes of injury. Kidney lacerations are also associated with fractures of the spine and ribs.

Small contusions and bruising are most common. Small lacerations will usually heal themselves. Hematoma will occur if the renal capsule is torn. These should be watched closely for signs of increase in size. When severe lacerations which extend into the kidney pelvis occur, massive bleeding can quickly lead to death.

At first, nursing care is mostly concerned with control of shock and hemorrhage. Whenever a person has been in an accident he should be observed for signs of injury to the kidney and urinary tract.

Ureteral Injuries

The most common injury to the ureters occurs during extensive gynecologic surgery, abdominal perineal resections, or cystoscopic manipulation.

Extravasation of urine into surrounding tissues occurs. The patient usually complains of pain in the flank and lower abdomen. A paralytic ileus may develop. Severe emesis often occurs. Urine may begin to drain through the incision in the abdomen or through the vagina.

Prompt surgical repair is usually very successful. If the injury is not detected until well into the postoperative period, nephrectomy may be required.

The nurse should be cognizant of ureteral injury as a complication in these procedures, and should observe the patient carefully and report any symptoms promptly to the surgeon.

Bladder Injuries

A bladder distended with urine can rupture when a direct blow is sustained. The bladder may also be punctured by bony splinters when the pelvis is fractured. Accidental surgical injuries also occur.

Rupture and perforation of the bladder cause urine to spill into the peritoneal cavity. Peritonitis and cellulitis occur rapidly and will be fatal unless prompt drainage and repair are instituted.

Pain low in the abdomen and hematuria, in addition to a history of an injury or blow to the abdomen, should always arouse the suspicion of bladder injury.

Nursing care, again, will be most concerned with control of shock and intensive observation for signs of complications.

Urethral Injuries

The urethra, as well as the bladder, may be injured in pelvic fractures. Instrumentation is also a common cause of injury. Falling astride an object with force is another cause of urethral lacerations and contusions.

Symptoms may be the same as in bladder perforation. Urethral strictures commonly occur in untreated urethral lesions.

RENAL PARENCHYMAL DISEASE

Glomerulonephritis

Glomerulonephritis is an allergic or autoimmune reaction of the glomeruli of the kidney to a streptococcal infection in the body. It usually occurs a few weeks after the infection. The exact mechanism is not clearly understood.

Acute glomerulonephritis is most often seen in children and young adults. Hematuria is almost always present. Edema, proteinuria, and decreased urine output frequently occur. Hypertension is often present, and headache and an increase in the blood urea nitrogen are common.

This disease is usually self-limiting, with full recovery. However, if oliguria occurs and continues for more than three days, severe and irreversible glomerular damage may occur. Sometimes dialysis is necessary to control uremia and hypertension while the kidney heals.

If recovery does not take place, the disease may develop into subacute or chronic glomerulonephritis. Hemoptysis and retinopathy are characteristic of subacute disease. Death from uremia or lung hemorrhage usually occurs within two years. The subacute disease may develop insidiously without the sudden features of acute glomerulonephritis.

Chronic glomerulonephritis may follow the acute disease or may develop many years later. In many cases it develops insidiously, with no history of an acute attack. There may be proteinuria and progressive hypertension for many years, or the disease may present with the symptoms of uremia, progressing rapidly to death.

There is no treatment that will heal the glomerular lesions. Treatment is directed toward preservation of renal function, by control of hypertension and infection, and alleviation of the symptoms of uremia with diet, drugs, and dialysis. Nursing care of patients with renal failure will be discussed in the next chapter.

Nephrotic Syndrome

The nephrotic syndrome is a set of symptoms that are caused by many different problems, most commonly glomerulonephritis or some systemic disorder such as diabetes or lupus erythematosus. The symptoms are heavy loss of protein in the urine, resulting in hypoalbuminemia and massive edema. There may also be a high blood cholesterol level. The prognosis depends on the underlying cause.

If the cause is a mild glomerulonephritis, found especially in children, treatment with steroids results in a 75 per cent five-year survival rate. In adults the nephrotic syndrome is usually just one of the stages in the progress toward chronic renal failure. When the nephrotic syndrome appears in a patient with systemic lupus erythematosus, death usually occurs within a year.

Hypertensive Nephropathy

Hypertension both causes and is caused by renal disease. Malignant hypertension is a set of symptoms in which diastolic pressure is 150 mm. Hg or more, papilledema is severe, and uremia occurs. The kidney is damaged by the depositing of fibrous material in the arterioles, which causes ischemia and sometimes infection. Severe headache, blurred vision, severe weight loss, and the symptoms of renal failure occur. Unless the hypertension is controlled, death results in a matter of months.

Hypertension may be caused by the types of renal disease in which there is decreased blood flow to the kidney, such as in vascular and parenchymal diseases. This is felt to be due to the excretion of renin, an enzyme that will raise the systemic blood pressure. Renin excretion is increased when renal ischemia occurs.

Control of hypertension is essential to prevent cerebrovascular complications and further damage to the kidneys. (See also Unit X.)

NEPHROTOXINS

There are many substances that will damage kidney tissue and function. Since the kidney receives 25 per cent of the cardiac output, it is especially

vulnerable to the effects of toxic substances carried in the blood stream.

Antibiotics are one of the many therapeutic agents that can cause damage to the renal tubules. Among these are the tetracyclines, neomycin, ampicillin, sulfonamides, kanamycin, cephaloridine, and colistin. Analgesics such as caffeine, aspirin, and particularly phenacetin, taken in large doses for extended periods, may also damage kidney tissue.

Heavy metals such as mercury and uranium will cause glomerular damage, as will poisoning with solvents, particularly carbon tetrachloride. Various insecticides also have been shown to cause renal lesions.

Treatment begins with withdrawal of the toxin and attempts to hasten removal from the body. If irreversible kidney damage has occurred, treatment will be that of a patient with renal failure, as discussed in Chapter 58.

CHAPTER 58

Nursing Care of the Patient in Renal Failure

THE UREMIC SYNDROME

Uremia literally means "urine in the blood." This term, and the term "uremic syndrome," are used to describe a set of symptoms that result from loss of renal function. This loss may be sudden or may develop over a long period; it may be self-limited or irreversible. Sudden loss of kidney function, such as occurs in damage from trauma, shock, toxins, or acute glomerulonephritis, brings on uremia rapidly and usually causes a severe deterioration of the patient's condition. Gradual loss of kidney function over an extended period may occur with glomerulonephritis, hypertension, chronic pyelonephritis, and other diseases.

When the loss of the kidney function is a gradual process, the patient may be able to function quite well for a long time in spite of his uremia.

SYMPTOMS

The uremic patient will be weak and easily fatigued. His skin may have a yellowish cast and itch severely. Often he has a poor appetite, with nausea, vomiting, and diarrhea. His breath may have an unpleasant odor. He may have high blood pressure and headache. He may be edematous and have congestive heart failure. He tends to bruise easily and may hemorrhage, especially from the gastrointestinal tract. Muscular twitching and numbness and tingling of the toes and hands may be present. As the uremia progresses, all the symptoms increase in severity. The patient usually begins to experience seizures and may have massive bleeding in the terminal stages. Death will ensue unless he regains his kidney function, or dialysis or renal transplantation is performed.

NURSING CARE

Nursing care will vary from patient to patient in the early stages of uremia, depending on the cause. However, when the uremia is severe there are general principles that can guide the nurse.

The patient invariably has disturbances of the gastrointestinal tract. His salivary flow is decreased, and he often has ulcerations of the mucous membranes of the mouth. He may be very thirsty and have an unpleasant taste in the mouth. Meticulous oral hygiene should be given hourly to combat these unpleasant symptoms. Because of the tendency for uremic patients to bleed, this care will have to be very gentle to avoid trauma.

Nausea, vomiting, and a poor appetite, sometimes a complete revulsion against food, frequently occur. The nurse should try to protect the patient from the sight and odors of food being served to others. Very small portions of those foods that seem most appealing to the patient should be offered.

Severe debilitating hiccoughs sometimes accompany uremia. Sedatives may be useful in controlling these.

Patients almost always become insomniac as uremia progresses. Severe fatigue, extreme restlessness of the legs, muscle cramps, and severe itching contribute further to this problem. The patient appears shaky, tense, and anxious; frightening hallucinations occur.

Symptomatic relief of each of these problems should be attempted. Keeping the skin clean and dry and experimenting with various lotions will sometimes provide relief of itching. Providing a footboard for the patient to press against will help to relieve the acute leg muscle cramps. A quiet, dark room of the desired temperature, a family member or friend to sit quietly with the patient, and soothing backrubs will sometimes induce badly needed sleep.

Unless treatment is instituted, the patient will inevitably become comatose, convulse, and die.

Because of the extreme unpleasantness of the symptoms of uremia and because no permanent relief of these symptoms is possible, those caring for the patient, as well as his family, may become very discouraged and tend to avoid contact with him as much as possible. Each nurse must explore this feeling within herself and try to recognize that she can do no more than offer measures of comfort to the patient. Helping the family to talk out their feelings about the situation and reassuring them as to the naturalness of these feelings will help them to offer support to the patient and avoid feelings of guilt for having abandoned him.

The advent of dialysis and transplantation in the last 10 years has fortunately reduced the number of patients with renal failure who die in uremia.

ACUTE RENAL FAILURE

Acute renal failure refers to the abrupt loss of kidney function caused by a variety of problems. Hemorrhage and circulatory failure from trauma or extensive surgery are common causes. Acute glomerulonephritis, vascular occlusions, and toxicity from drugs and other substances also produce acute renal failure.

The most common lesion is called acute tubular necrosis or ATN. The renal tubules are apparently injured more easily than the glomeruli. Usually, with time, healing will take place. In about 30 per cent of cases, however, the patient will succumb to uremia before the tubules regenerate. Careful conservative management greatly increases chances of recovery. Dialysis can prevent uremia until renal function is regained. The original illness, however, often causes the death of the patient even when the renal failure is controlled.

The first symptom of acute renal failure is a rapidly decreasing urinary output or oliguria. The hourly urine volume may fall to zero. The patient is considered anuric when the total 24-hour urine volume drops below 250 ml.

With anuria death may occur within 24 hours, but a person may live up to two weeks with no urine output.

One of the most serious results of anuria is hyperkalemia, or an excess of potassium in the serum, a result of the kidney's failure to excrete potassium. In addition, potassium is released in greater quantities from the body cells when acidosis is present. Acidosis occurs as a result of the kidney's inability to excrete hydrogen ions. The hyperkalemia is further increased by rapid catabolism of tissue, such as occurs with fever, severe infections, and trauma. Sometimes severe muscle weakness and circumoral numbness and tingling warn of hyperkalemia. Most often, however, cardiac arrest occurs with no warning symptoms unless ECG's are being monitored. The level of potassium in the serum should be measured frequently.

TREATMENT

Treatment of hyperkalemia includes dietary restriction of potassium intake. Cationic exchange resins, administered orally or by enema, will combine with potassium and allow its excretion in the stool. This process can lower the serum potassium level.

The administration of glucose and insulin, sodium bicarbonate, or calcium gluconate intravenously can temporarily prevent cardiac arrest in an emergency. Dialysis will remove the excess potassium from the serum.

As anuria continues, the end products of protein metabolism accumulate in the blood, and the BUN and serum creatinine rise. A diet high in calories and low in protein will help to control the accumulation of these toxic substances.

Control of fluid intake is very important during the oliguric phase of acute renal failure. Fluids should be limited to equal the urine output plus the 600 to 800 ml. of insensible loss that usually occurs in 24 hours.

Overloading the patient with fluid at this time can produce circulatory failure and death.

As uremia progresses, resistance to infection is impaired. When infection does occur it accentuates the uremia by increasing catabolism and causing further renal toxicity. Use of urethral catheters should be avoided because of their great potential for inducing infection.

Increasing urinary output signals the begining of recovery of renal function. This may occur within 48 hours or may require up to a month. Should the patient's renal function fail to return within this time period, he most likely has suffered irreversible kidney damage.

A period of diuresis usually lasts about a week. During this phase extremely large volumes of urine may be excreted. Electrolyte and fluid loss must be carefully monitored; prompt replacement of excessive losses is necessary, as death can result from depletion.

GENERAL NURSING CARE

The period of acute renal shutdown is very stressful to the patient and his family. One of these stresses is the fact that the renal failure is usually superimposed on another serious illness or injury. The uncertain prognosis for the patient is another source of stress. If it is necessary to treat the patient with dialysis, a great deal of fear may be aroused in patient and family if they are not adequately prepared. Allowing the patient and his family to talk about their anxieties and offering them as much information as they wish will help to support them through this crisis.

General physical care will be directed primarily toward those needs of the patient caused by his initial illness or injury. The degree of uremia experienced by the patient will also affect the kind of care he needs.

IRREVERSIBLE RENAL FAILURE

Irreversible or chronic renal failure can develop insidiously over a period of many years or can occur as a result of a bout of acute renal failure from which the patient fails to recover.

Chronic glomerulonephritis, polycystic disease, and repeated bouts of pyelonephritis are examples of disorders that gradually destroy the nephrons and finally result in irreversible renal failure. The end result for the patient is uremia and death, or treatment by dialysis or renal transplantation. Other systemic diseases such as hypertension, lupus erythematosus, arthritis, and polyarteritis nodosa may also produce irreversible kidney failure. Treatment of the renal failure will not prevent disability and death from the underlying disease.

The patient may have been seen by a physician for many years because of known chronic kidney disease. In this case, approaching renal failure may be noted by elevations in the serum creatinine and BUN, increasing anemia, and other abnormal laboratory test values.

Symptoms and Signs and Their Control

The person who has been unaware of his kidney disease may first notice an increase in the volume of urine. This may cause him to be awakened at night by the need to void. He also may experience an unusual thirst. These symptoms are caused by the kidneys' loss of ability to concentrate urine adequately. In an attempt to continue excreting the solutes, a large volume of dilute urine is passed. Now that the kidney does not have the ability to reabsorb water sufficiently, the patient may become severely dehydrated when he has vomiting and diarrhea, or for any reason that excessively limits his fluid intake.

Eventually the kidney also loses the ability to reabsorb electrolytes. This can result in what is sometimes called "salt washing," in which the patient voids urine containing very large amounts of sodium. This causes a severe sodium depletion, or *hyponatremia,* unless supplemental sodium is given. It is sometimes difficult to make a correct judgment of the amount of sodium the patient needs because his needs change with environmental changes. Excessive sodium intake can cause fluid retention, which leads to circulatory overload and congestive heart failure.

The best insurance that an adequate, but not excessive, sodium intake will be maintained is a well instructed patient. The nurse can ask the patient to weigh himself daily and teach him the relationship of daily weight loss or gain to his need for sodium. The patient should be taught to take his blood pressure daily and to use this as an additional indication of his need for sodium. He must be aware that edema represents a large sodium excess. He should understand that vomiting and diarrhea, or working or playing in a hot environment, can cause fluid and electrolyte loss that his kidney is unable to compensate for. Dehydration can quickly precipitate a crisis, causing the patient to become uremic.

Anemia produces fatigue and lethargy, and these are sometimes the initial symptoms that cause the patient to seek medical advice. The anemia of chronic renal failure is thought to be due to an inadequate production of erythropoietin by the diseased kidney. Erythropoietin is a substance that stimulates the bone marrow to produce red blood cells. It is also believed that the toxic substances that accumulate in the blood and cause uremia also cause a depression of the bone marrow. In general, the anemia becomes more severe as the degree of uremia increases.

Hypertension, if present, must be controlled to prevent further damage to the kidney. However, if the blood pressure is allowed to fall to very low levels, the renal blood flow is decreased, thereby further decreasing the excretion of solutes, which thus increases uremia. If antihypertensive drugs are used, the patient should be made knowledgeable in their use and alerted to the complications that can arise.

As the end products of protein metabolism begin to accumulate in the blood and the BUN and serum creatinine begin to rise, the patient is often placed on severe protein restriction. A popular diet, called the modified Giovanetti diet, which provides all essential amino acids while limiting protein to 10 Gm. in 24 hours, is often prescribed. There is controversy over the advisability of treating the patient by severe protein restriction. Some believe that allowing the patient to remain very well nourished, but instituting treatment by dialysis at an earlier time than might otherwise be necessary, is a better alternative. In this case, protein is usually restricted to 30 or 40 Gm. per day. In any restricted diet, vitamin supplements should be considered.

Another problem encountered by the patient is the development of *acidosis.* This is usually treated by the administration of sodium bicarbonate orally, unless a need for sodium restriction prevents it.

Hyperkalemia usually does not become a problem until the degree of uremia is very severe. As the level of uremia increases, bouts of gastrointestinal upset become frequent. The patient's resistance to infection is lowered. The patient is in a fragile state at this point. Any increased stress such as fever, nausea and vomiting, or surgery can tip the balance of his renal compensation, causing a life-threatening bout of uremia to ensue.

When the serum creatinine rises above 13 mEq. per liter and the glomerular filtration rate drops to 5 ml./minute, or when any of the symptoms of uremia become uncontrollable by conservative management, plans for dialysis should be made. If the patient cannot be treated by dialysis or transplantation, his care will be that of the patient with terminal uremia.

DIALYSIS

There are two major types of dialysis: peritoneal dialysis and hemodialysis. Each may be used to relieve the symptoms of renal failure temporarily until the patient regains his function; both are also used to sustain life in the person with irreversible kidney disease. In this case the dialysis must continue intermittently for the rest of the person's life. Dialysis is also used to overcome uremia and physically prepare the patient to receive a transplanted kidney. Dialysis is frequently necessary to keep the patient alive until a suitable donor kidney is found. If the transplanted kidney does not function adequately immediately, dialysis may be used to prevent uremia until the kidney functions sufficiently.

Dialysis, or diffusion, refers to the passage of particles (ions) from an area of high concentration to an area of low concentration across a semipermeable membrane, one with pores that are large enough to allow certain particles to pass through but too small to allow the passage of larger particles.

When two solutions are separated by a semipermeable membrane, solute particles will move toward the solution with the lesser concentration. Simultaneously water will move, by the process of osmosis, toward the solution in which the solute concentration is greater.

When dialysis is used as a substitute for kidney function, the semipermeable membrane used is either the peritoneal membrane (for peritoneal dialysis) or an artificial membrane (for hemodialysis). This membrane must have pores large enough to allow the passage of electrolytes, urea, and creatinine, but too small to allow the passage of blood cells and other protein molecules.

The two solutions used on opposite sides of the membrane are (1) the blood and (2) a specially prepared electrolyte solution called dialysate.

There are four basic goals of dialysis therapy:

1. Removal of the end products of protein metabolism (such as urea and creatinine) from the blood.
2. Maintenance of a safe concentration of the serum electrolytes.
3. Correction of acidosis and replenishment of the blood's bicarbonate buffer system.
4. Removal of excess fluid (water) from the blood.

It must be remembered that solute particles and water can move freely across the membrane in either direction between the blood and the dialysate. With this idea in mind it can be seen that if the patient's blood has a higher concentration of urea, creatinine, and certain electrolytes other than the prepared dialysate solution, these particles will move into the dialysate solution, thus lowering the level in the blood. Likewise, if the blood is deficient in a substance, such as bicarbonate, a higher concentration of this substance in the dialysate will cause it to move into the blood, raising the blood level.

Excess fluid can be removed from the blood by increasing the particle concentration of the dialysate with a solute such as dextrose. This increased particle concentration will cause water to move into the dialysate while, at the same time, the dextrose moves into the blood. The tendency is always toward an equalization of concentration of the two solutions.

PERITONEAL DIALYSIS

Peritoneal dialysis is used frequently to treat patients in acute renal failure. It is simple, requires very little equipment, and can be performed in any hospital setting.

Peritoneal dialysis is also used intermittently as a life-sustaining treatment for chronic renal failure. Patients are trained to perform the treatment at home. We will look mostly at the simplest form of peritoneal dialysis as performed in nonspecialized units in the community hospital. The principles are the same, but more sophisticated equipment and procedures are often used for patients who will be using this treatment for months and years as a substitute for their lost renal function.

The simplest form of peritoneal dialysis involves the placement of a catheter, by a physician, through the abdomen into the peritoneal space. Two liters of a sterile, commercially prepared dialysate solution is allowed to flow into the peritoneal space by gravity. The solution remains in the abdomen for about 20 minutes. The solution in the peritoneal cavity is in contact with the semipermeable peritoneal membrane. A large blood supply to the peritoneal membrane provides a solution for exchange of solutes and water. When the dialysate solution is permitted to flow out of the peritoneal cavity it has picked up urea and creatinine from the blood. Fresh solution is then introduced. As this process continues for many hours, the patient's blood is reduced in toxic substances and his electrolyte balance may be returned to a safe concentration. The dialysate solution will contain varying amounts of dextrose to alter the osmotic pressure, thus encouraging more or less water to leave the blood, depending on the patient's needs.

When dialysis is to be discontinued, the physician removes the catheter from the abdomen.

Nursing Responsibilities in Peritoneal Dialysis

With the exception of insertion and removal of the peritoneal catheter, peritoneal dialysis is entirely a nursing procedure.

Care of the patient receiving peritoneal dialysis is often complicated by the fact that the underlying illness that caused the renal failure is also threatening the patient's life. The patient and his family are likely to be very anxious and upset when they are told of the procedure. If the nurse performing the procedure lacks an understanding of the principles involved, it is unlikely she will be able to offer reassurance to patient and family. It is important for the nurse to realize, and impress on the family, that the dialysis itself is not a dangerous or hazardous procedure. The patient could, indeed, die during the procedure, but this would most likely be the result of his illness, not of the dialysis procedure itself.

Descriptions of specific procedures for peritoneal dialysis will be found accompanying the commercial dialysate solutions or will be prepared by the hospital where the procedure is performed. There are several major points, however, that should be kept in mind:

1. Insertion of the special peritoneal catheter and induction of fluid into the peritoneal cavity should be a meticulously sterile procedure. Diffuse peritonitis can occur as a result of contamination during this procedure.

2. The dialysate solution should be warmed to body temperature (by placing the bottle in a warm water bath) before it is introduced into the peritoneal cavity. The patient will feel great discomfort and may chill if this is not done.

3. A meticulously accurate record of the amount of solution introduced and the amount returned must be kept. The nurse should keep a record of each inflow and outflow, as well as a record of the total amount in and out. If the record shows 3 liters or more retained, the physician should be notified.

4. The patient should not experience pain during the procedure. If he does, the solution is either too hot or too cold or the catheter is not placed properly.

5. The patient's vital signs should be checked often. The nurse can expect a lowering of the blood pressure as the patient's blood volume is reduced. If excess salt and water are removed he may become severely hypotensive. The nurse should be alert to developing symptoms of depleted volume so that replacement of fluid can begin before there is a significant depletion.

6. The patient may eat and drink, within the restrictions imposed by his other problems, while he is undergoing peritoneal dialysis.

HEMODIALYSIS

Hemodialysis is also used to treat patients with either acute or irreversible kidney failure. Unlike peritoneal dialysis, hemodialysis does require specialized training for safe performance of the procedure.

There are several different pieces of equipment used for hemodialysis but they all operate in essentially the same way.

Hemodialysis Procedure

Hemodialysis involves allowing blood to flow from the patient's body into a membrane package and then returning the dialyzed blood to the patient. While the blood is within the external membrane compartment, the dialysate solution is delivered by a mechanical pump to flow on the outside of the membrane. Diffusion takes place between the blood and the dialysate solution.

Access to the patient's blood supply is obtained either by an external arteriovenous shunt or by an internal arteriovenous fistula.

The external shunt requires the surgical placement of two tubes, or cannulas, into the patient's forearm or leg (Fig. 58–1). One cannula is inserted into an artery and the other into a vein. The two tubes are brought out to the surface of the skin and connected together with a U-shaped segment called a shunt. Blood flows from the patient's artery through the shunt into the patient's vein. When he is to be attached to the hemodialyzer, or artificial kidney, a tube leading into the membrane compartment is connected to the arterial cannula. Blood then fills the membrane compartment and flows back into the patient by way of a tube connected to his venous cannula. Blood from the patient continues to flow through the membrane compartment for several hours. Dialysate solution is simultaneously pumped around the outside of the blood-filled membrane compartment. Fresh dialysate is utilized continuously, while used dialysate flows out and down a drain.

When the dialysis is to be discontinued, the flow of blood from the patient is stopped by clamping the arterial cannula. Remaining blood in the membrane compartment is returned to the patient by way of the venous cannula. The venous cannula is then clamped and the U-shaped shunt reapplied to connect artery to vein.

Creation of an internal arteriovenous fistula is also a surgical procedure, in which an artery in the arm is anastomosed to a vein in a sideways fashion. This creates an opening, or fistula, between a large artery and a large vein. The leaking of arterial blood into the venous system causes the veins to become engorged. These large veins may then be punctured, using 14- or 16-gauge needles. When the patient is to go on dialysis a needle is placed in the vein, using sterile venipuncture technique. Another needle is placed in a different vein or in an opposite direction to the first needle in the same vein. By use of a blood pump on the tubing leading to the hemodialyzer, arterial blood is pulled out of the vein by way of the fistula. Blood returns to the patient by a tube connected to the other needle.

Hemodialysis, as a treatment for irreversible renal failure, must be continued intermittently for as long as the patient lives. A typical schedule would be six to ten hours of treatment three days each week. This

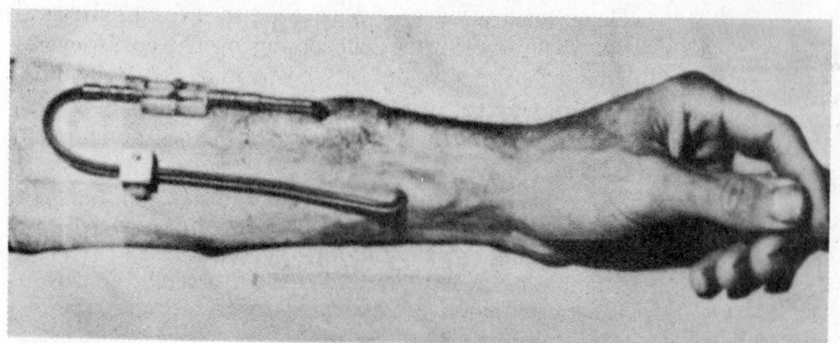

FIGURE 58–1. Cannula in place in wrist. (From Fellows, B. J.: *Nursing Clinics of North America, 1* (No. 4):579, 1966.)

schedule will vary with the size of the patient, the type of dialyzer used, the rate of flow of blood, the personal preference of the patient, and several other factors.

The membrane compartments of different hemodialyzers vary in the amount of blood they contain at any one time; however, none exceeds 700 ml. and some hold as little as 100 ml.

Nursing Care

A nurse should not care for patients undergoing hemodialysis until she has received special instructions. The following points can increase one's general knowledge of the nursing care required.

1. Anticoagulation of the blood is necessary throughout the procedure to prevent clots from forming and obstructing the blood flow.
2. The entire circuit through which the blood flows must be sterile. All connections must be made using aseptic technique. Bacteremia may result from contamination.
3. The entire blood circuit must be a completely closed system. Any break in the tubing or a minute hole in the membrane compartment will allow blood to escape. If this blood loss continues undetected, the patient can exsanguinate.
4. Dialysate concentration must be maintained within a certain safe limit. Dialysate concentrations that are excessively high or low can be fatal to the patient.
5. Monitoring devices with audible alarms to signal pressure changes, blood leaks, and dialysate concentration changes are an essential part of safe hemodialysis equipment.

Hemodialysis, and especially the lay term "artificial kidney," may provoke great apprehension in patient and family. This is further increased when the patient is actually hooked-up to the strange looking equipment. The patient and family can be helped to understand the purpose of the equipment. A calm nursing staff, unhurried and unpreoccupied, can do more than all the verbal reassurance to help the patient to relax.

It is not uncommon for the patient to feel quite grateful and optimistic at the start of his treatments. Usually he has felt poorly for some time and he views the treatment as a route to survival and a hope for feeling well again. It takes a few days or weeks for the full realization of the permanence of the treatment in his life to come into full focus. Depression during this period is expected. If the patient has sound psychologic coping mechanisms and help from those around him, he soon accommodates himself to this situation and plans his life realistically. The patient who handles stress poorly or who has little support from others sometimes never makes an adequate adjustment.

Home Dialysis

The ultimate rehabilitation for the patient who must spend a portion of every week of his life on an artificial kidney is for him to be able to perform the treatment for himself at home. One of the chief psychologic stresses of continued hemodialysis is the feeling of dependence evoked in the patient. When he has been trained to perform the treatment safely himself and is making all the routine treatment decisions on a day-to-day basis, his feelings of competence and independence are greatly enhanced. Also, the flexibility in his schedule that is achieved by home treatment is a great advantage. The cost of home treatment is about $3,000 per year as opposed to $21,000 or more per year for hospital-based dialysis treatment.

Home dialysis training programs for patients should be planned carefully. The patient needs assistance to help him to gain the technical and intellectual skills required and at the same time make a satisfactory emotional adjustment to his situation. Good family support is a great advantage to the patient on home hemodialysis. A nursing staff with a firm belief in the ability of most individuals to care for themselves is essential to the success of such a program. The nurse must be able to take pride in helping others become independent. The staff of a successful home dialysis program takes a very broad view of rehabilitation. Keeping the patient free of uremia is only the first essential step in his rehabilitation. Helping him to resume his former roles and to become as self-sufficient as possible should be the ultimate goal of the program.

RENAL TRANSPLANTATION

Renal transplantation, or renal homograft, is the surgical transfer of a human kidney from one individual to another. A normal person has two kidneys. However, a single healthy kidney can function as adequately as two kidneys. Because of this, kidneys are frequently transplanted from a living donor to a needy recipient.

Functioning kidneys are also removed from people immediately after death and transplanted into waiting recipients. New techniques of preserving the function of these cadaver kidneys has made it possible to wait for several hours until the most suitable recipient is found and also to transport the kidney from one geographical area to another.

The operative procedure consists of removal of the recipient's own kidneys, if they have not been previously removed. The donor kidney is placed in the iliac fossa and the renal vessels are anastomosed to the recipient's iliac vessels (Fig. 58–2). The surgical procedure is done swiftly to decrease the time the donor kidney is without a blood supply. Periods of ischemia longer than 30 minutes can damage the function of the newly transplanted kidney.

Usually the kidney begins functioning immediately. There is usually a period of diuresis for the first few days. Sometimes adequate functioning is delayed a few days. Hemodialysis may be performed intermittently until good function is established.

Rejection Reaction

The chief difficulty with transplantation is the homograft rejection reaction. When normal tissue from one individual is transplanted into an individual genetically dissimilar, a reaction sets in that will ultimately destroy the foreign tissue. Identical twins will not reject tissue transplanted between them because of their genetic similarity. A recipient will reject tissue from all other donors, though material from mothers, fathers, brothers and sisters will be accepted somewhat better than organs from genetically unrelated persons. Immunosuppressive therapy is necessary to prevent and to control the rejection reaction. This therapy is designed to block the patient's normal immune responses. Azathioprine (Immuran) and prednisone are the two chemical agents most widely used to suppress the rejection reaction. Serious side effects accompany the use of both drugs. The patient is very susceptible to infection while on immunosuppressive therapy.

The patient must be forever watchful for signs of rejection. Acute rejection episodes are handled by temporarily increasing the drug therapy. Symptoms of rejection are:

> Increased BUN and serum creatinine.
> Decrease in creatinine clearance.
> Decrease in urine volume.
> Elevated temperature and blood pressure.
> Weight gain.
> Restlessness and irritability.
> Tender, palpable kidney.

Nursing Care

Patients receiving transplants must be helped to realize that they will continue to need close medical supervision. It will be necessary for them to adhere faithfully to their prescribed medical regimen. They should be helped to prepare themselves emotionally for the event of rejection. Though development of realistic attitudes is necessary, the nurse should also stress the patient's positive progress. The staff can help the patient to develop an optimistic approach to life. As in all situations in which the patient must continue under medical supervision, independence should be encouraged.

Working with chronically ill patients can be tedious and emotionally taxing. The reward of seeing a person who has been ill for many years, and consequently dispirited, take on new life and health after transplantation can be very gratifying.

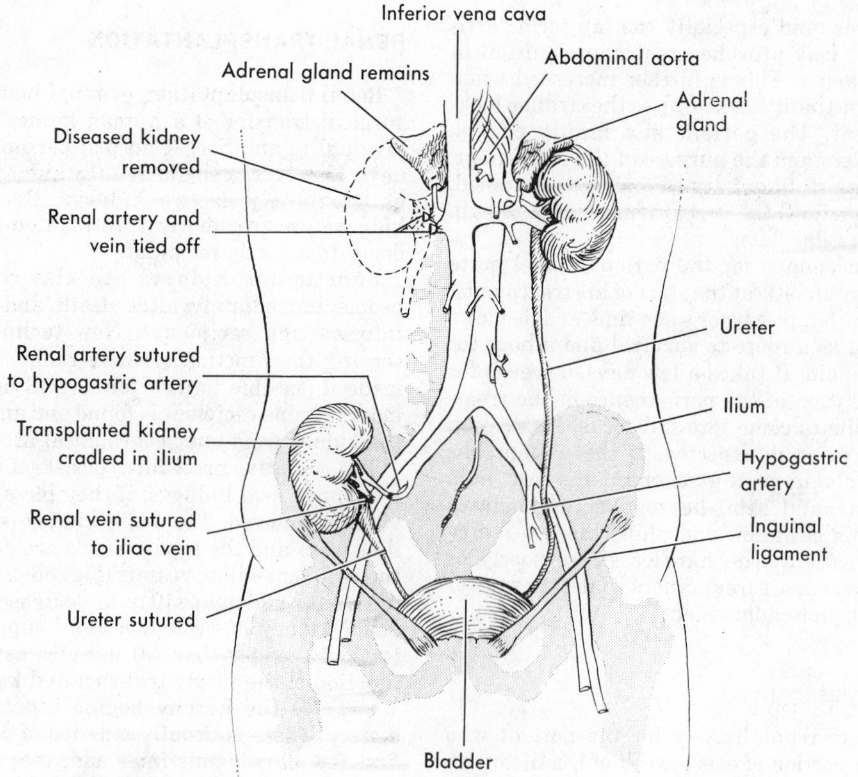

FIGURE 58–2. Transplanted kidney in place. (From Samartino and Preston: *In* Bergersen, B. S., et al. (ed.): *Current Concepts in Clinical Nursing.* St. Louis, The C. V. Mosby Co., 1967.)

References for Unit XI

1. Beeson, P. B., and McDermott, W. (eds.): *Cecil-Loeb Textbook of Medicine.* 13th ed. Philadelphia, W. B. Saunders Compny, 1971.
2. Blagg, C. R., et al.: Home hemodialysis: Six years' experience. *New England Journal of Medicine 283*: 1126, 1970.
3. Bois, M. S., et al.: Nursing care of patients having kidney transplants. *American Journal of Nursing 68*: 1238, June, 1969.
4. Cummings, J. W.: Hemodialysis: The pressures and how patients respond. *American Journal of Nursing 70*:70, Jan., 1970.
5. DeNour, A. K., Shaltiel, J., and Czaczkes, J. W.: Emotional reactions of patients on chronic hemodialysis. *Psychosomatic Medicine 30*:521, Sept.-Oct., 1968.
6. Dobbins, J., and Gleit, C.: Experience with the lateral position for catheterization. *Nursing Clinics of North America 6*:373, June, 1971.
7. Douglas, A. P., and Kerr, D.: *A Short Textbook of Kidney Disease.* London, Pitman Medical Publishing Co., Ltd., 1968.
8. Fulton, B. J. (ed.): Symposium on Patient Care in Kidney and Urinary Tract Disease. *Nursing Clinics of North America 4*:393, Sept., 1969.
9. Gutch, C. F., and Stoner, M. H.: *Review of Hemodialysis for Nurses and Dialysis Personnel.* St. Louis, The C. V. Mosby Co., 1971.
10. Hampers, C. L., Merrill, J. P., and Cameron, E.: Hemodialysis in the home—a family affair. *Transactions American Society for Artificial Internal Organs 11*:3, 1965.
11. Harrington, J. D., and Brener, E. R.: *Patient Care in Renal Failure.* Philadelphia, W. B. Saunders Company, 1973.
12. Kintzel, K. C. (ed.): *Advanced Concepts in Clinical Nursing.* Philadelphia, J. B. Lippincott Co., 1971, Chapter 13.
13. Miller, R. B., and Tossistro, E. R.: Current concepts: Peritoneal dialysis. *New England Journal of Medicine 287*:945, 1969.
14. Pendras, J. P., and Stinson, G. W. (eds.): *The Hemodialysis Manual.* Seattle, Edmark Corporation, 1970.
15. Quinton, W., Dillard, D., and Scribner, B. H.: Cannulation of blood vessels for prolonged hemodialysis. *Transactions American Society for Artificial Internal Organs 6*:104, 1960.
16. Read, M., and Mallison, M.: External arteriovenous shunts. *American Journal of Nursing 72*:81, Jan., 1972.
17. Rowson, L.: The lateral position in catheterization. *Nursing Clinics of North America 5*:189, March, 1970.
18. Sand, P., Livingston, G., and Wright, R. G.: Psychosocial assessment of candidates for hemodialysis program. *Annals of Internal Medicine 64*:602, March, 1966.
19. Scribner, B. H., et al.: The treatment of chronic uremia by means of intermittent hemodialysis: A preliminary report. *Transactions American Society for Artificial Internal Organs 6*:114, 1960.
20. Shaldon, S.: Independence in maintenance hemodialysis. Lancet *1*:520, 1969.
21. Shambough, P. W., et al.: Hemodialysis in the home—emotional impact on the spouse. *Transactions American Society for Artificial Internal Organs 13*: 41, 1967.
22. Shea, E. J., et al.: Hemodialysis for chronic renal failure. IV. Psychological considerations. *Annals of Internal Medicine 62*:558, 1965.
23. Short, M. J., and Wilson, W. P.: Roles of denial in chronic hemodialysis. *Archives of General Psychiatry 20*:433, 1969.
24. Smith, D. R.: *General Urology.* Los Altos, California, Lange Medical Publications, 1969.
25. Watson, J. E.: *Medical-Surgical Nursing and Related Physiology.* Philadelphia, W. B. Saunders Company, 1972.
26. Winter, C., and Roehm, M. M.: *Sawyer's Nursing Care of Patients with Urologic Diseases.* St. Louis, The C. V. Mosby Co., 1969.
27. Wright, G., Sand, P., and Livingston, G.: Psychological stress during hemodialysis for chronic renal failure. *Annals of Internal Medicine 64*:611, March, 1966.

UNIT XII

Nursing Patients Experiencing Disturbances of the Blood and Blood-Forming Organs

Introduction and Study Guide

Blood is part of the inner sea of body fluid which bathes, nourishes, and oxygenates every one of our cells and tissues. In addition, the blood carries cells and other substances which both protect the body from invading microorganisms and stop bleeding by inducing coagulation of the blood upon injury to a vessel. It is not surprising, then, that blood disorders affect any or all organs of the body and that the three problems basic to blood disease are *tissue hypoxia, susceptibility to infection*, and *hemorrhage*.

Because the manifestations of blood diseases are widespread and the causes are multiple, the nursing of patients with hematologic disorders is demanding and complex. The nurse must be knowledgeable in many diverse areas if she is to give competent care:

1. A knowledge of the *anatomy* and *physiology* of the hematologic system is needed to understand the numerous laboratory studies presented in this unit, the symptoms of different blood dyscrasias (a special term often used for blood disorders), and many of the therapies.
2. A review of *immune* and *autoimmune responses* (see Chapter 23) is necessary, because certain blood conditions are the result of antigen-antibody reactions.
3. Because some blood disorders are caused by deficiency states, principles of *nutrition* should be reviewed, including the roles of vitamins and iron in blood production.
4. A precise understanding of *drug action* is needed because many blood disorders are caused by drug toxicity. For instance, myelotoxins (drugs which damage bone marrow) cause the anemia of bone marrow failure; administration of oxidizing agents to persons with certain enzyme deficiencies causes hemolytic anemia, and other drugs can precipitate antigen-antibody reactions. It is important to learn which drugs fall into these three categories and to be aware of early clinical and laboratory indications of drug toxicity.
5. *Cancer nursing* is part of hematologic nursing. Many diseases discussed in this unit are caused by malignant changes within the blood-forming organs; e.g., the leukemias, Hodgkin's

disease, multiple myeloma, and possibly polycythemia vera. Consequently, a careful review of Unit VII is important (especially the sections on the psychologic impact of cancer, cancer chemotherapy, irradiation of tumor masses, radioisotope therapy, and general nursing care).

6. Some knowledge of *genetics* is necessary to educate and counsel patients with genetically transmitted blood disorders, e.g., sickle cell anemia, the thalassemias, and hemophilia.

7. It is necessary to be aware that patients with blood dyscrasias often have *psychologic problems* related to their disease because of prolonged pain and other discomforts. Most hematologic disorders are chronic in nature and many (particularly those that are malignant) are ultimately fatal. To help patients accept their disease and the prospect of a restricted existence and perhaps shortened life span, reconsider carefully Unit III, "Understanding the Experience of Illness," and attempt to apply mental health principles when planning patient care.

The following study guide will aid you in assimilating the information presented in this unit:

1. As you read this unit familiarize yourself with the following terms and concepts:

blood transfusion, ABO system of blood typing, Rh factor, universal donor, universal recipient, hemolytic transfusion reaction, "red shock," erythrocyte, erythropoiesis, hematopoiesis, hemoglobin, anemia, polycythemia, positive iron balance, extrinsic factor, intrinsic factor, leukocyte, leukopenia, agranulocytosis, leukocytosis, thrombocyte, thrombocytopenia, pancytopenia, myelotoxin, enzymopathy, chemical oxidant, hemolysis, hemolytic crisis, extracorpuscular defect, intracorpuscular defect, plumbism, hapten, dominant and recessive traits, heterozygous, homozygous, hemostatic mechanism, fibrinolysis, hematoma, hemarthrosis.

2. Acquaint yourself with the actions and untoward effects of the following drugs: ferrous salts (e.g., ferrous sulfate, ferrous gluconate), iron-dextran, or Imferon; cyanocobalamin (standard vitamin B_{12} preparation); vitamin K preparations (menadione sodium bisulfite [Hykinone], menadiol sodium diphosphate [Synkavite]); folic acid, hydrochloric acid; chelating agents (e.g., DTPA); myelosuppressant agents (e.g., radioactive phosphorus, nitrogen mustard, busulfan [Myleran]); alkylating agents (e.g., chlorambucil [Leukeran], triethylene melamine [TEM]).

3. Be aware of the nurse's responsibilities to the patient prior to and during these following special procedures: bone marrow biopsy, fecal and urinary urobilinogen tests, Schilling test (see pernicious anemia), blood administration, reverse isolation, venesection (see polycythemia vera), urea therapy (see sickle cell anemia), splenectomy, x-ray therapy, and radioisotope therapy.

CHAPTER 59

Introductory Concepts

REVIEW OF THE ANATOMY AND PHYSIOLOGY OF THE HEMATOPOIETIC SYSTEM

BLOOD: DEFINITION, FUNCTIONS, CHARACTERISTICS, AND FORMATION

Chapter 24 stated that the total body water (TBW) is divided into intracellular fluid and extracellular fluid. The extracellular fluid (ECF), in turn, is divided into *interstitial fluid* and *plasma.* Interstitial fluid occupies the tissue spaces, whereas plasma occupies the vascular space. Plasma, when mixed with blood cells (erythrocytes, leukocytes, and thrombocytes), is called *blood.*

Blood circulates continuously through the heart and vascular system. As the blood is propelled through the body by the heart's pumping action it performs many vital functions: It transports oxygen to the cells and carries carbon dioxide from the cells to the lungs for removal from the body. The blood also carries absorbed food products from the gastrointestinal tract to the tissues; at the same time, it removes metabolic wastes from tissues and carries them to the kidney, skin, and lungs for excretion. In addition, various hormones are conveyed by the blood from the endocrine glands (where they originate) to other parts of the body. Also, the blood protects the body from dangerous microorganisms by conveying leukocytes and antibodies to the site of infection, injury, or inflammation. Finally, the blood is instrumental in regulating body temperature by transferring heat from within the body to the small vessels supplying the skin, from which it can be released into the surrounding atmosphere.

Major characteristics of blood are as follows:

> *Color: Arterial* blood is bright red owing to the mixture of oxygen with hemoglobin within the red blood cells. *Venous* blood is dark red because of loss of oxygen from the hemoglobin.

> *Viscosity:* Blood is three to four times more viscous than water.

> *Reaction:* Blood has a slightly salty taste and a slightly alkaline reaction of pH 7.35 to 7.40.

> *Volume:* An adult has approximately 70 to 75 ml. of blood per kg. of body weight; thus, the average adult body contains around 5 to 6 liters of blood.

The organs involved in the formation of blood and its constituent cellular elements are the bone marrow, spleen, liver, and lymph nodes. Cells produced by these organs include erythrocytes, leukocytes, thrombocytes, plasma cells, and reticuloendothelial cells.

Blood Composition

Blood is formed by two components: plasma, which makes up 55 per cent of the blood; and solid suspended particles (blood cells and thrombocytes), which comprise the other 45 per cent of the blood.

Plasma, the liquid portion of the blood, is a straw-colored watery substance composed of:

> 92 per cent water

> 7 per cent proteins which include: (1) serum albumin, necessary for exerting colloid osmotic pressure (see Chapter 24); (2) fibrinogen, essential for hemostasis (blood coagulation); and (3) gamma globulin, which plays a vital role in the body's defense against microorganisms.

> Less than 1 per cent antibodies, nutrients, metabolic wastes, respiratory gases, enzymes, and inorganic salts.

The major *function* of plasma is the maintenance of blood volume within the vascular compartment.

The *particles* which travel suspended in the plasma include erythrocytes (red blood cells), leukocytes (white blood cells), and thrombocytes (platelets). Erythrocytes are principally involved in oxygen transport; leukocytes, in the defense of the body against microorganisms; and thrombocytes, in hemostasis. Each of these cellular types is discussed in detail in appropriate sections of this unit.

OVERVIEW OF ABNORMALITIES OF THE BLOOD AND BLOOD-FORMING ORGANS

Disorders of the blood and blood-forming organs are usually divided into diseases primarily involving: (1) erythrocytes; (2) leukocytes; (3) platelets; (4) reticuloendothelial cells; and (5) clotting mechanisms. The four basic physiologic disturbances characterizing hematopoietic disorders are as follows:

Decrease in Number of Cells (Cytopenia). When erythrocytes decrease, the result is *anemia,* a condition characterized by a reduction in the oxygen-carrying capacity of the blood. A *decrease* in leukocytes is termed *leukopenia,* while a reduction in granulocytes (one category of leukocyte) is called *granulocytopenia.* Patients with leukopenia and granulocytopenia suffer from a greatly increased vulnerability to *infection.* Finally, a decrease in the *thrombocyte* or platelet count is called *thrombocytopenia;* the hallmark of thrombocytopenia is *hemorrhage.*

Overproduction of Either Normal or Defective Cells. An abnormal increase in erythrocyte production is called *polycythemia;* an increase in the manufacture of abnormal, immature *leukocytes* is termed *leukemia;* the abnormal malignant proliferation of plasma cells results in a condition called *plasma cell myeloma* or *multiple myeloma.* These conditions (polycythemia, myelogenous and monocytic leukemia, and plasma cell myeloma) are usually classified as *myeloproliferative diseases* because the malignant overproduction of cells takes place within the *bone marrow.* When cellular overproduction occurs within the *lymphatic tissues,* the resulting conditions are classified as *lymphoproliferative disorders.* Examples include: (1) Hodgkin's disease (the malignant proliferation of one form of reticuloendothelial cell within the lymph nodes); (2) lymphatic leukemia (overproduction of lymphocytes within the lymph nodes which are released into the blood; and (3) lymphosarcoma (the abnormal proliferation of lymphocytes or lymphoblasts within the lymph nodes).

Defects in Coagulation Mechanism. This is caused by *depletion* or *absence* of one or more *clotting* factors. This group of disorders, which is characterized by persistent bleeding and hemorrhage, includes the hemophilias, hypoprothrombinemia, and disseminated intravascular coagulation.

Disorders of the Spleen. These include *enlargement of the spleen* (splenomegaly) and *splenic rupture.* Splenic rupture is usually the result of accidents or other trauma; splenomegaly occurs in association with numerous blood dyscrasias.

Generally *causative factors which can result in disorders of the hematopoietic system* include: hemorrhage, dietary deficiencies, malabsorptive disorders, infection, toxicity of drugs, malignant overproduction of cells, increased destruction of cells by an overactive spleen, genetic predisposition to faulty blood cell production, immunologic defects, and metabolic disturbances. In addition, a large number of blood disorders result from unknown (idiopathic) causes.

GENERAL PROBLEMS AFFECTING PATIENTS WITH HEMATOPOIETIC DISORDERS

As we have said, any disorder of the blood or blood-forming organs may adversely affect all organs and tissues; as a result, the major manifestations of blood disease are diffuse. Symptoms which characterize the majority of blood dyscrasias and their underlying bases include the following:

Symptoms	*Bases of Symptoms*
Chronic fatigue and dyspnea	Decrease in erythrocytes (anemias, leukemias, and hemorrhagic disorders) causes a reduction in the oxygen-carrying capacity of the blood
Increased susceptibility to infection	Decrease in mature circulating leukocytes (leukemia and leukopenia) decreases the number of cells available to combat invading microorganisms
Gastrointestinal symptoms (anorexia, weight loss, indigestion, sore mouth and tongue)	Decrease in gastric secretions (as seen in pernicious anemia); abnormal changes in mucous membrane cells; and the effects of certain drugs and extreme fatigue all contribute to the lack of desire or inability to eat
Hemorrhage and bleeding into tissues and joints (hemarthrosis) and from mucous membranes	Hemorrhage results either from a decrease in the platelet count (as a result of drugs, infections or autoimmune causes) or from absence of one or more clotting factors
Bone pain and deformity	Hyperactivity of bone marrow (seen in myeloproliferative disorders) and growth of bone tumors (seen in multiple myeloma) both produce bone pain and deformity
Jaundice (yellow discoloring of the skin and sclerae)	Rupture and hemolysis of abnormal erythrocytes (characteristic of hemolytic anemias and pernicious anemia) cause release of large amounts of bilirubin into the circulation, resulting in yellowing of the skin
Enlarged liver and spleen and hyperplasia of bone marrow	Caused by either: (1) congestion from overproduction of cells (e.g., polycythemia, leukemia, etc.); or (2) excessive demands upon these organs to destroy defective cells (e.g., hemolytic anemias)
Mental depression	Chronic depression results from the chronicity of most blood diseases and the fatigue and discomfort characteristic of these disorders

OVERVIEW OF DIAGNOSTIC TESTS AND THERAPEUTIC MEASURES

Blood disorders are primarily diagnosed in the laboratory. Although dozens of specific laboratory tests are used to diagnose individual hematologic disorders, the three major tests that are performed in all cases are: (1) the total blood count (erythrocyte, leukocyte, and platelet counts); (2) bone marrow biopsy; and (3) the blood film, i.e., a study of the morphology of blood cells within a peripheral blood smear.

Specific *clinical care* for patients with blood dyscrasias may involve either specific curative measures or palliative measures that relieve symptoms and prolong life. There are several general medical and nursing care measures that are used to treat the majority of patients with blood disorders. *Bed rest* is usually prescribed for persons suffering from severe anemias, hemorrhage, or bleeding diseases; rest counteracts the fatigue and weakness caused by the blood's decreased oxygen-carrying capacity. The *diet* in blood dyscrasias should be high in protein, iron, and vitamins. *Drug* administration is one of the nurse's most important responsibilities. Iron salts and vitamins B_{12} and K are given to correct deficiency states; anticancer agents are used to suppress the malignant proliferation of blood cells and reticuloendothelial cells. *Irradiation* and *radioisotope* therapy also play a vital role in the control of both myeloproliferative and lymphoproliferative disorders. *Reverse isolation* is a commonly employed procedure for patients with leukemia or with leukopenia from any cause. Isolation is needed to protect the patient with few mature, functioning leukocytes from overwhelming infection. *Special mouth care* is needed for patients with blood disorders because bleeding from the teeth and gums is extremely common.

The two operations that are performed on patients with hematopoietic diseases are: (1) *surgical excision of tumor masses* (performed in Hodgkin's disease and lymphosarcoma), and (2) *splenectomy* (performed to correct certain hemolytic and hemorrhagic disorders and to relieve symptoms in Hodgkin's disease and chronic lymphatic leukemia).

One form of therapy employed to treat *all* forms of blood disease is the *blood transfusion.* Transfusions are of great value in correcting many blood conditions, provided they are administered to the patient with full recognition of the dangers and complications involved. Because transfusions are a standard form of treatment for all blood disorders, they are discussed in a separate chapter rather than in relation to specific disease.

CHAPTER 60

Blood Transfusions and Reactions

INDICATIONS FOR TRANSFUSION THERAPY

A blood transfusion is the introduction of whole blood or blood components (serum, plasma, red cells, platelets) directly into the circulation for therapeutic purposes.* Blood transfusions may be used to: (1) quickly restore blood volume following hemorrhage, burns, or injuries to blood vessels; (2) combat shock; or (3) treat severe chronic anemia by increasing the oxygen-carrying capacity of the blood.

BLOOD GROUPS

The individual who gives his blood to a blood bank, hospital, or specific patient is called the *donor*, while the person who receives blood is called the *recipient.* It is mandatory that the donor's blood and the recipient's blood belong to *compatible* blood groups. If the donor and recipient belong to *incompatible* blood groups, antibodies in the recipient's plasma will agglutinate or clump the donor's erythrocytes, which contain certain specific antigens. When such an antigen-antibody reaction occurs during a blood transfusion it is called a *hemolytic transfusion reaction.*

*Solutions other than whole blood that are used to replace fluid losses resulting from hemorrhage or shock are discussed in Chapter 26.

Blood type is inherited from one's parents, as are eye color, hair color, and other features. The four major blood groups of clinical importance are *A, B, AB,* and *O,* according to the ABO system of blood typing originated by Karl Landsteiner in 1900.* In addition to belonging to one of the ABO blood groups, blood is classified as either *Rh positive* or *Rh negative.* The Rh factor was discovered by Landsteiner and Wiener in 1940. (See discussion below.) These scientists named the Rh factor after the rhesus monkeys used in their experiments.

Blood typing is based upon the type of *antigens* (agglutinogens) present in the erythrocytes as well as the type of *antibodies* (agglutinins) in the serum. Two *antigens* have been identified within the ABO blood classification: antigen A and antigen B (Table 60–1). Thus, persons with A type blood have A antigens in their red cells; those with B type blood have B antigens. Persons with AB blood have both A and B antigens, while those with O type blood do not have any antigens in their red cells.

There are also two types of *antibodies* in the ABO system: anti-A antibody and anti-B antibody (Table 60–1). As you can see, blood never con-

*Researchers have identified many other groupings and subgroupings in addition to the ABO classification. For more technical information on blood groups, consult a hematology textbook, medical laboratory manual, or a source in physical anthropology.

TABLE 60–1. SUMMARY OF INFORMATION: ABO BLOOD GROUPS

Blood Type	% of White Population	% of Black Population	Antigen (Agglutinogen) in Red Cells	Antibodies (Agglutinins) in Plasma	Incompatible Donor Blood	Compatible Donor Blood
A	38	30	A	anti-B	B, AB	A, 0
B	12	20	B	anti-A	A, AB	B, 0
AB	5	5	A and B	None (Universal recipient)	None	A, B, AB, 0
0	45	45	None (Universal donor)	Anti-A Anti-B	A, B, AB	0

tains both an antigen and its antagonistic antibody. For example, an individual with A type blood never has anti-A antibody within his serum; if he did, he could not survive because his blood cells would be completely destroyed. Instead, persons with A type blood have anti-B antibody; those with B type blood have anti-A antibody; those with AB type blood have no antibodies in their serum, and those with O type blood have both anti-A and anti-B antibodies.

Persons with O type blood are called *universal donors,* because their red cells do not contain any antigens that could be destroyed by antibodies within the recipient's blood upon transfusion. Persons with AB type blood are called *universal recipients* because their plasma contains no antibodies that could destroy the donor's red cells upon transfusion.

Refer again to Table 60–1. Observe that persons with A type blood can receive blood only from persons with the same blood type (A) or, in an emergency, from persons with O type blood, i.e., the universal donor. If a person with A type blood accidentally receives a transfusion of B or AB type blood, the anti-B antibodies present in his (the recipient's) serum rapidly agglutinate the red cells in the donor's B or AB type blood and a hemolytic transfusion reaction occurs. For the same reasons, persons with B type blood cannot receive a transfusion of A or AB type blood. The person with AB blood *can receive* blood from donors in all four blood groups because his serum contains no antibodies. Finally, persons with O type blood can *donate* their blood to recipients in all four blood groups because their erythrocytes do not contain any antigens. Note, however, that individuals with O type blood can receive blood or serum only from other persons with O type blood because their serum contains both anti-A and anti-B antibodies, which will agglutinate red cells in A, B, and AB type blood.

Rh BLOOD GROUPS

The Rh blood groups are of equal importance with the ABO groups because of their relation to hemolytic disease of the newborn and their significance in blood transfusion. The subject is quite complex, and different systems of terminology are in use.

According to the Fisher-Race theory, probably the most commonly accepted at present, the Rh blood groups are determined by a series of three closely linked genes, C, D, and E, with allelic forms c, d, and e. These genes occur in varied combinations in different races and in different parts of the world. Essentially these genes exist as antigens, and of them the D factor is the strongest antigen and of the greatest clinical significance. It is the presence or absence of the D antigen that determines whether a person is Rh positive or Rh negative. For example, persons with genotypes such as CDE, cDe, or CDe are all Rh positive, whereas those with genotypes cde or cdE are Rh negative. Approximately 85 per cent of the Caucasian population is Rh positive while the remaining 15 per cent is Rh negative. Almost 99 to 100 per cent of nonwhite persons are Rh positive. Persons whose erythrocytes carry this common antigen are often designated as having D(Rh_0) type blood, Rh_0 being one way of expressing the so-called Rh factor.

As in the case of the ABO blood types, persons who are *Rh positive* (i.e., whose erythrocytes carry an Rh or D antigen) never carry anti-Rh (anti-D) antibodies within their serum. In contrast to the ABO blood type, persons who are *Rh negative* develop anti-Rh antibodies in their serum gradually and only *after exposure* to Rh positive blood. For example, if a person with Rh negative blood is accidentally transfused for the first time with Rh positive blood, he will *not* have a transfusion reaction because his blood will not yet contain anti-Rh antibodies. However, because of the transfusion error, the Rh negative person becomes *sensitized* to the Rh antigen and consequently begins to develop antibodies against the Rh factor. Should this same person receive a *second* accidental transfusion of Rh positive blood, he will this time have a hemolytic reaction because he will have built up anti-Rh antibodies as a result of the first transfusion. Another example of a reaction between Rh-positive and Rh-negative blood is erythroblastosis fetalis, i.e., hemolytic disease of the newborn. (See Chapter 62.)

TYPING AND CROSSMATCHING

To prevent such serious errors and to insure that both the donor's blood and the recipient's blood are compatible *prior to transfusion,* blood from both persons is sent to the laboratory for a procedure called *typing* and *crossmatching.* First, laboratory technicians determine the blood type of the patient's and donor's blood; i.e., they test the blood for the presence of antigens A, B, and D (Rh_0). Next a major crossmatch is performed, i.e., serum from the recipient's blood and the donor's red blood cells are mixed together and incubated for 15 minutes. For the minor crossmatch the ingredients mixed are reversed and the recipient's cells and the donor's serum are incubated together. If no clumping of red blood cells occurs during either the major or minor crossmatch, the donor's blood and the recipient's blood are reported as compatible.

ADMINISTERING BLOOD SAFELY

Four major types of blood transfusions are:

Direct Transfusion. Blood is given directly from the donor to the recipient (rarely employed).

Indirect Transfusion. Blood is drawn from the donor, taken to the laboratory for testing, and is then later administered to the recipient. This method is most commonly used in hospitals today.

Exchange Transfusion. The recipient's blood, as it is being removed from his circulation, is simultaneously replaced by a donor's blood. Exchange transfusions are used to correct erythroblastosis fetalis.

Reciprocal Transfusion. Blood is drawn from a donor who is recovering from an infectious disease and is given to a recipient who has recently developed the same disease. The purpose of the transfusion is to *transfer antibodies* against the infectious agent from donor to recipient. In exchange, an equal amount of blood is drawn from the recipient and given back to the donor to replenish the donor's blood volume.

Although the administration of blood transfusions may be highly therapeutic—indeed, in some cases, lifesaving—transfusion therapy is also fraught with potential fatal consequences. For this reason there are numerous precautions that laboratory technicians, nurses, and doctors *must* observe both before administering a blood transfusion and during the transfusion.

Safe blood administration begins in the blood bank and laboratory. Blood donors must be in good health. Blood cannot be taken if a potential donor has suffered from infectious hepatitis, syphilis, a chronic disease such as tuberculosis, or serious allergies. Even if a potential donor is free of disease, the technician at the blood bank always checks his temperature, pulse rate, blood pressure, and heart and chest sounds. If the donor is in satisfactory physical condition, his blood is drawn into sterilized containers, properly labeled, and sent to the laboratory to be typed and crossmatched with the blood of a potential recipient. When it reaches the laboratory, the blood is stored immediately in the refrigerator at the proper temperature and is tested with properly sterilized equipment. Faulty refrigeration or the use of equipment contaminated by bacteria or chemicals may later result in a serious pyogenic transfusion reaction.

Blood is prepared for transfusion therapy in *units.* Each unit of blood (equivalent to 500 ml.) is contained in either a glass bottle or a plastic bag (Fig. 60–1). Tubing used to administer a blood transfusion closely resembles an intravenous set-up, except that the drip chamber contains a filter. Occasionally during a transfusion the filter must be changed if it becomes clogged with precipitates of fibrin, platelets, or leukocytes. Note in Figure 60–1 that the plastic bag is equipped with a second outlet for connecting the blood transfusion tubing, and also blood specimen tubing which contains a sample of the patient's blood which was used by the blood bank for typing and crossmatching tests. The needle used to administer blood has a larger gauge (18 gauge) than does the needle used to administer intravenous fluids (usually 21 gauge); the larger gauge is necessary because blood is more viscous than other intravenous fluids.

When blood is ordered for a patient, the nurse is largely responsible for its safe administration.

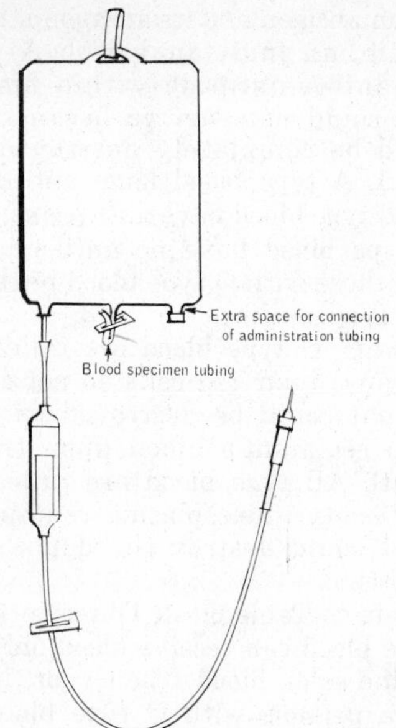

FIGURE 60–1. Basic blood transfusion equipment. (From Sutton, A. L.: *Bedside Nursing Techniques.* 2nd ed. 1969.)

Points to remember *prior* to starting a blood transfusion are as follows:

> With the help of a physician or another nurse, check the label on the blood container against whatever form the hospital uses to identify the patient and his blood type. A typical form is illustrated in Figure 60–2. Information to *check* and *double-check* on both the label and the identification form is as follows:

Check: *The patient's name, room, hospital number, the bottle number, the patient's blood group and Rh status, and the donor's blood group and Rh status.*

Make certain that the information on the blood label and the identification form correspond exactly. If there is any discrepancy in the data, *do not give the blood!* Notify the blood bank at once concerning the error.

Remember: *The administration of incompatible, mismatched blood is the major cause of hemolytic transfusion reactions.*

> If the blood is safe to give, administer it at room temperature or lower; do not give blood immediately after removing it from the refrigerator, as it will be too cold to introduce intravenously. On the other hand, do not allow blood to stand at room temperature for several hours before using because lukewarm blood is a good medium for bacterial growth. If blood must be held on the ward prior to administration, place it in the refrigerator until an hour or so before it is to be given.

> Never warm blood, because warming destroys certain vital factors within the blood and it also favors the growth of organisms.

Once the blood transfusion is started, stabilize the patient's arm on an arm board so that the needle will not be dislodged. During the first 15 minutes of the transfusion, administer the blood *very slowly* (20 to 40 drops per minute) because transfusion reactions (i.e., allergic, hemolytic, bacterial, etc.) typically occur during the first quarter hour after starting therapy. (See later discussion of causes and symptoms of transfusion reactions.)

> *Should a transfusion reaction occur, stop the blood at once and notify the physician.*

If symptoms of a transfusion reaction do not develop, it is then safe to administer the blood at the rate ordered by the physician (usually between 80 and 100 drops per minute). A unit of blood administered at this rate is usually completed within 1 to 1½ hours. In an emergency such as shock or hemorrhage, blood must be administered much more rapidly, e.g., a unit of blood may be given in 20 minutes or less. For rapid transfusions, use a 15-gauge needle and remove the clamp from the tubing so that the blood runs freely. When the patient is in critical condition, it is possible to administer a unit of blood within 8 to 12 minutes under pressure. In these cases, a pressure cuff (similar to a blood pressure cuff) is placed around a collapsible plastic blood container; when the cuff is pumped up, the bag is gently compressed and blood is quickly pushed into the patient's veins.

> *One major complication of administering blood under pressure is the infiltration of blood into the subcutaneous tissues. Carefully observe the injection site for signs of swelling.*

COMPLICATIONS OF TRANSFUSION THERAPY

The incidence of transfusion reactions varies from 0.2 to 10 per cent, although the exact frequency of untoward effects is unknown. Concerning this matter, Chaplin states:

> A conservative estimate would be that 2 per cent of all transfusions are accompanied by some sort of unfavorable response. Thus with 6 million units of blood administered annually in the United States, at least 120,000 recognizable reactions can be expected.[13]

As these conservative statistics indicate, blood transfusion is dangerous, and blood is administered only when absolutely necessary. It is particularly risky to give blood to an *unconscious* patient or to any individual who is anesthetized or heavily sedated. Because of their depressed consciousness, such persons are unable to complain of symptoms (e.g., dyspnea, cough, chills, headache) should they develop a transfusion reaction. Unless observable symptoms are noticed by the nurse, such persons could receive an entire unit of mismatched blood and, as a result, die from hemolysis and shock.

It is difficult to observe a reaction in the unconscious patient; it is also difficult to evaluate whether symptoms experienced by *any* patient during a transfusion are due to the *blood* he is receiving or to his *illness*. Many symptoms of transfusion reactions (dyspnea, apprehension, headache, vomiting) are the same as the symptoms caused by common disorders. Because it is the nurse who usually decides if a transfusion should be stopped, it is extremely important that she pause for a moment before terminating the transfusion to carefully evaluate the *total* situation.

The major complications of blood transfusion administration are: (1) hemolytic transfusion reactions, (2) bacterial reactions, (3) allergic reactions, (4) circulatory overload, and (5) the transmission of

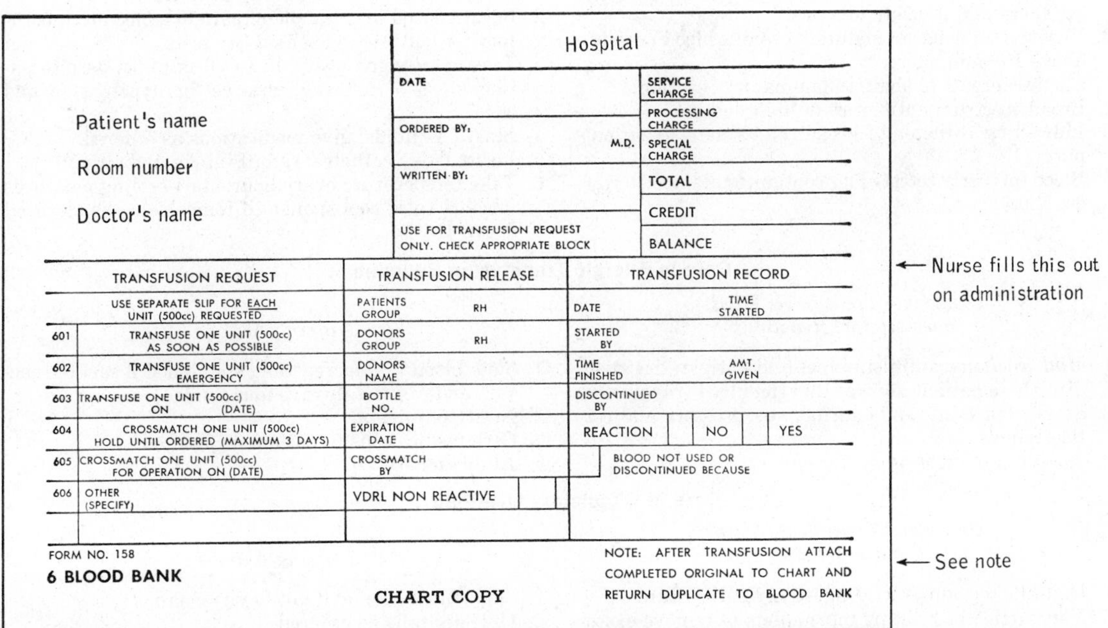

Hospital

Patient's name

Room number

Doctor's name

DATE	SERVICE CHARGE
ORDERED BY: M.D.	PROCESSING CHARGE
	SPECIAL CHARGE
WRITTEN BY:	TOTAL
	CREDIT
USE FOR TRANSFUSION REQUEST ONLY. CHECK APPROPRIATE BLOCK	BALANCE

	TRANSFUSION REQUEST	TRANSFUSION RELEASE	TRANSFUSION RECORD
	USE SEPARATE SLIP FOR EACH UNIT (500cc) REQUESTED	PATIENTS GROUP RH	DATE TIME STARTED
601	TRANSFUSE ONE UNIT (500cc) AS SOON AS POSSIBLE	DONORS GROUP RH	STARTED BY
602	TRANSFUSE ONE UNIT (500cc) EMERGENCY	DONORS NAME	TIME FINISHED AMT. GIVEN
603	TRANSFUSE ONE UNIT (500cc) ON (DATE)	BOTTLE NO.	DISCONTINUED BY
604	CROSSMATCH ONE UNIT (500cc) HOLD UNTIL ORDERED (MAXIMUM 3 DAYS)	EXPIRATION DATE	REACTION NO YES
605	CROSSMATCH ONE UNIT (500cc) FOR OPERATION ON (DATE)	CROSSMATCH BY	BLOOD NOT USED OR DISCONTINUED BECAUSE
606	OTHER (SPECIFY)	VDRL NON REACTIVE	

FORM NO. 158

6 BLOOD BANK

CHART COPY

NOTE: AFTER TRANSFUSION ATTACH COMPLETED ORIGINAL TO CHART AND RETURN DUPLICATE TO BLOOD BANK

FIGURE 60–2. Example of a typical blood transfusion form. (From Sutton, A. L.: *Bedside Nursing Techniques* 2nd ed. 1969.)

infectious agents. Pertinent information concerning the symptoms and care of patients with these complications is summarized here.

Hemolytic Transfusion Reaction

This complication is caused by the administration of *mismatched blood.* Hemolytic reactions, the most severe of all transfusion reactions, occur in approximately one out of every 5000 patients who are transfused. Reactions resulting from *ABO incompatibility* usually are evident within a few minutes after the transfusion is started. Reactions due to *Rh incompatibility* develop more gradually; also, as you recall, Rh reactions develop only after a patient who is Rh negative has been sensitized to the Rh antigen.

The pathologic chain of events in a hemolytic transfusion reaction is as follows: (1) antibodies in the recipient's plasma react with antigens carried in the donor's red cells; (2) the donor's cells agglutinate or clump together; (3) the clumped cells block the patient's capillaries, thus obstructing the flow of blood and oxygen to vital organs; (4) the clumped cells, after a few hours, are devoured by macrophages and the resulting hemolysis causes the release of free hemoglobin into the

Care in Hemolytic Transfusion Reaction

Drugs and Treatments Used to Counteract Reaction

1. Intravenous infusions of dextrose in water to counteract shock and promote diuresis.
2. Oxygen and epinephrine to treat dyspnea and wheezing.
3. Sedation to counteract restlessness and apprehension.
4. Indwelling catheter to accurately evaluate urine output.
5. Mannitol (an osmotic diuretic) to counteract oliguria. (See Chapter 26.)
6. Blood transfusion (with properly matched blood) to control shock.
7. Vasopressor drugs in event of severe shock (Chap. 26).

Nursing Actions

1. Discontinue blood immediately.
2. Notify physician and laboratory.
3. Return blood and sample of patient's blood to laboratory for another type and crossmatch.
4. Connect bottle of dextrose in water as ordered to blood or I.V. tubing to keep I.V. open.
5. Administer oxygen and other drugs as ordered.
6. Take vital signs every 15 to 30 minutes; observe for hypotension and shock.
7. Start intake and output record; observe for oliguria or anuria.
8. Insert Foley catheter and measure urine hourly.
9. Allay patient's anxiety.
10. Observe for effects of vasopressor drugs (Chap. 26).

Care in Bacterial Transfusion Reaction

Drugs and Treatments Used to Counteract Reaction

1. Intravenous infusions of dextrose in water to counteract shock and promote diuresis.
2. Vasopressor drugs to maintain systolic blood pressure above 100 mm. mercury.
3. Corticosteroids to abate inflammatory reaction.
4. Broad spectrum antibiotics in high dosages.
5. Indwelling catheter to properly evaluate urine output.
6. Blood (properly retested for contaminants) to counteract shock.

Nursing Actions

1. Discontinue blood and notify physician.
2. Return blood and sample of patient's blood to laboratory for culture and sensitivity tests.
3. Take vital signs every 15 to 30 minutes despite patient's "rosy" coloring; observe for hypotension and shock.
4. Start I.V. fluids; give medications as ordered.
5. Insert Foley catheter; record intake and output.
6. Take temperature every hour; start cooling measures (alcohol rubs, cool sponge) if temperature is elevated above 101°F.

Care in Allergic Transfusion Reaction

Drugs and Treatments Used to Counteract Reactions

1. *Mild reactions:* antihistamines and antipyretics given directly to patient and *not* into the blood transfusion.
2. *Severe reactions:* epinephrine, vasopressors and corticosteroids.
3. Appropriate *respiratory therapy.*

Nursing Actions

1. *Slow* blood if *mild* reaction; *stop* blood if *severe* reaction and connect intravenous fluids.
2. Notify physician.
3. Give medications to patient as ordered.
4. Allay anxiety.

Care in Circulatory Overload

Drugs and Treatments Used to Counteract Reactions

1. Digitalis to counteract congestive heart failure.
2. Venesection or rotating tourniquets to remove excess fluid from the general circulation. (See Unit X.)

Nursing Actions

1. Stop transfusion and notify physician.
2. Give digitalis as ordered.
3. Set up for venesection or rotating tourniquets.

plasma (hemoglobinemia) and the urine (hemoglobinuria); and (5) the free hemoglobin may plug the renal tubules, disrupt the work of the kidney nephron, and result in *renal failure.* In 10 per cent of cases, patients die from renal damage; in the remaining 90 per cent, the plugs of hemoglobin that close off the renal tubules disintegrate automatically and the patient recovers.

The principal manifestations of hemolytic transfusion reaction are chills, fever, hematuria, oliguria, jaundice, headache, backache, dyspnea, cyanosis, and chest pain. (See care summary, page 748.)

Bacterial Reactions

The most frequent cause of bacterial reactions (sometimes called "febrile reactions") is the administration of *contaminated blood.* Although approximately 2 per cent of bank blood is contaminated, the bacteria are usually harmless and do not cause symptoms. However, blood which is heavily contaminated with gram-negative bacteria causes the deaths of more than 50 per cent of the patients who receive it. Persons who receive grossly contaminated blood sometimes develop a dangerous condition called *red shock.* In contrast to other forms of shock, red shock is characterized by *flushing* rather than paleness of the skin, resulting from pronounced peripheral vasodilatation. Fortunately, today, as a result of modern aseptic blood banking techniques, severe reactions and fatalities due to blood contamination are rare.

The principal manifestations of bacterial transfusion reactions are fever, chills, lumbar pain, headache, malaise, bloody vomitus, diarrhea, and red shock (skin warm, dry, and pink due to peripheral vasodilatation). (See care summary, page 748.)

Allergic Reactions

It is not uncommon for a transfusion recipient to develop mild edema, hives, and bronchial wheezing in reaction to the blood; occasionally, however, allergic reactions are severe. (See also Chapter 23.) The exact cause of the allergy is unknown; in some cases the donor may have taken drugs or eaten certain foods to which the recipient is allergic. More severe reactions may include bronchospasm and severe dyspnea. (See care summary, page 748.)

Circulatory Overload

As you recall from Chapter 25, circulatory overload results when fluid is infused into the circulatory system either too rapidly or in too great a quantity. Patients who are particularly susceptible to overtransfusion are those who are elderly or debilitated, or who have limited cardiac reserve. Circulatory overload, particularly in the above cases, may precipitate the development of acute pulmonary edema and left-sided heart failure.

The principal manifestations of circulatory overload are cough, dyspnea, edema, tachycardia, hemoptysis, and frothy pink-tinged sputum. (See care summary, page 748.)

Transmission of Infectious Agents

Diseases that may be transmitted from donor to recipient via a blood transfusion include malaria, syphilis, and hepatitis. As stated earlier, potential donors are usually carefully screened before donating blood. Nevertheless, although the transmission of syphilis and malaria is rare, serum hepatitis is transmitted via the blood to one out of every 200 patients receiving a transfusion. *Hepatitis is a common complication of transfusion therapy* because donors with hepatitis may have such a mild form of the disease that they experience no symptoms whatsoever and consequently the disease remains undiagnosed. Fortunately 95 per cent of recipients who receive blood contaminated by the hepatitis virus develop only mild cases of the disorder. However, the remaining 5 per cent develop a severe liver condition called *postnecrotic cirrhosis* which often ends fatally. *

Patients who have suffered one transfusion reaction often develop reactions during subsequent transfusions; when administering blood to a patient who is reaction prone, remember to: (1) give the *entire* transfusion slowly; (2) observe the patient carefully for untoward symptoms throughout the transfusion; and (3) be prepared to terminate the transfusion immediately at the earliest sign of a reaction.

---

*Serum hepatitis and postnecrotic cirrhosis are discussed in Unit XVI.

CHAPTER 61

Nursing Patients with Disorders Primarily Affecting the Erythrocytes

THE NORMAL ERYTHROCYTE

REVIEW OF ANATOMY AND PHYSIOLOGY

The word *erythrocyte* is taken from the Greek terms *erythros* (red) and *kykos* (cell). Other terms used interchangeably with erythrocyte are "red blood cell" (RBC) and "red blood corpuscle," a phrase which means "little red body."

Red blood corpuscles are composed of two principal parts: (1) the supporting stroma and encircling membrane, which are responsible for approximately 2 to 5 per cent of the red cell's weight; and (2) the conjugated protein called *hemoglobin*, which is responsible for approximately 95 per cent of the red cell's mass.

Erythrocytes, along with leukocytes and thrombocytes, travel throughout the body as suspended particles in a river of plasma. As you recall, erythrocytes greatly outnumber both leukocytes and thrombocytes; thus, in a cubic millimeter of blood there are approximately 5 million erythrocytes, 250 thousand thrombocytes, and only 8 thousand leukocytes. In an adult human body, the total number of circulating erythrocytes approaches the fantastic sum of 35 trillion cells. Erythrocytes have a diameter which ranges between 6 and 9 μ, with 7.7 μ as an average. One micron is equivalent to one thousandth of a millimeter or 1/25,000 of an inch.

The *functions* of erythrocytes are threefold: the transport of oxygen from the lungs to the tissues and carbon dioxide from the tissues to the lungs, the promotion of normal hydrogen ion balance, and the maintenance of blood viscosity.

The *structure* of a red blood cell is admirably designed to enable it to carry out its most important function—oxygen and carbon dioxide transport. Normal erythrocytes, microscopic in size, are shaped like biconcave discs with rather thin centers and thicker outer edges. Such a shape gives the red cell two advantages: First, its biconcave shape provides a relatively *large surface area* for the efficient, rapid absorption and release of oxygen and carbon dioxide. Second, the biconcave discs have great *flexibility* and *elasticity*, which enable them to adapt their shapes to the diameter of the various blood vessels through which they circulate.

As discussed later, it is disastrous when disease causes erythrocytes to lose this biconcave shape and become spherical, elongated, or crescent-shaped. Abnormally shaped erythrocytes cannot carry the blood gases efficiently. Furthermore, these cellular anomalies are easily broken and fragmented as they travel through the smaller vessels; eventually these fragments jam together within the capillaries, thus blocking circulation to the tissues.

Structure and Function of Hemoglobin

Hemoglobin, the major constituent of the red blood cell, is composed of a simple protein called *globin* and a red-colored compound called *heme.* Heme is a complex molecule containing iron and the red pigment porphyrin, which gives blood its color. There are approximately 200 to 300 million molecules of hemoglobin within each erythrocyte.

The most important characteristic of hemoglobin is its ability to *combine chemically* with oxygen in a loose and easily reversed connection. The compound which results from the union of oxygen and hemoglobin is called *oxyhemoglobin.*

Oxyhemoglobin, which causes arterial blood to be bright red, is formed as the red blood corpuscles pass through the alveoli of the lungs. As the blood leaves the capillaries of the lungs and passes into the arteries, oxyhemoglobin releases its oxygen, which diffuses out of the blood vessels into the tissue fluid where it satisfies the oxygen requirements of cells and tissues. Once hemoglobin loses its oxygen, it is called *reduced hemoglobin.* Because venous blood contains reduced hemoglobin, it is dark red in color.

In addition to combining with oxygen, hemoglobin also combines with *carbon dioxide.* As carbon dioxide is released from the body's cells, it diffuses into the tissue fluid and then into the blood where it is picked up and carried by hemoglobin to the lung capillaries. In the lungs, carbon dioxide separates from hemoglobin and diffuses into the alveoli; from there it is exhaled into the atmosphere.

The third gas with which hemoglobin readily combines is *carbon monoxide*. When hemoglobin is combined with carbon monoxide, it is no longer able to transport oxygen to cells and tissues. Consequently the major pathologic alteration occurring in carbon monoxide poisoning is *tissue hypoxia*. The most common cause of carbon monoxide poisoning is inhalation within a closed area of fumes from auto exhaust systems, sewers, and gas or oil heaters. The victim of carbon monoxide poisoning may die from asphyxiation; if he lives, he may suffer permanent brain damage.

The numerous forms of hemoglobin, and the disorders affecting hemoglobin production, will be discussed later in this chapter.

Erythrocyte Production and Storage

During infancy *erythropoiesis* (i.e., red blood cell production) takes place within the marrow of both the long and short bones of the body. However, as the young child develops into an adult, the marrow of the long bones is replaced by fatty tissue. Consequently, in adulthood, erythropoiesis occurs only in the proximal ends of the femora and humeri and in the bones that form the ribs, sternum, skull, vertebrae, hands, and feet.

The bone marrow produces approximately 200 billion erythrocytes daily. Normal red blood cell production depends basically upon three factors: (1) the presence of normal genetic precursors for erythrocyte formation; (2) a healthy bone marrow which has not been damaged by drugs, toxins, and so forth; and (3) a proper diet that includes an adequate intake of iron, vitamin B_{12}, folic acid, protein, pyridoxine, and traces of copper. If any of these factors is missing or faulty, production of erythrocytes will be insufficient; the erythrocytes produced may be misshaped, overly fragile, excessively small or abnormally large; and hemoglobin production may be inadequate or defective.

The red blood cell has an average life span of approximately 120 days. Erythrocytes originally arise from primitive stem cells, called *hemocytoblasts,* located within the bone marrow; hemocytoblasts can evolve into either erythrocytes, leukocytes, or platelets. The differentiation of a hemocytoblast into an erythrocyte is stimulated by *erythropoietin*—a factor within the plasma which regulates red blood cell production. The evolving red blood cell finally loses its nucleus, leaves the bone marrow by a venous route, and enters the general circulation; it is now called a *reticulocyte.* Within the blood stream the young reticulocytes circulate for another four days; during this time they mature into adult erythrocytes.

The majority of erythrocytes are actively involved in the transport of oxygen and carbon dioxide; however, some erythrocytes are held in storage by the *spleen*—the body's blood reservoir. These "reserve corps" of erythrocytes are released by the spleen whenever the circulating red blood cell count begins to drop significantly below normal levels, e.g., during periods of great physical or emotional stress, during pregnancy, and during emergencies such as hemorrhage, shock, or carbon monoxide poisoning.

As the adult erythrocyte carries out its tasks, it is subjected to considerable stress as it squeezes and twists its way through the blood vessels; in time the aging cell becomes worn and fragile and eventually ruptures. At this point, hemoglobin leaves the cell and the withered remaining membrane is called a "ghost cell." Both the ghost cell and the hemoglobin it once contained are quickly phagocytized by macrophages within the liver, spleen, and red bone marrow. (See Chapter 22.) Hemoglobin, when phagocytized, breaks down into its globin and heme fractions. The *iron* of the heme fraction returns to the liver where it is reused in making fresh hemoglobin. The *porphyrin* molecules from the heme fraction are converted by the liver into *bilirubin,* an orange bile pigment. Bilirubin is excreted from the liver into the bile; it is finally excreted from the body in the feces and urine. During periods of severe red blood cell destruction (for example, in hemolytic anemia), large amounts of bilirubin are formed as a result of the massive breakdown of hemoglobin.

Under normal conditions the approximately 180 million aged erythrocytes that are destroyed every minute are replaced that same minute by approximately 180 million young erythrocytes. As a result, the population of red blood cells within the healthy body remains fairly constant. What happens, however, if the erythrocyte loss or destruction begins to *exceed* erythrocyte production? When the erythrocyte count becomes abnormally low, an inadequate amount of hemoglobin is available to carry oxygen to the tissues and, as a result, *hypoxia* develops. Hypoxia stimulates the release of erythropoietin, which then stimulates the bone marrow to produce more red blood cells (Fig. 61–

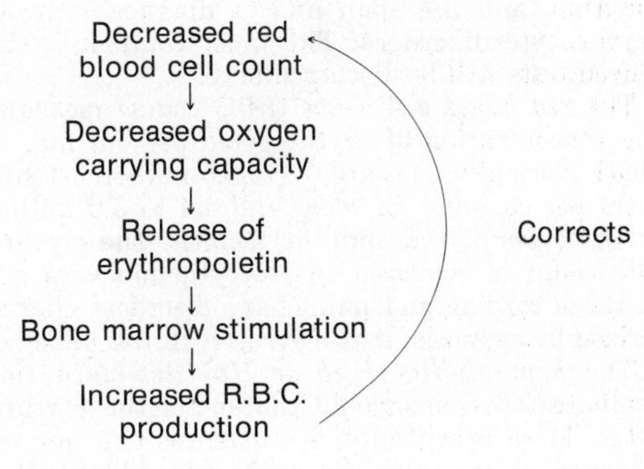

FIGURE 61–1. The homeostatic regulation of the red cell concentration in the blood. (After Langley, L. L., Cheraskin, E., and Sleeper, R.)

1). Because the healthy bone marrow is capable of producing six to eight times the amount of red blood cells which it normally produces, the red blood cell count increases so that erythrocyte production keeps pace with erythrocyte destruction. As a result of this homeostatic mechanism, erythrocyte concentration within the circulation remains remarkably constant.

ABNORMALITIES OF ERYTHROCYTE STRUCTURE, PRODUCTION, AND LIFE SPAN

CAUSES OF ABNORMALITIES

There are numerous diseases involving red blood cells. However, only two basic pathophysiologic developments underlie all erythrocyte disorders:

1. A *deficient number* of circulating red blood cells (*anemia*) due to one or all of the following: (a) insufficient erythrocyte production, (b) defective erythrocyte synthesis, (c) increased erythrocyte destruction, and (d) increased erythrocyte loss.
2. An *increased* number of circulating red blood cells (*polycythemia*) due to either: (a) a disorder of unknown etiology which is apparently similar to cancer, or (b) a compensatory mechanism which develops in response to tissue hypoxia (secondary polycythemia).

DETECTING ABNORMALITIES OF ERYTHROCYTES

A number of laboratory tests are used to detect abnormalities of erythrocyte production, structure, function, and life span and to diagnose various erythrocyte disorders. The most commonly employed tests will be discussed here.

The *red blood cell count* (RBC count) measures the concentration of erythrocytes per cu. mm. of blood. Normal values are 4.8 to 5.5 million erythrocytes per cu. mm. for *men,* and 4.4 to 5.0 million erythrocytes per cu. mm. for *women*. The erythrocyte count is *increased* in polycythemia vera and in those cardiac and pulmonary disorders characterized by cyanosis; it is *decreased* in the anemias.

The *hemoglobin (Hgb or Hb) determination* evaluates the hemoglobin content of the erythrocytes. More specifically, it measures the number of grams of hemoglobin per 100 ml. of blood. Normal values for *men* are 14.5 to 16.0 Gm./100 ml. blood, and for *women* 13.0 to 15.5 Gm./100 ml. blood. The hemoglobin content of the blood *increases* in polycythemia vera and in dehydration; it *decreases* in hemodilution of the blood as a result of fluid overload and in certain anemias, e.g., iron deficiency, pernicious, hemolytic, and hemorrhagic anemia.

The *hematocrit* (Hct) test, also known as the "packed red cell volume test," is sometimes used in place of the RBC count. To obtain a hematocrit reading, a sample of whole blood, usually 4 ml., is centrifuged until the erythrocytes separate from the plasma; the volume of red blood cells is then determined and expressed as either cubic milliliters of packed cells per 100 ml. blood or in volumes/100 ml. Normal values are 45-50 volumes/100 ml. of blood for *men,* and 40-45 volumes/100 ml. blood for *women*. The hematocrit is *increased* in polycythemia vera and in hemoconcentration resulting from fluid loss and dehydration; it is *decreased* in the anemias.

The *reticulocyte count* determines the effectiveness and speed of red blood cell production and the responsiveness of the bone marrow to a diminished number of circulating red blood cells. Specifically, this test measures the number of reticulocytes released from the bone marrow into the blood. The normal value is 25,000 to 75,000 reticulocytes per cu. mm. of blood, or 0.5 to 1.5 per cent of the total erythrocyte count, providing the erythrocyte count is within a normal range. An *increase* in the reticulocyte count indicates an abnormal increase in erythrocyte production, which is probably due to excessive red blood cell destruction (e.g., hemolytic anemia), or loss (e.g., hemorrhage). A *decrease* in the reticulocyte count may indicate bone marrow failure or pernicious anemia. This test is used routinely to check the efficiency of erythropoiesis in persons working with radioactive materials and to evaluate the effectiveness of treatment in cases of pernicious anemia and bone marrow failure.

Bone Marrow Biopsy Examination

This is an extremely important diagnostic procedure employed in the diagnosis of most blood dyscrasias (including aplastic anemia, the leukemias, pernicious anemia, and thrombocytopenia). Examination of the bone marrow reveals the number, size, and shape of red cells, white cells, and platelets as they evolve through their various developmental stages. Hematologists study the marrow cells for various maturational abnormalities.

Preparation of the patient for a bone marrow biopsy involves the following steps:

1. Explain to the patient the purpose of the procedure; tell him that a small piece of bone marrow will be taken from his sternum and sent to the laboratory for examination.
2. Ask the patient to sign a special permit prior to the biopsy. Although this procedure is not usually considered dangerous, accidental puncture of the pericardium can occur, especially if the pericardium is very thin.
3. Obtain an order for sedation if the patient appears to be extremely apprehensive.
4. Position the patient properly. The *sternum* is the site most commonly used; other sites are the iliac crest and the spinous process. For sternal puncture, place the patient on his back and put a small pillow lengthwise under the thoracic spine.

5. Shave and then cleanse the site of puncture with antiseptic solution. Drape the area with sterile towels.

The sternal puncture itself is performed by the doctor with the nurse's assistance. The *procedure* is as follows:

1. The physician injects the site with a local anesthetic.
2. Once the area is anesthetized, the doctor inserts a short, thick needle called a "sternal needle" through the bone cortex into the marrow space. He then removes the stylet from the needle, attaches a syringe to the needle and withdraws 1 to 2 ml. of marrow. At this point the patient may experience a slight sensation of pain.
3. The doctor ejects the specimen of marrow into a jar containing sodium oxalate, a preservative.

Aftercare following the procedure is as follows:

1. Apply a small sterile dressing to the site of puncture.
2. Make the patient as comfortable as possible.
3. Label the specimen jar and take it immediately to the laboratory.
4. If the patient experiences slight soreness over his sternum for three or four days following the procedure, tell him this is normal and no cause for concern.

Other Tests

The *blood film* is an examination of a blood smear to determine variations and abnormalities in erythrocyte size, shape, and hemoglobin content. Cells that are *normal* in size and shape are termed *normocytes;* cells which are *normal* in *hemoglobin content* are called *normochromic* (meaning normal color). Abnormalities of erythrocyte size, shape, and color are numerous; usually they indicate some form of anemia (Table 61–1).

Erythrocyte indices are *measurements* of erythrocyte size and hemoglobin content. These values are derived from the erythrocyte count, hemoglobin, and hematocrit and are obtained by laboratory study of a peripheral blood smear. The three erythrocyte indices, mean corpuscular volume (MCV), mean corpuscular hemoglobin (MCH), and mean corpuscular hemoglobin concentration (MCHC), are described in Table 61–2. The indices are extremely helpful in the diagnosis of various anemias.

The *erythrocyte fragility test* measures the rate at which erythrocytes become increasingly fragile and finally burst when suspended in a graded series of hypotonic saline solutions. The solutions range from 0.85 per cent saline solution (0.9 per cent is normal or physiological saline) to 0.30 per cent solution. Normal values are:

Hemolysis starts at 0.45 to 0.39 per cent saline solution.

TABLE 61–1. ABNORMALITIES OF THE ERYTHROCYTE

Cellular Abnormality	Characteristics of Abnormal Cell	Conditions Characterized by Abnormality
Anisocytosis	Erythrocytes vary in size from normal	Any of the anemias
Poikilocytosis	Erythrocyte abnormally shaped, (e.g., tear-shaped, club-shaped)	Any of the anemias; most bizarre shapes seen in the most severe anemias
Microcyte	Erythrocyte abnormally small ($<6\mu$)	Microcytic anemias, e.g., iron deficiency anemia, thalassemia major
Macrocyte	Erythrocyte abnormally large ($>9\mu$)	Macrocytic anemias, e.g., pernicious anemia, folic acid deficiency anemia
Hypochromic cell	Erythrocyte appears pale because of abnormally low hemoglobin content	Any of the anemias
Spherocyte	Erythrocyte relatively small and round rather than biconcave in shape	Thalassemia major; hemoglobin C disease
Schistocyte	Fragmented erythrocytes with extremely bizarre shapes, e.g., triangles, spirals	Hemolytic anemia
Sickle cell	Erythrocyte crescent- or sickle-shaped owing to presence of abnormal hemoglobin (hemoglobin S)	Sickle cell anemia
Target cell	Erythrocyte thin, with small amount of hemoglobin in center	Thalassemia major
Metarubricyte	Nucleated erythrocyte	Severe anemia

Hemolysis is completed at 0.33 to 0.30 per cent saline solution.

Fragility *increases* (that is, cells burst at a higher than normal saline concentration) in congenital hemolytic anemia and in hereditary spherocytosis; fragility is *normal* in acquired hemolytic anemias and is *decreased* in obstructive jaundice, that is, cells do not burst until a lower than normal concentration is reached.

The *erythrocyte life span determination* estimates the rate at which erythrocytes that are tagged with chromium-51 disappear from the circulation over a period of days or weeks; i.e., it measures the life span or survival rate of circulating red blood cells. This test is primarily employed in the differential diagnosis of the anemias. The procedure for measuring erythrocyte life span is somewhat complex. First, a blood sample is taken from the patient and the erythrocytes in the sample are tagged with chromium-51 (^{51}Cr), a radioisotope with a half-life of 77.8 days.* Next, one sample of the tagged erythrocytes is injected back into the patient and a second identical sample is injected into a healthy subject with a compatible blood type. Normally the half-life of an erythrocyte is 27 to 86 days. If the tagged erythrocytes have a shortened life span in *both* the patient and the normal subject it is assumed that the *cells* are defective. If the life span of the tagged erythrocytes is normal in the healthy subject but shortened in the patient, then it is known that the *patient* has an element in his blood that is destroying his erythrocytes early in their life cycle. The life span of erythrocytes in the various hemolytic anemias is only 6 to 12 days.

The *Coombs test* is used to: (1) detect certain antigen-antibody reactions between serum antibodies and red cell antigens; (2) differentiate between various forms of hemolytic anemia; (3) determine unusual or minor blood types; and (4) test for the possible development of erythroblastosis fetalis. The *direct Coombs test* is used to examine erythrocytes for the presence of antibodies (agglutinins) that damage erythrocytes but will not cause clumping or hemolysis. It is employed to cross match blood for blood transfusions, to test umbilical cord blood for the possible presence of erythroblastosis fetalis, and to diagnose acquired hemolytic anemia. The *indirect Coombs test* is used to identify antibodies to erythrocyte antigens in the serum of patients with a greater than normal chance of developing transfusion reactions. Both tests are agglutination procedures performed using a suspension of the patient's red blood cells.

The *fecal and urinary urobilinogen test* determines the amount of urobilinogen excreted in the urine and feces. Urobilinogen is a compound that results when bilirubin is broken down by intestinal tract bacteria (you recall that bilirubin results from the breakdown of hemoglobin following destruction of red blood cells). Normally 99 per cent of the urobilinogen formed is excreted in the feces and only 1 per cent is excreted in the urine. Normal values are:

Urinary urobilinogen: 1 to 4 mg. in 24 hours.
Fecal urobilinogen: 50 to 300 mg. in 24 hours.

Both urinary and fecal urobilinogen are increased in hemolytic anemia due to the excessive destruction of cells and resultant breakdown of large amounts of hemoglobin.

There is no special preparation for this test, and the procedure is very simple. The patient's urine is collected in a container either for a 24-hour period or for a two-hour period during the afternoon. Afternoons are used because urinary excretion of urobilinogen reaches its peak during the time span from midafternoon to early evening.

*See Unit VII for discussion of radioisotopes and their use in diagnosis.

TABLE 61–2. THE ERYTHROCYTE INDICES

Mean Corpuscular Volume (MCV)	Mean Corpuscular Hemoglobin (MCH)	Mean Corpuscular Hemoglobin Concentration (MCHC)
Measures average size or volume of individual erythrocyte	Measures hemoglobin content within erythrocyte of average size	Measures average hemoglobin concentration within 100 ml. of packed red cells
Formula for: $\frac{HCT}{RBC}$	Formula for: $\frac{HGB}{RBC}$	Formula for: $\frac{HGB}{HCT}$
Normal value: 87 ± 5 cu.μ	Normal value: 29 ± 2 μμg.	Normal value: 30–36 Gm./100 ml. packed red cells
MCV < 80 means abnormally small, i.e., *microcytic,* cells MCV > 94 means abnormally large, i.e., *macrocytic,* cells	MCH < 27 indicates hemoglobin deficiency *(hypochromic* cells) MCH > 32 indicates *macrocytic* cells with abnormally large volume of hemoglobin	MCHC < 32 indicates hemoglobin deficiency MCHC remains normal when MCH > 32 because cells are oversized, i.e., fewer cells can be packed together within 100 ml.

Nursing responsibilities are: (1) to note the exact times at which the urine collection is started and ended; and (2) to transport the total urine collected to the laboratory as soon as possible in order to prevent bacteria within the urine from converting urobilinogen to urobilin by oxidative processes.

THE ANEMIAS

DEFINITION AND INCIDENCE

Anemia is usually defined as "a decrease in the number of erythrocytes or a reduction in hemoglobin."[42] As you can see from this definition, anemia is *not* a disease in itself, but a *laboratory diagnosis* which takes many different forms; e.g., the cells may be microcytic, macrocytic, hypochromic, and so forth.

However, although anemia is not a specific disease, it is the *principal manifestation* of a number of abnormal conditions such as: deficiency states caused by a dietary lack of iron, vitamin B_{12}, folic acid, and so forth; (2) hereditary disorders of the erythrocyte; (3) disorders involving the hematopoietic tissues (bone marrow damage or a hyperactive spleen); and (4) bleeding from the gastrointestinal tract because of cancer, or hemorrhage from any organ as a result of trauma.

The *incidence* of anemia is extremely high. This is particularly true in underdeveloped countries where nutrition is poor, and in tropical regions where the hookworm (which sucks blood from the intestinal wall of its host) is endemic. Some epidemiologists calculate that at least one half of the world's population suffer from anemia at some time in their lives.

GENERAL CAUSES AND EFFECTS OF ANEMIA

Major Causes of Anemia

1. *Excessive blood loss.*
2. *Deficiencies and abnormalities of erythrocyte production.*
3. *Excessive destruction of erythrocytes.*

In turn, the three factors listed above may result from the following problems: bleeding due to trauma or cancer; dietary deficiencies; the ingestion or absorption of poisons or drugs that suppress the bone marrow; chronic infections; and genetic abnormalities that result in faulty erythrocyte genesis and/or structure.

We stated earlier that the major role of the erythrocyte is to transport oxygen to the tissues. Consequently, the major physiologic *effect* of anemia (which is a reduction in erythrocytes or hemoglobin) is to *reduce the capacity of the patient's blood to carry oxygen* to his tissues. This results in tissue hypoxia. *Tissue hypoxia* is the *basic underlying cause of all symptoms accompanying anemia.*

Symptoms accompanying anemia differ, depending upon the severity and chronicity of the anemia, the age of the patient, and whether the patient is afflicted with another malady. Patients with *mild* anemia (hemoglobin, 10 to 14 Gm.) are almost always asymptomatic unless they suffer, at the same time, from another disorder. If symptoms occur, they typically follow strenuous exertion. For example, following exercise, the patient may notice palpitations, dyspnea, and excessive diaphoresis due to the additional effort required by the heart and lungs to provide the body tissues with sufficient oxygen.

Patients with *moderate* anemia usually suffer from increased dyspnea, palpitations, and diaphoresis upon exertion as well as chronic fatigue, which occurs whether the patient is at rest or active.

When anemia is *severe,* patients appear pale and exhausted all the time; also, they complain of severe palpitations, sensitivity to cold, loss of appetite, profound weakness, dizziness, and headache. The severely anemic person (particularly if he is elderly) can eventually develop serious cardiac complications. Congestive heart failure (CHF) may arise as a result of increased demands upon the heart to beat faster and harder in order to transport more oxygen to the tissues. Angina pectoris may also develop, either alone or in conjunction with CHF. In severe anemia angina pectoris results from insufficient oxygenation of the myocardium.

DIAGNOSIS OF ANEMIA

Anemia is diagnosed on the basis of the various blood tests just described, the physical examination, and the patient's history. The three basic laboratory tests confirming the presence of anemia are the total erythrocyte count, the hemoglobin determination, and the hematocrit. To determine the *specific type* of anemia present, the hematologist (a specialist in the study of blood) examines both the patient's bone marrow specimen and the blood film. Also, he calculates the erythrocyte indices and, in some cases, the rate of erythrocyte destruction. In addition to ordering laboratory tests the physician also conducts a complete physical examination to determine the general state of the patient's health. Moreover, a careful medical and social history is helpful in determining the cause and the severity of the anemia.

Both doctor and nurse should question the patient about the following: his symptoms (presence of fatigue, dizziness, headache, sensations of "pins and needles" in the fingers and toes, etc.); the color of his urine and stools over the past weeks or months (tarry stools and/or brown, hazy or smoky urine indicate internal bleeding); the adequacy of his diet; his tolerance for exercise; medications he is taking or has taken in the recent past; whether he has been exposed recently to poisonous substances or insecticides; and whether he is or has been treated for chronic infections, cancer, renal disease, liver disease, bleeding ulcers, or hemorrhoids. Finally a family history is also useful. Some blood disorders are hereditary (e.g., hereditary spherocytosis); others are linked with race (e.g., sickle cell anemia) and place of birth (e.g., thalassemia major).

CLINICAL CARE OF THE PATIENT WITH ANEMIA

The goals of care for patients with anemia are to: (1) alleviate or control the causative factors; (2) relieve symptoms; (3) prevent complications; and (4) develop, for patients with chronic anemia, a realistic, practical, lifelong plan of care.

Therapy for the anemias ranges from specific treatment to purely symptomatic care. Therapy also varies in intensity and duration; some anemias can be cured within a few weeks or months, whereas others require lifelong treatment.

The anemias that respond best to *specific* treatment are those caused by deficiency states. For example, iron deficiency anemia is cured with iron preparations and diet, while pernicious anemia is controlled with injections of vitamin B_{12}. Other anemias (e.g., aplastic anemia due to bone marrow failure and some of the acquired hemolytic anemias) can often be successfully treated by discontinuance of a damaging drug or chemical agent. Anemia due to blood loss is usually corrected by investigation of the cause of the bleeding, medical and surgical control of the bleeding, and use of transfusions. Symptomatic care for *all* patients with anemias includes the following measures:

Rest. Rest is essential for lowering the patient's oxygen requirements and for reducing strain on the heart and lungs. Patients with *mild* anemia are rarely hospitalized and are usually fully ambulatory. However, these individuals should be encouraged to rest or nap frequently throughout the day, to shorten their working hours whenever possible, and to retire early. If the ambulatory patient experiences dizziness or lightheadedness while at work or at home, tell him to lie flat on a bed, couch, or floor for a few minutes; lying down without a pillow helps to relieve dizziness by increasing the circulation of blood and oxygen to the brain.

Patients with *severe* anemia are usually hospitalized and placed on bed rest until their blood picture improves. If the patient is extremely weak, help him to bathe, to turn, to eat his meals, and to care for his teeth or dentures. Also, to ensure sufficient rest, protect the severely anemic patient from frequent visitors, continuous telephone interruptions, and excessive noise. Planned rest periods are advisable.

Skin Care. Frequent turning is essential for patients with severe anemia if skin breakdown is to be prevented. Because of the reduction in circulating red blood cells, the tissues of the anemic patient do not receive adequate amounts of oxygen. Without preventative measures, the resultant tissue hypoxia can quickly lead to decubitus formation. (Nursing routines for preventing skin breakdown in bedridden patients are discussed in Chapter 27).

Diet. The diet in anemia should be high in protein, iron, and vitamins. These substances are essential for normal erythrocyte formation. Unfortunately patients with anemia may have little appetite for the nourishing foods that they need so badly. Anorexia often results from weakness and profound fatigue. Also, patients with pernicious anemia or iron deficiency anemia often have difficulty eating because of a sore mouth, tongue, or esophagus. The following measures are helpful in combating anorexia: (1) serve six small, easily digested meals a day instead of three large meals; (2) avoid hot spicy foods if the patient suffers from a sore mouth or throat; (3) give oral hygiene before and after the patient eats; and (4) feed the patient if he appears too exhausted to feed himself.

Anemic patients and their families need practical instruction on how to plan and prepare a nourishing diet at home. To teach patients about the dietary prevention and treatment of anemia, you can: (1) arrange for private consultation between the dietitian, the patient, and his family; (2) give the patient illustrated booklets on nutrition and meal planning and discuss them with him; (3) obtain for the patient appetizing recipes for foods high in iron, vitamin B_{12}, and other vitamins; (4) prepare several weeks of sample menus containing nutritious foods that the patient enjoys; and (5) arrange for a public health nurse to visit the patient at home for continued dietary supervision. *

Mouth Care. Special mouth care is a necessity for all patients with severe anemia because they often suffer from a sore mouth or tongue. Special oral hygiene measures include: (1) cleansing the teeth before and after meals with a soft-bristled toothbrush or applicators; (2) allowing the patient to rinse his mouth every two hours with mouthwashes that are cool and slightly alkaline; and (3) lubricating the lips frequently with mineral oil or petrolatum to prevent dryness or cracking.

Transfusions. Blood transfusions are not administered routinely to all patients with anemia because they can result in extremely dangerous reactions and complications. However, blood transfusions are valuable in the treatment of patients with anemia due to *acute* blood loss. The administration of several pints of blood is often lifesaving for the individual with a hemoglobin of less than 10 Gm. as a result of hemorrhage.

Blood transfusions may be used to treat patients with *severe chronic anemia* (hemoglobin less than 6 Gm.) who have responded poorly to other forms of therapy. However, in spite of its benefits, giving whole blood to persons with severe chronic anemia is extremely hazardous because of the potential complications mentioned in Chapter 60.

*Usually books on nutrition and sample menus and recipes can be obtained from the dietitian in your hospital or from the local public health department.

Patients who have a heart condition in addition to anemia are particularly vulnerable to circulatory and pulmonary complications.

To help alleviate the dangers of circulatory overload in the patient with cardiac complications, the doctor may order the administration of a small volume of *packed red cells* in place of whole blood. Additionally, the physician may attempt to reduce the patient's plasma volume *before* the transfusion by: (1) administering diuretics to promote the elimination of large amounts of water; or (2) by withdrawing an amount of plasma from the patient which equals in volume the amount of blood ordered for the transfusion.

As you administer blood to the patient with chronic anemia and heart disease, take the following precautions: (1) administer the blood *very slowly* to prevent overloading the heart and lungs; (2) check the patient's *pulse* every 15 minutes for tachycardia—an indication that the heart is overworking as a pump; (3) examine the patient's *neck veins* for fullness and monitor the *central venous pressure* (elevation of the central venous pressure over 10 cm. H_2O indicates a circulatory overload); (4) observe the patient for symptoms of *respiratory distress* and listen for the sound of *rales* in the patient's basilar lung regions; and (5) stop the transfusion at once and notify the physician if the patient's pulse becomes rapid (over 120 beats per minute), if the central venous pressure is elevated, or if the patient develops symptoms of pulmonary edema.

Oxygen Therapy. This is rarely ordered for patients with mild anemia. However, patients with *severe* anemia need oxygen because their blood is so greatly reduced in its capacity to carry this life-sustaining gas. In these cases the administration of oxygen helps to prevent tissue hypoxia and also lessens the work of the heart as it struggles to compensate for the deficiency of oxygen-carrying hemoglobin.

Protection of Patient. Protection of the patient from *chilling* and *burns* is an important nursing function. Because of poor circulation, patients with anemia typically complain of feeling cold and chilled. Warm clothing and blankets help anemic patients to feel more comfortable and consequently they rest and sleep better.

Avoid applying heating pads or hot water bottles to the patient with anemia, because his skin (which is poorly supplied with blood and oxygen) burns easily. Also, the patient may not be aware of any burning sensation.

The patient with pernicious anemia, in particular, suffers from a decreased sensitivity to heat. He may be severely burned by heating devices before he or the nursing staff becomes aware of his condition.

Isolation. Isolation of the patient from possible *sources of infection* is a necessity. Severely anemic patients are typically exhausted and debilitated and, consequently, develop infections easily. Do not care for patients with anemia if you have a cold or sore throat; also, do not permit infected visitors, patients, or other personnel to come into close contact with the patient. *Reverse isolation techniques* are needed to protect patients with aplastic anemia; these individuals suffer from leukopenia (a reduced leukocyte count) as well as anemia and are therefore particularly vulnerable to infection.

Classification of the Anemias

"Anemias are generally classified according to either the morphologic characteristics of the erythrocytes (i.e., normocytic, microcytic, etc.) or the etiology of the condition (i.e., hemolytic hemorrhagic, etc.). In many instances the etiologic method of classification is inappropriate since anemia is merely a symptom of an underlying pathophysiologic process whose nature and etiology may be obscure. Nurses should therefore be familiar with morphologic classification, which is in common usage because it is objective, descriptive, and independent of etiologic factors."[62]

Although our discussion of the individual anemias will consider them from an etiologic standpoint, a brief résumé of the more common morphologic categories usually employed is given first (below). You will recall that in earlier portions

MORPHOLOGIC CLASSIFICATION OF ANEMIAS

Type of Anemia	*Criteria*	*Clinical Examples*
Normocytic (normochromic)	MCV 80-94 c.μ MCHC >30%	Anemia of sudden blood loss, anemia of pregnancy, anemia of chronic disease, e.g., cancer, some hemolytic anemias
Macrocytic (normochromic)	MCV >94 c.μ MCHC >30%	Pernicious anemia, anemia in myxedema, folic acid deficiency, some hemolytic anemias
Microcytic (normochromic)	MCV <80 c.μ MCHC >30%	Anemia of chronic disease
Hypochromic microcytic	MCV <80 c.μ MCHC <30%	Iron deficiency anemia

of this chapter, particularly in Tables 61–1 and 61–2, the terms macrocytic and microcytic have already been introduced and the standards for applying these terms to cells, based on the mean corpuscular volume (MCV), were indicated. The mean corpuscular hemoglobin (MCH) and the mean corpuscular hemoglobin concentration (MCHC) "are the bases upon which the designations of normochromia, hypochromia, or hyperchromia are predicated."[62]

The etiologic classification given below, which we follow in this text, is used here because it is easier to relate patient care and teaching to the etiology of an anemia than to its cellular characteristics.

*ANEMIAS: ETIOLOGIC CLASSIFICATION**

I. Anemias Resulting from Excessive Blood Loss
   A. Acute posthemorrhagic anemia
   B. Anemia due to chronic blood loss
II. Anemias Resulting from Reduced Erythrocyte Production
   A. Anemias due to nutritional deficiencies
      1. Iron deficiency anemia
      2. Anemias due to deficiencies of vitamin B_{12} and folic acid (megaloblastic anemias)
         a. Pernicious anemia
         b. Other anemias due to vitamin B_{12} deficiency
         c. Anemia due to folic acid deficiency
   B. Anemia of bone marrow failure
III. Anemias Resulting from Excessive Erythrocyte Destruction (Hemolytic Anemias)
   A. Hemolytic anemias resulting from intracorpuscular defects
      1. Glucose-6-phosphate dehydrogenase (G6PD) deficiency
      2. Hereditary spherocytosis
   B. Hemolytic anemias mainly resulting from extracorpuscular abnormalities (acquired hemolytic anemias)
      1. Hemolysis due to trauma
      2. Hemolysis due to chemical agents and drugs (toxic hemolytic anemia)
      3. Hemolysis due to infectious agents
      4. Hemolytic disease secondary to systemic disease (secondary hemolytic anemia)
      5. Hemolysis due to isoimmune hemolytic reactions
      6. Hemolysis due to autoimmune disorders
      7. The paroxysmal hemoglobinopathies
IV. Anemias Resulting Both from Disturbances of Erythrocyte Production and from Increased Erythrocyte Destruction
   A. Anemias due to defective hemoglobin synthesis
      1. Hemoglobinopathies (e.g., sickle cell anemia)
      2. Thalassemias
   B. Secondary anemias (also called anemias of relative bone marrow failure or simple chronic anemias)

*Classification adapted from Holvey, D. N., et al. (eds.): *Merck Manual of Diagnosis and Therapy.* 12th ed. Rahway, N. J., Merck, Sharp & Dohme Research Laboratories, 1972, p. 250.

ANEMIAS RESULTING FROM EXCESSIVE BLOOD LOSS

Acute Posthemorrhagic Anemia

Definition, Etiology, and Symptoms. Acute posthemorrhagic anemia is a normocytic, normochromic anemia which develops following the rapid loss of large numbers of erythrocytes during a massive hemorrhage.

Common *causes* of acute bleeding are:

> Severed blood vessels due to trauma.
> Spontaneous rupture of an aneurysm.
> Hemorrhagic disorders.
> Erosion of an artery by a cancerous growth or ulcerative lesion.

The adverse *effects* of acute hemorrhage are due to the rapid decrease in blood volume and the reduced oxygen-carrying capacity of the blood which results from the loss of erythrocytes. The severity of the patient's symptoms as well as his prognosis depend upon: (1) the *rate* of bleeding; (2) the *site* of the hemorrhage; and (3) the *volume* of blood lost. A gradual loss of a large amount of blood is less threatening for the patient than the rapid loss of a smaller volume of blood.

The clinical manifestations of acute hemorrhage include: restlessness; dizziness; syncope; thirst; pallor; diaphoresis; rapid thready pulse; hypotension; rapid deep respirations, which later become shallow; severe headache; and disorientation. Disorientation indicates cerebral anoxia. In addition to these symptoms, internal hemorrhage into body organs and tissues causes fever, pain in the area of bleeding due to distention of tissues, and symptoms of organ displacement (e.g., hemothorax can result in a mediastinal shift). If internal or external hemorrhage remains uncontrolled, the blood pressure continues to drop and shock develops. Untreated, the shock becomes irreversible and death swiftly ensues.

Laboratory Findings. Following acute hemorrhage, the patient's blood picture is in a state of flux for several weeks. The erythrocyte count, hemoglobin, and hematocrit findings are completely unreliable for the first 24 to 48 hours following hemorrhage because *vasoconstriction* (a compensatory mechanism which occurs during shock) and *loss of plasma volume* mask the actual degree of erythrocyte and hemoglobin loss. In other words, the erythrocytes that remain following hemorrhage are concentrated within a smaller space and a smaller volume of plasma than normal. Consequently the erythrocyte, hemoglobin, and hematocrit appear deceptively high when, in fact, they may be dangerously low. However, after one to two days, extracellular fluid from the tissues and prescribed intravenous fluids enter the patient's vascular compartment and dilute the red blood cell concentration. As a result, the remaining (greatly diminished) erythrocytes circulate in a more normal amount of plasma; consequently the erythrocyte count, hemoglobin, and hematocrit reflect more accurately the degree of anemia present.

If there is no further bleeding, blood restoration begins within 4 to 5 days. The erythrocyte count and hemoglobin usually return to normal within a month to six weeks. During this period, large numbers of reticulocytes appear in the blood, sometimes accompanied by a few normocytes if the anemia is severe.

Clinical Care. Emergency treatment of patients with acute hemorrhage centers around controlling and stopping the hemorrhage, treating shock, and restoring the blood volume as rapidly as possible.

> *Blood transfusion is the treatment of choice if the patient's blood loss is greater than 20 per cent of his total blood volume.*

The patient is generally treated with intravenous infusions of plasma while his blood is being typed and crossmatched. Other supportive measures for the hemorrhaging patient are sedation, rest, and oral fluids if the patient can tolerate them and if he is not going to surgery.

Once the patient's blood volume has been restored and shock has abated, the next goal of care is to *replenish the iron stores* that were lost during hemorrhage. A nutritious diet helps the patient to overcome an iron deficiency; encourage the patient to eat foods high in protein, iron, and vitamins. If diet therapy proves inadequate, the doctor may order the administration of iron supplements.

Anemia Due to Chronic Blood Loss

The major *causes* of chronic blood loss are bleeding peptic ulcers, prolonged or excessive menses, bleeding hemorrhoids, and cancerous lesions within the gastrointestinal tract. The *results* of chronic bleeding are: (1) continuous loss of small numbers of erythrocytes, which are usually adequately replaced by the bone marrow; and (2) continuous loss of iron, which may result in a total depletion of the patient's iron stores. Because of the severe iron losses, the anemia of chronic bleeding is identical in symptoms and laboratory findings to *iron deficiency anemia* (see below). To treat anemia due to chronic blood loss, the physician must locate the site of bleeding, control the cause of bleeding, and correct the patient's iron deficiency with proper diet and iron supplements.

ANEMIAS RESULTING FROM REDUCED ERYTHROCYTE PRODUCTION

Anemias Due to Nutritional Deficiencies

We stated earlier that effective erythropoiesis depends upon the adequate intake and proper

assimilation of iron, vitamin B_{12}, folic acid, protein, pyridoxine, and traces of copper. Inadequate intake, defective assimilation, or excessive loss of any one of these factors will result in a deficiency of that nutrient followed by the development of anemia. The *most common* deficiency state is iron deficiency. Deficiencies of vitamin B_{12} and folic acid are also prevalent. Protein deficiency, also frequently encountered, is discussed in Chapter 25. Pyridoxine deficiency occurs infrequently in man; copper deficiency is extremely rare.

Iron Deficiency Anemia

DEFINITION AND INCIDENCE. Iron deficiency anemia is a chronic, microcytic, hypochromic anemia caused by either inadequate absorption or excessive loss of iron.

The *incidence* of iron deficiency anemia throughout the world is extremely high. It is the most prevalent of the anemias and it affects at least twice as many persons as all the other anemias put together.

The *distribution* of this condition is related to geographic location, economic class, age groupings, and sex. Viewed on a worldwide basis, iron deficiency anemia most commonly strikes persons in underdeveloped countries such as India where nutrition is extremely poor. This problem is also prevalent in tropical zones and in Southern United States, Mexico, and Puerto Rico, where blood-sucking parasites such as the hookworm are endemic.

The poor of all nations suffer far more frequently from iron deficiency than do the middle and upper classes. Also, women between the ages of 15 and 45 and young children are extremely vulnerable to iron deficiency. On the other hand, adult males and postmenopausal females are rarely troubled by this problem unless they suffer, at the same time, from conditions causing chronic blood loss. Population studies reveal that 10 to 30 per cent of all women suffer from iron deficiency, 10 to 60 per cent of pregnant women and young infants have this condition, while only 3 per cent of men have symptoms of iron lack.

IRON BALANCE. The adult human body contains approximately 50 mg. of iron per kg. of body weight. Total body iron ranges between 2 to 6 Gm., depending upon the size of the individual and the amount of hemoglobin his cells contain. Approximately two thirds of this iron is contained in hemoglobin ("essential iron"); the other third is stored in the bone marrow, spleen, and liver. If an individual develops an iron deficiency, his iron stores are depleted first, followed later by a reduction in hemoglobin formation.

We obtain iron from food, important dietary sources of iron being liver (the richest source), oysters, lean meats, kidney beans, whole-wheat bread, kale, spinach, egg yolk, turnip tops, beet greens, carrots, apricots, and raisins.

An adequate diet supplies the body with approximately 12 to 15 mg. of iron per day, of which only

5 to 10 per cent (0.6 to 1.5 mg.) is absorbed. The amount of iron normally absorbed daily is *just sufficient* to meet the needs of healthy men and older women past the childbearing age, but is *not* sufficient to supply the greater needs of menstruating and pregnant women, adolescents, infants, and children. Note in Table 61–3 that these five groups of individuals must have a higher daily intake of iron if iron deficiency is to be prevented. Fortunately if iron intake is inadequate during childhood or pregnancy or if bleeding develops, the gastrointestinal tract is capable of increasing the absorption of iron to around 20 to 30 per cent of the total daily intake of iron instead of only 10 per cent. In this way the body often compensates for diminishing iron stores due to inadequate iron intake or excessive iron loss.

Iron is *excreted* in urine, sweat, bile, and feces and from the skin as desquamated cells. Daily iron excretion is normally less than 1 mg. The normal monthly menses causes women of childbearing age to lose another 0.4 to 1.0 mg. of iron daily, or 12 to 30 mg. monthly. The only *abnormal* source of iron loss is *hemorrhage* or *chronic bleeding*. A chronic blood loss of as little as 2 to 4 ml. per day can result in iron deficiency anemia because 1 mg. of iron is lost in every 2 ml. of blood. To compensate for abnormal iron losses or an insufficient iron intake the body excretes less than 0.5 mg. of iron daily rather than the 1 mg. normally excreted.

In sum, the maintenance of a positive iron balance depends upon an intake of iron which is sufficient to meet the needs of the individual during the various phases of his or her life and to compensate for any abnormal iron losses. Iron balance is regulated first by controlled absorption of iron and secondly by controlled excretion of iron. In this way, the body compensates for mild degrees of iron deficiency. If iron deficiency is severe, pharmacologic iron supplements are necessary to restore positive iron balance.

ETIOLOGY OF IRON DEFICIENCY ANEMIA. Acute or chronic bleeding is the principal cause of iron deficiency anemia in adults. The major causes of excessive blood loss are *trauma, excessive menses* (more than 12 pads used per period), and *gastrointestinal tract bleeding;* the latter may result from peptic ulcers, hiatus hernia, gastritis, cancer, hemorrhoids, diverticuli, ulcerative colitis, or salicylate poisoning. Bleeding from the gastrointestinal tract is usually chronic in nature and occult (i.e., obscure or not readily apparent).

Blood donation, a form of blood loss, is also a source of iron depletion. Each time a blood donor gives a pint of his blood, he is losing 250 mg. of iron, provided his hemoglobin level is normal. To make up for this iron loss, the blood donor must increase his daily intake of iron by approximately 0.7 mg. for a full year following the blood donation.

A second cause of iron deficiency anemia is an *inadequate intake* of foods high in iron, as we have just discussed. Finally, iron deficiency anemia results when adequate iron is ingested but is *not absorbed* properly. Causes of defective assimilation of iron are:

> Chronic diarrhea.

> Malabsorption syndromes (e.g., celiac disease, tropical and nontropical sprue, cystic fibrosis).

> A high intake of cereal products coupled with a low intake of animal protein.

> Partial or complete gastrectomy, which causes a decrease in both the assimilation and absorption of food iron.

> Clay-eating (pica), a common practice of women and children in socioeconomically disadvantaged areas, which causes iron to precipitate as an insoluble substance within the intestinal tract.

SYMPTOMS. In mild cases of iron deficiency anemia, the patient is generally asymptomatic. However, in more severe cases he suffers from all the general symptoms of anemia discussed earlier,

TABLE 61-3. ESTIMATED DIETARY IRON REQUIREMENTS*

	Absorbed Iron Requirement (mg./day)	Daily Food Iron Requirement† (mg./day)
Normal men and nonmenstruating women	0.5–1.0	5–10
Menstruating women	0.7–2.0	7–20
Pregnant women	2.0–4.8	20–48‡
Adolescents	1.0–2.0	10–20
Children	0.4–1.0	4–10
Infants	0.5–1.5	1.5 mg./per kg.§

*Brown, E. B.: Hypochromic anemias. *In* Beeson, P. B., and McDermott, W. (eds.): *Cecil-Loeb Textbook of Medicine.* 13th ed. 1971.

†Assuming 10 per cent absorption.

‡This amount of iron cannot be derived from diet and should be met by iron supplementation in the latter half of pregnancy.

§To a maximum of 15 mg.

e.g., palpitations, dizziness, and sensitivity to cold. Later in the course of the disease, patients usually develop brittleness of hair and nails. In severe cases patients may experience dysphagia (difficulty in swallowing), stomatitis (inflammation of the mucosa of the mouth), and atrophic glossitis (tongue is inflamed and also smooth due to atrophy of papillae). This triad of symptoms is called the *Plummer-Vinson syndrome*. Despite the weakness and discomfort associated with iron deficiency anemia, patients rarely die from this condition unless severe cardiac complications develop.

DIAGNOSTIC TESTS. The diagnosis of iron deficiency anemia is based upon examination of the patient's blood and bone marrow. The *morphology* of the erythrocytes in this anemia is highly characteristic. The individual red blood cells are small (microcytic) and pale (hypochromic) because they are deficient in hemoglobin. The blood *hemoglobin* level is markedly reduced and may fall as low as 3.6 Gm./100 ml. However, the *total erythrocyte count* is usually only moderately reduced, rarely dropping below 3,000,000 cells per 100 ml. The MCV, MCH, and MCHC are all reduced. The *serum iron level* (normally between 50 and 150 μg. per 100 ml. of blood) may decrease to 10 μg. Finally, *hemosiderin* (an insoluble form of storage iron) is completely absent from the bone marrow.

Once the diagnosis of iron deficiency anemia is confirmed, studies are conducted to find the *cause* of the anemia. If gastrointestinal tract bleeding is suspected, the doctor orders a battery of tests to determine the approximate amount of blood lost daily, locate the site of bleeding, and pinpoint the lesion responsible for the blood loss. Diagnostic tests commonly employed in the study of gastrointestinal tract bleeding are x-rays of the gastrointestinal tract (G.I. series), stool examinations for occult blood, esophagoscopy, gastroscopy, and sigmoidoscopy. (See Unit XV for discussion of these procedures.)

CLINICAL CARE. Therapeutic goals for patients with iron deficiency anemia are: (1) to diagnose and correct the underlying cause of the anemia; and (2) to correct the iron deficit by means of medicinal iron preparations and a diet high in food iron.

Medicinal iron can be administered orally or parenterally; however, it is administered orally whenever possible. The drugs of choice for *oral* administration are:

> Ferrous sulfate, 0.2 Gm. (3 gr.) t.i.d. after meals.
> Ferrous gluconate, 0.3 Gm. (5 gr.) t.i.d. after meals.

It is important to administer oral iron preparations correctly. First of all, because iron salts are *gastric irritants*, they *should always be given following meals or a snack*. Iron preparations taken on an empty stomach cause dyspepsia, abdominal discomfort, and diarrhea. Second, undiluted liquid preparations of iron salts cause staining of the teeth; consequently, liquid iron preparations should be diluted well and administered through a straw. Third, whenever possible, give ferrous salts with *orange juice* because ascorbic acid helps to promote better iron absorption. Finally, warn the patient that iron preparations will change the color of his stools because iron is excreted in the bowel movements; emphasize that the tarry appearance of the feces is only a harmless side effect.

Parenteral iron therapy is administered to patients: (1) who have an intolerance to oral iron preparations, (2) who habitually forget to take their medications, or (3) who are continuing to suffer from blood losses. The following medication is the parenteral drug of choice:

> Iron-dextran (Imferon) I.M. 50 mg. stat, and then 100 to 250 mg. I.M. daily or every other day until the patient's hemoglobin is within normal range.

Iron-dextran causes darkening and discoloration of the skin around the injection site unless administered properly. When giving iron-dextran I.M., remember these points:

1. Use one needle to withdraw iron-dextran and another needle to administer it. Failure to change needles will result in staining of the patient's tissues.
2. When drawing up the medication, leave 0.5 ml. of air in the syringe.
3. Give the injection with a 2- or 3-inch, 19- or 20-gauge needle, *deep* into the upper outer quadrant of the buttock; never use the patient's arm or any other exposed area.
4. Use the "Z" tract injection technique (i.e., form the outline of a "Z" by pulling the subcutaneous tissue to one side) when giving the injection; this method prevents the medication from leaking into the tissues.
5. Make certain that the needle is not in a vein; then give the injection followed by the 0.5 ml. of air. The air removes iron-dextran from inside the needle's shaft, thereby preventing leakage of the drug as the needle is removed from the tissues.
6. Never massage the site of injection.
7. Encourage the patient to ambulate, because walking hastens drug absorption. However, caution the patient not to exercise vigorously or wear constricting garments or a girdle.
8. Throughout the course of injection therapy, observe for pain at the site of injection, the development of sterile abscesses, lymphadenitis, fever, headache, urticaria, hypotension, or anaphylactic shock. Fortunately, anaphylaxis is rare.

A favorable response to iron therapy typically occurs within 48 hours; the patient usually feels more energetic and less irritable and has a better appetite. Within 7 to 12 days following initiation of treatment, reticulocytes begin to flood the circulation. Under optimum conditions, the patient's hemoglobin is restored at a daily rate of around 0.3 Gm./100 ml. of blood. However, because iron stores are replenished at a slower rate than hemoglobin, patients must continue to take iron preparations for two or three months following return of their hemoglobin to normal.

PROGNOSIS. In the majority of cases, iron therapy is successful in reversing the symptoms of iron deficiency anemia. However, approximately one third of women and one fourth of men have a recurrence. In these cases, the anemia itself was evidently cured but not the underlying cause, e.g., severe bleeding, prolonged menses, etc.

Anemias Due to Deficiencies of Vitamin B_{12} and Folic Acid (Megaloblastic Anemias). *Vitamin B_{12}*, which contains cobalt, has two major functions: it is essential for normal red blood cell maturation, and it is necessary for normal nervous system function. Dietary sources of vitamin B_{12} are animal products such as liver, milk, and eggs; it is not contained in vegetables. Vitamin B_{12} is also produced by bacteria within the intestines of humans and animals. Other names for vitamin B_{12} are cyanocobalamin, anti-anemic factor and extrinsic factor, which means a factor of external origin. The *extrinsic factor* (i.e., vitamin B_{12} obtained from foods) cannot be absorbed by the small intestine unless a substance called the *intrinsic factor* (i.e., a factor of internal origin) is present. A condition called *pernicious anemia* develops when the intrinsic factor is missing.

Like vitamin B_{12}, *folic acid* (a B-group vitamin) is necessary for red blood cell formation and maturation. However, folic acid does not play a role in nervous system function. The major dietary sources of folic acid are green vegetables and liver.

Anemias due to deficiencies of vitamin B_{12} and folic acid are called *megaloblastic anemias* because they are characterized by the appearance of megaloblasts (large primitive erythrocytes) in the blood and bone marrow. Other common features of the megaloblastic anemias are: (1) the development of leukopenia and thrombocytopenia in addition to anemia; (2) oral, gastrointestinal, and neurologic symptoms; and (3) a favorable response to injections of either vitamin B_{12} or folic acid.

The underlying defect in the megaloblastic anemias is *disturbed synthesis of deoxyribonucleic acid (DNA)*, the basic substance composing chromosomes. Deficiencies of either vitamin B_{12} or folic acid evidently impede the formation of essential DNA precursors. As a result, maturation of erythrocytes, leukocytes, and platelets is defective.

The same basic *etiologic factors*—dietary inadequacies, impaired absorption, and metabolic disturbances—underlie both vitamin B_{12} deficiency and folic acid deficiency. In vitamin B_{12} deficiency the diet is deficient in meat and dairy products, and in folic acid deficiency vegetables are lacking in the diet.

As mentioned, the principal cause of impaired absorption of vitamin B_{12} is deficiency of the intrinsic factor. Folic acid absorption and utilization may be impeded by the administration of compounds known as folic acid antagonists, by the use of anticonvulsants, or by liver disease. Intestinal malabsorption of both vitamins can be due to any of a group of conditions such as sprue, celiac disease, steatorrhea, or surgical resection of the small intestine. Such additional conditions as tapeworm, excessive accumulation of intestinal bacteria, or intestinal diverticuli may also cause impaired absorption of vitamin B_{12}.

Metabolic disturbances such as hyperthyroidism, pregnancy, or cancer may lead to additional requirements for both these vitamins, thus producing deficiency states.

Because pernicious anemia is the most prevalent form of vitamin B_{12} deficiency in the United States and Canada, we discuss this formerly fatal condition in some detail. Other vitamin B_{12} deficiency anemias and folic acid deficiency anemia are considered briefly.

PERNICIOUS ANEMIA

Definition and incidence. Pernicious anemia is a chronic progressive, macrocytic anemia of adults, caused by a *deficiency* of the *intrinsic factor*. Major characteristics of pernicious anemia are: (1) abnormally large erythrocytes (macrocytic); (2) hypochlorhydria (deficiency of hydrochloric acid in the gastric juice); (3) neurologic and gastrointestinal symptoms; and (4) a fatal outcome without lifelong injections of vitamin B_{12}.

Although pernicious anemia is the most common of the megaloblastic anemias, it is not a common disease. Only 0.1 per cent of the population have this ailment.

Pernicious anemia mainly strikes men and women over 50. It most commonly affects blue-eyed persons of Scandinavian origin. However, pernicious anemia is occasionally seen in people under 35 and in blacks.

Etiology. Lack of the intrinsic factor (the basic defect in pernicious anemia) is caused by atrophy of the glandular mucosa of the gastric fundus. Unfortunately the exact factor or factors causing this mucosal atrophy and the associated hypochlorhydria remain unknown. However, the following theories of causation are gaining widespread acceptance. First, a *hereditary* basis for the disease seems likely but is currently unproved. Pernicious anemia does tend to "run in families." Prolonged *iron deficiency,* which can cause gastric atrophy, is a second possible predisposing factor. However, the most promising etiologic theory to date is that pernicious anemia is an *autoimmune disorder.* Ninety per cent of patients with pernicious anemia have autoantibodies which react specifically against parietal gastric cells, while 40 per cent of patients have antibodies to the intrinsic factor.

Unless controlled with vitamin B_{12}, pernicious anemia always develops following *total gastrectomy;* also, 15 per cent of patients develop pernicious anemia following partial gastrectomy or gastrojejunostomy for peptic ulcer.

Bases of symptoms. As stated earlier, vitamin B_{12} deficiency diminishes DNA synthesis; reduced DNA synthesis, in turn, results in defective maturation of cells. The cells most disturbed by defects in DNA synthesis are the more rapidly dividing body cells, i.e., cells of the bone marrow and gastrointestinal tract. Thus, consequences of vitamin B_{12} deficiency are *macrocytic anemia* and *gastrointestinal disorders.* Both these problems can be reversed with injections of vitamin B_{12}. Second, lack of vitamin B_{12} can alter the structure and disrupt the function of the peripheral nerves, spinal cord, and the brain. Thus, the third major consequence of this disorder is *disturbed nervous system function* and, in extreme cases, *permanent neurologic damage* occurs which cannot be reversed by treatment with parenteral vitamin B_{12}. Central nervous system symptoms develop in three quarters of patients.

More specifically, the symptoms of pernicious anemia and their bases are shown at the bottom of this page.

Patients with pernicious anemia have a high incidence of *benign gastric polyps* and *gastric carcinoma*. For this reason, persons undergoing treatment for pernicious anemia should be routinely examined for signs of gastric bleeding or obstruction due to tumor growth.

Untreated pernicious anemia terminates in death; *delayed* treatment results in *permanent disabilities*. In addition to the nervous system damage already mentioned, severe macrocytic anemia of long duration can trigger the development of congestive heart failure and angina pectoris in the elderly.

Diagnostic tests. Pernicious anemia is diagnosed on the basis of: (1) the presence of the triad of symptoms described above (anemia, gastrointestinal symptoms, neurologic disorders); (2) laboratory blood and bone marrow tests; (3) the absence of hydrochloric acid in the gastric juice; and (4) a favorable response to a "therapeutic trial" with vitamin B_{12}.

Laboratory findings which confirm a diagnosis of pernicious anemia include the following:

> *Erythrocyte count:* Erythrocytes are usually reduced to below 3 million RBC/100 ml.

> *Blood film:* Erythrocytes are oval and macrocytic and they contain an abnormally large amount of hemoglobin.

> *Bone marrow examination:* Bone marrow contains high numbers of megaloblasts (an abnormal form of erythrocyte maturation) but few normoblasts and normally maturing erythrocytes. The bone marrow also shows defects in the maturation of leukocytes.

> *Bilirubin:* Unconjugated bilirubin (a product of hemoglobin breakdown) is usually elevated due to hemolysis of defective erythrocytes.

> *Schilling test:* This measures the absorption of radioactive vitamin B_{12} (tagged with cobalt-60) both before and after parenteral administration of the intrinsic factor. This procedure is the *definitive test for pernicious anemia;* it is used to detect lack of the intrinsic factor, the basic defect in this disease.

The test is performed in two, and sometimes three, stages. If after the first stage, during which only vitamin B_{12} has been given, the patient's urinary excretion of the vitamin is in the normal range, pernicious anemia probably is not present and the test is terminated. If the excretion is abnormal, a second stage is performed in which intrinsic factor is given with the vitamin B_{12}. If the results of this are equivocal, a third stage is sometimes used to determine whether an alteration in intestinal bacteria is causing the malabsorption of the vitamin.

> *Gastric juice analysis* for the presence of free hydrochloric acid is another important test. Almost all individuals with pernicious anemia secrete gastric juice which has: (1) an abnormally low volume, (2) an abnormally high pH, and (3) no free hydrochloric acid. Furthermore, in pernicious anemia, gastric secretions remain scanty and the pH elevated even *after* the patient is given an injection of *histamine*—a substance which normally stimulates the flow of gastric juice.

> *Therapeutic trial with parenteral vitamin B_{12}.* For this test the patient is given I.M. injections of vitamin B_{12} for 10 days. If the patient has pernicious anemia he responds quickly and favorably to the medication; e.g., he has an increased sense of well-being and his blood picture improves. The diagnosis of pernicious anemia is confirmed if large numbers of reticulocytes appear in the blood 4 to 5 days following the vitamin B_{12} injection.

Clinical care. Patients with pernicious anemia need both immediate care and lifelong therapy with maintenance vitamin B_{12}.

During the *acute* phase of his illness, the patient may be treated with the following medications:

> *Cyanocobalamin* (the standard vitamin B_{12} preparation) 100 μg I.M. 2 to 3 times per week until 10 doses are given and a remission obtained.

Generally the patient responds quickly and dramatically to vitamin B_{12} injections. Within 24 to 48 hours he usually begins to feel less weak, irritable, and depressed, and he also starts to regain his appetite. Within 72 hours reticulocytes begin to increase, and by the end of the first week following initiation of therapy, the patient's total erythrocyte

Symptoms	*Bases of Symptoms*
Anemia: weakness; pallor; dyspnea; palpitations; fatigue	Reduced erythrocyte count (less than 3 million RBC/100 ml. blood) impairs oxygen-carrying capacity of blood
Gastrointestinal symptoms: sore mouth; smooth, beefy red tongue; weight loss; indigestion; constipation or diarrhea	Gastric lesion involves atrophy of gastric mucosa and causes reduced secretion of *hydrochloric acid* as well as intrinsic factor; HCl plays important role in chemical digestion of food
Neurologic symptoms: tingling, numbness of hands and feet; paralysis; irritability; depression; psychotic behavior	Lack of vitamin B_{12} causes degeneration of dorsal and lateral columns of spinal cord, peripheral nerve degeneration and even brain damage
Jaundice: pale yellow tinge to the skin	Rupture and hemolysis of abnormally large erythrocytes as they pass through capillaries

count is significantly higher. With improvement of the blood picture, patients with cardiovascular involvement usually experience a gradual lessening of cardiac symptoms. Unfortunately, although the function of the peripheral nerves may improve with treatment, any spinal cord or brain damage is almost always permanent.

> *Ferrous sulfate or ferrous gluconate,* 0.3 Gm. orally t.i.d. following meals, given if hemoglobin level fails to rise in proportion to increases in the total erythrocyte count.

As stated earlier, iron deficiency may play a role in the etiology of pernicious anemia; consequently an iron deficit, if present, must be corrected. Also, iron deficiency anemia can develop in the *course* of treating pernicious anemia. Injections of vitamin B_{12} can cause such a rapid regeneration of erythrocytes that the patient's iron stores become depleted. As a result of iron depletion, the hemoglobin level remains low even though the total erythrocyte count rises.

> *Hydrochloric acid* (HCl), well diluted in water, t.i.d. following meals.

Because patients with pernicious anemia suffer from achlorhydria, the oral administration of hydrochloric acid enhances digestion and helps to prevent dyspepsia. However HCl is usually given only during the first week or two of vitamin B_{12} therapy. Once the patient's condition improves, gastrointestinal tract complaints disappear. When administering HCl, remember:

HCl stains the teeth; always dilute this medication thoroughly in a glass of water and administer it through a straw.

> *Folic acid* 0.1 to 0.2 mg. daily.

Folic acid is sometimes given, in conjunction with vitamin B_{12}, to patients with a history of poor nutrition. However, folic acid can be a potentially dangerous drug when used to treat pernicious anemia, because it reverses the anemia and the gastrointestinal tract disorders, but it does *not* reverse the neurologic manifestations and may even intensify them.

Some physicians state that folic acid is *contraindicated* in the treatment of pernicious anemia; others point out that folic acid can probably be used safely if given in small doses.

In addition to medicinal therapy, a number of *supportive measures* may help to sustain the patient through the acute phase of his illness.

Blood transfusions. Generally blood transfusions are not necessary because patients with pernicious anemia respond quickly and favorably to vitamin B_{12} injections. Occasionally, however, a patient may suffer from anemia so severe that he is in danger of developing circulatory collapse and shock. In these extreme cases, blood transfusions may be lifesaving.

Nutritious diet. Encourage patients with pernicious anemia to eat foods high in iron, protein, and vitamins, e.g., fish, meat, milk, and eggs. Instruct the patient who has dyspepsia or a sore mouth to avoid foods which are either coarse, highly seasoned, or difficult to digest. If the patient's appetite is poor because of severe glossitis, administer oral hygiene both before and after meals to cleanse his mouth and ease discomfort.

Bed rest. If the patient has severe anemia, he is usually kept on bed rest until the acute phase of his illness is over and his blood picture improves. If progress is satisfactory the patient usually begins to ambulate within two to three weeks following the beginning of vitamin B_{12} therapy.

While the patient is on bed rest he needs special care because of the neurologic and mental disturbances associated with his illness. The individual who is confused or disoriented will need *side rails* on his bed to prevent falls; if the patient is extremely restless or delusional, a *Posey restraint* may be necessary. To prevent contractures, joint stiffness, muscle atrophy, and other complications of bed rest, do complete *range of motion exercises* with the patient at least three times daily. Footdrop can be prevented by using a *bedcradle* or *footboard* to lift the weight of bedclothes off the patient's feet. *Physical therapy* is usually ordered for persons with severe neurologic damage to prevent flaccid and spastic paralysis.

Once the patient begins to ambulate, protect him from falls, especially at night.

Patients with pernicious anemia often have great difficulty walking in the dark; instruct the hospitalized patient to ring for help should he need to get up at night for any reason.

Protection from burns. When applying hot compresses, hot water bottles, or heating pads, watch the patient carefully for reddening of the skin. Remember that persons with pernicious anemia have reduced sensitivity to sensations of heat and pain.

Maintenance therapy. Once the acute stage of the illness is past, the patient with pernicious anemia must enter a *lifelong program of maintenance therapy* with vitamin B_{12}. The nurse plays a vital role in educating patients with this disorder concerning the importance of continuous care. The typical *maintenance schedule* is as follows:

> *Cyanocobalamin* 200 μg. I.M. monthly or 100 μg. I.M. every 2 weeks. If the patient can be trusted to take his medications, the doctor may order *oral* vitamin B_{12} in doses of 500 to 1000 μg. daily.

In addition to lifelong drug therapy, patients with permanent neurologic disabilities need an intensive program of physical therapy and rehabilitation. All patients should be encouraged to see their doctors at least twice a year for a complete physical examination.

Prognosis. If therapy is adequate and uninterrupted, the patient can expect to feel free of the symptoms of anemia for the rest of his life; also he can be assured that the neuropathy will not progress further. However, should the patient fail to take vitamin B_{12} as ordered, symptoms of anemia will return and the neuropathy will worsen within two months to three years following interruption of therapy.

OTHER ANEMIAS DUE TO VITAMIN B_{12} DEFICIENCY. While pernicious anemia arises from lack of the intrinsic factor, another group of anemias results from *lack* of the *extrinsic factor* (vitamin B_{12}). Deficiency of the extrinsic factor may be caused by: faulty diet, defective absorption due to intestinal disease, or metabolic disturbances. Although the megaloblastic anemia which develops in these conditions is the same as that seen in pernicious anemia, hypochlorhydria and degenerative neurologic changes *do not occur.* Treatment of vitamin B_{12} deficiency depends upon the specific cause.

An *inadequate dietary intake* of vitamin B_{12} can be corrected by the oral administration of 25 μg. of the vitamin daily in conjunction with a more balanced diet. Diets deficient in vitamin B_{12} are rarely seen in the United States except among the very poor who cannot afford meat and among strict vegetarians; however, they are common in India and other underdeveloped countries of the world.

Poor absorption of vitamin B_{12} results from: (1) an overgrowth of bacteria within the intestinal tract due to intestinal stasis, (2) infestation with the fish tapeworm, or (3) one of the malabsorption syndromes. Bacteria, which proliferate within intestinal blind loops and diverticuli (small blind pouches which form in the walls of the colon), cause anemia by competing with the host for available vitamin B_{12}. This problem can be corrected by surgical removal of the pouches or blind loops and by administration of broad-spectrum antibiotics to control infection. The fish tapeworm, which is ingested in raw fish, also competes with its host for vitamin B_{12}. Treatment involves removal of the tapeworm and the temporary administration of vitamin B_{12} until the anemia is corrected.

To treat the anemia caused by malabsorption syndromes (e.g., sprue and celiac disease), the patient is given 100 μg. of vitamin B_{12} I.M. daily for 10 days, followed by 100 μg. of vitamin B_{12} monthly until the absorption dysfunction is corrected.

Supplemental vitamin B_{12} is given orally to individuals who have an increased need for the vitamin due to metabolic disturbances, e.g., pregnancy, hyperthyroidism, and so forth.

ANEMIA DUE TO FOLIC ACID DEFICIENCY

Etiology. Anemia associated with folic acid deficiency is very common. This condition has many causes, the majority of which are identical to the causes of vitamin B_{12} deficiency. Usually folic acid deficiency results from a *poor diet* lacking in such foods as green leafy vegetables, liver, citrus fruits, and yeast. *Chronic alcoholics,* because of their typically inadequate diets, are particularly susceptible to this problem; also, high levels of alcohol in the blood partially block the response of the bone marrow to folic acid, thereby interfering with erythropoiesis. Second, folic acid deficiency, like vitamin B_{12} deficiency, can develop in conjunction with *malabsorption syndromes* (e.g., sprue, celiac disease, steatorrhea, etc.). Also, certain drugs can impede folic acid absorption and utilization. For example, a serious anemia may develop in conjunction with the long-term use of anticonvulsant drugs (e.g., primidone, diphenylhydantoin, and phenobarbital); the administration of antimetabolites (e.g., folic acid antagonists, purine analogs, and pyrimidine analogs) to patients with cancer and leukemia; and the administration of certain oral contraceptives. Finally, folic acid deficiency is extremely common in women during the *third trimester of pregnancy;* at this time, expectant mothers have a six times greater than normal need for folic acid.

Bases of symptoms. Folic acid, like vitamin B_{12}, is necessary for the synthesis of DNA. Both vitamin B_{12} and folic acid deficiencies cause symptoms of megaloblastic anemia (fatigue, cardiac symptoms, slight jaundice) and gastrointestinal tract disturbances (dyspepsia, smooth beefy tongue, etc.); however, *unlike* pernicious anemia, a lack of folic acid does *not* cause neurologic manifestations.

Anemia due to folic acid deficiency has a slow and insidious onset. The patient usually appears quite ill and is often thin and emaciated. Because of the patient's malnourished, debilitated state, symptoms of folic acid deficiency (fatigue, weakness, dyspnea, etc.) are often obscured by other disorders. For example, the patient may suffer from deficiencies of iron, protein, minerals, and all the vitamins; also he may be in electrolyte imbalance. Some individuals additionally have neurologic symptoms owing to thiamine, calcium, or magnesium deficiencies; these problems are frequently linked with alcoholism. Cirrhosis of the liver and bleeding varices may further complicate the anemia.

Diagnostic tests. The megaloblastic anemia caused by folic acid deficiency is identical to that seen in pernicious anemia; it is diagnosed on the basis of blood film and bone marrow examination. Once the presence of a macrocytic anemia is confirmed, the physician must next decide whether the anemia is the result of folic acid or vitamin B_{12} deficiency. If folic acid deficiency is the cause: (1) the serum folate level is less than 4 nanograms (normal is 7 to 20 nanograms); (2) the Schilling test is normal; (3) hydrochloric acid is probably present in the gastric juice; (4) neurologic symptoms are absent; and (5) the patient responds favorably to a therapeutic trial of 50 to 100 μg. of folic acid I.M. daily for 10 days.

Clinical care. To treat anemia due to folate deficiency, the patient is given oral doses of folic acid (0.1 to 5 mg.) daily until his blood picture improves or until the cause of intestinal malabsorption is corrected. Patients with malabsorption syndromes may need parenteral folic acid initially, followed by maintenance therapy with oral doses.

Vitamin C is sometimes prescribed in addition to folic acid because it augments the role of folic acid in promoting erythropoiesis.

Anemia of Bone Marrow Failure

General Considerations. The anemia of bone marrow failure has several names, each of which is descriptive of some aspect of the disease, i.e., aplastic, hypoplastic, aregenerative, or primary refractory anemia. *Aplastic anemia* is the term most commonly used. The word "aplastic" means "having deficient or arrested development." Thus, aplastic anemia is a deficiency of circulating erythrocytes owing to the arrested development of red cells within the bone marrow.

Although aplastic anemia sometimes occurs alone (pure RBC aplasia), it is usually accompanied by *agranulocytosis* (a reduction in leukocytes, particularly granulocytes), and *thrombocytopenia* (reduction in thrombocytes or platelets). These three problems occur together because the bone marrow produces not only erythrocytes but leukocytes and thrombocytes as well. Consequently, if the bone marrow is abnormal for any reason or if it has suffered exposure to a myelotoxin (any substance which is toxic and damaging to bone marrow), production of erythrocytes, leukocytes, and thrombocytes slows greatly, and a deficiency of all three types of cells develops; this condition is called *pancytopenia* (i.e., depression of all cellular blood elements). Pancytopenia affects people of all ages; both sexes are equally susceptible. The incidence of aplastic anemia is approximately four cases per million population.

Etiology. In approximately one half of patients the etiology of aplastic anemia is *unknown;* the cause may possibly be associated with chromosomal aberrations or tumors of the thymus gland (thymomas). In the other 50 per cent, aplastic anemia or pancytopenia is clearly the result of exposure to a specific myelotoxin.

There are three groups of myelotoxins: (1) agents that *always* cause marrow damage when given in sufficiently large doses; e.g., radiant energy (x-rays, radium, radioactive isotopes of gold, phosphorus, etc.); benzene and benzene derivatives; and the alkylating agents and antimetabolites used to treat malignant tumors; (2) agents that are *occasionally* responsible for marrow failure; chloromycetin (the drug most commonly linked with aplastic anemia), sulfonamides, quinacrine, phenylbutazone, the anticonvulsants diphenylhydantoin and mephenytoin, and the gold compounds; and (3) suspicious agents that have been linked with aplastic anemia in *only a few cases,* e.g., streptomycin, tripelennamine, DDT, meprobamate, hair and aniline dyes, and carbon tetrachloride.

Why do the above agents cause the bone marrow to stop producing blood cells? Radiant energy inhibits mitosis or cell division. The antimetabolites employed in cancer chemotherapy block the synthesis of purines or nucleic acids. However, in the majority of cases, the exact mechanism by which the above agents cause marrow failure is unknown. Also, it is not known why certain drugs and chemicals cause a pancytopenia in some persons and not in others. To date, the most plausible reason is that some individuals are hypersensitive to certain drugs; consequently, the development of marrow failure in these cases is an *idiosyncratic reaction.*

Symptoms and Laboratory Picture. The onset of aplastic anemia may be insidious or rapid. In idiopathic or hereditary cases, the onset is usually gradual. However, when bone failure is the result of a myelotoxin, the onset may be explosive and the patient may quickly develop distressing symptoms.

The manifestations of pancytopenia are particularly severe because not only is the erythrocyte count reduced, but the leukocyte and platelet counts are lowered as well. Consequently the patient develops the following three conditions:

1. *Normocytic anemia.* The *erythrocyte count* is usually below 1 million/cu. mm. and the *reticulocyte count* is also low. The patient complains of progressive fatigue, lassitude, and dyspnea.
2. *Granulocytopenia.* The leukocyte count may be less than 2000/cu. mm. (normal is 6000 to 9000/cu. mm.). The patient suffers from an increased susceptibility to infection because, without leukocytes, his body cannot adequately battle bacteria and other invading organisms. (See Chapter 22.) If the leukocyte count drops below 1000 cells per cu. mm., the patient becomes vulnerable to severe fulminating bacterial infections.
3. *Thrombocytopenia.* The platelet count may fall to less than 30,000/cu. mm. (normal is 200,000 to 350,000/cu. mm.). Reduced thrombocyte levels usually cause bleeding into the skin and mucous membranes; if thrombocytes are severely reduced, the patient will hemorrhage.

The diagnosis of aplastic anemia and pancytopenia is based on the *hemogram* (which is "a graphic representation of the differential blood count"),[42] the patient's symptoms, a history of exposure to a myelotoxin, and a bone marrow examination. In pancytopenia, the bone marrow is fatty and it contains very few developing blood cells.

Clinical Care. The patient with pancytopenia is often critically ill; he needs prompt medical attention and skillful nursing care. The first step in halting the process of aplastic anemia is *immediate withdrawal of the offending agent or drug.* Any patient who is either undergoing radiotherapy or who is receiving a drug which is a suspected myelotoxin must be protected from marrow failure by frequent hemograms. The signal for withdrawal of the drug in question is a significant drop in the erythrocyte, leukocyte, or platelet count. Usually prompt termination of a suspicious agent is followed by a rise in the blood count. Unfortunately, in the case of chloromycetin, marrow failure may progress despite discontinuation of the antibiotic.

If aplastic anemia does develop, *blood transfusions* are the mainstay of therapy. However, transfusions are discontinued as soon as the bone marrow begins to produce blood cells. Repeated transfusions can result in hemosiderosis (an increase in tissue iron stores) and an enlarged spleen. *Corticosteroids* and *androgens* are sometimes prescribed on a trial basis to help to stimulate bone marrow function. Unfortunately, in a large number of cases, these drugs fail to restore bone marrow activity.

Splenectomy is considered when the patient has an enlarged spleen which is either destroying normal cells, or suppressing the development of blood cells within the bone marrow. However, for patients with decreased leukocyte and platelet counts, splenectomy is a dangerous operation because of the risk of infection and hemorrhage.

The prevention and treatment of *complications* resulting from pancytopenia is the final important aspect of therapy. The two major complications of this condition are *infections* (respiratory, urinary, etc.) and *bleeding*. The prevention of infection is largely a nursing responsibility. Patients must be isolated from other patients and from personnel with infections of any type. If the patient's white count drops below 1000 per cu. mm., strict reverse isolation is necessary.* To build resistance against infection, encourage the patient to eat foods high in vitamins and protein. If he has a sore mouth, administer oral hygiene before and after meals. Observe the patient carefully for signs that an infectious process is beginning, e.g., a rise in temperature, the "sniffles," a sore throat, severe anorexia, the appearance of ulcerations on mucous membranes, pain and burning upon urination, etc. When an infection develops the physician determines the causative organism and orders a specific antibiotic. Antibiotics are rarely administered prophylactically to patients with pancytopenia because such a practice encourages the development of drug-resistant organisms.

To control *bleeding* (which results from thrombocytopenia) corticosteroids are occasionally given to increase capillary resistance; also, the physician may order the administration of platelet-rich transfusions. Nursing measures and precautions which help to prevent episodes of bleeding are as follows:

> Caution the patient not to pick at his nose; advise him to use a soft toothbrush when cleaning his teeth, and an electric razor for shaving.

> Obtain orders for the *oral* administration of medications whenever possible; if you must administer a medication by injection, use an alcohol sponge to exert mild pressure over the injection site until bleeding has *stopped completely*.

> Carefully record the patient's bowel movements at the first sign of constipation and obtain an order for a stool softener or laxative if necessary. Hard stools or straining at stool can damage the rectal mucosa, thereby causing bleeding.

Prognosis. Over 50 per cent of patients with severe pancytopenia die, usually either from hemorrhage or from overwhelming infection. Death usually occurs within a few months following the onset of the anemia. Of the 40 to 50 per cent who survive, approximately 25 per cent die by the end of the third year following development of the condition; the other 25 per cent of patients either recover completely or remain semi-invalids for years. The prognosis for this condition is best when the myelotoxic agent is identified and discontinued *early* in the course of the disease.

*Reverse isolation procedures are considered in the discussion of leukemia. (See Chapter 62.)

ANEMIAS RESULTING FROM EXCESSIVE ERYTHROCYTE DESTRUCTION (HEMOLYTIC ANEMIAS)

General Considerations

As you recall, aged, dead, and defective cells are removed from the circulation by reticuloendothelial cells (located mainly within the liver, spleen and bone marrow). Normally erythrocytes survive in the circulation for approximately 120 days before removal. However, in hemolytic anemia, the rate of erythrocyte destruction is greatly accelerated. Thus, the three major hallmarks of hemolytic anemia are: (1) a shortening of the erythrocyte life span, (2) an abnormal increase in the numbers of erythrocytes destroyed by reticuloendothelial elements, and (3) failure of the bone marrow to produce sufficient erythrocytes to compensate for the vast numbers of red cells lost.

What are the causes of hemolytic anemia? Hemolysis of erythrocytes is the result of either: (1) an *intracorpuscular defect* within the erythrocyte itself, which is sometimes triggered by an extracellular factor (e.g., drugs, plasma components, or splenic hyperactivity), or (2) an *extracorpuscular factor* (a factor or mechanism *external* to the erythrocyte, e.g., infections, chemical, or physical agents).

Symptoms and Laboratory Findings

Hemolytic anemia may be acute or chronic; there are also chronic forms of hemolytic anemia punctuated by severe acute episodes of hemolysis called *hemolytic crises*.

The patient with hemolytic anemia suffers from all the general manifestations of *anemia* discussed earlier, i.e., lassitude, fatigue, and so forth. In addition, hemolytic anemia is characterized by symptoms listed and explained on the following page. In addition, some patients experience hemolytic crises. These are, in some cases, precipitated by the development of an acute infection. The major symptoms of hemolytic crisis are malaise, chills, fever, aches and pains in the abdomen or back, and red or black urine. The major complication of an acute hemolytic crisis is *acute renal failure* resulting from ischemic necrosis of renal tubules.

Laboratory findings diagnostic of hemolytic anemia usually include: normocytic anemia, reticulocytosis due to increased efforts of the bone marrow to compensate for excessive erythrocyte destruction, increased red cell fragility, shortened erythrocyte life span, hyperbilirubinemia, increased fecal and urinary urobilinogen, and hemoglobinemia in cases of massive intravascular hemolysis.

Clinical Care

The *treatment* of hemolytic anemia includes the following basic clinical steps:

> Pinpoint and *eliminate,* whenever possible, *causative factors* that precipitate episodes of hemolysis, e.g., infections, exposure to certain chemicals.

> Maintain *fluid and electrolyte balance.* Administer intravenous infusions as ordered, carefully check and record patient's intake and output.

> Maintain *renal function.* In cases of severe hemolysis, infusions of either sodium bicarbonate or sodium lactate are administered to alkalize the urine.

> *Combat anemia* and *shock* with the cautious administration of blood transfusions. Caution is necessary because the transfused cells will be rapidly destroyed if the patient has an autoimmune hemolytic disease. (See page 748.) If an autoimmune mechanism is responsible for hemolysis of cells, the patient is treated with steroids. When corticosteroids fail to halt hemolytic reactions in autoimmune disorders, splenectomy is usually the treatment of choice.

Hemolytic Anemias Due Mainly to Intracorpuscular Defects

Glucose-6-Phosphate Dehydrogenase (G6PD) Deficiency. G6PD is an important red cell enzyme; consequently G6PD deficiency can be defined as an *enzymopathy,* a *genetic defect* that involves the partial or complete deficiency of certain essential enzymes. The specific detrimental effect of G6PD deficiency upon erythrocytes is to make them more susceptible to hemolysis following ingestion of those drugs and foods classified as *chemical oxidants.*

An inherited sex-linked disorder, G6PD deficiency is a common problem, affecting at least 100 million persons in the world. Among Americans, G6PD deficiency affects about 10 per cent of American blacks and about 1.5 per cent of American Caucasians. It is also fairly common among people who live close to the Mediterranean, e.g., Greeks, Italians, Arabs. Individuals with this enzymopathy may remain completely asymptomatic throughout their lives since, typically, symptoms develop only following exposure to certain agents. Occasionally, however, Caucasians develop spontaneous attacks of hemolytic anemia which have not been precipitated by a known external factor.

G6PD deficiency causes hemolysis of red cells because erythrocytes require glucose for energy; the enzyme G6PD is responsible for approximately 10 per cent of the glucose metabolized by erythrocytes. When red cells are exposed to oxidative drugs and foods, the amount of glucose that the red cell must metabolize is greatly increased above normal. If a G6PD deficiency exists, the red cells are unable to adequately metabolize glucose and, consequently, they cannot cope with the oxidative effects of certain substances. As a result, hemolysis occurs. Because young, newly released erythrocytes contain a substantial amount of G6PD, only aging erythrocytes are destroyed upon exposure to causative agents.

Numerous oxidative drugs and foods produce hemolytic anemia in persons with G6PD deficiency, e.g., primaquine, quinine, aspirin, sulfonamides, phenacetin, vitamin K derivatives, chloramphenicol (Chloromycetin), the thiazide diuretics, and the fava bean.

Following exposure to any of the above agents, the individual with G6PD deficiency develops *acute intravascular hemolysis* lasting about 7 to 12 days. During this acute phase, the patient suffers from anemia and jaundice. Laboratory findings include moderate hemoglobinemia and hemoglobinuria, an elevated serum bilirubin, reticulocytosis, and the appearance of Heinz bodies (small particles of oxidized hemoglobin) within the red cell.

Symptoms of Hemolytic Anemia

Symptoms	*Bases of Symptoms*
Jaundice (yellowness of the skin and eyes)	Abnormally large amounts of bilirubin accumulate within the blood due to excessive destruction of erythrocytes
Splenomegaly, hepatomegaly, and hyperplasia of bone marrow	Reticuloendothelial elements within the spleen, liver, and bone marrow become hyperactive because of the increased demands upon them to phagocytize defective erythrocytes
Cholelithiasis (pigment gallstones)	Excessive accumulation of bilirubin due to destruction of erythrocytes leads to development of pigment stones within the gallbladder

Following the acute hemolytic stage, the patient's blood picture *automatically* begins to improve whether or not the offending drug is discontinued. The hemolytic reaction of persons with G6PD deficiency is self-limiting because, as mentioned, only *older* erythrocytes are destroyed when in contact with a chemical oxidant. However, if drug exposure continues for long, the patient will develop chronic hyperhemolysis until contact with the offending agent is finally terminated.

Treatment of this condition involves the identification and total removal of the drug or food precipitating the hemolytic reaction. Care of the patient during the week of acute hemolysis is purely symptomatic, i.e., rest, fluids, nutritious diet, and so forth.

Because drugs that precipitate hemolytic reactions in G6PD deficiency are common (e.g., aspirin, phenacetin), and because G6PD has a high worldwide incidence, screening tests for this enzymopathy should be a part of every public health program. Careful screening is particularly important for the black population. Tests must be performed when the patient is well or results are unreliable. It is important that persons be screened for G6PD deficiency before donating blood, because the administration of cells deficient in G6PD can be hazardous for the recipient.

Hereditary Spherocytosis (Congenital Hemolytic Jaundice, Congenital Spherocytic Anemia)

GENERAL CONSIDERATIONS. Hereditary spherocytosis is a common form of chronic hemolytic anemia found in all races and all ages. This condition is *inherited* as a simple mendelian dominant trait. Because the trait is *dominant,* a child can inherit hereditary spherocytosis if only one parent carries the abnormal gene.

The two most distinctive characteristics of hereditary spherocytosis are the appearance of large numbers of *spherical-shaped erythrocytes* ("spherocytosis"), and an *enlarged spleen. Spherocytosis* develops because the erythrocytes have a defective cellular membrane, extremely permeable to the influx of sodium ions. In order to curtail the flow of sodium ions through its defective membrane, the erythrocyte must increase its metabolic work and, consequently, its expenditure of glucose. Eventually glucose and cellular energy become depleted and sodium ions flow through the cellular membrane without resistance. Thus, the red cell interior becomes *hypertonic.* Intracellular hypertonicity, in turn, draws water to the cell, causing the erythrocyte to swell and become spherical in shape. Because spherocytes are thick and relatively inflexible, they are easily trapped within the splenic venous sinusoids, where they are devoured by phagocytes. As a result, the *spleen* becomes *greatly enlarged* owing to overwork, and the patient suffers from *anemia* and *jaundice* as a result of the massive hemolysis of red cells within the spleen.

SYMPTOMS AND LABORATORY FINDINGS. The symptoms of hereditary spherocytosis are the same as the general symptoms of hemolytic anemia discussed earlier, e.g., malaise, anemia, jaundice, gallstones, and splenomegaly. Splenomegaly is more pronounced in this condition than in any other form of hemolytic anemia. Because of the massive size of the spleen, patients with hereditary spherocytosis experience left upper quadrant fullness and abdominal pain. Occasionally *acute* abdominal pain develops as a result of splenic infarction. Persons with this disorder suffer from severe hemolytic crises, which are sometimes fatal.

Laboratory findings are distinctive and include: (1) spherocytes in the blood smear, (2) reticulocytosis, (3) lowered red cell count and hemoglobin values, and (4) increased osmotic fragility. Osmotic fragility is increased because the spherocyte has a smaller surface area than the normal biconcave erythrocyte and a larger cell content than normal because of the excessive inflow of water and sodium into the cell. As a result of these two factors, spherocytes rupture quickly when placed in hypotonic saline solutions because they cannot tolerate a further influx of water.

CLINICAL CARE. Although the administration of blood transfusions may benefit the patient in hemolytic crisis, the only treatment indicated in all cases of hereditary spherocytosis is splenectomy. Ninety per cent of patients who undergo splenectomy experience complete reversal of symptoms. Although spherocytes continue to circulate, these misshaped cells usually have a normal life span once the spleen is removed.

Hemolytic Anemias Due Mainly to Extracorpuscular Factors (Acquired Hemolytic Anemias)

The major extracorpuscular factors that can result in hemolytic anemia include: trauma, chemical agents and drugs, infectious agents, systemic diseases, isoimmune reactions, and autoimmune disorders.

Hemolysis Due to Trauma. Hemolytic anemia may develop swiftly following severe *burns.* Clinical findings include a large drop in the erythrocyte count, hemoglobinemia, and hemoglobinuria. Also, hemolysis of red cells sometimes occurs following replacement of defective heart valves with prosthetic valves or the repair of cardiac septal defects. Trauma to erythrocytes caused by either burns or surgery causes the cells to fragment. Fragmented erythrocytes (schistocytes) are quickly destroyed by phagocytes.

Hemolysis Due to Chemical Agents and Drugs (Toxic Hemolytic Anemia). Many drugs and chemicals can cause hemolysis of red cells. Chemical and drug reactions are generally due to one of the following factors: the *oxidant effects* of the drug or chemical, or an *immune reaction* precipitated by the drug.

Chemical oxidants vary greatly in their potency and consequently in their ability to destroy erythrocytes. Some chemical oxidants are relatively mild and cause hemolytic reactions in only a small segment of the world population (for example, persons with G6PD deficiency). Other chemical oxidants are so toxic that they cause hemolytic reactions in every person exposed to a sufficient dose of the substance, e.g., benzene, phenylhydrazine, nitrites, potassium chlorate, arsenic, colloidal silver, and lead. These powerful compounds are capable of damaging the red cell membrane. As a result, the cell becomes more fragile and is quickly destroyed.

One of the most common examples of hemolysis due to contact with a chemical agent is *lead poisoning (plumbism)*. Lead poisoning causes characteristic changes in the brain, nervous system, spinal cord, and digestive tract. Industrial workers who are daily exposed to lead vapors, mist, or dust may become victims of plumbism. Also, small children with *pica* (an abnormal desire to ingest substances that are not safe or fit to eat) develop lead poisoning when allowed to chew on furniture covered with lead-based paint. The symptoms of plumbism are illustrated in Figure 61–2. Treatment of this condition involves administering mild saline cathartics in order to promote the elimination of lead salts from the intestinal tract, followed by the giving of a chelating agent such as calcium disodium edetate.

An *immune* response, the second major cause of toxic hemolysis, is the result of an antigen-antibody

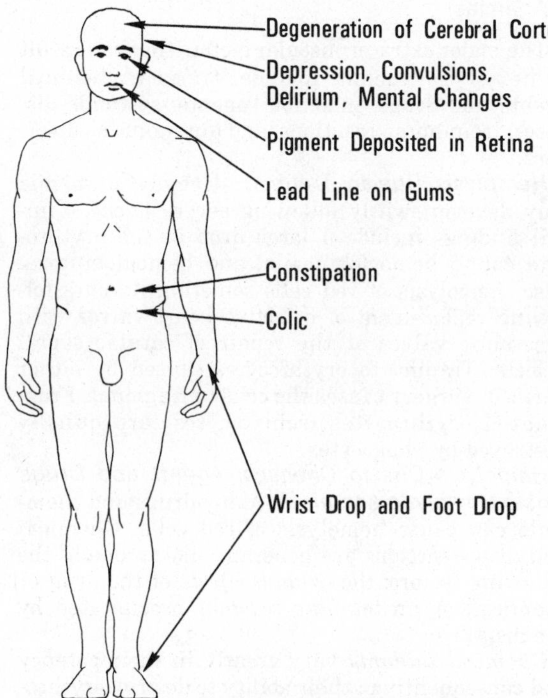

FIGURE 61–2. How lead poisoning affects man. (From Snively, W. D., Jr., and Beshar, D. R.: *Textbook of Pathophysiology.* Philadelphia, J. B. Lippincott Company, 1972.)

reaction. (See Chapter 23.) Drugs that can precipitate antigen-antibody reactions in susceptible individuals are quinine, quinidine, methyldopa, sulfonamides, phenacetin, and penicillin. The most common example of an immune response to a drug is the "penicillin reaction." Penicillin is a potentially dangerous drug because it is a hapten. As you recall from Chapter 23, a *hapten* is a substance that is normally nonantigenic but which has the capacity to combine with a body protein. When this combination takes place, the body protein is modified in such a way that it can act as a foreign antigen. As a result, the body builds antibodies that react with the altered body protein in an antigen-antibody reaction.

Finally, certain snake and spider venoms as well as some vegetable poisons (e.g., some mushrooms) cause hemolytic reactions that are frequently fatal.

Hemolysis Due to Infectious Organisms. Hemolytic anemia may develop as a complication of several different conditions caused by microorganisms, e.g., bacterial endocarditis, malaria, miliary tuberculosis, infectious hepatitis, infectious mononucleosis, and meningococcemia.

Infectious organisms can cause hemolytic anemia in three ways: by releasing toxins that act as hemolyzers, by entering the red cell and destroying it, and by promoting antigen-antibody reactions. For example, the organism may attach itself to the surface of the cell; as a result, the cell surface becomes so altered that it acts as a foreign antigen. In response to the altered red cell, antibodies form and an immune reaction takes place.

Hemolytic Anemia Secondary to Systemic Diseases. Hemolytic anemia sometimes complicates the following systemic conditions: Hodgkin's disease, leukemias, renal cortical necrosis, lymphomas, and systemic lupus erythematosus.

Hemolysis Due to Isoimmune Hemolytic Reactions. An isoimmune hemolytic reaction is an antigen-antibody reaction in which erythrocytes are destroyed by antibodies that have developed in response to antigens from another individual of the same species. One example of an isoimmune hemolytic reaction is the *transfusion reaction.* As you recall, the most severe transfusion reactions involve the hemolysis of the *donor* red cells by antibodies within the blood of the recipient.

Erythroblastosis fetalis, a disorder seen in the newborn, provides a second example of a hemolytic isoimmune reaction. This condition is the result of incompatibility between the blood of the fetus and the mother's blood, usually affecting the Rh blood groups. The sequence of events that leads to hemolysis of the baby's erythrocytes begins in utero. The fetus usually has Rh positive blood while the mother has Rh negative blood. When the fetus's Rh positive cells pass through the placenta into the mother's circulation, they are recognized by the mother's body as foreign antigens. As a result, the mother forms antibodies against the red cells of her child; these antibodies pass back through the placenta into the blood stream of the fetus where they rapidly destroy the baby's red cells. The bone marrow of the fetus, in turn, releases vast numbers of *erythroblasts* (very immature erythrocytes) which circulate in place of the erythrocytes that have been destroyed. If there are sufficient circulating erythroblasts and the fetus survives until birth, the treatment of choice is an *exchange* transfusion in which the fetus's Rh positive blood is replaced by Rh negative blood, thereby halting the hemolytic process.*

Hemolysis Due to Autoimmune Disorders. Autoantibodies, like isoantibodies, are capable of destroying red blood cells. Unlike isoantibodies, autoantibodies do not develop against an antigen from *another* individual of the same species; instead they arise in response to autoantigens which have developed within the body of the *individual himself.*

Autoimmune hemolytic anemia is a disorder of the immune mechanism in which the patient's immune system produces antibodies which agglutinate his *own red cells* in an antigen-antibody reaction. As a result, the agglutinated cells clump together and are phagocytized within the spleen.

This condition arises in two ways: First, it may develop *secondary* to other autoimmune disorders or following the administration of certain drugs. Autoimmune conditions sometimes complicated by hemolytic anemia include systemic lupus erythematosus and the lymphoproliferative diseases (leukemia, lymphosarcoma). Drugs that sometimes precipitate autoimmune hemolytic anemia include penicillin (which acts as a hapten), quinidine, quinine, and methyldopa. Second, this disease can develop spontaneously and without a history of prior autoimmune disease; this is known as *idiopathic autoimmune hemolytic anemia.* Possible causes include the emergence of forbidden clones (see Chapter 23), and an inherited capacity to produce more antibodies than the body needs for protection.

The symptoms of autoimmune hemolytic anemia differ little from those of other hemolytic anemias. Profound, sometimes fatal, sporadic *hemolytic crises* are common. Other complications include gallstones and thrombocytopenic purpura.

Autoimmune hemolytic anemia is mainly diagnosed on the basis of a positive Coombs test. As you recall, the Coombs test is a method for detecting whether the patient's red cells are coated with antibodies.

The *treatment* of secondary autoimmune hemolytic anemia includes treatment of the underlying autoimmune condition and termination of the use of any suspicious drugs.

The idiopathic form of the disease is treated with steroids, transfusions, and splenectomy when indicated. The *steroid* of choice is:

> Prednisolone (or its equivalent) 10 to 20 mg. 4 times daily until hemoglobin levels are normal.

Transfusions may give temporary relief from symptoms. However, they do not adequately restore the patient's erythrocyte level because the donor cells are often rapidly destroyed by the patient's antibodies.

Splenectomy is the treatment of choice if steroids fail to produce a remission or if the side effects of steroid therapy are too severe. Once the spleen is removed, recurrences of hemolytic anemia may develop, but they are far less severe than the hemolytic crises prior to surgery. Such minor hemolytic episodes are usually controlled by steroid therapy.

The Paroxysmal Hemoglobinurias. A "paroxysm" is an episode or occurrence of abrupt onset and termination. *Hemoglobinuria* means that hemoglobin is present in the urine. In sum, the term "paroxysmal hemoglobinuria" describes a rare and serious condition in which the patient suffers from acute episodes of intravascular hemolysis which result in the passage of hemoglobin into the urine.

Attacks of paroxysmal hemoglobinuria can be precipitated by: (1) *sleep* (paroxysmal nocturnal hemoglobinuria); (2) exposure to *cold* temperatures (paroxysmal cold hemoglobinuria); and (3) extreme *exertions,* as in marching for long distances (march hemoglobinuria). Because paroxysmal nocturnal hemoglobinuria is the most common of these three conditions, it is discussed in more detail.

PAROXYSMAL NOCTURNAL HEMOGLOBINURIA (PNH). This condition is a rare, severely incapacitating blood dyscrasia which most commonly strikes young men in their twenties. The exact cause of this disease remains a mystery. However, PNH evidently results from an unknown defect within the erythrocyte itself that makes the red cell vulnerable to hemolysis when in contact with components normally found in plasma (e.g., magnesium, properdin, and complement). Extrinsic factors that can precipitate hemolytic episodes include infection, menstruation, and the administration of iron or vaccines.

The anemia produced by PNH is both normocytic and normochromic. Symptoms are similar to those of other hemolytic anemias, e.g., jaundice, chronic fatigue, scleral icterus, splenomegaly. In addition to these manifestations, the patient's urine, following sleep, is often dark brown or the color of port wine because of acute hemolytic episodes. When hemoglobinuria continues for days or weeks, substantial losses of iron eventually result in the development of *iron deficiency anemia.* In severe cases of PNH, *complications* include leukopenia, thrombocytopenia, and thrombosis. Thrombi may develop following a severe hemolytic episode and commonly cause death.

Because PNH cannot as yet be cured, *treatment* is directed toward alleviation of symptoms. The treatment of choice is the administration of red blood cells that have been washed in saline. Whole blood transfusions are usually *not* given, because factors within the donor plasma may precipitate further hemolysis of the patient's erythrocytes. Also, iron salts are given to patients with iron deficiency anemia. Androgens are occasionally administered to promote erythropoiesis.

*More sophisticated techniques are being developed for the treatment of erythroblastosis fetalis. For information, consult a textbook of pediatrics.

Although an individual with this condition may live a normal number of years, the disease is *chronic,* and debilitating attacks of hemolytic anemia may occur throughout life. However, in many cases the patient is able to lead an active normal life between attacks.

ANEMIAS RESULTING FROM BOTH DISTURBANCES OF ERYTHROCYTE PRODUCTION AND INCREASED ERYTHROCYTE DESTRUCTION

Impaired Hemoglobin Synthesis

The Hemoglobinopathies. As mentioned earlier, each molecule of hemoglobin is composed of four molecules of an iron-porphyrin complex called *heme* and one molecule of a simple protein called *globin.* It is the *globin* portion of hemoglobin that is defective or deficient when hemoglobin synthesis is abnormal. In order to understand anemias due to defective hemoglobin synthesis, we must first review the basic structure of a globin molecule.

Each globin molecule is composed of two pairs of polypeptide chains; one pair of chains is called the "alpha" chain, the other pair, the "beta" chain (Fig. 61–3). Each alpha chain contains 141 amino acid residues, while each beta chain contains 146 amino acid residues, making 574 amino acid residues in all. The number and sequence of amino acids on the alpha chain is regulated by one gene called a "structural" or "regulatory" gene; another gene controls the amino acid sequence on the beta chain. The arrangement of amino acids on each pair of chains does not normally vary from person to person. *Any deviation* in the precise number or sequence of amino acid residues results in a disorder of hemoglobin synthesis.

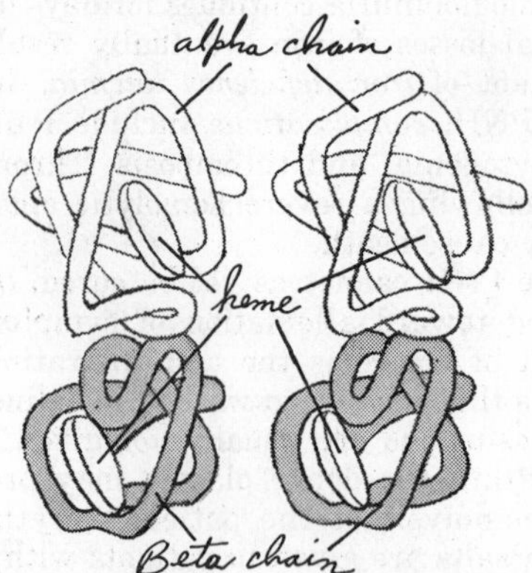

FIGURE 61–3. Structure of the hemoglobin molecule. (From Foster, S.: *American Journal of Nursing, 71*:1952, October, 1971.)

Hemoglobinopathies are a group of conditions characterized by the formation of abnormal hemoglobin. Specifically, they are due to abnormalities of the polypeptide chains forming the globin molecule. In the majority of cases, the beta chains are defective. The abnormalities of alpha or beta chains, resulting in defective hemoglobin, are generally caused by *minute variations* in the sequence of the amino acid residues composing the chains. As one author writes of sickle cell anemia (the most important hemoglobinopathy): "Of the 574 amino acid residues which compose the globin of a hemoglobin molecule, the substitution of only two [amino acid residues] causes 50 per cent of homozygous Hb S (sickle cell hemoglobin) carriers to expire before age 20 and is lethal to most of the remaining sufferers by middle age."[55] Thus, while the difference between normal hemoglobin and abnormal hemoglobin is minute, it is extremely important.

The three major forms of normal hemoglobin are hemoglobin A, hemoglobin A_2, and fetal hemoglobin (hemoglobin F); 97 per cent of the hemoglobin of a normal person is composed of hemoglobin A and 2 to 3 per cent is hemoglobins A_2 and F. *Variants* of hemoglobin A number over 100. They include hemoglobins C, D, E, G, H, I, J, K, L, M, N, O, P, Q, and S. Fortunately the majority of these abnormal hemoglobins are not detrimental to health and do not cause anemia or symptoms of any kind. In the United States the only abnormal hemoglobins that are of consequence are hemoglobin S (sickle cell hemoglobin), hemoglobin C, and hemoglobin D. These forms of abnormal hemoglobins produce a relatively mild disorder in persons who are heterozygous carriers of the trait (those who inherit the gene from only one parent), and profound sometimes fatal anemia in homozygous carriers (those who inherit the gene from both parents).

SICKLE CELL ANEMIA (Hb SS DISEASE) AND SICKLE CELL TRAIT. Sickle cell anemia is a chronic hereditary hemolytic disorder mainly affecting the black populations of the world and characterized by the presence of erythrocytes that mainly contain Hb S instead of Hb A; and that assume a sickle or crescent shape when exposed to lowered oxygen tensions (Fig. 61–4). Once they "sickle," these abnormal cells are easily destroyed by the thousands as they attempt to circulate through the body's smaller vessels.

Sickle cell trait is generally a relatively mild condition that may produce few or no symptoms. It is present in persons who are *heterozygous* for sickle cell hemoglobin.

Incidence and pathogenesis. As shown in Figures 61–5 and 61–6, whether a person will have sickle cell anemia, sickle cell trait, or neither, depends upon the genes for hemoglobin that he has inherited from each of his parents. Persons who are homozygous for Hb S are estimated to have erythrocytes that contain 80 to 100 per cent abnormal Hb S and only up to 20 per cent normal Hb A. The erythrocytes of persons with sickle cell trait contain approximately 25 to 40 per cent Hb S and 60 to 75 per cent Hb A.

Both sickle cell anemia and sickle cell trait are found almost exclusively among black people.

Within the United States alone, between 45,000 and 75,000 blacks have the disease, while 2.5 million blacks probably carry the sickle cell trait. Less than 1 per cent of nonblacks are heterozygous for Hb S and no nonblacks are homozygous. For this reason, one medical editorial points out the following sobering fact:

> The exclusiveness of sickle cell anemia to black persons has been the largest single hindrance to research, diagnosis and therapy. Likewise, the American black's struggle for identity and equality has spotlighted the indifference to sickle cell anemia as one of many social inequalities. Thus, a medical problem is a component of the larger emotional problems of racism, economics and politics.[55]

Sickle cell anemia develops as a result of a genetic mutation that is transmitted from parent to child. The underlying problem causing sickle cell hemoglobin at the molecular level is the substitution of valine for glutamic acid in the sixth place from the end (N-terminus) of each beta chain.

There are many theories to explain the phenomenon of the substitution of two valines for two glutamic acids, which causes the afflicted erythrocytes to assume the characteristic sickle shape. Murayama's theory of hydrophobic bonding is gaining widespread acceptance. In essence, Murayama's theory is that, when exposed to low oxygen tensions, the substituted valine* on each beta chain forms a hydrophobic bond with each alpha chain on an adjacent (second) molecule of Hb S. In turn, the two beta chains on the second adjacent molecule form hydrophobic bonds with the alpha chains on another (third) adjacent molecule of hemoglobin, and so forth. The final result of such bonding is the formation of a pathologic chain that causes the Hb S molecules to stack together and consequently twist the involved erythrocytes into a sickle shape.

*Valine is an amino acid that tends to form strong hydrophobic bonds (strong nonpolar bonds that prevent a molecule from reacting with molecules of water).

The exact mechanisms that precipitate sickling crises or "attacks," which take varying forms in different persons, remain somewhat unclear. However, two major factors are definitely linked with the sickling of cells; these are *hypoxia,* owing to low oxygen tensions, and an *elevated blood viscosity,* owing to an increased concentration of sickled cells.

Hypoxia develops in persons with Hb S whenever they are exposed to low oxygen tensions as a result of climbing to high altitudes, flying in nonpressurized planes, exercising strenuously, or undergoing anesthesia without receiving adequate oxygenation. Although both Hb S and Hb A have the same solubility when oxygenated, *deoxygenation* of the blood drastically affects Hb S. Thus, when normal hemoglobin is deoxygenated, it becomes only half as soluble as when oxygenated, whereas sickle cell hemoglobin becomes 50 times less soluble. According to various investigators, the decreased solubility of Hb S causes it to become more viscous and to crystallize, thereby deforming the shape of the cell. Also, as you recall, Murayama proposes that the forming of hydrophobic bonds upon deoxygenation may cause the characteristic sickling. In any event, the heavy concentration of misshapen cells during a sickling crisis makes the blood abnormally viscous; as a result, the circulation becomes extremely sluggish. If dehydration due to vomiting, diarrhea, excessive sweating, or the ingestion of diuretics is also present, the blood becomes even thicker and the pathologic situation is compounded. Because of the viscous blood, the sickle cells tend to pack together or "log jam" within the smaller blood vessels. As a result of this occlusion of the microcirculation, more severe hypoxia develops which, in turn, causes more

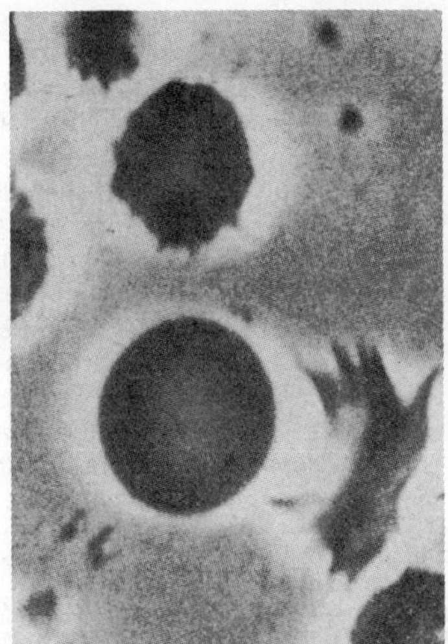
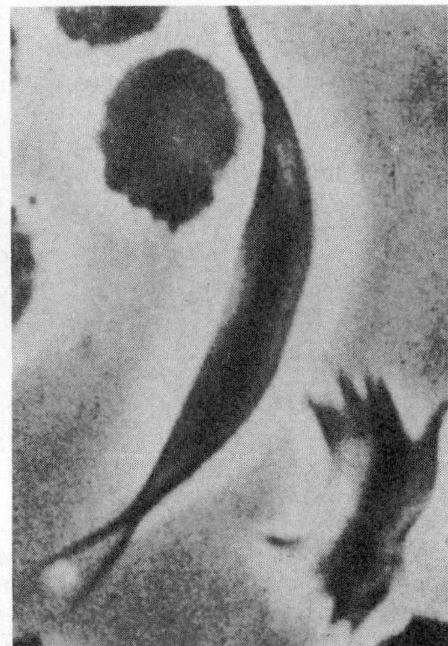

FIGURE 61–4. Comparison of a normal cell (left) and a sickle cell. (From Sickle Cell Anemia. *Medical World News,* p. 38, December 3, 1971.)

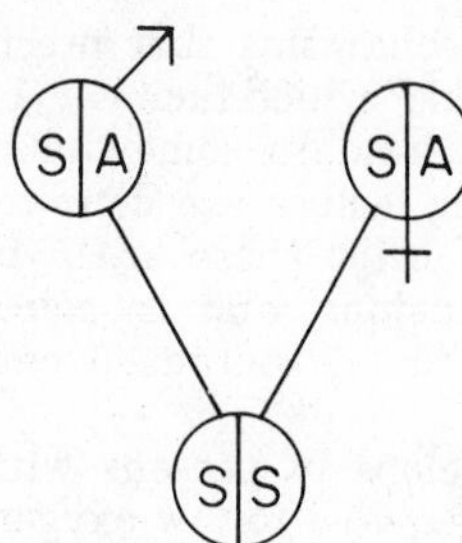

FIGURE 61–5. Inheritance pattern of homozygous sickle cell anemia (SS). (From Jackson, D. E.: *Nursing Clinics of North America* 7:727, December 1972.)

erythrocytes to sickle. A vicious circle thus develops. As the anoxia worsens, thrombosis and infarction develop and the surrounding tissues become necrotic. The organs most vulnerable to infarction and necrosis are the brain and kidneys, because of their constant demand for oxygen, and the bone marrow and spleen, because of their normally sluggish circulation.

Bases of symptoms. Sickle cell anemia usually manifests itself during childhood, but occasionally symptoms do not appear until the patient has reached adulthood. Young children who develop the disease fail to grow properly. They typically have spindly legs, a short trunk, and a tower-shaped skull because of hyperactivity of the bone marrow.

Symptoms, whenever they occur, are due to the following three underlying factors: hemolytic anemia resulting from the destruction of sickle cells; thrombosis and infarction owing to occlusion of the microcirculation by the sickled cells; and an elevated bilirubin owing to the release of hemoglobin, which results in gallstone formation (cholelithiasis). These three problems profoundly affect all the organs and tissues of the body with severe, often fatal consequences. Organs such as the spleen, liver, and penis are affected by the collection of sickled erythrocytes and undergo enlargement and, later, dysfunction. The interference with the circulation affects the brain, the kidneys, the heart, the lungs, and the skin. Leg ulcers are found in about 75 per cent of older children or adults with the disease. The proliferation of the bone marrow leads to osteoporosis and, later, osteosclerosis. These are only a few of the forms that symptoms may take in sickle cell anemia.

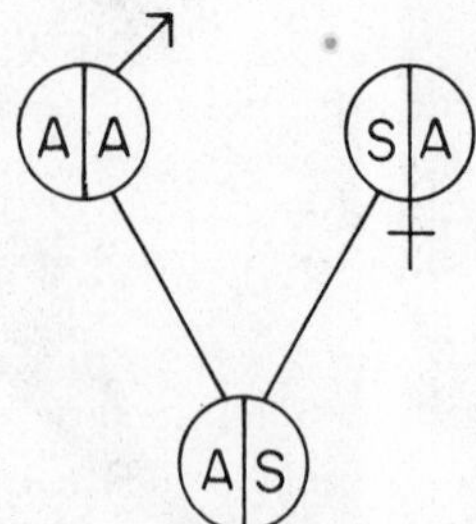

FIGURE 61–6. The inheritance pattern of sickle cell trait. AA represents the pair of genes for normal hemoglobin. SA represents the pair of genes for sickle cell trait. (From Jackson, D. E.: *Nursing Clinics of North America* 7:727, December 1972.)

Cerebral hemorrhage or shock claims the lives of many patients during childhood. However, some individuals manage to survive until they are 50 years of age or older. Death, when it comes, is usually the result of *uremia,* caused by progressive renal damage.

Diagnosing sickle cell anemia and trait. There are currently four laboratory procedures that are used to diagnose the presence of sickle cell hemoglobin in either homozygous or heterozygous carriers:

> *Stained blood smear.* Examination of a stained blood smear for the presence of sickle cells.

> *Sickle cell slide preparation* (sickle prep). Observation of a specimen of blood for the sickling phenomenon following deoxygenation of the blood. This test is accurate, but time-consuming to perform.

> *Sickle-turbidity tube test* (Sickledex). An excellent mass screening test for the detection of sickle cell hemoglobin. The patient's finger is pricked and the blood is mixed with Sickledex solution in a test tube. Five minutes later the specimen is observed for cloudiness. The presence of Hb S causes the Sickledex solution to become turbid, while solutions mixed with normal hemoglobin remain clear. Although this test indicates whether Hb S is present, it does not differentiate between sickle cell disease and the trait.

> *Hemoglobin electrophoresis.* Differentiates between sickle cell anemia and sickle cell trait. By means of an applied electric field, the various types of hemoglobin within a blood specimen are separated. If a blood specimen contains both Hb S and Hb A, the person has sickle cell trait; if only Hb S is present, the person has sickle cell anemia.

Clinical care. The treatment of sickle cell anemia consists chiefly of supportive care, e.g., rest, oxygen, I.V. administration of fluids and electrolytes, sedation, and the prescription of analgesics. In some cases the slow administration of packed red cells or partial exchange transfusions help to relieve severe anemic symptoms. Anticoagulants, steroids, and cobalt treatments have all been tried in the past without success in reversing the sickling process.

Recently a new, somewhat controversial treatment has been developed that seems to strike at the molecular basis of the disease. Urea therapy, which is based on Murayama's theory, is designed to unsickle cells by breaking the hydrophobic bonds which form between the alpha and beta chains of Hb S. The procedure is simple and inexpensive. Urea, which is normally found in the blood and is thus nontoxic to the body, is administered during sickle cell crises through a central venous catheter directly into the superior vena cava. According to advocates of this therapy, urea, once in the vascular system, diffuses into the sickle cells that are clogging the microcirculation, reverses the sickling process, and restores normal circulation by unclogging the afflicted venules, capillaries and arterioles.[21]

However, the intravenous administration of urea has several potential dangers. It causes extreme diuresis and may lead to dehydration. The urea solution may cause sclerosis and thrombophlebitis of the vessel through which the drug is administered. Urea also causes drowsiness, and if sedative analgesics are given as well, respiratory arrest may be produced.

For these reasons the treatment must be considered experimental at present. It is hoped that eventually some method may be developed for giving urea orally as a prophylactic measure to prevent sickle cell crises.

In addition to treating sickle cell crises, one must also treat the complications of sickle cell anemia. *Leg ulcers* are cleansed with warm saline soaks and an enzyme debridement agent (Biozyme, Elase, Panofil or Travase) and are then covered with a sterile dressing. The patient is placed on bed rest and his legs are elevated. A bed cradle is usually ordered to alleviate pressure on the legs. In cases of severe ulceration, skin grafts may be needed to close the wound. *Cholelithiasis* and/or *pathologic fracture* may require surgery. *Cardiac arrhythmias* can be treated by routine methods. Patients with eye disorders are referred to an ophthalmologist.

Educational aspects. Many blacks are totally unaware that they carry the sickle cell trait and that they can transmit this trait to their offspring. For this reason, mass screening tests for the detection of Hb S are being perfected for use among the black population. Persons having only the sickle cell trait may never be detected unless they are exposed to extremely low tensions (e.g., in mountain climbing or flying in a nonpressurized plane), which may cause sickling to occur. However, extremely hard work or exercise, or such stress as pregnancy, may cause the trait to be evidenced through collapse or other effects.

When counseling blacks about sickle cell anemia or sickle cell trait, it is important to include the following points in your discussion:

> Encourage black parents to have not only themselves but their children tested for the presence of Hb S.

> If a person does have sickle cell disease or trait, advise him how to prevent crises.

Warn the patient to avoid high altitudes or flying in unpressurized planes, because oxygen tension is lowered under these conditions. Also, caution the patient to guard against becoming dehydrated. Advise him to call his physician should he develop vomiting, diarrhea, a high fever, or any other cause of water loss.

> Encourage young black people who are carriers of Hb S to ask their physician for genetic counseling before marrying or having children.

> Warn young women with sickle cell anemia that pregnancy carries a very high risk for them; they may develop pulmonary and/or renal complications.

Other Variant Abnormal Hemoglobins. As stated earlier, the only abnormal hemoglobins that produce anemias of consequence within the United States are hemoglobins S, C, and D.

Homozygous hemoglobin C disease (Hb CC disease) is found in one out of every 6000 blacks; 2 to 3 per cent of American blacks carry the hemoglobin C trait. Individuals with Hb CC disease suffer from a fairly severe anemia that is accompanied by manifestations similar to those of sickle cell anemia, with the exception that their erythrocytes do not assume the sickle shape. Persons who carry the trait (i.e., they have A-C hemoglobin) usually remain asymptomatic. Treatment of the disease centers around the alleviation of symptoms; occasionally blood transfusions are required.

S-C hemoglobin disease is more common than Hb CC disease because so many blacks are heterozygous carriers of the sickle cell trait. Manifestations of this condition include sicklemia, anemia, hematuria, retinal hemorrhages, and aseptic necrosis of the femoral head.

Hb S-D disease is uncommon; apparently it affects both blacks and nonblacks. Symptoms are similar to those of sickle cell anemia, but less severe.

The Thalassemias. The thalassemias are a group of inherited chronic hemolytic anemias that predominantly affect persons with Mediterranean or Southern Chinese ancestry and are characterized by the production of extremely thin, fragile erythrocytes called *target cells.* Because the thalassemias were first discovered among people living around the Mediterranean, this group of conditions was named for the sea (*thalassos* meaning "sea"). The group has also been called Mediterranean anemia or Cooley's anemia. The thalassemias also affect American blacks and people from Central Africa and Southern Asia.

The severity of the anemia produced by the thalassemias depends upon whether the afflicted individual is homozygous or heterozygous for the thalassemia trait. *Thalassemia major* and *intermedia,* characterized by a *profound* anemia, appear in homozygotes. *Thalassemia minor* is characterized by a relatively *mild* anemia and develops in heterozygotes.

ETIOLOGY. You recall that hemoglobin is composed of two pairs of polypeptide chains called alpha chains and beta chains. Unlike sickle cell anemia, the polypeptide chains in the thalassemias are completely normal in structure. This group of disorders, instead, is characterized by an *insufficient amount* of polypeptide chains as a result of a genetic defect. Either alpha or beta chains can be affected by diminished synthesis. In *alpha thalassemia,* alpha chain synthesis is slowed; in *beta thalassemia,* beta chain synthesis is retarded.

Beta thalassemia is by far the most common form of the disease. For this reason, beta thalassemia is simply referred to as "thalassemia" or "classic thalassemia."

MANIFESTATIONS. The symptoms of thalassemia major are generally the same as those of other hemolytic anemias, e.g., jaundice, cholelithiasis, leg ulcers, enlarged spleen. However, one distinctive characteristic of thalassemia is a *pronounced bone hyperactivity* which results in thickening of the cranial bones. As a result of cranial bone hyperplasia, persons with this disorder have a *mongoloid* appearance or facies.

Laboratory findings in thalassemia (beta form) include the following:

> *Target cells* (abnormally thin fragile cells) and other bizarrely shaped erythrocytes appear in the circulation.

> The *serum bilirubin* and *fecal* and *urinary urobilinogen* are greatly elevated because of the severe hemolysis of abnormal cells.

> *Fetal* hemoglobin (Hb F) is greatly elevated; in some cases it rises to as high as 90 per cent.

> *Hb* A_2 (a normal variant of Hb A) is also elevated and may rise to as high as 6 per cent instead of the normal 1.5 to 3.0 per cent.

The high percentages of Hb F and Hb A_2 are evidently a result of the decrease in beta chains characteristic of this anemia, which forces the bone marrow to produce abnormally large numbers of *alpha chains, gamma chains* (which are normally made only during fetal life), and *delta chains*. The compensatory increase in fetal hemoglobin results from the combination of alpha and gamma chains, while the increase in Hb A_2 results from the combination of alpha and delta chains.

Thalassemia minor is usually asymptomatic with the exception of a mild anemia. Also, the blood smear of patients with this condition contains small, defective erythrocytes.

CLINICAL CARE. Transfusion therapy is the only treatment available today. Patients with thalassemia major are treated with transfusions of packed red cells which may be administered: (1) on a monthly or bimonthly basis (regular transfusion regimen); (2) whenever the patient's hemoglobin falls below 3–4 Gm./100 ml. (nonsystematic transfusion); or (3) every 15 days in order to maintain the patient's hemoglobin at 12–15 Gm./100 ml. (hypertransfusion regimen). When it becomes evident that transfused cells are being rapidly destroyed by the spleen (causing a severe hemolytic anemia), *splenectomy* is necessary.

Because patients with thalassemia must receive so many transfusions, they are in danger of developing an *iron overload*, which may eventually lead to myocardial hemosiderosis and resulting cardiac arrhythmias. Excessive iron can be removed from the blood to some extent by *chelating agents* such as diethylenetriamine pentaacetic acid (DTPA)—a drug still under investigation.

Thalassemia minor is generally so mild that patients do not require treatment. However, all persons who carry the thalassemia trait need genetic counseling.

PROGNOSIS. The outlook for patients with thalassemia major is usually poor. Children are retarded in their growth and development and many fail to live past puberty. Thalassemia minor, on the other hand, does not affect life expectancy.

Secondary Anemias

The secondary anemias, as the name implies, arise in association with other conditions such as chronic systemic diseases, (e.g., rheumatoid arthritis, malnutrition, leukemia, the lymphomas, multiple myeloma); chronic infections (lung abscess, empyema, pelvic inflammatory disease); acute and chronic renal disease complicated by uremia; cirrhosis of the liver; endocrine disorders (myxedema); and cancer.

The anemia accompanying cancer results from one of the following three factors: chronic blood loss, hemolysis of cells, or the development of space-occupying lesions within the bone marrow (myelophthisic anemia).

While the etiology of the secondary anemias varies with the underlying condition, all these anemias have two factors in common: the erythrocytes have a shortened life span, and the bone marrow, although functioning normally, is unable to produce enough red cells to compensate for erythrocyte losses. For this reason, the secondary anemias are also called "the anemias of *relative bone marrow failure.*"

The anemia which develops in these conditions may be moderate to severe, depending upon the underlying cause. *Treatment* involves correction of the underlying condition. Blood transfusions are sometimes given to patients with hemoglobin levels below 8–9 Gm./100 ml.

THE POLYCYTHEMIAS

Polycythemia is defined as an increase in both the *number* of circulating *erythrocytes* and the *concentration* of *hemoglobin* within the blood. In this condition, red blood cells may number as high as 8 to 12 million per cu. mm., and the hemoglobin concentration may rise to 8 to 25 Gm./100 ml. The three forms of polycythemia (polycythemia vera, secondary polycythemia, and relative polycythemia) are considered below.

Polycythemia Vera. Polycythemia vera is classified as a *myeloproliferative disorder* (meaning "overgrowth of bone marrow"). It usually develops in middle age and is particularly common among Jewish men.

Although the precise etiology of this disease remains unknown, it is believed to be a form of malignancy analogous to leukemia. The three major hallmarks of this condition are: (1) the relentless, unrestrained production of massive numbers of erythrocytes; (2) the production of excessive myelocytes (leukocytes within the bone marrow); and (3) an overproduction of thrombocytes. The overproduction of all three of these cell lines results in the following three pathologic consequences: an increase in the *viscosity* of the blood; an increase in the total *volume* of blood, which may be twice or even three times greater than normal; and severe *congestion* of all tissues and organs with blood. Because of these three problems the patient suffers from numerous symptoms. The most important symptoms of polycythemia vera and their causation are listed at the bottom of the page.

Thrombotic complications claim the lives of around 30 per cent of patients; another 10 to 15 per cent die from *hemorrhage.* Finally, for obscure reasons, approximately 15 per cent of patients die from either *myelogenous leukemia* or *myelofibrosis* accompanied by pancytopenia.

The goals of treatment in polycythemia vera are: (1) reduction of blood volume and viscosity; and (2) reduction of bone marrow activity. Methods of treatment are as follows:

> *Venesection* (phlebotomy regimen). Emergency treatment of the patient involves removal of 500 to 2000 ml. of blood until the hematocrit is 45 per cent. Once the hematocrit has been reduced, the doctor usually removes 500 ml. of blood from the patient every two to three months. Caution patients undergoing venesection to avoid foods high in iron (clams, oysters, liver, legumes) because a high iron intake somewhat counteracts the therapeutic effects of venesection.

> *Myelosuppressive agents.* The administration of radioactive phosphorus (^{32}P) sometimes produces remissions that last for six months to two years. (See also Chapter 35.) Other drugs useful for combating polycythemia are nitrogen mustard and busulfan (Myeleran).

> *Activity.* In order to prevent the development of thrombi as a result of circulatory stasis, encourage patients with polycythemia vera to ambulate if possible. Patients who are bedridden require frequent turning and passive exercise of their extremities.

> *Fluid balance.* To reduce the viscosity of the patient's blood, force fluids and carefully record intake and output.

Secondary Polycythemia. You recall that the major function of erythrocytes is to carry oxygen to the body tissues. Consequently, when the body's demand for oxygen increases for any reason, the bone marrow is forced to produce more erythrocytes to prevent tissue hypoxia. Whenever red cells must increase excessively as a compensatory response to *tissue hypoxia,* the condition is called *secondary polycythemia.*

Hypoxia that is sufficiently prolonged to cause polycythemia results from chronic lung disease (particularly emphysema), congenital heart disease, and prolonged exposure to altitudes of 10,000 feet or more. It is interesting that people who live in the Andes and other mountainous areas for prolonged periods are usually without symptoms of hypoxia because their blood has literally "thickened." These mountain dwellers produce high numbers of red blood cells, which increases the oxygen-carrying capacity of their blood and enables them to live and work at an altitude that would incapacitate a newcomer.

The *symptoms* and laboratory findings for per-

SYMPTOMS OF POLYCYTHEMIA VERA

Symptoms	*Bases of Symptoms*
Ruddy complexion and dusky redness of mucosa	Great volume of blood causes congestion of capillaries supplying skin and mucous membranes
Hypertension accompanied by dizziness, headache, and a sense of fullness in the head	Increased volume and viscosity of blood causes increased blood pressure
Congestive heart failure (shortness of breath, orthopnea, etc.)	Increased blood volume and viscosity increase work of the heart, leading to failure
Thrombus formation, particularly within vessels supplying the brain, heart, lungs, and lower extremities; cerebral vascular accidents, myocardial infarction, and gangrene of the feet can result	Increased viscosity of blood causes the circulation to slow, promoting thrombus formation; also, increased platelet count causes blood to clot more easily
Bleeding and hemorrhage in the gastrointestinal tract, oropharynx and brain, especially following minor accidents or surgery	Congestion and distention of capillaries, venules and arterioles causes rupture of the vessels, resulting in hemorrhage
Enlarged liver and spleen	Large numbers of erythrocytes collect within the liver and spleen; increased volume of blood within the portal circulation also causes organ congestion
Peptic ulcer (See Unit XV)	Gastric secretions are increased in polycythemia
Gout (painful swollen joints—usually of the big toe)	Increased cell production results in increased cell destruction; this leads to increased released nucleoprotein; one product of nucleoprotein breakdown is uric acid, and increased uric acid levels in blood cause gout

sons with secondary polycythemia are the same as for those with polycythemia vera, except that the leukocyte and thrombocyte counts are normal and splenic enlargement does not occur.

To *treat* secondary polycythemia, the physician must treat the underlying disease or condition causing hypoxia.

Relative Polycythemia. Whenever the body loses plasma without losing red blood cells, the concentration of erythrocytes increases *relative* to the amount of plasma contained within the vascular system. The *causes* of relative polycythemia are fluid loss and dehydration as a result of insufficient fluid intake, diarrhea, vomiting, burns, excessive administration of diuretics, and so forth. *Treatment* of this condition simply involves the re-establishment of fluid and electrolyte balance.

CHAPTER 62

Nursing Patients with Other Major Disturbances of the Blood and Blood-Forming Organs

NURSING PATIENTS WITH DISORDERS PRIMARILY AFFECTING LEUKOCYTES AND PLASMA CELLS

The leukocytes or white blood cells* are one of the body's major defenses against infectious and parasitic organisms. Normally leukocytes number between 5000 and 10,000/cu mm. A rise in the white cell count over 10,000/cu mm. is called *leukocytosis;* white cells usually increase in response to the entry of infectious organisms into the body. Conversely, a *decrease* in the white cell count below 5000/cu mm. is called *leukopenia;* leukocytes may decrease as a result of viral infections and exposure to drugs or myelotoxic agents.

Plasma cells, or plasmocytes, are mononuclear cells that are probably the primary producers of *gamma globulin;* they are formed within the bone marrow and lymph nodes. Pathologic conditions involving plasma cells are called *plasma cell dyscrasias.*

AGRANULOCYTOSIS

Agranulocytosis (granulocytopenia, malignant neutropenia) is an acute, potentially fatal blood dyscrasia characterized by profound neutropenia and a condition called "agranulocytic angina." *Neutropenia* is a reduction in the number of circulating polymorphonuclear neutrophils (granulocytes). "Agranulocytic angina" is an extremely painful and severe ulcerative infection of the oral mucosa and throat, accompanied by high fever and extreme weakness.

The most common cause of agranulocytosis is *drug toxicity* or *hypersensitivity*. There are two major groups of drugs that are capable of suppressing granulocyte production:

1. Agents that *always* produce neutropenia when given in sufficiently large doses over a period of time, e.g., nitrogen mustard and other anticancer drugs and therapies (radiation, radioisotopes, antimetabolites), and benzene.
2. Agents that produce neutropenia only in persons who are *particularly sensitive* to the drug, e.g., certain tranquilizers (Thorazine), antithyroid agents (propylthiouracil), anticonvulsants (diphenylhydantoin), and antibiotics (chloramphenicol).

Agranulocytosis may also develop during the course of certain diseases, e.g., tuberculosis, overwhelming infection, typhoid fever, malaria, and uremia.

Agranulocytosis occurs throughout the world, and particularly in areas where the drugs listed above are in common use. For as yet undiscovered reasons women are much more susceptible to this condition than are men. However, even among females, agranulocytosis is relatively rare.

The *symptoms* of agranulocytosis arise as a result of its characteristic severe neutropenia. You recall that neutrophils, which comprise 50 to 70 per cent of all circulating leukocytes, are one of the body's swiftest and most powerful lines of defense against invading microorganisms. Consequently, any decrease in neutrophils results in a severe increase in the body's susceptibility to bacterial invasion, particularly of the highly vulnerable mucous membranes of the throat and mouth.

Typically the onset of this acute disease is rapid. For the first two or three days the patient complains of severe fatigue and weakness. Next he develops a sore throat, ulcerative lesions of the pharyngeal and buccal mucosae, dysphagia, prostration, high fever, weak rapid pulse, and severe chills. Without prompt treatment with antibiotics the disorder is usually fatal within less than a week.

Diagnosis of agranulocytosis is based upon the following findings:

> *Leukopenia* (500 to 3000 WBC/cu. mm.) with an extreme reduction in polymorphonuclear cells (0 to 2 per cent).

> Bone marrow examination, revealing an *absence of polymorphonuclear leukocytes* or, in some cases, a maturational arrest of young developing cells.

> Cultures of the urine, blood, and ulcerative lesions

*The classification and function of both leukocytes and plasma cells are discussed more thoroughly in Chapter 22.

within the throat and mouth that are *positive for bacteria* (usually gram-positive cocci).

> A *history* of exposure to an offending drug plus all the above findings. Because many people medicate themselves with potentially dangerous drugs, it is important to investigate what drugs the patient takes as well as his drug sources.

The *clinical care* of patients with agranulocytosis involves the following steps:

> *Halt bone marrow arrest early.* Observe patients who are receiving potentially toxic drugs or anticancer therapy for extreme fatigue, the development of a sore throat or mouth, and fever. Check the patient's hemogram daily for a drop in the white blood cell count; immediately notify the physician should even a mild leukopenia develop.

> *Eradicate the infection.* The doctor will order a blood sample for culture and antibiotic sensitivity. The drug of choice is usually *penicillin.*

> *Guard* the patient from *further infection* while he is under treatment. Bed rest and a high protein, high vitamin, high caloric diet will prevent excessive weakness and debilitation. Place the patient in *reverse isolation* in order to reduce his exposure to infectious organisms.

> Give *meticulous mouth care.* To remove necrotic exudate from the oral and pharyngeal mucosa, irrigate the patient's mouth and throat with warm saline solution every 1 or 2 hours. An ice collar, anesthetic lozenges, and small doses of codeine or meperidine (Demerol) every 3 to 4 hours help to relieve the severe pain. Request soft bland foods and protein concentrates for the patient until his throat condition and dysphagia improve. The patient may also require sedation for sleep.

> *Relieve fever* with cooling measures (alcohol rub, tepid baths) and antipyretic drugs. Force fluids to 2500 ml. per day to prevent dehydration as a result of diaphoresis.

> *Prevent constipation.* Hard stools damage the intestinal and rectal mucosa and thus increase the risk of infection. Gentle enemas and stool softeners are usually ordered routinely.

> *Educate patients* to avoid medicating themselves without their doctor's consent. Explain the dangers of taking antibiotics or tranquilizers that have been prescribed for a friend or relative. Inform the patient that he may be hypersensitive to a drug that is safe for another individual.

With antibiotic therapy, many patients recover from agranulocytosis within two to three weeks. However, without antibiotics, the mortality rate from this condition is approximately 80 per cent.

THE LEUKEMIAS

Leukemia (which literally means "white blood") is a fatal neoplastic disease that involves the blood-forming tissues of the bone marrow, spleen, and lymph nodes. Its outstanding characteristic is the abnormal, uncontrolled, and destructive proliferation of one type of white cell (i.e., granulocyte, lymphocyte, or monocyte) and its precursors. Victims of leukemia and the lymphomas account for 6 per cent of all individuals suffering from cancer. Although leukemia strikes people of all ages, it is the leading cause of death among *children* between the ages of 4 and 14 (with the possible exception of congenital anomalies). Currently statisticians estimate that a total of 15,000 persons die of leukemia yearly and another 19,000 discover that they have leukemia.[12] For unknown reasons the incidence of leukemia appears to be on the rise. Indeed, there has been a 50 per cent rise in mortality from this disorder over the last 20 years.

Classification of the Leukemias

There are several forms of leukemia, each of which affects a different age group. Leukemias are classified according to the following criteria:

Course and Duration of Disease. *Acute* leukemia has a *rapid onset* and typically progresses to a fatal termination within days to months. The massive numbers of leukocytes produced are very immature and they accumulate extremely rapidly within the blood-forming organs, causing organ malfunction. The *chronic* leukemias have a *gradual onset* and a slower, more protracted course than the acute leukemias; in some cases the patient lives for five or more years. The white cells produced are more mature and consequently better able to carry out their task of defending the body against invading microorganisms. Acute leukemia is more common among children and young adults, whereas chronic leukemias tend to strike people between the ages of 25 and 60.

Type of Cell and Tissue Involved. Abnormal proliferation of one type of white cell (lymphocyte, myelocyte, or monocyte) occurs in both acute and chronic leukemias. Thus, there are six major types of leukemia: (1) acute lymphocytic leukemia, (2) acute myelocytic leukemia, (3) acute monocytic leukemia, (4) chronic lymphocytic leukemia, (5) chronic myelocytic leukemia, and (6) chronic monocytic leukemia. Variations of this classification are often employed. For example, the acute leukemias are sometimes classified as lymphoblastic, myeloblastic, or monoblastic because of the preponderance of immature cell forms in these categories of disease.

Lymphocytic leukemia is characterized by hyperplasia of lymphoid tissues, whereas myelocytic leukemia is characterized by hyperplasia of the bone marrow and spleen. Ninety per cent of all cases of leukemia (both acute and chronic) are lymphocytic, and only 10 per cent are monocytic and myelocytic.

Number of Leukocytes in Blood and Bone Marrow. Occasionally patients with acute leukemia have a normal or even *lower* than normal leukocyte count. In these instances the condition is called *aleukemic leukemia* or *subleukemic leukemia.*

Etiology, Pathogenesis, and Symptoms

As with other cancers, the exact etiology of leukemia is unknown. (See Unit VII.) There are several factors, however, associated to a greater or lesser degree with the development of leukemia. For example:

> Certain *viruses* have been proved to cause leukemia in cats, mice, and fowl. Possibly viruses may also cause leukemia in humans.

> *Ionizing radiation,* in a certain dosage, is definitely linked with the development of leukemia. For example, there is a high incidence of leukemia among radiologists and persons who work in nuclear fission installations. Surviving victims of atomic bombings at Hiroshima and Nagasaki have had an extremely high rate of leukemia, depending upon their degree of exposure to ionizing radiation.

> A *genetic* predisposition may also play a role. Studies show that the risk of developing leukemia is four times as high among siblings as it is among unrelated children. If one identical twin develops leukemia, there is one chance in five that the other twin will also be stricken. Finally, the rate of leukemia is thirty times as high among mongoloid children as among normal children under age 15.

> The *absorption* of *certain chemicals* may be linked with the development of leukemia, e.g., benzene, pyridone, and aniline dyes.

While the exact cause of leukemia remains elusive, the widespread and devastating effects of this malignant disease upon the body have been studied for years. The three major effects of leukemia are: (1) the *proliferation* of *high numbers of abnormal, immature leukocytes;* (2) the *accumulation* of these cells within the lymph nodes (e.g., lymphocytes accumulate within the lymph nodes; granulocytes, within the bone marrow); and (3) the eventual *infiltration* of these cells into tissues all over the body. These three developments, in turn, lead to other pathologic changes and many symptoms. Below are listed some major symptoms accompanying all forms of leukemia.

In sum, there is not an organ that is not eventually involved in the leukemic process. Hemorrhages into the retina may cause blindness, while hemorrhages into the brain tissue may cause a cerebral vascular accident. The lungs, mouth, throat, skin, and kidneys are all vulnerable to infection. Anorexia, nausea, and vomiting cause malnutrition. As you will see, the reactions to therapeutic measures cause further symptoms. It is no wonder that the victim of leukemia needs constant and meticulous nursing care and observation.

Diagnosis and Clinical Care

Leukemia, during its early stages, may be discovered by accident during a routine physical examination that includes blood work. An elevated leukocyte count with a "shift to the left" (a term indicating the presence of large numbers of immature neutrophils) usually alerts the physician to the possible presence of leukemia. Tests and symptoms that later confirm a diagnosis of leukemia include: (1) a differential leukocyte count in which one type of white cell is overwhelmingly predominant; (2) a bone marrow specimen that contains massive numbers of leuko-

Symptoms	*Bases of Symptoms*
Severe infections, e.g., ulcerations of the mouth and throat, pneumonia, septicemia	Although leukocyte count is high (15,000–500,000/cu. mm. or higher), leukocytes are immature or abnormal and consequently unable to fight and destroy microorganisms
Anemia accompanied by fatigue, lethargy, hypoxia, etc., and hemorrhage (gum bleeding, ecchymoses, petechiae, retinal hemorrhages) due to thrombocytopenia	Rapidly proliferating leukocytes evidently "crowd out" the developing erythrocytes and thrombocytes
Enlarged organs cause pressure on adjacent structures (e.g., splenomegaly, hepatomegaly, lymphadenopathy, bone marrow hypercellularity)	High numbers of white cells accumulate within the liver, spleen, lymph nodes, and bone marrow, causing distention of the tissues
Increased metabolic rate accompanied by weakness, pallor, and weight loss	Increased production of leukocytes requires large amounts of amino acids and vitamins. Increased destruction of cells leads to increased release of metabolic wastes which must be disposed of by the body
Uric acid stones which cause renal pain, obstruction, and infection	Large amounts of uric acid are released as a result of the destruction of mass numbers of leukocytes by antileukemic drugs
Renal insufficiency with uremia (a late development)	Abnormal leukocytes infiltrate into the kidneys
Central nervous system symptoms, e.g., headache, disorientation, convulsions (a late complication)	Abnormal white cells infiltrate into the brain and nervous system

cytes; (3) a blood smear that reveals many "blast" cells; and (4) the presence of anemia, bleeding tendencies, sternal tenderness, and organ enlargement.

The *treatment* of leukemia varies considerably with each form of the disease. However, the *goal of care* in all forms of leukemia is the same: to halt the destructive proliferation and infiltration of abnormal and immature leukocytes and to obtain a *remission* (i.e., lessening or cessation of symptoms) for as long a period as possible.

To date there is no lasting cure for leukemia. However, a number of measures are used to temporarily halt the malignant process, alleviate symptoms, and prevent complications, e.g., radiation therapy; radioisotope therapy; chemotherapy with antimetabolites, alkylating agents, and plant alkaloids; corticosteroid therapy; whole blood and platelet transfusions; antibiotics; bone marrow transplants; reverse isolation techniques; and supportive nursing care. When these measures are successful, patients may experience remissions which last for as long as 15 years.

Table 62–1 lists the various drugs used against different types of leukemia and also in Hodgkin's disease and other lymphomas (see below).

Varieties of Leukemia: Clinical Course and Clinical Care

Acute Leukemia. Acute leukemia is a disease of the young; its peak incidence occurs in children between the ages of 1 and 5.

The onset and manifestations of all forms of acute leukemia are somewhat similar. Typically there is a prodromal period during which the child experiences fatigue, headache, sore throat, night sweats, and shortness of breath. Following this, the patient develops acute symptoms of severe tonsillitis, ulcerations and sometimes gangrenous lesions within the mouth, bleeding from the gums and rectum, bleeding into the skin, and severe joint and bone pain. The lymph nodes, liver, and spleen enlarge, and severe anemia accompanied by debilitation and exhaustion develops. Eventually the patient's life terminates in either overwhelming infection or severe hemorrhage. Without therapy, the patient may die within a few days to a few months. With therapy,

TABLE 62–1. DRUGS USED AGAINST THE LEUKEMIAS AND LYMPHOMAS*

Acute lymphoblastic leukemia	Chronic myelocytic (granulocytic) leukemia	Hodgkin's disease and other lymphomas
Standard drugs	*Standard drugs*	*Standard drugs*
Methotrexate (formerly Amethopterin)	Busulfan (Myleran)	Cyclophosphamide (Cytoxan)
Mercaptopurine (Purinethol)	Chlorambucil (Leukeran)	Mechlorethamine (Mustargen; nitrogen mustard)
Prednisone (Deltasone, Meticorten, et al.)	Mercaptopurine (Purinethol)	Thiotepa (triethylenethiophosphoramide)
Cyclophosphamide (Cytoxan)	Triethylenemelamine (TEM)	Triethylenemelamine (TEM)
Experimental use†	*Experimental use†*	Vinblastine (Velban)
Vincristine (Oncovin)	Hydroxyurea (Hydrea)	Vincristine (Oncovin)
Cytarabine (Cytosar)	Colcemid (Demecolcine)	Procarbazine (Matulane)
Thioguanine	Dibrommannitol (DBM)	Prednisone (Deltasone, Meticorten, et al.)
L-asparaginase	**Acute myeloblastic (granulocytic) leukemia**	*Experimental drugs*
Carmustine (BCNU)	*Standard drugs*	Carmustine (BCNU)
Hydroxyurea (Hydrea)	Methotrexate (formerly Amethopterin)	Bleomycin
Daunorubicin (Daunomycin)	Mercaptopurine (Purinethol)	
Adriamycin	Cyclophosphamide (Cytoxan)	
Chronic lymphocytic leukemia	*Experimental use†*	
Standard drugs	Cytarabine (Cytosar)	
Prednisone (Deltasone, Meticorten, et al.)	Thioguanine	
Chlorambucil (Leukeran)	Daunorubicin (Daunomycin)	
Cyclophosphamide (Cytoxan)	Carmustine (BCNU)	
Triethylenemelamine (TEM)		

*The main drugs employed against the specific conditions named here are listed in the approximate order in which their utility is established for each condition. The generic or commonly accepted name of the drug is given first in each instance, followed in parentheses by the trade name(s) and/or synonym.

†Some of these drugs are experimental, some are approved for other uses.

some patients obtain a remission which lasts for more than a year, and survival for as long as five years is now sometimes achieved.

Examination of the blood of a patient with acute leukemia usually shows an elevated white count; sometimes, however, leukopenia is present. A bone marrow examination and blood smear are needed to differentiate acute leukemia from a severe infection, thrombocytopenia, or rheumatic fever (the latter disorder is also characterized by joint and bone pain).

The clinical care of persons with acute leukemia is structured to allow the young patient to continue to pursue as full a life as possible for as long as possible. When feasible, the patient should live at home, continue his studies at school, and engage in an active social life. To sustain the patient during his illness, the patient's family, teachers, and employers need information concerning the nature of leukemia—its symptoms, treatment, and prognosis.

The mainstay of therapy for acute leukemia is *chemotherapy*. (See Table 62–1.) In addition, patients also receive *blood transfusions* to correct anemia, *platelet transfusions* to prevent hemorrhage as a result of thrombocytopenia, specific *antibiotics* to combat infection, and a drug called *allopurinol* (Zyloprim) 100 mg. t.i.d. or q.i.d., to inhibit the formation of uric acid crystals within the renal tubules. When allopurinol is given, the patient should drink up to 1500 ml. of water per day in order to promote an adequate urine output.

Chronic Myelocytic or Granulocytic Leukemia (CML). This form of leukemia usually strikes individuals between the ages of 25 and 40. It is characterized by the abnormal proliferation of immature neutrophils, which flood the peripheral circulation, accumulate densely within the bone marrow, and infiltrate the liver, spleen, and other tissues.

The symptoms of CML are generally the same as those general symptoms discussed earlier (e.g., anemia, bleeding, and so forth). However, the outstanding characteristic of this particular form of leukemia is a *massive spleen,* which may grow so large that it fills the abdomen and part of the pelvis. The liver may also be greatly enlarged. In contrast to chronic lymphocytic leukemia, the lymph nodes tend to swell very little. Also, patients with CML suffer from severe pain in the long bones; this results from the engorgement of the marrow with abnormal leukocytes.

The most serious problem facing a patient with CML is *extreme vulnerability to infection.* The invasion of microorganisms poses a severe threat because the neutrophils, which comprise the majority of the body's leukocytes, are extremely immature. Moreover, the drugs used to treat CML tend to injure or kill the few normal circulating neutrophils, which further increases the patient's susceptibility to infection.

The onset of CML is usually insidious. For many months or even years the patient may complain of weakness and weight loss. The first specific sign may be a heavy sensation in the abdomen (due to the enlarged spleen) and a sense of extreme abdominal distention after meals. The patient may also suffer from sternal tenderness and mild lymph node enlargement. Bleeding problems due to thrombocytopenia do not usually develop for many years.

The *treatment* of CML includes the following measures:

> *X-ray therapy.* X-rays are either administered to the entire body or they are focused on the spleen or liver.

> *Radioisotope therapy.* Radioactive phosphorus (^{32}P) may be given in place of x-ray therapy; it yields results similar to total body irradiation. The advantage of radioisotope therapy is that ^{32}P produces almost no radiation sickness.

> *Chemotherapy.* The drug of choice in the treatment of CML is busulfan (Myleran), an alkylating agent. The starting dose is 2 mg. 2 to 4 times daily. Once the WBC count lowers to around 10,000, the drug is stopped or given periodically. The major toxic effect resulting from prolonged treatment with busulfan is *irreversible thrombocytopenia.*

Platelet counts should be performed daily on any patient receiving busulfan. Do not *give the drug if there is any drop in the platelet count.*

Other useful drugs are listed in Table 62–1.

Despite modern drug and x-ray therapy, CML is always fatal. Patients may live for three to five years following the onset of the disease whether or not they have received treatment. Death usually follows infection or an episode of either acute bleeding or thromboembolism.

Chronic Lymphocytic Leukemia (CLL). This form of leukemia is characterized by the uncontrolled proliferation of huge numbers of *lymphocytes,* which accumulate in the lymph nodes and lymphoidal tissues and eventually infiltrate the bone marrow, liver, and spleen. Although the cause of CLL is unknown, this neoplastic disorder appears related to the lymphomas (see below).

CLL principally affects older persons between 50 and 70 years of age. For unknown reasons, it is three times more common in men than in women.

The onset of CLL is insidious. Many patients are asymptomatic for years. Indeed 25 per cent of cases are diagnosed from a routine blood examination which reveals an elevated WBC (up to 600,000/cu. mm.), in which 80 to 98 per cent of the leukocytes are small, mature-looking lymphocytes.

Early symptoms of CLL are chronic exhaustion, anorexia, and swollen lymph nodes all over the patient's body. In some cases the patient may also have a slightly enlarged liver and spleen. Later, as the disease progresses, anemia, fever, susceptibility to infections, cachexia, and mild hemorrhagic tendencies develop. Leukemic infiltrations into the retina of the eye and the skin cause visual disturbances and skin lesions. Infiltration of lymphocytes into the ear or along the 8th cranial nerve can result in deafness, otitis media or Meniere's syndrome. Pressure of the enlarged lymph nodes upon various nerves causes pain and even paralysis. In approximately one third of all patients with CLL, mediastinal lymph node enlargement results in respiratory symptoms. Finally, during the last stages of this disorder, the patient's immune system may become involved in the disease process. Thus, two late complications of CLL are: (1) hemolytic anemia due to an autoimmune disorder; and (2) hypogammaglobulinemia—a condition which further increases the patient's susceptibility to infection.

The *treatment* of CLL centers around x-ray therapy and chemotherapy. Commonly used drugs include these *alkylating agents:*

> Chlorambucil (Leukeran) 0.1–0.2 mg./kg. daily in divided doses (administered following meals in order to prevent gastric irritation).

> Triethylenemelamine (TEM) 2.5 to 5 mg. daily (given before meals with 1 or 2 Gm. of sodium bicarbonate).

> Cyclophosphamide (Cytoxan) 50 to 100 mg. orally 1 to 3 times daily.

In addition, the patient is also given small daily doses of *corticosteroids*.

The complications of CLL also require treatment. Anemia usually responds to transfusion therapy and to doses of corticosteroids. Severe hemolytic anemia must sometimes be controlled by splenectomy. Antibiotics, which are always ordered on the basis of culture and sensitivity tests, are given to control infections. Patients with *recurring* infections due to low gamma globulin levels are treated with prophylactic doses of gamma globulin.

The prognosis for patients with CLL is poor. As in all forms of leukemia, the neoplastic process finally ends in death. However, in most patients drug therapy does promote remissions that last from 3 to 18 months. With repeated remissions, some patients live for 15 years or longer following the inception of chemotherapy.

General Nursing Care for Patients with Leukemia

The preceding discussions demonstrate that patients with leukemia suffer from multiple problems and from numerous symptoms involving every organ of the body. In addition, patients may develop *iatrogenic disorders*. For example, radiation therapy can cause radiation sickness, and the various antileukemic drugs may cause bone marrow depression, baldness, and uric acid accumulation. Finally, patients with leukemia also endure the same deep depressions and face the same fears that affect all persons dying of cancer.

Supportive nursing measures that alleviate some of the pain and depression accompanying leukemia and that also help to prevent complications are as follows:

Provide Adequate Rest. Encourage the ambulatory patient to sleep at least eight hours every night, and to take naps during the day as needed. As you recall, patients with leukemia experience an increased metabolic rate because of the massive overproduction of leukocytes; they also suffer from hypoxia due to anemia. Consequently, these individuals need additional rest because they are chronically fatigued and exhausted (a state that increases susceptibility to infection). In far advanced cases of leukemia, the patient may require sedation in order to sleep.

Control Pain. Leukemia produces many types of pain: bone pain, discomfort due to enlarged organs and lymph nodes, nerve pain, dysphagia due to ulcerations within the mouth and throat, and so forth. Because patients with leukemia often live for several years, it is best, at first, to alleviate the patient's pain with mild analgesics such as aspirin or propoxyphene (Darvon). Later in the course of the disease stronger analgesics (e.g., codeine or Demerol) may be required for pain control.

Provide Adequate Food and Fluid Intake. Patients with leukemia usually suffer from anorexia. An aversion to food may result from radiation sickness and/or painful ulcerations within the mouth and throat. Nevertheless, the patient needs a high caloric, high vitamin diet in order to prevent debilitation. Measures for relieving anorexia and discomfort associated with eating include the following: (1) give the patient small servings of soft bland foods that will not irritate his throat; (2) if the patient has mouth and throat ulcerations, have him gargle with an anesthetic solution immediately prior to eating; (3) when throat discomfort is severe, order nutritious cold or frozen foods such as ice cream, fruit sherbet, malted milk shakes, chilled fruit and vegetable juices, concentrated diet drinks that are high in protein, and so forth; (4) contact the dietitian if the patient continues to be dissatisfied with his diet; (5) relieve nausea by obtaining an order for administration of an antiemetic drug one half hour before mealtimes; and (6) if nausea and vomiting persist, obtain an order for intravenous infusion therapy.

In addition to eating an adequate diet, the patient with leukemia must also drink at least *3000 to 4000 ml. of fluid every day.* Fluids are needed to prevent dehydration resulting from fever and diaphoresis, and to dilute the high levels of uric acid that result from destruction of abnormal leukocytes by antileukemic drugs.

Administer Mouth Care. It is important to give mouth care to patients with advanced leukemia at least every two hours and prior to meals because painful ulcerations may be present in the mouth and throat. Also, old blood that has accumulated around the gums and teeth causes a nauseating taste and halitosis. Oral hygiene measures include the following: (1) use soft cotton applicators to clean the patient's mouth and teeth rather than a toothbrush, which may cause bleeding; (2) for cleansing purposes, use a solution of dilute hydrogen peroxide or lemon and glycerin rather than toothpaste; and (3) lubricate the patient's lips with petroleum jelly to prevent cracking and crust formation.

Control Temperature Deviations. High fever may accompany the infections that eventually strike all patients with leukemia. To control temperature elevations above 101°F., administer cooling sponge baths, alcohol rubs, and antipyretic drugs. It is also important to force fluids up to 4000 ml. per day.

Prevent Infection. The prevention of infection in leukemia patients is a major nursing responsibility. As you recall, severe infections develop because the majority of the patient's white cells are immature or abnormal, and because the anticancer drugs used to treat leukemia may produce a severe pancytopenia.

To decrease the threat of overwhelming infection, *observe* the patient continuously for restlessness, temperature elevation, sore throat, "sniffles," chills, skin lesions, and so forth. If these symptoms develop, notify the physician immediately so that appropriate antibiotic therapy can be started.

Check the patient's *blood studies daily* for indications of pancytopenia. If any degree of hematopoietic depression is present, place the patient in *reverse isolation.* Move the patient to a single room, and allow only persons who are in good health to visit or care for him. At this time explain to the patient that he is being isolated as a protective measure. If the pancytopenia worsens, wear a gown and mask when giving nursing care.

In a few institutions, patients with severe bone marrow depression are placed in a protective tent called a *Life Island*—a device that offers many advantages. Within the Life Island the patient is completely enclosed in a sterile environment. Also, he is totally protected from contact with outside microorganisms because all items (e.g., bedpans, trays, linens, etc.) are sterilized with ultraviolet radiation before they enter the tent. Caring for patients within this protective covering is convenient for nurses and doctors. No masks or gloves are required; the nurse simply places her arms into the long gloves that are attached to the sides of the Life Island to perform procedures. A final advantage of this device is that the patient (who is completely enclosed within the transparent tent) can freely visit with friends and relatives on the outside without fear of contamination.

Control Anemia and Hemorrhagic Tendencies. Transfusions of whole blood are administered to patients with hemoglobin levels less than 8 Gm./100 ml. of blood. Transfusions of platelets may also be given to control thrombocytopenia. In addition, bleeding or hemorrhage should be guarded against by: (1) protecting the patient from falls; (2) moving the patient gently; (3) applying steady pressure over an injection site following administration of a parenteral drug; and (4) preventing constipation and the passage of hard stools by requesting an order for a stool softener.

Psychologic Support. Whether or not the patient should be told he has leukemia is a vital question. (See also Unit III and VII.) Patients with this fatal disease often suffer from despair. Patients who know they have leukemia often need psychologic support throughout the difficult weeks, months or years following diagnosis. Fortunately most patients and their families are encouraged once they realize that the patient can lead an almost normal life during the periods of remission obtained by chemotherapy and radiotherapy.

Before patients are discharged, arrange for them to visit the social worker if there is a financial problem. Also, refer patients who face the prospect of long-term care to the local unit of the American Cancer Society for information concerning home nursing; housekeeping and cooking services; and purchase of wheelchairs, bandages, hospital beds, drugs, and so forth. Patients suffering from severe depression or other psychologic problems usually benefit from a psychiatric referral. It is the nurse's responsibility to report such symptoms of mental illness as withdrawal, constant weeping, inability to concentrate, total loss of appetite, insomnia, and threats of suicide so that the staff can take appropriate measures (i.e., referral to a psychiatrist, minister or priest, prescription of antidepressant drugs, occupational therapy, and so forth).

MULTIPLE MYELOMA (PLASMA CELL MYELOMA)

Multiple myeloma is a neoplastic condition characterized by: (1) the abnormal malignant proliferation of plasma cells; (2) the development within the bone marrow of either single or multiple tumors composed of abnormal plasma cells; and (3) bone destruction throughout the body, followed later by dissemination of the disease into the lymph nodes, liver, spleen, and kidneys.

This condition most commonly occurs in people over 40 years of age; it affects twice as many men as women. Although multiple myeloma was once considered a relatively rare disease, its incidence has increased in recent years and now approaches that of Hodgkin's disease.

The onset of multiple myeloma is usually gradual and insidious. Most patients pass through a long *presymptomatic period* which lasts from five to 20 years. During this phase of the disease, some individuals suffer from recurrent bacterial infections, particularly pneumonia. Increased susceptibility to infection is evidently linked to disturbances of antibody formation resulting from abnormalities of plasma cells.

Once symptoms finally appear they typically involve the skeletal system, particularly the pelvis, spine, and ribs. Some patients have backache or bone pain which worsens upon movement. Others suddenly suffer a pathologic fracture accompanied by severe pain. As time goes on, skeletal destruction increases and the patient may develop deformities of the sternum and rib cage. Some patients shrink 5 inches or more in stature as a result of shortening of the spine. Diffuse osteoporosis is also usually present, accompanied by a negative calcium balance. Drainage of calcium and phosphorus from the damaged bones eventually leads to the development of renal stones, particularly if the patient is immobilized.

In addition to bone destruction, multiple myeloma is characterized by disruption of erythrocyte, leukocyte, and thrombocyte production as a result of replacement of the bone marrow with plasma cells. Impaired production of these three cell forms causes: anemia, hemorrhagic tendencies as a result of thrombocytopenia, and increased vulnerability to infection owing to granulocytopenia.

Complications of multiple myeloma include both renal and neurologic disorders. The major neurologic complications are compression of the spinal cord by tumors, later followed by the development of paraplegia. Renal disease results from blockage of the convoluted tubules by particles of coagulated protein.

Diagnosis of multiple myeloma rests upon x-ray studies, a bone marrow biopsy, and laboratory examination of blood and urine. X-ray studies reveal diffuse lesions in the bone, widespread demineralization, and osteoporosis. The bone marrow contains large numbers of immature plasma cells. Normally plasma cells comprise only 5 per cent of the marrow cellular population, but in multiple myeloma, plasma cells make up between 30 and 95 per cent of the cell population. Because of the abnormal proliferation of plasma cells, blood studies generally reveal a high concentration of serum globulins, particularly of an abnormal type called M-type globulin. A final diagnostic sign of multiple myeloma is the appearance of an abnormal globulin in the urine that is called *Bence Jones protein.**

Once multiple myeloma is diagnosed, the treatment is purely symptomatic. The four major goals of care for persons with this fatal condition are as follows:

Reduce Tumor Mass. Radiotherapy and chemotherapy are currently used to reduce bone tumor size and growth. Tumors composed of plasma cells are usually radiosensitive; consequently only small doses of radiation are necessary to control symptoms and tumor size. The two alkylating agents which are used to treat multiple myeloma are melphalan (Alkeran) and cyclophosphamide (Cytoxan). (See also Chapter 35.) Alkeran has been the most successful drug to date in the treatment of multiple myeloma. The major toxic effect of Alkeran is *pancytopenia.* For this reason, observe the patient's hemogram daily for signs of bone marrow depression. Cytoxan, while helpful, is not consistently effective as Alkeran. Side effects of cytoxan include leukopenia, nausea and alopecia.

Control Pain. Patients with multiple myeloma suffer from severe bone pain and sometimes from spontaneous fractures. However, relief from pain can often be obtained by the administration of aspirin and codeine. Stronger analgesics are reserved for the final stages of the disease.

*In 1848 Henry Bence Jones identified a protein substance that is usually excreted in the urine of persons with multiple myeloma and other bone tumors.

Promote Adequate Ambulation and Hydration. You recall that multiple myeloma is characterized by osteoporosis and the resultant loss of calcium from the bones into the blood and urine. Calcium loss leads to hypercalcemia, hypercalciuria, renal stones, and potentially fatal renal damage. Osteoporosis and calcium loss always worsen if the patient is immobilized. (See Chapter 27.) To prevent complications, it is essential to move or to ambulate the patient frequently and to force fluids.

Ambulating patients with multiple myeloma is a major nursing challenge. Many patients, because of pain or fear of falling, prefer to remain immobilized in their beds. Analgesics and orthopedic supports and braces can be used to reduce the patient's pain and sense of insecurity. Because persons with multiple myeloma are particularly vulnerable to pathologic fractures, always accompany the patient when he is walking in order to prevent accidents and falls.

The administration of fluids is another important nursing responsibility. Patients with multiple myeloma require between 3000 and 4000 ml. of fluid per day. If fluid intake is adequate, patients have a 24-hour urine output of approximately 1500 ml. Sufficient fluid is needed not only to counteract the calcium overload but to prevent protein from precipitating in the renal tubules.

The necessity to ambulate and hydrate the patient with multiple myeloma cannot be stressed enough! As Osserman explains:

> Unless mobilization and hydration are accomplished by these measures, it is usually impossible to maintain a patient for the time required to accomplish a remission with chemotherapy.[45a]

Treat Complications. Anemia is treated with transfusion therapy. Infections are managed with antibiotics. To prevent recurrent infection, the doctor may order the administration of gamma globulin, 10 ml. I.M. every 2 weeks. Corticosteroids are prescribed for severe hypercalcemia accompanied by nausea and vomiting. Patients suffering from spinal cord compression must sometimes undergo a laminectomy.

Drug and x-ray therapy as well as excellent nursing care can extend the life of some patients with multiple myeloma for many years. However, patients usually die within 1½ to 2 years following diagnosis of the disease.

NURSING PATIENTS WITH DISORDERS PRIMARILY AFFECTING THE LYMPH NODES AND SPLEEN

THE LYMPHOPROLIFERATIVE DISORDERS (MALIGNANT LYMPHOMAS)

The lymphomas are a group of neoplastic tumors that chiefly affect lymphatic structures and are composed of either lymphocytes or reticulum cells. There are three major types of lymphomas: Hodgkin's disease,* the lymphosarcomas, and Burkitt's

*In some textbooks, Hodgkin's disease is not included in the lymphoma classification.

lymphoma (a disease affecting children who live in Central Africa).

Hodgkin's Disease

Definition and Incidence. Hodgkin's disease is a chronic, progressive, neoplastic disorder. It is initially characterized by enlargement of the lymph glands, spleen, and liver, followed later by the pathologic involvement of tissues and organs throughout the body. The cause of Hodgkin's disease is unknown.

A disorder of young adults, Hodgkin's disease principally occurs between the ages of 20 and 40. Among adults, men affected outnumber women by a ratio of 2:1; among children, boys are striken five times more often than are girls. Within the United States approximately 3400 persons die yearly from Hodgkin's disease.

Pathogenesis. You will recall that each neoplastic blood disorder is characterized by the abnormal proliferation of one particular type of blood cell. In Hodgkin's disease the proliferating cells are abnormal histiocytes (one category of reticuloendothelial cells) called *Reed-Sternberg* cells. As these atypical giant cells multiply, they eventually replace the normal cellular elements within the lymph nodes. In time, the structure of the lymph nodes is damaged and areas of necrosis and fibrosis develop.

Typically, Hodgkin's disease initially affects one lymph node and then travels to other lymph nodes throughout the body via lymphatic channels. In some cases, the neoplastic process may extend to other organs and structures. For example, nodules of varying size may appear in the liver and spleen; the vertebrae may be affected, resulting in vertebral collapse; and organs such as the ureters and bronchi may be invaded because of their close proximity to involved lymphatic structures.

Hodgkin's disease is often divided into categories or stages, classified according to the microscopic appearance of the involved lymph nodes, the extent and severity of the disorder, and the prognosis. One method of staging is shown in Table 62–2.

Bases of Symptoms. The first symptom of Hodgkin's disease is the painless enlargement of the lymph nodes caused by the massive proliferation of Reed-Sternberg cells. Later, as the disease disseminates throughout the reticuloendothelial system (a process which may be slow or swift), numerous and varied manifestations appear. The major symptoms of Hodgkin's disease and their bases are outlined on the following page.

During the late stages of the disease, the patient becomes severely anemic and cachexic. Also, as lymphatic obstruction worsens, large amounts of fluid accumulate in the patient's chest and abdomen. Eventually the patient dies in a state of shock and debilitation.

Diagnosis. *Lymph node biopsy* is the definitive examination for diagnosing Hodgkin's disease. When peripheral lymph node enlargement is present, one entire lymph node is removed and examined for the presence of Reed-Sternberg cells. However, some patients do not have enlarged peripheral lymph nodes but may simply notice pruritus, intermittent fever, and weakness. In these cases, Hodgkin's disease can often be diagnosed by x-raying the patient's chest for evidence of mediastinal or hilar adenopathy.

TABLE 62–2. STAGING OF HODGKIN'S DISEASE*

Stage†	Definition
0	No detectable disease due to prior excisional biopsy
I	Single abnormal lymph node
II	Two or more discrete abnormal nodes, limited to one side of diaphragm
III	Disease on both sides of diaphragm but limited to the lymph nodes, spleen, or Waldeyer's ring
IV	Involvement of bone, bone marrow, lung parenchyma, pleura, liver, skin, gastrointestinal tract, CNS, renal or sites other than lymph nodes, spleen, or Waldeyer's ring

*From Krupp, M. A., and Chatton, M. J.: *Current Diagnosis and Treatment.* Los Altos, California, Lange Medical Publications, 1972.

†All stages are subclassified as A or B to describe the absence or presence of systemic symptoms, respectively.

Blood studies typically reveal a normocytic normochromic anemia. Also, because of disturbances of the immune mechanism, patients with Hodgkin's disease are usually unable to react normally to skin tests for tuberculosis.

Clinical Care. While Hodgkin's disease is usually considered a fatal disorder, patients in stages I or II can sometimes be cured with wide-field megavoltage radiation. Doses of 3500 to 4000 roentgens (r) given over a 4- to 6-week period can possibly eradicate the disease for life, provided the neoplastic process has not spread beyond the lymph node chains, spleen, and nasopharynx. If sites other than the three listed above require irradiation therapy, the radiologist protects the vital organs (i.e., the heart, lungs, liver, bone marrow, kidneys) with tailor-made leaded shields in order to prevent permanent organ damage.

Unfortunately patients with stage III or IV disease cannot be cured by radiation therapy. However, they usually experience symptomatic relief when treated with radiotherapy and chemotherapy combined. See Table 62–1 for a list of drugs currently used for chemotherapy. Among the most commonly used drugs is nitrogen mustard.

> *Mechlorethamine* (nitrogen mustard), 0.4 mg./kg. body weight dissolved in physiologic saline and given intravenously either as a single injection within 5 minutes or in fractional doses over a 2-day period. In many cases the tumor masses begin to shrink and the patient's symptoms lessen within one to three months. Unless contraindicated, drug therapy is usually repeated every two months.

Despite the symptomatic relief that nitrogen mustard brings, many patients are unable to tolerate this drug because of its toxic effects. The most distressing and immediate side effect of nitrogen mustard is severe *nausea and vomiting,* which may last for hours. To reduce nausea: (1) give the medication in the evening following a light lunch and no dinner; (2) request an order for sedation and an antiemetic drug; and (3) keep the patient's room cool and quiet following administration of the agent. A second and more dreaded toxic effect of nitrogen mustard therapy is *pancytopenia,* which may develop within 10 to 14 days following the I.V. injection. If the patient's hemogram reveals any degree of leukopenia, anemia, or thrombocytopenia, nitrogen mustard therapy must be discontinued.

Combination chemotherapy is proving successful in reducing tumor masses with minimal toxic effects. The drug regimen currently used is "MOPP" and includes administration of mechlorethamine, vincristine, (Oncovin) prednisone, and procarbazine.

Surgery, a third form of therapy, is sometimes employed to remove tumors that are placing undue pressure upon an organ or nerve; e.g., surgical excision of a tumor that is pressing on the spinal cord will relieve pain and paralysis.

In addition to reducing the size of tumor masses, therapy is also directed toward the relief of symptoms. *Fever* is reduced with acetylsalicylic acid, 10 gr. every 4 hours, and the administration of cooling measures; *anemia* is controlled with transfusions; *pruritus* (an often intractable problem) is sometimes relieved by the administration of either colchicine or

SYMPTOMS OF HODGKIN'S DISEASE

Symptoms	*Bases of Symptoms*
Severe pruritus is an early sign	Cause unknown
Irregular fever usually present; typically, temperature is elevated for a few days and then drops to normal or subnormal for several days or weeks; continuous high fever may indicate impending death	Temperature elevation is apparently related to neoplastic involvement of the internal nodes or viscera
Splenomegaly and hepatomegaly	Dissemination of the disorder from the lymph nodes to other organs of the reticuloendothelial system
Jaundice	Obstruction of the bile ducts as a result of liver damage causes the pigment bilirubin to accumulate in the blood and discolor the skin
Edema and cyanosis of the face and neck	Enlarged lymph nodes may place pressure on the superior vena cava and cause edema of the areas which it drains
Pulmonary symptoms including cough, stridor, dyspnea, chest pain, cyanosis, and pleural effusion	Mediastinal lymph node enlargement, involvement of the lung parenchyma, and invasion of the pleura occurs in more than one half of patients
Progressive anemia accompanied by fatigue, malaise, anorexia, etc.	Erythrocyte life span is shortened, and erythropoiesis is unable to keep pace with erythrocyte destruction
Bone manifestations include pain, vertebral compression and, infrequently, fracture	Dissemination of the disease from the lymph nodes to the bones
Nerve pain	Compression of the nerve roots of the brachial, lumbar, or sacral plexuses
Paraplegia	Compression of the spinal cord resulting from extradural involvement
Laryngeal paralysis	Pressure of enlarged cervical nodes upon the cervical, sympathetic, and laryngeal nerves causes laryngeal damage
Increased susceptibility to infection	Impairment of immune mechanisms from unknown causes
Alcohol-induced pain: bone pain or pain around the mediastinum occurs immediately after drinking alcohol and lasts for 30 to 60 minutes	Cause unknown

chlorpromazine (Thorazine); *infections* are guarded against by reverse isolation techniques.

Prognosis. When untreated, patients with Hodgkin's disease have a life expectancy of approximately 5 years; the cause of death is either cachexia or obstruction of a vital organ. However, there is a 95 per cent cure rate for patients who are diagnosed in stage I or II of the disease and who are treated with intensive radiotherapy. Patients who are diagnosed in stages III or IV have a poor prognosis.

Lymphosarcoma

Like Hodgkin's disease, lymphosarcoma is a malignant condition of unknown etiology that primarily involves lymphatic tissues. This disease, which is neither common nor rare, develops in persons of all ages; however, it principally strikes middle-aged persons.

The earliest sign of lymphosarcoma is *painless lymphadenopathy,* which is usually unilateral. The first lymph nodes to enlarge are usually in the neck, although axillary or inguinal lymph nodes may sometimes enlarge initially. As the disease progresses, the neoplastic process spreads along lymphatic channels to other lymph nodes. Eventually lymphosarcoma invades the *bone marrow;* this is one of the outstanding features of this disease. Other organs that may be involved include the liver, spleen, skin, gastrointestinal tract, and nervous system. Pressure on these organs and organ obstruction, in turn, produce symptoms; e.g., abdominal pain, nerve pain or paralysis, and so forth. Other general problems that accompany lymphosarcoma include anemia, malaise, fever, weight loss, sweating, and pruritus.

The *diagnosis* of lymphosarcoma is based on *lymph node biopsy.* When the disease is present, destruction of lymph node architecture is evident, and normal cellular elements are replaced by huge numbers of lymphocytes or lymphoblasts. Once the diagnosis is confirmed, the patient is further evaluated in order to discern the stage of the disease. Staging for lymphosarcoma is the same as for Hodgkin's disease.

Like Hodgkin's disease, lymphosarcoma is treated with irradiation, chemotherapy and, occasionally, surgery. However, for patients with lymphosarcoma, irradiation is only a palliative rather than a curative measure, as it is in stages I and II of Hodgkin's disease. Irradiation is less successful in lymphosarcoma because: (1) lymphosarcoma tends initially to strike several sites at once, whereas Hodgkin's disease tends to limit itself to one site for a period of time; and (2) the dosage of radiation must be lower in lymphosarcoma than in Hodgkin's disease because the bone marrow, which is involved in lymphosarcoma, is easily injured by radiotherapy.

The drugs used to treat lymphosarcoma are the same as those used for Hodgkin's disease, e.g., cyclophosphamide (Cytoxan), vincristine (Oncovin), and prednisone.

On rare occasions, surgical excision of an involved lymph node is performed and is curative. For a successful operation, the disease must be discovered in its early stages and be limited to a single lymph node.

The prognosis for patients with lymphosarcoma is poor. Adults generally survive for about two years following the onset of the disease, while children under 16 usually die within less than one year.

INFECTIOUS MONONUCLEOSIS

Infectious mononucleosis (also known as "glandular disease" and the "kissing disease") is a benign self-limiting condition characterized by painful enlargement of the lymph nodes, lymphocytosis, and fever. The possible cause of infectious mononucleosis is a herpeslike virus called the Epstein-Barr virus (EBV). Although there is a possibility that the disease is transmitted by direct contact such as kissing, the exact mode of transmission remains unknown.

Primarily a disease of the young, infectious mononucleosis usually strikes children between the ages of 3 and 5 and young persons between the ages of 15 and 25. It has its greatest incidence among college students, medical students, and nurses. Although infectious mononucleosis usually occurs sporadically, it also sweeps in epidemic form through colleges and children's homes.

Although infectious mononucleosis is a relatively mild disorder, its effects upon the body are widespread. The lymph nodes enlarge; the blood picture reveals a lymphocytosis; the spleen may swell two to three times its normal size; liver function is sometimes impaired; and both the peripheral and central nervous systems may be involved in the disease process.

The onset of infectious mononucleosis follows an incubation period of uncertain length that is believed to extend from a few days to several weeks. The patient complains of fever, chills, malaise, severe headache, sore throat, and painful, swollen lymph nodes that are located mainly in the posterior, cervical, axillary, and groin regions. Ten to 15 per cent of patients develop a macular rash that closely resembles the rash seen in rubella. Splenic enlargement causes left upper quadrant pain. Nervous system involvement causes the severe headache. In rare cases, liver involvement may result in the development of a hepatitislike syndrome. When infectious mononucleosis is severe, the patient risks developing the following complications:

- Splenic rupture as a result of the infiltration of the spleen by massive numbers of lymphocytes.
- Streptococcal pharyngitis or Vincent's angina owing to secondary bacterial invasion of the throat.
- Guillain-Barré syndrome characterized by ascending paralysis, facial weakness, and mental disturbances. (See Unit VIII.)

The diagnosis of infectious mononucleosis is based upon the following three criteria: (1) the clinical picture (i.e., fever, lymphadenopathy, splenomegaly); (2) the blood picture, which includes a white count of 12,000 to 18,000 leukocytes per cu. mm., of which 60 per cent are large, atypical lymphocytes (known as Downey cells); and (3) a positive Paul-Bunnell heterophil test. The term *heterophil* means "having an affinity for more than one group or species."[22] In 1932 Paul and Bunnell discovered that the blood of patients with infectious mononucleosis contained antibodies that would clump or agglutinate the red blood cells of sheep. Normally human beings do not produce agglutinins against sheep erythrocytes; consequently, a positive heterophil test helps to confirm the diagnosis of infectious mononucleosis, though positive tests sometimes occur in other conditions.

There is no specific medical therapy for patients with this condition that will either alleviate or hasten the disease process. Infectious mononucleosis must simply run its course. However, it is possible to relieve the patient's symptoms and to provide comfort. Thus, the patient is confined to bed until his fever, malaise, fatigue, and headache lessen. Salicylates, cool sponge baths, and a large fluid intake are important measures for controlling fever. Warm saline throat irrigations are occasionally administered to very ill patients with beneficial results. Although steroids do not in any way alter or accelerate the course of the disease, these drugs tend to increase the patient's sense of well-being.

In addition to providing symptomatic relief, a second goal of care is to prevent and to treat complications. When caring for patients with infectious mononucleosis, remember the following points:

1. *Caution the patient against engaging in excessive activity; this may result in splenic rupture or a lowered resistance to infection.*
2. *Watch the patient closely for the two signs of splenic rupture: abdominal pain, and shock. Report these signs at once and prepare the patient for emergency surgery.*
3. *Isolate the patient from possible sources of bacterial contamination. If throat pain worsens, report this immediately so that appropriate antibiotic therapy can be started.*

Although complications sometimes develop, the prognosis for patients with infectious mononucleosis is generally excellent. The febrile phase of this disorder, which generally lasts from 2 to 4 weeks, is followed by a long convalescent period during which time the patient slowly regains his strength and energy.

THE SPLEEN AND ITS DISORDERS

The spleen, a glandlike organ that is located in the upper part of the abdominal cavity on the left side of the body, has long been an enigma. The ancients called the spleen "a dark organ . . . full of mystery." The spleen was once believed to harbor man's irritations, melancholy, and anger; thus, we still say that a person who expresses rage is "venting his spleen." Today, while we no longer regard the spleen as the site of negative emotion, we still fail to fully understand its physiologic role. As part of the reticuloendothelial system the spleen apparently performs a vital but not essential function in purifying the blood and protecting the body from various stresses. Known functions of the spleen include the following:

> Acts as a blood reservoir in animals and to a lesser extent in human beings. When the body is subjected to excessive stress (e.g., extreme exertion, bleeding, carbon monoxide poisoning), the spleen contracts and expels its store of erythrocytes into the circulation.

> Purifies blood and removes waste and infectious organisms.

> Acts as a primary source of antibodies in infants and small children; produces lymphocytes, plasma cells, and antibodies in adults.

> Performs extramedullary hematopoiesis (production of erythrocytes outside the bone marrow). The spleen normally produces red cells in the fetus. In adults, however, extramedullary hematopoiesis is *abnormal;* it occurs only in individuals with bone marrow depression and a resultant pancytopenia. If prolonged, extramedullary hematopoiesis leads to splenomegaly.

> Destroys red blood cells when they reach the end of their 120-day life span.

> Traps and destroys fragile or defective red blood cells (spherocytes).

Splenectomy

Despite the important functions listed above, the spleen can be removed (splenectomy) without harm to the adult patient. The role of the spleen can be completely taken over by other reticuloendothelial organs (e.g., the liver, lymph nodes, and bone marrow). However, because the spleen is a major source of antibody formation in children, pediatricians do not recommend splenectomy during the early years of a child's life. If splenectomy is absolutely necessary, the child must receive prophylactic antibiotics following surgery in order to prevent infection.

The most frequent indication for splenectomy is *rupture of the spleen* complicated by severe hemorrhage. Causes of splenic rupture include the following: (1) trauma, which can result from automobile accidents, penetration with a bullet or knife, a severe blow to the spleen, and so forth; (2) accidental tearing of the splenic capsule during surgery on neighboring organs; and (3) diseases of the spleen that cause softening or damage (e.g., infectious mononucleosis and malaria).

Hypersplenism is a second important indication for splenectomy. The term hypersplenism implies that the spleen is destroying, in excessive numbers, one of the cellular elements of the blood (i.e., erythrocytes, leukocytes, or platelets). Signs of hypersplenism include splenomegaly, anemia or leukopenia, and a compensatory increase in the production of the sequestered blood cells by the bone marrow. Overactivity of the spleen develops either as a primary condition of unknown origin or secondary to another disease. *Primary* hypersplenism occurs in idiopathic thrombocytopenic purpura and congenital spherocytosis. *Secondary* hypersplenism occurs in association with leukemia, the lymphomas, Hodgkin's disease, tuberculosis, and portal hypertension resulting from liver disease. Primary hypersplenism can be alleviated by splenectomy. However, splenectomy is simply a palliative measure for patients suffering from secondary hypersplenism, since the surgery has little or no effect on the course of the primary illness.

Once the indication for splenectomy is certain, the surgery itself is relatively simple unless the spleen is greatly enlarged or surrounded by adhesions. The pre- and postoperative care of patients is generally the same as that discussed in Unit VI. However, there are a few specific observations to remember when caring for patients following splenectomy.

> Observe the patient carefully for *hemorrhage* and *shock*. Patients with thrombocytopenic purpura suffer from bleeding tendencies as a result of their decreased platelet levels. Transfusions of platelets at the time of surgery may help to diminish the threat of hemorrhage but will not alleviate it. Also, accident victims may have suffered other serious injuries in addition to splenic rupture that may lead to shock and bleeding, e.g., fractured ribs, a head injury, broken limbs.

> Observe the patient for an *elevated temperature*. For unknown reasons, patients usually run a fever as high as 101° F. for 10 days or more following splenectomy. Usually this temperature elevation is *not* the result of infection, and consequently the patient does not benefit from antibiotic therapy. Occasionally, however, the fever is associated with complications such as pneumonia, wound infections, and so forth. For this reason, carefully observe the patient for *all* the symptoms of the various postoperative complications and do not simply rely upon temperature elevation as the major symptom heralding infection.

> Observe the patient for *abdominal distention* and *discomfort*. Removal of an enlarged spleen may cause the stomach and intestines to expand in order to fill the void. Abdominal distention can be relieved by application of a tight abdominal binder and the parenteral administration of neostigmine (Prostigmin).

NURSING PATIENTS WITH DISORDERS PRIMARILY AFFECTING PLATELETS AND CLOTTING FACTORS

HEMOSTASIS

Hemostasis is defined as the "arrest of the escape of blood by either natural (clot formation or vessel spasm) or artificial (compression or ligation) means."[42] The promotion and control of hemostasis depend upon the hemostatic mechanism, the fibrinolytic inhibitor mechanism, and natural anticoagulants circulating in the blood.

The Hemostatic Mechanism

The three components of the hemostatic mechanism are as follows:

Blood Vessels. Whenever there is bleeding as a result of injury or disease, the blood vessels supplying the damaged site *constrict;* vasoconstriction, in turn, slows the flow of blood to the injured area, thereby decreasing blood loss. Vasoconstriction is the result of reflex nervous system and muscular tissue reactions. *Serotonin* (a powerful local vasoconstrictor secreted by cells in the small intestine and absorbed by released platelets) also promotes blood vessel constriction upon injury.

Platelets or Thrombocytes. The precise meaning of the word thrombocyte is "clot cell"; however, platelets are not cells in the true sense of the word. They are tiny disc-shaped fragments derived from giant cells called *megakaryocytes* that are located in the bone marrow. Platelets perform three vital hemostatic functions: (1) they form a temporary clot by adhering to each other (aggregation) and to the vessel wall (adhesion); (2) they release incomplete thromboplastin which, along with other substances, aids in the formation of a permanent clot; and (3) they release a contractile protein that causes the soft permanent clot to contract, shrink, and grow firm. Hemostasis is largely controlled by platelets unless large blood vessels have suffered damage and bleeding is severe. In the case of hemorrhage, the coagulation factors must join with the platelets in the formation of a permanent clot. Normally the platelet count is 200,000-350,000/cu.mm. A decrease in platelets is called *thrombocytopenia,* while an increase is called *thrombocytosis.*

Coagulation Factors. The 12 coagulation factors are listed in Table 62–3 along with their sources, characteristics, and functions. Note that the factors are numbered with Roman numerals in order to coincide with the standard international nomenclature.

The exact manner in which the three components of the hemostatic mechanism work together to form a clot is not totally understood. However, physiologists recognize that the hemostatic mechanism—which is intricate and complex—occurs in the following three phases:

VASCULAR PHASE. Whenever the vascular epithelium is injured, bleeding from traumatized vessels is quickly reduced by means of the following phenomena: (1) the blood vessels reflexively constrict; and (2) blood flowing into the neighboring tissues forms a hematoma (tumorous mass of blood) which compresses the injured vessels, thereby lessening blood loss.

PLATELET PHASE. The intima of the blood vessels is normally covered with platelets and endothelial cells. Because both of these cellular elements are negatively charged, they consequently repel each other. However, when the epithelial lining of a vessel is torn, connective tissue containing *collagen* is exposed, which is *not* repellent to platelets. As a result, platelets adhere to the collagen cells and clump together, forming a soft friable plug capable of temporarily patching the rip in the vessel wall. In the process of forming the temporary clot, the platelet membranes rupture. As the platelets disintegrate, important substances are released which play a vital role in the third phase of blood coagulation.

COAGULATION PHASE. The third and final phase of blood clot formation takes place in three stages. In stage 1, *thrombokinase* (thromboplastin) is formed from the interaction of incomplete thromboplastin released from disintegrated platelets, calcium (factor IV), and coagulation factors V, VIII, IX, X, XI, and XII. Stage 2 is characterized by the formation of thrombin; and stage 3, by the formation of fibrin. An insoluble protein, fibrin is composed of dense interlacing threads that entrap erythrocytes and platelets. At this stage of the clot formation process, the platelets, by releasing a contractile protein, perform their final hemostatic function—shrinkage and retraction of the clot into a firm insoluble fibrin mass. In the process of retraction, a clear yellow substance called *serum* is squeezed from the clot; serum differs from plasma in that it does not contain clotting substances.

In some cases hemostasis is complete at the earlier stage and the formation of a permanent fibrin clot is not necessary; in other cases such clot formation is not sufficient to stop hemorrhage. For example, bleeding from a small pinprick can normally be terminated by a platelet plug, whereas more serious cuts require the interaction of the various coagulation factors. When an artery is severely traumatized

TABLE 62-3. COAGULATION FACTORS*

Factor	Name or Substance	Source, Characteristics, Function
I	Fibrinogen	Produced in the liver; protein present in plasma at an average level of 300 mg. %; when acted upon by thrombin, forms fibrin
II	Prothrombin	Produced in the liver, with vitamin K an essential part; present in plasma and measured according to its activity; when acted upon by thromboplastin, forms thrombin
III	Thromboplastin	Tissues and platelets (incomplete); plasma (complete); incomplete forms require factors V, VII, X; complete form is a product of interaction between factors VIII, IX, XI and platelets; acts upon prothrombin to form thrombin
IV	Calcium	Obtained from diet; present in serum levels of 4.8–5.2 mEq./l.; is an inorganic ion required in all stages of coagulation as an activator of enzyme activity
V	Labile factor	Derived from plasma globulin; found in normal plasma; used up in the clotting process; deteriorates rapidly at room temperature; accelerates conversion of prothrombin to thrombin
VI	Unassigned	In early studies, was thought to be the active form of factor V
VII	Stable factor	Produced in the liver; not consumed in clotting, therefore present in normal serum; stable to heat and storage; accelerates the conversion of prothrombin to thrombin
VIII	Antihemophilic globulin	Derived from plasma globulin; completely consumed in clotting; unstable at room temperature; essential to the formation of thromboplastin and conversion of prothrombin to thrombin
IX	Plasma thromboplastin component (Christmas factor)	Produced in the liver; not consumed during clotting; influences amount of thromboplastin generated
X	Stuart-Prower factor	Probably produced in the liver, with vitamin K essential; present in normal plasma and serum; stable at room temperature; similar to factor VII; essential to generation of thromboplastin and activity of prothrombin
XI	Plasma thromboplastin antecedent	Site of synthesis unknown; present in normal plasma and serum; stable; essential to formation of plasma thromboplastin
XII	Hageman factor	Site of synthesis unknown; relatively stable; activated on contact with glass; physiologic role not completely known
XIII	Fibrin stabilizing factor	Site of synthesis not known; high levels in plasma; deficiency associated with mild bleeding tendency, poor wound healing; maintains firm clot after formation.

*Modified from French, R. M.: *Nurses' Guide to Diagnostic Procedures.* 3rd ed. New York, McGraw-Hill Book Co., Inc., 1971.

or severed, surgical intervention with tourniquets, ligation or cautery is needed to halt hemorrhage.

Fibrinolysis (Clot Dissolution)

Once the tough fibrin clot has served its purpose (i.e., halting hemorrhage), it must be dissolved by the fibrinolytic or clot-lysis mechanism in order to prevent permanent thrombosis and occlusion of the injured blood vessel. The fibrinolytic mechanism is active in less than a day following the formation of a clot. The two substances involved in the lysis of a clot are *plasminogen* and *plasmin,* the active substance in fibrinolysis. Plasmin is a proteolytic enzyme capable of digesting such protein materials as fibrin, fibrinogen, and factors V and VIII. *Plasminogen,* a serum globulin, is the inactive precursor of plasmin. Plasminogen can be activated by a number of natural activators found in blood, urine, and so forth. In clinical practice the doctor may activate plasminogen and induce fibrinolysis in patients with pulmonary emboli by administering either streptokinase or urokinase intravenously.

Normally the fibrinolytic mechanism remains localized to the site of clot formation. Occasionally, however, the mechanism may become overactive (resulting in hemorrhage) or underactive (resulting in excessive thrombosis of blood vessels).

Control of Hemostasis

By what means is the coagulation system controlled so that it functions effectively when needed, but *only* when needed? First, as you recall, the normal epithelium does not attract platelets, nor does the normal blood contain activators of coagulation. Second, the blood contains natural anticoagulants that act continuously to inhibit coagulation, e.g., heparin, antithrombin, and antithromboplastin. Finally, the blood contains the proteolytic enzyme plasmin, which, upon activation, performs fibrinolysis and thereby clears the vessels of clots.

HEMORRHAGIC DISORDERS

Causes and Classification

Normal clot formation and lysis depend upon the presence of the following: (1) strong healthy blood vessels; (2) normal numbers of circulating platelets; (3) the 12 clotting factors; and (4) a well controlled fibrinolytic system. Conversely the four basic problems underlying hemorrhagic (bleeding) disorders are: (1) weak, damaged vessels that rupture easily or spontaneously; (2) platelet deficiency (thrombocytopenia) due to either hypoproliferation, excessive pooling or platelets in the spleen, or excessive platelet destruction; (3) deficiency or total lack of one of the clotting factors; or (4) excessive or insufficient fibrinolysis.

The major bleeding disorders can be classified as follows:

I. *Purpura* (extravasation of blood into the tissues and mucous membranes)
  A. Vascular purpuras
  B. Purpura due to platelet disorders
    1. Idiopathic thrombocytopenic purpura
    2. Secondary thrombocytopenias
II. Coagulation disorders
  A. Hemophilia
  B. Hypoprothrombinemia
  C. Defibrination syndrome

Diagnosis and Laboratory Studies

The diagnosis of hemorrhagic disorders rests upon the patient's medical and familial history, the physical examination, and a battery of specific laboratory tests for platelet and clotting defects. The patient's *history* usually offers numerous clues to the type of bleeding problem present and its cause. Questions typically included in the history-taking procedure are:

> How long has the patient had a bleeding problem? Since he was a child or only recently?

> Do any members of the patient's family have a history of bleeding episodes?

> Is bleeding linked with any specific event or procedure? For example, does severe bleeding occur following minor trauma? a tooth extraction? minor surgery? participation in contact sports? during shaving? during the menses in female patients?

> Does the patient have frequent nosebleeds? Does he have a history of bleeding into joints or cavities? Does he bruise easily?

> Does the patient have a history of hepatic, splenic, or renal disease? (These three conditions are often characterized by hemorrhagic manifestations.)

> How severe are the individual bleeding episodes and what is their duration? More precisely is there prolonged oozing of blood from a site or sudden massive hemorrhage? (Sudden hemorrhage is a far less common manifestation of bleeding disorders than is oozing of long duration.)

> Has the patient recently taken either anticoagulant drugs or drugs that tend to suppress bone marrow function (e.g., chloramphenicol, antineoplastic drugs)?

If the patient's history points to the presence of a bleeding disorder, the physician next examines the individual for the overt signs of bleeding. *Petechiae* (tiny hemorrhagic spots caused by intradermal or submucosal bleeding) are usually present in the vascular and thrombocytopenic purpuras. The presence of *ecchymoses* (large blotchy subcutaneous hemorrhagic areas), *hematomas* (blood tumors), and *hemarthrosis* (blood within the joints) is diagnostic of hemophilia. Patients who hemorrhage severely from several areas during a major surgical procedure or during childbirth may have a fibrinogen deficiency. In addition to examining the patient for evidence of bleeding, the physician also searches for evidence of cirrhosis of the liver (hepatomegaly, jaundice, and so forth) and splenomegaly.

The most crucial evidence for pinpointing the type and cause of a bleeding disorder is obtained from laboratory studies. Initially the physician usually orders the following four basic laboratory tests in order to detemine if the bleeding problem is due to a vascular, a coagulation, or a platelet defect: bleeding time, prothrombin time (one stage), platelet count, and partial thromboplastin time (PTT) (Table 62–4). Ninety-five per cent of all bleeding disorders are diagnosed by the PTT and prothrombin time. Once primary laboratory screening has been performed, the doctor may decide to order other more sophisticated tests of hemostatic function (Table 62–4).

General Clinical Care

Specific medical measures for treating the various hemorrhagic diseases differ. However, there are a number of general observations, precautions, and nursing actions that apply to all patients suffering from bleeding disorders. Important points to remember are:

> *Observe* the patient continuously for *signs of bleeding*. Examine his skin and the interior of his mouth for petechiae and ecchymosis. Observe stools for bright red blood as well as for the tarry appearance that indicates the passage of old blood. Observe urine for the smoky color that signals hematuria. Report and chart the development of nosebleeds, their severity and duration. Remember to observe for the subtle signs of *internal* hemorrhage, e.g., faintness, tachycardia, hypotension, confusion, disorientation, and air hunger.

> *Guard the patient from trauma.* If the patient is bedridden, turn him gently but frequently (every 1 to 2 hours). Assist weak or elderly ambulatory patients to the bathroom, particularly at night, in order to prevent bumps and falls. Caution the male patient to use an electric razor for shaving in order to avoid cuts. Also, to prevent bleeding of gums, instruct the patient to cleanse his teeth with a very soft toothbrush.

> *Prevent constipation.* Hard stools, straining at stool, and fecal impactions all traumatize the rectal and anal mucosa, causing bleeding. If constipation does develop, notify the physician. A gentle laxative, stool softener, or enema may be necessary.

> *Administer intramuscular injections with special care.* Remember to: (1) use a small needle, (2) apply pressure to the site of the injection for several minutes following administration of the medication, and (3) examine the injection site for continued bleeding several hours following the injection.

> *Instruct the patient to carry an identification card* with him at all times stating: (1) the patient's blood disorder, (2) the name of the patient's doctor or clinic, and (3) the patient's blood type.

PURPURA

Purpura is defined as the extravasation of small amounts of blood into the tissues and mucous membranes. As you recall, the smallest hemorrhages are called *petechiae,* while larger hemorrhagic lesions are called *ecchymoses*. These two forms of bleeding may result from either vessel damage or rupture (vascular purpura) or a platelet deficiency (thrombocytopenic purpura).

Vascular Purpura

The major characteristic of vascular purpura is easy rupture of the smaller blood vessels upon any undue pressure, with resultant bleeding into the tissues. The causes of vascular purpura are many, e.g., heredity, allergy, exposure to drugs and poisons, poor nutrition, infection, and hypertension. Major forms of vascular purpura include the following:

Familial Hemorrhagic Telangiectasia. This hereditary condition is characterized by episodes of nosebleed or gastrointestinal bleeding and telangiectatic lesions (small red lesions of the skin and mucous membranes resulting from dilated capillaries, arterioles, or venules). There is no cure for this condition. Severe gastrointestinal tract hemorrhage is treated with iron therapy and transfusions.

Anaphylactoid Purpura (Allergic Purpura). This form of vascular purpura evidently arises from an *allergic reaction* that damages the vascular epithelium. Its major characteristic is acute or chronic inflammation of blood vessels supplying the skin, joints, gastrointestinal tract, and kidneys. Symptoms include arthritic pains, abdominal pain, hematuria, gastrointestinal hemorrhage, fever, and malaise. Treatment is symptomatic. Steroids are often used to relieve distress. Typically, attacks of the disease automatically subside within 1 to 6 weeks; however, episodes of bleeding tend to recur over the years.

Toxic Purpura. This condition is characterized by damage to blood vessels following exposure to certain medications and poisons (e.g., snake venom). Treatment involves identification and cessation of the offending drug.

Symptomatic or Secondary Purpuras. These disorders arise secondary to other diseases and are not caused by intrinsic or inherited disorders of the vasculature. Conditions that can result in secondary purpura include: (1) serious tissue trauma arising from a blow or a burn; (2) arterial hypertension resulting in increased capillary pressure; (3) blood stream infections that damage the vascular epithelium (e.g., subacute bacterial endocarditis); (4) scurvy (the result of vitamin C deficiency), which causes increased capillary fragility; and (5) uremia and cachexia, which, for unknown reasons, result in vessel weakness. The alleviation of the secondary purpuras is based upon treatment of the primary disorders.

Purpuras Due to Thrombocytopenia

The term "thrombocytopenia" means a *reduction in platelets below 200,000 per cu. mm.* The two major problems that follow a serious reduction in the platelet count are: (1) spontaneous bleeding into the skin, mucous membranes, and internal cavities and organs; and (2) oozing of long duration from tiny lacerations and needle pricks. The two

TABLE 62–4. LABORATORY TESTS USED IN THE DIAGNOSIS OF HEMORRHAGIC DISORDERS

Name of Test	Purpose	Normal Values	Interpretation of Findings
Bleeding time (Bl time)	Measures rate of platelet clot formation after small puncture wound	3–8 minutes in adults	Bleeding over 10 minutes abnormal; prolonged bleeding occurs in vascular maladies, thrombocytopenia, and after aspirin ingestion
Platelet count	Measures number of circulating platelets in venous or arterial blood	250,000–450,000/cu. mm.	Low count results in prolonged bleeding time and impaired clot retraction; diagnostic of thrombocytopenia
Partial thromboplastin time (PTT)	Complex method for testing normalcy of coagulation process; employed to identify deficiencies of coagulation factors, prothrombin, and fibrinogen	39–53 seconds	Prolongation of time indicates coagulation disorder due to deficiency of a coagulation factor; not diagnostic for platelet disorders
Prothrombin time (Pro time)	Determines activity and interaction of factors V, VII, X, prothrombin, and fibrinogen; used to determine dosages of anticoagulant drugs	12–15 seconds (one-stage method)	Prolongation of time indicates: patient receiving anticoagulants; abnormally low fibrinogen concentration; deficiencies of factors II, VII, V, and X; presence of circulating anticoagulants as seen in lupus erythematosus; impaired prothrombin activity
Coagulation (clotting time)	Crude measure of coagulation process in venous blood; used to control heparin therapy	9–12 minutes (Lee-White method)	Prolonged time occurs in: severe coagulation problems; therapeutic administration of heparin
Thrombin time	Measures functional fibrinogen available, as shown by time needed to form fibrin clot	10–13 seconds	Prolonged time indicates: hypofibrinogenemia; presence in blood of excess heparin or other anticoagulants
Thromboplastin generation test (TGT)	Measures generation of thromboplastin; if result abnormal, second stage is done to identify missing coagulation factor	12 seconds or less (100%)	Abnormal values found in hemophilia
Fibrinogen level	Measures level of fibrinogen in plasma	200–400 mg./100 ml.	Abnormally low values may indicate liver disease, congenital afibrinogenemia, or acquired afibrinogenemia
Clot retraction	Indicates function and number of platelets; measures time needed for contraction of an undisturbed clot	Clot retraction begins within 2 hours and is finished within 24 hours	Clot retraction retarded in thrombocytopenia; clot is small and soft in thrombasthenia (functional disturbance of platelets)
Tourniquet test (Rumple-Leeds test; capillary fragility test)	Crude test of vascular resistance and platelet number and function; done by placing blood pressure cuff on arm for 5 minutes and then counting petechiae	No petechiae	Petechiae appear in thrombocytopenia and vascular purpura

principal types of thrombocytopenia are: idiopathic thrombocytopenic purpura (ITP), and secondary thrombocytopenia.

Idiopathic Thrombocytopenic Purpura (ITP). The major characteristic of this bleeding disorder is the *premature destruction of platelets.* Normally platelets survive within the circulation for 8 to 10 days; however, platelet survival in ITP is as brief as 1 to 3 days or less. Although the exact etiology of ITP is unknown, the majority of authorities currently support the *autoimmune theory* of causation. For unidentified reasons *autoantibodies develop* which either interrupt megakaryocyte development (which then results in reduced platelet production) or sensitize platelets, so that they become more vulnerable to destruction by the spleen.

Acute ITP is primarily a disease of children; 85 per cent of patients are under 8 years of age. Chronic ITP affects persons of all ages. It is more common among females.

The onset of this disorder is often sudden and acute, but in most cases, ITP is characterized by remissions and exacerbations which, in untreated cases, may occur for years. Symptoms include petechiae, ecchymosis, epistaxis, bleeding from the gums, and easy bruising. Women may have extremely heavy menses or bleeding between periods. *Complications* of ITP include:

> Cerebral hemorrhage, which proves fatal in 1 to 5 per cent of patients.
> Severe hemorrhages from the nose, gastrointestinal tract, and urinary system.
> Bleeding into the diaphragm, which can result in pulmonary complications.
> Nerve pain, anesthesia of extremities, and/or paralysis as a result of the pressure of a hematoma upon nerves or brain tissues.

Laboratory findings which confirm the presence of ITP include: (1) a platelet count below 100,000 per cu.mm.; (2) prolonged bleeding time *but* normal coagulation time (all coagulation factors are present and normal); and (3) increased capillary fragility as demonstrated by the tourniquet test.

The two basic treatments for ITP are steroid therapy and splenectomy. *Steroids* are given to patients suffering from severe bleeding of short duration; they are also administered preoperatively prior to splenectomy. The purpose of steroid therapy in ITP is to reduce the bleeding tendency and to elevate the platelet count; however, steroids are rarely able to produce a permanent cure. The steroid of choice for this condition is:

> Prednisone, 10–20 mg. 4 times daily.

The treatment of choice for patients with ITP is *splenectomy.* In 60 to 80 per cent of patients removal of the spleen results in a complete and permanent remission. No one knows exactly why splenectomy is so successful. If the autoimmune hypothesis is correct, removal of the spleen probably halts the premature destruction of sensitized platelets. Since young children often recover spontaneously from ITP, pediatricians do not usually recommend splenectomy until the child is at least 6 years of age.

Nursing care for patients with ITP is directed toward observing for and preventing internal hemorrhage, particularly *cerebral hemorrhage.* Patients with severe ITP are usually placed on *bed rest* in order to prevent excessive activity and consequent exhaustion. It is extremely important to observe for and to prevent: *constipation,* which is accompanied by straining at stool, and *upper respiratory infections,* which lead to coughing and sneezing.

> Remember: *Both straining at stool and coughing cause an increase in intracranial pressure, which can result in cerebral hemorrhage.*

The *prognosis* for patients with ITP is good. Seventy-five per cent of children and 25 per cent of adults with this disorder recover spontaneously without any treatment.

Secondary Thrombocytopenic Purpuras. Unlike idiopathic (primary) thrombocytopenic purpura, the secondary thrombocytopenias have identifiable causes. For example, these purpuras may arise secondary to viral infections, bone marrow failure, the defibrination syndrome, disseminated lupus erythematosus, lymphoproliferative disorders, and infectious mononucleosis. Drug hypersensitivity is another important cause of thrombocytopenia. Common offending drugs include quinidine, quinine, the sulfonamides, phenylbutazone, and chlorothiazide derivatives. Symptoms and laboratory findings are the same as those found in ITP.

Treatment

Treatment of these conditions centers around the total removal or at least partial alleviation of the underlying cause as well as the control of bleeding. All potentially toxic drugs must be identified and discontinued. Usually the platelet count begins to rise in a few days and is normal within a week following removal of toxic agents. To control bleeding the physician may order the administration of *corticosteroids.*

When hemorrhage is severe, *platelet transfusions* are usually given. Unfortunately the beneficial effects of platelet transfusions are short lived. Donor platelets received during the first transfusion may survive for 5 or 6 days; however, platelets received in each subsequent transfusion have a shorter life span; consequently, platelet transfusions can be employed only as a short-term emergency measure. Unlike ITP, *splenectomy* is usually *contraindicated* in the treatment of the secondary thrombocytopenias because splenic malfunction is not a causative factor in these disorders.

COAGULATION DISORDERS

The coagulation disorders are characterized by a *defect in the clotting mechanism* resulting from the depletion or absence of one or more of the clotting factors. The three important coagulation disorders discussed here are the hemophilias, hypoprothrombinemia, and disseminated intravascular coagulation (the defibrination syndrome.).

The Hemophilias

The hemophilias are relatively common disorders characterized by prolonged bleeding, particularly following accidental, surgical, or dental trauma. There are three major types of hemophilia: hemophilia A (classic hemophilia), hemophilia B (Christmas disease), and von Willebrand's disease. The major characteristics of these three disorders are compared in Table 62–5. Because *classic hemophilia* is by far the most common of the hemophilias (includes 80 per cent of all hemophilia cases), our discussion of symptoms and treatment refers only to this type.

Hemophilia A is classified as a childhood disorder; however, because of new developments in treatment that prolong life, this disease now extends into the patient's adult years. Manifestations of hemophilia A include the following:

> *Slow, prolonged, persistent bleeding* from cuts, scratches, and other minor traumas, which may finally result in massive, deadly hemorrhage unless medically controlled.

> *Delayed hemorrhage* following trivial injuries. Bleeding may not start from a site until hours or even days have passed following the moment of trauma.

> Severe *hemorrhaging* from the gums following dental extraction or even brushing the teeth with a hard toothbrush.

> Severe, sometimes fatal, *epistaxis* following injury to the nose, e.g., a blow or "punch" on the nose.

> Overwhelming *gastric hemorrhage,* which may be linked with gastric disorders such as ulcers.

> Recurrent *hematomas,* which may form in the deep subcutaneous tissue, intramuscular tissues, and around the peripheral nerves. If nerves are compressed by the hematomas, the patient suffers severe pain, anesthesia of the innervated part, and sometimes permanent nerve damage, paralysis, and muscular atrophy.

> Recurrent *hemarthrosis* (bleeding into the joints) is common in untreated cases and may result in serious joint deformity and permanent crippling. Hemarthrosis affects the knees, ankles, elbows, wrists, fingers, hips, and shoulders, in that order.

The five goals of treatment for patients with hemophilia are: (1) to stop topical bleeding as quickly as possible; (2) to raise the level of antihemophilic factor (AHF) in the patient's plasma, thereby temporarily supplying the missing factor causing hemorrhage; (3) to prevent crippling deformities from hemarthrosis; (4) to prevent unnecessary trauma; and (5) to educate the patient.

Topical bleeding can usually be temporarily controlled by applying pressure to the injured site, packing the area with Gelfoam or fibrin foam, and applying topical hemostatics such as thrombin. However, to permanently halt the bleeding episode, fresh plasma or fresh whole blood must be administered to the patient in order to supply vitally needed AHF.

Because AHF deteriorates quickly, the blood must be given to the patient within 6 hours following withdrawal from the donor.

In addition to whole blood and plasma, AHF levels may also be raised by the administration of commercial AHF concentrates, e.g., cryoprecipitate, Hemophil, AHF, and Fibro-AHG. Concentrates are also available for supplying factors VII, IX, X, and prothrombin. Commercial concentrates rich in the missing factors are also administered *prophylactically* to patients prior to dental extractions and surgical procedures.

There is one major *complication* linked with repeated transfusion and AHF therapy: about 5 per cent of hemophiliacs become sensitized to AHF and develop *autoimmune anticoagulants (Anti-AHF factor).* In this unfortunate circumstance, the patient is totally unable to respond to transfusion therapy and consequently hemorrhages to death.

Hemarthrosis is usually treated with AHF or whole blood administration, resting the joint (sometimes in a protective cast), and packing ice around the joint. Analgesics such as aspirin and corticosteroids are often given to reduce joint pain and swelling. If pain is severe, the doctor may be forced to aspirate blood from the joint. Once bleeding stops

TABLE 62–5. A COMPARISON OF THE THREE FORMS OF HEMOPHILIA

Form of Hemophilia	Etiology	Transmission	Major Laboratory Findings
Hemophilia A (classic hemophilia)	Inherited Factor VIII (antihemophilic globulin) deficiency	Transmitted as a sex-linked *recessive* trait; transmitted by females; occurs in males and, rarely, homozygous females	Coagulation time prolonged but bleeding time normal; factor VIII missing from plasma
Hemophilia B (Christmas disease)	Inherited Factor IX (plasma thromboplastin component) deficiency	Transmitted as a sex-linked *recessive* trait; transmitted by females; occurs in males and, rarely, homozygous females	Laboratory findings and symptoms same as in hemophilia A.
Von Willebrand's disease	Inherited Factor VIII deficiency and defective platelet dysfunction	Transmitted as an autosomal *dominant* trait to both sexes; occurs in both males and females	Both coagulation time *and* bleeding time prolonged; low factor VIII levels; platelet adhesiveness decreased

and the swelling is reduced, the patient is encouraged to move the joint. However, the patient should be cautioned not to put weight on an affected lower extremity until swelling completely subsides and muscle strength is normal.

Prevention of injury is dependent upon certain precautionary nursing measures as well as a willingness on the part of the patient to live sensibly with his disorder. Points to remember when caring for persons with hemophilia are as follows:

- Teach young patients to avoid all unnecessary sources of trauma, e.g., elective surgery, contact sports.
- Instruct patients to always inform doctors, dentists, teachers, and employers that they have hemophilia. Of course, the patient must also carry an identifying card.
- Should surgery or tooth extraction be necessary, request the patient to ask friends and family to donate blood so that a sufficient amount of blood is on hand.
- When administering intramuscular injections, always check the injection site every hour for *several days* following the injection.

Remember: *In hemophilia, bleeding and hemorrhage are often delayed for substantial periods of time following trauma.*

The *prognosis* for patients with hemophilia has greatly improved since the discovery of AHF. Formerly, 50 per cent of patients with this disorder died before they reached their fifth birthday. Today, death rarely occurs as a result of bleeding from minor trauma. Fatalities mainly follow the development of autoimmune anticoagulants (anti-AHF factors) and bleeding into the retroperitoneal space following internal hemorrhage.

Hypoprothrombinemia

The term "hypoprothrombinemia" means that the amount of prothrombin circulating in the blood is deficient. *Prothrombin* is a complex globulin protein produced in the liver and normally found in the blood. For prothrombin synthesis to take place, *vitamin K* (a fat-soluble vitamin) must be present in the liver to act as a catalyst.

Hypoprothrombinemia develops as a result of the following problems:

- *Vitamin K deficiency.* This fat-soluble vitamin is normally obtained in a balanced diet; also (in all but the newborn) vitamin K is synthesized by certain intestinal tract bacteria. Once ingested or manufactured internally, vitamin K, because it is fat-soluble, is dependent upon the presence of *bile* for absorption. When absorbed, vitamin K is ready to catalyze prothrombin synthesis within the liver cells. Vitamin K *deficiency,* then, is the result of: (1) improper diet; (2) gastrointestinal tract disorders which interfere with the absorption of vitamin K (e.g., malabsorption syndrome and obstructive jaundice due to bile duct obstruction); (3) liver damage that is so extensive that the liver cells cannot produce bile or synthesize prothrombin; or (4) prolonged sulfonamide or antibiotic administration which sterilizes the bowel, thereby halting the manufacture of vitamin K by intestinal tract bacteria.
- *Overdosage with Dicumarol.* Bishydroxycoumarin (Dicumarol) is an effective anticoagulant used to reduce the danger of clot formation in persons with heart disease and peripheral vascular disorders. Dicumarol acts by interfering with the conversion of vitamin K to prothrombin within the liver cells. If dosage is excessive, the patient's prothrombin time is prolonged (usually below 40 or 50 per cent). If the prothrombin time drops below 10 to 15 per cent, the patient is in danger of bleeding or hemorrhaging spontaneously.

The major manifestations of hypoprothrombinemia are: ecchymosis following minimal trauma, epistaxis, postoperative hemorrhage from the incision, hematuria, gastrointestinal tract bleeding, and prolonged bleeding from a venipuncture. The outstanding laboratory finding is a *prolonged prothrombin time.*

Treatment of hypoprothrombinemia is directed at the underlying cause. For example, vitamin K deficiency as a result of malabsorption is corrected by the administration of a parenteral preparation of vitamin K. The two drugs of choice are:

- Menadione sodium bisulfite (Hykinone) 5 mg. daily I.M.
- Menadiol (Synkayvite) 5 mg. daily I.M.

If Dicumarol overdose is the underlying problem, anticoagulant therapy is stopped and the patient is given the following drug in order to normalize the prothrombin time:

- Phytonadione (fat-soluble vitamin K; Mephyton) 5 mg. orally for minor bleeding problems and 10 to 15 mg. of Aqua-Mephyton I.V. for hemorrhage.

Finally, if the prothrombin deficiency is the result of liver disease, prothrombin can temporarily be replaced directly by transfusion therapy.

Disseminated Intravascular Coagulation (DIC)

The term "disseminated intravascular coagulation" means diffuse or widespread coagulation within arterioles and capillaries all over the body. DIC is a complex and important coagulation disorder characterized by two apparently conflicting sets of manifestations: (1) *diffuse fibrin deposition* within arterioles and capillaries all over the body with resultant *widespread clotting;* and (2) *hemorrhage* from the kidneys, brain, adrenals, heart, and other organs. The disorder is sometimes called the "defibrination syndrome."

Fifty per cent of persons stricken with DIC are expectant mothers with toxemia of pregnancy or other obstetric complications, while 33 per cent of patients suffer from terminal cancer. Although the cause of DIC is unknown, possibly its onset is linked with the entry into the blood of thromboplastic substances (e.g., in metastatic cancer, obstetric complications, shock, sepsis, tissue damage from burns or trauma, and snake bites).

The pathologic chain of events characterizing

DIC apparently is as follows: (1) certain disease states (toxemia of pregnancy, cancer, etc.) cause the release of thromboplastic substances which evidently promote the deposition of fibrin throughout the microcirculation; (2) as a result, microthrombi form in the brain, kidneys, heart, and other organs, causing microinfarcts and tissue necrosis; (3) red cells become trapped in the fibrin strands and are destroyed (hemolysis); (4) platelets, prothrombin, and other clotting factors are consumed in the process, which then leads to bleeding; (5) the excessive clotting activates the fibrinolytic mechanism, which causes the production of fibrin split products; these end products act to inhibit platelet clotting functions, which causes further bleeding.

The onset of DIC is usually acute; chronic cases of DIC characteristically develop in persons with cancer or in mothers who are carrying a dead fetus. Manifestations may be either mild or extremely severe. Symptoms include the following:

> Petechiae and ecchymoses on the skin, mucous membranes, heart lining, lungs, etc.

> Prolonged bleeding from a venipuncture.

> Severe, uncontrollable hemorrhage during surgery or childbirth.

> Oliguria and acute renal failure.

> Convulsions and coma, which may terminate in death.

Laboratory findings, in severe cases of DIC, indicate that the hemostatic mechanism has failed totally. A prolonged prothrombin time, very low platelet count, and incoagulable blood are typical findings.

The clinical care of a patient with DIC involves: (1) treatment of the basic problem (e.g., shock, delivery of a fetus, surgery for or irradiation of cancer); (2) the reversal of pathologic clotting; and (3) the control of bleeding and shock. To reverse clotting, the physician usually orders:

> Heparin I.V., 100 USP units per kg. of body weight every 4 to 6 hours.

Blood transfusions are administered to replace blood and lessen shock. Finally, human fibrinogen is sometimes given in cases of severe fibrinolysis; however, human fibrinogen is a dangerous medication because it can cause *hepatitis*.

The prognosis for patients with DIC varies. The condition may be self-limiting, or the patient may die from hemorrhage and organ damage within a few days.

References

1. Allen, J.: Recurrent infections in man associated with immunologic or phagocytic deficiencies. *Postgraduate Medicine 50*:89, November, 1971.
2. Asperheim, M. K., and Eisenhauer, R. A.: *The Pharmacologic Basis of Patient Care*. 2nd ed. Philadelphia, W. B. Saunders Company, 1973.
3. Baker, C. G.: Assessments of new methods of cancer therapy. *Postgraduate Medicine 48*:119, November, 1970.
4. Beutler, E.: Sickle cell anemia: How to detect and combat it. *Consultant 12*:21–3, April, 1972.
5. Blackburn, E. K.: Acute leukaemia. *Nursing Times 67*: 509, April 29, 1971.
6. Boggs, D. R., and Winkelstein, A.: *White Cell Manual, 1971*. Seattle, University of Washington Press, 1971.
7. Bouchard, R., and Owens, N. F.: *Nursing Care of the Cancer Patient*. 2nd ed. St. Louis, The C. V. Mosby Company, 1972.
8. Brown, D.: The history of blood transfusion. *Nursing Mirror,* June 14, 1968, p. 19.
9. Brown, E. B.: Hypochromic anemias. *In* Beeson, P. B., and McDermott, W. (eds.): *Cecil-Loeb Textbook of Medicine*. 13th ed. Philadelphia, W. B. Saunders Company, 1971.
10. Buckwalter, J. A.: Blood coagulation and transfusion. *In* Leichty, R. D., and Saper, R. T. (eds.): *Synopsis of Surgery*. St. Louis, The C. V. Mosby Company, 1968.
11. Bull, B. S.: Disseminated intravascular coagulation. *In* Conn, H. F. (ed.): *Current Therapy 1972*. Philadelphia, W. B. Saunders Company, 1973.
12. *'73 Cancer Facts and Figures*. New York, American Cancer Society, 1970.
13. Chaplin, H.: Transfusion reactions. *In* Beeson, P. B., and McDermott, W. (eds.): *Cecil-Loeb Textbook of Medicine*. 13th ed. Philadelphia, W. B. Saunders Company, 1971.
14. Cole, W. H. (ed.): *Chemotherapy of Cancer*. Philadelphia, Lea & Febiger, 1970.
15. Conley, C. L.: The hemoglobinopathies and thalassemias. *In* Beeson, P. B., and McDermott, W. (eds.): *Cecil-Loeb Textbook of Medicine*. 13th ed. Philadelphia, W. B. Saunders Company, 1971.
16. Control of haemophilic bleeding. *Nursing Mirror 130*: 43, March 6, 1970.
17. Diggs, L. W.: Screening tests for sickle cell anemia. *Postgraduate Medicine 51*:267, February, 1972.

17a. Dison, N. G.: *An Atlas of Nursing Techniques*. 2nd ed. St. Louis, The C. V. Mosby Company, 1971.

18. Does Rh stand for trouble? *Emergency Medicine 2*: 67, March, 1970.
19. Donovan, J.: Reverse barrier nursing. *Nursing Times,* June 16, 1967, p. 791.
20. Finch, C. A.: *Red Cell Manual*. Seattle, University of Washington Press, 1970.
21. Foster, S.: Sickle cell anemia: Closing the gap between theory and therapy. *American Journal of Nursing 71*:1952, October, 1971.
22. French, R. M.: *Nurses' Guide to Diagnostic Procedures*. 3rd ed. New York, McGraw-Hill Book Company, Inc., 1971.
23. Govoni, L. E., and Hayes, J. E.: *Drugs and Nursing Implications*. 2nd ed. New York, Appleton-Century-Crofts, Inc., 1971.
24. Hanebuth, L.: When your patient has multiple myeloma. *R.N. 34*:36, August, 1971.
25. Harker, L. A.: *Hemostasis Manual*. Seattle, University of Washington Press, 1970.
26. Hatcher, J.: Blood platelets. *Nursing Mirror 132*:37, July 2, 1971.

27. Hillman, R. S.: *Hematology Laboratory Manual.* Seattle, University of Washington Press, 1970.
28. Hoffbrand, A. V.: Pernicious anemia. *In* Conn, H. F. (ed.): *Current Therapy 1973.* Philadelphia, W. B. Saunders Company, 1973.
29. Holvey, D. N., et al. (eds.): *The Merck Manual of Diagnosis and Therapy.* 12th ed. Rahway, N.J., Merck, Sharp and Dohme Research Laboratories, 1972.
30. Jacobs, P.: Tumours of bone. *Nursing Times 68*:1572, December 14, 1972.
31. Jandl, J. H.: Intestinal malabsorption. *In* Beeson, P. B., and McDermott, W. (eds.): *Cecil-Loeb Textbook of Medicine.* 13th ed. Philadelphia, W. B. Saunders Company, 1971.
32. Krupp, M. A., and Chatton, M. J.: *Current Diagnosis and Treatment.* Los Altos, California, Lange Medical Publications, 1972.
33. Leukemia: A Report on Research. New York, American Cancer Society, 1971.
34. Livingston, B. M., and Krakoff, I. H.: L-Asparaginase—a new kind of cancer drug. *American Journal of Nursing 70*:1910, September, 1970.
35. MacBryde, C. M., and Blacklow, R. S. (eds.): *Signs and Symptoms: Applied Pathologic Physiology and Clinical Interpretation.* 5th ed. Philadelphia, J. B. Lippincott Company, 1972.
36. Malpas, J. S.: The functions of the spleen. *Nursing Times,* September 13, 1968, p. 1224.
37. Markson, J. L.: The anaemias: Introduction, Part 1. *Nursing Times 67*:1611, December 9, 1971.
38. Markson, J. L.: Pernicious Anaemia, Part 2. *Nursing Times 67*:1562, December 16, 1971.
39. Markson, J. L.: Haemolytic anaemia. Part 3. *Nursing Times 67*:1611, December 23, 1971.
40. Markson, J. L.: Aplastic anemia. Part 4. *Nursing Times 67*:1624–5, December 30, 1971.
41. Metka, R. J., et al.: *Nursing Care of Outpatients with Acute Leukemia.* (DHEW # (NIH) 72–94). Bethesda, Md., National Institutes of Health, November, 1971, pp. 1–22.
42. Miller, B. F., and Keane, C. B.: *Encyclopedia and Dictionary of Medicine and Nursing.* Philadelphia, W. B. Saunders Company, 1972.
43. Moore, C. V.: Diseases of the white blood cells and reticuloendothelial system. *In* Beeson, P. B., and McDermott, W. (eds.): *Cecil-Loeb Textbook of Medicine.* 13th ed. Philadelphia, W. B. Saunders Company, 1971.
44. Moore, C. V.: Hematologic and hematopoietic diseases: Introduction. *In* Beeson, P. B., and McDermott, W. (eds.): *Cecil-Loeb Textbook of Medicine.* 13th ed. Philadelphia, W. B. Saunders Company, 1971.
45. Moore, C. V.: The Anemias. *In* Beeson, P. B., and McDermott, W. (eds.): *Cecil-Loeb Textbook of Medicine.* 13th ed. Philadelphia, W. B. Saunders Company, 1971.
45a. Osserman, E. F.: Plasma cell dyscrasias. *In* Beeson, P. B., and McDermott, W. (eds.): *Cecil-Loeb Textbook of Medicine.* 13th ed. Philadelphia, W. B. Saunders Company, 1971.
46. Notter, D., et al.: *General Medicine.* Seattle, University of Washington School of Medicine, 1970.
47. Petty, T. L.: Pulmonary lesions that are not tubercular. *Consultant 11*:56, November, 1971.
48. Phelan, E. W.: *Radioisotopes in Medicine.* (Booklet in Understanding the Atom Series.) Washington, D.C., U.S. Atomic Energy Commission, Division of Technical Information, 1966.
49. Pochedly, C.: Sickle cell anemia: Recognition and management. *American Journal of Nursing 71*:1948, October, 1971.
50. Ratnoff, O. D.: Heritable disorders of blood coagulation. *In* Beeson, P. B., and McDermott, W. (eds.): *Cecil-Loeb Textbook of Medicine.* 13th ed. Philadelphia, W. B. Saunders Company, 1971.
51. Robbins, S. L., and Angell, M.: *Basic Pathology.* Philadelphia, W. B. Saunders Company, 1971.
52. Rodman, M. J.: Anticancer chemotherapy against the leukemias and lymphomas. Part 3. *R.N. 35*:49–50, April, 1972.
53. Rosenfield, R. E., et al.: Transfusion reactions. *In* Conn, H. F. (ed.): *Current Therapy 1972.* Philadelphia, W. B. Saunders Company, 1972.
54. Shanbrom, E.: Critique of lab medicine. *Medical Counterpoint.* December, 1971, p. 30.
55. Sickle Cell Anemia. *Medical World News,* December 3, 1971, p. 37.
56. Smith, S. E.: Drug therapy 1972: Drugs and the blood. Part 5. *Nursing Times 63*:383, March 30, 1972.
57. Snively, W. D., and Beshear, D. R.: *Textbook of Pathophysiology.* Philadelphia, J. B. Lippincott Company, 1972.
58. Stefanini, M.: Diffuse intravascular coagulation versus fibrinolysis. *Postgraduate Medicine 51*:215, April, 1972.
59. Sutton, A. L.: *Bedside Nursing Techniques in Medicine and Surgery.* 2nd ed. Philadelphia, W. B. Saunders Company, 1969.
60. Tolley, R. W.: Chemotherapy of solid tumors. *Postgraduate Medicine 48*:182, November, 1970.
61. Valentine, W. N.: Infectious mononucleosis. *In* Beeson, P. B., and McDermott, W. (eds.): *Cecil-Loeb Textbook of Medicine.* 13th ed. Philadelphia, W. B. Saunders Company, 1971.
62. Vaz, D. D. S.: The common anemias: Nursing approaches. *Nursing Clinics of North America 7*:711, December, 1972.
63. Waters, W. E.: Anaemia in women. *Nursing Mirror 134*:20, April 28, 1972.
64. Wessler, S., and Alexander, B.: A Guide to Anticoagulant Therapy. (Pamphlet prepared for the Committee on Medical Education of the American Heart Association.) New York, American Heart Association, 1970.
65. What is iron deficiency? *Nursing Mirror 130*:29, April 17, 1970.
66. Wheby, M. S.: Anemia due to iron deficiency. *In* Conn, H. F. (ed.): *Current Therapy 1973.* Philadelphia, W. B. Saunders Company, 1973.
67. Whitehead, J. A., and Chohan, M. M.: Paraphrenia and pernicious anemia. *Geriatrics 27*:148, May, 1972.
68. Whitehouse, J. M. A.: The leukaemias: Acute leukaemia. Part 1, *Nursing Times 68*:703–6, June 8, 1972.
69. Whitehouse, J. M. A.: Chronic leukaemias. Part 2. *Nursing Times 68*:737, June 15, 1972.
70. Wilson, P.: Iron-deficiency anemia. *American Journal of Nursing 72*:502–4, March, 1972.

UNIT XIII

Nursing Patients Experiencing Disturbances of Peripheral Vascular Function

Joan Luckmann, Marie Cowan, and Rosemary Pittman

Introduction and Study Guide

The study of peripheral vascular disease focuses upon disorders of the arteries, veins, and the lymphatics; it also focuses upon the tissue trauma that develops when the vascular system is damaged. More specifically, this unit covers diseases of the aorta, functional and organic diseases of the arteries and veins, and the anatomy and physiology relative to these disorders. Since the lymphatic system is closely related to the circulatory system, common lymphatic disorders are also discussed. Also, lower limb amputations are considered in this section because amputation may be necessary when peripheral vascular damage results in gangrene.

Although we discuss disorders of the aorta as well as conditions affecting the hands (e.g., Raynaud's disease and Raynaud's phenomenon), the primary emphasis in this unit is upon disease of the lower extremities. Also heavily stressed is the role of *atherosclerosis* in vascular disease. In Unit X we pointed out that atherosclerosis is a disorder of lipid metabolism which is characterized by deposits of fat-containing substances along the intima of blood vessels. Peripheral arterial disease must be looked at in relationship to atherosclerosis because the majority of arterial disorders are due to this important disease process. Atherosclerosis is a lifelong process and is not a single lesion or syndrome. The disease begins in infancy and progresses in episodic fashion over the individual's entire life.

Peripheral vascular diseases are an important group of disorders because they are so common. Few members of our population will escape some degree of vascular degeneration as they pass through the aging process. The majority of patients afflicted with vascular problems are middle-aged or older. They often suffer from other diseases that affect their vessels, e.g., diabetes, heart disease. Also, these patients are often depressed, and with good reason. Vascular diseases are usually chronic, painful, incapacitating and debilitating. Moreover, long-term medical care is costly, causing a severe strain on family finances. Patients with vascular disturbances need psychologic support as well as physical care.

The role of the nurse in caring for patients with peripheral vascular disease focuses heavily on patient education. Vascular conditions usually cannot be cured; however, extensive tissue damage can often be prevented by teaching the patient a number of simple measures for increasing his circulation. To reverse or at least to control the advance of vascular disease, nurse, doctor, and patient must all work closely together in developing a total plan of care that the patient will carry on at home and throughout his life.

Objectives for the student of this unit are as follows:

1. The student should be familiar with the definitions of the following words:

ischemia, intermittent claudication, rest pain, rubor, trophic changes, gangrene, aneurysm, acute arterial occlusion, thromboangiitis obliterans, functional vascular disease, Raynaud's phenomenon, bypass graft, varicosities, venous insufficiency, thrombophlebitis, phlebothrombosis, vein ligation, embolectomy, lymphadenopathy, lymphadema, lymphangitis.

2. At the end of the unit, the student should be able to do the following:

   a. Detect deviation from normal in the peripheral vascular system.

   b. Recognize the importance of taking the pulse in the posterior tibia and dorsalis pedis arteries and of comparing the limbs for symmetry; discover the patient's sensitivity to cold, nutritional damage as shown by lack of hair, tissue atrophy, and nail changes, and symptoms of numbness and pain on exercise or rest.

   c. Interpret to patient the pathologic changes that are occurring and assist him in understanding diagnostic tests and his treatment plan.

   d. Assist the patient in establishing a meticulous care plan for the affected limbs, as well as a plan for changing those life patterns that contribute to the exacerbation of his disease.

   e. Assist in establishment of the overall care plan for the patient.

3. The student should understand the pathophysiology of the peripheral arterial, venous, and lymphatic systems.

4. The student should understand the symptoms, diagnosis, and treatment of disease processes affecting these systems.

CHAPTER 63

Introductory Concepts

ANATOMY AND PHYSIOLOGY OF THE PERIPHERAL VASCULAR SYSTEM

The Structure of the Vascular System

Blood flow is essential to life. It is dependent upon the efficiency of the heart as a pump and the patency of the blood vessels. Circulation is influenced by viscosity, hydration, mechanisms affecting coagulation and fibrinolysis, local changes in the size of the vessels, as well as iatrogenic, inflammatory, and neurogenic processes.

Vessels are grouped into six categories: (1) the *aorta* and large *arteries,* which constitute a distribution system; (2) the *arterioles,* sometimes called the resistance vessels, which act as a regulating system; (3) the *microcirculation,* in which metabolites pass to and from the tissues across the endothelium of capillaries; (4) a collecting system of *veins* carrying blood to the heart; (5) the *larger veins* acting as a storage system; and (6) *lymphatic vessels,* which collect lymph from the tissues and return it to the blood at the junction of the internal jugular and subclavian veins.

The *anatomic pattern* of the blood vessels of the upper and lower extremities is similar. A large main artery (axillary, external iliac) enters the limbs and runs the length of the proximal segment (brachial, femoral). In the lower limb there is an additional major source of supply to the buttocks through the obturator and gluteal branches of the internal iliac artery. At the elbow or knee the main artery divides into two branches (radial and anterior and posterior tibial), which supply the forearm or leg and finally anastomose to form the plantar or palmar arch. From these arteries the digital arteries run to the fingers or toes. In sum, main arterial trunks give off branches, and each branch gives off further branches of arteries of smaller caliber until, from the smallest arteries, the blood passes into the arterioles and then into capillaries, where it nourishes the tissues. *Arterioles* are small thick-walled vessels with an overall diameter of about 0.2 cm. and are important regulators of the peripheral circulation. *Capillaries* are thin-walled vessels from 5 to 10 μ in diameter. Red blood cells must alter their shape to pass through the smallest of these vessels. From the capillaries the blood flows into the venules and then into the veins. The main venous drainage of the upper and lower limbs is similar and is through a superficial and deep set of veins. *Arteriovenous anastomoses* are special structures present only in certain sites. They are generally believed to regulate both local and general temperature.

Except for capillaries, all blood vessels are similar in *structure.* They consist of an outer layer of connective tissue (the *adventitia*), a middle coat (the *media*), and an endothelial lining called the *intima.* Between the media and intima there is a well-defined layer of elastic tissue named the internal elastic lamina. *Veins* have a thinner medial coat than the arteries, a greater proportion of white fibrous tissue, and less muscle and elastic tissue. Also, veins contain valves that direct the blood proximally. Finally, the walls of *capillaries* consist of two components: endothelial cells and a basement membrane surrounded by a pericapillary sheath of connective tissue.

Factors Regulating the Peripheral Vascular System

All arteries are contractile in that they can decrease (vasoconstriction) or increase (vasodilatation) their caliber in response to appropriate stimuli. The mechanism regulating vasomotor activity is complex, consisting of central nervous influences, chemical substances in the blood stream, and the autonomous action of the arterial wall itself.

Vascular Nerves. There is evidence that the *hypothalamus* is the chief regulating center for peripheral vasomotor activity, but the cerebral center also exerts some influence.

Arteries have a relatively rich nerve supply from the sympathetic nervous system. Stimulation of the sympathetic nerves causes vasoconstriction and sympathectomy causes vasodilatation. Evidence for the presence of sympathetic vasodilator nerves to the blood vessels of the skin is unsatisfactory, but there is good evidence that both constrictor and dilator nerves supply the muscles.

Hormonal and Chemical Control. There are three powerful substances within the blood that help to control the caliber of blood vessels; they are epinephrine, norepinephrine, and angiotensin II.* *Epinephrine* constricts superficial blood vessels, but in small doses dilates vessels supplying the muscles, brain, and heart. *Norepinephrine* constricts all blood vessels; it particularly affects the

---

*Epinephrine and norepinephrine are discussed in Unit XIX.

peripheral vessels. *Angiotensin* is a substance formed by the interaction of renin and a serum globulin fraction; it constricts arteries.

Local Regulatory Mechanisms. The following substances act locally on blood vessels, although they circulate in the systemic circulation:

> *Histamine* is a potent vasodilator of small blood vessels, although it may also constrict the large arteries.

> *Bradykinin* is one of a group of vasoactive peptides and is a powerful vasodilator, especially of cutaneous vessels.

> *Muscle metabolites* have a strong vasodilator action.

> *Acetylcholine* is another vasodilator substance, but its action is transient and is more apparent in the face and upper limbs than in the lower limbs.

> *Serotonin* is liberated from platelets that stick to the vessel wall in the injured area. It is a powerful constrictor of cutaneous arterioles but dilates capillaries.

> *Vasopressin,* often called the antidiuretic hormone (ADH), is secreted by the posterior pituitary and released into the blood stream by impulses in the nerves from the hypothalamus. In large doses, vasopressin elevates arterial blood pressure by action of the smooth muscles of the arterioles. Vasopressin is probably not secreted in amounts sufficient to produce appreciable vasoconstriction.

In addition, trauma to an artery causes it to constrict. Also, moderate *heat* dilates the arteries; *cold* constricts isolated segments of the artery, but after 10 to 15 minutes the cooled artery relaxes.

Vasomotor Reflexes. The principal vasomotor reflexes observed in the limbs are those concerned with regulation of *body temperature*. The degree of vasodilatation following the application of heat may be measured by recording skin temperature of fingers or toes, but accurate measurements of blood using a plethysmograph are preferable. In a normal person, indirect vasodilatation in the hands always follows when the trunk or the legs are placed in warm water.

Blood Flow

Understanding of blood flow to the different parts of the circulation is still limited. Within the systemic circulation, blood flows from the left ventricle into the aorta, to the arteries, arterioles, capillaries, venules, veins and, finally, into the right atrium of the heart, and so forth. Blood always flows in this direction because a *blood pressure gradient* exists within the vascular system. Because a fluid always flows from a high pressure area to a low pressure area, blood flows from the aorta (in which the blood pressure is around 100 mm. Hg) to veins (which have a blood pressure of only 1 to 6 mm. Hg) (Fig. 63–1).

Within the venous system, blood flow (which is against gravity) depends not only upon the blood pressure gradient, but also upon valves located within the veins and the pumping action of mus-

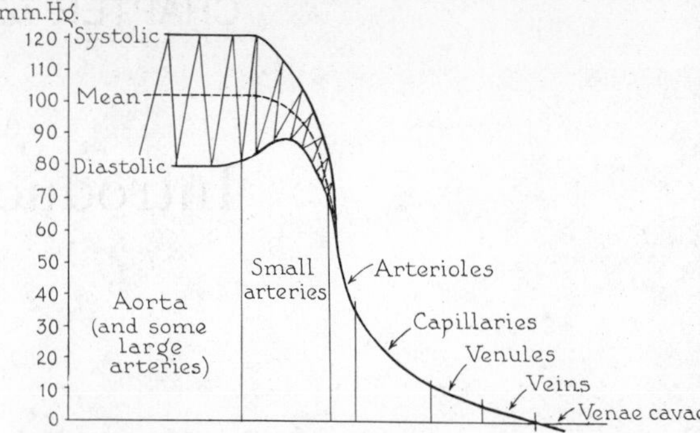

FIGURE 63–1. Diagram showing pressure gradients in different divisions of the circulatory system. (From King, B. G., and Showers, M. J.: Human Anatomy and Physiology. 6th ed. 1969.)

cles surrounding the veins. Venous blood flow is described in more detail in Chapter 65.

The flow of blood in the blood vessels is normally *laminar*. Within the blood vessels a thin layer of blood in contact with the vessel does not move. The next layer has a small velocity, the velocity being highest in the center of the stream. Laminar flow occurs at velocities up to a certain critical value. At or above this velocity, flow is turbulent. Streamline flow is silent, but turbulent flow creates sounds. Turbulence occurs more frequently in anemia because the viscosity of the blood is lower. Viscosity depends for the most part on the hematocrit. At any one time only 5 per cent of the circulating blood is in the capillaries, but in a sense it is the most important part because it is across the systemic capillary walls that oxygen and nutrients enter the interstitial fluid and carbon dioxide and waste products enter the blood stream.

The capacity of tissues to regulate their own blood flow is called *autoregulation*. The *myogenic theory of autoregulation* suggests that regulation probably results from the intrinsic contractile response of smooth muscle to stretch. As the blood pressure rises, the blood vessels are distended and the vascular smooth muscle fibers that surround the vessel contract. The blood vessel closes when the pressure of blood flowing through falls below 70.

ETIOLOGY AND PATHOPHYSIOLOGY OF PERIPHERAL VASCULAR DISEASE

All peripheral vascular diseases are characterized by disturbances of blood flow through the peripheral vessels that eventually result in damage to tissues of the extremities. As we stated before, blood flow is essential to life and health. The arterial flow of blood carries oxygen and nutrients to tissues; venous flow carries away cellular wastes; and lymphatic flow conveys tissue fluid back to the general circulation. When blood flow is inadequate, cells and tissues become malnourished because of oxygen lack and choked with wastes and excessive fluid as a result of venous or lymphatic stasis.

Basically, whether blood flow is adequate depends upon the following five factors:

> The efficiency of the heart's pumping action.
> The condition of the blood vessels (whether patent, dilated, or constricted).
> The rate of blood flow.
> The needs of the tissues for oxygen and nutrients as well as for removal of waste products.
> Nervous system activity.

The Role of the Heart

We stressed in Unit X that blood flow ultimately depends upon the continuous and efficient pumping of blood by the heart to all parts of the body. When, for any reason, the heart begins to fail as a pump, blood flow becomes abnormal. Recall that in left-sided failure, blood backs up into the lungs, causing congestion coupled with a decrease in cardiac output; these factors, in turn, reduce blood flow to the more peripheral vessels. When the right side of the heart fails, the patient suffers from severe venous congestion within the liver, gastrointestinal tract, and kidneys as well as edema of the ankles and lower extremities. Eventually, with failure of both the right and left pumps, the patient suffers severe malnutrition of tissues as a result of venous congestion and low cardiac output. In the end, the patient usually dies in severe shock and circulatory collapse.

The Role of the Blood Vessels

Arteries. To carry the blood adequately, arteries must be patent and they must be capable of dilating and constricting normally in response to thermal, hormonal, neural, and chemical stimulation. When arteries become obstructed or damaged, there is a decreased flow of oxygen and nutrients to the tissues, which leads to *ischemia* (a temporary and localized deficiency of blood to tissues), malnutrition of tissues, and, ultimately, tissue necrosis and gangrene. Causes of arterial narrowing and obstruction include the following: atherosclerosis and arteriosclerosis;* arterial thrombosis and emboli; damage due to chemical or physical agents; infectious processes; vasospastic disorders (also called functional disorders) which cause constriction of blood vessels, e.g., Raynaud's disease; and congenital malformation.

Whether the patient with arterial occlusion will develop tissue necrosis and gangrene depends upon the *extensiveness* of the block as well as upon the *speed* at which arterial obstruction develops. For example, total or near total occlusion of an artery by a thrombus or embolus is far more critical than is the partial narrowing of an artery as a result of arteriosclerotic changes. Likewise, the patient with an arterial obstruction which develops swiftly has a much poorer prognosis than does the patient with arteries which have gradually narrowed over the years. The gradual development of arterial disease is less dangerous because *collateral circulation* (the growth of new vessels to replace many of the damaged ones) has had an opportunity to develop.

Veins. The efficiency of veins in returning blood to the heart depends upon patency of the veins, competent valves within the veins, and adequate pumping action of the muscles surrounding the veins. Blood flow through the veins can be slowed by the following:

> *Defective valves,* which usually result either from *stretching* of the veins as a result of prolonged venous pressure or from *inflammation* of the veins. Defective valves eventually result in *varicose veins* (which are dilated, tortuous superficial veins) and in *venous insufficiency.* (See Chapter 65.)
> *Thrombus formation* within the veins, which may be caused by either stasis of blood flow, hypercoagulability of the blood, or damage to the endothelial lining of the veins.* Venous thrombi may or may not be accompanied by inflammation. The greatest danger when thrombophlebitis (thrombus formation with inflammation) or phlebothrombosis (venous thrombosis without inflammation) occurs is that the clot will break free of the vessel wall and travel as a deadly embolus to the heart, lungs, or brain.

Blockage of blood through the veins (whether caused by venous insufficiency, inflammation, or a blood clot) results in *increased venous pressure.* Increased venous pressure, in turn, causes the hydrostatic pressure to rise within the capillaries, which decreases the amount of fluid that the capillaries can reabsorb from the tissues. *Edema* results. Edematous congested tissues cannot receive the oxygen and metabolites which they need; also waste products, which cannot be transported back into the circulation, build up within the swollen tissues. The consequence of severe venous stasis is *malnutrition* of tissue. Malnourished tissue is highly susceptible to bacterial infection; consequently, patients with venous insufficiency are susceptible to *leg ulcers* and *cellulitis.*

Lymphatics. The lymphatic system drains intracellular fluid from the interstitial spaces and routes it back to the circulation. *Obstruction* of lymphatic flow can result from infection of lymphatic structures, trauma to lymphatic vessels, and blockage of the lymphatics by tumors. The most outstanding manifestation of lymphatic obstruction is *edema,* which is often massive in nature. Important disorders of the lymphatic system include localized lymphadenopathy, generalized lymphadenopathy, lymphedema, and tuberculosis of the lymphatic system.

Rate of Blood Flow

The rate of blood flow controls the amount of oxygen and nutrients that the tissues receive. When the blood flow through the vessels is seriously de-

*Atherosclerosis and arteriosclerosis are described at length in Chapter 51 as well as in Chapter 64.

*Thrombus formation is discussed in Chapters 27 and 47 as well as in Chapter 65 of this unit.

creased, the tissues which those vessels supply become ischemic and malnourished. Major causes of a decrease in the *rate* of blood flow include: (1) increased viscosity of blood as a result of polycythemia or dehydration; (2) atherosclerotic narrowing of the arteries; (3) spasm of the arterial walls as in hypertension; and (4) decreased pumping action of muscles surrounding the veins, which can result from immobility.

Metabolic Needs of Tissues

The needs of the tissues for blood and oxygen are *constantly changing,* depending upon the individual's activity level, his thermal environment, and his state of health. When the metabolic needs of the body *increase,* more blood flow to tissues is needed and the arteries normally *dilate.* When the metabolic needs of the tissues *decrease,* the needs of the tissues for blood also decrease and the vessels *constrict.*

Body tissues demand a *greater* than normal blood flow under the following conditions:

> *Increased physical activity* or strenuous exercise, which raises the needs of tissues for oxygen and the demands of the tissues for blood.

> The direct application of *heat* to a part of the body (e.g., a hot water bottle or heating pad), which results in arterial dilatation; an increased blood flow to the tissues exposed to the source of heat; and the consequent dissipation of excess heat.

> *Infection,* which leads to dilatation of the vessels supplying the involved tissues, resulting in more protective antibodies and leukocytes being conveyed to the infected site.

On the other hand, tissues require a *smaller* than normal blood flow under these circumstances:

> *Decreased physical activity* or rest, which lowers the tissue's needs for oxygen.

> *Chilling* of the body or direct application of cold (e.g., an ice pack) to a body part, which results in vasoconstriction, decreased blood flow to the chilled part, and the conservation of body heat.

Normally blood vessels, by dilating and constricting, are able to vary the amount of blood that the tissues of the extremities receive. However, sclerosed, obstructed, damaged, inelastic blood vessels are unable to dilate and constrict normally; consequently these vessels fail to supply tissues with the additional blood that they require when physical exercise increases, heat is applied, or infection develops. For this reason, patients with peripheral vascular disease experience pain in their legs upon walking, tissue damage when heat is applied directly to an extremity, and leg ulcers and cellulitis when infection develops.

Nervous System Activity

Blood flow also depends upon *sympathetic nervous system stimulation.* Stimulation of the sympathetic nervous system results in *vasoconstriction* and decreased blood flow to the tissues of the extremities. *Removal* of sympathetic nervous system stimulation by adrenergic blocking agents or by lumbar sympathectomy (an operation which interrupts sympathetic nerves) causes vasodilatation and increased blood flow to the extremities.

In sum, any factor that narrows, obstructs, or damages the blood vessels impedes blood flow. When blood flow slows, tissue nutrition decreases, cellular waste products increase, ischemia develops, and the danger of thrombus and embolus formation escalates. Without treatment, tissue damage may advance to the point of cellulitis, leg ulceration, or gangrene.

BASES OF SYMPTOMS

Patients with peripheral vascular disease all experience *ischemia.* Consequently, despite the wide variety of specific peripheral vascular disorders, patients with vascular problems suffer from many of the same symptoms. The most common nonspecific manifestations of peripheral vascular disease and their bases are listed on the opposite page.

CLINICAL CARE OF PATIENTS WITH PERIPHERAL VASCULAR DISEASE: OVERVIEW

As a general rule, patients with peripheral vascular disease suffer from one or more of the following problems: (1) decreased arterial blood flow to peripheral tissues; (2) venous stasis; (3) prolonged vasoconstriction; (4) vascular obstruction; (5) ischemic pain; and (6) tissue damage (either ulcerations, infections, or gangrene). Consequently the five major goals of care are as follows:

1. *Increase arterial blood flow to the extremities and increase venous return to the heart.*
2. *Promote vasodilatation.*
3. *Prevent and treat vascular obstruction.*
4. *Relieve ischemic pain.*
5. *Prevent tissue damage and infection and promote healing of ulcerated areas.*

Goal 1: Increase Arterial Blood Flow and Venous Return

The principal methods for augmenting the patient's circulation are proper positioning, prescribed exercise, and patient education.

Positioning. To safely position a patient with peripheral vascular disease, you must first learn whether his disorder is arterial or venous in nature. Patients with *arterial* blood disorders suffer from a deficit of oxygenated blood to their extremities. Because blood flows to *dependent* parts of the body (i.e., parts lower than the heart), position individuals with arterial disease so that blood flows toward their legs and feet. In serious cases of arterial insufficiency, the doctor may order the *head* of the patient's bed to be elevated on six-inch blocks so that blood from the heart flows more easily to the extremities whenever the patient is asleep or resting. In milder cases, patients can benefit from simply sitting for periods of time with their feet flat on the floor. Remind all patients with arterial insufficiency to avoid raising their feet above heart level unless this is specifically prescribed by their physician as an exercise measure. (See Buerger-Allen exercises below.)

In contrast to arterial disease, patients with *venous insufficiency* suffer from a pooling of deoxygenated blood in their extremities and poor venous return to the heart. To overcome the pull of gravity which further impedes venous return, instruct the patient with venous stasis to elevate his legs above heart level frequently and to avoid prolonged standing or sitting. Also, these individuals should sleep with the *foot* of the bed elevated on six-inch blocks.

Teach patients with either arterial or venous insufficiency to avoid standing in any one position for more than a few minutes because prolonged standing interferes with circulation.

Exercise. A moderate prescribed program of exercise and rest is a most helpful method for increasing the circulation. For example, the patient often benefits from taking short walks followed by periods of rest. Tell the patient to let pain be his guide to the amount of activity he should undertake. Pain in the extremities signals the patient that he is not receiving enough oxygen to the muscles

SYMPTOMS OF PERIPHERAL VASCULAR DISEASE

Symptoms	*Bases of Symptoms*
Intermittent claudication (severe pain in the calf muscles which occurs upon walking or exercise of the limbs, and which is relieved by rest)	Exercise increases the metabolic needs of tissues; damaged arteries are unable to dilate and supply the tissues with oxygen; evidently ischemia coupled with a build-up of lactic acid creates a painful muscle spasm which forces the patient to stop walking or exercising
Rest pain (pain in the extremities which occurs when the patient is resting)	Sudden blockage of a vessel by a thrombus or embolus or severe arterial disease may so reduce the blood supply to the tissues of the extremities that the patient experiences ischemic pain even at rest
Coldness and pallor of the extremities	An adequate blood supply gives the tissues a rosy hue; also, the warmth of the blood warms the extremities; when blood flow is deficient, the extremities feel cold and look pale; when a patient with peripheral vascular disease raises his legs above heart level, his extremities appear even whiter (blanching) because arterial blood flow is more critically reduced
Rubor (tissues of the extremities are reddish blue in color)	Rubor indicates peripheral vessel damage which is so severe that the vessels are no longer able to constrict, but remain *permanently dilated;* rubor typically develops after prolonged anoxia or exposure to severe cold
Cyanosis or blueness of the tissues	When the blood contains too little oxygen, the tissues turn a bluish color, indicating the presence of abnormal amounts of deoxygenated hemoglobin
Trophic changes (adverse changes in the skin and nails of the extremities; e.g., dryness, scaling of the skin, brittle toenails)	The word *trophic* pertains to nutrition; thus, trophic changes in peripheral vascular disease result from prolonged ischemia and malnutrition of tissues
Leg ulcers and cellulitis	Venous stasis is a consequence of venous insufficiency; stagnant blood pooling in the tissues of the extremities provides an excellent medium for bacterial growth and resultant infection and ulcerations
Gangrenous changes (death and decay of tissues of the extremities)	Severe and prolonged ischemia due to complete or almost total stoppage of blood flow to a part results in gangrene

and tissues of his legs. If a patient experiences severe discomfort in the calf of his leg after walking a block, then he should stop and rest before walking further.

A popular form of exercise for patients with vascular disorders is the *Buerger-Allen routine.*

> These exercises are divided into three parts. First, the patient lies on a bed or couch and elevates both feet on a special board for from a half minute to 3 minutes. A straight-backed chair may be used instead of the board, with the top of the chair back and the front of the seat resting on the bed or couch. The chair back or board should be padded with a pillow or other soft material.
>
> The patient then sits on the edge of the bed or couch with his legs spread out and relaxed and the heels resting on the floor. He bends the feet up and down as far as possible, and then turns the feet inward and outward. After this, he bends the toes up and spreads them, then down to close them. Each set of movements should be continued about 3 minutes. The feet should become entirely pink. If they should become blue or painful, the patient should lie down and elevate the feet until rested.
>
> Following this, the patient lies down with the legs horizontal and covered to keep them warm; he remains in this position for about 5 minutes.

Patients who cannot perform active postural exercises such as the Buerger-Allen routine or who have severe circulatory involvement of the lower extremities may benefit from using an *oscillating* bed. This electrically operated bed (also called the "rocking bed") rocks up and down in smooth continuous cycles of approximately three minutes each. The motion of the bed is such that the patient's feet are first raised about six inches above the horizontal position, and then lowered about 12 to 15 inches, then raised, then lowered, and so forth. This steady rocking motion provides the patient with continuous passive postural exercise.

If the doctor orders an oscillating bed for your patient, give the following instructions and care:

> Explain the purpose of the oscillating bed to the patient; reassure him that his circulation will improve with the use of the bed and that pain and discomfort in his legs will lessen.

> Show the patient how to operate the switch which rocks the bed; tell him to stop the bed for a short time should he develop dizziness or nausea—symptoms which are sometimes experienced when the bed is first used.

> Encourage the patient to operate the bed the majority of the time—both night and day, with the exception of mealtimes.

> Place a padded footboard at the foot of the bed to support the patient's feet.

Although exercise may help the majority of patients with vascular disorders, there are some patients for whom exercise is absolutely contraindicated. Patients who must not exercise are those with *leg ulcers, cellulitis,* or *gangrene.* As you recall, exercise and activity increase the metabolic needs of tissues and consequently tissue requirements for oxygenated blood. For this reason, patients with tissue breakdown or necrosis are placed on bed rest; even minimal activity raises the oxygen requirements of their tissues above that which their damaged arteries can provide.

Strict bed rest is also ordered for patients with *arterial or venous thrombosis.* Activity is dangerous because a thrombus could become detached and travel as an embolus to the heart, lungs, or brain.

Patient Education. Patients with peripheral vascular disease need special instruction in how to increase circulation to their extremities and prevent venous stasis. Four rules you should emphasize to all patients with vascular problems are as follows:

1. Avoid obesity; extra pounds exhaust the heart, decrease circulation, and increase venous congestion.
2. Avoid standing in any position for an extended period of time; prolonged standing promotes venous stasis.
3. Never wear constricting clothes: e.g., garters, girdles, tight belts, tight shoelaces.
4. Never cross the legs at the knee because this constricts the popliteal vessels.

Goal 2: Promote Vasodilatation

Dilated arteries have a greater capacity for carrying blood to the extremities. Measures which promote vasodilatation are listed below.

Warmth. Warmth can be both a blessing and a curse for patients with vascular disease. Warmth is beneficial for the patient only when it acts to insulate him against cold and chilling. For example, encourage the individual with vascular disease to set his home thermostat at around 70 to 72°F. If possible keep his hospital room comfortably warm. Remind the patient to wear gloves, scarves, and socks when going outside on a chilly day. If chilling occurs, tell the patient to have a warm drink or take a warm bath. It is also safe to apply a hot water bottle to the abdomen; this procedure causes reflex dilatation of arteries in the extremities, thereby increasing blood flow without untoward effects.

On the other hand, applying any source of heat *directly to the extremities* is especially dangerous.

The use of hot water bottles, heating pads, and hot foot soaks is strictly contraindicated unless specifically ordered by the physician.

As stated earlier, heat increases tissue metabolism. If the arteries are unable to dilate normally, blood flow to the extremities will be inadequate, and the tissues will become ischemic.

Prevention of Vasoconstriction. Factors that cause vasoconstriction are nicotine (which causes vasospasm), high emotion (which stimulates the sympathetic nervous system), and chilling. You can help patients to avoid the damaging effects of prolonged vasoconstriction in the following ways:

> Emphasize the dangers of smoking to the patient who uses tobacco. Encourage him to stop smoking completely.

The patient who realizes that smoking literally threatens his life and limbs may develop sufficient motivation to abstain permanently.

> Protect the patient, whenever possible, from upsetting, emotionally charged situations. Encourage the patient to try and relax, both mentally and physically. Counseling services may be indicated for very nervous, high-strung individuals.

> Prevent the patient from becoming chilled in the ways described above.

Vasodilators. Drugs that dilate the peripheral vessels either act *directly* on the smooth muscles of the arteries (e.g., papaverine hydrochloride) or by *blocking* the constricting effects of epinephrine and norepinephrine upon the nerve endings supplying arteries (adrenergic blocking agents, e.g., tolazoline [Priscoline] and phenoxybenzamine [Dibenzyline]). Alcohol, in moderation, is also an excellent vasodilator.

However, for vasodilators to work, arteries must still be capable of dilating. For this reason, vasodilators of any kind are of little benefit to patients with severely sclerosed and damaged vessels.

Sympathectomy. Sympathectomy is a surgical procedure in which sympathetic nerve fibers supplying the peripheral vessels are severed, causing relaxation of the arterioles and better blood flow. (See Chapter 52.) As is the case with vasodilators, sympathectomy is successful only in those patients in whom the vessels are still elastic enough to dilate. To determine how successful a sympathectomy might be, the doctor sometimes injects the vertebral sympathetic ganglia with alcohol, thereby temporarily interrupting sympathetic impulses to the extremities.

Goal 3: Prevent and Treat Vascular Obstruction

Any form of vascular obstruction hinders circulation—sometimes dramatically. Arteries can become clogged with accumulations of lipids, calcium deposits, complex carbohydrates, and fibrous tissue. Both arteries and veins can be obstructed by thrombi and emboli. How can vascular obstruction be prevented? As you recall from Unit X, the prevention of atherosclerosis and arteriosclerosis is still an engima because the precise causation of these conditions remains unknown. Researchers have suggested low cholesterol diets, exercise, control of obesity, avoidance of tobacco, and the development of a calm, rational attitude as possible preventative measures.

In contrast, methods for preventing venous thrombosis are more clear-cut. (See also Chapters 27 and 65.) Thrombus formation is usually caused by venous stasis, hypercoagulability of the blood, and/or injury to the venous wall. Preventative measures designed to counteract the above factors include: avoidance of *prolonged* bed rest; ample fluids to prevent dehydration and resultant hypercoagulability; range-of-motion exercises for the bedfast; proper positioning in bed (e.g., avoidance of use of the knee gatch and lateral recumbent position); and the use of anticoagulant therapy.

Unfortunately vascular obstruction may develop despite attempts to prevent it. When a vessel becomes partially or totally occluded, how is the condition treated? Severely sclerosed, obstructed arteries can be replaced with synthetic vessels; this procedure, called a *bypass graft,* is frequently used for femoropopliteal disease. (See Chapter 64.) Also, an *endarterectomy* may be performed to open clogged arteries and "ream out" obstructing atheromatous material. In cases of *acute arterial occlusion* owing to an embolus or thrombus, *embolectomy* (surgical removal of the embolus) is the treatment of choice.

Venous thrombosis, in contrast to acute arterial thrombosis, usually responds to more conservative treatment. Facets of care include: bed rest, elevation of the legs above heart level, elastic support hose, continuous warm moist packs, anticoagulant therapy and fibrinolytic drugs (drugs which dissolve thrombi), and dextran 70, which helps to prevent further thrombus formation. Thrombi can also be removed surgically from large veins (thrombectomy).

Goal 4: Relieve Ischemic Pain

The pain of ischemia is usually chronic and continuous in nature. For this reason, patients with peripheral vascular disease are often depressed and irritable. Pain limits their activities, disturbs their sleep, saps their energy, and demoralizes their spirits. Thus, pain must be relieved if the patient is to rest and to improve.

Any measure that increases circulation to the extremities will help to alleviate ischemic pain; e.g., warmth, proper positioning, the oscillating bed, vasodilators, avoidance of tobacco, and so forth. Also, pain can be subdued by the use of analgesics, although therapies that augment circulation are preferable.

Goal 5: Prevent Tissue Damage and Infection and Promote Healing of Existing Lesions

Because of their poor circulation, patients with peripheral vascular disease are highly susceptible to infections, ulcerations, and gangrene of the extremities. Moreover, once a lesion develops, it tends to heal poorly or not at all; without normal vessels and adequate blood flow, the damaged tissues fail to receive needed oxygen, nutrients, antibodies, and protective leukocytes, and the process of tissue damage continues. Consequently the prevention of circulatory complications cannot be stressed enough.

Patients must be taught to avoid injury to their extremities. For example, remind patients to check bath water with a bath thermometer instead of their toes and thus prevent burns; to wear shoes to avoid injury to the feet; to avoid creating open lesions by scratching flea or mosquito bites on the legs; to use mild soaps; and to rub soothing lotions or lanolin on hands, feet, legs, and arms to discourage dryness. Also teach patients to observe for trophic changes, e.g., dryness and cracking of the skin on the feet, thickening of the nails, and so forth. Such changes should be reported to the doctor promptly.

Foot Care

Foot care is particularly important to any person who has a problem with peripheral circulation, and preventive measures are easier to initiate than corrective ones.* Anyone working with a patient should ascertain whether he is wearing adequate footwear and hosiery, and whether nails and skin on the feet are cared for properly. Minor foot problems in peripheral vascular disease can easily become serious.

Corns and Calluses. A *corn* is a traumatic keratosis caused by friction and pressure of a shoe when a step is taken. Corns most commonly occur on the fourth or fifth toe, generally over a joint or bony prominence. The typical corn is conical, with its base on top and its apex reaching to deeper structures. Care consists of removing the keratosis with a scalpel or other instrument. Care should be taken not to cut too deeply. After the cornified layer is removed, regrowth may be inhibited by placing a U-shaped pad of felt directly behind the corn to eliminate or disperse the pressure.

A *callus* is a flat, ill-defined mass of keratotic material, usually found on the bottom of the foot under a bony protuberance. Pressure of a shoe and uneven walking are usual causes. Pressure can be alleviated with padding and protective devices and various types of inlays in the shoe. The overall care of the skin is very important. Lanolized cream keeps the skin soft and prevents cracks in dry, hyperkeratotic skin.

Ingrown Toenail. An ingrown toenail can be a serious problem in a person with impaired circulation. In one survey of 4600 patients almost 16 per cent had this problem.[20] As many as 46 causative factors have been cited by various authors. Three basic types of lateral nail problems are described: (1) incurvated nail, (2) ingrown nail, and (3) hypertrophic ungual labium. The patient may have one or more of these conditions.

The symptoms of a *simple incurvated nail* are tenderness, pain on walking, and pain on digital pressure. Prophylactic care consists in trimming the nail properly by cutting it straight across. Stockings and shoes should be long enough to allow for lengthening of the foot during weight-bearing.

Active treatment consists of removing the cellular debris and callus tissue from the margin of the nail gently with a probe. The nail groove should be packed so the nail plate grows forward and the soft tissue of the nail lip will not be impinged upon. The first packing should be done with cotton or lamb's wool after lubrication of the groove with an emollient ointment containing a topical anesthetic. The elderly person should not undertake this procedure and should be under supervision of a podiatrist, doctor, or nurse for the 3 or 4 months it takes the nail to grow the length of the toe plate.

The ingrown toenail or onychocryptosis is not so common but has more harmful results. If the lateral border of the nail is mutilated by improper trimming, a pointed sliver frequently remains attached. As the nail plate grows forward, pressure compresses the soft labium against the sharp point, which penetrates the skin. Treatment consists first of removing the sliver. After removal, warm boric acid soaks for 20 to 30 minutes every 4 hours may be instituted. A dry sterile dressing should be applied and a broad spectrum antibiotic prescribed. Rest in bed or hospitalization is advised. After the infection has cleared, the same treatment is used as described for the incurvated nail.

Hypertrophic ungual labium is a condition in which the nail lip is massively enlarged, frequently overriding a good portion of the nail plate. This is caused by irritation of the epithelium of the nail groove by the lateral nail margin as a result of repeated improper nail trimming. Confining footwear presses the lip against the nail border, producing irritation and chronic inflammation and leading to eventual permanent hypertrophy. Both ingrown toenail and incurvated nail lead to a hypertrophied lip if care is inadequate or lacking. Surgical intervention may be indicated if the condition is chronic and infection returns repeatedly.

Although the feet are most frequently the focus of trauma in vascular disease, the *legs* are also subject to tissue breakdown. Indeed, leg ulcers are a common complication of varicose veins. Varicose ulcers are treated with: bed rest, elevation of the feet above heart level, continuous warm moist compresses, antibiotics, special bandages, proteolytic enzymes such as streptokinase (Varidase) and trypsin (Tryptar), and skin grafting. As with all the complications of vascular disease, leg ulcers are far more easily prevented than cured. See Chapter 65 for details.

*The principles of foot care are described in Unit XIX, Chapter 95. Please refer to this section for basic information.

CHAPTER 64

Diseases of the Aorta and Arteries

DISORDERS OF THE AORTA

Structure of the Aorta

The aorta is the main artery of the body. It is divided into the ascending aorta, the arch of the aorta, and the descending aorta. The aorta is an elastic artery, composed chiefly of plates of elastic tissue remarkably able to withstand the systolic blood pressure and provide elastic recoil, although elasticity diminishes with age. The walls of the aorta contain pressor receptors which, when stimulated by a rise in blood pressure, lead reflexly to a fall in blood pressure and heart rate. The ascending aorta is about 3 cm. in diameter and has a course of about 5 cm. The root is dilated because of the three bulges in its wall, i.e., the sinuses of the aorta, each named for a cusp of the aortic valve.

The branches of the ascending aorta are the right and left coronary arteries. The ascending aorta continues into the arch, the branches of the arch of the aorta being the brachiocephalic trunk, the left common carotid artery, and the left subclavian artery. The thoracic aorta descends from the arch through the aortic opening in the diaphragm and becomes the abdominal aorta. The branches of the thoracic aorta may be classified as parietal and visceral. The parietal arteries supply the diaphragm and intercostal area; and the visceral, the bronchial, esophageal, pericardial, and mediastinal areas. The abdominal aorta divides into the right and left common iliac arteries.

Aortitis

Aortitis is inflammation of the aorta; primarily it damages the arch of the aorta. Causes include arteriosclerosis and syphilis.

By far the most common site of cardiovascular syphilis is the ascending portion of the aorta. In most cases involvement of the aorta produces only moderate dilatation of the ascending aorta (uncomplicated aortitis). However, it may lead to such complications as aortic insufficiency, aortic aneurysm, or narrowing or obstruction of the coronary ostia. These complications occur in 35 to 40 per cent of patients with syphilitic aortitis. The main finding is roentgenographic indication of dilatation and occasional calcification of the ascending aorta. This may also be produced by atherosclerosis in subjects over 50. If a patient under 45 has roentgenographic findings in the absence of other heart disease and has a history of syphilis and/or a positive serologic test, syphilitic aortitis should be suspected.

Serologic tests are positive in 75 to 95 per cent of patients with untreated syphilitic aortitis. The prognosis of treated uncomplicated aortitis is relatively favorable, since complications are prevented by treatment. Penicillin is the most effective agent.

Aortic insufficiency is the most frequent complication of syphilitic aortitis, occurring in approximately one third of the patients. Generally it becomes manifest 10 to 25 years after the primary infection, although in 7 per cent it may occur within the first five years. The prognosis is poor, as only 35 to 45 per cent survive 10 years after the diagnosis is made. If the patient is symptomatic, his chances for survival are much better.[13]

Aortic Aneurysms

An aneurysm is a sac formed by the dilatation of an artery as a result of localized weakness and stretching of the arterial wall. The following types of aneurysms are recognized: (1) *fusiform aneurysm,* a uniform, spindle-shaped dilatation of a segment of an artery; (2) *saccular aneurysm,* an outpouching from an artery caused by localized thinning and stretching of the medial coat; (3) *dissecting aneurysm,* a cavity formed by blood that has been forced between the layers of the arterial wall; and (4) *false aneurysm,* one resulting from a complete rupture or wounding of all coats of the artery, the blood then being retained by the surrounding tissues.

The most common *cause* of aneurysms is arteriosclerosis. Other causes are syphilis, congenital defects of the arterial wall, trauma, infectious arteritis other than syphilitic, periarteritis and other types of necrotizing arteritis.

Arteriosclerotic aneurysms usually develop at a site in the artery that is not surrounded by skeletal muscle or where the artery is subject to frequent bending during physical activity. Fusiform arteriosclerotic aneurysms occur most often in the aorta, especially the abdominal aorta, and in the iliac arteries. Saccular arteriosclerotic aneurysms are most often seen in the abdominal aorta and the popliteal arteries; they may also occur in the femoral artery. As noted below, aneurysms of the thoracic aorta presently are usually caused by arteriosclerosis rather than syphilis, and are usually fusiform rather than saccular. Aneurysms of arteriosclerotic type usually develop after the age of 60 years and are about 10 times as frequent in men as in women.

Thoracic Aortic Aneurysms. Syphilis was formerly the commonest cause of thoracic aortic aneurysms but is now second to atherosclerosis. The symptoms are variable and depend on the rapidity with which the aneurysm dilates and the effect of the pulsating mass on the surrounding structures. Most are asymptomatic unless large.

The thoracic aorta is the most common site of a *dissecting* aneurysm, with other arteries usually involved by extension of the dissection. The cause is not known, but a genetic predisposition is suggested. Hypertension is the most commonly associated clinical condition. Arteriosclerosis does not appear to be causally related, and syphilis appears to be a deterrent because it produces fusion of the layers of the aorta. Dissection usually begins in the medial layer and frequently extends partially around the aorta and occasionally completely around it. The most frequent cause of death in a dissecting aneurysm of the aorta is external rupture of the hematoma.

The clinical picture of dissecting aneurysm of the aorta is extremely variable.[20] Generally men outnumber women, and although the condition can occur at any time, it usually affects persons between 40 and 70 years of age. The onset is usually sudden; there is severe and persistent pain, described as "tearing" or "ripping." The pain usually begins in the anterior thorax but may be between or below the scapulae. It may begin high in the epigastrium or in some unusual site such as face or neck. If sudden collapse or syncope occurs, the pain can be absent.

The early symptoms in the patient are often pallor, sweatiness, and mild shock, with moderately or even markedly elevated blood pressure. Hypertension or a history of it has been found in about 70 per cent of patients. Blood pressure may be markedly different in both arms, and there may be lowered arterial pulsations and varying degrees of ischemia in one or more of the extremities. The heart rate may be moderately increased and there may or may not be murmurs. Abdominal tenderness may also be present. Because of the variable clinical picture, early diagnosis is not accurate in about 40 to 50 per cent of patients. The condition may be mistaken for acute myocardial infarction, cerebrovascular accident, acute abdomen, and acute peripheral arterial occlusion. Electrocardiograms, roentgenograms, and angiography may help in diagnosis and in localizing the dissection. The prognosis is poor in untreated patients and is unfavorably influenced by age, location of primary tear (ascending or arch portion of the aorta), hypertension, and other cardiovascular disease.[20]

The objectives of *surgical treatment* of dissecting aortic aneurysm are: (1) preventing further dissection, (2) eliminating the possibility of external rupture, (3) correcting aortic valve damage if present, and (4) restoring the patency of occluded vessels. Surgical mortality is high during acute dissection. In some treatment centers the acute stage is managed with drug therapy, followed in 2 to 3 weeks by corrective surgery. Drugs that reduce blood pressure and myocardial contractility are often used. The best treatment of aortic dissection is not clear at present.

Pain is the predominant symptom of *nondissecting* aneurysms of the thoracic aorta; it usually develops in the anterior chest and is frequently substernal, but sometimes it occurs in the back or shoulders. It is usually described as a steady ache and may be felt only when the patient is in the supine position. Obstruction of the superior vena cava or subclavian vein may occur; dysphagia, dyspnea, and stridor may be present, as may hoarseness and cough because of pressure on the recurrent pharyngeal nerve. Sometimes no physical signs develop. The electrocardiogram is not of value in making the diagnosis. The most helpful procedure is roentgenoscopy, and often the aneurysm is discovered only by x-ray. In arteriosclerotic aneurysms, deposits of calcium are frequently seen near the edges of the outline of the aneurysm.

The prognosis for persons with thoracic aortic aneurysms is not so poor as that for those with an abdominal aortic aneurysm. In a Mayo Clinic series, 68 per cent of patients survived three years; 50 per cent, 5 years; and 30 per cent, 10 years. Age greater than 50, a large aneurysm, and diastolic hypertension all affected the prognosis unfavorably.[20] Death is often caused by rupture of the aneurysm, which occurs in about a third of patients. Most thoracic aortic aneurysms require surgical treatment. However, patients with a chronic asymptomatic thoracic aneurysm resulting from trauma often recover without treatment.

Abdominal Aortic Aneurysms. The common cause of aneurysm of the abdominal aorta is arteriosclerosis. Syphilis is present in from 5 to 10 per cent of the patients, but arteriosclerosis is usually also present. Approximately 40 per cent of patients with abdominal aortic aneurysms have symptoms, abdominal pain being the most common. It may be persistent or intermittent and is most frequently felt in the middle or lower part of the abdomen at the left of the midline. Another frequent complaint is back pain, usually low in the back; this is frequently caused by rupture of the aneurysm. Less commonly an abdominal mass appears or abdominal throbbing occurs.

A pulsating abdominal mass is the most frequent and important physical sign. Determination of blood pressure in the arm and thigh of a patient in a supine position is of value in differential diagnosis. Normally the blood pressure in the thigh is higher than that in the arm by 15 mm. or more of mercury; however, in most patients with abdominal aortic aneurysm the systolic pressure in the thigh is abnormally low compared with that of the arm. However, normal comparative blood pressures in the arm and thigh do not rule out aneurysm. A systolic bruit can often be heard over the aneurysm. However, the best means of confirming the diagnosis is x-ray examination of the lumbar spine in the anteroposterior and lateral positions.

Newer surgical and grafting techniques now permit resection of abdominal aortic aneurysms and their replacement by grafts. A surgical mortality of approximately 5 per cent for elective resection and graft of abdominal aortic aneurysms has been reported, with the mortality higher (30 to 50 per cent) in surgical treatment of ruptured aneurysms. Survival rates are nearly twice as good for patients who have surgical treatment as for those who are not operated on.

Other Sites of Aneurysms. Aneurysms are found less commonly in the upper extremities than in the lower extremities. The most common sites in the lower extremities are the popliteal space and Scarpa's triangle.

Popliteal aneurysms are important causes of ischemic symptoms in the lower limbs. Although the patient may be aware of a swelling behind the knee, he seldom complains unless symptoms such as rest pain, coldness, or numbness develop. A peripheral aneurysm is differentiated from other swellings by the presence of expansile pulsation. Complications of popliteal aneurysms frequently occur and may lead to loss of an extremity or to death. The most dangerous complications are embolus distal to the aneurysm, leaking of the aneurysm, and pressure from the aneurysm on a neighboring vein or nerve. Thrombosis may occur, resulting in severe ischemia with development of gangrene and loss of the limbs. Surgical treatment is the only satisfactory method of dealing with aneurysms of the popliteal artery and should be done before complications occur.

Surgical Treatment of Aneurysms. Aortography is advised in patients suspected of having an aneurysm of the *ascending* aorta to establish the diagnosis and to assess the condition of the aortic valve, which may require graft replacement. Surgery usually involves resection of the aneurysm and replacement of the excised segment with a graft. Extracorporeal circulation with a pump oxygenator is sometimes employed. When the aneurysm has been opened a coronary cannula is inserted. A woven Dacron graft is sutured to the proximal and distal aortic segments, and the remaining wall of the aneurysm is approximated over the graft. Hospital mortality for resections of the ascending aorta, even when valve replacement is also required, is about 10 per cent.[20]

Aneurysms of the *transverse aortic arch* are rare with the decreasing incidence of untreated syphilis in the population. Because of the high surgical mortality, operation is advised only in those patients who experience symptoms and in whom the aneurysm is enlarging.

Aneurysms of the *descending* portion of the thoracic aorta usually occur just distal to the origin of the left subclavian artery. The cause is most often atherosclerosis, although this is also a common site for traumatic aneurysms. Since the aorta must be interrupted for the insertion of a graft, it is necessary to provide flow in the distal aorta to allow circulation to continue. Some form of bypass is instituted, using either the left atrial femoral artery or the femoral vein and femoral artery. After bypass is instituted, the aneurysm is incised and a woven Dacron graft is inserted and covered with the trimmed wall of the aneurysm. The current hospital mortality rate is about 10 to 12 per cent.[20]

Aneurysms involving the descending thoracic aorta plus the upper abdominal aorta are difficult to correct surgically because it is often necessary to reconstruct the celiac, mesenteric, and renal arteries. The operative mortality is high, but the risk may be justified because of the poor prognosis of patients with aneurysms in this area. A graft is attached to the side of the thoracic aorta proximal to the aneurysm and attached distally at the aortic bifurcation. Side branches are constructed from the main graft to the visceral arteries and the aneurysm is excised.

The *terminal aorta* distal to the origin of the renal arteries is a common site for aneurysm formation. Surgery is indicated for such an aneurysm if the patient is capable of withstanding an abdominal operation.

The excision of *popliteal* aneurysms is done preferably before the aneurysm becomes symptomatic or complicated. The results of operation are excellent in uncomplicated cases. The long-term effectiveness of the graft is determined by the extent of occlusion in the distal vessels. Patients with popliteal aneurysms have a high incidence of disease in the abdominal aorta and the iliac and femoral arteries.

Resection is generally indicated for aneurysms of the iliac and femoral arteries, with use of a prosthetic graft or an autogenous saphenous vein graft.[20]

PERIPHERAL ARTERIAL DISEASES

Peripheral arterial diseases can be divided into two groups: (1) conditions characterized by organic changes; and (2) conditions in which no organic changes develop. Organic changes are *present* in atherosclerosis and arteriosclerosis, thromboangiitis obliterans (Buerger's disease), acute arterial occlusion, and arterial embolism. Organic changes are *absent* in Raynaud's disease.

Atherosclerosis and Arteriosclerosis

Definitions and Etiology. The commonest form of arterial disease is atherosclerosis, atheroma, or arteriosclerosis. Some authors differentiate between arteriosclerosis and atherosclerosis by considering the latter to indicate focal changes, and using arteriosclerosis to refer broadly to "hardening of the arteries." Atherosclerosis rarely occurs in the absence of arteriosclerosis.

Atherosclerosis has been defined by the World Health Organization as a complex of changes in the intima of arteries consisting of "the focal accumulation of lipids, complex carbohydrates, blood products, fibrous tissue and calcium deposits and associated with medial changes." Atherosclerosis is a *generalized* arterial disease, and when it is present in the limbs, it is usually present elsewhere in the body. It chiefly affects the main arteries, often in a patchy manner. The branch arteries are unaffected except at their point of departure from the main artery, and the small arteries are also unaffected. Atherosclerosis is more common in the lower than the upper limbs, although it may be an important cause of vascular disturbance in the hands. The lesions cause narrowing of the arterial lumen and critically reduce blood flow, and thrombosis or aneurysm may result.

The etiology is uncertain. The condition is present to some degree in almost all adults and may develop to an advanced degree without ischemic complications, or an individual may have severe complications from a localized plaque. Various factors have been reputed to be associated with the condition; e.g., no population on a regular low-fat diet has been shown to have a high prevalence of the coronary heart disease. It is on this basis that cholesterol has been implicated as a causative factor, but this is not yet proved. Associated diseases such as diabetes and hypertension appear to accelerate atherosclerosis. Cigarette smoking is implicated by autopsy studies that show an increasing degree of coronary atherosclerosis with increasing age and the number of cigarettes smoked during life. Hormones, particularly estrogen, have a potent effect on atherogenesis. Obesity, physical inactivity, and emotional stress are all implicated as factors. Genetic factors seem to be important in combination with environmental factors. For further discussion of the etiology of atherosclerosis, see Chapter 51.

Incidence. Atherosclerosis is the most common disease in the elderly. It is the most frequent reason for death in persons over 65, and in the sixth and seventh decades kills ten times as many people as cancer. Over half of all persons between the ages of 60 and 70 will die of some manifestation of atherosclerosis, most commonly of the coronary arteries. About 50 per cent of patients with peripheral arterial insufficiency have other clinical signs of atherosclerosis.

Today, there is evidence that the incidence of atherosclerosis is increasing in the younger age group. As a group it contains a greater number of cigarette smokers than the general population.

Symptoms. The patient with chronic arterial occlusion due to peripheral arterial disease usually complains about *pain in the lower limbs* brought on by exercise and terminating when exercise ceases, although he may also have pain at rest. *Intermittent claudication* is the term applied to the symptom in which the patient experiences pain or discomfort in muscles after exercise but is relieved by rest. Symptoms associated with intermittent claudication are pain, coldness, or numbness. Signs are alterations in color or temperature; condition of skin, nails, tissue, and hair; condition of walls of arteries; auscultation or bruits; and absence of pulses.

Typically, pain occurs in the calf muscles after walking and disappears on rest. It can occur in muscles other than the calf but is frequently not recognized. Discomfort in the muscles of the thigh or buttocks is commonly attributed to sciatica or osteoarthritis of the hip joint. However, the pain of arthritis of the hip is generally more severe when the patient starts to walk after resting and improves as the patient continues to walk.[45]

Claudication is usually insidious in onset and generally occurs in men, although there is an increase in incidence in females after the menopause. If diabetics are excluded, only 10 per cent of patients are women. Usually claudication strikes males in their sixth or seventh decade.

Diagnosis and Assessment. The physician bases his diagnosis on the patient's symptoms (e.g., complaints of intermittent claudication, numbness of the legs), observable changes in the appearance of the limbs, palpation of the peripheral pulses, and a variety of diagnostic tests.

Signs observed by the doctor are alterations in color or temperature of the affected extremity. Nutrition of the limb may be inadequate, resulting in thickened and opaque nails, shiny and atrophic skin, decreased hair growth, dry or fissured heels, and loss of subcutaneous tissue in the digits.

The most important part of the examination is palpation of the peripheral pulses. Absence of a normally palpable pulse is the most reliable sign of occlusive arterial disease, since in the lower limb the femoral pulse in the groin and the posterior tibial pulse behind the medial malleolus are easily felt (Figs. 64–1 and 64–2). Comparison of pulses in both extremities is helpful. The popliteal pulse is often difficult to feel in obese or muscular patients. The position of the dorsalis pedis artery in the foot is variable and it is absent on one side in about 15 per cent of normal subjects, so that absence of the dorsalis pedis pulse is not a very reliable sign of arterial disease. When pulses are being palpated, it should also be ascertained whether the arterial wall is palpable, tortuous, or calcified. Auscultation over the main arteries is useful, as a systolic bruit usually indicates an atheromatous plaque.

There are a number of tests which can be performed as a part of the clinical examination of the patient. Five commonly used tests include: Oscillometry, skin temperature studies, angiography, exercise tests for intermittent claudication, and lumbar sympathetic block.

> *Oscillometry.* Alterations in the pulse volume are measured by placing a pneumatic cuff around the extremity at different levels, attached to an oscillometer (an aneroid system). The arterial pressure with each pulsation is transmitted via a sensitive diaphragm to a

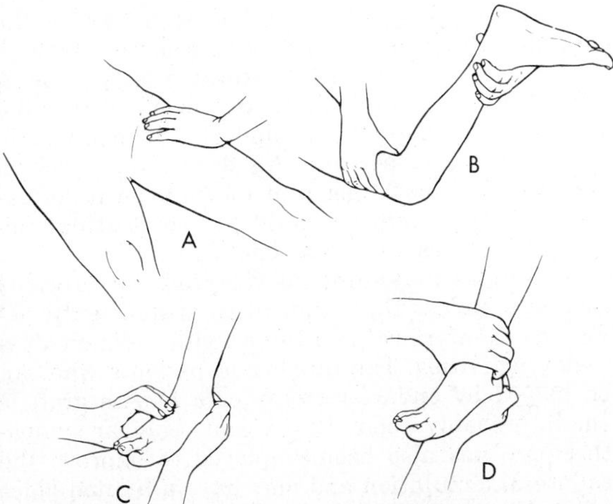

FIGURE 64-1. The method of palpation for pulsations in the peripheral arteries. *A*, Femoral artery. *B*, Popliteal artery. *C*, Dorsalis pedis artery. *D*, Posterior tibial artery. (From: Fairbairn, J. F., II, Jurgens, J. L., and Spittell, J. A., Jr.: *Peripheral Vascular Diseases.* 4th ed. 1972.)

needle attached to a dial. The reading is recorded in units called the *oscillometric index.* Abnormal findings help to pinpoint the level of arterial occlusion, but the results may vary in different patients and the information is not always conclusive.

> *Skin temperature studies.* These are done in various ways: (1) palpating and comparing skin warmth or coolness in opposing limbs; (2) the use of direct-reading skin temperature thermometers; (3) immersing one extremity in warm water, and observing for *rise* in skin temperature in other extremity, which should follow normally owing to reflex vasodilatation; (4) placing a hot water bottle on the patient's abdomen and observing extremities for reflex rise in skin temperature. Coldness of one or both extremities under normal room temperature implies poor circulation; the failure of the arteries in an extremity to dilate as described in (3) and (4) indicates arterial damage. However, these tests can be unreliable if the patient is anxious and, in general, are only of limited value in diagnosis.

> *Angiography (Arteriography).* Contrast dye is injected into the arteries and x-ray films are made of the vascular tree. The films may indicate abnormalities of blood flow due to arterial obstruction or narrowing. Disadvantages are the possibility of allergic reactions to the radiopaque dye, and the fact that the injection site may become irritated or thrombosed.

> *Exercise tests for intermittent claudication.* The patient walks or performs some other form of exercise until pain occurs; the length of time required for onset of calf pain following start of exercise is recorded. Claudication on exercise indicates the failure of damaged arteries to adjust the blood flow to the increased tissue requirements for oxygen.

> *Lumbar sympathetic block.* Local anesthetic is injected into the sympathetic ganglia, thereby temporarily blocking the sympathetic vasomotor nerve fibers supplying an ischemic limb. A decrease in limb pain and increase in skin temperature indicates that sympathetectomy could improve circulation to the extremities. A possible adverse reaction may be *shock* as a result of movement of the blood from the vital organs into the peripheral vessels.

Examination generally places the patient in one of three groups, depending on the area of the principal occlusion:

1. About 80 per cent of the patients with occlusive arterial disease of the lower limbs have disease in the femoropopliteal segments. The adductor region is the most common, followed by the popliteal artery just above the knee joint and the popliteal bifurcation.
2. The patients with aorto-iliac lesions make up about 15 per cent; here there is an occlusion in the common iliac artery or at the aortic bifurcation.
3. Patients with femoropopliteal lesions may also have one or more occlusions in the arteries of the leg, and the incidence of these combined lesions increases as the patient ages.

Prognosis. The significance of peripheral arterial occlusion is that it indicates the presence of atherosclerosis. Atherosclerosis of the coronary or cerebral arteries is more likely to cause death or disability than is intermittent claudication or other peripheral effects. Of patients with claudication, more than half die from myocardial infarction.[45]

Treatment. It is important to reassure the patient that his limbs are in no immediate danger and to give him some general information about necessary changes in his living habits.

The patient should be encouraged to walk and

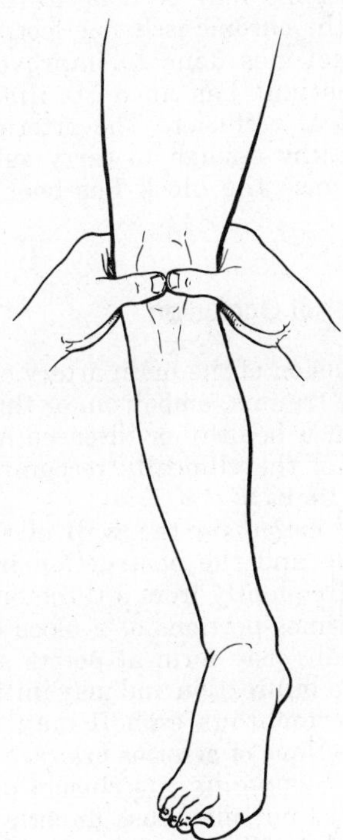

FIGURE 64-2. An alternative method for palpating pulsations in the popliteal artery. (From: Fairbairn, J. F., II, Juergens, J. L., and Spittell, J. A., Jr.: *Peripheral Vascular Diseases.* 4th ed. 1972.)

given a program of graduated walking. Overweight patients should be encouraged to reduce and to improve those dietary habits that contribute to overweight. There is no evidence that a special diet will alter the course of atherosclerosis once clinical evidence of it has appeared. Since smoking causes vasoconstriction of the extremities, the individual should be advised to give it up.

Meticulous care of the feet should be advised, using water of warm temperature, drying gently and thoroughly, using lubricants to keep the skin soft, and wearing clean cotton or wool socks daily. Shoes and slippers should be well fitted. Patients should never go barefooted. The patient should not wear constricting garters, foundation garments, or hosiery. Bed socks should be worn to bed and the bed warmed by an electric blanket rather than hot water bottles or heating pads.

Various *drugs* may be used in treatment of peripheral arterial disease. For a helpful tabulation of medications for this purpose, see the article by Jackson.[27] Drugs given are usually vasodilators, anticoagulants, and/or drugs that lower the serum cholesterol.

Drugs that cause dilatation of the peripheral blood vessels act as *adrenergic blocking agents* (such drugs as pentolamine and phenoxybenzamine); they interfere with the actions of epinephrine and norepinephrine when these substances are released at the nerve endings in the blood vessels, or they act directly on the smooth muscles in the walls of the blood vessels. There is some question about their effect when there is generalized atherosclerotic disease. Although the drugs are not toxic, there are unpleasant side effects such as facial flushing, tachycardia and palpations, nervousness and excitability, dizziness, shivering, nausea, and weakness. Since most patients do better when they are receiving treatment, even placebos, there may be merit in prescribing drugs which act directly on the blood vessels rather than adrenergic blocking agents which dilate mainly the cutaneous blood vessels and divert blood away from the muscles. *Alcohol* is a very good vasodilator and for occasional use is as good as any of the adrenergic blocking agents. *Vitamin E* has been used, and some patients seem to improve but probably no more than with a placebo. However, it is harmless.[45]

Although *anticoagulants* can be used effectively in patients with venous thrombosis, there is little evidence that they can reduce or prevent arterial thromboses, and they are generally not used unless there is some additional indication.

Finally, drugs *that lower serum cholesterol are sometimes ordered.* Although there is an association of atherosclerosis with a high concentration of cholesterol and lipid substances in the blood, there is no clear evidence that by the use of special diets and drugs the course of atherosclerosis will be modified. The safest method is to reduce the total fat intake in the diet and to replace saturated fat with oils rich in polyunsaturated fatty acids. A drug that has been found to lower serum cholesterol is clofibrate (Atromid-S). When given in a dose of 2 Gm. per day this drug reduces serum cholesterol 20 to 25 per cent in the majority of patients. Side effects are mild gastrointestinal upsets, drowsiness, and occasional skin rashes.

Patients should not be referred for *surgical treatment* unless the claudication is sufficiently severe as to interfere with life or with ordinary day-to-day activities. The number of patients who can be helped by endarterectomy or a bypass graft is small, probably about 10 per cent. Lumbar sympathectomy has also been employed to improve the collateral circulation and may have a limited place in some patients with intermittent claudication.

THE CHRONIC ISCHEMIC LIMB AND ITS CARE. Patients with a chronic ischemic limb have a disability that is usually of rather long duration. Such patients commonly have intermittent claudication, but their main complaint is either pain in the foot or areas of necrosis.

As mentioned previously, the care of the chronically ischemic limb should be meticulous, with careful attention to cleanliness and keeping the foot dry. Socks should be soft, preferably woolen, and well-fitted footwear should be worn. The feet should not be allowed to become cold. Localized areas of gangrene should be kept dry and should not be treated unless there is an infection. It is probably best for the patient to be up and about.

The pain of severe ischemia is difficult to relieve. When strong analgesics such as morphine are necessary, the patient should be prepared to accept amputation.

Sympathectomy may be done to relieve the circulation in the chronic ischemic foot. Arterial surgery is sometimes done to improve circulation when the patient has an aorto-iliac block or a femoropopliteal occlusion. The arteries in the leg must be healthy enough to carry sufficient blood to the foot once the block has been removed or bypassed.

Acute Arterial Occlusion

Acute occlusion of the main artery of a limb may be caused by trauma, embolism, or thrombosis and may occur in a healthy or diseased artery. About 90 per cent of the clinically recognized cases are in the lower limbs.

In *arterial embolism* the wall of the artery is often healthy and the obstruction in the artery comes most frequently from a thrombus within the heart. Sometimes portions of a blood clot, such as platelet emboli, may form at points of turbulence and lodge at a bifurcation and may initiate a thrombus, or atheromatous emboli may block small arteries. Infections of arteries are rare.

Signs and Symptoms. Occlusion usually has a dramatic onset but may pass unnoticed if the patient is seriously ill and confined to bed. Burning or aching pain in the tissues distal to the site of the occlusion is usually the first symptom, which rapidly increases in intensity and subsides slowly over a period of hours. Active or passive movement of the limb aggravates the pain. Occasionally the occlusion is painless and attention may be called to it by the appearance of the limb, or by numbness or paresthesias. The early symptoms are followed by a sense of coldness, numbness in the extremity, and muscle weakness. Arterial pulsation is absent or weakened distal to the site of the occlusion.

The circulatory changes that follow arterial occlusion, and that predict outcome, are complex and dependent on varied factors. In a normal artery normal blood flow is restored by collateral channels, but patients with acute arterial occlusion may have a weakened heart, and other factors such as immobility, anemia, or dehydration may be present.[45]

Treatment. The first decision is whether an operation should be performed to remove the occluding embolus or thrombus. Any surgery should be performed as quickly as possible. Patients can have a successful embolectomy performed under local anesthesia. If the patient is not seen until some hours have elapsed since the occlusion, the viability of the limb will determine if the operation can be performed.

The limb should be protected from pressure and other trauma and kept at room temperature, neither warm nor chilled. The best position for the limb is still in question, but probably a slight elevation is the most desirable.

If the decision is for medical treatment or there is a delay in procuring a surgeon, anticoagulants are generally started immediately. Heparin, 10,000 to 15,000 units as the initial dose followed by 10,000 units at eight-hour intervals, is recommended. If the patient has a cardiac condition the heparin should be given by a single intravenous injection rather than as a continuous drip to prevent overloading the circulation. Heparin should be continued for a minimum of 48 hours to seven days, after which a change to an oral anticoagulant may be made. It is the prevailing practice to treat all patients who have a definite source of embolism and who have made a satisfactory recovery from an acute episode of occlusion with long-term anticoagulant therapy for an indefinite period.

Aside from surgery, fibrinolytic agents may be used for removal of an occluding thrombus or embolus. At present two substances are available for use, streptokinase and urokinase. The drugs are expensive, difficult to monitor, and require some hours to clear the arterial lumen.

Prognosis. Because most of the patients have either a cardiac lesion or arterial disease their ultimate prognosis is uncertain and there is insufficient evidence to suggest significant improvement with long-term anticoagulant therapy.

Thromboangiitis Obliterans (Buerger's Disease)

In 1908 Buerger proposed the name thromboangiitis obliterans for an arterial disease which he felt was distinct from atherosclerosis in that acute inflammatory lesions and occlusive thrombosis of the arteries and veins were characteristic findings. The condition is sometimes called *Buerger's disease.*

The criteria accepted as favoring this diagnosis rather than atherosclerosis are the following:[45]

- The patient is a male of less than 40 years at the onset of the symptoms.
- The patient is a heavy cigarette smoker.
- Superficial thrombophlebitis may be present.
- Involvement of arteries of upper limbs or viscera is common.
- Arteriography reveals occlusive peripheral arterial disease.

Pain is the outstanding symptom. Intermittent claudication is a common complaint and occurs in almost all patients at some stage of the disease. It is frequently the first symptom noted by the patient and occurs most commonly in the arch of the foot. It is somewhat less common in the calf of the leg but may be noted in both sites. Rest pain with signs of persistent ischemia of one or more digits may be one of the first clinical indications. Coldness or sensitivity to cold may be an early symptom. Various types of paresthesias may occur. Pulsations in any or all the posterior tibial and dorsalis pedis arteries may be impaired or absent. In advanced cases the extremities may be abnormally red or cyanotic, particularly when dependent. The color changes are more significant if they involve only one extremity or only certain digits or portions of digits. Sometimes certain digits are colder than others on the same extremity.

Ulceration and gangrene are frequent complications and may occur early in the course of the disease. These lesions may appear spontaneously but often follow trauma. Gangrene usually occurs in one extremity at a time. Edema of the legs is fairly common in advanced cases. Changes in the nails and skin appear, and segmental thrombophlebitis affects the smaller veins in about 40 per cent of patients.

Diagnostic studies include leg arteriography, skin temperature determination, oscillometry, blood studies, and x-ray examinations. The clinical course of the disease is greatly influenced by whether the patient smokes, and if so, stops smoking. In the majority of patients who continue to smoke, the course of the disease is slowly and episodically progressive, with the development of first minor and later more extensive ulcerative gangrenous lesions after a period of months or years.

The *prognosis* as to survival of digits or limbs and the necessity for amputation depend on the stage of the disease when treatment is initiated, whether the patient continues to smoke, and whether he avoids major or minor trauma to the ischemic tissues. In a 10-year period, in one study,

6 per cent of the patients required amputations of fingers, 6 per cent amputation of toes, and 13 per cent amputation of a leg.[20] Patients in the study had a practically normal survival rate.

Treatment is generally pointed toward (1) arresting progress of the disease, (2) producing vasodilatation, (3) relieving pain, and (4) treating ulcers and gangrene. All patients are advised to abstain completely and permanently from use of tobacco in any form. The use of whisky or brandy may be of some value during periods of exacerbation. Exposure to cold should be avoided. Patients should be carefully instructed to prevent mechanical, chemical, and thermal injuries to the feet. Regional sympathetic ganglionectomy produces vasodilatation and may be of some value.

Amputation should be deferred until conservative treatment has been given a reasonable trial. It is almost always unwise to delay amputation of the leg when the gangrene extends well into the foot, and it should not be delayed if pain is severe and cannot be controlled or if severe infection or toxicity occurs. It is seldom necessary in these patients to carry an amputation above the knee.

Functional Vascular Disease

Raynaud's Disease. A confusion of terminology has existed in connection with this condition since its first description by Raynaud in 1862. The terms "Raynaud's disease" and "Raynaud's phenomenon" have both been used over the years, sometimes to describe the same set of findings. At present the consensus is that "Raynaud's phenomenon" should be used to refer to intermittent episodes of constriction of small arteries or arterioles of the extremities, causing changes in the color and temperature of the skin of the extremities. These local changes are not necessarily related to the status of the peripheral vascular system as a whole.[20] Raynaud's phenomenon may occur after trauma; for instance, after the use of high-speed vibrating tools under conditions of cold.[45] It may also be related to various neurogenic lesions, certain occlusive arterial diseases, and various other miscellaneous conditions.

The criteria for making the diagnosis of *Raynaud's disease* are:

> Intermittent attacks of pallor or cyanosis of the digits by exposure to cold or from emotional stimuli.

> Bilateral or symmetrical involvement.

> No evidence of occlusive disease in the digital arteries or any primary systemic disease to which the changes might be secondary.

> Gangrene which, when it occurs, is limited in large part to the skin of the tips of the digits.

> A history of symptoms for at least two years.

There are a large number of diseases associated with cold sensitivity of the Raynaud type categorized into intravascular disorders, e.g., cold agglutinins, diseases of the vessel walls such as thromboangiitis obliterans, occupational trauma and vascular injury, collagen disorders, and extravascular disorders. One of the first problems is establishing the diagnostic category for a patient with cold sensitivity.

Raynaud's disease is most likely to have an early age of onset, often commencing in the teens. The process will initially involve only the distal portion of one or more digits, although as the disease becomes more severe all the digits are involved. The feet are rarely as symptomatically involved as the hands. A careful history should be taken to elicit the possibility of other disease. On physical examination, normal-appearing fingers without ulceration suggest Raynaud's disease. Radial and ulnar pulses should be present and normal. Eighty per cent of patients with Raynaud's disease are women.

Reassurance of the patient that the condition is not likely to lead to a serious disability is desirable. Maintenance of warmth of the extremities and avoidance of smoking are important. Vasodilator drugs may be prescribed. Reserpine drugs, which decrease the store of norepinephrine in the peripheral arteries, have been tried and found to have few side effects. Although sympathectomy has been used in treatment, its effectiveness has not been conclusively demonstrated.

Acrocyanosis. In acrocyanosis the extremities tend to be blue and cold even when the environmental temperature is normal. Generally both hands and feet are affected and the changes are often found with increased sweating. The condition occurs most often in women.

Chilblains. Chilblains is a common vascular disorder due to cold in which the skin becomes discolored and there is pain, swelling, and itching. Acute chilblains occur mainly on the fingers and toes and consist of subcutaneous nodules over which the cyanosed skin is thinned and may break down into an indolent and painful ulcer. *Frostbite* occurs when tissues are frozen hard, and this happens when they are exposed suddenly to temperatures of −4°C. or lower.

Vasospasm of Disuse. The most common causes of long-term disuse of the limbs are anterior poliomyelitis, traumatic denervation, cerebrovascular accidents, and reflex sympathetic dystrophy.

At an early stage the arterioles of a limb with vasospasm from disuse will dilate fully when the subject becomes warm, but with long continued disuse and exposure to cold, atrophic changes proportional to the extent and duration of the disuse gradually occur. Natural wrinkles over the knuckles tend to smooth, fingers taper, the pulp atrophies, and the nails curve and thicken. Breaks in the skin due to minor trauma become painful and heal with difficulty. Over the limb as a whole the venules of the skin lose tone and become telangiectatic. Lymphatic drainage slows, and the legs in particular develop edema readily. Sympathectomy may effect an improvement in circulation in some patients, but it is simpler and more effective to keep the skin warm at all times.

Surgical Restoration of Primary Circulation

Arteries may be operated on when there is the possibility of removing the obstruction and restoring the patient to gainful employment or more enjoyment of living. Physician and patient may decide to attempt salvage rather than amputation.

Endarterectomy. Angiography is used to identify the exact nature and extent of disease. Endarterectomy is intended to open orifices of collateral arterial branches as well as segments of the main channel. Patches of autologous vein or Dacron may be necessary after removal of the atheroma. The surgery is generally fitted to the specific needs of the patient, and a combination of bypass and thromboendarterectomy may be required.

Bypass Graft for Femoropopliteal Disease. The repair of lesions in the femoropopliteal area is one of the principal concerns in vascular surgery today. The preferred method is an autogenous saphenous-vein bypass graft. Plastic prostheses have been used less because they have often failed to remain open. Knitted Dacron bypass grafts are used when it is difficult to obtain autologous tissues.

The method of selecting patients with femoropopliteal disease for grafting will affect the results, but one group reports overall long patency rates of 70 to 90 per cent with this method.[20] The operative risk is only about 1 per cent if the surgeon is a well-trained specialist; more attempts at surgical repair of this type of occlusion probably should be attempted.

PRE- AND POSTOPERATIVE CARE. Adequate circulating blood volume must be maintained to permit good perfusion throughout the period of arterial repair. Careful preoperative attention to the total body potassium stores is important, to prevent cardiac arrhythmias. Postoperatively, central venous pressure is monitored, and observation of kidney function is important. Every effort should be made to prevent thrombosis. The patient's legs should be elevated above the level of the heart. Anticoagulants are used during the operation and postoperatively if the patient's condition warrants.

CHAPTER 65

Diseases of the Veins and Lymphatics

This chapter provides an overview of the following general concepts: (1) the physiology of the veins pertinent to understanding their dysfunction; (2) the main causes of venous dysfunction; (3) the effects of venous dysfunction on the body; and (4) nursing interventions by which venous dysfunction can be eliminated or minimized.

PHYSIOLOGY OF THE VEINS

The functions of the veins are to serve as channels by which blood is returned from the capillaries to the heart, and to serve as reservoirs to hold varying volumes of blood without corresponding changes in venous pressure. The capacity of the venous system can be varied by venoconstriction, by valves in the veins, and by contraction of surrounding skeletal, visceral and respiratory muscles.

Blood flows from a higher pressure to a lower pressure. If the pressure in the venous system fell below the pressure in the right atrium the blood would not flow into the right atrium but would back up into the veins. The pressures in the right atrium and ventricle remain in a very narrow pressure range in spite of changes in blood volume. A discussion of factors which alter blood volume can be found in Chapter 47, Unit X.

Valves of the Veins. Veins which carry blood against the force of gravity are usually equipped with valves. Valves are most common in the lower extremities. The venae cavae, portal and pulmonary systems do not have valves. As long as blood flows continuously toward the heart, the valves are open. Should the blood reverse its direction of flow, the valves would close and occlude the vein.

Muscular Pumping Action. Veins depend largely upon the contractions of surrounding muscles for the flow of blood through them. Every time a muscle of the leg is contracted, the muscle is compressed against the veins of the leg, so that the veins are compressed. Blood tends to flow away from the areas of compression toward the heart. This pumping action is called the "muscle pump" or "venous pump." Thus, muscular contraction provides partial or complete emptying of both the deep and superficial leg veins. As the muscles relax, the valves of the veins close to prevent blood from flowing backward.

When a person is standing still the "muscle pump" does not work, and the venous pressures in the lower part of the leg rise. This increase in venous pressure causes an increase in the pressure in the capillaries; therefore, fluid is less readily resorbed from the tissues into the capillaries, and edema tends to develop. (See Chapter 24.)

Muscular pumping action, as occurs in walking, thus has two important functions: (1) it lowers the venous and capillary hydrostatic pressures, thereby preventing edema; and (2) it reduces the volume of blood contained within the veins of the legs.

Abdominal and Thoracic Pumping Action. *During inspiration, the flow of blood into the thoracic veins increases.* This increase in blood flow is caused by the negative intrathoracic pressure and the descent of the contracting diaphragm. The abdominal organs are displaced downward, causing an increase in abdominal pressure. Thus, during inspiration there is a greater pressure gradient between the thoracic and abdominal cavities. These external pressures compress the veins in the abdominal and thoracic cavities, causing the blood flow into the thoracic cavity to increase.

Effects of Posture on Blood Flow. *When a person is standing, less blood flows through the veins of the lower extremities* than when he is in a recumbent position. When a person stands up, the pressure in the veins is greater in the lower part of the body than in the upper part by an amount equal to the weight of a vertical column of blood from the level of the atrium multiplied by its density. An increase in pressure causes the veins to dilate, and blood tends to accumulate in the most dependent veins. In addition, the return of blood from the veins below the atrium is opposed by the force of gravity when the person is standing. If the feet are elevated above the heart in the supine position, blood flow to the heart is facilitated by the force of gravity.

Coagulation. Coagulation, or the clotting of blood, broadly consists of three phases: (1) the activation of the extrinsic or intrinsic pathway to activate prothrombin; (2) the transformation of prothrombin to thrombin by these factors; and (3) the conversion of fibrinogen to fibrin by thrombin. (See also Unit XII.)

There is a sequence of *blood clotting factors* that

leads to the formation of a thrombus. The relationships of these factors are:

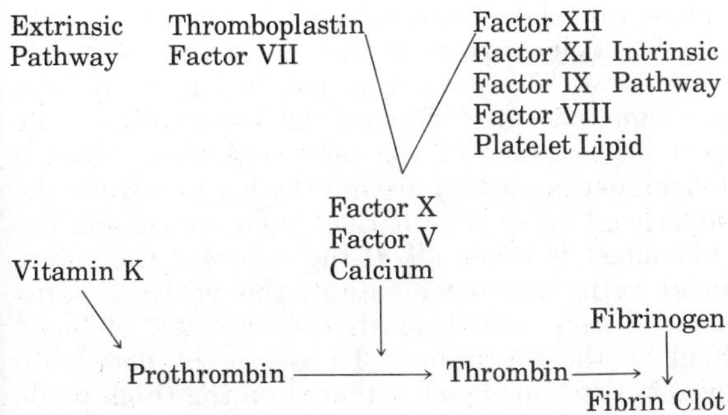

All the factors required for the intrinsic system are present in the circulating blood, whereas the *extrinsic system depends on the release of thromboplastin* from damaged cells of tissue, such as injury to the endothelium of the vein wall. It is not known how the intrinsic system is activated.

VENOUS INSUFFICIENCY

Venous insufficiency is the end result of incompetency of the valves of the veins.

Pathophysiology. Frequently the valves of the venous system are defective. This incompetency occurs when the veins have been overstretched by an excess of venous pressure for a prolonged period of time, as occurs in pregnancy, obesity, or an occupation that requires standing for long periods. The vein walls are weaker than those of the arteries. After prolonged periods of pressure they distend, preventing the leaflets of the valves from closing tightly and thus making them incompetent. Therefore, the valves will not block reverse flow in the dilated veins. Owing to this valvular incompetency there is venous stasis and increased venous pressure. The "venous pump," or the compression of the deep veins by skeletal muscle, cannot pump blood effectively to reduce the elevated venous pressure that results from the standing position. The high venous pressure results in increased hydrostatic pressure in the capillary, preventing reabsorption of fluid into the capillary from the tissues and promoting edema.

There may be an increase in permeability of the capillary walls, resulting in extravasation of red blood cells into the surrounding tissues. The red blood cells disintegrate, but they leave a deposit of hemosiderin which stains the tissues a characteristic brownish pigment. This pigment is usually noted on the distal third of the lower extremity and the malleolar areas.

Chronic edema of the subcutaneous tissue leads to inflammation, fibrosis, and atrophy. The edema prevents diffusion of nutrients from the capillaries to the skin cells. Microorganisms thrive and the patient sometimes develops cellulitis or stasis dermatitis. Finally, the skin dies and ulceration follows. Ulcers are characteristically located in the malleolar area.

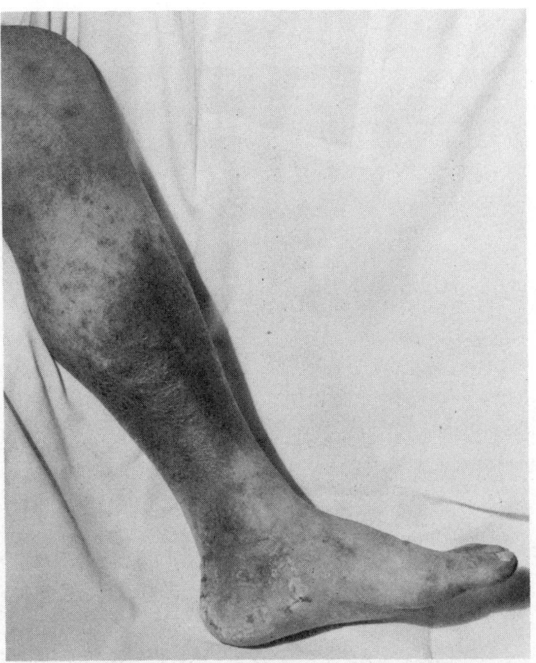

FIGURE 65–1. Pigmentation of leg resulting from chronic venous insufficiency of long standing. (From Fairbairn, J. F., II, Juergens, J. L., and Spittell, J. A., Jr.: *Allen-Barker-Hines Peripheral Vascular Diseases.* 4th ed. 1972.)

Often only one lower extremity is involved in venous insufficiency. It is chronically swollen, and the lower third of the leg may be indurated, discolored brown, scaly and ulcerated. Figures 65–1 and 65–2 show examples of pigmentation and stasis dermatitis resulting from chronic venous insufficiency.

Varicose Veins. Varicose veins are abnormally lengthened, dilated, tortuous, superficial veins. *Varicose veins are due to incompetent valves in the surface veins.* The greater and lesser saphenous veins and their tributaries are most commonly affected by varicosities.

The etiology of varicose veins may be primary or secondary to other disease conditions. Primary causes are congenital weakness of the veins, pregnancy, obesity, extreme height, and standing up for much of one's life. Varicose veins may be secondary to thrombophlebitis of the deep veins, acquired or congenital arteriovenous fistulas, and extrinsic pressure, such as from a tumor, on the inferior vena cava or iliofemoral veins.

ASSESSMENT OF PATIENT WITH VARICOSE VEINS. Many persons with dilated, tortuous skin veins have minimal or no symptoms, not even edema of the leg. The venous pump may not fail if only the superficial veins are incompetent. Other people may complain of diffuse dull aches, muscle cramps, and fatigability of muscles of the lower extremities. These symptoms are relieved by elevation of the leg, thus increasing the flow of blood back to the heart by gravity. Other patients with concomitant

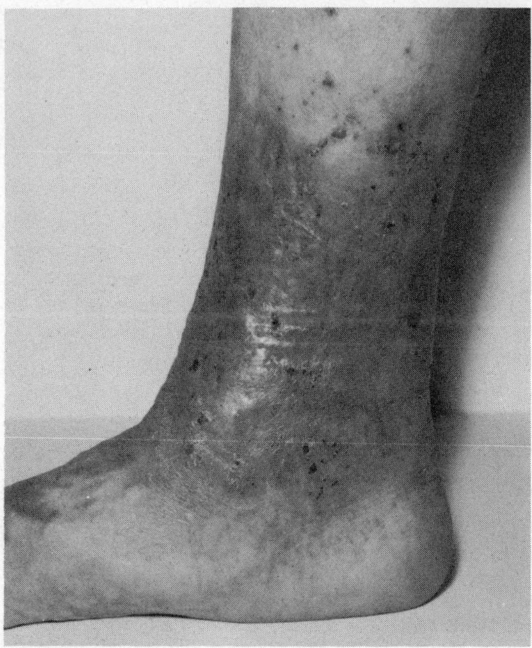

FIGURE 65–2. Stasis dermatitis with multiple excoriations of skin. (From Fairbairn, J. F., II, Juergens, J. L., and Spittell, J. A., Jr.: *Allen-Barker-Hines Peripheral Vascular Diseases.* 4th ed. 1972.)

venous insufficiency of the deep veins exhibit edematous, indurated, scaly, pigmented, and sometimes ulcerated extremities.

If the varicose veins represent a primary condition, the varicosities usually occur in both legs. If they are secondary to some other disease mechanism, the varicosities usually occur on one leg.

Incompetency of the deep and/or superficial veins can be *diagnosed* (1) by noting venous pressure changes during walking, (2) by the Trendelenburg test, and (3) by phlebography.

During walking, different venous pressures are noted between people with normal extremities and those with varicose veins. Normally there is a *marked decrease* in venous pressure in the saphenous vein during walking, indicating that muscular contraction has increased the flow of blood in the deep veins and allowed increased drainage of blood from the superficial to the deep veins. When exercise stops there is a *gradual return* of venous pressure to normal levels, indicating that the valves in the deep and superficial veins are closing and preventing backflow of blood. *Extremities with varicose veins have less of a decrease in venous pressure during walking and, upon cessation of walking, have a more rapid return to normal pressure.* Because of incompetent valves between the saphenous and deep veins, there is incomplete emptying of the saphenous veins during muscle contraction, and when walking ceases, the superficial veins, because of their incompetent valves, fill very rapidly.

Backward flow of blood through incompetent valves into the saphenous vein can be shown with the Trendelenburg test, also called the *retrograde filling test.* The patient is put in the recumbent position with his affected leg raised above the heart, thus emptying the veins (Fig. 65–3). Then a tourniquet is applied around the leg to occlude the superficial veins. The patient then stands and the tourniquet is taken off. If the valves of the superficial veins are incompetent, the varicose veins distend *very quickly* with the backflow of blood held by the tourniquet. To assess the deep vein system the tourniquet is placed on the thigh while the patient is standing, thus filling the veins. Then the patient is told to lie down with his legs elevated. The emptying of blood from the superficial veins indicates that the deep venous system is patent.

In phlebography, 50 ml. of angiographic contrast material is injected into the deep and/or superficial veins. Both normal and abnormal veins as well as the cusps of the valves can be visualized.

Nursing Intervention and Treatment. Patients with venous insufficiency cannot be cured but can be maintained in optimal health. The goals of nursing care are to promote the use of antigravity measures, to promote the use of elastic support hose, to reassure the patient, and to prevent leg ulcers.

Antigravity measures to increase blood flow from the veins to the heart include: (1) frequent elevation of the legs above the heart level; (2) avoiding prolonged standing or sitting, crossed legs, beds gatched at the knee, chairs that are too high for the patient's feet to touch the floor or that are too deep, placing pressure on the popliteal area; and (3) avoiding sources that would increase pressure above the legs, such as tight girdles and round garters. Note that blood flows from a higher to lower pressure, and if the intra-abdominal pressure is greater than the pressure in the extremities, there will be an impediment of venous flow and dilatation of leg veins. The patient should sleep with the foot of his bed elevated six inches by placement of blocks under the leg of the bed. He should spend at least one-third of every 24 hours with his feet and legs elevated.

Increased venous pressure on the surface of the leg can be counteracted by the compression of elastic support hose. Ideally this support should just balance the increased pressure. Thus, since in the standing position there is more pressure at the ankle than just below the knee, the stocking should be fitted individually to the patient's legs. Measurements are usually taken of the circumference at the ankle and calf, and from one inch below the knee or one inch below the groin to the bottom of the foot. Measurements are taken after the patient has been recumbent to reduce edema. Stockings that extend above the knee often bind the popliteal space and act as a tourniquet, especially when the knee is bent; knee length elastic stockings are preferable.

Many patients fear rupture of varicose veins with massive hemorrhage. This is an uncommon complication. Should it occur, the patient should be reassured that there is time to get to the hospital before he bleeds to death. Hemorrhage from the veins is not so threatening as from the arteries owing to the lower pressure and blood flow in the veins. In addition, hemostasis is achieved by vascular spasm, formation of a platelet "plug," blood coagulation, and the formation of fibrous tissue in the clot, thus closing the rupture in the vein.

VEIN LIGATION. When surgery of the superficial veins is being considered, the deep veins must be patent, as demonstrated by the Trendelenburg test; otherwise, the patient will have chronic edema and discomfort. The surgery consists of ligating the saphenous vein at the groin where it joins the femoral vein and stripping the saphenous vein system from the groin to the ankle. An incision is made in the ankle; a wire is threaded through the lumen of the vein from groin to ankle; then the wire together with the vein is pulled from the groin incision. The branches of the vein break off near their junction with the saphenous vein. Bleeding is minimal, especially if the legs are elevated during surgery. Some surgeons make additional incisions to remove varicosities of the smaller branches of veins. Other surgeons inject sclerosing solutions after surgery. Sclerosing solutions such as 5 per cent sodium morrhuate or 1 to 3 per cent sodium tetradecyl sulfate (Sotradecol) are injected into the vein, producing a localized phlebitis and thrombosis of the veins.

Following surgery, the legs are wrapped in elastic stockings and the foot of the bed is elevated above the heart. During the first week after surgery the patient is able to walk or to lie in bed with his feet elevated. He is not allowed to sit or stand. During the second week, the patient must keep his legs elevated about 18 out of 24 hours to avoid edema. During the third and fourth weeks, he can gradually resume his presurgical activity level.

TREATMENT OF VARICOSE ULCERS. Varicose ulcers can best be treated by bed rest with the feet elevated above the level of the heart. Continuous warm moist compresses of normal saline or boric acid help to eliminate infection, stimulate granulation, and relieve discomfort. If specific pathogens are isolated from the ulcer, appropriate antibodies may be ordered. Often the cellulitis that appears is a sterile inflammation.

In some instances an Elastoplast boot can be applied in order that the patient can be ambulatory. Other types of bandaging are Unna's paste boot and the zinc gelatin bandage. After one or two days of bed rest in order to decrease the edema, the boot is applied from the distal metatarsal level to the knee. At first it may be necessary to change the boot every three to four days because of edema and in

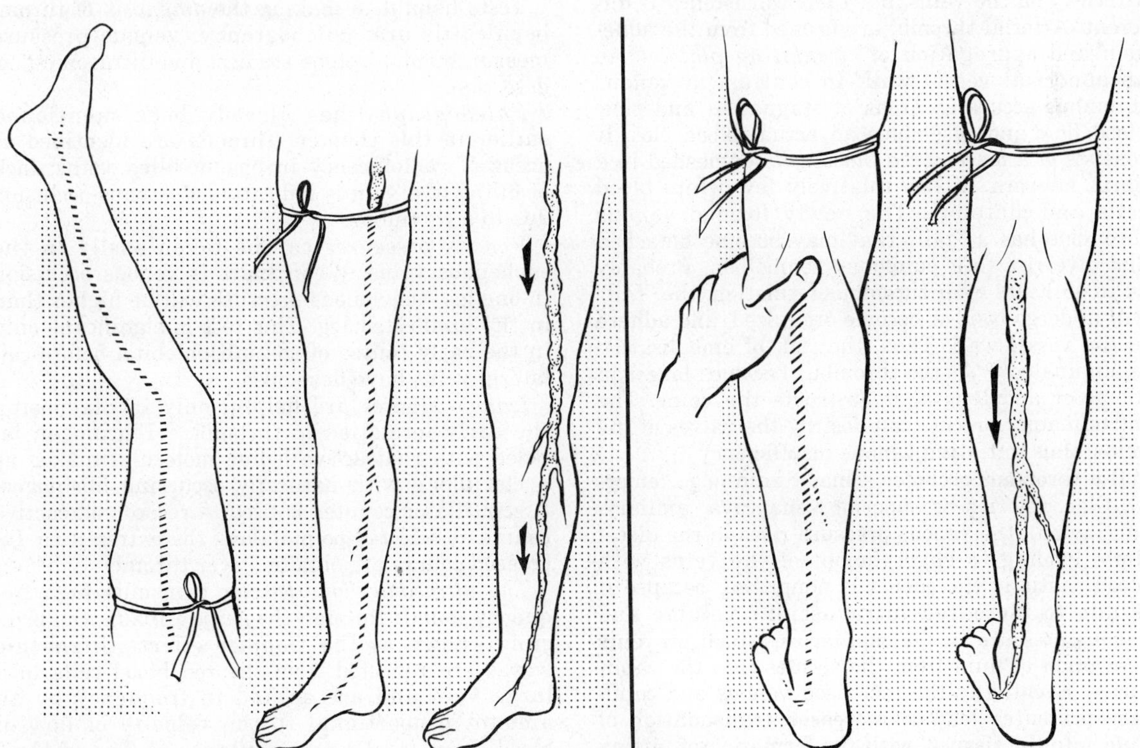

FIGURE 65-3. Representation of retrograde filling test. *Left Panel,* Great saphenous vein. *Right Panel,* Small saphenous vein. See text. (From Fairbairn, J. F., II, Juergens, J. L., and Spittell, J. A., Jr.: *Peripheral Vascular Diseases.* 4th ed. 1972.)

order to cleanse the ulcer. But as the edema decreases and the ulcer heals, the boot can be changed every week.

Healing can be hastened by applying skin grafts after the ulcer has become clean and granulation has started. If the arterial blood supply is not obstructed, healing usually occurs quickly.

Occurrence of leg ulcers should be prevented by the wearing of elastic support hose, elevation of the feet and legs a certain portion of each day, the avoidance of extremes of heat and cold and of too tight shoes and stockings, and the wearing of a foam rubber pad around the ulcer-bearing region, around and above the malleolus. This area tends to be very sensitive to trauma because the underlying venous insufficiency is still present.

THROMBOPHLEBITIS AND PHLEBOTHROMBOSIS

Thrombophlebitis is inflammation of a venous wall with clot formation. Phlebothrombosis is clot formation in the vein without or followed secondarily by inflammation. It is difficult to tell in some patients which condition came first; after several days, inflammation and thrombus are coexistent. Throughout this discussion, we shall use the term "thrombophlebitis" to designate this group of conditions.

Pathophysiology. Thrombi form in both the arteries and the veins, but their consistency is different. Arterial thrombi are formed from the adhesion and aggregation of *circulating platelets* to an abnormal vessel wall. In contrast, a venous thrombus occurs in areas of stagnation and slow blood flow and resembles an actual blood clot. It consists of a mass of *red blood cells* enmeshed in a fibrin network. It has relatively few white blood cells and platelets. The newly formed venous thrombus has a "tail" that may become detached and give rise to a pulmonary embolism. Probably 24 to 48 hours after thrombus formation, the "tail" will undergo lysis or become organized, and adhere to the vessel wall. Thus, the risk of embolization is eliminated.[60] As the thrombus becomes larger in diameter and length, it obstructs the veins. The inflammatory process can destroy the valves of the veins, thus initiating venous insufficiency.

If a thrombus occludes a major vein (e.g., femoral, iliac, inferior or superior vena cava, axillary, subclavian), the venous pressure rises in the distal limb, leading to engorgement of the veins with blood. Initially the edema is nonpitting because it is due to increased intravascular volume and venous pressure in the capillaries, which prevents resorption of fluid from the tissues into the capillaries. Eventually the increased venous and capillary pressures lead to increased transudation of fluid into the tissues, with the formation of pitting edema.[26]

Usually there is little functional disturbance as a result of thrombophlebitis of the superficial veins (saphenous) and the deep small veins (femoral, tibial, and popliteal). Abundant collateral venous channels usually evolve to relieve the increased venous pressure and volume.

The pathogenesis of thrombus formation is usually attributed to venous stasis, hypercoagulability, and/or injury to the venous wall (Virchow's triad). It is thought that at least two of the three conditions must be present for thrombi to form.[59]

Conditions that may cause *venous stasis* are varicose veins, obesity, surgery, pregnancy, *prolonged bed rest,* and congestive heart failure.

Conditions that may cause hypercoagulability are cancer; blood dyscrasias that raise the platelet count, decrease fibrinolysis, increase the clotting factors or increase the viscosity of the blood; and oral contraceptive (anovulatory) drugs. The processes leading to hypercoagulability are the least clearly defined among the triad of causative factors.

Conditions that may cause *endothelial injury* are I.V. injections, thromboangiitis obliterans (Buerger's disease), fractures and dislocations, and chemical injury from sclerosing agents, opaque media for x-ray, and certain antibiotics such as chlortetracycline.

The above divisions are not strict. For example, postoperative venous thrombosis is probably due to slow venous flow during bed rest as well as vein wall injury due to tight strapping during surgery and to the activation of clotting factors in the postoperative period.

Assessment of the Patient with Thrombophlebitis. Table 65–1 gives a summary of the causative factors and signs and symptoms of thrombophlebitis of the superficial and deep veins.

Tests helpful in making the *diagnosis* of thrombophlebitis are: phlebography, venous pressure measurements, isotope studies, and ultrasonic flow detection.

Phlebography has already been mentioned earlier in this chapter. Thrombi are identified as areas of radiolucency in opaque-filled veins; lack of filling of a vein is indicative of venous occlusion due to a thrombus.

Venous pressures can be taken easily in the saphenous veins. When there is venous occlusion in one leg, the venous pressure will be higher than in the unaffected leg. This test is significant only in the early course of thrombophlebitis before collateral veins have developed.

Isotope studies are helpful only in diagnosing the early formation of thrombi.[34] Fibrinogen labeled with radioactive iodine molecules makes up a clot along with naturally occurring fibrinogen. A scintillator counter is used to record radioactive counts at selected points along the extremities. Increased counts are obtained over thrombi.[26, 34, 40]

The ultrasonic flow detector transmits high frequency sounds through the skin, utilizing the principle known as the Doppler effect. Ultrasonic waves are reflected from the red blood cells in a large vein and are shifted in frequency by an amount proportional to the velocity of flow of blood. In normal persons velocity of flow of blood is increased during inspiration and decreased during expiration, as mentioned earlier in this chapter. If a deep vein such as the iliac vein is fully obstructed with a thrombus, then the ultrasonic detector transmits a continuous blood flow with no respiratory modulations. If the vein is partially obstructed, the instrument detects only poor respiratory modulations.[62] The instrument is used to study blood flow in the major arteries and veins.

Nursing Intervention and Treatment. The primary goals of clinical care are to prevent thrombi already formed from becoming emboli, and to prevent new thrombi from forming. Care measures include: (1) improving blood flow by physical means such as bed rest, elevation, elastic support hose; (2) applying warm moist packs; and (3) preventing hypercoagulability by drug therapy: anticoagulants, fibrinolytic drugs, and dextran. Superficial venous thrombosis usually requires anticoagulant therapy only when thrombophlebitis is extensive and threatens to involve the deep veins.

BED REST AND ELEVATION. Bed rest is indicated for four to seven days after the onset of thrombus formation in order to allow the "tail" to become firmly adherent to the vessel wall, thus decreasing the possibility of emboli. Bed rest also prevents fluctuations in pressure in the venous system that occur with walking.

Elevation of the legs above the level of the heart facilitates blood flow by the force of gravity. The increase of blood flow prevents venous stasis and the formation of new thrombi. Elevation of the legs also decreases venous pressure, thus relieving edema and pain. Elevation is best accomplished by raising the foot of the bed 6 to 8 inches on blocks. Use of pillows or gatching the bed too frequently results in elevation of the knee above the foot and interferes with proper flow.

ELASTIC SUPPORT HOSE AND EXERCISE. Elastic support is not required with adequate elevation of the lower extremities. When the patient walks, he must use elastic support hose or bandages. The elastic support compresses the superficial veins and, with walking, blood flow in the veins is increased and venous pressure kept to a minimum. *Standing and sitting are not allowed,* since they increase the hydrostatic pressure in the capillaries, promoting edema. Once the threat of embolization is over, walking and exercises in bed should be encouraged to decrease venous pressure and to promote blood flow by the contraction of muscles compressing the veins. A recommended exercise in bed is dorsiflexion of the feet against a footboard.

Sometimes pneumonic vascular compression (PVC) leggings will be ordered to aid blood flow.[25]

TABLE 65–1. CLINICAL APPRAISAL OF THROMBOPHLEBITIS

Veins	Causative Factors	Signs and Symptoms	Edema	Pulmonary Embolism	Venous Insufficiency
Superficial Veins: saphenous, median cephalic, median basilic	Varicose veins; I.V. injections; Buerger's disease; blood dyscrasias; cancer	Tender, indurated, red, visible palpable cord along vein; ovoid nodules in skin	Rare	Rare	Rare
Deep Small Veins: femoral, tibial, popliteal, pelvic	Postoperative; postpartum; prolonged bed rest; congestive heart failure; blood dyscrasias; cancer; oral contraceptives; fractures and dislocations	Increased muscle turgor over tenderness on affected vein; pressure; minimal or no venous distention; deep muscle tenderness; limb may be warmer than opposite limb; dorsiflexion of foot may cause calf pain (Homans' sign); occasionally fever—rarely exceeds 101°F.	Occasional edema may be masked and revealed by measuring circumference of extremities	Always a possibility	Rare
Major Deep Veins: femoral, ileal, axillary, subclavian, superior and inferior vena cava		No superficial signs of inflammation; cyanosis of extremity; venous distention of limbs	Usually	Always a possibility	Frequent

These leggings are attached by polyethylene tubing to an electric pump. Air is pumped into each legging alternately for one minute at a pressure of 40 to 45 mm. Hg. Use of these leggings is usually discontinued when the patient starts walking.

After thrombosis of a deep calf vein, the patient should wear elastic support for 6 to 8 weeks.

CONTINUOUS WARM MOIST PACKS. Warm packs around the involved area should be given initially for 20 hours out of every 24, decreasing the time as the condition improves. The purpose of the heat is to relieve venospasm, produce analgesia, and hasten resolution of inflammation.

ANTICOAGULATION THERAPY. Any increase in formed thrombi can be prevented with anticoagulants such as heparin or one of the coumarin derivatives. There is no evidence that heparin has any action on emboli already formed except to prevent propagation and platelet adhesiveness on the surface of thrombi.[17] Vascular occlusion that is resolved during heparin treatment is due primarily to the body's own mechanisms: thrombolysis, recanalization of the vein, and development of collateral vessels.

Heparin is thought to act by preventing the activation of clotting factor IX and inhibiting the action of thrombin in conjunction with a plasma cofactor.[17] Its effect can be determined by measuring the Lee-White clotting time. (See Unit XII.) The normal value is 5 to 10 minutes. A clotting time value may be determined before heparin injections in order to adjust the dosage. Propagation of emboli can be prevented if the clotting time is at least twice normal.

There are different opinions about the dosage and frequency of heparin administration for thrombophlebitis. Some authorities recommend 5000 units I.V. every 4 hours; others recommend 10,000 to 15,000 units I.V. every 4 hours for 48 hours, then reduced to lower levels (usually 5000 units); still others recommend 15,000 to 20,000 units subcutaneously every 12 hours. Heparin therapy is advised for varying lengths of time, from one day to seven days, based on the time when the thrombi present have become firmly adherent to the vein wall. Anticoagulation therapy is usually started with heparin and continued with coumarin.

Complications of heparin treatment are bleeding and arterial emboli. Bleeding is usually first observed in fresh surgical incisions, injection sites, or in the urine. As mentioned, arterial thrombi are formed from the aggregation of platelets, and since the primary hemostatic defense in heparinized patients is platelet aggregation, these patients are susceptible to arterial emboli.

The specific antidote to heparin is protamine sulfate 50 to 100 mg. I.V. or 1 mg/100 units of the last injected dose of heparin. Unfortunately, excess of protamine may prolong clotting.

Acetylsalicylic acid (aspirin) should never be given to patients receiving heparin. It may induce bleeding. Aspirin interferes with platelet aggregation, and thus hemostasis, in heparinized patients.

The *coumarin derivatives* inhibit hepatic synthesis of the four vitamin K-dependent clotting factors: factor II (prothrombin); factor VII (proconvertin); factor IX (Christmas); and factor X (Stuart-Prower).[32, 33] It is not known exactly how the coumarin derivatives interfere with these factors, but possibly it is by competitive inhibition with vitamin K or inhibiting the uptake of vitamin K at its site of action.[41]

The coumarins include acenocoumarol (Sintrom), bishydroxycoumarin (Dicumarol), ethyl biscoumacetate (Tromexan), phenprocoumon (Liquamar), and warfarin sodium (Coumadin).

The effect of the coumarin derivatives can be determined by measuring the prothrombin time, which is measured every day before coumarin is given. An effort is made to keep the prothrombin time at one and one half to two times the normal time (normal readings are 12 or 13 seconds by the Quick method and 13 to 17 seconds by the Link-Shapiro method). (See Unit XII.) The most serious complication from these drugs is bleeding: purpura, ecchymosis, hematuria, bleeding from the gums. The antidote for the coumarin derivatives is vitamin K (Mephyton, menadione, Hykinone, synkavite). If bleeding does occur, the drug is discontinued for a period of time.

The coumarin derivatives require a period of time before becoming effective. Therefore heparin, which is fast-acting, is used initially with a coumarin and then discontinued when the desired effect is achieved. Then therapy is continued with oral coumarin derivatives. Anticoagulation is usually continued approximately four weeks after an acute venous thrombosis and three to six months after pulmonary embolism (see below).

The following drugs should not be given with coumarin derivatives: (1) drugs that *inhibit* coumarin action (increased tendency to clot), i.e., the following hypnotics—the barbiturates, glutethimide (Doriden), and ethchlorvynol (Placidyl); (2) drugs that *potentiate* coumarin action (increased tendency to bleed) i.e., the anabolic steroids, chloral hydrate, chloramphenicol, glucagon, neomycin, phenylbutazone (Butazolidin), quinidine, and aspirin.[33, 41]

FIBRINOLYTIC DRUGS. Fibrinolytic drugs *dissolve thrombi.* Streptokinase and urokinase are fibrinolytics; Arvin is not, but removes plasma fibrinogen and renders the blood incoagulable. These drugs have been experimental; most of the clinical studies have been done on streptokinase.

Streptokinase is an enzyme derived from cultures of beta hemolytic streptococci. Its effect depends on the activation of plasminogen, which breaks down fibrin.[14] Complications involve bleeding and allergic reactions. The antidote for streptokinase is Epsikapron (aminocaproic acid).

Because streptokinase is highly antigenic, it must be given carefully, observing for symptoms of an allergic reaction and anaphylactic shock (hypotension, tachycardia, fever, chills, and rash). A typical dosage would be 600,000 units of streptokinase in 500 ml. of 5 per cent dextrose intravenously at a rate of 80 ml. per hour.[14] Other regimens have been reported using streptokinase initially, then heparin, followed by maintenance with warfarin sodium.[6]

DEXTRAN 70. Low molecular weight dextran (1) decreases blood viscosity, thus reducing hypercoagulability; (2) coats the vascular endothelium and blood elements, thus reducing contact factors which trigger coagulation; (3) reduces aggregation of blood cells; and (4) improves blood flow.[58] Best results are obtained when treatment is started four to eight hours after onset of symptoms of deep vein thrombosis or pulmonary embolism. The usual dose is 500 ml. of a 10 per cent solution every six hours intravenously. Because dextran also is antigenic and produces sensitive reactions, it is not widely used in treating venous thromboses.

SURGICAL MEASURES. Surgery is indicated if (1) anticoagulant therapy is not advised, (2) anticoagulant therapy is not effective (unusual), or (3) there is extreme thrombosis with impending gangrene. Thrombi can be successfully removed (thrombectomy) from major veins such as the subclavian, iliac, or femoral.

Embolus rarely complicates thrombectomy, but despite the use of heparin, thrombosis occasionally occurs, probably secondary to injury of the vein wall. There are two methods employed to disrupt the flow of blood and thus prevent pulmonary embolism: (1) Vein ligation traps the thrombus in the vein distal to the operative ligature. This procedure is usually done in massive iliofemoral thrombosis. (2) Plication of the inferior vena cava is done to partially interrupt blood flow, thus allowing normal flow but trapping emboli. This procedure is done by suturing parts of the vena cava or by insertion of a grid or umbrellalike prosthesis into the lumen of the vena cava. A frequent complication is the formation of new thrombi at the surgical site.[20] Figure 65–4 shows various techniques and devices for attempting to prevent fatal embolism without interrupting vena caval flow.

Complications. The three major complications of thrombophlebitis are venous insufficiency, pulmonary embolism, and postphlebitic neurosis.

Postphlebitic neurosis usually occurs in anxious, apprehensive women who have the misconception that their veins harbor clots that are going to break loose and move to the heart, causing sudden death. They refuse to bear weight on their extremities or to walk, so that disuse atrophy prolongs the disability. Often the nurse or doctor enhances the patient's fantasies by careless remarks.[21, 30, 34] For example, the use of the word "clot" in the presence of the patient tends to be more threatening than "thrombus" or "inflammation."

Prophylaxis. The prevention of thrombophlebitis and pulmonary embolism entails two problems: methods to prevent the formation of thrombi in the deep veins, and methods to prevent embolization after thrombi have formed. Prophylaxis,

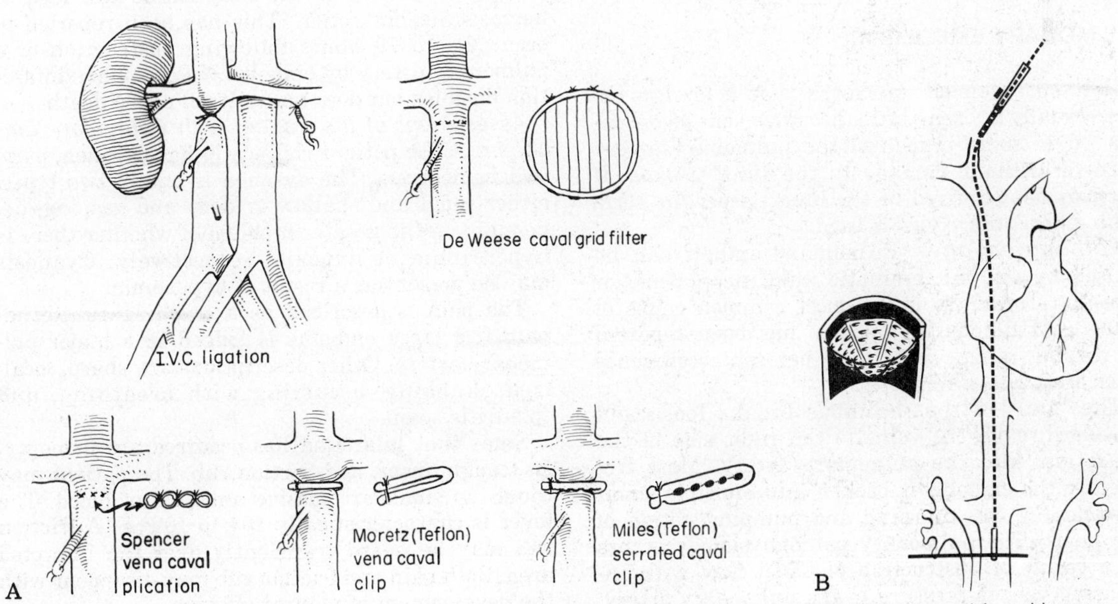

FIGURE 65–4. *A,* Drawings illustrating various surgical techniques available for preventing embolism from pelvic and lower extremity veins. Spermatic or ovarian vein ligation provides additional protection and is accomplished at time of vena caval procedure. *B,* Transvenous method of vena caval interruption using a caval prosthesis of umbrella design (Mobin-Uddin). Insert illustrates the opened umbrella. Both sieve-like and nonfenestrated prostheses have been used. (From Fairbairn, J. F., II, Juergens, J. L., and Spittell, J. A., Jr.: *Peripheral Vascular Diseases.* 4th ed. 1972.)

like treatment, is geared toward prevention of stasis of blood flow, injury to the endothelial wall and hypercoagulability.

Some preventative measures that can be taken or taught to the patient are:

Prevention of stasis

> Passive dorsiflexion of the foot and then active exercises in bed postoperative, postpartum, and for patients on prolonged bed rest.

> Tilting the surgery table head down by 15 degrees if the surgery warrants it.

> Electrical stimulation of the calf muscles and/or intermittent compression of the calf by pneumonic leggings during surgery.

> Early ambulation postsurgery and postpartum.

> Elastic support hose during and after surgery.

> Deep breathing exercises postoperatively to promote thoracic pumping action.

> Avoidance of tight garters and girdles.

Prevention of hypercoagulability

> Dextran 70 on day of surgery and one or two days postoperatively.

> Prophylactic coumarin therapy for elderly patients with hip fractures, obese patients undergoing gynecologic surgery, or patients with severe varicosities.

> Avoidance of taking the "pill" as a contraceptive.

> Avoidance of dehydration after surgery or prolonged bed rest.

Prevention of injury to the vein wall

> Avoidance of infiltration during intravenous therapy.

> Heel cushions during surgery to elevate the calves and avoid damage to the intima of the vein.

> Avoidance of gatch position in bed or putting pillows under calves postoperatively to avoid damage to endothelium of veins.

PULMONARY EMBOLISM

Pulmonary embolism means that a foreign object, usually a "tail" of a thrombus, has been deposited in some branch of the pulmonary artery with or without damage to the lung tissues. If necrosis has occurred in the lung tissue, the term "pulmonary infarction" is used.

Pathophysiology. Pulmonary emboli can be caused by air, fat, amniotic fluid, neoplasms, or thrombi. Thrombus is the most common cause of embolus. Pulmonary embolism has been reported in varying ranges of 4 to 60 per cent occurrence after deep vein thrombosis.

The "tail" of the thrombus breaks loose and travels through the veins to the right side of the heart and into the pulmonary artery. Most frequently the embolus is broken into multiple small particles by the churning and pumping action of the heart. The pulmonary pathophysiology occurs as a result of obstruction of blood flow with increasing venous pressure in the pulmonary artery, and perhaps the presence of reflex vasoconstriction as a result of thromboembolism. Serotonin, a vasoconstrictor, may be released from platelets, causing pulmonary hypertension.

Pulmonary embolism occurs abruptly. It may be severe to minor, depending on the size and number of the emboli. Of the patients who die, approximately one half die within a half hour of the onset, two thirds within one hour and three fourths within two hours. The mortality rate is approximately 38 per cent.[26]

Complete obstruction of a major pulmonary artery causes immediate death secondary to right ventricular failure (cor pulmonale), decreased stroke volume, poor diffusion of carbon dioxide and oxygen, and finally shock. Reduction of 50 to 60 per cent of the cross-sectional area of pulmonary arteries will cause respiratory and circulatory changes.[26] The obstruction due to the emboli causes increased pressure in the pulmonary artery. The "backward effects" are decreased emptying of the right ventricle, increased volume and pressure in the right ventricle, and increased volume and pressure in the great veins. The "forward effects" are decreased volume in the left atrium, decreased stroke volume, and stimulation of the baroreceptor reflex, thus maintaining arterial blood pressure and increasing contractility of the left ventricle for a period of time. Then shock ensues.

Obstruction of blood flow to the lung leads to poor perfusion and an increase in the dead space. Thus, initially the arterial pCO_2 is increased. (See Unit XIV.) Because of overcompensating hyperventilation, the arterial pCO_2 later becomes reduced. These patients have abnormal ventilation/perfusion ratios as a result of the obstructed blood flow to a ventilated portion of the lung. Frequently they develop arteriovenous shunts, leading to hypoxemia.

If there is a partial obstruction, the lung probably survives, and fibrinolysis resolves the emboli; resolution is slow (approximately two weeks, provided there is no cardiac or pulmonary disease).

Poor circulation to the lung tissue can lead to necrosis and infarction. This has been reported to occur 2½ to 79 hours following obstruction of a pulmonary artery by embolus.[26] Pulmonary infarction disables but does not in itself cause death.

Assessment of the Patient with Pulmonary Embolism. The patient classically has dyspnea, pain, and hemoptysis. The dyspnea is one of two types, either rapid and shallow or deep and gasping, depending on the greater problem of whether there is hypercapnia or hypoxia, respectively. Cyanosis may be present as a result of hypoxemia.

The pain is described as a crushing substernal pain if a large embolus is lodged in a major pulmonary artery. Other descriptions are sharp, localized, stabbing, occurring with breathing, and "pleuritis" pain.

Signs that infarction has occurred are hemoptysis, cough, fever, and friction rub. The patient may cough up small or massive amounts of blood. The fever is characteristically 101 to 102° F. A friction rub may be heard transiently over the infarcted area. Both pain and friction rub may disappear with the development of pleural effusion.

Shock (hypotension, tachycardia, cold, clammy extremities) and low arterial pCO_2 and pO_2 are ominous signs of massive emboli.

Pulmonary embolism can be *diagnosed* by chest

x-rays, electrocardiogram, blood enzyme levels, pulmonary angiograms, measurement of arterial blood gases, and radioisotope lung scan.

Chest x-rays show a wedge-shaped opacity if infarction is present. Other signs of pulmonary embolism are elevation of the diaphragm, decreased vascularity, and dilated pulmonary arteries.

The *EKG* shows an enlarged P wave, a prominent Q wave in Lead III with T wave inversion, depression of the S-T segment, and a T wave inversion in V_{1-3} in the presence of pulmonary embolism.[20, 39] There may or may not be right bundle branch block.

Blood enzymes show an elevation in the blood lactic dehydrogenase (LDH) level. There is usually no rise of serum glutamic oxaloacetic transaminase (SGOT). The serum bilirubin level rises in cases of increased pressure and blood volume in the great veins owing to right ventricular strain.

Pulmonary angiograms are the most effective means of diagnosing pulmonary emboli. This procedure is done by injecting radiopaque dye into the right atrium and pulmonary artery via a catheter threaded through a peripheral vein. Visualization of any filling defects of the heart and right pulmonary artery is done by taking sequential x-rays.

Arterial blood gases indicate an arterial hypoxemia (low pCO_2) and hypocapnia (low pCO_2) in massive pulmonary embolism. There may be a severe metabolic acidosis with a rise in lactic acid. The pH may be kept close to normal by hyperventilation.

Radioisotope lung scan is done by injecting intravenously particles of human serum albumin that have been labeled with radioactive iodine (^{131}I) or technetium (^{99m}Tc). These macro-aggregated particles are trapped in the pulmonary microvasculature and are distributed according to pulmonary flow. Both lungs are scanned with a scintillation counter and the amount of radioactivity counted gives an indication of obstruction to flow.

Nursing Intervention and Treatment. The general goals of the care of the patient with pulmonary embolism are: (1) anticoagulant and fibrinolytic therapy (refer to previous section); (2) prevention of formation of additional thrombi (refer to previous section); (3) treatment for shock, if warranted, giving vasoconstrictors such as levarterenol (Levophed) or metaraminol (Aramine) (see Chapter 26); (4) treatment of respiratory distress by continuous oxygen by nasal catheter or oxygen mask and positioning patient with the head of bed elevated at least 30 degrees to ease breathing (see also Unit XIV); and (5) allaying fear and apprehension.

The patient's fear is associated with the sudden onset of severe chest pain and his inability to breathe. The patient becomes anxious, restless, and apprehensive. Many times he will not reveal his innermost fears to others. Since sudden death can ensue from pulmonary embolism, the doctor may discuss the potential seriousness of the disease with the patient. The nurse's firm emotional support can be a stabilizing factor at this time. This support can effectively be shown by staying with the patient and honestly assuring him of the advances that have been made in the treatment of

pulmonary embolism. In addition, the nurse should give intensive care efficiently and unhurriedly and not display the emotional strain of caring for a seriously ill or dying patient.

There are three *surgical treatments* for pulmonary embolus: venous interruption by vein ligation to prevent the embolus from traveling to the heart (see previous section); vena cava plication to allow blood flow but to trap emboli (see previous section); and embolectomy.

An *embolectomy* is the surgical removal of emboli from the pulmonary arteries. Before the advent of the cardiopulmonary bypass, the procedure had an extremely high mortality rate. Even now embolectomy concurrently with anticoagulant therapy still carries a high risk,[42] partly because of possible misdiagnosis and partly because of the problems involved in operating on patients in profound shock.

DISORDERS OF THE LYMPHATIC SYSTEM

Review of Anatomy and Physiology

The lymphatic system is an offshoot of the collecting venous system with the function of returning to the circulation from the tissue fluid nearly all the protein and other macromolecules which cannot be directly resorbed into the blood capillaries. Specifically the functions of the lymphatic system are:

> The transport of lymph. Lymphatic vessels also transport viruses and bacteria, which may result in infection of the lymphatic channels *(tubular lymphangitis)* or of the lymph nodes *(lymphadenopathy)*. If the lymph nodes break down, the infection may enter the blood stream *(septicemia)*. Infection may be confined to the reticular lymphatics of the skin, as in erysipelas.

> Production of lymphocytes.

> Production of antibodies. Immune substances are extracted from lymphocytes.

> Phagocytosis, performed by the reticuloendothelial cells lining the sinuses of the lymph nodes.

> Hematopoiesis. Under pathologic conditions some blood cell formation may take place in the reticuloendothelial cells lining the sinuses of lymph nodes.

> Resorption of fluid and chemical substances that escape from the blood stream across the walls of blood capillaries.

> Absorption of fats and fat-soluble materials from the intestine.

The forces that govern the exchange between blood capillaries and tissue spaces regulate the *formation of lymph*. Any condition that increases the filtration of fluid from the blood capillaries may increase the flow of lymph. Filtration of fluid may be increased by:

> Increased capillary pressure as a result of increased venous pressure from venous obstruction.

> Conditions increasing permeability of the capillary wall, such as a rise in temperature, reduced oxygen supply, or the effect of certain drugs such as histamine.
> Increased metabolic activity from both muscular and glandular activity.
> Passive movement and massage.
> Hypertonic as well as isotonic solutions introduced intravenously.

It has been estimated that ordinarily an average of 200 million lymphocytes enter the blood stream from the lymphatic system per hour. In general, the lymphocyte count of the blood is greater in the young than in the old.

The lymphatic system has valves; it depends on the muscle pump for the movement of lymph against the force of gravity. The specific *factors affecting the movement of lymph* are:

> Compression of lymph vessels by surrounding structures, especially contracting muscles.
> Respiration.
> Propulsive action of smooth muscles in walls of lymphatic vessels.
> Arterial pulsations.
> Negative pressure in great vessels at the base of the neck.
> Peristaltic contractions of the intestines.
> Capillary blood pressure.
> Force of gravity.

The lymphatics originate as a fine network of small collecting capillaries in all tissues with a well-developed blood supply. They frequently anastomose and tend to travel in company with veins. The peripheral lymphatics join with larger lymphatics (the main lymphatic ducts) and pass through regional lymph nodes before entering the blood stream. The *main lymphatic ducts* include the right and left jugular trunks, the right and left subclavian trunks, the right and bronchomediastinal trunks, the right lymphatic duct, the intestinal trunks, the right and left lumbar trunks, and the thoracic duct. The *thoracic duct* is the main collecting duct of the lymphatics (Fig. 65–5). It carries lymph to the systemic venous system from the lower extremities, the perineum, and the pelvic and abdominal organs as well as the right half of the body above the sternal junction. Injury to this duct may result in considerable loss of fat, protein, and lymphocytes from the system.

The *regional lymph nodes* redistribute the fluid between the venous and lymphatic systems in response to the anatomic and functional state of the lymphatic and venous channels. Within the nodes particles such as microorganisms or neoplastic cells are filtered out of the lymph before it returns to the main blood stream. A lymph node is made up of (1) a connective tissue framework, (2) lymphoid tissue, (3) reticuloendothelial tissue, and (4) a system of sinuses. Lymph is conducted to the

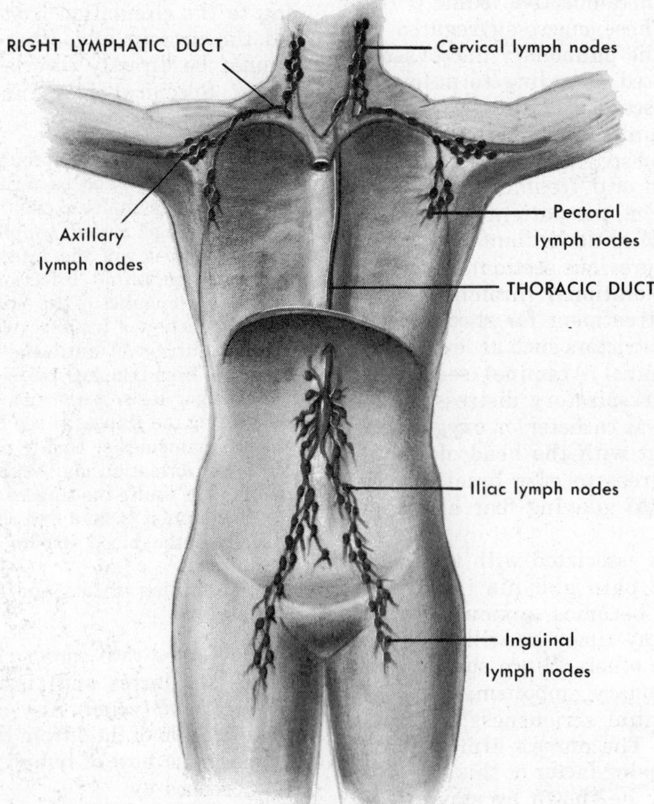

FIGURE 65–5. Lymph drainage of the body. (From Dienhart, C. M.: *Basic Human Anatomy and Physiology.* 2nd ed. 1973.)

node by afferent, and from it by efferent, lymphatic vessels (Fig. 65–6).

The amount of lymphoid tissue and the general distribution of lymph nodes are related to age. Growth is most rapid in infancy and continues at a high level throughout childhood, declining from puberty onward. The fact that the maximum development of lymphoid tissue occurs when acute infections are most common, and during the greatest growth period, indicates that it is part of the body's defense mechanism. Adenoid and tonsillar tissues, for example, reach their maximum at 3 to 5 years of age and become smaller thereafter.

Examination of the Lymphatic System

Although over 60 groups of lymph nodes are listed by anatomists, only three regional groups are usually examined: cervicofacial and supraclavicular, the axillary and epitrochlear, and the inguinal and femoral. The standard examination of the lymph nodes involves inspection and palpation. Usually lymph nodes cannot be felt in the adult, but enlarged nodes, perhaps as a result of some previous inflammation, are frequently palpable. Cervical nodes up to 1 cm. in diameter can always be felt in children up to 12 years of age. Palpable nodes are most common in the occipital, axillary, and inguinal regions. In adolescents and adults, palpable inguinal lymph nodes are common, probably because of the prevalence of recurrent infections of the feet. Femoral lymph node enlargement more often indicates a pathologic state. Any node, whether palpable or not, may show microscopic changes indicative of neoplasm.

Localized lymphadenopathy (lymph node enlargement) is usually due to either inflammation or cancer. Acute inflammation (lymphadenitis) causes enlarged, tender, rather soft nodes, sometimes associated with red streaks, indicating lymphangitis. Adenopathy due to cancer metastasis is usually hard, nontender, and somewhat fixed to the underlying structures.

Since the lymphatic system plays an important role in various diseases, its study by the injection of radiopaque material and roentgenographic visualization *(lymphography)* has become an important diagnostic tool. One purpose for which this method is especially valuable is the investigation of swelling in the lower extremities, which is often difficult to diagnose by other means.

Generalized Lymphadenopathy

Generalized lymphadenopathy means involvement of two or often three regionally separated lymph node groups in which enlargement results from a systemic disorder acting on lymphoid tissue. Sometimes infection may cause generalized lymphadenopathy in addition to a more pronounced localized swelling of regional nodes. Children often have more widespread lymph node enlargement in response to an infection than do adults. Generalized lymphadenopathy is usually due to inflammation or neoplasm. Viral infections (infectious mononucleosis, measles) and hypersensitivity reactions (serum sickness) are common causes of acute generalized lymph node enlargement. Such nodes are soft, movable, and slightly tender. Many chronic infections also may at times produce generalized enlargement.

Some forms of leukemia and malignant lymphoma cause generalized adenopathy. The *lymphoblastomas* are a common cause of the condition. They may produce progressive painless enlargements which at first may be localized. Later, enlargement may become generalized and the nodes become matted, firm, and fixed. *Leukemia* may or may not produce generalized lymphadenopathy; it is uncommon with the granulocytic form. In monocytic leukemia, lymph node involvement is limited to the cervicosubmandibular area and is usually the result of infection in the oropharyngeal area. Chronic lymphocytic leukemia often causes generalized lymph node enlargement; the nodes may feel nontender, freely movable, and rubbery. In acute leukemia, the nodes are frequently tender. In other instances generalized lymph node involvement may be primary, as in Hodgkin's disease, lymphosarcoma, and lymphatic leukemia.

Generalized lymph node enlargement may also be indicative of other diseases involving the hematopoietic system, such as sickle cell or hemolytic anemia.

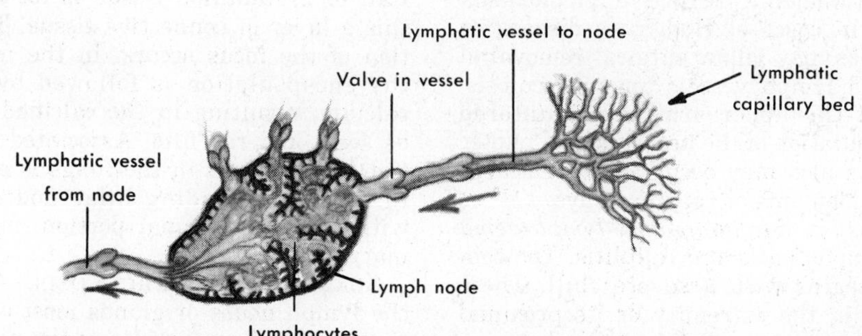

FIGURE 65–6. Lymphatic vessels and a lymph node. (From Dienhart, C. M.: *Basic Human Anatomy and Physiology.* 2nd ed. 1973.)

Lymphedema

Lymphedema is a swelling of soft tissues resulting from increased quantities of lymph. There are many causative factors in lymphedema, but the mechanism of its production seems to be the same in all instances.[20] Stasis of lymph occurs primarily as a result of obstruction, produced by either inflammatory or noninflammatory factors. When obstruction occurs, lymph vessels first dilate, and subsequently become incompetent. The lymph seeks new channels, and increased lymph in the tissues causes acute inflammation, thrombosis of the lymph vessels, more stasis of lymph, and fibrosis. The various types of lymphedema can be categorized according to their differing etiologies.

Lymphedema Praecox. Lymphedema praecox affects mostly females between the ages of 9 and 25 years (praecox means "early"). The swelling usually appears spontaneously and without known cause. The first indication may be a puffiness about the foot or ankle, particularly during menstruation, warm weather, and strenuous activity. Only one extremity may be involved. The edema usually progresses slowly up the leg until, in a period of months or years, the entire limb is involved.

Congenital Lymphedema. There are two types of congenital lymphedema: simple and hereditary. The simple type affects one member of a family; hereditary congenital lymphedema affects a sufficient number of blood relatives to indicate that a genetic defect is responsible. This condition is known as Milroy's disease. In simple congenital lymphedema a diffuse swelling involving all or part of a single extremity is present at birth. The swelling is firm and pits on pressure. It decreases greatly when the limb is elevated.[20]

Secondary Lymphedema. Secondary lymphedema can be either obstructive or inflammatory. *Obstructive lymphedema* may be the effect of occlusion of the lymph vessels as a result of metastasis to the lymph nodes of malignant disease of the breast, uterine cervix, uterus, vulva, prostate gland, bladder, testes, skin, or bones. The most common cause of obstructive lymphedema in men is carcinoma of the prostate, and lymphoma is the most common cause in women. Obstructive lymphedema also may occur in cases of Hodgkin's disease or lymphosarcoma, or may follow surgical removal of lymph nodes and lymph vessels for tuberculosis. Lymphedema of the upper arm is encountered after radical amputation of the breast. (See Chapter 93.) Lymphedema also may occur after treatment with radioactive elements or roentgen rays.

The characteristics of *inflammatory lymphedema* are recurrent lymphangitis and cellulitis. The condition usually begins with a severe chill. There may be distress in the extremity or its proximal lymph nodes. The temperature may be between 101 and 106° F. A small red area appears in the extremity and increases in size until the extremity is swollen, red, and tender. The lymph nodes are also swollen and tender. Chills may recur and high fever may persist for several days. The abnormal condition recedes slowly over four to fourteen days, and even after signs of inflammation have disappeared, swelling may be present. Single attacks may cause only minor swelling, but edema increases with successive attacks.

Medical treatment of all types of lymphedema, in order to be of value, must be carried out early. The longer the condition is uncontrolled, the more fibrosis develops and the less effective medical treatment becomes.

Diuretic therapy has greatly aided in the management of some patients. However, although the fluid portion of lymphedema can be removed in this way, any enlargement of the limb from tissue hypertrophy will not be affected; most patients will need to wear some type of elastic support. A specially fitted elastic stocking is most effective.

Patients with recurrent lymphangitis and cellulitis should receive appropriate antibiotic therapy in addition to the above measures.

When medical treatment alone does not control lymphedema, surgical treatment is considered. It is usually designed for one of two purposes: to improve lymph drainage, and to remove the markedly edematous and hypertrophied tissue. Postoperatively the limb should be supported with an elastic bandage for several months, and perhaps indefinitely.

Infectious Diseases Affecting the Lymphatic System

Tuberculosis. Tuberculosis is a clinically important disease and an important cause of death in many parts of the world. (See Unit XIV.) Tuberculosis has two important relationships to the lymphatic system: the primary complex, and glandular tuberculosis.

THE PRIMARY COMPLEX. The tubercle bacillus usually invades the body through the air passages or the intestines. The lungs are the site of infection in 70 to 80 per cent of cases, the intestines in 15 to 25 per cent, and other rare sites in 5 per cent. In each instance a primary complex is formed, consisting of a lesion at the site of entry and in the corresponding lymph glands.

When the bacillus reaches the lung alveoli an inflammatory reaction occurs, taking the form of a caseous bronchopneumonia. Around this area a wall of granulation tissue is formed, and outside this a layer of connective tissue. Thus, encapsulation of the focus occurs. In the majority of cases the encapsulation is followed by the deposit of calcium, resulting in the calcified focus that may be seen on x-ray film. Associated with the formation of this focus in the lungs is a similar process in the corresponding hilar nodes. These nodes, with the parenchymal portion, make up the primary focus.

GLANDULAR TUBERCULOSIS. Tuberculosis of the lymph nodes or glands most commonly affects the cervical lymph nodes of the neck. Tuberculous cervical lymphadenitis, also called scrofula, was much more common in the past than it is today. The infection usually is blood-borne. The most common method of invasion is through the lymphatic channels to the regional nodes, such as the submental, submaxillary, or superior deep cervical. Or the infection may proceed from abdominal or thoracic tuberculous lesions through the main lymphatic channels to the deep nodes in the posterior triangle of the neck. Tubercle bacilli that invade the cervical lymph nodes may be of the bovine or human type. At the present time, tuberculous cervical lymphadenitis is nearly always associated with tuberculosis elsewhere in the body, rather than being a localized condition.

The condition begins as a painless swelling, which may enlarge rapidly and may eventually develop into an abscess. Ulceration and a cutaneous sinus may follow. Isoniazid treatment is usually effective, but incision and drainage is used if necessary.

Other groups of lymph nodes that may occasionally be infected with tuberculosis include the mediastinal and tracheobronchial lymph nodes, the abdominal nodes, and, rarely, superficial nodes such as the axillary, inguinal, and epitrochlear.

Other Infections. Other infectious diseases affecting the lymph nodes are septicemia, cat-scratch disease, filariasis, rat-bite fever, scrub typhus, tularemia, lymphogranuloma venereum, bubonic plague, and chancroid. Most of these begin with a primary sore on the extremity; the patient then develops regional lymphadenopathy, fever, and systemic symptoms.

Septicemia, owing to hemolytic streptococci, is no longer seen frequently because of the use of sulfonamides and antibiotics. Red streaks up the extremity and enlarged nodes are signs that the infection is indeed spreading, and medical attention is needed.

Cat-scratch disease is a subacute, self-limited infectious disease characterized by malaise, granulomatous lymphadenitis, and variable degrees and patterns of fever. It is usually preceded by a cat scratch, from which a primary lesion develops followed by lymph node involvement. In about 25 per cent of the patients the lymph nodes suppurate. The infectious agent is unknown. Absence of bacteria in the pus and a positive reaction to the "cat-scratch antigen" help to establish the diagnosis.

Filariasis results from an infection by a nematode parasite. Early acute manifestations include fever, lymphadenitis, retrograde lymphangitis of extremities, orchitis, epididymitis, funiculitis, and abscess. Prolonged and repeated infection with obstruction to lymph flow often leads to hydrocele and to elephantiasis (massive enlargement) of limbs, genitalia, or breasts. Surgery may be necessary to treat the elephantiasis. The disease is endemic in most of the tropic regions of the world and is transmitted by a mosquito. Control is through elimination of mosquitoes. Diethylcarbamazine citrate (Hetrazan) is effective against the nematode worm and is often given to large populations.

Rat-bite fever is a term applied to two separate diseases, each transmitted by rat bite. One is caused by *Streptobacillus moniliformis,* the other by *Spirillum minus.* The spirillary form is more likely to have lymph node involvement. Usually there is a history of rat bite within 10 days, followed by a primary edematous lesion. There may be regional lymphadenitis, paroxysmal fever, a rash, polyarthritis, and leukocytosis. The bite wound, although apparently healed, later breaks down to leave an ulcer that runs a chronic course and occasionally develops into an abscess. Treatment is by tetracyclines or penicillin.

Scrub typhus is a rickettsial disease that begins with a primary skin ulcer that develops at the site of attachment of an infected mite, the transmitting vector. An acute febrile onset is followed by headache, conjunctival injection, and lymphadenopathy. The lymph nodes may enlarge to the size of acorns. Prophylaxis in endemic areas is by use of clothes and blankets impregnated with miticidal chemicals and by application of mite repellents to skin. Treatment is with tetracycline or chloramphenicol orally.

Tularemia is an infectious disease of wild animals and man, which is transmitted to humans from infected animals by insects such as ticks or deerflies. Onset begins with chills and fever. An ulcer appears at the site of original infection. In the glandular form of the disease, the regional lymph nodes become swollen and tender and then suppurate. Ulceration may occur. Prevention is by avoiding handling of carcasses except when wearing gloves and by thorough cooking of meat. Treatment is with streptomycin, tetracycline, or chloramphenicol.

Bubonic plague is a severe disease largely controlled today by immunization. It is transmitted by the bite of an infected flea or by handling of contaminated material. The most common type is characterized by acutely inflamed and painful swellings of the lymph nodes draining the site of the original infection. These swellings, called "buboes," most often affect the nodes of the groin.

Lymphogranuloma venereum and chancroid are discussed in Chapter 91.

CHAPTER 66

Nursing the Patient Undergoing an Amputation

Amputation is the surgical removal of all or part of an extremity. The most frequent indication for amputation of the *lower extremities* is *peripheral vascular disease.* Indeed, according to McCollough, "Recent major surveys of lower limb amputations have revealed that up to 85 per cent of civilian amputations being performed today are for complications of peripheral vascular disease."[35] Our aging population and the increased numbers of diabetics possibly account for this high incidence.

In contrast, the most common indication for amputations of the *upper extremities* is *severe trauma* due to electrical, chemical, and thermal burns; frostbite; armed conflict; war injuries; or explosions.[56] Only rarely are upper limb amputations performed to control peripheral vascular disorders.

Other reasons for amputating either upper or lower extremities include the following: malignant tumors; acute or chronic infections, e.g., chronic osteomyelitis, fulminating gas gangrene, trophic ulcers, and septic wounds; severe crushing wounds; and congenital deformities.

Faced with increasing numbers of amputees, the health professions have striven in recent years to improve the care of these patients. At one time, major goals of care were limited to removal of the injured or diseased limb and avoidance of infection and contractures. Today the goals have greatly expanded to include the *total rehabilitation* of the amputee, thereby insuring his return to full function and a normal active life. In Friedmann's words, attainment of full function includes "reconstructive amputation without procrastination, prompt healing of the stump, fast patient preparation to use a good artificial limb provided promptly, and training."[22]

Despite tremendous improvements in the care of amputees, the individual undergoing amputation still faces a severe—sometimes catastrophic—trauma that strikes not only the body but the mind and emotions as well. We live in a highly mobile society. Also, our society admires "the doer," the independent achiever, the individual who "gets around," and who "gets things done." Moreover, physical attractiveness is presented on every form of media as being almost essential for survival in a competitive world. The youthful, beautiful, intact body is upheld as the ideal to the United States public night and day on billboards, in magazines, and on television. For these reasons amputation signifies much more to the average person than simply the loss of a limb; it symbolizes the end of mobility and the loss forever of a whole, intact body and a satisfying self-image. These losses, in turn, cause the patient to fear further losses on the job market and in his family and social relationships. Is it any wonder, then, that a patient dreads amputation of a limb even though that limb may have pained and worried him for years?

To help the amputee to overcome his fears and anxieties and to return to full function is the major task of the nurse and the rehabilitation team. If the amputee is to reach these goals, the health team must design a total plan of care which is in keeping with the individual patient's personality and needs. Friedmann summarizes the "ideal" care plan when he states:

> Evaluating the patient's needs is central to good care, and should determine the total plan for that individual, which he understands, and in which he concurs. It includes the decision to operate, the type and timing of surgery, the postoperative care, fitting and training—physical, psychological, and vocational. This is what is necessary in treating the person rather than the diseased limb.[22]

SURGICAL EVALUATION OF THE PATIENT

When a surgeon evaluates a patient for possible amputation, he must decide upon: (1) whether to amputate; (2) the type of amputation (i.e., open or closed); (3) the level of amputation required; (4) the patient's rehabilitation potential; and (5) the type of postoperative prosthetic fitting and rehabilitative program desired. Let us briefly explore each of these problems.

The Decision to Amputate. The surgeon's decision whether to amputate depends primarily upon the patient's condition, results of tests of peripheral vascular function, and the general attitude of the surgeon and the patient toward amputation. First of all, an amputation is in order if the patient's life is in danger (e.g., in severe toxicity resulting from gangrene) or if the patient suffers from intractable limb pain. Also, the surgeon may amputate if his patient's ability to function is hopelessly impaired by a damaged extremity. Limb impairment may result from either severe injury, congenital deformity, or chronic ischemia resulting from extensive peripheral vascular disease.

Secondly, when peripheral vascular disease is the major indication for amputation, the surgeon orders diagnostic tests before making his final decision. Studies of peripheral function include oscillometry, tests for intermittent claudication, angiography, skin temperature studies, and palpation of the popliteal arteries. These tests were discussed in Chapter 64.

In addition, the decision to amputate is determined, in part, by the surgeon's attitude toward the procedure. Friedmann implies that amputation is equated in the minds of some doctors with failure, and that these surgeons may strive to save the patient's extremity "at all costs." On the other hand, Friedmann states, "When the surgeon views the problem as attempting to improve the overall function of his patient, he appreciates that proper amputation, and postoperative care, can restore the patient to a level of function only slightly different than the preamputation state."[22]

Like some surgeons, some patients may resist amputation even though it would greatly improve their function. For example, one of the authors (JL) once cared for a young woman whose hand had been horribly crushed and mangled in a wringer accident. This patient, even though her hand was deformed, painful, and useless, refused to consider amputation; unfortunately, she regarded amputation as a further form of mutilation. Finally, her doctors, after many months and great effort, convinced the young woman that a well-fitted, functioning prosthetic device would be superior to a hand that was useless and unsightly. The patient underwent surgery and prosthesis training and she eventually learned to accept her artificial hand as a functioning part of herself.

Type of Amputation. There are two types of amputation procedures: the open or guillotine amputation and the closed or "flap" amputation. The major indication for *guillotine amputation* is *infection.* The fact that the stump is not closed over with a skin flap allows the free drainage of purulent or infectious material. Patients undergoing an open amputation require antibiotic therapy and the use of strict aseptic technique whenever the incision is cleansed, the dressing is changed, and so forth. Once the infection is completely eradicated, the patient then undergoes *stump revision* or closure.

The *closed* or *flap* amputation is one in which the stump is closed or covered by a flap of skin sutured over the bone end of the stump. This type of amputation is performed when there is *no evidence of infection* and consequently no need for extensive open drainage. However, to prevent accumulations of blood and serous fluids, some surgeons elect to insert small drains into the incision site to prevent swelling of the stump. If a rigid dressing is applied during surgery, drains are not necessary because the dressing compresses the stump and alleviates swelling. (See discussion of the rigid dressing below.)

Level of Amputation. Specific amputation levels for the *lower extremities* are as follows:

> Amputation in the foot.
> Amputation at the ankle level (Syme operation).
> Below the knee (B/K) amputation.
> Knee disarticulation (bones separated at the knee).
> Hip disarticulation (amputation through the hip or pelvis, which is performed for malignant tumors, massive injuries, and extensive gangrene).

Specific amputation levels of the *upper extremities* are:

> Wrist disarticulation.
> Below-elbow amputation.
> Elbow disarticulation.
> Above-elbow amputation.

The level of amputation for either lower or upper extremities should never be higher than absolutely necessary. In the case of lower extremity amputations, the percentage of energy expenditure by the patient increases with each higher level of amputation as follows:[22]

> Unilateral B/K amputation: 10 per cent higher than in the nonamputee.
> Bilateral B/K amputation: 20 per cent higher than in nonamputee.
> Unilateral A/K amputation: 60 per cent higher than in nonamputee.

The surgeon tentatively decides upon the level of amputation prior to surgery. Circulation to the skin of the extremities must be adequate for the stump to heal satisfactorily. To evaluate circulatory status, the surgeon examines the patient's extremity for warmth and sensation; he may also order arteriography, oscillometry, and other procedures discussed earlier.

However, it is not until the patient is in the operating room that the surgeon makes his final decision concerning stump length. The selection of amputation level at that time is based upon the extent of bleeding from the incised skin edges. If skin bleeding is normal, then the amputation is performed at the level selected preoperatively. If skin bleeding is scant, then the surgeon is forced to operate at a higher level to ensure adequate postoperative healing.

Evaluation of Rehabilitative Potential. Ideally, patients should attain independent function with the use of a prosthesis. However, prosthetic rehabilitation requires patient cooperation, good coordination, and a tremendous expenditure of energy. Unfortunately some patients, because of age or disease, are unable to undertake prosthesis training. Conditions that prohibit prosthesis fitting and ambulation include the following:

> Severe neurologic disease.
> Disorientation, senility, psychosis, or severe mental retardation.
> Chronic heart failure accompanied by greatly reduced cardiac reserve.

Individuals burdened with these problems can usually hope for no more than wheelchair independence.

Postoperative Prosthetic Fitting and Rehabilitation. Prior to the 1960's, patients undergoing amputation faced the dreary prospect of months of stump wrapping and conditioning before they could be fitted with a prosthesis. This long delay (anywhere from three months to a year) created many complications for the new amputee. Joint contractures, weakness, intellectual deterioration, and emotional problems resulting from the immobilization greatly prolonged the patient's suffering and dependency as well as his hospitalization. Today, old-fashioned methods of protracted stump conditioning have been largely discarded. Patients are either fitted *immediately* with a prosthesis (immediate postsurgical prosthetic fitting), or prosthesis fitting is *delayed* a week or two until the stump wound is healed and the sutures are removed (conventional delayed prosthetic fitting). The surgeon must decide which type of prosthetic fitting is indicated prior to surgery, so that he can make the needed arrangements and explain the procedure to the patient.

Immediate Postsurgical Prosthetic Fitting

Immediate fitting of the patient with a prosthesis was first introduced in France in 1961. In 1963 this once radical technique was presented by the Polish surgeon Marion Weiss at the Sixth International Prosthetic Conference in Copenhagen. A year later, surgeons in the United States obtained a federal grant to further study the advantages and disadvantages of immediate prosthetic fitting. Despite early problems with stump abrasion and breakdown as a result of excessive early ambulation, this technique is now accepted by the medical profession as a highly useful procedure, and it is currently employed in medical centers throughout the world.

The program for immediate postsurgical prosthetic fitting typically involves the following aspects:[1, 22]

> *Myoplastic surgery.* Myoplasty is the plastic repair of muscles whereby severed muscles are reattached to one another and to the bone. It is employed during closed amputation in order to restore normal muscle tension, and to restore muscle and tendon sensory feedback loops which, in turn, make the stump sensitive and responsive to stimuli. A stump which acts as a sensory-motor end-organ enables the amputee to use his prosthesis more effectively, learn a more graceful gait, and regain his sense of balance. However, some authorities believe that the use of myoplastic techniques is unnecessary and even unwise in some amputations, and that they should be used only in young patients with adequate circulation. Sarmiento[48a] feels that myoplastic techniques in below-knee amputees with peripheral vascular disease are likely to lead to complications and increased morbidity.

> *Application of a total contact rigid dressing.* The rigid dressing, which is applied to the stump in the operating room, is one of the most important aspects of immediate prosthetic fitting. It consists of a plastic bandage that is wound over the various dressings covering the wound, i.e., nonadherent gauze, fluffs, sterilized stump sock, and felt pads, which act to cushion pressure points. The rigid dressing protects the stump from injury and it also prevents stump swelling by gently compressing the tissues. The socket of the distal end of the rigid dressing is designed to connect with a pylon, that is, an adjustable, rigid support whose proximal end is attached to the below-knee socket or to the knee unit of an above-knee prosthesis. The distal end is connected to a foot-ankle assembly (Fig. 66–1). The rigid dressing is usually changed three to four times before a permanent prosthesis is applied. Cast changes are necessary because, as the stump heals, it tends to shrink and is consequently no longer compressed by the original cast.

> *Early ambulation.* The real purpose of early ambulation with an immediate postsurgical prosthesis is to condition and prepare the patient's stump for later gait training.[22] The patient usually begins to ambulate the first postoperative day. Ambulation time is brief (3 minutes once or twice that day) and weight-bearing is strictly limited (see below).

> *Controlled progressive ambulation.* The patient ambulates a little more each day, depending upon his specific rehabilitation program and his tolerance of increased activity. At first, he simply stands at the bedside with help. Next he learns to walk between parallel bars. Gradually he progresses to crutches and then a cane. Finally the amputee is able to walk without assistance of any kind. This gait training period usually extends for approximately three months.

> *Limited weight-bearing.* Weight-bearing must be strictly limited during the first weeks of ambulation, be-

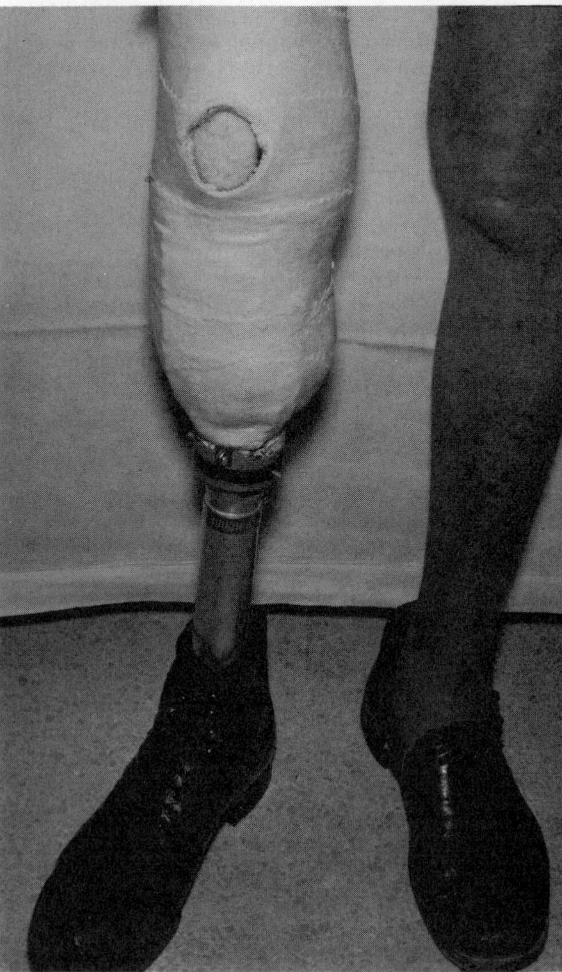

FIGURE 66–1. Immediate postsurgical prosthesis in place after below-knee amputation for occlusive arterial disease. Note rigid dressing, pylon, and foot-ankle assembly. (From Fairbairn, J. F., II, Juergens, J. L., and Spittell, J. A., Jr.: *Peripheral Vascular Diseases.* 4th ed. 1972.)

cause the wound is still healing. To learn to control weight-bearing, new amputees are placed on paired scales and told to note the amount of weight that they are placing on their prosthesis as compared with the unamputated limb. During the first two weeks following amputation, patients are instructed to *never place more than 20 to 25 pounds of weight* on the prosthetic limb.[1] As healing increases, weight-bearing increases. Because it is difficult for most patients to remember the "feel" of the proper weight, one hospital is now using a "beeper," which is placed between the prosthetic foot and the rigid dressing. The "beeper" is sensitive to pressure and it "beeps" to warn the patient whenever he exceeds his assigned weight-bearing capacity.[2]

> *Patient cooperation.* The patient is truly a prime member of the rehabilitation team. If immediate postsurgical prosthetic fitting is to be successful, the patient must be willing to limit weight-bearing, learn and apply the principles of stump and prosthesis care, and wholeheartedly enter into a program of progressive ambulation and gait training.

Benefits. Immediate prosthetic fitting offers the amputee many advantages. First of all, the patient adjusts better emotionally to his amputation if he awakens from surgery with a substitute limb already attached to his stump. In addition, the rigid dressing acts as a compression bandage, molding and shrinking the stump. This continuous sustained compression reduces stump edema, pain, phantom sensations, and contractures. Also, by alleviating the need for months of stump wrapping and preprosthetic conditioning, the rigid dressing shortens the patient's rehabilitation period and speeds his return to social and economic independence. Finally, the program of early progressive ambulation alleviates the complications of immobility, stimulates the circulation, and fosters a sense of hope and optimism in the patient and his family.

Indications and Contraindications. Immediate postoperative prosthetic fitting is almost always indicated for children and juveniles. It is also highly beneficial for individuals with below knee and below elbow amputations.

On the other hand, immediate fitting is contraindicated for the following patients:

> Above-knee amputees, because these patients are usually severely debilitated from the condition which resulted in amputation; e.g., diabetes, gangrene, osteomyelitis.

> Above-elbow amputees, because these individuals have usually suffered extensive trauma and are in poor or critical condition.

> Patients with incapacitating medical disorders; e.g., neurologic disease, severe heart disease, extensive vascular pathology, anemia, and hypoproteinemia.

> Patients who are unable or unwilling to control weight-bearing during the early postoperative period; e.g., confused, senile persons, patients who do not speak English, the psychotic, and the mentally retarded.

> Patients who have undergone vascular reconstruction or who have an infected stump.

In addition, immediate fitting should not be attempted in small hospitals with inadequate prosthetic facilities.

Conventional Delayed Prosthesis Fitting

Immediate prosthetic fitting is not always possible; however, authorities agree that every amputee

capable of eventually ambulating should receive a temporary prosthesis *as soon as possible* following surgery. Early prosthesis fitting and training benefits the patient psychologically. Also early ambulation prevents the complications associated with immobility; moreover, the pumping action afforded by walking reduces stump edema more effectively than does stump bandaging.

The timetable for patients undergoing delayed prosthesis fitting is approximately as follows:

> The patient returns from surgery with his stump dressed and covered with either Ace bandages or stump socks; note that the rigid dressing is generally not used for conventional delayed fittings.

> During the following one to two postoperative weeks, the patient's stump is wrapped in the manner shown in Figures 66–2 and 66–3; note the differences in technique from wrapping an above-knee stump and a below-knee stump.

> During the second or third postoperative week, the sutures are removed. If the stump has healed satisfactorily and no complications are present, the patient is then fitted with a provisional temporary prosthesis made of plaster of Paris or plastic. At this time the patient begins to ambulate; however, only partial weight-bearing is allowed.

> By the sixth week, the patient is allowed to put full weight on his prosthesis.

> By the tenth to twelfth week the patient is fitted with a permanent prosthesis provided progress has been satisfactory.

Which prosthetic fitting technique is generally more successful—the immediate or the delayed? Choice of technique depends upon the patient's needs and upon the surgeon's personal preference. On the one hand, the immediate technique is usually selected for young patients and for those who need the psychologic "lift" provided by immediate replacement of the amputated limb. Also, the use of the rigid dressing offers many advantages. On the other hand, delayed fitting may be preferred by some surgeons because it is generally safer. Wound disruption rarely occurs with delayed fitting because the wound must be almost completely healed before the patient can begin to ambulate. Further, the amount of rehabilitation time saved by using the more risky immediate fitting is only one to two weeks at most.[22] Finally, the use of immediate fitting techniques is limited to large medical centers where prosthetic experts are available.

CARE OF THE PATIENT UNDERGOING AMPUTATION OF THE LOWER EXTREMITIES

Preoperative Care

Psychologic Preparation. As we emphasized earlier, it is extremely difficult for the average person to accept amputation of one or more of his extremities even though it is absolutely necessary.

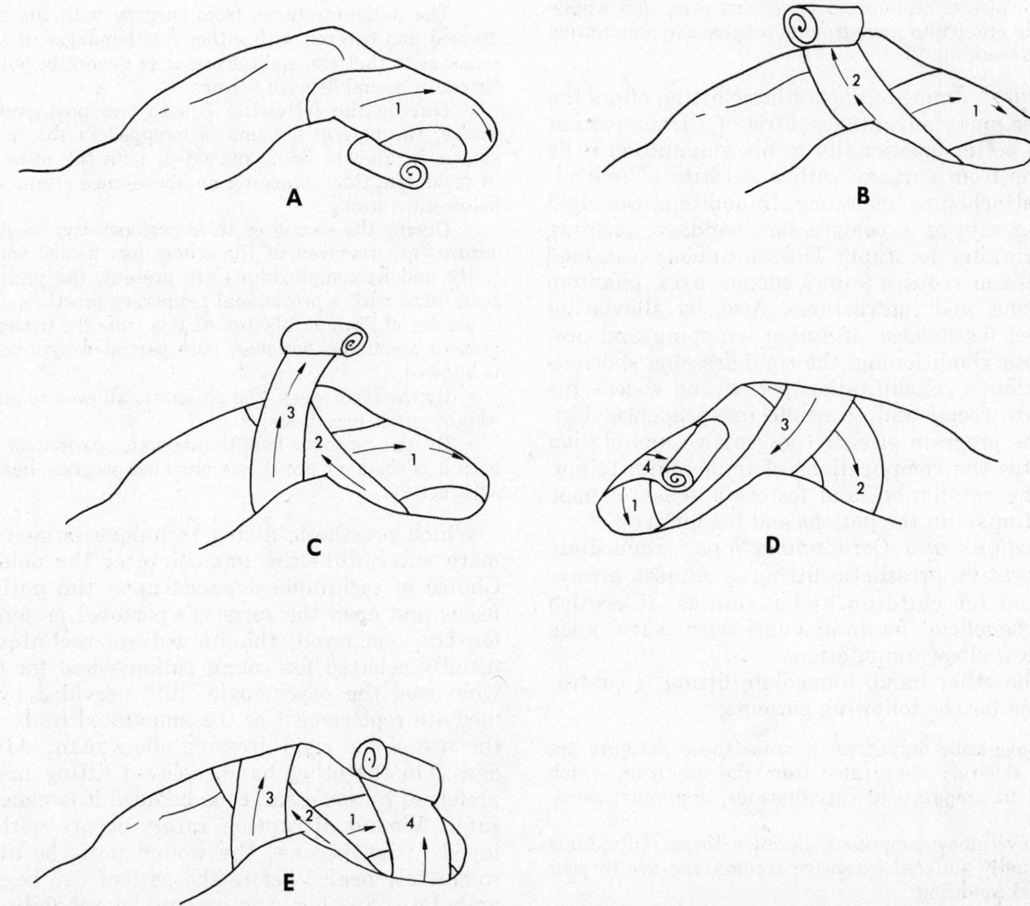

FIGURE 66–2. Bandaging a below-knee amputation stump. If a second bandage is needed, it should be started over the medial condyle, reversing the procedure shown. Anterolateral aspect: A, Start 4″ elastic bandage above lateral condyle. Enclose medial, distal end of stump. Apply pressure via bandage at distal end. Use diagonal, not circular, turns. Hold roll so it is upward for ease in unwinding. B, Bring roll around posterior aspect of calf, enclosing beginning of roll. Make turn around thigh above patella. Be sure there is *less* tension on bandage above knee than on end of stump. C, Turn No. 3 goes diagonally above knee and down to include medial condyle. Anteromedial aspect: D, Turns 3 and 4 continue to posterior aspect of calf. E, Turns 3 and 4 enclose lateral, distal end of stump. Continue to above knee as shown with turns 2 and 3. Finish enclosing end of stump using diagonal and figure-of-8 turns. Be sure greatest pressure is on end of stump. (Courtesy of Physical Therapy Department, Harborview Medical Center, Seattle.)

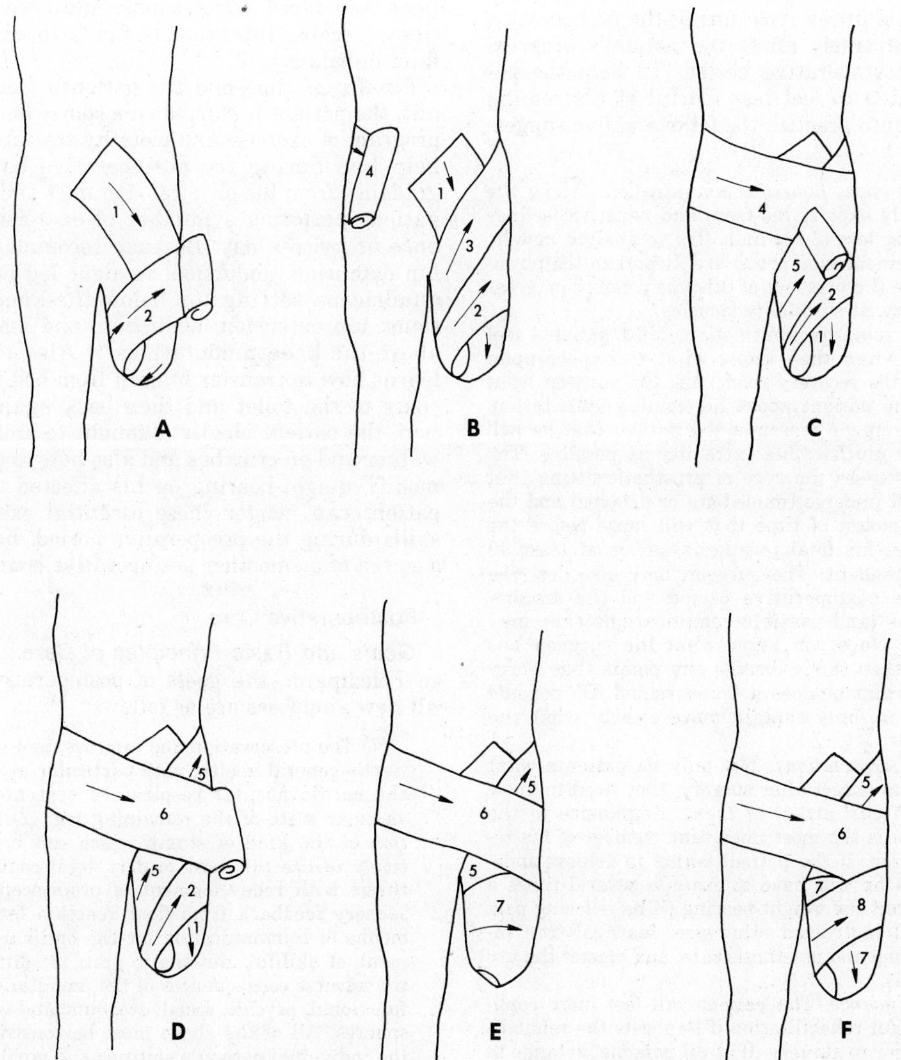

FIGURE 66–3. Bandaging an above-knee amputation stump. A, Use 6″ elastic bandage. Enclose medial, distal end of stump. Apply pressure via bandage to end of stump. Use diagonal, not circular, turns. B, Turn No. 3 must be high in groin and then turn made around waist to hold No. 3 in place. Do not pull hip into flexion. (A second 6″ roll may be needed.) C, Turn No. 5 must be high in groin and a loop made around waist again. D, See diagram. E, Enclose lateral, distal end of stump. (A 4″ roll may be needed.) Continue diagonal and figure-of-8 turns around stump. F, Continue turns to shape end of stump. (Courtesy of University of Washington Department of Prosthetics, from booklet *Prosthetics-Orthotics*.)

Amputation is dreaded because it destroys the patient's idealized body image, imposes both physical and social limitations, and temporarily (and sometimes permanently) disrupts his life style. In sum, amputation signifies a painful venture into a frightening unknown.

We know that fears and anxieties that remain unchallenged and unresolved during the preoperative period can adversely affect the patient's progress during the postoperative period. To help the potential amputee to feel less fearful of his coming surgery, put into practice the following five suggestions:

> *Establish open, honest communication.* Allow the patient to freely express his fears and negative feelings over the coming loss of his limb. Try to analyze how he perceives the amputation procedure. Report to the physician if you note the presence of extreme depression, great fear and anxiety, or suicidal tendencies.

> *Give and reinforce information.* Most patients feel less anxious when they know what to expect upon awakening in the recovery room. Ask the surgeon what he has told the patient about his coming amputation. Typically the surgeon reassures the patient that he will try to save as much of his extremity as possible. The doctor also discusses the type of prosthetic fitting that the patient will undergo (immediate or delayed) and the approximate amount of time that will lapse before the patient receives his final prosthesis and is at least 90 per cent independent. The surgeon may also describe the immediate postoperative period and the discomforts, problems, and possible complications that may accompany it. Once you know what the surgeon has said, you can then safely discuss any points that worry the patient or that he does not understand. Do not add any information; only explain more clearly what the doctor has said.

> *Establish expectations.* Not only do patients want to know what to expect after surgery, they need to know what the staff *will expect of them.* Emphasize to the patient that he is the most important member of his rehabilitation team. If the patient wants to achieve independence, then he will have to exercise several times a day, strictly limit his weight-bearing (if he is losing part of a leg) until instructed otherwise, learn all the intricacies of stump and prosthesis care, and master the use of his prosthesis.

> *Build confidence.* The patient will feel more confident of successful rehabilitation if he meets the rehabilitation team prior to surgery. If at all possible, arrange to introduce the patient to the physical and occupational therapy staffs, the prosthetist, and the vocational counselor; in some institutions the team also includes a social worker and psychologist.

> *Sustain hope and optimism.* Like the patient who faces mastectomy, laryngectomy, or permanent colostomy, the future amputee often feels that his social, vocational, and love life virtually end with his surgery. To counteract this hopeless outlook, it is extremely helpful to introduce the patient to other amputees who are mastering their prostheses and achieving independence.[49] The support, encouragement, and understanding of other amputees often provides the hope and courage that many future amputees so desperately need.

Physical Preparation. Physical preparation of patients for amputation focuses upon controlling or alleviating underlying illnesses and infections, correcting nutritional and fluid imbalances, and preparing the patient for postoperative ambulation by increasing his strength and endurance.

Thus, during the preoperative period patients with severe diabetes are brought under control with proper diet and insulin. Persons with ulcerated legs or osteomyelitis may be treated with antibiotics and bed rest. The debilitated person is nourished with foods high in protein; he may also be given supplements of vitamins and minerals. The severely anemic are treated with iron preparations and blood transfusions, and dehydrated patients receive intravenous fluids to correct their fluid imbalance.

Finally, if time and the patient's condition permit, the patient is started on a somewhat strenuous program of exercise and mobility training that will help him during the postoperative period. With guidance from his physical therapist and nurse, the patient performs a number of exercises at least once or twice a day. Bosanko recommends "active hip extension, abduction, straight leg raising, and quadriceps setting for below-the-knee amputations; hip extension, abduction, and adduction for above-the-knee amputations."[4] Also the patient learns how to transfer himself from bed to a wheelchair to the toilet and then back again. In addition, the patient ideally is taught to ambulate in a walker and on crutches and also how to control and modify weight-bearing on his affected side. If the patient can master these essential exercises and skills during the preoperative period, he is almost assured of a smoother postoperative course.

Postoperative Care

Goals and Basic Principles of Care. According to Friedmann, the goals of postoperative care for all new amputees are as follows:

> (1) The preservation and improvement of the patient's general health, with particular attention to the cardiovascular respiratory system and the vascular state of the remaining leg; (2) the creation of the kind of stump which can most effectively utilize the most modern total contact prosthesis with redevelopment of proprioception and sensory feedback from floor reaction forces as a means of communication for the optimal development of skillful, automatic gait; (3) diminishing the adverse consequences of the amputation in the functional, psychic, social, economic and vocational spheres. All of the above must be consistent with the individual patient's abilities and problems, and the conditions under which he must live and function.[22]

Basic postoperative goals are the same, but the actual postoperative care of amputees varies, according to whether the patient: (1) has been immediately fitted with a prosthesis while in surgery, (2) will be fitted at a later time, (3) is ineligible for prosthesis fitting for reasons cited earlier, or (4) has undergone a guillotine type of amputation because of infection. Let us begin by considering the first two groups.

In Table 66–1 we have compared and con-

TABLE 66–1. POSTOPERATIVE CARE: COMPARISON OF AMPUTEES UNDERGOING "DELAYED" PROSTHESIS FITTING AND "IMMEDIATE" PROSTHESIS FITTING

Type of Care	Delayed Prosthesis Fitting	Immediate Prosthesis Fitting
Stump care	Stump covered with dressings and Ace bandage or stump socks; note if Penrose drains were inserted during surgery to remove blood and serous fluid Observe dressings for signs of excessive bleeding; *always have large tourniquet on hand* to apply around stump in event of hemorrhage Reinforce or change dressings as ordered; wrap stump with Ace bandages as shown in Figures 66–2 and 66–3 or cover dressings with stump socks; *check bandages frequently;* they can slip and form a tourniquet around stump, occluding blood supply Sutures removed in 10 to 14 days if wound healing well; temporary prosthesis fitted at that time	Stump covered with dressings and rigid plastic dressing; Penrose drains usually not inserted because rigid dressing helps to prevent bleeding by compressing the stump Observe rigid dressing for signs of oozing; if oozing occurs, mark blood stain with a pen and observe stain every 10 minutes for increase in size; report excessive oozing at once Provide *cast care* as discussed in Unit XVII *Guard against cast slipping off stump* because edema and wound disruption rapidly develop; if slippage occurs, compress stump at once with tightly wrapped plastic bandage; *notify surgeon* Sutures usually removed in 10 to 14 days during first cast change; cast changed one to two more times thereafter, to compensate for stump shrinkage
Pain relief	Narcotics (Demerol and codeine) may be needed to control severe incisional and phantom pain (Unit IX)	Darvon usually sufficient for pain control because rigid cast greatly reduces pain and phantom sensation
Positioning	Elevate stump on pillow for 24 to 48 hours to hasten venous return and prevent edema; do *not* elevate for more than 48 hours or hip contracture may result	Elevation of stump for 24 hours usually sufficient; rigid cast acts to control swelling
Turning	Turn patient to prone position for short time first postoperative day and then 2 to 3 times daily to prevent hip contracture; have patient roll from side to side	Same; rigid cast, however, acts to prevent both hip and joint contractures and turning is not so essential
Exercises	Exercises to prevent contractures started as soon as possible (1st or 2nd day postoperative), including: active range of motion, especially of remaining leg; strengthening exercises for upper extremities; hyperextension of stump	Exercises not so essential because rigid dressing prevents contractures; also, early ambulation prevents all immobilization disabilities
Ambulation	Dangle and transfer to wheelchair and back within first or second postoperative day Crutch walking is started as soon as patient feels sufficiently strong (Unit XVII)	Dangle and ambulate patient in walker for short period first day Ambulate longer time each day; in physical therapy, patient uses parallel bars, then crutches, then cane
Psychologic support	Observe carefully for signs of depression or despondency; remind depressed patient that he will receive prosthesis when wound heals	Observe for depression; patients usually less depressed if they awaken with prosthesis attached

trasted postoperative care for patients undergoing immediate prosthesis fitting and those undergoing conventional delayed prosthesis fitting.

The third group of patients, which includes the elderly, senile, and debilitated, need continuous and conscientious nursing care throughout the postoperative period if their condition is not to worsen. These individuals may be seriously dehydrated and may consequently need intravenous fluids. Elderly and senile patients and those with neurologic conditions may be incontinent of both urine and feces; to prevent gross contamination of the stump wound, place a plastic material (such as Saran wrap) around the outside bandage and secure it with adhesive tape.

In addition, the elderly and debilitated are usually unable to perform active exercises; passively exercise these patients' limbs several times a day until strength increases. Take care to turn the debilitated amputee every one to two hours and have him cough and deep breathe frequently. Remember that patients in this group are highly susceptible to all the complications of immobilization. (See Chapter 27.) Observe these patients continuously for signs of hypostatic pneumonia, contractures, and bladder and kidney problems. Also, the new amputee who is old, ill, weak, and exhausted usually suffers from severe depression, which immobilizes him further.

Finally, there are the patients who undergo a *guillotine* amputation. As you recall, the indication for this type of amputation is *infection*. The stump is left open and unsutured to permit free drainage. To prevent retraction of the skin, traction is applied to the skin; either Buck's extension traction or a Thomas splint may be used. (See Unit XVII.) Infection is treated with bed rest and antibiotics. Once the infection is controlled, the patient returns to surgery for closure of the stump.

Postoperative Complications. What types of complications and problems can patients develop following amputation? Postoperative complications vary with the type of prosthetic fitting the patient receives. Persons who are scheduled for *delayed* prosthesis fitting are subject to the following preprosthetic complications:

> *Hemorrhage.* Some oozing and drainage is normal following amputation. However, excessive bleeding should be reported at once to the surgeon. Also, as stated in Table 66–1, always keep a large tourniquet at the bedside in event of massive hemorrhage.

> *Hematoma.* A hematoma is a tumorlike mass of coagulated blood that has escaped into the tissues or into a cavity. The surgeon can usually prevent stump hematoma by carefully clamping off vessels in surgery and by inserting drains into the wound.[56] Hematoma is a dangerous postoperative complication because it delays wound healing and it also provides culture media for infection-causing bacteria. To treat hematoma, the surgeon aspirates the blood from the tissues and firmly bandages the stump.

> *Stump edema.* A certain amount of stump edema is *inevitable* in patients who are not fitted with a rigid dressing in the operating room. However firm, correct stump bandaging may lessen not only the degree of stump edema, but also the problem of asymmetrical edema ("dumbbell" edema). Figure 66–4 shows detrimental and inadequate stump wrapping. In contrast, note the firm, smooth, proper stump wrapping shown in Figure 66–5.

> *Skin complications.* The major skin problems encountered following amputation include delayed healing of the surgical wound and necrosis of the incisional skin edges. Treatment of these problems may involve a return to surgery for stump revision.

> *Joint contracture.* Without the rigid dressing, the postamputation patient may develop various joint contractures, including hip joint flexion contracture, stump adduction contracture, knee flexion contracture, and footdrop. Contractures can be prevented by instituting the following nursing measures: (1) do not elevate the patient's stump on a pillow for more than 24 to 48 hours following surgery; (2) avoid positioning the stump in an externally rotated, abducted position; (3) prevent abduc-

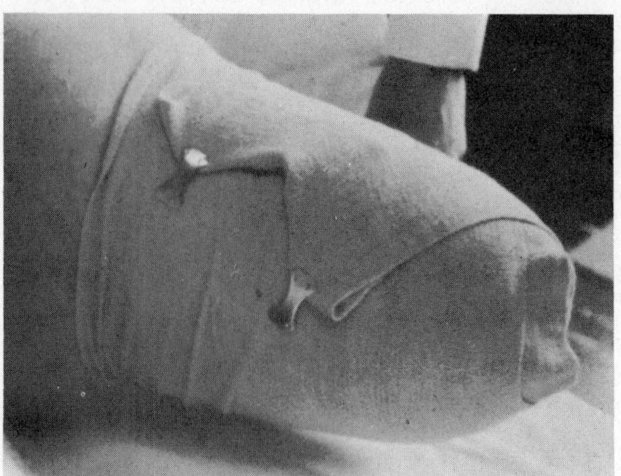

FIGURE 66–4. Inadequate stump wrapping. (From Thompson, R. G.: *Orthopedic Clinics of North America, 3*:323, July, 1972.)

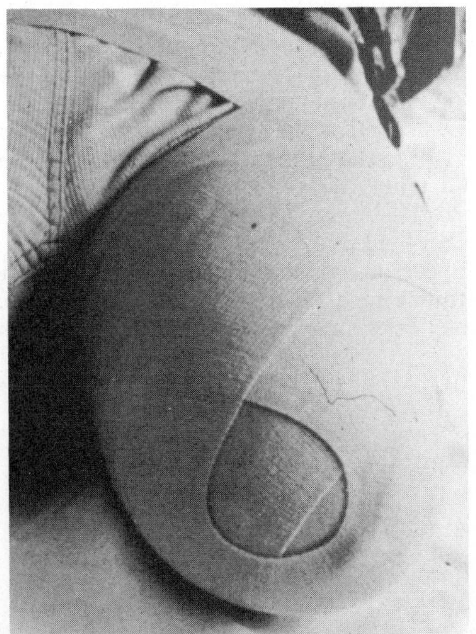

FIGURE 66-5. Proper stump wrapping. (From Thompson, R. G.: *Orthopedic Clinics of North America, 3*:329, July, 1972.)

tion contracture by adducting the stump on a scheduled basis; (4) put the patient through range-of-motion exercises (passive or active) at least three times a day; (5) position the patient in a prone position for several hours each day; and (6) place a footboard on the end of the bed to prevent footdrop of the remaining limb.

> *Phantom limb sensation.* The majority of new amputees experience the peculiar sensation that their amputated limb is still present. This sensation may or may not be painful; it may disappear within hours following amputation or it may continue for years. There is no cure or treatment for phantom limb sensation because the causation is not fully understood. However, it is helpful to warn patients about phantom limb sensation prior to amputation and to reassure them that these sensations are "normal."

> *Phantom pain.* Between 1 and 10 per cent of all amputees develop painful phantom limb sensation. The causation and treatment of phantom pain is discussed in Unit IX.

Patients who undergo *immediate* prosthesis fitting do *not* experience many of the complications listed above. Usually the rigid dressing compresses the stump sufficiently to prevent hemorrhage, hematoma, stump edema, and joint contracture. Also, incisional pain and phantom limb pain are often greatly lessened by the rigid dressing. However, serious complications may develop *because* of the rigid dressing and early ambulation program. First of all, the opaque rigid dressing makes it impossible for the surgeon and nursing staff to inspect the stump for beginning signs of skin breakdown, wound disruption, and so forth. Second, the rigid dressing can fall off the stump; this complication constitutes an *emergency* because stump edema forms in minutes and wound disruption may occur within half an hour following slippage of the cast (Table 66-1). Finally, too much weight-bearing during the first days of ambulation before the wound is healed may result in wound disruption and skin breakdown. Because of this grave danger, some doctors prefer delayed prosthesis fitting to the immediate technique.

Rehabilitation and Prosthesis Training

The purpose of postamputation rehabilitation is to help the new amputee to attain the highest level of independence of which he is capable. For elderly debilitated patients who cannot receive a prosthesis, the highest level of independence obtainable may be simply wheelchair independence. For the majority of new amputees, however, the goal of rehabilitation is to achieve at least 90 per cent independence with the use of a prosthesis.

The Prosthesis Prescription. Prostheses are prescribed by physicians and constructed by prosthetists who have ideally been examined and certified by the American Board for Certification of Prosthetists. Basically, lower limb prostheses are composed of the following four components: the socket, joints (hip and knee), suspension (suction system, pelvic band, waist belt, or leather thigh corset), and foot and ankle (Fig. 66-6). However, each of these four components can be modified in numerous ways to meet the needs of the patient. Describing the complicated task of prescribing a prosthesis, Friedmann explains as follows:

> To send a patient to a prosthetist with a "prescription" for an "above-knee prosthesis" is equivalent to sending a patient to a pharmacist with a prescription for "heart medicine." To illustrate the complexity of above-knee prosthetic prescription, there are at least fifteen varieties of feet and ankles. There are five types of friction, six of brake and six extension aids for prosthetic knees. There are eight types of socket designs and the same number of suspensions. . . . Prosthetically we fit not the stump but the individual.[22]

To tailor a prosthesis prescription to the individual, the physician must evaluate many factors. He must first consider the length and condition of the stump. He must also assess the patient's age, weight, agility, endurance, general state of health, finances, occupational goals, social and family situation, mental health, intelligence, and motivation to become independent. Motivation is one of the most important factors to be considered, because without sufficient motivation the patient will be unwilling to undertake the hard work and training that mastering a prosthesis requires. Sometimes the poorly motivated can be helped with psychiatric counseling. In other cases, motivation is increased when the patient meets other amputees who have mastered use of their prosthesis and achieved independence.

Adjustment to a Prosthesis. The new amputee must adjust to his prosthesis both physically and psychologically. *Physically,* the amputee must increase his strength and endurance with regularly scheduled exercise, because ambulating with a prosthesis requires a considerable expenditure of energy. Also, the patient must learn to control weight-bearing until his wound completely heals. In addition, the recent amputee must conscientiously practice ambulating with his new prosthesis until he develops a skillful automatic gait.

Psychologically, the patient must come to accept his new prosthesis as a part of himself if he is to become truly independent again. To fully accept the prosthesis, the patient must include the artificial limb in his body image. Because of deep-seated personal and social problems, psychologic adjustment to a prosthesis is often more difficult and may take longer than physical adjustment.

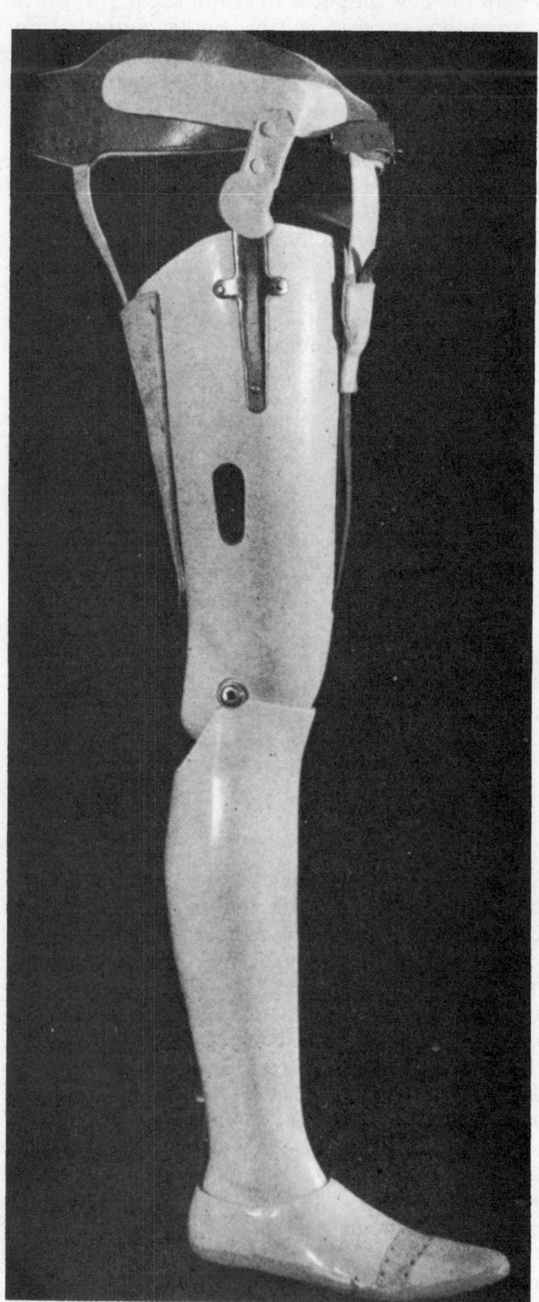

FIGURE 66–6. Conventional above-knee wood socket with hip joint and pelvic band; single axis knee and ankle. (Institute of Rehabilitation Medicine, New York University Medical Center, New York, N.Y.)

Postprosthetic Complications. Once the patient starts using his prosthesis he may develop skin complications and/or stump and generalized weakness. *Skin breakdown* on the stump is extremely serious because it interrupts prosthesis training and prolongs hospitalization. Specific skin complications include breakdown of the previously healed scar and blistering or ulceration of the stump. Diabetics are particularly susceptible to skin complications; also, peripheral neuropathy may obliterate the diabetic's awareness of stump pain.

The stump should be inspected hourly when the patient first begins to ambulate on his prosthesis. If skin irritation and abrasion develop, prosthesis use must be temporarily discontinued and the stump must be firmly wrapped in bandages until the skin irritation is alleviated. If ulcerations appear on the stump or the stump fails to heal, the patient may have to undergo surgical stump revision before he is able to resume prosthesis training.

Stump weakness and generalized weakness are problems that particularly plague elderly amputees and discourage them during prosthesis training. A carefully designed program of exercise will help to strengthen weak muscles and it will also increase the patient's general endurance level.

Stump and Prosthesis Care. Teaching the patient how to care for his stump and prosthesis in the hospital and at home is an important part of his rehabilitation program. When discussing *stump care* with the patient, emphasize the following points:

> The stump should be *inspected daily* for redness, blistering, or abrasions. A mirror can be used to examine all sides and aspects of the stump. Caution the patient against ever putting a Band-Aid on his stump; Band-Aids may irritate the skin and may cause sores and infection when they are pulled off.

> *Daily stump hygiene* is essential. The stump should be washed with a mild soap and then carefully rinsed and dried. Both soap left on the skin and dampness are very irritating and can eventually cause skin breakdown and infection. Also, nothing should be applied to the stump after it is bathed. Emphasize that alcohol dries and cracks the skin while oils and creams soften the skin too much for safe prosthesis use.

> *Woolen stump socks,* which are worn over the stump for cleanliness and comfort, must be washed in cool water and mild soap to prevent shrinkage. To prevent stretching, socks should be washed gently. Stump socks should be dried lying flat on a towel. If the socks tear, they must be replaced; the wrinkling caused by mending the socks is highly irritating to the skin.

> *Stump swelling* can be prevented by instructing the patient to put on his prosthesis the moment he gets up in the morning and keeping it on all day once the wound has healed completely. Emphasize that the more the patient wears his prosthesis, the more his stump will shrink.

The patient must also learn how to *care for his prosthesis.* Important points to stress are listed below:

> Sweat and dirt should be removed from the prosthesis socket daily. Tell the patient to wipe out the inside of the socket with a damp soapy cloth. To remove the soap, use a clean damp cloth; never pour water into the socket because the water may ruin the leather parts of the prosthesis and also rust the prosthetic joints. Remind the patient to dry the prosthesis socket thoroughly; a damp socket can irritate the skin and cause stump breakdown and infection.

> The patient should never attempt to adjust or mechanically alter his prosthesis. If problems develop, tell the patient to immediately consult his prosthetist for professional help.

> The prosthesis should be examined by the prosthetist for mechanical defects on a regular yearly basis.

CARE OF THE PATIENT UNDERGOING AMPUTATION OF THE UPPER EXTREMITY

Only 15 to 20 per cent of all amputations involve the upper extremities.[56] As we stated earlier, the major indication for upper extremity amputation is severe trauma; vascular disease is a rare causative factor.

Because of the trauma and shock that he has suffered, the patient who is undergoing upper extremity amputation requires extensive *preoperative care prior to surgery*. Blood transfusions, intravenous infusions, and antibiotics may all be necessary.

Psychologic preparation also is an extremely important aspect of care. Loss of a lower extremity is traumatic, but loss of an arm may be truly catastrophic. The functions of the arm and hand are highly specialized, and the loss of these functions threatens the patient in every aspect of his life. To obtain a slight sense of how incapacitating the loss of an arm is, place your dominant hand and arm in a sling for a full day. Note how frustrated you become when you cannot write with customary ease, carry a heavy package, use a can-opener, zip up the back of your dress, and so forth. Imagine how you would feel if you knew that your arm was to be *permanently* removed and that you would have to spend months relearning arm and hand functions with the use of a hook. It is not surprising, then, that these patients are deeply depressed prior to surgery and need constant psychologic support.

The *postoperative course* for upper extremity amputees depends upon whether the patient undergoes immediate prosthesis fitting or delayed fitting. As with lower limb amputations, there are several pros and cons for each type of prosthetic fitting procedure. Sarmiento points out that immediate fitting is useful for *below*-elbow amputees, but offers few benefits for those with above-elbow amputations.[49] Also, immediate prosthesis fitting may or may not offer psychologic benefits. Some patients may be relieved when they awaken from surgery with a prosthetic hook in place, whereas other patients may be frightened or repulsed by the hook.[22] In addition, the immediate fitting may be dangerous for the amputee who has suffered extensive injuries, because the opaque rigid cast prevents the physician and nursing staff from examining the stump.

If the patient does receive an *immediate* prosthesis, he returns from surgery with a rigid plaster of Paris dressing and a temporary prosthesis in place. The prosthesis socket is changed within 7 to 10 days after surgery. Two to three weeks postoperatively, the surgeon removes the sutures from the stump and changes the socket again. The patient receives his definitive prosthesis within four to eight weeks following surgery.

When delayed prosthesis fitting is chosen over immediate, the patient returns from surgery with his stump covered with soft dressings and an elastic bandage. Unlike the care of lower extremity stumps, an upper extremity stump is bandaged quite *gently* because compression of the traumatized area is to be avoided until healing takes place. The patient usually begins exercises the day following surgery. Within 10 to 14 days postoperatively, the patient's sutures are removed and he receives his temporary prosthesis.

The prescription for an upper extremity prosthesis is just as complicated as is a lower limb prosthetic prescription. A standard type of upper arm prosthesis is illustrated in Figure 66–7. Also note the cosmetic hands illustrated in Figure 66–8.

As with lower limb amputees, the individual who has lost an upper extremity must be highly motivated to master his prosthesis and achieve independence. Also, he must thoroughly integrate his prosthetic arm and hand into his body image.

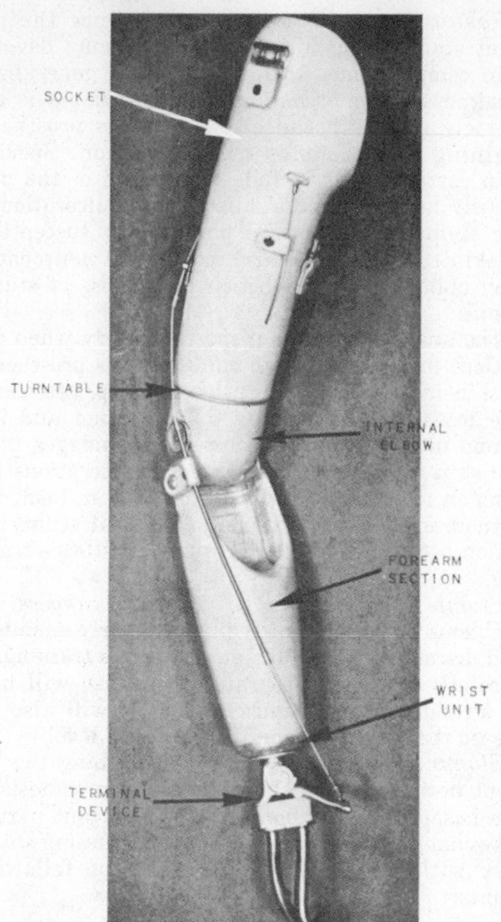

FIGURE 66–7. Standard above-elbow prosthesis. (From Stoner, E. K.: *In* Krusen, F. H., Kottke, F. J., and Ellwood, P. M., Jr.: Handbook of Physical Medicine and Rehabilitation. 2nd ed. 1971.)

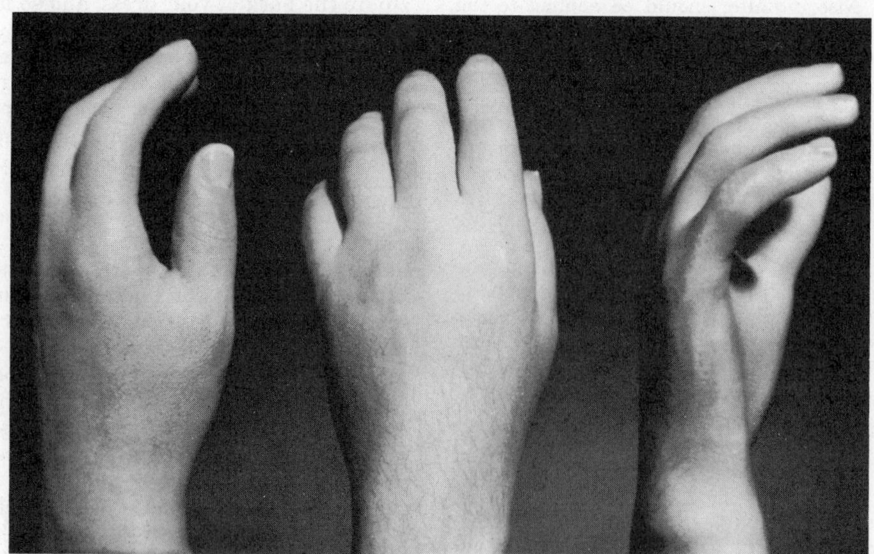

FIGURE 66–8. Cosmetic (nonprehensile) hand. (From Peizer, E., and Pirrello, T.: *Orthopedic Clinics of North America, 3*:397, July, 1972.)

References for Unit XIII

1. Alexander, A. G.: Immediate postsurgical prosthetic fitting: The role of the physical therapist. *Journal of the American Physical Therapy Association, 51*: 152, February, 1971.
2. Beeper keeps amputee on toes. *Journal of the American Medical Association, 209*:634, August 4, 1969.
3. Benenson, A. S.: *Control of Communicable Diseases.* Washington, D.C., American Public Health Association, 1970.
4. Bosanko, L. A.: Immediate postoperative prosthesis. *American Journal of Nursing, 71*:280, February, 1971.
5. Breslau, R. C.: Intensive care following vascular surgery. *American Journal of Nursing, 68*:1670–1676, August, 1968.
6. Brown, G.: Streptokinase therapy for pulmonary embolism. *Postgraduate Medical Journal, 49*:262, April, 1971.
7. Brown, N. L.: Prophylaxis of pulmonary embolism. *British Medical Journal, 2*:780–782, June 27, 1970.
8. Brown, N. L., et. al.: Prevention of recurrent pulmonary embolism. *British Medical Journal, 3*:382–386, August 16, 1969.
9. Burgess, E. M.: Immediate postsurgical prosthetic fitting: A system of amputee management. *Physical Therapy, 51*:139, February, 1971.
10. Chappell, M. B.: Pulmonary embolism. *Nursing Mirror, 132*:26–28, January 8, 1971.
11. Clarke, M. B., Kakka, V. V., and Flane, C.: Use of labelled fibrinogen in the detection and management of deep vein thrombosis. *British Journal of Radiology, 43*:829–830, November, 1970.
12. Clauss, R. H., and Redisch, W.: *Remediable Arterial Disease.* New York, Grune & Stratton, 1971.
13. Conn, H. L., Jr., and Horowitz, O.: *Cardiac and Vascular Disease.* Vol. II. Philadelphia, Lea & Febiger, 1971.
14. Davies, M.: Streptokinase therapy for deep vein thrombosis. *Nursing Times, 69*:211–212, February 15, 1973.
15. DeGowin, E. L., and DeGowin, R. L.: *Bedside Diagnostic Examination.* London, Macmillan & Company, Ltd., 1969.
16. DeWolfe, V. G.: Arteriosclerosis obliterans: Clinical diagnosis and treatments. *Geriatrics, 28*:93, September, 1973.
17. Deykin, D.: The use of heparin. *New England Journal of Medicine, 280*:937–938, April 24, 1969.
18. Deykin, D.: Warfarin therapy. *New England Journal of Medicine, 283*:691–694, September 24, 1970.
19. Deykin, D.: Warfarin therapy. *New England Journal of Medicine, 283*:801–803, October 8, 1970.
20. Fairbairn, J. F., II, Juergens, J. L., and Spittell, J. A., Jr.: *Peripheral Vascular Diseases.* 4th ed. Philadelphia, W. B. Saunders Company, 1972.
21. Foley, W. T., and Wright, I. S.: *Color Atlas and Management of Vascular Disease.* New York, Appleton-Century-Crofts, Inc., 1959.
22. Friedmann, L. W.: The prosthesis—Immediate or delayed fitting. *Angiology, 23*:518, October, 1972.
23. Ganong, W. F.: *Review of Medical Physiology.* 6th ed. Los Altos, California, Lange Medical Publications, 1973.
24. Gerhardt, J. J., et al.: Immediate post-surgical prosthetics: Rehabilitation aspects. *American Journal of Physical Medicine, 49*:3, February, 1970.
25. Hills, N. H., and Calnan, S. S.: Deep vein thrombosis after surgery. *Nursing Mirror, 135*:29–30, July 21, 1972.
26. Hurst, J. W., and Logue, R. B.: *The Heart, Arteries and Veins.* 2nd ed. New York, McGraw-Hill Book Company, 1970.
27. Jackson, B. S.: Chronic peripheral arterial disease. *American Journal of Nursing, 72*:928, May, 1972.
28. Jeglijewski, J. M.: Target: Outside world. *American Journal of Nursing, 73*:1024, June, 1973.
29. Johnson, B. J.: The hazards of immobilization: Effects on cardiovascular function. *American Journal of Nursing, 67*:781–782, April, 1967.
30. Juergens, J. L.: Venous thromboembolism. *Cardiovascular Clinics, 3*:234–246, 1971.
31. Kakkar, V. V., and Jouhar, A. J.: *Thromboembolism: Diagnosis and Treatment.* Baltimore, The Williams & Wilkins Company, 1972.
32. Koch-Weser, J., and Sellers, E. M.: Drug interactions with coumarin anticoagulants. *New England Journal of Medicine, 285*:487–498, August 26, 1971.
33. Koch-Weser, J., and Sellers, E. M.: Drug interactions with coumarin anticoagulants. *New England Journal of Medicine, 285*:547–558, September 2, 1971.
34. Mavor, G. E., et al.: Peripheral venous scanning with ^{125}I-tagged fibrinogen. *Lancet, 1*:661–663, November 25, 1972.
35. McCollough, N. C.: The dysvascular amputee. *Orthopedic Clinics of North America, 3*:303, July, 1972.
36. Miller, G. A. H.: Massive pulmonary embolism—Medical management. *British Medical Journal, 2*: 777–778, June 27, 1970.
37. Monks, B. E.: Venous thrombosis. *Nursing Mirror, 132*:40–41, June 4, 1971.
38. Mooney, V., et al.: Fitting of temporary prosthetic limbs immediately after amputation. *California Medicine, 107*:330, October, 1967.
39. Oakley, C. M.: Diagnosis of pulmonary embolism. *British Medical Journal, 2*:773–777, June 27, 1970.
40. O'Brien, J. R., and Kakkar, V. V.: Peripheral venous scanning with ^{125}I-tagged fibrinogen. *Lancet, 1*:909–910, April 22, 1972.
41. O'Reilly, R. A., and Aggeler, P. M.: Determinants of the response to oral anticoagulant drugs in man. *Pharmacological Reviews, 22*:35–96, March, 1970.
42. Paneth, M.: Surgical management of massive pulmonary embolism. *British Medical Journal, 2*:778–779, June 27, 1970.
43. Paulose, K. P., et al.: Diagnosis of pulmonary embolism, a correlative study of the clinical, scan, and angiographic findings. *British Medical Journal, 3*:67–71, July 11, 1970.
44. Peizer, E., and Pirrello, T.: Principles and practice in upper extremity prostheses. *Orthopedic Clinics of North America, 3*:397, July, 1972.
45. Richards, R. L.: *Peripheral Arterial Disease.* Baltimore, The Williams & Wilkins Company, 1970.
46. Roach, L. B.: Traumatic amputation. *Nursing '72, 2*: 40, November, 1972.
47. Rosenthal, H., and Rosenthal, J.: *Diabetic Care in Pictures.* 3rd Ed. Philadelphia, J. B. Lippincott Company, 1960.
48. Rushmer, R. F.: *Cardiovascular Dynamics.* 2nd ed. Philadelphia, W. B. Saunders Company, 1961.

48a. Sarmiento, A.: Recent trends in lower extremity amputation. *Nursing Clinics of North America, 2*: 399, September, 1967.
49. Sarmiento, A.: Postoperative management. *Orthopedic Clinics of North America, 3*:435, July, 1972.
50. Sasahara, A. A., and Foster, V. L.: Pulmonary embolism recognition and treatment. *American Journal of Nursing, 67*:1634–1641, August, 1967.
51. Schatz, I. J., et al.: Disability after real or alleged venous thrombosis. *Postgraduate Medical Journal, 31*:358–363, April, 1962.
52. Solnitzky, O. C., and Jegher, H.: Lymphadenopathy and disorders of the lymphatic system. *In* MacBryde, C. M. (ed.): *Signs and Symptoms*. Philadelphia, J. B. Lippincott Company, 1964.
53. Statham, L.: Pulmonary embolism. *Nursing Times, 68*:284–286, March 9, 1972.
54. Stoner, E. K.: Care of the amputee. *In* Krusen, F. H., et al. (eds.): *Handbook of Physical Medicine and Rehabilitation*. 2nd ed. Philadelphia, W. B. Saunders Company, 1971.
55. Strandness, D. E., Jr.: *Peripheral Arterial Disease*. Boston, Little, Brown and Company, 1969.
56. Tooms, R. E.: Amputation surgery in the upper extremity. *Orthopedic Clinics of North America, 3*: 383, July, 1972.
57. Wadsworth, T. G.: Postoperative deep vein thrombosis. *Nursing Mirror, 134*:28–29, January 28, 1972.
58. Wallach, R.: Dextran therapy for pregnancy-associated deep thrombophlebitis. *American Journal of Obstetrics and Gynecology, 112*:613–618, March, 1972.
59. Wessler, S.: The role of hypercoagulability in venous and arterial thrombosis. *Cardiovascular Clinics, 3*: 2–16, 1971.
60. Wessler, S.: Stasis, hypercoagulability and thrombosis. *Federation Proceedings, 22*:1366, 1963.
61. Wilson, A. B., Jr.: *Limb Prosthetics*. Huntington, New York, Robert E. Krieger Publishing Company, 1972.
62. Yao, S. T., Gourmos, C., and Hobbs, J. T.: Detection of proximal-vein thrombosis by Doppler ultrasound flow-detection method. *Lancet, 1*:1–4, January 1, 1972.

UNIT XIV

Nursing Patients Experiencing Disturbances of Respiratory Function

Introduction and Study Guide

The nurse participates in the care and rehabilitation of patients with both acute (short-term) and chronic (long-term) respiratory illnesses. These illnesses are common causes of disability. Respiratory illnesses are the most common type of acute disorder. For example, acute respiratory infections, e.g., "flu" and "colds," affect many persons annually, causing them to be confined at home. Respiratory allergies are a source of distress throughout the year to many persons. Chronic respiratory illnesses cause millions of Americans to lose work time, retire early and possibly eventually die. The incidences of chronic respiratory illnesses and lung cancer are increasing at alarming rates. Chronic lung diseases are second only to heart disease as a cause of death in this country. Lung cancer is the only form of cancer which is showing a rapid increase in incidence.

Many respiratory disorders are often preventable, e.g., chronic bronchitis, chronic obstructive pulmonary emphysema, lung cancer, tuberculosis, pneumonia and lung abscess. The nurse participates both directly and indirectly in the prevention of respiratory disorders. Her direct participation includes performing activities such as: (1) encouraging periodic deep breathing, coughing and turning among patients likely to develop atelectasis or pneumonia (e.g., postoperative patients, patients confined to bed rest); (2) preventing aspiration (e.g., in obtunded or paralyzed patients); (3) safely administering inhalation therapy and chest physical therapy (e.g., postural drainage) when indicated; and (4) performing suctioning to maintain a patent airway.

Indirectly a nurse may help to prevent numerous respiratory disorders through education. Topics on which the nurse may give information include: (1) hazards associated with pulmonary irritants, e.g., cigarette smoke, air pollutants; (2) dangers of foreign body aspiration, e.g., in children; (3) emergency care following airway obstruction or chest injuries; (4) methods of preventing spread of air-borne infections; (5) use of influenza vaccines; and (6) importance of early investigation and treatment of respiratory symptoms, e.g., cough, sputum production, shortness of breath. A nurse is often instrumental in urging persons with respiratory conditions to seek and to accept treatment. Early treatment of acute respiratory problems and an adequate period of convalescence following such illnesses are important to prevent the development of chronic disorders. A variety of teaching aids such as pamphlets are available without charge for use in patient-education programs. Throughout this unit examples of these aids are mentioned along with information about how to obtain them.

Respiratory care is important not only for patients with intrinsic respiratory disorders but also for patients who have other primary problems. For example, the first priority of emergency care in *any* situation is to maintain function of the lungs and heart, e.g., the airway is cleared and cardiopulmonary resuscitation is performed as indicated. During *any* surgery performed under general anesthesia the anesthesiologist maintains adequate respiration; following surgery the nurse maintains a patent airway and prevents postoperative pulmonary complications, e.g., atelectasis, pneumonia. *All* patients in intensive care units or confined to bed, regardless of their basic illnesses, are continuously cared for to prevent the development of respiratory complications associated with inactivity. An important part of *many* rehabilitative programs is to help patients to improve lung function. Prevention of respiratory complications is extremely important since these disorders can be fatal.

Increasingly, intensive respiratory care units are being established to provide skilled care for patients with serious respiratory conditions. Nurse clinicians, with advanced training and skills in respiratory care, are functioning effectively in these as well as other settings. The quality of nursing care given to seriously ill patients with respiratory disorders strongly influences the success or failure of treatment programs. Successful respiratory care requires the effective participation of a treatment team which basically consists of the physician, nurse, respiratory therapist (formerly called inhalation therapist), and physical therapist.

Pulmonary surgery has made tremendous advances in recent years. However, in spite of both medical and surgical advances, many patients suffer with and succumb to pulmonary conditions which cannot yet be successfully reversed or treated. In the future, lung transplantation (now successfully performed on laboratory animals) or insertion of artificial lungs may restore health to persons whose own lungs are irreparably damaged.

Occupational and community health nurses have important roles in the prevention and treatment of respiratory disorders. For example, occupational health nurses are active in helping employers find ways to protect workers from industrial substances which can cause respiratory disease, e.g., dusts, gases, fumes, sprays, liquids, bacteria, fungi. Community health nurses participate in home care and community education.

Disorders of the upper respiratory tract, i.e., nose, throat, pharynx and larynx, are presented in Unit XXII. Included in that unit are discussions of endotracheal intubation and tracheostomy. Acute pulmonary edema is discussed in Unit X; discussion of pulmonary embolism is in Unit XIII. This unit focuses on disorders of the pleurae, pleural spaces, tracheobronchial tree and lungs. Included in Chapter 67 is a brief overview of the anatomy and physiology of the respiratory system. Chapter 68 discusses diagnostic and evaluative procedures for assessment of the patient with a respiratory disorder. In Chapter 69 common nonspecific manifestations of respiratory disorders are considered, e.g., abnormal patterns of breathing, abnormal secretions, cough, hypoxia, pulmonary failure. Common respiratory therapeutic measures are reviewed in Chapter 70, e.g., factors of general importance as well as medications, pulmonary physiotherapy, and inhalation therapy. Chapter 71 considers in depth specific disorders of the pleurae, pleural spaces, tracheobronchial tree and lungs, e.g., pleurisy, pneumothorax, atelectasis, pulmonary tumors, pneumonias, tuberculosis, and chronic obstructive pulmonary disease. In Chapter 72 tracheobronchial, diaphragmatic and chest injuries are discussed. The unit's final chapter, Chapter 73, presents information about closed chest drainage and chest surgery.

Overview: Basic Types of Respiratory Disorders

The respiratory system is subject to a wide variety of disorders. Examples of some of these problems are briefly summarized below. In some conditions more than one causative factor is operative, e.g., infection and irritation are often coexistent.

TYPICAL EXAMPLES OF RESPIRATORY DISORDERS

Causative Factor	Examples of Disorders
Airway obstruction; aspiration	Chronic obstructive pulmonary disease (COPD); atelectasis; bronchiectasis; lung abscess; aspiration pneumonia
Allergic reactions	Bronchial asthma
Breakdown of alveolar walls	Pulmonary emphysema
Bronchopulmonary irritation	Pulmonary emphysema; lung cancer; chronic bronchitis; COPD; pneumoconioses ("dust diseases")
Bronchospasm	Bronchial asthma; COPD; chronic bronchitis; pulmonary emphysema
Infection	Influenza; pneumonia; pulmonary emphysema; pulmonary tuberculosis; pleurisy; thoracic empyema; bronchopleural fistula; lung abscess; bronchiectasis; atelectasis; bronchitis; tracheobronchitis; fungus infections; pulmonary infections caused by atypical organisms
Trauma	Penetrating chest injuries; nonpenetrating chest injuries (e.g., blunt or crushing injuries); pulmonary laceration; hemothorax; pneumothorax; flail chest; fractured ribs; tracheobronchial injuries; diaphragmatic injuries
Tumors	Benign pulmonary tumors; metastatic pulmonary tumors; primary malignant tumors (bronchogenic carcinomas)
Ventilation-perfusion abnormalities	May accompany various disorders; in some instances pulmonary capillaries are inadequately perfused with blood although alveoli are adequately ventilated; in other cases alveolar ventilation is impaired although blood flow is normal
Alveolar-capillary membrane permeability abnormalities	May develop with interstitial fibrosis and progressive granulomatous diseases; total area of the alveolar-capillary membranes may be reduced in disorders such as pulmonary emphysema, pneumoconiosis, and far advanced pulmonary tuberculosis

Table continued on following page.

TYPICAL EXAMPLES OF RESPIRATORY DISORDERS *(Continued)*

Causative Factor	Examples of Disorders
Arteriovenous (A-V) shunting	Hypoxia results from venous dilution of the arterial blood stream, or if large groups of alveoli are nonfunctioning and blood passes through pulmonary capillaries without gaseous exchange occurring
Restrictive pulmonary disorders	Expansion of the chest cage, diaphragm, or lungs may be limited by paralysis of the muscles of respiration, phrenic nerve paralysis, pulmonary fibrosis, kyphoscoliosis, pleural thickening, and scarring.

Study Guide

In preparation for studying this unit, review in appropriate textbooks: (1) normal *anatomy* and *physiology* of the tracheobronchial tree, lungs, muscles of respiration, and pleural space; (2) *pharmacologic agents* useful in treating respiratory disorders (e.g., antihistamines, antimicrobials, bronchodilators, cough medications, enzymes, gases, narcotic antagonists, respiratory stimulants, vasoconstrictors, and decongestants); and (3) *microbiology* of microorganisms which may produce diseases of the respiratory tract (e.g., *Mycobacterium tuberculosis, Haemophilus influenzae,* pneumococcus, staphylococcus, streptococcus, fungi, atypical organisms resembling tuberculosis).

As you proceed through this unit, refer back to other sections of this text as necessary for review. Possible areas of review include: *fluid-electrolyte imbalances*, especially respiratory acidosis and respiratory alkalosis (Chap. 25); mechanisms of *hypersensitivity* to more completely understand bronchial asthma (Chap. 23); the body's response to *injury* and *infection* (Chap. 22); *physiologic shock* (Chap. 26); nursing patients experiencing *surgery* (Unit VI) and *pain* (Unit IX) in association with chest injury, chest surgery and painful conditions involving the respiratory system; the body's response to *bed rest* and *immobilization* (Chap. 27); *disturbances of cellular function* as a review when studying lung cancer (Unit VII); and *cardiopulmonary resuscitation* (Unit X).

As you proceed through the unit, carry out the following:

1. **Summarize nursing responsibilities associated with bronchography, thoracentesis, sputum examination, gastric content analysis.**

2. State in your own words the value of blood gas analyses and auscultation, inspection, percussion and palpation of the chest.
3. List some observations of importance in assessing patients with respiratory disorders.
4. Summarize care of: (a) a dyspneic patient; (b) a patient experiencing hemoptysis; and (c) a patient in acute respiratory insufficiency or failure.
5. Identify ways in which nonproductive coughing can be minimized and productive coughing stimulated and made more effective.
6. State symptoms indicative of hypoxia.
7. Summarize nursing activities useful in promoting maintenance of a clear airway and removal of respiratory secretions.
8. State why oral hygiene is of importance in the presence of respiratory disorders.
9. List some pulmonary irritants which should be avoided by persons with respiratory problems.
10. Practice abdominal breathing so you will be able to effectively teach this exercise to patients.
11. Observe a patient receiving pulmonary physiotherapy (e.g., breathing exercises, postural drainage, clapping, vibrating). Review his condition and identify specifically how pulmonary physiotherapy is therapeutic.
12. Visit the respiratory therapy department or observe patients being treated with aerosolization, humidification, oxygen and positive pressure ventilation. Review these procedures with a qualified person. Identify hazards associated with oxygen therapy and positive pressure respirators. If medications are being given by IPPB, familiarize yourself with the medications and how they are prepared for administration.
13. State why a patient with chronic respiratory insufficiency and CO_2 retention should *not* be given high concentrations of O_2 even though his PaO_2 is low, i.e., why is the goal of treatment *not* one of attempting to rapidly raise the PaO_2 to "normal" by giving high concentrations of O_2?
14. Identify some hazards of deep tracheal suctioning and ways in which potential dangers may be avoided.
15. Summarize key points in the prevention of the following disorders and identify major patient-teaching points of importance in working with patients who have these disorders: atelectasis, lung abscess, bronchiectasis, pulmonary tuberculosis, lung cancer, pneumonia, influenza, chronic obstructive pulmonary disease, bronchial asthma, chronic bronchitis, chronic pulmonary emphysema, and pneumoconiosis.
16. Familiarize yourself with research reports which document the harmful effects of cigarette smoking and air pollution.
17. Describe the "atypical" organisms which produce pulmonary diseases similar to tuberculosis.
18. Name some fungus infections of the lungs, i.e., pulmonary mycoses, and review the etiology of these infections.
19. Identify some of the economic, social and emotional pressures patients with the following respiratory disorders may experience: lung cancer, pulmonary tuberculosis, bronchiectasis, chronic obstructive pulmonary disease, chronic bronchitis, or chronic pulmonary emphysema.
20. Describe how an open chest wound or chest surgery disrupts normal intrapleural pressure. What therapeutic procedures are used to restore normal intrapleural pressure?
21. Describe paradoxical motion, mediastinal shift and mediastinal flutter. How can these complications occur in chest injuries? What treatment is indicated?
22. Summarize factors of importance in pre- and post-operative care following chest surgery.
23. Make a drawing of three-bottle, closed chest drainage and state the purpose of each bottle. What is meant by closed chest drainage? What is meant by a water seal? Identify potential problems that can occur with closed chest drainage (e.g., the chest catheter is accidentally pulled out of the chest) and appropriate immediate care.

CHAPTER 67

Overview of Anatomy and Physiology of Respiratory System

> The lung is like a large sponge, the spaces of which are occupied by air, and the skeleton of the sponge is composed of thin partitions containing fine blood capillaries.[139]

Summarized below are some structures and functions of importance in the anatomy and physiology of the respiratory system. Consult Figure 67–1 as you review this system and refer as necessary to textbooks of anatomy and physiology.

The respiratory system consists of: nose, paranasal sinuses, pharynx ("throat"), larynx ("voice box"), trachea ("windpipe"), bronchi, and lungs. (Discussion of the nose, sinuses, pharynx, and larynx will be found in Unit XXII.)

ANATOMY

Trachea. Smooth, flexible, muscular, tube-like air passage about 3/5″ wide and 4 to 5 ″ long. Reinforced on sides and in front by 15 to 20 C-shaped rings of cartilage. Opening of the "C" faces posteriorly. Cartilage rings protect trachea and keep it open by preventing its collapse. The trachea extends from larynx to mainstem bronchi; it serves as passage to and from lungs. The inner surface is lined with ciliated epithelium.

Mainstem Bronchi (Right and Left). These are also called "primary" or "main bronchi." Two subdivisions of the trachea branch off from the tracheal bifurcation, and one mainstem bronchus enters each lung. These tubular passages conduct air between trachea and pulmonary bronchi. Walls contain cartilaginous rings and ciliated mucous lining. The right mainstem bronchus is shorter, wider and extends downward more vertically than the left. (Aspiration thus more frequently occurs into right main bronchus.)

Secondary Bronchi. These are also referred to as "bronchial tubes," "air tubes," and the "bronchial tree." Subdivisions of main bronchi spread in an inverted tree-like formation, branching through each lung field. These tubular passages convey air within the lung between the mainstem bronchi and bronchioles. There are lobar and segmental bronchi.

Bronchioles. These are the smallest subdivisions of bronchi; they conduct air from secondary bronchi into alveoli ("air sacs"). Segmental bronchi divide into smaller bronchioles within the bronchopulmonary segments. The final branches of bronchioles, i.e., terminal respiratory bronchioles, communicate directly with clusters of alveoli. The smooth muscle of bronchioles is supplied by both divisions of the autonomic nervous system: the sympathetic promotes relaxation, the parasympathetic promotes constriction.

Alveoli. Also called "air sacs" or "air spaces," these delicate, thin-walled, minute hollow chambers within the lungs are surrounded by networks of capillaries. Alveolar walls are only a single cell thick; they consist of a single layer of simple squamous epithelial tissue. Exchange of oxygen (O_2) and carbon dioxide (CO_2) occurs through these walls between air and blood. The combined surface of alveolar walls forms an extremely large surface for gas exchange. Alveoli usually always contain some air, even during the "rest" period between inspiration and expiration.

Respiratory Center. Located in the stem portion of the brain, i.e., medulla, immediately above spinal cord (Fig. 67–2), this center controls breathing. Normally the respiratory center is stimulated by the concentration of CO_2, and to a lesser degree by the amounts of O_2 in arterial blood. This mechanism is mediated by sensitive chemoreceptors located in the medulla and in the walls of the arch of the aorta and carotid arteries. Centrally, CO_2 and hydrogen ions in the cerebrospinal fluid stimulate central chemoreceptors. Stimulation of the respiratory center causes an increase in the rate and depth of breathing, thus blowing off excess CO_2 and reducing the blood's acidity. Peripheral chemoreceptor reflexes from the aortic and carotid bodies occur when the O_2 level drops. The respiratory center dispatches orders to the respiratory muscles, stimulating contraction. Nerve fibers extend down the spinal cord. In the cervical (neck) region of the cord these fibers continue via the *phrenic nerves* to innervate either side of the *diaphragm*. If one phrenic nerve is damaged, the diaphragm on the affected side is paralyzed in an elevated position.

GROSS ANATOMY

Thoracic Cavity. The thoracic cavity has 4 subdivisions: (1) *right pulmonary space,* which contains the right lung surrounded by visceral and parietal pleura; (2) *left pulmonary space,* which contains the left lung surrounded by visceral and parietal pleura; (3) *pericardial space,* which contains heart and pericardial sac; and (4) *mediastinal space,* the center of thoracic cavity, located between pulmonary spaces; this contains esophagus, trachea, and great blood vessels and heart.

Lungs (Right and Left). These main organs of respiration are located within the thoracic cavity on either side of the heart. Light, spongy, porous, elastic, cone-shaped organs, they inflate with inspiration of air and deflate (but do not completely collapse) with expiration. They extend from the diaphragm to just above the clavicles; i.e., the *base* of lung rests on diaphragm while the *apex* (top) extends above the first rib. The *hilus* or *hilum* is the notch or depression in the medial surface of the lung at which the mainstem bronchus, pulmonary blood vessels, and nerves join the lung. Sometimes the hilus is called the "root of the lung." Lungs are made of elastic tissues which have a tendency to recoil but are capable of stretching if a pulling force is exerted on them from outside or if they are "blown up" (inflated) from within. Normally the

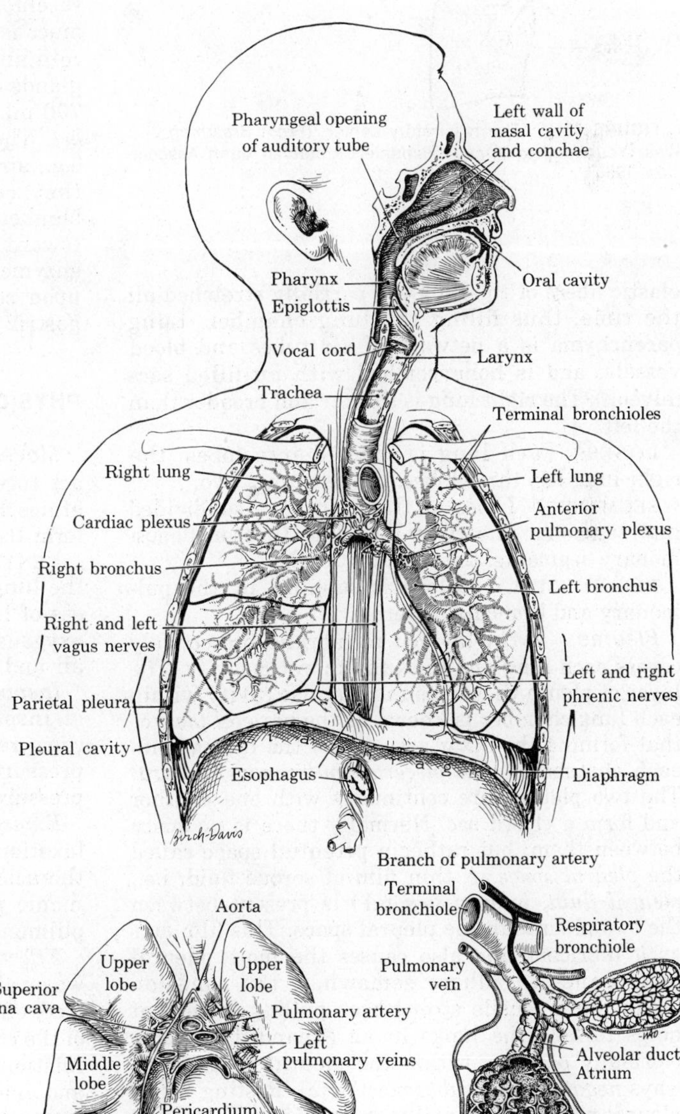

FIGURE 67–1. Organs of the respiratory system. (From *Dorland's Illustrated Medical Dictionary.* 25th ed. 1974.)

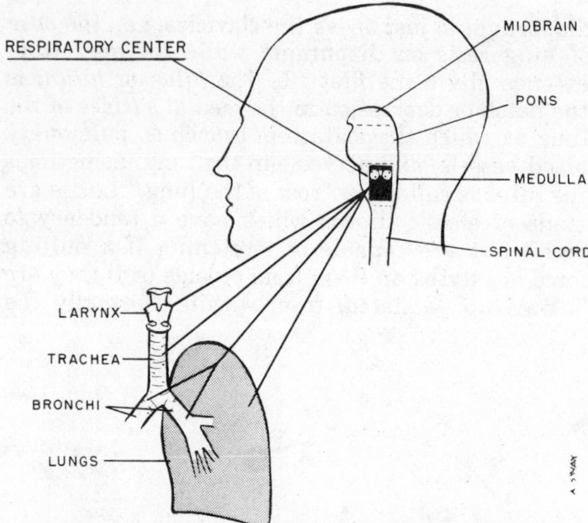

FIGURE 67–2. The respiratory center. (From *Breathing . . . What You Need to Know.* (Pamphlet) American Lung Association, 1968.)

elastic fibers of the lung are partially stretched all the time, thus filling the lung chamber. Lung parenchyma is a network of air tubes and blood vessels, and is honeycombed with air-filled sacs (alveoli). The right lung is shorter and broader than the left.

LOBES. Each lung is divided into lobes: the right lung has three lobes; the left lung, two.

SEGMENTS. Lobes of the lungs are subdivided into segments: the right lung has 10 bronchopulmonary segments; the left lung, eight.

BLOOD SUPPLY. Blood is supplied by the pulmonary and bronchial arteries.

Pleurae. A two-layered membrane protectively covers each lung and lines the thoracic cavity. The layer of pleura that lines the thoracic cavity within each lung chamber is known as the *parietal pleura;* that forming the outer covering of the lung within each chamber is the *visceral (pulmonary) pleura.* The two pleurae are continuous with one another and form a closed sac. Normally there is no space between them, but rather a potential space called the *pleural space.* A thin film of serous fluid, i.e., *pleural fluid,* (only a few ml.) is present between the two pleurae in the pleural space. This film acts as a lubricant and also causes the moist pleural membranes to adhere somewhat, the cohesion producing a tensile strength or pulling force that helps to hold the lungs in an expanded position. Normally *pressure* within the pleural space is always *negative* (i.e., *subatmospheric*). Resting intrapleural pressure is usually about 755 mm. Hg, but prior to inspiration it decreases to about 751 mm. Hg. A constant negative intrapleural pressure is essential for normal respirations. This pressure is another factor that prevents the lungs from recoiling and holds them expanded. Negative pressure exerts a sucking or pulling force.

Diaphragm. A muscular partition separating the thoracic and abdominal cavities, the diaphragm is innervated on either side by a phrenic nerve.

HISTOLOGY

Except for the pharynx, the respiratory tract is lined by specialized pseudostratified, columnar, ciliated epithelium. Each surface epithelial cell has 5 to 30 *cilia* attached to it. The cilia move automatically and rhythmically in waves of beating motion, propelling anything on their surface toward the pharynx for elimination from the body after swallowing. Cilia stroke approximately 250 times per minute. Beneath surface epithelial cells are three to four layers of replacement cells lying on a submucosa. Beneath the submucosa are tubular and racemose glands which supply both serous and mucous secretions. Goblet cells (intermixed with columnar epithelial cells) and the submucosal glands excrete a continuous flow of secretion (600–700 ml./24 hr.) which forms a viscid *mucous blanket.* The surface of this blanket catches particles, e.g., airborne particles of dust, pollens, bacteria, as they come in contact. The protective mucous blanket and its entrapped particles are transported toward the pharynx by ciliary action. Lysozyme, an enzyme within the secretion, destroys most bacteria upon contact. Residual bacteria are destroyed by gastric juices and hydrochloric acid in the stomach.

PHYSIOLOGY

Movement of Gases. The lungs and circulation act together to convey respiratory gases between atmospheric air and body tissues. The lungs perform their function by:

VENTILATION. Movement of air into and out of the lungs, along bronchial airways is a cyclic process of inspiration and expiration, bringing freshly oxygenated air into the lungs and removing "stale" air and CO_2.

Inspiration. This is characterized by contraction of inspiratory muscles, enlargement of thoracic cage, reduction in intrapleural and intrapulmonic pressures, and inflow of air until intrapulmonic pressure equals atmospheric pressure.

Expiration. Expiration is characterized by relaxation of inspiratory muscles, reduction in size of thoracic cage, increase in intrapleural and intrapulmonic pressures, and outflow of gas until intrapulmonic pressure equals atmospheric pressure.

Effective ventilation. This requires patent airways; elastic, expansile lungs and tracheobronchial tree; efficient, adequate musculoskeletal apparatus of the chest wall and related structures; and normal relation between amounts of air inspired per breath and amounts within lungs.

EXCHANGE OF GASES. Exchange of gases between the air and blood in the terminal alveolar capillary system is part of the process of *respiration* (Fig. 67–3). Specifically, respiration refers to the

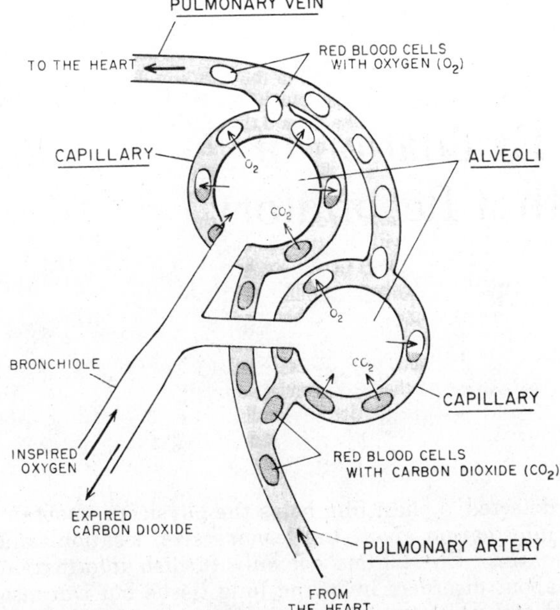

FIGURE 67–3. Action of the alveoli in the circulatory system. (From *Breathing . . . What You Need to Know.* American Lung Association, 1968.)

exchange of O_2 and CO_2 in the body: (1) within the lungs; (2) between the cells and their environments; and (3) in intracellular metabolism. (CO_2–O_2 transport is discussed in Chap. 25.) During respiration body tissues are supplied with O_2 for metabolism and CO_2 is released from the tissues.

Normal Body Respiration. This requires:

1. Adequate O_2 concentration in the alveoli.
2. Adequate amount of hemoglobin capable of combining with this O_2.
3. Transfer of O_2 from the alveoli in concentrations sufficient to saturate the blood adequately before it leaves the lung.
4. Transportation of the oxyhemoglobin thus formed to the tissues at a rate commensurate with tissue needs.
5. Availability of the body cells to use the O_2 supplied to them.

Gas Exchange. This occurs at two places within the body: the lungs (in pulmonary alveoli), and the tissues. Pulmonary gas exchange is effected by: *ventilation* (discussed previously); *perfusion* (i.e., supplying of the lungs with blood from the right side of the heart); and *diffusion* (i.e., the movement of O_2 and CO_2 between the gas phase (in alveolar air) and the blood phase (in capillaries).

Hydrogen Ion Imbalances. The lungs perform important functions in governing the body's hydrogen ion balance. This important homeostatic function is discussed in Chapter 25. Respiratory malfunctioning can cause serious hydrogen imbalances, e.g., respiratory acidosis and respiratory alkalosis. *Respiratory acidosis* is a serious result of *hypercapnia,* i.e., the retention of excessive amounts of CO_2. *Respiratory alklalosis* is a manifestation of *hypocapnia,* i.e., the excessive secretion (loss) of CO_2.

CHAPTER 68

Diagnosis and Evaluation of the Patient with a Respiratory Disorder

The nurse prepares the patient for respiratory diagnostic tests as ordered by the physician. She also discusses with the patient generally what the tests involve. Because anxiety influences respirations, it is especially important for the patient to be psychologically well prepared for diagnostic procedures and to be as relaxed as possible during them. Because pulmonary diagnosis may involve numerous diagnostic tests (some of which are acutely uncomfortable), the patient may become discouraged and irritable. Patients who are dyspneic tire easily and often require planned rest periods during the diagnostic process. When the nurse is present during tests she not only assists the physician but she also assists the patient by calming him, eliciting his cooperation and confidence, informing him of progress during the procedure, instructing him what to do (or not do) during the procedure, and appropriately offering praise and encouragement.

CHEST ROENTGENOGRAPHY

Common Chest X-ray Procedures

Chest x-rays are often taken for *screening* purposes, i.e., to detect pulmonary lesions such as tuberculosis, in large selected population groups. *Miniature films* or *microfilms* are typically used for screening purposes. The films are read by experts, and persons with suspicious findings are called back for larger chest films and other diagnostic tests. Chest x-ray screening programs not only help to detect pulmonary tuberculosis, but they also frequently call attention to other pulmonary problems and disorders involving the heart and other mediastinal structures, e.g., tumors, pulmonary bullae, cardiac disease, structural abnormalities. Some respiratory disease screening programs also include simple breathing tests (helpful in detecting such disorders as pulmonary emphysema) and tuberculin skin tests.

Routine chest x-rays are an important part of any complete physical examination. These routine films may demonstrate lesions in the chest which are asymptomatic and thus would otherwise go undetected in time for early treatment. When a lesion is detected, a chest film helps the physician to obtain information about the lesion's size, location, and nature. Chest films not only furnish information about disorders involving lung tissue but can also detect problems involving numerous related structures. For example, chest x-rays may reveal: (1) disorders of the soft tissues and bones of the chest wall; (2) abnormal diaphragmatic contours; (3) limited ranges of diaphragmatic excursions on respiration; (4) abnormalities in heart position, size, contour, and other abnormal mediastinal configurations; (5) tracheobronchial abnormalities; (6) pleural thickening; (7) fluid in the pleural space; and (8) grossly abnormal changes in the caliber or distribution of pulmonary arteries and veins.

Before chest x-rays are taken the patient is briefly told about the procedure and what his participation will entail. Clothing and metal objects are removed down to the waist and the patient is given a protective drape or gown. (Metal objects show up on the developed film and thus obscure the body structures in the area they cover.)

Chest x-rays may be taken at the patient's bedside or in the radiology department, depending on the patient's state of health. The films may be taken with the patient standing, sitting erect, or lying down. Most chest films are taken with the patient standing up. After he is correctly positioned the patient is usually instructed to take a deep breath and hold it while the "picture" is being taken. The maximal inspiration of air fills the lungs, thereby enabling a clearer view of pulmonary structures.

Although a variety of x-ray techniques may be employed in evaluating pulmonary disorders, the views most commonly taken are: a *postero-anterior* (PA or "flat plate") view taken with the x-ray beam passing from the body's posterior to anterior surface, *lateral* views taken through the right or left side of the chest, and various *oblique* views which are slanting or inclined at specified angles (Fig. 68–1). Additionally, a *lordotic* film may be taken to more clearly view the apices, i.e., the rounded upper portions of each lung which extend upward as high as the first thoracic vertebra. Of the oblique views the most common are the right and left anterior obliques; these permit views of structures obscured in the PA position and of the mediastinal

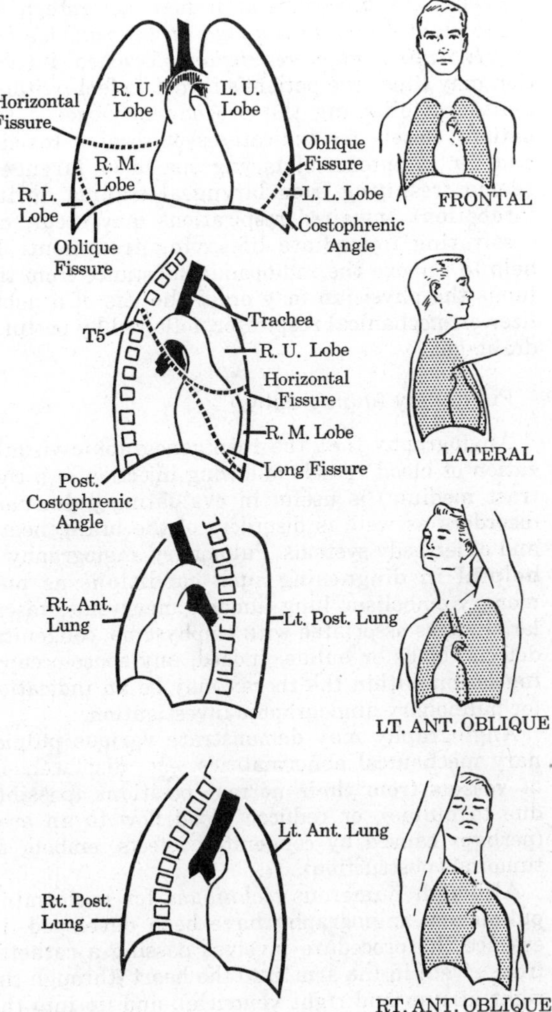

FIGURE 68–1. Pulmonary projections and relationships. (From *Merck Manual.* 12th ed. Rahway, N.J. Merck, Sharp & Dohme.)

contents. The recumbent lateral position (also called "decubitus") helps to localize fluid in the pleural space, i.e., pleural effusions.

Body Section Roentgenography; Stereoscopic Roentgenography

In addition to the x-ray views discussed above, special techniques of *body section roentgenography* may also be employed in pulmonary diagnosis. These techniques show detailed images of structures lying in a predetermined plane of tissue, while blurring the images of structures in other planes. It is thus possible to study areas normally concealed by overlying structures. These x-ray films of structures at selected layers of the body are obtained by various methods known by such names as *laminagraphy, planigraphy, stratigraphy,* and *tomography.* In performing body section roentgenography, numerous films are taken at differing planes of the chest until the area being studied is in clear focus. This technique is especially helpful in evaluating pulmonary densities, cavities, and tumors. *Stereoscopic roentgenography* (three-dimensional views) enables more accurate spacial localization of questionable areas than do the usual two-dimensional films.

Bronchography

A *bronchogram* is an x-ray of the tracheobronchial tree and lung taken after an opaque medium (a radiopaque oil or water-soluble dye) is instilled into a bronchus (via a tube passed nasally down into the trachea or via a bronchoscope). Bronchoscopes and bronchoscopy are discussed below. The opaque material coats and outlines the bronchial tree, thereby enabling visualization of this structure when the x-ray film is taken.

Because regurgitation and aspiration are potential dangers associated with bronchography, the patient receives special pre- and postprocedure care.

Prior to bronchography the following nursing activities are typically of importance: (1) instruct the patient to perform thorough oral hygiene the evening before and the morning of the procedure; (2) withhold oral intake for six to 12 hours (to prevent possible regurgitation and aspiration); (3) assist the patient with postural drainage as ordered the morning of the procedure (clearing the bronchi of secretions enables the radiopaque material to enter these areas and produce a more informative x-ray); (4) ask the patient if he has any loose teeth, capped teeth, dental bridges, or oral inflammations and chart their presence (loose teeth or dental prostheses can be broken off or dislodged and aspirated during the procedure); (5) remove and safely store removable dental structures; (6) report oral inflammations to the physician (it may be necessary for you to inspect the patient's mouth); (7) have the patient sign a consent permit if required by hospital policy; and (8) administer preprocedure medications as ordered. Inform the patient that the medications will reduce his awareness of his surroundings and thus help him to relax. Atropine may be ordered to minimize secretions and a short-acting barbiturate to sedate the patient and reduce the stimulating effects of anesthetic agents.

Although local anesthesia (cocaine, lidocaine, or tetracaine) prevents coughing and gagging when the tube is being passed (during bronchography or bronchoscopy), it can also cause serious (sometimes fatal) toxic reactions. Symptoms of *cocaine toxicity* include palpitations, excitation, rapid and bounding pulse, euphoria, elevated blood pressure, and rapid, deep respirations. These are symptoms of stimulation of the nervous system from above downward. Overstimulation is followed by depression of the nervous system in this same descending order. Unless symptoms of overactivity are promptly observed, reported, and treated, *fatal respiratory failure may occur.* Treatment may include artificial respiration, oxygen therapy, and the intramuscular or intravenous administration of a rapid-acting barbiturate, e.g., secobarbital sodium (Seconal).

Preparation of the patient for bronchography (or bronchoscopy) also involves giving appropriate *patient education* concerning the procedure itself, what is expected of the patient during the procedure, and any pre- or postprocedure restrictions (and the reasons for these restrictions).

Relaxation is important during intubation since the relaxed patient experiences less discomfort and the procedure can also be performed more rapidly and more successfully. The patient is reassured that he will be able to breathe at all times since the tubes passed into the trachea are hollow. It is desirable, however, if the patient can learn before the procedure to more consciously govern his breathing. For example, have him practice breathing through his mouth only, with his mouth open; then have him practice breathing through his nose only, with his mouth open.

Inform the patient that his throat will be anesthetized during the procedure to make him more comfortable and to prevent him from gagging. Tell him also that local anesthesia sprayed into the throat tastes bitter. Instruct him not to swallow this medication, but rather to spit it out into facial tissues or an emesis basin which will be provided.

Finally, tell the patient that he should not take anything by mouth following the procedure until he has been told it is safe to do so, i.e., until his gag reflex returns. Show him how his gag reflex will be tested.

Once the physician has properly positioned the bronchoscope or catheter in the trachea he introduces the radiopaque material. The patient is tilted into various positions, which causes the liquid material to run along the walls of the tracheobronchial tree, into the bronchi and bronchioles (Fig. 68–2). After a series of x-rays, postural drainage is used to help the dye to flow back out of the tracheobronchial tree so it can be expectorated. Postural drainage sessions should be supervised by the nurse while the patient is hospitalized. (Postural drainage is discussed on p. 910). It is desirable for as much dye as possible to be removed after bronchography. Some dyes are absorbed by the body within 12 to 24 hours; others may remain in the tracheobronchial tree for several months. Follow-up films are commonly taken. Surgery may be postponed for several months following bronchography if the physician believes that dye remaining in the tracheobronchial tree may jeopardize the patient's recovery. This precaution is particularly necessary if the dye used had an oil base.

Following bronchography the patient is not allowed oral intake until the nurse has ascertained that the local anesthesia has worn off and the patient's gag reflex has been restored. (See Unit VIII.) The gag reflex may return as soon as two hours following the procedure or it may not return for six to eight hours. *Post a sign on the patient's bed clearly stating intake restrictions.* Tracheal intubation may cause the patient's throat to feel irritated and sore following the procedure. Observe the patient closely for indications of cocaine toxicity and for symptoms of laryngospasm or laryngeal edema (resulting from laryngeal trauma during intubation). Impaired respirations may occur, necessitating immediate lifesaving treatment. To help to remove the radiopaque substance from the lungs the physician may order the use of a nebulizer or mechanical respirator, followed by postural drainage.

Pulmonary Angiography

Angiography (i.e., the roentgenographic visualization of blood vessels following injection of a contrast medium) is useful in evaluating pulmonary disorders as well as disorders of the brain, heart, and other body systems. Pulmonary angiography is helpful in diagnosing such conditions as pulmonary embolism, lung tumors, aneurysms, vascular changes associated with emphysema, congenital defects, blebs or bullae. Indeed, any space-occupying lesion within the thorax may be an indication for pulmonary angiographic investigation.

Angiography may demonstrate various pulmonary mechanical abnormalities, e.g., displacement of vessels from their normal positions (possibly due to bullae), or reduced blood flow to an area (perhaps caused by congenital defects, emboli, or tumorous obstruction).

Although numerous *techniques* for performing pulmonary angiography have been developed, in essence the procedure involves passing a catheter from a vein in the arm, into the heart (through the right atrium and right ventricle), and up into the pulmonary artery. Local anesthesia is used for the procedure. As the catheter is being progressively inserted pressures can be measured (e.g., in the right atrium, right ventricle, and pulmonary artery) and blood samples can be removed from various regions of the pulmonary circulatory system. Once the catheter is properly positioned a radiopaque substance is rapidly injected with a pressure injector and pulmonary x-rays are immediately taken and recorded on film or video tape (Fig. 68–3). Manual injection of the dye into a peripheral vein may produce satisfactory blood vessel visualization and is less hazardous than catheterization, but it is not routinely used because the pictures obtainable are limited in number and may be of poorer quality, and also a larger volume of contrast substance is necessary.

Complications associated with pulmonary angiography include: (1) mechanical problems associated with use of a catheter (e.g., local vascular problems, myocardial perforation with the catheter, or rupture, fragmentation, or perforation of the catheter itself); (2) pharmacologic problems (e.g., untoward allergic or toxic reactions to the contrast material or reactions to local anesthesia); and (3) cardiac complications (e.g., myocardial irritability caused by the catheter's presence in the heart's chambers). During the procedure the patient is

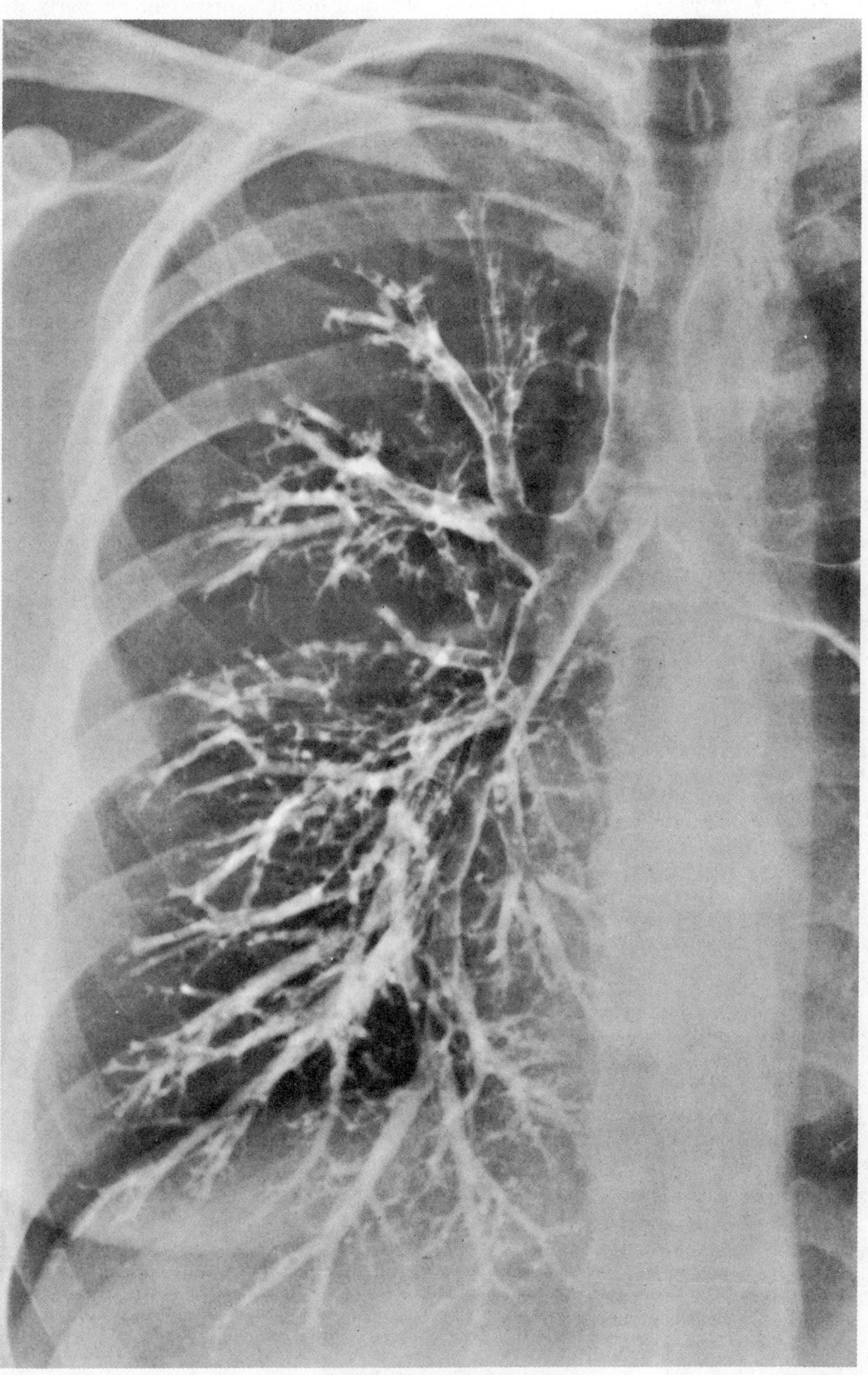

FIGURE 68–2. Right bronchial tree (frontal projection). Normal bronchogram of a 39 year old woman. (From Fraser, R. G., and Paré, J. A. P.: *Structure and Function of the Lung.* 1971.)

closely monitored by continuous electrocardiography for cardiac arrhythmias. (See Unit X.)

The patient is told before the contrast medium is injected into the lung that the injection may cause a temporary flushed, warm feeling. It is not uncommon for the injection to also provoke cough.

CHEST FLUOROSCOPY

Examination of the chest with fluoroscopic equipment enables the physician to view both lungs at the same time during the breathing process. Thus it is possible to actually view the dynamic activity of such cardiopulmonary mechanisms as cardiac action, diaphragmatic action, and lung expansion and contraction. By observing the movements of the thoracic wall and diaphragm during breathing, considerable information can be obtained about ventilation. Formerly it was not possible to have a permanent record of a fluoroscopic examination. Now, if desired, *spot films,* i.e., localized instantaneous x-rays, may be taken of questionable areas for later study. Modern special *image intensifier equipment* projects the fluoroscopic examination onto a *television screen* and may also record the entire examination on *film* for future study.

Sometimes mass roentgenographic surveys use techniques of *photofluorography* instead of routine

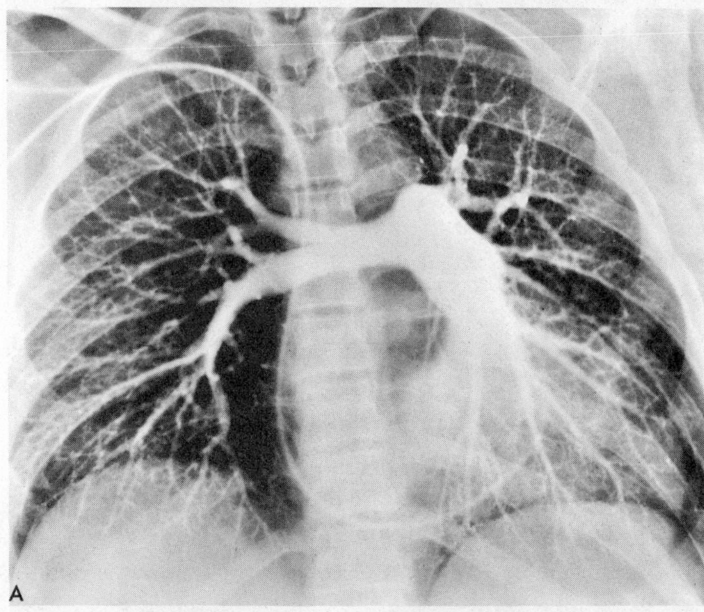

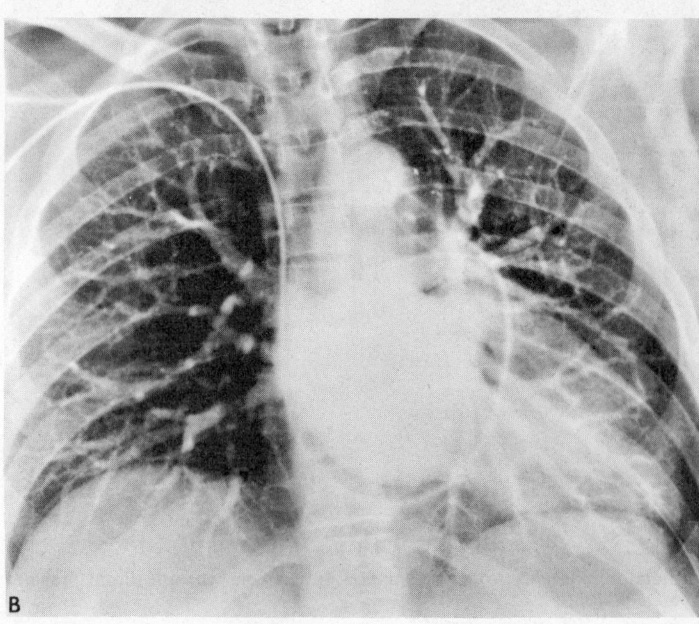

FIGURE 68–3. Pulmonary angiogram. *A,* Arterial phase; *B,* venous phase. (From Fraser, R. G., and Paré, J. A. P.: *Structure and Function of the Lung.* 1971.)

chest x-ray survey films; this is the photographic recording of fluoroscopic images on small films with the use of a fast lens.

The room may need to be darkened for *fluoroscopy*. The patient sits or stands in front of the fluoroscope. The procedure is painless. The physician gives the patient directions as he looks into the fluoroscope, e.g., "take a deep breath and hold it for a few seconds." To protect himself from unnecessary exposure to radiation the physician wears a lead-lined apron and gloves during the examination. If the nurse is present she also wears a protective apron. Properly maintained modern equipment minimizes radiation exposure.

LUNG SCINTIGRAPHY

Lung scintigraphy produces a graphic record of particles in the lung (as registered by a scintiscanner) following administration of a radioisotope. A scintiscanner is an apparatus used to record the concentration of a gamma ray emitting isotope in a tissue or organ. Lung scintigraphy may also be accomplished by using a scintillation camera. Lung scintiscanning may be carried out in different ways, e.g., radioaerosol inhalation, xenon-133 gas inhalation, and perfusion lung scan studies. (See also p. 878.)

Perfusion studies evaluate the perfusion of the lung with blood. Perfusion lung scanning procedures are performed by intravenous injection of macroaggregated albumin labeled with radioactive isotopes (e.g., ^{131}I or ^{51}Cr) and counting of the emissions of the radioactive isotopes with a scintiscanner. This determines the distribution of radio-

activity in the pulmonary vascular structures. The results are recorded on a diagram of the lungs, which then clearly shows which areas are well perfused with blood (indicated by a high uptake of radioactive substances) and which areas are poorly perfused (indicated by only small amounts of radioactive uptake). Areas of poor perfusion may result from emboli, tumors, or other disorders.

ENDOSCOPIC EXAMINATION OF THE TRACHEOBRONCHIAL TREE (BRONCHOSCOPY)

Bronchoscopy refers to the examination of the interior of the tracheobronchial tree through a *bronchoscope,* i.e., a long, slender, rigid, lighted tube containing mirrors. The scope is inserted through the mouth, pharynx, and trachea. Once it is properly positioned the physician can perform numerous procedures through this hollow tube. For example, he can see the trachea and mainstem bronchi and examine their surfaces for indications of disease or obstruction, e.g., tumor formation, ulceration. By passing other instruments through the scope the physician can obtain a tissue biopsy, apply medication, aspirate secretions for laboratory examination, aspirate a mucous plug causing airway obstruction, or remove aspirated foreign objects (Fig. 68–4). Bronchoscopy may be performed as an emergency or elective procedure.

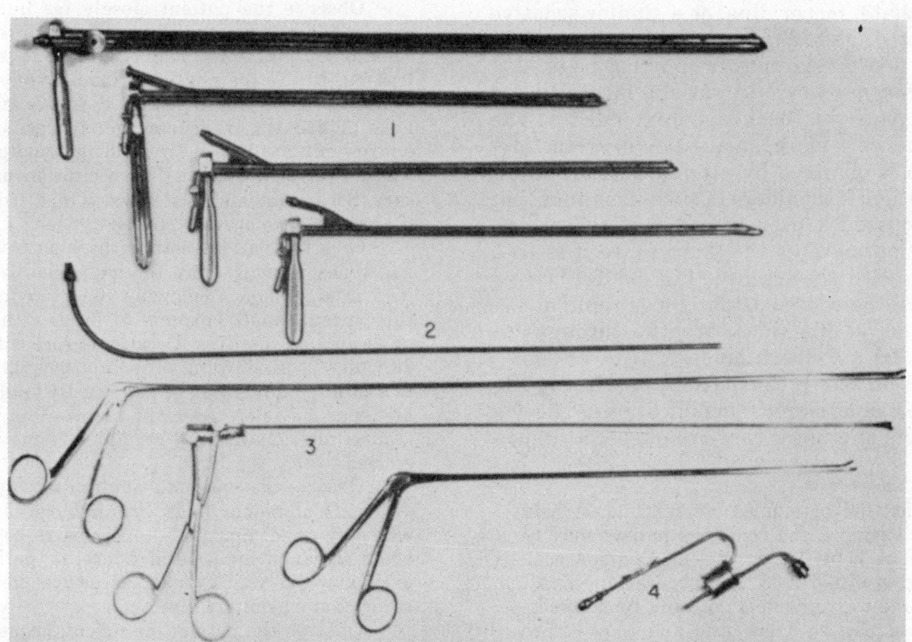

FIGURE 68–4. Instruments for bronchoscopy. **1,** Various sizes of bronchoscopes. **2,** Metal suction tip. **3,** Forceps used for biopsy and for removing foreign bodies. **4,** Suction trap used to collect secretions. (From DeWeese, D. D., and Saunders, W. H.: *Textbook of Otolaryngology.* St. Louis, The C. V. Mosby Co., 1968.)

Recently a flexible fiberoptic bronchoscope has been developed which is more versatile than the conventional rigid bronchoscope. The conventional bronchoscope permits only tunnel vision, but the fiberoptic instrument enables visualization of the segmental bronchi and their subsequent bifurcations, magnified, extremely sharp views of the endotracheal tree, and greater patient comfort during the examination. For a discussion of the fiberoptic bronchoscope see the article by Marici.[180a]

Bronchoscopy may be performed for either diagnostic or therapeutic reasons. It is routinely performed prior to bronchography. The procedure is uncomfortable for the patient and, as with other procedures involving intubation of the trachea, may cause the frightened patient to have brief feelings of suffocation.

Preparation of the patient for bronchoscopy is similar to that for bronchography, except for the following: (1) the procedure will be performed in a darkened room (often an operating room) so the doctor can more clearly see the structures lighted by the scope; (2) the patient should be told that the doctor and his assistants will be masked and gloved (reassure the patient that he is not going to have surgery performed at the time of the bronchoscopy); (3) he should also be informed that his eyes will be covered during the procedure to protect them (covering the patient's eyes also reduces anxiety caused from being able to watch the procedure); (4) postural drainage may not be ordered; (5) 30 to 60 minutes prior to the procedure morphine sulfate, meperidine, or a similar sedative may be ordered; and (6) a general anesthetic (e.g., intravenous anesthesia) may or may not be used.

During bronchoscopy the patient is positioned on his back with his neck hyperextended so the bronchoscope can more easily be inserted. Hyperextension is obtained by placing a small pillow under the patient's shoulders in such a manner that his head drops back over the edge of the pillow. Hyperextension elevates the pharynx so it is in a straight line with the trachea (Fig. 68–5). During the procedure the conscious patient is reminded to keep his arms at his sides, breathe through his nose, relax, and not clench his fists.

After bronchoscopy the patient is closely observed for possible serious complications. The following aspects of clinical care are of special importance:

> Position the patient as ordered and as indicated. For example, the conscious patient may be ordered to be kept flat or in semi-Fowler's position, lying on either side. If a general anesthetic was used and the patient is not fully conscious he is positioned flat, with his head and body turned to one side to prevent aspiration.

> Instruct the conscious patient with impaired swallowing to let saliva run from the side of his mouth (while lying on his side with a basin or tissues under his mouth) rather than attempt to swallow.

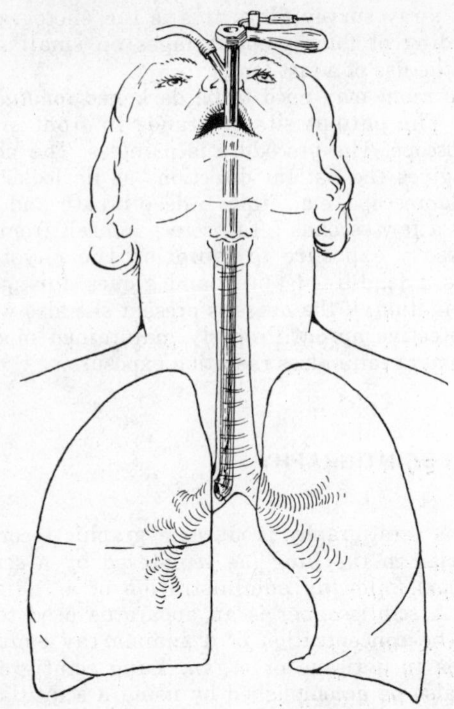

FIGURE 68–5. Diagram of a bronchoscope in place. **NOTE:** During bronchoscopy the patient's hair and eyes would be covered. (From De Weese, D. D., and Saunders, W. H.: *Textbook of Otolaryngology.* St. Louis, The C. V. Mosby Co., 1968.)

> Save all sputum expectorated for laboratory studies (cytology and culture). Copious amounts of sputum may be produced as a result of the trauma caused by passing the scope.

> Observe the patient closely for indications of impaired respiration. Laryngospasm or laryngeal edema (see Unit XXII) may occur due to laryngeal trauma. Notify the physician immediately of such symptoms as laryngeal stridor, dyspnea, and shortness of breath. Have emergency resuscitation equipment available (including tracheostomy tray). Provide emergency resuscitation as necessary. Set up and administer warm mist treatments if prescribed (to prevent laryngeal edema).

> Give the patient nothing by mouth until his gag reflex returns. Once the gag reflex is present (two to eight hours following the procedure) give the patient small amounts of fluids if he is not nauseated or vomiting. Because of sore throat and difficulty in swallowing after bronchoscopy, warm or soothing liquids may be more easily taken. A soft diet may be tolerated eight hours after the procedure; after 24 hours a regular diet may be prescribed.

> Observe the patient's sputum closely for indications of hemorrhage (frank blood) if biopsy was performed. Sputum is expected to be slightly blood streaked for several hours, or perhaps for one or two days; however, excessive bleeding is reported immediately.

> Observe the patient for subcutaneous emphysema (around the face and neck) and dyspnea. If present, immediately report these symptoms, for they indicate the serious (and fortunately rare)

complication of perforation of the trachea or bronchus. (Subcutaneous emphysema is discussed in Chapter 73.)

> Observe the patient closely for symptoms of toxicity caused by local anesthetic agents, e.g., cocaine, as described under Bronchography.

> Provide appropriate treatment if the patient has a sore throat. An ice collar may be used to minimize edema and soreness. Once the patient is able to swallow he may be given lozenges or soothing liquids to gargle.

> Inform the patient that sore throat, hoarseness, and voice loss related to bronchoscopy are only temporary.

> Instruct the patient not to attempt to clear his throat, to cough, or to talk. These actions cause further irritation to the throat and may disrupt clot formation at a biopsy site and precipitate hemorrhage. Provide pencil and paper and keep the patient's call signal handy for him. Smoking is restricted, at least for several hours following biopsy, because it can stimulate coughing and resultant bleeding. Because talking and smoking increase laryngeal irritation, these activities are typically restricted as long as hoarseness persists.

THORACENTESIS

Thoracentesis, also called thoracocentesis, refers to needle puncture through the chest wall into the pleural space for the purpose of removing pleural fluid (and/or possibly air). Thoracentesis may be performed for diagnostic or therapeutic reasons.

Therapeutically pleural fluid accumulations may be drained off to relieve lung compression and respiratory distress, or to remove excessive pleural fluid which could become infected and cause empyema. Thoracentesis may be therapeutically useful in treating such pulmonary disorders as pleurisy with effusion, empyema, hydrothorax, and hemothorax (see below).

Diagnostically, pleural fluid obtained by thoracentesis is subjected to careful study of its chemical, bacteriologic, and cellular composition. In the clinical laboratory the specimen's consistency, color, and the presence or absence of blood are noted. Evaluations are also made of glucose and protein content, specific gravity, white and differential blood counts, and the presence of bacteria and cells. Cellular composition may reveal the presence of neoplastic cells. Effusions characterized by lymphocytosis occur most often in patients with tuberculosis, lymphoma, or carcinoma.

Before thoracentesis the nurse prepares the patient psychologically, assembles necessary equipment, and properly positions the patient. Patient education includes briefly explaining the procedure, telling the patient that he can help by not moving during the procedure, and informing him that after the procedure he should have only minimal discomfort at the puncture site. If the patient moves suddenly during the procedure he can force the needle through the pleural space and injure the visceral (pulmonary) pleura and/or lung.

Equipment for thoracentesis includes: 5-ml. syringe and needle for local anesthesia, local anesthetic drug, 50-ml. syringe, 17-gauge aspirating needle, three-way stopcock, sterile tubing, hemostats, sterile specimen tube and collecting vial, sterile towels, materials for skin preparation, collodion, and small sterile dressing. A biopsy needle should also be on hand. (See below under Biopsy.)

It is important that the needle and syringe used for thoracentesis fit tightly to prevent atmospheric air from entering the pleural space. Since pleural exudates tend to coagulate easily, specimens are usually collected in tubes containing either sodium citrate or potassium oxalate.

Positioning is important. Thoracentesis is most effectively performed with the patient sitting upright (pleural fluid can then accumulate for removal at the base of the chest) with his neck and dorsal spine flexed and his arms and shoulders raised (this elevates and separates the ribs, thus ensuring less traumatic needle insertion). Have the patient sit on the edge of his bed with his feet supported on a chair. Then roll an overbed table in front of the patient, place a pillow or folded bath blanket on this table, and have the patient raise his arms and shoulders and lean over the padded surface, resting his head on the padding. Remain by the patient's side. Physically support the patient if he is very nervous or weak and have another nurse help the doctor.

If the patient cannot sit up for thoracentesis, turn him on his unaffected side and place his arm on that side up over his head.

Throughout the thoracentesis observe the patient's condition, reassure and advise him, assist the physician, and take the patient's pulse and respiratory rates several times. Tell the patient what is happening, e.g., when an injection will be made, so he is not startled into sudden movement. Observe the patient closely for shock, chills, pain, nausea, coughing, pallor, dyspnea, cyanosis, weakness, increased respiratory rate, or diaphoresis. Call the physician's attention to these symptoms.

Thoracentesis is performed aseptically with local anesthesia. The site of needle insertion for fluid removal is most often just below the angle of the scapula at the seventh intercostal space. At times the physician uses a chest x-ray for purposes of measuring the level at which he should perform the aspiration. He takes the lower tip of the scapula as a landmark and then measures how far the fluid is below this landmark. With the patient positioned as for the x-ray the physician then carries out the same measurements on the patient's back and performs the aspiration. If thoracentesis is performed too low, the liver or spleen may be punctured, causing serious aftereffects.

A small gauge needle and a 5-ml. syringe are used to locate the pleural space and to inject the anesthetic agent. Then a larger needle (17-gauge) is used for the fluid removal. This needle is attached to a three-way stopcock (to prevent air from entering the pleural space) and a 50-ml. syringe.

Hemostats (or artery clamps) may be used to hold the needle in place after insertion or to mark the desired depth of insertion.

As the needle passes through the parietal pleura (lining the walls of the parietal cavity), the patient may feel pressure or pain even though a local anesthetic has been injected.

Fluid in the pleural space is slowly and gently aspirated. Not more than 1200 ml. are removed at one time in order to reduce the dangers of circulatory collapse or acute pulmonary edema. Rapid removal does not provide sufficient time for the lung to reexpand and the patient may become short of breath, may cough, and may have chest pain. These symptoms indicate possible mediastinal shift toward the side of the thoracentesis. (See Chapter 72.) Precautions are taken to avoid tearing the lung and thus causing a pneumothorax during thoracentesis; for the same purpose, care is taken to maintain negative pressure. Excessive traction on the syringe plunger during fluid removal can cause lung puncture by drawing the lung forcefully against the needle point.

After the needle is removed, pressure is applied over the puncture site. The site is usually sealed with collodion and covered with a small sterile dressing. Specimens are sent immediately to the clinical laboratory. The patient may be positioned recumbent for an hour with his punctured chest side up. This position minimizes possible fluid seepage by gravity into the pleural space and allows the pleural puncture site to seal over. The nurse charts the procedure, including comments about the amount and character of fluid removed, and the patient's tolerance of the procedure, e.g., pulse, color, appearance, how he says he feels. She also notes and charts any relief that the patient may have obtained from the procedure, e.g., breathing more comfortably.

Following thoracentesis the nurse observes the patient for indications of *complications* or fluid reaccumulation in the pleural space. Specific observations include the following:

> Observe for symptoms of *shock,* e.g., faintness, falling blood pressure, weak rapid pulse, rapid respirations. Shock is a rare complication, but can result from fluid shifting into the pleural space from the vascular space. This shift decreases the circulating blood volume, thereby causing shock.

> Check the *puncture site* for indications of *leakage.*

> Observe for the following symptoms of possible *lung damage* (e.g., *pneumothorax,* p. 1002, or *tension pneumothorax,* p. 1002) or possible *reaccumulation of fluid:* (1) blood-tinged sputum or hemoptysis; (2) excessive, uncontrollable coughing or persistent cough; (3) indications of respiratory distress (e.g., dyspnea, cyanosis, tightness in the chest); and (4) subcutaneous emphysema.

> Watch for indications of *mediastinal shift* if large amounts of fluid were removed. Symptoms include those of cardiac distress or pulmonary edema (indicated by blood-tinged frothy sputum). These symptoms are caused by sudden shift of the mediastinal contents toward the side from which the fluid was removed.

> Observe for indications of *pyogenic infection* (due to contamination).

Frequently serum electrolyte blood studies are ordered after thoracentesis to guide planning for intravenous electrolyte replacement therapy. Replacement therapy is necessary if large amounts of fluid are removed since pleural fluid is isotonic. (See Chapters 24 and 25.)

A chest x-ray may also be ordered following thoracentesis to determine the effects of the procedure. The physician reading the x-ray looks to see if pleural fluid remains, air was accidentally introduced during the procedure, or mediastinal shift occurred, and if the lung is reexpanding satisfactorily to fill the space previously occupied by the fluid accumulation.

PULMONARY ECHOGRAMS

Reflected ultrasound, using the echo-ranging technique, can be useful in detecting and localizing pleural effusion. The ultrasound technique is not only useful diagnostically (in detecting pleural effusion which may not show up on chest x-rays or by thoracentesis), but it may also be of value in selecting sites for therapeutic pleural aspiration.

BIOPSY

Biopsy may be taken of various tissues during the process of investigating respiratory disorders. We have previously mentioned that biopsy may be taken of *tracheobronchial* structures at the time of bronchoscopy. Biopsies of *scalene* and *mediastinal nodes* may be performed (under local anesthesia) to obtain tissue for pathogenic analysis by culture, animal inoculation, or microscopic inspection.

Pleural biopsy was initially performed surgically through a small thoracotomy (open biopsy). Today pleural biopsy is most commonly performed with a special biopsy needle. Needle biopsy is a safe, simple, very useful diagnostic procedure of value in determining the etiology of many pleural effusions. The needle removes a small fragment of parietal pleura which is used for microscopic examination and culture. If bacteriologic studies are to be performed the biopsy specimen is obtained before chemotherapy is started. Pleural biopsy can easily be performed at the time of routine thoracentesis; thus, a biopsy needle, e.g., a Cope needle, should be available whenever pleural fluid is removed by thoracentesis.

In performing biopsy it may be necessary for the physician to make multiple needle insertions at different sites. Both the skin and pleura are injected with a local anesthetic. Then a small skin incision is made with a scalpel blade to facilitate insertion of the biopsy needle.

The specific diagnoses most frequently established from pleural needle biopsy specimens are tuberculosis, other granulomatous diseases, and tumors (primary or metastatic to the pleura). Disease processes that occur in the periphery of a lung often involve the parietal pleura and commonly are associated with pleural effusion. Thus, pleural biopsy is considered whenever there is radiologic evidence of fluid in the pleural space.[155]

The preparation and positioning of a patient for pleural biopsy is similar to that for thoracentesis. Rare complications include temporary pain resulting from intercostal nerve injury, pneumothorax, and hemothorax. Following the biopsy the patient is therefore observed closely for indications of these conditions, e.g., dyspnea. The danger of pneumothorax associated with needle pleural biopsy can be reduced by using special needles designed to obtain the specimen while the needle is being withdrawn, rather than upon insertion. Follow-up chest x-rays may be taken a few hours after the procedure. Possible hemothorax is indicated by a substantial increase in fluid in the pleural space. This finding indicates the need for immediate thoracentesis.

As with pleural biopsy, *lung biopsy* may be accomplished either by surgical exposure of the lung or by use of a needle. Tissue removed is examined microscopically and bacteriologically. Lung biopsies are most often performed to identify pulmonary tumors.

Needle puncture aspiration biopsy of chest lesions is performed under fluoroscopic monitoring. After the lesion is found on a chest film and localized under fluoroscopy, topical anesthesia is administered and a needle is inserted through the chest wall into the lesion. A small sample of cells is then aspirated for microscopic study and the needle is withdrawn. Aspiration biopsy may enable the definitive diagnosis of malignant neoplasms, granulomas, or other nonmalignant growths. Possible complications of needle aspiration biopsy of the lung are hemoptysis and pneumothorax. After the procedure the nurse examines the patient's sputum closely for evidence of blood and observes the patient for respiratory distress associated with possible pneumothorax.

Indications of complications following any biopsy are reported immediately to the physician.

SPUTUM EXAMINATION

Sputum is material coughed up from the lungs and tracheobronchial tree; it is different from postnasal secretions or saliva. When obtaining a sputum specimen, make sure the patient understands these differences so he will provide the correct specimen.

Sputum specimens may be collected for gross observation and evaluation or for such detailed laboratory analyses as those performed with microscopic smears or cultures.

Gross Sputum Evaluations

Bedside Sputum Observation. The physician may request that a patient be placed on "bedside sputum observation." Instruct the patient to col-

lect the sputum he expectorates in a container so the specimen's quantity, color, consistency, and odor can be evaluated periodically. Much can be learned about the patient's condition by this gross examination. For example, malodorous, yellow-green colored sputum is often indicative of infection; thick, tenacious sputum indicates the need for greater liquefaction of the tracheobronchial secretions. (See Chapter 69.) Appropriate orders can then be given, e.g., drug sensitivity cultures can be ordered to identify the appropriate medications to combat an infection or the patient can be encouraged to drink more fluids to liquefy secretions. Blood in the sputum may also be observed in bedside specimens. Provide clean collection containers daily after the physician has seen the specimen, or more often if the physician does not want to observe the specimen.

Quantitative Sputum Studies. These studies are conducted to determine the quantity of sputum produced over a given period of time, e.g., 24 to 72 hours. The total collected specimen is described in terms of its volume, weight, and character. Several containers may be necessary in collecting quantitative sputum specimens. Replace containers well before they are full.

Qualitative Sputum Studies. These studies determine the composition of secretions expectorated, i.e., whether they are pus, mucus, or saliva. When placed in a conical glass container the secretions separate into various layers..

Microscopic Sputum Evaluations

Sputum may be studied in the clinical laboratory for the presence of malignant cells, bronchial casts, pus, white blood cells, bacteria, or blood. Microscopically sputum may be examined following smear or culture.

Sputum Smear. In performing a smear in the laboratory a microscopic slide is smeared thinly with specimen matter so the material can then be studied microscopically. A special type of examination, often designated *cytology,* is performed on a smear when malignancy is suspected. Cytology or cytologic examination means the microscopic examination of cells shed from a body surface to look for indications of malignant change. Body materials used for cytology specimens may be not only bronchial secretions or bronchial washings, but also pleural fluid sediment. Specimens for cytologic examination must be taken to the laboratory immediately.

After a smear is made, appropriate stains may be applied to the slide. Staining characteristics help to identify various cell structures. For example, the high lipid content of the tubercle bacillus causes it to absorb and retain the red color of carbolfuchsin stain even when the slide is washed with acid-alcohol (i.e., the tubercule bacillus is an acid-fast organism). When viewed microscopically the bacilli then appear as red rod-shaped structures. (This is the Ziehl-Neelsen staining method). The presence of neutrophils (stainable by neutral dyes) and eosinophils (stained by eosin) is also noted in studying sputum slides. It is not uncommon for repeated smears to be ordered for several (three or four) successive days. One negative smear does not always mean that virulent organisms are not present.

Sputum Culture. Sputum cultures are used in diagnosing pulmonary infections. In performing laboratory cultures, microorganisms or living tissue cells are implanted or inoculated onto a special media which is conducive to their growth, e.g., agar. The specimens are then kept in special environments conducive to their growth and propagation, e.g., incubated at special temperatures. After sufficient growth is obtained on the culture, bacterial colonies are counted and the specific organism is identified. Subcultures can be made if desired. Some microorganisms are very slow growing. For example, it may take three to 12 weeks to obtain a positive culture of tubercle bacilli.

Both pathogenic and nonpathogenic bacteria may be found in sputum cultures with some lung diseases. Thus, after the physician has correlated all his findings he decides on the significance of a particular finding.

Specimens obtained for culture (bacteriologic examination) are always collected before the patient receives any bactericidal medications (e.g., antibiotics, sulfonamides), unless the culture is being taken to evaluate the effectiveness of medications already given. If bactericidal medications are given prior to the initial bacteriologic examination, it is impossible to obtain accurate antimicrobial drug sensitivity test results.

Antimicrobial drug sensitivity tests may be ordered to identify to which specific medications a patient's bacteria are sensitive, i.e., which antibiotics will be therapeutically effective. The collection procedure for a specimen for these tests is the same as that for any sputum culture, i.e., the specimen is protected so it is uncontaminated and so the organisms in the specimen remain viable.

Sputum Specimen Collection

Before obtaining a sputum specimen give the patient the necessary instructions. Tell him to be sure that he furnishes as a specimen only those secretions coming from below his larynx ("Adam's apple"). Next, help the patient to rinse out his mouth with *water.* Do not have him brush his teeth or use an antiseptic mouthwash. Antiseptic solutions affect the viability of microorganisms in the sputum specimen. Specimens are obtained by asking the patient to cough deeply, not just clear his throat. A deep, vigorous cough brings up a specimen from deep within the tracheobronchial tree. (See discussion of coughing in Chapter 73.)

It is desirable to collect sputum specimens when the patient first awakens in the morning. Secretions tend to pool and collect in the lungs during sleep and, thus, early morning coughing is likely to be more productive of sputum; also, a higher concentration of organisms tends to occur in secretions that accumulate at night. Give the patient the specimen jar the evening before the specimen is to be collected so he can expectorate mucus he brings up in the *first* cough upon awakening in the morning. At least one teaspoonful of sputum is necessary for laboratory examination.

Patients who have difficulty "raising" sputum may need to have a specimen collected with the help of a *heated aerosol.* In this procedure the patient inhales 10 per cent saline in distilled water from a heated nebulizer. The nebulizer is attached to compressed oxygen or air; thus, a fine mist of saline is produced. The production of secretions is stimulated by vapor condensation within the tracheobronchial tree; the patient can then more easily cough up these secretions.

Prior to the first heated aerosol sputum collection the patient is told that he will inhale a fine mist of warm saline and that this will help him to cough effectively so he can raise sputum. The patient is then shown how to: (1) place his mouth loosely over the nebulizer; (2) deeply inhale the mist vapor until coughing begins; and (3) cough effectively. (Aerosol treatments are discussed further in Chapter 70.)

Sputum specimens are collected in covered wide-mouthed jars or waterproof, disposable sputum cups or boxes. If a culture is to be performed the container's opening and inside must be sterile. Instruct the patient to expectorate directly into the center of the container without touching his mouth to the container. Also tell the patient to be careful that sputum does not contaminate the outside of the container.

Always keep sputum containers covered. This is not only esthetically desirable (because the odor and sight of sputum are offensive), but it also prevents spread of air-borne microorganisms from the sputum and prevents air contamination of the specimen. Cover the outside of glass containers with a paper towel held on with a rubber band. Sputum specimen containers should never become completely full. Provide extra containers as necessary. Sputum is sometimes collected in waxed paper cups (with lids) which are placed in metal holders. The holders are boiled often because their outsides are usually highly contaminated.

Provide tissues so the patient may cover his mouth when coughing up sputum and wipe his mouth after he expectorates the sputum specimen. Keep used tissues picked up and discarded. When the patient is coughing be certain you keep your head turned away from the direction of his cough to protect yourself from air-borne infections. Always wash your hands thoroughly after handling used tissues or sputum specimen containers. If a patient has suspected or known tuberculosis and has not been on chemotherapy, it may be desirable to wear a mask if you need to be present during the time the patient is coughing up the specimen. (See Chapter 71.)

If sputum is being obtained for laboratory study, the specimen should be promptly delivered to the laboratory bacteriology refrigerator and should not remain at the bedside. If it is not possible to *immediately* send the specimen to the laboratory after collection, refrigerate it on the ward, making sure it is clearly marked for identification. If a patient is in isolation the container's outside is considered to be contaminated and must be appropriately handled to prevent spread of infection.

GASTRIC CONTENT ANALYSIS (GASTRIC WASHINGS)

Some patients are unable to raise sputum for specimens, e.g., they are not producing enough sputum to raise or they are unable to cooperate enough to raise a specimen (unconscious, aged, young children, severely debilitated). In these patients pulmonary disease may be diagnosed or evaluated by examining gastric contents when the patient is in a fasting state. Gastric contents are aspirated for study through a nasogastric tube or a tube passed orally to the stomach. An analysis of gastric contents may reveal pathogenic organisms causing pulmonary infections, because these organisms are often swallowed.

Gastric aspiration is performed early in the morning before breakfast and before the patient arises (activity causes the stomach to empty its contents into the duodenum). The patient is given nothing by mouth for eight to 12 hours before the aspiration. The early morning hour is desirable because it is possible to aspirate secretions from the lungs, throat, mouth, and nose which have been swallowed during sleep.

Sometimes before the stomach contents are withdrawn, sterile water is instilled through the nasogastric tube. The stomach contents are withdrawn into a large syringe attached to the tube. The specimen is then transferred from the syringe into a sterile, covered laboratory container. Laboratory techniques used to study gastric contents include: guinea pig inoculation, culture, microscopic smear, and concentrate-flotation. Gastric content analysis is often performed on patients with suspected or proved tuberculosis. However, heated aerosol sputum collections are now replacing the need for gastric washings in many patients. This is fortunate since passage of a nasogastric tube is often an uncomfortable procedure, gastric analysis needs to be preceded by fasting, and gastric analysis can be performed only in the early A.M. Heated aerosol collections can be obtained at any time.

See Unit XV for further discussion of nasogastric intubation.

ANIMAL INOCULATION

Sometimes animal inoculation is necessary to differentiate between pathogenic and nonpathogenic organisms. The guinea pig, for example, is highly sensitive to tuberculosis. Specimens which may be used for guinea pig inoculation include: sputum, urine, ground-up or homogenized material from resected lung lesions, pleural fluid, or cerebrospinal fluid. At least two animals are used. Multiple subcutaneous inoculations of specimen material are made in the inguinal and axillary regions. Six to nine weeks after inoculation the animals are examined at autopsy for evidence of infection.

BLOOD TESTS

White Blood Cell (Leukocyte) Counts

A *total white blood cell count* (normally 6–9000/cu. mm.) and a *differential count* may help to diagnose respiratory inflammations, allergies, and infections. These tests may also help to distinguish between acute and chronic infections. The necessary blood sample is obtained from a venipuncture or a finger prick. White blood cells are discussed in detail in Chapter 22. Here we summarize only a few relevant points.

White blood cell counts usually increase with infections. Although *acute infections* usually produce a radical increase in circulating WBC's (i.e., leukocytosis), *chronic infections* may increase the total number of leukocytes only slightly. In fact, occasionally a marked decrease (i.e., leukopenia) occurs with tuberculosis or severe debilitation.

With acute infections, increases occur mostly in the *polymorphonuclear leukocytes*, i.e., the neutrophils, eosinophils (acidophils), and basophils. Most bacterial infections elevate *neutrophils*. These phagocytic cells normally form 50 to 70 per cent of the total WBC's; i.e., they are normally 3000 to 7000 per cu. mm. of blood. Allergic disorders, such as allergic asthma, elevate *eosinophils* (normally 50–400/cu. mm. or 0 to 1 per cent of WBC's). *Basophils* (normally 0–50/cu. mm. or 0 to 1 per cent of WBC's) may prevent coagulation in inflammatory conditions.

Chronic infections may increase the number of *mononuclear leukocytes,* i.e., lymphocytes and monocytes. *Lymphocytes* (normally 1500-3000/cu. mm. or 25 to 33 per cent of WBC's) increase with some bacterial infections. *Monocytes* (normally 285-500/cu. mm. or 4 to 6 per cent of WBC's) are typically increased in tuberculosis and chronic inflammatory conditions. These phagocytes are also increased during recovery phases of infections.

Red Blood Cell (Erythrocyte) Evaluations

Evaluations of red blood cells used in diagnosing and treating respiratory disorders include red blood cell count, hemoglobin concentration, hematocrit test, and erythrocyte sedimentation rate.

The hemoglobin in erythrocytes transports oxygen from the lungs throughout the body. Hemoglobin not only gives up oxygen to the cells but also carries carbon dioxide from the tissues back to the lungs. It is clinically important to determine not only a patient's *red blood cell count* (total number of RBC's) but also the amount of hemoglobin in the RBC's. Normal RBC counts for males are 4.8-5.5 million/cu. mm. of blood, and 4.4-5.0 million for females. *Hemoglobin concentration* for males is normally 14.5-16.0 Gm./dl. of blood, and 13.0-15.5 Gm./dl. of blood for females. Inadequate cellular respiration can occur if a patient's RBC count or hemoglobin concentration is deficient. It is also possible to measure the *per cent of oxyhemoglobin saturation,* i.e., the percentage of oxyhemoglobin saturated with oxygen. Normal arterial oxyhemoglobin saturation is 95 per cent; normal venous oxyhemoglobin saturation is 85 per cent.

Additional information about the number, capacity, and size of RBC's can be obtained by combining information about hemoglobin concentration with that obtained from a *hematocrit* test. This test determines the volume percentage of erythrocytes in whole blood. Normally RBC's comprise 45 to 50 per cent (expressed as volume per cent) of the volume of whole blood in males, and 40 to 45 volume per cent for females.

An *erythrocyte sedimentation rate* measures the rate of speed with which RBC's settle to the bottom of a volume of drawn blood. This test provides a rough measurement of abnormal concentrations of fibrinogen and serum globulins that accompany certain inflammatory or infectious disorders which destroy cells, e.g., tuberculosis and cancer. The normal values for this test vary with the method used to perform the test, e.g., Cutler, Westergren, Wintrobe. (RBC functions and laboratory evaluations are discussed more completely in Unit XII.)

C-Reactive Protein Test (CRPA)

A positive reaction (precipitate formation) occurs in the presence of tissue inflammation or destruction, such as that caused by widespread cancer or active tuberculosis. Normally C-reactive protein is not present in venous blood.

Lactic Dehydrogenase Level (LDH)

Lactic dehydrogenase (LDH) is an intracellular enzyme that affects the speed of intracellular metabolic processes. Blood serum LDH is normally 165 to 300 units. Five isoenzymes, or variants, of LDH have been identified. The isoenzyme which occurs in the lungs is LDH-3. Cellular injury or destruction of cells containing LDH causes the release of the enzyme into the blood stream. Elevated plasma concentrations of LDH thus may aid in diagnosing conditions causing cellular injury or destruction. Pulmonary infarction increases serum LDH-3. (LDH has also been discussed in Unit X.)

Blood Gas Analyses

"Blood gas studies" are measurements of oxygen, carbon dioxide, and hydrogen in the arterial and venous blood. These measurements are expressed as: pO_2 (partial pressure or tension of oxygen); pCO_2 (partial pressure or tension of carbon dioxide); and pH (hydrogen ion concentration). The pO_2 and pCO_2 are expressed as millimeters of mercury. The *arterial* blood gases are often referred to by the following symbols: $PaCO_2$, referring to arterial carbon dioxide pressure, and PaO_2, referring to arterial oxygen pressure.

It is helpful to measure the pH and pCO_2 in *venous* blood samples (these measurements are in fact replacing the test for CO_2 content) as part of total electrolyte examinations. However, venous samples are not used for pO_2 measurements, except for purposes of comparing the arterial and venous pO_2's.

Blood gas analyses are important in the care of critically ill and acutely ill patients, in caring for patients being mechanically ventilated (i.e., on respirators), in evaluating chronic pulmonary disorders (e.g., chronic obstructive pulmonary diseases), and as part of total electrolyte evaluations.

Blood gas measurements evaluate such factors as rate of cellular metabolism, tissue perfusion, ventilation efficiency, and the ability of hemoglobin to transport oxygen and carbon dioxide. They also reflect the state of buffer systems. Since the lungs are the principal regulators of acid-base balance, blood gas studies are important determinants of the state of pulmonary function.

Table 68–1 shows the most common terms used in blood gas analysis and the normal range of values for the various measurements.

In caring for acutely or critically ill patients and patients on respirators, *arterial* blood gas determinations may be made at frequent intervals. These samples may be taken from indwelling arterial catheters, e.g., an Angiocath in the radial, brachial, or femoral artery (Fig. 68–6), or by a femoral puncture performed by the physician. Indwelling catheters permit frequent drawing of blood specimens and reduce patient discomfort and danger associated with repeated punctures. *Venous* blood specimens may be drawn from a central venous catheter or, in special cases (e.g., open heart surgery), from a catheter in the pulmonary artery. Serial measurements are taken at frequent intervals, and changes and arteriovenous differences are carefully evaluated.

To obtain accurate test results, specimens for blood gas analyses must be correctly collected and handled. Unclotted blood is necessary, and specimens may be collected in a heparinized vacuum tube or a plastic syringe flushed with heparin. Small amounts of heparin will not significantly dilute the specimen; larger amounts would affect hematocrit readings if they are done on the specimen. In withdrawing the specimen care is taken to avoid getting any air bubbles into the sample,

TABLE 68–1. BLOOD GASES AND ACID-BASE BALANCE (TERMINOLOGY AND VALUES)

Term	Definition	Remarks	Normal Range (Mean)
Arterial O_2 saturation (SaO_2)	Ratio of oxygen content and capacity	Influenced by the S-shaped O_2-hemoglobin dissociation curve, with its steep slope between 10 and 50 mm. Hg Po_2 and flat portion between 70 and 100 mm. Hg Po_2	93–98% (97); rises to about 100% if breathing 100% O_2
Arterial O_2 tension (PaO_2)	Partial pressure of oxygen	In equilibrium with alveolar oxygen tension	80–104 mm. Hg (95); 600 mm. Hg if breathing 100% O_2
Arterial pH	Expression (negative logarithm) of the hydrogen ion concentration	Determined by the ratio of concentrations of bicarbonate ion and CO_2 (as dissolved CO_2, H_2CO_3, carbamino compounds), usually 20:1	7.38–7.44 (7.41)
Arterial CO_2 tension ($Paco_2$)	Partial pressure of carbon dioxide	Regulated by volume of alveolar ventilation; CO_2 retention (hypercapnia) always means *hypoventilation*	36–42 mm. Hg (39)
Total CO_2 content (or concentration) of plasma (venous)	Carbon dioxide obtainable from bicarbonate, dissolved CO_2, carbamino compounds, and H_2CO_3, measured anaerobically at the patient's Pco_2	Reflects both metabolic and respiratory disturbances; result is not a clear indicator of either	26–30 mEq./L. (28) 58–67 vol. % (64)
CO_2 combining power of plasma or serum "alkali reserve" (venous)	Total carbon dioxide content of plasma or serum when equilibrated at a Pco_2 of 40 mm. Hg	May be expressed as plasma bicarbonate by subtracting dissolved CO_2 (1.2 mEq./L.); reflects metabolic disturbances more reliably than respiratory	26–30 mEq./L. (28) 58–67 vol. % (64)
Serum or plasma bicarbonate (venous)	Bicarbonate ion concentration (HCO_3) Total CO_2 content minus H_2CO_3 and dissolved CO_2	Most important plasma buffer; level regulated by kidney; compensatory increase when CO_2 retention occurs, but abnormal levels primarily reflect metabolic disturbances	25–28 mEq./L. (26.5)

(Table continued on following page.)

TABLE 68–1. BLOOD GASES AND ACID-BASE BALANCE (TERMINOLOGY AND VALUES) *(Continued)*

Term	Definition	Remarks	Normal Range (Mean)
Standard bicarbonate of plasma (arterial or capillary)	Bicarbonate ion conc. measured at a P_{CO_2} of 40 mm. Hg in plasma of fully oxygenated blood	A term used by P. Astrup and associates for bicarbonate concentration corrected to reflect (HCO_3) concentration independent of respiratory changes, that is, of changes in arterial P_{O_2} and P_{CO_2}	22–26 mEq./L. (24)
Base excess concentration (arterial or capillary)	Expression of base excess in mEq./L. over the normal value (which is zero for blood with a pH of 7.4 and P_{CO_2} of 40 mm. Hg)	Astrup terminology; negative value indicates a base deficit or acid excess; independent of hemoglobin concentration; positive or negative values outside the normal range are more helpful in guiding therapy of metabolic than respiratory disturbances	−2.4 to +2.3 mEq./L. (0)
Respiratory acidosis	Excess of CO_2 resulting from inadequate alveolar ventilation	Degree of compensation depends upon the change in level of bicarbonate ion; this rises in the attempt to maintain the 20:1 ratio necessary for a pH in the normal range	Uncompensated, pH 6.8–7.37; compensated, pH 7.38–7.41
Respiratory alkalosis	Deficit of CO_2 resulting from alveolar hyperventilation	Does not have the life-threatening potential of respiratory acidosis; kidney responds by excreting bicarbonate	Uncompensated, pH 7.45–7.7; compensated, 7.41–7.44
Metabolic acidosis	Bicarbonate deficit, usually due to excess production of organic acids, excess loss of base, or retention of acids	Lung attempts to compensate by hyperventilation with removal of carbon dioxide; example, diabetic acidosis	Uncompensated, pH 6.8–7.37; compensated, pH 7.38–7.41
Metabolic alkalosis	Bicarbonate excess, usually due to excess loss of acids, excess intake of alkaline salts, or deficit of potassium	Retention of carbon dioxide by alveolar hypoventilation may improve acid-base balance; example, prolonged vomiting	Uncompensated, pH 7.45–7.8; compensated, pH 7.41–7.44

*National Tuberculosis and Respiratory Disease Association: *Chronic Obstructive Pulmonary Disease: A Manual for Physicians.* Copyright, 1965, Oregon Thoracic Society, 811 Southwest Washington Street, Portland, Oregon 97205 since the air would affect the blood gas measurements. A blood specimen of 2.5 ml. is adequate for most blood gas measurements; 0.5 ml. is sufficient for some gas analyzers. Some sources recommend placing the sample in a container of ice unless measurements are to be made immediately.

Blood gas norms differ for arterial and venous blood. It is thus important to always identify the origin of the blood sample on a specimen and when reading blood gas results.

Blood pH. Evaluation of the blood's pH gives important information on a patient's metabolic state and the effectiveness of his respirations. Blood pH levels are dependent on the amount of carbon dioxide in the blood. The pH is, thus, important in evaluating the blood's acid-base balance. Normally both venous and arterial blood are slightly alkaline. *Arterial* blood pH is about 7.41, while *venous* blood pH is about 7.36.

Carbon Dioxide Tension (pCO_2). The pCO_2 reflects the effectiveness of ventilation and varies with the amount (or partial pressure) of carbon dioxide in inspired air. The normal *arterial* pCO_2 ($PaCO_2$) is 36 to 42 mm. Hg; the normal *venous* pCO_2 is between 40 and 41 mm. Hg.

An elevated pCO_2 indicates *respiratory acidosis* or hypercarbia, i.e., excessive carbonic acid. An elevated pCO_2 may occur with underventilation because the CO_2 is not being effectively "blown off" by the lungs and, thus, the CO_2 builds up in the blood. Such underventilation may result from "splinting" the chest (breathing shallowly) because of pain upon breathing, e.g., pleuritic pain, incisional pain, pain from injured ribs.

Patients with chronic obstructive pulmonary diseases are often able to tolerate retention of increased amounts of CO_2 without showing symptoms of hypercarbia.

A low pCO_2 indicates *respiratory alkalosis* or hypocarbia. A low pCO_2 often results from hyperventilation, which causes the CO_2 to be blown off excessively. The pCO_2 decreases because the blood's CO_2 content is low. Hysteria and salicylate overdose are examples of conditions that can cause hypocarbia.

Oxygen Tension (pO_2). The pO_2 measures the effectiveness of the lungs in oxygenating the blood, i.e., the ability of the lungs to diffuse inspired oxygen across the alveolar membrane into the circulating blood. The normal *arterial* pO_2 (PaO_2) is 80 to 104 mm. Hg; however, patients with chronic obstructive pulmonary diseases may be able to tolerate an arterial pO_2 as low as 70 mm. Hg without showing symptoms of hypoxia. An awareness of this tolerance is highly important, since it is unnecessary (in fact, it can be fatal) to try to raise the pO_2 in these patients to within laboratory normal levels; the *patient's individual known normal* pO_2 becomes the guide for oxygen therapy in these patients.

The *arterial* pO_2 may be elevated by administering oxygen and by changing the patient's position. Position change can improve pulmonary ventilation and reduce the return of unoxygenated blood to the left atrium of the heart.

Because the pO_2 reflects the amount of oxygen passing from pulmonary alveoli into the blood, it is directly influenced by the amount of oxygen being inspired. When pO_2 measurements are being made to evaluate a patient's "normal" ventilatory effectiveness, the blood sample is taken before supplemental oxygen therapy is started. The pO_2 may also be determined once a patient is receiving oxygen therapy to evaluate the effectiveness of the therapy so necessary adjustments can be made.

As expected, the *venous* pO_2 is normally quite a bit lower than the arterial pO_2 since much of the blood's oxygen has been given up to the cells. Factors affecting venous pO_2 are tissue perfusion adequacy, blood volume (a low blood volume will be apparent from a low central venous pressure) the effectiveness of gaseous exchange, and cardiac output.

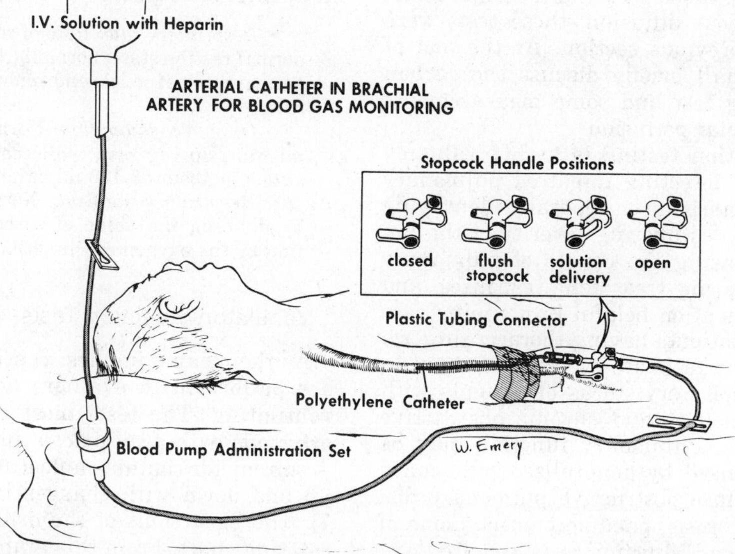

FIGURE 68-6. Catheter in place in brachial artery for blood gas monitoring. (From Kurihara, M.: *Nursing Clinics of North America* 3:65, March, 1968.)

For further discussions of the clinical significance of blood gas measurements and treatment of hydrogen ion imbalances (metabolic acidosis, metabolic alkalosis, respiratory acidosis, and respiratory alkalosis) see Chapter 24 and the article by Betson.[29]

Serum Electrolyte Analyses

Serum electrolyte analyses are frequently of importance in monitoring the fluid-electrolyte status of patients with respiratory disorders. Examples of two electrolyte imbalances that may be related to respiratory function are hyperpotassemia (potassium elevation) caused by chronic hypoventilation, and hyperchloremia (chloride elevation) caused by hyperventilation. (For further discussion of serum electrolytes and fluid-electrolyte imbalances see Chapters 24 and 25.)

PULMONARY FUNCTION TESTS

Basically the evaluation of pulmonary function involves two groups of measurements. The first group of tests evaluates the physical activities necessary to *mechanically ventilate* the lungs. These tests are sometimes said to be evaluations of the bellows actions of the lungs, i.e., the abilities of the chest wall, diaphragm, and lungs to move air in and out, and to *distribute* it to pulmonary alveoli. Tests belonging to this first group of measurements are called "ventilatory function tests" and they are discussed in this section.

The second group of pulmonary function tests are those that measure the effectiveness of *gaseous diffusion* across the alveolar capillary membrane and the effectiveness of *vascular perfusion* of the lungs by capillaries. Blood gas measurements assist in evaluating gaseous diffusion; these tests were discussed in the previous section. At the end of this section we shall briefly discuss the carbon monoxide diffusing test and some measurements of pulmonary vascular perfusion.

Pulmonary function testing is highly valuable in objectively: (1) detecting impaired pulmonary function, (2) characterizing or generally identifying the impairment, (3) estimating severity of the impairment, (4) following the course of pulmonary disease and evaluating treatment responses, and (5) providing information helpful in planning care and in caring for patients having thoracic surgery. Respiratory function tests are especially helpful in evaluating the respiratory status of patients with reduced lung capacities and chronic obstructive pulmonary disease. Pulmonary function may be seriously compromised by generalized pulmonary disorders, e.g., diffuse obstructive pulmonary disease, pulmonary fibrosis, pneumoconiosis. Some of the simpler pulmonary function tests are often employed for various screening purposes, e.g., periodic physical examinations, pre-employment health examinations, evaluating insurance and disability claims.

Some *limitations* of pulmonary function tests are:[87] (1) an etiologic or anatomic diagnosis is not directly given; (2) lesions are not precisely located; (3) a fairly large deviation from the predicted normal findings is necessary before the tests have meaning;(4) the tests lack the sensitivity necessary to identify early localized changes; and (5) misleading or useless test results can occur unless both the patient and the person performing the test give maximum cooperation and exertion.

The nurse participates in pulmonary function tests by helping to explain to the patient the general value of the tests, basically how the tests are performed, and what is expected of the patient during the tests. Patients with breathing difficulties are often apprehensive about having "breathing tests" performed. Many fear their air supply will be inadequate during the testing or that they will become too exhausted; others dread any anxiety-provoking situation, since anxiety usually increases their breathing difficulties. Pulmonary function tests may indeed be very tiring. Patients with breathing limitations often need planned rest periods during and after testing.

The nurse carries out any orders for physically preparing a patient for pulmonary function tests. Spirography (discussed below) generally requires no special preparation of the patient. During the test the patient is given necessary instructions, e.g., "take a deep breath," "exhale and try to push all the air out of your lungs," and so forth. If bronchospirometry is to be performed (see below), the patient is told that a flexible tube will be passed into his trachea ("windpipe") but that he will be able to breathe at all times through the tube. For bronchospirometry the nurse carries out pre- and postprocedure care similar to that previously discussed for bronchography. Pulmonary function tests are usually performed in a laboratory setting by a technician or physician.

The following information is of basic importance in understanding respiratory function:

> *Respiratory rate:* Rate of respirations during a normal resting state; normally 12 to 20 respirations per minute; exercise and emotions influence this rate.
>
> *Oxygen consumption:* Normally about 110-150 ml./min. during rest, while *carbon dioxide elimination* is about 88-120 ml./min.
>
> *Respiratory quotient:* Normally 0.8; obtained by dividing the value of carbon dioxide elimination by the oxygen consumption.

Ventilatory Function Tests

As their name implies, ventilatory function tests are performed to evaluate how well the lung is ventilating. The tests most commonly performed are made with a *spirometer* and a recording device. A spirometer contains a floating drum which moves up and down with changes in pressure (Fig. 68-7). The excursions of the drum are recorded on a rotating chart. From this graphic record it is possi

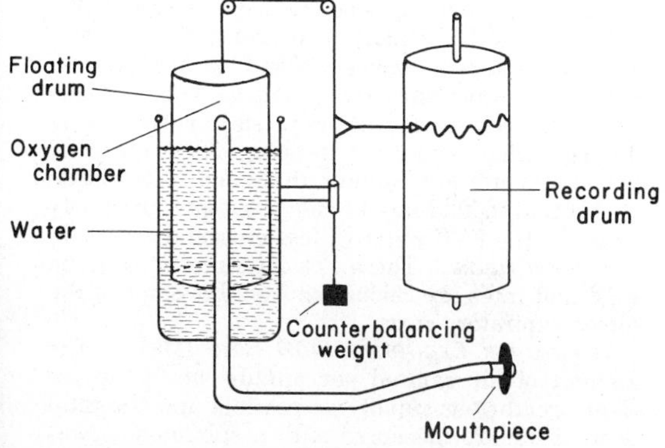

FIGURE 68–7. The spirometer. (From Guyton, A. C.: *Function of the Human Body.* 4th ed. 1974.)

ble to calculate the quantity of gas moved during each excursion of the drum.

Ventilation studies are performed with the patient breathing only through his mouth. To ensure mouth breathing a *nose clip* is often applied, and the patient is given time to adjust to the clip. A mouthpiece and connecting tube connect the patient's respiratory system and the spirometer.

No single factor adequately expresses pulmonary ventilation; rather a composite of values is necessary to give the full picture. The values most commonly measured in ventilatory function testing will be discussed below. Naturally the volumes of air inhaled and exhaled vary, depending upon such factors as weight, height, sex, age, activity, and the body's demands. Predicted normals for the various ventilation function tests are calculated for a given patient on the basis of the preceding factors. The examples of "normals" given in the following discussions are average for a normal young adult male (Fig. 68–8). Averages for the normal young adult female are often 20 to 25 per cent less than for a male.

> *Tidal volume* (VT or TV). Amount of air inspired or expired with each breath during quiet, normal breathing. This measurement is called "tidal" volume because it measures the flow of air coming in and out like the tides, i.e., the volume of air flowing in and out during one respiratory cycle. Sometimes VT is measured during exercise to evaluate dyspnea. (Exercise tests are discussed later.)

VT is normally about 500 ml. Of this, anatomic dead space gas (VD) equals about 150 ml. *Dead space air* refers to that air in the conducting airways from the nose and mouth down to the bronchioles. Air in the dead space does not exchange gases with the blood since it does not reach alveolar membranes. A dead space volume greater than one third of tidal volume indicates the need for an increase in total ventilation to prevent hypercarbia (alveolar hypoventilation).

> *Minute Respiratory Volume* (Vmin.). Also called *"minute ventilation,"* this is the total volume of air moved in or out of the lungs during one minute. The figure is obtained by multiplying the tidal volume (VT) by the respiratory rate per minute (f). Normal Vmin. = about 6000 to 7500 ml. A normal Vmin. may occur with emphysema, but a reduced Vmin. can occur with other pulmonary disorders. Minute ventilation can be subdivided into two divisions: (1) alveolar ventilation (about two thirds of the total air taken in one minute), and (2) dead space ventilation (about one third).

> *Inspiratory Reserve Volume* (IRV). Maximum amount of air that can be inspired from the end of a normal inspiration, i.e., the portion of the inspiratory capacity which is in excess of the tidal volume. Normal IRV = about 3000 ml.

> *Expiratory Reserve Volume* (ERV). Maximum amount of air that can forcibly be expired after a normal, quiet expiration. ERV is normally about 1000 ml.

> *Residual Volume* (RV). Amount of air remaining in the lung after maximum expiration. Also called *"residual air."* As long as the chest cavity remains closed the lung cannot be completely emptied of air. RV = about 1500 ml. RV and FRC (see below) are often measured simultaneously. The volume of residual air cannot be directly measured with a spirometer, but it can be measured by various other methods, e.g., having the patient inhale a gas such as helium and measuring its dilution in expired air, or by a "nitrogen washout" method, which measures the rapidity with which nitrogen in the lungs is washed out when a patient breathes 100 per cent oxygen. These measurements are possible because they are made on relatively insoluble gases which do not readily leave the alveolar gas to dissolve in lung tissue or the blood.

> *Total Lung Capacity* (TLC). Total amount of air in the lung after maximum inspiration. The TLC is the sum of all the primary lung volumes, i.e., residual volume (RV), inspiratory reserve volume (IRV), expiratory reserve volume (ERV), and tidal volume (VT). Thus, TLC = RV + IRV + ERV + VT. Another way of putting the same equation is TLC = RV + VC. The ratios between these usually are about as follows: the RV is 25 per cent of the TLC; the VC is 75 per cent of the TLC; normally the TLC is about 6 L. (i.e., 6000 ml.).

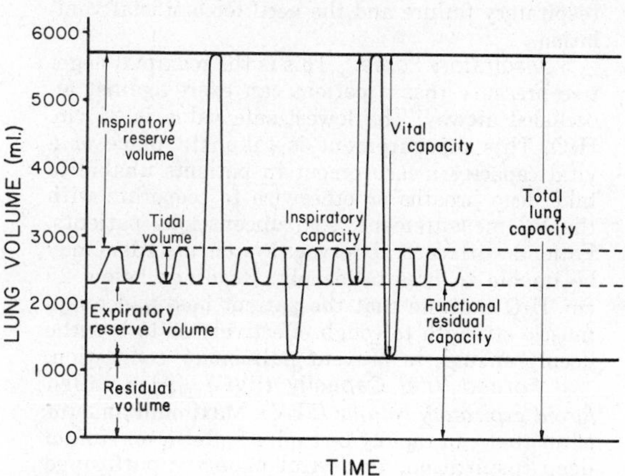

FIGURE 68–8. A spirogram, showing the divisions of the respiratory air. (From Guyton, A. C.: *Function of the Human Body.* 4th ed. 1974.)

This pulmonary function test, unlike others, is diagnostic of a specific disorder, i.e., emphysema. Emphysematous patients may have a TLC as high as 9 L. because of trapped air. TLC may be performed by either a gas dilution method or by using a body plethysmograph ("body box").

> *Vital Capacity* (VC). Maximum amount of air that can be completely expired following a maximum capacity, deep inspiration without forced or rapid effort. Simply stated, the VC measures a person's ability to take a deep breath. The VC is the largest volume measured. This measurement of total lung volume is normally about 4000 to 5000 ml. Results less than 3000 ml. indicate some respiratory insufficiency.

The VC is the sum of the tidal volume (V_T), the inspiratory reserve volume (IRV) and the expiratory reserve volume (ERV). Thus, $VC = V_T + IRV + ERV$. The VC and its subdivisions (V_T, IRV, ERV) are directly measured with simple volume recorders, e.g., spirometers.

Once the VC was the only breathing test. Today it is realized that the VC is of limited value by itself because of the wide range of individual variations which are "normal."

The VC can identify restricted lung volume. Usually the VC measurement relates closely to the MBC (see below). The VC can be affected by both pulmonary and nonpulmonary conditions. Almost all *pulmonary* disorders may reduce the VC, e.g., asthma, pulmonary fibrosis, bronchogenic tumor (and other space-filling disorders), tuberculosis, emphysema, pneumonia, airway obstruction, bronchiectasis, surgical pulmonary excision, pleural adhesion, and thoracic pain. *Nonpulmonary* conditions that reduce VC include: obesity, abdominal masses, neuromuscular disorders, ascites, depression of respiratory centers, and postoperative pain following abdominal surgery. These conditions all limit thoracic expansion or restrict breathing.

If a patient's VC is below 1000 ml. he needs encouragement to cough and deep breathe. An extremely low VC (e.g., below 700 ml.) indicates increased tissue resistance or decreased muscle strength. Typically the condition progresses to respiratory failure and the need for artificial venilation.

> *Inspiratory Force.* This is the maximal negative pressure that a patient can exert against an occluded airway. The lowest safe value is 25 cm. H_2O. This measurement is taken in place of a vital capacity measurement in patients unable to take deep breaths or otherwise to cooperate with the VC measurement, e.g., unconscious patients. Patients with central nervous system disorders may be unable to breathe deeply. Readings below 25 cm. H_2O indicate that the patient has inadequate muscle strength to cough effectively or to breathe deeply enough to prevent pulmonary congestion.

> *Forced Vital Capacity* (FVC). Also called *forced expiratory volume* (FEV). Maximum amount of air that can rapidly be expired after a maximum deep inspiration, i.e., vital capacity performed with expiration as forceful and rapid as possible. Three separate exhalations are measured, and the highest volume is recorded as the FVC. The recording is given in liters per second or as a FVC:VC ratio. This test is important in evaluating the mechanical factors in expiration and can indicate expiratory airway obstructive problems. The measurement may be significantly reduced in chronic lung diseases which cause air trapping. Although FVC measurements give almost the same information as MBC (the findings of the two tests are fairly similar), the FVC requires less muscular strength.

> *Flow Rates.* These are determined after the FEV and rates are calculated from the slope of the forced expiratory curve.

> *Maximal Expiratory Flow Rate* (MEF). The amount of air expired per minute while the patient breathes as rapidly as possible and the total expired air are measured with a spirometer. Normally MEF = about 400 L./min. MEF, like the timed vital capacity, indicates airway patency. MEF is reduced in pulmonary disorders associated with air trapping, e.g., emphysema.

> *Maximal Midexpiratory Flow Rate* (MMF). Also called *forced midexpiratory flow rate* (FEF 25 to 75 per cent), this is the rate of flow of air expelled during the middle portion of forced expiration. The mean rate of flow and the time required for expiration of the middle 50 per cent or middle two quarters of the total volume of expired air are measured by spirography. This flow rate has a very wide normal range and is reported as liters per second or liters per minute. A normal MMF is about 4.5 L./sec., with a range of 148-414 L./min.

Measuring the middle portion of the expiration excludes: (1) the early period of expiration (when airway obstructive diseases least affect breathing); and (2) the final period of expiration (when flow rate is greatly reduced even in normal subjects). MMF is the most useful indicator of expiratory airway obstruction (more so than FEV) and is also used to evaluate bronchodilator drug actions.

> *Maximal Inspiratory Flow Rate* (MIF). This is the amount of air inspired per minute while the patient breathes as rapidly as possible. MIF = 300 L./min.

> *Timed Vital Capacity* (TVC). Also called *timed forced expiratory volume* (FEV_T), this is the percentage of the vital capacity that can be expired in 1, 2, and 3 seconds. The subscript T indicates the time in seconds. For example, the measurement at one second would be indicated by $FEV_{1.0}$. Following maximum inspiration the patient is asked to expire the inhaled air as rapidly as possible into a spirometer. Normally about 81 to 83 per cent is expired in one second, 90 to 94 per cent in two seconds, and 95 to 97 per cent in three seconds. The measurement at one second is the most useful. Normally the total VC should be expired within six seconds.

The value of the VC measurement is greatly increased by timing the length of expiration, as is done in this test. The TVC is a highly useful test of pulmonary function. Patients with emphysema may have a normal untimed VC but an abnormal TVC. Values below the predicted normal indicate the severity of the expiratory airway obstruction. Increased airway resistance may cause some patients with chronic obstructive pulmonary diseases to take up to 10 to 12 seconds to exhale the VC volume.

> *Inspiratory Capacity* (IC). This is the maximum amount of air that can be inspired in one deep breath after a normal inspiration. $IC = V_T + IRV$. Normally IC = about 3500 ml.

> *Functional Residual Capacity* (FRC). This is the amount of air left in the lungs after a normal

resting expiration. FRC = ERV + RV. Usually the RV and FRC are measured simultaneously.

> *Maximum Breathing Capacity* (MBC). Also called *maximal voluntary ventilation* (MVV), this is the maximal amount of air that can be breathed in and out in one minute with maximal rates and depths of respiration. MBC is the best overall measurement of ventilation ability and can provide more accurate information about pulmonary function than any other single test. This test is a measure of pulmonary airway resistance and usually correlates well with complaints of dyspnea.

In some pulmonary disorders the vital capacity may be normal but the MBC is greatly reduced. MBC is lowered by reduced lung compliance and chronic obstructive lung disease.

MBC is calculated by having the patient breathe as deeply and rapidly as he can for 15 seconds. Typically the rate of breathing during this period varies from 50 to 70 per minute. The expired air is collected, the expiratory volume is measured, and a minute volume is figured by multiplying the volume of expired air collected (for the 15 seconds) by four. Normal MBC = about 125-150 L./min. As would be expected, this test is very fatiguing to perform, particularly for persons with respiratory impairment.

Patients may be ordered to be prepared for an MBC measurement as they are for a basal metabolic rate test. (See discussion of basal metabolic rate in Unit XIX.)

Exercise Tests. Some ventilation tests are done with the patient exercising as directed. During exercise, arterial blood specimens are taken for analysis of blood gases, and pulmonary function tests are performed. *Exercise tolerance tests* evaluate the amount of exercise a subject can experience before he becomes dyspneic. Patients with very low respiratory reserves may become dyspneic after walking only a few steps; some are dyspneic even at rest. Exercise tolerance may be tested by simply having the subject walk down a hallway and up and down a flight of stairs. It may more accurately be measured by having the patient pedal a stationary bicycle, walk a treadmill, or step up and down on a single stair step in the laboratory.

Bronchospirometry. In this procedure a special, flexible double-lumen rubber catheter with two balloons is passed into the anesthetized trachea. Under fluoroscopic monitoring the catheter is inserted into the left mainstem bronchus. The balloon around that portion of the catheter is then snugly inflated, so that air enters the left lung only through one lumen of the catheter. The other lumen opens into the trachea. Inflation of the balloon in the trachea seals the trachea off in such a manner that air from the right lung must pass through the catheter. Each of the two catheter openings is connected to a separate spirometer, so the air from each lung is measured separately. The two spirometers record on the same kymograph.

Bronchospirometric measurements are usually taken during both quiet breathing and hyperventilation; thus, it is possible to detect any air trapping resulting from partial bronchial obstruction. Bronchospirometry can determine the percentage of the total ventilation and oxygen absorption carried out by each lung. The left lung, which is smaller, normally contributes about 45 per cent of the total pulmonary ventilation and respiration function; the right lung contributes the remaining 55 per cent of ventilation and oxygen consumption.

The special techniques of *segmental bronchospirometry* enable catheterization of individual lung segments. Thus, the ventilation of these segments is individually studied and, when combined with gas analysis, provides additional information concerning the oxygen absorption and carbon dioxide excretion in the segment being evaluated.

Bronchospirometry is especially important preoperatively if a lung or portion of lung is to be removed. With this technique it is possible to determine if the patient would have adequate ventilatory and respiratory abilities if a lung or portion of lung were surgically removed. If a patient's respiratory reserve is borderline, the impact of possible surgery can be evaluated preoperatively, thereby preventing resection of more lung tissue than the patient could tolerate.

The pre- and postprocedure care of patients having bronchospirometry is similar to that discussed previously for bronchoscopy. Remember specifically to watch for cocaine reactions following the procedure and to give the patient nothing orally until his gag reflex returns. Discourage the patient from smoking prior to the procedure. *Contraindications* to performing bronchospirometry include the presence of bronchial lesions, recent hemoptysis, and recurrent colds or pneumonia.

Recently a new method of performing bronchospirometry during diagnostic bronchoscopy has been introduced. In this new procedure it is not necessary to insert a double-lumen endotracheal catheter, and the expired gas can be selectively collected from each lung through a special bronchoscope used during diagnostic bronchoscopy performed under topical anesthesia. The bronchoscope is fitted with an inflatable cuff. Once it is correctly positioned in the right or left mainstem bronchus (with the cuff inflated) a seal is obtained which enables measurement of air from one lung at a time.[262]

Radioactive Gas Function Tests. Significant advances in the study of regional pulmonary function have been made possible by the use of radioactive isotopes, multiple fixed or moving detectors, and scintillation cameras. For example, various aspects of pulmonary function can be evaluated by having a subject inhale a small amount of a relatively insoluble radioactive gas, e.g., xenon (Xe)-133. Radiation counters positioned over various portions of the chest can evaluate specific locations of uneven pulmonary ventilation; a high level of radioactivity occurs in well ventilated regions of the lung, while poorly ventilated regions are identified by a low level of radioactivity.

Aerosol inhalation scans are sensitive indicators of airway obstruction which can help to distinguish emphysematous, bronchitic, and mixed types of obstructive airway disease. These inhalation scans are useful counterparts to perfusion scans (discussed below). Aerosol inhalation scans also can help to evaluate response to treatment.[137]

Use of a scintillation camera and xenon-133 permits visualization of slowly ventilated spaces. The photographs (called "scintiphotographs") are examined for irregularities in distribution and clearance of radioactivity. (See also earlier discussion of lung scintigraphy.)

Tests of Pulmonary Circulation

Radioactive Gas Perfusion Tests. The use of radioactive gases has made possible evaluation of not only regional pulmonary function but also the regional distribution of blood flow, i.e., regional pulmonary perfusion. Capillary blood flow in the lungs can be measured by giving a radioactive tracer, e.g., xenon-133, intravenously. The xenon comes out of solution as it courses through the pulmonary capillaries, and it enters the alveolar gas. Radiation detectors then demonstrate a high concentration of xenon in areas well perfused with blood (i.e., those with good capillary blood flow); low concentrations of xenon occur in poorly perfused areas of the lung.

A *lung scan* may be useful in evaluating pulmonary perfusion when space-occupying disorders or pulmonary infarction are suspected (these conditions reduce perfusion). A lung scan is performed by intravenously injecting iodinated (^{131}I) serum albumin aggregated or technetium (^{99}mTc) serum albumin aggregated. These aggregates lodge in the pulmonary capillaries when injected, and scanning of the lung then permits detection and mapping of areas of impaired perfusion. The clumps of albumin collect in regions of the lung which have good blood flow and these areas thus show a high level of radioactivity. The clumps are not able to enter vessels obstructed by disease processes; thus, poorly perfused areas have a low level of radioactivity.

Plethysmography Perfusion Tests. Blood flow in the pulmonary capillaries can also be measured with a body plethysmograph, an airtight chamber large enough to hold a human subject. For this type of plethysmography the patient inhales a single breath of a mixture of oxygen and nitrous oxide while he is within the "body box". He then holds his breath for a few seconds. The flow of blood through the pulmonary capillaries is evaluated by studying the solubility of nitrous oxide in the blood. Excessive resistance to blood flow through the pulmonary capillaries thus may be identified.

Cardiac Catheterization. Cardiac catheterization is another important means of studying pulmonary circulation. During catheterization the pulmonary blood flow, pulmonary arterial pressure, and pulmonary end-capillary pressure may be determined. Evaluation may be made of changes that occur during exercise. Blood gas analyses may also be made of blood samples obtained during catheterization. (Cardiac catheterization is discussed in Unit X.)

Other Evaluations of Cardiopulmonary Circulation. Developing cardiopulmonary complications in critically ill patients may be detected by evaluating the *central venous pressure* (CVP) and by *pulmonary artery catheterization.* The CVP provides information about the filling pressure of the right ventricle and is useful in diagnosing right ventricular failure. (CVP is discussed in Unit X.) Pulmonary artery catheterization measures left-sided heart pressure and is valuable in diagnosing left ventricular failure, pulmonary edema, and pulmonary hypertension, all of which may develop without right ventricular failure. For details about pulmonary artery catheterization and significant findings consult Gernert and Schwartz's article, "Pulmonary Artery Catheterization."[101]

Carbon Monoxide Diffusion Tests

Three methods may be used to evaluate the diffusing capacity of the lungs (DL), i.e., the rate of gas exchange across the alveolar membrane. These three methods are the single-breath method, the rebreathing technique, and the steady-state technique. All three methods use carbon monoxide (CO) to measure the DL, because the blood's hemoglobin has a special affinity for CO such that CO combines with the hemoglobin more rapidly than does oxygen, and CO can be easily measured.

The *single-breath* CO test is performed by: (1) having the patient inhale a very low concentration of CO; (2) having him hold his breath for 10 seconds before exhaling; and (3) calculating the CO rate of diffusion by determining the difference between the CO concentration in the inspired air and that in the expired air. Normally the CO rate of diffusion is 25 ml./min./mm. Hg. Normally the rate at which CO disappears from the alveolar gas is directly proportional to its rate of diffusion.

The *rebreathing* CO test is performed by having the patient *rapidly* rebreathe for about 90 seconds from a bag containing a low concentration of CO and air. The diffusing capacity is then calculated.

The *steady-state* CO test is performed by having the patient breathe (at a normal rate) about 12 to 14 breaths of a mixture of air and a low concentration of CO. An arterial blood sample is then taken and a pCO_2 is obtained. From this the mean alveolar pCO is calculated. Normally the CO rate of diffusion with this test is 17 ml./min./mm. Hg.

Slow diffusion rates may result from the presence of abnormal fluids or thick, fibrosed alveolar membranes.

BASAL METABOLIC RATE

The basal metabolic rate (BMR) is the rate at which oxygen is taken in and utilized by the body's tissues while the subject is in a fasting state at complete rest. The rate is expressed as a percentage of a value established as normal for such a subject. The percentage indicates how far the rate varies above (plus) or below (minus) the average. The BMR is decreased in disorders which deprive tissues of substances regulating the rate of metabolism or which prevent adequate supplies of oxygen- or calorie-containing compounds. (BMR is discussed more completely in Unit XIX.)

AUSCULTATION

Auscultation is highly important in evaluating a patient's pulmonary status. Although the stethoscope was originally used only by physicians to listen to a patient's heart and lungs, today it is also widely used by nurses. By carefully auscultating patients' lungs, nurses may detect evidence of pneumonitis, congestive heart failure, or secretion accumulations. When a stethoscope is not available, abnormal respiratory sounds may be detected by listening with the ear against the patient's chest.

Pulmonary auscultation is best performed if the patient is encouraged to open his mouth and breathe deeply through it while the examiner listens to breath sounds by placing the stethoscope on various sections of the patient's back (Fig. 68–9). Pulmonary sounds (normal and abnormal) are most often relatively high pitched and easily auscultated. A few are very low pitched, however, and can be felt easier than they are heard. The examiner may thus gently place the palms of her hands against the patient's chest wall in an attempt to pick up the vibrations of these low-pitched sounds.

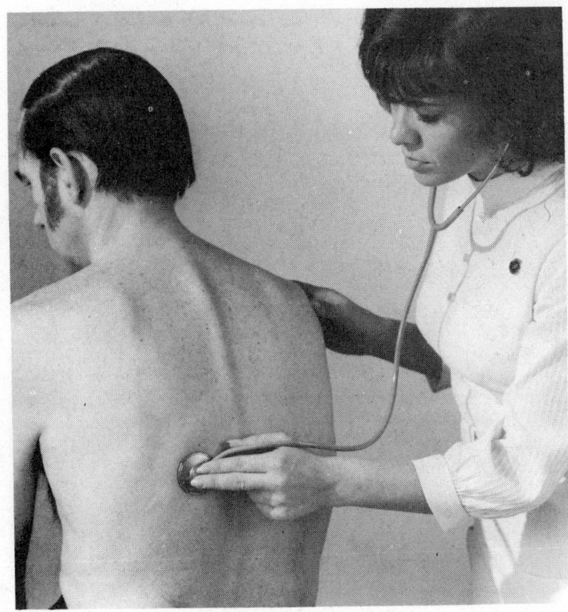

FIGURE 68–9. Auscultation. (From Littmann, D.: *American Journal of Nursing* 72:1238, July, 1972.)

Respiratory sounds are normally soft noises of a rustling or sighing nature, and are caused by air passing over the vocal cords. The sounds are modified by movement through the successively smaller and more numerous passages within the tracheobronchial tree. Pulmonary disorders may alter the pitch and other characteristics of breath sounds. Abnormal pulmonary sounds include noises described as groans, bubbles, squeaks, wheezes, and whistles. Abnormal respiratory sounds, e.g., bubbling sounds, most often result from secretions accumulated within the alveoli and air passages.

Bronchial asthma is characterized by squeaking noises resulting from spasm and narrowing of bronchioles. Pneumonitis and the pulmonary edema of congestive heart failure are characterized by *rales,* i.e., "fine, gentle, clicking sounds,"[172] produced by air moving through mucus in the alveoli. Rales have been described as being "much like the sounds generated by rolling a few strands of hair between the fingers just over or in front of the ear."[172] Other terms used to describe such sounds are *crepitation* or "crepitant rales." *Ronchi* are loud rales which result from air passing through mucus in the bronchial tubes. *Stridor* is a high-pitched, harsh, crowinglike sound that occurs from breathing air through a constricted trachea or larynx, e.g., in acute laryngeal obstruction. With experience in auscultation a *pleural rub* or *friction rub* may be heard upon inspiration when a rough, inflamed pleural surface rubs against the other pleural surface. (See discussion of pleurisy, p. 937.)

INSPECTION, PERCUSSION, AND PALPATION

In addition to auscultation, the chest may also be examined by inspection, percussion, and palpation. *Inspection* of the chest may reveal changes in its contour or mobility, e.g., both sides of the chest may not rise and fall evenly during inspiration and expiration. Intercostal ballooning or retraction in the intercostal spaces occurs when a patient has tremendous difficulty in ventilating his lungs and must exert extreme effort when trying to move air in and out of the lungs. Reduced chest wall movement on the affected side occurs with pneumothorax, atelectasis, and extensive parenchymal obstruction. Obviously if the nurse is going to properly inspect a patient's chest movements, she must lower his gown and compare both sides of the chest. In addition to the preceding observations, the rate and rhythm of ventilation are evaluated by inspection.

Percussion, (i.e., striking an area with short, sharp blows as an aid to diagnosing the condition of the parts beneath the blow by the sound ob-

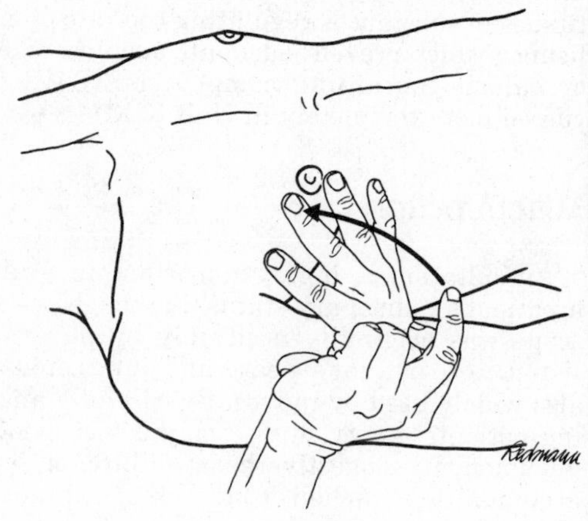

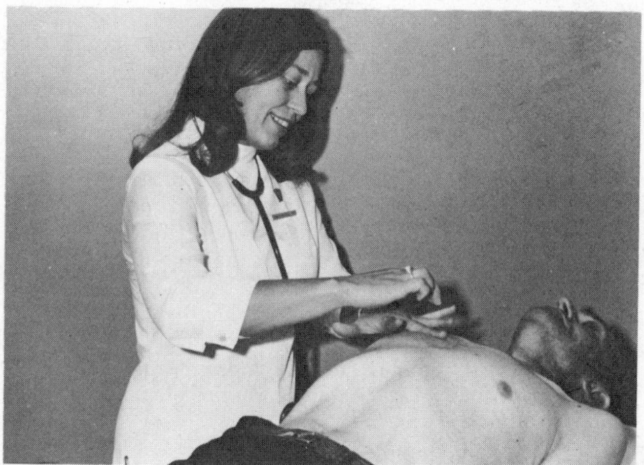

FIGURE 68–10. Percussion of the lungs. (From Traver, G. A.: American Journal of Nursing *73*:466, March, 1973.)

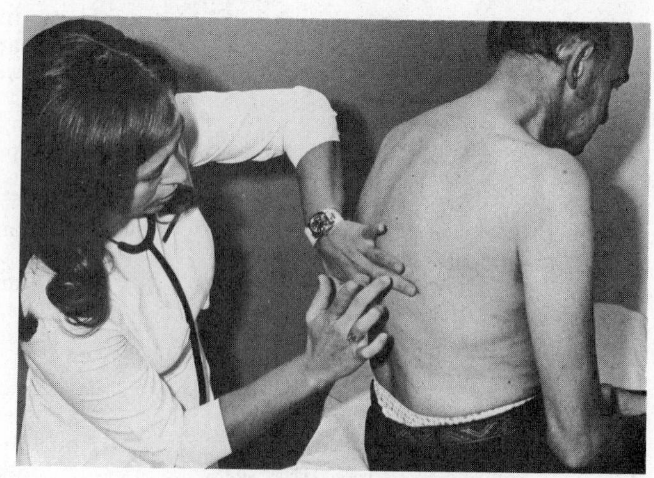

tained) may demonstrate changes in density in the lungs which are of significance (Fig. 68–10). Percussion over "normal" lung tissue produces resonance, i.e., intensification and prolongation of sound caused by the transmission of the sound vibrations to a cavity. When the density of lung tissue is increased, e.g., by the presence of fluid, percussion elicits dullness.

Palpation is the least useful method of physical examination of the chest. Palpation may detect *changes in muscle tone* and *fremitus,* i.e., a vibration or thrill perceptible upon palpation. A ronchal (or bronchial) fremitus is produced by air moving through a large, mucus-filled bronchus. A friction fremitus occurs when two dry surfaces rub together. Pleural fremitus is specifically a vibration of the thoracic wall felt when the pleural surfaces rub together, causing friction. Palpation may also be used to delineate areas of thoracic pain or masses.

Respiratory disorders may produce a variety of changes from normal functioning which may be detected by auscultation, inspection, percussion, and palpation. Many of these alterations are discussed throughout the unit. (See also article by Traver.[301])

SKIN TESTS

Skin tests performed in diagnosing and evaluating respiratory disorders include: tests to determine sources of hypersensitive (allergic) reactions, the Schick test to determine susceptibility to diphtheria, tuberculin tests to identify tuberculosis infection, and tests with other antigens to help in the differential diagnosis of fungus or nontuberculous mycobacterial infections.

Skin Tests for Allergies

Inhalant allergens (e.g., plant pollens and dusts) may cause seasonal hay fever, seasonal asthma, and allergic rhinitis. Skin tests may be performed to identify a patient's specific allergens. The patient may then be slowly hypersensitized against that particular allergen. (See Chapter 23.)

Schick Test

The Schick test is a measure of immunity to diphtheria. The test is performed by intracutaneously injecting a quantity of diphtheria toxin diluted in salt solution equal to one fiftieth of the minimal lethal dose. One thirtieth of a unit of antitoxin per cubic centimeter of blood is adequate to neutralize the toxin. If the subject receives less than this amount of antitoxin, the toxin is not neutralized and an area of inflammation appears at the site of the skin injection. Thus, lack of immunity to diphtheria is indicated by redness and edema at the injection site five to seven days following the injection.

Tuberculin Skin Tests

Tuberculin skin tests are used for diagnosis and case-finding for tuberculosis. (Tuberculosis is discussed in Chapter 71.) These skin tests identify persons who require further diagnostic investigation, i.e., positive tuberculin reactors who show sensitivity to tuberculin. Tuberculin skin tests are based on the fact that infection with *Mycobacterium tuberculosis* produces a specific sensitivity to certain chemical products of the organisms which are contained in culture extracts. These extracts are called *tuberculins.*

A *tuberculin reaction* is a delayed, acute, local, specific inflammation resulting from the injection of specified amounts of tuberculin. The intradermal injection of tuberculin in sensitized persons produces an area of *induration* (i.e., an abnormally hard place) 48 to 72 hours later which varies in size and intensity according to the individual's sensitivity and the amount of tuberculin injected. The degree of sensitivity is then determined by measuring the reaction. Let us emphasize that erythema (i.e., redness) may or may not surround the area of induration. Erythema without induration is without significance. (Reading or interpreting the tests is discussed later.)

A positive tuberculin reaction indicates that the individual being tested has, at some time during his life, been infected somewhere in his body by tubercle bacilli. The infection may have been minor and may no longer be active. A positive reaction does *not* provide definite proof of an infection and does *not* indicate whether the individual's infection is currently active or inactive. Further diagnostic tests are necessary to obtain this information. Note that a positive tuberculin skin test does *not* mean the subject was merely exposed to someone with active tuberculosis; it means that somewhere within his body the subject has a healed or active site of tuberculous infection.

Tuberculin tests are routinely given to children, young adults, persons known to have been exposed to tuberculosis, and persons with radiographic findings suggestive of tuberculosis (especially if sputum examinations are negative). The value of the tuberculin test as a screening procedure is increasing as the prevalence of tuberculosis in the population decreases; it is particularly valuable in identifying persons who require chemoprophylaxis.

Tuberculin converters are tuberculin reactors who are known to have been nonreactors within the previous 12 months (Chap. 71); those persons who do not have clinically detectable progressive disease are often given isoniazid prophylactically. Persons with positive tuberculin reactions who are proved to have clinically active tuberculosis by further diagnostic studies are given appropriate treatment.

With few exceptions, once acquired, definite sensitivity to tuberculin persists throughout life. The sensitivity may vary in intensity and temporarily may decrease or disappear in the course of certain severe illnesses. It may also decrease or disappear if chemoprophylactic treatment is given in the earliest stages of infection. Also, the skin reaction to tuberculosis is frequently abolished or reduced in intensity during the administration of corticosteroid drugs. A very small number of persons occasionally fail to react to tuberculin even after a natural infection or after administration of vaccine prepared from living or dead tubercle bacilli. Tuberculin sensitivity may also decrease in old age.

Although no direct or proportional relationship exists between the level of hypersensitivity to tuberculin and the extent or severity of the tuberculosis infection, the intensity of the tuberculin reaction is at times significant. For example, it appears that the greater the size of the tuberculin reaction, the greater the possibility that active disease exists or will appear in the subject and his close contacts. Generally, relatively high levels of sensitivity are found in persons with recently acquired infection, in those with caseous, nonpulmonary tuberculosis, and in persons in continuous contact with individuals with active tuberculosis but who are not themselves infected.

Test Procedures. Two kinds of tuberculin are currently widely used for tuberculin skin testing: *old tuberculin* (OT), which is obtained from heat-sterilized cultures of tubercle bacilli; and *purified protein derivative* (PPD), which consists of the protein of dead tubercle bacilli obtained from filtrates of autoclaved cultures of tubercle bacilli that have been grown on synthetic medium. *PPD is the preferred tuberculin preparation* because its strength is standardized and tests with the same dose are comparable. PPD and OT dilutions (in buffered diluents) can retain their potency for as long as six months if protected from contamination and kept refrigerated. Dilutions in physiologic saline should not be used after one week.

Contraindications to tuberculin testing include any rash, allergic dermatitis, scabies or current reactions to smallpox vaccinations. The nurse checks for these contraindications prior to administering a tuberculin skin test.

Before discussing specific techniques of tuberculin testing, consider the following points of importance in any skin testing procedure.

> Before giving the test, briefly explain the test procedure and its significance to the patient. Explain that a positive reaction does not mean active tuberculosis. Your explanation before the test may reduce a patient's anxiety if he develops a positive reaction.

> Keep tuberculin testing equipment separate from that used for any other injection. Tuberculin and other antigens (e.g., blastomycin, coccidioidin, and histoplasmin) are difficult to remove from glassware and other materials. Thus, bottles, syringes, needles, jet guns, and other equipment used for one antigen should not subsequently be used for another.

> Record any tuberculin test given. State the date the test was given; the type of test used; the type and dose of tuberculin administered; the date the test was read; and factual comments about any reactions to the test, e.g., millimeters of induration.

A *variety of techniques* are available for administering the tuberculin test. These include: the intracutaneous or intradermal (Mantoux) test, jet gun injection, multiple-puncture tests (e.g., Heaf, Sterneedle, Mono-Vacc, or tine), von Pirquet scratch test, and Vollmer patch test. Of all these techniques, *the method of choice for administering tuberculin is the Mantoux test* because it introduces a measured amount of tuberculin into the skin and produces the most consistent and reliable results. Jet injection and multiple-puncture techniques may be used for survey and screening purposes. Often a Mantoux test is subsequently per-

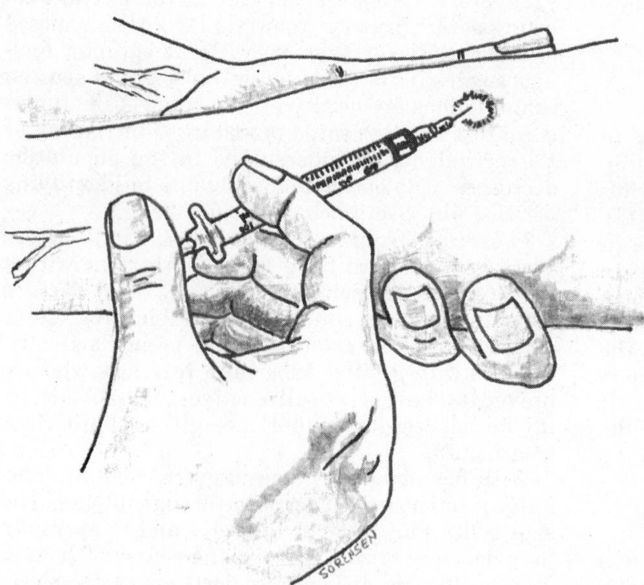

FIGURE 68–11. Mantoux tuberculin skin test. Note: skin is tightly stretched for the injection.

formed on persons who have reactions to these screening tests. The von Pirquet and Vollmer tests are not recommended because of relative unreliability.

Intradermal (Mantoux) Tuberculin Test. This test is routinely performed for differential diagnosis and survey by the intradermal injection of 5 tuberculin units (TU) of intermediate strength PPD (0.001 mg.). The injection is given into the upper third of the inner surface of the left forearm after the skin is cleansed with an alcohol sponge. When possible a disposable tuberculin syringe with an attached 26-gauge, ½-inch beveled needle is used. If a nondisposable tuberculin syringe is used, a very sharply beveled steel or platinum (25- or 26-gauge) needle is used. The needle bevel is held upward and the needle tip is inserted between the layers of the skin.

When the 0.1 ml. of PPD is properly injected into the skin a discrete, pale elevation of the skin resembling a mosquito bite is produced (Fig. 68–11). If this wheal is less than 6 mm. in diameter the injection is repeated, with another syringe, about an inch diagonally below the first. Skillful administration is necessary, so that the test material is injected intradermally rather than subcutaneously or outside the skin. A dressing is not applied over the injection site.

The Mantoux test is read 48 to 72 hours after the injection. The reading is made in good light, with the subject's forearm slightly flexed. The injection site is inspected visually and palpated. The site is observed from the side against the light as well as by direct light. Palpation is performed by gently stroking the area with the fingers. *A Mantoux skin test can be properly read only if the area is palpated;* merely looking at the puncture site is not sufficient. The diameter of the area of induration is measured transversely to the long axis of the forearm and is precisely recorded in millimeters. Erythema is also measured if present; however, as mentioned earlier, erythema without induration is insignificant. In some severe reactions necrosis may occur at the injection site; its presence is recorded.

An area of induration of 10 mm. or more is considered a *positive reaction.* Induration from 5 to 9 mm. in diameter is classified as a *doubtful reaction.* (Sometimes such a reaction indicates infection with unclassified atypical mycobacteria rather than the true tubercle bacilli.) Persons with doubtful reactions are routinely given further diagnostic tests. Induration of 4 mm. or less is considered to be a *negative* reaction.

Jet Injection Tuberculin Test. A jet gun delivers 5 TU of PPD intradermally under high pressure. As with the Mantoux test, the wheal produced should be 6 to 10 mm. in diameter. If it is less than 6 mm. the injection is repeated at another site. This test is read, recorded, and interpreted in the same manner as that discussed above for the Mantoux.

Multiple-puncture Tuberculin Tests. There are several different types of applicators for multiple puncture tests. All such tests are less accurate than the Mantoux because unknown amounts of tuberculin are administered and the reactions are less precisely defined and more difficult to measure. The tests are most often used for testing large groups of subjects. Multiple-puncture tuberculin tests puncture the skin either by pressing into the skin an applicator which has points on which tuberculin is dried (e.g., the tine test); or by puncturing the skin through a film of liquid tuberculin (e.g., the Sterneedle test). These techniques may introduce more than 5 TU of tuberculin because they all use concentrated tuberculin.

The time intervals between injection and reading vary with multiple-puncture tests according to the type of test given. Manufacturer's instructions must be followed carefully. Less skill is necessary to administer multiple-puncture tuberculin tests than to administer the Mantoux test; however, the subject's skin must be prepared and the test given and interpreted strictly.

Reactions to multiple-puncture tests may be in the form of discrete, separate papules at various puncture points, or coalescent reactions may occur in which several papules fuse together to form one larger reaction. The diameter of the largest single papule or the largest single coalescent reaction is measured as described for the Mantoux test.

Details of administering and reading multiple-puncture tuberculin tests can be obtained from the manufacturers of these products or from the American Lung Association. (Contact your local branch or write A.L.A., 1740 Broadway, New York, N.Y. 10019.)

Skin Tests with Other Antigens

Respiratory disorders caused by certain pathogenic fungi are sometimes diagnosed by skin tests. Three *fungal antigens* are currently commercially available for skin testing: coccidioidin, histoplasmin, and blastomycin. Reactions to these fungal antigens do not prove active disease, but rather suggest a possible diagnosis. Cross-reactions occur between fungal antigens.

CHAPTER 69

Common Nonspecific Manifestations of Respiratory Disorders

In order to properly assess a patient and give appropriate care the nurse must be familiar with some of the more common nonspecific indications of respiratory disorders. In Chapter 68 we discussed tests and activities used in the detection and evaluation of certain manifestations of respiratory disorders. We shall now consider a number of additional indications of respiratory disorders.

CONSTITUTIONAL SYMPTOMS

Among a variety of constitutional symptoms that respiratory disorders may produce are those indicative of: (1) *general debilitation,* e.g., anorexia, weight loss, fatigue, weakness, apathy, irritability; (2) *infection,* e.g., increased pulse rate, elevated temperature; and (3) *trauma,* e.g., symptoms of shock such as weak rapid pulse, drop in blood pressure.

ABNORMAL PATTERNS OF BREATHING

Breathing, or respiration, is difficult to evaluate because it can be voluntarily altered and is subject to emotional influences. In spite of this fact, much can be learned about the body's internal environment and respiratory disorders by assessing the nature of a patient's breathing.

The nurse strives to accurately observe, describe, and report abnormalities of breathing. This can be difficult since medical terminology is often inconsistent and many terms are not defined precisely or are used carelessly. Greater attempts must be made by all paramedical personnel to standardize definitions and to carefully describe the distinguishing characteristics of various patterns of breathing. If the nurse is uncertain about which terms to use, she should simply describe her observations in general terms, e.g., "The patient is breathing slowly and deeply." This is better than using inaccurate terminology.

The Terminology of Respiration

A variety of terms are used to describe breathing. Some of the commonest terms are clarified below (listed alphabetically):

Abdominal respirations: Breathing accomplished mostly by the abdominal muscles and diaphragm. Abdominal breathing can be highly effective. Often patients are taught abdominal breathing to increase the effectiveness of their ventilatory process, e.g., patients with diffuse obstructive lung disorders or following chest surgery.

Apnea: Temporary cessation of breathing.

Biot's respirations: A type of periodic breathing in which periods of tachypnea, and usually hypopnea, alternate abruptly with apnea. The irregular periods of apnea alternate with periods in which four or five breaths of uniform depth are taken. The duration of the periods is more variable than that in Cheyne-Stokes breathing, and Biot's breathing is viewed as an "irregular irregularity." It may occur with increased intracranial pressure, head injury, meningitis, encephalitis, brain abscess, and heat stroke.

Bradypnea: Slow breathing (less than 10 cycles/min.) with no significant changes in depth. Frequently occurs with increased intracranial pressure and following administration of depressing amounts of narcotics and sedatives.

Cheyne-Stokes respirations: The best known type of periodic breathing, characterized by rhythmic waxing and waning of the depth of respirations, with regularly recurring episodes of apnea or marked oligopnea. The periodicity of this type of breathing is fairly regular. A series of ventilations gradually increase in tidal volume and rate, then gradually decrease until they lapse into another apneic period. Cheyne-Stokes breathing occurs typically in severe heart failure, uremia, and coma caused by neurologic disorders.

Diaphragmatic respirations: Performed mainly by the diaphragm.

Dyspnea: Difficult, labored, or painful breathing. While dyspnea may be "normal" at times (e.g., as a result of extreme physical exertion), it may also be symptomatic of numerous disorders that interfere with adequate ventilation or perfusion of the blood with oxygen. The dyspneic patient is subjectively aware of his breathing difficulty and experiences such feelings as being smothered or unable to breathe.

Eupnea: "Normal," easy, quiet breathing. The normal adult respiratory rate is between 10 and 24 cycles/min.

Gasping: Rhythmic or irregular spasmodic inspiratory effort which is typically brief and maximal and terminates abruptly.

Hyperpnea: Abnormally deep breathing, i.e., an increase in tidal volume. Although rate may be increased to some degree, increased depth of breathing is the main abnormality. Occurs, for example, in well-conditioned athletes following strenuous exercise.

Hyperventilation: Increased minute ventilation. Abnormally rapid, deep, and prolonged breathing, e.g., caused by central nervous system disorders, drugs which increase sensitivity of respiratory centers, or acute anxiety. Often produces respiratory alkalosis; increased amounts of air enter the lungs, causing a reduction in CO_2 tension. Some experts prefer using "hyperventilation" to refer to increased minute ventilation (regardless of whether due to increased rate or to tidal volume) and "polypnea" when a striking increase occurs in both rate and depth of breathing. (Hyperventilation is discussed further below.)

Hypopnea: Greatly reduced depth of breathing with less striking reduction in rate. For example, may occur during sleep or following administration of narcotics or sedatives. Also, may result from poor posture or the partial paralysis of respiratory muscles.

Hypoventilation: Reduced minute ventilation. Abnormally low amounts of air enter the lungs. Causes an elevation of CO_2 tension. Some experts prefer using "hypoventilation" to refer to reduced minute ventilation (regardless of whether due to reduced rate or to tidal volume) and using "oligopnea" for states in which both rate and depth are reduced significantly. (Hypoventilation is discussed below.)

Interrupted respirations (cogwheel or wavy respirations): Jerky breathing pattern; the inspiratory and expiratory sounds are clearly split into two or more sounds rather than occurring as a normal continuous sound.

Kussmaul's respirations (air hunger): Paroxysmal dyspnea. Often precedes diabetic coma. While Kussmaul's breathing is sometimes an example of polypnea it is more often truly dyspneic.

Oligopnea: See hypoventilation.

Orthopnea: Inability to breathe except when the trunk is in an upright position. Dyspnea may or may not be present with the erect posture. Seldom occurs with primary pulmonary disorders; frequently accompanies heart failure. The erect posture reduces venous pressure and pulmonary congestion and thereby reduces resistance to breathing. Commonly the degree of orthopnea is described in terms of the number of pillows the patient needs to elevate his head so he can breathe, e.g., "two-pillow orthopnea" or "three pillow-orthopnea."

Paradoxical respirations: Breathing pattern in which a lung (or portion of lung) inflates during inspiration, i.e., acts opposite to normal. (Discussed further in Chapters 72 and 73.)

Periodic breathing: Respiratory arrhythmias in which the rate, depth, or tidal volume changes markedly from one interval to the next and the pattern of change is periodically reproduced, e.g., Cheyne-Stokes breathing, Biot's breathing.

Polypnea: See hyperventilation.

Rales: Gurgling, bubbling sounds, synchronized with breathing, which occur when the moving air passes over fluids in the tracheobronchial tree or lungs, for example, with pulmonary edema.

Shortness of breath (SOB): Quick respiration which is not necessarily dyspneic, i.e., difficult or painful. Indeed, at times SOB evokes a pleasurable affectual content, e.g., during erotic acts.

Stridor: Noisy respirations characterized by harsh whistling sounds caused by the forcing of air through a partially obstructed larynx or trachea in spasm.

Tachypnea: Rapid breathing (rate more than 24 cycles/min.) which does not significantly change the depth; occurs during periods of passion and states of fear.

Thoracic respirations: Breathing accomplished by the thoracic muscles, e.g., intercostal muscles and others.

Hyperventilation; Hypoventilation

At times both hyperventilation and hypoventilation may occur as normal compensatory states. For example, *hyperventilation* may replenish an oxygen deficit or lower excess acidity by increasing CO_2 excretion. Hypoxia, acidosis, or nervous impulses may all act to overstimulate the respiratory center into compensatory action.

In some persons attacks of hyperventilation occur during anxiety states. In such a situation hyperventilation does not seem to have an adaptive function because, as hyperventilation blows off CO_2, the blood becomes excessively alkaline and the patient experiences distressing symptoms, e.g., tingling and numbness of the arms, legs, and face; faintness; dizziness; and possibly tetany. These symptoms of acute alkalosis are reversible once normal blood acidity is restored, e.g., by breathing into a paper bag (and thus rebreathing some of the exhaled CO_2) or by inhaling an O_2-CO_2 mixture with 10 per cent CO_2. Once the acute episode is relieved the patient is helped to understand how anxiety contributes to hyperventilation and how he can try consciously to alter his breathing during periods of anxiety so hyperventilation will be minimized.

Hypoventilation produces symptoms that result from hypoxemia and CO_2 accumulations in the blood (i.e., not enough CO_2 is "blown off"). Symptoms may include rising arterial blood pressure and headache. The patient may also be somewhat disoriented even though he is alert. Some causes of hypoventilation include severe hypoxia or CO_2 narcosis (excessive CO_2), paralysis of respiratory muscles, injury or damage to the medulla, and depressant drugs, e.g., alcohol, many anesthetic agents, barbiturates, morphine. (Carbon dioxide narcosis is discussed in Chapter 70.)

Dyspnea

As previously indicated, dyspnea is a disturbing subjective feeling of breathlessness associated with sensations of ventilatory inadequacy. Dyspnea may be associated with hypo- or hyperventilation. Much of the sensation of dyspnea probably results from the sustained work of breathing (especially breathing against obstruction) necessary to try to maintain adequate gas exchange. Patients with moderate to severe difficulty in breathing typically become fatigued and mentally distressed from the increased physical and mental effort required. Dyspnea is a common clinical problem which requires skilled nursing care.

Numerous *respiratory problems* produce dyspnea, e.g., damaged lung parenchyma, airway obstruction, chest pain, reduced lung compliance, impaired alveolar-capillary gas exchange, overworked or weakened respiratory muscles. Specific respiratory disorders which may produce dyspnea include pleurisy, aspirated foreign bodies, and parenchymal as well as tracheobronchial lesions that cause inflammation and obstruction. Other examples are mentioned throughout this discussion. In addition to being caused by respiratory disorders, dyspnea may be *psychogenic* in origin or may result from *cardiac disorders* (e.g., cardiac insufficiency) or *anemia*. Changes in the blood's components may make the blood unable to effectively transport the respiratory gases.

Types of Dyspnea. There are various types of dyspnea. *Exertional dyspnea* is that induced by physical exertion or effort. This is the most common type and may occur with any condition that impairs ventilation, e.g., obstructive or restrictive pulmonary disorders, with diffusion defects, or from inefficient mechanics of breathing. Dyspnea is seldom produced by early pulmonary disease but is more common with chronic disorders, e.g., diffuse obstructive lung disease.

Cardiac dyspnea refers to dyspnea caused by heart disease. Left ventricular failure from aortic insufficiency or mitral stenosis may cause *paroxysmal dyspnea*. This type of dyspnea occurs in attacks, usually while the patient is sleeping at night but also during the daytime. Paroxysmal dyspnea may be relieved by having the patient sit upright and breathe deeply several times.

Some patients are dyspneic even when resting, i.e., *dyspnea at rest*. Dyspnea at rest does occur with chronic pulmonary disease but it is more typical of congestive heart failure. It may occur with diffuse pulmonary diseases causing alveolar-capillary block and in conditions in which secondary factors are superimposed on a reduced pulmonary reserve, e.g., in patients with both bronchitis and pulmonary emphysema. Marked dyspnea at rest also is produced by some acute pulmonary disorders, e.g., bronchial asthma, pneumonia, massive atelectasis, pneumothorax.

Clinical Care During Acute or Severe Dyspnea. Severe or acute dyspnea, e.g., during an asthmatic attack, is frightening for both patient and nurse. The patient struggles to breathe and is acutely uncomfortable. He is overwhelmed by feelings of panic, extreme anxiety, and fears of suffocation and death. The gasping patient may plead with the nurse, "Help me breathe! I can't get air!"

In order to work effectively with a dyspneic patient the nurse must have in mind a plan of care, be sensitive to her own reactions to extreme respiratory distress, and efficiently perform clinical actions directed at giving the patient relief. The nurse who panics when a patient develops acute dyspnea conveys her anxiety to the patient, thereby adding to his already devastating problems. Also, the anxious nurse's judgment may be impaired, increasing chances of error. For example, the nurse's overwhelming desire to terminate the dyspneic attack and calm the patient may cause her to administer excessive sedation or excessive oxygen. Both of these actions may have serious, possibly fatal consequences.

Activities important in caring for a dyspneic patient are summarized below:

> Maintain a clear airway; promote and assist effective ventilation and respiration; promote bronchodilation. Encourage the patient to practice controlled diaphragmatic breathing.

> Stay with the patient; maintain a positive, calm approach; allay the patient's stresses, anxieties, and fears; act in an efficient, quiet manner.

> Place the patient in the position that permits him to breathe most comfortably.

> Conserve the patient's energy for the work of breathing; anticipate his needs; promote rest, relaxation, and relief of tension. Do not excessively or unnecessarily increase his fatigue. Do not require the patient to talk or to move more than is minimally necessary. Do not excessively sedate or tranquilize the dyspneic patient.

> Thoughtfully interpret and carry out PRN orders, e.g., for O_2, sedatives, tranquilizers, bronchodilators. If in doubt about whether to use a PRN order, consult with the physician.

> Remove the cause of the dyspnea when possible. Carry out treatments directed at the underlying disorder responsible for the dyspneic attacks.

> Conduct procedures in such a way that they do not increase dyspnea, e.g., take rectal rather than oral temperatures, avoid use of heavy bedding over the patient's chest.

> Maintain a quiet environment that is relatively cool and moist.

> Protect the severely dyspneic patient from injury, e.g., by side rails. The patient's judgment may be poor because of his dire psychophysiologic state.

> Prevent fluid-electrolyte imbalances. Intravenous infusions may be necessary during severe attacks of dyspnea because the patient cannot take adequate food and fluids orally. Record intake and output.

> Make observations and evaluations of the dyspneic episode; report and use these observations and evaluations to plan and give clinical care directed at reducing the severity of the present dyspneic episode and preventing future periods of dyspnea if possible.

If the airway seems obstructed encourage the patient to cough productively; minimize ineffective coughing. Suction as necessary but not excessively. Suction removes air as well as secretions and thus can increase the problem of breathlessness. Efficiently administered IPPB, nebulizers, and other procedures and medications as ordered and as indicated to maintain ventilation and to clear the airway. Administer O_2 cautiously at a low rate if indicated. Prevent CO_2 narcosis. Dyspneic patients receiving oxygen by mask or tent may become anxious since these methods of O_2 administration increase the sense of suffocation. Dyspneic patients typically are most comfortable with O_2 administered per nasal cannula or catheter.

Do not leave the patient alone during an acute dyspneic attack. Often the mere presence of the nurse helps the patient to relax somewhat. Talk to the patient; give him instructions; tell him what you are doing. Listening helps to distract, relax, and rest the patient.

Assist the patient to a position which facilitates ventilation. Often, but not always, the preferred position is one with the head of the bed elevated. Respect the patient's preferences for positioning. He knows how he can breathe most comfortably, e.g., sitting upright, bending forward over a table, lying semi-upright. After you have helped the patient to assume the position of his choice, place pillows, supports, padding, and so forth, so he can maintain that position without fatigue or discomfort. Leaning forward facilitates use of the accessory muscles of respiration, e.g., abdominal, cervical, dorsal, pectoral muscles. These muscles are used during expiration, e.g., to expel trapped air.

During attacks of dyspnea remind the patient to practice controlled breathing. As stated, dyspnea usually causes the affected person to expend increased amounts of energy to breathe, and he often breathes more rapidly. Unfortunately these reactions only worsen the patient's condition by reducing the effectiveness of ventilation and by increasing O_2 requirements and airway obstruction. To prevent these detrimental effects, persons subject to dyspnea should be taught controlled breathing methods (e.g., diaphragmatic breathing) that reduce the effort necessary to breathe and improve the effectiveness of ventilation.

Observations important to make when a patient experiences dyspnea include: (1) notation of events which preceded the attack and what the patient was doing when the attack began; (2) patient's reaction to the attack and any accompanying symptoms, e.g., diaphoresis, emotional state, sputum, cough, color, pulse, rate and character of respirations; (3) severity of the attack and how long it lasted; and (4) responses to treatment. If episodes of dyspnea appear to be regularly recurrent, this observation should also be noted.

Following an acute attack of dyspnea ensure rest for the patient because he will be exhausted from the effort of breathing and the anxiety accompanying the attack. Also, the dyspnea may have caused him to lose sleep.

Because the dyspneic patient is commonly frightened, frustrated, fatigued, and uncomfortable, he may be short-tempered with persons caring for him. The nurse must be able to overlook abusive behavior and recognize and respond to the cause of the patient's behavior. Be certain that a dyspneic patient always has a call bell within easy reach. Respond rapidly to the patient's summons so he knows help is nearby when needed. Periodically "drop in" to visit the patient even though he has not called. These actions reinforce the feeling of being "looked after" in an anxious person.

Care in Chronic Dyspnea. The individual with chronic dyspnea, e.g., with emphysema or chronic obstructive lung disease, must be taught how to live with breathlessness. For example, teach the patient about the following factors which will help him to breathe most easily: dietary modifications, diaphragmatic breathing, improved breathing habits, breathing exercises, proper posture, isometric exercises, and room ventilation. Include family members in teaching sessions when appropriate.

Breathing exercises teach the dyspneic patient controlled breathing and breathing techniques that help him to ventilate his lungs more efficiently and easily. A detailed discussion of breathing exercises is given later in this unit.

General comfort measures can greatly help the dyspneic patient to relax and feel somewhat refreshed. Keep the patient in dry clothes and bed linens, and keep him as warm as is comfortable for him. Minimize feelings of suffocation by keeping the patient's environment open to circulating air. Frequent oral hygiene is of importance, especially if the patient is mouthbreathing. Massage of the upper back, neck, and shoulders helps to relieve physical tension resulting from labored breathing.

Adequate nutrition is required by the dyspneic patient because he is expending large amounts of energy and because his resistance against infection must be maintained. If the patient is overweight, respiratory requirements are increased and excessive work is placed on the heart; if he is underweight, expiration may be impaired because the diaphragm tends to flatten. Small, frequent feedings of nourishing foods and liquids are better than larger, less frequent intake. If the stomach is excessively full it distends, increasing pressure on the abdominal muscles and diaphragm; this impairs abdominal breathing. Advise the patient subject to dyspnea to avoid liquids and foods that are gas-forming, e.g., ice water, cabbage, onions, cauliflower, radishes, cucumbers, turnips, melons, and lima and navy beans. The administration of IPPB treatments before meals may minimize fatigue produced by eating. Nonetheless, even the minimal exertion necessary to eat may exhaust the dyspneic patient. Offer the patient assistance with eating as required.

Permit the dyspneic patient to help to plan his activity and treatment schedule, since his activity tolerance may vary at different times of the day. Two typical periods of increased dyspnea and fatigue are upon arising for the day and following meals, especially the last meal of the day. When he first gets up the patient's lungs are often congested by secretions that have pooled during the period of relative inactivity in bed. At the end of the day the patient is usually exhausted from the day's exertions.

The nurse closely observes the patient for evidence of increasing dyspnea or excessive fatigue upon exertion. Unnecessary invalidism is undesirable, but at times it is necessary to conserve the patient's energy by minimizing the number of activities he does for himself. Because of the beneficial effects of ambulation, it is encouraged as long as the patient can tolerate activity without producing excessive fatigue or dyspnea.

CHEST PAIN

Pulmonary disorders may produce pain in the following structures: chest wall (including its bony and cartilaginous structures), parietal pleura (the visceral pleura is insensitive to pain), bronchi, and trachea. The pain associated with pleural inflammation is often quite incapacitating if untreated and is worsened by changes in intrathoracic pressure, e.g., sneezing, coughing. (Pleurisy and pleural pain are discussed in Chapter 71.) Chest pain also commonly occurs with bronchogenic carcinoma, pneumonia, and tracheobronchial inflammations. The latter condition produces pain of a burning nature which patients frequently describe as a raw feeling in the lining of the throat and windpipe. Coughing aggravates this pain, but respirations do not worsen it. Chest injuries and chest surgery often produce moderate to severe pain. (See Chapters 72 and 73.) When administering pain-relieving drugs for any chest pain associated with respiratory disorders, be careful to prevent excessive depression of the patient's abilities to cough and breathe effectively. Narcotics are particularly hazardous.

Management of chest pain is discussed more completely as appropriate throughout this unit. The general problem of pain and pain management is discussed in Unit IX.

BRONCHOSPASM

Bronchospasm, that is, the spasmodic contraction of the walls of the bronchi, is a component of numerous respiratory disorders, e.g., asthma, chronic bronchitis, chronic pulmonary emphysema, foreign body aspiration. Reduction of the size of the bronchial lumina predisposes the patient to retention of secretions and infection, in addition to making ventilation of the lung more difficult. Severe bronchospasm is a life-threatening condition. Wheezing is a characteristic indication of bronchial narrowing. The specific treatment of bronchospasm is the administration of bronchodilators to open the airways by relaxing contracted muscles. Bronchospasm may also be reduced by preventing unnecessary irritation of the tracheobronchial tree, e.g., avoidance of irritating smokes, gases, and other air pollutants, avoidance of cold air, and prevention of unnecessary nonproductive coughing. Treatment of bronchospasm is discussed in greater detail elsewhere throughout this unit.

ABNORMAL SECRETIONS

The "normal" adult produces about 100 ml. of mucus daily. This mucus is produced by mucous cells and goblet cells lining the tracheobronchial tree. Mucus acts to entrap inspired particles and to moisten tracheobronchial membranes. Mucus is carried upward in the tracheobronchial tree by cilia lining the walls of the airway. Coughing and clearing the throat are other actions which move secretions into the pharynx.

Irritations or inflammation of the nasal mucosa or sinuses may cause *rhinorrhea,* i.e., copious mucus discharge from the nose. (Disorders of the nose and sinuses are discussed in Unit XXII.) Tracheobronchial or pulmonary irritations or infections often cause an increase in mucus production, and sputum frequently changes in consistency and/or color. *Sputum* is composed of mucus (from the tracheobronchial tree), leukocytes, epithelial cells, dirt, bacteria, and nasopharyngeal secretions. Saliva is not sputum. Certain pulmonary disorders produce sputum with specific characteristics. (See Table 69–1.)

Secretions may accumulate in the lower tracheo-

TABLE 69–1. SPUTUM CHARACTERISTICS IN RELATION TO SPECIFIC PULMONARY DISORDERS

Pulmonary Disorder	Sputum Characteristics
Abscess	Foul odor (anaerobic infection); large quantities
Asthma	Mucoid
Bronchiectasis	Periodic large quantities; separates into three layers while standing.
Bronchitis (chronic) or emphysema	Very tenacious; thick
Carcinoma (bronchogenic) or tuberculosis (advanced)	Contains frank blood
Edema	Frothy; large quantities; pink
Pneumonia (pneumococcus)	Sticky; small amounts; rusty or pink
Suppuration	Purulent; large quantities; yellow or green (bacterial infection)
Tracheobronchitis	Mucoid

bronchial tree as a result of an increase in secretion production, depression or failure of the normal tracheobronchial cleansing mechanisms, or both. Some possible detrimental effects of these accumulated secretions are: (1) airway obstruction; (2) prevention of normal alveolar gas exchange; (3) hypoxia (due to inadequate oxygenation of the blood); (4) respiratory acidosis (due to inadequate CO_2 elimination); and (5) pulmonary disorders such as atelectasis, tracheobronchitis, and bronchopneumonia. Hypoxia is particularly serious in patients with head injuries since hypoxia increases cerebral edema and thus elevates intracranial pressure. If secretions are retained in the lungs and tracheobronchial tree they easily become sites of infection since they provide an excellent medium for the growth of pathogens in a dark moist place. Retained secretions also may form mucous plugs which can obstruct airways, impair ventilation and respiration, and produce atelectasis, i.e., collapse of a portion of the lung. Atelectatic lung easily becomes infected.

The average diameter of the smaller bronchial tubes is less than that of a broom straw, thus they can easily be obstructed. Airways normally lengthen and widen during inspiration and shorten and narrow during expiration. If the airways are partially obstructed, air cannot bypass obstructions during expiration.

Various factors may prevent a patient with a respiratory disorder from being able to move his secretions effectively. For example, the patient may not be able to cough effectively because of postoperative pain, sedation, weakness, tracheostomy, or endotracheal intubation. Tracheostomies and endotracheal tubes not only reduce a patient's ability to cough, but they also increase secretion formation. The combination of these two factors is obviously dangerous and the tracheostomized or intubated patient must be closely observed to ensure maintenance of a patent airway. The cough reflex is weak in elderly persons, and respirations tend to be shallow.

A patient with thick, voluminous bronchopulmonary secretions may feel that he is suffocating and may panic when he experiences difficulty coughing up his secretions. Feelings of fear, anxiety, and panic further increase the patient's respiratory difficulties. Calmly the nurse attempts to reassure the patient and to enlist his cooperation as she carries out nursing activities that help to clear the patient's distressing, sometimes life-threatening, secretions.

Care of the Patient with Sputum Abnormalities

Activities important in helping to mobilize and to remove tracheobronchial secretions include:

> Coughing effectively and productively; breathing exercises.

> Suctioning.

> Humidifying inspired air.

> Maintaining body hydration, e.g., forcing fluids.

> Changing positions frequently. Causes secretions to move within the tracheobronchial tree and lungs; prevents pooling of secretions and stimulates coughing.

> Postural drainage.

> Chest percussion, clapping, tapping, vibrating. Increases force of expiration and moves secretions.

> Administering prescribed medications, e.g., bronchodilators, expectorants, proteolytic enzymes, mucolytic agents, nebulized detergents, heated aerosols.

> IPPB treatments. Increases inspired volume and increases diameter of bronchioles for more effective coughing.

>Tracheostomy. As mentioned above, tracheostomy is not without its hazards. However, when there are profuse secretions it is often desirable to perform a tracheostomy so that proper tracheobronchial hygiene can be performed. Tracheostomy is preferable to endotracheal intubation because secretions are usually more difficult to remove through endotracheal tubes.

Some patients find it helps to loosen mucus if they take a hot drink upon arising, inhaling the steamy vapor, sipping the drink, and holding the liquid momentarily in the mouth before swallowing.

Often secretion removal poses serious problems in giving clinical care. For example, a patient's secretions may be thick and tenacious and the patient may be unable to raise them, or his secretions may be so copious that he becomes fatigued by constantly trying to clear his tracheobronchial tree. A more forceful cough is necessary to dislodge dry, thick, or tenacious secretions (low in water content and high in viscosity) than thinner secretions. Secretions must be fluid enough that they can be moved up the tracheobronchial tree by effective coughing. Once in the pharynx, sputum may either be swallowed or expectorated.

Patients producing large amounts of sputum or having infected sputum, e.g., in tuberculosis, should be instructed to expectorate sputum into a sputum collection cup rather than swallowing it. The expectorated sputum is then available for observation and laboratory evaluation or it can be disposed of safely. Additionally, removal of sputum from the body prevents the infected material from entering the gastrointestinal tract and relieves the body of the need to dispose of the swallowed sputum. Large amounts of swallowed sputum reduce a patient's appetite. If a patient who is producing sputum cannot adequately protect you from contamination (e.g., by covering his mouth and nose when coughing) it may be advisable to mask the patient or to wear a gown and mask yourself. (See Chapter 71.)

Provide the patient who has a productive cough with ample tissues, a sputum collection cup, a paper bag (fastened to the bedside or a chair) for tissue disposal, and disposable hand wipes. Instruct the patient to protect others and to prevent contamination of his environment by covering his nose and mouth with several tissues when coughing or sneezing. Tell the patient to fold used tissues over before disposing of them in the toilet or tissue bag. The patient should wash frequently or use disposable hand wipes if he handles many contaminated tissues. (See Chapter 71.) Always provide equipment so the patient may wash before eating.

Impress upon the patient the importance of raising secretions from his lungs and tracheobronchial tree.

Teach him the proper methods of productive coughing. (See Chapter 73.) When caring for a patient who is producing abnormal secretions (rhinorrhea or sputum), periodically observe and chart the character and amount of secretions and the patient's response to treatments. Be certain to mention if the secretions have a foul odor.

Keep the patient as clean and comfortable as possible and maintain an orderly, pleasant environment. Used tissues are not only unsightly and often malodorous, but also are sources of contamination and should be removed from the bedside and properly disposed of. When a tissue collection bag becomes half full, remove, close securely, and dispose of it; then replace the bag. Always wash thoroughly after handling sputum-contaminated articles (e.g., tissues, tissue bags, sputum cups, soiled linens) and after giving mouth or nose care. Provide good room ventilation. Sputum produced with some pulmonary disorders is quite foul smelling.

Frequent mouth and nose care helps to minimize mouth and breath odors and the collection of thickened secretions in these areas. This care is especially important when a patient is mouthbreathing and/or is producing large quantities of sputum. Even though cleansing a patient's nose and mouth, and cleaning up expectorations, are activities that are often unpleasant to perform, they are an important part of total patient care (particularly when the patient has a respiratory disorder). The nurse must take care not to communicate to the patient any distasteful or repulsive feelings that she may have while performing these activities. Periodically examine the patient's oral and nasal mucous membranes for indications of lesions, inflammation, or other disorders. These inspections can easily be made while giving nose and oral care.

The unpleasant taste and odor of sputum often causes patients to have a poor appetite. Provision for frequent oral hygiene helps to refresh the mouth and may improve appetite. Chewing gum or sucking on hard candy between meals may also freshen the mouth. It is desirable to provide oral hygiene before as well as after meals. The sight of contaminated tissues and sputum collection cups may adversely affect appetite. Before serving trays be certain the bedside environment is picked up and sputum containers are out of sight.

Medications that may be prescribed for patients producing excessive or abnormal bronchopulmonary secretions include *expectorants, mucolytic enzymes,* and *detergent preparations*. Detergent and enzyme preparations may be given by aerosol. Sedatives and analgesics should be used judiciously to prevent oversedation and depression of the cough reflex.

Pulmonary congestion (or inflammation) causes the respirations to become more rapid and shallow. Respirations of this nature may indicate to the nurse that the patient needs to be encouraged or assisted to cough productively, or that he should be suctioned if he cannot clear his own airway. Noisy, moist respirations also indicate that secretions are accumulating in the lungs. Auscultate the patient's chest and observe his respirations before and after encouraging coughing or performing suctioning. Be certain to chart your observations. Contact the physician for necessary orders if a patient is having excessive difficulty in coughing up his secretions or if you are unable to clear his airway.

An obstructed airway is an emergency! The nurse must be familiar with the following cardinal indications of laryngeal and/or tracheal obstruction: gurgling and rattling respirations, stridor, cyanosis, rib retraction, and the use of accessory muscles of respiration. Occasionally oral fluids are regurgitated through the nose. The airway must immediately be cleared.

Hemoptysis

Hemoptysis is the expectoration of blood or blood-tinged sputum; it may vary in degree from slight amounts of blood in the sputum to large quantities of frank blood. Massive hemoptysis produces death, because the patient drowns in his own blood; death from obstruction occurs more commonly than death from exsanguination. Although hemoptysis can be fatal, it most typically is a nonfatal, self-limited disorder.

Conditions that most typically may produce hemoptysis are those which cause inflammation of the tracheobronchial tree, and/or erosion and necrosis of blood vessels and lung parenchyma. Hemoptysis may, thus, result from pneumonia or other acute respiratory infections (e.g., due to trauma of the tracheobronchial tree produced by repeated or severe coughing or other irritations) or from such other serious respiratory disorders as pulmonary infarction, aspirated foreign body, benign bronchial adenoma, crushing or penetrating chest injuries, bronchogenic carcinoma, tuberculosis, pulmonary abscess, or bronchiectasis. Nonrespiratory disorders that may produce hemoptysis include aortic aneurysm (in which the vessel has eroded into and ruptured into a bronchus), mitral stenosis (in which a blood vessel has ruptured within the congested pulmonary circulation), and congestive heart failure due to mitral stenosis. Sometimes disorders that cause a bleeding tendency or failure of the clotting mechanism produce hemoptysis.

Whatever the extent of hemoptysis, it is essential that the patient receive a thorough medical evaluation to determine the cause of the bleeding so appropriate treatment can be given. This investigative process may include history, general physical examination, chest x-rays, tomograms, bronchograms, bronchoscopy, and fluoroscopy.

When blood is expectorated, nursing observations of the expectorated material can be helpful in ascertaining the point of origin of the bleeding in the body and determining whether the blood is venous or arterial. Often it is desirable to save the specimen for the physician or laboratory to examine. Bloody secretions expectorated from the mouth can originate from such body areas as esophagus (e.g., bleeding esophageal varices), nose (e.g., epistaxis), nasopharynx, mouth, tongue, gums, lungs or tracheobronchial tree (hemoptysis), or stomach (hematemesis). Bleeding originating in the nose or nasopharynx often causes bloody discharge to appear in the nares, and sniffling usually precedes or accompanies the expectoration of blood. (See Unit XXII.)

Several points, as shown in the table below, help to differentiate hemoptysis from hematemesis and therefore should be considered when charting observations of expectorated bloody secretions.

Other symptoms of hemoptysis may include apprehension, salty taste in mouth, burning or bubbling feeling in chest, feelings of being smothered or drowning, and tickling sensation in throat.

Hemoptysis, especially if moderate to severe, is frightening for both patient and nurse. The nurse attempts to quiet and reassure the patient. She stays with him and gives him appropriate instructions. She tells the patient not to try to talk, to breathe slowly and deeply, and to expectorate (not swallow) the blood and secretions. The fearful patient tends to hyperventilate; this not only causes the lungs to be excessively active but also interferes with effective respiration.

One goal of clinical care is to provide rest for the affected lung tissue without unduly suppressing the protective cough reflex necessary to clear the airway. The patient with hemoptysis should immediately be placed on complete bed rest, kept warm, and positioned so that the drainage of blood from the bronchi is encouraged. A receptacle for expectoration is provided. When possible, codeine and sedatives are avoided in order to preserve those reflexes necessary to maintain a patent airway. However, if the patient is quite anxious, a sedative such as phenobarbital may be ordered. If violent coughing occurs, codeine may be prescribed in amounts which suppress but do not abolish the cough reflex. Morphine is contraindicated.

IPPB is contraindicated, but oxygen inhalations may be prescribed to relieve dyspnea or cyanosis. Suctioning is performed as necessary to clear the airway. A laryngoscope and bronchoscope should be available for the physician to perform deep suctioning if required. Hemoptysis can cause atelectasis and pneumonia if bronchi are obstructed by blood.

There is danger of spreading certain diseases within the lungs and tracheobronchial tree when hemoptysis occurs; e.g., tuberculosis may disseminate via hemoptysis and infect previously uninfected areas. When a patient with tuberculosis experiences hemoptysis he may be positioned on the infected side to prevent spread of the infection (via the blood) in the tracheobronchial tree.

Observe the patient's vital signs. Severe hemoptysis may produce shock as a result of blood loss. (See Chapter 26.) If shock appears to be developing, a blood transfusion and other measures may be employed. Formerly, in treating severe hemoptysis, an artificial pneumothorax was sometimes performed on selected patients in an attempt to rest lung tissue by temporarily collapsing the lung. Currently emergency surgery is occasionally performed in an attempt to save a patient's life, e.g., if prolonged severe hemoptysis occurs in a patient with cavernous tuberculosis. Thoracoplasty or resectional surgery may be indicated. When hemoptysis is believed to have resulted from defective blood coagulation, vitamin K_1, calcium gluconate, and blood transfusions may be ordered. Usually in treating hemoptysis infusions are administered slowly to prevent a rapid increase in blood volume and consequently an increase in bleeding.

Provide the patient with fresh linens as indicated, i.e., remove any blood-stained linen. Oral hygiene helps to freshen the patient's mouth. Following hemoptysis the patient may be placed on nothing by mouth orders for a while. If he is permitted oral intake, he may find cool liquids refreshing. Instruct the patient to avoid physical exertion until the physician gives his approval. Give only gentle back care to a patient who has recently had hemoptysis to prevent possibly reactivating bleeding.

COUGH

A cough is the sudden, noisy expulsion of alveolar air from the lungs, the air being under very high pressure. Coughing is usually a normal protective act that cleans the tracheobronchial tree (acting in cooperation with airway cilia) in an attempt to prevent aspiration and/or to remove irritants. Coughing may be a symptom of numerous thoracic and laryngeal disorders (acute, chronic, inflammatory, neoplastic).

Hemoptysis	*Hematemesis*
Source of bleeding: lungs or tracheobronchial tree	Source of bleeding: stomach
Secretions typically mixed with mucus or pus; bright red and foamy (because mixed with air); blood has liquid appearance and is alkaline	Expectorated material may contain food particles; blood may be dark red or black; blood which has had contact with gastric juices is typically clotted, dark colored (sometimes called "coffee-ground emesis"), and is acid
Coughing and/or wheezing usually precedes and/or accompanies expectoration	Retching, gagging, and nausea may precede vomiting of expectorated material
Chest pain sometimes occurs; patient may attempt to splint bleeding side	Pain may occur in abdominal or epigastric areas
Shock usually does not occur	Shock often occurs

Cough appears to be the most common symptom of respiratory disease. Cough is a protective mechanism in health, but it can become a disturbing phenomenon during disease; a nonproductive cough is both useless and damaging.

Generally coughing is an involuntary reflex act; however, it can be produced voluntarily. Although coughing can often be consciously inhibited, this voluntary control is limited. Reflex coughing results from the chemical or mechanical stimulation of receptors in the pharynx, larynx, or tracheobronchial tree or stimulation along the vagus nerve. Mechanical factors that commonly induce coughing include cooling, drying, irritation or inflammation of the tracheobronchial mucosa and/or lung parenchyma; foreign body or foreign particle aspiration; and accumulations of secretions within the tracheobronchial tree. The "cough center" is composed of a group of neurons in the brain's medulla. Impulses reach this center by way of the glossopharyngeal or vagus nerve.

A *chronic cough* is any cough that persists for a month or longer, even though the cough occurs only when getting up for the day or when lying down at the end of the day. Inhaled cigarette smoke is the commonest cause of chronic cough. All persons with chronic coughs should be medically evaluated, because this symptom may indicate a serious pulmonary or cardiac disorder that should be treated. Respiratory diseases that may produce chronic cough include tuberculosis, lung cancer, bronchiectasis, and bronchitis. Often people tend to overlook, minimize, or self-treat chronic coughs. These persons should be helped to realize that coughing is not itself a disease, but rather is symptomatic of other disorders. *"Short term"* coughs should always be investigated if they are accompanied by pain, shortness of breath, or production of blood-tinged sputum. Nonpulmonary disorders that may produce cough include otitis media, subdiaphragmatic irritation, congestive heart failure, and mitral valve disease.

In addition to the fatigue and loss of appetite that cough may cause in most persons, in some patients (e.g., with increased intracranial pressure or cardiac disorders) coughing causes dangerous muscular exertion or hazardous elevations in intrathoracic, intracranial, and blood pressures. These alterations may, in turn, precipitate such life-threatening problems as heart failure or aneurysm rupture. Severe episodes of coughing not only produce muscular soreness and pain, but have been known to fracture ribs.

Nursing observations concerning a patient's cough may be helpful in establishing diagnosis and treatment. Important observations to make and chart include:

> Factors that induce the coughing episode and measures that relieve coughing.

> Character of the cough, e.g., frequency, episodic, paroxysmal, productive or nonproductive, sound and depth (deep, shallow, whooping, rattling, dry, hacking, hard, croupy, racking).

> Time at which coughing episodes typically occur; e.g., "Patient coughed violently and productively upon awakening in the early A.M."

> Events apparently associated with or resulting from the coughing, e.g., nausea, vomiting, decreased appetite, interrupted sleep, fatigue, pain, changes in vital signs, dyspnea, anxiety.

Care of the Patient with a Cough

Effective clinical care of a patient with a cough is based on consideration of the patient's condition and the cause and character of the cough. When possible, cough is relieved by treating the underlying disorder. A patient who is coughing and expectorating is potentially infectious; therefore, personnel must take appropriate precautions when giving patient care. These precautions include: (1) instructing the patient to cover his mouth and nose with a tissue when coughing and to properly discard the tissue afterward; (2) teaching the patient how to correctly use sputum containers; (3) practicing appropriate self-protective measures, e.g., maintaining one's own level of health, wearing mask and/or gown if indicated, staying out of the direct line of a patient's cough, properly handling and disposing of contaminated sputum containers and tissues, and practicing thorough handwashing before and after caring for the patient. (See Chapter 71.)

Factors important in caring for patients with chronic coughs include: (1) minimizing respiratory irritants in the air (e.g., avoiding use of aerosol products, prohibiting smoking and use of powders); (2) providing uninterrupted rest periods; (3) administering appropriate medications (e.g., mucolytic enzymes, bronchodilators, expectorants); (4) relieving mucous membrane inflammation (e.g., by humidification of inspired air); (5) providing well-balanced meals; (6) forcing fluids to help to liquefy secretions; and (7) preventing respiratory infections.

Instruct the patient to cough purposefully when he needs to, i.e., cough only when necessary to raise secretions. With controlled coughing it is desirable for the cough to be gentle yet forceful enough to be productive. When coughing the patient should consciously contract his intercostal muscles and diaphragm. Teach the patient to fill his lungs with air before coughing; coughing with deflated lungs can trap sputum rather than expel it. Cough syrups or expectorants should not be taken unless prescribed. Secretions that have been loosened (e.g., by breathing steam, postural drainage) can be coughed up more comfortably. It is important to clear the lungs of secretions before bedtime, e.g., by steam inhalation followed by purposeful coughing.

When a patient's cough is excessive and ineffective (shallow, hacking, and nonproductive), he may be advised to try to voluntarily prolong the intervals between paroxysms of coughing. By consciously suppressing the cough and resting between paroxysms, he can then cough with greater force and greater productivity at less frequent intervals. Instruct the patient not to talk unnecessarily because talking may stimulate coughing, and tell him that swallowing inhibits coughing (provide fluids to sip on and hard candy to suck) and that mildly clearing the throat may eliminate the need to cough.

Sometimes medication is prescribed to mildly depress a nonproductive cough. Note: *cough depressants are typically inadvisable if a patient has a productive cough or if he has retained secretions.* Medications that depress the cough reflex act on the cough center in the medulla and are called *antitussive* medications. Prior to giving cough medications check the patient's respirations to see if they are "noisy." If rales are present encourage the patient to cough productively and clear the airway prior to administration of the medication. Also, instruct the patient not to take a drink soon after taking the medication, because the liquid swallowed will remove the soothing coating of cough mixture from the throat.

Often it is the nurse's responsibility to teach patients to breathe deeply and cough effectively. Periodic effective coughing and deep breathing not only help to prevent secretion accumulation within the tracheobronchial tree, but also provide the lung expansion necessary for efficient breathing. Patients who should receive coughing–deep breathing instructions include all patients who have respiratory disorders that increase secretion production, have retained bronchopulmonary secretions, have chest injuries, are going to have or have had thoracic or high abdominal surgery, or have restricted activity and are therefore subject to the complications of immobility. Effective, periodic coughing and deep breathing can often prevent complications which might otherwise develop from retained secretions and poor pulmonary aeration. Details of instructing the surgical patient in coughing are given in Chapter 73 of this unit.

To be effective, coughing and deep breathing sessions must be performed at prescheduled intervals, and between scheduled times if the patient's condition indicates. The patient should be told that coughing and deep breathing not only remove secretions from his lungs, but also expand the lungs and help air to circulate through them. Prior to coughing–deep breathing sessions the patient should either be turned from side to side or, if possible, placed in a modified Trendelenburg position. This helps to loosen secretions and increases the effectiveness of coughing. During the time the patient is actually coughing and deep breathing, position him with his head and chest upright if possible. This position facilitates maximal chest expansion. During coughing–deep breathing exercises observe the patient's condition carefully, provide rest periods, and give appropriate emotional support. Auscultate the patient's chest before and after he coughs and deep breathes so you can evaluate the effectiveness of the procedure.

A patient whose coughing produces pain (e.g., a patient with pleurisy or chest injury, or who has had chest surgery) usually tends to try to suppress coughing because it is painful. This may permit secretions to accumulate within the lungs and tracheobronchial tree. Such a patient benefits from mechanical support or "splinting" of his chest during vigorous coughing. Splinting is discussed in Chapter 73.

Sometimes it is necessary *to stimulate coughing* as in an acutely ill patient with retained bronchopulmonary secretions. Methods that may be employed to stimulate coughing include:

1. Direct external mechanical stimulation of the trachea by exerting finger pressure over the trachea.
2. Internal mechanical stimulation of the trachea by having the patient exhale forcefully and for as long as possible.
3. The use of suctioning, aerosols or nebulizers, or warm water.
4. Instillation of distilled water or sterile saline through a transcutaneous catheter inserted into the trachea (Fig. 69–1).

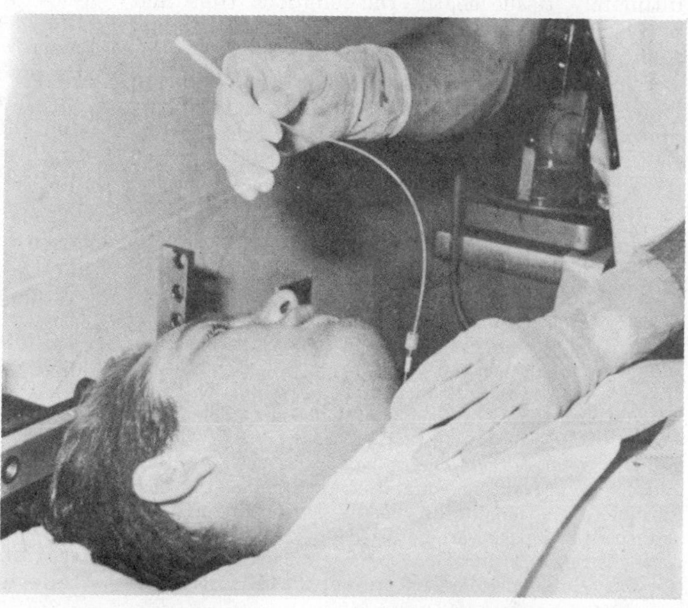

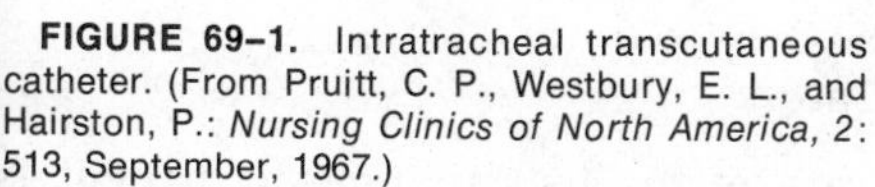

FIGURE 69–1. Intratracheal transcutaneous catheter. (From Pruitt, C. P., Westbury, E. L., and Hairston, P.: *Nursing Clinics of North America, 2*: 513, September, 1967.)

5. Endotracheal stimulation by a sterile catheter inserted through the nose into the trachea.

6. Endotracheal suctioning. (See discussion in Chapter 70.)

For a fuller discussion of the subject of cough stimulation see the article by Ungvarski.[306]

Before performing cough stimulation procedures be certain to prepare the patient physically and mentally. With practice, a cooperative patient may greatly increase the productiveness of these procedures. If techniques of mechanically stimulating coughing are correctly practiced, the necessity for endotracheal suctioning may be avoided or, at least, the frequency of suctioning may be reduced.

HYPOXIA AND ANOXIA

Definitions

In its broadest sense *hypoxia* refers to a deficiency of oxygen in body tissues. This condition has numerous internal and external causes (discussed further below) and may be acute or chronic. When the tissues are virtually without oxygen, the condition is correctly termed *anoxia*. In common practice, however, precise distinctions are not made between a deficiency and a total lack of O_2 and, therefore, the terms hypoxia and anoxia are frequently used interchangeably. *Hypoxemia* means a deficiency in the O_2 content of the blood (arterial blood usually). If correctly used, *anoxemia* would mean the complete lack of O_2 in the blood.

Effects of Anoxia

Anoxia produces irreversible tissue damage and, ultimately, tissue death. The length of time that passes before these changes occur varies, depending upon the affected tissue's metabolic rate. For example, brain damage occurs rapidly if the brain is anoxic for longer than 4 to 5 minutes. The heart and retina are also highly sensitive to O_2 deprivation.

Classifications

Hypoxia (or anoxia) may be classified as follows:[129]

> *Hypoxic (anoxic or arterial) hypoxia:* oxygenation of the arterial blood is deficient, even though the blood has a normal O_2-carrying capacity.

> *Anemic hypoxia:* Reduction in the blood's O_2-transporting capacity, i.e., hemoglobin deficiency. (See discussion of the anemias in Unit XII.)

> *Stagnant (circulatory) hypoxia:* Reduced capillary blood flow prevents adequate oxygenation of the body tissues, even though the blood's O_2 content and O_2-transporting capacity are normal.

> *Histotoxic (metabolic) hypoxia:* Impaired oxidative-enzyme cellular mechanisms prevent the cells from utilizing O_2. Even though the arterial blood may have a normal O_2 concentration, the cells may be hypoxic, e.g., if the cellular demand for O_2 is excessively high. Cyanide poisoning is an example of histotoxic hypoxia.

Clinical Manifestations

Clinical manifestations of hypoxia (anoxia) depend upon such factors as the severity and type of hypoxia, whether it is acute or chronic, and the prehypoxic physiologic adequacy of the involved tissues. Earliest indications of hypoxia include hyperventilation, tachycardia, and hypertension. Hypertension occurs because hypoxia induces increased sympathetic nervous system activity which causes tissue vasoconstriction and increased peripheral resistance. Other early symptoms of hypoxia are restlessness and possibly headache and slight confusion. Because of their relatively mild nature, the early symptoms of hypoxia may be overlooked except by the most careful of observers.

Although cyanosis is a classic sign of hypoxia, it is an unreliable indicator since it often does not appear until the hypoxia is far advanced, and, at times, may occur in the absence of arterial hypoxia. Oxygen saturations above cyanotic levels may exist in spite of severe tissue hypoxia. (Cyanosis is discussed below.) When hypoxia occurs in debilitated elderly patients or when it is of an advanced degree, the blood pressure falls to a hypotensive level and the heart rate markedly decreases (indications of failure of the sympathetic response).

The symptoms of *local hypoxia* depend upon the affected region of the body. For example, varicose veins may produce discoloration and ulceration of hypoxic tissues. Hypoxia of the lower extremities causes intermittent claudication. Angina pectoris results from myocardial hypoxia; hypoxia of the brain may result in attacks of syncope.

When hypoxia develops slowly and is *chronic*, the body often attempts to adapt physiologically by increasing the respiratory rate and increasing the blood's oxygen-transporting capacities. Bone marrow (which is sensitive to hypoxia) increases its production of RBC. The blood's oxygen-carrying power can be evaluated by the hematocrit and the hemoglobin level. Both may be elevated in chronic hypoxemia not caused by anemia. (See discussions of polycythemia below and in Unit XII.)

Clinical Care

Clinical care of the hypoxic (anoxic) patient is directed at relieving the underlying disorder, increasing O_2 supply, and maintaining effective ventilation of the lungs. The patient is kept at rest to minimize his oxygen needs. The effectiveness of O_2 therapy and the amount of O_2 indicated vary from patient to patient. (Oxygen therapy is discussed in Chapter 70.) Rest and the administration of relatively low concentrations of O_2 relieve many hypoxic individuals. However, O_2

therapy alone may be only slightly helpful in treating anemic, stagnant, or histotoxic hypoxia. Persons with these disorders require additional specific treatments. For example, respiratory stimulants (caffeine sodium benzoate, ethamivan) are employed when hypoxia results from the ingestion of poisons or depressant drugs. Vasodilators help to improve circulation and may relieve stagnant hypoxia. High O_2 concentrations are indicated at times to correct hypoxia resulting from diffuse, extensive pneumonia.

In the presence of impaired alveolar ventilation (indicated by an increased $PaCO_2$), treatment is directed at maintaining a patent airway and mechanically assisting ventilation. (Respirators are discussed in Chapter 70.)

It is important that the nurse develop skill in recognizing *early* indications of mild hypoxia so treatment can be started well before there is danger of tissue damage. Severe dyspnea and cyanosis usually indicate that serious hypoxia has developed. Hypoxia is particularly serious in patients with head injuries, since it increases cerebral edema and thus elevates intracranial pressure.

Because morphine and sedatives depress respiration they are contraindicated in the presence of significant hypoxia. If the nurse must administer these medications (e.g., to combat physiologic shock) she makes certain that equipment is at the bedside to assist ventilation if necessary and she observes the patient closely for indications of ventilatory impairment.

HYPERCAPNIA (CARBON DIOXIDE RETENTION)

The retention of CO_2, with pH below 7.35, produces respiratory acidosis. (See Chapter 25.) Pulmonary disorders may produce hypercapnia as a result of severe airway obstruction, e.g., secretions blocking large portions of the tracheobronchial tree or severe bronchospasm. If the arterial pCO_2 ($PaCO_2$) rises suddenly and markedly, the following symptoms may occur: tremor, altered mentation, headache, somnolence, or asterixis. With extremely high $PaCO_2$ levels (above 65 mm. Hg) the patient may need constant stimulation to breathe. Unless respiratory acidosis is corrected early, artificial ventilation is necessary.

Severe hypercapnia narcotizes the respiratory center in the medulla. When this happens the respiratory drive then originates from the peripheral chemoreceptors, i.e., carotid and aortic bodies. These chemoreceptors respond to the low PaO_2. High concentrations of oxygen must be avoided in treatment, or else this hypoxic respiratory drive will be suppressed. Controlled-flow oxygen therapy is given according to the patient's requirements, as indicated by his blood gases.

CYANOSIS

Cyanosis is a bluish discoloration of the skin, mucous membranes, and nail beds which occurs with changes in the circulating blood (rather than from pigmentary changes in the skin). Cyanotic discolorations may be gray, pale violet, blue, purple, or almost black. Although anoxemia is the most common cause of cyanosis, this discoloration may also result from other pulmonary or extrapulmonary factors, occurring singly or in combination. Pulmonary abnormalities that may produce cyanosis include insufficient alveolar ventilation, impaired diffusion from alveoli to capillaries, and abnormal perfusion-ventilation relationships. Pulmonary and extrapulmonary disorders that produce severe cyanosis include advanced chronic pulmonary disease, polycythemia, congestive heart failure, and some congenital cardiovascular defects.

As mentioned previously, *cyanosis is not an early indication of hypoxia.* In cyanosis resulting from a lack of O_2 in the blood the presence and depth of the cyanotic discoloration results from the amount of reduced hemoglobin (Hgb) present in the blood. Cyanosis does not appear until an excess of reduced Hgb is present, i.e., 5 Gm. or more of reduced Hgb/100 ml. of blood. A marked and even dangerous reduction of arterial O_2 tension (PaO_2) can occur before observable cyanosis appears. Cyanosis usually develops when the blood is about 85 per cent saturated with O_2 (PaO_2 about 50 mm. Hg).[142] In patients with anemic or histotoxic hypoxia, severe hypoxemia may occur without cyanosis. In contrast to this situation, only slight hypoxemia may produce cyanosis in a patient with polycythemia.

POLYCYTHEMIA

Disorders causing chronic pulmonary insufficiency (e.g., chronic obstructive pulmonary diseases) produce chronic hypoxemia (anoxemia). In turn, chronic hypoxemia often causes an impressive increase in the total erythrocyte mass, i.e., polycythemia. The polycythemia develops as a compensatory response to hypoxemia and represents the body's attempt to increase the blood's oxygen-transporting capacity by increasing the number of RBC. This compensatory response is not without its problems, however, because the increase in the number of RBC also thickens the blood, thereby increasing the likelihood of embolism and thrombosis and making it difficult for the heart to pump the thickened blood. Usually the disadvantages of the increased blood viscosity outweigh the advantage of increased O_2 capacity. Polycythemia is particularly dangerous in the patient who has cor pulmonale. (Polycythemia is discussed in Unit XII.)

PULMONARY OSTEOARTHROPATHY

Pulmonary osteoarthropathy is also called *secondary hypertrophic osteoarthropathy,* or sometimes is loosely referred to as simply *clubbing of the fingers and toes*. Although such clubbing is one manifestation of pulmonary osteoarthropathy (Fig. 69–2), there are others, e.g., arthralgia and subperiosteal proliferation in the long bones. These changes in bones and soft tissues of the extremities occur in chronic pulmonary as well as nonpulmonary disorders (e.g., congenital heart disease, hepatic cirrhosis) and may also occur as a congenital trait. Pulmonary conditions that may produce osteoarthropathy include bronchial carcinoma, pulmonary abscess, and bronchiectasis. Although the pathogenesis of pulmonary osteoarthropathy is not well understood, it is believed to result from increased vascularity developing in response to chronic hypoxia.

COR PULMONALE

Cor pulmonale (CP) refers to the chronic or acute enlargement of the heart's right ventricle, secondary to a disorder of respiration (e.g., neuromuscular disorders of the muscles of respiration) or disease of the lungs or pulmonary vasculature. Most commonly CP is chronic and results from chronic obstructive pulmonary diseases, e.g., pulmonary emphysema, chronic bronchitis. A massive pulmonary embolism may produce acute cor pulmonale. Heart failure may or may not accompany the condition. Acute pulmonary infections or other conditions that acutely increase arterial hypoxemia may produce acute, reversible episodes of CP in patients with chronic pulmonary disorders.

Factors operative in the development of CP and right-sided heart failure may include: (1) reduction in the size of the pulmonary vascular bed as a result of destruction of pulmonary capillaries or loss of large amounts of lung tissue; (2) increased resistance in the pulmonary vascular bed; (3) shunting of unaerated blood; and (4) the effect of reduced blood O_2 in causing pulmonary vasoconstriction and elevation of pressure in the pulmonary artery. The most common direct cause of CP is pulmonary arterial hypertension.

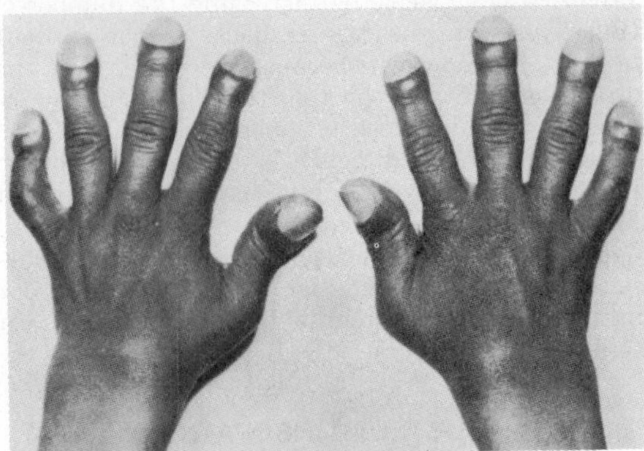

FIGURE 69–2. Clubbing of the fingers seen in pulmonary osteoarthropathy. (From Sedlock, S. A.: *American Journal of Nursing*. 72:1407, August, 1972.)

The hypertensive effect of arterial hypoxemia is increased by the respiratory acidosis that occurs with advanced chronic obstructive pulmonary disease. Arterial hypoxemia can induce an increase in cardiac output and produce a secondary polycythemia (which increases blood viscosity and volume). The hypoxemia thus exacerbates the effect of pulmonary hypertension.

Clinical indications of CP may include dyspnea, cyanosis, cough, substernal pain, syncopal attacks upon exertion, a loud pulmonic second sound (P_2), and a precordial systolic lift. In the presence of heart failure the patient develops orthopnea, peripheral edema, and distended jugular veins. With CP the chest x-rays demonstrate the enlarged pulmonary artery and right ventricle. In advanced CP there is evidence on the electrocardiogram of right ventricular hypertrophy.

Pulmonary hypertension may initially occur only when pulmonary blood flow is increased (e.g., with exercise or fever), but eventually it becomes continuous. Hypertrophy and dilation of the muscle of the right ventricle of the heart then develop and eventually heart failure occurs. Right-sided heart failure increases the work of the right ventricle and reduces cardiac output. Many patients with chronic obstructive pulmonary disease eventually die from heart failure when the overloaded heart reaches its limit of muscular compensation.

The *treatment* of congestive heart failure due to CP is complex and may include O_2 therapy, sodium restriction, rest, diuretics and digitalis. Digitalis toxicity must be closely watched for because it commonly occurs in patients with CP. (Heart failure and its management are discussed in Unit X.)

RESPIRATORY INSUFFICIENCY AND RESPIRATORY FAILURE

Respiratory insufficiency and failure are common clinical disorders. In simple terms, *respiratory insufficiency* means that respiratory function is inadequate to meet the body's needs *during exertion*. Exertional dyspnea is a common symptom of respiratory insufficiency and is caused by inability of the lungs to exchange gases efficiently during physical effort. *Respiratory failure* means that *even while resting*, respiratory function is inadequate; the lungs fail to maintain normal arterial blood gases because of thoracopulmonary or neuromuscular disorders that affect respiration. Focusing on abnormal blood gas levels as evidence of "respiratory failure" is analogous to identifying abnormalities of the blood urea as evidence of "renal failure." Most commonly, respiratory failure develops as a continuation of unrecognized or inadequately treated respiratory insufficiency.

In spite of the fact that respiratory insufficiency and failure have rather precise definitions, it is not unusual to find the terms used interchangeably. For example, instead of saying that a patient is in "respiratory failure," some physicians indicate the patient is in a "severe or extreme state of respiratory insufficiency." Possibly the two states can most easily be envisioned as existing on a continuum progressing from mild respiratory insufficiency to severe respiratory failure and death (if unrelieved by treatment).

> *Early recognition and treatment of respiratory insufficiency is imperative to prevent development of respiratory failure.*

Etiology

Respiratory insufficiency and failure may develop from a wide variety of conditions. Basically these conditions can be divided into three major groups: impaired ventilation, impaired diffusion and gas exchange, and ventilation-perfusion abnormalities and venous admixture (Table 69–2).

Some mechanisms operative in the development of respiratory insufficiency are illustrated in Figure 69–3.

Acute respiratory failure (ARF) most commonly results from chronic obstructive pulmonary disease complicated by conditions such as an exacerbation of bronchial infection, congestive heart failure, chest trauma (surgical or accidental), pulmonary embolism, or increased bronchospasm. In these situations a ventilation/perfusion disorder is added to the patient's pre-existing ventilatory disorder. ARF may occur in any person who develops disorders that acutely impair respiration, e.g., overwhelming pulmonary infections, reflex bronchospasm, acute left ventricular failure.

Chronic respiratory insufficiency or failure results from progressive diffuse degenerative disorders that cause destructive changes in alveolar and capillary structure, e.g., pulmonary emphysema, pulmonary fibrosis. Inadequate pulmonary ventilation typically causes the $PaCO_2$ to rise and the PaO_2 and pH to fall. When a patient's ventilatory disorder develops slowly his body is able to compensate gradually for the elevated partial pressure of CO_2 through elimination of chloride and the retention of base and bicarbonate. The CO_2 content is elevated and the serum chloride is low.

Frohlich observes that respiratory insufficiency often develops in two phases:[95]

> A period of adequate compensation occurs in which the patient compensates for abnormal gas exchange by increasing perfusion and/or ventilation. Increasing the car-

TABLE 69–2. DISEASE STATES PRODUCING RESPIRATORY FAILURE*

I. Impaired ventilation
   A. Chronic airway obstruction
      Emphysema, chronic bronchitis, asthma
   B. Restrictive defects
      1. Decreased lung expansion
         Interstitial fibrosis, pleural effusion, pneumothorax, fibrothorax
      2. Limited thorax expansion
         Kyphoscoliosis, multiple rib fractures, thoracic surgery, spinal arthritis
      3. Decreased diaphragmatic movement
         Abdominal surgery, ascites, peritonitis, severe obesity
   C. Neuromuscular defects
      Polio, Guillain-Barré syndrome, multiple sclerosis, myasthenia gravis, botulism, tetanus; brain or spinal injuries; drugs or toxic agents (e.g., curare, acetylcholinesterase inhibitors, colistin, kanamycin, streptomycin, neomycin)
   D. Respiratory center damage or depression
      Narcotics, barbiturates, tranquilizers, anesthetics; cerebral infarction or trauma; high flow, uncontrolled oxygen therapy

II. Impaired diffusion and gas exchange
   A. Pulmonary fibrosis
      E.g., sarcoidosis, Hamman-Rich syndrome, pneumoconioses
   B. Pulmonary edema
   C. Obliterative pulmonary vascular disease
      Thromboembolism with blood, fat, bone marrow, or amniotic fluid
   Anatomic loss of functioning lung tissue
      Pneumonectomy, tumor

III. Ventilation-perfusion abnormalities and venous admixture
   Emphysema, chronic bronchitis, bronchiolitis, atelectasis, pneumonia, thromboembolism, postperfusion syndrome and congestive atelectasis

*From Bigelow, D. B., et al.: *Medical Clinics of North America, 51*:323, March, 1967.

diac and pulmonary work in this way enables the maintenance of nearly normal blood gases. Patients with chronic obstructive pulmonary disease who are experiencing these increases in cardiopulmonary work are often referred to as *pink puffers*.

> The patient enters a phase of inadequate compensation in which alveolar hypoventilation develops as a result of increased resistance to breathing. This phase is characterized by severe hypoxia and CO_2 retention. Also, secondary polycythemia, cor pulmonale, and tissue edema frequently develop. Patients with chronic obstructive pulmonary disease in the phase of inadequate compensation are commonly described as *blue bloaters*.

Frohlich comments:

> The tempo of progression from the first to the second stage is highly variable, and indeed, the order in which they appear may vary. In addition, there seems to be no correlation between the degree of compensation and the severity of the patient's symptoms. In fact, many patients who are maintaining relatively normal blood gas tensions, although at the cost of a marked increase in respiratory work, are much more disabled than others who have chronic hypoxia and hypercapnia.[95]

The patient in chronic pulmonary insufficiency or failure may be able to compensate for his high $PaCO_2$ level for a while. However, this delicate balance can easily be upset if the patient experiences added stress. For example, the patient with chronic obstructive pulmonary disease (COPD) may be able to manage fairly well from day to day even though his blood gas levels are not "normal." But if he develops a respiratory infection (i.e., an added stress) he may rapidly develop acute respiratory failure in which his $PaCO_2$ levels continue to spiral upward while his pH levels decline.

Clinical Manifestations

Because respiratory insufficiency and respiratory failure both result from impaired alveolar gas exchange, the predominant clinical findings in these disorders are abnormal arterial blood gas values. The abnormalities that may be present are *hypoxemia,* indicated by a fall in the arterial oxygen pressure (PaO_2), and *hypercapnia* or hypercarbia, indicated by an elevated arterial CO_2 pressure ($PaCO_2$). For practical purposes it is possible to identify two clinical patterns distinguishable by the presence or absence of hypercarbia. Hypercapnia develops only when hypoventilation and/or ventilation-perfusion disorders are present. Hypoxemia without hypercapnia may occur when the pulmonary capillary bed is reduced or the alveolar-capillary membrane is thickened. Symptoms of hypoxia and hypercapnia are summarized in Table 69–3.

Symptoms vary, depending upon the underlying disorder and the severity and acuteness or chronicity of the pulmonary insufficiency or failure.

> "The clinical picture resulting from disturbances in the exchange of O_2 and CO_2, which may not be equally affected, depends partly on the preexisting state of the patient, especially his cardiopulmonary and renal status. His condition is affected not only by the level of blood gases, but also by the rapidity with which increased hypercapnia and hypoxemia develop. If CO_2 retention occurs slowly, there is time for the kidneys to excrete chlorides and reabsorb bicarbonate and sodium ions, thus maintaining the blood pH within normal range. If CO_2 accumulates too rapidly or in too great excess for the renal mechanisms to compensate, the pH falls below 7.38 and respiratory acidosis results.[200]

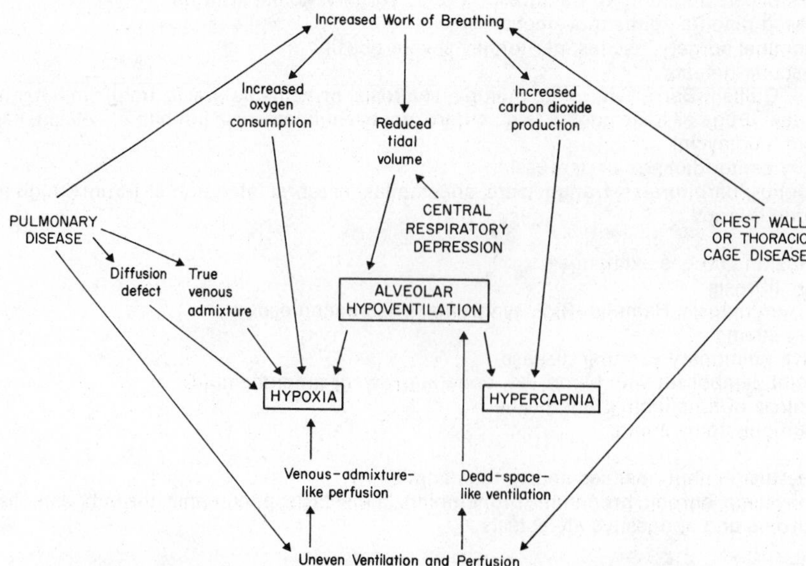

FIGURE 69–3. The mechanism of development of respiratory insufficiency. (From Cherniack, R. M., Cherniack, L., and Naimark, A.: *Respiration in Health and Disease.* 1961.)

The *early* cerebral manifestations of acute respiratory failure are anxiety, restlessness, dyspnea, and headache; *late* cerebral manifestations are somnolence, mental confusion, increased spinal fluid pressure, papilledema, and coma.

The following symptoms and signs indicate impending or actual *inadequacy of the muscles of respiration:*

> Gradual increase in blood pressure and pulse rates.
> Restlessness and irritability.
> Shallow, rapid respirations with flaring of the alae nasi, i.e., the cartilaginous expansions that form the outer, curving side of each nostril.
> Inability to repeat three or four numbers without pausing for breath.
> Use of the accessory muscles of respiration or purely diaphragmatic breathing.
> Absence of normal retraction of the lower intercostal spaces during inspiration.
> Asymmetry of movement of the thorax, particularly with deep respirations.
> Inability to sniff (an activity related to the diaphragm).

The nurse has an important role in observing for and promptly reporting symptoms of acute respiratory insufficiency or failure. *Early detection* of these disorders improves chances of providing effective treatment.

Diagnosis

In reaching a diagnosis the physician correlates clinical observations with knowledge of the patient's blood gases, pulmonary function tests, and the basic clinical disorder. Ultimately accurate diagnosis of respiratory insufficiency or failure requires demonstration of abnormal blood gas levels and pH values, since there are no specific physical symptoms upon which a purely clinical diagnosis can be made. The suggested figures for a diagnosis of pulmonary failure are a $PaCO_2$ of 50 mm. Hg or more, and a PaO_2 of less than 50 mm. Hg.

Laboratory tests are essential. Arterial blood is drawn as soon as possible for blood gas ($PaCO_2$ and $PaCO_2$) determinations. This procedure is usually repeated hourly until the patient's condition is stabilized. These laboratory evaluations monitor changes in alveolar ventilation and are the only methods for accurately identifying dangerous abnormal levels. On the basis of laboratory findings therapy is planned to correct respiratory acidosis and to ensure adequate oxygenation of body tissues.

Simple spirometric measurements may be performed at the bedside. Usually a chest x-ray, electrocardiogram, sputum culture and sensitivity, blood count, and determination of blood electrolytes are also ordered while emergency care is being given. The hematocrit is useful in detecting a reduced O_2-carrying capacity (anemia) or an excessive increase in the number of RBC (polycythemia). Although polycythemia may result from increased bone marrow activity in response to chronic hypoxemia, it may also be due to hemoconcentration resulting from dehydration.

Clinical Care

Treatment of *chronic pulmonary insufficiency* is basically symptomatic and supportive. Clinical care focuses on the underlying disorder, maintenance of effective tracheobronchial hygiene, prevention of infection, avoidance of bronchial irritation, and limitation of activity. (These aspects of care are discussed more completely in the section on chronic obstructive pulmonary diseases, Chapter 71.) The use of tracheotomy in the treatment of chronic pulmonary inadequacy is debatable. Possible advantages (reduction of dead space and resultant improved alveolar ventilation) are carefully weighed against potential hazards of infection and inspiration of dry, unfiltered air which has bypassed the upper respiratory passages. When there are acute complications, however, tracheotomy is often indicated in chronic obstructive pulmonary insufficiency.

Episodes of *acute respiratory failure* (ARF) often may be prevented by the early detection and treatment of mild respiratory insufficiency. When acute pulmonary failure does develop the patient is best cared for in an intensive care setting staffed by personnel who are skilled in observation and the performance of clinical care, which often involves the use of complex mechanical devices; experienced in dealing with respiratory emergencies; and aware

TABLE 69–3. CLINICAL MANIFESTATIONS OF RESPIRATORY FAILURE*

Hypoxia	Hypercapnia
1. Restlessness: impaired motor function and judgment	1. Headache
2. Confusion, delirium	2. Dizziness
3. Unconsciousness	3. Confusion
4. Hypotension	4. Unconsciousness
5. Tachycardia	5. Twitching
6. Central cyanosis	6. Miosis, engorged fundal veins, papilledema
7. Warm extremities (vasodilatation) ?	7. Hypertension
	8. Sweating

*From Bigelow, D. B., et al.: *Medical Clinics of North America, 51*:323, March, 1967.

of the pathophysiology of the disorder being treated. The intensive care unit should be equipped with the necessary therapeutic aids and monitoring equipment. The patient in respiratory failure is highly susceptible to infection and may therefore be cared for in an isolation setting at times, e.g., with discarded gown and mask technique.

Acute respiratory failure is a medical emergency which, without proper treatment, rapidly progresses to irreversible cardiorespiratory failure and death.

The chances of successfully managing a patient in acute respiratory failure have improved in recent years as a result of increased understanding of the physiologic changes characteristic of pulmonary failure, perfected methods of clinical care and the development of precise laboratory techniques for measuring blood gases. With the provision of excellent care, many situations may be reversed which initially appear hopeless.

Because untreated respiratory failure is a terminal event, questions often arise about the advisability of heroically treating a given patient. If the physician knows the patient and realizes that heroic treatment will at best only restore him to a miserable existence, the physician may decide to treat the patient in a conservative, routine manner, e.g., tracheostomy and IPPB continuous ventilation may not be employed. Factors that influence the physician's decision in this matter include the expressed wishes of the patient or family members and the patient's history prior to the episode of failure.

Clinical care of patients with acute respiratory failure is directed basically at relieving hypoxia, hypercapnia, hypotension, and dyspnea by maintaining respiration and supporting circulation as necessary. Essential aspects of the management of acute failure are summarized in Table 69-4.

In providing *intensive nursing care* for the patient in acute respiratory failure, do not leave the patient unattended. Observe carefully for indications of significant changes, e.g., worsening of hypoxia and/or hypercapnia. Frequently assess the patient's status, i.e., vital signs, level of consciousness, effectiveness of coughing. Chart and report appropriate observations.

Calm and reassure the patient while giving care. Hyperactivity increases O_2 requirements; relieve the patient's anxieties and fears as much as possible by acting in an efficient, reassuring manner and providing supportive mental care. If the patient experiences confidence in your ability to help him he may be able to relax somewhat and to breathe more comfortably and effectively.

Maintenance of Ventilation and Oxygenation. Position the conscious patient sitting upright in a supported, forward-leaning position. Instruct the patient how to breathe most effectively. Meticulously maintain a patent airway. Suction as necessary. Check for upper airway obstruction and relieve it if present. Prevent aspiration. If the patient is stuporous or unconscious insert an oropharyngeal airway to prevent airway obstruction and to facilitate secretion removal (until endotracheal intubation or

TABLE 69-4. MANAGEMENT OF ACUTE RESPIRATORY FAILURE*

1. Improve ventilation and oxygenation
   a. Insure clear airway by tracheal suction, oral or nasal endotracheal intubation, tracheostomy, mucolytic agents; combat bronchospasm by intravenous aminophylline, hydrocortisone, and nebulized bronchodilator
   b. Give oxygen for cyanosis or hypoxemia
   c. Humidification of O_2 or air, especially with tracheostomy or endotracheal tube
   d. Assist ventilation with IPPB device (cuffed tracheostomy tube when indicated); control ventilation with automatic cycling with or without muscle paralyzing agents
2. Treat cardiac and circulatory status
   Obtain history of recent medications, particularly digitalis, steroids; obtain ECG; treat congestive heart failure, arrhythmias, venesection if necessary for hematocrit of 60 or over
3. Combat bronchopulmonary infection
   Obtain sputum smear, culture and sensitivity tests; start antibiotic therapy; take chest x-ray film, by portable equipment if necessary, and compare with previous films.
4. Monitor laboratory values
   a. Arterial pH, pCO_2 (and O_2 saturation or pO_2 if available)
   b. Serum bicarbonate, sodium, potassium, chloride
   c. Hematocrit
5. Attend to fluid and electrolyte balance
   Chart fluid intake and output; intravenous fluids, usually glucose in water; supplement potassium intake if indicated; intravenous sodium bicarbonate if needed for refractory respiratory acidosis

Avoid use of opiates, barbiturates and excessive digitalis.

Avoid use of 100% O_2 given by close-fitting mask or cuffed tracheostomy tube.

*From *Chronic Obstructive Pulmonary Disease: A Manual for Physicians.* Portland, Oregon, Oregon Thoracic Society, 1965.

tracheostomy can be performed). Perform emergency resuscitation if indicated.

Assist with bedside bronchoscopy, tracheostomy, or endotracheal intubation when these procedures are indicated. Bedside bronchoscopy may be required to remove mucus plugs or foreign objects from the tracheobronchial tree. At the time of bronchoscopy, specimens may be obtained and sterile saline may be instilled (to liquefy secretions).

Prevent depression of the respiratory and cough centers by medications or excessive O_2. Sedatives and narcotics that depress these centers are typically contraindicated in the presence of acute respiratory insufficiency or failure. However, if they are ordered, use these medications cautiously and be prepared to mechanically support ventilation, to artificially stimulate coughing, to remove secretions via suctioning, or to administer ventilatory stimulants if ordered, e.g., nikethamide (Coramine), caffeine sodium benzoate, or ethamivan (Emivan).

Oxygen therapy is started immediately to correct hypoxemia; however, precautions must be observed to prevent depression of the respiratory centers and the development of CO_2 narcosis in the presence of hypercapnia. The danger of administering high concentrations of O_2 to hypercapnic patients has been discussed previously. Controlled concentrations of O_2 may be administered via a nasal cannula or Venturi mask. (See also p. 919.)

Ventilation must be improved immediately. Be prepared to help to initiate and supervise mechanical ventilation, e.g., with IPPB. Keep a respirator available at the bedside. (See discussion of respirators in Chapter 70.) Some patients do not require total ventilatory support but do benefit from IPPB treatments with low-flow O_2 every hour or so to improve ventilation and reduce the $PaCO_2$ level. Those in extreme respiratory failure require continuous IPPB treatment via endotracheal intubation or tracheostomy. For cooperative patients the physician may initially assist ventilation with a face mask. Intubation may thus be avoided if the patient shows clinical improvement or if his blood gas measurements improve after one hour. If it is necessary to intubate the patient, an endotracheal tube is generally inserted; later, tracheostomy is performed if indicated.

A variety of therapeutic measures may be used to mobilize, liquefy, and remove secretions. (See p. 889.)

Treatment of Fluid-Electrolyte Imbalances. Excessive administration of parenteral fluids must be avoided; however, dehydration needs to be relieved by replacement of lost fluids. Maintaining body hydration helps to thin secretions. Activities useful in guiding fluid replacement therapy include evaluation of serum sodium and hematocrit levels, measurements of fluid intake and output, notation of skin turgor, and recording of daily body weight.

Serious acid-base imbalances develop when an episode of acute respiratory failure occurs in a patient who has chronic respiratory failure. Respiratory acidosis usually develops, and metabolic acidosis may also occur if there is severe hypoxemia. *Severe* acidosis (pH below 7.15) is a life-threatening condition; sodium bicarbonate is immediately administered intravenously. After 15 minutes the pH is again checked and treatment is re-evaluated. It is not uncommon for alkalosis to develop *during the treatment* of respiratory failure. This may occur because bicarbonate levels are often elevated and bicarbonate excretion by the kidneys is slower than the excretion of CO_2 by the lungs (if the lungs are being mechanically ventilated).

The evaluation and treatment of electrolyte imbalances may be complicated by the effects of steroid and diuretic therapy and the presence of compensated respiratory acidosis and/or congestive heart failure. With compensated respiratory acidosis the patient may have a serum chloride level that is low in relation to bicarbonate and a low body potassium in spite of a normal serum potassium and, hence, a heightened sensitivity to digitalis. If congestive heart failure develops, the levels of sodium and potassium are commonly reduced because of dilution an increased blood volume.

Often potassium depletion is present in patients with chronic respiratory failure. If these persons develop acute respiratory failure the potassium depletion is seriously worsened and must be replaced. Potassium is usually not given early in the course of mechanical ventilation. When respiratory acidosis increases in severity rapidly, the pH falls, potassium leaves the cells, and total body potassium depletion may occur even though serum potassium is normal. These processes are reversed and the serum potassium may be low, once the respiratory acidosis is corrected. When normal ventilation is achieved, potassium may be replaced in the form of oral potassium chloride, because chloride depletion may also have occurred. (For complete discussion of fluid-electrolyte balance and imbalances see Chapters 24 and 25.)

Treatment of Complications. Prevent the complications of inactivity. (See Chapter 27.) Remember to give *total* patient care and not focus your attention exclusively on the patient's respiratory system. Prevent the infections that can be introduced if unclean inhalation therapy equipment or unsterile suction catheters are used.

If infection is present, e.g., tracheobronchial or pulmonary infection, administer antibiotics as ordered. In some instances antibiotics are ordered prophylactically, before culture and sensitivity reports are returned, to prevent superinfection. In treating patients who are critically ill, penicillin (or cephalothin) and kanamycin may be started; in less critical situations ampicillin or tetracyclines may be used. Often in chronic obstructive pulmonary disease, infection is the precipitating cause of the episode of respiratory failure.

Relieve bronchospasm if present by administering prescribed bronchodilators, e.g., aminophylline, 500 mg. in 500 ml. dextrose and water I.V. every 4 to 6 hours, and isoproterenol (Isuprel) 1:200, 0.5 ml. diluted with 3 ml. of water and administered every 2 hours by IPPB nebulization for

15 minutes. Adrenocortical steroids may be given for some bronchospastic or inflammatory pulmonary disorders.

Correcting hypoxemia and acidosis, improving ventilation, and reversing the basic causes of the acute episode of respiratory failure are typically the most effective methods of treating right heart failure, if present. Other therapeutic procedures are to digitalize the patient and administer diuretics as indicated once ventilation is established. Digitalis must be used cautiously because, as mentioned earlier, the patient may have a heightened sensitivity to digitalis.

Intestinal and gastric decompression may be necessary to relieve abdominal distention, which impairs ventilation by elevating the diaphragm.

CHAPTER 70

Common Respiratory Therapeutic Measures

GENERAL MEASURES*

Posture; Positioning. The patient with a respiratory disorder can usually breathe most comfortably if positioned with his head and chest elevated. The severely dyspneic patient often needs to sit completely upright; patients with less severe respiratory distress may find a semiupright position suitable. Elevation of the chest and head makes ventilation of the lungs easier by permitting the lungs and respiratory muscles to function without being cramped. Sitting with the shoulders slightly pulled back enables unrestricted movement of the diaphragm and, hence, facilitates diaphragmatic breathing. To position the patient correctly, place a pillow lengthwise behind his back and head. Do not flex the head forward with another pillow.

The patient who is weak or severely dyspneic (e.g., during an asthmatic attack) commonly finds it more comfortable if positioned upright with a padded overbed table in front of him to lean on. Place a pillow on the overbed table and encourage the patient to rest his head and arms upon the pillow while leaning slightly forward. Raise siderails if indicated and be certain the patient has call bell, sputum cup, and tissues within easy reach.

A person with a chronic respiratory disorder can breathe more effectively if he maintains correct posture at all times, i.e., while standing, sitting, or lying down. Encourage the patient to observe his posture in a mirror and to maintain a straight posture with shoulders pulled back.

Room Environment. Patients with respiratory disorders are generally most comfortable in a cool environment. Individual preferences concerning room temperature should be respected. Air-conditioning may facilitate respirations by keeping the air cool and fresh. Maintain an environment that is free of unnecessary air pollution, e.g., smoke, aerosolized room deodorant sprays. Adequate humidification of air is important to prevent drying of secretions.

Activity; Rest. Some respiratory disorders force the patient to modify his normal activity pattern. With many acute disorders, e.g., influenza, the patient may need to rest in bed for several days but may return to his usual level of activity upon recovering. Chronic respiratory disorders may make it necessary for the patient to gradually curtail or modify his activities. The patient may be advised to change to more sedentary work or to retire. Unless prohibited by the physician, ambulation and other activities are encouraged within the limits of a patient's abilities. Remaining as active as possible not only helps a patient's general morale but also prevents the complications that result from inactivity. (See Chapter 27.)

Although it is important for the patient with a respiratory disorder to be active, adequate rest is also necessary. Often it is difficult to obtain sufficient rest because of disruptive symptoms, e.g., dyspnea, cough. The nurse attempts to identify and to correct conditions that are inhibiting rest. For example, she positions the dyspneic patient in such a way that breathing is facilitated and she insures adequate room humidification if a hacking cough is present. When prescribed, cough depressant medications given prior to the night's rest help to ensure a quiet night. Often planned periods of uninterrupted rest during the day are helpful, since respiratory disorders can be especially fatiguing.

Oral Hygiene. Frequent oral hygiene is important when a patient has a respiratory disorder, because cleansing of the mouth temporarily removes the unpleasant taste and odor of sputum. Oral hygiene refreshes the patient and makes him pleasant for others to be around. Also, it may improve the patient's appetite and general feeling of well-being. When antiseptic mouthwashes are used, the number of pathogens in the mouth are reduced, thereby also reducing the possibilities of pulmonary infection.

Nutrition; Appetite; Hydration. As stated above, the patient with a respiratory ailment may have a poor appetite because of the unpleasantness of sputum production. Appetite may also be impaired because of dyspnea, fatigue, nausea or other unpleasant symptoms. To enhance the patient's appetite, maintain a pleasant environment (e.g., place sputum bottles out of sight, replace soiled linens) and offer oral hygiene and handwashing before and after meals. Smaller, more frequent servings of food are generally tolerated better than three large meals. Gas-forming foods are unde-

*Many of these points of general importance are discussed as appropriate in greater detail elsewhere in this unit.

sirable, since they may restrict ventilation by producing abdominal distention. A variety of nongasforming foods and liquids should be offered so the patient can select items that he enjoys.

Optimal hydration helps to liquefy bronchopulmonary secretions so they can be more easily removed (thick, tenacious secretions are difficult to cough up and expectorate), and to prevent constipation and fluid imbalances. The patient with tenacious secretions is encouraged to have a high fluid intake (3000 to 4000 ml. daily) and to be sure that a large amount of his fluid intake is water. Milk should be avoided since it tends to thicken mucus.

Frequently it is desirable to maintain an intake-output record. When appropriate the patient may participate in keeping this record. If the patient's activities are restricted, make certain that ample fresh fluids are within easy reach at the bedside. Emphasize to the patient the importance of maintaining hydration and instruct him to develop a regular daily routine for taking fluids to ensure that his intake reaches the prescribed amount. Fluid intake may need to be restricted in the presence of renal or circulatory insufficiency.

Infection Prevention and Control. Instruct the patient with a respiratory disorder to remember the following points of importance in preventing the development of new respiratory infections: (1) wear warm, dry, protective clothing if it is necessary to be outside in cold or damp weather; (2) avoid excessive exertion in very cold or humid environments; (3) maintain a balanced pattern of work, rest, and recreation; (4) avoid crowds during periods when respiratory infections are prevalent; (5) do not smoke; (6) follow the doctor's advice concerning influenza shots and antibiotics; (7) observe the sputum for indications of infection (e.g., increased amounts of sputum, change in color of sputum); and (8) consult the doctor if a new infection seems to be developing. The patient with a chronic respiratory problem should seek early treatment of any new, acute infection. Even those infections that appear "minor" must be treated vigorously to prevent the development of a progressive, serious superinfection.

The nurse has many opportunities while giving patient care to prevent the development of new infections and/or to control existing infections. Patients especially susceptible to the development of pulmonary infections include those who are: bedridden or otherwise immobilized, e.g., in traction, paralyzed; in respiratory failure; tracheostomized; and/or being treated with inhalation machines, antibiotics, antimetabolites, or corticosteroids.

Opportunistic infections are of increasing importance. These infections may be hospital-acquired (nosocomial) or drug-induced; e.g., superinfections may develop during the administration of antibiotics, or infection may develop in patients receiving antimetabolites or corticosteroids. Nosocomial infections include those that a patient may acquire from the use of contaminated equipment such as suction or urethral catheters or inhalation machines. The development of nosocomial infections from contaminated equipment indicates a serious error in technique.

To effectively control infections or prevent their development the nurse observes prophylactic measures such as:

> Observing isolation, gown, mask, and handwashing techniques as necessary to prevent cross-contamination.

> Turning and repositioning patients frequently while they are in bed; encouraging activity, coughing, deep-breathing to mobilize secretions.

> Maintaining a clear airway and preventing atelectasis. When suctioning is indicated it should be gently performed and carried out as a sterile procedure. Tracheostomy care should also be given aseptically and atraumatically.

> Sterilizing inhalation therapy equipment frequently, e.g., IPPB valves, tubes, humidifiers.

> Restricting the number of visitors or staff members who have contact with a patient who is susceptible to infections or who has a communicable infection.

> Protecting patients from persons with upper respiratory or other infections, i.e., from staff members, visitors, other patients.

> Locating patients within a ward in such a way that spread of infection is not promoted; overcrowding should be avoided and patients with communicable infections should be segregated from noninfected patients.

> Maintaining an optimal level of personal resistance and of resistance in patients, e.g., ensure adequate rest, nutrition, hydration.

> Teaching patients methods of preventing the spread of air-borne infections. For example, teach the patient to cover his nose and mouth with disposable tissues when sneezing or coughing.

> Observing closely for indications of infections in patients receiving antimetabolites or corticosteroids and the development of superinfections in patients receiving antibiotics.

> Administering antibiotics as prescribed. Specific antibiotic therapy is based on bacteriologic culture and sensitivity reports. At times broad-spectrum antibiotics are prescribed before culture sensitivity reports are available.

Avoidance of Pulmonary Irritants. Chronic pulmonary diseases, such as chronic bronchitis and pulmonary emphysema, represent a major health hazard that has become of increasing significance in the past few decades. The incidence of lung cancer has also increased markedly during the twentieth century. *Cigarette smoking* is related to the increase in deaths from these diseases and is the major cause of chronic bronchitis and lung cancer in the United States (Fig. 70–1). *Air pollution* may be an additional factor in the increased incidence of these devastating pulmonary disorders.

The one most important cause of respiratory irritation is cigarette smoking.

Experimental studies indicate that certain gases in cigarette smoke and polluted air may damage bronchopulmonary function in the following ways: (1) cilia are destroyed, thus impairing the removal of mucus via action of the cilia; (2) mucous cells enlarge (hypertrophy) and secrete excessive

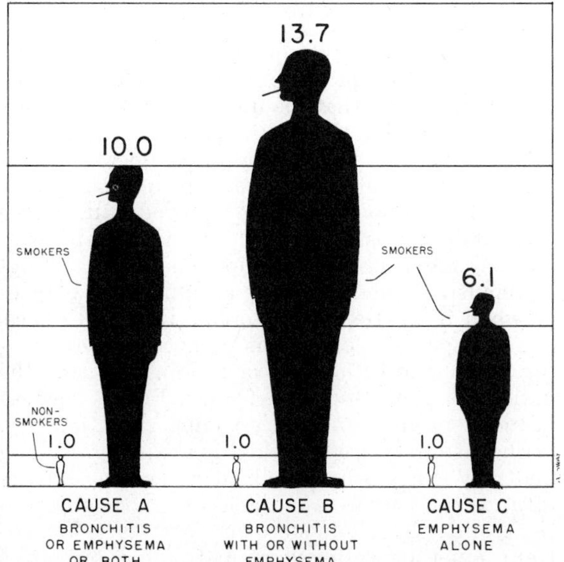

FIGURE 70–1. How heavy smokers compare with nonsmokers as victims of respiratory disease. (From *Breathing . . . What You Need to Know.* American Lung Association, 1968.)

mucus; (3) bronchial walls thicken and lose their elasticity; (4) alveolar-capillary membranes (through which O_2 and CO_2 exchange occurs) thicken; and (5) alveolar walls may rupture, producing large cavities in the lung parenchyma. These events cause numerous pulmonary problems. For example, reduced mucus flow, increased mucus production, and narrowing of the airways all contribute to *retention of secretions.* Retained secretions are an ideal site for the development of *infection.* Secretion retention and tracheobronchial irritation produce *coughing.* Narrowing and loss of elasticity of the bronchi produce *difficulties in moving air in and out of the lungs.* Expiration is usually abnormally prolonged and may be accompanied by wheezing sounds. Impaired lung capacity causes the patient to experience *dyspnea upon exertion.* Thickening of the alveolar membranes and breaking down of alveolar walls causes *impaired gas exchange.* Thickened membranes impede the transfer of gases across the membranes; normally alveolar membranes are extremely thin, delicate structures. Destruction of the alveolar walls not only reduces the amount of alveolar membrane surface available for gas exchange, but also reduces the blood supply coursing through the lungs because destruction of alveolar walls destroys the capillaries within the walls.

Cigarette smoking and air pollution are preventable situations; however, their prevention is not easily achieved. Habitual cigarette smoking is a practice that involves complex psychosocial-economic factors. The manufacturing and sale of cigarettes is financially a profitable business. Legislators are reluctant to prohibit by law behavior such as smoking.

Smoking is clearly contraindicated in the presence of bronchopulmonary and numerous other disorders involving the heart, blood vessels, stomach, trachea, and larynx. However, habitual smokers with such disorders often find it extremely difficult, perhaps impossible, to stop smoking. Nurses participate actively, but not judgmentally, in trying to help patients to stop smoking by providing encouragement and education. Educational materials designed for patient use may be obtained from agencies such as the American Heart Association, American Cancer Society, and the American Lung Association. Numerous opportunities arise for nurses to present factual information about cigarette smoking to patients as well as community members. Of course, nurses who refrain from smoking encourage others to make a similar individual decision. It is especially important for young people to be convinced that they should never begin to smoke.

A patient with a pulmonary disorder who smokes may believe that his condition will not improve if he discontinues cigarette smoking. He should be told that if he stops smoking he may prevent or at least slow down further deterioration of lung function, his cough should decrease, and his sputum production will decrease in amount. He should understand that if he cannot completely stop smoking it is certainly desirable to reduce the number of cigarettes smoked and to stop inhaling. However, smoking even one cigarette can worsen the symptoms of pulmonary disorders by causing bronchospasm and irritation of the mucosa of the tracheobronchial tree.

Smoking threatens health not only because of its relationship to lung cancer but also because it is a factor in other serious disorders. For example, smoking is known to be a factor in cardiac and circulatory disorders. Also, the mortality ratio of cigarette smokers compared with nonsmokers is high in other disorders such as oral cancer, peptic ulcer, and cancer of the larynx and esophagus.

During the process of breaking the habit of smoking the ex-smoker may be quite irritable and nervous. The physician may prescribe a tranquilizer as a means of helping the patient through this difficult time. He should be assisted to find ways of relieving his anxieties and tensions other than by smoking. For example, physical activities such as exercising or performing small repetitive motor movements (chewing gum, or handling a pen or pencil) may be helpful. Or the patient may obtain some relief by periodically inhaling deeply, as if he were smoking. Assistance, encouragement, and understanding given the patient by others during the withdrawal period can be very helpful. Even if the patient occasionally "slips" and "lights up," the overall progress he has made in cutting down on his smoking should be praised. The patient who is trying to stop smoking should not be treated like a child (e.g., "scolded") if he smokes. He is in the process of making a serious adult decision upon which his life may depend.

As mentioned before, some people cannot stop smoking. Psychosocial reasons that are difficult to identify, and that may be more important to the involved individuals than health and life, compel them to continue smoking. These people may become highly defensive about their smoking, even though they may inwardly be deeply distressed about being unable to control their own behavioral patterns. Feelings of guilt, depression, and loss of self-esteem often occur when such persons develop illnesses that they view as self-inflicted as a result of habitual smoking, e.g., lung cancer, chronic bronchitis.

Smoking can be viewed as both a private and a public concern, since cigarette smoke not only "pollutes" the body of the smoker but also contributes to general air pollution around the smoker and thus affects other persons. Increasing attempts are being made to permit nonsmokers to be segregated from smokers if they so wish.

General air pollution varies from time to time and from place to place. Public and governmental actions have in recent years been directed at minimizing air pollution. These activities require the continued support of concerned citizens. It has been clearly demonstrated that acute episodes of air pollution, e.g., in heavily industrialized communities, are associated with increased death and illness rates. These rates are particularly high among persons with chronic cardiac and pulmonary disorders. Persons with such disturbances who live or work in environments that have a high level of air pollution may be advised by their physicians to move or to change occupations.

There are *other pulmonary irritants* that should be avoided by persons with pulmonary disorders. Among these are airborne allergens, excessively cold or dry air, and some aerosolized products, e.g., spray deodorants, hair sprays. (See discussions elsewhere in this unit.)

Nurse-Patient Relationships. Chronic pulmonary disorders and cancer of the lung are examples of some respiratory conditions that may be especially difficult for patients to accept. As previously mentioned, patients with these disorders who have smoked heavily for a number of years often have feelings of guilt and anger about the possible association of their smoking habits with their illnesses. The nurse is *not* helpful in situations of this kind if she adopts a vituperative "you should have known better" attitude. Both nurse and patient must have realistic attitudes about the patient's condition and adopt realistic goals. For example, lungs that have been severely damaged, e.g., with chronic obstructive disease, cannot be permanently or markedly improved in function. However, some improved function may be possible, and that degree of improvement may be enough to make the patient feel better and increase his activity. An attitude of hopelessness on the part of nurse or patient is defeating. With encouragement and a sense of confidence, much can be accomplished, and symptomatic relief may be obtained even though the prognosis is guarded. The patient must feel that the nurse not only *gives* him care, but also that she cares *about* him.

Some symptoms caused by respiratory disorders may be disturbing for both patient and nurse. For example, the patient who is producing large amounts of foul-smelling sputum may feel unclean and be embarrassed. The nurse may have feelings of repulsion when handling contaminated articles or when the patient expectorates in her presence. Some respiratory conditions produce life-threatening feelings of suffocation or choking, causing the patient to panic and fight for air. Events such as acute respiratory failure, crushing chest injuries, or chest surgery are often highly anxiety provoking and may evoke concerns about dying. The nurse's attitude can help to calm the fearful, struggling patient while she administers necessary care. The patient must be relieved of disturbing anxieties whenever possible since these feelings worsen such bronchopulmonary symptoms as dyspnea and bronchospasm.

The patient's behavior may be influenced not only by psycho-emotional disturbances but also by physical factors. For example, metabolic imbalances such as abnormal blood gas levels may affect behavior. Fatigue, caused perhaps by the effort of breathing or lack of sleep, may cause the patient to be irritable and depressed. The nurse helps staff members and members of the patient's family to try to understand what the patient may be experiencing and to learn effective ways of being helpful.

Numerous serious problems must often be dealt with by a patient with a chronic pulmonary disorder: The patient may have socioeconomic concerns. Prolonged illness is expensive; the patient may need to pay for hospitalizations, physicians, and medications. Also, he may need to purchase or rent equipment, e.g., IPPB machine. Illness may not only force the patient to leave work but also may keep him from participating in social activities he enjoys. Infectious conditions such as tuberculosis may cause him to feel that a stigma has been placed on his life. Chronic respiratory disorders like emphysema impair normal sexual activity and thus remove the patient even further from his normal life pattern and his pre-illness self-image.

The patient with chronic pulmonary disease must learn to adapt to limitations imposed by his illness. He must accept that the goal of care is to *preserve* existing lung function, rather than to *restore* normal function. In this learning-adjustment process the patient can be helped by others, but he also must help himself. When an effective, therapeutic nurse-patient relationship exists, the nurse provides services both directly and indirectly beneficial to the patient. In addition to providing help within the boundaries of the nursing role, the nurse participates in making referrals to qualified persons who are of assistance in other ways, e.g., social workers.

Like many other illnesses, chronic respiratory disorders, lung cancer, or other pulmonary disorders may be denied by the affected persons until symptoms eventually force recognition of the illness. Once they do seek medical care, some patients hesitate to participate in the recommended therapy programs. These reluctant patients must be assisted to understand ways in which therapy will actually be of benefit. Emphasize that therapy is helpful even though improvement may not be rapidly apparent. Patient participation in many aspects of pulmonary therapy programs is essential. Self-care activities may include performing postural drainage and breathing exercises, forcing fluids, taking medications, and administering respiratory therapy. Praise patients who faithfully follow their recommended therapy regimens and encourage those who feel discouraged.

Respect for a patient's preferred activity schedule is especially important when caring for a patient with a pulmonary disorder. The dyspneic patient may require frequent rest periods and usually knows when he can most comfortably be active during the day. The patient who is producing large amounts of sputum may require pulmonary therapy techniques, e.g., postural drainage, before he can get out of bed in the morning. Nett and Petty[214] observe that patients with emphysema may develop ritualistic, compulsive tendencies concerning their bronchial hygiene and physical therapy programs. These tendencies should not be interfered with but rather should be viewed as useful and necessary for the patient.

PHARMACOLOGIC AGENTS

A variety of pharmacologic agents may be used to treat patients with pulmonary disorders. Some of the more common of these drugs are presented briefly in the following overview. Medications are discussed further throughout the unit in relation to specific conditions. Space does not permit detailed discussions of individual medications; consult a textbook of pharmacology for necessary details.

Antihistamines. Antihistamines are used to treat disorders caused by allergic reactions, e.g., bronchial asthma. Examples of antihistamines include brompheniramine maleate (Dimetane), chlorpheniramine maleate (Chlor-Trimeton), diphenhydramine hydrochloride (Benadryl), and tripelennamine citrate (Pyribenzamine). Drug hypersensitivity is discussed in Chapter 23.

Antimicrobials. Examples of antimicrobials used to combat pulmonary infections are tetracyclines, penicillin, cephalosporin antibiotics (cephalothin, Keflin), streptomycin, sulfonamides, and erythromycin. At times antibiotics are administered via aerosol to treat tracheobronchial infections, so that the particles of the drug may reach the air passages.

Bronchodilators. Bronchodilating agents are administered via several different routes: I.V., subcutaneously, rectally, orally, or by inhalation (by hand nebulizer, premeasured pressurized hand cartridge, or humidification in an IPPB device).

Bronchodilators are commonly divided into two groups: (1) sympathomimetic medications, e.g., epinephrine hydrochloride (Adrenalin), isoproterenol hydrochloride (Isuprel), and ephedrine sulfate; and (2) theophylline preparations, e.g., aminophylline. The above medications act *directly* on bronchial smooth muscle to relieve bronchospasm. Other medications *indirectly* improve bronchial function; antibiotics and adrenocorticosteroids are good examples. Antibiotics combat infections that tend to increase mucus production and thus block bronchi, and adrenocorticosteroids such as prednisone reduce inflammation, which causes bronchial walls to thicken and thereby reduces the size of bronchial lumina.

Cough Medications. *Antitussive agents* inhibit the cough reflex in the cough center. Examples are benzonatate (Tessalon), codeine phosphate (Methylmorphine), noscapine (Nectadon), dextromethorphan hydrobromide (Romilar), methadone hydrochloride (Amidon, Dolophine); dimethoxanate hydrochloride (Cothera), dihydrocodeinone bitartrate (Dicodid, Hycodan), carbetapentane citrate (Toclase), and levopropoxyphene napsylate (Novrad).

Expectorants aid in the expectoration of secretions. Examples are saturated solution of potassium iodide or ammonium chloride to liquefy mucus; tyloxapol (Alevaire), a mucolytic (i.e., mucus-dissolving) detergent used to "clean out" the tracheobronchial tree and lungs; acetylcysteine (Mucomyst) to reduce the viscosity of secretions; sodium ethasulfate (Tergemist), a mucolytic detergent used to liquefy tenacious mucus; glyceryl guaiacolate (incorporated in Robitussin) to increase flow of secretions and reduce viscosity of inflammatory exudate in tracheobronchial tree; hydriodic acid syrup to liquefy viscous sputum; ipecac syrup, a nauseant expectorant; and terpin hydrate, used to reduce abundant sputum. Mucolytic agents may be administered locally via nebulization.

Many cough medications are prepared in syrup form. By reducing local irritation these soothing syrups may reduce afferent nerve impulses which arise in the respiratory tract. Cough syrups may be made by adding various medications to demulcents or emollients that coat and protect the mucous membranes. Instruct the patient *not* to take water for a while after swallowing a cough medication. Swallowing water (or other liquids, foods, or medications) washes the medication off the pharyngeal mucosa, thus circumventing the desired local soothing effect.

Enzymes. Certain mucolytic or proteolytic enzymes, e.g., trypsin (Tryptar) and streptokinase-streptodornase (Varidase), may be used to help to liquefy thick purulent sputum by digestion or to debride the lesions of empyema.

Gases. Examples of gases that may be used

therapeutically are carbon dioxide (CO_2), a respiratory stimulant (generally contraindicated in the presence of respiratory failure, cardiac decompensation, or pulmonary edema); oxygen (O_2), used to correct hypoxemia (in some situations high concentrations of O_2 can produce the serious problem of CO_2 narcosis, see p. 919); and helium, an inert gas used as a vehicle for the administration of other gases, e.g., with O_2 or general anesthetics. Carbon dioxide (in 5, 7, or 10 per cent mixtures with oxygen) may be used to treat hiccoughs. Oxygen therapy is discussed later in this chapter. Light, inert helium (in an 80 per cent mix with oxygen) may be used to replace the nitrogen content of air; it is believed this provides a gas mixture that can be transported with less effort in the airways.

Narcotic Antagonists. Narcotic antagonists are used to overcome respiratory depression caused by narcotic drugs. Respiratory depression can be a serious side effect of narcotic analgesics, barbiturates, and numerous tranquilizers and nonbarbiturate sedatives. In some situations (e.g., chest injury, pulmonary failure) respiratory depression is a life-threatening complication. Examples of narcotic antagonists are nalorphine hydrochloride (Nalline) and levallorphan tartrate (Lorfan).

Respiratory Stimulants. Central nervous stimulants that increase the activity of respiratory centers include bemegride (Megimide), caffeine and sodium benzoate, carbon dioxide gas, doxapram hydrochloride (Dopram), ethamivan (Emivan), nikethamide injection (Coramine), and pentylenetetrazol injection (Metrazol).

Vasoconstrictors and Decongestants. Medications in this classification may be used to treat allergic reactions and are given by diverse routes, e.g., topically (as nosedrops, sprays, and aerosols), parenterally, and orally. Examples are cyclopentamide hydrochloride (Clopane), ephedrine sulfate, isoproterenol hydrochloride (Isuprel), and phenylephrine hydrochloride (Neo-Synephrine).

PULMONARY PHYSIOTHERAPY

Activities that are part of a pulmonary physiotherapy program include breathing exercises, productive coughing techniques, and postural drainage with vibration and cupping. Emphasis is placed on teaching the patient the above techniques so he can effectively participate in his care and continue it as long as necessary on an outpatient basis. Family members who will assist the patient with pulmonary physiotherapy at home are often included in teaching sessions. In many large hospitals and clinics, pulmonary physiotherapy is performed by physical therapists. However, in other settings not staffed with these specially trained persons, it is often the nurse's responsibility to perform and teach techniques of pulmonary therapy. Even when physiotherapists are available, the nurse often becomes involved in the program by providing continued patient teaching and supervision.

Pulmonary physiotherapy is useful in the treatment of numerous respiratory disorders, e.g., bronchiectasis, chronic obstructive pulmonary disease, pulmonary emphysema, chronic bronchitis, bronchial asthma, and following chest surgery and chest injury. The patient with a chronic pulmonary problem should be told that it may take several weeks before his physical therapy program produces noticeable improvement. For example, it may take several weeks of practicing breathing exercises before a patient feels he is able to breathe more comfortably and with less effort. If the patient expects rapid improvement he may become discouraged and not participate in his therapy schedule. *For pulmonary physiotherapy activities to be effective they must be performed routinely and diligently.*

As a patient learns the techniques of pulmonary physiotherapy he gradually realizes that *he can* relax and control his breathing; *he can* breathe more effectively during dyspneic periods (if he practices slow controlled breathing rather than breathing rapidly and forcefully); and *he can* feel generally better and improve his lung function by faithfully following his prescribed schedule of exercises and postural drainage.

Space does not permit detailed discussions of the techniques of pulmonary physiotherapy; breathing exercises and postural drainage will be discussed briefly. For additional detail consult specialized references. Helpful pamphlets include those listed in the references as Numbers 39, 111, 173, 202, and 204. Helpful articles include references 55, 88, 164, and 249. Secor's book[267] is another useful reference.

Breathing Exercises*

Breathing exercises improve pulmonary ventilation and help the patient to conserve energy. Therapeutic breathing exercises teach a patient to use more efficient, relaxed patterns of ventilation. Controlled slow abdominal breathing is emphasized. Many breathing exercises focus on helping the patient to learn how to use his diaphragm and abdominal muscles more efficiently during ventilation and how to exhale more completely. The most important breathing muscles are pictured in Figure 70–2. In order for breathing exercises to be most helpful the patient needs also to maintain the general muscle tone of his body by following a recommended program of regular exercises.

Prior to beginning breathing exercises the patient should attempt to clear his respiratory tract of secretions. The nurse helps as necessary, e.g., by suctioning or stimulating productive coughing. Aerosol treatments may be given immediately before the breathing exercises are started to relax

*See also discussion of a coughing–deep breathing regimen in Chapter 73.

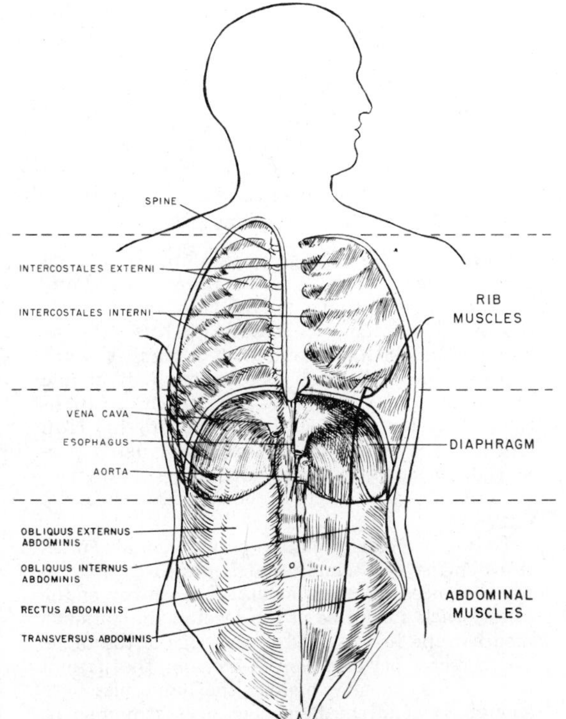

FIGURE 70–2. The most important of the breathing muscles. (From *Breathing . . . What You Need to Know.* American Lung Association, 1968.)

and open the air passages and to loosen tenacious mucus. Following aerosol treatments the patient is encouraged to cough effectively. Postural drainage may be employed to help to remove secretions. The nasal passages should also be cleared. If blowing the nose does not relieve nasal congestion, prescribed medications may be used to open nasal passages and shrink the nasal lining.

Many breathing exercises are performed with the patient lying flat (no pillow) on a firm surface. The ambulatory patient should perform most recumbent exercises on a carpeted floor rather than on a bed. Exercises cannot be effectively or comfortably carried out in tight, restrictive clothing.

Breathing exercise sessions are commonly scheduled two to four times daily, e.g., upon arising, before retiring and before meals, or in the late afternoon. The sessions should be relaxed and unhurried, with the patient resting as necessary. The length of the individual exercise periods is determined by the physician and by the patient's condition on any given day. Because the exercise sessions may sometimes last as long as an hour, it is often necessary for a patient to rearrange his usual routine to schedule time for physical therapy periods.

Abdominal ("Belly" or Diaphragmatic) Breathing. During abdominal breathing the abdomen visibly rises during deep inhalation and contracts during exhalation. With expiration the patient should feel his abdominal muscles tighten. Tightening the abdominal muscles helps the diaphragm to squeeze air out of the lungs. By placing one hand on his abdomen and the other on his chest, the patient can feel if he is breathing correctly while sitting up or reclining.

The basic position of the hands during breathing exercises is illustrated in Figure 70–3. Instruct the patient to always breathe in through his nose and to exhale by blowing gently out through slightly pursed lips (see below). Expiration should be a controlled, easy, comfortable act. During exhalation tell the patient to exhale air slowly while contracting his abdominal muscles. Pressure may be manually applied during exhalation by pressing on the upper abdomen or against the costophrenic angles. Complete exhalation is important. Teach the patient to relax the abdominal muscles while inhaling. Inhalation through the nose is desirable because nasal passages humidify and filter inspired air.

Once the patient has learned how to perform abdominal breathing effectively while flat on his back with his legs extended, he begins to practice it in other positions: lying flat on the floor with knees bent and thighs pulled toward the chest, lying on either side on the floor with knees bent and thighs pulled toward the chest, sitting on a chair, or standing. The patient also practices abdominal breathing while walking or exercising.

While abdominal breathing is initially an exercise that must be consciously performed, eventually it becomes unconscious and habitual. Controlled diaphragmatic breathing is particularly helpful to the patient with chronic obstructive pulmonary

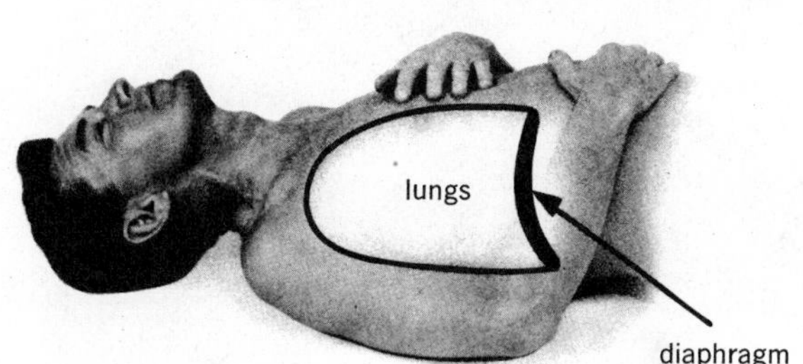

FIGURE 70–3. Basic position of hands during breathing exercises. The chest should move as little as possible. Note that the abdomen enlarges during inspiration and lowers during expiration. (From *Living with Asthma, Chronic Bronchitis, and Emphysema.* Northridge, California, Riker Laboratories, 1969.)

disease when he is exerting himself (e.g., climbing stairs) and during episodes of dyspnea. Gradually the patient learns to adjust his controlled breathing pattern to the rhythm of his body movements, e.g., walking. He develops a rhythm to his ventilation in which he takes at least twice as long to exhale as he does to breathe in. Some patients use a metronome to help them to establish this rhythm.

Various breathing exercises are directed at *forced exhalation,* forcing "trapped" air out of the lungs while using an abdominal breathing pattern. One method of forcing air from the lungs is as follows: while lying on his back the patient pulls his knees and thighs up tightly toward his chest *during exhalation* and then, after locking his hands over the tops of his knees, he pulls or squeezes his thighs down onto his chest, thus forcing accumulated air out of the lungs. A simpler method of forcing air from the lungs is to push on the chest with the flattened palms of the hands. Another exercise is to pull a band of material snugly around the chest while exhaling and relaxing the band during inhalation. Even tension should be applied during this exercise; the band of cloth should be a piece of tightly woven fabric (e.g., drapery pleating tape) that is at least 3 inches wide.

Pursed Lip Exhalation. In pursed lip exhalation the lips are positioned as if the patient were about to whistle (Fig. 70–4). Pursing the lips creates a resistance against the outflowing air. This resistance is desirable because it prevents collapse or narrowing of the airways during exhalation and helps to evenly distribute air throughout the lungs. As the patient exhales slowly he makes a soft blowing noise.

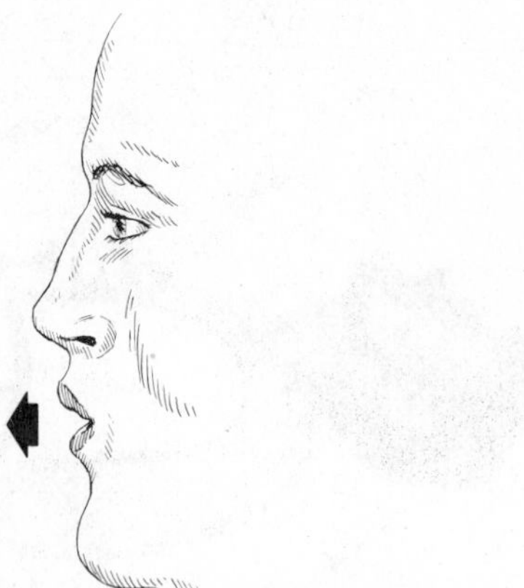

FIGURE 70–4. Pursing the lips has two advantages. Aside from increasing the pressure within the bronchus, it also prolongs the expiratory phase of breathing and converts the inefficient rapid panting into a slower respiratory rate which facilitates emptying the lung. (From Dirschel, K. M.: *Nursing Clinics of North America 8*(No. 4):617, December, 1973.)

Teach the patient to make a conscious effort to exhale slowly and as completely as possible. The patient may practice taking a deep breath, leaning forward from the waist and exhaling as completely as he can. Bending forward while walking also helps to make forced expirations possible.

While exhaling through pursed lips the patient can practice *blowing small objects* (Ping-Pong balls or pieces of chalk) around on a covered table top. A large table is necessary for this exercise. The top should be covered with a blanket which has its edges rolled up opposite the patient and on either side of the table. The patient positions himself at the edge of the table with his chin slightly above the table top. Then, using prolonged, smooth abdominal exhalations the patient tries to move the objects to the opposite side of the table.

To improve exhalation the patient can also practice blowing at a candle that is placed at increasing distances from his mouth. The height of the candle wick should be at the level of the patient's mouth while he is seated at the edge of the table. To correctly perform *candle blowing* the patient is instructed to blow against the flame just hard enough to bend the flame but not extinguish it. Slow, steady, prolonged exhalation is desirable. Initially the flame may be placed 6 inches from the patient's mouth. The distance is gradually increased 2 to 4 inches each day until the patient is able to carry out the exercise with the candle placed one yard away. Typically, candle blowing is practiced for 5 minutes at a time, once or twice each day.

Bubble blowing is another activity that improves ventilation. A blow bottle may be used for this exercise. The simplest blow bottle apparatus consists of a long glass tube extending beneath the water level in the bottle; the glass tube is connected to rubber tubing through which the patient blows. If a blow bottle is not available the patient may simply practice bubble blowing (for 3 minutes, 4 or 5 times daily) through a straw placed in a glass one third full of water.

All the above pursed-lip breathing exercises teach the patient to exhale in a slow, controlled manner while using muscles between the upper abdomen and lower thoracic rib cage.

Postural Drainage

Postural drainage clears the lungs of retained and infected secretions by using gravity to move the secretions instead of relying on the normal bronchial clearing mechanisms (which may be impaired as a result of injury or disease). The patient is placed in a position that gives maximum bronchopulmonary drainage by directing sputum from an involved peripheral area of the lung toward the hilum of the lung. Drainage of secretions to the more central portions of the tracheobronchial tree facilitates their expulsion by cough or by suction (if cough is ineffective). One controlled study by Lorin and Denning[176] demonstrated that postural drainage produced more than twice the volume of sputum produced by an equal period of coughing without postural drainage.

Postural drainage not only rids the lungs of infected material, and hence reduces sputum production and the absorption of toxic products, but also minimizes coughing and the development of atelectasis and bronchopulmonary infections. Additionally, postural drainage reduces the need for frequent, deep catheter aspiration in some patients.

Postural drainage is indicated in the treatment of numerous pulmonary disorders in which sputum production is copious and/or normal methods for clearing bronchopulmonary secretions are impaired, so that the patient cannot effectively cough and raise sputum. Examples of such disorders are chronic obstructive pulmonary disease (COPD), bronchial asthma, chronic bronchitis, pulmonary emphysema, bronchiectasis, pulmonary abscess, atelectasis, pneumonia, and following chest injury or chest surgery. Postural drainage is also used prophylactically to prevent secretion retention during prolonged artificial ventilation and in paralyzed or unconscious patients.

Postural Drainage Positions. Postural drainage can be accomplished by two major methods: (1) the patient remains for 5 to 15 minutes in one position without moving; or (2) the patient remains in one position for only a matter of seconds before he changes to another predetermined position. Space does not permit illustration or discussion of all the various positions that may be used to drain the various lobes and segments of the lungs. Some postural drainage positions are illustrated in Figure 70–5. Selection of the desired postural drainage position(s) is made after determining the area(s) of the lung(s) that require gravity drainage and after evaluating the patient's general condition and age. Skilled nurses learn to identify areas of the lung that should be drained by listening to the lungs to identify the location of rales and by palpating the chest for "rattles."

It is easier to remove secretions with postural drainage from the lower lobes of the lungs than from the upper pulmonary regions. This is generally fortunate, because man's usual upright position causes secretions to accumulate most often in the lower lung fields. Patients with extensive pulmonary impairment, e.g., those with COPD, may require drainage of all segments; these patients are placed in several drainage positions. If various positions are used for drainage, it is typical for the largest amount of secretions to be raised in the first head-low position used.

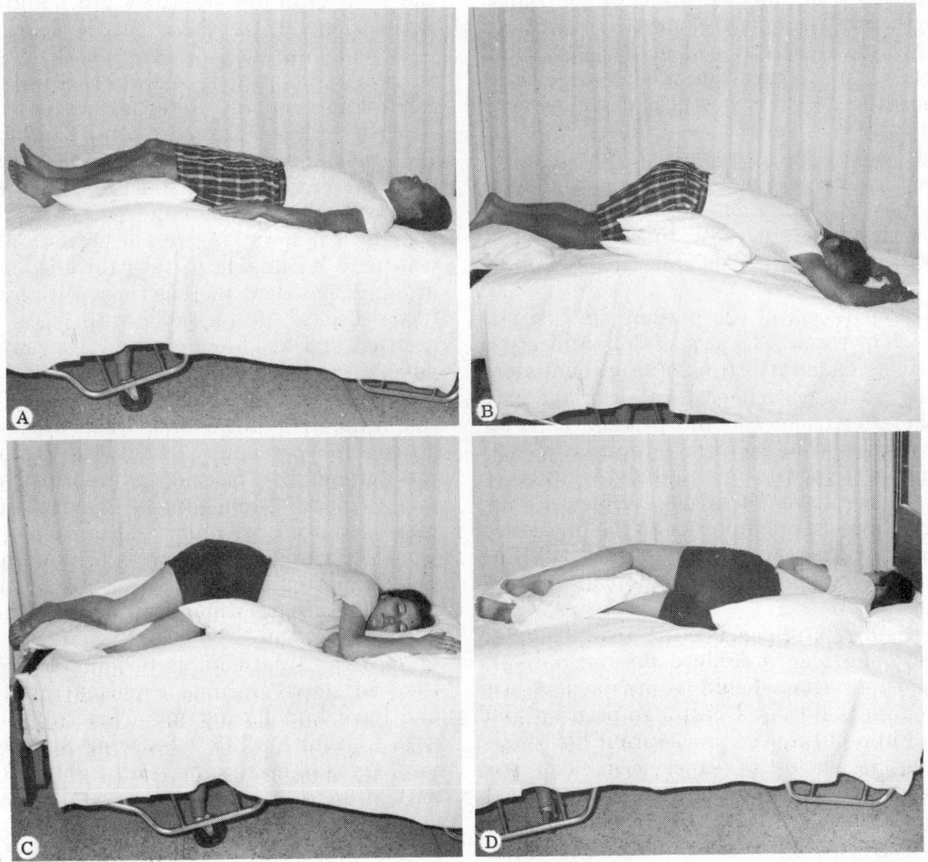

FIGURE 70–5. Some postural drainage positions. (From Krusen, F. H., Kottke, F. J., and Ellwood, P. M., Jr.: *Handbook of Physical Medicine and Rehabilitation.* 2nd ed. 1971.)

Procedure. In a hospital setting postural drainage may be carried out by using special equipment such as a tilt board, Stryker frame, or gatch bed. Another method is to elevate the foot of a bed on casters or on the seat of a sturdy chair. A common method is to elevate the knee-gatch of a gatch bed and position the patient with his head toward the foot of the bed and lying across the elevation in the bed, with his chest and head dependent. This "jack-knifed" position is most effective for draining the lower posterior lungfields (Fig. 70–5*B*).

It is desirable for a physiotherapist to provide the initial instruction for and supervision of postural drainage. However, when a physical therapist is not available a knowledgeable nurse performs these functions.

In preparation for the procedure the nurse identifies the affected area(s) of the lung(s) and familiarizes herself with the necessary postural drainage position(s) and the drainage pattern ordered by the physician. The nurse explains the routine to the patient and tells him his part in successfully performing the procedure. The patient is told that he will be positioned in such a way that the force of gravity, coughing, and deep breathing will help to drain secretions from affected areas of his lungs.

The length and frequency of postural drainage sessions are usually determined by the physician; however, the patient's condition may change these factors from time to time. Postural drainage may be ordered daily or several times a day, e.g., t.i.d., or every 4 hours. The procedure is particularly helpful upon awakening, before retiring, and prior to meals. Postural drainage sessions should be planned so they occur at least 45 to 60 minutes before meals and so they do not closely follow meals.

Physical preparation of the patient for postural drainage is important. The use of humidification procedures or the administration of bronchodilators or liquefying agents prior to postural drainage may increase the effectiveness of the procedure in removing secretions. Wait 10 to 15 minutes after administering bronchodilators and detergents to permit these medications to take effect. Other activities that may be helpful prior to the procedure are passively inflating the lung (e.g., with IPPB or an Ambu bag) or having the patient actively breathe deeply.

Because postural drainage is often an embarrassing and uncomfortable procedure for the patient, privacy and supervision should be provided. Assist the patient into the desired drainage position and remain with him during the procedure if his condition indicates he should be supervised. Some patients need to become accustomed to postural drainage positions. The time they remain in the desired position should be lengthened gradually until they can tolerate the drainage position for as long as 15 to 30 minutes, if so ordered. After positioning the patient correctly place a sputum container and a box of tissues within easy reach as well as a paper bag or wastebasket for discard of used tissues. Be certain the patient is protected from falling during the procedure. Assist him as he changes from side to side or from the supine to the prone position. If you must leave the patient unsupervised during this time be certain he has a call bell within easy reach.

While in the appropriate position(s) the patient should cough (a rapid firing of determined, easy little coughs) and deep breathe (exhaling slowly through the mouth). These activities enhance the removal of secretions and should be continued in each position (with rest periods as necessary) until no more sputum is produced. During postural drainage deep abdominal breathing helps to ventilate atelectatic regions of the lungs and encourages movement of secretions. If the patient cannot deep breathe and cough by himself, assistance should be given, e.g., inflate the lungs with a self-inflating (Ambu) bag and induce coughing. (Cough stimulation routines are discussed in Chapter 69.) A respiratory therapist may ventilate the patient during postural drainage. Perform clapping and vibrating of the chest wall during the drainage period as indicated by the patient's condition (see below). If the patient cannot cough up and expectorate his secretions, remove them with suction. Do not place such a patient in a postural drainage position until suction equipment is ready for use.

Closely observe elderly or weak patients during the time head-low positions are maintained. It is not uncommon for these positions to cause dizziness and faintness, or even shock or suffocation. Some patients cannot tolerate postural drainage or can tolerate it only if the positions are modified. At times, other treatments being administered, e.g., I.V. infusions, make it necessary to modify a postural drainage position. Modification of some positions may also be required because of injuries, e.g., head or spinal injuries or brain tumor. Patients who may be unable to tolerate head-low postural drainage positions include those with hypertension, heart disease, or unstable vital signs. The prone position and head-low position are contraindicated when a tracheostomy is present.

Postural drainage may evoke severe episodes of coughing. If a large bronchiole becomes blocked during the procedure (e.g., with a mucous plug) the patient may become severely dyspneic, weak, and cyanotic. Bronchoscopy may be necessary to remove the mucus plug. Sputum may or may not be raised while the patient is in the drainage position. Sometimes sputum is not raised until the patient resumes a normal position after the bronchial drainage session.

Once the treatment is terminated, help the patient to slowly resume a normal position in bed and have him lie flat for a few minutes. Remain with him for a while, observing his condition and vital signs to be sure he is all right. Encourage the patient to rest quietly to regain his equilibrium and strength before getting up or sitting upright. Following postural drainage, oral hygiene with an aromatic mouthwash is refreshing and should be offered.

After postural drainage has been completed, chart descriptions of the effectiveness of the procedure (e.g., type and amount of sputum produced) and how the patient tolerated the procedure. Be certain to report persistent dizziness or other symptoms.

Postural drainage procedures may need to be practiced at home by some persons, e.g., those with bronchiectasis, chronic bronchitis. Instruction is given in the hospital, clinic or home. The visiting nurse may initially supervise the procedure at home to be certain the patient understands the procedure and is performing it correctly. Encourage patients to practice postural drainage conscientiously when it is prescribed for them. Often patients neglect this procedure because it is "bothersome, time-consuming and uncomfortable."

Postural Drainage Exercises. Postural drainage exercises may be performed prior to positioning the patient for postural drainage. The exercises can help to mobilize secretions.

There are a variety of exercises in which the patient holds selected positions for 10 to 30 seconds and then repositions himself and briefly holds other positions. One such exercise is illustrated in Figure 70–6. This exercise is directed at promoting drainage from the upper lobes of the lungs. While in a sitting position the patient moves successively through several slightly different positions; each position is held 10 to 15 seconds.

Clapping; Vibrating; Tapping. Making rhythmic clapping and vibrating movements over the affected area of the chest (while it is being drained by gravity drainage) increases secretion removal, especially if secretions are dry and inspissated, i.e., thickened. These manual techniques are performed by physical therapists or nurses who have been given special training. Family members may be taught these techniques when they are important for a patient's home care. Clapping and vibrating does not mean pounding hard on the patient or roughly shaking him.

Clapping and vibrating are contraindicated in the presence of bleeding tendencies. Clapping is also contraindicated in the presence of pain, cardiac disorders, or acute inflammatory conditions, and if it increases bronchospasm.

Clapping is also called *"percussing"* or *"cupping."* The basic positions of the hands for clapping and vibrating are shown in Figure 70–7. Clapping the chest wall is accomplished by flexing and extending the elbows with the hands in a cupped position. The wrists and shoulders are relaxed. Cupping the hands makes the impact on the chest air-cushioned; thus, the procedure does not cause patient discomfort when correctly performed. Clapping is continued for 1 to 2 minutes over the involved area and is followed by vibration. Percussive action can dislodge mucous plugs, freeing them so they can be expelled by coughing. Clapping should be performed by skilled persons and only for short periods of time. The most congested areas of the lungs are the only areas percussed.

With her hands positioned for *vibrating,* the therapist tenses and contracts her hand, arm, and shoulder muscles—as if having a shaking chill. The movements are transmitted through the therapist's arms and hands to the patient's chest. As the vibratory movements are transmitted through the chest wall and underlying tissues they increase the turbulence and velocity of exhaled air in the smaller bronchi. Inspissated secretions are thus dislodged and moved to larger bronchi. From there

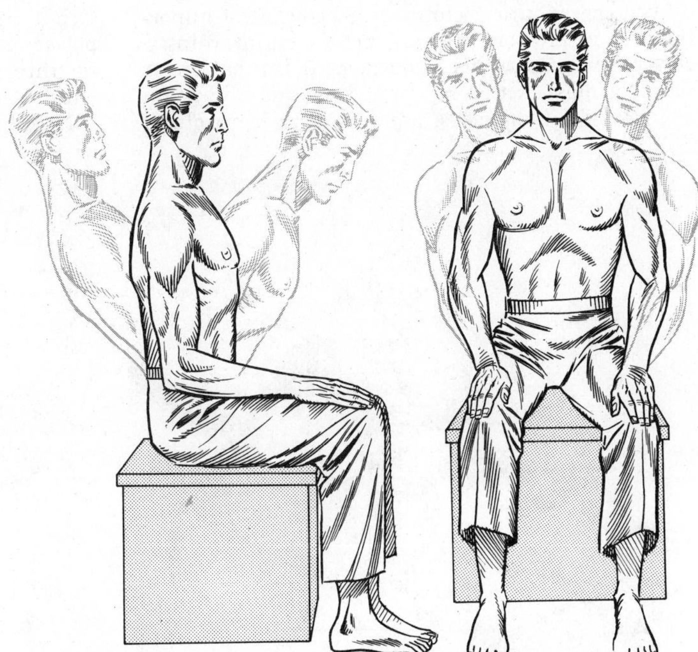

FIGURE 70–6. Postural drainage exercise to drain upper lobes. (From Secor, J.: *Patient Care in Respiratory Problems.* 1969.)

secretions can be expectorated. The movements should originate mainly in the shoulders rather than the hands or arms. The therapist presses her hands down on the patient's thorax as well as toward the body axis during the vibrations. Vibration is performed only while the patient exhales. Commonly it is performed during 4 or 5 deep exhalations. During vibration the patient should use abdominal breathing with pursed lip exhalation. Effective coughing is encouraged after the series of claps and vibrations. Vibration without preceding clapping may be used when pain contraindicates percussion, e.g., after chest injury or chest surgery.

A patient cannot effectively perform clapping or vibrating procedures on himself, but he can help to move secretions by making *tapping* movements on his chest. These movements, made with the fingertips of both hands, cause vibrations in the chest that help to dislodge secretions. Family members can also perform tapping.

For a good summary of a bronchial hygiene program using physiotherapeutic techniques, see the article by Foss.[88]

RESPIRATORY THERAPY

Techniques of respiratory therapy are of vital importance in the clinical care of patients with pulmonary disorders and in the prevention of pulmonary complications in other groups of patients. Respiratory therapy, formerly known as inhalation therapy, is a relatively recent area of clinical specialization. The scope of this field is rapidly enlarging owing to increasing knowledge and improved therapeutic techniques. Activities of importance in respiratory therapy include maintaining a clear airway, e.g., via endotracheal intubation or tracheostomy suctioning; providing humidification of inspired air or gases; administering aerosolized medications via nebulizers; administering oxygen or other gases; and assisting or completely controlling ventilation via respirators.

Respiratory therapy procedures should be performed by trained therapists or by nurses who have received advanced instruction in the techniques. Space does not permit detailed discussions in this text of the specialized procedures of respiratory therapy, but this section provides general descriptions of some of the more common procedures. For additional information consult with respiratory therapists and refer to textbooks and manufacturers' instruction materials prepared for use with specific types of equipment. Endotracheal intubation and tracheostomy are discussed in Unit XXII.

Nebulization; Humidification

Nebulization (Aerosolization). A nebulizer (atomizer) is a mechanical device that produces an aerosol, i.e., a suspension of solid or liquid particles in a gas. Particles of matter dispersed in the form of a fine aerosolized mist or spray are small enough that they do not settle out under the influence of gravity. The suspension of microscopic droplets can thus be inhaled into peripheral regions of the lungs and deposited directly onto the tracheobronchial mucosa.

Nebulizers may be used to deliver into the airways aerosolized sterile distilled water or isotonic saline solution, or aerosolized medications such as bronchodilators, antibiotics, corticosteroids, wetting agents, mucolytic agents, proteolytic enzymes, and pulmonary surfactants. Water or isotonic saline may be nebulized to humidify inspired air. (Humidification is discussed below.)

Nebulizers produce an aerosol by forcing air or oxygen through a solution. They may be powered in various ways, the simplest of which is manual compression of the rubber bulb of an atomizer. Other methods of powering nebulizers are by a power driven compressor, by compressed gas, or by an intermittent positive pressure breathing machine (see below).

Nebulization therapy may be ordered as a contin-

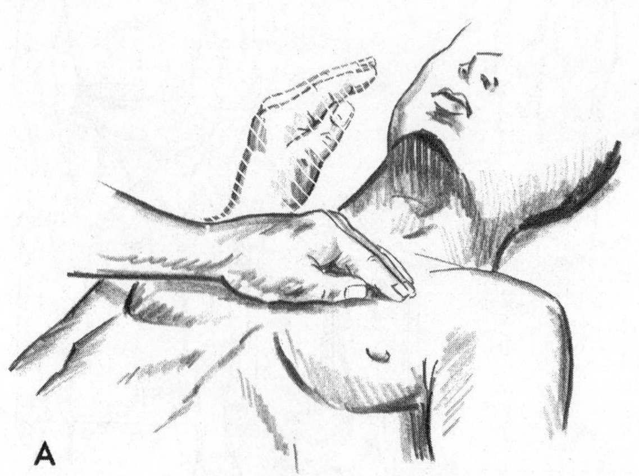

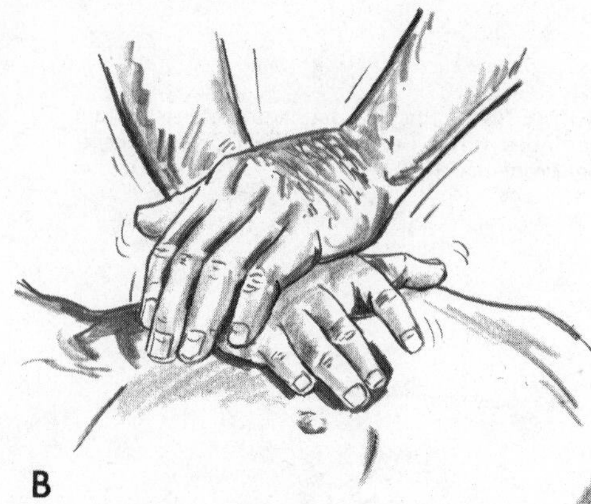

FIGURE 70–7. Positions of the hands for clapping (*A*) and vibrating (*B*). (After Kurihara.)

uous or intermittent procedure. For example, continuous nebulization may be required to humidify inspired air when treating patients in acute respiratory failure who are being artificially ventilated. Intermittent nebulization treatments may help patients with chronic obstructive pulmonary disease.

Intermittent aerosol treatments are commonly performed when the patient arises for the day, prior to meals, and before he retires for the night. Prior to administration of the aerosol the patient should attempt to clear his airway by coughing productively.

The nurse may teach a patient how to *self-administer* aerosol medications. If the patient is to mix his own medications (e.g., with water or saline solution) he must learn the correct mixing procedure. The patient also needs to learn how to assemble, take apart, and sterilize his nebulizing equipment. To correctly self-administer aerosolized medications (while sitting upright) the patient should follow these instructions:

> Hold the bowl of the nebulizer downward so the jet stream within the bowl remains vertical.

> Position the tip of the nebulizer nozzle well back into the open mouth.

> Do not close the lips around the nebulizer tip.

> Exhale slowly and as completely as possible through the mouth with the lips slightly pursed before inhaling the aerosolized medication.

> While deeply inhaling through the open mouth administer the medication, e.g., vigorously squeeze the bulb of a hand nebulizer, activate a compressed-gas hand nebulizer, or close the Y connector (if compressed gas is being used from a tank or wall outlet).

> Hold the completely inspired breath for 3 to 4 seconds to permit contact of the medicated spray with the lower respiratory tract.

> Slowly exhale through partially pursed lips. Pursing the lips increases airway pressure and carries the medicated spray to deeper levels of the lower respiratory tract.

The procedure should be repeated until the prescribed amount of medication has been used. When given by a nebulizer that is not hand-powered the aerosol treatment may take 10 to 15 minutes. During this time the patient should attempt to inhale and exhale evenly. The patient may need to rest periodically during the treatment. During rest periods the aerosol spray should be stopped so medication is not wasted.

Following aerosol treatments, postural drainage, chest percussion, and expulsive coughing may be employed. Nasal and oral hygiene should be performed and the aerosol equipment sterilized. Chart the effectiveness of the procedure and how it was tolerated by the patient. Observe for and report untoward effects from the procedure or from medications used.

Humidification. Humidifiers are devices that add moisture to the air. Humidifying inspired air is important in the clinical care of patients with respiratory disorders for the following reasons:

> Moist air can be ventilated within the respiratory system with less effort than dry air because moist air is lighter.

> Moist air prevents drying and irritation of the mucous membranes within the respiratory system.

> Moist air prevents drying and thickening of respiratory tract secretions and loosens these secretions so they can more easily be removed. By keeping secretions thin and liquid in nature, moist air makes them easier to raise. Dry thick secretions can form plugs and crusts within the tracheobronchial tree that can be life-threatening if they obstruct airways.

Extra moisture can be added to room air by relatively simple methods, e.g., placing a vaporizer or kettle of boiling water in a patient's room. Other methods of providing humidification include use of nebulizers (e.g., with IPPB machines), heated aerosols, high humidity tracheostomy collars, high humidity oxygen tents, and ultrasonic mist units of various sorts (e.g., to humidify room air or for use with tents, hoods, or masks). Bedside nebulizers and room humidifiers are more effective in treating disorders of the upper airways than disorders deeper within the bronchopulmonary system. These devices produce an aerosol output that is typically restricted to larger particle size; hence, the particles do not penetrate deeply within the lungs.

Vaporizers are especially helpful to patients with irritation of the nose, throat, or bronchi. Large electric vaporizers (which use a gallon size water jar) may be used in hospitals; smaller electric vaporizers (with pint or quart size jars) are available from drug stores for home use. A vaporizer produces steam by heating water placed in the water jar. The steam is then either directed toward the patient or is permitted to flow generally into the room.

When directing steam toward a patient be certain the vaporizer and flow of steam are far enough away from the patient to prevent accidental burns.

Sometimes the physician orders medicated steam inhalations, e.g., with menthol or tincture of benzoin. The aromatic medication is placed within a medicine cup in the vaporizer. If the vaporizer does not have an automatic shut-off device and if it is allowed to boil dry, it may start a fire. To prevent this, refill the water container when it becomes half empty.

If humidification is being obtained by simply boiling water on a hot plate in a pan or teakettle, be certain to place the apparatus at a safe distance from the patient and keep the water container more than half full.

Ultrasonic nebulization produces particles of such extremely small size that they may reach the pulmonary alveoli. These minute particles are produced when high-frequency sound waves vibrate through water or isotonic saline. Ultrasonic mists can be fanned as a "cold fog" into tents, i.e., high humidity tent therapy, or fog nebulizers can be attached to oxygen masks or thermal head hoods.

Mist therapy is sometimes ordered prior to IPPB treatments or postural drainage. Some patients tolerate mist therapy better than others. The high water content of the air used for mist treatments may *temporarily* contribute to a patient's feelings of shortness of breath; relief is usually obtained when the patient is able to clear his airway of water-laden secretions. It is important for a patient to be adequately prepared psychologically for mist treatments. Also, the patient should be closely supervised during these treatments until he becomes familiar with the procedure and experiences the benefits of mist therapy. Instruct the patient to cough effectively during and following the mist treatment. Charting should include a description of the patient's tolerance of the procedure (emotionally and physically) and the effectiveness of the treatment (e.g., amount of sputum produced). Complete charting helps the physician to determine the type and amount of mist that are of greatest benefit to the patient.

Adequate humidification is necessary during *artificial ventilation,* but excessive humidification must be avoided. Humidifying devices can cause problems in ventilatory therapy:[297] for example, continuous ventilation with fully humidified gas can cause a positive water balance (this can be a problem in oliguric patients); condensed water can partially obstruct the inspiratory tube of a pressure-limited respirator and thereby markedly reduce effective ventilation; and a bolus of water may be projected into the patient's tracheobronchial tree with the inspiratory phase of ventilation if water condenses in the tubes leading from the nebulizer to the patient.

Gases administered under pressure are very drying to respiratory tract mucosa. Unless *oxygen* is properly humidified when administered it will damage the respiratory mucosa, interrupt the normal formation and transportation of mucus, and result in the formation of thick secretions. Oxygen is a completely dry gas that takes up large amounts of moisture upon contacting the moist respiratory mucosa. Effective oxygen therapy, therefore, ensures that the inspired gas reaches the trachea fully saturated with water vapor at body temperature; it is usually bubbled through warm water before inspiration to increase its moisture content.

Humidification and warming of inspired air or air-oxygen mixtures is important following *tracheostomy (or endotracheal intubation)* whether or not the patient is using a respirator. Tracheostomy creates an artificial air passage that bypasses the upper airway (see Unit XXII); thus, the "new airway" is exposed to atmospheric air that is not warmed, moistened and filtered by upper respiratory mucosa. To compensate for loss of the normal functions of the upper airway, it is desirable to use a heated nebulizer immediately after tracheostomy is established. The object of this treatment is to project into the tracheostomy tube air-oxygen mixtures at body temperature that are saturated with water vapor. A relative humidity of over 100 per cent at about 37°C. is desirable.[232] If the temperature is in doubt, it should be monitored to prevent possible hyperthermia. High humidity tracheostomy collars are available that permit easy access for suctioning.

Following tracheotomy, warm moist air-oxygen mixtures are typically administered continuously for the first 2 to 3 postoperative days. A heavily saturated mist of inspired air can be produced in an ultrasonic fog tent or can be administered via tracheostomy mask. Room air can be moistened with steam or cold vapor. Humidification may also be enhanced by increasing the patient's water intake.

Usually the patient who has normal lungs is able to adapt within a few days to the upper airway bypass created by the tracheostomy. Gradually over this period of time the patient's respiratory system becomes accustomed to having more direct exposure to atmospheric conditions. Once this adaptation takes place it is possible to "wean" the patient away from nebulization.

Oxygen Therapy

Uses. Oxygen therapy, i.e., administration of O_2 in concentrations higher than those occurring in the ambient atmosphere, is beneficial in the treatment of numerous disorders. Examples of some conditions that may be treated in part by O_2 therapy include pulmonary or airway obstruction, pulmonary injury, pulmonary edema, shock, respiratory depression or failure (e.g., from drugs or paralysis), chronic respiratory insufficiency, acidosis, anemia, and cardiac disorders. In addition, supportive O_2 therapy is often given to unconscious or postanesthetic patients.

Oxygen is primarily used to correct hypoxia and to ensure adequate oxygenation, particularly of such vital structures as the heart and brain. However, O_2 may also be administered to displace other gases in the body, e.g., to treat caisson disease or subcutaneous emphysema, or to remove gases from closed intestinal loops, from the pleural space (following pneumothorax), or from the ventricles of the brain (following pneumoencephalogram).[267] Hypoxia has been discussed previously.

When hypoxia is accompanied by apnea or dyspnea it may be necessary to ventilate the patient artificially while administering O_2. Oxygen may then be administered by adding supplemental O_2 to an IPPB system driven by compressed air, or by an oxygen-driven IPPB device used with the air dilution setting. Methods of administration of O_2 are discussed further below.

Like a drug, O_2 should be given in amounts that are safe for the individual patient. In some instances high concentrations of O_2 can be fatal, while low concentrations can be lifesaving. Thus, it is *not* always true that if a little O_2 helps, a lot of O_2 will be even more helpful. Oxygen therapy prescriptions should be governed by blood gas levels, just as insulin prescriptions are governed by blood sugar levels. Recently, with the development of techniques that enable delivery of high O_2 tensions to patients, O_2 toxicity has become a major problem. This and other hazards of O_2 therapy are discussed further below.

Administration of Oxygen. Oxygen is supplied for administration either from a portable tank (cylinder) or from a wall outlet (which leads via pipes to a large stored O_2 supply). Oxygen can be administered by masks, nasal cannula, nasal catheter, face tent, regular (overbed) O_2 tent, funnel, ventilator, or tracheostomy. Much of the equipment used for O_2 administration is disposable. Some of the more common methods of administration are summarized in Figure 70–8. Additional details about O_2 administration procedures can be found in specialized references, e.g., Seedor's *Therapy With Oxygen and Other Gases,*[270] and Secor's *Patient Care in Respiratory Problems.*[267]

Regular (overbed) O_2 tents are not shown in Figure 70–8. In some settings these tents have become unnecessary with the development of more effective means of administering O_2—respiratory intensive care units, and air-conditioned hospital rooms. Sometimes O_2 tents are useful because they provide a cool environment. Although some patients find the tents uncomfortable, others prefer them. It is difficult, however, to maintain an accurate high concentration of O_2 within a tent and it is also difficult to have access to the patient if frequent nurse-patient contact is necessary. Periodically the O_2 concentration in the tent should be checked by the nurse with an *oxygen analyzer,* so that the rate of inflow can be adjusted to maintain the prescribed concentration.

The physician determines the method and concentration of O_2 to be administered after evaluating the patient. The rate of flow and percentage of O_2 to be given are individualized and are determined by the patient's response and blood gas reports. Success or failure of the gas exchange process is reflected by the amounts of CO_2 and O_2 in the arterial blood. Knowledge of arterial blood gas values is helpful because the arterial blood represents blood coming from the lungs, i.e., from the site of gas exchange.

Phipps and Barker offer the following advice concerning therapeutic O_2 concentrations:[228]

> The optimal concentration of oxygen is that which permits full use of the oxygen-carrying capacity of the arterial blood. In the sick or debilitated patient, increased physiological shunting is frequently present to such a variable degree that it is impossible to predict the arterial oxygenation that can be achieved by any given inspired concentration of oxygen. In general, a margin of safety is desirable and, as a rule, the optimal inspired concentration of oxygen is that which results in an arterial oxygen tension of approximately 100-150 mm. Hg with normal hemoglobin levels. Only in acute situations is a higher arterial oxygen tension desirable. In some cases of chronic obstructive pulmonary disease it may be necessary to regulate the inspired oxygen concentration very carefully to avoid respiratory depression. In such patients arterial oxygen tension of approximately 80 mm. Hg is optimal.

Some patients with chronic respiratory diseases need to have supplementary O_2 accessible in their homes; various types of O_2 equipment are available. Lightweight portable units with liquid oxygen can easily be carried with the patient while he is ambulatory or exercising. Ambulatory oxygen therapy is particularly useful in treating patients who have marked respiratory disability as a result of chronic obstructive pulmonary disease.[225]

The nurse must familiarize herself with the different methods of administering O_2. She should be able to supervise O_2 therapy and be able to detect malfunction of the apparatus in use. The percentages of O_2 delivered by most equipment are only approximate. The gas delivered to the patient should therefore be periodically monitored with an oxygen meter when the O_2 concentration must be closely governed. Oxygen is delivered in accurately measured amounts by some of the newer, more highly developed positive pressure respirators. A nurse responsible for oxygen therapy must familiarize herself not only with the equipment used to administer O_2 but also with the hazards of O_2 therapy and clinical indications of hypoxia, respiratory acidosis, CO_2 narcosis, respiratory alkalosis, and O_2 toxicity.

General clinical care measures of importance during O_2 administration include maintenance of a patent airway by correct positioning, suctioning, and productive coughing; mouth and nose care every 3 to 4 hours; periodic repositioning; skin care (if a mask is being used to administer O_2 the mask should be removed every 1 to 2 hours and the patient's face washed, dried, and soothed with a mild lotion); changes of equipment as necessary, e.g., tanks should be changed before they become empty, nasal catheters removed every 6 to 10 hours, cleaned, and reinserted in the opposite nostril after giving mouth and nose care; and appropriate patient teaching and reassurance given.

The first time O_2 is to be given to a patient, explain the procedure to him and familiarize him with the equipment to be used. Inform him of the benefits of oxygen therapy. Some patients (and their family members) are frightened by O_2 therapy and associate it with being near death. These attitudes need to be explored and realistically discussed. The dyspneic patient may initially fight an O_2 catheter or mask if the equipment adds to his feelings of suffocation. Remain with the patient long enough to help him to adjust to the equipment and to begin to feel the benefits of the O_2 being administered. Sometimes a patient becomes dependent on O_2 therapy and is afraid to have the treatment discontinued, even though the physician knows it is no longer necessary. The nurse, realizing the patient's deep concern, plans a program for gradually withdrawing the O_2 therapy while remaining with the patient and offering reassurance.

When it is advisable for a patient to receive O_2

Method	Max Per Cent Oxygen	Flow (L/min)	Comments
A. *Nasal catheter* 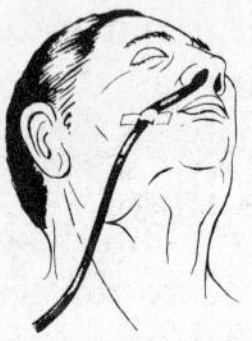	30–40%	6–8	Comfortable. Higher flows provide up to 40% oxygen, but can cause respiratory depression and drying of mucosa.
B. *Nasal prongs* 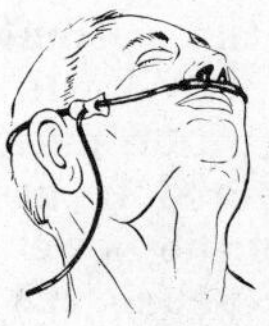	30–40%	6–8	Comfortable. Higher flows provide up to 40% oxygen, but can cause respiratory depression and drying of mucosa.
C. *T-piece* 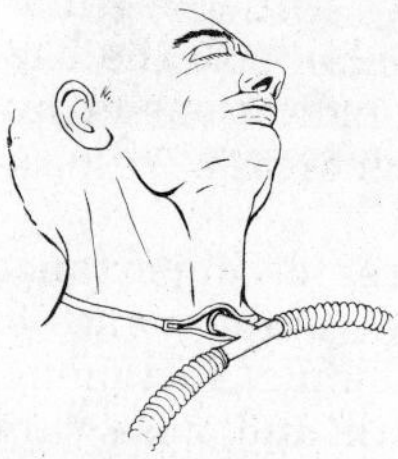	40–60%	4–12	Provides enriched oxygen mixtures and humidification. Used most often in weaning patients from ventilator assistance before endotracheal tube is removed.
D. *Face tent* 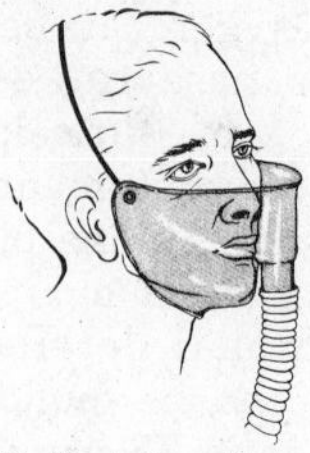	30–55%	4–8	Well tolerated. Good for supplying extra humidity.
E. *Venturi masks* 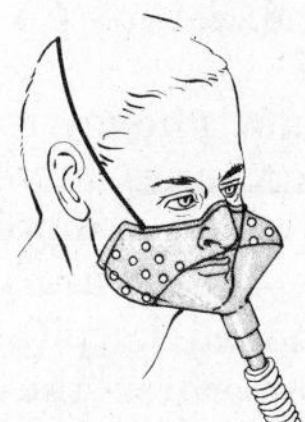	25–35%	4–8	Mask well tolerated. Accurate concentrations delivered.
F. *Mask without bag* 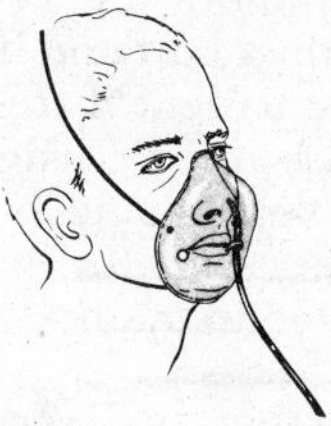	35–45% 45–55% 55–65%	6–8 10 10–12	Poorly tolerated. Significant CO_2 rebreathing possible at low flows. Highest percentage requires tight mask fit.
G. *Mask with bag* 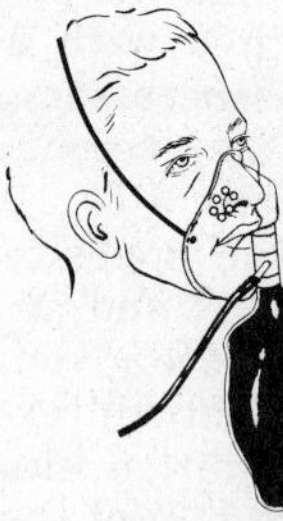	40–55% 50–60% 90 + %	6 8 8–12	Poorly tolerated. Significant CO_2 rebreathing possible at low flows. Highest percentage requires tight mask fit and a large bag.
H. *Pressure-regulated ventilator* 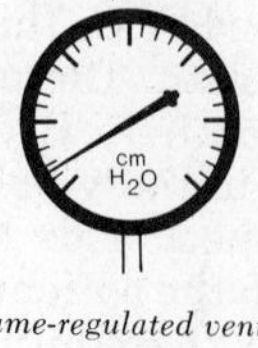	40–100%	Direct from supply	Oxygen per cent unpredictable
I. *Volume-regulated ventilator* 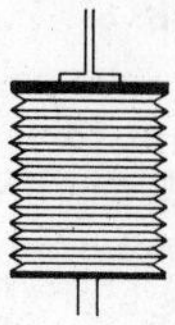	20–100%	Direct from fupply	Bennett MA1, Ohio 560 can be set to any desired per cent.

FIGURE 70–8. Methods of oxygen administration. (From Sanderson, R. G. (ed.): *The Cardiac Patient.* 1972.)

or IPPB therapy at home, the respiratory therapist, nurse, or doctor informs the patient and his family where to obtain the necessary equipment and how to use it correctly. The social worker may be helpful in arranging for the use of equipment and in offering advice about financing. Instructions for using respiratory therapy equipment should be given both verbally and in writing, and the patient and family members need to be supervised several times while performing the procedure. Visiting nurses may supervise use of equipment in the home.

HYPERBARIC OXYGENATION THERAPY. During hyperbaric oxygenation therapy the patient is given O_2 at increased atmospheric pressure while inside a large steel chamber that is pressurized by compressed air. At sea level the barometric pressure of ambient air is 760 mm. Hg (1 atmosphere), and the O_2 concentration is about 21 per cent. The partial pressure of inspired O_2 is therefore about 150 mm. Hg; this can be increased proportionately by giving the patient O_2 within a hyperbaric chamber at barometric pressures of 2 to 3 atmospheres. Increased amounts of O_2 are diffused into the blood.

During the last two decades the usefulness of hyperbaric oxygen therapy has been investigated. Patient care is given by attendants who also remain within the specially constructed chambers. Within the chamber the occupants pass through compression and decompression stages, and various problems may occur. For example, during decompression (a procedure necessary to prevent "the bends," as with deep sea diving), expanding gases, increased pressure, and release of dissolved nitrogen can cause problems such as abdominal distention, air embolism, middle ear pain, and joint pain. Fire is a serious potential hazard during hyperbaric oxygenation.

Hyperbaric oxygenation has not yet proved to be as clinically useful as was hoped. However, it has value as an adjunct to radiation for cancer, in cardiovascular surgery, and in treating anaerobic infections, carbon monoxide poisoning, arterial insufficiency in the legs, right-to-left cardiac anomalies, and diffuse overwhelming pneumonia, in which hypoxia cannot be corrected by 100 per cent O_2 at ambient pressure.

Hazards of Oxygen Administration

INFECTION. The use of contaminated equipment can infect the patient. Infecting organisms may be present in such places as suction catheters, tracheostomy or endotracheal tubes, connecting tubing, humidifier water, and masks. A few organisms, e.g., *Pseudomonas aeruginosa,* can even grow in some chemical disinfectants. The resultant infections are difficult to treat. To prevent infections of this nature, equipment must be properly sterilized and each person giving patient care must practice appropriate aseptic technique. Positive pressure oxygen equipment is particularly subject to contamination. Between use with patients the nurse should replace aerosol generators, tubing, manifolds, masks, and mouthpieces with sterilized equipment. These items should be changed daily when equipment is in continuous use on a given patient.

COMBUSTION. Oxygen does not itself burn but it supports combustion. Hence, fire is a potential hazard when O_2 is being administered. Flatter comments: "The greater the amount of oxygen present, the more easily fires start and the more rapidly they burn. . . . With the oxygen concentration increased above that of normal air, ignition becomes much easier, the rate of combustion is much faster, and extinguishment of such a fire may be extremely difficult."[86] The following *factors are of importance in preventing fires during O_2 administration:*

> Properly ground all electrical plugs and electrical equipment.

> Do not permit use of electric razors on the patient.

> Enforce no smoking rules; post no smoking signs. Remove the patient's cigarettes, pipe, cigars, and matches from his room.

> Do not permit open flames, frayed electrical wires, or extension cords within the patient's environment.

> Do not use oils (e.g., oily hair dressings, mineral oil as a lip lubricant), greases, or flammable solutions (e.g., alcohols, ether, antiseptic tinctures) on the patient. If lubricants are necessary use a product with a water base such as K-Y jelly.

> Never use oil on O_2 equipment. In pure O_2, fuels can ignite without a spark.

> Prevent static electricity. Electrical sparks can easily ignite fires in an O_2-enriched environment. Sparks from static electricity are also hazardous. Woolen blankets and other items that may produce static electricity should not be used during O_2 administration.

DRYING OF RESPIRATORY TRACT MUCOSA. As discussed previously, O_2 is a very drying gas when delivered into the respiratory system under pressure. To prevent hazardous drying and irritation of the respiratory mucosa, impaired ciliary action, and thickening of secretions within the respiratory tract, O_2 must *always* be humidified when administered. When O_2 is administered through a tracheostomy tube, special humidification is necessary so the gas mixture that enters the trachea is nearly saturated at body temperature. Oxygen can be passed through water or solutions (saline or medicated solutions) to humidify the gas before it is inhaled. Little O_2 is lost in the humidifying liquid because O_2 is only slightly soluble in water.

RESPIRATORY DEPRESSION; CO_2 NARCOSIS. Normally carbon dioxide (CO_2) stimulation governs the respiratory drive, and increased levels of CO_2 produce increases in the rate and depth of respiration (to "blow off" the accumulating CO_2). High flows of O_2 (5 to 10 liters per minute) usually can be given to patients who have hypoxemia and a *normal* $PaCO_2$ without increasing the $PaCO_2$. Increasing the $PaCO_2$ too much in these patients would remove the normal source of respiratory stimulation and thus reduce ventilation. While the above is true for most patients with "normal" lungs, it is not true for a large number of patients who often require O_2 therapy. For example, in patients with chronic respiratory insufficiency and *CO_2 retention* the use of high flows of O_2 may seriously aggravate respiratory acidosis.

> *It is dangerous to administer high concentrations of O_2 to patients who are chronically retaining CO_2, e.g., patients with chronic obstructive pulmonary disease. To do so may precipitate CO_2 narcosis and worsen respiratory failure by removing the* hypoxic stimulus *for respiration. Inhibition of the respiratory drive and further depression of breathing increases CO_2 retention and acidosis.*

It is paradoxical that the administration of high concentrations of O_2 can depress, rather than enhance, respirations in the presence of chronic CO_2 retention. This is called the "*oxygen paradox*" or "*carbon dioxide narcosis.*" Because the patient in CO_2 narcosis has no respiratory stimulus, he develops severe hypoventilation or apnea; his $PaCO_2$ level continues to rise to dangerous levels; he becomes semicomatose, then comatose; and he eventually dies unless properly treated. (The mechanisms of CO_2 narcosis were discussed in Chapter 25.)

Nevertheless, oxygen therapy is often indicated in treating chronic respiratory insufficiency. When a patient with chronic respiratory insufficiency and CO_2 retention requires O_2 therapy, the O_2 is administered cautiously in *low concentrations* (25 to 35 per cent) at a *low flow rate* (1 to 2 liters per minute) to prevent CO_2 narcosis. Oxygen administration of this kind is termed "low-flow" or "controlled-flow." Because the O_2 must be given with precision the therapy is guided by frequent blood gas monitoring. The goals of O_2 administration with such a patient become to preserve his hypoxic state (low PaO_2 level) and thus preserve the source of his respiratory drive, while also preventing an additional $PaCO_2$ buildup and increasing the transportation of O_2 in the blood to obtain adequate tissue respiration.

Recognition of the fact that the administration of high concentrations of O_2 causes some patients to develop CO_2 narcosis and become apneic led to the development of methods for administering O_2 by controlled methods. One effective method for giving controlled amounts of O_2 is to use a Venturi mask (Fig. 70–9). This disposable mask operates on the principle that an O_2 jet entering the mask sucks in a fixed proportion of air to dilute the O_2 down from 100 per cent but above the 21 per cent found in the air (Fig. 70–9). Three types of Venturi masks are available; each provides a different constant O_2 concentration—24, 28, or 35 per cent. These masks operate as follows: air is drawn into the tube by the jet of O_2; the O_2 concentration the patient receives is determined by the size of the openings through which air is drawn; and the streams of O_2 and air mix in the tube before entering the patient's airway. The O_2 is diluted to the various selected concentrations with reasonable accuracy.

It is also possible to obtain inspired O_2 concentrations of 24 to 30 per cent by administering O_2 flow through a two-pronged nasal cannula.

Good judgment, caution, and careful observation are necessary when initially administering O_2 to a patient whose history is unknown. Supervision is particularly important during the first 30 to 60 min-

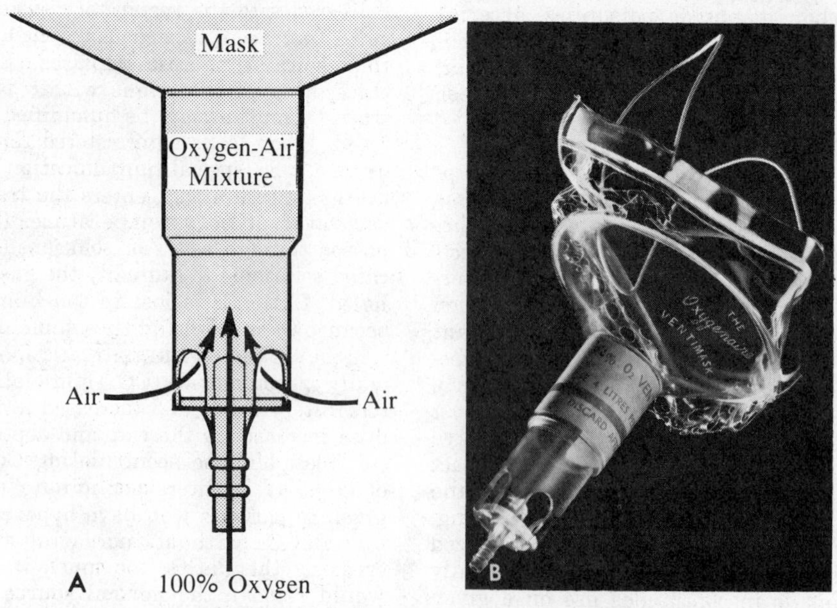

FIGURE 70–9. *A*, Venturi principle. *B*, Ventimask.

utes because apnea can occur, e.g., if the administration of O_2 abruptly removes the hypoxic respiratory stimulus. If this occurs the patient may "pink up and die." This phrase summarizes the following sequence of events: the patient's color may improve (as his blood PaO_2 level rises), but he hypoventilates, becomes increasingly stuporous, then comatose, loses his cough reflex, becomes apneic and dies. Correction of the hypoxemia "pinks up" the patient but proves to be fatal by removing his respiratory drive, and death occurs. Close observation and prompt treatment may break this fatal chain of events. Indications of the development of respiratory depression (e.g., reduced rate or depth of breathing, reduced levels of consciousness) or increasing hypercapnia signal the need to immediately lower the O_2 concentration, contact the physician, and prepare for IPPB therapy.

Once O_2 therapy has been started it should not be stopped if the patient's respiratory failure worsens and he becomes unconscious. To terminate O_2 administration under these circumstances may cause the PaO_2 to fall rapidly to dangerously low levels. Oxygen is removed more rapidly from the body than CO_2. The patient would therefore soon have a lower PaO_2 and a higher $PaCO_2$ than before the O_2 therapy was started. This must be avoided by continuing to give O_2 in amounts adequate to prevent serious tissue hypoxia while assisting ventilation.

The safest method of administering O_2 in the presence of CO_2 retention is via a positive pressure machine. However, not all patients require this form of O_2 therapy. If the patient is cooperative and alert, he may be given low-flow oxygen via mask, nasal prongs, or nasal catheter if he is closely observed and his blood gases are monitored. If this form of supplemental O_2 therapy does not adequately oxygenate the patient or if his condition deteriorates (e.g., $PaCO_2$ level remains elevated and respiratory depression occurs), ventilatory assistance with IPPB is indicated to increase ventilation and remove CO_2.

In treating severe respiratory insufficiency in patients with hypercapnia the patient should receive the lowest flow rate that relieves dyspnea. For the severely hypoxic patient this may mean he requires an initial high flow rate. In such a situation assisting ventilation with an IPPB apparatus delivering an air-oxygen mixture is safer than giving O_2 continuously in high concentrations.

Blood gas measurements are extremely important in guiding O_2 therapy. This is especially true in treating hypercapnic patients who are in respiratory failure. During the first few hours of oxygen therapy repeated PaO_2 measurements may be made.

Respiratory depression associated with the administration of O_2 may occur not only in the presence of chronic CO_2 retention, but also if a patient is under general anesthesia or is heavily narcotized.

OXYGEN TOXICITY. In some situations oxygen may be toxic to the *eyes, lungs,* and *central nervous system.*[214a] The likelihood of O_2 toxicity developing increases when O_2 is administered in high concentrations for prolonged periods of time or administered at greater than normal atmospheric pressure. The use of mechanical ventilators and hyperbaric oxygenation increases the possibilities of O_2 toxicity developing if high O_2 concentrations are administered continuously for prolonged periods of time. Cuffed endotracheal and tracheostomy tubes, mechanical ventilators, and hyperbaric oxygen chambers make possible the delivery of higher concentrations of O_2 at greater pressure; a patient's lungs thus may be subjected to almost a pure O_2 atmosphere.

If premature infants are exposed to excessive amounts of O_2 (e.g., 100 per cent O_2) for prolonged periods of time they will develop retrolental fibroplasia and irreversible blindness as a result of vasoconstriction of retinal blood vessels. Patients on respirators are most susceptible to pulmonary O_2 toxicity. In adults and children the administration of high concentrations of O_2 by a mechanical ventilator or via a cuffed tracheostomy or cuffed endotracheal tube can produce pulmonary damage after 24 to 48 hours of continuous administration. The pulmonary damage manifests itself basically by the development of atelectasis, exudation of protein fluid into alveoli, damage to and proliferation of pulmonary capillaries, and interstitial hemorrhage.[86] Early symptoms of the development of this disorder include cough, nasal congestion, sore throat, reduced vital capacity, and substernal discomfort (owing to tracheobronchitis). These symptoms are not produced by inhalations of 50 per cent O_2. Early symptoms of airway irritation may begin to appear when a patient has received 80 to 100 per cent O_2 continuously for 8 or more hours. Like medications, O_2 should be used conservatively and in safe dosages.

Convulsions may occur when O_2 is breathed at greater than normal atmospheric pressures. Central nervous system oxygen toxicity occurs with an oxygen tension of 1 to 2 or more atmospheres and is also related to the length of exposure time. Oxygen convulsions may occur in deep-sea divers or during treatment by hyperbaric oxygenation.

Oxygen toxicity is a serious problem. Measures important in the *prevention of oxygen toxicity* include:[86] alternating between air and O_2 breathing at prescribed intervals (lengthens the total time a patient may tolerate pure O_2 administration without harmful effects); administering no more than the prescribed concentration of O_2; and periodically inflating the lungs fully (helps to prevent or reverse the development of patchy atelectasis, which can result from breathing 100 per cent O_2). The conscious patient who is in control of his respirations should be asked to periodically inhale maximally. The patient whose respirations are being controlled with a respirator should periodically be "sighed." (See p. 928.) Pure O_2 is so rapidly absorbed that some areas of lung parenchyma collapse, producing atelectasis. Because O_2

concentrations of 70 to 100 per cent may be harmful if inspired for longer than a few hours, such concentrations should not be administered for long periods of time if adequate oxygenation can be obtained in other ways. The physician must carefully weigh the dangers of potential organ oxygen toxicity against the dangers of tissue hypoxia. If tissue hypoxia threatens, 100 per cent O_2 may need to be given.[228]

CIRCULATORY DEPRESSION. Phipps and Barker[228] note that circulatory depression may occur after O_2 administration. Circulatory rebound and collapse may occur when hypoxia is corrected if the preceding period of hypoxia caused marked activation of the sympathetic nervous system. To prevent severe circulatory failure the patient requires vigorous treatment, e.g., endotracheal intubation, oxygenation, and ventilatory support.

MECHANICAL RESPIRATORY AIDS

Indications and Types of Equipment

Some patients are unable to ventilate their lungs effectively. We have discussed previously the wide variety of disorders that may result in pulmonary insufficiency or pulmonary failure. These patients require immediate assistance, which includes either establishment of an artificial airway (e.g., by endotracheal intubation or tracheostomy) and mechanical ventilation of the lungs with a positive pressure ventilator, or mechanical ventilation of the lungs with a negative pressure respirator which does not require tracheal intubation.

As indicated above, there are basically two major types of respirators: those that administer *positive pressure,* and those that create *negative pressure.* The physician selects the type of respirator to be used on a given patient. More than 50 respirators are currently available. Examples of negative pressure respirators are the Emerson, Drinker, and Jefferson machines, as well as full-body and chest respirators. Respirators that administer positive pressure include the Air Shields, Bennett, Bird, Engstrom and Mörche machines. (Positive pressure ventilation will be discussed further below.) Positive pressure respirators are used to treat many disorders because negative pressure respirators isolate the patient and cause nursing care problems.[234] Nonetheless, negative pressure machines continue to have a place in the treatment of some disorders.

Negative pressure respirators (tank types such as the full-body respirator) are not effective in the treatment of persons with increased airway resistance but may be used for patients whose respiratory failure is the result of a neuromuscular disorder rather than internal pulmonary disease. *Respiratory failure from neurologic* disorders may occur in three general ways: *central respiratory failure* results from depression or destruction of the cells in the lower brainstem which integrate respiration; *peripheral respiratory failure* results from damage to the spinal motor pathways for breathing, their nerves, or the respiratory muscular structures themselves; or *airway obstruction* results from paralysis or sensory loss, which in turn causes the accumulation of foreign material and secretions in the lungs and tracheobronchial tree. Airway obstruction may occur with reduced states of consciousness or paralysis, which immobilize the expiratory muscles necessary for coughing, or the pharynx or larynx.

Impaired ventilation can be detected by measuring CO_2 tension (by arterial blood gas determinations) and also by evaluating the pH of arterial blood. The increase in CO_2 tension that hypoventilation produces causes the blood's pH to decrease. This indicates the patient is in respiratory acidosis. Blood gases are evaluated frequently when a patient is receiving mechanical respiratory assistance.

Principles of Nursing Care

Nurses caring for patients with inadequate ventilation must be familiar with clinical indications of respiratory distress (restlessness, apprehension, irritability, wakefulness, use of accessory muscles of respiration, pallor. increasing pulse rate, and increasing laborious respirations) and must have advanced training in the various types of mechanical respiratory aids that may be used to improve ventilation. Whenever possible patients are given respiratory assistance well before a crisis develops. This anticipatory care requires close observation and availability of necessary equipment.

Assisted ventilation is often initially alarming to conscious patients. The appearance of the machine may be frightening. Also, since respiration is vital, the patient may have fears that the machine will fail him and he will die. Psychologic preparation of a patient for use of a ventilator helps to ensure successful treatment. The patient who is inadequately prepared may panic and defeat the purpose of the ventilator by "fighting" the cycle of the machine and breathing ineffectively. As time permits, the patient is told how the apparatus will help him, what he will feel while on the machine, how he can cooperate, and the basic mechanics of the respirator. Because patients with respiratory difficulties are usually tense and apprehensive, the transition to the mechanical respiratory equipment needs to be carried out as smoothly and as calmly as possible. The nurse remains with a patient during assisted ventilation until the patient feels comfortable in using the machine. Frequent reassurance is helpful. A patient who is completely dependent upon mechanical ventilation is continuously supervised. A patient who requires continuous mechanical ventilation is best cared for in an intensive care unit where he can be constantly supervised by skilled personnel and where necessary equipment and drugs are available, e.g., intubation equipment, tracheostomy tray, oxygen equipment, suctioning apparatus, emergency medications.

Respiratory aids are often used in emergency

situations. They must therefore always be in working condition and be easily obtainable. Respirators in use should be checked frequently to ensure their proper operation. Since electrically operated equipment will cease to function if the cord plug becomes disconnected or if power failure occurs, precautions must be taken to ensure the continued ventilation of the patient. The plug should be taped in place to the wall outlet and should be checked periodically to be certain the connection is maintained. Also, cords should be placed so they are not underfoot, so that they will not cause accidents or be accidentally pulled loose. In the event of a power failure, equipment must be available to ventilate the patient manually until the respirator can be connected to an emergency electrical supply. A self-inflating (Ambu) bag with an expiratory valve should always be kept at the bedside of a patient being mechanically ventilated. Then emergency manual resuscitation (maintain a respiratory rate of 15/min.) can be given if the respirator fails to operate properly or if power failure occurs. Manual ventilation is also used at other times, e.g., if it is necessary to temporarily disconnect the respirator for tests or treatments or to change apparatus on the machine.

Modern mechanical ventilation is almost entirely automatic, but it is accompanied by various nursing problems, such as maintaining prescribed inspired O_2 concentrations, supplying adequate humidification, preventing trauma and infection, preventing mechanical problems such as loose connections and kinks in tubing that may interrupt proper functioning of the equipment, and maintaining patency of endotracheal and tracheostomy tubes.[86,260] (Endotracheal intubation and tracheostomy are discussed in Unit XXII.) The nurse must be able to ascertain if a patient is being inadequately ventilated and she must know appropriate actions to take. This means the nurse must recognize clinical indications of overventilation or underventilation of a patient and malfunction of the machine.

At times when patients are surrounded by a lot of machines it becomes easy to overlook "the person" being treated and instead focus attention on "the machines." This is indeed unfortunate. Patients who are dependent on ventilators require complete care which requires comprehensive planning and meticulous attention to detail.

Ventilation During Respiratory Paralysis

Respiratory paralysis is one cause of inadequate ventilation. Advancing severe polyneuropathy is one example of a condition causing respiratory paralysis. A variety of mechanical devices are available to aid respiration in the presence of inadequate ventilatory capacity due to respiratory paralysis. Among these aids are full-body (iron lung) tank respirator, rocking bed, cuirass or chest respirator, abdominal belt or pneumobelt, intermittent positive pressure breathing (IPPB) via mouth or tracheostomy, and respiratory aid by electric stimulation. Indications for use of these highly developed respiratory aids overlap.[42]

In the presence of acute respiratory paralysis the *full-body respirator* is most often used, since it can adequately substitute for completely paralyzed respiratory muscles at rest.[42] With this type of respirator the patient lies within a leak-proof metal tank-like structure with only his head exposed to the external atmospheric environment. The respirator provides the force required to ventilate the lungs. A full-body respirator limits the patient's activities because his body (from the neck down) is in a relatively restricted position within the tank. Nursing care is performed through portholes equipped with cuffs that can be closed tightly around the nurse's arms as she reaches within the tank, thereby maintaining the tank's airtight environment. Living in such a respirator is difficult psychologically and makes physical care more difficult to perform. Patients are therefore "weaned" to a partial respirator that fits over the chest as soon as possible.

In spite of its relatively formidable appearance, a body-respirator is a relatively simple mechanical apparatus that operates on the basic principle that air pressure within the body tends to equalize with the pressure of the external air. Within the respirator, periodic cycles of reduced air pressures are produced and cycles of inspiration and expiration occur because pressures tend to equalize. When negative pressure (subatmospheric pressure) is created outside the chest wall, i.e., within the tank, air at atmospheric pressure enters the lungs via the nose and mouth exposed to atmospheric air to equalize the pressure, i.e., inhalation occurs.

Respiratory aids that may be used in the presence of minor degrees of respiratory muscle weakness include the chest-abdomen respirator, chest respirator, and the oscillating ("rocking") bed. Chest respirators or rocking beds are less efficient than the full-body respirator or IPPB respirator; however, they may be adequate and more comfortable during limited periods of the day or night for some patients with incomplete respiratory paralysis. The full-body respirator produces larger tidal volumes per unit of pressure applied to the surface of the body than a chest respirator.

Chest and *chest-abdomen respirators* operate on the same principle as the body respirator. These respirators facilitate patient care and may be helpful during transition periods when the patient is being weaned from the body respirator. Chest respirators cannot be used for prolonged periods of time on some patients because they may not adequately aerate the lungs. Some patients may use two different types of respirators—chest respirator when sitting up and an oscillating bed when lying down.

The *oscillating bed* indirectly assists respiration by changing the position of the diaphragm. Inspiration occurs when the head of the bed rises and the abdominal viscera shift downward, causing the diaphragm to move downward. Expiration occurs when the head of the bed lowers and the abdominal viscera push against the diaphragm, elevating it. The rate of inspiration and expiration is adjustable by governing the bed's motions. When stopping the bed, be certain to stop it in a head-up position. Assist the patient to take fluids when the head of the bed is up; swallowing, talking, and coughing are accomplished when the head of the bed lowers.

In some countries intermittent positive pressure breathing (IPPB) is widely used to assist or to control breathing during both acute and chronic respiratory paralysis in place of full-body respirators or other equipment. Respirations may be helped, (during waking hours) in patients who have only moderate respiratory impairment by giving hourly assisted ventilation with a positive pressure breathing valve that cycles on demand. This treatment provides full, deep breaths and restores otherwise ineffective coughing mechanisms. Postural drainage enhances the treatment. Positive pressure ventilators are discussed in the following section.

Venous return to the heart is intermittently decreased by either IPPB or the intermittent application of negative pressure to the outside of the body in the full-body respirator. Both types of equipment intermittently raise the intrathoracic pressure above the level of the systemic venous return. The circulatory system can compensate for this intermittent reduction of venous return to the heart if a patient's cardiac reserve is normal. However, when respiratory paralysis coexists with circulatory embarrassment (e.g., due to valvular arteriosclerotic heart disease or blood loss), the cardiac output may fall to inadequate levels, and congestive heart failure develops.[42]

Respirator therapy must be conducted by skilled, confident persons who have had advanced instruction in the use of these machines. The degree of pressure and the rate of the cycle are usually determined by the physician. Excessive degrees of pressure are hazardous since they can damage pulmonary alveoli by producing inspirations that are too deep. A respirator is carefully adjusted to meet an individual patient's requirements.

Physical care varies with the type of respirator being used. For example, some requirements of a patient in a full-body respirator include *periodic* (scheduled) skin care to prevent irritation at the neck from the collar of the tank and to prevent decubitus in other regions of the body, repositioning to prevent hypostatic pneumonia, and passive exercises to maintain muscle tone and stimulate circulation. Complete care must be given, since the patient in a full-body respirator is totally dependent. Assist the patient to learn to cooperate with the respirator, e.g., to talk and swallow upon expiration. Because it is difficult for a patient to learn to swallow while in a respirator, keep suction equipment available. The confinement of a body respirator makes diversional therapy highly important. It is not uncommon for patients on respirators to feel discouraged and depressed. The patient needs to feel comfortable in talking openly about his feelings with a concerned, understanding person such as his nurse.

The physician determines when it is time to begin to *wean* a patient from respiratory assistance. During the gradual weaning process the patient is closely supervised and supplementary O_2 given if required. If respiratory distress begins to develop the patient is calmly returned to the respirator. A patient who has been in a full-body respirator may be gradually transferred to a portable chest respirator. Reassurance and understanding are essential during the weaning process. Some patients are fearful of leaving the security of the respirator and therefore appear overly dependent, but others may be excessively confident that they can manage alone.

Positive Pressure Ventilators (Respirators)

As their name implies, ventilators of this type intermittently produce positive pressure, i.e., pressure greater than atmospheric pressure, and use this pressure to deliver gas mixtures into a patient's airway. Intermittent positive pressure breathing (IPPB) is sometimes also called "intermittent positive pressure ventilation" (IPPV). IPPB has assumed an important place in respiratory therapy.

Bascially IPPB acts by forcing O_2 into the lungs and flushing accumulations of CO_2 from residual air spaces. These activities can reduce the arterial blood's CO_2 content ($PaCO_2$) if it is excessively elevated, and raise the O_2 concentration (PaO_2) to safe levels necessary for cellular metabolism. IPPB therapy improves ventilation by increasing tidal volume and minute volume and, thus, helps to overcome respiratory insufficiency; improves the effectiveness of coughing by forcing air past collections of secretions; promotes air flow into alveoli, thus producing more uniform distribution of alveolar aeration; reduces the work of moving air in and out of the lungs by minimizing energy expenditure; improves tracheobronchial drainage of secretions and thus helps to maintain airway patency; improves inspiration and is effective as a deep-breathing exercise; and may be used to administer aerosolized medications (with positive pressure the medications are delivered into peripheral regions of the bronchopulmonary system). Additionally, IPPB helps to humidify the respiratory mucosa. Because respirators deliver gas under pressure, they are all equipped with humidifying devices to prevent drying of respiratory tract mucosa.

Contraindications to IPPB treatment include recent pulmonary bleeding (hemoptysis), pneumothorax, hyperventilation states, and active tuberculosis.

Positive pressure ventilators may be used *continuously* or *periodically,* depending upon the patient's needs. IPPB therapy is commonly used during treatment and rehabilitative programs to improve pulmonary ventilation and/or to administer medications, and it is widely used to treat acute respiratory failure. IPPB is useful in treating patients who cannot spontaneously maintain an adequate tidal volume because of muscular exhaustion or central nervous system depression (oversedation, head injury, cerebral vascular accident, CO_2 narcosis). When continuous respiratory therapy is needed for more than 48 hours, an elective tracheostomy is usually performed. Endotracheal intubation may suffice for short periods. (Tracheostomy and endotracheal intubation are discussed in Unit XXII.)

IPPB is a safe method of administering O_2 to hypercapnic patients; excess CO_2 is efficiently eliminated by improved alveolar ventilation and respirations are safely maintained. IPPB may be used pre- and postoperatively to prevent or treat respiratory disorders, e.g., severe bronchospasm, secretion retention, hypoventilation. Postdischarge IPPB treatments at home are especially helpful in patients with secretion retention and severe bronchospasm. Most physicians recommend that a patient use rented equipment for several weeks before purchasing his own. During this trial time the value of the treatment can be appraised. Small compact IPPB machines that are easy to use are available (Fig. 70–10).

Types of Positive Pressure Ventilators. Two general types of mechanical ventilators provide IPPB: pressure-cycled, and volume-cycled. Most of these machines can provide either controlled or assisted ventilation, intermittently or continuously. Pressure-cycled ventilators are most commonly used for elective therapy. Volume-cycled ventilators are typically used when high pressures are necessary to inflate a patient's lungs or when prolonged ventilatory support is indicated. Both types of respirators commonly have a control for administering O_2 as prescribed. Some machines have only two O_2 settings (for 60 to 80 or 100 per cent O_2), whereas others make it possible to precisely mix O_2 in concentrations ranging from room concentration to 100 per cent.[66]

PRESSURE-CYCLED VENTILATORS. Also called "pressure-controlled" or "pressure-limited" ventilators, these include machines such as the Bird Mark 7 and Bennett (PR series) (Fig. 70–11). These ventilators are preset to deliver a specified amount of pressure (e.g., 10 to 30 cm. H_2O) of inspired air. Gas is delivered into the airway during inspiration until the inflow pressure equals the predetermined amount of pressure. When the preset pressure is reached in the airway, the machine is triggered to shut off momentarily and the patient exhales without assistance. With each inspiration the same pressure is reached. In the presence of increased pulmonary resistance it is necessary to increase the pressure required to deliver the gas. The amount of resistance with the system (including the lungs) governs to some extent the volume of gas delivered.

When using pressure-sensitive ventilators the total volume being expired is periodically measured by a *Wright respirometer* to ensure an adequate tidal volume; the machine is then adjusted as necessary, since the volume of gas that the patient receives is not always maintained at a constant level.

All models of pressure-cycled respirators have as primary controls:[66] a *pressure control* with a pressure gauge that governs the tidal volume delivered (commonly the control is set at 15 to 20 cm. H_2O), and a *sensitivity control* that determines how much negative pressure the patient's inspiratory effort must have to cycle the respirator. Other controls that pressure-cycled machines may have include:[66] (1) a *respirations control* or automatic cycling de-

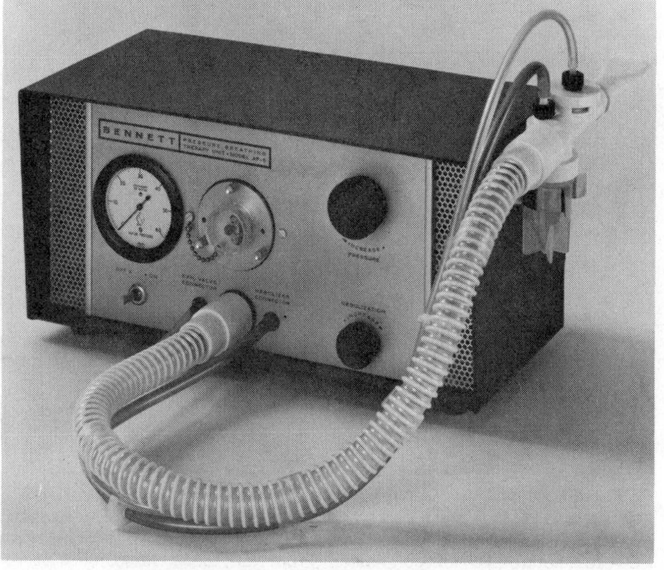

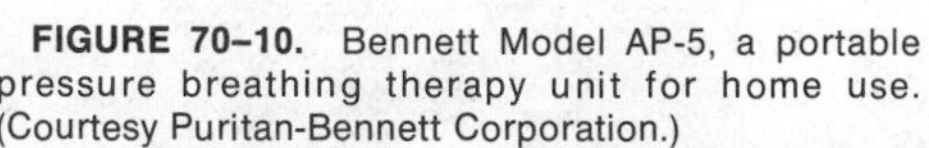
FIGURE 70–10. Bennett Model AP-5, a portable pressure breathing therapy unit for home use. (Courtesy Puritan-Bennett Corporation.)

vice, which ensures automatic ventilation if the patient's inspiratory efforts are absent or are too weak to trigger the sensitivity control; (2) *inspiratory flow-rate control,* which determines the length of the inspiration cycle (i.e., the rate of speed at which the amount of inspiratory pressure set on the pressure-control dial will be delivered); and (3) *negative-pressure control,* which can shorten expiration time by reducing pressure in the patient's chest. The negative-pressure control should be used only by physicians, since it can damage the lungs if incorrectly set.

VOLUME-CYCLED VENTILATORS. These are also called "volume-controlled" or "volume-limited" ventilators and include machines such as the Bennett MA-1, Emerson, Engstrom, Möerch, Ohio-560, and Air Shields (Fig. 70–12). These ventilators are used after the *volume* of inspired air to be delivered is preset. Within physiologic limits a predetermined total volume is delivered regardless of airway pressure. The patient receives air at whatever amount of pressure is required to deliver it within safe limits (see below). As stated before, volume-controlled ventilators may be used when a patient's airway resistance is too great (e.g., above 30 cm. H_2O) to maintain an adequate tidal volume. Patients with decreased pulmonary compliance ("stiff lungs") can best be treated by using newer machines whose advanced design makes it possible to sustain a positive pressure between the end of expiration and the beginning of inspiration.

Volume-cycled respirators are useful in the treatment of severe, chronic obstructive pulmonary disease (COPD); however, they must be used cautiously to prevent rapid overventilation of the patient. These machines may develop high inflation pressures, and they can produce pneumothorax by rupturing an emphysematous bleb, or can worsen air-trapping in the presence of COPD. To ensure safe and efficient delivery of air, a pressure cutoff valve attached to an audible alarm is built into volume-cycled ventilators. The maximum amount of pressure that can be used to ventilate the patient can thus be preset. If the patient begins to resist the machine or if he coughs or begins to accumulate secretions (which impede delivery of the predetermined volume of inspired air), the alarm sounds. The machine shuts off before the complete volume of air is delivered if the pressure needed to deliver the established volume is greater than that preset pressure limit.

A mouthpiece or mask can be used with pressure-cycled ventilators, but tracheostomy or endotracheal intubation is necessary for use of volume-cycled ventilators. (Pressure cycled ventilators may also be used on intubated patients.)

A pressure control is not required on volume-cycled respirators since the machine delivers air by volume rather than pressure. A *pressure indicator* is present, however, along with controls to govern *inspiratory time* (designated in seconds); *expiratory time* (designated in seconds); and *air volume* to be delivered (designated in milliliters).[66]

Assisted (Patient-cycled) and Controlled (Machine-cycled) Ventilation. With *assisted* ventila-

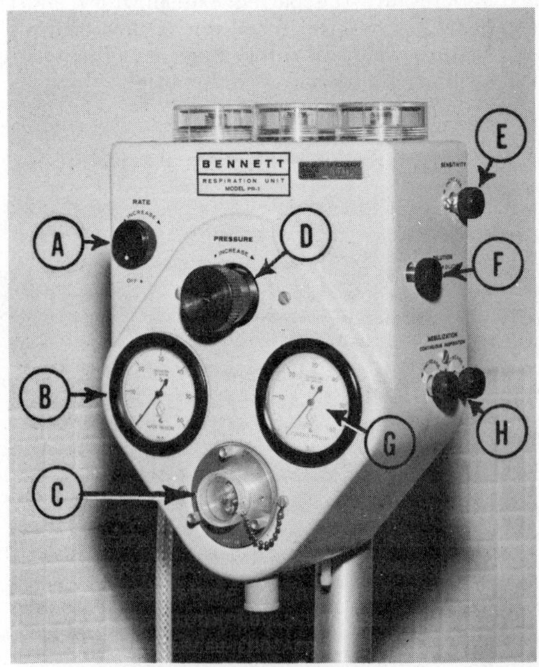

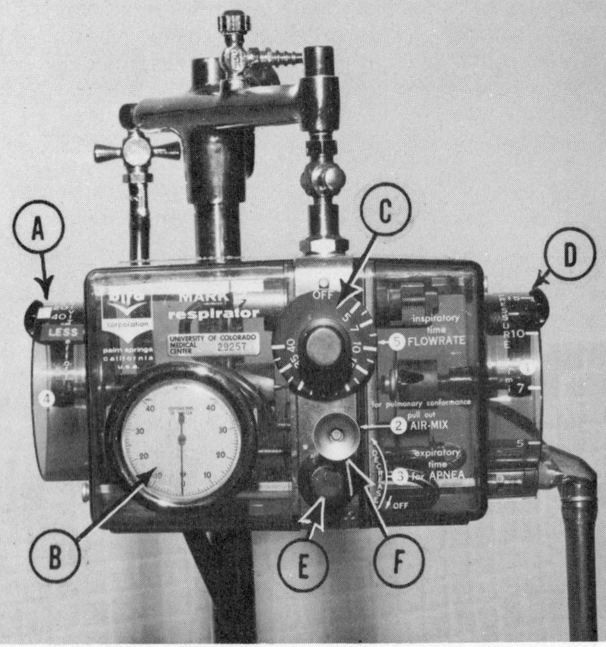

FIGURE 70–11. The Bennett PR-1 (left) has the following features: A = rate control; B = airway pressure indicator; C = flow-sensitive valve; D = pressure control; E = sensitivity control; F = oxygen diluter; G = machine pressure indicator; H = humidifier controls. The Bird Mark 7 (right) has: A = sensitivity control; B = airway pressure indicator; C = flow control; D = pressure control; E = rate control; F = oxygen diluter. (From Nett, L.: *Nursing Clinics of North America* 9:128, March, 1974.)

tion the patient's own inspiratory effort turns on ("trips") the respirator, thus initiating the mechanical inspiratory phase. The force of inspiration is then accelerated by the machine. Because some patients can make only weak inspiratory efforts, the respirator may be adjusted to respond to the individual patient's respiratory abilities. Thus, even a slight inspiratory effort may activate the positive pressure phase, causing the lungs to be rapidly inflated. When the flow of gas stops, the patient exhales with a gently forced expiration. The patient exhales without assistance from the machine. Some machines can be set to automatically trigger another inspiration if, after a period of delay, the patient does not spontaneously trigger the respirator. Setting the automatic cycling control thus safely assures ventilation if a patient's inspiratory efforts cease or become too weak to regularly trigger the machine.

When a patient is conscious and cooperative, assisted ventilation can be applied with a pressure-controlled IPPB machine using a tight-fitting mask or simple mouthpiece. If necessary, assisted ventilation can be used without interruption or periodically (e.g., 20 to 30 min./hr.) alternated with ambient pressure O_2 to correct hypoxia. Pressure-cycled IPPB machines are most commonly used for prolonged assisted ventilation.

Although the patient's own inspiratory efforts typically govern assisted ventilation, with *controlled* ventilation the patient's rate of ventilation is automatically cycled by the respirator at a predetermined number of cycles per minute. The respiratory cycle should allow three times as long for the lungs to deflate as was required to inflate them.

A tracheal airway (e.g., nasal or oral endotracheal tube, tracheostomy tube) and controlled ventilation are necessary for uncooperative, unconscious, or paralyzed patients. Cuffed tubes are used in the airway to prevent major air leaks. (Cuffed endotracheal and tracheostomy tubes are discussed in Unit XXII.) Humidification of inspired air and gases is imperative in treating the intubated patient. Also, a patent airway must be maintained by suctioning the patient as necessary, using sterile technique.

Some patients, who have spontaneous respirations, "fight" the respirator during controlled ventilation because they cannot synchronize their respirations with the machine's cycle. Ungoverned respiratory efforts that are out of phase with the respirator exhaust the patient and cause ineffective alveolar ventilation. If the nurse is unable to help the patient to relax and to breathe in cycle with the machine, she contacts the physician. When a patient is breathing out of cycle with the respirator, it is not advisable to overventilate him in an effort to reduce his spontaneous respiratory attempts. It is helpful to adjust the frequency of the automatic cycling to the patient's respiratory cycle when plac-

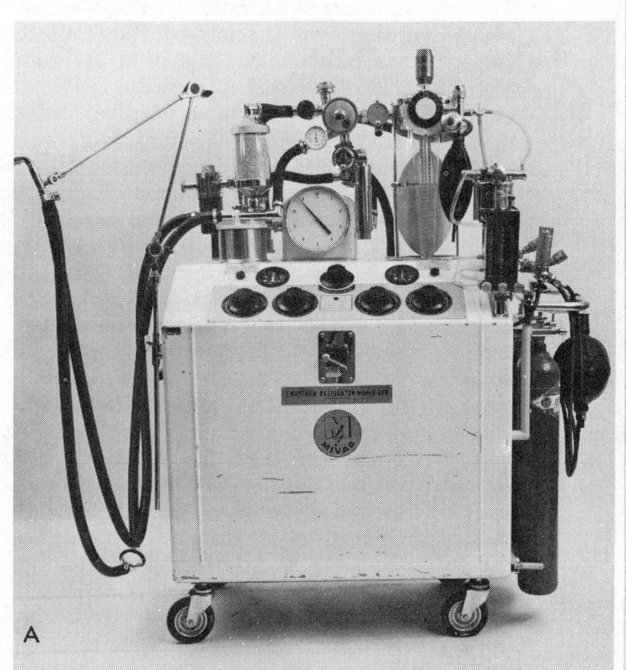

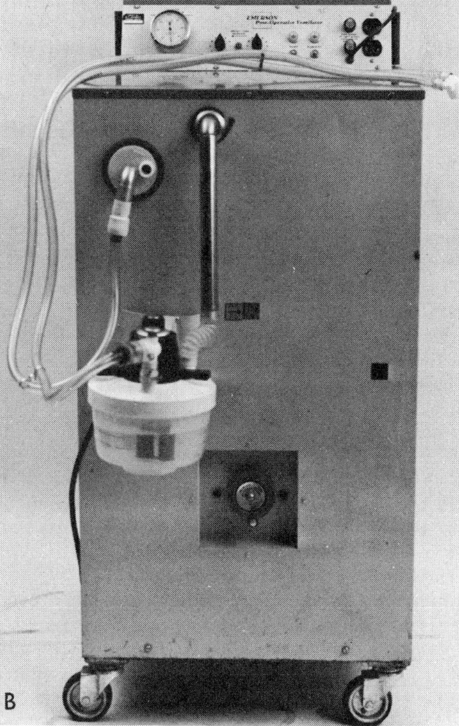

FIGURE 70–12. Engstrom ventilator. (From Gibbon, J. H., Jr., Sabiston, D. C., Jr., and Spencer, F. C.: *Surgery of the Chest,* 1969.)

ing the patient on the respirator and then gradually change the machine's automatic cycling to the desired frequency and stroke volume. When a tracheal tube is in place, a patient who is fighting the respirator may safely be sedated or narcotized to reduce his ventilatory efforts and successfully maintain automatic ventilatory control. Medications that may be given for this purpose are morphine, diazepam (Valium) and meperidine (Demerol). Some physicians administer small intravenous doses of *d*-tubocurarine (curare) to depress spontaneous ventilation. It is not safe to depress respirations in a patient who is not intubated. Breathing out of phase with the respirator or fighting the respirator may result from hypoxemia, low cardiac output, or inadequate alveolar ventilation.

Once a patient begins to ventilate spontaneously he is removed from continuous ventilation and given assisted ventilation.

A patient receiving continuous, controlled positive pressure ventilation is totally dependent and therefore requires constant supervision by skilled personnel. When a patient is initially placed on a ventilator he must be closely observed to evaluate effectiveness of the therapy and to prevent complications. Blood gases may be monitored and critical adjustments made on the mechanical apparatus. The most common serious complications that arise during the initial period of mechanical ventilation include rapid electrolyte changes; severe alkalosis, frequently with convulsions; and hypotension due to decreases in cardiac output. In an attempt to avoid these complications the initial ventilation may be limited to not more than 10 L./min., and repeated arterial blood gas determinations may be made to monitor the rate of ventilation. The respirator settings can then be adjusted to come close to a normal $PaCO_2$ over a period of several hours, and oxygen can be given to reach a desirable PaO_2 level.

Possible complications of continuous IPPB therapy include:[186, 228, 267]

> *Respiratory alkalosis* from continuous *hyperventilation.* Can occur if pCO_2 is blown off too rapidly before the kidneys can excrete proportional amounts of HCO_3. Can be corrected by periodically slowing the respiratory rate by 6 or 7 respirations per minute.

> *Gastric distention* and *paralytic ileus* from swallowed air. Can be relieved by gastric decompression. May be avoided by using a cuffed tracheostomy tube. If uncorrected, gastric distention can impair ventilation by elevating the left diaphragm and may cause *hypokalemia* and *hypotension.*

> *Gastrointestinal bleeding.* Observe for indications of bleeding from the gastrointestinal tract and report immediately.

> *Vomiting* and *aspiration.* If the patient vomits, remove him immediately from the respirator and apply suction. Aspiration can be fatal. Use of cuffed tubes may prevent aspiration; gastric decompression may prevent vomiting. Practice necessary precautions to prevent aspiration in patients who are obtunded or unable to cough or swallow.

> *Sudden ventricular fibrillation* and *death.* Can occur from rapid reversal of CO_2 tensions in patients with CO_2 retention who are ventilated to blow off excessive CO_2. Can be prevented by gradually returning a hypercapnic patient to desirable levels of volume pressure flows.

> *Progressive alveolar-capillary block.* Caused by prolonged ventilation (e.g., for months), which ruptures capillaries and causes hyalinization of the alveolar-capillary membrane. This serious complication necessitates progressive increases in volume and rate of ventilation and may eventually contribute to death.

> *Rupture of emphysematous bullae.* Caused by excessive inspiratory volumes or pressures. If rupture occurs, the treatment is that indicated for pneumothorax.

> *Diffuse atelectasis.* Caused by constant ventilation with normal or subnormal tidal volumes. Minute patchy areas of atelectasis tend to develop in patients being continuously ventilated at a set tidal volume. This complication can be prevented or minimized by keeping the patient in cycle with the machine, pulmonary physiotherapy, humidification, maintaining a patent airway, frequent turning, and periodic hyperventilation ("sighing") of the lungs, e.g., 5 to 10 deep breaths every 30 to 60 minutes.

> *Infection* due to the use of contaminated equipment or the patient's lowered resistance. Prevention of infection is highly important in a patient being continuously ventilated.[70]

> *Circulatory collapse* owing to impaired venous return to the heart. Immediately report indications of reduced cardiac output. As discussed previously, patients with impaired cardiac function may not tolerate prolonged positive pressure ventilation because of the decrease in venous return that occurs. Since abnormal intrathoracic pressures and venous return to the heart are detectable in the central venous pressure (CVP), the CVP may be frequently monitored. Usually the physician states the desirable CVP that should be maintained. (CVP is discussed in Unit X.)

Observe for early indications of complications and report their development so treatment can be started promptly.

Periodic or intermittent IPPB treatments may be given to a patient who is unable to cough effectively or who has pulmonary congestion or bronchospasm (Fig. 70–13). Prior to periodic IPPB treatments the patient should have postural drainage and cough productively or be suctioned. Periodic IPPB treatments may be given to assist with ventilation, relieve respiratory insufficiency, promote more effective coughing and removal of secretions, liquefy secretions, improve respiratory blood gas exchange, dilate bronchioles, and actively inflate the lungs more deeply.

IPPB may be used to give aerosolized medications to patients who cannot inhale deeply enough to take medications in this form by other methods such as a hand nebulizer. Medications may be administered by IPPB for their local effect on the respiratory tract. The IPPB machine's pressurized flow delivers medication deep into the tracheobronchial tree and distributes it widely throughout the lungs. Medications that may be administered by nebulization in this way include antibiotics as well as medications given to liquefy or loosen secretions (e.g., mucolytic agents) or to dilate the bronchi by relieving bronchial spasm or constriction. Make certain that the amount of medication in the nebulizer is adequate to last throughout the procedure. If the medication should run out before treatment is terminated the delivery of pressurized unmoisturized air by the machine would rapidly dry out the respiratory tract mucosa, producing harmful effects.

Have the patient breathe slowly at his own rate of comfortable ventilation. Observe the patient closely during the treatment for systemic effects from the medication used and for untoward effects of increased intrathoracic pressure on the heart's circulatory response (e.g., dizziness, nausea, or vomiting).

During the IPPB administration of aerosolized medications the patient should:[267]

> Sit upright to avoid air being forced into the stomach and to facilitate excursion of the diaphragm.
> Close lips tightly around the mouthpiece.
> Prevent air passage through the nose. (The patient may need to hold his nose or use a noseclip.)
> Exhale completely before attaching himself to the machine.
> Gently inspire to trigger the respirator.
> Relax.
> Remove the mouthpiece to cough.

Orders for periodic IPPB treatments should include identification of the types of machine to be used, delivery pressure, medications to be used and their dosage, and therapeutic procedures to be used following IPPB. Periodic treatments may be given three or four times daily for 15 to 20 minutes. Some acutely ill patients require hourly treatments. Commonly treatments are given at 15 to 20 cm. H_2O pressure. The patient is instructed how to obtain the greatest benefit from the IPPB treatments; for example, he is taught to practice slow diaphragmatic breathing with prolonged active respiration. Every few breaths the patient should inhale deeply and exhale down to his residual volume.

Clinical Care of the Patient on a Ventilator. Machine settings are specified by the physician to meet the individual patient's needs. The physician specifies the type of machine to be used, whether controlled or assisted ventilation is necessary, the volume and mixture of gases to be administered, and the settings, e.g., rate of respirations, volume, pressure, sensitivity. The physician also orders necessary monitoring, chest x-rays, and laboratory tests such as serum electrolyte levels, blood gases, and arterial pH to assess therapy.

A respirator is always tested before the machine is used on a patient. During this testing the O_2 level and humidification are evaluated and all tubings and connectors are examined for gas leaks. Prior to IPPB therapy remove poorly fitting dentures and dental bridges, which could be damaged or aspirated. Make certain the patient does not have gum, food, or pills in his mouth, which could be aspirated.

Do not attempt to use an IPPB machine unless you understand how to properly operate and care for the machine and the patient being artificially ventilated.

Space does not permit detailed discussion of IPPB therapy. The nurse who will be carrying out this type of inhalation therapy requires advanced specialized training. In addition to reading textbooks of respiratory therapy, hospital procedure manuals, and manufacturer's instructions, it is necessary to receive instruction from qualified individuals. In order to qualify to administer respirator therapy, a nurse should be familiar with appropriate theory, be skilled in the operation of respirators, and have had supervised practice in the use of respirators on patients. It is desirable for the nurse to try using a respirator herself so she can more completely understand the experiences of patients being mechanically ventilated.

Periodically the nurse checks the ventilating equipment. These periods of observation should include: (1) noting the various ventilator settings

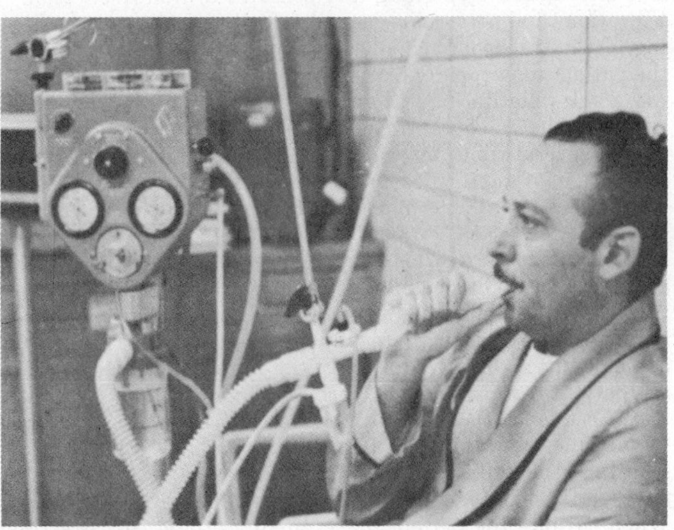

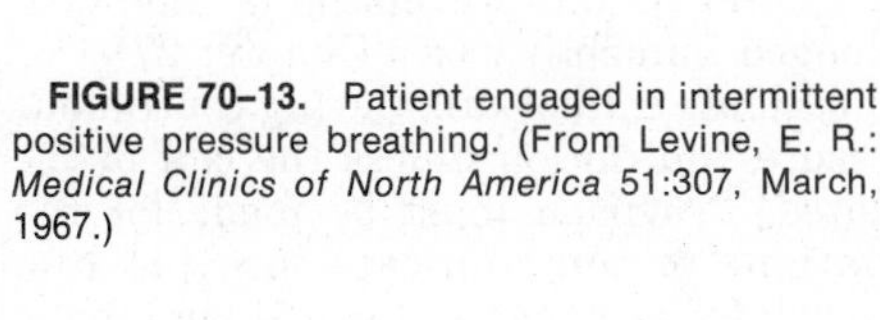

FIGURE 70–13. Patient engaged in intermittent positive pressure breathing. (From Levine, E. R.: *Medical Clinics of North America* 51:307, March, 1967.)

and gauge readings at the time of initial patient contact and comparing later observations with baseline observations to detect changes so that changes in the patient's condition or accidental dial changes will be readily detected; (2) making certain humidifiers are adequately filled; (3) watching the pressure gauge on the ventilator for oscillating movements (indicative of water condensation in the tubing which is impairing machine function—condensation should be frequently emptied from the tubing); and (4) checking the expiratory valve to be certain it moves freely (sticking valves cause a slow pressure drop during expiration and the conscious patient experiences distress—replace sticking valves immediately). The nurse also checks to be certain the tubing is free of kinks and tensions. An oxygen analyzer is used at intervals to check the O_2 concentration being delivered to the patient.

If the nurse observes that the patient is breathing out of phase with the ventilator or if she notes malfunctioning of the ventilator, she should immediately disconnect the machine, manually ventilate the patient with O_2 at a 10 L./min. flow (with a self-inflating bag), and have someone summon the respiratory therapist or physician.[197] Manual ventilation must be continued (squeeze the bag 15 times per minute) until help arrives and the patient is again being safely ventilated by machine.

Routinely, every hour around the clock, the following procedures are performed in sequence on patients being artificially ventilated:[197] (1) the patient is given 6 to 8 deep inflations ("sighed") with a self-inflating (Ambu) bag and O_2 at a flow rate of 10 L./min.; (2) the trachea is aspirated *if* secretions are present (aspiration is performed as often as necessary but only if required); and (3) the patient's position is changed.

A clean, patent airway is imperative for successful ventilator therapy. *Aspiration* is most effective if it is preceded by sighing and postural drainage. Vibrations and percussion may also facilitate clearing of the tracheobronchial tree. After suctioning, the patient may rapidly be reoxygenated by attaching a self-inflating bag to an O_2 source. With the use of high O_2 concentration the airway is ventilated several times by compressing the bag. Then the patient is reattached to the respirator. Special adaptors are available to attach the bag to tracheostomy tubes.[267]

The three basic *position changes* used are supine and left and right decubitus (complete 90 degree turns). With the physician's permission some of the hourly sighing, aspiration, and position changes can be omitted during portions of the night, so that the patient can have longer periods of undisturbed rest. Frequent repositioning is necessary not only to prevent complications of inactivity but also to facilitate adequate ventilation of the entire lung fields and secretion mobilization and removal. When turning the patient, have adequate help, so that the respirator parts attached to the patient can be kept properly aligned. Position the patient in such a manner that he has adequate chest expansion.

Hourly the nurse observes and records the patient's vital signs, pupils, level of consciousness, chest excursions (e.g., degree of chest expansion on both sides), muscle strength, reaction to the respirator, and color of the lips and nail beds. Temperature is usually taken every four hours. Both apical and radial pulses are taken. Reduced cardiac output and reduced venous return may cause an increase in the rate and a reduction in the volume of the pulse. Reduced venous return to the heart causes blood pressure to drop. Underventilation may initially cause the blood pressure to elevate before it gradually declines. Hypoxemia may produce reduced levels of consciousness.

The nurse should record hourly the tidal and minute volumes if the Wright respirometer is being used. The patient is observed closely for indications of hypo- or hyperventilation. For example, the nurse watches for indications of respiratory alkalosis such as vertigo, faintness, and numbness or tingling of the extremities. This condition can occur if the patient is being hyperventilated.

Phipps and Barker[228] identify the following clinical observations, which confirm *adequate ventilation* in a patient on a respirator:

1. Improvement in skin color or absence of cyanosis.
2. Rhythmic expansion of the chest with expiratory phase longer than inspiratory phase.
3. Normal pulse; a change in pulse rate may indicate decreased cardiac output due to the increase in intrathoracic pressure.
4. Stationary blood pressure; a drop of the blood pressure may reflect decreased cardiac output.
5. Absence of any abnormal neurologic signs.
6. Audible rhythmicity of respiration.
7. Normal function of respirator.
8. Absence of hyperventilation or hypoventilation.

Observations indicative of *inadequate ventilation* include hypo- or hyperventilation, absent inspiratory or expiratory cycle, impaired ventilatory excursion, or prolonged expiration with delay in inspiration.

Some *factors of importance in the general care* of a patient being artificially ventilated include: infection prevention; good skin, mouth, nose, and tracheostomy care (periodically deflate cuffed tubes to minimize tracheal damage); intake-output record (patients who cannot swallow are given I.V. or gastric tube feedings); and prevention of complications of prolonged immobility (see Chapter 27).

Intubated patients cannot talk during continuous positive pressure ventilation unless the cuff of the tube is deflated. Provision must be made for the conscious patient to communicate; provide him with a "magic slate" or paper and pencil, and make certain he always has a call bell. Attempt to anticipate the patient's needs, and talk to him when appropriate even though he cannot answer.

Continuous respirator therapy may be a frightening, depressing and costly experience for a patient and his family. During this difficult time the nurse strives to be helpful whenever possible to both patient and family. She also prepares family members for their initial visit with the patient and acquaints them with the value of the machine.

The physician decides when to begin *weaning* a patient from the respirator. Breathing efforts out of cycle with the machine sometimes indicate readiness to give up the ventilator. Usually a patient cannot be off the respirator for long if his vital capacity is less than twice his normal tidal volume.[228] The physician also evaluates the blood gases. It is helpful if the patient understands abdominal breathing patterns before he is weaned. Controlled abdominal breathing can help him to breathe more effectively without the respirator. During the weaning process the patient is gradually taken off the respirator for increasingly long periods as tolerated. For example, initially he may be off the respirator 3 or 4 minutes every half hour. Once this length of time is tolerated, the intervals of spontaneous respiration are increased.

If the patient was treated by a volume-controlled ventilator he may be transferred to a pressure-cycled machine before weaning begins. Once he is on the pressure-cycled ventilator the sensitivity can be progressively reduced, so that the patient gradually assumes greater responsibility for tripping the machine to initiate inspiration.

Typically it takes longer to wean a patient who has had prolonged controlled ventilation than a patient who required only short-term treatment. It is desirable to begin weaning as soon as the patient's physiologic measurements indicate he is ready. Early weaning is psychologically encouraging to the patient. Additionally, it enables restoration of normal muscle tone to the muscles involved in breathing. The early morning hours, when the patient is most relaxed and rested, are usually the most desirable for beginning weaning.

During periods of weaning humidified O_2 is provided when the patient is off the ventilator. If the patient is tracheotomized he is given warm, humidified oxygenated air via a Briggs adaptor attached to the tracheostomy tube during the time it is disconnected from the ventilator.

A patient who has received continuous automatic ventilation for a prolonged period of time may become highly dependent on the machine and may be fearful during the weaning process. It is helpful if the patient is cared for during the weaning procedure by a nurse he has confidence in and with whom he feels relaxed. A calm, relaxed atmosphere facilitates the transition from machine-controlled to patient-controlled breathing. Occasionally mild sedation helps the patient during the weaning process. The nurse remains with the patient while he is off the ventilator and observes for indications of poor tolerance such as a staring expression, increased, shallow respirations, diaphoresis, increased pulse rate, increased blood pressure (indicative of falling arterial pressure), decreased blood pressure (indicative of low cardiac output), gray pallor, a red flush rising from the neck to the face, or cyanosis. The patient's emotional responses are evaluated as well as his blood gases, tidal and minute volumes, and vital capacity. If the patient begins to show indications of needing mechanical ventilatory assistance he is rapidly, but calmly,

returned to the respirator. If the patient appears to be breathing too rapidly or too shallowly because of anxiety, the nurse talks with him and attempts to help him to practice slow, relaxed, controlled abdominal breathing.

Once the newly weaned patient is completely removed from mechanical ventilatory assistance, it is sometimes helpful to leave an easily operated respirator such as the Bird in the room for a day or so to give the patient the reassurance that it is available if needed. The patient may be taught to use the machine himself. Once complete weaning has taken place, continued observation of the patient's respiratory status is important for a few days to make certain that his spontaneous respirations are adequate.

SUCTIONING

Suctioning (aspiration of secretions) is a common nursing activity employed to remove secretions from the nose, mouth or tracheobronchial tree and to stimulate productive coughing. Suctioning of the nose and mouth is a relatively simple, safe procedure, details for which can be found in textbooks of nursing fundamentals. This discussion focuses on tracheal suctioning.

Tracheal Suctioning

Tracheal suctioning is also called "endotracheal" or "deep" suctioning. Suctioning of the trachea and proximal portions of each mainstem bronchus may be performed by passing a sterile catheter through the mouth ("orotracheal" suctioning), through the nose ("nasotracheal" suctioning), or through an endotracheal or tracheostomy tube. Physicians may orally pass suction catheters into the trachea via laryngoscopes. Nurses most commonly perform tracheal suctioning through the nose or via a tracheostomy tube. Suctioning through a tracheostomy is discussed in Unit XXII.

When properly performed, tracheal suctioning can be helpful and relatively painless and will promote the comfort (indeed, perhaps, save the life) of a patient in respiratory distress. If improperly performed, this procedure can be detrimental, painful, and possibly even fatal.

The various possible *complications* of tracheal suctioning are discussed throughout the following pages. Among these are infection, hypoxia, traumatic ulceration of mucosa, lobar collapse, perforation of a bronchial suture line, and sudden death. Use of contaminated equipment may introduce *infection*. *Hypoxia* results from prolonged suction, which aspirates the air from the patient's major airways. Brief suctioning periods, preoxygenation of the patient before beginning suctioning, and oxygenation during and following the suction process help to prevent this potential complication. *Lobar collapse* occurs when air cannot enter a portion of the lung. Suctioning may produce lobar collapse if a catheter is too large in diameter for the size of the airway being suctioned. It is important to carefully select a catheter of appropriate size for suctioning and not to force or wedge the catheter into a bronchus. (The diameter of the bronchus becomes smaller as it extends away from the trachea.) Caution is necessary when performing deep tracheal suctioning following pulmonary surgery because a suture line may be traumatized by the catheter, i.e., the catheter may be *accidentally pushed through a sutured bronchus.*

Continuous suctioning for 15 to 30 seconds can produce *sudden death.* Possible causes include:[297] prolonged suctioning, which causes anoxia and then *severe cardiac arrhythmias;* respiratory tract reflexes, which stimulate *bradycardia* and *bronchospasm;* and *distention of the heart with blood* from the superior vena cava and pulmonary artery. Critically ill patients should never be suctioned longer than 15 seconds, and it is safe to suction for that long *only* if the patient has been preoxygenated and is carefully monitored for indications of complications. It is generally safest to apply suction intermittently for no longer than 5 to 8 seconds.

Because it is a potentially hazardous procedure, deep tracheal aspiration should not be performed without advanced training in the procedure. In some settings the physician's permission is necessary for this procedure. *Techniques to mechanically stimulate coughing should be used before resorting to suctioning.* Techniques to mechanically stimulate coughing (e.g., direct external mechanical stimulation of the trachea and internal mechanical stimulation of the trachea produced by prolonged exhalation by the patient) are discussed on p. 893. Coughing is frequently stimulated by passage of a catheter through the nose or mouth.

Ungvarski comments as follows about the need for endotracheal suctioning:[306]

> It should be kept in mind that most patients, unless they are extremely debilitated, are quite capable, physiologically, of coughing up sputum into the pharynx and then expectorating or swallowing it. Therefore, the primary purpose of introducing a catheter into the trachea is not vigorous suctioning but, simply, tracheal stimulation with a catheter.
>
> Actual endotracheal suctioning need only be used for patients with tenacious secretions (which must be physically removed by suction) or impaired pulmonary function (which may interfere with the cough reflex), or for those who are extremely debilitated and too weak to bring up secretions even after vigorous coughing.

> *The goals of all suctioning procedures are to remove secretions and stimulate productive coughing without causing prolonged airway obstruction, infection, damage to delicate mucous membranes, or other complications.*

Factors of General Importance. *Observe patients closely for indications of the need to be suctioned,* such as noisy respirations, restlessness, and increased pulse and respiratory rates. Cyanosis is a late sign of upper airway obstruction. The conscious patient is usually aware of the need to be suctioned and can inform the nurse. Obtunded patients must be carefully observed and suctioned promptly when indicated. Keep operable suctioning equipment and ample suctioning supplies at the bedside of any patient who is unable to clear his tracheobronchial tree.

Patients who require suctioning often benefit from humidification of inspired air, since this tends to liquefy secretions and make them easier to remove by suction. Prior to suctioning, attempt to move secretions up into higher levels in the tracheobronchial tree by using postural drainage with percussion and vibration. To loosen tenacious, thick mucus the physician may order the nurse to instil a few milliliters of sterile water, normal saline, or sodium bicarbonate solution (5 per cent) into the trachea immediately prior to aspiration. Additionally, liquefying agents may be instilled through the catheter. The instillation of small amounts of sterile normal saline (1 to 2 ml.) may reduce the tendency of plastic catheters to stick to the walls of plastic intratracheal or tracheostomy tubes. The solution is inserted in this instance while the suction catheter is being passed.

As previously mentioned, infection is one hazard of suctioning. Nasal and oral suctioning is a clean procedure; wash your hands before suctioning. *Tracheal suctioning is a sterile procedure;** wear sterile gloves and use sterile solutions and catheters. Disposable gloves and catheters reduce the possibility of introducing infection into the lungs. Infection is risked each time a catheter is introduced into the tracheobronchial tree, since normally this is a sterile structure. *Always use separate equipment to suction the nose or mouth;* i.e., never suction the trachea with a catheter used previously for nasal or oral suctioning. Frequently exchange suction equipment kept at the bedside to prevent possible use of contaminated equipment.

Select an Appropriate Suction Catheter. Never use a closed-tip catheter, such as a urinary catheter, because it just pushes mucus plugs ahead of it. A coudé (bent) whistle-tip catheter is most successful for deep tracheal suctioning. The bend at the catheter's tip facilitates insertion into one of the mainstem bronchi. Soft plastic catheters are now available, and a transparent catheter is useful because suctioned material can be observed.

Catheter sizes used for suctioning vary, depending on the diameter of the orifice to be intubated,

*In some instances "clean technique" is used in caring for patients with permanent tracheostomies, e.g., the hands are thoroughly washed before suctioning.

e.g., nostrils, endotracheal or tracheostomy tube lumen, and so forth. Frequently No. 14 or 16 (Fr.) catheters are used for tracheal suctioning in an adult. The catheter should be one half to two thirds the diameter of the tube to be intubated. If the catheter's diameter is too small it may be impossible to remove thick secretions or mucous plugs. On the other hand, too large a catheter occludes the orifice's opening and causes excessive negative pressure, which may predispose to atelectasis or lobar collapse. It is most desirable to have available several sizes (Fr. Nos. 12, 14, 16, and 18) of sterile suction catheters for adult suctioning.

Prior to suctioning be certain the patient is well oxygenated. Some sources[278] recommend administering 100 per cent O_2 for 5 minutes to increase the patient's PaO_2 before suctioning. Because tracheal suctioning removes O_2, it lowers the PaO_2 and can trigger cardiac arrhythmias.

Evaluate a patient's pulse (for bradycardia) and his heart action (for indications of heart block) on a cardiac monitor if possible when preparing to suction and while suctioning. Monitor the patient throughout the suctioning procedure, observing for the following sequence of events, which may occur as a result of excessive suctioning, or in patients with a low PaO_2 or marginal cardiopulmonary reserve before suctioning:[142] initial tachycardia, followed by cardiac irritability and downward shifting of the natural pacemaker, i.e., premature contractions, nodal rhythm, resulting from myocardial hypoxia and acidosis; bradycardia; and, finally, asystole. If tachycardia occurs during tracheal suctioning, evaluate the severity of the symptom and proceed only if it is mild. *Discontinue suctioning immediately if bradycardia develops and ventilate the patient with high O_2 concentrations.* Report untoward effects of suctioning at once. The physician may then order medications (e.g., atropine sulfate) to assist with secretion removal or to control secretion production and/or recommend less frequent or less vigorous suctioning.

Perform the suction procedure gently; lubricate the catheter, insert it carefully, avoid excessive suction pressures, and do not move the catheter up and down within the trachea with poking or jabbing motions. Respiratory tract mucosa is easily damaged and is subject to edema, bleeding, ulceration, and infection. Rough or prolonged suctioning and excessive pressures traumatize tracheobronchial mucosa and may produce tracheobronchitis and perhaps its feared complications of tracheal or bronchial stenosis. Even with gentle suction technique the trachea's walls are irritated and traumatized slightly each time suction is performed. *Suction a patient as frequently as indicated but no oftener.* Excessive suctioning is not only traumatic but also stimulates production of increased secretions. Never insert a dry catheter into the trachea. Before insertion lubricate the catheter's distal end with sterile water, sterile normal saline, or a fine coating of a nonreactive, water-soluble lubricant, e.g., K-Y jelly. Release suction if you feel the catheter "grab" against mucous membranes; otherwise, the mucosa will avulse into the catheter openings.

Keep suction periods brief. Do not apply suction while inserting the catheter (Fig. 70–14). Application of suction during insertion causes suction on tracheal mucosa (thus irritating and traumatizing the mucosa) and unnecessarily takes away the patient's breath; remember that suction removes air as well as secretions. It is helpful if you hold your breath when suctioning the patient; this action will serve to remind you of how long the patient is without air during the procedure. As mentioned earlier, it is recommended that suctioning periods *never* exceed 15 seconds. *Prolonged suctioning may worsen respiratory insufficiency and produce hypoxia, asphyxia, and cardiac arrest.* Hypoxia may result from use of too large a catheter, use of suction that is too high, or not allowing the patient time to adequately ventilate between periods of suctioning[306] (Fig. 70–14). Overstimulation or prolonged irritation at the bifurcation of the trachea during deep endotracheal suctioning may produce multiple premature ventricular contractions, leading to cardiac arrest.[306] Prolonged suctioning results in asphyxia, since it prevents necessary respiratory exchange by continuing to suck air out of the lungs without providing input of a fresh supply of air.

Avoid excessive suction pressure. Adjust the suction to correspond with the nature of the secretions being removed. Use the lowest level of negative pressure that will be effective. Withdraw the catheter slowly while applying suction. During removal gently twirl or rotate the catheter between your thumb and forefinger. This exposes the catheter's openings to a greater tracheal surface area, enabling more effective removal of secretions.

If it is necessary to continue the suctioning procedure, *allow the patient to rest,* and administer O_2 if indicated for about three minutes before the next insertion. If the patient is on a respirator, ventilate him for a while and *administer O_2 before suctioning again.* At the termination of tracheal suctioning, again raise the patient's PaO_2 to presuctioning levels by administering high O_2 concentrations.

Be aware of patients for whom tracheal suctioning is particularly dangerous. Suction these patients only if absolutely necessary. Jacquette[142] identifies the following high risk situations: (1) PaO_2 below 70 mm. Hg (suctioning would further reduce the arterial O_2 tension); (2) large alveolar-arterial gradient* (indicates very low cardiopulmonary reserve); and (3) generally poor condition, e.g., inadequate oxygenation, hypotension, arrhythmias, acid-base imbalances.

*The alveolar-arterial gradient is normally a difference of about 50 to 55 mm. Hg. It represents the difference between the O_2 tension of alveolar air and of the arterial blood once respiration has occurred. Large alveolar-arterial gradients signify poor ventilation/perfusion ratio, poor ventilation of segments of the lung with air, and poor perfusion of pulmonary segments with blood.

Nasotracheal Suctioning Procedures. Nasotracheal suctioning is performed using sterile (preferably disposable) gloves, catheter, lubricant, and irrigating solutions. A catheter is inserted past the posterior oropharynx, around the epiglottis, through the vocal cords, and finally down into the trachea. The vocal cords open with inspiration.

Various problems can make it difficult to gain access to the trachea with a catheter; among these are presence of obstructing material in the nostrils, of swollen mucous membranes, and of nasal polyps or deviated nasal septum. Additionally, nasal passages are extremely tender; thus, pain is easily produced. Other problems that can occur are that the catheter may go into the esophagus if the patient swallows when the catheter reaches the epiglottis, or the catheter may coil in the nasopharynx instead of passing through the epiglottis.

The trachea bifurcates into the right and left mainstem bronchi. The right mainstem bronchus typically has a 15 degree angle to the vertical, while the left mainstem bronchus is angled at about 25 to 35 degrees. The more acute angulation of the left bronchus makes it more difficult to intubate than the right. Nonetheless, it is possible to intubate either mainstem bronchus during tracheal suctioning by angulation of the head and neck toward the side opposite the bronchus to be entered, using a suction catheter with a slightly curved tip, and rotating the catheter's tip so it points toward the bronchus to be entered.[297] To enter the right mainstem bronchus, position the patient partially on his right side, turn his head to the left, and point his chin up. Reverse these positions to enter the left mainstem bronchus.

Effective tracheal suctioning is a gentle yet swift procedure in which timing is important. The person performing the procedure works with deliberate, controlled actions. The suctioning procedure must be particularly well coordinated when a patient is attached to a respirator. If the patient has a cuffed endotracheal or tracheostomy tube, suctioning is performed, when possible, when the airway is deflated and the patient's position is changed, or when other treatments are given. By planning

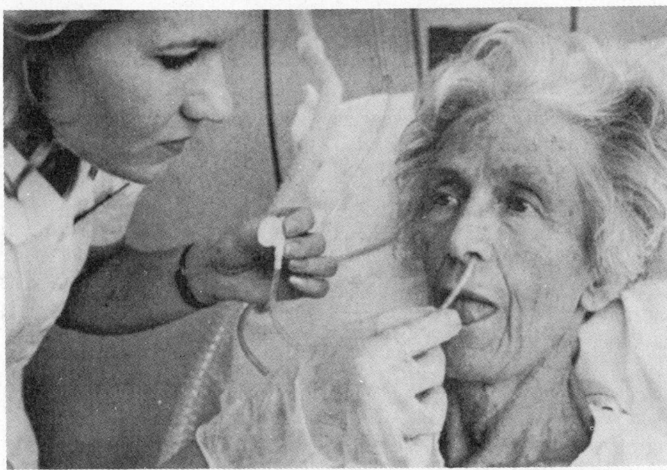

A

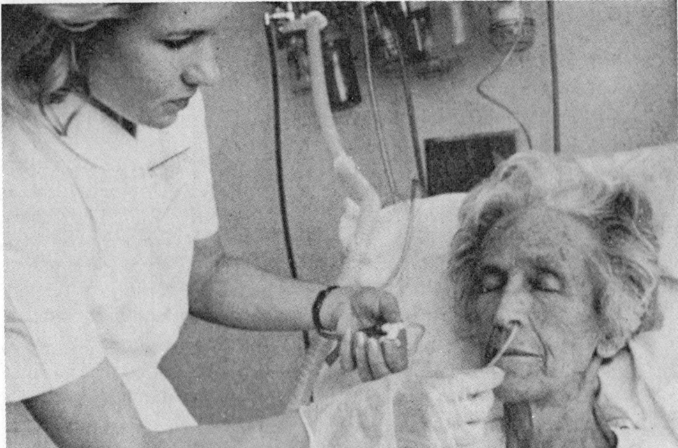

B

FIGURE 70–14. Precautions important with tracheal suctioning. *A,* Catheter is not attached to suction while it is being passed, but oxygen and suction tubing, placed across the pillow, are readily accessible for connection. *B,* Between suction attempts, the catheter is connected to oxygen and the patient rests. (From Jacquette, G.: *American Journal of Nursing, 71*:2362, December, 1971.)

nursing care activities so they coincide it is possible to provide the patient with more periods of undisturbed rest.

When performing tracheal suctioning on a patient with chest tubes, the tubes are temporarily clamped. This is done because violent coughing may be stimulated, and clamping the tubes limits dissipation of the effort and force of coughing.[297] If the tubes are not clamped, a significant reduction occurs in the peak negative and positive pressures, and energy is used during inspiration to draw water up the tubing (from the underwater seal) and to expel the air in the pleural space during expiration.[297]

Endotracheal suctioning is an uncomfortable, often frightening procedure for a patient. Once the catheter passes between the vocal cords the patient cannot talk because the cords cannot approximate. The catheter's presence in the trachea may make the patient highly anxious and acutely restless. The patient benefits from directions about what he should be doing to help during the procedure and from frequent reassurance. Often during tracheal suctioning the patient instinctively wants to pull at the catheter, especially when the cough reflex is stimulated. Cooperative patients can be asked to try to control this instinct.

Some patients tolerate tracheal suctioning better if they are given an analgesic half an hour before the procedure. Occasionally it is necessary to spray the nasopharynx and hypopharynx with a topical anesthetic in patients with extremely active gag reflexes. However, the use of an anesthetic is generally to be avoided because it depresses the cough reflex and increases the risk of aspiration if the patient vomits.[219]

In preparation for nasotracheal suctioning, place an emesis basin and tissues within easy reach for use when the patient expectorates. Have the patient blow his nose to clear the nasal passageways. With a flashlight inspect the patient's nostrils for possible obstructions (e.g., deviated nasal septum) before inserting the suction catheter. Select the least obstructed nostril for suctioning. If both nostrils appear free of obstruction, use them alternately for the different suctioning sessions so you do not excessively irritate one nostril. (Remember to chart which nostril was used.)

PROCEDURE. Nasotracheal suctioning may be accomplished as follows: (See Fig. 70–15)

> Position the patient sitting up, leaning slightly forward, with his back supported. The patient's face should look straight ahead, with his head extended and neck slightly flexed. If an assistant is present she should stand behind the patient.

> Have the patient extend his jaw, open his mouth widely and stick out his tongue. The assistant grasps the tongue with a dry 4 × 4 gauze. Pulling the tongue forward displaces the epiglottis forward and helps to prevent deflection of the catheter into the esophagus. (Once the catheter reaches the trachea the tongue is released and the patient can position his head more comfortably.)

> Note the position of the curved catheter tip in relation to the Y connector, so you will know in which direction the tip is pointed once it is out of sight. Also, predetermine approximately the amount of catheter that will be inserted when the tip reaches the vocal cords. This can be done by measuring from the tip of the patient's nose

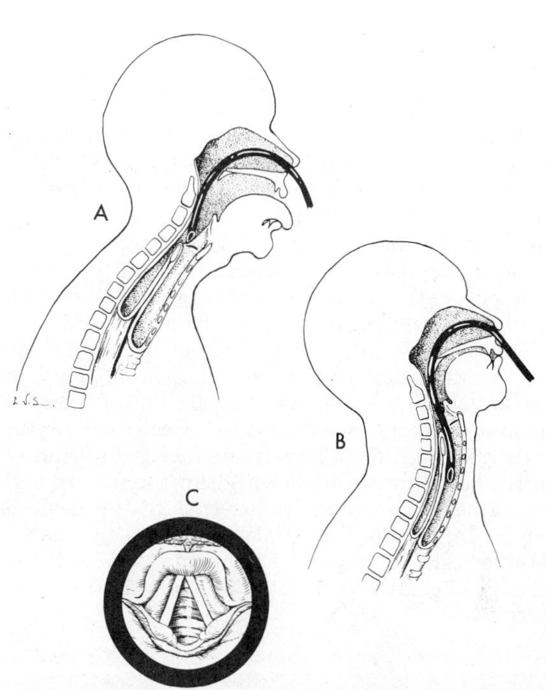

FIGURE 70–15. Technique of nasotracheal suctioning. *A*, Optimal position of head in order to direct catheter tip anteriorly into the trachea. The neck is flexed and the head is extended. The tongue is protruded (and held there by a gauze 4 × 4). *B*, After the catheter has been advanced into the trachea, the tongue is released and the patient's head may be more comfortably positioned. *C*, View of the vocal cords from above. The cords are most widely separated during inspiration. (From Sanderson, R. G. (ed.): *The Cardiac Patient.* 1972.)

to the lobe of his ear and then from there down the side of the neck to the "Adam's apple."

> Ask the patient to pant or breathe through his mouth. While he does this, gently insert the lubricated catheter through one nostril and into the hypopharynx. Advance the catheter slowly until the vocal cord level is reached. Make certain the tip of the catheter and the patient's head are properly positioned so the catheter will enter whichever mainstem bronchus you wish. Then ask the patient to take a deep breath (to open the glottis) and, as he does so, rapidly advance the catheter through the larynx into the trachea, unless resistance is met. To stabilize the position of the catheter and thus prevent its accidental withdrawal, hold the catheter near the patient's nose. Up to this time tracheal suction should not be applied.

> Apply suction by *intermittent* occlusion of the Y connector orifice or vent with the thumb for 5 to 8 seconds after any possible wedging of the catheter tip is corrected by withdrawing the catheter for 1 or 2 cm. Suction is applied only while the catheter is being withdrawn. During suctioning, listen for air sucking sounds at the level of the catheter tip. (If these sounds cease, or if the catheter tip feels as if it were stuck against the tracheal wall and is not easily withdrawn, stop suctioning.) While intermittently applying suction, progressively withdraw

the catheter a short distance until the entire length of the trachea is suctioned.

Allow the patient sufficient rest periods as you advance down each mainstem bronchus and as you suction that bronchus during withdrawal of the catheter. During rest periods the catheter may be left in place, but suction is not applied. If the patient appears anoxic, administer O_2 temporarily by mask or through the catheter. If indicated, instill 5 ml. of sterile water or sterile saline into each mainstem bronchus and repeat the suctioning.

Sometimes if the catheter cannot be inserted to the expected depth, a mucus plug is obstructing the lumen of the trachea. Instillation of a small amount of sterile water or normal saline is useful in such a situation to liquefy the mucus sufficiently for the suction catheter to withdraw the mucus, and the catheter can then be inserted to the desired depth. Injection of a mixture of acetylcysteine (Mucomyst) in normal saline may be ordered through the catheter to help to loosen and liquefy secretions.

Following tracheal suctioning, auscultate the chest to determine the effectiveness of the procedure. Repeat suctioning as indicated after letting the patient rest for at least 3 minutes and administering O_2. Chart the effectiveness of the procedure, the character and amounts of secretions removed, and the patient's tolerance of the procedure. Aspiration of blood-tinged mucus may indicate that suction has been too forceful and has damaged the mucous membranes.

EMERGENCY CARDIOPULMONARY RESUSCITATION

If a patient's respirations cease, immediately begin ventilation through the nose or mouth. Feel the carotid pulse after inflating the lungs a few times. If the pulse is not detectable, begin external cardiac compression in an attempt to restore circulation. Then continue both respiratory and circulatory resuscitation. If obstruction prevents artificial ventilation or if the airway cannot be cleared, emergency establishment of an airway is indicated to bypass the obstruction, i.e., tracheal intubation is indicated.[232] (Cardiopulmonary resuscitation is discussed in detail in Unit X. Mouth-to-neck resuscitation is discussed in Unit XXII.)

CHAPTER 71

Disorders of the Pleurae, Pleural Spaces, Tracheobronchial Tree and Lungs

DISORDERS OF THE PLEURAE OR PLEURAL SPACES

PLEURISY (PLEURITIS)

Inflammation of the pleura may be fibrinous (dry) or serofibrinous (wet). A wet pleurisy is accompanied by pleural effusion as a result of an abnormal increase of nonpurulent pleural fluid. In dry pleurisy the amount of pleural fluid does not increase.

Dry Pleurisy

This condition frequently accompanies pneumonia and other inflammatory pulmonary diseases, and may complicate such disorders as chest trauma, cancer, pulmonary infarction, chest wall infections, mediastinitis, and pericarditis. The size of the area affected may range from a small portion up to most of the pleural surface.

Dry pleurisy typically develops suddenly and is easily diagnosed by characteristic pleuritic pain and a friction rub, which can be detected by auscultation.

The *pleuritic pain* associated with dry pleurisy results from the rubbing together of the two inflamed pleural surfaces during breathing. The pain is caused only by inflammation of the parietal pleura, since the visceral pleura contains no pain receptors. Some patients with dry pleurisy have vague discomfort or pain only when coughing or breathing deeply, whereas others have severe, sharp stabbing pains that are aggravated by every respiratory movement. Often pleuritic pain is more severe during inspiration, which stretches the inflamed pleura. Pleural pain is commonly localized to one side of the chest..

The characteristic *pleural friction rub* results from the rubbing together of the congested, inflamed pleurae. If effusion develops, and fluid separates the pleurae, the friction rub ceases. A pleural friction rub most commonly is heard no sooner than 24 to 48 hours after the beginning of the pleuritic pain. The sounds of a pleural friction rub vary in intensity and are heard during both inspiration and expiration.

The patient with a dry pleurisy may have fever and malaise. Often pain causes him to breathe shallowly and rapidly. The breathing motions of the affected side may be observed to be limited since the patient may use accessory muscles to help him to breathe rather than fully expanding his lower chest. In an attempt to limit respiratory movements the patient may press the affected side of his chest with the palm of his hand while breathing or coughing, or he may lie on the affected side.

Treatment of dry pleurisy involves identifying and treating the underlying disease, placing the patient at rest, and providing symptomatic treatment directed at pain relief. In order to help to minimize the patient's pain the nurse may position the patient on his affected side to splint the chest; she may manually splint the patient's chest while he coughs (if he is unable to effectively assist himself in this manner). The correct method of splinting a patient's chest while he coughs is discussed on p. 1025. The patient on bed rest must be frequently turned and periodically encouraged to cough and deep breathe to prevent complications of inactivity. Since the patient's natural tendencies are to avoid coughing and to breathe shallowly, the lungs may be poorly aerated; thus, periodic expansion of lung tissue (by turning and deep breathing) and clearing of the tracheobronchial tree (by coughing and turning) are essential. Formerly a routine aspect of the treatment of pleurisy was to strap the patient's chest with strips of adhesive tape or bind it with a chest binder in an effort to minimize the pain associated with breathing. These methods of treatment are currently less commonly used because it is realized that they may detrimentally interfere with adequate aeration and respiration and foster the development of atelectasis and pneumonia.

Obtaining pain relief may require treating the patient with an antitussive medication (if a hacking, nonproductive cough is present) and analgesics. Some patients obtain sufficient pain relief from aspirin, but others require stronger analgesics, e.g., codeine, morphine, or meperidine (Demerol).

Narcotics are administered cautiously to prevent further reduction of coughing and ventilation (by depressing the cough and breathing centers of the brain). Applications of heat may be ordered over the painful area to provide comfort. Occasionally to relieve pleuritic pain it is necessary for the physician to block the intercostal nerves by the paravertebral infiltration of an anesthetic agent such as procaine 1 per cent.

Some physicians treat mild pleuritic pain by spraying ethyl chloride over the area of greatest pain for about one minute, and then spraying along the body's long axis through the entire area of pain in such a way that a line of frost about one inch wide is produced. This procedure often gives relief for one to 10 hours. Severe pleuritic pain may be treated with a series of subcutaneous injections of procaine hydrochloride solution (0.5 to 1.0 per cent). The injections are given in such a manner that they pass through the area of greatest pain with a 5-cm. margin on either side.[162]

Wet Pleurisy

As stated previously, wet pleurisy is accompanied by an abnormal increase in the pleural fluid. The fluid is nonpurulent. (If it is purulent, the disorder is called empyema. See p. 939). A wet pleurisy is also called *pleurisy with effusion* or *serofibrinous pleurisy*. As many as 5 liters of fluid may collect in the pleural cavity with pleural effusion.

Pleural effusion is actually a symptom (not a specific disorder) that may be produced by numerous conditions. It may develop with bronchial carcinoma, leukemias, lymphomas, breast cancer, trauma, acute pneumonia, pulmonary edema, pulmonary infarction, subdiaphragmatic abscess, cirrhosis of the liver, systemic infections, cardiac and renal diseases (e.g., congestive heart failure, nephrosis), and some of the collagen diseases (e.g., lupus erythematosus disseminatus, periarteritis nodosa). Pleural effusion most often results from cancer (in older persons) and tuberculosis (in younger persons).

The abnormal quantity of fluid in the pleural space (with pleural effusion) may be either an exudate or a transudate. *Exudates* are substances that have escaped from blood vessels; *transudates* are substances that have passed through a membrane or tissue surface.

The onset of pleurisy with effusion depends upon the underlying disorder and may be dramatically sudden or insidious. *Symptoms* may include dyspnea (possibly developing rapidly), pallor, fatigue, weight loss, prostration, high fever, pleural pain, and possibly a dry cough. Inspection of the side of the chest that has pleural effusion typically reveals distention and absence of movement during breathing. The area is commonly flat when percussed. Large collections of fluid in the pleural space will collapse the lung on the affected side, reducing pulmonary volume and vital capacity, and producing dyspnea and impaired pulmonary ventilation, and may cause embarrassment of the heart and mediastinal shift as a result of pressure on the heart and other mediastinal structures. (Refer to discussion of mediastinal shift on p. 1002).

Procedures used to *diagnose* pleurisy with effusion include history, physical examination, pleural biopsy, x-rays, reflected ultrasound, and exploratory thoracentesis. The etiology can be definitely established only by aspiration of some of the pleural fluid for laboratory investigation.

In the clinical laboratory a specimen of pleural fluid may be given a cytologic examination to detect cancer cells, and a bacteriologic examination in which Gram and acid-fast smears are done and cultures are made on appropriate media. Additional laboratory investigations include counts of erythrocytes and leukocytes, measurement of specific gravity and protein content, determination of glucose level, and examination for cholesterol crystals.

Bloody pleural fluid commonly occurs with carcinomatous effusions and may also occur following pulmonary infarction or with tuberculous effusions.

Small amounts of pleural effusion can be difficult to identify by x-rays. Generally 300 to 500 ml. of free pleural fluid must be present in the pleural space before this fluid is detected by a conventional erect roentgenogram, i.e., a routine posterior-anterior chest film. An x-ray taken with the patient in the lateral recumbent position is most useful in detecting small pleural effusions. Lateral decubitus films may help the physician to determine whether fluid or a thickened pleura is present. Recently, reflected ultrasound has proved useful in detecting and localizing even small amounts of pleural fluid.

Treatment of pleurisy with effusion is directed at the underlying disorder. Thoracentesis is always performed to establish diagnosis and to relieve any respiratory distress resulting from the presence of the space-occupying fluid. Pleural effusion caused by metastasized cancer often recurs and requires repeated thoracentesis. When large quantities of fluid accumulate after a thoracentesis, the physican may not repeat the chest tap but instead insert a small chest catheter (14 or 16 Fr.) and connect it to closed chest drainage without suction. The catheter may be left in place for three days. Catheter drainage enables easier pleural space drainage and fosters apposition of the visceral and parietal pleurae.

Nonpyogenic pleural effusions (i.e., sterile effusions) tend to absorb spontaneously if the patient is maintained on bed rest. Those effusions related to pyogenic infections are treated as an empyema (see below). If pleuritic pain is present it is managed as outlined in the discussion of dry pleurisy.

Observe patients with pleural effusion closely for indications of respiratory embarrassment. Report such findings at once so the physician can immediately perform thoracentesis and remove fluid that has reaccumulated and is compressing the lung on the affected side. Keep a thoracentesis tray available for emergency thoracentesis.

When a pleural effusion is neoplastic in origin the patient may be treated with x-ray therapy to the pleural space and by instillation of chemotherapeutic agents into the pleural space (after as much fluid is removed as possible). Agents that may be used include nitrogen mustard, mechlorethamine hydrochloride, quinacrine hydrochloride, or radioactive gold. When chemotherapy is used in this manner, the patient's position is changed every 15 minutes so the entire pleural space may have contact with the drug.

THORACIC EMPYEMA (PYOTHORAX, SUPPURATIVE PLEURISY)

Although the term "empyema" is frequently used to refer to the accumulation of pus in the *chest* it actually means the collection of pus in *any* body cavity. Hence, this section is correctly titled "thoracic empyema." For the sake of expediency, however, the term "empyema" is used in the remainder of this discussion to refer to thoracic empyema.

The accumulation of purulent exudate in the pleural cavity may occur in several ways. For example, empyema may be directly introduced (by penetrating chest wounds, chest surgery, or other penetrating therapeutic procedures) or it may result from the spread of infection from neighboring structures (e.g., lungs, mediastinum, chest wall). Also, empyema may complicate such disorders as pneumonia (especially staphylococcal pneumonia), tuberculosis, pulmonary abscess, or bronchiectasis.

Empyema is a serious disorder that fortunately occurs less often since the use of carefully selected antibiotic therapy. When it does develop, and is treated *early* with appropriate antibiotics, empyema can usually be effectively controlled.

The size of the area affected by an empyema varies from only a small area of inflammation to involvement of the whole pleural cavity. The exudate present varies in consistency from thin to thick pus. The appearance of the pleura may be essentially normal or, with long-term infections, may be grossly distorted and thickened.

When a *chronic* empyema develops it is usually a recurrent infection of the pleural space that results from the incomplete treatment of an acute empyema. Chronic empyema may be caused by such disorders as foreign body in the pleural space, bronchopleural fistula, tuberculosis, or osteomyelitis of a rib. Chronic empyema may be difficult to treat effectively, since the pleura often becomes extremely thick, and a tough exudate or fibrous tissue binds the lung to the chest wall. Enclosed in such an inelastic covering, the compressed lung cannot easily expand and contract to ventilate effectively. Pleural fibrosis with shrinkage may cause the involved side of the chest to appear shrunken. Scoliosis may develop along with the displacement of mediastinal structures as they are pulled toward the affected side. Multiloculated cavities filled with pus may be present between the chest wall and lung. Clubbing of the fingers often occurs with chronic empyema.

Empyema may be difficult to *diagnose,* since it may be obscured by symptoms of the primary disorder. All patients with pulmonary infection or chest injuries are closely observed for indications of empyema, and empyema is strongly suspected in patients with pulmonary infection who do not respond to treatment. Physical indications of empyema are the same as those of pleural effusion, e.g., dullness to percussion over the involved area. The severity of symptoms is variable, but typically a spiking fever is present. Pleural pain may occur. Some patients with empyema are chronically ill, with weight loss, malaise, and fever, whereas others are acutely ill, with a high fever and prostration.

In the process of establishing diagnosis special projection chest x-rays are usually taken in an attempt to identify the location(s) of accumulations of fluid. After the physical examination and x-rays are completed, the physician selects a site for thoracentesis. Thick pus is difficult to aspirate, and a large bore needle must be used. Diagnosis is confirmed by examining the pleural exudate removed by thoracentesis. In addition to evaluating the specimen's color, specific gravity, and cell count, Gram stains and aerobic and anaerobic cultures are performed. By means of culture the causative organisms are identified and their specific sensitivity to antibiotics is determined.

Treatment of empyema centers around complete drainage of the localized collection of pus and obliteration of the pleural space, and administration of antibiotics to clear the infection and prevent its spread. Antibiotics may be given systemically, or they may be instilled directly into the pleural space. Fibrinolytic enzymes (e.g., trypsin, streptokinase, streptodornase) may help to decrease the viscosity of the pus and dissolve fibrin clots. Intrapleural aspirations and instillations may be performed daily via thoracentesis or thoracotomy tube.

Some patients cannot be effectively treated with enzymatic debridement, intermittent aspirations and instillations of antibiotics. For example, these methods of treatment are ineffective if a multiloculated empyema is present. When these methods are impractical or ineffective, patients with empyema are treated with open or closed chest drainage through a large-diameter chest tube. *Closed chest drainage* may be used if the visceral pleura remains flexible (so the lung can re-expand and the pleural space will be obliterated once the pus-filled cavity is drained), and if the pus is relatively thin. The chest catheter may be inserted in a treatment room or at the bedside. *Open drainage* of thoracic empyema is possible only if there is no danger of collapse of the lung occurring when atmospheric pressure is allowed to enter the pleural space (i.e., through the incision in the chest wall and the drainage tube which is placed through that incision and left open to atmospheric pressure to drain). Open chest drainage may be employed if the empyema is localized within strong "walls" (boundaries) which bind the lung to the chest wall or which otherwise prevent collapse of the lung.

It is often necessary to remove portions of one or two ribs to place the chest drainage tube. With open drainage the tube is left in place and covered with a large absorbent dressing. Dressing changes are carefully performed, as necessary, to prevent introducing new infection and to prevent infection of the person changing the dressing (from the contaminated material on the dressing). The physician changes the tube periodically.

Patients with uncomplicated empyema are usually kept on bed rest as long as they have a fever. Care given the patient during the bed rest period is directed at preventing the complications of inactivity and helping the patient to overcome his infection. The nurse administers medications as prescribed and assists the physician with thoracentesis and instillations.

The patient who has a chest drainage tube is helped to be ambulant as soon as the physician gives his approval. Once able to be out of bed the patient may be assisted outdoors to rest in sunshine and fresh air if the weather permits.

Improvement is indicated by a reduction in pus production, general symptomatic improvement, and a fall in temperature.

In addition to medications and drainage of the pus-filled cavity, treatment also includes the performance of *breathing exercises* by the patient to help to ensure adequate lung expansion and pulmonary function. Breathing exercises are started as soon as the patient's temperature is normal. The patient is instructed to breathe deeply (perhaps every hour while awake) and to exhale against resistance (e.g., to blow into a blow bottle or a spirometer). Breathing against resistance increases intrapulmonary pressure, and helps to stretch the pleurae. Breathing exercises thus help to prevent the contraction and binding down of lung tissue in an unyielding fibrous encasement of thickened pleural tissue.

Patients with empyema should be observed for indications of pneumothorax (see below). Occasionally an untreated empyema drains spontaneously through the chest wall. *Complications* of empyema may also include brain abscess, meningitis, pericarditis, or endocarditis.

Patients with open chest drainage can often be discharged home and their treatment continued on an outpatient basis. Provision must be made for dressing changes at the patient's home. The patient and a family member or friend are taught how to properly change the dressing and dispose of contaminated items. A visiting nurse may visit the patient periodically to provide assistance as indicated and to inspect the wound.

Unfortunately, but characteristically, empyema tends to drain and heal slowly. Thus, drainage is usually necessary for a prolonged period of time. Sometimes the physician instills a radiopaque substance into the cavity to evaluate progress in the healing process. At times the physician orders the cavity to be irrigated periodically with a silver nitrate solution. The visiting nurse may perform these irrigations for the patient being treated at home. As the cavity heals the physician may slowly withdraw the drainage tube. The cavity must close before the drainage system can be discontinued. After the drainage tube is removed the chest wound is covered with appropriate dressings.

Some patients cannot be effectively treated even with tube drainage, e.g., if they have thick pus or extensive pleural damage. These persons require thoracotomy to resect the empyema cavity and surgically remove the binding fibrinous peel that tends to form in chronic cases. The latter procedure, i.e., stripping off the thickened membrane, is called "decortication" and is performed to permit reexpansion of the lung. (See Chapter 73.)

HEMOTHORAX

"Hemothorax" means a collection of blood (e.g., from severed or torn vessels) in the pleural space. The bleeding may occur following injury (e.g., pulmonary laceration, puncture by fractured rib) or chest surgery.

Symptoms of hemothorax may include chest pain, cyanosis, decreasing blood pressure, increased pulse and respiratory rates, dyspnea, decreased or absent breath sounds, and dullness over the affected side of the chest. Mediastinal shift may occur, i.e., displacement of mediastinal contents toward the unaffected side of the chest. In the presence of hemothorax the nurse observes the patient closely for indications of shock and/or respiratory distress.

Diagnosis of hemothorax is confirmed by chest x-ray and/or finding blood in the pleural space upon performing thoracentesis. *Treatment* is directed at evacuating the pleural space and completely reexpanding the lung. Treatment consists of needle aspiration (thoracentesis) or closed chest drainage via thoracotomy tube if thoracentesis is ineffective. When these measures are unsuccessful, surgery is indicated to control bleeding and evacuate blood and clots. Blood replacement may be indicated. A minor hemothorax may resolve without specific treatment. Often pneumothorax and hemothorax occur together, i.e., hemopneumothorax. (For additional discussion of hemothorax see Chapter 72.)

PNEUMOTHORAX

A pneumothorax is a collection of air or gas in the pleural cavity. This condition may develop in several ways. For example, pneumothorax may result from (1) *thoracentesis* (if the needle "nicks" the lung); (2) *thoracic surgery*, (in which the pleural cavity is entered); or (3) *accidental injury* (e.g., from a torn lung, fractured bronchus, or penetration of the chest wall). These causes of pneumothorax are discussed in appropriate sections of this unit. In the recent past a pneumothorax was artificially produced for therapeutic purposes by introducing measured amounts of air into the pleural space through a needle to collapse and rest lung tissue infected with tuberculosis. In modern treatment of tuberculosis artificial pneumothorax is almost never used.

Spontaneous pneumothorax may develop from air leaking from pulmonary alveoli or erosion of a disease process through the pulmonary pleura. For example, a large emphysematous bulla may rupture or a tubercular lesion may erode into the pleural space (Fig. 71–1).

An *open pneumothorax* exists when communication is present between the outside of the body and the pleural space, e.g., through an opening in the chest wall. With a *closed pneumothorax* there is no communication between the outside of the body and the pleural space; air enters the pleural space internally from ruptured alveoli or a bronchus. Closed pneumothorax is the more common. (See also Chapter 72.)

Indications of pneumothorax include sudden, sharp chest pain; cough; sudden shortness of breath with violent but futile respiratory effort; fall in BP; weak, rapid pulse; hyperresonance over the affected thoracic space; apprehension; anxiety; restlessness; diaphoresis; pallor or cyanosis; faintness; feeling of tightness in the chest; decreased or absent breath sounds over the collapsed lung; and cessation of normal chest movements on the affected side.

Respiratory insufficiency and other complications of a large pneumothorax may be rapidly fatal if not recognized and promptly treated. Untreated pneumothorax is a serious condition because it collapses lung tissue and may cause mediastinal shift. Indications of pneumothorax should be reported immediately to the physician. The *diagnosis* is definitely established by chest x-ray.

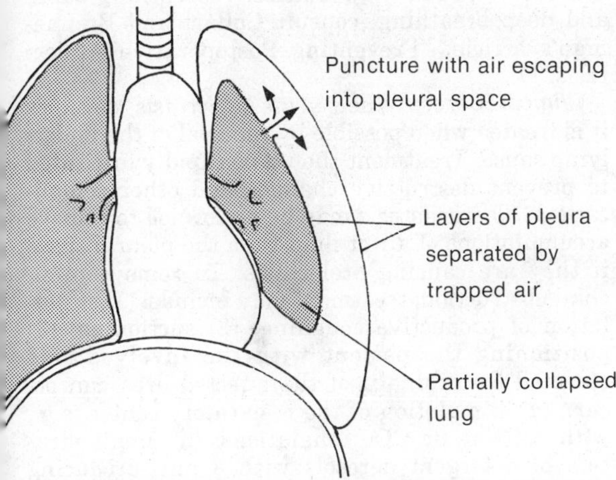

FIGURE 71–1. Spontaneous pneumothorax. (Modified from Knight, R. K.: *Nursing Times*, November 3, 1967.)

The following aspects of *clinical care* are important if a patient develops symptoms of a pneumothorax:

> Remain with the patient and keep him as calm and quiet as possible. Place him in a sitting position. Encourage him to try to control coughing and gasping.

> Without communicating undue alarm to the patient, have another nurse immediately notify the physician and bring thoracentesis equipment to the bedside so the physician can aspirate air as soon as he arrives, if indicated.

> Administer O_2 to relieve dyspnea if necessary. (Note: Administer O_2 cautiously in presence of chronic obstructive pulmonary disease or chronic respiratory insufficiency from other causes to prevent CO_2 narcosis).

> Evaluate pulse and respiratory rates for indications of shock, increasing respiratory distress, and mediastinal shift.

A small pneumothorax may require no specific treatment except restricted activity, mild cough suppression, and O_2 p.r.n. The air in the pleural space is gradually reabsorbed by the body. A larger pneumothorax may be treated by: (1) needle aspiration of the air with needle and syringe (thoracentesis); (2) insertion of a small polyethylene catheter through a needle and removal of air by a suction machine or with a syringe connected to a three-way stopcock; or (3) closed chest drainage, with or without suction, via an intercostal catheter (inserted under local anesthesia through a trocar). Closed chest drainage aspirates air and promotes lung reexpansion. Occasionally thoracotomy is necessary to treat pneumothorax adequately.

Following pneumothorax the patient is advised by the physician to avoid physical exertion until given permission to resume normal activities. The nurse observes the patient for indications of a persistent air leak or recurrent pneumothorax. With a spontaneous pneumothorax the air leaks occur most often in patients with chronic obstructive pulmonary disease because of their overinflated lung tissue, chronic cough, and heightened expiratory effort. During recovery from pneumothorax the physician periodically checks reexpansion of the lung with x-rays and possibly fluoroscopy.

BRONCHOPLEURAL FISTULA

A bronchopleural fistula is a persistent communication between the pleural cavity and the bronchial tree. Bronchopleural fistula is seen today in patients with "old" healed tuberculosis, particularly persons treated with artificial pneumothorax and no chemotherapy. Prior to the use of antimicrobial medications bronchopleural fistula also occurred commonly with other pulmonary disorders such as bacterial pneumonia, bronchiectasis, lung abscess, pulmonary infarction, and postpneumonic empyema.

Presently this complication is less common and more amenable to treatment. Surgical procedures are necessary to correct bronchopleural fistula, and may be employed to fill the pleural space, e.g., decortication, staged thoracoplasty.

DISORDERS OF THE TRACHEOBRONCHIAL TREE AND LUNGS

ATELECTASIS

Pathophysiology. "Atelectasis" refers to an area of lung tissue (or at times even a complete lung) that is collapsed, airless, and shrunken. An atelectasis may be complete or incomplete (partial) and may be an acute or chronic disorder.

Atelectasis occurs frequently in association with various pulmonary disorders, e.g., infections, pleural effusions, tumors; as a postoperative complication, e.g., following thoracic surgery or high abdominal surgery; and as a complication of immobility. It can often be prevented by efficient nursing care (see below).

The main cause of atelectasis is bronchial obstruction by secretions, tumors, bronchospasm, or foreign bodies. Within a few hours after a bronchus is obstructed the air is absorbed from the blocked lung tissue and the affected lung tissue collapses or shrinks. Trapped alveolar air is absorbed by the circulating blood. Frequently infection (e.g., pneumonia) and impaired regional circulation complicate atelectasis. If untreated, the airless, poorly perfused atelectatic area deteriorates into an infected, retracted, fibrotic portion of lung with bronchiectatic changes. (Bronchiectasis is discussed later.) If prompt treatment is given and the obstruction is removed before these destructive changes occur, air reenters the distal lung tissue and expands it, inflammation and infection subside, and effective circulation is restored.

Atelectasis can result not only from the internal obstruction of a bronchus but also from pressure applied to the outside wall of a bronchus, as by an enlarged lymph node or tumor, or to the outside of a lung, e.g., by an elevated diaphragm or accumulations of air or fluids in the pleural space or pericardial sac.

Symptoms. Symptoms of atelectasis are basically determined by the rapidity with which bronchial obstruction develops and by the presence or absence of secondary infection. Increased dyspnea and weakness are almost the only symptoms of a slowly developing atelectasis. A massive, rapidly developing collapse with infection typically causes sudden severe dyspnea, cyanosis, decreased blood pressure, tachycardia, shock, anxiety, and temperature elevation. Additionally, pain occurs on the affected side, and breath sounds and ventilatory excursions of the chest are reduced or absent. Ventilatory movements on the unaffected side may appear exaggerated as the patient struggles to breathe.

Percussion over the collapsed lung demonstrates dullness to flatness. X-ray examination reveals a solid lack of radiance of the airless area of the lung and diminished lung size. In the presence of large atelectatic areas the diaphragm is elevated on the affected side, the rib spaces are narrowed, and the heart, mediastinum, and trachea deviate *toward* the atelectatic area. (Note: Massive pleural effusion and spontaneous pneumothorax cause similar clinical symptoms, but with these disorders x-rays show the mediastinal structures pushed *away* from the affected side). Bronchoscopy may or may not reveal bronchial obstruction.

Prevention. As previously stated, atelectasis can often be prevented. Preventative measures include:

> Prevention of aspiration and maintenance of a clear airway by correct positioning and removal of bronchopulmonary secretions. Indications of bronchial obstruction include wheezing or a sharp, forced expiration. (See discussion of prevention of pneumonia, p. 952).

> Maintenance of effective aeration of the lung, e.g., by frequent deep breathing-coughing sessions.

> Use of IPPB (with air, not O_2) to improve ventilation and bronchial drainage.

> Turning and repositioning of patient every hour while he is obtunded or bedridden.

> Avoidance of large doses of sedatives and opiates, which depress cough reflex and respirations.

> Avoidance of tight dressings and restraints.

> Prevention of abdominal distention.

> Encouragement of mobility.

> Reduction of bronchospasm, e.g., by administering nebulized bronchodilators.

> Promotion of liquefaction of secretions by administration of aerosols of saline and water, humidifying inspired air, and maintaining body hydration.

> Avoidance of anesthetic agents with a long postanesthetic narcosis; avoidance of very high O_2 concentrations with too little nitrogen during anesthesia; and leaving the lung filled with air (not O_2) at the termination of operative anesthesia.

For a detailed discussion of the prevention of postoperative atelectasis following thoracotomy by the use of IPPB, blow bottles, rebreathing tubes and deep breathing, consult Collart and Brenneman's article, "Preventing Postoperative Atelectasis."[55]

Clinical Care. When *acute atelectasis* develops it is treated when possible by removal of the underlying cause. Treatment should be rapidly instituted to prevent destructive changes and other complications. Thoracentesis may be performed to remove accumulations of air or fluid from the pleural space if they are causing atelectasis. To remove bronchial obstruction, treatment may include: (1) stimulation of productive coughing; (2) suctioning; (3) positioning the patient with the involved side elevated (so drainage of the affected area can occur); (4) stimulation of the respiratory center, e.g., with caffeine or CO_2 inhalations; (5) administration of detergent aerosols with a mist-producing apparatus; and (6) bronchoscopy (to remove obstructions directly when they can be visualized in the tracheobronchial tree). Antibiotics are administered to treat or to prevent pulmonary infection. Once the obstruction is removed the patient is helped to regain normal lung function by IPPB, turning, coughing, and ambulation. *Chronic atelectasis* may be sucessfully treated by surgically removing the affected area—segment or lobe—and treating secondary infection.

INFLUENZA ("Flu," Grippe, Catarrhal Fever)

Epidemiology and Immunology. This acute, highly contagious respiratory disease is viral in origin. The influenza virus can be observed only with an electron microscope, since it is smaller than a bacterium.

Influenza may occur sporadically or in epidemics. Occasionally pandemics (i.e., epidemics spreading to all parts of the world) develop, characterized by a rapidly fatal pulmonary infection. In such fulminant fatal cases, dyspnea, cyanosis, hemoptysis, pulmonary edema, and death may result as soon as two days after onset of the illness.

An example of an influenza pandemic was that of 1918, which took the lives of more than 21 million persons. As a medical catastrophe this pandemic was second only to the Black Death in the 14th century. More recent examples of influenza pandemics are the 1957–58 ("Asian flu") infections, caused by a new mutant strain of Type A influenza virus, and the 1968–69 ("Hong Kong flu") illness. Typically, epidemics occur every one to four years and develop rapidly because of the brief (18 to 36 hours) incubation period. Locally, epidemics last for four to six weeks. Pandemics most typically return about every 30 to 40 years.

Immunologically four distinct types of the influenza virus can be recognized—Types A, B, C, and D. These are further subdivided into "families," e.g., Types A_1 and A_2 ("Asian"). Currently the types most frequently causing epidemics are Types A_1, A_2, B_2, and C. Type A typically produces epidemics about every two or three years; type B, every four or five years. Immunity is high for several months following an attack of influenza, but it then falls rapidly. Little cross-immunity occurs between types or families.

The influenza virus has a selective affinity for the respiratory tract's epithelial lining and causes inflammation of the airways, with patches of necrotic, sloughing epithelium. Influenza is basically an airborne infection, most commonly spread by droplet nuclei containing the virus. These infected droplet nuclei are spread by coughing, sneezing, kissing, and the use of towels, drinking glasses, and similar objects that have been freshly contaminated.

Symptoms. Following the incubation period the nonimmune infected person suddenly becomes acutely ill. Symptoms include prostration, fever (100 to 104°F.), severe headache, chills, weakness, generalized muscular aches and pains (most severe in the legs and back), anorexia, sore throat, anxiety, dry cough, coryza, sneezing, mild substernal distress, flushed face, and the formation of herpetic lesions on the mouth and lips. Temperature elevates rapidly and may remain high for two or three days in mild cases or four to five days in severe cases. Possible complications include secondary bacterial pneumonia, cardiovascular disease, cervical lymphadenitis, sinusitus, tracheobronchitis, and otitis media. Vasomotor collapse can occur with severe influenza.

Once the fever abates, the other acute symptoms rapidly disappear. However, fatigue, cough, weakness, and sweating may persist for several more days or, perhaps, weeks.

Treatment. Treatment is symptomatic and consists of measures such as bed rest (until 24 to 48 hours after fever abates), antipyretics and analgesics, light diet, increased fluid intake, mild codeine cough mixture, warm isotonic saline gargles, cool vapor or steam inhalations, humidification of inspired air, nasal instillations of 1 or 2 drops of 0.25 per cent phenylephrine in sodium chloride solution, and prevention of chilling and fatigue. General comfort measures, such as back rubs, oral hygiene, and sponges, can greatly reduce aggravating discomforts. Laxatives may be ordered. Observe the patient closely for indications of complications and report these immediately. As he improves the patient is gradually ambulated. Full activity out of bed is not permitted until easy fatigue, weakness, and dizziness have subsided. A convalescent period following recovery from acute symptoms is advisable to prevent relapse or secondary infection.

Persons with uncomplicated influenza usually recover without residual impairment. However, fatalities may occur, e.g., among pregnant women, the aged, diabetics, and persons with chronic lung disease or chronic cardiac disease. Most fatalities result from bacterial complications.

Control; Prophylaxis. Infected persons should be isolated and given instruction about measures they can take to minimize the spread of their airborne disease. (Methods of preventing the spread of droplet-nuclei infections are discussed more completely on p. 968.)

While most city dwellers cannot avoid some influenza infections, the severity of these infections may be minimized by the maintenance of an optimum level of general health, avoiding crowds during periods when the "flu" is prevalent, and attempting to stay out of the path of coughing, sneezing persons.

Polyvalent vaccines are now available against the prevalent types of influenza. When a new major antigenic mutation occurs in the virus, the new strain is isolated and incorporated into the vaccine. These influenza immunizations are recommended annually for persons most likely to succumb to influenza infections, e.g., debilitated, aged persons with chronic diseases. When epidemics are predicted, vaccination is recommended for other groups, e.g., pregnant women, persons performing vital public services.

Vaccination against influenza produces an immunity that lasts only one year. It is recommended that the primary vaccination and annual booster doses be given in the early fall. The primary immunization consists of two doses of the currently recommended vaccine given at a two-month interval. For adults the primary and booster dose is 1 ml. injected subcutaneously (not intradermally). Before administering the vaccine, inquire if the patient has a sensitivity to eggs, since the vaccine is made of virus propagated in chick embryos. Epinephrine should be kept available in case of a severe immediate reaction. (See Chapter 23.) Severe reactions are rare, but local or constitutional reactions are not uncommon. These can be minimized by giving the vaccine in divided doses at one- to two-day intervals. It takes about two weeks following vaccination for immunity to develop. A new vaccine is being studied which would require a smaller amount of virus and would produce a longer antigenic stimulus and greater antibody response. This vaccine contains an emulsified oil adjuvant and causes fewer reactions.

ACUTE BRONCHITIS; ACUTE TRACHEOBRONCHITIS

Pathophysiology. Bronchitis, i.e., bronchial inflammation or infection, may be either an acute or chronic disorder. (Chronic bronchitis is discussed on p. 989). Bronchitis may occur as a primary disorder or in company with numerous other pulmonary disorders, e.g., bronchiectasis, tuberculosis, chronic obstructive pulmonary disease, pulmonary emphysema. Bronchitis may be diffuse or localized and may be caused by infections or by physical or chemical agents, e.g., dust, fumes, smoke.

Acute tracheobronchitis is an acute inflammation of the mucous membranes of the tracheobronchial tree; usually the disorder is self-limited and does not permanently impair structure or function. If only the bronchi appear involved the condition is called "bronchitis"; if the trachea is also involved the condition is accurately called "tracheobronchitis." Tracheobronchitis is the more common disorder.

When tracheobronchitis results from an infection the condition is usually an extension into the trachea and bronchi of a general acute upper respiratory infection (URI). Temporary impairment of the self-cleaning mechanisms of the bronchi (e.g., cilia) permits bacterial invasion. Once bacteria invade the normally sterile bronchi, mucopurulent exudate and cellular debris accumulate. These accumulations must be expectorated.

Acute tracheobronchitis occurs most often during winter months. This disorder is only a mild illness for most persons, but it can be life-threatening in infants and small children (because their bronchi are easily obstructed) and in persons who have chronic pulmonary or heart disease or who are otherwise debilitated. *Prompt, thorough treatment of upper respiratory infection is important in the prevention of acute tracheobronchitis,* especially in the above described population. Acute tracheobronchitis may also occur with generalized infections such as chickenpox, measles, whooping cough, and influenza.

Symptoms. Acute tracheobronchitis is characterized by *early* symptoms of an acute URI (substernal tightness, chills, coryza, sore throat, muscle and back pain, and slight fever); *later* onset of cough, which is initially dry, irritating, and nonproductive and then progresses to become productive of mucopurulent to purulent sputum; and no x-ray densities and only a few pulmonary signs, e.g., musical rhonchi, wheezes. Persistent localized pulmonary signs may indicate serious complications. In uncomplicated cases, sputum cultures produce the common mouth organisms. At other times specific pathogens are demonstrated, e.g., pneumococci, beta-hemolytic streptococci. A temperature elevation (101 to 102°F.) may last three to five days in some of the more severe uncomplicated illnesses. Usually acute symptoms subside within two to five days; however, a cough may be present for as long as 14 to 21 days. Bronchospasm (which results from bronchial irritation) may cause the patient to be dyspneic, and sometimes may produce hypoxemia and hypoventilation. Secondary infections may include sinusitis and/or laryngitis.

Clinical Care. Clinical care is basically symptomatic and is similar to that given with any acute URI. Factors of importance include:

> Bed rest; steam (perhaps with menthol, oil of eucalyptus, or tincture of benzoin) or cool vapor inhalations; humidification of inspired air; expectorants, e.g., ammonium chloride; increased fluid intake (3000 to 4000 ml./day); moist heat applications to the chest wall; hot drinks (to stimulate productive coughing and relieve congestion); light or soft nourishing diet; antipyretic analgesic medications (to reduce fever and relieve malaise).

> Prevention of relapse or secondary infection. Protect patient from fatigue and chilling. Take precautions to prevent pneumonia. (See discussion on p. 952.) Encourage productive coughing and periodic deep breathing. Administer antibiotics if ordered.

> Relief of bronchospasm if present. Ephedrine, aminophylline and isoproterenol (Isuprel) are bronchodilators that may be prescribed. (See discussion of bronchodilators below).

> Prevention of spread of tracheobronchitis to others during period of communicability.

Antibiotics are not indicated initially if the causative organism is a virus. However, in the presence of bacterial infection antibiotics may be ordered if the patient is not rapidly improving or is more than mildly ill. A broad-spectrum antibiotic, e.g., tetracycline, may be ordered until sputum culture reports are available to guide specific antibiotic therapy. Antibiotics may be given in an attempt to prevent secondary infection in patients for whom severe acute infections could be fatal.

Cough depressants are not usually given, since it is important that the lungs be cleared of accumulated secretions. However, sometimes the physician mildly suppresses cough (e.g., with a codeine or another cough mixture) if the cough is unproductive and excessively fatiguing.

As can be seen, treatment of tracheobronchitis is generally conservative and is directed at preventing extension of the infection and the development of complications. Persons for whom tracheobronchitis can be serious are observed especially closely for indications of worsening of their conditions. It is advisable for the patient to observe a period of convalescence with reduced activity to ensure complete recovery.

BRONCHIECTASIS

Bronchiectasis is a disorder of the medium-sized bronchi characterized by *chronic dilatation* of these air passages and the destruction of bronchial elastic and muscular structures.

Pathophysiology. Bronchiectasis may affect the bronchial tube(s) uniformly (*cylindric bronchiectasis*), may produce irregular pockets (*sacculated bronchiectasis*), or may produce terminal bulbous enlargements at the end of the dilated tube (*fusiform* or *spindle-shaped bronchiectasis*) (Fig. 71–2). Cylindrical bronchiectasis is of doubtful clinical significance. The characteristic bronchial dilatations become apparent when a diagnostic bronchogram is performed (Fig. 71–3). The lower and middle lobes of the lungs are most often affected. Involvement varies, and may be bilateral or extensive.

The microscopic inspection of sections of bronchi affected with bronchiectasis reveals that the wall of the bronchus in the dilated sections has been replaced with scar tissue. The dilated bronchial sections may be surrounded by areas of pneumonia.

Etiology. Causes of bronchiectasis are *obstruction* and *infection*. Obstructions, e.g., mucus, pus, or foreign bodies, block the bronchi and eventually cause them to dilate. If the dilated bronchial walls become infected and damaged from the infection, the dilatation becomes irreversible. Bronchiectasis can also occur distal to an obstruction when infection develops beyond the point of obstruction.

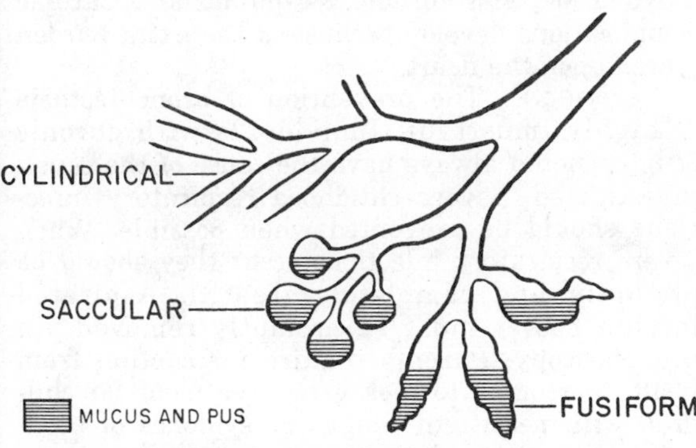

FIGURE 71–2. Bronchiectasis.

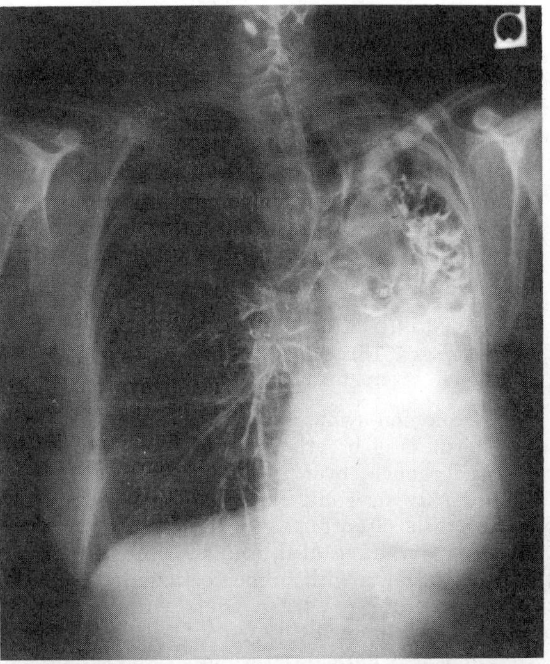

FIGURE 71–3. (Case IV). Bronchogram showing saccular bronchiectasis and destroyed left lung and normal right bronchial tree. (From Petty, T. L., and Mitchell, R. S., *Medical Clinics of North America,* No. 2, Vol. 51, March 1967.)

Bronchiectasis may be present at birth, but most often it begins in early childhood as an acquired disorder resulting from a pulmonary infection which complicates influenza, measles, or whooping cough, or is the result of foreign body aspiration. Bronchial obstructions leading to bronchiectasis also may occur as a result of such disorders as bronchial tumor, pulmonary tuberculosis, and cystic fibrosis (mucoviscidosis). Because children have bronchi that are small and soft, bronchial obstruction and damage can more easily occur at younger ages. However, since infection and bronchial obstruction do not routinely produce bronchiectasis, unknown intrinsic factors are believed to be important in its etiology.

Permanently damaged bronchial walls cannot move effectively and ciliary action is absent as a result of destroyed or damaged mucous membranes. Ectatic (i.e., distended) bronchi may collapse when intrapleural pressure is rapidly increased during cough. Because secretions cannot be adequately removed, infection subsequently occurs. Infected secretions then collect constantly in the bronchial dilatations. Changes in body position cause these secretions to flow into regions of healthy bronchial tissue. The infected secretions are raised from here as a result of ciliary action, bronchial wall movements, and coughing. Bronchial damage is more serious when it occurs in the lower regions of the lungs, since gravity cannot help to drain the affected bronchi, as would occur from the upper lung fields.

Symptoms. Bronchiectasis is basically characterized by:

> Chronic profuse discharge of thick sputum containing pus.
> Fetid breath.
> Hemoptysis. This occurs in about half the patients.
> Chronic, severe, frequent paroxysms of coughing.

Other common symptoms include fatigue, weight loss, shortness of breath upon exertion, and moist rales and rhonchi over the lower lobes. Sinusitis is frequently present. Patients with advanced bronchiectasis often appear weak, emaciated, and cyanotic, and have clubbing of the fingertips. Typically patients with bronchiectasis have a history of developing winter colds which usually progress to pneumonia.

Diagnosis. Characteristic history and symptoms are indicative of bronchiectasis. Bronchograms confirm the diagnosis. Bronchoscopy may be helpful in demonstrating bronchial obstruction and in identifying involved pulmonary segments. Persons with advanced bronchiectasis may show decreased ventilation when lung function studies are performed. Characteristic laboratory findings do not occur with bronchiectasis. Frequently a highly mixed bacterial content is revealed when sputum is microscopically examined.

Clinical Care. The treatment of bronchiectasis may involve both medical and surgical procedures. *Surgical resection* of involved portions of the lung (e.g., segment, lobe) is the only way by which bronchiectasis can be eliminated. However, not all patients are candidates for surgery. Pulmonary resection may be performed on young patients with recurring symptoms or persons up to age 60 who have severe symptoms, such as recurrent hemoptysis, caused by unilateral localized bronchiectasis. Segmental resections or lobectomies are most often performed, but sometimes pneumonectomies or bilateral procedures are carried out. (Care of the patient having chest surgery is discussed in Chapter 73).

The *medical management* and *general clinical care* of a patient with bronchiectasis focuses on the following activities:

> Periodic postural drainage, e.g., the first drainage upon awakening, the last at bedtime. Some patients with mild involvement require postural drainage only when they develop a cold; others with severe involvement require postural drainage several times a day. Patients with severe bronchiectasis may be positioned for several hours in a tipped-up position on a special bed. Some patients with severe disease are advised to permanently elevate the foot of the bed 4 to 6 inches.

> Treatment of complications with respiratory therapy is indicated for chronic respiratory insufficiency. Chronic sinus infections are treated appropriately. (See Unit XXII.)

> Liquefaction of sputum by keeping the patient hydrated, administering medications such as saturated solution of potassium iodide, and administering aerosol mucolytic agents.

> Bronchoscopic removal of bronchial obstruction and/or dilation of a stenosed bronchus.

> Avoidance of upper respiratory infections and air-polluted environments. The patient is advised not to smoke and to avoid dusty, smoky, or otherwise polluted atmospheres. The physician may advise the patient to live in a warm, dry climate. Tell the patient to avoid contact with persons who have influenza or respiratory infections and to contact his physician early if he develops symptoms of superimposed infection.

> Promotion of rest. Bed rest is often advised for persons with severe bronchiectasis and those with acute respiratory infections. The bronchiectatic person should avoid fatigue and chilling.

> Improve resistance to acute respiratory infections by encouraging a well-balanced diet and a program of balanced exercise and rest that is individualized for the patient's condition.

> Promotion of effective cough and deep breathing exercises. Instruct the patient how to cough productively. Deep breathing exercises improve alveolar ventilation and help to move secretions out of the inflated lungs.

> Frequent oral hygiene. Because of the copious sputum production, frequent oral hygiene is highly important. Always provide oral hygiene prior to meals.

> Administration of antimicrobial medications suppresses bacteria in the pockets of infection; reduces cough, sputum, and other symptoms; and treats the areas of pneumonia that occur around the bronchial dilatations.

Patient-family education is of importance in the care of a patient with bronchiectasis. The nurse participates actively in this instruction in a variety of settings, e.g., office, clinic, hospital and home. Whereas persons with severe bronchiectasis require year-round medical supervision, those with only mild involvement may need care only during and after acute respiratory infections. Persons who cannot be treated surgically and who are producing large quantities of sputum sometimes benefit from a permanent tracheostomy, which permits frequent suctioning.

Complications. Possible complications of bronchiectasis include chronic pulmonary suppuration, progressive pulmonary insufficiency, hemoptysis, amyloidosis, and chronic cor pulmonale. Cardiac complications develop because of the extra burden placed upon the heart.

Prevention. The prevention of bronchiectasis is highly important. Individuals with chronic coughs should always have the cause of the cough investigated. Severe childhood respiratory infections should be prevented when possible. When severe respiratory infections occur they should be promptly and completely treated. Aspirated foreign bodies must be promptly removed via bronchoscopy. Parents require instruction from health personnel to seek early treatment for children with persistent coughs or evidence of bronchial obstruction, before disease can become established.

Preventative measures are helping to reduce the incidence of bronchiectasis. Formerly a common disorder, today bronchiectasis occurs far less often because of the use of immunizations and antibiotics.

PULMONARY ABSCESS (Lung Abscess)

A pulmonary abscess is a localized collection of pus within a cavity that has been formed by the necrosis of surrounding inflammatory tissue and lung tissue. The areas of the lungs most often affected by abscess formation are the superior segment of the lower lobe or the lower part of the upper lobe. The right lung develops abscesses more often than the left. Multiple abscesses occur occasionally.

Etiology. Lung abscesses usually develop *secondary to localized bronchial obstruction,* which may occur from a neoplasm (e.g., bronchogenic carcinoma), from pneumonia, or following aspiration of secretions or foreign objects.

Pathology. Abscess formation represents an attempt by the body to wall off infection and inflammation and to keep it localized and encapsulated so it does not spread to adjacent structures. Early in the course of development of a pulmonary abscess, an area of consolidation (lobar or segmental) occurs. Gradually this consolidation assumes a round shape as a pus-filled cavity forms. For a while the abscess may remain somewhat isolated and not communicate with a bronchus. Eventually, however, most pulmonary abscesses erode and rupture into a bronchus.

When this has occurred, the patient begins to expectorate the contents of the pus-filled cavity as foul sputum. Satisfactory and rapid healing can occur if the abscess is able to drain freely and completely through its bronchial opening. If all the contents of the cavity are removed by drainage through the tracheobronchial tree, the cavity becomes air-filled and the walls of the abscess collapse and contract, eventually obliterating the cavity. However, if the cavity drainage is incomplete and prolonged, a chronic condition develops and healing is prevented by the retention of pus and the development of firm, fibrotic, epithelium-lined abscess walls.

Infrequently a pulmonary abscess perforates into the pleural space, rapidly producing an empyema and perhaps also shock and a bronchopleural fistula. Occasionally pulmonary abscesses erode into blood vessels, resulting in hemorrhage and possibly the transmission of infected emboli to the brain. These emboli develop into brain abscesses secondary to the pulmonary abscess.

Symptoms. The patient with a pulmonary abscess may be subacutely (but chronically) ill, or acutely ill, e.g., toxic, prostrate, febrile. Symptoms of pneumonia are often the first to appear, that is, sweats, chills, malaise, anorexia, fever (103°F. or higher), cough, dyspnea (if a large area is involved), and perhaps chest pain (if there is pleural involvement). Moist rales may be heard. Sputum is characteristically purulent (often dark brown) unless the abscess is totally walled off and does not have access to a bronchus for drainage. Hemoptysis may occur with a communicating lung abscess. A patient with a *chronic* pulmonary abscess develops anemia, weight loss, and clubbing of the fingers.

Diagnosis. Before a lung abscess perforates a bronchus (and begins to drain) it may be difficult to detect. Once bronchial drainage is established, the patient begins to expectorate large quantities of purulent sputum. The sputum may be streaked with blood, may contain pieces of gangrenous lung tissue, and may have a foul odor. This excessive sputum production may last for only several hours or may continue for several days. As the fluid drains out of the abscess, a cavity with a fluid level in it can be observed on the patient's chest x-ray. To establish diagnosis and obtain information necessary for proper treatment the physician usually: (1) performs a physical examination; (2) performs bronchoscopy to rule out tumor or foreign body and to obtain specimen; (3) orders serial x-rays and tomography; and (4) orders sputum and bronchoscopy specimens for bacteriologic and cytologic evaluation. Sometimes it is necessary to perform a needle aspiration of the abscess to obtain a specimen for laboratory examination.

Clinical Care. Treatment is aimed at maintaining effective drainage of the abscess and eliminating the infection. *Early treatment is important to prevent the development of a chronic condition.* Over three fourths of patients can be treated adequately without surgical procedures.

Drainage of the abscess is encouraged by the use of postural drainage. Often the physician requests that the patient's daily volume of sputum be measured and recorded. Decreasing amounts of sputum usually indicate effective treatment. The patient is also given instruction about how to cough productively so he will be able to raise and expectorate the purulent sputum collecting in his lung. Suctioning may help to keep the airway patent, and medications may be ordered to help the patient to raise sputum. If a patient is unable to cough effectively (e.g., if he is paralyzed or weakened) a tracheostomy may be necessary so sputum can be suctioned from the lung. Occasionally the physician must use a bronchoscope to aspirate thick, tenacious drainage.

Chemotherapy of a pulmonary abscess is started as soon as a specimen of the abscess contents has been sent to the laboratory for sensitivity tests and culture. The most effective antibiotic is generally penicillin. As a rule, large doses are administered to make certain effective tissue levels of the antibiotic are maintained in the abscess walls. Kanamycin or gentamicin may also be administered if a gram-negative organism is believed to be present. Generally a combination of medications is necessary, because various organisms are usually present. Typically, chemotherapy is continued for 6 to 8 weeks.

After a course of appropriate antibiotics, the symptoms resulting from suppuration of lung tissue are usually relieved. At this time the patient is reevaluated because the disappearance of these symptoms does not always mean that cure has been accomplished. Every attempt is made to prevent the abscess from developing into a chronic condition.

Bronchograms, and perhaps *planigrams,* are routinely performed several weeks after the ordinary chest x-ray has cleared. The results of these procedures are carefully evaluated to determine if adequate healing has occurred or if a persistent cavity or bronchiectatic changes are present.

Surgery is necessary if the causative organisms are resistant to chemotherapy or if residual cystic cavities or bronchiectasis is demonstrated. Resectional pulmonary surgery, e.g., lobectomy, pneumonectomy, is the procedure of choice. (See Chapter 73.)

PULMONARY TUMORS

Pulmonary tumors may be benign or malignant and primary or secondary. The most common pulmonary tumors are primary bronchogenic carcinomas. This means that *most* pulmonary tumors first arise within pulmonary structures rather than metastasizing to the lungs (i.e., most are not secondary tumors), arise specifically within the bronchial epithelium, and are malignant.

Benign and Metastatic Pulmonary Tumors

Very few nonmalignant pulmonary tumors occur. When they do, benign and metastatic (i.e., secondary) pulmonary tumors are generally asymptomatic. However, they sometimes cause symptoms as a result of local pressure. One exception is a benign bronchial adenoma, which typically bleeds and produces recurrent hemoptyses. Whenever possible, benign pulmonary tumors are surgically excised. When viewed by x-ray, these tumors often have clearly defined margins and smooth outlines. Benign pulmonary tumors may become malignant.

The lungs are the most common site of tumors that have metastasized from other organs. Metastatic tumors in pulmonary structures most often come from malignant tumors in the breast, stomach, prostate, kidney, thyroid, testis, or bone.[129] It is estimated that metastatic invasion of the bronchi occurs with approximately 25 per cent of all extrathoracic carcinomas.[255] This secondary bronchial carcinoma is difficult to differentiate from primary bronchial carcinoma because it produces similar x-ray densities, symptoms, and cytologic findings. The identification of malignant cells in sputum (or bronchial aspirate) only indicates malignant disease in the lung and does not clarify whether the cells are from primary or secondary disease.

Persons suspected of having primary lung cancers need to be thoroughly evaluated to rule out the presence of an extrathoracic carcinoma. The most definitive diagnostic procedure for confirming a diagnosis of metastatic bronchial carcinoma is the careful histologic examination of specimens of bronchial tissue obtained by biopsy or surgical resection. The diagnosis is clearly established by finding cells that are characteristic of extrathoracic carcinomas. For example, colloid-containing cells typify thyroid cancers, whereas clear and opaque cells typify renal cancers.[255] When possible, a patient may benefit from the removal of a metastatic lesion if it is a solitary lesion.

Primary Malignant Pulmonary Tumors (Bronchogenic Carcinomas)

Primary pulmonary tumors have a high rate of malignancy (98 per cent). Of those that are malignant, the vast majority arise from the bronchial epithelium (and hence are called "bronchogenic carcinomas"). The right lung is affected more often than the left. Centrally located pulmonary tumors occur more often than tumors in the peripheries of the lungs. The central location is, unfortunately, more frequently inoperable because of the tumor's proximity to the mediastinum. If untreated, bronchogenic carcinoma is usually fatal within 9 months.

Pathology. The most common type of primary pulmonary neoplasm is *squamous cell (epidermoid) carcinoma.* Squamous cell carcinomas develop in the main bronchi or larger bronchial branches. Generally they spread by direct extension and metastasize more slowly than other types. They occur most often in males and are almost always associated with cigarette smoking. Well-differentiated squamous cell carcinomas offer a better prognosis than less clearly differentiated types. The oat cell carcinoma is a poorly differentiated type of squamous cell carcinoma and has a very poor prognosis.

Other types of primary pulmonary carcinomas include *adenocarcinoma, bronchiolar (alveolar cell) carcinoma,* and *anaplastic or undifferentiated carcinoma.* The latter tends to metastasize early and most commonly occurs in males. Adenocarcinomas and bronchiolar carcinomas occur about three times more often in women than in men. Adenocarcinomas develop in the smaller bronchi, tend to be peripheral in location, and metastasize by all routes (particularly through the blood stream). Bronchiolar carcinoma is a rare, multinodular tumor that involves bronchiolar or alveolar linings.

Women tend to live longer than men following surgery for lung cancer. This sex difference in survival rates is partially related to the type of tumors women more commonly have, the extent of the disease, and the amount of surgery performed. Adenocarcinomas and bronchiolar carcinomas (more common in women) are usually confined to one lobe of the lung and are often treated surgically by lobectomy.[274]

Primary lung tumors may cause the malignant invasion of the brain, adrenal glands, liver, bones, and opposite lung. Mediastinal and cervical lymph nodes are often involved in spread of the tumor. The diaphragm and pleural cavity may also be affected by neoplastic extension.

Incidence and Etiology. *Lung cancer is the only form of cancer that is showing a rapid, almost epidemic increase.* Cancer of the lung now matches cancer of the colon and rectum as the site of greatest incidence. The mortality rate for lung cancer has increased steadily among women, and among men has increased more than 15 times in 40 years. The American Cancer Society estimated that in 1973 about 79,000 new cases of lung cancer would be diagnosed in the Unites States, and about 64,000 of these would be among men. It was also estimated that approximately 72,000 persons in this country would die from lung cancer in 1973, and about 58,000 of these would be males. *Lung cancer is the leading cause of male cancer deaths.*[8, 9] The incidence of lung cancer among females is increasing as greater numbers of women become habitual smokers over a prolonged period. Women smokers also have an increased mortality from heart disease. Primary lung cancer most often occurs between ages 40 and 70; the peak incidence is between ages 55 and 60.

Because early diagnosis (the time when cure is most possible) is difficult, the mortality rate associated with pulmonary cancer is high. The 5-year survival rate for lung cancer is currently below 10 per cent. About 91 per cent of persons who develop lung cancer die from it. *Cancer of the lung has one of the highest death rates of any cancer.* However, cancer of the lung (like other types of cancer) may be cured if detected *early* enough.

> *If cigarette smoking were eliminated, at least 75 per cent of the lung cancers occurring in the United States would be prevented!*

Cancer of the lung is a particularly tragic condition because it is largely a self-imposed, preventable disease caused most frequently by cigarette smoking. Bronchogenic carcinoma occurs 20 times more often among heavy smokers than among nonsmokers.

Cigarette smoke contains numerous chemical carcinogens (i.e., agents that assist the action of cancer-producing chemicals). The risk of developing lung cancer increases in proportion to number of cigarettes smoked, length of time an individual has smoked, how deeply the smoker inhales while smoking, and the age at which the smoking habit began.

Cigarette smoking causes progressive cellular changes of the kind that precede cancer. These cellular changes increase in degree as more cigarettes are smoked, and they diminish if the smoker stops smoking before invasive lung cancer develops. Additionally, it is statistically clear that a decrease in lung cancer death rates occurs among persons who stop smoking. This decrease is roughly proportional to the time elapsed since smoking was stopped.

Other irritating inhalants also appear to be significant in the development of lung cancer. These include chemical gases, dust, and other air pollutants. It is therefore of importance that air pollution be minimized or alleviated and that industrial workers exposed to irritants be given appropriate health supervision and protection in order to reduce the incidence of lung cancer.

The prevention of lung cancer also requires education concerning the importance of annual physical examinations that include chest x-rays and seeking medical evaluation promptly if any symptoms of lung cancer or any of "Cancer's 7 Warning Signals" appear. (See also Unit VII.)

The *nurse's role* in the prevention and early detection of pulmonary cancer includes: (1) encouraging persons with chronic cough or with a change in the character of a cough to seek medical evaluation; (2) encouraging persons who are habitual heavy smokers to have a chest x-ray every six months; (3) recommending medical evaluation to persons with recurring or chronic respiratory infections; (4) participating in community and other educational programs that present the facts about the harmful effects of smoking and other sources of air pollution; (5) informing persons in the community about local cancer detection clinics, symptoms that may indicate pulmonary cancer, and diagnostic tests used when pulmonary cancer is suspected; and (6) emphasizing the need for the early detection and treatment of all malignant lesions.

Symptoms. Pulmonary cancer is a "silent disease" in its earliest stages, giving no indication of its presence and often being undetectable by physical examination. Asymptomatic tumors developing in "silent areas" of the lung are detected only by chest x-ray. By the time symptoms begin to appear the cancer may have progressed beyond the point of cure. When symptoms of lung cancer do occur they may include blood in the sputum, chest pain, symptoms of a lingering pulmonary infection, and persistent cough. *All coughs or other evidences of respiratory infection which last longer than two to three weeks should be medically investigated,* particularly in heavy cigarette smokers.

The symptoms produced by pulmonary cancers vary, depending upon the location and size of the tumor. If the cancer begins in a bronchus, as it grows it tends to irritate and partially obstruct the bronchus. *The most common symptom of bronchogenic carcinoma is the development of a cough* or *a change in the severity or nature of a cough* (if chronic cough has been present). Tumors that block off a bronchus may cause numerous problems in the area distal to the stenosis or obstruction, e.g., atelectasis, dilating of bronchi beyond the block, abscess formation, bronchiectasis, or pneumonitis. Retained secretions may cause recurring episodes of pneumonia and/or bronchitis. These symptoms may also result from tumors compressing bronchi. The symptoms resulting from infection associated with bronchial obstruction or stenosis may be the symptoms, e.g., dyspnea, chills, fever, that initially prompt a person with pulmonary cancer to seek medical attention

Pulmonary tumors located near the pleura may produce pleuritic pain and bloody pleural effusion. Tumors located near the bottom of the lung may irritate the diaphragm and involve the phrenic nerve, producing referred pain along the top of the shoulder, as well as breathing difficulties. As tumors located at the top of the lung enlarge they may involve the ribs, the sympathetic nerve chain (producing pupil changes), or the brachial plexus (causing arm pain). Invasion of the mediastinal structures, e.g., esophagus, by tumor may produce ulceration, bleeding, and difficulty in swallowing. Obstruction of the superior vena cava or invasion of a portion of the heart may occur as a tumor extends within the thorax. Tumors which enlarge in such a direction that they press against the trachea produce tracheal symptoms. The recurrent laryngeal nerve may be involved, producing hoarseness and vocal cord paralysis.

Weakness, weight loss, anemia, and anorexia often occur with advanced lung cancer. These nonspecific systemic effects of malignancy are discussed more completely in Unit VII.

Various *systemic syndromes* often occur in association with lung cancer. Among these are *nonmetastatic* neuromuscular syndromes (occurring in patients with bronchogenic carcinoma), arthralgias and clubbing of the fingers and toes, and metabolic disorders such as hypercalcemia, polycythemia, inappropriate ADH secretion, Cushing's syndrome, and (in males) bilateral mammary gland hypertrophy. The destruction or removal of the primary cancer or performance of a bilateral adrenalectomy may correct adrenocortical hyperplasia caused by production of ACTH by the tumor.

Diagnosis. Procedures that may be used to diagnose lung cancer include: x-ray examinations; sputum cytology; mediastinoscopy; biopsy of scalene nodes or enlarged cervical or axillary lymph nodes (when mediastinal or hilar involvement is believed to be present); thoracentesis with evaluation of pleural fluid (if pleural effusion is present); bronchoscopy (with biopsy of the tumor and/or examination of bronchial washings); needle biopsy of the tumor (directly through the chest wall); lung scanning; pleural biopsy; and possibly thoracotomy and biopsy. (Diagnostic procedures are discussed in detail in Chapter 68.)

During the diagnostic investigation the physician not only establishes the location and type of tumor, but he also evaluates the operability of the tumor and the extent of its spread. The *ideal* means of detecting lung cancer early in persons who continue to smoke habitually (and have smoked for 15 to 20 years or longer) would be to periodically examine sputum specimens and perform bronchoscopy and to perform a yearly complete physical examination, with chest x-rays made every 3 to 4 months even though the individual is asymptomatic.[218]

The best *routine* means of detecting lung cancer early in the general public is to encourage people to have a large chest x-ray annually (preferably more often in persons who have smoked heavily for a number of years). As mentioned earlier, in asymptomatic persons who are harboring a lung cancer an abnormal chest x-ray is often the only change found during a routine physical evaluation. Such an x-ray may reveal such findings as thick-walled cavities, pleural effusion, small peripheral nodules, masses in the hilar region, lung infiltrations, atelectasis, pleural thickening, indications of pulmonary infection, bone erosion, or emphysematous dilatation of alveoli.

Pulmonary angiography is useful in diagnosing patients with bronchogenic carcinoma. To determine the hilar and mediastinal extent of the cancer, contrast visualization of the vena cava and pulmonary artery and veins is performed in both frontal and lateral projections. The pulmonary veins can be evaluated only by cineradiography, i.e., a motion picture record of successive images appearing on a fluoroscopic screen. Patients with lung tumors involving major pulmonary vessels have a poor prognosis following surgical resection. Therefore, often the angiographic demonstration of such involvement is sufficient to contraindicate attempts at surgical treatment.[45]

Treatment. Persons with resectable lung cancers are treated by *surgery*. It is possible, under favorable circumstances, for pulmonary cancer to be cured by complete surgical excision of affected tissue. The amount of lung tissue resected depends upon the extent of the disease. Although a lobectomy may suffice if the tumor is well localized, pneumonectomy is often required. Involved contiguous structures may also be removed. It appears that the careful block removal of the mediastinal lymph nodes draining the involved lobe or lung increases the chances of survival. This procedure is employed when the pulmonary nodes contain metastasis but the mediastinal nodes are free of metastasis. Some physicians believe that administering high voltage radiation to the tumor site and the adjacent pulmonary hilum prior to surgical resection minimizes the risk of metastasis. Sometimes irradiation shrinks previously inoperable tumors in such a way that surgery is then possible.

As with many other malignant tumors, the five-year survival rate increases if surgery is performed while the tumor is localized; the rate decreases if the tumor has spread to regional lymphatics and other structures.

Depending on the source of the figures, the percentage of patients with lung cancer having resectable tumors ranges from 25 to 50 per cent. Lung tumors sometimes prove to be inoperable at the time of surgical exploration. Some patients are unable to tolerate chest surgery because of severe cardiac or pulmonary conditions. Other contraindications include evidence that the cancer has metastasized either distantly (e.g., to the central nervous system or bone) or locally (e.g., as evidenced by pleural effusion, hilar lymph node metastases, obstruction of the superior vena cava, or laryngeal nerve involvement). Surgery may be performed on some persons with pericardial invasion or chest wall invasion if the involved area is technically resectable.

Some patients benefit temporarily from pulmonary surgery even though the total lung cancer cannot be resected. For example, such palliative resection may be performed if the patient has developed a lung abscess distal to an obstructed or stenotic bronchus.

Postoperative radiation therapy is usually given following pulmonary resection when metastases to adjacent structures are suspected. During radiation therapy unrecognized hypercalcemia (e.g., caused by parathormone production by the tumor) may be exaggerated or hyperuricemia may occur. When detected, these conditions are treated medically.

Palliative irradiation often helps to make patients with inoperable lung cancer more comfortable for a while. The objective of palliative therapy is to minimize or eliminate the acutely distressing aspects of the disease (e.g., pain, cough, shortness of breath) by producing a temporary regression of tumor size. Thus, the patient is more comfortable even though the lesion continues to progress. Palliative radiation may also somewhat prolong the patient's life; however, this is not the primary goal of the therapy. Severe blockage of the superior vena cava or innominate veins is an acutely distressing and potentially fatal complication of pulmonary cancer which causes respiratory embarrassment, distention of neck veins, cyanosis of the head and neck, and edema of the face and orbits of the eyes. Temporary relief may be given the patient by irradiation of the involved mediastinal region.

Palliative therapy for nonresectable pulmonary cancer may be provided by administering a course of supervoltage radiation carefully directed at the primary site and the mediastinal area of lymph node drainage. Another means of providing palliative therapy is the implantation of an isotope at the primary site, e.g., gold-filtered radon seeds or ^{125}I permanent implants. (See also Unit VII.)

Following pulmonary resection some physicians administer prophylactic long-range low-dose *chemotherapy*. For example, epidermoid cancers may be treated with cyclophosphamide (Cytoxan), 50 to 150 mg. per day (unless cystitis or leukopenia develops). A combination of medications may be given; e.g., vincristine (1 mg., I.V. once weekly) may also be given unless neurotoxicity develops.

Other antineoplastic drugs that may be used in chemotherapy of pulmonary cancer include mechlorethamine hydrochloride (nitrogen mustard) and triethylenemelamine (TEM). Sometimes chemotherapeutic agents are instilled locally through a bronchial arterial catheter. This method provides intensive local treatment, since the bronchial arterial system may be the major arterial supply to pulmonary neoplasms.[45]

Palliative chemotherapy may alleviate some distressing symptoms and provide a general improvement of a transient nature in some persons with extensive inoperable bronchogenic carcinoma. However, medical treatment of relapses is usually less effective than the first course of therapy, and remissions are usually of brief duration. (Chemotherapy of cancer is discussed in Unit VII.)

The prognosis of pulmonary cancer is very poor if cancer cells are found in a pleural effusion, because this means the cancer cells have spread into the lymphatics. When pleural effusion is detected, thoracentesis is performed. Once all the fluid is removed from the pleural space a sclerosing agent is instilled to stop this component of the cancer activity and to produce a pleural seal. Preparations that may be used for this purpose include radioactive gold, radioactive phosphorus, or a freshly prepared mixture of water and nitrogen mustard. Following the injection of one of these substances into the pleural cavity, the patient is turned in various positions to facilitate spread of the medication. Occasionally it is necessary to use closed chest drainage with high suction (e.g., 30 to 60 cm. of water) to accomplish complete drainage of the pleural effusion prior to instillation of the medication.

Any patient with primary pulmonary cancer, whether or not surgical resection has been performed, is carefully followed for evidence of metastases, e.g., to the brain, bones, contralateral lung. Patients are routinely scheduled for examinations each month for the first year and at longer intervals thereafter. Before discharge the patient is told to contact his physician if he develops additional symptoms, e.g., chest pain, dyspnea, hoarseness, dysphagia, or pain upon swallowing. These symptoms may indicate metastasis.

Nursing care of patients with terminal cancer is discussed on Unit VII; see also Chapter 15.

PNEUMONIAS

A "pneumonia" is an acute inflammation of the alveolar spaces of the lung that causes consolidation of lung tissue as alveoli fill with exudate. There are a variety of types of pneumonias, with different causative agents. Most pneumonias are caused by infection; however, some result from chemical irritants such as noxious gases. Generally pneumonias are referred to as "bacterial" or "nonbacterial," or they may be more precisely identified according to the specific etiologic agent, e.g., pneumococcal, Friedländer's, staphylococcal, rickettsial, fungal, mycoplasmal, or viral pneumonia. This classification, based on the etiologic organism, is the most commonly used.

At times pneumonias are designated in terms of their structural distribution. For example, bronchopneumonia involves only those alveoli in contact with bronchi; bronchopneumonias usually consist of diffuse patches of pneumonia scattered throughout both lungs. Another name for bronchopneumonia is "lobular pneumonia," i.e., pneu-

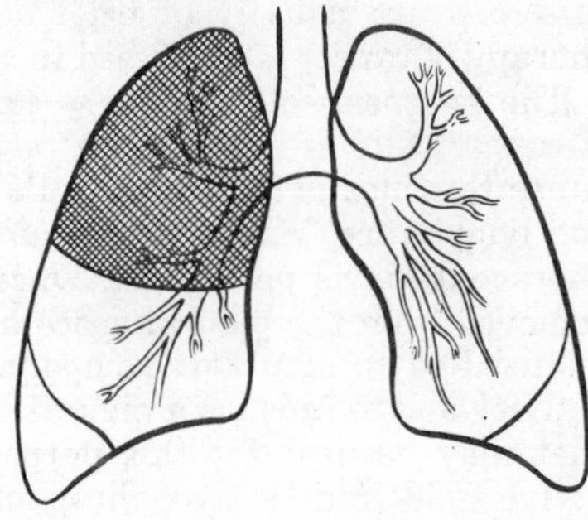

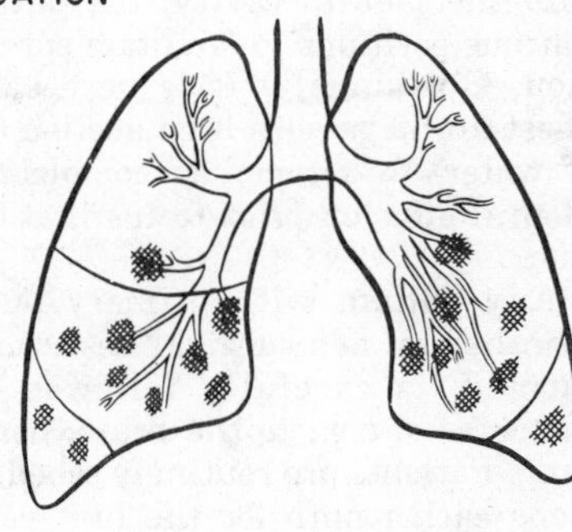

FIGURE 71–4. Two types of pneumonia, consolidation of one lobe (lobar) and patchy consolidation (lobular or bronchopneumonia). (Modified from *Introduction to Respiratory Diseases*, 4th ed. Copyright American Lung Association, 1969.)

monia involving only a portion of a lobe. A pneumonia that involves an entire lobe is termed "lobar pneumonia" (Fig. 71–4).

With any pneumonia it is essential that the etiologic agent be accurately identified so appropriate antimicrobial medications can be given. Sometimes mixed infections occur in which more than one type of organism is present. Reductions in the morbidity and mortality from pneumonias have occurred as a result of specific antimicrobial therapy; nonetheless, patients continue to die from pneumonia. Early diagnosis and vigorous therapy are therefore essential.

The clinical courses of the various pneumonias and their specific chemotherapeutic management may vary, but the general supportive care given is basically the same regardless of the etiologic agent. The recovery of patients seriously ill with pneumonia often depends on skilled nursing care.

Predisposing Factors. Numerous conditions and factors predispose an individual to pneumonia. Among these are chronic illness and debility, cancer, thoracic surgery, atelectasis, common cold and other viral respiratory infections, chronic respiratory infections and disorders, influenza, smoking, fibrocystic disease, malnutrition, cardiac failure, tracheostomy, exposure to noxious gases, exposure to cold, treatment with immunosuppressive agents, hypoventilation, hypostasis, impaired ciliary action in the tracheobronchial tree, impaired alveolar phagocyte function, depression of cerebral function, and aspiration.

Aspiration of secretions, liquids, foods, vomitus, pills, and so forth, can result from disorders which depress cerebral function, impair swallowing, and obliterate or depress the cough or epiglottal reflex. Examples of patients in danger of aspirating include persons who have had application of a local anesthetic to the throat or been under a general anesthetic, comatose or stuporous patients, and persons with central nervous system conditions that impair swallowing, e.g., bulbar paralysis. Comatose and stuporous patients hypoventilate and generally are inactive; these conditions promote retention of secretions in the lungs—an ideal medium for infection.

Pneumonia commonly develops among aged and debilitated persons. It most often occurs during those times of the year when upper respiratory infections are prevalent.

Prevention. Prophylactic administration of antibiotics is not effective in preventing pneumonia in predisposed individuals. Immunization against influenza is useful in preventing pneumonia that can complicate influenza.

Efforts directed at preventing pneumonia are most often those that maintain optimal respiratory function, prevent aspiration, and vigorously treat underlying diseases. Clinical states and medications that tend to suppress local bronchopulmonary defense mechanisms (e.g., ciliary action and pulmonary macrophages) are avoided when possible. Among these are hypoxemia, acidosis, narcotics, sedatives, and adrenocorticosteroids.

Many nursing activities focus on preventing pneumonia. Some of the more important of these are summarized below:

> Correctly position unconscious and semiconscious patients to prevent aspiration, e.g., postoperatively, or following strokes.

> Never administer food, fluids, or medications by mouth to comatose or stuporous patients or to patients who lack a gag reflex, e.g., those who have not recovered from a local throat anesthetic.

> Frequently turn and reposition patients who are immobilized.

> Encourage periodic coughing and deep breathing in patients who are recovering from surgery, are immobilized, or have retained pulmonary secretions.

> Maintain a patent tracheobronchial tree, e.g., by suctioning.

> Prevent overmedication with sedatives, narcotics, and cough-suppressive medications. Oversedation and respiratory depression predispose to secretion accumulation in the lungs.

> Observe for early indications of possible pneumonia; call symptoms to the physician's attention so early treatment can be instituted if necessary.

> Encourage prompt treatment of colds and "flu," especially in persons susceptible to pneumonia.

> Prevent spread of communicable respiratory infections by using appropriate medical asepsis and isolation. Keep the very young and very old away from close

contact with a person who has pneumonia. Encourage good room ventilation and minimize crowding. Properly clean inhalation therapy equipment to prevent spread of infection.

> Give frequent oral hygiene to dependent persons in your care.

> Observe necessary precautions that minimize the likelihood of aspiration when giving food or liquids to patients who are likely to aspirate. Make certain nasogastric tubes are correctly positioned in the stomach before administering a tube feeding or medication.

Bacterial Pneumonias

Most primary bacterial pneumonias are caused by *Diplococcus pneumoniae,* i.e., the pneumococcus. Other microorganisms that may cause bacterial pneumonias include *Staphylococcus aureus,* group A hemolytic streptococci, *Escherichia coli, Haemophilus influenzae,* Klebsiella-Enterobacter-Serratia group, *Francisella tularensis,* Proteus species, or Pseudomonas. Commonly aspiration pneumonias, hypostatic pneumonias (see Chapter 27), and "terminal" pneumonias are mixed infections. Often healthy carriers are responsible for infecting others. Pathogenic organisms that cause bacterial pneumonias are frequently present among the normal flora of the respiratory tract.

Because pneumococcal pneumonia is the most common type of bacterial pneumonia (accounting for 80 per cent or more of cases), and because it generally typifies pneumonias caused by all etiologic agents, this discussion focuses in detail on pneumococcal pneumonia.

Pneumococcal Pneumonia

Pathology. Pneumonia caused by pneumococci usually involves one or more lobes of the lung. Pneumococci are not the only organisms that cause lobar pneumonias. However, whatever the etiologic organism(s) may be, lobar pneumonias classically have the following four histologic stages: congestion, red hepatization, gray hepatization, and resolution. (Consult a textbook of pathology for details.)

Pneumococci initially reach the alveoli via the respiratory passages. During the course of the infection the sputum becomes rusty-colored because of the red blood cells which escape from the blood vessels and pass through the alveolar membrane. As alveolar fluids spill into the bronchioles they are eventually coughed up through the tracheobronchial tree. Inflammation of the mucous membranes of the bronchi, trachea, pharynx, and nose occurs. Thus, the entire respiratory system is involved. During the periods of consolidation (when the alveoli are filled with thick exudate), adequate gas exchange cannot occur in involved areas of the lungs; pulmonary ventilation and diffusion are impaired, and the blood oxygen tension is subnormal.

Symptoms. Pneumococcal pneumonia usually has a sudden onset, with shaking chills, high fever, cough, blood-flecked or pinkish (progressing to rust-colored) sputum, and "stabbing" chest pains (worsened by respiratory movements and, in some

instances, referred to the shoulder, abdomen, or flank). Chest pain is caused by pleuritic involvement. Occasionally gastrointestinal symptoms such as nausea, vomiting, diarrhea, and jaundice occur. Often herpes simplex is present and the cheeks are flushed. Frequently history reveals that the patient has had a recent respiratory illness, e.g., an upper respiratory infection was present for several days before the infection worsened and moved rapidly into the lower respiratory tract. The patient may experience a chill followed by fever at the beginning of pneumonia. Body temperature may rise within a few hours to 40.0 or 40.1°C. (104 to 106°F.).

Typically the patient with pneumonia appears severely ill and may be found lying on his affected side in an attempt to splint his painful chest. Toxic delirium often occurs with severe pneumonia, particularly in alcoholic patients. If conscious and alert the patient with pneumonia usually experiences aching pains, weakness, headache, and general malaise. Dyspnea is common and cyanosis may develop. Respirations are shallow. The nares flare with inspiration and the patient grunts with expiration. Marked tachypnea (30 to 45 respirations per minute) occurs. The pulse rate is also frequently increased, e.g., tachycardia may be present with 100 to 130 heart beats per minute. Abdominal distention and a pleural friction rub may also be present. Profuse perspiration is common.

Initially the cough tends to be dry, short, painful, and hacking. Later in the illness the cough becomes productive and pain decreases. Early in the course of pneumonia chest excursion on the affected side is diminished. Respiratory rales may be heard; breath sounds may be suppressed. Sputum is rusty during the earlier stages of the disease; it becomes yellow and mucopurulent during resolution. Sputum may be tenacious and difficult to expectorate.

Course of Illness. Patients with pneumococcal pneumonia who are treated early, vigorously, and appropriately usually respond well; 90 to 95 per cent survive. Without treatment the mortality rate is between 20 and 40 per cent. The higher mortality rates occur in patients over age 45 and those having complications or other diseases, e.g., heart failure. Untreated persons whose illness is uncomplicated usually experience resolution by *crisis* about 7 to 10 days after onset of the pneumonia. The crisis period, in untreated cases, is the period when the patient's temperature "breaks" and declines rapidly. Typically the temperature remains elevated until the crisis occurs.

Diagnosis. The presence of rusty sputum is practically diagnostic of bacterial pneumonia. In addition to the previously described symptom pattern, other key factors in the diagnosis of pneumococcal pneumonia include lung infiltration visible on x-ray, leukocytosis (20 to 35 thousand/cu.

mm.), and pneumococci present in the sputum and frequently also in the blood.

Sputum smears (Gram's stain) and cultures determine the bacterial etiology; blood cultures are also performed in bacteremic cases and are positive in about one fourth of the patients. Special laboratory procedures, i.e., the capsular swelling technique, may be used to type pneumococci. Types I to VIII most commonly occur in adults. Sputum from persons with pneumonia typically contains numerous pneumococci and red and white blood cells. The WBC count is usually elevated but it is sometimes normal or low; a low WBC indicates a poorer prognosis.

Sputum specimens for smear and culture and a blood culture should always be collected prior *to giving the patient any antimicrobial medications.*

It may be impossible to culture out, and hence identify, the infecting organism if antibiotics are started before the specimen is collected. When a good sputum specimen cannot be obtained, tracheal aspiration may be performed to obtain a specimen. (Be certain to collect sputum specimens in sterile containers.) Sputum cultures require at least 24 to 48 hours to grow.

X-ray findings with bacterial pneumonias vary, depending on the stage of the disease. For example, initially vague haziness appears in the involved area. Later, well defined areas of consolidation appear and pleural fluid may blunt the costophrenic angles. An electrocardiogram may be necessary to help the physician to evaluate the patient's cardiac status. Blood specimens may be collected for blood gas and electrolyte evaluations. Urinalysis is routinely ordered.

Clinical Care. Clinical care of any patient with pneumonia is basically directed at providing chemotherapy that will be effective against the specific etiologic agent, providing symptomatic or supportive care directed at relieving symptoms associated with the pneumonia, and preventing complications of pneumonia or treating these if present. Essential activities important in the clinical care of a patient who has pneumonia include:

> Observe and evaluate response to care.
> Observe for and treat complications.
> Carry out and/or assist with diagnostic procedures.
> Ensure adequate physical and mental rest.
> Prevent chilling and exposure to drafts.
> Prevent spread of infection.
> Give frequent oral hygiene and lip and nose care.
> Provide fluid-electrolyte replacements and treat imbalances.
> Provide appropriate diet.
> Promote good tracheobronchial hygiene to help the patient to breathe more comfortably and effectively.
> Administer specific chemotherapy and observe for side-effects or toxicity.
> Instruct the patient concerning convalescence and prevention of future respiratory infections.

OBSERVATIONS. When caring for a patient with pneumonia the nurse observes for indications of respiratory insufficiency or failure, shock, pulmonary edema, hyperthermia, spread of infection, atelectasis, pleurisy, abdominal distention, paralytic ileus, herpes simplex, fluid-electrolyte imbalances, and mental aberrations.

Shock and pulmonary edema are the most frequent causes of death in pneumonia. Pneumonia may precipitate congestive heart failure in elderly patients or patients with preexisting heart disease. Observe closely for *early* indications of complications and report pertinent symptoms *immediately*.

Space does not permit a detailed summary of all reportable symptoms; however, some are production of copious amounts of frothy sputum; increasingly labored respirations; temperatures below 98.6 or above 103°F.; marked alterations in pulse rate and/or blood pressure (abnormal increases or decreases); indications of increasing hypoxemia (e.g., marked restlessness, disorientation, cyanosis, and increasing pulse rate); and toxic delirium. The nurse also reports any situations for which she requires orders, e.g., abdominal distention, pleuritic pain.

Evaluate restlessness carefully and attempt to identify and relieve its cause when possible. The restless patient may require oxygen, suctioning, position change, dry linens, assistance to use the urinal or bedpan, relief from abdominal distention or pleuritic pain, encouragement to cough and deep breathe, or mild sedation. Also, evaluate hypotension carefully; it may indicate shock, bacteremia, or hypoxia.

The nurse also observes the patient's general response to therapy. One measure of the patient's condition and response is the temperature curve. The effect of antipyretics must be considered when evaluating the temperature curve.

Other measures that the nurse uses to evaluate a patient with pneumonia include periodic measurements of vital signs, intake and output; observations of the patient's respiratory movements, including inspection of the movements of both sides of the chest; inspection and palpation of the skin and abdomen; inspection and measurement of sputum; evaluation of cough, pain and sensorium; inspection of lips and mucous membranes; and evaluation of laboratory findings.

During the acute stages of pneumonia, vital signs are taken and recorded at least every four hours. If complications appear to be developing or if the patient's condition is otherwise changing rapidly, vital signs are taken more often. Because the patient with pneumonia is dyspneic and coughs frequently, rectal temperatures are taken to obtain more accurate readings.

REST. Ensure adequate rest, both physical and mental. Exertion and activity fatigue the patient and increase his oxygen needs. Bed rest is usually maintained and unnecessary activities are avoided until the infection begins to clear and respond to therapy. During the acute phase, complete bed rest is imperative except for the mildest of infections. Patients who respond rapidly to treatment may be permitted to be out of bed after having a normal temperature for two or three days. Longer periods of bed rest are necessary for patients with more severe or complicated illnesses. Check activity orders. Some patients are allowed to use the commode rather than bedpan while on bed rest. With improvement, activity is gradually increased but is interspersed with rest periods.

During the acute period of illness, soporifics, e.g., chloral hydrate or barbiturates, may be prescribed to help the patient to sleep.

Talking is fatiguing to a patient who is acutely ill and dyspneic. The nurse therefore minimizes "social" conversation and expresses her interest in the patient in other ways. Visitors may be restricted during the acute period of illness; those permitted are instructed to avoid excessive talking.

Keep the patient's environment pleasant and restful and provide planned, uninterrupted rest periods. Assist with personal hygiene as indicated by the patient's condition. During the period of bed rest turn the patient frequently and exercise his lower limbs. (See Chapter 27.) Place items needed by the patient, such as tissues, sputum cup, water, hand wipes, paper bag, call bell, within easy reach to minimize exertion.

The diagnosis of pneumonia is feared by some patients, especially older persons. Also, with severe infections various aspects of the illness itself may be highly anxiety provoking, e.g., dyspnea, pain, bloody sputum. The nurse strives to reduce the patient's fears and apprehensions by maintaining a calm, efficient manner and giving appropriate reassurance and explanations. Anxiety is carefully evaluated because it may indicate hypoxemia.

MAINTAINING WARMTH AND DRYNESS. Protect the patient from chilling and exposure to drafts and keep him comfortably warm, unless he is hyperthermic and cooling measures are being used. Flannelette sheets sometimes keep the patient more comfortable than cotton. To prevent possible chilling and unnecessary fatigue, omit a total bed bath while the patient is acutely ill; however, be certain to provide necessary skin care without chilling the patient. Frequently check the acutely ill patient to determine if his bed linens and/or gown are damp from perspiration; damp linens must be changed immediately.

PREVENTION OF SPREAD OF INFECTION. Because bacterial and viral pneumonias are communicable as long as the patient is febrile, appropriate precautions must be employed to prevent the spread of infection to others. The patient's room should be well ventilated to minimize air contamination. Instruct the patient to turn his head away from persons near him and to cover his nose and mouth with disposable tissues when sneezing or coughing. This helps to prevent infected droplets from becoming air-borne. After use, tissues should immediately be placed in a paper bag so they can later be burned. Provide disposable, covered sputum cups if sputum is copious or specimens are necessary. Change the paper bags used to hold contaminated tissues and sputum cups at least three times daily, as they become half full. Before disposing of sputum make certain the physician does not want a specimen saved or sent to the clinical laboratory. Always cover sputum containers before properly disposing of them.

Frequent handwashing is also of importance in preventing transmission of the infection. The nurse always washes after contact with the patient or with articles that could be contaminated. She also always washes prior to giving care to protect the patient from secondary infection. Persons with respiratory infections should not care for or visit the patient who has pneumonia.

To ensure medical asepsis it is often desirable for the nurse to cover her uniform with a gown when caring for patients who are acutely ill with pneumonia and who may be unable to properly protect the nurse.

Pneumococcal pneumonia is not highly communicable; however, the causative agent can be carried by a healthy person from one patient to another or to some other susceptible person. Staphylococcal pneumonia can also be spread by human carriers, in addition to apparently being spread by the inhalation of dust from dry sweeping or from bedding. The nurse should take care not to unnecessarily "flourish" or shake bed linens while giving care. Dust-laying sweeping compounds should be used and bedding should be treated with germicidal compounds as a preventive measure. Ultraviolet lights may be placed in strategic locations to decontaminate the air.

Specific isolation precautions are usually not necessary with most pneumonias; however, hospital policies vary. Some hospitals practice isolation during the acute phase of certain pneumonias, e.g., staphylococcal pneumonia, which has a tendency to cause periodic outbreaks in hospitals. It is always advisable during the acute phase to keep the patient away from other patients predisposed to pneumonia, such as patients who are seriously ill, elderly, debilitated, postsurgical, or those with chronic obstructive pulmonary disease. Single rooms are best during the acute period of illness.

Visitors need to be informed of necessary precautions if they visit an infectious patient.

ORAL HYGIENE; LIP AND NOSE CARE. Give frequent oral hygiene and lip and nose care. These nursing activities can make the patient more comfortable and are particularly important if he is febrile and dehydrated, has herpes simplex lesions, is mouth breathing, and/or is producing foul sputum. Oral hygiene may prevent spread of the infection to the ears, and is necessary to prevent stomatitis, i.e., inflammation of the oral mucosa. Lung abscess formation also may be prevented by frequent oral hygiene, since the most common cause of lung abscess is aspiration of anaerobic mouth flora. When giving oral hygiene be certain to clean the patient's tongue well and to lubricate his lips.

Dryness and crusting of the nares can be a minor, but distressing problem. Soothing creams or ointments may be applied around the nares. Crusts may be gently removed with swabs moistened in water or hydrogen peroxide.

MAINTAINING FLUID-ELECTROLYTE BALANCE. Fluid-electrolyte replacement must be provided. Maintain and evaluate the patient's intake and output record carefully for indications of imbalances and look for clinical symptoms of imbalances. (See Chapters 24 and 25.)

Fluid replacement is tailored to the individual patient's needs. Patients with pneumococcal pneumonia lose a great deal of fluid and salt because they usually perspire heavily. As mentioned earlier, vomiting and diarrhea sometimes occur. Also, patients with bacterial pneumonias often require increased hydration because of elevations in insensible fluid loss caused by fever and hyperventilation, and because pulmonary secretions are increased. Maintaining adequate hydration is important not only to prevent fluid imbalances, but also because it facilitates expectoration of bronchopulmonary secretions.

Frequently it is necessary to supplement hydration by mouth with intravenous fluids (75 to 150 ml. per hour). It is advisable to monitor the central venous pressure when replacing fluids in some patients (e.g., those with impending congestive heart failure) to prevent the development of pulmonary edema. (See Unit X.)

DIET. Intravenous fluids are sometimes ordered to provide nutrition as well as fluid intake for anorexic, nauseated or vomiting patients. Or, anorexic, dyspneic patients may best tolerate a liquid diet during the acute period of pneumonia. With improvement they progress to a soft-solid and then general diet. Patients with complications whose illness is prolonged may be given a high-protein, high-caloric diet with vitamin supplements. Increased metabolism and the loss of plasma and cells in the pneumonic exudate make it desirable for the caloric intake to be a minimum of 1200 to 1500 calories daily. Caloric intake can be increased by adding food concentrates to fluids, e.g., adding lactose to milk. Dyspneic, congested patients often have difficulty taking fluids and may find it fatiguing to drink. Unless contraindicated, salt intake may be increased in the diet of patients who are perspiring profusely, since sodium is lost via perspiration.

Some physicians prescribe a diet of solid food early in the course of the illness because they believe such a diet may prevent the possible complication of paralytic ileus. It is recommended that gas-forming foods be avoided to minimize the occurrence of abdominal distention and/or paralytic ileus.

RESPIRATORY CARE. Respiratory therapy is frequently necessary in the presence of pneumonia because effective ventilation and respiration may be impaired by the presence of inflammatory exudate in the alveoli, atelectasis, increased bronchopulmonary secretions, and secondary bronchospasm. Respiratory care is individualized. Elderly patients often have a diminished cough reflex and require intensive respiratory care to help them to remove secretions. Seriously ill patients and those with underlying pulmonary disease may develop severe hypoxemia and respiratory failure. The nurse participates actively in promoting good tracheobronchial hygiene and helping the dyspneic patient to breathe more comfortably and effectively.

Oxygen inhalation therapy may be required to help the patient to breathe more easily and to rest. Oxygen therapy may help to relieve restlessness and cough, prevent pulmonary edema, and also prevent or relieve abdominal distention. Indications for oxygen therapy include cyanosis, dyspnea, weakness, delirium, circulation disturbances, painful or labored respirations, and a pO_2 of 70 mm. Hg or lower. Oxygen is best administered to the patient with pneumonia via a nasal catheter or cannula (prongs) rather than by mask or tent. If oxygen tents are used they are used mainly for humidity control; the oxygen content is difficult to govern in an oxygen tent. The efficacy of oxygen therapy needs to be monitored periodically by determining blood gas levels. This is of special importance in patients with underlying chronic pulmonary or ventilatory disease in order to prevent suppression of respiration. (See previous chapters in this unit.) Arterial pO_2, pCO_2, and pH values are determined several times a day in seriously ill patients.

Some patients may require control with a *mechanical ventilator* to maintain effective respiration. In the presence of obvious *bronchospasm* the physician may order aminophylline (given intravenously over a period of several hours) and/or dyphylline (Lufyllin), and glyceryl guaiacolate administered orally. Because an adequate airway must be maintained it may be necessary to use *nasotracheal suction* (by sterile technique) and to *endotracheally intubate* the patient or perform *tracheostomy.* The latter procedures make it easier to remove by suction copious or thick secretions and they permit ventilation with a positive pressure breathing apparatus if necessary.

Effective coughing is necessary to remove secretions from the tracheobronchial tree. The patient is instructed how to cough effectively; if coughing is painful it may be helpful to splint the patient's chest. (See Chapter 73.) Ineffective coughing is discouraged since it tires the patient. Emphasize to the patient the importance of coughing up and expectorating (rather than swallowing) his infected sputum. Observe expectorated sputum and record your observations.

Respiratory physiotherapy, e.g., *percussion, clapping,* may be necessary to help to move tenacious secretions so they can be expectorated or removed by suction. Often supervised postural drainage (for 5 to 10 minutes three or four times daily) is necessary. *Intermittent positive pressure breathing* (IPPB) may be ordered two to four times daily.

Various substances (e.g., acetylcysteine, isotonic saline solution, or a bronchodilator such as isoproterenol) may be nebulized, depending upon the patient's needs.

Supervise planned coughing and *deep breathing sessions* and provide assistance as required. These sessions should be planned to coincide with periods when the patient is awakened for other care, such as administration of medications. During such sessions, protect yourself by having the patient cover his nose and mouth with tissues and by keeping your face away from his path of expiration. The frequency of planned coughing and deep breathing sessions depends upon the patient's condition. Deep breathing exercises help to prevent reductions in vital capacity and pulmonary compliance.

When hacking cough interferes with the patient's rest and is debilitating, the physician may prescribe medications to partially suppress (but not abolish) the cough. Excessive depression of the cough reflex dangerously encourages the retention of bronchopulmonary secretions and the development of atelectasis.

Although *cough suppressant medications* may be ordered early in the acute phase of illness (while the cough is typically painful and nonproductive), during the latter phase of pneumonia, expectorants may be prescribed. *Expectorants* help to clear the lungs and tracheobronchial tree of secretions and exudate. A cool-mist vaporizer may be used to help to liquefy secretions as well as to humidify inspired air.

ANTIMICROBIAL MEDICATIONS. Appropriate medications are selected after identification of the infecting organism(s); antibiotics to which the organism is known to be sensitive are prescribed. Generally the physician selects antibiotics that have as narrow a spectrum as possible, since the use of broad-spectrum antibiotics may lead to complicating superinfections.

Often it is necessary to begin antibiotic administration before the specific infecting organism can be identified by culture. In such cases the physician makes a presumptive diagnosis (based tentatively on the patient's history and physical examination and interpretation of a Gram stain of sputum and a capsular swelling test) and begins initial chemotherapy. Once laboratory results are available from blood and sputum cultures and the offending organism is precisely identified, the antibiotic therapy is changed if indicated. Except in mild infections, antibiotics are typically administered parenterally when treating pneumonia.

Pneumococcal pneumonia is generally best treated with crystalline penicillin G. This medication may be given intravenously in the presence of shock. Potassium penicillin V may be given orally to patients who are not severely ill and who do not have gastrointestinal symptoms. It may also be used when conditions preclude parenteral therapy or make it difficult. Currently all pneumonias are susceptible to penicillin.

Before the first dose of penicillin is given the patient's history is carefully reviewed for evidence of possible hypersensitivity to penicillin. An intravenous sensitivity test is advisable with a small amount of penicillin prior to giving the first dose. (See Chapter 23.) If the patient is hypersensitive to penicillin, or is suspected of being hypersensitive, he may be treated with another antibiotic such as erythromycin or lincomycin.

Administer antibiotics at the time ordered to maintain the desired blood level of medication. Observe the patient closely for indications of side-effects or toxicity of the antibiotics, e.g., diarrhea, vomiting, nausea, soft tissue reactions, pruritus, skin rash, or indications of anaphylactic shock. *Report indications of allergy or cross-allergy immediately.*

Patients with pneumococcal pneumonia who receive adequate chemotherapy early in the course of their illness have about a 5 per cent mortality rate. Fatalities usually occur in patients younger than two years of age and older than 45. Prognosis is less favorable and convalescence longer in the presence of the following conditions: involvement of two or more lobes; a positive blood culture; white blood count below 5000; blood urea nitrogen higher than 70 mg./100 ml.; endocarditis; meningitis; or underlying chronic disease.

If appropriate antibiotic therapy is started early enough, most patients respond favorably and symptoms begin to subside rapidly during the first two to three days of treatment. If this response does not occur, the physician reevaluates the patient for the presence of complications, possible drug fever, other disease, or superinfection.

Chemotherapy is continued in uncomplicated cases until bacteriologic evidence of infection has disappeared and an obvious improvement occurs clinically; prolonged chemotherapy is advisable in some destructive pneumonias (e.g., staphylococcal pneumonia) in an attempt to prevent relapse.

Complications of Pneumonia. Effective diagnostic and treatment methods have reduced the incidence of complications of pneumonia, but problems still occur. Some are life-threatening; therefore, the nurse observes closely for indications of delayed resolution of disease or the development of complications in persons acutely ill with pneumonia and she reports these observations promptly to the attending physician. Complications most frequently occur in aged patients, patients suffering from chronic illnesses, and patients who did not receive early, appropriate treatment. Both pulmonary and nonpulmonary complications may occur.

PULMONARY COMPLICATIONS. Pulmonary complications that may be associated with pneumonia include pulmonary edema, pulmonary abscess, atelectasis, respiratory failure, and superinfection with other bacteria as a consequence of therapy. Some patients infected with drug-resistant or highly virulent organisms experience a spread of the pneumonic activity or delayed resolution of the infection. These problems can usually be effectively managed by changing the prescribed medications to include agents to which the infecting organisms are sensitive.

NONPULMONARY COMPLICATIONS. Nonpulmonary complications that may occur with pneumonia include dry pleurisy, pleurisy with effusion, empyema, and various other infections, particularly septicemia, acute otitis media, acute sinusitis, septic shock, disseminated intravascular coagulation, herpes simplex, abdominal distention, paralytic ileus, mental aberrations, and hyperthermia.

Dry pleurisy fairly often accompanies pneumonia and may progress to *pleurisy with effusion. Empyema* necessitates total removal of the exudate by repeated thoracentesis or tube or open surgical drainage. At times antibiotics are instilled locally. Sterile pleural effusions usually require no treatment. However, all aspirated pleural fluid should be examined by smear and culture, so that early treatment can be started if an empyema is present.

Other extrapulmonary infections may accompany bacterial pneumonias. Among these are nephritis, peritonitis, pericarditis, endocarditis, meningitis, and purulent arthritis. These infections result from *septicemia,* i.e., invasion of the blood stream by bacterial toxins that are carried to other tissues or organs. Extrapulmonary infections require prolonged therapy with increased doses of specific antibiotics to which the infecting organisms are susceptible.

Acute *otitis media* and *acute sinusitis* may occur if the bacterial infection extends into the middle ear and sinuses.

Septic shock may occur in pneumonias in which treatment was delayed or is inadequate; those complicated by the presence of other debilitating illnesses; or those caused by highly virulent or drug-resistant organisms. Early symptoms of the peripheral vascular collapse occurring with septic shock include reductions in blood pressure, temperature, and level of consciousness; weak, rapid pulse; and cool, clammy skin. Measures that may be employed to treat septic shock are discussed in Chapter 26.

Patients with pneumonia who have underlying heart disease may experience *cardiovascular failure* associated with congestive heart failure. In such cases the physician evaluates the patient's heart size, peripheral edema, and CVP and prescribes appropriate treatment, e.g., digitalis and/or diuretics. (See Unit X.)

Disseminated intravascular coagulation may complicate some severe pneumonias. Full doses of heparin may be administered once the condition is identified. (See Unit XII.)

Herpes simplex (fever sores or cold sores) is a minor complication which frequently occurs, particularly with bacterial pneumonias. Treatment of these lesions in the vesicular stage may include applications of tincture of benzoin or spirits of camphor. Ointments may be prescribed once the lesions are encrusted.

Abdominal distention frequently complicates severe pneumonia and usually results from air swallowing by the severely dyspneic patient. It may also result from decreased peristalsis, which allows fluids and gas to collect in the intestinal tract. Abdominal distention is uncomfortable for the patient and, more seriously, may interfere with pulmonary expansion and further compromise respirations. It elevates the diaphragm and restricts diaphragmatic excursions, compressing the lower regions of the lungs. (See Unit XV.)

Paralytic ileus, i.e., absence of intestinal peristaltic action, may occur with severe pneumonia. To prevent this the nurse should: (1) record all bowel movements and report constipation; (2) observe the abdomen for tenderness, rigidity, or abdominal distention and report the occurrence of these symptoms; (4) report vomiting (with ileus the vomitus may contain fecal matter); and (4) periodically listen to the abdomen for bowel tones (in the absence of peristalsis no bowel tones can be heard). Enemas are usually not given in the absence of peristalsis because the fluid will be retained and will further increase abdominal distention unless the fluid is siphoned back. Treatment is basically decompression of the abdomen accomplished by insertion of a Miller-Abbott tube. (See Unit XV.)

Mental aberrations of various kinds may occur with pneumonia. Toxicity, hyperthermia, and oxygen deficiency each contribute to such abnormal mental states as confusion or disorientation, toxic delirium, or acute anxiety states. The nurse therefore periodically evaluates the patient's mental status and observes closely for indications of these complications. (Refer to Units III and VIII.)

Report mental aberrations to the physician and help family members to understand the basis for the patient's behavior. It is especially important that the patient not be restrained. The restrained patient may panic, become combative, and struggle against his restraints. Such exertion and anxiety can critically worsen the condition of the toxic, dyspneic patient. The physician carefully evaluates abnormal behavior in a patient acutely ill with pneumonia to be certain the symptoms are not caused by pneumococcal meningitis. If meningitis is suspected, a diagnostic lumbar puncture is performed.

When you give a patient sedatives or tranquilizers, remember to check his sensorium periodically and chart your observations. Avoid oversedation since it depresses the cough reflex and respiratory center.

Hyperthermia may also complicate pneumonia. Temperature elevations greater than 39.4°C. (103°F.) should be lowered by an electric fan, tepid sponges, alcohol sponges, or antipyretic medications. Some physicians order aspirin to be given according to the patient's temperature; others may order it to be given regularly every four hours. Antipyretics may help to relieve muscular aches and malaise in addition to reducing fever. Patients with extremely high temperature elevations may require hypothermia. (See Unit VIII.)

Convalescence. Pneumonia is a physically taxing illness; therefore, the patient may feel weakened and may fatigue easily for some time after acute symptoms have been relieved. The physician's instructions during the period of convalescence should be followed carefully. A fairly long period of convalescence is necessary for aged or chronically ill persons. Rest periods are usually advisable for a while even after only brief acute pneumonias. The physician decides when a patient can return to work. Prior to hospital discharge the nurse cautions the patient against overexertion and encourages him to keep follow-up medical appointments. During the period of convalescence the physician usually orders chest x-rays to evaluate clearing of the lung. Typically the patient is advised to continue deep breathing exercises for six to eight weeks after discharge.

Pneumonia tends to make the affected person susceptible to recurring respiratory infections. Therefore, the patient is advised about ways in which such infections can possibly be prevented and is told that he should seek early medical evaluation of any symptoms. Influenza vaccination may be recommended, since secondary bacterial pneumonias can occur with influenza.

Other Bacterial Pneumonias

Space does not permit detailed discussion of the various bacterial pneumonias. As stated earlier, the clinical courses and supportive treatments are generally similar to those of pneumococcal pneumonia. However, specific antibiotic therapy varies, depending on the infecting organism and its drug sensitivities. Summarized below are comments about the more common of these.

> *Streptococcal pneumonia* (most frequently caused by hemolytic group A organisms) is usually a complication of influenza or measles, but may follow scarlet fever or streptococcal sore throat. A large pleural effusion, often bloody, may occur early. Streptococcal pneumonia usually appears suddenly and is severe.

> *Staphylococcal pneumonia* (usually caused by coagulase-positive *Staphylococcus aureus*) may occur as a primary infection in the very young or aged, but otherwise most commonly develops as a complication of influenza. Also it may develop in hospitalized patients as a superinfection or as a complication of tracheostomy, immunosuppressive therapy, surgery, debility, or diseases affecting host defenses against infection. Staphylococcal pneumonia is a serious infection with a high mortality rate.

> *Pneumonia caused by Haemophilus influenzae* (most commonly by Types a and b) may occur in adults as a lobar pneumonia, bronchopneumonia or bronchiolitis. Recovery is typical. Sputum is characteristically tenacious and "apple-green" colored.

> *Friedländer's bacillus (klebsiellas) and other enterobacterial pneumonias.* Although any of the types of Friedländer's bacillus may cause pneumonia, the most common invaders are Types 1 and 2. Other organisms that can cause pneumonias similar to those caused by klebsiellas include *Escherichia coli,* Proteus species, Salmonella species, *Pseudomonas aeruginosa, Pseudomonas pseudomallei,* and anaerobic *Bacteroides* species. Prompt treatment of pneumonias caused by the preceding organisms is imperative; the mortality rate is particularly high if treatment is delayed beyond the second day of illness. These pneumonias cause critical illness.

Although pneumococcal pneumonia seldom causes any permanent damage to the lung, residual defects may result from other infections. Organisms such as staphylococcus, Friedländer's bacillus, tubercle bacillus, which cause the tissue in the center of the involved area to die, may leave abscess cavities and scarring of the lung. Also, when empyema develops it may cause permanent pleural thickening.

Primary Atypical Pneumonias

Primary atypical pneumonia (PAP) is a respiratory syndrome that may be caused by various agents (e.g., *Mycoplasma pneumoniae* or certain viruses) and usually differs from the "typical" bacterial pneumonias by having a more insidious, gradual onset and presenting with constitutional symptoms (e.g., headache, fatigue, fever), which may prevail over respiratory tract symptoms. Other common findings with PAP include x-ray evidence of infiltration but very few physical signs upon examination of the chest, white blood count that is normal or low (leukopenia), and gradually increasing cough with scanty sputum production and fever. Sputum is usually mucopurulent but occasionally may be blood-tinged.

Mycoplasmal Pneumonia. The *Mycoplasma pneumoniae* is also called the "Eaton agent." Mycoplasmal pneumonias occur year round and may have peak incidence in the summer. Often mycoplasmal infection causes severe frontal headaches. This type of pneumonia typically occurs in children and young adults. Death is rare, but sometimes the illness extends for several weeks. Cold agglutinins (autohemagglutinins for human type O erythrocytes) occur in at least 50 per cent of mycoplasmal infections and can be identified by a simple serologic test. *Mycoplasma pneumoniae* can be cultured from respiratory secretions.

Mild cases of mycoplasmal pneumonia usually do not require antimicrobial medications. Severe cases may be treated with erythromycin or tetracycline. General symptomatic care is the same as that indicated with pneumococcal pneumonia.

Viral Pneumonias. Viral pneumonias can be severe, even fatal illnesses (particularly with the virus of influenza A), but usually these infections are mild. Pulmonary involvement may not even be detected. Among the numerous agents that may cause viral pneumonias are adenoviruses, influenza and parainfluenza viruses, rhinoviruses, respiratory syncytial virus, herpes simplex, cytomegalovirus, and coxsackie-, echo-, and rheoviruses.

About 75 per cent of all acute pulmonary infections are viral pneumonias.[129]

Viral infections are indicated by the absence of respiratory pathogens when sputum is cultured. Commonly the diagnosis is made on the basis of clinical findings and serologic tests, since many hospital laboratories are not equipped to isolate viruses. Symptoms range from those of a common cold to respiratory insufficiency, which may progress rapidly. Prognosis is variable. Antibiotics are not indicated in the treatment of viral pneumonia. If the infection is an influenza A_2 viral infection, the patient may be given amantadine (Symmetrel) early in the course of the infection. Experimentally, cytomegalovirus and varicella pneumonias have been treated with inhibitors of normal DNA synthesis given parenterally, e.g., idoxuridine or cytosine arabinoside, and rhinoviral infections have been treated with the intranasal administration of interferon inducers, e.g., polyinosinic-polycytidylic acid (poly I:C). However, treatment of viral pneumonias is presently essentially symptomatic and is similar to that given for pneumococcal pneumonia.

Work is underway to develop effective *vaccines* against respiratory viruses, but these are difficult to prepare because of the numerous distinct antigenic serotypes. Possibly in the future vaccines will be available that can be administered via the respiratory route. This would be desirable, since vaccines administered in this manner would induce the formation of local antibodies that would control respiratory infections more effectively than circulating antibodies.

PULMONARY TUBERCULOSIS

Definition and Etiology. Tuberculosis is a reportable, communicable, infectious, inflammatory, and chronic disease that may occur in almost any part of the body. Because the lungs are most frequently infected, this discussion is chiefly limited to pulmonary tuberculosis.

Tuberculosis is caused by the *Mycobacterium tuberculosis,* which is the true "tubercle bacillus." Various atypical mycobacteria have recently been identified that resemble the true tubercle bacillus and produce diseases similar to true tuberculosis. (See discussion of atypical mycobacteria on p. 973.)

The *Mycobacterium bovis* (bovine tubercle bacillus) formerly caused numerous cases of tuberculosis in man as a result of the human ingestion of raw milk from infected cattle. Currently bovine tuberculosis has been practically eliminated in the United States because of the pasteurization of milk and tuberculin skin testing programs for cattle. (Infected cattle are destroyed.) Bovine tuberculosis continues to be a problem in other countries where similar public health programs are lacking and tuberculosis commonly occurs in cattle.

Mycobacterium avium produces a form of tuberculosis affecting birds and pigs, but it is only rarely virulent for human beings.

Unless otherwise stated, the discussion in this section is limited to the most common human form of tuberculosis, i.e., pulmonary tuberculosis resulting from infection by the *Mycobacterium tuberculosis.*

Characteristics of the Tubercle Bacillus. Tubercle bacilli are *rod-shaped, aerobic* (i.e., require oxygen to live), *nonmotile* (i.e., do not move), *gram-positive, acid-fast* microorganisms that *reproduce very slowly* within the human body (they divide approximately every 18 to 24 hours) and cannot reproduce outside the body (except under laboratory conditions). Tubercle bacilli have a high lipid content that contributes to their acid-fast staining characteristics.

Tubercle bacilli embedded in particles of dried sputum can lie dormant for months in dark places outside the body, but are rapidly destroyed when exposed to direct sunlight or ultraviolet rays. Within the body, tubercle bacilli may remain alive but dormant for decades; hence, reactivation of disease can occur years after an initial infection.

The tubercle bacillus can be destroyed by heat, e.g., burning, boiling for 5 minutes, autoclaving, pasteurization of milk; exposure to direct noonday sunlight for varying lengths of time, depending upon the strength of the sun's rays; contact with certain disinfectants (ordinary disinfectants are ineffective, coal tar preparations are most penetrating); and ultraviolet radiation (very effective).

Routes of Infection. Tuberculosis infections can occur by inhalation (most common); ingestion (relatively uncommon since reduction of bovine infections); direct infection, e.g., through a cut in the skin or mucous membranes (extremely rare); or prenatal infection (even more rare because the placenta is an effective barrier to tubercle bacilli). Because infection may result from ingestion of the bacilli, patients with pulmonary tuberculosis are cautioned to not swallow their sputum but rather to expectorate it; swallowed sputum can result in a spread of the infection to the gastrointestinal tract.

As indicated above, *the most common method of tuberculosis infection is from the inhalation of microorganisms.* Tubercle bacilli arise from infected persons and are present in the air as a result of coughing, sneezing, and expectorating. Infected minute droplet nuclei may then be inhaled into pulmonary peripheral alveoli. Droplet nuclei, transported by air currents, may remain suspended in the air for long periods of time. Large droplets are not inhaled into the alveoli because they tend to drop to the ground or be filtered out by the lung's protective mechanisms if inhaled. *Tuberculosis is,* thus, *essentially an air-borne infection* transferred from person to person via inhalation of infected droplet nuclei.

Pathology. If inhaled and implanted in healthy lung tissue bacillus-laden droplet nuclei can become a focus of infection. Infection is established if the bacilli survive and begin to multiply in the susceptible lung tissue. When tubercle bacilli infect the lung, the body's defensive mechanisms attempt to isolate and destroy the bacilli. Phagocytosis and lymphocytosis occur, and epitheloid cells and fibrous tissue attempt to wall off the infected area.

Tuberculosis infections are characterized by the formation of *tubercles*. Tubercles are gray translucent masses composed of small spherical cells that contain giant cells and are surrounded by a layer of epithelial connective tissue cells. The central portions of tubercles typically undergo a process of caseous degeneration (i.e., caseation), liquefaction, and cavitation.

Caseation is a necrotic process that is unique to tuberculosis. During the process of caseation the tissue changes into an amorphous cheeselike mass that consists of tubercle bacilli, dead white blood cells, and necrotic lung tissue. Large portions of caseous material may become encapsulated and form nodules that may be detected by x-ray. Caseous material is semisolid and gray-white in appearance.

At the peripheries of *caseous nodules* the tubercle bacilli and the body's white blood cells continue to battle in a zone of inflammatory reaction which consists of exudate, lymphocytes, multiplying connective tissue cells, and dilated capillaries. The center of the caseous nodule is avascular; thus, thrombosis formation occurs. Avascular, necrotic lung tissue that is sealed off in the lung and cannot be evacuated through the tracheobronchial tree provides an excellent medium for the bacilli. Tubercle bacilli located in caseous nodules live in an environment that is difficult to penetrate therapeutically, e.g., via the blood stream or tracheobronchial tree.

Eventually the caseous material in the center of the nodule tends to soften and liquefy. If erosion into a bronchus occurs, the liquefied material spills out into the tracheobronchial tree and is coughed up as *sputum*. Sputum may be highly infectious. Some of this infected material may spread throughout the lung or into the opposite lung via the tracheobronchial tree. As the liquefied material drains out of the nodule, an air-filled sac remains, i.e., a *cavity*.

All lesions do not progress to cavitation. Sometimes active inflammation subsides and some of the inflammatory products are removed by resolution, i.e., absorption of the inflammation. Some healing by resolution occurs, but most tuberculous lesions heal by scarring or fibrosis. Fibrous organization and healing occur, and the caseous lesions become encapsulated and gradually are infiltrated with deposits of calcium; *calcified lesions* are often visible by x-ray.

PRIMARY (FIRST) INFECTION. The first time an individual is infected with tuberculosis he is said to have a *primary infection*. Generally primary infections are located in the lower part of the upper lobe of the lung or near the pleura in the lower lobe. Although a primary infection may be only microscopic in size (and hence never even appear on x-ray), the following sequence of events typically occurs.

A small area of tuberculous pneumonic exudation develops in the lung parenchyma ("Gohn tubercle"); the center of this area quickly becomes caseous. Wandering white blood cells engulf the infecting mycobacteria and carry some of them to regional lymph nodes. Thus, the infection (although minute) is rapidly spread to the regional bronchopulmonary (hilar) lymph nodes. This regional adenitis in the hilar lymph nodes and the area of caseous pneumonia in the lung are referred to as a *primary complex* (Fig. 71–5).

Primary infections cause the body to develop a state of sensitivity that is manifest by a positive reaction to tuberculin skin tests. This development of tuberculin sensitivity in all body cells occurs three to 10 weeks after the primary infection and is maintained as long as living bacilli remain in the body (perhaps for life). This allergic reaction to tubercle bacilli or their proteins (tuberculins) is believed to be related to the continued presence of tubercle bacilli within caseous lesions (even though these lesions may be only microscopic in size).

Primary tuberculous infections often are never recognized because they usually are relatively asymptomatic. In the majority of cases body defenses are adequate to arrest primary infections, and they heal by fibrosis and calcification. Occasionally, however, the primary infection is not controlled, and the patient develops what is called *progressive primary tuberculosis*. In this situation the primary complex sites progress and worsen, possibly causing cavitation and spread of the active infection.

PROGRESSION OF TUBERCULOUS LESIONS. Basically tuberculous lesions can progress or extend in four ways: (1) by *local progression,* e.g., the local enlargement of a lesion by erosion through its capsule; (2) by *bronchogenic dissemination,* e.g., aspiration of infected material through the tracheobronchial tree into previously uninvolved areas of the lung(s); (3) by *lymphogenous dissemination,* e.g., spread to other areas of the body via the lymphatics; and (4) by *hematogenous dissemination,* e.g., infection spreads via the blood stream. Lymphogenous dissemination most commonly occurs during primary infections.

The most serious form of tuberculosis is *miliary tuberculosis*. This occurs when a tuberculous lesion extends into a sizable vascular channel, either artery or vein, or the thoracic duct. As a result of this erosion tubercle bacilli are shed into the passing blood or lymph stream and are disseminated to all organs of the body. Multiple small ("millet seed" size) lesions develop in many body tissues, e.g., brain, lungs. The chest x-ray is typically studded with countless small densities scattered throughout both lung fields. The patient with miliary tuberculosis is desperately ill. Before antituberculosis chemotherapy was available this condition was always fatal. Currently it may be effectively treated if diagnosed in time.

Tubercle bacilli spread through the lymph and blood may establish extrapulmonary sites of infection in the kidneys, genitalia, joints, brain, or other body tissues. *Extrapulmonary tuberculosis* is now much less common in the United States than formerly. When it does occur, prompt diagnosis and treatment are important, since chemotherapy can be effective in the early phases and may prevent deformity, disability, and fatality. Typically, extrapulmonary tuberculosis results from reactivated foci of tuberculosis, i.e., secondary tuberculosis, rather than from progressive primary disease. Space does not permit discussion

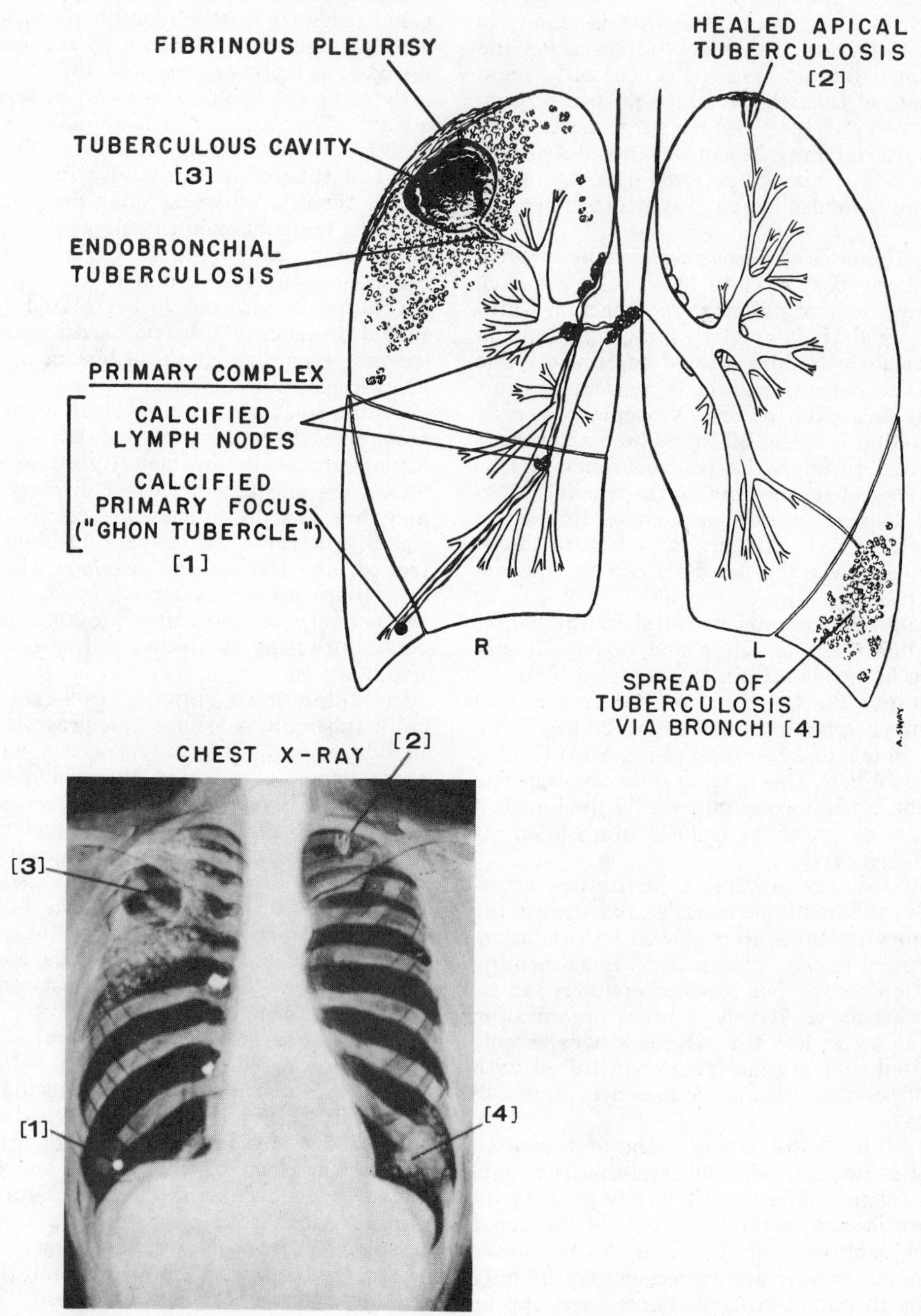

FIGURE 71–5. Chronic pulmonary tuberculosis. (From *Introduction to Respiratory Diseases*, 4th ed. Copyright American Lung Association, 1969.)

of specific types of extrapulmonary tuberculosis. However, concise discussion may be found in the booklet titled "Diagnostic Standards and Classifications of Tuberculosis," published by the American Lung Association.[206] The danger of infection from extrapulmonary tuberculosis is remote, since body discharges from the infected area(s) do not become airborne. However, thorough handwashing is naturally recommended after handling infected feces, urine, pus, and so forth, arising from sites of extrapulmonary infection.

REINFECTION (SECONDARY) TUBERCULOSIS. Reinfection tuberculosis is the most common form of clinical tuberculosis. A secondary infection with tuberculosis may occur exogenously or endogenously. *Exogenous reinfection* means that a new infection has entered the individual's body from outside. This type of reinfection rarely if ever occurs in the United States, but may occur in countries where tuberculosis is prevalent. In the United States most tuberculosis reinfection results from the postprimary progression of the first infection, i.e., *endogenous reinfection,* and represents reactivation of a previously dormant focus of tuberculosis.

Primary sites containing tubercle bacilli may remain latent for years and then reactivate if the patient's resistance becomes lowered. Because reinfection is possible (infection does not provide total immunity) and because dormant lesions may reactivate, *it is extremely important for persons who have had a tuberculosis infection to be reevaluated periodically for evidence of active disease.*

Reinfection pulmonary tuberculosis most commonly occurs in the upper regions of the lungs. Studies[72] indicate that tuberculosis reactivation tends to occur most often among persons at the lowest end of the socioeconomic scale, persons who live alone, and alcoholics. Other factors include inadequate chemotherapy of previous tuberculous infections, and the presence of such conditions as diabetes mellitus or peptic ulcer. (Predisposing factors are discussed further below.)

Classifications of Pulmonary Tuberculosis. Pulmonary tuberculosis infections are classified in the following ways:

> *Extent of disease:* Minimal, moderately advanced, or far advanced. This classification is made by examining chest roentgenograms and is periodically reevaluated following any therapy.

> *Status of clinical activity:* active; quiescent noncavitary and quiescent cavitary (terms applied to classes intermediate between active and nonactive); inactive noncavitary and cavitary; and activity undetermined (a temporary classification used for brief periods of observation or if inadequate bacteriologic or roentgenographic evidence has been accumulated to classify the disease in one of the preceding categories). The status of clinical activity is determined mainly from bacteriologic and roentgenographic findings and their duration. Periodic reclassifications are made as the clinical status of a patient's disease changes, e.g., from an active to an inactive status. *Active* pulmonary tuberculosis is typically a mixture of productive and exudative disease in which there are simultaneously present both progressive and retrogressive lesions.

> *Therapeutic status:* This classification is made by adding to the clinical status terms and dates that basically describe specific therapies used on the patient. For example: "Quiescent (since August 1973); chemotherapy (since November 1972); right upper lobe lobectomy (June 1973)."

The term *tuberculin convertor* is used to refer to persons who do not show roentgenographic or bacteriologic evidence of pulmonary tuberculosis, but in whom the tuberculin skin test converts from a known negative reaction to a known positive reaction, i.e., from less than 5 mm. of induration with a Mantoux skin test to 10 mm. or more.

Incidence. Before discussing some facts about the incidence of tuberculosis let us clarify some basic terms. *Morbidity rate* refers to the number of persons (per 100,000 population) who contract a disease, i.e., the ratio of diseased to well persons in a community for a given illness. *Mortality rate* refers to the number of persons (per 100,000 population) who die from a disease, i.e., the ratio of the number of deaths from a given disease to the total number of cases of that disease. During recent decades the mortality from tuberculosis has decreased markedly in the United States and, in spite of a population increase, morbidity is also declining. However, the number of new cases has declined less rapidly than the number of deaths (Fig. 71-6.) Tuberculosis was the leading cause of death in 1900. In that year tuberculosis caused 200/100,000 deaths in the United States; by 1967 this mortality figure had been reduced to 3.5/100,000. Similar declines have occurred in other countries that have relatively high standards of living. However, in impoverished areas high death rates from tuberculosis continue. Figure 71-7 shows the geographic areas of incidence of new cases in the United States.

Factors that have contributed to the dramatic reduction in tuberculosis mortality rates in the United States during the 20th century include: (1) implementation of case finding and isolation procedures; (2) early diagnosis and treatment; (3) provision for sanatorium care (much less common now than several decades ago); (4) improved standards of living; (5) elimination of bovine tuberculosis; (6) development of and enforcement of communicable disease laws; (7) widespread public education about tuberculosis; and (8) development of effective antituberculosis chemotherapy and precise techniques of surgical resection.

In discussing the incidence of tuberculosis it is important that the reader understand the difference between "tuberculosis infection" and "active clinical tuberculous disease." A positive tuberculin skin test indicates that an individual has had or has a tuberculous infection. It does not indicate whether that individual has active, overt clinical disease. An estimated 25,000,000 persons in the United States have been infected with tubercle

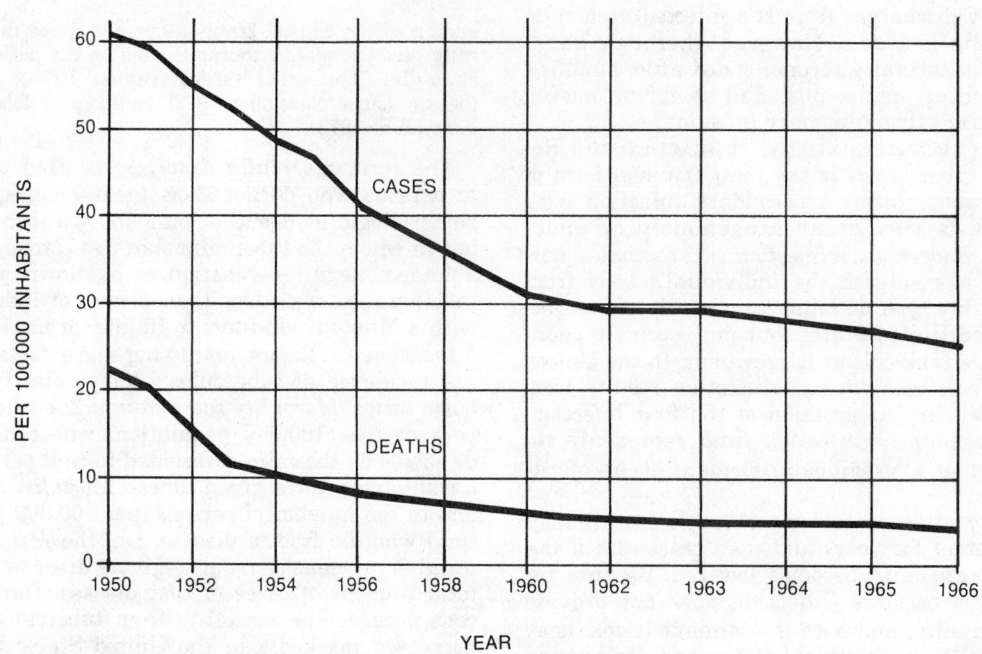

FIGURE 71-6. Tuberculosis morbidity and mortality in the United States 1950–66. (International Work in Tuberculosis. 1949–1964 WHO, Geneva, 1965.)

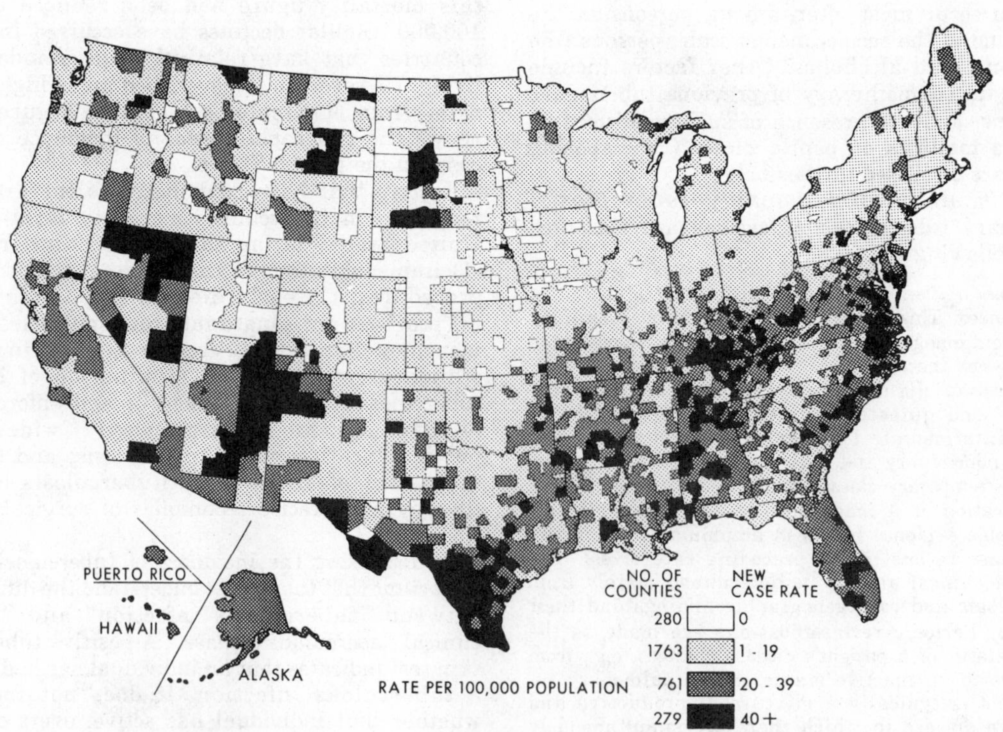

FIGURE 71-7. New active cases of tuberculosis per 100,000 population. (From Morbidity and Mortality, Vol. 19, 1970. U.S. Dept. of Health, Education and Welfare.)

bacilli sometime in the past.[302] Most of these infections have healed and will remain healed for the rest of the infected persons' lives. However, some of these infected persons will develop active disease. It is estimated that about 250,000 persons in the United States have active tuberculosis. The number of active cases throughout the world is probably between 15 and 20 million.

Many persons have adopted a complacent attitude toward tuberculosis and do not realize that this disease continues to be a serious public health problem in the United States and is a great problem in overpopulated, poor countries.

Predisposing Factors. The incidence of tuberculosis is high in overcrowded, poorly sanitized institutions. Increasingly, tuberculosis is becoming more common among city dwellers. It particularly affects those in cities who are in the lower socioeconomic groups, are poorly nourished, and have overcrowded, poorly ventilated living quarters.

Alcoholism, gastrectomy, and uncontrolled diabetes mellitus are examples of conditions that interfere with adequate nutrition and may cause reactivation of disease in previously infected individuals. Tuberculosis commonly affects males about twice as often as females. Nonwhites are over four times more susceptible, e.g., blacks and North American Indians are highly susceptible to tuberculosis. Tuberculosis thrives in catastrophic situations (e.g., war, large scale disasters), thus adding an additional burden to those unfortunate persons who are already suffering from the effects of the disaster.

Other important predisposing factors are the virulence of the organisms to which an individual is exposed and the length of exposure. Some organisms are more virulent than others. Infection with tuberculosis most often occurs from prolonged close associations with an individual who has active tuberculosis, but it is also true that many persons do not develop tuberculosis in spite of such associations.

In the United States an estimated 13 per cent of the population have a positive tuberculin skin test. Most of these persons are 45 years of age or older. Tuberculosis was formerly a disease affecting the young; currently this pattern has shifted and older persons are more commonly infected. This may be partially explained by the fact that lesions that have been controlled and inactive for a number of adult years reactivate during the later years of life when health may decline. Younger people of the present generation have benefited from health care programs that were not available during the youth of the now aged population. Infants and children below age five are quite susceptible to tuberculosis. The incidence also increases during puberty.

Tuberculosis infections are not inherited, but it is possible that some hereditary factor(s) causes some individuals to be more or less susceptible to infections than others. Silicosis appears to be the only pulmonary disease that promotes the development of active tuberculosis.

Persons who are going to receive prolonged adrenocorticoid therapy e.g., for arthritis, should be carefully evaluated prior to the administration of these medications to be certain no active tuberculosis infection is present. Also, during the course of steroid therapy the patient should be periodically evaluated for indications of active tuberculosis, since steroid preparations depress inflammation and antibody and lymphocyte production and thus may predispose to tuberculosis.

Although predisposing factors are important in determining the likelihood of infection with tuberculosis, no infection will occur unless tubercle bacilli enter the body.

Symptoms. Because of its typically insidious onset, tuberculosis infection may be actively present and progressing even though the patient is relatively asymptomatic. When symptoms do appear they may be both local and systemic.

Common *local symptoms* include cough and sputum production. Cough usually occurs with cavitary disease in which material drains into the bronchi, and it is therefore not typically an early symptom. The amount of sputum produced increases with progressive disease; it tends to be yellowish and mucoid. Less common symptoms are dyspnea, hemoptysis, and pleuritic pain (with pleural involvement). Occasionally hemoptysis is the first symptom. Rales may be heard over the affected lung. Sometimes the onset of tuberculosis is marked by symptoms indicative of influenza. Often patients feel as though they have a lingering cold or cigarette cough.

Constitutional symptoms are usually not indicative of pulmonary involvement and tend to be nonspecific, e.g., fatigue, night sweats, irritability, lassitude, rapid pulse rate, malaise, late afternoon low-grade fever, weight loss, anorexia, indigestion, and perhaps pallor. In women an early manifestation of tuberculosis may be irregularity or suppression of the menses. Vomiting may occur in advanced cases. Clubbing of the fingers occurs with many chronic pulmonary diseases, but it is not typical of tuberculosis.

Often persons with active tuberculosis appear amazingly well in spite of the fact that they may have far advanced disease with large tuberculous cavities in their lungs and other extensive lung damage. Some persons who have had active tuberculosis for long periods of time appear debilitated, but most persons with tuberculosis do not have this appearance.

Diagnosis. Individuals with active tuberculosis must be identified and properly treated not only for their own welfare, but also to prevent transmission of the disease to others.

Diagnostic procedures used to establish a diagnosis of tuberculosis *routinely* include complete medical and social history, complete physical examination, chest x-rays, tuberculin testing, and the bacteriologic examination of sputum or other specimens. Other diagnostic procedures may be performed, including photofluorography, bronchography, bronchoscopy, pleural biopsy, lung biopsy, and mediastinal and scalene node biopsies.

Routine laboratory tests include acid-fast smears and the planting of cultures to identify the specific organism(s) present. Drug-sensitivity cultures are also performed. Occasionally guinea-pig inoculations are made with urine. Several sputum specimens are taken before chemotherapy of any kind is started. Heated aerosol treatments may help to induce sputum for specimen purposes in persons who have difficulty raising sputum. Aspiration of fasting stomach contents may also be performed to obtain specimens for laboratory investigation. (Diagnostic procedures are discussed in detail in Chapter 68.)

The following three findings typically confirm a suspected diagnosis of pulmonary tuberculosis: a positive tuberculin skin test; appearance of areas of infection visible on chest x-rays; and the specific identification of the *M. tuberculosis* from cultured specimens. Because tubercle bacilli reproduce slowly, a minimum of three weeks is necessary to obtain a positive culture report and at least eight weeks for a negative report.

A positive reaction to a tuberculin skin test indicates that the individual has been infected with tuberculosis, but such a reaction does not indicate whether the infection is currently active or inactive. A positive tuberculin reaction merely indicates tissue sensitivity or allergy to tuberculin.

Positive tuberculin tests are usually followed by chest x-rays for evidence of active pulmonary tuberculosis. Usually even very small lesions can be seen because of the natural contrast furnished by air in the lungs. X-rays may be taken from several different positions. Calcified primary lesions or other healed lesions may be detected upon examination of the x-ray, as well as evidence of active disease, e.g., pulmonary infiltration, nodules, cavities, or other abnormalities such as pleural effusion.

A negative bacteriologic report does not routinely mean absence of active tuberculosis. Numerous sputum specimens may need to be examined before a positive specimen is located. Typically three or more specimens are meticulously examined to confirm the diagnosis. Some patients have a positive smear but a negative culture after they have taken antituberculosis medications for a while. This situation occurs because the organisms are still present in the patient's sputum (or whatever specimen is being observed) and thus can be identified on a smear, but they are too weak to reproduce and grow out on a culture. Often it is possible to identify disease caused by unclassified or anonymous mycobacteria only by culturing the organisms.

Because the tubercle bacillus may affect any body tissue, the symptoms of tuberculosis are highly variable, and depend upon the site of infection. Tuberculosis mimics over 100 other conditions and is compared with syphilis ("the great masquerader") in difficulty of diagnosis. Tuberculosis affecting the lung, for example, can be mistaken for such other conditions as cancer, fungus diseases, pneumonia, bronchiectasis, sarcoidosis, and emphysema. A differential diagnosis is made with care.

The erythrocyte sedimentation rate (ESR) is accelerated in active tuberculosis, paralleling the severity of the disease.

Clinical Management

TRENDS IN TREATMENT. Treatment methods for tuberculosis have passed through numerous modalities, and continue to be modified as new knowledge is gained. Prior to chemotherapy "open air" treatments and "rest cures" were advocated. Patients were often hospitalized for months, even years. Patients who recovered usually required long periods of rehabilitation. Such prolonged hospitalization often created physical, social, emotional, and financial problems for the patient.

Before chemotherapy and improved surgical and anesthetic techniques made pulmonary resectional surgery possible, various techniques were used to collapse and rest the affected lung. Some of these "collapse therapy" procedures were pneumothorax, pneumoperitoneum, oleothorax, phrenic nerve crush or nerve resection, extraperiosteal plombage, and thoracoplasty. Once pulmonary resectional procedures became possible (i.e., procedures which remove portions of lung), surgery was performed on many patients with tuberculosis. Resectional surgery shortened the hospital stay of many persons and at times made possible their discharge.

The discovery of effective chemotherapeutic methods of treating tuberculosis about 1944 revolutionized the treatment of this disease. Since that time the number of patients hospitalized for treatment of tuberculosis has dramatically decreased. Rehabilitation problems often are less complex than in earlier years. Hospitals and sanatoria which specialize in the treatment of tuberculosis are closing now that long-term hospitalization is typically unnecessary. Currently, patients with tuberculosis are often initially admitted to general hospitals for a period of time; then the majority of care is given on an outpatient basis, e.g., by clinics or private physicians. The period of hospitalization varies, but it is generally much shorter than that necessary in previous years.

Because patients with tuberculosis are increasingly being admitted to general hospitals (rather than specialized sanatoria) it is important that personnel in these hospitals be informed of current practices in managing tuberculosis.

There is an urgent need to expand outpatient services for persons with tuberculosis. The Public Health Service estimated in 1968 that only about 60 per cent of nonhospitalized persons with active tuberculosis had undergone current bacteriologic examinations and were receiving chemotherapy.[302]

HOSPITALIZATION. The initial hospitalization of new cases may be advantageous for the following reasons:[129] (1) complete clinical evaluation can be made; (2) early indications of drug toxicity can be detected; (3) a regimen for administration of medications can be accomplished; and (4) infectious patients, who might spread the disease if unhospitalized, can be isolated until chemotherapy renders them noninfectious. Weg comments: "The primary reason for hospitalization is to establish diagnosis rapidly and efficiently. . . . The least important reason for hospitalization today is isolation of the patient."[311]

During hospitalization the extent of the patient's disease is determined, his reaction to chemotherapy is evaluated, and laboratory reports are obtained. As with any hospitalized patient, care is not complete unless education is given during this period of time about the nature of the illness and its treatment. (See below.)

Chronic illnesses of any kind cause numerous problems for patients and for family units. Persons with communicable chronic diseases who must be confined to hospitals often suffer additionally because of their isolation. Time passes slowly and with difficulty for persons who prefer being at home and actively participating in their "normal," pre-illness life styles. During the time of hospitalization, occupational therapists and nurses can often help patients to participate in projects that are individually meaningful and help to make time pass more pleasantly.

Criteria upon which the decision to discharge a patient is based include:[311] (1) the patient's clinical well-being; (2) roentgenographic evidence that disease has stabilized or improved; (3) bacteriologic evidence that the number of acid-fast bacilli being excreted has been reduced; and (4) most important, the physician's judgment that the patient, his home situation, and his local outpatient care system will assure completion of the prescribed chemotherapy.

Typically, discharge is permitted when organisms can no longer be detected by a sputum smear, provided the patient understands the nature of his illness and the need for prolonged medication. Once discharged, the patient is followed closely as an outpatient. Initially smears and cultures are usually taken weekly. After the patient has three *consecutive* negative sputum cultures (i.e., cultures in which no tubercle bacilli appear), he is given permission to return to work. The intervals between outpatient visits are then gradually lengthened to one month and then three months.

HOME CARE. The majority of patients with tuberculosis are able to accept responsibility for their own care and most (perhaps all) of their treatment is carried out at home. Home care, rather than hospital care, is possible largely because antituberculosis medications effectively control transmission of tuberculosis. Hence, the presence of the patient in the home is not hazardous. Home care has reduced or eliminated many of the problems formerly created by prolonged hospital confinement. Public health nurses usually make frequent home visits to patients undergoing outpatient treatment for tuberculosis.

PATIENT EDUCATION. Frequently the nurse is the person responsible for providing patient education. Make certain your educational materials and comments are realistic and not outdated. Provide factual, current information about tuberculosis. Patient teaching materials of various kinds are available from local branches of the American Lung Association (formerly called the National Tuberculosis and Respiratory Disease Association). One pamphlet distributed by these agencies upon request was written by Dr. W. W. Stead and is titled "Understanding Tuberculosis Today: A Handbook for Patients." Educational materials should not merely be handed to the patient, but should be reviewed with him. The patient should be encouraged to ask questions and to discuss any related topics with the nurse or physician.

Tuberculosis tends to be a relapsing disease that may lie quiescent for years and then reactivate. It is not possible with present methods of treatment to totally "cure" a patient of tuberculosis; instead the patient's disease is considered to be "controlled." A patient with tuberculosis must understand that for the rest of his life he may carry in his body tubercle bacilli that are capable of causing reinfection, if his resistance is lowered. Often a patient can be helped to understand his illness better if it is compared with diabetes, in the sense that the condition may be controlled, but lifetime medical care and supervision are required.

Whether a person is merely infected with tuberculosis or has active disease, he must learn to understand the nature of his condition and his part in necessary care. For example, the infected person (i.e., with positive tuberculin skin test) needs instruction about what his tuberculin positive reaction means and the importance of periodic reevaluation (so that if his infection becomes active it may be treated promptly). The person with active disease requires instruction in the following areas: chemotherapy, protective precautions, complications, and follow-up care. Other information such as dietary instructions may also need to be given. If a patient is going to be treated surgically as well as medically, special instructions are given prior to and following chest surgery. (See Chapter 73.)

Patient-family teaching can often be conducted effectively in group sessions (in the hospital, clinic, or at home) with the patient and his family assembled together. Thus, all involved persons receive the same information and problems can be discussed openly.

Specific details important in patient education are presented throughout this discussion of tuberculosis.

PREVENTION OF DISEASE TRANSMISSION. The patient with active (communicable) tuberculosis requires information about how tuberculosis is spread and ways in which *he* can prevent the spread of his disease to others. Instead of expecting others to protect themselves from him, the patient must take the initiative and accept the responsibility for carrying out protective measures.

Major ways in which *patients* with communicable tuberculosis can prevent spreading their tuberculosis to others are summarized below:

> *Take antituberculosis medications regularly as instructed.* "Chemical isolation" is achieved by placing the patient on antituberculosis medications. Effective chemotherapy rapidly causes patients to become noninfectious even before alterations in smears or cultures occur, i.e., even though sputum remains positive. Patients taking antituberculosis medications are unlikely to transmit tuberculosis even though resistant organisms may still be present.

> *Cover the nose and mouth with several layers of disposable tissues when coughing, sneezing, or laughing.* Forceful respiratory activities may emit large numbers of droplet nuclei into the air unless the infected droplets are mechanically stopped at the nose and mouth by tissues. Used tissues should be promptly discarded in an appropriate place (i.e., down a toilet or into a paper bag for burning) and the patient should *wash his hands.*

> *Expectorate sputum into a disposable sputum container or tissues.* Since all sputum should be expectorated (and not swallowed), the patient requires tissues and a disposable sputum cup. He should be told how to use the sputum container properly, e.g., to avoid contamination of the edges and outside of the container and to wash after handling the container. Used sputum containers should be safely disposed of by filling them with sawdust and burning them.

> *Avoid close contact with others* until the physician advises such contact is safe. The physician decides whether a patient on home care should occupy a room by himself. If this is necessary for a period of time the public health nurse can help select the room best for the patient. The patient receiving home care should understand that he must be especially careful to adequately protect infants and children below age five from exposure to infection.

> *Ensure adequate air ventilation* with mechanical air circulators or by keeping windows open. Circulating air serves to dilute the amount of contaminated air, i.e., the numbers of infected droplet nuclei in a room.

Precautions are based on knowledge of whether a patient's tuberculosis is communicable. For example, evaluation is made of how long the patient has been receiving antituberculosis medications and whether his sputum is positive.

It the *hospital setting,* measures to prevent air contamination by tubercle bacilli and the cleansing or decontamination of infected air are the main means of protecting personnel from infection when caring for a person with communicable tuberculosis. Because tuberculosis is an airborne infection, *adequate room ventilation* is essential. Decontamination of the air can be achieved by the use of nonrecirculating air conditioning or ultraviolet lighting. Recirculated air is decontaminated by using ultraviolet lights in air ducts.

Ultraviolet light destroys the tubercle bacilli. These lights may be strategically placed in hospital areas in which newly admitted infectious patients are cared for and in areas where undiagnosed patients are treated, e.g., emergency rooms and admitting rooms. Irradiation of upper room air with ultraviolet light is the most effective method for decontaminating the immediate environment. This procedure can rapidly make room air noninfectious. Good ventilation is important, but it is usually much slower than ultraviolet light in reducing the concentration of airborne organisms.

In the recent past it was common practice for persons caring for patients with tuberculosis to attempt to protect themselves from infection by wearing masks, gowns, and hair coverings. It is now realized that these practices are generally unnecessary. Occasionally a patient who is unable to protect persons caring for him (e.g., by covering his nose and mouth when sneezing and coughing) may be masked during periods of close contact while direct, face-to-face, patient care is being given. Only certain types of masks are effective, e.g., the Ultra-Filter mask. Many masks permit the minute droplet nuclei (which transmit tubercle bacilli) to either pass through them or out around the edges and are thus ineffective. When masks are used they should be changed frequently, and used masks should always be discarded immediately. Always wash thoroughly after handling a patient's mask. Cooperative patients should not be masked, because this unnecessary action may needlessly increase their anxiety.

At times face masks must be worn by personnel, e.g., when having intimate contact with patients who are just beginning chemotherapy and who are unable (or unwilling) to take actions necessary to protect the nurse by wearing a mask, covering their noses or mouths when coughing, or properly disposing of sputum. Face masks should cover both the mouth and nose. After using a mask remove it carefully, discard it properly, and wash thoroughly. *Never* twirl a mask in the air and *never* allow a mask to dangle around your neck when it is not being used!

Gowns are no longer considered necessary in caring for patients with tuberculosis. However, gowns may be worn to keep one's uniform clean when caring for patients who are unable or unwilling to protect the nurse, e.g., by properly disposing of sputum, feces, emesis, and so forth.

Because tuberculosis is not transmitted by fomites (i.e., inanimate objects which can harbor pathogenic microorganisms and transmit them to others), special care is not necessary for personal belongings, linens, or eating utensils. Handwashing is an effective means of removing those organisms that might possibly be picked up from direct contact with infectious body discharges or from fomites. Dried secretions do not easily fragment and become air-suspended; those particles that may arise from surfaces and become airborne are too large to penetrate into the lung.

Frequent, thorough handwashing is desirable following and during patient care after handling highly contaminated articles, e.g., used tissues, sputum container. It is *always* advisable for a nurse to keep her nails short and clean and to avoid habits like nail chewing or habitually having her hands close to her face or in her hair. Hygienic measures routinely followed in caring for any patients are adequate when caring for patients with tuberculosis who have negative sputum.

Many misconceptions exist about the communicability of tuberculosis. These misconceptions unfortunately occur among some nurses who are not informed of recent well documented findings. It is the obligation of nursing personnel to participate whenever possible in the dissemination of correct information to co-workers, patients, visitors, family members, and members of the community as a whole. This important educative process can greatly help to reduce unnecessary isolation and fears associated with tuberculosis. The fears and anxieties which surround a diagnosis of tuberculosis are deeply rooted in past associations and practices. These concerns need to be discussed openly, factually, and comfortably.

GENERAL ASPECTS OF CLINICAL CARE. Tuberculosis is a diagnosis that is difficult to accept. Often persons with tuberculosis feel ashamed of their illness. Some say they feel "dirty" or that they are "being punished." Feelings of guilt commonly occur if a patient believes he has infected others. The diagnosis of tuberculosis raises many concerns. The nurse can be of help during the difficult period in which a patient and his family must adjust to this diagnosis. (See Unit III.)

A nurse's ability to be helpful to persons with tuberculosis is directly related to her own attitude toward tuberculosis. Because attitudes are communicated in many subtle ways, the nurse must evaluate carefully her feelings about and actions toward persons with tuberculosis.

Helping a patient to adjust to his diagnosis is an important aspect of the care of patients with tuberculosis, but other activities are also of clinical importance. These activities include:

> Preparing the patient for and assisting with diagnostic and investigatory procedures. Frequently the nurse participates in sputum specimen collections.

> Measuring the patient's vital signs and weight periodically.

> Evaluating the patient's apparent general state of health, appetite, and mental-emotional status.

> Administering antituberculosis medications as prescribed and observing for toxic effects from these medications.

> Evaluating the patient's sputum production.

> Managing cough and other related symptoms. As with other pulmonary disorders, sedatives and narcotics are used with great caution to prevent excessive depression of the cough and respirations. Because of the chronicity of tuberculosis special caution is required to prevent drug dependency.

> Performing cooling measures if the patient has a high body temperature, and providing dry linens if he perspires heavily.

> Observing for and treating complications such as pleurisy, hemoptysis, atelectasis, bronchopleural fistula, spontaneous pneumothorax, and airway disorders. Pulmonary impairment associated with obstructive airway disease is a common complication of advanced tuberculosis.

> Participating in designing and implementing a program of treatment and rehabilitation for the individual patient.

> Giving appropriate pre- and postoperative care if the patient is treated surgically.

It has been established (by numerous well-controlled studies) that once an effective program of chemotherapy has begun, a special diet, climate control, and prolonged bed rest are of no value in treating tuberculosis.[311] Rest is valuable as long as the patient is symptomatic, but with adequate chemotherapy prolonged rest appears to be unnecessary. A well-balanced diet is important for adequate healing and recovery from tuberculosis, but a special diet is unnecessary.

CHEMOTHERAPY OF ACTIVE TUBERCULOSIS. Tuberculosis is particularly difficult to treat medically because of pathologic changes associated with the disease process. For example, tissue tends to become ischemic and necrotic because blood vessels do not effectively perfuse involved tissue, and bronchioles and small bronchi become stenosed. Chemotherapy is also difficult because the bacilli may develop drug resistance and because there is currently no medication that can completely destroy the bacilli in the body. Medications used to treat tuberculosis are bacteriostatic, not bactericidal, i.e., they do not kill the organisms in the body. Antituberculosis medications act by hampering reproduction of the tuberculous organisms in various ways. For example, rifampin and ethambutol impair RNA synthesis, while isoniazid interferes with intermediary metabolism and DNA synthesis.

When prolonged effective chemotherapy can be administered to persons with newly discovered disease, the outlook for recovery is favorable. Prognosis is not so favorable for far advanced disease as for minimal or moderately advanced tuberculosis. As mentioned before, with chemotherapy most persons become noninfectious relatively quickly.

> *Chemotherapy of active tuberculosis requires uninterrupted, intensive, prolonged administration of medications to which the patient's specific organisms are sensitive.*

Interrupted chemotherapy or medications taken at doses too low to be therapeutically effective encourage the development of *drug-resistant strains of bacilli.* Drug-resistant organisms are mutants which develop as the bacilli reproduce. Some mutant organisms are resistant to some antituberculosis medications but remain sensitive to other medications.

In order for the chemotherapy of tuberculosis to be effective certain *basic principles of therapy* must be applied. Some of the more important principles are listed and briefly discussed below:[289]

> *Prior to starting any chemotherapy, adequate sputum specimens should be obtained* and sent to the laboratory for bacteriologic and biochemical studies. The results of drug-sensitivity and other tests form a baseline for continued therapy. The causative organisms, their susceptibilities and resistances must be accurately identified early in the course of therapy so medications can be selected to which the organisms are sensitive.

> *Multiple drug therapy (combination drug therapy) is always used in treating active tuberculosis.* Single drugs are never administered because this fosters the development of organisms that are resistant to the medication being administered. Combination drug therapy increases the number of organisms that will be incapacitated by the medications and speeds up recovery. Two, three, or sometimes more antituberculosis medications are given in combination.

> *New medications are always introduced in combination* if a drug treatment regimen appears to be ineffective. Single medications are never added to a failing treatment program for the above stated reasons.

> *Chemotherapy for tuberculosis is continued long after all radiographic, bacteriologic, and clinical evidence of active disease has vanished.* Typically drug therapy is given for a total of two years or longer in treating active tuberculosis. Tuberculosis heals very slowly and the disease process is likely to reactivate if chemotherapy is stopped prematurely. Some patients are advised to continue medication for the remainder of their lives.

> *Antituberculosis medications are most effective when administered in a single daily dose* rather than in divided doses throughout the day. Obtaining a single peak concentration of all the medications simultaneously each day has proved to be more effective than trying to maintain a sustained blood level by administering several doses during the day. The full dose of oral medications is, therefore, usually ordered to be taken on an empty stomach shortly after arising. Injectables are administered about one hour after oral medications so the peak concentrations of both the parenteral and oral medications will occur simultaneously.

Before drug therapy is started three sputum specimens (each a minimum of 5 to 10 ml.) are collected and rapidly stained. If results are negative, three more specimens are obtained.

Antituberculosis medications are commonly divided into "first-line" and "second-line" drugs. The first-line drugs (or primary medications) are those most effective and most commonly used. *First-line antituberculosis drugs* include isoniazid, streptomycin, para-aminosalicylic acid, ethambutol, and rifampim. *Second-line antituberculosis drugs* tend to have more frequent and more severe side-effects and generally are used only if a patient's organisms are resistant to the first-line medications. Examples of some second-line drugs are ethionamide (Trecator), pyrazinoic acid amide (pyrazinamide), cycloserine (Seromycin), capreomycin, viomycin (Viocin), and kanamycin (Kantrex). Some pertinent facts about antituberculosis drugs are summarized in Table 71-1. For additional details consult a textbook of pharmacology.

Patients with minimal or moderately advanced pulmonary tuberculosis are typically treated with two antituberculosis medications, e.g., isoniazid and ethambutol. Triple drug therapy is commonly used to treat patients with tuberculosis who are febrile and appear "toxic" or patients requiring re-treatment. Triple drug treatment is also used for patients with far-advanced pulmonary or extrapulmonary tuberculosis.

When *corticosteroids* are employed in treating tuberculosis they must *always* be given in combination with antituberculosis chemotherapy. Corticosteroids are generally used in tuberculosis only when the patient is in an overwhelming or life-threatening situation, e.g., tuberculous pneumonia or tuberculous meningitis. In these situations the anti-inflammatory and detoxifying effects of corticosteroids and corticotropin are helpful.

Frequently any symptoms of tuberculosis that a patient with active disease may have tend to disappear or abate after a few days of chemotherapy. It must be emphasized to the patient that he needs to continue taking antituberculosis medications long after his symptoms disappear. Since many patients with tuberculosis are treated on an outpatient basis, the responsibility for staying on the necessary medication regimen rests with the patient. *Patient education is a highly important aspect of tuberculosis chemotherapy.* Medications must be taken regularly, exactly as prescribed for as long as prescribed. The patient is advised to see his doctor if he feels his medication is upsetting him in any way, and is told not to stop taking his medication or to cut back on the number of pills taken.

Chemotherapy of outpatients may be supervised by clinic or public health nurses. These nurses evaluate the regularity with which medications are being taken, evaluate the patient's understanding of the importance of chemotherapy, observe for symptoms of drug toxicity, and attempt to provide motivation for the patient to continue taking medications as prescribed. Because therapy for tuberculosis is prolonged (and the patient must continue to receive medical supervision for the remainder of his life) long-term support and guidance are important aspects of caring for the patient.

When severe drug reactions occur the physician may decide to stop all drugs for at least 10 to 14 days. Drugs are then gradually reintroduced; first the patient may be given small doses of the least suspect single drug. Occasionally "desensitization" programs are necessary (under the cover of corticosteroids) when a drug is essential and alternative substitution with another drug is impossible.

When the medical treatment of tuberculosis fails, the failure can generally be attributed to errors in drug choice or dosage, initial improper use of multiple drugs, failure of the patient to take medications as prescribed, or cessation of chemotherapy prior to complete healing. Although it is relatively rare, a few persons are initially infected with drug-resistant organisms.

CHEMOPROPHYLAXIS. "Chemoprophylaxis" means the prevention of disease by chemical means. For example, many persons who are infected with tuberculosis may be prevented from developing active clinical disease if they take isoniazid (INH) prophylactically. INH is useful in tuberculosis prophylaxis because of its low cost, efficacy, and ease of administration.

Persons who may benefit from the chemoprophylactic administration of antituberculosis medications include:

> Tuberculin convertors who do not show evidence of clinically active disease, i.e., no x-ray evidence of tuberculosis and no positive laboratory tests that identify the presence of the tubercle bacillus in body secretions or tissues. Any child with a positive tuberculin test who is less than five years of age is considered to be a convertor and is treated chemoprophylactically. Additionally, the preschool friends or siblings of any child with a positive tuberculin test are given INH prophylactically (even though the tuberculin test has not converted).

> Persons who have been in close contact with individuals proved to have active tuberculosis.

> Individuals receiving long-term corticosteroid therapy.

> Persons with silicosis.

Chemoprophylaxis usually involves having convertors or high-risk individuals take INH daily for a minimum of one year. Medical supervision and follow-up are necessary with any chemoprophylactic program. Periodic chest x-rays and tuberculin tests are important in the follow-up program. It is particularly important that children at high risk or children who are convertors be under close medical supervision to detect active disease early if it develops.

SURGICAL TREATMENT OF PULMONARY TUBERCULOSIS. Although chemotherapy is the major method of treatment of tuberculosis, occasionally surgery is advisable if chemotherapy fails to effectively treat the disease or if chances of relapse are high. For example, pulmonary resection may be indicated in treating persons who have progressive disease caused by drug-resistant organisms which fails to respond initially to chemotherapy. Other persons who may benefit from resectional surgery are those with bronchopleural fistulas (resulting from tuberculous empyema) or with thick-walled, localized cavities that continue to shed organisms in spite of chemotherapy. Another indication for resection is repeated hemorrhaging from a tuberculous lesion. Some patients with tuberculosis benefit from decortication. (See Chapter 73.)

Patients with tuberculosis are carefully selected for surgical treatment. Not all persons require surgery and some cannot tolerate surgery even though it might be helpful. Surgery is never performed on patients with tuberculosis without providing preoperative multidrug antituberculosis

TABLE 71-1. ANTITUBERCULOSIS DRUGS*

Drug	Abbrev.	Usual Adult Dosage (Gm./day)	Route	Doses/Day†	Side-Effects in Addition to Drug Fever and/or Drug Rash
			Primary Drugs		
Isoniazid	INH	0.3	P.O., I.M.	1	Peripheral neuritis, hepatotoxicity, urinary retention, arthralgia.
Rifampin	RMP	0.6	P.O.	1	Nausea, vomiting, thrombocytopenia, neutropenia, or abnormal SGPT determinations. PAS ↓ GI absorption; intermittent therapy more apt to produce hypersensitivity.
Ethambutol	EMB	0.8–1.2 15 mg./kg.	P.O.	1	Rarely optic neuritis, almost always reversible; more apt to occur in patients with azotemia.
Streptomycin	SM	0.5 Gm./da. 1.0 Gm. 2–3 x/wk.	I.M.	1	Eighth cranial nerve (vestibular and auditory) toxicity; avoid when azotemia present; do not use with CM, KM, or VM.
Para-amino-salicylic acid	PAS	Free base 12 Na salt 12–16 PAS-C 6–8	P.O.	1–3	Anorexia, nausea, vomiting, diarrhea, hepatotoxicity; best to avoid in patients with history of peptic ulcer or irritable bowel.
			Secondary Drugs		
Ethionamide	ETA	0.5–1.0	P.O.	1–3	GI intolerance (nausea and vomiting), CNS (anxiety, agitated depression, psychosis), hepatotoxicity, musculoskeletal complaints and headache, alopecia, menorrhagia, enhanced SM 8th nerve toxicity.
Pyrazinamide	PZA	1.5–3.0 (25–35 mg./kg.)	P.O.	1	Hepatotoxicity, hyperuricemia with or without joint pain.
Capreomycin	CM	0.5–1.0/da. 1 Gm. 2–3 x/wk.	I.M.	1	Vestibular, auditory toxicity or nephrotoxicity; avoid with SM, KM, or VM.
Kanamycin	KM	0.5–1.0/da. 3–5 x/wk.	I.M.	1	Vestibular, auditory toxicity or nephrotoxicity; do not use with SM, VM, or CM.
Cycloserine	CS	0.5–1.0	P.O.	2–4	CNS toxicity (irritability, insomnia, psychotic reactions, and convulsions); concomitant use of sedatives, anticonvulsants, and especially pyridoxine may be advisable; always administer in divided doses; avoid in patients with azotemia.
Viomycin	VM	0.5–1.0/da. 1.0–2.0/2 x wk.	I.M.	1	Vestibular, auditory toxicity or hypokalemia; nephrotoxicity; not advisable with SM, KM or CM.

*Modified from Pitts, F. W.: Tuberculosis in Virginia, *Virginia Med. Monthly, 11*:1175–1179, 1972.

†Oral medications should be administered when stomach is empty; i.e., 1 hour before or 1 hour after meals or at bedtime.

chemotherapy to prevent spread of the disease at the time of surgery. (Chest surgery is discussed in Chapter 73.)

Tuberculosis Control Programs. Tuberculosis is a disease that could be eliminated through intensified public health control programs. Physicians, public health nurses, and clinic nurses are often active in providing health services necessary for tuberculosis case-detection and follow-up care. Groups active in tuberculosis control programs include local health departments, the United States Public Health Service (USPHS), and local organizations of the American Lung Association. Activities of importance in these control programs are summarized below:

> Intensified case finding directed at identifying every infected individual, e.g., conducting tuberculin test surveys and mass chest x-ray programs among high-risk groups.

> Long-range medical follow-up of individuals who have been treated for active tuberculosis and of persons suspected of having a tuberculosis infection. "Suspects" are persons with positive skin tests and x-ray indications of tuberculosis but who do not yet have provable active tuberculosis.

> Identification, evaluation, and follow-up of contacts of persons with active disease. Contacts are given skin tests and chest x-rays are taken. Medical follow-up is particularly important for the first year following exposure to active tuberculosis. Nurses frequently participate in identifying and following up persons who were in contact with a patient before his active tuberculosis was diagnosed.

> Dissemination of facts about tuberculosis.

> Provision of necessary diagnostic and long-term treatment facilities for all persons with active disease and provision of prophylactic treatment for convertors and high-risk individuals.

As the preceding discussion demonstrates, persons who are carefully followed in tuberculosis control programs include persons with active tuberculosis, those with inactive tuberculosis, i.e., those previously treated for active tuberculosis, persons with positive skin tests, convertors, and those considered to be at high risk of developing active infection. Persons considered to be at high risk of developing tuberculosis include: (1) persons who have had close association with someone with active disease; (2) infants and children under five years of age; (3) pregnant women and women in the childbearing years; (4) adolescents; (5) nonwhites of both sexes and all ages; (6) white men over age 45; (7) persons with strong tuberculin reactions, i.e., 12 mm. or more of induration; (8) persons with positive tuberculin reactions who are receiving long-term steroid therapy; (9) persons with silicosis, diabetes mellitus, or sarcoidosis; (10) chronic alcoholics, and (11) persons who have had a gastrectomy.

Case finding by means of *chest x-ray* screening is most successful among high-incidence groups in the population, e.g., close associates or contacts of active cases, low economic groups, and general hospital admissions. However, in order to avoid unnecessary exposure to radiation it is recommended that the *tuberculin test* (rather than the chest x-ray) be used as a preliminary screening tool. This is particularly important in screening children and young adults. Tuberculin tests are recommended as part of annual physical examinations. Persons who are at high risk of infecting children, e.g., school employees, should receive routine tuberculin tests followed by x-rays of positive tuberculin reactors.

The identification of tuberculin conversions in children is particularly important for the following reasons: (1) usually it is possible to locate and treat the person with active disease who infected the child (because children have relatively few associations with others, the problems of case finding are simplified); and (2) chemotherapy of the initial (primary) infection in the child prevents complications such as progressive primary tuberculosis or miliary tuberculosis.

Routine tuberculosis screening programs are usually conducted among foodhandlers, armed service personnel, and persons in large institutions. Routine admission chest x-rays are taken in many general hospitals, clinics, lodging houses, jails and among welfare clients and migrant farm workers. These routine chest x-rays are of value not only in detecting tuberculosis, but also other chest disorders, e.g., lung cancer.

Some persons with active tuberculosis refuse to accept treatment or to take the precautions necessary to prevent transmission of their disease to others. Unreliable persons of this nature seriously impede attempts to control and eventually eradicate tuberculosis. Occasionally legal action is necessary to commit these persons to hospital care. The problems of supervising the treatment of recalcitrant patients are especially difficult because of the long-term, uninterrupted period of drug therapy necessary to adequately treat tuberculosis.

Alcoholics under treatment for tuberculosis as outpatients often do not take their antituberculosis medications regularly, and if they are transient and move about from city to city a great deal, they often do not keep or make the necessary follow-up appointments for medical supervision. These circumstances favor the development of drug-resistant organisms. Skid row alcoholics tend to live in crowded, poorly ventilated surroundings which encourage the transmission of tuberculosis. Case finding among this segment of the population is difficult for many reasons, but it may be assisted by the use of routine jail admission x-rays. Ideally, when patients who are alcoholics are hospitalized for the treatment of tuberculosis, they should simultaneously receive treatment directed at the concomitant problem of alcoholism.

BCG (BACILLE CALMETTE GUÉRIN). BCG is a vaccine given in an attempt to produce increased resistance to clinical tuberculosis. BCG contains live, attenuated bovine tubercle bacilli incapable of producing active disease. Although BCG offers limited protection from tuberculosis, it is not completely prophylactic.

Considerable difference of opinion exists concerning the best method of administration. One method is to administer the vaccine intradermally (with a multiple puncture disc) to assure the administration of a controlled dose. Successful vaccination may be confirmed by demonstrating a positive tuberculin reaction six to eight weeks after vaccination. BCG is typically administered to young children and then may be repeated 12 to 15 years later. BCG can be given *only* to persons with a negative tuberculin skin test. It should *never* be given in the presence of active tuberculosis or skin disorders.

The advisability of using BCG is debatable, and practices vary from country to country. In the United States, BCG vaccination is seldom used, however, it is widely used in other countries, for example, France, England, and Denmark, as well as in developing countries which have a high incidence of tuberculosis.

Because BCG changes the tuberculin skin test from a negative to a positive reaction for varying lengths of time, it interferes with the usefulness of tuberculin testing case-finding programs and the goal of eventually having all persons in the United States be tuberculin negative. Attainment of this goal is highly important since endogenous reinfection is believed to cause most clinical tuberculosis in countries such as the United States.

The United States has effective methods of case finding, controlling, preventing, and treating tuberculosis. The battle against tuberculosis in this country is directed mainly at tuberculin reactors by providing them with chemoprophylaxis (especially if the reactors are persons who have a high risk of developing tuberculosis). It is therefore important to maintain the skin test as a means of case finding.

Most physicians in the United States believe that the risk of tuberculosis among nonreactors is too low to justify using BCG vaccination in that group, and that the vaccine possibly gives only a low level of protection. There is some evidence that certain persons who have been able to control primary tuberculosis infections have a heightened resistance to subsequent exposure, i.e., to *exogenous* reinfection. The protection in this instance is comparable to an acquired immunity.

Possible complications following the administration of BCG include local ulcers and (less commonly) lymph node abscess formation or suppuration. Research is still being conducted to try to develop a vaccine against tuberculosis that would be more effective than BCG.

PULMONARY DISEASE PRODUCED BY ATYPICAL ORGANISMS

Recently various atypical mycobacteria have been identified which produce in human beings pulmonary and lymph node disease similar to tuberculosis. It is debatable whether all these varied mycobacterial diseases should be called "tuberculosis" or "mycobacteriosis." Currently the practice is to reserve the term "tuberculosis" for those infections caused by the *M. tuberculosis* or *M. bovis,* (the so-called mammalian tubercle bacilli) or *M. avium.* Diseases caused by atypical mycobacteria, collectively termed the atypical mycobacterioses, sometimes are referred to by naming the particular species or group, e.g., "disease of the lung due to Battey bacillus." Although these diseases resemble tuberculosis they have different therapeutic and public health implications.

It is impossible to differentiate between typical and atypical acid-fast bacilli by means of smears performed in the clinical laboratory. However, the atypical organisms do differ in cultural characteristics from the "typical" forms of *M. tuberculosis.* Therefore, laboratory cultures are necessary for precise diagnosis. These culture results often are not available for two to three months after the patient has been started on antituberculosis chemotherapy. Once the physician realizes that the patient does not have tuberculosis he makes appropriate changes in chemotherapy according to the specific causative organism. Atypical organisms are frequently resistant to medications currently available, e.g., isoniazid, streptomycin, and para-aminosalicylic acid. When a patient is discovered to have atypical organisms, drug susceptibility tests are usually made with both primary and secondary drugs (see preceding discussion of antituberculosis medications) to identify the most effective drug combination.

Infections with atypical organisms are common; however, only a few actually produce disease. Person-to-person transmission of atypical infections or disease has not been proved. Thus, patients with atypical microorganisms are treated in open wards and are not considered to be infectious. Atypical organisms are widely distributed in nature, e.g., in water, vegetable matter, soil, and raw milk. Also, they may be recovered from the gastric contents and sputum of healthy persons.

It is believed that a weak reactivity to tuberculin skin testing frequently indicates a subclinical dormant infection with atypical mycobacteria. When clinical infection with these organisms occurs it tends to be more apparent in persons who have some other chronic lung damage, e.g., silicosis, chronic bronchitis, emphysema.[289]

Summarized below are some facts about the four groups of atypical mycobacteria:

> Group I: *M. kansasii* and *M. marinum (balnei).* Also called photochromogens. Yellow pigment develops rapidly only after exposure to light during growth phase. Most reported cases in the U.S. are from Texas, Kansas, and Illinois. These infections respond to antituberculosis medications less well than *M. tuberculosis* infections, but they do show some susceptibility to the usual antituberculosis drugs in higher doses.

> Group II: *M. scrofulaceum* and *M. aquae.* Also called scotochromogens. Yellow to orange pigmentation appears without exposure to light. Occurs in soil in most areas of the U.S; also commonly found in water. Seldom produces pulmonary disease in man. Often found

as harmless saprophytes in sputum. May produce scrofula in children. Drug treatment may give enough inhibition to permit surgical excision of the nodes if they are fluctuant or draining.

> Group III: *M. intracellularis* (Battey bacillus), *M. avium,* and *M. xenopei.* Also called nonchromogens. White or ivory appearance; no pigment produced when exposed to light. Found in soil and in tissues of certain domestic animals, e.g., cattle, swine. Battey infections are more common in the southeastern U.S., especially Florida and Georgia. Typically these infections are difficult to treat because the organisms usually are highly resistant to the usual concentrations of all antituberculosis medications. Some patients respond to a five-drug program of prolonged treatment but must be closely observed for the numerous side-effects that can occur. If the disease cannot be controlled it produces widespread pulmonary disease which slowly progresses until death occurs from cor pulmonale and pulmonary insufficiency. Some patients with localized disease may have surgical resection (e.g., lobectomy) performed if they have adequate pulmonary function. (Group III organisms which do not produce disease in man include *M. terrae* ["radish" bacillus], *M. gastri,* and *M. trivale* ["V" subgroup]).

> Group IV: *M. fortuitum.* Organisms in this group are also called "rapid growers." The only pathogen in the group is *M. fortuitum.* Only rarely causes pulmonary disease.

PULMONARY MYCOSES (FUNGUS INFECTIONS)

It is not uncommon for the respiratory tract to be infected with fungi (molds). Some fungus infections are increasing in incidence. The mode of infection, immunologic status, and best means of prevention have not been identified for most fungus infections of the lungs. However, specific drug treatments are available and have improved the prognosis of many fungus infections. Without chemotherapy some fungus infections, e.g., blastomycosis, may be progressive and fatal.

The fungicidal antibiotic, *amphotericin B,* has been especially valuable in reversing the prognosis of many fungus infections which were previously critical. The patient is hospitalized for the administration of this medication because cautious administration and close observation for toxic effects are necessary. Be certain to follow the manufacturer's directions carefully when preparing infusion solutions of amphotericin B, and consult a textbook of pharmacology for discussions of the procedure for administering this medication, dosage, toxic effects, and so forth. Saline solutions should not be used, since saline precipitates this medication.

Because of the specificity of treatment for pulmonary mycoses, it is essential that an accurate *diagnosis* be made so the proper chemotherapy can be given. Precise diagnosis may be difficult because mycotic diseases involving the lungs commonly produce clinical symptoms and radiologic findings indistinguishable from those produced by bacteria (e.g., tuberculosis), viruses, or carcinoma. The diagnosis of a mycosis depends upon either actually isolating the organism from sputum, gastric washings, spinal fluids, blood, urine, bone marrow, joint fluid, skin and mucous membrane lesions, prostatic secretion, bronchial aspirates, or biopsy specimens or demonstrating specific measurable immunologic changes in host response.

Skin tests with commercially available antigens are possible only for histoplasmosis, coccidioidomycosis and blastomycosis. Of these, the test which has the greatest diagnostic value is the test for coccidioidomycosis. *Before* skin tests are applied to a patient suspected of having a systemic mycosis, 15 to 20 ml. of venous blood should be drawn for serum separation. If the skin tests have been applied before the blood serology sample is drawn, be certain this information and the date and result of the test are sent with the serum specimens.

Often it takes two to eight weeks for some fungi to be isolated and specifically identified from clinical materials. When cultures have not been performed or are negative, the physician may make a diagnosis based on correlating the morphology of the organism with skin tests, serologic reactions, and residential and occupational data. In contrast to viral and bacterial diseases, it is possible to diagnose fungus diseases with a high degree of reliability by examining specially stained tissue sections. Although the tissue reaction to the fungus is not diagnostic, the distinctive morphology of the fungus may permit a skilled histopathologist to make a specific etiologic identification.

Two relatively common pulmonary fungus infections are histoplasmosis and coccidioidomycosis. Both these disorders are fairly clearly localized geographically.

Histoplasmosis. Histoplasmosis is also called "histo," cave fever, or cytomycosis. This chronic granulomatous disease of the reticuloendothelial system principally affects the lungs and occasionally spreads by hematogenous dissemination. The causative fungus is *Histoplasma capsulatum.* This disorder occurs most commonly in the East and Midwest, particularly in the Ohio and Mississippi river valleys. More than 30 million Americans are believed to have been infected, but few fatalities occur. Histoplasmosis does not appear to be transmitted from man to man, but rather the fungus spores grow in moist, dark protected soil such as that found in old chicken houses, pigeon lofts, belfries, and bat-infested caves. The fungus is lightweight enough to float when infected dust is stirred up and is small enough to be inhaled.

In the lungs the fungus causes pathologic changes which closely resemble those of tuberculosis, e.g., tubercle formation, central caseation, scarring, cavity formation, and calcification. Symptoms vary (from flu-like to more serious symptoms), depending upon the degree of exposure. Treatment of the more severe infections may include administration of amphotericin B and/or surgical removal of sections of lung imbedded with spores.

Public health nurses in rural areas are active in

the prevention of histoplasmosis by urging farmers to keep farm buildings clean and dry and reminding them to wet down the floor before sweeping out farm buildings (to prevent dust from rising). Chicken droppings should always be wetted down before chicken houses are cleaned out. Storm cellars should be kept clean and dry. Of course, it is desirable to avoid bat-infested belfries and caves. Persons raising pigeons should be advised how to properly care for these birds and clean their lofts.

Coccidioidomycosis. Other terms for coccidioidomycosis are "the bumps," San Joaquin valley fever, and desert fever. This granulomatous disease, caused by the fungus *Coccidioides immitis,* produces acute and chronic pulmonary lesions. In the United States coccidioidomycosis occurs almost exclusively in the Southwest. The primary form of this disorder is typically a benign, acute, self-limited respiratory disease. The progressive form is a chronic (possibly fatal) infection involving not only the lungs but other structures such as skin or bone. Disease is produced in man by the inhalation of dust which is contaminated with spores. An animal reservoir may occur in some rodents. The only effective medication is amphotericin B.

Other Pulmonary Mycoses. Four other generalized fungus infections involving the lungs, which are relatively less common and less well localized geographically, are:

> *Blastomycosis:* A chronic granulomatous infection caused by *Blastomyces dermatitidis,* which has a predilection for the skin and lungs.

> *Cryptococcosis* (torulosis): A generalized granulomatous infection caused by *Cryptococcus histolyticus,* with a predilection for the meninges and lungs.

> *Actinomycosis* ("lumpy jaw"): A chronic granulomatous infection caused by *Actinomyces bovis,* which is characterized by abscess formation with numerous draining sinus tracts, e.g., through the chest wall.

> *Nocardiosis* (streptothricosis): A chronic granulomatous disease caused by *Nocardia asteroides,* which produces numerous abscesses and sometimes sinus tracts.

CHRONIC OBSTRUCTIVE PULMONARY DISEASE (COPD)

Chronic obstructive pulmonary disease (COPD)* is a term applied to respiratory disorders that involve persistent obstruction of bronchial airflow. COPD is a *functional* category (rather than a specific disease). This means that the patient has *persistent* airway obstruction that is a chronic problem and tends to slowly and progressively worsen. Various diseases may be associated with COPD, e.g., pulmonary tuberculosis, bronchiectasis, silicosis, pulmonary fibrosis. However, *the conditions that most frequently give rise to COPD are bronchial asthma, chronic bronchitis, and anatomic pulmonary emphysema.*

Numerous diseases of the respiratory tract, including those referred to as COPD, produce similar physiologic alterations and symptoms. These similarities may make an accurate diagnosis difficult. Figure 71–8 illustrates the relationship of asthma, bronchitis, and emphysema. Each disorder can occur alone or in combination with another; each may or may not be associated with COPD. *Bronchitis and emphysema coexist most frequently.* Bronchial asthma and emphysema rarely coexist without bronchitis. The coexistance of asthma and bronchitis is called "asthmatic bronchitis."

In England the terms "chronic bronchitis" and "emphysema" are used synonymously. However, in England chronic bronchitis is the diagnosis most commonly used when a patient has combined chronic bronchitis and emphysema (and possibly also bronchial asthma). In the United States it has been more usual for emphysema to be diagnosed as the more important component of such combined disease, and the presence of bronchitis has tended to be ignored. Currently, attempts are being made to focus on the common problem of COPD rather than emphasizing one

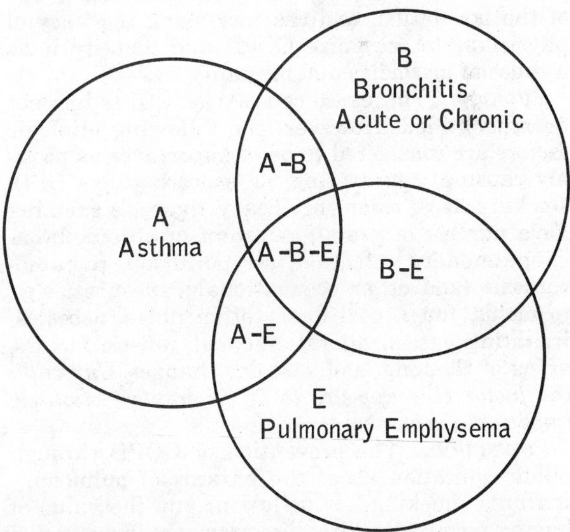

FIGURE 71–8. The relationship of emphysema to asthma and bronchitis can be illustrated by the overlapping rings. Each should be considered a separate disease entity which can occur alone or in combination with another. Symptoms and physiological findings may or may not differentiate one from the other; consequently they are frequently misdiagnosed. The occurrence of two entities in the same individual should not imply that one has produced the other. (From Tomashefski and Pratt: Pulmonary emphysema. *Medical Clinics of North America, 51*:269, March, 1967.)

*Other terms which have been used to refer to this group of conditions include: diffuse obstructive pulmonary syndrome (DOPS); diffuse obstructive lung disease (DOLD); chronic obstructive lung disease (COLD); chronic obstructive pulmonary emphysema (COPE); obstructive airway disease; obstructive ventilatory syndrome; obstructive ventilatory disease of the lungs; and chronic obstructive bronchopulmonary disease.

predominant diagnosis, since a more definitive diagnosis is not necessary for treatment.

> *COPD is the most common chronic pulmonary disorder. Like bronchogenic carcinoma, the prevalence and death rates from COPD have markedly increased during recent years.*

Incidence. United States Public Health Service statistics show that chronic obstructive pulmonary diseases are on the increase at alarming rates. Statistics are difficult to obtain for the overall incidence of COPD in the United States because of confusion and varying interpretations of pertinent definitions. However, it is estimated that between 2 and 17 million persons in the United States have some degree of bronchial asthma, chronic bronchitis, or emphysema.[113] *Chronic airway obstruction is the second most common cause of admission to hospitals.*[214] In addition to producing suffering and death, COPD causes serious socioeconomic problems. In 1958 the Social Security Administration indicated that COPD ranked second only to heart disease as the cause of permanent disability in men over age 40 who were covered by Social Security work disability allowances.

Factors believed to be of importance in the increasing incidence of COPD include the increasing incidence of habitual cigarette smoking, increasing survival rates of patients because of improved treatment procedures, the increasing age of the population, and the increasing tendency of physicians to recognize COPD and identify it as a cause of morbidity and mortality.

Etiology. The exact cause(s) of COPD has not been identified. However, the following etiologic factors are considered to be of importance as possibly causing, aggravating, or exacerbating COPD: smoking (most commonly heavy cigarette smoking for a number of years), recurrent or chronic bronchopulmonary infection, air pollution, pneumoconiosis (and other occupational exposures, e.g., to molds, fungi, coal dust, cotton fibers, asbestos, irritating gases), allergic factors, genetic factors, aging of the lung, and vascular changes. *Currently the factor that appears to be of greatest etiologic importance is smoking.*

Prevention. The prevention of COPD through public education about the hazards of pulmonary irritants (smoking, air pollution) and the value of having respiratory disorders promptly investigated and treated is important, since the early detection of COPD is difficult, and affected persons are unable to recognize the development and progression of this disorder. Haas and Cardon comment, "By the time a patient is seen in the physician's office with the symptomatic triad of dyspnea, intermittent cough and easy fatigability that follows even minimal physical effort—which prompted the patient to seek professional help—the structural damage to his lungs may be so far advanced that he no longer has the necessary cardiopulmonary reserve to fulfill his physiologic needs."[113] Persistent coughs (including those referred to as "smoker's cough" or "morning cough") should always be evaluated *early* and treated. Periodic physical examinations (e.g., annually) are important in the prevention or early detection of COPD.

Symptoms. Early symptoms of COPD develop insidiously and progress slowly; a common triad that occurs with COPD is dyspnea (especially upon exertion), intermittent cough, and fatigue following exertion. These symptoms may begin as only a slight shortness of breath, a mild morning cough, and a bit of fatigue, e.g., from walking upstairs. Because of the mild nature of the symptoms, the affected person commonly does not seek medical evaluation. Gradually, however, symptoms worsen and the patient develops COPD which, even in its mild to moderate forms, is a distressing chronic illness.

In its more severe forms, COPD is a crippling condition which increasingly causes the victim to struggle for air. COPD typically causes a forced exhalation which is always noticeable with chronic anatomic pulmonary emphysema, occurs in some patients with chronic bronchitis, and is present during an attack of bronchial asthma. Wheezing, weight loss, general debilitation, and abnormal blood gas levels are other common symptoms of COPD. Pulmonary function tests demonstrate retardation of expiratory flow, which, if progressive, causes dyspnea, hypoxemia, and hypercapnia.

Pathology. The pathologic changes that occur with bronchial asthma, chronic bronchitis, and anatomic pulmonary emphysema are distinct; frequently there are also various pathologic aspects of these disorders that overlap. The separate changes most typical of each of these conditions are presented in discussions of the specific disorders.

Summarized below are some features characteristic of the *natural history of progression* of COPD. (See also Figure 71–9.)

> Thick bronchial secretions, swollen bronchial walls, and unequal alveolar ventilation result from infectious or allergic processes.

> Some alveoli may become hyperinflated; others become atelectatic.

> Thoracic excursion is reduced by chronic bronchial obstruction, air trapping, and thoracic overdistention.

> Gradual destruction of lung parenchyma and loss of the lung's elastic contractility (ability to recoil) occurs. These factors cause an increased (less negative) intrapleural pressure, which contributes to the collapse of bronchioles and poorly supported bronchi.

> The weight of the abdominal viscera lowers the diaphragm because of the lung's weakened elastic recoil.

> Tidal volume, vital capacity, and the inspiratory reserve necessary for effective coughing are diminished by the reduced thoracic excursion.

> Increased work of breathing occurs, fatiguing the patient and perhaps confining him to chair or bed. In order to breathe, the patient involuntarily employs the accessory muscles of respiration, uses his shoulder girdle and abdominal muscle groups, and purses his

lips to help the diaphragm with inspiration and expiration.

> Eventually the patient develops permanently reduced alveolar ventilation, carbon dioxide retention, hypoxia, and chronic respiratory acidosis owing to the syndrome of bronchial obstruction, alveolar air trapping, patchy atelectasis, and chronic muscle fatigue.

> As the patient's condition worsens, hypoxia debilitates him by weakening the myocardium, interfering with renal function, increasing capillary permeability, and causing polycythemia, anorexia, and weight loss.

> Increasingly the patient's body buffers are consumed by attempts to compensate for chronic respiratory acidosis.

> The patient's ability to meet life's stresses is reduced. Recurrent episodes of pulmonary infections (e.g., acute bronchitis, pneumonia) may eventually cause cor pulmonale, respiratory failure, coma, and death.

Most patients with COPD who are persistently hypoxic have an increase in their hematocrits beyond the normal range. (See "Polycythemia," Unit XII.) The association of hypoxemia, polycythemia, and cor pulmonale occurs most often in those persons with COPD who have severe chronic bronchitis. Because of their appearance, these individuals have been described as *"blue bloaters"* (abbreviated as "BB"). Persons with dyspnea caused by severe emphysema, who do not have accompanying cyanosis or indications of congestive heart failure, have been described as *"pink puffers"* ("PP").[82, 200] (See Tables 71–2 and 71–3.) These two contrasting types of chronic airway obstruction are distinguishable by clinical criteria alone. This classification is therefore useful in the early identification of COPD, before laboratory measurements of physiologic function are made.

Detection of COPD. Because many patients in a nurse's care may have COPD (and therefore require special care to make them more comfortable while preventing possible complications), *the nurse must be able to assess patients in such a manner that she can detect COPD.* One cannot rely on the Kardex or the patient's chart for the identification of COPD, because often only the primary diagnosis or impression may be available. In emergency situations no chart or Kardex information may be available. The nurse must, therefore, be capable of rapidly making her own assessment. Essential changes produced by COPD are summarized in Table 71–4. Many of these key observations are discussed further in this text. Refer also to Sedlock's article.[269] Awareness that a patient has COPD is especially important to prevent CO_2 narcosis when giving O_2 therapy.

Complications. Complications of COPD include carbon dioxide narcosis, acute respiratory failure, metabolic alkalosis, uncompensated respiratory acidosis, bronchopulmonary infections, cor pulmonale (observe for digitalis toxicity when digitalis is prescribed to treat cardiac failure), spontaneous pneumothorax (due to ruptured pulmonary bleb or bullae), arteriosclerotic and hypertensive heart disease (because many patients with COPD are middle-aged or elderly), pulmonary thromboembolic disease (especially if significant polycythemia is present), and peptic ulcer.

Because almost one fourth of patients with COPD are estimated to have a peptic ulcer at some time, the nurse observes closely for indications of this complication (especially if a patient is receiving steroid or anticoagulant therapy). Symptoms of peptic ulcer include abdominal soreness, hematemesis and epigastric pain. Abdominal pain may diminish the patient's appetite and contribute to weight loss. Among the factors that may predispose to the development of peptic ulcer are increased gastric secretion, psychosomatic influ-

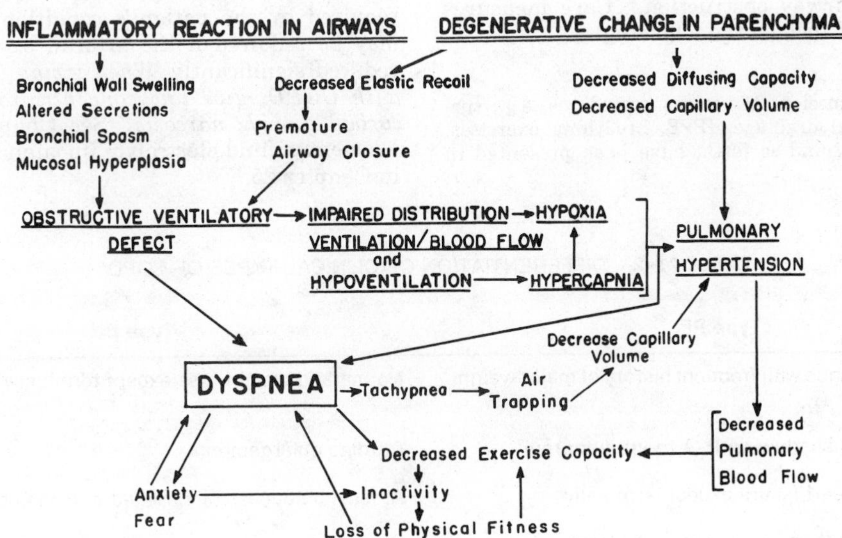

FIGURE 71–9. The nature of chronic obstructive lung disease. (From Miller, W. F.: *Medical Clinics of North America, 51*: 349, March, 1967.)

ences, CO_2 retention, and reduced arterial oxygen saturation.

Clinical Care of Patients with COPD. Providing appropriate, comprehensive clinical care for the patient with COPD is highly challenging and may tax the nurse's knowledge, ingenuity, and patience. Meticulous attention to detail is essential. The nurse's expertise is necessary in making clinical judgments and in skillfully performing nursing procedures. Additionally, the nurse must provide the emotional care required by a chronically ill, dyspneic patient.

Clinical care attempts to maintain existing lung function, prevent additional irreversible lung damage and loss of pulmonary function, promote symptomatic relief (with bronchodilators, antibiotics, tranquilizers, IPPB therapy), and provide a vigorous program of total rehabilitation (through patient education, postural drainage, breathing training and retraining exercises with added oxygen, and vocational training or retraining).

Basically the treatment of obstructive pulmonary disease is directed at restoring and maintaining patency of the peripheral bronchial tree. This means that therapeutic procedures are employed to: (1) remove viscid and inspissated secretions from occluded bronchioles; (2) improve ventilation, enlarge air passages, and reduce resistance to the flow of gases into and out of the alveoli (by reducing in thickness the walls of bronchioles that are swollen by cellular infiltration and submucosal edema); and (3) alleviate respiratory acidosis and hypoxia by improving alveolar exchange of CO_2 and O_2 and decreasing the work of breathing.

Summarized and discussed below are factors of importance in the care of all patients with COPD regardless of the basic disorder. Clinical care is directed at the problem of chronic, diffuse, irreversible airway obstruction.* Care measures to be discussed include the following:

> Cleanse and dilate the tracheobronchial tree. Promote bronchial drainage.
> Assist ventilation and respiration.
> Remove, avoid and/or minimize bronchial irritants.
> Control chronic respiratory infection and prevent acute infections.
> Observe for and treat complications, e.g., prevent heart failure.
> Provide patient-family education, general supportive and emotional care, stimulation routines, and total rehabilitation.
> Provide long-term supervision and care.

CLEANSING AND DILATING TRACHEOBRONCHIAL TREE; PROMOTING BRONCHIAL DRAINAGE. Assist with postural (gravity) drainage and other techniques of pulmonary physiotherapy to stimulate peristalsis in small peripheral bronchi so sputum will be moved centrally to larger airways where it can be coughed up, or removed by suction if necessary. Promote effective coughing and deep breathing. Some patients with COPD cannot cough effectively, so cough stimulation routines are necessary. Suction as indicated to remove secretions. Promptly remove liquefied secretions, if the patient cannot do so himself, to prevent suffocation. Maintain hydration to thin secretions and encourage appropriate physical activity (e.g., ambulation) to move secretions. Force fluids as indicated. Maintain humidification of inspired air, e.g., with ultrasonic nebulizer. Administer medications ordered to cleanse and dilate the tracheobronchial tree, e.g., bronchodilator aerosols, mucolytic (mucus-dissolving) aerosols, wetting agents, detergents, expectorants, systemic bronchodilators, antibiotics, steroids.

Bronchospasm commonly occurs with COPD. Normally bronchi have a tremendous ability to change the size of their lumina; damaged bronchi may require bronchodilator medications to relax the smooth muscle surrounding the bronchi. Figure 71–10 demonstrates bronchial changes that occur with acute bronchial asthma.

ASSISTING VENTILATION AND RESPIRATION. Administer respiratory therapy (IPPB, oxygen) as required by the patient's condition. Oxygen (O_2) may be required if the arterial oxyhemoglobin is reduced significantly. *When giving O_2 to a patient with COPD, give low concentrations to prevent carbon dioxide narcosis.* (See Chapter 70.) Management of fluid-electrolyte imbalances is discussed in Chapter 25.

*Detailed discussions of various procedures, e.g., suctioning, postural drainage, IPPB, breathing exercises, oxygen therapy, and so forth, have been presented in Chapter 70.

TABLE 71–2. DIFFERENTIATION OF CLINICAL TYPES OF COPD*

Type PP	Type BB
Thin in appearance with frequent history of major weight loss	No marked weight loss except terminally
Narrow cardiac shadow on P–A roentgenogram	Cardiac enlargement
No history of heart failure except terminally	At least 3 successfully treated episodes of heart failure
Hematocrit less than 55 per cent; no history of phlebotomy	Hematocrit greater than 60 per cent; 10 or more phlebotomies

*Modified from Filley, G. F.: *Medical Clinics of North America, 51*:283, March, 1967.

TABLE 71-3. CLINICAL FINDINGS IN TWO CONTRASTING PATIENTS WITH COPD*

	E.A.	L.S.
Age	48	40
Onset	Dyspnea and cough at 33	Cough without dyspnea at 30
Course	Dyspnea rapidly progressive, cough slight, 30 lb. weight loss	Dyspnea moderate, cyanosis severe, ankle edema
On admission	Complete disability, depressed, unrelenting downhill course	Ambulatory, frequent phlebotomies with relief
Type	PP	BB

*Modified from Filley, G. F.: *Medical Clinics of North America, 51*:283, March, 1967.

TABLE 71-4. DETECTION OF CHRONIC OBSTRUCTIVE LUNG DISEASE*

Primary Changes	Secondary Changes
Chest	*Blood Pressure*
Increased A-P diameter ("barrel chest"); chest fixed in inspiratory position; expanded lower rib margin; due to air trapping and enlargement of lungs with loss of ability to recoil	Pulsus paradoxus (reduction of arterial pulse during inspiration); due to effect on cardiac filling from accentuated respiratory effort; during inspiration increased negative intrathoracic pressure occurs
Enlarged accessory muscles of respiration; use of these muscles and abdominal muscles during ventilation to help force air out of lungs	*Red Blood Cells*
Prolonged expiratory time; due to air trapping and collapse of airways upon expiration	Polycythemia develops in response to hypoxia
Expiratory wheezing (high-pitched, whistling sound); due to bronchospasm	*Heart*
Rhonchi (loud snoring sounds or low-pitched rattling sounds at end of expiration); due to mucus in airways	Right ventricular strain and enlargement (cor pulmonale); due to pulmonary hypertension which results from hypoxia and acidosis; liver engorgement, peripheral edema also occur; evidence of cor pulmonale; apical sound in epigastric area; right ventricular lift or thrust; loud P_2; tall, pointed P waves; and right axis deviation
Decreased breath sounds; due to reduced air flow, pleural effusion, or lung parenchyma destruction	
Fingernails and Hands	*Blood Vessels*
Clubbing; vertical fingernail ridging	Venous engorgement (which elevates venous pressure); results from impeded venous return to heart (due to elevated pressures in right side of heart and altered intrathoracic pressure); indications of venous engorgement; jugular venous distention; hepatojugular reflux; peripheral edema; pleural effusion (typically right-sided); or ascites
Hyperemia; due to excess blood supply as CO_2 build-up causes arteries to dilate	
Fine; twitching of extremities; asterixis ("metabolic flap"); due to hypoxemia, hypercapnia	*Electrolytes*
Neurologic	Low serum chloride and elevated serum CO_2; resulting from retention of bicarbonate ions (in an attempt to buffer additional carbonic acid formed by excess CO_2) and excretion of chloride ions in their place
Restlessness, agitation, lethargy, coma, headaches (during night or upon arising), nightmares, difficulty sleeping; due to alterations in O_2, CO_2, and hydrogen levels; brain sensitive to changes	

*Modified from Sedlock, S. A.: *American Journal of Nursing, 72*:1407, August, 1972.

Oxygen may need to be administered quite often to the patient with COPD. Some patients require oxygen during any exertion. Lightweight, portable oxygen equipment may be used during ambulation or when the patient is out of bed. At times it is necessary to give total ventilatory support to the patient with COPD. (See discussion of respiratory insufficiency and respiratory failure, Chapter 69.) Provide appropriate supportive care during periods of severe dyspnea and acute exacerbations.

Provide patient education concerning breathing exercises and methods of improving breathing effectiveness. Fatigue is a major enemy of persons with COPD since it adds to breathing problems. To avoid fatigue the patient must learn to plan his activities carefully and thereby budget his energy. Restful sleep is also important. Emotional stress and unpleasantness impair sleep and increase fatigue. Advise the patient not to take sleeping pills or tranquilizers without his doctor's explicit order, because these medications tend to depress respirations during sleep. Constipation should be prevented, since the full bowel pushes against the diaphragm, impeding diaphragmatic movement. Measures helpful in relieving dyspnea are discussed in Chapter 69.

REMOVING, AVOIDING AND/OR MINIMIZING BRONCHIAL IRRITANTS. Smoking is clearly contraindicated in the presence of COPD, but often it is difficult for the patient to give up this habit. Smoke-filled rooms and activities that send dust into the air should be avoided. Dust-producing articles (e.g., feather-filled bedding) and strong cooking odors (e.g., smoke from frying, barbequeing) can also irritate the respiratory tract.

Instruct the patient with COPD to avoid inhaling excessively cold air (cover the mouth and nose with a scarf when outside in very cold weather). The inhalation of extremely cold air may precipitate bronchospasm. Excessive heat should also be avoided since it increases oxygen requirements. Sudden temperature changes (hot or cold) are undesirable.

The avoidance of specific allergens (foods, pollens, animal danders) to which the patient is known to be sensitive is particularly important in extrinsic bronchial asthma. This point is discussed more completely in the section on bronchial asthma on p. 982.

Advise the patient to avoid using powders and aerosolized commercial products (e.g., spray deodorants, hair sprays), and to stay away from air-polluted environments, since air pollutants may cause bronchospasm. The physician may advise occupational changes if the patient works in a polluted environment. Some patients benefit from the use of a home air conditioning unit equipped with an effective filter system. Maintenance of a high relative humidity in the home (40 to 50 per cent) is also helpful, particularly during the winter.

In some cases the physician advises the patient to move to a climate that has minimal shifts in humidity and temperature. Very warm, dry climates are as undesirable as those that are very cold or very humid. High altitudes are also undesirable; they worsen hypoxia. Commonly persons with COPD can live more comfortably at altitudes between 300 and 600 feet. However, some people prefer altitudes up to 3000 feet. Flying in pressurized aircraft at high altitudes should not give the patient added respiratory distress.

Nosedrops should be used only if prescribed, since some over-the-counter products contain oils that may damage the lungs.

Excessive, forceful coughing irritates the tracheobronchial tree. Although productive coughing is essential to clear the tracheobronchial tree of secretions, nonproductive coughing should be controlled. The patient should try to avoid situations that may produce a coughing spell.

INFECTION CONTROL AND PREVENTION. Control *chronic* respiratory infections and prevent *acute* respiratory infections in the patient with COPD, since infections cause further lung damage and deterioration of lung function. In addition to possibly structurally damaging the lung, infections increase mucus production and further restrict ventilation. Also, drug-resistant infections can become a problem. An acute respiratory infection can be fatal to the patient with COPD.

Acute pulmonary infections constantly threaten the patient with COPD because of the patient's lowered resistance. In an attempt to minimize the severity of acute infections some physicians prescribe daily prophylactic doses of antibiotics during cold damp months or if the patient has been exposed to an acute respiratory infection. Upper respiratory infections often precipitate attacks of asthma and chronic bronchitis.

The lung in COPD is always chronically infected; it is impossible to completely rid the lung of bacteria. The goal of therapy in such a situation becomes one of suppressing the bacteria rather than eliminating them. This may be accomplished by giving the patient intermittent doses of antibiotics, e.g., on any two consecutive days of the week. Encourage the patient to stay on the prescribed routine.

Instruct the patient concerning the following actions, which are of importance in preventing infections: (1) avoid close contact with persons who have respiratory infections or "flu"; (2) avoid crowds during times of the year when respiratory infections most commonly occur; (3) maintain a high resistance (e.g., by getting adequate rest and relaxation, eating a nourishing diet high in vitamin C, and avoiding stressful situations and exposure to temperature extremes, dampness, and drafts); and (4) practice frequent thorough oral hygiene.

Influenza vaccines are usually advised prophylactically as a precaution against the development of severe acute infections. Chronically infected tonsils and obstructive adenoids may be removed and sinus infections treated.

Teach the patient to observe his sputum for indications of infection, e.g., increased sputum production or changes in color (from clear or white to gray, yellow, or brown). Other symptoms of acute infection include excessive drowsiness, chest pain, chills, increased dyspnea, cyanosis, leukocytosis, and increased tightness in the chest. Instruct the patient to seek medical care promptly if an acute infection appears to be developing.

During periods of acute infection continuous daily antibiotic treatment is usually indicated. Before the results of sputum culture and sensitivity tests are available, broad-spectrum antibiotics may be prescribed.

Excessive, unproductive coughing is usually mildly suppressed in the patient with COPD because it traumatizes the respiratory system and thus increases the susceptibility of this system to infections.

COMPLICATIONS. Observe for indications of worsening of the patient's condition such as increased sputum production, cough, dyspnea, or wheezing, cyanosis, edema, and mental confusion. In order to evaluate the patient's condition, daily charting for the hospitalized patient with COPD should include notation of: sputum (amount, character); coughing (amount, productivity); skin, mucous membrane and nail bed color; amount of dyspnea and/or wheezing; appetite; and mental state. Notations of the patient's weight are made as requested by the physician or as indicated. Right-sided heart failure (cor pulmonale) is a chronic problem with COPD. Heart failure is controlled by rest, salt restriction, diuretics, and heart muscle strengthening medications. (See Unit X.)

PATIENT-FAMILY EDUCATION; GENERAL SUPPORTIVE AND EMOTIONAL CARE; REHABILITATION. Include family members at appropriate times during patient teaching sessions. Carefully evaluate and meet learning needs. Areas that may need to be covered include: explanation of the basic respiratory disorder; preventative measures; activity adaptations; and such treatment procedures as medications (actions, side-effects, methods and times of administration), dietary restrictions, pulmonary physiology (postural drainage, breathing exercises, exercise retraining programs, effective coughing techniques) and respiratory therapy techniques (oxygen administration, aerosol, and IPPB administration).

Establish individualized programs to help each patient to achieve and attempt to maintain his optimal level of activity. Assist the patient to accept realistic long-term goals and to be as comfortable and independent as his condition permits. Help him to adapt his daily activities to his respiratory limitations without encouraging unnecessary passivity or invalidism. The more active the patient can be (without excessively increasing dyspnea), the better he will feel generally and the stronger he will be. Activity also minimizes complications that tend to accompany inactivity. (See Chapter 27.) Physical activity tolerance varies from patient to patient, and a given patient's tolerance may vary from day to day or even within the same day.

The rehabilitation of patients with COPD can be as successful as that of patients with neuromuscular and skeletal disabilities. Rehabilitative procedures will not reverse the permanent structural pulmonary damage caused by COPD, but they can teach the patient ways to live with his limited cardiorespiratory reserve, and they can prepare him for employment or self-care attuned to his mental and physical capacities. Successful rehabilitation programs involve participation by the patient, his family, physician, nurses and other paramedical personnel. A multidisciplinary approach is desirable.[113]

It is estimated that with proper rehabilitation techniques about half of the people who are already disabled by respiratory disease can be restored and improved enough that they can return to work or at least to self-care. Most patients with chronic respiratory diseases are able to pursue some form of regular employment. Vocational retraining may be necessary to enable the patient to perform work that is compatible with his respiratory limitations. Some communities have COPD rehabilitation programs sponsored by hospitals, clinics, or local agencies of the American Lung Association. Social workers and employees of state rehabilitation services may be helpful if the physician recommends a change of employment to avoid bronchial irritants or to reduce physical exertion. Social workers may also be able to make appropriate referrals to help to obtain equipment necessary for home care, to relieve socioeconomic problems, or to obtain total care if indicated. Over a period of years costs of equipment, oxygen, medications, and hospitalizations are considerable.

Numerous informational materials are available (pertaining to bronchial asthma, chronic bronchitis, pulmonary emphysema, and COPD) from the Chronic Respiratory Diseases Branch, Division of Chronic Diseases, Public Health Service, Washington, D.C. 20201 and the local branch of the American Lung Association. An illustrated manual (which is helpful to patients when used with their physician's supervision), titled *Essentials of Living With Pulmonary Emphysema* is available from the Institute of Physical Medicine and Rehabilitation, New York University Medical Center, 400 East 34th Street, New York, New York 10016. The manual is 50 cents per copy. For the same price a guide to self-care titled *Living With Asthma, Chronic Bronchitis and Emphysema* can be obtained from Riker Laboratories, Inc., Northridge, California. Public Health Service Publication No. 1726, titled *If You Have Emphysema or Chronic Bronchitis,* is available (for 15 cents) from the Superintendent of Documents, U.S. Government Printing Office, Washington, D. C. 20402.

LONG-TERM SUPERVISION AND CARE. The patient with COPD requires long-term follow-up care which may involve community nurses as well as personnel in hospital or clinic outpatient departments. The visiting nurse is helpful in: (1) assessing the home situation; (2) giving or supervising home care; (3) helping the patient to adapt treatment procedures (e.g., dietary restrictions, humidification, postural drainage, oxygen administration) to the home environment; (4) suggesting ways in which the home environment can be modified to minimize energy expenditure; (5) making needed referrals; and (6) counseling, teaching, and emotionally supporting the patient and family. Family support, encouragement, and participation in the care of a family member with COPD can greatly help the patient to improve. Family members often require assistance in increasing their acceptance and tolerance of the problem.

Because of the distressing nature of COPD it is not uncommon for a patient with this disorder to become discouraged and depressed. COPD may force the patient to make numerous changes in his life style and to abandon pleasurable activities. Emotional support must be realistic, sensitive, flexible, and freely given.

It is essential that the patient not neglect any aspects of his treatment regimen. In general, the patient can most thoroughly follow his prescribed treatment program if he establishes and adheres to a scheduled routine. The nurse can help the patient to construct a timetable that lists in order the various recommended treatment activities and when they should be performed.

The patient with COPD commonly experiences his greatest difficulty upon arising. It may take an hour or longer before the routine activities of the day can be started, e.g., grooming, eating, dressing. The patient may need to get up earlier or arrange to start work later than he formerly did to allow time for his necessary morning treatments, e.g., aerosolized bronchodilator, IPPB, oxygen, steam inhalation, postural drainage, breathing exercises.

Factors adversely affecting *prognosis* include: (1) cor pulmonale, particularly if one or more episodes of congestive heart failure have occurred; (2) polycythemia; (3) impaired gas exchange (low diffusing capacity); and (4) severe ventilatory impairment with hypoxemia and hypercapnia.

BRONCHIAL ASTHMA

Definition. Although chronic bronchitis and pulmonary emphysema both produce continuous airway obstruction, bronchial asthma produces obstruction of an intermittent nature (unless complicated with COPD). The word "asthma" comes from the Greek word for "panting" and refers to *attacks* of shortness of breath (dyspnea). The asthmatic patient experiences recurrent *paroxysms* of dyspnea that characteristically are of a wheezing type, produced by obstruction of air flow in the bronchioles and smaller bronchi.

Thus, bronchial asthma is typically an *intermittent* or *reversible* type of obstructive lung disease in which the widespread narrowing of bronchial lumina changes in severity over brief periods of time either spontaneously or as a result of treatment. Bronchial asthma is also characterized by an increased responsiveness of the tracheobronchial smooth muscle and mucous glands to various stimuli. Some patients have mild, uncomplicated asthma that produces symptoms only occasionally, whereas others have chronic, severe asthma. Persons who have had asthma for years commonly develop anatomic pulmonary emphysema and cor pulmonale; bronchitis and bronchiectasis are other possible complications.

Asthmatics classified as having COPD have some degree of *persistent* airway obstruction. Persons who have both asthma and bronchitis, in addition to persistent (although variable) airway obstruction, are said to have "chronic asthmatic bronchitis" and are classified as having COPD.

Bronchial asthma is not due to cardiovascular disease. The condition called *cardiac asthma* (due to left ventricular failure) also produces wheezing respirations. The clinical management of this condition is entirely different from that of bronchial asthma and is not discussed here.

Etiology. Bronchial asthma has basically two forms:

> *Extrinsic asthma* is caused by external agents such as dust, lint, insecticides, mold spores, pollens, food items, synthetic drugs (e.g., aspirin), animal danders, and feathers. This form is best understood and is a reaction to specific allergens. (See Chapter 23.) In many cases the history of hypersensitivity to external agents can be confirmed by skin testing. Most commonly extrinsic asthma develops in children or young adults (prior to age 40) and the attacks gradually become more frequent and of longer duration. Sometimes when affected children reach adolescence they recover completely; others experience a worsening of their condition at adolescence. Adults with extrinsic asthma less commonly experience spontaneous recovery.

> *Intrinsic asthma* is also called "infectious" or "infective asthma"—an unsuitable phrase which incorrectly implies that asthma can be communicable. Intrinsic asthma, in which the specific cause frequently cannot be identified, is difficult to understand. Often the precipitating cause is predominantly infection in the upper (nose, sinuses) or lower (bronchi, lungs) respiratory tract. Enlarged adenoids, nasal polyps or spurs, or sinus infections may be present. Intrinsic asthma may begin at any age, but most commonly develops after age 40. It develops into a lifelong chronic condition in which attacks gradually increase in frequency and severity. The condition often merges into asthmatic bronchitis; at times emphysema coexists.

The basic cause of bronchial asthma is an inherited tendency (called *atopy*) to develop a hypersensitivity reaction of the antigen-antibody type. The reaction is manifested physically by bronchospasm and skin wheals. Usually patients with asthma (extrinsic or intrinsic) give a family medical history which includes hypersensitivity (e.g., asthma, rhinitis, eczema) as well as a personal medical history of allergic disorders such as eczema, urticaria, dermatitis, or hay fever. When both parents have allergies, 75 per cent of their children will also be allergic.

Extrinsic asthma results from the sensitization of an atopic person to specific allergens, so that exposure to even minute amounts of those allergens precipitates an acute asthmatic attack. The main component of the attack is the production of histamine in the cells of the bronchial mucosa. Allergic disorders of the respiratory tract are most commonly caused by such inhalant allergies as pollens (particularly the ragweed family), household dusts, and animal danders.

With intrinsic asthma the respiratory tract reacts to infections, but it is usually not possible to prove the presence of sensitivity to specific infecting organisms by skin tests. Also, a correlation does not exist between the development of reinfections and attacks of asthma. A theory of etiology which focuses on probable hypersensitivity to bacteria has been proposed to explain why intrinsic asthma occurs; however, evidence for this theory is not convincing. It is not uncommon for patients who have had extrinsic asthma to later develop intrinsic asthma.

Secondary factors may perpetuate asthmatic attacks and may profoundly influence the severity and frequency of these attacks. Examples of these factors are emotional stress, fatigue, endocrine changes (menopause, pregnancy, puberty, menstruation), environmental changes (in humidity and temperature), and exposure to noxious fumes (paints, chemicals, smoke). These factors precipitate symptoms by upsetting the delicate balance maintained between the patient and his allergic environment.

Patients with extrinsic asthma commonly smoke cigarettes and have chronic bronchitis (with or without pulmonary emphysema). Any of these conditions may produce dyspnea, wheezing, hypersecretion of mucus, and severe, paroxysmal episodes of coughing. "Asthmatic" attacks occurring in persons with chronic bronchitis and/or emphysema may indicate that the patient is experiencing an acute exacerbation of his established chronic airway obstruction. Such a condition can progress rapidly to hypoxia, hypercapnia, and respiratory acidosis.[203]

Pathology. Pathologically a bronchial asthma attack is characterized by: (1) bronchi plugged with thick, tenacious, slightly cloudy mucus; (2) bron-

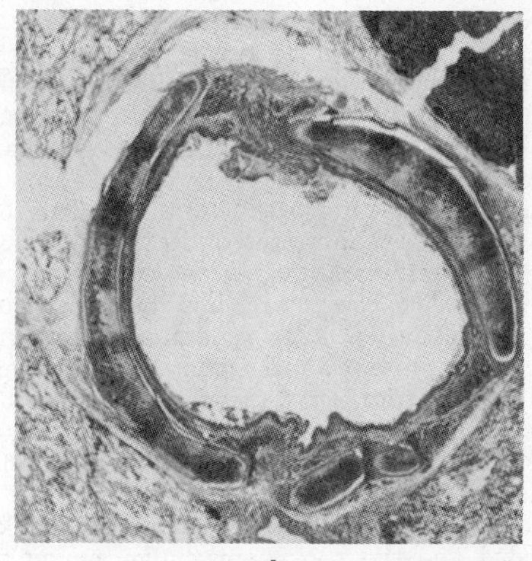

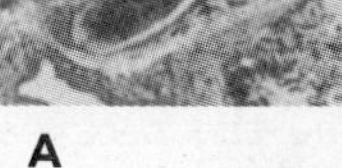

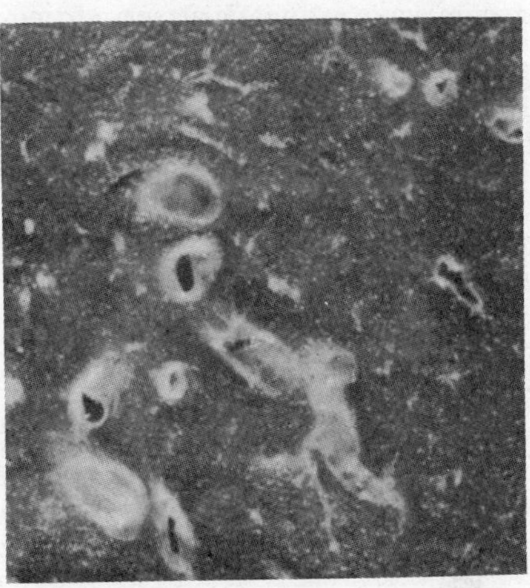

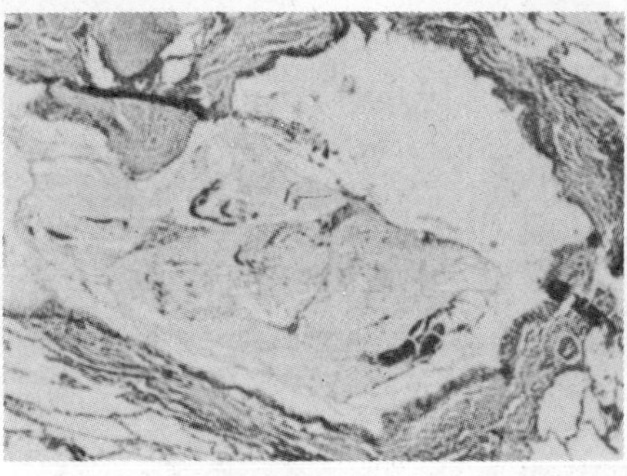

FIGURE 71-10. A, Cross-section of normal bronchus, containing cartilage, smooth muscle, glands, and intact epithelium. B, Close-up view of cut surface of asthmatic lung, showing plugs of mucus in bronchi. C, Low-power (35×) microscopic view of bronchus similar to that in B, showing mucus plug and epithelial changes typical of asthma. (From *Asthma*, published by American Lung Association, 1973.)

chial walls contracted (owing to spasm or increased bronchial smooth muscle tone) and thickened (as a result of acute inflammation and edema); (3) hyperactive mucous glands; and (4) hyperinflation of alveoli, alveolar ducts, and respiratory bronchioles. Note that breakdown of the alveolar walls is *not* characteristic of asthma, as it is with anatomic pulmonary emphysema (see p. 992), and that mucous glands are *not* increased in number (as with chronic bronchitis).

The following pathophysiologic events typically occur during an asthmatic attack: airway resistance is increased; residual volume of the lung is increased; abnormal intrapulmonary gas-mixing occurs; CO_2 is retained; and arterial O_2 saturation is decreased. Respiratory alkalosis (arterial pH ↑ 7.45) may occur early if there is hyperventilation, or respiratory acidosis (arterial pH ↓ 7.35) may develop as a result of airway obstruction.[194] Respiratory function tests are often normal between asthmatic attacks. However, ventilatory impairment remains with some patients, especially persons who have had asthma for a number of years.

During an acute asthmatic attack, air movement is impaired during expiration because of constricted edematous bronchial lumina, which are filled with excess secretions (Figs. 71–10 and 71–11). Characteristically a wheeze occurs and

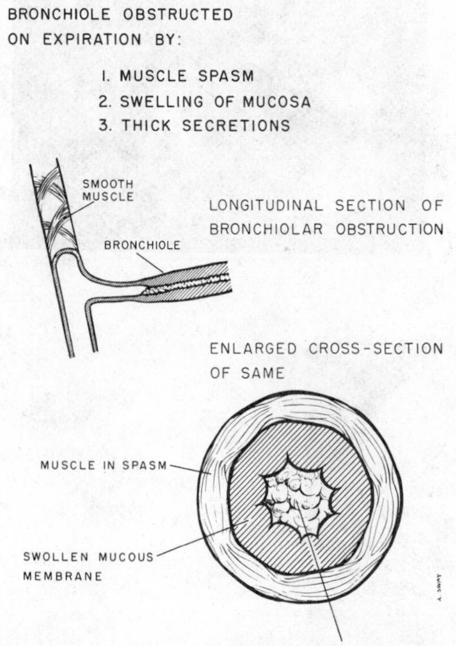

BRONCHIOLE OBSTRUCTED ON EXPIRATION BY:

1. MUSCLE SPASM
2. SWELLING OF MUCOSA
3. THICK SECRETIONS

SMOOTH MUSCLE

BRONCHIOLE

LONGITUDINAL SECTION OF BRONCHIOLAR OBSTRUCTION

ENLARGED CROSS-SECTION OF SAME

MUSCLE IN SPASM

SWOLLEN MUCOUS MEMBRANE

THICK SECRETIONS

FIGURE 71–11. Bronchial asthma. Two views of an obstructed bronchiole, showing how it may be completely blocked by secretions, swollen membranes and muscles in spasm during an attack of asthma. (From *Introduction to Respiratory Diseases*, 4th ed. Copyright American Lung Association, 1969.)

expiration is prolonged. The wheeze is produced as air is forced through the constricted bronchi. The lungs appear hyperextended and voluminous. The alveoli are greatly distended. As the attack worsens, a temporary emphysema-like situation occurs with air trapping and ballooning. Air trapping occurs after air enters the alveoli because the bronchial lumina narrow during the expiratory effort. Air trapping not only distends alveolar walls, but also weakens them.

In allergic forms of asthma the local bronchial reaction is due to antigen-antibody combination. In addition to the tissue changes already mentioned, increased capillary permeability occurs and increased numbers of eosinophils appear in the tissues, peripheral blood, and secretions.

Symptoms. As stated, asthmatic attacks are paroxysmal and vary in frequency, intensity, and duration. Most commonly the attacks are of short duration. Between attacks the patient may be asymptomatic, or some symptoms may persist, especially upon exertion or during extremes in emotion.

Attacks frequently begin suddenly, without warning, when the patient is at rest. Typically the patient suddenly becomes short of breath and feels as if he is suffocating or drowning. He sits up or stands up and leans forward. Devoting all his energy to breathing, the patient struggles to try to breathe slowly and deeply. Expiration is prolonged. Wheezing is most pronounced during expiration and can often be heard at some distance from the patient. Respirations are difficult, but the rate is frequently normal. Most often the patient is pale rather than cyanotic. However, cyanosis may occur with severe attacks.

Cough and sputum production commonly occur. Rales are easily auscultated. Initially the cough is dry and minimal, but as the attack increases in severity the cough becomes more pronounced and productive of large amounts of sputum. If infection is present the sputum is mucopurulent. Often termination of the attack is indicated by severe coughing and the expectoration of thick, tenacious sputum followed by a feeling of relief and clearing of the airways.

During severe attacks the chest is markedly distended and the neck veins bulge, owing to increased intrathoracic pressure caused by air trapping in the lungs. The increase in negative intrapleural pressure is also indicated by marked retraction of the intercostal, supraclavicular, and suprasternal spaces. The chest appears fixed in the inspiratory position, and accessory muscles of respiration are used in an attempt to increase the effectiveness of ventilatory efforts. Profuse perspiration often occurs as a result of increased sympathetic innervation, indicating the stress to which the patient is being subjected and the effort he is expending. After a severe attack the patient's chest may be quite sore.

Symptoms may subside in less than an hour, may persist for several hours, or may last for several days if status asthmaticus develops. *Status asthmaticus* is an acute episode of bronchospasm that is distressing to the patient and is not relieved by conventional bronchodilator therapy. This is a serious, exhausting condition of sustained shortness of breath that is intractable to ordinary treatment methods and produces respiratory insufficiency and hypoxia. These attacks may last for days without relief and may terminate in death. (Treatment is discussed later in this section.)

Other types of acute asthmatic attacks are seldom fatal. They are, however, serious, frightening, and exhausting experiences. Acute asthmatic attacks may be dangerous in persons with cardiac disorders and in elderly persons. *During asthmatic attacks sudden death from respiratory exhaustion may occur, especially if sedatives are administered unwisely and too freely.*

Diagnosis. The differential diagnosis of bronchial asthma is usually made easily from: (1) a history of recurrent, paroxysmal attacks of dyspnea, cough, wheezing and production of mucoid sputum; (2) a family or personal history of allergy; (3) prolonged expiration with wheezing noises and musical rales; and (4) eosinophils in the sputum or blood.

Asthma does not produce characteristic chest x-ray findings. Pulmonary function studies are unnecessary for diagnosis; however, if performed, they may indicate that between attacks some air trapping continues (producing an increased volume of residual air). Often patients with extrinsic asthma have elevated serum levels of immune globulin E (IgE). Arterial hypoxemia (low PaO_2) may be present during severe attacks in which acute bronchospasm develops.

"All that wheezes is not asthma" is a phrase to remember during the process of establishing a differential diagnosis. Other conditions that produce symptoms similar to asthmatic attacks include heart failure (cardiac asthma), pulmonary embolism, endobronchial tuberculosis, obstructive pulmonary emphysema, bronchogenic carcinoma, and bronchial obstruction due to a foreign body.

Although it is relatively easy for the physician to make a differential diagnosis of bronchial asthma, it is more difficult to diagnose the specific etiology of the asthmatic attacks. When possible, a careful search is made to identify the causative agent. A thorough history is taken and includes exploration of familial susceptibility, environmental exposure, and secondary modifying factors such as psychogenic stimuli. Often the nurse can be of assistance in the compilation of such a history. Skin testing is employed to attempt to identify specific extrinsic allergens. (See Chapter 23.) The patient is also investigated for evidence of respiratory infections. Every patient with asthma is investigated for both *sensitization* and *infection,* because patients are often affected by both external allergens and infective factors.

Prevention of Asthmatic Attacks. Clinical care of the asthmatic is directed at providing immediate relief from acute attacks, reducing chronic symptoms (wheezing, coughing, shortness of breath), and minimizing the frequency of attacks. Often the nurse participates in teaching the patient with asthma ways in which he can try to prevent asthmatic attacks. Long-term care, directed at controlling the causes of attacks, may include treatment of infection, emotional disorders, and allergies.

When *specific allergens* are identified as precipitating extrinsic asthmatic attacks, the patient is instructed about possible ways to avoid these allergens. Specific hyposensitization is also commonly performed by the physician. Food extracts are not used for hyposensitization. Foods to which the patient may be sensitive include milk, eggs, chocolate, wheat, and shellfish. Examples of medications to which the asthmatic may be sensitive include acetylsalicylic acid (aspirin), antibiotics, horse serum, and iodine preparations. (See also Chapter 23.)

When disorders such as chronic sinusitis, nasal polyps, and tonsillitis are present and are believed to contribute to asthmatic attacks, these conditions are treated appropriately. Currently tonsils and adenoids are less often removed than formerly because of their recognized importance in the immune response.

If *infection* is believed to contribute to asthmatic attacks, care is directed at preventing recurrent respiratory infections and instructing the patient to see his doctor promptly if he thinks he is developing an infection.

Commonly *vaccines* are beneficial in chronic intrinsic asthma. Stock catarrhal vaccines are used cautiously because asthmatics may be highly sensitive to them. Autogenous vaccines may be prepared (from nasopharyngeal cultures or sputum cultures) and injected weekly. Some physicians give combinations of equal parts of stock and autogenous vaccine to protect the patient against bacteria commonly acquired with respiratory infections as well as those bacteria that the patient is known to harbor.

The patient with asthma must also learn to avoid or to minimize *secondary factors* that can precipitate attacks of asthma, e.g., fatigue, emotional stress. Psychotherapy may be useful in helping the patient to maintain an optimal state of mental well-being. Sometimes small amounts of tranquilizers or sedatives are prescribed to help the patient to relax and feel calmer. Observations concerning the patient's activities immediately prior to an attack may be helpful in identifying factors that precipitate an attack. Such observations should be charted; they may help to prevent future attacks. During intervals between attacks the patient should avoid violent exertion (which produces dyspnea), but may benefit from mild, general exercise such as walking or golfing.

Persons with asthma should be informed of the importance of maintaining adequate *hydration.* Some asthmatic attacks are precipitated by dehydration of the mucous membranes. The asthmatic person should drink 3000 to 4000 ml. of fluids per day, unless contraindicated by cardiac or renal disease.

Changes of climate (e.g., moves to warmer, drier climate) are sometimes recommended for the patient with severe asthma that is refractory to usual medical treatment. The benefits to be derived from climatic changes vary, depending upon the specific etiology of the patient's asthma. Permanent moves should not be made until the patient has had a trial residence to determine the beneficial effects of such a change. It may be desirable for the patient to avoid fog, smog, and extremely cold weather.

Some patients benefit from the use of air conditioners equipped with special devices to filter out pollens. Keeping environmental air humidified may also be helpful. Some types of "air purifiers" are ineffective. The patient who is advised by his physician to purchase an air conditioner can benefit from reading the pamphlet, *Room Air Conditioners, How to Choose the Model Best Suited for Your Needs*. This pamphlet can be obtained by writing the National Better Business Bureau, 230 Park Avenue, New York, N.Y. 10017.

Persons with asthma are commonly targets of advertising programs which exploit their illnesses by inaccurately claiming the ability to give relief from asthmatic attacks if only the sufferers will purchase some gadget, book, or medicine. The patient with asthma who is tempted to obtain relief by purchasing items advertised on television, radio, or in the newspapers can obtain reliable information about his condition and its proper treatment by reading the pamphlet, *Asthma, Hay Fever and Other Allergies*. This pamphlet can be obtained free from the Allergy Foundation of America, 801 Second Avenue, New York, N.Y. 10017.

The development of status asthmaticus and many of the deaths that occur from asthma are believed to be preventable by providing appropriate treatment and by impressing on the patient the need to precisely follow at home the medical regimen prescribed. Asthma causes approximately 8000 deaths annually.[194]

Clinical Care During and Following Acute Asthmatic Attacks. During an acute asthmatic attack the goals of care are to maintain efficient respiratory function while relieving bronchial spasm and promoting the expulsion of secretions.

MEDICATIONS. Relaxation and dilatation of the bronchi may be accomplished by administering medications such as epinephrine and its derivatives (e.g., isoproterenol), aminophylline and its derivatives (e.g., oxtriphylline), ephedrine, antihistamines, or corticosteroids. Bronchodilators may be administered orally, intravenously, or subcutaneously; some are inhaled, e.g., isoproterenol hydrochloride (Isuprel, Aludrine) and isoetharine (Bronkosol).

Most asthmatic attacks initially respond to *epinephrine (Adrenalin)* 1:1000 solution, subcutaneously. The medication may be repeated after 5 to 15 minutes when necessary. The patient and his family members may require instructions about how to administer the medication by the subcutaneous route. In acutely ill patients, epinephrine 1:1000 may be administered intravenously—cautiously and very slowly because of vasoconstricting effects. (Monitor pulse rate and blood pressure during administration.) Epinephrine is also available for administration by nebulizer (two or three deep inhalations at the beginning of an attack). For prolonged activity it may be given intramuscularly in preparations in oil or glycerin. Check orders carefully to be certain you have the correct preparation, the prescribed concentration and amount, and that you are administering the medication via the correct route.

The vasoconstricting effects of epinephrine often cause the patient to become pale and to experience such side-effects as palpitation, tremor, nervousness, anxiety, tachycardia, and insomnia. Epinephrine must be used cautiously in the presence of severe hypertension, hyperthyroidism, or heart disease.

Observe closely for indications of drug toxicity and side-effects during and after administration of medications to combat acute asthmatic attacks.

Isoproterenol (Isuprel), an epinephrine derivative, is available in tablets for sublingual use or can be used via nebulizer. Generally inhalation of this medication produces fewer cardiovascular side-effects. Instruct patients to use aerosol bronchodilators only as prescribed. Their overuse may lower PaO_2 and produce bronchospasm.

If the asthmatic attack does not respond to epinephrine, then *theophylline ethylenediamine (aminophylline)* may be given very slowly intravenously in saline (taking about 10 minutes to inject) or by intravenous drip. Aminophylline can be fatal if injected too rapidly. Observe the patient closely for the following untoward symptoms while he is receiving aminophylline: sudden decrease in blood pressure accompanied by headache, faintness, dizziness, and palpitation. The patient may self-administer aminophylline via a rectal suppository or in solution as a retention enema. Aminophylline in the form of a rectal suppository may cause anorectal irritation. Patient-family instruction may be necessary concerning proper insertion of a rectal suppository or the administration of a retention enema.

Antihistamines do not often relieve asthma, as they do hay fever. Adults are usually not helped by antihistamines, particularly during severe asthmatic attacks. However, the *corticosteroids* and *corticotrophin (ACTH)* are among the most useful therapeutic agents for the temporary control of severe or intractable asthma, e.g., status asthmaticus. It is not known exactly how steroids interrupt an asthmatic attack. Corticosteroids are used only when other agents are unsuccessful, because of their serious side-effects. Corticosteroids are contraindicated in the presence of diabetes, tuberculosis (active or inactive), and peptic ulcer. Because of the dramatic relief corticosteroids may give to patients with asthma, patients may become overly dependent on these medications. Occasionally physicians maintain some patients on long-term therapy with prednisone or a similar corticosteroid. Sometimes, in borderline situations, the use of an inhaler, e.g., Decadron Medihaler, provides the beneficial effects of corticosteroids with a minimum of side-effects. In order to properly use the inhaler the patient is told that this inhaler must be used *regularly,* as prescribed, rather than for immediate relief.

Numerous combination preparations are available for treating asthmatics, e.g., ephedrine hydrochloride or sulfate, aminophylline, and a sedative such as phenobarbital. The actions of *ephedrine* are similar to those of epinephrine but are milder. Since ephedrine taken by itself often evokes anxiety and tachycardia, it is desirable to give it in combination with medications that minimize these stimulatory effects. Ephedrine, epinephrine, and isoproterenol all reduce bronchospasm by relaxing the smooth muscle that lines the larger bronchioles and bronchi.

Sedatives are contraindicated in the treatment of severe asthma. Nervousness in the patient with severe asthma is frequently caused by hypoxemia; the respiratory depression produced by sedation aggravates this. In addition, sedatives may depress the cough reflex. However, sedation is used at times in treating mild cases to counteract the overstimulation that bronchodilator medications sometimes produce. In a situation of this kind, phenobarbital or diazepam (Valium) may be administered orally. *Narcotics* are generally contraindicated because they depress respirations; however, at times they are used cautiously provided respirators are available if needed to mechanically support respiration. Morphine not only depresses respiration but also causes bronchoconstriction.

The asthmatic patient may be given *mildly sedative cough mixtures* such as antihistamine mixtures with codeine or elixir of terpin hydrate with codeine to relieve excessive, nonproductive cough. *Expectorants,* (ammonium chloride or potassium iodide) may loosen thick, tenacious bronchial secretions.

Infections that may be present are treated specifically when possible with *antibiotics* and *sulfonamides* to which the infecting organisms are known to be sensitive. Recurrent infections are common. Tetracyclines may be given before laboratory culture and sensitivity results are available. Although penicillin is a useful antibiotic for gram-positive infections, it does (like horse serum) often tend to produce serious and sometimes fatal allergic reactions in asthmatics. Moreover, cross-allergenicity exists between the penicillins and the newer semisynthetic derivatives, e.g., ampicillin and oxacillin.

> *Penicillin and other related medications, e.g., ampicillin and oxacillin, must be used cautiously in asthmatic patients because of possible serious allergic reactions.*

A sensitivity test is performed prior to administering the first dose of penicillin when penicillin is ordered.

Patients with asthma are given medications for *home use* during attacks. Because asthmatic attacks tend to vary in their severity and their response to chemotherapy, medications given the patient for home use may include (in the order to be used if necessary): (1) an adrenergic aerosol; (2) an oral preparation of ephedrine and/or theophylline; and (3) a theophylline preparation for rectal insertion.

CARE MEASURES. Summarized below are activities of importance in the clinical care of a patient *during* an acute asthmatic attack:

> Administer medications (bronchodilators) promptly to provide relief as soon as possible after the onset of attack.

> Observe for toxic affects of medications as well as therapeutic effects.

> Position the patient so he can breathe more comfortably (Fig. 71–12); manually assist ventilation if indicated.

> Maintain clear airway; suction if indicated.

> Offer appropriate reassurance; provide constant care (do not leave patient alone during acute attack).

> Maintain quiet, restful environment; restrict visitors; minimize environmental irritants (e.g., remove feather pillows, prohibit smoking and flowers, maintain effective air conditioning); maintain emotional atmosphere in which patient feels comfortable expressing his anxieties. Some patients are admitted to the hospital temporarily during an acute attack and are placed in an area where environmental control of allergies can be maintained.

> Minimize patient's exertion and fatigue by anticipating his needs and providing assistance, e.g., with eating, drinking, as necessary. Discourage unnecessary talking.

> Evaluate frequently: rate and character of respirations; pulse; color of nail beds, mucous membranes and skin (observe for cyanosis); amount of perspiration; fre-

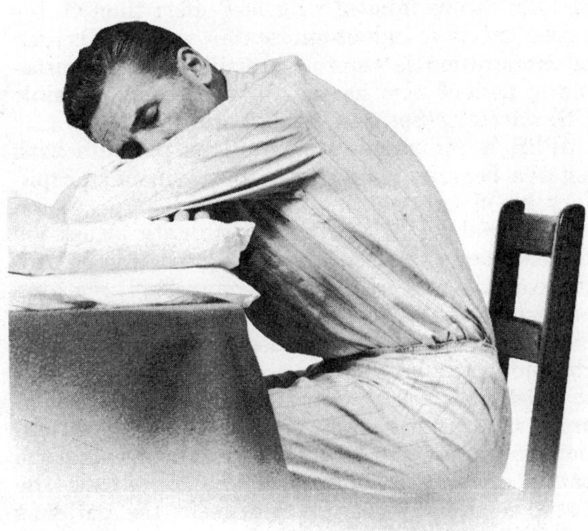

FIGURE 71–12. A comfortable position during an asthma attack. (From *Living with Asthma, Chronic Bronchitis, and Emphysema.* Riker Laboratories, 1969.)

quency and character of cough; amount and character of sputum (color, viscosity); emotional state; activity (e.g., restlessness); and physical stamina (fatigue, exhaustion). Monitor vital signs every four hours, or more frequently if indicated. Observe for indications of untoward side-effects of therapy, e.g., arrhythmia, tachycardia, nausea and vomiting.

> Evaluate patient frequently for indications of need for respiratory therapy, (e.g., indications of hypoxia, respiratory insufficiency). Provide oxygen therapy as indicated and ordered.

> Provide humidification of inspired air (steam, cool vapor).

> Prepare for and assist with emergency care, e.g., bronchoscopy, tracheostomy.

> Observe for and report indications of infection, congestive heart failure, or other complications.

> Control excessive, unproductive cough without depressing respiratory reflexes.

> Use sedatives cautiously if ordered and indicated.

> Observe for indications of fluid-electrolyte and acid-base imbalances; provide appropriate care to prevent or correct. Maintain hydration and nutrition. Record intake and output. If indicated, force fluids to thin secretions.

> Protect against chilling; keep patient dry if diaphoretic; prevent drafts.

The administration of oxygen during an asthmatic attack is usually not necessary if the bronchodilator medications are effective. However, it may be necessary during severe, prolonged attacks. Observe for indications of hypoxia—progressively rising pulse rate, restlessness, confusion, cyanosis. If respiratory insufficiency appears to be developing, oxygen may be ordered by nasal cannula, nasal catheter, IPPB, or mask. Occasionally an oxygen tent is used because it provides an allergen-free and air-conditioned atmosphere. At times oxygen with helium is cautiously administered to the cyanotic patient to relieve hypoxia. Helium can be inhaled with less effort than O_2 because it has a lighter molecular weight. Oxygen administration is carefully regulated if the asthmatic patient also has COPD to prevent possible CO_2 narcosis. (See Chapters 25 and 70.)

IPPB is contraindicated in some patients with asthma because it decreases the pulmonary capillary blood volume and thus decreases perfusion and arterial pO_2.[194] During an asthmatic attack the patient may obtain some relief by practicing breathing exercises that enable him to control his breathing pattern and breathing efficiency.

It has long been recognized that patients with chronic bronchial asthma are unusually sensitive to emotional factors. Some patients appear to improve significantly when given reassurance, attention and optimistic treatment. Realizing that the patient may be frightened of another attack, the nurse stops in frequently and keeps the patient's call bell within his easy reach. If the patient signals, his summons is answered quickly. At night it is reassuring to some patients to keep the room dimly lighted. Attempt to maintain an atmosphere that promotes relaxation. The nurse and the patient's family members should realize that asthmatic attacks that may be precipitated by emotional factors *cannot* be controlled or stopped "if only the patient makes up his mind to do so." Because of the stressful nature of severe asthmatic attacks some patients are reluctant to leave the security of the hospital environment.

Following an acute asthmatic attack:

> Attempt to identify and report any conditions you observed that may have precipitated the attack.

> Ensure a period of undisturbed rest because the patient is usually exhausted. Expectorants may be given to help to remove tenacious secretions. Postural drainage with clapping and vibrating may be ordered to help to clear the tracheobronchial tree. Ample fluid intake is important following an attack to prevent dehydration.

> Provide appropriate patient-family teaching based on identified needs. Areas emphasized may include: (1) describing the nature of asthma; (2) clarifying diagnostic tests, e.g., skin tests, and desensitization procedures; (3) preventative measures, e.g., prevention of respiratory infections, environmental control to avoid irritants, minimizing emotional strain, dietary restrictions, fluid intake; (4) care during an attack, e.g., medications used (their names, purposes, dosages, frequency of administration, undesirable side-effects, routes of administration) and how to administer them (e.g., injections, suppository insertion, aerosols); (5) pulmonary physiotherapy (e.g., breathing exercises, effective coughing, postural drainage); (6) any necessary activity restrictions; and (7) need for long-term medical supervision, follow-up care, long-term planning, rehabilitation procedures, and maintenance therapy. Advise the patient not to spend his money on advertised medications or quack remedies, and that he should not take *any* medications without his doctor's permission. If the patient has known drug allergies, encourage him to wear a bracelet or tag that states his allergy.

Treatment of Status Asthmaticus. Status asthmaticus is a *medical emergency*. It is frequently caused by respiratory infection but may also occur as a result of a medication (e.g., acetylsalicylic acid), severe stress (worry, fatigue), persistent exposure to an allergen, withdrawal of previous corticosteroid medication, dyspnea (e.g., due to exposure to air pollutants, the presence of emphysema or the occurrence of complications such as myocardial failure).

The use of antimicrobial and corticosteroid medications has improved the treatment of patients with status asthmaticus. Commonly the patient is admitted to the hospital where he can be placed under environmental control, can rest away from anxious relatives, and can benefit from close supervision and intensive diagnostic and treatment procedures.

Once the patient is hospitalized for the treatment of status asthmaticus the initial orders typically include the following:

> Bed rest in orthopneic position. This promotes rest and relieves dyspnea.

> Cover pillows with allergen-proof covers; eliminate pollen contact, dust factors, and other irritating inhalants (e.g., smoke); give no acetylsalicylic acid, penicillin, or opiates. This prevents exposure to allergens and medications to which patient may be sensitive. Avoid overuse of medications such as sedatives and narcotics, *which cause respiratory depression.*

> Soft (5 Gm. salt) diet; force fluids; monitor intake and output. Maintain hydration and nutrition. Food allergens to which the patient is known to be sensitive are eliminated from the diet. I.V.'s may be given slowly to maintain adequate hydration until sufficient oral intake is possible. During prolonged I.V. administration, serum electrolytes are monitored and adjusted.

> Sputum for culture and drug-sensitivity tests (guide to future specific antimicrobial treatment). Specimen is taken prior to giving first dose of antimicrobial drugs.

> Tetracycline, 250 mg. Q.I.D. (*Immediate antimicrobial treatment* is started before sputum culture reports are returned because respiratory infection often precipitates status asthmaticus).

> Dexamethasone, 4 mg. I.M., stat. Prednisone, 10 mg. Q.I.D. for eight doses; then 5 mg. Q.I.D. (*Corticosteroids are very effective* in treating status asthmaticus. Infusions of hydrocortisone are given separately from other infusions.)

> Bronchodilators, e.g., aminophylline, 0.5 Gm. suppository, stat. (repeat twice daily as necessary); 0.25 Gm. I.V., very slowly, on special order. Or epinephrine, 1:1000, 0.5 ml. SC for acute asthmatic attack, every 4 to 6 hours as necessary. Or Tedral tablet, T.I.D. (*combination of bronchodilator and mild sedative*).

> Saturated solution of potassium iodide, 1.0 ml. T.I.D. (expectorant).

> Chloral hydrate, 0.5 to 1.5 Gm., if necessary for sleep. (*Use minimal effective dose to ensure rest without depressing respiratory reflexes.)*

> Chest roentgenogram, stat, (necessary to make differential diagnosis). Roentgenogram of nasal sinuses (to locate foci of infection).

> Electrocardiogram, stat. If present, heart failure is appropriately treated.

> Complete blood count and urinalysis.

> Blood for urea nitrogen, CO_2, sodium, potassium, chloride, sugar, sedimentation rate. Arterial blood gases are followed carefully if asthma is severe, and IPPB is administered if values are progressively abnormal. Arterial blood gas values are determined as soon as possible and are repeated every 30 to 60 minutes until the patient is clearly improved. An elevated or rising $PaCO_2$ is serious.

At times patients in status asthmaticus die. The causes of death are most commonly pneumonia, impaired respiratory function, cardiac failure, or acidosis. Unfortunately, oversedation is also too frequently a factor. The nurse observes the patient in status asthmaticus closely for early indications of the development of these complications. When administering medications she guards against oversedation. If in doubt about whether a medication should be given, she checks with the attending physician. Remember, it is more desirable to preserve the patient's respiratory reflexes, even though he may be somewhat restless, than to depress these reflexes by oversedating the patient so he can "rest quietly."

Surgical Treatment of Asthma. Bronchoscopy and tracheostomy may be lifesaving during an asthmatic attack. Occasionally *bronchoscopy* is necessary to aspirate secretions trapped in the tracheobronchial tree or to irrigate the airways. Secretions blocking the airways may seriously impair alveolar oxygen and carbon dioxide exchange and may produce atelectasis and respiratory insufficiency. *Tracheostomy* facilitates repeated secretion aspiration, irrigation of the airways, humidification, and IPPB therapy when indicated.

Numerous surgical procedures have been suggested to treat patients with chronic bronchial asthma; however, these procedures are typically unsuccessful. Various functional types of surgery have attempted to relieve bronchospasm by inhibiting nervous influences traveling via the sympathetic or parasympathetic (vagal) system, or both. Recently another procedure, *glomectomy* (removal of the glomus, i.e., carotid body) has been attempted in the management of asthma and emphysema. The beneficial effects of this procedure have not been confirmed.

CHRONIC BRONCHITIS

Definition and Incidence. Chronic bronchitis is a chronic inflammation of the tracheobronchial tree with recurrent cough and sputum production. Chronic bronchitis is more precisely defined as a *clinical* disorder characterized by the hypersecretion of bronchial mucus, and accompanied by a chronic or recurrent productive cough. The symptoms must occur for a minimum of three months a year for at least two consecutive years before the condition can be accurately diagnosed as chronic bronchitis. Also, other possible causes of the symptoms must be excluded.

Chronic bronchitis is almost always associated with heavy cigarette smoking. Heavy smokers have a very high incidence of chronic bronchitis.

Chronic bronchitis occurs principally among middle-aged or elderly men, particularly in city dwellers and heavy cigarette smokers, as stated.

The prevalence and activity of chronic bronchitis increase during periods of fog and cold, wet weather. It is thus not suprising that there is an extremely high incidence of chronic bronchitis in England—a foggy, highly industrialized country. An estimated 25 per cent of all male illnesses in England are believed to result from chronic bronchitis, and in Great Britain chronic bronchitis is the third commonest cause of death. Accurate statistics are not available concerning the incidence of chronic bronchitis in the United States, but it is known that *chronic bronchitis is a leading cause of disability in this country and its incidence continues to increase.*

As stated in the discussion of COPD, both chronic bronchitis and pulmonary emphysema are present in the vast majority of patients with COPD. These conditions present similar clinical features, appear to have a common etiologic basis, and are treated by essentially the same procedures. Chronic bronchitis commonly precedes and complicates pulmonary emphysema. Nonetheless, some patients with chronic bronchitis, at autopsy, have almost no structural pulmonary emphysema, and some patients with terminal destructive pulmonary emphysema have almost no bronchitis.

Etiology. Chronic bronchitis develops in response to irritation, e.g., from cigarette smoke, air pollution (toxic industrial gases, irritating dusts, smokes, chemicals), and infections (low-grade chronic pulmonary infections, pneumonia, influenza). Possibly heredity is important. Other factors that promote the progression of chronic bronchitis include inadequate bronchial drainage; narrow, compressed or constricted bronchi; inadequate circulation; pulmonary fibrosis; and mechanical distortions. In addition to commonly occurring with pulmonary emphysema, chronic bronchitis also frequently accompanies pulmonary tuberculosis, chronic bronchial asthma, pulmonary fibrosis, chronic sinusitis, bronchiectasis, and kyphoscoliosis.

Onset. Chronic bronchitis is a serious, progressive, potentially fatal illness with an insidious onset. Some patients with chronic bronchitis never experience more than a chronic or recurrent cough productive of mucoid sputum (which may persist for years without causing respiratory distress), whereas others suffer progressive breathlessness, repeated pulmonary infections, and eventually succumb to respiratory failure. Commonly chronic bronchitis progresses over a period of years and the illness is punctuated with periodic acute exacerbations. Bronchopneumonia is a frequent complication of acute exacerbations.

Many people neglect chronic bronchitis until it is in an advanced stage. The bronchitic individual's medical history typically includes: habitual cigarette smoking; a habitual morning cough (commonly ascribed to smoking); and an increasing tendency to expectorate for progressively longer periods after every cold. Gradually the duration of cough and the amount of sputum produced increase over the years until these symptoms are steadily present. These changes often occur gradually without special awareness on the patient's part.

This pattern of insidious development is indeed unfortunate because if the patient followed relatively simple precautions and received vigorous treatment when his bronchitis was of a mild degree, permanent lung damage might be limited. Unhappily, chronic bronchitis often becomes increasingly severe and eventually becomes merely a part of progressively fatal disorders, e.g., cor pulmonale, pulmonary emphysema. Oswald observes, "The person with a cough and sputum through most of the winter months and an annual absence of about two weeks from acute infections and breathlessness probably has reached the stage of irreversible bronchial damage."[220]

Prevention. Like lung cancer, pulmonary emphysema and some other respiratory disorders, *chronic bronchitis can often be prevented* by relatively simple precautions. Since chronic bronchitis seldom occurs among nonsmokers, the prevention of this disorder is possible to a large extent by the elimination of cigarette smoking. Attempts are also made to try to prevent or alleviate air pollution and occupational exposure to fumes and dust. The nurse plays an important role in the prevention of chronic bronchitis by providing instruction about the hazards of cigarette smoking and air pollution, and by encouraging persons with symptoms of respiratory disorders to seek early evaluation and treatment.

Pathology. Pathologically chronic bronchitis is characterized by chronic inflammation of the bronchial wall, mucosal edema, and hypertrophy, hypersecretion, and hyperplasia of bronchial mucous glands and epithelial mucous goblet cells. The increase in the size and number of mucous glands and cells is noticeable clinically by the increased production of sputum. Additionally, there is usually some emphysema (enlargement of the air spaces caused by breakdown of the alveolar walls).

Chronic bronchitis causes the bronchi to appear thick and inelastic. The bronchial surface may be dry or covered with mucus and pus, and is dark red in color. Cilia are absent. The epithelium, mucous glands, and muscular layers are deformed. Diverticula ("pockets") in the bronchi result from the openings of enlarged mucous glands. Bronchiectasis is frequently present in the form of cylindrical bronchial dilations.

Because of degenerative changes in the bronchi (e.g., destruction of cilia), the patient's normal mechanisms for removing sputum, bacteria, and so forth, from the lungs are ineffective and he must cough increasingly in order to try to clear his lungs. Ineffective bronchial drainage promotes the retention of pus and mucus and the obstruction of air passages. Hence, repeated pulmonary infections occur frequently, and the mucous membranes are usually chronically inflamed and infected. Bronchospasm may aggravate the various dysfunctions associated with chronic bronchitis. Narrowing of the smaller airways produces dyspnea, wheezing, and impaired gas exchange.

It is not unusual for chronic bronchitis to progress to COPD with structural destruction of the alveolar walls and alveolar capillary bed. These irreversible lung changes may cause serious obstructive problems. Chronic bronchitis with obstruction may produce the following lung function findings: *increased* residual lung volume, and *reduced* vital capacity, maximum breathing capacity, and timed vital capacity (slow retarded expiration). Increased resistance to airflow is the first change in pulmonary function caused by chronic bronchitis. This produces some degree of alveolar hypoventilation; i.e., even though the tidal volume may be normal, the O_2 and CO_2 exchange is insufficient. Obstructed expiratory air flow may result from bronchial scarring, bronchial spasm, mucus obstructing the bronchi, and thickening of bronchial walls (from edema and inflammation). All these factors reduce the size of the lumina of the bronchi. Air trapping in the alveoli and bronchioles results from obstruction of air flow during expiration.

As chronic bronchitis progresses, hypoventilation is indicated by an increased arterial pCO_2 and reduced pO_2. Pulmonary hypertension, cor pulmonale (right ventricular hypertrophy), right heart failure, and respiratory failure often develop.

Symptoms. Commonly the symptoms of chronic bronchitis worsen during cold, damp weather. Persistent cough and sputum production are principal symptoms. Often more than one ounce of odorless sputum is produced daily; it may be white (mucoid), gray, mucopurulent, or purulent. Microscopic examination of sputum reveals many kinds of bacteria. Organisms most commonly isolated include the influenza bacillus, pneumococci, staphylococci, streptococci, and Friedländer's bacillus. Occasionally sputum is blood-tinged following severe coughing. Usually sputum is tenacious. The cough may be loose, rattling, and constant or paroxysmal, with severe spasms lasting several minutes. Commonly the cough is worse in the morning and the evening. Chest expansion is usually reduced. Bronchial exudate may produce rales that are sonorous and moist, squeaking or wheezing. The patient may experience a sensation of heaviness in his chest.

Usually the patient's nutritional state is well maintained. In fact, he may be overweight.

Acute episodes of infection tend to occur several times each winter. During these episodes the patient becomes febrile. Between these episodes the patient with chronic bronchitis is characteristically afebrile, with no change in his WBC or ESR. Attacks of bronchopneumonia may cause a sudden worsening in the patient's condition.

During periods of acute exacerbations the patient may suddenly develop severe, potentially fatal hypoxia, hypercapnia, acidosis, and cor pulmonale. These abnormalities may not be present between periods of exacerbation; however, gradually, with progression of the disease, the patient may develop chronic hypoxia, hypercapnia and cor pulmonale.

With progression and worsening of chronic bronchitis the patient develops: obstructive symptoms (e.g., he uses accessory muscles for ventilation and purses his lips during prolonged expiration); symptoms of hypoxia and hypercapnia; increasing dyspnea of an asthmatic nature; wheezing respirations; and incapacitating paroxysms of coughing. The patient's color is usually dusky or cyanotic. Emphysema may gradually be superimposed and obstructive symptoms predominate. Exertional dyspnea gradually curtails the patient's physical activity. Dyspnea does not usually occur in uncomplicated chronic bronchitis, but appears with COPD. Death may result from irreversible respiratory failure or may occur during an acute, possibly reversible, exacerbation.

Diagnosis. Chronic bronchitis is easily *diagnosed* from the history of a chronic, productive cough. Ventilatory function and respiratory gas exchange tests are performed to evaluate the severity of the condition, and the patient's respiratory system is carefully examined to establish a differential diagnosis and to detect other serious pulmonary disorders. The volume of sputum raised per day may be measured to evaluate severity of the disorder.

An ordinary chest x-ray does not demonstrate characteristic abnormalities in the presence of chronic bronchitis, but bronchograms will show the following characteristic changes: diverticula, cylindrical dilations, "accordion-like" irregularities,[208] and small round terminal expansions of the bronchial tree. Routine bacteriologic sputum examination seldom provides the physician with information of value; cytologic examination of the sputum, however, may be useful. For example, some "purulence" may be caused by eosinophils. This indicates to the physician that he should investigate and treat allergic aspects of the disorder.[220]

Clinical Care. Clinical care of the patient with chronic bronchitis (and pulmonary emphysema) is basically the same as that previously discussed for patients with COPD. Care focuses on reducing or controlling symptoms, e.g., improving ventilation and respiration, relieving bronchospasm; minimizing progression of disease by reducing bronchial irritation; preventing additional tissue damage by preventing acute episodes of pulmonary infection; and preventing or controlling complications. Success of therapy rests largely upon the nurse's ability to skillfully give and coordinate the necessary clinical care and the patient's ability to thoroughly perform aspects of self-care that are essential for him to function at an optimal level.

Discussed below are some factors of particular importance in the clinical care of patients with chronic bronchitis (and pulmonary emphysema).

> *Minimize bronchial irritation,* e.g., by removing or reducing chemical irritants and by avoiding acute respiratory infections. Reduce exposure to general air pollution and occupational atmospheric hazards. It is imperative that smoking be stopped. Job changes may be necessary. The patient may be advised by his physician to live in a mild climate. A home air-conditioning unit with an effective filtration system may help to minimize bronchial irritation. A relatively high humidity should be maintained in the home, especially during cold months. Nasal breathing (rather than mouth breathing) is encouraged, so inspired air can be normally warmed, filtered, and humidified in the nasal passages. Known allergens should be avoided. (See discussion of allergens in previous section on bronchial asthma.) Cold drinks may precipitate coughing. Also, coughing may be precipitated by rhinitis and postnasal drip. Antihistamines may be given to control these nasal and postnasal problems. Codeine phosphate or a comparable antitussive may be used to mildly suppress nonproductive, irritating cough.

> *Control chronic respiratory infections and promptly treat intercurrent acute infections,* e.g., with antibiotics, expectorants, bronchodilators. The patient should seek medical care at the *beginning* of *any* respiratory infection or "flu." If sputum becomes purulent, antibiotics may be indicated.

> *Relieve bronchospasm and combat air trapping.* Bronchospasm may be relieved with ephedrine sulfate or related drugs, or isoproterenol hydrochloride (Isuprel, Aludrine) in solution by nebulization. Isoproterenol and ephedrine may be used together. Aminophylline may also be used to relieve bronchospasm. Antihistamines may help to relieve bronchial inflammation. Persistent bronchospasm that cannot be relieved with simple bronchodilators and physiotherapy may be treated with a course of corticosteroids to reduce bronchial inflammation. Many bronchitics are helped during winter months by taking as little as 5 to 10 mg. of prednisone a day, and they have no problem stopping the drug once winter passes.

> *Prevent or minimize acute intercurrent respiratory infections* by having annual influenza injection, by avoiding exposure to colds and "flu" at home or in public, and by maintaining an optimal level of general health. Undue emotional strain should be avoided. The patient should maintain a desirable weight. During winter months the patient may prophylactically be given either penicillin or a broad-spectrum antimicrobial medication to reduce the severity and length of disability if infection occurs. Such maintenance antibiotic therapy does not reduce the *frequency* of intercurrent acute respiratory infections. The upper airways are carefully inspected for evidence of treatable conditions (e.g., infected sinuses, nasal polyps, deviated nasal septum) to restore nasal patency and/or minimize the possibility of subsequent pulmonary infections.

> *Minimize dyspnea* by breathing retraining. An electrocardiogram is performed for diagnostic purposes, and obesity and hypertension are reduced if present. Commonly a triad of chronic bronchitis, obesity, and hypertension occurs.

> *Facilitate raising of sputum and clearing of air passages; support ventilation and respiration.* A saturated solution of potassium iodide may be ordered to help the patient to raise mucus. The IPPB inhalation of isoproterenol for one minute followed by a mucolytic agent for 10 minutes T.I.D. can often effectively remove sticky sputum. Frequently a physiotherapist can best perform this treatment, following it with postural and breathing exercises. The patient is taught how to effectively cough, perform breathing exercises, and perform postural drainage. He must *meticulously* follow a pattern of thorough tracheobronchial and oral hygiene and must force fluids to prevent dehydration and drying of secretions. Steam, mist, or other inhalants may help the patient to clear his air passages. Nebulization with warm normal saline may be employed to moisten the respiratory mucosa. Postural drainage is especially important if bronchiectasis is also present.

IPPB (using either O_2-air mixtures or air, and combined with bronchodilator aerosols) may be useful if marked bronchial obstruction is present and ventilatory capacity is reduced. These treatments may be given for 15 to 30 minutes several times per day. If oxygen therapy is necessary it is given cautiously to prevent CO_2 narcosis.

PULMONARY EMPHYSEMA

Definitions and Types. The word "emphysema" comes from the Greek word *emphysan* meaning to "puff up with air." Emphysema is actually a *pathologic diagnosis* only, not a clinical diagnosis. In the United States the term "emphysema" has been overused and misused as a clinical diagnosis. "Emphysema" means that destruction of lung tissue has occurred and an *anatomic* alteration of the lungs is present, characterized by an abnormal enlargement (overinflation) of the distal air spaces (alveoli) accompanied by destructive changes of the alveolar walls, e.g., rupture of the alveolar walls and destruction of the alveolar capillary bed.

Pulmonary emphysema is not a single entity but rather is primarily a defect in the alveolar walls that may result from various diseases. Several types of pulmonary emphysema have been differentiated pathologically.

Primary emphysema, which commonly occurs after years of chronic bronchitis, may be pathologically classified as either *centrilobular,* i.e., beginning in the center of the lung lobules and producing destructive changes in the region of the respiratory bronchiole; or *panlobular* (or panacinar), i.e., occurring throughout the lung and characterized by the generalized dilatation of air spaces of secondary lobules.* The centrilobular type is the most common and has a predilection for the upper portion of the lungs; panlobular emphysema occurs most often in the lower lungs. *Secondary* emphysema occurs as a result of any condition that causes scarring or fibrosis in the lung. This type of pulmonary emphysema is pathologiccally classified as the *paracicatricial* (or traction) type and is characterized by alveolar wall destruction and alveolar overdistention adjacent to fibrotic pulmonary lesions. The focal air cysts produced are generally called "blebs," "bullae," or "pneumatoceles." Usually the smaller lesions are referred to as "blebs," whereas the larger air cysts (over 1 inch in diameter) are called "bullae."

Paracicatricial emphysema and the lobular types of emphysema, e.g., centrilobular or panlobular, may occur within the same lung. When large, thin-walled air spaces (bullae) are created by the destruction of numerous alveoli and interlobular septa, a bronchial communication is commonly present which acts like a check valve and causes air trapping.

The type of pulmonary emphysema under discussion in this section is chronic destructive pulmonary emphysema associated with obstructive lung disease. This discussion does *not* pertain to: (1) *senile or atrophic emphysema,* a decreased state of pulmonary elasticity which normally occurs with aging and is accompanied by only minimal impairment of function; (2) *compensatory emphysema,* the simple and nonobstructive overinflation of lung which occurs as lung tissue expands to fill a space produced by the contraction or surgical removal of another pulmonary segment or lobe; (3) *nondestructive overinflation of alveoli* secondary to a check-valve, air-trapping type of bronchial obstruction (produced by tumors, secretions, or foreign bodies obstructing a bronchial lumen or occurring during acute bronchial asthmatic attacks); (4) *skeletal emphysema,* associated with distortion and immobility of the thorax due to kyphosis; or (5) *subcutaneous, mediastinal, or interstitial emphysemas,* which

*Secondary lobules consist of three to five terminal bronchioles and their associated respiratory tissue.

are not pulmonary disorders but result from injuries that cause air leakage into other body tissues or spaces.

Incidence

Emphysema is by far the most common chronic lung condition and is the major cause of pulmonary disability. Emphysema occurs more often than tuberculosis and lung cancer combined.[315]

According to the United States Department of Health, Education, and Welfare, more than 10 million persons in this country have frank emphysema, and more than 20 million others have some form of COPD (e.g., bronchitis, asthma) bordering on emphysema.[38] Chronic bronchitis and emphysema most often occur in cold, damp climates among white males who are middle-aged or older (50 to 70). The incidence of these disorders is increasing among females, however, presumably due to increasing habitual cigarette smoking among women. Currently women are affected in a ratio of less than one to every 10 men. Emphysema is 50 per cent more common among whites than blacks.

Most persons over age 40 who have asthma and chronic bronchitis also have pulmonary emphysema. *Chronic bronchitis and emphysema are the fastest rising causes of death in the United States. Only heart disease surpasses emphysema as a major cause of disability.*[315]

Etiology. We have previously discussed factors of *etiologic* significance in the development of COPD and chronic bronchitis. These factors are of importance also in the development of emphysema. Emphysema is believed to often be a late result of chronic bronchial irritation or infection. It is estimated that more than 90 per cent of persons with pulmonary emphysema smoke heavily; however, emphysema can also occur among nonsmokers. Persons with emphysema often live where air pollution is a constant problem. Possibly a genetic factor is also important in the etiology of emphysema.

Prevention. Measures of importance in the prevention of pulmonary emphysema are the same as those discussed previously pertaining to the prevention of COPD and chronic bronchitis. Because preventative measures may be unsuccessful, efforts are directed also at the early detection of emphysema and related pulmonary disorders.

Pathology. Chronic pulmonary anatomic emphysema is characterized by breakdown of the alveolar walls, alveolar ducts, and respiratory bronchioles. This results in a reduction in the total number of alveoli and the formation of enlarged air spaces in the lung as several alveoli coalesce and form one larger space.

At the time of autopsy or surgery the lungs do not collapse when the chest is opened (normal lungs collapse when atmospheric pressure enters the chest). Grossly, emphysematous lungs appear enlarged, dry, relatively bloodless, and pale. Commonly they contain numerous superficial blebs (air blisters) of different sizes along the margins of the lungs. When cut, the lung surface contains numerous large air spaces which are so enlarged they are visible with the naked eye. Microscopically it can be seen that the alveolar walls are thin, stretched out and, frequently, broken down. The alveoli appear ragged, disrupted, and distended and have lost their elasticity. Instead of multiple minute alveoli honeycombing the lung parenchyma, large air cysts haphazardly occur.

Commonly the bronchi show evidence of chronic bronchitis or atrophy. With atrophy the bronchial walls become thin and dilated and collapse easily. Other pathologic changes typical of chronic bronchitis are frequently also present.

With emphysema a vicious circle of events becomes established that increases the patient's susceptibility to respiratory irritation and infection and allergic reactions. Some events that perpetuate the circle of repeated pulmonary infection include: (1) increased mucus formation; (2) collapse of bronchi during expiration (trapping air, mucus, and germs); (3) ineffective coughing (due to impaired forceful expiration); (4) narrowed bronchial lumina; (5) destruction of cilia (loss of a normal mechanism for cleansing the tracheobronchial tree); (6) mouth breathing (which dries out pulmonary secretions, making them more difficult to expel; and (7) mucus retention (retained mucus serves as a medium for bacterial growth). Infections increase tissue damage in the already damaged lung, thus setting the stage for reinfection.

Destruction of alveolar walls results in the destruction of portions of the pulmonary capillary bed located in the alveolar walls. Thus, the total alveolar surface area of the lungs, where gas exchange occurs, is reduced. Air trapping and the reduction in the number of alveoli (with the subsequent reduction in the blood supply available for gas exchange) produce ventilation and perfusion imbalances that are typically indicated by an elevated $PaCO_2$ and a reduced PaO_2.

The resultant hypoxia causes numerous responses throughout the body. For example, hypoxia produces vasoconstriction and thus further decreases pulmonary blood flow. (Refer back to Chapter 69 for a discussion of the effects of hypoxia.)

Pulmonary hypertension develops because of the reduction in space that has occurred in the pulmonary vascular bed. Eventually the patient develops cor pulmonale and right-sided heart failure.

The altered O_2–CO_2 exchange that occurs with emphysema produces changes "from the bronchial tree to the heart."[263] These changes and the adjustments they require the patient to make are discussed clearly in detail by Schwaid in her article, "The Impact of Emphysema."[263]

Symptoms. Pulmonary emphysema (like chronic bronchitis) has an insidious onset and the illness is often denied until the condition is far advanced. In the earlier stages patients with emphysema commonly attempt to treat themselves with home remedies or over-the-counter patent medicines. Eventually symptom progression forces the patient to seek medical help. Commonly emphysema becomes disabling when the patient is between 45 and 55 years of age.

The major symptom of pulmonary emphysema is shortness of breath, resulting from collapse of the airways upon expiration. Exertional dyspnea is an early symptom, but eventually the patient may become dyspneic even when at rest, especially during episodes of acute bronchial disease. Persistent dyspnea forces the patient to work increasingly harder to move air in and out of his lungs. The greatest difficulty is experienced in exhaling. Although expiration is normally an involuntary action, it becomes an active muscular effort for the emphysematous person. Expiration is prolonged and deflation of the lungs becomes increasingly difficult. The patient must actually "squeeze" the air out of his lungs by producing a positive pressure in the chest. This pressure may collapse the air passages during expiration. Commonly during expiration the neck veins increase in prominence and the patient breathes through his mouth, pursing his lips (to help to keep the air passages open). Wheezing may be audible during expiration. Inspiration is usually short and rapid.

Wheezing and rales occur in proportion to the amount of bronchitis present. When percussed the lungs give an exceptionally resonant note. Breath sounds are faint. Respirations tend to be shallow and rapid. The patient may breathe as frequently as 25 to 30 times per minute and still not get enough oxygen. The patient with established emphysema often has some cyanosis (i.e., blueness of the fingernail beds, lips, ear lobes, and skin) and clubbing of the fingertips. The face may be pale or may be ruddy to ruddy-cyanotic. (The latter reflects anoxia and compensatory polycythemia.)

Gradually changes occur in the shape and size of the chest as a result of pulmonary overdistention and air trapping. Eventually the patient develops a characteristic "barrel-shaped" chest in which the chest appears hyperinflated, i.e., rounded chest and back (dorsal kyphosis), ribs in a more horizontal position, and enlarged anteroposterior diameter of the chest (Fig. 71–13). The chest is then rigid and fixed in an inspiratory position and the lungs are chronically hyperexpanded. A reduction occurs in the normal rise and fall of the chest during ventilation; the entire thorax tends to move vertically as a unit. The ribs become fixed at their joints, and the work of breathing increases greatly. The patient experiences a feeling of tightness in his chest. Diaphragmatic movement is absent or severely impaired and the diaphragm becomes flattened. The flattened diaphragm depresses the liver.

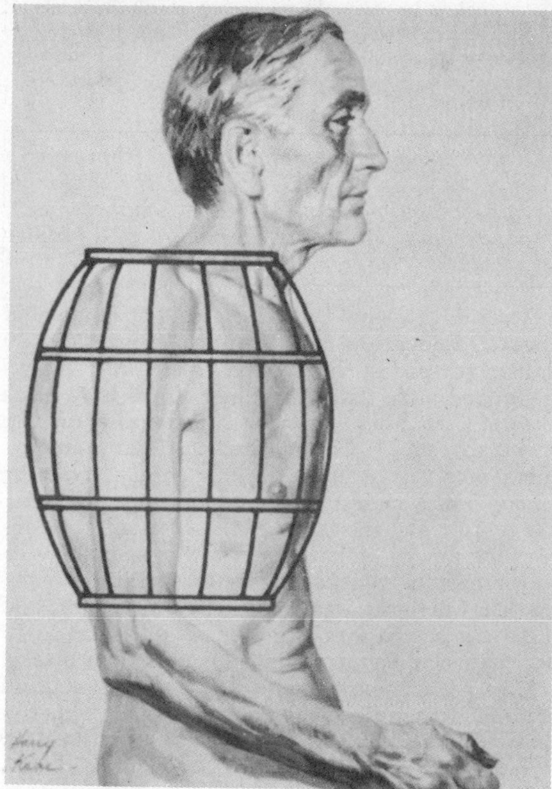

FIGURE 71–13. The common "barrel chest" condition of the patient with emphysema. (Knoll Pharmaceutical Co.)

The rigid chest cage forces the patient to overuse his abdominal and upper intercostal muscles and also to use the accessory muscles of respiration (sternocleidomastoids, scaleni, pectorals) to ventilate his lungs. The muscles in the chest and upper neck are held taut to help with ventilation. Even during quiet ventilation the neck muscles are used. The neck appears to be shortened because the neck muscles are tense and contracted. Typically the patient sits leaning forward with his hands on his knees and his shoulders elevated (Fig. 71–14). This position helps to elevate the diaphragm. During expiration the patient sometimes manually presses on his diaphragm. The patient with emphysema speaks in short jerky sentences and usually appears anxious and gaunt. Even minor physical exertion may produce extreme respiratory distress and fatigue.

In addition to dyspnea, a chronic productive cough is another frequent symptom of emphysema. Even though the cough is productive, it is usually inefficient and only small amounts of sputum are raised. Morning paroxysms of coughing commonly occur that produce thick, viscous sputum. Cough is typically spasmodic, fatiguing, hard, and initiated by even minimal exertion (e.g., talking). Severe episodes of coughing may produce nausea and vomiting. Intercurrent acute respiratory infections and cold, damp weather aggravate the cough.

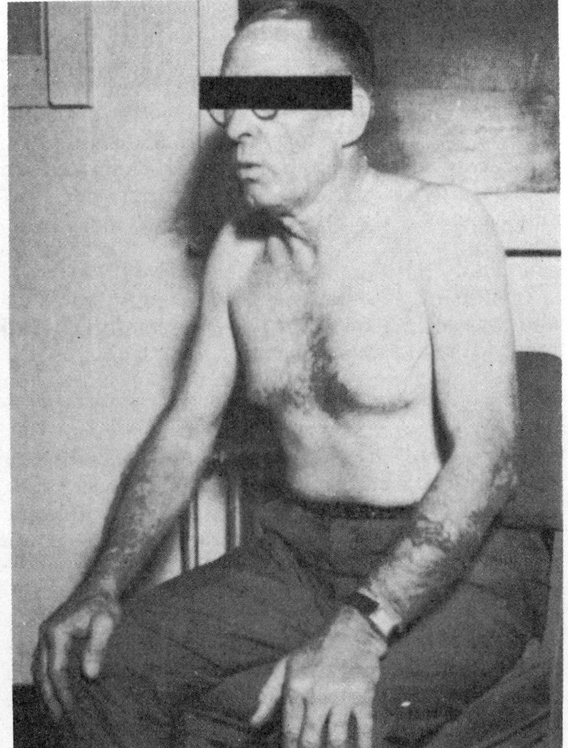

FIGURE 71-14. Clues to emphysema. Note posture: leaning forward, arms on knees, to elevate the diaphragm. Pursed lips help keep air passages open while exhaling. Muscles in neck, upper chest are taut as they help in work of breathing. (From Whatley, J. L.: Battle for breath. *Today's Health,* February, 1967.)

Symptoms of right-sided heart failure (e.g., peripheral edema, venous distention) may be present with advanced emphysema. Prior to the development of heart failure, dyspnea may be relieved by lying down flat. However, once heart failure develops, dyspnea becomes continuous and is unrelieved by reclining. Persons with advanced emphysema have a rapid heart rate.

Hypoxia, respiratory acidosis, and the increased muscular effort necessary for ventilation produce lethargy, anorexia, weakness, and weight loss. Respiratory function is severely impaired in advanced emphysema. Deficient oxygenation of the brain and high CO_2 levels in the blood may produce mental changes, e.g., impaired memory, poor judgment, confusion, lethargy, possibly coma. With severe ventilatory insufficiency the patient may experience impairments of sensorium and headache; papilledema, miosis and asterixis (flapping tremor) are observable.

In patients with pulmonary emphysema death most usually results from heart failure (caused by cor pulmonale), an acute bronchopulmonary infection, or respiratory failure. Other complications that can be fatal include spontaneous pneumothorax, pulmonary thromboembolism, or peptic ulcer. Deaths from emphysema have reportedly increased fourfold in the past decade.

Diagnosis. History and *physical examination* demonstrate many of the characteristic symptoms discussed above, e.g., exertional dyspnea with an insidious onset, wheezing, prolonged expiration, chronic productive cough, barrel chest, use of accessory muscles of respiration. Medical history frequently includes heavy smoking for a number of years and repeated pulmonary infections which have increasingly left the patient short of breath upon exertion.

Chest x-ray may appear normal until emphysema is in its advanced stages (Fig. 71-15). With advanced emphysema x-ray findings may include: (1) overaeration of the lungs (i.e., on x-ray lung parenchyma does not appear normally darkened); (2) increased vascularity at lung peripheries; (3) abnormal heart size and position; (4) increased anteroposterior chest diameter; (5) enlarged lungs; (6) low flat diaphragm images; (7) widening of the rib spaces; and (8) large cysts that appear as ringlike or annular translucencies. The latter changes are referred to as "vanishing lung."

Fluoroscopy may reveal difficulty with expiration, low, flat diaphragms that move poorly during ventilation, and limited rib motion during inspiration.

Scintillation scanning and *pulmonary angiog-*

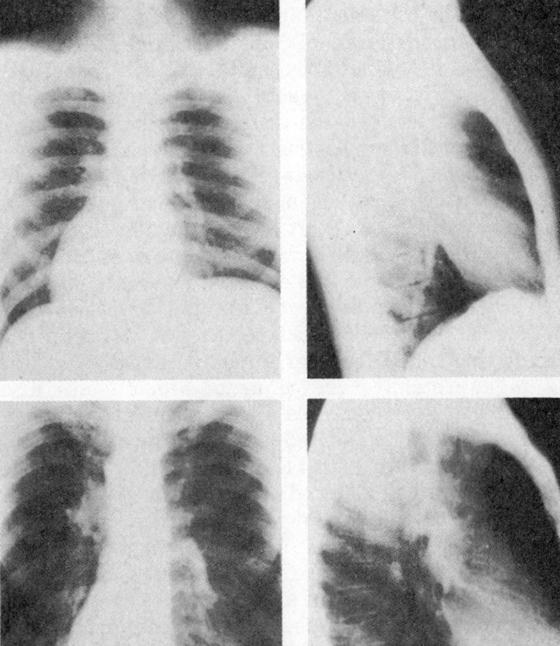

FIGURE 71-15. Lungs of healthy adult (top row) compared with lungs of patient with moderately severe emphysema. Top x-rays show normal degree of darkness; diaphragm is "domed"; rib interspaces are not widened; and heart outline is not enlarged. Bottom x-rays show increased blackening due to excess retained air; diaphragm is flattened; rib interspaces are widened; and lateral view shows "barrel chest." (From Whatley, J. L.: Battle for breath. *Today's Health,* February, 1967.)

raphy help the physician to evaluate the non-affected areas of the lungs (especially helpful if pulmonary surgery is being considered). Radioactive gas studies of ventilation-perfusion relationships show that patients with pulmonary emphysema have abnormalities of both perfusion and ventilation. Bronchograms usually demonstrate a characteristic "tree in winter" effect, in which the smaller "branches" and "foilage" are not outlined. Also, bronchograms show changes in the bronchi typical of chronic bronchitis.

Pulmonary function tests are useful in confirming a diagnosis of pulmonary emphysema and evaluating the condition. Characteristic findings are reduced maximal breathing capacity, reduced forced expiratory volume, slow maximal midexpiratory flow, increased residual volume, and reduced expiratory reserve volume. The vital capacity may be normal even with extensive disease; however, the timed vital capacity is commonly reduced. Exercise tolerance tests may produce severe, frightening respiratory distress.

If equipment is not available to measure pulmonary function it is possible to roughly evaluate lung function in the following ways: First, see if the patient can blow out a lighted match that is held 6 inches from his open mouth. The match must be blown out by exhaling air forcefully through the open mouth, i.e., without pursing the lips. If this "match test" cannot be performed, severe ventilatory obstruction is generally present. The second test consists of timing (with an ordinary watch that has a second hand, or with a stop watch) the rate at which the total vital capacity can be exhaled with maximum effort. Normal emptying time is 3 seconds; moderate obstructive disease is present if emptying time is 5 to 6 seconds. Severe obstructive disease is present if emptying time is greater than 7 seconds.

Measurements are made of *blood gases* and blood pH (acid-alkali balance). Arterial oxyhemoglobin saturation is reduced. Ventilatory insufficiency results in alveolar hypoxia and, hence, the blood's PaO_2 is reduced. Also, because the lungs cannot effectively blow off CO_2, the $PaCO_2$ increases (hypercapnia). Although this developing respiratory acidosis can be compensated for at first by the retention of bicarbonate by the kidneys, eventually this compensatory mechanism fails (indicated by falling of blood pH) and the respiratory acidosis worsens progressively. Blood pH may remain normal, even in the presence of respiratory acidosis, until failure of the compensatory mechanisms occurs. To buffer increased amounts of carbonic acid the serum bicarbonates are elevated.

As a result of secondary polycythemia, the red blood cell count and packed cell volume (sedimentation rate) may be increased. The white blood cell count is normal with emphysema; however, it is elevated in the presence of acute infections.

An electrocardiogram may be performed to evaluate the patient's cardiac status.

Clinical Care. Clinical care for patients with pulmonary emphysema is basically similar to that previously discussed for COPD, chronic bronchial asthma, and chronic bronchitis. Similarities in care occur because bronchospasm is a problem common in all these disorders. (Refer back to previous sections as necessary. Specific procedures, e.g., oxygen therapy, postural drainage, are discussed more completely in Chapter 70.)

Treatment of emphysema is basically palliative and focuses on helping the patient to maintain tidal respiration (without excessive effort) during the greatest possible range of exercise. To accomplish this goal, efforts are directed at preventing and/or minimizing pulmonary infections, improving pulmonary circulation and ventilation, and reducing bronchial spasm and edema and hypersecretion of mucus. Techniques of pulmonary physiotherapy are employed to make the maximum use of the respiratory muscles. Also, intermittent positive pressure breathing is frequently used and medications are given to reduce airway obstruction. The patient must work hard to maintain an optimal level of activity in spite of increasing rigidity of the chest wall in a position of expansion. Because pulmonary emphysema forces the affected individual to make numerous life changes, emotional care is highly important.

Plan nursing care of the emphysematous patient in such a manner that the patient's breathlessness will not be excessively worsened. Provide frequent rest periods. In writing about his own experiences as a victim of emphysema W. R. Jones comments:

> Anyone working with this breathless part of the population should have some physical realization of how these people must live and breathe. Take a *full* deep breath, then let out only *one-third* of it, and continue to breathe out while retaining that *two-thirds* of the original breath for the better part of a day. Each breath will be only partial; the retained portion becomes essentially toxic, and every tissue of your body takes the rap. If you do this conscientiously, you will be breathing somewhat in the manner of a patient with emphysema—except that he will do this about 20,000 times a day and over 7,000,000 times a year.[150]

ASSISTING VENTILATION. IPPB may be used alone or combined with oxygen or drug therapy (administered through the machine in nebulized form). The physician specifies the pressure to be applied by the IPPB device and the composition of the air to be forced into the lungs. Oxygen may be administered diluted, undiluted, or mixed with medications (e.g., bronchodilators). Intermittent pauses in the pressure make it possible for the patient to exhale.

The indiscriminate prolonged administration of O_2 at ambient pressure to patients in respiratory acidosis may remove the final remaining stimulus to respiration (i.e., hypoxia), and therefore produce hypoventilation, increasing acidosis, respiratory failure, and coma. Although oxygen therapy is often necessary for the patient with emphysema, it is used with great caution to prevent CO_2 narcosis and at low flow rates, 2 to 3 liters per minute nasally. The patient is observed frequently for indications of CO_2 narcosis. (See Chapters 25 and 70.) When oxygen therapy is started the PaO_2, $PaCO_2$ and arterial blood pH are monitored. When monitoring is not available, IPPB ventilatory assistance is also used (15 to 30 minutes every 1 to 4 hours) until the patient is clinically improved. IPPB or a tank respirator can be helpful in removing retained CO_2 by hyperventilating the patient. IPPB is a safe way to give O_2 because it also ensures adequate ventilation and removes CO_2. If severe respiratory depression appears to be developing (e.g., from CO_2 narcosis, excessive administration of narcotics, or sedatives), respiratory stimulating medications may be indicated, e.g., N,N-diethylvanillamide (ethamivan).

An external portable body respirator, called an "extrathoracic assisted breathing device" (ETAB), is sometimes used to assist with ventilation. This device is especially useful in emphysema because it helps the patient to exhale by forcing air out of the lungs.

Patients who give their own IPPB or oxygen treatments at home must be warned that the excessive use of O_2 can be dangerous and may actually suppress breathing rather than making breathing easier. By comparing oxygen to a drug that must be used only as prescribed, the patient may be helped to realize that excesses can be dangerous.

It is essential that the patient with emphysema be well hydrated (to prevent dehydration and to thin secretions) and that optimum tracheobronchial hygiene be maintained by postural drainage, expectorants, aerosols, and humidification of inspired air. Suctioning is performed as necessary. Some patients benefit from tracheostomy, since this procedure reduces the dead space and facilitates suctioning and IPPB ventilation. (Care of the patient with tracheostomy is discussed in Unit XXII).

CONTROLLING COUGH. Mild cough depressants are indicated if cough is very fatiguing or nonproductive; sedatives and narcotics are contraindicated since they depress respirations. Ineffective coughing is discouraged since it worsens the patient's disorder by enlarging emphysematous cystic spaces, slowing down even further the escape of air from the alveoli, and compressing normal lung tissue. Coughing produces a sudden increase in intrabronchial pressure, which is not evenly distributed throughout the emphysematous lung. This pressure increase, associated with unequal airway resistance in the bronchi, may increase alveolar damage.

BREATHING EXERCISES. Breathing exercises and exercises that strengthen the abdominal muscles and facilitate more complete exhalation are taught to the patient with emphysema. The patient learns to become aware of his diaphragm, how to use the diaphragm more effectively during ventilation (by developing a slow, relaxed pattern of abdominal breathing), and how to maintain the diaphragm's optimal mechanical efficiency. During exercise the patient may benefit from long-term oxygen therapy administered from lightweight portable containers of liquid oxygen. An elasticized abdominal support ("abdominal belt") may be prescribed for the patient to wear since emphysema flattens the diaphragm. By pushing the diaphragm back up into the thorax the belt facilitates expiration if the patient cannot learn efficient abdominal breathing control with breathing exercises. The support exerts pressure upward from below the umbilicus. Breathing exercises, improved posture, and mild physical exercise help the patient to combat respiratory insufficiency as a result of reduced lung compliance and restricted pulmonary excursion.

OTHER MEASURES. Allergic responses increase bronchospasm and must therefore be prevented or controlled by desensitization to known allergens. (Refer back to discussion of bronchial asthma.) Bronchodilators are administered to relieve bronchospasm and increase airway patency. Adrenal corticosteroids, e.g., prednisone, may be required if other measures fail to relieve bronchospasm.

COMPLICATIONS. Observe the patient closely for the development of possible complications of emphysema, e.g., spontaneous pneumothorax (as a result of rupture of a bleb or bulla), acute respiratory infections, peptic ulcer, anemia, cor pulmonale, respiratory failure. *Early* treatment of these conditions is imperative and may be started as a result of the nurse's alert observations. Because acute respiratory infections can be fatal in the presence of emphysema, every attempt is made to prevent or minimize them, e.g., by annual influenza immunizations. The patient should know the danger signals of infection and see his doctor if they begin to develop. Antibiotics are given to control chronic infections and to treat acute infections. Some patients require prolonged antimicrobial therapy. When specific bacterial sensitivity cannot be determined, tetracycline may be given. Cor pulmonale and respiratory failure are late complications. Emphysema is the most common cause of chronic cor pulmonale and chronic pulmonary insufficiency. (Treatment of patients with respiratory insufficiency or respiratory failure was discussed earlier in this unit.)

REHABILITATION AND EMOTIONAL CARE. The nurse focuses rehabilitation on helping the emphysematous patient (and his family) to learn ways of controlling his symptoms and minimizing their effects. Self-care is encouraged for as many activities as possible, for as long as possible. The patient must learn to live within his limitations and to routinely follow recommendations made by his physician and other health services personnel. Patient teaching may be difficult if the patient is severely hypoxic, because mental acuity may be reduced.

Chronic destructive pulmonary diseases, such as COPD and pulmonary emphysema, create numerous *emotional* and *socioeconomic problems* for patients and their families. Progressive invalidism is both emotionally and financially burdensome, requiring changes in life patterns and withdrawal from many of the normal activities of daily life. Often patients with these disorders pass through periods of denial of their illnesses, before their obvious loss of health forces them to seek help. Even then many patients are unable to stop smoking or to comply with other recommendations, even though they are told that the prohibited activities worsen their physical disorders.

Obviously, crushing psychologic problems occur with diseases that are as devastating as pulmonary emphysema and COPD. *Total* patient care must include recognition of psychopathologic reactions in addition to awareness of pathophysiology. Suicide occurs fairly commonly in men with emphysema.[214] (For additional discussion read bibliography numbers 214, 263, and 265).

SURGICAL TREATMENT. Some patients with pulmonary emphysema benefit from the *surgical resection* of large, solitary bullae (confined to one area of the lung) or the removal of nonfunctioning pulmonary tissue. Bullae may compress the normal lung tissue next to them. Breathing efficiency is improved by the removal of nonfunctioning lung tissue in some persons. Only selected patients with emphysema are candidates for surgical therapy. Surgical procedures that attempt to improve pulmonary blood circulation or cut nerves to make breathing easier (i.e., carotid body surgery or glomectomy) have not been successful.

PULMONARY EMBOLISM AND PULMONARY INFARCTION

Refer to Unit XIII for a discussion of these topics.

PNEUMOCONIOSES ("DUST DISEASES")

The word "pneumoconiosis" is a very general term which simply means that dust is retained in the lungs. Disease-producing dusts typically cause a fibrous tissue reaction in the lungs and produce symptoms such as shortness of breath, chronic cough, and mucus production. Disease-producing dusts tend to be those associated with certain occupations. The familiar dusts of smoke-filled cities, gravel or dirt roads, and household dusts do not produce pneumoconioses.

Silicosis is the best known of the pneumoconioses because it is the most common and most crippling. Silicosis was formerly called silicotuberculosis; other common names for silicosis include "stonecutter's disease," "miner's phthisis," "potter's asthma" and "grinder's rot." Silicosis results from the occupational inhalation of dust containing free silica. This disorder may occur in mining, granite cutting and polishing, foundries, sandblasting, pottery manufacturing, and concrete breaking. Silicosis produces fibrous pulmonary nodules or diffuse pulmonary fibrosis, which may increasingly impair lung function. Silicosis develops in direct proportion to the percentage and concentration of silica and the duration of exposure.

Symptoms of advanced silicosis may include shortness of breath upon exertion, cough, wheezing, expectoration of dark gray to black sputum with pulmonary infections, and chest pains. Chronic bronchitis and pulmonary emphysema often occur with advanced silicosis. *The main complication of silicosis is pulmonary tuberculosis.* Multiplication of tubercle bacilli appears to be stimulated by the cellular toxicity of silica. Silicosis causes irreversible lung damage. *Treatment* of advanced cases is similar to that previously described for COPD, e.g., IPPB, bronchodilators, and the antimicrobial treatment of intercurrent infections. Treatment of chronic bronchitis and pulmonary emphysema have also been discussed.

Examples of other pneumoconioses include:

- *Anthracosilicosis,* caused by inhalation of a combination of coal dust and silica.
- *Asbestosis,* caused by inhalation of asbestos fibers.
- *Bagassosis,* caused by inhalation of dust from pressed sugar cane stalks.
- *Baritosis,* caused by inhalation of dust from barium sulfate.
- *Berylliosis,* caused by inhalation of beryllium dust (a metal that is inert except in sensitized individuals).
- *Byssinosis,* caused by inhalation of cotton dust.
- *Farmer's lung,* caused by inhalation of dust from moldy hay.
- *Siderosis,* caused by inhalation of dust of iron oxide.
- *Stannosis,* caused by inhalation of dust of tin oxide.

Of the above pneumoconioses the following are benign, i.e., they do not cause pulmonary fibrosis, impaired lung function or increased susceptibility to tuberculosis: bagassosis, baritosis, byssinosis, farmer's lung, siderosis, and stannosis.

Because pneumoconioses result from occupational exposures to certain dusts, the *prevention* of these disorders is often possible. Most pneumoconioses can be prevented by the implementation of safety practices designed to reduce hazardous dust levels. Nurses in public health and occupational health positions are active in the prevention and early detection of pneumoconioses.

CHAPTER 72

Injuries to the Chest

"The thorax presents a fairly large exposed portion of the body that is particularly vulnerable to impact forces. Grave thoracic injuries are becoming more frequent; injuries to the thorax and vital structures contained in the thoracic cavity cause more severe and fatal injuries than do head and facial injuries. Chest injury is a major killing injury, necessitating urgency of treatment."[267]

CAUSES AND TYPES OF INJURIES

Accident prevention is highly important in reducing the number of chest injuries, since these injuries often result from falls, the use of machines, and the use of potentially lethal weapons, e.g., knives, guns. Chest injuries frequently result from automobile accidents in which the driver is thrown against the steering wheel and the occupants are thrown against the dashboard or front seat. The nurse can contribute to accident prevention in many settings by participating in safety education programs and encouraging enforcement of safety precautions, e.g., slip-proof mats in bathtubs and showers, seat belts and shoulder straps in automobiles. Some chest injuries result from seemingly innocuous activities. For example, the ribs may be fractured from the strain of severe coughing or sneezing.

Normal respiratory function requires integrity of the tracheobronchial tree, lungs, diaphragm, pleurae, and thoracic wall. Additionally, the heart and cardiovascular system must be intact. These various structures may be damaged by chest injuries. The major dangers associated with chest injuries are punctured organs deep within the body (e.g., heart, lungs) and internal bleeding. As with other injuries, chest injuries range from relatively minor bumps and scrapes to severe crushing or penetrating injuries that are rapidly fatal because of cardiopulmonary damage.

Chest injuries may be of a penetrating or nonpenetrating (blunt) nature. Blast injuries, e.g., caused by explosions, may rupture pulmonary alveoli and vessels. Hemorrhage and asphyxiation then often cause death. Crushing chest injuries may fracture ribs and seriously compress and damage the lungs and heart. Penetrating chest wounds (e.g., from bullets, knives, flying shrapnel, or splinters) may cause an open chest wound that permits atmospheric air to enter the pleural space and disrupt the normal mechanisms of ventilation. Additionally, penetrating chest wounds may seriously damage the lungs, heart, and other thoracic structures.

Head injuries frequently coexist with chest injuries and may modify the treatment of the chest injury. The patient with a concomitant head injury must be protected from anoxia, which may result from an inadequately treated chest injury. Therefore, a tracheostomy may need to be performed even though it may not be necessary for treatment of the chest injury.

GENERAL MANAGEMENT OF THE CHEST-INJURED PATIENT

After the chest-injured patient is given emergency care, he is examined more thoroughly and a chest x-ray is taken to specifically identify and evaluate injuries. An electrocardiogram is also performed to ascertain possible cardiac injury. A complete history is helpful to the physician as he attempts to rapidly evaluate the extent of the patient's injury.

The nurse may help to obtain information of importance concerning the accident from the patient or witnesses. It is beneficial to know:[100] the identity, velocity, and pathway of the wounding agent; the type and speed of the vehicle; and, if the patient was in a car, whether he was restrained by seat belts or thrown by the impact. Information of this nature helps the physician to assess injury to regional as well as distant anatomic structures.

A thorough physical examination of the chest (front and back) with the patient completely undressed is performed to look for indications of injury. Subtle changes or physical findings can be highly important in evaluating the chest-injured patient.

Geiger[100] summarizes some of the important basic techniques used for the physical diagnosis of chest injuries.

> *Inspection and observation:* (1) Determine the level of consciousness, emotional state, or degree of apprehension; (2) note the color of mucosa, nail beds, and the presence and degree of cyanosis or pallor; (3) evaluate the respiratory pattern and rate, and the use of accessory muscles of respiration; (4) note the status of cervical pulses and veins; (5) determine whether injury is closed or contused and search for wounds of entrance and exit; (6) note character and amount of sputum or tracheal secretions.

> *Palpation and percussion:* (1) Determine equality

and amplitude of pulses; (2) determine cardiac size and location of apical impulse; (3) evaluate chest expansion and check for areas of hyperresonance or dullness; (4) determine areas of tenderness or pain, abnormal mobility of ribs or sternum, tracheal shift, or crepitation.

> *Auscultation:* (1) Evaluate breath sounds; (2) assess cardiac sounds; (3) determine blood pressure in both arms and legs, when indicated.

Treatment of chest injuries may include closed chest drainage and/or thoracotomy. (Both topics are discussed in Chapter 73.) Thoracotomy is necessary for only about one out of 10 chest-injured patients. Whether or not chest surgery is necessary, much of the clinical care given the chest-injured patient is similar to that given postoperatively following chest surgery. (Refer to Chapter 73 as necessary.) Some general activities of importance in caring for any chest-injured patient are discussed briefly below.

Maintain Patent Airway. This can be done by correctly positioning the patient to prevent aspiration, suctioning as necessary, and turning and "coughing" the patient at least hourly. The airway may be obstructed by mucus, bone fragments, broken teeth or dentures, blood and/or vomitus.

Ensure Adequate Ventilation. Some patients require oxygen, endotracheal intubation, tracheostomy, assisted ventilation, or full mechanical ventilation. Carefully evaluate blood gas reports and the patient's general respiratory status, e.g., rate of respiration, chest movements, dyspnea. The head-elevated position makes breathing easier and is usually the most comfortable position for the conscious chest-injured patient. (Positioning and care of unconscious patients is discussed in Unit VIII. Tracheostomy and endotracheal intubation are discussed in Unit XXII.)

If a patient does not ventilate normally after the upper airway is established, or if his condition continues to deteriorate without an obvious cause, undetected injuries may be present, e.g., hemothorax, pneumothorax, flail chest, ruptured bronchus, cardiac tamponade, ruptured thoracic aorta.[279] Immediately notify the physician of the patient's condition so further evaluation can be made. (Treatment of complications is discussed below.)

Assist with Diagnostic and Therapeutic Procedures as Indicated. Thoracentesis, bronchoscopic aspiration, chest drainage tube insertion, tracheostomy, or endotracheal intubation may need to be done. *Maintain effective functioning of equipment* such as that used for respiratory therapy and closed chest drainage.

Replace Blood Loss and Prevent or Treat Shock. Shock often accompanies chest injuries and should be closely observed for and treated early. (See Chapter 26.) Upon admission of the patient a blood sample is taken for typing and cross-matching, so that blood loss can be replaced. Until these laboratory results are available the patient is given a blood substitute, such as plasma or dextran. Examine the patient carefully for external bleeding and estimate blood loss. Observe also for symptoms of internal bleeding: pallor, restlessness, cold clammy skin, low blood pressure, empty veins, and rapid thready pulse. Internal bleeding may result from injuries to the thoracic or abdominal viscera, torn muscles, or fractures. Bleeding into the pleural space may be of a large amount (e.g., 2 or more liters) but can usually be rapidly detected. Hemorrhage into areas such as the chest wall, as from torn intercostal muscles, is more difficult to detect. A liter of blood can accumulate between the chest wall muscles within the chest wall planes without producing much swelling.

Immediately call to the physician's attention any indications of hemorrhage. The volume of blood replacement is determined by the physician after he evaluates clinical findings, laboratory reports (e.g., hemoglobin, packed cell volume), and central venous pressure. Rapid blood replacement is essential in the management of thoracic injuries. As Clarke observes:

> Blood loss acquires an additional significance when respiration is impaired by damage to the lungs and chest wall. The loss of a pint of blood may be critical in a patient already hypoxic because of crippled ventilation, for not only is oxygen transport impeded, but the diminution in cardiac output associated with haemorrhage may lead to systemic capillary vasoconstriction and poor tissue perfusion. This gives rise to a metabolic acidosis in addition to the respiratory acidosis associated with lung trauma.[53]

Prevent, Observe for and Treat Other Complications. Observe the patient closely for symptoms of cardiopulmonary dysfunction. Report immediately symptoms indicative of complications, e.g., dyspnea, sudden sharp chest pain, blood-streaked sputum, agitation. Because indications of complications may not appear immediately, continued close observation is essential for the newly injured patient. Observe for symptoms of previously undetected injuries, e.g., fractures, abdominal injuries.

Prevent complications associated with inactivity as discussed in Chapter 27. Promote effective tracheobronchial secretion movement and removal. Supervise and encourage periodic coughing, deep breathing, turning, and exercise. Instruct the patient to make a conscious effort to breathe deeply during normal respiration since he will tend to breathe shallowly to minimize pain. Encourage productive coughing because it removes sputum and other tracheobronchial secretions and prevents them from pooling and becoming potential sources of infection and obstruction. Administer antibiotics as prescribed to combat pulmonary infection, which may result from trauma and infected secretions.

Control Pain Without Causing Excessive Depression of Respirations or Cough. Cautiously administer analgesics as indicated. Analgesics help the patient by making deep breaths and coughing more comfortably possible, minimizing pain, and permitting periods of rest and relaxation. Pain associated with coughing may be minimized by "splinting" the patient's chest when he coughs. (See Chapter 73.) Atropine, morphine, and barbiturates are contraindicated because they cause respiratory depression. Mild sedation and frequent small doses of meperidine (Demerol) may control pain. Nerve blocks may also be helpful.

Maintain Fluid-Electrolyte Balance and Nourishment. When administering I.V.'s to the chest-injured patient remember the possible danger of pulmonary edema and watch for symptoms of this complication. Pulmonary edema can occur if impaired pulmonary circulation is overloaded with fluid. Maintain an accurate intake and output record to guide fluid replacement. I.V. feedings are given until it is safe for food to enter the stomach. Oral intake may be temporarily contraindicated because of abdominal injury, nausea, surgery, or impaired consciousness. Once it is no longer necessary to keep the stomach empty, unconscious patients are given nasogastric tube feedings and conscious patients are started on a light diet.

Attempt to Calm the Patient and Enlist his Cooperation. The chest-injured patient may be in extreme cardiopulmonary distress and therefore highly fearful and anxious. Efficient, skillful actions on the part of calm, reassuring attending personnel can help the patient to relax somewhat and breathe more effectively.

Figure 72-1 illustrates some treatment procedures that may be utilized in the clinical care of the chest-injured patient. Intensive nursing care is essential for the severely injured patient.

COMPLICATIONS OF CHEST INJURIES

Severe trauma to the chest may produce numerous complications. Among these are:

> Hemothorax, pneumothorax (open or closed), hemopneumothorax.

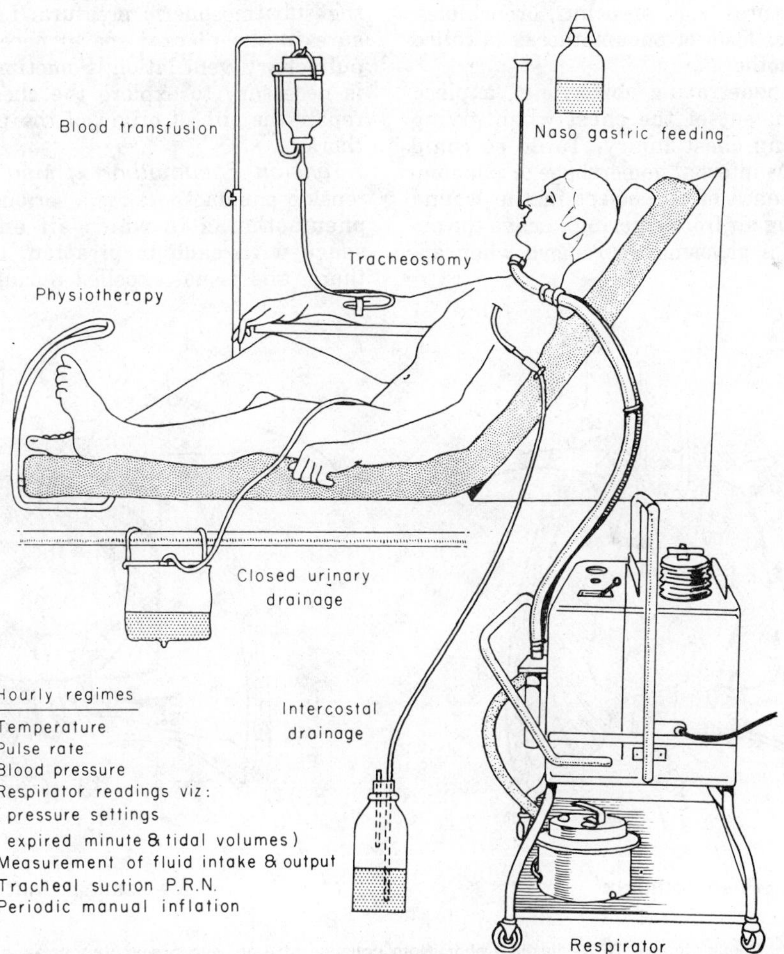

FIGURE 72-1. Some treatment procedures which may be utilized in the clinical care of the chest-injured patient. (From Ambiavagar, M.: *Journal of Postgraduate Medicine, 43*:256, April, 1967.)

> Mediastinal flutter, mediastinal shift.
> Lung compression, lung laceration.
> Fractured ribs, flail chest, paradoxical motion.
> Subcutaneous emphysema, mediastinal emphysema.
> Injuries to the diaphragm and/or mediastinal contents, cardiac tamponade.
> Wet-lung syndrome.
> Shock, severe pain, dyspnea.
> Tracheal and/or bronchial tears.

Hemothorax; Pneumothorax; Hemopneumothorax

Chest injuries frequently cause hemothorax (blood in the pleural space), *pneumothorax* (air in the pleural space), or *hemopneumothorax* (both blood and air in the chest cavity). These conditions were briefly discussed in Chapter 71. Blood in the chest cavity results from pulmonary lacerations or torn intercostal blood vessels. Air may enter the pleural space directly through a hole in the chest wall ("open" pneumothorax) or diaphragm, or it may escape into the pleural space from a puncture or tear in one of the internal respiratory structures, e.g., bronchus, bronchioles, alveoli. The latter form of pneumothorax is called a "closed" pneumothorax.

Never pull a penetrating object, e.g., a piece of steel or wood, out of the chest when giving first aid following chest injury. To do so could precipitate serious internal hemorrhage or pneumothorax (the presence of the object in the wound may be preventing air from entering). Leave the object in place for a physician to remove when appropriate.

Indications of pneumothorax include hyperresonance on percussion, diminished breath sounds, and pain. Chest x-rays may reveal a slight shift of the trachea away from the affected side and retraction of the lung back from the parietal pleura. If the physician suspects a pneumothorax (but the patient's respiratory distress is so severe that there is not enough time for x-ray confirmation), he may insert an 18-gauge needle into the second interspace in the midclavicular line. Aspiration will then demonstrate whether free air is present.

Accumulations of blood, fluids, and air in the pleural space cause positive pressure to build up in that area. (Remember: negative pressure normally exists in the pleural space.) As the pressure build-up increases it begins to collapse the lung and impair respiratory exchange; the patient becomes dyspneic and frequently goes into shock (Figure 72–2).

Immediately following chest injury *emergency thoracentesis* may be performed to remove accumulations of air, blood, or secretions. These emergency needle aspirations may prevent death from cardiopulmonary failure. Next, a catheter may be placed in the pleural space and connected to *closed-chest drainage.* The catheter permits the continuous escape of air, secretions, and blood and helps the lung to reexpand by reestablishing the subatmospheric pressure (i.e., negative pressure in the pleural space) necessary for normal pulmonary ventilation. Sometimes a *thoracotomy* is necessary to explore the chest and surgically repair the site of origin of the pneumo- or hemothorax.

Tension Pneumothorax; Mediastinal Shift. A tension pneumothorax is a serious valvular type of pneumothorax in which air enters the pleural space with each inspiration, becomes *trapped* there, and is not expelled during expiration. The

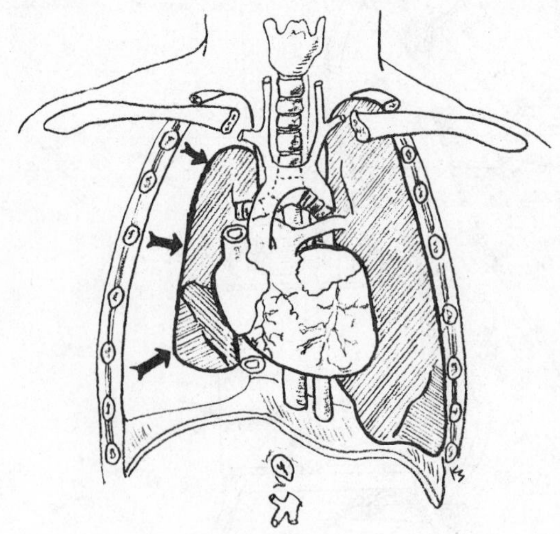

Pneumothorax

A

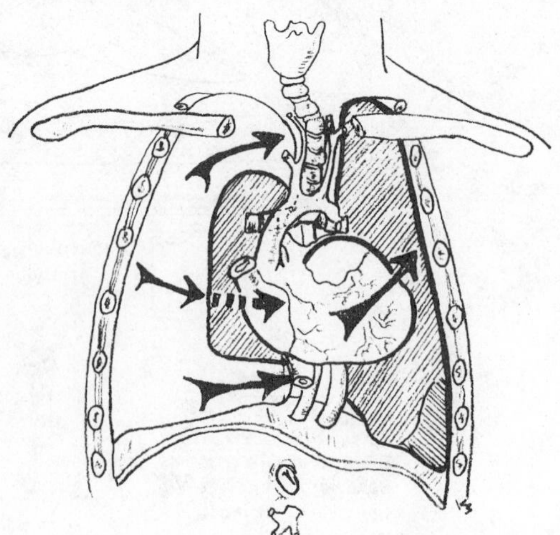

Mediastinal Shift

B

FIGURE 72–2. A, Pneumothorax. B, Mediastinal shift. Note collapse of lung with pneumothorax as air gathers in pleural space. With mediastinal shift, in addition to collapse of the lung, the mediastinal contents are displaced against unaffected side of chest.

trapped air continues to build up pressure in the chest as the amount of air accumulating in the pleural space increases with every inspiration.

If untreated, as the intrapleural pressure or tension increases it *collapses the lung* on the affected side and then may cause a *mediastinal shift* (Fig. 72–2). A "mediastinal shift" means that the contents of the mediastinum (heart, trachea, esophagus, great vessels) are pushed or "shifted" toward the unaffected side of the chest. Mediastinal shift may cause compression of the lung in the direction of the shift (i.e., the lung opposite the pneumothorax) and compression, traction, torsion, or kinking of the great vessels (e.g., vena cava), thus dangerously impairing blood return to the heart.

Tension pneumothorax produces serious circulatory and pulmonary impairment which can rapidly be fatal. Tension pneumothorax is a high priority surgical emergency that must be promptly diagnosed and treated.

Symptoms of *tension pneumothorax* include: marked dyspnea; subcutaneous emphysema (trapped air escapes into the subcutaneous tissue of the chest wall causing the tissue to swell up and feel spongy); cyanosis; acute chest pain; shift of the trachea to the opposite side; tympany on percussion, hyperresonance, and reduced or absent breath sounds on the affected side; increased pulse and respiratory rates; feeling of pressure within the chest; and decreased movement of the affected side of the chest on inspiration.

Indications of *mediastinal shift* include cyanosis, severe dyspnea, deviation of the larynx and trachea from their normal midline position in the neck toward the side of the chest opposite the pneumothorax, and a change either medially or laterally in the heart beat's position of maximum impulse (normally near the midclavicular line in the fifth interspace). Some symptoms of mediastinal shift are similar to those produced by congestive heart failure, e.g., displacement of the trachea to one side, distended neck veins, dyspnea, and increased pulse and respiratory rates. Because no blood is available for cardiac output, the patient's blood pressure cannot be obtained in the presence of severe mediastinal shift. A suspected mediastinal shift may be confirmed by x-ray or by directly measuring intrapleural pressure with an open-end "U" manometer. Laryngeal and tracheal deviation can be detected by gentle palpation as well as by x-ray.

The *immediate treatment* of a tension pneumothorax is to convert the tension pneumothorax into an open pneumothorax (a less serious disorder) by providing an escape route for the air or fluid in the pleural space on the affected side. This can be accomplished most easily and rapidly by simply inserting a needle into the pleural space. If thoracentesis equipment is available (instead of merely a needle), lifesaving treatment may be prompt thoracentesis using a three-way stopcock in the anterior 2nd intercostal space at the midclavicular line. As the trapped air rushes out, tension is relieved and the lung reexpands. Once the lung has been expanded, closed chest drainage (often with suction) is instituted. This permits air and fluid to leave the pleural space, but will prevent them from reentering.

Antibiotics are usually given because of the danger of empyema resulting from leakage of pulmonary secretions into the pleural space.

Open Pneumothorax; Mediastinal Flutter. An open pneumothorax occurs with *"sucking" chest wounds.* In this type of wound the traumatic opening in the chest wall is large enough that air moves freely *in and back out* of the chest cavity during ventilating movements (Fig. 72–3). This abnormal movement of air through the chest wound produces a "slurping" or "sucking" noise that *is audible if the environment is quiet.*

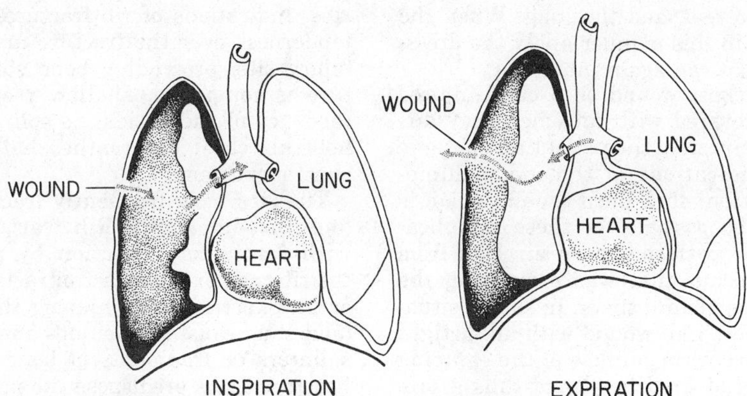

FIGURE 72–3. Open pneumothorax, i.e., "sucking" chest wound. (From Grant, H., and Murray, R.: *Emergency Care.* Robert J. Brady Co., 1971.)

To prevent possibly fatal complications from open pneumothorax, the opening in the chest wall must immediately be covered, thus preventing the abnormal passage of air.

Open sucking chest wounds may result not only from accidental injuries but also from surgical trauma. For example, if a chest drainage tube is accidentally pulled out of the chest, the remaining puncture incision in the chest wall may become a sucking wound.

When an open sucking chest wound is detected the emergency treatment is to securely cover the wound immediately with anything present. An airtight covering usually prevents a tension pneumothorax from developing and preserves ventilation of the opposite lung. Time is not wasted to obtain a sterile gauze petrolatum dressing (the ideal covering for such a wound) if such a dressing is not immediately available. Instead, at the scene of an accident the wound may be temporarily covered with a folded scarf or handkerchief, or possibly the heel of the examiner's hand.

In the hospital or clinic setting if you discover a sucking chest wound, immediately cover it with whatever is at hand, e.g., a towel, until someone else can bring a petrolatum dressing. Never leave the patient unattended while you go off to find the proper dressing. Administer appropriate first aid treatment, stay with and reassure the patient, and continue to apply pressure over the chest opening while you summon help. When your summons is answered ask that the physician be notified and that a proper dressing or other needed equipment be brought to you. When possible, fix the temporary dressing firmly in place with several strips of wide tape.

If the patient with an open pneumothorax is conscious and cooperative he can assist you. Instruct him to take a very deep breath and then to try to blow it out while keeping his mouth and nose closed. This pushing effort against a closed glottis helps to push air out through the chest wound and helps to reexpand the lung. When the patient assists you in this manner apply the dressing before the patient can again inhale.

After a sucking chest wound on a chest-injured patient has been covered with an emergency airtight dressing, remain with the patient and observe him closely for indications of tension pneumothorax and mediastinal shift until the physician is present. It would be possible for these complications to occur if the patient had an air leak from the lung or a bronchus that was permitting the escape of air into the pleural space. In such a situation, closing the chest wall wound with an airtight dressing would prevent the outflow of the escaping air (from the lungs or bronchus), and thus a previously open pneumothorax would be converted into a tension pneumothorax. Although it is dangerous to have air moving in and out of the pleural space with each respiration (open pneumothorax), it is far more dangerous to have a situation in which air moves only into the pleural space and cannot move back out (tension pneumothorax). If the patient appears to be developing tension pneumothorax after sealing of the wound, immediately unplug the seal (Fig. 72–4).

Once the physician is in attendance he usually orders chest films to determine the amount of air in the pleural space and displacement of thoracic structures. Closed chest drainage may be necessary to remove the air and allow the lung to reexpand if it is collapsed. A closed chest drainage system permits air to move out of the pleural space but not into it. If the patient is in severe respiratory distress, the physician may need to perform emergency procedures, e.g., thoracentesis. Be certain that equipment he might require is available at the bedside when the physician arrives.

In addition to *dyspnea* and *collapse of the lung* on the affected side, the patient with an open pneumothorax may experience *mediastinal flutter*. This complication results from the rush of air in and out of the thoracic cavity on the affected side. With inspiration the mediastinal structures and collapsed lung are pushed toward the injured side. Then, with expiration, these structures move back toward the unaffected side. These fluttering back and forth movements of the vital structures produce severe cardiopulmonary embarrassment which is fatal if not treated promptly.

Because infection can complicate an open pneumothorax, antibiotics are usually prescribed.

Hemothorax. To confirm a diagnosis of hemothorax the physician may aspirate blood by inserting a needle into the 8th interspace. To drain intrathoracic accumulations of blood the physician inserts two large caliber chest tubes—one anteriorly, the other posteriorly. The tubes may then be connected to a single water-sealed drainage bottle to maintain closed chest drainage. Thoracotomy is indicated if bleeding continues for an abnormally long period of time or if the patient is losing large quantities of blood.

Fractured Ribs

Chest injuries frequently fracture one or more ribs. Indications of rib fractures include pain and tenderness over the fracture area, bruising at the injury site, protruding bone splinters if the fracture is compound, shallow respirations, and the tendency of the patient to splint his chest, i.e., to hold his chest or breathe shallowly to minimize chest movements.

The ribs most frequently fractured are numbers four through eight. Rib fractures can interfere with respiratory function by producing pain as the rib cage expands or contracts during breathing, or by puncturing or injuring the pleura and lung (and thus causing pneumo- and/or hemothorax) if splinters or fragments of bone penetrate inward. Fractured ribs predispose the patient to atelectasis and pneumonia because pain causes the patient to breathe shallowly and prevents him from coughing effectively. Secretions therefore accumulate, obstructing bronchi and becoming a focus of infection. Shallow breathing also reduces lung compliance, i.e., causes "stiff" lungs. All these problems can be combated by frequent coughing, deep breathing, and position changes. Adequate pain coverage and splinting the chest during coughing and deep breathing help the patient to carry out these painful but vital activities more comfortably.

Care in Rib Fractures. Pulmonary function may be inhibited if more than two ribs are fractured. Severe crushing injuries to the rib cage seriously interfere with the mechanics of respiration. The pain from multiple rib fractures may cause the newly injured patient to go into shock. In an attempt to prevent shock, nerve blocks may be performed (e.g., by injecting procaine) in the intercostal nerves above and below the fractured ribs or by continuous segmental thoracic extradural nerve blocks. Pain relief obtained in this way makes it possible for the patient to breathe deeply, cough, and move about. Pain caused from simple fractures of only one or two ribs may be relieved by injecting a local anesthetic at the fracture site itself. Analgesics may be ordered for pain relief.

Analgesics are administered cautiously to the chest-injured patient. Narcotics may worsen respiratory depression and may depress the cough reflex (particularly in older persons).

Pain must be managed cautiously, e.g., with mild sedatives and small frequent doses of meperidine (Demerol).

Formerly the affected side of the chest was immobilized if a patient had fractured ribs and no visceral damage was present. Immobilization was accomplished by "strapping" the ribs with strips of adhesive tape, an Ace bandage, or chest binder. This was done to try to reduce pain upon ventilation. Today strapping is condemned since it is realized that by restricting deep breathing strapping can cause complications such as hypoxia, hyperventilation, hypercapnia, pneumonia, or atelectasis.

Bone splinters from fractured ribs may cause pneumothorax or hemothorax by puncturing the lung and pleura. Chest x-rays are carefully reviewed for indications of these complications. The nurse watches for symptoms of pneumothorax or hemothorax and reports them promptly if they appear. Bright red sputum may be coughed up by the patient if the lung has been penetrated.

Fractured ribs are generally treated conservatively unless the lung or pleura has been penetrated.

Stove-in Chest; Flail Chest; Paradoxical Motion

Severe crushing chest injuries that compress the rib cage often produce a "stove-in" chest, in

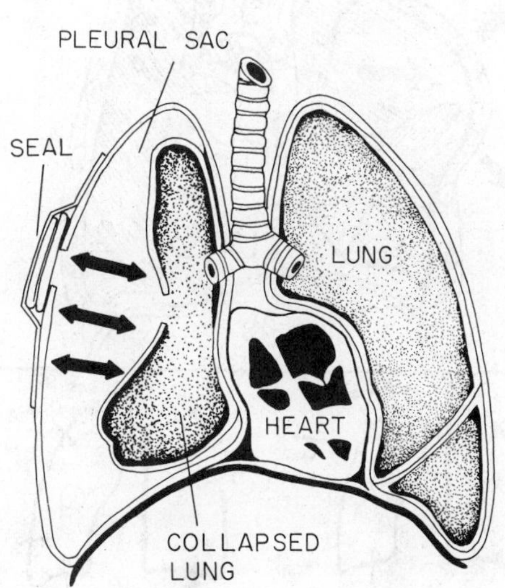

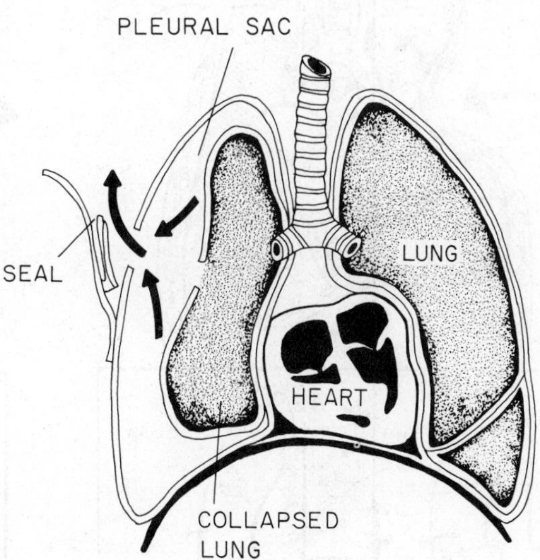

FIGURE 72-4. Correction of tension pneumothorax caused by covering open pneumothorax. (From Grant, H., and Murray, R.: *Emergency Care.* Robert J. Brady Co., 1971.)

which the ribs are pushed in on the lung, and a "flail chest," which disrupts the normal bellows action of the thorax by causing paradoxical motion. (Note: Paradoxical motion may also result from surgical removal of several ribs, as in thoracoplasty, or from diaphragmatic paralysis, which impairs the action of the thoracic bellows.)

With stove-in chest it is common for a fractured rib end to tear the pleura and lung surface, thereby producing hemopneumothorax. Both sides of the chest may be involved. Also, with a stove-in chest it is common for several *adjacent ribs to be fractured in two or more places.* These double-line fractures produce a flail slab of the chest wall (i.e., flail chest) which no longer has bony or cartilaginous connections with the rest of the rib cage. Lacking attachment to the thoracic skeleton, the section of chest wall between the fractures "floats" and moves independently during ventilation.

In flail chest the detached portion and its underlying lung tissue move *paradoxically* in opposition to the remainder of the chest cage and lungs. Paradoxical respirations permit little movement of gases during inspiration and expiration. During *paradoxical motion* the flail portion of the chest and its underlying portion of lung are "sucked in" upon inspiration (instead of expanding normally outward) and they are ballooned out ("blown out") upon expiration (instead of collapsing normally inward) (Fig. 72–5). Severe cardiovascular disturbances and respiratory insufficiency progressing to hypoxia and carbon dioxide retention can result from these maverick actions unless rapid treatment is instituted.

> *Flail chest is one of the most critical of all chest injuries. The majority of patients who die from thoracic trauma in traffic accidents die from the effects of flail chest.*

Loss of rigidity of the thoracic cage makes it impossible for the lungs to expand fully. Paradoxical motions neutralize the normal respiratory excursions of the chest wall and not only move air up and down in the trachea but also shunt stale air back and forth from one lung to the other.[53] During inspiration some already used air ("pendulum air") may move from the affected to the nonaffected lung and thus further reduce effective ventilation. Upon inspiration some air is sucked from the flail portion of the lung into the expanding regions of both lungs. During expiration some expiratory air is pushed into the flail portion of

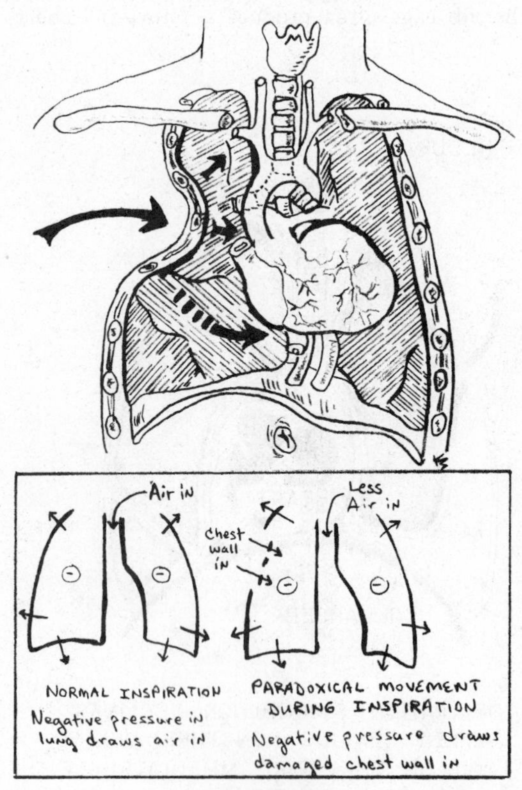

FIGURE 72–5. Paradoxical motion.

lung which is blowing out. These exchanges of stale air further reduce the effectiveness of respiration.

Paradoxical motion not only severely impairs normal breathing but also makes effective coughing impossible; therefore, secretions collect in the lung and eventually drown the untreated patient if he does not first die from respiratory failure. Secretions tend to be copious and thick and often are blood-tinged. Additionally, the mediastinal structures tend to swing back and forth during ventilatory movements. With a large area of paradoxical motion, these "swings" may seriously affect circulatory dynamics, producing elevated venous pressure, impaired filling of the right side of the heart, and decreased atrial blood pressure.

Severe cardiac or pulmonary failure causes a high mortality rate in persons with crushing chest injuries. Pulmonary edema, pneumonitis, and atelectasis often develop rapidly when the chest is crushed because fluids tend to increase and collect at the injured site.

In sum, paradoxical motion causes ineffective respiration (resulting in diminished O_2 absorption and CO_2 accumulation), accumulation of pulmonary secretions, and impaired filling of the right side of the heart as a result of a lowering of the intrapleural negative pressure, which eventually progresses to right-sided heart failure and death.[22]

Symptoms and Diagnosis. The patient with untreated flail chest suffers extreme distress as he desperately tries to ventilate in spite of the excruciating pain. Hypoxia is worsened as the effort necessary to try to breathe further depletes the diminished available oxygen supply. The patient is usually cyanotic and severely dyspneic. His respirations are typically rapid, shallow, and grunty. Large amounts of tracheobronchial secretions are produced. Shock commonly occurs and the patient may be hemorrhaging from the lungs or major vessels. Symptoms of paradoxical respirations include breathlessness or dyspnea with tachycardia as well as obvious paradoxical chest movements.

The patient who has sustained blunt trauma to the thorax and abdomen should be disrobed for emergency evaluation to observe for flail chest. Flail chest and paradoxical motion may result from sternal and rib fractures or from costochondral separations which cannot be detected by x-ray. Commonly the 3rd to the 9th ribs are fractured at the necks posteriorly and also in the midaxilla. Paradoxical motion is frequently present soon after injury; however, sometimes it does not develop for several hours.

> *When multiple rib fractures are present, observe the patient's chest movements closely for paradoxical motion. Report this complication immediately.*

Clinical Care. Clinical management of flail chest may include:

> Intensive nursing care.

> Suction to maintain airway. When tracheal aspiration fails to maintain a clear airway the physician must perform bronchoscopy.

> Tracheostomy or cuffed endotracheal tube to maintain airway and to assist ventilation.

> IPPB and oxygen.

> Control of shock, hemorrhage, and pain. Control of hemorrhage helps to treat shock and hypoxia. Pain may be managed by nerve blocks and meperidine. Carefully evaluate agitation and restlessness to determine whether they are caused by pain or hypoxia.

> Prevention and treatment of infection. Administer antibiotics. Turn, cough, and deep breathe the patient to prevent pneumonia. Prevent aspiration.

> Relief of abdominal distention.

> Promotion of pulmonary reexpansion.

> Stabilization of flail portion of chest wall (internally or externally) to eliminate paradoxical motion. (See emergency management, Fig. 72–6.)

Rapid, effective treatment of flail chest and continued close supervision and nursing care are mandatory. As an emergency measure, e.g., at the scene of an accident, while waiting for help to arrive apply pressure with a firm pad or the palm of the hand over the flail portion of the chest wall. Even though the underlying lung is compressed, the patient's respiratory distress will be somewhat relieved by stopping the paradoxical motion. Another means of applying pressure is to simply turn the patient onto his affected side.

In the hospital various treatments may be used to externally or internally stabilize a portion of flail chest and thus prevent paradoxical motions during ventilation. *External* stabilization may be obtained by applying skeletal traction to the chest wall to pull the chest wall outward. In this procedure a small incision is made with the patient under local anesthesia and the flail ribs are grasped by towel clips, special clamps, or stainless steel wires. Weights (about 5 lb.) and pulleys are then attached to the clamped instruments or to the wires, and the flail portion of the chest is thereby pulled outward and prevented from collapsing. The traction is usually necessary for two to three weeks. At the end of this time the chest wall is generally rigid again. External fixation of flail chest is less helpful than internal pneumatic stabilization.

Internal stabilization of a flail chest may be achieved surgically or by intubating the patient with a cuffed tracheostomy or endotracheal tube and then providing positive pressure ventilation through the tube with a volume-controlled respirator.

The patient with a flail chest has lost the mechanical ability to maintain adequate ventilation (since he lacks maximal negative pressure in the pleural space). The treatment of choice is therefore to perform a tracheostomy and institute intermittent positive pressure ventilation. These actions immediately expand the lungs, reduce hypoxia and hypercarbia, restore adequate ventilation, decrease paradoxical motion, remove pendulum air, relieve pain by decreasing movement of the fractured ribs, provide an avenue for suctioning and cough stimulation, and combat the development of atelectasis, pneumonia, and pulmonary edema. Also, the use of a mechanical respirator provides fixation of the chest wall by internal pneumatic stabilization. By this means the lungs are inflated by an IPPB apparatus and "the loose segment is held outward on a cushion of expanded air."[53] This stabilizes the chest in the inflation position and keeps the fractured ribs properly aligned for healing.

A tracheostomy is performed because it is necessary to maintain the IPPB treatment for at least six to 14 days. The patient is commonly managed initially with an indwelling endotracheal tube. As an emergency procedure an intravenous relaxant medication may be administered, an endotracheal tube is passed, and the patient is manually ventilated with an Ambu bag or anesthetic machine. Once the endotracheal tube is in place and the patient's condition permits, a tracheostomy is performed under controlled conditions which minimize the possible hazards of this procedure. Frequent evaluations of blood gases and electrolytes are necessary with IPPB treatment to maintain effective respiration and combat possible fluid-electrolyte imbalances. A variety of factors may produce metabolic and respiratory acidosis in chest-injured patients (Fig. 72-7). Frequent roentgenograms are also necessary to evaluate the chest.

If a thoracotomy (chest wall incision) is necessary for other problems, e.g., diaphragmatic rupture, persistent bleeding, the surgeon may fixate the fractures internally while he has the chest open. Operative fixation of a flail chest may be achieved by applying various devices to stabilize the flail portion of the chest wall, by passing sutures through the intercostal muscles, or by passing wires through holes drilled in the ribs if the intercostals are too damaged to hold stitches. Operative fixation of the flail chest segment is necessary when an air leak is present, e.g., from lacerated lung, or positive pressure ventilation may cause a tension pneumothorax in spite of the use of closed chest drainage.[53]

Subcutaneous Emphysema

Frequently fractured ribs and other chest injuries cause air to escape into the subcutaneous tissues. This may also occur after thoracic surgery. The escaped air may then travel through the tissue for some distances under the skin; the presence of air causes the affected areas to puff out. (The word "emphysema" means a swelling or inflation caused by the presence of air.) If the skin is gently palpated over the air-expanded areas a crackling sensation may be noted (crepitus).

Although various areas of the body may be affected, some of the regions that may appear most

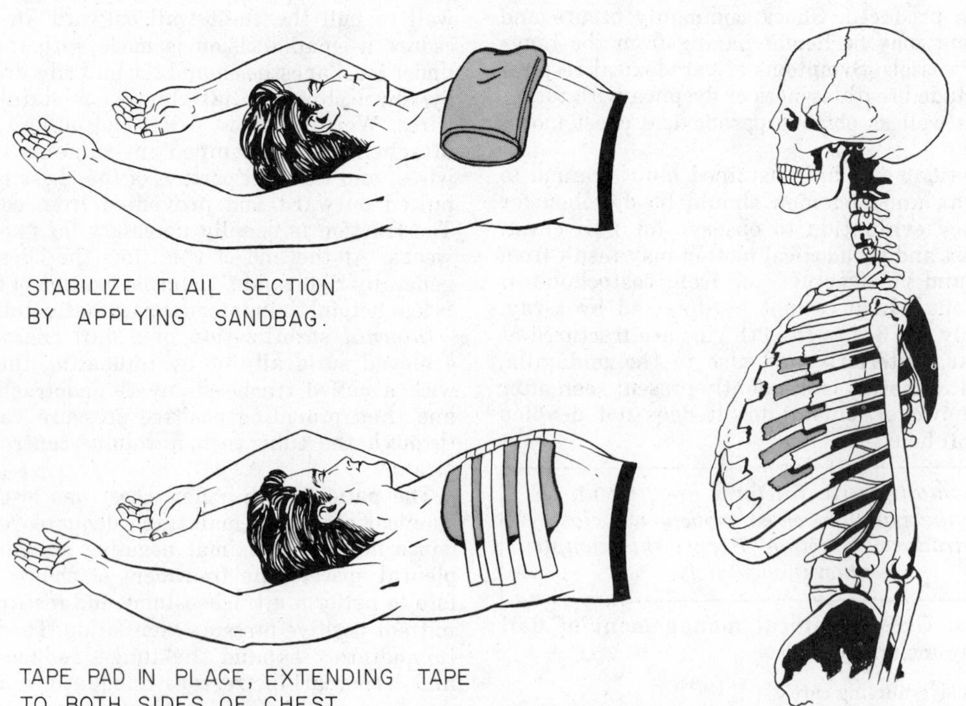
STABILIZE FLAIL SECTION
BY APPLYING SANDBAG.
TAPE PAD IN PLACE, EXTENDING TAPE
TO BOTH SIDES OF CHEST.

FIGURE 72-6. Emergency management of flail chest. (From Grant, H., and Murray, R.: *Emergency Care.* Robert J. Brady Co., 1971.)

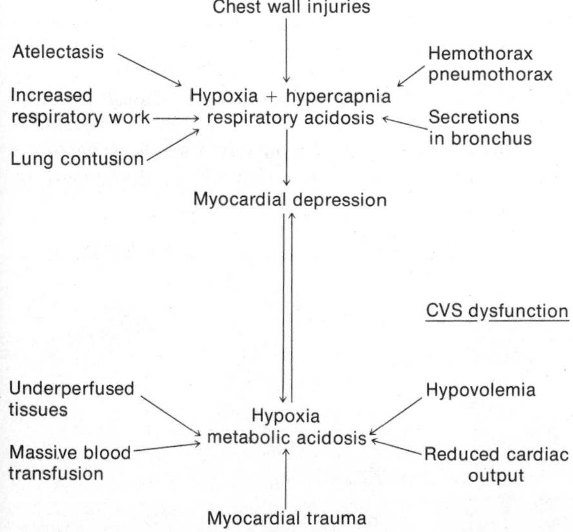

FIGURE 72-7. Factors producing metabolic and respiratory acidosis in chest injuries. (Modified from Reid and Baird, 1965.)

grossly distorted by subcutaneous emphysema are the face, neck, and scrotum. Because of the bloated look of the face and neck, the patient's appearance may be alarming and visitors should be forewarned and given a simple explanation of the condition. Usually subcutaneous emphysema is not serious; however, the patient should be closely observed for respiratory distress if the neck is quite swollen.

The source of the air leak into the tissues may close spontaneously or may require treatment. Subsequently the body gradually absorbs the air from the subcutaneous tissues.

Mediastinal Emphysema

Mediastinal emphysema (i.e., the presence of air in the mediastinal tissue) is a serious form of emphysema which can be rapidly fatal. The pressure produced in the mediastinum may prevent cardiac filling and emptying.

Cardiac Tamponade

Cardiac tamponade is acute compression of the heart resulting from the collection of blood or fluid in the pericardial sac. This may occur following either blunt or penetrating chest trauma. Bleeding into the pericardium may be caused by rupture of the heart or coronary vessel. Even a small quantity of blood in the pericardial cavity will embarrass cardiac action and lead to cardiac arrest unless treatment is given promptly.

Rapid pericardiocentesis can be lifesaving. The removal of as little as 10 to 20 ml. of blood may relieve symptoms, and the patient's vital signs may immediately improve. As long as the patient continues to improve the physician withdraws as much blood as he can easily obtain. An 18-gauge needle is inserted through the xiphocostal angle to aspirate the pericardial sac. The patient is closely observed for repeated episodes of tamponade and several pericardiocenteses may be necessary. Usually thoracotomy is performed after tamponade has been relieved so the cardiac wound can be repaired surgically.

Cardiac tamponade is suspected when an injured patient is received in the emergency room in shock without evidence of blood loss. In some instances tamponade does not appear until one or two hours later. The nurse must therefore closely observe the chest-injured patient for symptoms of cardiac tamponade. These symptoms include high central venous pressure, narrowed pulse pressure (with or without cyanosis), paradoxical pulse, distant and muffled heart sounds, declining blood pressure, decreased pulse pressure, dyspnea, and reduced consciousness owing to impaired cerebral circulation. Electrocardiographic monitoring is advisable, and an aspirating needle and syringe should be readily available to prevent myocardial injury. Once the pressure of the accumulated fluids in the pericardial sac is relieved, the heart can again attempt to function normally.

Wet-Lung Syndrome

The wet-lung syndrome (also called "traumatic wet lung") develops with most serious chest injuries. The syndrome consists of (1) impaired ability to cough and thus clear the airway and help to reexpand a collapsed portion of lung; (2) airway obstruction; and (3) atelectasis of portions of the affected lung or complete collapse of the lung. Impaired coughing results from mechanical damage to the chest and chest pain. Airway obstruction is caused by blood and/or increased tracheobronchial secretions. Atelectasis results from airway obstruction.

The patient experiencing wet-lung syndrome manifests cyanosis (caused by poor oxygenation of the blood) and noisy, dyspneic respirations (caused by secretion and blood in the tracheobronchial tree and obstructed airway passages). Treatment centers around aspiration of the tracheobronchial tree with a catheter since the patient cannot cough effectively. Aspiration may be performed via bronchoscope or tracheostomy if necessary.

Mechanical, hemodynamic, and neurogenic factors appear to combine to produce traumatic wet lung. The result is increased production of bronchial secretions with a reduced ability to expel them, increased permeability of alveolar capillaries, and disturbed pulmonary ventilation ratio.[5] The wet-lung syndrome may be prevented by the early use of a mechanical respirator in the injured patient.

Shock

The chest-injured patient may require large quantities of blood to treat hypovolemic shock. When possible, surgery is delayed until the blood volume is restored. Although shock is frequently the result of hypovolemia, in the chest-injured patient it may also be caused by pericardial tamponade, flail chest, respiratory obstruction, or tension pneumothorax. Central venous pressure readings are carefully interpreted, since cardiac tamponade can be hidden by hypovolemia with a normal venous pressure; i.e., in the presence of hypovolemia the CVP may be normal even though cardiac tamponade is present. Once the physician correctly identifies the etiology of a patient's shock, treatment is rapidly administered. (Shock is discussed in Chapter 26.)

CHAPTER 73

Chest Surgery

The specific thoracic conditions that may be treated surgically have been discussed in Chapters 71 and 72. Successful thoracic surgery depends not only on the skills of the operating team, but also on competent professional nursing care during the pre- and postoperative periods. The nurse caring for a chest surgery patient must be familiar enough with the anatomy and physiology of the chest that she can recognize alterations from the normal that have resulted from the patient's underlying disorder and the operative procedure he has undergone. Also, the nurse must be able to recognize changes from the chest's normal structure and function that occur if postoperative complications develop. Such basic knowledge forms the framework upon which the nurse plans and administers personalized patient care directed at an uncomplicated recovery from the operative procedure. Much of the clinical care given chest surgery patients is *preventive care* directed at averting the numerous complications that can develop following thoracic surgery. (Emphasis in this chapter is primarily on pulmonary surgery. Surgical procedures performed on the heart are discussed in Unit X. Refer to Unit VI for a general discussion of nursing care given patients undergoing surgery.)

PREOPERATIVE CLINICAL CARE

Prior to thoracic surgery the patient is prepared both physically and psychologically. Additionally, a thorough evaluation is made of his cardiopulmonary and general physical status. A great deal of time is spent during the preoperative period in teaching the patient ways in which he can effectively participate in his care during the postoperative period.

PREOPERATIVE PHYSICAL EVALUATION AND PREPARATION

Evaluation is made during the preoperative period of the patient's vital signs, general health, state of nutrition and hydration, and general cardiopulmonary status. When possible, attempts are made prior to surgery to improve the patient's hydration and nutritional status to optimal levels. For example, fluids may be forced to help to thin bronchopulmonary secretions, and a high-calorie, high-protein, increased vitamin diet may be given. Additionally, problems detected during the preoperative work-up, such as cardiac disorders, are evaluated and given appropriate treatment. When conditions are observed that contraindicate surgery (e.g., acute respiratory infection or skin lesions), they are called to the surgeon's attention.

Smoking causes bronchopulmonary irritation, increases tracheobronchial secretions, decreases oxygen saturation, and increases carboxyhemoglobin in the blood. Because oxygen saturation and minimal secretion production are important during and following thoracic surgery, *the patient is advised not to smoke* during the pre- and postoperative period. This advice is often extremely difficult for the patient to follow if he is a habitual smoker, since anxiety about his condition may increase the desire to smoke.

During the preoperative period the patient is given frequent thorough oral hygiene with antiseptic mouthwashes to reduce the number of pathogens in the upper respiratory tract. This is of importance prior to thoracic surgery because the mouth is a major entrance to the lower respiratory tract. If when the nurse gives oral hygiene care to the patient, she notes infected teeth or lesions in the mouth, she reports these findings to the surgeon.

If a patient has a known pulmonary infection, broad-spectrum antibiotics are usually ordered prior to surgery to minimize the number of pathogens. Postural drainage may also be prescribed (e.g., if an abscess, bronchiectasis, or retained secretions are present) to promote drainage from the lung of infected matter. (Postural drainage was discussed in Chapter 70.) Usually the patient is placed on a sputum observation routine preoperatively and his sputum is observed, measured, and recorded every 8 or 24 hours. Sputum specimens are sent to the laboratory as ordered. Patients with impaired pulmonary function may be treated preoperatively with antibiotic and bronchodilating medications and intermittent positive pressure breathing equipment. Supervised breathing exercises help to improve respiratory efficiency prior to thoracic surgery.

Preoperative Tests

Special tests may be ordered prior to thoracic surgery and include sputum examination, pulmonary function tests, bronchospirometry, chest x-rays (including tomograms), bronchoscopy, bronchogram, electrocardiogram, and possibly cardiac catheterization. Prior to a pneumonectomy or left lobectomy it is especially important to study the distribution of pulmonary function between the two lungs to determine if the patient can tolerate the proposed loss of lung tissue without becoming a "pulmonary cripple"; bronchospirometric studies are thus routinely performed. (Pulmonary diagnostic tests and procedures are discussed in Chapter 68). *Routine preoperative tests* are also ordered.

Immediate Preoperative Physical Preparation

Immediate physical preparation of the patient, beginning the day before surgery, may or may not include an enema and postural drainage. Thorough oral hygiene is routinely performed the morning of surgery. When atropine is ordered preoperatively (to minimize secretion formation), it should not be given until postural drainage has been completed (if ordered for the morning of surgery). Because it is important to minimize secretions in the tracheobronchial tree during thoracic surgery, patients about to undergo thoracic surgery may be ordered to receive larger preoperative doses of atropine than patients scheduled for surgical procedures involving other areas of the body. (See Unit VI for discussion of other aspects of the immediate preparation of a patient for major surgery.)

PREOPERATIVE TEACHING AND PSYCHOLOGIC PREPARATION

During the preoperative period the patient about to undergo thoracic surgery is given emotional and intellectual preparation for the experience. The physician discusses with the patient and his family reasons why the proposed surgery will be helpful. Often patients and family members are reluctant to ask a physician questions or to express to him their emotional concerns about surgical procedures. Frequently the nurse is helpful in these areas. The nurse answers those questions posed by the patient or family members that are within the scope of her profession. She appropriately refers to other qualified persons those questions or concerns that others can discuss more competently.

Patients are naturally apprehensive about having surgery performed on vital organs like the lungs. Preoperative emotional support is therefore of major importance. Because pulmonary surgery involves surgery on the "breathing apparatus" it is not uncommon for patients to express concern about being unable to breathe effectively following surgery.[234]

> *Teaching the patient preoperatively how he can effectively help himself during the postoperative period is especially important before chest surgery.*

The nurse discusses with the patient what will be happening to him during the early postoperative period, and how he will participate in his recovery. These aspects of patient education are carefully planned by the nurse and are carried out in detail. Notes are made in the patient's chart of teaching sessions, e.g., what was generally discussed, whether the patient appeared to understand the discussion, what procedures were demonstrated, whether the patient correctly redemonstrated exercises, and so forth.

Unless it is explained to the patient *before* surgery that he will be surrounded by a lot of equipment (e.g., chest drainage, oxygen, ventilator), when he awakens from the anesthetic, he will tend to think that the equipment is present because his condition is poor. It must, therefore, be emphasized preoperatively that it is *routine* procedure to use various types of equipment following surgery to help the patient to recover more rapidly. Family members should also be prepared for what will be happening to the patient following surgery, so they are not unnecessarily frightened by the equipment and procedures.

Tell the patient preoperatively that he will not be able to have long periods of rest for several days following surgery. For example, for the first 24 postoperative hours he will be awakened hourly to deep breathe, cough, and change his position. On subsequent days he may be awakened every four hours, day and night, to ambulate, exercise, cough, and deep breathe.

Preoperatively teach the patient how to effectively deep breathe, cough, and carry out exercises that are important postoperatively. Teach him leg exercises to prevent thrombi from forming in the calves of the legs, and arm and shoulder exercises on the operative side to maintain normal range-of-motion and correct posture. Breathing exercises are also important for effective pulmonary function. When available, a physical therapist may do the preliminary teaching for these activities. The nurse, however, is often responsible for supervising activity sessions. Be certain to familiarize yourself with the physician's preference for the patient's activity program. Some physicians order specific exercises.

Tell the patient that coughing and deep breathing are important following chest surgery not only because these activities help to move secretions out of the lung, but also because they help to reexpand the lung (which is temporarily collapsed when the thoracic cavity is opened during surgery), and help to force air and drainage out of the chest cavity when drainage tubes are used. (Note: Of course, if an entire lung is going to be removed [pneumonectomy], there will be no lung tissue to reexpand postoperatively on the operated side. Nonetheless, coughing and deep breathing are highly important to prevent complications in the remaining lung.) Inform the patient that the most important single activity for him to perform following surgery is to *cough up sputum.*

Tell the patient the frequency with which he will perform various postoperative activities and that he will be assisted and given medications to make him more comfortable while performing these activities. Emphasize, however, that not all discomfort can be removed postoperatively with medications and that the patient is expected to be active (deep breathe, cough, exercise, turn, sit up, ambulate) in spite of moderately severe pain.

Practice sessions (for coughing, deep breathing, exercising) are important during the preoperative period. Supervise the patient during these practice sessions until he can correctly perform the activity. Remember to give encouragement and praise.

Other areas important to include during preoperative patient teaching sessions include:

> Evaluating the patient's understanding of the anatomy of the thorax and of the surgical procedure he is to undergo. Provide appropriate instruction as indicated.

> Telling the patient that his vital signs may be monitored or taken frequently during the postoperative period. It is desirable to show the patient monitoring equipment that may be used and to explain briefly the function of the equipment. If the patient's vital capacity will be measured by the nurse following surgery the patient should be familiarized with this procedure.

> Informing the patient that various equipment will be used following surgery to help him to breathe more comfortably and effectively. For example, oxygen will probably be given nasally, and other inhalation therapy equipment such as a nebulizer or respirator may be used. Appropriate teaching is given concerning this equipment. If it is known preoperatively that a tracheostomy will be performed, the patient is prepared for this procedure. (Tracheostomy is discussed in Unit XXII.)

> Informing the patient of the reasons for suctioning and closed chest drainage (if chest drainage tubes will be used). Basically the patient is told that suctioning helps to remove secretions from his lungs, and that because chest surgery normally causes fluids to accumulate inside the chest postoperatively, chest tubes will help to drain off this fluid and air from the chest cavity.

> Telling the patient that he will be turned frequently (every 1 to 2 hours) and may sit up and ambulate soon after surgery. Explain that these activities are not only good for his general condition, but that they also help to move secretions out of the lungs and help to reexpand lung tissue.

> Preparing the patient for the fact that he will probably be receiving intravenous feedings and may have a central venous pressure apparatus as part of routine care. A cut-down may be performed on a leg vein during surgery (to ensure a route for intravenous therapy if shock occurs).

> Discussing with the patient the fact that he will have moderately severe pain postoperatively and encouraging him to discuss his pain with the nurse. Tell him he will be given medications to reduce the pain.

COMMON THORACIC SURGICAL PROCEDURES

During thoracic surgery endotracheal anesthesia is usually administered. In fact, thoracic surgery became routinely possible only after the endotracheal method of anesthesia was perfected. This form of anesthesia makes it possible for the anesthetist to maintain effective functioning of the unoperated lung during the operative procedure. Once the pleural space is entered, the lung on the operative side collapses due to the entrance of air under atmospheric pressure. (Anesthesia is discussed in Unit VI.)

EXPLORATORY THORACOTOMY

As its name indicates, exploratory thoracotomy is an operation performed in order to "explore" the thorax to locate sources of injury or bleeding, or to inspect and take a biopsy of suspected carcinoma. The biopsy may be of a lymph node or a section of the lung or may be a wedge resection (to be discussed). Exploratory thoracotomy may be accomplished through either a posterolateral parascapular incision or an anterior incision through an intercostal space. With either approach, the incision is of major size, the pleura is opened, and the ribs are spread to clearly expose the entire lung and hemithorax for inspection. Usually closed chest drainage is necessary postoperatively.

RESECTIONAL PULMONARY SURGERY

Resectional pulmonary surgery refers to those surgical procedures in which a lung or portion of a lung is removed. The various types of resection procedures differ in the amount of lung tissue removed. Closed chest drainage is not routinely used following pneumonectomy (removal of an entire lung), but it is always used following other pulmonary resections.

Pulmonary resections are performed either via a posterolateral parascapular approach (through the 4th, 5th, 6th, or 7th intercostal space) or via an anterior approach (through the 3rd, 4th, or 5th intercostal space). Typically the anterior approach causes less disability and pain. Pulmonary resections are used to treat numerous conditions, e.g., chronic localized infections, cysts, bronchiectasis, pulmonary tuberculosis (unhealed by chemotherapy), bronchial adenoma, bronchogenic carcinoma.

Resectional operative procedures commonly performed on the lung are briefly discussed below:

> *Pneumonectomy:* Removal of an entire lung, e.g., in the presence of bronchogenic cancer, extensive (unilateral) tuberculosis, bronchiectasis, or lung abscess. In order to remove a lung the surgeon severs and sutures the mainstem bronchus at its bifurcation and the large pulmonary artery and veins. A pleural flap is sutured over the bronchial stump as an added precaution against postoperative air leakage through the stump. Once the lung is removed the thoracic cavity is an empty space. To help to reduce the size of this cavity

the surgeon severs or crushes the phrenic nerve on the affected side; this paralyzes the diaphragm in an elevated position.

Closed chest drainage is generally not used after pneumonectomy because the surgeon wants fluids to accumulate in the empty thoracic space. Eventually the thoracic space fills in with serous exudate which consolidates, preventing extensive mediastinal shift of the heart and remaining lung. Sometimes the surgeon places a chest tube and *leaves it clamped* upon completing pneumonectomy. He may use this tube during the postoperative period as an avenue for inspecting for frank bleeding and measuring and regulating pressure in the thoracic space. (It is desirable to leave a slightly negative pressure in the closed thoracic space.) Some physicians use a pneumothorax apparatus to measure the intrathoracic pressure and to add or remove air in order to maintain the pressure at the desired level. Pneumonectomies are most often performed to remove lung cancer.

> *Lobectomy:* Removal of a lobe of the lung, e.g., when disease (bronchiectasis, abscess, tumor, fungal infection, tuberculosis, cyst, or bleb) or injury is confined to one lobe. Any of the lobes of the lungs can be removed. (Remember: The right lung has three lobes; the left lung, two.) The bronchus leading into the removed lobe is sutured. Following pulmonary resection some compensatory, nonpathologic emphysema occurs as the remaining lung tissue overexpands to fill in the portion of the thoracic space previously occupied by the resected tissue. Closed chest drainage is used postoperatively.

> *Segmental resection (segmentectomy):* Removal of one or more segments of the lung when the disorder is limited to only the segment(s) resected, e.g., bronchiectasis, tuberculosis. (Remember: The lobes of the lungs are divided into parts called "segments." The right lung contains 10 segments and the left has eight.) By delicate dissection the surgeon identifies and ligates the appropriate segmental bronchus, pulmonary artery, and vein. The remaining lung tissue then overexpands to fill the space occupied by the removed segment. Closed chest drainage is used postoperatively.

> *Wedge resection:* Removal of a small, localized area of disease (e.g., tuberculosis) near the surface of the lung. The portion removed is triangular (wedge-shaped) and is only part of a segment. Because the area resected is so small, pulmonary structure remains relatively unchanged after healing. The area to be removed is isolated by clamps and then resected. Sutures and chest drainage tubes are then placed.

When performing pulmonary resectional surgery, the surgeon is careful to remove no more lung tissue than necessary and thus save as much functional tissue for the patient as possible and minimize postoperative disruption of lung structure.

DECORTICATION

Decortication is the removal or "stripping off" of a thick fibrous membrane or "peel" that sometimes develops over the visceral pleura. Such a membrane interferes with the lung's normal ventilatory movements; it may develop as a result of empyema or the prolonged presence of blood or fluid in the pleural space. The lung may become constricted and "trapped" by an infection or organized clot.

During the blunt dissection necessary to remove the membrane, numerous lung leaks are inevitably created. Postoperatively it is necessary to have at least two chest catheters present to accomplish closed chest drainage. If the surgery is to be successful it is necessary for the decorticated lung to be rapidly and completely reexpanded. Closed chest drainage with suction is used to help the lung to reexpand rapidly and fill the pleural space. If the fibrinous membrane has restricted the lung for some time, the lung may not effectively reexpand even after the peel is removed. In such instances, once the surgeon is convinced that the lung cannot expand sufficiently (even though "freed" from its restrictive cover), a thoracoplasty may be performed.

THORACOPLASTY

A thoracoplasty is a plastic operation on the thorax in which ribs or portions of ribs are removed to reduce the size of the thoracic space. Removal of ribs weakens the chest wall and permits atmospheric pressure (pushing against the outside of the chest) to collapse the weakened portion. When thoracoplasty is performed, the periosteum is stripped from the ribs before the ribs are removed. The periosteum is left in place in the chest wall and eventually a bony substance re-forms which holds the chest wall in that area in a collapsed position. Although the surgeon attempts to remove the desired ribs while remaining outside the pleural space, the pleura is sometimes inadvertently entered. When this occurs, closed chest drainage or aspiration is necessary postoperatively to reexpand the lung.

Before it became possible to resect the lung or portions of it, thoracoplasty was frequently used as an extrapleural form of collapse therapy to treat cavitary pulmonary tuberculosis. Currently it is seldom used for this purpose, but may be used to close a chronic empyema space, or to help to reduce the thoracic space before or after resectional surgery. (Note: This procedure is not routinely performed with resectional surgery, but only when clearly indicated.) Prior to pneumonectomy, for example, a thoracoplasty (called a "preresection" or "tailoring" thoracoplasty) may be performed to minimize chances of a postresectional mediastinal shift. This procedure may also be performed prior to other resectional surgeries if the surgeon believes the remaining portions of a patient's lung will not be able to expand enough following the resection to fill the pleural space or that they may overstretch and become pathologically emphysematous. Following some resections a "postresection" thoracoplasty is necessary if the remaining portions of lung fail to adapt themselves to the pleural cavity.

Some of the earlier thoracoplasties were quite disfiguring because the surgical procedures interfered with the shoulder girdle in such a way that the shoulder on the operated side drooped noticeably below the "normal" shoulder, the scapula sank medially against the mediastinum, and the chest on the operated side appeared markedly "caved in." Newer surgical procedures have greatly reduced these problems, since the shoulder girdle is not disrupted and the number of ribs removed is fewer; generally no more than three ribs are removed. The removal of many ribs at one time is incompatible with continued life, because the soft, unstable chest wall that results goes into paradoxical motion. Paradoxical motion seldom occurs following modern thoracoplasty.

POSTOPERATIVE CLINICAL CARE

Chest surgery is traumatic; many of the aftereffects and complications are therefore similar to those that follow chest injuries (Chapter 72). MacVicar and Mendelsohn observe that following chest surgery (or chest injuries) patients may develop "important and dangerous physiological and biochemical alterations" that basically result from "inadequate pulmonary ventilation and/or inadequate pulmonary or systemic blood circulation."[178] During the postoperative period the basic aim of care is, therefore "to obtain and maintain respiratory and circulatory efficiency and to prevent physiological and biochemical alterations that may result from inadequate pulmonary ventilation and tissue perfusion."[178]

As previously stated, opening the thoracic cavity permits atmospheric air to enter the pleural space (which normally has negative pressure) and collapse the lung. Special postoperative care is thus necessary to reestablish negative pressure in the pleural space and to reexpand those portions of lung remaining. During the postoperative period much nursing attention is directed at maintaining effective closed chest drainage; keeping the patient's airway patent, e.g., by assisting the patient with the necessary deep-breathing and coughing regimen, and by suctioning; and ensuring good lung expansion by positioning the patient so his chest cage and diaphragm are unrestricted and by encouraging deep breathing.

In general, following thoracic surgery the patient is kept on a "mobilization" and "stir-up" regimen for several days—coughing, deep breathing, sitting up, ambulating, turning, exercising. The necessary care typically demands that the patient be active during the early postoperative period. Well-meaning but inexperienced nurses sometimes hesitate to insist that patients be active at this time. For example, such "sympathetic" nurses may permit patients to sleep through periods when they should be awakened to cough or deep breathe; or they may tell patients that exercises can be "skipped this time." These attitudes of misplaced sympathy are a grave disservice to patients.

Sensitivity to a patient's postoperative anxieties is also necessary during the stressful postoperative period. The nurse attempts to discuss the patient's concerns and to offer appropriate reassurance and encouragement. The skillful nurse also inspires confidence in the patient when she is self-confident while giving postoperative care. Such self-confidence comes, in part, with familiarization with routines and equipment used postoperatively.

COMPLICATIONS FOLLOWING THORACIC SURGERY

Numerous complications can occur following thoracic surgery. Among these are the following: respiratory insufficiency, hypoxia, anoxia, function loss; hyperventilation, CO_2 retention, hypercapnia; mediastinal shift; paradoxical motion; pneumothorax; hemorrhage, hemothorax; shock, hypotension; cardiac arrhythmias, myocardial infarction; respiratory arrest, cardiac arrest; pulmonary embolism, thrombophlebitis; residual pleural space; bronchopleural fistula; atelectasis, pneumonia; infections, e.g., wound infection, empyema; adrenal exhaustion; gastric dilatation, abdominal distention, paralytic ileus; subcutaneous emphysema; and acute pulmonary edema. Many of these complications result from inadequate ventilation or inadequate circulation.

Following thoracic surgery *inadequate ventilation* (causing alveolar hypoventilation) may occur because of: (1) airway obstruction (caused by retained bronchopulmonary secretions); (2) atelectasis; (3) incisional pain and discomfort from chest tubes (causes the patient to breathe shallowly and ineffectively); (4) depression of the central nervous system (e.g., caused by narcotics, sedatives, anesthetic agents, and muscle relaxants); (5) preexisting disease of lung parenchyma; (6) compression of lung tissue (caused by pneumothorax, hemothorax, abdominal distention, or phrenic nerve injury); (7) reduction of the amount of lung tissue available for aeration; (8) paradoxical respirations; or (9) bronchiolar narrowing or spasm. Alveolar hypoventilation produces hypoxia and hypercapnia and lowers the ventilation-perfusion ratio.

Circulatory insufficiency (indicated by hypotension) following thoracic surgery may result from: hypovolemia caused by blood loss or fluid depletion (when hypovolemia causes low cardiac output the shock syndrome develops); cardiogenic disorders (e.g., underlying myocardial disease causing arrhythmias, hypotension, myocardial infarction); and neurogenic causes (e.g., pain-induced hypotension).[178] Circulatory insufficiency produces hypoxia, acidosis, and ischemia of the vital organs.

Physical indications of possible complications include low systolic blood pressure (below 90), temperature elevation (above 99°F. or 37.2°C.), indications of hemorrhage through the incision, bloody chest drainage, pallor, dyspnea, cyanosis, increased pulse rate, increased respiratory rate, and acute chest pain. Specific symptoms associated with some of the more common specific complications are discussed more completely in the following pages.

Respiratory Insufficiency; Hypoxia; Hypercapnia

These disorders have all been discussed in Chapter 69 and can all develop following thoracic surgery. The nurse giving postoperative care must be particularly alert to *early* indications of the development of these complications so appropriate treatment can be given promptly. Some postoperative factors leading to hypoxemia are illustrated in Figure 73-1.

Tension Pneumothorax; Mediastinal Shift; Paradoxical Motion

These complications have also been previously discussed in detail (Chapter 72). Tension pneumothorax can result from postoperative air leakage through pleural incision lines if closed chest drainage fails to function properly. A large pneumothorax (or hemothorax) causes mediastinal shift. Also, mediastinal shift can easily occur following pneumonectomy if the patient is incorrectly positioned. If three or more ribs have been removed, paradoxical motion may occur with respirations.

Hemorrhage; Hemothorax; Hypovolemic Shock

Blood loss during major thoracic surgical procedures may be greater than that lost during most general surgical procedures because the blood vessels dissected within the thorax are of large caliber (and a technical accident can produce considerable blood loss in a brief period of time); the incision is quite large and tends to have considerable capillary oozing; and adhesions and tissue planes within the thorax are generally quite extensive and vascular.

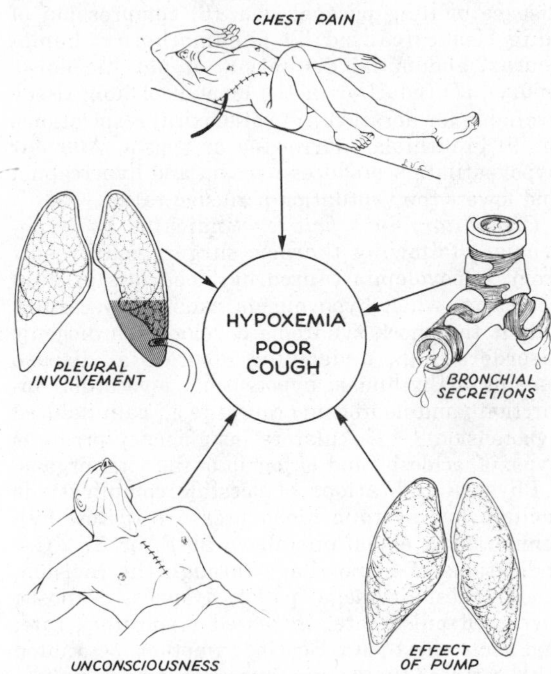

FIGURE 73-1. Postoperative factors leading to hypoxemia. (From Thomas, A. N.: *In* Sanderson, R. G., *The Cardiac Patient: A Comprehensive Approach*. 1972.)

Periodically check the dressing or incisional area (if a dressing is not present) for evidence of bleeding or drainage. Record findings, noting if the dressing is dry or the type and amount of drainage. Examine drainage in the closed chest drainage system for evidence of bleeding, and periodically evaluate the patient's pulse and blood pressure for indications of hypovolemic shock, i.e., an increasing pulse rate or a drop in blood pressure (lower than the preoperative blood pressure). Manifestations of hemorrhage into the pleural space include bloody chest drainage, unstable blood pressure, increased pulse, dyspnea, and other symptoms of pulmonary collapse.

Since progressive oliguria or anuria is another late symptom of shock, the patient's urinary output should be evaluated carefully each hour during the immediate postoperative period. The nurse also observes for changes in the sensorium that may indicate shock. Laboratory tests that may be employed to detect hypovolemia include a hematocrit and a determination of blood volume by means of radioactive albumin or dye-dilution techniques.

When a patient shows indications of hemorrhaging, have intravenous solutions, blood replacements, and plasma expanders readily available. The rate of fluid replacement can best be governed by continuously monitoring the central venous pressure. When managing postoperative shock in a patient who has undergone thoracic surgery the Trendelenburg position is generally contraindicated since it causes the diaphragm and abdominal contents to elevate and, thus, restrict ventilation. Hemothorax may be treated with needle aspiration or closed chest drainage. Occasionally surgery is necessary. (Hemothorax was discussed in Chapter 72.)

As previously mentioned, not all hypotensive patients are in hypovolemic shock; shock may also develop as a result of cardiogenic or neurogenic causes.

Cardiac Arrhythmias; Myocardial Infarction

A high percentage of patients who require thoracic surgery have underlying cardiac disease. Thus, the cardiovascular system is carefully evaluated prior to surgery so patients can be managed safely during and following surgery. High-risk patients with underlying cardiac disease may have continuous electrocardiographic (ECG) monitoring during the postoperative period. Cardiac effectiveness can be severely limited by arrhythmias or myocardial infarction postoperatively. Cardiac arrhythmias occur fairly often following thoracic surgery. The arrhythmia that occurs most often is atrial fibrillation; however, any of the arrhythmias may occur. Cardiac arrhythmias and myocardial infarction must be promptly treated since they may be life-threatening. (See Unit X.)

Respiratory Arrest; Cardiac Arrest

These grave complications and their clinical management are discussed in detail in Unit X. Following thoracic surgery the nurse must be prepared to give appropriate emergency cardiopulmonary resuscitation.

Pulmonary Embolism

Pulmonary embolism (producing obstruction of the pulmonary artery) is a serious potential complication following pulmonary surgery. Observe the patient closely for indications of this infarction of lung tissue. Symptoms of pulmonary embolism and infarction are variable, depending upon the location and degree of infarction. Symptoms may include dyspnea, pleuritic or crushing substernal pain, fever, hemoptysis, symptoms of right heart failure, hypoxia (producing metabolic acidosis), engorgement of neck veins (especially on inspiration), rapid and deep or shallow respirations, and symptoms associated with circulatory collapse, e.g., tachycardia, hypotension, pallor, apprehension, sense of impending doom, nausea, sweating, weakness, and breathlessness. (Pulmonary embolism is discussed in Unit XIII.)

Residual Pleural Space

If a persistent pleural space develops from inadequate reexpansion of lung tissue, additional surgery such as a thoracoplasty may be required.

Bronchopleural Fistula

Bronchopleural fistula can result postoperatively from: (1) inadequate closure of the bronchus at the time of pulmonary resection; (2) inadequate blood supply to the bronchial stump, with resultant necrosis and "blow out" of the stump; (3) infection at the point of the bronchial amputation, with resultant "blow out" of the suture line; and (4) alveolar or bronchiolar tears on the surface of the remaining lung. When a bronchopleural fistula occurs, air escapes into the pleural space and is forced into the subcutaneous tissues around the incision, producing subcutaneous emphysema, and/or infection occurs in the pleural space as a result of tracheobronchial secretions draining into the pleural space. Additional surgery may be necessary to correct bronchopleural fistula.

Atelectasis; Pneumonia

Maintenance of a patent airway is a primary goal of clinical care following thoracic surgery. If airway obstruction is allowed to develop, atelectasis typically results. Atelectasis, in turn, causes two major complications of thoracic surgery—hypoxia and hypercapnia. Also, once atelectasis occurs, pneumonitis soon develops. Airway obstruction is indicated by restlessness, inadequate chest expansion, stridor, cyanosis, dyspnea, and noisy respirations. Indications of massive atelectasis include increased rate of respirations, rapid pulse, elevated temperature, profuse perspiration, and cyanosis.

If atelectasis is suspected the physician may order oxygen therapy, and the nurse may be asked to assist with bronchoscopic aspiration. Numerous therapies are employed in the treatment of pneumonia, e.g., antibiotics, IPPB, aerosol mixtures, mucolytic agents, chest physiotherapy, intratracheal suctioning and irrigation, CO_2 inhalation, bronchoscopy, tracheostomy, blow bottles, rebreathing tubes, and intercostal nerve blocks. Generally the development of postoperative atelectasis indicates that the patient's nursing care was inadequate and that all the necessary measures were not performed to maintain airway patency. (Atelectasis and pneumonia were discussed in Chapter 71.)

Infections

Prior to the use of more thorough preoperation preparation of the patient, and the advent of definitive antibiotic chemotherapy, pulmonary and pleural infections commonly occurred following thoracic surgery. Currently routine prophylactic antibiotic coverage is *not* used with thoracic surgery. Antibiotics are administered if infected areas were surgically entered or if an infection is known to exist in the wound, pleurae, or tracheobronchial tree. Whenever possible, antibiotics are selected after sensitivity studies have identified the specific medication to which a patient's organisms are sensitive.

Postoperative infection may be prevented by aseptic suctioning technique, aseptic technique when caring for the closed chest drainage system (e.g., when emptying the fluid collection bottle), administration of antibiotics as ordered, hygienic nose, mouth and skin care, and maintenance of a patent airway. If empyema occurs, additional surgery may be needed.

Adrenal Exhaustion

Patients who have had long debilitating illnesses prior to surgery may experience adrenal exhaustion postoperatively because of the stress of surgery. The nurse watches the patient for early indications of hypoadrenalism. (See Unit XIX.) Treatment includes administration of adrenocortical steroids.

Gastric Distention

Gastric distention may result from air swallowing as well as from depression of gastric motility as a result of anesthesia. Additionally, insufflation of anesthetic gases into the stomach may occur during surgery. Observe for gastric distention by inspecting and percussing the patient's abdomen. Abdominal distention is not only uncomfortable but is also potentially dangerous following thoracic surgery because the enlarged abdomen elevates the diaphragm and, thus, impairs the patient's ventilatory movements, which may already be precariously limited. Gastric dilatation most commonly occurs following surgical procedures on the left hemithorax, and occurs early in the postoperative period. An upright chest x-ray establishes the diagnosis.

When gastric dilatation occurs, the physician may order nasogastric suction to accomplish gastric decompression. The tube is left in place until gastrointestinal motility returns and the patient is taking adequate oral intake. Neostigmine (Prostigmin) may be prescribed to stimulate peristalsis and facilitate flatus expulsion. Ambulation and exercising also help the patient to expel flatus.

Subcutaneous Emphysema

Observe the patient for subcutaneous emphysema around his incision and in his chest and neck. To evaluate the rate of progression of the emphysema the nurse periodically marks the patient's chest with a skin-marking pencil at the outer periphery of the emphysematous tissue. If subcutaneous emphysema reaches the level of the patient's neck, measurements are periodically made of the neck's circumference.

Subcutaneous emphysema commonly occurs following thoracic surgery and usually is not dangerous (except in infants). However, a *progressive increase* in the amount of subcutaneous emphysema occurs if the patient's chest drainage tubes are not functioning effectively. Progressive emphysema is particularly serious when it occurs following pneumonectomy, because it may signify air leakage through the bronchial stump. If the rate of increase is rapid, the surgeon is notified. The treatments necessary may include: (1) insertion of a new thoracotomy tube; (2) the addition of suction to the closed chest drainage system (or increasing the amount of suction if it is currently in use); or (3) aspiration of the mediastinum. Occasionally it is necessary to return the patient to surgery to repair a bronchial stump. Severe subcutaneous emphysema of the neck may require tracheostomy. Areas of subcutaneous emphysema may be tender and therefore should be handled gently and palpated no oftener than necessary. Severe subcutaneous emphysema may be quite uncomfortable for the patient.

Acute Pulmonary Edema

Circulatory overload resulting in acute pulmonary edema is a potential threat following any resectional procedure because the operated lung does not immediately reexpand following surgery, and pulmonary tissue was extirpated during the operative procedure. Both of these factors cause a reduction in the size of the pulmonary vascular bed.

Fortunately acute pulmonary edema does not often occur following thoracic surgery. However, when failure of the left ventricle does occur as a result of surgery, it most typically develops following pneumonectomy or in patients who had congestive heart failure preoperatively. Acute pulmonary edema may occur rapidly following removal of one lung, not only because of the drastic reduction in the pulmonary circulatory system, but also because of the increased permeability of capillaries caused by hypoxia. *Acute pulmonary edema is a life-threatening complication.* Therefore, during the postoperative period the nurse directs her efforts at *preventing* this complication. *Remember:*

> *Following thoracic surgery never administer intravenous fluids at a rate exceeding 40 gtts./min. (unless specifically ordered otherwise) because of the possibility of precipitating circulatory overload and causing pulmonary edema.*

The possibility of overloading the vascular system and precipitating acute pulmonary edema following thoracic surgery can be reduced by carefully evaluating intake and output and by monitoring the central venous pressure (CVP) during the early postoperative period. Regulation of the rate of flow of intravenous fluids is determined by evaluating the CVP. (See Unit X.) Usually the surgeon specifies that if this pressure reaches a given level the nurse should limit the patient's fluid intake and notify him immediately. The CVP reflects the ability of the heart to pump the blood and the pressure under which the blood is returned to the superior vena cava or the heart's right atrium. Venous return to the right atrium is influenced by respiratory movements and intrathoracic pressure alterations. Resistance to the outflow of blood from the right side of the heart (causing elevation of the CVP) may result from the reduction in the pulmonary vascular compartment following resectional surgery (see also below).

The symptoms of pulmonary edema include copious frothy sputum, rales, dyspnea, cyanosis, and gurgling respirations. Observe the patient closely for these symptoms while he is receiving intravenous infusions, report their occurrence immediately, and reduce at once the flow rate of the infusion. If pulmonary edema occurs, obtain a rotating tourniquet set-up. Diuretics and parenteral digitalis may be prescribed.

ROUTINE POSTOPERATIVE CARE FOLLOWING THORACIC SURGERY

Specific orders are individualized after thoracic surgery, but certain routines are frequently followed. Some of the more common aspects of postoperative clinical care are discussed in this section.

Immediate Care

Upon receiving the patient in the recovery room or intensive care unit the nurse: (1) institutes oxygen therapy and suction as indicated; (2) positions the patient according to his condition; (3) evaluates and records vital signs (pulse, blood pressure, central venous pressure, temperature, and respirations); (4) makes certain that thoracotomy tubes are correctly attached to the prescribed type of closed chest drainage apparatus (with or without suction, as ordered); (5) examines the dressing or incision area (a dressing may not be present) for bleeding and/or drainage; (6) examines the patient for evidence of subcutaneous emphysema; (7) checks the rate of flow of intravenous blood or fluid replacements; (8) evaluates the sensorium of the conscious patient; (9) observes and auscultates the patient's chest for indications of complications (e.g., retraction of the rib cage during ventilatory movements, paradoxical respirations, ease or difficulty of ventilation, presence of stridor or rales); and (10) evaluates other factors indicative of the patient's general condition (skin, nail bed, and mucous membrane color; skin texture; respiratory pattern; body position; movement or lack of movement of facial muscles and extremities). Observations are made as frequently as the patient's condition warrants.

Equipment

Equipment that must be available and in good working condition during the immediate postoperative period following thoracic surgery typically includes apparatus for suctioning, closed chest drainage, measuring CVP, thoracentesis, inhalation therapy (oxygen, mist), and intravenous therapy. The nurse should have a stethoscope.

Equipment for *emergency care* that should be readily available includes Ambu type bag, respirator, tracheostomy set, laryngoscope, bronchoscope, endotracheal tubes, needles, syringes, vasoconstrictors, heart stimulants, and intravenous solutions.

Vital Signs

Typically, for the first two or three postoperative hours, the vital signs are taken every 15 minutes. Thereafter, if the pulse rate and blood pressure have started to stabilize at the preoperative level, vital signs are taken every 30 minutes for several hours and then hourly throughout the operative night. The blood pressure is closely evaluated for 24 to 36 hours postoperatively because it may fluctuate during this period. The patient with a persistently low blood pressure is closely observed because this finding may be caused by cardiac disorders, hemorrhage, pain, hypoxia, or an inadequate circulating fluid volume. During the postoperative period the patient is also closely observed for respiratory distress.

Central Venous Pressure Readings

As previously mentioned, the CVP is important following thoracotomy and is measured continuously or at least frequently. The nurse observes the CVP for sudden increases or decreases. Since the CVP measures the heart's ability to adequately accept and put out the circulating blood volume, an elevated CVP signals impaired venous return to the heart. (See also Unit X.)

When indicated, the CVP catheter may be used for such additional activities as drawing blood for laboratory tests, intravenous infusions, drug administration, and performing phlebotomy.

Fluids and Nutrition

During or immediately following surgery the patient is given a blood transfusion followed by whatever intravenous fluids the surgeon orders. As discussed, intravenous feedings and blood transfusions must be run slowly (unless specifically otherwise ordered) to prevent overloading of the vascular system, with resultant pulmonary edema. Once the patient is fully conscious, is not nauseated, and is generally doing well, he is usually permitted to have clear fluids. He then progresses to a soft and then a general diet as tolerated. Fluid intake is increased, also as tolerated, and is encouraged during the postoperative period, since fluid intake helps to liquefy tracheobronchial secretions so they can be more easily expectorated. Record intake and output and evaluate for imbalances.

Pain Management

Following thoracic surgery knowledgeable pain management is imperative. Unless the patient is adequately medicated the extreme pain and discomfort of the first few postoperative days may indirectly result in complications. On the other hand, if the patient is overly medicated with narcotics his cough reflex and respirations will be depressed, again setting the stage for the development of complications.

Pain may cause the patient to experience neurogenic hypotension, as pointed out earlier. Also, if the patient is not given adequate pain relief, he is unable to perform the essential postoperative activities of coughing, deep breathing, turning, exercising, sitting up, and ambulating. The patient in severe pain breathes shallowly and rapidly (in other words, ineffectively), and tries to avoid moving his chest. Also, he resists other movements. As a result of this inactivity secretions are retained and the lung does not properly reexpand. Atelectasis and pneumonia rapidly ensue. These complications may be fatal. When possible, medicate the patient prior to deep-breathing, coughing, and exercise sessions so he can participate more effectively.

In addition to the physical consequences of inadequate pain coverage the patient also suffers emotional anguish and is fearful. Obviously the nurse contributes greatly to the patient's total well-being by skillfully helping to relieve postoperative pain. Medications are, of course, not the only means of reducing pain. For example, correctly positioning and turning the patient are comfort measures that also provide relief (see below). (See also discussion of pain in Unit IX.)

During the first few days of postoperative care the patient may require frequent medication for pain relief. Commonly morphine or meperidine hydrochloride (Demerol) is prescribed. Some physicians do not prescribe morphine following thoracic surgery because of its depressing effects on the respiratory and cough centers; therefore, the medication of choice is meperidine. In addition to giving pain relief, meperidine also appears to dilate the bronchi. The opiates tend to have the opposite detrimental effect of producing bronchospasm and thickening secretions.

If narcotics are ordered following chest surgery, they are used sparingly. Sometimes dosages smaller than usual are ordered so the medication can be administered more frequently without depressing the respiratory centers in the brain. Medications that have analgesic-potentiating properties, such as hydroxyzine (Atarax, Vistaril) may be prescribed to be given in combination with small doses of narcotics. Following the administration of narcotics, closely observe the patient's respiratory rate and quality for indications of depression.

Following thoracic surgery the patient's chest is often extremely painful not only because of the trauma of the surgery, but also because of the presence of large chest drainage tubes. Sometimes severance of intercostal nerves at the time of surgery produces postoperative sensations of pain, numbness, or heaviness in the operative region. Usually these sensations are temporary. At the time of surgery some surgeons inject the intercostal nerves with a local anesthetic, e.g., procaine, to minimize pain during the immediate postoperative period. Occasionally performance of an intercostal nerve block is necessary postoperatively for pain relief.

Positioning; Turning

Following chest surgery the supine position is often the position of choice while the patient is unconscious. *Generally the Trendelenburg position is contraindicated* because it causes the abdominal organs to push against the diaphragm (and hence restrict lung excursions), and also because it creates pressure on the mediastinal contents. Such pressure decreases venous return and cardiac output. In some patients postoperative hypotension results from venous pooling of blood in the legs. This hypotension may be alleviated by applying elastic bandages to the legs or elevating the legs without elevating the hips.

Typically following thoracic surgery the patient remains flat until his vital signs have stabilized and he has regained consciousness. Then he is often positioned in a semi-Fowler position (head of the bed elevated 30 to 45 degrees). This position is desirable because it causes the diaphragm to drop down in a normal position (thus enhancing lung expansion); it makes possible ventilation with the least effort by the patient; and it facilitates drainage through the chest catheters. When moving the patient from a supine to a semi-Fowler position, elevate his head gradually.

Check positioning orders carefully for each patient. If these orders are unclear, clarify them before positioning the patient. Be certain you know if the patient is permitted to lie on the operated side or if the surgeon prefers that he be on his unoperated side or back. *Correct positioning is especially important following pulmonary resection. Following lobectomy* it is generally permissible to use full lateral turning on both sides. This permits expansion of the lung tissue on both the operated and unoperated sides. Occasionally the surgeon specifies that the patient is not to lie on the operated side. Lying on the operated side may also be forbidden *following segmentectomy or wedge resections* because the surgeon wants to foster expansion of the remaining pulmonary tissue. *If the patient has a sternum-splitting incision,* he may be positioned on his back or either side (the back position is most comfortable).

Following pneumonectomy extreme lateral turning is avoided because the mediastinum is not held in place by lung tissue on both sides; typically the patient is permitted to turn only one quarter of the full lateral position to prevent mediastinal shift and compression of the remaining lung. Generally the patient is allowed to lie on the operated side for brief periods, e.g., to permit back care. Then, if his pulse and blood pressure remain stable while he is turned, he may be turned on either side 24 hours following surgery. Some surgeons permit the patient to be positioned only on his back or on the operated side. The patient is turned hourly from one position to the other.

As the preceding discussion demonstrates, it is necessary to check positioning orders for each patient.

When helping the patient to move about, e.g., to slide up in bed or to sit up, support the back of his head and assist him from his unoperated side, e.g., do not tug or pull on the arm on the operated side. In many hospitals a piece of muslin or a rope (with a handle) long enough for the patient to grasp is tied securely to the foot of the bed. The patient is instructed to grasp this "pull rope" when pulling himself up to the sitting position or lowering himself to lie flat, during his later convalescence. Also, be careful not to exert traction on the chest tubes. While in bed the patient may find it comfortable to have a pillow under his neck and head; a pillow under the back may be uncomfortable.

Turn the patient every one or two hours to mobilize and promote drainage of secretions within the tracheobronchial tree and the drainage of air and fluids from the pleural space (if closed chest drainage is employed). Allowing the patient to remain in one position for too long predisposes to thrombus formation (because it slows blood flow) and may cause inadequate aeration of part of the lungs. Turning improves circulation generally since it causes muscles to squeeze on blood vessels. Position changes also have favorable effects on the patient's general comfort. When changing the patient's position, reposition him so he maintains good posture and body alignment, and so his thoracic movements are unrestricted. If the thorax cannot move freely to ventilate and expand the lungs, alveolar hypoventilation and its serious consequences occur. Also, when positioning the patient, be certain his chest and drainage tubes are correctly placed and are not kinked or compressed.

Patients usually have very sore, aching chests after chest surgery. If ribs have been resected, the patient's rib cage may remain sore for weeks. The large rib-spreading retractors used during surgery also make the chest cage very sore. Gentleness in handling the patient is essential.

Ambulation

As with other types of surgery, early ambulation following thoracic surgery helps to reduce postoperative complications since it improves ventilation, circulation, and the patient's morale. Even though the patient may be reluctant, ambulation is usually encouraged as soon as vital signs are stable postoperatively. It is thus not unusual for patients to ambulate on the evening of surgery or the morning of the first postoperative day. Closed chest drainage does not prevent the patient from getting out of bed, sitting up in a chair, or walking about. Some physicians order ambulation every four hours, around the clock, to prevent vascular stasis and its related complications. Patients with limited cardiovascular reserve or heart disorders may not be able to ambulate as soon as other patients whose general state of health is better.

Exercises

Exercising is another important aspect of postoperative care following thoracic surgery. As stated previously, exercises to be performed postoperatively are taught to the patient during the preoperative period whenever possible so the patient can become familiar with them and practice them at a time when he is not in acute discomfort. Postoperatively the exercises ordered by the surgeon are reviewed with the patient and are performed with assistance or under the supervision of the nurse and/or physical therapist. Nonvigorous exercises of the arms, trunk, and lower extremities begin soon after surgery.

Goals. Postoperative exercises following thoracic surgery are directed at:

- Preventing collapse of lung tissue, atelectasis, and impaired ventilation. Breathing exercises and abdominal breathing (see Chapter 70) are performed to reexpand the lung, improve ventilation, obtain maximal pulmonary function, and help the patient to cough more effectively. Abdominal breathing helps to minimize pain associated with ventilation.
- Preventing musculoskeletal and circulatory disorders. Complete range-of-motion (ROM) exercises are performed while the patient is confined to bed to prevent the complications of bed rest (see Chapter 27) and to preserve body postural symmetry.
- Preventing ankylosis of the shoulder and stiffness and contractures of the arm on the operated side. Exercising the arm and shoulder on the operated side is directed at maintaining normal joint range-of-motion, reeducating injured or unused muscles, and minimizing postoperative discomfort (see below).
- Preventing a generally depressed mental state. Exercising improves the patient's general feeling of well-being.

Following thoracoplasty and pneumonectomy it is particularly important to maintain correct body alignment when positioning the patient and to have the patient practice maintaining good posture. The prevention of postoperative scoliosis is especially important following pneumonectomy.

Preparation. Prior to exercise sessions, encourage the patient to cough productively to clear his tracheobronchial tree. This ensures more effective oxygenation during the exercise activities. Provision of adequate pain coverage prior to exercise sessions has previously been discussed.

Tolerance. During periods of exercising the patient is closely observed for indications of dyspnea, shortness of breath, or fatigue. The patient's ability to tolerate his exercise program is evaluated and recorded so his exercise program can be increased or modified according to his abilities. Care is taken to not fatigue the patient and to not perform exercises beyond the point of pain. Exercising is restricted if a patient has persisting dyspnea or shortness of breath, and the surgeon is notified of the patient's condition. It takes time for a patient's exercise tolerance to increase, because the body must gradually adjust to its reduced respiratory capacity following resectional surgery; the greater the amount of lung resected, the longer the period of adjustment.

Exercises are introduced in an orderly sequence and are increased in number as the patient's tolerance improves. Exercises are first performed with the patient lying in bed, later while sitting up and, finally, while standing. Planned rest periods are important during exercise periods. The activity tolerance that a patient has two to three months after discharge is about the maximal level that will be attained. Some patients find that this level is below their exercise capacity level before surgery.

Arm and Shoulder Postoperative Exercises. Following thoracic surgery the arm and shoulder on the operative side are actively or passively taken through a full range of motion several times daily to prevent a "frozen" shoulder. *Passive* exercises on the operated arm and shoulder are usually initiated four hours following recovery from anesthesia. Exercises may be performed twice every four to six hours through the first 24 postoperative hours. Some surgeons believe that in order to prevent the dysfunction syndrome the arm and shoulder on the operated side should be exercised through a full range of motion approximately 20 times every two hours. Remember to support the patient's arm when performing passive exercises.

Active exercising is encouraged as soon as the patient's condition permits and the surgeon gives approval. Often on the first or second postoperative day the patient begins actively exercising his arm and shoulder. He should be supervised to be sure the exercises are performed correctly. Preoperatively the physical therapist should measure the patient's joint range of motion; postoperatively the goal of physical therapy is to return the patient to this preoperative level of function.

Postoperative arm and shoulder exercises help to prevent the formation of adhesions between the muscles incised during surgery. During thoracotomy an incision is made across two separate layers of muscle. Normally these layers glide smoothly over one another. However, after each layer has been cut across and then sutured, the two layers tend to adhere at the suture lines postoperatively. Adhesions joining the two layers of muscle will quickly form unless the muscles are repeatedly exercised.

The muscles typically transected by thoracotomy incisions include the trapezius, latissimus dorsi, rhomboideus major, and serratus anterior. These muscle groups form the shoulder girdle and maintain the posture of the trunk. Unless these injured muscles are restored to efficient functioning, porstural deformities result from the overdevelopment of similar muscle groups on the other side of the body. Postoperatively some exercises are directed at hyperextending the arms with resistance (to strengthen the latissimus dorsi), adducting and flexing forward the upper extremities (to maintain shoulder girdle motion), and adducting the scapula (to strengthen the trapezius).

If you are unfamiliar with a surgeon's preferences for an exercise program following thoracotomy, it is advisable to obtain the necessary details from him. Some specific arm and shoulder exercises commonly prescribed following thoracic surgery include:

> Elevate the shoulders (thus elevating the clavicle and scapula). Hunch the shoulders forward and then pull them back as far as possible.

> Raise the elbow upward, keeping the elbow as close to the ear as possible and then extend the arm straight out at the level of the shoulder.

> Extend the arm up and back, then out to the side and back, and finally down at the side and back. This exercise extends and abducts the arm.

> Sit erect in an armchair and grip the arms of the chair in such a manner that pressing down on the palms of the hands will raise the body straight up in the chair. Next, while slowly inhaling, press down on the palms of the hands, pull in the abdomen and stretch up from the waist until the elbows are completely extended. After briefly holding this position, slowly exhale while slowly lowering the body back into the chair. This exercise depresses the shoulder in addition to exercising the lungs.

> Place the hands on the small of the back and attempt to push the elbows and shoulder blades toward one another. This exercise adducts and elevates the scapula.

> Reach over the head and push the arm in an upward and outward manner. This exercise rotates the scapula, fixing it against the rib cage.

> Place the arm bent at the elbow so the hand lies on the stomach (Fig. 73-2, *A*). Then grasp the arm at the

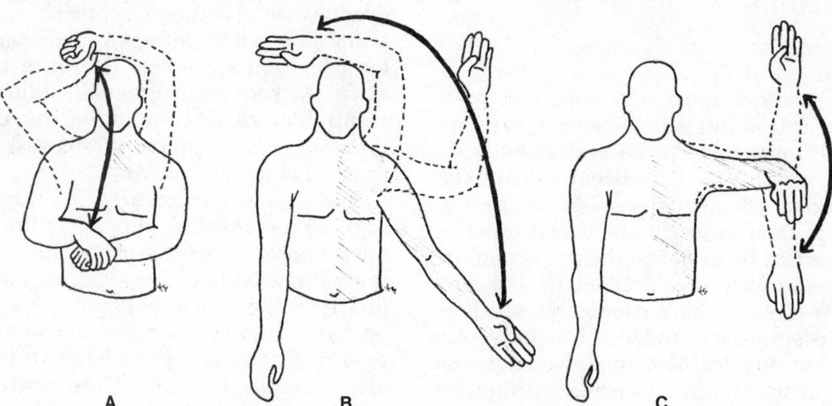

FIGURE 73-2. Some arm and shoulder exercises commonly prescribed following thoracic surgery. See text for discussion.

wrist (the patient can do this himself by using his "good" arm and hand) and raise the arm in an arc up off the abdomen and up directly over the top of the head. Return to the beginning position. This exercise flexes the operative arm. (This exercise can be performed while the patient lies flat on his back in bed, as well as while sitting or standing erect.) Instruct the patient to inhale while raising his arm and to exhale while lowering it. This adds a breathing exercise to the arm exercise.

> Place the arm at the side, palm up, and raise the arm in an arc sideward up to the top of the head (Fig. 73-2, *B*). Return to the starting position. (These exercises can be performed while the patient is in bed by sliding the arm on the mattress.) Again, have the patient inhale while raising his arm and exhale while lowering it. This exercise abducts and adducts the shoulder.

> Place the arm to the side at shoulder level with the elbow bent at a right angle. Then rotate the shoulder by moving the arm in an arc so it goes back (to touch the bed with the back of the hand), and then forward (to touch the bed with the palm) (Fig. 73-2, *C*). This exercise rotates the shoulder outward and inward.

Throughout the postoperative period the patient is encouraged to further exercise his arm on the operated side by making a conscious effort to use that arm in the daily activities of eating, reaching for things, grooming himself, and so forth. Placing the bedside stand on the operated side encourages the patient to reach with his affected arm. Also, it is desirable for the patient to pull himself up to a sitting position by using the arm on the operated side to grasp the pull rope.

Expectedly, patients are reluctant to carry out postoperative exercises after surgery because of pain and other discomforts. However, the patient must realize that if the arm and shoulder are not exercised, they will become stiff, and painful contractures will develop. Thus, some pain and discomfort must be tolerated during the postoperative period in order to avoid future disability and discomfort.

Respiratory Therapy

Routinely following chest surgery the patient receives supportive oxygen therapy, follows a deep-breathing, coughing regimen (with his chest "splinted" by the nurse), and is suctioned as indicated. Postural drainage may or may not be ordered. When ordered, postural drainage should be continued as scheduled until the cough is nonproductive and the patient is ambulatory. Techniques of chest percussion and vibrating are not used in the early postoperative period because of the presence of the wound.

Various other techniques of respiratory therapy may be ordered to mobilize tracheobronchial secretions following thoracic surgery. These include humidification or steam inhalations, inhalations of an aerosol mist to thin tracheobronchial secretions, inhalation of high concentrations of carbon dioxide to force deep breathing, tracheal instillations of solutions, e.g., saline, through a small plastic tube (placed percutaneously) to produce coughing, and the use of intermittent positive pressure breathing (IPPB) or blow bottles to cause pulmonary expansion and improve ventilatory volume. IPPB treatments may be prescribed with such medications as isoproterenol (Isuprel). Consult Chapter 70 for discussion of most of these procedures.

Evaluation. Following thoracic surgery the patient's respiratory status is carefully evaluated, since temporary or permanent changes from normal respiratory function may result from thoracotomy. Usually the changes in ventilation and respiration that result from surgery are basically unilateral. Evaluation of the effectiveness of ventilation and respiration in a patient following chest surgery includes the following actions:

> Expose the patient's chest periodically to observe the rise and fall of both sides of the chest during ventilatory movements. (Following pneumonectomy the chest wall on the operated side is obviously not expected to move since the entire lung has been resected.) Decreased movement on one side of the chest during inspiration is one indication of possible pneumothorax.

> Auscultate the chest and carefully evaluate the quality of respirations; e.g., rales indicate congestion. Observe the patient closely for indications of respiratory distress. After pneumonectomy the removal of an entire lung may lower the patient's vital capacity and the patient may easily become dyspneic.

> Measure and record the tidal and minute volumes as requested by the surgeon.

> Obtain blood specimens or assist the physician in obtaining these for blood gas evaluation.

Postoperatively, to detect hypoventilation, hypoxia, and hypercapnia, the patient's arterial blood gases and pH are periodically analyzed and his ventilatory efficiency is evaluated by measuring tidal ventilation. The latter measurement is made with a spirometer, which may be attached to a cuffed tracheostomy or endotracheal tube or may be used with a nose clip and mouthpiece or face mask. The nurse may be asked to measure the patient's ventilatory capacity. Additionally, the patient's pulse and respiratory rates and blood pressure are carefully evaluated and he is closely observed for indications of respiratory insufficiency such as cerebral indications of hypoxia and hypercapnia, e.g., irritability, restlessness, disorientation, or (more seriously) stupor and coma; decreased respiratory excursion; retraction of the rib cage; and dyspnea, stridor, rales, or rhonchi. (See discussion of respiratory insufficiency and failure, Chapter 69.) The patient with respiratory insufficiency may require oxygen therapy, assisted ventilation, and a tracheostomy. Rarely, the reduction in alveolar surface following resectional surgery causes respiratory acidosis as a result of the retention of increased quantities of carbon dioxide.

Oxygen Therapy. The administration of oxygen during the immediate postoperative period ensures adequate oxygenation during the time that the patient's ventilation may be reduced from anesthetic depression, lethargy, and pain. Also, it is during the immediate postoperative period that the lung is the most fully collapsed. Collapse of the lung and resection of pulmonary tissue reduces the alveolar-capillary surface, where exchange of respiratory gases occurs. This situation corrects itself as remaining lung tissue reinflates, or, following pneumonectomy, as the body adjusts to the loss of one lung.

Nasal oxygen (6 to 8 L./min.) is routinely administered by cannula or catheter until the patient recovers from anesthesia, or longer if respiratory insufficiency is present. Some surgeons order oxygen therapy for the first 24 hours postoperatively and then P.R.N. Sometimes it is possible to relieve a patient's restlessness by administering oxygen nasally or into a tracheostomy. Routinely the nasal method of administering oxygen is preferred to mask administration following thoracic surgery, since the mask interferes with suctioning, coughing, and expectorating.

Usually patients adapt quite rapidly to their altered pulmonary capacities. Because oxygen therapy impairs ambulation and effective coughing, it is usually discontinued as soon as possible. (Oxygen therapy is discussed in Chapter 70.) Nasal oxygen is administered if the patient is able to breathe effectively without assistance; a respirator is generally necessary if the patient's respirations are ineffective.

Coughing and Deep-breathing Regimen. The most important activities that the postoperative thoracotomy patient can perform are coughing and deep breathing. As discussed earlier, this fact is emphasized during preoperative teaching, and the patient is instructed in the correct procedures for performing these activities. Also, the patient is informed that he will be expected to cough and deep breathe at least every one to two hours during the first 24 to 48 postoperative hours.

Following chest surgery coughing and deep breathing are important because they help to move tracheobronchial secretions out of the lung, assist with reexpanding the lung, improve pulmonary circulation, prevent "stiffness" of the lung, and help to force air and fluid out of the pleural space through chest drainage tubes.

Coughing is a protective mechanism by which foreign material is expelled from the air passages. Coughing loosens secretions and forces them into the upper respiratory tract, from which they may be expectorated or suctioned. Adequate ventilation cannot be obtained unless the airway is clear of secretions. *Deep breathing* expands the lung tissue surface, thereby increasing the area for respiratory exchanges (O_2 and CO_2) to occur across the alveolar membranes. Deep breathing also improves pulmonary circulation, because lung expansion decreases intrapleural pressure and this, in turn, stimulates the flow of blood to the lungs. If the lungs are not periodically stretched by deep breathing they tend to become progressively stiffer and more difficult to inflate.

These activities are especially important following thoracic surgery. If the lung is not promptly reexpanded, adhesions may form in the pleural space and keep the lung compressed. Infections may develop if secretions accumulate in the pleural space, collapsed lung, or tracheobronchial tree. Accumulations of secretions in the tracheobronchial tree also may cause obstruction, atelectasis, and ventilatory insufficiency.

Any patient with a chest incision and chest drainage tubes has a natural tendency to avoid coughing and deep breathing because of the pain caused by these motions. However, it is necessary for the patient to force himself to cough and breathe deeply in spite of moderately severe pain and discomfort if postoperative complications are to be avoided. The nurse's assistance and encouragement are necessary to keep the patient on an effective coughing and deep-breathing regimen. The nurse helps the patient to perform these important activities by giving verbal encouragement and instruction; reminding the patient when it is time to cough and deep breathe; providing appropriate pain medication to help to alleviate the chest pain associated with coughing and deep breathing; administering treatments ordered to help to loosen secretions and to increase the efficiency of the coughing and deep breathing; and properly positioning the patient and splinting his chest (see below).

Coughing and deep-breathing routines are started once the patient regains consciousness and are usually continued every hour (or oftener) for the first 24 postoperative hours. Turn the patient, take his vital signs, administer medications, and perform other necessary nursing care when awakening him hourly to cough and deep breathe; then it is not necessary to reawaken him later for these activities. In addition to coughing, the patient is instructed to take five to 10 deep breaths hourly. After the first 24 hours it is usually sufficient if the patient coughs and deep breathes every two to four hours. The routine varies, however, according to the patient's condition.

Effective coughing cannot occur if the patient's body alignment is poor, e.g., if he is slumped down or curled up in bed. The most effective coughing is achieved with the patient sitting erectly upright. Thus, as soon as the patient's blood pressure is stable he is assisted to sit up in bed and cough.

Often patients are afraid to deep breathe and cough following thoracic surgery because they fear they may "split open" their incisions or damage their lungs. These fears can be abated by patiently yet firmly reassuring the patient that the coughing and deep-breathing regimens are actually helpful. The patient is also reassured by having the nurse manually splint his incision. (Splinting is discussed later.)

Pain, fatigue, and fear may cause the patient to merely clear his throat rather than cough effectively. Also, he may tend to breathe shallowly rather than deeply. The nurse tactfully reminds the patient to deep breathe and to cough in the manner he practiced preoperatively, e.g., to inhale deeply enough that the chest expands and the "voice box is shut off," then to let pressure build up in the chest, and finally to suddenly let the air out by coughing with his mouth and throat open. Keeping the glottis tight increases the intrapulmonary pressure. Before coughing it is helpful if the patient takes several deep breaths.

Additional details important in the proper coughing and deep-breathing routine are as follow: (1) give the patient two tissues to cover his mouth and nose when exhaling or coughing; (2) tell the patient to expand his chest by breathing in deeply enough so that his chest wall will move your hands as they rest lightly on the rib cage; (3) instruct the patient to relax his abdomen while breathing in, so his abdomen will expand while his chest expands; and (4) once the expansion is complete, have the patient forcibly cough while consciously tightening his abdomen and squeezing down his rib cage.

Because pain coverage is best 20 to 30 minutes after the patient is given his pain medication, schedule coughing and deep-breathing sessions at those times when possible. Remember that the less pain the patient experiences the more effectively he can cough and deep breathe; remember also the hazards of overmedicating the patient.

After the patient coughs several times, listen to his chest with a stethoscope. If the breath sounds are still "wet," let the patient briefly rest and then help him to cough again. Encourage him to cough until his chest sounds clear of secretions. Sips of warm water sometimes help a patient to cough more effectively.

Occasionally a patient momentarily loses consciousness (syncope) during the deep-breathing and coughing regimen. This may occur because: (1) cerebral ischemia develops because of the fact that the activities increase intrathoracic pressure and thus impede venous return to the heart and reduce cardiac output; and/or the blood's carbon dioxide content is suddenly reduced because hyperventilation "blows off" large quantities of CO_2 from the lungs.[178] Usually the patient recovers within a few minutes, since syncope is typically a self-limited disorder.

Splinting the Chest. The nurse splints a thoracic incision (or a painful chest) by placing her hands anteriorly and posteriorly around the incised area* (Fig. 73-3). (Be certain you wash prior to and after handling the patient.) When splinting a chest keep the palms of your hands open and your fingers together (separating your fingers could cause uncomfortable uneven pressure or squeezing). Apply firm even pressure over the incision without restricting chest expansion. Next, instruct the patient to cover his nose and mouth with tissues and tell him you are ready for him to take a deep breath and cough.

Note in Figure 73-3 that the nurse has positioned herself on the side of the patient opposite to his incision and she is standing so her head is behind the patient's chest. This protects her by keeping her out of the path of the patient's cough, and it also permits her to listen to the chest during the coughing. Because she has her hands on the patient's chest the nurse can feel if the patient expands his chest as he should while taking a deep breath.

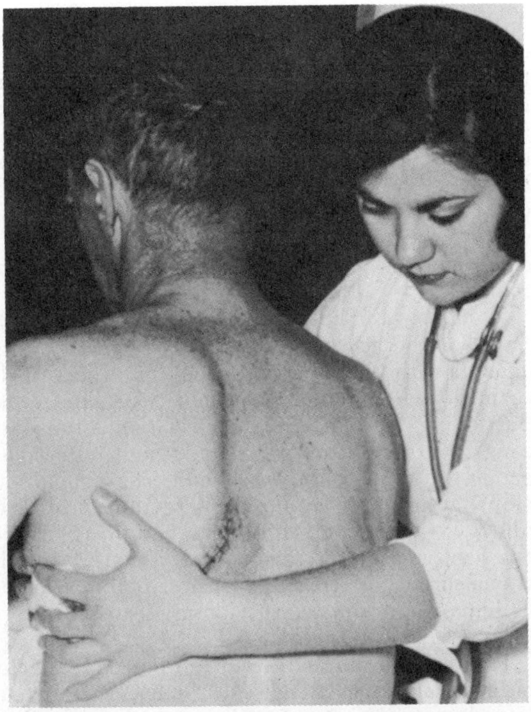

FIGURE 73-3. Correct position for "splinting" a patient's chest. See text. (From MacVicar, J., and Mendelsohn, H. J.: *In* Meltzer, L. E., Abdellah, F., and Kitchell, J. R. (eds.): *Concepts and Practices of Intensive Care for Nurse Specialists.* Philadelphia, The Charles Press, 1969.)

Good body mechanics are important when you splint a patient's chest, so that neither you nor the patient experiences fatigue from the position assumed and so the patient feels securely supported but not painfully squeezed. Proper splinting does not depress the sternum and does not restrict the normal excursions of the diaphragm (by holding the lower part of the rib cage, i.e., the last five pairs of ribs). The diaphragm contributes over half to the ventilatory process and thus must be free to move. During inspiration the diaphragm flattens out and the sternum elevates. While properly splinting the chest incision the nurse helps to depress the rib cage during the expiratory phase of ventilation. This application of pressure during the expiratory phase helps the patient to expel secretions.

Correctly splinting a patient's chest, as described, provides security for him in addition to reducing his discomfort when coughing and deep

*Splinting may also be performed by supporting beneath the incision with one hand and exerting downward pressure on the shoulder of the affected side with the other hand.

breathing. Splinting decreases stretching of a chest incision and thus minimizes pain during the forceful ventilatory movements of deep breathing and coughing. For the first few postoperative days the chest is splinted by the nurse during deep-breathing and coughing sessions. However, the patient is soon able to splint his operated side with one hand and to cover his mouth with the other while coughing and deep breathing, and thus independence is gained for the performance of this routine.

Suctioning. The nurse caring for patients who have had thoracic surgery needs to become familiar enough with chest auscultation that she can determine when a patient should be suctioned. Suctioning is performed when a patient's lungs are congested and he is unable to cough effectively enough to remove the secretions. Pharyngeal suctioning helps to remove secretions from the pharynx and also stimulates coughing. Endotracheal suctioning removes secretions from the tracheobronchial tree and also stimulates an excellent cough reflex. Suctioning is discussed in Chapter 70.

During the immediate postoperative period orders may be written for the patient to be suctioned at least every two hours and then P.R.N. Sometimes a tracheostomy is necessary to facilitate maintenance of a clear airway.

> *Following pulmonary resectional surgery there is the potential danger of accidentally traumatizing or actually pushing the suction catheter through a bronchial suture line while performing deep tracheal suctioning.*

In some settings deep tracheal suctioning is performed only by physicians. Certainly it should never be performed by a nurse who is unskilled in the procedure. The possibility of breaking through the bronchial suture line is greatest when pneumonectomy has been performed, because the suture line is at the tracheal bifurcation. With other resectional procedures, e.g., lobectomy, it is usually considerably more difficult to break the suture line since the suction catheter would have to make two turns before reaching the bronchial stump.

A mucous plug blocking one of the bronchi may cause a patient to become confused and cyanotic and to develop a rapid respiratory rate and tachycardia. Suctioning is necessary. In some instances the physician can remove the mucous plug only by suctioning through a bronchoscope.

The airway of the unconscious patient is carefully maintained with suctioning, correct positioning, and other appropriate measures to maintain its patency. (See Units VI and VIII.)

Postural Drainage. Postural drainage in the Trendelenburg position may or may not be ordered to be routinely performed during the postoperative period. Do not carry out this procedure unless you have a specific order from the surgeon to do so. Some surgeons do not want their patients placed in a head-low position following thoracic surgery because they believe it is too difficult for the patient to breathe while in that position. If you do perform postural drainage following chest surgery, be certain to observe the patient closely for respiratory distress during the procedure, and be certain to use only those positions authorized by the surgeon for a given patient. Do not leave the patient unattended during postural drainage sessions. (Postural drainage is discussed in Chapter 70.)

Chest X-Rays

Chest x-rays are often taken daily for several days following thoracic surgery so the surgeon can evaluate the patient's progress. The surgeon looks at the chest x-ray for indications of pulmonary expansion or collapse; infection in the pleural space, lung parenchyma, or tracheobronchial tree; atelectasis; or air or fluid collections in the pleural space. Treatment is then planned in accordance with the needs of the patient.

CLOSED CHEST DRAINAGE

As previously mentioned, during chest surgery atmospheric air enters the pleural space through the thoracotomy. This causes the lung to collapse on the operated side. Following thoracotomy it is thus generally necessary to use closed chest drainage to foster and permit the drainage of air and/or fluid from the pleural space and to prevent their reflux (i.e., backward or return flow); to help to reexpand remaining lung tissue by reestablishing negative pressure; and to prevent shifting of the mediastinum and collapse of lung tissue by equalizing pressure.

The nurse has numerous responsibilities associated with the use of closed chest drainage, e.g., to maintain proper functioning of the apparatus and to periodically observe the chest drainage.

Closed chest drainage means simply that the drainage system used is closed to atmospheric pressure. As explained in the following pages, various types of apparatus may be used. The classic form of closed chest drainage is a water-seal bottle (a one- or two-bottle set-up may be used). Controlled mechanical suction may or may not be applied to a water-seal set-up. When suction is used, two or three bottles are attached together and connected to a suction source such as a wall suction outlet or a portable suction motor.

In some settings bottle drainage systems have been replaced with newer equipment of simpler design and maintenance, e.g., Pleur-Evac units (discussed later). However, the nurse must still understand the water-seal forms of bottle chest drainage because she may need to set up and use these systems in settings where the newer equipment is not available. Additionally, an understanding of the principles of bottle chest drainage is basic to understanding any type of closed chest drainage equipment.

The nurse caring for a patient with closed chest drainage must: (1) understand the principles and purposes of chest drainage; (2) understand the specific apparatus being used so she can tell when it is functioning correctly, when it is malfunctioning, and, if possible, how to correct malfunctions, (3) understand necessary precautions of importance; and (4) detect early symptoms of impending complications in the patient, e.g., tension pneumothorax. It is necessary to be prepared for emergencies by keeping available a thoracentesis tray and an extra set of bottles, connectors, tubing, and so forth.

Before caring for a patient on closed chest drainage be certain to familiarize yourself with the apparatus being used. Literature describing some closed chest drainage systems and their functions is available from the distributors of commercial equipment. Hospital procedure books are another source of information. Explain the basic purposes of closed chest drainage to the patient and his family. Also, inform them of necessary precautions they should know. Show the patient how to be careful of the drainage tubes and other apparatus when he is moving about so he does not kink or pull on tubing. Place a sign on the patient's bed which clearly cautions visitors and others not to handle the chest suction equipment and to be careful not to accidentally displace any of it.

Uses and Objectives

Closed chest drainage is used in the treatment of empyema and pneumothorax (e.g., following chest injuries or spontaneous pneumothorax), and postoperatively after thoracic or thoracico-abdominal surgery. Although it appears somewhat formidable initially, the apparatus for closed chest drainage is actually quite simple. Regardless of the type of apparatus used, all have the same objectives: to remove fluid and/or air from the pleural space; to reduce the size of the pleural space; to reestablish normal negative pressure in the pleural space; to promote reexpansion of the lung with apposition and cohesion of the parietal and pulmonary pleurae (so normal ventilation is restored); and to prevent reflux (i.e., backward or return flow) of air and/or fluid back into the pleural space from the drainage apparatus.

Insertion of Chest Catheters

Usually chest catheters are inserted in an operating room at the time of chest surgery. However, in some emergencies and in treating such disorders as empyema, a chest catheter may be inserted in a treatment room or at the bedside. (Chest catheters are sometimes also called "chest drains," "thoracotomy tubes," or "chest tubes.")

In the course of pulmonary surgery, the surgeon incises the parietal pleura, and thus enters the pleural space. Atmospheric air then rushes into the pleural space. As a result, the lung recoils to its unexpanded size and remains compressed, and the cohesion of the parietal and pulmonary pleurae is disrupted. Chest surgery thus causes the patient to have a pneumothorax on the operated side.

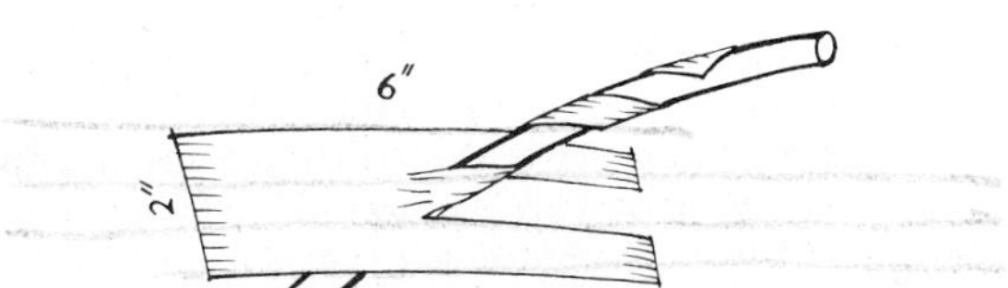

FIGURE 73–4. Tape attached to chest catheter to provide additional support on outside of chest dressing. (From Sutton, A. L., *Bedside Nursing*. 2nd ed. 1969.)

During chest surgery the anesthetist carefully manages pulmonary function for the patient. As the surgeon prepares to close, the anesthetist mechanically expands the operated lung. The surgeon positions chest drainage catheters within the chest and then closes the chest wall while the anesthetist inflates the lung.

When the chest wall is closed, pressure within the pleural space is initially atmospheric. Additional air may continue to escape into the pleural space for a while through openings in the pulmonary pleural incision. Although the pleura is sutured it takes time for it to heal. The trauma of surgery causes serosanguineous fluid to collect in the patient's chest until healing occurs. Unfortunately this fluid is a good culture medium and may thus predispose to infection. Also, the fluid may cause pleural thickening, which reduces pulmonary compliance and reduces the lung's ventilatory and diffusion capacities by "stiffening" the lung. Closed chest drainage (via the chest catheters) is therefore used postoperatively to remove air and serosanguineous fluid from the pleural space.

Following resectional surgery (except pneumonectomy) two catheters are usually placed in the chest. One of these (the "upper" or "anterior" tube) is placed anteriorly through the second intercostal space to permit the escape of air rising in the pleural space. The other catheter (the "lower" or "posterior" tube) is placed posteriorly through the 8th or 9th intercostal space in the midaxillary line to drain off serosanguineous fluid accumulating in the lower portion of the pleural space. The lower tube may have a larger diameter than the upper to enhance free drainage. Chest catheters may be brought out of the chest wall through stab wounds or through the incisional line. Although the catheters are secured to the patient's skin with suture, the tubes also may be taped to the outside of the dressing, as shown in Figure 73–4 to provide security against displacement.

The two chest catheters may be joined to each other with a glass Y-junction (and then attached to one water-seal drainage set), but it is preferable to leave the two catheters separate and to attach them to two separate water-seal drainage systems. This makes it possible to monitor the air and fluid drainage from each tube and then to remove the nondraining tube without disrupting the rest of the system. Flexible drainage tubing connects the chest catheter with the drainage apparatus. Usually the catheters are connected to the drainage apparatus before the patient leaves surgery.

Factors Affecting Chest Drainage

Various factors may affect the removal of air and fluid through the chest drainage system.

Location of Chest Drainage Apparatus. The apparatus for closed chest drainage must always be located at a level *lower than the patient's chest* (unless for some reason the catheters are clamped). Drainage by gravity is thus maintained, and air and fluid are not forced back into the pleural space. The drainage apparatus may be located in a box or special rack (fastened to the patient's bed or on wheels at the bedside) or taped securely to the floor so it will not accidentally be knocked over. The preferred arrangement is the rack attached to the bed, because the danger of breaking, elevating, or upsetting the bottles is reduced. If drainage bottles are on the floor, be careful not to lower a high-low bed or side rails onto the bottles. Keep the drainage bottles about two to three feet below the patient's chest.

When moving the patient from surgery to the recovery room the tubing may be *double clamped* and the drainage apparatus may then be placed on top of the patient's bed while he is being transported. After the patient is situated in the recovery room the apparatus is lowered below the level of the patient's chest and then the clamps are opened. *Never open clamps on the drainage tubing if the apparatus is above the level of the patient's chest or the fluid in the drainage bottle will run down or be siphoned into the patient's pleural cavity.*

Position of the Patient. Positioning following chest surgery has been discussed. Positioning orders must be followed carefully. Frequently a semi-Fowler position is used. If the patient can be positioned on the side that has the chest catheters coming out of it, position him in such a way that he is not lying on (and compressing or kinking) the catheters or tubing, since this not only impairs drainage and causes retrograde pressure (which forces drainage back into the pleural cavity) but also greatly increases the patient's discomfort. When the patient is in a lateral position place a small sandbag or folded towel on either side of the tubing to prevent the patient's body weight from compressing the tubing.

Placement and Length of Drainage Tubing. Drainage tubing (connecting the chest catheters with the drainage apparatus) should be neither too short nor too long. Attach the tubing to the edge of the patient's mattress bedding in such a way that it falls in a straight line to the drainage apparatus with no dependent loops. Dependent loops of tubing that contain fluid obstruct flow and create back pressure, thus impairing drainage of air or fluid. Drainage tubing may be secured to the bedding in various ways. For example, place a rubber band or strip of adhesive tape around the tubing and then pin the other end of the rubber band or tape to the mattress. Or, make a trough in the drawsheet around the drainage tube, then pull the two sides of the trough up on either side of the tube and pin them together. Do not pin the tubing so tightly in the trough that it is constricted or cannot be moved. Sandbags, small pillows, or folded abdominal pads can also be positioned around the tube to make a trough.

From the mattress to the patient the tubing length should be adequate for the patient to turn and sit up without pulling on the chest catheters. Coil excess tubing flat on the bed. Excessive tubing length adds to problems with tangling and kinking of the tube. Each time the patient is turned or otherwise moved, check chest catheters to be certain they are not displaced, and check drainage tubing to be certain it is properly positioned.

Maintaining Patency of Drainage Tubing. Frequently check the patency of the drainage tubing and chest catheters. Make certain the patient is not lying on the tubing and that it is not otherwise kinked or compressed. Also, make sure the tube is not internally plugged, e.g., with blood clots. The flow of drainage fluids can easily be observed through clear plastic tubing. A glass adapter in rubber tubing makes observation of drainage possible. Also, observe the fluid collecting in the drainage bottles. *If the tubing is not patent, drainage of air and fluid from the pleural space is impossible.*

Sometimes when there is a great deal of bloody drainage from the chest, e.g., in the early postoperative period following chest surgery, drainage tubes are "milked" every 30 to 60 minutes. *"Milking" a drainage tube* means the tubing is gently compressed in the direction of the drainage apparatus (away from the patient) to remove air, fluid or blood clots. The tubing is gently clasped in the nurse's hand and then (with her other hand stabilizing the tube so it will not have traction on it and be displaced) the hand is slid over the tubing in a direction *away from* the chest and *toward* the drainage system. (Alcohol sponges held in the hand make it possible to slide more easily down the length of the tubing). ("Milking" is also called "stripping.") Another way to milk a chest tube is to clasp one hand around the tube as close to the chest as possible and squeeze the tube against the palm of the hand, and then proceed similarly downward, hand over hand toward the drainage apparatus. Some plastic chest tubes have a built-in bulb device for milking. Because milking the tubing changes intrapleural pressure and can be painful if performed too vigorously, the nurse is as gentle as possible during the procedure.

Taping the portion of the drainage tubing that enters the drainage bottle to a piece of tongue blade prevents kinking of the tube in this area, and is another way of maintaining tube patency.

The accumulation of blood, fluid, or air in the pleural space may eventually compress the lung, with the possibility of tension pneumothorax or mediastinal shift occurring. Therefore, if malfunction of the drainage apparatus occurs, the nurse tries to immediately correct the problem and to observe the patient closely for *early* symptoms indicative of complications. The *early* detection of tension pneumothorax, for example, can prevent mediastinal shift if appropriate treatment is given promptly.

The nurse notifies the physician immediately if these complications are suspected. While waiting for the physician to come, the nurse attempts to locate and correct the cause of any problems within the chest drainage system. Perhaps a relatively simple action corrects the malfunctioning system, e.g., straightening a kinked tube or setting upright a water-seal bottle that has been knocked over accidentally. Sometimes milking the tube will dislodge a blood clot that is obstructing the tube. Occasionally it is necessary for the physician to irrigate the chest catheters to remove obstructions.

Maintaining an Airtight Drainage System. Closed chest drainage systems must be kept airtight (closed to atmospheric air). To accomplish this, *bottles in the drainage apparatus are sealed with tight-fitting stoppers and all connections are taped.* If air leaks into the drainage tubing it enters the pleural space and thus not only defeats the purposes of the drainage system, but can possibly cause complications such as tension pneumothorax. When the drainage system is not airtight it is impossible to reestablish negative pressure in the pleural space because atmospheric air continues to enter the pleural space through the air leak. Obviously if tubes in the drainage system are accidentally disconnected or if bottles in the apparatus are broken, the drainage system is no longer airtight.

Controlling the Amount of Suction. When suction is used it must be maintained at the level ordered by the physician to most effectively drain off air and fluid from the pleural space. Suction control is discussed in the section on mechanical chest suction below.

Infection Prevention with Chest Drainage

When properly used, closed chest drainage helps to prevent infections in the pleural space by removing serosanguineous fluids. However, unless careful aseptic technique is used in caring for chest catheters and the drainage system, infection may be introduced into the pleural space. *Observe strict asepsis whenever you are changing the apparatus or any of its connections.* If you disconnect the tubes, maintain a sterile field. Be certain to protect the tubes' open ends with sterile dressings. Always wash your hands thoroughly before and after caring for chest tubes. Because an infection can occur along the tube tract, chest catheters are usually not used for more than five to seven days.

Activity with Chest Drainage

The patient with water-seal chest drainage can sit up in bed, get in and out of bed, and ambulate without clamping his chest catheters as long as: (1) the water-seal bottle is kept upright (so the long glass tube in the bottle is kept below the fluid level in the bottle); (2) the bottle is kept lower than the chest; and (3) all connections remain intact. Be careful not to exert traction on the tubings. Various arrangements are used for keeping the patient's chest bottles with him while he moves around. If suction is to be maintained during ambulation the patient can walk only the few steps permitted by the length of the tubing.

Sometimes the physician orders a patient's chest catheters to be double clamped and disconnected while he is ambulatory. However, *if air drainage has been occurring the tubes are never clamped because of the danger of tension pneumothorax.* With the tubes clamped, the air would continue to accumulate in the pleural space, thus exerting increasing pressure since there would be no means of escape.

Encourage the patient on closed chest drainage to *frequently cough and deep breathe.* In addition to clearing the bronchi of secretions these activities promote lung expansion and the expulsion of air and/or fluid from the pleural space (by increasing intrapulmonic and intrapleural pressures.

Clamping Chest Drainage Tubing

Rubber-shod clamps are routinely kept at the bedside of any patient on closed chest drainage. The clamps are 6- to 8-inch, strong hemostats with protective rubber placed over their tips. Two clamps are kept available for each chest catheter so each catheter can be *double clamped* (for extra safety) if clamping is necessary. When not in use, clamps should be stored in an easily visible place where they are readily available. They can be kept clamped to the bottom sheet at the head of the bed when the patient is in bed. When the patient is out of bed the clamps are usually kept clamped to the patient's bathrobe. Do not tape the clamps to the bed or they will be too difficult to release for emergency use. Also, do not leave the clamps merely lying on the bedside stand or in a drawer; if you do it is likely that they will not be there when you need them or they will be hidden by other articles. When clamps are attached to linens, be careful they are not accidentally sent to the laundry.

There are times when clamping a patient's chest tubes is definitely contraindicated. Clamps are currently not used on chest tubes as frequently as they formerly were.

> *Except for those emergencies in which clamping is clearly indicated, do not clamp chest drainage tubes without an order to do so.*

Occasionally it is necessary to *briefly* clamp a chest tube to locate a source of malfunction in the apparatus. Sometimes an order is given to clamp a patient's chest tubes for a few minutes while he is being transported to another area of the hospital, e.g., x-ray. However, usually the tubes are not clamped when the patient is moved, but rather care is taken to keep the drainage system below the level of the patient's chest and the drainage system is transported with him.

The best time to apply clamps to a chest catheter is following an expiration. The clamps should be removed again as soon as possible. Never cover

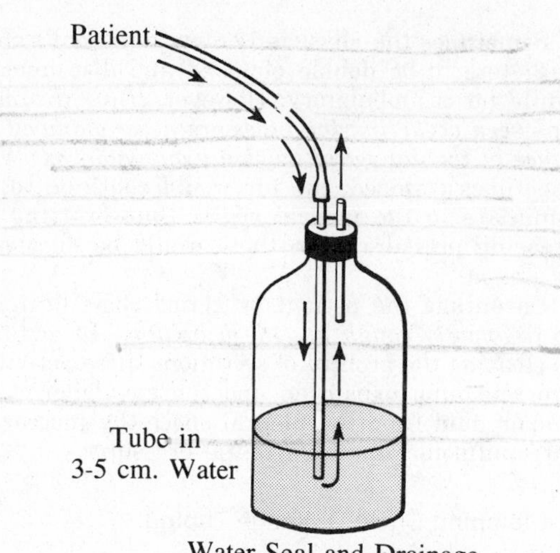

FIGURE 73–5. One-bottle system for closed chest drainage. (From Secor, J.: *Patient Care in Respiratory Problems.* 1969.)

the clamps with bedding while they are in use. If they are left clamped on the chest tube and are covered up they are easily forgotten and may not be released when they should be.

One-Bottle Water-Seal Apparatus

Basic Set-up. This, the most simple apparatus for establishing closed chest drainage, consists of: (1) a sterile bottle that contains about 100 ml. of sterile normal saline or sterile water; (2) a tight-fitting rubber stopper with two holes in it (the stopper is placed in the opening of the bottle and is taped securely in place); and (3) two hollow tubes (inserted through the holes in the stopper and taped into place once they are positioned). One tube is short and acts as an *air vent;* the other tube is longer and acts as a *water-seal* (Fig. 73–5).

> *Water-seal drainage acts as a one-way valve, permitting the unidirectional flow of air and fluid out of the pleural space, but permitting none to enter from the drainage system.*

The longer tube in the water-seal apparatus is placed so it extends into the solution in the bottle and terminates about 3 to 5 cm. below the fluid level. The other end of the long tube (i.e., the end outside the bottle) is attached to the patient's chest drainage tubing. Once attached to the patient's drainage tubing *the end of the long tube in the bottle must always be kept below the fluid level in the bottle.* If this end of the tube is above the fluid level, atmospheric air passes through the bottle's air vent (short tube), into the open end of the long tube, through the drainage tubing, and into the pleural space.

A "water-seal" means simply that the water in the bottle seals off the atmospheric air, preventing atmospheric pressure from entering the chest drainage tube and thus from entering the pleural space. Atmospheric air enters the air vent in the water-seal bottle, but it cannot penetrate the surface of the water and enter the end of the long tube under the water. Similarly, air and fluid can escape from the pleural space by passing through the long tube in the bottle and into the fluid in the bottle. Air escaping from the chest then bubbles up through the fluid in the bottle (because air is lighter than water), and escapes out of the bottle by passing through the air vent. The fluid in the water-seal bottle is not drawn up into the chest tube because the fluid is heavier than air and is thus held down in the bottle by gravity. Thus, water-seal drainage creates a *closed drainage system* that permits air and fluid to escape out of the pleural space but also prevents outside air or fluid from entering the pleural space. (Of course if the bottle is accidentally raised higher than the level of the patient's chest, the force of gravity will cause the fluid to run down the tube into the chest).

The one-bottle water-seal chest drainage apparatus does not produce suction, but rather operates by gravity. This system may be used following pneumonectomy (where suction is not necessary to expand the remaining lung tissue since the lung was removed) and in treating empyema. It may also be used following resectional surgery or open chest wounds if the physician does not think mechanical suction is necessary.

How to Tell if the Drainage Apparatus Is Functioning Properly. It is the nurse's responsibility to make certain the water-seal apparatus is functioning properly. The evaluations she makes to determine this are discussed further below.

OBSERVATION OF THE WATER-SEAL TUBE. As previously discussed, pressure changes occur during respiration. During inspiration, fluid is sucked up into the tube a few centimeters because of the decreased intrapleural pressure. Conversely, during expiration the heightened intrapleural pressure forces the fluid back down the tube. When you observe this *fluctuating or oscillating movement of fluid* up and down in the long tube in the water-seal bottle, you know that the drainage tubes are patent and the apparatus is functioning properly because it is reflecting the patient's ventilatory movements.

Fluctuation of fluid in the water-seal tube stops when the lungs have reexpanded (this point is discussed further below) or if the tubes are kinked or obstructed. If fluctuation does not occur check to be sure the tube is not kinked or compressed; try milking the tube to remove possible obstructions; and change the patient's position and have him cough and deep breathe. If these measures fail to restore fluctuation, notify the physician.

OBSERVATION OF THE AIR-VENT TUBE. Make certain that the short *air-vent tube is kept open* to the atmosphere to permit the escape of intrapleural air from the bottle. If this tube is stopped up, any intrapleural air being expelled into the bottle is trapped in the collection bottle and thus increases pressure within the bottle. If this pressure becomes great enough it prevents drainage of air and fluid from the pleural space and can produce tension pneumothorax and mediastinal shift.

OBSERVATION OF THE FLUID IN THE WATER-SEAL BOTTLE. Watch for bubbling in the water-seal bottle. The bubbling is caused by air passing out of the pleural space and up through the liquid in the bottle. *Intermittent bubbling* is not abnormal; in fact, it indicates that the water-seal drainage is accomplishing one of its purposes, i.e., the removal of air from the pleural space. Intermittent bubbling may occur with the patient's normal expirations, since expiration increases intrapleural pressure and forces air through the tube.

Continuous bubbling during both inspiration and expiration may indicate that air is leaking into the drainage system. Obviously this situation must be corrected, since air entering the system is also entering the pleural space. Attempt to locate the source of the *air leak* and repair it if you can. Begin by inspecting the chest wall where the catheters are inserted. If a chest catheter appears to be loose, gently squeeze the skin up around the catheter or apply sterile petrolatum gauze around the area of insertion and see if this stops the continuous bubbling in the bottle. If this does not stop the leak, check the tubing inch by inch and all connections. You may find a break in the tubing or a loose connection that can be sealed with tape. If you still cannot locate the leak it may be necessary to replace the drainage bottle with another sterile water-seal bottle.

Rapid bubbling (in the absence of an air leak) indicates that considerable loss of air is occurring, e.g., from an incision or tear in the pulmonary pleura. The physician should be notified immediately so he can take appropriate steps to prevent collapse of the lung or mediastinal shift. Thoracentesis may be necessary.

When assigned to care for a patient on water-seal drainage, it is important to know if the patient is a "bubbling" patient, i.e., a patient who has air in his pleural space which has been bubbling up in the water-seal bottle. Knowing this enables you to observe for significant changes in his drainage pattern. For example, you can note if intermittent bubbling changes to constant bubbling, or if a patient who has not been bubbling begins to bubble. Also, knowledge about a patient's "bubbling status" prepares you to give appropriate emergency care if anything goes wrong with the drainage apparatus.

Notify the physician of any accidents involving closed chest drainage.

What to do if the water-seal bottle is broken. If the bottle is broken you know that atmospheric air will enter the pleural space through the drainage tubing. This can be prevented by immediately clamping the chest catheter. It must be realized, however, that clamping the catheter also prevents air (or fluid) from leaving the pleural space; thus, clamping a chest catheter is not always the procedure of choice.[195]

If a water-seal bottle is broken and the patient is known to have been bubbling (i.e., it is known that air has been coming out of the pleural space), the chest tube is not clamped but is left open until it can be attached to a new water-seal bottle. (A second water-seal bottle should always be kept available.) Even though an open pneumothorax will occur, this is far less serious than a closed tension pneumothorax, which will compress the lungs and progress to a mediastinal shift. If the bottle breaks and it is known that the patient has not been bubbling, the nurse immediately clamps the chest catheter. She then wipes the exposed ends of the catheter with an antiseptic solution and reconnects them to another sterile water-seal bottle.[68]

It can be seen that in such an emergency an evaluation is rapidly made of the extent to which exposure of the pleural space to atmospheric air would disrupt therapy, and of the pros and cons of shutting off airflow into and out of the chest cavity with clamps. The nurse must be prepared to make such a decision and immediately take appropriate action. Obviously it is necessary to know whether the patient has been bubbling air *before* the bottle is broken, since there is no way to observe this once the bottle is broken.

Once a patient's chest tubes are clamped observe him closely for symptoms of tension pneumothorax and mediastinal shift.

If you have applied clamps to a chest tube after a water-seal has been broken (or for some other reason) and you notice the patient is beginning to experience respiratory distress before he can be reconnected to a water-seal apparatus (e.g., he is breathing rapidly and shallowly, is apprehensive, and is becoming cyanotic), he is probably suffering from tension pneumothorax and possibly mediastinal shift. Immediately release the clamps on the chest catheter and call for the physician. It is best to open the clamps and thus create an open pneumothorax, since at least with an open pneumothorax air can move both in and out and is not trapped in the pleural space building up pressure.

What to do if the chest tubing accidentally is disconnected. A tube that is accidentally disconnected should simply be reconnected and the system observed to be certain it is functioning. Taping the tubing at the site of the disconnection should prevent another similar accident.

What to do if the water-seal bottle is accidentally kicked over. If this happens the water-seal breaks and atmospheric air begins to enter the pleural space. To correct this situation simply return the bottle to the upright position, thereby reestablishing the water-seal. Once the water-seal is again functioning instruct the patient to take one or two deep breaths to force out of the pleural cavity any air that may have entered while the water-seal was broken.

What to do if the water-seal bottle is accidentally elevated to the level of the patient's chest. Elevation of the bottle to this level causes any fluid in the tubing to flow back into the pleural space. Immediately lower the bottle to reestablish the drainage system.

What to do if the water-seal bottle is accidentally elevated above the level of the patient's chest. This is serious, since fluid in the bottle will be siphoned or flow by gravity into the pleural space. If much fluid enters the pleural space from the drainage bottle, the patient's lung may be collapsed on the affected side and he may have a mediastinal shift. Lower the bottle at once and contact the physician immediately.

Measuring and Observing Chest Drainage

The air being removed from the pleural space escapes through the water-seal bottle's air vent, but the fluid is simply evacuated into the collection bottle and stays there. Expiration causes intrapleural pressure to rise higher than the pressure exerted by the water on the end of the water-seal tube, and fluid (and air) is forced from the pleural space into the bottle. As drainage collects in the water-seal bottle of a one-bottle set-up, more pressure is required to force the fluid down in the submersed water-seal tube upon expiration in order to permit the escape of fluid and air from the pleural space. *The depth to which the water-seal tube is immersed below the fluid in the bottle determines the pressure exerted by the water.*

To reduce the amount of pressure that the drainage must overcome, the long water-seal tube may be periodically pulled up in the bottle as fluid accumulates. Thus, less of the tube is under the fluid in the bottle. (Remember never to pull the end of the tube above the fluid level line.) Of course, it may be necessary to change the drainage bottle as it fills. Be certain it is never allowed to become so full that it covers the opening of the air vent.

Because it is important to know the amount of drainage coming from the pleural space and its rate of accumulation, a piece of tape is placed on the bottle so levels can be noted. This record helps the physician to determine the amount of blood loss and the rate of flow of drainage from the pleural space. These facts are important in planning blood replacement therapy and in evaluating the patient's status. Patients with excessive drainage may need to be returned to surgery for exploration to determine the cause.

The *marking tape* is applied when the apparatus is first set up. As mentioned, usually 100 ml. of sterile saline or sterile water is initially placed in the water-seal bottle. A mark is then made on the tape indicating this fluid level. Above the initial fluid level mark, the tape is marked at intervals representing additional 50-ml. accumulations. The times at which these various marks are reached by the draining fluids are marked on the tape opposite the drainage level mark.

Carefully measure and record chest drainage. It is not unusual for as much as 500 to 1000 ml. of drainage to occur in the first 24-hour period following chest surgery. Between 100 and 300 ml. of drainage may accumulate during the first two hours; following this, the amount of drainage should lessen.

Chest drainage is normally grossly bloody immediately following surgery, but it should not continue to be so for more than several hours. If the drainage remains frankly bloody for an abnormal period of time or if bleeding recurs after it has obviously stopped, contact the surgeon. Blood loss is evaluated by observing the rising level in the fluid collection bottle. If the patient's blood pressure drops and his pulse is rapid, *hemorrhage* is suspected. The drainage collection bottles are checked for a rise in the fluid level. If the level has not risen, the tubes are checked for patency. The physician is always immediately notified since the patient may be bleeding rapidly within his chest.

Replacement of a One-bottle Chest Drainage Apparatus. Periodically the drainage collection bottle must be replaced with another sterile set-up. Usually water-seal bottles are changed only if the physician orders them to be or if they are broken or malfunctioning. The person changing the bottles must be qualified to do so.

A physician or nurse may change a one-bottle water-seal apparatus in the following manner. (1) First assemble the necessary equipment: two clamps and a sterile water-seal bottle set up as the original bottle was with 100 ml. of sterile normal saline or sterile water, a labeled measurement tape on the side of the bottle, and a snug stopper with two tubes (one short, one long) properly positioned. (2) Double clamp the chest catheters close to the patient's chest to prevent air from entering the pleural space through the disconnected tubing. (3) Disconnect the bottle to be replaced and attach the new set, making certain the connections are airtight and that the end of the long tube in the bottle is below the fluid level. (4) Be certain the bottle is located lower than the patient's chest. (5) Unclamp the patient's chest catheter (be sure you remove *both* clamps) and make certain the system is functioning properly before leaving the patient. Do not clamp the chest catheters until you have everything ready to complete the replacement. Keeping the catheters clamped for too long may permit air and fluid to accumulate to dangerous levels in the pleural space.

Two-Bottle Water-Seal Drainage

Basic Set-Up. With a two-bottle water-seal apparatus one bottle collects drainage and the other bottle is the water-seal bottle. In this set-up the *empty drainage bottle* is between the patient and the *water-seal bottle* (Fig. 73–6). The empty drainage bottle: (1) has a strip of tape applied to the side of the bottle to record the rate and quantity of drainage; (2) is sealed off at the top with a snug-fitting rubber stopper; and (3) has two short tubes that pass through holes in the stopper. Each tube extends into the bottle for about one inch. One of these short tubes is attached to the drainage tubing coming from the patient; the other is attached (with a small section of tubing) to the underwater tube of the water-seal bottle. Because drainage does not pass into the water-seal bottle in this set-up, the strip of tape on the outside of the water-seal bottle is marked only to indicate the initial level of the sterile saline or sterile water. As with the one-bottle water-seal apparatus, the air vent of the water-seal bottle must be left open to atmospheric air.

A two-bottle water-seal apparatus makes it easier to observe the amount and character of drainage from the patient's chest (since the drainage does not mix with the water or saline in the water-seal bottle). Also, the two-bottle set-up makes it easier to control the pressure within the system, and thus makes it easier for fluid and air to leave the pleural space. As mentioned earlier, when a one-bottle drainage apparatus begins to fill up with drainage fluid, the level of fluid in the underwater tube rises unless the tube is gradually pulled up as the fluid level increases. The higher the level of fluid in the tube, the more pressure is required to push the column of fluid down. Thus, air or fluid attempting to leave the pleural space must exert more pressure. This problem is solved by having a separate bottle for drainage collection.

Except for the differences just discussed, the one- and two-bottle water-seal systems perform similar functions in similar ways. The fluid in the underwater tube fluctuates with inspiration and expiration when the system functions properly, and air escapes from the air vent in the water-seal bottle.

How to Tell When Water-seal Drainage Is No Longer Necessary

The physician determines when to remove water-seal drainage. As mentioned, one indication that evacuation of intrapleural air and fluid is completed and the lung has reexpanded is the cessation of fluid fluctuation in the long tube of the water-seal bottle. The reexpanded lung blocks the catheters' openings in the pleural space, and thus

the fluctuations of intrapleural pressure during inspiration and expiration are no longer transmitted to the water-seal apparatus. When the lung is completely reexpanded, no air or fluid passes through the chest catheters.

Usually the lung is fully reexpanded after two or three days of chest drainage postoperatively. Generally chest catheters are left in place for 24 hours after all air drainage and significant fluid drainage has stopped. Chest catheters may not be removed if the chest is draining more than 50 to 75 ml. of fluid daily. The sooner the tubes can be removed, the better, since their presence often contributes to the patient's postoperative pain and inactivity. Also, the longer the tubes are in place the greater the risk of infection. In treating empyema, chest drainage tubes may be used for longer periods of time than following chest surgery.

To confirm his impression that the lung has reexpanded the physician auscultates and percusses the patient's chest and orders a chest x-ray. If he is convinced that it is safe to remove the chest catheter the physician then proceeds to do so. Although both chest tubes may be removed at the same time, it is more common for the upper chest tube to be left in place for a while longer than the lower. (Removal of chest catheters is discussed later.)

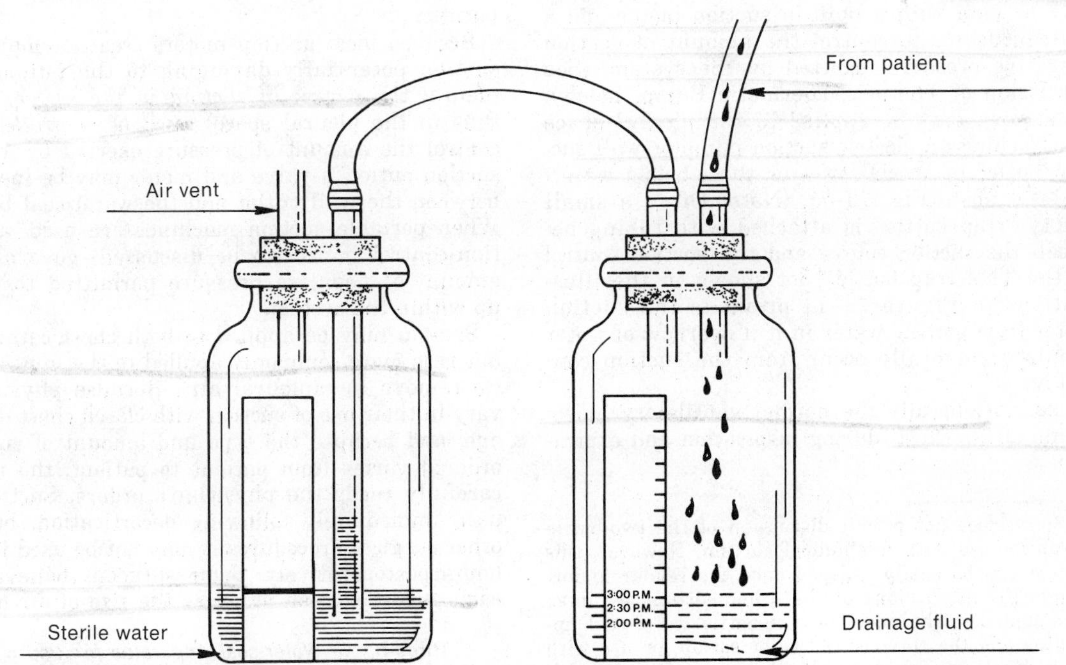

FIGURE 73–6. Two-bottle water-seal drainage. (After *Closed Drainage of the Chest,* U.S. Public Health Service Publication No. 1337, May, 1965.)

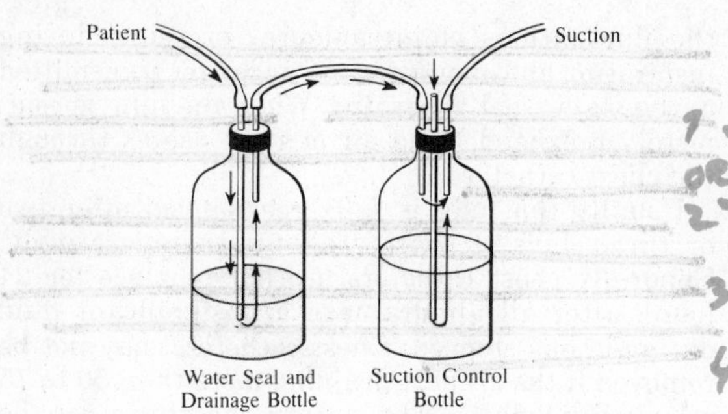

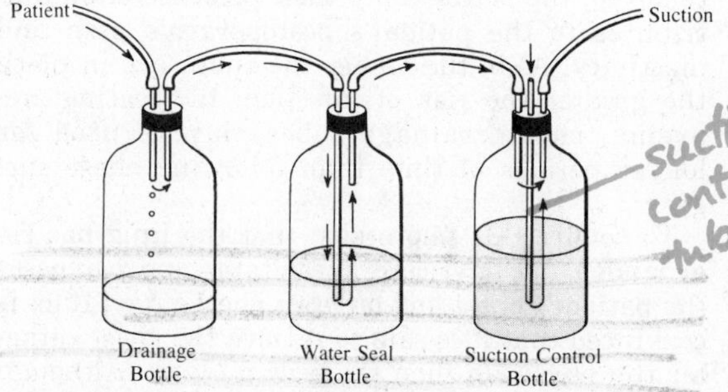

FIGURE 73–7. *A,* Two-bottle system for closed chest drainage with suction; *B,* three-bottle system. (From Secor, J.: *Patient Care in Respiratory Problems.* 1969.)

Mechanical Suction Closed Chest Drainage

Mechanical suction can be applied to the chest in various ways. For example, a special apparatus may be used with a built-in suction motor and a built-in device to control the amount of suction (negative pressure) exerted by the system. (See discussion of Thoracic Thermotic Pump, below). Or suction may be applied to the pleural space by attaching an electric suction pump or wall suction outlet to special two- or three-bottle water-seal set-ups* (Fig. 73–7). (Note: Often a small empty "trap bottle" is attached with tubing between the suction source and the suction control bottle. This trap bottle [not shown in the illustrations in Figure 73–7] prevents the suction motor from getting water in it if overflow of water should accidentally occur from the suction control bottle.)

Uses. Generally the normal ventilatory movements of the chest (during inspiration and expiration), coughing, and deep breathing adequately pump air and fluid from the pleural space and re-expand the lung, along with simple water-seal drainage. However, when these activities and gravity drainage are not adequate to promote re-expansion of the lung and emptying of the contents of the pleural space, a suction apparatus of some type is necessary. Continuous gentle suction may be used when a patient's cough and respirations are too weak to force air and fluid out of the pleural space through the chest catheters. Suction may also be applied to closed chest drainage in the treatment of empyema. Additionally, suction may be used if air is leaking into the pleural space faster than it can be removed by a water-seal apparatus (e.g., if there is considerable air leakage through the pulmonary pleura) and/or to speed up the removal of air or fluid from the pleural space.

There are two ways to provide chest suction. Occasionally the physician attaches a chest catheter to a needle and then inserts the needle into a *vacuum blood donor bottle* (500 ml. capacity). This set-up provides very mild suction. More often, a *mechanical suction pump* is used, e.g., a Moe, Emerson, or Stedman pump or suction from a wall outlet.

The suction motor establishes and maintains suction (negative pressure) throughout the closed drainage apparatus and within the pleural space because the motor continually removes air from within the system (including air drawn into the system from the pleural space). As air is removed, the system's capacity increases and the pressure within it falls. The negative pressure thus created actively pulls or sucks air and fluid from the pleural space. The evacuated fluid collects in a bottle (in some set-ups this is the water-seal bottle, as will be discussed); the air drawn out of the pleural space is forced out of the system, with air from the system itself, through the motor's exhaust apparatus.

Because most suction motors create amounts of suction potentially damaging to the pulmonary pleura, the *degree of suction in the system* (and thus in the pleural space) *must be controlled.* To control the amount of pressure exerted by a wall suction outlet, a valve and meter may be inserted between the wall outlet and the water-seal bottle. When portable suction machines are used, a suction-control bottle (to be discussed) governs the amount of negative pressure permitted to build up within the system.

Suction may be applied to both chest catheters, but is is more commonly applied to the upper tube (to remove intrapleural air). Because physicians vary in their use of suction with closed chest drainage, and because the type and amount of suction ordered varies from patient to patient, the nurse carefully reads the physician's orders. Suction is used immediately following decortication, but in other surgical procedures it may not be used for 24 hours postoperatively. Some surgeons believe the early use of suction enlarges the size of air leaks.

Three-bottle Water-seal Apparatus for Use with Mechanical Suction. The three-bottle suction set-up consists of: (1) a drainage collection bottle

*Space does not permit discussion of the two-bottle set-up for use with mechanical suction. However, this system can be easily grasped once the reader understands the discussions of the other set-ups we have presented, i.e., the one- and two-bottle water-seal apparatus and the three-bottle water set-up for use with mechanical suction. A two-bottle set-up for use with mechanical suction is illustrated in Figure 73–7.

(the bottle closest to the patient); (2) a water-seal bottle (the middle bottle); and (3) a suction control bottle (connected to a suction source). (Refer back to Figure 73-7.) The set-up is the same as the two-bottle water-seal apparatus previously discussed, except that attached to the water-seal bottle's former air vent opening is the third bottle. The drainage and water-seal bottles are connected to each other as previously described.

SUCTION CONTROL BOTTLE ("BREAKER BOTTLE"). In a three-bottle water-seal apparatus for use with mechanical suction the purpose of the third bottle is to control the amount of pressure in the system. The suction control bottle contains water and a tight-fitting stopper with *three openings* in it. The stopper is taped to the bottle; all connections are also taped to prevent air leaks. Two short tubes are passed through two of the openings in the stopper. These tubes extend into the bottle about 1 inch. One tube is joined with flexible tubing to the former air vent of the water-seal bottle; the other short tube is connected with flexible tubing to the suction motor. Passing through the third opening in the stopper is a third tube much longer than the other two. One end of this is open to the atmosphere; the end in the bottle extends below the water level. This tube is the *suction control tube.*

The depth to which the suction control tube is inserted below the fluid level in the bottle controls the amount of pressure within the system. The physician orders how far he wishes this control tube to be kept below the fluid level. For example, if the physician wants to limit the suction on the pleural space to 10 cm. of water* (approximately the normal intrapleural pressure during inspiration), he orders the tube to be kept submerged 10 cm. below the fluid level in the suction control bottle. Then, regardless of the amount of negative pressure from the suction machine, the amount of negative pressure in the three-bottle system (and hence in the pleural space) will not exceed 10 cm. of water.

The level of water in the open tube of the suction control bottle sinks in proportion to the amount of negative pressure in the apparatus when the suction source is turned on. For example, if there are 10 ml. of water between the tip of the tube under the water and the water level, 10 cm. of water is the amount of negative pressure in the system. The water in the control tube would thus sink to the bottom of the tube when the suction source is turned on in order to reach this amount of negative pressure. If the amount of negative pressure in the system begins to increase (i.e., the pressure in the system falls below that for which the suction control tube is set), air is drawn into the system through the control tube and the suction breaks at the 10 cm. of water level. Excessive degrees of negative pressure are thus not permitted to build up in the system. As much air is pulled in as is needed to raise the pressure back up to the set level. It is important that the upper end of the suction control tube be kept open to atmospheric air for the apparatus to function properly.

The initial water level in the suction control bottle should be marked on a piece of tape placed on the side of the bottle. (Marking tapes needed for the drainage and water-seal bottles have been discussed.) It is the nurse's responsibility to periodically check the suction control tube to be certain it is submerged the prescribed distance beneath the fluid level in the bottle.

HOW TO TELL IF THE APPARATUS IS FUNCTIONING PROPERLY. Proper functioning of the suction control bottle is indicated by the periodic emptying of the fluid in the control tube, and by bubbling through the water of the air being drawn into this tube. In order to govern pressure within the system, the water in the suction control bottle bubbles almost constantly as outside air is drawn into the system.

Absence of bubbling in the suction control bottle means the system is not properly functioning and the correct suction level is not being maintained.

Possible reasons for malfunctioning of a mechanical suction apparatus include air leaking into the pleural space or into the drainage apparatus, and mechanical problems in the pump. The most serious problem would be air leaking into the pleural space. Therefore, check for this problem first by briefly clamping off the chest drainage tube and then observing the suction control bottle. If you see the bottle bubbling, you know that nothing is wrong with either the drainage apparatus or the pump; the problem is therefore an air leak into the pleural space around the chest tubes. If you cannot effectively seal off this air leak, e.g., with petrolatum gauze, notify the physician immediately. If the suction control bottle fails to begin to bubble when the chest catheter is clamped, you know the problem is in the drainage connections or the pump. Check the system carefully, looking for loose connections, air leaks around bottle tops, or air leaks in the tubing, e.g., split tubing. Also, make certain the tubing is not kinked and that it is correctly positioned and there are no dependent loops. Because the chest catheter remains clamped during this inspection, observe the patient closely for indications of tension pneumothorax. As soon as you have corrected the problem with the system, the suction control bottle's fluid will begin to bubble. Then immediately remove the clamps on the chest catheter. If the suction motor appears to be causing the problem, i.e., the suction control bottle does not function properly after you have checked all the tubing and all connections, obtain another pump at once.

When the water in the suction control bottle fails to bubble and the nurse cannot identify and correct the source of difficulty, she contacts the physician. It may be that the amount of suction in the system needs to be increased if air is rapidly leaking from the pleura. If the physician decides this is the cause of the system's malfunctioning, he will order the amount of suction to be increased so the escaping air can be more rapidly removed from the pleural space. To increase the

*In some settings the usual suction applied postoperatively is 20 to 30 cm. of water. At times the suction has been increased as necessary up to 90 cm. of water without proving harmful.[178]

amount of suction, water is added to the suction control bottle. Thus, the distance is increased between the tip of the tube and the water level in the bottle and the suction is proportionally increased.

In a mechanical suction arrangement (unlike the simpler water-seal set-ups discussed earlier) the fluid level in the long water-seal tube *does not* fluctuate with the ventilatory movements of the patient's chest because the suction holds the fluid level in the tube at a fixed level. Thus, you do not have the fluctuating of this fluid column to indicate proper functioning of the system or, conversely, the absence of fluctuation to indicate malfunction. However, as with the simpler water-seal arrangements discussed previously, *continuous bubbling in the water-seal bottle does indicate an air leak in the system.*

To detect an *air leak* in a closed-chest mechanical suction apparatus, first look for observable defects in the mechanical suction system and make certain all connections are taped. If the system continues to malfunction begin to look for a leak by clamping the tubing briefly. Start at the chest catheter end of the tubing and work your way toward the apparatus. If you place a clamp between the leak and the water-seal bottle, and the continuous bubbling in the water-seal bottle stops, you know the leak is located between the end of the catheter and the water-seal bottle. Thus, when you have been able to place a clamp at a point between the air leak and the water-seal bottle you will be able to identify the area of the leak because the continuous bubbling in the water-seal bottle will stop.

Periodically, to see if the system is operating properly (e.g., to make certain the tubing is not obstructed), the mechanical chest suction apparatus may be modified so it becomes a simple water-seal system for a few moments. (Note: It is also modified in this way when the physician wants to check to see if the lung has reexpanded and the chest suction can be discontinued.) Once the system has been converted to a simple water-seal system, the underwater tube in the water-seal bottle is observed. (Remember that fluctuation of the fluid in this tube indicates normal functioning, whereas cessation of this fluctuation occurs when the tubes are clogged or the lung has reexpanded.)

To modify the mechanical apparatus so it becomes a simple water-seal apparatus, the suction motor is turned off and the section of tubing running to the motor is disconnected and left open to atmospheric air. (If you prefer, disconnect the tube between the water-seal bottle and the suction control bottle.) Leaving this tubing open provides an air vent so any intrapleural air can escape from the system. If the tubing is not disconnected when the motor is off, the intrapleural air may build up in the system and cause a tension pneumothorax. (As stated earlier, when the motor is running and the tubing is connected, the intrapleural air escapes through the motor's exhaust system.) While the suction is briefly interrupted, the fluid level in the water-seal tube is observed for fluctuations.

Removal of Chest Catheters

When chest catheters are to be removed, premedication for pain is usually given about one half hour before the procedure, since removal of the catheters is moderately painful. After premedicating the patient, the nurse assembles equipment for the physician, e.g., sterile scissors, a knife or suture set to cut the suture; sterile petrolatum gauze and a 4 × 4 gauze square to cover the wound; and three 2-inch wide strips of tape about 6 inches long.

The patient is positioned sitting on the edge of the bed or lying on his unoperated side. After clipping the stitches the physician quickly removes the catheters. Removal is accomplished either during expiration or at the end of a full inspiration to prevent air from being sucked back into the pleural space while the drain is being pulled out. Following removal of the chest catheter the wound may be closed with skin clips or covered with petrolatum gauze. A dressing is then firmly applied over the wound and is secured with wide strips of tape. The wound heals in a few days. Usually a chest x-ray is ordered following removal of chest tubes.

Be certain to check the areas of the catheter skin incisions for air leakage for the first few hours after the catheter has been removed. Observe for subcutaneous emphysema of surrounding tissues. Also, closely observe the patient during this time for indications of respiratory distress that could be caused by loss of negative intrapleural pressure or tension pneumothorax. Notify the physician immediately so he can reinstitute closed chest drainage if indicated.

Alternate Equipment for Chest Drainage

Some newer pieces of equipment for chest drainage and suction will be mentioned briefly here.

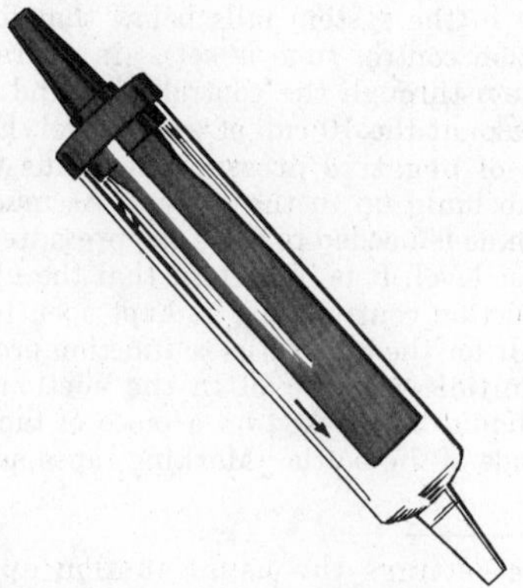

FIGURE 73–8. B-P Heimlich Chest Drainage Valve. (Courtesy of Becton, Dickinson & Co., Rutherford, N.J.)

Flutter Valve. A flutter valve can be used to replace underwater drainage bottles in closed chest drainage apparatuses (Fig. 73–8). The B-P Heimlich Chest Drainage Valve is presterilized, disposable, and about 7 inches long. When inserted between a chest catheter and a drainage collecting apparatus the valve permits the unidirectional flow of air and fluids from the pleural space into the collection apparatus, but it does not permit the reflux of air or fluid back into the chest.

The flutter valve itself is actually a single piece of wide, thin rubber tubing which is open at the end of the valve attached to the chest catheter and then is compressed at its other end so its flattened sides remain in contact with each other. Fluids draining from the intrapleural space thus can enter the open end of the tubing and pass out through the flattened ends of the valve, but they cannot reenter the flattened sides of the tubing because the two sides remain in contact with each other. The valve offers minimal resistance to the passage of air or fluids leaving the intrapleural space. The piece of rubber tubing is enclosed in a clear plastic case, which makes it easy to observe the passage of fluids, blood, and so forth, through the valve. Also, the expansion and contraction of the valve leaflets (caused by changes in the intrapleural pressure associated with ventilatory chest movements) can be observed. The flutter valve functions in any position; thus, the patient may assume any position.

Water-seal systems that use bottles are not only cumbersome but also tend to restrict the patient's mobility and are frequently the cause of accidents and a great deal of anxiety for both patient and staff. The plastic flutter valve is safer for the patient and easier for the nurse. It enables greater freedom of movement for the patient, a factor of importance in the postoperative course of chest surgery patients, who tend generally to want to be less active than is desirable. With the valve the patient can be comfortably ambulatory if the drainage tubing is connected to a portable plastic bag.

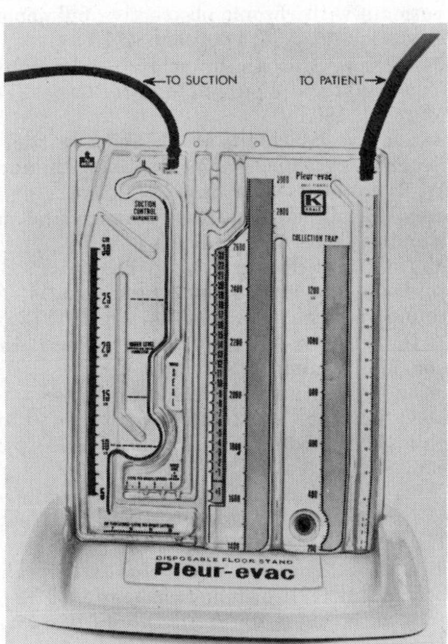

FIGURE 73–9. Pleur-evac. (Courtesy of Deknatel, Inc., Queens Village, N.Y.)

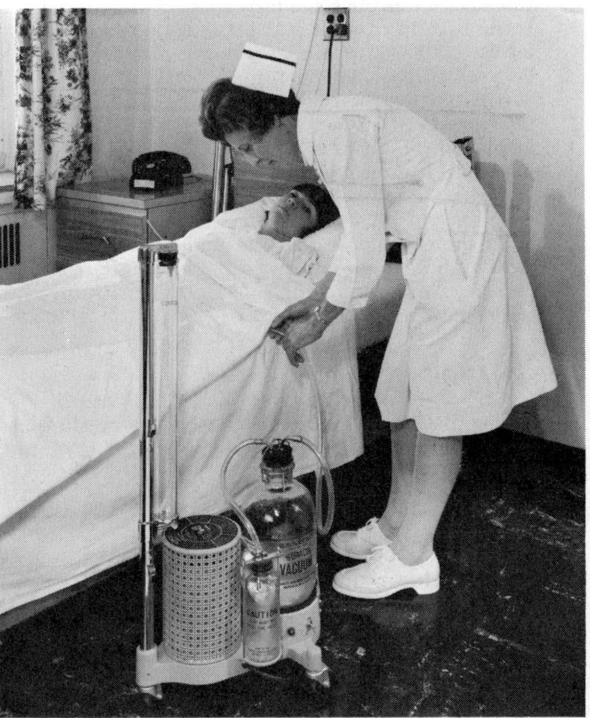

FIGURE 73–10. Gomco Thoracic Thermotic Pump for closed chest drainage. (Courtesy of Gomco Surgical Manufacturing Corp., Buffalo, N.Y.)

Since it functions in the same manner as a water-seal bottle, the flutter valve can be attached to chest suction if necessary.

Pleur-Evac. The Pleur-Evac is a presterilized, disposable plastic apparatus that duplicates in principle the three-bottle closed chest drainage system (Fig. 73–9). Within the one apparatus there are three separate chambers which: (1) collect drainage (the chest catheter attaches to this chamber which has a a self-sealing diaphragm at the bottom for sterile removal of specimens); (2) provide a water-seal (1 to 2 cm. of water are added to this chamber to form the water-seal); and (3) provide suction control (this chamber is filled with water to the desired height, e.g., 10 to 25 cm.). Tubing is attached from the suction chamber to the suction source. The Pleur-Evac may be placed in a floor stand or attached to the bedside. (For additional details consult the manufacturer's information sheet.)

Some of the newer equipment designed for closed chest drainage simplifies the nurse's responsibilities in caring for the equipment. However, the same high level of patient care and observation is necessary and the nurse must understand the basic principles of closed chest drainage.

Thoracic Thermotic Pump. This pump, manufactured by Gomco, is especially designed to create a controlled amount of suction for the purpose of removing air and fluid from the pleural space (Fig. 73–10). The apparatus contains a manometer (bubble type), with a long manometer tube which functions similarly to a suction-control bottle tube in a water-seal bottle set-up modified for use with suction. Either water or mercury may be used in the manometer. Mercury is used if suction greater than 25 cm. of water is desired. (Mercury is 13.6 times as dense as water. For example, 10 cm. of water equals 0.74 cm. Hg or 7.4 mm. Hg). If even greater suction is required, two pumps can be attached to the chest catheter with a Y connector. A water-seal can be set up as part of the drainage apparatus. The pump has an off-on switch and a high-low switch. (For details concerning this equipment consult the manufacturer's instruction booklet.)

DISCHARGE

Before discharge following chest surgery the patient is advised as to the care regimen that he should practice at home. Specifically, he is usually instructed to continue the routines of oral hygiene, nutrition, rest, deep-breathing, coughing, and exercising that he followed in the hospital just prior to discharge. Naturally these activities are modified by the surgeon according to the patient's individual needs during his recovery. Additionally, the patient is advised to avoid activities or environments that irritate the tracheobronchial tree and could cause severe coughing episodes. For example, the patient may be advised not to smoke, not to use aerosol products (e.g., spray deodorants), to avoid dusty areas, and to avoid exposure to persons who have upper respiratory infections. The patient should be told to contact his physician if he develops symptoms of an upper respiratory infection or other ailments.

Plans for returning to work activities are individualized and are made with the physician's and social worker's guidance. Some persons are able to return to work within a few weeks after thoracic surgery, whereas others need occupational counseling because a change of occupation is necessary; still other patients are unable to work.

References for Unit XIV

1. A New NTA-ATS Statement: Infectiousness of tuberculosis. *Bulletin National Tuberculosis Association 53*:6, November, 1967.
2. Adams, W. E.: Current concepts of surgical management of carcinoma of the lung. *Diseases of the Chest 51*:233, March, 1967.
3. Affronti, L. F., Fife, E. H., and Grow, L.: Serodiagnostic test for tuberculosis. *American Review of Respiratory Disease 107*:822, May, 1973.
4. Ahlstrom, P.: Raising sputum specimens. *American Journal of Nursing 65*:109, March, 1965.
5. Ambiavagar, M.: Treatment of respiratory failure following chest injuries. *Journal of Postgraduate Medicine 43*:256, April, 1967.
6. Ambiavagar, M., et al.: Intermittent positive pressure ventilation in the treatment of severe crushing injuries of the chest. *Thorax 21*:359, July, 1966.
7. Ambrus, L., and Warnecke, J.: The emphysema patient: An approach to conditioning exercises. *Physical Therapy 47*:369, May, 1967.
8. American Cancer Society: *1973 Cancer Facts and Figures.* (Pamphlet.) New York, American Cancer Society, Inc., 1972.
9. American Cancer Society: *Answering the Most-Often-Asked Questions About . . . Cigarette Smoking and Lung Cancer.* (Pamphlet.) New York, American Cancer Society, Inc. 1965.
10. American Thoracic Society, Committee on Therapy: Principles of respiratory care. *American Review of Respiratory Diseases 95*:327, February, 1967.
11. Andrewes, C. H.: The common cold: Prospects for its control. *Medical Clinics of North America 51*: 765, May, 1967.
12. Ashenburg, N. J.: The effects of air pollution on health. *Nursing Outlook 16*:22, February, 1968.
13. Austrian, R.: Answers to questions on "Pneumonias." *Hospital Medicine 4*:41, February, 1968.
14. Ayres, S., et al.: Respiratory management of the critically ill patient. *New York State Journal of Medicine 68*:2871, November, 1968.
15. Bailey, A. J.: Lung cancer and smoking. *Canadian Nurse 61*:285, April, 1965.
16. Barham, V. Z.: Tuberculosis care—1971: Changing the attitudes of hospital nurses. *Nursing Outlook 19*:538, August, 1971.
17. Barrett, N. R.: The pleura. *Thorax 25*:515, September, 1970.
18. Baskfield, M. M.: Preoperative and postoperative care of the patient with cancer of the lung. *Nursing Clinics of North America 21*:609, December, 1967.
19. Bass, H., et al.: Exercise training: Therapy for patients with chronic obstructive pulmonary disease. *Chest 57*:116, February, 1970.
20. Bates, D. V.: Chronic bronchitis and emphysema. *New England Journal of Medicine 278*:546, March 7, 1968.
21. Bates, D. V., Macklem, P. T., and Christie, R. V.: *Respiratory Function in Disease.* Philadelphia, W. B. Saunders Company, 1971.
22. Bates, M.: Crush injuries: Nature and causes. *Nursing Times 63*:455, April 7, 1967.
23. Baum, G. L., Schwarz, J., and Barlow, P. B.: Sarcoidosis and specific etiologic agents: A continuing enigma. *Chest 63*:488, April, 1973.
24. B.C.G. *Bulletin National Tuberculosis Association 53*:8, January, 1967.
25. Beeson, P. B., and McDermott, W. (eds.): *Cecil-Loeb Textbook of Medicine.* 13th ed. Philadelphia, W. B. Saunders Company, 1971, pp. 865–946.
26. Beland, I. L.: *Clinical Nursing: Pathophysiological and Psychosocial Approaches.* 2nd ed. New York, The Macmillan Company, 1970.
27. Belinkoff, S.: *Introduction to Inhalation Therapy.* Boston, Little, Brown and Company, 1969.
28. Bendixen, H. H., et al.: *Respiratory Care.* St. Louis, The C. V. Mosby Company, 1965.
29. Betson, C.: Blood gases. *American Journal of Nursing 68*:1010, May, 1968.
30. Bhattacharya, S. K., and Polk, J. W.: Management

of postpneumonectomy space. *Chest 63*:233, February, 1973.

31. Bibler, D. D., Jr., and Merendino, K. A.: Nonpenetrating chest trauma in the geriatric patient. *Geriatrics 22*:119, October, 1967.
32. Bigelow, D. B., et al.: Acute respiratory failure. *Medical Clinics of North America 51*:323, March, 1967.
33. Black, A. J., and Light, R. W.: Alternate day steroid therapy in diffuse pulmonary sarcoidosis. *Chest 63*:495, April, 1973.
34. Blalock, J. B., and Ochsner, J. L.: Management of thoracic trauma. *Surgical Clinics of North America 46*:1513, December, 1966.
35. Bocles, J. S.: Status asthmaticus. *Medical Clinics of North America 54*:493, March, 1970.
36. Bouchard, R.: *Nursing Care of the Cancer Patient.* St. Louis, The C. V. Mosby Company, 1967.
37. Bradford, J. K., and DeCamp, P. T.: Bronchiectasis. *Surgical Clinics of North America 46*:1485, December, 1966.
38. Bradley, J.: Emphysema: Are nurses prepared? *RN 31*:41, January, 1968.
39. Breathing Exercises for Home Use. (Pamphlet.) New York, Breon Laboratories, Inc., 90 Park Avenue, (10016) 1967.
40. Brooks, W.: Replacing ritual with reason in tuberculosis isolation. *American Journal of Nursing 69*: 2410, November, 1969.
41. Brown, E. B.: Hyposensitization therapy in respiratory allergy. *Modern Treatment 3*:845, July, 1966.
42. Brown, J. R., and Opitz, J. L.: Treatment of neuropathies. *In* Vinken, P. J., and Bruyn, G. W. (eds.): *Handbook of Clinical Neurology*. Vol. 8. New York, American Elsevier Publishing Company, Inc., 1970.
43. Brummer, D. L.: Oxygen therapy in cardiopulmonary disease. (Committee on Therapy, American Thoracic Society.) *American Review of Respiratory Diseases 101*:811, 1970.
44. Brunner, L. S., et al.: *Textbook of Medical-Surgical Nursing*. 2nd ed. Philadelphia, J. B. Lippincott Company, 1970.
45. Buckingham, W. B., Cugell, D. W., and Kettel, L. J.: Pulmonary angiography in lung diseases. *Journal American Medical Association 200*:122, June 19, 1967.
46. Buescher, E. L.: Respiratory disease and the adenoviruses. *Medical Clinics of North America 51*: 769, May, 1967.
47. Burgess, A. M.: A comparison of common methods of oxygen therapy for bed patients. *American Journal of Nursing 65*:96, December, 1965.
48. Burrows, B.: Pulmonary diffusion and alveolar-capillary block. *Medical Clinics of North America 51*:427, March, 1967.
49. Burrows, B., and Earle, R. H.: Course and prognosis in chronic obstructive lung disease. *New England Journal of Medicine 280*:397, February 20, 1969.

49a. Bushnell, S. S.: *Respiratory Intensive Care Nursing.* Boston, Little, Brown & Co., 1973.

50. Caldwell, W. L., and Bagshaw, M. A.: Indications for and results of irradiation of carcinoma of the lung. *Cancer 22*:999, November, 1968.
51. Chapman, J. S.: The atypical mycobacteria: Their significance in human disease. *American Journal of Nursing 67*:1031, May, 1967.
52. Cherniak, R. M., Cherniak, L., and Naimark, A.: *Respiration in Health and Disease.* 2nd ed. Philadelphia, W. B. Saunders Company, 1972.
53. Clarke, D. B.: The management of thoracic injuries. *Journal of Postgraduate Medicine 43*:639, October, 1967.
54. Clayton, L. B.: Respiratory disease—How much of a problem? *Bulletin National Tuberculosis Association 53*:5, April, 1967.
55. Collart, M. E., and Brenneman, J. K.: Preventing postoperative atelectasis. *American Journal of Nursing 71*:1982, October, 1971.
56. Committee on Therapy, American Thoracic Society: Current status of surgical treatment of pulmonary emphysema and asthma. *American Review of Respiratory Diseases 97*:486, March, 1968.
57. Committee on Therapy, American Thoracic Society: Therapy of pleural effusion. *American Review of Respiratory Diseases 97*:479, March, 1968.
58. Comroe, J. H., Jr., et al.: *The Lung*. 2nd ed. Chicago, Year Book Medical Publishers, Inc., 1962.
59. Conn, H. F. (ed.): *Current Therapy 1974*. Philadelphia, W. B. Saunders Company, 1974.
60. Crocco, J. A., et al.: Massive hemoptysis. *Archives of Internal Medicine 121*:495, June, 1968.
61. Crofton, J.: The chemotherapy of bacterial respiratory infections. *American Review of Respiratory Diseases 101*:841, 1970.
62. Davenport, F. M.: Prospects for the control of influenza. *American Journal of Nursing 69*:1908, September, 1969.
63. Davis, D. F.: A review of detection methods for the early diagnosis of lung cancer. *Journal of Chronic Diseases 19*:819, August, 1966.
64. Davis, L. (ed.): *Christopher's Textbook of Surgery.* See Sabiston.
65. Deenstra, H., and Van Ditmars, M. J.: Sarcoidosis. *Diseases of the Chest 53*:57, January, 1968.
66. DeMeyer, J. A.: Emphysema: Effective positive-pressure breathing therapy. *RN 31*:46, January, 1968.
67. Diener, C. F., and Burrows, B.: Occupational disability in patients with chronic airway obstruction. *American Review of Respiratory Diseases 96*:35, July, 1967.
68. Dittbrenner, M., Sr., and Hebert, W. M.: Regimen for a thoracotomy patient. *American Journal of Nursing 67*:2072, October, 1967.
69. Downie, P.: Lung function tests and their application in industrial pulmonary disease. *Occupational Health 18*:297, November-December, 1966.
70. Dyer, E. D., and Peterson, D. E.: Safe care of IPPB machines. *American Journal of Nursing 71*: 2163, November, 1971.
71. Early, M.: The gaseous exchange process: Nursing implications. *In* Kintzel, K. C. (ed.): *Advanced Concepts in Clinical Nursing*. Philadelphia, J. B. Lippincott Company, 1971.
72. Edsall, J., Collins, J. G., and Gray, J. A. C.: The reactivation of tuberculosis in New York City in 1967. *American Review of Respiratory Disease 102*:725, November, 1970.
73. Edwards, P. Q.: Tuberculosis today. *Chest 63*:465, April, 1973.
74. Egan, D.: *Fundamentals of Respiratory Therapy.* 2nd Ed. St. Louis, The C. V. Mosby Company, 1973.
75. Egan, D. F.: Inhalation therapy in the general hospital. *G.P. 33*:99, March, 1966.
76. Emphysema: Postural drainage and breathing exercises. *RN 31*:44, January, 1968.

77. Evans, A. S.: Clinical syndromes in adults caused by respiratory infection. *Medical Clinics of North America 51*:803, May, 1967.
78. Fagerhaugh, S. Y.: Getting around with emphysema. *American Journal of Nursing 73*:94, January, 1973.
78a. Fahy, A.: Enemies in the dust. Occupational respiratory diseases. *Bulletin National Tuberculosis Respiratory Disease Association 58*:14, June, 1972.
79. Farber, S. M., and Wilson, R. H. L.: Chronic obstructive emphysema. *Clinical Symposia 20*:35, April-June, 1968.
80. Feldman, S. A. (ed.): *Tracheostomy and Artificial Ventilation.* London, Edward Arnold, Ltd., 1967.
81. Ferguson, T. B., and Burford, T. H.: The changing pattern of pulmonary suppuration: Surgical implications. *Diseases of the Chest 53*:396, April, 1968.
82. Filley, G. F.: Emphysema and chronic bronchitis: Clinical manifestations and their physiologic significance. *Medical Clinics of North America 51*:283, March, 1967.
83. Filley, G. F.: *Pulmonary Insufficiency and Respiratory Failure.* Philadelphia, Lea & Febiger, 1967.
84. Fingerhut, A. G., Chin, F. K., and Shultz, E. H.: Radical radiation therapy for cancer of the lung. *Chest 60*:244, September, 1971.
85. Fishman, S. I.: Pulmonary emphysema. *New York State Journal of Medicine 67*:2573, October 1, 1967.
86. Flatter, P. A.: Hazards of oxygen therapy. *American Journal of Nursing 68*:80, January, 1968.
87. Foley, M. F.: Pulmonary function testing. *American Journal of Nursing 71*:1134, June, 1971.
88. Foss, G.: Postural drainage. *American Journal of Nursing 73*:666, April, 1973.
89. Fox, W.: Changing concepts of the chemotherapy of pulmonary tuberculosis. *American Review of Respiratory Diseases 97*:767, May, 1968.
90. Francis, T., Jr.: Epidemic influenza: Immunization and control. *Medical Clinics of North America 51*: 781, May, 1967.
91. Fraser, R. G., and Paré, J. A. P.: *Structure and Function of the Lung.* Philadelphia, W. B. Saunders Company, 1971.
92. Freedman, S. O. (ed.): Symposium on treatment of respiratory allergy. *Modern Treatment 3*:813, July, 1966.
92a. Freedman, S. O.: Tuberculin testing and screening: A critical evaluation. *Hospital Practice 7*:63, May, 1972.
93. Friedman, A. H.: The patient with chronic obstructive lung disease and his care at home. *Nursing Clinics of North America 3*:437, September, 1968.
94. Friedman, R. M.: Inferons and virus infections. *American Journal of Nursing 68*:542, March, 1968.
95. Frohlich, E. D. (ed.): *Pathophysiology: Altered Regulatory Mechanisms in Disease.* Philadelphia, J. B. Lippincott Company, 1972.
96. Frouchtman, R.: Psychosocial aspects of bronchial asthma. *Diseases of the Chest 53*:227, February, 1968.

97. Fuerst, E. V., and Wolff, L.: *Fundamentals of Nursing.* 4th ed. Philadelphia, J. B. Lippincott Company, 1969.
98. Gaensler, E. A.: "Idiopathic" pleural effusion. *New England Journal of Medicine 283*:816, October 8, 1970.
99. Garner, J. S., and Kaiser, A. B.: How often is isolation needed? *American Journal of Nursing 72*:733, April, 1972.
100. Geiger, J. P.: Diagnosis of chest injuries. *Hospital Medicine 7*:109, October, 1971.
101. Gernert, C. F., and Schwartz, S.: Pulmonary artery catheterization. *American Journal of Nursing 73*: 1182, July, 1973.
102. Gibbon, J. H., Jr., Sabiston, D. C., Jr., and Spencer, F. C.: *Surgery of the Chest.* 2nd ed. Philadelphia, W. B. Saunders Company, 1969.
103. Ginsberg, F.: Inhalation therapy techniques require these procedures for patient safety. *Modern Hospital 108*:130, June, 1967.
104. Goff, W. F.: What to do when foreign bodies are inhaled or ingested. *Postgraduate Medicine 44*: 135, October, 1968.
105. Goldbarg, A. N., Krone, R. J., and Resnekov, L.: Effects of cigarette smoking on hemodynamics at rest and during exercise. Normal subjects. *Chest 60*:531, December, 1971.
106. Grant, H., and Murray, R.: *Emergency Care.* Washington, D. C., Robert J. Brady Company, 1971.
107. Grater, W. C.: Diagnosis and treatment of acute asthma after 40. *Geriatrics 22*:146, September, 1967.
108. Griffith, E. W.: Nursing process: A patient with respiratory dysfunction. *Nursing Clinics of North America 6*:1, March, 1971.
109. Grimes, O. F.: Neuromuscular syndromes in patients with lung cancer. *American Journal of Nursing 71*: 752, April, 1971.
110. Griner, P. F.: Treatment of acute pulmonary edema: Conventional or intensive care? *Annals of Internal Medicine 77*:501, October, 1972.
111. Guyton, A. C.: *Function of the Human Body.* 4th ed. Philadelphia, W. B. Saunders Company, 1974.
112. Haas, A.: Essentials of living with pulmonary emphysema: A guide for patients and their families. (Pamphlet.) Patient Publication No. 4. New York University Medical Center, Institute of Rehabilitation Medicine, 1963.
113. Haas, A., and Cardon, H.: Rehabilitation in chronic obstructive pulmonary disease. *Medical Clinics of North America 53*:593, May, 1969.
114. Haas, A., and Rusk, H. A.: Rehabilitation of patients with obstructive pulmonary diseases. *Postgraduate Medicine 39*:612, June, 1966.
115. Hanamey, R.: Teaching patients breathing and coughing techniques. *Nursing Outlook 13*:58, August, 1965.
116. Hanchett, E., and Johnson, R. A.: Early signs of congestive heart failure. *American Journal of Nursing 68*:1456, July, 1968.
117. Hargreaves, A. G.: Emotional problems of patients with respiratory disease. *Nursing Clinics of North America 3*:479, September, 1968.
118. Harkins, H. P.: Aspiration pneumonia. *Hospital Medicine 4*:52, November, 1968.
119. Harrison, T. R., et al. (eds.): *Principles of Internal Medicine.* 6th ed. New York, McGraw-Hill Book Company, 1970.
120. Hasenfus, J. L.: Report of the World Conference on Smoking and Health. *Journal Maine Medical Association 58*:234, November, 1967.
121. Hedges, J. E., and Bridges, C. J.: Stimulation of the

cough reflex. *American Journal of Nursing 68*:347, February, 1968.
122. Heimlich, H. J.: A flutter valve to replace underwater drainage bottles. *Journal of American Medical Association 192*:262, April 19, 1965.
123. Helmholz, H. F., Jr., Stillwell, G. K., and Sessler, A. D.: Disorders of respiration (pulmonary function); Chest physical therapy. *In* Krusen, F. H., Kottke, F. J., and Ellwood, P. M., Jr. (eds.): *Handbook of Physical Medicine and Rehabilitation.* 2nd ed. Philadelphia, W. B. Saunders Company, 1971.
124. Helming, M. G.: Nursing care of patients with chronic obstructive lung disease. *Nursing Clinics of North America 3*:413, September, 1968.
125. Helming, M. G. (ed.): Symposium on nursing in respiratory diseases. *Nursing Clinics of North America 3*(No. 3), September, 1968.
126. Henriksen, J. D.: Physical medicine rehabilitation of asthma, bronchitis, and emphysema. *Life and Health 83*:18, February, 1968.
127. Hinshaw, H. C.: *Diseases of the Chest.* 3rd ed. Philadelphia, W. B. Saunders Company, 1969.
128. Hohle, B. M.: The atypical mycobacteria: Patient care at home. *American Journal of Nursing 67*: 1033, May, 1967.
129. Holvey, D. N., et al. (eds.): *The Merck Manual.* 12th ed. Rahway, N. J., Merck, Sharp and Dohme Research Laboratories, 1972.
130. Hopewell, P. C.: Chemoprophylaxis for the prevention of tuberculosis. *American Review of Respiratory Diseases 97*:721, April, 1968.
131. Hopkins, W. A., and Turk, L. N., III: The current treatment of severe chest injuries. *Southern Medical Journal 62*:243, March, 1969.
132. Horwitz, O.: Tuberculosis risk and marital status. *American Review of Respiratory Disease 104*: 22, July, 1971.
133. Huse, W. F.: The least you should know about chest injuries. *Consultant 8*:42, September, 1968.
134. Hyde, R. W.: Clinical interpretation of arterial oxygen measurements. *Medical Clinics of North America 54*:617, May, 1970.
134a. . . . In managing chest trauma. *Emergency Medicine 3*:116, February, 1971.
135. Ingraham, H. S.: What it will take to eradicate tuberculosis in the United States. *Bulletin National Tuberculosis Association 53*:12, March, 1967.
136. Inouye, W. Y., Berggren, R. B., and Johnson, J.: Spontaneous pneumothorax: Treatment and mortality. *Diseases of the Chest 51*:67, January, 1967.
137. Isawa, T., Wasserman, K., and Taplin, G. V.: Lung scintigraphy and pulmonary function studies in obstructive airway disease. *American Review of Respiratory Disease 102*:161, August, 1970.
138. Itkin, I.: The pro's and con's of exercise for the person with asthma. *American Journal of Nursing 66*:1584, July, 1966.
139. Jack, G. D.: Chest injuries: A graded therapeutic regime. *Nursing Times 63*:1398, October 20, 1967.
140. Jacob, S. W., and Francone, C. A.: *Structure and Function in Man.* 2nd ed. Philadelphia, W. B. Saunders Company, 1970.
141. Jacobs, E. M., and Denault, P. M.: *Neurology for Nurses.* Springfield, Ill., Charles C Thomas, 1964.
142. Jacquette, G.: To reduce hazards of tracheal suctioning. *American Journal of Nursing 71*:2362, December, 1971.
143. Jeffis, L., and Baker, C.: Nasopharyngeal and tracheal suctioning. *American Journal of Nursing 67*:2361, November, 1967.
144. Jodoin, G., et al.: Early effects of asbestos exposure on lung function. *American Review of Respiratory Disease 104*:525, October, 1971.
145. Johansen, J. L.: Taking the mystery out of water-sealed chest drainage. *RN 23*:40, January, 1960.
146. Johnson, R. F., and Hopewell, P. C.: Chemotherapy of tuberculosis. *Annals of Internal Medicine 70*: 359, February, 1969.
147. Johnson, T. M., McCann, W., and Davey, W. N.: Tuberculous: bronchopleural fistula. *American Review of Respiratory Disease 107*:30, January, 1973.
148. Jones, J. C., et al.: Long-term survival after resection for bronchogenic carcinoma. *Journal of Thoracic and Cardiovascular Surgery 54*:383, September, 1967.
149. Jones, J. M.: Tuberculosis: Present day concepts of management. *Hospital Medicine 3*:76, June, 1967.
150. Jones, W. R.: Living with emphysema. *Nursing Outlook 15*:53, September, 1967.
151. Joyner, C. R., Herman, R. J., and Reid, J. M.: Reflected ultrasound in the detection and localization of pleural effusion. *Journal of American Medical Association 200*:129, May, 1967.
152. Katz, S.: Don't surrender to lung cancer. *Consultant 7*:40, June, 1967.
153. Kearns, B.: Tracheostomy suctioning technique. *Canadian Nurse 66*:44, February, 1970.
154. Kelly, H. B.: Tuberculosis care—1971: Patient population and treatment choices. *Nursing Outlook 19*:541, August, 1971.
155. Kettel, L. J., and Cugell, D. W.: Pleural biopsy. *Journal of American Medical Association 200*: 141, April 24, 1967.
155a. Kilburn, K. H., Kilburn, G. G., and Merchant, J. A.: Byssinosis: Matter from lint to lungs. *American Journal of Nursing 73*:1952, November, 1973.
156. Killen, D. A., and Gobbel, W. G., Jr.: *Spontaneous Pneumothorax.* Boston, Little, Brown and Company, 1968.
157. Kinney, M.: Rehabilitation of patients with COLD. *American Journal of Nursing 67*:2528, December, 1967.
158. Kirby, W. M. M. (ed.): Symposium on modern management of respiratory disease. *Medical Clinics of North America 51*(No. 2), March, 1967.
159. Kirschner, P. A.: A coordinated surgical approach to diagnosis and treatment of lung cancer. *Chest 57*:214, February, 1970.
160. Koonz, F. P.: Nursing in tuberculosis. *Nursing Clinics of North America 3*:403, September, 1968.
161. Kristensen, H. S., et al.: Treatment of severe respiratory insufficiency in diffuse chronic disease by tracheostomy and intermittent positive pressure ventilation (IPPV). *Postgraduate Medical Journal 43*:244, April, 1967.
162. Krupp, M. A., and Chatton, M. J.: *Current Diagnosis and Treatment.* Los Altos, California, Lange Medical Publications, 1972.
163. Kurihara, M.: Assessment and maintenance of adequate respiration. *Nursing Clinics of North America 3*:65, March, 1968.
164. Kurihara, M.: Postural drainage, clapping and vibrating. *American Journal of Nursing 65*:76, November, 1965.

165. Larson, E. L.: The patient with acute pulmonary edema. *American Journal of Nursing 68*:1019, May, 1968.
166. Lawther, P. J., Waller, R. E., and Henderson, M.: Air pollution and exacerbations of bronchitis. *Thorax 25*:525, September, 1970.
167. Lebovitz, J. J.: Pleural effusion: Causes and management. *Consultant 11*:23, December, 1971.
168. LeRoux, B. T.: Bronchial carcinoma. *Thorax 23*:136, March, 1968.
169. Lester, W.: Tuberculosis: An urban problem. *Annals of Internal Medicine 68*:947, April, 1968.
170. Levine, E. R.: Inhalation therapy—Aerosols and intermittent positive pressure breathing. *Medical Clinics of North America 51*:307, March, 1967.
171. Levine, I.: Tuberculosis risk in students of nursing. *Archives of Internal Medicine 121*:545, June, 1968.
172. Littmann, D.: Stethoscopes and auscultation. *American Journal of Nursing 72*:1238, July, 1972.
173. Living with Asthma, Chronic Bronchitis, and Emphysema. (Pamphlet.) Northridge, California, Riker Laboratories, 1963.
174. Lloyd, J. W.: Chest injuries and their management. *Nursing Mirror 124*:iv, September 8, 1967.
175. Longo, A. M., Moser, K. M., and Luchsinger, P. C.: The role of oxygen therapy in the rehabilitation of patients with chronic obstructive pulmonary disease. *American Review of Respiratory Disease 103*:690, April, 1971.
176. Lorin, M. I., and Denning, C. R.: Evaluation of postural drainage by measurement of sputum volume and consistency. *American Journal of Physical Medicine 50*:215, October, 1971.
177. Lourenco, R. V. (ed.): Inhaled aerosol symposium. *Archives of Internal Medicine 131*:21–166, January, 1973.
178. MacVicar, J., and Mendelsohn, H. J.: Chest surgery. *In* Meltzer, L. E., Abdellah, F., and Kitchell, J. (eds.): *Concepts and Practices of Intensive Care for Nurse Specialists*. Philadelphia, The Charles Press, 1969.
179. Mannsell, K., Pearson, R. S. B., and Livingstone, J. L.: Long-term corticosteroid treatment of asthma. *British Medical Journal 1*:661, March 16, 1968.
180. Manson, R. M., et al.: Respiratory tract and mediastinum. In *Current Diagnosis and Treatment*. Los Altos, Calif., Lange Medical Publications, 1972.
180a. Marici, F. N.: The flexible fiberoptic bronchoscope. *American Journal of Nursing 73*:1776, October, 1973.
181. Martin, C. J., et al.: Tuberculosis, emphysema and bronchitis. *American Review of Respiratory Diseases 97*:1089, June, 1968.
182. Martin, C. J., Katsura, S., and Cochran, T. H.: The relationship of chronic bronchitis to the diffuse obstructive pulmonary syndrome. *American Review of Respiratory Disease 102*:362, September, 1970.
183. Masferrer, R.: Role of patient instruction in improving IPPB treatments. *Inhalation Therapy 14*:17, April, 1969.
184. Mausner, J. S.: Cigarette smoking among patients with respiratory disease. *American Review of Respiratory Disease 102*:704, November, 1970.
185. McArdle, K. H.: The patient and the Bennett. *Nursing Clinics of North America 1*:143, March, 1966.
186. McCallum, H. P.: The nurse and the respirator. *Nursing Clinics of North America 1*:597, December, 1966.
187. Medina, J. R., et al.: Use of the scintillation anger camera and xenon (Xe-133) in the study of chronic obstructive lung disease. *Journal of American Medical Association 208*:985, May 12, 1969.
188. Meyers, J. A.: The changing face of tuberculosis—A lifetime study. *Postgraduate Medicine 44*:166, October, 1968.
189. Miller, W. F.: Treatment of chronic pulmonary emphysema. *Postgraduate Medicine 39*:230, March, 1966.
190. Miller, W. F.: Pulmonary function tests. *Hospital Medicine 4*:88, May, 1968.
191. Miller, W. F.: Aerosol therapy in acute and chronic respiratory disease. *Archives of Internal Medicine 131*:148, January, 1973.
192. Mitchell, R. S.: Control of tuberculosis. *New England Journal of Medicine 276*:905, April 20, 1967.
193. Moghissi, K.: Laceration of lung following blunt trauma. *Thorax 26*:223, March, 1971.
194. Moody, L.: Asthma: Physiology and patient care. *American Journal of Nursing 73*:1212, July, 1973.
195. Morgan, C. V., Jr., and Orcutt, T. W.: The care and feeding of chest tubes. *American Journal of Nursing 72*:305, February, 1972.
196. Moyer, J., and Oaks, W. (eds.): *Pre- and Post-Operative Management of the Cardiopulmonary Patient*. New York, Grune & Stratton, 1970.
197. Murphy, E. R.: Intensive nursing care in a respiratory unit. *Nursing Clinics of North America 3*: 423, September, 1968.
198. Murray, J. F.: Shock lung. *California Medicine 112*: 43, February, 1970.
199. Mushin, W. W., et al.: *Automatic Ventilation of the Lungs*. 2nd ed. Philadelphia, F. A. Davis Company, 1969.
200. National Tuberculosis and Respiratory Disease Association:* *Chronic Obstructive Pulmonary Disease: A Manual for Physicians*. New York, 1965.
201. National Tuberculosis and Respiratory Disease Association: *Principles of Respiratory Care*. New York, 1967.
202. National Tuberculosis and Respiratory Disease Association: *What You Can Do About Your Breathing*. New York, 1967.
203. National Tuberculosis and Respiratory Disease Association in Cooperation with the Allergy Foundation of America: *Asthma: A Practical Guide for Physicians*. New York, 1968.
204. National Tuberculosis and Respiratory Disease Association: *Breathing . . . What You Need to Know*. New York, 1968.
205. National Tuberculosis and Respiratory Disease Association: *Cleaning and Sterilization of Inhalation Equipment*. New York, 1968.
206. National Tuberculosis and Respiratory Disease Association: *Diagnostic Standards and Classification of Tuberculosis*. New York, 1969.
207. National Tuberculosis and Respiratory Disease Association: *Air Pollution Primer*. New York, 1969.
208. National Tuberculosis and Respiratory Disease Association: *Introduction to Respiratory Diseases*. 4th ed. New York, 1969.
209. Nealton, T. F., Jr., and Sandler, S. C.: The treatment of respiratory failure with continuous venti-

*Now designated as American Lung Association.

latory support. *Surgical Clinics of North America 47*:1207, October, 1967.
210. Nett, L. M., and Petty, T. I.: Acute respiratory failure. *American Journal of Nursing 67*:1847, September, 1967.
211. Nett, L. M., and Petty, T. I.: Respirator controls. *American Journal of Nursing 67*:1852, September, 1967.
212. Nett, L. M., and Petty, T. I.: Effective treatment for emphysema and chronic bronchitis. *Journal of Rehabilitation 33*:10, September-October, 1967.
213. Nett, L. M., and Petty, T. I.: A new IPPB device for bronchial hygiene. *American Journal of Nursing 68*:2570, December, 1968.
214. Nett, L. M., and Petty, T. I.: Why emphysema patients are the way they are. *American Journal of Nursing 70*:1251, June, 1970.
214a. Nett, L. M., and Petty, T. I.: Oxygen toxicity. *American Journal of Nursing 73*:1556, September, 1973.
215. Newman, R., et al.: Rifampin in initial treatment of pulmonary tuberculosis. *American Review of Respiratory Disease 103*:461, April, 1971.
216. Noehren, T. H.: Is positive pressure breathing overrated? *Chest 57*:507, June, 1970.
217. Ochsner, A.: Lobectomy or pneumonectomy. *Surgical Clinics of North America 46*:1255, October, 1966.
218. Ochsner, A., Jr., and Ochsner, A.: Cancer of the lung: Recognition and management. *Surgical Clinics of North America 46*:1411, December, 1966.
219. Ochsner, J. L., and Keller, C. H.: Removing bronchial secretions. *Nursing Clinics of North America 2*:521, September, 1967.
220. Oswald, N.: Modern day treatment of chronic bronchitis. *Geriatrics 22*:125, July, 1967.
221. Paez, P. N., et al.: The physiologic basis of training patients with emphysema. *American Review of Respiratory Diseases 95*:944, June, 1967.
222. Palva, T., Viikari, S., and Inberg, M.: Pulmonary carcinoma: Mediastinoscopic criteria for curative resections. *Diseases of the Chest 56*:156, August, 1969.
223. Petty, T. I.: Why not take inhalation therapy seriously? *Chest 57*:403, May, 1970.
224. Petty, T. I., and Ashbaugh, D. G.: The adult respiratory distress syndrome. *Chest 60*:233, September, 1971.
225. Petty, T. I., and Finigan, M. M.: Clinical evaluation of prolonged ambulatory oxygen therapy in chronic airway obstruction. *American Journal of Medicine 45*:242, August, 1968.
226. Petty, T. I., and Nett, L. M.: *For Those Who Live and Breathe with Emphysema and Chronic Bronchitis*. Springfield, Ill., Charles C Thomas, 1967.
227. Petty, T. I., et al.: A comprehensive care program for chronic airway obstruction. *Annals of Internal Medicine, 70*:1109, June, 1969.
228. Phipps, W. J., and Barker, W. L.: Respiratory insufficiency and failure. *In* Meltzer, L. E., Abdellah, F. G., and Kitchell, J. R. (eds.): *Concepts and Practices of Intensive Care for Nurse Specialists*. Philadelphia, The Charles Press, Publishers, Inc., 1969.
229. Pierce, A. K., and Sanford, J. P.: Bacterial contamination of aerosols. *Archives of Internal Medicine 131*:156, January, 1973.
230. Polk, J. W.: Treatment of pulmonary histoplasmosis. *Diseases of the Chest 56*:149, August, 1969.
231. Prather, J. R., et al.: Initial and late management of penetrating chest wounds. *Medical Times 96*: 1013, October, 1968.
232. Proctor, D. F., and Safar, P.: Management of airway obstruction. *In* Safar, P. (ed.): *Respiratory Therapy*. Philadelphia, F. A. Davis Company, 1965.
233. Programmed instruction: Respiratory tract aspiration. *American Journal of Nursing 66*:2483, November, 1966.
234. Pruitt, C. V., Westbury, E. L., and Hairston, P.: Nursing care of patients with surgery of the chest. *Nursing Clinics of North America 2*:513, September, 1967.
235. Public Health Service: *Closed Drainage of the Chest*. Washington, D.C., U.S. Department of Health, Education, and Welfare, May, 1965. Public Health Service Publication No. 1337.
236. Public Health Service: *Management of Chronic Obstructive Lung Disease*. Washington, D.C., Department of Health, Education, and Welfare, May, 1966. Public Health Service Publication No. 1457.
237. Public Health Service: *If You Have Emphysema or Chronic Bronchitis*. Public Health Service Publication No. 1726, Chronic Respiratory Disease Control Program, Arlington, Virginia 22203.
238. Pulley, H. C.: Precedents in pollution control. *American Journal of Nursing 66*:2711, December, 1966.
239. Purcell, R. H., and Chanock, R. M.: Role of mycoplasmas in human respiratory disease. *Medical Clinics of North America 51*:791, May, 1967.
240. Rankin, J., et al.: Pulmonary granulomatoses due to inhaled organic antigens. *Medical Clinics of North America 51*:459, March, 1967.
241. Ream, C. R.: Tuberculosis in the general hospital. *Public Health News 50*:182, August, 1969.
242. Rees, H. A.: Management of status asthmaticus. *Journal of Postgraduate Medicine 43*:225, April, 1967.
243. Reiman, H. A.: Viral versus bacterial and other pneumonias. *Hospital Medicine 4*:36, September, 1968.
243a. Reitz, M., and Pope, W.: Mouth Care. *American Journal of Nursing 73*:1728, October 1973.
244. Report of the Committee on Fungus Diseases and Subcommittee on Criteria for Clinical Diagnosis, American College of Chest Physicians: The diagnosis of pulmonary mycoses. *Chest 60*:82, July, 1971.
245. Report of the Committee on Fungus Diseases and Subcommittee on Therapy, American College of Chest Physicians: Chemotherapeutic agents for the pulmonary mycoses. *Chest 60*:260, September, 1971.
246. Revolution in chest drainage. *RN, 31*:50, March, 1968.
247. Ribando, C. A., and Grace, W. J.: Pulmonary aspiration. *American Journal of Medicine 50*:510, April, 1971.
248. Riding, W. D., and Ambiavagar, M.: Resuscitation of the moribund asthmatic. *Postgraduate Medical Journal 43*:234, April, 1967.
249. Rie, M. W.: Physical therapy in the nursing care of respiratory disease patients. *Nursing Clinics of North America 3*:463, September, 1968.
250. Robley, S. H.: *Emphysema and Common Sense*. West Nyack, N.Y., Parker Publishing Company, Inc., 1968.
251. Rodman, M. J.: Drugs for respiratory tract infections. *RN 34*:55, September, 1971.

252. Rodman, T.: Management of tracheobronchial secretions. *American Journal of Nursing 66*:2474, November, 1966.
253. Rodman, T., and Sterling, F. H.: *Pulmonary Emphysema and Related Lung Diseases*. St. Louis, The C. V. Mosby Company, 1969.
254. Rosa, U. W., Prolla, J. C., and da Silva Gastal, E.: Cytology in diagnosis of cancer affecting the lung. *Chest 63*:203, February, 1973.
255. Rosenblatt, M. B., Lisa, J. R., and Collier, F.: The diagnosis of secondary bronchial carcinoma. *Geriatrics 22*:135, September, 1967.
256. Ross, J. K., et al.: Mediastinoscopy. *Thorax 25*: 312, May, 1970.
257. Rossi, N. P., and Soper, R. T.: Thoracic and pulmonary surgery. *In* Liechty, R., and Saper, R. T. (eds.): *Synopsis of Surgery*. St. Louis, The C. V. Mosby Company, 1968.
258. Rowland, J. A.: How about smoking? *Nursing Outlook 19*:422, June, 1971.
259. Rutherford, A. M.: Inhalation therapy in the recovery room. *Nursing Clinics of North America 3*:497, September, 1968.
259a. Sabiston, D. C.: *Davis-Christopher Textbook of Surgery*. 10th ed. Philadelphia, W. B. Saunders Company, 1972.
260. Safar, P. (ed.): *Respiratory Therapy*. Philadelphia, F. A. Davis Company, 1965.
261. Sander, O. A.: Silicosis, the preventable occupational lung disease. *Bulletin National Tuberculosis Association 54*:7, February, 1968.
262. Sanderson, D. R., Dawson, B., and Wang, J. K.: Bronchospirometry during diagnostic bronchoscopy. *Chest 60*:225, September, 1971.
263. Schwaid, M.: The impact of emphysema. *American Journal of Nursing 70*:1247, June, 1970.
264. Schwartz, J. L., and Dubitzky, M.: One-year follow-up results of a smoking cessation program. *Canadian Journal Public Health 59*:161, April, 1968.
265. Scott, B. H.: Tensions linked with emphysema. *American Journal of Nursing 69*:538, March, 1969.
266. Seabury, J. H.: Pulmonary ventilation and respiration; Tests of respiratory function. *In* Sodeman, W. A., and Sodeman, W. A., Jr.: *Pathological Physiology*. 4th ed. Philadelphia, W. B. Saunders Company, 1967.
267. Secor, J.: *Patient Care in Respiratory Problems*. Philadelphia, W. B. Saunders Company, 1969.
268. Secor, J.: The patient with emphysema. *American Journal of Nursing 65*:74, July, 1965.
269. Sedlock, S. A.: Detection of chronic pulmonary disease. *American Journal of Nursing 72*:1407, August, 1972.
270. Seedor, M. M.: *Therapy with Oxygen and Other Gases*. New York, Teachers College Press, 1966.
271. Segal, M. S., and Weiss, E. B.: Current concepts in the management of the patient with status asthmaticus. *Medical Clinics of North America 51*: 373, March, 1967.
272. Sentman, A. D.: An education program for the pulmonary handicapped. *Hospitals 41*:87, September 1, 1967.
273. Seremetis, M. G.: The management of spontaneous pneumothorax. *Chest 57*:65, January, 1970.
274. Sex difference in lung cancer survival rates. *Nursing Mirror 31*:26, January, 1968.
275. Shafer, K. N., et al.: *Medical-Surgical Nursing*. 5th ed. St. Louis, The C. V. Mosby Company, 1971.
276. Shaw, R. F., et al.: An assessment of the tuberculin tine test. *Diseases of the Chest 51*:162, February, 1967.
277. Sheffer, A. L., and Valentine, M. D.: The treatment of bronchial asthma. *Medical Clinics of North America 53*:239, March, 1969.
278. Shim, C., et al.: Cardiac arrhythmias resulting from tracheal suctioning. *Annals of Internal Medicine 71*:1149, December, 1969.
279. Shires, T.: Initial care of the injured patient. *The Journal of Trauma 10*:940, 1970.
280. Smith, D. W., Hanley Germain, C. P., and Gips, C. D.: *Care of the Adult Patient*. 3rd ed. Philadelphia, J. B. Lippincott Company, 1971.
281. Smoking. *American Review of Respiratory Diseases 96*:613, 1967.
282. Snider, G. L., and Soleh, S. S.: Empyema of the thorax in adults: Review of 105 cases. *Diseases of the Chest 54*:410, November, 1968.
283. Soffer, A.: The nursing profession and management of cigarette smoking problems. *Chest 60*:1, July, 1971.
284. South, J.: *Tuberculosis Handbook for Public Health Nurses*. 4th ed. National Tuberculosis Association, 1965.
285. South, J.: Impediments to TB eradication. *Nursing Outlook 15*:50, September, 1967.
286. South, J.: Public health nursing services in tuberculosis control programs. Part 1. *Nursing Outlook 15*:46, January, 1967; Tuberculosis clinic services. Part 2. *15*:66, February, 1967.
287. Spencer, R.: Helping your asthmatic patient to breathe. *RN 34*:36, April, 1971.
288. Stead, W. W.: Care of tuberculosis patients in the 1970's. After the sanatorium, then what? *Chest 60*:309, October, 1971.
289. Stead, W. W.: Tuberculosis and atypical mycobacterioses. *In* Conn, H. F. (ed.): *Current Therapy 1973*. Philadelphia, W. B. Saunders Company, 1973.
290. Stead, W. W., et al.: The clinical spectrum of primary tuberculosis in adults. *Annals of Internal Medicine 68*:731, April, 1968.
291. Steele, J. D.: The surgical treatment of pulmonary tuberculosis. *Annals of Thoracic Surgery 6*:484, November, 1968.
292. Stephen, C. R.: Guidelines for respiratory management. *AORN Journal 17*:97, March, 1973.
293. Stromberg, M. F.: Preparation for respiratory disease nursing. *Nursing Outlook 19*:741, November, 1971.
294. Sullivan, H. J.: Bronchogenic carcinoma: The true story. *Geriatrics 28*:140, March, 1973.
295. Sutton, A. L.: *Bedside Nursing Techniques*. 2nd ed. Philadelphia, W. B. Saunders Company, 1969.
296. Teixeira, J.: The present status of thoracic surgery in tuberculosis. *Diseases of the Chest 53*:19, January, 1968.
297. Thomas, A. N.: Respiratory care. *In* Sanderson, R. G.: *The Cardiac Patient*. Philadelphia, W. B. Saunders Company, 1972.
298. Thomas, P. A., Lynch, R. E., and Merrigan, E. H.: Incidence of contralateral pulmonary atelectasis after thoracotomy: An evaluation of preventive after care. *Diseases of the Chest 51*:288, March, 1967.
299. Thompson, L. F.: The hazards of immobility—Effects on respiratory function. *American Journal of Nursing 67*:783, April, 1967.
300. Tomashefski, J. F., and Pratt, P. C.: Pulmonary emphysema: Pathology and pathogenesis. *Medical Clinics of North America 51*:269, March, 1967.

301. Traver, G. A.: Assessment of thorax and lungs. *American Journal of Nursing 73*:466, March, 1973.
301a. Traver, G. A., (ed.): Symposium on care in respiratory disease. *Nursing Clinics of North America 9*:97–207, March, 1974.
302. Tuberculosis in the United States . . . An Overview. (Pamphlet.) Washington, D.C., U. S. Department of Health, Education, and Welfare. Public Health Service, 1969.
303. Turck, M.: Current therapy of bacterial pneumonias. *Medical Clinics of North America 51*:541, March, 1967.
304. Turner, H. G.: The anatomy and physiology of normal respiration. *Nursing Clinics of North America 3*:383, September, 1968.
305. Ujiki, G. T., and Shields, T. W.: Newer trends in the diagnosis and treatment of bronchogenic carcinoma. *Surgical Clinics of North America 51*: 183, February, 1971.
306. Ungvarski, P.: Mechanical stimulation of coughing. *American Journal of Nursing 71*:2358, December, 1971.
307. Urban, B. J., and Weitzner, S. W.: Avoidance of hypoxemia during endotracheal suction. *Anesthesiology 31*:473, November, 1969.
308. von Magnus, P., Engbaek, H. C., and Jespersen, A.: Tuberculosis and BCG. *Medical Clinics of North America 51*:753, May, 1967.
309. Waligara, B. M., Sr.: The effect of nasal and oral breathing upon naso-pharyngeal oxygen concentrations. *Nursing Research 19*:75, January-February, 1970.
310. Watson, J. E.: *Medical-Surgical Nursing and Related Physiology*. Philadelphia, W. B. Saunders Company, 1972.
311. Weg, J. G.: Treatment and Control of Tuberculosis. (Pamphlet.) New York, National Tuberculosis and Respiratory Disease Association, 1972.
312. Weg, J. G.: Tuberculosis and the generation gap. *American Journal of Nursing 71*:495, March, 1971.
313. Weiss, W., and Flippin, H. F.: Treatment of nonspecific primary lung abscess. *Archives of Internal Medicine 120*:8, July, 1967.
314. Wellon, H., et al.: Prognostic factors in malignant tumors of the lung. *The Annals of Thoracic Surgery 5*:228, March, 1968.
315. Whatley, J. L.: Battle for breath. *Today's Health 45*: 42, February, 1967.
316. Winter, P. M., and Lowenstein, E.: Acute respiratory failure. *Scientific American 221*:23, November, 1969.
317. Winterbauer, R. H., et al.: Recurrent pneumonia. *Annals of Internal Medicine 70*:689, April, 1969.
318. Wolf, J.: Management of the patient with inoperable bronchogenic carcinoma. *Medical Clinics of North America 51*:563, March, 1967.
319. Woolf, C. R., and Suero, J. T.: The respiratory effects of regular cigarette smoking in women. *American Review of Respiratory Disease 103*:26, January, 1971.
319a. Youngman, P. M. E.: Chest injuries. *Nursing Mirror 134*:30, April 21, 1972.
320. Zelch, J. V., et al.: Aspiration biopsy in diagnosis of pulmonary nodule. *Chest 63*:149, February, 1973.

UNIT XV

Nursing Patients Experiencing Disturbances of Digestive Function

Shirley Harlow

Unit Introduction and Study Guide

The writer of the book of Proverbs in the Bible said, "A dry crust eaten in peace is better than steak every day along with argument and strife."[57] This ancient bit of wisdom is still true today. One of the purposes of this unit is to make the student aware of the influence of the emotions on the functioning of the gastrointestinal tract.

A second purpose is to make the student cognizant of the types of disease entities that occur within the digestive system —abnormalities in structure, secretion and motility, tumors, infections, perforations, injuries, and vascular abnormalities— along with recognition of the effect that each of these may have.

A third purpose of this unit is to enable the student to understand the various tests and devices that are used in the diagnosis of disorders of the gastrointestinal tract and to know the nurse's responsibilities to the patient and to the physician prior to, during, and following these examinations.

The student should also know the various abnormalities in function that are created by the surgeon in his attempt to help the patient. The nurse not only must understand the alteration in function that has occurred and its effect upon the patient's physiology, but also must understand the effect it has upon the individual's life.

The fifth purpose of this unit is to familiarize the student with the common manifestations of abnormal function (symptoms) which occur in the gastrointestinal tract, their cause, and the rationale for the treatments used to correct them.

The following study guide is prepared to help you to achieve these objectives. Knowledge of these terms and procedures will help you to meet the objectives listed above.

1. Before you begin your reading ask yourself the following questions: What would I do if I had a severe stomach ache? What do I do when I am constipated or have diarrhea? What would I recommend to a friend who was complaining of abdominal pain, rectal bleeding, excessive gaseousness, vomiting, diarrhea, or other symptoms of malfunction of the gastrointestinal tract? What would I say to a friend who said he had a stomach ulcer?

2. Familiarize yourself with the following prefixes: entero-, gastro-, oro-, ano-, colo-, ileo-, endo-, herni-.

3. Familiarize yourself with the following suffixes: -otomy, ostomy, -orrhaphy, -itis, -oscopy.

4. Practice putting the prefixes in No. 2 with the suffixes in No. 3 to make words.

5. Familiarize yourself with these words: friable, diverticulum, polyp, herniation, prolapse, obstruction, perforation, peritoneum, gland, enzyme, hormone, digestion, absorption.

6. Following your reading try to answer the following questions:

a. What is hunger? What causes satiety?

b. What is the specific digestive function of each of the organs of the digestive system?

c. Consider the relationship of structure to function for each organ, including the protective mechanisms and physiologic processes taking place at each level.

d. What kinds of symptoms might be expected with disorders at various levels of the gastrointestinal system?

e. How do the various disorders of the gastrointestinal system affect the nutritional status of the individual?

f. How is the gastrointestinal system, and each of its component parts, controlled?

g. What are the common surgical procedures that are performed at each level of the tract? What problems does the patient face in adjusting to the changes in function created by each of these procedures?

h. What lay workers are very helpful, if not essential, in meeting the needs of the patient with an "ostomy"? Where would you find such a worker in your local community? Where would you refer a patient? Where can patients go in your local community to secure equipment to use with an "ostomy"?

i. What diagnostic tests are used for gastrointestinal disorders? What are the nursing responsibilities for each? What preparation does the patient need for each? What follow-up care?

j. What are the various dietary modifications that are ordered for patients with diseases of the gastrointestinal tract? What is the rationale for each? What are the modifications for a patient with an "ostomy"? Why?

k. What is an "acute abdomen"? What observations should a nurse make of this patient? Why?

l. When is hyperalimentation a useful treatment? What are the major nursing responsibilities in relation to this treatment?

CHAPTER 74

Review of the Anatomy and Physiology of the Digestive System

The digestive tract, sometimes also called the alimentary canal, is a hollow muscular tube that extends from the mouth to the anus and has as its principal function the provision of the body with fluids, nutrients, and electrolytes. It is lined with secreting cells and glands and has accessory organs, all of which contribute to this function of providing the body with the materials it needs to function. Normally the digestive tract is the only source of intake for the body. Raw materials, taken in through the mouth, after proper chemical conversions are used by the body in all its functions. See Figure 74–1 for the structural arrangement of the tract and the names of the parts. The portion of the tract from the stomach to the anus is the gastrointestinal tract, where the major digestive activity takes place, but this term is often loosely applied to indicate the entire digestive apparatus.

A secondary function of the tract is to dispose of the waste residues from this digestive process. Only wastes from this tract are eliminated from it, as wastes from body metabolism are excreted by other routes such as the lungs, kidneys, and skin.

ACTIVITIES OF THE TRACT

The activities of the tract are (1) the secretion of electrolytes and enzymes to be used in the breakdown of the materials ingested, and (2) the movement of ingested products through at the proper rate to ensure (3) complete digestion of the food and (4) absorption of the end products into the blood stream.

MOTILITY

There are two types of movements in the gastrointestinal tract: mixing and propulsive. These are produced by rhythmic contractions of the smooth muscle fibers which lie in the stomach and gut. These fibers vary somewhat from one segment to another because of their different functions, but they usually consist of an outer longitudinal layer, an inner circular layer and a thin layer in the deeper portion of the mucosa. The mixing movements, sometimes called segmentation contractions, consist of rhythmic contractions between individual segments alternating with contractions occurring at the mid-point of each segment. A propulsive movement, called *peristalsis,* consists of a wave of contraction which moves forward, forcing the contents of the tube ahead of it. This type of movement occurs in all smooth muscle tubes of the body and can go in either direction from the point of stimulation; however, in the bowel the waves usually move analward.

Distention of a local segment of the bowel is the usual stimulus for the initiation of a peristaltic wave, but one can also be stimulated by any irritation of the mucosa or by the presence of a specific chemical substance. Nervous stimulation occurs by means of the intramural nerve plexuses, which lie within the layers of the bowel wall beginning at the esophagus. These are known as the myenteric plexus (Auerbach's) in the outer layer and the submucosal plexus (Meissner's) in the inner layer. These nerves maintain the continuous tone of the bowel and also stimulate movements. The control is almost entirely through the vagus nerves. In general, stimulation of the parasympathetic fibers causes increased activity, while stimulation of the sympathetic fibers decreases activity.

SECRETIONS

There are two general types of secretions in the digestive tract: mucous secretions, which are produced from the mouth to the anus, and digestive secretions composed of enzymes and electrolytes, which are produced from the mouth to the end of the ileum. Mucus is produced to protect and to lubricate the walls of the tract and to ease the passage of food and partially digested products. Digestive juices are secreted to break down the various foods for absorption.

DIGESTION AND ABSORPTION

The digestive process is the breaking of food by digestive juices into compounds which are small enough in size and in the right chemical form for absorption. They are absorbed into the blood stream by diffusion and by active transport. Glandular secretions and fluids that are ingested are also absorbed from the small bowel.

CONTROLS ON INGESTION

Hunger is the body's expression of its need for nutrients. In animals and in small infants hunger controls ingestion, but humans also have an appetite which is learned and which is not necessarily related to the body's need for food and fluids. Frequently we eat because we enjoy the taste sensations we derive from eating rather than because our bodies have a hunger for that particular nutrient. Satiety is the feeling we have when our hunger and/or appetite has been satisfied.

THE MOUTH, PHARYNX, AND ESOPHAGUS

THE MOUTH

The first act of digestion is chewing. This occurs immediately upon entry of the food into the mouth and not only prepares the food for swallowing but meets a psychologic need. The teeth, tongue, walls of the cheeks, and palate all participate in this activity, which is controlled by reflex activity through the fifth cranial nerve and is stimulated by the presence of food in the mouth. The functions of chewing are to break the food products into smaller

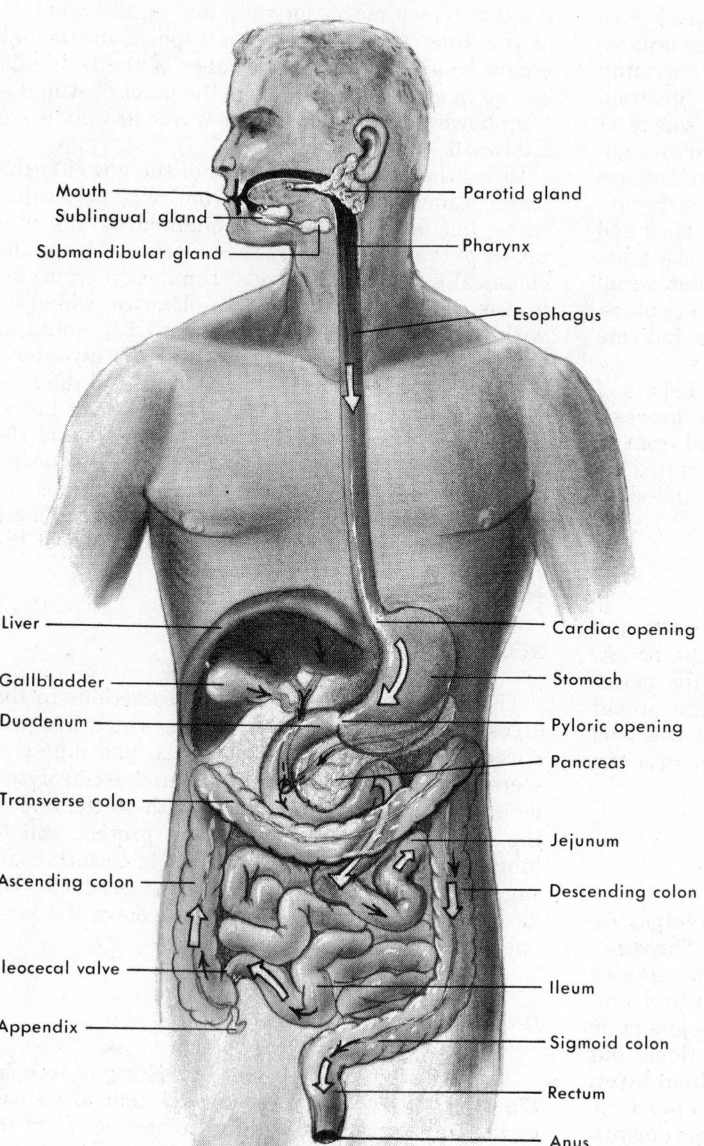

FIGURE 74–1. The digestive system. (From Jacob, S. W., and Francone, C. A.: *Structure and Function in Man.* 2nd ed. 1970.)

portions; to break down the fibrous coverings so as to provide access for the digestive enzymes to the food particles; and to prevent traumatizing the mucous membrane lining of the esophagus by making the food smoother.

Saliva acts to lubricate and to soften the food mass and to dissolve the readily soluble components of the food, thus stimulating the taste buds and increasing the enjoyment of the food. It contains the enzyme ptyalin (amylase), which acts to hydrolyze starches by splitting off maltase. If allowed to function long enough, amylase will break starches down to maltose.

Maintenance of dental health is important, since pressures ranging from 25 to 275 pounds are exerted during the chewing process, depending upon the nature of the food and the teeth involved. Artificial dentures are not so efficient in chewing as are natural teeth and can contribute to malnutrition, because poorly chewed foods are not so readily utilized in the digestive process.

SWALLOWING (DEGLUTITION)

After a mouthful of food, which is now called a bolus, has been sufficiently chewed, it is swallowed. The quantity in each bolus is approximately 5 ml. and consists of particles 2 mm. in size. The act of deglutition, which consists of three phases, is extremely complex. The first phase, called the voluntary, occurs when the food is pressed by the tongue against the palate, forcing it backward toward the pharynx. From this point on the process is involuntary. The second stage of swallowing, called the pharyngeal, begins with a wave of peristalsis, which was initiated by the voluntary act and causes a number of things to occur simultaneously. As the bolus is forced between the tonsillar pillars, the soft palate draws upward to close the posterior nares, respirations cease momentarily, the vocal cords approximate, and the larynx pulls upward, covering the vocal cords and stretching the opening of the esophagus. This causes the relaxation of the upper esophageal (hypopharyngeal) sphincter and begins the third stage, in which the peristaltic wave forces the bolus down the esophagus by the force of muscle contraction, by the momentum produced, and by the force of gravity. The time it takes for the bolus to reach the stomach depends upon its consistency and the individual's body position. Fluids tend to arrive ahead of the peristaltic wave, and the more solid masses may arrive after it. The bolus travels faster when the individual is in a vertical position.

THE ESOPHAGUS

Peristaltic waves in the esophagus are stimulated by primary and secondary means. Primarily the act of swallowing activates them reflexly through the glossopharyngeal nerves. Secondary stimulation of esophageal peristalsis occurs from dilatation of the lower half of the organ and is probably reflex in origin.

All glands in the esophagus are mucus secreting. The function of mucus is lubrication of the bolus to promote its passage and protection of the esophageal mucous membrane from trauma due to passage of partially chewed food products.

THE STOMACH

FUNCTIONS

The stomach is a muscular organ which has as its main function the storage, mixing, and liquefaction of the bolus of food into chyme, which it discharges slowly into the duodenum. The main digestive function of the stomach is the first stage of protein breakdown and the digestion of the connective tissues of meat to make these cells more accessible to the enzymes of the small bowel. Digestion of starches, which was begun in the mouth by the action of ptyalin, continues in the stomach in the center of the bolus and can continue for as long as 30 minutes or until the mixing function of the stomach allows the acid contents of the stomach to contact the ptyalin, inactivating it. Digestion of fats in the stomach is minimal and probably limited to butterfats. Other than alcohol, there is very little absorption in the stomach.

ACTIVITY

When the bolus arrives in the stomach, secretion of digestive juices has already begun in response to the stimulus of smelling, tasting, and chewing the food. This is known as the cephalic stage of digestion. The gastric stage of digestion is stimulated by the presence of food in the stomach and is regulated both by nervous stimulation via the parasympathetic fibers of the vagus nerve and hormonal stimulation through secretion of gastrin by the gastric mucosa. Gastrin is absorbed into the blood stream and then stimulates motility and secretion by the stomach.

The stomach empties slowly, accommodating itself to the ability of the duodenum to receive and act upon the materials. Tonic contraction of the musculature of the stomach causes the pressure within it to remain almost constant whether it is empty or full. This is accomplished by expansion and contraction of the fundus as the stomach fills and empties. Mixing of the chyme and emptying of the stomach occur by means of slow mild rhythmic peristaltic waves which begin about every 20 seconds at the fundus and continue over the antrum to the pylorus. These waves gain in strength as they progress, becoming very vigorous at the pylorus. A few milliliters of chyme are forced through the pylorus with each peristaltic wave and the remainder is propelled back into the stomach, further

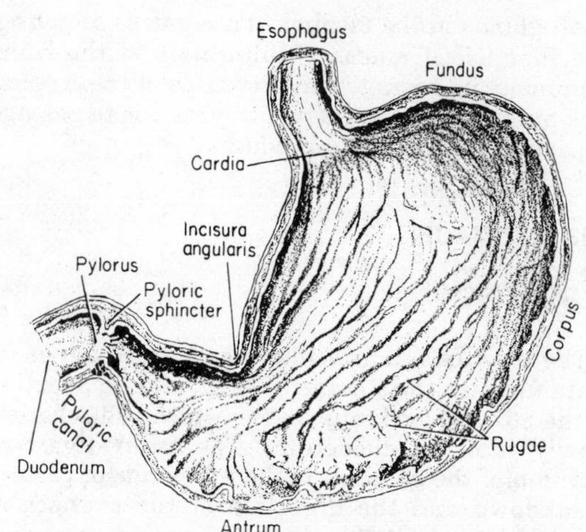

FIGURE 74–2. Physiologic anatomy of the stomach. (From Guyton, A. C.: *Textbook of Medical Physiology.* 4th ed. 1971.)

mixing the mass. The rugae of the walls of the stomach also contribute to the mixing by digging deeply into the chyme with each wave. As the stomach empties, the tone of the fundus maintains a constant internal pressure.

SECRETIONS

Gastric juices that contribute directly to the digestive process include mucus, hydrochloric acid (HCl), pepsin, small amounts of lipase, and the intrinsic factor. Pepsin is the most active factor in the digestive processes of the stomach, acting to break down proteins to polypeptides, proteoses, and peptones. The hydrochloric acid is essential to provide the acid medium that is necessary for the function of pepsin. (See Tables 74–1 and 74–2 for the names and actions of the various types of digestive secretions.)

RATE OF EMPTYING

Factors that influence the rate of emptying of the stomach include: the fluidity of the chyme, the amount in the stomach, and the receptivity of the small bowel. The enterogastric reflex and enterogastrone, the hormone secreted by the small bowel, both act to inhibit the emptying of the stomach. Practically any stimulation of the duodenum—distention, presence of acid, hypotonic or hypertonic substances, and the presence of any carbohydrate, fat, or protein product—will cause the enterogastric vagus reflex arc to slow gastric motility and secretions. Fat in contact with the duodenal mucosa causes release of enterogastrone, which is absorbed into the blood stream and causes inhibition of both secretions and motility of the stomach within a few minutes. The presence of carbohydrates in the small bowel also causes the release of enterogastrone, but to a lesser extent.

THE SMALL BOWEL

The small bowel is only about 10 feet long and 1 inch in diameter, but the secreting and absorbing surfaces are very large owing to the presence of circular folds involving the mucosa and a portion of the submucosa and fingerlike projections called villi (Fig. 74–3). The functions of the small bowel are to complete digestion of foodstuffs and to absorb the products of this digestion. The waste residues are moved on into the colon.

MOTILITY

Movements of the small bowel are mixing, or segmental, and peristaltic. The peristaltic waves are a continuation of the waves initiated in the stomach and propel the chyme along the gut. It normally moves forward at an average rate of about 1 cm. per minute and remains in the small bowel between 3 and 10 hours. Mixing movements of the small bowel consist of the alternate contraction of circular muscle fibers. These mixing movements, in addition to mixing the chyme, also bring it into closer contact with the glands and juices for better digestion and into closer contact with the villi for absorption.

A *peristaltic rush* is a powerful peristaltic wave which begins in the duodenum and passes to the ileocecal valve in a few minutes. Its purpose is to relieve the intestine of an irritating substance. It can be caused by any intense chemical or mechanical irritation or by extreme distention.

DIGESTIVE ACTIVITY

Digestive secretions of the small bowel are numerous and each has a specific function (Table 74–1). The small bowel also secretes two hormones which enter the blood stream and stimulate the pancreas to release its digestive secretions (Table 74–2). When the digestive functions are completed and the end products are ready for absorption, the following transformations have occurred:

Carbohydrates	changed to:	monosaccharides, disaccharides (few)
Proteins	changed to:	amino acids, dipeptides (minute quantity)
Fats	changed to:	fatty acids, monoglycerides, diglycerides, and triglycerides (few)

These products are absorbed along with water and electrolytes by diffusion and by active transport. Carbohydrates and proteins are absorbed by active transport along with sodium in a mutually depen-

TABLE 74–1. THE DIGESTIVE ENZYMES

Enzyme	Source	Action and Products
Ptyalin (amylase)	Parotid and submaxillary glands	Hydrolyzes starch to maltose
Pepsin	Chief cells of gastric mucosa	Breaks down dietary protein into proteoses, peptones, and polypeptides
Gastric lipase	Gastric mucosa	Digests butterfat
Enterokinase	Duodenal mucosa	Activates trypsin
Peptidases	Intestinal glands	Split polypeptides into amino acids
Sucrase, maltase, isomaltase, lactase	Intestinal glands	Split disaccharides into monosaccharides
Intestinal lipase	Intestinal glands	Splits fats into glycerol and fatty acids
Trypsin	Pancreas	Splits proteins to peptides and amino acids
Chymotrypsin	Pancreas	Splits proteins and polypeptides
Nucleases	Pancreas	Split nucleic acids
Carboxypeptidase	Pancreas	Splits polypeptides into smaller peptides
Pancreatic lipase	Pancreas	Hydrolyzes fat into glycerol and fatty acids
Pancreatic amylase	Pancreas	Splits starches into maltose and isomaltose

TABLE 74–2. THE GASTROINTESTINAL HORMONES

Hormone	Source	How Stimulated	Action
Gastrin	Mucosa of gastric antrum	Distention by food; action of certain food extractives (e.g., protein, alcohol); vagal stimulation	Stimulates secretion of HCl by parietal and chief cells of gastric glands
Enterogastrone	Intestinal mucosa	Fats, sugar, and acid in small intestine	Inhibits gastric secretion and motility
Secretin	Duodenal mucosa	Gastric contents entering duodenum	Stimulates secretion of pancreatic fluid
Pancreozymin	Duodenal mucosa	Products of protein digestion in duodenum	Stimulates secretion of enzyme-rich pancreatic juice
Cholecystokinin	Duodenal mucosa	Fat in duodenum	Contraction of gallbladder

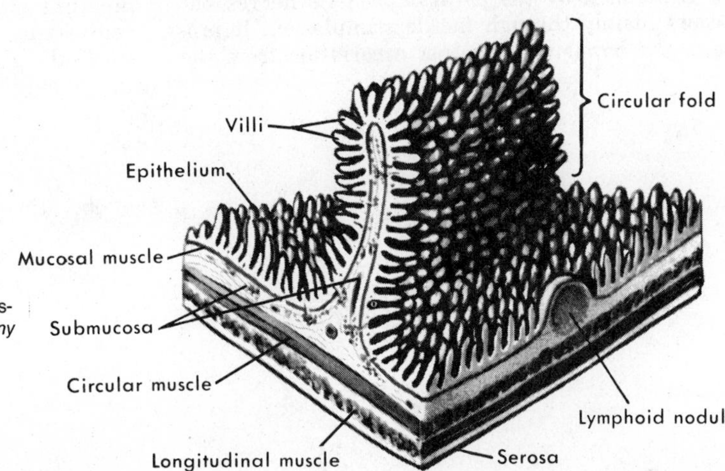

FIGURE 74–3. Section of wall of small intestine. (From Dienhart, C. M.: *Basic Human Anatomy and Physiology.* 2nd ed. 1972.)

dent relationship in which neither material is transported without the other. The active transport of carbohydrates and amino acids is called a secondary type of active transport. Fatty acids are absorbed by diffusion, whereas most of the electrolytes are absorbed actively. Water diffuses by osmosis as a result of these other transport systems.

Digestion and absorption from the small bowel is very efficient. The chyme obtained from the terminal ileum contains no digestible carbohydrates, very few lipids, and only 15 to 17 per cent nitrogen-containing substances, most of which are bacterial or desquamated epithelial cells and the remains of digestive secretions.[55]

THE COLON, RECTUM, AND ANUS

The major function of the colon is absorption of water and electrolytes in the proximal half and storage of the feces in the distal half until defecation occurs. Anatomically the colon is larger in diameter than the small bowel and does not contain villi. The only secretion is mucus, and the cells are columnar absorbing cells and goblet cells.

MOTILITY

The movements are, as in the small bowel, mixing and propulsive. The mixing movements, sometimes called haustral contractions, facilitate absorption by exposing all the fecal matter to the musosal surfaces. The propulsive movements or mass movements occur three or four times a day and are initiated by distention of the colon walls and by the gastrocolic or duodenocolic reflex. These reflexes are strongest after the first meal of the day.

SECRETION

The mucous secretion of the large intestine can be stimulated by the parasympathetic nerves but occurs mainly through tactile stimulation. It protects the bowel wall against excoriation from the fecal mass and from bacterial activity, and counteracts the effects of acid formation from this bacterial action. Mucus also provides adherent qualities for the feces.

ABSORPTION

Absorption of sodium, chloride, and water occurs in the large bowel and reduces the volume of chyme from 500 ml. in the cecum to 100 ml. of fluid in the feces. The colon is capable of absorbing 90 per cent of the sodium and water presented to it.

BACTERIAL ACTION

Bacterial action in the large bowel causes the formation of gases, which provide bulk and help to propel the feces. These organisms also synthesize some important nutritional factors such as vitamin K, thiamin, riboflavin, vitamin B_{12}, folic acid, biotin, and nicotinic acid.

DEFECATION

Feces are three fourths water and one fourth solid matter. The organic constituents include undigested food residues, digestive secretions and enzymes, dead cells, bile pigments, and mucus. Thirty per cent of the mass consists of bacteria and another 30 per cent is fat. The nature of the diet does not change the contents of the stool except for the amount of cellulose present.

The defecation reflex is stimulated by distention of the rectum. This occurs when feces and gas are propelled into the rectum from the descending colon during a mass peristaltic movement. This distention sets the defecation reflex in motion as the pressure within the rectum rises and the internal and external sphinctors are relaxed. The individual may voluntarily suppress this defecation urge by contracting the striated muscles of the pelvic floor and the external sphincter. This slows the motility of the bowel. If the individual elects to defecate when the reflex is set in motion, he augments pressure within the colon by increasing the intra-abdominal pressure. This is done by lowering the diaphragm and contracting the abdominal muscles. The diaphragm is lowered by contracting the chest muscles on an inflated lung while the glottis is closed.

CHAPTER 75

Disorders of the Gastrointestinal Tract: Diagnostic Tests and General Treatment Measures

The major function of the gastrointestinal tract is the digestion and absorption of nutrients needed by the body for proper functioning. To accomplish this the tract carries these nutrients along at a rate consistent with proper digestion and absorption. The mucous membrane lining, the glands which lie within it, and the accessory organs secrete digestive juices and enzymes which act chemically upon the foods and liquids to digest them. After this has taken place, the end products are absorbed into the blood stream and taken to the liver and other portions of the body for storage and use.

Abnormalities and disease conditions that occur in this tract manifest themselves through interference with one or more of these functions. These conditions may interrupt the continuity of the muscular or mucous layers, harm the tissues of the tract by damage to the blood or nerve supply, interfere with the flow of chyme through the tract, or hamper digestion of the material while it is in the gut. These abnormalities can be of mechanical, infectious, traumatic, neoplastic, vascular, nervous, or emotional origin.

COMMON CAUSES OF DYSFUNCTION OF THE GASTROINTESTINAL TRACT

OBSTRUCTION TO FLOW OF CHYME

Motility of the gut can be stopped, slowed, or increased by an abnormality of the nervous system regulatory mechanism, and it can be interrupted by interference with the blood supply to the gut. Nervous system abnormalities usually result from some general toxic or traumatic condition. Interruption of the central nervous system, as by transection of the spinal cord, does not interfere with peristalsis, since that is mainly regulated by the intramural plexuses (Auerbach's and Meissner's).

Blood supply is necessary to a viable tissue and is essential to the health of the organ. Any local interruption of blood supply is an emergency.

Tumors

Neoplasms may be either intra- or extraluminal. Since the chyme is liquid, a tumor must be relatively large to interfere with its flow through the tract. Total obstruction of gastrointestinal flow is a late symptom of tumor growth. Both benign and malignant tumors can cause such an interruption. Malignant tumors also cause other problems, since they invade the tissues and metastasize.

Loss of Structural Integrity

There are both developmental and acquired conditions that interfere with the structure of the bowel enough to impede flow through the tract. *Strictures* occur in the esophagus as a result of trauma, especially from drinking extremely hot foods or caustic substances. Strictures also occur in the lower tract, but here they are more often the result of healing of scars from ulcerations or surgical procedures. Bands of *adhesions* (scar tissue) from surgical operations sometimes cause constriction of the lumen when they encircle a loop of bowel. This is a common cause of bowel obstruction.

A *herniation* (protrusion through an abnormal opening) can occur in many portions of the tract. As the gut squeezes out through the internal or external opening, there is apt to be interference with the flow within it or with the blood supply to the herniated segment. The more common types of hernias are hiatus, inguinal, femoral, umbilical, and incisional. They are named by the location of the herniated portion.

The gastrointestinal tract has two structural deformities that occur within its wall; one is an outpouching, and the other an invagination. The outpouching, called a *diverticulum,* may involve all layers of the bowel wall but usually occurs through a weakness in the muscular layer. These occur more commonly as the individual ages, since the muscle fibers gradually lose their tone. A *polyp,* or inward growth, involves the inner mucosal layers of the bowel wall. These may be large or small, single or multiple. Polyps are particularly dangerous in the bowel, as they tend to become malignant. A large polyp can obstruct the lumen of the bowel by occupying space; it can also become twisted on its pedicle and strangulate.

Trauma

Any type of trauma may occur—from blunt blows, knife and stab wounds to gunshot perforations. Trauma is apt to cause bleeding or contusions and may open the bowel lumen. Since bowel secretions contain digestive enzymes, they are very irritating to the peritoneal cavity. The bowel also contains bacteria, so whenever the lumen of the bowel is opened to the peritoneal cavity, there is danger of infection. A physical insult, the presence of chemical or infectious agents, or their sequelae, are apt to cause cessation of bowel motility.

Infections

Bacteria are normally present in the lumen of the bowel, and since all food is potentially contaminated, foreign organisms can be ingested. Most of these organisms are destroyed in the highly acid medium of the stomach, but some may survive and, if pathogenic, cause disease. Worms of many kinds, amoeba, and other parasites are commonly acquired when tourists visit certain tropical countries.

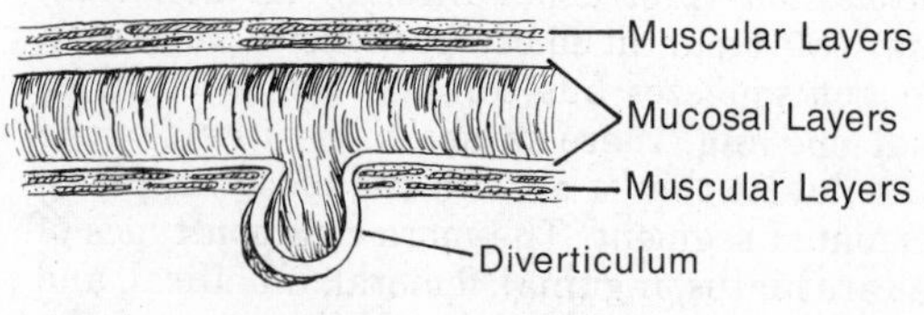

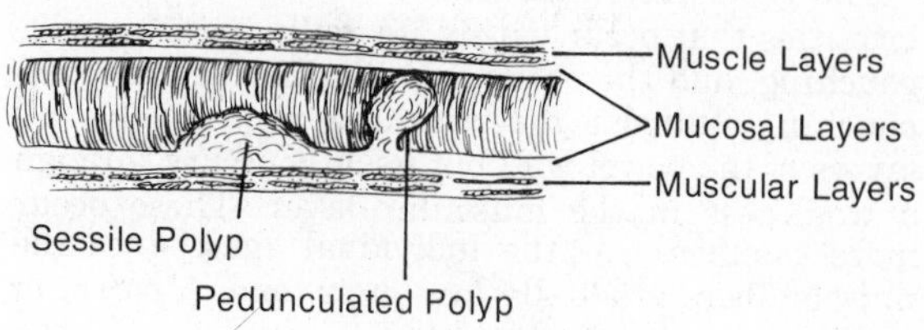

FIGURE 75–1. Diverticulum vs. polyp.

Toxins released from some bacteria, such as those which cause staphylococcal food poisoning, are very irritating to the lower tract. This type of condition usually causes diarrhea and vomiting in the body's effort to remove the offending substance. The major problem in these conditions is electrolyte balance, since digestive juices are not resorbed completely because of the increased rate of passage.

INTERFERENCE WITH DIGESTIVE FUNCTION

Mechanical

Whenever the forward progress of chyme through the bowel is stopped, a chain of events is set in motion. Peristalsis usually increases in intensity and rate in an effort to overcome the obstruction. Pressure within the lumen of the bowel increases as gases and fluids begin to accumulate. Increased pressure within the lumen of the bowel causes the secretory function of the small bowel to increase without an increase in the absorptive process; thus, the problem is rapidly compounded. The patient can go into shock as a result of these fluid shifts.

Secretory Dysfunction

Inadequate or excessive amounts of some of the digestive juices will cause interruption in the digestive function, especially if the pH level is altered, since the acidity of the environment must be within very narrow limits for most of these enzymes to function. Diagnosis of the cause of these problems can be quite difficult. Tests are made of the levels of various substances in various portions of the bowel and symptoms are considered.

An increase in the acidity of the stomach and duodenum is probably the main reason for the development of peptic ulcers. Excessive amounts of digestive juices can digest the mucosa because they overpower the normal protective mucous layer.

DIAGNOSTIC MEASURES

Since disease can occur any place in the gastrointestinal tract, diagnostic measures attempt to locate the level of the problem and identify the nature of the abnormality. The general methods of diagnosis are x-ray, endoscopy or viewing the inside through a lighted tube, analysis of the secretions from various parts of the tract, biopsies, cytologic studies, and radionuclide uptake tests.

X-RAYS

Since x-rays show shadows of the relative densities of the structures photographed, the inside of the gastrointestinal (GI) tract cannot be visualized unless a contrast medium is ingested or instilled into it. A flat plate (x-ray taken without contrast media) will show only general shadows, fluid levels, and gas. The usual terms given for x-ray studies of the gastrointentinal tract are: upper GI or barium meal, and lower GI or barium enema. The two together are known as a GI series.

Upper GI

In an upper GI study, the patient drinks barium sulfate, which is a white chalky, radiopaque substance. It is frequently flavored to increase its palatability. As the patient swallows the substance, the swallowing mechanism is studied by fluoroscope to detect the presence of abnormalities. Pictures are taken as the barium passes through the esophagus to show structural and/or functional problems. In the stomach the barium outlines the walls and shows the presence of ulcer craters and filling defects that could be caused by tumors. The emptying time of the stomach is observed. Barium is usually followed through the small bowel with x-rays to determine its rate of passage and to look for structural abnormalities.

Lower GI

The large colon is studied with barium given per rectum. Sufficient barium is given to distend the bowel and show any abnormality in structure or a space-occupying tumor mass. Follow-up pictures are taken after the patient eliminates the barium to determine the efficiency of emptying the colon.

Preparation of the Patient

Preparation of the patient for a gastrointestinal x-ray study includes explaining the procedure to him so he will understand what is happening and what the physician hopes to learn from the test. The upper GI or barium meal must be done on an empty stomach, so food and fluids are withheld for several hours. Since barium becomes solid when moisture is absorbed from it, a laxative is given following the test to empty the large bowel before a barium impaction can form. The normal diet is resumed after the x-ray study if there are no contraindications to it.

Enemas must be given before a lower GI study to empty the bowel of all feces. Any retained fecal matter will cause a filling defect to show on the x-ray and confuse the diagnosis. Since fecal matter is constantly entering the right colon from the cecum, the small bowel is emptied too, usually by means of a purgative such as castor oil, which is given the night before the test. Sometimes the patient is given only liquids the night before the test. Breakfast can usually be eaten the morning of the x-ray because the procedure will be completed before the food reaches the large bowel. Following the procedure, a cleansing enema is given if the follow-up x-ray shows retained barium.

ENDOSCOPY

Endoscopy is the visualization of the inside of a body cavity by means of a lighted tube. In the GI tract the esophagus, the stomach, and sometimes the duodenum are visualized by means of a tube inserted through the mouth, whereas the rectum, sigmoid colon, and recently even the transverse and right colon are visualized via a tube inserted through the anus. Flexible scopes that utilize glass fibers for their lens systems are used for these examinations. The scopes are equipped in various ways. Many are equipped with a camera to enable the physician to obtain color photographs which can be studied closely after the examination (Fig. 75–2). These scopes are increasing in versatility. In addition to being able to visualize the appearance of the mucosa and look directly for pathologic lesions, the physician can also obtain a biopsy specimen with some or do washings to secure specimens for cytologic examination.

Nursing Responsibilities

The physician frequently prefers to examine these cavities when they are empty. Because of this and because of the danger of aspiration, the patient who has a gastroscopy usually fasts several hours before the examination. Since enemas alter the appearance of the mucosa, some physicians do not want them given in preparation for examination of the bowel. Materials retained in these cavities can be aspirated during the examination to improve visibility. The rectosigmoid is empty immediately after defecation, so a suppository may be ordered prior to the examination to stimulate defecation. When the patient has a condition in which there is extreme irritation of the bowel with numerous bowel movements, no preparation is used.

Most patients find the intrusive entry of the gastrointestinal system by a lighted tube a traumatic experience. The musculature of the tract tends to react with spasms, causing the patient crampy pain; it is uncomfortable to swallow a tube and embarrassing to have the rectum entered. Thus, the patient who is undergoing these examinations needs understanding support from the nurse and clear explanations of what to expect and why the test is being performed.

The patient who has had a gastroscopy may have received a local anesthetic to the posterior pharynx to ease discomfort from the introduction of the tube; following the examination, he should receive no food or fluids until this has worn off. (See care of the patient after bronchoscopy, Unit XIV.) All endoscopy patients should be given an opportunity to rest following the examination and should be observed for bleeding and swelling or dysfunction of the involved area. Cramping of the bowel may occur briefly following these examinations.

ANALYSIS OF SECRETIONS

Analysis can be made of the contents of the gastrointestinal tract for the presence or absence of digestive juices, bacteria, or parasites. Secretions can be secured at the time of endoscopy examination or, as is more common, by the insertion of a tube into the stomach or small bowel. Stool specimens and rectal aspirations are also used.

Gastric Analysis

The contents of the fasting stomach are aspirated and analyzed for free and total acid. If none is found, some means of stimulating the stomach may be used such as a meal of crackers or bread (Ewald meal), ingestion of alcohol or caffeine, or the injection of histamine. Aspirations are made through a stomach tube at intervals after the injection of the stimulus. Gastric acidity is typically high in the presence of duodenal ulcers and low when the patient has pernicious anemia (see Table 75–1).

Insulin is given to test the stomach's response to vagal stimulation in the Hollander test. Insulin given intravenously causes a drop in blood sugar which stimulates the vagus nerve. Blood sugar determinations and aspirations of the gastric secretions are done. In a normal stomach a drop in blood sugar does not cause a significant rise in gastric acidity. This test is frequently done after vagotomy to see if the surgical procedure was successful in reducing the vagal stimulation of gastric acidity.

The tubeless gastric analysis is done by having the patient ingest Diagnex Blue or azuresin (the dye azure A in an exchange resin). Acid in the stomach displaces the dye from the exchange resin. The dye thus released is then absorbed by the bowel mucosa and excreted in the urine. The amount of dye excreted indicates the amount of acid available. The test is done on an empty stomach and consists of having the patient empty his bladder, giving him an agent that stimulates gastric acid and the dye. At the end of the test, the bladder is emptied again and the urine tested for the dye. The total quantity of dye excreted in this time period is analyzed and an estimation made of the amount of acid in the stomach.

Tubercle bacilli may be present in the stomach of a person with active pulmonary tuberculosis because mucous secretions from the lungs are normally carried by ciliary action to the pharynx where they are propelled to the stomach. Therefore, gastric washings are sometimes taken of patients who do not raise sputum and in whom a diagnosis of pulmonary tuberculosis is difficult to obtain. Gastric washings are taken the first thing in the morning and analyzed for the presence of acid-fast bacilli.

Analysis of Stools

Stool cultures are taken in the presence of diarrhea or dysentery. Various parasites ranging from the microscopic protozoa and amebae to fairly large organisms such as worms are possible causes. Stool cultures are also done for bacteria and viruses.

The specimen must be sent to the laboratory for examination while it is still warm. Stools for chemical analysis are usually examined for the total quantity expelled, so the complete stool is sent to the

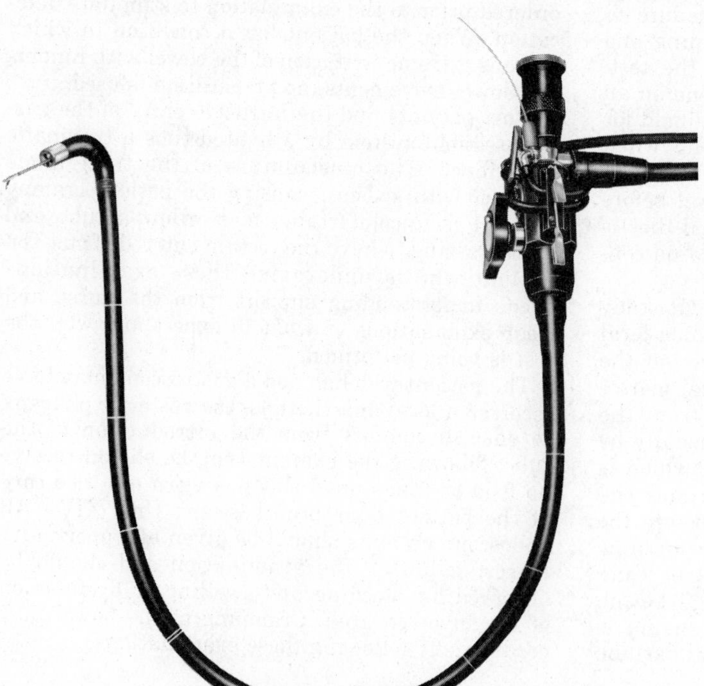

FIGURE 75–2. Fiberscope for gastric examination. (Courtesy of American Cystoscope Makers, Inc.)

TABLE 75–1. GASTRIC ACID LEVELS*

	Hydrochloric Acid Secretion (Average Values)		
	Basal (mEq/hr.)	*Maximal Histamine (mEq/hr.)*	*Nocturnal (mEq/12 hr.)*
Normal	2	20	18
Gastric ulcer	4	20	8
Duodenal ulcer	8	35	60

*Adapted from Beeson, P. B., and McDermott, W.: *Cecil-Loeb Textbook of Medicine.* 13th ed. 1971.

laboratory rather than a small sample from it. Analysis for fat content is frequently made, as well as for some of the other dietary products and digestive secretions. An unusually high content of fat in the stool could mean inadequate absorption from the small bowel.

Blood is another factor commonly sought in the stool. This examination is done on a very small sample and is frequently performed by the guaiac test. The patient is sometimes on a meat free diet for three days before these specimens are collected because of potential false positive results as a result of meat ingestion.

Examination of Small Bowel Secretions

Samples of secretions from the small bowel are sometimes analyzed for digestive enzymes and for bile.

Biopsy and Cytology

Specimens for cellular examination are secured during endoscopy examinations by means of biopsy forceps or by taking scrapings of cells. In addition, by means of special apparatus attached to rubber or plastic nasogastric tubes, gastric and small bowel biopsies may be secured and washings done for cytologic studies. A nasogastric tube is passed into the segment of interest and, when the location of the tube has been checked by x-ray, the apparatus is operated to secure the specimen and the tube is withdrawn.

RADIONUCLIDE UPTAKE

The uptake of substances such as vitamin B_{12} (Schiller test) and fat is sometimes studied by tagging the substances with a radioactive isotope (radionuclide) to assess the degree of absorption of these factors.

BLOOD EXAMINATIONS

Analysis of the blood through hematologic studies and electrolyte determinations gives information concerning the general status of the patient.

NURSING RESPONSIBILITIES FOR SPECIMEN COLLECTION

The nurse must know what specimen is to be collected and in what manner. She must know whether the whole specimen or only part of it is to be sent to the laboratory and whether it must be sent immediately (as a warm stool) or if it should be kept in the refrigerator. She should know the purpose for any specimen sent to the laboratory and collect it accordingly. She should also make sure that the patient understands what is being collected, how, when, and why so he can cooperate with the test. The nursing assistants must also understand how the specimen is to be collected and when. A specimen that is inadvertently discarded or improperly collected sometimes makes it necessary for the patient to undergo the entire test a second time.

TREATMENT MEASURES

DECOMPRESSION

Decompression is the removal of fluid and air from the gastrointestinal tract via a nasogastric tube attached to suction. Since any obstruction to the flow of chyme through the bowel causes many problems in homeostasis, patients with potential problems are frequently intubated, as well as those who have already developed symptoms of obstruction. Decompression may be used preoperatively and is almost universally used in the postoperative patient who has had surgery on the gastrointestinal tract.

Purpose

The purpose of decompression is to relieve the pressure caused by intestinal contents and gases that remain in the bowel because of some obstruction; it can also be used in diagnosis. Postoperatively it is used to remove secretions that cannot pass because of swelling and edema in the area of surgery.

Types of Tubes

There are two types of tubes used to achieve decompression. Short tubes are used for the stomach and duodenum and long tubes for the remainder of the tract. Short tubes are the Levin and the Rehfuss, both rubber, and the newer plastic nasogastric tubes. These tubes are long enough to extend into the stomach but not into the bowel. The Rehfuss tube is sometimes threaded just through the pylorus to aspirate duodenal contents.

The long tubes are intended to extend the length or a portion of the length of the small bowel, so are between 6 and 10 ft long. The more common ones are the Miller-Abbott, Cantor, and Harris. These tubes all have one thing in common, namely, some means of attaching a heavy substance, usually mercury, to allow peristalsis of the bowel to propel the tube through the tract. (See Table 75–2 and Figure 75–3 for details concerning these tubes.) The tube is threaded from the nose into the stomach and then through the pylorus, where peristaltic activity of the bowel carries it to the desired area.

Sometimes it is quite difficult to get the tube to pass through the pylorus. The patient is instructed to lie on his right side. The physician frequently guides the tube through the pylorus under fluoroscopic visualization. Once the tube has passed into the duodenum, it is advanced an additional 2 to 4 inches every hour or half hour (as ordered by the physician) to give it slack so peristalsis can carry it along. When it has reached the desired location, it is taped securely into place to prevent further advancement.

Suction

Only low pressure suction is used because excessive negative pressure within the stomach or bowel might cause the mucosa to be sucked into the openings on the tube, impairing the effectiveness of the suction. Intermittent electrical suction is commonly used. Since mucus tends to plug the openings of these tubes, it is often necessary to irrigate them to maintain or check their patency. The plastic Salem sump has a second lumen which is open to air, preventing the development of excess negative pressure because the extra lumen brings air into the cavity continuously. This tube will not function effectively if attached to intermittent suction because the second lumen must be kept free of secretions by constantly aspirating air.

Insertion of Tubes

Nasogastric tubes are inserted through the nose or mouth into the stomach. The procedure of inserting these tubes is frequently very frightening to the patient. The nurse must be understanding, gentle, and helpful to the patient by her explanations and manner. The explanation of what will be done should be adapted to the patient's need. Some wish to know all the details, whereas some prefer only brief instructions, as too much information increases their anxiety.

The tube is gently inserted through the nares into the posterior nasal pharynx and allowed to bend downward into the oral pharynx. It is well to have the patient swallow once the tube has rounded this curve because the sphincter at the proximal end of the esophagus remains closed except during swallowing to prevent the introduction of air into the stomach during respiration. During swallowing the larynx rises, stretching the cricopharyngeus muscle and causing it to relax. Resistance might be felt at this sphincter when the tube is first inserted, but the sphincter will relax as the patient swallows. Swallowing also encourages the tube to enter the esophagus rather than the trachea. Swallowing water, if it is allowed, lubricates the tube, making it easier to pass. After passing the sphincter, the tube is advanced fairly rapidly until it is in the stomach. Its presence in the stomach can be verified by several means: by aspiration of gastric contents, by listening with a stethoscope to hear air pass into the stomach as it is rapidly instilled into the tube with a syringe, or by holding the end of the tube under water to see if air comes out (as it will if the tube is in the lungs).

Nursing Management of the Patient with Nasogastric Tube in Place

Maintaining his comfort while the tube is in place is of utmost importance to the patient. The

TABLE 75–2. GASTRIC AND INTESTINAL TUBES

	Length	Size (French)	Lumen	Other Characteristics
Short Tubes				
Levin type	50″	12, 16, 18	Single	
plastic				
rubber				
Rehfuss		12, 14	Single	Metal tip
Salem sump	48″	12, 14, 16, 18	Double	Sump type suction
	36″	10		
Long Tubes				
Cantor	10′	16	Single	Mercury-weighted
Harris	6′	14, 16	Single	Mercury-weighted
Miller-Abbott	10′ 6″	12, 14, 16, 18	Double	Mercury-weighted

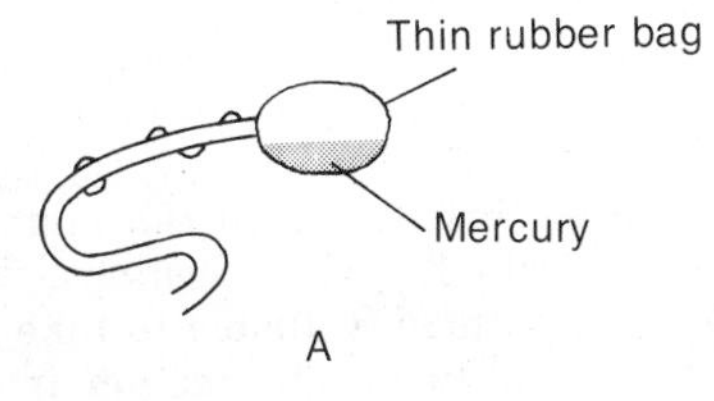

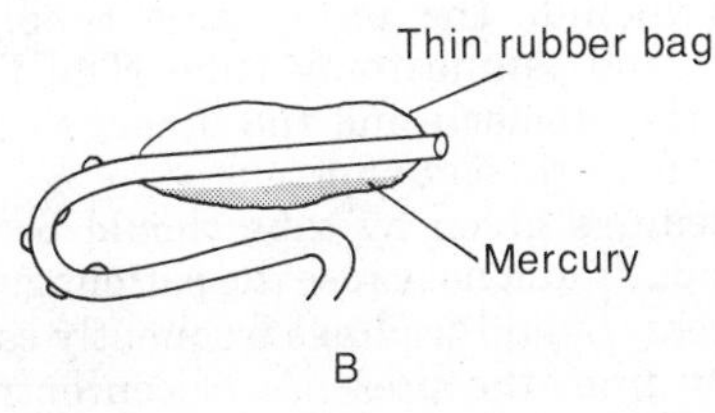

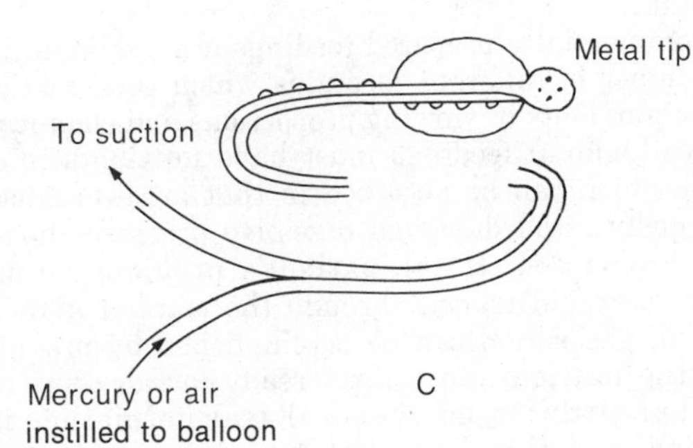

FIGURE 75-3. Three types of long intestinal decompression tubes. *A,* The Cantor tube. Mercury is instilled before insertion of tube. Suction is done along the sides. *B,* The Harris tube. Mercury is instilled before insertion. Suction is at the end and sides. *C,* The Miller-Abbott tube. Mercury instilled after insertion. Suction is at end and side.

external nares may become sore from crusted secretions around the tube or from pressure. The tube should be gently cleansed to remove crystals which form from dried mucus. Water-soluble lubricants can be used on the tube and the external nares. The tube should be taped in such a manner as to prevent pressure. The patient's mouth is usually dry because of the absence of chewing, which is the normal stimulus to salivary secretions, and because of mouth breathing, which results from the presence of the tube. Frequent oral hygiene will increase the patient's comfort by removing debris and stimulating salivation. The teeth should be brushed even though the patient is not eating because bacterial action continues in the mouth and gingival stimulation is still needed. Sometimes the patient is allowed to chew gum or suck on sour candies or ice chips to aid in stimulating salivation.

Patients frequently complain of a sore throat from the presence of the tube. Anesthetic lozenges or gargles may be ordered for this. Sometimes the patient needs only the reassurance that this is a common feeling from the presence of the tube.

The material aspirated via the tube should be observed frequently for color, odor, and quantity, and any changes should be reported to the physician. Contents of the suction bottles must be measured to maintain an accurate count of fluid intake and output. It is important to record what area of the digestive tract the measured contents came from, because the electrolyte content of the small bowel is entirely different from that of the stomach. Sometimes samples of these secretions are sent to the laboratory for analysis. After the volume of the total specimen has been measured and thoroughly mixed, a small portion is sent for analysis.

It must be remembered that any irrigating solution that is instilled into this tube is counted as intake for the patient. An accurate record must be kept of how much is instilled and how much aspirated from the tube during irrigations. Solution that does not return during an irrigation will be returned in the suctioned fluids later so must be included as intake. Normal saline is frequently the irrigating solution of choice because water, a hypotonic solution, can increase the loss of electrolytes through osmotic action if too much of it is instilled. If the tube is irrigated often, this can be a significant factor.

SURGICAL INTERVENTION

Surgical intervention is intended to restore the ability of the gut to propel the digestive materials through. Thus, many procedures involve repairing a structural abnormality, for example, reducing a herniation, releasing adhesions, or patching a perforation. Removal of a neoplastic growth or other pathologic condition such as an ulcer or polyp is also common. The removal of lesions frequently involves making changes in the route by which the chyme flows. Sometimes large segments are bypassed or a short circuit is created as segments are removed. After resections are done, the lumina of the various portions are sutured together by side-to-side, side-to-end, or end-to-end anastomoses.

In some instances it is necessary to divert the fecal stream to the surface of the abdomen, either to temporarily rest the portion distal to it or because the diseased portion extends to the anus and it is not possible or desirable to make an anastomosis there. In these instances a colostomy (opening of the colon onto the abdomen) or an ileostomy (opening of the ileum to the surface of the abdomen) is done. (See sections on colostomy and ileostomy below.)

Cecostomy

Following surgical procedures on the large bowel, there is swelling and impaired function for a few days. During this time the vast quantities of digestive juices (7 to 10 liters) continue to be secreted and, if they are not diverted, the patient may become very distended. A nasogastric tube is sometimes inserted into the stomach, but since most of this fluid is secreted in the small bowel, a tube is frequently inserted surgically into the cecum (cecostomy) to decompress this portion of the bowel. The tube is attached to a drainage bottle and drained by gravity. Irrigations are usually necessary, as this tube tends to become plugged with fecal material.

GENERAL NURSING PROBLEMS

Nursing care of patients with disease of the gastrointestinal tract is aimed at keeping the intestinal contents flowing freely through the gut, keeping tubes open, and maintaining the patient's electrolyte and nutritional balance. Since nutrition, eating, and elimination have deep emotional implications for many people, malfunction in these areas can cause deep distress to the patient. Cancer is a frequent diagnosis, and this disease in itself causes great emotional distress. Patients need support and understanding from the nurse, who must remember that people frequently express their concerns indirectly by their behavior rather than by words.

Eating is a social activity and when a person is unable to do this normally or his diet is severely restricted, some other means of meeting this need is necessary. The nurse can help by letting the patient express his frustration and feelings about restrictions and by making sure he understands his condition and the reasons for the restrictions.

Elimination is viewed as a very important function by many people, and many feel that a bowel movement every day is essential to good health. For this reason patients tend to become quite upset when they have a disturbance of elimination. Patients who do not understand what normal elimination is and how it is achieved need even more instruction to understand the alterations that occur.

Many people feel that elimination is a shameful subject and are embarrassed to be in the hospital for such a problem. The nurse can help these people by her manner of acceptance of their condition and by making sure they understand what is happening to them. She should avoid doing or saying anything in front of a visitor that might embarrass the patient.

Some special procedures for feeding patients and providing for their elimination processes when disease has interfered with normal functioning will be discussed next.

Gavage

Feedings instilled into the stomach through a tube are called gavage feedings. They are given when the patient is unable to take foods normally owing either to an obstruction in the esophagus or to the inability to swallow. They are sometimes used temporarily after esophageal surgery. Tubes used include the nasogastric tube, gastrostomy tube, and jejunostomy tube. The first two lead into the stomach and the other, as the name implies, is in the jejunum.

Feedings given by tube should be balanced nutritionally and not cause the patient gastrointestinal distress. Liquid feedings frequently cause diarrhea, either from the presence of concentrated ingredients or from improper storage, which allows organisms to grow or toxins to form. Liquid feedings can also cause constipation because of their lack of bulk.

Commercially prepared feedings are available in a number of different formulas which contain the basic nutrients in varying proportions and chemical states. Jejunal feedings must have nutrients in a form which can be absorbed in that area, because the gastric and duodenal digestive processes have been bypassed. If the patient's problems stem from too rapid transit through the tract, a higher rate of absorption can be accomplished by providing the nutrients in a form ready for absorption, so that little or no chemical transformation is needed, and the short time the chyme is in the small bowel is used to better advantage.

For convenience to the patient and also for ease of preparation, the regular diet of the hospital or the family at home can be liquefied in a blender, diluted to proper consistency, and given by tube. This is done only when the patient does not have special dietary needs. When chewing is important to the patient's mental state or when his digestion needs the stimulation, he may want to chew the food and spit it out. It can then be placed in the feeding or discarded.

Several methods are used to administer tube feedings. They can run through a syringe or funnel which is attached to the tube or by drip from a bottle or bag (Murphy drip). Feedings can also be pumped through the tube at a set rate. Pumps are frequently used when the feeding is given continuously during the day and night.

For the patient in the home, feedings given at intervals through an Asepto syringe are common. When feedings are given in this way they should be allowed to run in by gravity and the bulb or plunger used only to start the flow when necessary; discomfort and nausea from too rapid filling result. The feeding should be at, or slightly below, body temperature. Heat will coagulate a feeding made from milk and eggs, and hot liquids could burn or irritate the gastric mucosa. Cold starts unfavorable gastric reactions by causing vasoconstriction, which reduces the flow of gastric digestive juices.

The patient should receive 2500 to 3000 ml. of fluid through the tube daily. Water is given prior to the feeding to make certain the tube is patent and to help to start the flow of the feeding solution. Following the feeding, the tube is cleansed by instilling from 50 to 100 ml. of water. Air can be prevented from entering the tube during the feeding by keeping the syringe full and by pinching the tube while more fluid is added. Fluids can be instilled between meals as indicated.

Most patients are sensitive about taking food in this manner and would prefer privacy while receiving feedings. Other patients in a ward usually do not like to watch this type of feeding while they eat their own food. Some patients enjoy joining others at the family dinner table to participate in the social exchanges even though they cannot eat. Others cannot tolerate watching other people eat normally. Thus, arrangements as to timing and location for eating and tube feedings, both in the hospital and in the home, should be made to the satisfaction of everyone involved.

TOTAL PARENTERAL ALIMENTATION (HYPERALIMENTATION)

Many patients with disorders of the gastrointestinal system are unable to ingest or digest sufficient nutrients to maintain themselves in a state of positive nitrogen balance or anabolism. These patients include those who have debilitating diseases such as malabsorption of the bowel, inflammatory diseases of the bowel or who for some reason are unable to eat adequate amounts, infants with major congenital abnormalities in the digestive tract, and patients who have excessive metabolic needs because they are losing vast quantities of protein-laden body fluids daily as a result of extensive burns or draining wounds. These patients are all candidates for total parenteral alimentation or hyperalimentation, which is the intravenous administration of hypertonic solutions of glucose plus nitrogen (amino acids and polypeptides) and other nutrients sufficient to achieve tissue synthesis and anabolism in patients with normal or excessive nutritional needs.

Until recently this has not been practically feasible because the amount of nutrients needed to achieve anabolism, dissolved in the volume of fluid that the body can tolerate daily, produces a solution which is so hypertonic it causes phlebitis, clotting, and local swelling of the blood vessel used for the infusion. For instance, intravenous fluids of 2500 ml. per day of 5 per cent glucose supply about 500 calories and no amino acids; this same volume of 10 per cent glucose would supply only 1000 calories, which is still below the basal caloric requirements of the resting adult and would contain no protein. A solution containing sufficient calories and protein, when diluted enough for toleration by the body, would be from 12 to 15 liters.

This problem has been circumvented two ways. The most common is by the insertion of a catheter into the superior vena cava via the right or left subclavian vein (Fig. 75–4). The hypertonic solution is rapidly diluted by the large amount of blood flowing through this vein. The other ap-

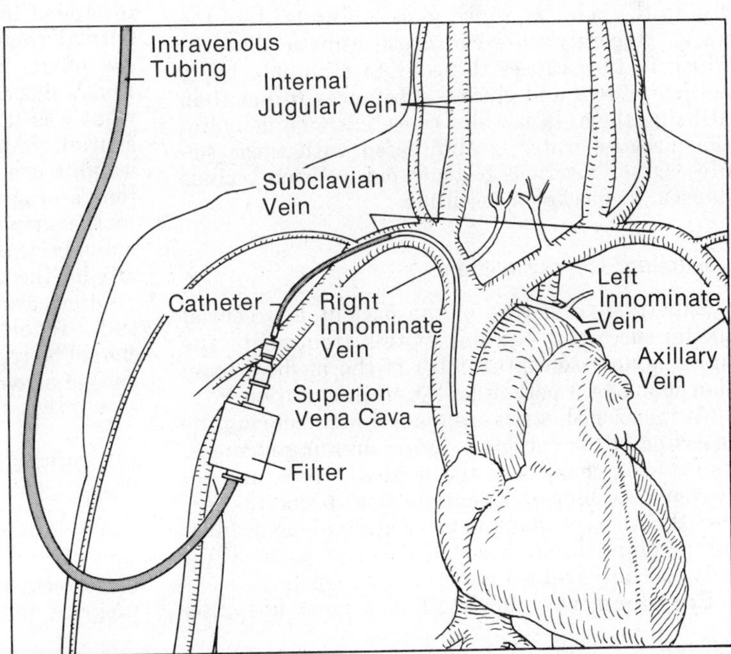

FIGURE 75–4. Insertion of catheter into superior vena cava via right subclavian vein.

proach is to make an external arteriovenous fistula, as is done in renal dialysis. (See Unit XI.) The solution is infused into the plastic fistulous tract and is mixed and diluted there before it comes into contact with the patient's vein. Both methods have proved successful in large numbers of patients.

Complications

Infection is the major complication from this therapy. This can occur through the entry site of the catheter or by seeding of the indwelling catheter from blood-borne bacteria or from the solution that is infused. Rigid aseptic technique must be used during insertion, changing, and care of the catheter and its tubing and in the preparation of the solution (see below). In order to minimize the possibility of infection occurring from the solutions, they are mixed under rigid aseptic control in a closed location to minimize contact with airborne particles. Mixing under a laminar flow, filtered air hood is recommended if one is available. Because concentrated glucose solutions are an excellent media for bacterial growth, no more than a 24-hour supply should be prepared in advance. A filter is commonly used in the intravenous tubing to trap bacteria and particles.

Among the complications that can occur during the insertion of the catheter are those from accidental perforation of the pleura, injury to the brachial plexus or the artery, and an air embolism. Other problems are from the infusion of a hyperosmolar solution of high glucose content. When the solution is instilled too rapidly, blood sugar levels rise to the point at which glucose "spills" into the urine. Hyperglycemia can cause osmotic diuresis, which in turn causes the body to eliminate badly needed protein and glucose substances rather than utilizing them. It can also cause extreme dehydration because water is eliminated with these solutes. Other reactions to too rapid infusion include nausea, headache, or lassitude.

Nursing Responsibilities

Expert nursing care of the patient is essential to the successful outcome of this treatment. The nurse is an essential member of the medical team that manages a patient on hyperalimentation.[21]

As mentioned, strict aseptic technique during the insertion of the catheter, during dressing changes, and during changes in the bottles, filters, and intravenous tubing is essential. Most hospitals that use the therapy have developed rigid procedures for accomplishing these duties, and some allow only specially trained nurses to do them.

Procedures vary in detail, but most hospitals change the tubing and filters routinely every 24 to 48 hours and the dressings around the catheter insertion site every 2 to 3 days. The skin is cleansed with a substance such as acetone or ether to remove oils, since they harbor bacteria; this also breaks down the cellular walls of the bacteria. The skin is then cleansed with an antiseptic solution such as iodine and an antibiotic ointment is applied to the insertion site. After cleansing and application of a sterile dressing, tape is used to form an occlusive dressing that will be impervious to air and small amounts of moisture. A mask should be worn by all those near the wound to prevent the introduction of organisms from the nasal pharynx.[9]

Since too rapid a flow of the solution will cause hyperglycemia and too slow a flow will fail to instill the needed nutrients, it is vital that close attention be given to regulation. It is important that the flow rate not be increased in speed even though it is behind schedule. Many institutions use a pump to regulate the flow and to eliminate the changes in rate of flow that occur with alterations in the patient's activity and position.

It is essential that no air enter the system. This can easily occur when the catheter is in the vena cava since changes in thoracic volume, as from taking a deep breath, cause changes in the pressure within this vein. If this occurs while the catheter is open during a tubing change or during insertion, air could be sucked into the system, causing an air embolus that might be fatal. This possibility is avoided by having the patient in slight Trendelenburg (head down) position when the tube is being manipulated or by having the patient perform the Valsalva maneuver of increasing intrathoracic pressure by bearing down during the brief periods during which the tube is open.

Nursing observations are concerned with the patient's electrolyte balance, the presence of infection, untoward reactions to the hyperosmolar infusion, weight gain, and tissue repair. Accurate records of intake and output, including all the abnormal routes that are employed, are absolutely essential. The physician will monitor the patient's blood electrolytes, but an accurate count of what was taken and what was excreted is still essential. Blood pressure measurements and daily weights are frequently ordered to monitor the patient's progress. The presence or absence of sugar in the urine is usually tested every six hours to make certain the infusion is not running too rapidly for the body to metabolize the glucose.

Other observations of nausea, vomiting, lassitude, fever, and any other abnormal response should be reported, as they might indicate the presence of a complication.

COLOSTOMY

A colostomy, which is the opening of some portion of the colon onto the abdominal surface, is performed when it is impossible for the feces to progress through the colon and out the anus because of some pathologic condition. Temporary colostomies are done to divert the fecal flow away from an area of inflammation or around an operative area. A permanent colostomy is created as a means of elimination when the rectum or anus becomes nonfunctional as a result of disease or a traumatic condition.

When only one loop of bowel is open on the abdominal surface, the patient has a single-barreled colostomy because there is only one stoma. A double-barreled colostomy is one in which both loops, the distal and proximal, are open on the abdominal wall (Fig. 75–5). A single-barreled colostomy is permanent if the bowel distal to it has been resected, while a double-barreled colostomy may be permanent or it may be closed at a later time, depending upon the disease present. A temporary colostomy is done most commonly at the midpoint of the left colon or the transverse colon, whereas a permanent colostomy is usually close to the end of the descending colon. Since the function of the large bowel is absorption, the stools are more formed and the colostomy is easier to manage when it is nearer the terminal (left) colon than in the transverse or right colon.

Management

The immediate postoperative care is the same as for any abdominal surgery patient, with the addition of watching for spillage through the colostomy if it is open. Fecal contents are highly contaminated with bacteria, so care should be taken to keep these secretions away from the surgical incision. When creating a temporary colostomy, the surgeon usually brings a loop of bowel out through a wound which is separate from the surgical incision and keeps it from slipping back by placing a glass rod beneath it (Fig. 75–6). Two or three days postoperatively the bowel will be opened, usually with a cautery. Since there are no sensory nerve endings in the bowel wall, this procedure is painless to the patient, except for some cramping pain, which may occur if the trauma stimulates contractions.

The surgeon will usually indicate which loop is the proximal and which the distal. This is not always immediately obvious until feces begin to flow, since the loop is sometimes reversed as it is brought through the abdominal wall.

Emotional Response by Patient

The patient who has a colostomy usually has some difficulty adjusting to it. Feces are associated in most people's minds with "dirt" and shame, and bowel movements become a private function quite early in life. Depending upon the individuals's attitude toward his own excretory functions, his knowledge about colostomies prior to his surgery and his ability to adjust to stressful situations, the patient's reactions may range from apparently easy acceptance to a total withdrawal from social contacts. Some individuals refuse to look at the stoma and have a great deal of difficulty accepting its presence, while others take it in stride and immediately begin to help care for it.

The nurse must make a careful assessment of the patient and his mental acceptance before attempting to teach him. Discussion with the family to find out the patient's general reactions to life's stresses will give much needed information. The type of relationship between a husband and wife is important to understand also. Which partner is the dominant figure? which the dependent one?

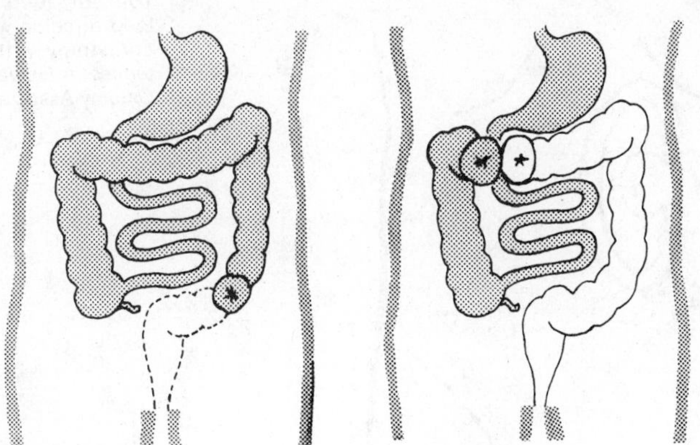

FIGURE 75–5. The location of colostomy stomas. Left, single-barreled colostomy. Right, double-barreled colostomy. (From *Colostomies: A Guide*, published by the United Ostomy Association, Los Angeles.)

Teaching must be paced to the patient's acceptance of the colostomy as well as his ability to perform the tasks of management. The patient with a temporary colostomy will also need to learn how to care for it, as these are usually kept for several months. If he is physically able to do so, an adult usually prefers to care for the colostomy without involving his spouse or another family member more than absolutely necessary. However, a husband or wife should be knowledgeable about the colostomy and the care it needs. He or she must also learn to accept this mode of elimination as a way of life for the mate; lack of acceptance by the spouse makes the patient's problem even greater.

Control of Elimination

Elimination can be handled in two ways: Natural elimination patterns of the body can be utilized, with the patient wearing a bag to collect the feces whenever they come, or an attempt can be made at control by irrigations. If the colostomy is in the transverse or right colon, wearing a bag will be necessary, as the feces are still quite liquid in these areas. When irrigations are not used, then the attempt at control is made by adjusting the diet so as to obtain a stool of the desired consistency. Some people prefer to have rigid dietary regulation and not be bothered with irrigations, and some people are not physically or emotionally able to cope with the irrigation procedure. Few people are able to regulate a colostomy well enough by diet alone to avoid wearing a bag over the stoma.

When regulation by irrigation is attempted, irrigation is done daily or every two to three days, depending on the patient. In this way the patient hopes to empty his colon and to have little if any passage of stool until the next irrigation. This method also necessitates control of the patient's diet to avoid laxative foods which might cause an unexpected evacuation.

A colostomy irrigation, which is very similar to an enema, can be done at any time of day that is convenient for the patient. The purpose of the irrigation is not to "wash out" the colon but to distend it sufficiently to stimulate peristalsis, which will cause the evacuation to occur. Most patients can stimulate evacuation of the bowel with a relatively small amount of water (200 to 300 ml.). Since there is no sphincter on a colostomy, the fluid tends to return as it is instilled.

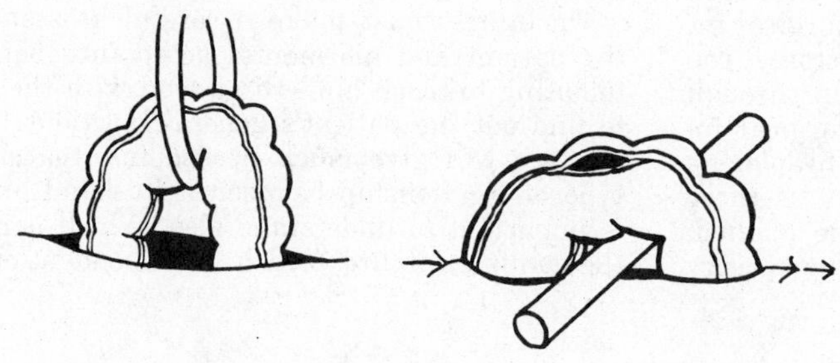

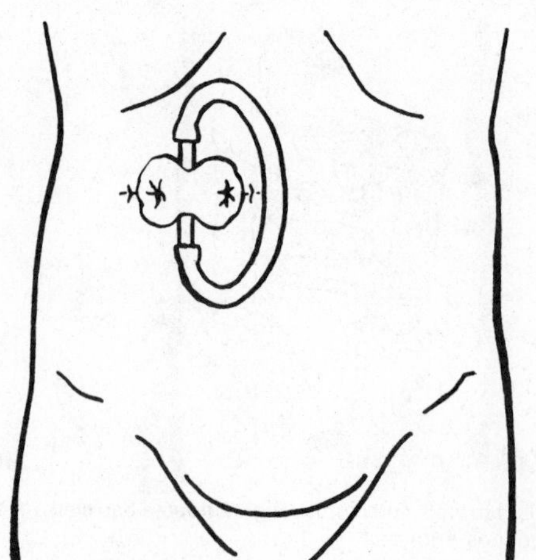

FIGURE 75–6. Loop colostomies. Top left, loop of colon; top right, loop of colon with rod. Bottom, loop colostomy with rod. (From *Colostomies: A Guide*, published by United Ostomy Association, Los Angeles.)

The rectal tube or catheter that is used to instill the fluid is inserted about 3 inches. Care should be used in inserting it to avoid perforation of the bowel; if any resistance is encountered, some solution should be instilled to distend the bowel ahead of the tube and thus ease its insertion. Frequently the bowel makes a turn shortly below the abdominal wall, and there may be a constriction owing to an attachment made during surgery, so the patient must become familiar with the contour of his bowel and learn to insert the tube without undue poking, which might damage the delicate mucous membrane. The temperature of the solution should be at or very slightly below body temperature, since warmer solutions tend to cause the bowel to relax. Every colostomy is different, and some people may need to use more solution than this or to insert the tube farther to avoid backflow. Each patient must learn the best method to manage his own bowel.

There is a large assortment of commercial equipment available for irrigating a colostomy. Most physicians have a set purchased for the patient while he is hospitalized which he takes home with him. The expense of these sets varies widely, and the type of apparatus used is largely a matter of personal preference. The patient should be referred to a surgical supply house in his locality so he can see the variety of sets available and make his own selection. It is usually best that he use the set he starts out with until he is familiar with his colostomy and its problems and the problems of irrigating it before he invests in a new apparatus.

In an emergency a temporary irrigation set can be made from a plastic bread wrapper and a rubber canning ring (Fig. 75–7). Many people already own an enema bag, and with the addition of a glass connector an irrigating catheter can be attached. The rigid rectal tube that comes with these sets should not be used on a colostomy because of the danger of trauma to the bowel wall.

Stoma bags are not necessary if the colostomy is regulated, but before regularity is achieved, for a few hours after irrigations, or when the patient has a bout of diarrhea, most people prefer to wear a bag to protect their clothing. Surveys have shown that a high percentage of patients with colostomies wear a bag at least part of the time. Bags can be held in place by a belt worn around the abdomen or they may be attached to the abdominal wall by an adhesive substance. Some bags are made with a karaya gum ring which adheres to the abdomen when held with a belt (Fig. 75–8). However, the use of a belt increases the incidence of prolapse of the bowel with herniation as a result of pressure of the ring around the stoma. Even though a person does not usually wear a bag, he will probably want to keep some on hand for use during bouts of diarrhea.

Mucous secretions from the bowel make some protection over the stoma necessary when the patient does not wear a bag. A piece of tissue or a thin gauze square with a piece of plastic over it to retain the moisture is usually sufficient. Commercial pads with a moisture-proof backing are available.

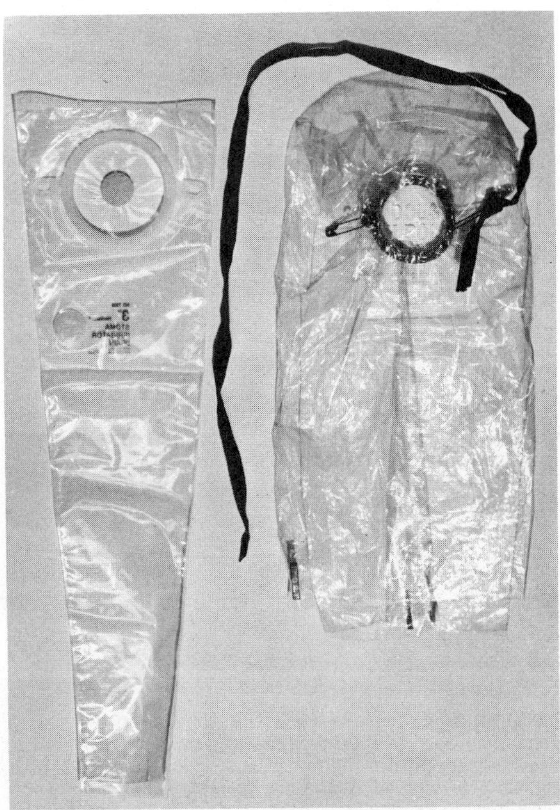

FIGURE 75–7. Disposable colostomy irrigation equipment. The bag on the left is commercially made. Note the wedged circle through which the irrigating catheter is inserted. The home-made irrigator (right) is made by creating a hole near the closed end of a plastic bread bag and wrapping the plastic around a rubber canning ring to form a snug bond. A belt to hold the apparatus close to the abdomen can be threaded through safety pins that pierce the rubber ring. A small hole can be made for insertion of the irrigation catheter. The bag is discarded after use. As with most other irrigating equipment, the patient uses these bags as he sits on the stool with the open end of the bag between legs to direct the returning flow into the toilet.

Diet

Diet is of utmost importance in the management of a colostomy, because both the consistency of the stool and the presence of gas depend on the type of foods ingested. Each individual is different and must find out for himself what he can and cannot eat. In general, the foods that bothered him before the surgery will be troublesome, and roughage, fresh fruits, and dried prunes and other laxative or bulk-forming foods will need to be taken judiciously. On the other hand, if the individual eats a totally constipating diet, he will have problems with hard stools. The patient must find out for himself what balance of foods creates the best consistency of stool with the least amount of gas.

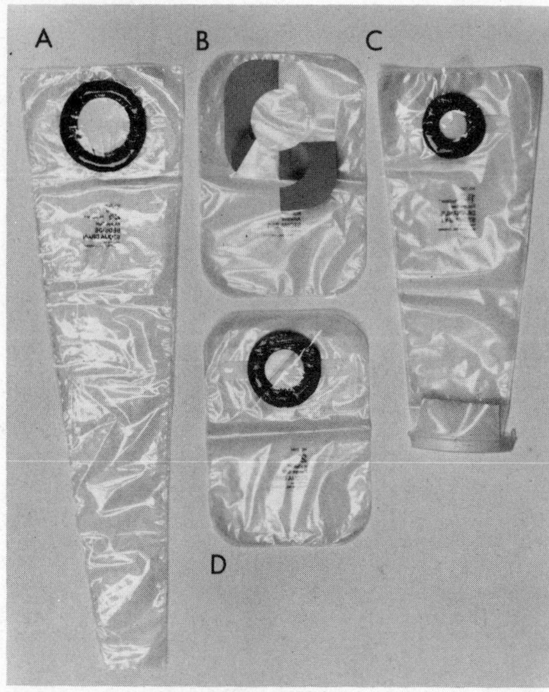

FIGURE 75–8. Types of stoma bags. A, C, and D have karaya rings. Note the difference in size to fit stomas of varying sizes. Bag B adheres to the skin after the backing (partially folded back in picture) is removed. Bags A and C are open at the bottom to allow them to be emptied and left in place, while B and D are closed at the bottom and not intended for continued use.

Special Problems

Diarrhea, as already mentioned, is a serious problem for colostomy patients and can create havoc in the best managed life style. The person should contact his physician for instruction concerning medications that can be taken to slow the motility of the bowel. Many people keep such medications on hand and use them at the first indication of trouble.

Two further problems can result from diarrhea: *excoriation of the skin* from the digestive juices that have not been resorbed, and *electrolyte imbalance* when the condition persists. The individual should be encouraged to continue taking water and possibly plain tea when diarrhea begins, but it is usually best to take no food until bowel motility has returned to normal.

When *hard stools* are present, it is difficult to evacuate the bowel and may be difficult to get water into the colostomy for irrigation. Fecal impactions can also occur. Oil instilled directly into the stoma at bedtime or several hours before irrigation will usually help this situation. Only a small amount is needed; the individual might try 5 to 10 ml. first and await the results before trying more. Too much oil will cause the colostomy to leak oil after irrigation. Sometimes the physician has the patient take the stool softener dioctyl sodium sulfosuccinate to hold more fluid in the feces.

Gas is an embarrassing problem since the individual has no control over its passage and has no sensations to tell him he is about to pass it. The noise of the passage of gas and the resultant odor can cause him to avoid social situations. Charcoal and bismuth subcarbonate are thought by some to help and can be taken orally with the physician's approval. Deodorants are available for placement in the bag, but the most satisfactory method of control is dietary. Since each individual is different, the person will have to find out by trial and error which foods cause him problems. In general, nuts, cabbage, sauerkraut, broccoli, corn, and cauliflower are gas-forming foods. Swallowing air by eating too rapidly and chewing gum can also be causes for intestinal gas.

Strictures of the stoma occur because the rectus muscles of the abdominal wall tend to close over any artificial opening made through them. Some physicians routinely teach their patients to dilate the stoma daily or before each irrigation. The person uses a glove or finger cot with lubricant and inserts a finger into the opening to stretch it. This tends to be painful, so the patient needs to understand the purpose and importance of really dilating the stoma to the required width by sufficient penetration of the finger. Other physicians feel that the passage of a formed stool is sufficient dilatation.

Regular cleansing of the skin around the stoma is necessary to prevent irritation. A light dusting with talcum powder or karaya powder will usually prevent or heal excoriations due to the constant presence of moisture.

Patient Adjustment

The person who has a colostomy can lead a completely normal life. He can engage in all the sports and social activities he enjoyed before his surgery. He can travel, but he must allow extra time in the itinerary for stoma care in strange situations. Many people do these things without difficulty. There are no restrictions in dress except that a change of undergarments should be carried in case of accidental soiling.

There is no physical reason why the person cannot enjoy normal sexual relationships. Psychologic barriers because of the supposedly "dirty" opening on the abdomen of one partner may cause some problems, but with love, patience, and understanding, and with good hygienic practices on the part of the person with the colostomy, there need be no problem. However, it may take several months after surgery before a couple manages to reestablish a satisfactory relationship.

The above paragraphs may make the adjustment of the colostomy patient sound easy, but the average person has many problems in achieving this level of rehabilitation. Depression is common and "management" of anything as unpredictable as the human intestine is very difficult, if not impossible, without a sphincter. The ultimate resolution of difficulties is the patient's problem, and he needs much support and knowledgeable advice as he learns to live with the situation. Some cities have established "ostomy" rehabilitation clinics to help these patients with their problems. A fairly new paramedical worker called an enterostomal therapist is trained to work with these patients and with medical personnel caring for them. These therapists help nurses to develop and to implement care plans that provide a smooth transition from the hospital to the home and to the rehabilitated life.

In most large communities there is an "ostomy" club. These clubs are beneficial, as people share their concerns with others who understand and exchange "solutions" to their common problems. Information concerning the local colostomy club can be acquired from a local hospital, the local cancer society office, or from the United Ostomy Association, Incorporated, 111 Wilshire Boulevard, Los Angeles, California 90017.

ILEOSTOMY

An ileostomy is the opening of the ileum onto the abdominal surface. The colon may or may not be resected. The most frequent reason for doing an ileostomy is the treatment of ulcerative colitis, but the operation is also done as a treatment for regional enteritis (Crohn's disease), multiple polyposis, cancer of the bowel, and sometimes as a temporary diversion of the fecal stream. The vast majority of ileostomies are permanent.

The major difference between an ileostomy and a colostomy is the consistency of the fecal stream. The feces are liquid in the terminal ileum and contain digestive enzymes which can digest the skin. There is no way to regulate the fecal flow, so the only method of control is for the individual to wear a collection bag over the stoma.

The patient returns from surgery wearing a temporary bag which adheres to his skin. It is very important to make sure that secretions do not leak from this bag, as they will cause a skin burn which keeps the bag from sticking and causes further leakage and further burning. Prevention of leakage is especially important while the surgical incision is healing. Karaya powder is used when excoriations occur, as it aids healing and also helps to seal the bag snugly about the stoma. The patient will receive his permanent appliance before he leaves the hospital and must know how to apply it. He should practice this in a situation as closely resembling his own bathroom as possible.

There are a number of appliances on the market, but none is perfect. The patient should seek help until he finds one which fits him, does not leak, and which he can wear at least one day (and preferably 3 to 5 days) without changing. He should know the names and locations of local surgical supply companies from whom he can purchase this equipment and receive help in procuring a properly fitting appliance.

Since no control over the fecal flow is possible, there is little reason for dietary control. These patients may find that some foods cause them to have excessive problems with gas and with odor and may have to make some minor dietary adjustments. The major difficulty this patient has is with skin care, so his biggest problem is in achieving a good fit between the appliance bag and the skin.

When the patient develops diarrhea from any source, he must seek medical care because he can rapidly go into a state of acute electrolyte imbalance owing to the excessively rapid loss of digestive juices. Family members as well as the patient must be aware of this ever-present danger.

As mentioned, the most common reason for doing this surgery is an inflammatory condition of the bowel (Chapter 79). The average patient has usually had the bowel disorder for a number of years before deciding to have surgery and is in a poor state of nutrition. He frequently has many emotional problems as a result of his condition and has decided upon surgery as the lesser of two evils. The surgical procedure in which the colon is resected is a great physiologic shock to an already malnourished body, and the ileostomy is an equally great shock to a patient in a depressed emotional state. When the patient awakens after surgery and realizes what has been done to him, he is frequently very depressed. A research study found that even though the nature of the surgery was discussed with patients preoperatively, they "were shocked and horrified after surgery when they realized what the operation entailed."[38]

Recently a new procedure for coping with ileostomy drainage has been developed. A reservoir for storage of fecal drainage is created by forming a pouch from a portion of the small bowel. The open end of this pouch is threaded between the rectus muscles to form a seal and then opens onto the abdomen. Fecal material, retained within this pouch, is irrigated out two or three times a day when the patient inserts a small irrigating catheter through the tract. This procedure seems to have merit because it gives the patient more control over his bowel elimination.

In caring for this patient the nurse must remember that he or she has had an emotionally draining disease and that the decision to have this type of surgery was not made lightly. This person needs patient understanding and reassurance that the ileostomy will be "manageable" and that he can still live a normal life. Many of these patients are irascible, and consequently many nurses find them difficult to care for.

Members of ostomy clubs visit these patients in many communities. Patients in the previously mentioned study reported that a preoperative visit by one of the members was helpful in reassuring the patient that a person still looked normal after undergoing this surgery. Visits are made only on the invitation of the physician, so in many instances the person is not seen preoperatively. However, a visit from an ileostomy patient is helpful after surgery too, because the patient can identify with another person who has the condition better than he can with the doctors and nurses who have had no personal experience with the problems involved.

The family of the ileostomy patient has as much of an adjustment to make as the patient does, and at the same time they must understand what the patient is going through and accept his sometimes unpredictable behavior. Nurses can do much in the way of helping the family by listening to their reactions and interpreting the patient's problems to them. The family relationship problems are very similar to those of a colostomy patient, except that they tend to be more intense.

It should be assumed from the beginning that the patient will learn to manage the stoma and bag as soon as he is physically able to do so; this is as necessary to the ileostomy patient as learning to use his prosthesis is to the amputation patient. The patient, to achieve a satisfactory adjustment, should have an appliance which fits snugly, does not leak or cause odor or skin irritation, and stays in place for several days. He should be able to change the bag himself without undue problems or undue expenditure of time. He should be able to eat a balanced diet to his liking and live a normal life—socially, vocationally, recreationally, and sexually. These are the goals of nursing care.

CHAPTER 76

Abnormalities of the Mouth and Oropharynx

DENTAL DISORDERS

Since dental care and dental hygiene are provided by workers in these disciplines, we shall discuss only conditions that the nurse needs to understand when caring for the sick person and when functioning as a health teacher and case finder.

One aim of dentistry is to preserve the natural teeth in good health as long as possible, because a dental prosthesis is almost never as functional as the natural teeth. Proper mastication of food is dependent upon functional dentures and is necessary to efficient digestion.

Decay and periodontal disease are the major causes of tooth loss. Plaque has been cited as the major cause of both caries (decay) and periodontal disease and is also the initial stage in the formation of calculus.

> "Dental plaque is a soft mass of proliferating bacteria with a scattering of leukocytes, macrophages and epithelial cells in a sticky polysaccharide-protein matrix that adheres to the teeth, from which it can only be detached by mechanical cleansing. It is transparent and colorless and escapes detection unless it absorbs pigment from within the oral cavity or is stained in the dental office by disclosing solutions or wafers available for that purpose."[20]

Food affects plaque because bacterial enzymes liquefy food debris after a meal and utilize some of these ingredients along with saliva in plaque formation. The polysaccharide dextran is the major component of the intercellular matrix that envelops the plaque bacteria and attaches them to each other and to the tooth surface. Dextran can be formed from any carbohydrate but is formed most readily from sucrose. Plaque formation is increased by the addition of sucrose to the diet.

CARIES

Dental decay is a common condition. Its etiology is multifaceted and involves the resistance of the tooth enamel, the nature of the plaque, including its bacteria, and the diet ingested by the individual. Of these factors, the dental plaque is probably the most important. The most commonly accepted theory today is that acids produced by bacteria in the plaque begin to decalcify the inorganic tooth enamel when the pH goes as low as 5.5. However, plaque also offers some protection, since it has buffering qualities. Acid-producing cariogenic bacteria and carbohydrates must both be present in order for decay to develop. Any carbohydrate in the mouth stimulates acid production by bacteria, but sucrose seems to be the most effective form. The longer carbohydrate remains in the mouth after ingestion, the longer it takes for the pH to return to normal levels; therefore, increased frequency of ingestion causes an increased acid level in the mouth for longer periods of time and an increase in cavity production. The only treatment for caries is prevention (see below).

PERIODONTAL DISEASE

The early form of periodontal disease is gingivitis, inflammation of the gingiva. The late form of the disease is periodontitis or pyorrhea. In *periodontitis* the inflammation extends from the gums into the periodontal pockets, resulting in loosening of the teeth as their supporting structures are destroyed (Fig. 76–1).

Gingivitis is manifested by bleeding of the gums from minor trauma. There is usually some alteration in color of the gingiva and there may be swelling, but pain is not a prominent symptom. It is characterized by inflamed gingiva, with the formation of pockets which gradually deepen and eventually cause destruction of the underlying tissues and separation of the gingiva from the tooth.

PREVENTIVE MEASURES AND ORAL HYGIENE

The only method of control of periodontal disease and caries is prevention. Since dental plaque is thought to be instrumental in the production of both these conditions, control measures focus on its removal. Since plaque cannot be removed without friction, rinsing the mouth is ineffective alone. Toothbrushing, the use of dental floss, interdental cleansers, and water irrigation under pressure are the most important means of oral hygiene. The friction measures dislodge the plaque and debris and rinsing removes it.

Research has shown that reducing the carbohydrate content of the diet reduces the amount of decay that occurs. Since this is difficult to accomplish in the average person, other approaches have been to incorporate agents in the dentifrice that will either neutralize the acid or destroy the bacteria. This approach has not shown very promising results. The use of mouthwashes is of dubious value because their effect wears off in from one half to three hours, depending upon the strength of the solution; also, microorganisms tend to develop resistance to the solutions. To be most effective they should be used at least twice a day, and the brand should be changed routinely to prevent bacteria from building up resistance.[47]

DENTAL EMERGENCIES

A patient sustaining an injury that *fractures a tooth* must be seen by a dentist, as entry of bacteria into the pulp canal of the tooth can cause infection.

Postextraction hemorrhage can be either primary, occurring within an hour or two of the extraction and usually caused by dislodging of the clot, or secondary, probably caused by infection in the socket or a loose clot. Both types of hemorrhage can be treated in an emergency situation with the application of local pressure. A sterile gauze pad, applied over the extraction site with the patient biting upon it, frequently brings about hemostasis. Sometimes biting on a moistened tea bag is a successful home remedy since pressure is achieved and the tannic acid in the tea helps to promote hemostasis. Any continued bleeding should be treated by a dentist.

Emergencies such as deep *lacerations of the gums* and *fractures of the jaw* should be treated by a surgeon. Lacerations bleed freely owing to the excellent blood supply. Local pressure is the best first aid treatment.

In any wound of this nature, care should be taken to remove debris from the mouth gently to prevent accidental aspiration. This can be accomplished by gentle irrigation or, if possible, gentle rinsing by the patient.

EXTRACTIONS AND DENTURES

Local application of ice for alternate half-hour periods will help to prevent swelling after a tooth

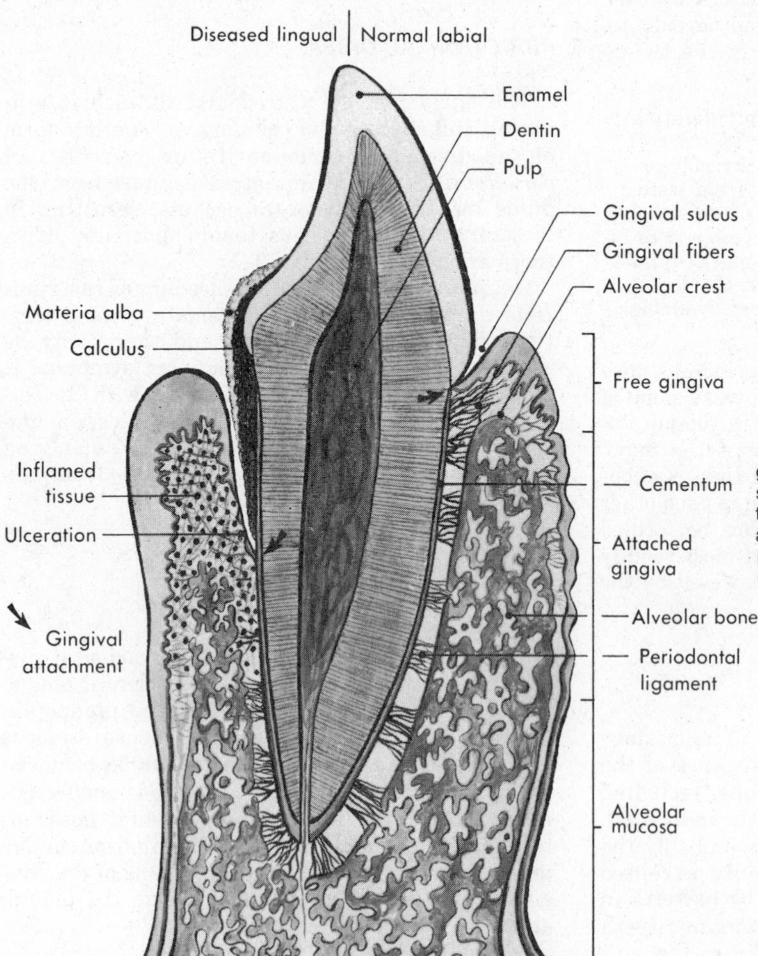

FIGURE 76–1. Periodontal disease. Diagramatic representation of a tooth. The right side illustrates normal healthy tissues. Note, on the left side, the destruction of alveolar bone and periodontal fibers which hold the tooth in place. (Courtesy Department of Dental Hygiene, University of Washington School of Dentistry.)

extraction. Patients should eat only bland soft foods and avoid vigorous rinsing of the mouth. Frequent gentle oral hygiene will make the patient feel better.

Extractions are sometimes done in the hospital when the patient has complicating medical conditions or when a full denture extraction is to be done. Immediate insertion of the denture helps to prevent postoperative swelling and provides a covering for the open operative area, but makes subsequent fitting of the denture more difficult. Patients with a history of rheumatic heart disease are usually given penicillin to prevent a flare-up from the transient bacteremia that follows an extraction.

Regardless of the claims of dental adhesive products in television advertisements, artificial dentures never function as well as natural teeth. Patients with dentures usually need added time to chew foods properly. Since many individuals have dentures at the age when the gastrointestinal tract is less able to cope with improperly masticated food, this has an important influence on the total nutrition of the individual. Many people have poorly fitting dentures that are uncomfortable. Tissues of the mouth and jaw change during the lifetime, especially after the removal of teeth, so dentures may need to be modified to achieve proper fit and efficiency. Undoubtedly many persons with dentures have not visited a dentist regularly for proper maintenance of the denture.[7] Nurses should encourage patients to seek dental aid to achieve better mastication.

Persons who wear dentures should massage the gums twice daily when dentures are out of the mouth for cleansing. This stimulates circulation of the underlying tissues.

Since many individuals are sensitive about wearing dentures, partially because the dentures change their appearance, and partially because they equate dentures with aging, the nurse must be tactful in her mention of them. Some individuals do not wish to be seen by anyone, including their spouse, unless the dental appliance is in place.

ORAL INFECTIONS

STOMATITIS

Stomatitis is an inflammation of the mouth; inflammation of the tongue is glossitis; and of the gums, gingivitis. These may be of infectious origin or a symptom of systemic disease. Stomatitis is commonly caused by mechanical trauma such as from jagged teeth, biting the cheeks, and mouth breathing; by chemical trauma owing to foods and drinks or sensitization to contactants such as mouthwashes and dentifrices; or by infection with organisms such as viruses, streptococci, borrelia, yeasts, and molds.

A person who has a sore mouth has little interest in eating, has excessive salivation, and may have a foul breath. Treatment, in addition to removal of the cause, consists of frequent soothing oral hygiene and topical medications, which are sometimes applied in mouthwashes. A soft bland diet is usually necessary.

Aphthous Stomatitis (Canker Sore)

There is no agreement as to the etiology of these lesions, which are ulcers of the mouth and lips. Factors which have been suggested include emotional stress, trauma, vitamin deficiency, food and drug allergy, endocrine imbalance, viral infections; some consider them a manifestation of herpes. There is much evidence that they occur as a result of hypersensitivity. They heal spontaneously in from one to two weeks. Topical or systemic steroids shorten the healing time, and the routine administration of steroids has suppressed their recurrence in susceptible individuals.

HERPES SIMPLEX

By the age of five years, 90 per cent of the population have had an infection, usually asymptomatic, of primary herpes simplex. The majority of the cases of recurrent herpes simplex take the form of herpes labialis (fever blister, cold sore). The lesions occur as clear vesicles, which are most frequently located at the mucocutaneous junction of the lips and face. They heal without scarring in about a week. People differ greatly in their susceptibility to the blisters. Some develop them following very short exposure to sunlight or heat or after a very short period of fever. Given sufficient stimulus, almost every adult will develop one.[3]

Unless the ulcer is secondarily infected, antimicrobial treatment does not affect the progress of the ulcer. The only treatment is symptomatic; local ointments and anesthetics may soothe the lesions. Some think that repeated vaccinations prevent the occurrence of these lesions, but research studies have not validated this.

VINCENT'S ANGINA

Formerly thought to be very contagious and frequently called "trench mouth," this infection is a gingivitis that is manifested by ulcers that are covered with a pseudomembrane. It is caused by fusiform bacteria and spirochetes that are resident in most people's mouths. It is now thought to be brought on by poor oral hygiene, nutritional deficiencies, local tissue damage, and debilitating diseases. There are acute, subacute, and chronic forms, depending upon the severity of the symptoms. The acute form manifests itself by the sudden onset of a sore mouth, spontaneous bleeding of the gums, the presence of a membrane, and a foul odor. Treatment is the removal of the devitalized tissues and correction of the underlying cause by such measures as rest, bland diet, and vitamins. Pain medications and peroxide mouthwashes are also used to promote patient comfort.

ORAL TUMORS

LEUKOPLAKIA

Leukoplakia is an area of hyperkeratinization which is yellow-white or gray-white in color, occurs in any region of the mouth, is of varying sizes and shapes, is usually elevated with a roughened or leathery surface, and has clearly defined borders. This lesion is caused by chronic irritation of the mucosa by physical, thermal, or chemical means, and is sometimes related to systemic factors such as poor nutrition or syphilis. These lesions are frequently precancerous and sometimes cover an already malignant lesion. They should be watched carefully, and a biopsy should be taken if there is any question about the lesion or if it changes in character. Any irritating cause should be eliminated. Since these lesions can be readily seen in the mouth, the nurse should be alert for their presence and report them.

CANCER

The death rate for cancer of the mouth is much greater than it should be considering the incidence of this disorder and the availability of the oral cavity for inspection and case finding. The majority (90 per cent) of the malignant lesions in the mouth are squamous cell carcinomas, of which 70 per cent occur on the lips, lateral border of the tongue, and floor of the mouth.

Cancer of the tongue has the poorest prognosis because of the extensive vascular and lymphatic supplies to this organ and probably also because its vulnerable position exposes it to all manner of trauma inflicted from within the mouth.

The lesions ulcerate early, tend to be fixed and hard, and typically are not painful. Any lesion in the mouth which does not heal in two weeks should be examined by a competent physician, especially in persons over 55 who have a history of smoking and the use of alcohol.

Etiologic factors seem to be poor oral hygiene with bacterial irritation, physical trauma as from jagged teeth or improperly fitting dentures, or chemical and thermal trauma from tobacco, alcohol, and hot or spicy foods. Malnutrition, syphilis, and cirrhosis have also been found to be present in a large number of patients with this condition.

The cancer spreads primarily by local extension and to regional lymph nodes, but rarely invades the venous system to form distant metastases. The condition is diagnosed positively only by biopsy. Cytologic study has been shown to be of significant value in screeening, but unfortunately is not used widely enough to have reduced the mortality rate. Cytologic examination, when used as a diagnostic aid, is performed on any suspicious appearing mucosa and is followed by biopsy when the reports show questionable cells. Cancer of the mouth, even when completely cured, tends to recur in another primary lesion. A study showed a significant increase in the incidence of recurrence in patients who continue to smoke after the first lesion is treated.[42]

Treatment is primarily by surgical excision or by radiation, depending upon the location and type of cell.

BENIGN TUMORS

The most common benign tumors of the mouth are fibromas, lipomas, neurofibromas, and hemangiomas. As with benign tumors in other parts of the body, they cause problems for the patient mainly by occupying space and by pressure. They can usually be excised when they cause the patient functional or cosmetic problems.

DISORDERS OF THE SALIVARY GLANDS

INFLAMMATION

The most common inflammation of the salivary glands is parotitis, that is, inflammation of the parotid glands, or surgical mumps. However, any of the salivary glands can become inflamed. This is probably usually the result of inactivity of the gland caused by certain medications and lack of oral feeding. As secretions of the salivary glands diminish, oral bacteria have an opportunity to invade and multiply. Good oral hygiene to keep the bacterial count of the mouth as low as possible is probably the best preventive measure in addition to keeping the patient well hydrated and stimulating secretions of the glands by various means such as sucking on hard candies or chewing.

CALCULUS

Stones, or calculi, usually form in the salivary glands as a result of inactivity of the gland combined with a metabolic condition favoring precipitation of salts. As with stones in other locations, a focus or nidus is necessary for stimulating the precipitation of the salt. Irritation from the stone causes local inflammation, swelling, and pain when the gland is called upon to secrete, as during chewing. Treatment is local excision. Stones occur most commonly in the submaxillary glands, probably because this duct is longer and the secretions are more viscous and alkaline than those from other glands.

TUMORS

Most tumors occurring in the salivary glands are benign. The most frequent malignant tumor is adenocarcinoma; cancer occurs more often in the submaxillary glands than in the parotids. Enlargement is the main symptom of both types of tumors, with the malignant ones growing more rapidly than the benign. Pain occurs when expansion within the capsule of the gland creates pressure on sensory nerves.

Some of the malignant tumors spread predominantly by means of the lymphatics and some by means of the veins. Some are radiosensitive. The decision as to type of treatment will be made on the basis of the type of cell and the extent of growth or spread.

LUDWIG'S ANGINA

This is a fairly rare condition in which infection from the mouth, usually from an infected tooth, spreads into the soft tissues below the chin and around the submaxillary glands. The patient has a fever, local swelling, and tenderness. The treatment is by antibiotics and local heat. If the infection is not checked, the patient can suffer acute respiratory distress as a result of pressure on the adjacent trachea and pharynx. The nurse should observe the patient for respiratory problems (see Unit XIV) and notify the physician before the condition becomes acute.

ORAL SURGERY

In addition to procedures involving the teeth and gums, surgery done in the oral cavity includes the repair of injuries and the removal of tumors. Any portion of the oral cavity, including the sinuses and nasal structures, can be affected. (See Unit XXII for nasal and sinus conditions.) Removal of malignant tumors frequently involves a fairly wide local excision of tissue along with removal of associated lymph nodes. Since removal of these structures can interfere with talking, chewing, and swallowing and frequently results in a cosmetic defect, the rehabilitation of these patients following surgery can be quite a challenge. Various types of trauma also frequently result in a cosmetic defect and may cause problems in eating and speaking. Prosthetic devices are available to replace some of the hard tissue structures such as the hard palate and to seal off openings into the sinuses. These improve the appearance and aid in chewing and swallowing with varying levels of effectiveness.

GLOSSECTOMY

The removal of the tongue has vast implications for the patient, since the tongue is the major organ of taste and speech and is active in chewing and swallowing. The most common reason for removal of this organ is carcinoma. Because the tongue is a very vascular organ and has excellent lymphatic drainage, the prognosis is poor even following removal early in the disease process. Following surgery the patient's speech is difficult to understand.

MANDIBULECTOMY

Cancer occurring on the floor of the mouth or near the lower jaw sometimes requires removal of a portion of the mandible to achieve adequate excision. This results in a very noticeable cosmetic defect and also presents a problem in achieving adequate mastication. As with other oral surgery for cancer, it is usually done in conjunction with a radical neck dissection.

RADICAL NECK DISSECTION

Since death from cancer of the oral cavity most frequently comes from pressure on the trachea, esophagus, blood vessels, and nerves in the neck as a result of spread of the tumor into the cervical lymph nodes, a radical neck dissection is frequently done on patients with this condition. (See Unit XIV.)

MANDIBULAR FRACTURES

Trauma to the face or jaws sometimes results in fractures. As with fractures elsewhere, the segments must be immobilized in order to maintain alignment while healing takes place. Immobilization is accomplished by internal fixation with screws and plates or by wiring the teeth together. Wires are placed between the teeth and the two jaws are held together by means of rubber bands stretched between the upper and lower jaws. These can easily be removed in case the patient experiences difficulty such as choking or vomiting. The patient will be unable to chew while these wires are in place, so will be fed a liquid diet. Oral hygiene is important and, with the exception of the exterior surfaces of the teeth, can be done only by frequent rinsing or irrigation of the mouth. The diet is monotonous in consistency, and the patient tends to experience constipation because of a lack of bulk, but since these fractures heal fairly rapidly, the jaw immobilization usually lasts only from four to five weeks.

NURSING MANAGEMENT IN ORAL SURGERY

The nursing care needed by this patient is determined by the extent of the procedure, the location of the incisions, whether a tracheostomy has been done, and whether the patient is able to talk and swallow. Catheters are frequently used under the skin flaps to eliminate the need for large bulky dressings. These will be attached to some source of suction. Dressings vary from none at all to large bulky ones. There may be packing present in the mouth, nose, or sinus cavities.

Airway

Maintenance of an airway is the most critical need for these patients. If the surgical procedure has been extensive, most of them will have a tracheostomy to prevent respiratory difficulty as a result of edema and swelling of the oral and pharyngeal structures. Patients are positioned in a sitting posture after surgery to promote venous and lymphatic drainage. They may have a dusky appearance about the face resulting from venous congestion rather than from poor aeration. Checking the color of the fingers and toes will show whether proper oxygenation is being achieved. Restlessness and apprehension in this patient may be symptoms of air hunger rather than pain. (See Unit XIV for nursing care of the tracheostomy patient.)

Nutrition

Normal eating may be difficult because of swelling, the location of suture lines, or because swallowing is impossible. A nasogastric tube, which is placed during surgery, is frequently used to provide nourishment. If it is accidentally dislodged, it should not be replaced without checking with the physician because of potential damage to the suture lines. Sometimes a gastrostomy is done for feeding purposes; occasionally the patient is able to drink a liquid diet.

Pain

Pain is not as much of a problem for these patients as their appearance would indicate. Frequently mild analgesics are all that is needed to keep them comfortable. Swelling is the cause of most of the discomfort.

Oral Hygiene

Mouth care gently and frequently given is mandatory for these patients. Some centers use a gentle spray to cleanse the tissues instead of irrigations or cotton-tipped applicators. Solutions frequently used are physiological saline, weak hydrogen peroxide, and weak sodium bicarbonate. Antibiotic solutions or dilute mouthwashes may also be ordered. Suction tips used to aspirate the irrigating solutions from the mouth should be handled with care to prevent trauma to the exposed sutures. Gentle care given frequently is essential to patient comfort and infection-free healing.

Saliva

When the patient is unable to swallow, the management of his saliva becomes a problem. A wick placed in his mouth with the other end in an emesis basin is one way of collecting it when the patient is in bed. The basin should be emptied frequently, as the pan is apt to spill in the bed and because of the odor that results from decomposing saliva.

Complications

Hemorrhage. This can occur in the first few hours after surgery or several days postoperatively and can be massive because of the large vessels that supply this area. Local pressure is the best method of meeting this emergency until the physician can be reached. Usually the repair will have to be done in the operating room.

Infection. When this occurs there may be severe pain. Frequent oral hygiene is a preventive measure. Local medications may be used to treat a wound infection from anaerobic organisms, and systemic antimicrobial therapy may be employed.

Emotional Reactions of the Patient

Patients who undergo radical oral surgery and, to a lesser extent, those who have minor procedures done have a number of adjustments to make. We are all influenced by our physical appearance, and when this is altered, especially when the contours of the face and jaws become abnormal, the patient feels conspicuous and different. The head and neck are publicly visible, so deformities are evident to others. In addition to disfigurement, this patient also has normal fears about surgery and about having cancer, and he frequently experiences difficulty in breathing and communication.

Fear, anger, and grief are normal reactions to his situation. He probably has generalized fears of the future, the outcome of his condition, and his ability to live normally, as well as specific fears of rejection by others, of being alone, of being unable to communicate his needs, and of the occurrence of sudden complications. Anger at the general situation, his loss, and his helplessness to control it are part of the grieving process. It is necessary for him to go through this as he learns to accept his situation and reconstructs his life style.

The nurse must recognize these problems and give support to the patient as well as to his family members as they attempt to work through the situation. The family may need explanations concerning the necessity for the patient to grieve and the normality of his reactions to the situation. They will probably also experience the same emotions.

When the patient is unable to communicate, the problem is to help him express his needs and feelings adequately. The nurse can provide paper for him to write down his thoughts and his needs and should check on him frequently so he will know that he is not alone. A call bell should always be placed conveniently and should be answered promptly. Much communication can be accomplished by sign language and a few written words. The sensitive nurse can communicate her compassion and concern to the patient and find out from writing and from nonverbal replies to her verbal questions what his specific needs and problems are. Her manner should communicate to the patient that she accepts him as he is.

The patient's inability to eat normally is another factor for him to accept and may be the one he feels safe in complaining about. The nurse must remember that his complaints are probably directed at his general situation rather than at her as a person.

An attempt should be made to help this patient begin to meet others by walking about the hospital corridors. This type of patient is usually up and about quite soon after surgery, and social encounters and physical activity are both good for him.

CHAPTER 77

Abnormalities of Deglutition and of the Esophagus

Review of Anatomy and Physiology

The esophagus is a hollow muscular tube that is collapsed in its resting state. It is composed of striated muscle in the upper portion and smooth muscle in the lower. There is a sphincter mechanism at both ends of this tube, and there are areas of natural narrowing where the aorta and left mainstem bronchus pass it. These four narrowed areas are also the points at which disease processes most frequently occur (Fig. 77–1).

The esophagus is innervated by the 10th and 11th cranial nerves and also has sympathetic nervous fibers from the cervical and thoracic areas. Its intrinsic nervous control comes from the intramural plexus (Auerbach's) in the mucosal layer. Although pressure within the esophagus is lower than pressure within the stomach, stomach contents do not normally regurgitate into the esophagus because of pressure at the cardiac sphincter. The act of swallowing initiates a wave of peristalsis, or contraction, which moves down the esophagus to the stomach. This contraction is preceded by a wave of relaxation. Food from the esophagus is propelled into the stomach by this peristaltic wave, gravity, and the opening of the cardiac sphincter during the wave of relaxation.

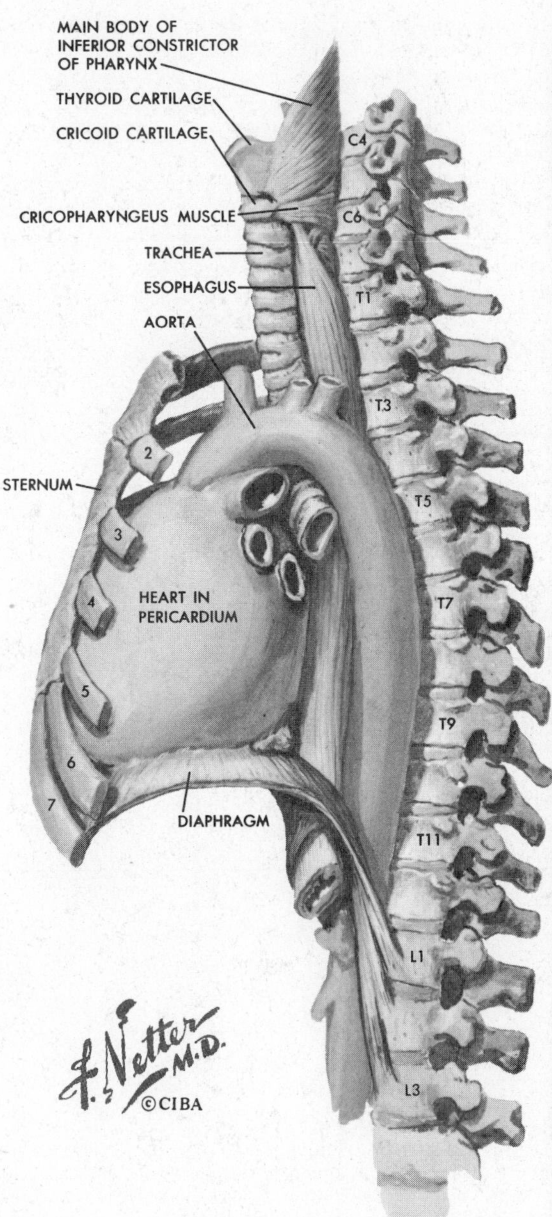

FIGURE 77–1. Relationship of esophagus to adjacent structures. ©Copyright 1959 CIBA Pharmaceutical Company, Division of CIBA-GEIGY Corporation. Reproduced, with permission, from THE CIBA COLLECTION OF MEDICAL ILLUSTRATIONS by Frank H. Netter, M.D. All rights reserved.

Symptoms of Disorders

Dysphagia, or difficulty in swallowing, is the most prominent symptom of any disorder of the esophagus. This may be difficulty in initiating the act, pain in relation to the act, or a feeling that the food is meeting resistance and sticking or pausing as it passes a particular portion of the esophagus.

Heartburn or *pyrosis* is another common symptom of esophageal disease. The term is frequently used by patients to describe very different sensations, so it is important to find out what this term means to the patient who uses it. It usually means substernal midline burning, which tends to radiate, generally in waves, upward to the neck. It is important to find out if the symptom is amplified when the patient lies down or bends over.

Esophageal regurgitation is the bringing of gastric contents up into the mouth without eructation and without the propulsive wave of reverse peristalsis present in vomiting. This tends to occur when stomach contents have refluxed into the esophagus or when the esophagus does not empty into the stomach.

Causes of Swallowing Problems

Swallowing is a highly complex act and causes of difficulty are numerous. Most problems are due either to some mechanical obstruction or to neuromotor malfunction.

Constriction of the passageway by congenital defects or such acquired conditions as tumors, inflammation, strictures, or hiatus hernia will cause difficulty in passing food masses that are larger than the constricted area. The patient usually first experiences difficulty in swallowing solids and then liquids when the problem is mechanical.

Motor dysfunction is usually caused by a problem in the reflex coordination of the act or in muscle function. In neuromotor disorders it is usually equally difficult to swallow solids and liquids. Neuromuscular disorders that can upset this delicately balanced act of swallowing include scleroderma, polymyositis, and diabetes mellitus. Myasthenia gravis can reduce the force of the propulsive wave.

DISORDERS OF THE ESOPHAGUS

STRUCTURAL

Congenital Anomalies

Several anomalies can occur during the embryonic development of the esophagus in its separation from the trachea. The two principal types of anomalies are atresia and fistula, which occur in several different forms. These become evident shortly after birth since the infant is unable to swallow without either regurgitating the fluid or aspirating it into the lungs. The most common types of anomalies are pictured in Figure 77–2. All of these require prompt surgical repair if the infant is to survive. Consult a pediatrics nursing text for the details of diagnosis, treatment, and nursing care.

Diverticuli

A diverticulum is a pouch opening out from a hollow viscus. They occur in the esophagus at the pharyngoesophageal sphincter, in the midesophagus at the level of the bifurcation of the bronchus, and in the region near the diaphragm. The second two are called traction diverticuli, are relatively rare, and frequently cause no symptoms.

A pulsion diverticulum, also called Zenker's diverticulum, is seen most often in males over 50 years of age. It occurs on the posterior wall of the pharynx above the upper border of the cricopharyngeus muscle and results from excessive pressure during swallowing, usually the result of the pharynx contracting before the sphincter relaxes. The sac gradually enlarges and descends into the superior mediastinum. The major symptom is the sensation of a foreign body in the throat and dysphagia for both solids and liquids.

As the diverticulum enlarges, it gradually alters the alignment of the esophagus and pharynx so that the most direct route from the pharynx is into the diverticulum rather than down the esophagus, causing an increasing volume of food to enter the diverticulum. Complications are malnourishment from inadequate intake and tracheal aspiration as a result of regurgitation from the sac on lying down. Perforation of the sac results in contamination of the mediastinum with potentially grave sequelae. This could occur during the passage of a nasogastric tube or esophagoscope.

Strictures

Strictures may be of inflammatory, traumatic, or congenital origin. Esophagitis, radiation, and corrosive burns are the most frequent causes. Treatment includes removal of the cause, if possible, and performing dilatations. Surgical excision may be necessary.

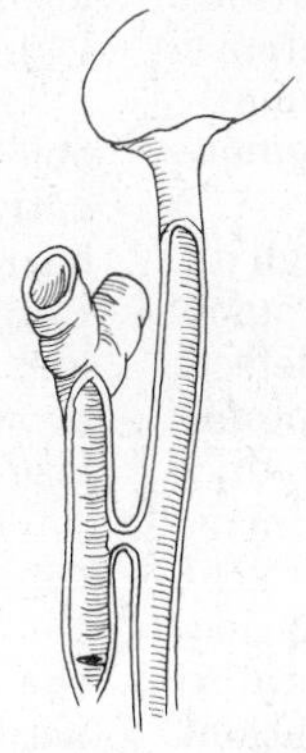

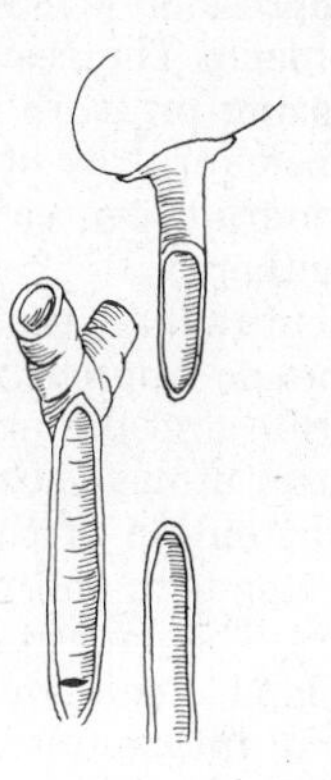

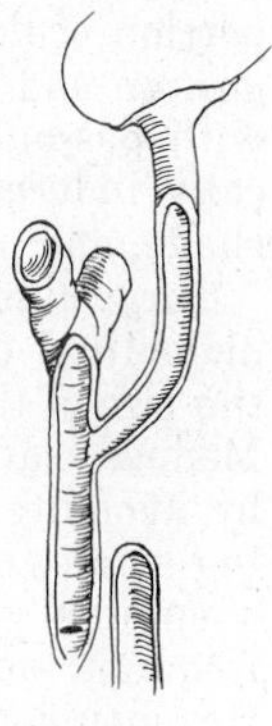

FIGURE 77–2. The most common forms of tracheoesophageal fistula and esophageal atresia. *A,* Atresia of the upper portion of the esophagus with a fistula connecting the lower portion of the esophagus to the trachea. *B,* Esophageal atresia without tracheal involvement. *C,* Fistulous connection of a normal trachea and esophagus (H-type fistula). (From Davis, L. A.: *Nursing Clinics of North America,* September, 1973.)

Achalasia

This condition is sometimes called cardiospasm or aperistalsis. It is caused by failure of swallowed food to enter the stomach and results in esophageal dilatation. It is probably due to the lack of a normal peristaltic wave, so that no stimulus for opening the cardiac sphincter occurs. A distended esophagus can cause pressure on the trachea, producing dyspnea and cough, and on the great vessels and heart, resulting in cardiac problems. Tracheal aspiration of foods retained in the esophagus occurs when the patient lies down.

The most probable cause of the condition is degeneration of innervation, either from the vagal motor nuclei or the myenteric plexus (Auerbach's). The interruption varies from mild to complete. Since innervation is destroyed, the only treatment is to dilate or cut the sphincter. This must be done extensively enough to allow the food to pass through but not so much as to allow the gastric contents to reflux back into the esophagus and cause esophagitis. In addition to dilitation, nonsurgical treatment includes helping the patient to learn to relax and to live with the condition.

Hiatus Hernia

This is a diaphragmatic hernia in which a portion of the stomach is herniated through the esophageal hiatus of the diaphragm. It can occur from sudden penetrating or compressive trauma or it can develop through congenital or acquired weaknesses in the diaphragm. In both the congenital and acquired weaknesses, intra-abdominal pressure, as from obesity, pregnancy, ascites, and physical exertion, can cause the abdominal contents to herniate upward through the defect.

Symptoms of the disorder, which vary from none at all to acutely severe, come mostly from esophageal reflux of gastric contents. The extent of symptoms is determined by the size of the hernia and the amount of compression placed on the herniated portion of the stomach. The resulting venous congestion and increasing pressure cause interference with passage of food into the stomach. Traumatically induced herniation can cause shock, hemorrhage, and pneumothorax.

Surgical treatment reduces the hernia through an abdominal or thoracic approach, depending upon the size of the hernia and the nature of the defect. Medical management aims to control the symptoms by avoiding overdistention of the stomach, reducing acidity of the stomach, and reducing the intra-abdominal pressure. The patient is instructed to eat frequent, small, bland meals and to take antacids. He should take no anticholinergic drugs because they delay emptying of the stomach. The patient should also avoid coughing and activities that involve bending forward. The patient usually has the head of his bed elevated to help to prevent esophageal reflux during sleep.

NEOPLASMS

Benign

There are very few benign lesions of the esophagus and most of these are asymptomatic. Leiomyoma accounts for more than half of those that do occur.

Malignant

Cancer of the esophagus occurs predominantly in men over 50 and accounts for only 2 per cent of cancer deaths. The mortality rate for carcinoma of the esophagus in white males in this country has remained constant since 1930, while the incidence among nonwhite males has risen from 1.3 to 10.2 per 100,000 male population between 1934 and 1966. Nonwhite males acquire this disease at an average age of 55.2 as opposed to 62.3 for white males. The reason for these differences is not clear. The worldwide incidence of the disease varies from country to country and from one area of a country to another. The ratio of incidence between males and females also varies from location to location. The etiology is unknown, but study is being made of the environmental differences between the locations with a low and high incidence. It is generally agreed that smoking and the ingestion of alcohol are related to the development of this disease.

The prognosis of cancer of the esophagus is very poor, with a low five-year survival rate. The reasons for this are the early lymphatic spread and late development of symptoms. The tumor growth causes a reduced amount of flexibility in the normally very distensible esophagus, causing most of the symptoms. The first symptom is typically dysphagia, but this usually does not occur until the tumor involves the whole circumference of the esophagus. By the time this symptom is reported to the physician, the tumor has frequently invaded the deeper layers of the esophagus and sometimes even adjacent structures such as the bronchus.

Tumors occur in any part of the esophagus, but the majority are in the lower two thirds. Diagnosis is made by barium swallow, esophagoscopy, cytologic examination, and direct biopsy.

Treatment is mainly surgical, with the major objective being to enable the patient to continue eating. Even when the tumor is small enough to be resected, a cure is not achieved. Cobalt radiation produces palliation by reducing tumor size and slowing growth, but it tends to cause fistulas to develop. Dilatations can be done to maintain the size of the lumen.

Various approaches have been used to maintain continuity of the esophagus and to allow the patient to eat normally after resection of the tumor: the stomach may be brought up into the mediastinum after the esophagus is shortened by a resection; a segment of the colon may be implanted to replace the resected portion; an artificial prosthesis may be inserted in the lumen; or a channel may be made to the exterior above and below the resected portion and an exterior tube used to connect them. None of these approaches is very satisfactory, but they have all achieved the purpose of allowing the patient to continue to eat normally for a longer period of time. When these approaches are impossible, a gastrostomy is usually done to maintain the patient's nutrition.

TRAUMA

The major traumatic conditions that affect the esophagus are chemical burns, foreign bodies, and injuries from external forces or from examination with an esophagoscope. Chemical burns occur from the ingestion of acids or alkalies and sometimes from the ingestion of highly spiced foods. Thermal burns can result from drinking extremely hot liquids. Foreign bodies are most apt to lodge in the natural narrow spots of the esophagus. Possible results of trauma are perforation with a resultant contamination of the mediastinum and stricture formation as healing occurs.

Vascular Disorders

Esophageal varices are the major disorder of vascular origin. Since these are the result of pressure in the portal system, they are discussed with liver conditions in Unit XVI.

Inflammatory Disorders

Esophagitis is an inflammation of the mucosa and submucosa that is usually caused by the reflux of gastric juices into the lower esophagus. The most prominent symptoms are heartburn; intolerance of spices, alcohol, and caffeine; and regurgitation, sometimes with vomiting. The patient may also experience dysphagia. Esophagitis is usually associated with hiatus hernia, but it can also occur independently. It is due to failure of the cardiac sphincter of the stomach to maintain enough pressure to prevent gastric contents from entering the esophagus.

Treatment is aimed at preventing the gastric juices from damaging the esophageal mucosa by the use of oral antacids, a bland diet, avoiding eating before lying down, and sleeping with the head of the bed elevated. Surgical approaches are intended to reduce the acidity of the stomach, as by a vagotomy, or to reduce reflux by tightening the sphincter muscle.

NURSING CARE OF THE PATIENT WITH A DISORDER OF THE ESOPHAGUS

Even though conditions that affect the esophagus differ widely in etiology, the symptoms are similar, varying mostly in intensity and time of occurrence. Difficulty in swallowing and discomfort due to regurgitation of gastric contents are the major symptoms presented by these patients. Nursing care needs, which are determined in large measure by the symptoms, are related to maintaining nutrition because of the swallowing difficulties, preventing complications resulting from malnutrition, and minimizing discomfort, since regurgitation and inability to eat cause both physical and psychologic pain. Nursing care will be discussed on the basis of the symptoms that may be presented by the patient.

DYSPHAGIA

This symptom varies from a mild feeling that food is sticking in the throat or esophagus to the total inability to consume foods or fluids. The patient who is admitted to a health care facility because of difficulty in swallowing should be closely observed by the nurse, since diagnosing the cause is one of the major aims of care. The nurse should record what kinds of foods the patient tolerates best —solids or liquids, hot or cold food—and whether he swallows better when he is alone or when he is in a social group, and if the time of day makes a difference in his ability. These observations will aid the physician in his determination of the cause, which might be psychogenic, neurologic, muscular, or a space-occupying lesion.

The patient who has a tumor within the lumen of the esophagus will experience increasing difficulty in taking food. More complete chewing and a diet that is thinner in consistency will aid in swallowing for a while. He should be encouraged to take only small amounts of food and to chew them thoroughly before attempting to swallow. Helping him to relax during meals by making him physically comfortable and by avoiding emotional stress will also be helpful.

The patient with acute dysphagia is frequently malnourished and may have problems as a result of altered electrolyte and metabolic balances within the body. Thus, he is a very good candidate for the complications of debilitating disease such as decubitus ulcer and pneumonia. He is particularly prone to develop respiratory complications from aspirated materials.

APHAGIA

Many problems ensue when the patient is unable to swallow anything, even liquids, because of a tumor or stricture in the upper esophagus. Since saliva and other nasopharyngeal mucous secretions must go somewhere, the patient can easily choke and must spit frequently or he drools. Constant wiping of saliva from his lips can cause irritation, with cracking of the skin and open lesions. Since it is impractical to collect this quantity of secretions in tissues, he should carry a receptacle to receive them. As most people find the sight of a jar of expectorated saliva repugnant, it is helpful if it is covered or made of opaque material and has a screw lid. This jar should be emptied fairly often, because of the odors which result from the presence of decomposing bacteria, pus, blood, and saliva. An exudate may be present, resulting from bacterial growth and necrosis of the devitalized tissues in the tumor mass.

When the tumor mass or stricture is in the lower two thirds of the esophagus, the patient's symptoms will come from distention of the esophagus and regurgitation.

The patient should have frequent oral care to maintain a tolerable taste in his mouth. A pleasant tasting mouthwash, a mild bicarbonate solution, or a physiological saline solution can be used. Diluted hydrogen peroxide is effective against anaerobic organisms and is sometimes mixed half and half with a mouthwash. The mouth should be rinsed often, and care taken to keep it in as healthy a condition as possible. Some patients chew food and expectorate it. This also helps to maintain the health of the oral tissues.

Gastrostomy. When surgical methods of providing a route from the mouth to the stomach fail, a gastrostomy is frequently done. Occasionally a nasogastric feeding tube is left in place. In either method, the patient must consume his diet through a tube, which means he does not derive pleasure from eating and chewing and all food that is ingested must be in liquid form. (See Chapter 75 for Gavage.)

A gastrostomy is made by suturing the anterior wall of the stomach to the abdominal surface and tightly suturing either a valve prosthesis or a tube (frequently a Foley catheter) into the opening. The tube prevents leakage of the acid gastric juices onto the abdominal wall, and the attachment between the wall of the stomach and the abdomen prevents the leakage of gastric contents into the abdominal cavity.

The skin about the opening should be washed with a gentle soap and thoroughly dried twice daily, or whenever secretions leak. Protective ointments such as zinc oxide can be applied to the skin for lubrication and protection from secretions.

Intake of nutrients and fluids through the gastrostomy is essential to this patient's continued life. Members of his family should also know how to manage the feedings. Frequently these patients remain at home, and nursing supervision will aid the family in coping with problems that arise. In addition to routine health supervision, the nurse should check facets of care related to the gastrostomy such as urinary and bowel elimination. An inadequate urine output might mean that the patient is getting insufficient fluids via the gastrostomy tube or that his kidneys are overloaded with nitrogenous products. Constipation could indicate an inadequate fluid intake, or it could result from the liquid feedings. Diarrhea can be caused by improper storage of the feedings, or it could be due to the formula used in the feedings.

The nurse should check for evidence that the tube is patent and that the patient is using proper technique in caring for it and that he is consuming a well balanced diet.

Since a gastrostomy, if done for cancer, is a palliative measure, the patient and his family will need support from the nurse, as for any dying patient. (See Chapter 15 for care of the dying patient and Chapter 35 for care of the terminal cancer patient.)

Discomfort

Heartburn is the usual symptom of regurgitation of stomach contents into the esophagus. Its origin is not certain, but is thought to be due to irritation of the esophageal mucosa by the acid secretions of the stomach. Antacids help by neutralizing the acid secretions. Emptying of the esophageal contents into the stomach is sometimes facilitated by having the patient maintain an upright position for several hours after meals and by helping him to relax. Of course, the cause of the retention of food in the esophagus may alter the approach to treatment.

When the esophagus is occluded and swallowed food is retained, discomfort comes mainly from the distention and the shortness of breath caused by pressure on the lungs. Little can be done except to help the patient to relax and to encourage him to ingest smaller amounts at one time. Dilatations of the stricture and sometimes surgery are the treatments of choice.

OBSERVATIONS TO BE MADE ON PATIENTS WITH ESOPHAGEAL PROBLEMS

In addition to the observations of the patient's ability to swallow, the nurse should also observe and report the patient's general nutritional status and his state of hydration. His weight should be checked. Sometimes the patient is able to obtain sufficient foods and fluids even when he encounters great difficulty in swallowing. Other patients may need supplementary fluids and nourishment.

Pain—its type, duration, location, and the time of its onset—is a significant factor, as is the presence of gaseousness as evidenced by eructations, abdominal distention with tympanites, and flatulence. Does the patient retain the food he eats? Does he regurgitate it, or is it vomited? If he vomits it from the stomach with propulsive waves, is this accompanied by nausea?

The patient's acceptance of the condition and his general mental state are important in evaluating his acceptance of some of the potential treatment measures. His family and their helpfulness to him as well as their emotional stability are also important factors to assess.

PRE- AND POSTOPERATIVE NURSING CARE

In addition to the usual factors involved in nursing care of the surgical patient there are some specific things to consider when a patient has esophageal surgery, but they depend upon where in the esophagus the problem is located and the patient's nutritional status. A gastrostomy may be done to enable the patient to take a high protein, high caloric diet preoperatively, since a poorly nourished patient is not a good surgical risk. In most surgical procedures the patient should be prepared for a chest incision and be taught about chest tubes and coughing, as are other thoracic surgical patients. (See Section XIV for care of the thoracic surgical patient.)

Depending upon the procedure to be done, the patient's prognosis will vary from excellent to very poor. The surgical procedure may offer a hope of cure, as in a pulsion diverticulum or benign stricture, or it may offer only palliation, as in surgery for cancer of the esophagus. Procedures that are done for incompetency and overcompetency of the cardiac sphincter are only partially successful. The nurse should find out from the surgeon what the probable survival results will be before discussing anticipated surgery with the patient. He should not receive, even indirectly, an expectation of results that are impossible to achieve.

After surgery the patient will probably have both chest and gastric suction and an incision that extends from the thoracic region to the abdomen. A tracheostomy may be present. A nasogastric tube is usually placed in the stomach during surgery and attached to suction to remove fluids and drainage from the surgical site and to divert food and fluids away from the surgical anastomosis until healing has taken place. It should not be removed or adjusted, because the suture line might be damaged by trauma from the tube. It will remain in place postoperatively until enough healing has occurred to allow food and fluids to pass without danger of the formation of a fistula into the mediastinum.

In the immediate postoperative period, *maintenance of patency of the chest, tracheostomy, and gastric tubes* is the most important nursing responsibility. The major goal of care in the convalescent surgical period is to aid in the healing of the esophageal suture lines by keeping the gastric suction open and functioning. This prevents tension from distention and keeps the tubes free from secretions, fluids, and food which might leak into the mediastinum, creating a fistulous tract and causing infection. The patient may be kept flat in bed immediately after surgery to prevent pulling and tension on the suture line when an anastomosis has been created in the esophagus.

This patient should be observed for respiratory complications and for the occurrence of a fistula and/or infection. Mouth care is important in the prevention of both of these complications. Routine postoperative measures such as leg and arm and breathing exercises are also extremely important.

Patients who are not allowed to eat for 10 days to 2 weeks after surgery may have a gastrostomy for feeding purposes, or if a nasogastric tube is left in place, a diet may be instilled through it.

After an oral diet has been resumed, the patient who has had his stomach brought up into the thoracic cavity may experience discomfort because of the presence of a full stomach within the chest. Procedures in which the cardiac sphincter has been eliminated or made incompetent may leave the patient with heartburn from esophageal reflux of gastric acid. Remaining upright after meals, sleeping with the head of the bed elevated, and taking antacids will help to control these symptoms.

When the patient resumes oral feeding, he will begin with clear water and gradually progress to soft foods as his ability to swallow develops. A high esophageal anastomosis may create difficulties for the patient in relearning to swallow.

CHAPTER 78

Abnormalities of the Stomach and Proximal Duodenum

ANATOMY AND PHYSIOLOGY

Digestion, which has started in the mouth, continues in the stomach by the action of saliva in the center of the bolus. Gastric secretions begin the next phase of digestion, by breaking down connective tissues and beginning the digestion of proteins, as described earlier in this unit. There is very little absorption within the stomach. Alcohol and acetylsalicylic acid are the two most important chemicals absorbed there. The chief functions of the stomach are to mix the chyme and to regulate the flow of gastric contents into the upper intestine. The rate of emptying depends upon the volume ingested, the thoroughness with which it has been chewed, and the nature of the ingested food. Fats and foods that have been poorly chewed are retained longer.

SYMPTOMS OF DYSFUNCTION

Symptoms of dysfunction are caused by excessive gastric secretions (which feed upon the stomach mucosa), by excessive motility, or by retention of gastric contents. The most prominent symptoms are pain, acid eructations and belching, nausea, vomiting, hemorrhage, and diarrhea.

Pain, the most characteristic symptom, is caused mostly by acid in contact with eroded stomach mucosa resulting in chemical irritation of nerve endings. It is also caused by stretching and sudden contractions of the stomach, which results in a stretching of the nerve terminals. This can be caused by increased motility and increased smooth muscle tension, as found in an obstruction.

Anorexia or loss of appetite occurs in various diseases such as hepatitis and is also present in mental depression. Hunger is caused by a number of stimuli, including contraction of the empty stomach. When the stomach empties slowly, one normal stimulus of the hunger sensation is missing and anorexia can result.

Nausea is produced by any condition, such as unpleasant stimuli or distention, that increases tension on the walls of the stomach, duodenum, or lower end of the esophagus. *Vomiting* can follow nausea or occur without it. Vomiting is caused by stimulation of the emetic center, which is in the medulla near the sensory nucleus of the vagus. It is influenced by the chemoreceptor trigger zone as well as by nerve impulses and can be excited by (1) direct mechanical stimuli, as in increased intracranial pressure; (2) chemical stimuli from bloodborne metabolites or toxic substances; and (3) afferent nerve impulses through the vagus, glossopharyngeal, vestibular, and possibly even the splanchnic nerves. In most people higher center impulses such as those caused by unpleasant odors, subjects, and sights can also stimulate vomiting. Drugs of the phenothiazine derivative group, such as chlorpromazine (Thorazine), promazine (Sparine) and prochlorperazine (Compazine), depress vomiting caused by chemoreceptor stimulation.

Bleeding results from local trauma or irritations that cause erosion or ulceration of the mucosa. *Diarrhea* can be caused by increased peristalsis resulting from an increased gastrocolic reflex or from the effort of the stomach and intestines to eliminate a local irritant. *Belching* and *flatulence* are caused predominantly by swallowed air. Frequently the individual attempts to belch to relieve a vague feeling of distress in the stomach. When attempting to belch with the mouth closed, the person sometimes adds more air to the stomach than he removes. Air is swallowed easily during eating and drinking, especially by nervous persons who ingest food rapidly.

FUNCTIONAL DISORDERS

Gastric functions are mediated largely through central nervous system activities. The central nervous system is strongly influenced by stimuli from social, environmental, and psychologic influences; these factors also affect the individual's gastric response. The stomach mirrors the emotions.

INDIGESTION (DYSPEPSIA)

Since the factors influencing digestion are so numerous, dyspepsia can be due to emotional problems, to disease of the gastrointestinal system, to disease processes elsewhere in the body, or to such things as eating too rapidly, chewing inadequately, eating during a period of emotional upset, poorly cooked foods, or ingestion of foods known as gas formers. Food allergy may be responsible. Symptoms usually occur from altered gastric secretion or motor activity. They include a feeling of fullness,

TABLE 78–1. CAUSES OF ALTERED GASTRIC MOTILITY AND SECRETION

Increased Motility	Decreased Motility
Hunger	Marked distention (overeating)
Prospect of appetizing food	Ingestion of fats
Pleasant sensory stimuli	Smoking
Moderate distention	Physical fatigue
Alcohol	Unpleasant sensory stimuli
Coffee	Pain
Hostility	Fear
Anxiety	Shock
Resentment	Depression
	Sadness
Increased Secretion	**Decreased Secretion**
Sight, smell, and taste of food	Depression
Prolonged anxiety, guilt, conflict, hostility, or resentment	Release of enterogastrone
Presence of food in stomach	pH of 1.5 or lower

nausea, belching or eructations, heartburn, and flatulence. Table 78–1 lists causes of altered motility and secretion.

ANOREXIA NERVOSA

This is a psychoneurotic state that usually occurs in females in their late teens and early twenties. The patient develops amenorrhea as a result of a block to the release of neurohumoral impulses from the hypothalamus, preventing the release of luteinizing hormone from the pituitary. No other glandular failure is evident. A distaste for food develops and the patient refuses to eat. Treatment, after the patient has gained some weight, is psychotherapy. Gentle persuasion to encourage the patient to eat is the preferred method of achieving weight gain, but this is difficult to accomplish and sometimes tube feedings are used. Vomiting is common when the patient is fed by force.

OVEREATING (OBESITY)

The presence of an excess of adipose tissue in the body is termed obesity. It is caused by a caloric intake that exceeds the energy expenditure. Although it can be the result of a metabolic dysfunction, it is usually due merely to an intake that is greater than the body's needs. A number of metabolic abnormalities are present in obese persons, but they are probably the result of the obesity rather than the cause. Obesity tends to run in families, but this is probably the result of appetite and food patterns learned in the home rather than an inherited dysfunction. The average person balances his intake with his needs, and his weight remains fairly constant throughout most of his adult life. A weight gain frequently accompanies aging because activities become more sedentary and the individual frequently does not adjust his intake to meet these lowered needs. Since weight tends to be self-sustaining, vigilance is needed to maintain losses that are achieved.

Treatment is basically dietary. A number of diets are advocated but, at the present time, there is no basis for recommending one over another, except that a diet that is maintained over a long period of time must supply necessary nutrients for the continued health of the individual. Starvation can be tolerated for repeated periods of 10 to 15 days if fluids and vitamins are provided; it results in an average weight loss of one pound per day. Complications include postural hypotension, anemia, cardiac irregularities, and a decreased uric acid excretion with a hyperuricemia, which is reversed when the fast is halted and may then result in uric acid neuropathy and retention of sodium and water. It is best that the individual be hospitalized when this method of therapy is used.

Drugs. Appetite depressant drugs from the amphetamine group are sometimes used at the beginning of a diet. They are effective for only a few weeks and may cause problems because of their stimulating effects. More importantly, it is sometimes difficult to withdraw the person from their use because they are addictive.

Exercise. As a method of weight loss this is not of practical value because of the amount of exercise needed to lose one pound; however, any added activity increases the energy output and increases the caloric deficit of a patient who is following a weight loss dietary regimen. In some sedentary patients a little planned activity without any alteration in dietary habits can make the difference between a diet that maintains weight and one that achieves a small weight loss. Any obese patient who is on a calorie-restricted program should have a planned, gradually increasing program of energy output to aid in weight loss and to tone muscles.

Surgery. The surgical approach to treating obesity is an attempt to reduce the ability of the body to absorb nutrients that are ingested. This is done by short-circuiting the small bowel. Trial has shown that the best results from this type of surgery are obtained when a shunt is created by severing the jejunum 14 inches from its beginning and anastomosing this end to the terminal ileum 4 inches above the ileocecal valve. This leaves the patient with 18 inches of small bowel. The weight loss after operation averages 11 pounds per month for six months and then six pounds per month the second six months, 4½ pounds per month the second year, and 2 pounds per month the third year. When the patient reaches his optimal weight he tends to maintain it. When the short circuit has been removed surgically and the bowel returned to normal, patients have regained their former weight.[48] Postoperatively the patient may have diarrhea for a period of time because of induced malabsorption. This surgery should be reserved for the extremely obese person, weighing 300 or more pounds, for whom weight loss is essential to the maintenance of health. Before the surgery is done, a psychiatric evaluation should be made, as patients who have been meeting emotional needs or escaping problems by their excessive weight may have other problems after a weight loss.

Complications. Atherosclerosis and its associated ischemic heart disease are caused by the altered metabolism of obesity. Hypertension and left ventricular hypertrophy occur as a result of pumping blood through an enlarged vascular bed. Diabetes mellitus is four times more common in the obese individual.

INFLAMMATIONS

ACUTE GASTRITIS

The acute form of gastritis may be manifested by nausea and vomiting, hemorrhage, pain, malaise, anorexia, or headache and is usually due to ingestion of a corrosive, erosive, or infectious substance. Aspirin, acute alcoholism, and food poisoning are common causes. This type of gastritis is usually of short duration unless extensive damage is sustained by the gastric mucosa. Treatment is to remove the cause and treat the condition symptomatically. Vomiting frequently responds to some of the drugs of the phenothiazine group given orally or intramuscularly; pain usually responds to antacids. If hemorrhage is severe enough, a transfusion may be necessary.

CHRONIC GASTRITIS

This condition is seen in three different forms: Superficial gastritis causes a reddened, edematous mucosa with hemorrhages and small erosions. Atrophic gastritis occurs in all layers of the stomach, with a decreased number of parietal and chief cells. This form of gastritis is seen frequently in association with gastric ulcer and gastric cancer and is invariably present in pernicious anemia. Hypertrophic gastritis produces a mucosa that is dull and nodular in appearance and has irregular, thickened, or nodular rugae. Hemorrhages are frequent. Chronic gastritis usually heals without scarring but can go on to hemorrhage and the formation of an ulcer. Symptoms of chronic gastritis are vague and may be absent. The patients are apt to have a loss of appetite, a feeling of fullness, belching, vague epigastric pain, and nausea and vomiting. Most patients learn to avoid foods that cause symptoms. Antacids sometimes give symptomatic relief.

ULCERATIONS

An ulceration is a sharply circumscribed area in which there is loss of tissue. Peptic ulcers are caused by excessive acid and occur in the stomach, proximal duodenum or, occasionally, in the lower esophagus. Many authorities now question that peptic ulcers are one disease entity and feel that a gastric ulcer is not the same condition as a duodenal ulcer and that gastric ulcers may be of different types. The incidence, etiology, and treatment of these lesions are different, but the symptoms are quite similar.

Even though gastric secretions are capable of breaking down any living tissue, the stomach mucosa is not ordinarily digested by them because they are adequately diluted, neutralized, and buffered before they can harm the mucosa; also, the mucosa is thickly covered by a protective layer of mucus. An alteration in either of these defense systems can cause autodigestion to occur. Another protective mechanism is the rapidity with which the gastric mucosa normally heals. In addition to peptic and gastric ulcers, stress ulcers, sometimes called Cushing's; Curling's, which occurs in conjunction with severe burns; and drug-induced ulcers also occur.

ETIOLOGY

Peptic, Duodenal and Gastric Ulcers

Duodenal ulcers and some prepyloric gastric ulcers are caused by an increased quantity or an increased level of acidity of the gastric juice, which apparently overcomes the mucous blanket. Hypersecretion of acid continues between meals when there is no stimulus for secretion. The cause of this is unknown, but in duodenal ulcer it is thought to be of vagal origin because a vagotomy reduces it.

Gastric ulcers are not associated with excessive acid levels, and theories as to their origin vary and include one which proposes that excess acid is secreted by the stomach but is resorbed by an abnormal diffusion of hydrogen ions through the mucous membrane, damaging the mucous barrier. Another theory suggests that destruction of the mucous blanket occurs from the reflux of alkaline duodenal contents. There is a variation in the number of parietal cells in relation to the location of the ulcer. The normal stomach is estimated to have 0.92 billion, while the stomach with a gastric ulcer has 0.65 billion, and the one with a duodenal ulcer has 1.72 billion. It is felt that vagal stimulation causes this increase in the parietal cell mass.

Psychogenic influences have been shown to affect the development of peptic ulcers. This is more true for the duodenal than the gastric ulcer. The tensions and strains of life cause an increase in the tonus of the vagus nerves, involving both the motor and secretory fibers. The secretions increase and the friability of the mucosa also increases. Those who live under stress, such as those with responsible managerial positions, are more prone to this disorder. However, prolonged psychotherapy has not proved to be of any help.

Stress and Drug-induced Ulcers

Other ulcerations are associated with irritations to the stomach from the ingestion of drugs, especially aspirin, alcohol, and some spices. Prolonged psychologic or physiologic stress produces a so-called stress ulcer, which is thought to be due to increased secretion of gastric juices as a result of prolonged vagal stimulation. Menguy[40] described this condition, which causes superficial gastric erosions and is frequently manifested by massive gastric hemorrhage, as an acute gastric mucosal lesion. The patient characteristically has multiple lesions, usually small, which may give the appearance of "oozing blood." The etiology is not certain and may be excessive acid or an alteration in the protective ability of the mucous barrier. Brooks,[6] observing patients who had gastric hemorrhage following organ transplant surgery, found organisms growing in the aspirated gastric contents when the pH rose. He instilled antibiotic solutions into the nasogastric tubes and in two patients the pH dropped and in six patients the bleeding stopped. This suggests some interesting avenues for future research into this subject in which there are many questions, many opinions, and very few definite answers.

SYMPTOMS

The most common and typical symptom is chronic and periodic *pain*, which has been variously described as gnawing, aching, burning, and boring. It occurs from one to four hours after eating and may also occur in the middle of the night. The pain is sharply localized in the epigastrium to the left of the midline. Sometimes it occurs as heartburn. Periods of remission, which may last from a few months to a period of years, are common. Pain of this nature is pathognomonic of a peptic ulcer.

Weight loss, probably from a reduced intake of food, is typical, but some persons gain weight from excessive eating to neutralize the pain. Other symptoms relate to the development of complications. *Bleeding* from erosion through a blood vessel is common. It may occur as a massive hemorrhage or it may be occult from slow oozing.

Longstanding disease causes scarring from repeated ulcerations and repeated healing. Scarring, when it occurs at the pylorus, frequently causes pyloric obstruction, which is manifested most often by pain at night as a result of the retention of acid. Pyloric obstruction can also lead to *vomiting.*

Perforation occurs when an ulcer erodes through the muscularis and is manifested by sudden, sharp, severe pain which begins in the midepigastrium and, as peritonitis develops, spreads over the entire abdomen, which then becomes hard and rigidly board-like.

INCIDENCE

Ulcers are more common in men than in women, and this is particularly true for duodenal lesions. Both gastric and duodenal ulcers occur at all ages, but peptic ulcers have the highest incidence in the 45 to 55 year old group. The possible presence of a hereditary factor in the development of an ulcer, which has been suspected for years, has recently gained some credence. A relationship has been shown between the individual's ABO blood group and the site of occurrence of an ulcer. For instance, Johnson[27] found an association between blood group A and certain types of gastric ulcer. Also, the parietal cell mass, and consequently the rate of gastric acid secretion, are felt by some workers to be genetically determined.[55a] Hereditary factors cannot be considered without also considering other factors that might influence the incidence, such as dietary habits, emotional reactions, and economic and occupational status, which are frequently similar among family members. Gastric ulcers are more apt to occur in the impoverished social groups, in the elderly, and in the poorly nourished.

DIAGNOSIS

Ulcers are diagnosed by the symptoms, by x-ray evidence and, when indicated, by gastroscopy. The differentiation between the types of ulcer is sometimes difficult. The time lapse between eating and the onset of pain may help to pinpoint the location of the ulcer. Pain relieved by antacids or food is typical of duodenal ulcer. Acid determinations may be done on aspirated gastric juices, but the results are frequently not very helpful because individual variations tend to obscure the typical findings in each type of ulcer.

COMPLICATIONS

Hemorrhage varies from minimal, which is manifested by occult blood in the stool, to massive, in which the patient vomits bright red blood—hematemesis. The usual symptoms of GI bleeding are either vomiting coffee-ground material or passing tarry stools. Acid digestion of blood in the stomach results in a granular dark emesis, whereas the complete digestion process results in a black stool. If the patient bleeds rapidly enough, he can be prostrated and go into shock. It is important to locate the area of bleeding so treatment can be started.

Observations as to the color, consistency, and quantity of emesis and stools and the time of their passing will help the physician to make this decision. A nasogastric tube may be inserted and lavage with iced water or saline carried out to slow or to stop the bleeding; gastroscopy may be done to view the bleeding area, or a string test may be performed. In this test the patient swallows a measured string that is viewed for staining after its removal to help to locate the level of the bleeding

Perforation is usually a surgical emergency, since anterior wall perforation, unless it is walled off by the omentum, causes a chemical peritonitis. Surgical treatment is usually limited to closure of the perforation by patching it with a bit of omentum and cleansing the peritoneal cavity. The mortality is high in this condition, approximating 10 to 15 per cent. If the perforation occurs on the posterior gastric wall, it may erode through to adjacent organs and be sealed off, causing few symptoms. Pancreatitis usually results when a perforation erodes into that organ.

Obstruction, manifested by vomiting, occurs at the pylorus and is due to scarring, edema, and inflammation, or a combination of these. When vomiting persists, the patient is apt to go into alkalosis as a result of losing large quantities of acid gastric juice in the emesis. A patient who vomits persistently is usually hospitalized to receive intravenous fluids fortified with electrolytes. Before stenosis causes complete obstruction, the patient will probably experience gradually increasing difficulty in emptying his stomach and have feelings of fullness, with a loss of appetite and weight loss. The treatment is surgical release of the scar.

THERAPEUTIC REGIMEN

The goals of treatment for a patient with an ulceration are to prevent complications and to allow the ulcer to heal. Gastric mucosa has great regenerative powers, and ulcers frequently heal when the etiologic agent is removed. Mental, physical, and gastric rest is frequently sufficient therapy. Since psychogenic influences in the development of this condition are great, the patient needs emotional support while he identifies the stressors in his life and learns either to eliminate them or to cope with them. In many cases the biggest problem is the patient's inability to admit that he has stress or that it is a problem.

Much of the therapeutic regimen is aimed at relieving symptoms. This means eliminating factors that stimulate secretions, especially smoking, alcohol, coffee, and ulcerogenic drugs such as aspirin, steroids, and indomethacin. Antacids are administered to neutralize excess acidity; they seem to work even when excess acidity has not been shown to be present.

Medical

Traditionally, diet and antacids have been the principal method of managing an ulcer. Milk and cream formed the basis of the diet and were taken every hour, with antacids given on half hour in between. Currently this has fallen into some disfavor. Many authorities feel that eliminating strong secretagogues, roughage, gas-forming foods, and highly seasoned foods is sufficient. The patient should avoid any food that causes him pain, and this varies with the individual. Some physicians feel that six small meals are desirable, whereas others prefer the normal three-meal routine, but both groups agree that antacids are essential between meals. This provides a fairly continuous neutralization of the excess acid and also coats the mucous lining of the stomach to provide protection.

Medications

The ideal antacid is one that decreases the acidity, is effective for a prolonged period of time, is pleasant to take orally, is not constipating or cathartic in effect, and is not absorbed to cause systemic effects. There is no perfect antacid. Calcium carbonate is a potent antacid but is constipating. Magnesium carbonate and magnesium oxide are also potent antacids but are laxative; they are sometimes prescribed to counteract the constipating effects of calcium carbonate. Frequently the patient takes them alternately or balances dosages of each to produce a stool of the desired consistency. Aluminum hydroxide, phosphate, and carbonate, in doses of 15 to 30 ml. hourly, are less effective, since they only partially neutralize the acid. The magnesium and aluminum preparations are more palatable. Sodium bicarbonate is a potent antacid, but its effects are very brief and it is absorbed systemically. New products are on the market that are mixtures of aluminum and magnesium products with some calcium carbonate. Pharmaceutical firms have attempted to produce an antacid with ideal qualities by mixing these drugs. Table 78–2 lists the more commonly used antacids.

Other medications used are anticholinergics, sedatives, and ataractic drugs. Anticholinergics interfere with the transmission of nerve impulses at the neuro-effector junctions of the postganglionic nerves. They suppress both vagal and antral secretion mechanisms and produce what is sometimes called a medical vagotomy. The problem with these drugs is that they do not suppress acid secretion in response to food as well as they do the basal flow of secretion, and in order to achieve sufficient suppression of secretion a large enough dosage is necessary to cause intolerable side effects such as dryness of the mouth, blurring of vision, constipation and, sometimes, urinary retention owing to bladder atony. They also reduce the motility of the stomach, causing a feeling of fullness because of slowed emptying. There are many drugs of this nature on the market, but none is used for total therapy.

Sedatives frequently used are phenobarbital, 15 to 300 mg. 4 times daily, and ataractic drugs, including prochlorperazine (Compazine 5 mg.) and methaminodiazepoxide (Librium 5 to 10 mg.).

Instruction of Patient

Patient cooperation, which results from patient education, is the cornerstone of treatment. The patient must understand the pathogenesis of the ulcer and the significance of the pain. He should realize that healing takes place rapidly when the irritating effect is removed. He must understand what caused his condition to develop and what must be done to lessen the stimulation so a cure can occur and be maintained. He must discover what substances cause him to have pain because they stimulate the secretion of gastric juices, and he must be willing to eliminate them from his diet until healing has occurred. Later he will probably be able to resume use of some of them in moderation. He must understand the importance of continuing his medical regimen, even though his pain is gone, until healing is completed. He will need and should receive instruction and understanding support from the medical and nursing personnel who work with him during the course of his disease.

Nursing Responsibilities

Nursing management depends upon the physical state of the patient. Observing and reporting symptoms that might indicate the presence of a complication and symptoms that will help in pinpointing the diagnosis are among the most important nursing functions. These were mentioned in the preceding discussion. Symptoms should be recorded accurately and reported to the physician immediately when indicated.

The nursing goal is to help the patient to achieve total rest—physically and mentally. This is done by strictly maintaining the medical regimen and arranging the patient's environment to promote physical and mental relaxation. Interacting with the patient and helping him to accept and to maintain the prescribed dietary and drug regimen is chiefly a nursing function. Listening to him attentively is important, because the nurse is in a strategic position to help the patient to understand himself and his situation.

Nursing staff must be alert for factors that interfere with the patient's rest. Certain visitors may cause the patient to become agitated. Some patients attempt to do their normal work routine from the hospital bed; one patient moved his secretary and her typewriter into his hospital room. Obviously such actions as these are not conducive to mental or physical rest. Sometimes the nurse's ingenuity and tact are stretched to their limits in attempting to deal with these patients in a constructive manner.

SURGICAL TREATMENT OF GASTRIC ULCER

Surgery of the stomach is done (1) to reduce the acid-secreting ability of the stomach, (2) to remove a malignant or potentially malignant lesion, or (3) to treat a surgical emergency that develops as a complication of peptic ulcer disease.

When medical management of an ulcer fails,

TABLE 78–2. GASTRIC ANTACIDS

Official Nonproprietary Name		Properties	Synonyms or Trade Names	Dosage
Aluminum hydroxide gel U.S.P.	C	Slowly reactive as antacid	Amphojel, Creamalin	5 to 30 ml.
Aluminum phosphate gel N.F.	C	Slowly reactive as antacid	Phosphalgel	15 ml.
Calcium carbonate, precipitated U.S.P.	C	Chalky taste	Precipitated chalk, Titralac	1 to 2 Gm.
Dihydroxy aluminum aminoacetate, N.F.	C	Less constipating and faster acting than aluminum hydroxide	Alglyn, Robalate	500 to 1000 mg.
Magaldrate (monalium hydrate)			Riopan	400 to 800 mg.
Magnesium carbonate N.F.	L	High neutralizing action; forms CO_2		600 mg.
Magnesium oxide U.S.P.	L			250 to 1500 mg.
Magnesium trisilicate U.S.P.	L	Slower onset of action		1 to 4 Gm.
Milk of magnesia U.S.P.	L	Some systemic action	Magnesium hydroxide, magnesia magma	5 to 30 ml.
Polyamine-methylene resin	L	May cause mild bulk laxative action; low neutralizing action	Resinat, Carboresin	500 to 1000 mg.
Potassium bicarbonate U.S.P.		Systemic action		500 to 2000 mg.
Sodium bicarbonate U.S.P.		Systemic action	Baking soda	100 to 4000 mg.

C = constipating action; L = laxative or cathartic action.

surgical intervention is indicated. Most chronic, recurring ulcers are eventually treated surgically.

The possibility of cancer in a gastric lesion is a generally accepted indication for surgery. When an ulcer does not respond to intensive medical therapy and a definite diagnosis cannot be made by x-ray and gastroscopy, surgery is done to remove the lesion and to make certain it is not malignant.

Emergencies such as acute obstruction, perforation, and acute intractable hemorrhage are usually treated by surgical intervention as soon as possible. Hemorrhage, as mentioned, sometimes responds to medical management, but when medical approaches such as cooling and neutralization of the acid do not stop the bleeding, the situation is a surgical emergency if the patient's life is to be saved.

Goals of Therapy

Since excess acidity is the cause of many ulcerations, the goal of surgery is to reduce the acidity and thus allow the ulcer to heal. The surgical procedure may or may not remove the ulcer itself. In the presence of obstruction the second goal is to reestablish the patency of the lumen of the bowel by removing or relaxing the pyloric scar formation or by creating a new exit from the stomach.

Types of Surgery

The approaches for reducing acidity of the stomach surgically are (1) severing nerves that stimulate the acid-secreting cells, and (2) removing the acid-secreting portions of the stomach.

A *vagotomy* is done to eliminate the acid-secreting stimulus to gastric cells. The number of branches of the vagus nerve removed is dependent upon how much reduction in secretory ability is desired. When an insufficient number of nerves are removed, the ability of the stomach to secrete tends to regenerate with time. Since the vagus nerve also stimulates motility, the stomach is relatively atonic following this surgery and empties slowly. In order to prevent this and the resultant feeling of fullness, belching, and weight loss, a pyloroplasty or gastroenterostomy is usually done in conjunction with the surgery to enhance emptying (Fig. 78–1).

An *antrectomy* or *subtotal gastrectomy* is done to reduce the acid-secreting portions of the stomach. An antrectomy removes the cells that secrete gastrin and thus delays or eliminates the gastric phase of digestion by withdrawing that source of stimulation for acid release. In a subtotal gastric resection, the removal of 60 to 80 per cent of the stomach eliminates the acid-secreting cells. The extent of reduction of acid is determined by the amount of stomach removed. A vagotomy is sometimes done in conjunction with either of these procedures (Fig. 78–1). It must be remembered that pancreatic secretions and bile continue to be secreted into the duodenum even after gastrectomy and are necessary for digestion, so a route must be preserved for them to reach the chyme.

Complications

When a high level of gastric acid secretions remains after a gastroenterostomy or gastric resection, a *marginal* ulcer can develop where the gastric acids contact the operative site, either at the site of the anastomosis or in the jejunum. This ulceration can cause scarring and obstruction of the passages; hemorrhage and perforation can also occur.

Afferent loop syndrome is the name given to a complication in which the duodenal loop is partially obstructed after a Billroth II resection and the pancreatic secretions and bile which fill it after a meal are unable to reach the jejunum. The loop becomes distended, and painful contractions occur as effort is made to propel these secretions. When they finally enter the jejunum, the excessive pressure forces them back into the stomach and vomiting occurs. The patient experiences pain, nausea, and distention after meals, which is relieved by vomiting; the vomit usually contains bile.

Several *problems of nutrition* develop from removal of the stomach; these include a deficiency in vitamin B_{12} and folic acid, a disordered calcium metabolism, and reduced absorption of calcium and vitamin D. These are caused by a shortage of the intrinsic factor resulting from the resection, and inadequate absorption owing to rapid entry of food into the bowel. In the Billroth II gastric resection there is a reduction in the secretion of pancreatic juices and bile because the stimulus of food passing through the duodenum is missing.

The *dumping syndrome* occurs after gastric resection because of the rapid entry of ingested food into the jejunum without proper mixing and without the normal digestive processes of the duodenum having been accomplished. Early manifestations, which occur 5 to 30 minutes after eating, are the vasomotor disturbances of vertigo, sweating, pallor, palpitation, diarrhea, nausea, and the desire to lie down. The patient's blood pressure and pulse may either rise or fall. The late manifestations, which occur two to three hours after eating, are caused by a release of excessive insulin, which follows a rapid rise in the blood sugar resulting from the rapid entry of high carbohydrate food into the jejunum. The early manifestations are thought to be due to rapid movement of extracellular fluids into the bowel to convert the hypertonic material that entered very rapidly into an isotonic mixture. This rapid fluid shift decreases the circulating blood volume, causing the symptoms.

The treatment of the dumping syndrome is to decrease the amount of food taken at one time and to give a high-protein, high-fat, low-carbohydrate diet. Gastric emptying can be delayed by not taking fluids with meals and by eating in a recumbent or semirecumbent position or by lying down after meals. Sedatives and antispasmodics are given to

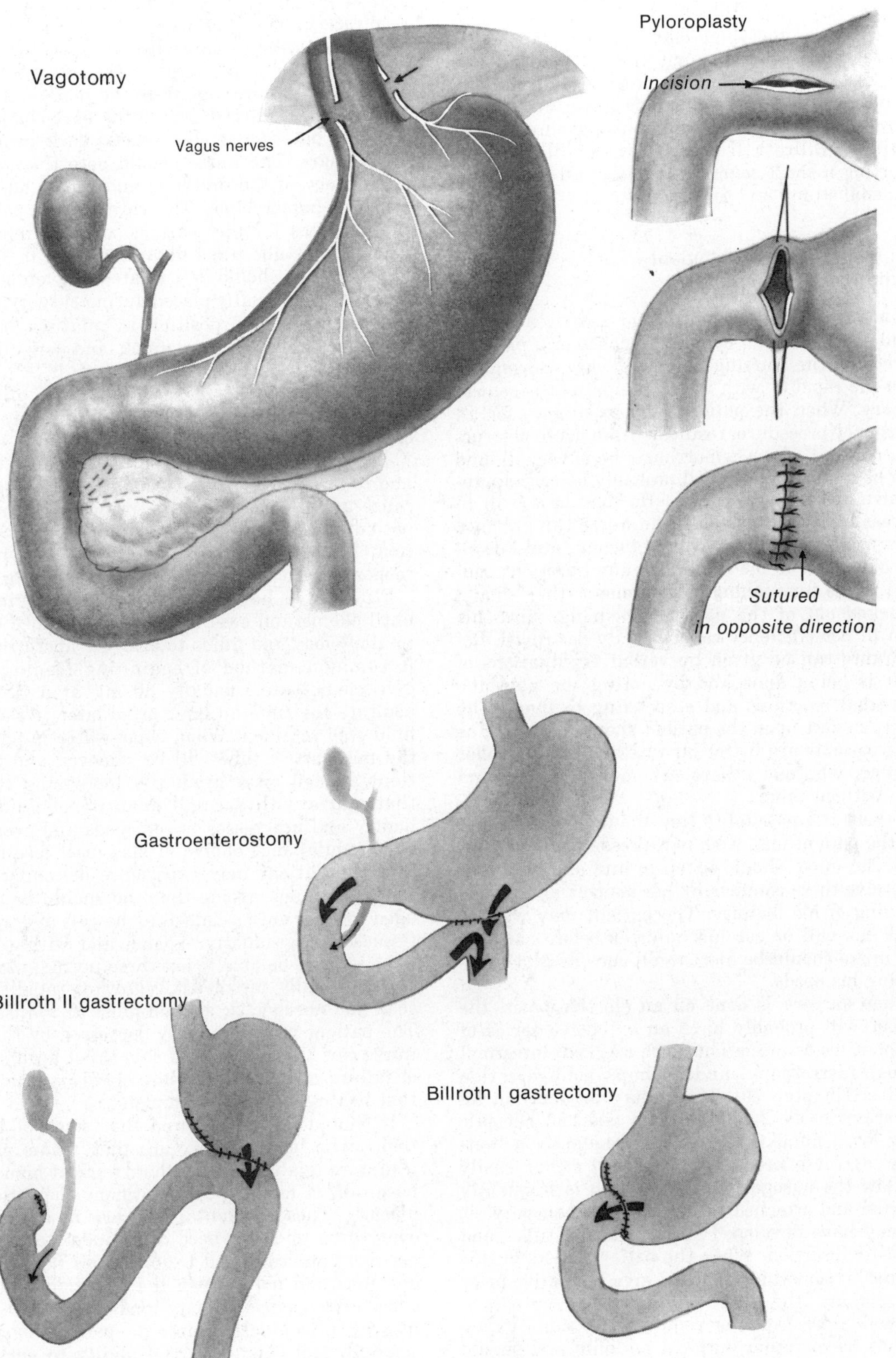

FIGURE 78–1. Gastric surgical procedures.

delay gastric emptying. This syndrome frequently occurs soon after surgery and subsides in six months to a year. When it continues, surgical attempts to relieve the symptoms have included reducing the size of the gastroenterostomy or converting a Billroth II resection to a Billroth I by inserting a short segment of jejunum between the duodenal stump and the stomach.

Nursing Care of the Patient Who Has Gastric Surgery

Since surgical intervention for gastric and duodenal conditions can be an emergency or a planned procedure, the nursing care will vary, depending upon the rapidity with which the patient is sent to surgery. When the patient goes to surgery for an emergency procedure, resulting from acute obstruction, perforation, or hemorrhage, he is very ill, and both he and his family will probably be very apprehensive about his condition. He may be too ill to express his apprehensions. The nurse can enhance his sense of security by calm, efficient, and knowledgeable care. If the nurse has any questions concerning the functioning of equipment, they should be asked out of the patient's hearing, since his faith in her efficiency can be easily destroyed. Reassurance can be given by verbal explanations of what is being done and by noting the patient's nonverbal reactions and responding to them. The family's effect upon the patient should be noted, as some patients are better off with a family member present, whereas others are more relaxed and calm without them.

If there is a possibility that the diagnosis is cancer, the patient may wish to express his fears about this. The nurse should listen to him and help him to resolve these conflicts by her support and understanding of his feelings. The patient may wish to check his will or see his minister before surgery. The nurse should be alert to all cues he gives concerning his needs.

When surgery is done on an elective basis, the patient will probably have an extensive series of preoperative examinations such as gastrointestinal series, gastroscopy, and perhaps acid-secretion studies (Chapter 75). These may be done on an outpatient basis. A patient who has had a peptic ulcer for a number of years is frequently a "veteran" at these procedures and will either easily swallow the nasogastric tube, which is frequently inserted and attached to suction before surgery, or he may have developed strong fears of tubes and resist its insertion. When the patient reacts in this manner, it sometimes helps to give a sedative prior to insertion of the tube.

Preoperative teaching requires the same explanations as for other surgical patients and should also include an explanation that gastric suction will be present after surgery and that fluids will be given by intravenous infusion until the gastric surgical site is healed. Discussing the need for deep breathing is especially important for this patient because of the high abdominal incision, which causes increased discomfort from deep breathing and is an added hazard for the development of respiratory complications.

Postoperative nursing observations, in addition to those made on all surgical patients, include the observation of drainage from the nasogastric tube. It may be bright red during the early hours after surgery, but this should become dark by the end of 24 hours. The nurse should note the color and consistency of the drainage and report any occurrence of hemorrhage. The care of this patient is the same as for any patient with an indwelling nasogastric tube. (See details of care in Chapter 75.) The tube should be irrigated only on a specific order, as it is usually placed during surgery and the surgeon knows its position in relation to suture lines and can tell how much and what kind of fluid can safely be instilled through it. A nonfunctioning tube should be reported to the physician, as distention of the operative area by gas and fluids can have drastic sequelae.

The patient must be encouraged to deep breathe and to move, even though this may be difficult because of the location of the incision. Keeping the patient comfortable with the judicious administration of pain medications will allow him to be more cooperative in deep breathing and coughing.

Fluids will be given by intravenous infusion until edema and swelling have diminished enough to allow food and fluids to pass the operative area. A common method of beginning feedings is to give clear water, usually 30 ml. at a time, and aspirate the tube an hour or so later to see if the fluid was retained. When clear water is tolerated, the nasogastric tube will be removed and the patient started on a gradually increasing regimen that starts with a small quantity of fluid given hourly and progresses to soft foods and eventually to a regular diet of five of six small feedings. At first the patient may experience discomfort if he takes too much at one time; he should be encouraged to take only as much as he can tolerate. The tissues will gradually expand, and within a year or so he may be able to eat three normal meals.

Occasionally the diet is begun too rapidly or too soon and nasogastric suction must be re-instituted. The patient is usually very depressed by this. The nurse can assure him that this is not an indication of failure of the surgery but merely an indication that healing is not yet complete.

It should be remembered that some of the patients who have surgery are those same patients who were unable to leave their work at home when hospitalized for medical treatment of peptic ulcer disease. These patients, who are in a hurry for everything to occur, need calm understanding and need to be encouraged to let nature heal them in her time and not to rush the situation. Convalescence after gastric surgery tends to be slow, and it may be three months before the patient regains his strength and even a partial ability to eat in the manner he feels is acceptable.

When complications such as the afferent loop

syndrome or the dumping syndrome occur, the patient should be allowed to express his displeasure at the situation. (Remember that the patient probably held high expectations for the surgical result.) He can frequently be taught how to control these symptoms by the measures mentioned previously.

Patient teaching includes helping him to learn to live with the residual deficiencies resulting from the surgery, helping him with his diet or referring him to the dietitian for assistance as necessary, and helping him to understand the need for continued medical supervision. He should be made aware that his convalescence may be fairly long.

NEOPLASMS

The incidence of cancer of the stomach has diminished steadily in the United States during the last two decades. The reason for this is unknown. Despite the reduction in incidence, it was the fourth ranked cause of death from cancer among males in the United States in 1968 because of the low cure rate.

Little is known about its etiology, but it is twice as common in men as in women, more common in the American black than in American whites, and it occurs more frequently in persons who have pernicious anemia. It often occurs in conjunction with atrophic gastritis. Worldwide mortality varies greatly, being high in Japan, Bulgaria, Poland, and Chile, but low in the United States, El Salvador, Nicaragua, Thailand, the Phillipines, and Australia. The reasons for these differences are unknown, but studies are being done of the variations in diet in these countries.

Summarizing what is now known about gastric cancer and drawing what conclusions are possible Kirsner states:[34]

> Gastric carcinoma thus may be regarded as an acquired disease, developing in an abnormal gastric mucosa and probably arising on the basis of cellular reaction to continued injury, presumably from unknown chemical carcinogens.

SYMPTOMS AND DIAGNOSIS

Cancer of the stomach is seldom diagnosed in an early stage because the symptoms occur late and then, unless hemorrhage or perforation occurs, are vague and indefinite. They depend upon where in the stomach the tumor occurs. If it is near the cardia, the patient may experience dysphagia from early involvement of the esophagus; if it is near the pylorus, he may have symptoms from obstruction. The major symptoms are weight loss and a vague indigestion or feeling of fullness or mild discomfort that is so insidious that the patient does not recognize it as an abnormality or seek medical aid. Discomfort may be brought on, or relieved, by food. Anemia from blood loss is a common symptom, and occult blood is present in the stools of 45 per cent of persons with this condition. The presence of a palpable mass, ascites, or bone pain from metastasis may be the first symptom.

When the cancer causes ulceration, differentiating it from a benign gastric ulcer can be difficult, but upper gastrointestinal x-rays and fluoroscopy used together with gastroscopy diagnose about 95 per cent of the cases correctly. Cytology as an aid to diagnosing gastric lesions is thought to be valuable by some and worthless by others. Most authorities agree that, to rule out cancer, surgery should be done for any gastric lesion that does not improve after two weeks of intensive medical therapy.

METASTASIS AND PROGNOSIS

Cancer of the stomach is spread by direct extension into the pancreas; by lymphatic spread, which occurs early; or by hematogenous spread to the liver, lungs, and bones, which occurs at varying times. The occurrence of spread by these routes depends upon the location of the tumor and the type of growth it undergoes, since some penetrate, some ulcerate, and some spread along the tissue planes.

The overall prognosis is poor, with a five-year cure rate for all patients of between 5 and 10 per cent. When curative surgery is done at an early stage this five-year survival rate is from 30 to 35 per cent. When surgery is done and metastases are found, the rate is only 7 per cent. This explains the high death rate for this low-incidence cancer.

TREATMENT

Surgery is the only treatment that affects the progress of the disease favorably. Unfortunately, because of the usually late diagnosis, this is more often palliative than curative. Gastrectomy, either partial or complete, depending upon the location of the tumor, is the usual procedure. Ideally all local growth and the associated lymph nodes are removed. When extensive growth makes resection impractical or impossible and the pylorus is obstructed, palliation is often achieved with a gastroenterostomy. (See Fig. 78–1.)

Radiation therapy has not proved helpful and response to chemotherapy is not consistent. Occasionally a patient has an excellent response to the administration of fluorouracil (5-FU).[46]

POSTOPERATIVE NURSING CARE

Patients with cancer of the stomach are frequently malnourished and anemic. They should be protected from secondary infections as well as from the various complications of debilitating conditions. When a total gastrectomy has been done, the patient will probably have chest drainage because the thoracic cavity is usually entered in order to do a total resection. The nasogastric tube will have very little drainage because most secretions normally come from the stomach.

Postoperative progress will be similar to that with a subtotal gastrectomy but is usually much slower. As with other gastric surgery, the first feeding will be clear water. Feedings will be increased gradually until the patient is on five to six small meals a day. The patient should be taught to chew his food well, since the mixing and liquefying functions of the stomach have been lost. When a good surgical response is achieved, a high-protein, low-carbohydrate, moderate-fat diet is tolerated well. Some patients are not noticeably improved by surgery and may be unable to tolerate or digest even small amounts of food satisfactorily.

Because of the loss of the intrinsic factor, this patient will need injections of vitamin B_{12} to maintain his hemoglobin. Balanced nutrition is important. The nurse should encourage the patient to eat a well-balanced diet that is not too high in bulk because of his limited capacity. He may need instructions on what foods to include.

Other nursing responsibilities in cancer of the stomach are in case finding by recognizing the vague symptoms and encouraging people to seek medical assistance for vague gastric complaints that persist or for changes from the patient's normal digestive habits. These patients usually undergo many diagnostic tests and need nursing support and instructions concerning these tests.

CHAPTER 79

Disorders of the Large and Small Bowel

The major function of the small bowel and of the proximal half of the large bowel is digestion of food substances and absorption of the end products, while the function of the left colon is storage of the feces until defecation occurs. The small bowel is narrower in diameter and longer than the large bowel. The arterial supply and venous drainage are so divided that the small bowel and right colon to the midpoint of the transverse colon receive blood from the superior mesenteric artery, whereas the remainder of the colon and the rectum receive blood from the inferior mesenteric artery. The venous drainage is divided the same way. Peristaltic activity in the small bowel is much more active than that in the large bowel, which is relatively inactive except during the mass movements that are stimulated by distention of the rectum.

SYMPTOMS AND PROBLEMS

Symptoms that occur in this area depend upon which function—motility, digestion or absorption—is disturbed and upon the cause of the disturbance. The major symptoms of dysfunction are pain, tenderness, hemorrhage, distention, nausea and vomiting, constipation and diarrhea, abdominal masses, and abnormal constituents in the feces.

Obstruction to the flow of chyme in either portion causes increased peristalsis, pain, and distention, but the symptoms occur sooner and will be more intense in a small bowel blockage than in the large because of the differences in size and normal activity in the two segments. The large volume of secretions from the small bowel add to the distention; the only secretion from the large bowel is mucus.

Hemorrhage

Bleeding may be caused by trauma or by ulceration or inflammation that erodes through a blood vessel. It is usually manifested by blood in the stools rather than by emesis and varies from a minute quantity that is invisible except by testing (occult blood) to larger quantities that cause the stools to be any gradation of color from bright red to tarry black. Since color comes from the digestive processes acting upon the blood, the amount of color change can be used to determine roughly the level of the bowel in which bleeding occurs. The rapidity with which the chyme passes through the bowel will also affect this. When the patient is passing bloody stools, the nurse should note the number of stools passed in any certain time period and what color changes occur between early and late specimens. For instance, slow bleeding from the duodenum might not increase peristalsis and could be manifested by a tarry stool; if the rate of bleeding or the rate of peristalsis increased, the patient could have subsequent stools that become brighter. The knowledge that previously black stools have changed to bright bloody ones and are now occurring every half hour is a fact that will help the physician in making his diagnosis or in determining what tests to make to confirm his diagnosis.

Pain

Pain is caused by stimulation of the nerve endings in the muscular or submucosal layers of the bowel and by an increase in tension; it may also be influenced by the rate of tension change. It is manifested in various places, including the involved portion of the bowel, another previously diseased area, or a nearby somatic portion of the body. Previous surgical procedures will also influence the location at which pain is felt.

Obstruction of the blood supply to the intestine is another cause for pain. This can be from acute occlusion of the mesenteric artery or from partial occlusion, which causes intermittent pain when digestion is taking place because of the increased need for blood at that time. Acute occlusion can occur in the major artery or one of the smaller branches. Partial occlusion causing intermittent pain is sometimes called intestinal angina.

Nausea and Vomiting

When this symptom originates in the bowel, it is usually due to an obstruction of the forward motility of peristalsis. Nausea occurs from distention of the duodenum.

Constipation and Diarrhea

Usually fast propulsion of intestinal contents through the bowel results in diarrhea, unless it is compensated by a longer period of residence in the large bowel; however, increased peristalsis in the small bowel usually affects forward motility within the large bowel also.

Irritant action of various constituents of intestinal contents is the usual cause for increased activity. This can result from the presence of abnormal bacteria or parasites or from highly irritating organic acids that are formed by bacterial actions, made possible by an abnormal absorptive process.

Constipation results when peristaltic activity is slowed or stopped or when the intestinal flow is blocked by mechanical obstruction. Another cause for constipation is inadequate stimulation of mass movements in the rectum or the voluntary suppressive action of the patient to overcome the urge to defecate.

Abdominal Masses

Palpation of abdominal masses is more useful in finding lesions in the large bowel than in the small bowel. The amount of abdominal adipose tissue will also affect the ease of palpation.

Abnormalities in Fecal Content

The presence of nonabsorbed factors such as fats in the stool indicates malabsorption. Other abnormal constituents that may aid in diagnosis are bacteria, parasites, pus, blood, and abnormal quantities of mucus from the colon.

INFLAMMATIONS

Inflammations occur in any portion of the bowel and can be caused by an organism, by toxins produced by an organism, by infiltration of the bowel wall by granulomatous processes, by injury from radiation, and by drugs. All types of organisms can be involved, from viruses to large parasites. Almost any abnormal constituent in the bowel can cause an inflammatory process to develop.

INFLAMMATIONS USUALLY TREATED MEDICALLY

BACTERIAL, PARASITIC, AND CHEMICAL IRRITATIONS

Gastroenteritis

This is a general name for a condition that affects the small bowel predominantly and is manifested by abdominal cramps, diarrhea, and vomiting. It can be caused by a number of different agents, with viruses and bacteria being common causes. Staphylococcal food poisoning, in which the irritating factor is the toxin produced by the organism, may occur when foods such as cream-filled pastries, custard pies, processed meats and potato salad are allowed to remain at room temperature for a period of time before they are eaten. The staphylococcal organisms multiply and form a toxin which, when ingested, causes a violent gastroenteritis in two to four hours. Bacterial and viral food poisoning usually develop 10 to 16 hours after ingestion of contaminated food.

Many organisms "pass through" a community during a year, and transitory epidemics of gastroenteritis are common. These infections are temporarily quite disabling, depending upon the intensity of the symptoms, but they are of short duration and usually are not serious, except in infants, the very elderly, and weakened debilitated individuals. Fluid and electrolyte imbalances occur easily in these persons because of the lowered efficiency of their compensatory mechanisms.

Bed rest with nothing by mouth until vomiting has stopped is the best treatment. Fluids such as broth, ginger ale, and lemonade, which contain nutrients and electrolytes, are given as soon as possible to replace losses. Sometimes antibiotics are given if the infecting organism is identified and the condition is persistent.

Dysenteries

The conditions that fall into this category affect the large bowel and are manifested by an intense diarrhea. Most are caused by amebic and bacterial organisms such as *Entamoeba histolytica* and shigella bacilli. Cholera also causes dysentery-like symptoms. These organisms are carried in the large bowel by infected individuals and transmitted by ingestion of contaminated foods and drinking water. Dysentery develops commonly in countries where there is crowding, where sanitary conditions are poor, and where the temperature is high enough for the organisms to incubate easily. The major manifestation is a profuse diarrhea, and the resultant fluid loss is the greatest problem. As with gastroenteritis, dysentery can be very serious in the debilitated, the aged and the very young.

Parasitic Infestations

The intestinal tract may be infested with any of several species of parasitic worms. These include the Ascaris (roundworms), the Enterobius (pinworms), the *Trichinella spiralis* (causing trichinosis), and various species of tapeworms. These parasites are found in all parts of the world, and are often encountered in the poorer regions of the United States. Worm infestations can cause serious and even fatal disease if the parasites are not eradicated from the intestinal tract. Fortunately most of these parasites are susceptible to treatment with compounds such as piperazine (Antepar). Trichinosis, formerly the most difficult of the group to treat, is now often effectively treated by thiabendazole.

REGIONAL ENTERITIS (TERMINAL ILEITIS, GRANULOMATOUS JEJUNO-ILEITIS, CROHN'S DISEASE)

This disease was first described in 1932 by Crohn. Originally it was thought to affect only the terminal ileum, but it has been found in segments of the alimentary tract from the mouth to the anus. It is a chronic, relapsing disease that is characterized by involvement of the whole thickness of the bowel wall. It is typically present in several separated segments and is grossly visible and sharply demarcated from normal tissue. There is an edematous, heavy, reddish purple area; there may be granular spots. The disease causes a narrowed lumen, ulcerations, abscesses, and fistulas and their complications.

The etiology is unknown, though it has been suggested that the disease may be related to an altered immunologic reactivity. It has an equal incidence in the sexes and occurs at all ages, but 50 per cent of the cases occur between the ages of 20 and 30. There is a high incidence of familial occurrence, a high incidence in Jews, and a low incidence among blacks.

Symptoms result from the inflammatory reaction, the obstructive problems, and dysfunction of the bowel. Treatment is mainly symptomatic and is aimed at maintaining good nutrition for the patient so he can lead a productive life. Other therapies include surgery, which is used only to treat the complications, (since removal of the diseased portion of the bowel has resulted in a 50 per cent incidence of recurrence), antibiotics to control infectious processes, and anti-inflammatory drugs for patients who fail to respond to general supportive measures.

IRRITABLE COLON

An irritable colon is a chronic noninfectious irritation that is thought to be caused by an increased spasticity of the colon. It can be manifested in a number of different ways, including frequent liquid stools, scanty, small hard stools, and abdominal cramps that are brought on by eating coarse or raw foods, since these increase the spasticity. The condition occurs in people who are tense, anxious, and emotionally labile. Its major danger is that it mimics a number of other conditions and the patient may undergo unnecessary surgery, or the presence of a serious illness may not be recognized. Among the disorders simulated are infections of the colon, food allergies, ulcerative colitis, carcinoma of the colon, diverticulitis, gallbladder disease, and even angina pectoris and myocardial infarction.

NURSING CARE

In caring for a patient with an inflammatory condition of the bowel, the nurse must remember that the patient is losing fluids at an abnormally rapid rate or by an abnormal route and, thus, electrolyte imbalance and inadequate nutrition are potential problems. These patients experience a great deal of discomfort from nausea, frequent liquid stools, abdominal cramping, and generalized debility from inadequate intake. The goals of nursing should be to promote the patient's comfort and to maintain adequate nutrition and hydration.

If the condition is actually or suspected of being caused by a microorganism, the nurse should take care to wash her hands, the patient's hands, and all the utensils used if the patient vomits or defecates. Handwashing and preventing contamination of the uniform to avoid taking the organisms to another patient are basic factors of good nursing.

The following discussion of nursing care of patients with diarrhea and nausea is applicable to all patients with these conditions, and not just to persons with an inflammatory bowel condition.

Diarrhea

Prompt emptying of the patient's bedpan or commode is essential to his peace of mind and frequently the comfort of others in the room, as liquid stools are usually very malodorous. Washing the patient after defecations and gently drying and lightly dusting the area with a nonirritating powder will help to prevent excoriation from the stools, which may be very irritating to the skin about the anus. Sometimes patients have involuntary stools and are unable to position themselves on a commode or bedpan in time. They should not be censured or ridiculed for this; rather, the nurse should by her manner and words make the patient feel that this is not his fault and that he need not be embarrassed about it. He should, of course, be cleansed immediately and his bed linens changed.

Intake of fluids and foods should be encouraged. Sometimes eating stimulates the gastrocolic reflex and brings on another stool, so many of these patients fear eating. Very small feedings may avoid this problem. Foods should be bland and easily digested to promote absorption during the short period the food remains in the bowel.

Nausea

The patient who is vomiting should be kept as physically comfortable as possible. Removing the emesis basin promptly, rinsing his mouth, cleansing his teeth, and keeping the physical unit attractive, aired, and clean will help to eliminate the psychogenic and physical influences that perpetuate vomiting. He especially needs to have a pleasant taste in his mouth and to have the odor and sight of the vomitus removed.

He should not be forced to eat, as this frequently promotes more vomiting. He should be the judge of when he can tolerate food. However, sometimes these patients need encouragement because they are afraid to eat.

Broth, ginger ale, and weak tea are frequently the first foods tolerated. Fluids that contain electrolytes are preferred to clear water. The first foods should be bland and easily digested. Strong secretagogues should be avoided. When vomiting continues for more than 24 to 48 hours, intravenous fluids will usually be given to maintain fluid balance.

Medications

Antispasmodics, binding agents, sedatives, and antiemetics may be given to help to control the patient's symptoms of nausea and vomiting.

Observations

Included in the observations made on the patient who is vomiting or has diarrhea should be the presence of pain or tenderness in the abdomen, including its location, intensity, duration, type, and timing in relation to the diarrhea or vomiting. The presence of cramping of the bowel and tenesmus, which is the feeling of cramping pain and discomfort that occurs in the lower abdomen when one is straining to defecate, should also be reported. Whether these are relieved by the passage of a stool is also pertinent.

The characteristics of the stool should be reported and recorded and include the color, volume, odor, quantity, and the presence of any abnormal constituents such as mucus, blood, undigested food, foam, pus, oil, and other matter such as worms. The physician may wish to have the stool saved for his inspection.

Emesis should also be described completely as to color, odor, consistency, the presence of undigested food particles or drug particles, and the volume. Other things to observe about the patient who vomits include the nature of the vomiting process. Does the vomitus come up slowly and easily or is it propelled out forcibly? Does the patient have warning that he is about to vomit? Is the vomiting accompanied by nausea? Does the emesis relieve the symptoms and for how long? The patient should also be observed for signs of fluid imbalance. (See Chapter 25.)

INFLAMMATIONS USUALLY TREATED SURGICALLY

Appendicitis

Even though today almost all lay people are familiar with the disease entity appendicitis, it was not until 1886 that its cause was identified and surgical removal advocated as the treatment of choice. Prior to this the treatment had been to wait for the appendix to rupture and then to treat the resulting abscess. Remember that this was long before the days of antibiotics; it is small wonder few survived the disease.

The *symptoms* are classic and begin with *acute abdominal pain,* which comes in waves. In the beginning it may be merely a discomfort that makes the patient feel as though passing flatus or having a bowel movement will give relief. Unfortunately many individuals take a laxative during this period. The pain typically starts in the epigastrium or periumbilical region and shifts to the right lower quadrant as the inflammatory process spreads to involve the serosal layers of the bowel and brings the inflammation into contact with the peritoneum. (See the section on peritonitis below.) The pain now becomes steady rather than intermittent, and the patient guards the area by lying still and drawing his leg up to relieve tension on the abdominal muscles. The exact location of pain depends upon the location of the appendix.

Other symptoms include vomiting, which begins after the pain starts, loss of appetite, a low-grade fever, coated tongue, and bad breath. A mild leukocytosis is usually present, with the white blood cell count between 10,000 and 15,000.

There are several causes for inflammation of the appendix, including a fecolith which occludes the lumen. This is the only cause many laymen are aware of, and the stories children are told about not eating cherry pits because they may cause appendicitis have some basis in fact because such foreign objects can occlude the lumen of the appendix. Fibrous disease conditions in the wall of the bowel and external occlusion by an adhesion may also cause appendiceal inflammation.

Treatment is removal of the appendix within 24 to 48 hours of onset of the symptoms; when this is done the mortality rate is less than 0.5 per cent. Delay usually causes rupture of the organ and resulting peritonitis. A frequent cause for delay in surgery is difficulty in diagnosis or the late arrival of the patient for medical aid. Older people may have very few symptoms and frequently do not seek aid until after perforation has occurred. In very young children diagnosis can also be difficult. Many diseases mimic appendicitis, including mesenteric adenitis, ovarian cyst, cholelithiasis, renal or ureteral calculi, diverticulitis, Meckel's diverticulum, and pneumonia.

Meckel's Diverticulum

This is an outpouching of the bowel, a vestige of embryonic development found on the ileum within 100 cm. of the cecum. It may be lined with gastric mucosa or contain pancreatic tissue and sometimes develops a peptic ulcer that may bleed or perforate, or it may become inflamed and mimic appendicitis. It is sometimes attached to the umbilicus by a fibrous band and may be the focus around which the bowel twists, causing an obstruction. Treatment is surgical excision.

Diverticulosis, Diverticulitis

A diverticulum is an outpouching of the mucosa and may or may not be covered by muscular tissue. Diverticula occur at any point in the gastrointestinal tract but are most common in the sigmoid region of the colon. Acquired diverticula are caused by increased pressure within the lumen, which causes the tissue to balloon out between the muscle fibers. This usually occurs at spots where blood vessels pass through the bowel wall. The presence of diverticula is referred to as diverticulosis.

Unless complications develop from its presence, a diverticulum is no problem to the patient. Complications are perforation, hemorrhage, and inflammation (diverticulitis). Perforations are frequently walled off by the omentum and heal over without surgical intervention. Patients who have periodic bouts of pain from diverticulitis are usually encouraged to eat either a high- or low-residue diet and take bulk laxatives and are given antispasmodics to relax the bowel. Many can avoid attacks by this routine. Antibiotics are frequently given during periods of inflammation. Complications include abscess formation in the pelvis with development of a fistula to the bladder or other adjacent structures.

Peritonitis

The peritoneum covers all the organs in the abdominal cavity and lines the cavity. It is highly permeable, and constituents of the blood pass through it freely. For this reason peritoneal dialysis can be used in renal failure (Unit XI). Stimulation of the parietal portion that lines the abdominal and pelvic cavities causes sharp, well-localized pain since it is well supplied with somatic nerves. The visceral peritoneum is relatively insensitive.

Peritonitis can be primary or secondary, acute or chronic. The major sources of inflammation are from the gastrointestinal tract, from the external environment, and through the blood stream. In the female the uterine tubes penetrate the peritoneum, providing a potential route from the outside. The peritoneum is able to produce an inflammatory reaction and to wall off a localized process and thus combat an infection if the stimulus is not too massive or if the source of infection does not continue. For instance, a perforation, as of a gastric ulcer, that continues to drain contaminants into the peritoneal cavity will overcome the ability of the peritoneum to localize and combat the inflammatory process.

Symptoms of peritonitis vary, depending upon the cause. Pain is universal and may be either localized or generalized. A well-localized pain that causes rigidity of the abdominal muscles and increased pain from any pressure or motion of the abdomen is almost pathognomonic of peritonitis. The patient is usually nauseated and vomiting and may have a low-grade fever. Bowel sounds are absent and respirations are usually shallow because the patient attempts to avoid the pain caused by any motion of his body.

Systemic Effects. The circulatory system undergoes great stress from several sources: The infectious process causes an increased amount of circulating blood volume to be detoured to this area to combat the process. The peristaltic activity of the bowel ceases, with a resultant retention of fluids and air within its lumen and consequent increased pressure that causes increased secretion of fluid into the bowel. The circulating blood volume is thus reduced.

The inflammatory process causes an increase in the oxygen requirements at a time when the patient has a decreased ability to ventilate because of pain and an elevated diaphragm caused by increased abdominal pressure. These fluid shifts and respiratory alterations can pose grave problems in fluid and electrolyte management of the patient.

Treatment. If possible the cause is eliminated surgically, but sometimes the process has progressed so far that the patient is in no condition for surgery. Intravenous fluids for replacement of electrolyte and protein losses are essential. Usually a long tube is inserted through the nose into the intestine to reduce the pressure within the bowel. Positive pressure respiratory treatments may help to achieve adequate ventilation.

The patient may be placed in a semi-Fowler's position or have the head of the bed elevated four to six inches on blocks to promote the flow of drainage to the pelvic region where it can localize in an abscess and be drained or be resolved by body defenses.

NURSING CARE OF THE PATIENT WITH AN ACUTE SURGICAL INFLAMMATION OF THE BOWEL

The patient who has an acute inflammatory process of the bowel is very ill, usually is in a great deal of pain, frequently is vomiting, and needs expert medical and nursing care. In the early stages the diagnosis of the problem is of prime concern. The nurses' responsibilities therefore, in addition to making the patient comfortable, include making observations that will aid in diagnosing the condition.

Specific nursing measures for the patient in pain, who is vomiting, and who has gastrointestinal decompression are mentioned elsewhere in this text. The patient needs gentle handling to avoid increasing his pain, and complete care to conserve his strength and to promote rest. Supportive nursing measures such as bathing, mouth care, and frequent position changes, and comfort measures such as backrubs, if tolerated, are important, as are the therapeutic measures that include careful attention to the maintenance and flow of intravenous fluids, gastrointestinal suction, and catheter drainage. Observations to help the physician include the patient's description of the pain, the vital signs, and other signs of systemic malfunction such as skin condition, the position the patient assumes for comfort, and general patient responses, including his alertness and mental perceptiveness. Analgesics are usually not given because they may mask symptoms that might help in making a diagnosis.

The postoperative care of patients who have undergone surgery to treat these inflammatory conditions has been covered in Unit VI.

ULCERATIVE COLITIS

This is a condition of unknown cause that involves the mucosa and submucosa of the colon. It consists of congestion, edema, and minute ulcerations that ooze blood and eventually develop into abscesses. The edema may lead to extreme friability of the mucosa, so that bleeding occurs from any minor trauma. The general manifestations of this disorder are frequent stools that contain pus, blood, and mucus and may or may not contain liquid feces; weight loss; anorexia, and an intermittent mild fever.

The condition has three typical types of onset: In one it is gradual, beginning with malaise and vague abdominal discomfort which develops into attacks of crampy abdominal pain, with the passage of blood, pus, and mucus. The desire to defecate is great, and the patient experiences severe tenesmus. Stools are apt to be scanty and hard. In another type the onset is abrupt and manifested by bloody diarrhea, fever, anorexia, and weight loss that becomes progressively worse. The stools are sometimes liquid and sometimes hard, depending upon which portion of the colon is involved. The patient usually has abdominal tenderness, and the rectum and anus are spastic. Signs and symptoms tend to fluctuate, with remissions and exacerbations. The third general type also has an abrupt onset, but the course is rapid and fulminating, and unless successful treatment is achieved, the patient can die of toxicity or shock from the sequelae.

Ulcerative colitis occurs at all ages but is most common among young adults. It is more common among Jews, and less common among blacks than among whites. One of the problems in identifying the etiology may be that the condition can be caused by several disease entities and does not necessarily have a single causative factor. A number of theories exist, including the possibility that the disease is of bacterial origin, since a number of patients have had a history of a bacterial infection prior to the onset of the condition. Allergic reactions have been suspected, because remission sometimes occurs when the patient eliminates milk from his diet. It is thought by some to be due to an altered immunity, because colon antibodies have been found in patients with the condition. These antibodies may cause the disease, perpetuate it, or may result from the tissue damage caused by the disease. A number of the theories of etiology depend upon the assumption of a specific vulnerability of the bowel to certain stimuli. The bowel may be hypersensitive to trauma or other stimuli, and the inflammation of the mucosa may result from the release of histamine or some other substance in response to these stimuli.

Many have implicated emotional instability as a factor in the disease. Patients with ulcerative colitis have been described as dependent, immature, and hypersensitive to criticism; many are known to have different inward feelings than their outward appearance would indicate. One theory states that there is an increased cholinergic stimulation induced by emotional stress or some other agent and an increased tissue vulnerability to this stimulation. This has not been substantiated in all studies. However, all researchers do agree that emotional stress does influence recurrences of the disease.

Complications

Local tissue involvement causes rectal complications such as hemorrhoids and anal fissures, and such bowel complications as local abscesses, perforation, and stenosis from healing lesions. As a result of the physical manifestations of the conditions, patients develop anemia and malnutrition owing to malabsorption and iron deficiency. They may also be deficient in vitamins K and G, with resulting bleeding tendencies. They develop weakness, anorexia, weight loss, and sometimes a stomatitis resembling that of vitamin deficiencies. Cancer of the colon is more common among patients with this condition than among the general population; the incidence is greatly increased among those who develop ulcerative colitis before the age of 16 and those who have had the condition more than 10 years. The five-year survival for the colitis patients who undergo surgery is also much lower than for other patients with cancer of the colon.

Treatment

The aims of treatment are to maintain the patient's nutritional status, give symptomatic relief, prevent complications, and restore blood volume.

A high-protein, high-caloric diet is given in an attempt to restore normal nutritional levels. This is not always well ingested or tolerated. Eating tends to increase the diarrhea and the anorexia with nausea and vomiting that are frequently present. These patients tend to have definite ideas about what they want to eat and, probably because of the miserable symptoms of the disease, they tend to vent their aggressions on the diet. If the patient can be given a self-selected diet it will probably be more beneficial than attempting to give the low-residue, bland, high-caloric, high-protein diet that is usually ordered and is accepted so poorly. Foods the patient wants tend to be better tolerated than those he is given. Fluids, electrolytes, and blood are replaced as indicated to maintain the patient's homeostasis.

Antibiotics may be given to control secondary bowel inflammations.

During acute exacerbations the patient is put

on bed rest and given anticholinergic drugs to relieve the abdominal cramps and to help to control the diarrhea. In an attempt to control diarrhea, tincture of opium and paregoric are sometimes given on a routine basis instead of after each stool, as in other conditions.

The patient needs a great deal of emotional support. The physician usually attempts to establish an open relationship with the patient, and the nurse also should be aware of the patient's reactions and encourage him to express his feelings. He should be allowed to develop a positive self-image and helped to accept himself as he is.

Surgical Treatment

When medical management fails and when the condition proves intractable, surgical treatment is usually indicated. Surgical intervention varies, but the most common procedure is the surgical excision of the entire colon, rectum, and anus and the creation of a permanent ileostomy. Sometimes the rectum is retained and at a future time the ileum is attached to it, but this has not proved too successful. The entire colon is usually removed, as toxic products are absorbed from it even when it is nonfunctional and symptoms of general toxicity may continue if it remains.

Another indication for surgical intervention is the probability of the presence of a carcinoma of the colon. Some surgeons recommend colectomy for all patients who have had this condition for more than 10 years because of the high cancer incidence in these persons. Since a permanent ileostomy is a serious consequence, most surgeons do not consider this an adequate indication for surgery. However, such patients should be examined frequently for the possibility of cancer even when they are in a period of remission of the disease.

HERNIATIONS

The classic definition of a hernia is a "protrusion of a viscus from its normal cavity through a congenital or acquired aperture." This definition limits a hernia to a situation in which there is a protrusion, but in normal usage a patient who has a weakness in the abdominal musculature through which a viscus or other abdominal structure periodically penetrates is considered to have a hernia, whether or not it is protruding.

Hernias may penetrate through any defect in the abdominal wall, through the diaphragm, or through some internal structure within the abdominal cavity. For this discussion only the more commonly seen types of hernia will be mentioned.

CAUSES

Two things must be present for a hernia to occur: a defect in the integrity of the muscular wall, and increased intra-abdominal pressure. Defects in the muscular wall may be developmental, owing to an inherited tendency such as weakened collagen tissues or a wide space at the inguinal ligament, or may be caused by trauma.

Intra-abdominal pressure is most commonly increased from pregnancy or obesity. Heavy lifting also causes increased pressure, as do coughing and traumatic injuries from blunt pressure. When two of these factors coexist, along with some tissue weakness, a hernia can easily occur. Increased pressure without a weakness is not likely to cause a hernia. Weaknesses, in addition to being present from birth, are acquired as part of the aging process as muscular tissues become infiltrated and replaced by adipose and connective tissues.

TERMINOLOGY

When the contents of the hernia sac can be replaced into the abdominal cavity, the hernia is said to be *reducible. Irreducible* and *incarcerated* are terms used to refer to a hernia that cannot be reduced. When the blood supply to the herniated segment of bowel is cut off by pressure from the hernia ring, the bowel becomes *strangulated.* Incarcerated hernias usually become strangulated sooner or later. This is a surgical emergency, because unless the bowel is released it soon becomes necrotic owing to lack of blood supply. A *hernia ring* is the ring of muscular tissue through which the bowel protrudes.

TYPES

The most common hernias, which will be discussed here, are the inguinal, both direct and indirect, femoral, incisional, and umbilical (Fig. 79–1). The hiatus hernia was discussed with conditions of the esophagus.

Indirect Inguinal

This herniation occurs through the inguinal ring and follows the spermatic cord through the inguinal canal. It is far more common in males because of the space allowed for the descent of the testes. These hernias have a high incidence among infants and young persons, after which the incidence drops, then rises again among persons in their 50's, and then tapers off. These hernias can become extremely large and frequently descend into the scrotum.

Direct Inguinal

This hernia passes through the abdominal wall in an area of muscular weakness and not through a canal, as do the indirect inguinal and the femoral. It is more common in the elderly and is the result of a gradually developed weakness in an area that is congenitally deficient iin the number of fibers present.

Femoral

The femoral hernia occurs through the femoral ring and is more common in females than in males. It begins as a plug of fat in the femoral canal that enlarges and gradually pulls the peritoneum, and almost inevitably the urinary bladder, into the sac. There is a high incidence of incarceration and strangulation in this type of hernia (Fig. 79–1).

Umbilical

There are three kinds of umbilical hernias, two of which occur in infants. One of these is a surgical emergency at the time of birth, because abdominal viscera protrude through the umbilicus with the cord and, unless surgery is done to replace them and repair the associated defect of the abdominal wall, necrosis occurs along with the normal umbilical cord necrosis. The more common type of umbilical herniation at birth is due to an abnormality of the muscular structures about the cord. It frequently gradually disappears owing to pull of the muscles and fascia across the defect, and heals in the months following birth; the usual treatment has been to keep the herniated area in position with a small strip of adhesive tape during this time. However, some authorities now feel that the hernia will heal whether or not it is kept reduced.

The third type of umbilical hernia, the adult type, is acquired and is more common in women. It is due to increased abdominal pressure and occurs in obese persons and women who have had several pregnancies. It is due to a defect of the umbilicus that has persisted from birth.

Incisional

This type of hernia occurs at the site of a previous surgical incision. It is the result of inadequate healing of the incision because of a postoperative problem such as infection, inadequate nutrition, extreme distention, obesity, or other factors. The incidence of this type of hernia is increasing, probably because of the higher number of surgical procedures being performed.

NURSING CARE

The care the patient needs after hernia repair is dependent upon the location of the hernia and the type of anesthesia used. The hernias in the inguinal region are usually repaired under a spinal or local anesthetic, and the patient is allowed to ambulate as soon as he has recovered from the immediate effects of the anesthesia and the surgical procedure. The patient should be checked to make certain he voids after returning from surgery. A full diet is given as soon as the patient

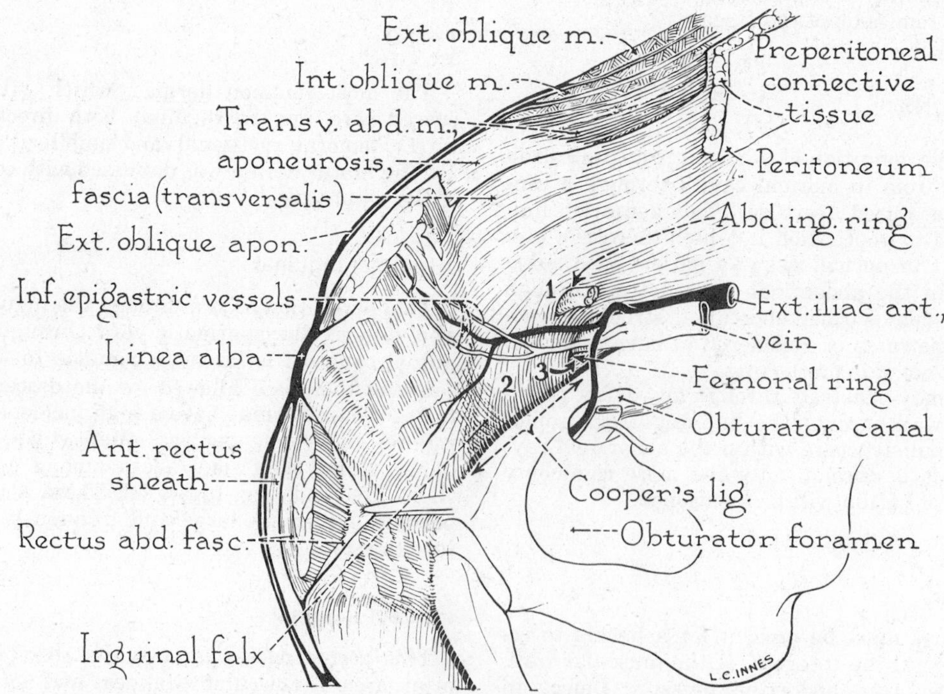

FIGURE 79–1. Anatomical sites of the development of inguinal and femoral hernias. Numbers indicate sites of (1) indirect inguinal hernia, (2) direct inguinal hernia, (3) femoral hernia. (From Davis, L.: *Christopher's Textbook of Surgery.* 9th ed. 1968.)

tolerates food, which is usually soon after recovery from the anesthesia. A general anesthesia is commonly used for hernias in the upper abdomen, and the postoperative progress is thus slower.

The patient can be assured that during the immediate postoperative period there is no chance of his hernia breaking open again. Some patients hesitate to become active because of this fear. Obese patients make slower progress, heal more slowly, and may need more encouragement to participate in postoperative activities.

INTESTINAL OBSTRUCTIONS

Any impairment to the forward flow of the intestinal contents, whether by partial or complete stoppage or a reversal of the flow, is known as an intestinal obstruction. It can be caused by mechanical, vascular, or nervous disorders.

PATHOPHYSIOLOGY

With the onset of an obstruction, fluids and air collect proximal to the site of the problem. This causes a temporary increase in peristalsis as the bowel attempts to force the material through the obstructed area. Within a few hours the increased peristalsis ends and the bowel becomes flaccid, thus decreasing the pressure within the lumen and slowing the process caused by the obstruction. Increased pressure within the bowel causes a decrease in the absorptive ability of the bowel, which increases the fluid retention still further. Soon the intraluminal pressure causes a reduction in venous return, which increases venous pressure. This, in turn, increases the capillary permeability and allows plasma to extravasate into the bowel lumen and also into the peritoneal cavity. The bowel wall becomes permeable to bacteria, and bowel organisms enter the peritoneal cavity. Increasing pressure in the bowel wall soon slows the arterial blood flow, causing necrosis to develop.

Normally 7 to 8 liters of electrolyte-rich fluid are secreted by the bowel and most of it is resorbed. During an obstruction this fluid is partially retained within the bowel and partially eliminated by vomiting, thus causing a severe reduction in circulating blood volume which results in hypotension and a diminished renal and cerebral blood flow. Since fluid is lost without blood cells, the hematocrit and hemoglobin increase, thus increasing the potential for vascular occlusive disorders such as coronary, cerebral, and mesenteric thrombosis. These complications are especially likely to happen in elderly patients, who tend to have atherosclerotic narrowing of these vessels, making thrombosis more likely.

MECHANICAL FACTORS THAT CAUSE OBSTRUCTION

Adhesions

This is probably the commonest cause of intestinal obstruction. Adhesions always form following abdominal surgery, but for an unknown reason some people develop massive ones. Irritants that remain in the abdomen following surgical procedures enhance the formation of adhesions. These fibrous bands of scar tissue can become looped over a portion of the bowel and either be the focus about which a volvulus occurs (see below), or be the band that mechanically obstructs the bowel by external pressure. The presence of multiple adhesions increases the potential of this occurring.

Hernia

An incarcerated hernia may or may not cause an obstruction, depending upon the size of the hernia ring. However, the potential for obstruction is always present in any hernia. A strangulated hernia is always obstructed, because the bowel is not functional when its blood supply is cut off.

Volvulus

This is a twisting of the bowel that frequently occurs about a stationary focus in the abdominal cavity. It can occur in either the large or small bowel and sometimes releases without surgical intervention. When decompression with a long tube is accomplished successfully, a small bowel volvulus may relax as the pressure against the proximal end of the loop is relieved. A large bowel volvulus sometimes releases when a barium enema is given as the advent of pressure distal to the obstruction equalizes the forces on both sides of the loop.

Intussusception

This is a telescoping of the bowel upon itself and is most common in infants, occurring at the ileocecal junction, with the small bowel telescoping inside the large bowel. In adults it is usually associated with a tumor of the large bowel which telescopes into the bowel distal to it from peristaltic activity. In infants, barium enema sometimes causes intussusception to release, making surgery unnecessary unless the process was present long enough to cause irreversible damage to the bowel wall.

Tumors

In the large bowel, this is the chief cause of obstruction. The process develops slowly and, because of the large lumen of the bowel may be quite advanced before a fecal mass becomes lodged at the constricted site and precipitates an acute obstructive process.

NEUROGENIC FACTORS THAT CAUSE OBSTRUCTION

A paralytic ileus, also called an adynamic obstruction, is caused by a lack of peristaltic activity. The cause is a reflex paralysis and can be due to a number of different pathologic processes. It commonly occurs following abdominal surgery as the bowel ceases to function for a period of time, which may vary from a few hours to several days. Procedures in which the bowel is handled extensively and procedures in the retroperitoneal area are quite apt to cause a postoperative problem. Treatment is aspiration of the secretions by gastric suction until the bowel begins to function.

Infections of the abdomen and sometimes of the thoracic cavity, such as lobar pneumonia, peritonitis, or pancreatitis, are frequent causes of an ileus of infectious origin. The other common cause is electrolyte imbalance, especially hypokalemia.

VASCULAR FACTORS THAT CAUSE OBSTRUCTION

Interruption of blood supply to any body part causes pain to occur and function to cease. Blood is supplied to the bowel by way of the celiac and superior and inferior mesenteric arteries. These vessels have anatomotic intercommunications at the head of the pancreas and along the transverse bowel.

Complete Occlusion (Mesenteric Infarction)

Any occlusion of arterial blood supply to the bowel, as in mesenteric thrombosis, will effectively stop bowel function. This is usually caused by an embolus, and the extent of symptoms is determined by the size of the vessel that is occluded, the extent of bowel without blood supply, and the rapidity with which the occlusion occurs. An acute occlusion will, at its onset, cause intense abdominal pain without signs of advanced intestinal obstruction because the pain is caused by ischemic tissue rather than the results of obstruction. As the process advances, symptoms of gangrene of the bowel develop, such as fever, leukocytosis and shock.

Acute mesenteric obstruction is a surgical emergency and has a high mortality rate—approximating 75 per cent. Sometimes an embolectomy can be done to restore circulation. Necrotic segments of the bowel must be resected, so early surgical intervention is essential.

Partial Occlusion (Abdominal Angina)

This is usually due to atherosclerosis of the mesenteric arteries which is quite common though asymptomatic, and is found in 33 per cent of routine autopsies. Pain may develop 15 to 30 minutes after eating, as an increased need for oxygenation occurs during the digestive process. Originally pain may occur only on ingestion of a large meal, but as the arterial process enlarges, it may occur even after ingestion of a small meal and eventually become almost continuous. Symptoms are caused only when the interruption of blood supply is sufficient to compromise the function of the bowel and may include, in addition to pain after eating, a change in bowel habits, nausea and vomiting, and weight loss because the patient restricts his intake owing to the discomfort experienced when food is ingested. Vascular or by-pass grafts can sometimes be done to improve the blood supply to the affected portion of the bowel.

TREATMENT

The major objective in treating bowel obstruction is to relieve the cause and thus eliminate the problem. However, the cause is not always immediately obvious. The diagnosis of the cause of an acute abdominal condition may be quite difficult and frequently is made in surgery. It is important to make as specific observations as possible to aid the physician in his diagnosis. In the vast majority of the vascular and mechanically caused obstructions the only treatment is surgical intervention to remove the cause. In adynamic ileus, drugs are not effective in stimulating bowel activity, and the best treatment is rest and prevention of distention by use of gastric suction. The bowel will respond when recovery from the physical insult is complete.

TUMORS

Both benign and malignant tumors occur in all portions of the bowel, but their incidence varies greatly from one area to another. Malignant tumors are uncommon in the small bowel, being less than 1 per cent of all malignant neoplasms of the alimentary tract. Few benign tumors are found in this region either, but this may be due mostly to their lack of symptoms. In the large bowel, carcinoma is the most common tumor, and 80 per cent of these occur in the distal portion, from the sigmoid to the anus.

BENIGN

In the small bowel various kinds of benign tumors are found. Polyps are the most commonly found benign tumor of the large bowel. A *polyp* is a lesion that projects into the lumen of the bowel. If it has a stem, it is known as *pedunculated;* if there is no stem, it is called *sessile* (Fig. 75–1). These lesions can be either benign or malignant, but the term polyp usually refers to the benign form. Some types of polyps are precursors of cancer and can be considered to be premalignant tumors. The symptoms of benign tumors may be quite similar to those of malignant tumors. Also, benign tumors, in both the large and small bowel, may be the cause of an intussusception. The major dangers they present are in masking a malignant tumor and serving as the focus for a bowel obstruction. Some benign tumors bleed profusely and cause symptoms of abdominal discomfort. These are usually removed surgically.

MALIGNANT

Small Bowel

Malignant tumors of the small bowel are rare, occur in younger people than do malignant tumors of the large bowel, and are twice as common in men as in women. The majority are in the second portion of the duodenum, and they spread to the liver and local lymph nodes. The symptoms are pain and, depending upon the site, biliary obstruction, malabsorption, or bowel obstruction. They frequently bleed but are seldom palpable.

Surgery is the only treatment that offers any hope of cure, but even when diagnosis is made early and a resection is done, prognosis for five-year survival is only about 20 per cent. With late diagnosis or early spread to the liver, the five-year survival rate is about 5 per cent.

Large Bowel

In both men and women cancer of the colon and rectum is the second most frequent cause of death from cancer in the United States, being rated behind only cancer of the lung in men and of the breast in women. It affects males and females in equal numbers, but carcinoma of the colon is more common in women, whereas carcinoma of the rectum is more common in men. The incidence of malignant lesions varies from one portion of the bowel to another, with the greatest incidence occurring in the portion most accessible to examination (Fig. 79–2). The death rate has decreased only slightly in the last two decades. Considering the possibilities for early diagnosis with a resultant improvement in mortality figures, this would seem to indicate that many people still do not avail themselves of the knowledge currently available concerning the diagnosis and treatment of this condition.

Symptoms. Symptoms vary according to the area in which the tumor is found, but include bleeding, changed bowel habits, abdominal pain, weight loss, anorexia, and nausea and vomiting. In general, tumors in the small bowel and right colon are more likely to cause abdominal pain and nausea and vomiting, while those in the left colon and rectum are more likely to cause an alteration of bowel habits and passage of blood or mucus and a feeling that the bowel is not empty after defecation. The symptoms differ, also depending upon the type of growth that is involved. Polypoid, cirrhous, ulcerating, annular, and colloid growths may occur in the bowel.

When the tumor occludes the bowel, symptoms

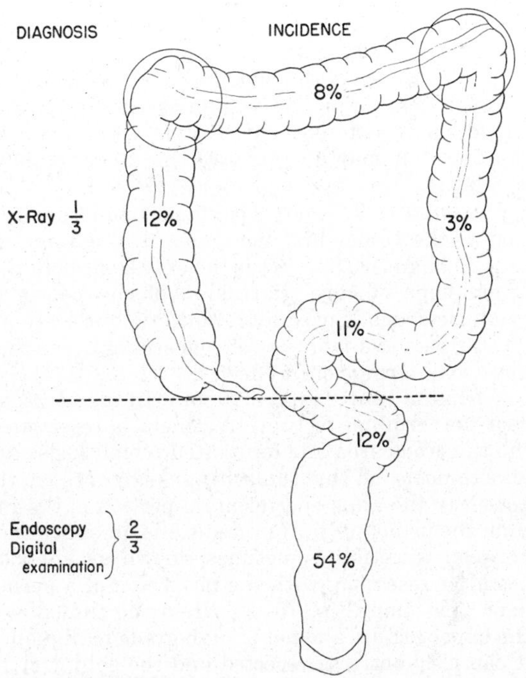

FIGURE 79–2. The incidence of carcinoma in various portions of the large bowel. (From Davis, L.: *Christopher's Textbook of Surgery.* 9th ed. 1968.)

of an obstruction result. Tumors in the right colon are unlikely to cause obstruction because of the large lumen of the bowel and the liquid quality of the feces. Tumors in the left colon and rectum frequently cause obstructive symptoms (Fig. 79–3).

Diagnosis. One third of the malignant tumors of the distal colon and rectum can be felt with the examining finger. This makes the digital rectal examination one of the more important diagnostic methods. X-rays of the colon show either a filling defect or a stricture when cancer is present. By use of the sigmoidoscope one half of the tumors can be seen. Many authorities feel that all individuals over 40 should have a sigmoidoscopy done as part of a routine yearly physical examination. Fiberoptic flexible scopes for examining the colon are now gaining general use, and they can reach even into the right colon, extending the diagnostic capabilities of the physician greatly. Cytologic examination is used in some medical centers, but, as with stomach tissues, authorities do not agree on its usefulness. More than 90 per cent of the patients who have noninvasive lesions and who survive surgery live five years following the surgery. This would indicate the importance of early diagnosis in improving the mortality figures for this condition.

Spread. Tumors of the bowel spread by direct extension to a nearby organ, as to the stomach from the transverse colon; by lymphatic and hematogenic channels; and into the peritoneal cavity by seeding or implanting of cells. The urinary bladder, ureters, and reproductive organs are frequently involved by direct extension, and the formation of a fistula between the bladder and the bowel or between the bowel and vagina is not uncommon. Blood-borne extension goes most frequently to the liver but may also involve the lungs, kidneys, and bones.

Treatment. This is dependent upon the location of the tumor and how advanced it is at the time of diagnosis. Surgery is the only treatment that offers hope of cure. Perfusion of the pelvis by cytotoxic drugs is used after surgery, but there are no statistics available as yet concerning chemotherapy's long-term overall effect.

When the cancer is at any point in the bowel except the terminal rectum, treatment is resection of the tumorous area and associated lymph nodes and anastomosis of the remaining segments of the bowel. In the anus and terminal portion of the rectum, the usual surgical procedure is an abdominal-perineal resection, sometimes known as anterior-posterior resection, with the formation of a permanent colostomy (Fig. 79–4). When the tumor is in the upper rectum and not of high grade malignancy, it can frequently be resected and the sphincter retained.

Occasionally, in some medical centers, a procedure called a "pull through" is done. This consists of loosening the bowel through an anterior incision and then literally pulling it through the rectal sphincter. Thus, the tumor is eliminated and the sphincter is retained. This is usually employed when the growth is extensive, the hope of cure is small, and the physician does not wish to inflict a colostomy on the patient in addition to his other problems.

Nursing Care. The patient who is suspected of having cancer of the colon may be admitted to the hospital for x-ray and sigmoidoscopic examinations, or these may be done on an outpatient basis. The patient will probably be apprehensive about both the test procedures and their outcome. If his lesion is in the rectum, the physician may have told him of the probability of a colostomy being done. The average patient has had almost no contact with others who have a colostomy and has only vague ideas concerning it. Usually the preconceived ideas he has are erroneous and include the notion that the colostomy will be "awful." In the preoperative period the nurse should give the patient some positive information about a colostomy. However, before he is told anything some knowledge should be gained about his general acceptance of life's traumatic situations. Too much information or the wrong type of information can cause more anxiety than it relieves.

There should be a consultation between the doctor and nurse to assess the probability of a colostomy's being done, the patient's probable acceptance, and what should be explained to him and his spouse. He should be prepared for a colostomy only if there is a strong possibility that one may have to be done. Always remember that the patient may decide that his condition was inoperable if one is not performed after he has been told of the possibility. See Chapter 75 for care of the patient who has a colostomy.

A nursing function, in addition to caring for a patient with potential or diagnosed cancer, is to aid in case finding. Some patients will not go to a physician who routinely performs a sigmoidoscopy during a physical examination. The nurse is in a good position to interpret the importance of the

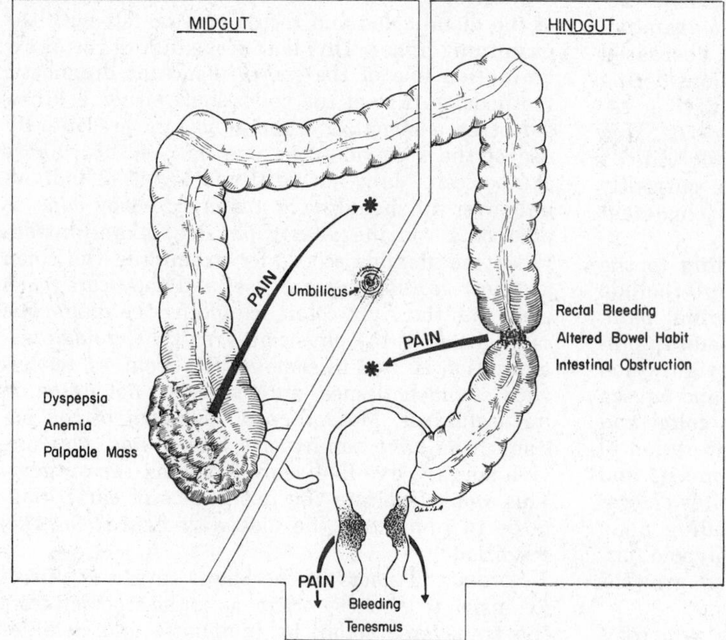

FIGURE 79–3. Symptoms of carcinoma in the right and left colon. (From Davis, L.: Christopher's Textbook of Surgery. 9th ed. 1968.)

examination in diagnosis and thus cure of debilitating conditions. Much teaching should be done among the general public concerning the importance of the symptoms of rectal bleeding and a change in bowel habits. If more patients presented themselves to the doctor at the first sign of such symptoms, more patients would survive.

NURSING CARE OF PATIENTS WHO HAVE HAD BOWEL SURGERY

Care of patients with bowel surgery varies according to whether or not the lumen of the bowel was opened during the surgical procedure. The repair of hernias and the release of some types of bowel obstruction do not require that the bowel be opened, whereas the resection of a tumor in the lumen of the bowel or the resection of a portion of the bowel will necessitate its opening.

PREOPERATIVE CARE

Patients who have the bowel opened will probably enter the hospital a day or so before surgery for bowel preparation. This includes a low-residue or liquid diet to reduce the fecal contents of the bowel and the administration of antibiotics either by mouth, parenterally, or occasionally by means of rectal or colostomy instillation. Enemas to cleanse the bowel are mandatory. The objective is to make the inside of the lumen of the bowel as clean and bacteria-free as possible. When the surgical procedure is done as an emergency, preparation is of necessity brief and the patient has a higher probability of developing postoperative complications and infection.

Preoperative management may include gastrointestinal decompression with either a long or short tube. See Chapter 75 for care of a patient receiving this therapy.

The preoperative teaching is dependent upon the nature of the proposed surgery but will always include such things as what to expect postoperatively in the way of therapy, and the various measures such as deep breathing and leg exercises that are designed to prevent complications. The type of anesthetic used and duration or presence of intravenous infusions and gastric suction will vary.

POSTOPERATIVE CARE

Depending upon the extent of the surgical procedure and the type of anesthesia used, the patient may be up immediately after surgery and walking down the hall, as in a herniorrhaphy done with a local anesthetic, or he may be severely ill for several days, e.g., patients who have had large portions of the bowel resected.

An important problem in any type of bowel surgery is the return of bowel function. The passage of flatus rectally indicates that peristalsis is returning. The presence of peristalsis can also be determined by using a stethoscope to listen for bowel sounds. Gastric suction is frequently used until peristaltic activity returns. It is usually several days before food and fluids are taken orally. Diet is resumed progressively beginning with liquids and advancing as the patient tolerates food. The presence of abdominal cramps is common, as is distention of the bowel. Distention is uncomfortable for the patient and, if too extreme, not good for new suture lines. Some surgeons routinely use a cecostomy when large bowel surgery is done in order to decompress the bowel and prevent tension on sutures. The insertion of a rectal tube for 20 to 30 minutes will be of help if there is gas in the rectum, but the insertion of any tube into the rectum should be done only with the physician's consent and instructions, especially if the anastomosis of the bowel is in that area. Frequently the physician sutures or tapes a rectal tube in place when rectal sutures are present. Like a cecostomy

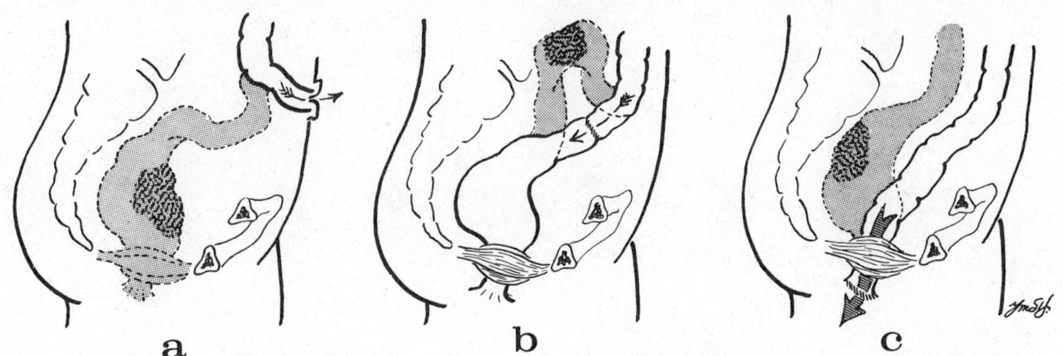

FIGURE 79-4. Diagrams illustrating the alternative approaches to resection of malignant tumors in the rectosigmoid segment: *a*, combined abdominoperineal resection with permanent abdominal colostomy (Miles' operation); *b*, anterior resection with primary anastomosis; and *c*, proctosigmoidectomy with "pull-through" and anastomosis and preservation of external sphincter muscles. Shaded areas represent the resected segments (but do not necessarily indicate the actual extent of resection). (From Berk, J. E., and Haubrick, W. S.: *In* Bockus, H. L.: *Gastroenterology.* 2nd ed. Vol. II. 1964.)

tube this tube should be kept open; it is usually irrigated periodically with water.

Drains are often left in the incision, and frequent dressing changes are needed postoperatively. The character and volume of drainage should be noted carefully in addition to the odor. Should the drainage in any way suggest a developing infection, a culture should be taken to identify the organism and thus give information about what antibiotic will be effective and the possible necessity for isolating the patient. Isolation precautions should be used on all dressings from any draining wound, both to protect the wound from infection and to prevent the spread of organisms that may be present.

It may be several weeks before the patient regains his strength after major bowel surgery. When segments have been removed from the bowel, the patient's bowel habits may be altered for a time until the body readjusts to the situation. He will probably have many questions, especially after returning home. Draining wounds occasionally develop into chronically draining fistulas, and it is not uncommon for dressings to have to be changed at home by the patient or a family member. The nurse should make sure that the patient understands any dietary and activity restrictions and the proper technique for changing dressings. The patient should know whom he can call if he has difficulty or needs help after returning home. A public health nurse's visit can add much to the patient's peace of mind and can also identify problems that might not otherwise be known.

CHAPTER 80

Disorders of the Rectum and Anus

The major function of the rectum is storage of the feces until evacuation takes place. Entry of feces into the rectum distends its walls and causes mass peristaltic movements to occur and, ideally, at this time the patient cooperates and encourages defecation. Many of the disorders that occur in the rectal area result from constipation and failure of the patient to empty the rectum when the mass peristaltic movements occur.

SYMPTOMS

At the mucocutaneous border of the anal canal, the mucous membrane changes to skin that has cutaneous somatic nerve endings. Lesions of the external anal canal are exquisitely painful. The two most common symptoms are bleeding and pain. Drainage of mucus and fecal matter and irritation of the skin from organisms can cause intense itching. Hemorrhoids and skin tags may protrude from the anal opening and there may be drainage of pus from abscesses.

DEVELOPMENTAL, STRUCTURAL AND VASCULAR DISORDERS

HEMORRHOIDS

Hemorrhoids, sometimes called piles, are a very common affliction of mankind. They are probably caused by man's upright position, and the pressure it causes on the anorectal veins; they have their greatest incidence during the most active years of adulthood, from 20 to 50 years. Hemorrhoids may be either internal or external and consist of dilated veins which lie under the mucous membrane. Internal hemorrhoids are varicose dilatations of veins of the superior hemorrhoidal plexus. They occur above the mucocutaneous border and are covered by mucous membrane. External hemorrhoids are dilatations of the inferior hemorrhoidal plexus, are below the mucocutaneous junction, and are covered by anal skin. As these vessels dilate, they stretch the overlying mucous membrane and skin and eventually protrude down the anal canal to prolapse outside. Figure 80–1 illustrates the venous drainage of this area.

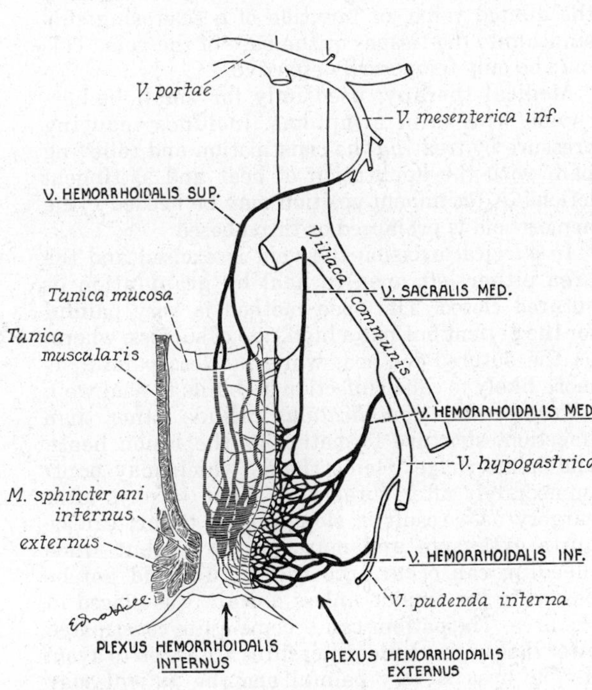

FIGURE 80–1. Venous drainage from the rectum and anus. Note the dual return to both the portal and caval systems providing for collateral venous circulation through the hemorrhoidal plexuses. (From Bockus, H. L.: *Gastroenterology.* 2nd ed. Vol. II, 1964.)

Internal hemorrhoids are frequently caused by portal hypertension, while both types can be caused by the many anastomoses between the plexuses and the lack of valves in the veins of the superior hemorrhoidal plexus which leads into the portal vein.

Several precipitating causes contribute to the acute enlargement of hemorrhoids. These include both constipation and diarrhea, each of which causes straining, which increases pressure within the veins. Congestive heart failure and its resultant increased venous pressure can cause hemorrhoids to develop, as does portal hypertension.

The primary *complications* of hemorrhoids are bleeding, strangulation, and thrombosis. Trauma to the vein during defecation can cause enough bleeding to produce an iron deficiency anemia. Blood oozes or may even spurt out following a bowel movement. Thrombosis, or clotting of the blood within the hemorrhoid, can occur at any time and is manifested by intense pain. Prolapsed hemorrhoids may come out during defecation and spontaneously return; they may have to be replaced by the patient; or they may be prolapsed at all times. A strangulated hemorrhoid is a prolapsed one in which the blood supply is cut off by the anal sphincter. The blood within it becomes clotted and thombosis occurs. This is a very painful condition, with extreme edema and inflammation present. Cold applications and elevation of the buttocks may allow the prolapsed hemorrhoid to reduce itself spontaneously.

Three *treatments* are commonly used for hemorrhoids: medical management, surgical excision of the dilated veins, or injection of a sclerosing substance into the tissues at the base of the vein. This may be only temporarily effective.

Medical therapy, used only for small hemorrhoids with mild symptoms, includes reducing pressure by treating the constipation and relieving pain with the application of heat and astringent lotions. A recumbent position may be needed if the hemorrhoid is prolapsed or thrombosed.

In surgical excision the vein is excised and the area either left open to heal by granulation or sutured closed. The open method is very painful for the patient but has a high rate of success, whereas the sutured method, while far less painful, is more likely to cause infection and fails to heal well.

Postoperative complications include, other than infection, stricture formation as the lesion heals, and hemorrhage. Hemorrhage, which may occur immediately after surgery or about 10 days after surgery as a result of sloughing of tissue, can be quite extensive and may not be evident since bleeding can occur into the rectum and not be passed to the outside unless a drain was placed in the area. The patient can become quite constipated after the surgery unless measures are taken to avoid it. The area is very painful and the patient may avoid defecating to avoid the pain he is sure will accompany passage of a stool. This can result in the formation of a hard stool (which may traumatize the area) or a fecal impaction. Most surgeons give the patient bulk laxatives and order enemas or mineral oil to promote passage of a stool. The patient is usually not allowed to leave the hospital until he has had a bowel movement. The nurse should check the stool, since some patients pass only a very small particle of feces in the first bowel movement. Rectal dilatations are frequently given at intervals after surgery to dilate the area and to prevent stricture formation; however, it is preferable for the patient to have a well-formed stool daily to dilate the area naturally.

Nursing Care

A patient who has a rectal condition is frequently sensitive and embarrassed about his condition and needs matter of fact care from the nurse. The importance of keeping the stool soft but formed to help to prevent the formation of strictures should be stressed as well as the importance of keeping the area clean. The patient should be encouraged to wash the anal area after defecation and to pat it dry rather than irritate the tissues by cleansing with dry paper. Local moist heat on a washcloth or a piece of cotton applied directly to the anal opening for a few minutes is soothing, cleansing, and healing for a sore area. Heat should not be applied in the immediate postoperative period because of the possibility of hemorrhage. Most physicians order sitz baths to be taken three or four times a day or as the patient desires, beginning 12 hours after surgery. These cleanse the area as well as apply localized heat.

Postoperative complications include urinary retention. The proximity of the bladder and the tenderness in the area sometimes make urination difficult. The patient should be carefully checked for voiding after surgery, as well as for hemorrhage. Reestablishing bowel habits is another postoperative problem. A diet high in bulk and including sufficient fluids should be encouraged. This patient may need instruction on the relationship of diet and fluid intake to bowel regularity, the physiology of defecation, and the importance of establishing a routine.

PILONIDAL CYST

This is a cyst usually containing hair, which becomes infected, forms an abscess, and then a sinus tract. It occurs at the base of the sacrum and is most common in young adults, especially males. It has traditionally been thought to be caused by abnormal embryologic development, but recently theories have been advanced which suggest that it results from hairs that penetrate the skin and cause sinus tracts to form. Rubbing of clothing and from chairs can cause hairs in this area to become embedded and then infected. Acute pain and swelling result, followed by a discharge.

Treatment is surgical excision of the abscess formation. The period of healing is quite long. If the infectious process is not completely removed the patient may have a recurrence of the condition. Removing the hairs in this area is a good measure to help to prevent recurrence after healing has occurred.

INFLAMMATIONS

RECTAL FISSURE (FISSURE-IN-ANO)

This is an ulceration of the skin of the anal canal that is actually a longitudinal crack in the skin. It occurs as a result of stretching of the tissue and possibly from the trauma of a hard or excessively large stool passing through the area. The skin is torn as the mass passes and leaves a long open area which is very tender and which tends to reopen at the time of the next defecation. Severe burning follows defecation because of the presence of mucus, fecal matter, and general irritation of the open area. Severe muscle spasm of the sphincter may accompany the condition. The patient may try to avoid having a stool, which of course only aggravates the condition.

Treatment is surgical excision of the tract so it can heal if local dilatations, cleansing, and ointments do not help. The patient should be taught to achieve a soft stool, have a defecation daily, and cleanse the area after defecation, preferably with warm water. Sitz baths aid healing and may relieve pain.

RECTAL FISTULA (FISTULA-IN-ANO)

A fistula is a sinus tract that develops between two body cavities or between a body cavity and the outside. A rectal fistula is a tract that goes from the anal canal to the skin outside the anus or from an abscess to either the anal canal or the perianal area. It is usually preceded by the formation of an abscess.

A fistula may heal over temporarily and then open up periodically to drain. It is a chronic condition for which surgery is the only cure. The tract is surgically excised and the area cleansed and left open to heal by granulation. It may take some time to heal and will be very painful during this time. The patient needs to be encouraged and taught the importance of cleanliness in caring for the wound.

RECTAL ABSCESS

Rectal abscesses form in several positions; Figure 80–2 illustrates the common ones. Many of the abscesses of this area begin as cryptitis (inflammation of the anal crypts), with the formation of cysts that extend through the tubular ducts into the submucosal spaces. These abscesses may also originate from abrasions of the local tissues, with the entry of a virulent organism.

The treatment of these conditions is drainage of the abscess and surgical excision of any associated fistulas. It may take two stages of surgery to accomplish the needed resection.

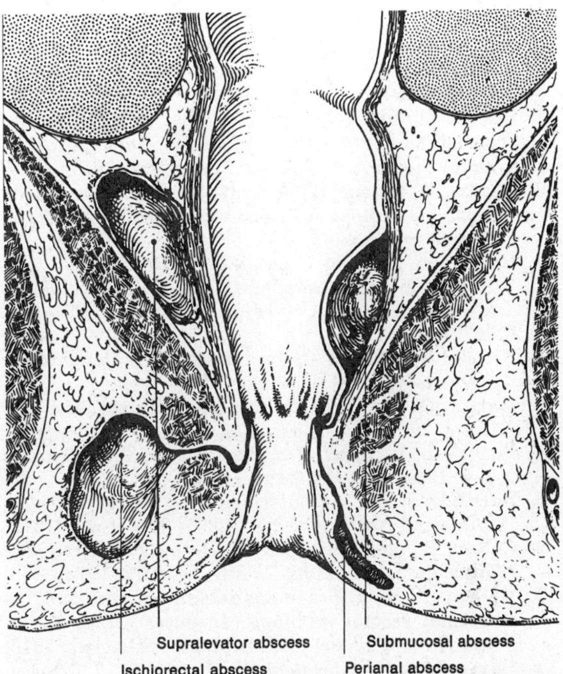

FIGURE 80–2. The anal canal and common locations of rectal abscesses. (From Nigro, N. D., Common Rectal Emergencies. *The American Family Physician,* 6:98–107, November, 1972.)

TUMORS

Carcinoma and melanoma both occur at the anus but both are relatively rare. They spread by local extension into the perirectal spaces and then to the inguinal nodes. Treatment is excision of the anus with an abdominal-perineal resection (Fig. 79–4).

Cancer of the anal canal or lower rectum can coexist with other rectal conditions and the patient may falsely attribute bleeding to a hemorrhoid instead of the more serious condition. Many cancers are overlooked until they are quite large and until the prognosis is poor. A physician should investigate all cases of rectal bleeding, even though it can easily be attributed to hemorrhoids or some other local rectal condition. The nurse should encourage all persons who experience rectal bleeding to consult a physician and have the origin of the bleeding investigated.

See Chapter 79 for treatment and nursing care of a patient with cancer of the rectum; the treatment for anal cancer is the same.

References for Unit XV

1. Adson, M. A., and Akwari, O. E.: Management of gastrointestinal dysfunction after gastric surgery. *Surgical Clinics of North America 51*:915–926, August, 1971.
2. Beahrs, O., and Adsen, M. A.: Ileal pouch with ileostomy rather than ileostomy alone. *American Journal of Surgery 125*:154–158, February, 1973.
3. Beeson, P. B., and McDermott, W. (eds.): *Cecil-Loeb Textbook of Medicine.* 13th ed. Philadelphia, W. B. Saunders Company, 1971.
4. Brantigan, O., and Cocco, A. E.: Recognition and management of esophagitis, a pathophysiologic disease. *American Surgeon 39*:134–141, March, 1973.
5. Brooke, B. M. (ed.): Crohn's disease. *Clinics in Gastroenterology,* Vol. I, No. 2, 1972.
6. Brooks, D. K.: Organ failure following surgery. *Advances in Surgery 6*:302–304, 1972.
7. Burket, L. W.: *Oral Medicine.* 6th ed. Philadelphia, J. B. Lippincott Company, 1971.
8. Burnside, I. M.: Accoutrements of aging. *Nursing Clinics of North America 7*:291–301, June, 1972.
9. Colley, R., and Phillips, K.: Helping with hyperalimentation. *Nursing '73 3*:6–17, July, 1973.
10. Dailey, T. H.: Office management of common intestinal stomal problems. *Diseases of the Colon and Rectum 13*:401–403, September-October, 1970.
11. Davis, L. (ed.): *Christopher's Textbook of Surgery.* 9th ed. Philadelphia, W. B. Saunders Company, 1968.
12. Dudrick, S. J., and Rhoads, J. E.: Total intravenous feeding. *Scientific American 226*:73–80, May 1972.
13. Dudrick, S. J., and Ruberg, R. L.: Principles and practice of parenteral nutrition. *Gastroenterology 61*:901–910, December, 1971.
14. Elwyn, D. H., and Greenstein, A. J.: A critique of parenteral alimentation with respect to amino acid metabolism. *American Journal of Gastroenterology 58*:242–258, September, 1972.
15. Falconer, M., et al.: *The Drug, The Nurse, The Patient.* 5th ed. Philadelphia, W. B. Saunders Company, 1974.
16. Fischer, J. E., et al.: Hyperalimentation as primary therapy for inflammatory bowel disease. *American Journal of Surgery 125*:165–175, February, 1973.
17. Fox, S. R.: The surgical treatment of obesity. *AORN Journal 16*:56–58, July, 1972.
18. Gibbs, G., and White, M.: Stomal care. *American Journal of Nursing 72*:268–271, February, 1972.
19. Given, A., and Simmons, S. J.: *Nursing Care of the Patient with a Gastrointestinal Disorder.* St. Louis, The C. V. Mosby Co., 1971.
20. Glickman, I.: Periodontal disease. *New England Journal of Medicine 284*:1071–1077, May 13, 1971.
21. Grant, J. A. N.: Patient care in parenteral hyperalimentation. *Nursing Clinics of North America 8*: 165–181, March, 1973.
22. Grant, J. A. N., Moir, E., and Fago, M.: Parenteral hyperalimentation. *American Journal of Nursing 69*:2392–2395, November, 1969.
23. Gutowski, F.: Ostomy procedure: Nursing care before and after. *American Journal of Nursing 72*:262–267, February, 1972.
24. Guyton, A. C.: *Medical Physiology.* 4th ed. Philadelphia, W. B. Saunders Company, 1971.
25. Happenie, S. D.: *Colostomy: A Second Chance.* Springfield, Illinois, Charles C Thomas, 1968.
26. Harris, R. S. (ed.): *Art and Science of Dental Caries Research.* New York, Academic Press, Inc., 1968.
27. Johnson, J. B.: Gastric ulcers: Classification, blood group characteristics, secretion patterns and pathogenesis. *Annals of Surgery 162*:996–1004, December, 1965.
28. Judd, E. S.: Selection of treatment for patients with duodenal ulcer disease. *Surgical Clinics of North America 51*:843–850, August, 1971.
29. Katona, E. A.: Learning colostomy control. *American Journal of Nursing 67*:534–541, March, 1967.
30. Keele, C. A., and Neil, E.: *Samson Wright's Applied Physiology.* 12th ed. London, Oxford University Press, 1971.
31. Keough, G., and Niebel, H. N.: Oral cancer detection —A nursing responsibility. *American Journal of Nursing 73*:684–686, April, 1973.
32. Kerr, D. A., and Ash, M. M.: *Oral Pathology.* 3rd ed. Philadelphia, Lea & Febiger, 1971.
33. Keusch, G.: Bacterial diarrheas. *American Journal of Nursing 73*:1028–1032, June, 1973.
34. Kirsner, J. B.: The stomach. *In* Sodeman, W. A., and Sodeman, W. A., Jr.: *Pathologic Physiology, Mechanisms of Disease.* 4th ed. Philadelphia, W. B. Saunders Company, 1967.
35. Knoebel, L. K.: Movements of the digestive tract. Secretion and action of digestive juices: absorption. Energy metabolism. *In* Selkurt, E. E. (ed.): *Physiology.* Boston, Little Brown and Company, 1962.
36. Lenneberg, E.: Role of enterostomal therapists and stoma rehabilitation clinics. *Cancer 28*:226–229, July, 1971.
37. Lenneberg, E., and Mendelssohn, A. N.: *Colostomies: A Guide.* United Ostomy Association, 1971.
38. Lenneberg, E., and Rowbotham, J. L.: *The Ileostomy Patient.* Springfield, Illinois, Charles C Thomas, 1970.
39. Levine, P., and Grayson, B. H.: Safeguarding your patients against periodontal disease. *RN 36*:38–41, July, 1973.
40. Menguy, R.: Gastric ulceration. *Advances in Surgery 6*:103–139, 1972.
41. Miller, J., and Kazmer, N.: Endoscopy review. *AORN Journal 16*:146–156, November, 1972.
42. Moore, C.: Cigarette smoking and cancer of the mouth, pharynx and larynx. *J.A.M.A., 218*:553–558, October 25, 1971.
43. Morrey, L. W., and Nelsen, R. J. (eds.): *Dental Science Handbook.* American Dental Association and The National Institute of Dental Research. Washington, D.C., U.S. Government Printing Office, 1970.
44. Morrissey, J. F.: Gastrointestinal endoscopy. *Gastroenterology 62*:1241–1268, June, 1972.
45. Nasset, E. S.: Physiology of the digestive system. *In* Mountcastle, V. B. (ed.): *Medical Physiology.* St. Louis, The C. V. Mosby Company, 1968.
46. Nelson, R. S.: Tumors of the stomach. *In* Conn, H. F. (ed.): *Current Therapy 1973.* Philadelphia, W. B. Saunders Company, 1973.
47. Nolte, W. A.: *Oral Microbiology.* 2nd ed. St. Louis, The C. V. Mosby Company, 1973.
48. Payne, J. H., and DeWind, L. T.: Surgical treatment of obesity. *American Journal of Surgery 118*:141–147, August, 1969.
49. Redman, B. K., and Redman, R. S.: Oral care of the critically ill patient. *In* Bergersen, B. S., et al. (eds.): *Current Concepts in Clinical Nursing.* Vol. I. St. Louis, The C. V. Mosby Company, 1967.
50. Rodman, M. J., and Smith, D. W.: *Pharmacology and*

Drug Therapy in Nursing. Philadelphia, J. B. Lippincott Company, 1968.

51. Rosillo, R. H., Welty, M. J., and Graham, W. P., III: The patient with maxillofacial cancer II. Physiologic aspects. *Nursing Clinics of North America 8*:153–158, March, 1973.
52. Rowbotham, J. L.: Colostomy problems—Dietary and colostomy management. *Cancer 28*:222–225, July, 1971.
53. Scribner, J. J., Cole, J. J., Christopher, T. G., Vizzo, J. E., et al.: Long term total parenteral nutrition. *J.A.M.A. 212*:457–463, April 20, 1970.
54. Secor, S. M.: Colostomy rehabilitation. *American Journal of Nursing 70*:2400–2401, November, 1970.
55. Selkurt, E. E. (ed.): *Physiology.* Boston, Little, Brown and Company, 1963.

55a. Sleisenger, M. H., and Fordtran, J. S.: *Gastrointestinal Disease.* Philadelphia, W. B. Saunders Company, 1973.

56. Sodeman, W. A., and Sodeman, W. A., Jr.: *Pathologic Physiology, Mechanisms of Disease.* 5th ed. Philadelphia, W. B. Saunders, 1973.
57. The Living Bible, Paraphrased. Wheaton, Tyndale House Publishers, 1971.
58. Turell, R. (ed.): *Diseases of the Colon and Anorectum.* Philadelphia, W. B. Saunders Company, 1969.
59. Usher, F. C., and Matthews, J.: Surgery, treatment of choice for hernia. *American Journal of Nursing 64*: 85–87, September, 1964.
60. Wayler, T., and Klein, R. S.: *Applied Nutrition.* New York, The Macmillan Company, 1965.
61. Welty, M. J., Graham, W. P., III, and Rosillo, R. H.: The patient with maxillofacial cancer, I. Surgical treatment and nursing care. *Nursing Clinics of North America 8*:137–151, March, 1973.
62. Zuidema, G. D., and Klein, M. K.: A new esophagus. *American Journal of Nursing 61*:69–72, September, 1961.

UNIT XVI

Nursing Patients Experiencing Disturbances of the Liver, Biliary Tract, and Pancreas

Joyce V. Zerwekh

Introduction and Study Guide

The liver, biliary tract, and pancreas are located together in the upper abdominal cavity. They all function to facilitate digestion and utilization of foods; in addition, the liver is vital to various other bodily processes. Disease of one organ is often manifested by a sign or symptom in an adjacent organ. Though disorders of each are very different, some common clinical problems will be noted.

A variety of nursing challenges are involved. Manifestations of severe hepatic and pancreatic damage demand complex, intensive nursing care. Chronic progressive disorders of liver and pancreas cause lifelong limitations and necessitate long-term nursing planning and involvement. Gallbladder removal (cholecystectomy) is one of the most common situations encountered in surgical nursing. Drug and alcohol dependency are implicated in disorders of high incidence: hepatitis, cirrhosis, and pancreatitis. In such cases, a patient's goals often conflict with nursing plans to maximize his health, and communication then becomes the greatest therapeutic tool.

This unit will review anatomy and physiology, discuss tools and information necessary for assessment, present a summary of pathophysiologic dynamics and clinical care in problems commonly seen, and then discuss in turn the specific disorders of each organ.

The reader may find the following guide helpful to study:

1. Before beginning reading, clarify for yourself the following: inflammation; necrosis; peritonitis; immune process; clotting process; diuresis; mechanisms of edema; mechanisms of shock; renal failure; complications of bedrest; dynamics of pain; functions of carbohydrate, protein, fat, and fat-soluble vitamins.
2. As you study, familiarize yourself with these terms:
   hepatitis, cirrhosis, jaundice, icterus, ascites, esophageal varices, hepatic encephalopathy, vascular spiders, liver flap or asterixis, pancreatitis, cystic fibrosis, Australian antigen, steatorrhea.
3. You will need to understand the effects of the following medications:
   diuretics, antibiotics, barbiturates, narcotics, corticosteroids, albumin, neomycin, vitamin K.

CHAPTER 81

Normal Liver, Biliary, and Pancreatic Structure and Function

LIVER AND BILIARY STRUCTURE AND FUNCTION

The liver is located in the upper abdomen and is enclosed by the rib cage, except for a lower margin. The liver lies just below the diaphragm, with the lungs extending over its upper portion. The lower portion of the liver provides a roof over the stomach, pancreas, and intestines. Most of the liver is blanketed by peritoneum, as is the adjacent gallbladder. The gallbladder is a pear-shaped sac that rests directly beneath the right lobe of the liver. The liver is involved in so many physiologic processes that new ones are continually being proposed and discovered. It facilitates multiple metabolic reactions and the production of many substances, filters blood, and secretes bile which is then stored and concentrated by the gallbladder.

Three major vessels carry blood to and from the liver. A third of the incoming blood is arterial; the *hepatic artery* carries oxygenated blood from the aorta. Two thirds of the incoming blood is venous; the *portal vein* carries blood from the stomach, spleen, and intestines to be filtered by the liver. Figure 81–1 illustrates the origin of blood flowing into the portal system; increased pressure in the sys-

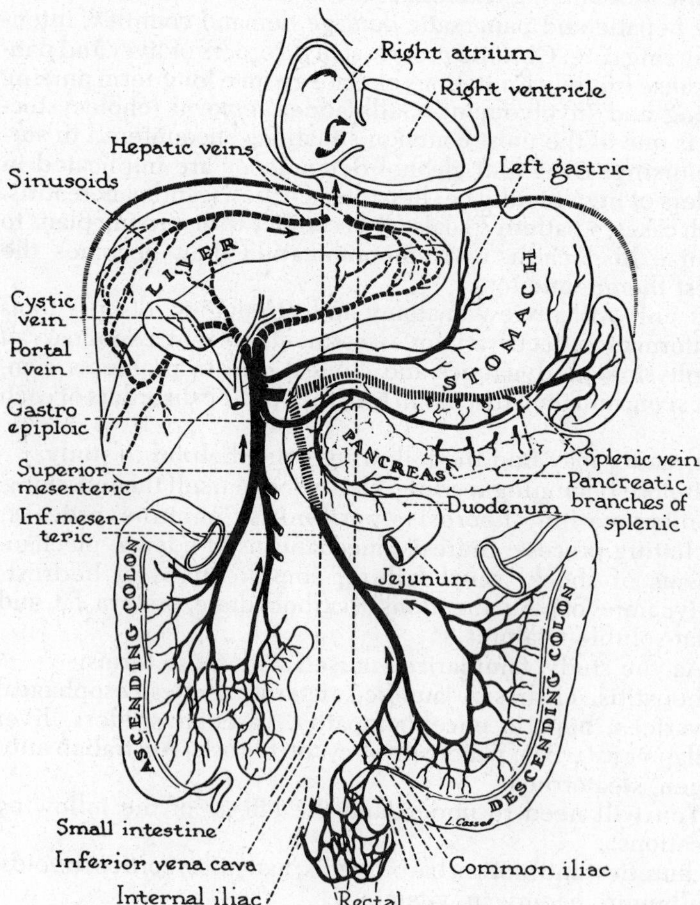

FIGURE 81–1. The portal system of veins. The transverse colon and small intestine have been partially removed and the organs separated in order to show the vessels. (From King, D. G., and Showers, M. J.: *Human Anatomy and Physiology.* 6th ed. 1969.)

tem is a common manifestation in liver disorders, with serious consequences involving vessels where portal blood originates. These consequences will be discussed in Chapter 83. The *hepatic vein* carries all blood leaving the liver to the inferior vena cava.

Bile secreted by the liver is carried by a system of extrahepatic ducts to the gallbladder and then to the duodenum. The right and left hepatic ducts join to form the common hepatic duct, which joins the cystic duct coming from the gallbladder to form the common bile duct. The common bile duct courses under the duodenum and through a short portion of the head of the pancreas before joining the pancreatic duct in the ampulla of Vater. The sphincter of Oddi controls passage into the duodenum.

The functional hepatic unit is the liver lobule (Fig. 81–2), in which cell groups are centered around a central vein. Incoming portal and arterial blood follows minute branches until it reaches a network of passageways called hepatic sinusoids. Blood passes into the sinusoids through the liver lobule from its rim to the hub which is the central vein; each cell is exposed to the sinusoid blood. The sinusoids are lined by special reticuloendothelial cells, the Kupffer cells, which are central to the liver's filtration function, as will be discussed later. Minute bile channels, the canaliculi, also come in contact with each hepatic cell; they course in the opposite direction, from the hub of the lobule to its rim, where they drain into bile ducts (cholangioles) of increasing size, eventually reaching the left and right hepatic ducts.

PRODUCTION OF BILE

The secretion of bile is a major function of the liver, while the sole function of the biliary tract (bile ducts and gallbladder) is to transport, store, and release the bile into the duodenum as needed. The multiple processes involving bile production by the hepatic cell will be discussed first. Basic components of bile include bilirubin, bile salts, cholesterol, lecithin, fatty acids, electrolytes, and water. Though bilirubin (bile pigment) is merely a metabolic end-product with no active physiologic role, its tendency to color whatever medium it is in becomes an indicator of a variety of disorders of hepatic cells and biliary tract. Bilirubin is produced initially in the reticuloendothelial system through the breakdown of hemoglobin (Fig. 81–3). Bound to albumin, it is carried by the circulation to the liver and conjugated to form bilirubin glucuronide. With the other components of bile, it enters the intestine where it is converted by bacteria to urobilinogen. Some is eliminated as the brown-colored fecal urobilin, some is absorbed by the portal circulation and recycled back to the liver, and a small amount is absorbed into the general circulation and carried to darken the urine as urinary urobilin.

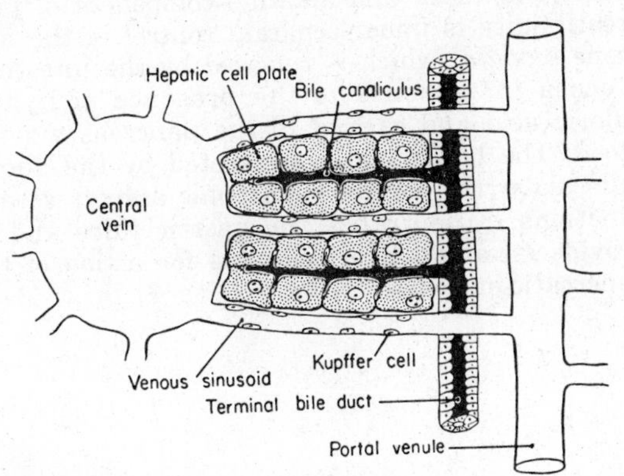

FIGURE 81–2. Basic structure of the liver lobule, showing the hepatic cellular plates, the blood vessels, and the bile ducts. (From Guyton, A. C.: Textbook of Medical Physiology. 4th ed. 1971.)

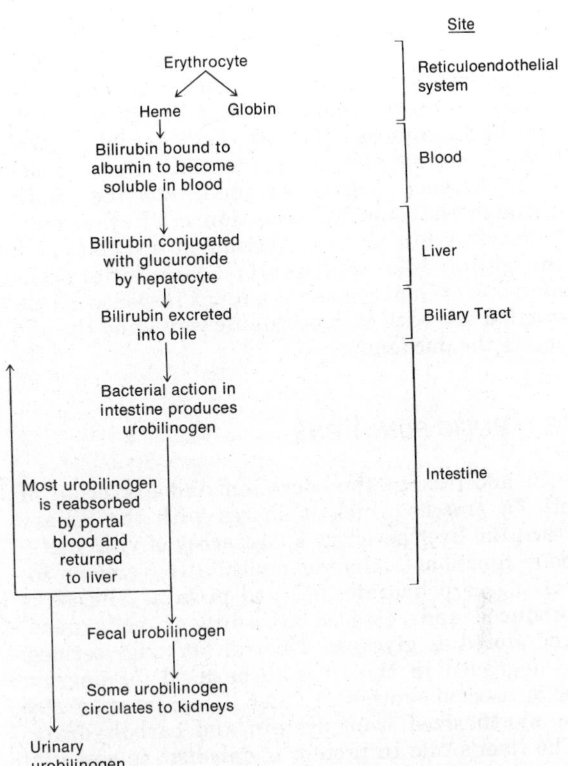

FIGURE 81–3. Bilirubin metabolism and excretion.

Bile salts are the physiologically active component of bile; they increase fat solubility and have a detergent action that breaks up fat into tiny particles and thus facilitates passage through the intestinal wall. Bile salts are synthesized from cholesterol. With lecithin and cholesterol, they exist in bile as molecular aggregates which serve to keep the water-insoluble cholesterol in solution; when this delicate balance is interrupted, gallstones form in the biliary tract. Cholesterol seems to be physiologically inert in bile, and is therein excreted as a metabolic end-product.

Bile is continually being secreted by the hepatic cells, moves through the biliary ducts, and is usually stored and concentrated by the gallbladder, which absorbs an immense quantity of water and electrolytes. The prime variable that controls release of bile is the presence of fat in the small intestine, which initiates the mucosal secretion of the hormone cholecystokinin and its subsequent circulation to the gallbladder to stimulate contraction. The sphincter of Oddi relaxes as a reflex response to contraction and with each peristaltic wave, and the bile enters the duodenum.

METABOLIC FUNCTIONS

In addition to the secretion and excretion of bile, a process which it shares with the biliary tract, the liver performs a vast array of vital metabolic functions including multiple conversions involving carbohydrate, fat, and protein. Glucose is produced and released according to body need, and stored as glycogen. Neutral fat (triglycerides) is degraded in the liver to be used for energy, or is used to synthesize other lipids; fat may also be synthesized from protein and carbohydrate. The liver's role in protein metabolism is essential to survival. Most degradation of excess amino acids begins in the liver with deamination, the removal of the amino group (NH_2). The ammonia released is then converted into urea and excreted by the kidneys. The plasma proteins, except gamma globulin, are synthesized in the liver. These include albumin, essential to maintaining plasma osmotic pressure, and several important clotting factors including prothrombin and fibrinogen. Other metabolic functions of the liver include the storage of vitamins, the storage of iron as ferritin, the conjugation and excretion of adrenal and gonadal steroids, and the detoxification of multiple foreign substances.

BLOOD STORAGE AND FILTRATION

Finally, the liver has a circulatory function, that is, to store blood in the sinusoids which drain in the event of systemic blood loss. The sinusoid Kupffer cells filter the circulation by phagocytosis of colon bacteria and debris carried to the liver in the portal blood.

PANCREATIC STRUCTURE AND FUNCTION

The pancreas stretches retroperitoneally, with its head in the concavity of the duodenum and its tail against the spleen. The liver lies above, and the stomach passes close to the anterior surface. It functions both as an endocrine gland, secreting insulin and glucagon directly into the blood stream from the islets of Langerhans scattered throughout the organ with greater concentration in the body and tail, and as an exocrine gland, secreting multiple digestive enzymes into a system of ducts which empty into the duodenum. It is this exocrine function which is the focus of the present discussion. Endocrine function and disorder are discussed in Unit XIX.

The exocrine functional unit is the secreting acinus, composed of a central area surrounded by pyramidal epithelium containing zymogen granules, considered to be enzyme precursors. The pancreatic acini are arranged in lobules. From each acinus, channels extend to a main lobular duct and finally to the main pancreatic duct and its accessory duct which extend the length of the gland. The main pancreatic duct enters the duodenum at the ampulla of Vater, where it is joined by the common bile duct. A short common channel may be present before the sphincter of Oddi, which controls the release of pancreatic juice and bile into the duodenum.

Normally, 1200 to 3000 ml. of pancreatic juice are produced daily; it is a clear alkaline solution carrying three major types of digestive enzymes. Pancreatic *amylase* hydrolyzes carbohydrate to yield disaccharides; pancreatic *lipase* hydrolyzes fat to yield glycerol and fatty acids; and *trypsin* is representative of the group of proteolytic pancreatic enzymes which split proteins. Trypsin is activated in the bowel and functions as a catalyst to initiate a chain of other proteolytic enzymes. Within the acini, a special trypsin inhibitor is stored to prevent that enzyme from digesting pancreatic tissue.

Outpouring of digestive enzymes into the pancreatic juice is under the control of the vagus and of the hormone *pancreozymin,* released by the intestinal mucosa in response to the presence of chyme and carried to the pancreas via the blood. The water and alkaline component of pancreatic juice is under separate control of the hormone *secretin,* which is released by the intestinal mucosa in response to the presence of hydrochloric acid and carried to the pancreas via the blood. The bicarbonate is secreted by the ductal cells under the control of carbonic anhydrase and functions to neutralize the gastric juice and to provide an alkaline pH suitable for action of the pancreatic enzymes.

CHAPTER 82

Assessing Abnormalities of Liver, Biliary, and Pancreatic Function

The purpose of this chapter is to overview the disorders most common in the liver, biliary tract, and pancreas, and to identify specifically the information needed and tests used to gather enough data to determine the identity and course of these illnesses.

OVERVIEW OF ABNORMALITIES

Listed below are the most common of these disorders, together with a brief definition of each, and some of the typical clinical problems encountered.

PATHOLOGY AND CAUSATIVE FACTORS

Pathologic changes in these disorders are multiple and vary widely. They may be broadly categorized into three types: inflammatory, fibrotic, and neoplastic. Hepatitis, pancreatitis, and cholecystitis show evidence of acute and chronic inflammation of involved tissues. Fibrotic changes occur with cirrhosis and with inflammatory diseases which have become chronic. Primary tumors, benign or malignant, of these tissues are rare.

Factors implicated in pathogenesis vary from viruses to alcoholism to gallstone formation. Hepatitis is the only inflammatory process attributed to a virus; though the hepatitis virus is still to be isolated, multiple viruslike particles have been demonstrated. The relationship between alcoholism and cirrhosis and pancreatitis is timeworn, but the underlying mechanisms that actually cause disease remain hypothetical. Gallstone formation usually underlies cholecystitis and sometimes pancreatitis, but the processes underlying stone formation are incompletely understood, as are the processes whereby stones precipitate inflammation. The etiology of each disorder will be further discussed in separate sections, but the underlying mechanisms remain open to considerable dispute.

MEDICAL ASSESSMENT

PHYSICAL EXAMINATION

Physical examination for the purpose of determining the presence of liver, biliary, or pancreatic disease involves exhaustive exploration of the entire body. In particular, *palpation of the abdomen,* especially the liver and spleen, is definitive. The pancreas is not palpable. Deep palpation is essential to evaluate tenderness, a common complaint with inflammatory processes of these organs. Since

Disorder	Definition	Typical Clinical Problems
Hepatitis	Inflammation of liver due to viral infection transmitted by fecal-oral (type A) or blood (type B) route	Fatigue, anorexia, nausea, vomiting, jaundice, pruritus, abdominal pain, bleeding tendencies
Cirrhosis	Chronic liver disease with impaired function due to extensive scar tissue; usually associated with alcoholism	Ascites, bleeding tendencies, ruptured esophageal varices, anemia, alcoholism, malnutrition
Cholecystitis	Inflammation of gallbladder usually associated with presence of gallstones (lithiasis)	Abdominal pain, nausea and vomiting, jaundice, fever, bleeding tendencies
Pancreatitis	Inflammation of pancreas often associated with alcoholism or biliary tract disease	Abdominal pain and vomiting; hypovolemia and shock in acute episodes; hyperglycemia; incomplete digestion and vitamin deficiency; steatorrhea and diarrhea in chronic cases

the peritoneum is often involved, the presence of localized peritoneal irritation is determined by rapidly removing the examining hand, which as a consequence rapidly jerks the peritoneum. If it is inflamed, pain is severe with this maneuver and *rebound tenderness* is thus established.

The liver edge is palpated in the right upper quadrant just below the ribs; inhalation and hand pressure over the posterior ribs bring the liver closer to the examiner's hand as he evaluates it for tenderness, size, presence of masses, and consistency (scarring or swelling). The spleen is palpated in the left upper quadrant just below the ribs; the same maneuvers as described with the liver bring it closer to the examiner's hand. Enlargement of the spleen is common in cirrhosis as a result of congestion from portal hypertension.

In addition to palpation, comprehensive inspection is essential. Inspection of the abdomen reveals ascites (fluid-filled abdomen) and prominent venous collateral networks common to cirrhosis. Systemic signs such as jaundice, weight loss, the enlarged breasts and reddened palms of cirrhosis, are among a long list of manifestations to be seen.

DIAGNOSTIC PROCEDURES

Common tests of liver, biliary, and pancreatic function are summarized in Table 82-1 on page 1122.

Radiologic Techniques

Cholecystogram (Gallbladder Series). This is a test for gallbladder disease done by visualizing the gallbladder. Telepaque or another organic iodine dye is given 12 hours before the test. Be sure to check whether the patient is allergic to iodine or seafood before giving the dye. The allergic effects of the dye may include nausea and vomiting, diarrhea, abdominal pain, and rash; anaphylaxis also is possible.

The patient is given a low-fat evening meal to avoid gallbladder contraction, and is NPO or on fluid restriction in the morning. The bowel is cleansed with enemas, and sometimes a cathartic is given.

The dye is conjugated in the liver, excreted into bile as an opaque medium, and outlines the gallbladder. The test takes about an hour; sometimes a high-fat meal is given after the procedure to test gallbladder contraction. Gallbladder disease is indicated by poor or no visualization of the bladder, presumably because biliary obstruction prevents passage of the dye into the gallbladder. Occasionally stones are visualized as shadows within the opaque medium. The test results are accurate only when gastrointestinal and liver function allows absorption and conjugation of the dye.

Cholangiogram. This procedure is used to visualize the bile ducts. Cholografin or another organic iodine dye is used, and again iodine allergies should be considered. Possible allergic reactions include dyspnea, tachycardia, sweating, nausea and vomiting, and chills. The dye burns intensely on injection. Prior fluid restriction is observed and the bowel is cleansed beforehand.

The dye usually is given intravenously but may be given through percutaneous puncture when obstructive jaundice prevents the flow of dye through the bile. Occasionally the dye is also introduced directly into the ducts during surgery, or into a T-tube postoperatively. Other than drug reactions, the main danger is from bleeding and bile peritonitis, which sometimes complicate percutaneous cholangiography.

Duct obstruction is directly visualized by the failure of the opaque dye to pass a certain point in the bile ducts.

Other Procedures Using Contrast Media. Procedures in which contrast media are injected into the portal and related vessels include: celiac angiography, hepatoportography, splenoportography, and umbilical venography. The pancreatic vessels are studied using pancreatic angiography. In all these procedures, Hypaque or another organic iodine dye is injected into a vessel, then flows to the vessels being studied and outlines them. The solution burns intensely for a few seconds after injection. Possible allergic reactions to iodine should be watched for, and the I.V. site should be observed for edema or thrombosis.

These procedures determine the patency of vessels supplying the organ in question and disclose the presence of lesions that may distort the vasculature. They are used particularly in cirrhosis in order to detect esophageal varices.

Radioisotope Scanning of the Liver. Iodine-131 rose bengal, ^{198}Au colloidal gold, or technetium is administered intravenously and a scintillation detector is passed over the abdomen. These gamma-emitting isotopes are concentrated in functional liver tissue, with lesions appearing as filling defects. (See Unit VII for details on radioisotope scanning.)

Measures of Portal Pressure and Flow

These are minor surgical procedures performed in the operating room. They are often combined with the injection of contrast media. They require standard preoperative and postoperative care, with special observation of the incisional site for hematoma.

The principal procedures are transhepatic puncture, umbilical-portal or hepatic vein catheterization, and percutaneous splenic pulp manometry. In the last-mentioned procedure, a manometer is inserted into the spleen through a needle placed between two of the lower ribs. Careful observation for bleeding is important afterward.

These procedures measure portal vein pressure and flow, indicate the severity of portal hypertension, and guide decisions as to appropriate treatment measures. The indirect calculation of sinusoid pressure helps to determine the location of obstruction and thus identify the underlying disorder.

Analysis of Digestive Juices

Duodenal drainage is done through a nasogastric tube in a fasting patient. For a period of one to six hours the tube is left in the duodenum. Magnesium sulfate is inserted to stimulate bile flow and the secretions are aspirated. It may be followed by the *secretin test,* in which secretin is given intravenously, possibly followed by pancreozymin, and the secretions are again aspirated.

These procedures are currently reserved for patients allergic to iodine who cannot undergo cholecystography or cholangiography. Disproportions in the bile and pancreatic juice fractions indicate obstruction to ductal flow. The presence of cholesterol crystals indicates lithiasis. The secretions are analyzed for volume, bicarbonate, enzyme, and biliary content.

Peritoneoscopy

A peritoneoscope is inserted through an abdominal stab wound to permit direct visualization of the liver and peritoneum. The patient is NPO and is sedated before the procedure. A local or general anesthetic may be used. Structural changes can be visualized, thus aiding in the diagnosis of cirrhosis or cancer.

Liver Biopsy

Liver biopsy is usually performed at the bedside and is frequently used to gain specific information regarding tissue changes, thus to facilitate differential diagnosis or provide data regarding the course of illness. Nursing responsibilities are multiple. Prothrombin time should be evaluated first. Vitamin K may be given intramuscularly several days beforehand to increase prothrombin synthesis and to reduce the chance of hemorrhage. Written permission is given by the patient only after thorough explanation of the procedure in language he can grasp. Prior to the procedure, baseline vital signs are obtained, the patient fasts for several hours, and sedation is given at least one half hour beforehand.

The procedure itself is brief. The skin is cleansed and anesthesized with a local anesthetic and, while the supine patient holds his breath, a needle is introduced in the eighth or ninth right intercostal space or subcostally. The needle is rotated in the liver to cut off a tissue specimen, the specimen is aspirated, and the needle is withdrawn. To prevent tearing of the liver, it is vital that the patient understand and be capable of holding his breath for about 10 seconds, not moving until the procedure is completed. He is instructed to take several deep breaths and to hold on exhalation; once the needle is removed, he is immediately instructed to breathe. After the procedure, the patient remains immobile and on his right side for several hours, the length of time determined by medical judgment.

Complications of needle biopsy of the liver are rare but dangerous. Hemorrhage due to penetration of a blood vessel is possible, and vital signs are taken frequently (every 15 minutes initially) until evaluated as stable. Dressings are checked frequently for local bleeding, and a pressure dressing is applied if necessary. Accidental puncture of a bile duct is also possible, and a patient's complaint of severe abdominal pain may indicate bile peritonitis.

Paracentesis

Paracentesis or peritoneal tap is performed to analyze fluid accumulations in the peritoneum (ascites). It is usually done at the bedside; the nurse is actively involved in care. The patient is instructed and must give written permission beforehand. To avoid puncture of the bladder, he must void immediately prior to the procedure. He is then positioned sitting upright on the edge of the bed with his feet resting on a stool and his back well supported. Following cleansing of the skin and infiltration with local anesthetic, a trocar is inserted aseptically through a small stab wound below the umbilicus and fluid slowly drained through a catheter into a collection bottle. Many complications threaten with paracentesis. The greatest danger is hypovolemia as circulatory fluid rapidly shifts into the peritoneal cavity to replace that lost. Vital signs and peripheral circulation are noted frequently during and following the procedure. Other manifestations of reduced systemic circulation, renal failure, and hepatic coma owing to reduced tissue perfusion should be anticipated. Because of the high protein concentration of ascitic fluid, salt-poor albumin is often infused over the 24-hour period following the procedure. Infection (peritonitis) and bleeding due to trauma of vessels are occasional complications; complaints of abdominal pain must be carefully assessed.

NURSING ASSESSMENT

Nursing assessment of these patients focuses particularly on gathering complete data on nutrition and elimination, fluid balance and circulation, skin, and comfort status. In conditions associated with alcohol or drug abuse, sensitive psychosocial and environmental assessment is vital. Presenting clinical problems are thoroughly explored at the time of the patient's admission, and a baseline nursing diagnosis of functional level is established. Ongoing evaluation of the status of problems may lead to an ever-changing diagnosis.

TABLE 82–1. LABORATORY TESTS OF LIVER, BILIARY, AND PANCREATIC FUNCTION

Measurement	Normal Value	Procedure	Interpretation
1. Biliary excretion			
a. Serum bilirubin		Blood drawn without special patient preparation	
Direct (conjugated)	<0.2 mg.		Direct bilirubin increased with impaired biliary excretion, causing conjugated fraction to accumulate in plasma
Indirect (not conjugated)	<0.8 mg.		Indirect bilirubin increased with increased erythrocyte hemolysis
Total	<1 mg.		Total bilirubin measures direct and indirect
b. Urine bilirubin	0	Simple urine collection	Urine bilirubin measures conjugated bilirubin only and is increased with impaired bile excretion
c. Urine urobilinogen	0–4 mg./24 hr.	24 hr. or 2 hr. afternoon collection placed in brown refrigerated bottle with sodium carbonate	Urinary urobilinogen decreased with impaired bile excretion. Increased with erythrocyte hemolysis
d. Fecal urobilinogen	40–280 mg./24 hr.	Entire stool to laboratory	Fecal urobilinogen decreased with impaired bile excretion; increased in erythrocyte hemolysis.
e. Serum cholesterol	150–250 mg./100 ml.	Blood drawn after low cholesterol diet for 12 hr.	Cholesterol elevated when excretion blocked by bile duct obstruction, but reduced when severe liver damage reduces ability to synthesize it
2. Carbohydrate metabolism			Pancreatic digestive enzyme released with breakdown of acinar cells; serum elevations over 300 U. indicate pancreatitis; elevations not directly correlated with severity; urinary levels elevated longer (about 1 week); over 300 U./hr. indicates pancreatitis
a. Serum amylase	80–160 U./100 ml.	Blood drawn without special patient preparation	
b. Urine amylase	<260 U./hr.	2, 12, or 24 hr. urine collection with no preservative unless specified	
3. Protein metabolism			
a. Total protein	6–8 Gm./100 ml.	Blood drawn without special patient preparation	Less plasma proteins synthesized in liver damage; albumin synthesis consequently reduced, but increased serum gamma globulins produced by plasma cells
b. Serum albumin	3.5–5.5 Gm./100 ml.	Same as above	
c. Serum globulin	2.5–3.5 Gm./100 ml.	Same as above	
d. Prothrombin time	12–15 sec. = 100%	Same as above	Prothrombin time prolonged with decreased synthesis owing to liver cell damage or decreased vitamin K absorption (fat-soluble) when bile duct obstruction reduces bile in intestine; vitamin K essential to synthesis of prothrombin

TABLE 82–1. LABORATORY TESTS OF LIVER, BILIARY, AND PANCREATIC FUNCTION (*Continued*)

Measurement	Normal Value	Procedure	Interpretation
e. Blood ammonia	<75 mcg./100 ml.	Blood drawn without special patient preparation	Reduced synthesis of urea from body ammonia in severe hepatocellular damage produces elevated blood ammonia
f. Flocculation tests			
Cephalin	0 or 1+	Blood drawn without special patient preparation	Hepatocellular disease indicated when precipitation occurs in sera mixed with thymol or cephalin-cholesterol; alterations in serum protein fraction cause reaction
Thymol turbidity	0–5 U.	Blood drawn on patient with fat restriction 12 hr. beforehand	
g. Serum methemalbumin	Absent	Fluid from peritoneal or pleural tap analyzed	Product of hemoglobin digestion elevated when blood released into body fluids, as in hemorrhagic pancreatitis
4. Fat metabolism			
Serum lipase	<1.5 U.	Blood drawn on fasting patient	Pancreatic digestive enzyme released with breakdown of acinar cells
5. Metabolism of foreign substances			
a. BSP excretion	<0.4 mg./100 ml. <5% retention in 1 hr.	Control blood taken from patient fasting for 12 hr.; Bromsulphalein given, blood drawn at 30 min. and 1 hour or once at 45 min.	Dye retained with diminished hepatocellular ability to remove it from the blood and excrete it
b. Indocyanine green excretion	500–800 ml./sq.m.body surface/min.		
6. Serum enzymes			
a. SGOT	5–40 U./ml.	Blood drawn without special patient preparation	Serum glutamic oxaloacetic transaminase, serum glutamic pyruvic transaminase, and lactic acid dehydrogenase released from damaged hepatic cells; levels not directly correlated with degree of damage; elevations noted in other conditions, particularly myocardial infarction
b. SGPT	5–35 U./ml.		
c. LDH	Varies with units used		
d. Alkaline phosphatase	Varies with method	Blood drawn without special patient preparation	Increase in biliary obstruction, probably due to continued hepatic production with excretion blocked
7. Tests for Australian antigen including agar gel diffusion, counterelectrophoresis, complement fixation, passive hemagglutination, and radioimmunoassay	Negative	Blood drawn without special patient preparation	Multiple techniques identify Australian antigen indicating viral hepatitis B (serum)

CHAPTER 83

Clinical Problems Commonly Encountered with Liver, Biliary, and Pancreatic Disorders

This chapter will focus on those manifestations of disease which actually give a patient functional trouble and cause problems which lead him to seek health care. The problems discussed are among the most common requiring medical and nursing intervention; a thorough acquaintance with their underlying dynamics and derived clinical interventions will effectively prepare the student to plan and provide care in many situations. The approach used is problem-oriented rather than disease-centered. Disease-centered data necessary to complete student knowledge of how to plan for specific conditions are included in the chapters following.

JAUNDICE

Jaundice or icterus is the yellow pigmentation of the skin due to accumulations of bilirubin pigment. *The degree of jaundice is best seen in the sclera of the eye.*

CAUSATIVE FACTORS AND DIFFERENTIAL DIAGNOSIS

There are two common causes of jaundice:
1. Red blood cell destruction.
2. Impaired excretion of bile.

1. *Red blood cell destruction* occurs in hemolytic anemias when the rapid rate of erythrocyte hemolysis results in excessive accumulations of unconjugated bilirubin. The skin becomes jaundiced and, as the liver conjugates and excretes the excessive amount of pigment, greater than normal quantities of urobilinogen become present in urine and feces. Diagnosis is made on the basis of increased indirect (unconjugated) serum bilirubin values, absence of bilirubin in the urine (unconjugated bilirubin is water insoluble), and increased urobilinogen levels.

2. *Impaired excretion of bile* may be caused by failure of the hepatic cells to release conjugated bilirubin or by obstruction of intrahepatic or extrahepatic bile ducts. Resultant stagnation of bile in the hepatic cells and bile ducts is termed *cholestasis.* Through undefined channels, the pooling bile components are absorbed into the blood stream. Both reduced hepatic cell secretion and inflammatory ductal obstruction[9] have been implicated in the jaundice of hepatitis. Extrahepatic obstruction is caused by gallstones (cholelithiasis) or neoplasm.

The jaundice of hepatitis and that of common bile duct obstruction have many manifestations in common, as well as other manifestations that differentiate the two types. Common symptoms include increased levels of direct (conjugated) serum bilirubin, since it returns to the plasma when excretion is blocked; increased indirect serum bilirubin for unclear reasons; increased bilirubin in urine owing to high blood concentrations; reduced fecal urobilinogen, since it does not reach the intestine; increased alkaline phosphatase and cholesterol serum levels, since they cannot be excreted as normal into the bile; increased serum bile salts with consequent deposition in the skin to cause pruritus; and prolonged prothrombin time owing to reduced absorption of fat-soluble vitamin K. Hepatitis is differentiated from extrahepatic blockage by demonstration of reduced hepatic cell function (diminished serum proteins, increased release of enzymes as a result of cellular damage). Extrahepatic obstruction to biliary excretion is more complete and may be differentiated from hepatocellular jaundice by higher alkaline phosphatase and cholesterol levels, more extreme pruritus, and the almost complete absence of fecal urobilinogen. Percutaneous cholangiography will visualize the site of obstruction by injection of opaque media directly into the extrahepatic ducts.

CLINICAL INTERVENTION TO RESOLVE JAUNDICE OR ALLEVIATE SYMPTOMS

Jaundice can be reduced only by elimination of the underlying disease. (See Chapter 61 for discussion of therapy in hemolytic anemia.) Extrahepatic biliary obstruction can be treated solely by surgical removal of obstruction. Final differentiation between choledocholithiasis (stone in the common bile duct) and tumor can only be made during the surgical exploration of the common bile duct, a procedure termed choledochostomy. If carcinoma, most commonly affecting the head of the pancreas, is found, a palliative anastomosis of the gallbladder to the jejunum is done to bypass the common bile duct. Resolution of jaundice in hepatitis relies on time as the prime therapeutic agent. Treatment is symptomatic.

Jaundice is a warning sign of disease, but of itself does not cause physical injury. Therapy will reduce accompanying complaints. Pruritus, believed to be caused by accumulation of bile salts in the skin when biliary excretion is obstructed, can be merely irritating or can drive the patient to distraction and to tearing at his skin until excoriation develops. Oral cholestyramine resin provides some relief by binding bile salts and promoting intestinal elimination. Anabolic steroids can be palliative, but they aggravate jaundice.[18] Antihistamines provide some help.

A highly visible sign of illness, jaundice may have considerable emotional impact and may impair body image. Each day the person may fearfully study his eyes in hope of improvement, and may ask every staff member who walks in, "Do you think my color is any better?" Jaundice becomes a stigma, and the isolated hepatitis patient may associate it with his separated status. His feelings need acknowledgement, and ongoing explanation reduces unfounded fear. The patient may become preoccupied with physical appearance; his sense of ugliness may be compensated for by helping him to maintain an otherwise satisfying appearance.

ASCITES

CAUSATIVE FACTORS

Three underlying pathophysiologic forces interact to cause the development of ascites (fluid accumulation in the peritoneal cavity): *portal hypertension, lowered plasma colloidal osmotic pressure,* and *sodium retention.* This combination of events occurs most commonly in cirrhosis.

Portal hypertension, elevated pressure in the portal vein, is seen when pathologic processes cause *obstruction to flow of blood out of the sinusoids.* Most commonly, this occurs in cirrhosis, in which the block is believed to be either parasinusoidal[29] or postsinusoidal, and in congestive heart failure, in which increased central venous pressure causes damming of flow of blood. Backup of blood in portal veins causes splenic congestion and enlargement, development of collateral channels to bypass the liver, and ascites. Clinical implications of the first two will be discussed later. Mechanisms by which portal hypertension causes ascites are still being debated. Most authors emphasize consequent increased venous hydrostatic pressure in the preportal vessels of the peritoneum, with fluid under pressure forced out into the peritoneal cavity. Some authors state that large quantities of lymph drain through lymphatic channels from the congested sinusoids and under pressure, leak into the peritoneal cavity. It would seem that both mechanisms are involved in

producing fluid accumulations, and increased hydrostatic pressure is basic to both.

Lowered plasma colloidal osmotic pressure occurs with *reduced hepatic synthesis of albumin,* which is synthesized exclusively in the liver and is the major substance maintaining fluid in the blood vessels. When portal hypertension is also present, two factors combine to move fluid from the vessels into the peritoneal cavity: reduced colloidal osmotic pressure and increased hydrostatic pressure.

Finally, *sodium retention* contributes to water retention and therefore ascites volume. Reduced sodium excretion is attributed to *increased aldosterone* in the blood; presumably aldosterone is not being metabolized by the damaged hepatic cells and so accumulates. In addition, pooling of blood in the peritoneum results in diminished renal perfusion, stimulation of the renin-angiotensin mechanism, and consequent stimulation of increased aldosterone production. Thus more aldosterone is being made and less is broken down. (See Chapter 24 for sodium and aldosterone relationships.)

Remember the three mechanisms underlying ascites formation:
1. Portal hypertension resulting in increased plasma and lymphatic hydrostatic pressure.
2. Hypoalbuminemia resulting in decreased colloidal osmotic pressure.
3. Hyperaldosteronism resulting in increased sodium retention.

DIAGNOSIS

Ascites is diagnosed by inspection of the fluid-filled abdomen, percussion for dullness, and tapping of massive ascites to produce fluid waves. When these signs are accompanied by other manifestations of disease associated with ascites, usually cirrhosis, identification of the problem is validated. Paracentesis is performed to permit analysis of ascitic fluid and determination of volume, and peritoneoscopy is occasionally used to visualize the liver. Serum albumin and sodium levels are usually obtained and will be used to determine therapy. Portal circulation is usually not evaluated unless another complication of portal hypertension, bleeding esophageal varices, is present. (See Bleeding, p. 1126, for discussion of varices.)

CLINICAL INTERVENTION

Five goals guide reduction of symptoms due to abdominal pressure from ascites:

1. *Evaluate extent of ascites accumulation.* Ascites is evaluated on an ongoing basis after diagnosis to determine the pathologic course and the effectiveness of therapy. *Daily weights* provide a sensitive monitor of fluid retention and loss. Meas-

urements of *abdominal girth* provide a gross estimate of progress or regression of abdominal swelling. A patient with ascites faces long-term medical management and the need for ongoing adjustments in therapy. He must be taught the importance of assessing his weight and measuring his abdomen and immediately report rapid gain in pounds and inches to his physician. Be sure that the patient will have access to a scale or all your teaching will be hypothetical!

2. *Control sodium and water retention through dietary restriction and diuretics. Dietary restrictions* needed to reduce salt and water retention are initially based on 24-hour urine collections to estimate sodium chloride loss. The clinician will then prescribe intake equalling but not exceeding that loss. "Ascites formation ceases when *no* Na is ingested. It follows, therefore, that the low Na diet is a cornerstone for the treatment of ascites."[26] Restrictions vary from 3 Gm. sodium daily with mild ascites to 200 mg. for patients with large collections of fluids. (See Chapter 25 for Sodium Restricted Diets.) Such diets can be quite unpalatable, and ongoing consultation with dietitians is essential. Patient understanding and motivation must be high to follow low-sodium diets over a period of time. Fluid restrictions of 1000–2000 ml./day are sometimes imposed when body weight increases despite severe sodium restrictions.

Diuretics are added to treat ascites when dietary restriction alone is not providing effective control. This occurs when the primary causal factors in ascites—portal hypertension and hypoalbuminemia—are severe. The kidneys stop excreting sodium, and even the minimal sodium of a restricted diet results in retention of ascitic fluid. The use of diuretics is based on the fact that they stimulate the kidneys to increase their reduced sodium and water excretion. Two diuretics are usually combined. A combination of spironolactone or triamterene, both of which have potassium-retaining properties, with thiazides, ethacrynic acid, or furosemide can be adjusted carefully to balance potassium losses.

Occasionally potassium chloride supplementation is necessary. Fluid and electrolyte levels are watched very carefully during the first few days of diuretic therapy. Hypokalemia, with alkalosis, as well as hyperkalemia, and hyponatremia, are possible. Too rapid diuresis can precipitate oliguria and uremia owing to diminished circulatory volume, and the development of hepatic encephalopathy is not unusual. The student may wish to refer to Chapter 25 to review mechanisms of the fluid and electrolyte imbalances which threaten. Ongoing diuretic therapy necessitates the patient's understanding of drug therapy and the needed combinations to achieve balance.

3 and 4. *Increase albumin levels when hypoalbuminemia is severe and remove fluid by paracentesis.* When diet and diuretic therapy fail to control ascitic accumulations, intravenous albumin and paracentesis may benefit the patient. Salt-poor albumin is given, and expanded blood volume should initiate diuresis; the patient must be observed carefully for concomitant signs of pulmonary edema. Occasionally ascitic fluid is reinfused to expand volume.

Though it used to be standard therapy, paracentesis is now indicated only when fluid accumulations are large and disabling and all else has failed. Only small amounts are removed to avoid the risks of fluid shift and protein loss, but multiple complications are still possible. The fluid removed rapidly reforms, and the patient is right back where he started.

5. *Relieve symptoms due to pressure of ascites.* Gross distention may force the diaphragm upward and restrict lung expansion. High Fowler's position will maximize respiratory effectiveness. Skin circulation is also compromised by pressure within the abdomen and by inadequate cellular perfusion due to interstitial edema. Turning and positioning are vital to prevent prolonged external pressure and breakdown.

BLEEDING

CAUSATIVE FACTORS

Bleeding tendencies may be present in viral hepatitis, cirrhosis, and biliary obstruction. There are two fundamental causes of bleeding: reduced clotting factors, and ruptured esophageal varices.

Reduced clotting factors involve reduced prothrombin synthesis as well as reduction of other components necessary to clotting. Hypoprothrombinemia will occur when bile duct obstruction prevents passage of bile into the small intestine; resultant reduced fat absorption causes reduced absorption of fat-soluble vitamins, of which vitamin K is one. Vitamin K is a necessary catalyst for the synthesis of prothrombin in the liver. Hypoprothrombinemia will also occur when liver cells are so severely damaged that they cannot synthesize adequate amounts of prothrombin; this situation occurs in cirrhosis and in severe cases of hepatitis. Hypoprothrombinemia due to hepatic damage is differentiated from that due to reduced vitamin K absorption by the administration of vitamin K parenterally; a rapid return to normal prothrombin time indicates the problem is due to biliary obstruction. Many other clotting factors can be deficient with liver cell damage. The platelet count will sometimes be reduced owing to destruction by an enlarged spleen. "Fibrinogen, even though it is made wholly in the liver, is uncommonly deficient except in massive liver necrosis."[9]

2. *Ruptured esophageal varices* (swollen, dilated esophageal veins) produce massive hemorrhage as a dreaded complication of cirrhosis. They develop as a consequence of portal hypertension. Basically, pathologic obstruction to flow of portal blood through the liver, as mentioned under Ascites (p. 1125), causes backup of blood into the veins that deliver blood to the portal vein (Fig. 81–1). These veins develop an elaborate system of collateral channels to bypass the liver. Collateral channels underlie

several manifestations of cirrhosis which will be discussed later; *the development of collateral portal channels in the esophagus* is the focus here.

"The varices presumably result from the greater volume of blood under higher pressure which these collateral veins must carry when cirrhosis is present."[9] Rupture of esophageal varices can occur with any increase in portal hydrostatic pressure, such as with increased intrathoracic or intra-abdominal pressure or with increased blood volume. Blood loss under such pressure is rapid and great. Direct trauma by food and irritation by gastric juices have also been implicated.

DIAGNOSIS

Bleeding tendencies due to hypoprothrombinemia or thrombocytopenia are identified through blood tests such as prothrombin time or platelet count. Prothrombin time is routinely evaluated with patients being worked up for biliary and liver disease, and is included in intermittent evaluations of those with an identified disorder. These patients need to be watched carefully and need to be aware themselves of the implications of ready bruising, epistaxis, bleeding from oral mucosa, menorrhagia, hematuria, melena, and hematemesis. They should be taught to avoid trauma to tissues incurred by rough physical exercise, forceful noseblowing, or use of a toothbrush with hard bristles.

The gastrointestinal tract is the most common site of bleeding in patients with cirrhosis. Bleeding from gastric and duodenal ulcers must be distinguished from bleeding from esophageal varices. In known cirrhosis with developed collateral channels and distended spleen, varices are very likely. The blood from varices is bright red and appears suddenly and unexpectedly in large quantities; blood from stomach and duodenum tends to be darker and is usually preceded by severe dyspepsia. If bleeding is effectively reduced by use of a Sengstaken-Blakemore tube (see below), it is assumed to be due to varices. Once bleeding is under control, barium swallow and endoscopy with flexible fiberscopes permit indirect and direct visualization of varices. To evaluate the portal system, contrast media may be injected into vessels and portal pressure and flow may be measured.

CLINICAL INTERVENTION TO RESTORE HEMOSTASIS

Hemostasis in liver and biliary disease is achieved in four ways:

1. *Restore clotting factors.* When hypoprothrombinemia has been identified, parenteral vitamin K is given with the hope that reduced fat absorption due to reduced bile excretion has been at least a partial cause. When hepatic damage is the sole cause of reduced prothrombin synthesis, vitamin K will not help, and prothrombin itself has not been isolated for therapy. In such a case, fresh plasma or whole blood will be effective in replacing clotting factors for short periods. When the problem is reduced platelets, platelet transfusions are possible.

2. *Lavage bleeding gastric ulcers using cold fluid.* Ice water or saline is instilled through a nasogastric tube; the resulting vasoconstriction will reduce blood flow from peptic or duodenal ulcers, but will have little impact on hemorrhaging varices.

3. *Apply pressure to ruptured varices.* A *Sengstaken-Blakemore tube* (Fig. 83–1) provides pressure with balloons directly over the bleeding varices and in the cardia of the stomach to compress supplying veins. It usually controls the massive bleeding while in place. Occasionally ice water is circulated through the balloon to promote vasoconstriction.

4. *Lower portal pressure.* Temporary lowering of portal pressure is achieved by the administration of *posterior pituitary hormone* (pituitrin, Pitressin). It is believed to constrict afferent arterioles and thus reduce portal blood flow to cause portal hypotension. Systemic side effects include fluid retention, myocardial ischemia, and stimulation of uterine and gastrointestinal contraction (cramping and diarrhea).

Permanent lowering of portal pressure is achieved

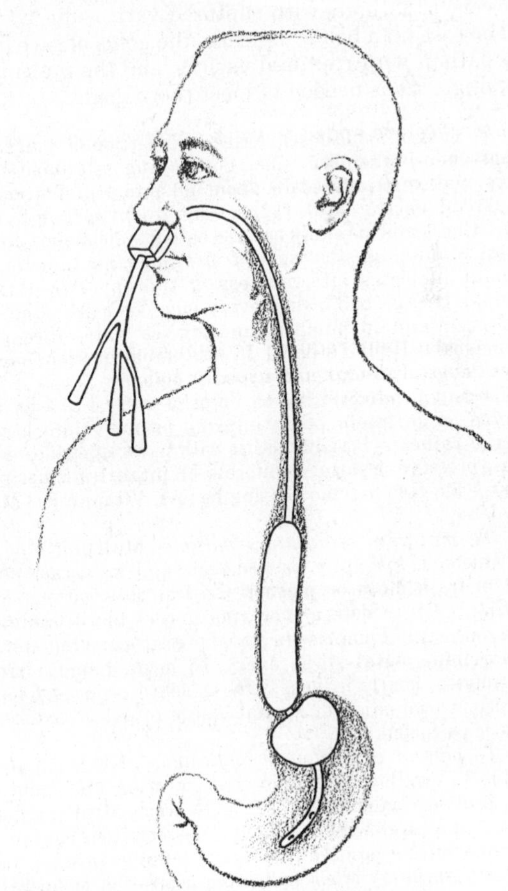

FIGURE 83–1. Intubation for esophageal compression. (From Nealon, T. F., Jr.: *Fundamental Skills in Surgery.* 2nd ed. 1971.)

by surgical procedures which shunt blood away from the portal system. Most commonly performed are portacaval and splenorenal shunts. The *portacaval shunt* lowers portal pressure by anastomosing the portal vein and the inferior vena cava; blood flowing into the portal system is then carried into the vena cava. The liver and the obstructions within it that had caused the portal hyperension are bypassed. The *splenorenal shunt* lowers portal pressure by anastomosing the splenic vein and the left renal. Blood flowing into the portal vein through the splenic vein (Fig. 81–1) is diverted into the renal vein and thus bypasses the obstructing liver. Splenectomy is necessary to allow splenorenal anastomosis. Portal shunts definitely stop bleeding, but the overall survival of cirrhotic patients is not much enhanced owing to multiple complications. Patients are considered good surgical risks in the *absence* of jaundice, severe ascites, encephalopathy, and severe hypoalbuminemia.

Special Care for Esophageal Varices

1. *Ruptured bleeding esophageal varices* comprise an acute physiologic and emotional crisis, and nursing care is intensive and complex. Sixty-seven per cent of patients with ruptured varices die.[31]

The care plan below indicates the goals of care for the patient with ruptured varices, and the multiple nursing actions needed to meet these goals.

> *To achieve hemostasis.* Assist in insertion of deflated Sengstaken-Blakemore tube. Positioning is guided by x-ray. Balloons inflated to about 30 mm Hg. Traction is placed on the tube to prevent downward movement. Check and maintain ordered ballon manometer pressures. Monitor gastric suction drainage for bleeding; amount indicates effectiveness of therapy. Maintain traction. Iced gastric lavage every hour, or more often if ordered. Maintain pump circulating ice water through esophageal balloon if ordered. In case of malfunction, have extra Sengstaken-Blakemore tube on hand.

Pitressin or pituitrin in I.V. Volutrol every 1 to 4 hr. if ordered, or maintain pump infusing pituitrin into local arterial catheter. Possibly assist with paracentesis to decrease pressure on portal collaterals. Maintain transfusions of *fresh* blood to provide clotting factors. Vitamin K I.M., if ordered.

> *To maintain circulatory volume.* Multiple blood transfusions, including packed cells and an occasional unit of fresh blood or plasma. Critical observation, including: CVP to detect overexpansion of blood volume with concomitant increase in portal pressure and therefore hemorrhage; vital signs every 15 min.; hematocrit, electrolytes; hourly urines, BUN to detect reduced renal perfusion; evaluation of mental status to detect reduced hepatic perfusion.

> *To prevent respiratory complications.* NPO, patient unable to swallow. Frequent expectoration and mouth care, oral suction of saliva. Frequent tracheal suctioning to prevent aspiration of blood and clear secretions. Oxygen and intermittent positive pressure breathing. Observe for sudden respiratory crisis indicating aspiration or airway obstruction due to upward balloon displacement from pull of traction when gastric balloon ruptures. Check for esophageal balloon in oropharynx and then deflate. Remove tube if still indicated.

> *To prevent esophageal erosion.* Periodically deflate balloons every 8 to 12 hours; some physicians will leave balloons fully inflated for two to three days.

> *To prevent hepatic coma.* Cathartics, enemas, neomycin as ordered. Restraints as necessary in patients with encephalopathy.

> *To prevent nasal breakdown.* Keep nostrils clean and lubricated. Maintain padding (foam rubber) in position.

> *To provide patient and family comfort.* Calm environment. Family frequently included in intensive care environment. Ongoing explanation given; touch used. Acknowledgment of the dreadful situation of literally being gagged and "hung up" by the tube; honest information on how long the situation is likely to last. Judicious use of p.r.n. pain medication with consideration of how drug is detoxified.

> *To prepare patient for emergency portal shunt if indicated.* Measures to improve prothrombin levels, reduce ascites, increase albumin levels, reduce encephalopathy, reduce anemia, and overcome concurrent infection may be necessary.

> *To provide postoperative care after shunt.* Standard postoperative abdominal measures with special attention to respiratory measures and circulatory monitoring. Observe for and prevent encephalopathy. Prevent edema due to increased inferior vena cava hydrostatic pressure by elevation of bed and use of elastic stockings. Maintain heparin if infused through regional catheter to prevent portal thrombosis at site of anastomosis.

2. *Asymptomatic esophageal varices* are frequently visualized when the cirrhotic patient is thoroughly evaluated. "Recognizable hemorrhage (hematemesis, anemia with guaiac positive stools) occurs, at some time, in at least 40% of patients with varices."[17] The risk of preventive surgery is too great, and the patient must live with the threat of bleeding. He and his family should be advised to develop a plan of action for such an emergency.

Certain behavior will decrease his chance of bleeding: avoiding aspirin and alcohol, which irritate the mucosa; avoiding constipation so that straining at stool will not increase intra-abdominal pressure; avoiding heavy lifting; treating coughs to avoid increased intrathoracic pressure; and avoiding eating large meals which may temporarily increase portal pressure.[29] Food should be chewed well in small portions to avoid trauma to mucosa. Antacids may be ordered to neutralize irritating gastric acid. Occasionally dietary sodium restrictions and diuretics may be prescribed to keep plasma volume, and therefore portal pressure, low.[17]

No matter what the preventive measures, the odds are still stacked against the patient with varices; his behavior and response to therapy will reflect a variety of ways of coping with the awareness that he could hemorrhage at any moment. That is quite a threat for anyone!

HEPATIC ENCEPHALOPATHY

CAUSATIVE FACTORS

Hepatic encephalopathy (disordered brain function) occurs with severe liver cell injury or when portal blood bypasses the liver through collateral channels which develop physiologically in response to portal hypertension or as shunts created surgically. In either case, *blood ammonia levels increase* when the liver cell is no longer able to remove ammonia from the blood and convert it to urea. The origin of the ammonia is absorption from the intestine, where it is produced by bacterial action on amino acids and urea. *Any process that increases protein in the intestine, such as increased dietary protein or gastrointestinal bleeding, will cause elevated blood ammonia.* Increased blood ammonia has a toxic effect on the brain, which results in nervous system and psychiatric disturbance. Since blood level does not predict severity of toxic symptoms, other factors are believed to be involved. Electrolyte and acid-base imbalances, constipation, tissue hypoxia, uremia, infectious processes, and central nervous system depressants may contribute to encephalopathy.

ASSESSMENT

Manifestations of hepatic encephalopathy progress from early prehepatic coma with mild mental confusion to deep hepatic coma. Critical observation and interviewing are essential in all susceptible patients. Memory, attention, concentration, and rate of response become impaired and worsen with depression of function. Handwriting and speech are evaluated for change. Personality changes with labile feeling states are often seen. As the syndrome progresses, *level of consciousness is slowly depressed,* and confusion becomes more severe. Flapping tremor ("liver flap" or asterixis) is elicited when the patient is asked to dorsiflex his hand with the rest of the arm resting on the bed. At this time, delta waves on the electroencephalogram (EEG) are characteristic. Finally, coma follows and may deepen until there is no pain response and the reflexes, including corneal, are completely absent.

Fluctuations in level of depression are common. The nurse, who is with the patient over time, is the best person to see a change in level of mental functioning. Early detection greatly improves the patient's chance of recovery. Nursing progress notes are relevant when they describe behavioral change vividly as raw data ("Patient states pigeons are pecking at his bedclothes") rather than as a vague generalization that has a different meaning for each reader ("Patient seems more confused"). As the patient progresses into coma, ongoing neurologic checks by the nurse are essential to determine level of consciousness. (See Chapter 38 for checks usually performed on comatose patients.)

Some patients develop hyperventilation with *respiratory alkalosis.* A characteristic odor on the breath, *fetor hepaticus,* is attributed to the presence of volatile sulfur compounds. Throughout the course of this syndrome, serum ammonia levels, electrolytes, blood gases, and hepatic function (bilirubin, albumin, prothrombin, enzymes) are monitored to determine degree of imbalance and extent of hepatic injury and failure to function.

CLINICAL INTERVENTION

Four goals guide therapy in hepatic encephalopathy, prehepatic coma and coma:

1. *Reduce protein in intestine.* This is accomplished by *reduction of dietary protein.* If no other precipitating factors are present, this alone may eliminate symptoms. Protein may be eliminated entirely with an intake of fruit juices and intravenous fluids, or it may be restricted to 20 to 40 Gm. In the patient chronically susceptible to coma, a long-term low protein diet (50 to 60 Gm.) may impose severe strain on self-control. Patient understanding and motivation are essential for cooperation. Gastrointestinal bleeding resulting in accumulations of protein in the intestine must be identified and treated to reverse the progression of symptoms. Constipation must be reversed. As behavioral manifestations worsen, *cathartics* and *enemas* will be prescribed to hasten exit of protein material from the intestine.

2. *Reduce bacterial production of ammonia.* This is commonly accomplished by the administration of neomycin in large oral doses; neomycin is not absorbed into the circulation and therefore exerts a powerful effect on the intestinal bacteria responsible for ammonia production. Undesirable side effects due to the depletion of intestinal flora include diarrhea and vitamin K deficiency. *Neomycin is commonly combined with protein restriction and bowel cleansing in the treatment of late prehepatic coma and coma.* It may be prescribed in maintenance doses with low-protein diet in the patient with a tendency to chronic recurrence of coma. Lactulose, a 5-carbon sugar, is sometimes administered in these cases. It has been demonstrated to decrease ammonia production by lowering the pH of the bacterial environment.

3. *Eliminate imbalances: fluid and electrolyte, uremia, hypoxia, infection, sedation.* Hypovolemia often precipitates hepatic coma by reducing hepatic cellular perfusion. Therapy during coma requires intravenous intake. Therefore, achieving, maintaining, and monitoring fluid balance are essential to prevent further hepatic injury as well as reduced renal perfusion with uremia. Accumulating urea breaks down to form more ammonia. Intravenous volume must be delivered evenly over a period of time. Vital signs and central venous pressure are monitored frequently; often hourly urine determinations are essential. Electrolyte and acid-base disturbances may precipitate hepatic coma or develop during coma. Laboratory tests indicate the replacement therapy necessary.

Hypoxia may precipitate hepatic coma due to hypoxic damage to the hepatic cell; both therapeutic and preventive management of the patient will include attention to respiratory measures such as maintaining a patent airway, oxygenation, and intermittent positive pressure breathing. Concurrent infection, with protein accumulating from tissue catabolism, must also be treated, and the patient is particularly vulnerable to hospital-acquired infections. Careful attention must be paid to the prevention of cross infection. Finally, depressants may precipitate coma, and must be avoided during therapy. Sedation during agitation occurring in prehepatic coma must be provided by agents, such as phenobarbital, which are excreted through the kidney instead of the liver.

4. *Maintain function in the unconscious patient.* Complications possible in the immobile patient lacking reflexes are numerous, and their prevention requires intensive nursing. (See Chapter 38 for care of the comatose patient.)

Therapy usually alleviates hepatic coma, though the patient may succumb to circulatory or respiratory complications, infection, or delirium and convulsions. There is a high mortality among patients who progress into coma with hepatic failure. Many dramatic measures, such as peritoneal dialysis and exchange transfusions which remove and then replace approximately 80 per cent of the person's blood, have been developed to reduce toxic levels in hopes of regeneration of cells. Corticosteroids and antimetabolites improve laboratory values, but whether they halt degeneration is questionable. In the most advanced research centers, liver transplant may be tried when there is complete hepatocellular failure in a young, otherwise healthy, patient.

INTOLERANCE TO SEDATION

The patient with hepatic damage responds adversely to sedation. Reasons remain unclear. The explanation is often given that the drug accumulates to toxic levels when the damaged liver cells fail to metabolize and excrete it, but elevated levels may not be demonstrated during drug reactions.[5] It has been postulated that the brain of the patient with hepatic damage is oversensitive to the effects of these drugs; underlying dynamics remain undefined.[5] Precise information on routes of drug metabolism is also lacking.[5] Opiates, short-acting barbiturates, and major tranquilizers are believed to be metabolized primarily in the liver, and are avoided as therapeutic agents. In the absence of drugs, nursing measures become the major means of achieving rest and comfort for these patients. Phenobarbital, believed to be excreted primarily through the kidney, is the agent of choice if medication is indicated.

ALCOHOL AND DRUG ABUSE

Alcoholism and parenteral drug abuse precipitate many disorders discussed in this unit. They also become ongoing clinical problems, as therapy is limited and prognosis often grim when the patient is unwilling to give up the cause of disorder. Increasingly, both alcohol and drug abuse are being seen in the same person.

Alcoholism is characterized by physiologic dependency manifested by withdrawal symptoms when ethanol intake is eliminated, development of tolerance to increasing quantities, blackout spells, and psychologic dependency when the person drinks despite social or medical contraindications.[8] Alcoholic hepatitis, Laennec's cirrhosis, and pancreatitis are commonly associated with alcoholism.

Drug abuse may rarely precipitate toxic hepatitis if hepatic toxins are ingested over time, and commonly precipitates viral hepatitis if needles contaminated with infected blood are shared without intervening sterilization. The injected agents that most commonly are involved in producing viral hepatitis are the opiates, amphetamines, and barbiturates.

CLINICAL INTERVENTION

Clinical goals focus on (1) maintaining physiologic function, and (2) facilitating rehabilitation.

Maintaining physiologic function involves sustaining the patient through the crises of the presenting disease and preventing drug-associated crises, particularly withdrawal. Withdrawal from alcohol and barbiturates induces a variety of problems ranging from vomiting to hallucinations to convulsions. These must be avoided by sedation appropriate to the drug and dosage used. In hepatic disease, the agents are carefully chosen to avoid those which are detoxified through the liver.

Facilitating rehabilitation may be divided into two phases. The first phase emphasizes attaining the highest possible level of physical health despite the patient's ongoing habit. Approaches include dietary teaching, teaching procedures for sterilizing of needles, hygiene measures, and periodic follow-up. This interim phase is fraught with frequent disappointment, as the patient often retreats defensively from medical intervention.

The second phase emphasizes attainment of a drug- or alcohol-free state. This is a realistic goal only when the patient is motivated toward change, when he acknowledges the problem and seeks a solution. Motivation may develop during a crisis such as illness, but can be sustained only by grappling with those forces which originally determined the problem: social pressures, loneliness, uncertainty about the future, alienation, impulsiveness, and noncomformity,[6] among others. Individual psychotherapy, group therapy, communal therapy, and family therapy help the patient to work through these forces. The hospital nurse actively uses nondirective techniques to help him explore his need to change and suggests possible community resources and therapeutic approaches that might meet his need. She must understand that he will not change unless he can envision a meaningful alternative to the alcohol or drug experience; alternatives often seem terribly limited in today's distressed society. The self-destructive appearance and behavior of the patient often scare and repel the nurse; the extent to which she can be helpful may be determined by her ability to recognize her own feelings and to reach beyond them to the suffering individual.

CHAPTER 84

Disorders of the Liver

VIRAL HEPATITIS

EPIDEMIOLOGY

Two epidemiologically distinct types of viral hepatitis have been identified, type A and type B. Since pathologic changes demonstrated in tissue, as well as the signs and symptoms of the patient, are nearly identical, the two types have traditionally been difficult to distinguish.

Type A hepatitis is commonly known as *infectious hepatitis* (IH). Primary means of transmission is through *ingestion of infected fecal material;* therefore, the disease has a low incidence in places where standards of sanitation are high. Occasional outbreaks occur when water becomes contaminated; shellfish from contaminated waters have occasionally been vehicles of infection. Most victims are children and young adults. Though epidemics tend to occur in waves, the cases in the United States appear to be plateauing at a low level.[23] In addition to fecal-oral transmission, parenteral transmission through the blood of the infected person is also possible. Infectious hepatitis is also called *short incubation hepatitis;* jaundice and elevated cellular enzymes appear one month after exposure and last about three weeks. The person is considered to be infectious from three weeks prior to developing jaundice to three weeks afterward.[21] Infection confers an individual immunity specific to type A.

Type B hepatitis is commonly known as *serum hepatitis,* but this incorrectly implies a single means of parenteral transmission through the blood of infected persons. "At present it seems quite definite that type B hepatitis is at least occasionally contact-associated through ingestion or inhalation of blood. The extent of person-to-person transmission in the general population and the role of the fecal-oral route remain to be defined."[23] Oral-oral transmission has also been suggested. In 1965 a viruslike particle, Australian antigen, was demonstrated to be present in most cases of serum hepatitis. Australian antigen may be a viral component; its exact relationship to the infectious agent is unknown. Simple laboratory tests (see Table 82–1) are now available to screen blood products for hepatitis B antigen (HBag) and to differentiate hepatitis B from A.

Serum hepatitis is also called *long incubation hepatitis.* Serum enzymes do not elevate until two months after exposure, and jaundice appears after about three months; manifestations usually last for several weeks. The time the person is considered infectious varies and lasts as long as Australian antigen can be identified in his serum.[21] Four per cent of patients are positive six months after symptomatic recovery and therefore become carriers.[23] Infection confers individual immunity specific to type B. The number of cases and the number of carriers of hepatitis B are increasing in the United States, attributable largely to the increasing incidence of parenteral drug abuse. The disease is a rising threat to the public health.

CONTROL

Hepatitis in the community is reduced as sanitation is maintained and parenteral drug abuse with use of contaminated equipment decreases. Gamma globulin affords immunity to those known to be exposed. Standard gamma globulin must be given within two weeks of exposure to hepatitis A to prevent symptoms. Standard gamma globulin has no effect on hepatitis B, but new gamma globulin preparations with higher titers against Australian antigen appear to be effective in modifying clinical manifestations.

Hepatitis in the home is controlled by thorough understanding by the patient and all members of his household of how the disease is contagious. Most essential is that he wash his hands after defecation. Separate toilet facilities are best when feasible; otherwise, disinfection after each use must be arranged. Food preparation and handling by the patient must be strictly avoided. His dishes should be disposable or kept for individual use; his sheets, underwear, and pajamas should be laundered separately. Kissing may result in oral transmission. Needles shared without sterilization practically guarantee infection of fellow drug users.

Hepatitis in the hospital is controlled by isolation barriers to fecal and parenteral spread. A private room is not necessary for a responsible adult.[33] Gowns and gloves are worn by all staff having direct patient contact. All articles potentially contaminated with blood or feces must be handled with special precautions, disinfected, or discarded. Separate toilet or portable commode is essential. Linens are isolated. Dishes are disposable. Rigorous handwashing following patient care is the most important barrier to contagion. All these precautions require thorough explanation to the patient. Nevertheless, he will often express dismay or anger at being treated as "unclean"; staff must be careful that medical isolation does not lead to social isolation.

Rigid controls must be applied to reduce the incidence of *iatrogenic hepatitis* transmitted by parenteral therapy. Infected blood and protein fractions have been an ongoing problem. Careful screening of donors, and discouragement of the practice of paying the poor, down-and-out person who has no resources left to sell except his own blood and is more likely to be infected with either type of hepatitis owing to living conditions, reduce the incidence of transfusion-borne infection. New screening tests for antigen will eliminate the use of blood infected with hepatitis B, but there as yet remains no test for A. Kidney dialysis patients are subjected to a high risk of hepatitis, and rigid precautions are necessary to protect these extremely vulnerable people. Physicians and nurses must be careful of any breaks in their own skin; also, oral ingestion through casual hand-mouth transmission by such activities as cigarette smoking, nail biting, and eating and drinking without strict handwashing has been implicated. Finally, inadequate sterilization or unsafe disposal (throwing needles in the wastebasket so that the housekeeping maid punctures herself when picking up the waste) of instruments contaminated with blood must be eliminated to protect staff and other patients.

BASES OF SYMPTOMS

Common symptoms of hepatitis and their pathophysiologic explanation are identified below:

DIAGNOSIS

Observation and interview yield the symptom pattern seen above. Enlarged and tender liver is noted on palpation. Laboratory tests reveal altered bile pigment levels. Serum enzymes (SGOT and SGPT) are elevated, BSP excretion and flocculation tests are abnormal, albumin is slightly reduced, and serum globulin is elevated. Before jaundice appears, symptoms must be differentiated from other viral illnesses such as influenza, and abdominal pain must be differentiated from that due to other cases such as appendicitis or cholecystitis. When jaundice occurs, the cause must be distinguished from extrahepatic obstruction. (See discussion under Jaundice, Chapter 83.)

CLINICAL INTERVENTION

Acute viral hepatitis is commonly benign and little therapy is needed as it follows its course. Long periods of *bed rest* have commonly been prescribed, but the ambulatory treatment necessitated in Viet Nam and in rising numbers of drug abusers in the United States has indicated that activity in the young patient does not affect course and mortality. The best guide to activity restriction is the *avoidance of fatigue.*[27] The patient should be instructed to rest when he feels like it. Initially he will probably want to stay in bed continually. Bed rest during the acute phase in the older patient may prevent complications; research in this population is lacking.

Dietary recommendations have varied widely. Adequate caloric intake is essential, and creative feeding approaches that take into consideration the problems of nausea, vomiting, and anorexia are needed. Antiemetics offer little relief. Intravenous dextrose is necessary if caloric intake falls too low.

Symptoms	Bases of Symptoms
Jaundice, clay stools (no pigment), darkened urine (bilirubin and urobilinogen)	Impaired excretion of conjugated bilirubin into intestine results in elevated serum levels, staining of skin (jaundice), reduced bile pigment in feces, high levels of conjugated bilirubin excreted into the kidneys, and elevated urinary urobilinogen, because small amount of urobilinogen still produced in intestine and reabsorbed into blood is excreted through kidney instead of liver
Pruritus	Bile salt accumulation in skin
Abdominal pain in right upper quadrant	Stretching of Glisson's capsule due to swelling of inflamed liver
Fever	Release of pyrogens in inflammatory process
Fatigue and weakness	Reduced energy metabolism by liver
Anorexia, nausea, vomiting	Possibly visceral reflexes reduce peristalsis. Postulated changes in stomach or bowel
Bleeding tendencies in severe cases	Reduced prothrombin synthesis by injured hepatic cell. Reduced fat-soluble vitamin K absorption due to reduced bile in intestine

A balanced diet is encouraged, and vitamin supplementation is introduced if this cannot be accomplished. Diets low in fat or large doses of vitamin B are sometimes ordered but have not been shown to be effective.

Corticosteroids and antimetabolites are being used for their nonspecific anti-inflammatory effects and possible other actions which alleviate the symptoms and improve the biochemical status of patients with severe acute hepatitis or hepatitis which persists into a chronic phase. Reduction in progressive disease has not been demonstrated.[32]

Drug therapy is reduced to a minimum. Those drugs known to be toxic to the liver (see Hepatic Toxic States) are eliminated. Sedatives and opiates are used with particular caution.

PROGNOSIS

Recovery from hepatitis is usually complete and uneventful. Less than 1 per cent of persons progress rapidly into a *fulminant hepatitis* that results in hepatic failure and, usually, death.[18] A small number develop a subacute hepatic necrosis that results in fatal hepatic failure or postnecrotic cirrhosis. (See Hepatic Encephalopathy, Chapter 83 for intervention in hepatic failure.)

Occasional cases become chronic and are treated with long-term steroids and antimetabolites to suppress symptoms. Immune mechanisms are probably involved in this chronic progressive destruction of the liver lobule, which may lead to cirrhosis. One form of chronic hepatitis is called *cholestatic hepatitis;* those manifestations due to biliary obstruction (jaundice, pruritus, high serum cholesterol and alkaline phosphatase) are severe. It may progress to terminal *primary biliary cirrhosis.*

HEPATIC TOXIC STATES

Many drugs are toxic to the liver and produce manifestations similar to those of viral hepatitis. Carbon tetrachloride ingestion results in a reversible syndrome which progresses to cirrhosis only with repeated exposures. Jaundice may develop with the administration of certain sex hormones, including contraceptives. Use of the popular inhalation anesthetic, halothane, is followed rarely by hepatic necrosis and failure. Occasional hypersensitivity reactions to a wide variety of therapeutic agents may result in reversible viruslike syndromes; chlorpromazine (Thorazine) is the most common.

The toxic effects of excessive alcohol ingestion accompanied by malnutrition may result in fatty liver, alcoholic hepatitis, and cirrhosis. Fatty liver is an apparently benign and reversible accumulation of fat in liver cells. Though all alcoholics have fatty livers, only a minority have alcoholic hepatitis and cirrhosis. Alcoholic hepatitis may be relatively benign or may cause widespread necrosis leading either to scar tissue and cirrhosis or to progressive hepatic failure and death.[22]

CIRRHOSIS

PATHOLOGY AND ETIOLOGY

Cirrhosis is the final stage of many types of liver injury. The cirrhotic liver varies in appearance, but a nodular consistency with bands of fibrosis (scar tissue) is prominent. Since pathology varies and causes are difficult to demonstrate, classification of types of cirrhosis is uncertain. Most cirrhosis is classified as *Laennec's* or *portal cirrhosis* and is associated with alcoholism. (See Hepatic Toxic States for related variables.) Cirrhosis may also be posthepatic (or postnecrotic) as a sequela to toxic or viral hepatitis; biliary, associated with intrahepatic cholestasis; or cardiac, owing to congestive heart failure.

BASES OF SYMPTOMS

Common manifestations of advanced cirrhosis and their pathophysiologic explanation are identified on the following page.

Biliary cirrhosis is distinct from the above symptom pattern; it develops from cholestatic hepatitis and is probably a disturbance of immune mechanisms. Manifestations are primarily those of chronic severe biliary obstruction: jaundice, pruritus, bleeding, and bone demineralization due to reduced fat-soluble vitamin and calcium absorption. Xanthomas, skin lesions composed of cholesterol deposited because of high serum levels, may develop. Treatment is symptomatic; prognosis is fatal after several years.

DIAGNOSIS

The cirrhosis patient frequently presents with critical problems such as ascites, gastrointestinal bleeding, or encephalopathy. The disease often progresses quietly until such an emergency occurs. Hepatomegaly (enlarged liver), splenomegaly (enlarged spleen), vascular changes, or abnormal laboratory tests may be the first indicator in the patient who is seen for another complaint. The patient may also be seen for hepatitis or other disabling complaints.

Inspection and interview reveal the presence of at least several of the symptoms listed above. Palpation reveals a firm (scarred), lumpy (nodular), usually enlarged liver. Splenomegaly may be present if portal hypertension is severe. Identification of ascites, bleeding with esophageal varices, and hepatic encephalopathy are discussed in Chapter 83. Laboratory tests indicate impaired hepatocellular function: elevated serum enzymes (SGOT, SGPT, LDH), abnormal flocculation tests, reduced BSP dye excretion, hypoalbuminemia, and elevated prothrombin time. Anemia, leukopenia, or thrombocytopenia may be a result of splenomegaly. Liver biopsy is considered essential to definitive diagnosis of cirrhosis and its follow-up.

CLINICAL INTERVENTION

Two goals guide care of the patient with cirrhosis:

1. *Maximize liver function.* Though cirrhosis is a progressive degenerative disorder, certain actions will at least minimize trauma and maximize regeneration. Thereby, the course of the illness can possibly be slowed and life prolonged. *Diet* should provide ample protein to rebuild tissue, at least .5 Gm./lb. or 75 Gm. daily in a 150-lb. person.[19] Enough carbohydrate must be given to sustain weight and spare use of protein for energy—about 20 cal./lb. or 3000 cal. daily in a 150-lb. person.[19] Fat restriction is no longer considered necessary. Small frequent meals will expedite consumption of sufficient quantities in an anorexic patient. A maintenance multivitamin preparation is usually prescribed, and therapeutic levels are given in severe malnutrition. Vitamins A, D, E, and K are given in cases of fat malabsorption. Severe malabsorption may necessitate intravenous vitamins with calcium gluconate supplemented.

Intake of all hepatotoxins must be eliminated. The alcoholic must stop drinking completely; "with continued alcoholism no medical or surgical measures will significantly prolong his life."[18] The problem of alcoholic motivation is discussed in Chapter 83. All known hepatotoxic drugs must be removed from therapeutic regimens, and the drug abuser must understand that certain drugs may further damage his liver. Dosage of all drugs thought to be metabolized by the liver must be lowered. Sedatives and opiates are avoided.

Infection must be prevented by adequate rest, diet, and environmental control. Prior to antibiotics, infection was the major cause of cirrhosis mortality. *Rest* is often prescribed for the cirrhotic, but the amount is debatable. During periods of acute mal-

SYMPTOMS OF CIRRHOSIS

Symptoms	Bases of Symptoms
Emaciation, ascites (Chapter 83)	Malnutrition; portal hypertension, hypoalbuminemia, and hyperaldosteronism
Lower leg edema	Hypoalbuminemia, hyperaldosteronism, and pressure of massive ascites obstructing venous return from legs
Prominent abdominal wall veins	Collateral vessels bypass scarred liver to carry portal blood to superior vena cava
Esophageal varices (Chapter 83)	Collateral veins in esophagus bypass scarred liver to carry portal blood to superior vena cava. Portal hypertension causes dilatation
Hemorrhoids	Internal hemorrhoidal veins dilate with pressure of portal hypertension
Palmar erythema, amenorrhea, atrophy of testicles, enlarged breasts, parotid hypertrophy, spiders (vascular lesions resembling small spiders)	Probable abnormal hormone metabolism in liver, resulting in manifestations of estrogen excess, androgen deficit[9]
Bleeding tendency, especially gastrointestinal (Chapter 83)	Hypoprothrombinemia, thrombocytopenia; portal hypertension and esophageal varices; peptic ulcers common in alcoholics
Anemia	Gastrointestinal blood losses; erythrocyte destruction by pooling in enlarged spleen; folic acid deficiency due to dietary inadequacy
Renal failure	Rapidly failing hepatic function; occasionally precipitated by volume depletions[2]
Infections	Leukopenia due to enlarged overactive spleen. Hypoproteinemia; bacteria in portal blood bypass liver so not removed by Kupffer's cells
Encephalopathy and coma (Chapter 83)	Ammonia, no longer removed by liver, accumulates to levels toxic to brain
Initial or recurrent symptoms of hepatitis	Chronic viral, toxic, or alcoholic hepatitis progressing to cirrhosis may have inflammatory exacerbations

function, rest will reduce metabolic demands on the liver and increase circulation. Long-term planning should include counseling the patient to rest frequently and to avoid unnecessary fatigue. In postnecrotic and posthepatic cirrhosis, *corticosteroids* may be given to reduce manifestations and improve liver function.

2. *Control disabling symptoms.* Ascites, bleeding esophageal varices, and hepatic encephalopathy progressing to coma are discussed in depth in Chapter 83. These three are the most feared complications of cirrhosis and frequently the cause of death. Renal failure and infection can also be mortal complications. See Unit XI for identification and care of the person in renal failure.

PROGNOSIS

The new cirrhotic who immediately eliminates alcohol intake may recover completely with maximum liver regeneration.

The course of the patient with chronic damage who eliminates intake of alcohol and other toxic chemicals and maximizes his nutrition may be slow and prolonged over many years, permitting a meaningful life occasionally interrupted by hospitalization for control of disabling symptoms. Death will eventually ensue, usually precipitated by ruptured varices or hepatic coma.

TRAUMA TO THE LIVER

From 30 to 35 per cent of abdominal injuries involve the liver. The injury may be *open,* owing to penetrating objects, in which case the peritoneal cavity is drained and a T-tube (see Chapter 85, Surgical Intervention) inserted. A *closed* injury, consequent to a blow on the abdomen, is more common. Usually a *transcapsular rupture* (torn Glisson's capsule) is involved, and there is hemorrhage into the peritoneum. Emergency surgery involves ligating vessels, suturing tears, application of pressure, and resection of the liver if necessary. Massive doses of antibiotics are given, and the patient is closely monitored postoperatively for cardiovascular and respiratory complications. Infrequently a *subcapsular* rupture occurs and a hematoma develops, causing right upper quadrant tenderness, and must be opened and drained if it becomes large.[16]

LIVER PARASITES

The liver may be invaded by amebae, tapeworms, or flukes. In schistosomiasis, liver flukes gain entry through skin immersed in infested waters and eventually lodge in the liver to cause fibrosis and presinusoidal obstruction leading to portal hypertension. Since hepatic function usually is not impaired significantly, portacaval shunt eliminates the main problem—bleeding from esophageal varices.[18]

CARCINOMA OF THE LIVER

Primary carcinoma is rare, causing about 2 per cent of all cancer deaths.[1] It frequently follows prolonged cirrhosis and is suspected when the condition of the patient suddenly begins to deteriorate. Massive hemorrhage into the peritoneum is often the first indication. A mass may be palpable in the right upper quadrant. Liver scan and angiography are used to validate diagnosis. Irradiation, regional chemotherapy, and hepatic resection have been tried but their value has not been proved. In general, treatment is palliative.

Metastatic cancer of the liver occurs frequently and is indicative of a grave prognosis. Laboratory and clinical manifestations do not occur until malignant change is far advanced. Jaundice owing to intrahepatic obstruction and portal hypertension caused by invasive obstruction to blood flow may develop. Radiation and chemotherapy are used to prolong life a few more months, but general care is palliative.

CHAPTER 85

Disorders of the Gallbladder and Bile Ducts

BILIARY TRACT TERMINOLOGY

It may be helpful to present first a list of the rather confusing terms used in discussing disorders of the biliary tract.

- chole—pertaining to bile
- cholang—pertaining to bile ducts
- cholangiography—x-ray of bile ducts
- cholangitis—inflammation of a bile duct
- cholecyst—pertaining to gallbladder
- cholecystectomy—removal of gallbladder
- cholecystitis—inflammation of the gallbladder
- cholecystography—x-ray of gallbladder
- cholecystostomy—incision and drainage of gallbladder
- choledocho—pertaining to common bile duct
- choledocholithiasis—stones in the common bile duct
- choledochostomy—exploration of common bile duct
- cholelith—gallstone
- cholelithiasis—presence of gallstones

CHOLECYSTITIS WITH CHOLELITHIASIS

ETIOLOGY

Gallstones in the bile ducts or gallbladder are usually present in cholecystitis. They are composed of cholesterol, bile pigment, and calcium in varying proportions. The reasons for their precipitation are still uncertain. Excess cholesterol or impaired excretion of bile acid which normally solubilizes cholesterol is implicated in cholesterol stone development. It is still unclear whether stones or inflammation occurs first. Most authors hypothesize a chain of events beginning with *obstruction* of the cystic duct or gallbladder outlet, *edema* due to circulatory stasis, and *chemical inflammation* due to stasis of bile which is irritating because of altered components. Usually no infecting organisms are found. The inflammatory process contributes to stone formation by altering bile metabolism and providing waste materials around which crystals may develop.

BASES OF SYMPTOMS

Symptoms occur with interference to flow of bile. The common symptoms of cholecystitis and cholelithiasis are listed below with their pathophysiologic explanation.

DIAGNOSIS

Cholecystitis usually causes pain, gastrointestinal disturbances, and fever as described below. These

Symptom	Basis of Symptoms
Abdominal pain, most commonly right upper quadrant or epigastric. Often radiates to back	In cholelithiasis, ductal spasm when a stone moves from gallbladder into ducts may cause waves of pain (biliary colic); in cholecystitis, pain may be steady owing to inflammation, and increases in severity with peritoneal extension
Nausea and vomiting	Distention of bile ducts initiates impulses to vomiting center
Fat intolerance	Contraction of inflamed gallbladder to release bile to digest fat often precipitates pain
Fever and leukocytosis	Response to inflammation
Jaundice	In cholelithiasis, obstruction to common bile duct causes increased serum bilirubin; in cholecystitis, edema sometimes obstructs the duct enough to increase bilirubin levels

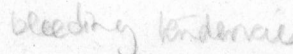

must be distinguished from many other inflammatory processes, including hepatitis and pancreatitis. Acute cholecystitis may subside or progress to abscess formation or peritonitis; chronic cholecystitis is manifested by repeated intermittent attacks.

Cholelithiasis is demonstrated by cholecystography and cholangiography. Duodenal drainage reveals crystals or particles. See Chapter 82 for discussion of these procedures. When stones cause obstruction, jaundice may be present. Prothrombin time may be elevated with reduced vitamin K absorption. Differential diagnosis of jaundice is discussed in Chapter 83. Final diagnosis of cholelithiasis is made when the stone is found during choledochostomy or after cholecystectomy.

MEDICAL INTERVENTION

Four goals guide care of the person with acute cholecystitis:

1. *Relieve pain*. Meperidine (Demerol) in small frequent doses is the drug of choice. Morphine is believed to increase spasm of the sphincter of Oddi. Phenobarbital may be given for sedation and to relax smooth muscle. Nitroglycerin sublingually also reduces pain and may relax smooth muscle. Medication is combined with nursing measures to allay discomfort. (See Unit IX.)

2. *Relieve vomiting and reduce gastric stimulus*. A nasogastric tube is usually passed and attached to suction. This relieves distention and vomiting and eliminates the gastric juices that stimulate cholecystokinin.

3. *Maintain fluid and electrolyte balance*. This is achieved by intravenous solutions and careful monitoring of fluid output and serum electrolyte levels.

4. *Eliminate infection*. Some physicians will prescribe broad-spectrum antibiotics, particularly if the acute process does not subside in 24 hours. Any infection superimposed on the chemical inflammation will thus be eliminated.

Administration of bile acid (chenodesoxycholic acid) has been employed to restore the proper bile acid : cholesterol ratio to dissolve cholesterol stones in research studies.[30] This therapy may greatly reduce the need for surgery in the future if its adverse effects on the liver can be controlled.

SURGICAL INTERVENTION

If manifestations of acute cholecystitis persist beyond 48 hours, most surgeons recommend immediate surgery to avoid complications. Prothrombin time is determined and vitamin K given preoperatively if indicated. If the attack subsides sooner, the patient is usually advised to return to the hospital for elective surgery in four to six weeks. He is maintained on a low-fat, high-protein diet.

In 90 per cent of patients, cholecystectomy is the surgery performed; the cystic duct and artery are ligated and the gallbladder is removed from its hepatic attachments. When jaundice is present, the common bile duct is probed, palpated, and irrigated and stones are removed. Two general goals guide care following cholecystectomy and choledochostomy: prevention of postoperative complications; and identification of complications.

Preventing postoperative complications involves thoughtful postoperative measures to avoid those problems that are common to all major abdominal surgery. (See Units VI and XV.) Respiratory therapy and rapid mobilization are vital. Return of bowel sounds is monitored. Distention is often prevented by use of a nasogastric tube; provision of nutrition and fluids begins with intravenous solutions and progresses to oral ingestion of liquids and solids with return of peristalsis. Ambulation and return flow enemas aid in releasing flatus. Fowler's position and initially generous narcotic dosage allay pain and facilitate movement. Owing to copious irritating drainage from the Penrose drain usually inserted in the gallbladder bed, incisional dressings must be reinforced and changed often, with careful skin care provided.

After choledochostomy, a T-tube prevents spillage of bile into the peritoneum and maintains ductal patency in the presence of edema from trauma due to surgery or stones. The T-tube is sutured into the common duct, with arms toward the hepatic duct and the duodenum; its length is brought out in a stab wound near the incision and sutured to the skin. T-tubes may be attached to continuous bedside gravity drainage, or collapsible bags may be attached at the dressing site to drain only bile overflow. Tension on long tubing and obstruction by kinking must be avoided. Drainage is carefully measured; 200 to 500 ml. daily is normal initially and will decrease as more bile enters the intestine. Continuing large amounts indicate obstruction. After a few days the T-tube may be clamped during meals to aid digestion of fat. It is left in place about 10 days and removed when T-tube cholangiogram indicates abscence of obstruction.

Identifying complications unique to biliary tract surgery involves early recognition of the implication of symptoms. *Jaundice* indicates injury to ducts or obstructing stones not removed during surgery.[10] *Failure of stools to return to normal brown* color of urobilin also indicates continuing obstruction to bile flow. As noted above, *excessive T-tube drainage* may be an indication of obstruction; occasionally it means that a biliary fistula has developed.[10] Excessive bile losses may necessitate recycling the patient's bile drainage and administering it to him in a medium such as fruit juice. *Fever and severe abdominal pain* with guarding may indicate bile peritonitis resulting from seepage of bile at the sutures or slippage of the T-tube, or occasionally it may mean that direct trauma to the pancreas has caused pancreatitis.[10] *Bleeding* after cholecystectomy may indicate reduced prothrombin levels as a result of decreased vitamin K absorption.

In poor-risk patients, cholecystostomy, wherein a catheter is sutured into the lumen of the gallbladder and brought out through a stab wound to drain the gallbladder, is performed until patient condition permits cholecystectomy. The catheter may not be removed for weeks or months; often the patient goes home with the tube or with the resultant sinus tract draining. Large losses may necessitate recycling of bile for oral intake, as with excessive T-tube drainage.

PROGNOSIS

Cholecystitis followed by cholecystectomy is generally not considered to be a serious threat to life, but the rate of complications does increase with age. Postoperative convalescence necessitates no special precautions other than the avoidance of excessive fatigue.

CARCINOMA OF THE GALLBLADDER

Cancer of the gallbladder is quite rare. The most common type is adenocarcinoma associated with chronic gallstones. It is preventable by early cholecystectomy.[19] Early symptoms are indistinguishable from cholecystitis with cholelithiasis; pain, weight loss, and a right upper quandrant mass are late symptoms. Prognosis remains dim, with little gained by radical surgical excision.

CHAPTER 86

Disorders of the Pancreas

PANCREATITIS

ETIOLOGY

Pancreatitis is associated with multiple causal factors; most commonly implicated are *excessive alcohol intake* and *biliary tract disease*. It is hypothesized that alcohol either has a direct toxic effect on the pancreas or causes backup of pancreatic juice into the pancreas. This would occur when alcohol in the stomach stimulates acid flow which induces secretin and therefore pancreatic juices. Since alcohol is also known to increase sphincter of Oddi resistance, obstruction to flow occurs, and secretions accumulate. Biliary tract disorder might precipitate pancreatitis through many mechanisms. A biliary stone in the ampulla of Vater would cause pancreatic duct obstruction and backup of pancreatic juice. Cholecystitis might be implicated either by reflux of irritating altered bile components into the pancreatic duct to cause chemical inflammation or by lymphatic channels carrying some sort of inflammatory toxins.[3, 12] None of these explanations has been validated. Pancreatitis is also occasionally associated with hyperparathyroidism, with consequent hypercalcemia and precipitation of calcium from pancreatic juice into the ducts, and with operative trauma.

BASES OF SYMPTOMS OF ACUTE PANCREATITIS

Underlying acute manifestations is the process of autodigestion, in which enzymes are activated and released into the pancreas. It is still unknown how trypsinogen is converted to trypsin and thus catalyzes activation of other enzymes. Activated enzymes erode into surrounding tissue, breaking down protein structures and causing fat necrosis and liquefaction. The disease is classified as either edematous, which is usually self-limiting, or hemorrhagic, which is a medical crisis with 50 per cent mortality.

Below are the common symptoms encountered with hemorrhagic pancreatitis and the current concepts of pathophysiologic cause.

SYMPTOMS OF CHRONIC PANCREATITIS

Chronic pancreatitis involves progressive degeneration of both acinar and islet functions of the

Symptoms	Bases of Symptoms
Extreme epigastric or umbilical pain, extending into back and flank	Edematous distention of pancreatic capsule, local peritonitis due to enzyme release into peritoneum, ductal spasm; stimulated by increased secretion of enzymes by eating
Persistent vomiting	Pain induces stimulus to vomiting center; intestinal peristalsis reduced owing to localized peritonitis
Abdominal distention	Paralytic ileus of small bowel loop due to localized peritonitis
Fever	Release of pyrogens by tissue breakdown
Shock	Kinin, a vasodilator, activated by trypsin; inflammatory fluid lost into peritoneum; activated elastase dissolves elastic fibers of blood vessels to cause hemorrhage into peritoneum; multiple other factors implicated
Hypocalcemia, usually mild, though tetany is possible	Calcium may be deposited in areas of fat necrosis
Impaired glucose tolerance	Some degree of islet involvement
Jaundice	Common bile duct obstruction by pancreatic edema

pancreas due to scarring and calcification of tissue after repeated attacks of acute pancreatitis. Dull pain alternates with severe pain, vomiting, fever, and jaundice as in acute pancreatitis. Eventually hyperglycemia becomes a clinical problem with manifestations of diabetes. Digestive enzyme secretion is so severely reduced that malnutrition and weight loss, coupled with severe elimination problems, become evident. Abdominal distention with flatus and cramps is accompanied by frequent foul fatty stools (steatorrhea).

DIAGNOSIS

The patient with acute pancreatitis usually is first seen in acute pain with the manifestations detailed above. Pain or digestive disturbance may motivate the chronic patient to seek help. The pancreas is never palpable, but a pseudocyst, a pocket created by chronic obstruction to accumulating secretions, may occasionally be felt.

Diagnostic tests are nonspecific. Elevated serum amylase and lipase are cardinal signs, but they may be caused by other acute gastrointestinal disorders, and are not directly correlated with the severity of the disorder. Serum amylase rises in a few hours and lasts about three days; urinary amylase remains elevated longer. Lipase rises in 24 hours and lasts up to 10 days. Enzymes may be normal with reduced functioning tissue in chronic pancreatitis. Plain x-rays may show reduced bowel motility, calcifications, and adhesions. Angiography indicates vascular changes. Cholangiography and/or cholecystography show biliary changes which may be either causes or consequences of pancreatic disorder. Paracentesis frequently reveals bloody fluid, high in amylase and methemalbumin from hemoglobin digestion.[13] Rarely, the secretin test is performed (see Table 82–1).

CLINICAL INTERVENTION IN ACUTE PANCREATITIS

Treatment of the milder edematous pancreatitis may require only analgesics, but acute hemorrhagic pancreatitis necessitates intensive measures. The following goals direct intervention:

Maintain circulatory volume and replace fluid and electrolyte loss. Shock and anuria are the main causes of death.[7] Colloid and large volumes of electrolyte solution are administered; central venous pressure and urine output are carefully monitored hourly. Intravenous mannitol is given when hourly urine output drops, and the response is noted. Electrolyte serum levels are monitored and replacements determined accordingly; calcium gluconate is often indicated. The patient should be observed for the increased neural excitability of tetany. (See Chapter 25.)

Alleviate pain. Frequent doses of meperidine (Demerol) are indicated rather than morphine and its derivatives, which increase sphincter of Oddi spasm. Extensive nursing measures are applied to relieve the severe pain. (See Unit IX.)

Reduce pancreatic stimulus. Multiple approaches are involved here. *Fasting* and insertion of a nasogastric tube connected to intermittent suction reduce acid stimulation of secretin. Three types of medication reduce pancreatic secretion: The anticholinergics, Pro-Banthine especially, oppose vagal stimulation and, in effect, reduce pancreatic secretion and relax the sphincter of Oddi. They are very commonly given, but contraindicated in the presence of intestinal ileus or tachycardia, which they aggravate. Antacids are administered every two hours in mild cases, and the person convalescing from a severe attack will progress to hourly antacids once he is free of pain and has normal peristalsis. Azetazolamide (Diamox) is occasionally administered to prevent carbonic anhydrase from catalyzing secretion of bicarbonate into pancreatic juice. With regression of symptoms, the patient is placed on a diet that avoids pancreatic stimulus: low fat, no alcohol, no caffeine to stimulate gastric acid.

Prevent or treat infection. Organisms readily multiply in necrotic tissue, and a broad-spectrum antibiotic that is secreted by the liver into the biliary tract is often administered.

Prevent hyperglycemia. Blood glucose is determined frequently, and fractional urine specimens may be tested for sugar and acetone. Insulin is given intravenously as indicated, especially if the patient is receiving glucose infusion.

Other measures are occasionally used to treat acute pancreatitis. These include peritoneal dialysis and unproven enzyme inhibitors. Surgery is indicated when diagnosis is doubtful, when biliary tract disorder is suspected, or when a pseudocyst requires drainage.

CLINICAL INTERVENTION IN CHRONIC PANCREATITIS

Therapy focuses on (1) reducing pancreatic stimulus, (2) alleviating fat indigestion, and (3) treating diabetes.

Reducing pancreatic stimulus is accomplished by a low-fat diet with avoidence of alcohol and caffeine; meals should be small. The dietary regimen in itself may prevent recurrence of chronic attacks after the initial acute episode. Oral antacids to reduce gastric acid stimulus to pancreatic juice secretion are frequently taken by the patient with chronic disease.

Alleviating fat indigestion is accomplished by several approaches.. Up to 4 Gm. of pancreatic extracts, such as Pancreatin or Viokase, are taken with each meal. Fat losses in stool should diminish. Medium-chain triglyceride (MCT) losses may be replaced. Finally, supplementary fat-soluble vitamins and calcium are given.

Treating diabetes involves dietary and insulin control. See Unit XVIII for care of the patient experiencing diabetes.

Surgery for the patient with chronic disease is occasionally tried to revise the biliary or pancreatic ducts or sphincter of Oddi to reduce pressure and promote free flow of pancreatic juice.

Prognosis in chronic pancreatitis is good if acute attacks decrease in frequency; replacement therapy for chronic fat indigestion permits a fairly normal life. If the patient continues to drink, prognosis is grim, with repeated attacks eventually causing death from shock or renal failure.

CYSTIC FIBROSIS

The child with cystic fibrosis suffers a multiple exocrine gland disorder manifested particularly by inability of sweat glands to conserve salt; inability of pancreas to secrete enzymes to digest fat, with consequent steatorrhea and malnutrition; and pulmonary disorder caused by increased viscosity of mucous gland secretions. The patient is given extra salt during hot weather, pancreatic extract and a low-fat diet are introduced, and intensive respiratory care is provided as needed. He rarely survives to adulthood, usually because of pulmonary complications. See a pediatric textbook for details.

PANCREATIC CARCINOMA

This malignancy accounts for 5 per cent of cancer deaths.[1] It usually begins in the head of the pancreas and rapidly invades the remainder, the lymph nodes, the liver and biliary tract, and the duodenum. Jaundice, pain, and weight loss are the most prominent symptoms and occur only after extension has occurred. A right upper quadrant mass is palpable in later stages. Diagnostic tests used are the same as those for pancreatitis; only exploratory laparotomy results in certainty of diagnosis. The prognosis is grim; the patient seldom survives a year. Care is symptomatic. Procedures to bypass obstructing common bile duct extensions and thus alleviate jaundice and pruritus include choledochoduodenostomy, choledochojejunostomy, and cholecystojejunostomy. Surgical measures to interfere with pain pathways, such as sympathectomy, may allay the persistent pain. (See Unit IX.) The Whipple procedure, which removes the head of the pancreas, the duodenum, and a portion of the gallbladder and stomach, is associated with a high risk of mortality.

References for Unit XVI

1. American Cancer Society: *'73 Cancer Facts and Figures*. New York, American Cancer Society, 1973.
2. Baldus, W.: Renal failure in advanced liver disease. *In* Popper, H. and Schaffner, F. (eds.): *Progress in Liver Diseases. Vol. IV*. New York, Grune & Stratton, 1972.
3. Banks, P. A.: Acute pancreatitis. *Gastroenterology, 61*:382, September, 1971.
4. Bielski, M. T., and Molander, D. W.: Laennec's cirrhosis. *American Journal of Nursing, 65*:82, August, 1965.
5. Breen, K., and Schenker, S.: Hepatic coma: present concepts of pathogenesis and therapy. *In* Popper, H. and Schaffner, F. (eds.): *Progress in Liver Diseases*. Vol. IV. New York, Grune & Stratton, 1972.
6. Cisin, I. H., and Calahan, D.: Some correlates of American drinking practices. *Recent Advances in Studies of Alcoholism: An Interdisciplinary Symposium*. Washington, D.C., U.S. Government Printing Office, 1971.
7. Creutzfeldt, W.: Pancreatitis. *In* Conn, H. (ed.): *Current Therapy 1973*. Philadelphia, W. B. Saunders Company, 1973.
8. Criteria Committee, National Council on Alcoholism: Criteria for the diagnosis of alcoholism. *Annals of Internal Medicine, 77*:249, August, 1972.
9. Davidson, C. S.: *Liver Pathophysiology, Its Relevance to Human Disease*. Boston, Little, Brown & Company, 1970.
10. Dowdy, G. S.: *The Biliary Tract*. Philadelphia, Lea & Febiger, 1969.
11. Garb, S.: *Laboratory Tests in Common Use*. New York, Springer Verlag, 1971.
12. Geokas, M.: Acute pancreatitis. *California Medicine, 117*:25, August, 1972.
13. Geokas, M., et al.: Acute pancreatitis. *Annals of Internal Medicine,* 76:105, January, 1972.
14. Guyton, A. C.: *Textbook of Medical Physiology*. Philadelphia, W. B. Saunders Company, 1971.
15. Hayter, J.: Impaired liver function and related nursing care. *American Journal of Nursing, 68*:2374, November, 1968.
16. Hellstrom, G.: Traumatic liver injuries. *In* Popper, H. and Schaffner, F. (eds.): *Progress in Liver Diseases,* Vol. III. New York, Grune & Stratton, 1970.
17. Iber, F. L.: Management of the patient with esophageal varices. *Modern Treatment, 7*:1320, November, 1970.
18. Jeffries, G. H.: Diseases of the liver. In Beeson, P. and McDermott, W. (eds.): *Textbook of Medicine*. Philadelphia, W. B. Saunders Company, 1971.
19. Jones, D. P.: Cirrhosis. In Conn, H. (ed.): *Current Therapy 1973*. Philadelphia, W. B. Saunders Company, 1973.
20. Kowlesser, O.: Diseases of the pancreas. In Beeson, P. and McDermott, W. (eds.): *Textbook of Medicine*. Philadelphia, W. B. Saunders Company, 1971.
21. Krugman, S., and Giles, J.: The natural history of viral hepatitis. *Canadian Medical Association Journal, 106*:442, February 26, 1972.
22. Lesesne, H., and Fallon, H.: Alcoholic liver disease. *Postgraduate Medicine, 53*:101, January, 1973.
23. Mosley, J.: Viral hepatitis: a group of epidemiologic entities. *Canadian Medical Association Journal, 106*:427, February 26, 1972.
24. Netter, F. H.: *The Ciba Collection of Medical Illustrations*. Vol. 3, *Digestive System*. Part III,

Liver Biliary Tract and Pancreas. New York, Ciba Pharmaceutical Products, 1957.

25. Priest, R. J.: Cholecystitis and cholelithiasis. In Conn, H. (ed.): *Current Therapy 1973*. Philadelphia, W. B. Saunders Company, 1973.
26. Reynolds, T. B.: Origin and treatment of ascites in liver disease. *Warren-Teed GI Tract, 2*:12, October–December, 1972.
27. Schaffner, F.: Treatment of viral hepatitis. *Canadian Medical Association Journal, 106*:505, February 26, 1972.
28. Sleisenger, M. H.: Diseases of the gallbladder and bile ducts. In Beeson, P. and McDermott, W. (eds.): *Textbook of Medicine*. W. B. Saunders Company, 1971.
29. tenHove, W., and Leevy, C.: Hepatic circulation and portal hypertension. *Postgraduate Medicine, 53*:135, January, 1973.
30. Thistle, J.: Gallstones: pathophysiology and dissolution. *Postgraduate Medicine, 53*:65, January, 1973.
31. Tumen, H. J.: Pitfalls in the management of advanced cirrhosis. *Hospital Medicine, 7*:64, April, 1971.
32. Tygstrup, N.: Anti-inflammatory treatment of chronic active liver disease. In Popper, H. and Schaffner, F. (eds.): *Progress in Liver Diseases*, Vol. III. New York, Grune & Stratton, 1970.
33. United States National Communicable Disease Center: *Isolation Technics for Use In Hospitals*. Washington, D.C., U.S. Government Printing Office, 1970.

UNIT XVII

Nursing Patients Experiencing Disturbances of Musculoskeletal Function

Introduction and Study Guide

Care of patients with musculoskeletal disorders requires a team approach directed at identifying and meeting individual patient needs, preventing complications, and minimizing the handicapping effects of disability. The nurse caring for patients with these disorders not only must be familiar with the anatomy and physiology of bones and muscles but also must be knowledgeable about which nerves and blood vessels are located near specific bones and the muscles they supply. Such knowledge is essential to identifying nerve and blood vessel injuries which may coincide with musculoskeletal injuries or which can develop as a complication of treatment procedures, e.g., casting.

Surgical treatment of bone, muscle, and joint disorders may involve the combined efforts of an orthopedic surgeon, a vascular surgeon, a neurosurgeon, and a plastic surgeon. For example, in the treatment of an open (compound) fracture, in which the broken bone protrudes through the skin, the orthopedic surgeon realigns the bone, while a vascular surgeon may reconstruct the limb's blood supply. A neurosurgeon may also be necessary if the broken bone has torn or otherwise severely traumatized nearby nerves. A fractured or dislocated limb may be correctly realigned and heal without deformity, but the limb will be useless if its nerve supply is not restored, and it will be lost if it is not adequately perfused with blood. For example, amputation may be necessary if a dislocated knee is not reduced early, because the arterial blood supply may be irreparably compromised. The successful reimplantation of extremities which are traumatically severed is sometimes possible with the coordinated efforts of a surgical team. For example, an orthopedist realigns and reconnects severed bones, while vascular and neurosurgeons do the same with blood vessels and nerves. A plastic surgeon may also participate, e.g., by performing necessary skin grafting, cosmetic surgery, or hand surgery.

Advances are constantly being made in the diagnosis and treatment of musculoskeletal disorders. For example, it is now possible to perform endoscopic examination of some joints, e.g., knee, by inserting an instrument (arthroscope) through which the interior of the joint can be visualized and photographed. A porous ceramic material ("ceramic bone") is being tested for possible use in the surgical replacement of bone.[180] Experiments are being made to determine whether heating fractured bones hastens the healing process.[66] Recently it has become possible to totally replace hips, knees, and elbows which are seriously damaged, e.g., because of arthritic changes. Silicone joint implants can also be made in the hands or feet to replace diseased or destroyed joints.

Musculoskeletal disorders may cause short-term or long-term periods of illness. However, with the exception of simple uncomplicated injuries, many musculoskeletal problems are of a chronic nature or require long-term care. Rehabilitative care may be implemented by a team consisting of doctors and nurses specializing in physical medicine, as well as a physical therapist, occupational therapist, social worker, psychiatrist, and prosthetist (a specialist who constructs and applies prostheses). Spiritual help is obtained according to an individual patient's expressed preferences. Nurses who specialize in orthopedic care are active in providing patient care in clinics and hospitals. Community health nurses bring nursing care into the home setting when appropriate.

As indicated above, the treatment-rehabilitative processes used with musculoskeletal disorders may extend over long periods of time. Some patients require several surgical procedures. Pain, immobility, and changes in self-image often cause patients with musculoskeletal disorders to become discouraged and depressed. Because of her prolonged contact with patients, the nurse can frequently be of assistance during periods of distress and can help keep hope and motivation at high levels. Occupational therapy not only helps patients to occupy time meaningfully during recovery-rehabilitation periods but also enables patients with musculoskeletal disorders to improve or maintain muscle strength, coordination, and dexterity. Successful rehabilitation is not possible without careful planning and scheduling of activities. Rehabilitation cannot be a haphazard process which one simply "hopes" will occur.

It is necessary for the orthopedic nurse to possess some "mechanical know-how" and knowledge of basic physics. Of necessity, orthopedic settings contain a multitude of equipment. In addition to the equipment routinely found on hospital wards (e.g., dressings, catheters, gloves, medications, bath basins, linens), orthopedic wards commonly require special linens and an abundance of pillows, cushions, sand bags, padding, binders, elastic bandages, elastic stockings, and tape. Other equipment includes:

> *Casting equipment,* e.g., casting materials, cast dryer, cast cutter.
> *Bracing and splinting equipment,* e.g., leg braces, padded foot splints.
> *Traction equipment,* e.g., metal bars, ropes, pulleys, weights.
> *Transfer equipment,* e.g., sliding board, mechanical lift, overhead sling, Davis roller.
> *Occupational therapy* and other adaptive or recreational equipment.
> *Transportation equipment,* e.g., wheelchairs, crutches, canes, walkers, stretchers.

Because musculoskeletal disorders affect the locomotor and structural systems of the body, they often make it difficult for the affected individual to support himself and move about. It is therefore necessary for orthopedic settings to be amply equipped with devices to help a patient support himself and move about, e.g., handrails in the hallways, grab bars by toilets. Mirrors in hallways help patients observe their posture-walking habits and learn correct habits. Special frames (e.g., Foster frame, Stryker frame) or CircOlectric beds are sometimes employed to more effectively care for a patient with a musculoskeletal impairment. (See Unit VIII for discussions of special frames, CircOlectric beds, and wheelchairs.)

A nurse can greatly benefit a patient with musculoskeletal problems by skillfully using comfort and positioning items, e.g., padding, cushions, special wheelchair attachments. While giving care to the orthopedic patient, the nurse spends a great deal of time on making him comfortable, e.g., changing the patient's position, padding a brace that "rubs," adjusting a wheelchair or a traction set-up, giving skin care, relieving muscle spasms, administering pain medications.

Similarities exist between some neurologic disorders (see Unit VIII) and some musculoskeletal disorders. For example, both can cause impairment or loss of body motion; both are commonly long-term illnesses; and both require prevention of the complications of immobility (see Unit V, Ch. 27) in their treatment and extensive rehabilitative services.

Impaired or lost musculoskeletal abilities must be regained or compensated for whenever possible. The orthopedic nurse patiently assists the patient as he works to regain musculoskeletal function, e.g., to bend his knees, to use his fingers, to stand up and walk. It is difficult to be dependent and unable to move. Relearning processes are time-consuming; however, learning musculoskeletal activities can take place only if the patient is given the supervised opportunity to "try" by himself. It is imperative that the patient have confidence in persons caring for him and that accidents, e.g., falls, be prevented. As in any setting, the nurse must constantly be safety conscious. Also, when handling or supporting a patient who has a musculoskeletal disorder, the nurse needs to remember to (1) be gentle, (2) provide adequate support, and (3) avoid sudden movements. Handle the patient as carefully as you would a large pane of glass. Also, always keep in mind positions and movements which are contraindicated for a specific patient. Careless or contraindicated movements or positioning may cause unnecessary pain, tissue trauma, and the disruption of delicate bone, nerve, or blood vessel healing processes. Once you cause a patient unnecessary or unexpected discomfort, it is difficult (perhaps impossible) to regain his confidence. To assist most effectively a disabled person (e.g., to sit up, walk, get into bed), help him on his affected side. You can thus best contribute to his strength and you will avoid traumatizing affected tissues, e.g., by grasping or pulling on them.

The successful orthopaedic nurse is a good teacher who helps a patient (and his family) learn about his condition and its treatment. Additionally, the nurse teaches the patient how to live most effectively with his disorder during the recovery-rehabilitation period of illness. The patient is helped to understand and correctly use and care for equipment which is to be part of his self-care. Also, he is helped to accept his need for the equipment and the benefits of using assistive devices. Assistive devices used on or by a patient should (1) help, not hinder, the patient; (2) be physiologically tolerated; (3) permit function with reasonable body alignment; and (4) be cosmetically as acceptable as possible. In situations in which assistive devices may be permanently necessary, e.g., wearing of a brace, or when a patient must adapt to permanent cosmetic deformity, it may take a substantial period of time for the patient to adjust to changes in his body image (see Unit III, Ch. 14). In the home setting, a community health nurse may work with the patient and his family to help the patient continue to return to or maintain a maximum level of function and to make necessary adaptations in the home environment.

The nurse caring for patients with disorders of bones, joints, and muscles must be highly observant and diligently attentive to details of patient care. *Much orthopedic nursing care is of a preventative nature.* Activities of special importance include:

> Maintaining proper body alignment during periods of bedrest to promote correct posture and the return of effective balance once bedrest is no longer needed.

> Performing or supervising range-of-motion exercises to maintain joint mobility and other exercises to maintain muscle strength.

> Ensuring correct positioning and support to prevent ischemia, nerve damage, muscle spasms, contractures, atrophy, and other deformities, e.g., foot drop. While deformities may be easily prevented, often they are extremely difficult or impossible to correct. Support must be given to painful, weak, or casted body areas.

> Performing periodic neurovascular checks to observe for indications of nerve or circulatory impairment.

> Giving frequent skin care to prevent skin breakdown.

> Checking traction set-ups to be certain that traction is being correctly applied.

> Observing indications of special complications, e.g., fat embolism, shock lung. Observing patients in casts for indications of complications, e.g., infection, pressure.

> Assisting with ambulation and other self-care activities.

> Relieving pain.

As discussed previously, because many patients with musculoskeletal disorders are limited in their ability to move or to support themselves, the nurse often helps with positioning and transporting activities. The nurse on the orthopedic service must practice good body mechanics or she may injure herself as she performs these assistive services. Casts and braces can be very heavy, thus adding to a patient's total weight and easily throwing him off balance.

This unit consists of four chapters. Chapter 87 presents a brief overview of musculoskeletal anatomy and physiology and musculoskeletal disorders. Chapter 88 focuses on diagnostic procedures used to investigate the musculoskeletal system and clinical problems and therapeutic measures common with musculoskeletal disorders. In Chapter 89 musculoskeletal injuries are discussed. The final chapter, Chapter 90, presents other musculoskeletal disorders. Neuromuscular disorders and spinal and skull injuries and their treatment are discussed in Unit VIII. Amputations are discussed in Unit XIII. Mandibular fractures are considered in Chapter 76 of Unit XV, and fractures of the ribs in Unit XIV.

Answering the following *study questions* and performing the activities suggested below will help you more comprehensively to study this unit:

I. On separate blank cards (or small pieces of paper) define each of the following terms as you study the unit. Use the completed cards for review purposes.

abduction
adduction
amphiarthroses
ankylosis
arthritis
arthrodesis
arthrograms
arthroplasty
arthroscope
arthrotomy
articular
bursa
bursitis
Bryant's traction
"cast syndrome"
closed reduction
compound fracture
crutch palsy
diarthroses
dislocation
eversion
extension
fat embolism
flexion
fracture
gelation
genu varus
genu valgus
haversian system
internal fixation
inversion
kyphosis
laminograms
lordosis
lupus erythematosus
multiple myeloma
"muscle splinting"
myositis
open reduction
orthopedics
osteoblasts
osteomalacia
osteomyelitis
osteoporosis
periarteritis nodosa
pronation
scleroderma
scoliosis
simple fracture
sprain
striated muscle
supination
synarthroses
synovectomy
synovial fluid
synovitis
tendon
tendonitis
Volkmann's ischemic contracture

II. Answer the following questions.

1. Where does hematopoiesis occur in the bones?
2. Where is yellow marrow located in bones?
3. How can flexion contractures be prevented?
4. What are some physiologic benefits of heat and massage in the treatment of musculoskeletal disorders?
5. What is the difference between active and passive exercises?
6. During correct usage of crutches, where should the patient rest his weight, i.e., on the handbars or axillary bars of the crutches?
7. What are the "Five P's" and what is their significance in the care of patients with postoperative or casted extremities?
8. What is the difference between skin traction and skeletal traction?
9. What are the symptoms of fat embolism?
10. Why is it important to prevent external rotation of the hip following hip surgeries such as pinnings or arthroplasties?

III. Perform the following activities:

1. Use a textbook of nursing fundamentals to review (1) basic principles of body mechanics, (2) basic techniques for lifting and moving patients and assisting with ambulation, (3) principles of bandaging and massage, and (4) range-of-motion exercises and hot and cold applications.
2. Identify the major bones of the upper and lower extremities. While studying the unit, review individual bones, muscles, and other anatomic structures as necessary. Give examples of a hinge joint, ball and socket joint, and gliding joint.

3. Review the evaluation of pain and clinical care of patients in pain as discussed in Unit IX. Also, review as necessary Units VI and VII and Sections One and Two of this text.
4. Use a textbook of pharmacology to review medications used in the treatment of musculoskeletal disorders, e.g., muscle relaxants, analgesics.
5. Review the following diets: (1) high-protein, (2) high-vitamin, and (3) low-purine.
6. List some specific effects of prolonged musculoskeletal pain on bones, muscles, tendons, and joints.
7. List some physiologic effects of heat, massage, and exercises.
8. Summarize general observations of importance when inspecting a patient's traction set-up.
9. List potential complications which may occur postoperatively following orthopedic surgery.
10. Identify factors of importance in first aid for a fracture victim.
11. Summarize factors of importance in the clinical care of patients with the following disorders: (1) fractured femur, (2) cancer of the bone, (3) rheumatoid arthritis, (4) gout, and (5) collagen diseases.

CHAPTER 87

Introductory Concepts

OVERVIEW OF NORMAL ANATOMY AND PHYSIOLOGY OF THE MUSCULOSKELETAL SYSTEM

Space does not permit a detailed review of the normal structure and function of the musculoskeletal system; however, the following summary in outline form will help orient the reader. Consult textbooks of anatomy and physiology for additional detail as required.

I. *Musculoskeletal System:* Includes bones, joints, muscles, and related connective tissue.

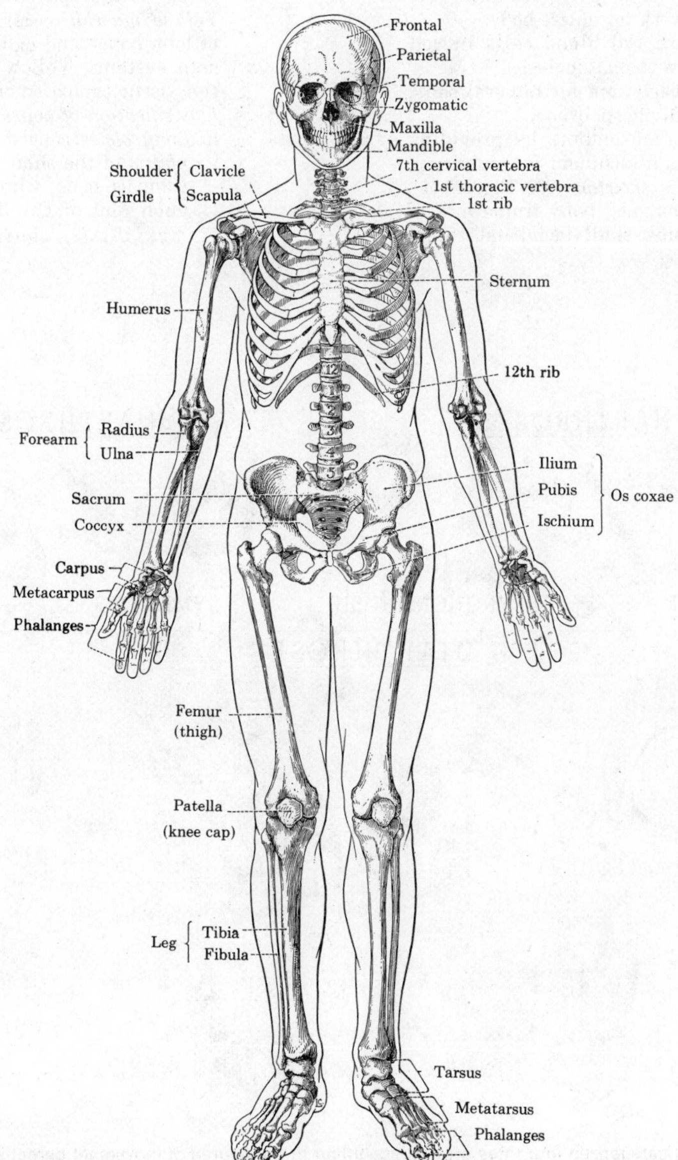

FIGURE 87–1. Anterior view of human skeleton. (From *Dorland's Illustrated Medical Dictionary.* 25th ed. 1974.)

Can be divided into (1) skeletal system (bones), (2) articular system (joints), and (3) muscular system (muscles).

A. *Skeletal System.* Bone tissue is nourished by the *haversian system,* a network of minute canals traversed with blood vessels. Bone tissue is constantly being created and reabsorbed. The rate of activity of these two processes (i.e., the *deposition* of new bone by osteoblasts and the *reabsorption* of bone) determines skeletal bone size and strength.
   1. *Functions* of the skeleton (a joined framework of 206 bones).
      a. Protect vital organs and other soft tissues.
      b. Support surrounding tissues and serve as a framework for entire body.
      c. Manufacture red blood cells in red bone marrow (hematopoiesis).
      d. Provide storage area for mineral salts, e.g., calcium, phosphorus.
      e. Assist body movements by providing leverage and attachment for muscles.
   2. *Divisions of the skeleton* (see Fig. 87–1).
      a. *Axial skeleton,* i.e., bony framework of head and trunk: skull (facial and cranial bones); vertebral column; ribs; hyoid bone; sternum.
      b. *Appendicular skeleton,* i.e., bony framework of arms and legs: upper extremities (scapula, clavicle, humerus, ulna, radius, hand, i.e., carpals, metacarpals, phalanges); lower extremities (pelvic bone, femur, patella, tibia, fibula, foot, i.e., tarsals, metatarsals, and phalanges).
   3. *Histology of bone.* Histologically bone is of two types: (1) *compact,* i.e., strong and dense with closely spaced lamellae (concentric layers of mineral deposits); or (2) *cancellous,* i.e., spongy in appearance with more widely spaced lamellae. Between layers of lamellae are small cavities, i.e., *"lacunae."* Suspended in tissue fluid within each lacuna is an *osteocyte,* busy making new bone. Osteocytes are mature, bone-forming cells. *Red marrow,* which has a hematopoietic function (manufactures red and white blood cells), is located in the spaces of cancellous bone. *Yellow marrow* occurs within the shafts of long bones and extends into the haversian systems. Yellow marrow is connective tissue composed of fat cells.
   4. *Classification of bones* according to shape.
      a. *Long bones* consist of a *shaft* (the *diaphysis* of the shaft is basically made of compact bone, while the flared part at each end of the diaphysis, i.e., the *metaphysis,* consists of cancellous

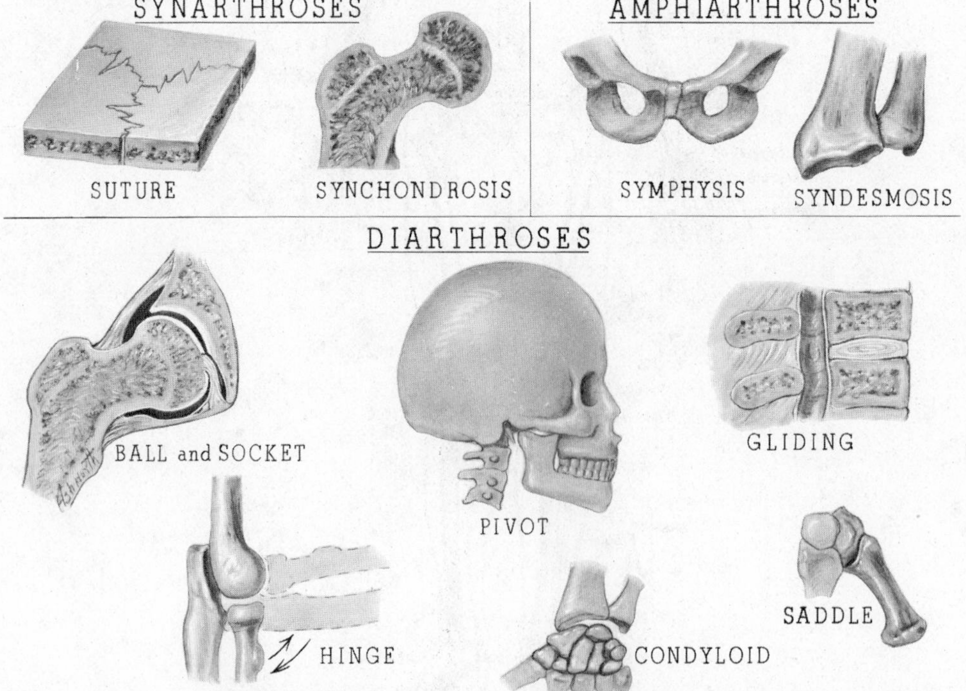

FIGURE 87–2. Joints are categorized into three groups, according to the degree of movement permitted. Each of these groups is, in turn, subdivided with respect to the structural components of individual joints. (From Jacob, S. W., and Francone, C. A.: *Structure and Function in Man.* 3rd ed. 1974.)

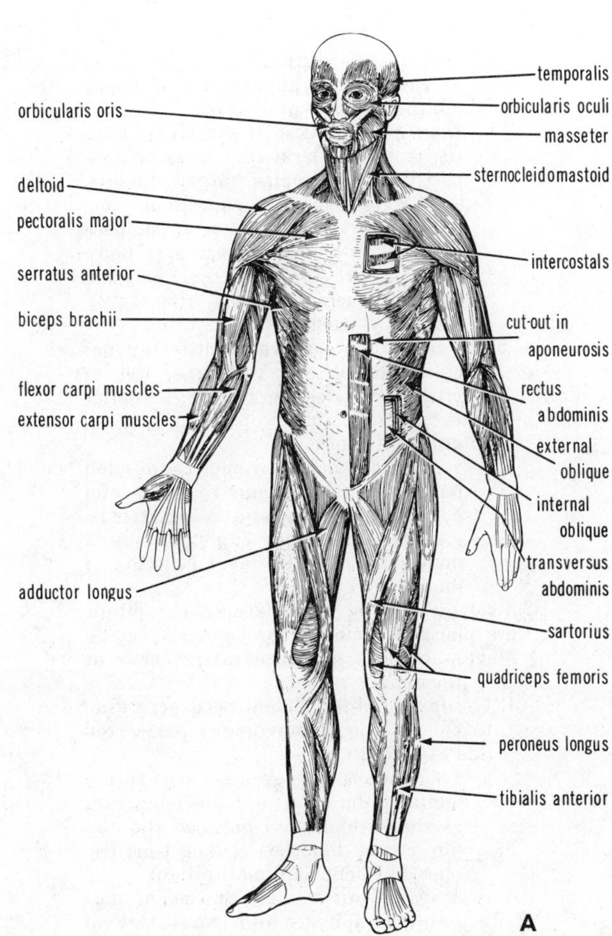

FIGURE 87-3. Principal muscles. *A,* Anterior view. *B,* Posterior view. (From Memmler, R. L., and Rada, R. B.: *The Human Body in Health and Disease.* 3rd ed. Philadelphia, J. B. Lippincott Company, 1970.)

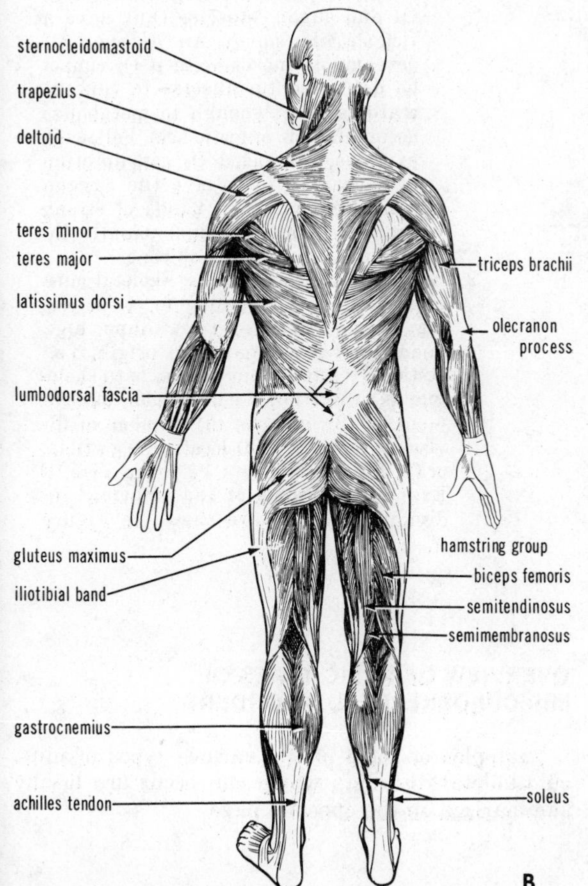

bone) and two extremities, each termed an *epiphysis*. Examples of long bones are the humerus and radius.

b. *Short bones* consist of cancellous bone tissue covered by a thin layer of compact tissue. Examples: carpals, tarsals.

c. *Flat bones* consist of cancellous bone encased in two flat plates of compact bone. Flat bones protect soft body parts or provide large surfaces for muscle attachments, e.g., ribs, skull, scapula, portions of pelvic girdle.

d. *Irregular bones* are of differing peculiar shapes, e.g., vertebrae, ossicles of the ear. Irregular bones are similar in structure and composition to other groups of bones.

e. *Sesamoid bones* are small, rounded bones located adjacent to joints and encased in tendon and fascial tissue, e.g., patella ("knee cap"). Sesamoid bones increase the lever-function of muscles.

B. *Articular System.* Articulations, i.e., joints, are places of union of two or more bones. Movement does not necessarily occur at such junctions.

1. *Groups of joints.* Categorized according to the degree of movement permitted (see Fig. 87-2).

a. *Synarthroses:* no movement, e.g., suture joints of the skull and the temporary cartilage connection between the epiphysis and diaphysis of long bone (replaced by bone with maturation).

b. *Amphiarthroses:* slight movement, e.g., pubic symphysis and connection of ligaments where radius articulates with ulna.

c. *Diarthroses* (synovial joints): freely movable to permit changes of position and motion. Consist of (1) an articular cavity (lined with synovial membrane which produces synovial fluid for joint lubrication and cartilage nourishment) enclosed by a capsule of fibrous articular cartilage; (2) ligaments reinforcing the capsule and helping to limit motion; and (3) cartilage covering the ends of opposing bones (cartilage makes a smooth surface so bone ends can glide over one another). Articular disks are located between the articular cartilage of some synovial joints to help buffer forceful impacts. Muscles help stabilize joints and maintain firm contact of articular surfaces. Synovial joints are classified by the shape of the articulating end of the involved bones (see Fig. 87-2 for types of joints).

Some kinds of movements occurring at synovial joints include protraction, retraction, eversion, inversion, flexion, extension, abduction, adduction, rotation, supination, and pronation.

C. *Muscular System:* Muscles make up 40 to 50 per cent of the body's weight. By *contraction* they produce movement of the body as a whole or of its parts.

1. *Types of muscle.*

a. *Cardiac muscle:* involuntary muscle found only in the heart. Is striated crosswise and longitudinally.

b. *Smooth muscle:* involuntary muscle found in hollow structures (such as digestive tract, blood vessels, and urinary bladder) and other areas, e.g., eye. Not striated. Controlled by autonomic nervous system.

c. *Striated (skeletal) muscle:* voluntary muscle of the skeletal system. Composed of combination of muscle and connective tissue. Muscle fibers are arranged in bundles *(fasciculi)* held together by connective tissue. Groups of bundles are similarly bound together, and entire muscle is encased in tough sheath of connective tissue. The *muscle sheath* contains blood and lymph vessels and nerve fibers. Nerve fibers (each supply perhaps over 100 individual muscle cells) carry impulse-messages to muscles. Endings of motor nerve fibers are called *motor end plates or myoneural junctions.* A continuous flow of stimuli maintains *muscle tone,* i.e., keeps muscles partially contracted in a state of readiness for action. To generate heat and power, muscle cells require large amounts of O_2 and sugar. Muscles thus have a rich *vascular supply.* An *"oxygen debt"* develops during exercise if O_2 cannot be delivered to muscles in concentrations great enough to metabolize accumulations of lactic acid. Following exercise, increased O_2 consumption is necessary to relieve the oxygen debt. *Tendons* (i.e., bands of strong inelastic fibrous tissue) usually indirectly attach muscle to bone.

2. *Individual skeletal muscles.* Skeletal muscles are named according to (1) action, e.g., flexor, extensor; (2) shape, e.g., quadrilateral, pennate; (3) origin, i.e., stationary attachment of muscle to skeleton; (4) insertion, i.e., movable attachment of the muscle; (5) number of divisions, e.g., "tri"; (6) location, e.g., tibia; or (7) direction of fibers, i.e., transverse.[113] Examples of some of the principal individual muscles are shown in Figure 87-3.

OVERVIEW OF BASIC TYPES OF MUSCULOSKELETAL DISORDERS

Examples of some of the various types of musculoskeletal disorders which can occur are briefly summarized on the opposite page.

Causative Factors	Examples of Disorders
Infection	Osteomyelitis (bone infection); tuberculosis of bones and joints.
Inflammation	Arthritis (joint inflammation); bursitis (bursa inflammation); osteitis (bone inflammation); myositis (muscle inflammation); synovitis (synovial membrane inflammation).
Trauma	Fractures; sprains; strains; dislocations; traumatic arthritis.
Tumors	Multiple myeloma; osteogenic sarcoma; giant-cell tumor; metastatic bone tumors (tumors arising from tissues other than bone).
Degeneration	Osteoarthritis (hypertrophic degeneration of joints).
Neurogenic muscular impairments	Myasthenia gravis and muscular dystrophies (see Unit VIII).
Metabolic	Arthritis associated with gout; osteoporosis.
Vitamin deficiency	Osteomalacia (vitamin D deficiency in adults results in softening of bones due to impaired calcium and phosphorus metabolism).
Autoimmune	Rheumatoid arthritis; collagen or "connective tissue" diseases (e.g., systemic lupus erythematosus, periarteritis nodosa, scleroderma).
Unknown	Osteitis deformans, i.e., Paget's disease (chronic bone disease characterized by enlargement, softening, and deformity of certain bones).

CHAPTER 88

Diagnostic Procedures, Clinical Problems, and Therapeutic Measures

DIAGNOSIS AND EVALUATION OF ORTHOPEDIC DISORDERS

Orthopedic History and Examination

The *orthopedic history* includes evaluation of the onset and course of the presenting illness as well as general information about the patient. Past history, family history, and social history are also included. Important factors include previous symptoms, onset and duration of present symptoms, progression of symptoms, and extent of disability. Musculoskeletal disorders may produce symptoms of neurologic involvement, deformity, pain, or loss of joint motion. Some musculoskeletal disorders are aggravated by motion of the part, weather change, or weight-bearing. These factors are evaluated along with the effect of rest on the ailment. The physician seeks to determine not only what aggravates the disorder but also what relieves it. Previous treatments and their effects are carefully scrutinized. A nurse's descriptive charting of symptoms may be helpful in the diagnostic process, e.g., precise descriptions of pain characteristics.

During the *orthopedic examination* subjective physical findings are considered (e.g., tenderness to palpation, presence of muscle weakness) as well as objective observations (e.g., signs of redness, limb lengths, and circumferences). Subjective findings are under the patient's voluntary control; because these findings may be feigned by some patients, subjective findings must be carefully evaluated.[221]

Both a general and a local orthopedic examination may be given. During the *general* orthopedic examination, the examiner inspects general appearance; posture; gait and body mobility; body alignment; body contours; body attitude; carriage; muscle strengths; limb lengths and circumferences; joint motion; cervical, thoracic, and lumbar spines; and the relationships of various body parts to one another, e.g., relationship of feet to legs and hips to pelvis.

While observing a patient's movements and gait, the physician watches for[6] *gait patterns* associated with specific disorders; objective evidence of *discomfort;* evidence of *joint stiffness* or *muscle weakness; lack of coordination;* and *deformities.*

Observation of a patient's stance may reveal *spinal deformities:* (1) *kyphosis,* i.e., abnormally increased roundness of the thoracic curve; (2) *scoliosis,* i.e., an obvious lateral deformity of the spine; and (3) *lordosis,* i.e., abnormal increase in the lumbar curve. Other abnormalities which may be noted are *genu varus,* i.e., "bowed" legs, and *genu valgus,* i.e., "knock-knees" (see Fig. 88–1). (Note: The terms "varus" and "valgus" refer to the direction in which the apex of a deformity lies in relationship to the midline; i.e., a "varus" deformity is one in which the apex of the deformity points away from the midline, while a "valgus" deformity is one in which the apex of the deformity points toward the midline. These terms may be used in any body region to describe the direction of a deformity.)

Other deformities that may be detected during orthopedic examinations are (1) equinus and calcaneal deformities of the foot; (2) claw hammer, or mallet toes (see Fig. 88–2); (3) finger deformities, such as mallet finger, boutonniere deformity, swan-neck deformity, or claw-finger deformity. Many orthopedic deformities can be surgically corrected.

The *local* orthopedic examination focuses primarily on the site of the specific complaint. Comparisons are made between the affected and nonaffected sides of the body. For example, if the patient's disorder is in his right arm, the examiner compares the right arm with the left arm. The local orthopedic examination utilizes inspection and palpation and evaluation of range of motion and joint position. Joint motion is measured in degrees of a circle (see Fig. 88–3). Also, measurements are made (with a tape measure) of limb circumference to identify hypertrophy or atrophy of a part.

Aspects of neurologic examination which may be included in the local orthopedic examination are evaluation of (1) the integrity of cutaneous sensation; (2) strength of muscle power; and (3) quality of superficial and deep tendon reflexes.[85] (Evaluation of cutaneous sensation and tendon reflexes has been discussed in Unit VIII.) Two methods of grading muscle power are commonly used. One method is to grade numerically from "0" through "5"; 0 represents the weakest end of the scale while 5 is the strongest. The second

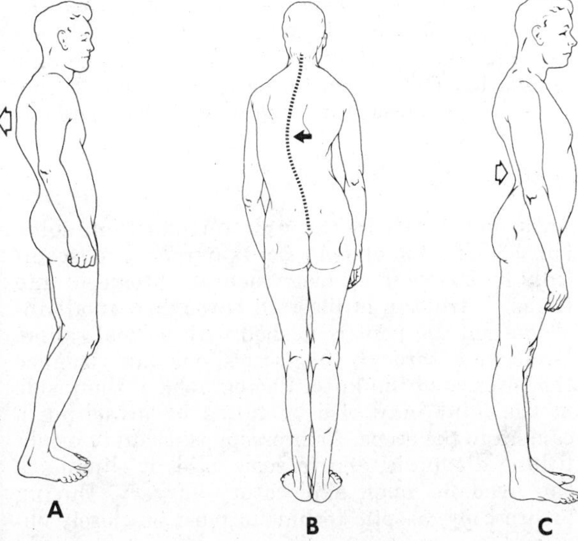

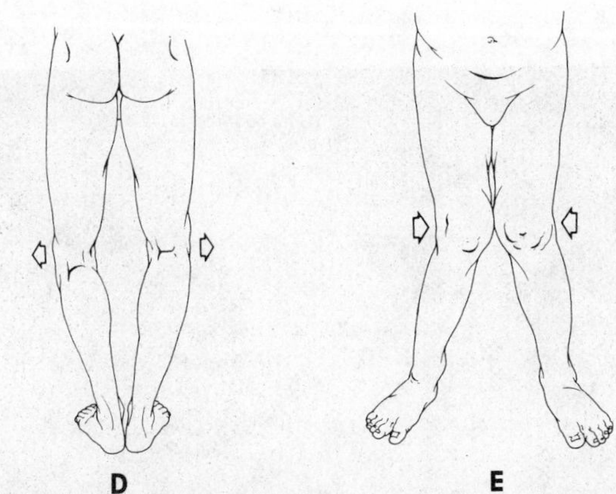

FIGURE 88–1. *A*, Kyphosis; *B*, scoliosis; *C*, lordosis; *D*, genu varus; *E*, genu valgus. (From *Manual of Orthopaedic Surgery.* Chicago, American Orthopaedic Association, 1972.)

method of grading muscle strength is to use the following grades (comparable to grades 0–5): (a) zero; (b) trace; (c) poor; (d) fair; (e) good; and (f) normal.

Examination of patients following musculoskeletal trauma is discussed in Chapter 3.

X-Rays

Roentgenography is the technique most commonly used to help establish the diagnosis of musculoskeletal disorders. X-rays are often viewed not only by the attending physician but also by a radiologist. The most useful x-rays are typically the *anteroposterior* and *lateral* films. Visualization of bone in both of these planes is desirable whenever possible. Some special x-ray studies which may be used with orthopedic patients include (1) *myelograms* (see Unit VIII); (2) *arthrograms* (see Fig. 88–4), i.e., x-rays taken following the injection of radiolucent gases or radiopaque dyes into joints (used to outline masses or soft tissue defects); (3) *sinograms*, i.e., x-rays taken after sinuses are injected with radiopaque dyes (to delineate the course of the sinuses and tissues involved); and (4) *laminograms (planograms)*, i.e., x-rays which clarify details of structures which are otherwise hidden by overlying radiopaque bone. Laminography or planography is also called *"body section roentgenography."* Special techniques used in this type of roentgenography permit detailed visualization of images of structures which lie in a predetermined plane of tissue, while images of structures lying in other planes are blurred or detail is otherwise eliminated. Body section roentgenography is useful in locating small cavities, for-

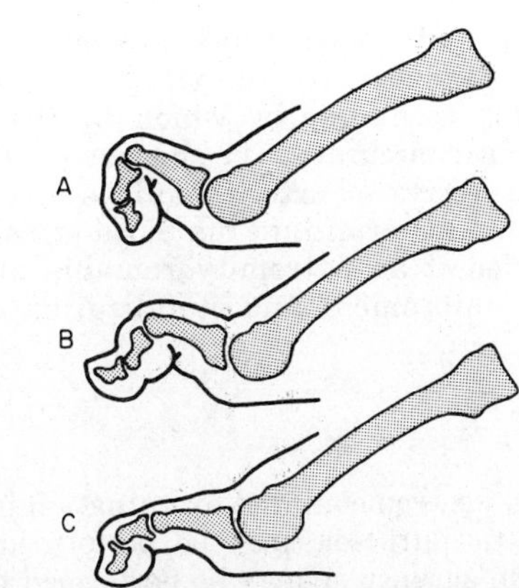

FIGURE 88–2. Common toe deformities. *A*, Claw toe; *B*, hammer toe; *C*, mallet toe. (From *Manual of Orthopaedic Surgery.* Chicago, American Orthopaedic Association, 1972.)

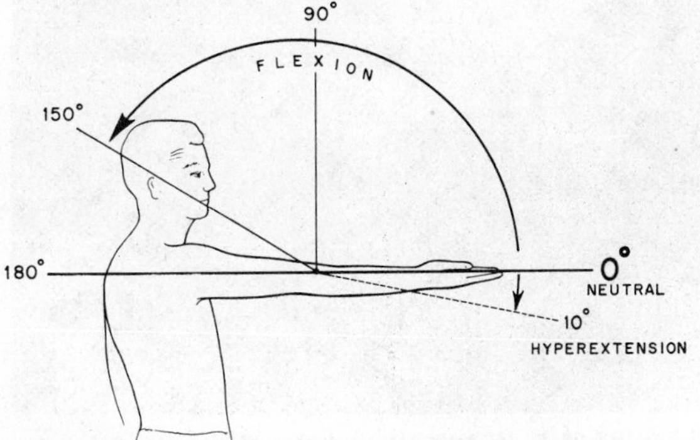

FIGURE 88–3. Joint motion is measured in degrees of a circle. (From Gartland, J. J.: *Fundamentals of Orthopaedics.* 1965.)

eign bodies, and lesions which are overshadowed by opaque structures. *Scanography* is another special x-ray technique by which the lengths of long bones can accurately be measured. *Arteriography,* i.e., x-rays of arteries following injection of radiopaque material into the blood stream, may be performed if an extremity remains pulseless following realignment and stabilization of fractures.

Biopsy

A biopsy, i.e., removal and examination of tissue for diagnostic purposes, may be performed at the time of open surgery or may be performed through a special needle or bore which does not necessitate a surgical incision. The latter types of biopsies are called aspiration, punch, or needle biopsies. Special needles which may be used for needle biopsies in diagnosing musculoskeletal disorders include the Craig needle for bone and the Vim-Silverman needle for soft tissue lesions. Once tissue is obtained by biopsy, it is histologically examined by a pathologist. Often the histologic evaluation of biopsied tissue is necessary to confirm the diagnosis of musculoskeletal disorders.

Arthroscopy

As mentioned in the unit introduction, some joints (e.g., knee) may be examined endoscopically by inserting an instrument (arthroscope) into them. A trochar is inserted through a small incision and the joint is flushed with normal saline. By looking through the "scope" one can visualize the interior of the knee. Photographs of the inside of the joint may also be taken by attaching a camera to the scope. Arthroscopy is useful in establishing diagnosis, and in some cases it eliminates the need for open exploratory surgery. During arthroscopy, aseptic technique must be closely observed.

Laboratory Tests

Laboratory tests may be employed in orthopedic patients[6] (1) to help establish diagnosis; (2) to preoperatively screen the functional capacity

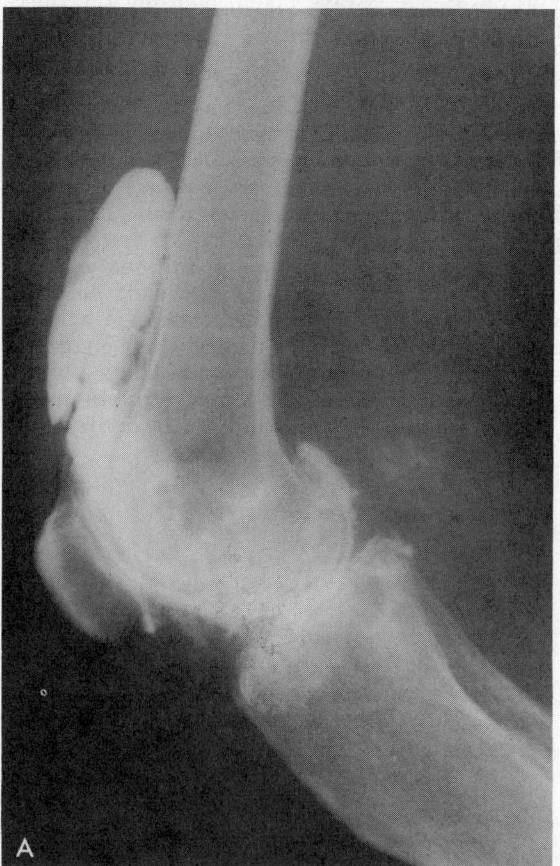

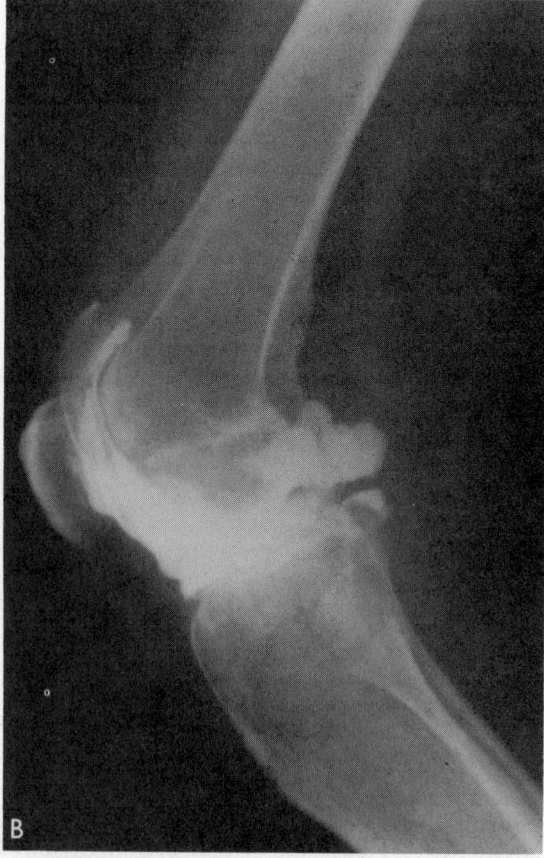

FIGURE 88-4. *A,* Arthrogram of knee showing a large suprapatellar pouch with many nodular filling defects. *B,* Three months after synovectomy the arthrogram shows a small smoothly outlined suprapatellar pouch. (From Taylor, A. R., and Ansell, B. M.: *Journal of Bone and Joint Surgery* 54-B:110, 1972.)

of other body systems; and (3) to monitor various physiologic processes following injury or surgery. *Post-traumatic* and *postoperative* laboratory monitoring is extremely valuable in the prevention or early detection and treatment of complications, e.g., shock, acidosis, alkalosis, dehydration, pulmonary embolism, pulmonary edema. Serial determinations may be made of glucose levels or prothrombin times, and determinations may be made of electrolyte balance, blood volume, and fluid balance. *Preoperative* laboratory studies are discussed briefly later in this chapter.

Diagnostic laboratory tests[6] in orthopedic patients may include analysis of (1) cerebrospinal fluid (to identify infections, neoplasms, and degenerative processes); (2) synovial fluid (to distinguish inflammatory from degenerative types of arthritis); (3) muscle enzymes (to distinguish between muscle weakness due to atrophic results of denervation and dystrophic diseases of the muscle itself; and (4) mineral metabolism (levels of calcium, phosphorus, and alkaline phosphates are measured to establish or rule out various specific musculoskeletal disorders).

The most important inorganic constituents of bone are calcium and phosphorus, so that *calcium and phosphorus ion levels* in the serum and urine reflect skeletal metabolic activity. The normal blood value for calcium is 8.5–10.5 mg./100 ml. and for phosphorus 3.0–4.5 mg./100 ml. The average adult urinary excretion of calcium is between 100 and 200 mg./day. About 600 mg./day of phosphorus is excreted in the urine with an ordinary intake. Plasma levels of phosphorus and the daily urinary excretion of phosphorus are both more variable than values for calcium; phosphorus levels vary depending upon time of day and intake.

Evaluations of calcium and phosphorus are useful in differentiating diseases which cause changes in skeletal density, e.g., osteoporosis, renal disease, osteomalacia, rickets, parathyroid or thyroid hyperactivity. *Alkaline phosphatase* levels are used to assess osteoblastic activity, i.e., formation of new bone. Alkaline phosphatase is an enzyme necessary for mineralization of the organic bone matrix.

In addition to the laboratory tests discussed above, bacteriologic studies (e.g., smears and cultures) may be employed to identify bacteria causing infections.

Other Diagnostic Tests

Joint aspiration, electromyography, and radioisotope skeletal surveys are other tests which may be of value in diagnosing some musculoskeletal disorders. *Aspiration,* e.g., of the knee joint, may be performed to obtain a specimen for diagnostic purposes as well as to instill medications or relieve pain. Blood, synovial fluid, or pus may be aspirated from joints. Local anesthesia may be used for the aspiration. Aseptic technique is imperative. *Electromyography* is of value in evaluating lower motor neuron lesions. This procedure, which measures the electrical potential change associated with skeletal muscle contraction, is discussed in Unit VIII. *Radioisotope skeletal surveys,* e.g., with a whole-body profile scanner using radioactive strontium (^{85}Sr), are useful in detecting localized bone disease, e.g., bone cancer.

COMMON CLINICAL PROBLEMS WITH ORTHOPEDIC DISORDERS

Pain

Disorders of the bones, joints, and muscles commonly produce discomfort and pain. Because of the chronicity of many of these disorders, chemotherapeutic pain management must be carefully planned to prevent drug dependency. Whenever possible, in lieu of administering analgesics and other medications, the nurse uses a wide variety of activities to relieve or prevent pain, e.g., changes of position, applications of heat or cold, massage, and relief of pressure from casts or traction.

General measures used to reduce pain and inflammation associated with *rheumatic disorders* include (1) resting the affected joint or extremity, e.g., by bedrest or the application of splints or casts; (2) employing physical measures, e.g., heat (dry or moist), massage, therapeutic exercises; and (3) chemotherapy, e.g., aspirin (analgesic, anti-inflammatory), phenylbutazone (Butazolidin), oxyphenbutazone (Tandearil), indomethacin (Indocin), corticosteroids (administered systemically or injected intra-articularly, i.e., into the joint), muscle relaxants. Specific management of various rheumatic disorders is discussed as appropriate in other sections of this unit.

Not only may *orthopedic disorders* cause pain, but also *pain may result from some treatment procedures.* For example, prolonged pressure over bony prominences (e.g., from a cast, traction, or malpositioning) may cause "burning" pain which should be immediately relieved by appropriate measures, e.g., cutting the cast to relieve pressure over the painful area, or correcting the traction setup or the patient's position to relieve the pain-producing, skin-damaging pressure. Areas especially susceptible to prolonged pressure include the tuberosity of the tibia, the heel, and the head of the fibula on the lateral side (see Unit V, Ch. 27).

Following *musculoskeletal surgery,* pain management is a priority in postoperative clinical care. Orthopedic surgical procedures can be extremely painful. Causes of pain and discomfort must be carefully evaluated so that appropriate relief can be given. Pain-relieving measures are similar to those just mentioned.

Generally severe musculoskeletal pain causes a patient to be restless and to frequently change his position. Also, the patient attempts to protect the anatomic region from which the pain arises by (1) *muscle splinting,* i.e., active (often involuntary) muscle contraction which immobilizes the part; and (2) *pseudoparalysis* of the part not accompanied by loss of sensation. Muscle splinting differs from muscle spasm in that relaxation of the affected muscles occurs at rest (see below). Prolonged pain in bone, muscle, tendons, or joints, with resultant muscle splinting and pseudoparalysis, may lead eventually to osteoporosis in the affected bone and possibly in adjacent bones. Joint contractures also may develop. Tables 88–1 and 88–2 summarize the characteristics of pain in musculoskeletal tissues, and also the patterns of pain experienced in various types of joint disorders (see also Unit IX).

Muscle Spasms

Muscle cramps or spasms often produce discomfort and pain in persons with musculoskeletal disorders. Powerful involuntary muscular contractions shorten the flexor muscles and cause extreme pain which may be incapacitating. These contractions may be stimulated by ischemia and hypoxia of muscle tissue, e.g., due to mechanical compression of blood vessels.

Muscle spasms are a prominent and distressing symptom of *myositic-fibrositic disorders* and many *articular disorders*. In an attempt to relieve skeletal muscle spasms, the physician may order heat applications and massage and may prescribe muscle relaxants, e.g., chlormezanone (Trancopal), carisoprodol (Rela, Soma), methocarbamol (Robaxin), orphenadrine (Norflex), chlorzoxazone (Paraflex), or mephenesin. Usually muscle relaxants are not very potent.

Patients confined to bed commonly experience muscle spasms in the calves of their legs which cause the toes to plantar flex and the feet to forcefully extend and invert. Muscle spasms of this nature are frequently experienced by persons with *advanced arteriosclerosis* and usually occur in positions which create pressure in the popliteal space.

Nursing care activities that may prevent leg cramps include: (1) frequent position changes; (2) use of a bed cradle to prevent the weight of bed linens on the feet and legs; (3) insuring adequate warmth; (4) avoidance of heavy sedation (sedation reduces spontaneous movements during sleep); (5) positioning which prevents pressure on the popliteal space and minimizes external compression of calf muscles; and (6) active or passive exercise as recommended by the physician. Medications which may be prescribed to treat

TABLE 88–1. CHARACTERISTICS OF PAIN IN MUSCULOSKELETAL TISSUES*

Tissue	Characteristics
Bone	Slow pain; ache; poorly localized; often throbbing Aggravated by forces of all attached muscles, aggravated by torque (applied manually) and percussion Causes pseudoparalysis of all attached muscles Tenderness, but localization of tenderness mediocre
Muscle belly	Mostly slow pain at rest; aching, some fast pain on contraction Aggravated directly by contraction of affected muscle and by passive stretch Poor subjective localization Affected muscle protected by pseudoparalysis Tenderness with good localization Wasting in pain of long duration, plus osteoporosis in activated bones, plus joint contracture.
Tendon, ligament, fascia	Mostly slow pain at rest; some fast pain on contractile force; localization poor; tender, and localization of tenderness is good
Bony attachments of tendon, ligament, fascia	Mixed slow and fast pain; localization good; protected by pseudoparesis or pseudoparalysis; tenderness accurately localized
Hyaline cartilage	Totally insensitive
Synovia	Slow pain; ache; poorly localized May produce the gelation phenomenon.

*From Frost, H. M.: Musculoskeletal pain, In *Facial Pain.* Alling, C. C., III (ed.), Philadelphia, Lea and Febiger, 1968, p. 159.

benign muscular cramps may include Benadryl, quinine sulfate, and Myanesin. When a muscle cramp does occur in the calf of the leg, it may be relaxed by causing the vigorous contraction of the opposing muscle group. This maneuver, called "reflex inhibition," involves forcefully dorsiflexing the foot and toes while pressing downward on the top of the foot (e.g., with the heel of the opposite foot or the hand). When correctly performed, the ankle of the affected leg should be at an angle of about 90°. Motor nerve impulse transmission is thus prevented to the calf muscles.

Contractures

As mentioned previously, joint contractures may develop in painful limbs if these extremities are maintained for long periods of time in pain-reducing positions. The patient with a painful limb, e.g., arthritic shoulder and arm, must be encouraged to exercise the affected extremity as prescribed by the physician to maintain maximum range of motion. A patient's natural tendency in such a situation is not to move the limb (since movement may produce pain) but rather to hold it in the position which causes the least discomfort, e.g., a painful arm may be held flexed close to the body. Prolonged inactivity may cause positional deformities and stiffness, not only in affected limbs but also in uninvolved parts of the body, unless frequent position changes, correct repositioning, and exercises are faithfully carried out.

In *flexion contractures* the patient cannot extend the affected extremity. Flexion contractures will develop in bed patients who are not given proper preventative care. Poor posture in bed and a sagging mattress contribute to the development of joint contractures, particularly *hip flexion contractures.* Following fracture of the hip, contractures may develop if the patient is permitted to (a) flex and adduct his hips; (b) flex the knees; or (c) maintain an equinus position of the feet for prolonged periods of time. Continuous support of the knees of any patient in a flexed position causes *knee flexion contractures.* The hamstring muscles of the posterior thigh (whose tendons pass under the knee) contract over a relatively short period if the knee is continuously flexed.

Absence of proper foot support, e.g., against a padded footboard, encourages *"foot drop,"* especially in patients with muscular weakness. If the foot is permitted to rest unsupported, the muscles in the anterior leg stretch, and the tendon of the calf muscles shortens.

TABLE 88–2. SOME JOINT PAIN PATTERNS*

Lesion	Pattern
Acute distention by fluid	Slow pain; ache; mediocre localization; joint held in attitude of greatest fluid volume; pronounced splinting of motion by active muscle contraction; active and passive motion markedly limited; tenderness pronounced and well localized; dramatic relief by aspiration or drainage of joint
Hypersensitive synovia and/or capsule	Splinting of motion by active muscle contraction; comfortable at rest in any attitude once it is produced; gelation phenomenon exists Slow pain, ache, poor localization Synovia usually tender Always pain with motion; usually no pain under load without motion Relieved by intra-articular local anesthetic
Bone pain due to irregular joint surface	Comfortable at rest in any attitude Motion under major load much more painful than motion while free of load Load without motion is painless No tenderness Slow pain; ache; poorly localized Referral and radiation are common Usually not relieved by intra-articular local anesthetic
Bone pain due to subchondral expansile noxious lesion	Worse at night; aggravated by load but not by motion without load; often helped temporarily by motion without load
Gelation	"Stiffens" at rest, hurts for a few minutes when activity resumes but then improves as long as activity is maintained
Prolonged pain	Muscle wasting; local osteoporosis; joint contracture or diminished range of passive motion

*From Frost, H. M.: Musculoskeletal pain, In *Facial Pain.* Alling, C. C., III (ed.), Philadelphia, Lea and Febiger, 1968, p. 161.

Contractures will develop in the *pectoral muscles* and other muscles close to the *axilla* if a patient is permitted to assume a posture for prolonged periods in which he holds his arms close to his sides, flexes his elbows at right angles, and drops his wrists. Contractures in these positions may develop following cerebrovascular accidents or in any patient who lies in bed for long periods.

Kerr[123] observes: "We all tend to allow the desperately ill patient to remain in any position in which he appears comfortable because it seems a waste of his limited strength to disturb or move him. . . . Such mistaken kindness and consideration may permanently deform the patient if he survives." There is commonly a tendency not only not to "disturb" patients who are desperately ill, but also not to require patients who are in pain to move about or change their positions. These tendencies are not generally in the best long-range interests of persons who are ill and suffering. The skillful nurse can, with compassion and understanding, perform necessary position changes and exercises even for persons who have a natural reluctance to move about. It is indeed tragic when preventable contractures are allowed to develop, since contractures may seriously interfere with successful rehabilitation. For example, post-amputation contractures may prevent the use of a prosthesis.

Volkmann's ischemic contracture (see Fig. 88–5) is a serious, deforming, crippling condition of the hand and forearm which may develop as a complication of a fracture about the elbow joint or forearm bones. Vascular obstruction following reduction of the fracture may result from a position of extreme flexion or tight bandages. Vascular obstruction in this instance is indicated by absence of a radial pulse, and this finding should be immediately reported, before massive infarction of muscle tissue can occur. After such infarction, muscle is slowly replaced with fibrous tissue, and tendons and nerves become restricted by scar tissue. Although it most commonly involves the arms, Volkmann's ischemic contracture may also develop in the lower extremities as a complication of fractures of the femur and tibia. Immediate treatment of suspected ischemia includes the release of constricting bandages and the elevation of the extremity. Emergency surgery may be necessary if relief of the ischemia does not occur within 1–2 hours.

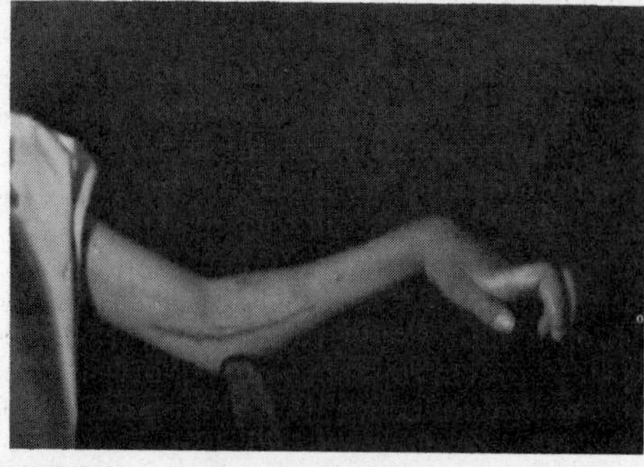

FIGURE 88–5. Volkmann's contracture after fracture of the elbow. (From O'Donoghue, D. H.: *Treatment of Injuries to Athletes.* 2nd ed. 1970.)

THERAPEUTIC MEASURES COMMONLY USED IN THE TREATMENT OF ORTHOPEDIC DISORDERS

Rest

Rest is an important aspect of the treatment of many musculoskeletal disorders. Following trauma, a period of rest promotes healing and minimizes inflammation, swelling, and pain. In the management of rheumatic diseases, rest of the affected joints or extremities helps reduce pain and inflammation. At times bed rest is advisable. Immobilization of affected joints may be achieved by the application of splints or casts. Splints prevent joint deformities in addition to minimizing pain by relieving muscle spasms.

Physical Therapy

Physical therapy is an integral part of the total care of persons with musculoskeletal disorders. The goals of physical therapy are variable but may include maintenance or improvement of range of joint motion, dexterity, and muscle strength; reduction or relief of pain and swelling; relief of muscle spasms; prevention of complications of inactivity (see Unit V, Ch. 27); and teaching of self-care and ambulation techniques. In many settings specially trained physical therapists are available to implement physical therapy. The nurse assumes the responsibility for performing many aspects of physical therapy in the absence of registered physical therapists.

Some of the more common techniques of physical therapy employed in the care of patients with musculoskeletal disorders include application of heat, administration of massage, and assistance with exercises. Space does not permit detailed discussions of these physical therapy processes; however, they are discussed briefly in following pages.

Heat. Heat may be applied in several ways, e.g., hot packs, hot soaks, hot paraffin applications, infrared radiation, whirlpool baths, diathermy. Commonly the application of heat is followed by exercise or massage. Among the physiologic effects of heat are softening of fibrous tissue, sedation, increased edema and arterial blood supply, and reduction or relief of pain.[128] Heat may relax muscle, relieve pain, and induce vasodilation (this, in turn, improves local blood supply and nutrition). Heat may be applied either dry or moist and may be directed *locally* (e.g., at a single joint) or *systemically.*

Methods of applying *moist heat* include the

Hubbard tank (for application to multiple joints) and whirlpool baths, hot compresses, or hot paraffin (wax) applications (for local applications). Diathermy and ultrasound may be used in treating nonarticular rheumatic disorders, but generally they are not applied to acutely inflamed joints. Most commonly *dry heat* is applied by using hot air, heat lamps, or heating pads.

Massage. Massage may relieve pain, stretch fibrous tissue, and reduce edema (because the stroke is toward the heart with the hand, thus improving return circulation).[128] Massage relaxes muscles, improves muscle tone, and increases blood flow. It may relieve muscle spasms in many muscular and fibrotic inflammations. Note that acutely inflamed joints should never be massaged.

Exercises. Prescribed exercise varies in type, depending upon an individual patient's needs. It may be (a) *active* (the motion is performed by the patient); (b) *passive* (the motion is performed by another person for the patient); or (c) *active-assistive* (the patient actively performs as much of the motion as he can, with the help of another person as needed).

Exercises are often categorized according to the type of muscular activity required. *Isotonic* exercises are the "normal" type of exercise in which motion of a part takes place, involving shortening of the muscle and muscle contraction. With *isometric* exercise, also called static exercise or muscle-setting exercise, there is active contraction and relaxation of muscles without movement of the joint that is normally mobilized by these muscles. *Resistive* exercises are those in which motion of a part takes place against the resistance of another person or of the person's own antagonistic muscles. Pulleys and ropes may be used for resistive exercises. *Range of motion* (ROM) exercises are those in which a joint is moved through its full range of motion, that is, the full extent to which it is capable of being moved. ROM exercises may be active, passive, or active-assistive.

Therapeutic exercises have numerous benefits. Among these are maintenance or restoration of adequate joint activity; prevention of muscular atrophy and other deformities; building or maintaining muscular bulk and strength; maintaining or improving joint range of motion; building endurance; and stimulating circulation.

In some instances exercises are directed specifically at "building up" those muscles necessary for use with ambulation, e.g., the quadriceps muscles may be strengthened by having the patient straighten his knee while sitting. Bed exercises help prepare a patient for ambulation. These exercises may include (a) joint ROM exercises, active or passive, to preserve joint motion; (b) deep breathing exercises (see Unit XIV) to stimulate circulation and promote effective lung function; (c) quadriceps setting to stabilize the knees; (d) gluteal and abdominal muscle tightening to improve trunk stability; (e) lifting exercises to increase strength in the biceps; and (f) push-up exercises to increase strength in the triceps.

In addition to the previously discussed activities, the physical therapist (or nurse) may teach patients: *transfer techniques,* e.g., bed to wheelchair; *wheelchair usage;* application of *braces* or other appliances; usage of *crutches, canes,* or *walkers;* or usage of other self-care equipment. Some of these activities are discussed in Unit VIII. Crutch walking and the use of canes, walkers, and braces are discussed below.

Crutches. Crutches must be selected which are of proper length for the individual patient. Space must be present between the axilla and the top of the crutch. If the crutches are too long, the patient cannot get his arms up over them or they cause excessive pressure and rubbing in the axilla.

> *Excessive axillary pressure from crutches may cause nerve damage (to branches of the brachial plexus) and arm paralysis or numbness, i.e.,* crutch palsy *or* crutch paralysis.

Emphasize to the patient that he can injure himself in the above manner if he permits excessive axillary pressure to occur while using crutches. If too short, crutches slip out from under the patient's arm, possibly causing him to fall.

To measure a patient for crutches if he cannot stand up, either (a) subtract 16 inches from his total height, or (b) have the patient lie supine (arms at sides, walking shoes on) and measure from the axilla to a point level with the bottom of the heel of the shoe and about 6–8 inches laterally from the foot.

Not only should crutches fit comfortably under the patient's arms, but also the *hand grip* should be at a height comfortable for use. The hand bar should be of such a height that the patient can almost completely extend his elbow without the axillary bar causing pressure on the axilla. The patient should be able to stand erect when using his crutches (not "hunch" over), and he should be able to comfortably extend his arms with his hands grasping the hand grip. The patient should carry his weight on his hands (not his axillae), with his wrists in hyperextension while crutch-walking. When possible a physical therapist selects crutches for a patient. A variety of crutches are available, e.g., some are adjustable, some are made of wood, others are made of metal. Crutches must always be fitted with pure rubber suction tips to prevent the crutches from sliding out from under the patient when he puts his weight on them. Some crutches are fitted with shoulder or hand pads or both to minimize pressure on the axillae or hands.

Crutch-walking is a permanent method of ambulating for some patients; for others, crutches are only required temporarily.

Preparation for crutch-walking may involve (a) instruction (by illustration and demonstration) and measuring for crutches; (b) obtaining flat, properly fitting, oxford shoes which give good foot support and have heels and soles which will not slip (it is not safe to walk with crutches in stocking feet, slippers, or high heeled shoes); (c) exercises to strengthen arm and shoulder muscles; and (d) use of parallel bars in front of a mirror.

Exercises taught in preparation for crutch usage may include use of sawed-off crutches on the bed for straight elbow push-ups; or sitting upright in bed (or over the edge of the bed) and pressing both palms on the mattress while straightening the elbows and lifting the body weight up enough (on the hands) that the buttocks are lifted off the bed. Additionally, the patient may lift sandbags while lying on his back, and/or he may perform push-ups while lying on his abdomen. These exercises strengthen the triceps (extensor muscles of the upper arm). Also, straight-elbow push-ups help the patient learn how to bear weight on the palms of his hands. While standing between parallel bars, the patient learns to stand erect and swing forward by pushing down on his hands and swinging his body.

The patient is told by his physician whether or not he may place weight on his affected side, e.g., he may be permitted *full weight-bearing* or only *partial weight-bearing,* or he may be instructed to be *non-weight*-bearing while crutch-walking. While walking on crutches, the patient should practice (a) maintaining an erect posture; (b) looking forward, not downward, i.e., "eyes up" and "head up"; and (c) taking short steps of equal length. The patient should wear slacks or trousers to learn crutch-walking, rather than a bathrobe. Robes are cumbersome (crutches may catch in them), and they prevent viewing of the body posture.

Beginning by standing up in a tripod position (i.e., feet 6–8 inches apart and crutches about 4 inches ahead and 4 inches to the side), the patient can learn the gait for walking which is best suited to his situation. *Basic gaits* are (a) *swing-through,* i.e., simultaneously advance both crutches and swing body through so the feet assume a place ahead of the crutches; (b) *two-point,* i.e., simultaneously advance right foot and left crutch, then left foot and right crutch; (c) *three-point,* i.e., while keeping weight off of the affected limb, stand on the strong leg and advance both crutches, then swing the strong leg ahead through the crutches; and (d) *four-point,* i.e., in individual sequence the left crutch, right foot, right crutch, and then left foot are placed down and ahead. The swing-through gait may be used in the presence of complete leg and hip paralysis, e.g., paraplegia, and when a patient is attempting to move quickly, e.g., to avoid danger. However, this gait should be avoided unless necessary because it fosters hip and leg atrophy. The three-point gait is used in the absence of one leg or when weight-bearing on an affected leg is to be avoided or minimized. Encourage the patient to tighten his abdominal and gluteal muscles while walking.

During practice crutch-walking sessions, or if a patient on crutches at other times appears to be in need of assistance, stand behind the patient and hold him securely by his belt or have one person walk in front of and another behind the patient. *Be prepared to support the patient if he begins to fall.* Patients who are elderly, poorly coordinated, weakened, or who have impaired balance require especially close supervision while using crutches. A patient using crutches should be told that if he feels he is falling (while walking unassisted), he should try to throw his crutches away to the side and try to relax and fall limply. These actions can help minimize possible injury. As a patient develops skill and confidence in using crutches, he is taught to get up and sit down in a chair and to go up and down stairs with crutches.

People on crutches are vulnerable to accidents. Staff members on orthopedic services must therefore be especially careful to keep floors litter-free and dry to prevent patients on crutches from tripping or slipping. Additionally, doors must be slowly and cautiously opened (to prevent toppling over a patient on crutches on the other side of the door), and patients on crutches must be given plenty of room when walking past them (to avoid accidentally kicking away a crutch). Falls can be tragic and often can be prevented by safety-conscious staff members. Also, falls may be avoided by teaching patients on crutches to watch out for hazards such as slippery, littered, highly polished, or uneven floor surfaces; throw rugs (scatter rugs); electric wire cords; or untied shoe laces. Rubber crutch tips should be inspected periodically and soft or worn tips replaced.

In preparation for teaching crutch-walking and for assisting patients who are on crutches, you could practice using crutches. Try each of the gaits previously described. Think about how you could most effectively teach crutch-walking, then practice with an associate.

Canes. A cane is used on the side opposite the impaired leg. Body weight is thus maintained by the weak leg and cane while the strong leg is moved forward. The cane should be of such a length that the patient can extend his elbow and bear his weight on the hand grasping the cane. In addition to having a pure rubber suction tip, the cane should have a curved handle with a comfortable grip.

Walkers. Walkers of various kinds are available to help patients ambulate. Walkers may be used prior to crutches for some persons, e.g., postoperatively if a patient has joint disease. In preparation for using a walker, patients may practice resistance exercises while in bed to strengthen the triceps muscles. Other instruction may include methods of properly bearing weight on the hands and assistance on parallel bars (to help reestablish balance and resume a normal walking gait). Some walkers have underarm supports similar to those found on crutches. As with crutch-walking, to prevent accidents while patients are using walkers be certain floors are dry and free of litter and that supportive shoes are worn. It is desirable for patients to be dressed while using walkers, since bathrobes may easily become entangled and cause falls.

Braces. Braces and other orthopedic devices, e.g., corsets, may be worn as part of the treatment of musculoskeletal disorders. Orthopedic appliances are made by an *orthotist* (also spelled "orthetist") and are individually designed for each patient. Often a physical therapist helps a patient learn to apply, use, and care for his braces. A patient may have difficulty adjusting to new braces because they may rub, pinch, or otherwise not fit correctly. Additionally, braces are often heavy and may cause a person unaccustomed to them to feel clumsy or off balance. It is not uncommon for a patient to initially dislike the change in his appearance which is caused by wearing a brace (see discussion of self-image, Unit III, Ch. 14).

Braces must be correctly applied and cared for. It is essential that braces fit correctly and comfortably. Braces must not rub or chafe the skin or cause other irritations, e.g., excessive pressure. The patient who wears braces is taught to make frequent skin inspections to be certain that no skin damage is being caused by the appliances. A mirror should be used to visualize those areas which could not otherwise be seen. If the patient has impaired sensation (e.g., numbness to pain and pressure) in the braced portion of his body, these visual self-inspections of the skin are of particular importance, since they are the primary means by which the patient can detect problems caused by his braces. In the hospital the nurse makes these skin inspections at first, and she charts and reports indications of skin damage. Poorly fitting appliances are then padded (perhaps with lamb's wool or felt pads), or other adjustments are made, e.g., a strap may be loosened. Often it is necessary initially for the orthotist to redesign and refit new braces. Periodic adjustments in braces may also be necessary later, e.g., if the patient loses or gains weight, regains function, or if the structure of the braces changes with long-term use.

Encourage the patient who wears braces to report areas of discomfort. If the patient is made to feel that he is unnecessarily "complaining" or "causing trouble" by reporting such discomfort, he may hesitate to report essential observations and suffer needlessly. If a brace does not fit comfortably and correctly, the patient will become discouraged and his condition may be worsened. The apron, ties, or belts of a brace (or corset) must be smooth when the appliance is being worn, and not be wrinkled or twisted next to the skin. Buckles, stays, or hinges should not poke against the skin or cause excessive pressure. The appliance must be fitted with proper snugness, neither too loose nor too tight. Frequent skin care is of obvious importance. If a patient is capable of giving this care to himself, he is taught how to do so correctly. Other patient teaching may include care of the brace, e.g., oiling joints, applying saddle soap to leather parts, replacing worn ties. Injury may be prevented by carefully inspecting the brace at regular intervals for indications of the need for service.

The nurse may be of great assistance to a patient during the time necessary for him to learn how to use a brace. By maintaining a helpful, encouraging, enthusiastic attitude during this time, a nurse can help a patient to view his brace as a device which is of benefit to him, rather than as an uncomfortable, unsightly encumbrance.

Casts

Major *purposes* of casting include (a) immobilization, support, and protection of a part during healing processes (e.g., healing of fractures once they are reduced and properly aligned or healing following surgery); (b) prevention of deformities (e.g., with arthritis); and (c) correction of deformities (e.g., scoliosis). The ideal plaster cast, used for immobilization, should (a) be meticulously molded "like a glove" to the contour of the casted part; and (b) include "the joint above and the joint below" the affected part. Use of a cast following surgery or in the treatment of a fracture often makes it possible for a patient to be more active during the healing process than he could be if the disabled part were immobilized by traction. The use of a leg cast, for example, enables a patient to be ambulatory (and possibly weight-bearing) once the physician permits. While several types of casting materials are available, plaster of Paris is commonly used.

Plaster of Paris. Plaster of Paris (anhydrous calcium sulfate) is a chalky white powder made by a process which removes water from gypsum. In the process of making plaster of Paris, crystals of gypsum are broken up and reduced to powder form, and intense heat is applied to remove the water from the crystals. A chemical process of rehydration occurs when plaster of Paris is placed in water. The exothermic reaction which takes place during this recrystallization or "setting" period generates heat which can be felt in the newly applied cast. It is important that the heat generated in a newly applied cast be permitted to dissipate into circulating air. If the cast is covered with blankets or placed on a pillow or mattress during the period of most intense heat formation (e.g., the first 10–15 minutes following cast application), the patient could be burned, or (if the cast is large, e.g., a body cast) he could experience symptoms of heat prostration. The amount of heat given off by a setting cast is affected by factors such as the temperature of the water in which the plaster is immersed for rehydration and the amount of plaster used.

Plaster of Paris *bandages* come in individually wrapped, precut rolls of crinoline impregnated with plaster. The bandages are available in varying widths, e.g., from 2 inches to 8 inches. Plaster is available in various setting speeds, e.g., extra fast (2–4 minutes), fast (5–8 minutes), and slow (10–18 minutes). The strength of a completed cast is determined by the number of layers of plaster used. Commonly a cast consists of 5–7 layers of plaster bandage in unreinforced areas. Plaster of Paris *splints* of varying sizes are also available. Splints may be applied by themselves (and held in place with elastic or other bandages when dry), or they may be used to strengthen and reinforce areas of casts which require additional support, e.g., areas of stress, such as the axilla, groin, back of knee.

A plaster cast becomes firm (i.e. "sets") rapidly, but takes a while to actually dry. During the setting process, the plaster reacts with water, and long slender crystals develop which interlock through the layers of gauze. Movement during this setting process disrupts these formations and weakens the cast. A newly set plaster cast is called a "*green*" cast. In a green cast, excess unbound water accumulates in pockets in the crystalline lattice work. This water adds to the weight of the cast during the green stage. Eventually the unbound water evaporates, leaving a mature cast. A cast attains its full strength once evaporation occurs of all the water in the cast in excess of that water needed for crystallization. Within mature plaster are numerous pockets of air which (a) lighten the weight of the cast; (b) make the cast permeable; and (c) permit the skin to "breathe."[221]

Preparation For Casting. Prior to cast application, the procedure is explained to the patient, and the skin is prepared over the part of the body to be casted. If a fracture is to be reduced before the cast is applied, the patient may be given a narcotic; a general or local anesthetic may then be administered. *Skin preparation* may include cleansing with soap and water; gentle but thorough drying; application of alcohol; or dusting with a borate or stearate of zinc talcum powder. Some physicians recommend gently rubbing the skin with alcohol to increase skin tone. The skin is closely examined while it is prepared, and lesions, unremovable dirt, or foreign particles are noted and called to the physician's attention.

After the skin is prepared to receive the cast, it may be protectively covered with stockinette or padding. *Stockinette* is a soft knit material which is available in bias-cut (for circumferential wrapping) or tubular form (to completely encircle a body part, like a footless stocking, without seams). Stockinette comes in rolls of various widths, e.g., to cover an arm, leg, or body. Tubular stockinette is always cut longer than the expected finished cast length, so the excess portions can be pulled over the rough cast edges.

Before applying tubular stockinette, some physicians place one or two narrow strips of bandage or 3-inch strips of flannel lengthwise over the area to be casted. These strips are cut long enough that they extend well beyond the end of the finished cast. The strips may then be grasped at each end and pulled back and forth under the cast during the convalescent period to give the skin a gentle friction rub. (Caution the patient to keep the free ends outside the cast, so the strips do not become wadded up or "lost" inside the cast. Also tell the patient to move the strips gently so he does not traumatize underlying skin.)

Materials which may be used for *padding* under a cast include sheet wadding, Webril, sponge rubber, or felt. The skin may be treated with a liquid adhesive, e.g., tincture of benzoin, prior to the application of padding, or padding may be applied directly over the skin or over a covering of stockinette. When used, padding is commonly placed over bony prominences, and may be held in place with crepe paper bandage or narrow strips of adhesive to give better conformation to body structures.

> *When stockinette or padding is applied under a cast, it* must be smooth *on the skin before the plaster cast material is applied. Wrinkled or wadded material under a cast invites trouble, e.g., pressure areas and skin breakdown.*

Physicians vary in their usage of stockinette or padding under casts; some use more than others. In general, casts are not as heavily padded as they once were. While stockinette and padding does protect the skin, nerves, and blood vessels close to the surface of the body, it also tends to make a cast somewhat looser in its fit than if the cast were applied directly against the skin. Thus padding defeats the purpose of some casts. At times casts are applied directly against the skin (without underlying stockinette or padding) when the physician wants a cast to fit exceptionally close to the body surface.

If a plaster splint is to be applied without a cast, the extremity is usually covered with sheet wadding before the splint is placed, and external wrappings (e.g., with elastic bandage) are placed after the plaster begins to cool, e.g., 5–15 minutes following application.

Casting Equipment. A cast may be applied in a physician's office, clinic, emergency room, or at a patient's bedside. Portable carts ("*cast carts*") are usually available in hospitals and clinics. These carts contain equipment necessary for casting and are taken to wherever the patient is when the cast is to be applied. However, in a hospital the more common procedure is to take the patient to a specially equipped "*cast room*" for cast application.

Equipment which may be used during casting includes buckets; plaster of Paris splints and bandages; walking heels or irons; metallic splints; wooden sticks; stockinette, sponge rubber, sheet wadding, or Webril; a plaster knife; cast saw; bandage scissors; tape; lubricant; and plaster shears. Sterile dressings (for wounds) may also be needed.

Lining water buckets with plastic liners helps keep the buckets clean and makes it easier to dispose of plaster sediment in the water after the casting is completed. *Never empty plaster-laden water into an ordinary sink,* because the plaster sediment will solidify and plug the plumbing. If a sink with a plaster trap is not available, wait for sediment to settle into the bottom of the plastic-lined bucket, then carefully drain off the water from the top of the bucket while flushing the drain with large quantities of water. Throw the plastic bag, with its plaster sediment, into the garbage. The physician and persons helping him apply a cast need to be protectively covered so their clothing will not be soiled with plaster. If the patient is clothed, his clothing should also be covered.

Applying a Plaster Cast. One or two large buckets (containing tepid water) are necessary to saturate the plaster bandages and splints. Setting time is influenced by the type of plaster used and the temperature of the water used to soak the bandages. Warmer temperatures speed up the setting procedure, while colder water temperatures slow down setting time.

A nurse or technician assists the physician by submerging two rolls of plaster bandages vertically ("on end") in a bucket of water. Inserting a thumb under the loose end of a bandage before placing it in water makes it easier to grasp the free end when the wet bandage is ready for use. Once all air bubbles stop coming from the rolls, one roll of bandage is grasped in both hands (one hand over each end to prevent the escape of plaster from the ends) and is turned on its side and lifted above the water level. The hands are slightly squeezed or twisted in opposite directions, at the same time they are gently moved towards each other. These movements form a bulge in the center of the bandage and gently expell excess water. Then both hands are used to slightly flatten the roll. (Plaster bandages should not be forcefully "wrung out.") After 3–4 inches of the bandage are unrolled, it is handed to the physician when he is ready, and another roll is placed in the water bucket.

A roll of plaster bandage should be slightly sloppy wet when handed to the physician for use. Do not prepare several rolls of plaster ahead; instead pace the preparation of individual rolls to the physician's pace in applying the cast. Plaster of Paris bandages and splints may be ruined (and must be discarded) (a) if permitted to soak too long; (b) if prepared too far in advance of their use (they harden rapidly); or (c) if squeezed excessively dry.

As mentioned earlier, additional strength may be given to a cast by attaching splints or braces to the cast as it is being formed. Splints of various kinds are available (e.g., basswood or plaster of Paris splints), or reinforcements of steel or wire may be used. To remove excess water from plaster splints during their preparation, gently rub the splint along the rim of the cast bucket or draw the splint between the index and middle finger while exerting a slight squeezing pressure.

If a large cast is being applied, it may be necessary to change the water in the cast buckets if excessive sediment accumulates and begins to adhere to new rolls of plaster. Plaster residue in the dipping water (from previous use) causes the freshly dipped plaster to set too slowly and produces lamination and weakness of the cast.

During application of a cast, the physician positions the patient, and assistants help hold the patient in the desired position until the cast has started to set. It is important to hold the patient precisely as the doctor wishes so the casted structures will remain properly aligned. When supporting newly casted areas for the physician (while he works on other areas), hold the cast on open palms. Never grasp or pinch the wet cast with your fingertips because they will make indentations in the cast.

Throughout the casting procedure the physician works to apply a smooth, strong, correctly positioned cast. The cast is continuously rubbed with moderate pressure exerted by an open hand and molded during application, until the cast is completely set. Rubbing smooths the layers and edges of the plaster bandage together by spreading the plaster evenly throughout the layers of gauze. Like a sculptor, the physician molds the cast to bony prominences and other body contours. To function effectively and safely, the cast can be neither too loose nor too tight. Because the patient will live in the cast for some time, every effort is made to apply a cast which will be comfortable as well as therapeutic.

Because casting must be done in an uninterrupted, fairly rapid manner, it is easy for the patient to be overlooked while everyone concentrates on properly applying the cast. The nurse can be helpful during the casting process by periodically talking with the conscious patient and providing minor comforts, e.g., making certain the patient is not unnecessarily exposed and that he is kept as warm as possible. Reassurances that "all is going well" help to relax the patient. The nurse encourages the patient to relax and hold still during application of the cast. If the patient tenses his muscles the cast will not fit properly once he relaxes. The application of a large cast is especially fatiguing for the patient, and he may easily become tense and irritable. The patient should be informed that the heat he feels during the setting process of the cast is normal and will subside after 10–15 minutes.

If a leg cast is to be used for bearing the patient's weight during ambulation, it is fitted (during the green stage) with a *walking heel* or *walking iron* on the plantar surface (see Fig. 88–6). The "walker" bears the patient's weight and prevents wear on the bottom of the cast.

Early in the "green stage" of the cast the physician trims off excess plaster with a knife. Also, if the physician expects excessive swelling following application of the cast, he splits the completed cast longitudinally through all layers to relieve pressure which would otherwise dangerously accumulate within the confines of the cast (see below). As soon as casting is complete, the patient's skin is cleaned (e.g., with a weak solution of vinegar or damp sponge) to remove excess plaster while it is still damp. Unless removed, these pieces of plaster will dry and may fall under the cast and cause skin damage. Following application of a cast, an x-ray is commonly taken to ensure correct bone alignment. Subsequent x-rays are taken whenever a cast is removed or applied.

"Windowing" and Bivalving a Cast. Cutting "windows" in casts and bivalving casts are two techniques commonly used to relieve or prevent

excessive accumulations of pressure in casted body areas, or to permit access to or visualization of certain body areas. *Windows* may be cut (in dried casts) for any of the following reasons: (a) to prevent uncomfortable abdominal distention (e.g., in a body cast or hip spica); (b) to permit taking of the radial pulse (e.g., with an arm cast to check circulation in the involved arm); (c) to inspect areas of discomfort or areas in which tissue damage is suspected; or (d) to remove drains postoperatively or otherwise tend a surgical wound. (When a window is present observe the skin exposed for indications of complications, e.g., edema, discoloration).

Bivalving a cast means splitting it along both sides. A cast may be bivalved (a) to permit room for tissue swelling; (b) so half of it can be removed to facilitate giving care and during the taking of x-rays; (c) during the time a patient is learning to gradually adjust to being without a cast; or (d) to make a half-cast which can be used as an intermittent splint (e.g., to prevent deformities). Once a cast is bivalved, either half of it can be removed easily (without disturbing alignment) to inspect the body surface and give necessary care, e.g., the "top half" of the cast may be removed while the patient lies on his back and remains in the "bottom half" of the cast, and visa versa. The doctor may order both halves of the cast removed periodically, e.g., to permit exercising. When reapplying a bivalved cast, be certain to handle the patient carefully and take care not to pinch skin between the two cast halves. Once the halves of the cast are properly fitted on the patient, they are secured in place, e.g., with straps.

Types of Casts. The body and extremities can be casted in numerous different ways. In this section some of the more common types of casts are described and illustrated. A short arm cast, a long arm cast, and a hanging arm cast are illustrated in Figure 88-7, along with potential pressure points in a casted arm.

Short arm casts may be used in the treatment of stable fractures of the finger metacarpals, carpals, or distal radius and stable wrist sprains. *Finger splints* may be attached to short arm casts, extending from the plaster in the palm. Finger splints are used to stabilize ligamentous injuries of phalangeal and metacarpal phalangeal joints, phalangeal fractures, and unstable finger metacarpal fractures. A *long arm cast* may be used to treat stable injuries of the elbow joint; stable fractures of the distal humerus; fractures of one or both bones of the forearm; unstable ligamentous injuries of the wrist joint; and unstable fractures of the carpal bones.

The purpose of a *hanging arm cast* is for the weight of the hanging cast to exert gentle traction on the humerus while the patient is upright. To accomplish this, the patient should remain erect or semi-erect with the casted arm hanging in position at *all* times. This includes sleeping while sitting upright. A hanging arm cast may be used to treat some shoulder injuries, displaced fractures of the surgical neck of the humerus, or spiral or comminuted fractures of the humeral shaft. The joints above or below the fractured humerus are not immobilized with a hanging cast.

A *Velpeau dressing* is made of plaster bandage or cloth, and splints the arm to the chest (see Fig. 88-8). The elbow is flexed, the forearm is against the abdomen, and the forearm is supported in a sling type of support. Skin-to-skin contact must be avoided, e.g., between the trunk and arm, to prevent skin irritation and maceration. Because skin care is impossible under the dressing, the dressing needs to be changed frequently. Superficial skin irritation often occurs. The dressing is seldom left on continuously for longer than 3–4 weeks. The Velpeau dressing immobilizes the shoulder girdle (including the scapula, clavicle, and humerus and their mutual joints) and is used to treat ligamentous injuries to the shoulder joint or acromioclavicular joint, and fractures of the scapula, clavicle, or humerus.

Figure 88-9 illustrates a short leg cast, a long leg cast, and a long leg cylinder cast, as well as areas of the leg which are especially vulnerable to pressure when casted.

A *short leg cast* (SLC) may be either non-weight-bearing or weight-bearing. All toes should

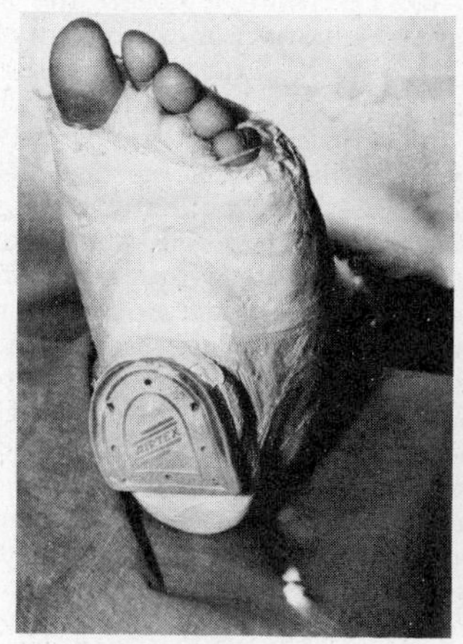

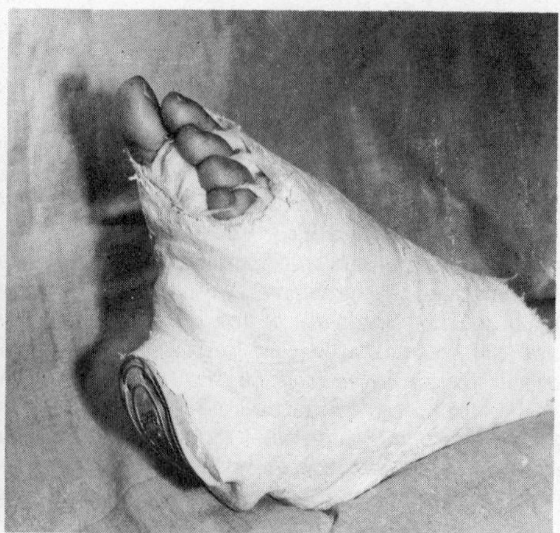

FIGURE 88-6. Plaster-of-Paris shoe with walking rubber heel. In this instance the cast was applied following surgery of the forefoot. (From Joplin, R. J.: *Surgical Clinics of North America 49*:861, 1969.)

be visible to check for complications and to permit movement. The knee joint is freely moveable. The ankle joint is at 90°, and the heel is neither inverted nor everted. Compression of the peroneal nerve may cause serious complications (e.g., foot drop) in any leg cast and must be prevented. If the cast is to be weight-bearing, a walking heel or iron is applied. An SLC may be used to treat stable ankle fractures and stable ligamentous ankle joint injuries; stable fractures of the metacarpals; fractures of the calcaneus, talus, navicular, cuboid, and cuneiforms; and subluxations and dislocations of the tarsal bones.

The *patellar tendon weight-bearing cast* is a special type of short leg weight-bearing cast which extends higher on the leg than the typical SLC. This cast is used to treat unstable fractures of the tibia and fibula.

A *long leg cast* (LLC) is similar to a short leg cast on the bottom but extends over the knee joint to terminate at the groin. If the LLC is to be weight-bearing, a walking heel or iron is incorporated into the cast. Long leg casts are used to treat stable injuries to the knee joint and distal femur and unstable fractures of the tibia, fibula, and ankle joint. A *long leg cylinder cast* (LLCC) is similar to an LLC except that the foot and ankle are not casted and the cast may not extend as high on the upper leg. The position of the knee is variable. This cast is used in the treatment of stable injuries of the distal femur, proximal tibia, or knee joint.

Two types of *body casts* are used: (1) Minerva jacket; and (2) body jacket. Body casts are used to immobilize the spine to relieve degenerative disorders and to promote healing of surgical spinal fusions and unstable spinal injuries. Body casts are sometimes fitted (then bivalved and removed when dry) several days before surgery. The cast is then sent to surgery so it can be reapplied when the operation is complete. This is easier than fitting the cast at the end of long, delicate surgery. Additionally, preoperative fitting makes it possible for the patient to identify areas of discomfort in advance of surgery, and these can be corrected.

A *Minerva jacket* covers the frontal and occipital regions of the skull and extends over the neck, chest, back, abdomen, and iliac crests. The face, ears, buttocks, pubic area, and extremities are exposed or they will develop pressure necrosis. With a *body jacket* the head, shoulders, and extremities are free, and the cast extends from the upper chest over the trunk to the pubis. The iliac crests are covered; the buttocks and perineal area are exposed. Some body jackets also include the thighs and pelvis (to more effectively reduce motion in the lumbar spine) or the cervical spine (to more completely immobilize the thoracic spine). Body casts may be used to immobilize the spine in a position of hyperextension to treat compression fractures. Body casts should not be applied too tightly because room must be provided for changes in the size of the chest cage (with breathing) and abdomen (with eating and abdominal distention).

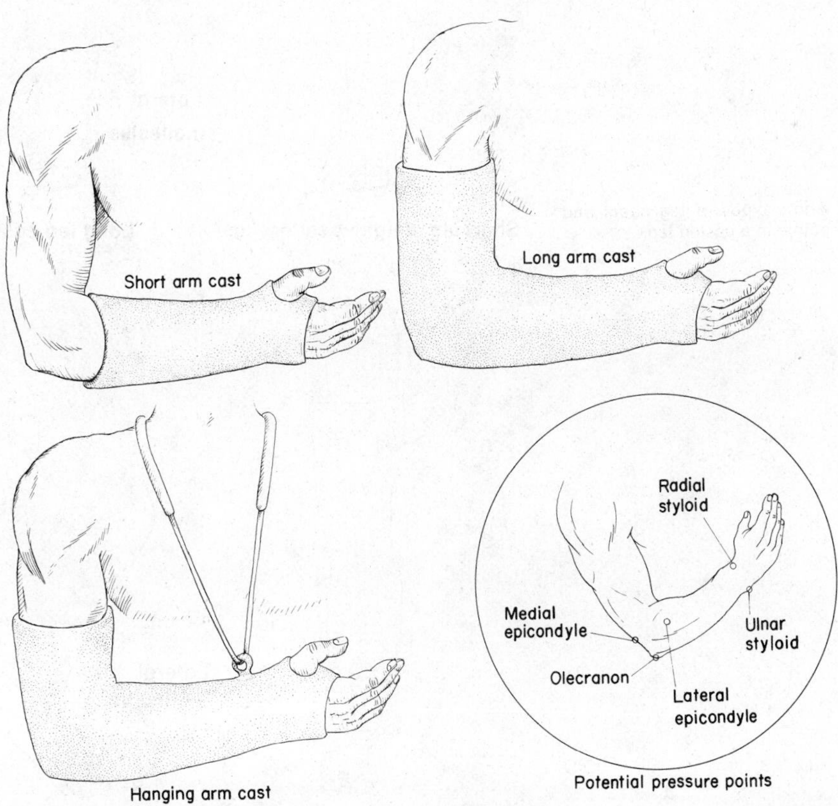

FIGURE 88–7. Some types of arm casts and potential pressure points in a casted arm.

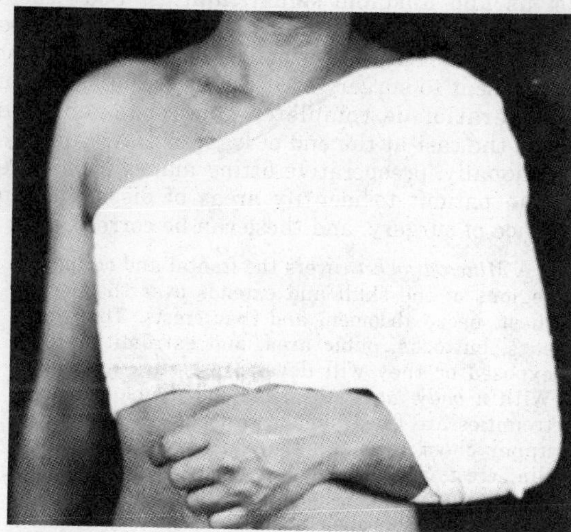

FIGURE 88–8. Velpeau dressing. Plaster-of-Paris is applied over the dressing for the treatment of some conditions. (From Gartland, J. J.: *Fundamentals of Orthopaedics*, 1965.)

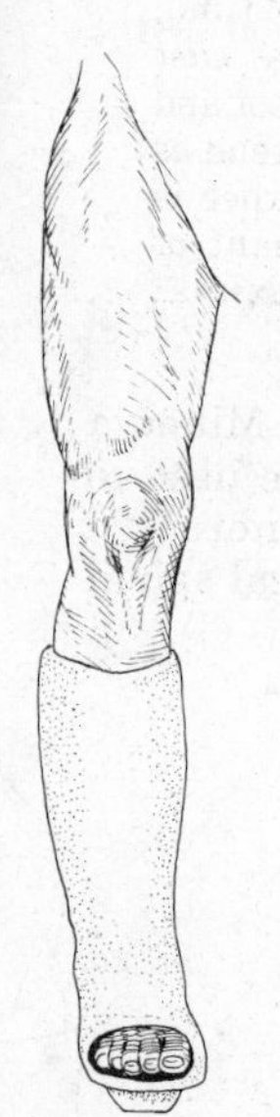

FIGURE 88–9. Some types of leg casts and potential pressure points in a casted leg.

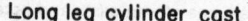

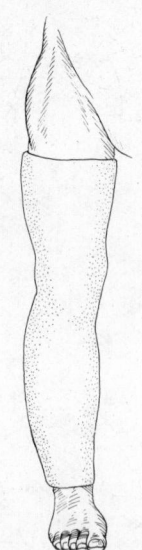

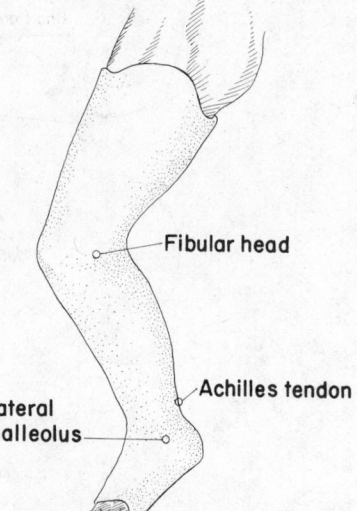

A *turnbuckle cast* is a special type of body cast most commonly used to correct abnormal lateral spinal curvatures, e.g., scoliosis. As Figure 88–10 demonstrates, a turnbuckle and hinges are incorporated into the cast. Periodically the physician makes adjustments on the turnbuckle which change the angle of the cast (and hence of the underlying spine). Even though adjustments of the turnbuckle are made gradually each day over a period of several days, each manipulation of the turnbuckle cast creates new pressure areas and thus requires meticulous, attentive nursing care directed at the prevention or early detection of cast complications. Care must be taken when moving the patient not to displace the turnbuckle apparatus. Also, *never* use the turnbuckle as a handle to lift or support the casted patient.

Spica casts may be applied to the hip, shoulder, or thumb joints. The word "spica" refers to a figure-eight or spiral, having turns that cross one another. With a spica cast, the casted appendage is immobilized to the main part of the body or extremity. To immobilize the affected joint, the bandages are applied in a spiral manner, e.g., around the thumb and the hand or an extremity and the trunk.

A *shoulder spica cast* (see Fig. 88–11) is a combination of a body jacket and long arm cast joined together. Indications for use of a shoulder spica include unstable fractures of the shoulder girdle and humerus; unstable elbow joint injuries; and dislocations of the shoulder girdle.

A *hip spica* extends from midtrunk (just below the nipple line) down the entire length of one leg on the affected side (often including the foot). It may or may not extend down to above the knee on the unaffected side. The cast has an opening around the buttocks and perineal region for purposes of elimination and cleanliness. Hip spica casts may be (a) single (includes trunk and one complete extremity); (b) one and one-half (includes trunk, one lower complete extremity, and the other lower extremity to the knee); or (c) double (includes trunk and both complete lower extremities, i.e., a body jacket and two long leg casts). Hip spica casts may be used to treat congenital dislocation of the hip or to immobilize reconstructive surgeries (e.g., following hip fusions or osteotomy of the knee) or injuries to the pelvis, hip joint, femur, or (sometimes) knee. Shoulder or hip spica casts may be reinforced by plastering a stick or bar (abduction bar) between the extended portion of the cast (e.g., leg or arm) and the main body of the cast (e.g., trunk). Never lift a spica cast by these reinforcing devices.

A *thumb spica* is a short (below the elbow) arm cast which includes the thumb. The spiral bandaging is between the thumb and hand. Only the tip of the thumb is exposed. Thumb spica casts are indicated in treatment of fractures of the carpal navicular, fractures of the thumb metacarpal and phalanges, and ligamentous thumb joint injuries.

Drying Casts. Casts take variable lengths of time to dry. While some casts dry completely in

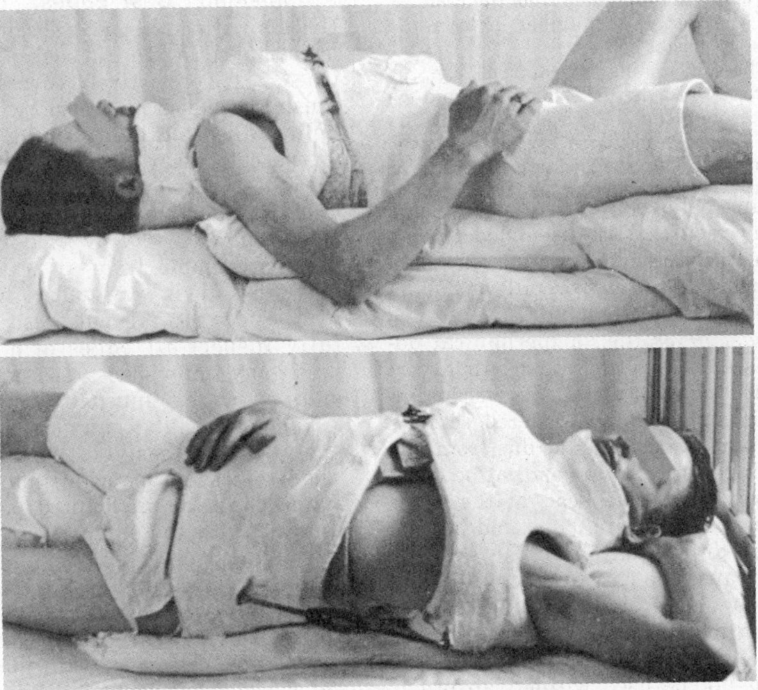

FIGURE 88–10. Turnbuckle cast used for forcible correction of scoliosis. The turnbuckle and hinges are incorporated into the plaster. Each time the turnbuckle is adjusted, new points of pressure tend to appear. Prevention of pressure areas and skin breakdown may be difficult. (From Larson, C. B., and Gould, M.: *Orthopedic Nursing.* 7th ed. St. Louis, The C. V. Mosby Company, 1970.)

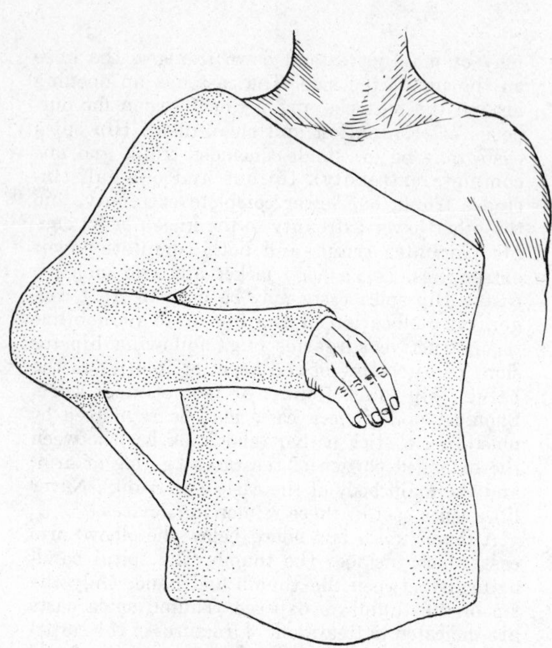

FIGURE 88–11. Shoulder spica cast.

only a few hours, others may take several days. Factors influencing drying time include:

> Type of material used for casting.
> Amount of water to be evaporated from the cast.
> Thickness of the cast, e.g., number of layers of plaster bandage, use of plaster splints.
> Condition of the surrounding environment, e.g., humidity, temperature, air circulation. A damp, humid environment delays drying. The circulation of warm, dry air around a cast enhances moisture evaporation from a wet cast and hence speeds up the drying process.

Many physicians believe that cast drying can best occur if the green cast is suspended from a frame (so air can freely circulate around the cast). Others prefer supporting the cast on pillows during the drying process.

Sometimes a *cast dryer* (i.e., a mechanical device which circulates heated air like a hair dryer) is used to promote drying of a cast, but more commonly the cast is simply left uncovered so it is exposed to room air. A cast should dry from the inside out. It is important that a cast not be dried out too quickly with excessive heat, or the inner portions of the cast may remain damp and become moldy. Also, rapid drying may burn the skin beneath the cast or cause the cast to crack. If a cast dryer is used, it should be placed about 18 inches away from the cast and moved frequently so the entire surface area of the cast is gradually dried. A cast dryer should not be used without an order. Hemorrhage may be caused by applying heat to a freshly operated area.[123] Never use a heat lamp to dry a cast.

Excessive heat or prolonged exposure to heat may cause skin to burn under a cast.

As mentioned earlier, heat is generated during the initial setting period of a cast (i.e., the period of recrystallization). This heat formation typically causes anxiety; however, the patient will be less anxious if he understands why heat is developing and if he is prepared to expect this "normal" reaction. If the patient with a large body cast or hip spica cast is acutely uncomfortable during this period, an ice bag may be applied to his head or a fan may be used to circulate air around his head. Do not direct the fan on the cast. In extremely warm weather the patient may be made more comfortable if given a cooling bath or if circulation of room air can be improved. It is necessary, however, to protect the patient from direct exposure to drafts.

During the green period of the cast (while the cast is still damp and water is evaporating from it), the patient may feel cold and chill easily. Be certain to provide adequate covering for him at this time, while leaving the casted area exposed. If a patient is in shock and has a large cast, it may be desirable to avoid excessive chilling by covering some portions of the cast and rotating the exposed portions during the drying process.

A dry cast is (a) odorless; (b) resonant when percussed; (c) white and somewhat shiny in appearance; and (d) feels similar to the surrounding room temperature. A cast which still retains moisture is (a) musty smelling; (b) dull on percussion; (c) gray and lusterless in appearance; and (d) feels cool to touch (except during the early period of intense heat formation).

"Finishing" Cast Edges. One of the first activities performed once a cast is completely dry is to make certain *all* edges of the cast are "finished," i.e., protectively covered. Some physicians finish the edges of a cast (while applying it) by pulling the stockinette lining out over the edges of the cast and securing the stockinette against the outer portion of the cast with plaster. *Unfinished, rough plaster edges may cause damage to surrounding skin by friction.* Also, as pieces of plaster crumble from an unfinished edge, they may work their way under the cast and produce skin lesions. To prevent these complications, carefully inspect *all* edges of a newly dried cast; finish any unfinished areas; and pad any finished areas which feel unusually rough or bumpy.

Cast edges also may be finished by placing "petals" of adhesive tape over the cast edges. These adhesive tape petals may be cut either oval-shaped or pointed. Pointed petals are applied to the cast with the single point on the outside and the double points on the underside of the cast. When applying petals make certain the tape inside the cast is secured to the cast lining and not the patient's skin. The application of adhesive tape to the skin can cause skin maceration. Press the outer edges of the tape firmly against the cast. You may moisten a strip of plaster of Paris and secure it over the outer edges of the adhesive tape to prevent the edges from rolling.

The edges of a leg cast are particularly likely to cause skin irritation (e.g., at the top of a long leg cast or at the ankle of a cylindrical cast). These edges may be covered with moleskin to make a soft edge.

With body casts, hip spica casts, or long leg casts, it is necessary to protectively cover those areas of the cast near the buttocks and perineal region to prevent dampness and soilage. Waterproof material (e.g., 4-inch strips of thin plastic material) can be *smoothly* placed under the cast edges and taped to the exterior surface of a dry cast. The material must be smoothly applied because wrinkles will promote pressure damage of the skin. Some sources recommend waterproofing the cast by painting it (when thoroughly dry) with shellac, varnish, white lacquer, or cellulose acetate, or by applying a plastic spray. When painting or spraying a cast, be certain to protectively cover exposed body surfaces, e.g. perineal areas, with a towel. *The entire surface of a cast should not be coated with an air-impervious substance* or the skin beneath cannot properly "breathe" and may macerate. Remember that the porous nature of plaster permits the evaporation of moisture from the skin.

Change and reinforce bindings on the cast edges as indicated to protect the patient and maintain a strong cast. Change protective plastic or respray or repaint the cast with waterproofing substances as necessary to maintain cleanliness.

Skin and Cast Care. Skin care (e.g., washing and drying the skin, applying emollient lotions, inspecting the skin, turning the patient frequently) is an extremely important part of caring for any patient wearing a cast. The nurse not only *provides* skin care but also *teaches* the patient how to care for his skin (if he is able) and tells him ways to avoid skin damage. Areas of skin subjected to irritation or pressure can easily develop into decubitus ulcers and therefore require prompt, special attention. Notify the physician of the development of areas of skin irritation or pressure. (For a discussion of the effects of immobility on the skin and related area, see Unit V, Ch. 27.)

It is essential that the buttocks be adequately exposed with a hip spica or body cast so the patient will not become soiled or damp while using the bedpan, and so that adequate skin care can be given. Damp, soiled casts become malodorous and may mold or break. Dampness also causes skin irritation.

Frequently inspect *all* exposed areas of skin, especially around the edges of the cast, and all body pressure areas, e.g., back of the head, ears, elbows, iliac crests, sacrum, heels. Look for friction rubs, swelling, and discoloration, e.g., redness, blanching, cyanosis. A mirror can be used to look inside the cast as far as possible. When using a mirror, pull the skin taut away from the cast and shine a light down inside the cast. Teach the patient how to inspect his skin and the importance of these observations.

Each time the patient is turned, make certain to (a) brush away loose pieces of plaster; (b) inspect the exposed skin on which the patient has been lying; (c) give appropriate skin care to those areas; (d) smooth out linens on which the patient will be lying; and (e) inspect exposed cast edges. When giving skin care, dip your fingers in alcohol and reach up under the edges of the cast as far as you can. While inspecting the cast edges (for rough places or plaster breakdown), reach up under the edges of the cast as far as you can and remove plaster crumbs.

> *It is not safe to insert any foreign object under a cast or to scratch the skin under a cast.*

Instruct the patient not to poke *any* objects under his cast and not to try to scratch vigorously under the cast. Rigid objects placed under a cast create pressure areas and therefore predispose to skin breakdown, infection, and decubitus ulcer formation. Children are particularly likely to poke objects (e.g., coins, buttons, toothbrushes, small toys) under their casts. Often itching under a cast is extremely uncomfortable (especially in hot weather), and a patient is tempted to slip a knitting needle, wooden back scratcher, pencil, or some other object under the cast to scratch his skin. Explain to the patient that scratching under a cast is prohibited because (a) the skin may be broken and infection develop; (b) the scratching movements disturb the smooth padded surface under the cast and make wrinkles that may contribute to skin breakdown; and (c) the "scratcher" may become lost under the cast and cause pressure and skin breakdown. Also, explain that scratching the skin when it itches usually provides only temporary relief and often causes itching and discomfort to worsen. *If a foreign object becomes caught under the surface of a cast, the physician should be immediately notified.*

Tell the patient not to pull stockinette or padding out of his cast. Explain that these materials are placed under the cast to protect the skin and that their removal not only exposes the skin to the plaster surface but also loosens the cast. Petaling a cast or fixing the turned-back stockinette to the outside of the cast helps secure the inner lining and padding.

Keep the fingers or toes (and their nails) clean in a casted extremity. This can most easily be accomplished by using an applicator dipped in alcohol. Cleanliness is not only refreshing to the patient but also permits better visualization of the toes and fingers and removes potentially infectious materials. To prevent drying and scaling of the fingers or toes on a casted extremity, they should be bathed, covered lightly with oil, and massaged at least daily.

It is important to maintain in good condition the skin of *uncasted* body areas as well as those regions which are casted. As a patient pushes himself about in bed, he may irritate the skin on exposed elbows and heels. These and other exposed pressure areas should be inspected regularly for indications of skin breakdown and appropriate skin care should be frequently given. Powdering the skin is generally not advisable, since powder tends to cake and produce skin irritation.

While giving skin care, *inspect the condition of the cast* and *check its fit*. Excessively loose casts may need replacing. Sometimes casts are somewhat loose in the morning but fit more securely later in the day, e.g. after a casted leg has been dependent during ambulation. Call to the physician's attention areas of a cast which are deteriorated, cracked, molding, soft, or broken. Loose bracing bars should also be reported. The physician may reinforce weakened or soiled areas of the cast by applying fresh plaster at the bedside.

Positioning the Patient. A patient with a cast can easily become off balance and fall off a stretcher. When a casted patient is being transported on a stretcher, make certain he is secured to the cart with safety straps. Supervise transfer procedures, e.g., from stretcher to cart, to make certain the transfer team exercises care when moving a newly casted patient. Post a sign on the patient's bed stating that he has a damp cast and must be handled and positioned cautiously. Once the patient is in bed, make sure he is positioned in correct alignment.

Handle a damp cast carefully so that you do not accidentally make finger or thumb impressions in the cast. Lift the cast by cupping your hands and sliding them, palms up, under the cast rather than by grasping the cast with a pinching motion. Unwanted indentations in a cast can cause pressure and decubitus formation on the underlying skin once the cast dries.

A casted extremity should be elevated to minimize swelling. Elevation of a casted limb is especially important for the first 24–48 hours after casting.

By promoting drainage, elevation of a dependent part stimulates circulation and reduces edema (and thus pressure within the cast). Elevation of casted extremities often may be done with pillows, but sometimes ropes, weights and pulleys, or slings are used. Placing the newly casted area on pillows also protects the cast from pressure and flattening while drying. Support a damp cast on pillows which have rubber or plastic undercovers. A cast should not rest on a hard surface while drying, or continuous pressure will cause it to adapt itself to the contour of the surface, e.g., become flattened. Once a cast is completely dry, it can safely be placed on a hard surface if the patient so desires (e.g., a casted arm may rest on a table), but generally it is still most comfortable if the casted area rests on pillows.

Place supportive pillows along the entire length of a casted area. This is of special importance while the cast is drying. To prepare a bed to receive a patient with a green body cast, place three pillows crosswise on the bed. Make certain the pillows are placed side by side touching each other so that no spaces occur between them; i.e., make certain the cast is completely supported so areas of weakness will not develop during the drying period. To prepare a bed for a patient with a wet hip spica cast, place one pillow crosswise at the waist and two pillows lengthwise under the casted leg. If both legs are casted, use two pillows for each leg. It is generally desirable to place a small pillow or folded flannelette sheet under areas such as the popliteal space or lumbar region to maintain the desired body contour of the cast. Be careful that excessive pressure is not applied over bony prominences and weight-bearing areas, e.g., shoulders, buttocks, hips, heels, during the drying process.

Place pillows in such a way that they help the patient to feel "securely" rather than "precariously" positioned. To prevent a casted limb from rolling off a pillow, e.g., while the patient is up in a wheelchair, it is generally wise to secure the limb to the pillow, e.g., by pinning a towel across the limb and onto the pillow, or by placing a tie around the limb and pillow. If a casted extremity falls off a pillow, it not only may cause unnecessary pain, but also may break the cast. A damp cast may be moved by pulling gently on the pillows on which the cast rests, with the cast lightly supported while being moved.

Firm orthopedic mattresses or mattresses with fracture boards beneath them are generally used for persons wearing casts. A sagging mattress will tend to deform a green cast and may crack a dry cast.

A patient with a hip spica or body cast must be carefully positioned on the bedpan in such a manner that he is not uncomfortable and so that soilage of the cast will not occur during elimination. With the patient turned onto his unaffected side, place a pad or small plastic-covered pillow just behind the bedpan and place a pillow under the patient's back and shoulders so his upper body will be level with or slightly higher than his hips and the bedpan. *Slightly* raise the head of the bed (to prevent expelled fluids from running up under the back of the cast), but do not raise the head of the bed so far that the front edge of the cast causes abdominal discomfort. Elevation of the head and shoulders to use the bedpan is generally permissible unless the patient is in shock or is hemorrhaging, or has a spinal injury. When the patient is finished using the pan, remove it carefully to avoid spillage and gently but thoroughly cleanse the perineal region and buttocks.

If a body or spica cast is still green, do not place pillows under the shoulders and head, because the pillows push the patient forward against the front of the cast, deforming the cast and producing pressure on the chest and abdomen. When a patient uses the bedpan and he has a hip spica cast (body cast or long leg cast) which is still green, the head of the bed may be elevated on shock blocks rather than raising just the top half of the bed by elevating the headrest.

A casted leg should not remain dependent. Keep the leg elevated to the level of the body to avoid swelling. If swelling is already present, it is necessary to elevate the leg higher than the heart, e.g., the foot higher than the knee, the knee higher than the hip to reduce swelling. To avoid placing excessive pressure on the back of the heel, a patient with a leg cast should be positioned with his foot extending over the edge of the pillow. To prevent foot drop, make certain the plantar surface of an uncasted foot has adequate support while the patient is supine. Protect the toes of a casted foot from pressure caused by bed clothing when the patient is supine. Also, prevent outward rotation of the casted leg. Correct body alignment must be maintained. When a patient with a leg cast (or hip spica cast) is lying prone, he should have a pillow beneath the casted leg under the dorsum of the foot to prevent pressure on his toes. An alternative method of preventing pressure on the toes is to position the prone patient with his foot over the end of the mattress.

Turning the Patient. Unless it is contraindicated, the patient with a green cast is turned periodically so that more of the casted area is exposed to air during the drying process. The physician may specify when a patient can first be turned and how often he should subsequently be turned. When a large cast has been applied (e.g., body cast), the physician may specify that the patient is not to be turned until the evening of the day the cast was applied. Thereafter the turning orders may specify that the patient is to be turned from front to back and vice versa every two hours. Position changes are important during the drying period not only to promote drying but also to prevent pressure damage in structures immobilized in the cast. However, if a patient is turned too soon, a wet cast may be bent or otherwise damaged.

Turning is made easier (for patient and staff members) if the patient was given turning instructions and was able to practice turning with help *prior to* application of the cast. This patient teaching should be given again when the patient is first turned in his cast. Frequent position changes are essential while a patient is in bed to prevent complications of immobility (see Unit V, Ch. 27).

Plaster casts are heavy and inflexible. Thus, they not only may limit a patient's activities but also may cause serious accidents. A patient wearing a cast is naturally more clumsy than he would normally be, and, therefore, more susceptible to accidents, e.g., falls. Keep the patient's environment as safe as possible, e.g., keep bed wheels locked so the patient will not slip and fall as he gets out of bed. Straps are placed around a bivalved cast, when the patient is being turned, to secure the two sides of the cast together.

Have adequate help to move and position the casted patient. Do not attempt to turn a patient with a heavy cast by yourself. *Always* have at least one other person to help you, and always have someone on each side of the bed. Three or four persons may be needed to turn a patient in a body or hip spica cast. Wet casts are particularly heavy.

The weight of a cast may throw a patient off balance as he turns over in bed or starts to sit up; therefore side rails should be kept up. Side rails can also help the patient to turn and move about in bed more easily by giving him something to grasp. An overhead frame with a trapeze bar often helps a casted patient to be more active and self-sufficient. For example, the patient with a large cast may be able to lift his body up (by grasping the trapeze bar) so the bedpan can be slid under him more comfortably or so that skin care can be given or bed linens smoothed out or changed. Use of a trapeze also helps prevent the patient from chafing the skin on his elbows as he tries to push himself about in bed.

> Never *use cast braces or turnbuckles to lift a casted patient. These devices are not placed in casts to serve as handles. They may easily be broken, dislocated, or pulled out of casts.*

Never lift hip spica casts by the ankle, foot, or abduction bar (between the legs). This is true not only while the cast is damp but also when it is dry. *To correctly turn a patient in a hip spica cast,* do as follows. Move the patient to the side of the bed. Slide him on the bed or on pillows toward the side of his fractured or operated limb. Move the patient by slipping your hands beneath his buttocks and pulling him toward you. At the same time, have another person slide and support the patient's shoulders and head, while a third person does the same with the legs. (All upper bedlinens should be fanfolded to the foot of the bed and the patient protectively draped. If a head pillow is present, it should be removed before turning the patient.) While the patient is on one side of the bed, prepare the unoccupied side to receive him, e.g., smooth or change sheets and place pillows. When he is ready to be turned, the patient places his arms at his sides or over his head. The arms should *never* be placed over the head if the patient has a dorsal or cervical spinal injury. If the patient keeps his arms at his sides when being turned, place a folded towel between his arm and the cast (on the side toward which he will be turned) so his arm will not be pinched when the weight of the cast rolls over it. Then roll the patient onto the freshly prepared pillows and pull him back to the center of the bed. The patient rolls on his uninvolved side. During the turning process the casted limb is supported in the air.

> *As a general rule, always turn a casted patient away from his injured or operated side, i.e., keep weight off the fractured or operated side.*

The turning process should occur with one smooth movement, rather than in jerky, piecemeal movements, and the patient should feel securely supported. When turning a patient with a hip spica, be certain to support the casted limb inside the thigh and at the knee and ankle. Provide adequate support along the entire length of a cast so excessive strain does not occur on the casted area. Always support the areas of greatest strain, e.g., joints. Once the patient is turned, position him comfortably in good body alignment and place pillows along the length of the cast to provide support.

Weight-bearing and Ambulation. Extremity casts set rapidly, in 10 minutes, but may not be completely dry for two days. Weight-bearing is typically not permitted for at least 24 hours after application of the cast. Pain may be experienced when a casted leg is lowered into a dependent position for the first few times, e.g., when the patient first begins to stand up and walk. Prepare the patient for this. Explain that the pain is not unusual and that it results from blood rushing into the leg as the leg is lowered. Lower the leg for only short periods of time at first and then gradually lengthen the periods of dependency. Once the leg becomes accustomed to complete circulation the pain subsides. Also, tell the patient that his cast will feel very heavy at first, but that he will adjust to this added weight. Weak, aged, and debilitated patients often find the weight of a cast to be extremely fatiguing and may tire rapidly when up for the first few times. Observe such patients closely and avoid excessive fatigue and accidents.

If a patient has a walking cast, he should keep his leg elevated when not ambulatory. The leg may not swell while the patient is walking because intermittent weight-bearing that occurs with walking acts as a pump, circulating the blood and forcing venous return. However, once the patient stops walking and stands still, or sits down with his leg dependent, it will swell.[123]

A casted arm should be kept elevated when the patient is out of bed. Most commonly this elevation is achieved by placing the arm in a *sling*. Remember the following points: (a) support the entire arm, including the elbow, wrist and hand (permitting wrist drop encourages neurovascular complications); (b) when the arm rests in the sling, the fingers should be higher than the elbow (to minimize edema); (c) secure the sling at the back of the neck with two pins (do not tie a knot over the cervical vertebrae; do not place pins over the cervical vertebrae; use two pins to ensure secure fastening of the sling); and (d) secure the elbow flap with pins so the elbow is well supported and the arm will not slip out of the sling. Periodically inspect and readjust the sling so it is comfortable and correctly positioned. Placement of a pad at the back of the neck between the sling and the skin may prevent skin irritation and pressure.

If a sling is awkward while the patient is sitting up, the arm may be elevated on a pillow. To prevent the arm from falling off the pillow place a tie around both arm and pillow. Precautions such as these take but a moment to observe and may spare the patient further pain and injury. Also, they contribute to the patient's feelings of security and thereby promote mental relaxation (an important component in the recovery process).

Remember to properly position and support *uncasted* extremities so they will remain in good condition. For example, an uninvolved leg should be kept in correct alignment (to prevent foot drop, external rotation of the leg, and hyperextension of the knee) and exercised prophylactically (to maintain muscle tone and to prevent stiffness of joints and development of contractures).

Exercises. Exercising is important while a patient is in a cast. Appropriate exercises help prevent complications during periods of immobility, enhance healing, and facilitate the rehabilitation process following cast removal. Typically the patient is taught to *exercise the joints above and below the cast.* Thus the patient in a long arm cast is usually advised to exercise his shoulder, thumb, and fingers. With a casted arm it is generally important to exercise the shoulder (if it is outside the cast) because (a) the shoulder joint can rapidly become stiff or "frozen"; and (b) the shoulder must support the weight of the cast. Often there is a tendency to hold the shoulder immobile on the affected side even though it is not casted. Teach the patient to periodically lift the casted arm up over his head. Also, teach the patient with an arm cast to frequently move each finger.

A patient with injury to the shoulder or humerus should *not* exercise the involved arm or shoulder unless specifically directed to do so by his doctor. Shoulder motion should be limited with a hanging arm cast. Maintain the hanging position of this cast at all times.

The patient in a long leg cast should exercise his hip joint and toes. Exercising toes and fingers stimulates circulation and increases venous return.

Isometric exercises (isometric muscle contractions) of the muscles immobilized by the cast usually are not routinely performed without the physician's approval. However, when the physician permits, the patient learns isometric exercises and may be advised to practice them at least hourly while awake.[221] Explain that these exercises do not actually cause the limb to move or joints to bend, but they cause muscles to contract.

Teach the patient isometric exercises first on the unaffected limbs. Ask the patient to observe how the exercises contract the muscles without moving the limb. The patient with a casted knee may be taught to try to push down with his knee inside the cast. This exercise (quadriceps setting) tightens the leg muscles. It may be helpful, when teaching the patient this exercise, if you place your hand beneath the knee and instruct the patient to try to push his knee down onto your hand. In a casted arm, opening and closing the hand (to make a fist) provides isometric exercising of the arm muscles.

Isometric muscle exercises help to maintain

muscle strength and muscle mass. Thus they combat the weakness and disuse atrophy which tend to develop in unused muscles. All forms of exercising help a patient to retain command of his muscles, i.e., help him remember how to send nerve impulse messages through the central nervous system to control movements.

The patient confined to bed may be taught other exercises to prevent complications and to prepare him for future activities, e.g., crutch walking. These exercises may include gluteal setting, abdominal tightening, and deep breathing.

To maintain the muscle tone and mobility of uncasted structures, the unaffected joints should be put through their full range of motion several times daily. Uncasted structures often have to perform "extra duties" to relieve casted areas, and therefore they should be maintained in optimum condition. Encourage the patient to actively exercise by himself. Participation in self-care activities indirectly provides additional exercise for a patient.

Complications. A patient wearing a cast requires professional observation and care, particularly for the first day or two following cast application. A cast does not surround a patient in a haven of protective safety. Although a cast may provide protective and therapeutic functions, it may also create and then hide from view serious complications. Complications in a casted part may be caused by such factors as (a) swelling of the casted part; (b) application of a cast that is too tight; (c) indentations in the plaster; (d) wrinkles in underlying padding; (e) foreign objects pushed under the cast; (f) vascular or nerve damage sustained during injury or treatment, e.g., surgery, fracture reduction, or the formation of vascular emboli or thrombi.

Pressure upon casted structures can cause irreparable damage to skin, muscles, blood vessels, or nerves. Because a cast is inflexible, it makes certain movements impossible and can dangerously cause pressure on and constriction of underlying structures. Serious complications can develop quite rapidly in a casted limb. As a result of the development of complications, a limb may be paralyzed or anesthetized for life. Loss of blood supply or innervation jeopardizes a limb, and in some instances amputation of the limb is necessary. The development of "cast syndrome" (see below) in a patient with a body cast can be fatal if untreated.

Below are summarized some of the complications most frequently seen in a casted patient, and the symptoms indicative of these complications. These symptoms and their detection and evaluation are discussed further in following paragraphs.

1. *Impaired blood flow* producing soft tissue ischemia, e.g., due to pressure in casted extremity. Possible symptoms include:

Pulselessness in extremity
Inadequate capillary refill in nail beds
Pallor, blanching, or cyanosis of skin
Pain of various types
Coldness of skin
Swelling; painful edema peripheral to cast
Paresthesias
Hypesthesia
Anesthesia (numbness)
Motor paralysis of previously functioning member

2. *Nerve damage,* e.g., due to pressure on a nerve as it passes over a bony prominence. Possible symptoms include:

Pain, increasing, persistent, and localized
Hypesthesia
Anesthesia (numbness)
Feelings of deep pressure
Paresthesias
Motor weakness or paralysis not previously present

3. *Infection, tissue necrosis,* e.g., due to skin breakdown. Possible symptoms include:

Musty, unpleasant odor over cast and/or at ends of cast
Drainage through cast or cast opening
Sudden unexplained body temperature elevation
"Hot spot" felt on cast over lesion

4. *"Cast syndrome,"* occurs with body casts. Possible symptoms include:

Prolonged nausea
Repeated vomiting
Abdominal distention
Vague abdominal pain

Constriction of a casted limb may result (a) from application of a cast that is too tight; (b) from swelling of the limb after a properly fitting cast has been applied; or (c) from blood-saturated dressings under the plaster which will not expand if underlying tissue swells. Constriction of the limb may reduce or prevent arterial and venous circulation. *Gangrene* may develop in an ischemic limb which has inadequate arterial blood flow. *Swelling* and *vascular engorgement* typically develop in a limb in which venous return is impaired but the arterial blood flow continues. Blood flow may also be obstructed by the presence of an embolus or thrombus within a blood vessel (e.g., from thrombophlebitis or fat embolism).

A limb may have its arterial blood flow completely interrupted for 2–4 hours without residual effects.[221] Therefore, with early treatment, circulatory embarrassment to a limb need not cause irreversible damage. However, *early* recognition and treatment are essential.

Volkmann's ischemic contracture (discussed earlier in this chapter) is a permanent deformity which can develop in a casted arm unless vigilant preventative care is given. Indications of developing Volkmann's contracture include diminished or absent radial pulse; swelling of the hand and fingers; and bluish discoloration of the hand, fingers, and fingernails. Observe a patient with a casted arm closely for these symptoms and report them immediately if they begin to develop so the cast can be cut and blood flow can be restored to the ischemic tissues before irreparable damage occurs.

A cast can cause *nerve damage* by compressing a superficial peripheral nerve (e.g., the common peroneal nerve in the region of the knee) against underlying bone (e.g., the neck of the fibula). Nerve damage disrupts the transmission of nerve impulse messages back and forth through the nerve. As a result, structures distal to the damage are not adequately innervated, and their function is impaired, i.e., they develop *anesthesia* and *paralysis.* For example, destruction of the common peroneal nerve (located on the lateral side of the leg below the head of the fibula) causes loss of sensation on the foot's dorsolateral aspect and paralysis (loss of ability to extend the toes or dorsiflex the foot, i.e., "foot drop"). While nerve damage is sometimes reversible (incomplete), in other cases the damage is irreversible. Irreversible paralysis may develop within 24 hours.

Bony prominences are subcutaneous and have only minimal protection from overlying soft tissues. Pressure from a cast over these prominences produces localized *tissue ischemia* by compressing the skin and subcutaneous tissue (with their local veins and arterioles) against the bone. If this pressure continues, the ischemic tissue eventually breaks down and becomes necrotic, i.e., a *decubitus ulcer* (pressure sore) develops. While pressure areas may be painful initially, the pain subsides once death of the tissue devitalizes the nerves in the region. Areas of skin slough, thus become anesthetic (i.e., without pain or other sensations) soon after the local sensory nerve endings are destroyed. Pain may last only a few days. While it is present the pain is typically of a localized burning nature. *Remember:* cessation of pain does not mean "all is well." Instead it often means that a lesion has developed which is anesthetized but worsening.

> *Cast-related complications (e.g., paralysis, pressure sores, and the results of ischemia) are all* preventable. *The nurse plays an important role in the prevention of these disabling disorders.*

Because the nurse is most commonly the professional person who is with a newly casted patient, it is her responsibility to observe the patient closely and report early indications of complications at once. Immediately following casting, a patient should be evaluated for indications of cast complications every 10–15 minutes for the first four hours. If no abnormalities are present, the observations may be made at 30-minute intervals for the following 4 hours, and then every hour for the next 4 hours. If all is well at the end of this time, the observations may be made once during each shift.

Evaluate the patient's general condition. Report nausea, chills, vomiting, rash, and fever. These symptoms may indicate complications under the plaster. If the patient has been given an anesthetic or has had surgery, give appropriate postanesthesia and postoperative care (see Unit VI, and the last section of this chapter). Watch for symptoms of delayed shock, e.g., sudden weakness, faintness, pallor, dizziness, diaphoresis, alterations in pulse and blood pressure (see Unit V, Ch. 26).

Observe the patient closely for indications of complications caused by nerve compression, circulatory impairment, or skin damage. Paralysis and skin necrosis may develop within the first 24 hours. Make frequent observations of parts distal to the cast, e.g., toes and fingers. A patient wearing a cast which positions a limb in acute flexion (e.g., to treat a fractured elbow) is particularly likely to develop circulatory impairment and must therefore be observed especially closely.

> *Evaluation of a casted patient for indications of cast-related complications should be conducted in a planned, orderly manner so that significant findings are not missed.*

Establish a pattern for your observations and always carry observations out sequentially. For example, in a casted extremity evaluate (1) skin color; (2) skin temperature; (3) vascular return; (4) sensation; (5) swelling; and (6) active motion. One helpful way of remembering some of the significant symptoms of cast-related complications is the mnemonic of *the "5 P's":* (1) *P*ain; (2) *P*allor; (3) *P*ulselessness; (4) *P*aresthesia; and (5) *P*aralysis.

The nurse uses her senses of touch, sight, smell, and hearing to evaluate a patient with a cast. The observations made should be explained to the patient. Patients who are sent home with casts must be taught how to make routine observations for developing complications. They should be instructed to contact their physician immediately if untoward symptoms begin to develop.

A. *Tactile observations:* Feel the *temperature of the skin* in areas distal to a cast, e.g., hand, foot, fingers, toes. Compare the patient's skin temperature on his casted side with the other side of his body. Abnormal skin temperatures should be immediately reported. Remember that ice bags applied to the sides of the cast will contribute to coolness in the casted limb. Arterial insufficiency causes coolness (and pallor) in exposed fingers and toes.

Check *peripheral pulses* and compare the pulse in the casted arm with that in the opposite normal limb. Impaired arterial blood flow to a limb causes loss of the peripheral pulses. Check the radial pulse at the wrist (of a casted arm) or the dorsalis pedis pulse on the dorsum of the foot (of a casted leg). Casts may be windowed over these areas to permit palpation of the pulse. Notify the doctor at once of pulselessness.

Evaluate the patient's awareness of *pinpricks* and *light touch.* Hypesthesia (hypoesthesia) and anesthesia are indications of serious damage to the limb. "Hypesthesia" means an abnormally reduced sensitiveness of the skin; "anesthesia" refers to total loss of feeling or sensation.

Have the patient shut his eyes while you touch each finger or toe on a casted extremity. Ask him to tell you when he can feel the touch and have him identify which finger or toe he thinks you are touching. With a pin, gently touch the surface of the skin to identify areas of numbness. Specifically search for indications of damage to the peroneal nerve (in a casted leg) and the median, ulnar, and radial nerves (in a casted arm).

> *Peroneal nerve:* check for sensation in the web space dorsally between the great and second toes. Report loss of sensation immediately. As stated previously, peroneal nerve damage can result in foot drop.

> *Median, ulnar, and radial nerves:* check volar surface of index finger for innervation by the median nerve; test volar surface of little finger for ulnar innervation, and dorsal surface of web space between thumb and index finger for radial innervation.

When evaluating sensory losses, review the chart to see if these losses were present before the cast was applied.

Feel the *surface* of the cast. Place the palm of your hand on the cast and move it over the entire surface of the cast. This inspection is made to identify areas of the cast which feel appreciably warmer than other areas, i.e., "hot spots." Often areas of tissue necrosis or infection will cause the overlying area of cast to feel warmer. Evaluate with particular care the cast sections which are over pressure points.

B. *Visual observations:* Note the *color of the skin* distal to the cast. Observe for indications of circulatory impairment, e.g., pallor, blanching, cyanosis. Compare the skin color around casted areas with skin color in other parts of the body. Compare the color of the skin in the casted extremity with the opposite extremity (when held in the same position). Cyanosis results from impaired venous return (e.g., due to soft tissue constriction) and may be a late indication of impaired circulation. Increasing cyanosis, accompanied by persistent pain or paresthesias, requires immediate relief. Pallor or blanching may indicate arterial insufficiency, e.g., due to thrombosis or vasospasm. Freshly oxygenated blood is not reaching the part when arterial blood flow is impaired.

> The *blanching test* is a useful measurement of circulatory effectiveness of particular importance in evaluating a patient with an extremity cast. The test evaluates capillary refill in the nailbed of a casted limb. With your thumbnail briefly (and gently) compress the nail of the patient's thumb (on a casted arm) or the great toe (on a casted leg). You will be able to see color leave the compressed area. Then quickly release the pressure and observe the speed with which color returns to the blanched area (as the capillaries, which had blood squeezed out of them, refill with blood). Compare the capillary refilling on the casted limb with the patient's unaffected side. If color returns too rapidly, it may indicate venous congestion. Sluggish return of color may be indicative of circulatory obstruction producing arterial insufficiency.[123] However, it is possible for capillary refill to be relatively normal in the nailbeds even though a limb is pulseless.

Ask the patient to *move his fingers or toes* on the casted limb. Movement should typically be easy and painless, unless the patient has an injury to the hand or foot which restricts motion. Motor paralysis of the fingers or toes may be present owing to primary nerve damage, or the patient may be unable to move because of pain. Painful motion usually indicates an excessive degree of swelling and should be reported. Even gentle passive motion of the fingers or toes of an ischemic limb produces extreme pain. Extension of the digits is especially painful. Motor paralysis is a late symptom of ischemia. When motor paralysis results from primary nerve injury, other symptoms of vascular insufficiency are not present.[221]

All five toes should be observable on a casted foot, and all five fingers on a casted hand. Observe *each* finger or toe separately, e.g., for abnormal skin color, paralysis, loss of sensation, skin lesions, and swelling. If the cast covers fingers or toes, report this to the physician so he can modify the cast for purposes of future observations.

Inspect the skin all around the cast edges for evidence of *skin damage or swelling.* Injury to an extremity and the subsequent treatment of the injury (e.g., reduction, surgery) usually produce swelling which progresses for the first 12 to 24 postinjury or postoperative hours and may be greatest for the first 24–48 hours. While mild swelling, i.e., edema, of exposed fingers and toes is not unusual (particularly if the casted limb is in a dependent position), moderate or severe swelling associated with pain and discoloration is abnormal. Edema should not be painful and should not be greater than plus 2. When a casted part swells markedly, mechanical constriction occurs of the structures within the cast, and severe complications result. Swelling causes the cast to feel tight. Edema may obstruct blood flow so much that blood moves ahead in vessels only when the heart contracts. This may cause a throbbing sensation which may be painful. Report increasing edema, accompanied by pain or other symptoms, e.g., paresthesia, numbness.

Measures effective in preventing or relieving excessive swelling include[123] (a) elevating full length of the cast higher than the heart; (b) exercising the fingers and toes to stimulate circulation; and (c) placing ice bags beside (not on) the cast. If excessive swelling and pressure persist in spite of therapeutic measures, notify the physician immediately and bring to the bedside equipment which he may require to bivalve the cast, e.g., cast cutter. Pressure caused from edema must be relieved by cutting the cast before irreversible damage occurs. In the absence of edema, pressure against the skin caused by the edge of a cast may be relieved by changing the patient's position or by loosely padding the area which is causing the patient discomfort.

Observe the surface of the cast for indications of

wound drainage (stains) or *bleeding.* Inspect the cast closely at areas covering known wounds (e.g., surgical incisions or accidental wounds) and over all pressure points (for indications of damage to underlying skin). Often it takes longer for wound drainage and bleeding to seep through a cast than it does for it to pass through other dressings. When an area of drainage or bleeding becomes visible, it should be circled with an indelible pencil, and notation should be made (on the edge of the circle) of the time and date of the observation. Charting should include the size of the drainage area and the character of the drainage. Repeated observations are made to determine if the area of drainage is enlarging. If the area enlarges, recircle and relabel it on the cast and make notations on the chart. Always call areas of drainage or bleeding to the physician's attention. The physician may decide to remove a circle of cast ("window the cast") over draining areas to examine the wound directly. Complete cast removal may be necessary if excessive hemorrhage occurs.

Observe the patient wearing a body cast for *abdominal distention.* It may be necessary to have an opening cut over the patient's abdomen to relieve pressure from distention and listen for bowel sounds. Additionally, if the physician orders, a nasogastric tube may be inserted for decompression. *"Cast syndrome"*[178] is a potentially fatal complication which can develop in a patient with a body cast. The syndrome is characterized by prolonged nausea and repeated vomiting secondary to gastric and duodenal dilatation. Abdominal distention and vague abdominal pain may also occur. If untreated, the patient develops severe hypokalemic alkalosis and hypovolemia and eventually dies. While gastrointestinal dilatation may have various causes, when it occurs as part of the cast syndrome the pathogenesis is mechanical compression of the fourth portion of the duodenum by the superior mesenteric artery. Total bowel obstruction may develop once the edematous duodenum dilates so much that it cannot continue to propel its contents into the jejunum. Treatment includes intestinal decompression, fluid and electrolyte replenishment, and removal of the cast. In some cases surgical intestinal anastomosis is necessary.

C. *Olfactory observations:* Place your nose close to the cast and smell for odors indicative of tissue necrosis and infection. It is not unusual for casts to develop a somewhat "sour" smell after a period of time. This odor is produced by perspiration and the normal amount of sloughing of the skin's outer layers. Pathologic tissue necrosis emits a musty offensive odor which can easily be detected and which is much more unpleasant and strong than the typical odor of a cast which has been on for some time. With experience, the nurse can easily identify abnormal odors *if* she takes the time to smell the cast each day. Cast odor may take several days to appear. Areas of the cast which must be evaluated especially carefully in this manner are around the edges of the cast and over any "hot spots" or areas of discoloration on the cast. A musty odor may be the only indication of skin necrosis or infection (e.g., gas bacillus infection) beneath a cast. However, also evaluate the patient for other indications of infection, e.g., elevated temperature, elevated white blood count.

D. *Auditory observations: Listen, listen, listen* to the patient's comments about how he feels and investigate *all* reports which are indicative of developing complications! Many patients have sufferred serious irreversible complications from casts because no one listened and appropriately responded to their "complaints." Negligence of this sort is inexcusable. Pay attention to what patients tell you and evaluate what they say. Ask for further clarification when necessary. Make additional observations of your own and make appropriate responses.

Ask the casted patient if he notices any unusual feelings (paresthesias) such as tingling, prickly, or burning sensations in the casted area. Ask if he has pain. Evaluate pain carefully in an attempt to identify its cause: is it incisional pain or is the pain caused from excessive swelling within the cast? See if changes of position will relieve pain or swelling before resorting to the administration of analgesics.

Do not administer pain medication to a patient wearing a cast until the cause of the pain has been evaluated.

Sustained pain is indicative of pressure-related complications. A well-defined, single area of burning sensation or pain should always be reported for immediate investigation.

Pain is the main symptom of circulatory impairment from a cast.[221] The pain is not localized and is usually burning or cramping in nature. The amount of pain is greater than that expected to occur from the surgery or injury. A fractured extremity typically becomes progressively painless once it is properly immobilized. Constant, undiminished pain which is present for as long as *four* hours after a patient recovers from anesthesia should be viewed with suspicion. If the pain remains unchanged after *six* hours the physician is notified and an immediate investigation is made of the cause of the pain. The patient is not given narcotics until the safety of the extremity is established. Pain is an important diagnostic symptom in this situation, and should not be suppressed or masked until a thorough evaluation is made of the patient's condition.

All personnel working with casted patients should be knowledgeable about potential complications of casts and should see that indications of these complications are reported at once to persons who will provide help to the patient. *All* patients wearing casts should be encouraged to report any abnormal symptoms, and each patient should be given a *complete* cast inspection at least once each day (more often in the newly casted patient). Findings from these inspections should be charted. These records not only serve as guides for future care but also may provide useful evidence in court in malpractice or negligence suits.

Notify the physician *immediately* of any indications of complications in a casted patient so appropriate action can be taken immediately. Waiting to tell the doctor "the next time he comes by" may cause the patient to suffer serious complications which could have been prevented by prompt therapy.

Often when symptoms of complications are present the physician decides to bivalve (split) the patient's cast to relieve pressure or to inspect the limb. *The cast and underlying padding must be cut completely down to the skin to properly bivalve a cast.* It is not sufficient to merely cut through the top layers of the cast, because the pressure is being exerted by those layers of bandages and casts which are directly against the skin. If cast pressure was the cause of the patient's symptoms, he will experience immediate relief of pain when the cast is opened. If pain persists, the physician continues his investigation to determine the cause of the pain. It may be necessary to return the patient to surgery. When bivalving is performed to relieve pressure, be certain to elevate the limb after bivalving is accomplished to aid in the reduction of swelling.

Nutrition. Increased roughage content in the diet of a patient with limited activity may help him maintain normal bowel elimination. The patient in a body cast or hip spica cast may need to avoid gas-forming foods if they tend to create abdominal distention. A general, well-balanced diet promotes wound healing.

Psychologic Adjustments. Patients wearing casts frequently find it difficult to become accustomed to the physical restraint imposed by confinement in plaster. In addition to restricting mobility and natural movements, casts often create other discomforts, e.g., itching, fatigue (from the weight of the cast). It is not unusual for persons with casts (especially large casts, such as body casts, hip-spicas, etc.) to become irritable, tense, discouraged, or depressed.

Physical tension may be relieved by activity and massage. Patients should be encouraged to practice self-care as much as possible and to follow their physician's orders for exercises and activity. The nurse, occupational therapist, and physical therapist combine their professional efforts to help patients engage in meaningful activities during the rehabilitative-recovery period. Activities are individually selected to meet a given patient's needs, physically and emotionally. The individual patient's interests and life style are evaluated, and he is encouraged to participate in activities which are of interest and benefit to him. When a nurse understands the problems which a patient may be experiencing during his recovery, she can more accurately interpret his behavior and help others (e.g., family members) so they do not unnecessarily contribute to the patient's burdens.

Self-Care. It is desirable for a casted patient to perform as much self-care as he can so that he will move about (indirectly exercise) and maintain feelings of independence and self-esteem. Remember that a cast limits motion. Thus, if you want a patient to be able to perform various self-care activities, you must make certain he is able to reach the items he needs. Attempt to anticipate the patient's needs and then unobtrusively perform activities which the patient cannot manage for himself, e.g., cutting meat. Have a call bell within easy reach at all times. When the patient with a cast is able to be dressed, he may require instruction about how to put on his clothes most easily. Some casts restrict the wearing of certain types of clothing, and clothing must be modified to be worn over the cast.

Discharge. Some patients are sent home with green casts. Others are kept in the hospital until their casts are dry and then are discharged if no symptoms of complications have appeared. Still others remain hospitalized as long as they are casted.

The patient who is sent home with a cast should be provided with explanations of proper cast care and cast observations. Include family members in these teaching sessions when possible. Printed instructions for the patient will give him something accurate to refer to once he is home. Anxious persons often have difficulty remembering details, and if the patient is sent home soon after the cast is applied, he may be too overwhelmed by the injury and its treatment to remember detailed instructions. Illustrations can be valuable teaching aids for both literate and nonliterate persons.

Instructions should include not only details of immediate cast care during the drying period (if the cast is wet), but also information about care of the dry cast. Tell the patient to keep the casted extremity elevated and to keep the cast dry and protected. A stocking or piece of stockinette may be worn to keep the exterior of the cast clean and to keep toes or fingers warm. If the cast is to be worn for some time, the exterior sometimes may be painted with shellac, plastic spray, or varnish (once it is dry) to help keep the surface clean. If the cast surface becomes soiled, it may be cleaned by using a damp (not soaking wet) cloth and some scouring powder.

If the patient has a casted leg he should be told whether or not he can place weight on the affected limb. A weight-bearing cast must be completely dry before weight is placed on it. When crutches are necessary, they are fitted to the patient and he is given instruction in their use before discharge.

Make certain the patient understands the symptoms of complications he should watch for and that he knows how to notify his doctor if any complications appear to be developing. Emphasize that symptoms such as severe pain, burning, numbness, tingling, swelling, skin discoloration (e.g., blueness), paralysis, and pallor should be reported *im-*

mediately day or night. Provide instruction for activity, e.g., move toes and fingers for several minutes every one-half hour. Also, supply the patient with information about when and where he is to see his doctor for his next scheduled appointment. Between appointments the patient should report by telephone indications of deterioration of the cast, e.g., cracking or softening.

Cast Changes. Changes are commonly necessary when a cast no longer fits, e.g., due to weight loss, weight gain, muscular atrophy. Sometimes it is necessary to change a patient's cast more than once, to provide additional treatment, or to inspect the involved area. Between changes the patient's skin is cared for according to the physician's specifications. Sometimes the doctor orders calamine lotion with Benadryl to be applied before recasting to relieve or prevent itching. Frequent observations should be made for the first day or two following cast changes, just as with a newly casted patient. These observations are especially important if the angle of the cast has been changed (e.g., with a body cast or turnbuckle cast) because new pressure areas may appear and rapidly cause severe neurovascular damage.

Cast Removal. The length of time a patient continues to wear a cast varies depending upon the type and extent of injury, disease, or surgery and the rate of healing.

Removal of a cast is usually accomplished with an electric cast cutter, which resembles a small electric saw with a circular blade. Because of its appearance and the noise it produces, a cast cutter is often frightening to the patient. Explain to the patient that the fine toothed blade does not whirl around and cut like a saw blade, but rather the blade breaks the plaster by oscillating or vibrating rapidly back and forth. The vibrations separate the plaster by shaking it. Reassure the patient that he will not be cut by the blade, since the blade stops when it reaches stockinette or padding material. Bandage scissors are then used to cut open these final layers of the cast. When a cast cutter is used, the patient may feel sensations of heat, vibrations, or pressure, but no pain. Instruct the patient to hold still while the cutter is being used. Because a cast cutter scatters plaster dustings around, it is necessary to remove the cast on a surface which is protected and can easily be cleaned. A vacuum apparatus may be used to suction up the plaster dust.

A cast may also be removed manually by drawing the blade of a plaster knife or hand saw along the outside of the cast and then cutting the cast with heavy plaster shears or wedging the cut open with a spreader. Cast cutting is sometimes made easier by applying acetic acid (vinegar) along the cutting line to soften the plaster.

The time of cast removal is frequently a time of mixed anxiety and anticipation for the patient. To keep the patient's expectations realistic, he should be told before the cast is removed generally how the casted area will look and feel. The skin under a casted area is commonly mottled and covered with yellow-brown scales or crusts of dead skin, oil, and exudate. The muscles may appear flabby and slightly atrophied (disuse atrophy). If an incision underlies the cast, it will be exposed, possibly for the first time. Additionally, a casted extremity will not "feel like new" when the cast is removed, but rather it will be stiff and weakened from inactivity. New aches and pains may appear with movement following cast removal as muscles and tissues are subjected to new stresses and strains. Finally, removal of the weight of the cast will cause the body to feel lighter, e.g., a limb may feel as if it were floating.

Handle the limb gently when removing it from the cast. The patient may be physically quite tense and fearful of motion and pain. Provide adequate support, especially under joints, and avoid quick or jerky movements. Joints tend to be unstable initially when the rigid support of a cast is removed. It is necessary to continue to protect and support the weakened limb for a while. This may be accomplished in various ways, e.g., by the use of pillows, elastic bandages, crutches, or a splint, brace, sling, or cane. The patient will initially be most comfortable if he is positioned in a way similar to the position maintained while casted.

Opinion varies concerning management of the skin following removal of a cast. Some physicians believe that the caked exudate on the skin serves a protective function, and they recommend gradually cleansing the skin over a period of several days by general soaking. Other physicians recommend scrubbing off the exudate, e.g., with pHiso-Hex or Betadine. If scrubs are ordered, they should be gently performed so as not to traumatize the skin or be painful to the patient. The underlying new skin is highly sensitive. Whether or not the exudate is removed, the skin is lubricated with cocoa butter, a lanolin solution, mineral oil, A & D ointment, or some other emollient to help soften and remove the crusts. A soft cotton wrap or elastic bandage may then be applied. If Ace bandages are recommended, they should be used only during the daytime. During the day the bandages need to be periodically removed and reapplied to prevent excessive constriction. Care must be taken not to pull the bandages taut when applying them. Advise the patient not to pick at or scratch his skin.

Rehabilitation. Rehabilitative instructions are given by the physician and are individualized according to the patient's condition. If a leg has been casted, the patient is told if he can be weight-bearing and how much ambulation is permitted. If an arm has been casted, the patient is instructed as to how he should use his arm, e.g., how much weight he can safely lift. Reassure the patient that with exercise and use he will overcome muscle atrophy and the weakness and stiffness present when the cast is removed.

The physical therapist often participates in rehabilitative care following cast removal, e.g., by teaching and supervising graded active exercises (to stimulate circulation and increase muscle strength and joint range of motion) and by carrying out other prescribed activities, e.g., whirlpool baths, massage. It is undesirable to force joints and muscles during the period of recovery (e.g., by passive stretching exercises, resistive exercises, or forced movements) because placing excessive demands on stiff, weakened limbs will only cause further impairment of motion by increasing fibrosis and excessively engorging the area with blood. Commonly the patient is advised to move the limb actively within limits of stiffness or pain, but not to force movement.

Following cast removal, edema and swelling tend to occur for a while when the involved limb is placed in a dependent position. With increased activity and improvement in muscle tone and circulation, these problems will gradually lessen. However, until they subside the limb should be kept elevated most of the time (higher than the heart) while the patient sits or lies down. Sometimes the physician recommends the use of elastic bandages or stockings during ambulation to minimize swelling. Support stockings may be more effective than the bandages, but they are costly and the patient must be measured for a proper fit. Encourage ambulation because intermittent weight-bearing acts as an effective venous pump. Inform the patient that dependent edema will gradually lessen.

Traction

Therapeutic traction is accomplished by exerting a pull (on the head, body, or limbs) in two directions, i.e., the pull of the traction and the pull of countertraction. The *traction force* commonly consists of weights. The *countertraction* force may be either (a) the weight of the patient's body (as it rests on and tends to slide down an inclined surface, such as a tilted bed); or (b) other weights. When traction (pull) is applied in one direction it is necessary to have an equal traction (countertraction) in the opposite direction.

When traction is properly applied, the patient is centered in his bed and the affected part is held properly aligned by a constant pull. The patient will be immobilized in the center of the bed when traction and countertraction are equal. The direction of pull when applied to long bones is in line with the bones' long axes; it is in line with the spinal column when applied to the head or pelvis. As indicated, countertraction may be obtained by elevating the bed in such a way that the patient's body weight opposes the pull of the traction. Commonly the bed is elevated or tilted under the part which is in traction; e.g., the foot of the bed may be elevated when traction is applied to the lower extremities. If the bed is not properly tilted, the countertraction achieved is inadequate and the patient tends to slide in the direction of the traction force rather than away from it. This defeats the purpose of the traction apparatus, and an effective stretch cannot be obtained on the injured part. With some types of traction, countertraction can be applied with ropes, pulleys, and weights pulling in a direction opposite to that of the traction (see below).

Methods of Applying Traction. Traction may be applied (a) *manually,* by pulling on the part with the hands; (b) *mechanically,* by exerting a pull on the part with ropes and pulleys; (c) with special devices inserted in *casts* (plaster traction); or (d) with *braces.*

Manual traction may be applied by a physician for various therapeutic purposes, e.g., correction of a dislocation or reduction of a fracture. With the physician's permission and direction, nurses may apply manual traction (a) when a patient, with an injury requiring continuous traction, is being transported or repositioned in bed; or (b) when casts or traction are being initially applied or changed. Manual traction is applied with a firm steady pull rather than a sudden jerking motion. Manual traction may be used when giving emergency care to an injured person, e.g., to immobilize the injured part during transportation.

Mechanical traction can be applied (e.g., with special halters, splints, bandages, ropes, pulleys, and weights) to either the skin (*skin traction*) or bones (*skeletal traction*) (see below).

Plaster traction may be accomplished by the use of turnbuckle casts or hyperextension casts. Also, skeletal traction can be applied by fixing the ends of Kirschner wires or Steinmann pins in plaster when applying a cast. Skeletal traction obtained in this way provides a fixed type of traction which maintains the position of the extremity and yet permits the patient to move around without disturbing the alignment of the traction.[123] (Turnbuckle casts and body casts were discussed in the previous section.)

Traction may also be applied with special *braces,* e.g., hyperextension braces. (Braces were discussed earlier in this section.) In sum, traction can be applied manually or mechanically, as well as by using casts or braces. The remainder of this discussion pertains to mechanical traction.

Uses. Therapeutic traction may be applied to the neck, extremities, or pelvis. It is most commonly used to align fragments of broken bones and to maintain proper alignment until bone union develops. Traction used to reduce fractures is most frequently used on the extremities. The application of traction overcomes the injured limb's tendency to shorten (due to muscle spasm) and holds the limb constantly in a position of corrective extension with the ends of the fractured bone aligned. Other uses of therapeutic traction include (a) relief of painful muscle spasms; (b) correction and prevention of deformities; (c) stretching adhesions; and (d) immobilization or distraction (i.e., pulling apart) of diseased or painful joints. Traction may be used in the treatment of painful arthritis, sore muscles and ligaments, dislocations, degenerated or ruptured intervertebral disks, and spinal cord compression.

General Care of the Patient in Traction. The major *disadvantage*[220] of traction is that it requires a long period of recumbency, and the patient typically must remain hospitalized during treatment. *Advantages* of traction include (a) greater potential for exercising joints and muscles than is possible with casting; and (b) avoidance of surgically induced bone devascularization and infection (if surgery is not required prior to application of traction). Any type of traction must permit some movement of the patient in bed and be only minimally uncomfortable.

The nurse caring for a patient in traction should know (a) the nature of the patient's injury; (b) the purpose of the traction; (c) how the traction device accomplishes its purpose; (d) movements and positions which are permitted and those which are contraindicated; and (e) potential complications associated with the use of traction and their prevention.

When caring for a patient in traction remember to maintain (a) alignment of the injured part; (b) general body alignment (the pull of the traction tends to move the patient out of positions of good alignment); (c) alignment of the traction apparatus; and (d) range of motion in as many joints as possible.

Before a patient is placed in traction, he should be prepared psychologically as well as physically. Because of its formidable appearance, a traction set up may look to lay persons like an implement of torture rather than a helpful, therapeutic device. Explain to the patient (and his family) the purposes of traction and reasons why he must remain in certain positions for long periods of time. Make sure the patient is informed of contraindicated movements or positions. Tell him that if he moves into contraindicated positions he will defeat the purposes of the traction and may disrupt healing processes. When a patient is first placed in traction he should be told that traction will help his muscles begin to relax after a few hours and he will begin to feel more comfortable. A patient placed in traction to treat a fracture should feel progressively better after traction is applied. The doctor should tell the patient how long he will be in traction.

Three factors of importance in therapeutic reduction traction are[220] (1) the extremity should be supported and stretched in a direction which will properly align bone fragments (traction is exerted on the distal fragment to align it with the proximal fragment); (2) the extremity should not be overstretched (overstretching results in excessive distraction of bone fragments); and (3) stretching forces must remain constant (in amount and direction) until bone union occurs. The amount of weight applied in treating a fracture with traction may be gradually reduced by the physician as the injured bone heals.

In order to conserve space only some of the more commonly used types of mechanical traction will be discussed and illustrated here. Traction techniques for the arm, hand, and forefoot are omitted entirely. The intricacies of actually setting up specific types of traction are not discussed. Commonly persons with special training in setting up traction are available in hospital settings, or the physician assists with setting up the equipment. Detailed manuals discussing specific pieces of traction equipment and various traction set-ups are provided by manufacturers. Additionally, it is helpful to consult books on traction or orthopedics for details.

Equipment. Bed boards and firm mattresses are necessary components of any traction bed in order to prevent uncomfortable and incorrect positioning of the patient. A *Balkan frame* is used with some traction set-ups. The metal frame is fastened to the corners of the bed and consists of an overhead rectangular structure (about the size of the edges of the bed) which is supported by uprights. This frame serves as the basic overhead structure from which other parts of the traction set-up may be suspended or to which they may be attached, e.g., crossbars, clamps, pulleys. Basic traction set-ups can be modified in numerous ways to meet a patient's individual therapeutic needs. Strong, light-weight aluminum equipment is available which requires little maintenance. Commonly octagonal poles are preferable to round poles because the latter tend to slip at clamped joints under stress.

Traction carts are available in most hospitals. These carts contain basic equipment necessary to position and care for a patient in traction. The large pieces of traction equipment, e.g., splints, trapezes, frames, poles, pulleys, are commonly stored in a *traction room.* Traction carts and traction rooms easily become disheveled unless everyone using them participates in neatly storing unused equipment.

Periodically inspect a patient's traction set-up to ensure that the apparatus is accomplishing its purpose and that the equipment is as safe as possible. Some factors of importance to note during inspection of a traction apparatus are summarized below:

> *Ropes, knots,* and *pulleys:* Braided nylon cord (⅛-inch thick) is commonly used as a traction rope. Traction ropes must be of adequate strength to support the weights without breaking. The rope should be discarded after use. Prior to cutting lengths of traction rope, wrap the rope with adhesive tape where the cut is to be made. Then cut through the rope. The tape prevents raveling of the rope ends. Traction ropes must be of proper length and contain no unnecessary knots which can catch in the pulleys. If the ropes are too short, the weights may be pulled up against the pulleys; if the ropes are too long, the weights may rest on the floor.

Traction ropes should be kept free of the bed and bedding. The ropes should feel taut and ride easily over pulleys. Traction ropes should not touch the patient or rub together. Ropes passing over the foot of the bed should not touch the mattress or the bed. Make certain the ropes do not slip out of the wheel grooves of pulleys. See that frayed rope is replaced with fresh rope to prevent accidental breakage of the rope.

Ropes and pulleys should be unobstructed, freely movable, and in straight alignment. Pulleys should not squeak. All pulleys should be lubricated with silicone spray or a small amount of mineral oil *before* they are

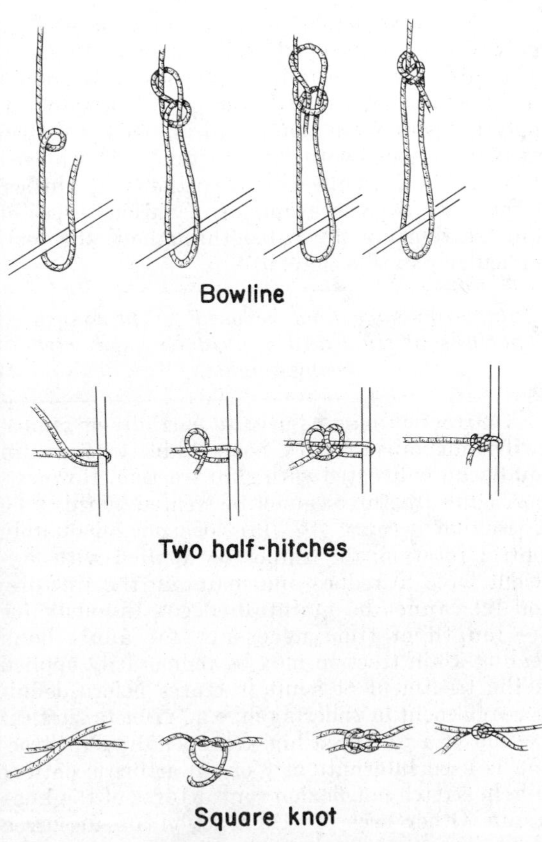

FIGURE 88–12. Types of knots.

threaded with ropes. Once the traction is set up, the pulleys should not be lubricated unless the physician is present to readjust the amount of traction weight. Lubrication changes the balancing forces because it alters the friction.[278]

Pulleys should be free of the supporting equipment. They should be placed out on traction arms far enough that weights hang free of the bed.

Examine knots frequently to make certain they are secure. Knots used with traction equipment should not slip. Three types of knots which may be used are illustrated in Figure 88–12. The *bowline* may be used to hang some weight carriers. It makes a loop which will not slip. *Two half-hitches* may be used to secure a rope to a pole or a ring. *Square knots* will firmly hold two pieces of rope together. Some sources recommend taping the ends of knots with small strips of adhesive tape to make them more secure.[221]

> *Clamps* and *weights:* Check clamps to make certain they are tightened securely. Traction weights may be made of metal or bags of sand or shot. Weights should hang free so they will maintain an even, constant pulling force in a straight line. Weights should not rest on the bed, floor, a chair, or other weight systems. Also, they should not have added weight placed on them by bed linens. If weights are resting on the floor, it is because the rope is too long or the patient has slipped too far in the direction of the pull. Keep weights visible so they are not displaced. Weights should be securely fastened to the rope (e.g., knots should be covered with adhesive tape) so they will not slip off or accidentally be jarred off.

Weights should not hang over any part of the patient to prevent their falling and injuring him. If necessary the traction apparatus should be modified so the weights will hang freely away from the patient.

Always check the traction apparatus after a patient has moved to make certain the patient is correctly repositioned and that the force of the traction is being properly applied. The patient must be aligned so the traction pulls in a straight line.

Do not bump or jar the bed or traction equipment, thus causing weights to swing. This can easily happen when equipment projects beyond the edges of the bed and not only is uncomfortable and disturbing to the patient but also can injure you.

If you detect adjustments that need to be made on the traction equipment (e.g., changing a frayed rope) and you know how to make the necessary adjustments, ask the physician's permission to do so. Also, ask if he wants traction to be maintained manually until the mechanical traction is reapplied.

Continuous or Intermittent Traction. Traction may be required either *continuously* or *intermittently,* depending upon a given patient's specific disorder. The physician specifies if the patient's traction is to be continuous (i.e., pull constantly applied) or intermittent (i.e., pull may be relieved periodically). The pull of traction is relieved by lifting the traction weights. Typically continuous traction is necessary in the treatment of fractures or dislocations. Traction may be applied intermittently in arthritis (e.g., to reduce flexion contractures) or in the treatment of low back disorders (e.g., to reduce pain and muscle spasm). Traction is always assumed to be continuous unless the physician specifies that the traction may be relieved periodically. Orders for intermittent traction should state precisely the length of time traction may be removed.

Running or Suspension Traction. Mechanical therapeutic traction may be either (1) running traction; or (2) suspension traction. *Running traction* (also called "straight" traction) exerts a direct pull on the affected part without a hammock or splint to give balanced support. Running traction exerts a pull in one plane and may be unilateral or bilateral. There are both skin and skeletal types of running traction. Buck's extension and Bryant's traction are examples of running traction.

Suspension traction (also called "balanced" traction) exerts a pull on the affected part and also supports the extremity in a hammock or splint which is held in place by balanced weights attached to an overhead bar (see Fig. 88–13). With suspension traction the countertraction is supplied by a system of ropes, pulleys, and weights rather than by the patient's body. With this form of traction the pull of the traction remains the same even when the patient moves. The suspension apparatus gives countertraction which takes up any slack caused in the traction by the patient's movements. As the patient lifts himself up off the bed, the weights attached to the traction apparatus move down (thus maintaining the original line of pull). For example, when suspension traction is applied to a leg, the leg and splints should rise when the patient elevates his hips. Thus, an extremity placed in suspension traction "floats," suspended (or balanced) in the traction apparatus.

Suspension traction permits greater range-of-motion and activity than standard running traction. It makes it easier to care for a patient and improves the patient's comfort and general well-being. By increasing circulation to the affected part and by decreasing prolonged pressure on weight-bearing areas, suspension traction reduces the possibilities of complications developing.

Suspension traction may be used with either skeletal or skin traction, and with any splint or hammock type of traction. Examples of suspension traction are Russell's traction and the use of a Thomas splint with a Pearson attachment. Suspension traction may be set up on a CircOlectric bed or from a Balkan frame. The traction must be maintained continuously to be effective.

Skin Traction. Skin traction is a nonsurgical procedure which indirectly applies traction on the underlying skeletal system and other structures, e.g., muscles. Skin traction may be applied (a) by fastening traction strips (e.g., strips of moleskin or adhesive tapes) to the extremities with woven bandage or bias-cut stockinette; or (b) by encircling a part with a special halter, corset, or sling. Traction strips are used with Buck's extension, Bryant's traction, and Russell's skin traction (see below). (Russell's traction may also be applied directly to the skeleton.) A halter may be used to apply traction to the head, and a corset or sling may be used to exert traction on the pelvis. A special anklet or bandage may be used with a splint to apply temporary traction to an ankle. If countertraction is needed with skin traction, it is achieved by using the patient's weight on the tilted surface of the bed. (Specific examples of various types of skin traction are presented throughout the text, particularly in this chapter.)

Skin traction cannot be used for prolonged periods of time and cannot be used with heavy weights.

Skin traction may be used to partially or temporarily immobilize a part. Some stable fractures in adults can be treated with skin traction. However, most adult fractures cannot be treated by this type of traction because it[221] (a) does not adequately control rotation; (b) cannot be applied with sufficient force to reduce and maintain the fracture; and (c) cannot be maintained continuously for the length of time necessary for adult bone healing. Skin traction may be temporarily applied in the treatment of adult fractures before definitive treatment is undertaken, e.g., prior to surgical fixation of a fractured hip. Occasionally skin traction is used intermittently on an arthritic patient to help stretch out flexion contractures of the knee or hip. Other uses of skin traction are discussed as appropriate throughout the text.

A variety of tapes for skin traction are available commercially, under such names as Fas-trac, Flex-foam, Foam-trac, and Trac-grip. These products are usually accompanied by information about recommended skin preparation and use of the tapes.[123] Some physicians use strips of moleskin or adhesive tape instead of commercial products for skin traction tapes.

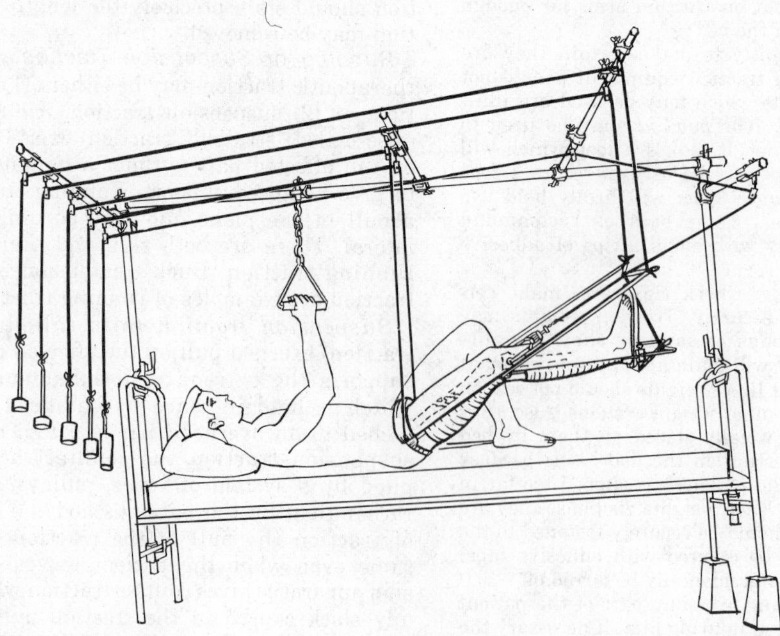

FIGURE 88–13. Proximal tibial traction with balanced suspension. (From Schmeisser, G., Jr.: *A Clinical Manual of Orthopedic Traction Techniques.* 1963.)

Traction tapes cannot be applied to skin which is irritated or damaged; otherwise skin breakdown may occur under the tape. Also, skin tapes cannot be applied over areas which may subsequently be operated on, because skin damage from the tape increases the possibility of postoperative infection.

Opinions differ concerning *skin preparation* for the application of skin traction. Some physicians believe the skin should be shaved (especially if the patient is quite hirsute) or that tincture of benzoin should be applied or both. Others believe that shaving the skin denudes it (inviting skin damage when the traction strips and overlying bandage are applied) and that the application of tincture of benzoin is unnecessary or undesirable. Still other physicians paint the extremity with an Ace adherent and cover it with stockinette before applying the traction strips and covering bandage. It is necessary to check skin preparation orders carefully to comply with these varying practices. Proponents of benzoin claim that it is helpful because it minimizes itching of the skin, promotes the adhesion of materials to the skin, disinfects the skin, and generally keeps the skin in better shape and the patient more comfortable when skin traction is applied. If shaving the skin is ordered, it must be carefully performed so the skin is not denuded, irritated, or cut.

Traction tapes should not encircle a limb or they may compromise circulation and cause skin damage. The tapes are placed lengthwise on opposite sides of the limb. The tapes must not be so wide that they completely surround the limb. The traction tapes extend beyond the length of the limb and are attached to a spreader bar, which is attached to the pulley-weight apparatus. The pull of the traction is in line with the free ends of each tape.

With an indelible felt pen, place a mark on the skin adjacent to the proximal ends of newly applied tapes. Slippage of the tapes can then easily be identified by the appearance of skin between the line and the edge of the tape.

After the traction tapes are applied, they are covered with an encircling bandage to hold them securely in place. Wrapping the extremity in elastic or other outer bandages helps adhesive strips to adhere and prevents any type of traction tape (adhesive or nonadhesive) from slipping out of place. Limbs must be adequately supported once skin traction is applied.

The amount of traction that can safely be applied is determined by the *skin's tolerance to traction and friction* rather than by the strength of the traction tape material. Only 5 to 7 pounds of longitudinal force can safely be applied to the skin. Three to four weeks is the maximum length of time for which skin traction can be applied.[221]

Skin traction applied to the leg may cause pressure on the Achilles tendon at the back of the ankle or over the malleoli or the peroneal nerve below the knee (at the neck of the fibula) on the lateral side of the leg or both. Skin traction applied to the arm may cause pressure damage to the ulnar nerve at the elbow. *Bony prominences must be protectively padded* prior to the application of skin tapes or the traction force will rapidly cause skin breakdown or damage to superficial nerves or both. Prominences which should be padded on the arm include the lateral and medial epicondyles, the olecranon, and the styloid process of the ulna. On the leg the head of the fibula and the lateral and medial malleoli should be padded.

Bandages and tapes must be smoothly applied. Wrinkles irritate the skin and cause pressure damage. Some physicians request that the outer bandages be rewrapped periodically. Frequently inspect the condition of the skin around the tape and bandage edges. Look for and report pimples, irritation, abrasions, reddened areas, maceration, and purulent discharge. Also, check the condition of tapes and bandages. Slipping tapes and loose bandages should be called to the physician's attention.

The possibilities of *complications* developing increase with (a) application of excessive weights; (b) failure to adequately pad bony prominences and areas having superficial nerves, and (c) application of a bandage which is tightly wrapped. Complications which may occur with skin traction include (a) skin necrosis (caused by the shearing force of the tape); (b) nerve damage (caused by pressure on superficial nerves); and (c) impaired venous and arterial circulation (caused by twisting of a limb in traction or constriction from tight bandages). After applying elastic bandages, inspect the foot or hand frequently for indications of circulatory impairment or nerve damage. Make the first evaluation a few minutes after the bandages are applied and then subsequently make periodic evaluations. During your evaluations make certain the patient is correctly aligned with the pull of the traction.

As mentioned earlier, some types of traction have pieces of equipment which encircle a body part, e.g., head halter, pelvic traction corset, anklet, or a ring or half-ring on an arm or leg traction splint. The pull of the traction may then be exerted on the encircled body part. The skin under *encircling devices* is especially prone to breakdown from pressure and friction, and must be given vigilant preventative skin care.

Skeletal Traction. Skeletal traction is accomplished by surgically first inserting metal wires (Kirschner wires) or pins (Steinmann pins) through bones or by anchoring metal tongs (e.g., Crutchfield, Barton, or Vinke tongs) in the skull. The traction apparatus is then attached to the metal insertion. Skeletal traction applied to the skull is discussed in Unit VIII.

Kirschner wires and Steinmann pins are round stainless steel rods which are typically inserted (with a drill) perpendicular to and completely through bones. A traction bow is then attached to the wire or pin and the traction force is applied to the bow (also called spreader, stirrups, or

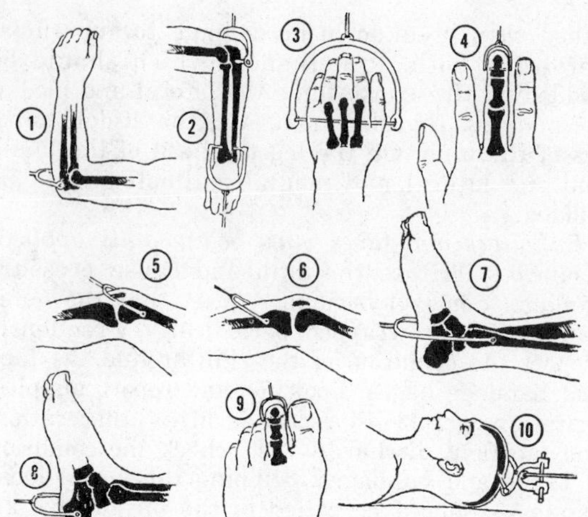

FIGURE 88–14. Sites for skeletal traction. 1, Below the olecranon, 2, below the olecranon together with a pin through the distal ends of the radius and the ulna; 3, through the middle three metacarpals; 4, through the distal phalanx of the fingers; 5, through the supracondylar area of the femur; 6, through the upper end of the tibia; 7, through the lower end of the tibia and fibula; 8, through the os calcis; 9, through the distal phalanx of the toes; 10, skull traction. (From DePalma, A. F.: *The Management of Fractures and Dislocations.* Vol. 1. 2nd ed. 1970.)

calipers). Figure 88–14 shows common sites of insertion of skeletal traction. The site of insertion of the pins, wires, or tongs determines precisely the location to which the traction force will be applied.

Note that wires and pins are not inserted through joints. The physician attempts to place the wire or pin in such a way that only skin, subcutaneous tissue, and bone are penetrated, e.g., he tries to avoid muscles, tendons, arteries, and nerves. Skeletal pins should not pass through a fracture hematoma. Also, the pins cannot be inserted through skin which is infected, abraded, or has a rash.

Bone infection (osteomyelitis) can develop with skeletal traction. This is a serious complication.

The procedure of inserting skeletal pins or wires must be performed with aseptic technique to prevent postoperative infection. Skin preparation for skeletal traction is the same as that prior to any orthopedic surgical procedure (see below). Skeletal pins or wires are inserted under either local or general anesthesia. The procedure requires a signed surgical consent from the patient.

Skeletal traction can be used for relatively long periods of time and can be used with heavier weights than skin traction. It is highly effective in treating fractures in bones surrounded by large muscle masses (e.g., femur) and in reducing unstable dislocations and fracture-dislocations. Other disorders which are commonly treated with skeletal traction are unstable spinal cord injuries and displaced fractures of the pelvis. The proper application of skeletal traction typically causes the patient with a fracture to become increasingly comfortable as it reduces muscular spasms and holds fractured bones in alignment.

Skeletal traction provides excellent traction because it applies force directly to the bone, making it possible not only to exert a longitudinal pull on the bone, but also to control rotation.[221] With skeletal traction, as much as 20–30 pounds of pull may be exerted, and the traction may safely be applied for several months. The pull is exerted via a fixed system of ropes, pulleys, weight carriers, and weights. Special equipment which may be used to apply skeletal traction to the lower extremities may include a Thomas splint (or a variation of this splint), with or without a Pearson attachment or Böhler-Braun frame.

During application of skeletal traction, neurovascular evaluations should be made frequently. The neurovascular status of the part should be evaluated and recorded prior to pin insertion so that a basis of comparison between the pre and post pin insertion is available.

Periodic inspections of the skeletal traction apparatus are essential. Sometimes the sharp ends of the wires or pins extend beyond the bow. Place corks or adhesive over these protruding ends to prevent bed linens from catching on the sharp points and to prevent scratching of the patient's skin or that of persons giving care. If a tong becomes accidentally displaced and it catches soft tissue, the patient experiences severe pain. The physician should be notified immediately. Loose wires or pins should also be called to the attention of the physician at once because movement of the extremity causes the wire or pin to cut into the bone and may introduce infection from outside (into the pin tract and along the tract into the bone).[123]

The insertion points of skeletal wires, pins, or tongs may become infected. Observe skin around these sites frequently for indications of infection, e.g., odor, redness, drainage. Take care that these stab wounds do not get wet, e.g., when bathing the patient. Opinions vary about the management of the insertion points. Some doctors cover the stab wounds with small sterile dressings and do not want the dressings to be disturbed unless there is evidence of infection. Therefore, do not change dressings or otherwise tend the wounds without specific orders. Some experts[139] state that infections may result from overzealous dressing and cleansing of these wounds and that daily wound inspections are not necessary. Others[123] emphasize that the areas around pins, wires, and tongs should be kept clean and dry and not be covered with collodion, dressings, or accumulations of serum exudate. Several sources recommend that each insertion point should be inspected daily and drainage should be aseptically removed by cleaning the site with solutions as specified by the surgeon. They maintain that if the opening to the insertion tract becomes sealed off (e.g., with accumulations of drainage), an ideal medium is developed within the tract for the growth of bacteria. Infection may then proceed inward internally along the tract and affect the bone.

Also, to prevent infection, instruct the patient who has skeletal traction not to touch the skin around the insertion points of wires, pins, or tongs.

When a skeletal wire (or pin) is to be removed, prepare the surrounding skin according to the physician's instructions. Iodine, alcohol, and ether may be used to sterilize the exposed wire end on the outer portion of the limb. The physician then removes the wire by (a) depressing the skin around that end of the wire and cutting the wire beneath the surface of the skin; and then (b) pulling the wire through from the opposite side of the limb. The insertion and exit incisions on the skin may then be covered with small sterile dressings.

Specific Types of Traction

PELVIC TRACTION. A pelvic traction belt or bilateral Buck's extension (see below) may be used to relieve low back pain which is not caused by spinal fracture or dislocation. (Spinal injuries are discussed in Unit VIII.) While these forms of traction do not apply adequate force to directly affect the paravertebral muscles or the vertebral articulations, they may bring relief from pain by keeping the patient recumbent and relatively inactive through enforced bedrest. The patient must be kept in straight alignment with the traction so the force will be effectively applied.

Pelvic traction (see Fig. 88–15) is accomplished with an encircling device, i.e., a belt applied just above and surrounding the iliac crests. The belt is attached to a spreader bar and pulley system. Traction is applied to the lumbar spine. Note in Figure 88–15 that the backrest is slightly elevated and the hamstring muscles are relaxed by placing pillows beneath the knees. Some physicians do not use pillows beneath the legs, but instead elevate the foot of the bed in a gatch position. If the backrest is excessively elevated, the patient will slide

down in bed. An overhead trapeze is generally provided so the patient can lift himself up. The pelvic belt must fit snugly to secure adequate traction. Pelvic traction should not increase a patient's back or leg pain. If it does so, notify the physician.

BUCK'S EXTENSION. This is a relatively simple form of skin traction which exerts a straight pull on the affected leg. One or both legs may be put in Buck's extension, depending upon the requirements of a given patient. Buck's extension may be used to immobilize a limb for a short time (e.g., a fractured hip prior to internal surgical fixation) or to reduce muscle spasm. Other uses include treatment of arthritis, hip dislocations, tuberculosis of the hip, pelvic injuries, and fractures of the upper or lower leg. Persons for whom Buck's extension is *contraindicated* include those with allergies to adhesive tape; diabetic gangrene; stasis dermatitis; arteriosclerosis; or serious varicosities or varicose ulcers. Buck's extension can be applied only in amounts of traction which the skin can safely tolerate. These relatively small amounts of weight are inadequate to treat some conditions, e.g., fractures with extensive overriding of bone fragments. In such situations, the patient must be treated by other means, e.g., another form of traction (skeletal traction) which can exert greater amounts of force.

Buck's extension (see Fig. 88–16) can be applied in varying ways. Details of application can be found in many of the reference sources listed at the end of this unit. Essentially the application of Buck's extension is as follows: (a) the skin is prepared according to the physician's instructions; (b) traction strips are smoothly applied to the

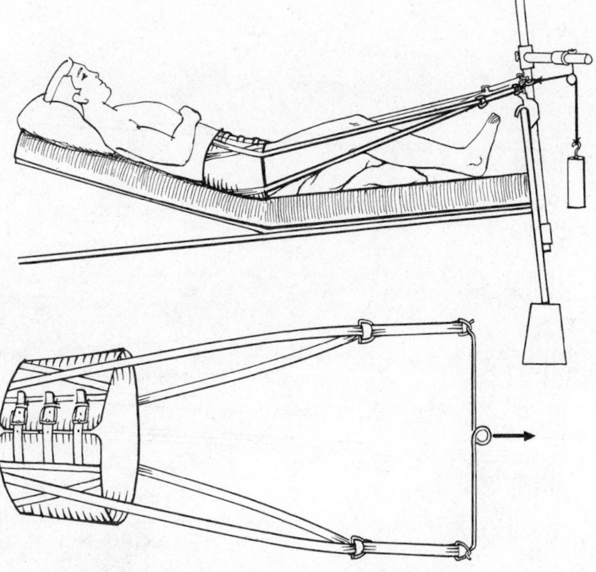

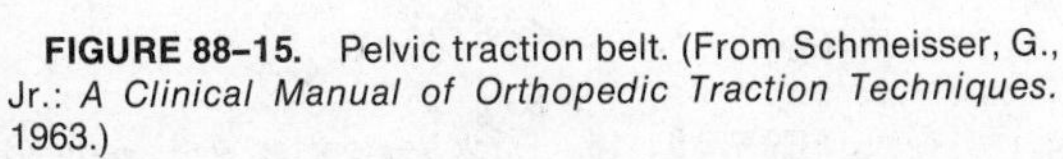

FIGURE 88–15. Pelvic traction belt. (From Schmeisser, G., Jr.: *A Clinical Manual of Orthopedic Traction Techniques.* 1963.)

lateral and medial aspects of the thigh and leg; (c) the strips are secured in place by smoothly bandaging the leg with elastic bandage or circular gauze; (d) the ends of the strips (which extend beyond the foot) are attached to a spreader or footplate; and (e) the traction rope (with its system of pulleys and weights) is attached to the spreader or footplate. Countertraction may be obtained by elevating the foot of the bed.

During application of the traction strips, the knee may be held slightly flexed to prevent hyperextension when the traction is applied. If the strip or bandages cover the head of the fibula (on the lateral side of the leg), the area is protectively padded before it is covered to prevent damage to the peroneal nerve, which is close to the surface of the leg in this region.

The traction strips are not attached to the skin over the malleoli or the foot, but rather they extend unattached from a point above the malleoli on down past the foot to the spreader. If the traction strips are made of an adhesive substance, the sticky side of the tape is covered with another piece of the material (sticky side to sticky side) to prevent the strip from adhering to the malleolar region or the foot.

Spreader bars or blocks (sometimes blocks of wood are used for spreaders) must be of correct width. If spreaders are too narrow, the traction tapes will rub against adjacent areas of skin, e.g., malleoli. If spreaders are too wide, they will pull the traction tapes away from the skin.

BRYANT'S TRACTION. This form of skin traction is occasionally used to reduce fractured femurs or to reduce hip dislocations in very young children. Bryant's traction (also called "gallows traction") is a *dangerous* type of traction in which both of the child's legs are suspended vertically, with the hips flexed at 90° and the knees extended. The buttocks just clear the bed. Owing to the hazards associated with Bryant's traction, it is seldom used today. Because of the position of the legs, Bryant's traction compromises circulation, and also it may damage the popliteal vessels (posterior to the knee) by hyperextending the knees. Currently Bryant's traction is sometimes used in very young infants as a primary stage of reducing dislocated hips. (Management of hip dislocations and other orthopedic disorders affecting children is discussed in pediatric nursing textbooks.)

RUSSELL'S TRACTION. This form of traction is frequently used in treatment of fracture of the shaft of the femur. Also, it is sometimes applied bilaterally to treat low back pain. It may be applied as either skin or skeletal traction. Skin traction may adequately treat femoral fractures in children; however, adults usually require skeletal traction. Russell's traction creates a forward and upward pull on the leg by applying vertical traction at the knee at the same time a horizontal force is exerted on the tibia and fibula. The knee joint can be bent and the patient can move about with relative ease with Russell's traction.

The patient lies supine with his hip and knee moderately flexed. The lower leg should remain parallel to the floor. If skin traction is used it is applied to the lower leg (beginning just below the head of the fibula to prevent peroneal nerve damage) as with Buck's extension. If skeletal traction is used it is applied with a wire or pin through the calcaneus ("heel bone"). This applies force along the long axis of the leg. This distal femur may then be brought anterior by either (a) placing a sling under the distal thigh (or behind the knee); or (b) inserting a pin in the distal femur. Russell's traction apparatus may be set up with either a single pulley to apply traction to both the heel and distal femur (called "single Russell's") or a double system of independent pulleys. With the latter method, called a "split Russell's," one pulley arrangement applies force on the heel and the other governs the distal femur. The knee gatch is raised and the lower leg may be supported on a pillow with the heel protected. Some physicians place a thin pillow lengthwise under the thigh. A countertraction force may not

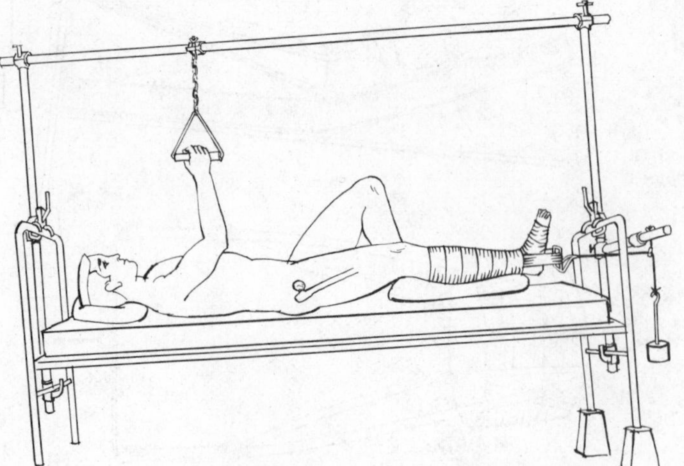

FIGURE 88–16. Buck's extension with overhead trapeze. (From Schmeisser, G., Jr.: *A Clinical Manual of Orthopedic Traction Techniques.* 1963.)

be required, but if it is it can be obtained by elevation of the foot of the bed on shock blocks.

With Russell's traction the peroneal area is exposed, but the popliteal area may be subjected to pressure. If the sling is applied behind the knee or if it impinges on the popliteal area, precautions must be taken to prevent pressure damage. A heavy piece of felt (covered with stockinette) may be placed in the sling as protective padding. Check the popliteal area daily for indications of skin damage, and report abnormal findings to the physician. Also, pressure on the popliteal vessels and immobility can cause thrombophlebitis. Notify the physician immediately of indications of this complication. Provide a foot support to prevent foot drop.

It is important that the patient not move up or down in bed because such movements alter the direction of the proximal pulley system (and hence the result and force). Note the patient's position in bed when the traction is first applied and periodically check his position so the original position can be maintained.[221] When moving the patient up in bed do not lift the weights. Pulling the patient up in bed against the pull of the traction does not increase the traction on the legs or produce pain; rather, the amount of pull remains constant.[123] Elevation of the head of the bed reduces the amount of traction; however, the physician may give permission for the head of the bed to be slightly elevated. Find out precisely the maximum amount of elevation permitted.

RING LEG SPLINTS; PEARSON ATTACHMENT. Various ring leg splints are available, e.g., Thomas, Hodgen, Keller-Blake. The original ring leg splint was the *Thomas splint*. A Thomas splint in balanced traction with a Pearson attachment is illustrated in Figure 88–18.

The Thomas splint may be applied either in balanced or fixed traction, and may be used alone or in combination with a Pearson attachment. A Thomas splint consists of (a) two rods on either side of the limb, which converge distally to conform to the limb; (b) a large ring which connects the two rods proximally and encircles the upper thigh when in place; and (c) a crossbar which connects the two rods distally. The crossbar is located beyond the foot when the splint is in place. Thomas splints are available with either full rings or half-rings. When a half-ring Thomas splint is used, the ring portion is placed over the anterior thigh. Thus, the patient does not have to sit on the ring. Separate Thomas splints are available for use on the right or left legs.

Thomas splints may be used (a) to *immediately* splint and *temporarily* immobilize femoral and humeral fractures; and (b) for the *long-term* management of femoral fractures. A Thomas splint extends from the groin to beyond the foot, in a straight line from the femur.

Before a Thomas splint (or one of its variations) is applied, slings are attached to the splint rods to support the leg. Slings may be made of strips of muslin or canvas; they must not slide or stretch when the splint is in place. The sling material must be smooth to prevent skin pressure damage from wrinkles.

A Thomas splint makes it possible to maintain two separate lines of pull on the same extremity, e.g., fractures can be aligned in the femur as well as the lower leg of the same extremity. With "fixed" traction, the distal end of the Thomas (or Keller-Blake splint) is attached to a fixed point at the foot of the bed and does not move with the patient.

Attachment of a *Pearson attachment* to a straight ring splint makes it possible to flex the knee and move the lower leg if desirable. Slight flexion of the knee prevents subsequent joint instability by preventing stretching of the posterior knee capsule and ligaments. With balanced suspension traction, the knee can be moved actively and passively if the physician desires.

A Pearson attachment looks like a small Thomas splint, except that instead of having a proximal ring, the proximal end of the rods each have a clamp. The Pearson attachment is fastened to the

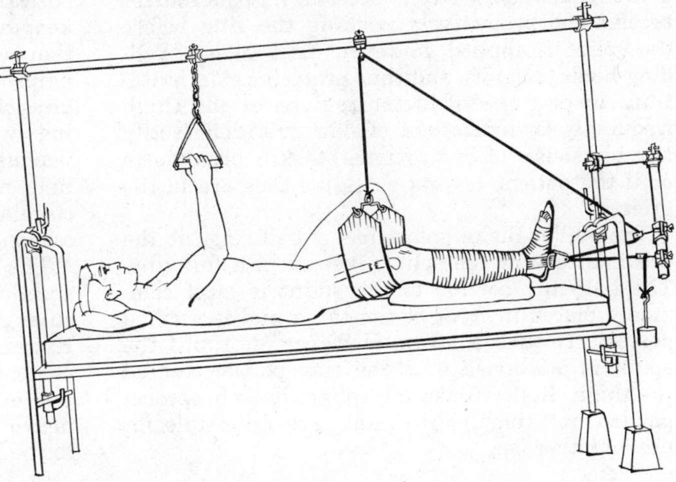

FIGURE 88–17. Russell's skin traction (single) with overhead frame and trapeze. (From Schmeisser, G., Jr.: *A Clinical Manual of Orthopedic Traction Techniques.* 1963.)

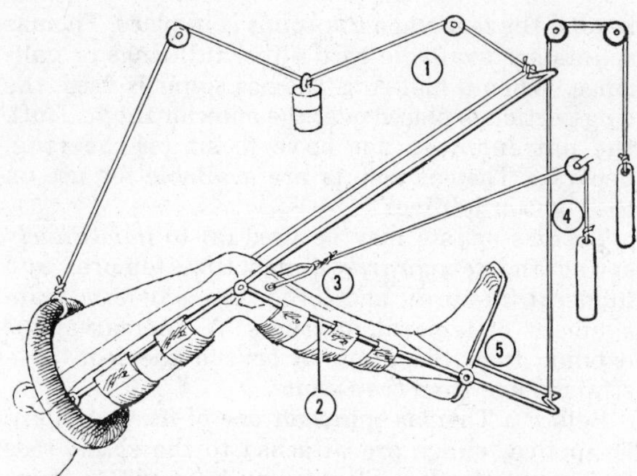

FIGURE 88–18. Thomas splint with Pearson attachment using balanced suspension traction. 1, The limb is suspended in balance in a Thomas splint by a system of cords and weights. 2, A Pearson attachment permits motion of cords and weights designed to exert continuous traction in the line of the femur. 5, Foot plate (this is essential to prevent footdrop). (From DePalma, A. F.: *The Management of Fractures and Dislocations*. Vol. 1. 2nd ed. 1970.)

Thomas splint at the patient's knee joint by fastening these clamps onto the rods of the Thomas splint. Hinges are built into the clamps. Thus the Pearson attachment can move independently of the long leg splint.

Typically the Thomas splint is elevated at a 45° angle to the bed and the leg is flexed at 45°.[139] The lower leg rests horizontal to the mattress in the Pearson attachment. A Thomas splint with a Pearson attachment may be used with either skin or skeletal traction. Sometimes Buck's extension is applied below the knee. The ring of a Thomas splint must fit snugly in the perineum (against the ischium); however, it should not cause excessive pressure in the groin. The ring makes it difficult for the patient to use a bed pan and keep the ring dry. Frequent skin care is necessary. Some sources recommend protectively padding the ring before the splint is applied; however, most do not. Padding holds moisture and thus promotes skin irritation. Inspect the adductor regions of the thigh frequently for indications of skin irritation. Notify the physician of indications of skin breakdown or if the patient reports excessive pressure in the groin.

The Keller-Blake splint has a half-ring, at the proximal end of the splint, instead of a full ring. The half-ring portion of the splint is most commonly placed in front of the thigh and is secured posteriorly with a strap. However, at times the splint is positioned with the ring portion behind the thigh. Keller-Blake leg splints have neoprene-padded half-rings. The splints are reversible for use on either leg.

Complications. Prime goals in the care of any patient in traction are to prevent complications which (a) can develop from prolonged immobility and recumbency; and (b) can result from the traction equipment being used. Details about complications of immobility (their development, recognition, and prevention) are presented in Unit V, Chapter 27. Traction equipment can produce complications similar to those which may result from casting, e.g., skin breakdown, neurovascular damage. These complications and their recognition are discussed in detail earlier in this chapter. Refer back to these previous discussions as necessary.

Summarized below are some of the potential complications which may develop in a patient immobilized by traction:

- Hypostatic pneumonia; atelectasis.
- Constipation; fecal impaction; abdominal distention.
- Urine retention; kidney stones.
- Impaired circulation; edema; thrombophlebitis; phlebothrombosis; emboli, e.g., pulmonary embolism, fat embolism (see below).
- Disorientation (see Unit III).
- Nerve damage; motor weakness or paralysis; foot drop; wrist drop.
- Hyperextension of the knee; outward rotation of the leg.
- Disuse osteoporosis; muscle atrophy; contractures; joint stiffness.
- Wound infection, e.g., with skeletal traction, infected decubitus ulcers, or infection in traumatic open wounds or surgical incisions.

The patient in traction is given intensive *preventative care* and is *evaluated frequently* for indications of developing complications. Symptoms indicative of complications are promptly reported to the physician, so *early* treatment can be started.

Investigate all *symptoms indicative of developing complications and all complaints stated by a patient in traction.*

Various techniques of pulmonary physiotherapy and respiratory therapy are used to prevent respiratory complications in the patient immobilized by traction (see Unit XIV, Ch. 70). These activities, e.g., breathing exercises, IPPB treatments, are basically directed at promoting lung expansion and keeping the tracheobronhcial tree free of secretion accumulation. Maintaining a high fluid intake helps prevent problems with elimination. Some physicians have their patients wear elastic stockings while in traction to help prevent problems of venous stasis in the legs. Therapeutic exercises help minimize disuse osteoporosis and stimulate circulation. Additionally, exercises combat muscle atrophy, contractures, and joint stiffness.

The patient in traction requires frequent inspections to identify skin breakdown or neurovascular damage or both. Skin care is discussed below. Extremities in either skin or skeletal traction are particularly vulnerable to neurovascular damage. For example, as mentioned previously, peroneal nerve damage may occur with traction applied to the leg, e.g., Buck's extension.

Below is a summary of some areas which may be subjected to pressure (and hence develop pressure damage to skin or nerves) during therapeutic traction of particular extremities or body areas.

1. Pressure areas in traction of arm:

> Axilla.
> Anterior soft tissues of elbow joint.
> Bony prominences around elbow, e.g., olecranon, lateral epicondyle, medial epicondyle.
> Bony prominences around wrist, e.g., styloid process of ulna.
> Dorsum of hand.
> Volar (palm) surface at base of hand.

2. Pressure areas in traction of leg:

> Greater trochanter (upper outer thighs).
> Popliteal space; hamstring tendons at back of knee.
> Outer aspect of head of fibula (lateral upper calf) where peroneal nerve is superficial.
> Bony prominences around ankle, e.g., lateral malleolus, medial malleolus, Achilles tendon.
> Back of heels.
> Soft tissues at front of ankle and top of foot.

3. Pressure areas in traction of trunk:

> Borders of scapulae (shoulder blades).
> Prominences of spine.
> Iliac crests (upper edges of pelvic bones.
> Sacral areas (tail bone).

To detect neurovascular damage examine distal portions of extremities in traction for symptoms such as coolness, swelling, discoloration, paralysis, or anesthesia. Ask the patient if he is experiencing pain or paresthesias. (See previous discussion of cast complications.) Circular bandages must be carefully applied in such a manner that they will not become excessively tight. Pressure points need ample protective padding. Rewrap circular elastic bandages periodically as specified by the physician. These bandages easily wrinkle and become misplaced.

If symptoms of neurovascular damage appear in an extremity in skin traction and you cannot contact the doctor and do not have permission to unwrap the bandages, do as follows: (a) snip the bandage at the point of pressure; (b) anchor the traction above (to maintain the pull of traction); and (c) notify the doctor of the situation and your actions as soon as he can be reached.[123]

Observe wrapped extremities for indications of constriction due to swelling. Swelling is most likely to occur during the first 24-48 hours following fracture. The toes or fingers should be visible for observation. Indications of constriction were discussed in detail in the section on cast complications.

Skin Care. The patient in traction is highly susceptible to skin breakdown because he is usually not permitted to turn off his back or have traction released. The underside of the body is thus subjected to sustained pressure for a prolonged period, and skin care is difficult to administer effectively. *Skin care must be given frequently.* Check with the physician concerning the positions which a given patient may safely assume for skin care. If the patient is permitted to turn slightly, this facilitates giving skin care. If he cannot turn, skin care may be given while the patient raises himself for brief periods by using an overhead trapeze. Similarly, bed linens can be smoothed and changed, or the bed pan may be placed or removed while the patient lifts himself up with a trapeze.

A patient should not try to hold himself up with a trapeze for such long periods of time that he becomes fatigued. Instead, he should raise himself for shorter periods more frequently. Instruct the patient to lift himself up periodically merely to "rest" his buttocks and permit circulation to enter the compressed areas of skin on which he is lying most of the time. Remember it will take a while for some patients (e.g., elderly persons) to learn how to use trapezes effectively. They will gradually develop the muscular skills, strength, and coordination needed to lift themselves up with their arms. Some patients need assistance and support while lifting themselves.

When a patient is first learning to use a trapeze, instruct him to grasp the bar firmly and lift himself *straight up* off the bed. The body should not be twisted sideways. Teach the patient to place his feet (or uninjured foot) *flat* on the bed to help push himself up while pulling on the trapeze. Discourage pushing with the back of the heels, since these areas can develop pressure and friction damage. Synchronize your movements to those made by the patient, e.g., when he raises up, reach under the buttocks and give skin care.

Often skin care can most effectively be given to a patient in traction by two persons working together. One person may help the patient lift himself up on a trapeze and help hold him in an elevated position, while the other gives skin care. If the patient requires no lifting assistance, the two attendants can give skin care from either side and thereby speed up the process. If a patient cannot use a trapeze, one person presses down on the mattress while the other gives skin care by sliding her hand under the patient.

Periodically use a flashlight to inspect the skin on the patient's back and buttocks while he lifts himself up. A mirror will help you inspect areas difficult to view directly. Look for indications of skin pressure or breakdown. Give extra skin care to areas which show indications of developing complications. While giving care inspect the patient's skin carefully with your hands. Development of an increased acuteness of your sense of touch will help you to locate lesions which you cannot see and to detect crumbs and wrinkles in bed linens. Ask the patient to report wrinkles or other sources of irritation and pressure which he feels beneath him.

Immediately report if the patient notices paresthesias, burning, or pain under skin traction bandages.

Skin breakdown may result from contact of the skin with the traction equipment (e.g., bows, spreader blocks, ropes) or may result from irritation caused by friction against bedding, traction tapes, or bandages. Pressure necrosis may develop rapidly. Inspect skin at the edges of traction strips. Examine areas covered with adhesive materials or bandages for indications of skin necrosis or infection. Look for drainage through adhesive dressings and elastic bandages and smell the areas to detect odors indicative of infection and drainage.

Meticulous preventative skin care is required for areas of skin which are in contact with adhesive bandages or other pieces of traction equipment, especially when contact occurs over pressure points. The nurse should familiarize herself with areas of potential skin damage associated with specific types of traction. For example, the ring of a Thomas splint may traumatize skin in the groin and gluteal fold. Skin traction applied to the lower leg may cause damage to skin on the ankle malleoli. When skin traction is applied to the leg, look for pressure over the dorsum of the foot and the heel if bandages or tapes appear loose. The traction weights may pull the bandages or tapes down in these areas and cause pressure damage to the skin.

The patient with one leg in traction may develop skin breakdown on the heel of his other foot if he pushes with this heel when he lifts himself up in bed. A patient's elbows may become sore from rubbing on the sheets during attempts to push himself up. Use of an overhead trapeze helps the patient lift himself without pushing on his elbows. Remember to frequently examine and give appropriate skin care to *all* pressure points upon which the patient rests while recumbent, e.g., back of the head, shoulder blades, elbows, iliac crests, sacrum, back of the heels. Cleanse the fingers or toes of extremities which are in traction. (For details of care to prevent skin damage in an immobilized patient, review Chapter 27, Unit V.)

Bedding. Without interfering with the effectiveness of the traction it is often desirable to cover an affected limb (or limbs) to prevent chilling. This may be accomplished in various ways, e.g., wrapping the limb in cotton batting or a lightweight blanket. Coverings should not press on the footplate with leg traction. Make certain that ropes and pulleys are free of bedclothes. Split linens, which fit around the top of an extremity in traction, can be used to keep the rest of the patient's body warm. Linen changes can be made either by working from the top toward the bottom of the bed or by working from the unaffected side toward the affected side. Be careful not to jerk the patient by catching linens on the traction equipment.

Positioning; Turning; Release of Traction. Check the doctor's orders to determine if a patient can turn or if traction can be removed periodically. Also, identify contraindicated positions.

> *Never lift or change traction weights without a doctor's orders. Do not remove traction or increase or decrease the amount of the weights without specific orders.*

With the physician's permission some patients, e.g., with arthritis or low back pain, are permitted to be relieved of traction for short periods. Patients with pelvic traction, for example, may have bathroom privileges. However, continuous traction is necessary with other disorders, e.g., when traction is being employed to immobilize a new fracture. If the doctor states that the traction may be removed periodically, lift and reapply weights gently so the patient is not subjected to the sudden release from traction or to the sudden reapplication of tension. Always tell the patient when you are going to remove or reapply the tension. Never "drop" a weight when reapplying traction, but gradually lower the weight so the patient does not undergo sudden, extreme stress.

> *Never change the heights of elevating blocks ("shock blocks"), knee rests, or backrests of patients in traction without the physician's permission.*

A patient in traction should not roll over onto his sides or have the position of his bed changed without his physician's permission. Twisting, turning movements disturb the alignment of body structures being immobilized by the traction. Turning on the side changes the line of pull even with balanced traction.

Some patients in traction are restricted in the amount the headrest can be elevated, since raising the head of the bed disrupts the line of pull in arm and cervical traction and the amount of pull in leg traction. Changing the position of the bed (e.g., elevating the backrest of a patient who has been kept in a flat position) may make effective traction impossible by disrupting the line of the pull. If elevation of the headrest is permitted, the physician should specify how far the bed can be elevated and still maintain adequate countertraction. Raising and lowering the headrest (when permitted) not only increases the patient's comfort but also minimizes pulmonary complications by promoting drainage of the tracheobronchial tree. A patient who may have his headrest up and down at his request should be positioned *completely flat* at least half the time to prevent hip flexion contractures. Explain the importance of this positioning to the patient to enlist his cooperation. With many types of traction, hip flexion contractures are also prevented by maintaining 20° of hip flexion between the thigh and the bed.

If the doctor gives permission for the patient to turn slightly (e.g., for back care and linen changes), make certain you know which side he may turn toward, e.g., the patient with a fracture may be permitted to turn slightly toward the side of the fracture. With the physician's permission a patient with a limb in traction may be turned slightly toward the limb which is in traction. Turning away from the traction set-up would obviously not be possible. A patient in traction cannot assume a prone position unless he is on an orthopedic frame or CircOlectric bed.

When the patient moves about (e.g., lifts himself up by the trapeze, turns for back care, or slides up in bed), someone should steady the traction equipment while another person assists the patient or provides other care, e.g., places a bed pan or gives skin care. In some cases it is advisable to manually exert a slight pull on the traction during these times. As mentioned before, suspension traction maintains the affected limb in good alignment when the patient lifts himself up (e.g., with a trapeze) and thus may permit greater activity.

Help the patient to be as comfortable as possible while he is on his back. Even slight changes of position can be relaxing. Make frequent evaluations of the patient's position in bed and his body alignment. The patient should be centered in the bed. If he slips toward the pull of the traction, he must be repositioned or the effectiveness of the traction may be compromised, e.g., footplates or spreaders may be pulled against the foot of the bed or against pulleys.

Some patients in traction should not be pulled up in bed since movement alters the traction pull. For example, a patient with arm traction cannot be moved up in bed once traction is applied. Thus, he must be properly centered in the bed (e.g., so his hips and knees fit the gatched areas of the bed) *before* traction is applied. Position must subsequently be checked periodically. If repositioning in the bed is necessary, it must be done with the physician's help. We have mentioned previously that bed position must also be precisely maintained with Russell's traction.

Maintain correct body alignment and effective traction. Exercise special precautions to prevent foot drop. When traction is applied to a leg, a foot plate may be applied to prevent foot drop. An alternative method of preventing the equinus position is the application of a wide strip of adhesive tape to the bottom of the foot. The free end of the tape extends beyond the toes and may then be attached to a small rope, pulley, and weight (or to another piece of the traction apparatus) to hold the foot upright. Prevent rotation of the leg and splint. The leg should not rub against the rods of the splint. The heel should not rest on the bed or pressure necrosis will develop. Sometimes the foot is left free for exercising.

Remember to care properly for extremities which are *not* in traction as well as those which are immobilized. For example, keep *both* legs in straight alignment; prevent hyperextension in both knees; and maintain both feet in a natural position (without inward or outward rotation). If the patient appears to be developing abnormalities (e.g., hip flexion contractures, hyperextension of the knee, foot drop, wrist drop), take appropriate corrective action and call the defect to the attention of the doctor. If a patient's leg is in traction, his foot should never rest against the foot of the bed. This prevents effective traction.

Often it is difficult to place a patient on the bed pan while he is in traction. As discussed, the foot of the bed may be elevated for countertraction. This elevation causes expelled liquids to tend to run up beneath the patient while he is on the bed pan. Another problem is that the patient must be kept in proper alignment while on the bed pan and while moving off the bed pan.

When possible, a *fracture bed pan* (i.e., a small, flat bed pan with a tapering slope from front to back) is used for a patient in traction. However, a large bed pan is necessary for enemas. Some women can void into a female urinal or kidney basin. The patient will be more comfortable on a bed pan if a folded bath blanket or small plastic-covered pillow is placed at his lower back to slightly elevate that area. Placement of a pad behind the bed pan prevents expelled liquids from running up the patient's back. When permitted, placing a pillow under the back and shoulders keeps the patient more level with the bed pan. The physician may permit the backrest to be elevated slightly for bed pan use. Place and remove the bed pan carefully so you do not traumatize the skin on the buttocks or spill contents of the pan. Damp linens under the patient must be immediately removed and replaced with clean ones, since dampness promotes maceration of the skin.

Patients with injuries which prevent use of an overhead trapeze (e.g., upper extremity injuries, spinal injuries) or which make it difficult to place a bed pan (e.g., unstable pelvic fractures) may be placed on special orthopedic frames (Bradford frames) which have an opening for placement of a bed pan beneath the patient without lifting him. If the patient can use a trapeze, the bed pan is placed and removed while the patient raises his hips off the mattress.

Do not place any pillows under a limb in traction without the permission of the physician. If pillows are permitted, the doctor should place them the first time so the limb is positioned as he wants it, with effective traction. Some physicians do not want *any* pillows placed under a limb in traction because they believe it increases the chances of thrombosis. If pillows are used they should be firm so they will provide adequate support and will maintain alignment of the limb with the traction apparatus. Do not support just a portion of an extremity, but rather provide support along its entire length. When placing a pillow under the lower leg, make certain the heel is free of the bed. Elevation of the heel should not hyperextend the knee.

Exercises. Consult with the physician concerning exercises for a patient in traction. Maintenance of general muscle tone and joint mobility not only prevents complications but also speeds up the patient's rehabilitative progress once the traction is removed and mobility is permitted. Commonly the physician advises the patient to put every joint (except those immediately above and below fractures) through a full range of motion several times each day. Deep breathing exercises and abdominal setting exercises are routinely instituted as soon as the patient is placed in traction. The patient is often placed on an exercise program that will prepare him for crutch walking if indicated. (See discussions of exercises and of crutches earlier in this chapter.) Typically when pain and swelling are sufficiently reduced, the physician permits muscle-setting exercises (e.g., quadriceps setting) over the injured part of an extremity, and once callus formation is visible on x-ray, limited range of motion exercises are initiated in the joints immediately above and below fractures. Since one advantage of traction is that it may permit greater movement of the affected limb, the amount of exercise advised by the physician should be performed.

Other exercises may include gluteal tightening; push-up exercises with the arms (while sitting up); ankle exercises (e.g., foot circling); and flexion and extension exercises of the unaffected leg. The patient in leg traction often tends to lie with his unaffected leg flexed. To prevent shortening of the flexors he should be reminded to exercise this leg and to extend it periodically.

Self-care and Diversion. Lying on one's back in traction is tiring, and the patient usually welcomes diversion, e.g., visitors, occupational therapy projects, visits from the staff or patients. Television sets may be elevated so they can be viewed while the patient remains on his back. The use of prism glasses may enable the patient to read more easily while flat. Also, mirrors may be placed in ways which help enlarge the patient's view of his surroundings. The patient's immediate environment should be kept neat and attractive.

Prolonged immobilization may induce disorientation in some patients, especially older persons. Prolonged immobilization also fosters discouragement, depression, and difficulty sleeping at night. Evaluate the patient's mental attitude and sensorium periodically. Inform the physician if a patient appears disoriented or seriously depressed, or if he is sleeping poorly (see Unit III). Make every attempt to keep the patient meaningfully involved in daily activities. If the patient remains awake during the day, he may be able to sleep for longer periods at night.

Encourage self-care as much as possible for a patient in traction, since it provides stimulation and exercise. The patient should do as much of his bath as he can and any other self-care activities, e.g., feeding, exercises. Explain to the patient that self-care is an important part of his treatment and that you are not having him do things for himself simply to reduce the work load of the staff. Place items which the patient may require within easy reach and make sure he has a call bell at all times to summon help as needed. Consciously strive to minimize the discomforts of the dependency which traction imposes on a patient. Attempt to anticipate the patient's needs, e.g., it may be difficult to cut food while lying flat. Also, teach the patient ways of helping himself.

Removal from Traction. When the patient is finally removed from traction he will probably find that he is quite weak and possibly unsteady. If a limb has been immobilized in traction, it may show some muscle atrophy (appear thin) and be weak and unstable. Additionally, orthostatic hypotension is commonly present if the patient has been in a head-lowered position. To combat hypotension the patient is helped to gradually resume a sitting (and later standing) position. The head of the bed is elevated progressively higher. Raising the bed to a full sitting position may require several sessions. Physical support is given when the patient first sits on the edge of the bed or moves out of bed. Safety precautions, such as supporting the patient until you are confident that he can support and balance himself, can prevent falls which may otherwise result from weakness or faintness.

Before the traction is finally released, the patient should be told how he might expect to feel once the traction is released. Explanations should be given about why the patient may feel faint or weak, and why his joints may be stiff or unstable. The physician's plan for rehabilitative activities (to help regain strength and function) is discussed with the patient and reassurances are given that after following the prescribed exercise-activity program for a while the patient soon should feel stronger. The physician should talk with the patient about activities and movements which are permitted and those which are contraindicated. Weakened limbs may require support at the joints. Crutches may be required for a while.

Orthopedic Surgery

While the majority of orthopedic patients can be treated successfully without surgery, many do undergo surgery. Orthopedic surgical procedures are usually not emergency surgeries but rather are performed electively. Thus, there is usually time to prepare patients physically and psychologically for surgical experiences.

Giving patients and their families appropriate *psychologic support* pre- and postoperatively is an integral aspect of the clinical care provided with orthopedic surgery. Prior to surgery some patients have had long, fatiguing, painful periods of illness. For example, some patients with degenerative joint diseases may be ill for long periods before reconstructive surgery is performed. Commonly such persons face surgery with mixed feelings of hope and dread. They are hopeful that surgery will reduce their pains and increase their mobility; they are fearful that surgery will merely add to their burdens of suffering and disability.

Physician and nurse attempt to realistically discuss with patients the expectations of surgical procedures and to help patients adjust their lifestyles to accommodate permanent disabilities when necessary. Patients who have required numerous operations may well be discouraged and depressed as they face still other procedures. Financial concerns may also be overwhelming. Some orthopedic surgical procedures cause significant changes in body image which may be difficult for patients to accept (see Unit III). In addition to providing direct patient care services during pre- and postoperative periods, the nurse also provides indirect services by helping to refer patients to other persons who are qualified to give specialized help, e.g., social workers, psychiatrists, clergy.

As with any surgery, patients should be told preoperatively how they can expect to feel and where they can expect to be when they awaken from general anesthesia, e.g., "You will awaken in a recovery room with a cast on your arm. A nurse will be nearby to help you as you need her."

Preoperative Preparation. The general preparation of a patient for surgery is discussed in Unit VI. This discussion focuses specifically on preparation for othopedic surgery.

Pre- and postoperatively it is important to maintain adequate levels of hydration in patients immobilized for prolonged periods. Adequate hydration helps prevent some complications of immobility, e.g., renal complications (see Unit V, Ch. 27).

Preoperatively, antibiotics may be ordered for some patients, e.g., those with a history of osteomyelitis. Other preoperative orders typically include orders to increase fluid and carbohydrate intake and orders for preoperative skin preparation and sedation. Barbiturates may be ordered the evening before surgery or the morning of surgery. Breakfast is withheld prior to general anesthesia. While inhalation anesthesia is commonly used for orthopedic procedures, in some cases spinal, rectal, or local anesthesia may be employed. A mild cathartic or enema may or may not be ordered preoperatively.

In addition to ordering routine preoperative laboratory tests (e.g., urinalysis, bleeding and clotting time, blood count, Hgb estimation), the orthopedic surgeon may also order evaluations of the blood sedimentation rate and serum calcium, phosphorus, and phosphatase.[139] The latter tests are useful in evaluating metabolic bone changes. Many diseases of coagulation cause joint disorders. Bleeding tendencies must be carefully evaluated preoperatively in the presence of such joint disorders.

Prior to orthopedic surgery special precautions are taken to minimize the possibility of postoperative infection. Bone is more susceptible to infection than soft tissue. If infection of the bone, i.e., osteomyelitis, develops, it is difficult to treat and may result in permanent disability, e.g., chronic infection or stiffness of the joint. Also, in the presence of infection, bone union will not occur. To prevent infection, careful attention must be given to preoperative skin preparation, operating room technique, and postoperative dressing changes and reinforcements.

While specific preoperative skin preparation procedures for orthopedic surgery may vary from place to place, the underlying principles are similar. Orthopedic skin "preps" are meticulously performed in a nontraumatic manner. If ordered, cleansing enemas are given prior to skin preparation. Skin "preps" may be performed in the patient's room, emergency room, or operating room. Final preparation of the operative site is always carried out in the operative suite.

Specific procedures for preparing the operative site and the antiseptic solutions used vary, depending upon the surgeon's preferences and hospital policies. In the recent past 72- or 48-hour sterile orthopedic skin preparations were commonly performed. Currently these practices are being replaced by less rigorous preparations, e.g., mild soap and water scrubs followed by careful skin shaving or preps similar to those used for general surgery. The surgeon's preoperative skin preparation orders are carefully followed.

When casted areas are to be operated on, it is usual for the cast to be removed several days before surgery. This allows adequate time for skin inspection and preparation. During skin preparation the skin is carefully inspected, and any skin lesions or abrasions observed are reported to the surgeon. If there are skin infections, the surgeon may postpone surgery until the infection has been adequately treated. Shaving is gently performed to prevent denuding or breaking of the skin and to ensure complete removal of hairs. Hair is difficult to disinfect. Time is spent removing grime from the hand or foot and thoroughly cleaning and then clipping the fingernails or toenails. It may be necessary to soak the hand or foot to clean it thoroughly. Persistent grime or evidence of lesions around the nails or both are reported to the surgeon.

In surgery, open traumatic wounds, e.g., compound fractures, are carefully cleansed since each is potentially contaminated. The prep is carried out under aseptic conditions (masks, sterile gowns, gloves) and is commonly performed by the surgeon. During the prep the open wound is covered with sterile gauze while the area surrounding the wound is cleansed with solutions. Care is taken to prevent the solutions used during this time from entering the open wound. After the surrounding area has been cleansed, the dressing is removed from the open wound, and fresh sterile solutions are used to flush the open wound of dirt, debris, and bacteria. Following preparation of the wound it is debrided, i.e., "dead" or devitalized tissue is removed. Thorough wound debridement and removal of every particle of foreign material is imperative to prevent postoperative infection. During bone surgery care is taken by the operative team to prevent tearing of their sterile gloves as they handle sharp bone fragments.

Orthopedic Surgical Procedures. Orthopedic surgical procedures may be performed to reconstruct or replace diseased or injured structures or to correct deformities. Orthopedic surgery encompasses a variety of specific surgical procedures, including reduction of fractures, reconstructive procedures, replacement procedures, tendon repair (realigning severed ends, lengthening, shortening, transferring). Orthopedic surgical procedures may be performed on bone or soft tissues. Examples of orthopedic bone procedures include arthrodesis, arthroplasty, arthrotomy, bone grafting, and osteotomy. Soft tissue surgical procedures include tendon transplantation, tendon lengthening, tenotomy, and capsulotomy.

Below are descriptions of some of the more common orthopedic procedures:

> *Tenotomy:* the cutting of a tendon, for example, to correct club foot.

> *Tendon lengthening:* procedure to lengthen a tendon without disrupting its continuity.

> *Tendon transplantation:* procedure by which a tendon from a normal muscle is moved to another location so it can assume the function of a damaged muscle.

> *Capsulotomy:* surgically incising a joint capsule.

> *Synovectomy:* excision of a synovial membrane, e.g., at the knee. May be used to treat arthritic joints.

> *Osteotomy:* cutting bone to correct bone or joint deformities.

> *Arthrotomy:* incising a joint for exploration or removal of diseased tissue.

> *Arthrodesis* (artificial ankylosis or fusion): repairing a joint by fusing the joint's surfaces. Fusing the bones together makes the joint permanently immobile. Such procedures may be used to treat spinal disorders, i.e., spinal fusion (see Unit VIII), or to stabilize painful joints or knee (Fig. 88–19) and ankle joints that have become unable to support weight. In the latter instances, arthrodesis minimizes pain caused by rubbing together of irritated joint surfaces, and it facilitates weight-bearing. Thus, arthrodesis commonly produces a stiff but stable and painless joint once the bones of the joint have fused, i.e., grown together. Frequently arthrodesis is accomplished surgically by removing the articular hyaline cartilage and placing bone grafts across the surface of the joint. In some instances metallic internal fixation devices are placed.

> *Arthrolysis:* loosening adhesions in an ankylosed (i.e., abnormally immobile) joint.

> *Arthroplasty:* plastic surgery on injured or diseased joints to reestablish a movable joint. Arthroplasties may be performed in differing ways, e.g., the bones of the joint may be surgically reshaped, and soft tissue or a metallic interposition device may be placed between the reshaped bone ends to help reestablish motion, or joints or parts of joints may be replaced with prostheses made of metal or other materials (see below).

> *Bone grafting:* pieces of cancellous or compact bone are surgically transplanted to other locations in the body. Grafts or transplants of bone may be (a) *autogenous,* i.e., obtained from the person into which they are being transplanted; (b) *homogenous,* i.e., obtained from another individual of the same species; or (c) heterogenous, i.e., obtained from animals of another species. Autogenous bone transplants are the most successful. Bone transplants or grafts may be used to (a) establish bony joint fusion; (b) fill in gaps or defects in bone; or (c) facilitate the healing of fractures which are difficult to heal otherwise.[85]

A variety of other surgical procedures may be used in orthopedic practice, e.g., *excision of calcium deposits* from joints, *removal of* the *tophi* (i.e., chalky deposits of urates) produced by gout, *excision of rheumatic nodules,* and surgical *removal of exostoses,* i.e., bony growths projecting outward from bone surfaces.

Reconstructive surgical procedures are commonly performed on persons beyond middle age. Degenerative bone and joint diseases, e.g., arthritis, cause pain and deformity by eliminating the smooth surfaces of bones inside joints. *Silastic implants* may be used to replace diseased knuckles. In the *hip* joint the head of a diseased femur may be replaced with a *prosthetic device.* Recently it has become possible to *replace the total hip,* i.e., the acetabulum as well as the head of the femur, with a Vitallium or other prosthesis. *Total knee and elbow replacements* can also be performed on selected patients, and replacement procedures on still other body parts are being done on a limited basis. Procedures such as these restore useful function and relieve pain.

During surgery implants are handled carefully.

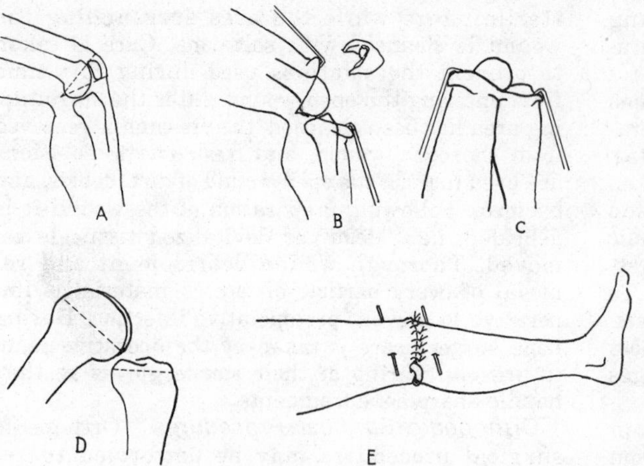

FIGURE 88–19. Steps in simple technique of knee fusion. *E* shows drain in place and pins in place for desired compression apparatus. (From Mead, N. C.: *Surgical Clinics of North America, 45*:208, 1965.)

Implants are subject to erosion postoperatively if they are marred or scratched when implanted.

Postoperative Care. General postoperative care is discussed in Unit VI. Following bone and joint surgery a prolonged period of immobilization is usually necessary to permit adequate healing. Immobilization may be achieved in various ways, e.g., special orthopedic frames (Stryker, Foster, CircOlectric beds), casts, or traction. Care of patients in casts and traction has been discussed in the preceding sections of this chapter. Management of pain following orthopedic surgery was discussed earlier in this unit. Muscle spasms may occur postoperatively following orthopedic procedures; see discussion earlier in this chapter.

As with any postoperative patient, much of the clinical care given the postoperative orthopedic patient is directed at *preventing complications* which may result from (a) the surgical procedure; (b) pre-illness pathology; or (c) immobilization. Since complications cannot always be prevented, the patient is closely observed for *early* indications of developing complications so that prompt treatment may be instituted. *Postoperative complications* to be watched for following orthopedic surgery include the following:

> *Shock.* As with other surgery, shock may occur during the early postoperative period. Patients especially prone to shock during surgery include (a) elderly hypertensive patients who have been on prolonged antihypertensive drug therapy; and (b) patients who have received corticosteroid therapy, e.g., persons with arthritis who are undergoing reconstructive joint procedures. It is important that a complete drug history be obtained preoperatively so adequate preventative precautions can be taken to ensure safety during and following surgery. (Shock is discussed in Unit V, Chapter 26.)

> *Thrombophlebitis* is indicated by such symptoms as pain, swelling, redness or heat in the extremity, e.g., calf of the leg. The common necessity for prolonged periods of immobilization, plus the nature of orthopedic surgical procedures, makes thrombophlebitis with subsequent pulmonary embolization a particularly common complication in postoperative orthopedic patients. Preventative actions are indicated pre- and postoperatively to reduce the likelihood of these serious complications. (Thrombophlebitis and pulmonary embolism are discussed in Unit XIII.)

> *Pulmonary embolism and fat embolism.* Fat embolism, i.e., embolism of a globule of fat, may follow bone surgery or bone injuries, e.g., multiple long bone fractures. (Fat embolism following fracture is discussed in Chapter 89. Treatment is also briefly discussed in that section. See also Unit XIII.) Symptoms of fat embolism vary depending upon the area in which the embolus lodges, whether in the brain or lung or peripherally. Indications of cerebral fat embolism may include pupillary changes, muscular twitching, and altered states of consciousness (see Unit VIII). Among the symptoms of fat embolism in the lungs are tachycardia; pallor followed by cyanosis; hypoxia; petechiae over the chest and shoulders; disorientation; and rapid, dyspneic breathing. When an embolus lodges in an extremity, the affected area typically becomes pale and numb and feels cold to touch. The patient may become faint and experience nausea and vomiting. Shock may develop. Gangrene of the extremity may develop unless the vascular obstruction caused by the embolus can be relieved. *Pulmonary embolism* typically develops much later in the postoperative period than fat embolism, perhaps as much as 10–24 days postoperatively. Indications of pulmonary embolism include sudden severe chest pain. Sudden death may occur. Fat embolism and pulmonary embolism, e.g., from blood clots or air, are serious complications which must be given emergency treatment. The alert, competent nurse who recognizes early indications of these complications and who participates effectively in obtaining and initiating emergency care can play a significant role in saving the lives of patients with these complications.

> *Urine retention* or *abdominal distention* or both are other complications which may develop following orthopedic surgery. Treatment of these disorders has been discussed in other sections of this text.

While observing for indications of the above complications, the nurse also evaluates the postoperative orthopedic patient for early symptoms of other potential complications, e.g., infection, hemorrhage, pneumonia, atelectasis, mechanical obstruction of circulation (e.g., from a tight cast), or neurologic damage.

Neurovascular complications are most likely to develop following the reduction of open fractures, but they may also occur postoperatively with other disorders. Frequent neurovascular checks are made by the nurse during the postoperative period. Neurovascular damage may be indicated by the presence of any of the following *"five P's":* (1) Pain; (2) Pallor; (3) Pulselessness; (4) Paresthesia; and (5) Paralysis. The presence of any of these previously discussed symptoms in an operated extremity should be immediately reported. (Neurovascular complications are discussed in detail in the earlier discussion of casts.) During the evaluative process the nurse makes comparisons between the operated and unoperated extremities. In order to accurately identify possible postoperative neurovascular damage, the nurse must be knowledgeable about the patient's history of previous injuries or other presurgery disorders or disabilities. For example, a patient may fall and break an arm that has been paralyzed for years. In this situation, postoperative paralysis of the operated arm (following open reduction of the fracture) would not be an abnormal finding indicative of postsurgical complications.

Orthopedic surgeries are often lengthy procedures. Therefore postoperatively it is not uncommon for a patient to feel stiff and sore from lying relaxed on the operating table for a long period. During surgery care is taken to prevent neurovascular injuries by correctly aligning and supporting the patient's body and extremities. Postoperatively, periodic back care (including massage) can greatly contribute to the patient's comfort.

Following orthopedic surgery it is important to know (and hence avoid) contraindicated positions, movements, or activities for individual patients.

Position, turn, and exercise the patient as ordered during the postoperative period. To ensure healing in correct alignment and to prevent musculoskeletal complications, frequently check the posture and positioning of orthopedic patients while they are confined to bed. Often beds on orthopedic services are equipped with special firm mattresses to promote comfort and correct body alignment during periods of prolonged immobilization. If orthopedic mattresses are not available, bed boards may be placed under the mattress.

Operated extremities are typically elevated during the postoperative period to minimize or prevent edema. Remember to support extremities along their entire length. Do not simply place a pillow under the heel or knee, for example. Do not assume that adequate pillow support is unimportant because the leg or arm is in a cast. Unless casted body areas are properly supported, excessive strain is placed on the cast and it may crack, and also the patient may feel extremely uncomfortable. For example, the patient in a hip spica cast will be acutely uncomfortable if the head of his bed is raised without also placing support under the cast to the sacrum. Flexing the upper body in this manner would cause the cast edges to press into the abdomen.

Check *dressings* frequently during the postoperative period. Report postoperative drainage when it occurs in previously sterile wounds. Use sterile forceps and sterile dressings to reinforce saturated dressings; use of these sterile techniques minimizes the chance of infection being introduced into the wound via capillary action. Dressing changes must be done carefully on orthopedic surgical wounds to prevent introduction of infection. Principles of asepsis are meticulously followed: (a) each patient should have an individual dressing tray, (b) clean wounds should be dressed before contaminated wounds, (c) dusting or sweeping or bed linen changes should never be performed during dressing periods, and (d) the patient and attendants should be masked during dressing changes.[139] Infected patients should always be segregated from those who are free of infection. Chart and report staining of casts, e.g., from seepage of blood, or serous or purulent drainage. Include in your charting measurements of the dimensions of the stained area (e.g., "a circle of drainage about 1 inch in diameter") so these measurements can be used as a baseline when future observations are made to determine if drainage has stabilized or is increasing.

Mobilization during the postoperative period is of special importance following surgery on patients with joint disease. Without adequate mobilization the affected joints will rapidly become stiff and immobilized. Postoperative orders for activity must be conscientiously followed. The skillful nurse uses her resourcefulness to encourage self-care following orthopedic surgery. Often patients with orthopedic disorders are reluctant to move because they are fearful that movement will be painful or damaging. Gently and patiently the nurse helps the patient to learn activities which can safely be performed with a minimum of discomfort. The nurse helps the patient to understand the importance of moving as the doctor has ordered. She points out that while some discomfort is necessary during the postoperative period, the immediate discomfort caused while moving is only temporary and will prevent later problems of greater disability and discomfort, e.g., loss of movement and painful contractures.

Early *ambulation* is desirable postoperatively but sometimes cannot be started until the physician determines that adequate bone healing has occurred. Soft tissues heal more rapidly than bone. Thus, while a patient's skin incision may be healed, it must be remembered that underlying bone may not be healed. It is not uncommon for periods of convalescence to be prolonged following bone injury or bone surgery. A long period of healing is especially necessary for weight-bearing structures. Check the physician's orders carefully to determine if weight may be placed on the affected limb while standing or walking. Commonly the patient is ordered to stand (rather than sit) when first getting out of bed postoperatively. Be certain to have adequate help when getting the patient out of bed. Acutely aware that his musculoskeletal structure is impaired, the patient is fearful of falling and being unable to protect himself from injury.

Postoperative *rehabilitation* programs for orthopedic patients may include occupational therapy, prosthetics (for amputees), bracing, and physical therapy, e.g., gait training, muscle re-education, exercises, heat applications, massage. During convalescence it is of prime importance to keep the patient mobilized and engaged in safe self-care practices. The patient must realize that he shares responsibility for his progress and recovery with staff members, i.e., others will not rehabilitate him, but rather he works with others to rehabilitate himself. His role is active rather than passive. By participating meaningfully in his treatment-recovery program, the patient actively influences his levels of motivation and performance. Of course, it is necessary for the patient to be taught those self-care activities which he is expected to perform.

After hospital *discharge* the patient continues to be seen by his physician and other members of the health care team as necessary. Home visits may be made by a community health nurse. The patient should be familiar with self-care activities which he is to perform and he should also be informed of contraindicated activities and indications of complications.

CHAPTER 89

Musculoskeletal Injuries

INTRODUCTION

Musculoskeletal injuries are relatively common occurrences. Nurses frequently care for patients who have sustained these injuries.

Many musculoskeletal injuries result from *home accidents.* Examples of home accidents include (a) dropping or lifting heavy objects; (b) slipping in a wet bathtub, or on a wet or highly polished floor; (c) tripping over hoses, rugs, pets, telephone cords, or light cords; and (d) falling from ladders or chairs, down stairs, or when getting out of bed.

The increased use of *motor-driven vehicles* has greatly increased the incidence of musculoskeletal injuries, particularly whiplash injuries to the neck and fractures (sustained by pedestrians, cyclists, and automobile occupants). High-impact accidents (which throw a pedestrian some distance or which forcibly hurl automobile occupants against the steering wheel, ceiling, floor, or dashboard of the car) often cause multiple system injuries in addition to musculoskeletal injuries.

Musculoskeletal injuries may occur with participation in *sports, physical fitness programs,* or *self-defense programs.* For example, contact sports such as football may cause sprains, strains, or fractures when participants collide. Boxers may break their hands or sustain broken jaws. Sprinters may fracture the spine of the ilium as a result of the violent muscle contraction experienced at the beginning of a sprint. Each sport may have its own unique injuries, e.g., tennis elbow, jogger's heel.[227] The knee is highly susceptible to sports injuries (see article by Drain[61]). Persons practicing karate may suffer from the HIT syndrome of the hand ("HIT" stands for hypertrophic infiltrative tendinitis).[83]

Some *occupations* are associated with various possible musculoskeletal injuries. Nurses, for example, can injure their backs if they lift patients incorrectly (see article by Davis[52]). Infantry soldiers may suffer fractures in the metatarsals of their feet as a result of long hikes or marches. (These fractures are called fatigue, stress, or march fractures.) Persons employed in various hazardous occupations are likely to sustain musculoskeletal injuries.

Some forms of musculoskeletal trauma occur quite *unexpectedly* during relatively "normal" activities. For example, during a wide yawn the jaw may dislocate, or during violent coughing a rib may fracture. Persons with some diseases (e.g., cancer of the bone, osteoporosis) may sustain fractures spontaneously in the absence of preceding trauma. These fractures (called "pathologic fractures") are discussed later.

Age may also be a factor in musculoskeletal injuries. As a group, older persons are susceptible to fractures. Their vision and hearing may be impaired, increasing the possibilities of accidents. Atrophy of bone, occurring as part of the aging process, may also increase susceptibility to fracture, e.g., fracture of the femur (commonly referred to as "hip fracture"). Additionally, aged persons may be poorly coordinated, have a decline in postural ability, and have difficulty walking. The abilities to stand erect and walk are learned abilities in human beings, i.e., they are not goverened by built-in neural mechanisms. A newly hatched bird may walk out of its eggshell, but a human being does not attain full control of stance until he is in his twenties. With age the level of proficiency progressively deteriorates.

Finally, aged persons may have disorders which predispose them to musculoskeletal injuries, e.g., "drop attacks," cerebral ischemia, osteoporosis, cancer of the bone, arthritis, "dizziness," postural hypotension, muscular weakness, or neurologic disorders which affect locomotion. While disorders such as these predispose a person of any age to injury, the elderly person may be particularly at risk because of other concomitant factors already discussed, e.g., processes which accompany aging. Older women are especially prone to fractures, e.g., Colles' fracture or fractured femur. Men most commonly sustain fractures in their younger years, up to age 45.

Musculoskeletal injuries range in severity from relatively minor soft tissue injuries to severe, crushing fractures.

EXAMINATION AND EMERGENCY CARE OF THE PATIENT WITH MULTIPLE SYSTEM INJURIES

As mentioned earlier, the patient who has been injured in an automobile accident commonly suffers not only from musculoskeletal trauma, but also from multiple system injuries. Prompt evaluation of the patient's injuries and rapid treatment of these injuries (in the order of their importance) is essential. The *respiratory* system is evaluated first for indications of apnea, obstruction, and ineffective respirations, e.g., due to open sucking wound, tension pneumothorax, hemothorax, hemopneumothorax, or flail chest (see Unit XIV).

Once an adequate airway is established the, *circulatory system* is evaluated and treated. The heartbeat is checked by auscultation, palpation, and electrocardiograph monitor, and the patient is examined for indications of shock. External cardiac massage may be necessary until an effective heartbeat can be resumed (see Unit X). Hemodynamic shock may result from external or internal bleeding. The patient in acute shock is monitored by pulse and blood pressure and central venous pressure readings. Also, the urinary output is measured hourly by catheter. To treat hemodynamic shock, access is immediately made to a vein (by needle or cannula) and saline, lactated Ringer's, or plasma is infused rapidly until blood pressure is restored. Once a blood sample has been typed and cross-matched, correctly matched blood is administered to restore a normal blood volume. (Shock is discussed in Unit V, Ch. 26.) After treatment for shock is initiated, a systematic investigation is made as follows to identify *internal bleeding:*[6]

> *Thorax:* intrathoracic bleeding may be confirmed by needle aspiration. Treatment may require closed chest drainage or surgical repair or both.

> *Abdomen:* intra-abdominal bleeding is indicated by the presence of muscle spasm and the absence of bowel sounds. Blood may be aspirated by quadrant taps with a needle. Emergency exploratory surgery is necessary if free blood is demonstrated in the peritoneal cavity. Common abdominal injuries are ruptures of the liver, spleen, and intestines.

> *Urinary tract:* although usually not itself an emergency, genitourinary bleeding can indicate other serious injuries, e.g., closed pelvic fractures. Bladder catheterization is immediately performed. Pelvic bones are cancellous and highly vascular. Fracture of these bones can cause the pelvis to fill rapidly with 25–50 per cent of the blood volume. Bladder rupture is treated by prompt surgery.

> *Central nervous system:* commonly CNS bleeding does not produce shock. In the presence of skull fracture, emergency craniotomy may be necessary to treat epidural hemorrhage.

> *Extremities:* acute shock is often caused by concealed hemorrhage from multiple major fractures. For example, 30 minutes after fracture of the femur, 25 per cent of the blood volume may be contained in the adult thigh.

Early evaluation is necessary of patients with possible *skull* or *spinal injuries*. Persons with suspected cervical spine injuries must be protected (by manual or mechanical traction) against further cord damage until definitive x-ray studies can be done. Emergency reduction of vertebral fractures or dislocations is not necessary unless cord injury is detected. Prompt surgery is indicated for head injuries in which there are depressed or open skull fractures or expanding hematomas. Upon admission to the hospital, baseline evaluations are established (e.g., for level of consciousness and localized neurologic deficits), and close observation is maintained for indications of increased intracranial pressure (see Unit VIII).

During the administration of emergency care, *fractures of the extremities* are temporarily disregarded (except for the shock they may produce), because they are seldom immediately life-threatening even where they are multiple. Once lifesaving emergency care has been administered, attention is directed at giving emergency care to injured extremities. Bleeding is controlled by external pressure, and impaired circulation is corrected by manipulation or traction. All suspected fractures are splinted until they receive definitive treatment or until it is established (by x-ray) that a fracture is not present. Air splints (inflatable plastic devices which permit taking of x-rays with the splint in place) are commonly used to temporarily immobilize suspected fractures. Patients with suspected fractures must be moved carefully, e.g., when being transferred to x-ray, to prevent pain and additional tissue damage. Open wounds are examined with aseptic technique (masks and gloves are worn) and covered with sterile dressings. Since the incidence of osteomyelitis increases with every hour of undebrided contamination, open fractures must be debrided and sterilely dressed as soon as possible.[6] First aid following fractures is discussed more completely on p. 1207.

The nurse assists the doctor as he evaluates the multiply injured patient and gives emergency care. During this time nursing activities may include taking vital signs, providing for the patient's comfort, reassuring the conscious patient, obtaining necessary medications and equipment, charting, obtaining blood samples, arranging for x-rays. The nurse may also help by obtaining a history of the injury from witnesses to the accident, police, or ambulance attendants. Pain medication may be ordered immediately. Nothing is given by mouth until the physician gives his permission.

Seriously injured patients should be moved as little as possible. When the patient reaches the emergency room he should remain on the ambulance carrier or stretcher until the doctor states he may be moved. Leave splints in place. When it is necessary to remove the patient's clothing, do so as gently as possible, with a minimum of tugging and pulling. Cut off clothing that cannot be easily removed. Remove other clothing by starting on the uninjured side. Keep the injured part as motionless as possible.

EXAMINATION OF THE PATIENT WITH MUSCULOSKELETAL TRAUMA

Injured extremities are routinely kept elevated and are observed frequently for indications of complications, e.g., neurovascular damage. (Observations were discussed in the section on cast complications, Chapter 88.) Temporary splints should not be removed by the nurse unless the physician orders their removal.

Patients with suspected musculoskeletal trauma are examined thoroughly by the physician for evidence of injury. Commonly missed orthopedic injuries include[7] shoulder dislocations; torn supraspinatus tendon (in shoulder); fractured medial epicondyle (in elbow); fracture-dislocation of forearm (fracture is easily identified, but dislocation may be missed); fractured scaphoid (associated with wrist injury); dislocated lunate (wrist); fractured neck of femur (hip); slipped upper femoral epiphysis (associated with hip injury); locked knee (i.e., a knee which may bend fully but lacks some normal extension, e.g., the last 3–4° of extension); dislocated patella; and ruptured Achilles tendon.

A brief history which gives some details of a patient's accident can be extremely helpful to the physician when he examines the patient. The nurse can help obtain such a history from the patient or from persons bringing the patient to the hospital, office, or clinic. If possible, persons who witnessed the accident should wait to talk with the physician. Details of how an injury was sustained can help the physician to identify possible injuries because he is knowledgeable about structures commonly injured as a result of specific traumatic forces. For example, a fall on an outstretched hand may transmit stress to the clavicle, humerus, radius, or ulna.

Indications of traumatic damage to the musculoskeletal system include swelling, subcutaneous bleeding (ecchymosis or "black-and-blue" marks), instability of an extremity, crepitation (the sensation felt or heard by the examiner when two ends of fractured bone move against one another, like the sound of loose gravel); and indications of neurologic or circulatory impairment or both.

Injured extremities are gently and thoroughly examined. Commonly 15–30 minutes following injury *swelling* appears. Initially the edema is soft and compressible. Once examination of the extremity is completed, continued swelling is treated by applying continuous external pressure, e.g., with an air splint. *Ecchymoses* ("black-and-blue" marks) reflect bleeding subcutaneously. Depending upon the depth of the bleeding, the ecchymoses may appear soon after injury or perhaps not for several days. Ecchymoses usually indicate major tissue damage or fracture. Bleeding within a joint (*hemarthrosis*) commonly occurs following tearing of intra-articular structures. After several days the blood may seep from the injured joint into subcutaneous tissues. Joint swelling which develops more slowly is generally due to a reactive synovial effusion. Joint aspiration may be performed to determine whether blood is present.

When the initial examination of an injured limb reveals swelling and ecchymosis, the physician gently moves the limb to determine the presence or absence of *instability*. Instability indicates either a fracture or significant ligament rupture. As he examines the unstable, swollen, ecchymotic limb, the physician attempts to elicit localized *crepitation*. Crepitation is indicative of fracture.

As a final part of his initial examination of the injured limb, the examiner rapidly evaluates the *neurologic and circulatory status* of the extremity, e.g., for evidence of injury to major arteries and nerves. It is important that this evaluation be made *before* any treatment (even splinting) is given. Thus, it can accurately be determined in the future whether neurocirculatory damage resulted from the injury or occurred later as a result of treatment, possibly during reduction of the fracture or as a result of the application of a splint or cast.

Upon completion of the examination, the unstable limb is temporarily splinted until more complete care can be given. Temporary splinting of the limb is important because it enhances the patient's comfort and immobilizes the fracture. Splinting prevents additional soft tissue damage, rubbing together of the ends of the fracture, and poking through the skin of the ends of the fractured bone. Splinting also helps reduce muscle spasms.[6] (See also first aid treatment of fractures later in this chapter.)

Pain medication (morphine, Demerol) is usually ordered promptly once the physician sees the patient with a musculoskeletal injury. Fractures often cause severe pain, and pain medications may have to be given intravenously. Cold, local applications (ice bags) may also be ordered.

CONTUSIONS

A contusion is a soft tissue injury resulting from a blunt force or blow. Local hemorrhage occurs and the skin, subcutaneous tissue, and deep soft tissues may also be damaged. Several days after injury the affected area develops ecchymosis. As the blood in the bruised area is absorbed, the discoloration changes to brown, then yellow, and finally the skin resumes its normal color. In addition to discoloration, a contusion typically produces well-localized tenderness and swelling.

Sometimes a *hematoma* develops, i.e., a sac filled with effused blood. This may occur when a major blood vessel in a muscle is injured; brisk bleeding results. The blood in the hematoma eventually clots and may then be gradually resorbed. It may take several months for the hematoma to disappear. Occasionally the physician may decide to evacuate the hematoma by aspiration or to remove the sac surgically.

Immediate *treatment* of a contusion may include (a) application of cold; (b) elevation of the part; and (c) application of a bandage. Some sources recommend massage and the application of heat to enhance resorption of the blood once a clot has formed.

STRAINS

Strains are produced by overstretching of tendons or overuse of muscles. Strains may be *acute* (e.g., occurring during unaccustomed vigorous exercise) or *chronic* (e.g., developing after the repetitive overuse of muscles). The terms "strain" and "sprain" should not be used interchangeably, since they refer to two different types of injuries.

With an acute strain the patient experiences sudden, severe incapacitating pain (e.g., while running). The acute pain subsides, but the area remains locally tender. Discomfort may be elicited by passively stretching the affected part. Swelling occurs rapidly. Ecchymosis may appear after several days.

With a chronic strain symptoms do not appear for several hours following the overactivity. Onset of symptoms is gradual. Commonly the affected parts feel stiff and sore and may exhibit diffuse generalized tenderness when palpated. Swelling, ecchymosis, and loss of function do not occur.

Chronic strains require no specific *treatment,* but the patient may be made more comfortable by local applications of heat. Acute strains require rest and possibly splinting. Immediately following injury, ice packs may be applied for 24–48 hours to reduce swelling. Heat may then be used if it enhances the patient's comfort. Surgical repair may be necessary if a muscle is completely ruptured. During the healing process (which takes 4–6 weeks) movement of the injured part should be minimal. Activity should never be so great that it produces symptoms, e.g., swelling, pain. After mature scar tissue has formed, the part is gradually and progressively exercised. During rehabilitation overactivity must be avoided.

SPRAINS

A sprain results from the forcible hyperextension or wrenching of a joint associated with tissue damage. The capsule and ligaments may be incompletely torn, and the synovial lining may be disrupted, resulting in hemarthrosis, i.e., bleeding into the joint. Sometimes a sprain results from a dislocation which reduces itself but leaves a damaged joint. Sprains are often caused by sudden twisting injuries.

Following injury tenderness to palpation develops which is well localized at first and later becomes more diffuse. Other symptoms include swelling, severe pain, discoloration, decreased motion (limitation of joint motion and function), and disability. Disability may not be very severe initially after the injury occurs, but may be extensive 2–3 hours later. X-rays may demonstrate soft tissue swelling but no evidence of bone or joint injury.

Immediate *treatment* includes elevation of the injured joint and the application of ice. (Do not have the patient hold the affected part in a dependent position and soak it in hot water.) The joint may then be immobilized by either (a) splinting the joint in a position of comfort and applying a compressive bandage, e.g., Ace bandage; or (b) application of a plaster cast (if the sprain is severe). Casting (a) prevents tissue damage resulting from chronic edema; (b) alleviates pain; and (c) controls swelling. If an Ace bandage is used, it is applied gently, not tightly. A mature scar forms in connective fibrous tissue in 4–6 weeks. Immobilization of the injured part for 3–4 weeks is usually adequate. Following complete healing the joint should be actively exercised.

A "*whiplash*" *injury* of the cervical spine is a sprain of ligamentous tissue around bones and joints in the neck. Commonly the injury results from an automobile accident in which the car in which the person was riding was struck from the rear. The impact (rapid acceleration) suddenly and forcibly hyperextends the spine. Then the spine is acutely flexed during rapid deceleration (when the force of the impact ceases). A cervical sprain is treated by immobilizing the neck with a cervical collar.

DISLOCATIONS; SUBLUXATIONS

A *dislocation* is present when a bone is displaced from its normal joint position and the articulating surfaces lose contact. The displaced bone may impede blood supply; tear ligaments; rupture blood vessels; damage nerves; and rupture muscle attachments. With a *subluxation* the joint's articulating surfaces are only partially separated. Dislocations and subluxations disrupt the joint by tearing the capsule and ligaments. Often these disorders are accompanied by a fracture of the joint surface.

Dislocations may result from trauma or may occur spontaneously as a result of diseases affecting joints. Some dislocations, especially of the hip, may be present at birth.

Deformity may or may not be visible with dislocations or subluxations. Dislocation may change the length of the affected extremity. Localized joint pain and loss of function (i.e., mobility) may be present. A dislocation partially immobilizes a joint, and thus differs from a fracture. (A fracture site typically has abnormal free movement.) X-rays demonstrate the abnormality, i.e., complete or partial separation of the articulating surfaces (Fig. 89–1).

Some dislocations reduce themselves, leaving a sprain. Others must be therapeutically reduced by a physician. Prior to treatment the neurovascular supply to parts distal to the injury must be carefully evaluated and deficits noted. Once x-ray establishes the diagnosis, the dislocation or subluxation is reduced.

Prompt treatment is necessary to prevent complications, which include (a) ischemia or aseptic necrosis (resulting from impaired blood supply to parts distal to the dislocation); and (b) impaired

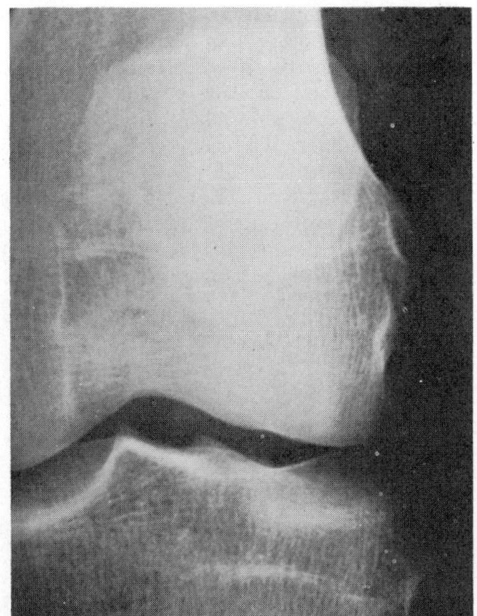

FIGURE 89–1. Anteroposterior view of dislocation of the patella or kneecap. (From O'Donoghue, D. H.: *Treatment of Injuries to Athletes.* 2nd ed. 1970.)

nourishment of the hyaline cartilage on the articulating surfaces of the injured joint (normally this tissue is nourished by synovial fluid, but disruption of the joint impairs the nourishment process).

Reduction is most often accomplished without surgery ("closed reduction"), but in some cases surgery ("open reduction") is indicated, e.g., with some knee injuries which completely rupture ligaments. When reduction is accomplished by closed manipulation, the physician pulls on the joint with a gradual steady pull rather than a quick forceful jerk. Anesthesia may consist of a local or regional block or a general anesthetic.

Following reduction of a dislocation or subluxation, the joint is immobilized by application of a splint or cast or by placing the patient in mild traction. Immobilization may be maintained for 3–6 weeks. Adjacent joints which are not immobilized are actively exercised during the period of healing. Once the affected joint is removed from immobilization, active motion is encouraged, e.g., voluntary muscle contraction. Passive stretching can be harmful.

FRACTURES

A fracture is a disruption of the normal continuity of bone. Commonly a fracture is accompanied by soft tissue injury in surrounding tissues. While some fractures are life-threatening (because of associated hemorrhage and shock), most are not.

CAUSES

Most fractures result from accidents, e.g., automobile accidents, blows, falls, twisting, crushing injuries. As discussed below, some fractures result from disease processes which weaken bone.

Fractures may result from[123] (a) *direct force,* in which the fracture occurs at the point of contact; (b) *torsion,* in which the fracture occurs at a point remote from the location of the force (e.g., a forceful twisting of the foot may break bones in the leg); (c) *violent contractions* of highly developed muscles (e.g., forcibly throwing an object produces powerful muscle contractions which can fracture the humerus); and (d) *various disease processes* that cause fractures, in the absence of trauma, by weakening bone structure. The latter type of fractures are termed *pathologic* or *spontaneous fractures.* These fractures result from disorders such as osteoporosis (increased porosity of bone), particularly in the lumbar spine or hip; Cushing's syndrome; malnutrition; complications of cortisone or ACTH therapy; osteogenesis imperfecta (congenital disorder affecting formation of osteoblasts); or metastatic or primary bone tumors (tumors decalcify bone). These various disorders cause bone tissue to collapse or break easily.

TYPES

There are more than 150 different types of fractures which are classified in various ways. Some of the more common types of fractures are described briefly in following paragraphs. (Refer to Fig. 89–2.)

The following terms are useful in establishing generally the *severity* of a fracture:

> *Open (compound) fracture:* A break in the skin is present over the fracture site and the wound communicates from the skin (externally) to the fractured bone (internally). Because of this communication with the external environment, an open fracture is potentially infected. The wound may result (a) from external trauma (e.g., bullet) which penetrated through the skin and fractured underlying bone (direction of the injuring force was from outside the body moving inward); or (b) from the ends of a broken bone penetrating out through the skin when the fracture occurred (see Fig. 89–2). The ends of the broken bones may or may not be visible in the skin wound. Sometimes they push through the skin at the time of impact and then are withdrawn back under the surface of the skin.

> *Closed (simple) fracture:* An uncomplicated fracture in which the skin is intact over the fracture site, e.g., broken bone does not protrude through the skin (Fig. 89–2). Because there is no communicating wound, infection is not introduced into the fracture at the time of injury.

> *Complete fracture:* The fracture line extends entirely through the bone substance; i.e., the periosteum is disrupted on both sides of the bone. Two fragments of bone are present on either side of the fracture line.

> *Incomplete (partial) fracture:* The fracture line extends only part way through the bone substance, i.e., the bone continuity is not completely disrupted. Also sometimes called a *willow, greenstick,* or *hickory stick* fracture (Fig. 89–2). Like bending a green stick to the breaking point, one side breaks but the other merely bends.

> *Impacted fracture* (also called "*telescoped fracture*"): One bone fragment is forcibly driven into another adjacent bone fragment.

> *Comminuted fracture:* There is more than one fracture line, and the bone fragments are crushed or broken into several pieces. A *butterfly fracture* is a type of comminuted fracture in which the fragments resemble a butterfly, i.e., on each side of the main fragment are two fragments resembling wings.

> *Displaced fracture:* The bone fragments are separated at the fracture line.

> *Complicated fracture:* The fracture is associated with injury to surrounding structures, e.g., adjacent organs, nerves, blood vessels, joints. For example, a fractured rib may penetrate adjacent lung tissue.

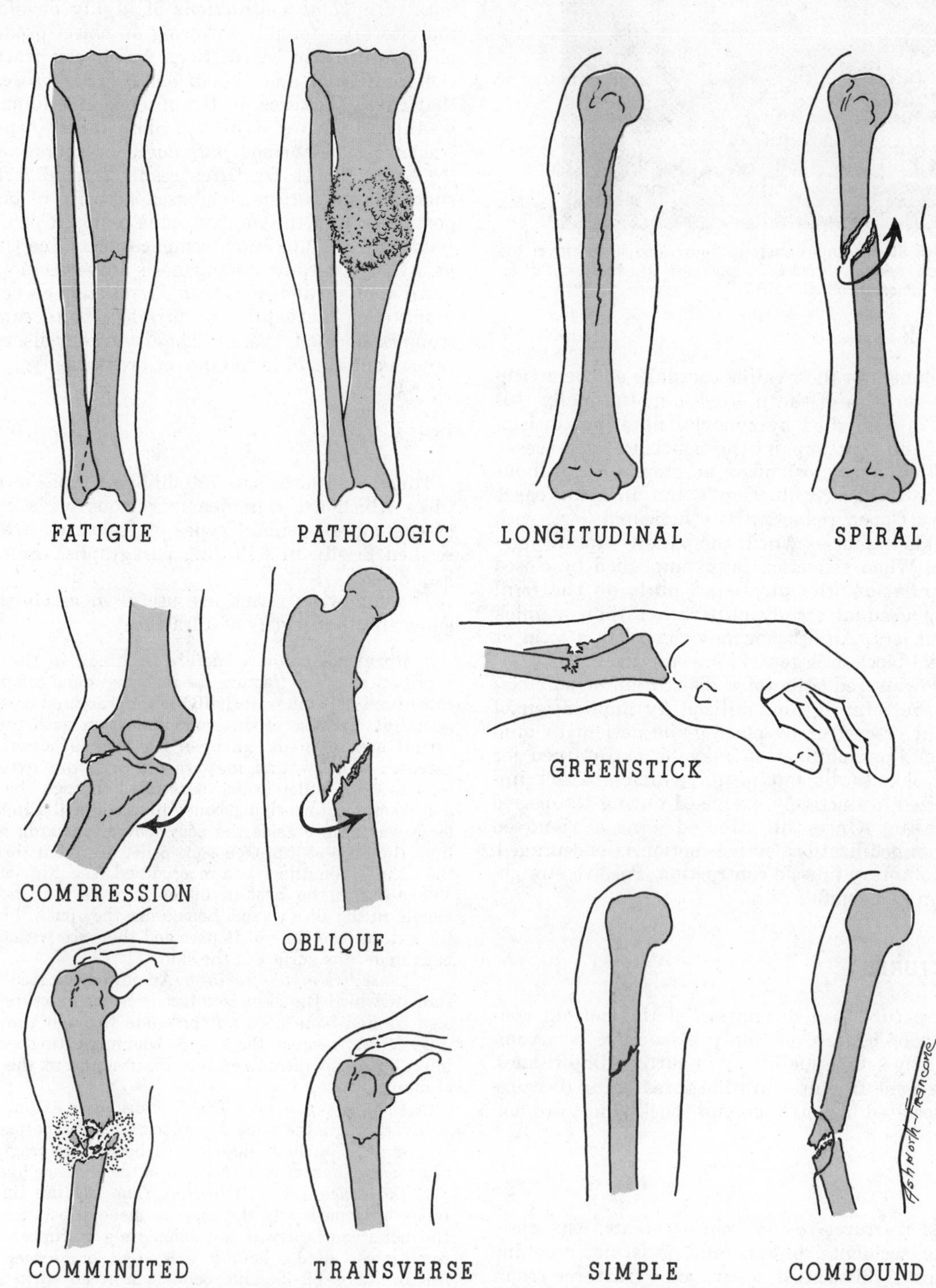

FIGURE 89–2. Types of fractures. (From Jacob, S. W., and Francone, C. A.: *Structure and Function in Man.* 3rd ed. 1974.)

Terms used to describe fractures may be used in combination to provide a more complete description. For example, a patient may have a closed, complete fracture which is displaced.

When a fracture of an extremity divides a bone into two fragments, the fragments are referred to as the *proximal (uncontrollable) fragment* and the *distal (controllable) fragment.* The proximal fragment is that section of the bone which is nearest to the body. This fragment cannot be manipulated or moved when the fractured bones are being "set" (i.e., correctly aligned) because of its muscle attachments and location. The distal fragment (farthest away from the body) can be manipulated or moved therapeutically to realign it with the proximal fragment.

Summarized below are some terms used to describe the *direction of fracture line* in relation to the affected bone's longitudinal axis.

> *Linear fracture:* line of the fracture runs parallel to the bone's long axis.

> *Longitudinal fracture:* line of the fracture extends in a longitudinal direction.

> *Oblique fracture:* line of the fracture is at an oblique angle (about a 45° angle) to the shaft (axis) of the bone.

> *Spiral fracture* (also called a *"torsion fracture"*): line of the fracture forms a spiral which encircles the bone. Results from a twisting force, e.g., in sports such as football or skiing.

> *Transverse fracture:* line of the fracture is straight across the bone, i.e., at a right angle to the bone's axis.

Fractures are also classified according to the *force* that produces the fracture. Some of these terms include angulation fracture, avulsion fracture, blowout fracture (results from blow that fractures the floor of the orbit of the eye), compression fracture, fatigue or march fracture (fracture of metatarsals due to long marches), and missile fracture.

Fractures are often named for the *physician* who first described them. Two common examples are:

> *Colles' fracture:* A common type of fracture in which the distal portion of the radius is fractured within one inch of the articular surface. Colles' fracture is typically characterized by a "silver fork" deformity (see Fig. 89-3) caused by dorsal displacement of the distal fragment with dorsal and radial deviation of the wrist and an abnormal radioulnar articulation.

> *Pott's fracture:* This fracture occurs at the distal end of the fibula and often is associated with rupture of the internal lateral ligament or chipping off of a piece of the medial malleolus or both. The tibiofibular articulation is seriously disrupted. Frequently the foot is displaced outward.

Finally, another method of classifying fractures is in terms of their *anatomic location.* The site of *long bone fractures* is indicated by visualizing the bone as divided into thirds and then stating the location of the fracture, e.g., in the proximal, middle, or distal third.

Fractures involving or close to *joints* are described as:

> *Articular fractures* (also called *"joint fracture"*): The fracture involves the surface of a joint.

> *Extracapsular fracture:* The fracture is near a joint but does not enter the joint capsule.

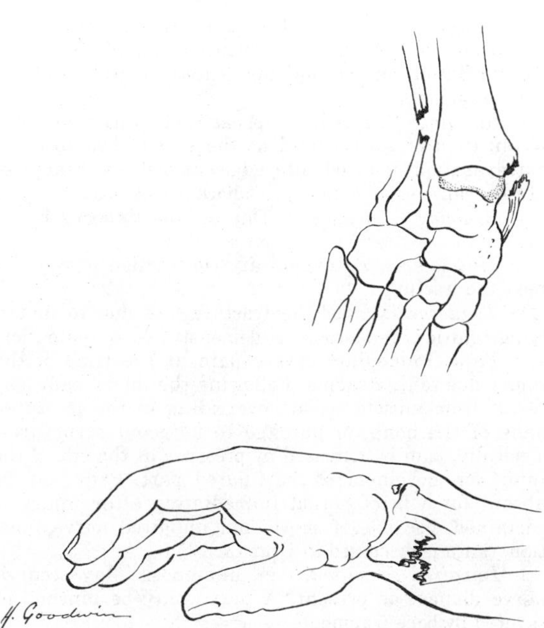

FIGURE 89-3. *A,* Colles' fracture. *B,* Pott's fracture. (From *Dorland's Illustrated Medical Dictionary. 25th ed. 1974.*)

> *Intracapsular fracture:* The fracture is within a joint's capsule.

Fractures involving *major bones* may be classified in special terms. For example, fractures of the *humerus* may be identified as follows:

> *Condylar fracture:* A small fragment of bone (including the condyle) is separated from the inner and outer aspect of the humerus.

> *Supracondylar fracture:* The fracture is at the distal end of the humerus.

> *Transcondylar fracture:* The fracture is at the level of the condyles of the humerus (or just above or below the condyles) and partially within the capsule.

SYMPTOMS

Numerous factors influence the symptoms which a given fracture may produce, e.g., the site, severity, and type of fracture and the amount of damage to other structures. Some fractures produce almost no symptoms and would not be detected if routine x-rays were not taken to evaluate injuries. Symptoms which may occur with a fracture are briefly summarized below. Various combinations of symptoms may be present.

> *Deformity:* Changes in alignment and contour, such as (a) angulation, rotation, or shortening of a limb; (b) depression of bone; or (c) altered curves. To identify subtle deformities compare the injured limb with its uninjured counterpart on the opposite side. Shortening of the injured limb occurs with fractures of long bones

(e.g., humerus) because the muscles attached above and below the fracture site contract in a state of muscle spasm. Strong muscle pull may cause overriding of the bone fragments.

> *Swelling:* Edema may appear rapidly as a result of localization of serous fluid at the site of fracture and extravasation of blood into adjacent tissues. Fractures always cause some damage to adjacent soft tissues.

> *Bruising (ecchymosis):* Due to subcutaneous bleeding.

> *Muscle spasm:* Involuntary contraction of muscles near the fracture.

> *Tenderness:* Over the fracture site due to underlying injuries. Tenderness is demonstrated by palpation.

> *Pain:* Immediate severe pain at the time of the injury due to the trauma. Following the injury pain may result from muscle spasm, overriding of the fractured ends of the bone, or damage to adjacent structures. Typically, pain is increased by pressure at the site of the injury or movement of the injured part. Pain may be absent for a brief period immediately after injury is sustained, because of shock and impaired nerve function. (Pain is discussed in Unit IX.)

> *Impaired sensation,* e.g., numbness: May occur if nerve damage is present. A nerve may be pinched or severed by bone fragments.

> *Loss of normal function:* May result from instability of the fractured bone or from pain or muscle spasm or both. Paralysis may be caused by nerve damage.

> *Abnormal mobility:* Movement of a part which is normally immobile may occur due to instability when long bones are fractured.

> *Crepitus:* Grating sensations or grating sounds may be felt or heard if the injured part is moved. Crepitus results from broken bone ends rubbing together.

> *Shock:* May result from blood loss, i.e., hypovolemic shock, or other factors such as severe pain or extensive soft tissue damage. (Shock is discussed in Unit V, Ch. 26.)

> *Abnormal x-ray or fluoroscopic findings:* X-ray or fluoroscopy is used to confirm the diagnosis by showing the location of the fracture and the direction of the fracture line. Findings vary according to the site and type of fracture.

If a fracture is suspected the injured part should be kept at rest until a physician can evaluate the condition. Do not attempt to elicit symptoms (e.g., crepitus, abnormal mobility) by moving the injured part. Movement can cause additional damage, such as displacement of fragments, injury to adjacent structures, or establishment of an open fracture.

X-rays of fractured bones should be taken in two planes and should include the joint above and the joint below (so dislocations or subluxations can be identified if present). X-rays are typically taken in anteroposterior and lateral projections. X-rays are commonly taken prior to reduction, following reduction, and then periodically during the healing process. The physician may show the patient x-rays of his fracture as he discusses with him the treatment plan. It is helpful to the patient to know about how long his injury will incapacitate him so he can make realistic plans concerning transportation, work, and finances.

FRACTURE HEALING

The body's general responses to injury and infection are discussed in Chapter 21 (Unit V). The following discussion focuses on physiologic processes active in bone healing. Unlike many specialized tissues, bone can regenerate. Healing of fractures thus takes place by the formation of new bone tissue (to reunite bone fragments) rather than by the formation of nonspecialized fibrous scar tissue. Fractures usually heal by passing through the following stages:

> *Hematoma formation:* Bleeding occurs into the fracture site immediately following the fracture. Inflammatory exudate also appears. The blood comes from vessels ruptured within the bone as well as from tears in the periosteum (covering the bone) and adjacent soft tissues. A hematoma forms surrounding the area of the injured bone and filling the cleft of the fracture. After 24 hours the main blood supply increases to the fractured bone ends. Also, new capillaries are starting to grow into the blood clot. The clot becomes bound together by fibroblasts. As the blood in the hematoma clots (coagulates), a loose, delicate mesh of fibrin forms around the fracture site. The fibrin mesh protectively encloses the damaged area of bone and also acts as a scaffold for the ingrowth of capillary buds and fibroblasts. Within 24 hours the blood clot begins to organize. Unlike most hematomas, the hematoma which surrounds a fracture is not resorbed during healing. Instead it undergoes changes and develops into granulation tissue.

> *Granulation tissue formation:* Gradually cells and new capillaries invade the hematoma. Within a few days the blood clot is replaced by granulation tissue. Two days after the injury, red blood cell and tissue debris is being removed by phagocytosis. Simultaneously the periphery of the clot is invaded with fibroblasts (from the medullary cavity, periosteum, and adjacent connective tissue). Thus the reparative process is started as fibroblasts form a *soft tissue callus* surrounding the fracture site.

> *Callus formation:* Six to 10 days after the injury the granulation tissue changes and a *provisional callus* or *procallus* is formed. Newly formed cartilage and bone matrix (derived in part from the periosteum and endosteum of the adjacent bone margins) disperse through the soft tissue callus and increase in numbers until the provisional callus is established. The provisional callus is a large, loosely woven mass of bone and cartilage which is considerably wider than the bone's normal diameter. The provisional callus extends beyond the fracture line for some distance, thus serving as a temporary splint to the injury. The provisional callus usually reaches its maximal size at about 14–21 days in an uncomplicated fracture. This mass is subsequently remodeled according to Wolff's law, which basically states that the structure of a bone is determined by its function, e.g., the stresses and strains placed upon it.

> *Ossification.* With the deposition of calcium salts, a permanent callus of rigid bone eventually forms. Calcification first forms an external callus (between the periosteum and cortex), next an internal callus (medullary plug), and finally an intermediate callus (between the cortical fragments). During the third to tenth weeks of healing, callus is converted into bone. The formation of bone firmly binds together the fractured ends and healing is complete. While the provisional callus can effectively hold the bone fragments together temporarily, it is not strong enough to hold up if subjected to strains or if made to bear weight. Gradually the provisional callus is increasingly strengthened by the formation of

true bone as calcium salts are deposited. At the same time, the callus is remodeled by osteoblastic and osteoclastic activity. In effect, excess bone is chiseled away from the callus and the excess bone is absorbed. Muscle and weight-bearing stresses imposed on the bone govern the remodeling process. During the healing process the external callus is absorbed (by rarefying osteitis), and the intermediate callus consolidates into hard sclerosing osteitis and becomes permanent callus.[171]

Effective bone healing is facilitated by achieving close, accurate approximation of the fractured ends and then immobilizing the structure in this position of proper alignment, by pinning, traction, or casts, until healing occurs. Movement and irritation at the fracture site impair callus formation. During the healing process it is important for the injured part to have adequate circulation. Circulation not only brings oxygen, nutrients, and calcium to the callus but also removes debris from the callus. To promote effective circulation the limb may be elevated (to reduce edema), and the patient is mobilized as soon as possible. Early mobilization promotes not only effective circulation but also a favorable nitrogen balance. A callus must be protected from strain or the delicate healing processes will be interrupted and the bone may refracture.

Fractures normally heal more rapidly in children than adults. Bone union typically occurs in 4–6 weeks in children, 6–8 weeks in adolescents, and 10–18 weeks in adults. Some healing processes may continue for as long as a year. With successful healing the bone is eventually well consolidated, as strong as it was before injury, and contains fat and marrow cells. The healing process is monitored by periodic x-rays. Healing time is affected by the type of bone injured and the specific nature of an injury. Non–weight-bearing bones may heal more rapidly than weight-bearing bones. Larger bones heal more slowly than smaller bones. Dense bone (which is not highly vascularized) heals more slowly than cancellous, vascular portions of bone, e.g., ends of long bones. Flat bones typically heal rapidly. The patient's general physical condition may also influence healing, e.g., a poor general condition or malnutrition impairs healing. To facilitate healing the patient's diet should be high in vitamins, protein, iron, and calcium.

Unfortunately all fractures do not heal in the usual sequential manner described above. *Nonunion* of a fracture is said to exist when the healing processes at the fracture site stop before bony union develops. In this situation healing processes will not resume without treatment. *Delayed union* refers to a fracture which does not heal in the predicted usual healing time. Additional treatment is not always necessary in a case of delayed union for complete healing to eventually occur.

Factors which may contribute to nonunion or delayed union of a fracture include (a) infection; (b) inadequate circulation; (c) inadequate immobilization; (d) distraction of bone fragments (e.g., fragments held apart by excessive traction); (e) displacement of bone fragments (e.g., soft tissue interposed between fragments); and (f) accidental loss of the hematoma, e.g., through an open wound or at the time of surgery. Additionally, some congenital disorders cause nonunion. As mentioned earlier, adequate circulation is highly important in the healing process. *Aseptic necrosis* of the head of the femur may occur if a fracture impairs circulation to the femur's head. Tissue distal to the fracture then dies from lack of circulation.

Surgery is sometimes performed in an attempt to correct nonunion, e.g., a graft of bone may be applied to the bone fragments to provide a bony union ("bridge") between the fragments. If satisfactory union cannot be achieved, the patient may need to wear a brace or be on crutches indefinitely.

FIRST AID TREATMENT

A detailed discussion of the first-aid treatment of fractures is beyond the scope of this text. The reader is advised to consult specialized texts that focus on emergency care, e.g., the first aid manual published by the American Red Cross.

The immediate care given persons who have head or spinal injuries is highly important. This care is discussed in Unit VIII. Penetrating rib fractures may be life-endangering injuries. Emergency care of a patient with a punctured lung is discussed in Unit XIV.

Several *principles* are of outstanding importance in the emergency management of a patient with a known or suspected fracture. Among these principles are the following:

> Take no actions which can cause harm to the patient.

> Organize bystanders, e.g., direct someone to call for help, ask others to direct traffic around the scene of the accident, and keep crowds back away from the patient.

> Move the patient no more than absolutely necessary. Ensure correct handling and transportation of the patient to be moved (unless he is in danger) until he has received necessary care at the scene of the accident.

> If a fracture is suspected but is not obvious, treat the patient as if he were fractured.

> Consider the patient's total condition, i.e., do not focus only on the fracture site and overlook other disorders such as shock.

> Keep the patient as comfortable as possible while giving emergency care.

> Do what you safely can, but do not act beyond your qualifications, e.g., do not try to reduce a fracture or dislocation.

> Expose the fracture site to search for evidence of skin breakage.

> Dress open wounds, e.g., compound fractures, before applying a splint.

> Splint the injured site *before* permitting the patient to be moved (no matter how short the distance he is to be moved). Remember the motto: "Splint them where they lie."

> Inspect and carefully prepare a splint *before* it is applied (e.g., apply padding if necessary) to make certain

the application of the splint will not cause additional damage, e.g., pressure damage.

> Do not try to "push back" any exposed portions of bone, e.g., ends, fragments, or splinters of bone.

> Elevate the injured extremity when possible (a) to minimize circulatory congestion and edema (swelling); and (b) to control hemorrhage.

> Make certain the patient is taken directly to a facility where he will receive prompt definitive treatment.

Movement of a fractured limb before the limb is immobilized may cause irreparable damage, e.g., bone fragments may move about and sever a nerve or blood vessel. If it is *absolutely* necessary to move the patient before a splint can be applied (e.g., to move him to safety), support the injured extremity both above and below the site of the fracture and have someone apply gentle traction during transportation (i.e., maintain a slow, steady pull on each side of the fracture site while moving the patient).

Do not allow the patient to try to get up or sit up until he has been evaluated to identify possible injuries. Also, do not permit other persons to hastily move the patient. When it is time to move the patient make certain that persons helping to transport him know actions they should (and should not) take *before* starting to move the patient. Coordinated, safe movements are imperative. One person should control the injured (splinted) extremity while the patient is moved.

Do not focus exclusively on the fracture and neglect to care for other disorders, e.g., shock, hemorrhage. Remember to evaluate the patient's mental-emotional status and give appropriate care. The person who has suffered a traumatic injury may be highly anxious or in a state of emotional shock.

Fractures may elicit fears of permanent deformity or crippling. The patient's emotional shock (resulting from the impact of the injury process) may be greatly intensified if he views his deformity, for example, a limb that is abnormally positioned. The nurse who is unaccustomed to seeing fractures also may initially find it distressing to view the disfigurement caused by injuries such as fractures. Such a nurse must take care not to convey her own discomfort to the patient.

Expose the site of the injury. If necessary, gently cut or tear away overlying clothing without moving the limb. If it is necessary to cut clothing, try to do so along a seam, so the clothing can later be repaired if the patient desires. Remove rings, bracelets, watches, and so forth from an injured arm as soon as possible before swelling prohibits their removal.

Splinting. Immobilization of a fractured limb is highly important. Prompt application of a splint is useful because immobililization accomplishes the following:

> Prevents additional damage, by preventing movement of bone fragments. Movement of fragments can damage adjacent structures or can convert a closed fracture into an open fracture. Bones in the arms and legs lie very close to the surface of the skin. Rough, splintered bone ends can easily penetrate the skin if carelessly handled. Movement of the fracture can also convert a simple fracture into a comminuted fracture, and can sever nerves or blood vessels and injure other soft tissues.

> Minimizes and/or prevents pain, muscle spasm, shock, and hemorrhage. Fractures are often extremely painful. A patient may feel much more comfortable after a splint is applied and muscle spasm is overcome. Severe, unrelieved pain can contribute to shock.

> Minimizes deformity (e.g., angulation or overriding of the injured limb) which severe muscle spasm causes.

> Permits blood to clot at the fracture site. As discussed, clotting and formation of a hematoma is of importance in the body's natural healing process.

A variety of commercial splints are available, e.g., inflatable plastic (air) splints, wooden splints, molded aluminum splints, soft wire splints, scored cardboard splints, and special metal splints (e.g., Thomas splints). If commercial splints are not available, splints can be *improvised* from numerous materials, such as pillows, folded blankets, rolled-up newspapers, padded boards or sticks, golf clubs, heavy magazines, baseball bats, or tongue depressors.

Rigid splints should always be long enough that they immobilize the entire bone and can be secured well above and below the fracture site. When applying a splint, apply slight traction. A splint should be securely applied but should not be so tight that it impedes circulation. The splint should immobilize the joints above and below the fracture. Also, a splint should be properly padded (if necessary) before application to protect soft tissues.

Air splints (i.e., plastic inflatable splints or pneumatic splints) are useful because the clear plastic permits visualization of underlying structures to note skin condition and color of the limb, and x-rays can be taken through the splint. Air splints are easy to apply, may help control bleeding, and provide good support. A bulky, absorptive sterile dressing should be applied over compound fractures before application of the splint. Because the splint will deflate if punctured, it must be protected from sharp objects both inside and outside.

Air splints are available in various shapes; some are rectangular, others are boot-shaped. Some have zippers or other fasteners. Air splints cannot be used to immobilize fractures of the femur or humerus, since they would not immobilize the joint above the fracture. However, they are of value in splinting fractures of the forearm or lower leg.

If an air splint is applied outside in cold weather and the patient is then transferred into a warm area, the air in the splint expands. To prevent excessive pressures from forming in the splint, it may be necessary to remove some air.[90] The proper amount of pressure in an air splint should be about 30 mm. Hg. When firm manual pressure is applied to the plastic of an inflated splint, the tension of air should be such that the plastic can be dimpled about ½ inch.

When indicated, *traction splints* are extremely useful because they can overcome the severe muscle spasms that fractures produce in some large muscles. Hip, femur, and lower leg injuries should be traction splinted if possible. The immediate application of traction may prevent muscle spasm and relieve pain.

> *For a fracture in the shaft of a long bone, traction may be applied manually until the splint is securely positioned.*

When applying traction, remember that it is being applied to align the fracture and immobilize the bone fragments, not to reduce the fracture. To apply traction, grasp the extremity firmly with one hand over the break and the other further down the limb (e.g., grasping the hand or foot). Ask another person to apply countertraction by holding the patient firmly, e.g., grasping the joint above the fracture site. Then pull with a slow, steady motion on the part distal to the fracture. Do not pull quickly and forcibly and do not attempt to overcome firm resistance if it is encountered. Sudden jerks can damage blood vessels, nerves, or soft tissue. Do not apply excessive traction; apply just enough to support and immobilize the fracture in a position of proper alignment. *Once you initiate traction do not release it.* Maintain traction until the splint is secured or until the patient receives appropriate care.

When traction is indicated it can best be applied before muscles in the injured limb go into spasm, i.e., involuntarily contract. It is difficult to apply traction to a spastic limb. Immediately following a fracture the surrounding muscles are flaccid for 10–40 minutes. The muscles then go into spasm. Muscular spasms may interfere with circulation of blood and lymph. Additionally, they are painful and may increase deformity by pulling bone fragments further out of alignment.

Space does not permit discussion of the application of splints to various sites. Figure 89–4 illustrates a method of immobilizing hip or femur injuries, using a padded board splint. Fractures of the foot or ankle can be immobilized by securing a pillow around the back of the ankle and bottom of the foot (Fig. 89–5). Figure 89–6 illustrates immobilization of a fractured humerus.

Compound Fractures. Apply a sterile dressing (if available) to the site of a compound fracture. If a sterile dressing is not available, cover the wound with a piece of clean white cloth if possible. Control bleeding by applying local pressure over the dressing. Remember that even though bone is not exposed, a compound fracture may be present if the skin is open over the fracture site. If bone is initially visible but later pulls back under the skin (e.g., due to muscle spasm or during application of a splint), pin a note on the patient's clothing which tells the doctor that the bone was exposed.

It is generally agreed that compound fractures should not have traction applied to them since with traction any exposed bone fragments may be pulled back under the skin. This could damage underlying structures; cause the interposition of muscle, nerve, or blood vessels between fragment

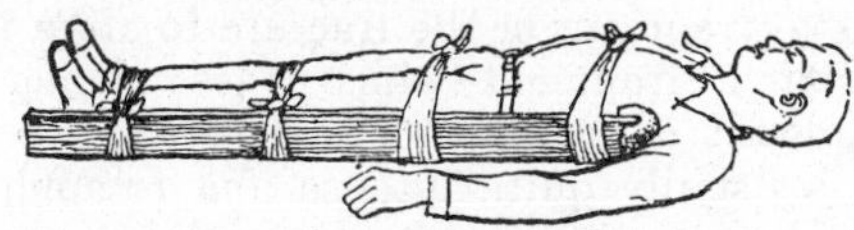

FIGURE 89–4. To immobilize a fracture of the hip or femur, bandage both limbs together to a board extending from the axilla to the foot on the injured side. (From DePalma, A. F.: *The Management of Fractures and Dislocations.* Vol. 1. 2nd ed. 1970.)

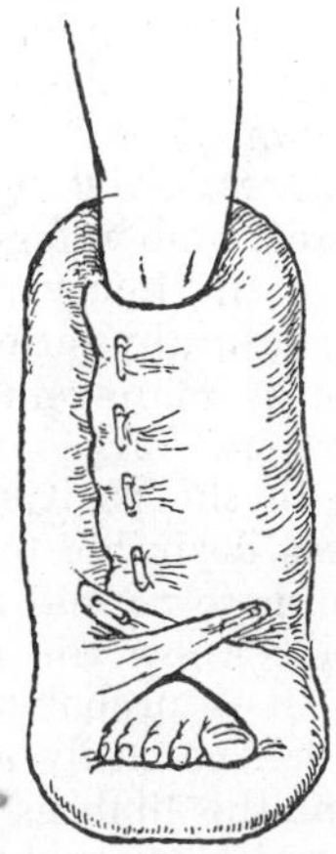

FIGURE 89–5. For fractures of the ankle and foot, apply a pillow splint snugly around the lower leg, ankle, and foot. (From DePalma, A. F.: *The Management of Fractures and Dislocations.* Vol. 1. 2nd ed. 1970.)

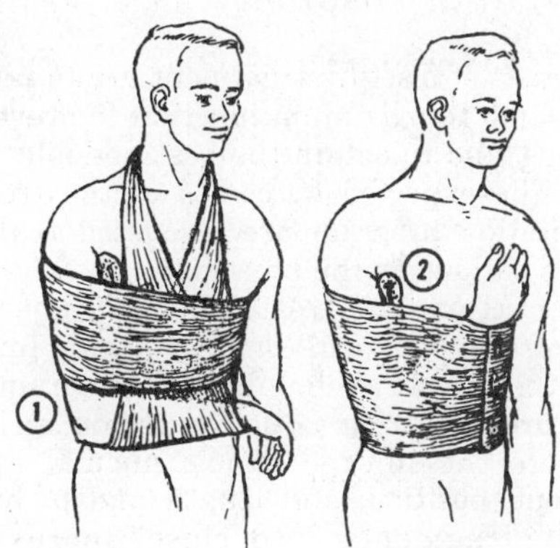

FIGURE 89–6. For fractures of the humerus and elbow, (1) apply a swathe and sling or (2) bandage the arm to the side (place a small pad in the axilla). (From DePalma, A. F.: *The Management of Fractures and Dislocations.* Vol. 1. 2nd ed. 1970.)

ends; and/or introduce contaminated material (e.g., hairs, pieces of dirt) into the wound. *Splint the limb in the position in which it is found.*

Angulated Fractures; Joint Injuries. "Angulation" of a fractured limb refers to deformity of the limb caused by the injury displacing the extremity into an unnatural position. Opinion varies about the emergency management of angulated fractures. While some surgeons prefer that the limb be splinted in the position of angulation, others believe it is desirable for the limb to be gently moved into more normal alignment.[123] Unless you happen to know the attending physician's preference, it is probably best to align a limb only if this can be easily accomplished, and otherwise to splint the limb as found. Fractures of the extremities which are only slightly angulated may easily be immobilized in place; however, severely angulated fractures (e.g., in which a limb is at a right angle from its normal position) may make it difficult to transport the patient.

> *If a joint is injured do* not *attempt to straighten the injured part. Immobilize the limb as found.*

Some sources[90] recommend straightening any severely angulated fracture which can be safely straightened, e.g., fractures of the upper and lower extremities *except* for fractures of the shoulders, elbows, wrists, or knees. Straightening fractures involving joints may cause permanent nerve damage because of the close proximity of major nerves and blood vessels.

A word about *dislocated joints.* They should be immobilized when giving emergency care, but do not attempt to straighten or reduce any dislocation. To do so may damage nerves and blood vessels adjacent to the joint.

TREATMENT OF FRACTURES

The *goals* of fracture treatment are to return the injured limb to maximum function to prevent complications, and to obtain the best possible cosmetic result. The expected outcomes of the treatment-rehabilitation program are discussed realistically with the patient by the physician.

Most fractures are treated by *reduction* and *immobilization. Physical therapy* is an important part of the recovery-rehabilitation program.

Fracture reduction is performed in an attempt to restore the injured bone's normal anatomic alignment, position, and length and to bring the fracture fragments into close approximation to one another so that healing will be promoted. Reduction of a fracture is sometimes called "setting" the bone. It is not always possible to bring fracture fragments back into near-perfect anatomic alignment for healing. In some instances the bone fragments must heal with minor shortening or angulation. Repeated attempts at reduction are undesirable.[221]

Fractures may be reduced in three basic ways: (1) by *reduction traction;* (2) by *manipulation* ("closed reduction"); or (3) by *operative procedures* ("open reduction"). These techniques are described further on. Some fractures are treated with a combination of procedures, e.g., traction may be applied for a while before open reduction is performed. Early reduction is important. Reduction minimizes pain and muscle spasm and promotes healing.

Both closed and open reduction procedures are painful. Therefore, anesthesia is administered. Anesthesia also helps muscles relax. Reduction procedures may be performed under local anesthesia, nerve blocks (e.g., spinal anesthesia or brachial or axillary nerve blocks), or general anesthesia. (See discussion of nursing patients experiencing surgery, Unit VI.)

Not all fractures require reduction. For example, an undisplaced fracture does not require reduction (because the bone fragments are already correctly aligned). In such a case splinting may be advisable, however, to prevent future displacement. Likewise, it is futile to reduce a fracture if it is impossible to hold the position of reduction once reduction is achieved, e.g., with a fractured calcaneus ("heel bone").[97] A few fractures, such as those of the distal phalanges, cannot even be adequately splinted and are treated by simply keeping the part at rest until adequate healing occurs.

As we have emphasized throughout this chapter, fractures often injure adjacent soft tissues, e.g., nerves, tendons, muscles, blood vessels, subcutaneous tissue, fat, skin. The treatment of a fracture thus includes the treatment of related injuries. For example, seriously injured major nerves and vessels require surgical repair. Laceration of an artery and severance of a major nerve are surgical emergencies. Injured soft tissues become swollen and edematous. If edema fluid is allowed to solidify, it causes pain, adhesions, and stiffness. The fluid must therefore be removed before it can solidify. Removal of edema fluid can be facilitated by[97] (a) *elevation* of injured parts; (b) *bandaging;* and (c) *activity*. Uninjured joints which are not immobilized should be actively exercised. Muscular activity helps to pump away edema fluid. Active function helps prevent fibrosis and stiffness in injured muscles and affected joints. Various techniques of physical therapy enhance recovery.

Reduction Traction. Traction techniques have been discussed in detail in Chapter 88. With reduction traction considerable pull is exerted on the distal fragment of the fracture to align it with the proximal fragment (which is less manageable). The amount of traction needed to achieve alignment is usually quite intense and is applied for only a short period of time. Once the fracture has been reduced, the amount of weight applied with the traction set-up is reduced to the smallest amount which will maintain proper alignment and apposition of the bone fragments. As previously mentioned, excessive traction is undesirable during the healing process because it may pull the fragments of bone apart and thereby impede healing.

It is desirable for traction to be applied to the injured limb *before* muscle spasm begins. Prompt application of therapeutic traction may prevent muscle spasm and pain, in addition to maintaining alignment of the fractured bones.

Closed Reduction (Manipulation). The physician performs closed reduction by manually applying traction to lock the ends of the fragments together and thus restore normal bone alignment (see Fig. 89–7). A surgical incision is not performed. The three basic maneuvers used during manipulation are (1) traction and countertraction; (2) angulation; and (3) rotation. Manipulation requires skill and tactile sensitivity. It is a scientific process which reverses the causal force of the fracture. Following closed reduction x-rays are taken and usually a cast is applied.

Open Reduction. After a surgical incision is made, the fracture is aligned under direct vision. At the time of surgery various *internal fixation devices* may be applied to the bone to maintain alignment. These devices consist of metallic screws, plates, pins, wires, nails, or rods which may be placed through bone fragments, fixed to the sides of the bone, or (with rods) inserted directly into the bone's medullary cavity. When both screws and a plate are inserted, they must be made of the same metal to avoid a possible electrolytic reaction. The insertion of skeletal pins and wires for use in maintaining skeletal traction has been discussed earlier in this unit.

While internal fixation devices initially help immobilize a fracture and prevent deformity, they are not a substitute for bone healing. Thus, if proper bone healing does not occur, the metallic structures eventually succumb to stress and they loosen or break, thereby failing to rigidly support the weakened bone.

The major *disadvantage* of open reduction is the possible introduction of infection into the bone because surgery converts a closed fracture into an open fracture.[85] Other *potential hazards* include[221] (a) impaired circulation (open reduction reduces blood supply to the bone, because dissection divides small blood vessels around the bone, and periosteal elevation damages periosteal vessels); (b) accidental injury to major nerves or blood vessels during surgery; and (c) additional damage to bone or adjacent structures caused by the metallic fixation devices implanted during surgery. Because open reduction is not without potential problems, the decision to treat a fracture by this procedure is carefully made.

For some fractures, open reduction is the treatment of choice. For example, *surgery is necessary to treat* compound fractures; fractures accompanied by serious neurovascular injuries; fractures with widely separated fragments; and fractures which have soft tissue interposed between bone fragments. Also, open reduction is typically performed with fractures of the femur and fractured joints. Comminuted fractures may be treated by internal fixation; however, severely comminuted fractures usually do not respond well to internal fixation because enough firm bone is not available to hold the metallic devices, or because the extensive dissection necessary to perform the surgery compromises blood supply to the injured site. Additionally, bone which has a lot of osteoporosis does not respond well to treatment by internal fixation.

To accomplish reduction the patient may be placed on a special fracture table rather than a standard operating table. Fracture tables help hold the patient in position and are particularly useful in procedures such as hip nailing and procedures to be followed by cast application.

X-rays may be taken during and following open reduction to evaluate alignment of the fractured bone. Upon completion of surgery the patient may be placed in traction or a cast may be applied.

Care of the patient undergoing surgical treatment is discussed in Unit VI and in Chapter 88.

Immobilization. Healing fractures must be immobilized until the physician decides that adequate clinical union of the bones has developed. Immobilization prevents movement of the fragments and thus promotes healing, prevents possible overriding or displacement of fragments due to muscle spasm, minimizes pain, and prevents the interposition of soft issue between the fragments. Immobilization may be accomplished by application of casts, splints, or bandages, or by application of traction. Casts and traction (their uses,

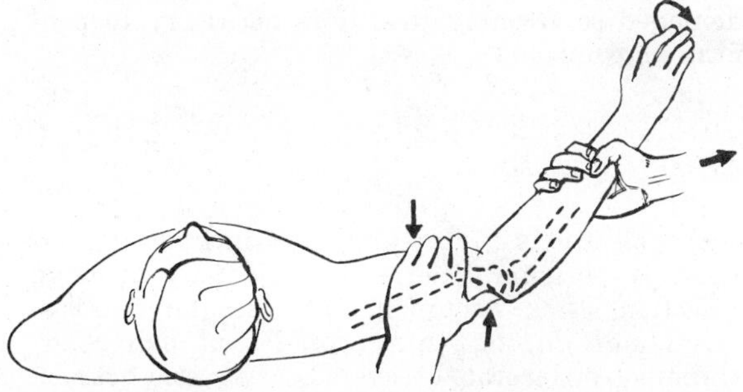

FIGURE 89–7. Closed reduction. Manipulative reduction of supracondylar fracture. (From Schmeisser, G., Jr.: *A Clinical Manual of Orthopedic Traction Techniques.* 1963.)

application, complications, and appropriate clinical care) are discussed in Chapter 88. The body's general responses to bed rest and immobilization, and clinical care of immobilized patients to prevent complications of immobility are discussed in Chapter 27.

Excessive immobilization in the treatment of fractures is undesirable since it contributes to muscle atrophy and impaired circulation. It is therefore important that the movement of adjacent structures (joints, muscles) not be unnecessarily restricted when immobilizing a fractured part.

Compound Fractures. The treatment of compound fractures presents special problems because of the possibility that bacteria and foreign objects may have been introduced when the injury was sustained. Every attempt must therefore be made to prevent subsequent infection. With prompt aseptic cleansing of the wound and surgical treatment, infection can frequently be prevented. Antibiotics are commonly prescribed.

Because an open fracture predisposes the patient to possible *tetanus,* the patient may immediately be given tetanus antitoxin (if he has not been previously immunized) or a booster dose of tetanus toxoid (if he has been immunized). Before tetanus antitoxin is administered, an intracutaneous test dose is given.

Compound fractures are surgical emergencies. The patient should be operated upon within 4 to 6 hours after injury. The sooner surgery can be performed, the better it is for the patient. During surgery the surgeon removes or flushes away (with sterile solutions) bacteria and foreign particles. Surgical treatment also includes cutting away (debridement) of all devitalized tissue. After reducing the fracture and repairing soft tissue injuries the surgeon either closes the wound primarily (with sutures) or leaves the wound unsutured to be closed several days later with secondary sutures or skin grafts. The latter procedure may be the treatment of choice if treatment has been delayed or when a wound is grossly contaminated. The open wound may be loosely packed, as with petrolatum gauze, and covered with a compression dressing. The surgeon subsequently tends the wound and may leave orders for treatments he wants the nurse to administer. At times extremities with compound fractures are damaged so severely that it is necessary to perform amputation.

COMPLICATIONS

Complications of fractures may include arterial damage, peripheral nerve damage, fat embolism, infection, shock, nonunion, and avascular necrosis.

Arterial damage may consist of contused, thrombosed, lacerated, severed, or spastic vessels, as a result of injury associated with the fracture. Vessels may also be constricted by bandages or casts which are excessively tight. Vessels that are highly vulnerable are the popliteal artery (with fractures near the knee joint or dislocations of the knee) and the brachial artery (with supracondylar fractures of the humerus). Impairment of circulation in the brachial artery can produce Volkmann's ischemic contracture. Indications of arterial damage include variable or absent pulse, swelling, pallor or patchy cyanosis distal to the fracture, continuing blood loss, pain, a large fracture hematoma, poor capillary return, poorly filled veins in a cold extremity, and paralysis or anesthesia distal to the fracture (in the absence of known neurologic injury). The nurse observes the fractured extremity closely for indications of these complications and reports symptoms promptly. Emergency treatment may involve splitting or removing tight encircling casts or bandages, elevation or change of position of the part, reduction of fractures or dislocations, or explorative surgery.

Peripheral nerve damage may result from the injury or from pressure over nerves by casts, bandages, or traction equipment. Indications of peripheral nerve damage and the detection of this complication has been previously discussed. Nerves which are particularly susceptible to injury by broken bones or dislocations include the ulnar nerve in medial epicondylar injuries of the elbow; the radial nerve in fractures of the middle and lower humeral shaft; the circumflex nerve in shoulder dislocations; the sciatic nerve in posterior hip dislocations; and popliteal nerves in knee dislocations. When nerves are severed in association with open fractures, immediate surgery is indicated. Commonly nerves recover following reduction if they are merely temporarily stretched, compressed, or contused at the time of fracture or dislocation.

Symptoms of *fat embolism*[102, 182, 191] have been described earlier in this unit. The patient may be treated in the high Fowler's position. Oxygen is given at once to reduce local anoxia and reduce the surface tension of the fat globules. Other respiratory support may be indicated, e.g., intratracheal tube, tracheostomy, respirator. Oxygen therapy is governed by monitoring the arterial oxygen tension. Various other treatments may be employed, directed at treating or preventing shock and heart failure. Opinion varies concerning management of fat embolism. Treatment may include the administration of alcohol intravenously (5 per cent dextrose-5 per cent ethanol solution); corticosteroid hormones; blood and fluid replacements (to treat shock); digitalis; aminophylline, heparin; and low molecular weight dextran (40,000). A variety of specific treatments have been reported. Among these are hypothermia; Pluronic F 68 (a nonionic detergent); decholin (an emulsifying agent); and antihyperlipemic drugs.

Laboratory tests in the presence of fat embolism may show a sudden drop in hemoglobin, fat in the urine or in sputum, a low arterial oxygen tension, and elevated free fatty acids. The most valuable single diagnostic test is a cryostat test which demonstrates fat droplets in frozen sections of blood clots.

Fat embolism can occur at the scene of an accident, in the emergency room, in surgery, or at the bedside, precipitating cardiorespiratory insufficiency and cardiac arrest. Most frequently it occurs with multiple fractures of long bones, but may also occur with some other disorders (e.g., fatty liver, burns, diabetes, pneumonia) and poisonings. Sometimes it develops in injuries without fractures. Emboli may lodge in the brain, heart, or lung, producing life-threatening situations.

Some physicians believe that fat emboli may be prevented by proper splinting, careful transportation, and gentle handling of patients with fractures. These actions also reduce shock in persons with fractures.

Infection may result from contamination of open fractures or can be introduced at the time of surgery. Compound fractures may be complicated by the development of *tetanus* or *gas gangrene.* Gas gangrene infections may develop in deep, grossly contaminated wounds. Gas gangrene is caused by anaerobic bacteria (various species of *Clostridia*). These organisms produce a characteristic cellulitis in which gas is present under the skin. Indications of infection with this contagious organism are precipitous drop in hemoglobin, temperature elevation, rapid pulse, pain, sudden local puffiness (with discoloration of tissues), and a thin, watery exudate which is extremely foul smelling. Crepitation may be felt, upon palpation of the skin, due to the presence of gas bubbles in muscles and subcutaneous tissues.

Treatment of gas gangrene involves opening the wound widely to admit air and permit drainage. Generous and multiple incisions are made through the skin and fascia. Sutures and any gangrenous material are removed and the wound is irrigated. Transfusions may be indicated. Anti-infective agents are administered, e.g., antitoxin with penicillin G or a tetracycline. A cephalosporin and erythromycin are other anti-infectives which may be helpful. If massive gangrene develops amputation is necessary.

Shock is another potential complication of fractures. As stated previously, most musculoskeletal injuries are not life-threatening. However, some are because of shock resulting from the injury. A fractured femur can be a life-threatening injury because severe shock can result from the amount of blood lost from the circulation into tissues. Fractures of the tibia and fibula may also be serious injuries. With open fractures of these bones as much as half of the blood supply may be lost. Traumatic or hypovolemic shock may also occur with fractures of the spine, thorax, and pelvis.

Nonunion and *avascular necrosis* of fractured bone are complications which were discussed previously in relation to healing.

FRACTURES OF THE FEMUR

Space does not permit discussion of the specific treatments of various types of fractures. Most fractures are treated by the application of casts or traction, and details of these methods of treatment have been presented in Chapter 88. Treatment of fractures of the femur has been selected for additional discussion for the following reasons: (a) fractures of the adult femur require treatment by hospitalization (nursing care is therefore important); (b) fractures of the femur commonly occur in older persons (nurses thus frequently care for patients with these disorders); and (c) fractures of the femur are often treated by open reduction with internal fixation (care of patients undergoing internal fixation has not been discussed).

Fractures of the Proximal End of the Femur. Fractures of the proximal end of the femur (the end of the femur which engages with the acetabulum in the innominate bone to form the "hip joint") are classified as either intracapsular or extracapsular. *Intracapsular* fractures are those occurring within the "hip" joint and capsule (a) through the head of the femur (capital fracture); (b) just below the head of the femur (subcapital); and (c) through the neck of the femur (transcervical). *Extracapsular* fractures are those outside of the joint and capsule, occurring through the femur's greater or lesser trochanter or in the intertrochanteric area, i.e., pertrochanteric and intertrochanteric fractures. Extracapsular fractures are located in that portion of the femur which is distal to the neck of the femur and which extends about 2 inches below the lesser trochanter. Figure 89–8 illustrates an intracapsular fracture of the femur and an intertrochanteric fracture of the femur.

Elderly women with osteoporosis are especially prone to fractures of the proximal end of the femur sustained during a fall. Even accidents which appear relatively minor can fracture the femurs of elderly persons. Because these injuries are common among the elderly, x-rays of the hip are routinely taken when a person of advanced age falls or is in an accident. With impacted fractures of the hip a patient may be able to bear weight and perhaps even walk for a short time after he is injured. However, the more typical fracture of the femur, with displacement, immediately incapacitates the patient, and he lies with his painful injured leg shortened, adducted, and in a position of external rotation. The greater trochanter may be felt, displaced in the buttock.

Clinical management of hip fractures in an elderly patient is often complicated by the presence of other coexisting medical disorders which are common among the aged, such as diabetes or cardiac, peripheral vascular, or neurologic disorders. In order to give effective "total patient care," the nurse must be aware of these coexisting problems as well as the location (type) of fracture and methods being employed to treat the fracture.

Treatment programs vary, depending upon the patient's general condition, length of time since the fracture was sustained, and the type of fracture. Some patients are placed in traction for short periods of time prior to open reduction of the fracture. Temporary distraction, via traction, disengages bone fragments and prevents muscle spasm until the patient is ready for surgery. Elderly patients often cannot tolerate prolonged immobilization and therefore may not be able to withstand methods of treatment which require long-term immobilization in traction or hip spica casts. Fractures of the femur are commonly treated by various surgical methods of *internal fixation,* e.g., insertion of pins or nails; fixation of screw plates; or implantation of a prosthesis to replace the head and neck of the femur. Internal fixation generally makes early mobilization possible soon after surgery. This is especially important for older persons who are susceptible to the complications of immobility (see Unit V, Ch. 27). Some patients with femoral fractures are treated by the application of *traction* (e.g., *Russell's traction*) or *casts* (e.g., *hip spica casts*). These procedures and related care are discussed in Chapter 88. Discussion here focuses on treatment by *internal fixation.*

The surgeon performing internal fixation of a femoral fracture has a variety of metallic fixation devices to choose from. In deciding upon the best method of fixing a given fracture, the surgeon considers the angle and location of the line of the fracture. He then selects the fixation device which will most securely hold the fragments of the fracture and which will cause the least disruption of the bone. Fixation devices are made of metals such as stainless steel or Vitallium.

Pins and nails are inserted through the trochanter and femoral neck and then on into the head of the femur (Fig. 89–8, *C*). Plates may be fixed with screws to the shaft of the femur. A *hip prosthesis* consists of a ball and intramedullary stem. The head and neck of the femur is surgically removed, and the stem of the prosthesis is then inserted into the shaft of the femur. The ball portion of the prosthesis then replaces the head of the femur in the acetabulum. Prostheses may be used in treating intracapsular fractures which are difficult to reduce, comminuted or prone to nonunion or the development of aseptic necrosis.

During surgery, when internal fixation is being performed, x-rays or fluoroscopy may be used periodically to guide in placement of the fixating devices. Also, sometimes the surgeon places bone grafts around the fracture line in an attempt to facilitate healing by stimulating bone growth. The grafts may be taken from the patient's tibia or iliac bones.

Among the *complications* which may occur with fractures of the proximal portion of the femur are the following:

> *Shock and hemorrhage:* May occur immediately following injury or during the early postoperative period.

> *Complications of immobility* (see Unit V, Ch. 27): In spite of attempts to prevent these complications, they may rapidly develop, especially among the elderly. Some can be fatal, e.g., pneumonia, thrombophlebitis, pulmonary embolism.

> *Delayed healing, nonunion:* Commonly intracapsular fractures heal more slowly than extracapsular fractures because they may have an impaired blood supply. Nonunion frequently occurs with subcapital fractures treated by nailing. Nonunion may result from poor approximation of the fragments, movement of the fragments, or impaired blood supply.

> *Aseptic necrosis of the head of the femur:* This is a frequent complication following fractures of the proximal femur and traumatic dislocation of the hip. These injuries may jeopardize the blood supply which is delivered to the head of the femur primarily by the posterior retinacular arteries.

> *Deformities; malposition of the femur; secondary arthritis:* Displacement of fragments can produce deformities. Some fractures are difficult to align correctly, and the femur may be malpositioned. The trauma of the injury and surgery may produce secondary arthritic changes in the joint.

> *Postoperative problems with the internal fixation devices:* Internal fixation devices may weaken and break or migrate out of position, causing soft tissue damage. It is therefore sometimes necessary to again perform surgery to remove or replace the damaged or deviant structure.

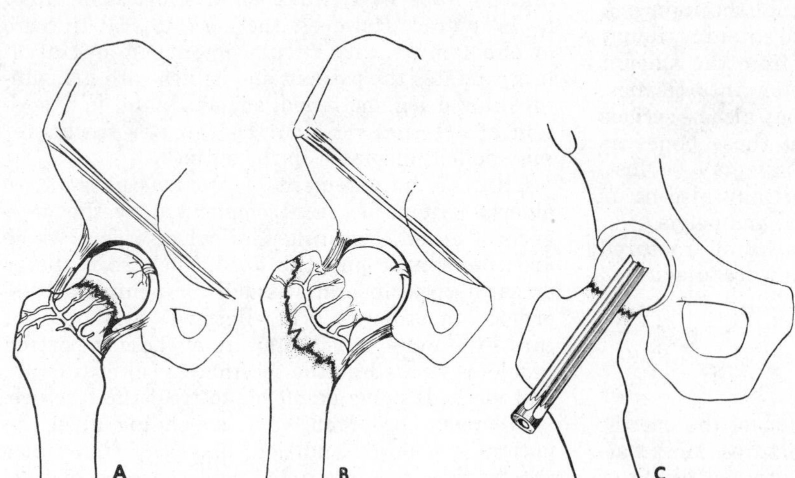

FIGURE 89–8. Fractures of the femur. *A,* Intracapsular fracture. *B,* Intertrochanteric or extracapsular fracture. *C,* Intracapsular fracture with nail inserted for reduction. (From Warren, R., et al.: *Surgery,* 1963.)

Postoperative care can be adequately given only when the nurse is familiar with the type of operative procedure performed, the presence of coexisting disorders, and the physician's specific orders for the patient. Because postoperative management is variable from patient to patient, it is necessary to check orders carefully to be certain that nursing care given a specific patient conforms with that prescribed.

General postoperative care is discussed in Unit VI. See Chapter 88 for a discussion of general postoperative care following orthopedic surgery. Discussion here focuses on aspects of care of special importance following insertion of internal fixation devices in the hip. Some patients are placed in casts or traction for a while following surgery. The application of traction for a few days may help overcome muscle spasm. Care of patients in casts and traction is discussed in Chapter 88.

Early in the postoperative period, dressings and linens are checked frequently for drainage and bleeding. Remember to check not only the hip dressing but also dressings over other areas if bone grafts were taken. A Hemovac (low suction drainage device) may be present to prevent fluid accumulation in the operative wound. Injections of narcotics may be required at first to control pain. Later the patient may be given non-narcotic analgesics. A light sedative may be prescribed to facilitate sleep. Respiratory therapy treatments are commonly administered to stimulate coughing. To prevent thrombophlebitis the doctor may have the patient's legs wrapped with elastic compression bandages to minimize venous stasis and dependent edema and to support venous circulation.

The patient often not only is weakened (from the trauma of his accident and surgery) but also is commonly elderly. Therefore it is frequently necessary for the nurse to consider special aspects of geriatric care when caring for a patient with a fractured hip. For example, a patient of advanced age may have a reduced tolerance to drugs. Thus caution is exercised to prevent oversedation or excessive doses of pain medications. It may be advisable to run IV's more slowly to prevent overloading the circulation and straining the heart. Overloading the circulation is dangerous in a patient with limited cardiac reserve. An elderly patient may be more prone to the development of cardiac failure, shock, respiratory depression, and such complications of immobility as disorientation, urinary stasis, skin breakdown, hypostatic pneumonia, thrombophlebitis, and contractures. *Prevention of the complications of immobility* (e.g., by helping the patient to frequently turn, cough, deep breathe, exercise, and take fluids) *is particularly important in an aged patient* (see Unit V, Ch. 27). Skin breakdown can rapidly develop. Nutritional problems are common with an elderly patient. Healing is retarded if the patient does not eat adequate protein, vitamins (e.g., B,C,D), and calcium. Supplements may be indicated. Siderails help the disabled older person to move about in bed, and they are a protection for a patient who can easily become confused.

As you care for the patient postoperatively, observe closely for indications of shock, hemorrhage, infection, paralytic ileus, confusion, fat embolism, thrombosis, dislocation of the hip joint, aseptic necrosis, and nonunion. Watch for indications of *dislocation of the hip,* e.g., sharp hip pain or "abnormal" positions of the operated leg (leg shortened and externally rotated). Report these symptoms at once. If dislocation has occurred, as determined by x-ray and physical examination, the patient must be returned to surgery. Also, report excessive *temperature elevations.* They may indicate wound infection, urinary tract infection, pneumonia, or other complications. *Thrombophlebitis* is another possible complication; report lower quadrant pain or pain or tenderness in the calf. *Inadequate reduction* or *avascular necrosis of the head of the femur* may produce pain or muscle spasm during the postoperative period. Report these symptoms if they seem excessively prolonged. Avascular (aseptic) necrosis following hip pinning causes pain, muscle spasm, and limping. Continued weight-bearing can crumble the bone. Early treatment is important. The patient may be taken to surgery where the pins and head of the femur may be removed and replaced with a prosthesis. *Nonunion* may be treated with insertion of bone grafts.

> *Following hip surgery check the physician's orders carefully concerning position and activity restrictions. Usually it is necessary to prevent adduction and external rotation of the leg and acute hip flexion.*

The nurse caring for a patient with a hip injury or hip surgery *must* be familiar with the following terms:

> *Adduction:* meaning to "bring toward," drawing toward a center or median line. For example, moving one leg toward the midline of the body while the patient lies flat with both legs straight together, i.e., swinging the leg inward across the other leg.

> *Abduction:* meaning to "take away," drawing away from a center or median line. For example, moving one leg out away from the midline of the body while the patient lies flat with both legs straight together, i.e., swinging the leg out, away from the other leg.

> *Internal rotation:* meaning to twist, or rotate toward the midline of the body.

> *External rotation:* meaning to twist, or rotate away from the midline.

While the terms "adduction" and "abduction" are very similar in their spellings, their meanings are completely different. These differences are extremely important when applied to patient care. *Adduction, external rotation, or acute flexion of the hip can dislocate a hip before it is healed.* Check the position of the operated leg frequently to make sure the hip, knee, and foot are aligned as ordered. Know the restrictions of position and activity for a given patient. Teach the patient activities and positions which are desirable and talk with him about those which are undesirable. Tell him *why* some positions are contraindicated.

Handle the operated leg gently. Tell the patient what you are going to do and how he can be of help. A *trapeze* is usually placed on the patient's bed to help him move about. Teach the patient how to correctly use the trapeze.

As a general rule, *avoid extremes of position* for a patient following hip surgery. Keep the leg *abducted,* i.e., out to the side, at all times—when patient lies flat, while turning, and when patient lies on his side. *Never* adduct the leg past the neutral point or you may dislocate the head of the femur or prosthesis out of the acetabulum. To help maintain abduction a pillow is sometimes placed between the legs when the patient is supine. This serves as a reminder not to cross the legs.

Check to see if the head of the bed can be elevated. If this is permitted, find out how high it can be safely raised. Some patients can have the bed raised 35 to 40°. *Avoid acute flexion of the hip.* This would be caused by excessive elevation of the head of the bed. If the head of the bed can be elevated, instruct the patient not to lean further forward, e.g., to reach for something lying on the foot of the bed. This would additionally increase flexion of the hip.

Often a patient's operated leg tends to lie in slight external rotation when he is on his back. To *prevent external rotation* while the patient is supine, place a trochanter roll beside the external aspect of the thigh. Also, a covered sandbag may be placed beside the outer aspect of the lower leg. The sandbag should not press against the neck of the fibula (location of the peroneal nerve) or against the external malleolus. To prevent external rotation teach the patient to "toe in" or keep his toes pointed "straight up at the ceiling" while lying on his back.

Turn the patient only with a doctor's order. Most commonly following hip surgery the patient is permitted to be turned to the unoperated side. Some patients following hip pinning are permitted to turn to either side. After some types of hip surgery (e.g., total hip replacement, discussed in Chapter 90), no turning is permitted for several days. Checking orders is of obvious importance.

When helping a patient to turn following insertion of an internal fixation device in the hip, remember to avoid adduction and extremes of motion, prevent strain on the hip, and maintain proper alignment of the leg and hip.

Never turn a patient onto his operated hip unless you have a specific order. Typically the patient is turned every two hours during the postoperative period, from his back to his unaffected side, then onto his back again. When turning the patient onto his unoperated side place one pillow between the patient's thighs and another between his lower legs and feet. The pillows help keep the operated leg in a position of abduction and in a straight line with the trunk. One nurse gently rolls the patient toward her, onto his unaffected side. She does this by reaching across the patient and holding his shoulder and buttock on the operated side. Another nurse supports the operated leg in abduction during the turning by supporting the leg full length (on the pillows) at the same level as the trunk. Once the patient is on his side, keep the hip and knee in the same plane elevated on pillows. Unless pillows are between the legs, the operated leg (uppermost leg) will drop down into adduction. While the patient is on his side the physician may permit the knee of the operated leg to be flexed at right angles to the hip. Before leaving the patient make certain the leg is securely positioned so it will not accidentally become misplaced by falling off the pillows.

If the patient is permitted to turn onto his operated side, roll him gently toward you after placing pillows between the legs. The bed acts as a splint for the injured leg. If the patient is not allowed to turn on either side, he may be able to lift straight up on the trapeze periodically for back care and linen changes.

Check with the surgeon to see if the operated limb should be elevated on a pillow. If elevation is ordered, support the entire leg. Sometimes the leg is elevated in traction. When traction is not used the leg is always supported when the patient is turned (as discussed), and is not elevated when the patient is on his back.

Postoperative orders following insertion of a prosthesis usually depend upon the operative approach taken through the joint capsule. Positioning must prevent straining this incision line. Strain on the joint capsule incision can cause the prosthesis to dislocate and push out through the weakened capsule. Commonly with an *anterior* surgical approach the operated limb is rotated internally and is either in a neutral or abducted position. The patient may be permitted to sit up unless the capsule was removed. With a *posterior* approach the leg is positioned in slight abduction and external rotation. (Yes, *external* rotation—a change from the "typical" positioning.) Also, with the posterior approach the patient is kept relatively flat.

Help the patient to *get out of bed* and *sit in a chair* as soon as the doctor permits. This may be on the first postoperative day. Do not rush or hurry the patient during this activity. Remember an elderly patient may become confused if hurried. Give directions slowly to the patient, tell him what he can do to help and tell him whether or not he can bear weight on the operated leg. Commonly weight-bearing is not permitted early in the postoperative course. If the patient experiences postural hypotension a tilt table may be useful in helping him gradually resume an upright position.

When helping the patient get up in a chair, first select a proper chair. A straight-back, relatively high chair with arms is best. Do not select a low, soft chair. Place the chair on the patient's unoperated side. The chair should be facing the head of the bed and parallel to the bed. To help the patient get up, roll him onto his unoperated side and have him flex his leg. (He may be unable to flex the operated leg's knee.) Then gently swing the patient around into a dangling position. Support the injured leg while swiveling the patient. Let the patient rest a moment sitting up. Then, if he is not to bear weight on the operated leg, have him stand up on his "good" leg and pivot on that leg and sit down. Support the patient during this transfer and remind him not to put weight on his operated leg. Weight-bearing before it is permitted can refracture bone, or displace or break the internal fixation device. Elderly patients often forget easily and tend to bear weight on both legs unless frequently reminded not to do so. Some patients need to be lifted from their beds to chairs. If there is a choice, it is better for a patient to stand and pivot rather than be lifted.

The position of a patient's bed should not be too low when he gets up following hip surgery. He can get up with less strain and less bending of the hip if the bed is somewhat elevated. Make certain that casters on the bed are locked so the bed will not slip away from under the patient as he gets up. Likewise, elevated toilet seats are desirable when the patient has bathroom privileges.

Commonly when a patient first gets up in a chair, his operated leg is extended and supported (elevated). Make certain the leg is securely supported. Later, when the physician permits, the leg is lowered into a dependent position. The first few times the leg is lowered, observe it for swelling and discoloration. Once the operated leg is lowered, the patient should sit with his hips even with his knees. Tell the patient not to cross his legs but to remember to "keep both feet on the floor." Crossing the legs adducts the operated leg and can dislocate the hip.

Assist with *exercises* as soon as they are ordered. Exercises may include quadriceps-setting, gluteal-setting, breathing exercises, exercises for the upper extremities (to prepare the patient for crutch walking), and exercises for unoperated extremities, e.g., to flex and extend the knee and ankle of the unoperated leg to stimulate circulation. Most exercises are started on the day following surgery. The patient may also be instructed to flex and dorsiflex the foot on the operated leg and to begin moving the knee on the operated leg. Moving the knee is done with the patient lying on his side so he can flex his knee while keeping his hip extended. Other specific exercises may be prescribed as the patient progresses.

Patient-family teaching facilitates the recovery process. The patient may become discouraged with the slow rate of healing which occurs in some persons. Encouragement, emotional support, diversion, and self-care can help the patient pass through periods of discouragement. Elderly patients may feel they will not recover. Many fear hip fractures because they know of friends or family members who suffered these accidents and succumbed to them. These deep, real concerns should be discussed if the patient wishes to do so. Teaching a patient positive actions he can take to help himself gives the patient independence and motivation to recover.

Instruct the patient about how to correctly use a trapeze and siderails to help himself move about. Also, teach the patient exercises he can do. Be sure you remember to tell the patient when and how many times specific exercises should be performed. Once the patient can get up, teach him to stand and pivot on his uninjured leg when transferring to a chair. Giving praise and recognition of progress can greatly help lift the patient's spirits. Teach family members methods of helping the patient; they can be helpful by reminding the patient to cough, deep breathe, take fluids, and exercise. Also, talk with family members about positions contraindicated for the patient. Instruct the patient not only about actions he can take to enhance his recovery but also about actions which will be harmful. For example, the patient should know which positions it is unsafe to assume, and he should understand *why* these positions are undesirable.

The doctor determines when the bone is healed enough for *ambulation* to begin. He also specifies when the patient can begin to bear weight on the injured leg. Progress of bone healing is carefully followed by periodic x-rays. Parallel bars and a walker may be used before crutches. Walkers are

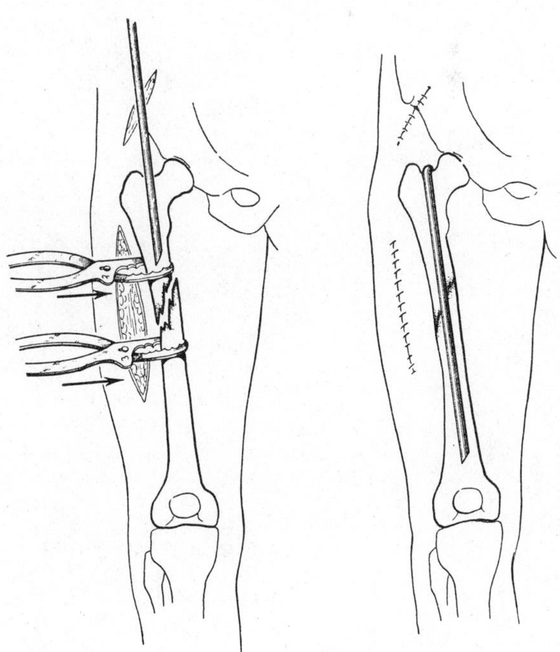

FIGURE 89–9. Treatment of fracture of mid-shaft of femur by fixation with intramedullary nail. (From Warren, R., et al.: *Surgery.* 1963.)

especially helpful for elderly persons. Some older patients are not taught crutch walking because they are not strong enough or well enough coordinated to safely use crutches.

Follow-up care is important after discharge. The physician continues to evaluate the patient's progress via x-rays and physical examinations. Visiting nurse services provide valuable home services for the elderly patient living alone.

Fractures of the Shaft of the Femur. This type of fracture most often results from severe violence and occurs in a young or middle-aged patient. The injury commonly produces marked displacement and deformity, and extensive soft tissue damage with swelling. It is of extreme importance that the leg be protectively immobilized during transportation of the patient, as with a Thomas splint. Often blood loss at the time of injury is considerable and the patient goes into shock.

If the fracture is relatively simple and the patient is in good general condition with no skin damage, the fracture may be treated by open reduction and insertion of an intramedullary rod to maintain fixation. This technique enables early ambulation (with guarded weight-bearing) and early discharge.

Intramedullary fixation of the shaft of the femur by the insertion of an *intramedullary nail* is illustrated in Figure 89–9. Postoperatively a compression dressing is applied. X-rays of the femur are taken on the first postoperative day to evaluate the fixation. The patient is mobilized in bed, and gradual movement of the knee and hip joints is encouraged. After several days (when the physician believes fixation is adequate), the patient begins to ambulate on crutches. If the patient has a transverse fracture which demonstrates adequate fixation, he may be permitted to partially bear weight on the fractured leg early in his recovery period. Sutures are usually removed about 8 days after surgery.

Persons with fractures of the shaft of the femur often are placed in *traction* (e.g., Russell's traction or ring leg splints) to counteract muscle spasms in the powerful thigh muscles. Spasm of these strong muscles can cause the bone fragments to become displaced and override each other. Traction may be used *temporarily* prior to intramedullary nailing. *Continuous* skeletal traction (for 10 to 16 weeks) may be necessary to treat complicated fractures, fractures occurring in a patient whose general condition is poor, or fractures in a leg which has other injuries. Frequent x-rays are taken to check alignment of the fragments. It is important to prevent overpull with traction because this distracts the fragments and impairs healing. The joints and quadriceps are actively exercised early. After 16 to 20 weeks, partial weight-bearing on crutches is usually permitted, and full weight-bearing is permitted after about 6 months.

Supracondylar and Condylar Fractures of the Femur. These fractures of the distal end of the femur may be treated by reduction with continuous skeletal traction and manipulation, or by internal fixation with rods, nails and plates, or screws. These fractures can tear or compress the sciatic nerve or popliteal artery.

CHAPTER 90

Arthritis and Other Musculoskeletal Disorders

ARTHRITIS

The terms "*rheumatism*" and "*rheumatic diseases*" embrace a variety of disorders, all of which are characterized by pain and stiffness referable to the musculoskeletal system. "*Arthritis*" refers to those types of rheumatic disease in which an abnormality of the joint itself is producing the symptoms. As discussed later, there are different types of arthritis. Forms of *nonarticular rheumatic disease* are those in which symptoms result from pathologic changes in structures related to or contiguous to the joints (not within the joint itself). These structures include fibrous tissue, muscles, tendons, tendon sheaths, bursae, and nerves. Some of these disorders are described briefly below:

> *Fibrositis* (also called "muscular rheumatism"): inflammation of connective tissue in any location, but especially of that around joints and in or near tendons, muscle sheaths, or other fascial layers of the locomotor system.

> *Bursitis:* inflammation of a bursa, a fluid-filled small sac which facilitates joint movement by making it possible for muscles and tendons to glide over ligaments or bones. Major bursae are located in the shoulder, elbow, knee, and hip; smaller joints also have bursae.

> *Tendonitis:* inflammation of a tendon.

> *Myositis:* inflammation of voluntary muscle tissue.

> *Peritendinitis:* inflammation of a tendon sheath.

> *Synovitis:* inflammation of a synovial membrane.

> *Tenosynovitis:* inflammation of a tendon and the tendon sheath; most commonly of the hands, wrists, ankles, or feet.

Discussion in this section focuses on diseases of the joints. The American Rheumatism Association publishes a detailed classification of diseases of the joints. The following classification by Robinson is somewhat abbreviated and modified from the more detailed classification but it is adequate for our purposes:

1. Polyarthritis of unknown etiology
   a. Rheumatoid arthritis (atrophic arthritis)
   b. Juvenile rheumatoid arthritis (Still's disease)
   c. Ankylosing spondylitis
   d. Psoriatic arthritis
   e. Reiter's syndrome
2. "Connective tissue" disorders
3. Rheumatic fever
4. Degenerative joint disease (osteoarthritis, osteoarthrosis, hypertrophic arthritis)
5. Arthritis associated with known infectious agents
6. Traumatic and/or neurogenic disorders
7. Gout and pseudogout
8. Tumor and tumor-like conditions[213]

Space does not permit discussion of all of these disorders. Included in the following pages are discussions of rheumatoid arthritis, osteoarthritis, gout, and certain connective tissue disorders (systemic lupus erythematosus, polyarteritis nodosa, scleroderma, polymyositis, and dermatomyositis).

Joint diseases have occurred in man and other animals for millions of years. Evidence of degenerative joint disease or osteoarthritis has been identified in the skeletal remains of dinosaurs living 100 million years ago. Signs of arthritis have been found in skeletons of prehistoric man, and in Egyptian mummies.

Today arthritis is the number one crippling disease in the United States, affecting in some form at least 50,000,000 Americans. Of this number at least 17,000,000 require medical care. The suffering caused by arthritis is immeasurable. In 1966, in the United States, lost wages and medical bills attributed to arthritis amounted to more than $3.6 billion.[254] Some arthritis develops in almost anyone who lives long enough. Few victims of arthritis have the money or insurance to afford the necessary periods of long hospitalization, surgery, medications, and physical therapy which are of importance in the treatment of crippling types of arthritis.

It is still not known what causes arthritis or how to cure it, but it is possible in many cases to prevent or correct its crippling effects. A variety of medications may be used to treat arthritis, and recently developed surgical techniques can restore function and relieve pain in many cases. Physical therapy is valuable in the treatment of arthritis as a means of relieving pain and preventing deformity. All of these treatment techniques are discussed in detail further on.

Both *acute* and *chronic* forms of arthritis occur. Acute exacerbations may occur with chronic forms, and acute types of arthritis may progress into subacute or chronic stages. Two basic pathologic processes affect the joints with any arthritic disorder: *inflammation,* and *degenerative changes.* Inflammation may be exudative or proliferative or a combination of both types. The degenerative changes which take place within involved joints depend essentially on the ability of articular cartilage to repair itself. In any given patient varying degrees of inflammation and degeneration may be present.[213]

RHEUMATOID ARTHRITIS

Rheumatoid arthritis is the most virulent form of arthritis. Women are affected three times more frequently than men. While rheumatoid arthritis can occur at any age, it most commonly affects young adults. The usual age at onset is 20 to 40 years. Rheumatoid arthritis is a chronic, systemic disease in which inflammatory changes occur throughout the body's connective tissues. Commonly the smaller, peripheral joints are involved in a pattern of symmetric distribution. The articular and periarticular structures are progressively destroyed by a chronic proliferative inflammation which replaces involved structures with granulation tissue. As the disease destroys the joints internally, the patient suffers with pain, stiffness, and swelling. Unexplainable remissions and exacerbations occur. Physical and emotional stresses are often associated with the onset of rheumatoid arthritis.

An estimated 5 million persons in the United States have rheumatoid arthritis. The incidence of rheumatoid arthritis appears to be about the same in the United States and Canada; the disease is relatively rare in tropical climates. Arthritis is even more common in Great Britain than in the United States.

Etiology. In spite of intensive research efforts the etiology of rheumatoid arthritis currently remains unknown. Hypotheses are many and varied. Among theories under investigation are those which speculate that the disease may be caused by an undefined virus or some other microorganism (e.g., *Mycoplasma*), by metabolic aberrations, or by immunologic mechanisms. The role of the immune response in the mediation of tissue injury is being given careful consideration (see Unit V, Ch. 23). Possibly there is a genetic basis for a predisposition to rheumatoid arthritis. It is possible that this disease is caused by several factors.

Pathology. If unarrested, the joint pathology in rheumatoid arthritis passes through four stages: (1) synovitis; (2) pannus formation; (3) fibrous ankylosis; and (4) bony ankylosis (see Fig. 90–1). The involved joint(s) becomes inflamed with a proliferative type of inflammation that is initially localized in the joint capsule, primarily in the synovial membrane (*synovitis*). Edema and congestion thicken the tissue. A *pannus* is a layer of granulation inflammatory tissue which eventually develops, derived from the synovial membrane. The pannus extends over the surface of the articular cartilage into the interior of the joint. It appears reddish and rough and adheres tightly to

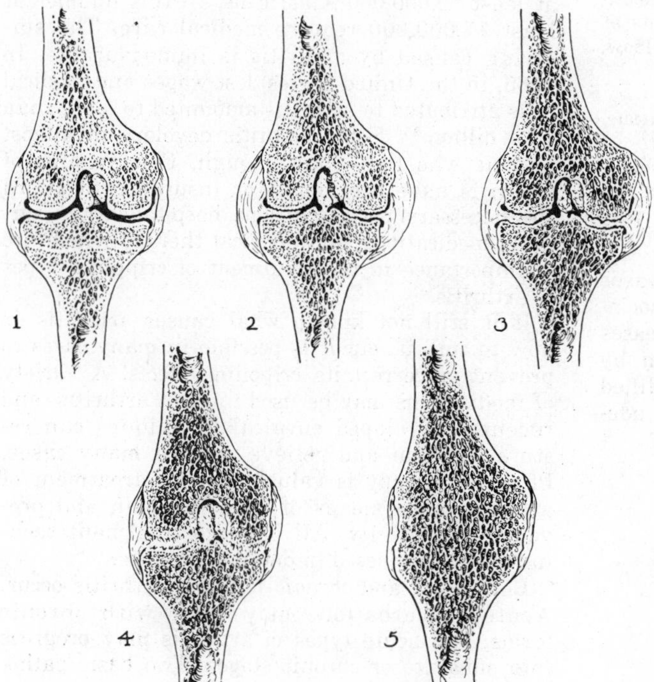

FIGURE 90–1. Sketches showing the joint pathology in rheumatoid arthritis. (1) Inflammation of the joint capsule with synovitis; beginning proliferative changes. (2) Progression of inflammation with pannus formation; beginning destruction of cartilage and mild osteoporosis. (3) Advanced synovitis with extensive pannus, cartilage destruction, and osteoporosis. (4) Inflammation subsided; fibrous ankylosis. (5) Bony ankylosis. (From Sodeman, W. A., and Sodeman, W. A., Jr.: *Pathologic Physiology: Mechanisms of Disease.* 5th ed.)

the underlying cartilage. The pannus formation erodes and destroys the cartilage by interfering with cartilage nutrition. The articular cartilage is then slowly destroyed by invasion, lysis, and starvation. Additional destruction may occur as granulations from the pannus develop on contiguous areas and in subchondral bone. The joint capsule and subchondral bone are thus progressively damaged. *Fibrous ankylosis* (with subluxation and distortion of the affected joint) then occurs as the granulation tissue becomes invaded with tough fibrous tissue and is converted to scar tissue (which inhibits or prevents joint motion). *Bony ankylosis* (firm bony union) may then develop as the fibrous tissue becomes calcified and changes into osseous tissue.

Other changes occur in addition to the above described joint changes. The muscles, bones, and skin adjacent to an affected joint become somewhat atrophic, and the skin becomes tight, thin, and glossy in appearance. The most characteristic histologic lesions of rheumatoid arthritis are *subcutaneous nodules*. These nodules, which may be present for weeks or months, most commonly develop over bony prominences, especially near the elbow (see Fig. 90–2).

While joint involvement is the most obvious manifestation of rheumatoid arthritis, other body tissues are also affected. Rheumatoid arthritis is a *systemic* disease, attacking connective tissues throughout the body. Nonarticular connective tissue may be diffusely involved; degenerative lesions may be present in *collagen* in the lungs, heart, muscles, blood vessels, pleura, or tendons. (Collagen is a scleroprotein present in the body's connective tissue.) *Vasculitis* may occur in the eyes, nervous system, and skin, producing ischemia and thrombosis.

Clinical Description. As mentioned, rheumatoid arthritis is characterized by remissions and exacerbations. Some patients experience a relatively brief period of illness lasting only a few months, and then may have their symptoms completely disappear for several months or possibly several years. Even in well-established chronic arthritis, the patient typically has periods in which the disease activity is heightened and other periods in which he is relatively comfortable. Tendencies toward remission tend to be greatest, however, early in the course of the disease. Each attack tends to be more stubborn than that which preceded it. Occasionally permanent spontaneous remission occurs, but this is not usual. Generally rheumatoid arthritis progresses, producing some degree of deformity. According to one source,[70] 10 years after onset 15 per cent of patients are likely to be bedridden, 35 per cent may be ambulatory but unable to earn a living, and 50 per cent may be capable of self-care and be employable.

Rheumatoid arthritis may begin abruptly, but more commonly develops insidiously. Prodromal symptoms include vague articular pain and stiffness, malaise, weight loss, and vasomotor disturbances such as paresthesias (numbness and tingling of the hands and feet). Typically pain and stiffness worsen markedly following strenuous activity. These symptoms are usually most

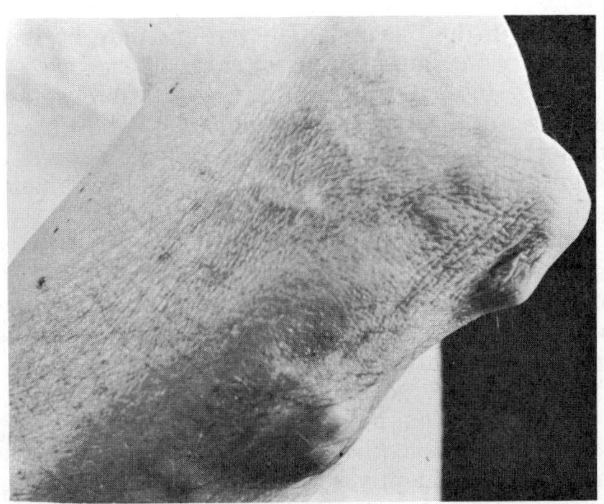

FIGURE 90–2. Rheumatoid nodules in olecranon bursa and over upper portion of ulna in a patient with classic rheumatoid arthritis. (From Beeson, P. B., and McDermott, W. (eds.): *Cecil-Loeb Textbook of Medicine.* 13th ed.)

prominent in the morning and subside during a day of moderate activity. Affected joints not only are stiff and painful, but may be swollen, red, tender, and warm.

Other findings which may occur with rheumatoid arthritis include: subcutaneous nodules, enlarged spleen, enlarged lymph nodes, anorexia, low-grade fever, weakness, mental depression, and early afternoon fatigue. With advanced disease, ocular manifestations and joint deformities may be present. Atrophy of the muscles and skin around the involved joints may be noticeable. Flexion contractures result from spasm of flexor muscles around inflamed joints and reflex relaxation and atrophy of the antagonistic extensor muscles.

The onset of rheumatoid arthritis often coincides with disturbances which tend to deplete physical or emotional reserves or both, e.g., emotional strain or worry, exposure, overwork, or acute infections.

When rheumatoid arthritis develops *insidiously,* the patient usually experiences pain (on use) and stiffness in one or several joints, followed by swelling. Muscle aching may be present in any part of the body. The temperature may be normal or only slightly elevated. While almost any joint of the body may be initially affected, within several weeks the smaller joints of the hands and feet are typically involved. With an *acute onset* of rheumatoid arthritis, numerous joints suddenly become painful and swollen. The patient experiences chills, prostration, and fever.

Pain produced by rheumatoid arthritis is variable in intensity and tends to be most persistent upon use of the involved joint. Stiffness is often the most constant symptom, tending to be greatest upon arising in the morning. The patient may be most limber in the late morning or early afternoon.

The joints of the hands, knees, elbows, and ankles are most commonly involved. The characteristic appearance of the hands is shown in Figure 90–3. Usually the patient has a weakened grip and is unable to make a tight fist.

The typical patient with rheumatoid arthritis appears undernourished and chronically ill. He may also appear anemic. Eighty percent of patients have a hypochromic, normocytic anemia because of the effect of rheumatoid arthritis upon blood-forming organs.

In addition to a physical examination, *laboratory findings* help establish a diagnosis of rheumatoid arthritis. Frequently serum protein abnormalities are present. Many patients with rheumatoid arthritis have in the serum of their blood *"rheumatoid factors"* (RF), which are large antibody-like protein molecules. In 90 per cent of cases of rheumatoid arthritis, the erythrocyte sedimentation rate (ESR) is elevated. The ESR and C-reactive protein are elevated during both acute and chronic phases. As mentioned earlier, a hypochromic, normocytic anemia is common. Usually the WBC is slightly elevated or normal; however, leukopenia may be present (e.g., with splenomegaly).

The presence of RF supports the theory that rheumatoid arthritis is a disorder of immunity. It is believed that RF are produced in response to alterations in the connective tissues' gamma globulin. While RF are not specific for rheumatoid arthritis (they are found in numerous granulomatous and infectious diseases), a high RF titer helps confirm the diagnosis of rheumatoid arthritis when symptoms and history of the typical clinical syndrome are present. Treatment influences the RF titer, which commonly falls as inflammatory activity in joints decreases. Typically a high RF titer is indicative of a poor prognosis and is associated with progressive disease, vasculitis, nodules, and pulmonary involvement.[106] A variety of serologic techniques are used to assess the RF titer. The F2 latex fixation test is one such test; usually it is positive in 60 to 75 per cent of cases. Even higher percentages of positive reactions occur with tests which are more sensitive. False-positive reactions may occur.

It is helpful for the physician to *aspirate* some *synovial fluid* ("joint fluid") for examination. The fluid is always abnormal in rheumatoid arthritis. The abnormalities reflect the varying degrees of inflammation within the joint. The fluid is generally opaque and sterile with reduced viscosity. From 3000 to over 50,000 WBC's/cu.mm. are present.

X-rays may show only soft tissue swelling early

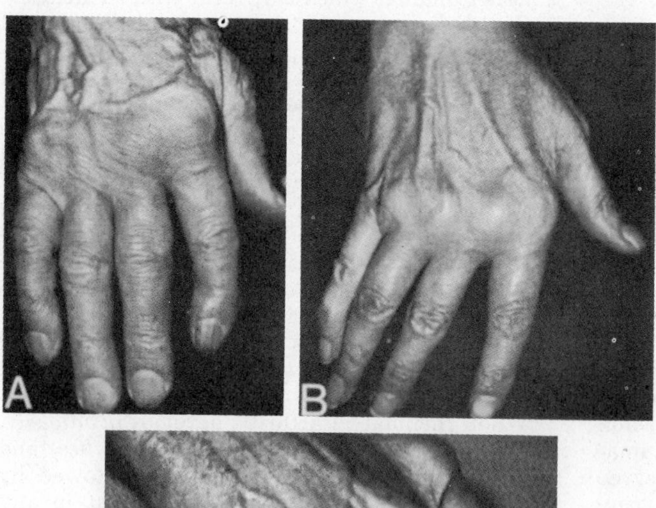

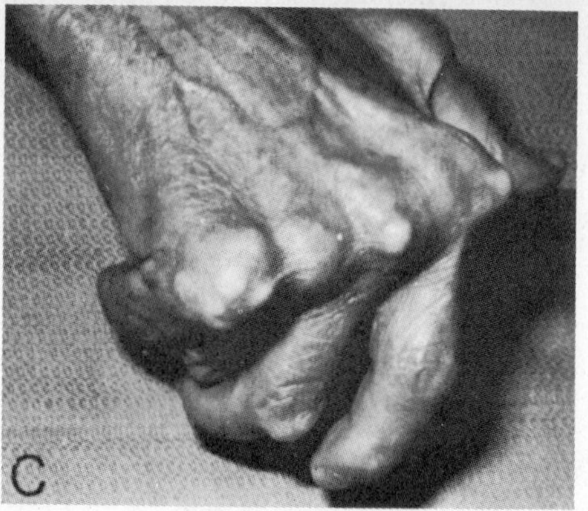

FIGURE 90–3. Metacarpophalangeal deformities in rheumatoid arthritis. *A,* Stage one demonstrates moderate synovitis of the metacarpophalangeal joints with normal finger alignment. *B,* Early ulnar drift with displacement of the extensor tendons. *C,* Advanced ulnar drift with volar dislocation of the proximal phalanges. (From Nalebuff, E. A.: Metacarpophalangeal surgery in rheumatoid arthritis. *Surgical Clinics of North America 49*:825, 1969.)

in the course of rheumatoid arthritis. Other changes appear later with progression. These changes include osteoporosis around the involved joint, erosion of the cartilage at the periphery of the joint surface, joint space narrowing (due to erosion of cartilage), and bony cysts (from invasion of granulation tissue). After several years the degenerative changes of secondary osteoporosis are apparent.

Because of its chronic and sometimes crippling nature, rheumatoid arthritis is a *difficult diagnosis for a patient to accept.* At the time that the physician discusses the diagnosis with the patient, he should attempt to discuss realistically how the illness may affect the patient's life. Because of the variable nature of rheumatoid arthritis, it is difficult to discuss with accuracy the expected rate of progress. It should be emphasized to the patient that many persons with rheumatoid arthritis continue to lead active productive lives and that with early, intensive treatment only slight modifications in life style may be necessary. Patients who cannot or will not accept their limitations and modify their lives accordingly do more poorly than those who are able to do so. Arthritis does not need to be a "hopeless" disease; however, if treatment is delayed or avoided it typically progressively worsens. A relatively small number of persons with rheumatoid arthritis (10 to 15 per cent) are completely incapacitated, i.e., confined to a bed or wheelchair, in spite of treatment.

Treatment. Rheumatoid arthritis is usually best treated by a conservative approach, e.g., with salicylates, rest, and physical therapy. Some patients are treated initially with a period of hospitalization. An important part of a successful treatment program involves *teaching* the patient about the nature of his illness and about the best methods of treatment. Victims of arthritis often tend to try "quack" cures in hopes of obtaining relief. Patients who do not understand the nature of rheumatoid arthritis are especially vulnerable to claims made by manufacturers of "quack remedies." According to the Arthritis Foundation, more than $400,000,000 per year is spent by arthritics on worthless or harmful treatments, devices, or "cures."

Early, active therapy before the establishment of fibrosis or bony ankylosis is most successful. *Treatment goals* include preservation of function, reduction of pain and inflammation, and prevention or correction of deformities. It is desirable if the patient with rheumatoid arthritis can be seen by both a rheumatologist and an orthopedic surgeon. Preventive surgery can be highly beneficial when performed in earlier stages of the disease.

Individually prescribed treatment-rehabilitation programs are essential in the treatment of rheumatoid arthritis. Because rheumatoid arthritis is a chronic disorder, the patient requires long-term medical supervision. Prescriptions are changed from time to time as the patient's condition varies. In addition to receiving prescriptions for medications, the patient should be given *written* prescriptions concerning rest and activity (e.g., exercises).

Since the patient is the central figure in his treatment-rehabilitation program, he must be accurately advised about how he can help himself. For example, exercises should be supervised until it is clear that the patient can correctly perform them without causing additional trauma to involved joints. The patient must also be able to take medications as ordered and treat himself with applications of heat or cold if ordered. The importance of exercising, taking medications, resting, and performing other aspects of treatment on a *regular* basis, as advised by the physician, is emphasized during patient-family education sessions. The patient needs to be familiar with reportable side effects of medications which he is taking.

Patient education should include discussion of factors which will not be curative so he will not waste his money on ineffective "quack" cures (e.g., tonics, diets, vibrators). Also, the patient should be informed of local assistance programs which may be of help to him. For example, the Arthritis Foundation provides clinical research and treatment centers, information services, group physical/hydrotherapy programs, home living assistance programs, and a limited number of patient care grants. Helpful patient education booklets are available from local chapters of the Arthritis Foundation (National headquarters are located at 1212 Avenue of the Americas, New York, N.Y. 10036.)

A community nurse can help a patient with rheumatoid arthritis plan modifications in his activities and home environment which make it easier to perform activities of daily living. Physical therapists have many helpful suggestions about work simplification techniques. Social workers can help the patient to meet problems created by reduced income and high medical expenses. Psychiatric and religious counseling may be of benefit to the patient as he adjusts to the chronicity and disabilities of his illness.

While some persons with rheumatoid arthritis find it necessary to change their type of employment, many are able to continue their jobs. Those individuals who need to make job changes may be helped by the State Department of Vocational Rehabilitation if vocational retraining is needed.

Family members need to be included in the treatment-rehabilitation program so they understand the nature of a patient's illness and so they can participate in his care. Both the patient and his family should understand that much disability and deformity can be prevented with vigorous, early therapy and adherence to prescribed treatment programs.

To facilitate the following discussion, methods of treatment are divided into six sections: (1) rest; (2) activity; (3) heat and cold; (4) diet; (5) medications; and (6) surgery.

REST. Both systemic and emotional rest are part of the basic treatment of rheumatoid arthritis. It is important to remember that rheumatoid arthritis is not merely a disorder of the joints, but rather it is a systemic disease. It is equally important to remember that illnesses must be approached as somatopsychic disorders (see Unit IV).

The amount of *systemic rest* necessary varies depending upon the severity of the patient's disease at any given time. With extensive systemic and articular involvement, complete bedrest is indicated. Complete bedrest is anti-inflammatory. As a general rule, the more acute the disease or the greater the number of joints involved, the greater is the benefit of bedrest. With mild rheumatoid arthritis, 2 to 4 hours of rest daily (in addition, of course, to the usual amount of rest at night) may be adequate. Commonly the prescribed amount of rest is continued until the patient has maintained a level of significant improvement for at least two weeks. The physician may then modify the prescription.

In order for *bedrest* to be effective, the bed must be firm and the patient must be correctly positioned to prevent deformities (foot drop, fixation of the joints in extension, flexion contractures). Foot boards, splints, sandbags, and other devices are used to maintain proper body alignment.

The patient with rheumatoid arthritis should *not* be positioned in such a manner that hip and knee flexion contractures are encouraged. For example, pillows should not be placed under the knees, and the patient should not be permitted to remain for long periods of time with his head and knee rests elevated. Frequent position changes are important. To prevent hip flexion contractures, at least 2 to 3 times per day the patient should lie prone for ½ hour. To prevent flexion deformities of the neck, the patient should be advised to use only a small pillow beneath his head if he requires a pillow.

During periods of bedrest the patient should be positioned much of the time flat on his back with affected joints in positions of extension. Extension is important to combat the joints' tendencies to be pulled into flexion contractures. Only a small pillow or folded towel should be under the patient's head. A small pillow may be placed under the ankles to straighten the knees. The arms should be positioned (palms upward) with small pillows or folded towels under the elbows or wrists to maintain extension. Sandbags and trochanter rolls are used as necessary to maintain proper body alignment. This supine position should be maintained periodically for at least 10 hours each day while the patient is on complete bedrest. Because it is not the position of greatest comfort, the patient must be helped to realize the reasons for maintaining a position of extension.

Attention must be intensively directed at *preventing complications of immobility* when a patient's activities are reduced, e.g., during bedrest, and if the patient is confined to a wheelchair. For a detailed discussion of the complications of immobility and their prevention see Unit V, Chapter 27.

Emotional factors are of paramount importance in rheumatoid arthritis, although current thinking tends to place less emphasis than formerly on emotional factors in the basic etiology.[13a] Once the disease is established, emotional problems can trigger exacerbations. The patient requires emotional support from all persons involved in his care and from family members. The physician attempts to help the patient understand the importance of *emotional rest* in his illness. It is helpful to evaluate the patient's emotional reactions to his diagnosis and illness (see Unit III). It is also necessary to try to understand a given patient's personality. The hospital nurse can provide significant insights into these factors because of the length of time she may spend with the patient. Additionally, persons working with the patient in his home (visiting nurse, or visiting occupational or physical therapist) can evaluate the home situation and family relationships and offer appropriate assistance.

Providing *rest for joints* involved with rheumatoid arthritis helps reduce articular inflammation. Weight-bearing joints may be rested by complete bed rest. *Splints* may also be applied to more completely rest inflamed joints. Splints also relieve pain (by relieving spasm) and prevent or reduce deformities. For example, a posterior knee extension splint not only keeps the knees in full extension but also properly positions the ankles. Plaster is the least expensive material for making these splints. Plastic materials of various sorts (e.g., Plastazote) are easier to use for making small splints, e.g., for the hands and wrists. Some physicians use dynamic splinting (see Fig. 90–4), with rubber bands and springs, in an attempt to reduce deformity and increase function. Splints commonly require frequent periodic adjustments to keep them fitting comfortably (they must not damage the skin) and effectively.

Splints must be removable for exercises and other treatments, such as heat applications. To prevent fibrous ankylosis the joints are periodically exercised; for example, splinted joints may be carried through a full range of motion once or twice daily. With improvement, some patients require splints only at night or perhaps not at all for a while.

ACTIVITY. Prescribed amounts of activity help the patient with rheumatoid arthritis to attain and maintain optimum levels of function and independence. Activity also helps the patient to feel more comfortable mentally.

A person with a chronic illness often tends to think more about his body than he would if he were well. While paying attention to his physical needs can be helpful during illness, excessive preoccupation with himself is unhealthy. To prevent excessive self-concern with his body and illness, the patient needs to become involved in other meaningful interests and activities, such as self-care and occupational therapy. The physician should be informed if a patient shows a sustained

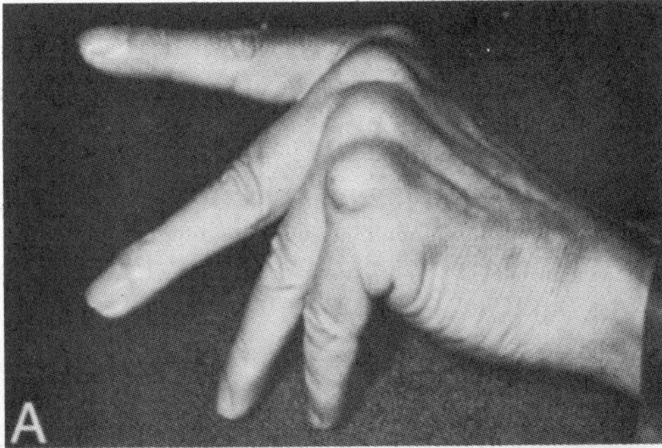

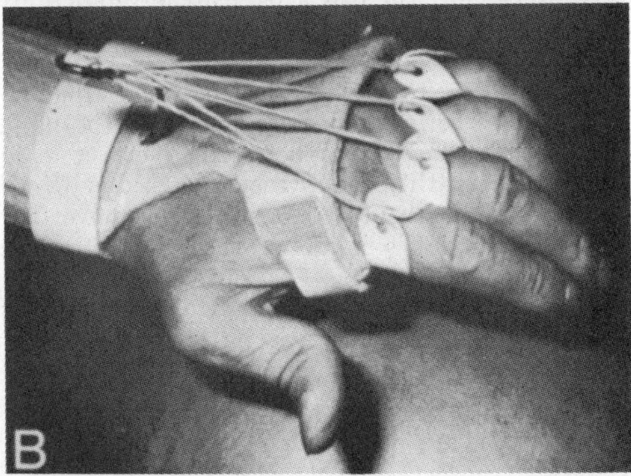

FIGURE 90-4. Dynamic splints are useful in both the preoperative and postoperative care of the rheumatoid hand. *A*, Patient with loss of active finger extension secondary to displacement of extensor tendons. *B*, Note improved postoperative posture of hand with dynamic splint. (From Nalebuff, E. A.: Metacarpophalangeal surgery in rheumatoid arthritis. *Surgical Clinics of North America 49*:796, 1969.)

tendency toward excessive self-preoccupation. Psychiatric counseling may help relieve the patient's anxieties.

Acutely inflamed joints are extremely painful when moved. The patient is thus often reluctant to move even though he may know that he requires some activity. *Occupational therapy* provides an excellent means of encouraging purposeful movements and makes "exercising" seem less burdensome.

> *Handle affected joints gently, keeping them supported during movement. Avoid sudden, jarring movements.*

Encourage *self-care* and activity as permitted by the physician. Do not attempt to rush or hurry the patient. Remember, he may be experiencing pain with every movement and his joints may be stiff and difficult to move.

Physical therapy is of importance in the treatment of rheumatoid arthritis[184] because it prevents and corrects deformities, controls pain, strengthens weakened muscles, and improves function. Deformities are prevented and corrected by a vigorous positioning program and an active exercise program. Knee and elbow deformities are sometimes corrected by progressive casting. Pain is controlled by teaching the patient methods of regulating his activities in ways which will not increase pain. Psychologic support also is freely given to help the patient continue with his treatment program in spite of some pain. Isometric exercises and progressive resistance methods of isotonic strengthening exercises against maximal force are employed to strengthen weakened muscles. Function is improved by identifying the individual patient's needs and helping him to learn more effective methods of daily living.[184] A variety of *self-care appliances* are available to help the patient with rheumatoid arthritis maintain a maximum level of independence. These include such things as eating utensils with special handles, long-handled "reachers" and combs, specially elevated chairs and toilet seats, and so forth.

Continuous immobilization can cause increasing pain in the patient with rheumatoid arthritis. Exercise (moving the painful joints) can actually relieve pain. This important fact should be explained to the patient. Often a patient hesitates to move because he fears that movement will intensify his pain. The patient may find it helpful to take aspirin ½ hour before exercising, but if he does he must be cautioned not to overexercise (because his pain threshold will raised by the aspirin).

Isometric exercises are important in maintaining muscle function even when splints are applied. When there is only slight joint activity, *isotonic* exercises are best performed. *Exercises are the most important single part of the physical therapy program* for a patient with rheumatoid arthritis. Rest and therapeutic exercise must always be kept in proper balance. Because fatigue is a common symptom, the patient's tolerance to exercise must be carefully evaluated. Overactivity can inflame affected joints. Exercises should be performed within the limits of pain tolerance. Some specific exercises which the physician may instruct the patient to learn are illustrated in the booklet "Home Care Programs in Rheumatoid Arthritis."[257] Deep breathing exercises are also helpful to the patient with rheumatoid arthritis. These are discussed in Unit XIV.

During exercises the patient may experience some pain which persists for a short time. This is not unusual; however, pain which lasts for several hours following exercises may indicate that the exercises are excessive and need to be modified. The patient's reaction to exercises is carefully evaluated, as mentioned, and increased pain or excessive fatigue are reported. The physician may then decide to change the exercise program.

Knapp[132] observes that resistance exercises to strengthen finger flexors (e.g., squeezing a rubber ball) should not be prescribed for persons with rheumatoid arthritis, since these exercises only increase the deformities commonly found in arthritic hands, e.g., ulnar drift of the fingers.

When correctly performed, *massage* may help relieve pain and muscle aching. Joints which are actively inflamed should *not* be massaged, because massage may aggravate inflammation. The patient should be told this because he may have a tendency to "rub" inflamed, aching joints. Massage should be given over surrounding muscles, not over the joints. Most family members cannot be taught to skillfully perform massage. If massage is necessary to relieve pain, it is best performed by a skilled physical therapist.

Emphasize the importance of *proper posture* to the patient. Teach him to look at his posture in a mirror and to make conscious attempts to sit and stand erect, to "think good posture." Show the patient illustrations of correct and incorrect posture.

When the patient begins *ambulation,* care is taken to avoid aggravation of flexion deformities by weight-bearing. Until these contractures are corrected, the patient may require supports (crutches, braces) during ambulation. Supportive shoes are of importance when the patient is out of bed. Properly fitted shoes help support the feet and also make ambulation safer. Some patients require corrective shoes or molded shoes. The patient with arthritis should not be permitted to wear soft slippers while out of bed.

The arthritic person with involvement of his hips or knees or both is most comfortable if he sits on a straight-backed armchair which is elevated 3 to 4 inches more than ordinary chairs. This added height prevents excessive hip and knee flexion and makes it easier for the patient to get up and down. Similarly, elevation of the toilet seat may also help the patient to get up and down more easily. "Grab bars" placed on or beside the toilet provide additional help. It is also best if the patient's bed is somewhat raised. For example, if the patient must transfer from his bed to a wheelchair, the bed should be elevated to the height of the wheelchair.

It is not unusual for a person with arthritis to find that his knees become stiff after he sits for a while. Instruct him to flex and extend his knees several times before trying to stand up. This "limbering up" will help the patient to arise more easily and to feel steadier when he does get up. Similar periodic flexions and extensions of the knees while seated may make prolonged periods of sitting more comfortable by helping to eliminate stiffness.

HEAT AND COLD. Applications of heat are frequently used in the treatment of rheumatoid arthritis. *Heat applications* have an analgesic effect and help relax muscles. Heat may also relieve joint stiffness and swelling. Exercises can usually be performed more effectively if preceded by the application of heat. Various forms of heat therapy may be used: moist heat, dry heat, diathermy, ultrasound.

Whirlpool baths are quite effective. They permit active exercising in the bath with minimal resistance. Home models are available (e.g., Jacuzzi or Vibrabath) and may be useful when prolonged treatment is indicated. Hot packs, paraffin baths, and warm tub baths or showers are commonly used methods of applying heat in the treatment of rheumatoid arthritis. Hot towels can be wrung out and wrapped around painful knees. Painful hands can be immersed in paraffin baths.

The patient can be taught to perform paraffin baths at home as follows: (a) in the top of a double boiler melt 4 pounds of paraffin wax and 2 ounces of mineral oil; (b) use a candy thermometer to maintain a temperature of about 130°F.; (c) dip the hands (one at a time) in and out of the warm mixture (allow the wax to cool between dippings); and (d) after dipping 6 or 7 times slip the hands into plastic bags placed between layers of folded towels. After the hands rest, covered with the warm wax, for about 20–30 minutes remove them from the plastic bags. Peel off the wax and replace it in the double boiler for reuse at the time of the next treatment. When performed the first thing in the morning, the patient may obtain considerable comfort from this procedure and may be able to move his hands with greater ease. Coats of melted wax can be painted (with a brush) on joints which cannot easily be submerged.

Because paraffin is flammable, it must be heated with caution when a gas appliance or other open flame is used. Advise the patient not to pour the wax or any water with wax drippings down the drain, because when the wax solidifies it will clog plumbing. If accidentally spilled or excessively heated, hot wax can seriously burn the patient. A thermometer must be used, and the patient must be able to read it correctly. Advise the patient to exercise caution during paraffin treatments to prevent accidents. If a patient cannot safely manage paraffin baths (or other treatments) at home, visiting nurse services may be of value.

The physician may order some patients to use dry heat from an electric heating pad, hot water bottle, or infrared heat lamp. Infrared radiation is an effective method of applying heat therapeutically. Most drugstores have the necessary equipment available at reasonable prices.

Some patients with rheumatoid arthritis obtain relief from *cold applications* (e.g., crushed ice packs) which induce local anesthesia. Regardless of the manner in which heat or cold is applied, the skin must be protected appropriately from possible trauma. (Details of the application of hot and cold treatments can be found in textbooks of nursing fundamentals and hospital procedure books.)

DIET. No specific dietary measures have been identified which are effective in the treatment of rheumatoid arthritis. A well-balanced general diet is therefore usually indicated. If a patient is overweight he may be placed on a weight-reducing diet to relieve his joints from the need to support excessive amounts of weight. Also, the overweight patient is less likely to exercise effectively.

MEDICATIONS. While numerous drugs are available for use in treating rheumatoid arthritis, aspirin remains the single drug most widely prescribed. No medication is available which will cure rheumatoid arthritis. The patient should be informed that during the course of his treatment the doctor may prescribe various medications. Patient and physician work together to identify which medications are most effective in treating the patient's disease process. The patient needs to be informed of side effects which should be reported. Detailed descriptions of medications used with rheumatoid arthritis are presented in textbooks of pharmacology.

Aspirin or sodium salicylate. Salicylates form the backbone of drug therapy in rheumatoid arthritis. These medications have analgesic and anti-inflammatory properties. Additionally they are relatively safe and inexpensive. Aspirin is available in various forms: plain tablet; soluble tablet; enteric-coated (Enseal or Ecotrin); with buffer added; and as a suppository. Some physicians believe the enteric-coated and buffered tablets offer little advantage; others believe they are helpful. Commonly the patient is allowed to take the type which he feels best helps him.

Aspirin should be taken with food because of its possible irritating effects on the stomach. It may be prescribed after meals, with an antacid, or with milk. Usually the medication is prescribed (in writing) in doses sufficient to produce mild symptoms of drug intoxication, e.g., reduced hearing, tinnitus, or gastrointestinal upset. Once those symptoms are produced, the dose may then be reduced slightly. The physician works closely with the patient in an attempt to get the patient to take as much aspirin as he can tolerate. Toxic doses in elderly patients produce acidosis with ataxia and slurred speech. When toxic doses are suspected, a serum salicylate level is obtained.

One method of prescribing aspirin is to order 3–9 Gm. (10–30 tablets) per day in four divided doses with meals (3 regular meals and a bedtime snack). The largest dose is usually ordered with the bedtime snack in an attempt to provide good early morning blood-tissue salicylate levels, and thus minimize morning stiffness. An average dose is 4.2 Gm. (14 tablets) per day: 3 tablets with each of 3 meals and 5 tablets with a bedtime snack. Enteric-coated tablets may be prescribed at night because of their 6- to 8-hour delay in dissolving.

Indomethacin (Indocin). This is a relatively new analgesic anti-inflammatory medication which appears to be no more effective in treating rheumatoid arthritis than the salicylates. Its efficacy is believed to be similar to that of phenylbutazone. Numerous untoward effects may occur with indomethacin, e.g., headache, nausea, vomiting, anorexia, peptic ulcer, abdominal pain, diarrhea, depression, giddiness, mental confusion, psychosis. Possibly this medication is less toxic than the butazones. Indomethacin shows some antipyretic activity. If gastrointestinal bleeding occurs, medication must be stopped. Patients with significant central nervous system symptoms should be warned not to engage in hazardous occupations or drive. Indomethacin should be taken with food and is usually started at a low dosage and gradually increased at weekly intervals until the patient is taking 100–200 mg. a day.

Phenylbutazone (Butazolidin) and oxyphenbutazone (Tandearil). These drugs have anti-inflammatory and analgesic properties but are not used as major drugs in treating rheumatoid arthritis because of their serious toxic effects and because their usefulness in treating this disorder appears limited. Toxic effects include peptic ulcer, agranulocytosis (bone marrow depression), dermatitis, stomatitis, and sodium and water retention. When used, the dosage is commonly 100 mg. three or four times a day or less frequently. Weekly white blood counts and hemoglobin determinations are made for the first few months and thereafter at monthly intervals. The patient is advised to stop taking the medication and see his physician if he develops symptoms such as sore throat, melena (darkening of the feces due to blood pigments), or skin rash.

Pure analgesics. These medications may be necessary (in addition to analgesic anti-inflammatory drugs) to control pain. Analgesics which may be prescribed include propoxyphene hydrochloride (Darvon); acetaminophen (Tyelenol); and codeine. Narcotics are commonly not used because of addicting properties. (See Unit IX for discussion of pain.)

Other medications which may be used in the treatment of rheumatoid arthritis are gold compounds, antimalarials, and adrenocorticosteroids. Immunosuppressive drugs (e.g., azathioprine [Imuran] and cyclophosphamide [Cytoxan], developed as anticancer drugs) are being used on an investigational basis (see Unit V, Ch. 23, and Unit VII).

Gold compounds. The mode of action of gold salts (chrysotherapy) in the treatment of rheumatoid arthritis is not known; however, they are used in treating selected patients. Commonly they are given with salicylates to patients who (a) are not favorably responding to conservative treatment; and/or (b) should not be given corticosteroids. Gold compounds are believed to be most effective when given early during the acute stage of rheumatoid arthritis; however, they may also be given to some patients with long-standing disease. Colloidal gold has proved to be ineffective; water-soluble gold compounds are used. Gold compounds do not produce a dramatic effect, but rather are slow acting. They are relatively safe if given cautiously with supervision. This form of treatment is contraindicated in patients with past or present renal or hepatic disease, acute systemic lupus erythematosus, blood dyscrasias, or drug allergies. Toxic reactions include dermatitis, purpura, stomatitis, agranulocytosis, bronchitis, hepatitis, aplastic anemia, nephritis, photosensitization, and nitroid reaction, i.e., acute sensitivity reaction similar to that which can occur after the ingestion of nitroglycerin (flushing, dizziness, sweating, weakness, nausea, vomiting, syncope). Medication is stopped if any of these symptoms appear. The patient should be warned against exposure to strong light, and the skin and mucous membranes should be inspected (before each injection) for dermatitis or purpura. The urine is examined for protein and microscopic hematuria, and every two weeks evaluations are made of the WBC, hemoglobin, and differential white count. If indicated, the physician also orders liver function tests or platelet counts.

Aqueous preparations of gold compounds used in treating rheumatoid arthritis are gold sodium thiomalate (Myochrysine) and gold sodium thiosulfate. Myochrysine is most commonly used and is given intramuscularly at weekly intervals. A typical dosage schedule is (a) 10 mg. first week; (b) 25 mg. second week; and (c) 50 mg. weekly thereafter until a total dose of 1 Gm. is given without improvement, or an adequate response occurs or toxic reactions appear. If the patient shows a good response he may continue to receive 50 mg. every two weeks and then (with continued improvement) be given injections every 3 or 4 weeks indefinitely.

Antimalarials. Chloroquine (Aralen) and hydroxychloroquine (Plaquenil) are antimalarials sometimes used in treating rheumatoid arthritis. Like gold compounds, these medications are slow acting. Antimalarials can be administered orally, but many physicians believe their toxic effects outweigh possible beneficial effects. Accumulations of these agents in pigmented tissues, particularly the eye, may produce partial or complete loss of vision. When antimalarials are used, the patient should have ophthalmologic examinations 3–4 times a year to detect early retinopathy. If detected early, ocular damage is usually reversible. However, some patients have developed irreversible retinal degeneration. Other possible toxic reactions are blanching of hair, nausea, vomiting, rash, leukopenia, and toxic psychosis.

Adrenocorticosteroids. These anti-inflammatory medications are important in the treatment of rheumatoid arthritis, but are not a substitute for other forms of comprehensive treatment. Adrenocorticosteroids do not change the natural progression of the disease, even though they often produce dramatic and immediate symptomatic relief. Examples of these medications are cortisone, prednisone, hydrocortisone, prednisolone, triamcinolone, methylprednisolone, and dexamethasone. Side effects of adrenocorticosteroids can worsen some features of rheumatoid arthritis; prolonged usage can create toxic side effects which are more problematic to treat than the rheumatoid arthritis. Severe rebound phenomena may follow withdrawal of these drugs.

Adrenocorticosteroids may be given after a thorough, sometimes prolonged evaluation of less hazardous medications. They may then be prescribed for patients (a) who should not be given gold compounds; and/or (b) have active, progressive disease which has not favorably responded to conservative treatment. The medication is given in the smallest amount which will permit functional improvement. Efforts are made after several weeks to reduce the dose. Morning stiffness may be relieved by giving 5 mg. of prednisone orally at bedtime.

It is *not* advisable to (a) give the medication on alternate days; (b) give large "loading doses" followed by a rapid dosage reduction; or (c) give daily oral doses of more than 7.5 mg. of prednisone or equivalent.

Adrenocorticosteroid dosages must be increased during major stressful situations, e.g., surgery. The patient should, therefore, carry a card which states that he is receiving steroid therapy. Such a card will advise medical personnel of the patient's condition if he is injured or requires emergency surgery.

Intra-articular injections of corticosteroids are helpful in temporarily suppressing inflammation in specific joints. These treatments are most effective with acute inflammations of smaller joints. Fluid is removed from the joint prior to injecting the medication. If there is suspicion that a joint is infected, corticosteroids are never injected. Frequent injections cannot safely be made into the same joint because of the possible development of a Charcot joint–like syndrome. Prior to injection the site is sprayed with ethyl chloride or is injected with lidocaine (Xylocaine). Hydrocortisone has commonly been used for intra-articular injections. Other longer-acting intra-articular steroids have now been developed, e.g., prednisolone tertiary-butylacetate (Hydeltra-T.B.A.) and triamcinolone acetonide (Kenalog). Some long-acting preparations may suppress inflammation for as long as 12 months.

SURGERY. Many excellent surgical procedures can be implemented to correct ankylosed and deformed joints. Surgical procedures used in the treatment of arthritis are discussed below.

OSTEOARTHRITIS

Osteoarthritis is also known as degenerative or senescent arthritis. This is a common disorder of unknown etiology. Predisposing factors appear to include aging, joint trauma, and obesity. Women are affected more often than men. Osteoarthritis may first appear in women at the time of menopause, or symptoms may be markedly accentuated at this time if they have previously been present. Certain forms appear to be familial. Older persons are most commonly affected. The weight-bearing joints and terminal interphalangeal joints of the fingers are characteristically involved. Almost all persons over age 45 have some form of osteoarthritis. It is, therefore, the most common joint disorder.

Figure 90–5 illustrates the progression of joint abnormalities in osteoarthritis. The process is initiated by loss of matrix components from the cartilage. Erosion of the cartilage follows. A proliferative response at the joint margins then produces an outgrowth of cartilage and bone. These outgrowths are called "*osteophytes*" or "*spurs.*" The earliest and more severe degenerative changes most typically appear in the spine and weight-bearing joints of the lower extremities. Characteristic hypertrophic spurs cause swellings called "*Heberden's nodes*" in the terminal interphalangeal finger joints.

Unlike rheumatoid arthritis, osteoarthritis is *not* a systemic disease, but rather a local joint disorder. Also, osteoarthritis is not deforming and is not crippling unless the hip joint is involved. It is important that the patient understand which type of arthritis he has.

The patient with osteoarthritis usually does not appear ill and is commonly obese. *Symptoms* usually do not appear before age 40 unless involved joints have been subjected to trauma. Commonly the onset is insidious and gradual. Aching pain is the most common symptom. Other symptoms are limitation of motion or contractures, and muscle spasm. Unlike rheumatoid arthritis, pain is most pronounced after exercise. Pain may occur with use; however, night pain and morning stiffness may also occur. Constitutional symptoms do not occur. Flexion contraction of the hip and loss of ability to extend the knee may be disabling symptoms. Pain at rest may be caused by muscle spasm. The severity of symptoms and the degree of degenerative joint changes are often not correlated. Therefore a patient with minor degenerative changes may be quite uncomfortable, while a patient with advanced changes may have few or no symptoms. Affected joints may appear normal but may be locally tender. Creaking, grating, and crepitus are often detectable in osteoarthritic joints. Occasionally bony enlargement is prominent. Ankylosis does not occur; however, limitation of motion is common.

X-ray abnormalities are commonly apparent, but laboratory findings indicative of inflammation are absent, e.g., the erythrocyte sedimentation rate is normal.

Osteoarthritis progresses slowly; therefore, even though there is no "cure" for this disorder, joint function may be maintained more effectively than with other types of arthritis. Treatments such as weight reduction, medications, physical therapy, and orthopedic procedures may completely relieve the discomforts of osteoarthritis for some patients.

Weight reduction relieves the strain on affected joints (weight-bearing joints) in obese patients. Acetylsalicylic acid (aspirin) is the most effective *medication.* Indomethacin (Indocin) or phenylbutazone (Butazolidin) may be used if conservative treatment with salicylates fails. Patients who are unable to take aspirin may tolerate acetoaminophen (Tylenol). Muscle spasm may be relieved with diazepam (Valium), methocarbamol (Robaxin), meprobamate (Equanil), or chlorphenesin carbamate (Maolate). Systemic corticosteroid therapy is not given for osteoarthritis, but intra-articular injections (e.g., of hydrocortisone acetate) may be helpful in treating selected joints (e.g., knee).

Physical therapy is of major importance in the management of osteoarthritis. Heat, massage, and prescribed exercises help relax muscles and relieve aching and stiffness. Moist heat tends to be more effective than dry. Sometimes involved extremities are splinted. Overactivity must be avoided. Good posture is stressed. Pain in the hands may be relieved by contrast baths, e.g., the hands are submerged in warm water for 4 minutes, then in cold water for 1 minute. The process is repeated for 15 minutes two or three times daily. Nerve root pressure in the neck may be relieved by a cervical collar or traction. Progression of osteoarthritis may be delayed by minimizing use of involved joints; however, total rest produces muscle atrophy and must be avoided.

Orthopedic procedures such as total hip replacement may provide dramatic relief for patients with severe osteoarthritis. Surgical procedures used in treating arthritis are discussed next.

SURGICAL TREATMENT OF ARTHRITIS

Surgical procedures are gaining increasing importance as part of the treatment-rehabilitation programs used with arthritis. A variety of different procedures may be performed to relieve general

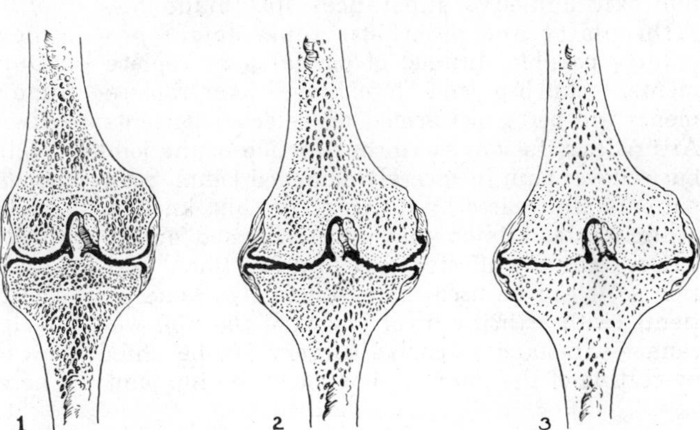

FIGURE 90–5. Sketches showing progression of the joint abnormalities in osteoarthritis. (1) Early degenerative changes in cartilages. (2) More extensive cartilage degeneration and early hypertrophic changes of bone at joint edges. (3) Late stage with almost complete destruction of articular cartilages, irregular subchondral bone surfaces, underlying eburnated bone, and extensive hypertrophic spur formation at margins of the joint. (From Sodeman, W. A., and Sodeman, W. A., Jr.: *Pathologic Physiology: Mechanisms of Disease.* 5th ed.)

symptoms (e.g., pain), improve function, and correct deformities. Not too many years ago surgery was used only late in the course of arthritis, after severe joint destruction or deformity had developed. Preventative surgery (e.g., to prevent deformities) is now used during early phases of treatment. Surgery may be performed with active arthritis. (Orthopedic surgery was discussed generally in Chapter 88 of this unit.)

Among the numerous types of surgical procedures which may be used in the treatment of arthritis are tendon transfers and osteotomy. (See definitions in Chapter 88.) *Tendon transfers* can prevent progressive deformity which would be caused by muscle spasm. Nodules or bony tumors (exostoses) may be surgically removed, and established flexion contractures may be surgically relieved. *Osteotomy* may improve the function of deformed joints or limbs. For example, osteotomy of the femoral neck may give symptomatic relief by changing the position of the head of the femur (when it is being subjected to impact stress against the acetabulum). Femoral osteotomy performed for rheumatoid arthritis of the hip has been less successful than with osteoarthritis. With rheumatoid arthritis the femoral head frequently collapses.[238]

Synovectomy (e.g., of the elbows, wrists, fingers, knees) has proved of value in treating rheumatoid arthritis by helping to maintain joint function. Early surgical removal of the synovium helps prevent recurrent inflammation. With rheumatoid arthritis, joint destruction begins in the synovial tissue and then proceeds to involve bone, cartilage, and other structures.

Surgical correction of problems due to osteoarthritis may reduce abnormal stresses within joints and delay the progression of early disease. Joint instability or malalignment may be corrected, or loose bodies or torn cartilages may be removed. Persons with advanced joint destruction and intractable pain may benefit greatly from surgical procedures such as *arthrodesis* or *arthroplasty* (with or without replacement of joint parts with prostheses). The development of effective, nontoxic adhesive substances has made new arthroplasty and prosthetic replacement procedures possible. Instead of partial joint replacements, "total hip" and "total knee" joint replacements are being performed on selected patients. Arthrodesis (fusion) sacrifices function of the joint but relieves pain in severely damaged joints. Some patients are treated by fusion of the hip, knee, or other joints. Fusion may be performed on the wrists tc fix the affected part in a functional position so it can be used more effectively. Some patients (with arthritic involvement of the hip) who cannot withstand extensive surgery are benefited by cutting of the muscles that move the hip joint. This "hanging hip" procedure maintains reasonable function while providing symptomatic relief.

Numerous silicone rubber implants have been developed for use in reconstructive surgery of the extremities in treating deformed hands and feet. Such implants are used to replace finger joints and the great toe, ranging up to implants to replace joints as large as the shoulder joint.

Arthroplasties of the hip and knee have been selected for further discussion because these procedures are gaining increasing importance and require comprehensive nursing care.

> *Following surgery on joints or bones, postoperative positioning and exercise orders must be precisely followed.*

Hip Arthroplasty. A severely involved arthritic hip can be the most disabling joint disorder for a patient. Severe hip pain can interfere with sleep; prevent the patient from walking; produce narcotic addiction; and impair or totally prevent sexual function. The most common resultant hip deformity is that of adduction and flexion which, in turn, produces or worsens deformity of the knee.[42a] As indicated previously, disabling osteoarthritis of the hip may be surgically treated by major procedures such as arthrodesis (fusion) or arthroplasty. Arthrodesis of the hip is contraindicated with rheumatoid arthritis because (a) the disease is generalized, and (b) often the other hip becomes involved. Arthroplasty may be performed for rheumatoid arthritis or osteoarthritis to relieve pain and restore joint motion.

Two types of arthroplasties of the hip can be performed: (1) *hemiarthroplasty,* in which only one joint component is replaced; and (2) *total hip replacement,* in which both components of the joint are surgically replaced. (Postoperative care following hip surgery was discussed in detail in the section on fractures of the femur, Chapter 89.)

HEMIARTHROPLASTY. Hemiarthroplasty may be performed not only to treat arthritic joints but also in the early stages of necrosis of the head of the femur or in the presence of post-traumatic pseudarthrosis of the femoral neck. Either the head of the femur or the acetabulum may be separately replaced. *Replacement of the head of the femur* with a metal prosthesis has been discussed in Chapter 89.

Another technique involves *remodeling the head of the femur and the acetabulum* and positioning a movable metal (Vitallium) cup between them. During surgery, ankylosed spongy bone is removed. The interposition of the metal between the newly shaped joint surfaces prevents ankylosis of the joint. Postoperatively, following *cup (mold) arthroplasty,* the patient is often placed in suspension traction to maintain abduction. (Suspension traction was discussed in Chapter 88.) Abduction and internal rotation of the operated leg are important following cup arthroplasty because they help maintain the head of the femur and the cup in the acetabulum. Continuous abduction may be necessary for about 6 weeks. (When the head of the femur is replaced with a prosthesis, continued abduction is usually necessary for only 3 weeks.)[123]

Permitting the operated leg to move into adduction before adequate healing has occurred can ruin the arthroplasty.

On about the fourth postoperative day, muscle setting exercises are started, e.g., quadriceps-setting, gluteal-setting. The physician may permit the backrest to be gradually elevated several days after surgery. The amount of elevation permitted by the physician should not be exceeded because excessive flexion of the hip joints may be intolerable. Once the patient can tolerate sitting up, care must be taken to prevent flexion contractures of the hip and knee. Prolonged periods of sitting up must, therefore, not be allowed. The bed should be flat (with hips and knees extended) for periods of time equal to those in which the head is elevated with the hips flexed. Also, the patient should sleep with his bed flat.

After about 3 weeks, traction is usually removed. The physician may then order the patient to lie prone periodically (to stretch the flexors) and to begin roller skating exercises (to strengthen abductors). These exercises are accomplished by placing a smooth wide board across the foot of the bed and placing a roller skate type of apparatus on the patient's foot in such a manner that the rollers are beneath the heel. By pulling on ropes attached to pulleys, the patient can then swing the affected leg in an arc across the board. He first abducts the limb as far as he can without assistance, then pulls the rope to passively abduct the leg further (just to the point of pain). He then returns the leg to a normal midline position. During abduction of the operated leg the nurse may hold the hip of the unoperated leg to prevent compensatory adduction.

During the recovery period, care is taken to prevent adduction and external rotation of the hip joint. One method of preventing accidental external rotation is to place a trochanter roll alongside the outer upper leg. This roll of material helps prevent a rolling outward of the thigh and leg (and thus the hip). The hip is maintained in abduction while turning the patient and helping him sit up on the edge of the bed.

About 4 weeks following surgery (possibly earlier), the patient is permitted to stand without putting weight on the operated leg. Naturally the patient will be weak after being in bed for such a long period of time. He must be well supported when he first sits and stands, and the upright position must be assumed gradually. The patient then is helped to use crutches until the physician gives permission for him to ambulate bearing weight. Stationary bicycle exercises (and other exercises that promote flexion and extension of the hip joint) help prepare the patient for ambulation, by strengthening muscles and increasing hip and knee joint motion. Exercises must be faithfully performed for many months to attain and maintain maximum function of the remodeled hip joint.

Following hemiarthroplasty complications may develop such as pain caused by the bony head of the femur or the acetabulum rubbing against the prosthesis, or loosening of the prosthesis.

Some physicians prefer cup arthroplasties (rather than total hip replacements) in treating younger arthritic patients because of the uncertain durability of total replacements. However, the results of cup arthroplasty are less predictable,[238] and longer periods of hospitalization and rehabilitation are required. Total hip replacements are increasingly popular.

TOTAL HIP REPLACEMENT. Cup arthroplasty is being rapidly replaced by total hip arthroplasty in the treatment of rheumatoid arthritis and osteoarthritis (except in treating very young patients). Total hip replacements are typically used if the destructive process involves both the acetabulum and femoral head. Bilateral surgery may be performed during the same procedure or several weeks apart. Infection is a contraindication to total hip replacement.

With total hip arthroplasty the femoral head and acetabulum are both replaced by prostheses (see Fig. 90-6.) The prostheses are cemented into the bone with a plastic cement called methyl methacrylate. Total hip replacements have been widely used in Great Britain and Canada for about a decade but were slower in coming into use in the United States because the use of acrylic bone cement was restricted by the Food and Drug Administration (FDA). Until recently permission from the FDA was required for procedures using methyl methacrylate.

Several different total hip prostheses are available, e.g., Charnley-Müller, Bechtol, McKee-Farrar, Ring, and Trapezoidal-28. Commonly the acetabulum is implanted first during the operative procedure. The location and degree of angulation of this part of the prosthesis are precisely determined, since these factors decide the position of the femoral head and neck piece. The acetabular prosthesis may be made of high-density polyethylene plastic, while the femoral prosthesis is made of metal, usually stainless steel. The bone cement has been used for many years as a dental filling material but only recently has been used in orthopedics. Bone cement is not an adhesive or glue, but instead acts as a filler, filling in all the tiny irregularities in the prepared surfaces of the bone. The cement thus securely locks the parts of the prosthesis in place.

Preoperative teaching is highly important when total hip replacement is to be performed. During this time of preoperative education, the patient is told that he may need to remain on his back for several days. Also, he is taught how to correctly use a trapeze to lift himself for back care during the period of recumbency. The operative procedure and its goals are discussed, and the patient is taught exercises he will do postoperatively, e.g., quadriceps-setting exercises, gluteal-setting

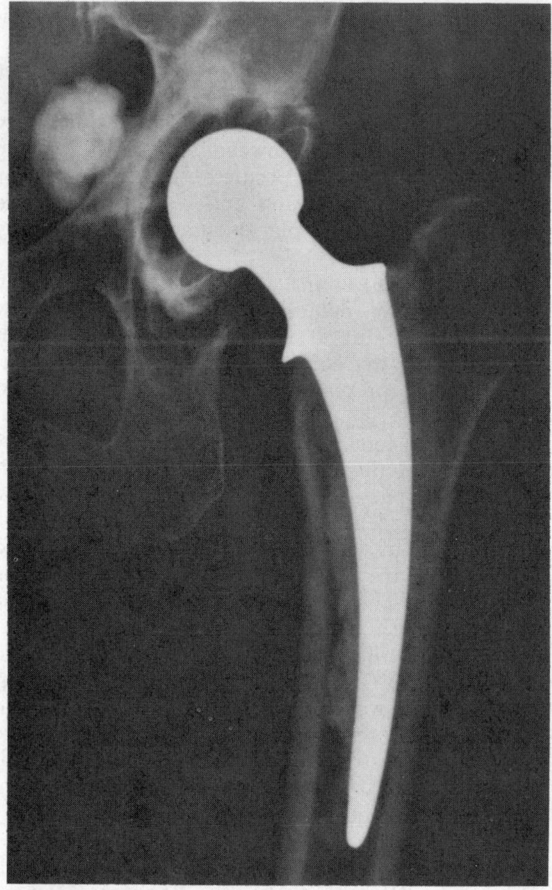

FIGURE 90–6. Charnley-Müller prosthesis in place six months after hip replacement. (From Galante, J.: Total hip replacement. *Orthopedic Clinics of North America* 2:144, 1971.)

exercises, and isometric hip extension and abduction exercises. Upper extremity strengthening exercises may also be taught, in preparation for crutch walking or use of a walker.

Postoperative care is discussed generally in Unit VI and in Chapter 88 of this unit, and postoperative care following hip surgery is discussed in Chapter 89. Care of patients in casts or traction also is discussed in Chapter 88. The following discussion emphasizes only selected aspects of postoperative care which are important following total hip replacement. For detailed discussions of nursing care with these procedures, refer to Eyre[72] and Graves.[93]

Postoperatively following total hip replacement the patient is commonly placed immediately in his own bed, and Buck's extension or Russell's traction is applied (Chapter 88). The patient may not be permitted to turn to either side for several days because of the possibility of dislocating the operated hip. While some surgeons do not permit any turning for 3–7 days, others permit turning onto the uninvolved side as early as the evening of surgery. During turning hip abduction *must* be maintained with pillows. Turning following hip surgery has been previously discussed.

Postoperatively the affected leg is maintained in an abducted position in straight alignment while the patient is recumbent. A sling support is used with Russell's traction, and the leg may be positioned on a pillow from mid-calf to mid-thigh. The surgeon may order the legs wrapped with Ace bandages to prevent thrombosis. A hip spica dressing may be applied in the operating room to provide compression and help prevent tissue separation and hematoma formation. Hemovacs are usually in place in the wound immediately following surgery for wound drainage. Some surgeons routinely give antibiotics and dextran therapy. At times, instead of Russell's traction a posterior splint is used. In some settings the patient is cared for on a CircOlectric bed.

Exercises, e.g., quadriceps-setting, are encouraged as ordered during the early postoperative period. Muscle strengthening, as of the gluteal muscles, helps prevent dislocation since muscular control replaces the function of the hip capsule. Dislocation of the prosthesis and infection are major possible complications during the early postoperative period. Indications of these complications are immediately reported.

With some procedures the greater trochanter (with the attachment of the abductor muscles) is transferred, e.g., moved distally on the femur to increase the efficiency of the abductor mechanism. When such a transfer is made the greater trochanter is usually held in its new position by wires. The transfer must be protected until it heals in place (e.g., 4–6 weeks). In this situation, progressive abduction exercises are limited by the transfer. Excessive exercise may cause nonunion or fracture of the osteotomy site. The surgeon's orders concerning movement and positioning must be precisely followed.

Following total hip replacement the patient may be kept flat for several days, or the surgeon may specify that the bed can be elevated. For example, some surgeons state that the bed can be elevated 45–60° immediately following surgery and 90° on the first postoperative day. Others specify 35° on the second postoperative day and progressively thereafter until a comfortable level is reached. During the time the patient is supine he should receive back care every two hours. Back care is given while the patient turns (if turning to the unoperated side is allowed) or while he raises straight up on an overbed trapeze (if turning is prohibited). It is helpful if the patient lies on a sheepskin and wears sheepskin booties to protect his skin while supine.

Nerve function and circulation checks are initially made every hour (for the first 24 hours) and then every 2 hours (for the next 24 hours). Thereafter they are made as frequently as the patient's condition warrants. Pink-tinged sputum may appear postoperatively and is believed to result from some part of the cement being excreted through pulmonary alveoli. This is not considered to be dangerous but should be noted in charting.

Position checks are made frequently while the patient is in bed. External rotation of the leg may be prevented with sandbags. The patient may be dangled on the fourth to seventh day after surgery. Abduction must be maintained while helping the patient to sit up. Progressive ambulation then follows, e.g., use of parallel bars, crutches or walker, and finally a cane. The surgeon may recommend partial weight-bearing initially or may permit full weight-bearing on the operated leg.

Physical therapy may be started on the fifth or sixth postoperative day. In addition to helping the patient ambulate, physical therapy may include Hubbard baths, use of powder boards, and gentle active assisted range-of-motion exercises in sling suspension (within the pain-free range). Until discharge, the patient continues to work on exercises which increase range of motion and muscle strengthening of the hip.

On the fifth or sixth postoperative day, the physician may order the patient to lie prone twice a day for 20–30 minutes to prevent hip flexion contractures. This practice may be continued at home after discharge.

The total period of hospitalization for total hip replacement is usually 2–3 weeks. The patient is often discharged with the assistance of only a light cane while walking. Total hip replacement produces dramatic results. Patients are commonly surprised to find their pain relieved and movement increased so markedly and rapidly.

Prior to discharge the patient should be given written instructions for home care, including detailed exercise prescriptions and activity limitations. The patient may be advised to continue to place a pillow between his knees (while lying down) for several weeks, to prevent adduction while turning. He may be advised never to sit for longer than one hour continuously; he should stand, stretch, and take a few steps periodically to prevent hip flexion contractures. Hip flexion should not exceed 90° or the operated hip may dislocate. Therefore, the patient must learn to put on his shoes and stockings without acutely flexing. Additionally he should sit in a straight chair with a straight back and use a raised toilet seat. Rocking or reclining chairs and low toilet seats cannot be used following total hip replacement because of the possibility of dislocation of the prosthesis. Bicycle exercises may be used to supplement the home program once the patient has gained adequate hip flexion range.

Additional instructions which the physician may give at the time of discharge may include the following: (a) avoid crossing the legs for 3 months; (b) continue to wear support hose for 6 weeks following surgery; and (c) sexual activity and driving may be resumed in 6 weeks. Extremes of flexion, adduction, and internal rotation must be permanently avoided.

Knee Arthroplasty. Like the hip joint, the knee joint may be partially replaced (*hemiarthroplasty*) or totally replaced. Hemiarthroplasty may consist of the replacement of the femoral condyles or tibial plateau, using McKeever and MacIntosh prostheses. This discussion focuses on total knee replacement.

Total knee replacement has been under development for over 20 years. This type of surgery is still in a stage of development and is undergoing rapid changes. Numerous different prostheses have been developed for use in *total knee arthroplasty*. The first hinged knee prosthesis was developed and used by Walldius. The Walldius prosthesis is still in use. Other prostheses based on a similar principle include those by Shires, Young, Macausland, and Von Hellens. Another well-known total knee prosthesis is the McKee prosthesis. Recently attempts have been made by Gunston and Freeman-Swanson to design a smaller knee prosthesis. These new joints permit more natural movement because gliding occurs between the two joint surfaces rather than simply hinge movement.

The recent use of methyl methacrylate (acrylic bone cement) in reconstruction of the knee has helped resolve many technical problems by making it possible to securely fix prosthetic components into bone tissue. Acrylic bone cement is now used during the implantation of numerous types of knee prostheses. Two such procedures are the geometric total knee arthroplasty and the polycentric total knee arthroplasty. In these procedures diseased arthritic surfaces of the femoral condyles and tibial plateaus are removed and replaced by durable prosthetic components that are firmly fixed to the bone. Once in place, the components permit simulation of normal knee motions.

Space does not permit detailed discussions of the various techniques of total knee replacement and the postoperative care necessary following each technique. The nurse is advised to consult specific postoperative orders carefully and clarify with the surgeon any questions she has. Discussed briefly below is postoperative care related to the Walldius knee hinge and the polycentric type total knee arthroplasty.

The Walldius knee hinge was designed for use without bone cement but now may be cemented into the medullary cavities of the femur and tibia. Originally the prosthesis was made of acrylic, but this proved to be not strong enough. The prosthesis was later modified in stainless steel and is now constructed of a cobalt-chrome alloy. *Postoperatively* Walldius uses a full-leg padded plaster cast with the knee in extension for 3 weeks. Then sutures are removed and exercises started. Once the patient can perform a straight leg raise, he is started walking with full weight-bearing.

Other surgeons using the Walldius prosthesis prefer changing plaster at two weeks (to remove sutures) and then applying a groin to ankle cast with the foot free. The patient is permitted weight-bearing at this time to combat osteoporosis. At the sixth week postoperatively the cast is split for exercises and discarded at 8 weeks. While some patients rapidly regain movement it may take others as long as 12 months to reach maximum range. *Physical therapy is highly important* in reconstructive surgery of the knee.

Possible postoperative *complications* include infection; fat embolism; peroneal nerve palsy; skin breakdown; medical complications; technical failure; synovial herniation; loosening of the prosthesis; and stress fracture.

Postoperative care following the polycentric type of total knee arthroplasty is essentially as follows:[47a]

> A compression dressing immobilizes the knee in maximum extension immediately following surgery. On the third postoperative day the dressing is removed and a posterior plaster shell is applied for use during ambulation and as a resting splint at night.

> Re-education of the quadriceps muscles begins with isometric quadriceps setting on the first postoperative day. As pain decreases and voluntary muscle control improves, exercising progresses to active straight leg raising. Both ankles are actively exercised to prevent thrombophlebitis.

> After the compression dressing is removed, gentle active assistive range of motion exercises are started and a progressive exercise program is continued until discharge to increase muscle strength and range of motion in the operated knee.

> Once the patient has 90° of knee flexion and good voluntary control of his quadriceps muscle (can actively straight-leg raise and initiate active knee extension against gravity), ambulation is started.

> A posterior splint may be used during early gait training, e.g., in parallel bars and on crutches. Weight-bearing on the operated leg may be permitted to tolerance or the point of pain.

> The patient is discharged with detailed instructions for a home exercise program.

Flexion contractures can develop with total knee replacement. To prevent this complication the patient's knee is kept extended at all times while he is in bed. A trochanter roll is used in bed to prevent external rotation. Swelling can also be a problem; therefore the leg is usually kept elevated with a pillow under the ankle. This position also promotes full extension with the aid of gravity. Whirlpool baths may help the patient obtain adequate flexion and full extension of the knee.

GOUTY ARTHRITIS

Primary gout is a familial metabolic disorder of purine metabolism which results in abnormal amounts of urates in the body. Purines are products of the digestion of certain proteins. Inability to properly metabolize purines results in an excessive accumulation of uric acid in the blood's plasma (i.e., hyperuricemia). As a result of this, urate crystals may be precipitated and deposited throughout the body. These deposits of crystals then initiate local irritation and an inflammatory response. Hyeruricemia may result from[232] (a) increased production of urates caused by the abnormal metabolic degradation of purines; (b) a reduced excretion of urates; or (c) a combination of both of these factors. Hyperuricemia may occur without gout.

Acute attacks of gouty arthritis may accompany other disorders (e.g., disorders of the hematopoietic system such as polycythemia or leukemia). These attacks are called "*secondary gout*" and usually do not have tophi (see below) or a familial history of gout.

The main clinical problem with gout is arthritis. Early in the course of the illness, a recurring acute arthritis occurs which is usually monarticular, i.e., involves one joint. Later a chronic, deforming arthritis develops. About 95 per cent of patients with gout are men over age 30. If gout develops in women it usually does so after the menopause.

Gout is characterized clinically by acute periodic episodes of pain, swelling, and inflammation in a joint. The joints of the foot (great toe, instep, or ankle) are most often affected; however, any joint may be involved.

Histologically gout is characterized by the formation of *tophi*. A tophus is a nodular deposit of sodium acid urate crystals with an associated foreign body reaction. Tophi may occur in various regions of the body, such as periarticular tissue, bone, tendon, cartilage, kidneys, and subcutaneous tissue. About 10–20 per cent of patients with gouty arthritis have uric acid kidney stones.

During acute gouty arthritis, urates may be demonstrated in synovial tissues, producing synovitis. It is this severe joint synovitis that causes the functional disturbances characteristic of an acute attack of gouty arthritis. The attack usually occurs suddenly, most often involving the great toe's metatarsophalangeal joint. However, other joints may be affected. While the attack typically involves only one joint, at times several joints may be involved during the same attack.

The involved joint(s) is usually intensely painful, swollen, and extremely tender. The skin over the joint feels warm and tense and appears dusky red or purple. Other symptoms commonly occur, e.g., headache, tachycardia, fever, malaise, anorexia. The patient may be completely incapacitated. Commonly he is unable to move the inflamed joint and cannot stand the weight of linens over the affected part. During recovery, pruritus and local desquamation may occur as edema subsides.

Early attacks end rapidly, usually after only a few days or a week or two. Inflammation completely subsides and the affected joints return to normal functional and anatomic states. Following the initial acute attack the patient may be asymptomatic for months or years. Eventually other attacks occur. Gouty arthritis may become chronic so that the patient is disabled by symptoms and progressive loss of function. Gross deformities are then apparent, and x-rays reveal punched-out areas in the bone called "radiolucent urate tophi."

Following repeated acute attacks of gouty arthritis tophi may be detected in the cartilage of the ears and on the hands, olecranon, feet, and prepatellar bursae. Large urate deposits develop in and around joint structures. These deposits and the accompanying inflammatory changes may severely damage articular cartilage and subchondral bone; fibrous or bony ankylosis of the joint may develop.

Laboratory findings with gout include (a) elevated WBC and sedimentation rate during acute attacks; (b) elevated blood uric acid (unless uricosuric medications are being taken); (c) presence of crystals of sodium urate in material aspirated from a tophus or in joint fluid.

Early diagnosis and treatment of gout are important. The emphasis of treatment has shifted from the simple treatment of recurrent attacks to permanent medical supervision and treatment directed at preventing not only acute attacks but also progressive disability (e.g., from erosion of bone and joint cartilage and progressive renal dysfunction). Progressive renal dysfunction is the greatest threat to life. With early, sustained treatment almost all patients can live full productive lives without disability. Treatment is also beneficial to persons with advanced disease, e.g., joint function can be improved, tophi can be resolved, and renal dysfunction may be improved or arrested. The severity of gout is greatest in patients whose clinical symptoms first appear before age 30.

Acute attacks may be terminated by administering medications such as (a) colchicine; (b) phenylbutazone (Butazolidin); (c) indomethacin (Indocin); or (d) corticotropin (ACTH). Additionally the treatment of acute attacks includes bedrest (continued for at least 24 hours following subsidence of the attack) and analgesics, e.g., codeine. Some patients receive added relief from hot or cold compresses; others find compresses intolerable. Fluids are forced to reduce precipitation of urate in the kidneys and to combat dehydration. A soft diet is usually prescribed.

Between attacks treatment is directed at (a) reducing the frequency and severity of recurrent acute attacks; and (b) minimizing the deposition of urate in tissues, i.e., by lowering the serum urate level to a range which will resolve any crystalline deposits of monosodium urate which are present and will prevent further deposition of these crystals.

Therapeutic factors of importance in obtaining the above goals include:

Medical Management. Daily administrations of colchicine have preventative actions (i.e., reduce frequency of acute attacks) and may be continued indefinitely. Also, uricosuric drugs may be given, e.g., probenecid (Benemid), sulfinpyrazone (Anturane), or salicylates. Uricosuric medications block the tubular reabsorption of filtered urate in the kidneys and thus reduce the metabolic pool of urates by increasing uric acid excretion. Salicylates cannot be given with any other uricosuric drug because they antagonize the action of other uricosuric agents. The patient should be told not to take salicylates if he is taking other uricosuric drugs. Another method of ongoing treatment is the administration of the xanthine oxidase inhibitor allopurinol (Zyloprim). Thus drug inhibits uric acid formation. In selected patients allopurinol is used in conjunction with uricosuric drugs. Fluid intake should be at least 3 L. per day when uricosuric drugs are being taken, and attempts are made to keep the urine alkaline (to prevent formation of urinary calculi). The patient is taught to test his urine and may be advised to take sodium bicarbonate tablets and ingest alkaline-producing foods and liquids.

Dietary Management. Rigid dietary restrictions are emphasized less than the proper ingestion of uricosuric medications with increased amounts of fluids. The patient is informed of the importance of avoiding acidity and dehydration. Restriction of the purine content of the diet may be temporarily recommended until the serum urate concentration returns to normal. Then dietary restrictions are usually no longer necessary because drugs are effective. Foods high in purine include liver, kidney, sweetbreads, anchovies, sardines, and meat extracts. A moderate ingestion of alcohol does not appear to precipitate acute attacks of gout or be otherwise harmful. However, the patient should avoid foods or alcoholic beverages which precipitate attacks and should practice moderation.

With advanced gout large tophi may be removed surgically to correct deformity and reduce the load on renal function. Some patients with renal involvement require hemodialysis.

CONNECTIVE TISSUE DISORDERS

Connective tissue disorders are commonly called *"collagen diseases."* These diffuse diseases are discussed generally in Unit V, Ch. 23. A variety of disorders are referred to as collagen diseases. Rheumatoid arthritis is a member of this group and has been discussed earlier in this chapter. Other possible collagen diseases are rheumatic fever, nonthrombocytopenic purpuras, glomerulonephritis, systemic lupus erythematosus, polyarteritis nodosa, scleroderma, and dermatomyositis. The last four of these disorders are discussed briefly in following sections.

As a group, collagen diseases (a) produce widespread changes in collagenous connective tissue; (b) cause a wide variety of symptoms referable to almost every organ; (c) may be autoimmune in etiology; (d) are difficult to diagnose; (e) have no cure; and (f) cannot be prevented. General treatment measures used for autoimmune conditions include corticosteroids, ionizing radiation, and salicylates.

Frequently with collagen diseases the anatomic, immunologic, and histologic findings overlap from one disease to another. While serologic tests may help in the process of establishing the differential diagnosis of the various collagen diseases, these tests are not specific. The diseases do tend to differ in their prognosis, clinical patterns, and response to treatment.

Systemic Lupus Erythematosus (SLE). This serious inflammatory disease of unknown etiology occurs mainly in young women and produces symptoms referable to multiple organ systems. SLE diffusely involves the vascular and connective tissues of multiple organs, producing inflammation and biochemical and structural changes. Usually the most important abnormalities occur in the viscera; however, pathologic changes exactly like those with rheumatoid arthritis may also occur in the joints, fascia, tendons, and bursae. The rheumatic symptoms are commonly less severe than with classic rheumatoid arthritis. Also, the prognosis of SLE is poorer than that of rheumatoid arthritis because of the greater visceral pathology.[232] Commonly death results from failure of a vital organ, e.g., renal failure.

Several abnormal serum protein fractions and antinuclear antibodies may be found with SLE; these findings suggest that an autoimmune mechanism occurs with this disease. Characteristic histologic findings are the so-called lupus erythematosus (LE) cells and extracellular masses called "hematoxylin bodies." However, the LE cell may be found in many diseases and may or may not be demonstrated with SLE. Most patients with SLE have a mild to moderate normochromic, normocytic anemia. The sedimentation rate is usually high, a mild leukopenia is often present, and the serum globulin may be increased.

The clinical pattern and prognosis with SLE are highly variable. The illness may develop rapidly with an acute fulminant course which may produce death within a few weeks, or it may develop insidiously and become a chronic illness subject to remissions and exacerbations. The chronic pattern is more common and with proper steroid therapy the patient may live for many years.

Acute clinical findings may include[70] fever; prostration; delirium; convulsions; psychosis; coma; musculoskeletal aches and pains; "butterfly rash" on the face; pleural effusion; basilar pneumonia; generalized lymphadenopathy; pericarditis; tachycardia; gallop rhythm; hepatosplenomegaly; and nephritis.

Clinical findings which may occur with *chronic* SLE are variable, depending upon the organ systems involved, but may include[70] fever; malaise; weight loss; cutaneous discoid LE lesions; erythema of exposed surfaces; generalized lymphadenopathy; severe hemolytic anemia; thrombocytopenic purpura; hypersplenism; pericarditis; tachycardia; gallop rhythm; peripheral vascular syndromes (e.g., Raynaud's phenomenon, gangrene); ulcerative lesions of the mucous membranes; abdominal pains; nausea; vomiting; anorexia; bloody stools; hepatic dysfunction; hepatomegaly; focal glomerulitis progressing to glomerulonephritis; myalgia; arthralgia; neuritis; hemiplegia; psychosis; convulsions; and coma.

Nursing care is supportive and is determined by the organ systems involved and the prescribed medical therapy. Corticosteroids or corticotropin are commonly prescribed in the treatment of SLE. These medications produce variable, sometimes highly favorable effects. If corticosteroid therapy does not produce an adequate response, purine antagonists (e.g., mercaptopurine) or alkylating agents (e.g., nitrogen mustards, cyclophosphamide) may be tried. These drugs are immunosuppressive agents. Physical therapy, salicylates, and other analgesics may be prescribed to reduce musculoskeletal discomforts. Other disorders, e.g., anemia, pneumonia, renal disease, are given appropriate treatment. Commonly a high-caloric, high-vitamin diet is prescribed. The patient is advised to avoid excessive exposure to ultraviolet radiation (e.g., sunlight) and excessive fatigue. Bedrest is necessary during exacerbations.

Polyarteritis Nodosa. This collagen disease produces diffuse inflammation and necrosis in the walls of small to medium sized arteries. While arterial lesions may occur in any organ, the structures most often involved are muscles, kidneys, heart, liver, gastrointestinal tract, and peripheral nerves. Aneurysms or thrombosis may develop. Muscle biopsy of painful areas demonstrates vasculitis. Laboratory findings may include leukocytosis; mild normocytic anemia; eosinophilia; and an elevated sedimentation rate and serum globulin level. Urinary findings may include hematuria; proteinuria; pyuria; and casts.

Like SLE, the symptoms and course of polyarteritis nodosa are highly variable. It is not uncommon, however, for polyarteritis nodosa to run a fulminating course which proves fatal within a few months. Clinical findings may include fever; weakness; malaise; weight loss; hypertension; renal disease; musculoskeletal aches and pains; peripheral neuritis; variable skin lesions; angina; congestive heart failure; nausea; melena; abdominal pain; hematemesis; bronchial asthma; and bronchial pneumonia.

Treatment of polyarteritis nodosa is mainly supportive and symptomatic. Corticosteroids may be helpful.

Scleroderma. This collagen disorder is also called "diffuse scleroderma" or "systemic sclerosis." The word scleroderma means "hard skin." In this chronic disorder the connective tissue proliferates in the skin and in numerous internal structures. Insidious symptoms may be present for years (e.g., sweating of the hands and feet, stiffness of the hands), and eventually the toes and fingers become fixed in position and the skin becomes thick and hard. As areas of skin become increasingly involved, ulceration, calcification, pigmentation, or depigmentation may occur. Eventually skin over the entire body may be involved, producing a variety of disorders. For example, sclerodermatous constriction of the thorax may impair effective breathing and, as a result, pulmonary complications may develop. Numerous other disorders may occur, such as difficulty swallowing, impaired gastrointestinal mobility, cardiac and renal disorders, osteoporosis of bone, and destruction of distal phalanges.

Scleroderma typically progresses slowly. When death occurs it often results from infection or renal or cardiac failure. Supportive, symptomatic treatment is given. Low molecular weight dextran may be administered. Corticosteroids are typically not helpful.

Dermatomyositis; Polymyositis. These collagen diseases affect mainly the skin and voluntary (striated) muscles. When skin changes are the prominent feature, the illness is called "dermatomyositis"; when muscle weakness is the principal clinical feature, it is termed "polymyositis."[266] With either form, the onset is most commonly insidious, and the disease may progress over a period of years, crippling the patient. Treatment is basically symptomatic and supportive. Corticosteroids may be quite helpful. Biopsies may demonstrate inflammatory, degenerative muscular changes and variable dermatitis. Serum enzyme levels, e.g., SGOT, are elevated. Creatinuria parallels muscle destruction. Creatine is formed in the muscle, passes into the blood, and is excreted by the kidneys. The serum globulin level and sedimentation rate may be increased, and a mild normocytic anemia may be present.

The symptoms of dermatomyositis and polymyositis are variable but among them are desquamation; pigmentary changes; diffuse erythema; calcification; weakness; fatigue; weight loss; mild fever; multiple gastrointestinal ulcers; muscular tenderness; and aching. Muscular involvement may cause dysphagia or respiratory embarrassment. Emergency restoration of the airway may be necessary. The proximal muscles of the upper and lower extremities and the flexor muscles of the neck are most commonly affected. Muscle contractures and loss of function may occur. During the active inflammatory phase of the disease, range of motion exercises are important to prevent these complications.

BONE TUMORS

Primary bone tumors (originating in the bone) may be benign or malignant. Primary malignant bone tumors are rare, comprising only about 1 per cent of all forms of cancer.[23] Benign tumors of bone most commonly include osteomas, chondromas, giant-cell tumors, cysts, and osteoid-osteomas. Benign tumors are usually well circumscribed, grow slowly, and seldom spread. Primary malignant bone tumors tend to be extremely malignant and metastasize early, often to the lung. Examples of primary malignant bone tumors are osteogenic sarcoma (most common); Ewing's sarcoma; multiple myeloma (also called plasma cell myeloma or plasma cell leukemia); reticulum cell sarcoma; and angiosarcoma. Some authorities consider multiple myeloma to be a disorder of the blood-forming organs (bone marrow) rather than a primary tumor of the bone (see Unit XII).

Certain tumors tend to occur at certain ages. For example, osteogenic sarcomas appear in children, adolescents, and young adults (below age 25); giant cell tumors occur between ages 21–35; and multiple myeloma most commonly occurs between ages 50 and 70.

Metastatic (secondary) bone tumors are relatively common, and may come from primary lesions in the breast, lungs, prostate, kidney, ovary, or thyroid. Carcinomas tend to metastasize to bone more commonly than sarcomas. Prognosis with metastatic bone lesions is poor.

Symptoms of bone tumors are swelling, pain, restricted motion, aching, and fracture (due to weakening of the bone). Bone pain may be quite severe and is commonly persistent. Pain may occur before metastases become detectable in x-rays. Diagnosis may be made by using x-rays, biopsies, or frozen sections. Many bone tumors produce characteristic radiologic appearances. Whenever malignant tumors are suspected, chest films are routinely taken to look for pulmonary metastases and a skeletal radiologic survey is conducted to locate additional bone lesions. The precise identification of tumor type is extremely important. Therefore, biopsy (via aspiration needle or incision) is mandatory.

Bone tumors may be treated by chemotherapy, irradiation, and surgery. (Treatment of cancer is discussed in Unit VII.) Radical surgery may be required for primary malignant bone tumors. A major portion of an involved limb may be amputated or possibly completely disarticulated. In some cases an interscapulothoracic amputation is required for upper extremity lesions or a hemipelvectomy for lesions involving the lower limbs. (Amputation is discussed in Unit XIII.) Metastatic bone lesions are treated by palliative measures. Symptomatic relief may be obtained from irradiation and chemotherapy.

OSTEOPOROSIS

Osteoporosis is a common disorder of bone metabolism in which the mass of bone is decreased. Both mineral and protein matrix components are reduced. This reduction in bone density occurs in approximately one fourth of all elderly persons, most frequently in women between the ages of 50 and 70. In this disorder bone resorption occurs faster than bone formation takes place over a prolonged period. Osteoporosis may occur (a) with a deficit of estrogen (in postmenopausal women); (b) with catabolic hormone excess (e.g., with Cushing's disease); (c) with long-term administration of high amounts of corticosteroids; (d) with prolonged immobilization; and (e) as a result of other disorders such as liver disease. Osteoporosis is most common in fair-skinned, light-weight, postmenopausal women.

Osteoporosis can be detected with x-rays. Blood calcium, phosphorus, and phosphatase are normal.

Symptoms, particularly with postmenopausal women, usually begin with pain in the weight-bearing vertebrae. Because the involved bone tissue loses its density and tensile strength, fractures and kyphosis may occur. Even slight trauma may fracture brittle, osteoporetic bone. Multiple vertebral fractures may cause a loss of height.

Physical activity and exercises are important in the treatment of osteoporosis. Postmenopausal women may be treated with cyclic estrogen administration. Large doses of calcium, vitamin D, or fluoride have been tried, as well as calcitonin (which inhibits bone resorption). Currently high doses of calcium and treatment with fluoride are considered to be investigational, and calcitonin has not been adequately evaluated. Androgen and other anabolic steroid therapy is not advised.

OSTEOMYELITIS

Osteomyelitis, i.e., bone infection caused by pyogenic microorganisms, is most commonly produced by *Staphylococcus aureus*. Infection may reach the bone directly (e.g., via compound fracture), through the blood stream, or by direct extension from infections in adjacent structures.

Local symptoms of acute bone infection are sudden pain in the affected bone; tenderness over the bone; heat; redness; swelling; painful movement; and involuntary restriction of movement. General symptoms with acute severe bone infection may include sharp rise in temperature; chills; rapid pulse; marked leukocytosis; elevated ESR; and possibly positive blood cultures. Evidence of bone infection may not appear for some time on x-rays.

Early diagnosis of osteomyelitis is extremely important because chronic osteomyelitis can be a serious, disabling disorder. With early treatment, the chances of effectively controlling acute osteomyelitis are quite good. Once osteomyelitis is suspected, an antibiotic is given as soon as blood count results are available. The physician does not wait for other laboratory or x-ray evidence. A penicillinase-resistant penicillin is usually given initially. Later, after laboratory reports are obtained and the causative organism identified, medication may be changed. It is important that the medication reach the bone before necrosis occurs. With delayed treatment, bone necrosis develops and the antibiotic cannot enter the dead bone to combat the infectious organisms effectively.

Infected bone is placed at rest by cast or traction, and the patient is maintained on bedrest until evidence of active infection disappears. If an abscess is present it is evacuated and an appropriate antibiotic is instilled into the cavity daily. The medication is also given systemically. Sometimes a catheter is placed in the wound and is used for continuous drip instillation of an antibiotic solution or for irrigation of the wound. A closed irrigation and drainage system with low pressure suction is another procedure that may be used in treating osteomyelitis. If chronic bone infection develops, the wound is widely exposed and all infected dead bone is carefully removed. Immobilization and antibiotics are also used as discussed above. Drug-resistant organisms can develop which make treatment exceedingly difficult. Fortunately chronic osteomyelitis is now much less common than in previous years.

Strict aseptic technic must be practiced when changing dressings over open wounds. If a patient is placed in isolation the nurse must meticulously follow isolation technic. Because infected bone may be extremely painful, the patient must be handled gently.

Every attempt is made in orthopedic practice to *prevent* osteomyelitis. If indications of bone infection do appear they are immediately reported.

OSTEOMALACIA

Osteomalacia is a disorder in which adult bone becomes softened as a result of disturbed calcium and phosphorus metabolism. These metabolic disturbances result from a vitamin D deficiency due to inadequate dietary intake of vitamin D, to the body's failure to absorb or use vitamin D, or lack of exposure to ultraviolet rays. With inadequate vitamin D, the effect of the parathyroid hormone on bone resorption is decreased, and calcium absorption is decreased. Secondary hyperparathyroidism occurs in response to the resultant hypocalcemia. This has little effect on calcium absorption but does increase the kidney's phosphate loss. Both calcium and phosphorus are consequently low. Parathyroid hormone is believed to stimulate osteoblastic differentiation. The increased number of osteoblasts increases alkaline phosphatase. However, the osteoblasts do not form large amounts of bone, and mineralization is defective in the bone that is formed.

Osteomalacia is characterized by widespread decalcification and softening of the bones, especially those in the spine, pelvis, and lower extremities. The bones become deformed (bent, flattened) as they soften. Osteomalacia develops insidiously and may be identified by reduced calcium and phosphorus levels, rachitic bone deformities, bone pain and tenderness, and x-ray changes (such as pseudofractures or possibly cyst formation). Biopsy may help establish diagnosis. A similar disorder occurs in children and is called *rickets*.

Treatment of osteomalacia may involve large amounts of vitamin D and dietary measures to insure adequate intakes of calcium and phosphorus, e.g., eggs, milk, vegetables, fish. Calcium salts and phosphate supplements may also be given.

SCOLIOSIS

"Scoliosis" means a lateral curvature of the spinal column from its normal vertical anatomic position. Scoliosis may develop from various disorders (e.g., rickets, neuromuscular disorders, vertebral disorders), but 90 per cent of the time it is idiopathic (without known cause). While scoliosis may develop at any age, it most frequently develops in children 10–12 years of age. With idiopathic scoliosis, girls are affected 10 times more frequently than boys. The type of treatment used depends upon the cause and the severity of the deformity. Corrective exercises may be used. Other treatment methods include use of braces (Milwaukee brace), casts (Risser localizer cast, turnbuckle cast), plastic body jackets, or surgery (the Harrington operation which consists of spinal instrumentation and fusion). Casts and braces are discussed in Chapter 88. For a discussion of the Harrington operation, refer to Boegli.[21] Detailed discussions of scoliosis may be found in pediatric texts and orthopedic texts.

References for Unit XVII

1. Adams, J.: Foot problems in adults. *Postgraduate Medicine 42*:1, July, 1967.
2. Ainsworth, T. H.: Immediate full weight-bearing in the treatment of hip fractures. *Journal of Trauma 11*:1031, December, 1971.
3. Alba, I. M., and Papeika, J.: The nurse's role in preventing circulatory complications in the patient with a fractured hip. *Nursing Clinics of North America 1*:57, March, 1966.
4. Allgire, M. J.: *Nurses Can Give and Teach Rehabilitation.* 2nd ed. New York, Springer Publishing Company, 1968.
5. Altemeier, W. A.: The significance of infection in trauma. *AORN Journal 15*:92, March, 1972.
6. *Manual of Orthopaedic Surgery.* Chicago, American Orthopaedic Association, 1972.
7. Apley, A. G.: Commonly missed orthopaedic injuries. *Journal of Postgraduate Medicine 43*: 568, September, 1967.

7a. Arden, G. P.: Total knee replacement. *Clinical Orthopaedics and Related Research 94*:92, July-August, 1973.

8. Aronoff, P. M., Davis, P. M., Jr., and Wickstrom, J. K.: Intramedullary nail fixation as treatment of subtrochanteric fractures of the femur. *Journal of Trauma 11*:637, August, 1971.
9. Ashton, H.: Effect of inflatable plastic splints on blood flow. *British Medical Journal 2*:1427, December 10, 1966.
10. Austen, K. F.: Connective tissue diseases ("collagen diseases") other than rheumatoid arthritis: Introduction. *In* Beeson, P. B., and McDermott, W. (eds.): *Cecil-Loeb Textbook of Medicine.* 13th ed. Philadelphia, W. B. Saunders Company, 1971.
11. Austen, K. F.: Periarteritis nodosa (polyarteritis nodosa). *In* Beeson, P. B., and McDermott, W. (Eds.): *Cecil-Loeb Textbook of Medicine.* 13th ed. Philadelphia, W. B. Saunders Company, 1971.
12. Ballinger, W. F., Treybal, J. C., and Vose, A. B.: *Alexander's Care of the Patient in Surgery.* 5th ed. St. Louis, Mo., C. V. Mosby Company, 1972.
13. Bame, K.: Halo traction. *American Journal of Nursing 69*:1933, September, 1969.

13a. Baum, J.: Rheumatoid arthritis. *In* Conn, H. F. (ed.): *Current Therapy 1973*. Philadelphia, W. B. Saunders Company, 1973.

14. Beaumont, E.: Wheelchairs. *Nursing '73 3*:49, November, 1973.
15. Beetham, W. P., Jr.: The management of the collagen diseases. *G.P. 31*:113, February, 1965.
16. Berk, R. N.: Liquid fat in the knee joint after trauma. *New England Journal of Medicine 277*: 1411, December 28, 1967.
17. Bitenc, I.: Hip arthroplasty. *Canadian Nurse 60*:463, May, 1964.
18. Blair, S.: Tumors of bones and muscles of the lower extremities. *Surgical Clinics of North America 45*:247, February, 1965.
19. Bland, J. H. (ed.): Symposium on rheumatoid arthritis. *Medical Clinics of North America 52*: 477, May, 1968.
20. Blount, W. P., and Bolinske, J.: Physical therapy in the nonoperative treatment of scoliosis. *Physical Therapy 47*:919, October, 1967.
21. Boegli, E. H., and Steele, M. S.: Scoliosis: Spinal instrumentation and fusion. *American Journal of Nursing 68*:2399, November, 1968.
22. Bonner, C., et al.: Tips on choosing and using crutches, canes and walkers. *Patient Care 2*:17, October, 1968.
23. Bouchard, R.: *Nursing Care of the Cancer Patient.* St. Louis, Mo., C. V. Mosby Company, 1967, Chapter 7.
24. Bovill, E. G., Horowitz, B. G., and Pollock, S. F.: The incidence of major arterial laceration accompanying fractures of long bones. *California Medicine 107*:261, September, 1967.
25. Boyes, J. H.: *Suture Technics for Wounds of the Hand.* Booklet published by Ethicon, Inc., Somerville, N. J., 1970.
26. Bray, A. P., and Thomas, J. R.: Severe fat embolism syndrome following multiple fractures. *Nursing Times 65*:109, January 23, 1969.
27. Brodsky, I., et al. Treatment of multiple myeloma. *Geriatrics 22*:140, March, 1967.
28. Brooks, S. M.: *Integrated Basic Science.* 2nd ed. St. Louis, Mo., C. V. Mosby Company, 1966.
29. Browler, P., and Hicks, D.: Maintaining muscle function in patients on bed rest. *American Journal of Nursing 72*:1250, July, 1972.
30. Brunner, L. S., et al.: *Textbook of Medical-Surgical Nursing.* 2nd ed. Philadelphia, J. B. Lippincott Company, 1970.
31. Brunner, N. A. *Orthopedic Nursing: A Programmed Approach.* St. Louis, Mo., C. V. Mosby Company, 1970.
32. Butt, W. P., and McIntyre, J. L.: Double contrast arthrography of the knee. *Radiology 92*:487, March, 1969.
33. Calabro, J. J., and Maltz, B. A.: Current concepts on ankylosing spondylitis. *New England Journal of Medicine 282*:606, March 12, 1970.
34. Cannon, B., and Murray, J. E.: Reflections on skin

grafting in hand repairs. *Journal of the American Medical Association 200*:663, May 22, 1967.

35. Casagrande, P. A., and Turner, R.: Total knee replacement. *Clinical Orthopaedics and Related Research 89*:150, November-December, 1972.
36. Casscells, S. W.: Arthroscopy of the knee joint: A review of 150 cases. *Journal of Bone and Joint Surgery 53-A*:287, March, 1971.
37. Charnley, J.: Postoperative infection after total hip replacement with special reference to air contamination in the operating room. *Clinical Orthopaedics and Related Research 87*:167, September, 1972.
38. Charosky, C., Bullough, P., and Wilson, P.: Total hip replacement failures. *Journal of Bone and Joint Surgery 55-A*:49, January, 1973.
39. Ciuca, R., Bradish, J., and Trombley, S. M.: Range-of-motion exercises, active and passive: A handbook. *Nursing '73 3*:25, December, 1973.
40. Clark, W. S.: Arthritis and rehabilitation. *Journal of Rehabilitation 31*:10, September-October, 1965.
41. Clary, B. B., and Couk, D. E.: Experience with the MacIntosh knee prosthesis. *Southern Medical Journal 65*:265, March, 1972.
42. Clawson, D. K., and Dunn, W.: Management of common bacterial infections of bones and joints. *Journal of Bone and Joint Surgery 49-A*:164, January, 1967.

42a. Clayton, M. L.: Care of the rheumatoid hip. *Clinical Orthopaedics and Related Research 90*:70, January-February, 1973.

43. Cole, W. H., and Puestow, C. B.: *Emergency Care*. 7th ed. New York, Appleton Century Crofts, 1972.
44. Collins, D. K., and Johnston, R. C.: Comparative evaluation of the results of cup arthroplasty and total hip replacement. *Clinical Orthopaedics and Related Research 86*:102, July-August, 1972.
45. Conaty, J. P., and Nickel, V. L.: Functional incapacitation in rheumatoid arthritis: A rehabilitation challenge. *Journal of Bone and Joint Surgery 53-A*:624, June, 1971.
46. Committee on Injuries, American Academy of Orthopaedic Surgeons: *Emergency Care and Transportation of the Sick and Injured*. Menasha, Wisconsin, George Banta Company, Inc., 1971.
47. Committee on Trauma of American College of Surgeons: *An Outline of the Treatment of Fractures*. 8th ed. Philadelphia, W. B. Saunders Company, 1965.

47a. Convery, F. R., and Beber, C. A.: Total knee arthroplasty. *Clinical Orthopaedics and Related Research 94*:42, July-August, 1973.

48. Covalt, N. K.: *Bed Exercises for Convalescent Patients*. Springfield, Ill., Charles C Thomas, Publisher, 1968.
49. Cozen, L.: *An Atlas of Orthopedic Surgery*. Philadelphia, Lea and Febiger, 1966.

49a. Current surgical nursing: Symposium. *Nursing Clinics of North America 8*:107, March, 1973.

50. Dahlin, D. C., and Ivins, J. C.: Fibrosarcoma of bone: Study of 114 cases. *Cancer 23*:35, January, 1969.
51. Dandy, D. J.: Fat embolism following prosthetic replacement of the femoral head. *Injury 3*:85, 1971.
52. Davis, P. R.: The nurse and her back. *Nursing Times 63*:1403, October 20, 1967.
53. Dee, R.: Total replacement arthroplasty of the elbow for rheumatoid arthritis. *Journal of Bone and Joint Surgery 54-B*:88, February, 1972.
54. Dehne, E.: The weight-bearing principle in treatment of lower-extremity fractures, 1885–1972. *Journal of Trauma 12*:539, June, 1972.
55. del Bueno, D. J.: Recognizing fat embolism in patients with multiple injuries. *RN 36*:48, January, 1973.
56. De Nardo, G. L., et al.: Radioisotope skeletal survey. *Journal of the American Medical Association 200*:621, April 10, 1967.
57. Derian, P. S.: Fat embolization—Current status. *Journal of Trauma 5*:580, September, 1965.
58. DiStefano, V., and Nixon, J. E.: Steroid-induced skin changes following local injection. *Clinical Orthopaedics and Related Research 87*:254, September, 1972.
59. *Dorland's Illustrated Medical Dictionary*. 24th ed. Philadelphia, W. B. Saunders Company, 1965.
60. Doyle, J. R.: Dupuytren's contracture: Etiology and principles of treatment. *California Medicine 110*:292, April, 1969.
61. Drain, C. B.: The athletic knee injury. *American Journal of Nursing 71*:536, March, 1971.
62. Drury, J. H., Jr.: Handbook of range-of-motion exercises. *Nursing '72 2*:19, April, 1972.
63. Dunn, A. W.: Senile osteoporosis. *Geriatrics 22*:175, November, 1967.
64. Dupont, J. A., Charnley, J., Jr.: Low-friction arthroplasty of the hip for the failures of previous operations. *Journal of Bone and Joint Surgery 54-B*:77, February, 1972.
65. Durbin, F. C.: Affections of the toes. *Practitioner 201*:749, November, 1968.
66. Eagleson, W. M., et al.: The effect of heat on the healing of fractures. *Canadian Medical Association Journal 97*:274, August 5, 1967.
67. Eaton, P., and Heller, F.: Therapeutic nursing care of orthopedic patients. *Nursing Clinics of North America 2*:429, September, 1967.
68. Eckert, C.: *Emergency Room Care*. Boston, Little, Brown and Company, 1967.
69. Engel, A., and Burch, T. A.: Chronic arthritis in the U. S. health examination survey. *Arthritis and Rheumatism 10*:61, February, 1967.
70. Engleman, E. P., Giansiracusa, J. E., and Chatton, M. J.: Arthritis and allied rheumatic disorders. *In* Brainerd, H., Margen, S., and Chatton, M. J.: *Current Diagnosis and Treatment*. Los Altos, Cal., Lange Medical Publications, 1969.
71. *Nursing Care of the Patient in the O.R.*. Ethicon, Inc., Somerville, N. J., 1973.

71a. Evarts, C. M. (ed.): Symposium on interposition and implant arthroplasty. *Orthopedic Clinics of North America 4*:233, April, 1973.

72. Eyre, M. K.: Total hip replacement. *American Journal of Nursing 71*:1384, July, 1971.
73. Fairbank, T. J.: Deformities of the arches of the foot and related conditions. *Practitioner 201*:742, November, 1968.
74. Falconer, M. W., et al.: *The Drug, The Nurse, The Patient*. 5th ed. Philadelphia, W. B. Saunders Company, 1974.
75. Felstein, I.: Rheumatoid arthritis. *Nursing Mirror 126*:28, 31 May, 1968.
76. Finsterbush, A., et al.: Recent experiences with intravenous regional anesthesia in limbs. *Journal of Trauma 12*:81, January, 1972.

76a. Foss, G.: Body mechanics: Use your head and save your back. *Nursing '73 3*:25, May, 1973.

77. Foss, G.: Breaking the architectural barrier with crutches, wheelchairs and walkers. *Nursing '73 3*:17, October, 1973.
78. Foss, G.: The "how to's" of bed positioning. *Nursing '72 2*:14, August, 1972.
79. Francis, S. M.: Nursing the patient with internal hip fixation. *American Journal of Nursing 64*: 111, May, 1964.
80. Freyberg, R.: Rheumatoid arthritis: The natural history, diagnosis, prognosis and management. *Medical Times 95*:742, July, 1967.
81. Frost, H. M.: Musculoskeletal pain. *In* Alling, C. A., III (ed.): *Facial Pain*. Philadelphia, Lea and Febiger, 1968.
82. Furey, J. G.: Complications following hip fractures. *Journal of Chronic Disease 20*:103, February, 1967.
83. Gardner, R. C.: Hypertrophic infiltrative tendinitis (HIT syndrome) of the long extensor. *Journal of the American Medical Association 211*:1009, February 9, 1970.
84. Garner, J. H., and Peltier, L. F.: Fat embolism: The significance of provoked petechiae. *Journal of the American Medical Association 200*:226, May, 8, 1967.
85. Gartland, J. J.: *Fundamentals of Orthopaedics*. Philadelphia, W. B. Saunders Company, 1965.
86. Gerifacts: Prevalence of osteoarthritis. *Geriatrics 42*: 104, March, 1967.
87. Gerifacts: Rheumatoid arthritis. *Geriatrics 42*:70, February, 1967.
88. Ginsberg, M., Miller, J. M., McElfatrick, G. C.: The use of inflatable plastic splints. *Journal of the American Medical Association 200*:190, April 10, 1967.
89. Gordon, P. C.: The probability of death following a fracture of the hip. *Canadian Medical Association Journal 105*:47, July 10, 1971.
90. Grant, H., and Murray, R.: *Emergency Care*. Washington, D.C., Robert J. Brady Company, 1971.
91. Grant, W. R.: Aids to mobility: Walking aids, Wheelchairs, and Hoists. *Physiotherapy 52*:146, 1966.
92. Grattan, E., and Hobbs, J. A.: Injuries to hip joint in car occupants. *British Medical Journal 1*:71, January 11, 1969.
93. Graves, S., and Vincent, S.: Total hip replacement is a family affair. *RN 34*:35, June, 1971.
94. Gray, K. D.: O.R. sterility for total hip replacement. *AORN Journal 16*:72, October, 1972.
95. Griffin, W., Anderson, S. J., and Passos, J. Y.: Group exercises for patients with limited motion. *American Journal of Nursing 71*:1742, September, 1971.
96. Haas, H.: Osteoporosis. *Geriatrics 22*:100, December, 1967.
97. Hadfield, G.: Casualty fractures. *Journal of Postgraduate Medicine 43*:647, October, 1967.
98. Harris, E. D., Jr.: Systemic sclerosis (scleroderma). *In* Beeson, P. B., and McDermott, W. (eds.): *Cecil-Loeb Textbook of Medicine*. 13th ed. Philadelphia, W. B. Saunders Company, 1971.
99. Harris, W. H., and Heaney, R. P.: Skeletal renewal and metabolic bone disease. *New England Journal of Medicine 280*:193, January 23, 1969.
100. Hartman, J. T., and Phalen, G. S.: Needle biopsy of bone. *Journal of the American Medical Association 200*:113, April 17, 1967.
101. Heaney, R. P.: Diseases of bone. *In* Beeson, P. B., and McDermott, W. (eds.): *Cecil-Loeb Textbook of Medicine*. 13th ed. Philadelphia, W. B. Saunders Company, 1971.
102. Herfort, R. A.: *The Surgical Relief of Pain in Arthritic Disease*. Springfield, Ill., Charles C Thomas, 1967.
103. Herndon, J. H., Riseborough, E. J., and Fischer, J. E.: Fat embolism: A review of current concepts. *Journal of Trauma 11*:673, August, 1971.
104. Hollander, J. L. (ed.): *Arthritis and Allied Conditions*. 7th ed. Philadelphia, Lea and Febiger, 1966.
105. Hollinshead, W. H.: *Functional Anatomy of the Limbs and Back*. Philadelphia, W. B. Saunders Company, 1969.
106. Holvey, D. N. (ed.): *The Merck Manual*. 12th ed. Rahway, N.J., Merck & Company, Inc., 1972.
107. Hoover, S. A.: Job-related back injuries in a hospital. *American Journal of Nursing 73*:2078, December, 1973.
108. Hoppenfeld, S.: *Scoliosis*. Philadelphia, J. B. Lippincott Company, 1967.
109. Hudson, O. C.: When to operate for hip fracture in the aged. *Geriatrics 20*:206, March, 1965.
110. Hygiene and the full body cast. *American Journal of Orthopedics 9*:141, July, 1967.
111. Jackson, J. P.: Internal derangement of the knee-joint. *Physiotherapy 52*:229, 1966.
112. Jackson, R. W., and Abe, I.: The role of arthroscopy in the management of disorders of the knee. *Journal of Bone and Joint Surgery 54-B*:310, May, 1972.
113. Jacob, S. W., and Francone, C. A.: *Structure and Function in Man*. 3rd ed. Philadelphia, W. B. Saunders Company, 1974.
114. Jebsen, R. H.: Use and abuse of ambulation aids. *Journal of the American Medical Association 199*:63, January 2, 1967.
115. Jeffreys, T. E.: The hand in rheumatoid arthritis. *Nursing Mirror 123*:viii, February 17, 1967.
116. Jones, G. P. (ed.): Symposium on orthopedic and surgical nursing. *Nursing Clinics of North America 2*:383–435, September, 1967.
117. Kane, W., et al.: Halo-femoral pin distraction in the treatment of sciolosis. *Journal of Bone and Joint Surgery 49-A*:1018, July, 1967.
118. Katz, S., et al.: Long term course of 147 patients with fracture of the hip. *Surgery, Gynecology and Obstetrics 124*:1219, June, 1967.
119. Keim, H. A.: Scoliosis. *Ciba Clinical Symposia 24*:No. 1, 1972.
120. Keiser, R. P.: Treatment of scoliosis. *Nursing Clinics of North America 2*:409, September, 1967.
121. Kendall, H., and Kendall, F.: Developing and maintaining good posture. *Physical Therapy 48*: 319, April, 1968.
122. Kern, F. C., and Poole, L.: Transfer techniques. *Nursing '72 2*:25, July, 1972.
123. Kerr, A. H.: *Orthopedic Nursing Procedures*. 2nd ed. New York, Springer Publishing Company, Inc., 1969.
124. Kersley, G. D.: Antimalarials and the connective tissue diseases. *Nursing Times 63*:691, May 26, 1967.
125. Kessler, F. B.: The nurse in hand surgery. *AORN Journal 15*:44, June, 1972.
126. Kessler, I.: Silicone arthroplasty of the trapeziometacarpal joint. *Journal of Bone and Joint Surgery 55-B*:285, May, 1973.
126a. Kettelkamp, D. B., and Leach, R. B. (guest eds.): Symposium: Total knee replacement. *Clinical Orthopaedics and Related Research 94*:2–256, July-August, 1973.

127. Kirk, J. A., and Kersley, G. D.: Heat and cold in the physical treatment of rheumatoid arthritis of the knee. *Annals of Physical Medicine 9*:270, August, 1968.
128. Knapp, M.: Aftercare of fractures. *In* Krusen, F. H., Kottke, F. J., and Ellwood, P. M. Jr.: *Handbook of Physical Medicine and Rehabilitation.* 2nd ed. Philadelphia, W. B. Saunders Company, 1971.
129. Knapp, M.: Orthotics (bracing). *Postgraduate Medicine 43*:241, March, 1968.
130. Knapp, M.: Orthotics: Bracing the lower extremity. *Postgraduate Medicine 43*:225, April, 1968.
131. Knapp, M.: Orthotics: Bracing the upper extremity. *Postgraduate Medicine 43*:215, June, 1968.
132. Knapp, M.: Rheumatoid arthritis. *Postgraduate Medicine 42*:A-99, November, 1967.
133. Knocke, L.: Crutch walking. *American Journal of Nursing 61*:70, October, 1961.
134. Krusen, F. H., Kottke, F., and Ellwood, P. (eds.): *Handbook of Physical Medicine and Rehabilitation.* 2nd ed. Philadelphia, W. B. Saunders Company, 1971.
135. Kurth, J. S.: Correct application of the Thomas splint and Pearson attachment. *Nursing '73 3*:20, July, 1973.
136. Laine, V. A.: Early synovectomy in rheumatoid arthritis. *Annual Review of Medicine 18*:173, 1967.
137. Lamont-Havers, R. W.: Arthritis quackery. *American Journal of Nursing 63*:92, March, 1963.
138. Lane, P.: A mother's confession: Home care of a toddler in a spica cast. What it's really like. *American Journal of Nursing 71*:2141, November, 1971.
139. Larson, C. B., and Gould, M.: *Orthopedic Nursing.* 7th ed. St. Louis, Mo., C. V. Mosby Company, 1970.
140. Leach, R. E., and Torgerson, W. R.: The management of metastatic disease in the skeletal system. *Surgical Clinics of North America 47*: 757, June, 1967.
141. Leddy, J. P., Grantham, S. A., and Stinchfield, F. E.: Hip-mold arthroplasty and postoperative infection. *Journal of Bone and Joint Surgery 53-A*:37, January, 1971.
142. Licht, S., and Kamenetz, H. L. (eds.): *Orthotics Etcetera.* New Haven, Elizabeth Licht, Publisher, 1966.
143. Licht, S., and Kamenetz, H. L. (eds.): *Rehabilitation and Medicine.* New Haven, Elizabeth Licht, Publisher, 1968.
144. Lichtenstein, L.: *Bone Tumors.* 4th ed. St. Louis, Mo., C. V. Mosby Company, 1972.
145. Lockie, L. M.: How to recognize and treat gout. *Postgraduate Medicine 43*:98, June, 1968.
146. London, P. S.: General complications of fractures. *Nursing Mirror 119*:ii, November 20, 1964.
147. Lowman, E.: Clinical management of disability due to rheumatoid arthritis. *Archives of Physical Medicine and Rehabilitation. 48*:136, March 1967.
148. Lowman, E.: Connective tissue diseases. *In* Krusen, F. H., Kottke, F. J., and Ellwood, P. M., Jr.: *Handbook of Physical Medicine and Rehabilitation.* 2nd ed. Philadelphia, W. B. Saunders Company, 1971.
149. Lowman, E., and J. Klinger. *Aids to Independent Living.* New York, McGraw-Hill, 1969.
150. Lutwak, L.: Osteoporosis: A public health problem. *American Association of Industrial Nurses Journal 14*:21, September, 1966.
151. MacGinnis, O.: Rheumatoid arthritis—my tutor. *American Journal of Nursing 68*:1699, August, 1968.
152. Mahoney, R. F.: *Emergency and Disaster Nursing.* 2nd ed. New York, Macmillan Company, 1969.
153. Marcove, R. C., and Miller, T. R.: Treatment of primary and metastatic bone tumors by cryosurgery. *Journal of the American Medical Association 207*:1890, March 10, 1969.
154. Marmor, L.: *Surgery of Rheumatoid Arthritis.* Philadelphia, Lea and Febiger, 1967.
155. Marmor, L., and Treace, J.: A new balanced suspension. *Clinical Orthopaedics and Related Research 85*:146, June, 1972.
156. Marmor, L., et al.: Rheumatoid arthritis—surgical intervention. *American Journal of Nursing 67*: 1430, July, 1967.
157. May, C. M.: Wheelchair patient for a day. *American Journal of Nursing 73*:650, April, 1973.
158. Mayer, J.: Nutrition and gout. *Postgraduate Medicine 45*:277, May, 1969.
159. McCarthy, B., et al.: Subclinical fat embolism: A prospective study of 50 patients with extremity fractures. *The Journal of Trauma 13*:9, January, 1973.
160. McEwen, C.: Editorial: Synovectomy and the rehabilitation of the patient with rheumatoid arthritis. *Journal of Bone and Joint Surgery 53-A*: 621, June, 1971.
161. McKee, G. K.: Replacement hip surgery. *Nursing Times 63*:984, July 28, 1967.
162. Acrylic glue gains favor in total hip replacement. *Journal of the American Medical Association 209*:638, August 4, 1969.
163. Artificial thumb joint restores motion. *Journal of the American Medical Association 207*:845, February 3, 1969.
164. Fluoride protects against bone loss. *Journal of the American Medical Association 200*:31, May 1, 1967.
165. Prosthesis replaces entire hip joint. *Journal of the American Medical Association 207*:1445, February 24, 1969.
166. Setting long bones: Search for vascular injuries saves limbs. *Journal of the American Medical Association 201*:29, August 21, 1967.
167. Meek, R. N., Woodruff, B., and Allardyce, D. B.: Source of fat macroglobules in fractures of the lower extremity. *The Journal of Trauma 12*: 432, May, 1972.
168. Meltzer, M.: The management of musculoskeletal pain. *In Diagnosis and Management of Pain Syndromes.* 2nd ed. Finneson, B. (ed.), Philadelphia, W. B. Saunders Company, 1969.
169. Memmler, R. L., and Rada, R. B.: *The Human Body in Health and Disease.* 3rd ed. Philadelphia, J. B. Lippincott Company, 1970.
170. Meyer, S.: *Functional Bandaging Including Splints and Protective Dressings.* New York, American Elsevier Publishing Company, 1967.
171. Michele, A.: Principles of fracture care. *American Journal of Orthopedics 9*:34, February, 1967; *9*:54, March, 1967.
172. Mikkelsen, W. M., and Robinson, W. D.: Physiologic and biochemical basis for the treatment of gout and hyperuricemia. *Medical Clinics of North America 53*:1331, November, 1969.
173. Miller, B. F., and Keane, C. B.: *Encyclopedia and Dictionary of Medicine and Nursing.* Philadelphia, W. B. Saunders Company, 1972.

174. Monteirio, L. A.: Hip fracture—A sociologist's viewpoint. *American Journal of Nursing 67*:1207, June, 1967.
175. Nagle, W. C.: Grease gun injury of a hand. *American Journal of Nursing 69*:1264, June, 1969.
176. *Rehabilitative Aspects of Nursing.* (A programmed instruction series.) Part I. Physical Therapeutic Nursing Measures: Unit 1, Concepts and goals (1966); Unit 2, Range of joint motion (1967). New York, National League for Nursing.
177. Naylor, A.: *Fractures and Orthopedic Surgery for Nurses and Physiotherapists.* 6th ed. Baltimore, Williams and Wilkins, 1968.
178. Nelson, J. P., Ferris, D. O., and Ivins, J. C.: The cast syndrome. *Postgraduate Medicine 42*:457, December, 1967.
179. Neufeld, A. J.: Surgical treatment of hip injuries. *American Journal of Nursing 65*:80, March, 1965.
180. Ceramic "bone" tested. *American Journal of Nursing 69*:1408, July, 1969.
181. Newton, M.: Surgery in arthritis of the lower extremity. *Surgical Clinics of North America 45*: 201, February, 1965.
182. Nice, W.: An increasing problem—fat embolism syndrome: Diagnosis and treatment. *Journal of the Kansas Medical Society 69*:45, February, 1968.
183. Nice, W., Huaman, A., and Young, I.: Fat embolism syndrome: Diagnosis and treatment. *AORN Journal 17*:197, January, 1973.
184. Nickel, V., Kristy, J., and McDaniel, L.: Physical therapy for rheumatoid arthritis. *Physical Therapy 45*:198, March, 1965.
185. Nickel, V., et al.: The halo. *Journal of Bone and Joint Surgery 50-A*:1400, October, 1968.
186. O'Brien, J. P., et al.: Halo pelvic traction. *Journal of Bone and Joint Surgery 53-B*:217, May, 1971.
187. O'Riordan, C., et al.: A prospective study of wound infections on an orthopedic service. *Clinical Orthopaedics and Related Research 87*:188, September, 1972.
188. Pearson, C. M., et al.: Rheumatoid arthritis and its systemic manifestations. *Annals of Internal Medicine 65*:1101, November, 1966.
189. Peers, J.: The care and handling of orthopedic implants. *RN 28*:66, October, 1965.
190. Peltier, L.: A brief history of traction. *Journal of Bone and Joint Surgery 50-A*:1603, December, 1968.
191. Peltier, L.: The diagnosis and treatment of fat embolism. *Journal of Trauma 11*:661, August, 1971.
192. Perez, C. A., Bradfield, J. S., and Morgan, H. C.: Management of pathologic fractures. *Cancer 29*: 684, March, 1972.
193. Perry, J., and Nickel, V.: The halo. *Journal of Bone and Joint Surgery 50-A*:1400, October, 1968.
194. Peszczynski, M.: Why old people fall. *American Journal of Nursing 65*:86, May, 1965.
195. Petrello, J. M.: Temperature maintenance of hot moist compresses. *American Journal of Nursing 73*:1050, June, 1973.
196. Potter, T. A., and Nalebuff, E. A. (eds.): Symposium on the surgical management of rheumatoid arthritis. *Surgical Clinics of North America 49*: No. 4, August, 1969.
197. Powell, M.: *Orthopaedic Nursing.* 6th ed. London, E. & S. Livingstone, Ltd., 1968.
198. Powers, J. A.: Meniscectomies in women. *Journal of the American Medical Association 208*:663, April 28, 1969.
199. Principles of lower extremity bracing. *Physical Therapy 47*:September, 1967.
200. Continuous cold applications for athletic injuries. *Journal of the American Medical Association 207*:962, February 3, 1969.
201. Ralston, E. L.: *Handbook of Fractures.* St. Louis, Mo., C. V. Mosby Company, 1967.
202. Ranalls, J.: Crutches and walkers. *Nursing '72 2*: 21, December, 1972.
203. Rankin, T. J., and Good, A. E.: Corticosteroid injection of small joints by hypospray. *Arthritis and Rheumatism 9*:611, August, 1966.
204. Reckling, F. W., and Peltier, L. F.: Acute knee dislocations and their complications. *Journal of Trauma 9*:181, March, 1969.
205. Rheumatic diseases. *Postgraduate Medicine 45*: January, 1969.
206. Rheumatoid arthritis. *Medical Clinics of North America 52*:May, 1968.
207. Ring, P. A.: Complete replacement arthroplasty of the hip by the ring prosthesis. *Journal of Bone and Joint Surgery 50-B*:720, November, 1968.
208. Ring, P. A.: Fractures of the pelvis. *Nursing Times 61*:732, May 28, 1965.
209. Ring, P. A.: Replacement of the hip joint. *Annals of the Royal College of Surgeons of England 48*:344, June, 1971.
210. Robbins, S. L.: *Pathology.* 3rd ed. Philadelphia, W. B. Saunders Company, 1967, Chapters 8 and 31.
211. Roberts, J. M.: New developments in orthopedic surgery—Fractures. *Nursing Clinics of North America 2*:386, September, 1967.
212. Robinson, M., and Van Volkenburgh, S.: Intermaxillary fixation: Immediate postoperative care. *American Journal of Nursing 63*:71, January, 1963.
213. Robinson, W. D.: Diseases of the joints. *In* Beeson, P. B., and McDermott, W. (eds.): *Cecil-Loeb Textbook of Medicine.* 13th ed. Philadelphia, W. B. Saunders Company, 1971.
214. Rodman, M. J.: Drugs for rheumatic disorders. *RN 31*:55, September, 1968.
215. Rosenthal, D., and Moloney, W. C.: Treating multiple myeloma. *Postgraduate Medicine 44*: 143, October, 1968.
215a. Rothberg, J. S. (ed.): Symposium on chronic disease and rehabilitation. *Nursing Clinics of North America 1*:352, September, 1966.
216. Rotstein, J.: *Simple Splinting–The Use of Light Splints and Related Conservative Therapy in Joint Diseases.* Philadelphia, W. B. Saunders Company, 1965.
217. Rowe, J. W., and Wheble, V. H. A.: *Concise Textbook of Anatomy and Physiology Applied for Orthopedic Nurses.* Baltimore, Williams and Wilkins, 1967.
218. Salter, R. B.: *Textbook of Disorders and Injuries of the Musculoskeletal System.* Baltimore, Williams and Wilkins, 1970.
219. Schechter, D. E.: Osteoarthritis of the hip in the aged. *Geriatrics 22*:149, November, 1967.
220. Schmeisser, G. J.: *A Clinical Manual of Orthopedic Traction Techniques.* Philadelphia, W. B. Saunders Company, 1963.
221. Schneider, F. R.: *Handbook for the Orthopaedic Assistant.* St. Louis, Mo., C. V. Mosby Company, 1972.
222. Schur, P. H.: Systemic lupus erythematosus. *In* Beeson, P. B., and McDermott, W. (eds.): *Cecil-Loeb*

Textbook of Medicine. 13th ed. Philadelphia, W. B. Saunders Company, 1971.
223. Seegmiller, J. E.: Goals in gout. *Postgraduate Medicine 45*:99, January, 1969.
224. Shands, A. R., and Raney, R. B.: *Handbook of Orthopaedic Surgery*. 7th ed. St. Louis, Mo., C. V. Mosby Company, 1967.
225. Shaw, B. L.: The nursing challenge of lupus: The uncertain killer. *RN 31*:32, September, 1968.
226. Sheafer, K. N., et al.: *Medical-Surgical Nursing*. 5th ed. St. Louis, Mo., C. V. Mosby Company, 1971.
227. Siegel, I. M.: Jogger's heel. *Journal of the American Medical Association 206*:2899, December 23–30, 1968.
228. Slocumb, C. H., et al.: Some unusual manifestations of rheumatoid arthritis. *Postgraduate Medicine 42*:309, October, 1967.
229. Smith, D. W., Hanley Germain, C. P., and Gips, C. D.: *Care of the Adult Patient*. 3rd ed. Philadelphia, J. B. Lippincott Company, 1971.
230. Smith, L. H., Jr.: Disorders of purine metabolism. *In* Beeson, P. B., and McDermott, W. (eds.): *Cecil-Loeb Textbook of Medicine*. 13th ed. Philadelphia, W. B. Saunders Company, 1971.
231. Smyth, C.: Newer drugs for arthritis. *Postgraduate Medicine 44*:77, July, 1968.
232. Sodeman, W. A., and Sodeman, W. A., Jr.: *Pathologic Physiology: Mechanisms of Disease*. 5th ed. Philadelphia, W. B. Saunders Company, 1974.
233. Soika, C. V.: Combatting osteoporosis. *American Journal of Nursing 73*:1193, July, 1973.
234. Sorenson, L., et al.: *Ambulation: A Manual for Nurses*. Minneapolis, American Rehabilitation Foundation, 1966.
235. Stauffer, R. N.: Total hip replacement: First year's experience. *Archives of Surgery 103*:668, December, 1971.
236. Stern, M., and Grant, S. S.: Fifty total hip replacements. *Clinical Orthopaedics and Related Research 86*:79, July-August, 1972.
237. Stiles, P. J.: Internal fixation of fractures in patients with diffuse malignant disease. *Nursing Mirror 125*:i, October 6, 1967.
238. Stiles, P. J.: Surgical treatment of rheumatoid arthritis. *Nursing Mirror 126*:20, 7 June, 1968.
239. Stillwell, G. K.: Therapeutic heat and cold. *In* Krusen, F. H., Kottke, F. J., and Ellwood, P. M., Jr.: *Handbook of Physical Medicine and Rehabilitation*. 2nd ed. Philadelphia, W. B. Saunders Company, 1971.
240. Stinchfield, F. E., and A. C. Chamberlin. Arthroplasty of the hip. *Journal of Bone and Joint Surgery 48-A*:564, April, 1966.
241. Strange, F. G. St. C.: Pinning under local anaesthesia for the treatment of subcapital fractures of the femoral neck. *Injury 1*:100, October, 1969.
242. Suiter, R. D., and A. J. Bianco, Jr.: Fractures of the femoral shaft. *Journal of Trauma 11*:238, March, 1971.
243. Sullivan, C. R.: Fractures of the pelvis: Fundamentals of management. *Postgraduate Medicine 39*:45, January, 1966.
244. Surgery of the lower extremity. *Surgical Clinics North America 45*:No. 1, February, 1965.
245. Swanson, A. B.: Disabling arthritis at the base of the thumb. *Journal of Bone and Joint Surgery 54-A*:456, April, 1972.
246. Swanson, A. B.: Flexible implant arthroplasty for arthritic finger joints. *Journal of Bone and Joint Surgery 54-A*:435, April, 1972.
247. Swanson, A. B.: Implant arthroplasty for the great toe. *Clinical Orthopaedics and Related Research 85*:75, June, 1972.
248. Sweetman, R. (ed.): *Will's Fractures, Dislocations, Sprains*. 2nd ed. London, J. and A. Churchill, Ltd., 1969.
249. Talbott, J. H.: *Gout*. 3rd ed. New York, Grune and Stratton, Inc., 1967.
250. Talbott, J. H.: Gout. *Medical Clinics of North America 54*:431, March, 1970.
251. Tambakis, A. P., and Weinsaft, P.: Fractures of the femoral neck: A ten-year review. *Geriatrics 22*:122, August, 1967.
252. Taylor, A. R., and Ansell, B. M.: Arthrography of the knee before and after synovectomy for rheumatoid arthritis. *Journal of Bone and Joint Surgery 54-B*:110, February, 1972.
253. Temporary tendons aid hand injuries. *Nursing Mirror 125*:xvi, November 3, 1967.
254. *Arthritis–The Basic Facts*. New York, The Arthritis Foundation, 1970.
255. *Arthritis Quackery*. New York, The Arthritis Foundation, 1970.
256. *Gout: A Handbook for Patients*. New York, The Arthritis Foundation, 1966.
257. *Home Care Programs in Arthritis: A Manual for Patients*. New York, The Arthritis Foundation, 1969.
258. *Osteoarthritis: A Handbook for Patients*. New York, The Arthritis Foundation, 1967.
259. *Rheumatoid Arthritis: A Handbook for Patients*. New York, The Arthritis Foundation, 1966.
260. *The Truth about Aspirin for Arthritis*. New York, The Arthritis Foundation, 1970.
261. The Foot. *Physiotherapy 53*: April, 1967.
262. Thomas, B. J.: Nursing care of patients with cancer of the bone. *Nursing Clinics of North America 2*:459, September, 1967.
263. Thomas, B. J., and Alexander, C.: Psychological aspects of physical trauma. *AORN Journal 15*:45, February, 1972.
264. Thomas, S.: Fat embolism—A hazard of trauma. *Nursing Times 65*:105, January 23, 1969.
265. Turek, S. L.: *Orthopaedics: Principles and Their Application*. 2nd ed. Philadelphia, J. B. Lippincott Company, 1967.
266. Tyler, H. R.: Polymyositis and Dermatomyositis. *In* Beeson, P. B., and McDermott, W. (eds.): *Cecil-Loeb Textbook of Medicine*. 13th ed. Philadelphia, W. B. Saunders Company, 1971.
267. Wagner, M. M.: Assessment of patients with multiple injuries. *American Journal of Nursing 72*:1882, October, 1972.
268. Wainwright, D.: Annotation: Fractures of the neck of the femur. *Injury 1*:89, October, 1969.
269. Walike, B. C.: Rheumatoid arthritis—Personality factors. *American Journal of Nursing 67*:1427, July, 1967.
270. Walike, B. C., Marmor, L., and Upshaw, M. J.: Rheumatoid arthritis. *American Journal of Nursing 67*:1420, July, 1967.
271. Warren, J. D.: The early management of fractures. *Applied Therapeutics 8*:614, July, 1966.
272. Watson, J. E.: *Medical-Surgical Nursing and Related Physiology*. Philadelphia, W. B. Saunders Company, 1972.

273. Williams, R. C.: Osteoarthritis and rheumatic disease. *Postgraduate Medicine 42*:334, October, 1967.

274. Williams, R. C.: Recent concepts in the treatment of arthritis and rheumatic disorders. *GP 36*:129, November, 1967.

275. Wilson, E. S., Jr., and Katz, F. N.: Stress fractures. *Radiology 92*:481, 1969.

276. Young, C. G., and Barger, J. D.: *Introduction to Medical Science*. St. Louis, Mo., C. V. Mosby Company, 1969, Chapter 18.

277. Young, J. R., et al.: Restless leg syndrome. *Geriatrics 24*:167, April, 1969.

278. *The Traction Handbook*. Warsaw, Indiana, Zimmer Manufacturing Company, 1971.

UNIT XVIII

Nursing Patients Experiencing Disturbances of the Integumentary System

Rosemary Pittman

Unit Introduction and Study Guide

The integumentary system is the exterior organ that is commonly taken for granted, but is vital in the emotional and physical health of the individual. Care of the skin has long been the responsibility of nurses, and prevention of disease and maintenance of its integrity are important functions that the nurse may assume. In this unit, major problems of the skin and its appendages are presented. This includes major and minor skin problems, trauma and burns. The breast as a modified sebaceous gland is considered part of this system, and carcinoma of the breast is presented in some detail.

Basically the material covers: (1) review of the anatomy and physiology of the skin and breast; (2) the natural history of the presenting disturbances; (3) the major treatments commonly in use; and (4) nursing concerns.

The nurse's role involves being able to understand the above for the purpose of referring the patient to the doctor for early care if indicated by her assessment, preventing complications or recurrences, and assisting the patient in understanding and following the medical regimen by instructing him and being involved in his care. Nurses in schools, industry, emergency rooms, doctors' offices, outpatient rooms and in home visits are particularly likely to be the patient's first contact with the health care system. Many patients will present minor concerns to the nurse, which they do not believe are important enough to take up the doctor's time. It is very important, therefore, that the nurse be knowledgeable in this early assessment. Patients frequently do not understand or do not follow the prescribed treatment. Again it is the nurse who can assist the patient in comprehensive follow-through.

To aid in the study of this material, the following guide is presented:

A. *Skin Disease:* Upon completion of this unit, the nurse should be able to:
   1. Explain to a patient how the integrity of the skin is maintained;
      a. that the skin has a normal ecologic flora;
      b. that there is more flora in moist intertriginous areas;

c. that bacteria grow less readily on a dry surface;
d. that any break in the integrity of the skin results in proliferation of organisms and that simple cleansing and exposure to air is best for minor wounds.

2. Adjust the cleansing of the skin to the patient's age and condition, and realize that excessive soap destroys the protective film of the skin and changes the pH.
3. Explain to a patient the cause, symptoms, course and common treatment of any skin condition.
4. Explain to a patient proper care of hair and nails.
5. Counsel the patient concerning early gentle meticulous attention to any skin condition and refrain from using the neighbors' medications and switching treatments rapidly.
6. Assess the patient's skin problem and refer a potentially serious condition for early expert medical care.
7. Help the patient to understand and follow the treatment.
8. Involve and teach the patient self-care and monitoring of his disease.
9. Assist the patient with problems of itching and disfigurement.
10. Describe a skin condition in acceptable technical terms.

B. *Trauma:* The nurse will be able to:
1. Explain the process of wound healing to the patient.
2. Assess the wound for further referral.
3. Suture minor wounds or assist the doctor with suturing.

C. *Burns:* The nurse will be able to:
1. Understand the major problems of emergency care of burns.
2. Describe to the patient the rationale for burn wound care, prevention of infection and skin grafting.
3. Observe early signs of complications such as burn shock, acidosis, Curling's ulcer and infection.
4. Establish a nursing regimen for management of burn patients.
5. Realize the importance of involvement of the total family and care team in care of the severely burned patient.

D. *Cancer of the Breast:* The nurse should be able to:
1. Realize the importance of early detection of lumps and utilize every opportunity to teach the patient about self-examination of the breast.
2. Recognize and manage the profound psychologic problems that may arise from breast biopsy through terminal cancer.
3. Realize the importance of arm edema and prevention of this complication.
4. Explain the rationale for treatment of advanced mammary cancer.

CHAPTER 91

Diseases of the Skin and Its Appendages

INTRODUCTION

The extent of the problem of skin disease is difficult to determine, because many patients with skin disease do not seek medical care and treat their complaints with home remedies and patent medicine. Because of their chronicity and lack of dramatic complications, disorders of the integumentary system are relatively unnoticed except by the victim. Dermatitis causes considerable occupational disability, a high percentage of workmen's compensations claims being awarded for skin disease. The economic cost of skin disease is considerable. Military skin disease ranked first in outpatient services in Vietnam in 1966 and fourth as a cause of total disabilities among all diseases, excluding trauma.[1*]

Consultation for acne is one of the most common reasons for seeking medical care. Having a smooth unblemished skin is valued in our culture, as is obvious from the new mother's concern about the baby's rash as well as the schoolteacher's referral of all skin eruptions to the school nurse. Millions of dollars are spent every year on cosmetic preparations. Cutaneous stimulation may play an important part in psychologic development, and the individual with a chronic skin disease may be deprived of his share of this means of human relating.

Many skin diseases are overtreated and mistreated, and the nurse needs to be aware of those conditions that can best be treated by the dermatologist at the onset. Minor vesicular eruptions between the toes and scabies are examples of conditions that can safely be treated by the nurse with the doctor's approval or consultation. More and more paraprofessionals are working with patients, and the nurse may spend considerable time teaching these individuals about care and treatment of minor skin disorders, prevention and first aid.

Nurses are frequently regarded as a source of information concerning disorders of the skin, since individuals may think the situation too minor to bother the doctor with. People are frequently concerned about the causes of rashes and eruptions and the handling of insect bites, sunburn, "cold" sores, acne, damaged nails, falling hair, etc. Frequently, the nurse has to decide when cuts should be referred for suturing. At present, nurses are, in fact, expected to do minor suturing in health stations, outpatient clinics and isolated areas.

ANATOMY AND PHYSIOLOGY OF THE INTEGUMENTARY SYSTEM

In order to understand the numerous malfunctions of the integumentary system, it is important to have a good understanding of the anatomy and physiology of the skin and its appendages. A review of this system is included to provide a basis for nursing action.

The skin is divided into three main parts—the epidermis, the dermis and the subcutaneous tissue. The skin comprises about 15 per cent of the body weight.[6] The thickness of the skin varies from 1.5 to 4 mm., the epidermis being uniformly thin (0.06 to 0.1 mm.) over most of the body except on the scalp, the palms and the soles.[7]

The Epidermis

Two cell types, melanocytes and keratinocytes, make up the majority of the epidermal cells (Fig. 91–1). The epidermis is stratified into four or five

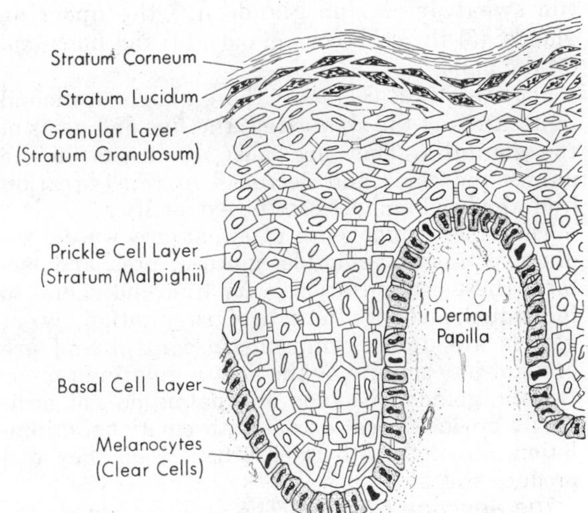

FIGURE 91–1. Diagram of epidermis. (From Lewis, G. M., and Wheeler, C. E., Jr.: *Practical Dermatology*. 3rd ed. 1967.)

*References for Chapter 91 appear on page 1276.

layers (the basal cell layer, the prickle layer, the granular cell layer and the cornified layer). The cells in the basal layer evolve into cells of the cornified layer as they make their way to the surface. This tough protective covering acts as a barrier to the loss of water and electrolytes, providing a homeostatic internal environment for other organs. The epidermis is also resistant to electrical current and corrosive chemicals. Its dry external surface impedes the growth of microorganisms. Normal mitotic activity and desquamation insure replacement of the epidermis in about 28 days.[7]

The ability of the outer layer of the epidermis to absorb water varies directly with the humidity. When submerged in water, this layer can absorb four times its weight in water.[7] The flexibility of the skin depends on desirable water content of the outer layer. Fluctuations in the water content are adjusted by the interstitial water of underlying tissues. This water is continually moving through the skin to the outside and is called *insensible* perspiration. In a 24-hour period, 500 to 600 ml. of body water will escape in this way.[7] The skin barrier is easily permeated by gases, with the exception of carbon monoxide. Substances penetrate more easily with increased skin temperature, in lipid solutions and with increased water in the epidermis. The application of these facts can be used clinically to enhance drug penetration of the skin.

Differences in the amount of pigment among ethnic groups result from the rate and quality of production of melanin. A melanocyte-stimulating hormone (M.S.H.) has been isolated from the pituitary gland.[7]

The epidermis invaginates into the dermis and forms the following appendages (Fig. 91–2): (1) the sweat or eccrine glands; (2) the apocrine glands; (3) the sebaceous glands; (4) the hair; and (5) the nails.

Eccrine Sweat Glands. These glands are found in all areas of the skin except the lips and parts of the genitalia. They are most numerous on the palms and soles and decrease in concentration from the head and neck to the extremities.

The chief components of sweat are water, sodium, potassium, chloride, glucose, urea and lactate. These concentrations vary from individual to individual, and with the rate of perspiration. Sweat glands are under sympathetic control and are brought into activity by the heat-regulating center. Eccrine glands in hands and palms do not ordinarily produce sweat except with emotional stimulation, although with intense heat even they will produce sweat.[14]

The Apocrine Glands. The apocrine glands are large sweat glands whose ducts open into hair follicles to which they are attached and rarely open onto the surface of the skin, as do the eccrine

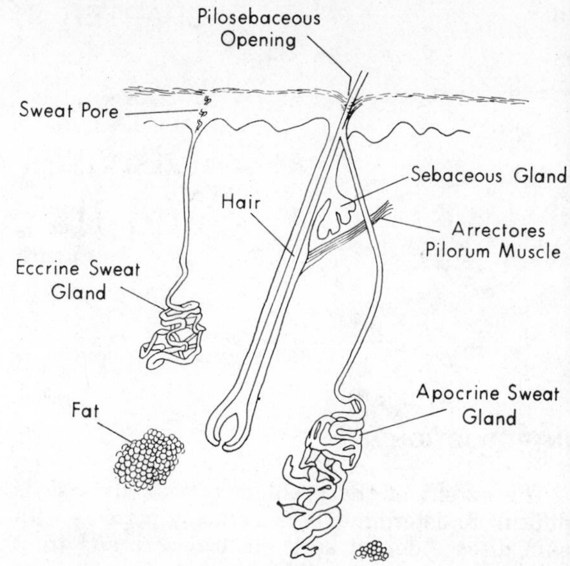

FIGURE 91–2. Diagram of skin and epidermal appendages. (From Lewis, G. M., and Wheeler, C. E., Jr.: *Practical Dermatology,* 3rd ed. 1967.)

glands. They are found in the axillae, anogenital areas, nipple and areola, but do not develop fully until puberty. They are also found in the external ear, producing wax, and on the eyelids, where cystic blockage may occur.[12] They are adrenergic, respond to emotional stimulation and produce milky and distinctly alkaline sweat.

Sweating is a major function of the skin because of its role in the regulation of body temperature by evaporative cooling. Each liter of evaporated sweat is capable of removing 540 cal. of heat from the body.[6] Under dry hot conditions, a man may lose 6 liters of sweat in 24 hours (average 1.5 liters).[14] Abnormality of sweating plays an important role in cystic fibrosis. These patients cannot tolerate salt restriction or periods of excessive sweating, because of the high concentration of sodium in the sweat.[6]

Sebaceous Glands. The sebaceous glands develop from, and are continuous with, hair follicles which may or may not possess a hair. Occasionally they open directly onto the skin surface. Their secretion, sebum, results from degeneration of the cells plus an accumulation of fat. The activity of these glands is under hormonal control, being increased by androgens and suppressed by estrogens. There are natural changes in the activity of the sebaceous glands during the life cycle, varying from the dry skin of the baby when the sebaceous glands are small, to puberty, when there is an increase in the size of the glands, especially those of the face, chest and back. After puberty, the sebum output remains at a high level until menopause and old age, when the skin tends to return to a preadolescent level. In males, it is the androgenic hormones of the testes that are responsible for the increase at puberty. With increasing age, the androgenic output continues to fall and the production of sebum decreases. In females, androgenic hormones are produced by both the ovaries and the adrenals.[5]

The Hair. Hair is a keratinized structure which grows out of a tubular invagination of the epidermis called a hair follicle. Most of the hair is associated with sebaceous glands and this combination is spoken of as the pilosebaceous unit. Hair goes through cyclic changes: growth (anagen), atrophy (catagen) and rest (telogen).[5] Healthy human hair on the scalp has a growth period of two to five years. Melanocytes are present in the bulb of the hair and are responsible for its pigmentation. Hair follicle muscles are immediately beneath the sebaceous glands and, when innervated by adrenergic fibers, cause "goose bumps," a vestigial function which serves fur-bearing animals by increasing their thermal insulation.[5] There are about 100,000 follicles on the human scalp and they grow in a mosaic pattern. Old hairs are lost at the rate of about 50 a day. The health of the hair depends on the health of the individual. The visible hair is a dead structure.

Hair may be classified as being under control of the female or male sex hormones, or as not being under hormonal control. Scalp, eyebrows and eyelashes are nonsexual; aural and nasal hair is under control of androgens, as are the beard and mustache. Body hair on the chest, shoulders, back and abdomen is male sexual and is androgen dependent. Axillary hair is probably independent of adrenal androgen.[14] Extremity hair is under mixed control and heredity plays an important part in extremity hirsutism. Pubic hair is divided into upper and lower areas, the upper border of pubic hair being androgen dependent.

Nails. Human nails are hard keratinized epidermal structures. The nail plate grows continuously and, under normal conditions, persists through life. It is usually replaced if injured, unless matrix is destroyed, in which case it is permanently lost and replaced by the stratum corneum of the epidermis. If the matrix is damaged, the nail grows in a distorted manner or is split.[8] Nails are produced from follicles, represented on one side by the nail bed and on the other side by the nail fold. The body of the nail, the nail plate, grows forward from the nail fold and covers the nail bed. The paronychium is the soft tissue surrounding the nail border.

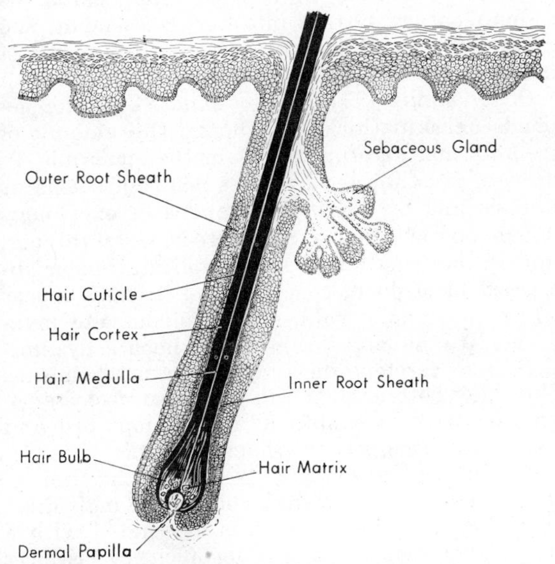

FIGURE 91–3. Diagram of pilosebaceous apparatus. (From Lewis, G. M., and Wheeler, C. E., Jr.: *Practical Dermatology.* 3rd ed. 1967.)

The average growth rate of nails is 0.1 mm. daily. It takes 100 to 150 days for a fingernail to reproduce itself and about three times as long for a toenail to do so. Nail growth is accelerated by biting and by warm weather. Nails function to protect the toes and fingers, especially the delicate sense of touch located in the ends of the fingers. Also, they assist in picking up small objects and provide clues to internal disorders.

Dermis

The dermis is the connective tissue layer of the skin which supports the epidermis and separates it from the cutaneous adipose tissue. The dermis is divided into papillary and reticular areas. It serves as a source of nutrition for the epidermis. The papillary part interdigitates with the epidermis and contains blood vessels and some nerve elements. The reticular part contains connective tissue fibers (elastin and collagen), cellular elements, blood vessels, nerves and lymphatics. Collagen, a fibrous protein, forms the greatest part of the substance of the dermis. Although it is present in every organ system, approximately one half of the total collagen in the body is in the skin.[6, 12]

Apart from sensory information derived from sight and hearing, the major part of our sensory apparatus is in the skin. The sensory fibers responsible for pain, touch and temperature form a complex dermal network.[5] There are four types of sensation: pain, touch, cold and warmth. Pain may be caused by physical, chemical or mechanical stimulation. Touch stimuli are received from hair follicles and intervening skin. Itching arises from terminal nerve endings close to the skin surface. (Itching does not occur when the epidermis is absent.) Temperature sense is probably gained through the free sensory nerve endings in the epidermis.

Bacterial Flora

The normal bacterial flora on the human skin includes the following: *coagulase positive staphylococci, coagulase negative staphylococci, group A hemolytic streptococci, nonhemolytic streptococci, diphtheroids, mycobacteria,* and *pseudomonas organisms.*[14] A damaged area of skin can be a source of entry for infection. Some persons have large numbers of resident bacteria on the skin and others have small numbers. The number for the individual remains relatively constant from month to month unless disturbed. The axillae, groin, perineum and areas of occlusion and intertrigo constantly harbor large numbers. Persons with oily moist skin have a larger number of organisms and more are present on the skin in warm wet weather than in cold dry weather. Body odor is influenced by bacterial flora. Resident gram-positive bacteria operate on apocrine sweat to produce the characteristic odor of the axilla.

Although the skin is constantly bombarded by potentially pathogenic bacteria, infection seldom occurs. Continuous exfoliation of the skin removes organisms. Bathing and rubbing may also remove organisms, as may drying. The normal pH of the skin, which is 4.2 to 5.6, retards the growth of some organisms.[14] Streptococci are more affected than staphylococci by acid pH. Fatty acids in the surface film are fungostatic or bacteriostatic for certain organisms. Certain organisms may exert an inhibitory defense on other organisms, and leukocytes in the epidermis may contribute to defense against invasion by microbes.[6] A damaged area of skin can be a source of entry for infection.

THE CLASSIFICATION OF SKIN LESIONS

Because the nurse is assuming more responsibility in the primary care setting, as the first person who sees the patient, she needs to become increasingly skillful in the observation and description of dermatologic conditions. One method of describing lesions is to classify them according to size (Watt and Jillson).

A. *Primary Lesions:*
  1. Macule: A flat circumscribed discoloration of the skin or mucous membrane up to 1 cm. in the largest diameter. A macule is not raised above the skin and cannot be felt. If the lesion is greater than 1 cm., it is called a "patch."
  2. Papule: A raised solid lesion up to 1 cm. in size. Lesions that are greater than 1 cm. in their longest diameter are called "plaques."
  3. Nodule: A raised solid lesion that can be felt to be deeper in the skin than a papule. If greater than 1 cm. in its longest diameter, it is called a "tumor".
  4. Vesicle: A fluid-filled superficial elevated lesion of the skin or mucous membrane less than 1 cm. in diameter. If it is larger, it is called a "bulla."

  Some other lesions of varying sizes are:

  5. Pustule: A vesicle or bulla containing pus.
  6. Wheal: Irregularly shaped, elevated, changing lesion of the skin or mucous membrane due to edema.
  7. Telangiectasia: A fine, often irregular, red line produced by a dilatation of a normally invisible capillary.

B. *Secondary Lesions:*
  1. Plaques: Usually result from a confluence of papules developing into flat-topped elevated layers, e.g., psoriasis.
  2. Scales: Dry or greasy masses of dead tissue from the horny layer. They may be dry and silvery, as in psoriasis, or greasy and yellow, as in seborrheic dermatitis.
  3. Erosion: Frequently a ruptured bulla or vesicle. A moist demarcated depressed area due to loss of partial or full thickness of epidermis.
  4. Ulcer: Irregularly shaped excavation resulting from necrosis of tissue including complete loss of dermis. Each ulcer has a shape, floor, base, edge or secretion. All ulcers leave a scar when they heal.
  5. Scars: Scars are the result of damage to the dermis.
  6. Lichenification: A dry leathery thickening of the skin with increased skin markings. The thickening of the epidermis is a result of excessive rubbing of the skin in chronic dermatitis.
  7. Fissure: A deep linear split through the epidermis into the dermis.

Nursing Functions in Skin Diseases

The extent of the nursing process depends on the setting. In occupational health, school nursing, community health, doctors' offices and in those settings where nurses assume the triage role, their judgments concerning appropriate actions are very important. In a dermatologist's office, and in the hospital where the more acute and serious conditions are seen, their functions may be somewhat different.

Many skin diseases are chronic, and the knowledgeable concern for and support of patients with these diseases extends over a considerable period of time. In this day of increasing specialization, it is easy to focus on the primary complaint and difficult to maintain a generalized awareness of the total patient in dynamic interaction with his environment.

Assessment. Observation and history are the main tools of assessment. Observation involves education, awareness and practice. Before the nurse can synthesize an educated appraisal of the integumentary system into her assessment, she must observe and describe the skin in patients of different ages and with different conditions.

Observations. (1) *Color of skin:* Skin color depends on skin thickness and on the amount of melanin and keratin present in the epidermis. In disease, it is affected by the amount of edema or fibrosis and by either endogenous or exogenous pigmentary substances. Skin is reddened if thinner, and if there is cutaneous vasodilatation or increased hemoglobin concentration. It may appear white in anemia, cold, shock, edema and myxedema. It may be yellow owing to hepatic dysfunction, high carotene diet, myxedema or chemicals. Skin may be blue owing to increased deoxyhemoglobin, methemoglobin or sulfhemoglobin and gray-brown from silver or hemosiderin.[2]

(2) *Texture and dryness:* Texture of the skin reflects the age and working habits of the individual. Increased thyroid hormone is associated with a fine, warm, moist skin, and insufficiency produces a dry, puffy and coarse skin. The patient may be perspiring. The location should be described. Is the skin chapped, dry, greasy, scaly or wrinkled?

(3) *Observation of nails:* Color of nails, condition—whether soft, hard, ridged, discolored, thickened, bitten—corns and calluses should be noted.

(4) *Hair:* Note color and whether it is thin, dull, lifeless, thick or glossy. Note the distribution of hair.

(5) *Rashes, injuries or lesions:* Most of these areas and characteristics will be swiftly observed by the nurse in her initial history or admission of the patient. The history will give further clues for investigation. If the patient gives a history of skin disorder, the nurse may ask to see the eruption. An accurate description of any skin condition at the initial encounter is helpful in ascertaining progress. A small clear plastic ruler is useful for ascertaining the size of the circumscribed lesion. The description should include the distribution or site of the eruption. Distribution may provide initial clues to diagnosis, since skin diseases occur in characteristic distribution, e.g., involving only the hairy areas of the body, the trunk, the limbs, etc. Common dermatoses have fairly characteristic distribution patterns. The configuration may be described as grouped, single or linear, since lesions or groups of lesions have certain configurations. The character of the lesion itself may then be noted, i.e., macular, papular, vesicular, acute, chronic, weeping, inflamed, etc. The color of the lesion may be helpful. Symptoms (itching, painful, burning) should be elicited.

History. After the description of the current disorder, further history will need to be taken. Has the patient seen a doctor for the condition and how recently? Was the doctor a dermatologist? What did the doctor say the skin condition was, and what should be done? Did it help? If the answer to the last question is no, the nurse then inquires how the patient carried out the doctor's recommendation, and assesses a tentative reason for treatment failure. Of course, some patients who do not follow the prescribed medical regimen get better.

What home remedies or other treatment have been used? Many people have items in the medicine cabinet that were used for other conditions, or have gotten some neighborly or drugstore advice. Patients frequently under- or overtreat skin conditions.

If the diagnosis of the condition is known and the condition is chronic, the nurse needs to ascertain the patient's knowledge about the condition and its management, and how the patient feels about the skin disease and treatment. This question may be answered indirectly by careful attention to verbal tones, monosyllabic answers, changing the subject, avoidance, etc. What do the patient's actions concerning his treatment imply? Does the patient have any other serious systemic diseases? What tensions are there at home and work? Are there financial problems?

It is probably best to elicit the history by following the patient's leads, and then later comparing information obtained with a systematic guide (see suggested form) to see if all necessary information has been obtained, especially at the outset when the interviewer wishes to establish a good rapport. Listening carefully to the patient and following tangential leads may give more relevant information than a systematic interview with the nurse's eye on the blank spaces on the form rather than on the patient.

DERMATOLOGIC ASSESSMENT HISTORY

Name:

Presenting complaint (Use patient's words):

How does it bother you? (Elicit symptoms and their duration. Use questions such as: When did it start? Does it come and go? Is it wet or dry? Does it itch? Did it spread?)

What have you done for it? (Has the patient seen a doctor? What kind? What did the doctor say the condition was, and what was prescribed? Did it help? If it did not, what did the patient do? How did he carry out the doctor's recommendations? What did he understand about them? What drugstore or home remedies were used and with what effect? If he has not seen a doctor, what are the reasons?)

Observation of the lesion (Describe distribution, character and configuration):

General history:

Tensions (Clues may be elicited from the following questions): How do you sleep? Eat? What is your job and how has it been going? Who is in your family? How are they? What do you do when you aren't working?

General: Do you or your family have any serious systemic diseases? Record general observations concerning skin, hair, nails, etc.

The nurse always needs to include in the history of women a question about breast examination, and to urge its importance.

Patient Participation in Care. Following assessment, an important function of the nurse is to obtain the participation of the patient as an equal in planning his care. Granted, the nurse and doctor both bring special competencies to the situation; however, the patient should exercise decision-making and responsibility for his own care. This means education of the patient concerning his condition and treatment. More patients can learn to monitor their own symptoms and treatment by learning what causes exacerbations or improvement. Many skin diseases are chronic and, if the patient is hospitalized, it is probably owing to management failure.

Education of the Patient. Education of the patient requires that the nurse assume the role of learner, since every patient has much to teach the nurse. With maximum patient input, the nurse can gauge more astutely the particular area of need, and flexibly individualize her nursing functions. Patients need to know the rationale for treatments and their role in making them effective. Striking the proper balance of treatment is the art of medical care, since overtreatment and undertreatment are common problems.

Realism is always the best policy in dealing with the patient. Giving the patient all the information she can provide about the disease helps him to eliminate misconceptions. The patient may need to know what the disease is not, as well as what it is. He needs meticulous directions about his care. Discouragement is easy and reinforcement to persist with treatment is necessary as the patient may wish to change treatment every few days.

The nurse may assume the role of patient advocate, arbitrator, and intermediary for the inarticulate. Patients hesitate to reveal their ignorance or worries, for fear of being considered stupid, inadequate, or complaining. On the other hand, advocacy does not mean taking over for the patient, but encouraging and supporting the patient to speak for himself.

Psychologic Needs of the Patient. Awareness of the psychologic needs of the patient is particularly important in disorders of the skin, given the value of a smooth unblemished skin in our society. While the patient may be complaining or silent, the nurse needs to maintain an open mind about the meaning of the patient's behavior. Behavior is meaningful, but inferences must be confirmed with the patient and supported by recorded observation. If patients fail to follow through with treatments, there is a reason or reasons, and these may be tangential to the immediate skin disorder. Many skin diseases are aggravated by psychologic factors, and some decision must be made as to the importance of these factors to the skin condition, and the possibility of change. Again change is the prerogative of the patient, when he becomes aware of the possible contributing factors. Patience in dealing with slow progress and discouragement with a chronic condition are difficult patient problems.

Serious skin diseases can pose severe psychologic handicaps. The individual who focuses his attention excessively upon his chronic skin problem has less energy and desire to invest in relations with other people. An accepting sympathetic attitude on the part of the nurse and doctor is important in assisting this patient with social contacts.

Self-inflicted injuries to the skin, compulsive excoriations and delusions of parasitosis (acarophobia) are conditions that generally need psychiatric care. Other conditions such as pruritus vulvae may have a large functional component.

Special Nursing Care Problems. PRURITUS. Pruritus is defined as an *unpleasant* cutaneous sensation which produces the desire to scratch. Itching is a common complaint of individuals with skin disease.

Stimulation of the nerve endings is brought about by chemical, thermal, mechanical and electrical stimuli, both internal and external. Even after the initial itching stimuli have subsided, the area seems to remain in a state of increased excitability and vicious cycles of increasingly violent itching and scratching may develop. The nerve endings mediating the itching sensation are made more sensitive by increased capillary dilatation. Heat thus increases the symptoms, while cold and vasoconstriction decrease it. Corticotropin and adrenal corticoids have a dramatic effect because of their anti-inflammatory action.

Tissue anoxia due to venous stasis results in itching and is relieved when blood flow becomes adequate. The perception of itching may be elicited not only by peripheral mechanisms but centrally. The perception of itching has an integrating center in the hypothalamus and the excitability of this center can be influenced by drugs. Thomas Lewis and his associates advanced the theory that itching is due to the release of histamines or a histamine-like substance, whatever the stimulus may be. Rothman and Shapiro are of the opinion that this applies only to allergic and anaphylactic reactions.[10]

Presence or absence of the symptom of itching is of considerable value in the diagnosis of certain diseases. There are many skin manifestations of cutaneous syphilis, tuberculosis and leprosy that do not evoke itching. Nevi and benign and malignant neoplasms of the skin can be ruled out when itching is present. Itching may be established when scratch marks are present, but patients' statements are not necessarily reliable. Like the absence of sleep, the presence of itching tends to be exaggerated. A patient may complain of itching associated with a rough area or an elevated lesion, where rubbing or handling may set up an itching cycle.

One must ask the patient if he is disturbed in his sleep by itching and wakes up at night and finds himself scratching. Can the patient forget his itching in the daytime when his attention is distracted? Can he stop scratching easily when he makes up his mind to do so? Does itching arise only in certain situations, such as warm environment, cold weather, etc.? Itching may be classified as "obligate itching" only if it disturbs the patient's sleep.

CLASSIFICATION OF OBLIGATE, FACULTATIVE AND NONITCHING DISORDERS*

A. *Obligate Itching Disorders:*
   1. Pediculosis, scabies and related mite infestations, insect bites and other external injuries resulting in urticarial wheals

*From Rothman, S., and Shapiro, A. L.: Itching (pruritus). *In* MacBryde, C. M. (ed.): *Signs and Symptoms.* 4th ed. Philadelphia, J. B. Lippincott Company, 1964, pp. 900–921.

2. Contact dermatitis (both primarily toxic and allergic) caused by exposure to chemical or physical agents
3. Urticaria and toxic eruptions
4. Neurodermatitis, prurigo, strophulus (miliaria)
5. Pruritus due to pregnancy, liver diseases, lymphoblastoma, malignant internal neoplasms, kidney insufficiency
6. Dermatitis herpetiformis
7. Lichen planus

B. *Facultative Itching Disorders* (with great variety in intensity, largely depending upon the degree of inflammation):
1. Asteatosis (xerosis, dry skin)
2. Pruritus due to diabetes
3. Psoriasis
4. Seborrheic dermatitis
5. Pityriasis rosea
6. Skin infections due to pyogenic organisms and fungi
7. Local anoxia due to varicose veins, tight clothing, etc.
8. Mechanical irritation

C. *Nonitching Disorders:*
1. Developmental anomalies
2. Atrophies, degenerations and hyperplasias
3. Benign neoplasms
4. Malignant neoplasms
5. Dermotropic virus infections
6. Chronic infectious granulomas (tuberculosis, syphilis, etc.)
7. Lupus erythematodes
8. Pigmentary anomalies
9. Trophic and deficiency diseases
10. Diseases of sweat glands, sebaceous glands, hair follicles and nails

Of importance for the nurse to remember are the following:

1. There is a marked variation from individual to individual in response to the itch stimulus, as there is to the pain stimulus (see Unit IX).

2. Some skin diseases produce itching and others do not.

3. Itching is worse at night.

4. Areas most frequently affected by itching are around body openings. Pruritus ani, pruritus vulvae and otitis externa are the most common.

5. The epidermis becomes dry and brittle with age. The majority of cases of dermatitis in the aged are due to irritants superimposed on dry, already itchy skin. Aged skin dehydrates and chaps more readily than younger skin; the alkalinizing effects of soap aggravate this condition.

General nursing activities to relieve itching fall into the areas of temperature control, diversionary activities, alleviation of anxiety and stress, and carrying out the treatment regimen. Observation of when the patient scratches, how long and the way he scratches may be helpful in setting up some kind of a plan with the patient to reduce trauma from itching. Obviously the patient should have his nails cut short, and could use a soft brush for stroking, or gentle firm pressure on the itching area if this relieves it. The itching is rarely alleviated except when the patient traumatizes his skin. The itching cycle is activated, and the more he scratches, the more he itches, unless pain intervenes.

Baths of various kinds may relieve the itching:

> Two tablespoons of liquor carbonis detergens, Zetar, Alma-Tar, Balnetar or Dometar may be added to a tub of water. Tar baths are used chiefly in the treatment of psoriasis.

> Potassium permanganate bath solution 1:10,000 may be used in infected weeping dermatoses. However, it stains the skin, so it is infrequently used as a general measure.

> Dial or pHisoHex baths may be used for pyodermas.

> Oil baths are often helpful if the skin is dry. These can be prepared by adding ½ to 1 oz. of Lubath, Alpha-Keri, Geri bath or Nivea oil to the tub. Eczematous skin may be relieved by mixing ½ cup oilated Aveeno with a bath oil. Mineral oil, olive oil or peanut oil will also work. One must be careful that the patient is not allergic to any of these mixtures. Bath water should be at body temperature and the patient should not stay in the tub too long. With oil and colloidal baths, one must be extremely careful that the patient does not slip.

> Cornstarch baths may be used—½ to 1 lb. of starch to a pot of very hot water. This makes a gel which is then put into a tub of water in which the patient immerses himself for about 15 minutes. The bath should be body temperature.

> Oatmeal bath: Put old-fashioned cereal in a cloth bag and cook it in boiling water for a half hour. Put cooking water and bag in tub of water. Squeezing the bag presses out soothing gelatinous starches. The commercial preparation Aveeno oatmeal (½ to 1 cup to a tub of water) is much easier to use.

> Soyaloid is a preparation made from soybeans and is used for soothing baths. Aveeno and Soyaloid can be used to both soothe and clean.

Baths have the advantage of not cooling the patient as much as extensive wet dressings. However, they are often not used because of the amount of time required for supervision. Antipruritic lotions, creams or ointments may be applied after the bath.

Antipruritic lotions are:

> Quotane lotion contains menthol and quotane, a relatively nonsensitizing topical anesthetic.

> Cetaphil lotion, 0.125 to 0.5 per cent menthol, may be added for antipruritic effect.

> Hydrocortisone lotion: Hydrocortisone in 0.125 to 0.5 per cent concentration may be added to lotions for its anti-inflammatory effect.

> Phenol: 0.5 to 1 per cent can be added to calamine lotion or calamine liniment, Schamberg's lotion or Wises' lotion.

Shake lotions are aqueous suspensions of powdered solids which, on evaporation of water, leave a thick deposit of powder on the surface of the skin. These are applied to vesicular or slightly exudative surfaces, and may be applied with a soft paintbrush or the bare hand. An *emulsion,* which is a shake lotion containing oil, is less drying and has less tendency to cake on the surface.

Ointments and *creams* are in water-washable ointment bases or are not freely water-washable. Some examples of water-base ointment bases are Unibase, Acid Mantle, Cetaphil and Neobase. Examples of water in oil bases are yellow and white petrolatum, lanolin, cold cream, Nivea Cream, Aquaphor and Eucerin. Phenol, 0.5 to 1 per cent, or menthol, 0.125 to 1 per cent, may be added to almost any base. Boric acid ointment (2.6 to 5 per cent) is mildly bacteriostatic and fungistatic. Its use over extensive areas is contraindicated because of the danger of possible absorption and renal damage.

Hydrocortisone and related preparations are effective and safe anti-inflammatory agents for use on the skin, and do relieve pruritus.

Cool *wet compresses* may be used for localized itching. If the area becomes dry from the compresses, a teaspoonful of Alpha-Keri or other oil may be added to the compress fluid. Acute eczematous eruptions are frequently treated with *wet compresses* for their soothing and anti-inflammatory effects. These are often helpful in cleansing the skin as well as in getting rid of old crusts. Solutions used could be normal saline, Burow's solution (aluminum acetate) diluted 1:10 or 1:20, or milk of magnesia diluted equally with water. These should be applied to light coverings of gauze (four to eight layers) at body temperature, and are not to be covered with other materials to prevent maceration. A schedule is useful, i.e., compresses should be applied for a half hour, and removed for a half hour the first day or two. As the acute eruptions subside, the intervals can be decreased to several times a day. Handy packets of Burow's solution available commercially are Bluboro and Domeboro, each diluted in 8 to 16 oz. of water.

Soaks of mild antiseptic solutions may be used for acute or weeping conditions or infections in the extremities for 15 minutes or so several times a day. Soaks may be used for acute athlete's foot. Between soaks, drying lotions (suspensions of inert powders in water) are helpful in drying weeping eruptions as well as being soothing and antipruritic.

Individuals with dry skin should avoid hot soapy baths, and the oil film on the skin can be replaced with such preparations as Nivea cream, Lubriderm, Eucerin, etc.

Nursing activities planned to relieve anxiety and reduce stress are highly important in a patient with skin disease, since the doctor may be reluctant to prescribe medications in many patients with serious skin problems. Seeing that the room is cool with the proper amount of humidity, that the patient has sufficient covering, but not too much, is important. It is necessary to find out his usual sleep pattern, and to see that this is provided. TV or reading material at bedtime may assist him in falling asleep. He may be in the habit of having a light snack. If he wishes to talk, the nurse may be able to help the patient work out some stress situation. In all situations, observation as to when scratching occurs or is aggravated is essential.

DISFIGUREMENT. The patient with a chronic noticeable skin disease may be acutely sensitive and may wish to isolate himself. In the hospital, it is advisable to inform roommates, if any, that the disease is not contagious. It may be of assistance to have the "right kind" of roommate. For example, one with hordes of staring visitors would not be acceptable. The nurse needs to be keenly aware of the effect of a roommate on a patient with skin disease. Mutual temperature requirements need to be ascertained. If the patient with a skin disorder is getting cool compresses, he needs a warm room. If he has severe itching, he needs a cool room. Patients can be therapeutic for each other, and this needs to be carefully considered.

If the patient has severe problems of disfigurement, the nurse needs to be aware of the patient's tendency to isolate himself and avoid others. The nurse thus needs to prepare and provide adequate staffing. Planned friendly interaction cannot be taken for granted, as staff may provide only essential services. If the patient has the expectation of being rejected, he may behave in a way that causes this to take place. Such patients are acutely sensitive to expressions and comments about other patients. It is as important to provide a therapeutic milieu for this type of patient as any other, and the patient may need an interactive group or referral to the psychiatric consultant or social worker for assistance. Certainly he is going to be stared at, and has to learn to deal with this problem.

Opaque coverings may be used to cover some areas of disfigurement. Ths opaque coverings, Covermark and Spotstik, are manufactured by Lydia O'Leary. Use of these products should be checked with the physician.

The nurse, faced with the problem of assisting a patient with a visible disability, has to help him realize the existence of other values. Devaluations due to damaged appearance will be lessened to the extent that the person feels surface appearance to be less important than other factors such as kindness, wisdom, effort and cooperativeness. Individuals should be encouraged to think of their remaining assets and values rather than using a comparative frame of reference.

Important areas to be remembered in the care of skin disease are the following:

1. The importance of seeking early referral to a dermatologist in order to get started on a good management program if the disease is chronic or if the condition does not improve under minor simple treatment.

2. The individual with a skin condition needs careful directions and reinforcement concerning the importance of using the recommended treatment as directed, and promptly returning or reporting to the nurse or doctor if the expected progress does not ensue. It is a good idea to have the patient repeat to you exactly how she is going to manage the treatment to be sure the directions are understood, and to caution the patient about trying anything else. It is also necessary to find out exactly whether the patient will have all the neces-

sary ingredients for carrying out the treatment. The nurse must spend enough time to help the patient with any emotional feelings connected with the treatment. Demonstration is always desirable.

3. Serious skin diseases are frequently chronic problems, and principles of chronic disease management apply to these diseases as well. The management has to be integrated into the total life pattern, and the patient has to find his unique and best way of managing his disability. The nurse can help the patient by her awareness of the totality of the situation.

4. Nurses are in an especially favorable position to teach the importance of good skin care and the management of any break in prevention of disease.

DISEASES OF THE APPENDAGES

Common disorders of the nails, hair, scalp and several glands are presented here.

Diseases of the Nails

Paronychia. This is an inflammation of the tissue surrounding the nail plate. Acute paronychia (whitlow) is a rapidly developing, painful red swelling around the nail. Acute infection usually follows an injury or a "hangnail." It may spread around the nail and, if neglected, a cellulitis or lymphangitis may develop. Approximately half the cases are due to monilia (*Candida albicans*). Chronic paronychia is frequently found in middle-aged women who have their hands continually in water. It is approximately three times as common in patients with diabetes as in the general population.

If neglected the lesion may have to be incised surgically and the patient given antibiotics and warm wet packs. The most important point in preventing recurrence is to keep the area scrupulously dry. Squeezing the affected area aggravates the condition.

The nurse should urge attention to any injury around the nail to prevent infection, and stress the importance of gentleness in manicuring. If a hangnail is not infected, the filament may be flattened and secured with flexible collodion. If an infection occurs or a person is prone to chronic paronychia, a finger cot or gloves should be used to keep hands dry.

Ingrown Toenails (Unguis Incarnatus). This is a penetration of the edges of the nail plate into the surrounding tissues, resulting in a painful inflammation and infection. Ingrown toenails usually have two etiologic factors, a special familial configuration of the nail and use of tight ill-fitting shoes. Obesity, flat feet and short nails favor development.

Progress can be arrested by raising the toenail from its bed by means of a small pledget of cotton under the free edge of the nail, thus relieving pressure on the lateral edge. The nail should be trimmed to allow the lateral part to grow forward. The elderly have difficulty in reaching their toes, in seeing them and in handling the trimming instruments. Therefore, a nurse with special training or a podiatrist should trim the toenails if there is any problem. Nursing observation of predisposing factors and education of the patient concerning prevention are desirable.

Hypertrophy of the Nails (Onychaxis). This is usually associated with change in shape, color and texture of the nail. The hypertrophy is in all directions and is more frequent on the toes. The affected nail may be thickened, raised, elongated or green or black in color. In some cases, the nail tissue becomes like the horn of an animal. The subungual space and nail bed are often filled with a horny accumulation. This hypertrophy is frequently observed in elderly individuals with such conditions as peripheral neuritis, heart disease, hemiplegia or other chronic diseases. Patients with hypertrophied nails should be examined by a physician if this has not been done. Surgical removal of the hypertrophied nails with an electric drill and hand clippers is local treatment and has to be repeated at intervals. This is best done by a podiatrist. A massage with warm olive oil induces some improvement in patients with hypertrophied nails. Nurses can teach patient about care of the feet, urging physical examination and referral to a podiatrist.

Brittleness of the Nails. This is a common disorder of the nails, in which they are soft and split. The exact etiology is not known. Individuals are commonly concerned about this and wish to know what to do about it. Evidence is somewhat controversial, but one dermatologist recommends 7 gm. daily of gelatine for about 15 weeks as a result of a controlled experimental trial.[5]

Clubbing. This is a secondary condition that may be observed in patients with chronic cardiac and pulmonary conditions. The nails, as well as the ends of the fingers and toes, are enlarged. The nails appear lustrous, are curved in shape and hard and thickened, but without change in color. Local hypoxia is thought to produce the change.

The effects of other skin diseases on the nails are discussed under specific diseases.

Diseases of the Hair and Scalp

Seborrheic Dermatitis. Seborrheic dermatitis is a common, chronic, recurrent condition frequently associated with an oily skin and scalp. It is often seen in patients with acne vulgaris and rosacea. Tension and diet may be associated with flareups, although the cause of this disorder is not known. The lesions are greasy, scaly red patches affecting the scalp, the eyebrows, the nasolabial and postauricular areas, the chest and skin folds. The lesions may become secondarily infected and show eczematous changes.

For mild cases, shampooing with a detergent shampoo several times weekly and application of scalp lotion for slight scaling are recommended. With heavier scaling, an ointment or steroid lotions and creams may be applied. Mild bland baths daily for 15 minutes may be helpful in widespread eruptions. All external irritants, excess heat and excess perspiration will aggravate the disorder. Rubbing and scratching also aggravate the condition and may produce infection. If a patient has oily skin or hair, urge frequent shampooing and reassure the patient that his condition can be controlled with care. The patient should be cautioned about overtreatment.

Rosacea. This is a chronic disorder which usually occurs in middle age or later. It tends to localize in the middle third of the face (the flush area). In mild cases there is vasodilatation of the capillaries of the cheek and nose but, in more severe cases, papules and pustules may appear as well. The condition can be quite disfiguring and, when there is a gross hyperplasia of the sebaceous glands of the nose, the person may be unfairly accused of being a "rumpot." The condition affects females in the fourth and fifth decades who have a labile vasomotor system. Enlargement of the nose is seen more often in males. Treatment is directed toward avoiding anything that contributes to facial hyperemia, such as alcohol, hot foods or excessive sun exposure. Hair should be shampooed frequently to reduce oiliness. Topical medications may be prescribed or antibiotics may be given if there is pustule formation. Cosmetic surgery may be of benefit if there is a nose problem. Since the disease may be somewhat embarrassing and disfiguring, the nurse needs to encourage the patient to express his feelings and concerns and to obtain and continue treatment. Cosmetic surgery may be encouraged if the patient is very concerned about his nose.

Acne Vulgaris. *Consultations for acne are more frequent than for any other skin disease.* Acne is a disease of the sebaceous glands that affects adolescents and young adults. It may be divided into noninflammatory and inflammatory types. Noninflammatory acne is characterized by open and closed whiteheads and blackheads (comedones), consisting of compact masses of keratin, sebum and bacteria dilating the follicular duct. In inflammatory acne, the skin is inflamed and there are papules, pustules and nodulocystic lesions with a tendency for destructiveness and scarring (Fig. 91–4). The lesions are found in areas of greatest concentration of the sebaceous glands—the face, neck and upper trunk.

CAUSAL FACTORS. Three factors are thought to contribute to acne: (1) hormonal stimulation; (2) obstruction of sebum flow onto the skin surface; and (3) possibly, the presence of *Cornynebacterium acnes*. Severe cystic acne is thought to have a familial tendency. Sebaceous glands are very sensitive to androgenic stimulation, and females, even with relatively low levels of androgens, have as much trouble with acne as males. Inflammation around comedones, because of leakage of some irritating components of sebum, is believed to initiate the other lesions of acne. From the clinical point of view, the most important type of comedo is the closed comedo or "whitehead." They are the main precursors for highly inflamed nodular lesions. Careful attention should be directed to expressing their contents. The whiteheads can be felt by running the finger over them and, since each opening is small, it has to be enlarged with a sharp pointed scalpel blade before the comedo extractor is applied.[15]

TREATMENT. Many types of treatment have been employed. Estrogens decrease sebum production and offset androgenic stimulatory effect. All authorities are not agreed on its value. Topical preparations to promote desquamation and peeling of the superficial cell layers of the stratum corneum and improve the flow of sebum onto the skin surface are universally advised. The first step is thorough cleansing of the skin several times a day. A mild sunburn or ultraviolet light to produce a mild erythema may be used. Patients generally improve in the summer. One authority recommends tetracycline to decrease the number of acnes on the skin. Blackheads can be extracted with a comedo extractor, and whiteheads picked with a Bard-Parker knife and extracted. Although there is wide public belief in the value of diet control, most doctors believe that no special dietary restrictions are necessary, although the individual should be encouraged to eat an adequate and well balanced diet.

NURSING IMPLICATIONS. Young people should be taught in late preadolescent years about the natural course and care of acne. The school and office nurse may be in a particularly strategic position to assist in the management and prevention of severe acne. Frequent washing of oily hair and skin is desirable, as is a hairdo in which the hair is not touching the face. Parents may be taught the use of the comedo extractor, extracting only those blackheads that come out easily, and doing 10 or so at one sitting. Squeezing, rubbing and picking should be discouraged. The patient should be encouraged to eat a well balanced diet, avoid undue stress, fatigue and perspiration, and get out into the sunlight.

Because an ultraviolet light may be prescribed for home use, the patient's understanding of the use of the ultraviolet lamp should be reviewed. Does he always wear dark glasses? Does he always have someone else time the exposure, in case the timing mechanism does not work or he falls asleep? Does he measure the distance from the lamp with a yardstick so he is always the same distance. The amount of ultraviolet light recommended is the amount that will produce a mild erythema in 24 hours.

The nurse may need to give psychologic support to young people with acne, since they are particularly sensitive about their body image at this time. Acne may disturb relationships with the adolescent's peer group and undermine his self-confidence by irrational fears of its association with such problems as masturbation and sexual development. The adolescent may use acne as an excuse to avoid anxiety-arousing social relationships. A sympathetic and understanding relationship with a doctor or nurse can help the vulnerable young person through this difficult time.

Alopecia Areata. This refers to the idiopathic, usually rapid loss of one or more multiple patches of hair from any part of the scalp. This may take place within 24 hours. The etiology is obscure, though some emphasis is directed toward psychogenic relationships. Postpartum loss of hair by diffuse thinning occurs two to four months after delivery but, as a rule, the hair is completely restored after six months. The duration of alopecia areata is unpredictable. The duration of the initial attack may last up to six months for one third, and up to one year for half, of the population.

Psychologic support and a bland topical placebo preparation may be used. Use of hairpieces should be considered. The patient should be allowed to express fears concerning his condition. Attempt to

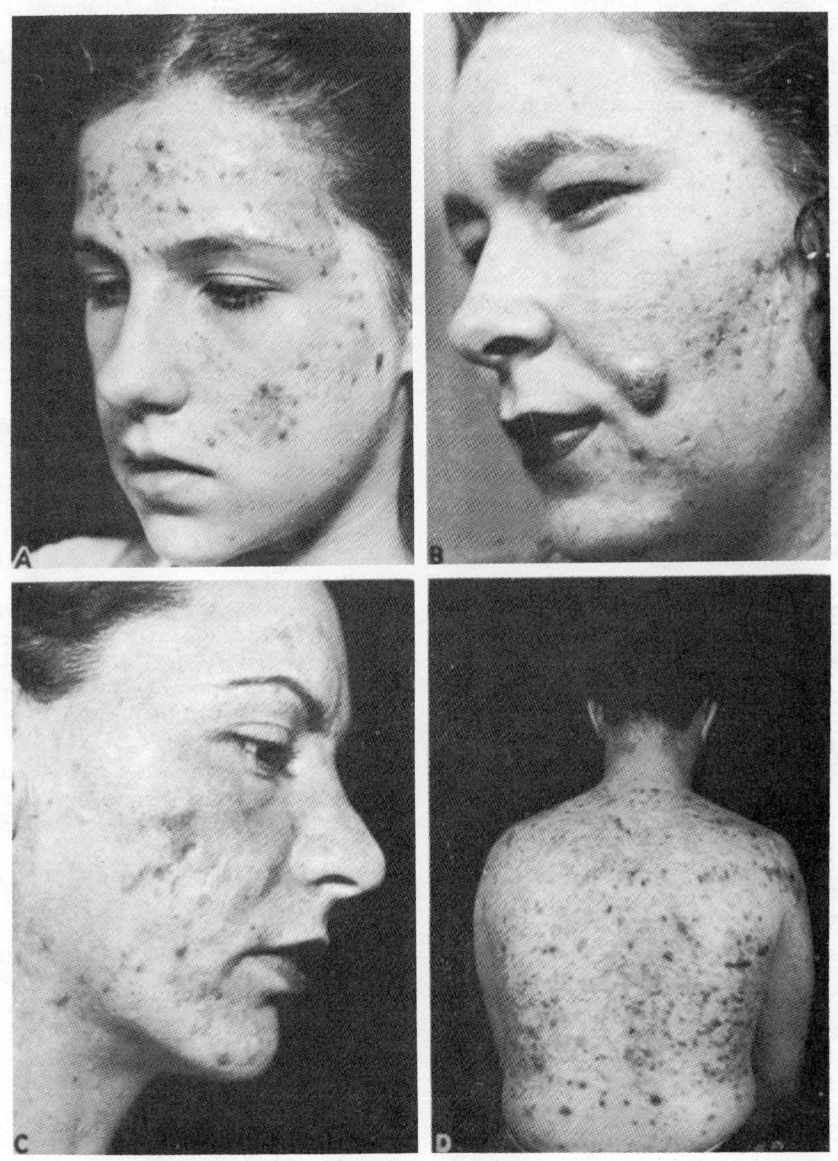

FIGURE 91–4. Acne vulgaris. *A*, Moderately severe, with comedones, papules, and pustules. *B*, The formation of cysts is a complication. *C*, Permanent scars may be sequelae if acne is neglected. *D*, Extensive distribution of cysts, pustules, and scars. (From Lewis, G. M., and Wheeler, C. E., Jr.: *Practical Dermatology.* 3rd ed. 1967.)

resolve any underlying problem by referral if necessary.

Hirsutism (Hypertrichosis). Essential hirsutism is usually due to heredity rather than disease. Hormonal imbalance should be considered in all but the mildest cases. This condition is marked by an increase in the amount of coarseness or darkness of body or facial hair. It causes greatest worry when the hair is on the face.

Normal menstrual history is important in ruling out endocrine hirsutism. Treatment involves dealing with any endocrine disorders. Electrolysis will permanently remove hair. Some hair may be removed merely by shaving, bleaching or depilating. However, such hair removal is not permanent.

Changes in hair are evident in aging, and scalp hair is lost with increasing maturity in both sexes. Axillary, pubic and eyebrow hair also change, generally decreasing. Hormonal changes are more important in the study of hair distribution than aging as such. All areas that are hairy in men may become hairy in women under pathologic conditions.

Diseases of the Sweat Glands

Hyperhidrosis (Excessive Perspiration). An abnormal increase in perspiration is seen most frequently during stress situations in predisposed individuals. Most frequently affected are the axillae, palms, soles and face, and it most frequently occurs in adolescents and young adults. Other signs may point to a labile sympathetic nervous system, such as tachycardia, vasomotor instability and cold, clammy hands.

Treatment includes soaking the feet in 1:1000 solution of potassium permanganate 20 minutes daily. Antiperspiration powders are used several times daily, as well as antiperspirants. Successful use of a 10 per cent solution of glutaraldehyde, a tanning agent, has been reported.

Patients are embarrassed by this condition and may withdraw from physical contact and be less socially active. The nurse needs to assist the patient in coping with this condition and in not withdrawing from social contact. The patient may wear cotton underwear and socks and change these daily.

Sebaceous Cysts. These are round, smooth, globular, cutaneous or subcutaneous tumors arising from the sebaceous glands and are found on the face, neck, scalp, back and genitalia. They are caused by occlusion of a sebaceous gland or cystic dilatation of a sebaceous gland. Treatment is excision to include the epithelial wall; otherwise the cyst will probably re-form.

Epidermoid Cyst (Wen). This is difficult to distinguish from a sebaceous cyst, but it is a nevoid structure with an epidermal lining. Treatment is the same. It appears to be an inherited disorder, transmitted as an incomplete dominant trait.

DISEASES DUE TO PARASITES AND INSECTS

The nurse in any setting may have frequent occasions to see patients with insect bites or parasitic infections. *The second most common source of referrals to the school nurse after upper respiratory infections is skin disease.* Vagabonds and individuals who have had to live in communal facilities without clean clothing and washing facilities may suffer from parasitic disease, such as scabies and pediculi. The incidence of these conditions has increased in recent years among young people in communes and other informal living arrangements.

Scabies. Scabies is an infection caused by a crab-shaped mite whose penetrations into the skin are visible as papules and vesicles, housing males and nymphs, or as tiny linear burrows, containing females and their eggs. The condition causes severe itching, especially at night. The itching is at first intermittent, then continuous, and may persist for days after treatment. The lesions appear between the fingers, in the flexures of the wrist and anterior axillary folds, on the penis and the buttocks, and around the waist, lower abdomen and areolae of the nipples (Fig. 91–5). The skin above the neckline is rarely affected, because the mite avoids the cold. Transmission is by direct contact and, to a limited extent, from soiled sheets and undergarments.

TREATMENT. The most satisfactory treatment is to take a hot bath and apply 25 per cent benzyl benzoate emulsion over the entire skin and leave it on for 48 hours and then wash it off. After two days with no treatment, the procedure is repeated. A soothing lotion such as calamine may be applied for the pruritus. It is important not to overtreat. Individuals are likely to be uncomfortable for some weeks; they should not take this as an indication that the disease is still active. All potential cases in the family should be treated at the same time.

NURSING IMPLICATIONS. School nurses need to remember that some people may consider scabies a stigma, and may need to be reassured that it is *easy* to get and can easily be eliminated.

Pediculosis. Pediculosis means infestation by lice. There are three types: (1) pediculosis capitis (head louse); (2) pediculosis corporis (body louse); and (3) phthirus pubis (pubic louse).

Lice are oval and gray, about 2 to 4 mm. long, and wingless with six legs. Pubic lice are the smallest and body lice the largest. The female lays several eggs called "nits," each one being glued to hair. A larva is hatched in 6 to 10 days and becomes a fully grown louse in one or two weeks. Lice live on blood which they suck from the skin.

PEDICULOSIS CAPITIS. Examination of the hair will disclose the nits. They are firmly fastened to the hair and cannot be removed with the fingers but can, with difficulty, be removed with the nails or a fine comb. Since the louse attaches the nit near the scalp, the duration of the infestation may be gauged by how far the nit is from the scalp.

Two per cent DDT emulsion is rubbed into the hair or 10 per cent dusting powder shaken into it, being careful to keep it out of the eyes. The emulsion is left on the head overnight and washed off the next day. The hair need not be cut. All individuals in a family or friendship group should be examined, especially if they share hats, combs or beds.

PEDICULOSIS CORPORIS. The louse lives in clothes and only leaves them to have a meal off the skin. Scratch marks that are secondarily infected and pruritus may be the only signs. Pediculosis corporis is generally associated with unhygienic living conditions, and is frequently found in the lower strata of society. It is sometimes called "vagabond's disease."

Treatment consists of sterilization of the clothing by laundering and pressing with a hot iron. Dusting the seams of the clothing with 10 per cent DDT powder or 10 per cent lindane powder may be useful. Unless these actions are taken, the condition will return.

PEDICULOSIS PUBIS. Transmission is generally by close personal contact, usually sexual inter-

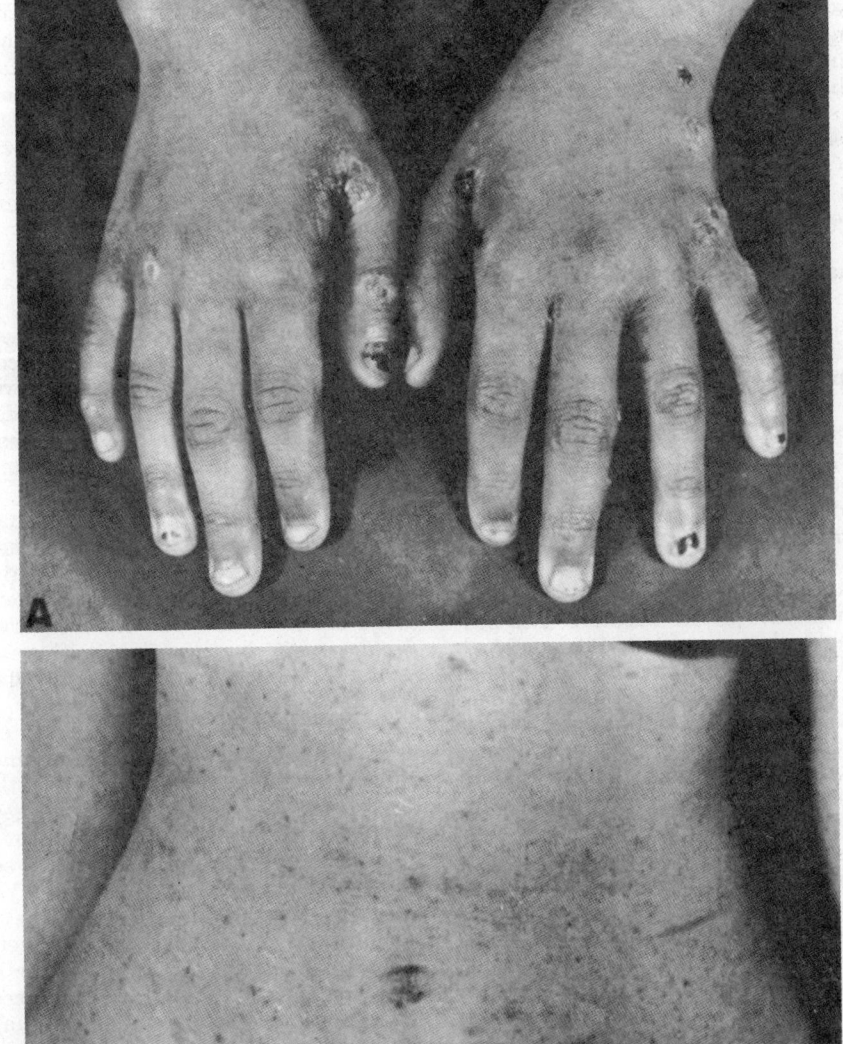

FIGURE 91–5. Scabies. *A.* Interdigital burrows and excoriations, with some secondary pyoderma. *B,* Excoriations over abdomen and lesions in the umbilicus. (From Lewis, G. M., and Wheeler, C. R., Jr.: *Practical Dermatology.* 3rd ed. 1967.)

course. It should be looked for in cases of pruritus ani and vulvae. There may be reddish brown dust on the underclothing from the excreta of the insects. Dusky gray macules 1 to 3 cm. in diameter may be observed on the thighs, trunk and axillae, as a result of the insect's saliva.

Treatment consists of 2 per cent DDT cream or 25 per cent benzyl benzoate emulsion or Kwell on two successive days.

Nursing implications. School nurses should have witnesses to identify lice, since an occasional parent becomes highly indignant. The nurse needs to be aware that any person who has been living in unsanitary conditions may be infested with lice. Teaching the individual how to clean his clothing and surroundings, as well as the importance of getting contacts examined and treated, is the usual role of the nurse.

Nurses are frequently queried concerning the bites or stings of insects; bedbugs, fleas, spiders, mosquitoes, bees, wasps and chiggers are common problems.

Fleas. Humans are attacked by dog and cat fleas only when the customary host is absent. Many people are relatively immune or become so. The legs are chiefly attacked. The bite produces a hemorrhagic spot surrounded by an itchy wheal. It is necessary to get rid of the fleas by spraying with 5 to 10 per cent DDT; carpets, upholstered furniture, sleeping places of pets and the pets themselves should be treated. A lotion for itching may be applied to the legs several times a day.

Bedbugs. The bedbug (*Cimex lectularius*) lives in cracks and crevices in the room and usually comes out at night to acquire food. The bugs may be picked up in motion picture theaters. The bedbug has a disagreeable strong odor if squashed. Bites are usually found in the morning, grouped in twos or threes around the buttocks or ankles. There is a wheal with a central punctum. Local antipruritic treatment may be given and the environment should be rid of bedbugs. Since DDT resistant bedbugs have been reported, it may be necessary to get a professional fumigator.

Chiggers. Several species of reddish mites are found throughout the world. They are common in the southern United States but extend at least to the Canadian border. They are found on grass and bushes. The mite attaches itself to the legs or thighs and punctures the skin to obtain blood. Dermatitis consists of papules with surrounding urticaria, excoriations and subsequent pustules. There may be marked erythema and itching. The mite leaves the skin of its own accord, so treatment is directed toward relief of itching. Insect repellent on wrists and ankles may help in prevention.

Spiders. The most significant poisonous spiders in the United States are the brown fiddleback (recluse) spider and the black widow. The bite is often unobserved and only discovered with the onset of swelling, pain and redness. Onset of acute symptoms depends on the location of the bite and the amount of venom. Dizziness, weakness, sweating, abdominal pain and cramps, and muscle cramps may occur. The bites of either of these spiders may produce local necrosis at the site of bite, more severe necrosis being produced with the bite of the brown recluse.

TREATMENT. Antivenin is given parenterally for neutralization of the toxin of the black widow. Adrenocorticosteroids and 10 per cent calcium gluconate are given for muscle spasm and hypotension. Prompt administration of corticosteroids is indicated for the brown recluse bite.

PREVENTION. Care is indicated in working with old lumber, and in unused sheds and places where such spiders reside. Wearing of heavy gloves and protective clothing is advised. Individuals suspected of having a poisonous spider bite should seek immediate medical attention. These poisonous spiders avoid light and bite only in defense. The black widow is recognized by a black or orange marking on the underside. The brown recluse is small, light to dark brown with a light fiddle-shaped mark on its head. The black widow is found universally throughout the United States and southern Canada, and the brown recluse primarily east of the Rockies.

Mosquitoes. The mosquito bite produces a small erythematous wheal-like papule with or without a visible central punctum. The bites are generally on the exposed areas of the skin. Itching is relieved by topical adrenocorticosteroid ointments every one to two hours, to which 0.25 per cent menthol and phenol has been added.

PREVENTION. Mosquitoes are less attracted to individuals in light clothing. Commercial insect repellents are helpful for a short time but are diluted by perspiration, so they have to be reapplied every one to two hours. Preparations should contain 20 per cent of the chemical N,N-diethylmetatoluamide.[14] Two commonly effective preparations are Deet and Off. Children should not have smallpox vaccinations during the season of mosquitoes, as bites may become inoculated with the vaccine.

Bee and Wasp Stings. The bee or wasp sting produces pain, local inflammation and edema. Ordinary treatment is to remove the stinger if stung by a honey bee. Generally, bumblebees and wasps do not leave the stinger. Bee poison is acid, and ammonia and sodium bicarbonate should be applied after extraction of the stinger. Wasp poison is alkaline or neutral and should be treated with lemon juice or vinegar and cool wet compresses. An individual who is allergic to the sting may go into anaphylactic shock, and may need to be given intramuscular epinephrine (see Chapter 25). Individuals known to be allergic to bee stings need to have an emergency kit available and someone able to administer emergency treatment when they are around bees. A generalized reaction, urticarial or otherwise, is an indication for desensitization with polyvalent insect extract, a prolonged procedure carried out over a period of several years.

NURSING IMPLICATIONS. Nurses are frequently in a position to give advice concerning first aid for bee stings, and to educate persons who are allergic to the danger and advise their desensitization. Wearing shoes and light protective clothing and being careful to avoid contact with bees help to avoid bee stings. To remove the stinger, unless the individual is in distress because of a generalized reaction, scrape it off gently with a knife blade, the side of tweezers or a finger nail. The sac or stinger should not be grasped since this forces remaining venom into the skin, but should be teased sideways.

BACTERIAL DISEASES

The flora of the skin is normally colonized with many potentially pathogenic organisms, the major bacteria being the staphylococcus and the streptococcus. A local area of infection is accompanied by a rapid increase in number of bacteria on the skin which serve as a source of continuing infection. The incidence of staphylococcal infections decreases with increasing age. Women have more lesions in the axillae, the pubic area and, in lactating women, the breast. Males have infections more frequently on the upper extremities, buttocks, upper thighs, neck and chest.

More than half of the general population harbor staphylococci in the external nares. A damaged area of skin quickly becomes a focus of "staph." Certain strains are dermotropic and colonize and flourish in the layers of the corneum. Phase type 71 is frequently found in impetigo. Phase type 80/81, the hospital infection strain, is dermotropic, readily transmissible, and more virulent than other strains.[14] Once the skin is colonized, the incidence of pyodermas in the individual and his contacts increases considerably.

Impetigo. Impetigo occurs primarily in children. The disease is characterized by intraepidermal vesicles which progress to pustules and are soon overlaid with gummy honey-colored crusts. The size of the lesion varies, but is roughly circular. The causative organism may be either a streptococcus or staphylococcus, or both. Acute glomerulonephritis can be an uncommon complication in children.

TREATMENT. Treatment consists of debriding the lesions, eliminating the infection and preventing fissuring and drying. Compresses of Burow's solution or powders of aluminum acetate (1 tablet or powder to 1 pint of cool water) may be used to soften the crust. The lesions are allowed to air dry and an antibiotic ointment such as bacitracin, neomycin, gramicidin or polymixin B may be used. Many doctors prefer not to use antibiotics systematically, for fear of producing resistant organisms. A bland emollient may be used to prevent drying and fissuring.

PREVENTION. Early recognition and treatment are desirable. Hexachlorophene soaps such as Dial may be used by the rest of the family to prevent spread, and careful separation of towels and such articles is necessary. Handwashing after handling the lesions is a must. Lesions near the nose are *dangerous* in *adults,* and probably need systemic treatment to avoid spread. General teaching about the methods of control and demonstration of care of the lesions may be indicated.

Erythrasma. Erythrasma is a low-grade infection involving the intertriginous areas and moist areas of the body. Recent studies show the causative organism to be a diphtheroid, causing slightly inflamed, dry, slowly spreading, slightly scaling, circumscribed macular patches. The condition may be diagnosed by the coral red fluorescence under the Wood's lamp. Safeguard soap is effective against the condition. The doctor may administer erythromycin or tetracycline. Recurrence is not uncommon. About 10 per cent of older people may be found to have the condition.

Cellulitis. This is a more serious infection of the dermis and subcutaneous tissue by streptococci. Red streaks and enlarged regional nodes are indications of the infection. Pronounced constitutional symptoms are common. If the infection is recurrent, permanent lymphedema may result. Treatment consists of rest and immobilization of the infected area. If there are constitutional symptoms, the patient should be hospitalized and treated with systemic antibiotics.

Erysipelas. This is an acute streptococcal cellulitis usually occurring on the face. The lesion is warm with a raised advancing area of erythema and a definite border. Elderly persons are particularly susceptible. Constitutional symptoms accompany the disease and systemic treatment is necessary.

Furuncle (Boil). A boil or furuncle is an acute painful infection of a hair follicle caused by *Staphylococcus pyogenes*. A carbuncle is a conglomerated mass of boils. The onset is quite sudden, with the skin becoming red, tender and hot around a hair follicle; the center becomes yellow with pus and soon forms a core which may be extruded spontaneously or with gentle manipulation.

TREATMENT. Recurrent boils are sometimes a symptom of underlying disease, such as glycosuria. Thus, persons with boils should be urged to have a complete medical examination. Systemic antibiotics are frequently prescribed, particularly broad-spectrum antibiotics like tetracycline. Patients are advised to bathe with hexachlorophene soaps. A bandage is useful only to protect the boil from trauma, unless it is draining.

The patient must take precautions to prevent the rest of family from obtaining the disease by isolating towels, linen and clothing, burning dressings and washing hands with hexachlorophene soap after handling. Family members should also use hexachlorophene soap. The patient should keep moist skin areas dry with antiperspirants or alcohol lotions, since dryness inhibits growth of bacteria.

NURSING IMPLICATIONS. In all bacterial skin diseases, the nurse needs to emphasize scrupulous cleanliness in the family. Dial soap and prompt care of any slight trauma are important.

Syphilis. Syphilis is presented here because of its cutaneous manifestations in the secondary phase. Syphilis is an infectious systemic venereal disease caused by the spirochete *Treponema pallidum*. It is usually acquired through sexual contact.

From 2 to 10 weeks after the initial contact, the primary lesion (chancre) will appear at the site of the first contact with the spirochete. The chancre is a small moist ulcer that has a raised edge and may be painless. At this stage of the disease, a blood test may not be positive, and a darkfield examination must be made from material from the chancre. If untreated, the chancre will disappear in one to four weeks. Serologic tests for syphilis will be positive four to six weeks after first infection with the spirochete. Infection without the appearance of a chancre is fairly frequent.

EARLY (SECONDARY) SYPHILIS. The cutaneous lesions of secondary syphilis appear six weeks to six months after the chancre or original infection. There may be associated systemic symptoms of malaise, fever, headache and mild sore throat with the eruption. The lesions may follow different patterns of distribution and may be macular, papular, scaling or pustular (Fig. 91–6). They rarely itch.

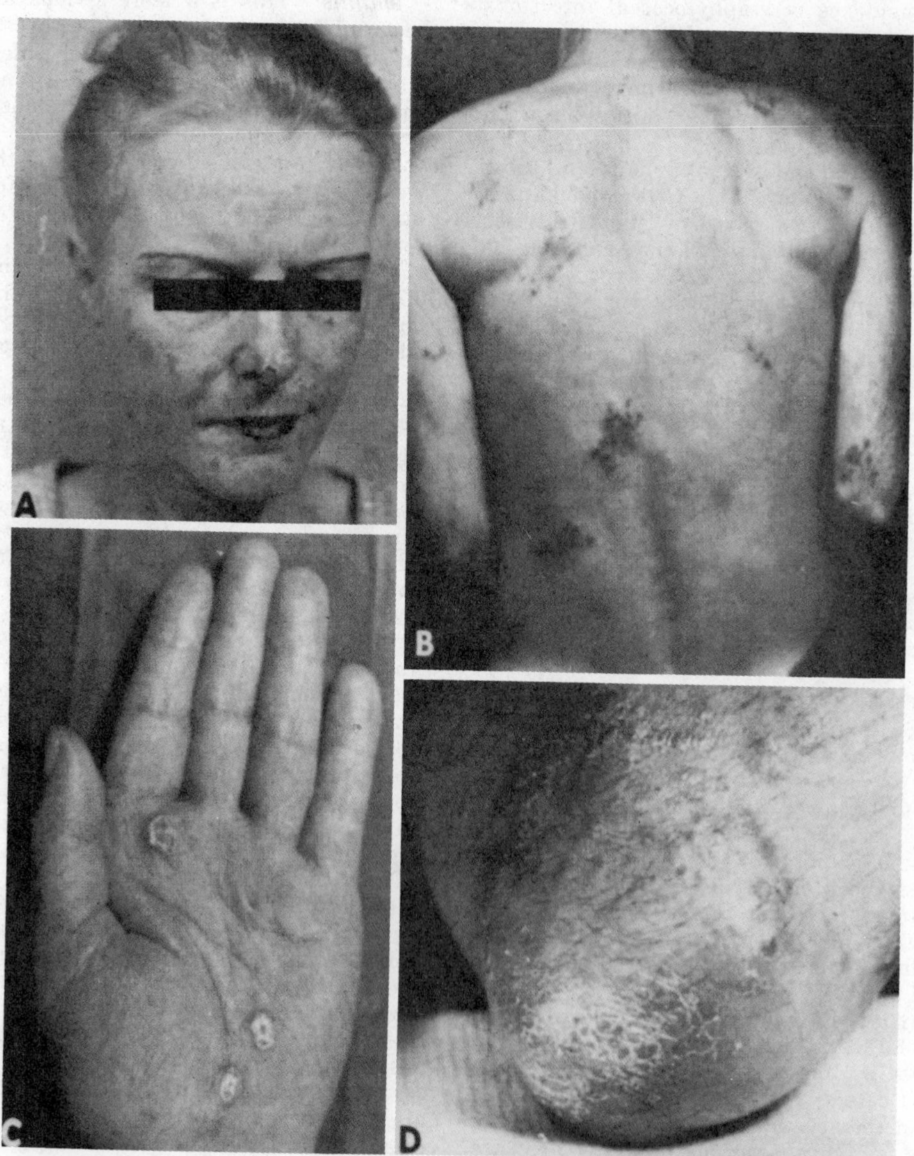

FIGURE 91–6. Early syphilis. *A*, Lesions are erythematous and might be mistaken for seborrheic dermatitis. *B*, Corymbose (grouped papular) eruption is an uncommon expression. *C*, Large papulosquamous lesions of the palm simulating psoriasis. *D*, Although unilateral involvement is more typical for late syphilids, such lesions may be observed early in the course of the disease, when inadequate therapy has been administered. (From Lewis, G. M., and Wheeler, C. E., Jr.: *Practical Dermatology.* 3rd ed. 1967.)

Lesions characteristically appear on the palms and soles. Any suddenly appearing, generalized eruption should call to mind the possibility of secondary syphilis. All secondary lesions are highly infectious.

After the disappearance of the signs of early syphilis, a latent stage ensues with potentially damaging effect on multiple organs if untreated (see Unit VIII).

TREATMENT. Syphilis is treated with penicillin intramuscularly, or with other oral antibiotics if penicillin is not tolerated.

NURSING IMPLICATIONS. There are many nursing implications in the detection and treatment of venereal disease and contacts. However, for present purposes, the nurse needs to have a heightened awareness of the potential in any painless, slow-healing sore, and of the need for referral of any patient with a suddenly appearing generalized eruption with lesions on the palms and soles of the feet.

VIRAL DISEASES

A virus is an ultramicroscopic organism. Viruses are often divided into those containing ribonucleic acid (RNA) and those containing deoxyribonucleic acid (DNA). Useful antiviral agents include the following:[14]

> Idoxuredine (IDU, Stoxil) and cytosine arabinoside. By preventing certain aspects of DNA synthesis, these agents inhibit propagation of the virus without interfering with normal cellular activity.

> Thiosemicarbazones (methisazone). These agents inhibit replication of the virus and prevent its maturation. This is useful in vaccinia and early smallpox.

> Interferon. Interferon is a protein produced by cells that have harbored viruses. This agent is active against all known viruses.

> Immune globulin. Vaccinia immune globulin (VIG) is prepared from blood of adults taken four to six weeks after primary vaccination. This agent is used in treating smallpox vaccination complications.

> Amantadine. An amine that is useful in influenza, rubella and some tumor viruses.

Herpes Simplex. This lesion, often called cold sore or fever blister, is caused by two types of herpes virus, hominis type, I and II. Type I is the more common and causes most of the common herpes lesions. Most of the primary infections occur in childhood and are subclinical.

Herpes is characterized by a cutaneous viral infection which starts out with burning, tingling and itching in the area, soon followed by multiple, grouped tiny vesicles on an erythematous base. Generally after 48 hours, crusting occurs. The lesion most frequently occurs on the lips and face and around the mouth. It normally runs a course of about 7 to 10 days and is troublesome to the 1 per cent of individuals in whom it is recurrent.

Type II virus is less common and is responsible for the majority of genital herpetic lesions. It is transmitted through sexual contact and causes the severe disseminated herpes infection of the newborn.[7] Herpes virus can invade preexisting skin lesions, and patients with existing dermatitis should avoid persons with herpetic or, in fact, any infectious skin lesion. Herpes simplex may be irritated by one or numerous "trigger" mechanisms, such as sunlight, fever or menses.

TREATMENT. During the acute stages, cold compresses may help. If applied frequently, 70 per cent alcohol will dry the lesion. Very potent adrenocorticosteroids applied every half hour will abort most cold sores.[14] IDU can be used topically in treatment of herpes simplex. It must be applied frequently—about every half hour. Inoculation with smallpox vaccine has not been found to be of any value. If the herpes is recurrent, detection and elimination of the trigger factor should be initiated.

Herpes zoster, or shingles, an acute virus infection of the central nervous system which causes cutaneous lesions, is discussed in Unit VIII.

Warts (Verrucae). Warts are caused by papovavirus hominis. They are moderately contagious and autoinoculable, and may affect any part of the body. There appears to be tremendous individual variation in susceptibility. They have an unpredictable course and eventually disappear without any treatment.

Among the varieties of warts are the *common wart* (verruca vulgaris), usually occurring on the hands and fingers, the *plantar wart,* which appears on the sole of the foot, and the *venereal wart* (condyloma acuminatum), seen in the mucous membranes or skin of the genital organs and the perianal region.

TREATMENT. Treatment of unobtrusive warts is not advised. One of the most frequent methods of removing bothersome warts is electrodissection and curettage under local anesthesia. Refrigeration is another useful method. The application of solid carbon dioxide to the lesion several times will produce a blister which frequently removes the wart. Salicylic acid preparations are helpful but probably less so than the previously mentioned treatment. For plantar warts, in addition to curettage and freezing, salicylic acid or cantharadin may be applied to the wart. Venereal warts are treated by podophyllin, 20 to 25 per cent in tincture of benzoin, applied to the warts and washed off in four to six hours. Patients should be warned against transfer to the eyes as it produces severe conjunctivitis.

FUNGUS DISEASES

A fungus is a saprophytic or parasitic plant that possesses cells lacking true chlorophyll. *Ringworm* is a general term applied to fungus, or mycotic, infections of keratinized areas of the body, hair, skin and nails. Various genera and species of fungi known collectively as the dermatophytes are causative agents. Microsporum, Epidermophyton and Trichophyton are the three important genera. Contraction of an infection depends a great deal on individual susceptibility and individual factors such as moisture and warmth.

Ringworm of the Scalp (Tinea Capitis). The infection begins as a small papule and spreads peripherally, leaving scaly patches of alopecia. Infected hair becomes brittle and breaks off easily. Occasionally boggy, raised and suppurative lesions called "kerion" develop. Examination of the scalp under a Wood's lamp may be helpful in detecting the presence of a fungus, as there will be a bright green fluorescence of infected hair. There is a higher incidence in children than in adults, and males are infected more frequently than females.

INFECTIOUS AGENT. Various species of Microsporum and Trichophyton. It is important to determine the genus and species for prognosis. *Microsporum canis* causes a self-limited, moderately contagious infection contracted from dogs or cats and passed from child to child. Infection with *Microsporum audouini,* transmitted from man to man, generally runs a chronic course and ends by puberty. The Trichophyton infections are relatively rare. Infected hairs on clothing, barber clippers or combs or the backs of theater seats may also be sources of infection. The incubation period is 10 to 14 days.

TREATMENT. Griseofulvin, an antibiotic, is the most effective treatment for all forms. The hairs over the infected area should be kept clipped to prevent spread to other children. Topical treatment may be given while the systemic drug is taking effect, as the condition is communicable as long as infectious lesions and viable sores are present.

NURSING IMPLICATIONS. The school and office nurse will most likely be involved in following children with tinea capitis. In school, it may be necessary to examine an entire class under the Wood's lamp, and to instruct parents and teachers about the source of infection and prevention of spread. Fortunately, the advent of griseofulvin makes this a less arduous task.

Ringworm of the Body (Tinea Corporis). A cutaneous infection of areas other than the scalp, bearded area or feet, this characteristically appears as flat, spreading, ring-shaped lesions. The periphery is reddish, vesicular or pustular, and may be dry and scaly or dry and crusted. As the lesions progress peripherally, the center often clears and appears normal.

Treatment is with griseofulvin. Griseofulvin may cause phototoxicity, urticaria, headaches and nausea. It produces exacerbation of porphyria (an uncommon metabolic disease) and antagonizes warfarin, necessitating an increased dose of that anticoagulant if being taken. Phenobarbital reduces the efficacy of the drug and should not be taken concurrently.[14] Topical treatment is satisfactory if there are few lesions. A specific topical antifungal agent, tolnaftate tinactin liquid, may be applied sparingly three times a day.

Ringworm of the Foot (Tinea Pedis). Scaling or cracking of the skin, especially between the toes, or blisters containing a thin watery fluid, are so characteristic that most people recognize "athlete's foot." In severe cases, vesicular lesions appear on various parts of the body, especially the hands. These dermatophytids ("id" reaction) do not contain the fungus and constitute an allergic reaction to fungus and spores.

TREATMENT. In the acute stage, bland treatment is desirable. Rest and foot soaks of 1:8000 potassium permanganate solution may be given for five minutes two to three times a day. As the condition becomes chronic, corticosteroid creams, half strength Whitfield's ointment, or Desenex may be applied.

PREVENTION. Plenty of ventilation should be given the feet, and being barefoot on the beach for an extended vacation may help clear up the condition. The person should wear well ventilated shoes and clean lightweight socks. Dusting between the toes with antifungal powder may help prevent a recurrence. The "id" reaction on the hands may clear up when the infection on the feet has been cured, or it may not.

Ringworm of the Nails (Tinea Unguium). This is a chronic infection involving one or more nails on the hand or foot. The nail gradually thickens, becomes discolored and brittle, and an accumulation of caseous-appearing material forms beneath the nail, or the nail becomes chalky and disintegrated. It is treated by scraping off as much of the affected nail as possible and applying an ointment containing salicylic acid or one of the higher fatty acids, propionic acid or undecylenic acid. Griseofulvin by mouth is the treatment of choice.

Tinea versicolor is a very superficial infection of the skin caused by the fungus *Malassezia furfur.* The lesions consist of asymptomatic patches which filter out the sunlight, producing white or light patches on a tanned skin. Almost any type of mild antifungal preparation is temporarily effective, but recurrences are common. The infection fluoresces under a Wood's lamp, giving a whitish, yellow or brown color. The patient should be examined under a Wood's lamp both before and after treatment.

Fungus infections among the *elderly* usually occur in the diabetic. Tinactin, which is not irritating like the peeling agents, can often be helpful with applications two to three times a week. Yeast infections or moniliasis between the toes can cause problems. Mycolog cream is effective in most cases. Good cleansing and careful drying are important.

ECZEMA AND DERMATITIS

More than half of all skin diseases are included in this heading. Both terms are used to describe a condition that exhibits some of the following symptoms: (1) edema and swelling; (2) discrete or grouped vesicles, changing to weeping and crusted lesions and/or papules and scaling; and (3) itching or burning with scratching or rubbing leading to lichenification of the skin.

General Nursing Care in Dermatitis. Dermatitis can be divided into two types, based on what the nurse sees and feels: that is, acute and chronic.

In *acute* dermatitis, one sees erythema, pruritus or burning, edema, bullae, and/or weeping. In *chronic* dermatitis, erythema, lichenification, dryness, scaling, fissuring and a feeling of roughness may be present. Both conditions may be secondarily infected. Treatment is based on whether the condition is chronic or acute (see Table 91–1 below). Acute dermatitis is generally treated with intermittent moist compresses which produce evaporation. This results in cooling, thus reducing itching, burning and redness, and produces drying. Intermittent compressing results in effective debridement. After the acute symptoms have subsided, the lesion can be treated as a chronic dermatitis.

Chronic dermatitis is commonly treated by a topical application of a dilute concentration of a fluorinated steroid sparingly applied several times a day to reduce inflammation and diminish itching and dryness. In some patients, an oral antihistamine will help with the itching. If the specific cause can be found and eliminated, this will of course aid in patient recovery, but since in many cases no specific cause is discovered, care must be consistent, gentle and persistent.

Some specific forms of dermatitis will be discussed below.

Atopic Dermatitis (Allergic Eczema, Neurodermatitis). Atopy is used to describe the following: (1) a history of infantile atopic eczema; (2) a familial tendency for asthma, hay fever, rhinitis and urticaria; (3) hypersensitivity to protein; and (4) unusual reaction to heat, cold and emotional tensions. (See Fig. 91–7.)

Atopic dermatitis may appear soon after birth with skin lesions on face, neck, scalp and diaper area. The disease may clear at about four years of age but may become clinically apparent as the person gets older. The antecubital and popliteal areas are commonly involved. Pruritus is the main complaint. The involved sites are usually dry, excoriated and erythematous, and the skin exhibits lichenification. The disease tends to improve in the summer and generally disappears around the age of 30.

TREATMENT. The most important treatment principle is control of the pruritus. If the process is acute and localized, wet compresses of Burow's solution (1 tablespoon to 1 pint of water) may be used three times daily for 10 minutes. If the process is generalized, a cool brief tar or colloidal bath may be advised. Regular application of an adrenocorticosteroid cream three times daily is one of the most effective treatments. For localized areas, steroid creams should be used every three to four hours under occlusive pliable dressings. Alternative topical medication is a vioform or coal tar ointment under a dressing at night. Since this is a chronic disease, dermatologists are reluctant to use systemic steroids.

NURSING IMPLICATIONS. (1) General measures for pruritus. (2) Encourage the individual to get adequate rest and relief from nervous tensions and pressure. Working may be less nerve-racking than staying at home with the children. The individual should not be compulsive about housework and should use as many labor-saving devices as possible. (3) The person should avoid vaccination or any person with a vaccination or with herpes simplex to avoid Kaposi's varicelliform eruption. This is a generalized infection and, if the infection is due to smallpox vaccine, early administration of hyperimmune gamma globulin may be necessary and may be obtained through local health departments. School nurses or nurses working in immunization clinics need to be especially mindful of the total family and should inquire if any other children have eczema. (4) Irritating clothing such as woollens should be avoided. Nothing must be applied that will irritate the skin. Detergents and household cleaners should be avoided. The patient

TABLE 91–1. SUMMARY OF NURSING CARE IN DERMATITIS

Acute		**Chronic**	
Signs and Symptoms	*Treatment*	*Signs and Symptoms*	*Treatment*
Erythema	See Vesicles weeping	Erythema	Topical steroids sparingly
Pruritus	See Vesicles weeping; plus oral antihistamines	Pruritus	Topical steroids sparingly; oral antihistamines
Infection	Appropriate oral antibiotics	Infection	Appropriate oral antibiotics
Vesicles/weeping	Intermittent compresses	Lichenification/dryness	Emollients frequently

From Scotvold, M. J.: The Management of Dermatitis.

should avoid being chilled or overheated. Emotional support and encouragement are necessary because of the disfigurement and the smelly ointments necessary to control the itching.

Contact Dermatitis. This condition is characterized by redness, edema, vesicles, bullae and itching. It is caused by irritant subjects coming into contact with the skin. There are two types—primary dermatitis and allergic dermatitis. A *primary* dermatitis is caused by an irritant capable of producing a dermatitis in almost any skin. Prevention of recurrence is by avoiding the irritant by means of special clothing, washing after exposure or barrier creams.

Allergic dermatitis is caused by sensitizers. The number of exposures to substances which will produce the rash varies from a few to many. The cause is an allergen to which the patient is specifically and often highly sensitive. There is a wide

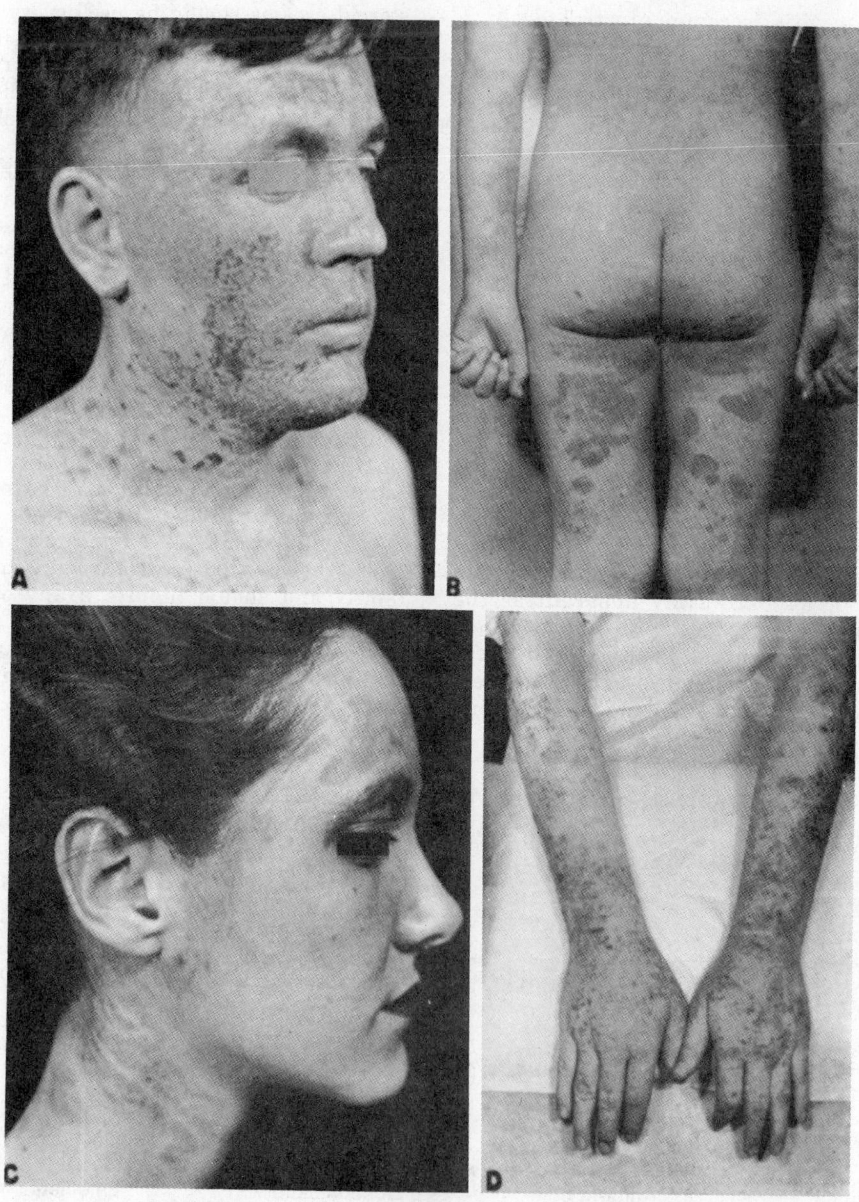

FIGURE 91–7. Atopic eczema. *A,* The disease usually begins early in life and is intermittently present for many years. *B,* Widespread patchy and confluent eruption; the intense pruritus may interfere with sleep. *C,* Traumatization of the skin causes lichenification in plaques. *D,* Scratching may induce superficial pyogenic infection with vesiculation and occasional pustules. (From Lewis, E. M., and Wheeler, C. E., Jr.: *Practical Dermatology.* 3rd ed. 1967.)

variety of possible agents, but generally a few for each patient.

Agents may be divided into the following classes: (1) clothing; (2) cosmetics; (3) household articles; (4) occupational; (5) plants; and (6) medicines.

CLOTHING. The first location of the eruption is important. Offending clothing will cause dermatitis in the area covered by it. The irritation is generally caused by a dye in the clothing. The feet may be affected by dye, glue or leather in shoes. After a time, the acute infection tends to spread to other areas, even without additional exposure to the causal agent. The exact mechanism of this spread is not known.

COSMETICS. Perfume, deodorants, nail polish, lipstick, hair dyes, shampoos and hair sprays may all cause dermatitis; the causal agent can usually be determined from the site and history of use of any new product.

HOUSEHOLD PRODUCTS. Detergents are the most common cause. They defat the skin and may cause a persistent rash that is hard to treat, since it is difficult for women to keep their hands out of water.

OCCUPATIONAL. Almost any substance used in industry, such as paints, dyes, cement, can cause dermatitis. Industry, however, usually requires protective clothing, etc.

PLANTS. Poison ivy dermatitis is probably the most common allergic eczema in the United States. Common antigens are also present in poison oak, poison sumac, Japanese lacquer tree, cashew nut, mango fruit and Gingko tree. A resinous, sticky, saplike substance in all parts of the plant from roots to leaves is the source of the reaction. No one is immune to it and, although a person does not react on the first exposure, he may become sensitized and have a reaction the next time. The individual can become affected by directly touching the stem or leaves or by touching trails of the sap that have adhered to clothing, tools, the fur of pets, or from particles in the air. The diagnosis is made on the basis of history of exposure, and the finding of linear arrangement of the eczematous vesicles. This linearity is due to a brushing motion over the extremely antigenic plant. The way to cope with these plants is to learn to recognize and avoid them.

TREATMENT. If exposure has occurred, the oil can be washed off with soap and water if this is done immediately. Application of a drying alcoholic shake lotion or calamine lotion is sufficient in mild cases. To ease the itching, a cold wet dressing made of Burow's solution (1 part to 10 parts of water for adults and 1 part to 20 parts of water for small children) or Epsom salts (1 tablespoon to a quart of water) may be used. The dressings may be covered with plastic wrap. For intense reactions, potent topical steroid ointments are frequently applied every two hours. Systemic adrenocorticosteroids may be given if the case is severe and there are no contraindications.

For highly sensitive individuals who must be exposed to poison ivy, a prophylactic desensitization may be carried out by daily ingestions of small measured amounts of Rhus oleoresin. The poison ivy plant may be eliminated by weed-killer sprays, fuel oil, etc.

Erythema Nodosum. This is an acute inflammatory condition characterized by red tender nodules on the anterior portion of the legs and thighs, usually varying in size from 6 to 8 mm. and maybe larger. There may be associated fever and joint pains. The lesions appear in crops and there are frequent recurrences. As the lesions fade after a varying length of time, they begin to resemble old bruises. In a large number of cases, the cause remains undetermined. The condition occurs most frequently in young women. There is an underlying systemic cause in more than 50 per cent of the cases.[14] It is an important initial sign in sarcoidosis, since 30 per cent of individuals with that disease have the condition. The most common cause in North America is the streptococcus. Allergic reactions to drugs can produce this condition while the drugs are being taken. A thorough physical examination is indicated. Treatment is symptomatic.

Exfoliative Dermatitis. This condition is characterized by a more or less sudden episode of generalized erythema with a scaling of the cutaneous surface in either fine scales or larger sheets. It may begin without obvious cause, or may occur secondarily to some other skin disorder or follow administration of a drug. Itching may be severe. This is a severe disease and can have a fatal outcome. The patient is in acute distress since the total skin area is affected, and there is considerable water and protein loss from the skin. Control of heat regulation is poor, and the patient is susceptible to infection.

TREATMENT. The patient is taken off his present drugs. Fluid and electrolyte balance must be maintained and infection prevented, necessitating nursing care similar to that given in burn cases. Anti-inflammatory agents may be applied externally, and adrenocorticosteroids given as a lifesaving procedure.

Urticaria (Hives). This is a common pruritic condition characterized by transient wheals or welts of varying size. The trunk is the usual site of involvement, although they may appear anywhere on the body. If they involve the lips or eyes, there may be just a generalized swelling. Hives develop quickly, often in large numbers, and disappear in a few hours without sequelae. There is generally not much difficulty in determining the cause of an acute onset, but it may be more difficult in chronic or delayed cases. The latter may be due to allergic response to a food such as fish, nuts, eggs, wheat, milk, chocolate, strawberries and pork. Drugs are common offenders, as are inhalants, infections, systemic diseases, bites and chemicals. It is even possible that urticaria may be psychogenic.

TREATMENT. It is important to eliminate the cause. Skin tests are not very helpful because the patient's skin is very reactive. Antihistamine drugs may be helpful. Colloidal baths or some lotion such as Cetaphil or any oil-in-water type that can be easily washed off, with 0.025 to 0.050 per cent menthol, may be soothing. Epinephrine (0.3 ml. of 1:1000 solution) may be lifesaving in an emergency and may relieve the urticaria in any situation.

Erythema Multiforme. This is a toxic eruption characterized by symmetrical distribution of macules, papules and vesicles (Fig. 91–8). The lesions may have elevated circular borders, a depressed inner ring and central erythema or fluid-filled bullae. The disease varies in severity from a mild form without symptoms to a generalized serious bullous disease accompanied by fever and prostration. The etiology is unknown.

The disease may follow any of five general patterns. It may be idiopathic and self-limited, lasting from four to six weeks. It may result from drug eruptions. It may be associated with the last half of pregnancy, with internal disease or viral infections, or rarely with various kinds of internal cancer.

TREATMENT. Systemic adrenocorticosteroids will relieve the disease or shorten the course if no infection or underlying cause is found. Local treatment depends on the type of lesions.

Pityriasis Rosea. This is a self-limited disease of unknown etiology that has peaks of occurrence during the spring and fall. Characteristically, a single oval lesion develops first, called a herald patch. From several days to two to three weeks later, an eruption develops on the trunk and extremities in the direction of lines of cleavage of the skin. Lesions are rarely seen on exposed areas and they are usually confined to the trunk. Individual lesions are fawn colored with a pink or reddish edge. Each lesion is covered by a fine scale attached at the edge. Itching varies from severe to practically none. Spontaneous cure regularly occurs in six to eight weeks. Ultraviolet exposure will shorten the disease course. Treatment is ordinarily unnecessary unless there is severe itching.

Drug Reactions. Adverse reactions to drugs are more often seen in the skin than in any other organ, and are most common in patients with serious illness who receive a number of drugs. The following considerations regarding drug allergy are important:

> The drug may have been used before without untoward reaction.

> After the first reaction to the drug, only a small dose is required to cause a recurrence.

> Drugs may produce different reactions in different people and many drugs produce similar reactions.

> The risk is directly related to the number of drugs the patient is taking.

> Drug reactions persist.

Some drugs may produce an inflammatory reaction in the skin when light is present. These may include the sulfonamides, phenothiazine and some tetracyclines. *Fixed drug reactions* recur specifically at previously affected areas. The eruption is usually a purplish red, round or oval plaque with a sharply defined border. They are more common in the extremities. Some drugs likely to produce fixed eruptions are barbiturates, salicylates and antipyrine.

TREATMENT. Most drug eruptions disappear when the causal agent is discontinued. A relapse may be caused by taking a very small amount of the drug. Fluids should be forced to speed up the elimination of the drug. The patient should be advised of the sensitivity and the necessity of informing any physician who may be prescribing medication.

Lichen Planus. Lichen planus is a chronic, pruritic, inflammatory, papular eruption of the skin and mucous membranes of unknown etiology. The disease begins insidiously with the individual appearance of a discrete shiny flat-topped papule. The lesions are usually found on the front of the wrists or forearms, ankles, thighs and abdomen. They are seldom found on the scalp, face, palms and soles. Mucous membranes are affected in 25 per cent of all cases. In about 10 per cent of the cases, the nails will be involved, with thinning or increased longitudinal ridging. Most of the cases occur in adult life. Women are more likely to develop the disease than men. Nervous strain is regarded as a secondary factor.

TREATMENT. The patient is generally taken off all drugs, and a substitute given for essential drugs. Adrenocorticosteroid cream under occlusive dressings may be used for localized lichen planus. In cases of hypertrophic lichen planus of the legs, a firm occlusive dressing of an Unna boot type, changed weekly, relieves the pruritus and flattens the lesions over a period of weeks. Grenz radiation may be prescribed. Systemic administration of adrenocorticosteroids may be helpful in suppressing the disease when patients have generalized disease. A lotion for itching may be advised.

NURSING IMPLICATIONS. The nurse may be the first one to notice or be told about the first lesions of lichen planus. Since early care and discontinuation of medication are important, a high level of awareness of skin lesions is necessary.

Psoriasis. Psoriasis is a common skin disease found in people in good health. The disease affects about 5 per cent of the population and commonly begins in the second and third decades and runs a variable course. Psoriasis is definitely familial and is classified genetically as an irregularly dominant trait with incomplete penetrance. This is a chronic disease characterized by sharply demarcated lesions of a deep red color covered by thick overlying silvery scales. There is a marked frequency of lesions in certain areas of the body, such as the scalp, regions over the elbows and knees, and the lower part of the back. However, no portion of the skin is free from the disease. It is common to observe pitting and discoloration of the nails with an accumulation of detritus under the free edge of the nails.

Psoriasis is extremely variable in its duration and course. A single lesion may persist for a lifetime or many lesions may be present. Some patients are never free of the disease while others have long remissions. Most patients are better in the summer.

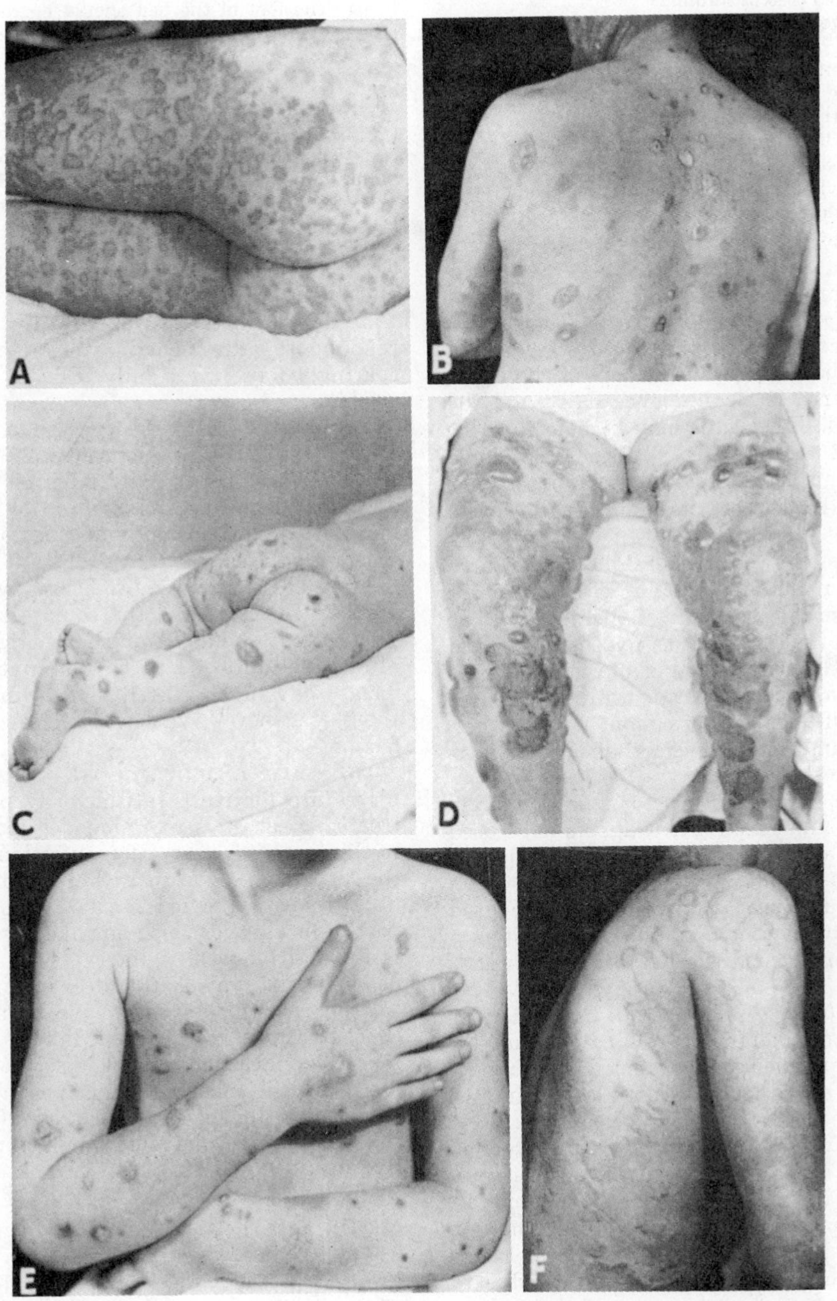

FIGURE 91–8. Erythema multiforme. The clinical appearance varies in location, form and chief presenting component. *A*, Multiple erythematous plaques with tendency to coalescence., *B* and *C*, Similar, discrete erythematous, vesicular lesions appearing in crops but in different locations in adult and child. *D*, Large bullae predominate and coalescence is the rule. *E*, Some of the erythematous plaques are topped by vesicles. *F*, Configurate and serpentine, superficial, erythematous areas produced by extension and coalescence of discrete lesions. (From Lewis, G. M., and Wheeler, C. E., Jr.: *Practical Dermatology.* 3rd ed. 1967.)

TREATMENT. General principles of treatment are:

> The physician has to establish the necessity of continual adherence to the treatment plan.
> No treatment should produce trauma to the skin, as this may result in new psoriatic lesions since they tend to form in the area of skin trauma.
> Slow inactive thick lesions should be treated aggressively.
> Acute recent spreading lesions should be treated gently.
> Tar and dithranol compounds should be used very cautiously in flexural and anogenital areas because of the irritating potential.
> When topical steroids are discontinued, some other preparation should be used to maintain therapeutic effect because of possible rebound.

Therapy is directed at slowing down epidermal turnover time and reducing pruritus. Topical application of steroids with plastic wrap occlusion may be prescribed for as many hours of the 24 as possible. The area is cleaned once daily and the cream reapplied. The plastic may be held in place with articles of clothing, socks, etc., by occlusive plastic gloves on the hands, and plastic shower caps for the scalp. The air must not be allowed to dry the areas.

Regular exposure to ultraviolet light (one to three times weekly), avoiding production of erythema or burning, is desirable. Grenz ray therapy may be used for lesions that are difficult to control by local therapy alone. Grenz radiation is a form of ionizing radiation with a spectrum between ultraviolet and roentgen rays. It has no permanent effects when used correctly and has a beneficial effect on superficial psoriatic lesions.

Methotrexate, an antifolic acid drug, is one of the most important and effective new agents to be used in severe psoriasis. It is applied under occlusion as indicated for steroids.

Many different drugs and treatments are used in the treatment of psoriasis, but because it is a long-term, chronic condition, caution is emphasized.

Stasis Dermatitis and Ulceration. Stasis dermatitis is a very common problem related to an underlying venous insufficiency. It is identified with varicose veins with or without varicose ulcers (Fig. 91–9).

One of the earliest indications of chronic venous insufficiency is ankle edema, usually occurring at the end of the day. After a time, patches of tan pigmentation appear on the lower third of the leg. The pigment is hemosiderin resulting from extravasation of blood through capillary walls due to increased venous pressure. A patchy erythema may develop which may be dry or oozing and vesicular. Secondary infections may occur and a characteristic subcutaneous induration may develop. The final stage is associated with atrophy and fibrous scarring of the area. At any stage of this process, an ulcer may develop in the devitalized area.

Hypostatic ulcers are very slow in healing and, since the skin is easily irritated, bland nonsensitizing applications must be used. The basis of treatment of venous insufficiency is the prevention of orthostatic edema. The following suggestions are offered for those patients who must be managed conservatively:

> Strict avoidance of standing or sitting in one position for a long period of time.
> Regular 15- to 20-minute rest periods during the day when the legs can be maintained at a level well above the heart. The foot of the bed should be raised 6 inches or more.
> Proper instruction in the wearing of an adequate support for the limb. This can best be achieved by the application of a 3-inch elastic bandage from the base of the toes to just below the knee, or an individually fitted heavy elastic stocking. If surgery is not feasible, the individual may have to wear these supports indefinitely.
> If obesity is present, a weight reduction diet should be instituted.

TREATMENT. This depends on the stage of development.

1. Early lesions which are dry and localized respond to adrenocorticosteroid cream applied sparingly four times daily. Elastic support is desirable.
2. Subacute (moist) lesions are treated with cool compresses of Burow's solution 1:20 dilution for 15 minutes three times daily followed by air drying, and steroid ointment. Elevation of the leg for 15 minutes three times daily and use of elastic stockings are advised.
3. Severe lesions require bedrest with the foot of the bed elevated, and the compresses and cream. The patient should wear the elastic support only after he is allowed to be ambulatory. Systemic drugs may be indicated, depending on whether there is generalized dermatitis or secondary infection.

TREATMENT OF VARICOSE ULCER. Varicose ulcers are far more satisfactorily prevented than treated. Bedrest is recommended. Steps are taken to eliminate infection. After infection is eliminated, the leg may be covered with a commercially available gelatin-zinc oxide paste (modified Unna's boot), allowing for some shrinkage when dry. This is replaced at weekly intervals at first, and then at longer intervals as the ulcer heals.

Other treatments used have been high oxygen concentrations in the immediate region of ulcer, topical application of gold leaf, oral zinc sulfate, etc. Surgical consultation is recommended, since the earlier the chronic venous insufficiency of the limb is corrected, the more satisfactory is the operative result.

LUPUS ERYTHEMATOSUS

Lupus erythematosus is usually classified as one of the "collagen" diseases. These are a group of diseases of connective tissue characterized by widespread inflammation of tissue and deposits of fibrinoid material in various parts of the body. Lupus erythematosus takes two forms: localized, or discoid, and systemic. The disease is considered here because both forms have skin manifestations.

Discoid Lupus Erythematosus. This term refers to a chronic skin eruption which is not life-threatening, whereas systemic lupus erythematosus is a serious disease often terminating fatally. Views differ as to whether these are two different diseases or whether the discoid type is the benign end of the disease spectrum.

Discoid lupus begins with scaling erythematous macules over the nose, cheeks, forehead and temples, the so-called "butterfly" distribution. It may start with a small lesion and gradually involve more areas on the neck, ears and scalp. Exposure to sunlight may precipitate the appearance of new lesions and aggravate those already present. Antibiotics should be avoided, since they disseminate the disease process.[12]

TREATMENT. Fluorinated adrenocorticosteroid under a plastic dressing may be used; chloroquine, an antimalarial drug, also has been found to be a satisfactory treatment. Patients may need to avoid sunlight and use a sunscreening agent.

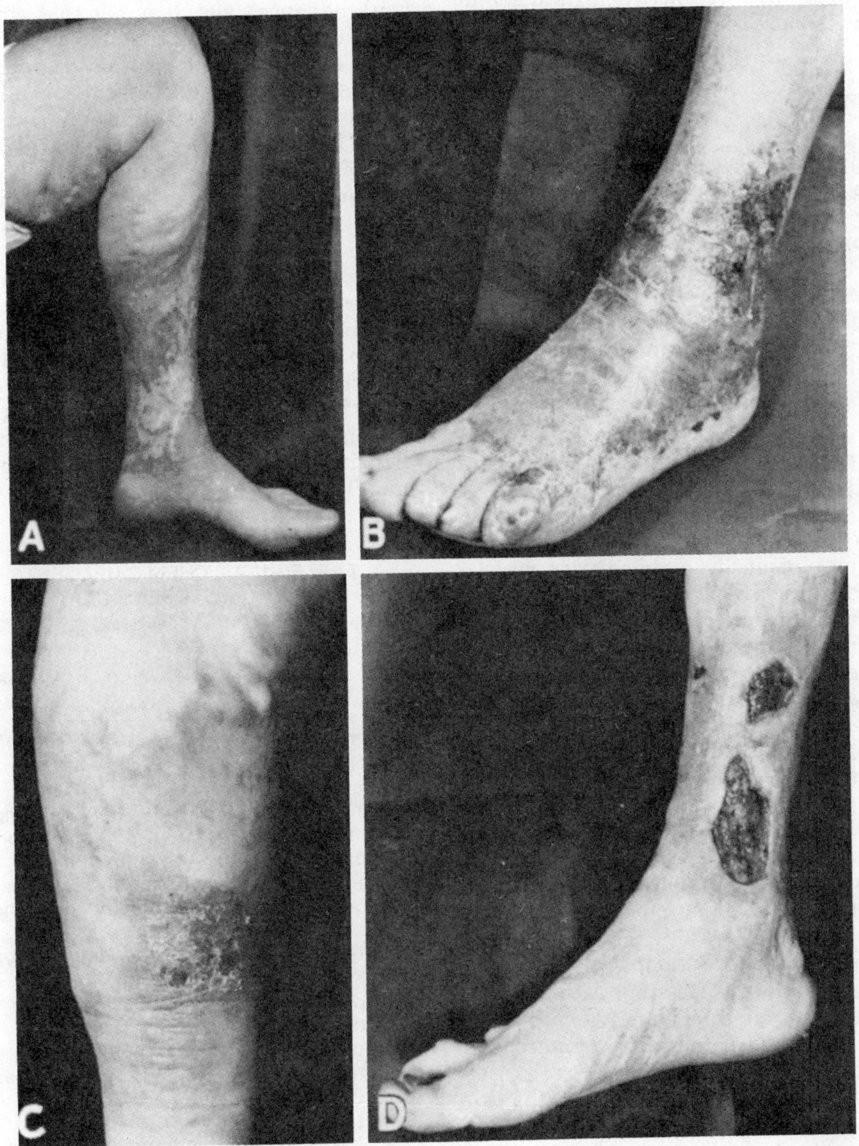

FIGURE 91–9. Stasis dermatitis (eczema) and stasis ulcers. *A*, Inactive and latent status in case of long standing; pigmentation and scar tissue represent healed lesions. *B*, Diffuse eczematous eruption; varicosities, heredity, middle age, and occupation (standing) are usual etiologic factors. *C*, Patchy eruption; varices are usually apparent. *D*, Ulcers are often furthered by trauma and infection in a setting of stasis dermatitis. (From Lewis, G. M., and Wheeler, C. E., Jr.: *Practical Dermatology.* 3rd ed. 1967.)

Systemic Lupus Erythematosus. This is considered an autoimmune disease, and patients with this condition have a very reactive antibody system. Antigen-antibody reactions lead to petechial skin lesions, skin ulcers, glomerulitis or widespread vasculitis, arthritis, pericarditis and pleuritis. The L.E. test, seen in blood smears, is positive in about 60 per cent of patients. The disease is more prevalent in women than men, and occurs between 10 and 50 years of age. Progressive renal failure is one of the most common causes of death.

Glucocorticosteroids are effective in reducing systemic symptoms but frequently produce side effects. Other drugs are presently being studied for their action in suppressing the inflammatory response.

PEMPHIGUS

Pemphigus is a rare disease of unknown etiology, although it is suspected of being an autoimmune disease. Large bullae appear in crops on the skin and mucous membranes. If untreated, the disease is frequently fatal. Large amounts of steroids are given until remission occurs. Symptomatic treatment is given for the skin lesions. Fluid balance and nutrition must be maintained and secondary infection prevented. Patients frequently have side effects from the high doses of steroids.

SKIN CONDITIONS DUE TO HEAT AND SUNLIGHT

Prickly Heat (Miliaria Rubra). This condition is characterized by pinpoint or pinhead-sized vesicles and papules with pricking and burning sensations, generally occurring under clothing and in individuals working in tropical climates or in conditions of excessive heat. Obstruction of outflow of sweat occurs at the sweat pore. Continued secretion of sweat results in its escape into the epidermis. This condition is frequently seen in infants.

Treatment is by avoiding sweating and by allowing circulation of air with looser, cooler clothing. Air conditioners and fans should be used when available. Cool baths and steroid sprays may be helpful. Topical ointments that are occlusive should be avoided. Once the tendency to prickly heat is established, it persists.

Skin Conditions Due to Sunlight. Exposure to sunlight is not an unmixed blessing. Although sun is necessary for life on this planet, exposure to ultraviolet radiation is potentially dangerous to people with white skin.

Sunburn is an inflammatory response of the skin to the ultraviolet radiation. The skin defends itself against this by producing more melanin. Tanning therefore provides the best protection against sunburn. Ultraviolet radiation can be reduced to as much as 90 per cent by a good tan.[7] Individuals incur more ultraviolet radiation at the mountains or beach because of the reflected radiation from sun or snow. The longer the pathway through the atmosphere, the less ultraviolet radiation. Sunbathing is therefore safer in the early morning and late afternoon.

Long-term exposure to ultraviolet radiation can cause damage to the skin. The damage in the dermis attributed to aging is in reality the result of chronic exposure to the sun and to short-wavelength ultraviolet light, as can be evidenced by comparing aging skin from the buttocks with skin from exposed areas. The alterations in connective tissue give the skin the coarse wrinkled appearance of aging. Undue exposure to the sun undoubtedly predisposes the skin to cancerous and precancerous growth (see below).

Lentigo Senilis. This common skin condition called "liver spots" seldom occurs before the fourth or fifth decade. The spots increase in numbers with advanced age. It is felt that chronic sunlight exposure is an important factor in their development. They have no relation to internal disease.[16]

Cheilitis. Because of the prominence of the lower lip, people with chronic sun damage may have lesions confined to the lower lip. These appear in the warm season as a result of exposure to the sun. A sunscreen like A-fil sun stick should always be used by those sensitive to sun damage when outdoors.[16]

Topical or systemic photosensitizers produce abnormal reactions to sunlight or artificial light. A number of internal diseases are characterized by abnormal reactions to light. In diagnosing dermatitis that is first affected or is limited to exposed areas, and that worsens in summer with outdoor exposure and is intensely pruritic, the possibility of photosensitivity must be considered (see Tables 91–2 and 91–3).

TABLE 91–2. CHEMICAL AGENTS CAUSING PHOTOSENSITIZATION

Substance	Reaction
Topical Photosensitizers and Usual Types of Reactions	
Bithionol	Erythema
Tetrachlorosalicylanilide	Erythema
Coal tar preparations	Erythema and pigmentation
Perfumes	Pigmentation
Laundry whiteners	Erythema
Parsnips and celery	Vesiculation and bullae
Lime and citrus fruits	Erythema and vesiculation
Ingested Chemicals Producing Photosensitivity	
Phenothiazines	Chloroquine
Tetracyclines	Quinine
Griseofulvin	Psoralens
Sulfonamides	Sulfonylureas
Chlorothiazide	Gold
Barbiturates	

Modified from Stewart, W. D., Danto, J. L., and Maddin, S.: *Synopsis of Dermatology.* 2nd ed. Chicago, The C. V. Mosby Company, 1970.

TABLE 91-3. SKIN DISEASES ADVERSELY AFFECTED BY SUNLIGHT

Albinism and vitiligo	Porphyria
Hartnup syndrome, a rare genodermatosis	Psoriasis (benefited by moderate sun exposure but made worse by sunburn)
Herpes simplex	Xeroderma pigmentosum
Lupus erythematosus	
Pellagra	

*Modified from Stewart, W. D., Danto, J. L., and Maddin, S.: *Synopsis of Dermatology.* 2nd ed. Chicago, The C. V. Mosby Company, 1970.

Sunburn. Varied burns of the skin result from intense and prolonged exposure to ultraviolet rays. First, second or third degree burns may occur, although the first two are more common.

TREATMENT. For mild first degree burns, bland creams or corticosteroid creams may be applied several times daily. Second degree burns characterized by blister formation should be treated by the doctor if extensive. A prolonged soak in a tub of cold water can be tried. Cold wet compresses or a water-miscible ointment can be applied to the affected areas. Fluids should be forced. Aspirin can reduce the general discomfort.

PREVENTION. Avoidance of sun exposure during the hours of intense short-wavelength ultraviolet light, that is, between 10 A.M. and 3 P.M., is important in all ages. Whenever possible, one should wear adequate clothing and gradually develop a tan. If untanned skins must be exposed to sun rays, sunscreens may be useful.

Precancerous Conditions. There is a direct relationship between the changes of chronic sun exposure and the development of precancerous or cancerous growths on the skin. The use of sun screens by individuals with marked skin change can be helpful (A-fil or Block-Out). Topical chemotherapeutic agents are being used. One of the most often used is 5-fluorouracil. This topically applied antimetabolite has been used by persons with actinic keratoses. The individual applies the medication with the fingers to the entire face and neck twice daily after washing, taking care to avoid the eyelids and lips. Erythema develops. The application is generally continued for two to three weeks on the face and for six to eight weeks on the hands and arms. The patient needs to be seen by the doctor every 7 to 10 days. This treatment produces photosensitivity and the patient has an unsightly appearance and some local discomfort during treatment, but it has been fairly successful in clearing the skin of precancerous lesions.

MALIGNANT TUMORS OF THE SKIN

Basal Cell Epithelioma. This is the most common type of skin cancer. The average age of onset is 57.3 years. It accounts for approximately 65 per cent of all skin cancers.

The most common variety begins as a papule that enlarges peripherally. It soon develops a central depression, becomes crusted and may bleed easily. The central area may become depressed, leading to ulceration and the classic rodent ulcer. The border may be translucent and elevated with a smooth shiny appearance on which fine telangiectatic vessels may be found. The lesion tends to be asymptomatic. Ninety per cent of the cases occur between the hairline and the upper lip. This is a locally invasive cancer that destroys underlying and adjacent tissue. It rarely metastasizes.

The major causative factor is prolonged sun exposure. The greatest natural protection is pigmentation. The tumor occurs more frequently in males, blonds and redheads. The incidence is increasing in the younger age group because of greater sun exposure.

TREATMENT. The three equally effective treatment modalities are (1) electrodesiccation and curettage; (2) x-ray therapy; and (3) surgical excision. The initial treatment of the lesion should be aggressive enough to be curative and patients should be checked at six-month intervals for evidence of recurrence.

Squamous Cell Carcinoma (Epidermoid Carcinoma). These lesions often come from keratoses due to exposure to ultraviolet, but may lack the pearly border of the basal cell epithelioma. Instead, one sees a flesh-colored nodule that may ulcerate. It enlarges more rapidly and can produce metastases. Squamous cell carcinomas arise on the mucous membrane from the chronic irritation of pipe smoking, dentures and teeth, and on the glans penis in uncircumcised males. However, squamous cell carcinomas are most often found on the lower lip, ears, neck and dorsum of the hands. They are more likely to metastasize if they are on the ears, cheek or temple areas, and particularly on the mucous membranes.

TREATMENT. The most satisfactory treatment includes surgical excision or irradiation by superficial or deep x-ray, radium or cobalt therapy.

Melanoma. Melanoma is the most malignant primary cutaneous tumor. This tumor is increasing in the Western world, with the greater exposure of light-skinned persons to sunlight.

A *nevus* is a tumor arising from cells present during the embryonic period. Cells composing it are called nevus cells. These cells in adults are present in collections in the dermis and epidermis, having migrated to these locations during the developmental period. They form growths of various sizes and degrees of brown pigmentation and are commonly referred to as "moles." Nevus cells wholly in the dermis characterize a benign lesion. Nevus cells lining the dermal-epidermal junction, usually in circumscribed nests or clusters, characterize a *junction nevus,* and lesions with these active junction nevus cells are the ones that may eventuate into a malignant melanoma. Pigmented nevi of the palms, soles, genitalia and mucous membranes are almost always junction nevi, as are flat or slightly elevated dark brown or black nevi. Lesions of the mucous membranes as well as those subjected to continual trauma or rubbing should probably be removed prophylactically.

Most invasive malignant melanomas arise from a previous pigmented junction nevus. The change from benign to malignant produces few warning symptoms. The incidence of the tumor is higher in females than in males and hits a peak around the menopausal years. One third of the lesions occur on the face and neck and one third on the lower extremities.

A biopsy of a potentially malignant melanoma should consist of total excision and microscopic examination of the whole lesion. Treatment of a malignant melanoma consists of adequate surgical excision with removal of regional lymph nodes. Arterial regional perfusion with new cytotoxic agents shows some promise in treatment.

SKIN LESIONS AS INDICATORS OF SYSTEMIC DISEASE

Diabetes. In diabetes, *pruritus* is the presenting symptom in 12 per cent of the cases. Diabetics have increased susceptibility to skin infections, both bacterial and fungal. Recurrent furuncles and carbuncles are usually found on the neck, axillae or vulvae. Paronychia, felons, cellulitis, styes, erythemas and widespread pyodermas are frequently seen as presenting signs. Frequently, the above-mentioned lesions are surrounded by an *erythematous halo.* Moniliasis is very common in diabetes, and all diabetic women have vulvovaginitis. Itching as a symptom of other systemic diseases has already been discussed under pruritus.

Pigmentation Disorders. Hyper- and hypopigmentations may occur and are of importance to the nurse in that she may be the first to see the condition and can provide this information for the doctor. *Hyperpigmentation* may be intensification of color at sites which are normally pigmented. Patchy brown to black pigmentation can be seen in many conditions not always related to systemic disease. A generalized or localized gray, slate or blue color may be concurrent with a disease process or may result from administration of drugs. A generalized yellow color may appear in jaundice, carotinemia, and after taking atabrine, an antimalarial drug. The skin may have a yellow cast in myxedema, uremia and pernicious anemia. Atabrine and carotene do not usually color the sclera. Much of skin color depends on blood flow through the skin and the status of blood in the vessels.

Disorders in which there is generalized *hypopigmentation* are albinism, hypopituitarism, hypothyroidism and phenylketonuria. Patchy hypopigmentation may be present in vitiligo, Addison's disease, burns, trauma and numerous other conditions.

Bleeding into the skin as a result of systemic disease may take the form of petechiae, purpura, ecchymoses and easy bruising. The appearance of any of these conditions needs to be reported and invgestigated if the underlying cause is not known.

References

1. American Public Health Association: *The Control of Communicable Diseases in Man.* Washington, The American Public Health Association, 1970.
2. Finch, C.: *A Patient Oriented Approach to General Medicine.* 1972.
3. Glick, A. W.: Basic soothing dermatologic therapy. *Cutis,* November, 1971.
4. Henderson, J.: *Emergency Medical Guide.* 2nd ed. New York, The Blakiston Division, McGraw-Hill Book Company, 1969.
5. Jarrett, A., Spearman, R. I. C., and Riley, P. A.: *Functional Dermatology.* Philadelphia, J. B. Lippincott Company, 1966.
6. Lewis, G. M., and Wheeler, C. E., Jr.: *Practical Dermatology.* Philadelphia. W. B. Saunders Company, 1967.
7. Odland, G. F.: *The Skin: A Description of the External Organ and Its Common Afflictions.* Seattle, University of Washington Press, 1971.
8. Pardo-Costello, V., and Pardo, O. A.: *Diseases of the Nails.* 3rd ed. Springfield, Ill. Charles C Thomas, 1960.
9. Reisner, R.: Rational therapy of acne vulgaris. *Cutis,* February, 1971.

9a. Rice, A. K.: Common skin infections in school children. *American Journal of Nursing,* 73:1905–1909, November, 1973.

10. Rothman, S., and Shapiro, A. L.: Itching (pruritus). *In* MacBryde, C. M. (ed.): *Signs and Symptoms.* 4th ed. Philadelphia, J. B. Lippincott Company, 1964, pp. 900–921.
11. Shafer, K. N., et al.: *Medical Surgical Nursing.* 5th ed. St. Louis, The C. V. Mosby Company, 1971.
12. Solomons, B.: *Lecture Notes on Dermatology.* Philadelphia, F. A. Davis Company, 1965.
13. Spoor, H. J.: Cosmetic dermatology. *Cutis,* November, 1971.
14. Stewart, W. D., Danto, J. L., and Maddin, S.: *Synopsis of Dermatology.* 2nd ed. St. Louis, The C. V. Mosby Company, 1970.
15. Strauss, J. S., and Pochi, P. E.: Acne vulgaris. *In* Yaffee, H. S. (ed.): *Newer Views of Skin Disease.* Boston, Little, Brown and Company, 1966.
16. Tindall, J. P.: Geriatric dermatology. *In* Chinn, A. (ed.): *Working with Older People.* Vol. IV, Clinical Aspects. Washington, D.C., U. S. Government, Department of Health, Education, and Welfare, 1971.
17. Tompkins, R. K.: Dermatological manifestations and systemic manifestations of diabetes mellitus. *Cutis,* March, 1972, p. 33.
18. Weigand, D. A., and Olson, R. L.: *Cutaneous Medicine.* Case Studies. Flushing, N. Y., Medical Examination Publishing Company, 1971.
19. Wilentz, J., and Berger, R. O.: Hippie dermatology. *Cutis,* July, 1972, p. 42.
20. Wright, B.: *Physical Disability. A Psychological Approach.* Evanston, Ill., Harper & Row, 1960.

CHAPTER 92

Trauma and Burns

The anatomy of the skin was reviewed in Chapter 91. One of the most frequent troubles that besets man is trauma, and the skin is the recipient of the major portion of this buffeting. In general, those tissues most likely to be injured have the greatest power of repair. The epidermis, for example, regenerates very well, probably better than any other tissue in the body. In most superficial wounds, such as minor burns and abrasions, the only tissue lost is the superficial layer of the epidermis. This is healed by acceleration of the normal process of maturation of basal cells. (Wound healing is also discussed in Chapter 22.) The phenomenon of blistering, unique to man, may have a protective function for this rapid multiplication of basal cells. The fluid from the blister, if left alone, is absorbed quite rapidly. When there is a large patch of epidermis lost, repair is by a process of epithelial migration from the edges of the wound and from any epithelial remnants left in the dermis.

THE BASIS OF WOUND HEALING

The healing of a deeply incised wound is divided into three phases: (1) Traumatic inflammation: Immediately after a deep wound, the edges become sealed together by a fibrous clot. Very soon the capillaries along the wound edge become dilated and the wound becomes swollen and red. (2) The destructive phase: This phase is continuous with the first phase and is concerned with removing dead and dying tissue and blood from the wound. Leukocytes and macrophages move into the wound and ingest all dead and dying tissue. During these two phases of four to six days no repair takes place. (3) The third phase is the *proliferation phase*. New capillaries sprout off the sides of existing ones. Fibroblasts then appear and proceed to lay down collagen, and the tensile strength of the wound rapidly increases. The process is thought to last for 4 to 14 days. Fibroplasia reaches its peak at 14 days, following which there is a general shrinkage and maturation of connective tissue in the wound.

A wound may heal by *first intention* or *second intention*. First intention healing is primary healing of a noninfected incised wound whose edges are brought together accurately. Second intention healing is the slow healing of a large defect by grannulation tissue and by epithelialization from the wound tissues. When there is a large skin defect, the aim is to speed reepithelialization by suturing the gap or covering it by means of a *skin graft* for the following reasons: (1) Until the wound is covered with epithelium, collagen formation in the deeper layers is poor; (2) bacterial contamination may be prevented; (3) fluid loss is lessened; and (4) painful dressings are not required.

Healing is a predictable process but can be disturbed by such factors as protein deficiency, which is associated with poor wound healing in man. Anemia delays healing by tissue anoxia, and lack of vitamin C, essential for formation of collagen, also delays healing. Metabolic diseases such as diabetes, liver failure and uremia, as well as aging, all affect wound healing. Steroids may have some effect on normal healing since they are anti-inflammatory in nature and inflammation is part of the process of wound healing. Lack of blood supply to an area, infection, hemorrhage and retained foreign bodies may impede healing. Absence of immobilization delays the healing process. Wounds of limbs unite better if the limb is splinted, and raw areas heal more quickly if left alone than if dressings are frequently pulled off and changed.

THE CARE OF CLOSED WOUNDS

Wounds may be classified as open or closed. The most common type of closed wound is a *contusion,* a bruise from a direct blow causing injury to the skin and underlying tissue. The degree or extent of the injury is in direct proportion to the force of the blow or degree of violence exerted against the tissue. Contusions are diagnosed by swelling and tenderness.

Treatment consists of cold wet compresses. An ice bag or fresh water aids in preventing further leakage of blood into the tissue from the broken blood vessels. The injured part should be put at rest. After 24 hours, heat may be applied to enhance absorption. If the contusion does not begin to improve within 24 hours or increases in size, the individual should see a physician.

A common and painful example of a contusion is hitting the fingertip with a hammer. The bruise occurs under the nail and, since the nail bed contains many small blood vessels, a little pool of blood accumulates under the nail and in a few days the nail turns black and the finger may become painful. The nail may be saved by prompt draining of the accumulated blood from beneath the nail by drilling a small hole into the nail. If the nail starts to heal, it should be kept in place with tape until the new nail pushes it off as it grows. The old nail will protect the nail bed and the new nail will look better.

THE CARE OF OPEN WOUNDS

Abrasions (Scrapes). An abrasion is an irregular superficial open wound of the skin in which the outer layers are scraped off. There is usually not much bleeding, but many nerve endings are exposed, making the wound painful and prone to infection. If the injury occurs where grease or gravel may be ground into the wound, the individual may get a permanent tattoo as well as infection if the foreign material is not removed.

Abrasions require careful tedious cleaning. A petroleum jelly dressing can be applied for comfort. If left exposed to the air, an eschar will form and provide proper protection.

Incised Wound. This is a wound cleanly cut by a sharp instrument. This tidy wound has no bruising or crushing of the wound margin. It tends to gape and bleed freely.

Stab or Puncture Wound. This wound is deeper than it is long and is caused by such objects as knives, pins and spikes. The entrance wound may be surprisingly small, but there may be damage to important deep structures and concealed blood loss.

Perforated or Penetrating Wound. These are puncture wounds caused by forcing bodies which may lodge in or pass through the tissue.

Laceration. This is an untidy wound caused by tearing, destruction and disruption of the tissues. A lacerated wound is unlikely to heal well. Immediate management is directed toward control of bleeding and the prevention of infection. Foreign matter may be flushed out with hydrogen peroxide after cleansing around the wound with antiseptic soap and water. Superficial lacerations which are not large and deep can be drawn together with a "butterfly" strip. A strip of ½ inch wide adhesive tape may be folded back on itself, and broad nicks cut at the folded end on each side to make the butterfly.

Patients with dirty wounds should be given prophylactic treatment against tetanus. The nurse has an important role in educating all individuals concerning the importance of tetanus immunization. Individuals who have been immunized within the past four years should be given a booster dose of toxoid. The reason for keeping individual tetanus immunity at a safe level is to avoid the problem of sensitivity to tetanus antitoxin. Human hyperimmune serum may be given if the individual has a history of reaction. If there is no history of allergic reaction and the patient needs tetanus antitoxin, sensitivity tests must be given prior to administration of the antitoxin.

MINOR SUTURING OF WOUNDS

In some areas, the nurse may have the option of doing minor suturing, if she has been prepared and supervised by the doctor. The patient will probably arrive at the site with the wound covered. Traumatic wounds are all contaminated to some degree.

After bleeding has been controlled, the first aim should be to prevent infection. The nurse should discard the bandage and cover the wound with a sterile pad after observation. History and observation of the extent and location of the injury will help her decide the necessity of securing medical assistance. In face or hand lacerations and wounds involving repair of deep nerves, blood vessels and tendons, the patient should be sent to a doctor.

Preliminary steps are as follows:

Step 1: Clean the surrounding skin with soap and water or a detergent. The cleansing should continue until no more material can be removed or seen. Follow this with a wash with sterile water or saline. If the wound is to be sutured, it is covered with a sterile pad while anesthesia is applied.

Step 2: Anesthesia. The patient should be questioned about allergy to anesthetic agents. Circumferential injection of 1 per cent procaine or lidocaine is satisfactory. To infiltrate the area, raise a skin wheal with a 25-gauge needle. Insert a longer 22-gauge needle through the wheal to infiltrate the deeper area desired. Not only the skin but all the deeper tissues implicated by the wound must be infiltrated. Injection must be made in sites away from and towards the wound. The drug begins to act in 5 to 15 minutes and its duration of action is 45 to 90 minutes.

Step 3: Cleaning the wound proper. Sterile gloves may be used and the dressing again discarded. The wound may be flushed with sterile saline and foreign bodies extracted with sterile forceps.

Exploration, Identification and Excision. Using dissecting forceps and skin hooks, the wound should be opened and all foreign bodies removed. Contused or frayed skin edges must be pared. In general, the walls of the wound are all cut back about 2 mm. All loosened and very bruised tissue is excised. This is best done with a knife rather than scissors. Hemostasis should be by pressure without any ligature if possible. If larger vessels require ligation, the doctor will do this, using the very finest size catgut. If nerves, tendons or damaged muscles are present, the doctor will wish to do the suturing himself. The nurse may test the viability of muscle by color, evidence of bleeding and contractility of the muscle when it is pinched.

In suturing in a deep field, the tissue should be grasped with a forceps. When working on skin, forceps with teeth should be used. While holding the tissue with a forceps, insert the needle. To insert the curved needle (a quarter of the distance from the eye end of the needle), a turning force may be exerted on the needle holder.

The sutures should not be tied with excess tension but only approximated so that a square knot may be tied. The wound is closed layer by layer as exactly as possible. Dead space must be obliterated if possible. Skin edges are opposed by 000 or 0000 nonabsorbable sutures placed very close together and as near the edge of the skin as possible. Clips are used only in areas where the blood supply is excellent, and require removal within 48 hours. Inter-

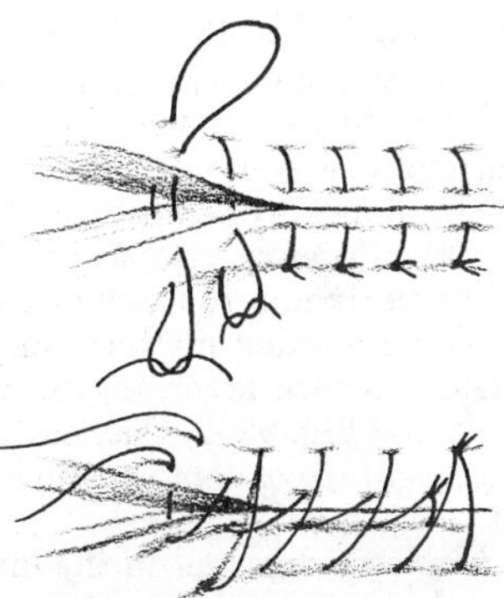

FIGURE 92-1. Vertical mattress suture. (From Nealon, T. F., Jr.: *Fundamental Skills in Surgery.* 2nd ed. 1971.)

rupted and vertical mattress sutures are used (Fig. 92-1).

A no-touch technique may be achieved by using a sterile towel and by placing those parts of the instruments that touch the wound on the towel.

Instruments necessary:

Dissecting forceps, one with and one without teeth
Suture scissors
Scissors with blades curved on the flat
Gillies skin hooks
Needle holder
1 Bard Parker scalpel with handle No. 3
2 scalpel blades Nos. 10, 11 or 15
1 tissue forceps 4½ inches
1 straight skin needle
1 medium curved cutting edge needle
1 medium curved taper point needle
Suture material

Minimal trauma needles are available. In these, suture material is threaded into the needle beforehand. Suitable lengths of fine silk or other nonabsorbable material can be threaded on curved needles beforehand. Curved needles are necessary for the deep parts of the wound and straight needles should only be used for the skin. The point of the needle may be tapered or it may have a cutting edge. The cutting edge needle is used for suturing skin and a needle with a tapered tip is used in deeper tissues.

Wound Care. If the wound edges are perfectly opposed and not disturbed or manipulated, adhesion of wound edges is achieved in some six hours and infection cannot enter. Dry skin is more resistant to infection than moist, and friction adds to the chance of infection. Unless signs of distress occur, a dressing should be left alone until the sutures are removed. For a wound of minimal extent, a simple dry dressing is applied and held in place by ventilated strapping. Dressings should be removed only if there is hematoma, drainage, indications of infection or unexplained fever. Reassurance of the patient and instructions concerning care and return should be given to the patient. It is advisable to keep the wound dry.

Removal of Sutures. Skin sutures are generally left in for 7 to 10 days, or longer if in an area where there is a lot of movement. The dressing is removed and the skin cleaned with ether. To remove a suture, the knot is seized in a hemostat and sufficient traction is exerted to raise the stitch from the skin. Employing a fine, pointed scalpel, the suture is severed flush with the skin. It is important that no part of the stitch above the skin level enter and contaminate the stitch tract. After removal of all sutures, it is not necessary to cleanse the wound. It should be left dry and a vapor-permeable dressing applied.

BURNS

Incidence. Accidental injuries involving burns are usually acquired in one of two ways—(1) by involvement in an uncontrolled fire or explosion or (2) through contact of some part of the body with a hot object, liquid, acid or other substance with a flame. The former is the more common cause of death, and the latter, of nonfatal injury.

Fires and explosions are the third leading cause of accidental deaths in the United States, causing about 7200 deaths annually, a rate of 4.0 per 1000 persons. This has been relatively stable in the last 10 years. Burns are the leading cause of deaths from nontransport accidents in children one to four years of age, and the second leading cause in children 5 to 14 and persons 45 and over. There are about 270,000 persons in the United States with impairments due to uncontrolled fires and explosions. The injury rate is the inverse of the mortality rate for individuals 15 to 24 years old.

The death rate for nonwhite persons is more than three times that for white persons everywhere in the United States, and is greatest under age five. Under age one, the rate for nonwhites is more than seven times the rate for whites. The death rate is highest for Indians and second highest for blacks. More than 80 per cent of these deaths occur in homes. Burns are unevenly distributed geographically, being 20 to 30 per cent more frequent in the South and West.

Deaths and injuries from fires and explosions are usually caused by one of the following: (1) fire from cooking or heating sources; (2) smoking and the use of matches; (3) electrical deficiencies or improper use of electrical equipment or utilities; (4) fire in rubbish or trash; (5) flammable liquids or grease.

Prevention. Doctors and nurses faced with the problem of treating burns have every reason to be motivated to work on the problem of prevention. The causes of burns are complex. Frequently they happen to the dependent young in situations where there is inadequate supervision. The high incidence in the nonwhite points to a relationship with poverty. Parents who are emotionally disturbed or lack money for child care need emergency resources where help can be secured. The nurse, in working with patients or children, can be alert to those cues indicating inability to adequately protect the child. In the home, the community health nurse has an even better opportunity to help the family to "burn-proof" the home and to establish a family escape plan in case of fire.

Education concerning first aid care may also be helpful. The school nurse can work for incorporation of fire prevention and first aid in the school curriculum. As a citizen, the nurse can bring dangerous appliances, clothing, etc. to the public attention and encourage citizen action. The elderly need to take special safety precautions, and the cigarette-smoking drinker is another special problem.

First Aid. The only treatment that has been found to materially decrease the degree or depth of a burn is immediate immersion or covering of the burned area with cool or cold water as soon as possible after the burn. This decreases the temperature, lessening the amount of tissue damage by the burn. Actually, nothing should be done for a patient except to wrap him in clean sheets and a blanket and to transfer him to the nearest hospital for a physician's care. No clothing should be removed, no ointment applied, and no sedation given.

Evaluation of Burns. It is important to classify a burn as soon as it is first seen in order to determine the type of treatment that will be needed. A superficial burn of 1 to 12 per cent may be treated in the emergency room or doctor's office with home care provided thereafter, including visits to the doctor's office as required. A superficial burn of up to 15 per cent may receive oral replacement therapy in the hospital. A deeper burn of this extent should be regarded as serious and should always have hospital care.

There are in general two methods for appraising the percentage of body surface burned: the Rule of Nines, first proposed by E. J. Pulaski and C. W. Tennison, and a more precise method devised by Lund and Browder. In the Rule of Nines, the body is divided into areas which equal 9 per cent of total body surface. The head and neck represent 9 per cent; the anterior and posterior trunks each represent 18 per cent; the upper extremities each represent 9 per cent, and the lower extremities each represent 18 per cent. The perineum represents 1 per cent.[2]

The Lund and Browder method computes percentages of body surface according to relative age (see Table 92–1 and Fig. 92–2). The doctor attempts to gauge the percentage of depth of the burn as well as the extent.

The depth of a burn depends on the intensity and the duration of the heat. In a hot water burn, the body temperature cools the heat from the hot water and generally results in a superficial second degree burn. The body cannot rapidly cool heat from a flame burn. It usually results in deep second degree or third degree burn.

Crews[7] classifies burns as follows:

> A *first degree* burn has redness of the skin without blister formation.

> A *superficial second degree* burn causes blisters to burn with redness in and around the blistered areas. This is usually caused by contact with a hot or boiling liquid.

> A *deep second degree* burn is one in which all is destroyed but the deeper layers of the dermis. Certain areas of clothing burns will cause deep second degree burns.

> A *third degree* burn causes complete destruction of the skin. The burned skin has a brownish leathery appearance.

> A *fourth degree* burn has not only destroyed the full thickness of the skin but structures underneath the skin as well.

> A *char burn* is a destruction of the body area involved by charring. The area is black. Deep electrical burns are char burns and usually produce toxins which endanger life.

Methods of Treatment. Minor burns not requiring hospitalization are less extensive first degree burns and superficial second degree burns of less than 15 per cent and deep second degree burns of less than 6 per cent or small spots of third degree burns. The extensive first degree burn may be

TABLE 92–1. CONTRIBUTION OF VARIOUS BODY AREAS TO TOTAL BODY SURFACE AT DIFFERENT AGES, BY PER CENT*

Area	Birth	1 Year	5 Years	10 Years	15 Years	Adult
Head	19	17	13	11	9	7
Neck	2	2	2	2	2	2
Anterior trunk	13	13	13	13	13	13
Posterior trunk	13	13	13	13	13	13
Buttocks	5	5	5	5	5	5
Genitalia	1	1	1	1	1	1
Upper arms	8	8	8	8	8	8
Forearms	6	6	6	6	6	6
Hands	5	5	5	5	5	5
Thighs	11	13	16	17	18	19
Legs	10	10	11	12	13	14
Feet	7	7	7	7	7	7

*From Artz, L. P., and Moncrief, J. A.: *The Treatment of Burns.* 2nd ed. Philadelphia, W. B. Saunders Company, 1969, p. 91. (Adapted from Lund, C. C., and Browder, N. C.: The estimation of areas of burns. *Surgery, Gynecology and Obstetrics,* 79:352, 1944.)

treated in the doctor's office or in the emergency room by cleaning with pHisoHex, debriding ruptured blisters and those that might rupture, and bandaging with an inner layer of Furacin gauze. Individuals with such burns should have tetanus prophylaxis and the doctor will probably prescribe antibiotics for several days. The patient should keep a daily temperature record and notify the physician of any rise.

Most burns of any extent require hospitalization and receive the cleansing and debriding treatment but are treated by the "open" method. If the depth of the burn is not yet determined, the patient may stay in the hospital for a couple of days and then be discharged with the closed method of treatment. Patients with deep second degree burns or third degree burns of less than 15 per cent may be given saline solution, if tolerated (1 teaspoon salt, ½ teaspoon soda per quart of water). If the patient cannot take oral fluids, intravenous therapy may be started.

Patients with superficial second degree burns of greater than 30 per cent or third degree burns of lower than 15 per cent should be started on intravenous electrolyte and colloid replacement and hourly intake and output of fluids.

The outcome of treatment of burns is related to the extent and degree of depth of the burns. In the elderly, the chances for survival are much less. Any patient who survives will have to be covered with his own skin. Homografts are only a temporary solution and a three-week interval must elapse before skin can be taken from the same donor site. Infection, antibiotic resistance, supporting nutrition and the patient's will to live are all important factors in recovering.

Admission to the Hospital. The patient may be taken immediately to the intensive care unit or operating room, if there is no special burn unit in the facility, or to a private room on the surgical floor.

Of first concern in the severely burned patient is survival and maintenance of vital functions. If respiratory distress is present, an airway must be established. An endotracheal tube or tracheostomy may be necessary. The following information should be obtained as soon as possible:

> When and how the burn occurred: Fluid therapy for the first 24 hours is based on the number of hours after the burn. Associated injuries must be considered. A patient burned in an automobile accident may have other injuries.

> Identification of cause and circumstances of burn: Was it a flash explosion, scald, chemical or electrical burn? Was it accidental or intentional?

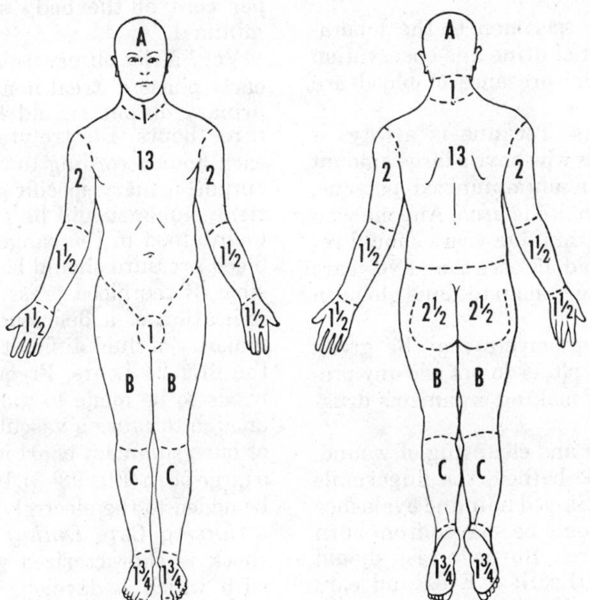

Relative Percentage of Areas Affected by Growth

	Age in Years					
	0	1	5	10	15	Adult
A—½ of head	9½	8½	6½	5½	4½	3½
B—½ of one thigh	2¾	3¼	4	4¼	4½	4¾
C—½ of one leg	2½	2½	2¾	3	3¼	3½

FIGURE 92-2. Lund and Browder charts. These charts permit a rather accurate method for determining percentage of body surface involved. (From Artz, C. P., and Moncrief, J. A.: *The Treatment of Burns.* 2nd ed. 1969.)

> Prior treatment: What kind of first aid was given? Has patient been given medication or fluids? Amount and kind. Has tetanus prophylaxis been given?

> Relevant past history: Heart disease, renal disease, diabetes, ulcers, and allergies will influence treatment. Were there any other contributing causes, such as alcoholism, epilepsy or psychiatric disorders?

Procedure for the Early Treatment of Major Burns in Treatment Room or Operating Room

1. A cutdown may be performed and a plastic cannula inserted by aseptic technique. One of the best areas is the cephalic vein in the shoulder area. Cutdowns are not used frequently in many hospitals.
2. Continuous infusion of 5 per cent glucose in lactate Ringer's solution. Morphine sulfate, 0.1 mg./lb. for children and 10 mg. total for adults diluted in 3 to 5 ml. of saline, may be injected into the vein over a period of two to three minutes to allay apprehension and relieve pain. Extreme restlessness in burn patients may be due to hypovolemia and hypoxia rather than pain from severe burn injury, and gastric dilatation may occur.
3. Nothing by mouth. Paralytic ileus is often a complication.
4. Foley catheter-urine specimen to the laboratory. Hourly measurement of urine and observation of pH, specific gravity and presence of blood are vital.
5. Tetanus prophylaxis. Tetanus is always a potential danger in patients who have a large amount of dead tissue present. In unimmunized persons, hyperimmune tetanus globulin is used. Anyone who has had tetanus toxoid within five years should receive a booster dose of toxoid. If more than five years have passed, hyperimmune human tetanus globulin should be used.
6. Antibiotics and streptomycin may be given prophylactically. Some hospitals do not use any prophylactic drugs for fear of making organisms drug-resistant.
7. Intravenous sedation and cleansing of wound. The whole body should be bathed, the fingernails trimmed and the hair cut. Singed hair and eyelashes should be clipped. Hair should be shaved from burn wound and surrounding area. Burned areas should be gently washed with pHisoHex. Eyes and ears should be checked to see if special treatment is necessary. Photographs should be taken if possible.
8. The patient should be transferred to a bed on clean sheets and a cradle placed over him. It will be necessary to change the sheets because of dampness. Electrical heaters may be placed on either side of the bed to keep the patient warm.
9. Strict isolation technique must be instituted from time of admission until grafting is done. Personnel must use gowns and masks and wash their hands scrupulously for those procedures not requiring sterile gloves.
10. The patient is placed in a supine position during shock phase of treatment. Later, if burns are circumferential, he is rotated in a circular bed or a Stryker frame to allow the back to dry. The crust becomes fairly firm after two to three days of exposure to the air.
11. Burned hands are treated by the closed method. Each finger is wrapped separately with Furacin gauze and the fingers separated with plain gauze. The hand is placed in a position of function. In deep neck burns or inhalation burns, a tracheotomy may be done after the initial vital procedures have been carried out and before edema becomes a problem. These patients should also be treated with humidifiers and oxygen therapy.

Sedation in large burns should be minimal and should be administered intravenously. The patient has to learn to live 24 hours a day with discomfort. Tranquilizers are of great aid to the adult while he is adapting to being a burn patient.

Blood chemistry, blood count and urinalysis specimens should be taken on admission. Blood should be typed and cross-matched. Chest x-rays, electrocardiograms and blood urea nitrogen should be obtained in the elderly and when indicated.

Sulfamylon is a recently introduced topical agent that has been used successfully in many institutions. Sulfamylon in a 10 per cent water base is applied with a gloved hand once a day or as necessary to keep a good quantity on the surface. Mortality rates from burns of 40 to 50 per cent have been reduced from 61 to 20 per cent. With burns of over 50 per cent of the body surface, success has been minimal.

Very strict observation of the patient during the early phase of treatment is required. An adequate urinary output should be obtained within two to three hours. Electrolyte mixture may be ordered each hour according to the previous hour's urinary output, urinary specific gravity, etc. In an adult patient, fluids should be given so that the output is maintained in the range of 20 to 30 ml./hour. The blood pressure should be charted every hour if possible. If the blood pressure is low, it is usually an indication of a deficiency in plasma volume. The majority of fluid difficulties are encountered during the first 24 hours. Frequent adjustment in intake needs to be made to make up for the loss but not enough to cause a vascular overload. A metabolism or burn summary chart is a necessity when treating a large burn (Fig. 92–3). Intravenous vitamins should be added to the electrolyte solution every day.

Nursing Care During the Shock Phase. Burn shock is characterized primarily by the slowness with which it develops. The adult patient is frequently alert and able to give an intelligent history of the accident when admitted.

SYMPTOMS OF BURN SHOCK. The nurse is an important member of the team in the observation and management of the patient, and must be alert to indications of shock. Burn losses are such that the body can respond to them initially. It is only after the body has exhausted its protective defenses that shock is manifest. The body is quick to preserve the blood volume and its constituents by vasoconstriction, increased heart rate, decreased cardiac output, decreased blood flow, oliguria and output of protective

TIME OF BURN

NAME							DAY POST BURN INJURY				WEIGHT		HEIGHT		PERCENTAGE OF BURN					DATE		
TIME	T	P	R	BP	CVP	HCT	ELECTROLYTE INSERTION SITE	HOURLY / TOTAL	COLLOID INSERTION SITE	HOURLY / TOTAL	D5W INSERTION SITE	HOURLY / TOTAL	URINE HOURLY / TOTAL	SPEC. GRAVITY	HEM	ph	PO or NG IN HOURLY / TOTAL	TYPE	NG OUT or EMESIS HOURLY / TOTAL	STOOL	HEM	REMARKS
3							*lactated ringers rt. arm*		*albuminsol rt. subclavian*				100/100	1.030	+	6			0/0			*10 mgm morphene sulfate IV push*
3^{15}	97	120	30	110/70	4	56	//	100/100	//	100/100			0/100						0/0			*0.5 Tet. Toxoid*
3^{30}							//	200/300	//	300/400	*rt. subclavian*		0/100						0/0			
4		120	28	120/72	6		//	200/500	//	0/400	//	100/100	50/150	1.029	+	7			120/120			*5 mill. units penicillin IV push*
4^{30}							//	300/800	//	100/500	//	0/100	0/150						0/120			
5	98	116	24	120/72	7		//	200/1000	//	0/500	//	200/300	30/180	1.024	0	7			100/220			
6	98	110	24	120/70	7	50	*D-5 lactated ringers*	200/1200		0/500		100/400	40/220	1.024	0	7			0/220			

FIGURE 92–3. Burn summary sheet. (From Jacoby, F. G.: *Nursing Care of the Patient with Burns*. St. Louis, The C. V. Mosby Co., 1972.)

stress hormones such as epinephrine, antidiuretic hormones and aldosterone. The wound edema is caused by damaged capillaries which have lost water, sodium chloride and plasma into the damaged areas. Large replacement solutions must be given before shock sets in.

THIRST. Nearly every burn patient complains persistently of thirst. Burned patients are not permitted to drink anything for the first 48 hours in burns of severe or undetermined extent. Renal excretion of water is drastically decreased shortly after burning so that water intoxication can easily occur. Clinically, water intoxication shows itself by apathy, tremors, loss of visual acuity, headache, diarrhea, oliguria, vomiting and, finally, generalized seizures and death.

RESTLESSNESS. Restlessness is always likely to be present in severely burned patients. It is important to observe whether it increases or regresses as the treatment continues. Increasing restlessness is likely to be a sign of inadequate resuscitation.

DELIRIUM, COMA OR SEIZURES. Delirium or coma is an especially serious sign within the first 96 hours if there has been no head injury, since it probably results from inadequate cerebral blood flow. Seizures can result from cerebral ischemia and may be a sign of increasing shock. Alcoholics can be expected to develop delirium tremens during the first hours after burning. Many patients are drunk when they are burned and it is helpful to elicit this from friends or family or from the history.

BLOOD PRESSURE AND PULSE. The badly burned patient should be left supine for at least 48 to 72 hours to eliminate unnecessary postural stress. The supine person can tolerate a deficit of 20 to 25 per cent of his blood volume with little or no change in pulse or blood pressure. The blood pressure may be unobtainable with a pneumatic cuff, since there frequently are burns on all limbs. Central venous pressure may be monitored in some instances. Blood pressure and pulse should approach a normal rate as treatment progresses.

CYANOSIS. Unburned skin should be pressed for capillary filling. A warm pink skin with normal capillary filling time indicates a circulation that is physiologically intact. Most patients with severe burns have pale cool skin for some hours owing to the compensatory cutaneous vasoconstriction. This is not a serious symptom unless it persists. Cyanosis in an acutely burned patient may be due to (1) a circumferential eschar—if it is thoracic or abdominal, it may cause general cyanosis; (2) cardiovascular decompensation with stasis of blood in the peripheral tissues; (3) ventilatory insufficiency due to injury to the respiratory tract.

OLIGURIA. Urine flow is scanty or absent. The first urine may be chocolate brown or red owing to hemoglobin pigment released into the plasma by the destroyed red blood cells. In adults, a flow of at least 30 ml./hour is a reasonably safe indication that the kidneys are functioning. Renal shutdown is a serious problem.

RESPIRATION. Tachypnea may be present but the character of the respiration should be normal unless there is some problem. Pulmonary injury may be detected by prolongation of the expiratory phase of respiration.

FLUID DEFICIT AND REPLACEMENT FORMULAS

Burned parts immediately and inevitably swell. The blisters may contain fluid, and fluid may ooze from debrided areas, but most of the fluid is in the tissues around and beneath the wound.

Metabolic acidosis develops within a few hours after burning. Treatment of the acidosis may be expected to reduce the possibility of pulmonary venous engorgement.

Monafo[20] has evaluated the various fluids used in burns and believes hypertonic lactated saline solution is best. The HLS solution is given by mouth as well as intravenously whenever possible, up to 100 ml./hour depending on the size of the patient.

In addition to observing for signs of shock and coordinating the management of treatments, the nurse is responsible for seeing that the patient is as comfortable as possible. Medication for pain may be given intravenously. Burned limbs are elevated on pillows. The establishment of normal urinary flow and fluid replacement is the first step in survival.

Numerous formulas have been proposed and used for fluid and electrolyte replacement in burns, and each of them has its advocates. We include here three typical burn formulas for use during the first 48 hours after injury, adapted from Artz and Moncrief's book *The Treatment of Burns.*[2]

THE EVANS FORMULA. The Evans formula was introduced in 1952. The fluid requirements during the first 24 hours are as follows:

Colloids: 1 ml./kg./per cent of body surface burned.

Physiologic saline solution: 1 ml./kg./per cent of body surface burned.

Nonelectrolytes: 2000 ml. of 5 per cent dextrose in water, or correspondingly less in children.

Evans recommended one half these amounts of colloids and electrolytes during the second 24-hour period. He was the first to warn that, in a burn involving more than 50 per cent of the body surface, fluid requirements should be estimated as though only 50 per cent of the body surface had been burned.

THE BROOKE FORMULA. The Brooke formula, developed at Brooke Army Medical Center, and published in 1953, is a slight modification of the Evans formula. It estimates the following fluid requirements for the first 24 hours following injury:

Colloids (blood, dextran or plasma): 0.5 ml./kg./ per cent of body surface burned.

Lactated Ringer's solution: 1.5 ml./kg./per cent of body surface burned.

Water requirement (dextrose in water): 2000 ml. for adults, children correspondingly less.

The second 24-hour period requirements for colloids and lactated Ringer's solution are about one-half those for the first 24 hours. In applying this formula to burns larger than 50 per cent, requirements must be calculated as though only 50 per cent had been burned. Usually it is not necessary to give more than 10 liters of fluid during the first 24 hours to any patient, regardless of the extent of the burn. If, in a burn of more than 50 per cent in a large patient, fluid therapy based on a 50 per cent restriction fails to prevent signs and symptoms of circulatory failure, therapy must be cautiously increased. One half of the estimated fluid requirement for the first 24 hours is usually given in the first eight hours, one fourth in the second eight hours and one fourth in the third eight hours.

THE MGM FORMULA. The Massachusetts General Hospital formula favors a therapeutic approach in which plasma with only a very small amount of added saline is used. In adults, this formula calls for the following fluids:

For the first 24 hours:

1. *125 ml. plasma/per cent of burn.*
2. *15 ml. saline/per cent of burn.*
3. *2000 ml. 5 per cent dextrose in water.*

For the second 24 hours:

1. *One half of the first 24-hour requirement of plasma and saline.*
2. *2000 ml. 5 per cent dextrose in water.*

For children, a more precise allowance for surface area is necessary, and it is recommended that 90 ml. of plasma and 10 ml. of saline for each per cent of burn times the surface area in square meters be used to calculate the colloid and electrolyte requirements. In addition, an amount of 5 per cent dextrose in water is given according to the calculated normal fluid needs of the child.

Burn Wound Care

The skin can be considered an effective barrier between man and his environment. Until a new skin cover is provided, the patient is in serious jeopardy from overwhelming infection. Effective treatment of the wound is just as important as shock prevention because, after 18 to 24 hours, the wound will become densely colonized with pathogenic bacteria if untreated. Unfortunately if the bacterial count is reduced, other organisms such as *Candida albicans* (a fungus) or Pseudomonas proliferate. The resistance to bacterial infection is decreased markedly for the first week after injury.

Infection. Infection is controlled by removal of the eschar and necrotic material, by wound cleansing, and by the use of topical agents to inhibit bacterial growth. Except for *Staphylococcus aureus* and β-hemolytic streptococcus, the majority of wound organisms are gram-negative (*E. coli,* Proteus, Enterobacter, Klebsiella, Aerobacter and Pseudomonas). The bacteria of the normal flora do not cause disease unless accidentally introduced into normally protected regions of the body.

Each region of the body has a characteristic flora. The bacteria that populate the skin include mainly corynebacterium, micrococci, nonhemolytic streptococci, and mycobacteria (see Chapter 91). Moist areas harbor yeast and other fungi. *Pseudomonas aeruginosa,* an anaerobic gram-negative organism, requires organic compounds as an energy source and is able to establish infection only in individuals with a severely lowered natural resistance. Yeasts and Candida are dominant and important when more susceptible bacteria of the normal flora are suppressed. They may invade the blood stream and result in fatal sepsis.

Polymixins and gentamicin are the most effective antimicrobial agents used against Pseudomonas. Normal flora of the intestinal tract may also invade burn wounds (gram-negative *E. coli, Aerobacter aerogenes* and *Proteus vulgaris*). Kanamycin and nitrofurantoin are most effective drugs against Proteus. If invasion by yeast is suspected, nystatin and amphotericin B are the most effective drugs.

The nurse can use the tabulation found below in observing for signs of infection.[12]

Systematic measures against infection are generally taken in the following order: antibiotic therapy; vaccine therapy; whole blood; hyperalimentation; and supportive measures.

	Staphylococcus aureus	**Pseudomonas**	**Candida albicans**
Appearance of wound	Dissolution of granulation	Patchy black necrosis	Dry, flat, yellow or orange, granular
Course	Insidious, 2–6 days	Rapid, 12–36 hours	Chronic
Disorientation	Severe	Mild or absent	None
Temperature	Hyperpyrexia	Hypothermia	Normal to low
WBC	Usually increased	Usually depressed	Normal to increased
Ileus	Severe	Severe	None
Hypotension	Insidious, followed by oliguria	Sudden, with oliguria	None
Mortality	0–10%	50–60%	90%

The use of Pseudomonas vaccine therapy in all significantly burned patients causes the incidence of Pseudomonas infections to drop. If invasion with yeast is suspected, treatment with nystatin and amphotericin B is most effective.

The course of infection may be as shown in the table at the bottom of the page.

The use of exposure treatment in an environment of 32° C. (90° F.) and 20 to 30 per cent relative humidity without systemic antibiotics seems to be strikingly successful. The method seems to have dramatically improved mortality and provided rapid drying of the burn and a smaller weight loss.[14]

Specific measures that the nurse can take to decrease infection are: avoid undue contamination; use strict control over hand washing; use protective clothing and masks, sterile instruments and gloves when touching the wound; and thoroughly clean Hubbard tanks. Whether the wound is treated by an open or closed method is not the key factor, since in the closed method the moist warm environment promotes growth but limits bacteria from outside, but in the open method drying inhibits bacterial proliferation. Coverage of the wound by skin grafting will eliminate virtually all bacteria within 24 hours.

Curling's ulcer is a complication of severe burns. The incidence of Curling's ulcer increases with increasing burn size to a maximum of 40 per cent in burns of 70 per cent or more of the total body surface.[22] Preexisting sepsis has been shown to be an additive stress predisposing the burn patient to development of Curling's ulcer. Gastric distention is an early sign in some cases; ileus, bleeding and a drop in hematocrit are more acute signs. The time from the onset of infection to the evidence of Curling's ulcer formerly averaged about 4.5 days. Since the advent of sulfamylon therapy, the mean postburn onset of Curling's ulcer has increased from 10 to 15 days, reflecting the control of the bacterial complication in burn wounds. The most frequent initial complication is a gastrointestinal hemorrhage. Curling's ulcer is one of the most frequent life-threatening complications in burn patients.[22] Nurses can be particularly alert for signs of gastric distress in severely burned patients whose wounds have become infected.

The Use of Silver Compounds. Silver has been shown to be an effective agent in inhibiting the growth of both gram-positive and gram-negative bacteria. Commonly used treatments are: 0.5 per cent aqueous silver nitrate solution; colloidal silver complex; and silver sulfadiazine.

SILVER NITRATE TECHNIQUE. A plastic washbasin is filled with warmed 0.5 per cent silver nitrate solution. Precut and rolled dressings 6 feet in length are soaked in the solution and then applied to all burned areas. The dressings are held in place with bias cut stockinette, secured with safety pins, and the patient is covered with dry sheets and at least one dry cotton blanket. The dry covers are important and must be changed when they become wet. The dressings are kept soaking wet. If kept wet, reepithelialization will take place within the 15th to 40th day.

During the first 7 to 14 days, the dressings need be changed only once daily. After the eschar begins to liquefy and separate, three or four daily dressings may be necessary. As soon as treated parts are exposed to sunlight, the eschar darkens and turns brown or black or blue, depending on the depth of the burn and the amount of sunlight. Hard blue-black eschars on wounds dressed with solution for more than a week indicate a probable subdermal burn. If infection is controlled, these will remain in place for weeks, until they finally separate from the granulating adipose tissue. If the adipose tissue is burned, the eschars will begin to separate a few days after the injury. If this occurs, they must be removed promptly as liquefied fat is an excellent medium for bacterial growth.

Eschars of intradermal burns are brown or brown black and begin to separate after 7 to 10 days.

THE COURSE OF BURN INFECTION AND ITS TREATMENT

Initial:	0–7 days	β-hemolytic streptococcus	Penicillin
Autolytic:	8–21 days	*Staphylococcus aureus*	Staphycillin Erythromycin Novobiocin
Granulating:	22–30 days	Pseudomonas	Gentamicin Colymycin Carbenicillin
Grafting:	31 days to coverage	β-hemolytic streptococcus Yeast	Penicillin Chloramphenicol Nystatin Amphotericin B

DANGERS OF USE. Sodium, potassium and other minerals and water-soluble vitamins are leached into the dressing. Patients must be continually monitored by blood and urine tests, and mineral and vitamin supplements are given regularly.

Silver nitrate stains everything that it touches. Special rooms, linen, etc. are necessary.

Colloidal silver complex drastically reduces mineral losses into the dressing. It is relatively unstable and is more expensive. Where this has been used, wounds do not convert to full thickness injury, skin grafts are reduced and the patient has less trauma, since wounds not contaminated by bacteria have no odor, do not bleed freely at dressing change and are relatively painless. The patient can use the injured part with little pain so that muscle atrophy and contractures are reduced. Patients have little sign of systemic illness and eat well and lose relatively little weight.

Silver sulfadiazine is now used as a 15 per cent ointment in a water-soluble base which is simply smeared over the burned areas. To date, the drug does not appear to cause acid-base disturbances and is not painful to apply, although cutaneous sensitivity could still occur.

Sulfamylon (Mafenide Acetate 10 Per Cent). This is one of the two most effective treatments of major burn wounds, because of its simplicity and apparent effectiveness. Sulfamylon is a topical sulfonamide drug intended to prevent burn wound sepsis, the major factor contributing to mortality of severely burned patients. In patients with intact subcutaneous vasculature, peak concentrations occur two hours after application, or up to four hours in avascular areas. Sulfamylon is effective against *Pseudomonas aeruginosa, Staphylococcus aureus* and *Aerobacter aerogenes.*

The drug is applied in cream form daily with a gloved hand (Fig. 92–4). Sulfamylon has the consistency of soft butter, and burns and stings for 15 minutes to an hour because it is hygroscopic and draws water out of the tissue. The cream must be applied so the wound cannot be seen. To remove the cream, the patient is put in the Hubbard tank or whirlpool and inspected and any necrotic tissue debrided (Fig. 92–5). This is frequently done in the physical therapy department in hospitals without a burn unit.

The danger is that patients may develop metabolic acidosis, and this may be correctable at times only by stopping Sulfamylon treatment. Patients may develop an allergy, and a range of 5 to 15 per cent of patients may develop such conditions as generalized maculopapular eruption, pain on application, and interference with wound healing.

Gentamicin is an antibiotic which is effective against gram-negative bacteria including many strains of Pseudomonas. It has been reported to be used primarily when established invasive wound sepsis occurs.

Removal of Burn Eschar. Dead or heavily contaminated tissue must be removed daily. This must be done with great delicacy and care as well as with maximum speed. Explaining the reason and instilling a forward-looking attitude may be helpful. A matter-of-fact attitude that this has to be done must be assumed by the nurse, but still the patient must sense the nurse's concern with the daily ordeal and the desire to do everything possible to ease the patient's discomfort. Distraction such as television may be helpful in some cases. The patient has to be watched carefully for signs of fainting.

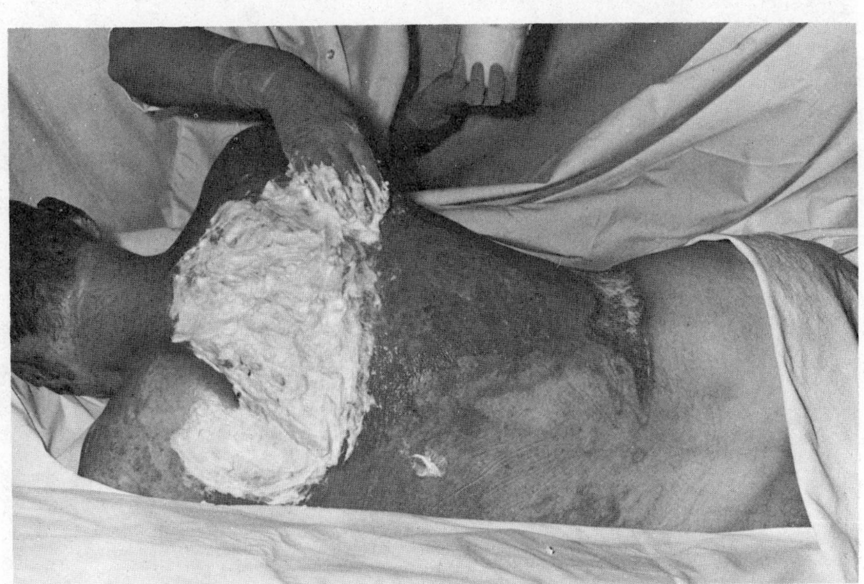

FIGURE 92-4. Photograph of back of patient with deep second-degree burn being treated with Sulfamylon. The Sulfamylon cream is put on in a thick layer with the gloved hand. (From Artz, C. P., and Moncrief, J. A.: *Treatment of Burns.* 2nd ed. 1969.)

Grafting

Skin grafting should be begun as early as possible. Grafts fall into three classes: allografts or homografts—skin taken from cadavers of the same species; xenografts—skin from other species; autografts—skin from the individual himself.

Homografts are frequently used as a dressing for the wound. The graft is taken off before tissue rejection occurs and another homograft is applied, or an autograft if available. Homografts may be applied two or three times a day until large islands of epithelium appear and then an autograft can be applied.

Skin may be transferred from one part of the body to another either as a free graft or as a flap (see below). A free graft is a piece of skin which is completely detached from its donor area and placed on the area to be grafted. It depends for its survival on the blood supply and nutrition of the recipient area. It will not survive if placed on compact bone, bare cartilage, tendons or on heavily irradiated tissue.

Free grafts are classified as follows: (1) Thiersch grafts; (2) split thickness grafts; (3) Wolfe full thickness grafts; and (4) pinch grafts. A *Thiersch* graft is a thin sheet of skin consisting of the epidermis and the superficial part of the dermis. This term is applied only to the thinnest type of grafts. The donor areas will usually heal in 7 to 10 days. *Split thickness grafts* are grafts that take more dermis than a Thiersch graft but less than a Wolfe graft. When cut into small squares, they are known as "postage stamp" or patch grafts, and are used to cover extensive granulating surfaces. The donor area will usually heal in 10 to 14 days. The *Wolfe graft* consists of the full thickness of the skin with no subcutaneous fat. The donor area does not heal spontaneously. Pinch grafts are small, full-thickness pieces of skin. They are particularly resistant to infection and grow in areas of poor blood supply. They leave an unsightly pitted donor area which cannot be used again. The Tanner Vanderput mesh graft has multiple slices in the graft, allowing it to be opened to three times its original size.

Biologic Dressings. A frequently used way to clean up a site and prepare it for grafting is by the use of biologic dressings which are changed every two to three days. Biologic dressings prevent loss of water and protein from the wound. They decrease pain in open wounds, permit increased mobility of the area and decrease bacterial growth on the wound surface, and appear to enhance growth of epithelium.

Xenografts are most readily available and require less time and effort. Porcine xenografts have been shown to have no immunologic properties. They are placed carefully on the wound without wrinkles and trimmed to fit the raw area, and allowed to remain in place one to three days. If the wound is large and very dirty, the patient is placed in a Hubbard tank every day or two. When the xenograft comes off, a new one is placed after the patient comes out of the

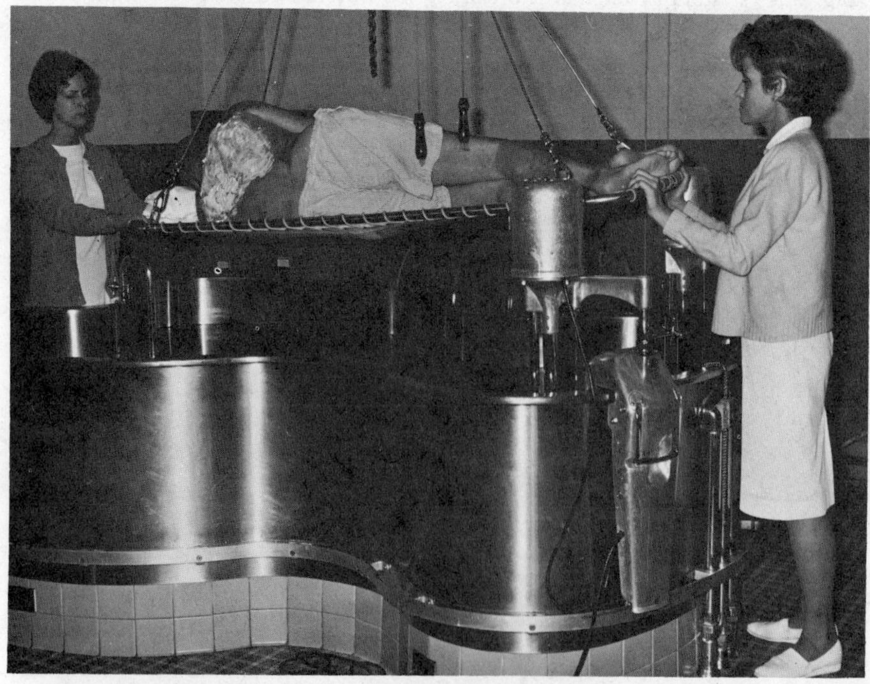

FIGURE 92–5. One of the best ways to remove Sulfamylon cream each day is by immersing the patient in the Hubbard tank. Here a patient with Sulfamylon on his back is shown being placed in the tank to remove the cream. This permits the patient active movement. (From Artz, C. P., and Moncrief, J. A.: *The Treatment of Burns.* 2nd ed. 1969.)

tank. Pig skin has also been used over mesh autografts.

Porcine xenografts are of value in: (1) preparation of the recipient site for grafting; (2) second degree burns as a cover for mesh grafts; and (3) protection of large open wounds until autografts are available.[3]

When a free graft is placed on a raw surface, it usually adheres in a few minutes, but this adhesion is easily broken down by any moving of the graft sideways. After 72 hours, the graft will have "taken" and will survive unless a severe infection or shearing force occurs. Free grafts can be left exposed to the air as long as nothing is allowed to rub them off. A thick graft is more likely to maintain its normal color and is more durable. A thin graft is more likely to contract but also is more likely to survive because it is easily permeated by tissue fluid. There is usually pain and temperature sensation within three months.

The Grafting Procedure. In a general hospital, the grafting procedure is done in the operating room. When large amounts of skin are needed, as for a burn, any surface of the limbs and trunk may be used as a donor area. The largest surface available is the medial aspect of the thigh. The physician gives priority to grafting of the hands and face and areas that will help the patient to be self-sufficient.

Skin for burn coverage is usually cut with a dermatome. The greatest care should be taken to prevent infection, so rigid skin preparation is usually prescribed. The Padgett dermatome depends on the efficiency of an adhesive cement for successful skin cutting. For successful adhesion of the cement, no moisture or grease must be allowed near the dermatome or drum. Both skin and drum are cleaned with ether. The cement is painted onto the skin and onto the drum and allowed to become tacky. The skin adheres to the drum which is slowly rotated as the graft is cut by to-and-fro movements of the blade (Fig. 92–6). The electrical dermatome permits removal of callibrated skin grafts without requiring use of adhesive cement.

The donor site is draped aseptically and is anesthetized with the use of lidocaine injected intradermally and subcutaneously. After 10 to 20 minutes, the skin grafts are cut with the dermatome. An assistant provides appropriate traction and positioning of the skin. The grafts are placed in a basin of balanced solution after they are cut. The grafts are then smoothed out, epidermal side down, on sterile wrapping paper. A paper template is cut out leaving a few millimeters of paper beyond the graft edge, and the graft is laid on the wound at the selected site using the edge of the paper as a handle. If grafts are exposed, the entire area should be covered. If there is not enough skin, one should use homografts.

Nurses on the ward may apply the graft and are responsible for rolling it regularly with a sterile applicator to express any fluid to the edge. If it is a whole graft, a nick may be made in the center and the fluid expressed through the opening. If the patient is treated by the open method, he may be put in the Hubbard tank within 72 hours. If the graft is washed off by this agitation, it is already dead. Grafts may also be cared for by the closed method with dressings and silver nitrate. Dressings are changed in 18 to 24 hours.

Some physicians believe the donor area should be dressed before the graft is applied, and others favor putting wet sterile saline dressings on the wound and dressing the site after the oozing stops. The donor site may be covered with fine meshed hot packs. These large packs are later removed, leaving only the fine mesh gauze as a covering for the donor area. This is allowed to remain in place until it automatically detaches itself, usually between two and three weeks later. Monafo applies a single layer of

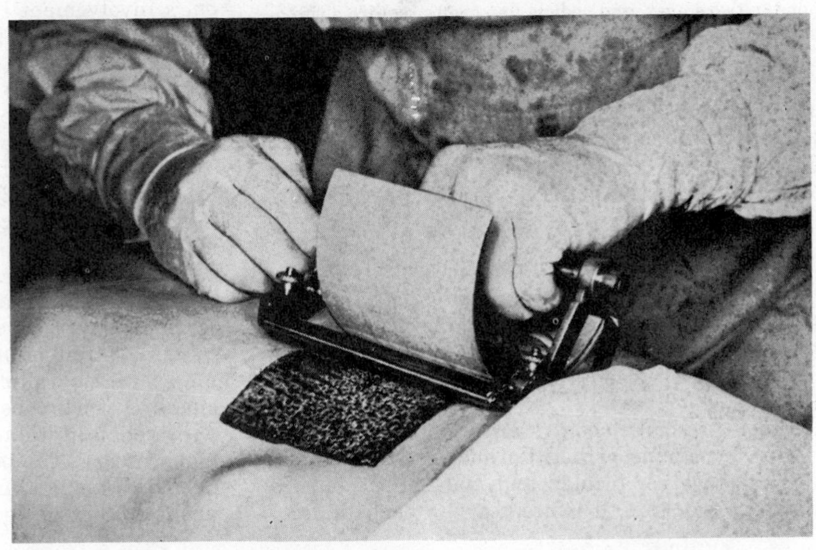

FIGURE 92–6. The Padgett dermatome in action. A full drum of skin measures 10 by 20 cm. This dermatome is particularly useful in removing skin for coverage of areas of motion. (From Artz, C. P., and Moncrief, J. A.: *The Treatment of Burns.* 2nd ed. 1969.)

porous polyurethane foam 1/16 inch in thickness. The site may be treated with wet silver nitrate dressings as is the burn wound, or topical antiseptic cream may be smeared over the polyurethane and renewed as needed.

Reconstructive and Plastic Procedures. Persistent attention to preserving the range of motion, and splinting in functional positions, are important in preventing significant contractures. Much less effort and expense are required to prevent contractures than to correct them surgically.

Reconstructive surgery may be either functional or cosmetic. Plastic surgery is generally one of the following procedures:

> *Z-plasty.* This procedure elongates the line of contracture and distributes the tension in the scar. Adjacent soft tissue must be sufficiently pliable. If the underlying muscle and tendon are contracted, prolonged immobilization in extension in a plaster cast may be necessary.

> *Thick, split-thickness skin grafts.* If Z-plasty is not applicable, thick, split-thickness grafts are probably best and should be as thick as possible to prevent recurrent postoperative contracture. Physical therapy and splinting may be necessary in the extremities.

> *Full-thickness free skin grafts.* These are used at times on the face and on the hands in small areas, e.g., resurfacing of the eyelids.

> *Adjacent flaps and distant flaps.* These are occasionally used in reconstruction of the axilla and in coverage of exposed bone. Cosmetic surgery is done to restore destroyed parts such as ear, nose, mouth or eyebrows, or to remove disfiguring scars. The pedicle flap takes in the full thickness of the skin and subcutaneous fat. It is left attached to both the recipient and donor areas until a sufficient blood supply to the recipient site is established. This graft is used in areas where a free graft could not be used, and to restore lost features, contour or bulk. These may be local flaps rotated to the wound from a near area or distant flaps brought from a farther area in stages. A sliding graft is a single stage graft where the skin flap is rotated over the recipient area and sutured to it. The donor area may be covered with a split thickness graft. Flap grafts are done in two stages, and pedicle flap grafts require a three-stage procedure.

The immobilization necessary for these extensive procedures is distressing for the patient and the nurse, and the nurse must be ingenious in creating distractions or comfort devices. She also must be alert to the condition of the graft, color, infection, etc.

Nutrition

The extensively burned patient offers problems that never cease until skin grafting is complete. The continuous discomfort of extensive burns and daily dressings or treatments may ruin the patient's appetite.

Frequent small feedings are probably best. The doctor, nutritionist or dietitian and nursing staff need to work together to plan and manage the burned patient's nutrition. It is necessary to keep an accurate account of everything the patient eats. Patients need a high carbohydrate-protein diet and, in spite of all efforts, patients generally continue to lose weight until they are grafted. Special attention to the patient's likes and dislikes and involvement of the family in providing special foods in accord with the overall plan are helpful. In some cases, nutritional needs must be met by tube feedings or parenteral hyperalimentation.

Emotional Problems of Burned Patients

Special nurses are frequently assigned to severely burned patients in general hospitals and, in those instances when they are not, it is desirable to have one person responsible for overall nursing care, to whom he relates well and whom he can consider his nurse. Sufficient attention and reinforcement must be given to the burn patient for good behavior; that is, he should not get attention only when he is complaining. However, the patient should not be reinforced for not complaining because of the importance of early monitoring and treatment of problems.

The severely burned patient faces a catastrophe of major proportions and perhaps a fatal outcome. Any individual facing such a severe crisis needs support, and the caring of significant persons can be crucial in recovery. The will to live is nourished by the concern of others who wish the patient to get well. For those individuals who do not have such persons, the role of the hospital team is doubly important.

It is important that the team caring for the patient know what the individual was like in health, and talk to his family and friends about him. How did he cope with crisis prior to the illness? Was he a fighter? Did he give up easily? Is he the "grin and bear it" type? Is he a perfectionist? Each person needs at least one person to whom he can relate closely during this ordeal and this might be any one caring for him.

Hopefully the patient will have confidence in all members of the team, including the doctor planning his major medical management. The nurse's role in coordinating, implementing and planning for hour-to-hour care of the patient is important. However, no matter how staffing is managed, *everyone's* involvement and planning together is important. If the hospital has a public health nurse assigned to the unit, she can assist in marshalling family and friends in assisting with recovery. A psychiatrist, psychologist or social worker may be helpful in early planning for care.

The major problems faced by the patient relate to (1) fear of death; (2) fear of disfigurement; (3) prolonged physical discomfort; and (4) prolonged surgical procedures and long convalescence.

The patient will go through the process of grieving over his loss. This may take many forms. *Denial* is a common way of warding off anxiety and temporarily blocks off troublesome emotional reactions. Denial may serve as a protective function for the patient, enabling him to cope. If it persists so that it interferes with rehabilitation, psychiatric intervention may be necessary. The patient may deal with his anger by *depression,* and he may need to be helped to talk about this and move on to constructive effort. *Regres-*

sion and *dependency* is a culturally accepted aspect of the sick role. The treatment for exaggerated dependency is a gentle push by the total team. Sometimes the patient is passively stubborn and sometimes overtly angry and resistive, but in time he will see that moving on is in his best interest.

Some patients are furiously unaccepting of their situation and will vent their hostility on physician, hospital personnel, friends and family. These others may become defensive and retaliatory, setting up a vicious circle that allows the patient to say honestly that he is being mistreated. Correct handling involves early recognition of this situation and termination by a united effort of the health team and family to get the patient to recognize and verbalize his anger and channel it into rehabilitation.

The nurse needs to be aware that the patient's complaints may not be his major concerns and may be only symptomatic of his fear of death, suffering, loss of others in his life or worry over his future. "Emotional support" is a term rather frequently used. This may be differentiated from a reaction which involves the release of pent up feelings which have been induced by a specific conflict situation. In emotional support, there is a taking in of emotional strength and coping capacities from the supporter. Patients with strong passive-aggressive behavior toward staff tend to reject emotional support because of a somewhat pathologic need to maintain their sense of independence. Often the rejection is ambivalent, with the patient sometimes resisting the help offered to him. Some patients need support despite their superficial rejection of it.

Patients frequently demonstrate an unwillingness to accept advice or suggestions. What they actually seem to want is an opportunity to find their own solutions, utilizing only the strengths of the supporter. Emotional support is the process of temporarily borrowing from the strengths of the supporter for the purpose of tension reduction, which leads to problem-solving behavior on the part of the supported.

In order to give emotional support, it is necessary to have this strength to give. It is important that everyone working with the patient work together and give each other support in order that they may sensitively and compassionately meet the needs of the patient. Caring for a burned patient is emotionally taxing, and ways of giving the helping personnel sustenance must be considered.

When the patient is ready to face his disfigurement, he will indicate it; he should not be forced to do so prematurely. Depending on the individual, group and one-to-one relationships in the hospital setting should be encouraged.

The patient should be involved in his plan of care. He has to accept the role of "co-manager" of his disability. If he needs to increase calories or increase fluids, the problem should be brought to him and his help in figuring out how to do this encouraged. The nurse may help him chart a graph at the bedside so he can see his own progress.

Discharge Planning

In a study of selected burn patients who had gone home, certain findings indicated how the patient might be prepared for discharge. Patients were found to have some difficulty with insomnia when they first went home, and medication was sometimes helpful during this adjustment. The patient had to learn how to handle his deformity and answer questions. As time went on, progressive desensitization to the burn injury occurred and the patients in the study eventually were generally found to be successful in their adjustment.[1]

However, the need for preparing the patient for the kinds of problems faced on discharge seems indicated, either individually or in a group. Including the family in a predischarge session is important, so that they know the stages to be expected in transition. If the hospital has a public health nurse coordinator, she should be involved in discharge planning, and a referral to the health department may be indicated in most instances.

References

1. Andreasen, N. J. C., Norris, A. S., and Hartford, C. E.: Incidence of long term psychiatric complications in severely burned adults. *Annals of Surgery,* 174: 785–793, November, 1971.
2. Artz, C. P., and Moncrief, J. A.: *Treatment of Burns.* 3rd ed. Philadelphia, W. B. Saunders Company, 1974.
3. Artz, C. P., Rittenbury, M. S., and Yarbrough, D. R., III: An appraisal of allografts and xenografts as biological dressings for wounds and burns. *Annals of Surgery,* 175:934–938, June, 1972.
4. Ballinger, W. F., Rutherford, R. B., and Zuidema, G. D.: *The Management of Trauma.* 2nd ed. Philadelphia, W. B. Saunders Company, 1973.
5. Beal, J. M., and Eckenhoff, J. E.: *Intensive and Recovery Room Care.* New York, The Macmillan Company, 1969.
6. Blakemore, W. S., and Fitts, W. T., Jr. (eds.): *Management of the Injured Patient.* New York, Harper & Row, 1969.
7. Crews, E. R.: *A Practical Manual for the Treatment of Burns.* Springfield, Ill., Charles C Thomas, Publisher, 1964.
8. Douglas, D. M.: *Wound Healing.* Baltimore, The Williams & Wilkins Company, 1963.
9. Epstein, E. H. (ed.): *Skin Surgery.* 3rd ed. Springfield, Ill., Charles C Thomas, Publisher, 1970.
10. Hartford, C. E.: The early treatment of burns. *Nursing Clinics of North America,* 8:447–455, September, 1973.
11. Henderson, J.: *Emergency Medical Guide.* New York, Blakiston Division, McGraw-Hill Book Company, 1969.
12. Hummel, R. P., MacMillan, B. C., and Altemeier, W. A.: Typical and systemic antibacterial agents in the

treatment of burns. *Annals of Surgery,* 172:370–384, September, 1970.
13. Iskrant, A. P., and Joliet, P. V.: *Accidents and Homicide.* Cambridge, Harvard University Press, 1968.
14. Jackson, D. M.: Burns as a special problem in trauma. *Journal of Trauma,* 10:991-996, November, 1970.
15. Jacoby, F.: Current nursing care of the burned patient: a review. *Nursing Clinics of North America,* 5:563–575, December, 1970.
16. Jacoby, F.: *Nursing Care of the Patient with Burns.* St. Louis, The C. V. Mosby Company, 1972.
17. Krupp, N. E.: Psychiatric implications of chronic and crippling illness. *Psychosomatics,* 9:109–113, March-April, 1968.
18. McFarlane, D. A., and Thomas, L. P.: *Textbook of Surgery.* Edinburgh and London, F. and S. Livingstone, Ltd., 1968.
19. Minckley, B.: Expert nursing care for burned patients. *American Journal of Nursing,* 70:1888–1893, September, 1970.
20. Monafo, W. W.: *The Treatment of Burns, Principles and Practice.* St. Louis, Warren H. Green, Inc., 1971.
21. Nealon, T. F., Jr.: *Fundamental Skills in Surgery.* Philadelphia, W. B. Saunders Company, 1971.
22. Pruitt, B. A., Jr., Foley, F. D., and Moncrief, J. A.: Curling's ulcer: a clinical–pathology study of 323 cases. *Annals of Surgery,* 72:523–535, October, 1970.
23. Rosello, R. H., and Fogel, M. L.: Emotional support. *Psychosomatics,* May–June, 1970.
24. Shafer, K. N., Sawyer, J. R., and McCluskey, A. M.: *Medical-Surgical Nursing.* 5th ed. St. Louis, The C. V. Mosby Company, 1971.
24a. Stinson, V.: Porcine skin dressings for burns. *American Journal of Nursing,* 74:111-112, January, 1974.
25. Taylor, S., Cotton, T., and Murray, J. G.: *A Short Textbook of Surgery.* Philadelphia, J. B. Lippincott Company, 1967.

CHAPTER 93

Diseases of the Breast

The principal concern of this chapter will be breast cancer, a topic in which nurses, who are predominantly female, feel a strong interest. The nurse can identify closely with the patient with breast cancer, and nurses should feel an obligation to encourage all women to learn self-examination of the breast and to undergo regular physical check-ups.

Before turning to the topic of cancer, let us review the anatomy and physiology of the breast.

ANATOMY AND PHYSIOLOGY

The breast is a modified sebaceous gland, an appendage of the skin. The mammary gland extends vertically from the 2nd to the 6th rib and horizontally from the sternum to the midaxillary line. It lies entirely within the superficial fascia of the anterior chest wall. The largest part of the breast rests on the fascia of the pectoralis major fascia and the rest on the fascia of the serratus anterior. The nonlactating breast weighs about 150 to 250 gm., and the lactating breast weight may be between 400 and 500 gm.

The mammary gland is made up of 12 to 20 lobes subdivided into lobules and these in turn are composed of acini. The lobes are arranged like the spokes of a wheel around the nipple. Each lobe is drained by a duct, 12 to 20 of which open on the nipple. Each duct opens independently of each other on the surface of the nipple and has a dilated ampulla just before its opening (Fig. 93–1).

The breast is fixed to the overlying skin and underlying pectoral fascia with fibrous bands (Cooper's ligaments). A fascial cleft on the undersurface of the breast allows for mobility of the breast.

The nipple is located in the 4th intercostal space. Its base is surrounded by a circular pigmented area called the areola. Pigmentation at any age is in-

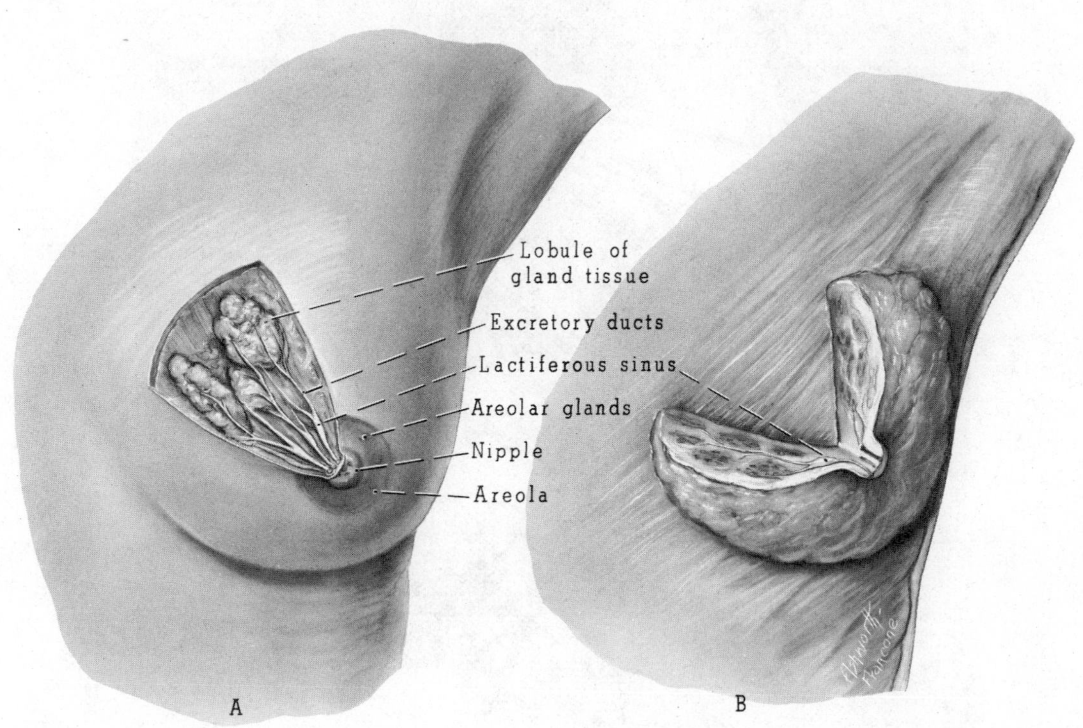

FIGURE 93–1. The female breast. *A*, The skin has been partly removed to show the underlying structures. *B*, A section has been removed to show the internal structures in relation to the muscles. (From Jacob, S. W., and Francone, C. A.: *Structure and Function in Man*. 3rd ed. 1974.)

creased by the administration of estrogen. The areolar epithelium contains some small hairs and three types of glands—sebaceous glands, sweat glands and accessory mammary glands. The sebaceous glands (Montgomery's glands) enlarge during pregnancy and lactation to lubricate the nipple.

The parenchyma of the breast consists of the ductular, lobular and acinar epithelial structure. The stroma of the breast is made up of fibrous and fatty tissue. In the absence of pregnancy, obesity determines the size of the breast. The central and upper portion is mostly glandular and the periphery mostly fatty. The large amount of glandular tissue in the upper outer quadrant probably accounts for more cancer occurring in that area.

The two main sources of blood supply to the breast are the lateral mammary artery and the lateral thoracic artery. These arteries form an extensive network of anastomoses over the breast. The main veins follow the arterial pattern. The veins are a key to the lymphatic pathways which, in general, follow the pathways of the veins. The superficial veins over the breast are often dilated over an area which contains disease. Tumors, malignant or benign, need an increased blood supply, and the prominent superficial veins are indicative of the need. The lymph drainage of the breast consists of three parts: (1) cutaneous or superficial; (2) areolar; and (3) glandular or deep. Figure 93–2 shows the principal routes of lymphatic drainage from the breast.

The nerve supply is derived from the anterior and lateral branches of the 4th to 6th intercostal nerves.

There are three types of physiologic changes affecting the breast—those related to growth and development, to the menstrual cycle, and to pregnancy and lactation.

Estrogen and progesterone act synergistically with the pituitary growth hormones, prolactin and corticotropin, to produce the development and function of the mammary gland. Estrogens are responsible for the growth of the mammary gland and of the periductal stroma, whereas progesterone promotes the development of the lobular and acinar structures. In women with normal menstrual cycles, the cyclic secretion of estrogen and progesterone is responsible for the female breast structure. During pregnancy there is a high increase in these hormones and in the pituitary hormones, resulting in an increase in the vascularity of the breast and in the

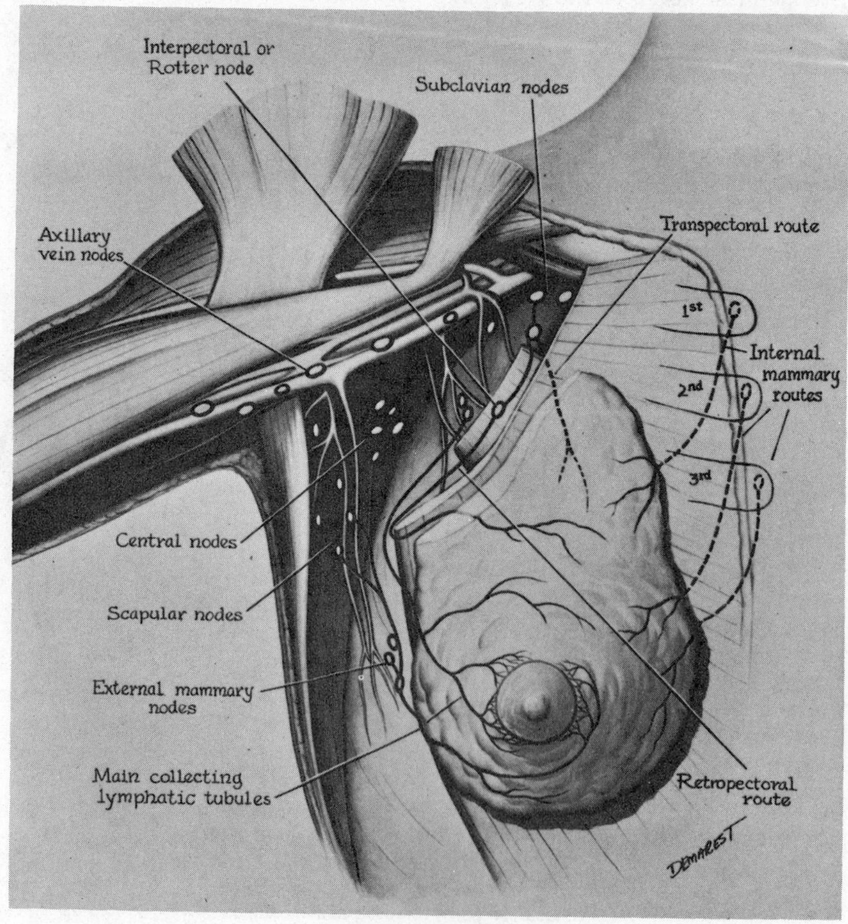

FIGURE 93–2. Axillary and internal mammary lymphatic routes from the breast. (From Haagensen, C. D.: *Diseases of the Breast.* 2nd ed. 1971.)

permeability and dilatation of the lymphatics of the breast.

With the termination of pregnancy, prolactin initiates lactation. Prolactin and corticotropin help maintain lactation, but the "letting down" of milk is a more complex response involving the mother's subjective response and the mechanical stimulation of suckling. Suckling causes release into the blood stream of the pituitary hormone, oxytocin, which causes the mammary acini to contract and release milk into the duct system.

After the menopause, the ovaries cease producing the cyclic secretion of estrogen and progesterone. Estrogens are then produced by the adrenals through stimulation from the anterior pituitary. There is a continuous involution of the breast with loss of the glandular elements and atrophy.

DIAGNOSIS OF BREAST LESIONS

Ninety per cent of breast cancers are detected by the woman herself. Many more would be detected earlier if *regular self-examination of the breast* were practiced. Nurses have the opportunity to encourage and educate the patient concerning this important procedure. This examination may be done in the following manner:

> The woman should lie down and put one hand behind her head. With the flat of the other hand, she should gently check all parts of both breasts. The operation should then be repeated sitting up, with the hand still behind the head. The breasts should be checked once a month after the menstrual period, and after the menopause on a monthly basis.

Women may not go to the doctor even if they feel a lump because of lack of education that the disease is curable. The patient may also be afraid of the mutilating effects of mastectomy and the effect on the emotional relationship with her husband.

Early diagnosis is of prime importance and the patient should be encouraged to see her physician at the first suspicion of a breast lump. Every nodule in the breast should be removed for histologic examination before mastectomy is performed. Patients with the smallest cancers and the least spread to the lymph nodes have the most favorable prognosis.

It should be emphasized that a substantial number of breast abnormalities in women are not cancer. The following are the most common causes of breast lesions in the order of frequency: (1) fibrocystic disease; (2) cancer; (3) adenofibroma; (4) intraductal papilloma; and (5) duct ectasia.

Mammography. Radiographic techniques for detecting breast cancers are being perfected, and the refinement and wider use of these methods have been encouraged by the American College of Radiology and the Cancer Control branch of the United States Public Health Service. The yield in various studies varies from two to four cases of breast cancer per 1000 women having mammograms, that is, x-rays of the breast. The ultimate goal is to use mammography with surveys of high-risk groups of women such as those with nodules, cystic disease, previous breast cancer, familial incidence, etc. Mammography is the only way that breast cancer can be detected before signs and symptoms develop. It is not a substitute for physical examination, but the two are mutually complementary.

Some newer techniques are thermomastography and xerography. Thermomastography measures the infra-red emission of the human breast and is a direct function of surface temperature; thermograms can be portrayed on a photographic film. In xerography, the x-ray image of the breast is secured on a selenium-coated metal plate. It results in a picture with much better definition than with mammography, and all tissues of the breast including the skin can be portrayed with a single exposure, thus exposing the patient to less radiation. This technique is expected to be the procedure of choice when the equipment is improved, because xerograms will be easier to make and interpret than mammograms.

Certain laboratory studies are being done in the hope of finding a practical way of detecting breast cancer in high-risk patients as well as finding it in a preclinical stage. Such studies include determination of certain steroids in the urine, sex chromatin status of the buccal musosa, determination of the estriol urinary excretion quotient, and studies of serum glycoproteins. Further studies with these methods are being conducted. Recent improvement in saving patients seems to be due to finding more early lesions rather than to improvement in treatment. At the present time, mammography seems to offer the best chance of detecting cancer of the breast in an early presymptomatic stage.

Symptoms and Classification. Tumors due to cancer are more likely to be solitary and unilateral, while benign breast lesions are likely to be multiple and bilateral. Cancers tend to be irregular and poorly outlined. Tenderness is common in benign lesions but uncommon in cancers. Cysts are clear on transillumination but cancers are always opaque.

Mobility, attachment and fixation are terms used by the physician to describe certain physical signs. *Mobility* indicates movement of a lesion within the breast (especially characteristic of fibroadenoma). Mobility is never found in tumors due to cancer, but is a common symptom in benign disease. *Attachment* means adherence to skin or nipple with skin dimpling, edema or nipple retraction or elevation. *Fixation* is used to indicate inability to move the tumor on the chest wall. Nipple changes such as retraction, elevation and ulceration are very uncommon in benign lesions. Although discharge is usually due to intraductal papilloma, it can be due to cancer.

Skin changes such as dimpling, color change and ulceration are commonly due to cancer. The ordinary breast cancer may be roughly classified as follows:[16]

> *Early.* Solitary, unilateral, hard, painless, solid, irregular, poorly outlined, nonmobile lump usually located in the upper outer quadrant of the breast, and opaque to transillumination.

> *Moderately advanced locally.* Axillary nodes, nipple retraction or elevation, skin dimpling, nipple discharge.

> *Far advanced locally.* Signs of local inoperability. Superclavicular nodes, fixation of axillary nodes, fixation of tumor to chest wall, edema (peau d'orange or redness over more than a third of the breast), edema of the arm, ulceration of the skin, satellite nodules.

> *Distant metasis.* Inoperable. Parietal, osseous or visceral.

The International Classification of Cancer describes a method of evaluating the stage based on the T (primary), N (nodes), and M (metastases) system (Table 93–1).

BENIGN DISORDERS OF THE BREAST

Fibrocystic disease is the most frequent lesion of the female breast. It accounts for over 45 per cent of all biopsied female breast lesions.[13] The exact cause of this disease remains unknown, although some evidence indicates a hormonal imbalance. It improves during pregnancy and lactation. The disease occurs during the reproductive years and disappears with the menopause. Nodularity, tenderness and cysts may be present. The lesions may change in size and are much more labile than carcinomas or adenofibromas. Cysts are generally aspirated rather than formally biopsied. However, if there is any question, a biopsy is done. Haagenson reports having successfully aspirated 10,000 cysts and avoided an operation each time.[8] Others have equally good records.

Adenofibroma is the third most common tumor of the breast, exceeded only by carcinoma and cystic disease. Adenofibroma is a disease of youth. In a study of 496 cases, the mean age of the patients was 21 years. These tumors are usually well outlined, rounded, discoid or lobulated, and may be soft but more often have a rubbery firmness. Relative movability of the adenoma in the breast tissues is one of its most distinctive characteristics. Excision is the only effective treatment.

Papilloma. Intraductal papillomas are neoplasms growing in the terminal portion of a duct (solitary) or throughout the duct system of a sector of the breast (multiple). Most are of the solitary type. Papillomas within the nipple itself are rare. With few exceptions, solitary intraductal papillomas are not precancerous lesions.

The symptom of intraductal papilloma is usually a serous, serosanguineous or bloody discharge from the nipple. Frequently, no tumor mass is palpable although a small soft tumor in a central or periareolar portion of the breast is usually present. It is necesary to excise the lesion and have the tissues examined. Some doctors recommend doing this on a permanent paraffin section rather than on a frozen section because of the difficulty in determining whether the lesion is benign or malignant.

Duct ectasia or comedomastitis is a disease of the ducts in the subareolar zone. It is a disease of the aging breast and is most common in or near the menopause. It usually occurs in women who have had children and who have nursed them. The patient may have a thick, sticky nipple discharge, and burning pain, itching and inflammation. Some doctors treat this conservatively at first, but if indicated the major central ducts of the breast may be excised. There is no demonstrated association with carcinoma.

CARCINOMA OF THE BREAST

Breast cancer occurs more often and causes more deaths than any other form of cancer. In order of

TABLE 93–1. ABRIDGED TNM* SYSTEM OF CLASSIFICATION OF CARCINOMA OF THE BREAST†

Symbol	Description
T_1	Less than 2 cm. No skin fixation
T_2	2 to 5 cm. Skin tethered or dimpled No pectoral fixation
T_3	5 to 10 cm. Skin infiltrated or ulcerated Pectoral fixation
T_4	More than 10 cm. Skin involvement not beyond breast Chest wall fixation
N_0	No nodes
N_1	Axillary nodes movable Not significant Significant
N_2	Axillary nodes fixed
N_3	Supraclavicular nodes Edema of arm
M_0	No metastases
M	Metastases including skin involvement beyond breast and contralateral nodes
Four Clinical Stages Designated by TNM Symbols	
Stage I	$T_1 N_0 M_0$ $T_2 N_0 M_0$
Stage II	$T_1 N_1 M_0$ $T_2 N_1 M_0$
Stage III	$T_1 N_2$ or $N_3 M_0$ $T_2 N_2$ or $N_3 M_0$ $T_3 N_0, N_1, N_2,$ or $N_3 M_0$ $T_4 N_0, N_1, N_2,$ or $N_3 M_0$
Stage IV	Any combination of T and N symbols including M

*T = tumor; N = nodes; M = metastases.

†From Rubin, P.: Current Cancer Concepts, Carcinoma of the Breast, Stage I, Surgical Spectrum. American Cancer Society, 1973. (Adapted from Copeland. Copyright 1973, American Medical Association.)

frequency as a cause of death in women, it stands fifth. In the United States there are 71,000 cases each year, with 32,650 estimated deaths in 1973. Most cases are found in women over the age of 45, and the incidence increases with age (Fig. 93–3). Epidemiologic studies reveal that cancer occurs more often on the left side than on the right, and in the outer quadrant rather than the inner, and occurs more often in women who have not borne or breast fed infants.

The overall group with increased risk of breast cancer includes women over 40; unmarried, childless women; those who have not nursed; women whose first pregnancy was after 25 years of age; those with an early menarche and prolonged menstrual history; women with fibrocystic disease of the breasts; those who have had cancer of the uterus; women with one breast removed for cancer; those with a positive family history; fat and hypothyroid women; Caucasians; women living in the western world, in highly developed countries and in the upper socioeconomic group; Jewish women; and in women of certain other races and countries (incidence is highest in Denmark and lowest in Japan).

Surgical Treatment. The diagnosis of breast cancer has been discussed above. The selection of the best therapeutic procedure for a patient with breast cancer is based on the stage of the disease and the individual patient. There is no noteworthy difference in survival rates with any given procedure, and survival seems more closely related to earlier diagnosis than to more extensive therapy.

In most centers throughout the world, the standard *radical mastectomy* is the procedure of choice for operating on invasive cancer. The radical mastectomy means the removal of the entire breast, the pectoralis major and minor muscles, the deep pectoral fascia, with the subclavicular or superior apical nodes, the pectoral nodes and the axillary nodes. There are many modifications of radical mastectomy.

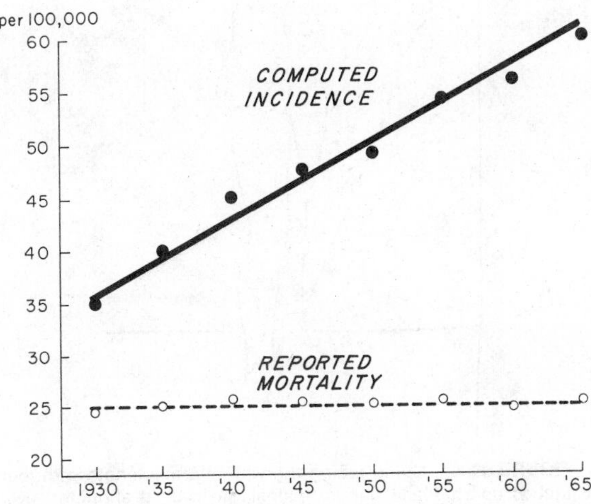

FIGURE 93–3. Computed age adjusted incidence rates for breast cancer in females in Connecticut compared with age-adjusted mortality rates for breast cancer in the United States (Schneiderman: Biometry Branch, National Institutes of Health in Haagensen, C. D.: *Diseases of the Breast.* 2nd ed. 1971.)

Recently, a less extensive type of procedure that removes one quarter to one third of the breast has received considerable publicity and has been advocated by surgeons and lay persons who deplore the mutilating effects of a radical mastectomy. This procedure is sometimes called a "lumpectomy." Leis[16] states that the 10-year survival rate is much lower then that with radical or modified radical mastectomy for the same types of cancer. He feels it is applicable only to a small percentage of patients with early, small and peripherally located cancers.

PREOPERATIVE CARE. Cancerphobia is a prevalent condition in American society. Persons with cancer often die of other causes, but there is still an aura of pain and early death associated with the word. Cancer of the breast is doubly threatening to women in this culture, since the breast is a symbol of sexuality and femininity. Even this failure to exercise self-examination may be related to latent fears.

The nurse who first is in contact with a patient has to assess where her patient is in this potentially frightening experience. A supportive family and doctor are of great help to any person undergoing this crisis, but there are many individuals who do not have ideal support. The patient needs a person to whom she can relate and who will evaluate her preparation for the events to follow. The assembly line hospital care with many people going in and out of the room is not conducive to meeting the emotional needs of any patient. The nursing staff should not leave the emotional preparation of this patient to a fortuitous relationship that might occur, but should plan so that the patient has the opportunity to talk about her surgery and to feel that someone cares about her.

Nurses and doctors share the dread of cancer with the rest of society, and the nurse must have had the opportunity to explore her own feelings about cancer of the breast before she can most satisfactorily help the patient. The nurse also needs to be as knowledgeable as possible about all aspects of care and of the particular doctor's plan so that she can answer the patient's questions.

The patient must be informed of the total care plan and the rehabilitative efforts that she will need to fully participate in to insure adequate recovery. The preoperative physical routine will be in accordance with the guidelines of the particular physician. The general preoperative routine is similar to that for most operations except for the fact that the patient does not know generally when she goes to surgery how extensive the operation will be. In some cases, the surgeon does the biopsy of the lesion and the nodes and then does the surgery later after he gets a complete pathology report.

Skin preparation may involve having the operative area washed with pHisoHex several days before admission to the hospital, and later, shaving, along with the usual preparation. If a skin graft is to be done, the donor areas will also have to be prepared.

POSTOPERATIVE CARE. Rest for the patient and early food and fluid intake are immediate objectives. Upon awakening, the patient is quick to feel if the breast has been removed. The possibility of a cure and the fact that there was no spread, if this is true, should be emphasized. Early ambulation and resumption of activity is the usual procedure with mastectomy patients. Exercises will be prescribed by the physician. The American Cancer Society provides a book, *Help Yourself to Recovery,* which lists exercises that the physician may prescribe.

The "Reach to Recovery" program of the American Cancer Society is a rehabilitation program for women who have had breast surgery, and is designed to help them meet their psychologic, physical and cosmetic needs. Upon authorization of the doctor, volunteers from this program visit the hospital and give information and help as follows:

1. Reach to Recovery kit, ball, book, rope and a temporary prosthesis.
2. Explanation and demonstration of the exercises prescribed.
3. Suggestion for bra comfort.
4. Explanation of various breast prostheses.
5. Suggestions for clothing adjustment.
6. Where indicated, a discussion of personal problems.
7. The volunteer's phone number is left with the patient so that help is always available.

When told by the doctor that she is ready to be fitted with a prosthesis, the patient may visit the ACS office, and further information is given concerning clothing, particularly bathing suits.

When the nurse or doctor cannot meet these needs fully, a volunteer who has gone through these problems can be of great assistance.

Edema. Nearly all patients will have some degree of arm edema following radical mastectomy. It is the only significant postoperative complication of this operation.

Early postoperative *arm exercises* are recommended. The patient is instructed to keep the arm at the side for the first week and to avoid any attempt at abduction. Bed exercises should be started within 24 hours. The patient is instructed in hand and wrist movements and in flexion and extension of the elbow at hourly intervals. She is encouraged to feed herself, comb her hair and wash her face, being careful not to abduct the arm.

When wound healing is well established, abduction and external rotation of the upper arm are begun in the recumbent position. At about the 10th to 12th day, the patient is started on exercises in the erect position, consisting of pendulum swings to improve shoulder function (Fig. 93–4), forward and lateral elevation of the arms, overhead pulley suspension to obtain full elevation, and wall climbing (Fig. 93–5).

The arm should be compressed postoperatively with an elastic bandage, to be followed by a custom-fitted pressure gradient elastic sleeve to avoid the changes of edema during the period needed for regrowth of lymphatic pathways. Ordinarily, patients have a transient slight increase in diameter of the arm following surgery. This kind of edema usually produces an increase of less than 3 cm. and ordinarily disappears with the restoration of arm function. Edema is considered a true complication when it is severe enough to make the patient socially unpresentable and gives her a feeling of tension and discomfort.

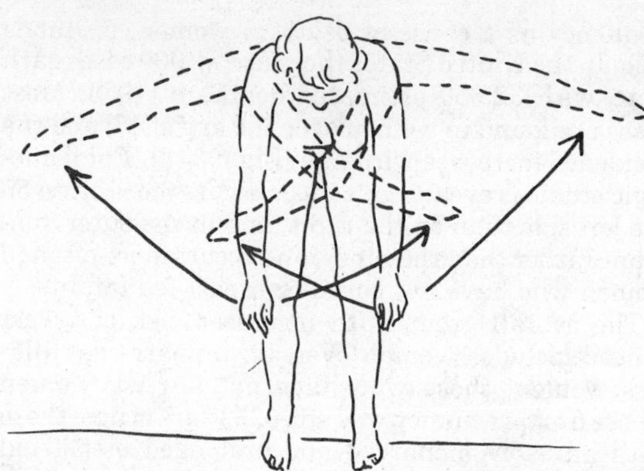

FIGURE 93–4. Stand with feet 8 inches apart. Bend forward from the waist allowing arms to hang toward the floor by gravity. Swing both arms together describing an arc from one shoulder to the other. Do not bend elbows. Stand and allow arms to fall to side. (Wolf, E. S.: *Nursing Clinics of North America.* December, 1967.)

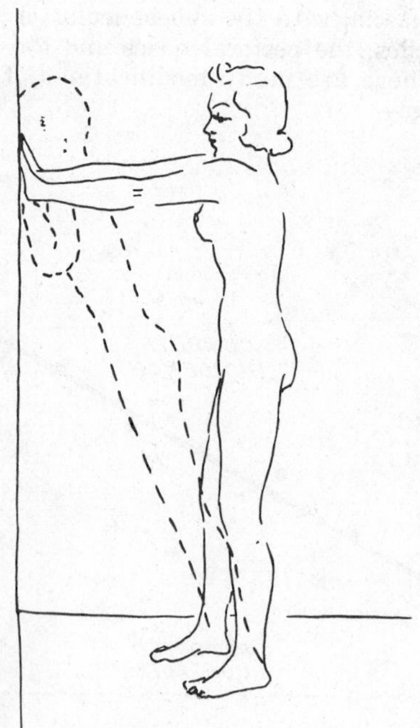

FIGURE 93–5. Stand facing the wall at arm's length with feet 8 inches apart. Place hands against the wall at shoulder level parallel to each other. Slowly flex the elbow, bending the trunk forward until forehead touches wall. Straighten elbows slowly until body is upright. Repeat. Note: Keep head, trunk, and legs in straight line. (Wolf, E. S.: *Nursing Clinics of North America,* December, 1967.)

Secondary edema resulting from infection in the arm is more frequent, and patients may have some permanent edema following an infection. If wound healing is normal, adequate collateral lymphatic circulation usually develops within a month. Common sources of infection result from necrosis of skin flaps or imperfectly obliterated dead space in the axilla. Postoperative radiation to the axilla frequently increases the frequency and degree of edema of the arm.

The patient must be told she is vulnerable to secondary edema for the rest of her life and that trauma may lead to infection and edema. Burns, cuts, abrasions and paronychia are the most frequent sources of infection. Obesity is an important factor in reducing edema. "Wearing a custom-made elastic sleeve extending from the wrist to the shoulder during the day, when the patient is up and about, is the most useful method of limiting and improving edema of the arm in its chronic stage."[10] Haagensen also advises that spironolactone, a diuretic, may be tried in moderate doses in combination with the elastic sleeve. He also advocates skin grafting and meticulous aftercare in securing wound healing and avoiding the triad of tension on the skin flaps, necrosis and infection.

Included in the opposite column is a sample of the type of instruction sheet that may be given by the physician to postmastectomy patients.

Treatment of Advanced Cancer

Radiation Therapy. The value of radiation in early stage I and II carcinoma continues to be argued. There seems to be no difference in survival rate in these patients treated by radical mastectomy alone, with therapy given when complications arise, when compared with patients who were given pre- or postoperative radiation.

Radiotherapy is the preferred treatment in locally advanced stage III cancer either alone or combined with a simple mastectomy in certain cases. Radiation is used for palliation in regional and distant metastases. Radiotherapy finds its most useful indication in the treatment of bone metastases from cancer of the breast. Early radiotherapy to metastatic lesions of the vertebrae rapidly eliminates pain and avoids collapse of the vertebrae and subsequent paraplegia. It may prevent a fracture or help recalcify one that has already occurred.

For irradiation of neoplasms from external sources, roentgen rays generated at voltages between 85 kv. and 35 mv. and gamma rays from radium 226, cobalt 60 and cesium 137 are used clinically. The energy and penetrating power of ionizing radiation increases as the photon wavelength decreases. Between 400 and 800 kv., there is reduced absorption of radiation in bone, less damage to the skin at the portal of entry, better tolerance of the vasculoconnective tissue, greater radiation at a depth relative to the surface dose, and reduced lateral scatter of radiation in the tissues. Ionizing radiation of sufficient energy to have these characteristics is termed *supervoltage radiation.*

Early and late radiation reactions may occur. Early reactions occur during or soon after treatment and include systemic effects and transient local changes in irradiated tissues. Radiation sickness may start with a few days of headache followed by anorexia, nausea and vomiting. The probable cause is absorption of breakdown

HAND CARE

After a radical mastectomy, an arm may swell because lymph nodes and lymph vessels were necessarily removed and the body is therefore less able to combat infection in this extremity.

Make every effort to avoid all cuts, scratches, pin pricks, hangnails, insect bites, burns, and the use of strong detergents as these can lead to serious infection with increased swelling.

Some "DO NOT'S":

DO NOT hold a cigarette in this hand

DO NOT carry your purse or anything heavy with this arm

DO NOT wear a wristwatch or other jewelry on this arm

DO NOT cut or pick at cuticles or hangnails on this hand

DO NOT work near thorny plants or dig in the garden

DO NOT reach into a hot oven with this arm

DO NOT permit injection in this arm

DO NOT permit blood to be drawn from this arm

DO NOT allow your blood pressure to be taken on this arm

Some "DO'S":

DO wear a loose rubber glove on this hand when washing dishes

DO wear a thimble when sewing

DO apply a good lanolin hand cream several times daily

DO wear your "Life-Guard Medical Aid" tag engraved with "CAUTION—LYMPHEDEMA ARM—NO TESTS—NO HYPOS"

DO contact your doctor if your arm gets red, warm or unusually hard or swollen

DO return for a check-up and re-measurement for a new sleeve in two months

DO show this Hand Care Sheet to your surgeon

Reprinted through the courtesy of the CLEVELAND CLINIC Department of Physical Medicine and Rehabilitation.

products of the irradiated tissues. Radiation sickness can be prevented or minimized by adjustment of the treatment to the response of the individual patient. The warning signals indicate that the limits of the patient's constitutional toleration to radiation therapy are near.

Early tissue reactions of significance include those of the skin and mucous membranes. Skin reactions were common with use of low or medium voltage x-ray, but with supervoltage irradiation, maximum ionization occurs below the epidermis, and skin reactions are usually avoided because the tolerance of other structures limits the dose. The radiosensitivity of mucosal epithelium is greater than that of underlying connective tissue and underlying small vessels. By observing the mucosal reaction, it is possible to avoid damage to the vasculoconnective tissue, the basis of later complications.

Late radiation reactions are generally proportional to the incidence and severity of early reactions. Late changes of atrophy, telangiectasia, epilation and fragility are permanent in skin and mucosa.

Since advanced cancer therapy is on an outpatient basis, the nurse in the doctor's office or cancer treatment unit will have the most opportunity to talk with the patient about her fears and to attempt to help her to see cancer as similar to other chronic diseases that one must learn to live with and treat as symptoms arise. The patient needs to be informed of the effects of radiation therapy. Skin changes may vary from a mild erythema to a severe reaction, with pain and weeping. Strong soaps and ointments or creams should not be used, and the skin should not be exposed to the sun. Cornstarch may be used several times a day to keep the skin dry. Vitamins A and D ointment or plain lanolin might be applied. If the skin has broken down or is painful, the doctor will prescribe appropriate treatment. For systemic effects of fatigue or lethargy, nausea and digestive upsets, patients should eat frequent small meals and get plenty of rest.

Hormone Therapy. About 40 to 50 per cent of breast cancers are hormone-dependent. That is, their growth is dependent on the hormonal environment that was present when the cancer began. Hormonal treatment is palliative, and produces an appreciable increase in comfort and survival time for a fair number of patients. The average life expectancy for a woman with disseminated mammary cancer without treatment is about 9.5 months. Hormonal treatment will increase survival and comfort in about 40 per cent of the patients.[15]

The hormonal environment may be changed by the ablation of endocrine organs or the addition of exogenous hormones. Ablative hormonal therapy involves castration, adrenalectomy or hypophysectomy. In the premenopausal woman, the cancer develops in an environment of estrogen and progesterone from the ovaries. Surgical or radiation *castration* is the procedure generally used in this group of patients. Most clinicians prefer to use castration as a therapeutic approach in premenopausal women with stage I and II breast cancers.

In the menopausal woman, the cancer develops in an unbalanced hormonal environment of estrogen from the adrenals and, in some cases, from the ovaries. *Bilateral adrenalectomy* may be performed to remove another source of endogenous estrogens. *Hypophysectomy,* the removal of the anterior pituitary, removes the source of the adrenocorticotropic hormones as well as hormones that may directly stimulate the breast. Patients with these operations require daily cortisone replacement to maintain life. Any lapse in the administration of cortisone may cause the patient to go into adrenal crisis, manifested by hypotension, elevated temperature, nausea, vomiting, diarrhea, abdominal pain and weakness. There may be mood swings as the cortisone is being regulated. The patient and those caring for him need to be aware of the need for cortisone replacement and the need for increased dosage in stress, infection, accidents, etc. Patients also may require replacement of the adrenal salt-regulating hormone. Florinef acetate, 0.1 mg. every other day, is usually given.

A woman should carry identification papers indicating the type of surgery she has had and the type of replacement therapy required. An identification emblem bracelet to alert others to the medical problem can be purchased from Medic Alert Foundation International, Turlock, California.

The administration of testosterone propionate produces relief from pain, a feeling of well-being and a gain in weight. The chief unfavorable effects are virilization, hoarseness, hirsutism, acne, a ruddy complexion and increased libido.

Breast cancer in a postmenopausal woman develops in an environment without estrogen or progesterone, so initial treatment after the fourth postmenopausal year could be with estrogen or estrogen and progesterone. Diethylstilbestrol is usually given in 15-mg. dosage daily. Deep pigmentation of the nipple and areola is the most obvious outward sign that full estrogen effect has been achieved. Breasts may become engorged and uterine bleeding may occur. In any patient with extensive bone metastases, hypercalcemia may be precipitated by the administration of estrogen. Hypercalcemia may occur in patients with metastatic breast cancer either spontaneously or after administration of hormones. It is estimated that 10 per cent of patients with mammary cancer die of hypercalcemia. The kidney, heart and lung are damaged by deposits of calcium, although this can be reversed by withdrawal of the hormones and the administration of steroids.

If the nurse is thoroughly familiar with the rationale for treatment, she can be much more effective in assisting the patient and family in their problems.

Chemotherapy. Chemotherapy of breast cancer is a nonspecific treatment. Therefore, it has an effect on normally functioning cells such as those of the bone marrow and the epithelium of the gastrointestinal tract. It is important that the nurse be aware of the potentially serious side effects of such treatment.

The principal types of chemotherapeutic agents used are alkylating agent and antimetabolites, but other drugs such as antibiotics and various alkaloids also have been used. The most common agents currently employed are listed in Table 39–2, along with information as to dosages and side effects. For detailed information about the nursing care of patients receiving these chemotherapeutic agents, see Chapter 35.

All of the chemical agents used today are toxic to the patient and are generally used after hormonal manipulations, except when life-threatening metastases occur. Six to 12 weeks are required before maximum benefits are apparent from hormonal therapy, but hormonal therapy offers a higher rate of remissions which last longer. An objective remission rate in 20 to 30 per cent of cases with disseminated mammary cancer may result from use of antitumor agents. 5-FU seems to be the drug of choice at the present time.

In the administration of drugs, an initial loading of the system is given to the level of mild toxicity. From this point, maintenance dosage is given. If the WBC falls below 3000 or other toxic effects develop, the drug is discontinued. Gastrointestinal symptoms, bleeding, dermatitis and alopecia may occur. Death can occur from bone marrow and liver failure.

The nurse is largely responsible for educating the patient concerning the correct dosage and administration of the drug, and for helping the patient to tolerate the milder side effects while being alert for more serious symptoms.

EMOTIONAL PROBLEMS AFTER MASTECTOMY

It is important to obtain a complete history on every woman admitted to the hospital for breast cancer biopsy, and to attempt to assess the woman's adjustment and preexisting family problems. Such questions as "Tell me about your family" and "Who is taking care of things while you are in the hospital?" are nonthreatening and may help the nurse understand the patient. The nurse needs to know whom she can talk to in the family about their feelings, about the crisis and about plans for supporting the patient. This is only possible in a situation where the hospital and private physician encourage the nurse's participation in a family-centered approach.

TABLE 93–2. CHEMOTHERAPEUTIC AGENTS MOST COMMONLY USED IN THE TREATMENT OF BREAST CANCER

	Brand Name	Generic Name	Route of Administration	Dosage	Toxicity
Alkylating agents	Thiotepa	Triethylenethiophosporamide	I.V.	0.2 mg./kg./day for 4 days	Bone marrow depression
	Cytoxan	Cyclophosphamide	P.O.	50–200 mg./day	Bone marrow depression, alopecia, cystitis, jaundice
	Melphalan	Phenylalanine mustard	P.O.	2–6 mg./day initially 2–4 mg./day maintenance	Bone marrow depression
Antimetabolites	Fluorouracil, 5-FU	5-Fluorouracil	I.V.	10–15 mg./kg./day 3–5 days 5–7.5 mg./kg./ for 3–5 alternate days	Gastrointestinal, bone marrow depression, alopecia
	Methotrexate	Methtrexate	P.O.	0.5 mg./kg./day	Gastrointestinal, liver damage, bone marrow depression
Others	Oncovin	Vincristine	I.V.	0.02–0.05 mg./kg./weekly	Gastrointestinal, peripheral neuritis, bone marrow depression
	Velban	Vinblastine	I.V.	0.1–0.15 mg./kg./ weekly	Gastrointestinal, bone marrow depression, alopecia

From Haagensen, C. D.: *Diseases of the Breast.* Philadelphia, W. B. Saunders Company, 1971, p. 770.

The sexual history of the patient is most appropriately handled when the nurse has the confidence of the patient. However, since the breast is an important aspect of sexuality in our culture, someone needs to consider its importance in this context, preferably the whole team.

The patient who has a mastectomy may use a number of defense patterns in adapting to stress. Not all patients will perceive or handle stress in the same way. Displacement, projection, denial, hope and prayer, stoicism-fatalism or a combination of these defenses may be used. Patients who lose a breast may adapt in the same way they would to any loss. Phantom breast symptoms are not uncommon. Of 203 women with unilateral mastectomy, 33.5 per cent reported phantom symptoms in the missing breast. Premenopausal women demonstrated significantly greater incidence of this phenomenon.

Losing a breast does not make its full impact until the patient goes home. Many women are surprised at the amount of pain and discomfort, marked fatigue, slow healing of the incision, their swollen arm and jittery feelings. Such mundane things as how to find a comfortable position in bed may be a problem. The patient has to decide whether to hide the lesion from her family or to let them see it. The defect may be camouflaged by an appropriately fitted brassiere or a special bathing suit or evening dress, but doubts and fears about her sexual attractiveness may affect even the most secure woman.

The patient may relax from one check-up to the next, but in many instances new symptoms cause the patient to realize she is suffering from advanced cancer. In a study of 60 private hospital patients suffering from fatal cancer, it was found that anxiety and depression were common. About a quarter of the patients reported financial and family problems precipitated by the disease.

To give the patient hope, the nurse must understand and appreciate her difficulties. The practical role for the nurse is to help the patient set expectations that failure will be overcome. By setting short-term goals, the patient may see that she has a choice as to how she faces each small crisis. If she feels that she will not be abandoned and that she will have help in avoiding excessive pain and in "working through" dying, the patient may be better able to live and enjoy each day. Social workers, if available, and pastors can also be sources of ongoing strength. Certainly, the ongoing adjustment will be facilitated by a family and health professionals who understand and care.

Each new development may precipitate aspects of the grieving process such as anger, depression and regression. New symptoms may be overexaggerated, and every new ache and pain may set off the alarm button. The patient needs someone to whom she can talk about these fears. Hopefully, the public health nurse or the nurse in the doctor's office or cancer unit will be the person who can help the patient to realistically handle the new symptoms. Mastectomy groups also can provide a place where patients can talk about their problems. When the disease becomes terminal, the patient needs to be encouraged in self-help as long as possible to give her a feeling of worth. Nurses and others working on a cancer unit need a great deal of help in handling their own feelings and in learning how to interact in a supporting and realistic way with the patient.

BREAST CANCER AND PREGNANCY

Breast cancer is uncommon in pregnancy since most breast cancers occur over the age of 40. The average incidence is about 3 in every 10,000 pregnancies.[15] The overall poor prognosis thought to be associated with pregnancy is probably due to lack of early diagnosis. The pregnant woman should practice breast self-examination and should have a careful breast examination by her doctor at office visits. All true three-dimensional lumps should be biopsied. Thickening should be studied by soft tissue mammography. The prognosis for the pregnant woman is as good as for the nonpregnant woman if there is no axillary node involvement. Radical mastectomy is indicated for operable cases. In pregnant patients with disseminated mammary cancer, abortion combined with castration is of benefit, with use of radiation therapy and chemotherapy as needed for palliation. The nurse can be of benefit to pregnant patients in informing them that lumps may not be due to pregnancy and that early treatment, if they are suspicious, is as important and effective as in other patients.

THE NURSE'S RESPONSIBILITY IN CANCER DETECTION

Cancer of the breast is a major concern to women and to the medical and nursing profession. Breast examination by the patient can be taught to all women at some time during their stay in the hospital, as well as to individuals in other settings. This needs frequent reinforcement to become a pattern with the individual. After a suspicious lump is detected, the woman may still delay going to the doctor. Women who are upset or depressed or who have serious problems neglect medical attention for various reasons. Much more attention must be given to the routine inclusion of breast examination by physicians in their contacts with patients, as well as by the nurse and other paraprofessionals working with the patient. High-risk individuals should be especially attentive to the possibility of cancer. Since at the present time, getting the patient under care at the earliest possible time offers the best chance of cure, every avenue should be used to insure regular breast examination.

References

1. Ackerman, L. A., and Regato, J. A.: *Cancer, Diagnosis, Treatment and Prognosis*. St. Louis, The C. V. Mosby Company, 1970.
2. Baltruch, H.-J. F.: Einige Psychosomatische Aspekte der Krebskrankheit unter Berucksichtigung Psychotherapeutischer Gesichtspunkte. *Zeitschrift fur Psychosomatische Medizin und Psychonalyse, 15*(1): 31–36, January, 1969.
3. Barckley, V.: Enough time for good nursing. *Nursing Outlook, 12*:44–48, April, 1964.
4. Buschke, F., and Parker, R. G.: *Radiation Therapy in Cancer Management*. New York, Grune & Stratton, 1972.
5. Egan, R. L.: Mammography. *American Journal of Nursing, 66*:108–111, January, 1966.
6. Fitzpatrick, G.: Caring for the patient with cancer of the breast. *Bedside Nurse*, February, 1970.
7. Francis, G. M.: Cancer: The emotional component. *American Journal of Nursing, 69*:1677–1681, August, 1969.
8. Gribbons, C. A., and Aliapoulios, M. A.: Treatment for advanced breast carcinoma. *American Journal of Nursing, 72*:678–682, April, 1972.
9. Gros, C., Brun-Valery, L., Israel, L., and Durand de Bousingen: Approche Psychosomatique des Affections Mammaires. *Revue de Medecine Psychosomatique et de Psychologie Medical, 11*(2):239–240, 1969.
10. Haagensen, C. D.: *Diseases of the Breast*. 2nd Ed. Philadelphia, W. B. Saunders Company, 1971.
11. Harrell, H. C.: To lose a breast. *American Journal of Nursing, 72*:676–677, April, 1972.
12. Klagsbrun, S. C.: Cancer, emotions and nurses. *American Journal of Psychiatry, 126*(9):1237–1244, 1970.
13. Klagsbrun, S. C.: Communications in the treatment of cancer. *American Journal of Nursing, 71*:944–948, May, 1971.
14. Koenig, R. R.: Fatal illness: A study of social service needs. *Social Work, 4*:85–89, 1968.
15. Leis, H. P., Jr.: *Diagnosis and Treatment of Breast Lesions*. New York, Medical Examination Publishing Company, 1970.
16. Leis, H. P., Jr.: Surgical approach to breast cancer. *New York State Journal of Medicine*, August 1, 1973.
17. Livingston, R. B., and Carter, S. K.: *Single Agents in Cancer Chemotherapy*. New York, IFI/Plenum Data Corporation, 1970.
18. Marcus, S. L., and Marcus, C. C. (eds.): *Advances in Obstetrics and Gynecology*. Baltimore, The Williams & Wilkins Company, 1967.
19. Quint, J. C.: The impact of mastectomy. *American Journal of Nursing, 63*:88–92, November, 1963.
20. Rubin, P.: Current Cancer Concepts, Carcinoma of the Breast, Stage I, Surgical Spectrum. American Cancer Society, 1967.
21. Weinstein, S., Vetter, R. J., and Sersen, E. A.: Phantoms following breast amputation. *Neuropsychologica, 8*(2):185–197, April, 1970.
22. Zislis, J. N.: Rehabilitation of the cancer patient. *Geriatrics, 25*(3):150–158, 1970.

Nursing Patients Experiencing Disturbances of Endocrine and Metabolic Function

Introduction and Study Guide

Only within the last 50 years has endocrinology been regarded as a bona fide part of internal medicine. Before that time the study of glands and hormones appeared more linked with ritual and magic than with science and medicine. Patients with endocrine disorders were regarded as fascinating "oddities" rather than as people with treatable physiologic disturbances.

Today endocrinology is an exciting, highly respected, rapidly expanding area of study and practice. Because of the explosion of knowledge, nursing patients with endocrine disorders is now more challenging than ever. It is the nurse who must teach the patient about his disease and how to live successfully with it; also, nurses often conduct the newest complicated diagnostic studies and administer the latest potentially dangerous hormonal drugs. If the nurse is to succeed in these endeavors, she must be, above all else, knowledgeable. Thus it is essential not only to obtain a basic understanding of the endocrine system and its disorders but also to keep abreast of new discoveries in the field as well. To aid you in the basic study of endocrinology we suggest using the following guide:

1. Familiarize yourself with the definitions of the following terms: endocrine gland, exocrine gland, hormone, tropic hormone, target gland, insulin, glucagon, carbohydrate catabolism, carbohydrate anabolism, juvenile diabetes, maturity-onset diabetes, fractional urines, lipodystrophies, hyperglycemia, hypoglycemia, ketoacidosis, diabetic coma, insulin reaction, microangiopathy, diabetic retinopathy, thyroxine, thyroid-stimulating hormone (TSH), protein-bound iodine, euthyroid, hypothyroidism, hyperthyroidism, goiter, thyroiditis, thyrotoxicosis, exophthalmos, hyperparathyroidism, hypoparathyroidism, osteitis fibrosa cystica, nephrocalcinosis, adrenal medulla, adrenal cortex, catecholamines, steroids, corticoids, pheochromocytoma, hypocorticism, hypercorticism, virulism, pseudohermaphroditism, neurohypophysis, adenohypophysis, hyperpituitarism, hypopituitarism, gigantism, acromegaly, dwarfism, hypophysectomy.
2. Set up a program of instruction for a diabetic patient in

the hospital: (a) help the patient draw up a week of menus from the American Diabetic Association food lists; (b) teach him how to give himself an injection of insulin; (c) instruct him concerning foot care and the care of cuts and abrasions.

3. Learn the signs of underdosage and overdosage of the following hormonal drug preparations: insulin, thyroid hormone, cortisone, hydrocortisone, fludrocortisone, deoxycorticosterone, vasopressin tannate.

4. Summarize the preoperative and postoperative nursing care of patients undergoing the following surgeries: thyroidectomy, parathyroid gland resection, unilateral adrenalectomy, bilateral adrenalectomy, hypophysectomy.

CHAPTER 94

Introductory Concepts

NORMAL ANATOMY AND PHYSIOLOGY OF THE ENDOCRINE SYSTEM

THE ENDOCRINE GLANDS

The word "gland" is derived from the Latin *glans,* meaning "acorn." The word is thus an appropriate symbol of the powerful effect that minute bodies such as the pituitary have on the total function of the body.

There are two types of glands: exocrine glands and endocrine glands. *Exocrine glands* release their secretions through *ducts,* either inside the body or onto the skin. Examples of exocrine glands include the salivary, sebaceous, and sweat glands; the liver, gastric, and intestinal glands; the pancreas (which is also in part endocrine gland); the prostate; and the mammary and lacrimal glands. In contrast, the *endocrine glands* discharge their secretions (which are called hormones) *directly* into the blood stream rather than through ducts. The endocrine glands include the islands of Langerhans in the pancreas; the gonads; the adrenal, pituitary, thyroid, and parathyroid glands; thymus; and the pineal gland (see Fig. 94-1.) Although each endocrine gland has its own unique independent functions, the various glands are also *interdependent.* Thus the release of hormones from one gland influences the release of hormones from other glands and vice versa. The influence of the endocrine glands upon each other helps to maintain optimum hormonal levels, thereby promoting homeostasis.

HORMONES AND THEIR FUNCTIONS

The term *hormone* is derived from the Greek term *hormon,* which means "to set in motion." Hormones set in motion the various processes that govern our lives—physical and intellectual growth, puberty, reproduction, metabolism, personality development, reactions to stress from both the external and internal milieu, and the maintenance of homeostasis. Although hormones themselves do not initiate the above processes, they act as chemical envoys, creating an intricate chain of communication which links one body system with another, thereby controlling and integrating the body's functions. In its communicative and integrative roles, the endocrine system resembles the nervous system. However, the nervous system sends its messages more swiftly than do the endocrine glands; also neural effects are more rapid in onset, shorter-lived, and more localized.

In terms of their *chemical nature,* hormones are classified as follows:

> Amines (epinephrine, norepinephrine).
> Amino acids (thyroxine).
> Peptides (vasopressin, or antidiuretic hormone).
> Proteins (pituitary growth hormone, parathyroid hormone).
> Steroids (aldosterone, cortisol, androgenic hormones).

The major specific *functions* of each of the endocrine glands and its hormones are delineated in Table 94–1. Note that each of the endocrine glands affects organs and tissues which are far removed from its location in the body; e.g., oxytocin, which is released from the posterior lobe of the pituitary gland located in the brain, causes uterine contractions. Also note that several glands (the thyroid, gonads, and adrenal cortex) are under control of the "master" pituitary gland. The pituitary hormones which govern the secretion of hormones from other glands are called *tropic* hormones. On the other hand, the glands which are influenced by tropic hormones are called *target* glands. As explained later, the target glands also control the secretion of tropic hormones from the pituitary gland by means of negative feedback.

CHARACTERISTICS OF HORMONES

Although each endocrine gland possesses its own unique attributes, all endocrine glands share in common the following characteristics:

> Endocrine glands secrete hormones *cyclically* and in response to certain body and environmental rhythms. For example, estrogen levels rise and fall in a predictable fashion during the menstrual cycle. Also, blood levels of adrenocortical hormones are low in the early morning, rise during the day, and then drop back to lower levels at night.

> Endocrine glands control the *rate* of cellular activities; they do not in themselves initiate biochemical changes.

> Hormones are secreted in *minute* concentrations; however, even tiny amounts of a hormone can have far-reaching effects on body structure and function.

HORMONAL REGULATION

The release of hormones from their parent glands is controlled by both chemical and neurologic factors.

Chemical Control. Hormonal blood levels are controlled in part by *negative feedback*.* Thus a rise or fall in the blood level of one hormone can cause an increase or decrease in the blood level of another hormone. For example, we explained in Unit I that an increased secretion of adrenocortical tropic hormone (ACTH) from the anterior pituitary gland stimulates a rise in the blood level of cortisol from the adrenal cortex, which in turn causes a drop in the blood level of ACTH, and so forth. In addition, blood levels of substances *other than hormones* affect hormonal secretion. For example, you recall from Unit V, Chapter 25, that the calcium level in the blood regulates the release of parathormone (PTH) from the parathyroid glands. Also the release of insulin from the islets of Langerhans in the pancreas depends upon blood glucose levels.

Neurologic Control. Both the autonomic nervous system and central nervous system aid in hormonal regulation. The central nervous system reacts to stimuli of all types from both the external and internal milieu. These reactions are transmitted to the hypothalamus (a vital part of the autonomic nervous system), which in turn conveys impulses to the pituitary gland. Pitui-

*Negative feedback systems are discussed in Unit I.

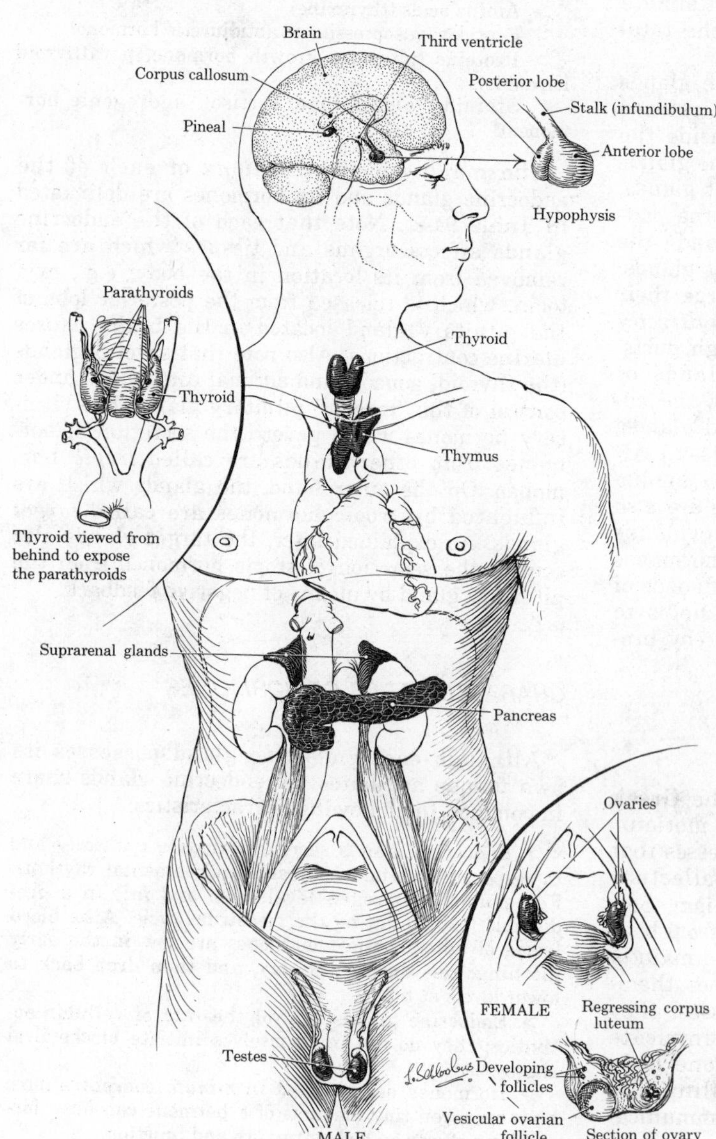

FIGURE 94–1. Diagram of the endocrine system. (From *Dorland's Illustrated Medical Dictionary.* 25th ed., 1974.)

tary hormonal secretions next stimulate appropriate target glands, which results in the release of more hormones.

In addition, two endocrine glands—the adrenal medulla and the posterior pituitary—are of neural origin and are actually a part of the autonomic nervous system. Should these two glands be destroyed or removed, their functions are completely taken over by the nervous system.

ABNORMALITIES OF THE ENDOCRINE SYSTEM: AN OVERVIEW

In essence, endocrine diseases result from hormonal imbalance. Traditionally, endocrine disorders have been classified as arising from either a deficiency or an overabundance of a particular hormone or hormones. However, this way of viewing endocrine disease constitutes a gross oversimplification of a highly complex subject. As Christy points out: "In the light of the discoveries made during the last two decades, it is no longer enough to think of endocrine disease simply as too much or too little hormone."[14] For this reason,

TABLE 94-1. FUNCTIONS OF ENDOCRINE GLANDS

Gland	Hormone	Action of Hormone
PITUITARY		
Anterior lobe	Thyrotropic hormone (TSH)	Stimulates thyroid gland
	Somatotropic hormone (STH)	Stimulates growth
	Gonadotropic hormones (LH, FSH, LTH)	Affect growth, maturity and functioning of primary and secondary sex organs
	Adrenocorticotropic hormone (ACTH)	Stimulates cortex of adrenal glands
	Melanophore-stimulating hormone (MSH)	Stimulates adrenal cortex; affects pigmentation
Posterior lobe	Vasopressin	Decreases production of urine
	Oxytocin	Stimulates uterine contractions
THYROID	Thyroxine Triiodothyronine	Stimulates metabolism (catabolic phase)
	Thyrocalcitonin	Lowers plasma calcium and phosphates
PARATHYROID	Parathyroid hormone	Regulates blood calcium level
ADRENAL		
Cortex	Hormones divided into three main groups:	
	Glucocorticoids	Tend to increase amount of sugar in blood
	Mineralocorticoids	Tend to increase amount of blood sodium and decrease amount of potassium in blood
	Androgens (male hormones)	Govern certain secondary sex characteristics All corticoids important for defense against stress or injury to body tissues
Medulla	Epinephrine (Adrenaline): "fight or flight" hormone	Elevates blood pressure; converts glycogen to glucose when needed by muscles for energy; increases heartbeat rate; dilates bronchioles
OVARIES	Estrogens and progesterone	Stimulate development of secondary sex characteristics Effect repair of endometrium after menstruation
TESTES	Testosterone	Essential for normal functioning of male reproductive organs Stimulates development of male secondary sex characteristics
ISLANDS OF LANGERHANS OF PANCREAS	Insulin	Promotes metabolism of carbohydrates

Christy suggests using the following comprehensive clinical classification:*

1. *Primary hyperfunction of endocrine glands:* major causes include benign tumors and hyperfunctional states which are not linked with tumor growth. Malignant hormone-secreting tumors are uncommon.
2. *Primary hypofunction of endocrine glands:* causes include congenital absence of the gland, tumor growths which destroy the gland, and infections. In addition, some authorities speculate that certain hypofunctional disorders of the thyroid, parathyroid, and adrenal glands may be autoimmune in nature.
3. *Secondary failure of endocrine glands:* hypofunction of the gonads, thyroid, and adrenal cortex may develop secondary to *pituitary* insufficiency.
4. *Functional disorders of the endocrine glands:* endocrine disease develops not only secondary to pituitary disorders but also as a consequence of nonendocrine disease. For example, hyperparathyroidism may complicate renal failure, and hyperaldosteronism may develop secondary to cirrhosis of the liver.
5. *Failure of an end-organ to respond to a hormone:* for example, the bones may fail (for unknown reasons) to grow linearly despite the administration of human growth hormone.
6. *Production by an endocrine gland of an abnormal or unusual hormone:* these congenital disorders are classified as *inborn errors of metabolism.* Examples include congenital adrenal hyperplasia and goitrous cretinism.
7. *Production of a hormone by a nonendocrine organ:* ectopic secretion of hormones by nonendocrine tumors is a fairly common cause of glandular hyperfunction. Tumors which are most frequently linked with ectopic syndromes are cancers of the lung, thymus, and pancreas.
8. *Iatrogenic endocrine disease:* causes include (a) the prescribed administration of hormones either for hormonal replacement therapy or as a pharmacologic method for controlling inflammation, obesity, infertility, and so forth; (b) surgical removal of a gland; and (c) destruction of a gland by irradiation.

NONSPECIFIC SYMPTOMS OF ENDOCRINE DISEASE

The manifestations of endocrine disease are numerous and varied. Nonspecific symptoms which may develop in some endocrine disorders include the following:

> Growth abnormalities: growth may be delayed, stunted (dwarfism), excessive (gigantism), or inappropriate (acromegaly).
> Weakness and exhaustion.
> Appetite changes (polyphagia or anorexia).
> Blood pressure abnormalities (hypertension or hypotension).
> Polyuria and polydipsia.
> Renal colic and stones.
> Tetany, paresthesias, and muscle cramps.
> Bone and joint disease.
> Untoward changes in appearance.
> Abnormal skin pigmentation.
> Hirsutism.
> Personality changes (patients may be nervous and restless or lethargic, depending upon the nature of the imbalance).
> Sexual disturbances (loss of potency in men and infertility in women).

NURSING CARE OF PATIENTS WITH ENDOCRINE DISEASES: OVERVIEW

Patients with endocrine disorders endure many problems and experience multiple needs. For example, they may suffer from a loss of self-esteem due to their often grotesque appearance; they may experience family problems and rejection from loved ones due to personality changes; they may feel exhausted, debilitated, disgusted, and totally unable to cope with the stresses of life. Moreover, these persons must endure numerous exacting diagnostic tests, and some face the possibility of undergoing dangerous surgery; others are faced with the often bitter realization that they must permanently change their diet, activities, and life style. How can the nurse help these patients cope with such serious problems?

First of all, the nurse must offer genuine emotional support to both the patient and his family. This is not always easy to do because patients with endocrine diseases may be either lethargic, agitated, forgetful, depressed, or even frankly psychotic. Patients may also be afraid of the final consequences of their disease, and their fear may be manifested toward others in the guise of anger, hostility, rejection, and so forth. It is important to recognize that the patient's behavior, however bizarre, is probably a symptom of his illness and that his personality will return to normal with treatment.

Secondly, the nurse is usually responsible for collecting specimens for laboratory tests. It is essential to begin and end all tests on time, to preserve specimens correctly, and to instruct the patient and other ward personnel concerning their role in conducting tests.

Thirdly, the nurse is responsible for administering hormones to patients with hormonal deficiencies. When giving a particular hormone, always know the symptoms of underdosage and overdosage. The dosage of hormones must often be readjusted to meet the changing needs, tempos, and stresses of a person's life, or serious imbalances occur. For example, a diabetic must increase his insulin dosage if he increases his food intake or develops an infection.

Finally, the nurse must act as a teacher. Most patients with endocrine disorders undergo a lifelong program of therapy. It is her task to teach patients the basics of self-care, e.g., dietary requirements, self-administration of drugs, personal hygiene, and the signs of hormonal imbalance. With help and guidance, the majority of patients with chronic endocrine disorders can learn to regulate their lives and successfully live with their disease.

*Classification adapted from Christy,[14] p. 1720.

CHAPTER 95

Nursing Patients with Endocrine Disorders of the Pancreas

PHYSIOLOGY OF THE PANCREAS

The pancreas, a large, fish-shaped organ which lies behind and inferior to the stomach and liver, is both an exocrine and an endocrine gland. You recall that the *exocrine* role of the pancreas is carried out by cells within the walls of the tubular and acinar units of the gland; these cells secrete enzymes which catabolize the *digestion* of *proteins, carbohydrates,* and *fats* (see Unit XVI, Ch. 81).

The *endocrine* functions of the pancreas are controlled by the *islets of Langerhans;* the islets, which are differentiated into alpha and beta cells, are scattered throughout the pancreatic tissues. The two hormones (insulin and glucagon) secreted by the islets play a vital role in the control of carbohydrate metabolism. *Insulin,* which is synthesized by the beta cells, is a powerful *hypoglycemic* agent; i.e., it acts to lower blood sugar levels by promoting the passage of glucose into the cells. Conversely, *glucagon,* which is synthesized by alpha cells, is a *hyperglycemic* agent; i.e., it raises blood sugar by promoting the conversion of glycogen (the principal form in which carbohydrates are stored in mammals) to glucose within the liver. In the section below and throughout this chapter, we will study the effects of these powerful hormones more closely.

HORMONAL FACTORS REGULATING CARBOHYDRATE METABOLISM

The hormones which play a role in the regulation of carbohydrate metabolism include the following: (a) insulin, (b) glucagon (c) adrenocorticotropic hormone (ACTH), (d) corticosteroids, (e) epinephrine, and (f) thyroid hormone. The role of each hormone is considered below.

Insulin and Glucagon. The two principal hormones controlling carbohydrate metabolism are insulin and glucagon, both of which are simple proteins. *Insulin,* the hypoglycemic factor, plays a key role in carbohydrate, fat, and protein metabolism; more specifically, it performs the following functions:

> Stimulates the active transport of glucose into muscle and adipose tissue cells. When insulin levels are inadequate, glucose remains outside of the cells, which in turn causes the blood sugar concentration to rise above normal. The exact means by which insulin promotes intracellular transport remains unknown.

> Regulates the rate at which carbohydrates are burned by cells for energy.

> Promotes the conversion of glucose to glycogen for storage, but inhibits the conversion of glycogen to glucose.

> Promotes the conversion of fatty acids into fat which can be stored as adipose tissue, but inhibits the breakdown of adipose tissue, the mobilization of fats, and the conversion of fat to glucose.

> Stimulates protein synthesis within the tissues, but inhibits the conversion of protein into glucose.

In sum, insulin actively *promotes* those processes which *lower* blood sugar levels (e.g., the transport of glucose into cells and the conversion of glucose to glycogen) and *inhibits* those processes which *raise* blood sugar levels (e.g., the conversion of glycogen, fats, and proteins into glucose).

The *rate* of insulin secretion by the beta cells is regulated by the amount of sugar in the blood. When the blood sugar level *rises,* the islet cells are stimulated to release increased amounts of insulin into the blood, which accelerates glucose transport into the cells and glucose conversion into glycogen. As the blood sugar level *falls,* insulin release from the islets slows until the blood sugar drops below normal. If food is absorbed, the islets again release insulin, and so forth.

When insulin secretion is *deficient,* the blood sugar level remains abnormally high, and *diabetes mellitus* eventually develops. When insulin is secreted or administered in *excessive* amounts, blood sugar levels drop dangerously low and *insulin shock* develops.

In contrast to insulin, *glucagon* promotes a *rise* in blood sugar, whenever glucose levels drop too low. Glucagon causes hyperglycemia by promoting (in some obscure fashion) the conversion of glycogen to glucose. Glucagon imbalance (excess or deficiency) is rare.

To illustrate the opposing but complementary roles of insulin and glucagon, consider what happens to your blood sugar when you eat a meal. Note in Figure 95-1 that when you have breakfast at 8:00 in the morning, around 8:15 your blood sugar starts to rise and insulin release begins. By approximately 9:00 A.M. the blood sugar level will have reached its peak, and insulin secretion will stop shortly afterwards. By 10:00 A.M. your blood sugar will have dropped back to a low normal, because insulin will have promoted glucose transport into the cells and glucose conversion into glycogen and fatty deposits. If you are unable to eat again until noon or 1:00 P.M., the body (with the aid of glucagon) will convert glycogen back to glucose, and this glucose will then be used by the cells for in-between meal energy. If you are fasting and cannot eat until 8:00 that evening, your body will obtain energy by converting adipose tissue into glucose.

What factors are necessary for the production of insulin and glucagon? Production of these essential hormones is dependent upon the following three requirements:

> A *healthy pancreas* with actively functioning alpha and beta cells.

> A diet adequate in protein; remember that both insulin and glucagon are simple protein substances.

> Normal *potassium* (K^+) levels; for unknown reasons, hypokalemia (abnormally low K^+ levels) results in diminished insulin production.

When either insulin or glucagon production is inadequate to meet the body's needs, the missing hormone may be administered *parenterally*. These two hormones cannot be given orally because they are both inactivated within the gastrointestinal tract by proteolytic enzymes.

Other Hormonal Factors. Although insulin and glucagon play the predominant roles in carbohydrate regulation, the following hormones also influence blood sugar levels:

> Adrenocorticotropic hormone (*ACTH*) and the *glucocorticoids* of the adrenal cortex raise the blood sugar by stimulating the conversion of fat and protein into glucose. These hormones are released whenever the body is subjected to stress or blood sugar levels drop abnormally low.

> *Epinephrine,* another hormone released under stress, stimulates a rise in blood sugar by promoting the conversion of glycogen to glucose.

> *Thyroid hormone* can raise or lower the blood sugar. Under normal conditions, thyroid hormone (like insulin) promotes the utilization of glucose for energy. However, under starvation conditions, thyroid hormone promotes the conversion of fats and proteins to glucose for energy.

NORMAL CARBOHYDRATE METABOLISM

Carbohydrates (which are compounds of carbon, hydrogen, and oxygen) are the body's *preferred fuel* as well as its most immediate source of energy. The metabolism of carbohydrates involves a number of intricate chemical processes which are dependent upon the presence of insulin, glucagon, and, to a lesser extent, the other hormones discussed above. In review, carbohydrate metabolism, like all forms of metabolism, has a destructive phase (catabolism) and a constructive phase (anabolism). *Carbohydrate catabolism* is the process by which the body breaks carbohydrates down into smaller molecules and uses the energy which is released in the process. The three major forms of carbohydrate catabolism are listed below.

1. *Glycolysis,* the initial process in carbohydrate catabolism, is the breakdown of sugars into simpler compounds. As a result of glycolysis, a molecule of glucose is split, and its energy is partially released.
2. The *Krebs cycle,* which completes the mechanism of carbohydrate catabolism, is a series of chemical changes which results in the total breakdown of the glucose molecule into carbon dioxide, water, and energy.
3. *Glycogenolysis*—the conversion of glycogen to glucose—takes place whenever blood sugar

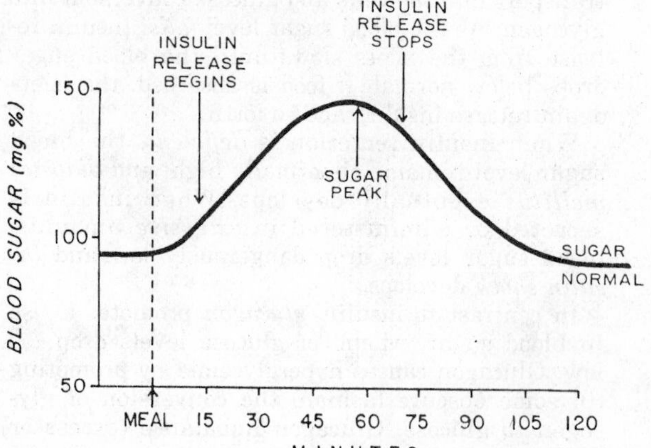

FIGURE 95-1. The effect of insulin upon blood sugar following meals. (From Crampton, J. H., et al.: *Instructions for the Diabetic Patient.* 9th ed. Seattle, Washington, The Mason Clinic, 1966.)

levels drop abnormally low. As stated earlier, this process depends upon the presence of glucagon.

Carbohydrate anabolism, on the other hand, is a process by which molecules of carbohydrate, fat, or protein are chemically converted into glycogen and stored principally within the liver. The process of anabolism, unlike catabolism, does not release energy but instead uses the body's energy. The two biochemical processes which are involved in carbohydrate anabolism are as follows:

1. *Glycogenesis* (the reverse of glycogenolysis) is the conversion of glucose, fructose, or galactose into glycogen; as you recall, this process depends upon the release of insulin.
2. *Glyconeogenesis* is the transformation of fats and proteins (i.e., noncarbohydrate materials) into glucose or glycogen for use by cells as fuel. This process is employed by the body as an emergency measure whenever carbohydrates are not available for use as fuel.

In sum, carbohydrate metabolism involves (a) the active transport of glucose into the cells and the release of energy; (b) the storage of that glucose which is not immediately needed for energy as glycogen and as fat; (c) the conversion of glycogen back to glucose whenever blood glucose drops; and (d) the conversion of fats and proteins to glucose or glycogen, whenever these two carbohydrate substances are depleted and energy is needed.

It is apparent from this discussion that carbohydrate metabolism is intricately linked with protein and fat metabolism. Carbohydrates, proteins, and fats can all be burned by the body for energy. However, as we emphasized earlier, carbohydrates are the body's *preferred* source of fuel. This means that the body will always burn carbohydrates rather than fats and proteins, provided (a) carbohydrate intake is adequate; (b) sufficient insulin is present to spark the passage of glucose into the cells; and (c) reserve stores of glycogen are present. However, carbohydrates *cannot* be used for fuel whenever (a) the blood glucose is low and glycogen stores have been depleted (e.g., during starvation diets); or (b) when the body is unable to utilize its available glucose due to lack of insulin (e.g., in diabetes mellitus). In these cases, the body is forced to obtain its fuel by converting first fats and then proteins to glucose. As you will learn later, fats are only partially metabolized in the absence of normal carbohydrate metabolism. As a result of faulty fat metabolism, ketone bodies and acetone bodies accumulate in the blood, thereby lowering the pH. Without medical intervention, these acidic substances can eventually precipitate diabetic acidosis and coma.

HYPOFUNCTION OF THE ISLETS OF LANGERHANS (DIABETES MELLITUS)

BASIC CONSIDERATIONS

Diabetes mellitus is a disorder of carbohydrate metabolism due to an insulin deficiency; it eventually results in (a) disturbances of protein and fat metabolism with symptoms of ketosis and acidosis; and (b) severe vascular lesions which can lead to blindness, heart disease, peripheral vascular disease, and neuritis.

The term *diabetes* is derived from a Greek word which means "something which goes through," or a *siphon;* thus the term "diabetes" is applied to diseases which are characterized by *polyuria* (overproduction of urine).* The term *mellitus* is taken from the Latin *mel,* which means "honey," thereby describing the "honeyed" or sweet taste of the urine. The urine is "sweet" in diabetes mellitus because, in the absence of sufficient insulin, sugar accumulates in the blood and eventually spills into the urine.

The exact *cause* of diabetes mellitus is unknown. However, diabetes mellitus inevitably develops in the face of a *persistent insulin deficiency.* What causes insulin deficiency? Insulin deficiency may result from one or more of the following three factors:

1. *Beta cell damage:* the beta cells which secrete insulin may be destroyed or injured by either pancreatitis, pancreatic tumors, or possibly by exposure to certain cytotoxic chemicals.
2. *Insulin inactivation:* although insulin production is normal, the insulin secreted is inactivated by circulating antibodies or altered by insulin antagonists. Little is known to date about insulin antagonists except that they are substances which combine with insulin and in some way block or alter its effect on glucose metabolism.
3. *Increased insulin requirements:* obesity, hyperthyroidism, acromegaly, hyperadrenocorticism, pregnancy, infection, and stress are all conditions which increase the body's need for insulin by raising the blood sugar. When the blood sugar remains persistently high (especially in a diabetes-prone person or a diagnosed diabetic), the islet cells eventually exhaust themselves in their effort to produce sufficient insulin to handle the blood sugar overload.

There are two recognized types of diabetes: *juvenile diabetes* and *adult-onset diabetes.* These two disease forms are compared and contrasted in Table 95–1.

INCIDENCE AND PREDISPOSING FACTORS

Diabetes mellitus is currently the most significant endocrine disorder, and is a major cause of death in the United States. Even when diabetes does not kill, it can produce major permanent disabilities, such as blindness, severe vascular in-

*Diabetes *insipidus,* which is characterized by the excretion of large amounts of dilute urine, is described on p. 1385.

sufficiency, and so forth. Moreover, diabetes is a widespread disease; the exact numbers of persons whom it affects is as yet undetermined. The American Diabetic Association claims that 4,200,000 people in the United States have diabetes (approximately one out of every 50 persons); 1,600,000 persons have *undiagnosed* diabetes; and 5,600,000 individuals are *potential* diabetics.[34]

The four groups of persons who are particularly susceptible to diabetes include the following:

1. *Older individuals:* Although diabetes may develop at any age, it particularly affects those between the ages of 40 and 60. Once a person turns 65, he has a 50 per cent chance of becoming a diabetic before he dies.[44]

2. *Obese persons:* As illustrated in Figure 95–2, the chances of developing diabetes are truly substantial if one is both over 40 and overweight. Obese people are probably more susceptible to diabetes because the excess food which they consume forces the islets of the pancreas to produce massive amounts of insulin, which eventually causes beta cell exhaustion.

3. *Women:* Mothers who have had many children are more likely to develop diabetes than men or women who have never been pregnant. The stress and metabolic demands of pregnancy increase the need for insulin secretion. The grand multipara (the woman who has had seven or more children) may eventually develop beta cell exhaustion. Moreover, a woman who gives birth to a heavy baby (over 10 pounds) is more than 30 times as likely to develop diabetes as the woman whose infant has a normal birth weight.

4. *Persons with diabetic relatives:* Note in Table 95–2 that the risk of developing diabetes is greatly increased when one has relatives with diabetes; indeed, if both parents have diabetes, their offspring stand a 100 per cent chance of becoming diabetic themselves. The exact mode of inheritance for diabetes is not yet known.

Diabetes also strikes the young; 4 out of every 10,000 children under 15 are diagnosed as diabetics.[25]

Over the last decades, the incidence of diabetes in the United States has been steadily increasing. Every year more than 250,000 new cases of diabetes are discovered. Diabetes is on the rise for a number of reasons. People live longer today than in the past; consequently there is a large population of older persons who are more susceptible to diabetes. Also diagnostic tests for diabetes are improving, and public awareness of the disease is growing. Finally, treatment with insulin has lowered the mortality rate among those people with juvenile diabetes; as a result, young diabetics marry and pass the disease on to their offspring, which further increases the already swelling rolls of diabetic patients.

PATHOPHYSIOLOGY AND BASES OF SYMPTOMS

Insulin, as emphasized, directly regulates the rate of carbohydrate metabolism and indirectly influences fat and protein metabolism. Consequently, an insulin deficiency, due to beta cell damage, obesity, overwhelming stress, and so forth, inevitably triggers a chain reaction of unto-

TABLE 95–1. A COMPARISON OF JUVENILE DIABETES AND ADULT-ONSET DIABETES

Factors	Juvenile Diabetes	Adult-Onset Diabetes
Age at onset	May occur at any age; usually appears before age 15	Usually occurs in obese persons over age 40
Synonyms	Growth-onset diabetes, labile diabetes, brittle diabetes, insulin-dependent diabetes	Maturity-onset diabetes, senile diabetes, mild diabetes
Possible etiology	*Absolute* deficiency of insulin caused by deficiency of pancreatic islets	*Relative* insulin deficiency possibly cuased by insulin antibodies, by insulin antagonists, or by excessive demands for insulin due to obesity, persistent stress, etc.
Severity	Very severe; little or no circulating insulin may be present	Usually mild; some circulating insulin almost always present
Therapeutic control	Insulin injections and careful planning of diet essential	Insulin injections often unnecessary; condition controlled by diet and oral hypoglycemic agents
Sequelae	Vascular and neural damage inevitably develops	Same

ward events. First of all, glucose is not conveyed from the extracellular fluid to the intracellular compartment. Without glucose for energy, the cells become *energy-depleted* and must oxidize fats and proteins drawn from adipose tissue and muscle stores. The resultant breakdown of tissue composed of fat or amino acids causes *wasting* of tissue, a *negative nitrogen balance* (due to protein breakdown), and *ketosis* (due to fat breakdown).

Glucose, which is locked outside the cells without the "insulin key," begins to accumulate and eventually raises the blood sugar level to about 160–180 mg./100 ml. (hyperglycemia). The elevated blood sugar (which exerts a strong osmotic force) pulls cellular water into the blood, which results in *cellular dehydration* (see Ch. 24). As the blood sugar level rises, glucose eventually spills into the urine, causing *glycosuria*. The osmotic pull of glucose within the urine prevents the reabsorption of water within the kidney tubules, causing *extracellular dehydration*. Finally, these pathologic developments result in the following *four cardinal symptoms of diabetes:*

Symptom	Bases of Symptoms
Polyuria (frequent urination)	Water is not reabsorbed by the renal tubules because of the osmotic activity of glucose.
Polydipsia (excessive thirst)	Polyuria causes severe dehydration, which in turn causes thirst.
Weight loss (juvenile-onset only)	Because glucose is not available to the cells, fat and protein stores are broken down and used for energy.
Polyphagia (excessive hunger)	Tissue breakdown and wasting causes a state of starvation which compels the stricken individual to eat voraciously.

In addition to the four cardinal symptoms, persons with diabetes may develop other distressing problems. One of the most severe complications of diabetes is *metabolic acidosis;* this condition arises in untreated diabetics and in those patients whose condition remains uncontrolled by insulin and diet (see later in this chapter).

A second serious complication of diabetes is *chronic hyperlipemia* (excessive fats in the blood). Chronic hyperlipemia coupled with hyperglycemia results in the premature development of vascular lesions both in the coronary arteries (*atherosclerosis*) and in the peripheral arteries and arterioles (*peripheral arteriosclerosis*). Vascular degeneration may, in turn, affect the kidneys, causing *nephropathy,* and the eyes, resulting in diabetic *retinopathy* and *blindness*. In addition, a persistently high blood sugar may eventually cause either a painful or painless *neuropathy*.

Finally, patients with diabetes are easy prey for *microorganisms* and *fungi* because of the high sugar content of their blood and urine. Also diabetics, because of their poor circulation, suffer from *retarded healing* of infections and wounds.

DIAGNOSTIC TESTS

Diabetes mellitus is diagnosed on the basis of the following findings:

> A family history of diabetes.

> A medical history of obesity, multiple pregnancies, and easy susceptibility to infection.

> Presence of the cardinal symptoms of polyphagia, polydipsia, polyuria (the three P's), and weight loss.

> Laboratory findings which include glucosuria, mild ketonuria, hyperglycemia, decreased glucose tolerance, and a high serum cholesterol.*

The two major forms of diagnostic tests for diabetes include blood tests and urine tests for glucose and acetone.

Blood Tests. The major blood tests which are employed to diagnose the presence and severity of diabetes include (a) fasting blood sugar; (b) postprandial blood sugar; (c) oral and intravenous

*The serum cholesterol test is discussed in Unit X, Chapter 48.

OUT OF EVERY **20** DIABETICS OVER 40 YEARS OF AGE,

17 WERE OVERWEIGHT BEFORE ONSET

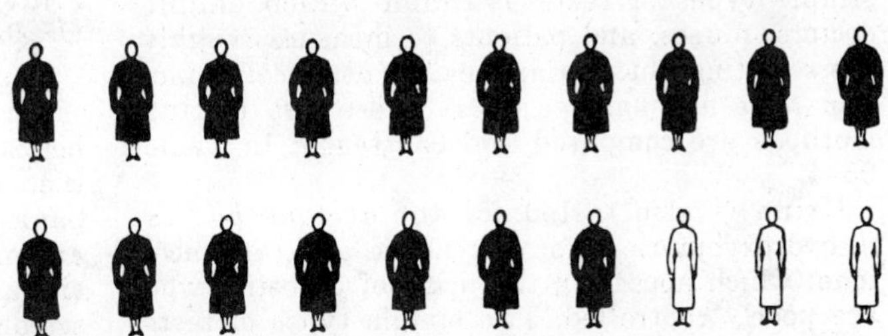

FIGURE 95–2. Incidence of overweight before onset of diabetes. (Used by permission of Metropolitan Life Insurance Company.)

TABLE 95–2. PROBABILITY OF DEVELOPMENT OF DIABETES IN RELATION TO KNOWN DIABETES IN RELATIVES

Probability Per Cent	Diabetic Relatives
100	Identical twin or both parents
80	One parent, a sibling, and a grandparent via the nondiabetic parent
65	One parent and a sibling of the nondiabetic parent One parent and a parent of the nondiabetic parent
50	One parent and one sibling
40	One parent and first cousin on the nondiabetic parent's side
35	Two grandparents (not spouses)
25	One sibling
20	Two grandparents (spouses) or one parent One grandparent Uncle or aunt First cousin

From Spencer, R. T.: *Patient Care in Endocrine Problems.* Philadelphia, W. B. Saunders Company, 1973, p. 142.

glucose tolerance tests (GTT); and (d) tolbutamide (Orinase) tolerance test. These blood tests are described in Table 95–3. Instruct the patient taking these tests to ingest only the food and drugs which he receives from the hospital staff. Explain to your patient that food and certain medications can distort test results.

Urine Tests. Three common nursing procedures related to diabetic care are (a) collecting urine specimens at specified times, (b) testing the urine for sugar and acetone, and (c) teaching patients methods for testing their own urine. Let us first consider urine tests for *sugar*.

As we stated earlier, when the blood sugar level rises to abnormal heights, the excess glucose eventually spills into the urine. There are two simple types of tests available which enable doctors, nurses, and patients to measure roughly the resulting glucosuria; they are *chemical reduction tests* and *enzyme tests*. These two testing methods are compared and contrasted in Table 95–4.

Urine is also tested for the *acetone bodies* (β-hydroxybutyric acid, acetoacetic acid, and acetone) which appear in the urine of diabetics who are poorly controlled. Two simple types of tests are available: the *Ketostix test* and *Acetest*. To perform these tests, place a drop of urine on an Acetest tablet or insert a Ketostix stick in the urine specimen. Wait for the time period indicated on the instructions and then compare the color of the tablet or stick with an accompanying color chart.

Urine testing may be ordered for a variety of reasons. There are three different types of urine specimens: (a) the single specimen, (2) fractional urine specimens, and (3) 24-hour specimens. Briefly, these tests are used for the following reasons:

1. The *single* specimen of urine for glucose testing is often ordered as a *screening procedure* for diabetes. If sugar is found in the patient's urine, the doctor will order further blood and urine tests to confirm or rule out the diagnosis.
2. *Fractional urines* for glucose and acetone are performed by nurses or patients at specified times throughout the day, usually before meals and at bedtime. The results of the urine tests are often used to determine the patient's insulin dosage for the day (see below); test results also indicate whether or not the diabetic's condition is being adequately controlled by diet and medication. Because accuracy is necessary, the specimen collected for testing should *not* contain urine which has been in the patient's bladder all night or even for several hours. Stagnant urine will *not* accurately reveal the amount of glucose in the urine at the *time of the test.* To assure accuracy, have the patient void ½ hour before the test, drink some fluid, and then void again. Urine from the second voiding can then be used with confidence for testing.
3. *24-hour urine specimens* are ordered to determine *quantitative sugar* or the amount of glucose which a patient loses over a 24-hour period. At the beginning of the 24 hours, the patient is asked to void and the urine is discarded. Thereafter, all urine voided is saved in a gallon jug. At the end of the 24 hours, the patient is again asked to void, the urine is poured into the jug, and the jug is sent to the laboratory. Normally, the urine is sugar-free.

STAGES OF DIABETES

The four recognized stages of diabetes are suspected diabetes, prediabetes, chemical or latent diabetes, and overt diabetes. These stages are compared in Table 95–5.

PREVENTION AND EARLY DETECTION OF DIABETES

As we stated earlier, the number of new diabetics diagnosed yearly is rising. Health agencies (i.e., public health departments, insurance companies, and the American Diabetic Association) are attempting to control diabetes through professional and public educational programs, mass screening tests, and research.

Basically, the control of diabetes centers around *prevention programs* and *early case finding* of diabetics who are still in the early stages of the disease. The *prevention* of diabetes rests primarily upon public education. Through educational campaigns, Americans are gradually becoming aware of the dangers of obesity, diabetes being but one such danger. Persons with prediabetes are being taught to adhere to low-calorie, low-carbohydrate diets in order to prevent the eventual surfacing of overt diabetes. Because diabetes is hereditary, doctors and public health nurses are encouraging known diabetics married to each other to adopt children rather than to have their own children who will also suffer from diabetes.

Since diabetes cannot always be prevented, health agencies are striving to diagnose diabetes in its early, less dangerous stages. Persons who should always be examined for diabetes include (a) the obese; (b) anyone suffering from excessive thirst, hunger, urination, and weight loss; (c) women over 40; and (d) mothers who have given birth to several overweight babies.

The laboratory tests used for mass screening include (a) the Dextostix blood test for blood glucose, which uses blood from a pinprick; (b) postprandial blood sugar; and (c) urine tests for glucose. Of these three tests, urine tests for glycosuria are considered the least accurate and least specific for diabetes.

Mass testing must be followed by further testing of all persons with suspected diabetes. Individuals with an elevated blood sugar or glycosuria should be referred to their physician for careful evaluation of their health status. It is important to emphasize to possible diabetics that early treatment of this disease can prevent many of its serious complications.

CLINICAL CARE

Introduction. To date, there is no cure for diabetes. Consequently, the overall goal of care for diabetic patients is *control* or *regulation* of their disease rather than cure. When diabetes is successfully regulated, the diabetic is able to avoid complications while continuing to live a normal useful life.

Essentially diabetic control depends upon the proper interaction of the following three factors: (1) diet; (2) insulin or hypoglycemic pills; and (3) exercise. The *diet,* which is low in calories and carbohydrates, is prescribed on the basis of the patient's size, weight, age, and occupation (i.e., sedentary, moderately active, very active). *Insulin,* which must be present in sufficient amounts for proper carbohydrate metabolism, is either produced by the patient himself or administered via injections when production is inadequate. Ideally, it is best if diabetics are able to regulate their disorder by dietary control alone. However, the majority of juvenile diabetics and approximately one quarter of maturity-onset diabetics require insulin injections for the rest of their lives. In addition, one third to one half of maturity-onset diabetics take oral hypoglycemic agents (e.g., Orinase, Diabenese) in addition to controlling their diets.[14]

Finally, the diabetic must regulate his *exercise* or activity so that the rate of energy expenditure is in balance with the injection and utilization of carbohydrate. For instance, if the patient exercises less than usual, he will require either a lighter diet or more insulin; if he exercises more than usual, the diabetic will need to either eat more food or lower his insulin. Thus any variance in one factor will necessitate adjustment of the other two factors.

What are the major *criteria* for good control of diabetes? Generally diabetes is considered under control when the following conditions are met:[15]

> The fasting blood sugar is normal.

> The blood sugar is no higher than 180 mg./100 ml. 2 hours after breakfast and no more than 200 mg./100 ml. 2 hours after lunch.

> The urine is negative for sugar and acetone before breakfast and dinner.

> 24-Hour collections of urine contain below 5 Gm. of sugar.

> The patient has optimal weight and enjoys good health.

More specific criteria of "control" are related to the chemical severity of the diabetes and the strictness of control necessary. Haunz writes that diabetic patients can be placed into one of five groups, which are based on the severity of the diabetes, Group 1 being the least serious category and Group 5 the most severe [24] (see Table 95–6).

While all authorities agree that diabetes *must* be controlled if the diabetic is to avoid complications, exactly what constitutes a workable program of control remains debatable. As in the treatment of all chronic disorders, the patient's age and basic personality patterns must be considered when drawing up a treatment regime. For example, an adolescent with "brittle" diabetes may rebel if his diet and activities are too strictly controlled; rebellion, in turn, may result in the patient's self-destructive refusal to comply with *any* restrictions on diet or activity. On the other hand, an obsessive-compulsive person may ritualize his diabetic regime to the point that it totally dominates his life. An anxious individual may worry so much about his diabetes that the accumulated stress actually alters his blood sugar! Therefore it is essential to investigate the patient's habits and attitudes toward his illness before deciding on the exact degree of control necessary. The program which is tailored as much as possible to the individual diabetic's personality is most likely to prove successful over the years.

The Diabetic Diet. Despite the discovery of insulin in 1921 and oral hypoglycemic agents during the 1950's, *diet* still remains the most important aspect of the diabetic treatment regime. The twofold purpose of the diabetic diet is to curtail the ingestion of excess carbohydrate and to correct or avoid obesity.

The most important factor in the success of a diabetic diet is the patient's wholehearted willingness to adhere to his prescribed diet.

If the diabetic maintains his diet and controls adult-onset weight, he will not need to take insulin or oral hypoglycemic agents. As we emphasized earlier, it is ideal to control diabetes with diet alone, thereby eliminating the need for medication. However, for the following reasons, this ideal is not always attainable:

> Diabetic diets are *expensive*. Foods high in carbohydrate (i.e., spaghetti, macaroni, bread, sweets) tend to cost far less than foods with a high protein and fat content (e.g., meats, butter, milk). Consequently, without financial aid, diabetics from the lower economic classes sometimes cannot afford the foods on a diabetic diet even though they wish to cooperate.

> The *older* diabetic may resist dieting. Lifelong food habits are difficult to change. Food is associated in the minds of many persons with love, memories of childhood, religious rituals, ethnic holidays, and special personal occasions, such as birthdays, weddings, and so forth. Adherence to a diet, especially during holidays, may make the patient feel deprived, rebellious, and unwilling to continue dieting.

> The *adolescent* diabetic may resent any diet which forces him to eat differently from his peers; for example, a young person may find it difficult to eat low-calorie, low-carbohydrate foods while his friends drink

TABLE 95–3. BLOOD TESTS FOR DIABETES MELLITUS

Measurement and Purpose	Restrictions (Food, Water, Activity)	Procedure
Fasting blood sugar (FBS): determines amount of glucose in blood when patient fasting	No food for 12 hours prior to test (usually 8 P.M. to 8 A.M.); water allowed	Blood drawn from venipuncture and sent to laboratory
Postprandial blood sugar: measures blood sugar following a meal	None	Patient given meal with approximately 100 Gm. carbohydrate; venous blood drawn 2 hours after meal
Oral glucose tolerance test (GTT): determines patient's response to a measured dose of glucose	No food for 12 hours prior to test or during test; water allowed; no smoking, coffee, or tea allowed during test; these substances alter body's response to carbohydrate. *Minimize activity* (e.g., walking) which alters glucose metabolism; *minimize stress* because epinephrine and cortisone released raise blood sugar by promoting gluconeogenesis	High carbohydrate diet for 3 days prior to test; NPO for 12 hours before test; weigh patient; obtain fasting blood and urine specimens; administer 100 Gm. glucose by mouth diluted in lemon juice; obtain blood and urine specimens ½, 1, 2, 3, 4, and 5 hours after dose of glucose; mark all specimens with time obtained and take to laboratory
Intravenous glucose tolerance test: performed when patient unable to drink or tolerate oral glucose	Same as oral GTT	High carbohydrate diet for 3 days prior to test; NPO 12 hours before test. Weigh patient; obtain fasting blood and urine specimens; administer 50 ml. of 50% glucose in distilled water I.V. over 2-minute period; take blood and urine specimens every ½ hour for 2 hours
Tolbutamide (Orinase) test: tests insulin production in cases of questionable diabetes or prediabetes	NPO for 12 hours prior to test; water allowed	Venous blood drawn for FBS; 1 Gm. of sodium tolbutamine given I.V. in 20 ml. of normal saline; blood for FBS drawn at intervals of 15, 30, 45 minutes and 1, 1½, 2, 2½, and 3 hours

endless bottles of soda pop and eat all the candy and potato chips they desire. Adolescence in our culture is already a time of crisis and stress. Needless to say, being a diabetic *and* an adolescent may cause the patient to rebel against his parents, his doctor, and his diet.

> Highly *neurotic persons* are sometimes compulsive eaters. Satisfying the urge to eat may be more important to such individuals than the need to control their diabetes. To prevent complications, the obese compulsive eater will need to seek psychiatric help.

Because diabetes is a chronic disease, weight reduction in the obese patient must be *permanent.* Many persons (including nondiabetics) do not have the necessary self-discipline for permanent weight maintenance. According to reports from private and public hospitals, only 5 to 40 per cent of diabetic patients are successful in their weight control programs.[24]

When patients cannot or will not adhere to their prescribed diabetic diets, the doctor is then forced to prescribe insulin or oral hypoglycemic agents in order to maintain the patient's blood sugar within normal limits and thereby prevent symptoms. However, as Haunz points out: ". . . the use of insulin or oral agents becomes a highly undesirable therapy of concession. It is safe to say that this is the predicament in which the vast ma-

TABLE 95-3. BLOOD TESTS FOR DIABETES MELLITUS (*Continued*)

Findings	Untoward Effects	Precautions
Normal: 80–120 mg./100 ml. serum; *abnormal:* 200 mg./100 ml. or more diagnostic of diabetes mellitus	None	None
Normal: Same as normal findings above (see Fig. 95-1)	None	None
Normal: blood glucose climbs to peak of 140 mg./100 ml. in first hour and returns to normal by 2nd or 3rd hour; *abnormal:* blood glucose *does not* return to normal by 2nd or 3rd hour; all urine specimens *positive for glucose*	Transitory weakness, sweating, and dizziness may develop during 2nd and 3rd hour	Diuretics, glucocorticoids, estrogens, and oral contraceptives may distort test findings; these medications should be omitted prior to testing. Test should *not* be performed on patient with initial FBS of over 200 mg./100 ml.
Normal: blood sugar returns to normal by end of 2 hours; *abnormal:* blood sugar remains elevated over 2-hour period. *Note:* I.V. test *not* as reliable as oral GTT	Patient may feel facial warmth and dizziness during I.V. administration	Same as oral GTT
Normal: fasting blood sugar levels fall by 30% within 30 minutes following tolbutamine injection; *abnormal:* FBS level fails to fall by 30% within 30 minutes following injection; this failure indicates limited insulin production	Signs of hypoglycemia (see pp. 1330–1331)	Test should not be used in cases of suspected hypoglycemia or hyperinsulinism; severe hypoglycemic crisis could result

TABLE 95-4. METHODS OF URINE TESTING FOR SUGAR

	Chemical Reduction Method	Enzyme Method
Basis of Test	Substances used for testing contain metallic ions (e.g., copper and bismuth). When urine containing glucose is heated, the ions are reduced. Due to ion reduction, precipitation occurs, and the urine changes color, depending upon the amount of glucose present.	Substances used for testing contain an enzyme called glucose oxidase. When urine containing glucose contacts glucose oxidase, a color change occurs which varies with the amount of glucose present.
Types of Tests	(a) Benedict's test (used only in laboratories today). (b) Clinitest tablets (Ames Company).	(a) Test Tape (Eli Lilly and Company). (b) Clinistix (Ames Company).
Procedure	Clinitest: (a) Place in test tube 5 drops urine, 10 drops water, and 1 Clinitest tablet. (b) Allow solution to boil. (c) When boiling stops, wait 10 seconds and compare color of urine to color chart accompanying set-up. (d) *Blue* color indicates negative result, *yellow* moderately positive for sugar, and *orange* highly positive for sugar.	(a) Dip a tape (Tes Tape) or enzyme strip (Clinistix) into the urine. (b) Wait one minute. (c) Compare tape or strip with color chart accompanying set-up to evaluate if acetone or glucose is present.
Specificity of method	Reaction not specific to glucose alone; test also detects galactose, lactose, fructose, maltose, salicylates.	Reaction occurs *only* in the presence of glucose.
Advantages	Inexpensive; reasonably reliable; colors of urine easily differentiated.	Extremely simple to use; easy to transport tape or tablets when traveling; reacts positively only to glucose.
Disadvantages	More difficult to use than enzyme methods; equipment somewhat cumbersome; positive reactions can occur in presence of substances other than glucose.	Expensive; less reliable than Clinitest; positive reactions occur in presence of even tiny amounts of glucose; difficult to differentiate colors.
Sources of Error	Tablets become inactive if exposed to air; keep bottle tightly closed. Administration of vitamin C may cause a false-positive reaction.	Tes-Tape deteriorates in 4 months, Clinistix strips within a few months. Use only fresh testing materials. Administration of vitamin C and the diuretic Mercuhydrin may cause a false-negative reaction.

TABLE 95-5. THE STAGES OF DIABETES

Stage of Diabetes	Symptoms	Laboratory Findings
Prediabetes	None	None
Suspected diabetes	Symptoms only during stress (trauma, infection, pregnancy)	Temporary hyperglycemia during stress periods
Chemical or latent diabetes	No symptoms	Abnormal GTT; postprandial hyperglycemia
Overt diabetes	Symptoms of diabetes; ketoacidosis may occur	Elevated FBS; abnormal GTT

jority of obese diabetics and their well-meaning physicians find themselves today."[24] What nurses can do to reverse this undesirable situation is discussed on pp. 1324 to 1325.

TYPES OF DIABETIC DIETS. There are two types of diabetic diets: (1) the qualitative diet, and (2) the quantitative diet. The *qualitative* diet is prescribed for persons with mild (Grade I diabetes) (see Table 95-6). Patients on the qualitative diet must be taught to (a) avoid adding sugar to their coffee, cereal, and so forth; (b) avoid foods sweetened with sugar, e.g., jellies, jams, cakes, ice cream; (c) limit foods which are high in starch (e.g., spaghetti, macaroni, bread); (d) test their urine daily for sugar and acetone 2 hours following dinner; and (e) make an appointment for a postprandial blood sugar every 3 months to insure that the diet is adequate.

> *Caution patients on a qualitative diet to call their physician should they develop an infection or undergo surgery or accidental trauma; during these times mild diabetics may need a stricter diet and possibly medication.*

The stricter *quantitative* diet is prescribed for Grades II through V diabetes. There are two methods for preparing quantitative diets; they are as follows:

Exchange measured diet. This highly practical diet is followed by the majority of diabetics today, and is advocated as the diet of choice by the American Diabetic Association. The exchange method is based upon the premise that foods which contain the same food value can be exchanged with one another without altering the patient's basic dietary prescription. For example, note in Table 95-7 that foods are categorized into six basic lists or groups: (1) milk exchanges; (2) vegetable exchanges; (3) fruit exchanges; (4) bread exchanges; (5) meat exchanges; and (6) fat exchanges. Note further that the foods in each lists contain the same number of calories, as well as the same amounts of protein, fat, and carbohydrate. For instance, all the foods within the milk exchange contain 12 Gm. of carbohydrate, 8 Gm. of protein, 10 Gm. of fat, and 170 cal. Thus a patient may drink 1 cup of whole milk or ½ cup of evaporated milk or 1 cup of buttermilk made from whole milk and still receive the same amount of calories, carbohydrate, protein, and fat. As you can see, the exchange diet provides the patient with considerable variety and choice. It is also less cumbersome than the weighed diet because the patient can measure his food and liquids with household measures (i.e., measuring cups, tablespoons) and can estimate the size of meat and fruit portions (e.g., 1 slice cold cuts, 1 medium peach).

Fixed weighed diet. This form of quantitative diet is much more accurate than the exchange measured diet, but it is also more cumbersome and tedious. As the name implies, the diabetic weighs his food (drawn from a list of meats, fish, vegetables, and fruit) in grams on a food scale. The diet is "fixed" in that the amounts of milk, fat, bread, and cereal do not vary from day to day. For most diabetics, weighing food is unnecessary and time-consuming.

TABLE 95-6. METHODS AND CRITERIA FOR CONTROL OF DIABETES

Group	Diet	Insulin	Oral Hypoglycemic Agents	Criteria for Control
Group 1 ("Grade I" diabetes)	"Qualitative" diet; sugar restricted	None	None	Weight normal No glycosuria FBS under 100 mg./100 ml. Postprandial blood sugar less than 150 mg./100 ml.
Group 2 ("Grade II" diabetes)	"Quantitative" diet; all food measured	None	None	No glycosuria FBS less than 120 mg./100 ml. Postprandial blood sugar under 160 mg./100 ml.
Group 3 ("Grade III" diabetes)	"Quantitative" diet	30 Units of insulin or less	Oral agent may be given in place of insulin	Minimal glycosuria FBS below 130 mg./100 ml. Postprandial blood sugar below 125 mg./100 ml.
Group 4 ("Grade IV" diabetes)	"Quantitative" diet	More than 30 units insulin required daily	None	Same as Group 3
Group 5	"Quantitative" diet	None	Combined therapy with a sulfonylurea and phenformin (DBI)	Same as Group 3

TABLE 95-7. AMERICAN DIETETIC ASSOCIATION (ADA) EXCHANGE LISTS*

LIST 1. MILK EXCHANGES
Carbohydrate—12 grams; protein—8 grams; fat—10 grams; calories—170

	Measure	*Grams*
Milk, whole	1 cup	240
Milk, evaporated	½ cup	120
Milk, powdered	¼ cup	35
Skim milk*	1 cup	240
Powdered skim milk (nonfat dried milk)*	¼ cup	35
Buttermilk (made from whole milk)	1 cup	240
Buttermilk (made from skim milk)*	1 cup	240

*Add 2 fat exchanges.

LIST 2. VEGETABLE EXCHANGES

A. These vegetables may be used as desired in ordinary amounts. Carbohydrates and calories negligible.

Asparagus	"Greens"	Lettuce
Broccoli	Beets	Mushrooms
Brussels sprouts	Chard	Okra
Cabbage	Collard	Pepper
Cauliflower	Dandelion	Radishes
Celery	Kale	Rhubarb
Chicory	Mustard	Sauerkraut
Cucumbers	Spinach	String beans
Escarole	Turnip	Summer squash
Eggplant		Tomatoes

B. Vegetables: 1 serving equals ½ cup equals 100 grams. Carbohydrates—7 grams: protein—2 grams; calories—36

Beets	Peas, green	Squash, winter
Carrots	Pumpkin	Turnips
Onions	Rutabaga	

LIST 3. FRUIT EXCHANGES
Carbohydrate—10 grams; calories—40

	Measure	*Grams*
Apple	1 sm (2″ diam.)	80
Applesauce	½ cup	100
Apricots, fresh	2 medium	100
Apricots, dried	4 halves	
Banana	½ small	50
Berries: strawberries, raspberries, blackberries	1 cup	150
Blueberries	⅔ cup	100
Cantaloupe	¼ (6″ diam.)	200
Cherries	10 large	75
Dates	2	15
Figs, fresh	2 large	50
Figs, dried	1 small	15
Grapefruit	½ small	125
Grapefruit juice	½ cup	100
Grapes	12	75
Grape juice	¼ cup	60
Honeydew melon	⅛ (7″ diam.)	150
Mango	½ small	70
Orange	1 small	100
Orange juice	½ cup	100
Papaya	⅓ medium	100
Peach	1 medium	100
Pear	1 small	100
Pineapple	½ cup	80
Pineapple juice	⅓ cup	80
Plums	2 medium	100
Prunes, dried	2 medium	25
Raisins	2 tbsp.	15
Tangerine	1 large	100
Watermelon	1 cup	175

LIST 4. BREAD EXCHANGES
Carbohydrate—15 grams; protein—2 grams; calories—68

	Measure	*Grams*
Bread	1 slice	25
Biscuit, roll	1 (2″ diam.)	35
Muffin	1 (2″ diam.)	35
Cornbread	1 (1½″ cube)	35
Flour	2½ tbsp.	20
Cereal, cooked	½ cup	100
Cereal, dry (flake and puffed)	¾ cup	20
Rice or grits, cooked	½ cup	100
Spaghetti, noodles, etc., cooked	½ cup	100
Crackers, graham (2½″ sq.)	2	20
Oyster	20 (½ cup)	20
Saltines (2″ sq.)	5	20
Soda (2½″ sq.)	3	20
Round, thin (1½″ diam.)	6	20
Vegetables		
Beans and peas, dried, cooked	½ cup	100
Baked beans, no pork	¼ cup	50
Corn	⅓ cup	80
Parsnips	½ cup	125
Potatoes, white, baked, boiled	1 (2″ diam.)	100
Potatoes, white, mashed	½ cup	100
Potatoes, sweet, or yams	¼ cup	50
Sponge cake, plain	1 (1½″ cube)	25
Ice cream (omit 2 fat exchanges)	½ cup	70
Popcorn	1 cup	

LIST 5. MEAT EXCHANGES
Protein—7 grams; fat—5 grams; calories—73

	Measure	*Grams*
Meat and poultry (med. fat) (beef, lamb, pork, liver, chicken, etc.)	1 oz.	30
Cold cuts (4½″ sq., ⅛″ thick)	1 slice	45
Frankfurter	1 (8-9/lb.)	50
Fish: cod, mackerel, etc.	1 oz.	30
Salmon, tuna, crab	¼ cup	30
Oysters, shrimp, clams	5 small	45
Sardines	3 medium	30
Cheese, cheddar, American	1 oz.	30
Cottage	¼ cup	45
Egg	1	50
Peanut butter*	2 tbsp.	30

*Limit to one serving per day unless adjustment is made to balance carbohydrate content.

LIST 6. FAT EXCHANGES
Fat—5 grams; calories—45

	Measure	*Grams*
Butter or margarine	1 tsp.	5
Bacon, crisp	1 slice	10
Cream, light, 20%	2 tbsp.	35
Cream, heavy, 40%	1 tbsp.	15
Cream cheese	1 tbsp.	15
French dressing	1 tbsp.	15
Mayonnaise	1 tsp.	5
Oil or cooking fat	1 tsp.	5
Nuts	6 small	10
Olives	5 small	50
Avocado	⅛ (4″ diam.)	25

*From Haunz, E. A.: Diabetes mellitus in adults, *In Current Therapy 1973.* Conn, H. F. (ed.), Philadelphia, W. B. Saunders Company, 1973, pp. 373, 374.

CALCULATING THE DIABETIC DIET. The balanced diabetic diet should contain the following nutrients: (a) calculated quantities of carbohydrates, proteins, and fats; (b) normal amounts of vitamins and minerals, and (c) no more than 100 Gm. of fat, principally drawn from the polyunsaturated fat group. When the doctor prescribes a diabetic diet, he must consider the following factors:

> The patient's *ethnic, religious, and cultural background;* e.g., if the patient is an Italian, some allowance must be made for eating slightly starchier foods and drinking an occasional glass of wine with dinner. When such allowances are not made, the patient may eventually reject his diet completely.

> The patient's *height* and *weight.* If the patient is overweight for his height, the doctor will prescribe a low-calorie reducing diet. If the patient's weight is satisfactory, the doctor will prescribe a maintenance diet. The *basal* caloric *requirement* (i.e., the caloric requirement in the resting state) for the maintenance of one's ideal weight is 10 cal. per lb. ideal weight. Thus the woman who ideally weighs 120 lb. will need 120 × 10 or 1200 cal. a day to maintain her weight when *at rest;* note below that calories must be added to the basal calorie requirement to compensate for the patient's activity level.

> The patient's *occupation* and *normal activity level.* Patients who have sedentary occupations (e.g., typist) will require fewer calories than a person with a moderately active occupation (e.g., floor nurse) or a strenuous job (e.g., manual laborer). To calculate total daily calories, the physician adds 25 per cent of the basal caloric requirement to the total daily caloric allowance of the sedentary person, and 50 to 75 per cent of the basal requirement for more active patients. For example, a typist who ideally weighs 120 lb. and whose basal caloric requirement is 1200 cal. per day will require 300 more calories daily (25 per cent of 1200) and thus a total daily requirement of 1500 calories.

> *Distribution of carbohydrate, protein, and fat in the diet.* Normally the diabetic diet contains approximately 40 per cent carbohydrate, 20 per cent protein, and 40 per cent fat. Using the exchange system, the ADA has developed nine different diabetic meals which are based upon the patient's daily caloric requirements. For example, a 1200-cal. diet calls for 125 Gm. of carbohydrate or 500 cal. (125 × 4); 60 Gm. of protein or 240 cal. (60 × 4); and 50 Gm. of fat or 450 cal. (50 × 9).*

> *Meal distribution.* For a mild diabetic who does not require insulin, the physician usually distributes the food exchanges between three daily meals. However, the diabetic patient who takes insulin will need mid-afternoon and evening snacks to prevent insulin shock.

A typical meal plan based upon the exchange method for a hypothetical patient called Mrs. L. Jones is shown in Table 95–8.

*Recall from Unit V, Chapter 25, that 1 Gm. of carbohydrate is equivalent to 4 cal., 1 Gm. of protein to 4 cal., and 1 Gm. of fat to 9 cal.

TABLE 95–8. TYPICAL MEAL PLAN*

Write or paste your meal plan on this page

*MEAL PLAN FOR Mrs. L. Jones

Carbohydrate 168 Protein 85 Fat 55 Calories 1300

YOUR FOOD FOR THE DAY

Amount	Kind of Food	Choose From
2 cups	MILK	List 1
Any Amount	VEGETABLE EXCHANGES A	List 2A
1	VEGETABLE EXCHANGES B	List 2B
4	FRUIT EXCHANGES	List 3
3	BREAD EXCHANGES	List 4
8	MEAT EXCHANGES	List 5
3	FAT EXCHANGES	List 6

Divide this food as follows:

YOUR MEAL PLAN

Breakfast:
1 Fruit Exchange
1 Bread Exchange
1/2 c Skim Milk
1 Meat Exchange
1 Fat Exchange

Lunch or Supper:
1 Bread Exchange
3 Meat Exchange
1/2 c Skim Milk
1 Fat Exchange
1 Fruit Exchange
1 Vegetable A Exchange

Mid Afternoon:
1 Fruit Exchange

Dinner or Main Meal:
1/2 Bread Exchange
4 Meat Exchange
1 Vegetable A Exchange
1 Vegetable B Exchange
1 Fruit Exchange
1 Fat Exchange

1/2 C Skim Milk

Bedtime Meal:
1/2 c Skim Milk
1/2 Bread Exchange

*From *Meal Planning with Exchange Lists.* Prepared by American Diabetes Assoc., Inc. and the American Dietetic Association.

Note that this diabetic diet is relatively low in calories; note also that the various exchanges are listed for the entire day as well as for each individual meal. Because this patient takes insulin, she requires mid-afternoon and bedtime snacks.

Two possible breakfast menus for Mrs. Jones drawn from the ADA exchange lists could include the following foods:*

Exchange	Breakfast No. 1	Breakfast No. 2
1 fruit exchange	½ cup orange juice	1 cup berries
1 bread exchange	1 muffin	1 slice toast
Skim milk	½ cup skim milk	½ cup skim milk
1 meat exchange	1 egg (hardboiled)	1 poached egg
1 fat exchange	1 teaspoon butter (for muffin)	1 slice crisp bacon

There are many other combinations of breakfast foods which you could plan for this patient, as well as many appetizing lunches and dinners. Remember, the more varied the exchanges, the more enjoyable the patient will find eating and the more likely she will be to adhere to her diet.

BASIC DIABETIC DIETARY RULES. Usually it is either the nurse or dietitian who must instruct the diabetic patient concerning his diet. When you have this responsibility, be certain to emphasize to your patient the following rules and patient guidelines:

> Accurately measure all foods with household measures; i.e., the cup, tablespoon.

> Vary the different exchanges so that the daily diet is interesting and palatable.

> Weigh in at least twice a week, at the same time, in the same amount of clothing and on the same scale. Report to the doctor changes in weight of over 3 lb.

> Do not add sugar, syrup, honey, jelly, or jam to foods, and do not add sugar when cooking.

> Do not use fruits which are packed in heavy syrup; use only water-packed fruits, artificially sweetened candies, gelatin desserts, beverages, and so forth. However, it is expensive and unnecessary to buy "dietetic foods."

> Use only pure canned or frozen fruit juices, and avoid the purchase of fruit "drinks" because these usually contain sugar.

> Drink only certain approved "diet" pops. Among these are: Canada Dry Low-Calorie Sodas, Fresca, Diet Shasta, Sugar-Free Dr. Pepper, and Tab. Since the banning of cyclamates by the Federal Food and Drug Administration (FDA), other diet drinks contain too much sugar for use by diabetics.

> Do not drink excessive amounts of coffee, because caffeine causes the blood sugar to increase significantly.

> Alcohol may sometimes be used moderately; however, do not drink more than 2 oz. of liquor a day. If a mix is desired, combine liquor with either water or nonsweetened mixers. However, always consult the physician for his policy concerning the ingestion of alcohol.

> Eat *all* of the food prescribed; this is particularly important when insulin or oral hypoglycemic agents are also prescribed. If unable to finish a meal, always compensate for the uneaten portion of food by eating a comparable amount of calories and nutrients as a snack later in the day.

*From *Meal Planning with Exchange Lists*. Prepared by American Diabetes Association, Inc., and the American Dietetic Association.

> If a meal is delayed, drink a glass of milk or eat a cracker while waiting in order to avoid an insulin reaction.

> When dining out in restaurants, order standard foods (e.g., a broiled steak, baked potato) and avoid casseroles, gravies, fried foods, and sweetened desserts.

Insulin Therapy. As we stated earlier, the *principal action* of insulin is to lower the blood sugar by (a) promoting the transport of glucose into the cells, and (b) inhibiting the conversion of glycogen, fats, and proteins into glucose.

Insulin injections are necessary when either (a) the patient's beta cells are so severely damaged that he cannot manufacture sufficient insulin (e.g., in "brittle" juvenile diabetes and cancer of the pancreas); and (b) the patient (usually an obese maturity-onset diabetic) is unable to adhere to a low-calorie, low-carbohydrate diet, and consequently needs additional insulin to metabolize the excessive carbohydrates.

It is important to remember that any person who takes insulin may develop an insulin (hypoglycemic) reaction or insulin "shock" owing to an overdose of insulin or the omission of a meal or part of a meal. Insulin reactions are discussed below.

TYPES OF INSULIN. There are seven different types of insulin which are grouped according to their speed of action in the body; they include the following:

A. Rapid-acting insulins
   1. Crystalline zinc insulin (regular insulin)
   2. Semilente insulin
B. Intermediate-acting insulins
   1. Globin zinc insulin
   2. Neutral protamine Hagedorn insulin (NPH insulin)
   3. Lente insulin
C. Slow-acting insulins
   1. Protamine zinc insulin (PZI)
   2. Ultralente insulin

These various insulins are compared and contrasted in Table 95–9. While the basic action of all seven types of insulin is the same (i.e., the reduction of blood sugar), note that the various insulins differ in appearance, in time span of action, and in the time period during which an insulin reaction is most likely to occur.

For patients who are difficult to control, two different insulins are sometimes mixed together and administered in an injection. For example, doctors often order NPH insulin or PZI insulin mixed with regular insulin in order to provide for both the patient's immediate needs and his day-long requirements. Likewise, Lente, Semilente, and Ultralente insulins may be mixed with each other; also Lente insulin and regular insulin can be mixed. Insulins, once mixed, should be used at once and never stored. (See Fig. 95-3.)

INSULIN DOSAGE. Insulin dosage is highly vari-

TABLE 95–9. A COMPARISON OF INJECTABLE INSULIN PREPARATIONS

Type of Insulin	Appearance	Indications	Time Span of Action	Time of Administration	Time When Insulin Reaction May Occur
Rapid-acting:					
1. Crystalline (regular)	Clear	Poorly controlled "brittle" diabetes; infections, trauma, and surgery (as temporary supportive measure); ketoacidosis and coma; fractional urines indicating glycosuria or acetonuria	Onset: 1 hour or less; "peak" (hours): 2–4 hours; duration: 6–8 hours	Before breakfast, lunch, dinner. and bedtime if fractional urine indicates glucosuria or acetonuria	Before lunch if given in the morning; before bedtime if given prior to evening meal. Reactions prevented by eating meals on time
2. Semilente	Cloudy	Patients allergic to crystalline insulin	Onset: 1 hour; "peak" hours: 4–10 hours; duration: 12–16 hours	Usually 30 to 45 minutes before breakfast	Before lunch
Intermediate-acting:					
1. Globin	Clear	Rarely used today	Onset: 2–4 hours; "peak" hours: 6–12 hours; duration: 18–24 hours	30 minutes to 1 hour before breakfast	Late afternoon
2. NPH	Cloudy	Patients who can be controlled by one dose of insulin daily	Onset: 2-4 hours; "peak" hours: 6–12 hours; duration: 24–48 hours	Usually 30 minutes to 1½ hours before breakfast	Late afternoon; during the night
3. Lente	Cloudy	Patients allergic to NPH insulin	Onset: 2–4 hours; "peak" hours: 6–12 hours; duration: 24–48 hours	30 minutes to 1½ hours before breakfast	Late afternoon; during the night
Slow-acting:					
1. Protamine Zinc (PZI)	Cloudy	Rarely used today except in patients uncontrolled by other insulins; used to prevent hyperglycemia during night	Onset: 3–6 hours; "peak" hours: 12–20 hours; duration: 24–36 hours	Before breakfast	Between 2 A.M. and breakfast
2. Ultralente	Cloudy	May be mixed with Semilente to obtain a satisfactory 24-hour action curve	Onset: 8 hours; "peak" hours: 12–24 hours; duration: 36+ hours	Before breakfast	Between 2 A.M. and breakfast

able; it ranges from as low as 5 U. per day for the patient with occasional glucosuria to thousands of units daily for the patient who is insulin resistant. Insulin dosage is regulated, first of all, by the *requirements of the individual.* For example, the "brittle" juvenile diabetic has a greater insulin requirement than does the maturity-onset diabetic. Also, the insulin requirement always increases when a patient is seriously ill, develops an infection, undergoes surgery, or suffers trauma.

Secondly, insulin dosage is based upon the patient's *response* to his insulin injections. The patient's response, in turn, is measured by blood glucose tests and urine tests for sugar and acetone. Because diabetics vary widely in their response to insulin, the doctor initially determines dosage by trial and error. The process of regulating the patient's insulin dosage may require from 1 to 3 weeks. For example, the admitting orders for a newly diagnosed patient whose diabetes is not complicated by ketosis or acidosis may be approximately as follows:

Intermediate insulin (either NPH or Semilente insulin can be used), 20 U. A.C.
Fractional urines QID
Fasting blood sugar daily
Daily postprandial blood sugar 2 hours following lunch
Regular insulin for glucosuria to be given on the following schedule:

1+ .... no insulin
2+ .... 5 U.
3+ .... 10 U.
4+ .... 15 U.
Positive acetone ..... add 5 U. insulin

Guided by the patient's blood sugar levels and urine tests, the physician next increases the dosage of NPH insulin by 4 to 6 U. daily until the patient's blood sugar level stabilizes and he no longer requires supplemental doses of regular insulin. In some cases, the doctor may prescribe mixing an intermediate insulin or long-acting insulin with a short-acting insulin for better control.

ADMINISTRATION OF INSULIN. Administered correctly, insulin is a life-saving drug for the severe diabetic; administered incorrectly, insulin may cause complications ranging from tissue damage to lethal hypoglycemia (insulin shock). To administer insulin properly, you will need to study the following subject areas: (a) insulin concentrations; (b) insulin syringes; (c) insulin storage; (d) preparation for administration; (e) site selection and rotation; (f) insulin administration; and (g) self-injection of insulin.

Insulin concentrations. Insulin dosage is always prescribed in *units;* this means that all types of insulin (crystalline, NPH, Lente, and so forth) are commercially prepared in 10-ml. vials which contain either 40, 80, or 100 U./ml. Thus U-80 insulin contains 80 U. of insulin per ml., and is *twice* as strong a preparation as U-40 insulin, which contains 40 U. of insulin per ml. U-100 insulin is a new preparation which may eventually replace both U-40 and U-80 insulins. The concentration of an insulin preparation is always clearly marked on the bottle—U-40 insulin in *red* and U-80 insulin in *green.*

Insulin syringes. Administer insulin in an *insulin syringe* which corresponds in calibration to the concentration of insulin in the vial.

Remember: *To prevent dangerous error, administer U-40 insulin in a U-40 syringe, U-80 insulin in a U-80 syringe, and U-100 insulin in a U-100 syringe.*

Needles used to administer insulin include (a) 25 or 26 gauge (½–¾ inch long) stainless steel needles, or (b) the more expensive 25 to 26 gauge disposable needles. However, Burke points out that an obese diabetic patient may need a 1–1½ inch needle for best results.[10] Teach patients who will give their own insulin to discard any needles which have dull or rough points.

Storage. Insulin must be refrigerated but *never frozen.* Once opened, insulin vials should be stored in their boxes to protect them from contamination and from exposure to strong light. Discard any bottle of insulin which (a) is older than the expiration date printed on the bottle; (b) has sat open but unused for several weeks; or (c) contains granules or clumped particles.

Preparation for administration. Always observe the following safety rules when preparing insulin:

> Carefully check the label on the insulin bottle against the doctor's order for both the *type* of insulin and the *dosage* ordered; also check the bottle for the *concentration* of insulin (U-40, U-80, U-100), the *expiration* date, and the *appearance* of the insulin (i.e., clear, cloudy, or containing abnormal precipitation).

> Prepare insulin at room temperature; the administration of cold insulin may possibly be one factor in the development of lipodystrophy (see p. 1332). Insulin should be removed from the refrigerator several hours before preparation time.

> Use an insulin syringe which corresponds to the concentration of the insulin you are administering.

> Before drawing up NPH, Lente, Semilente, Ultralente, or PZI insulins, roll the bottle between the palms of your hands until the insulin is thoroughly mixed. Do not shake the bottle.

> If you must mix two types of insulin (e.g., NPH or PZI with regular insulin), follow the procedure illustrated in Figure 95–3.

> Before giving insulin to the patient, *always check the insulin you have prepared with another nurse.* Double check the information on the medication card against both the label on the insulin bottle and the amount of insulin in the syringe.

Remember: *Administering an overdose of insulin or the wrong type of insulin could kill the patient.*

> Before giving insulin, also double check the *patient's identity*. Patients are often drowsy in the early morning hours before breakfast and may answer to any name. As an added precaution, ask the patient to tell you his name as well as checking the patient's armband.

> Do not give insulin to the patient who is NPO prior to surgery or a special diagnostic procedure without first consulting the physician.

Remember: *If the patient does not eat for a long period but still receives his usual dose of insulin, he will develop an insulin reaction.*

Site selection and rotation. The diabetic patient may need to receive or give himself insulin injections for the rest of his life. Over time, the repeated use of only a few sites for injections results in either *atrophy* or *hypertrophy* of the tissues at the injection site (see p. 1331). These abnormal tissue changes result in poor absorption of the injected insulin with consequent loss of control. To prevent tissue changes, it is important to choose the site for injection carefully and *rotate sites systematically*. The sites for injections should be (a) easily accessible (use thighs, abdomen, upper back, buttocks, and upper arms); (b) relatively insensitive to pain (avoid the midline of the body where there are numerous nerve endings); and (c) relatively normal in appearance and to touch (avoid areas already damaged by hypertrophy or atrophy).

Once the sites for injection have been chosen,

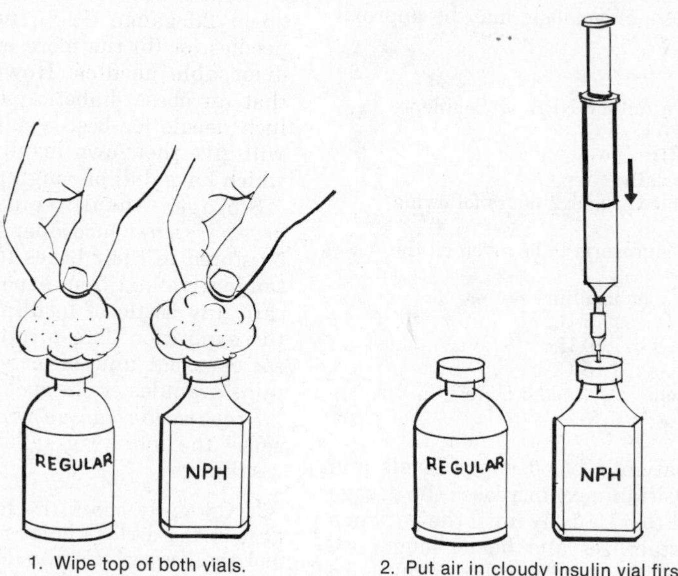

1. Wipe top of both vials.

2. Put air in cloudy insulin vial first.

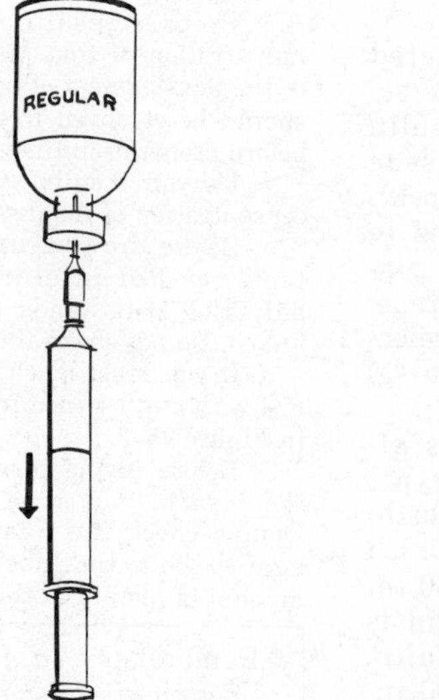

3. Withdraw regular insulin into syringe, then cloudy insulin.

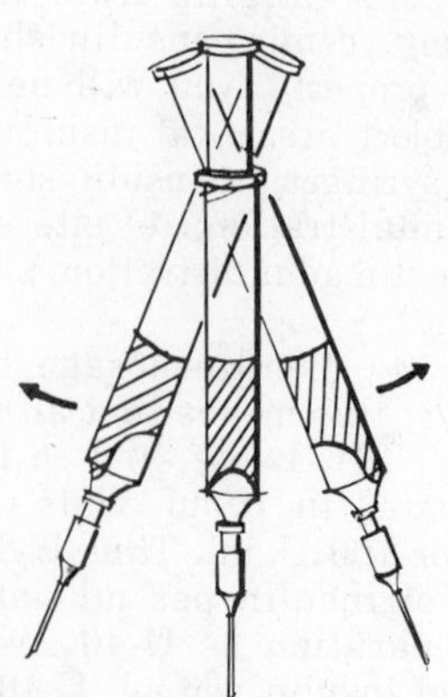

4. Put air bubble in syringe and mix.

FIGURE 95-3. The technique of preparing two types of insulin in one syringe. (From Sutton, A. L.: *Bedside Nursing Techniques in Medicine and Surgery.* 2nd ed. 1969.)

you must rotate them *systemically* so that the same site is not injected more often than once every 6 to 8 weeks. To plan the patient's site rotation, first of all construct a map of the sites you will use (see Fig. 95–4). Note in Figure 95–4 the large number of sites available. When you or the patient daily inject each site, check that site off on the map. Emphasize to the patient the importance of adhering to a definite injection plan to avoid eventual tissue damage.

Insulin administration. There are three methods for injecting insulin. Two of these methods are illustrated in Figure 95–5. In both these technics, the injection is given subcutaneously with a 25 gauge, ½ inch needle at a right angle to the skin. These two technics differ in that the skin is stretched taut in one method and pinched up into a fold in the alternate method.

Some authorities believe that the traditional methods of insulin injection pictured in Figure 95–5 result in slowed absorption of insulin; also they may cause adverse tissue changes—scarring if injected into fat and irritation if injected into the muscle. Consequently, some sources recommend that insulin be injected "deep *between* the layer of fat and muscle" to insure better absorption and reduce tissue irritation[10] (see Fig. 95–6). This method of injection involves the following three steps:

1. Grasp the skin and fat and lift the tissue away from the muscle, thereby forming a pocket at the base of the fold.
2. Inject with a long enough needle to pass through the fat (a 1–1½ inch needle may be needed for the obese patient).
3. Inject the insulin into the pocket between the fat and muscle at a 20 to 45° angle (this angle is almost parallel to the skin).

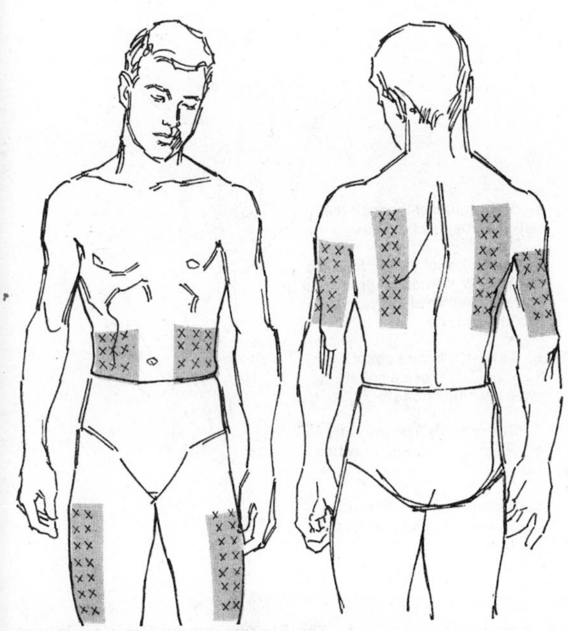

FIGURE 95–4. Sites for insulin injection. (From Burke, E. L.: *American Journal of Nursing 72*:2194, 1972.)

While this technic is not new (it has been used since the 1920's), it is now beginning to receive more recognition for its value in preventing lipodystrophy.

Self-injection of insulin. The majority of patients who take insulin learn to give their own injections. It is principally your responsibility to instruct diabetic patients in the technic of preparing insulin and giving injections to themselves. Teaching patients about insulin and other aspects of diabetic care is described later in this chapter.

Equipment which the diabetic patient will need to purchase for home use includes (a) insulin of the type prescribed, (b) absorbent cotton, (c) approved syringes (may be either glass or disposable), (d) needles (2 rustless 25 gauge hypodermic needles or disposable needles), (e) 70 per cent ethyl or 91 per cent isopropyl alcohol, and (f) a pan and large strainer for boiling and sterilizing nondisposable syringes and needles. The major steps involved in the self-injection technic are shown in Figure 95–7. Note in part 5 the patient is giving himself an injection deep into the pocket between the fat and muscle.

The actual process of learning to give an injection to oneself is usually quite traumatic. For this reason, Sutton suggests using a "surprise attack technic" for the patient's first self-injection. Simply prepare the insulin, walk up to the patient, and tell him he is going to help you give his injection today. Next let the patient cleanse his skin with an alcohol sponge; then hold his hands as shown in Figure 95–8 while you give the injection. After checking for blood by pulling back the plunger, let the patient push the plunger in and withdraw the needle from the skin himself.[46]

When instructing patients in self-injection technics, emphasize the following points to them:

> Always purchase an extra bottle of insulin, an extra syringe, and extra needles; extra equipment is needed in case the insulin bottle or glass syringe breaks.

> Wash hands thoroughly before preparing an injection.

> Use only sterile syringes and needles. To resterilize equipment following use, boil the syringe, plunger, and needle in a pan of water for 10 minutes. When traveling, use disposable syringes; also it is permissible to sterilize the syringe parts and needle by covering them with alcohol for 5 to 10 minutes.

> Always clean the top of the insulin bottle before inserting the sterile needle and withdrawing the insulin.

> Prepare the insulin injection as shown in Figure 95–7 and administer it in the manner recommended by the physician.

> Rotate sites systematically according to a definite plan.

> Following the injection, break the needle and

syringe when using disposable equipment. When using nondisposable equipment, place the needle in a dish of alcohol to prevent it from becoming plugged. Also wash the syringe parts in clear water or alcohol.

> When taking insulin, carefully follow the diet prescription. Do not alter the diet without consulting the doctor. If for some reason a meal is postponed and the insulin injection has already been given, drink a glass of orange juice. Always have hard candy or lump sugar handy in the event of a hypoglycemic reaction.

> Consult the physician if nausea, vomiting, fever, or infection develops. Nausea and vomiting decrease one's need for insulin, whereas fever and infection increase insulin requirements.

> Urine must be tested for sugar and acetone at least once daily. When ill, urine should be tested every 3 to 4 hours, and the physician should be consulted concerning the results.

> Be thoroughly familiar with the early symptoms of hypoglycemia and hyperglycemia and the treatment for each (see below).

COMPLICATIONS OF INSULIN THERAPY. Insulin therapy may result in one or more of the following six complications: (1) hypoglycemia, (2) hyperglycemia, (3) tissue hypertrophy or atrophy or both, (4) erratic insulin action, (5) insulin allergy, and (6) insulin resistance. These problems are briefly considered below.

Hypoglycemia. An abnormally low blood sugar (hypoglycemia) develops when the blood glucose

1. With thumb and index finger of one hand, stretch the skin away from clean area selected for injection and cleanse area with an alcohol swab. Using a circular motion, wipe injection area from the center out toward the edge of injection site.

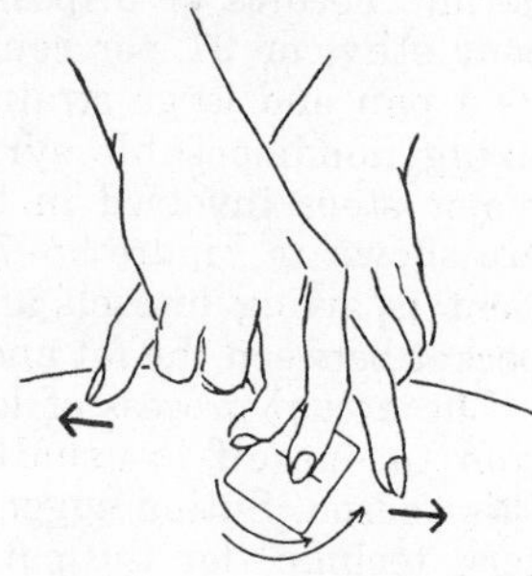

3. Release pressure on skin and use freed hand to hold syringe while other hand pulls back slightly on plunger.
If blood appears in bottom of syringe barrel, pull unit out of skin slightly — 1/16 to 1/8 inch — to remove needle tip from blood vessel. Pull back slightly on plunger again. If more blood appears, select new injection site. Replace the needle if you do this because the first one is contaminated.

2. Keeping skin stretched, grasp syringe firmly near its tip with other hand, taking care not to touch sterile needle.
Quickly thrust needle straight into injection site, as illustrated. Thrust needle in up to its hub.

ALTERNATE METHOD TO STEP 2.
2a. If injection is to be made into an area with only a thin layer of fat, pinch a fold of skin between fingers, rather than stretching skin. This will keep needle from penetrating into a muscle.
Taking care not to touch sterile needle, grasp syringe firmly near its tip.
Quickly thrust needle straight into injection site, as illustrated. Thrust needle in up to its hub.

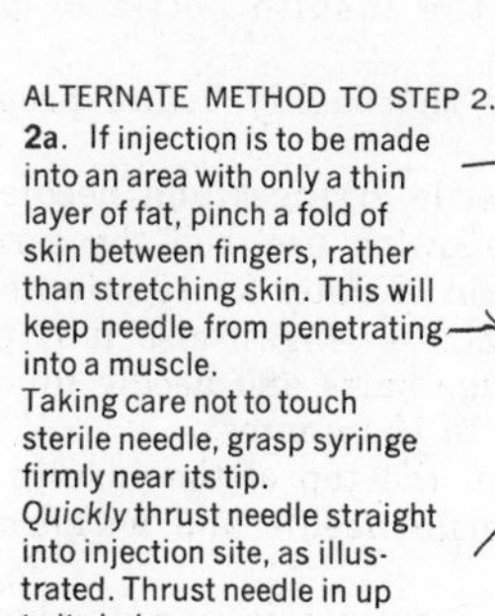

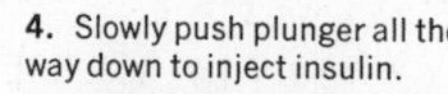

4. Slowly push plunger all the way down to inject insulin.

5. Hold alcohol swab close to needle hub. Withdraw syringe and attached needle rapidly, in a straight line.

6. As needle comes out of skin, quickly place alcohol swab over injection site.

7. Briefly apply firm pressure on alcohol wipe over injection site.

8. Record injection site and do not use it again for at least 14 days.

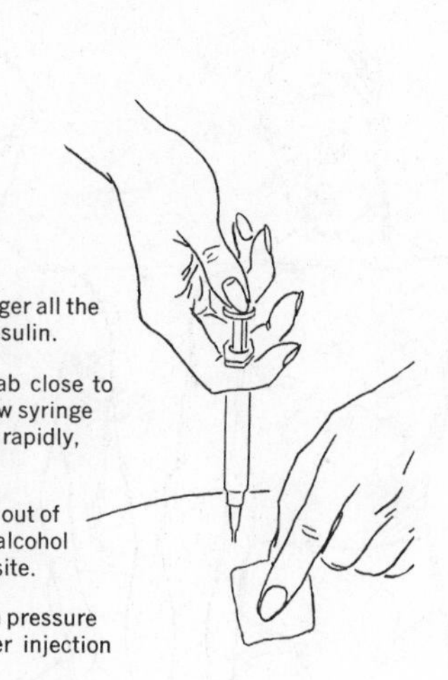

FIGURE 95–5. Insulin injection technique. (From Asperheim, M. K., and Eisenhauer, L. A.: *The Pharmacologic Basis of Patient Care.* 2nd ed., 1973.)

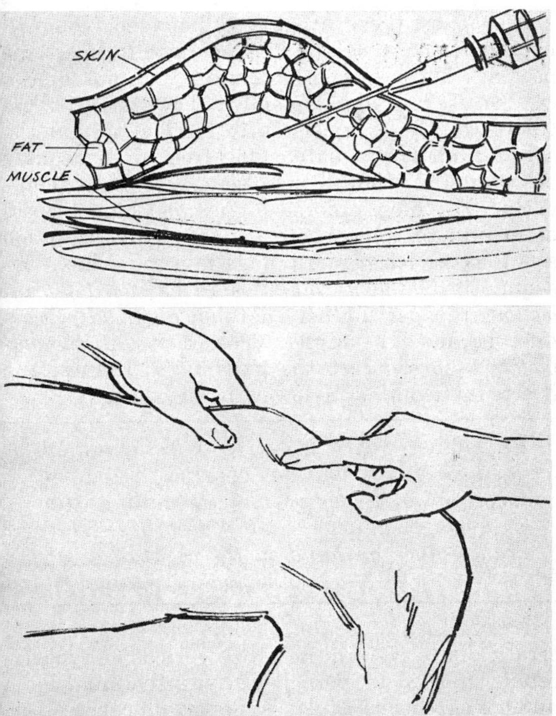

FIGURE 95–6. Injecting insulin between the muscle and fat. (From Burke, M. L.: *American Journal of Nursing 72*:2195, 1972.)

level drops to 60 mg./100 ml. or less (Folin and Wu method). In diabetes, hypoglycemic reactions are usually caused by an overdose of insulin or overzealous exercise—both of which remove glucose from the blood. Details concerning the symptoms and treatment of hypoglycemia are discussed later in this chapter.

Hyperglycemia. In this disorder there is an elevated blood glucose of 100 mg./100 ml. or more. When the blood sugar levels rise extremely high (300–800 mg./100 ml.), the patient enters a state of ketoacidosis which may proceed to coma. Hyperglycemia and ketoacidosis are discussed later in this chapter.

Tissue hypertrophy or atrophy. Tissue hypertrophy, which is sometimes termed an "insulin tumor," is "a thickening of the subcutaneous tissues at injection sites."[10] On the other hand, *atrophy* is a "loss of subcutaneous fat or depression at the site of injection."[10] A hypertrophied area may feel lumpy and hard, or soft and spongy. Tissue changes due to atrophy may be slight, causing only a dimpling of the tissues, or they may

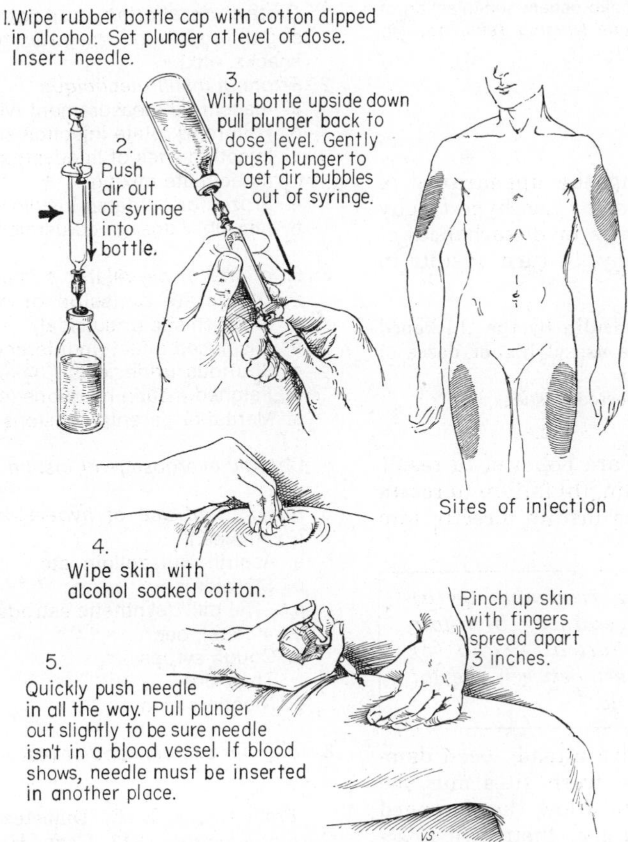

1.Wipe rubber bottle cap with cotton dipped in alcohol. Set plunger at level of dose. Insert needle.
2. Push air out of syringe into bottle.
3. With bottle upside down pull plunger back to dose level. Gently push plunger to get air bubbles out of syringe.
Sites of injection
4. Wipe skin with alcohol soaked cotton.
Pinch up skin with fingers spread apart 3 inches.
5. Quickly push needle in all the way. Pull plunger out slightly to be sure needle isn't in a blood vessel. If blood shows, needle must be inserted in another place.

FIGURE 95–7. How to administer insulin; sites of injection. (Dowling, H. F., and Jones. T.: *That the Patient May Know.* 1959.)

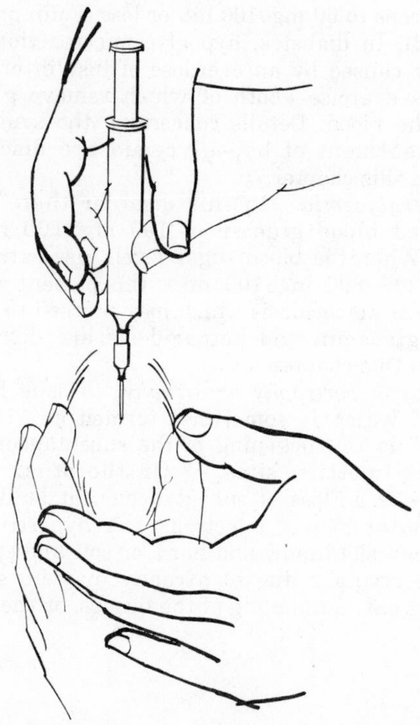

FIGURE 95–8. Teaching the diabetic patient self-injection of insulin. (From Sutton, A. L.: *Bedside Nursing Techniques in Medicine and Surgery.* 2nd ed. 1969.)

be more extensive, causing the appearance of large craters. Both tissue atrophy and hypertrophy are classified as *lipodystrophies* or disturbances of fat metabolism. Lipodystrophy, in turn, results in the following problems:

> Decreased absorption of insulin by the thickened tissues, which necessitates the use of higher doses of insulin to prevent hyperglycemia.

> Loss of sensation in the affected tissues.

Atrophy and hypertrophy are believed to result from (a) the use of cold insulin, (b) failure to rotate sites, and (c) injection of the insulin directly into the fat or muscle.

To prevent lipodystrophy, remember to (a) use insulin at room temperature; (b) rotate the injection site systematically; and (c) inject insulin into a pocket between the fat and muscle.

If the patient's tissues have already been damaged by repeated injections, fresh sites must be used for a period of time to allow the damaged areas to heal. Patients who give their own injections normally use their abdomen, thighs, and arms. When these areas are damaged, you will need to teach a neighbor or relative to inject the patient's buttocks and back until the injured sites can be used again. Remember, however, that patients who have consistently used abnormal tissues for injection usually suffer from an inadequate absorption of insulin. In these cases, the patient's doctor may have ordered higher and higher doses of insulin to compensate for the poor absorption and to cover for sugar spillage into the urine. Consequently, when *normal tissues are used for injection,* the patient may develop an *insulin reaction,* because the higher dose of insulin is *completely absorbed* into the undamaged tissues, and it acts immediately to lower the blood sugar.

Remember: *When injecting a fresh undamaged site with insulin, observe the patient for signs of hypoglycemia (trembling, diaphoresis, headache, and irritability). Have orange juice on hand in the event of an insulin reaction.*

Erratic insulin action. Some patients respond erratically to insulin (i.e., with periods of hypoglycemia followed by periods of hyperglycemia) for a number of reasons. The most important causes of erratic insulin action are listed in Table 95–10.

TABLE 95–10. CAUSES OF ERRATIC INSULIN ACTION*

1. *Dietary dereliction* (surreptitious overeating, free sugar ingestion, irregular feedings, omission of snacks, etc.)
2. *Errors in insulin technique*
   a. Inaccurate measurement (visual ?)
   b. Failure to rotate injection sites
   c. Injecting sites of lipodystrophy
   d. Inadequate mixing
   e. Frozen or outdated insulin
   f. Improper dosage adjustment ("insulin timing")
3. *Emotional or psychiatric conflicts*
   a. Deliberate omission or overdosage of insulin (masochistic or suicidal)
   b. Misplaced affect (indifference or obsessed)
   c. Spurious urine tests ("faked" vs. spoiled tablets)
   d. Feigned insulin reactions (especially children)
   e. Marital or parental tensions
4. *Chronic overdosage of insulin* (Somogyi effect)
5. *Intermittent use of hyper- or hypoglycemic drugs* (Examples:)
   a. Aspirin, Butazolidin, etc.
   b. Steroids
   c. "The pill" (synthetic estrogen mestranol)
   d. Alcohol, beer
   e. Cough syrups
   f. Thiazides
   g. Nicotinic acid
6. *Irregular exercise and/or rest periods*

*From Haunz, E. E.: Diabetes mellitus in adults, *In Current Therapy, 1973*. Conn, H. F. (ed.), Philadelphia, W. B. Saunders Company, 1973, p. 379.

Insulin allergy. Patients who develop allergies during insulin therapy are sensitive either to the protein component of insulin (particularly with pork-containing insulins) or to the alcohol used for cleansing and sterilization. Localized allergic reactions to insulin occur frequently, but systemic allergic reactions are rare.

Symptoms characteristic of local reactions include itching, redness, and burning at the site of injection. Fortunately, the majority of allergic reactions are self-limiting in nature. For example, allergic symptoms may appear during the first day or so of insulin therapy and then disappear 1 to 2 weeks later.

Treatment of local allergic reactions varies with the cause and severity of the reaction. For example, if the patient is sensitive to pork-containing insulin, the doctor may prescribe beef insulin for a period of time; also new "single-peak" neutral insulins are now appearing on the market which are hypoallergic. If the patient is allergic to alcohol, the patient will need to either boil his syringes or use disposable equipment; also Zephiran chloride can be used to cleanse the skin prior to injections. When allergy is severe, the doctor may order an *antihistamine* drug such as diphenhydramine (Benadryl) to be given until the allergy disappears. If all the above therapeutic methods fail, the doctor must then attempt to *desensitize* the patient to insulin so that insulin can be used both on a daily basis and in emergencies (e.g., diabetic acidosis). The desensitization program involves injecting the patient several times a day with diluted insulin solutions. Over time, the physician increases the amount of insulin in the daily injections until the patient tolerates his prescribed insulin dosage without allergic symptoms.

Insulin resistance. The patient who is insulin resistant must take more than 100 U. of insulin per day to control his diabetes. The exact etiology of insulin resistance is unknown; it may be caused by specific insulin antagonists within the blood or by circulating antibodies which are destructive to insulin. Some authorites classify the degree of resistance to insulin as follows:[44]

> Mild resistance—80 to 125 U. required per day.
> Moderate resistance—126 to 200 U. required per day.
> Severe resistance—more than 200 U. required per day.

To treat insulin resistance, the doctor may first attempt to give the patient a pork-based insulin; pork insulin is very similar in chemical structure to human insulin, and its use is sometimes sufficient to overcome the patient's insulin resistance. If the use of pork insulin fails, the physician must then order as high a dosage of insulin as is needed to control his patient's diabetes. Consequently, dosages may range from as low as 80 U. per day to as high as thousands of units per day. There are special preparations of U-500 insulin available for those patients who require 500 or more units daily.

Patients who are being treated for insulin resistance must be carefully watched for signs of either hyperglycemia or hypoglycemia (see below). *Hyperglycemia* is a signal that the patient needs a higher dosage of insulin than he is receiving to overcome his insulin resistance. On the other hand, *hypoglycemia* and shock nay occur quite suddenly when the insulin resistance barrier is broken and the high doses of insulin are abruptly absorbed. For this reason patients being treated for insulin resistance require at least biweekly blood tests and careful nursing observation and supervision.

Oral Hypoglycemic Agents. As we mentioned earlier, insulin must be administered parenterally because it is destroyed by gastrointestinal tract enzymes. To date, scientists have never succeeded in developing an oral form of insulin. However, there are oral agents available (called oral hypoglycemic agents) which are capable of lowering the blood sugar. Oral hypoglycemic agents are mainly prescribed for *mild* diabetics who are unable to control their condition with diet alone.

There are two classifications of oral hypoglycemic agents: (1) the sulfonylureas, and (2) the biguanides (see Table 95-11.) The *sulfonylureas* (a form of sulfa preparation) lower the blood sugar by stimulating the pancreatic beta cells to release insulin. For this reason the sulfonylureas can be prescribed only for *adult-onset* diabetics whose beta cells are still capable of producing insulin. Thus the average candidate for the sulfonylureas can be described as follows: (a) is over 40 years old; (b) has been a diabetic for less than 10 years; (c) cannot be controlled by diet alone; and (d) can be controlled with less than 20 U. of insulin daily.

Major sulfonylureas are tolbutamide (Orinase), chlorpropamide (Diabinese), acetohexamide (Dymelor), and tolazamide (Tolinase). These drugs can occasionally produce hypoglycemic reactions. Warn patients not to ingest large amounts of aspirin when taking the sulfonylureas because aspirin tends to increase the hypoglycemic effect of these agents. Also instruct patients taking oral agents to notify their physician at once should they develop an infection or febrile illness. When ill, the diabetic has a greater need for insulin; consequently he will probably need temporary insulin injections as well as his usual oral agent.

The *biguanides* are still being studied for their exact mode of action. These drugs, by some mysterious means, are capable of lowering the patient's blood sugar in the absence of beta cell function. Many theories have been advanced to explain the effectiveness of the biguanides but none have been fully accepted. The biguanide most commonly used is phenformin; phenformin is marked in a short-acting form (DBI) and a long-acting capsule (DBI-PT). Phenformin is sometimes given in conjunction with insulin to increase the latter's effectiveness. Instruct patients to always take the biguanides with meals in order to prevent nausea, vomiting, and diarrhea.

While the oral hypoglycemic agents have their place in diabetic therapy, we must emphasize again that diabetes should ideally be controlled by diet alone. Instruct patients that oral tablets must never be considered a substitute for their prescribed diet.

Exercise. Moderate, planned exercise can be highly beneficial for the diabetic patient because exercise (like insulin) acts to lower the blood sugar by oxidizing carbohydrates. Also exercise aids in weight reduction and proper weight maintenance. On the other hand, unplanned highly strenuous exercise can cause a dangerous hypoglycemic reaction unless the patient ingests additional carbohydrate. Unplanned exercise can be particularly dangerous for patients who take insulin or oral agents. When instructing patients concerning exercise, take care to include the following points in your discussion:

> While the doctor is initially planning the treatment regime, the patient should follow his usual activity schedule so that diet and insulin dosage are in balance with activity level.

> Once insulin dosage has been determined, the patient should eat additional food if he exercises more than usual; the equivalent of a bedtime snack is generally adequate.

> If the patient still experiences a mild hypoglycemic reaction after eating a snack, then he must consume more food when performing that particular activity. If, on the other hand, his urine test is positive for sugar or acetone, then he has eaten more than necessary for a certain activity.

> Stress that, with time and practice, the patient will gradually learn how much energy is consumed in various activities, and he will be able to regulate his diet accordingly.

THE COMPLICATIONS OF DIABETES

Acute Complications

KETOACIDOSIS AND COMA. The two major hallmarks of diabetes mellitus are *hyperglycemia* and *ketosis*. As stated earlier, hyperglycemia results when glucose cannot be transported to the cells because of a lack of insulin. You will recall that, without available carbohydrates for cellular fuel, the liver converts its glycogen stores back to glucose, and gluconeogenesis increases. Unfortunately, however, these maneuvers only aggravate the situation by raising the blood sugar even higher.

As the need for cellular fuel grows more critical, the body begins to draw first on its fat stores and then on its protein stores for energy. Excessive amounts of fat are mobilized from adipose tissue cells and transported to the liver. The liver, in turn, accelerates the rate at which it produces

TABLE 95–11. ORAL HYPOGLYCEMIC AGENTS USED IN THE TREATMENT OF DIABETES*

Type and Name of Drug	Mechanism of Action	Side Effects
Sulfonylurea compounds Tolbutamide (Orinase) Chlorpropamide (Diabinese) Acetohexamide (Dymelor) Tolazamide (Tolinase) Carbutamide (not licensed in the United States because of frequent allergic reactions)	Stimulate production of insulin by pancreatic beta cells (action is potentiated by sulfanilamides, salicylates, phenylbutazone, probenecid, monoamine oxidase inhibitors, and propranolol)	Malaise, fever, minor skin eruptions, anorexia, weakness, lethargy, dizziness, paresthesias, pounding headache, tinnitus, intolerance to alcohol (excessive surface vessel sensitivity to alcohol, causing flushing), hypoglycemia, hypothyroidism (after long use), weight gain Toxic: cholestatic jaundice, liver impairment, blood dyscrasias (all rare)
Phenethyl biguanide Phenformin (DBI) (DBI–TD) Metformin	Unknown—appear to have a peripheral site of action. Do not stimulate beta cells, but some endogenous insulin appears to be necessary for successful treatment	Nausea and vomiting, diarrhea, slight tendency to weight loss, lactic acidosis (phenformin) No severe hypoglycemic reactions known Toxic: impaired liver and kidney function (phenformin)

*From: Spencer, R. T.: *Patient Care in Endocrine Problems.* Philadelphia, W. B. Saunders Company, 1973, p. 147.

ketone bodies (ketogenesis) for catabolism by the tissue cells. As fat metabolism increases, the liver may produce *too many* ketone bodies for the cells to catabolize, which results in the accumulation of ketone bodies in the blood (ketosis) and the spillage of ketone bodies into the urine (ketonuria). *Metabolic acidosis* develops whenever the rate of ketogenesis is so great that (a) the pH of the blood falls to as low as 6.9, and (b) the CO_2 combining power of the blood is 9 mEq. per liter or less (see also Unit V, Ch. 25). When acidosis is severe, the patient may lose consciousness. Loss of consciousness in the diabetic due to metabolic acidosis is termed *diabetic coma.*

Etiology and prevention of ketoacidosis. Acidosis is primarily a complication of juvenile-onset diabetes. Common precipitating causes of diabetes acidosis include (a) taking too little insulin; (b) omitting doses of insulin; (c) overeating; (d) an increased need for insulin due to surgery, trauma, or pregnancy; and (e) insulin resistance due to the development of insulin antibodies.

The development of this grave complication can be almost entirely prevented by careful patient teaching. To prevent diabetic coma, patients must be taught to (a) take their insulin or oral hypoglycemic agents faithfully as prescribed; (b) if taking insulin, perform fractional urines at least twice daily when in good health and 3 to 4 times daily when ill or under stress; and (c) schedule regular monthly appointments with their physician for urine tests, review of weight gains or losses, and so forth. Remind patients to call their physician should they develop any of the following: (a) an infection or febrile illness; (b) anorexia, nausea, or vomiting; (c) ketonuria which persists for more than 12 hours; or (d) any of the signs and symptoms of acidosis. Emphasize that conscientious adherence to their therapy program and early treatment of mild ketosis are the patient's greatest weapons against development of diabetic coma.

Pathophysiology. When insulin is lacking and carbohydrates cannot be used for energy, ketosis and acidosis represent the final stages in the body's struggle for fuel. The process of burning fats for fuel in the absence of carbohydrates gives rise to four pathologic events: (1) incomplete lipid metabolism, (2) dehydration, (3) lactic acidosis, and (4) electrolyte imbalance. Let us briefly consider each area.

Incomplete lipid metabolism. First, let us review a few facts about normal fat metabolism. The three ketone bodies (beta-hydroxybutyric acid, acetoacetic acid, and acetone) are the intermediate products of fat metabolism. In the nondiabetic, ketone bodies are quickly used by cells for energy as needed, swiftly disarmed by the body's buffer systems, oxidized, and finally excreted as CO_2 and water.

In the diabetic, however, fat metabolism and the production of ketone bodies are greatly accelerated owing to the unavailability of carbohydrates. As production speeds, the increase in ketone bodies eventually exceeds the body's capacity to oxidze them for energy. When ketone bodies are not oxidized and excreted as CO_2 and water, these intermediate products of fat metabolism soon begin to escape into the urine. Once the numbers of ketone bodies overwhelm the kidney's capacity to excrete them, they accumulate in the blood.

In the meanwhile, to defend itself against the rising ketosis, the body brings into play its three lines of defense against H^+ excess (see Ch. 25). As you recall, the first line of defense is *buffering.* Thus acetoacetic acid unites with sodium bicarbonate to form carbonic acid acetoacetate—a weak acid. The lungs excrete carbonic acid as carbon dioxide, and the kidneys excrete sodium acetoacetate in the urine. The phosphate buffer system is also active in the buffering of other ketone bodies. At the same time the *respiratory system* (the second line of defense) becomes activated, and acetone as well as carbonic acid in the form of CO_2 and H_2O are blown off in the breath. Owing to this defense, respirations increase in depth and rate (Kussmaul respirations), and the breath has a "fruity" acetone odor. The *renal* system (the third line of defense) attempts to excrete between 30 and 100 Gm. of ketone bodies every day to control ketoacidosis. Also the ammonia mechanism is activated, which promotes the removal of excess H^+.

Unfortunately, in uncontrolled ketoacidosis, the rising tide of ketone bodies eventually overwhelms the body's defenses against H^+ excess. With depletion of its alkaline reserves and failure of its respiratory and renal defenses, the body finally succumbs to its acid overload, and diabetic coma ensues.

Dehydration. Patients suffering from ketoacidosis are losing fluids from several sources. First of all, severely ill diabetics excrete large amounts of urine in an attempt to eliminate excessive amounts of glucose and ketone bodies. Secondly, acidosis causes severe nausea and vomiting, which results in further losses of fluid and electrolytes (notably sodium and chloride). Finally, water is lost in the breath as the patient attempts to blow off excessive acetone and CO_2. Severe dehydration resulting from these fluid losses may be followed by the complications of *hypovolemic shock* and *lactic acidosis.*

Lactic acidosis. When water losses are critical, the patient's blood volume falls, with resultant *hemoconcentration.* Hemoconcentration, in turn, impedes blood circulation, causing a severe generalized tissue anoxia accompanied by the production of large amounts of lactic acid. The rise in lactic acid within the blood adds more H^+ to the body's already overwhelming acid load.

Electrolyte imbalance. As the pH of the blood decreases in acidosis, the rapidly accumulating H^+ moves from the extracellular fluid (ECF) to the intracellular fluid (ICF). The movement of H^+ into the cells propels the movement of K^+ out of the cells into the ECF. As a result, the cells are deficient in K^+, but there is excessive K^+ in the serum (hyperkalemia). If the patient is severely dehydrated, hemodilution coupled with oliguria due to renal involvement causes the serum K^+ levels to rise higher. Hyperkalemia, in turn, results in muscle weakness, paralysis, and respiratory or cardiac arrest.

In addition to K^+ losses, the patient in metabolic acidosis also loses excessive amounts of sodium, phosphate, chloride, and bicarbonate in the urine and vomitus.

Bases of symptoms. Diabetic acidosis has many easily recognized symptoms. The major manifestations of this complication and their bases are as shown in the opposite column.

Clinical care. Severe diabetic acidosis is an emergency! The patient must receive immediate intelligent medical and nursing care or he will die in coma.

The primary goal of care in diabetic acidosis is "to shift the metabolism from a fat to a carbohydrate substrate and thus restore carbohydrate utilization."[12] Secondary goals include (a) reversal of shock, (b) correction of fluid and electrolyte imbalances, and (c) correction of those factors which precipitated the development of acidosis in the first place.

When the diabetic patient is first admitted in probable diabetic coma, he is generally rushed immediately to the intensive care area of the hospital where he can receive continuous expert nursing care. If the patient has only mild ketoacidosis and is fully conscious, he is placed on a general medical ward. Initial orders for the critically ill diabetic generally include the following:

> NPO (unless patient is still conscious).
> I & O.
> Vital signs q. 15 minutes until stable.
> Foley catheter stat to drainage. (If patient is unconscious, a foley catheter will insure adequate measurement of urine output; also the patient may suffer from bladder distention.)
> Sulfisoxazole diethanolamine (Gantrisin), 1 Gm. I.M. b.i.d. (Gantrisin is given prophylactically to prevent dangerous bladder infections resulting from catheterization).
> EKG stat (an electrocardiogram helps to detect potassium levels).
> Start a record of all important findings and measurements to be kept constantly updated.
> 1000 ml. isotonic saline with B-complex vitamins I.V. stat.
> Blood glucose stat (it is important to obtain the patient's blood glucose level *before* giving insulin. Diabetic patients in coma may be suffering from *either* ketoacidosis or profound insulin shock. Without knowing the blood sugar level, the physician could make the fatal error of giving more insulin to a patient already critically ill from an insulin overdose).
> Stat plasma ketone and acetone, plasma carbon dioxide combining power, blood pH, serum sodium, potassium, and chloride, leukocyte count (to determine presence of infection), hematocrit (to determine degree of hemoconcentration), and urea nitrogen (BUN)—to determine level of kidney function. (For comparison of normal blood values and values in ketoacidosis, see Table 95-12.)

Once the patient's laboratory results are reported, definitive treatment begins. A fairly standard program of care for the patient in diabetic coma is described below.

Symptoms	*Basis of Symptoms*
Polyuria (early symptom)	Large amounts of glucose, ketone bodies, and protein must be excreted by the kidney; osmotic effect of sugar attracts water and promotes diuresis
Thirst (early symptom)	Polyuria causes loss of ECF, which causes water to be drawn from the cell, thereby promoting cellular dehydration
Nausea and vomiting	Cause of vomiting not known; nausea results from electrolyte imbalance due to glucosuria and ketonuria
Dry mucous membranes and cracked lips; hot, flushed skin	Severe dehydration; flushed appearance is due to acidosis
Weight loss	Dehydration is one cause; also patient is unable to use carbohydrate for energy, and consequently must burn protein and fat reserves
Abdominal pain and abdominal rigidity (similar to "acute abdomen")	No known cause; possibly associated with either dehydration or sodium deficit
Kussmaul respirations (deep rapid breathing)	When the alkaline reserve is depleted and the body can no longer buffer the excessive ketone bodies, the lungs attempt to blow off the overload of acetone as well as excess CO_2, which decreases the amount of carbonic acid in the blood, thereby raising the pH
Acetone odor of the breath	Excess acetone is being blown off through the lungs
Weakness, paralysis, and paresthesia	Either K+ deficiency or excess can produce neurologic problems
Soft eyeballs	Dehydration
Chest pain	May be due to excessive chest motion caused by Kussmaul respiration
Hypotension and shock (a late symptom)	Profound dehydration eventually leads to hypovolemic shock and circulatory collapse
Oliguria or anuria (late symptoms)	A dreaded complication arising secondary to severe dehydration and shock; decreased circulating fluid volume lessens blood flow to the kidney, resulting in renal shutdown
Coma or stupor (late signs)	Electrolyte imbalances, profound shock, and the rapidly lowering pH all contribute to loss of consciousness

Insulinization. Insulin dosages vary, depending upon the patient's condition and the level of his blood sugar. In the majority of cases, the physician prescribes between 300 and 500 U. of regular crystalline insulin I.V. within the first 24 hours. Insulin is not given subcutaneously during this period because the patient's subcutaneous tissues are dehydrated and poorly perfused with blood, owing to dehydration and hypovolemic shock. As long as shock persists, insulin administered subcutaneously will tend to accumulate within the tissues rather than enter the general circulation. Then once dehydration is relieved, all of the insulin trapped in the subcutaneous tissues may suddenly enter the blood as one massive dose, thereby causing insulin shock. For this reason, insulin must be administered I.V. until the patient's condition improves.

During the period when insulin is being given, laboratory studies should be ordered every 2 hours so that insulin is administered only on the basis of current laboratory work.

Correction of salt and water losses. As mentioned, dehydration resulting in hypovolemic shock, acute tubular necrosis, and uremia is a major cause of death in diabetic acidosis. The typical patient in diabetic coma loses an amount of water equivalent to 10 per cent of his body weight, and he also loses approximately 40 Gm. of sodium.[12] Consequently, intravenous infusions of isotonic saline (0.9 per cent sodium chloride) are started immediately upon admission. Typically, 1000 ml. of isotonic solution is given I.V. during the first hour, followed by 2000 to 3000 more ml. of solution over the next 24 hours.

Once the patient is fully conscious (usually 6 to 12 hours following initiation of treatment), encourage him to drink as much fluid as possible. Drinking broth is quite beneficial because broth contains needed sodium chloride. Remember to record the patient's intake *accurately*.

If the patient is being sufficiently hydrated, skin turgor improves, weight increases and the hematocrit drops to normal levels.

Reversal of shock. If the patient is in circulatory collapse, the physician will order either blood, plasma, or plasma volume expanders, such as dextran, to be administered alternately with normal saline solutions. Also combinations of col-

TABLE 95–12. NORMAL BLOOD VALUES CONTRASTED WITH THOSE FOUND IN KETOACIDOSIS AND TYPE OF BLOOD SPECIMEN REQUIRED*

Blood	Normal Value	Ketoacidosis	Type of Specimen Required
Glucose	60–90 mg./100 ml.	300–800 mg./100 ml. common, may be higher. Lower levels indicative of adequate renal reserve.	Oxalated blood
Urea nitrogen	10–16 mg./100 ml.	50–200 mg./100 ml.	Oxalated blood
Ketones		50–200 mg./100 ml.	Oxalated blood
Acetone		4+ in undiluted or diluted plasma or serum	
Carbon dioxide	20–28 mEq./L.	2 to 9 mEq./L.	Oxalated blood
pH	7.4	6.9–7.3	
Sodium	132–142 mEq./L.	Variable Tend to be normal or low Depends upon degree of hydration	
Potassium	3.5–5 mEq./L.	Variable Depends upon degree of hydration	
Chloride	98–106 mEq./L.	Variable Depends upon degree of hydration	
Leukocyte count	7000–9000 cells per cu. mm.	15,000–25,000 per cu. mm.	
Hematocrit	36–47 Vol.%	Above 50% with hemoconcentration	Oxalated blood

*From Beland, I., et. al.: Metabolic crisis. *In Concepts and Practices of Intensive Care for Nurse Specialists.* Meltzer, L. E. (ed.). Philadelphia, The Charles Press, 1969, p. 196.

loids and saline solution may be administered to raise the serum levels of both sodium chloride and plasma protein.

Correction of pH. Sodium bicarbonate or 1/6 molar lactate is administered to patients with a pH of 7.0 or below or a carbon dioxide combining power of 15 mEq. per liter or less. Replacement therapy should ideally cause an increase in the blood pH from between 7.2 and 7.4.

Restoration of potassium balance. As you recall, K^+ leaves the cells in untreated ketoacidosis, and hyperkalemia develops; however, *once treatment starts,* the patient may develop a transitory but dangerous *hypokalemia* with weakness, extreme dyspnea, and even cardiac arrest. Hypokalemia develops because (a) K^+ reenters the cells along with glucose once insulin is administered; and (b) K^+ is washed out in the urine once dehydration is relieved and renal function reestablished. There is some disagreement among clinicians concerning K^+ administration. However, general agreement exists on the following points of care:

> Observe the patient continuously for signs of hyperkalemia (bradycardia, cardiac arrest, weakness, flaccid paralysis, oliguria) or hypokalemia (weakness, flaccid paralysis, paralytic ileus, cardiac arrest) or both. Hyperkalemia will be present upon admission and approximately during the first 4 hours after the start of therapy. Hypokalemia usually develops during the period of 8 to 24 hours following initiation of therapy.

> Carefully monitor the patient's ECG. Flattening or inversion of T waves and prolonged Q-T intervals indicate hypokalemia, while peaking of T waves, loss of P wave, and a disrupted QRS complex indicates hyperkalemia (see Unit X, Ch. 48).

> K^+ administration is usually started 4 or more hours after the patient's admission or once the blood level of glucose has fallen to 200 mg./100 ml. or less.

> If the patient is conscious, always give K^+ orally rather than intravenously because oral administration is safer. Usually the doctor orders Liquid Potassium Triplex, 8 ml. every 3 to 4 hours. Also, if the patient is not vomiting, force fluids which are high in potassium; e.g., broth, tea, skim milk, orange juice, bananas osterized in milk.

Prevention of hypoglycemia. Once insulin therapy is started and the patient's blood sugar has dropped to 300 mg./100 ml., 5 to 10 per cent glucose in water must be given intravenously to prevent hypoglycemia. The blood sugar level usually begins to drop within 4 to 6 hours following insulinization. To cover for the glucose and thereby prevent sugar spillage into the urine, a small dose of crystalline insulin is either added to the I.V. glucose bottle or given subcutaneously.

Several days of intensive therapy may be needed to correct severe ketoacidosis. Moreover, it may take 10 days or longer to restore fluid, electrolyte, and nitrogen balance in the critically ill patient. Once the patient is fully conscious and alert, it is important to explore with him and his family the reasons why ketoacidosis developed and to correct any faulty health practices. As we emphasized earlier, ketoacidosis is entirely preventable provided the patient is both knowledgeable and willing to adhere to his therapeutic program.

HYPOGLYCEMIA (INSULIN) REACTION. Most diabetics who take insulin experience a hypoglycemic reaction at one time or another. Because insulin reactions are so common, it is important to instruct your patients concerning (a) why reactions occur; (b) when reactions are most likely to occur; (c) the early symptoms of hypoglycemia; (d) the danger of severe or repeated reactions; and (e) the early treatment and prevention of insulin reactions.

First of all, hypoglycemic reactions result from (a) an overdose of insulin or (rarely) tolbutamide; (b) omission of meals or eating less food than prescribed; (c) overexertion without compensating with the ingestion of additional carbohydrates; and (d) nutritional and fluid imbalances due to nausea and vomiting.

The *time period* during which an insulin reaction is most likely to occur depends upon the type of insulin given. You will recall from Table 95–9 that short-acting insulins tend to produce reactions before lunch and bedtime, intermediate-acting insulins 2 or 3 hours before dinner, and long-acting insulins between 2 A.M. and breakfast.

Early symptoms of an insulin reaction include headache, weakness, irritability, lack of muscular coordination, and apprehension. (Note in Table 95–13 differences in rate of onset, symptoms, signs, and urinalysis between diabetic coma and insulin reactions. Also, because epinephrine is released whenever the blood sugar drops abnormally low, the patient usually becomes diaphoretic. In addition, patients who take protamine zinc insulin may behave in a bizarre, even psychotic fashion.

When you care for diabetic patients at night, always check your sleeping patients for diaphoresis, because sweating may be the only *observable symptom of insulin shock. Don't just visually observe the patient; actually* feel *his bed clothing for moistness.*

When hypoglycemia is allowed to continue unchecked, the patient eventually becomes comatose. If hypoglycemia is severe or attacks are habitual, the patient not only is in danger of dying but also may suffer from *permanent brain damage* if he survives. Brain damage resulting in memory loss, lessened learning ability, and even paralysis can develop because the brain is deprived of needed glucose when the blood sugar is low. In this respect, hypoglycemic shock is more dangerous than diabetic coma; in ketoacidosis, the brain can still use available glucose, even in the absence of insulin. For this reason, some physicians actually prefer that their patients spill a little sugar into their urine (trace or 1+ sugar) rather than risk repeated insulin reactions.

The *treatment* for hypoglycemia depends upon whether the reaction is mild or severe. To reverse *mild* hypoglycemia, instruct the patient to drink a glass of orange juice mixed with two teaspoons of sugar, or to eat some lump sugar or candy whenever he feels diaphoretic or shaky. Also instruct patients to carry lump sugar or candy upon their person at all times so that they can guard against insulin shock when away from home. Finally, be certain that the patient obtains a diabetic identification tag or bracelet and an identification card from his doctor or the ADA (see Fig. 95–9). Sometimes diabetics who are suffering an insulin reaction behave as if they are intoxicated or mentally disturbed. By carrying proper identification, the diabetic protects himself from being arrested at a time when he desperately needs emergency care.

The patient with *severe* hypoglycemia who is unconscious needs *intravenous glucose immediately;* usually the patient is slowly given 20–50 ml. of 50 per cent glucose I.V. Once the patient fully regains consciousness, ask him to drink sugar water or orange juice to raise his blood sugar.

> *Never attempt to force an unconscious or semiconscious patient to drink liquids, because he will aspirate the fluid into his lungs!*

Two other emergency drugs which are used to treat severe hypoglycemia are:

> Glucagon, 1 mg. given intravenously.
> Epinephrine (Adrenaline), 0.5–1 ml. of 1:1000 solution administered subcutaneously.

Both glucagon and epinephrine help to raise the blood sugar by promoting the conversion of glycogen reserves within the liver back to glucose. Unfortunately, these drugs will reverse hypoglycemia only in those cases in which glycogen reserves are still available. If the patient is critical and has been in coma for some time, he will probably have already utilized his glycogen stores, and he therefore will respond only to the administration of I.V. glucose.

Once the patient fully recovers from his episode of hypoglycemia, it is essential to reassess his program of care. In some cases, insulin reactions

TABLE 95–13. COMPARISON OF CLINICAL FEATURES OF INSULIN REACTIONS AND DIABETIC COMA*

Clinical Feature	Insulin Reaction	Diabetic Coma
Onset	Sudden or gradual (minutes to hours)	Slow (days)
Causes	Delayed mealtime Omission of meal Excessive exercise Insulin overdosage	Neglect of treatment Intercurrent disease
Symptoms	Nervousness Weakness Sweating Hunger Blurred or double vision Abnormal behavior Unconsciousness Convulsions	Thirst Headache Nausea Vomiting Abdominal pain Dim vision Constipation Drowsiness Shortness of breath
Signs	Pallor Shallow respiration Sweating Pulse normal Eyeballs normal	Florid face Air hunger Loud, labored breathing Dry skin Rapid pulse Soft eyeballs Acetone breath Loss of consciousness
Urinalysis:		
Sugar	Usually absent, especially in second voided specimen	Positive
Acetone	Negative	Positive
Diacetic acid	Negative	Positive
Response to Treatment	Rapid; occasionally delayed	Slow

*From Rosenthal, H., and Rosenthal, J.: *Diabetic Care in Pictures.* 3rd ed. Philadelphia, J. B. Lippincott Company, 1960, p. 141.

I Am a Diabetic and Take Insulin

If I am behaving peculiarly but am conscious and able to swallow, give me sugar or hard candy or orange juice slowly. If I am unconscious, call an ambulance immediately, take me to a physician or a hospital, and notify my physician. **I am not intoxicated.**

My name ____________________

Address ____________________

Telephone ____________________

Physician's name ____________________

Physician's address ____________________

Telephone ____________________

FIGURE 95–9. Identification card which should be carried by all diabetics who take insulin.

develop because the patient is careless about preparing his insulin dosage, or he fails to eat or exercises excessively. Talk to patients who are careless about the dangers of repeated insulin reactions and stress the importance of conscientious adherence to the doctor's orders. In other cases, hypoglycemia develops because the prescribed insulin dosage is too large or the patient's dietary intake is too small. Under these circumstances, the doctor will alter the patient's regime until hypoglycemic reactions cease. As we stated earlier, some physicians prefer to lower insulin dosage to the point at which the patient experiences a continuous *mild* hyperglycemia, thereby preventing any possibility of insulin shock.

Chronic Complications. Because diabetes is a long-term disease, diabetics suffer from a myriad of chronic complications. Major chronic disorders associated with diabetes are vascular degenerative changes, neuropathy, ocular disturbances, kidney diseases, infections, and tuberculosis. These complications principally strike the *blood vessels* and *nerves* and mainly damage the heart, extremities (particularly the feet), the eyes, and the kidneys.

PREMATURE VASCULAR DEGENERATIVE CHANGES. Diabetes is inevitably associated with severe vascular degenerative changes. Lesions of the blood vessels not only strike diabetics at an earlier age than nondiabetics but also tend to produce more severe pathologic changes in diabetics than in the general population. Basically diabetics are prone to two types of vascular disease: (1) severe atherosclerosis, and (2) microangiopathy.

Severe atherosclerosis. As you recall from Unit X, atherosclerotic lesions cause hardening and degeneration of the walls of the *large* arteries; among diabetics, early atherosclerotic changes are probably caused by the high glucose and lipid levels which are characteristic of diabetes. Atherosclerosis, in turn, leads to the premature appearance of *coronary artery disease* (i.e., angina pectoris and myocardial infarctions) among large numbers of young diabetics. In addition, atherosclerosis results in reduced blood supply to the *feet,* causing intermittent claudication, cold feet, paresthesias, foot infections, inadequate healing of foot lesions, and ulceration and gangrene of the extremities. Lesions of the extremities may become so severe that the patient faces amputation of his toes, foot, or leg. To decrease the development of foot infections and lesions, it is important to teach diabetics the principles of *good foot care.* Instructions for the care of the feet are outlined on the opposite page.

Microangiopathy. While atherosclerosis is common among the general population, destruction of the *small blood vessels* is a major hallmark of diabetes. The specific characteristic of microangiopathy in diabetes is thickening of the basement membrane of the capillaries. Small vessel involvement is apparently caused by a specific defect which is linked to the diabetic gene. Moreover, pathology of the capillaries may appear at an earlier age than the chemical and clinical symptoms of the diabetes itself.

The widespread effects of microangiopathy can be disastrous if not controlled. The two organs which are most seriously affected are the *eyes* and the *kidneys.* Vascular degeneration within the retina can cause microaneurysms, retinal hemorrhages, and eventual blindness. Small vessel changes within the kidney eventually result in intercapillary glomerulosclerosis.

NEUROPATHY. Diabetics may develop both temporary and permanent neurologic problems during the course of their illness. Major causes of diabetic neuropathy include vascular insufficiency, vitamin B deficiency, and high blood sugar levels, all of which can lead to metabolic disturbances within the neuron itself. The three major forms of diabetic neuropathy are discussed below.

Peripheral nerve degeneration. This common form of diabetic neuropathy tends to develop in stages. During its earliest stage, the patient usually suffers from temporary episodes of pain and tingling in the extremities (particularly the feet). In later years the pain tends to grow more nagging and constant; also discomfort is particularly troublesome at night. Finally, 10 or 15 years following development of diabetes, the patient may experience a *painless neuropathy* characterized by an *inability to perceive pain.*

Painless neuropathy is an extremely dangerous condition. Patients may be totally unaware of injury–particularly of the lower extremities.

Instructions in the Care of the Feet for Persons With Diabetes Mellitus or Vascular Disturbances

Hygiene of the Feet

(1) Wash feet daily with mild soap and lukewarm water. Dry thoroughly between the toes by pressure. Do not rub vigorously, as this is apt to break the delicate skin.

(2) When feet are thoroughly dry, rub well with vegetable oil to keep them soft, prevent excess friction, remove scales, and prevent dryness. Care must be taken to prevent foot tenderness.

(3) If the feet become too soft and tender, rub them with alcohol about once a week.

(4) When rubbing the feet, always rub upward from the tips of the toes. If varicose veins are present, massage the feet very gently; never massage the legs.

(5) If the toenails are brittle and dry, soften them by soaking for ½ hour each night in lukewarm water containing 1 tbsp of powdered sodium borate (borax) per quart. Follow this by rubbing around the nails with vegetable oil. Clean around the nails with an orangewood stick. If the nails become too long, file them with an emery board. File them straight across, and no shorter than the underlying soft tissues of the toe. Never cut the corners of the nails. (If the patient goes to a podiatrist for this attention, he should tell him that he has diabetes.)

(6) Wear low-heeled shoes of soft leather which fit the shape of the feet correctly. The shoes should have wide toes that will cause no pressure, fit close in the arch, and grip the heels snugly. Wear new shoes ½ hour only on the first day and increase by 1 hour each day following. Wear thick, warm, loose stockings.

Treatment of Corns and Calluses

(1) Corns and calluses are due to friction and pressure, most often from improperly fitted shoes and stockings. Wear shoes that fit properly and cause no friction or pressure.

(2) To remove excess calluses or corns, soak the feet in lukewarm (not hot) water, using a mild soap, for about 10 minutes, and then rub off the excess tissue with a towel or file. Do not tear it off. Under no circumstances must the skin become irritated.

(3) Do not cut corns or calluses. If they need attention it is safer to see a podiatrist.

(4) Prevent callus formation under the ball of the foot (a) by exercises, such as curling and stretching the toes several times a day; (b) by finishing each step on the toes and not on the ball of the foot; and (c) by wearing shoes that are not too short and that do not have high heels.

Aids in Treatment of Imperfect Circulation (Cold Feet)

(1) Never use tobacco in any form. Tobacco contracts blood vessels and so reduces circulation.

(2) Keep warm. Wear warm stockings and other clothing. Cold contracts blood vessels and reduces circulation.

(3) Do not wear circular garters, which compress blood vessels and reduce blood flow.

(4) Do not sit with the legs crossed. This may compress the leg arteries and shut off the blood supply to the feet.

(5) If the weight of the bedclothes is uncomfortable, place a pillow under the covers at the foot of the bed.

(6) Do not apply any medication to the feet without directions from a physician. Some medicines are too strong for feet with poor circulation.

(7) Do not apply heat in the form of hot water, hot water bottles, or heating pads without a physician's consent. Even moderate heat can injure the skin if circulation is poor.

(8) If the feet are moist or the patient has a tendency to develop athlete's foot, a prophylactic dusting powder should be used on the feet and in shoes and stockings daily. Change shoes and stockings at least daily or oftener.

(9) Exercises to increase circulation should be prescribed by a physician.

Treatment of Abrasions of the Skin

(1) Proper first-aid treatment is of the utmost importance even in apparently minor injuries. Consult a physician immediately for any redness, blistering, pain, or swelling. Any break in the skin may become ulcerous or gangrenous unless properly treated by a physician.

(2) Dermatophytosis (athlete's foot), which begins with peeling and itching between the toes or discoloration or thickening of the toenails, should be treated immediately by a physician or podiatrist.

(3) Avoid strong irritating antiseptics such as tincture of iodine.

(4) As soon as possible after any injury, cover the area with sterile gauze. Sterile gauze in sealed packets may be purchased at drug stores.

(5) Elevate and, as much as possible until recovery, avoid using the foot.

*From Krupp, M. A., and Chatton, M. J.: *Current Diagnosis and Treatment.* Los Altos, California, Lange Medical Publications, 1972, p. 648.

One of the authors (J. L.) once witnessed a dramatic example of the dangers of painless neuropathy. Her patient, a 50-year-old woman with *undiagnosed* diabetes, was admitted to the hospital one evening with a huge ulcerated lesion on her heel. Only that morning, the patient had gone with her family to a county fair where she had walked (without pain) for most of the day. Before she left for the fair, the woman had noted a small blister on her heel but had disregarded it. That evening, when the patient removed her shoe, she was horrified to discover that the tiny blister had grown into a large gaping sore. It took many weeks following admission for the lesion to heal and for the patient to be brought under control. Throughout her hospitalization, the patient faced the definite possibility that her foot might have to be amputated.

You can see from this example how important it is to instruct diabetic patients to visually and manually inspect their feet for blisters, sores, cuts, ingrown nails, and so forth. Emphasize to older diabetics that their ability to perceive pain may be diminishing and that they must rely upon their senses of touch and sight to protect them from injury. Also point out that even trivial injuries (particularly of the feet) require medical care to prevent the development of severe complications.

Other neurologic lesions. There are two rare forms of diabetic neuropathy: lesions of the autonomic nervous system and cranial nerve lesions. Symptoms of autonomic nerve damage include diarrhea or constipation, urinary incontinence or retention, decreased sweating, orthostatic hypotension, and impotence in the male. Symptoms of cranial lesions include facial grimacing and twitching of the eyes.

OCULAR DISORDERS. Diabetes is the second leading cause of new cases of blindness in the United States today.[19] The most common eye complications affecting diabetics include blurring of vision, cataracts, and diabetic retinopathy.

Blurred vision is usually caused by an abnormally elevated blood sugar; consequently, once the patient's diabetes is brought under control, vision clears. Advise patients to wait until control is established before obtaining new prescription lens.

Cataracts, the second type of ocular disturbance, strikes a proportionately greater number of diabetics than nondiabetics. (A cataract is a clouding or opacity of the lens of the eyes, see Unit XXI). Fortunately, in more than 95 per cent of cases, cataracts can be surgically removed from the eyes and vision restored.[33]

The third entity, *diabetic retinopathy,* is a major cause of blindness among diabetics. As mentioned, one of the severe complications of diabetes is microangiopathy or vascular degeneration of the small vessels supplying the eyes and kidneys. The *retina,* which is the most essential structure of the eye, has the highest rate of oxygen consumption of any tissue in the body. Consequently, if the retina is deprived of oxygen-carrying blood owing to destruction of its capillaries, tissue anoxia swiftly develops. In addition, the weakened damaged vessels frequently rupture, causing retinal hemorrhage. Hemorrhage is followed by the growth of new capillaries into the vitreous and by the formation of retinal scar tissue. Finally, contraction of the scar tissue can result in retinal detachment.

While all diabetics apparently inherit the tendency to develop microangiopathy, fortunately not all diabetics develop retinal disorders. Many diabetics live with their disease for 30 or 40 years without developing ocular complications. When retinopathy does occur, it tends to develop slowly and insidiously. Diagnosis of this condition is based upon direct ophthalmoscopic observation of vascular changes within the retina.

Unfortunately, no therapy currently exists which is guaranteed to cure this condition; it may progress to permanent blindness—either partial or total. The advance of diabetic retinopathy can sometimes be slowed by instituting and maintaining good diabetic control. Also, a few patients are benefiting from hypophysectomy (surgical removal or destruction of the pituitary gland) (see Ch. 97). Destruction of the pituitary gland alleviates the secretion of the following four pituitary hormones, all of which act to raise the blood sugar and consequently have a diabetogenic effect: growth hormone, corticotropin, thyrotropin, and luteotropin. In the absence of these hormones, diabetes is easier to control, and the progression of retinopathy slows or halts. Following hypophysectomy, the patient will need hormonal replacement therapy throughout his life.

KIDNEY DISEASE. Diabetics are highly susceptible to kidney infections—particularly *recurrent pyelonephritis.* Female diabetics are far more susceptible to renal infections than are males. One source estimates that one half of all women who have had diabetes for 10 or more years have suffered from at least one kidney or bladder infection during that time.[15] Fortunately, the majority of diabetics with renal infections are successfully treated with sulfonamides, antibiotics, and the urinary antiseptics.

A second and far more devastating form of kidney disease is diabetic *nephropathy.* A consequence of microangiopathy, nephropathy is characterized by damage and eventual obliteration of the tiny capillaries which supply the glomerulus of the kidney. Damage of the glomerular capillaries, in turn, leads to a complex of symptoms (intercapillary glomerulosclerosis, nephrosis, gross albuminuria, and hypertension) called the *Kimmelsteil-Wilson syndrome.* With worsening of the nephrosis, chronic renal failure ensues. Unless the patient can be maintained with hemodialysis, he eventually dies in *uremia.* Indeed, uremia causes more than 50 per cent of deaths among juvenile-onset diabetics.

As in the case of diabetic retinitis, there is as yet no cure for diabetic nephropathy. However, severe renal damage and uremia can usually be forestalled by strict diabetic control.

INFECTIONS. Diabetics are highly susceptible to infections of all types, and infections, once they occur, are extremely difficult to treat. Infected areas heal slowly because the diabetic's vascular system is usually damaged and unable to carry oxygen, antibodies, and lymphocytes to the injured site. Also infections increase the diabetic's need for insulin and predispose him to the possibility of ketoacidosis. Areas which are particularly subject to infection include the neck, axillae, and groin. In addition, obese diabetic women may develop raw infected areas under their breasts.

Diabetic patients need careful instruction in how to prevent and treat infections and skin injuries. Important points to stress when teaching diabetics skin care include the following:

> Even *slight injuries* can become infected; e.g., scratches, small cuts, hangnails, slivers under the skin, and so forth.

> Carefully cleanse areas which are slightly injured with soap and water. Do not use antiseptics which contain iodine, phenol, bichloride of mercury, oil of mustard, cantharidin, or salicylic acid, because these substances tend to burn the skin. After cleansing, apply a sterile gauze bandage. Avoid using adhesive tape because it irritates the skin.

> Report serious injuries and infections to the physician immediately; e.g., boils, carbuncles, ulcers, burns, abscesses, blisters, deep cuts.

> Exercise caution when using heat lamps, hot water bottles, and heating pads, particularly in the presence of painless neuropathy.

> Avoid the use of irritating household cleaning fluids, powders, and disinfectants unless protective gloves are worn.

TUBERCULOSIS. Diabetics are twice as prone to the development of tuberculosis as are nondiabetics. Advise diabetic patients to have chest x-rays at least twice a year.

NURSING DIABETIC PATIENTS WHO UNDERGO SURGERY

Undergoing surgery is a stressful experience for anybody. For the diabetic patient, surgery imposes several additional stresses. For example, surgery interrupts the patient's usual treatment regime; the diet must be temporarily changed and insulin dosage readjusted. Furthermore, diabetics are highly susceptible to infection, and the surgical incision itself opens a new portal for infectious agents. Also postoperative healing in diabetics is particularly slow owing to the degeneration of the vascular system.

To offset these problems, diabetic patients require special care both preoperatively and postoperatively. Specific clinical care varies, depending upon whether the patient has maturity-onset diabetes or juvenile diabetes and also upon whether the surgery is elective or emergency.

The goal of *preoperative care* for diabetic patients is to *thoroughly regulate their diabetes* before taking them into the operating room. Patients with "brittle" diabetes may need to be hospitalized for several days or even weeks prior to elective surgery in order to stabilize their condition and thereby decrease surgical risk. If the "brittle" patient needs *emergency* surgery, the surgeon must sometimes make the painful choice between operating on a poorly controlled diabetic or postponing an emergency operation while attempting to control the diabetes. In either case, the patient will need constant monitoring of vital signs, frequent laboratory studies, and vigilant nursing care.

In contrast to the "brittle" diabetes, patients with well-controlled *maturity-onset* diabetes usually undergo surgery with only slightly more risk than nondiabetics. Typically, preoperative preparation for these patients includes the following:[24]

> The omission of food, water, insulin, or oral hypoglycemic agents on the morning of surgery.

> Early morning scheduling of the surgery so that the patient's diet and insulin regime are interrupted as little as possible.

> Preoperative laboratory tests, including fasting and postprandial blood sugars, urine tests for sugar and actone, CO_2 combining power, and blood urea nitrogen; also an EKG and chest x-ray.

> A blood sugar determination performed and reported to the physician within 1 hour before the operation. Haunz points out that the preoperative blood sugar is vital because it prevents the possibility of the patient (who has been NPO since midnight) developing hypoglycemia while in surgery. If the blood sugar level is low, then the patient will require an intravenous infusion of 5 per cent glucose in water prior to the induction of anesthesia.[24]

Once the patient arrives in surgery, his management depends, once again, upon the severity of his diabetes and the extensiveness of the surgery. The patient with *mild* diabetes who is undergoing minor surgery usually does not require either insulin or intravenous glucose until he returns to the recovery room. If the patient is undergoing major surgery or he has moderate or severe diabetes, he is then given an intravenous infusion of 1000 ml. 5 per cent glucose in saline or water while in surgery. To "cover" the I.V. glucose, a prescribed dosage of crystalline insulin (usually around 12 U.) is added to the I.V. bottle.

Following surgery, the goals of *postoperative care* are to stabilize the patient's condition, reestablish control of the diabetes, prevent wound infection, and promote wound healing. Important postoperative clinical measures are as follows:

> Intravenous infusions of 5 per cent dextrose in water and regular insulin are administered until the patient is able to take oral nourishment.

> Once the patient can eat, he is usually placed on a *4-meals-a-day feeding plan.* The patient returns to his normal 3-meals-a-day plan as soon as his diabetes is under control.

> Blood sugar levels are usually ordered 3 times daily, and fractional urines for sugar and acetone 4 times daily.

> Regular insulin is administered on the basis of urine tests. The patient returns to his preoperative insulin type (i.e., NPN, lente, and so forth) and dosage once diabetic control is reestablished.

> Catheterization is avoided if at all possible in order to prevent bladder infections.

> Wound dressings are changed with meticulous sterile technic in order to prevent wound infection.

EDUCATING THE DIABETIC PATIENT FOR LIFELONG SELF-CARE

Throughout our discussion of diabetes, we have stressed the importance of patient education. We have indicated strongly that the success of any diabetic regime depends almost entirely upon the patient's willingness to adhere to his care plan.

Essentially, learning to be a diabetic is like any other form of learning; it requires that the "student" (a) obtain a grasp of unfamiliar factual material (e.g., the nature of diabetes, insulin, and so forth); (b) learn to perform certain procedures (e.g., urine testing); and (c) permanently change certain behavior patterns (e.g., eating habits, recreational activities, and so forth). Like any student, the diabetic needs scheduled classes; planned instruction; reading materials which are geared to his educational level; demonstrations of procedures (e.g., urine tests and insulin preparation); and the opportunity to perform these procedures himself with supervision.

Diabetics may be instructed either individually or in groups, depending upon the policy of the individual hospital or clinic and the number of staff members available for teaching. One advantage of group instruction is that diabetics have an opportunity to meet other diabetics and to discuss mutual problems and feelings.

When it becomes your responsibility to instruct diabetics for lifelong self-care, you will, first of all, want to review the important principles of learning. For instance, we know that students learn more easily when they are rested and alert, when the environment is quiet, when instruction is given at the patient's level of education and new terms are defined, and when assimilation of new knowledge is periodically tested.

Next, you will wish to plan your course of instruction and obtain the necessary teaching aids. Trayser in her article, "A Teaching Program for Diabetics," suggests planning classes which cover the following five topics:[49]

1. What is diabetes?
2. Complications of diabetes.
3. Diet and diabetes
4. Blood and urine testing in diabetes
5. Medications used in diabetes

Helpful teaching aids for your classes include instructional charts and free pamphlets which can be obtained from the ADA; diabetic identification cards; copies of *ADA Forecast* and *ADA Forecast Reprints;* "A Cookbook for Diabetics"; "Learning about Diabetes: A Programmed Course of Instruction"; urine testing apparatus; samples of various types of insulin; insulin syringes calibrated for 40, 80, and 100 unit insulin; alcohol and alcohol sponges; and a pan and strainer for boiling injection equipment.* It is also helpful to give patients a price list, drawn from local pharmacies, for the various items they will need to purchase.

Throughout each session, you will want to test your patient to make certain that he is grasping all the key points concerning diabetes and its care. Ask questions frequently. Have the patient perform urine testing and insulin preparation and injection until he can do so with ease. At the end of your course, stress the importance of continued medical supervision; emphasize that the patient will need to schedule periodic medical examinations for the rest of his life.

You may wish to close your class with the thought that learning is a continuing process and that your classes have presented only the most basic facts about diabetes. Hopefully, your patients will continue to read and learn about their disorder and to keep abreast of new developments in the field. Knowledge and self-confidence go hand in hand. The more the patient knows about diabetes, the easier it will be for him to control his disorder and to live a normal, productive life.

HYPERFUNCTION OF THE ISLETS OF LANGERHANS (HYPERINSULINISM)

Hyperinsulinism (excessive secretion of insulin by the pancreas) is classified as either organic or functional. *Organic* hyperinsulinism is usually caused either by *hyperplasia* (overgrowth) of the islets or by an *adenoma* of the pancreas which secretes excessive amounts of insulin.

Because oversecretion of insulin causes an abnormally low blood sugar, the *symptoms* of hyperinsulinism are identical to those of hypoglycemic shock, previously discussed (e.g., hunger, weakness, tremor, sweating, personality changes). Repeated or prolonged attacks of hypoglycemia may ultimately result in progressive and irreversible neuropathy and myelopathy, retinal hemorrhages, cerebral vascular accidents, permanent personality changes, and intellectual damage.

Emergency treatment of acute hypoglycemic attacks is the same as that for an insulin reaction, i.e., immediate administration of sugar in any quickly utilized form (sugar lumps, orange juice).

**ADA Forecast* is a bimonthly magazine which is published by the ADA for diabetics. Currently a subscription costs $3.00 per year. "A Cookbook for Diabetics" and "Learning about Diabetes" are also published by the ADA and can be purchased for $1.00 and $2.00 respectively. The address of the American Diabetes Association is 18 East 48th Street, New York, N.Y. 10017.

However, to permanently alleviate organic hyperinsulinism, the patient must undergo *surgery*. The operation involves either removal of the insulin-secreting tumor or resection of hyperplastic pancreatic tissue. In a few cases, partial or total pancreatectomy is necessary (see Ch. 86).

Functional hyperinsulinism develops with far greater frequency than does the organic form. In this case, the exact cause of insulin hypersecretion is unknown. However, functional hyperinsulinism frequently strikes *tense, anxious persons* who also have various manifestations of autonomic nervous dysfunction, e.g., neurocirculatory asthenia and excessive diaphoresis. Secondly, this disorder may possibly be a forerunner of *diabetes mellitus*. According to some investigators, a large majority of persons diagnosed with functional hyperinsulinism later develop diabetes. Theoretically, individuals who secrete excessive amounts of insulin in response to carbohydrate ingestion could eventually develop beta cell exhaustion and permanent insulin deficiency. Finally, functional hyperinsulinism sometimes follows *gastrectomy*. When the stomach is removed, ingested carbohydrates pass directly into the small bowel (the "dumping syndrome") and are absorbed. The sudden resultant hyperglycemia causes excessive insulin release with symptoms of hypoglycemia appearing 1 to 2 hours later (see Unit XV).

The goal of care in functional hyperinsulinism is to control and prevent the symptoms of hypoglycemia. Methods of treatment include the following:

> *Psychological counseling:* Tense, nervous persons may find relief from symptoms by learning to relax more fully and more frequently. The help of a psychiatrist may be needed in extreme cases.

> *Diet:* A high-protein, low-carbohydrate diet reduces the amount of stimulus to the pancreas to secrete insulin. Carbohydrates ingested should be of the slowly assimilated variety (e.g., bananas and vegetables).

> *Medications:* Sedation may help the anxious person relax. Also anticholinergic drugs may be used to control the "dumping syndrome."

> *Follow-up:* Patients with functional hyperinsulinism should be examined at least every 6 months for the signs of overt diabetes mellitus. Early diagnosis of diabetes helps prevent the development of later complications.

CHAPTER 96

Nursing Patients With Disorders of the Thyroid and Parathyroid Glands

THE THYROID GLAND

NORMAL ANATOMY AND PHYSIOLOGY

The thyroid gland is a shield-shaped organ located in the neck below the larynx. It consists of two lobes, located on either side of the trachea, and connected by a thin isthmus which stretches over the trachea's anterior surface. Each of the lobes is composed of irregular lobules, while the lobules themselves consist of multitudes of tiny sacs called *follicles.* The follicles are filled with a jelly-like, iodine-containing substance called *colloid,* which is mainly composed of *thyroglobulin* —the storage form of the hormone *thyroxine.*

Thyroxine is one of the three hormones secreted by the thyroid gland—triiodothyronine and thyrocalcitonin being the other two. A derivative of the amino acid tyrosine, thyroxine is composed largely of *iodine.* The major role of thyroxine is to *regulate body metabolism* so that oxygen consumption and heat production keep pace with the body's needs and activities. By controlling body metabolism, thyroxine also aids in regulating growth and development (both physical and mental); carbohydrate, fat, and protein metabolism; reproduction; vitamin requirements; and resistance to infection. Too much thyroxine causes a dangerous speeding of metabolism and high rate of oxygen consumption. Conversely, too little thyroxine results in a sluggish metabolism, a slowing of both physical and mental function in the adult, and a tragic retardation of growth and development in the child. As Boyd states:

> Thyroid secretion appears to act as a general and necessary stimulant without which there can be no health or vigor of the body, no flash and speed of the mind. Someone with a turn for the picturesque has remarked that thyroxine converts the sluggish toad into the lively frog.[9]

Production of this remarkable hormone depends upon the ingestion of sufficient amounts of protein and iodine and upon the release of a vital anterior pituitary hormone called *thyroid-stimulating hormone* (TSH), or thyrotropic hormone. TSH, as the name implies, stimulates the thyroid gland to produce thyroxine from iodine and tyrosine. TSH release is controlled by a *negative feedback system* in which low serum levels of thyroxine stimulate the increased secretion of TSH, and high serum levels of thyroxine inhibit TSH secretion, thereby promoting a steady state of hormonal production and release.

Thyroxine production is also dependent upon a number of environmental factors. Situations which speed thyroxine production are physiologic and psychologic stress, and prolonged exposure to cold. Factors which depress thyroxine secretion are excessive intake of dietary goitrogens (see below), ingestion of certain drugs (sulfonamides, salicylates, phenylbutazone, and *para*-aminosalicylic acid), and exposure to prolonged heat.

Once produced, thyroxine combines with protein and is then stored within the thyroid follicles as *thyroglobulin.* Whenever the body's circulatory thyroxine levels drop too low, thyroxine is released from thyroglobulin into the blood. Within the blood, thyroxine combines with a plasma protein and is carried to organs and tissues in the form of *protein-bound iodine.*

Triiodothyronine, a second thyroid hormone, is much more potent and is five times as active as thyroxine. Thyroxine is converted to triiodothyronine whenever heat production and body metabolism drop abnormally low.

Thyrocalcitonin, the third thyroid hormone, is a polypeptide. Discovered recently (during the 1960's), thyrocalcitonin is capable of lowering both plasma calcium and plasma phosphates. Apparently it serves no other function.

ABNORMALITIES OF THYROID FUNCTION

There are many terms to describe normal and abnormal states of thyroid function. *Euthyroid* is a word which signifies *normal* thyroid function and secretion. Thyroid *abnormalities* are basically of three types: (1) enlargement of the thyroid (goiter), (2) hyperfunction (hyperthyroidism), and (3) hypofunction (hypothyroidism).

Enlargement of the thyroid gland may or may not be associated with abnormalities of hormone secretion. An enlarged thyroid may result from either (a) lack of iodine (simple goiter), (b) inflammation (thyroiditis), or (c) benign or malignant tumors. Enlargement may also appear as part of the clinical picture of hyperthyroidism, especially Graves' disease.

Hyperthyroidism is a condition characterized by overactivity of the thyroid gland, hypersecretion of thyroid hormone, and increased body metabolism and heat production. Persons suffering from severe hyperthyroidism may become overactive to the point of mania and psychosis. Conversely, *hypothyroidism* is charactered by *underactivity* of the thyroid, hyposecretion of thyroid hormone, and decreased body metabolism and heat production; in its most extreme form—myxedema coma—body metabolism slows almost to the point of death.

ASSESSMENT OF THYROID FUNCTION

A number of tests are available for the assessment of thyroid function. They include the following: (1) basal metabolic rate (BMR); (2) protein-bound iodine (PBI); (3) radioactive iodine (^{131}I) uptake and excretion tests; (4) triiodothyronine (T_3) resin uptake test; (5) thyroid stimulating hormone (*thyrotropin,* TSH) test; (6) Achilles tendon reflex recording; (7) serum cholesterol; and (8) serologic studies. The purposes of each of these diagnostic studies, as well as of factors which interfere with testing, are briefly considered below. Details concerning patient preparation, the procedure, after-care of the patient, and normal and abnormal findings for the most important tests are outlined in Table 96–1.

Basal Metabolic Rate (BMR). The basal metabolic rate is an indirect measure of the amount of oxygen which is consumed by the body under basal conditions during a given time, i.e., while the patient is in a state of complete mental and physical relaxation. Factors which can alter test results include inadequate rest prior to the examination, anxiety and emotional stress, a noisy environment, and the prior ingestion of almost any drug. The BMR, once the major test of thyroid function, is now being largely replaced by newer, more sophisticated diagnostic technics.

Protein-Bound Iodine (PBI). Protein-bound iodine is a test of thyroid function which measures the amount of iodine attached to protein molecules within the blood. You recall that, when thyroxine is released from the thyroid gland into the serum, the iodine within the thyroxine becomes bound to protein molecules and consequently circulates as protein-bound iodine rather than as free thyroxine. Thus, while free thyroxine within the serum cannot yet be measured, it is possible to *estimate* the amount of thyroxine released into the blood by determining the PBI.

A large number of factors can distort the PBI test results, producing either a false high or a false low. The worst offenders are commonly used drugs, as well as the radio-opaque, iodine-containing, injectable contrast media used in various diagnostic x-ray studies. When preparing a patient for this test, it is essential to ask him or his family the following questions:

> Has the patient recently taken any of the following drugs or used any of these agents, all of which may produce a spurious *elevation* of the PBI?[21]

Barbiturates
Barium sulfate (used in GI series and barium enema)
Estrogens
Gargles
Iodine-containing drugs
Lithium carbonate
Metrecal
Some mouthwashes
Oral contraceptives
Perphenazine
Some suntan lotions

> Has the patient recently received any of the following drugs which produce falsely *low* test results?[21]

ACTH
Androgens
Cortisone-like drugs
Diphenylhydantoin (Dilantin)
Gold salts
Isoniazid
Mercurial diuretics
Para-aminosalicylic acid (PAS)
Reserpine
Salicylates (including ASA)
Sulfonamides
Thiazides
Some vitamin preparations

> Has the patient undergone a bronchogram, histosalpingogram, or spinal myelogram within the last two or three years? Or a cholecystogram, cholangiogram, or arteriogram within the last six months? The iodine-containing contrast media used in the performance of these procedures could possibly obscure PBI and radioiodine test results for up to 20 years.

> Have any antithyroid medications (carbimazole, methimazole, propylthiouracil, or methylthiouracil) which act to suppress thyroid function been prescribed recently?

> Has the patient suffered recently from a biliary tract obstruction which may falsely elevate protein-bound iodine levels?

> Has the patient received any intravenous solutions through a catheter prior to testing? The catheters which are used to administer I.V. solutions contain iodine which can falsely raise PBI results.

Radioiodine Uptake Test (^{131}I Uptake). This important test for estimating thyroid function and diagnosing thyroid disease was discussed in Unit VII. As you recall, the body cannot distinguish between radioactive or "tagged" atoms of iodine and nonradioactive iodine; consequently the thyroid takes up radioactive iodine and processes it in exactly the same manner as it does regular iodine. Furthermore, radioiodine is excreted in the urine just as is ordinary iodine. Thus by using a scintillation scanner, it is possible to measure the amount of radioactive atoms of iodine which are concentrated in the thyroid following the administration of a radioactive iodine preparation. In addition, the laboratory may measure the patient's urine output of radioactive iodine following the test.

As with the PBI, there are many factors which can distort findings. Careful questioning of your patient concerning the following drugs, procedures, and activities will ensure more accurate test results.

> Has the patient taken any iodine-containing drugs within the last 30 days? Any estrogens which can cause a false high?

> Has the patient within the last decade or longer undergone x-ray studies of the gallbladder, ureters, bronchi, uterine tubes, or heart?

> Within the last 2 weeks, has the patient been eating principally sea foods? Seafood is so rich in iodine that ^{131}I uptake could show a falsely high reading. Be certain to inform the physician if the patient answers "yes" to any of these questions.

Triiodothyronine (T_3) Resin Uptake. Triiodothyronine (like thyroxine) circulates in the plasma attached to protein molecules and to red blood cells. However, triiodothyronine tends to bind itself far more readily to protein molecules than to erythrocytes; indeed, only when there are few protein molecules available does triiodothyronine link itself to circulating red cells.

In this test a specimen of the patient's serum is incubated with (a) a specific amount of radioactive triiodothyronine, and (b) particles of resin, which act as an absorbent material in place of erythrocytes. If thyroid function is low or if serum protein levels are high, resin uptake of T_3 will be depressed. On the other hand, if thyroid function is increased above normal or serum protein levels are low, resin uptake of T_3 will be elevated. While this test is helpful, it has the disadvantage that test findings may reflect *either* abnormal thyroid function or abnormal serum protein levels.

Thyrotropin Test (TSH). The TSH test is used to make a *differential* diagnosis between *primary* hypothyroidism (a condition originating in mal-

TABLE 96–1. THYROID FUNCTION TESTS

Test	Patient Preparation	Procedure
Basal metabolic rate (BMR)	NPO 10 hours prior to test; 8 hours sleep night before test. No smoking morning of test. Omit early morning care of in-patient. Reassure patient that test is simple, painless, and harmless.	Patient lies on comfortable cot in quiet, cool room. He breathes pure oxygen through mouth from tube linked to oxygen container. Nostrils are clamped and mouthpiece is moistened with water to prevent dryness of mucous membranes from inhaling oxygen. BMR machine measures and records amount of pure oxygen used during a specified time period.
Protein-bound iodine (PBI)	No food or water restrictions. Question patient concerning drugs recently taken and diagnostic procedure using iodine-containing contrast media undergone in the past (see text).	Sample of venous blood drawn and sent to laboratory
Radioactive iodine uptake test (^{131}I uptake)	No food or water restrictions. Reassure patient that doses of radioiodine used for tests are extremely small and not harmful. Question patient concerning past history of drug ingestion and diagnostic tests (see text).	Patient receives capsule containing tracer dose of ^{131}I. 24-Hour urine specimen is started at time of drug administration. After 24 hours, scintillation counter is placed over thyroid gland to measure exact amount of radioactivity emitting from the gland. 24-Hour urine specimen is labeled and sent to laboratory for analysis
Triiodothyronine (T_3) resin uptake	No food and water restrictions. No special preparation.	Blood sample drawn from patient and sent to laboratory for incubation with T_3 and resin particles.
Thyrotropin test (TSH)	No food or water restrictions.	^{131}I uptake and PBI performed. Thyrotropin given by injection. ^{131}I uptake and PBI repeated 24 hours following TSH administration.

function of the thyroid gland itself) and hypothyroidism *secondary* to pituitary malfunction.

You recall that thyrotropin is a hormone, secreted by the anterior pituitary gland, which stimulates the thyroid gland to secrete thyroid hormone. Normally, when a patient receives large doses of TSH, his thyroid gland will function at its highest possible level in secreting thyroid hormone; consequently PBI and ^{131}I uptake levels will be elevated. However, if the patient has *primary* hypothyroidism, a dose of TSH will have *no* effect upon PBI and ^{131}I uptake test results; i.e., no amount of TSH will be able to increase thyroid function if the gland is in a state of hypofunction

due to disease. On the other hand, if the patient suffers from hypothyroidism *secondary* to anterior pituitary gland insufficiency, an injection of TSH *will raise* PBI and ^{131}I uptake test results, because the thyroid gland is normal and capable of responding to TSH when it is available.

Achilles Tendon Reflex Recording. The Achilles tendon reflex test is a measurement of the ankle jerk when the strong tendon at the back of

TABLE 96-1. THYROID FUNCTION TESTS *(Continued)*

After-care	Normal Findings	Significance of Abnormal Findings
None	Findings are recorded as % deviation from normal, (+10 to −10 %).	Greater than + 10 % is a sign of hyperthyroidism; greater than −10 % is a sign of hypothyroidism.
None	3.0–8.0 mcg./100 ml. of serum.	Low concentration of protein-bound iodine indicates hypothyroidism; excessive concentration of protein-bound iodine indicates hyperthyroidism.
None	15–35% uptake. Urine excretion: 40–80% ^{131}I within first 24 hours.	(1) *Uptake results:* early high peak in ^{131}I uptake indicates hyperthyroidism; persistent low ^{131}I uptake indicates hypothyroidism. (2) *Urine excretion:* excretion less than 40% indicates hyperthyroidism; excretion greater than 80% indicates hypothyroidism.
None	Men: 11–19%; women: 11–17%.	Depression of resin uptake of T_3 may indicate hypothyroidism; elevation of resin uptake of T_3 may indicate hyperthyroidism.
None	Not relevant.	

the heel is tapped with a special instrument. Persons with hyperthyroidism tend to experience a more rapid tendon reflex; individuals with underactive thyroid glands and diabetes, and pregnant women have a slower jerking reflex and a prolonged relaxation time.

Serum Cholesterol. Serum cholesterol is *not* a specific test of thyroid function, because its levels are influenced by many other factors beside thyroid hormone levels. Nevertheless, the serum cholesterol tends to be relatively elevated in myxedema and hypothyroidism, possibly because these conditions are accompanied by a marked tendency toward atherosclerosis. Persons with hyperthyroidism usually have a relatively low serum cholesterol (see also Unit X, Ch. 48).

Serologic Tests. Many thyroid disorders are presumed to have an autoimmune basis, e.g., Hashimoto's thyroiditis, myxedema, and Graves' disease (a form of hyperthyroidism). Consequently serologic tests are performed in order to determine if the patient's blood contains any antithyroid antibodies.

ENLARGEMENT OF THE THYROID

Enlargement of the thyroid may be caused by the following three disorders: (1) simple goiter, (2) thyroiditis (inflammation of the goiter), and (3) tumors of the thyroid (benign and malignant). Each of these conditions is briefly considered below.

Simple Goiter (Nontoxic Goiter, Nodular Goiter). As stated earlier, the thyroid gland needs iodine in order to manufacture and secrete its hormones. If an individual fails to ingest sufficient amounts of iodine in his diet or if the production of thyroid hormone is suppressed for any other reason, the thyroid enlarges in an attempt to *compensate* for hormonal deficiency. Thus goiter essentially "is an adaptation to the deficiency of thyroid hormone."[28] Enlargement of the gland occurs in response to increased pituitary secretion of TSH; as you recall, TSH stimulates the thyroid to secrete more thyroxine when blood thyroxine levels are low. Eventually, in its attempt to respond to TSH and meet the body's needs, the gland may become so large that it compresses structures in the neck and chest, causing respiratory symptoms and dysphagia.

TYPES OF GOITER. There are two major forms of simple goiter: endemic goiter and sporadic goiter. *Endemic goiter* is principally caused by *nutritional iodine deficiency.* It tends to occur in "goiter belts," which are geographic areas characterized by soil and water deficiency in iodine; major "goiter belts" within the United States are the Midwest, Northwest, and Great Lakes Region. Endemic goiter typically occurs in the winter and fall; it is twice as prevalent among women as men. Also, because the need for thyroid hormone is particularly great during growth spurts, pregnancy, and lactation, goiter commonly develops among adolescents, pregnant women, and nursing mothers residing in iodine-deficient regions.

Sporadic goiter is not restricted to any geographic area. Major causes include:

> *Genetic defects* resulting in faulty iodine metabolism.

> Ingestion of huge amounts of *nutritional goitrogens* (goiter-producing agents which inhibit thyroxine production), e.g., rutabagas, cabbage, soybeans, peanuts, peaches, peas, strawberries, spinach, and radishes, all of which contain goitrogenic glycosides.

> Ingestion of *medicinal goitrogens,* e.g., thioureas (propylthiouracil), thiocarbamides (aminothiazole, tolbutamide), and iodine in large doses (some persons take iodine-containing solutions as a tonic).

DIAGNOSIS AND TREATMENT. Typically the patient with goiter seeks medical advice when his goiter grows large enough to distort the appearance of his neck. Also, the patient may complain of respiratory distress and difficulty swallowing if the goiter is very large. In addition to the patient's appearance and complaints, diagnosis of simple goiter is confirmed by the patient's history (he may reside in a "goiter belt" or have ingested large amounts of goitrogens) and by laboratory tests (^{131}I uptake is usually high, while the PBI and BMR are normal). Typically the patient with simple goiter is euthyroid; symptoms and laboratory signs of hypothyroidism seldom appear, because the gland enlarges to the point where it produces normal amounts of thyroxine.

The *goals of treatment* for simple goiter are to halt further enlargement of the thyroid and to promote regression of the gland. Because enlargement is a compensatory reaction to iodine deficiency and consequent suppression of thyroxine secretion, patients with simple goiter are treated with preparations of iodine and thyroid hormone. *Iodine* is administered either in the form of strong iodine solution (Lugol's solution) or saturated solution of potassium iodide (SSKI drops). Dosage is usually 5 drops of iodine solution given daily in ½ glass of water. Drugs of choice for *thyroid hormone replacement* include desiccated thyroid, sodium–L-thyroxine, and L-triiodothyronine. Dosage is based upon the age of the patient; children and elderly patients receive smaller doses than adults.

When administering thyroid preparations, watch the patient carefully for symptoms of *thyrotoxicosis,* i.e., tachycardia, increased appetite, diarrhea, sweating, agitation, tremor, palpitations, shortness of breath. If any of these symptoms develops during thyroid therapy, notify the physician at once so that he can reduce the dosage. Also the patient must be carefully observed for *further enlargement* of the gland, as well as for growth of *nodules* within the thyroid tissues; these signs are particularly dangerous because they may indicate cancer of the thyroid.

While patients with small or moderately large goiters may respond successfully to drug therapy, those with large goiters may need to undergo a subtotal thyroidectomy (see p. 1358). In such cases, surgery is indicated for cosmetic reasons and also to alleviate respiratory problems. Surgery is also performed on patients with possible malignancy of the thyroid. Cancer is suspected whenever the thyroid gland contains a single nodule, and also when there has been no decrease in the size of the goiter despite 3–6 months of thyroid and iodine therapy.

PREVENTION OF SIMPLE GOITER. Endemic goiter can be completely prevented by the use of *iodized salt.* The bare minimum adult iodine requirement is 50 μg. iodine per day; however, an adequate iodine intake guaranteed to prevent goiter is 200–300 μg. per day. Iodized salt, which has been used in the United States since 1924, contains one part iodine per every 100,000 parts of salt. Thus the average person, who ingests approximately 6.2 Gm. of salt a day, is also ingesting 474 μg. of iodine daily *if* the salt is iodized. The problem is that many Americans are unaware of their need for iodized salt as a goiter preventative; indeed, it is possible that fewer Americans are using iodized salt today than during the 1950's.[28] Also many modern foods are being processed with the cheaper, noniodized, bag salt rather than with iodized salt. As a result of public misinformation and new food processing methods, the potential for developing simple goiter today is as great or greater than in the past. To correct this problem, Malovinovic suggests that *all* salt to be used for human or animal consumption should be iodized. He points out that the use of iodized salt by persons with normal thyroid glands is in no way harmful to them.

Nurses can play an important role in educating the public to use iodized salt. Many persons strongly believe that *any* additive to food or water is harmful; e.g., groups lobbied for years against fluoridation of water even though there was ample evidence that fluorine prevents tooth decay. It is the nurse's task to help change outmoded attitudes and dispel irrational prejudice with scientific facts. The need for iodized salt in the diet as a goiter preventative cannot be overemphasized.

Thyroiditis. Thyroiditis simply means inflammation of the thyroid gland; it appears in three basic forms: (1) acute suppurative thyroiditis, (2) subacute granulomatous thyroiditis, and (3) chronic thyroiditis.

Acute suppurative thyroiditis is a rare condition caused by bacterial invasion of the thyroid gland. This disorder usually responds to antibiotic therapy and to incision and drainage of the infected gland.

Subacute granulomatous thyroiditis is a self-limited inflammatory condition which is believed to be caused by a *virus.* Although no etiologic agent has as yet been identified, subacute thyroiditis usually follows in the wake of rheumatic fever, streptococcal infections, and mumps. *Symptoms* include high fever, extreme tenderness of the neck over the thyroid gland, severe pain which sometimes radiates to the jaws and ears, fatigue, and malaise. Thyroid function usually remains normal. *Treatment* is based upon the severity of the disease. Patients with *mild* cases usually respond adequately to rest, fluids, and acetylsalicylic acid to relieve pain. *Severe* subacute thyroiditis may be treated with (a) corticosteroids to reduce inflammation, (b) propylthiouracil (see below) to reduce glandular tenderness, (c) desiccated thyroid to suppress TSH secretion and thus shrink the gland, and (d) low-dosage x-ray therapy if other measures are unsuccessful. Even without treatment, many patients with subacute thyroiditis experience a spontaneous remission within one week to several months following the appearance of symptoms.

Chronic thyroiditis (Hashimoto's thyroiditis), a long-term inflammatory disorder, is the most common form of thyroiditis. It strikes females 30 times more frequently than males, and particularly tends to affect women during the menopause.[38] Like myxedema and Graves' disease, chronic thyroiditis is believed to have an autoimmune basis; genetic predisposition may also play a role in its etiology. *Symptoms* of chronic thyroiditis include painless enlargement of the gland, respiratory distress, and dysphagia due to pressure of the swollen gland upon surrounding structures. *Diagnosis* is based upon (a) needle biopsy of the thyroid, which reveals typical tissue changes; and (b) serologic tests, which reveal the presence of circulating antithyroid antibodies.

The course of Hashimoto's thyroiditis varies: (a) a few cases remit spontaneously; (b) many patients' conditions remain stable for years; (c) hypothyroidism and myxedema develop in approximately one third of cases owing to the gradual atrophy of the gland. It has been suggested but not fully confirmed that cancer may develop in some cases. *Treatment* is directed toward reducing the size of the thyroid and preventing hypothyroidism. Thus patients are given desiccated thyroid to prevent hypothyroidism as well as to suppress TSH secretion and thus reduce gland size. In stubborn cases, x-ray therapy is occasionally used to shrink the gland. Corticosteroids are also useful on a short-term basis for reducing thyroid inflammation and swelling. In a few cases, the patient may be forced to undergo a partial thyroidectomy for relief of symptoms. However, surgery is used only as a last resort, because removal of part of the thyroid increases the risk of myxedema. If surgery is absolutely necessary, the patient will need to take thyroid hormone for the rest of his life.

Thyroid Tumors. Benign adenomas and malignant thyroid tumors constitute the third cause of thyroid enlargement. The *benign adenomas* are mainly composed of follicles; consequently they are called *follicular adenomas.* While these tumors may affect persons of any age, they are mainly discovered in the thyroids of young adults. Typically, benign adenomas are soft and multinodular. Like other benign tumors, most thyroid adenomas are usually well encapsulated and consequently do not spread out or extend into other tissues. When the patient is given tracer doses of ^{131}I, these tumors readily take up the radioiodide; consequently benign adenomas are said to have "hot nodules."

Benign adenomas are usually not dangerous, although they may grow large enough to cause respiratory symptoms by pressing against the trachea. Occasionally, however, *malignant transformation* occurs, and the benign nodules become cancerous. While no one knows the exact incidence of malignant transformation, one study estimates that it occurs in 14 per cent of patients with benign thyroid tumors.[38]

Malignant tumors of the thyroid are fortunately fairly rare; thyroid cancer accounts for around 0.5 per cent of cancer deaths. It mainly develops in persons between the ages of 40 and 60, and it strikes twice the number of women as men.[38]

Thyroid carcinoma seems to develop most frequently in persons who have received large doses of radiation to the head and neck. Also, malignant transformation of benign nodules can apparently follow prolonged stimulation of the thyroid gland by the pituitary hormone TSH.

The major *symptom* of thyroid cancer is the appearance of a hard, painless nodule in an enlarged thyroid gland; the nodule itself is typically solitary, rapidly enlarging, and "cold" (i.e., it does *not* take up radioactive iodine). Also, the patient's lymph nodes are sometimes palpable. In long-standing cases, the patient may suffer from respiratory difficulty and dysphagia due to pressure of the enlarged thyroid against structures in the neck.

The are four major types of thyroid cancer: (1) papillary adenocarcinoma, (2) follicular adenocarcinoma, (3) medullary carcinoma, and (4) anaplastic carcinoma. The incidence, symptoms, treatment, and prognosis of each of these thyroid cancers are compared in Table 96-2.

DISORDERS OF THYROID HORMONE PRODUCTION

The thyroid gland can produce either too little hormone or too much. The hypometabolic hypoactive state associated with a deficiency of thyroxine or triiodothyronine or both is called *hypothyroidism*. The hypermetabolic, overactive state associated with an excess of thyroxine or triiodothyronine or both is called *hyperthyroidism*. Both conditions affect the heat and energy-producing mechanism, the circulatory system, the muscular system, the nervous system, and other endocrine glands; hyperthyroidism often produces an effect exactly opposite to that of hypothyroidism.

Treatment of these two conditions can also be sharply contrasted. The goal of care in *hypothyroidism* is to increase the patient's metabolism by correcting the thyroid hormone deficiency; thus the major form of treatment is *thyroid hormone administration*. Conversely, the goal of care in *hyperthyroidism* is to slow the patient's racing metabolic state by correcting the thyroid hormone excess. The three methods for reducing thyroid hormone secretion include (1) *surgical removal* of part of the thyroid (subtotal thyroidectomy); (2) *drug therapy* with antithyroid preparations; and (3)

TABLE 96–2. TYPES OF THYROID CANCER: INCIDENCE, CHARACTERISTICS, TREATMENT, AND PROGNOSIS

Type	Incidence	Characteristics
Papillary adenocarcinoma	Mainly affects persons in their 40's. Comprises 61% of thyroid cancers	Slow-growing tumor. Palpable nodules appear within thyroid. Spreads to regional nodes in approximately 50% of cases.
Follicular adenocarcinoma	Comprises 18% of thyroid cancers. Mainly affects persons in their 50's.	Composed of well-developed follicles. Rarely spreads to regional lymph nodes. Tends to adhere to trachea, muscle, skin, and great vessels of neck, causing dyspnea and dysphagia.
Medullary carcinoma (amyloidic carcinoma)	Comprises 6% of thyroid cancers. Mainly affects persons in their 50's.	Tumor may be hereditary and familial. Tends to secrete calcitonin, ACTH, and serotonin. Tends to invade surrounding structures.
Anaplastic carcinoma	Comprises 15% of thyroid cancers. Mainly affects persons between 60 and 80 years.	Highly malignant. Grows extremely rapidly. Widespread metastasis within one year.

irradiation of the thyroid with radioiodine. Let us now pursue the study of each of these conditions in more detail.

Hypothyroidism. There are two major forms of hypothyroidism: (1) cretinism, and (2) myxedema. *Cretinism* is a severe hypothyroid condition of infancy which is caused by a deficiency of thyroid hormone synthesis during fetal life or soon after birth. Causes of cretinism include the following:

> Severe iodine deficiency in the diet of the mother; this is particularly common in the Alps and Himalayas.
> Inborn errors of iodine metabolism and of thyroxine or triidothyronine synthesis or both.
> Congenital absence of the thyroid or anatomic malformation.

The two major hallmarks of cretinism are *defective physical development* and *mental retardation.* As William Osler once wrote of the cretin:

> No type of human transformation is more distressing to look at than an aggravated case of cretinism. The stunted stature, the semi-bestial aspect, the blubber lips, retroussé nose sunken at the root, the wide-open mouth, the lolling tongue, the small eyes half closed with swollen lids, the stolid expressionless face, the squat figure, the muddy dry skin, combine to make the picture of what has been termed "the pariah of nature."[9]

The tragic syndrome of cretinism can be partially reversed if the infant is treated immediately upon diagnosis with daily doses of desiccated thyroid. It is unfortunate that, even with early treatment, the child remains mentally deficient even though physical and sexual development may unfold normally.

In contrast to cretinism, *myxedema* results from a deficiency of thyroid hormone synthesis in the adult. Distinguishing features of myxedema are (a) slowed body metabolism due to decreased oxygen consumption by the tissues, (b) pronounced personality changes (lethargy, apathy), and (c) the appearance of generalized interstitial edema—thus the term myxedema.

The *etiology* of myxedema may be traced either to pathologic changes within the thyroid gland itself (*primary* hypothyroidism) or to disorders of the pituitary gland which disturb thyroid gland function (*secondary* hypothyroidism). The development of *primary* myxedema may possibly have an autoimmune basis; studies show that 98 per cent of patients with newly diagnosed myxedema and 70 to 80 per cent of patients with myxedema of long duration have circulating thyroid autoantibodies within their blood.[38] Further, you recall that myxedema may appear during the course of chronic (Hashimoto's) thyroiditis, which is also an autoimmune disorder. Finally, primary myxedema sometimes develops as an iatrogenic result of treating hyperthyroidism. Thus myxedema may follow (a) thyroidectomy without sufficient thyroid hormone replacement therapy, (b) destruction of the thyroid gland by overzealous radioiodine therapy, and (c) overuse of antithyroid drugs.

TABLE 96–2. TYPES OF THYROID CANCER: INCIDENCE, CHARACTERISTICS, TREATMENT, AND PROGNOSIS (*Continued*)

Treatment	Prognosis
Surgical resection of part of gland and removal of involved lymph nodes.	Excellent if cancer restricted to thyroid gland. Surgical resection usually curative.
Surgical resection, usually of one lobe and the isthmus.	Prognosis good but inferior to that of papillary adenocarcinoma.
Total thyroidectomy. Radical neck resection necessary if metastasis present.	Poor. Mean survival time approximately 6.6 years.
Surgery to prevent respiratory obstruction.	Extremely poor. Typically results in death within one year.

Secondary hypothyroidism may follow (a) the development of destructive pituitary tumors, (b) pituitary insufficiency, and (c) postpartum necrosis of the pituitary gland. Without the stimulating effect of TSH, the thyroid gland atrophies and ceases to function.

Myxedema is principally a disease of older persons and of women. Thus it mainly strikes people in their 60's, and it affects five times as many women as it does men.

The *symptoms* of myxedema depend upon whether the degree of hypothyroidism is mild or full-blown. Patients with mild myxedema (the most common form) may be asymptomatic; in other cases, they may suffer from vague complaints which are so ordinary that they often escape detection, e.g., mild sensitivity to cold, lethargy, dry skin and hair, forgetfulness, and some weight gain. On the other hand, individuals with the rarer full-blown myxedema develop a multitude of striking symptoms. The patient slows drastically in both physical and mental reactions and appears abnormally fatigued and apathetic; for example, he may sit for hours in one place without moving or responding to persons or things around him. Indeed, the person with myxedema must often be taken to the doctor by a friend or relative because he is too complacent and apathetic to seek help for himself.

The patient's physical appearance also changes (see Fig. 96–1). In a large number of cases, obesity develops; features become coarse; hair grows in dry and sparse; skin feels dry, flaky, and inelastic. The patient also looks puffy and edematous due to the infiltration of fluid into the interstitial tissues. In addition, the patient suffers from a severe intolerance to cold due to his decreased metabolic rate; ability to sweat markedly diminishes. Constipation and fecal impactions due to slowed peristaltic action and lack of normal physical activity constitute serious problems. Susceptibility to infection increases markedly. Finally, patients with myxedema become dangerously hypersensitive to narcotics, barbiturates, and anesthetics.

> Remember: *Even an average dose of a narcotic, barbiturate, or anesthetic agent may result in the death of a myxedematous patient!*

Diagnostic tests for myxedema confirm the clinical picture of hypometabolism and depressed thyroid activity. The BMR is below 30 per cent owing to decreased oxygen utilization by the body tissues. ^{131}I and PBI test results also are abnormally low. In addition, the serum cholesterol is markedly elevated—a factor which undoubtedly contributes to the later development of cardiac problems.

Complications of myxedema principally affect the heart. Long-term myxedema patients are particularly subject to the rapid development of arteriosclerosis, coronary heart disease, angina pectoris, myocardial infarction, and congestive heart failure. *Acute organic psychosis* is a second complication of severe hypothyroidism. Patients with "myxedema madness" typically suffer from paranoia and delusions. Finally, a few patients with severe myxedema may develop *myxedema coma.* This critical condition is characterized by hypoventilation, hypothermia, and respiratory acidosis. Without emergency treatment with injectable thyroid hormone preparations, myxedema coma is usually terminal.

The *goals of care* in myxedema are to correct thyroid hormone deficiency, reverse symptoms, and prevent further heart and arterial damage. To permanently reverse hypothyroidism, the patient *must take thyroid hormone preparations for the rest of his life.* Thyroid drugs available include thyroxine (Synthyroid), triiodothyronine (Cytomel), or desiccated thyroid which is a combination of thyroxine and triiodothyronine. Dosage varies with the severity of the patient's hypothyroidism and the degree of heart disease present.

Persons with cardiac complications must be initially started on *small doses* of thyroid hormone; large doses could precipitate heart failure or

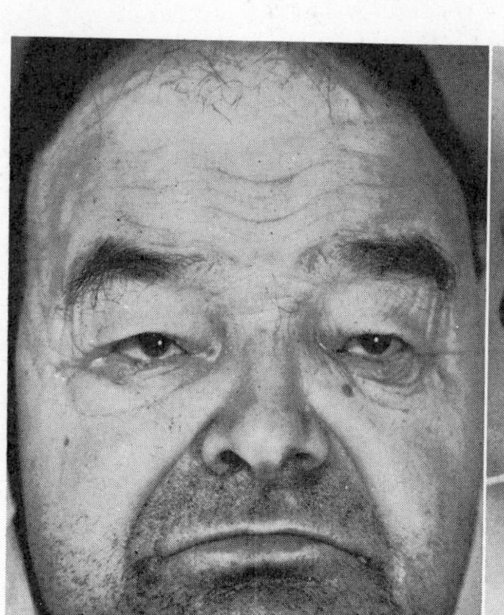

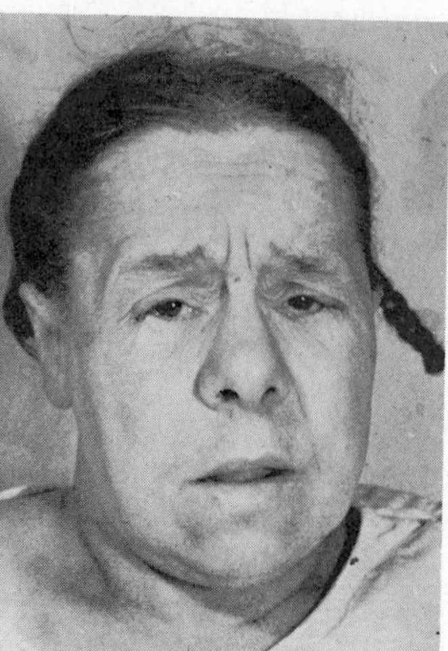

FIGURE 96–1. Typical facial appearance of myxedematous patients. (From Williams, R. H.: *Textbook of Endocrinology.* 4th ed. 1968.)

myocardial infarction by increasing body metabolism, myocardial oxygen requirements, and consequently the work of the heart. When administering thyroid hormone to a myxedematous patient with heart disease, watch the patient carefully for anginal pain, dyspnea, orthopnea, and so forth. If any new cardiac symptoms appear, notify the physician immediately; *do not* give the hormone until the doctor reappraises the patient's condition.

Once the patient has adequately responded to thyroid hormone therapy, he is placed on a maintenance dose of 1–3 grains of thyroid hormone daily.

Nursing patients with myxedema is very rewarding because these patients respond so dramatically to hormone replacement therapy. To assess the patient's progress and prevent complications, take time to make the following observations and perform the following measures.

> Observe the patient's level of physical and mental activity. With thyroid hormone therapy, the patient should gradually become more energetic and more interested in his surroundings.

> Observe daily for a lessening of the patient's edematous, puffy appearance. Note intake and output records; urine output should significantly increase during the course of thyroid therapy. Obtain the patient's daily weight; as activity increases and edema decreases, the patient should experience a significant weight loss.

> Observe the patient's sacrum, coccyx, elbows, scapula, and so forth for signs of redness or tissue breakdown. Remember that edematous tissues are particularly prone to decubitus ulcer formation (see Unit V, Ch. 27). Place the patient on a strict turning schedule and on an alternating pressure mattress. If the patient has cardiac complications, obtain help in moving him so that you don't place a greater strain on his already overburdened heart.

> Avoid sedating the patient if at all possible. If a sedative or narcotic must be given, administer no more than one half to one third the usual dose and then observe the patient carefully for signs of respiratory depression or coma.

> Provide the patient with a comfortable, warm environment. Remember that hypothyroidism sharply increases sensitivity to cold. If necessary, give the patient extra clothing and warm blankets.

> Observe the patient's appetite; typically he is placed on a low-calorie diet until his weight stabilizes at a normal level.

> Prevent constipation and fecal impactions. As the patient's hypothyroidism reverses and his heart condition improves, encourage him to be more active. Also remind him to drink at least 6–8 glasses of water every day and to eat foods which contain roughage, e.g., apples, lettuce. In stubborn cases, patients may need to take a stool softener or mild cathartic.

> Once the patient is mentally alert, teach him the importance of taking thyroid hormone *daily* for the rest of his life. Also give him a written list of the symptoms of thyroid deficiency or excess so that he will know when his dosage needs readjustment by his physician.

With early thyroid hormone replacement therapy, the prognosis for patients with severe hypothyroidism is excellent. Moreover, as long as the patient continues to take thyroid hormone daily, he should never again experience the depressed hypometabolic state of myxedema.

Hyperthyroidism (Thyrotoxicosis). Hyperthyroidism is a highly prevalent endocrine disease. Like the majority of thyroid conditions, hyperthyroidism is predominantly a disorder of females; it affects women four times as frequently as it does men. It has a particularly high incidence among young women between the ages of 20 and 40.

Graves' disease (toxic diffuse goiter, exophthalmic goiter) is the major cause of hyperthyroidism. The three principal hallmarks of Graves' disease include (1) enlargement of the thyroid gland (goiter); (2) hyperthyroidism; and (3) exophthalmos (abnormal protrusion of the eyes). Less commonly, hyperthyroidism is caused by a functioning toxic adenoma; in these cases, the patient may fail to demonstrate the many toxic symptoms associated with Graves' disease. Also overtreatment of myxedema with thyroid hormone may result in hyperthyroidism. Very rarely a pituitary adenoma causes hyperthyroidism by secreting excessive amounts of TSH. Because the most common as well as classic picture of hyperthyroidism is caused by Graves' disease, our discussion will center upon this condition.

ETIOLOGY OF GRAVES' DISEASE. For generations, physicians have linked the appearance of Graves' disease with periods of emotional stress in the patient's life. However, evidence for the theory that psychologic upheavals cause Graves' disease is meager. It is far more likely that Graves' disease, like Hashimoto's thyroiditis and primary myxedema, is an *autoimmune disorder.* Around 60–80 per cent of patients with Graves' disease have circulating autoantibodies which react against thyroglobulin.[16] Moreover, "long-acting thyroid stimulator" (LATS), a gamma globulin, has been discovered circulating in the serum of around 80–90 per cent of hyperthyroid patients.[38] There is still much to learn about LATS and its role in the causation of Graves' disease. Evidently LATS is an autoantibody which reacts against a "component of the thyroid cell membranes," somehow stimulating enlargement of the thyroid gland and secretion of excess thyroid hormone. Apparently, LATS is not involved in the development of exophthalmos.

SYMPTOMS AND DIAGNOSTIC TESTS. Because *hyperthyroidism* is caused by an excess secretion of thyroid hormone rather than by a deficiency, the clinical picture of Graves' disease is, in many ways, directly opposite that of myxedema. Thus the patient is extremely nervous, agitated, and irritable. Despite a ravenous appetite, the patient loses weight owing to the quickened metabolism. Because of the high levels of circulating thyroid hormone, the patient's bodily processes literally "speed up"; loose bowel movements, heat intolerance, profuse diaphoresis, tachycardia, incoordination due to tremor, and an accelerated circulation to the tissues causes the skin to become warm, smooth, and silky; also the hair appears smooth and soft.

Moreover, the patient's emotions are adversely affected by the turbulent activity within his body. Moods may be cyclical, ranging from mildly euphoric states to extreme hyperactivity to delirium. The excessive hyperactivity, in turn, leads to extreme fatigue and depression which is then followed by episodes of overactivity, and so forth. As a result of the patient's chaotic emotional state, family life and social relationships may deteriorate rapidly, which further accentuates the patient's emotional disturbance.

Goiter, the second characteristic of Graves' disease, is due to hyperplasia and hypertrophy of the thyroid cells; cellular overgrowth results in the release of excessive amounts of thyroid hormone into the blood. The gland may enlarge up to three to four times its normal size.

Exophthalmos, the third and final major manifestation of Graves' disease, has an obscure etiology. It may possibly result from oversecretion of a hormone called exophthalmos-producing substance (EPS), released by the anterior pituitary gland. The patient who suffers from exophthalmos has protruding eyeballs and a fixed stare due to the accumulation of fluid in the fat pads which lie behind the eye balls. Because the eyeballs are surrounded by unyielding bone, edema of the fat pads forces the eye balls forward out of their sockets, producing the typical facies of exophthalmos (see Fig. 96–2). In severe cases, the patient may be unable to close his eyelids and must have his lids taped shut to protect his eyes. Without treatment, severe exophthalmos can progress to corneal ulceration or infection and loss of vision.

Graves' disease is *diagnosed* on the basis of the patient's often striking physical appearance (enlarged neck, protruding eyeballs, agitated expression); his symptoms of restlessness, weight loss, and so forth; and laboratory findings. Typically the patient's BMR is *high,* which indicates that his tissues are utilizing excessive amounts of oxygen. Also the PBI, 24-hour radioiodine uptake, and T_3 resin uptake are all elevated, although they may occasionally be within the normal range. Serum cholesterol levels are usually depressed.

SPECIFIC TREATMENT MEASURES. The goals of treatment for patients with Graves' disease are to curtail the excessive secretion of thyroid hormone, to return the patient to a euthyroid state,

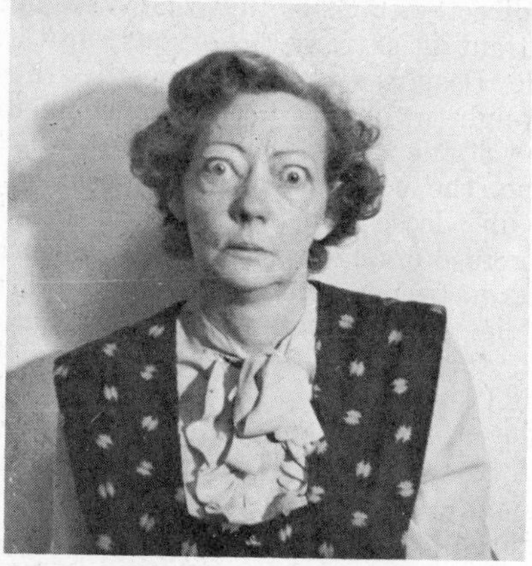

FIGURE 96–2. Hyperthyroidism. (From Guyton, A. C.: *Textbook of Medical Physiology.* 4th ed. 1971. Courtesy of Dr. Leonard Posey.)

and to prevent and treat complications. The three major forms of therapy include (1) antithyroid drug therapy, (2) surgery, and (3) radioiodine therapy. Choice of treatment is based upon (a) the patient's age, (b) the size of the goiter, and (c) whether or not other medical problems exist. Below, we have briefly pursued each of these clinical methods.

Antithyroid drug therapy. This form of treatment is recommended for patients who are under 18 and for pregnant women. The major drugs used to control hyperthyroidism include (1) propylthiouracil, (2) methimazole (Tapazole), and (3) iodine (Lugol's solution or saturated solution of potassium iodide). Adrenergic blocking agents are also administered as adjunctive therapy.

Propylthiouracil is the antithyroid drug of choice. It corrects hyperthyroidism by blocking thyroid hormone synthesis. The usual dosage of 100 mg. orally every 8 hours ameliorates Graves' disease within 4–8 weeks; however, several months may pass before symptoms completely vanish. Once the patient is euthyroid, he is given a maintenance dose of 50–55 mg. of propylthiouracil daily. While propylthiouracil is an ideal drug in many ways, it produces toxic reactions in approximately 9 per cent of patients.

The most serious toxic effect of propylthiouracil is *agranulocytosis* (see Unit XII, Ch. 62). A white blood count should be taken prior to initially administering the drug. Instruct nonhospitalized patients to report a sore throat, fever, or rash immediately to their physician so that further WBC tests can be performed and the patient's condition evaluated. Other less severe drug reactions include mild allergies (rash and pruritus). Rarely, the patient develops hepatitis or drug fever.

Methimazole (Tapazole) acts upon the thyroid gland in a way very similar to propylthiouracil, so that this drug can often be given to patients who are allergic to propylthiouracil. Unfortunately, methimazole also produces agranulocytosis in a small percentage of patients.

Iodine therapy is prescribed for two reasons: (1) to reduce the vascularity of the thyroid gland prior to subtotal or total thyroidectomy; and (2) to treat "thyroid storm" (see complications of Graves' disease, below). Iodine preparations *temporarily* act to prevent release of thyroid hormone into the circulation by increasing the amount of thyroid hormone stored within the gland. However, the stored thyroid hormone is eventually released back into the circulation, once again producing hyperthyroidism. For this reason, iodine preparations are usually only given for a 10- to 14-day period prior to surgery. If iodine is given for a longer period, or if it is given alone (i.e., not in combination with propylthiouracil), the thyroid gland may "escape" prior to thyroidectomy. The term "escape of the thyroid" means that the iodine is no longer capable of maintaining thyroid hormone storage; as a result, thyroid hormone floods the circulation, and hyperthyroidism returns in a more severe form than before.

The iodine drug of choice is saturated solution of potassium iodide (SSKI); the usual dose of SSKI is 5 drops in water 3 to 4 times daily. Lugol's solution is also used, but it is more expensive than

SSKI, and it tends to inactivate antithyroid preparations within the bowel.

Adrenergic blocking agents are sometimes given as adjunctive therapy to control overactivity by the sympathetic nervous system, thereby lessening such distressing symptoms as tachycardia, tremor, and nervousness. Drugs of choice include reserpine, guanethidine, and propranolol.

Surgery. Surgery has been performed since the early 1880's to treat hyperthyroidism. Ideally, patients selected for surgery are fairly young and free from any condition which would make them poor operative risks (e.g., diabetes, heart disease, renal disease, drug allergies).

Preoperative preparation for a subtotal thyroidectomy is extremely important. The patient should be euthyroid prior to the operation if possible. Thus preoperative care for patients with Graves' disease includes (a) the administration of antithyroid drugs to suppress secretion of thyroid hormone, and (b) the administration of iodine preparations to reduce the size and vascularity of the organ, thereby diminishing the chance of hemorrhage. The patient should be adequately rested, at optimum weight, and in good health before entering the operating room. Adequate preoperative preparation may take as long as 2 to 3 months.*

Well-prepared patients with Graves' disease stand a reasonable chance of being cured by surgery. Only 4–19 per cent of patients are reported to suffer a recurrence of hyperthyroidism, while another 15 per cent may develop hypothyroidism.[23] Rarely, vocal cord paralysis or hypoparathyroidism or both develops.

Radioiodine therapy. Therapy with ^{131}I is principally prescribed for middle-aged and elderly patients. This form of treatment offers many advantages: it is economical, simple to administer, and it can be prescribed on an outpatient basis. Radiotherapy is contraindicated in pregnant women and is rarely used for individuals of childbearing age.

The rationale behind ^{131}I therapy for Graves' disease is simple. You recall that the thyroid gland is unable to distinguish between regular iodine atoms and radioiodine atoms. Consequently, when the patient receives a dose of ^{131}I, his thyroid gland picks up the radioiodine and concentrates it just as it would regular iodine. As a result, some of the cells which concentrate iodine and make thyroxine are destroyed; thus thyroid hormone secretion diminishes, and the signs of hyperthyroidism and goiter disappear. However, because radioiodine destroys thyroid cells, one of the major possible complications of ^{131}I therapy is *myxedema.* Also radiotherapy has been theoretically linked with the possibility of malignant growths developing in tissues adjacent to the thyroid.

^{131}I is administered orally in the form of a "radioactive cocktail." Dosage is determined both by the size of the gland and by the thyroid's degree of radiosensitivity (see Unit VII, Ch. 35). Once the patient receives his "cocktail," he may then go home unless the dosage is extremely large; in the latter case, the patient must be placed in isolation for the half-life of ^{131}I, which is 8 days. The symptoms of hyperthyroidism are dispelled within 6 to 8 weeks following the administration of ^{131}I in more than 80 per cent of cases. The remaining 20 per cent of patients will require a second or (in rare cases) a third dose of radioiodine.[35] Patients should continue to have regular medical check-ups once they become euthyroid, because hypothyroidism may develop several years following radiotherapy. Should the patient become hypothyroid, he will need lifelong hormonal replacement with thyroid preparations.

GENERAL SYMPTOMATIC CARE. No matter which treatment the hyperthyroid patient receives (drug, surgery, radiotherapy), he needs expert nursing care to help him cope with his distressing symptoms. Provide an environment which is *restful* both mentally and physically. Ideally the patient with Graves' disease should be on bedrest, particularly if he is being prepared for surgery. Helping patients who are hyperthyroid to relax is a true challenge. Assigning the patient to a private room may help him to rest, and it will also prevent him from agitating other patients with his restless activities. Explain to friends and relatives that the patient's bizarre, difficult behavior is only temporary and should steadily improve with treatment. Caution visitors to avoid discussing upsetting topics with the patient until he feels better and calmer. Attempt, yourself, to maintain a quiet, understanding manner when working with the patient; accept his irritation and emotional outbursts for what they are—expressions of his disease.

Ask the occupational therapy department for assistance; the occupational therapist may be able to provide the patient with simple activities designed to distract him from his symptoms, e.g., putting together a puzzle with large pieces, molding clay, watching TV, and so forth. For the very restless patient, obtain an order for a sedative (e.g., phenobarbital) or for one of the adrenergic blocking agents discussed earlier.

Provide a well-balanced *diet.* The patient with Graves' disease is usually extremely hungry due to his increased metabolism. Indeed, he may require six full meals a day to satisfy his appetite. However, you recall that these patients lose weight rapidly despite huge meals; also they usually are in a state of negative nitrogen balance. Therefore, encourage patients to eat foods which are highly nutritious and contain ample amounts of protein, carbohydrates, and minerals. Discourage ordering foods which increase peristalsis and resultant diarrhea; e.g., highly seasoned, bulky, or fibrous foods. Weigh the patient daily and report weight losses of more than 3 lb. If the patient continues to appear malnourished despite an ample diet, obtain an order for supplemental vitamins—particularly vitamin B complex.

*Pre- and postoperative care for patients undergoing thyroidectomy are discussed further on pp. 1358 to 1359.

Provide a *cool* environment. Remember that patients with Graves' disease suffer from heat intolerance. When making the bed, omit the plastic draw sheet as it tends to cause diaphoresis. Use only a lightweight sheet for the top cover. Provide the patient with light, loose pajamas; if the patient is diaphoretic, he will need frequent changes of bedsheets and night clothes.

TREATING COMPLICATIONS OF GRAVES' DISEASE. The three major complications of Graves' disease are (1) exophthalmos, (2) heart disease, and (3) thyroid storm.

Unlike the manifestations of goiter and hyperthyroidism, exophthalmos does not necessarily regress with treatment; in fact, occasionally the removal of thyroid secretion greatly worsens exophthalmos. Possibly removal or destruction of thyroid tissue aggravates the patient's eye condition because the pituitary gland is no longer controlled by thyroxine secretion, and consequently it secretes even more excessive amounts of EPS. Exophthalmos is generally treated with the following specific drugs and procedures:

> *Thyroid hormone* is administered orally if the patient continues to have progressive exophthalmos following treatment. Possibly thyroid preparations act to control pituitary secretion of EPS.

> *Corticotropin* (ACTH) or prednisone is given in large doses to reduce inflammation of the periorbital tissues. Unfortunately steroids produce many undesirable side effects, including acute psychoses.

> *Estrogen* therapy is occasionally of value in postmenopausal women.

> *Methylcellulose eye drops,* ¼ per cent four times daily, help reduce eye irritation.

> *Surgical decompression* of the *orbits* is performed when all other measures fail to correct the exophthalmos; this procedure may save the patient's vision when eye changes are severe.

There are also a number of general nursing measures which help to reduce eye discomfort and prevent corneal ulceration and infection; they are as follows:

> Instruct patients with exophthalmos to wear dark glasses; warn them to avoid getting dust or dirt in their eyes.

> When the patient cannot close his eyelids easily or at all, have him wear a sleeping mask (which can be bought in drug stores) or lightly tape his eyes shut with scotch tape. In severe cases, the physician may be forced to suture the patient's lids closed.

> Elevate the head of the bed at night and have the patient restrict his salt intake to relieve edema.

> Encourage the patient to exercise the extraocular muscles daily by having him direct his eyes from the upper left to the upper right to the lower left to the lower right and so forth several times around. Exercise of the eye muscles seems to improve eye function.

Heart disease, the second complication of Graves' disease, poses a serious threat. Tachycardia almost always accompanies thyrotoxicosis; atrial fibrillation may also appear. Congestive heart failure is found among older persons with longstanding thyrotoxicosis. The treatment of these cardiac complications is discussed in detail in Unit X.

Thyroid storm is a sometimes fatal, acute episode of thyroid overactivity characterized by high fever, severe tachycardia, delirium, dehydration, and extreme irritability. Once a commonly occurring crisis, thyroid storm seldom develops today, thanks to modern treatment technics. However, it can develop when a patient with Graves' disease undergoes severe sudden stress, develops an infection, or enters labor; also it strikes patients who have not been adequately prepared for thyroid surgery. Recently, some investigators are linking the etiology of thyroid storm with adrenal insufficiency.

Because it is an emergency, thyroid storm requires heroic treatment measures for control. The high fever is combated with hypothermia or ice packs; dehydration is relieved with intravenous fluids. To block thyroid hormone secretion, the doctor orders an oral or parenteral antithyroid drug, followed 1 hour later by potassium iodide. Corticosteroids are administered if there is any possibility that the patient is suffering from adrenal insufficiency. Sometimes large doses of propranolol (Inderal) are given to block sympathetic nervous stimulation and relieve cardiac arrhythmias; the use of Inderal is still investigational.

THYROIDECTOMY

Thyroidectomy (removal of the thyroid gland) may be either total or partial. *Total* thyroidectomy is performed to remove thyroid cancer; patients who undergo this operation must take thyroid hormone on a permanent basis. *Subtotal* thyroidectomy is employed to correct hyperthyroidism and extreme cases of simple goiter. Approximately 5/6 of the gland is removed. Because 1/6 of the functioning thyroid tissue is left intact, hormonal replacements are not necessary.

PREOPERATIVE CARE. As emphasized earlier, patients must be carefully prepared for thyroidectomy or complications will ensue (e.g., thyroid storm and hemorrhage). Criteria for successful preparation of patients for thyroid surgery include the following:

> The patient is *euthyroid* before entering the operating room; tests of thyroid function are within the normal range.

> Signs of thyrotoxicosis are greatly diminished or absent; the patient appears rested and relaxed.

> Weight and nutritional status are normal; any weight losses suffered earlier have been regained.

> Cardiac problems are under control; pulse rate is normal; electrocardiogram tracings taken before surgery show no dangerous arrhythmias.

To help him meet these four criteria, the patient facing thyroidectomy is treated with antithyroid drugs, iodine preparations, bedrest, nutritious diet, and supplemental vitamins. As we stated earlier, thorough preparation may take months. However, once armed with good health and adequate weight, the patient can undergo surgery with confidence that his operation will be successful and his symptoms alleviated permanently.

POSTOPERATIVE CARE. The immediate goals of postoperative care following thyroidectomy are (a) to decrease strain on the patient's suture line; (b) to relieve discomfort from sore throat and tracheal irritation; (c) to prevent pooling of respiratory secretions; and (d) to prevent and/or relieve the complications of thyroidectomy.

The major complications which may follow thyroidectomy include: (1) hemorrhage; (2) respiratory obstruction due to edema of the glottis, bilateral laryngeal nerve damage, or tracheal compression from hemorrhage; (3) weakness and hoarseness of the voice due to damage of one laryngeal nerve; (4) hypocalcemia and tetany resulting from accidental removal of one or more of the parathyroid glands; (5) thyroid storm.

Typical postoperative orders accompanied by rationale and important associated nursing actions are outlined in Table 96–3. Note that you will need to assemble several pieces of equipment at the patient's bedside before he returns from surgery, e.g., blood pressure cuff and stethoscope, sandbags or additional pillows, a suction machine, tracheostomy set, oxygen, humidifier, and rectal thermometer; ampules of calcium gluconate should also be on hand in the medicine cabinet or on the emergency tray.

Hoarseness and weakness of the voice may occur if there has been unilateral injury of the pharyngeal nerve during surgery; this condition is usually temporary. The patient's voice should be assessed by asking him to state his name as soon as he fully recovers from anesthesia. Have him speak every 30 to 60 minutes thereafter, and carefully note any voice changes. If hoarseness or voice weakness is present, reassure the patient that the problem will probably subside in a few days. Discourage him from unnecessary talking because overuse of vocal cords prolongs hoarseness.

Muscular twitching and hyperirritability of the nervous system indicates *tetany;* hypocalcemia develops if one or more of the parathyroid glands are accidentally removed during surgery. Symptoms may develop in from 1 to 7 days after surgery. Report immediately any muscular spasms or twitching; have calcium gluconate ampules on hand. (The care of patients with tetany is discussed in Unit V, Ch. 25, and later in this unit.)

Once the immediate postoperative period and its dangers have passed, turn your attention next to patient instruction. Important areas to cover are as follows:

> Teach the patient how to support the weight of his own head and neck when sitting up in bed. Show him how to place his hands at the back of his head when flexing his neck or moving. Usually the patient is able to perform this maneuver by the second postoperative day.

> Once sutures have been removed (usually on the second to fourth postoperative day), instruct the patient in range of motion neck exercises to prevent contractures. With the surgeon's permission, teach the patient to flex his head forward and laterally to hyperextend his neck and to turn his head from side to side. Have the patient perform these exercises several times every day.

> To diminish scarring of the neck, have the patient apply cold cream or other lubricant daily to the incision once sutures are removed.

> If a total thyroidectomy has been performed, instruct the patient concerning the self-administration of thyroid medications.

> Make an appointment for the patient for a follow-up visit in the hospital clinic or doctor's office following discharge. Emphasize to the patient that he must see his physician at least twice a year for the rest of his life in order to avert any possible complications (e.g., hypothyroidism, hypoparathyroidism, or recurrent hyperthyroidism).

THE PARATHYROID GLANDS

The parathyroid glands are four small glands which are either near to, attached to, or embedded in the thyroid gland. The hormone secreted by the parathyroid gland is a polypeptide substance called parathormone (PTH). The *functions* of PTH are as follows:

> Controls calcium and phosphate metabolism (see Unit V, Ch. 24).

> Increases the breakdown and resorption of bone, thereby maintaining normal serum calcium levels.

> Maintains an inverse relationship between serum calcium and phosphate levels, thereby fostering normal excitability of nerves and muscles.

The regulation of PTH release depends upon a feedback relationship between the level of serum calcium and the level of PTH in the blood (see Fig. 25–4, p. 236). Note that, when serum calcium is elevated, PTH secretion decreases, resulting in the increased excretion of calcium ions in the urine and a lowering of the serum calcium. Conversely, when serum calcium levels are low, PTH secretion increases, resulting in the decreased excretion of calcium ions in the urine and an increase in the level of serum calcium.

DISORDERS OF THE PARATHYROID GLANDS AND THEIR DIAGNOSIS

There are two major disorders of the parathyroid glands. The parathyroid glands may secrete *too much hormone* (hyperparathyroidism), or they may secrete *too little hormone* (hypoparathyroidism). *Hyperparathyroidism* is characterized by the following findings:

Increased bone resorption
Elevated serum calcium levels
Depressed serum phosphate levels
Hypercalcinuria and hyperphosphaturia
Decreased neuromuscular irritability

Conversely *hypoparathyroidism* has the following characteristics:

- Decreased bone resorption with increased bone density
- Depressed serum calcium levels
- Elevated serum phosphate levels
- Hypocalcinuria and hypophosphaturia
- Increased neuromuscular activity which may progress to tetany.

Laboratory studies of parathyroid function and malfunction include the following: total serum calcium, qualitative urinary calcium (Sulkowitch test), quantitative urinary calcium (calcium deprivation test), serum phosphorus, serum alkaline phosphatase, and radioimmunoassay of parathormone. In Table 96–4 these tests are briefly characterized and compared.

Hypersecretion of the Parathyroid Glands (Hyperparathyroidism). Hyperparathyroidism is a disorder caused by *overactivity* of one or more of the parathyroid glands. It is classified as either primary, secondary, or "tertiary." *Primary* hyperparathyroidism is a rare, potentially curable condition which develops within the parathyroid glands themselves. Ninety per cent of cases of primary hyperparathyroidism arise from a *single adenoma* (a benign epithelial tumor composed of glandular tissue); 8 per cent of cases result from *hyperplasia* and *hypertrophy* of the four glands; while 2 per cent develop from *carcinoma* of a single gland.[25] *Secondary* hyperparathyroidism is caused by a *compensatory oversecretion* of PTH in response to the hypocalcemia caused by chronic renal disease, rickets, osteomalacia, and acromegaly. "Tertiary" hyperparathyroidism is associated with the ectopic secretion of parathormone by cancerous tumors located in the lungs, kidneys, and so forth.

PATHOPHYSIOLOGY AND SYMPTOMS. You recall that the normal function of PTH is to control and increase bone resorption, thereby maintaining the proper balance of calcium and phosphorus ions within the blood. What happens then when PTH secretion is excessive? Excessive circulating PTH creates the following pathologic changes:

> *Bone damage:* Oversecretion of PTH causes excessive *osteoclast* growth and activity within the bones. Osteoclasts are large multinuclear cells which are ac-

TABLE 96–3. POSTOPERATIVE ORDERS, RATIONALE, AND ASSOCIATED NURSING ACTIONS FOLLOWING THYROIDECTOMY

Postoperative Order	Rationale	Associated Nursing Actions
1. Vital signs q. 15 minutes until stable; then q. 30 min. for next 12 hours.	Following thyroidectomy, hemorrhage and respiratory obstruction may develop. Elevated pulse and hypotension indicate hemorrhage and shock. Dyspnea, crowing respirations, and retraction of neck tissues indicate respiratory obstruction.	Check dressing after checking vital signs. Observe for bleeding at front, sides, and *back* of neck. Examine back of patient's neck and shoulders for bleeding because blood tends to drain posteriorly. Check dressing for tightness; uncomfortable tautness may indicate bleeding into tissues. Loosen dressing and call surgeon immediately.
2. Semi-Fowler position when conscious; support head and neck with pillows and sandbags; ambulate second day as tolerated.	Immobilization of head and neck is essential to prevent flexion and hyperextension of neck with resultant strain on suture line; semi-Fowler position is used for comfort.	Place sandbags on either side of patient's head for immobilization and maintenance of good alignment. Warn patient not to extend or hyperextend neck; reassure him that sandbags will prevent him from moving his head too much. Gently rub back of patient's neck to relieve tension. Support patient's head and neck when moving him, or changing his position.
3. Fluids by mouth as tolerated; if nausea or vomiting, notify surgeon. Soft diet second day P.M.	Patient who is nauseated or vomiting is given I.V. fluids; otherwise, oral fluids are started as soon as patient is fully conscious.	Maintain intake and output record for 2 or 3 days. Observe patient for difficulty in swallowing; normally this problem lasts for only a day or two postoperatively. Weigh patient once he starts full diet; weight lost during early postoperative period should be regained.

tive in promoting resorption of bone. Because of increased bone resorption, calcium drains from the bones into the blood, causing *hypercalcemia*. Thus the bones suffer *demineralization* due to calcium loss. In time, the bones may become so fragile that they break easily with even mild trauma, causing pathologic fractures. Also, as the uncontrolled osteoclast proliferation continues, the entire skeleton may become filled with cystic lesions; without treatment of hyperparathyroidism and without replacement of calcium losses through diet and medication, the patient eventually develops a severe bone disease called *osteitis fibrosa cystica* (Von Recklinghausen's disease of bone).

> *Hypercalcemia:* An increased serum calcium level is the consequence of bone resorption due to excessive PTH secretion. Hypercalcemia eventually results in *hypercalciuria* (spillage of excess calcium into the urine). Also, because of the high serum calcium levels, calcium eventually precipitates as calcium phosphate into the lungs, muscles, heart, and eyes. In addition, hypercalcemia causes gastric ulcers, possibly because excess serum calcium acts to increase gastric secretions.

> *Kidney damage:* You recall that an inverse relationship exists between serum calcium and serum phosphorus. Consequently, as serum calcium rises, serum phosphorus drops, and *hyperphosphaturia* (increased phosphate levels within the urine) develops. As serum calcium continues to rise, excessive amounts of both phosphorus and calcium are excreted and lost from the body. Because high amounts of both calcium and phosphate are being processed by the renal system, calcium phosphate is deposited within the renal tubules, causing a kidney condition called *nephrocalcinosis*. Also *kidney stones* composed of calcium phosphate are found in the urine of approximately 80 per cent of patients with primary hyperparathyroidism. Stones develop because calcium salts are generally insoluble in urine.

Patients with hyperparathyroidism may be asymptomatic, with the exception of hypercalcemia, as demonstrated by laboratory tests. Other patients suffer from a myriad of symptoms arising from skeletal damage, renal involvement, and hypercalcemia.

Manifestations of *bone disease* range from backache, joint pain, and bone pain to pathologic fractures of the spine, ribs, and long bones. In longstanding cases, deformities and bending of the bones due to osteitis fibrosa cystica develop.

Symptoms of *renal* involvement include polyuria and polydipsia; the appearance of sand, gravel, or stones within the urine; azotemia; and

TABLE 96-3. POSTOPERATIVE ORDERS, RATIONALE, AND ASSOCIATED NURSING ACTIONS FOLLOWING THYROIDECTOMY (*Continued*)

Postoperative Order	Rationale	Associated Nursing Actions
4. Meperidine (Demerol), 50 mg. q. 3–4 hours p.r.n. for pain in throat area.	Demerol and morphine sulfate are both used during early postoperative period to relieve pain and promote rest.	Do not give narcotics to patients with respirations below 12 per minute or to patients with respiratory congestion; consult physician for further orders.
5. Cough and deep breathe q. ½ hour; suction mouth and trachea if necessary.	Pooling of mucous secretions in trachea, bronchi, and lungs will cause respiratory obstruction with resultant atelectasis and pneumonia. Secretions must be raised to prevent respiratory complications.	Instruct patient to cough and deep breathe as he was taught during preoperative period. If patient cannot raise secretions, gently suction mouth and trachea. Do not oversedate patients with profuse respiratory secretions; also give narcotics judiciously.
6. Tracheostomy set and oxygen on hand in room.	Acute respiratory obstruction due to hemorrhage, edema of glottis, laryngeal nerve damage, or tetany is an emergency; equipment for establishing an airway and administering oxygen must be available for immediate use.	Continuously observe patient for signs of airway obstruction, e.g., increasing restlessness, tachycardia, apprehension, cyanosis, crowing respirations, and retraction of neck tissues. Report any of these signs to surgeon immediately.
7. Continuous steam inhalation until chest clear.	Humidification of the air promotes easier breathing; moistness of air also helps to liquify mucous secretions.	Keep patient's door closed so that the moist air is retained in his room.
8. Rectal temperature q. 4 hours for 24 hours, then orally.	One of the first signs of thyroid storm is an elevated temperature.	Carefully observe patient for signs of thyroid storm: elevated temperature, extreme restlessness, agitation, and tachycardia. Report any elevation over 100° rectally or 99° orally.

hypertension due to renal damage. Without treatment, renal insufficiency may progress to fatal renal hypertension and uremia.

Hypercalcemia mainly produces gastrointestinal tract symptoms, e.g., thirst, nausea, anorexia, constipation, ileus, and abdominal pain. Often patients have a history of peptic ulcer or gastrointestinal bleeding. Psychiatric symptoms (listlessness, depression, paranoia) are also associated with high levels of serum calcium. Finally, calcium may form calcifications within the eyes, impairing vision.

The diagnosis of hyperparathyroidism mainly rests upon laboratory and x-ray findings. Serum calcium is elevated, while serum phosphate is depressed; urine calcium and phosphate are both high. In addition, alkaline phosphatase is elevated among the 25 per cent of patients who have associated bone disease. Also, patients with skeletal damage have the following characteristic x-ray findings: diffuse demineralization of bones, bone cysts, subcortical bone absorption, and loss of the lamina dura about the teeth.

CLINICAL CARE. Primary hyperparathyroidism is always treated *surgically;* the parathyroid tumors which are causing hypersecretion of parathormone are located and removed. Usually only the diseased parathyroid glands are resected. However, if all four glands are hyperplastic, 3½ glands are removed. Fortunately one half of a parathyroid gland is sufficient to maintain normal levels of circulating parathormone.

The goals of *preoperative care* for hyperparathyroid patients undergoing surgery are (a) to reduce hypercalcemia, (b) to prevent further renal damage,

TABLE 96–4. DIAGNOSTIC TESTS OF PARATHYROID FUNCTION: PURPOSE, WARD PROCEDURE, NORMAL RANGE, AND INTERPRETATION OF ABNORMAL FINDINGS

Test	Purpose	Ward Procedure
Total serum calcium	Measures amount of ionized and nonionized calcium in serum.	Venous blood to laboratory.
Qualitative urinary calcium (Sulkowitch test)	Measures roughly amount of calcium in urine. Used as a quick method for diagnosing if tetany is due to hypoparathyroidism.	Collect urine specimen and send to laboratory.
Quantitative urinary calcium (calcium deprivation test)	Measures exact amount of calcium in a 24-hour urine specimen following a period of calcium deprivation.	Low-calcium diet for 3–6 days prior to test; 24-hour urine specimen collected and sent to laboratory.
Serum phosphorus	Measures amount of inorganic phosphorus in the serum.	Venous blood to laboratory.
Serum alkaline phosphatase	Measures amount of alkaline phosphatase in serum. Aids in diagnosing bone and liver disorders.	Venous blood to laboratory.
Radioimmunoassay test	Measures level of PTH in serum.	Venous blood to laboratory.

and (c) to treat and prevent complications, e.g., pathologic fractures, peptic ulcers, and so on. Actions which promote these goals include the following:

> *Force fluids* to at least 3000 ml. per day. Dehydration is dangerous for these patients, because it both increases the serum calcium level and promotes the formation of renal stones. Encourage the patient to drink cranberry juice and prune juice, because these acid-ash fruit juices make the urine more acidic. Higher urinary acidity helps prevent renal stone formation, because calcium is more soluble in an acid urine than in an alkaline urine.

> *Phosphate or sodium phytate* (Rencal) may be ordered to lower reabsorption of calcium by the gastrointestinal tract. Also the hormone *calcitonin* is being experimentally used in some cases to lower serum calcium. The benefits of calcitonin therapy are still debatable.

Encourage a *low-calcium, low-phosphate diet* to correct hypercalcemia. Explain to the patient that the omission of milk and milk products from his menu may help alleviate some of the distressing gastrointestinal symptoms. If the patient suffers from peptic ulcers, he will need to substitute other types of protein feedings for milk and milk products.

> *Prevent constipation* and *fecal impaction* resulting from hypercalcemia. Help the patient to be as active as possible, depending upon the extent of his bone disease. If constipation continues despite these measures, obtain an order for a stool softener or laxative.

> *Strain all urine* for gravel and stones; save any specimens of abnormal urine for the physician to examine. Also observe the urine for blood and the patient for renal colic (see Unit XI, Ch. 57).

> Protect the patient from accidents. If bone involvement exists, the patient may develop pathologic fractures from even small bumps or minor falls. Keep the patient's bed in the low position and use siderails. If he is

TABLE 96–4. DIAGNOSTIC TESTS OF PARATHYROID FUNCTION: PURPOSE, WARD PROCEDURE, NORMAL RANGE, AND INTERPRETATION OF ABNORMAL FINDINGS (*Continued*)

Normal Range	Interpretation of Abnormal Findings	Remarks
4.8 to 5.2 mEq./liter or 8–11 mg./100 ml.	Elevated in hyperparathyroidism; depressed in hypoparathyroidism, tetany, rickets, nephrosis, and osteomalacia.	Normally 50% of total serum calcium is ionized. Ionized calcium is the only form of calcium utilized by the body. Amount of ionized calcium available decreases in alkalosis.
Fine white precipitate should form when Sulkowitch reagent is added to urine specimen.	Absence or decreased density of precipitate indicates low serum calcium and hypoparathyroidism.	Drugs which falsely elevate serum calcium levels include Vitamin D, parathyroid injection, and dihydrotachysterol.
75–175 mg. of calcium per 24 hours.	Elevated in hyperparathyroidism; depressed in hypoparathyroidism.	Foods high in calcium include milk, cheese, molasses, turnip greens, and dandelion greens.
4.0 to 5.4 mEq./liter.	Elevated in hypoparathyroidism, uremia, alkalosis, and Bright's disease; depressed in hyperparathyroidism, rickets, osteitis, and osteomalacia.	Serum phosphorus is normally around one half that of serum calcium. There is an inverse relationship between serum calcium and serum phosphorus. Drugs which falsely elevate serum phosphorus levels include Dilantin, heparin, Pituitrin, and vitamin D.
2.0–5.0 Bodansky units.	Elevated in hyperparathyroidism, osteomalacia, rickets, healing fractures, pregnancy, and following ingestion of large amounts of vitamin D.	Alkaline phosphatase is an enzyme normally present in small amounts in serum. Some drugs causing false elevations of alkaline phosphatase levels include allopurinol, some androgens, colchicine, erythromycin, methyldopa, some oral contraceptives, procainamide, and tolbutamide.
Less than 0.6 Mug. per ml.	High concentrations indicate hyperparathyroidism.	Still an experimental procedure. In near future, will probably be definitive test for hyperparathyroidism.

weak or has joint or skeletal disease, always assist him to ambulate.

> If the patient has heart disease, administer digitalis very cautiously.

Individuals with hypercalcemia are hypersensitive to digitalis and may quickly develop toxic symptoms.

During the *postoperative* period, new problems arise, some of which are the reverse of those found preoperatively. During the *immediate* postoperative period, nursing care is similar to that following thyroidectomy; i.e., observe the patient carefully for hemorrhage, airway obstruction, injury to the recurrent laryngeal nerve, tetany, and so forth. In addition, watch the patient for signs of *hormonal imbalance.*

First of all, *mild tetany* due to the drop in serum calcium is *expected* following removal of parathyroid tissue (see Ch. 25). Typically, the uncomfortable tingling of the hands and around the mouth which follows parathyroid resection usually disappears without problem. However, if tetany persists or is severe, calcium gluconate is administered I.V. to relieve symptoms.

Secondly, hyperparathyroid crisis, a rare complication, may be precipitated by the surgery. This severe disorder is characterized by a *rise in serum calcium* to 30 mg./100 ml. or more. Extreme hypercalcemia, in turn, produces manifestations ranging from dyspnea, weakness, nausea, vomiting, and headache to collapse and coma. Hyperparathyroid crisis is reversed by the administration of phosphorus and fluids I.V. in order to foster calcium excretion, thereby lowering the serum calcium level.

Patients with *bone disease* require additional therapy following surgery. Because removal of the parathyroid glands reduces bone resorption and because bone rebuilding proceeds at a rapid rate, the patient can develop the "hungry bones" syndrome. This syndrome is characterized by hypocalcemia and severe tetany resulting from the rapid utilization of calcium by the bones. To prevent low serum calcium levels due to bone recalcification, the patient should eat foods high in calcium. Tetany is treated with injections of calcium gluconate. To maintain adequate calcium levels, oral calcium preparations are usually given for months until the skeletal tissues have been rebuilt. Finally, patients are encouraged to ambulate as soon as possible following surgery because weight-bearing speeds the recalcification process.

PROGNOSIS. If hyperparathyroidism is surgically treated early in its course, the chance for total recovery is good. Bone pain may disappear within three days following removal of parathyroid tissue, and bone lesions may heal completely. Unfortunately, serious renal disease tends to be progressive and is not reversible with surgery.

Hyposecretion of the Parathyroid Glands (Hypoparathyroidism). Hyposecretion of the parathyroid glands produces a syndrome which is opposite that of hyperparathyroidism; thus serum calcium levels are abnormally low, serum phosphate levels are abnormally high, bone density increases, and pronounced neuromuscular irritability (tetany) develops.

The causes of hypoparathyroidism are either iatrogenic or idiopathic. *Iatrogenic causes* of hypoparathyroidism include (a) accidental removal of one or more of the parathyroid glands during thyroidectomy, (b) infarction of the parathyroid glands resulting from an inadequate blood supply to the glands during surgery, (c) and strangulation of one or more of the glands by postoperative scar tissue. *Idiopathic* hypoparathyroidism (like myxedema, Graves' disease, and Hashimoto's thyroiditis) may possibly be an *autoimmune* disorder with a genetic basis. This type of hyperparathyroidism is far less common than the post-thyroidectomy form. It strikes children nine times as frequently as adults, and it affects twice as many women as men.

PATHOPHYSIOLOGY AND SYMPTOMS. As stated before, parathormone normally acts to increase bone resorption, which in turn maintains proper serum calcium levels. The hormone also regulates phosphate clearance by the renal tubules, thereby maintaining the correct inverse balance between serum calcium and serum phosphate. Consequently, when parathyroid secretion is reduced, bone resorption slows, serum calcium levels fall, bone density increases, calcifications form in varied organs (e.g., eyes, basal ganglia), and severe neuromuscular irritability develops. Also without sufficient PTH fewer phosphorus ions are secreted by the distal tubules of the kidney, renal excretion of phosphate decreases, serum phosphate levels rise, and more phosphate ions (along with calcium ions) are deposited in the bones.

The *symptoms* of hypoparathyroidism are mainly caused by low serum calcium levels. *Acute* hypoparathyroidism (caused by accidental damage to parathyroid tissues during thyroidectomy) is characterized by greatly increased neuromuscular irritability, resulting in tetany. You recall from Unit V that patients with tetany experience painful muscle spasm, irritability, grimacing, tingling of fingers, laryngospasm, and arrhythmias. Chvostek's sign (signifying hyperirritability of the facial nerve) and Trousseau's sign (carpal spasms of the fingers and hands following application of a pressure cuff to the arm) are present. In some cases, tetany is so severe that tracheostomy is required to correct acute respiratory obstruction due to laryngospasm.

Chronic hypoparathyroidism (which is usually idiopathic in nature) causes lethargy, thin patchy hair, brittle nails, dry scaly skin, and personality changes. Paradoxically, the low serum calcium levels may result in the formation of ectopic calcification in the eyes and basal ganglia; thus, the patient may develop cataracts and permanent brain damage accompanied by psychoses or convulsions. In addition, severe persistent hypocalcemia adversely affects the heart, causing arrhythmias and eventual heart failure. When hypoparathyroidism develops in infancy or early childhood, the patient may suffer from malformed teeth, poor physical growth and development, and mental retardation.

The symptoms of hypoparathyroidism are always more severe in patients who have an *elevated serum pH* (alkalosis) due to any cause (e.g., ingesting antacids, hyperventilating from emotional causes). Symptoms worsen because (a) only *ionized* calcium (which comprises around 50 per cent of total calcium) can be utilized by the body; (b) when the pH of the blood rises, the amount of ionized calcium drops, even though total serum calcium remains the same; (c) with even less ionized calcium available to the body, the symptoms resulting from hypocalcemia become more severe until the alkalosis is corrected.

The *diagnosis* of hypoparathyroidism is based upon the following:

> Presence of a positive Chvostek's sign and Trousseau's sign.

> Laboratory findings of low serum calcium, high serum phosphate, and a low or absent urinary calcium.

> X-ray studies which show increased bone density and possibly calcifications of the basal ganglia.

> Eye examinations which may reveal the early development of cataracts due to the formation of calcifications within the eyes.

CLINICAL CARE IN ACUTE HYPOPARATHYROIDISM. One cannot live without parathormone. Thus acute hypoparathyroidism (with its major manifestation of acute tetany) is a *life-threatening disorder*. The goals of *emergency* care are (1) to elevate serum calcium levels as rapidly as possible, (2) to prevent or treat convulsions, and (3) to control laryngeal spasm and consequent respiratory obstruction.

First of all, to quickly elevate serum calcium levels, the patient is given 10 per cent calcium gluconate solution in an intravenous infusion (see Ch. 25, p. 237). While administering calcium gluconate, instruct the patient to inhale his own carbon dioxide by breathing into a paper bag. The inhaled carbon dioxide causes a mild respiratory acidosis which serves to elevate the amount of *ionized* calcium in the blood.

If these measures fail to control tetany and the patient begins to convulse, the doctor will next order a sedative such as phenobarbital as well as an anticonvulsant drug, e.g., Dilantin. To help prevent convulsions, place the patient in a quiet room and keep the lights low to promote rest (see Unit VIII). Finally, be prepared for the possibility that the patient with tetany may suffer laryngeal spasm and respiratory obstruction.

Always have an endotracheal tube *and* tracheostomy set *close at hand when caring for patients with acute tetany.*

Once the patient's condition has stabilized and the dangers of tetany have passed, he is given *oral* calcium salts in order to maintain normal serum calcium levels.

CLINICAL CARE IN CHRONIC HYPOPARATHYROIDISM. The goal of maintenance therapy for patients with chronic hypoparathyroidism is to maintain the serum calcium level at no lower than 10 mg./100 ml. To achieve this goal, the following measures are taken:

> Instruct the patient to eat a diet high in calcium but low in phosphorus; remind the patient to omit cheese and milk products from his diet because these nutrients have a high phosphorus content.

> Give the patient *aluminum hydroxide gel* (Amphogel) as ordered before meals. Aluminum salts are helpful during the initial treatment of hypoparathyroidism because they help reduce phosphate absorption by the gastrointestinal tract, thereby raising blood calcium levels.

> Administer *oral calcium salts* (either calcium gluconate, calcium lactate, or calcium chloride) as ordered. Calcium supplements may be obtained in either tablet or solution form, depending upon the patient's preference. Oral calcium administration is usually discontinued if the patient responds successfully to the vitamin D preparations described below.

> Administer prescribed *vitamin D* preparations. You recall from Chapter 24 that the absorption of calcium is dependent upon the presence of vitamin D. Indeed, vitamin D is capable of totally replacing parathyroid hormone in the body, thereby raising blood calcium levels to normal. Commercially available forms of vitamin D include calciferol (vitamin D_2), cholecalciferol (vitamin D_3), and dihydrotachysterol (Hytakerol). Although calciferol is a more reliable and less expensive drug than Hytakerol, all three forms of vitamin D are effective in correcting hypocalcemia. They are all obtainable as either tablets or oily liquids. Also all forms are slowly assimilated by the body; therefore, warn the patient that it may take a week or longer for symptoms to improve.

> Rarely you may be asked to administer *parathormone injections* to prevent tetany. Parathyroid hormone is infrequently used for a variety of reasons: (a) tolerance to it develops and it cannot be used with full beneficial effects for more than a week; (b) it must be injected at least daily and preferably 3 to 5 times daily for maximum effectiveness; and (c) it has not yet been manufactured in a preparation which is consistently stable. Consequently when parathormone injections are ordered, they are replaced by vitamin D preparations as soon as possible.

> Emphasize to the patient the importance of *lifelong* follow-up medical care. Instruct the patient to have his serum calcium level checked by his physician at least three times a year—*every year*. Normal blood serum calcium levels must be maintained to prevent complications. If either hypercalcemia or hypocalcemia develop, the doctor will have to adjust the patient's treatment regime to correct the imbalance.

PROGNOSIS. The patient may fully recover from the effects of hypoparathyroidism if his condition is diagnosed *early*, before the advent of serious complications. Unfortunately cataracts and brain calcifications, once formed, are irreversible.

CHAPTER 97

Nursing Patients With Disorders of the Adrenal and Pituitary Glands

THE ADRENAL GLANDS

NORMAL ANATOMY AND PHYSIOLOGY

The adrenal glands (or suprarenal glands) are two small but vital endocrine structures which cap the top of the kidneys. Each adrenal gland is composed of two distinct structures, each with its own function, which are merged into one powerful glandular organ. The inner core of the adrenal gland is called the *adrenal medulla* while the outer shell of the gland is called the *adrenal cortex*. Although both structures contribute to the individual's survival and well-being, only the adrenal cortex is essential for life.

The Adrenal Medulla. The adrenal medulla, which is a part of the sympathetic nervous system (sometimes called the sympathoadrenal system), releases two potent hormones called epinephrine (Adrenaline) and norepinephrine. The secretion of these two *catecholamines* is controlled by the hypothalamus. (Catecholamines are compounds composed of a catechol and an amine; their actions simulate the sympathetic nervous system.) The effects of both epinephrine and norepinephrine upon the body are identical to those of the sympathetic nervous system; for this reason they are called "sympathomimetic agents." Like the sympathetic nervous system, these medullary hormones enable threatened individuals to either fight or flee when faced with danger.

The primary actions of *epinephrine* during situations of stress are as follows: (a) converts glycogen within the liver into glucose, thereby raising the metabolic rate, which in turn temporarily raises the individual's energy level; (b) boosts the oxygen-carrying capacity of the blood; and (c) increases cardiac output. It is the release of epinephrine which produces the cold sweat, pounding heart, deep rapid breathing, and wide-eyed, "keyed up" alertness which we all experience in times of emergency.

The primary action of norepinephrine is to produce extensive *vascular constriction,* thereby causing a marked rise in blood pressure. Note, however, in Table 97–1 that norepinephrine has several of the same general effects upon the body as epinephrine, e.g., increases the pulse rate, dilates the pupils, inhibits the gastrointestinal tract.

Overactivity of the adrenal medulla can be life-threatening. Overactivity is usually caused by a catecholamine-producing tumor called a *pheochromocytoma.* Pheochromocytomas, in turn, produce marked hypertension, hypermetabolism, and hyperglycemia owing to the oversecretion of epinephrine and norephinephrine. This condition can usually be cured by surgical removal of the tumors.

While overactivity of the adrenal medulla is dangerous, *underactivity* or loss of this gland rarely causes problems. As implied earlier, the adrenal medulla is *not* an essential structure. Should the medulla be destroyed by disease or surgically removed, its loss is compensated for by the sympathetic nervous system.

The Adrenal Cortex. The adrenal cortex, unlike the adrenal medulla, is *absolutely essential for survival.* If this vital structure is removed or destroyed, death automatically follows within a few days.

The adrenal cortex releases numerous steroid hormones called *corticoids. Steroids* are molecules with a nucleus composed of four interlocking rings containing carbon atoms. Three of the rings hold six carbon atoms apiece, while the fourth ring contains five.

Corticoids may be classified into three groups according to their specific functions: thus one group regulates sodium and electrolyte balance; the second group regulates carbohydrate, fat, and protein metabolism; while the third group is linked with sexual characteristics. As Boyd helpfully reminds us:

> For those of weak memory or mentality, the three functions [of the hormones of the adrenal cortex] may be represented by the letter S: salt, sugar, and sex. To the more sophisticated they are the mineralocorticoids, the glucocorticoids and the androgens (masculinizing hormones).[9]

MINERALOCORTICOIDS. The mineralocorticoids (which include aldosterone, desoxycorticosterone, and corticosterone) regulate electrolyte balance by promoting sodium retention, secondary water retention, and potassium excretion. The principal mineralocorticoid is *aldosterone,* which was discussed more fully in Unit V, Ch. 24. You will recall that the major functions of aldosterone are to conserve sodium and to maintain the blood and extracellular fluid volume, thereby sustaining normal blood pressure and cardiac output. When the mineralocorticoids are deficient (as in Addison's disease), the patient suffers from hyperkalemia, hypotension, decreased cardiac output, and (in acute cases) severe shock. On the other hand, *excessively high levels* of mineralocorticoids (hyperaldosteronism) result in hypertension due to sodium and water retention and hypokalemia.

GLUCOCORTICOIDS. The glucocorticoids derive their name from the fact that they act to regulate blood sugar by conserving body glucose and promoting gluconeogenesis. The major steroids composing the group are cortisol (the principal glucocorticoid), cortisone, and corticosterone, the latter being also a mineralocorticoid. Release of these potent hormones has the following effects upon the body:

> *Glucose metabolism:* Protein and fat molecules are converted within the liver to glucose (gluconeogenesis), which raises the blood sugar; for this reason, the glucocorticoids are said to have an "anti-insulin" effect. Indeed, excessive glucocorticoid secretion can eventually produce diabetes mellitus.

> *Protein metabolism:* Protein tissue catabolism increases. Amino acids are transported into the extra-

TABLE 97-1. COMPARATIVE EFFECTS OF EPINEPHRINE AND NOREPINEPHRINE*

Epinephrine	Norepinephrine
Cardiovascular System	
Constricts superficial blood vessels. In small doses dilates muscle, brain, and coronary vessels, thus shunting blood supply to organs essential for "flight or fight"	Constricts all blood vessels, especially peripherally, causing greatly increased peripheral resistance
Raises blood pressure	Markedly hypertensive
Increases cardiac output	Tends to decrease cardiac output because of increased peripheral resistance
Increases pulse greatly	Increases the pulse, but not greatly
Constricts the spleen, shunting stored red blood cells into general circulation	
Increases coagulability of the blood	
Respiratory System	
Increases rate and depth of respirations	
Dilates bronchi	
Nervous System	
Stimulates the central nervous system, increasing alertness and producing a feeling of fright, excitation, and impending doom	
Dilates the pupil	Dilates the pupil
Inhibits the gastrointestinal tract	Inhibits the gastrointestinal tract
Metabolism	
Increases the nonesterified fatty acid level of the blood	Increases the nonesterified fatty acid level of the blood
Promotes the conversion of glycogen to glucose	
Increases body metabolism	Increases body metabolism slightly

*From Spencer, R. T.: *Patient Care in Endocrine Problems.* Philadelphia, W. B. Saunders Company, 1973, p. 52.

cellular fluid and then to the liver where they are converted to glucose. Excessive secretion of the glucocorticosteroids causes tissue wasting. On the other hand, the glucocorticoids promote the use of amino acids to repair tissue damage during and following periods of stress.

> *Fluid and electrolyte balance:* Sodium retention, secondary water retention, and potassium excretion all increase. Overabundance of glucocorticoid secretion results in hypervolemia and hypertension due to sodium and water retention. Note that these effects of the glucocorticoids are similar to those of the mineralocorticoids.

> *Inflammation and immunity:* The glucocorticoids suppress both the normal inflammatory response to tissue injury and the protective immune response to invasion by infectious agents. As you recall from Unit II, Chapter 5, Selye calls the glucocorticoids *anti-inflammatory corticoids* (A.C.'s) because he evidently believes that the suppression of inflammation as a response to stress is the glucocorticoid's major role. In some cases, the suppression of inflammation can be beneficial. For example, patients with arthritis (inflammation of the joints) obtain relief from severe pain with cortisone injections. On the other hand, too much cortisone or other glucocorticoid impedes healing, decreases antibody formation, lowers the numbers of circulating eosinophils and lymphocytes, and lowers resistance to infection.

> *Stress:* Resistance and adjustment to stress of all kinds is dependent upon the presence of glucocorticoids. Selye points out that during the "alarm reaction" to stress (stage 1 of the General Adaptation Syndrome) large amounts of both adrenal and glucocorticoids are released into the blood stream. These hormones, if secreted in sufficient amounts, enable the individual to cope with stress provided the stressor is not overwhelming, e.g., severe burns over the majority of the body. Conversely, insufficient production of glucocorticoids (as seen in Addison's disease) *decreases* resistance to stress; such patients may die in profound shock following relatively minor traumas unless they quickly receive an injection of cortisol.

SEX HORMONES. The adrenal cortex secretes very small quantities of *androgens* (masculinizing hormones) and *estrogens* (female sex hormones). Normally, adrenal secretion of the sex hormones is considered physiologically insignificant because both androgens and estrogens are secreted in large amounts by the gonads. However, when production of sex hormones by the adrenal glands is excessive, symptoms result. For example, excessive release of androgens causes virilism, while excessive release of estrogens causes sodium and water retention (see discussion later in this chapter).

DISORDERS OF THE ADRENAL MEDULLA

There are two important disorders of the adrenal medulla: (1) *pheochromocytoma*—a tumor which results in hyperactivity of the gland, and (2) *neuroblastoma*—a malignant tumor which is a major cause of death in children.*

Pheochromocytoma. The pheochromocytoma is a small tumor (usually less than 200 Gm.) which is composed of pheochromocytes. Pheochromocytes are the cells which compose the tissues of the sympathoadrenal system; pheochromocytes are also called *chromaffin cells* because they stain a dark color with chromium salts. In 80–90 per cent of cases, pheochromocytomas arise within the adrenal medulla; occasionally, however, they develop from the chromaffin tissues forming the sympathetic paraganglia.

These tumors are typically benign; less than 5 per cent of pheochromocytomas are malignant. However, these miniature growths can produce severe symptoms and even death owing to the excessive amounts of epinephrine and norepinephrine which they secrete. An estimated 800 persons within the United States die yearly from undiagnosed pheochromocytoma.[25] Fortunately, when pheochromocytomas are discovered early in their development, they are usually curable.

This relatively uncommon tumor growth usually affects children and middle-aged women. In some cases they apparently have a hereditary basis. Also, in a small percentage of cases, these tumors appear in association with neuroectodermal diseases and with medullary cancer of the thyroid gland. The two events which apparently precipitate the development of pheochromocytoma are pregnancy and stress.

BASES OF SYMPTOMS. Symptoms experienced by the patient with pheochromocytoma result from the excessive secretion of epinephrine and particularly norepinephrine by the tumor. The outstanding symptom of pheochromocytoma is *hypertension,* which may be either persistent, fluctuating, intermittent, or paroxysmal in nature. Typically the patient suffers from attacks in which he experiences not only high blood pressure accompanied by a pounding headache, but numerous other manifestations of sympathetic overactivity; e.g., sweating, apprehension, palpitations, nausea, and vomiting. Moreover, remember that the release of catecholamines results in the conversion of glycogen into glucose within the liver; consequently hyperglycemia and glycosuria usually appear during attacks. Such manifestations may develop spontaneously, or they may be precipitated by emotional stress, physical exertion, or position change.

When attacks are acute, the patient appears to be in a shocklike state due to the excessive adrenalin released; i.e., diaphoresis is profuse, the pupils are greatly dilated, and the extremities are cold. Also, the patient may develop a cerebral vascular accident or sudden blindness as a result of severe hypertension. Without early treatment, permanent cardiovascular damage develops, and death may follow cerebral hemorrhage or cardiac failure.

DIAGNOSIS. The clinical picture of the patient with pheochromocytoma resembles that of several

*For a description of neuroblastoma, consult a pediatrics textbook.

other disorders; e.g., diabetes mellitus (elevated blood sugar and glycosuria), essential hypertension (elevated blood pressure, headaches), hyperthyroidism (increased metabolic rate, diaphoresis, agitation, rapid pulse, emotional outbursts), and psychoneurosis (emotional instability). Because pheochromocytoma is potentially curable, the importance of early and accurate diagnosis cannot be stressed enough. Current methods of diagnosis include the following:

> *History and physical examination:* The patient may complain that he has suffered attacks of symptoms (such as those just described) for weeks, months, or even years. Upon examination, you may note that the patient's blood pressure sharply rises whenever he changes position, exerts himself, or becomes emotionally upset. Also, in long-standing cases, the patient may already have developed the complications of hypertension: e.g., visual disturbances, symptoms of heart disease (dyspnea, exhaustion, edema), and manifestations of kidney damage (albuminuria, proteinuria, and an increased blood urea nitrogen).

> *Pharmacologic tests:* The two types of pharmacologic tests that confirm the presence of pheochromocytoma are (1) provocative tests, and (2) blocking tests. Although rarely ordered any more, these tests were formerly the major procedures used for establishing a diagnosis. In the provocative tests, a drug is administered that increases the secretion of epinephrine and norepinephrine, thereby provoking hypertension in the patient with a tumor. In the blocking test, the drug phentolamine, which acts to lower blood pressure, is administered. If the pressure reaches a designated low level, the diagnosis is positive. Today, both tests have been almost totally replaced by assays of urinary catecholamines and their metabolites, the latter tests being far more reliable and safer than the pharmacologic tests.

> *Chemical tests (hormonal assays):* As stated, chemical tests are rapidly replacing the more dangerous and inaccurate pharmacologic tests. The two hormonal assay tests available are (1) assay of urinary catecholamines, and (2) assay of urinary VML (vanillylmandelic acid, or 4-hydroxy-3-methoxymandelic acid), the principal metabolite of the catecholamines.

Assays of catecholamines may be performed on a single voided urine specimen, on a 2- to 4-hour specimen, and on a 24-hour urine specimen. The normal range of urinary catecholamines is up to 14 μg./100 ml. of urine. In pheochromocytoma, catecholamine levels are elevated.

Assays of urinary VML levels are performed on 24-hour urine specimens only. Prior to testing, advise the patient to avoid chocolate, tea, vanilla, and all fruits for at least 2 days before urine collection begins. Also remind the patient not to take any drugs for 3 days prior to testing. Finally, when collecting urine for 24-hour hormonal assays of VML or other hormones, proceed with care or test results will be inaccurate. Rules to remember when collecting these specimens are:

1. Ask laboratory personnel how urine is to be preserved over the 24-hour period (i.e., refrigeration, use of a special collecting bottle, or addition of hydrochloric acid to the collecting prior to beginning the test).
2. Accurately time collections; have patient begin test with an empty bladder and also empty his bladder just at the end of the test.
3. Remind patient to void *before* defecating so that urine is not contaminated by feces.

Normally, the amount of VML is under 7 mg./24 hours. Urinary VML is elevated in pheochromocytoma.

> *Direct assay of catecholamines in the blood:* The normal range of the catecholamines in the blood is as follows:

Epinephrine, 0.48 to 0.51 μg./liter
Norepinephrine, 1.55 to 3.73 μg./liter

Blood catecholamine levels increase in pheochromocytoma.

> *X-ray examinations:* Presence of an adrenal medullary tumor can often be confirmed by various x-ray techniques; e.g., arteriography, intravenous urogram, venography, and retroperitoneal pneumography.

> *Miscellaneous nonspecific laboratory tests:* In the presence of pheochromocytoma, the basal metabolic rate is elevated, blood sugar is elevated, and glycosuria usually appears.

CLINICAL CARE. There is only one form of treatment for pheochromocytoma—*surgical excision of the tumor.* While surgery may completely cure the patient (provided the growth is discovered before cardiovascular damage becomes permanent), the operation is not without its dangers. Sjoerdsma warns that there are two serious hazards. "First, excessive discharge of pressor hormones may occur during induction of anesthesia or during manipulation of the tumor leading to extreme rises in blood pressure and *cardiac* arrhythmias. Second, following resection, the blood pressure may fall precipitously to shock levels."[42]

During the *preoperative* period, the goal is to prevent further attacks of acute paroxysmal hypertension, thereby decreasing the risk of further damaging the cardiovascular system. Important general measures include (a) promotion of rest and relief from emotional tension; (b) sedation; (c) high vitamin, mineral, and caloric diet; (d) the omission of such stimulating beverages as coffee and tea; and (e) frequent monitoring of vital signs. In some cases, the doctor may order the administration of antihypertensive drugs, such as reserpine.

One or two days prior to surgery, phentolamine (Regitine) is usually given in doses of 50 mg. every 2 to 4 hours to block the vasoconstricting effects of epinephrine and norephinephrine.

Check the blood pressure frequently (every 30 minutes) following administration of phentolamine because the blood pressure may become unstable.

If the dose of Regitine is too great, blood pressure may drop radically. If adrenergic hormone levels remain high, blood pressure will continue to rise.

Following surgery, the patient enters a critical period ranging from 24 to 48 hours, during which time constant nursing observation and care is needed. During the *immediate postoperative period,* observe the patient closely for signs of *shock* and *hemorrhage.* Following removal of the tumor, profound shock may develop because catecholamine blood levels drop dramatically; hypotension may persist for 24 to 48 hours postoperatively. Also hemorrhage can occur because the adrenal glands are highly vascular organs.

To combat postoperative shock, take the following actions:

> Administer norepinephrine as ordered (usually 4 to 12 mg. per liter) intravenously at a rate sufficient to maintain the patient's blood pressure within a safe range. Check the patient's blood pressure as frequently as is necessary to regulate the norepinephrine drug (every 2 to 14 minutes).

> Carefully measure the patient's hourly urinary output. If the patient excretes less than 15 ml. in one half hour or 30 ml. in an hour, notify the physician. Oliguria may signify the development of profound shock and consequent renal shutdown.

> Give intravenous fluids as ordered to maintain the blood volume and combat shock. Blood, plasma, dextran, and glucose in water are all employed for this purpose.

> Observe the patient for signs of hemorrhage. Check the dressing every half hour for bloody drainage. If the patient is bleeding internally, he may develop an abdominal hematoma with resultant paralytic ileus. Symptoms of paralytic ileus include abdominal pain, distention, severe nausea, and vomiting.

> When administering medication for incisional pain, monitor the patient's blood pressure frequently. Remember that narcotics, particularly Demerol, produce hypotension as a side effect.

> If cortical tissue was resected during surgery, observe the patient closely for signs of adrenal cortical insufficiency (see below). Total removal of one affected adrenal gland necessitates the temporary administration of corticosteroid drugs. Replacement therapy with corticosteroids is discontinued once the remaining adrenal gland has hypertrophied and consequently secretes sufficient corticosteroids to compensate for the resected gland. However, if *both* adrenals have been removed, the patient must take corticosteroids for the rest of his life.

Once the critical immediate postoperative period is over, the majority of patients pass through an uneventful convalescence. Patients who will be taking corticosteroids upon discharge will need instruction concerning their administration and side effects (see below).

DISORDERS OF THE ADRENAL CORTEX

The major disorders of the adrenal cortex are characterized by either glandular hypofunction or hyperfunction. Underactivity of the adrenal cortex (*hypocorticism*) results in a deficiency of glucocorticoids, mineralocorticoids, and adrenal androgens, while overactivity (*hypercorticism*) results in excessive production of the corticosteroids. The majority of conditions arise because of the excessive secretion of only one of the three cortical hormones.

Adrenal Cortical Hypofunction (Hypocorticism). Hypofunction of the adrenal cortex is usually caused by a disorder originating within the adrenal gland itself (primary adrenal cortical insufficiency). However, in other cases, adrenocortical insufficiency develops *secondary* to hypopituitarism, prolonged administration of corticosteroids, or adrenal infarction (secondary adrenocortical insufficiency). Primary adrenocortical insufficiency may be either chronic or acute.

CHRONIC PRIMARY ADRENOCORTICAL INSUFFICIENCY (ADDISON'S DISEASE)

Incidence and etiology. Chronic primary adrenocortical insufficiency was named Addison's disease in honor of Thomas Addison who first described this condition more than a hundred years ago. A clinically rare disorder, Addison's disease strikes only four out of every 100,000 persons. However, because symptoms of adrenal insufficiency appear late in the disease (only after 90 per cent of the adrenal parenchyma has been destroyed), untold numbers of persons possibly suffer from undiagnosed Addison's disease.

The causative factors in Addison's disease have changed in recent years. At one time, the majority of cases developed as a complication of chronic tuberculosis. Today, less than half of cases are caused by tuberculosis, and approximately 70 per cent of cases are considered *idiopathic* in origin. However, since 50 to 67 per cent of patients with idiopathic Addison's disease have circulating autoantibodies which react specifically against adrenal tissues, it is possible that this condition may have an *autoimmune* basis.[38] Also, a few cases of Addison's disease are caused by neoplasm, amyloidosis, and deep fungi.

All age groups and both sexes are susceptible to adrenal insufficiency.

Bases of symptoms. As stated earlier, the adrenal cortex is essential to life. Untreated Addison's disease is ultimately fatal because it destroys the adrenal cortex, thereby causing severe deficiencies of the vital adrenocortical hormones. As a result of this condition, the adrenal glands become shrunken and contracted. Although the adrenal medulla continues to function normally, the cortex eventually collapses. Over time, once-functioning cells atrophy and die, and the cortex becomes a mass of fibrous nonfunctioning scar tissue. Finally, the cortex no longer produces adequate amounts of aldosterone, cortisol, and androgens, and symptoms appear.

Aldosterone deficiency causes numerous *fluid and electrolyte* imbalances. Recall that aldosterone *normally* promotes the conservation of sodium (and consequently water) and the excretion of potassium. When aldosterone is deficient, *sodium excretion increases,* which results in the following unfortunate chain of events: (a) water excretion increases, (b) extracellular fluid volume becomes depleted (dehydration), (c) hypotension develops, (d) cardiac output decreases, and (e) the heart becomes smaller owing to its diminished work load. Eventually hypotension may become so severe and heart action so weak that the patient dies in circulatory collapse and shock. Secondly, while excessive sodium ions are being excreted, excessive potassium ions are being retained in the body. Potassium levels of more than 7 mEq./liter result in arrhythmias and possibly cardiac standstill.

Glucocorticoid deficiencies cause widespread *metabolic disturbances.* Remember that the glucocorticoids promote gluconeogenesis (the conversion of fat and proteins into glucose within the liver) and are thus said to have an "anti-insulin" effect. Consequently, when glucocorticoids are deficient, gluconeogenesis decreases with resultant *hypoglycemia* and liver glucogen deficiency. The patient grows weak and exhausted and suffers from anorexia, weight loss, nausea, and vomiting. Secondly, *emotional disturbances* develop, ranging from mild neurotic symptoms to deep depression. In addition, *resistance to even minor stress diminishes* when glucocorticoids are deficient. Surgery, pregnancy, injury, infection, or salt loss due to profuse diaphoresis during hot weather can cause the patient to go into Addisonian crisis. Finally, cortisol deficiency stimulates the pituitary gland to secrete greater amounts of ACTH and melanocyte-stimulating hormone (MSH)* (see Fig. 97-1). Increased MSH secretion results in *increased pigmentation* of the skin and mucous membranes. As a result, patients with Addison's disease have an "eternal tan" and a peculiar bronzed appearance.

Androgen deficiency fails to produce symptoms in men because the testes supply the male with adequate amounts of sex hormones. However, females are dependent upon the adrenal cortex for an adequate secretion of androgens. For this reason, women with Addison's disease have less axillary and pubic hair growth than do women with normal adrenal function.

*Melanocytes are epidermal cells which synthesize melanin—the dark pigment which colors the hair, skin, and parts of the eye.

The *onset* of Addison's disease is usually insidious, and the patient experiences mild fatigue, languor, irritability, weight loss, nausea, vomiting, and postural hypotension weeks or months before the disease is diagnosed. As the disease progresses, symptoms intensify. Addison himself vividly describes the manifestations of this debilitating and potentially fatal condition:

> The patient in most of the cases I have seen, has been observed gradually to fall off in general health; he becomes languid and weak, indisposed to either bodily or mental exertion; the appetite is impaired or entirely lost; . . . the pulse small and feeble . . . excessively soft and compressible; the body wastes . . . slight pain or uneasiness is from time to time referred to the region of the stomach, and there is occasionally actual vomiting . . . it is by no means uncommon for the patient to manifest indications of disturbed cerebral circulation. . . . We discover a most remarkable, and, so far as I know, characteristic discoloration taking place in the skin,—sufficiently marked indeed as generally to have attracted the attention of the

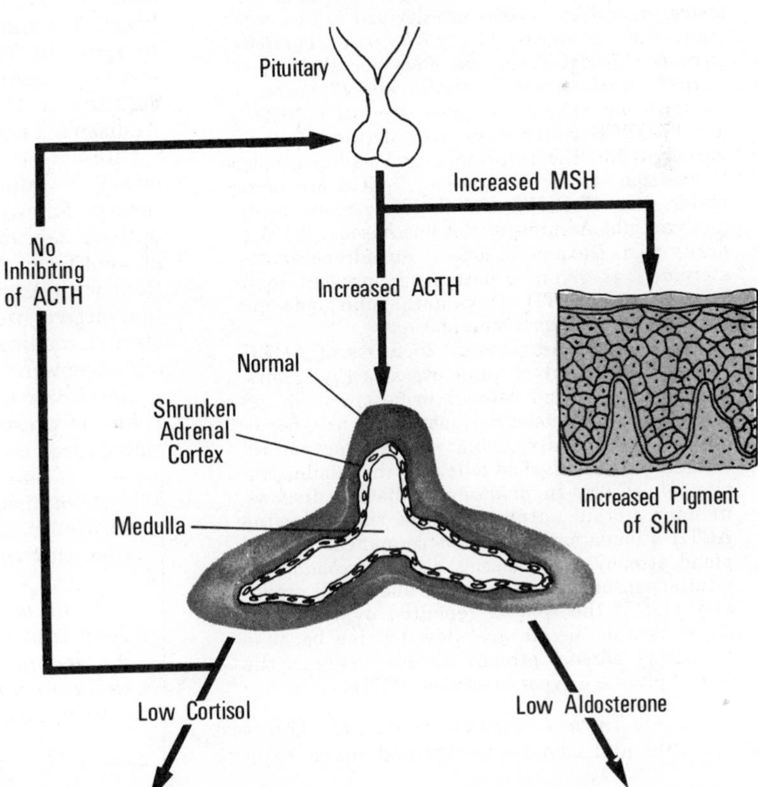

FIGURE 97-1. Causation of increased skin pigmentation in Addison's disease. (From Snively, W. D., and Beshear, D. R.: *Textbook of Pathophysiology.* Philadelphia, J. B. Lippincott Company, 1972, p. 192.)

> patient himself, or of the patient's friends. . . . It may be said to present a dingy or smoky appearance, or various tints or shades of deep amber or chestnut brown. . . . The body wastes . . . the pulse becomes smaller and weaker, and . . . the patient at length gradually sinks and expires.[26]

Without early diagnosis and treatment, the patient with Addison's disease lives in the constant (often unrecognized) danger of fatal Addisonian crisis should he be subjected to almost any stress. Acute Addisonian crisis is characterized by sudden profound asthenia; severe abdominal, back, and leg pain; hyperpyrexia followed by hypothermia; peripheral vascular collapse; coma; and finally renal shutdown.

Diagnostic studies. Addison's disease is primarily diagnosed on the basis of blood and urine hormonal assays. Dangerous provocative tests such as the *salt withdrawal test* are no longer used. Modern definitive tests of adrenocortical hypofunction include the following:

1. *The 8-hour intravenous ACTH test:* This is the most reliable diagnostic test for Addison's disease. The procedure is as follows:

Day one: (a) Start 24-hour urine specimen for measurement of 17-ketosteroids (17-KS) and 17-hydroxycorticosteroids (17-OHCS) or 17-ketogenic steroids (17-KGS). The *17-ketosteroids* (17-KS) are the excretory metabolites of the *androgenic* (male) *hormone.* In men two thirds of 17-KS are derived from the adrenals and one third from the testes; in women, 17-KS are derived exclusively from the adrenals. The *17-hydroxy corticosteroids* (17-OHCS) are excretory metabolites of *cortisol, corticosterone, cortisone,* and *11-hydroxycorticosterone.* The *17-ketogenic steroids* (17-KGS) are 17-OHCS which have been artificially converted within the laboratory to 17-ketosteroids. Conversion is helpful because 17-KGS are more stable than 17-OHCS and therefore more easily analyzed. (b) Administer dexamethasone, 0.5 mg. orally t.i.d. Dexamethasone is an adrenocortical steroid; it is given to patients to prevent toxic reactions to ACTH. Dexamethasone does not seriously alter urinary steroid levels.

Day two: (a) Administer 25 units of ACTH dissolved in 500 ml. of saline over exactly 8 hours. (b) Collect a second 24-hour urine specimen. (c) Continue to administer dexamethasone as ordered.

Results: Normally, urinary steroid output increases three- to fivefold following the administration of ACTH. In *primary* Addison's disease, urinary steroid output *does not* rise following ACTH stimulation because of permanent adrenal gland atrophy. In Addison's disease *secondary* to pituitary insufficiency, 17-OHCS and 17-KS gradually rise if the test is repeated over several days. Steroid levels are slow to rise because temporary adrenal atrophy always occurs in the face of pituitary hyposecretion of ACTH.

2. *Plasma cortisol response to ACTH:* This test is reliable and can be performed more rapidly than the 8-hour I.V. ACTH test. First of all, the patient's blood is drawn in the fasting state and examined for plasma cortisol levels. Next, 25 U. of ACTH is given I.M. Thirty minutes later a second blood sample is drawn. If the plasma cortisol level in the second blood specimen fails to rise by at least 10 μg./100 ml., Addison's disease is probably present.

3. *Thorn test* (4-hour corticotropin test): Today the Thorn test has been largely replaced by the two tests which we just described. The object of the Thorn test is to measure the *eosinophil count* following an I.M. injection of ACTH. Normally, glucocorticoids owing to their immunosuppressive action, cause the eosinophil count to fall to 20 to 30 per cent of the initial count of 200 per cu. mm. If the patient has Addison's disease, the injection of ACTH does not stimulate glucocorticoid secretion, and it consequently fails to cause the expected decrease in the eosinophil count.

4. *Water excretion test (Robinson-Kepler-Power):* This test of diuresis following ingestion of a large amount of water is sometimes used as a screening procedure. First ask the patient, who is NPO, to void and discard the urine. Next, give the patient 1500 ml. of tap water and ask him to drink it within 15 to 30 minutes. Finally, collect all the patient's urine for the next 5 hours and send it to the laboratory. Normally, the patient will void more than 1000 ml. following the water ingestion. Patients with Addison's disease excrete less than 800 ml. because adrenocortical insufficiency reduces the body's ability to handle the stress of an additional water load.

5. *Laboratory findings:* Addison's disease is characterized by a low serum sodium ($<$ 130 mEq./liter) and a high serum potassium ($>$ 5 mEq./liter). Other important laboratory findings are summarized in Table 97–2. Also autoimmune antibodies to adrenal tissue are sometimes found circulating in the blood of patients with idiopathic Addison's disease.

Clinical care in chronic adrenocortical insufficiency. Addison's disease was once fatal within months following diagnosis. Fortunately, this grim outlook has totally changed since the manufacture of synthetic corticosteroid drugs. Today, the patient with Addison's disease can hope to live a normal active life *provided* he religiously takes his steroid medications (see Table 97–3) daily without exception.

Cortisone or *hydrocortisone* (both glucocorticoids) is prescribed daily to correct the metabolic imbalances created by adrenocortical insufficiency.

> *Administer oral cortisol preparations with meals or antiacids to lessen gastric irritation and the possible development of peptic ulcer.*
>
> *Administer* parenteral *cortisol preparations* deep *into the gluteal muscle and* not *into the deltoid muscle; cortisol injected into the subcutaneous tissue can cause sterile abscesses, atrophy of tissues, and abnormalities of pigmentation.*

TABLE 97–2. LABORATORY FINDINGS SUGGESTING ADDISON'S DISEASE*

Blood chemistry	Low serum Na† (< 130 mEq./liter) High serum K (> 5 mEq./liter) Ratio of serum Na:K (< 30:1) Low fasting blood sugar (< 50 mg./100 ml.) Decrease in CO_2 combining power (< 28 mEq./liter) Elevated BUN (> 20 mg./100 ml.)
Hematology	Elevated hematocrit Low WBC count Relative lymphocytosis Increased eosinophils
X-ray	Evidence of: Small heart Calcifications in the adrenal areas Renal tuberculosis Pulmonary tuberculosis

*From Holvey, D. N., et al. (eds.): *The Merck Manual of Diagnosis and Therapy.* 12th ed. West Point, Pa., Merck Sharp & Dohme Research Laboratories, 1972, p. 1160.

†Na = sodium; K = potassium.

Carefully observe the patient for signs of Cushing's syndrome—the eventual consequence of long-term cortisol therapy. Also incorporate the nursing actions described in the section on Cushing's syndrome into your plan of daily care; e.g., check daily weight, blood pressure, intake, and output (see below).

Fludrocortisone acetate (Florinef) is also given daily or every other day for its sodium-retaining action. *Deoxycorticosterone (Cortate, DOCA-A),* a mineralocorticoid, is used to correct electrolyte imbalance and hypotension and to maintain plasma volume levels within the normal range. If DOCA-A or Florinef is unavailable, 5–20 Gm. of *sodium chloride* may be substituted on a daily basis.

Finally, the debilitated, malnourished patient often benefits from injections of *testosterone;* this androgenic agent has a protein anabolic effect, and it also imparts a sense of vitality and well-being.

In addition to drug therapy, there are also gen-

TABLE 97–3. MAJOR ADRENOCORTICAL DRUG PREPARATIONS: ACTION, USES, SIDE EFFECTS

Drug	Action	Uses	Side Effects
Cortisone acetate	Glucocorticoid, mineralocorticoid, anti-inflammatory, anti-immunologic, antianabolic.	Replacement therapy for Addison's disease. Control allergic reactions. Suppress inflammatory reactions. Treat mesenchymal or collagen disorders. Suppress immunologic response in organ transplants.	Overdosage produces Cushing's syndrome and its symptoms (see p. 1375). Abrupt withdrawal of drug may cause headache, nausea, and vomiting, and papilledema.
Hydrocortisone	Similar to cortisone except glucocorticoid and anti-inflammatory activity is substantially greater.	Replacement therapy for Addison's disease. Management of inflammatory skin, joint, and eye conditions.	Same as cortisone acetate.
Fludrocortisone acetate (Florinef)	Glucocorticoid and mineralocorticoid action.	Replacement therapy for Addison's disease.	*Mineralocorticoid effects:* hypertension, edema due to sodium retention, muscle weakness, and arrhythmias due to hypokalemia. *Glucocorticoid effects:* same as for cortisone acetate.
Deoxycorticosterone (cortate, DOCA-A)	Mineralocorticoid.	Replacement therapy for Addison's disease and Simmond's disease. Management of severe burns and surgical shock.	*Mineralocorticoid* effects: same as for Florinef. *Glucocorticoid* effects: none.

eral measures used to correct Addison's disease. When caring for patients with this disorder, be certain to include the following procedures in your plan:

> Check vital signs on a regular basis. Report to the physician drops in blood pressure below the patient's baseline blood pressure.

> Observe the patient for signs of increased physical vitality and emotional well-being. With therapy, the listlessness and exhaustion which shadow the individual with Addison's disease should gradually lessen and disappear.

> Prevent exposure to infection. Report "sniffles," sore throats, bladder infections, and so forth at once to the physician. Remember that the person with Addison's disease cannot tolerate even minor stress. Because infection always imposes additional stress upon the body, untreated infections may culminate in Addisonian crisis.

> Record intake and output. With the administration of steroids, water loss should lessen and output normalize.

> Weigh the patient daily. Weight gain usually occurs as a result of sodium and water retention due to the steroid drugs.

> Observe carefully for signs of sodium and potassium imbalance (see Ch. 25). If steroid replacement therapy is inadequate, sodium loss and potassium retention will continue. If the dosage of steroids is too high, excessive amounts of sodium and water will be retained, and potassium will be excreted in inordinate amounts.

> Encourage a high-carbohydrate, high-protein diet. Ask the dietitian to order six small feedings a day for the patient rather than three large feedings.

> Construct a plan for teaching the patient self-administration of steroid drugs. Your plan should include the following points: (a) oral administration of drugs; (b) self-injection technics; (c) the action of the prescribed hormones; and (d) signs of overdosage and underdosage. Emphasize to the patient who takes glucocorticoids that he must call his doctor for an increase in dosage when undergoing situations involving stress; e.g., emotional upheavals, dental extractions, minor surgery, or upper respiratory tract infections. In addition, dosages of mineralocorticoids may need to be temporarily raised if the patient is diaphoresing profusely for any reason; e.g., as a result of "heat spells," strenuous physical exertion, fever. Finally, while steroids are usually administered orally, remind the patient that he will need to give the drugs intramuscularly if he is nauseated or vomiting.

> Prior to discharge, obtain for the patient an identification bracelet and an emergency kit which he must carry with him at all times. The identification bracelet should carry the patient's name as well as the names and telephone numbers of his doctor and closest relative. Also, on the bracelet, Liddle recommends engraving the following inscription:[26] I have adrenal insufficiency. In any emergency involving injury, vomiting, or loss of consciousness, the hydrocortisone in my possession should be injected under my skin, and my physician notified. The hydrocortisone (100 mg. of hydrocortisone phosphate solution) is kept in a prepared syringe within the emergency kit along with sterile alcohol sponges. Also the emergency kit may contain notes concerning the patient's drug prescription, dosage schedules, and so forth.

> Remind the patient to make biyearly appointments with his doctor, even when he is in good health. Like diabetes mellitus, the control of Addison's disease is a lifelong responsibility.

Clinical care in acute adrenal insufficiency (Addisonian crisis). Acute adrenal insufficiency is characterized by a critical deficiency of glucocorticoids, severe hypotension, hyperkalemia, and vascular collapse. Thus the development of Addisonian crisis constitutes a medical emergency which must be treated rapidly and vigorously. The three major goals of care are to (1) reverse shock, (2) restore blood circulation (the patient usually suffers from a deficit of at least 20 per cent of his extracellular fluid volume), and (3) replenish the body with needed steroids.

Upon admission, the patient is rapidly infused with 1000 ml. of physiologic saline to which has been added 100 mg. of a water-soluble glucocorticoid (hydrocortisone phosphate or hydrocortisone sodium succinate). The dosage of the prescribed glucocorticoid is then lowered to 50 mg., and it is administered (either I.M. or I.V.) every 6 hours during the first day of the crisis, every 8 hours of the second day, and then gradually reduced thereafter. In addition, the doctor may order plasma, oxygen, and vasopressor drugs to counteract persisting hypotension. Also, if an infection triggered the crisis, antibiotics or sulfa drugs are given. Throughout this emergency period, the nurse is responsible for (a) monitoring blood pressure, (b) administering the intravenous infusions and medications, (c) measuring hourly urinary output and reporting oliguria (a sign of shock), and (d) guarding the patient from further emotional and physical stress. In addition to observing for signs of shock, you must also watch for symptoms of overhydration and overdosage with glucocorticoids, e.g., generalized edema due to fluid retention, hypertension, flaccid paralysis resulting from hypokalemia, psychoses, and loss of consciousness (see Table 97–3).

With rapid, efficient treatment, Addisonian crisis usually passes within a few hours; the patient's condition stabilizes, and the convalescent period begins. While convalescing, the patient begins to take water and food by mouth. Also corticosteroids are given orally and the dosage is gradually reduced to maintenance levels.

SECONDARY ADRENOCORTICAL INSUFFICIENCY. Secondary adrenocortical insufficiency develops in response to the following four conditions:

> Bilateral adrenalectomy.

> Hemorrhagic infarction and necrosis of the adrenal glands; adrenal apoplexy may develop as a complication of meningococcal septicemia or anticoagulant therapy.

> Hypopituitarism resulting in the decreased secretion of ACTH by the pituitary gland, which in turn results in the decreased secretion of cortisol and androgens by the adrenal gland.

> Suppression of the hypothalamic-pituitary secretion of ACTH due to either (a) the pharmacologic administration of corticosteroids, or (b) the oversecretion of corticosteroids by an adrenal tumor. In both these

cases the adrenal glands shrink, atrophy, and become filled with lipids. However, because the level of circulating corticosteroids is high, these patients do not develop symptoms of adrenocortical insufficiency *unless* steroid therapy is discontinued suddenly or the tumor is resected. Fortunately, if corticosteroid drug therapy is terminated gradually and if the dosage of medication is slowly reduced each day, the adrenal glands usually return to normal function.

Clinically, patients with secondary adrenocortical insufficiency suffer from the symptoms of cortisol and androgen deficiency; aldosterone continues to be secreted in sufficient amounts. Also, as in Addison's disease, these persons are subject to the development of acute crises when exposed to various stresses.

Treatment involves the administration of glucocorticoids in the same manner as for Addison's disease. Mineralocorticoids are not given except after bilateral adrenalectomy. The patient, as in Addison's disease, should be instructed to carry an identification card and emergency kit with him at all times in event of an acute crisis.

Adrenocortical Hyperfunction (Hypercorticism). Hyperfunction of the adrenal cortex results in the excessive production of either glucocorticoids, mineralocorticords, or androgenic steroids. The three major conditions classified under hypercorticism and the type of steroid overproduction which predominates are as follows: (1) Cushing's syndrome (glucocorticoid oversecretion), aldosteronism (aldosterone oversecretion), and (3) adrenogenital syndrome (adrenal androgen oversecretion). All three of these conditions appear more frequently in women than in men.

CUSHING'S SYNDROME

Etiology and incidence. Cushing's syndrome was first described by Dr. Harvey Cushing in 1932. It results from overactivity of the adrenal gland with consequent *hypersecretion* of *glucocorticoids*. Hypersecretion of glucocorticoids is caused by one of the following pathologic conditions:

1. A cortisol secreting *adrenal tumor* (primary Cushing's syndrome). Adrenal tumors are responsible for approximately 30 per cent of cases of Cushing's syndrome (sometimes called primary Cushing's syndrome). The majority of tumors (85 per cent) are benign, while 15 per cent are malignant. Primary Cushing's syndrome is diagnosed in approximately one out of every 10,000 hospital admissions.

2. *Hyperplasia* of the *adrenal cortex* caused by overproduction of adrenocortical-stimulating hormone (secondary Cushing's syndrome). Bilateral adrenal hyperplasia due to excessive ACTH stimulation accounts for approximately 60 per cent of cases of Cushing's syndrome (sometimes called secondary Cushing's syndrome). Sources of excessive ACTH secretion are two in number:

1. *Pituitary hypersecretion:* Pituitary tumors cause approximately 10 per cent of cases of Cushing's syndrome.[26] The tumors, which are usually benign, are either small basophil adenomas or large chromophobe adenomas. However, there are numerous cases of pituitary hypersecretion of ACTH in which no tumor can be located; to date there is no satisfactory explanation for this phenomenon. In any case, when pituitary hypersecretion of ACTH (due to either a tumor or unknown causes) results in excessive secretion of glucocorticoids, the condition is usually referred to as *Cushing's disease* rather than Cushing's syndrome. Cushing's disease is discovered in approximately one patient out of every 2000 patients admitted to the hospital.

2. *Ectopic hypersecretion of ACTH:* ACTH-secreting tumors located in organs far removed from the pituitary gland are a major cause of Cushing's syndrome. This particular form of the syndrome is sometimes called the *ectopic ACTH syndrome*. The tumor which is most frequently linked with ectopic ACTH syndrome is the bronchogenic oat-cell carcinoma.

In addition to being caused by adrenal tumors (primary Cushing's syndrome), pituitary hyperfunction (Cushing's disease), and ectopic ACTH-secreting tumors (ectopic ACTH syndrome), Cushing's syndrome also results from the prescribed administration of synthetic glucocorticoids; this complication is called *iatrogenic Cushing's syndrome*. Prolonged administration of cortisone results in temporary atrophy of the adrenal glands and in the typical symptoms of Cushing's syndrome.

Bases of symptoms. The function of the glucocorticoids was described at the beginning of this chapter. When Cushing's syndrome develops, all the normal functions of the glucocorticoids become exaggerated, and the classic picture of the patient with Cushing's syndrome as shown above emerges (see Fig. 97–2). Exaggeration of the normal functions of the glucocorticoids results in the following problems:

> *Persistent hyperglycemia* which may eventually result in the development of diabetes mellitus.

> *Protein tissue wasting* and the excessive deamination of amino acids which results in (a) the stunting of linear growth in children, (b) weakness due to wasting of muscle, (c) capillary fragility resulting in ecchymosis, and (d) osteoporosis due to wasting of the bone matrix. Osteoporosis may grow so severe that the patient develops pathologic fractures upon even mild trauma. Also compression fractures of the osteoporotic spine leading to kyphosis and height loss are not uncommon.

> *Potassium depletion* leading to hypokalemia, arrhythmias, muscular weakness, and renal disorders.

> *Sodium and water retention* which causes edema and hypertension. Hypertension, in turn, eventually predisposes the patient to left ventricular hypertrophy, congestive heart failure, and strokes.

> *Abnormal fat distribution* (in conjunction with edema) which results in a moon face, cervical-dorsal fat pad on the patient's neck (called a "buffalo hump"), and truncal obesity with slender limbs. Also pink striae appear on the breasts, axillary areas, and legs. Striae develop when the skin in a particular area is unduly stretched by large accumulations of fatty tissue. Changes

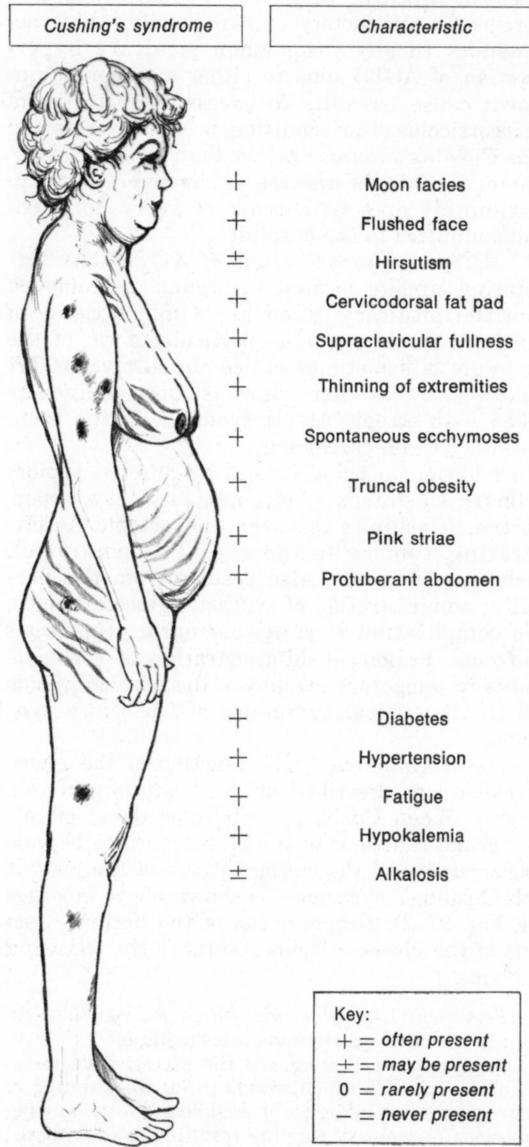

FIGURE 97–2. Findings in Cushing's syndrome. (From Meloni, R. C.: Obesity of Cushing's disease? *American Family Physician* 5:93, 1972.)

in appearance following the development of Cushing's syndrome as well as after therapy are striking.

> *Increased susceptibility to infection* and *lowered resistance to stress* make the patient vulnerable to microorganisms of all types. Because the inflammatory response is suppressed, the patient develops very few symptoms even in the face of a severe infection. Also, once infection or injury occurs, the healing process is greatly retarded.

> *Increased production of androgens* may occur, giving rise to mild virilism in women. Manifestations of virilism include acne, thinning of the hair, and hirsutism (abnormal growth of hair).

> *Mental changes* resulting from increased levels of glucocorticoids and ACTH include mood swings, euphoria, and depression; some patients develop a frank psychosis.

Diagnostic studies. Although the patient with Cushing's syndrome usually displays a highly characteristic array of symptoms, precisely performed diagnostic studies are nevertheless essential. First of all, Cushing's syndrome must be differentiated from (a) obesity compounded by diabetes mellitus and hypertension, and (b) the adrenogenital syndrome (see below). Secondly, once a diagnosis of Cushing's syndrome is established, then the physician must decide whether the causative factor is hyperplasia of the adrenal glands or an adrenal tumor. Important diagnostic measures are listed below.

Laboratory tests. Laboratory data diagnostic of Cushing's disease reflect the hyperglycemia, fluid and electrolyte disturbances, and immunosuppressive actions which are so characteristic of excessive glucocorticoid secretion. Thus, in Cushing's syndrome, *glucose tolerance* is lowered and *glycosuria* may be present. The *white count* is elevated to over 10,000, but the total eosinophil count is depressed to less than 50 cells per cu. mm. and lymphocytes are reduced to fewer than 20 per cent. *Urinary 17-hydroxycorticosteroids* are elevated and *blood corticosteroids* are high.

Special diagnostic tests. Three special tests which are extremely valuable in confirming a diagnosis of Cushing's disease are as follows:

1. *Plasma cortisol:* Normally the diurnal pattern for plasma cortisol is an elevated level in the earlier morning (10 to 25 μg./100 ml.), followed by a gradual decline until evening, at which time, the level is less than 10 μg./100 ml. Individuals with Cushing's syndrome have elevated plasma cortisol levels in the morning, and furthermore they do not experience a normal decline in cortisol levels as the day proceeds.
2. *ACTH stimulation test:* This test is performed in three parts. First, a 24-hour urine specimen is collected, and the level of 17-ketosteroids and 17-hydroxycorticosteroids are measured. Next the patient is given intramuscular injections of ACTH over a 1- to 3-day period. Finally, a second 24-hour urine specimen is collected and sent to the laboratory. Normally, the *second* urine specimen will have a corticosteroid level which is more than triple that of the first specimen. However, if the patient has Cushing's disease, the corticosteroid level of the second urine specimen will be ten times that of the first specimen owing to adrenal hyperactivity.
3. *Cortisone suppression test:* This test is mainly employed to differentiate between Cushing's syndrome (caused by an adrenal tumor), Cushing's disease (caused by pituitary oversecretion of ACTH), and ectopic ACTH syndrome (caused by ectopic ACTH-secreting tumor).

Steps in the suppression test are as follows:

(a) 24-hour urine specimens (used to establish a baseline) are collected for 2 days and are examined for urinary steroids; (b) on the third and fourth days, the patient is given 0.5 mg. dexamethasone (a derivative of fludrocortisone) every 6 hours for 2 days; (c) during the two days of dexamethasone administration, 24-hour urine specimens are again collected and examined for steroid content.

The action of dexamethasone is to *suppress* the *pituitary secretion* of *ACTH*. Thus, normally by the second day of dexamethasone administration, the levels of urinary ketogenic steroids and hydroxycorticoids drop more than 50 per cent below those of the baseline urine specimen. However, if the patient has Cushing's disease (which is a *pituitary* disorder), urinary 17-OHCS will decrease, but *less* than the normal 50 per cent below baseline unless the dosage of dexamethasone is raised to 2 mg. daily. This is because the diseased pituitary tends to be relatively resistant to the action of dexamethasone unless dosage is high. On the other hand, patients with either Cushing's syndrome (due to an adrenal tumor) or ectopic ACTH syndrome *fail to respond at all* to dexamethasone; i.e., levels of 17-OHCS do not decrease during the test because dexamethasone has no effect upon the adrenals or upon ectopic ACTH-secreting tumors.

Clinical care. Liddle states:

> The prime therapeutic objectives in Cushing's syndrome are to reduce cortisol levels to normal and to irradicate any associated tumors. Secondary objectives are to avoid producing hormonal deficiencies and to avoid making the patient chronically dependent upon medication.[26]

The form of therapy prescribed depends, first of all, upon whether the patient has true Cushing's syndrome (due to an adrenal tumor), Cushing's disease, or ectopic ACTH syndrome. Secondly, therapies differ, depending upon whether the causative lesion is benign or malignant.

As you can see in Table 97–4, the main form of therapy for all three subvarieties of Cushing's syndrome is *surgery;* drugs are prescribed only as palliative measures for the treatment of inoperable cancer. Current drugs in use are as follows:

- *o,p'*-DDD [2,2-bis(2-chlorophenyl-4-chlorophenyl)-1,1-dichloroethane]* This cytotoxic agent is still under investigation. It acts to inhibit the production of glucocorticoids by the adrenal glands, but leaves aldosterone production intact. Side effects include minor gastrointestinal tract disturbances, skin rash, lethargy, and ataxia. *o,p'*-DDD is the least toxic of all the adrenocorticolytic drugs.
- *Aminoglutethimide* (Elipten): Like *o,p'*-DDD, aminoglutethimide is an investigational drug which decreases cortisol production; it is also an anticonvulsant. Side effects include transient leukopenia, mild respiratory depression, drowsiness, ataxia, gastrointestinal disturbances, and skin rashes.
- *Metyrapone* (Metopirone): This drug acts to decrease cortisol production by selectively inhibiting 11-beta-hydroxylation in the adrenal cortex. It is rapid-acting and may produce therapeutic effects in one day. Side effects are transient vertigo and nausea.

Care of the patient undergoing adrenocortical surgery. During the *preoperative* period, the patient with Cushing's syndrome needs expert nursing care. The crucial problems of hypertension, edema, possible heart disease, diabetes mellitus, increased susceptibility to infection, decreased resistance to stress, and emotional lability must all be brought under control. Important nursing actions during this time include the following:

- Promote mental and physical rest. Obtain orders for sedatives or hypnotics as necessary.

*Cytotoxic agents and cancer chemotherapy are discussed in Unit VII, Chapter 35.

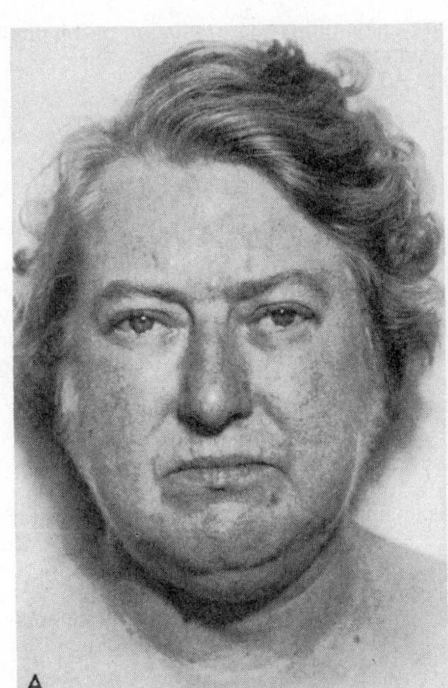

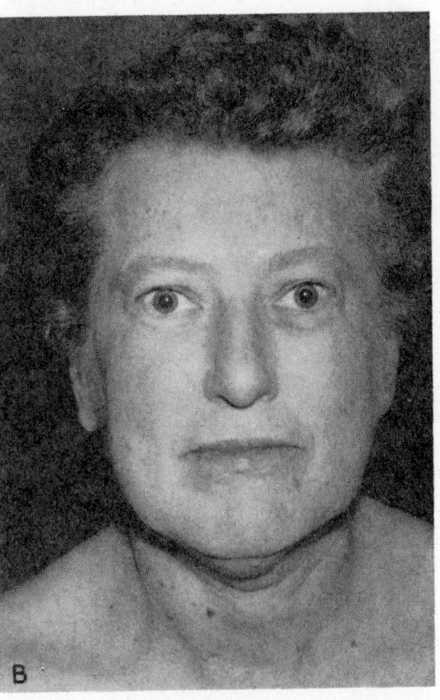

FIGURE 97–3. *A,* Face of a patient with Cushing's syndrome due to bilateral hyperplasia of the adrenals. This 45-year-old patient underwent a two-stage bilateral total adrenalectomy. *B,* Disappearance of all signs and symptoms 8 months after the second adrenalectomy, during which patient received complete substitution therapy. (From Williams, R. H.: *Textbook of Endocrinology.* 4th ed., 1968.)

> Encourage a diet which is low in calories, carbohydrates, and sodium, but has ample protein and potassium content. Such a diet will promote weight loss, reduction of edema and hypertension, control of hypokalemia, and rebuilding of wasted tissue. Special diets are required for the patient with frank diabetic mellitus (Ch. 95) or gastric ulcers (Unit XV).

> Check vital signs on a scheduled basis. Observe the patient carefully for signs of severe hypertension, e.g., elevated blood pressure readings, headache, failing vision, irritability, and dyspnea.

> Weigh the patient every morning at the same time and on the same scales. If sodium intake is decreased, the patient's weight should decrease and edema lessen.

> Test the patient's urine for sugar and acetone daily. Positive fractional urine specimens may indicate the development of overt diabetes mellitus.

> Protect the patient from exposure to infectious organisms. Isolate the patient from hospital personnel, family members, or other patients with contagious disorders. Unfortunately infections, once they develop, give little indication of their presence.

Remember: *Because glucocorticoids suppress the immune and inflammatory reactions, the patient with Cushing's syndrome may experience very mild symptoms even though he has actually developed a severe infection.*

For this reason, even a slight temperature or a little drainage from a cut or wound must be considered serious. Almost without warning, it is possible for a superficial bacterial infection to develop into a severe cellulitis followed by bacteremia. Furthermore, due to the patient's decreased resistance to stress, infections are extremely difficult to treat, and they tend to linger and smolder despite therapy.

> Guard the patient from falls and other accidents. Remember that individuals with Cushing's syndrome have osteoporosis and a resultant tendency to develop pathologic fractures even upon mild trauma. Therefore be careful to keep the patient's bed on "low." Also raise the siderails if the patient is restless or mentally disturbed. Steady the patient (who is obese and often uncoordinated) when he ambulates.

> Attempt to understand the patient's mood swings and depressions. Most people with Cushing's syndrome are understandably upset by the rather grotesque changes in their appearance due to the disease; they may also be alarmed by the bizarre emotional feelings

TABLE 97–4. THERAPIES PRESCRIBED FOR CUSHING'S SYNDROME

Condition	Responsible Lesion	Therapies	Remarks
Cushing's syndrome	Unilateral adrenal tumors (benign or malignant); bilateral adrenal tumors	*Adrenalectomy* (surgical excision of the adrenal gland containing the tumor); total bilateral adrenalectomy (surgical incision of both adrenal glands)	Adrenalectomy for a benign unilateral tumor usually curative Bilateral adrenalectomy must be followed by lifelong administration of *cortisteroids* to prevent Addison's Disease
	Adrenal carcinoma with widespread metastases	Chemotherapy: *o,p'*-DDD, aminoglutethimide, and metyrapone used to promote remission in patients with inoperable cancer	Chemotherapy largely unsuccessful; drugs used highly toxic
Cushing's disease	Pituitary tumor (or unidentified lesion) which secretes excessive amounts of ACTH	Irradiation of the pituitary gland	Irradiation successful in 25% of cases; therapeutic effects not apparent for months following initiation of therapy
		Total bilateral adrenalectomy (corrects adrenal hyperplasia due to excessive ACTH stimulation)	Total bilateral adrenalectomy must be followed by lifelong replacement therapy with a glucocorticoid and mineralocorticoid
		Hypophysectomy or subtotal destruction of the pituitary by either cryosurgery, yttrium implant, proton beam, or localized high-dosage irradiation (see p. 1386)	Hypophysectomy results in panhypopituitarism; all hormonal secretions dependent upon pituitary stimulation must be replaced for rest of patient's life (i.e., glucocorticoids, thyroid hormone, gonadal steroids, antidiuretic hormone)
Ectopic ACTH syndrome	Extra-adrenal malignant tumor	Surgical removal of the ectopic malignant tumor. Chemotherapy: used to control hypercorticism and promote remission in patients with inoperable cancer	Surgery rarely successful because metastasis usually occurs prior to diagnosis; chemotherapy purely palliative.

which they experience. It helps to explain to the patient that his appearance and moods should gradually return to normal with treatment.

> On the morning of surgery, administer a glucocorticoid preparation (usually intramuscularly) as ordered. A water-soluble cortisol preparation (diluted in an I.V. infusion) is also administered throughout the surgical procedure. Cortisol protects the patient from developing acute adrenal insufficiency during adrenalectomy. Even if only one adrenal gland is being removed, temporary support with glucocorticoids is still necessary; this is because the "normal" gland may have atrophied in response to the excessive secretion of glucocorticoids by the tumorous gland. Usually the normal remaining adrenal gland begins to secrete corticosteroids again at some point following surgery.

During the immediate *postoperative* period, major goals are to (a) prevent shock, (b) prevent infection, (c) sustain adequate cortisol levels, and (d) control pain and abdominal discomfort. Important nursing actions include (a) observing for signs of shock (hypotension, rapid weak pulse); (b) taking and recording vital signs at least every 10 to 15 minutes; (c) measuring the patient's urine hourly and observing for oliguria (a sign of shock and renal shutdown); (d) administering intravenous fluids, pressor amines, and corticosteroid preparations as ordered; (e) encouraging coughing, turning, and deep breathing to prevent dangerous respiratory infections; and (f) employing meticulous sterile technic when changing or reinforcing the dressing in order to prevent wound infection.

Because the abdominal approach is usually preferred, some patients will also require nasogastric suction until peristalsis returns to normal and nausea and vomiting diminish.

Once the patient becomes a convalescent, he will then need instruction in the self-administration of replacement hormones. As stated earlier in Table 97-4, the patient who undergoes either total bilateral adrenalectomy or hypophysectomy will need to take cortisol preparations for the remainder of his life. On the other hand, if only one adrenal gland has been removed, 15 to 20 mg. of cortisone is given daily until the remaining adrenal gland begins to function normally. Usually the maintenance dose of cortisone can be discontinued within 6 to 12 months.

PRIMARY HYPERALDOSTERONISM (CONN'S SYNDROME). In review, aldosterone is the most powerful of the mineralocorticoids. Its primary role is the conservation of sodium. Important secondary roles are water conservation and promotion of potassium excretion.

Hypersecretion of aldosterone due to an adrenal lesion results in *primary* hyperaldosteronism. In contrast, *secondary* hyperaldosteronism arises as a consequence of edematous disorders (cardiac failure, cirrhosis of the liver with ascites, the nephrotic syndrome); it also develops in hypertension due to destructive renal artery disease.

The major cause of primary hyperaldosteronism is a *benign aldosterone-secreting adrenal tumor* called an *aldosteronoma*. Although multiple tumors are sometimes found, the causative factor in 90 per cent of cases is a *single* adenoma.[38] Rarely, Conn's syndrome develops as a consequence of adrenocortical carcinoma.

The exact incidence of Conn's syndrome is unknown. However, the aldosteronoma is the most frequently diagnosed functioning adrenal tumor. Also, according to Haunz, primary aldosteronism possibly accounts for 20 per cent of cases of hypertension; however, other authorities believe that hypersecretion of aldosterone causes fewer than 5 per cent of cases.[25] Conn's syndrome strikes females twice as often as males, and it appears most frequently among middle-aged individuals.

Hypersecretion of aldosterone results in sodium and water retention and excessive potassium excretion. The two major hallmarks of primary hyperaldosteronism are *hypertension* and *hypokalemia.* Hypertension possibly results from edema of the arteriole walls; edema acts to narrow the arterioles, thereby raising the blood pressure. Without treatment, the patient eventually develops all of the complications of chronic hypertension, e.g., visual disturbances, heart failure, renal damage, and cerebral vascular accidents.

Hypokalemia, the second major manifestation of Conn's syndrome, results from excessive urinary excretion of potassium (see Ch. 25).* Hypokalemia, in turn, causes *muscle weakness* because potassium loss reduces normal neuromuscular irritability. In addition, the excessive excretion of K^+ causes *polyuria.* A large urinary output coupled with an increased number of sodium ions in the blood results in *polydipsia* (excessive thirst). Finally, hypokalemia leads to *metabolic alkalosis* due to (a) the shifting of H^+ into the cells in exchange for K^+ and (b) the exchange of hydrogen ions within the tubular cells for sodium ions from the tubular urine (see Fig. 97-4). Metabolic alkalosis causes a decrease in ionized calcium levels, which results in tetany and respiratory suppression (Ch. 25).

Oddly enough, despite sodium retention, patients rarely develop overt edema. Although extracellular fluid increases moderately, excessive water is usually excreted in the urine along with the potassium ions. Also the kidneys, over a period of time, tend to physiologically "adjust" to the excessive secretion of aldosterone, so that water excretion reaches an equilibrium with sodium intake. The ability of the kidneys to eventually "escape" from the sodium- and water-retaining action of aldosterone is sometimes referred to as the "renal escape phenomenon."[26]

Diagnosis of primary hyperaldosteronism is based upon the following laboratory findings: low serum potassium, mild elevations of serum sodium, alkalosis, and elevated urinary aldosterone levels. In addition, x-ray studies may reveal cardiac hypertrophy resulting from chronic hypertension. The aldosteronomas themselves are too tiny to be exposed by x-ray examination.

The three *goals of treatment* for patients with primary hyperaldosteronism are to (1) reverse hypertension, (2) correct hypokalemia, and (3) prevent kidney damage. In two thirds of cases, hypertension is completely reversed by removal of the aldosterone-secreting tumor. Indeed, the majority of patients have normal blood pressure readings by the third postoperative month. *Hypokalemia* is corrected by the administration of potassium salts. Unfortunately the *renal complications* resulting from long-term hypertension tend to be progressive. For this reason, it is important for patients with primary hyperaldosteronism to be diagnosed and treated *early* in the course of the disease.

ADRENOGENITAL SYNDROME. The adrenogenital syndrome is a rare condition which is characterized by *virilism* resulting from the excessive secretion of *androgenic steroids* from the adrenal cortex.

In the majority of cases, the androgenic syndrome is a *congenital* disorder. In essence, the cause of prenatal androgenic syndrome is an inherited enzyme deficiency which leads to a number of pathologic consequences. Note in Figure 97–5 that, without the missing enzyme, adequate amounts of cortisol cannot be synthesized. As you recall, cortisol, by means of negative feedback, normally acts to regulate the secretion of ACTH from the anterior pituitary gland (see Ch. 3). Thus, without the inhibitory effects of cortisol, pituitary secretion of ACTH is not suppressed, and blood levels of ACTH are consequently elevated. Excessive secretion of ACTH results in hyperplasia of the adrenal glands and the hypersecretion of sex steroids. Finally, the excessive production of androgenic steroids results in *masculinization* of the afflicted individual.

While the adrenogenital syndrome is primarily a congenital syndrome, it does occasionally develop during adulthood. This form of the disease is due to either a benign or malignant *adrenal tumor*. It is possible that in some fashion these tumors cause enzyme deficiencies.

The symptoms of the adrenogenital syndrome differ, depending upon the age or sex or both of the patient. The female infant may be born with *pseudohermaphroditism* ("masculinization of the female external genitalia").[23] Older girls and women with adrenal tumors may develop hirsutism, enlargement of the clitoris, balding, atrophy

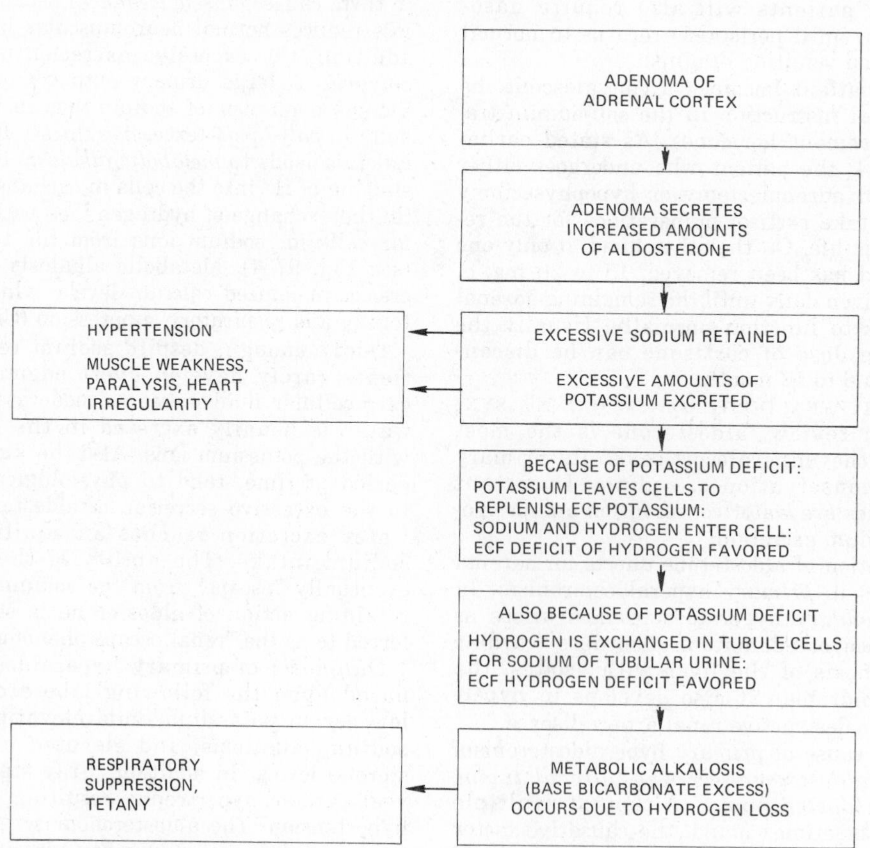
SEQUENCE OF EVENTS:
PRIMARY ALDOSTERONISM
ADENOMA OF ADRENAL CORTEX
ADENOMA SECRETES INCREASED AMOUNTS OF ALDOSTERONE
EXCESSIVE SODIUM RETAINED
EXCESSIVE AMOUNTS OF POTASSIUM EXCRETED
HYPERTENSION
MUSCLE WEAKNESS, PARALYSIS, HEART IRREGULARITY
BECAUSE OF POTASSIUM DEFICIT:
POTASSIUM LEAVES CELLS TO REPLENISH ECF POTASSIUM:
SODIUM AND HYDROGEN ENTER CELL:
ECF DEFICIT OF HYDROGEN FAVORED
ALSO BECAUSE OF POTASSIUM DEFICIT
HYDROGEN IS EXCHANGED IN TUBULE CELLS FOR SODIUM OF TUBULAR URINE:
ECF HYDROGEN DEFICIT FAVORED
METABOLIC ALKALOSIS (BASE BICARBONATE EXCESS) OCCURS DUE TO HYDROGEN LOSS
RESPIRATORY SUPPRESSION, TETANY

FIGURE 97–4. Sequence of events; primary aldosteronism. (From Snively, W. D., and Beshear, D. R.: *Textbook of Pathophysiology.* Philadelphia, J. B. Lippincott Company, 1972, p. 194.)

of the breasts, and a masculine body build. Masculinizing changes in boys and men are not nearly as dramatic as they are in females. For example, a male patient may only grow a heavier beard and develop larger male genitalia. Young male children may be sexually precocious for their age.

Other manifestations (depending upon the specific type of enzyme deficiency) may include either *salt wasting* accompanied by hypotension and dehydration or *excessive salt and water retention* accompanied by hypertension. In addition, many patients (particularly women) suffer from mental disturbances due to their abnormal appearance.

Diagnostic findings which confirm the adrenogenital syndrome include elevated 17-ketosteroids and an elevation of urinary and plasma testosterone. In some cases, the physician discovers a palpable adrenal or ovarian tumor.

Treatment of the adrenogenital syndrome depends upon the cause. Children with prenatal adrenogenital syndrome are given cortisol preparations in order to (a) correct the cortisol deficiency, and (b) inhibit the production of ACTH by the anterior pituitary gland which, in turn, reverses adrenal hypertrophy and overproduction of androgenic steroids. In addition, these patients should take the same precautions as persons with Addison's disease, i.e., wear an identification bracelet and carry an emergency kit which contains an ampule of hydrocortisone. On the other hand, if an adrenal tumor is causing masculinization, the tumor must be removed surgically. Malignant tumors must be discovered early and removed before metastasis occurs.

THE PITUITARY GLAND

NORMAL ANATOMY AND PHYSIOLOGY

The pituitary gland (also called the hypophysis cerebri) is a tiny organ which is securely cradled within a small recess in the sphenoid bone called the *sella turcica* (Turk's saddle). It is composed of a posterior and an anterior lobe which are separated and connected by a small, rather poorly developed, intermediate lobe.

The *posterior* lobe is called the *neurohypophysis* because it is of *neural* origin rather than glandular origin. An extension of the hypothalamus, the posterior lobe evidently does not produce any hormones itself; instead it simply stores and releases antidiuretic hormone (ADH) and oxytocin (a hormone which stimulates uterine contractions). Both these hormones are manufactured by the hypothalamus.

In contrast, the *anterior* lobe (called the adenohypophysis) is a *glandular* structure.* It is composed of three basic cell types: (1) eosinophils, (2) basophils, and (3) chromophobes. As a gland, the adenohypophysis synthesizes and releases vital hormones (see Table 97–5). Of the seven hormones, only the *growth* hormone (STH) acts directly upon the body's tissues. The other six hormones stimulate the "target" glands governed by the pituitary (thyroid, adrenals, gonads), thereby *indirectly* influencing body growth, structure, and function as well as intellectual and sexual development. As you have learned in earlier chapters, the "target glands" depend upon the stimulation of the pituitary gland to synthesize their own hormones. If stimulation is excessive and too much of one pituitary hormone is released, the "target" gland involved becomes overactive in response; e.g., too much adrenocorticotropic hormone from the pituitary stimulates the adrenal cortex to hypertrophy and produce excessive amounts of cortisol, thereby causing Cushing's disease. Conversely, if pituitary production of one or more hormones is inadequate, the target gland which depends upon that hormone for stimulation becomes hypoactive in response; e.g., insufficient

**Adeno* is a Greek word element meaning *gland.*

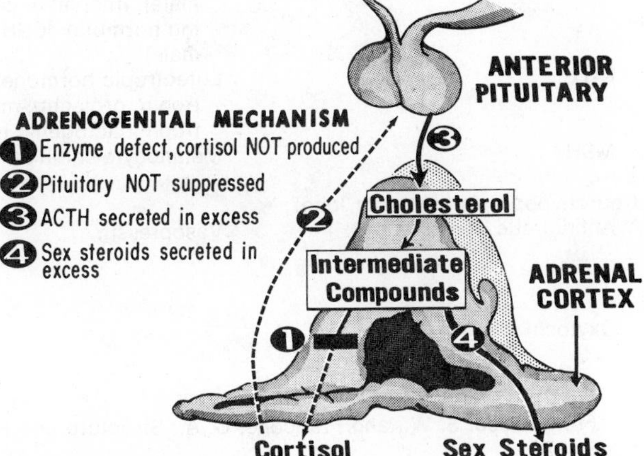
ANTERIOR PITUITARY
ADRENOGENITAL MECHANISM
1 Enzyme defect, cortisol NOT produced
2 Pituitary NOT suppressed
3 ACTH secreted in excess
4 Sex steroids secreted in excess
Cholesterol
Intermediate Compounds
ADRENAL CORTEX
Cortisol
Sex Steroids

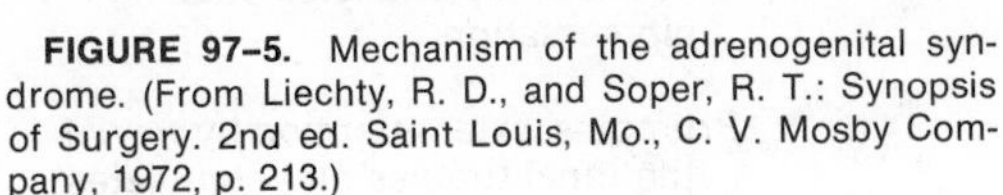
FIGURE 97–5. Mechanism of the adrenogenital syndrome. (From Liechty, R. D., and Soper, R. T.: Synopsis of Surgery. 2nd ed. Saint Louis, Mo., C. V. Mosby Company, 1972, p. 213.)

production of adrenocortical-stimulating hormone (ACTH) can cause secondary adrenocortical insufficiency. When one considers the powerful influence of the anterior pituitary directly upon other glands and therefore indirectly upon the body as a whole, it is no wonder that the pituitary gland is often described as the "master gland."

If the pituitary controls growth as well as the activities of other glands, what then controls the pituitary? To help answer that question, review Figure 97–6. Note that the hypothalamus (an absolutely essential portion of the brain) lies above the pituitary, and is connected to the master gland by the hypophyseal (pituitary) stalk. The hypothalamus continuously receives messages from the internal milieu and the external world via the nervous system. In turn, the hypothalamus transmits these messages to the pituitary gland via the pituitary stalk. In response to stimulation from the hypothalamus, both lobes of the pituitary gland release their hormones into the blood stream as needed to maintain the individual in a state of homeostatic balance.

Disorder of the pituitary gland predominately develop in the anterior lobe. Major causes of pituitary disease include (a) functioning tumors, (b) nonfunctioning tumors, (c) pituitary thromboses, (d) genetic disorders, and (e) trauma. The three principal pathologic consequences of pituitary disorders are (1) hyperpituitarism, (2) hypopituitarism, and (3) local compression of brain tissue by expanding tumor masses.

DISORDERS OF THE ANTERIOR LOBE

Hyperpituitarism. Hyperpituitarism is defined as the oversecretion of one or more of the hormones secreted by the pituitary gland. The major cause of hyperpituitarism is a *secreting pituitary tumor,* which is typically a benign adenoma. More specifically, there are three major types of pituitary tumors, each of which represents an overgrowth of one of the basic cell types comprising the anterior pituitary gland, i.e., eosinophils, basophils, and chromophobes. Important characteristics of each type of tumor are as follows:

> *Eosinophilic tumor:* a secreting tumor which produces excessive amounts of growth hormone (STH) and possibly prolactin (LTH). Eosinophilic tumors tend to develop in males who are between the ages of 20 and 50. Although they are rarely malignant, these benign adenomas can produce gigantism in children and acromegaly in adults.

> *Basophilic tumor:* a secreting tumor which can produce excessive amounts of adrenocortical-stimulating hormone (ACTH), thyroid-stimulating hormone (TSH), follicle-stimulating hormone (FSH), luteinizing hormone (LH), and possibly melanocyte-stimulating hormone (MSH). Typically only ACTH is synthesized in excessive amounts. As you recall, excessive secretion of ACTH by the pituitary causes *Cushing's disease.* Like

TABLE 97–5. HYPOPHYSEAL HORMONES

Name and Source	Synonyms	Function
Adenohypophysis (anterior lobe)		
TSH	Thyroid-stimulating hormone; thyrotropin	Stimulates thyroid growth and secretion
ACTH	Adrenocorticotropic hormone; corticotropin	Stimulates adrenocortical growth and secretion
STH	Growth hormone; somatotropin	Accelerates body growth
FSH	Follicle-stimulating hormone	Stimulates growth of ovarian follicle and estrogen secretion in the female and spermatogenesis in the male
LH	Luteinizing hormone (in the female); interstitial cell-stimulating hormone, ICSH (in the male)	Stimulates ovulation and luteinization of ovarian follicles in the female and production of testosterone in the male
LTH	Luteotropic hormone, luteotropin, prolactin, mammotropin, lactogenic hormone	Maintains the corpus luteum and stimulates secretion of milk
MSH	Melanocyte-stimulating hormone	Stimulates melanocytes causing pigmentation
Neurohypophysis (posterior lobe)		
Antidiuretic Hormone (ADH)	Vasopressin	Promotes water retention by way of the renal tubules and stimulates smooth muscle of blood vessels and digestive tract
Oxytocin		Stimulates contraction of smooth muscle in the uterus

*From Jacob, S. W., and Francone, C. A.: Structure and Function in Man. 3rd ed. Philadelphia, W. B. Saunders Co., 1974.

the eosinophilic tumors, basophilic tumors are rarely malignant.

> *Chromophobe tumor:* most common of the pituitary tumors. This benign adenoma may or may not secrete hormones. Secreting chromophobe tumors probably elaborate ACTH and growth hormone, thereby causing hyperpituitarism. On the other hand, nonsecreting tumors may cause hypopituitarism by growing so large in size that they eventually obliterate the pituitary gland (see Hypopituitarism.)

Pituitary tumors produce both systemic effects and local manifestations. *Systemic* effects include (a) excessive or abnormal growth patterns (due to overproduction of STH), and/or (b) overstimulation of one (or more) of the target glands, which results in the release of excessive thyroid, sex, or adrenocortical hormones. *Locally,* pituitary tumors produce symptoms because the bony cranium which houses the tumor cannot expand to accommodate a growing space-occupying mass. Local manifestations include blindness due to pressure on the optic chiasma, headaches, and somnolence.

Major disorders arising from hypersecretion of one or more of the pituitary hormones include the following:

> *Gigantism and acromegaly:* Both of these disturbances of growth arise from an oversecretion of *growth hormone* (STH). Gigantism, which is an overgrowth of the *long bones,* develops in *children* before the age at which the epiphyses of the bones close. Individuals suffering gigantism may grow as tall as 8 or 9 feet. On the other hand, *acromegaly* is a disease of *adults* which develops following *closure* of the epiphyses of the long bones. As implied by its name, acromegaly (*acro* is the Greek word element for "extremity") is marked by both increases in bone thickness and hypertrophy of the soft tissues. Victims of full-blown acromegaly have a grotesque appearance; note in Figure 97-7 the gradual coarsening of the patient's features over the years, as well as the prognathism (protrusion of the jaw), wide hands, and broad, spadelike fingers which characterize the final stages of the disease. In addition, persons with acromegaly develop local manifestations due to compression of brain tissues by the causative tumor; e.g., headache, diplopia, blindness, and lethargy. In far-advanced cases, victims may suffer from associated hormonal disturbances, e.g., diabetes mellitus, goiter, Cushing's disease, disturbances of libido, and menstrual disorders. The treatments of choice for both gigantism and acromegaly are either surgical hypophysectomy or supervoltage irradiation of the pituitary. Prognosis depends upon the age at which oversecretion of STH develops and is diagnosed. Obviously, because changes are irreversible, the earlier the problem is discovered, the more likely the patient is to benefit from therapy.

> *Cushing's disease:* As you recall, Cushing's disease is one form of Cushing's syndrome. It results from oversecretion of ACTH by a basophilic tumor, which in turn results in the oversecretion of adrenocortical hormones.

> *Sexual disturbances:* Excessive secretion of gonadotropic hormones from pituitary tumors produces sexual precociousness in children. Treatment of choice is surgical removal of the tumor.

Hypopituitarism. In contrast to hyperpituitarism, *hypopituitarism* is a *deficiency* of one or more of the hormones produced by the anterior lobe of the pituitary. When both the anterior *and* posterior lobes are failing to secrete hormones, the condition is referred to as *panhypopituitarism.*

The five important *causes* of hypopituitarism are as follows:

> *Hypophysectomy* (removal or destruction of the pituitary): This procedure is sometimes performed as a palliative measure for persons with diabetic retinopathy or cancer of the breast.

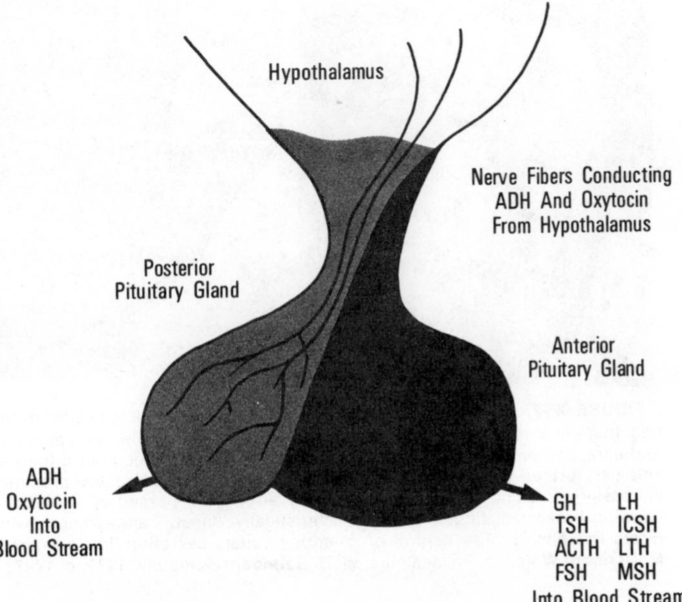

FIGURE 97–6. The relationship between the hypothalamus and the pituitary gland. The posterior pituitary gland (neurohypophysis) stores antidiuretic hormone (ADH) and oxytocin. The anterior pituitary gland (adenohypophysis) secretes hormones to stimulate growth (GH), the adrenal cortex (ACTH), ovarian follicles (FSH), corpus luteum (LH), testicular interstitial cells (ICSH), milk production (LTH), and melanocytes (MSH). (From Snively, W. D., and Beshear, D. R.: *Textbook of Pathophysiology.* Philadelphia, J. B. Lippincott Company, 1972, p. 184.)

> *Nonsecreting pituitary tumors:* The are two types of nonsecreting pituitary tumors which cause hypopituitarism: the *nonfunctioning chromophobe adenoma* and the *craniopharyngioma.* Because these tumors expand and therefore occupy space, they eventually compress and obliterate pituitary tissues, thereby diminishing the secretion of pituitary hormones.

> *Hereditary transmission of an autosomal recessive gene:* When a child is born with congenital hypopituitarism, he inherits a deficiency of growth hormone and is consequently destined to be dwarfed in stature. Victims of *hypophyseal dwarfism* are normally proportioned and have normal intelligence.

> *Postpartum pituitary necrosis:* Hypopituitarism develops following postpartum hemorrhage and circulatory collapse. The radical drop in blood pressure following the baby's delivery evidently causes multiple pituitary thrombi and subsequent necrosis of the gland due to tissue anoxia.

> *Functional disorders:* Functional hypopituitarism develops whenever the pituitary gland is inadequately nourished. Causes of this problem include starvation, severe anemia, and gastrointestinal tract disorders which reduce the absorption of nutrients.

Because of the pituitary's enormous functional reserve, manifestations of hypopituitarism usually do not appear until almost 75 per cent of the pituitary has been obliterated by tumors, thromboses, and so forth. Symptoms depend upon the age at onset of the disorder as well as upon the hormones which are deficient. Specific disorders resulting from pituitary hyposecretion include the following:

> *Dwarfism:* Severely stunted growth results from either (a) congenital lack of growth hormone, or (b) the development of space-occupying intracranial tumors, meningitis, or brain injury during early childhood. Dwarfism, if diagnosed early, can be sucessfully treated with injections of human growth hormone. Unfor-

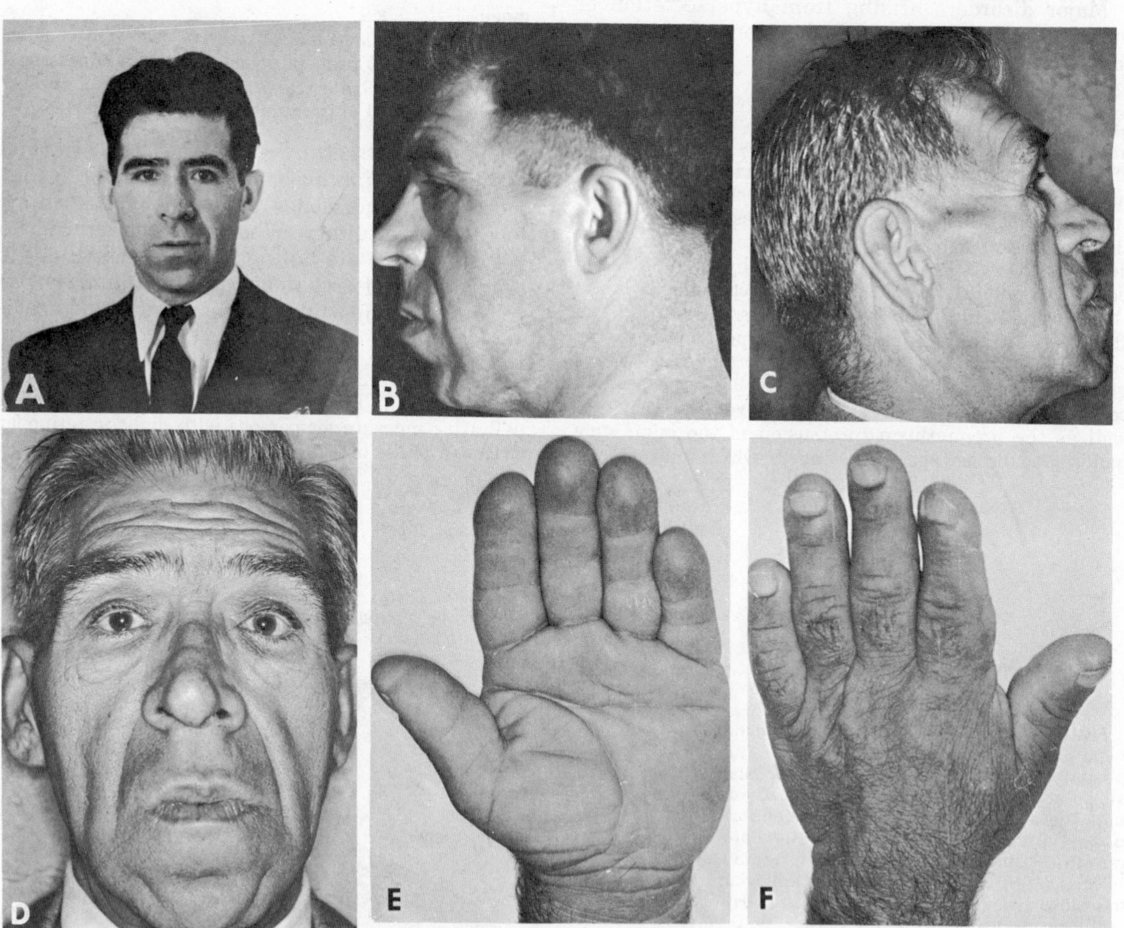

FIGURE 97–7. Evolution of acromegaly. *A,* Age 38, within a year after onset of the disease. *B,* Age 55, after two courses of radiation therapy to sella; disease has progressed with moderate coarsening of features: thickening of lips, enlargement of nose and ears, and prognathism. *C, D,* Age 64, 26 years after onset, after a third series of x-ray treatments to sella; nose and ears have enlarged further, supraorbital ridge and zygoma have become more prominent, and jaw is more prognathous, frontal view shows increasing wrinkling of the skin (temporary atrophy is a result of x-irradiation). *E, F,* Age 64, volar and dorsal aspects of hand, showing broadened fingers and characteristically "meaty" appearance owing to the gross increase in the soft tissue, not bone. (From Reichlin, S.: The control of anterior pituitary secretion, In *Cecil-Loeb Textbook of Medicine.* 13th ed. Beeson, P. B., and McDermott, W. (eds.), Philadelphia, W. B. Saunders Company, 1971, p. 1747.)

tunately human growth hormone is currently available for only a few patients. Methods of commercially producing synthetic growth hormone are under investigation.

Secondary adrenocortical insufficiency: Adrenocortical insufficiency can follow diminished synthesis of ACTH by the pituitary gland, which in turn causes diminished secretion of adrenocortical hormones by the adrenal cortex.

> *Myxedema:* Because the synthesis of thyroid hormone is dependent upon the production of thyroid stimulating hormone (TSH) by the pituitary, therapeutic ablation or pathologic destruction of the pituitary can cause myxedema unless the patient is treated with thyroid extract (see Ch. 96).

> *Sexual and reproductive disorders:* Deficiencies of the gonadotropins (LH, LTH, and FSH) can produce sterility, diminished sexual drive, and decreased secondary sexual characteristics. Women who suffer from lessened FSH and LH synthesis develop infertility and amenorrhea. Men who lack FSH and LH experience diminished spermatogenesis and testicular atrophy. The hypogonadism which follows hypophysectomy or destruction of the pituitary gland by disease leads to permanent sterility which cannot be corrected by hormonal replacement therapy.

The *treatment* of hypopituitarism is based upon (a) alleviation, if possible, of the causative factor (e.g., tumors), and (b) permanent replacement of the hormones secreted by the target organs. If the patient suffers from a pituitary tumor, therapeutic ablation of the pituitary gland is the treatment of choice.

Drugs used for permanent hormonal replacement include (a) corticosteroids for correction of secondary adrenocortical insufficiency, (b) thyroid hormone for treatment of myxedema, and (c) sex hormones to correct hypogonadism. To date, tropic hormones are not used because of their expense and ineffectiveness when used on a long-term basis. Also as stated earlier, human growth hormone (HGH) is used to correct hypophyseal dwarfism.

DISORDERS OF THE POSTERIOR LOBE (NEUROHYPOPHYSIS)

Unlike the adenohypophysis, the neurohypophysis is rarely destroyed by disease. Even if the posterior lobe becomes damaged or is surgically destroyed along with the anterior lobe, hormonal deficiencies do not develop because oxytocin and ADH continue to be synthesized by the hypothalamus. On the other hand, if the hypothalamus is damaged, deficiencies of oxytocin and ADH will develop even if the neurohypophysis is healthy and intact.

The major posterior lobe disorder is *ADH deficiency* (diabetes insipidus). In addition, inappropriate secretion of ADH may occur in conjunction with lung cancer, head injuries, pituitary tumors, encephalitis, poliomyelitis, and myxedema. Oxytocin imbalances have not been documented; for further information concerning oxytocin, consult an obstetrics textbook.

Diabetes Insipidus. Diabetes insipidus, like diabetes mellitus, is characterized by the passage of excessive amounts of urine. However, the urine of patients with diabetes mellitus contains large amounts of sugar, whereas the urine in diabetes insipidus is highly dilute and contains no sugar. The fundamental cause of diabetes insipidus is a *deficiency* of the *antidiuretic hormone (ADH)*. You recall from Unit V, Chapter 24, that the major functions of ADH are to: (a) promote water reabsorption by the kidney, and (b) control the osmotic pressure of the extracellular fluid. Thus, when ADH production decreases excessively, water is *not* reabsorbed by the kidney tubules, and consequently the stricken individual secretes large amounts of dilute urine.

Causes of ADH deficiency are categorized in the following way:[25]

A. *Vasopressin deficiency*
   1. The pituitary gland is itself defective due to familial or idiopathic causes (primary diabetes insipidus).
   2. The gland is destroyed by tumors in the hypothalamopituitary region, trauma, infectious processes, vascular accidents, or metastatic tumors from the breast or lung (secondary diabetes insipidus).

B. *"Nephrogenic" diabetes insipidus:* Due to an inherited defect, the kidney tubules are unable to reabsorb water. Also this condition may develop secondary to potassium depletion or pyelonephritis.

Diabetes insipidus may arise slowly, or it may appear suddenly following injury or infectious disease.

> *The two major manifestations of diabetes insipidus are increasing polyuria and polydipsia.*

The patient may drink and excrete from 5 to 40 liters of fluid per day! Because it is so dilute, the urine has a low specific gravity of between 1.001 and 1.006 (normal:1.003—1.030). Unless the patient continues to drink fluid almost continuously, he is in danger of developing severe dehydration and hypovolemic shock.

The symptoms of diabetes insipidus are controlled in 90 per cent of cases by the administration of *vasopressin tannate* (Pitressin tannate), 0.5–1 ml. in oil I.M. Pitressin typically alleviates polyuria and usually polydipsia for 24–72 hours.

> *When administering vasopressin tannate, always shake the bottle well before drawing up the drug to insure adequate suspension of the hormone in the oil.*

In addition to parenteral preparations, posterior pituitary hormone is also available in the form of a *snuff* which the patient can inhale two or three times daily. Although the snuff is less expensive than the oil suspension, unfortunately it is irritating to the nasal mucosa. Secondly, persons with mild diabetes insipidus often benefit from treatment with the *benzothiadiazine diuretics;* the thiazides are often capable of decreasing urine volume by > 50 per cent. Finally, individuals with diabetes insipidus secondary to a known causative factor (e.g., a tumor) may be cured by *surgical resection* or *irradiation* of the pituitary. When an infectious process is the cause, *antibiotic therapy* may correct not only the primary infection but also the ADH deficiency.

NURSING CARE OF THE PATIENT UNDERGOING HYPOPHYSECTOMY

Removal of the pituitary gland is performed for the following reasons:

> To slow the growth and expansion of endocrine-dependent malignant neoplasms of the breast and ovaries.
> To slow the metastatic spread of cancer cells to other sites.
> To halt the advance of diabetic retinopathy (see Ch. 95).
> To correct Cushing's disease (which is caused by a pituitary tumor).

Methods used for ablating the pituitary gland include (a) yttrium-90 implantation, (b) irradiation, (c) cryohypophysectomy (destruction of the pituitary by the use of extreme cold), (d) pituitary coagulation with radiofrequency, (e) transphenoidal microsurgical hypophysectomy, and (f) total or partial surgical removal of the gland.[45]

Surgical removal of the pituitary is a frightening prospect for patients and their families because it involves manipulation of the brain. Consequently it is essential to provide the patient with emotional support and comfort throughout the preoperative period. Let the patient know what he can expect to experience following surgery. Tell him that his vital signs will be checked three or four times an hour immediately following the operation. Advise him that he will have an indwelling catheter and an I.V. needle in his arm, and his head will be wrapped in dressings which may feel tight and uncomfortable; also his eyes may be swollen and black due to ecchymosis.

On the day prior to surgery, the patient usually receives his first injection of cortisol. A glucocorticoid is given to help the patient better endure an operation which will result in loss of adrenocortical function. Also at this time the patient's head is prepared for brain surgery according to the surgeon's instructions. Usually it is necessary to shave only a small area at the front of the head.

Postoperative care following hypophysectomy is the same as for a craniotomy (see Unit VIII, Ch. 40). Immediately following surgery, remember to check for the signs of cerebral edema and rising intracranial pressure (elevated blood pressure, low pulse rate, pupil changes). Also, because tropic hormones are no longer being produced, watch for signs of target gland deficiencies, e.g., adrenal insufficiency and hypothyroidism. In addition, the patient may temporarily suffer from diabetes insipidus due to ADH deficiency. Finally, observe the patient carefully for the signs of *meningitis*—a complication of brain surgery. Report any elevation of temperature, severe headache, irritability, and so forth.

Drug replacement of cortisone is started during surgery, and it is continued for the rest of the individual's life. Some patients may also require thyroid hormone replacement as well as the administration of sex hormones. Also, a few patients will require posterior pituitary hormone replacements to control polyuria. It is a major nursing responsibility to educate the patient who has undergone hypophysectomy in the technic of safe self-administration of hormones. Also, because of the many hormonal imbalances which can potentially develop due to hypophysectomy, be certain to advise the postoperative patient to obtain a medical check-up at least every 6 months and whenever symptoms of imbalance appear.

References for Unit XIX

1. Anthony, C. P.: *Textbook of Anatomy and Physiology.* 6th ed. St. Louis, Mo., C. V. Mosby Company, 1963.

1a. Ashkar, F. S.: A better outlook in thyroid cancer. *Consultant 12*:148, January, 1972.

2. Asimov, I.: *Words of Science and the History Behind Them.* New York, New American Library, 1969.

3. Asperheim, M. K., and Eisenhauer, L. A.: *The Pharmacologic Basis of Patient Care.* 2nd ed. Philadelphia, W. B. Saunders Company, 1973.

4. Aurbach, G. D.: Parathyroid, *In Cecil-Loeb Textbook of Medicine.* 13th ed. Beeson, P. B., and McDermott, W. (eds), Philadelphia, W. B. Saunders Company, 1971.

5. Beahrs, O. H.: Carcinoma of the thyroid gland, *In Current Therapy, 1973.* Conn, H. F. (ed.), Philadelphia, W. B. Saunders Company, 1973.

6. Beland, I., et al.: Metabolic crisis, *In Concepts and Practices of Intensive Care for Nurse Specialists.* Meltzer, L. E. (ed.), Philadelphia, The Charles Press, 1969.

7. Bell, M.: Pre-operative teaching and post-operative care of the hypophysectomy patient. *Neurosurgical Nursing 4*:165, December, 1972.

8. Bloodworth, J. M. B.: Diabetes mellitus and vascular disease. *Postgraduate Medicine 53*:84, March, 1973.

9. Boyd, W.: *An Introduction to the Study of Disease.* 5th ed. Philadelphia, Lea and Febiger, 1962.

0. Burke, E. L.: Insulin injection: The site and technique. *American Journal of Nursing 72*:2194, December, 1972.
1. Burrell, Z. L., and Burrell, L. O.: *Intensive Nursing Care*. St. Louis, Mo., C. V. Mosby Company, 1969.
2. Carozza, V.: Ketoacidotic crisis: Mechanism and management. *Nursing '73*, May 13, 1973.
3. Caso, E.: Diabetic meal planning, *In Nutrition: A Book of Readings*. Brennon, R. (ed.) Dubuque, Iowa, William C. Brown Company, 1967.
4. Christy, N. P.: Diseases of the endocrine system: General considerations, *In Cecil-Loeb Textbook of Medicine*. 13th ed. Beeson, P. B., and McDermott, W. (eds), Philadelphia, W. B. Saunders Company, 1971.
5. Crampton, J. H., et al.: *Instructions for the Diabetic Patient*. 9th ed. Seattle, Washington, The Mason Clinic, 1966.
6. DeGroot, L. J.: Diseases of the thyroid, *In Cecil-Loeb Textbook of Medicine*. 13th ed. Beeson, P. B., and McDermott, W. (eds), Philadelphia, W. B. Saunders Company, 1971.
17. Diabetes Instruction Course. Seattle, Washington Diabetes Association, 1970.
18. Diabetic ketoacidosis. *Emergency Medicine 5*: 103, February, 1973.
19. Fact Sheet on Diabetes. New York, American Diabetes Association, Inc., February 20, 1973.
20. French, R. M.: *Nurses' Guide to Diagnostic Procedures*. 3rd ed. New York, McGraw-Hill Book Company, 1972.
21. Garb, S.: *Laboratory Tests in Common Use*. 5th ed. New York, Springer Publishing Company, Inc., 1971.
22. Govoni, L. E., and Hayes, J. E.: *Drugs and Nursing Implications*. 2nd ed. New York, Appleton-Century-Crofts, 1971.
23. Holvey, D. N., et al. (eds.): *The Merck Manual of Diagnosis and Therapy*. 12th ed. West Point, Pa. Merck Sharp & Dohme Research Laboratories, 1972.
24. Haunz, E. A.: Diabetes mellitus in adults, *In Current Therapy, 1973*. Conn, H. F. (ed.), Philadelphia, W. B. Saunders Company, 1973.
25. Krupp, M. A., and Chatton, M. J.: *Current Diagnosis and Treatment*. Los Altos, California, Lange Medical Publications, 1972.
26. Liddle, G. W.: Adrenal cortex, *In Cecil-Loeb Textbook of Medicine*. 13th ed. Beeson, P. B., and McDermott, W. (eds.), Philadelphia, W. B. Saunders Company, 1971.
27. Liechty, R. D., and Soper, R. T.: *Synopsis of Surgery*. 2nd ed. St. Louis, Mo., C. V. Mosby Company, 1972.
28. Matovinovic, J.: Simple goiter, *In Current Therapy, 1973*. Conn, H. F. (ed.), Philadelphia, W. B. Saunders Company, 1973.
29. Meal Planning with Exchange Lists. Pamphlet, American Diabetic Association, Chicago, and American Diabetes Association, Inc., New York. Revised, 1956.
30. Melick, R. A.: Hyperparathyroidism, *In Current Therapy, 1973*. Conn, H. F. (ed.), Philadelphia, W. B. Saunders Company, 1973.
31. Meloni, R. C.: Obesity or Cushing's disease? *American Family Physician 5*:93, June, 1972.

Chapter 97—Nursing Patients With Disorders of the Adrenal and Pituitary Glands

32. Metheny, N. M., and Snively, W. D.: *Nurses' Handbook of Fluid Balance*. Philadelphia, J. B. Lippincott Company, 1972.
33. Miller, B. F., and Keane, C. B.: *Encyclopedia and Dictionary of Medicine and Nursing*. Philadelphia, W. B. Saunders Company, 1972.
34. Nickerson, D.: Teaching the hospitalized diabetic. *American Journal of Nursing 72*:935, May, 1972.
35. Pittman, J. A.: Hyperthyroidism, *In Current Therapy, 1973*. Conn, H. F. (ed.), Philadelphia, W. B. Saunders Company, 1973.
36. Reichlin, S.: The control of anterior pituitary secretion, *In Cecil-Loeb Textbook of Medicine*. 13th ed. Beeson, P. B., and McDermott, W. (eds.), Philadelphia, W. B. Saunders Company, 1971.
37. Robbins, J.: Thyroiditis, *In Current Therapy, 1973*. Conn, H. F. (ed.), Philadelphia, W. B. Saunders Company, 1973.
38. Robbins, S. L., and Angell, M.: *Basic Pathology*. Philadelphia, W. B. Saunders Company, 1971.
39. Robin, N. I.: Hypothyroidism, *In Current Therapy, 1973*. Conn, H. F. (ed.), Philadelphia, W. B. Saunders Company, 1973.
40. Rosenthal, H., and Rosenthal, J.: *Diabetic Care in Pictures*. 3rd ed. Philadelphia, J. B. Lippincott Company, 1960.
41. Rosner, W., and Christy, N. P.: Cushing's syndrome, *In Current Therapy, 1973*. Conn, H. F. (ed.), Philadelphia, W. B. Saunders Company, 1973.
42. Sjoerdsma, A.: Sympatho-adrenal system, *In Cecil-Loeb Textbook of Medicine*. 13th ed. Beeson, P. B., and McDermott, W. (eds.), Philadelphia, W. B. Saunders Company, 1971.
43. Snively, W. D., and Beshear, D. R.: *Textbook of Pathophysiology*. Philadelphia, J. B. Lippincott Company, 1972.
44. Spencer, R. T.: *Patient Care in Endocrine Problems*. Saunders Monograph in Clinical Nursing—4. Philadelphia, W. B. Saunders Company, 1973.
45. Stowe, S. M.: Hypophysectomy for diabetic retinopathy. *American Journal of Nursing 73*:632, April, 1973.
46. Sutton, A. L.: *Bedside Nursing Techniques in Medicine and Surgery*. 2nd ed. Philadelphia, W. B. Saunders Company, 1969.
47. Tracht, M. E.: Thyroid function evaluation. Part 1. *Consultant 13*:145, April, 1973.
48. Tracht, M. E.: Thyroid function evaluation. Part 2. *Consultant 13*:80, May, 1973.
49. Trayser, L. M.: A teaching program for diabetics. *American Journal of Nursing 73*:92, January, 1973.
50. U 100 Insulin. *Nursing Clinics of North America 8*: 369, June, 1973.
51. Willey, L. (ed.): Diabetic out of control. *Nursing '73 3*:10, May, 1973.
52. Williams, S. R.: *Nutrition and Diet Therapy*. St. Louis, Mo., C. V. Mosby Company, 1969.
53. Williams, R. H.: *Textbook of Endocrinology*. 5th ed. Philadelphia, W. B. Saunders Company, 1974.

UNIT XX

Reproductive System

Introduction and Study Guide

Unless symptoms are acute, disorders of the reproductive system are frequently not brought to the attention of the doctor. In the male, the urinary and reproductive systems are closely related anatomically, and disease in one system frequently affects the other.

Societal attitudes have affected the role of the nurse. Quite frequently male nurses or aides are expected to cope with the more intimate details of nursing care, and male patients may be reluctant to discuss their symptoms and problems with a female nurse. The nurse can play an educative and counseling role in dealing with wives and patients. With knowledge, respect, technical skill and a sincere desire to help, the nurse can overcome the patient's reticence, thus helping to uncover early symptoms, and can assist in appropriate action on the family's part.

Chapter 98 will discuss the anatomy, function and dysfunction, diagnosis and nursing care of the male reproductive system. For an exhaustive treatment of the subject, one should consult a good textbook on urology, since this unit deals with only the most common problems.

At the end of her study of this chapter, the nurse should be able to:

> Identify the anatomic features of the male reproductive system.
> Identify signs and symptoms of common dysfunctions.
> Interpret the rationale for diagnostic tests and treatments to patients and families.
> Utilize knowledge of dysfunctions in teaching patients and their families.
> Examine the psychologic aspects of dysfunction of the male reproductive system and provide opportunity for the patient to receive adequate counseling.
> Organize safe nursing care in dysfunctions of the male reproductive system.

Gynecology is the branch of medicine that deals with diseases of the female reproductive tract. The gynecologist uses the tools of both medical therapy and surgery in treating disorders of the reproductive tract; however, he does not operate on the breast. It is estimated that the average gynecologist sees about 25 to 30 outpatients for each inpatient treated; the most common problems observed are vaginal discharges, abnormal vaginal bleeding and psychosexual problems. Preventive medicine is emphasized in management of such patients.

In nursing practice, the focus is very similar. The nurse is likely to see patients, in every setting, with minor (e.g., office gynecology) gynecologic problems, or patients who wish to receive preventive instructions. Two examples follow: (a) the patient with uncontrolled diabetes mellitus, with concurrent vaginitis; and (b) the elderly lady with atrophic vaginitis who is being treated by the public health nurse. Thus, even the nurse who is not working primarily with gynecologic patients needs to be well informed about prevention and treatment of these disorders. Although gynecologic problems may occur at any age, this discussion concentrates on the adult patient or client. This unit is designed to increase the nurse's knowledge about problems of the female reproductive tract.

Chapter 99 reviews the anatomy of the female reproductive tract, the physiology of menstruation, "sex" hormones, menopause and menstrual abnormalities. Chapter 100 discusses inflammatory and infectious problems, including leukorrhea, vaginitis, vulvitis, cervicitis, pelvic inflammatory disease and venereal diseases. Chapter 101 considers benign gynecologic problems, including tumors of the lower genital tract, fistulas, uterine displacement and relaxation of the pelvic organs, while Chapter 102 deals with malignancy of the lower genital tract. Since many of the diagnostic and treatment modalities are common to more than one condition, they, along with related nursing care, are discussed in Chapter 103. The last chapter discusses birth control and associated problems and includes ectopic pregnancy, infertility, contraception, birth control measures, sterilization and abortion.

This unit does not systematically discuss sexuality or the nurses' and clients' feelings about such subjects as sexuality, morality and femininity. However, comprehensive nursing care requires that each nurse consider her own feelings and those of the client regarding these intimate and often private feelings. For this reason, the nurse is asked to consider these short study guide questions as she reads each section of this unit.

1. How does the gynecologic condition or problem discussed affect sexuality and reproductive function?
2. How might I feel if my wife (if a male nurse) or I (if a female nurse) had a similar problem?
3. What other feelings might someone else experience with such a problem?
4. How can I evaluate the client's feelings and provide appropriate care?

CHAPTER 98

Disorders of the Male Reproductive System

ROSEMARY PITTMAN

The structures of the male reproductive system include the penis, the prostate, the scrotum, the testis, the epididymis, the vas deferens, the seminal vesicles and the ejaculatory ducts (Fig. 98–1).

THE PENIS

Anatomy and Function

The penis is primarily a sexual organ with a urethral pathway for elimination of urine and the ejaculate through the urethral meatus. Erection is caused by engorgement of the cavernous structures with blood as a result of varied stimuli. The penile shaft is composed of three columns of erectile tissue bound together by heavy fibrous bands. The two lateral columns are the cavernosa penis and the ventral column containing the urethra is the corpus cavernosum. The expanded proximal portion of the glans is known as the corona and its junction with the corpora cavernosa is the coronal sulcus; a flap of skin, the prepuce or foreskin, covers the glans. The skin of the penis is dark, nonhair-bearing, thin and loose, allowing considerable distention.

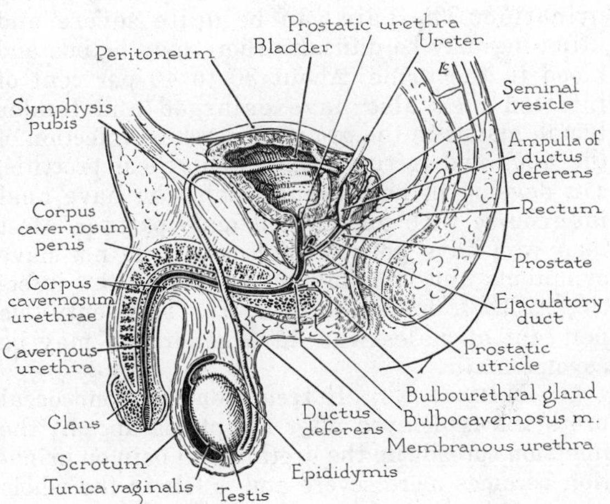

FIGURE 98–1. Diagrammatic sagittal section of the male pelvis, showing the genital organs and their relation to the bladder and urethra. (From King, B. G., and Showers, M. J.: *Human Anatomy and Physiology.* After Turner: General Endocrinology.)

There is wide variation in the normal size of the penis. Striking discrepancies between penile size and age may indicate hypoplasia or hyperplasia. Penile hypoplasia is a manifestation of eunuchoidism occurring before puberty, or a feature of intersexuality. The distinction between a hypoplastic penis with hypospadias and a hyperplastic clitoris may be difficult to make without surgical or histologic examination. Usually, penile hyperplasia is seen only before normal puberty and is commonly caused by tumors of the pineal gland or hypothalamus, tumors arising from the Leydig cells of the testis or tumors of the adrenal gland.

Inspection and Palpation

The most common disorders of the penis can be discovered by inspection and palpation. In boys, these are redundancy, adhesions, phimosis, paraphimosis, posthitis and balanitis, ulceration of the external meatus, herpes, chafing, scabies, pediculi, verrucae and syphilis. Early circumcision eliminates the problem of redundancy of the prepuce. If circumcision is not performed, the mother should be taught to retract the prepuce at an early age. The condition is important only when the prepuce cannot be retracted. It has been believed that irritant debris may cause penile cancer, since Jews who have been neonatally circumcised almost never have penile cancer; however, many practicing pediatricians are not convinced that past research indicates the need for circumcision for religious reasons. Adhesions existing at birth may be separated by preputial retraction or by stretching so that the prepuce can be freely retracted.

Dysfunctions

Paraphimosis. A tight foreskin, once retracted, may become edematous thus impeding the circulation of the glans, with resultant swelling. Manual replacement may be attempted but surgical incision may be necessary.

Herpes Progenitalis. A small group of vesicles with an erythematous base is frequently found on the glans or prepuce. These may rupture, producing superficial ulcers, heal in about a week or serve as a point of entry for other organisms. Treatment consists of local cleanliness, although tetracycline has sometimes been used.

Herpesvirus Hominis Type II. This may produce a penile lesion of clear vesicles much like a cold sore. If a man with the lesion has sexual contact, the woman may become infected. There is no known cure and, during the acute stage, the disease is very painful. Symptomatic treatment with pain medicine and local cortisone may be used. If a child is delivered when the woman has the disease, it definitely will not survive. Because of the severity of the infection in women, men with a herpes infection on the penis should abstain from intercourse. After a herpes infection, women thought to be more susceptible to cancer should have a pap smear every year. Intercourse should be avoided by the male while he has a herpes lesion.

Penile Ulcers. SYPHILITIC CHANCRE. This is the primary lesion of syphilis and commonly occurs on the corona or the inner side of the prepuce. It begins as a silvery papule that gradually becomes a superficial ulcer containing the treponema pallidum. The chancre is painless, usually round and with a smooth, slightly raised border. The regional lymph nodes may also be moderately enlarged. The ulcer is extremely contagious and the organisms may penetrate the unbroken skin. The diagnosis may be confirmed by a dark-field microscopic examination, since the lesion appears before the serology becomes positive. (Syphilis is discussed in more detail on p. 1417.)

CHANCROID. Another type of lesion producing a penile ulcer is the chancroid or soft chancre caused by the bacillus *Hemophilus ducreyi.* The border is irregular, the center is necrotic, and there is profuse suppuration. In some cases, the regional lymph nodes become swollen, tender and suppurative. Chancroid is much more universally prevalent than syphilis. It is a predominantly local and regional disease of rather superficial nature, contacted generally during coitus and fostered by poor genital hygiene. Most cases are adequately treated by cleansing, by protecting the lesions and by using sulfonamides that have no masking effect on the appearance of syphilis.

Lymphogranuloma Venereum. This is caused by a rickettsialike organism, *Miyagawanella lymphogranulomatosis,* and is another venereal disease involving the lymphatic system. The initial lesion on the penis is frequently overlooked. This infection manifests itself in a variety of ways: bubo formation, ulceration, elephantiasis of the genitalia, and rectal stricture. Diagnosis is aided by a skin test with Frei antigen. The disease, which occurs throughout the world, especially in tropical and subtropical areas, is endemic in the southern United States and affects the most sexually promiscuous. The course of the disease is often long and disability is great, but the disease is essentially nonfatal. It is communicable when active lesions are present. Specific treatment varies with the stage of the disease. Sulfadiazine is the drug of choice in the bubo phase; tetracyclines may be orally administered for proctitis and other ulcerative lesions.

Condyloma Accuminatum. Venereal warts occur on the corona or in the retroglandular sulcus. In the presence of moisture, secondary infection results in ulceration. Excessive growth and ulceration must be distinguished from carcinoma by biopsy. *Condyloma latum,* a flat and warty growth, is a secondary syphilid and is highly contagious. Treatment consists of proper hygienic measures. Circumcision may be required and, for the smaller clusters, local cauterization by either electrocoagulation or the application of a 2 per cent alcoholic solution of podophyllin may be necessary.

Gonorrhea. In North America, gonorrhea is presently an epidemic disease affecting 2,000,000 Americans each year. A man has a 20 to 50 per cent chance of contracting gonorrhea from a single sexual exposure to an infected partner. The risks of gonorrhea transmission during oral-genital or anal intercourse are not known exactly but they probably are the same as with vaginal intercourse. Chances of getting an infection increase with repeated exposure to an infected partner.

SYMPTOMS. Most men notice symptoms three to five days after the infecting sexual contact. It may be up to 17 days, however, before symptoms occur. At first, a thin clear mucus appears at the meatal opening. Within a day or two, the discharge becomes heavy, thick and creamy. It is usually white but may be yellow or green. The lips of the meatus become swollen and stand out from the glans. Most men feel pain and a burning sensation in the penis or at the meatus during urination. The pain can be quite severe and urinating may be difficult. There may be pus and blood in the urine. About 30 to 40 per cent of infected men also have enlarged and tender lymph glands in the groin. Gonorrheal infection of the anus and rectum, called gonorrheal proctitis, can develop in homosexual men who have anal intercourse with an infected male partner. Most men who have gonococcal proctitis do not have symptoms and can unknowingly give the infection to their male partners. Ten to twenty-two per cent of males who have gonorrhea may be asymptomatic.

COMPLICATIONS. If treatment of gonococcal urethritis is delayed after symptoms appear, the infection spreads up the urethra and pain on urination becomes more severe and is felt in the whole penis.

After about two weeks, symptoms of urethritis begin to disappear on their own. However, the man can still infect his sexual partner. After two to three weeks of untreated infection, the bacteria invade the posterior urethra and the prostate gland and a prostatic abscess may develop. In about 20 per cent of men who remain untreated for more than a month, the bacteria spread down the vas deferens and reach the epididymis, causing gonococcal epididymitis. If the infection is not treated, testicles will become involved and the man will become sterile.

TREATMENT. The regular treatment is with 4.8 million units aqueous procaine penicillin G intramuscularly, with 1.0 Gm. probenecid orally, preferably given 30 minutes prior to injection. The injection is divided into two doses and given in different sites. Oral treatment is with ampicillin 3.5 Gm. orally with 1.0 Gm. probenecid orally at the same time.

For patients in whom penicillin is contraindicated because of allergy or in whom penicillin or ampicillin has been ineffective, spectinomycin 2.0 Gm. intramuscularly may be given in males or tetracycline 1.5 Gm. orally, then 0.5 Gm. orally four times daily for four days (a total of 9.5 Gm.) may be administered.

Posthitis and Balanitis. These are inflammations of the prepuce and glans penis caused by irritation and invasion by some organism. The initial treatment is cleansing with mild soap and water, followed by application of a drying powder to minimize moisture. Antibiotic therapy will help to control local infection. Circumcision may be necessary.

Stricture of the urethral meatus is usually a congenital malformation.

Urethritis. This is manifested by redness, edema and eversion of the edges of the meatus. A variable amount of pus may be discharged from the urethra. Lymph channels in the dorsum of the penis, as well as the inguinal lymph glands, may be tender and palpable. Micturition and erection may be painful. The cause is difficult to determine. Gonorrhea must be excluded by slide and culture, as it is the most common cause. Nonspecific urethritis may be part of a triad, along with conjunctivitis and arthritis in Reiter's disease. Fifty per cent of nonspecific urethritis has been found to be associated with *Chlamydia trachomatis*. Treatment is with 500 mg. tetracycline four times a day for a week. The female sex partner should also be treated. If symptoms recur, the individual should be treated for 21 days with 250 mg. tetracycline four times a day.

Common Congenital Defects. HYPOSPADIAS. In the fetus, the urethral meatus may develop so that it occurs on the ventral surface of the glans, on the shaft or at the penoscrotal junction. This is one of the most common urogenital anomalies and requires early attention, the treatment depending on the location. In *epispadias,* the urethral meatus opens dorsally on the glans, on the shaft or at the penoscrotal junction.

Priapism. This is a prolonged, persistent penile erection without sexual desire, usually accompanied by pain. Local mechanical factors such as thrombosis, hemorrhage, neoplasm or inflammation in the penis may be the causes. It is associated with leukemia and sickle cell anemia. Treatment is difficult and frequently unsuccessful.

Impotence. Impotence is the inability to achieve and maintain erection necessary in the performance of coitus. The two main mechanisms connected with erection are vascular and neurologic. There are various etiologic factors, although the most frequent seems to be psychogenic. The following types of causes have been cited: congenital; inflammatory: prostatitis, seminal vesiculitis, peripheral neuritis; neurologic; endocrinologic: diabetic neuropathy, bilateral testicular failure; vascular aortic obstruction; neoplastic; traumatic, iatrogenic (radical perineal prostatectomy) accidental injury; and psychogenic. Impotence is common in diabetes and may manifest itself preclinically. Drugs may have an effect on potency, such as ganglionic blocking agents in hypertension; reserpine, alcohol, narcotics and tranquilizers may all interfere.

In any case of impotence, it is important to obtain a comprehensive history and do a physical examination to exclude other than psychogenic causes. Problems of sexual performance contribute largely to the anxiety states of the elderly male. Impotent males are susceptible to quack medication and therapies advertised by word of mouth or in the back of certain magazines. Our culture tends to deprecate sexual activity in the aged; an elderly man is likely to be thought perverse or at best comic if he is interested in satisfying his sexual needs, and an elderly woman even more so. Poor health may reduce sexual activity but does not necessarily eliminate it. The individual should have a frank discussion with his doctor about whether he should continue sexual activity and about realistic guidelines regarding changes in habit that may be necessary. Patients need to be reassured that transurethral surgery or genital manipulation does not cause impotence.

When impotence occurs to a significant degree, the man and his sexual partner must be treated simultaneously. The secret of successful management is not to treat the symptoms at all since an erection cannot be voluntarily obtained. The three principal goals are: (1) removal of the man's fears about his sexual performance; (2) reorienting of his involuntary behavioral pattern so that he becomes an active participant; and (3) allaying of the woman's fears about her partner's sexual performance. It is necessary to reestablish communication between the partners and to treat the relationship.

Cancer. Cancer of the penis is essentially skin cancer. The glans and the prepuce are usually the parts affected. Carcinoma of the penis is often related to the presence of chronic infection in the area. Circumcision seems to help in preventing the development of cancer. The treatment is excision of the affected area. Sometimes it is necessary to amputate the penis partially or totally.

THE PROSTATE

Anatomy and Function

In childhood, the prostate is a small gland but, in puberty, grows to the size of a walnut. It lies in the pelvis about 2 cm. posterior to the symphysis pubis. It is inverted so that the base is superior and the apex inferior. The basal surface is overlain by the bladder, and the posterior prostatic surface is in close contact with the rectal wall and is the only surface of the prostate subject to palpation (Fig. 98–2). The prostate urethra runs through the prostate. A shallow median furrow divides the lower part of the prostate into the right and lateral left lobes. The middle lobe is created by the ejaculatory ducts from either side, which pierce the prostate and converge in the urethra.

In the normal adult male, the prostate measures about ¾ × 1½ × 2 inches. The structure is a network of branching glands which manufacture a prostatic secretion. The glands are embedded in muscles which contract during ejaculation to eject prostatic secretion. This secretion goes through the ejaculatory ducts. The sole function of the prostate is to manufacture this secretion. This secretion aids the passage of spermatozoa and helps to keep them alive, supplying them with an emergency food supply if needed.

Dysfunctions

Chronic Prostatitis. This is probably the most common chronic infection in men over 50 years of age. It has been reported that 35 per cent of all men over 50 years have chronic prostatitis. In the prostatic secretion, staphylococci are the most frequently found organisms. Chronic infection of the seminal vesicles accompanies prostatitis. It is generally a nonspecific infection and has an extremely varied symptomatology. Many patients with a mild infection have no symptoms. There may be a persistent urethral discharge, usually appearing at the meatus in the morning or during the day when a long time elapses between voidings. There is frequency of urination with mild urgency, dysuria and burning on voiding. A dull ache may be felt; referred pain may occur anywhere below the diaphragm. It is often felt when the patient first arises in the morning and may wear off during the day. There is frequently sexual dysfunction. Treatment consists of general hygienic measures, chemotherapy, attack on the distant primary focus of infection, eradication of complications and local therapy. Prostate massage is accomplished by stroking the posterior surface of the prostate toward the midline. The fluid is milked from the urethra and examined under the microscope. In prostatitis, the fluid contains many leukocytes.

The prognosis is not very encouraging, although approximately 50 per cent of cases will be cured and 25 per cent will markedly improve.

Benign Prostatic Hypertrophy. Benign enlargement develops in 1 of 10 40-year-old men and increase in frequency with advanced age. The cause is not known, although the common opinion is that the condition is the consequence of an endocrine disturbance.

Most patients present with varying degrees of urinary obstruction, although benign hypertrophy is usually slow in developing and may persist for a long time without creating a major problem. As the person becomes older, he may assume that his frequency of urination will increase. However, reduction in both the size and force of the urinary stream is abnormal and necessitates an examination. The urinary stream first lacks force, then becomes weak and dribbling. The individual feels unable to empty his bladder and has to strain to urinate or has to urinate more frequently. Blood in the urine may be another symptom and is more common in benign hypertropy than in cancer.

As the prostate enlarges, there is a danger of complete obstruction of urination, which may be precipitated by the person's being chilled and by his having a drink. Obstruction is a painful emergency which can be treated by insertion of a catheter. If the retention is of long standing and there is over 1000 ml. of urine in the bladder, it is wise to remove the urine gradually, about 100 ml. an hour.

Infection in an enlarged prostate causes exacerbation of the symptoms in addition to the problems of urinary infection. During the later stages of prostatic disease, the kidneys may be damaged owing to the backing up of urine into the kidney, causing uremic poisoning.

DIAGNOSIS. The disorder is diagnosed by: (1) general physical examination, including a rectal examination; (2) laboratory examination of blood, urine and renal functions; (3) x-ray examination,

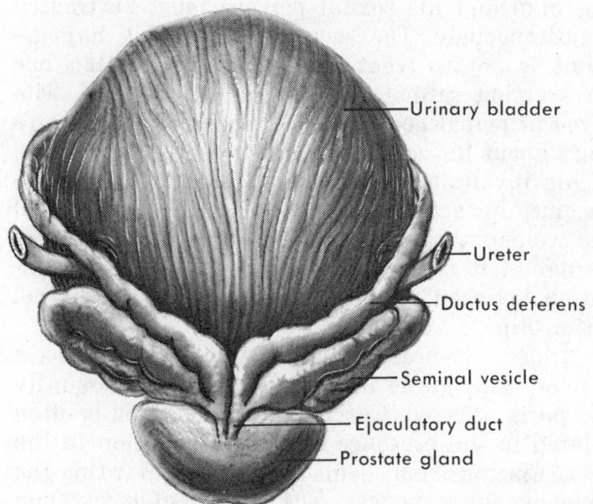

FIGURE 98–2. The bladder, seminal vesicles and prostate gland—posterior view. (From Dienhart, C. M.: Basic Human Anatomy and Physiology. 2nd ed., 1973.)

including intravenous pyelography and excretory cystography; and (4) instrumental examination, including catheterization, cystourethroscopy and biopsy.

Most patients are vague and unsure about what an enlarged prostate is and may be afraid of the tests and their results. Since many of the patients are facing the increasingly debilitating effects of age, a complete explanation of each step of the procedure is helpful. The patient may be shown a picture of the reproductive organs and prostate, and the effects of enlargement upon the excretion of urine can be explained. If the patient sees such a picture, he can better understand how the doctor can determine the size and consistency of the glands and the seminal vesicles. The patient may be placed in the knee-chest position or bent over the table. The nurse may explain that relaxing and taking slow deep breaths may make the procedure easier. Prostatic secretion may be obtained during the rectal examination and examined under the microscope for pus cells which indicate infection. The urine may be normal in asymptomatic cases or may show infection by the presence of red or white cells, albumin and bacteria, or an alkaline reaction.

Renal function tests may be done if the prostatic symptoms indicate the need. Normal ranges in blood chemistry tests most often used in urology are shown in Table 98–1. Excretory urography, phenosulfophthalein excretory tests, specific gravity test, radioisotope renograms and renal radioscintillation scanning are tests used in further diagnosis.

The instruments used in urology include certain urethral catheters and sounds. The catheters are used to (1) relieve urinary obstruction, (2) obtain urine for diagnosis and (3) test for residual urine and bladder lavage or medication. If a catheter is to be left indwelling, a retention catheter of the Foley type is generally used. This catheter is kept in the bladder by an inflatable balloon filled with 5 ml. of water (Fig. 98–3).

The cystoscope is indispensable in both the diagnosis and treatment of urologic disease. It is a metal instrument with optical systems that provide a magnified illuminated image of the bladder. The cystoscopic examination is a valuable diagnostic procedure. The examination should be done by a urologist certified by the American Board of Urology. Some indications for cystocopy are: (1) to

TABLE 98–1. NORMAL RANGE OF BLOOD CONCENTRATIONS OF FUNCTIONAL CONSTITUENTS AND EXCRETORY SUBSTANCES*†

Calcium	9.5–10.5 (10) mg./100 cc.	4.8–5.2 (5.0) mEq./L.
Sodium	317–340 (329) mg./100 cc.	138–148 (143) mEq./L.
Potassium	16–21 (18.2) mg./100 cc.	4.0–5.4 (4.7) mEq./L.
Chloride	355–390 (370) mg. Cl/100 cc.	100–110 (104) mEq./L.
Phosphate		
Adults	3.0–4.5 (3.8) mg. P/100 cc.	1.7–2.6 (2.2) mEq./L.
Children	5.0–8.0 (6.5) mg. P/100 cc.	2.9–4.6 (3.8) mEq./L.
Bicarbonate (HCO_3)	57–62 (60) cc.	25–28 (27) mEq./L.
Plasma Proteins		
Total (including fibrinogen)		6.5–8.0 (7.3) gm./100 cc.
Albumin (Howe method)		4.0–5.5 (4.5) gm./100 cc.
Globulin (Howe method)		2.0–3.0 (2.5) gm./100 cc.
Fibrinogen		0.2–0.4 (0.3) gm./100 cc.
Hemoglobin		
Male adults		14–18 (16) gm./100 cc.
Female adults		12–16 (14) gm./100 cc.
Total nonprotein nitrogen		10–30 (20)
Whole blood		20–40 (32)
Urea nitrogen		8–28 (12)
Whole blood		5–23 (11)
Uric acid		3.0–5.0 (4.0)
Whole blood		3.0–5.9 (4.5)
Creatinine		0.6–1.1 (0.8)
Whole blood		0.7–1.5 (1.2)
Serum Enzymes		
Alkaline phosphatase—Bodansky		
Adults		2.0–4.9 units/100 cc.
Children		5–15 units/100 cc.
Prematures		10–20 units/100 cc.
Acid phosphatase—Bodansky		0.0–1.0 units/100 cc.
Acid phosphatase—King and Armstrong		1.0–5.0 units/100 cc.
Glucose (Folin-Wu method)		80–120 (100)

*Average value is in parentheses; values are for plasma and in terms of mg./100 cc. unless otherwise specified.

†From Leader, A. J., and Carlton, C. E.: Urologic diagnosis and the urologic examination. *In* Campbell, M. F., and Harrison, H.: *Urology.* 3rd. ed. Philadelphia, W. B. Saunders Company, 1970.

determine the source of urinary bleeding; (2) to determine the cause of unexplained urinary symptoms; (3) to determine the source of pyuria; (4) to catheterize the ureters for the purpose of localizing the infection and therapy; (5) to obtain biopsy specimens; and (6) for follow-up examinations. The nurse may assist the patient by explaining the procedure and the fact that it will be done under local or general anesthesia.

CATHETERIZATION OF THE MALE. Initially, the prepuce is widely retracted and the glans and meatus are washed with surgical soap solution. The distal end of the catheter should be covered with a good surgical lubricant such as KY jelly. The catheter is gently inserted and pushed forward. As it meets the resistance offered by the external sphincter, increased but gentle pressure is maintained until the catheter again moves forward. Once past the sphincter, the catheter usually passes into the bladder. The person inserting the catheter should wear sterile gloves. Absolute asepsis is necessary in the catheterization. Prepackaged sterile packs are generally used for the procedure and contain sterile drapes, cotton balls, lubricating jelly and catheters.

Hypertrophy alone is not an indication for surgery; only deteriorating function makes it imperative. The indications for surgery are: (1) Upper tract dilatation and renal failure; catheter drainage and stabilization of renal function are necessary before surgery. (2) Presence of a nonemptying bladder diverticulum. (3) Vesical calculus, indicative of longstanding vesical neck obstruction that results in vesical decompensation. (4) A residual urine of 60 ml. or more, also indicative of longstanding obstruction and vesical detrusor complication. (5) Severe and prolonged hematuria from congested prostatic vessels. (6) Acute urinary retention. Severe symptoms are less pressing indications of the need for surgery. Prostatectomy must be done early before decompensation occurs. This is especially important in the patient with coronary artery disease, whose condition can be expected to deteriorate.

The surgical approaches that can be used are: (1) A transurethral resection for a benign gland estimated to weigh 30 to 40 Gm. or less. This offers direct pinpoint control of bleeding. (2) Retrograde or suprapubic surgery for enucleating larger glands and for correcting associated disease. (3) Perineal approach in the elderly person who is not an ideal surgical candidate, who has a large prostate and in whom retention of potency is not a determining factor. (4) Transsacral surgery for patients who have had previous operations or injury resulting in rectourethral fistulas or other lesions involving the rectum.

Transurethral Resection. The TUR, generally accepted as the method for removing minor obstructive lesions, is the most widely used of all prostatic surgery. A resectoscope is inserted through the urethra and the enlargement is scraped out. The resectoscope has two parts: an insulated sheath which prevents damage to the urethra after the instrument is inserted; and a working element, a movable loop of tungsten wire which cuts tissue with a high frequency cur-

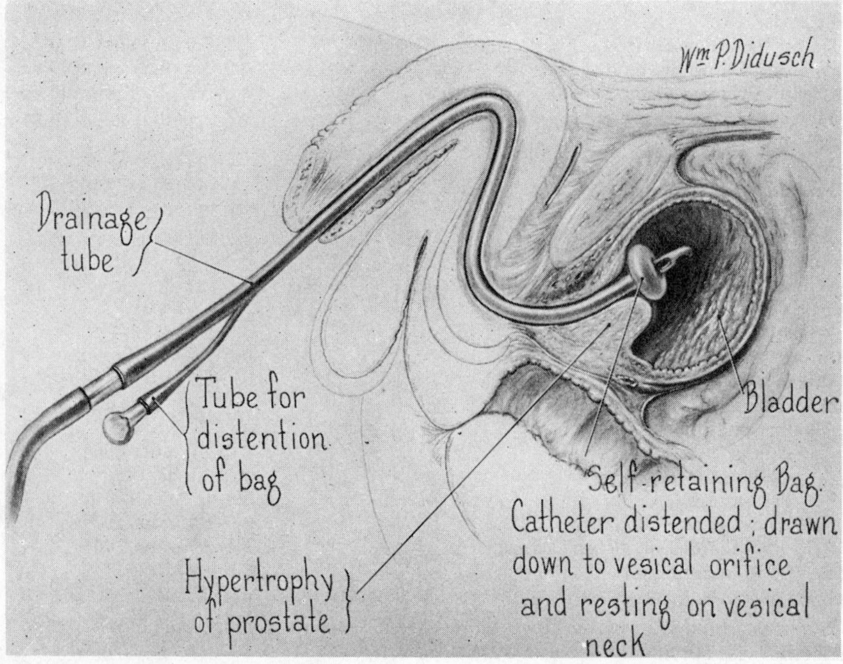

FIGURE 98–3. Demonstrating the use of the self-retaining catheter of the Foley type. (Courtesy of American Cystoscope Makers, Inc.)

rent that is turned on by a foot pedal. The surgeon operates the cutting loop by looking through a telescope; the field is illuminated by a bright electric light. Irrigating fluid can be shot in and out through the instrument, and the debris falls back into the bladder and is washed out. Hospitalization is usually short and convalescence more rapid than with other types of surgery.

In punch prostatectomy, a cold knife is used to remove the enlargement. Tissue is punched out piece by piece with a circular hollow blade. Healing is more satisfactory than when tissue is burned. However, burning is not eliminated, as bleeding is controlled by electric current. The patient returns to the ward with a uretheral catheter and an intermittent catheter irrigation system.

PREOPERATIVE NURSING CARE. This includes: (1) facilitation of the patient's and family's understanding of anesthesia, surgery and procedures; (2) relieving the patient's and family's anxiety about the outcome with reasonable information; (3) meticulous attention to asepsis in catheterization, etc.; (4) encouragment of good fluid and dietary intake during hospital stay prior to surgery. (5) For specific preoperative preparation, the patient should take a shower twice daily, using a detergent soap. The skin should be shaved in the area of the operative field. A tap water enema is usually given the night before. Patients are generally given a soporific drug the night before, and the preoperative medication is given according to the needs of the individual patient.

POSTOPERATIVE CARE. During immediate recovery, the blood pressure, pulse and respiration should be observed every 15 minutes until stable. One risk due to transurethral resection is accidental perforation of either the bladder wall or the capsule of the prostate. If this is not recognized during the operation, the patient's condition will rapidly deteriorate; he will have abdominal pain, signs of shock, some rigidity of the abdominal muscles and a rise in his pulse rate. This complication requires further surgery—a suprapubic cystotomy.

The type of irrigation system used after surgery depends on the individual physician. *Closed irrigation* is designed to permit constant or intermittent flow of washing fluid without the hazard of breaking aseptic technique. It is commonly used following a TUR when there may be considerable bleeding and possible obstruction of the system by blood clots. One method utilizes a glass Y tube attached to the catheter. One limb of the Y is attached to drainage and the other to a reservoir of fluid suspended from a pole. The fluid may be allowed to flow continuously or used as needed. Another method is the use of a three-way catheter (Fig. 98–4). The nurse must ascertain whether or not the catheter is functioning by watching the free oscillations of the fluid in the inverted Y tube at the foot of the bed in response to the patient's cough. Sluggish movement of this column of fluid, along with a slow drip into the collecting bottle, indicates the need for bladder irrigation. This condition must be observed early before the bladder has become distended.

The fluid intake of the patient may generally

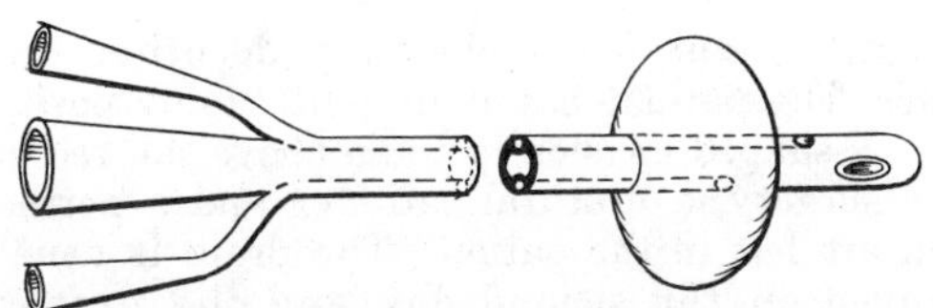

FIGURE 98–4. The Foley-Alcock three-way catheter. (From Sutton, A. L.: *Bedside Nursing Techniques in Medicine and Surgery.* 2nd ed., 1969.)

be maintained orally, since he seldom has a general anesthetic. The patient may have a soft diet on the day of surgery, with a general diet thereafter.

Patients recovering satisfactorily will experience little pain and do not require narcotics. The day after surgery, the catheter can be attached to a urinary leg bag to encourage early ambulation of the patient. The urethral catheter is usually removed on the third postoperative day. Following this, the patient may have a soapsuds enema if needed and a hot bath. He is encouraged to maintain a large fluid intake, is supplied with several glass bottles and is instructed to use a separate one for each voiding. The doctor can immediately observe the volume and appearance of the urine with each act of voiding. If it becomes necessary to reinsert the catheter should the patient be unable to void or voids poorly, it may be removed again the following day for another trial. If this proves unsuccessful, reoperation may be necessary. Patients who live nearby may remain in the hospital for four to eight days, but those living far away should remain for 14 days, since the danger of secondary hemorrhage is generally not over until then. At home, the patient is encouraged to rest and to exercise only moderately. Abstinence from sexual activity for at least four weeks is emphasized, and the patient should be encouraged to continue his large fluid intake until his first checkup.

Urinary tract infection is very common following a TUR but ordinarily clears up six to eight weeks postoperatively.

Retrograde or Suprapubic Prostatectomy. This is the procedure by which the gland is removed through the bladder after extraperitoneal incision of the superior wall. This procedure is used when the obstructing tissue is estimated to weigh more than 60 Gm., if the patient is going to a part of the country where adequate urologic care is not available, or if the patient has sizeable diverticula of the bladder and significant bladder neck obstruction.

Perineal Prostatic Surgery. This is used in suspected early carcinoma of the prostate or for removal of prostatic calculi. It probably interferes with active sex life more than do other techniques. The patient is put in a lithotomy position and a V-shaped incision is made above the rectum. After surgery, a urethral catheter and a perineal drain are left in the patient. The drain is usually removed on the second day and the urethral catheter is left in until the stitches are removed on about the seventh day and the area has been dry for a couple of days.

Retropubic Prostatectomy. The retropubic approach is used in all types of prostatic diseases. With the patient in a modified Trendelenburg position, an incision 2 to 5 inches long is made above the pubis, and the prostatic capsule is excised. On the patient's return to bed, the catheter is connected to a bedside KCH bottle by sterile tubing. The patient is generally allowed out of bed the next day and the catheter and drain removed the third day.

Prostatic Cancer. Prostatic cancer is the second most common cause of death from cancer in the male. The rate for the white population in 1964 was 16.6 per 100,000 and, for the nonwhite population, 18.9 per 100,000. Epidemiologic variables in prostatic cancer were studied, with data from the California and Alameda County Tumor Registries. The statistically significant data included an (< 0.05) excess of familially associated carcinoma, a history of venereal diseases, coital frequency, the number of sexual partners before and after marriage and the use of contraceptive agents in the prostatic cancer cases as compared with the controls.

Blacks have the highest incidence of prostatic carcinoma, and Chinese and Japanese, the lowest. The five-year survival rate for prostatic carcinoma was 64 per cent (1955 to 1965) for all stages of the disease. The median age at diagnosis was 72.8. There were four times as many cases of the disease in persons 65 and over. An increasing tendency to diagnose prostatic cancer at an earlier stage was shown. The number of cases treated by surgery remained relatively constant at approximately 60 per cent, those treated by irradiation being 2 per cent and those by irradiation and surgery, 2 per cent. The number of patients receiving chemotherapy alone had increased from 19 per cent (1942 to 1954) to 28 per cent from 1954 to 1969. Survival rates were slightly higher between 1945 and 1965. There was a 10-year absolute survival rate of 16 per cent between 1955 and 1969.

Most prostatic cancers are adenocarcinoma. The doctor suspects prostatic carcinoma on rectal examination. Symptoms at a stage prior to spread are not characteristic of the disease. Late in the disease, rectal findings include a hard, irregular or nodular gland. Cystoscopy may be used to determine whether or not surgery is indicated. A pelvic x-ray examination is essential, since the bones of the pelvis and spine are the most frequent sites of metastasis. Serum acid phosphatase determination aids in finding whether or not the cancer has spread, since the value is frequently elevated in metastatic carcinoma. It is almost never elevated in benign prostatic hypertrophy.

Operable prostatic cancers will be found more frequently if routine rectal examinations are done on all men over 50 years of age. The prognosis has been studied and, of 86 patients with localized cancers, one-third lived for 15 years or longer without any evidence of cancer and without any postoperative endocrine therapy.

Prostatic carcinoma can be divided into four stages: *Stage A,* in which the lesion is occult, small, well differentiated and located within the gland; *Stage B,* in which the lesion is completely limited to the prostate and may be large or small; *Stage C,* in which the lesion invades the capsule and partially invades the areolar tissue around the base of the seminal vesicles, with no evidence of distant metastases; *Stage D,* in which the lesion has vascular and lymph node metastases.

A radical prostatectomy is associated with a small but significant degree of incontinence and a considerable degree of impotence. If the patient is an acceptable surgical risk and is willing to accept the disadvantages of a total prostatectomy, then this procedure is the treatment of choice. Total perineal prostatectomy has the highest cure rates.

In perineal surgery, some preoperative bowel preparation is necessary, such as enemas containing neomycin. Postoperatively, the patient returns from surgery with a urethral catheter. Its retention in the bladder is necessary for urinary drainage and as a splint for the urethral anastomosis. The catheter is usually left in place for two weeks. The patient should have fewer bladder spasms and should not have much bleeding. The amount of urinary drainage on the dressing should rapidly decrease. A tissue drain is generally removed in 24 to 48 hours. A suprapubic drain will remain longer. Since perineal surgery may affect the perineal muscles, the patient may suddenly become incontinent. This may be avoided by having the patient start perineal exercises a day or two after surgery. Exercises should be continued even after control of the anal sphincter returns. Perineal exercises consist of contracting the abdominal, gluteal and perineal muscles while breathing normally. The patient may be asked to contract his muscles as he would if his need to void was very urgent and there was no place to go. Unless the urethral sphincter has been damaged, the patient who has done the exercises will usually regain urinary control more readily when the catheter is removed.

Irradiation can cure some patients with carcinoma of the prostate. There is strong evidence that a 5 mg. daily dose of diethylstilbestrol, once a favored treatment, carries a significant risk of death due to cardiovascular disease. Endocrine therapy is advisable in patients with advanced prostatic carcinoma. Remission can be induced and patients may remain comfortable for two to three years or longer. The use of Cyproterone acetate, a steroid exhibiting both endogenous and exogenous androgenic action, is thought to be as effective as estrogen and does not cause painful, enlarged breasts. In stage C of the disease, bilateral orchiectomy may be done to remove all testicular stimuli to continued prostatic growth. Prosthetic implants are available for esthetic reasons. Stilbestrol or TACE (chlorotrianisene) may be given. X-rays of the chest, lumbar spine and pelvis should be taken at six-month intervals.

Radiation as a form of treatment has certain benefits. It does not cause impotence and does not have the psychologic implications of castration, nor is there the likelihood of increased risk of death due to cardiovascular complications.

THE SCROTUM

Anatomy and Function

The scrotum is a bilocular sac containing the testicles and portions of the duct system of the male genital tract. The sac hangs from the root of the penis, the left side being lower than the right because the left spermatic cord is longer. The skin of the pouch is bisected by a median raphe extending from the ventral aspect of the penile shaft under the entire sac to the anus. Internally, the two halves of the pouch are separated by a dartos tunic. Each half contains a testis with its epididymis and spermatic cord.

The testis is a smooth, solid, oval structure suspended in the scrotum by the spermatic cord. The testis has 600 to 1200 seminiferous tubules with a combined length of almost a mile. The upper end of the testis is capped by the head of the epididymis and the body of the epididymis is attached to the posterior surface of the testis. The apex of the epididymis at the lower end of the testis becomes continuous with the vas deferens that joins other vessels to form the spermatic cord. The spermatic cord consists of the vas deferens, arteries, veins, nerves and lymphatic vessels held together by spermatic fascia. The cord goes through the inguinal canal, and the vas deferens continues in the abdominal cavity, passing behind the bladder and anterior to the rectum to join the duct of the seminal vesicle and becoming the ejaculatory duct. The spermatic cord is movable for protection from trauma and facilitates optimum spermatogenesis.

The scrotum is examined by inspection and palpation. Because of the rugae, the walls may be inspected by spreading the layers between the fingers. Transillumination will help to distinguish most structures in the scrotal sac.

The seminal vesicles are paired 5 cm. long structures that are closely parallel to the bladder. The ejaculatory ducts separate the posterior and median lobes of the prostate and empty into the urethra. The seminal vesicles secrete a portion of the ejaculate and may contribute to the nutrition and activation of the sperm. Surgically, the seminal vesicles seldom require consideration without simultaneous removal of the prostate. Tumors of the vesicles are rare.

External Conditions. The scrotal skin is very thin and contains a large number of apocrine glands that tend to form cysts. It is in constant contact with the clothes and the skin of the thighs. It has many rugae that inhibit proper ventilation and so is subject to collecting moisture and to rubbing. The scrotum is prone to many infections by all organisms as well as to diseases indigenous to tropical areas. Nonvenereal disorders such as erysipelas, abscesses, fistulas and gangrene may occur in the scrotum. Venereal diseases such as chancroid, granuloma inguinale, lymphogranuloma venereum and syphilis may all manifest symptoms in this area. Parasites such as scabies and lice may also infect the scrotum. Many of the common skin diseases such as fungal infections, contact dermatitis, drug eruptions, eczema, lichen planus, herpes progenitales and psoriasis may spread to the scrotum. Cancer of the scrotum does occur but is rare.

Itching and intertrigo may be severe if the genitalia are affected because of heat, friction and moisture. Obesity and tight clothing aggravate the condition. The cause of the condition must be found and good local hygiene and use of dusting powder such as cornstarch may improve the condition.

The five most common disorders that give rise to a scrotal mass of short duration are (1) mumps orchitis, (2) epididymitis, (3) tumor, (4) tuberculosis and (5) torsion.

Mumps Orchitis. This is a complication of mumps in about 18 per cent of cases which rarely occurs before puberty. Onset of the orchitis is usually four to six days after the appearance of the parotitis, although it may occur without it. In about 70 per cent of the cases, it is unilateral. Impotence and sterility are frequent sequelae. Signs and symptoms are nausea, vomiting and chills, followed by some testicular swelling. The gland is swollen, tender and usually extremely painful. Treatment includes bed rest, scrotal support and hot or cold applications. Mumps orchitis usually subsides in 7 to 10 days.

Epididymitis. Epididymitis is the most common of all the intrascrotal infections. Organisms usually reach the epididymis from established infection in the urine, urethra, prostate or seminal vesicles. Postoperative epididymitis may complicate all varieties of prostatectomy and urethral catheterization weeks or months after an operation, with recurrent episodes. In cases not responding to antibiotics, removal of the epididymis under local anesthetic is advised in the older age group. Routine use of modern antibiotics and improved surgical technique have reduced the incidence from 20 to 4 per cent.

Torsion of the Spermatic Cord. The peak incidence of torsion is in puberty, although it may occur at any age. Most patients, just before the onset of symptoms, have engaged in some physical exercise such as playing basketball, shoveling snow or riding a bicycle. The presenting symptom is intrascrotal pain radiating to the corresponding groin area. Palpation reveals a tender irregular edematous mass in the scrotum. There is pain only during the first hour or two, followed by marked tenderness of the testicle, nausea, vomiting and scrotal edema. One testicle may be twisted and drawn up much higher. Elevation and support of the scrotum for an hour does not help the pain in torsion, although it relieves it in epididymitis. The leg of the involved side is often held in flexion. This is an emergency and, if surgery is performed within 6 to 10 hours, a 70 per cent salvage rate is achieved. Only 20 per cent of testes are preserved if more than 10 hours have elapsed.

Inflammation of the spermatic cord may involve primarily the vas deferens or one of the other major structures of the cord. The vast majority of infections occur as a result of complications of prostatitis and especially involve the prostate and seminal vesicles.

Varicocele. Varicocele refers to any abnormal dilatation and tortuosity of the veins of the pamponiform plexus within the scrotum. A varicocele is secondary to an altered venous physiology of the blood supply of the testicle. It is generally believed that 10 per cent of young men have a varicocele. The age incidence is usually between 15 and 25 years of age at the time of onset and generally occurs on the left side. Varicoceles often disappear or become asymptomatic after sexual intercourse.

The most distressing disturbance associated with varicoceles is subfertility with regard to the motility and number of the sperm. This effect on spermatogenesis is due to vascular changes. The symptoms vary according to individual toleration of discomfort, but the main complaint is a dragging, pulling or dull pain in the area of the scrotum. The diagnosis is made by physical examination of the scrotum where the dilated and tortuous veins are readily palpable in the standing position (usually likened to feeling a bag of worms). If the onset is sudden or if the lesion is present on the right side, a complete study is indicated because of the possibility of retroperitoneal disease or pathologic obstructive lesions affecting the venous drainage of that area. The treatment of varicocele is usually conservative, with surgery reserved for more severe cases. Surgical ligation is superior to other types of surgery for varicocele and can restore fertility.

Cystic Diseases of the Scrotum. Sebaceous cysts of the scrotal skin are not uncommon. The tunica vaginalis may be distended with fluid under several conditions. If the contents are straw colored and uninfected, the lesion is called a *hydrocele.* A hydrocele is a common urologic finding usually secondary to an abnormality in the lymphatic drainage of the testicle, and is said to be present in 1 per cent of all male admissions to general hospitals. Ninety per cent occur after the age of 21. The hydrocele may be chronic, idiopathic primary or secondary and symptomatic. Symptoms depend on the size of the mass and the amount of tension created by the fluid within the sac (Fig. 98–5). Aspiration is a helpful palliative in certain elderly, poor-risk patients but rarely leads to cure of the hydrocele. Surgical incision is popular today and present-day technique is successful in probably all cases of primary hydrocele.

Treatment of acute secondary or symptomatic hydrocele is generally conservative, either for relief of symptoms or for aspiration. The patient is prescribed bed rest, with the scrotum elevated. Aspiration is used for the relief of pain or to obtain fluid and to clarify the diagnosis by allowing the scrotal contents to be palpated. Treatment is aimed at the underlying disease which may be orchitis or epididymitis. A spermatocele is an intrascrotal cyst resulting from a partial obstruction of the tubular system that transports sperm. Treatment is unnecessary for smaller cysts, although they may cause discomfort.

The Testis, Epididymis and Their Adnexa and Tunic. The testes are involved in the propagation of the species by producing spermatozoa and elaborating hormones, whereas the rest of the genital tract is concerned with the maturation, protection, nutrition and reactivity of the sperm. The scrotum regulates the environmental temperature around the testes.

During fetal development, either or both of the testes may be arrested in the abdomen, in the

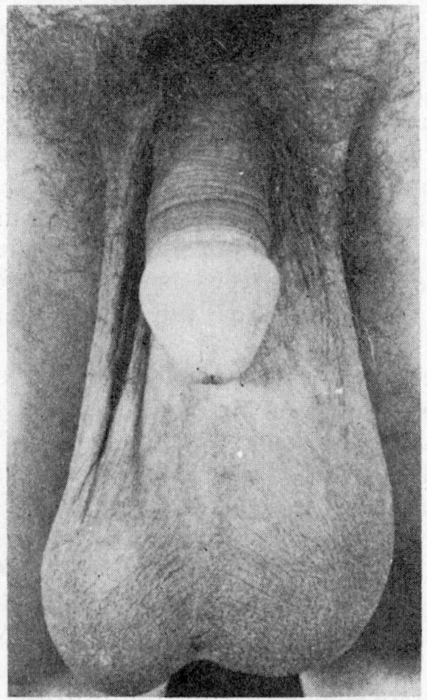

FIGURE 98–5. Hydrocele. Left hydrocele of moderate size with the testicle in a posterior and somewhat inferior position. The cystic hydrocele mass above the testicle was translucent to light. (From Campbell, M. F., and Harrison, J. H.: *Urology,* 3rd ed., 1970.)

inguinal canal or at the puboscrotal ring, a condition known as *cryptorchism.* When the testis remains in the abdomen, it cannot be palpated. In the inguinal canal or at the puboscrotal junction, the testis can be felt but is frequently smaller than might be expected. A maldescended testis is frequently associated with a congenital inguinal hernia on the same side. Bilateral maldescent may result in sterility. In bilateral cryptorchism, steps to correct the condition should be begun by three or four years of age. The administration of chorionic gonadotropin makes it unnecessary to wait until puberty to see if the testicle will descend. Early surgery is preferred, since maturation of the testis starts at about five years of age.

When the testes fail to secrete testosterone, puberty does not occur and *enuchoidism* develops. The genitals and prostate remain infantile, the voice is high-pitched, axillary and pubic hair are scanty and no beard hair develops. Skeletal proportions are abnormal. Medical advice should be sought if puberty seems delayed and secondary sexual characteristics are not developing.

Cancer. Both benign and malignant neoplasms that are found in the testis are diagnosed only by biopsy. The testis is usually enlarged, harder with softer cystic regions, and heavier than with orchitis or a hydrocele. The presence of metastatic lesions elsewhere would indicate that a nodule in the testis might be malignant. The rarity of testis tumor is the greatest obstacle to early diagnosis. Orchiectomy is usually the first step in its treatment.

NURSING CONCERNS IN HUMAN REPRODUCTIVE DYSFUNCTION

The nursing responsibilities in diseases of the male reproductive system demand that the nurse be highly aware of symptoms and psychologic problems resulting from dysfunction of the reproductive system, and thus encourage the patient and his family to seek early diagnosis and treatment. The nurse must recognize the need for rectal examination of all men over 40 in order to help prevent the high incidence of death from cancer of the prostate. The nurse can help the individual and his family to differentiate between the normal impairments of age and signs of dysfunction. Frankness concerning sexual history is important in discussing with the patient and his family what may be expected after surgery. Both husband and wife need to speak openly with the doctor or nurse concerning sexual adequacy.

Special care and respect need to be given to patients who are in the hospital for genital manipulation and surgery. These patients are likely to feel somewhat embarrassed and threatened by this invasion of the most private aspects of their lives. Encouraging decision making and showing interest in the patient as a person, while always important, are especially necessary in this situation.

Competence in management of the technical aspects of care and scrupulous attention to asepsis, combined with preparation and instruction concerning tests, routines and upcoming procedures or treatments, give the patient added reassurance in these awkward circumstances.

References

1. Baumrucker, G. O.: *Transurethral Prostatectomy Techniques, Hazards and Pitfalls.* Baltimore, Williams & Wilkins Company, 1968.
2. Campbell, M. F., and Harrison, J. H.: *Urology.* Vols. I and II. Philadelphia, W. B. Saunders Company, 1970.
3. DeGowin, E. L., and Degowin, R. L.: *Bedside Diagnostic Examination.* 2nd ed. London, The Macmillan Company, 1971.
5. Gordon, H. L., Scott, F. B., Carlton, C. E., and Beach, P. D.: *Current Controversies in Urologic Management.* Philadelphia, W. B. Saunders Company, 1972.
6. Jaffe, J. W.: Common lower urinary tract problems in older persons. *Working with Older People.* Vol. IV, Clinical Aspects of Aging. U. S. Department of Health, Education, and Welfare. Rockville, Md., July, 1971.
7. Krain, L. S.: Epidemiological variables in prostatic cancer. *Geriatrics, 28*:93–98, May, 1973.
8. Kaufman, J. J.: Urologic factors in impotence and premature ejaculation. *Medical Aspects of Human Sexuality, 1*:43, September, 1967.
9. Kunin, C. M.: *Detection, Prevention and Management of Urinary Tract Infections.* Philadelphia, Lea & Febiger, 1972.
10. Masters, W. H., and Johnson, V. E.: *Human Sexual Inadequacy.* Boston, Little, Brown and Company, 1970.
11. Mellenger, G. T. (ed.): *Urologic Surgery.* The Surgical Clinics of North America. Philadelphia, W. B. Saunders Company, 1965.
12. Mitchell, J. P.: *Urology for Nurses.* Bristol, John Wright and Sons, Ltd., 1965.
13. Tucker, E. C.: Clinical evaluation and management of the impotent. *Journal of the American Geriatric Society, 19*:180, February, 1971.
14. Weyrauch, H.: *Life After Fifty. The Prostatic Age.* Los Angeles, The Ward Ritchie Press, 1967.
15. Winter, C. C., and Barker, M. R.: *Nursing Care of Patients with Urologic Disease.* 3rd ed. St. Louis, C. V. Mosby Company, 1972.

CHAPTER 99

The Menstrual Cycle and Related Disorders

JUDITH ATWOOD

A thorough understanding of the anatomy and physiology of the female reproductive tract is essential for the nurse giving care to a variety of female clients. She has the opportunity to use this knowledge both in helping patients with problems in this area and in teaching the prevention of disorders of the reproductive tract. In addition, she may speak to a variety of groups about the female reproductive system, e.g., school children.

To help the nurse to gain this understanding, this chapter provides a review of the anatomy, a review of the menstrual cycle, a discussion of the menopause, and some consideration of menstrual abnormalities.

ANATOMIC AND FUNCTIONAL CONSIDERATIONS

Internal Female Genital Organs

The *ovaries* are located in the posterior lower pelvis, on both sides of the uterus, below the Fallopian tubes. They are contained in the posterior surface of the broad ligaments and are supported by several other ligaments which connect to the abdominal wall and to the uterus. The ovaries are approximately the size, shape and weight of an almond. Their surfaces are slightly lobulated and pale. Each ovary is composed of a cortex (the outer portion) and a medulla (inner portion). Follicles, each containing a developing ovum, grow and mature in the stromal part of the medulla, close to the abundant blood supply and the lymphatics. Mature follicles (those which are ready to erupt and discharge mature ova) and primary follicles (those which have not yet started growing) are found in the cortex.

At birth, there are some 200,000 to 400,000 follicles, each of which contains an oocyte (early stage ovum). They decrease in number as puberty approaches and gradually disappear at about the time of menopause.

The ovaries manufacture hormones which stimulate sexual desire, prepare and maintain the uterus for implantation, and have additional effects elsewhere in the body.

The *Fallopian tubes* (uterine tubes) connect the uterus to the ovaries. They are the usual site of fertilization (if it occurs) and convey either the fertilized or the unfertilized egg to the uterus. The tubes are approximately 4 inches long and are relatively thin. Each has four subdivisions: (1) Nearest to the ovary is the fimbriated end which has small fingerlike projections that "cup" over the ovary like a funnel; (2) next to this is the ampulla which makes up the major portion of the length of the tube and is where fertilization usually occurs; (3) following this is the isthmus, a narrow, short, wavy portion of the tube adjacent to the uterus; and (4) last is the straight intramural (interstitial) portion which passes through the uterine wall.

Cilia, or hairlike structures, which are part of the interior of the tubes, undulate to sweep the ovum toward the uterus. The walls of the tubes have a serosal covering, a muscular layer and a mucus lining; the latter contains the cilia. The tubes are supported by ligaments and supplied by blood from the uterine and ovarian vessels.

The *uterus* is a hollow, thick-walled, muscular organ which looks like an inverted pear. It is about 2 inches long, 2 inches at the widest portion, 1 inch wide at the cervix and between 1 and 2 inches thick. It is situated in the pelvic cavity slightly below and between the Fallopian tubes, almost at right angles to the vagina. The bladder is above and in front of it, and the rectum behind it. The uterus is attached to the bladder in front. It is separated from the rectum behind by a pouch (the "cul-de-sac of Douglas") which normally maintains the integrity of the two organs. It is normally movable in all directions.

The uterus is divided into three anatomic areas: (1) the fundus, (2) the corpus and (3) the cervix. The *fundus* or dome is the area between the insertion of the tubes. The *corpus* or body is the largest portion and is separated from the cervix by a slight constriction called the isthmus. The corpus is normally two times larger than the cervix in the adult, whereas in the newborn this relationship is reversed. The *cervix* attaches to and projects into the vagina for a short distance. The cervical opening into the vagina is termed the "external os" while the opening into the uterus is called the "internal os." The canal itself contains, among other things, glands which produce a mucin secretion.

The uterus has three functional layers: (1) the parametrium, (2) the myometrium and (3) the endometrium. The *parametrium* is the thin peritoneal and fascial covering of the uterus. The *myometrium,* which makes up the bulk of the uterus, is the muscular portion and is itself composed of three layers of mostly involuntary muscles. Blood supply to the myometrium comes from the uterine branch of the hypogastric artery and from collaterals from the ovarian and vaginal arteries; it is then distributed to the rest of the uterus but particularly to the endometrium. The *endometrium* has a type of epithelium, the superior two-thirds of which has a cyclic response to hormones, whereas the basal one-third does not. Menstrual flow begins here and it is at this site that the fertilized ovum is implanted.

The uterus assumes its position in the body cavity through the action of *six ligaments* and the *pelvic floor.* Innervation is provided by both the sympathetic and the parasympathetic divisions of the autonomic nervous system.

The *vagina* is a musculomembranous canal which connects the uterus, through the cervical opening, to the external genitalia. It has three layers: (1) the epithelium, (2) the fibrous connective tissue and (3) the muscular layer. The upper third of the vagina is attached to the cervix. At

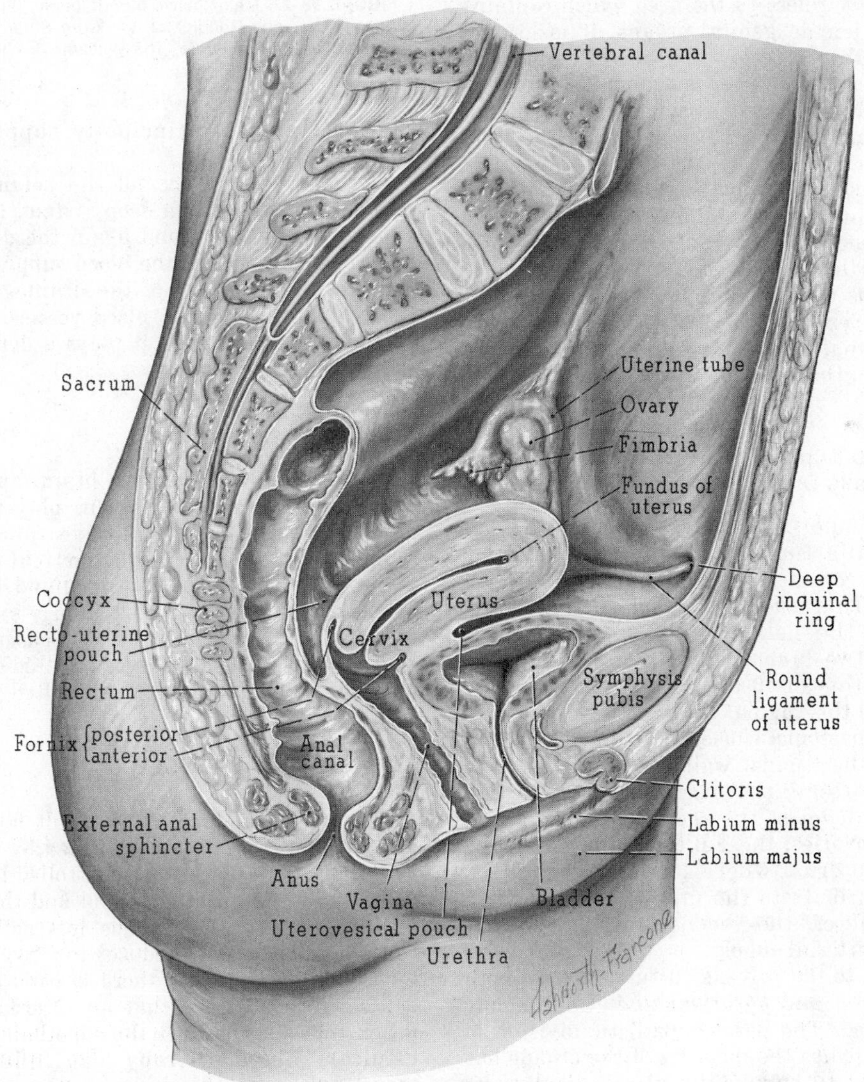

FIGURE 99–1. Female reproductive organs (*side view*). (From Jacob, S. W., and Francone, C. A.: *Structure and Function in Man.* 3rd ed. 1974.)

the level of attachment, there is a shallow space in front called the "anterior fornix." In addition, there are two "lateral fornices" and a deep "posterior fornix." The mucosa of the vaginal wall folds over in a rugal pattern which, in addition to the elasticity of the organ, allows it to be very distensible. The rugal pattern and the elasticity diminish with age during the menopausal and postmenopausal years. The bladder and the urethra are anterior to the vagina, and the rectum is posterior to its lower two-thirds. Thus, the vagina can easily become infected from urethral or rectal secretions, and vice versa.

External Female Genital Organs

The *perineum* refers to the area which contains the external female genital organs. It is located between the thighs, below the pelvic diaphragm and in front of the rectum and anus. The organs contained in this area play a role in sexual stimulation and in maintaining the integrity of the body from foreign materials.

The *vulva* contains the labia majora, the labia minora, the clitoris, the vaginal opening (with the hymen), sebaceous glands, the urethra, Skenes' ducts and Bartholin glands. The "vestibule" is the area of mucous membrane containing the urethral and vaginal openings, and is bounded by the labia minora. The anal region is posterior to this and is separated from the vulva by the perineal body.

Pelvic Blood Supply, Innervation and Lymphatic Drainage

The most important *blood supply* to the external genitalia comes from the internal iliac artery (the hypogastric), a division of the common iliac artery. This artery branches to supply the pelvic floor, the pelvic walls and the pelvic viscera. The two branches which are of primary relevance to this discussion are: (1) the uterine artery and (2) the vaginal artery. The former provides a rich, anastomotic network to the uterus, and the latter to the vaginal walls. In addition to the hypogastric artery, the ovarian artery (which arises at the level of the renal artery) supplies blood to the ovaries, the Fallopian tubes and the body of the uterus (where it joins the uterine artery to contribute to the uterine blood supply). In both instances, the venous drainage roughly parallels the arterial supply.

Innervation to the pelvic structures is from both the *sympathetic* and *parasympathetic* autonomic nervous system. The parasympathetic division of the system supplies the majority of the organs but does not seem to supply the uterus itself. The sympathetic system supplies most of the organs through a complex series of plexuses and branches.

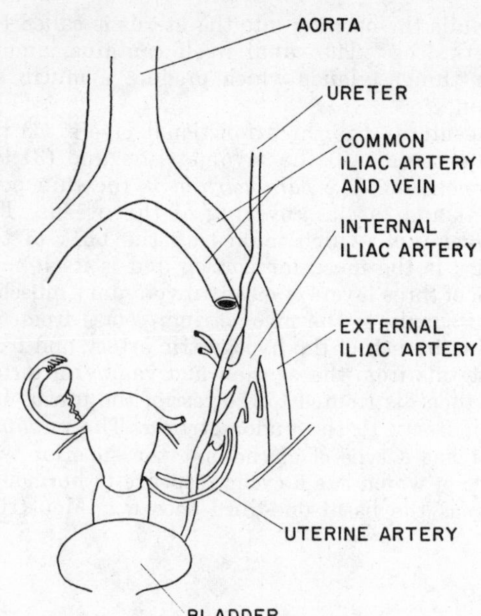

FIGURE 99–2. Major pelvic blood supply. (From Dilts, P. V., Greene, J. W., and Roddick, J. W.: *Core Studies in Obstetrics and Gynecology.* Baltimore, The Williams & Wilkins Company, 1971.)

The perineum is principally supplied by the pudendal nerve.

The *lymphatic system* of the pelvis is divided into a superficial and a deep system. It is a richly anastomotic network and again the drainage system roughly parallels the blood supply. There is a definite intermingling of the drainage from both the lymphatics and the blood vessels. This is important to recognize, as it plays a definite role in the spread of cancer.

Distant Structures

The hypothalamus (in the brain) and the pituitary gland (also in the brain) play roles in the regulation of the reproductive function of the genital organs and, more particularly, in the menstrual cycle. The thyroid gland and the adrenals may be involved, particularly in dysfunction of the menstrual cycle. Full discussion of these structures is beyond the scope of this chapter, and appropriate Units should be consulted.

THE MENSTRUAL CYCLE

The menstrual cycle of an adult female can be divided into two phases, separated by the event of ovulation. Both phases are controlled by hormones secreted by the pituitary gland and those secreted by the ovary itself. It is the interaction between these hormones that produces the "typical, normal menstrual cycle." Also, there is experimental evidence which suggests that an interdependent relationship exists between the hypothalamus and the pituitary gland, thereby also influencing the menstrual cycle. This is in keeping with the fact that the central nervous system is known to control the function of many glands and to adjust their function in relation to stimuli provided by the body environment. In addition to the influence on the pituitary by the hypothalamus, other areas of the brain have been identified that also seem to influence pituitary function and hence, potentially, the menstrual cycle. The menstrual cycle can then be conceptualized as a "hypothalamic-pituitary-ovarian cycle."

The Proliferative Phase

In the *ovary,* after the menstrual flow has begun, primary follicles (which contain an oocyte) and follicular cells begin to develop under the influence of FSH (follicle stimulating hormone) from the anterior pituitary gland. The cells surrounding the ovum, termed "thecal" and "stromal" cells, produce estrogens. The level of estrogen produced by these cells begins to rise and signals the pituitary to inhibit further production of FSH and to stimulate secretion of LH (luteinizing hormone). Then the two pituitary hormones act together to stimulate the further production of estrogens which, in turn, further inhibit the release of FSH from the anterior pituitary. The LH hormone becomes the dominant one and stimulates further maturation of the follicle. About two days before ovulation, one follicle, now called the "Graafian follicle," reaches full maturity. The reason why one particular follicle is chosen is unknown. The remaining follicles undergo degeneration (called "follicle atresia"). The Graafian follicle migrates to the cortex of the ovary. There it ruptures through the wall into the abdominal cavity and is picked up, usually by the fimbriated ends of the tubes.

In the *uterus,* changes are occurring primarily in response to the estrogen from the developing follicle. At the end of a menstrual flow, the endometrium of the uterus (which contains surface epithelium, glands, connective tissue, spaces and blood vessels) is very thin, much of it having in essence been "sloughed off" during the menses. Then estrogen begins the process of creating a new surface layer, stimulating growth of the glands and the stroma and changing the blood vessels which become progressively more coiled. The *cervix* also undergoes changes, the most important being that the amount of mucus secretion greatly increases just prior to ovulation. At the time of ovulation, mucus secretion is maximal and is a clear fluid which is receptive to sperm.

The *vagina* also undergoes changes. Estrogen causes proliferation and thickening of the vaginal epithelium, a change that is maximal at the time of ovulation. This whole phase of the cycle is thus dependent on the ratio of FSH to LH.

Ovulation

Increasing levels of estrogen cause a decrease in the secretion of FSH, thus allowing an LH flood which occurs over a 24-hour period and produces ovulation as well as begins the luteinizing process of the follicle cells. *Ovulation* occurs between 12 and 15 days before the onset of the next menstrual period.

The Secretory Phase

During ovulation, the ovarian follicle collapses and there is a temporary drop in the production of estrogens. Some hemorrhage occurs into the center of the ruptured follicle (where a clot forms quickly) and also occasionally into the abdomen where it irritates the wall and produces the characteristic transient pain that some women experience with ovulation. Occasionally this pain is mistaken for appendicitis.

Shortly before ovulation, the thecal and granulosa cells which line the follicle begin to hypertrophy and proliferate. This process is enhanced by the LH flood which occurs with ovulation. The clot, which formed in response to the hemorrhage when the follicle ruptured, is replaced with yellowish luteal cells containing lipids. These cells produce progesterone and eventually form the corpus luteum, or "yellow body," in response to stimulation from LH. As the corpus luteum is formed, increasing amounts of progesterone and some estrogen are produced.

Full maturity of the corpus luteum is attained about nine days after ovulation. If pregnancy does

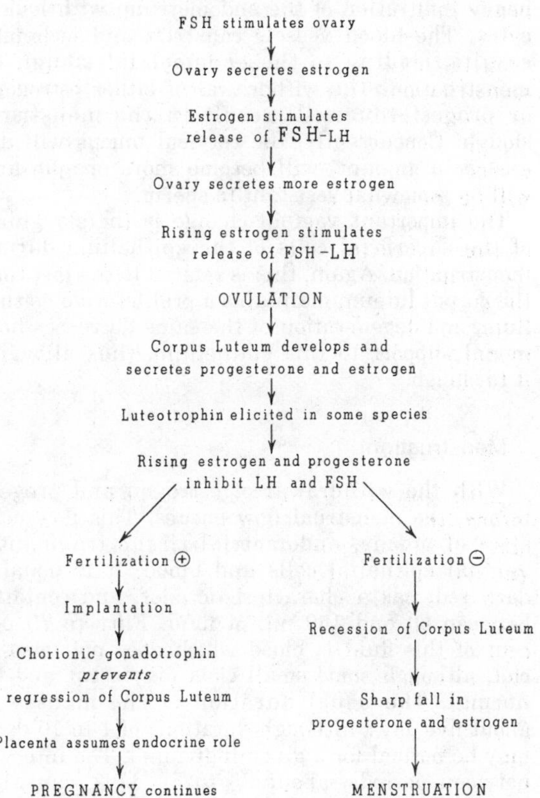
FSH stimulates ovary
Ovary secretes estrogen
Estrogen stimulates
release of FSH-LH
Ovary secretes more estrogen
Rising estrogen stimulates
release of FSH-LH
OVULATION
Corpus Luteum develops and
secretes progesterone and estrogen
Luteotrophin elicited in some species
Rising estrogen and progesterone
inhibit LH and FSH
Fertilization ⊕
Implantation
Chorionic gonadotrophin
prevents
regression of Corpus Luteum
Placenta assumes endocrine role
PREGNANCY continues
Fertilization ⊖
Recession of Corpus Luteum
Sharp fall in
progesterone and estrogen
MENSTRUATION

FIGURE 99-3. Diagram of the menstrual cycle. (From Tepperman: *Metabolic and Endocrine Physiology.* Year Book Medical Publishers, 1962.)

not occur, the corpus luteum begins to degenerate on or about the fourth or fifth day before the onset of the next menstrual period, with a concurrent drop in progesterone and estrogen production. The LH and FSH ratio are changed again and the pituitary is stimulated to increase its production of FSH to begin the cycle again.

The changes occurring in the uterus are intimately associated with and dependent on those occurring in the ovaries. Primarily under the influence of estrogens, proliferation of the endometrium peaks about two days before ovulation. During the secretory phase, the progesterone, in addition to the estrogen, promotes the secretory activity of the endometrium. This is characterized by edema of the stromal part of the endometrium, changes and enlargement of the glands, coiling and tortuosity of the arteries, and hypertrophy of the connective tissue. The endometrium is ready then for implantation of the fertilized ovum. This development peaks about seven or eight days after ovulation, which is the most favorable time for implantation.

If implantation does not occur, degeneration of the corpus luteum, with its concurrent decline in progesterone and estrogen production, causes retraction and degeneration of the endometrium. Two to three days before the menses, there is a heavy infiltration of the endometrium with leukocytes. The blood vessels constrict and ischemia results, leading to the endometrial slough or menstruation. The withdrawal of either estrogens or progesterone will result in the menstrual slough. Concurrently, the cervical mucus will decrease in amount, will become more opaque and will be somewhat resistant to sperm.

The important vaginal change is the sloughing of the superficial cells of the epithelium during menstruation. Again, this is related to the fact that the corpus luteum maintains a proliferative epithelium, and degeneration of the same decreases hormonal support to this epithelium, thus allowing it to slough.

Menstruation

With the withdrawal of estrogen and progesterone, the menstrual flow ensues. This flow consists of mucus, endometrial tissue fragments, vaginal epithelial cells and blood. It is usually dark red, has a characteristic odor, and contains between 60 and 150 ml. of fluid. Fifty to 75 per cent of this fluid is blood which does not usually clot, although some small clots may occur and be normal. The usual duration of the menses is about five days, although durations of 1 to 10 days may be normal for a given individual. The interval between periods, about 25 to 32 days, can also vary considerably and be normal. Most women develop a characteristic pattern, although there are normal women whose patterns are unpredictable. The menstrual pattern can be altered by climate changes, emotionally traumatic experiences, stress and acute or chronic illness.

The important menstrual abnormalities to be suspicious of are intermenstrual bleeding and prolonged, heavy bleeding. Either of these two problems should be investigated by a physician because, although they may not indicate an abnormality, they can be symptoms of more serious disorders, e.g., cancer.

The amount of bleeding can be assessed approximately by knowing that the average saturated perineal pad contains between 30 and 50 ml. of fluid and by keeping track of the number of pads used in 24 hours.

In the normal woman, the blood lost during the menstrual flow slightly decreases the hemoglobin level. If the woman already has iron-deficiency anemia, this loss aggravates the anemia. In addition to the medical therapy which the physician may have prescribed, the nurse should assess the nutritional status and patterns of the woman and counsel her appropriately. (Anemias are discussed in Unit XII).

Some women experience minor discomfort befor and/or during the menstrual flow (this is discussed more fully later in this chapter). It is important for the nurse to remember that attitudes about menstruation are formed during the early years of life. The nurse may be asked to present information to young people during these formative years. Two factors are important in giving such a presentation. One, and probably most important, is consideration of the nurse's own attitudes, beliefs and background so that she can be sure that her own "house is in order." The second is the awareness and understanding of the myriad of old wives' tales about menstruation. Questions may be asked by the children which reflect the cultural beliefs of the children's family. These questions require tactful but honest answers by the nurse. In any such presentation, the normalcy of the menstrual function should be stressed.

THE SEX HORMONES: OTHER FUNCTIONS

Before consideration of the menopause, some of the additional roles of the sex hormones should be discussed. Estrogen and, to a lesser extent, progesterone both have effects on the body besides those discussed in association with the normal adult menstrual cycle. In fact, the menopause is often considered as an "estrogen deficient state."

Estrogens (steroids) are manufactured primarily by the ovarian follicular cells, but a small amount is produced by the adrenal glands. The additional effects produced by estrogenic stimulation are primarily those seen at the time of puberty. These include: growth of the breasts, particularly fatty tissue deposition and pigmentation; fat deposition in the vulva; growth of pubic and axillary hair; growth and broadening of the bony pelvis; vaginal epithelial changes; and growth of the internal and external genitalia. Thus, the typical contours of the adult female are acquired.

In addition to the effects cited above, estrogens have an influence: (a) on maintaining positive nitrogen balance; (b) on calcium and phosphorus metabolism and retention of calcium in the bones; (c) on retention of sodium chloride and hence on sodium and water balance; (d) on the control of blood proteins and lipids; (e) on the vascular and skeletal systems; and (f) on thyroid function, insulin production and adrenal function. Because the exact nature of all these relationships is not always clear, there is some controversy regarding treatment with estrogen supplementation during the menopausal and postmenopausal years.

Progesterone also plays a role in sodium and water balance, although a minor one. It also influences nitrogen balance as well as breast function and body temperature during the menstrual cycle.

THE MENOPAUSE

A transitional phase called "the climacteric" heralds the onset of the menopause, some time between the ages of 45 and 50. Over a period of one to two years during the climacteric, the monthly menstrual flow occurs less frequently, is irregular and the flow is diminished in amount. After there have been no periods for one year, the "menopause" is said to have occurred. (Note: many people refer to the climacteric as the menopause.) During this transitional time, both ovulatory and anovulatory periods occur. Occasionally unplanned pregnancy results if women are not informed that contraception should be continued until the menses have been absent for at least six months.

The climacteric may be induced by surgical removal of the reproductive organs (including the ovaries) or pelvic irradiation in a woman of any age. In these instances, because of the rapidity of onset, unless replacement hormones are given, many women have a greater tendency for the accompanying signs and symptoms to be severe. Delayed onset of the climacteric, or that occurring at an age later than 50, is associated with a higher incidence of pathologic conditions and should be investigated by a physician.

The climacteric, with its gradual decline in ovarian function, leads to a relative estrogen deficiency state. This is only a "relative" deficiency state because, in addition to the estrogen produced by the adrenals, the ovaries apparently continue to produce estrogens in diminished amounts for up to 10 years. The pituitary gland, in response to the lowered estrogens, secretes gonadotropins, leading to a continuous elevation of the blood gonadotropin level. Therefore, the menopause is sometimes referred to as an "excess gonadotropin period" rather than an "estrogen deficiency state." In any event, many changes occur during this time of life which are related to a rebalancing of physical, hormonal and chemical patterns.

Approximately 85 per cent of all women experience some symptoms during the climacteric. However, only 25 per cent of these are distressed enough to consult a physician. The most prominently and consistently seen symptoms are those of the vasomotor group. Hormonal imbalances probably account for their occurrence. Hot flushes (involving the head, neck and upper thorax) and excessive perspiration especially at night are the primary vasomotor symptoms. Combined with the irregularity and final cessation of the menses, these represent the classic symptoms of the climacteric.

A myriad of other symptoms can occur which may or may not be related to the climacteric changes. These include: insomnia, headaches, palpitations, nervousness, apprehension, depression and other emotional symptoms, e.g., feelings of futility and uselessness. Emotional problems are severe in a small number of women; some of these women develop involutional melancholia and require psychotherapy.

Estrogen deficiency leads to other changes, in many instances a reversal of the changes which began at puberty. These do not all occur at the time of the climacteric; in fact, they often become evident many years later. These changes include: a redistribution of fat; a tendency to gain weight more readily; arthralgias and muscle pain; loss of elasticity in the skin; atrophy of the external genitalia; loss of subcutaneous fat within the labial folds; thinning of vaginal and vulvar mucosa; and atrophy of breast tissues. The vaginal changes may cause atrophic vaginitis (discussed in the next chapter). One of the last changes may lead to the development of osteoporosis with the presence of the "dowager hump" and loss of height. (Moreover, osteoporosis can contribute to the higher incidence of fractures, such as those of the hip, in this stage of life.) A tendency toward hypothyroidism (and less frequently, to hyperthyroidism) may result owing to the changes in glandular interrelationships.

Additionally, increasing evidence supports a relationship between estrogens and the function of the cardiovascular system. The statistical incidence of atherosclerotic vascular disease and its sequelae (coronary artery disease, stroke and hypertension) is much higher in postmenopausal women. It equals the incidence in men.

Clinical management of the patient who is having difficulty with the menopause is highly individualized and is based on an accurate assessment of the woman and her needs. Several types of drugs may be used, but regardless of what else is done, *patient education* and *reassurance* are always indicated.

Sedatives and *tranquilizers* may be prescribed and can be helpful with some of the symptoms, e.g., insomnia, nervousness and other emotional manifestations. *Hormonal substitution* with estrogens may also be used on a short-term basis to relieve the classic vasomotor symptoms of hot flushes and excessive perspiration. In some cases, these hormones also give some relief from other symptoms including palpitations, nervousness and other more typically emotional manifestations. Estrogens also help to relieve the pain from climacteric arthralgias and arthritis.

It is possible for the physician to demonstrate that the patient is estrogen deficient by doing a "maturation index." This is a test done on a smear of cells from the vaginal wall. Estrogen deficiency causes a shift in the types of predominant cells. Substitution therapy for a few months up to about two years is frequently undertaken with satisfactory relief of the symptoms, and then is discontinued gradually after the transitional phase of climacteric has ended.

Estrogen may at times be used to treat late manifestations of estrogen deficiency in some patients. These can include osteoporosis and atrophic vaginitis with or without urethritis. In osteoporosis, the estrogens seem to help maintain calcium in the bones, preventing further collapse of the vertebral column and further reduction in the patient's height. The latter is a good index of the success of therapy. With atrophic vaginitis and its attendant symptoms of burning, pruritus and discharge, a short course of estrogens will cause reepithelialization of the mucosa and, combined with other measures, may relieve the problem.

Much more controversial is the role of estrogen in the prevention of atherosclerosis and its sequelae and, consequently, in the appropriate uses of replacement therapy. There is increasing evidence that estrogens help to protect the woman from many cardiovascular problems before menopause. With this evidence, some physicians advocate treating all women with estrogens during the entire menopausal phase of life, or approximately for 38 years. Others feel that only those women with some form of atherosclerotic disease or those with a strong family history of these types of problems should be treated. Many physicians still feel that lifetime substitution therapy is not indicated except in a few unusual cases, because the long-term effects of estrogens have not been clearly defined, nor has it been completely proved that estrogens and the incidence of cancer are unrelated. In fact, when the patient has an estrogen dependent neoplasm or has been treated for one, estrogens are contraindicated.

As mentioned before, one of the more important aspects of the therapy is patient education and reassurance. The nurse can play a substantial role in both of these areas. In order to do so, she must plan to spend some time with the patient both as a sympathetic listener and in gathering information about the woman's life style and interests. In this way, she can help the patient to make realistic plans for the future. Among the considerations which the nurse should keep in mind in both her assessment and teaching are:

> The symptoms of the climacteric can be managed.

> The woman should understand the physiology of the menopause, and misconceptions should be clarified.

> The climacteric and its more common symptoms are normal and limited to the transitional phase.

> Overfatigue and other environmental factors can aggravate the symptoms.

> A normal sex life is still possible.

> Physical activity (including participation in sports) and development of new interests may help to alleviate tension and anxiety.

> Attention to nutrition and diet can prevent weight problems and feelings of fatigue.

> Annual medical check-ups including a "Pap test," can prevent or detect early cancer.

> This phase of life is often as long as the child-bearing years and the woman can be useful socially as well as to her family.

> A general improvement in health habits can cause the woman to feel better and to have a more optimistic outlook.

Regardless of the treatment plan devised, it is important for the nurse to help the patient to understand the plan and to adapt it to her needs. If drugs are prescribed, the nurse may be the one who teaches the patient about the drugs and their side effects, with special emphasis on the need for the patient on estrogen therapy to check with her physician should she experience vaginal spotting and/or bleeding. Although withdrawal bleeding can occur, postmenopausal bleeding may also be a sign of cancer and should be investigated.

MENSTRUAL ABNORMALITIES

Commonly encountered menstrual disorders include: abnormal uterine bleeding: premenstrual tension syndrome; and dysmenorrhea.

Dysmenorrhea

"Dysmenorrhea" literally means "pain with menses" and should be considered in two categories, primary and secondary. Primary dysmenorrhea is essential in nature and the etiology of the problem is not really known, although hormonal, intrinsic and psychologic factors usually are thought to participate in its development. Secondary or acquired dysmenorrhea is associated with pelvic disease; however, a cause-and-effect relationship cannot always be demonstrated.

The incidence of some form of pain with menstruation varies widely but occurs in about one-third of all women. Not all of these women have symptoms severe enough that they consult a physician. However, dysmenorrhea still remains one of the most common symptoms of gynecologic disorders seen in the gynecologist's office. Additionally, it is an economic problem, as it is one of the most common causes of absenteeism for women.

Primary or *idiopathic dysmenorrhea* usually does not occur until several years after the menarche, when ovulatory cycles occur more regularly. Anovulatory cycles rarely, if ever, cause primary dysmenorrhea. Usually the pain has its onset at the beginning of the menstrual flow or a few hours before, and lasts for intervals varying between a few hours to one or two days. It is generally most severe during the first day and gradually tapers off. During the maximal pain, the flow is scanty and increases as the pain diminishes. The pain is spasmodic and cramping in nature and is compared by some to the pain of labor. It occurs in the lower abdomen and occasionally may radiate into the groin, thighs and vulva. It may be accompanied by malaise, nausea and vomiting, chills, headache, diarrhea, flushing and the premenstrual tension syndrome. The pain occurs most commonly in the younger reproductive years, although it may persist into later years, particularly in the absence of delivery of an infant. In any event, dysmenorrhea is self-limited in nature, a fact that should be considered when treating a woman with this problem.

Despite the lack of firm knowledge of the etiology of primary dysmenorrhea, several factors are related. These include: psychologic factors; a low pain threshold; obstruction of the flow (as seen with cervical stenosis); vascular ischemia to the uterine musculature; and probably some hormonal imbalance. Factors which aggravate the condition include: a sedentary occupation, poor posture, poor personal hygiene, and constitutional illnesses such as anemia. Therefore, improving the health status and health habits is always indicated, and the nurse can be most helpful to the patient with regard to the latter.

There is an increased incidence of pain in high-strung, sensitive girls. It is not uncommon to find that these girls feel that menstruation is unhealthy or dirty. Although difficult to assess, fear and ignorance seem to contribute to enhancing the pain. The nurse, in her assessment of the health status of an individual, may observe clues which help her to understand the part that these various elements play in pain, and may be able to cautiously instruct such an individual. It is easy to assign the psyche total responsibility for pain with menses. However, this leaves too many factors unexplained. While the psyche cannot be considered the sole cause of menstrual pain, it is equally wrong to ignore its contribution to it. In treating the patient, the psychologic health status of the individual must be considered.

Treatment of primary dysmenorrhea presupposes that organic disease has been ruled out. Clinical care must be tailored to fit the individual. However, empathy and an understanding attitude on the part of the health care team members are always indicated.

Immediate treatment of a mild to moderate attack includes resting for one or two hours, aspirin, hot beverages and the application of heat to the lower abdomen. This regimen suffices for many and allows them to soon continue their usual activities. The nurse may assist the patient who finds this regimen satisfactory by suggesting that taking aspirin and perhaps hot beverages before the attack becomes acute may abort the attack. Therefore, at the first sign of pain or discomfort, the woman may be able to prevent further problems.

Other drugs that may be prescribed by the physician include: antispasmodics; vasodilators; tranquilizers; mild doses of psychic energizers; and occasionally, for very severe pain, narcotics in the form of codeine. Great caution should be taken with some of these drugs because of their addictive potential. The nurse may be the one who teaches the patient about the drugs. She should stress that the drugs alone should not be relied on, but that other measures designed to decrease or prevent the pain should also be continued. These include: (a) regular exercise for those with sedentary occupations; (b) waist-bending types of exercises just before the onset of the period; (c) improving posture when indicated; (d) improving dietary habits when indicated; (e) avoiding constipation; and (f) avoiding overfatigue and overexertion during the period preceding the flow itself. If the pain is mild, remaining active and interested in one's activities may also help.

With increasing frequency, hormones in the form of oral contraceptives are being prescribed to induce anovulatory cycles to prevent pregnancy as well as to treat dysmenorrhea. When the latter is the only goal, therapeutic trials of three to six cycles with the drug may be employed to see if the pattern of dysmenorrhea can be broken. If pain persists while the patient is following the pill regimen, it may mean that some underlying disease is responsible. In any event, after the therapeutic trial has been discontinued, caution should be exercised in evaluating the results, as ovulatory and anovulatory cycles coexist in some patients.

Additional treatment measures to which the physician may resort to eradicate dysmenorrhea are: (a) dilatation of the cervix (which may give up to six months' relief in some patients) and (b) presacral neurectomy (which is employed very rarely but may produce results in some patients).

Secondary dysmenorrhea characteristically appears somewhat suddenly, with the patient having a history of previously painless periods. The pain often starts two to three days before the menses appear and radiates into the entire abdomen, the small of the back and down the legs. It tends to be more constant and congestive in nature, without sharp cramps, and continues throughout the period and even for a short time thereafter.

It is usually associated with pelvic disease such as tumors, inflammatory problems, endometriosis, a fixed malpositioned uterus and other problems. When possible, it is treated by removing the cause either medically or surgically. In others, treatment must be palliative. In either case, the nurse's role is to see that the patient receives medical attention and to provide supportive care based on the treatment plan designed by the physician.

Premenstrual Tension Syndrome

This syndrome not uncommonly occurs in the patient who also has dysmenorrhea. However, it can occur as a separate entity, as can dysmenorrhea. In either case, for treatment purposes, it is more helpful to consider it separately.

The syndrome is characterized by some combination of the following symptoms: backache, abdominal distention, edema, headache, painful breasts, nervousness, restlessness, tremors, irritability, faintness and insomnia. The symptoms may be mild. In its severest form, the patient may closely approach a psychotic state with striking personality changes, and may be suicidal.

The syndrome may be difficult to recognize and the etiology is not well understood. Hormonal imbalances leading to fluid retention combined with emotional tension and disturbances have, however, been implicated in the etiology. With these hormonal imbalances, the patient may become somewhat hypoglycemic and feel weak and faint. This is exacerbated by poor dietary intake. One clue which frequently helps to establish the diagnosis is the appearance of a significant weight gain 2 to 10 days before the onset of menstruation.

Assessment and treatment are again aimed at the general health habits of the individual, the specific symptoms and the psychologic health of the individual.

General health habits, such as the consumption of excess coffee, alcohol, salt and nicotine, may exacerbate some of the symptoms. These agents should be decreased or eliminated during the latter half of the menstrual cycle.

Psychologic health problems and environmental stresses may respond to mild pharmacologic agents such as tranquilizers and/or energizers; however, these should be used only in conjunction with spending time with the patient for the purpose of listening to and trying to help the patient to find ways to modify the environment appropriately.

The premenstrual edema, abdominal bloating, headaches, breast tenderness, irritability and depression may respond to diuretic therapy during the second half of the cycle. This may be accompanied by a mild sodium restriction, or the latter alone may suffice. The nurse can assist the patient in working out a satisfactory diet with the sodium restriction and to recognize the need for potassium supplementation with many of the diuretics. Potassium supplementation almost always can be accomplished with increased dietary intake by eating bananas, drinking orange juice, and the like.

Abnormal Uterine Bleeding

Abnormal uterine bleeding includes a variety of menstrual disorders which are always symptomatic of underlying disease. All patients with any of the following symptoms should be seen by a physician for diagnosis of the cause and, in many instances, for a treatment program.

Amenorrhea

The *absence of menses* can be either primary amenorrhea or secondary amenorrhea. "Primary amenorrhea" refers to failure of menstrual periods to appear by the age of 18. Further discussion of this topic is beyond the scope of this book, and the reader is referred to books and articles dealing specifically with congenital abnormalities and sterility.

"Secondary amenorrhea" refers to failure to menstruate after regular menstrual cycles have been established. The most frequent causes in the young female of reproductive age are physiologic and include pregnancy and breast feeding. The other two instances in which amenorrhea is normal are before menarche and after menopause.

With these exceptions, amenorrhea presents a diagnostic challenge because of the numerous potential causes. It can be related to tumors or other abnormalities of the endocrine glands including the adrenal, the thyroid, the pituitary gland and the ovaries. Disease of the vagina and uterus can cause it, as can the so-called "hypothalamic causes" such as emotional stress, psychoses or fear of pregnancy. Chronic debilitating diseases, severe anemias, uncontrolled diabetes mellitus, tuberculosis, chronic nephritis, malnutrition and obesity may also cause or worsen secondary amenorrhea. Some drugs, including the contraceptive agents and phenothiazines, may cause either scanty or absent menses.

Thus, the primary nursing role is to assist the patient in procuring the needed medical attention. In addition, the nurse may wish to assess recent changes in the patient's life style or general health picture, so that she may be better able to assist the patient with appropriate counseling and teaching once the diagnosis has been established. It is important for the nurse to remember that dietary and general hygienic factors may be overlooked in the therapeutic plan, and assessment of these areas with appropriate intervention may help to ensure success of the medical therapeutic plan.

Dysfunctional Uterine Bleeding (DUB)

Use of this term implies that there is *an endocrine abnormality which causes improper regulation of the menses.* Unfortunately, DUB has been used by some to imply any abnormal bleeding associated with menstruation. Therefore, the nurse will need to pay close attention to how the term is being used in her particular situation.

Dysfunctional uterine bleeding is commonly manifested by an episode of profuse bleeding, but may also present as chronic hypermenorrhea (prolonged, excessive menses) or chronic polymenorrhea (excessive menses). Blood loss, both acute and chronic, is frequently a concurrent problem and requires evaluation and treatment as needed.

Other causes of abnormal uterine bleeding, beyond dysfunctional uterine bleeding, include: (a) those associated with reproductive problems, e.g., ectopic pregnancy and incomplete abortions; (b) those associated with diseases of the pelvic organs, e.g., tumors and inflammatory processes; and (c) those associated with disease of other body systems, e.g., blood dyscrasias and hypertension. Some of these problems will be discussed in succeeding chapters, while others have been covered in preceding chapters.

Menorrhagia

This term means *"excessive bleeding at the time of a normal period."* In the early reproductive years, it is commonly associated with endocrine problems and blood dyscrasias. Later, it is more commonly associated with tumors (including carcinoma) or inflammation of the uterus or ovaries. As has been pointed out, assessing the actual amount of blood loss can be a problem, especially because many women are unable to give a reliable history of loss and tend to either minimize or exaggerate it. Asking them to compare the number of pads used during the abnormal period with the number used during a normal cycle can be helpful. In a more controlled setting, it may be valuable to weigh the pads before and after use to estimate the blood loss. In addition, the usual tests for anemia may be performed.

Metrorrhagia

Bleeding between periods may occur in the form of spotting or as outright bleeding. The common causes are similar to those responsible for menorrhagia. Additionally, ectopic pregnancy, spotting with ovulation and "breakthrough bleeding," (which sometimes occurs with contraceptive pills) may be considered. In the latter instance, the dosage needs to be adjusted. The nurse should remember that irregular spotting may be the only early sign of cervical cancer.

SUMMARY

Each of these problems can indicate serious diseases and should be investigated. In the older female, these symptoms are not uncommonly associated with malignancy of the reproductive tract and, with early diagnosis and therapy, the results can be quite favorable. The individual treatment is related to the cause and, in many instances, will be discussed in succeeding chapters.

CHAPTER 100

Inflammatory and Infectious Problems

JUDITH ATWOOD

The female reproductive tract maintains its integrity through a variety of naturally occurring defense mechanisms. Inflammation and infection of the genital tract occur when organisms overcome the natural defenses or when these defenses have been disrupted. Most often, some combination of the two factors is responsible for the problem. Therefore, the usual treatment of problems is based not only on elimination of the cause, but also on increasing the resistance of the host. While the nurse may assist in the former by administering antibiotics and the like, she can play a particularly important role in improving host resistance by carefully assessing the health habits of the patient and modifying those which may predispose her to future problems.

The specific types of disorders presented in this chapter include leukorrhea, the most common symptom of these disorders; vaginitis and its more common causes; vulvitis and related causes; cervicitis; pelvic inflammatory diseases; venereal diseases; and nursing care. The most common causes of pelvic inflammatory disease today are venereal diseases; for this reason, this chapter ends with a presentation of the various types of common venereal diseases, with emphasis on those that are a major public health problem.

COMMON SYMPTOMS

Leukorrhea

"Leukorrhea" refers to any discharge from the vagina which is not bloody. The endocervical glands secrete a clear exudate which keeps the vaginal mucous membranes moist and clear. As it passes through the vagina, it may become cloudy and acquire a slight odor because of the addition of desquamated epithelial cells, leukocytes and normal vaginal flora. The amount of discharge normally varies from one woman to the next and, during the menstrual cycle, it is greatest at ovulation and just before the menses begin. Pregnancy, sexual stimulation and oral contraceptives also tend to increase the amount of discharge.

When there is a change in the amount (other than as mentioned above), color, character or odor of the discharge, it may indicate that something is wrong. Most of the inflammatory and infectious problems subsequently discussed are accompanied by a pathologic leukorrhea. The leukorrhea can be copious, malodorous and an abnormal color. It frequently leaks from the vagina, causing irritation and/or redness of the vulva and surrounding areas. It may also be accompanied by burning and frequence of urination, anal discomfort and pain in the lower abdominal region.

Vaginitis

Before discussing vaginitis and its causes, it is important to review the defense mechanisms protecting the vagina. A potential cavity, the vagina has normal flora which includes streptococci, staphylococci, diphtheroids, Doderleins' bacilli and other organisms which live in a symbiotic state with certain fungi. The pH of the adult vagina is acidic because of lactic acid which is formed from the glycogen, and this also contributes to its integrity.

Vaginitis or inflammation of the vagina occurs when there is a change in the normal flora, when the pH becomes more alkaline, when the invading organism is virulent, or when some combination of these three conditions occurs. It is a common problem experienced by most women at some time in their lives. It can be caused by a variety of insults including: congestion of the pelvic organs; mechanical irritation (foreign objects, e.g., tampons); chemical irritation (e.g., strong douches); vaginal infections; overmedication especially with antibiotics (destruction of flora); and long-term steroid therapy.

Vaginitis is almost inevitably characterized by a change in the normal vaginal discharge, which usually becomes profuse, odoriferous and purulent. It can be a stubborn, discouraging problem, and should be treated early and vigorously to avoid chronicity. Treatment is aimed at the cause, but attention to the overall health status of the individual is mandatory to ensure complete success. Rest and sleep, appropriate nutrition and exercise and meticulous personal (particularly perineal) hygiene are all factors which can affect the success of the treatment program.

A pelvic examination is performed to diagnose vaginitis and may be painful for the patient. Also, there may be some bleeding during or after the examination. The patient should be told this and provided with a perineal pad.

Simple Vaginitis. Simple vaginitis occurs when the resistance of the host is low, and may be seen in a variety of settings. The normal vaginal flora changes, and overgrowth of staphylococci, streptococci or contamination of the vagina with *Escherichia coli* may result. The symptoms include a profuse, yellow, mucoid discharge which may cause vulvar irritation and urethritis. The latter will be further irritated by voiding and defecating.

Treatment may include: systemic or local antibiotics, restoration of the normal vaginal environment with douches of a weak acid (one tablespoon of white vinegar in one quart of warm water), and beta lactose in the form of a suppository to stimulate the growth of bacilli. Sulfonamide creams may also help. In addition, after elimination, thorough gentle cleansing of the perineum from front to back should be done by the nurse, or by the patient if she is properly instructed. Sitz baths may relieve local irritation.

Atrophic (Senile) Vaginitis. Atrophic vaginitis occurs in the postmenopausal years when the atrophic, thin mucosa and thin alkaline, vaginal secretions provide an environment conducive to invasion by pyogenic bacteria (as in simple vaginitis). The symptoms include a discharge which may be blood-flecked, burning in the vagina, itching of the vagina and vulva, dyspareunia (painful intercourse) and, if secondary infection is present, burning with urination and vulvar excoriation.

Treatment is similar to that used for simple vaginitis. In addition, short-term local or systemic estrogen therapy or cortisone intravaginally may help to relieve the symptoms.

Trichomonas Vaginitis. Trichomoniasis is a common minor disorder which affects 25 per cent of all women and is caused by a protozoan, *Trichomonas vaginalis.* The initial source of the infection is unknown, but it is known that the organism prefers an alkaline climate and that changes in the vaginal flora make the woman more susceptible. The organism is transmitted sexually from one partner to another, making treatment of both partners necessary to effect a cure. The organism does not affect the uterus and tubes.

The symptoms may be minor and are usually so in the male. In the female, they include a heavy white or yellow, frothy, slightly malodorous discharge which can irritate the vulva, causing itching, burning, excoriation and maceration of the vulvar tissues. The vaginal mucosa is reddened and slightly edematous, and some women may experience dyspareunia. If the infection extends to involve the urethra, the woman may experience frequency and burning with urination. Anal involvement also may occur either asymptomatically or with a slight discharge. Bladder and anal involvement are more common when the infection has become chronic. Symptoms during the chronic phase tend to be minimal. The infection may be difficult to cure and remissions are not uncommon.

The diagnosis is established by obtaining a vaginal smear and looking for the organism under the microscope. The speculum used to perform the examination should be inserted without lubrication to avoid destroying the organism. The patient should be instructed not to douche before the examination which may be uncomfortable or painful. Reassurance and a calm attitude may help to allay the patient's anxiety and minimize the discomfort of the examination. Several infections may occur simultaneously, so other specimens may be obtained at the time of examination.

As with other problems, treatment is directed toward the offending organism and toward increasing the resistance of the host. Flagyl (metronidasole) is used with good results in many patients. Additional therapy can include: Floraquin tablets vaginally; Carbasone suppositories rectally (arsenic compound); Chlortetracycline in gelatin capsules; Argyrol or sulfonamides (bladder involvement); sexual abstinence or condoms; douches; sunshine, rest, good nutrition; tampons to absorb the discharge; good perineal hygiene; and proper douche technique.

Treatment should be continued through the menstrual period, as the vagina is more alkaline during this time of the cycle. With extensive cervical involvement, especially due to chronic or repeated infections, conization or removal of part of the cervix may be necessary. After therapy has been completed, both sexual partners should be reevaluated and treated again if necessary.

Monilial Vaginitis. Moniliasis is caused by a fungus, most commonly *Candida albicans,* and has a higher incidence in pregnant women, in women with uncontrolled diabetes mellitus, in those taking oral contraceptives, and in those who have taken long-term steroids or antibiotics. It also occurs in others. The source of the infection is unknown. The symptoms are similar to those of trichomoniasis. The discharge is characteristically thick or watery, white or yellowish, and curdlike. The vaginal mucosa is diffusely reddened and frequently covered with white patches which can be removed, although removal may cause bleeding.

Diagnosis is made by examining a smear of the white patches or exudate under the microscope. Cultures may also be obtained as indicated.

Mycostatin (nystatin), an antifungicide, is given systemically and, at times, in suppository form to treat this infection. Douches may be used except during pregnancy and attention is paid to strict perineal hygiene measures to avoid recontamination. In some instances, jellies, acid gels and/or gentian violet may be used locally in conjunction with, or instead of, nystatin. The gentian violet causes staining of the clothing, so perineal pads should be used and old clothing worn. The organism can lie dormant in the vagina until the environment is appropriate, thereby making the infection difficult to cure and tending to recur readily.

Vulvitis

Vulvitis is caused by direct irritation of the vulvar tissues or by extension of irritation from the vagina to the vulva. Many problems can cause vulvitis. Among the more common are skin disorders, inflammatory problems, infection, kraurosis, leukoplakia and vulvovaginitis.

The most common symptom related to vulvitis is *pruritus*. Common causes of this can include: senile atrophy; irritation secondary to vaginitis; uncontrolled diabetes mellitus (with high urine sugar); pediculosis and scabies; allergies; psychologic problems; cancer; ulcerative, glandular or skin lesions; systemic conditions; urinary incontinence; and poor perineal hygiene.

Treatment is based on determination of the cause. If the cause cannot be determined or the itching is severe, the following may provide some relief: calamine lotion; hot compresses; sitz baths; wearing light, nonrestrictive clothing; wearing well washed and rinsed cotton underclothing; avoiding feminine hygiene sprays; cleansing the vulva well especially after elimination; and keeping the vulva dry with cornstarch, hydrocortisone ointment and anesthetic sprays. Heavy sedation and a vulvectomy may be done in severe cases.

Skin disorders involving the vulva include many of those mentioned previously as well as chemical burns, irritation with harsh soaps, herpes, psoriasis, folliculitis and eczema. All are treated by removing the cause when possible and by promoting excellent perineal hygiene. Two causes deserving of special consideration include the mite *Sarcoptes scabiei,* and the louse *Phthirus pubis.* Both cause vulvar irritation and are transmitted through sexual contact, through infested bedding and from toilets. Both the patient and his environment must be treated to get rid of the organisms and their eggs.

Bartholinitis and inflammation of the other glandular structures of the vulva and of the cervix can be caused by a variety of organisms including the gonococcus, streptococci, staphylococci and *E. coli.* The infection moves in a retrograde fashion and involves the duct, resulting in edema and eventually in obstruction. The drainage from the inflamed gland cannot escape, causing swelling and abscess formation. Cellulitis develops in the surrounding tissues, producing more pain and systemic symptoms. The abscess may rupture spontaneously or may require incision and drainage to relieve the symptoms. After the acute episode, occlusion of the duct due to fibrosis and scarring will lead to retention of the secretions and dilatation of the duct which then becomes a cyst. The cyst is palpable, mobile and usually not painful. It is usually asymptomatic, except for symptoms related to its size, such as dyspareunia or pain on walking.

In addition to drainage of the abscess, treatment is with systemic antibiotics specific for the causative organism. Local heat may be helpful in promoting drainage. A cyst may require removal of the entire gland or marsupialization of the cystic duct.

The last two conditions to be discussed are *leukoplakia vulvae* and *kraurosis vulvae,* both of which affect the vulvar epithelium. The former is characterized by areas of thickened gray patches of epithelium scattered over the vulva and the perineum. Cracked areas in these patches set up an ideal medium for infection which can lead to ulceration and maceration of the involved areas. Eventually these areas may become malignant. Kraurosis can also become secondarily infected and is characterized by bright red, smooth, almost transparent, vulvar epithelium. It is most common in postmenopausal women and, with progression of the condition, the vulvar tissues shrink with constriction of the vaginal opening. Both disorders cause itching and soreness or pain, or may be asymptomatic. Both are diagnosed according to their appearance but, in the case of leukoplakia, a biopsy should be done to rule out cancer. Infection in both disorders is treated with the appropriate systemic antibiotic, and other manifestations are treated symptomatically as previously discussed.

Cervicitis

The cervix is a barrier that prevents the spread of infection from the lower to the upper genital tract. Constant exposure to potential pathogens introduced at intercourse, by douching, by trauma from instruments, surgical procedures, childbirth and other sources may result in inflammation of the cervix. This, in turn, can serve as a focus for the development of infection, both acute and chronic. If the infection is chronic, erosion will occur and repeated insults may lead to an abnormal healing process which is potentially malignant. Thus, evaluation of chronic cervicitis includes looking for a cancerous lesion.

Acute (and ultimately chronic) cervicitis is usually caused by streptococci, staphylococci, *E. coli* and the gonococcus. These organisms invade the inflamed cervical face or lacerated areas and spread from the epithelium to the endocervical glands. Here congestion and edema occur and later a discharge may be present. This is usually thick, viscid and white; with the vaginal pH more alkaline, propagation of the infection occurs readily. If the infection is minor or chronic, the patient may be asymptomatic or may have minimal symptoms.

If infection is acute, treatment should be prompt and vigorous to prevent spread (see PID) or chronicity. Identification of the organism from cultures or smears will allow appropriate antibiotic administration to begin. Chronic cervicitis may require cauterization or conization (removal of the affected part) of the cervix. After cautery, a vaginal discharge may be present which will last for up to three weeks. Care after conization is similar to that given after a D & C (see Chap. 103).

Nursing Care

In addition to the nursing care already discussed, the nurse's primary role is that of a teacher of these patients. She should assess the patients' understanding of the various measures prescribed and hence her ability to carry them out. Many women have never been taught to give intravaginal medications, to use the bathtub to take Sitz baths, or to douche properly. Particular attention should be paid to the latter, as many women douche or use feminine hygiene sprays to get rid of the unpleasant symptoms of a vaginal disorder which, in fact, should be treated. The nurse can help the woman to understand the importance of the symptoms and that overzealous douching can be harmful as it can destroy the vagina's natural resistance, thus making her more susceptible to infection. Feminine hygiene sprays can be dangerous, as they are frequently irritating. Lastly, the nurse can help the patient to understand the relationship between her general health and gynecologic problems.

Pelvic Inflammatory Disease

"Pelvic inflammatory disease" (PID) refers to ascending pelvic infections after they involve the upper genital tract (beyond the cervix). The gonococcus, staphylococci, streptococci and other pyogenic organisms are common causes of PID. The symptoms are those of a generalized infection. They include: general malaise, fever, chills, anorexia, nausea, vomiting and general aching. In addition, the patient usually experiences acute, sharp and severe aching on one or both sides of the abdomen or pelvis. This

pain is aggravated by defecation, and is accompanied by a heavy, purulent discharge which has a foul odor (the latter depends on the organism). The rapidity of onset of PID depends on the virulence of the infecting organism, the status of the pelvic organs and the general health status of the woman.

The infection, once introduced, travels along several routes (see Fig. 100-1). Tuberculosis, a rare cause of PID, travels through the blood and affects the Fallopian tubes and sometimes the ovaries, uterus and pelvic peritoneum. The symptoms are those of PID combined with those of pulmonary tuberculosis (see Unit XIV). It is treated with antituberculosis drugs, and the excreta are contaminated until the drugs have become effective.

The gonococcus and staphylococcus spread along the uterine endometrium to the Fallopian tubes where they cause an acute salpingitis (inflammation of the tubes) and thus the characteristic symptoms. The tubes become partially occluded and may drain pus, leukocytes and other debris into the pelvic cavity, causing pelvic peritonitis, or the material may form a pocket around the ovary, causing a tubo-ovarian abscess. The streptococci spread in a similar fashion, except that they tend to travel via the uterine or cervical lymphatics across the parametrium to the tubes or ovaries. Here they cause pelvic cellulitis and sometimes thrombophlebitis of the major pelvic veins, with the inherent danger of embolic episodes.

The third route is from the pelvic cavity itself. Organisms such as *E. coli* may be extruded from a ruptured viscus, causing peritonitis.

Treatment of the acute phase of PID may require hospitalization. Antibiotics appropriate for the of-

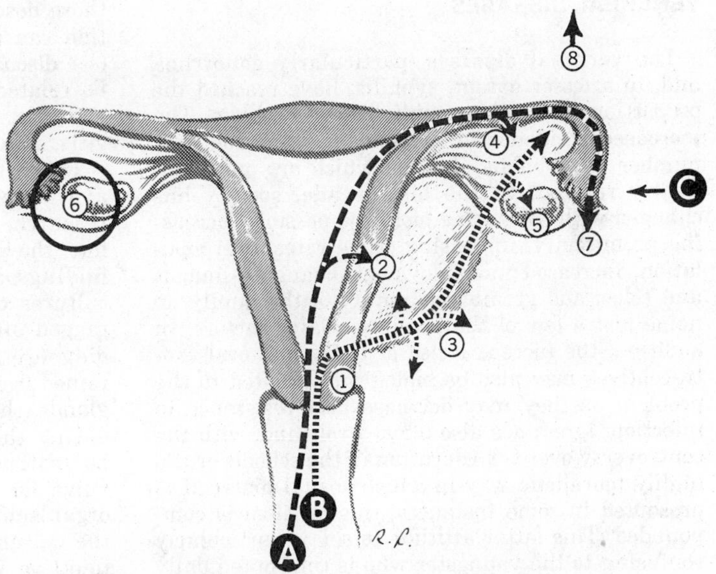

FIGURE 100-1. The routes of spread of PID: (A) staphylococcus, gonococcus; (B) streptococcus; (C) *E. coli*. (1) Endocervicitis. (2) Endometritis. (3) Parametritis. (4) Salpingitis. (5) Oophoritis. (6) Tubal ovarian abscess. (7) Pelvic abscess. (8) Systemic spread. (From Behrman, S. J., and Gosling, J. R.: *Fundamentals of Gynecology.* 2nd ed. New York, Oxford University Press, 1966, p. 173.)

fending organism are given in maximal doses. The woman is placed in semi-Fowler's position to promote downward drainage. Heat to the lower back or abdomen or Sitz baths may decrease the pain as do analgesics and sedatives. Douches should be avoided to prevent spreading the infection. The amount, color, odor and appearance of the vaginal discharge are recorded and frequent perineal cleansing should be done. Depending on the organism, the patient may be isolated. After treatment, she should avoid intercourse until the drainage is gone, and until her physician gives permission to resume sexual activity. If abscesses form, they may need to be drained if they do not do so spontaneously. One of the most important factors that the nurse must consider in caring for a patient with PID is how the patient feels about the disease and about herself. As PID is often caused by venereal diseases, there may be guilt feelings about contracting the illness, along with other related family problems. In any event, the nurse will need to be sympathetic and understanding and to carefully examine her own attitude about such problems.

Chronic PID can occur if the acute phase of the illness does not respond to therapy or if therapy is inadequate. The symptoms include chronic pelvic discomfort, disturbances of menstruation, constipation, malaise and periodic recurrence of the acute symptoms. Sterility, one of the more serious complications, is the result of destruction of part of the tubes and loss of their patency. It is usually irreversible.

Treatment is aimed at removing the offending organism and improving the general health status of the woman. If treatment is unsuccessful, removal of the pelvic organs may be necessary.

VENEREAL DISEASES

The venereal diseases, particularly gonorrhea and, to a lesser extent, syphilis, have reached the proportions of a major public health problem. The increased incidence of these diseases is due to a number of problems, some of which are only incidently related. In the last decade, society has changed with increasing mobility, possibly increasing promiscuity, increasing crime rates, overpopulation, increased unemployment, changing images and roles, and greater instability of the family, to name just a few of the possibly related factors. In addition, the increased use of IUD's and oral contraceptives may also be biologically related to the problem as they may decrease host resistance to infection. Ignorance also plays a role and, with the controversy over sex education in the schools or the highly moralistic way in which sexual material is presented in some instances, this problem is compounded. This latter attitude to sex is particularly confusing to the youngster who is confronted daily by the "glamorous" approach to sex advocated by the media. Only recently have the media and other organizations begun to deal with education about sex and venereal diseases in a manner calculated to appeal more to, and hence educate, the young.

The nurse needs to be well informed about sex and venereal diseases, and to separate morality from the educational process if she is to help combat these major public health problems. The following information is presented to provide some of the basic facts about these diseases. The nurse working with patients who have these diseases or who are at high risk of contracting them may wish to consult other textbooks to increase her knowledge on this subject.

Gonorrhea

Gonorrhea (also called whites, the drips, the strain, clap and the dose) is the most common reportable communicable disease in the country today. There are a number of reasons for this, one of which is that up to 90 per cent of infected women are asymptomatic or only mildly symptomatic, thus providing a large pool of carriers. Caused by the organism *Neisseria gonorrhoeae,* the incubation period of the disease in women is not definitely known but is thought to be between two and seven days. The infection is transmitted sexually in almost all cases, the exceptions being that a child may develop it when in close contact with the discharge from her infected mother, and medical personnel who have lacerations may develop it if they are not careful in disposing of infected discharges. However, these instances are rare, as the organism does not survive very long outside the body.

The initial infection may involve the vestibular glands, the urethra, the anus and the endocervix. The adult vagina is resistant to the infection, although the prepubertal child's is not. Symptoms, when present, can include a red, swollen and sore vulva; a minor, purulent, yellow discharge; dysuria; frequency; pruritus; and a rectal discharge. The Bartholin glands (and other vestibular glands) may be involved, with symptoms such as those described earlier in this chapter. The infection can progress to pelvic inflammatory disease (see discussion of PID) and the first symptoms may be related to this problem. Sequelae can include arthritis, joint inflammation, endocarditis, meningitis, skin lesions and sterility.

There are no blood serology tests currently available to establish the diagnosis (although research is being done to develop one). Therefore, the diagnosis is based on the history, physical findings and identification of the organism on cultures or smears. Occasionally, the fluorescent tagged antibody method is used to establish the diagnosis. The cultures or smears should be obtained from the cervix, the urethra, the vestibular glands, the ducts and the anus. They can be done during the menstrual period. The woman should be instructed not to void, douche or clean the vulva for two hours before the examination. The organism may disappear after a short time and the cultures may thus be sterile even though the infection is still present. The nurse should know that syphilis and gonorrhea may coexist and that the diagnostic tests differ. This is important, as many patients erroneously believe that the blood study that was done for syphilis also rules out gonorrhea.

Gonorrhea is treated with large doses of a short-acting penicillin. The dosage scale for women is larger than that used to treat men. If the patient is allergic to penicillin, or the organism is penicillin resistant, alternate antibiotics can be used successfully. After treatment is completed, repeat cultures should be taken. Those who have been exposed to the infection are also treated with large doses of penicillin to avoid its development. It is important to note that the doses are much greater than those used to combat other infection, as some patients may believe that an antibiotic taken for another problem will cure venereal disease.

Syphilis

Syphilis (bad blood, lues, pox, syph), while less common than gonorrhea, has potentially severe late complications including blindness, insanity, paralysis, heart disease and death. It is caused by *Treponema pallidum* and is transmitted through sexual intercourse, although rarely infection of an open wound is possible. Syphilis can occur alone or in conjunction with other venereal diseases, and has an average incubation period of one to four weeks. There are four stages of the infection: primary, secondary, latent and tertiary.

The *primary stage* is characterized by the development of a small, painless chancre (ulcerative lesion) or group of chancres which have a serous discharge that is highly contagious. Local lymph glands may swell. The chancre is usually located on the genital organs and is seldom seen in the female. It heals spontaneously in about 4 to 10 weeks and the disease progresses to the secondary stage.

The *secondary stage* appears about two to four weeks after the chancre disappears, and lasts for two to four years. The symptoms, which may be intermittent, include a macular or papular rash, fever, malaise, headache, weight loss, sore throat, muscle and joint aching, and lymph node enlargement. If the rash becomes infected, pustules develop and, with chronic irritation, these areas may develop into condyloma lata. The latter tend to grow together and have a moist surface. They, along with the fluid exudate from the rash, are contagious. The symptoms disappear and may recur intermittently.

The *latent phase* is asymptomatic. It occurs approximately two or more years after the appearance of the primary lesion and can last for up to 50 years.

The *tertiary phase* is rare, but devastating. The complications developed at this time are irreversible. There may be an ulcer (a gumma) which is usually located on the vulva but can appear elsewhere. Other manifestations may include: chronic inflammation of the bones and joints; cardiovascular problems including valvular involvement and aneurysms; skin lesions; and central nervous system problems including insanity, slurred speech, ataxic gait, paralysis, judgment loss and senility. While this stage is not infectious, if the disease is not treated, it may be terminal.

The diagnosis is based on a careful history, a search for the characteristic findings and laboratory studies. Once lesions have appeared, they can be scraped, and organisms may be located with the darkfield microscope technique. The VDRL, a nontreponemal blood test, will not be positive until the organism has been present in the body for four to six weeks and, at times, remains positive after treatment. In addition, it may be falsely positive in the presence of some febrile illnesses, autoimmune diseases and collagen diseases. In these instances, the treponemal tests such as the FTA-ABS test may be helpful, although once they are positive they remain so, and therefore are not useful in evaluating the success of therapy. In the late stage, the spinal fluid may be examined for characteristic findings.

Treatment is accomplished with large doses of long-acting penicillin or another antibiotic if the individual is sensitive to penicillin. In the last stage, the treatment is prolonged. Contacts are treated in the same manner as those with an early infection.

Other Venereal Infections

There are three other venereal diseases which will be discussed briefly as they are more commonly found in the tropics and their incidence in the United States is low. *Granuloma inguinale* is a chronic infection which occurs more commonly in those with poor hygienic habits. It is characterized by the development of papular lesions on the genitalia which become ulcerated and cause tissue destruction. It is treated with antibiotics and may be difficult to differentiate from cancerous lesions. Discovery of Donovan's bodies in the lesions establishes the diagnosis.

Chancroid is caused by *Hemophilus ducreyi* and is also associated with poor hygiene. A pustular ulcer develops, leading to ulceration of the vulva. This is often very painful but may heal spontaneously. The diagnosis is difficult to establish, and treatment is with antibiotics.

Lymphogranuloma venereum is caused by a virus and may cause systemic symptoms. It is characterized by the development of a small pustule followed by involvement of the lymphatics along with vulvar edema. Eventually ulceration and extensive scarring may occur with marked deformity of the external genitalia. The diagnosis is based on the results of a variety of tests and treatment is with sulfonamides or antibiotics.

Nursing Care

This section could be more appropriately titled "health care," as nurses have made broad and valuable contributions to the attempts to eradicate these pandemic infections. The focus of the attack on venereal diseases has been twofold: to educate the public about these diseases, and to identify and treat more of those who are infected. These goals have provided direction to a wide variety of community and national programs in which health care professionals have collaborated with lay people. In some instances, the nurse has played a pivotal role by helping to identify the needs of the public as well as by helping to meet them. In doing so, nurses have stepped out of more conventional roles and been more facile in working as team members, thus making it impossible to provide a fixed approach to nursing care.

Success in meeting the above objectives has made it mandatory for health care personnel to examine their own attitudes toward sexuality and sexual behavior, and to become more open-minded in approaching clients or potential clients. While the individual's own moral values are important in guiding his own behavior, it has been found that these attitudes interfere with the exchange of information that must occur between the client and the health care worker. This biased attitude can be either obvious, when the client feels he is not being heard or accepted and thus will not give information, or more subtle, when the professional fails to detect clues given by the client, which should be followed up. Thus, mutual acceptance or trust is implicit in a successful relationship and requires tolerance of each other's personal, sexual and moral standards.

Besides actually treating the client, which she often does, the nurse also obtains information from the patient as well as gives him information about his disease. Both jobs are difficult, but the former may require that the health care personnel be extremely skilled at interviewing. Skilled epidemiologists spend many hours in this type of interviewing and they can often provide valuable clues as to how to deal successfully with these patients. The information to be obtained (not necessarily by the nurse) includes: a comprehensive sexual history; a history of sexual contacts; a history of previous infections, their treatment and test results; a history of parental infections; a history of recent use of antibiotics; a history of allergy to antibiotics (including manifestations); and a history of any signs or symptoms.

After the organism or organisms have been identified, the patient is usually treated with large doses of penicillin intramuscularly. Before administering the injections, the nurse should again check for penicillin allergy. The patient should then be observed for a short time to be sure she does not react badly to the drug. Additionally, the nurse may suggest that the patient do mild exercises to decrease the pain at the site of the injection.

The third important aspect of the treatment program is educating the patient. There are many myths about venereal diseases and many patients need solid factual information so they can avoid reinfection. The following should be included in the instructions: modes of transmission; incubation periods; signs and symptoms; asymptomatic problems; methods of treatment; consequences of lack of treatment; and consequences of repeated infections.

More specifically, examples of the questions patients may ask include:

Q: Will treatment protect me from getting this again?

A: No, immunity to reinfection is rare if it indeed exists.

Q: Can I resume my sex life?

A: It is better to wait for a few days or a week to be sure that the infection is gone.

Q: Do I have to come back?

A: We would like to see you again in ________ to be sure that you are cured (especially with the resistant strains of gonorrhea).

Q: Since I didn't have any symptoms this time, how will I tell if I have this again?

A: When you have your periodic "Pap" test with the gynecologist, you can ask him to check you for gonorrhea and syphilis too. (Modify this answer for the male patient.)

These are only a few of the questions which the patient may ask or be curious about but fail to ask. In all of her contacts with the patient, the nurse should continuously assess the patient's understanding of the infection and provide information as needed. To do this well, the nurse will need to extend her knowledge beyond what is possible to cover in this text.

Moreover, the nurse will need to extend her knowledge about the kind of information that various types of people want if she is to participate in community education programs about venereal diseases. These lectures are more in demand and requests may come from various groups including men's groups, women's groups, schools, the Boy Scouts, the Girl Scouts and others. To meet the needs of each requires versatility and understanding of the type of information needed, as well as an appreciation of the learner's maturity.

In summary, the nurse who works with patients who have contracted a venereal disease will find a variety of needs which she can fulfill besides the administration of drugs used to treat these patients. Because sexuality is such a private matter, the nurse will need to examine her attitudes toward sexuality and to be nonjudgmental in her approach to such patients. In this way, nurses can provide a valuable service in educating and comforting the patient during what may be a very distressing and guilt-ridden period in his life. Through these person-to-person contacts, we can hope to rid society of the many problems caused by venereal diseases.

CHAPTER 101

Benign Gynecologic Conditions and Problems

JUDITH ATWOOD

One important consideration in caring for the patient with a benign tumor of the genital tract is the malignant potential inherent in several of these tumors. Despite the fact that the malignant potential is frequently very low, patients are often concerned about the possibility of having a malignancy. These are important concerns to take into account when planning care. Malignant changes are often asymptomatic until late in the course of the disease after metastasis has occurred. (See Unit VII for further discussion of cancer.) In addition to benign tumors of the lower genital tract, several conditions involving the organs in this area are discussed, e.g., endometriosis and fistulas. These conditions bear a close relationship to sexuality and the reproductive function of the affected woman. Therapy may involve disruption of one or both of these functions, and it is important for the nurse to consider these factors in planning individualized care.

The last part of the chapter discusses pelvic relaxation and displacement. Again the areas of sexuality and reproductive function must be considered in planning care to meet a patient's needs. Moreover, pelvic relaxation and/or displacement may be caused by malignancies, may be aggravated by malignancies, or may be the result of treatment to eradicate malignancies.

BENIGN TUMORS OF THE LOWER GENITAL TRACT

Benign tumors of the lower genital tract (below the cervix) are relatively uncommon and may result from chronic inflammation or from a variety of other causes. Benign tumors are classified as either cystic or solid tumors. In Chapter 100, some of the cystic tumors were discussed. These included granulomas from syphilis, granuloma inguinale and lymphogranuloma venereum. One of the glandular cysts discussed was the Bartholin cyst. None of the solid tumors have been or will be individually discussed because they occur infrequently. Suffice it to say that they (solid tumors) are tumors which involve either endometrial or supporting tissues. Both types of tumors have a low malignant potential. Further details about particular types of tumors can be obtained from specialty textbooks.

Questions which the nurse may need to answer in caring for a patient with a benign tumor of the lower genital tract include: (a) the malignant potential of the tumor, (b) the type of symptoms produced by the tumor, (c) the type of therapy planned, and (d) the expected results of therapy. If symptomatic, many of these tumors are surgically excised. Nursing care is then similar to that given after any minor surgical procedure, with special attention to aseptic perineal care to maximize healing. (See Chapter 103 for nursing care related to specific gynecologic procedures.)

BENIGN CONDITIONS INVOLVING THE UTERUS

Uterine Myomas. *Uterine myomas are the most common tumors of the female genital tract,* occurring in more than 25 per cent of all women over 35. Frequently these benign tumors are asymptomatic. Symptoms which do appear are generally related to the size (very small to very large), location (see below), or number of tumors (they tend to be multiple). Additionally, abnormal bleeding, often hypermenorrhea, may be present. This is true because myomas are thought to be hormone (estrogen) dependent, growing slowly during the reproductive years (except during pregnancy) and atrophying after menopause.

The myomas are known by a variety of *names* (some of which are not technically correct) related to the tissues involved. Some of these are fibroids, fibromas, fibroleiomyomas, leiomyomas, fibromyomas, and fireballs. These tumors are made up of connective tissue and muscle in varying proportions.

Myomas may be *classified according to location,* those occurring in the body of the uterus being most common. There are six types:

> *Intramural*—in the uterine wall, surrounded by myometrium. These tend to increase the size of the uterus and may cause bleeding and dysmenorrhea.

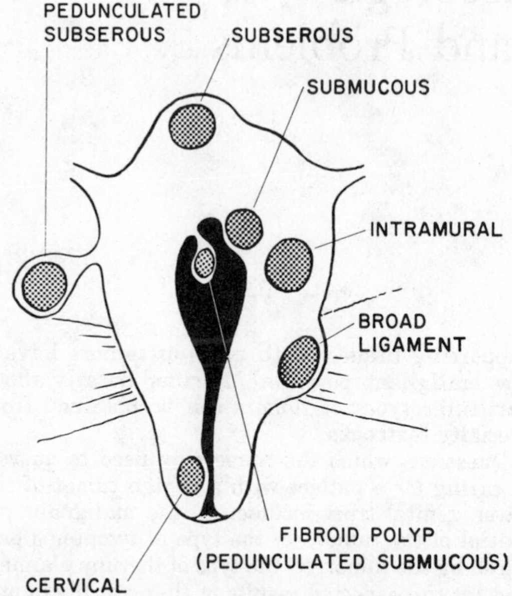

FIGURE 101–1. Diagram showing some locations of myomas. (Modified from Dilts, P. V., Greene, J. W., and Roddick, J. W.: *Core Studies in Obstetrics and Gynecology.* Baltimore, The Williams & Wilkins Company, 1971.)

> *Submucous*—directly under the endometrium, involving the endometrial cavity. These may cause prolonged bleeding and cramps and may become pedunculated (grow on a stalk) and protrude through the cervix.

> *Subserosal*—on the outer surface (under the serosa) of the uterus. These tend to become pedunculated, "wander" (see below), and are likely to be multiple and large with symptoms such as backache, constipation, and bladder problems.

> *Wandering or parasitic*—occurs when a myoma which is pedunculated twists on its pedicle and "breaks off." It then attaches to other tissues, particularly the omentum to obtain a blood supply.

> *Intraligamentary*—implants on the pelvic ligaments and may displace the uterus or involve the ureters.

> *Cervical*—occurs infrequently. May obstruct the canal.[7]

Secondary changes can occur in myomas (all six categories). Types of changes can include:

> *Hyaline degeneration*—occurs when the tumor outgrows its blood supply.

> *Cystic degeneration*—tends to follow hyaline degeneration. The tumor becomes liquefied and ultimately cystic.

> *Calcification*—more common in large tumors.

> *Infection*—more common in submucous tumors.

> *Sarcomatous (malignant) degeneration*—rare. It should be suspected in rapidly enlarging tumors, in recurrent tumors, and when hemorrhage occurs in the presence of a known tumor.

> *Red (carneous) degeneration*—usually occurs during pregnancy. This type may be accompanied by acute pain over the area of the myoma, fever, tachycardia, nausea, vomiting, and abdominal rigidity.

> *Fatty degeneration*—rare.

> *Acute torsion of the pedicle*—leads to acute disruption of the blood supply, with gangrenous changes in the myoma and symptoms of an acute abdomen. (See Red carneous degeneration above.)[7]

Symptoms occur in only about 50 per cent of patients with myomas. Large tumors may cause a mass or general enlargement of the lower abdomen with associated pelvic heaviness. Abnormal bleeding, which may be present, is usually due to both the hormonal effects and the increased surface area available to bleed. When excessive bleeding is present, the physician may do a dilatation and curettage to rule out the presence of a malignancy. Anemia may be present owing to blood loss. With infection or torsion of a pedicle, pain may be present and is frequently severe. Otherwise, little pain is experienced with myomas except for dyspareunia, which occurs with cervical myomas, and occasionally dysmenorrhea. Pressure on surrounding organs may cause retention of urine, constipation, varicosities, pelvic discomfort, and edema. Additionally, abortion and infertility occur somewhat more frequently in patients with myomas, but it is difficult to tell whether the myomas cause these problems or vice versa.

The *treatment* plan is formulated by considering the symptoms, the patient's age, the location and size of the tumor(s), the onset of complications, and the patient's desire to have additional children. If the patient is nearing menopause and the uterus is smaller than 12 weeks' gestation in size, the physician may elect to follow the patient closely (every three to six months) and simply allow the menopause to "solve the problem." Although malignant degeneration is rare, should such a woman show a rapid increase in the size of the myomas, more definitive therapy is necessary. Younger, asymptomatic women may also require no therapy. However, when definitive therapy is indicated, it typically includes myomectomy (removal of the tumor without the uterus) if the tumor is small, or hysterectomy (removal of the uterus). Irradiation has been used rarely if the patient is unable to undergo surgery.

Endometriosis. Endometriosis is characterized by the presence of aberrant endometrial tissue outside the uterine cavity; while this tissue is usually confined to the pelvic cavity, extrapelvic locations have been found. Several theories as to the cause of this condition have been offered, but to date none has provided a satisfactory explanation. What is known is that the aberrant tissue is hormone dependent and subject to the same cyclic changes that occur in normal endometrial tissue. The highest incidence of this condition occurs in women between the ages of 25 and 45 who have never been pregnant and who are in the higher socioeconomic groups.

Aberrant endometrial tissue may be found in: (a) ovaries (most common location), (b) tubes, (c) ligaments, (d) cul-de-sac, (e) bladder or rectum, (f) rectovaginal septum, (g) appendix, and (h) bowel. Moreover, it may be found in the uterus itself, where it causes "adenomyosis" (see below).

Rarely, the tissue may be found outside the pelvis in surgical scars, the lungs, the extremities, or other areas.

Because aberrant endometrial tissue responds to hormonal stimulation, it may bleed. This can cause problems, particularly when there is no outlet for the blood. When this occurs, typical "chocolate cysts" may develop on the surface of the ovaries. Because of this "menstruation" property, the disease may be considered to be self-limited. With regression of ovarian function during the menopause, the tissue atrophies. It also regresses during pregnancy. Therefore, women who desire children are encouraged to become pregnant. Malignant changes are possible, though rare.

Because of the variety of locations which may be affected, the *symptoms* are often bizarre and vague, and the woman is thought to be neurotic. Also since the disease progresses slowly, there may be no symptoms. Characteristically the symptoms, if present, are exacerbated and sometimes incapacitating during the menstrual period. Symptoms can include: secondary dysmenorrhea starting before the menses, general discomfort, a "boring" pain, backache, rectal pain, and persistent lower abdominal discomfort throughout the cycle. Others symptoms are dyspareunia, menstrual irregularities, infertility without tubal obstruction, and severe pain if a cyst ruptures. Implants on the ureters may obstruct them; those involving the rectum may be associated with bleeding and obstruction. In any event, the symptoms do not necessarily coincide with the amount of disease present.

Definitive *therapy* for endometriosis is removal of the uterus, ovaries, tubes, and as many implants as possible. Those women with significant disease eventually come to this type of therapy if the menopause does not intervene. Other types of therapy which may be used in the interim, or with patients with less severe disease, are the induction of a state of "pseudopregnancy" with antiovulatory drugs, and more conservative surgery. Antiovulatory drugs (in larger doses than used for contraception) are given for six to nine months and may alleviate the symptoms for a period of time after they are discontinued. However, side effects can include irregular bleeding, nausea, vomiting, depression, and fatigue. "Conservative surgery" refers to the removal of as much of the aberrant tissue as possible. In addition to the care given the patient undergoing one of the forms of surgery, the nurse can assist the patient by (a) reinforcing the physician's explanation of the expected results of treatment, (b) dispelling false fears or hopes, and (c) stressing the importance of regular check-ups and the need to report any abnormal bleeding.

Adenomyosis. Adenomyosis, or "internal endometriosis," is a condition caused by invasion of the myometrium by endometrial tissue. This disorder is more common in older women who have had children. It can be diffuse or be localized in the form of a tumor (adenomyoma). The uterus is enlarged and if the disease is extensive, the process may extend to involve adjacent organs.

Bleeding and even hemorrhage are characteristic *symptoms* of the disease. Hypermenorrhea with dyspareunia is the most common combination of symptoms. Since the condition can occur in combination with endometriosis or with myomas, the symptoms may be diffuse. Endometrial adenocarcinoma may develop in the uterus and present the same general symptoms. Therefore, the possibility of cancer is ruled out before a therapeutic course is chosen. Otherwise, the treatment is similar to that given for endometriosis. Nursing considerations are also comparable, except that patients with extensive disease may have significant bleeding with resultant anemia. Therefore, part of the nurse's teaching responsibilities may be related to the care of patients with anemia. (See Unit XII.)

POLYPS

Polyps (they may be called fibroid polyps) are pedunculated tumors which arise from the mucosa and extend into the opening of a body cavity. They are found primarily in the endometrium (uterus) and in the cervix. Cervical polyps may cause bleeding after intercourse and are subject to infection. Those in the uterus may cause hypermenorrhea, intermenstrual bleeding, and bleeding after menopause. They occasionally undergo malignant changes, particularly in postmenopausal women. Since cervical and endometrial polyps frequently co-exist, when cervical polyps are seen or felt, uterine polyps should be searched for.

OVARIAN TUMORS

Ovarian tumors may be roughly classified as non-neoplastic (physiologic) and neoplastic. Neoplastic tumors are either benign (the topic of this chapter) or malignant, and may have hormonal effects. Non-neoplastic tumors are solid or cystic. All of the neoplastic tumors and some of those that are non-neoplastic are subject to surgical removal. Surgery is indicated because of the potential interference with function of the pelvic organs caused by both types. Fortunately, the physiologic, and particularly the cystic, tumors are more common.

There are a number of different types of ovarian tumors which are benign and rare. To obtain specific information about individual types of tumors, specialty literature should be consulted. The following information is presented to help the nurse gain a general understanding of the implications of benign ovarian tumors.

Many ovarian tumors are asymptomatic until they become large enough to cause pressure *symptoms,* thus making early detection of malignancies difficult. Some smaller tumors may cause symptoms owing to their location. Symptoms related to location and/or size can include: painful defecation, constipation, dyspareunia, vague aching, heaviness, and sterility. Later symptoms include abdominal distension with dyspnea, peripheral edema, and anorexia. Pelvic pain may be present, particularly if the tumor is growing rapidly. If the tumor produces hormones, there may be menstrual irregularities and masculinizing or feminizing effects.

Complications of ovarian tumors include: hemorrhage into a cyst, with rupture and possibly infection; torsion of a cystic pedicle which may cause the former; and malignant changes. The first two complications cause symptoms similar to those previously discussed under uterine myomas. Malignancy is suspected when there is a sudden rapid growth of a tumor, if the tumor is bilateral, or if it is large. The incidence of malignancy is higher in postmenopausal women.

Treatment is based on the type of tumor present. Cysts tend to regress in size and are therefore a type of tumor that allows the physician to watch the reproductive aged patient closely during one or two menstrual cycles. Tumors which are growing rapidly, those that disrupt the function of the pelvic organs or the ovary, those which are bilateral, and neoplastic tumors are removed surgically with or without the ovary. Therefore, surgery includes removal of the tumor, removal of the ovary (ies), or removal of the ovaries, tubes, and uterus. Nursing care is related to the type of surgery. If the patient is managed conservatively, the nurse should stress the importance of close follow-up. (Refer to Chapter 103 for a discussion of the types of surgery and related nursing care.)

BENIGN FALLOPIAN TUBE TUMORS

Tubal tumors are extremely rare and may be cystic or solid.

FISTULAS

Fistulas are an extremely distressing and common problem in the genital and urinary tracts. They occur (a) when there is an abnormal opening between two adjacent organs (b) as a result of the spread of a malignant lesion, (c) after irradiation for cancer, (d) after pelvic or radical surgery, and (e) after a prolonged and difficult labor and delivery. The latter was formerly the most frequent cause, but improved labor and delivery techniques have changed this. Infrequently, in addition to the above causes, fistulas may result from venereal and other inflammatory diseases.

Fistulas are classified by location; there are two general types: (1) vaginal fistulas and (2) urinary tract fistulas. Urinary tract fistulas are not the focus of this discussion, although much of the following information is relevant to this type of fistula. Vaginal fistulas include vesicovaginal (bladder), ureterovaginal (ureter), urethrovaginal (urethra), and rectovaginal (rectum) fistulas.

All of the above vaginal fistulas cause some similar *symptoms*. Urine or flatus and feces leak into the vagina. Excoriation and irritation of the vaginal and vulvar tissues occur. Severe infection may result from this irritation. Rectovaginal fistulas may cause an offensive odor which is particularly unpleasant. The patient experiences wetness and the sensation of feeling "dirty."

In addition to the physical symptoms, fistulas tend to be among the most psychologically distressing problems which women face. Patients with these disorders frequently become social recluses, causing great disruption to their family relationships and other social activities. Often they fail to consult a physician until the problem has become severe, and even then they are reluctant to discuss it.

Diagnosis and treatment may be difficult. *Treatment* varies with the location, extent, cause, and general condition of the patient. Small fistulas may heal spontaneously after one to three months. However, surgical excision is frequently required. Surgery is not always successful in curing the problem, and, for this reason, it is extremely important that the patient be in optimal condition before it is attempted. A waiting period of about six months is required while the inflammation and tissue edema subside. Treatment during this time is directed toward avoiding infection by performing thorough perineal hygiene and improving the overall health status of the individual. A temporary colostomy may be done to treat a rectovaginal fistula. (See Unit XV for colostomy care.)

During the waiting period prior to surgery and again after surgery, the nurse can help the patient to learn to minimize the symptoms and to care for herself. Perineal hygiene measures include cleansing the perineum about every four hours (with sterile materials after surgery), sitz baths, douches, and perineal pads (which should be changed frequently). Deodorizing and comforting measures may include using vitamin A and D ointment, deodorant powders, heat lamps, and various types of weak acid or weak base irrigating solutions (depending on the pH of the urine). The latter solutions are poured over the perineum. Deodorizing douches (e.g., Clorox, 1 tsp. per 1 quart water) may also be ordered. The patient should be cautioned to avoid using excessive pressure when giving the douches because the water pressure may force the solution through the fistula tract, thereby causing infections. Some patients inadvisably restrict their fluid intake in an attempt to decrease drainage. This may actually increase the size of the fistula and cause infection.

Occasionally the patient with a rectovaginal fistula may be given an enema to clean the bowel and temporarily decrease the drainage. When an enema is permitted, a soft rubber catheter should be used. The catheter should be gently inserted above and away from the fistula tract.

After surgery, care is directed toward two objectives: (1) *avoiding stress on the repaired area,* and (2) *preventing infection.* A Foley catheter may be in place postoperatively to drain the bladder. Care must be taken to keep the catheter *draining at all times* and to provide enough fluid for the patient so that *internal catheter irrigation* is accomplished. The catheter should not be routinely irrigated (externally), but if this is essential, minimal pressure should be used. Strict asepsis is essential in addition to maintaining dependent drainage. Some patients have a suprapubic catheter and the same precautions are used. A few patients may have an ileal conduit (see Unit XI). Following bowel surgery, the first stool may be purposefully delayed with liquid diet and other measures. Several days later, the patient is given stool softeners and laxatives. The patient should be cautioned not to strain at stool. Enemas should be avoided.

The nurse should remember that expert nursing care, including the above measures, is extremely important, since successful surgery may not result even under optimal conditions. This is particularly true if the patient has extensive tissue damage from tumors or irradiation.

UTERINE DISPLACEMENT

Normally the uterus flexes anteriorly about 45 degrees and is movable, and the cervix points downward and posteriorly. Uterine displacements include anterior displacement, lateral displacement, posterior displacement (retrodisplacement), and downward displacement (prolapse). Of these, posterior and downward displacement are the most important and are the focus of the discussion below.

Posterior Displacement. Retrodisplacement includes retroflexion and retroversion. Retroversion occurs when the uterus is tilted posteriorly and the cervix is pointed anteriorly. If the tilt is mild, the retroversion is said to be "first degree"; if the fundus is in the hollow of the sacrum, it is said to be "third degree." Retroflexion is said to be present when the body of the uterus is bent backwards on the cervix. The cervix may maintain a normal position in the vagina.

Retrodisplacement is caused by congenital or acquired weakness of the pelvic support structures. These structures can be injured during surgery, during childbirth, by tumors, by inflammatory diseases, by endometriosis, and by other problems. The majority of patients with these problems are asymptomatic, and *symptoms,* when present, do not necessarily correlate with the amount of displacement. Backache (accentuated by standing a long time or occurring during the menses), secondary amenorrhea, infertility, a sense of pelvic pressure, and dyspareunia may be present. Pelvic congestion and adhesions may be the cause of some of these symptoms because the uterus is less mobile.

Treatment is directed toward the underlying cause if it can be determined. In other instances, particularly post partum, the patient may be helped by exercise therapy. Assumption of the knee-chest position for a few minutes several times each day may correct mild retrodisplacement. In other cases, the physician may elect to insert a vaginal pessary. After the uterus is manually placed in a normal position, the pessary is inserted. The pessary should maintain the uterine position by holding the cervix posteriorly, thus allowing the uterus to fall forward. After insertion, the patient should not be aware of the pessary. Before leaving the physician's office, the patient should be checked to see that the pessary stays in and that she is able to void. A pessary irritates the vaginal mucosa; therefore, the patient should be instructed to douche regularly to remove excess vaginal debris. Four to six weeks following insertion of the pessary, the patient should return to the physician and let him know if the symptoms have been relieved. At that time the physician checks to see that the pessary is not excessively irritating to the tissues, changing or removing it if indicated. If left in place too long, a pessary may cause cervical erosion and adhere to the mucosa. The nurse should be sure that the patient understands the need for periodic check-ups. Occasionally, retroversion may be corrected by a surgical procedure called a "uterine suspension." More often, this procedure is not done alone but rather is performed in combination with another surgical procedure to correct another problem.

Prolapse of the Uterus or Downward Displacement. Uterine prolapse or downward displacement of the uterus into the vagina may be caused by weakening of the pelvic supports, including ligaments, fascia, and muscles. In addition, uterine prolapse may result from childbirth injuries, loss of elasticity due to aging, congenital weaknesses, or increased intra-abdominal pressure (e.g., from tumors or occupations requiring heavy lifting). When the pelvic floor relaxes, the uterus "sags" into the vaginal canal or through it to the outside of the body.

Prolapse or descent of the uterus occurs in three stages:

1. First degree—uterus decends into the vaginal canal and the cervix reaches but does not go through the introitus.
2. Second degree—body of the uterus is still within the vagina, but the cervix protrudes through the introitus.
3. Third degree (also called "procidentia" or "complete prolapse")—the entire uterus and the cervix protrude through the introitus with inversion of the vaginal canal.

During the descent of the uterus, other structures may be "pulled" down or out of position. These structures include the bladder, the rectum, and the urethra. The disorders resulting from such displacements, e.g., cystocele, rectocele, are discussed below.

The development of complete prolapse usually occurs over a period of time. Once the cervix has protruded through the vaginal outlet, it is subjected to constant irritation with the attendant

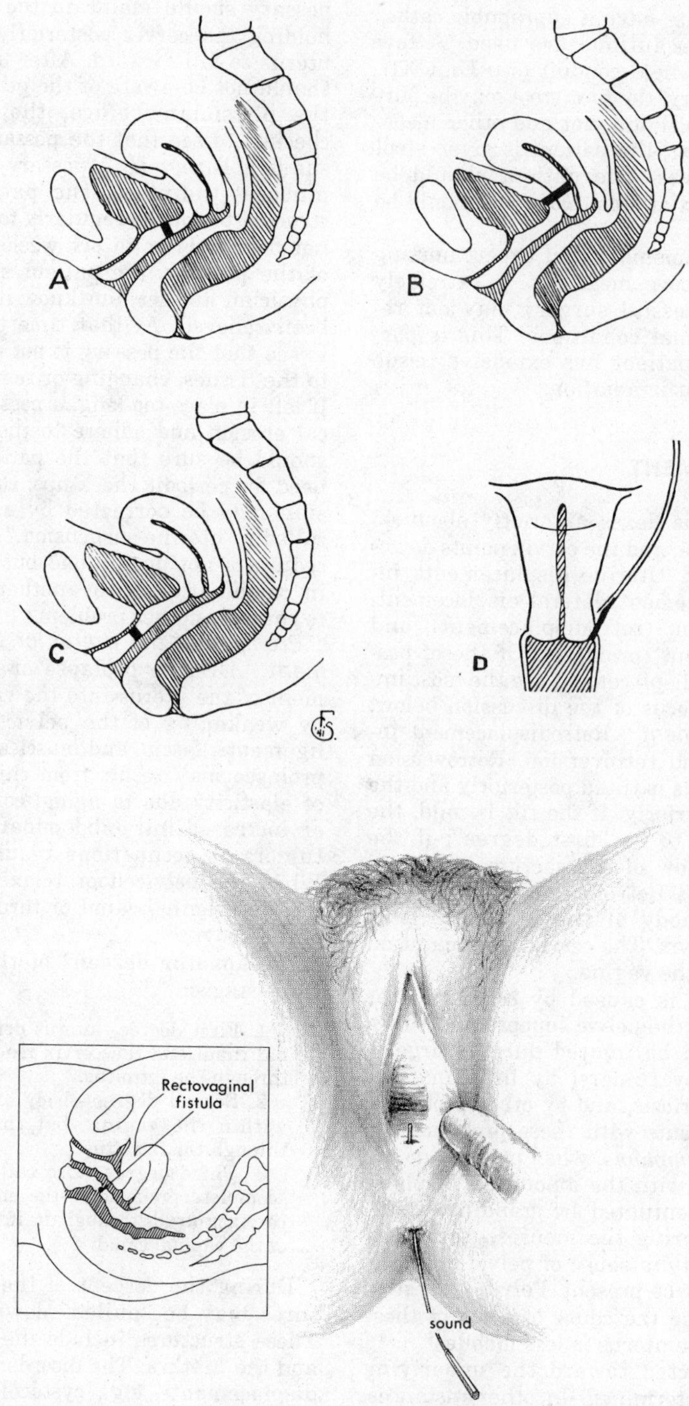

FIGURE 101–2. Diagram of chief varieties of urinary fistula. *A*, Vesicovaginal; *B*, vesicouterine; *C*, urethrovaginal; *D*, ureterovaginal. (*A* to *D* from Novak, E. R., Jones, G. S., and Jones, H. W.: *Gynecology.* Baltimore, The Williams & Wilkins Company, 1971. *E* from Miller, N. F., and Avery, H.: *Gynecology and Gynecologic Nursing.* 5th ed. 1965.)

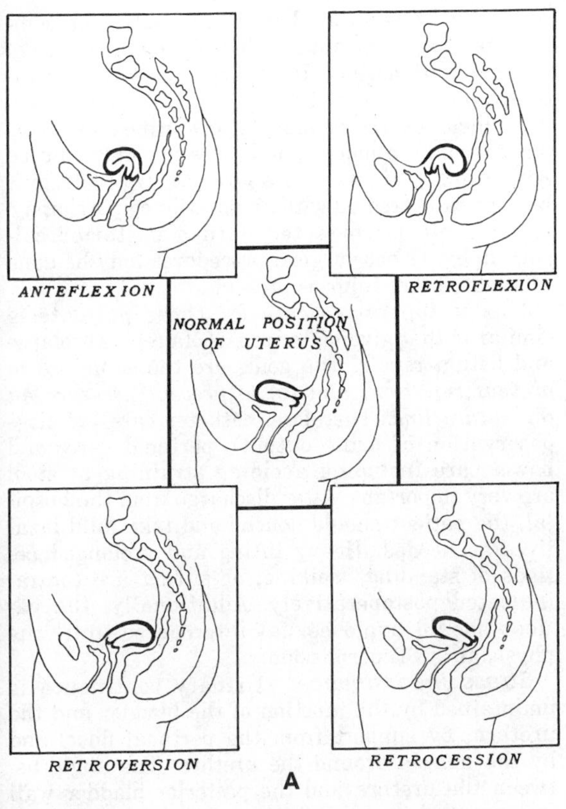

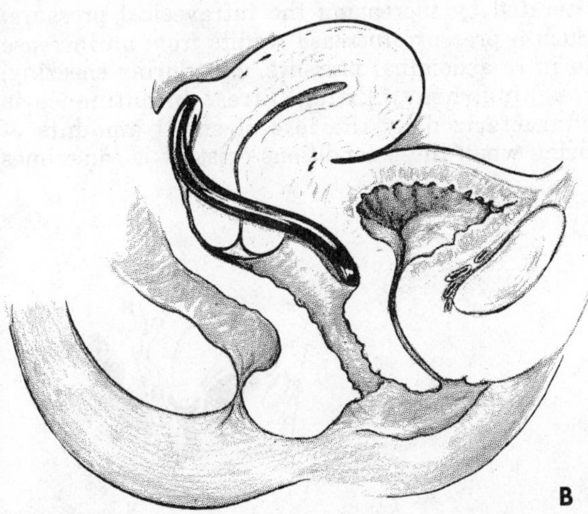

FIGURE 101–3. *A*, Degrees of posterior uterine displacements; *B*, pessary treatment. (From Miller, N. F., and Avery, H.: *Gynecology and Gynecologic Nursing*. 5th ed. 1965.)

tissue changes. Malignant degeneration is always possible. Also, the vaginal mucosa is subjected to drying, trauma, and irritation once it is outside the body.

Symptoms do not necessarily correlate with the amount of prolapse. However, most patients with a significant degree of prolapse are aware that "something is coming down in there." Additionally, patients may complain of dyspareunia; vague abdominal problems including a feeling of pressure, dragging and heaviness; backaches; and bladder and/or bowel problems if there is an associated cystocele or rectocele. Stress incontinence may be present.

Better than *treatment* is prevention, particularly through improved obstetric care (this has already decreased the incidence of prolapse). The nurse can assist in preventing uterine prolapse by (a) encouraging pregnant patients to seek qualified obstetric care, and (b) teaching patients after delivery to alternately tense and relax their

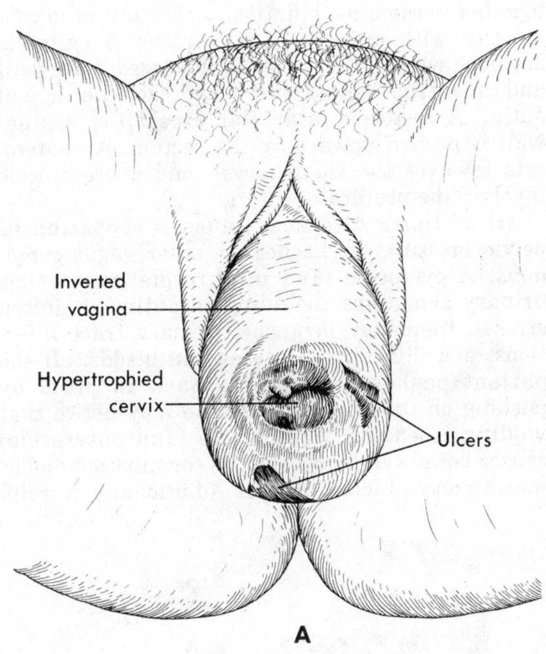

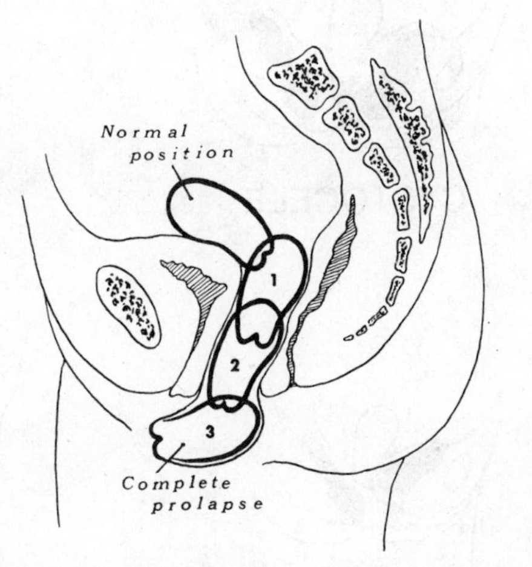

FIGURE 101–4. Uterine prolapse. *A*, Complete prolapse of the uterus, showing hypertrophy and ulceration of the cervix. *B*, Course followed by the uterus as it descends: 1 and 2, incomplete prolapse; 3, complete prolapse. (From Miller, N. F., and Avery, H.: *Gynecology and Gynecologic Nursing*. 5th ed. 1965.)

gluteal muscles and the muscles of the pelvic floor (can she stop the urinary stream?). In some instances prolapse is treated with pessaries (see above). The third method of treatment is surgical. Various surgical procedures may be employed. One procedure is vaginal hysterectomy with anterior and posterior colporrhaphy (repair of vagina and underlying fascia). Nursing care is related to the form of therapy. (See Chapter 5.)

Cystocele, Rectocele, Urethrocele and Enterocele. Caused by problems similar to those resulting in uterine prolapse, these conditions occur together in some combination, separately, or in conjunction with prolapse of the uterus. A cystocele develops when the bladder is displaced downward and causes the vaginal wall to approach the vaginal outlet. A rectocele is similar except the vaginal wall is pushed upward by the rectum. An enterocele involves the small bowel, and a urethrocele involves the urethra.

All of these disorders cause a sensation of pelvic pressure, backaches, or other vague *symptoms.* A cystocele (and urethrocele) may cause urinary symptoms including incontinence (often stress), frequency, urgency, urinary tract infections, and difficulty emptying the bladder. If the patient pushes the bladder back in place by pushing on the vaginal wall, she may notice that voiding is easier. A rectocele (and enterocele) causes bowel symptoms such as constipation and/or incontinence of feces and gas. Additionally, a rectocele may be associated with incomplete or complete tearing of the anal sphincter. Complications of these conditions include infection, cervical ulceration, hemorrhoids, and cystitis.

Perineal exercises may be prescribed as *treatment* for mild problems, and a pessary may be used with some patients (see above). A cystocele may be surgically treated with an anterior colporrhaphy. A rectocele is corrected with a posterior colporrhaphy. Other surgical procedures may be done related to other injuries present.

The postoperative care for these patients is similar to that given after repair of uterine prolapse and fistula repair. The goals are the same: (a) *to prevent infection,* and (b) *to prevent pressure on the suture line.* Therefore, catheter care (or close observation of urine output), perineal care, and bowel care including avoiding straining at stool are very important. After discharge from the hospital, the patient should douche and take mild laxatives as needed. Heavy lifting and prolonged periods of standing, walking, or sitting are contraindicated postoperatively. Additionally, the patient should avoid sexual intercourse until the physician gives permission.

Stress Incontinence. Urinary continence is maintained by the junction of the bladder and the urethra, by support from the perineal floor, and by the muscle around the urethra. The angle between the urethra and the posterior bladder wall is acute and is obliterated by the process of voiding. With stress incontinence, this angle is obliterated by increasing the intravesical pressure. Such a pressure increase results from an increase in intra-abdominal pressure, e.g., during sneezing, coughing, heavy lifting. Stress incontinence is characterized by the loss of small amounts of urine when these conditions exist. It is sometimes

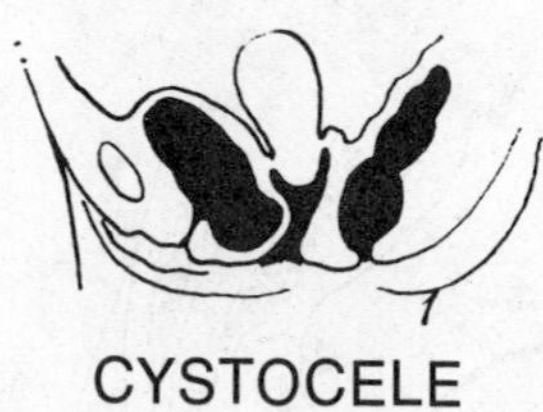

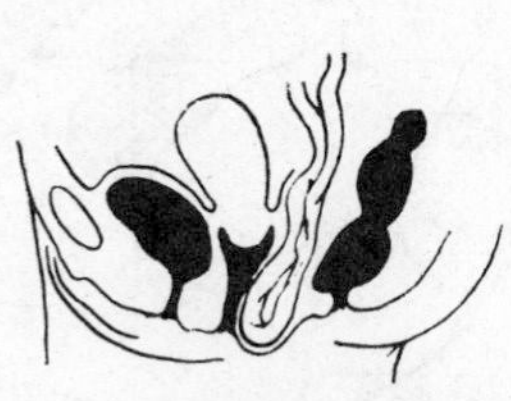

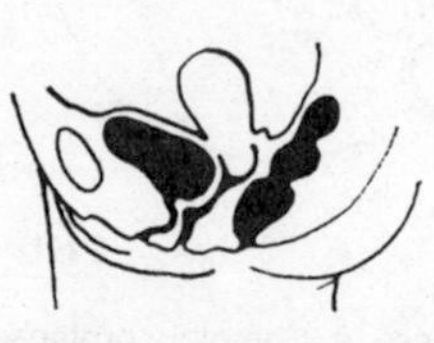

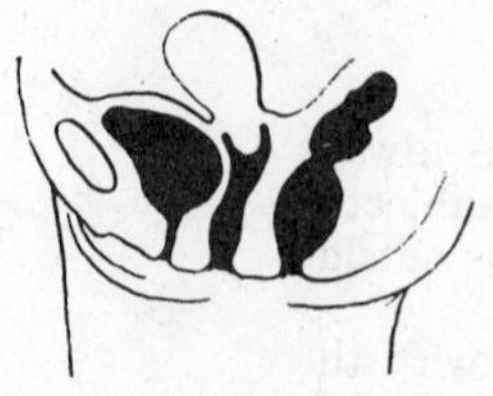

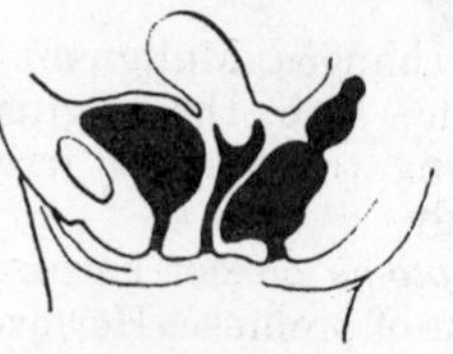

FIGURE 101–5. Sagittal view of normal pelvis compared to defects of cystocele, urethrocele, enterocele, and rectocele. (Modified from Dilts, P. V., Greene, J. W., and Roddick, J. W.: *Core Studies in Obstetrics and Gynecology,* Baltimore, The Williams & Wilkins Company, 1971.)

difficult to distinguish stress incontinence from other types of incontinence. Stress incontinence is due to many of the same problems that cause the previously discussed conditions and is usually made worse by the menopausal decrease in tissue elasticity. It can be caused by a cystocele, or can occur after a cystocele has been repaired.

Prevention is the most efficient care. Perineal exercises as previously discussed can help to cure mild cases. Surgical procedures done to correct this condition usually attempt to elevate the urethra and reestablish the normal angle between the urethra and the posterior bladder wall. Many of these procedures are the so-called sling operations. After surgery, the nurse should carefully observe the urinary output and take catheter precautions, if the patient has a catheter. If there is no catheter or it has been removed, the patient may find it easier to bend forward and put her feet on a support to loosen the abdominal muscles when trying to void.

CHAPTER 102

Cancer of the Female Genital Tract

JUDITH ATWOOD

Over the years, early diagnosis and treatment of cancer of the genital tract has improved the prognosis for patients with this problem. However as Dilts et al. state, ". . . carcinoma of the female genital tract steadily continues as one of the more deadly malignancies."[24] This is true because not all women present themselves for care in the early stages, nor do they avail themselves of good preventive care on a yearly or more frequent basis. Therefore, one of the major concerns today is to *promote preventive care;* this requires that nurses be well informed about genital tract malignancies in order to maximize their many contacts with women who have a myriad of fears which prevent them from seeking care.

This chapter, Chapter 103, the unit on cancer (Unit VII), and the unit on surgery (Unit VI) are all designed to help increase the nurse's knowledge of the many considerations involved in planning and delivering care to women with malignancies. This chapter contains a discussion of the various types of malignancies, their symptoms, how they are diagnosed, and types of medical treatment employed. Chapter 103 discusses the nursing care related to the various gynecologic procedures used in diagnosing and treating not only malignant conditions but also other specific problems. The unit on cancer is designed to increase the nurse's understanding of malignant properties of lesions and the type of treatment used with the appropriate nursing care considerations. Additionally, the emotional response of the patient is discussed extensively. The unit on surgery gives the same type of coverage.

The nurse is therefore directed to the appropriate units for consideration of those topics most useful to her. To facilitate her understanding of this chapter the following definitions are provided:

1. Sub-total hysterectomy—removal of the uterus without the cervix.
2. Total hysterectomy—removal of the uterus and the cervix.
3. Panhysterectomy—removal of the uterus, the cervix, the fallopian tubes, and the ovaries.
4. Vaginectomy—removal of the vagina.
5. Wertheim's operation—a panhysterectomy, a partial vaginectomy, and dissection of the lymph nodes in the pelvis.
6. Lymphadenectomy—excision of lymph nodes.
7. Intracavity irradiation—radiation source placed within a cavity of the body, e.g., the uterus.
8. External irradiation—radiation source is outside the body.
9. Exenteration operation—Wertheim operation, total vaginectomy, removal of the bladder with diversion of the urinary system, and resection of the bowel with colostomy.
10. Anterior exenteration—above operation except bowel is not resected.
11. Posterior exenteration—above operation except bladder is not removed.
12. Chemotherapy—treatment of a disease with drugs; in this instance treatment of cancer with drugs specific to the type of lesion.

CARCINOMA OF THE VULVA

Usually of the squamous cell type, vulvar carcinoma is a form of malignancy found primarily in women over 50 years of age. Although relatively rare, it may follow chronic leukoplakia or other conditions causing chronic irritation of the vulvar tissues. The early symptoms (pruritis, minimal soreness of the vulva, and tissue irritation with some bleeding) may be ignored by the patients, as these symptoms differ little from those experienced with the earlier, nonmalignant lesion. As the disease progresses, the symptoms may include edema of the vulva and pelvic lymphadenopathy. Moreover, secondary infection may cause a foul smelling discharge. Distant metastasis, infection, and general disability are the usual causes of death when the disease is extensive.

The early malignant lesion may be of the in situ variety, or it may be invasive. If invasive, extensive local spread occurs, particularly into the lymphatic channels, both deep and superficial. If of the in situ type, a simple vulvectomy (resection of the vulva) may be adequate treatment. However, more often a radical vulvectomy with superficial and deep lymph node dissection is indicated. Because the vulvar resection is of necessity extensive, some type of plastic repair procedure may be needed to close the excised area. The surgery may be done in either one or two stages. In either instance, both the patient and the nurse may find that the mutilation of this area is very unpleasant to look at. The nurse should be particularly careful that her response to the patient does not increase the patient's distress. Irradiation is not generally used in this area, since the tissues do not tolerate it well. The prognosis is poor with invasive lesions.

CARCINOMA OF THE VAGINA

Primary invasive carcinoma of the vagina is a rare lesion. Primary in situ vaginal malignancy is also rare, but when it occurs, it is usually part of an in situ vulvar lesion. Metastasis or secondary carcinoma may result from several causes, e.g., trophoblastic disease (discussed later in this chapter). Secondary carcinoma is also rare. Primary invasive carcinoma tends to involve the anterior, the posterior, or both of the vaginal walls, with resultant complications such as fistula formation. The signs and symptoms include vaginal discharge and bleeding, presence of a mass in the vagina, and pain. The usual treatment consists of radiation therapy, both externally and intravaginally. Despite active therapy, the prognosis is generally poor, and the complications tend to be quite bothersome.

CARCINOMA OF THE CERVIX

Carcinoma of the cervix is the most common genital tract malignancy in women, being several times more common than carcinoma of the endometrium (uterine body). The majority of the cervical carcinomas are of the squamous cell type (about 95 per cent), although adenocarcinoma does exist and is more difficult to diagnose. The squamous cell carcinoma usually begins at the squamocolumnar junction near the external os of the cervix, while adenocarcinoma involves the endocervical glands.

Potentially, 100 per cent of the patients with early cervical cancer (that is, before it becomes invasive) can be cured. For this reason, one of the most important roles of the nurse is encouraging women to have annual check-ups including a Papanicolaou smear ("Pap" test). Although there is no general agreement among authorities as to the age when these check-ups should begin, it is safe to say that all women over 30 should be checked. There is general agreement that prevention of invasive cervical carcinoma may be accomplished by early diagnosis and treatment while the cancer is still confined to the pre-invasive stage. There is also general agreement that 5 to 10 years may elapse between the pre-invasive and invasive stages, and that cervical cancer is rare before the age of 20, occurring more frequently between the ages of 30 and 50. Moreover, several factors have been identified which seem to correlate with the incidence of cervical carcinoma, and the presence of several of these conditions might indicate that the woman should be followed earlier than 30 years of age, as her risk is higher. These factors include early marriage; early, frequent intercourse (before age 20); multiple sexual partners; multiple pregnancies, postpartum lacerations; untreated chronic cervicitis; and heredity. Although these factors do not cause cancer, and in fact early marriage may in reality relate to the frequency of sexual contact, there seems to be some increased risk that these patients are more prone to develop cervical carcinoma. In any event, the nurse should make every effort to see that each woman understands the importance of and reason for annual Pap tests. Moreover, knowledge does not necessarily mean that the woman will follow through and obtain the test, so the nurse must also consider the woman's motivation when working with patients. Perhaps stressing the positive outcomes resulting from early diagnosis and treatment will help increase motivation.

Cancer of the genital organs is grouped into several stages according to an international classification developed by the World Health Organization. This classification and treatment of the various stages along with five year survival rates are included in Table 102–1. Stage O, the pre-invasive stage or carcinoma in situ of the cervix, involves the epithelial tissue, usually through the full thickness of this tissue. Asymptomatic, the malignant changes are frequently discovered by routine Pap smears, a cytologic test which is done on the discharge from the vaginal pool in the posterior fornix, and on cells obtained by scrapping the cervix. An early lesion may be present but is often difficult to distinguish from other benign lesions. If this lesion is present, a biopsy should be performed (as described later in the chapter).

From this early in situ stage, the malignancy may spread into the stroma of the cervix, over the epithelial surfaces of the cervix to the vagina and/or the uterus, into the parametrial tissue (tissue around the broad ligament), along the lymphatic pathways to the pelvic wall, and eventually into the pelvic blood vessels. Extension within the pelvis will eventually lead to fixation of the pelvic organs: involvement of the blood vessels may precipitate hemorrhage; invasion of nerve tissue will lead to pain, and invasion of the rectum and/or bladder leads to the development of fistulas or obstruction of these organs. Distant metastases are late events and may occur in a variety of organs including the liver, lungs, and bones. General debilitation (cachexia) and emotional deterioration are common, and death occurs from a variety of problems, usually within two to four years after the onset of invasive carcinoma. These events can include death from the following conditions: pulmonary metastasis with pneumonia or other sequelae, peritonitis due to gastrointestinal obstruction and perforation, hemorrhage due to erosion of major blood vessels, or urinary tract obstruction (usually from blockage of the ureters) and subsequent uremia.

There are no symptoms early in the course of cervical carcinoma. When symptoms develop, a vaginal discharge and bleeding occur first. Metrorrhagia, postmenopausal bleeding, and polymenorrhea may be present. However, early bleeding may be in the form of spotting or contact bleeding from trauma to the cervix secondary to sexual intercourse, douching, or other such causes. This early minimal bleeding increases in amount and duration as the disease progresses and usually means that the disease process involves the lymphatics. Postmenopausal bleeding is of particular importance, as in about 50 percent of cases this type of bleeding heralds the onset of some form of genital cancer.

The discharge is usually watery and becomes dark and foul smelling as the disease advances. With infection of the neoplastic area, the discharge becomes more profuse and malodorous. Moreover, the concurrent bleeding adds to the unpleasantness. Other symptoms which develop are related to the areas involved in the malignant process. These include pressure on the bowel and/or bladder, bladder irritation and rectal discharge, symptoms of ureteral obstruction, heavy aching abdominal pain, and fistula formation when the malignancy has eroded through the walls of adjacent organs. Pain is a late symptom and usually becomes a difficult problem with the onset of the general wasting (cachexia) that accompanies the terminal stage of cancer.

In the presence of a suspicious appearing lesion, or a positive Pap test, the physician will obtain a *cervical biopsy* to determine if the patient has carcinoma. This frequently allows the diagnosis to be established early, when the prognosis for eradicating the malignancy is good. It is important for the nurse to instruct the patient who is going to have a Pap smear to avoid douching before the test. Additionally, the nurse may assist with the biopsy procedure, which, if done in the office, is a minor one, causing little discomfort to the patient. The procedure is relatively painless because the cervix has few nerve endings. Prior to the biopsy, the physician may do a *Schiller test.* This consists of cleaning debris off the cervix and then painting the tissue with an iodine preparation. Abnormal tissue which is glycogen depleted will not stain. The biopsy is then performed by removing a bit of tissue from various areas, including all of those which are not stained. Sometimes, in addition to the latter procedures, the physician looks through a *culposcope* (which is an instrument which magnifies the area) so that he may inspect the tissue more closely, and be guided in obtaining the tissue from appropriate areas.

The biopsy may be obtained in the operating room, in some instances, by doing a *cold conization.* This procedure involves obtaining a cone-shaped

TABLE 102-1. WORLD HEALTH ORGANIZATION INTERNATIONAL CLASSIFICATION (CARCINOMA OF THE CERVIX)

Stage	Extent	Treatment	Prognosis For 5-year Survival (%)
Stage O (pre-invasive)	Carcinoma in situ (also called pre-invasive intraepithelial); focal in nature, confined to epithelial layer of cervix	Cervical conization; total hysterectomy with partial vaginectomy	95–100*
Stage I (invasive—Stages I to IV)	Confined to cervix, but has invaded into cervical tissue; small lesion may be present	Wertheim's hysterectomy; irradiation	75–85
Stage IIa	Has extended to vaginal mucosa but not to lower one third	Irradiation; Wertheim's hysterectomy	65–75
Stage IIb	Has extended to parametrial tissue (tissues around the broad ligament) but not to pelvic wall, or has extended to corpus of uterus	Irradiation	50–65
Stage III	Has reached pelvic wall or lower one third of vagina	Irradiation	20–30
Stage IV	Has invaded bladder and/or rectum or distant metastasis	Irradiation; surgery, e.g., exenteration	1-10

*Statistics are compiled from a variety of references. Those most generally agreed upon are used.

section of the cervix with a knife. This provides more tissue for analysis, thus increasing the chance that any area of invasive carcinoma will be identified, since invasive and in situ carcinoma may coexist in the same patient. Such a procedure may also be the only type of therapy needed if analysis of the tissue demonstrates that a wide area of normal tissue surrounds the excized malignancy. The end result is that the patient retains the capacity to reproduce (fertility may be decreased, however), which in some instances is an important consideration. However, it is *extremely* important that the patient recognize the necessity for close follow-up care, including serial Pap tests, since conization is not always adequate therapy. With evidence of recurrent cancer, or if reproduction is not an issue, a total hysterectomy with removal of part of the vaginal cuff is a safer type of treatment.

The nursing care following conization is similar to that following any type of minor vaginal surgery but also includes that given after a vaginal or abdominal hysterectomy for other problems. It is important for the nurse to remember, however, that this is a patient with cancer, in addition to a gynecologic disorder. Therefore, this is a patient who is likely to be undergoing a stress response to the knowledge that she has a potentially lethal disease and that the treatment for the disease will alter her reproductive status. The emotional responses to cancer and the nurse's function in helping the patient to cope with them are discussed more fully in Unit VII. One of these responses, that of denial, may have serious implications for the patient who has had a cervical conization. Should she feel quite well after the procedure and fail to obtain adequate follow-up care, she could remain uncured. Without frightening the patient, the importance of adequate follow-up care must be stressed.

Early invasive carcinoma is treated by removing or destroying the involved areas and lymphatic drainage in addition to the adjacent uninvolved tissue. This is done with external and/or internal irradiation or surgery. At times, both types of therapy are used in the same patient. Stage I cervical cancer is frequently treated by panhysterectomy, partial vaginectomy, and dissection of the pelvic lymph nodes. If the disease has spread to the parametrial tissues and/or to the pelvic wall, surgery is less valuable, and irradiation is the usual treatment of choice. However, irradiation is not always effective in sterilizing the involved lymph nodes. Advanced cases are irradiated except in rare instances, when a partial or total exenteration may be done. The latter carries with it a high surgical mortality rate.

Some patients will become terminally ill despite vigorous therapy. In this instance, the treatment goals change and are directed toward promoting physiologic and psychologic comfort, and relieving pain. The latter may be accomplished through the use of conventional drug therapy, including narcotics, sedatives, and, at times, sedation. When these agents do not produce the desired results, palliative irradiation (which also helps to achieve hemostasis when this is a problem) or selective nerve blocks may help. In some instances, various neurosurgical procedures, including cordotomy (destruction of spinal sensory pathways), give some relief. Other procedures may become necessary, e.g., a colostomy to relieve a bowel obstruction. The patient's course may be complicated by a variety of problems including fistulas, bowel and bladder obstruction, persistent pain, and cachexia. Death results within a relatively short time after the onset of the terminal phase of the illness. (See Unit VII for discussion of the care of the dying patient.)

CARCINOMA OF THE ENDOMETRIUM (UTERUS)

Endometrial carcinoma is the second most common genital malignancy, being second only to cervical carcinoma. Like cervical carcinoma, if endometrial carcinoma is diagnosed early, the prognosis is relatively good. Unlike cervical malignancy, the cell type is usually adenocarcinoma (involving the glands), and is more common in older females, the average age of patients being 57. It is a relatively slow growing tumor and metastasizes late. However, once it has spread to the cervix, increased the size of the uterus, or spread outside the uterus, the prognosis is seriously altered, being somewhat grim. Although the relationship is indirect, women who are obese, hypertensive (or have cardiovascular problems), diabetic, or have not had children seem to have a higher incidence of endometrial carcinoma. Moreover, women with a history of abnormal bleeding before menopause and/or menstrual abnormalities at the time of the menopause also have a higher incidence of this type of cancer.

The adenocarcinoma is either a diffuse process involving much of the endometrium (and glands) or is restricted to a smaller area (involving fewer glands). The tumor tissue tends to be well differentiated, but this is less important in determining the prognosis than is the extent of the spread. Lymph node involvement is less common and occurs later than with cervical carcinoma.

This malignancy tends to be slower in spreading to other organs and may cause uterine bleeding before extensive spread has occurred. Most commonly, the carcinoma invades the uterus itself, entering into either the cavity or the myometrium from where it can progress to involve other peritoneal structures including the lymphatics and blood vessels. From there, it can spread to the vagina, through the lymphatics, to other areas and occasionally to distant structures such as the brain and lungs. The carcinoma may extensively invade the uterus itself, causing it to become enlarged. Moreover, the extension of the cancerous process may occur along the endometrial surface to either the cervix or the tubes and ovaries. After invasion of the cervix, further spread resembles that seen with cervical carcinoma. Death may result from problems similar to those seen with cervical malignancy.

The Pap test is not reliable in ruling out endometrial carcinoma; thus, it is usually discovered only after the first symptom has appeared. This first symptom is generally some type of abnormal uterine bleeding. Most frequently it is postmenopausal bleeding, since the average patient is in this stage of her reproductive life. Less frequently, the patient may experience some type of watery discharge as her first symptom. On occasion, abnormal tissue is present in the cervix or in the vaginal pool, and the patient has a suspicious Pap test. As with cervical carcinoma, pain occurs relatively late, and other symptoms are related to invasion and/or metastasis to other organs. The diagnosis is established by the physician by doing a dilatation and curettage to obtain tissue for analysis by the pathologist.

The treatment is similar to that employed with cervical carcinoma. Early endometrial carcinoma is treated by removing the uterus (with the cervix), the fallopian tubes, the ovaries, and a part of the vaginal cuff. This may be preceded by irradiation either externally (e.g., with cobalt) or internally (e.g., with intracavity radium and a cervical source in some instances). Another form of treatment which may be used in some situations, particularly with recurrent disease, is progesterone therapy. A variety of synthetic progesterone agents may be used in large doses.

CARCINOMA OF THE FALLOPIAN TUBES

Primary tubal carcinoma is extremely rare, and is a malignacy of older women. Like ovarian carcinoma, symptoms do not appear until late in the course of the malignancy. Secondary metastases (those from other primary metastases) are somewhat more common and are generally from ovarian or uterine sites. Usually tubal carcinoma is treated with surgery; the prognosis is poor.

CARCINOMA OF THE OVARY

Fortunately, ovarian carcinoma is rare, since it is exceedingly lethal. Malignancy in the ovary can occur at any age, but is more frequent in women between the ages of 40 and 65. Carcinoma can arise from the ovarian tissue itself, from malignant transformation of previously benign processes, or as a result of metastasis from another primary site, such as the breast, the urinary tract, the gastrointestinal tract, and from adjacent pelvic malignancies. The tissue type is usually either adenocarcinoma or squamous cell carcinoma. Ovarian carcinoma is associated with an increased incidence of infertility and a high familial incidence.

Ovarian carcinoma tends to grow and spread silently (without symptoms) until it causes pressure on adjacent organs or abdominal distention. This is the primary reason why it is such a lethal disease. When the pressure phenomena finally appear, the malignancy has usually spread to the tube, uterus, and ligaments, and the potential is great for rapid spread to the opposite ovary and its associated tissues. Moreover, it may have invaded bowel surfaces, including the omentum and other organs. The pelvic blood vessels may become involved, with resultant distant metastasis.

The *symptoms*—abdominal distension, urinary frequency and urgency, constipation, ascites with dyspnea, bleeding from the uterus, and ultimately pain—do not occur until the malignancy is well established, and frequently not until it has spread. The patient will eventually develop many of the symptoms of terminal cancer, e.g., cachexia, anorexia, nausea, vomiting, and weight loss, if the malignancy is not diagnosed early, usually in its asymptomatic phase. Early diagnosis is best accomplished by routine pelvic examination. The examiner may palpate a mass in the ovarian area and if it is a suspicious one will elect to do a laparotomy to establish the diagnosis. If the mass turns out to be a malignancy, the standard treatment will be carried out: a panhysterectomy. If early spread is suspected, this will either regress with removal of the primary tumor or be treated by postoperative irradiation. In some cases, even in the face of advanced disease, the physician may elect to remove as much of the malignancy as possible, not to cure the patient but rather to make her more comfortable. This procedure is usually followed by palliative irradiation. Chemotherapy may also be used for palliation, especially in the face of extensive ascites. Compounding the problems faced by an already sick patient, complications such as hemorrhage and/or infection of the tumor mass are not uncommon. Though not a true complication, the rapid onset of a surgical menopause in younger patients will produce various uncomfortable sequelae of the menopause. Estrogens are used to treat the latter problem if not contraindicated by the type of malignancy.

GENITAL TRACT SARCOMAS

Constituting a very small percentage of the genital tract malignancies in women (about 2 to 5 per cent), sarcomas are most commonly found in the uterus and ovaries. Uterine myomas are one type of tumor which may undergo sarcomatous degeneration, although this is rare in relation to the total incidence of myomas in women. Sarcomatous lesions tend to develop in younger women (20 to 30 years old) and grow very rapidly. They metastasize, particularly to the lungs, and may result in death from pulmonary causes. Treatment usually includes wide excision of the involved area and normal surrounding tissue, at times followed by irradiation. The prognosis is poor.

TROPHOBLASTIC DISEASE*

There are two or three types of trophoblastic disease, depending on which classification is used. Trophoblast refers to a type of embryonic tissue which aids in deriving nourishment for the development of the embryo from the decidual lining of the uterus. Additionally, these cells help produce human chorionic gonadotropins (H.C.G.) and estrogens. The types of disease are: (a) hydatidiform mole, (b) chorioadenoma destruens, and (c) choriocarcinoma. More recent classifications tend to distinguish between hydatidiform mole, invasive mole, and choriocarcinoma, the latter being called chorionepithelioma. Due to current therapeutic measures, however, invasive mole or chorioadenoma and choriocarcinoma or chorionepithelioma are difficult to distinguish from each other, as no tissue is obtained for analysis.

Many articles on this disease have been included in the references at the end of this unit to aid those who wish to review the literature for further information.

All of the entities are quite rare, the most common being the mole, which occurs in one out of every 2000 to 2500 pregnancies. Of these moles, about 80 to 85 per cent are benign; the remainder develop into one of the malignant conditions. Although they can occur during any of the reproductive years, they are more common in either the early or late years. It is distressing but not uncommon to have a very young patient with a so-called molar pregnancy. The signs and symptoms of a mole include: (1) intermittent bleeding in the first trimester which sometimes contains some of the characteristic grape-like tissue (such tissue should be sent to the pathologist for analysis); (2) excessively rapid growth of the uterus; (3) absence of fetal heart tones, a fetal skeleton, and fetal movement; and (4) spontaneous abortion at about 14 to 18 weeks of gestation. There is a high association with bilateral ovarian cysts, hyperemesis gravidarum, and toxemia, particularly during the first or early in the second trimester.

The diagnosis of a mole is made from a specimen submitted to pathology, obtained either by spontaneous passage or by dilatation and curettage. A persistently elevated H.C.G. level in blood or urine is highly suggestive and is considered by many to be diagnostic. When the diagnosis is uncertain. ultrasound, angiography of the uterine vessels, and pelvic x-rays (which shows absence of a fetal outline) may help to clarify the problem, but these measures must be used with caution lest there be a viable fetus present. Moles are treated by evacuating the uterus. This may be done with a Pitocin drip, by dilatation and curettage, or by hysterotomy (incision into the uterus). The follow-up care is of particular importance and must be meticulous. H.C.G. titer levels are followed frequently and usually return to normal within a week of evacuation of the uterus. During the early care, the titers are followed weekly, then every other week, and finally monthly for a year to be sure that metastatic invasion has not occurred. In some centers, patients are also treated with a course of chemotherapeutic agents (e.g., methotrexate) in an effort to insure that invasion has not occurred.

Chorioadenoma destruens is a neoplasm of the chorion with grossly visible invasion of the myometrium and sometimes of the adjacent tissues. It is often referred to as invasive mole. Metastases rarely occur, and the disease is often benign. It was previously treated with hysterectomy; however, drugs (e.g., methotrexate) are the treatment of choice today. For this reason, an absolute diagnosis is difficult to obtain, since tissue studies cannot be done.

Choriocarcinoma is a malignant neoplasm of the chorion characterized by its tendency to metastasize early, rapidly, and widely. It is an extremely malignant, necrotic tumor with its usual primary site in the uterus. The primary site may also occur in the ovaries or in the testes in men, but these forms of the disease are associated with a grim prognosis.

The clinical course is capricious and, without intervention, rapid. Without therapy, choriocarcinoma is often fatal within 6 to 12 months, although a few patients may experience spontaneous disappearance of the disease without therapy. The presenting symptoms may include heavy vaginal or abdominal bleeding or may be related to metastasis, e.g., the patient may present with lung problems. Death occurs as a result of respiratory embarrassment, hemorrhage into the tumor, and so forth. The prognosis is directly related to the duration of the illness and to the H.C.G. titer level on admission. If the duration has been short and the titers low, then, with careful management of the patient's drug regimen, she may have an excellent prognosis. Metastases occur to the following organs: (1) lungs, (2) vagina, (3) brain or central nervous system (these respond poorly to treatment), (4) liver (responds poorly), (5) kidney, and (6) spleen. Metastasis to the lungs is the most common occurrence and responds quite well to the drug program. The tumor is not radiosensitive.

Methotrexate is the drug of choice in treating trophoblastic disease. For this very malignant tumor, it is given in very high doses with one to two week rest periods between courses of therapy. The response of the patient is measured by various laboratory studies and by serial H.C.G. determinations. When the H.C.G. titer level has returned to

* The author adapted this section from a lecture by Dr. Douglas Der Yuen and from experience caring for patients with trophoblastic disease under the care of Dr. David Figge. Both these doctors are from the Department of Obstetrics and Gynecology at the University of Washington.

normal for about two courses of therapy, the patient is discharged and followed closely as an outpatient.

Nursing care of these patients is extremely challenging and requires extensive planning. In addition to the daily need for psychologic support through what is often a long therapeutic period, the patients are extremely ill because of the toxic effects of the drugs used. The nurse must be a keen observer and able to revise and improvise to meet the many needs of the patient. The drug side effects, which are discussed in Unit VII, are potentially life threatening, thus making meticulous attention to all details of care important in order to avoid losing the patient to the therapy.

SUMMARY

Consideration of each of the types of malignancy discussed in this chapter makes it apparent that the key elements in treating malignancies of the female genital tract are early discovery and prevention of the more serious forms of these diseases. The nurse in her various contacts with patients in a wide variety of settings is in an excellent position to help educate and motivate women to meet this goal.

CHAPTER 103

Diagnostic and Treatment Modalities and Related Nursing Care

JUDITH ATWOOD

In earlier chapters of this unit the importance of early diagnosis and treatment of gynecologic problems is stressed. This chapter discusses some of the more common diagnostic and treatment modalities used to accomplish these goals of early diagnosis and treatment. However, before proceeding with such a discussion, consideration of the psychologic impact of disease of the genital organs and manipulation of them during diagnostic testing and treatment is pertinent.

The functions of the genital organs are symbolic to many people in a wide variety of ways. In addition to sexual and reproductive functions, some women associate normalcy of these organs with femininity. For these women, disease, its diagnosis, and treatment may have a major impact on self-concept; such women may experience great difficulty in accepting care. For others, the whole process may be annoying at best, but if the disease is relatively minor, no major psychologic impact is felt. However, the overt reaction of the woman patient will not necessarily correlate with either her intimate feelings or the seriousness of the condition. For this reason, it is extremely important for the nurse to assess the patient's psychologic status and reaction. In doing do, however, the nurse must be sensitive and careful not to intrude or force the patient to disclose information that she might later wish she had not discussed. Moreover, she should remember that the patient herself may not really understand her own response. In any event, the nurse, by being a sensitive listener, may be able to provide considerable support for the patient, thus lessening the potential trauma she may experience. This is particularly true if the patient feels that her physician does not or is unable to understand her.

Some of the specific, nontherapeutic feelings that patients may experience include fear, humiliation, guilt, embarrassment, and anger. These feelings have been implicated by many women as part of the reason why they fail to have yearly examinations. The opportunity to ventilate these feelings to an empathetic listener may help the patient to cope more easily with the situation. Moreover, aiding a patient in this manner may encourage her to come in for care or insure that she will seek adequate follow-up or preventive care. Ventilation sessions may also provide the nurse with an opportunity to clarify misconceptions which the patient may have either about her diagnosis or proposed treatment. Since discussion of problems involving reproductive organ is a private matter, many patients have never had an opportunity to acquire reliable information. Some examples of the more common misconceptions which the nurse may encounter include:

1. Removal of the uterus means induction of the menopause.
2. A radical hysterectomy (without vaginectomy) means that one's sex life is terminated.
3. Removal of reproductive organs makes a woman less womanly.
4. Removal of one ovary produces sterility.
5. A suspicious Pap test positively establishes the diagnosis of malignancy.

Although reassurance that the above statements are incorrect may help the woman, such reassurance does not end the patient's need to talk to someone, nor does it necessarily always correct the patient's misinformation. The nurse must continue to assess the patient's needs and may find that repetition of factual information is necessary. In addition, every effort to maintain the patient's privacy, to understand her emotional liability, and to listen to her expression of her needs must continue. The nurse should remember that the goal for the patient who is having difficulty in handling her feelings is to help her to cope in the most healthy manner possible. This is a continuous process attended with ups and downs and does not mean that the patient should remain tranquil and not express her feelings.

THE GYNECOLOGIC EXAMINATION

The gynecologic history and pelvic examination are two major screening modalities used by physicians in determining the presence of problems involving the genital tract of women. Currently, nurses are also being trained to use these modalities to screen patients and identify those who need the physician's special attention. While these nurses are providing a service to both the physicians and the patients, the focus of this discussion is on more conventional nursing roles. In addition, it is important to recognize that a specialized examination is only a portion of a total health assessment of a woman. This fact should be stressed, since many women do not recognize this.

The History. The gynecologic history is designed to provide information for the physician as to potential problems which the patient may have. In this way it guides the physical examination. It has several components which are listed in Table 103–1.

TABLE 103–1. COMPONENTS OF THE GYNECOLOGIC HISTORY*

The Menstrual Cycle
Age at onset of menarche
Length of cycle
Interval between cycles
Regularity of cycle
Amount and type of flow
Date of last menstrual period (L.M.P.)
Associated symptoms (e.g., pain, intermenstrual bleeding, etc.)
Marital and Sexual History
Medications
Contraceptives
Hormones
Others
Obstetric History
Number of pregnancies and outcome of each
Complications of pregnancy and delivery and/or abortion
Previous Surgery and Illness
Gynecologic
Other major surgery or illness
Bowel and Urinary Assessment
Associated Organ Review (e.g., endocrine)
Presenting Problem

*Adapted from Behrman and Gosling.[7]

The Pelvic Examination. When the patient calls to make an appointment for a pelvic examination, she should be instructed to avoid douching for 24 hours before she is seen. Just before the examination begins, the patient should void and empty her bowels. The urine is frequently sent for examination and so she should be given appropriate instructions regarding its collection. The nurse should then instruct the patient to remove sufficient clothing to allow examination of both the abdomen and perineal structures. In some settings, the physician also examines the breasts; in this instance, asking the patient to disrobe completely and wear a gown is easier. The patient is assisted in assuming the desired position on the examining table. Frequently this is the dorsal recumbent or lithotomy position (Fig. 103–1), although either the Sims' (side lying) or knee chest position may be used. The most important considerations in appropriate assumption of the lithotomy position are the following: (1) the buttocks should be flush with the end of the table (or end of the table leaf if there is one), and (2) the legs should be placed in and taken out of the stirrups simultaneously. A triangular drape is used, and the legs should be well protected. (Consult a basic nursing text for a discussion of this type of drape.) The following equipment should be ready for use by the physician: (1) an appropriate size speculum, (2) materials with which to obtain smears and cultures (e.g., a Pap test), (3) long forceps and cotton balls, (4) a good light source, (5) water-soluble lubricant, and (6) appropriate size gloves. Additionally, equipment to perform a biopsy or cauterization should be in the room, thus avoiding the necessity for the nurse to leave the room if these procedures should be indicated. The examination consists of four parts:

1. Inspection of the external genitalia.
2. The speculum examination.
3. The bimanual examination.
4. The rectal examination.

Inspection of the external genitalia is usually carried out first. Abnormalities including discharge, areas of inflammation, outlet relaxation, etc. are noted.

After examining the external organs, the physician (using gloves) inserts the *speculum* without lubricant (which would interfere with the accuracy of the various smears). Insertion can be facilitated by running warm water over the speculum. Through the speculum the physician inspects the vaginal walls and the cervix. Smears, such as the Pap smear as well as others, are obtained. The speculum is then removed slowly, observing the vaginal surfaces during removal.

Next, a *bimanual* examination is usually conducted. One or two of the physician's fingers are inserted into the vagina and the other hand is placed on the abdomen. The organs are palpated between the fingers and the abdominal hand (Fig. 103–2).

Lastly, a *rectal* examination is performed in some patients. With insertion of one finger into the rectum, the rectal tissues can be evaluated for such things as hemorrhoids, and the posterior aspect of the genital organs can be evaluated between the vaginal finger and the rectal one.

For the most part, the examination in women who have no pathologic conditions causes no discomfort. Exceptions which may produce some discomfort include palpation of the tender ovaries during the bimanual examination, and the rectal examination. The nurse should anticipate this and ask the patient to bear down during the rectal examination and to breathe deeply through her mouth during the palpation of the ovaries. The latter helps to relax the abdominal muscles and may facilitate the whole examination if the patient is tense. After the examination is completed, any indicated instructions should be given. In many instances, this is the nurse's responsibility.

Although the pelvic examination is done rapidly, and usually with minimal patient discomfort, it is quite common to hear women discuss this type of examination in a manner which points out how much they dread this procedure. Fear and embarrassment regarding the necessary exposure of private organs and private matters, as well as fear of what may be found, may make certain patients reluctant to submit to such an examination. Even those who undergo the examination may fail to give a completely frank history. A kind and matter-of-fact attitude on the part of the nurse and physician may help alleviate part of this distress. Proper draping, explanation of the examination, and explanation of the types of questions asked may also help. In any event, failure to attain a satisfactory patient relationship can hinder obtaining a satisfactory examination.

On occasion, the physician may find a suspicious mass or other problem during the office examination. In some instances, he will then admit the patient to the hospital for an examination under anesthesia in the operating room. The examination is conducted mostly as described with the addition of anesthesia and sterile conditions. Such an examination is also conducted before some of the various other special tests done in the operating room and before some types of surgery.

SPECIAL TESTS

Cytology. Most frequently, cytology refers to the *Papanicolaou smear* when the term is used in gynecologic testing. However, this is not a strict definition, as clinical cytopathology is the study of cells obtained from a variety of sources; therefore, there are many different types of specific studies used.

Papanicolaou Smear. This test is based on the fact that both normal and abnormal cells from the lining of the various organs (e.g., uterus, cervix) exfoliate and pass into both cervical and vaginal secretions. By making a smear of these secretions, early cellular changes can be detected before they become clinically apparent. The Pap test is the most useful in diagnosing cervical carcinoma and may be up to 95 per cent accurate in detecting this lesion in its early stages. It is much less accurate (about 40 per cent) in detecting endometrial carcinoma. The smears are read by a clinical cytologist and frequently reported as follows:

Class I – no abnormal or atypical cells present
Class II – atypical, but no evidence of malignancy
Class III – suggestive, but not conclusive for malignancy
Class IV – strongly suggestive of malignancy
Class V – conclusive for malignancy

Classes II to IV should be followed up with further testing. However, it is important to remember that

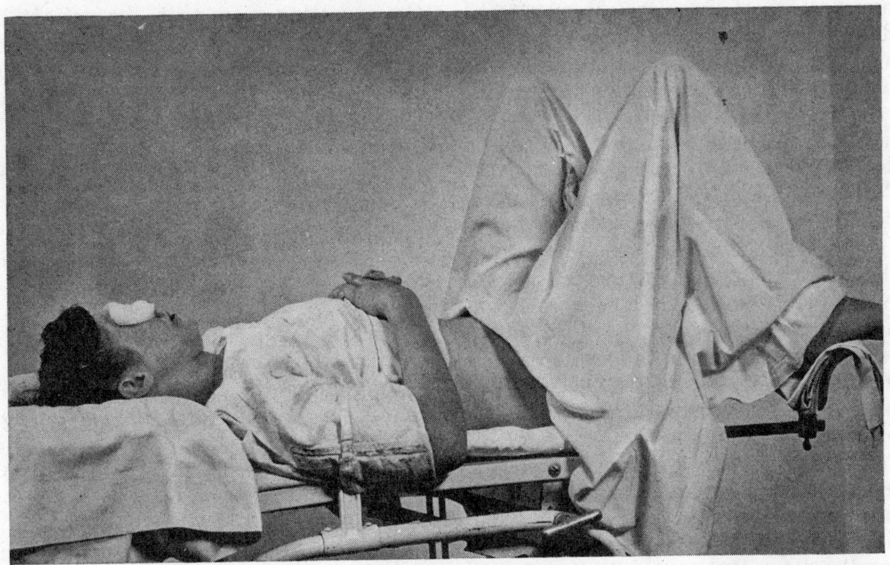

FIGURE 103–1. Patient ready for examination. (From Delp, M. H., and Manning, R. T. (eds.): *Major's Physical Diagnosis.* 7th ed. 1968.)

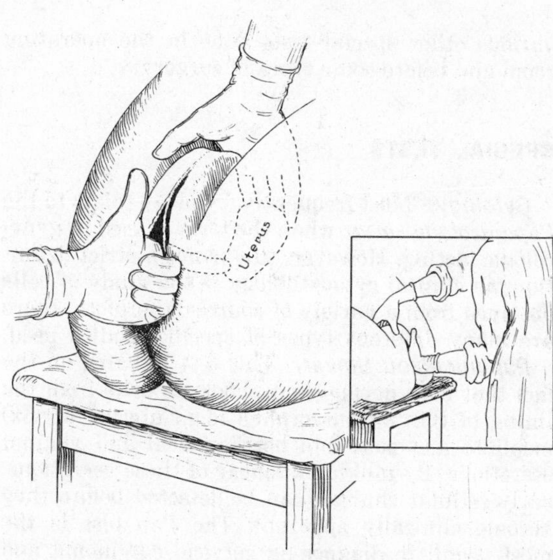

FIGURE 103–2. Method of performing bimanual examination (vaginoabdominal). (From Miller, N. F., and Avery, H.: *Gynecology and Gynecologic Nursing*. 5th ed. 1965.)

a suspicious test does not necessarily mean that the patient has a malignancy. Many patients falsely correlate a suspicious test with the presence of malignancy and become quite frightened. The Pap test may be used to follow some abnormality, and in this instance, patients are at times taught to obtain their own specimens.

The technique for obtaining the smear varies with the desires of the physician performing the test and with those of the cytologist reading it. The following describes one of the more common techniques for obtaining specimens. A small amount of the secretions found in the vaginal pool located in the posterior fornix and of the secretions extruding from the cervix are obtained using an Ayre spatula. These secretions are smeared separately on clean and dry slides. The slides are marked with "C" for cervix and "V" for vaginal pool. Immediately after the smears are made they are fixed, using either a commercial spray or fixative solution. It is important to fix the secretions before any drying occurs, as drying will distort the cells and make the reading either difficult or impossible. Lubricant is not used on the speculum for the same reason. The procedure is usually painless. After the examination is completed, the nurse should inform the patient how to obtain the results.

Endometrial Smear. Many of the same principles apply in obtaining an endometrial smear. The test differs in that the cervix must be dilated under sterile conditions to obtain the specimen. The procedure is usually done during the first 12 hours following the onset of the menses. At this time, the cervix is somewhat easier to enter. Dilatation of the cervix may cause some cramping which is usually relieved by analgesics and heat application to the lower abdomen.

Cervical Biopsy and Cautery. These procedures are frequently performed on an outpatient basis. A biopsy may be done at the time when a cervical lesion is noted or delayed until about one week after the menstrual period when the cervix is least vascular. Multiple biopsies are usually obtained at specified sites (frequently those identified by doing a Schiller test) with special biopsy forceps. The material is "fixed" appropriately, and then attention is directed toward achieving hemostasis. This is often accomplished using cautery. A lubricated lead plate is placed beneath the patient in contact with her skin. The actual cauterization is then performed. An unpleasant odor results from the burning tissue, and the patient may experience some discomfort. After the procedure is completed, vaginal packing is inserted and the patient rests for a short time before going home. She should be instructed to avoid any strenuous activity for the next 24 hours. Additional instructions include: (1) leave the packing in until the physician gives permission for it to be removed (usually 12 to 24 hours), (2) report excessive bleeding to the physician immediately, (3) abstain from coital activity and douching until otherwise instructed by the physician, and (4) avoid using tampons until the physician gives his permission. The patient should also be made aware of the fact that she will have a foul smelling, grey-green discharge beginning about four days after the procedure and lasting for about three weeks.

Cervical Conization. Conization is the removal of the diseased part of the cervix by taking a cone-shaped section of the structure. A special knife is used, and the procedure is generally done in the operating room under anesthesia. The postoperative care is similar to that employed after a "D. and C." A discharge may be expected after about four days and is frequently blood tinged.

Culdoscopy. This procedure is usually done in the operating room with the patient in the knee-chest position. Instrument visualization of the structures in the cul-de-sac is accomplished through an incision in the posterior fornix of the vagina. Through this incision, a tubular instrument with an attached light source is passed into the cul-de-sac. Preparation for the procedure is similar to that done for minor vaginal surgery, and post-procedural care is simple, since the incision heals rapidly. Douching and sexual activity are avoided for about one week (until the physician tells the patient that these activities may be resumed). Complications can include infection, hemorrhage and, rarely, air embolism.

Culdocentesis. This procedure may be performed in the office or in the operating room. It is similar to culdoscopy except that a needle is inserted through the posterior fornix into the cul-de-sac to drain this area.

Posterior Culpotomy. Similar to culdoscopy, this procedure involves making a horizontal incision into the posterior fornix for the purpose of allowing an examining finger to be slipped into the cul-de-sac. In this manner the various structures can be palpated.

Culposcopy or Culpomicroscopy. A magnifying instrument is used to examine the cervical epithelium. In the hands of an expert, epithelial abnormalities can be identified quite readily.

GYNECOLOGIC SURGERY

There are a number of types of gynecologic surgery procedures and, for this reason, several different ones have been chosen for discussion here. By consolidating the information discussed in this unit and chapter with that presented in the unit on surgery, the student should be able to predict the type of nursing care required for procedures which are not subsequently discussed. Moreover, the general pre- and postoperative care considerations are not included in order to avoid repeating the information discussed in the general surgical unit. An example of a surgical procedure involving each of the major genital organs or areas follows.

Vulvectomy. Radical vulvectomy involves the removal of a large amount of tissue including the clitoris, the labia, the perineal subcutaneous tissues, vulvar glands, and extensive dissection of the femoral and inguinal lymphatics. Pre-operatively, preparation of the skin in the perineal and lower abdominal areas is done, and the patient herself should be prepared to face a prolonged healing period with an unpleasant appearing and uncomfortable wound. However, after healing has progressed, skin grafts which are performed at the time of the initial surgery or delayed until later usually produce a somewhat more aesthetic result. Moreover, sexual function is often retained.

There are several operative approaches, and the procedure is done in either one or two stages, depending on the pre-operative condition of the patient. After surgery, there are also several approaches to care. The patient has essentially two wounds, one in the perineal area, and one in the groin. The perineal wound may be covered with a bulky pressure dressing which should be secured with a T-binder, or the area may be left without a dressing. The groin wound may also be covered or left uncovered. In the latter situation, drains in the wound are usually connected to suction. In both instances the wounds frequently have drains, and care must be exercised to avoid disloding them. Wound care is done with either hydrogen peroxide or sterile saline and is usually followed by a heat lamp treatment or sitz bath after the sutures are removed. The care must be meticulous in order to avoid infection with delayed healing. Because the drainage may be extensive, the dressings should be changed frequently.

Bowel and bladder care is important in these patients. Feces from the bowel may contaminate the wound; therefore, both constipation and diarrhea should be avoided. A retention catheter is inserted into the bladder at the time of surgery which, of course, involves the area of the urinary meatus. If the catheter is dislodged postoperatively, the extensive edema in the area makes it extremely difficult to replace. Some patients have a suprapubic catheter. Even when the surgeon orders the catheter removed, the patient may experience difficulty in voiding. Postoperative bladder infections are not uncommon, particularly since the catheter is usually left in place for an extended period. Every effort should be made to avoid this sequela.

Pain is another problem in the postoperative stage. Heavy, taut sutures are used to close the wounds and are left in place for two to three weeks. Therefore, many patients require longer periods of analgesics to control the pain. Additionally, pain may be alleviated by careful positioning of the patient in bed. Frequently, a low Fowler's position or a side-lying position with pillow support of the lumbar area and between the legs helps to decrease discomfort in the patient. The upper leg should be bent and kept slightly forward. The knees should not be gatched in order to avoid stasis in the perineal area and thrombophlebitis, one of the complications of this procedure. Hourly leg exercises and frequent position changes will also help to avoid thrombophlebitis and other complications. The patient is usually ambulated two or three days after surgery. Standing in one position should be avoided, both in the hospital and at home, because of the potential for pelvic congestion.

The surgery causes mutilation of the perineal area and is accompanied by a high incidence of complications in the postoperative period. For these reasons (and others), the patient usually requires extensive care and psychologic support. After discharge the patient generally still has not completed her recovery phase and therefore needs instructions in self-care. This type of patient can benefit from follow-up in the community by a public health nurse.

Vaginal Surgery. Several types of vaginal surgery have been discussed previously, including such vaginal repair procedures as those done for prolapse and fistulas. These discussions present the major points to be considered in caring for patients who have undergone vaginal surgery.

Dilatation and Curettage. Dilatation refers to widening the cervical opening with a dilator, and curettage, to scraping the lining of the uterine cavity with a curette. This is an extremely common gynecologic operation which, without complications, is relatively minor in nature. The most common indication for the operation is abnormal bleeding.

Preoperatively, the patient should restrict her food and fluid intake. The perineal area is prepared for surgery, and a perineal shave may or may not be done, depending on the wishes of the surgeon. Some surgeons also order an enema before surgery.

Postoperatively, the patient returns to the ward with a sterile perineal pad in place, and she may also have vaginal and cervical packing. The latter two are usually removed within the first 24 hours, and the perineal pad should be changed as needed. During the first few hours after surgery, the patient should be carefully watched for excessive vaginal bleeding. Voiding should be assessed and may be difficult particularly if the patient has vaginal packing which exerts pressure on the urethra. The patient is usually only somewhat uncomfortable, with cramping being the major complaint, especially if a pack is left in the cervical canal. Mild analgesics such as aspirin and codeine should relieve this discomfort. Pain which is not relieved with these measures should be reported to the physician, since occasionally the uterus is perforated by the curette during the procedure.

The patient is most commonly discharged the day after surgery and instructed to: (1) avoid strenuous activity for about one week, (2) avoid douching and sexual activity until the physician gives his consent, and (3) expect a vaginal discharge during the healing phase after the procedure. The subsequent menstrual period is not usually affected.

Hysterectomy. Hysterectomy, or removal of the uterus, is done either through the vagina or through the abdominal wall. The vaginal approach is used when vaginal repair is to be done at the same time, while the abdominal approach is used in the presence of large tumors, or if the ovaries and tubes are to be removed at the same time as the uterus. In the past, a partial hysterectomy was done and involved leaving the cervix in site. However, except in rare instances today, only total hysterectomy, or removal of the uterus and the cervix, is performed.

Preoperative preparation includes either a standard perineal or abdominal preparation and shave. A vaginal douche and enemas may or may not be given. Postoperatively the patient has either an abdominal dressing and perineal pad or a sterile perineal dressing (pad). These dressings should be checked relatively frequently for bleeding during the early postoperative phase. The perineal pad will normally have a moderate amount of serosanguineous drainage on it.

Fluids and foods are restricted for a time and then resumed cautiously, since the majority of patients are nauseated or vomit early. If extensive handling of the viscera has been necessary, some physicians will order a nasogastric tube to be inserted and left in for several days or until the bowel sounds return to normal. A rectal tube may help to relieve "gas pains." Frequently a Fleet enema is given several days postoperatively, as the patient may have difficulty defecating.

Abdominal distention may be present, particularly if a large tumor was removed or if the surgery was extensive. Some physicians will order a scultetus binder for this distention.

If the circulation has been interfered with, the patient may develop thrombophlebitis. The same types of precautions as discussed under vulvectomy should be taken to avoid this sequela. Most patients are ambulated the day following surgery.

One of the more serious complications which should be watched for is accidental ligation of the ureter. For this reason, any low back pain or decrease in output should be reported to the surgeon. Many of the patients have an indwelling bladder catheter for the first few days postoperatively, as operative handling of the bladder and associated structures can predispose to problems with voiding postoperatively. In any event, postoperative voiding should be checked, as retention is rather frequent. Other bladder complications including development of fistulas and infection are not uncommon. Other potential complications include: (1) embolism, (2) lung complications, (3) incisional or peritoneal infections and pelvic abscesses, (4) evisceration, and (5) late hemorrhage (about 10 to 14 days after surgery).

At the time of discharge, the patient should be instructed to:

1. Avoid sexual activity and douching until further notice.
2. Wear a girdle and/or do abdominal strengthening exercises.
3. Avoid heavy lifting for about two months.
4. Avoid any activities which increase pelvic congestion for several months, e.g., dancing, horseback riding.
5. Avoid constrictive clothing for several months.
6. Report any bleeding to the physician.
7. Return for follow-up care at a specified interval.

The effects of surgery upon a patient's menstruation should be understood by her before surgery. She should know that removal of both the uterus and cervix, i.e., total hysterectomy, will result in the cessation of menstruation.

A hysterectomy is a major operation and is associated with a great deal of anxiety in some patients. All patients have the right to receive supportive care; however, those who are extremely distressed may require more extensive care. It is important for the nurse to continually assess the patient's psychologic responses and to help the woman to cope in a healthy manner with her emotional responses. It is not unusual for women who have had a hysterectomy to experience periodic "crying spells;" these periods are often helpful for the woman. However, the nurse should be alert to signs and symptoms that the woman is having more than a usual amount of difficulty in coping, and she should bring this to the attention of the physician.

Removal of the Ovaries and Fallopian Tubes. Bilateral salpingectomy (removal of the tubes) and oophorectomy (removal of the ovaries) are often done in conjunction with a hysterectomy. The procedure is abbreviated "BSO" in many institutions, and if the menopause has not already occurred, this procedure will induce it. With the exception of care directed toward treating the unpleasant side effects of abrupt induction of the menopause, the postoperative care is similar to that given after abdominal hysterectomy or other abdominal procedures. An important fact which the nurse should keep in mind is that this procedure is attended by abrupt hormonal changes which may be manifested by unusual (psychologic) behavior by the patient.

RADIATION THERAPY

Irradiation of the pelvic organs is similar to irradiation done elsewhere in the body. The pertinent nursing care is discussed extensively in Unit VII. Other aspects of care are discussed under the appropriate disease classifications.

CHEMOTHERAPY

Chemotherapy is discussed in Unit VII. That discussion applies to the care of the gynecologic patient who is receiving chemotherapy. With the exception of the patient with trophoblastic disease (see Chapter 102) who receives chemotherapy as a primary form of treatment, most types of chemotherapy have proved to be relatively useless in treating gynecologic illness. When this treatment is resorted to, the care is complicated by the fact that the patient is usually quite ill and debilitated.

TERMINAL CARE

While care of the terminally ill patient has been discussed elsewhere (see Unit VII), one fact should be pointed out. Patients with terminal gynecologic tumors usually do not die until late in the course of their illnesses. This is true because many of the tumors do not metastasize to vital organs early, and thus the terminal event is something like renal failure. Therefore, nursing care of these patients must be carefully planned and must take into account the relative longevity of the patient.

SUMMARY

The preceding discussion has focused on some of the diagnostic and treatment modalities used in treating problems involving the female genital tract. It should be noted that the associated care can frequently be predicted if the nurse has a sound knowledge of principles discussed in this and previous chapters.

CHAPTER 104

Birth Control and Related Disorders

JUDITH ATWOOD

The topic of controlling birth is not a new one, having been a matter of concern to individuals for many years. However, what is relatively new is the concern of the society as a whole about such social issues as population control, the rights of women, and ecology. Intimately linked to these three issues is the rapid increase in medical technology which has markedly increased the life span of individuals while decreasing the infant mortality rate. Thus, as our world population has grown, concern has been expressed, first by scientists, ecologists, and demographers and then by large groups of society and the mass media. One solution to the population problem which has received much attention is the restriction of children by couples to two per each family unit. This solution has, of course, pointed up the need for adequate methods to restrict conception and a great deal of effort has been expended to perfect such methods. In addition to the work done on contraceptive methods, there has been increasing discussion concerning abortion and sterilization. More recently, these two areas have become linked with the women's liberation movement and in a broader sense, with the rights of women in general. There has been and continues to be much controversy concerning the rights of individuals to obtain sterilization on demand, but more particularly, concerning the right of women to control their own destiny, a right which some link with the issue of abortion on demand.

Abortion on demand has been particularly controversial, with all levels of society involved in the discussion. As a result of Supreme Court action and certain state legislation, increasing numbers of nurses have been confronted with patients needing care after an abortion. This is a particular problem for those nurses who find such a duty distasteful or immoral. This attitude, coupled with the frequently stated professional values of respecting the individuality of the patient and her right to make decisions, may cause the nurse to find herself in a double bind. Many hospitals have partly solved this conflict by having only those who choose to do so care for post-abortion patients. However, this solution is not totally satisfactory, as extenuating circumstances may prevail. For this reason, every nurse may come into contact with an abortion patient and she must consider how she can best cope with such an eventuality. Moreover, nurses and other health care personnel must work together to avoid allowing differing feelings to cause intrastaff conflict and thus diminish the quality of care given to the patients.

Within the broad category of birth control can be considered those methods which are voluntary and those which are involuntary. In addition to voluntary measures, some individuals suffer from conditions which promote involuntary "birth control." Three of these conditions are infertility, ectopic pregnancy, and spontaneous abortion; these are discussed in this chapter along with the methods more conventionally thought of as birth control measures.

ECTOPIC PREGNANCY

Implantation of the fertilized ovum outside the uterine cavity is called an ectopic pregnancy. Usually the implantation occurs in the ampulla of the fallopian tube, although other tubal sites are possible. Moreover, implantation may rarely occur in the cervical os, the ovary, or the abdomen. A small number of abdominal implantations have been reported to be carried to term. Delivery is accomplished by laparotomy in such cases.

Approximately one of every 250 to 300 pregnancies are ectopic in nature and many of these patients have been pregnant before. In addition, patients who have experienced one ectopic pregnancy are more likely to have another.

The *causes* of ectopic pregnancy or faulty implantation are many. Blockage of the fallopian tubes or abnormal tubal peristalsis impedes or slows down the passage of the ovum through the tube, thus promoting tubal fertilization. Adhesions, other residuals of inflammatory problems, large myomas, endometriosis, and other causes of tubal distortion or disease may also result in delayed passage of the ovum through the tubes. Once implantation has occurred in one of the tubes, one or more of the blood vessels eventually erode and bleeding results. Usually the fetus dies. The process of growth and erosion may continue through the tubal wall with bleeding into the abdominal cavity. Blood collects in the abdominal cavity and in the cul-de-sac, the latter site giving rise to a pelvic hematocele. In other situations, the fetus extrudes through the end of the tube or is retained in the tube.

The diagnosis may be very difficult to establish, as the clinical picture resembles other conditions, and not infrequently the patient is not yet aware that she is pregnant. Somewhat more frequently the typical presumptive signs of pregnancy are present.

The signs and symptoms of an acute tubal rupture are usually rapid in onset and the patient is suddenly acutely ill. She may go into shock if the blood extruded rapidly into the abdominal cavity is sufficient in amount. Early complaints (often before the onset of shock, if it occurs) may include intermittent pain localized on the involved side. The pain gradually increases in intensity. An episode of sharp, localized pain may follow, and then, as the tube ruptures, the pain becomes generalized and involves the lower abdomen. This latter type of pain is presumably due to blood entering the peritoneal cavity and irritating the peritoneal membranes. The pain may be referred to the shoulder. The patient may double over, vomit, and go into hypovolemic shock rapidly, as manifested by the classic signs and symptoms. This represents an emergency, and may present a particular problem if the diagnosis is still in doubt. Surgical intervention is usually undertaken as soon as the patient's condition is stabilized. It is sometimes preceded by culdocentesis in an attempt to find blood in the cul-de-sac and establish the diagnosis. The surgical intervention involves removal of the fetus and control of the hemorrhage. This frequently means a salpingectomy.

In less acute situations, the patient continues to have intermittent pain. In addition to the abdominal pain, she may experience pain on defecation because of the blood in the cul-de-sac (an excellent diagnostic cue). Five to seven days after the onset of the pain, vaginal bleeding may occur. This is presumably due to the death of the fetus with subsequent loss of hormonal support of the uterine lining which is then shed. Earlier bleeding in the form of spotting may also have been present. Again, the treatment is surgical, although the need for urgency is diminished.

Nursing care of a patient who loses an ectopic pregnancy depends on the condition of the patient and how she feels about the loss. If the diagnosis is in question, nursing observations are extremely important in helping to establish one. If the diagnosis has been determined, observations are more critical in the early identification of problems. The care may involve rapid preparation of a patient for surgery, helping the physician control shock, and other such acute measures. As these patients usually have a major abdominal operation, postoperative care is similar to that given to other patients who have undergone this type of surgery. It is important to assess the patient's emotional response to the whole experience and to help her to cope with the process as well as she can. This involves understanding the physician's interpretation of the potential effects on the patient's ability to have future normal pregnancies, and the extent of the surgery done. The more serious postoperative complications include hemorrhage and peritonitis.

INFERTILITY

Infertility refers to the inability of a couple to conceive after 12 months of adequate exposure without the use of contraceptives. Sterility implies the absolute inability to procreate, e.g., the woman who has had a hysterectomy cannot have children. Infertility is seldom caused by a single factor. Contrary to the opinion held by many lay people, factors involving the male partner's ability to reproduce are almost as frequently the cause (about 40 per cent) as are those factors involving the female partner's ability to reproduce (about 50 per cent). A smaller percentage of couples are unable to reproduce owing to factors involving the couple as a unit (about 10 per cent). Not infrequently, a single cause for infertility cannot be identified, and the cause is presumed to be multiple factors. In any event, an infertility work-up must involve both partners. The problem is not uncommon, as only about 10 per cent of all marriages are barren, and between 20 and 50 per cent of couples can be helped.

Since minor and major health problems can contribute to infertility, the evaluation usually begins with an assessment of the general health status of the two individuals. The work-up may be difficult, time consuming, and expensive. Couples seeking such evaluation are wise to choose their physician carefully, seeking out a specialist, particularly one with expertise and interest in the problem of infertility. In many instances the work-up will involve using the services of more than one specialist, e.g., a gynecologist, a urologist, an endocrinologist, and at times, a psychiatrist.

A comprehensive list of the various *causes* of infertility is beyond the scope of this discussion. However, the following list should demonstrate the complexity of the evaluation of the female partner only:

> loss of organ patency, e.g., tubal adhesions and occlusion

> glandular malfunction, e.g., pituitary, thyroid, adrenal
  (1) impairment of ovarian function
  (2) loss of secretory endometrium

> ovarian failure, e.g., polycystic ovarian disease

> organ infection, e.g., with changes in pH of cervical and vaginal secretions

> organ displacement, e.g., uterus

> obesity and debilitating diseases

> marital, sexual, psychologic maladjustment and ignorance
> psychologic stress

The evaluation itself may "cure" the patient who presumably has a psychologic cause for infertility. It is thought that the decrease in tension is a major contributing factor. For this reason, as well as others, it is very important for the couple and the physician to have a satisfactory relationship. Other health team members should also relate well with the couple if they are to contribute to the care.

In addition to the extensive work-up, there are several special tests which may be performed to evaluate the cause of infertility in a woman. Some of these are discussed below.

Basal Body Temperature Record. This test is done in an effort to document ovulation and the development of a secretory endometrium. Other tests done before or in conjunction include cervical and serial vaginal smears, analysis of the urine for pituitary gonadotropins and an endometrial biopsy on about day 21 or 22 of the cycle.

The basal body temperature is one of the cheapest tests used to determine when ovulation occurs. The woman takes a daily rectal temperature before arising, smoking, drinking, eating, or moving about, i.e., in a "basal state." This is charted on a graph (see Fig. 104–1); such records are kept for several months. At approximately midcycle, the basal temperature drops slightly, followed by a rise of 0.5 to 0.7 degree under the influence of progesterone. Ovulation is thought to occur just before, at the time, or just after the low temperature. The temperature charts may be somewhat confusing and the doctor should help the patient to interpret them. Those patients who wish to become pregnant should have intercourse during this time while those who wish to avoid pregnancy should practice abstinence (the rhythm method of birth control.)

Rubin Test. This is one of several tests used to evaluate tubal patency. Carbon dioxide or compressed air is introduced into the uterus and through the tubes into the peritoneal cavity under pressure. The amount of pressure is measured with a mercury manometer, the pressure being measured when gas is heard, via a stethoscope, swishing through the abdomen. If the pressure is less than 180, then the tubes are open; if it is over 200, they are considered to be closed. If the finding is between these two values, the test results are less conclusive and some other type of test is usually indicated. Atropine may be given to minimize tubal spasm. After the test, an x-ray may be taken to see if there is gas under the diaphragm.

After the test is completed, the patient should rest for about three hours. She may experience cramping pain, dizziness, shoulder pain, vomiting, and nausea. These symptoms are minimized by having her lie on her abdomen with her pelvis higher than her head (either the knee chest position or Trendelenberg position) so that the gas will rise in her pelvis. One additional value of the test is that it may treat a partial tubal obstruction by "blowing" it out.

Hysterosalpingography. This is an x-ray study of the uterus and tubes. An aqueous radiopaque substance is injected into the genital tract and

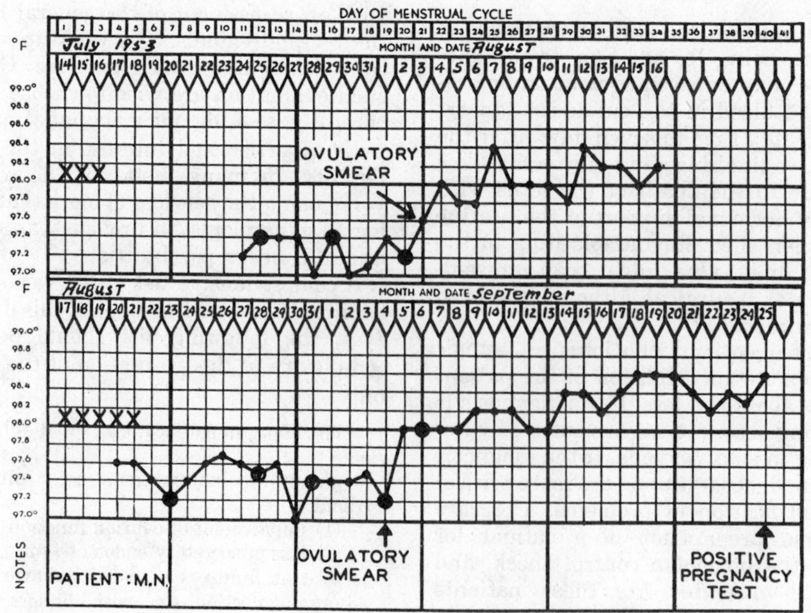

FIGURE 104–1. Basal body temperature chart. Upper curve represents type obtained with normal ovulatory cycle. Lower curve reveals first an ovulatory response, followed by leveling off due to pregnancy. (From Miller, N. F., and Avery, H.: *Gynecology and Gynecologic Nursing*. 5th ed. 1965.)

x-rays are taken to see the outline of the various structures. Among other things, the patency of the tubes and the presence of uterine pathology can be determined. The patient is usually asked to take a laxative the night before the test, and sometimes an enema the day of the test. This is to prevent distention and gas shadows which make the x-ray films difficult to read. The patient may experience some discomfort after this test and should be watched for the appearance of dye sensitivity. The symptoms of dye sensitivity are similar to those of an allergic reaction to other substances, and the discomfort is similar to that experienced after the Rubin test.

Sims-Huhner Test. Usually done at about the time of ovulation, cervical and vaginal pool secretions are aspirated and a smear is made. These secretions are obtained at a specified time after the woman has had intercourse. The time may be one hour or several hours, depending on the instructions of the physician. The secretions are then checked for the presence of viable spermatozoa. Failure to find any sperm suggests faulty intercourse technique, while failure to find any viable sperm in the cervical or vaginal secretions, or both, implies that the environment is not conducive to them. Vaginal infections with a resultant change in pH are one cause of the latter problem. The patient should wear a perineal pad, and avoid douching or bathing before coming to the office for the test. Moreover, it is helpful if she remains on her back with her hips elevated for about one half hour after intercourse.

The *treatment* of infertility depends on the cause. Some of the more common treatments are presented below.

As already mentioned, insufflation of the tubes may open them. If this does not occur, plastic operations are sometimes done to restore patency. It is unfortunate that this surgery is frequently unsuccessful and, in fact, may result in tubal pregnancy.

At times improving the general health of the patient may help. This is particularly true if the patient has either a debilitating disease or a chronic one. Improving the patient's emotional outlook also helps, as previously stated.

Still other patients may receive hormonal therapy. One drug, Clomid (clomiphene), may be given to stimulate the oocyte to mature. An artificial gonadotropin such as Pergonal may be given to stimulate the hypothalamic-pituitary-ovarian cycle. This latter drug may result in ovarian cyst development. Both drugs may cause multiple pregnancy.

It is important to remember that an infertility evaluation and treatment program may be very time consuming. Thus, no matter what the outcome, patients undergoing such a process should be allowed to talk, and they should receive proper support.

CONTRACEPTION AND BIRTH CONTROL

For every 100 women who are proved fertile and who do not use some means of contraception, about 80 of them will become pregnant in one year. Family planning, therefore, is seen as a duty by some in our society. There is increasing need for the distribution of information about contraceptives and for the contraceptives themselves. The nurse of today is expected to be well informed about the various techniques for contraception and how they are used. She should keep up to date on the latest developments in this field and know the community resources so that she can refer people who wish to obtain contraceptives. One such resource in most communities is Planned Parenthood. In addition, she should be able to provide literature to those who request it.

The choice of a contraceptive is usually made either by the client or by the client and consulting physician. The contraceptive chosen should be effective, in keeping with the patient's moral views, aesthetically acceptable, easy to use, and one that can be used consistently. More importantly, it should reflect the choice of the patient, who hopefully is then motivated to use it. With some methods of contraception, the patient should also choose an alternative method to be used in emergencies; e.g., the patient who forgets to take several of her "pills" may use foam and have her partner use a condom. None of the methods presently available is totally effective, although all are more effective than nothing. Some of them have side effects which can be quite serious. However, it should be remembered that pregnancy is a great risk to some people and frequently exceeds the risk from the form of contraception chosen for these individuals.

Coitus Interruptus. The "withdrawal" method is presumably the oldest form of birth control known to man. As ejaculation becomes imminent, the man must quickly withdraw his penis from the vagina in order that the spermatozoa be deposited outside the woman's body. Moreover, care must be taken to avoid depositing seminal fluid on the vulva where it could conceivably enter the vagina. Withdrawal requires that the male partner be highly motivated as well as aware of, and in control of, ejaculation. Many men feel that this method makes coitus less enjoyable, as there is a need for conscious control of the male impulse of deep penetration at the time of ejaculation which is contrary to the desire for self-abandonment.

Coitus interruptus is certainly better than no birth control method. However, the pregnancy rate can be relatively high and it is possible to have "accidents." Moreover, the contribution of the Cowper's glands to the seminal fluid may contain sperm which may be deposited in the vagina prior to ejaculation. Also, the first few drops of the ejaculate contain many of the total deposit of spermatozoa.

Spermicidal Preparations. There are a number of different types of creams, jellies, foams, aerosols, suppositories, and tablets which are chemicals with a spermicidal action. Of these, the jellies, creams, and foams are usually the most effective. All must be inserted into the vagina before intercourse. It is important to tell the patient who plans to use one of these preparations to read the instructions and follow them carefully. The patient should also receive the following information. Various types of preparations are inserted at different times before intercourse, depending on the properties of the agent; e.g., tablets need time to melt and should be inserted earlier than some of the other preparations. The patient should avoid douching for about six hours after intercourse, since the spermicidal preparation should not be washed away before that time. If coitus occurs more than once in a short interval it is important to check to see if another application of the product is necessary. Vigorous intercourse can force most of the agent out of the vagina, thus negating its action.

These products are considered to be quite effective when used properly. Some are viewed as being better than others. They are frequently used in combination with another form of contraception, such as a condom or diaphragm. Alone or with one of these other methods, the spermicidal agents provide additional lubrication for coitus. They tend to be messy.

All of these preparations can be bought without a prescription. They are inexpensive and easy to use. There are virtually no side effects, with the possible exception of irritation, particularly in the male.

Condoms. Condoms are widely used and provide a mechanical barrier for the spermatozoa, as well as for the organisms causing some venereal diseases. They are readily available, relatively inexpensive, and do not require a prescription. When properly used, they are highly effective.

Condoms are made from a variety of synthetic materials and have a ring around the top. They must be put on the penis after the male has an erection, and, for this reason, many men consider them a nuisance. Additionally, some men feel that they lessen the sensation during coitus.

As the male loses his erection after intercourse, the condom may not retain its fit and semen can leak into the vagina. Also, if the male fails to grasp the ring of the condom as he removes his penis from the vagina, the condom may come off in the vagina. The third way that semen can leak into the vagina is rupture or perforation of the condom. This latter event can frequently be avoided by using condoms which have a built in dead space to collect the ejaculate. They are slightly more expensive.

Condoms are frequently used with one of the spermicidal agents which is inserted in the woman's vagina at the appropriate time. This provides lubrication as well as additional protection against pregnancy.

Douches. Douches under high pressure may actually force spermatozoa into the uterus. They are not an effective birth control method.

The Rhythm Method. This is the only form of birth control which is approved by all religions in some circumstances. It is based on abstinence from coitus during ovulation. Ovulation is most frequently said to occur about 14 days before the next menstrual period, and only once each month or cycle. An ovum is said to live about 24 hours unless it is fertilized, and spermatozoa supposedly live about 72 hours. Unfortunately, all of these postulates are not necessarily true. However, they are the basis for using a period of abstinence as a form of birth control.

The primary problem with using the rhythm method is pinpointing the event of ovulation. This is most commonly done using the basal body temperature records (described earlier in the chapter). Many physicians request that the patient keep these records for six months to one year. From these records they use a formula to calculate the "safe period" for intercourse. This usually means abstinence for about eight days each month during approximately midcycle.

As can be readily seen, to be effective, the couple using this method must be highly motivated. In addition, the woman's cycle must be relatively regular. Variations in the cycle can be caused by stress, illness, fever, medications, travel, and other such events. However, despite all of these potential pitfalls, the rhythm method is quite effective for some couples.

Diaphragm. The diaphragm, another means of mechanical contraception, fits over the cervical os. It must be fitted to the woman by her physician and is made from a synthetic material or rubber with a flexible ring or coil around the outside. The woman inserts some spermicidal agent in the dome of the diaphragm, folds it over and inserts it sometime before retiring. It is then removed and cleaned the following morning. Some women may then reinsert it the subsequent day, repeating the routine. In any event, the diaphragm should not be removed for at least six hours after intercourse. In addition to using the spermicidal agent in the dome, women may also use the same agent intravaginally before intercourse for extra protection.

The diaphragm is not difficult to insert. However, the woman may find it cumbersome at first. For this reason, no woman should ever leave the physician's office without being carefully checked to see that she can insert it and remove it. She should also be taught to check its position.

The size of the diaphragm should be checked several months after it is initially used, with every pregnancy, and periodically to be sure that it is still appropriate.

If properly inserted, neither partner should be aware of a diaphragm. Well-fitting diaphragms are effective in preventing pregnancy in the majority of well-motivated women. A few with uterine descent or other pathology may not be able to use this type of contraceptive.

Intrauterine Devices (IUD). IUD's were used for camels as early as Biblical times. They were used to prevent pregnancy, especially while crossing the desert. They were first used in humans in the late 1800's but did not become popular until more recently. An IUD is an object of varying shape which is placed in the uterus to prevent pregnancy.[55] The mechanism of action of the device is not really known, although it has been postulated that it either interferes with implantation or causes rapid contraction of the tubes so that the ovum is transported through too rapidly to be fertilized.

IUD's are made in a variety of shapes and sizes, and from a variety of materials. Nurses should be familiar with the types used in their community. Such information should include knowledge of the side effects, rate of complications, and other characteristics of the particular device. No effort has been made here to discuss the various brands available, as this is an area of rapid development.

An IUD is inserted and removed by a physician. Insertion involves sounding the uterus for size and placement and then inserting the IUD through the cervix with a plunger or inserter. This may be done as a sterile out-patient procedure. Many IUD's have strings attached to them which are left in the vagina in order that the presence of the device can be validated. The patient is taught to check these strings frequently, and especially after a menstrual period. Insertion may cause discomfort, including cramping. Patients are encouraged to rest after the insertion and may be given an analgesic. Some women, frequently those who have never been pregnant, may not be able to retain an IUD or have it inserted. Thus, another type of contraception must be used.

Complications of these devices include expulsion of the device, cramping, spotting, heavy bleeding with menstrual periods, an increase in vaginal discharge, and rarely, perforation of the uterus. They are quite effective, although the pregnancy rate is somewhat higher than that for the contraceptive pill.

While the IUD is in place, the patient should have her usual annual examination. At this time some physicians will remove the IUD and replace

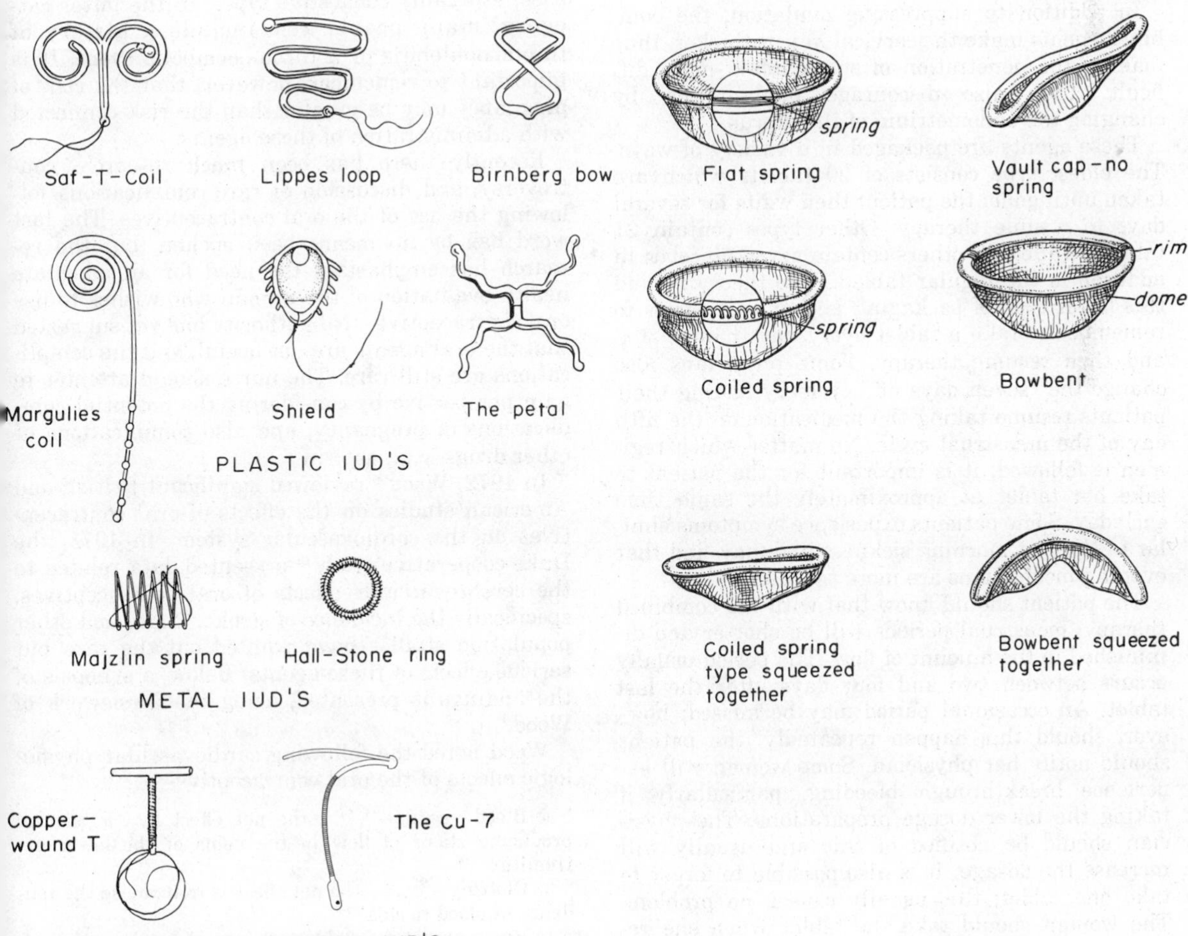

FIGURE 104-2. Birth control devices. *A*, Intrauterine devices; *B*, diaphragms. (From Hubbard, C. W.: *Family Planning Education*. St. Louis, The C. V. Mosby Company, 1973.)

it. About 20 per cent of women fitted with an IUD find them unacceptable either because of cramping or because of other side effects. These women are usually better advised to use some other form of birth control.

Oral Contraceptive Agents. Oral contraceptive agents, or the "pill," are the most effective method of birth control available today, short of sterilization. They are synthetic steroid preparations which are designed to suppress ovulation by inhibiting the production of pituitary gonadotropins. There are several types of preparations; however, the combined agents are the most effective and therefore the most commonly used. (This discussion will focus on these agents.) The combined agents consist of synthetic estrogens and progesterone. The other two types of agents are the sequentials, which contain a progesterone preparation only in the last seven tablets, and the "mini" pill, which is a very low dosage agent. Both of these types of contraceptives have an associated higher risk of pregnancy and are used infrequently. The "mini" pill is currently being studied in many agencies.

In addition to suppressing ovulation, the combined agents make the cervical mucus thicker, thus making the penetration of spermatozoa more difficult. They also discourage implantation by changing the endometrium of the uterus.

These agents are packaged in a variety of ways. The oldest type consists of 20 tablets which are taken until gone; the patient then waits for several days to resume therapy. Other types contain 21 tablets, while still others contain seven placebos in addition to the regular tablets. The theory behind this latter type of packaging is that it is easier to remember to take a tablet every day than to stop and then resume therapy. Some physicians also change the "seven days off" cycle by having their patients resume taking the medication on the fifth day of the menstrual cycle. No matter which regimen is followed, it is important for the patient to take her tablet at approximately the same time each day. Some patients experience symptoms similar to those of morning sickness and may find that evening medications are more satisfactory.

The patient should know that with the combined therapy, menstrual periods will be shorter and diminished in the amount of flow. The period usually occurs between two and four days after the last tablet. An occasional period may be missed; however, should this happen repeatedly, the patient should notify her physician. Some women will experience breakthrough bleeding, particularly if taking the lower dosage preparations. The physician should be notified of this and usually will increase the dosage. It is also possible to forget to take one tablet; this usually causes no problem. The woman should take the tablet when she remembers the omission. Should she forget more than one, however, she should notify her physician and/or use an alternative method of contraception for the rest of the cycle. However, the chances of pregnancy with the combined type of therapy remain low.

Minor and annoying side effects are experienced by many women as they begin taking oral contraceptives. These effects are rarely serious in an otherwise healthy woman. They include: nausea, vomiting, enlargement and tenderness of the breasts, minor depression, vaginal spotting, weight gain, headache, changes in libido, and changes in amount and quality of vaginal discharge. Some patients actually feel better on an oral contraceptive regimen. This is particularly true if they have experienced primary dysmenorrhea, a condition which is frequently relieved by oral contraceptives. Patients who are taking oral contraceptives are, however, more likely to develop trichomonas or yeast infections which may be very difficult to treat.

The relative contraindications to the administration of oral contraceptives include: varicosities, a history of convulsions, liver disease, diabetes mellitus, migraine headaches, and hypertension. Absolute contraindications include a history of a hormonally dependent carcinoma, hypertension which is exacerbated by these agents, a history of a neurologic vascular event, and some types of heart disease, especially congestive types. In the latter category, many people also include a history of thrombophlebitis or a thromboembolic event. It is important to remember, however, that the risk of pregnancy may be greater than the risk connected with administration of these agents.

Recently there has been much research, controversy, and discussion of rare complications following the use of the oral contraceptives. The last word has by no means been spoken, but the research has emphasized the need for an adequate health evaluation of the woman who wishes to use oral contraceptives. No authority has yet suggested that the oral agents are not useful, and the complications are still rare. The nurse should attempt to gain perspective by considering the potential complications of pregnancy, and also complications of other drugs, e.g., aspirin.

In 1972, Wood[96] reviewed significant British and American studies on the effects of oral contraceptives on the cardiovascular system. In 1973, the Duke cooperative study[19] presented data related to the cerebrovascular effects of oral contraceptives, specifically the incidence of stroke. These and other population studies have pointed out the rare but serious effects of these agents. Below, a synopsis of the findings is presented, using the framework of Wood.

Wood noted the following cardiovascular physiologic effects of the oral contraceptives:

> Blood vessels—" . . . the net effect . . . is that of producing stasis of flow in the veins of the lower extremities."[96]

> Clotting—" . . . the net effect is to increase the tendency of blood to clot."[96]

> Renin-angiotensin-aldosterone system—"the net effect is an increase in angiotensin and thus aldosterone with a potential exaggeration of hypertension."[96]

Clinically the following conclusions have been drawn from the various studies and cited by Wood and the Duke study.[19,96]

> Thromboembolism – the incidence of this problem was cited as being 12 times as high as that in a comparable population not taking these agents in the British studies. The incidence of thrombophlebitis was eight times as high.[90] These problems are frequently manifested clinically by pulmonary emboli and deep vein thrombosis. Wood concluded that these data demonstrated that these agents were not suited to patients suffering from some forms of heart disease.[96]

> Varicose veins – since the physiologic effect of these agents was venous dilatation of the legs, Wood concluded that those patients with varicosities who could use another type of birth control ought to do so.[9]

> Migraine headaches – those suffering from migraine are better treated with another type of birth control measure, according to Wood.[96]

> Cerebrovascular disorders – The Duke population study revealed that the incidence of thrombotic stroke was nine times greater in those on oral contraceptive agents than in matched controls.[19] The evidence for a correlation between hemorrhagic stroke and oral contraceptives was less conclusive. The study did not report the incidence of other risk factors for stroke (e.g., diabetes mellitus) in either the study group or the control group.[19] Vessey, in an editorial commenting on this study, stated: "Although the increase in risk of thrombotic stroke among women using oral contraceptives has been found to be large in this study, in relative terms, *it must be remembered that the absolute risk to the individual woman is extremely small* (italics mine).[89] He cited this risk at about five deaths per one million users per year.[43,89]

> Hypertension – there is evidence that, in some women, hypertension may be exacerbated with these agents. The changes occur early and reverse soon after the oral contraceptives are discontinued.

Summarizing the collected data, Wood pointed out the need for individual evaluation. He stated: "As in all branches of medicine, the physician must balance these risks against other potentially more substantial risks."[96]

STERILIZATION

Sterilization is the termination of the reproductive capacity of either a man or a woman. In the case of the male partner, sterilization through vasectomy is an easier procedure than any of the methods currently employed in women. Vasectomy is gaining increasing popularity. In women, incidental sterilization can be accomplished through several of the procedures discussed in Chapter 103. The most common procedure to produce sterility without other untoward effects in women is tubal ligation. This procedure is done without disruption of either ovulation or the menstrual function. However, with these two functions present, failure of the tubal procedure can result in pregnancy. The patient and her husband should be aware of this, as the tubes may recanalize or in other ways allow for pregnancy.

Recently the laws governing sterilization have become more liberal and increasing numbers of patients are taking advantage of this. Despite the legal status in a given state, the woman and her husband should both understand the potential effects of any proposed procedure before they consent to its being done.

Tubal ligation can be done vaginally or through the abdomen; the latter approach is used more commonly. When done vaginally, it is usually in combination with a vaginal repair procedure. Abdominally, it is performed through an incision in the lower abdomen or through a laparoscope. The fallopian tube is freed from surrounding tissues and a loop is brought up. The loop is ligated and either the area around the ligation is crushed or the ligated segment is excised. In some instances metal clips have been used in an experimental effort to provide temporary sterility. The more common techniques for tubal ligation are the Pomeroy and Irving techniques.

In the healthy woman, tubal ligation is associated with few complications. However, complications, if they do exist, may include pulmonary embolism, hemorrhage, infection, and tubal pregnancy.

ABORTION

As noted in the beginning of this chapter, the topic of abortion is one which arouses many and conflicting emotions in people. It is not uncommon to discover that many people have stereotypes of emotions which they feel the patient ought to experience. Conflicting emotions may be present in the staff when such stereotyped responses are absent. When the nurse-patient interaction breaks down, it is often because the nurse has failed to separate her own emotions from those of the patient and from those she expects the patient to experience. This is true of patients who have experienced an induced or a spontaneous abortion. It is very important for the nurse to keep in mind how easy it is to confuse these emotions and to attempt to understand this process carefully so that the care that she provides will be psychologically therapeutic for the patient.

Abortion may be defined as the spontaneous or induced expulsion of the products of conception before the fetus is legally viable. Viability as defined legally varies between 20 and 28 weeks of gestation and between 500 and 1000 gm. of weight. Miscarriage is the lay term for a spontaneous abortion. After the viable period has been reached and before term pregnancy is reached, there is a period when expulsion of the fetus is termed premature labor. The incidence of spontaneous abortion is somewhere between 10 and 15 per cent of all pregnancies, while the incidence of induced abortion is quite high, figures being very difficult to produce. With spontaneous abortion, the incidence of either fetal or maternal abnormalities is also quite high.

A number of classifications of types of abortion are presented below. First, a review of the major symptoms is pertinent. These include the presence of pregnancy with its signs and symptoms, spotting and then vaginal bleeding, cramping pain which becomes intense during the actual separation of the fetal tissues, and low back pain which frequently accompanies dilatation of the cervix and heralds the onset of inevitable abortion.

Threatened Abortion. This condition is thought to be present when the patient shows early labor-like signs, including a small amount of bleeding. The cervix is not dilated. The patient is put to bed immediately for about 24 hours, after which her activity is restricted. Sedation may be used. Cathartics and vaginal examinations are avoided. Hormones such as progesterone preparations may be given to maintain implantation, although their use is controversial. If abortion is successfully averted, the patient is asked to report any subsequent symptoms immediately.

Inevitable Abortion. Inevitable abortion is said to occur when the symptoms of threatened abortion have progressed to the point where expulsion is unavoidable. The symptoms usually include bleeding, cramping, and dilatation of the cervix.

Complete Abortion. When inevitable abortion results in the expulsion of all of the products of conception, complete abortion results. The uterus is emptied of both the fetus and the placental tissues in their entirety.

Incomplete Abortion. This type of abortion is said to occur when the patient continues to bleed after the fetus and other tissues have been expelled. It is usually due to retention of part of the placenta and is treated either with drugs, such as oxytocin, or by dilatation and evacuation (D and E) of the uterus under anesthesia.

Septic Abortion. A septic abortion usually results when tissue is retained and then becomes infected. It is associated with symptoms such as abdominal pain or tenderness, fever, a foul discharge, and laboratory evidence of infection. It is treated with antibiotics in large doses and D and E. Occasionally the serious complication of septic shock may occur with septic abortion.

Missed Abortion. This disorder is present when a dead fetus weighing less than 500 gm. is retained in the uterus for more than four weeks. It can occur after the administration of progesterone preparations to maintain a threatened fetus. It is characterized by the disappearance of signs and symptoms of pregnancy. It is usually treated by evacuating the uterus.

Habitual Abortion. Three or more consecutive abortions without an intervening successful pregnancy constitute the criteria for habitual abortion. The abortion usually occurs early in the course of the pregnancy. The treatment of such a condition is based on discovery of the cause, which may be a complex process. One cause which has received attention is an incompetent cervical os. In this instance, a purse string suture may be placed in the cervix until labor begins. At time of delivery, it is important that the patient let the medical team know that such a suture is in place. Habitual abortion is usually manifested by the painless onset of dilatation of the cervix, with rupture of the membranes and expulsion following quite rapidly. If bleeding and pain are present, they are late symptoms.

Therapeutic and Criminal Abortion. The distinction between these types of abortion is a legal one and is not very clear, owing to the changing laws. In a practical sense, criminal abortion is frequently associated with a clandestine and often unsafe abortion.

Abortion may be induced in a variety of ways, and since the popularity of openly induced abortion is increasing, a review of the major points about some of the types of induction is presented here. The least common way of aborting a fetus is hysterectomy, which is discussed in Chapter 103. Three other more common techniques are hysterotomy, curettage, and saline abortion. Hysterotomy is simular to a cesarean section and is discussed in obstetric textbooks.

Suction curettage is a popular method of inducing early abortion before 12 weeks of gestation. The cervix is dilated and "cleaned out" with a suction curettage which is much safer than the older, more conventional type of curettage. The procedure takes only a few minutes and complications are quite rare.

Saline abortion is usually done between 14 and 20 weeks of gestation and involves the replacement of amniotic fluid with hypertonic saline. The amniotic fluid is withdrawn through a spinal needle which has been placed through the fetal membranes. The saline is injected through the same needle and results in the death of the fetus within about one hour of the injection. Labor usually begins within 24 hours and the products of conception are expelled. When carefully done on appropriately selected patients, the procedure results in few complications. If the saline is injected into the intravascular spaces, the patient will experience hypernatremia with an increase in the intravascular volume. If this happens, it occurs during the injection or right after and should be treated with dextrose in water intravenously to reverse the hypernatremia. Hypernatremia may also result from leakage of the saline into the peritoneal cavity and is treated in the same fashion. If the saline is inadvertently injected into the bladder, sloughing of the epithelium may occur. This is treated with immediate bladder irrigation with normal saline. An occasional patient may develop water intoxication secondary to the administration of oxytocics to induce labor. This is treated with lactated Ringer's solution intravenously or with another electrolyte preparation. The other two complications of saline abortion are amniotic fluid embolism and retained placental tissues, the latter being treated with curettage.

The nursing care is often complicated by the emotional responses of the patient and/or nurse. In addition, the ward climate and the physician's attitude will affect the care given. Other than the emotional aspect, the care is similar to that given to a patient in labor.

SUMMARY

This chapter has, in a limited way, discussed the more controversial aspects of gynecology. Unfortunately, the scope of the presentation does not permit extensive discussion of the controversies or of the solutions which have been presented to alleviate these controversies. However, there are many excellent articles and books in the nursing and other literature which devote themselves to such a discussion. The nurse will find these topics and others presented earlier easily available.

References for Chapters 99 to 104

1. Alford, D. M. (ed.): Symposium on the woman patient. *Nursing Clinics of North America, 3:*193, June, 1968.
2. Anderson, N. J.: Vulvectomy: Nursing care. *American Journal of Nursing, 60:*668, May, 1960.
3. Arnold, E.: Individualized nursing care in family planning. *Nursing Outlook, 15:*26, December, 1967.
4. Association for the Study of Abortion, Inc. 120 West 57th Street, New York, New York, 10019.
5. Association for Voluntary Sterilization, Inc. 14 West 40th Street, New York, New York, 10018.
6. Behrman, S. J.: Management of infertility. *American Journal of Nursing, 66:*552, March, 1966.
7. Behrman, S. J., and Gosling, J. R. G.: *Fundamentals of Gynecology.* 2nd ed. New York, Oxford University Press, 1966.
8. Brewer, J. I., and DeCosta, E. J.: *Textbook of Gynecology.* 4th ed. Baltimore, The Williams and Wilkins Company, 1967.
9. Brewer, W. J., Molbo, D. M., and Gerlbie, A. B.: *Gynecologic Nursing.* St. Louis, C. V. Mosby Company, 1966.
10. Brewer, J. I., Gerlbie, A. B., Dolkart, R. E., Skom, J. H., Nagle, R. G., and Torak, E. E.: Chemotherapy in trophoblastic disease. *American Journal of Obstetrics and Gynecology, 90:*566, November, 1964.
11. Brown, W. J.: V.D.-Acquired Syphilis. *American Journal of Nursing, 71:*713, April, 1971.
12. Brunner, L. S., Emerson, C. P., Ferguson, L. K., and Suddarth, D. S.: *Textbook of Medical-Surgical Nursing.* 2nd ed. Philadelphia, J. B. Lippincott Company, 1970.
13. Buxton, C. L.: One doctor's opinion of abortion laws. *American Journal of Nursing, 68:*1026, May, 1968.
14. Calame, R. J.: Ureterovaginal fistula as a complication of radical pelvic surgery. *Archives of Surgery, 94:*876, June, 1967.
15. Celano, P. J., and Sawyer, J. R.: Vaginal fistulas. *American Journal of Nursing, 70:*2131, October, 1970.
16. Chalfant, R. L.: Diagnosis and treatment of cancer of the uterus. *Nursing Forum, 4:*67, 1965.
17. Choyce, J. M., and Cronenwett, L. R.: Saline abortion. *American Journal of Nursing, 71:*1754, September, 1971.
18. Cianfrani, T., and Conway, M. K.: Ectopic pregnancy. *American Journal of Nursing, 63:*93, April, 1963.
19. Collaborative Group for the Study of Stroke in Young Women: Oral contraceptives and increased risk of cerebral ischemia and thrombosis. *New England Journal of Medicine, 288:*871, April, 1973.
20. Connell, E. B.: The pill and the problems. *American Journal of Nursing, 71:*326, February, 1971.
21. Copenhaver, E. H., and Iliya, F. A.: Treatment of urinary stress incontinence—A current appraisal. *Surgical Clinics of North America, 45:*765, June, 1965.
23. Delp, M., and Manning, R. T. (eds.): *Major's Physical Diagnosis,* 7th edition. Philadelphia, W. B. Saunders Company, 1968.
24. Dilts, D. V., Greene, J. W., and Roddick, J. W.: *Core Studies in Obstetrics and Gynecology.* Baltimore, The Williams and Wilkins Company, 1971.
25. Educational Broadcasting Corporation: *V.D. Blues.* New York, Avon Books, 1972.
26. Eichner, E.: Progestins. *American Journal of Nursing, 65:*78, September, 1965.
27. Fischman, S. H.: Choosing an appropriate contraceptive. *Nursing Outlook, 15:*28, December, 1967.
28. Fitzpatrick, G. M.: *Gynecologic Nursing.* New York, The Macmillan Company, 1965.
29. Fleshman, R. P. (ed.): Symposium—The young adult in today's world. *Nursing Clinics of North America, 8:*1, March, 1973.
30. Fonseca, J. D.: Induced abortion: Nursing attitudes and action. *American Journal of Nursing, 68:*1022, May, 1968.
31. Funnel, J. W., and Raaf, B.: Before and after hysterectomy. *American Journal of Nursing, 64:*120, October, 1964.
32. Ganong, W. F.: *Review of Medical Physiology.* Los Altos, California, Lange Medical Publications, 1967.
33. Glynn, R.: Vaginal pH and the effect of douching. *Obstetrics and Gynecology, 20:*369, September, 1962.
34. Goldzieher, J. W.: Incidence of side effects with oral or intrauterine contraceptives. *American Journal of Obstetrics and Gynecology, 102:*91, September, 1968.
35. Gonzales, B.: Voluntary sterilization. *American Journal of Nursing, 70:*2581, December, 1970.
36. Goodman, L. S., and Gilman, A.: *Pharmacological Basis of Therapeutics.* 4th ed. New York, The Macmillan Company, 1970.
37. Goodrich, S. M., and Wood, J. E.: Peripheral venous distensibility and velocity of venous blood flow during pregnancy or during oral contraceptive therapy. *American Journal of Obstetrics and Gynecology, 90:*740, November, 1964.
38. Gusberg, S. B.: Cancer in situ of the cervix: Treatment as preventive medicine. *American Journal of Nursing, 64:*76, April, 1964.
39. Guttmacher, A. F.: Family planning: The needs and the methods. *American Journal of Nursing, 69:*1229, June, 1969.
40. Guyton, A. C.: *Textbook of Medical Physiology.* 4th ed. Philadelphia, W. B. Saunders Company, 1971.

41. Hall, R. E. Therapeutic abortion, sterilization, and contraception. *American Journal of Obstetrics and Gynecology, 91:*518, February, 1965.
42. Howie, P. W., Prentice, C. R. M., Mallinson, A. C., Horne, C. H. W., and MoNical, J. P.: Effect of combined oestrogen-progesterone contraceptives, oestrogen, and progestogen on antiplasmin and antithrombin activity. *Lancet, 2:*1329, December, 1970.
43. Inman, W. H. W., and Vessey, M. P.: Investigation of deaths from pulmonary, coronary, and cerebral thrombosis and embolism in women of childbearing age. *British Medical Journal, 2:*193, April, 1968.
44. Inman, W. H. W., Vessey, M. P., Westerholm, B., and Engelund, A.: Thromboembolic disease and the steroidal content of oral contraceptives: A report to the Committee on Safety of Drugs. *British Medical Journal, 2:*203, April, 1970.
45. Iorio, J.: Culdoscopy: Nursing care. *Nursing Outlook, 12:*35, September, 1964.
46. Iorio, J.: *Principles of Obstetrics and Gynecology for Nurses.* 2nd ed. St. Louis, The C. V. Mosby Company, 1971.
47. Kinsey, A. C.: *Sexual Behavior in the Human Female.* Philadelphia, W. B. Saunders Company, 1953.
48. Kirkendall, L. A.: *Premarital Intercourse and Interpersonal Relationships.* New York, The Julian Press, Inc., 1961.
49. Kistner, R. W., Gore, H., and Hertig, A. T.: Carcinoma of the endometrium: A preventable disease. *American Journal of Obstetrics and Gynecology, 95:*1011, August, 1966.
50. Lane, M. E.: Emotional aspects of contraception. *Bulletin of American College of Nurse-Midwives, 15:*16, February, 1970.
51. Lenz, P. E.: Women, the unwitting carriers of gonorrhea. *American Journal of Nursing, 71:*716, April, 1971.
52. Leroux, R. (ed.): Abortion. *American Journal of Nursing, 70:*1919, September, 1970.
53. Lewis, G. C., Jr.: Cancer in situ of the cervix: Screening and diagnosis. *American Journal of Nursing, 64:*72, April, 1964.
54. Mangen, Sister F. X.: Psychological aspects of nursing the advanced cancer patient. *Nursing Clinics of North America, 2:*649, December, 1967.
55. Manisoff, M. T.: Intrauterine devices. *American Journal of Nursing, 73:*1188, July, 1973.
56. Marshall, J.: A field trial of the basal body temperature method of regulating births. *Lancet, 2:*8, July, 1968.
57. Marshall, M. H., and Caillouette, J. C.: Septic abortion. *American Journal of Nursing, 66:*1042, May, 1966.
58. Martin, C. E.: Marital and coital factors in cervical cancer. *American Journal of Public Health, 57:*803, May, 1967.
59. Masters, W. H., and Johnson, V. E.: *Human Sexual Response.* Boston, Little, Brown and Company, 1966.
60. Mathews, R.: VD: TLC with the penicillin. *American Journal of Nursing, 71:*720, April, 1971.
61. Maudsley, R. F., and Robertson, M. B.: Common complications of hysterectomy. *Canadian Medical Association Journal, 92:*908, April, 1965.
62. McCary, J. L.: *Human Sexuality.* Princeton, D. Van Nostrand Company, Inc., 1967.

63. McEwen, D. E.: Estrogen replacement therapy at menopause. *Canadian Nurse, 63:*34, February, 1964.
64. McGowan, L.: New ideas about patient care before and after vaginal surgery. *American Journal of Nursing, 64:*73, February, 1964.
65. Menaber, J. S.: When menstruation is painful. *American Journal of Nursing, 62:*94, July, 1962.
66. Miller, N. F., and Avery, H.: *Gynecology and Gynecologic Nursing.* 5th ed. Philadelphia, W. B. Saunders Company, 1965.
67. Moidel, H. C., Sorensen, G. E., Giblin, E. C., and Kaufmann, M. A.: *Nursing Care of the Patient With Medical-Surgical Disorders.* New York, McGraw-Hill Book Company, 1971.
68. Montagu, G. B.: Psychiatric illness after hysterectomy. *British Medical Journal, 2:*91, April, 1968.
69. Munnell, E. W.: The changing prognosis and treatment in cancer of the ovary. *American Journal of Obstetrics and Gynecology, 100:*790, March, 1968.
70. Neubardt, S.: *Contraception.* New York, Pocket Books, 1968.
71. Newt, M.: Feminine hygiene. *American Journal of Nursing, 64:*100, December, 1964.
72. Novak, E. R.: Benign ovarian tumors. *American Journal of Nursing, 64:*104, November, 1964.
73. Novak, E. R., Jones, G. S., and Jones, H. W.: *Gynecology.* Baltimore, The Williams and Wilkins Company, 1971.
74. Peterson, E. P., and Behrman, S. J.: Laparoscopic tubal sterilization. *American Journal of Obstetrics and Gynecology, 110:*24, May, 1971.
75. Planned Parenthood-World Population. 515 Madison Avenue, New York, New York 10022.
76. Poller, L., Thomson, J. M., Tabiowo, A., and Priest, C. M.: Progesterone oral contraception and blood coagulation. *British Medical Journal, 1:*554, March, 1969.
77. Rutledge, F.: Cancer of the vagina. *American Journal of Obstetrics and Gynecology, 97:*635, March, 1967.
78. Sabiston, D. C., Jr. (ed.): *Davis-Christopher Textbook of Surgery.* 10th ed. Philadelphia, W. B. Saunders Company, 1972.
79. Shafer, K. N., Sawyer, J. R., McCluskey, A. M., Beck, E. L., and Phipps, W. J.: *Medical-Surgical Nursing.* 5th ed. St. Louis, C. V. Mosby Company, 1971.
80. Siegler, A. M.: Tubal sterilization. *American Journal of Nursing, 72:*1625, September, 1972.
81. Smith, D. W., Hanley-Germain, C. P., and Gips, C. D.: *Care of the The Adult Patient.* Philadelphia, J. B. Lippincott Company, 1971.
82. Stephens, G. J.: Mind-body continuum in human sexuality. *American Journal of Nursing, 70:*1468, July, 1970.
83. Steward, M. J.: Testing home tests for cervical cancer. *American Journal of Nursing, 65:*75, December, 1965.
84. Taylor, E. S.: *Essentials of Gynecology.* 4th ed. Philadelphia, Lea and Febiger, 1965.
85. TeLinde, R. W., and Mattingly, R. F.: *Operative Gynecology.* 4th ed. Philadelphia, J. B. Lippincott Company, 1970.
86. Thornblad, I.: Hormonal ablative therapy for the premenopausal patient with advanced cancer. *Nursing Clinics of North America, 2:*659, December, 1967.
87. U.S. Food and Drug Administration, Advisory Committee on Obstetrics and Gynecology: Report on oral contraceptives. Washington, D.C., U.S. Government Printing Office, 1966.
88. U.S. Food and Drug Administration, Advisory Committee on Obstetrics and Gynecology: Second report on oral contraception. Washington, D.C., U.S. Government Printing Office, 1969.

89. Vessey, M. P.: Oral contraceptives and stroke. *New England Journal of Medicine, 288:*906, April, 1973.
90. Vessey, M. P., and Doll, R.: Investigation of relation between use of oral contraceptives and thromboembolic disease: A further report. *British Medical Journal, 2:*651, June, 1969.
91. Warren, J. C.: Hormone therapy in the post-reproductive years. *Bedside Nurse, 3:*21, May, 1970.
92. Watson, J. E.: *Medical-Surgical Nursing and Related Physiology.* Philadelphia, W. B. Saunders Company, 1972.
93. Weir, R. J., Biggs, E., Browning, J., Mack, A., Naismith, L., Taylor, L., and Wilson, E.: Blood-pressure in women after one year of oral contraception. *Lancet, 1:*467, March, 1971.
94. Willson, J. R., and Ledger, W. J.: Complications associated with the use of intrauterine contraceptive devices in women of middle and upper socioeconomic class. *American Journal of Obstetrics and Gynecology, 100:*649, March, 1968.
95. Willson, J. R., Ledger, W. J., and Andros, G. J.: The effect of an intrauterine contraceptive device on the histological pattern of the endometrium. *American Journal of Obstetrics and Gynecology, 93:*802, November, 1965.
96. Wood, J. E.: The cardiovascular effects of oral contraceptives. *Modern Concepts of Cardiovascular Disease, 16:*37, August, 1972.
97. Woods, J. W.: Oral contraceptives and hypertension. *Lancet, 2:*653, September, 1967.
98. Zahaurek, R.: Therapeutic abortion and cultural shock. *Nursing Forum, 10:*8, 1971.

UNIT XXI

Nursing Patients Experiencing Disturbances of the Eye and Ear

Introduction and Study Guides

Eye

Sight is man's most dominant sense. We live primarily in a visual world. It is estimated that 90 per cent of our information reaches our brain by way of the eyes. Ocular disorders are common and can pose serious problems for the person experiencing them. It is thus not surprising that patients with ocular disorders are frequently anxious.

The nurse has an important role in detecting ocular disorders and referring patients for medical evaluation. Practices vary concerning treatment of disorders of the eye; we shall discuss some of those more commonly accepted. We have concentrated on those disorders that are particularly important.

Ophthalmology refers to the sum of knowledge concerning the eye and ocular diseases. Much confusion exists concerning terminology related to occupations in the field of eye care. Some important terms are clarified below:

> *Ophthalmologist* or *oculist* refers to an M.D. who has taken special training in care of the eye and management of ocular disorders, and who is qualified to give complete eye care, i.e., refraction and medical and surgical therapy.

> *Optometrist* (*or O.D.*) does *not* have a medical degree, but is qualified to measure the refractive error of the eyes *without* the use of eyedrops. The optometrist cannot diagnose or treat ocular or systemic disease.

> *Orthoptist* is a medical technician who assists an ophthalmologist in examining and caring for patients with disorders of ocular movement. An orthoptist may direct ocular exercises.

> *Optician* is a technician who grinds and fits lenses according to the prescription given to him.

> *Ocularist* is a technician who makes ophthalmoscopic prostheses, e.g., artificial eyes.

Study Guide for the Eye

1. Review anatomy, physiology, pharmacology, and nursing fundamental procedures in greater detail as necessary, in addition to content included in Chapter 105.
2. What are some common ocular symptoms and their significance?
3. List common ocular emergencies and in your own words state major principles of ocular first aid.
4. What are some common groups of ocular medications, and what are the major functions of each group? Be certain you know the differences between

mydriatics and miotics; name some examples of each, some conditions they are used for, and some contraindications to their use.

5. Why should atropine never be put in an eye unless ordered by a physician? How should eyedrops and eye ointments be administered?

6. Define the following: diplopia, amblyopia, cycloplegic, scotoma, photophobia, hyphema, iridocyclisis, ophthalmia, enucleation, proptosis, exenteration, nystagmus, emmetropia, presbyopia, exophthalmos, ptosis, hordeolum, chalazion, ectropion, dacryocystitis, iritis, panophthalmitis.

7. What is accommodation? What is binocular vision? Diagram and explain the rays of light converging in the normal eye, the myopic eye, and the hypermetropic eye. Illustrate and explain how lenses correct myopia and hyperopia.

8. Common specific disorders that should receive special emphasis as you study include strabismus, conjunctivitis, ophthalmia neonatorum, trachoma, keratitis, corneal ulcer, corneal opacity, retrolental fibroplasia, retinal detachment, glaucoma, cataract, errors of refraction, trauma, and enucleation. What are major symptoms of a cataract? of glaucoma? of detached retina? Where are cataracts formed? Why do patients need a corrective lens following cataract surgery?

9. Identify major nursing functions related to intraocular surgery.

10. Familiarize yourself with services for the blind in your community.

Ear

The ear is a complex, extraordinarily delicate sense organ which consists of two functional units: the *acoustic* apparatus, concerned with the exteroceptive sense called "hearing"; and the *vestibular* apparatus, concerned with the special proprioceptive sense involved with posture and equilibrium. The acoustic apparatus is innervated by the cochlear nerve; the vestibular apparatus is innervated by the vestibular nerve. Collectively these two nerves form the eighth cranial nerve (also called the vestibulocochlear, acoustic, auditory, or statoacoustic nerve). The ear translates sound of between some sixteen to twenty thousand cycles per second into nerve impulses. Although the ear can perceive sound waves up to sixteen thousand cycles, 250 to 6000 cycles covers most of the speech range. Much is known about how the ear works, but the phenomenon of hearing (which involves auditory centers in the brain) has long been one of the mysteries of physiology.

The nurse's role in the prevention, detection, and treatment of hearing and vestibular disorders is highly diversified. Such disorders are common and may occur at any age. By teaching others how to properly care for their ears, the nurse works to prevent aural damage. Also, she encourages persons with aural disorders to seek appropriate medical evaluation and help. Infections of the ear and related structures can have serious complications, and should thus receive early treatment before irreparable damage occurs. In many settings the nurse participates in the case-finding of persons with hearing disorders and in the rehabilitation of these individuals. In the physician's office, clinic, and hospital the nurse contributes to the medical and surgical treatment of aural disorders.

Chapter 106 focuses on some of the more common diagnostic procedures used to investigate disorders of the ear; the more common types of aural disorders; and the usual treatment of these problems. General ear care, protection of the ear, and common nursing procedures related to ear care are also discussed. Ear surgery and rehabilitation of the deaf individual are considered only briefly.

Otology refers to the sum of knowledge concerning the ear and ear diseases. An *otologist* is a physician who has specialized in studying and treating aural disorders. An *otolaryngologist* treats ear problems, but is also a specialist in problems of the throat and nose. *Audiology* refers specifically to the study of hearing. An *audiologist* is a person who specializes in the evaluation of individuals who have hearing problems and in the rehabilitation of these individuals. Generally the audiologist has an M.A. or Ph.D. degree and not an M.D. degree.

Study Guide for the Ear

1. *Review* anatomy, physiology, pharmacology, and nursing fundamentals procedures in greater detail as necessary, in addition to content included in Chapter 106. You may find it helpful to draw an anatomic picture of the ear (cross section, horizontally). Label the significant parts in addition to stating the major function of each part.
2. *Define* the following terms in your own words: otoscope, tuning fork, audiogram, furuncle, otitis media, mastoiditis, myringotomy, myringoplasty, tympanoplasty, otosclerosis, stapedectomy, fenestration, cold caloric test, presbycusis, conductive hearing loss, sensori-neural hearing loss, cerumen, vertigo, tinnitus, and nystagmus.
3. *Review* Meniere's syndrome and acute labyrynthitis. These disorders were discussed in Unit VIII.
4. *Familiarize* yourself with services for the deaf in your community. Familiarize yourself with various hearing aids by examining different types, if possible.

CHAPTER 105

Disorders of the Eye and Related Structures

BASIC ANATOMY AND PHYSIOLOGY

The eye and its adnexa represent a complex anatomical structure. Included within the small space of these structures are examples of almost all the tissues found in the rest of the body. Additionally the eye contains avascular structures not duplicated elsewhere in the body, e.g., cornea, lens, and vitreous. Physiologically the eye is also complex.

Specific details of the anatomy and physiology of the eye and related structures are discussed as appropriate throughout this chapter. The following outline summarizes basic facts which will help orient you to the anatomy and physiology of the eye and related structures as a whole. Study this outline and the associated illustrations carefully.

I. *Description of the eyes* (see Fig. 105–1): The eyes are a pair of spherical organs located in bony cavities (*orbits*) in the front of the head. The eyes are the body's organs of vision. The orbits protectively surround each eye completely except for a relatively small area which is anteriorly exposed. The eyes are each about 1 inch in diameter, have a clear circular window (*cornea*) in front to allow entrance of light, and have *muscles* originating at the back of the orbit which are inserted around the outer circumference, thereby supporting the eye and enabling it to be rotated in various directions to view the environment. From the back of each eyeball, an *optic nerve* passes through the posterior portion of the orbit, carrying impulse messages to the brain from the eye's light-sensitive tissues in the *retina*.

II. *Protection of the eye:* The eye is protected by:
   - A. The *bony skull orbit,* which dorsally surrounds the eyeball, and *pads of fat* lying under each eyeball over the base of the orbit.
   - B. The *eyelids* (*palpebrae*) and *eyelashes* which close over the eye.
   - C. The *lacrimal apparatus,* i.e., lacrimal gland and its ducts and passages, which produces tears to wash over the eye's surface, thus lubricating the eye and washing off foreign particles.
   - D. A delicate mucous membrane (*conjunctiva*) which lines the eyelids and is also reflected over the eyeball's exposed surface.

III. *External structures of the eye:* orbital cavity; extrinsic ocular muscles; eyelids and eyelashes; conjunctiva; lacrimal apparatus.

IV. *Internal structures of the eye:*
   - A. *Three separate coats or "tunics" of the eyeball:*
     1. *Outer fibrous protective layer* composed posteriorly of the *sclera* and anteriorly of the *cornea.* The sclera is white and opaque, i.e., "the white of the eye," and is composed of firm, tough connective tissue. The cornea, or "window of the eye," is a forward continuation of this outer fibrous protective layer and is transparent and colorless.
     2. *Middle vascular layer* called the "choroid coat" consists of the *choroid* posteriorly, the *ciliary body* and *iris* anteriorly. The choroid is highly vascular and darkly pigmented, thus preventing internal reflection of light. The ciliary body enables the lens to be flexible, thus increasing visual acuity. The iris is a diaphragm with a circular opening in the center, i.e., *pupil,* which regulates the amount of light admitted to the eye's interior. With strong light and near vision, the pupil contracts; with dim light and far vision, the pupil enlarges. The choroid, ciliary body, and iris are also collectively called the *uveal tract.*
     3. *Inner nervous layer* called the "*retina*" includes some ten different layers of nerve cells, including those photosensitive receptive end-organs called rods and cones. The retina translates light waves into neural impulses.
        - a. *Rods:* receptors concerned with twilight vision. Rods are sensitive to dim light.
        - b. *Cones:* receptors concerned with daylight and color vision. Cones are more sensitive to light than rods.
   - B. *Refracting media:*
     1. *Cornea* (previously mentioned).
     2. *Aqueous humor,* a watery fluid filling the eyeball's *anterior chamber,* i.e., cavity in front of the lens. This fluid not only serves as a refracting media but also helps maintain a slight forward curve in the cornea.
     3. *Lens,* i.e., *"crystalline lens,"* a biconvex crystalline body enclosed in a transparent elastic capsule suspended by suspensatory ligaments. The shape of the lens changes to properly focus the image.
     4. *Vitreous humor,* a jellylike material filling the posterior cavity of the eye behind the lens. The vitreous humor not only serves as a refracting medium but also maintains the eyeball's spherical shape.

V. *Muscles of the eye:*
   - A. *Intrinsic muscles:* the iris; the ciliary body.
   - B. *Extrinsic muscles:* four straight (rectus) muscles, i.e., superior, inferior, lateral, and medial; two oblique muscles, i.e., superior and inferior.

VI. *Nerve supply to eye:*
   - A. *Optic nerve* (second cranial nerve) carries visual impulses, received by the rods and cones, to the brain. The sclera has an opening posteriorly thru which the optic nerve enters the eyeball. Within the eyeball the nerve spreads out over the

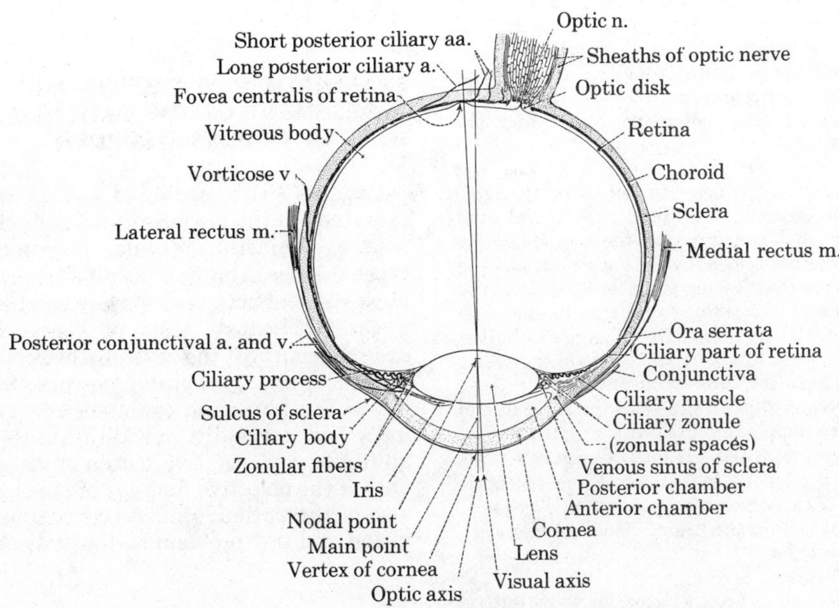
Optic n.
Short posterior ciliary aa.
Sheaths of optic nerve
Long posterior ciliary a.
Optic disk
Fovea centralis of retina
Vitreous body
Retina
Vorticose v
Choroid
Sclera
Lateral rectus m.
Medial rectus m.
Posterior conjunctival a. and v.
Ora serrata
Ciliary part of retina
Ciliary process
Conjunctiva
Sulcus of sclera
Ciliary muscle
Ciliary body
Ciliary zonule
(zonular spaces)
Zonular fibers
Venous sinus of sclera
Iris
Posterior chamber
Anterior chamber
Nodal point
Cornea
Main point
Lens
Vertex of cornea
Visual axis
Optic axis
HORIZONTAL SECTION THROUGH RIGHT EYE

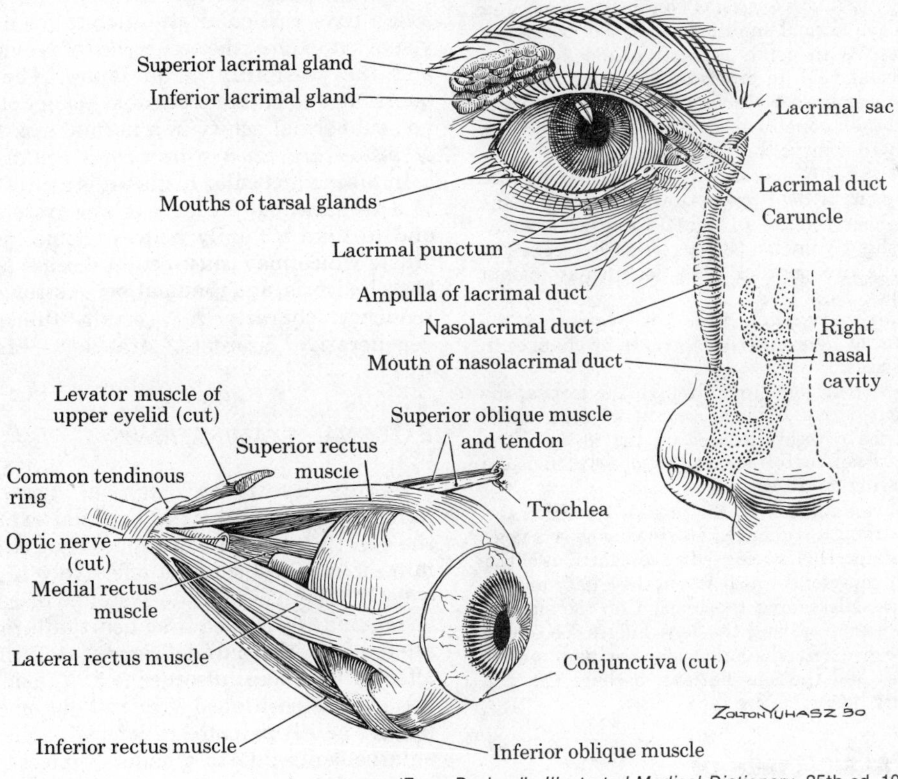
Superior lacrimal gland
Inferior lacrimal gland
Lacrimal sac
Lacrimal duct
Caruncle
Mouths of tarsal glands
Lacrimal punctum
Ampulla of lacrimal duct
Nasolacrimal duct
Right
nasal
cavity
Moutn of nasolacrimal duct
Levator muscle of
upper eyelid (cut)
Superior oblique muscle
and tendon
Superior rectus
muscle
Common tendinous
ring
Trochlea
Optic nerve
(cut)
Medial rectus
muscle
Lateral rectus muscle
Conjunctiva (cut)
ZOLTON YUHASZ '80
Inferior rectus muscle
Inferior oblique muscle

FIGURE 105–1. The eye and related structures. (From *Dorland's Illustrated Medical Dictionary.* 25th ed. 1974.)

posterior two thirds of the globe's inner surface, thus forming the thin layer of the retina.

B. *Ophthalmic nerve* (a branch of the fifth "trigeminal" cranial nerve) carries impulses of pain, touch, and temperature from the eye and its surrounding structures.

C. *Motor nerves:* oculomotor, trochlear, and abducens.

VII. *Sensory pathway for vision* (summary): The *rod* and *cone* receptors, which are sensitive to light, initiate *nerve impulse messages* which travel over the *optic nerves.* Upon entering the cranial cavity the optic nerves meet, forming the *optic chiasma.* The optic chiasma is the crossing point for fibers from the medial halves of the retinae. That is, in the optic chiasma the optic nerve fibers from the medial halves of the retinae cross to the opposite side of the brain, while those from the lateral halves of the retinae remain uncrossed. Thus fibers from the right half of each eye carry impulses to the brain's right occipital lobe, and fibers from the left half of each eye carry impulses to the left occipital lobe. From the optic chiasma the optic nerves continue, as *optic tracts,* to the cerebrum. Within the brain, visual *impulses are interpreted as sight.*

VIII. *Reflexes of the eye:*

A. *Light reflex:* pupil becomes smaller when light is flashed in the eye (see Unit VIII).

B. *Accommodation reflex:* pupil becomes smaller when gaze is shifted from distant to near object.

IX. *Physiology of binocular vision* (summary): Binocular vision is the normal simultaneous use of both eyes, which results in depth perception and enables a larger visual field. In order for binocular vision to occur, images must be brought to focus on identical points on the two retinae. The coordinated processes necessary to achieve this goal include:

A. *Convergence of visual axes,* i.e., the coordinated movement of the two eyes toward fixation of the same near point, e.g., together the two eyeballs turn slightly inward to focus on close objects. The eyeballs are parallel when looking at distant objects.

B. *Regulation of pupil size,* i.e., regulating the amount of light entering the eyes by changes in pupil sizes.

C. *Refraction of light rays* through the cornea, the aqueous humor, the lens, and the vitreous humor until the rays are focused on the retinae. The rays are bent or refracted as they pass thru media of varying densities.

D. *Accommodation,* i. e., the process by which the lens strength is changed for viewing objects near or distant. This is achieved by contractions of the ciliary muscle. For near vision the ciliary muscle contracts, lessening the tension on the suspensory ligaments, and the lens bulges, becoming more convex. For distant vision the ciliary muscle relaxes and the lens flattens, because the suspensory ligaments are taut.

OVERVIEW: BASIC TYPES OF OCULAR DISORDERS

In addition to being the site of numerous *primary* disorders, the eye also *secondarily* reflects multiple disorders located elsewhere in the body (discussed further on). There are many possible ways of classifying primary disorders of the eye and related structures. One way is to list them according to the structures which they basically affect, as we have done in Table 105–1. The list of disorders is by no means all-inclusive, but rather lists some of the more common problems for comparison.

EXAMINATION OF THE EYE AND ASSESSMENT OF THE PATIENT WITH AN OCULAR DISORDER

Patients with ocular disorders are generally examined in the physician's office or clinic. Patients with eye injuries or ocular emergencies of other types may be seen in a hospital emergency service. Most cases of acute eye disease can be diagnosed by a careful history, tests of visual function, and examination of the eye with relatively simple instruments, e.g., ophthalmoscope, tonometer, slit lamp. The physician examines the eye both externally and internally, in addition to testing the eye's ability to perform. Evaluation of vision is made not only of the objective findings of the examination but also of the patient's subjective comments about his vision and any problem he has noticed.

HISTORY

When taking an ophthalmic history, the physician pays particular attention to the nature of the visual symptoms, the occurrence of previous trouble, and the possibility of an injury. The patient is questioned to obtain a possible history of *amblyopia,* i.e., subnormal acuity in a normal eye. *Pain or loss of vision are always important ocular symptoms.*

In taking an ocular history it is also of importance to determine the presence of any systemic diseases and to take a family history. Some systemic disorders which may cause ocular disease are diabetes, thyrotoxicosis, and rheumatism. A strong hereditary tendency characterizes certain tumors, various degenerative disorders, strabismus, and myopia.

EXTERNAL EXAMINATION

Eyelids, Eyelashes, Lacrimal Apparatus, Conjunctiva. As part of the external examination of the eye, the physician examines the *eyelids* to determine if (a) the lids close effectively to protect the eyes; (b) the lids indicate systemic disease (e.g., lid edema may be caused from heart failure, nephrosis, allergy, or thyroid deficiency); (c) the lids are affected by a local disorder (e.g., tumor); or (d) the lids are malpositioned (e.g., roll out or roll in). The lids are gently palpated to determine the presence of enlargements due to glandular infections and are inspected for crusting or scales.

The *eyelashes* are observed to see if they are properly placed or if the eyelashes abnormally turn in toward the eye, thereby irritating the cornea.

A portion of the *lacrimal gland* may be observed beneath the retracted upper lid when the patient looks down. The region of the "tear sac" is examined for swelling. By pressing on the lacrimal sac (inside of the lower inner orbital rim), the physician can check for obstruction of the nasolacrimal duct and can express any infected material which may be present.

The *conjunctiva* consists of the palpebral conjunctiva (which lines the posterior lid surface) and the bulbar conjunctiva (which covers the eyeball up to the limbus, i.e., the junction of the cornea and sclera). The palpebral conjunctiva is examined by everting the eyelid; the bulbar conjunctiva is examined by widely separating the lids and having the patient look up, down, and toward either side. The conjunctival surfaces of the eyelids are inspected for any change in color, smoothness, or thickness and for the presence of secretions or foreign bodies.

Cornea. Superficial corneal irregularities are searched for by oblique moving illumination, with a small flashlight directed at the eyeball from the side. Corneal abrasions are difficult to see unless they are stained with a drop of sterile 2 per cent fluorescein solution. This stains abrasions a bright greenish color. Dropper bottles of fluorescein solution easily become contaminated with *Pseudomonas aeruginosa* and are thus unsafe. Therefore, individually packaged strips of filter paper are used which are saturated with fluorescein solution, dried, and sterilized. For use, the drug strip is wetted with a drop or two of sterile saline or sterile water, or the paper is touched to the patient's lower cul de sac so his tears will dissolve the fluorescein and disperse it over the eyeball. The paper is momentarily placed in the lower fornix, and the patient is directed to shut his eyes and then quickly look up and down to distribute the stain. Excess stain may be washed out of the eye with sterile saline solution. Then, if a corneal abrasion is present, it is clearly marked by the stain.

The *corneal reflex* is a test of corneal sensitivity (an activity governed by the fifth cranial nerve). The nurse frequently performs this test on patients with neurologic disorders and altered states of consciousness (as discussed in Unit VIII). If the eyelids do not completely close to protect the cornea, or if the corneal reflex is absent (e.g., in an unconscious patient), the unprotected cornea may become dry and injured–possibly resulting in blindness.

Eye care is not only of importance in unconscious patients; it also should be performed on all patients with *corneal anesthesia* or *facial palsy* and on all patients *following section of the 5th cranial nerve.* Conscious patients with the preceding conditions are taught to frequently and regularly inspect their eyes each day for signs of irritation or the presence of foreign bodies, e.g., eyelashes, cinders. Such persons must learn to live with their anesthetized,

TABLE 105–1. EXAMPLES OF DISORDERS OF EYE AND RELATED STRUCTURES

Areas Involved	Examples of Disorders
Eyelids	Blepharitis (inflammation of lid margin); chalazion (cystic dilation of meibomian gland); edema; hordeolum (sty); positional defects of lids (e.g., entropion, ectropion, ptosis); trichiasis (eyelashes turning in against cornea); tumors; virus infections
Lacrimal structures	Dacryocystitis (inflamed tear sac); hyposecretion of lacrimal fluid (dry eye); hypersecretion of lacrimal fluid (lacrimation); tumors
Bony orbit and eyeball	Orbital fractures; inflammatory diseases of orbit; lesions of orbital bones; tumors; displacement of eyeball (e.g., enophthalmos, exophthalmos, proptosis); hyperopia (error of refraction due to short anteroposterior diameter of eyeball); myopia (error of refraction due to long anteroposterior diameter of eyeball)
Extraocular muscles	Strabismus or "squint" (deviations of eye); diplopia (double vision); nystagmus (rhythmic involuntary oscillation of eyes); ophthalmoplegia (paralysis of eye muscles)
Conjunctiva, cornea, sclera	Conjunctivitis (inflammation of conjunctiva); subconjunctival hemorrhage; trachoma (blinding viral infection); keratitis (corneal inflammation); keratoconus (cone-shaped distortion of central cornea); corneal opacity; astigmatism (various irregularities in corneal curvature which cause optical distortion); scleritis (inflammation of sclera); ophthalmia neonatorum (acute purulent conjunctival infection in newborn); tumors
Uveal tract (iris, ciliary body, choroid)	Uveitis (inflammation of uvea); iritis (inflammation of iris); choroiditis (inflammation of choroid); cyclitis (inflammation of ciliary body); choroidocyclitis (inflammation of choroid and ciliary process); choroidoiritis (inflammation of choroid and iris); tumors
Retina	Retinitis (inflammation of retina); retinal hemorrhages; retinal detachment; retrolental fibroplasia (destructive overgrowth of retina in premature infants placed in high concentrations of oxygen); tumors
Lens	Opacity of lens (cataract); loss of elasticity of lens (presbyopia)
Ocular chambers and humors	Increased intraocular pressure (glaucoma)

deinnervated corneas and protect their vision. Protective glasses or goggles may be advisable when out of doors or performing tasks hazardous to their vision, e.g., sanding, working in areas with heavy dust in the air, chopping wood. These persons should be particularly careful when using aerosol products that spray does not get into their eyes, e.g., hair spray, deodorant sprays. Additionally, these patients are instructed to (a) frequently blink the affected eye to help it cleanse itself; (b) never rub the affected eye because this could seriously damage the cornea, particularly if a foreign body is present; (c) avoid irritating the cornea when pulling on clothing and from contact with cold compresses, washcloths, sheets; (d) to irrigate the eye and use protective drops or ointments as prescribed; and (e) to always wash their hands before examining the eye or performing eye care (see Unit VIII).

Pupil. Pupils are normally equal in size, are perfectly round, and visibly constrict during accommodation and when exposed to light. Each of these characteristics of the normal pupil is evaluated during the ocular examination. It is important for the nurse to be familiar with normal and abnormal pupillary findings and how they are obtained. In the hospital setting the nurse often evaluates the pupils of neurologic patients (see Unit VIII).

> *Enlargement of the pupil is called* mydriasis; *constriction of the pupil is called* miosis. Mydriatics *are drugs which enlarge the pupil;* miotics *are drugs which constrict the pupil.*

It is always important to know if either a mydriatic or miotic has been used on the patient's eye before the eye is examined. Irregularity of the *contour* of the pupil is always an abnormal finding. It may indicate such disorders as trauma, central nervous system syphilis, congenital defects, or iritis.

The *reaction to accommodation* is tested by holding one fingertip directly in front of the eye being tested, about 4 inches from the eye. The patient is then asked to look alternately at the fingertip and at the far wall directly beyond the finger, thus using both near and distant vision. *Direct pupil reaction to light* refers to constriction of a pupil when it is receiving increased illumination. Such a light reflex should not be checked by approaching a flashlight from straight ahead, but rather by bringing the light in from the side. *Consensual pupil reaction* refers to constriction of the pupil in the eye opposite the eye being illuminated. Such a pupillary reaction normally occurs, even though the opposite eye does not receive an increase in illumination.

Placement of the Eyeball in the Orbit. The physician may use a special instrument called an *"exophthalmometer"* to measure the height of the summit of the cornea of each eye, from the outer margin of each eye's orbital rim in the skull. The physician thus determines the placement of the eye in the orbit, e.g., whether the eye is pushed forward (exophthalmos, proptosis) or is sunken (enophthalmos). If an exophthalmometer is not available, the doctor may measure with a millimeter ruler.

Extraocular Muscles. The mobility of the eyeball is assessed to determine if the two eyes move together and whether the visual lines meet at the object of fixation. The physician tests the ability of both eyes to follow a test object smoothly and synchronously as it is moved to various positions of gaze (see Fig. 105-2). Deviations in mobility are investigated to ascertain whether there is loss of motion in any direction (paralysis or paresis) or a disorder of muscle balance, either latent (*heterophoria*) or obvious (*strabismus*).

Straightness of the two eyes is tested by observing the reflection of a light upon the cornea. A flashlight is held directly in front of the examiner's eyes, and the patient is asked to direct his gaze at the light. Normally reflection of the light symmetrically occurs in the two pupils. If one eye deviates, the light reflex is asymmetric.

Some patients' eyes develop a rhythmic twitching motion, called *"end-positional nystagmus,"* when looking to the side. In this benign condition the quick portion of the movement is always in the direction of the gaze and is followed by a slow drift back. *Pathologic nystagmus* is that in which the quick component of the movement is always in the same direction, regardless of the direction of the

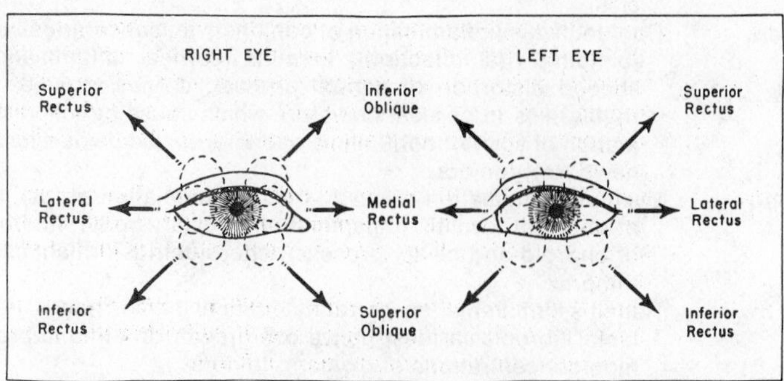

FIGURE 105-2. Diagram showing the muscles acting predominantly in the six cardinal directions of gaze. The six cardinal directions of gaze are; (1) right; (2) left; (3) up and right; (4) up and left; (5) down and right; and (6) down and left, (From Allen, J. W. (ed.): *Diseases of the Eye.* 24th ed. Baltimore, The Williams & Wilkins Co., 1968.)

patient's gaze. Nystagmus may be defined as "rhythmic involuntary oscillation of the eyes due to abnormal innervation or to lifelong reduced vision."[40] The movement of the eyeball may be horizontal, vertical, rotary, or mixed, i.e., of two varieties. The direction of the nystagmus is designated by the direction of the quick component of the movements. Nystagmus is closely related to the oculovestibular mechanisms and concerns the function of the vestibular nerve (discussed in the section pertaining to the ear). There are numerous kinds of nystagmus of which end-positional nystagmus is but one.

Visual Fields. (See also p. 1465). The integrity of the visual pathways may be roughly determined by testing the peripheral extent of the field of vision. Such an examination is made by *confrontation testing*. Peripheral vision refers to indirect vision or indistinct vision. Peripheral vision is highly important for safety and guidance. With confrontation testing the patient is directed to cover one eye and look steadily straight ahead. The examiner then takes a small object, e.g., pen, and slowly moves it. Beginning by holding the object beyond the limits of the field of vision, he gradually advances it centripetally (i.e., toward the center of the patient's gaze) to the point at which the patient first says he can see the object approaching from the periphery. The visual field may be altered by central nervous disorders, e.g., brain tumors or syphilis, and by ocular disorders, e.g., glaucoma. Normally the visual field of each eye is such that the patient can see about 60° nasalward, 50° upward, 90° temporally, and 70° downward.

Intraocular Pressure. The intraocular pressure is routinely examined in all patients over age 40 and in all others known to have, or suspected to have, a pressure increase.

> *Measurement of intraocular pressure is important because elevated intraocular pressure (called "glaucoma") may cause blindness by slowly destroying nerve fibers. (Glaucoma is discussed later in this chapter.)*

The physician may *crudely* estimate intraocular pressure by gently applying alternating pressure (with the forefinger of both hands) over the upper sclera. This is accomplished through the upper lid while the patient looks down. A *precise measurement* of intraocular pressure is obtained by *tonometer measurement* (Fig. 105-3). The tonometer is not applied to the eye until the eye is anesthetized. Next, with the patient lying flat and his eyes directed upward, the lids are gently separated without pressing on the eyeball. The tonometer is placed gently on the center of the upturned cornea and allowed to rest there by its own weight. Different weights are then superimposed, depending on the degree of suspected alteration in tension. The tonometer's needle deflects to indicate a certain number which the physician then translates, with an accompanying scale, into a definite number of millimeters of mercury. The normal intraocular pressure varies, but averages around 16.1 mm. Hg. (using Schiötz tonometers).

The tonometer cannot be boiled or autoclaved but

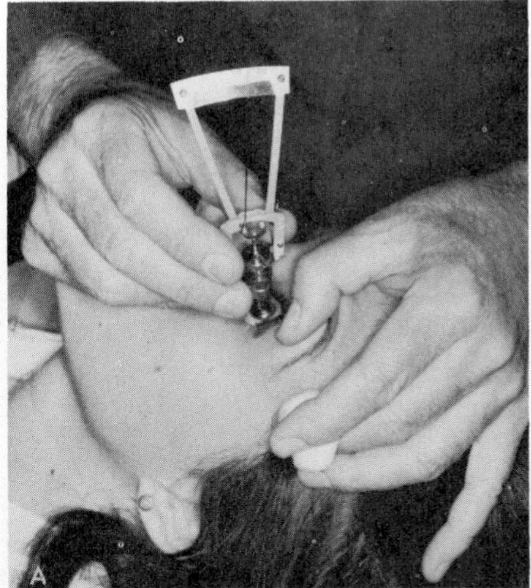

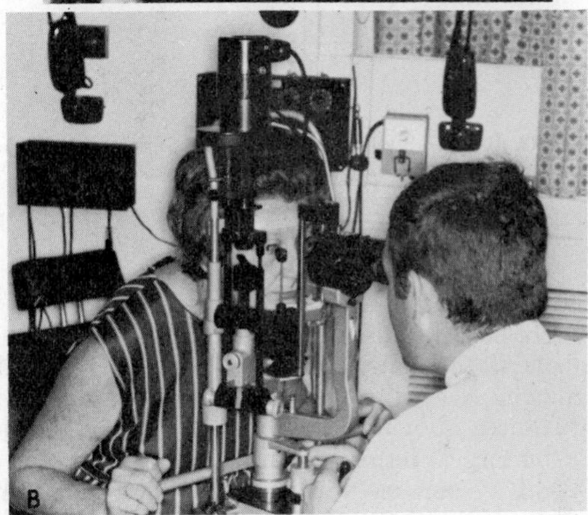

FIGURE 105-3. *A,* Schiötz tonometer, more commonly used. *B,* Applanation tonometer, used for research and verification. (From Scheie, H. G., and Albert, D. M.: *Adler's Textbook of Ophthalmology.* 8th ed. 1969.)

may be cleansed with soap and water or wiped off with solutions which are not irritating to the cornea, e.g., with benzalkonium chloride. Some sources recommend sterilizing the foot plate of the tonometer with a flame.

Visual Acuity. Havener comments: "*The most rewarding single test of ocular function is the evaluation of visual acuity.* Reduced acuity will betray the presence of a great variety of diseases as well as the need for refractive correction. Determination of visual acuity should be a part of every complete physical examination."[40]

Visual acuity is examined in one eye at a time while the patient is comfortably seated. The eye not being tested is kept covered with an opaque card.

Distant visual acuity is measured with a standardized *visual acuity chart,* e.g., *Snellen's chart* (Fig. 105-4). The nurse may be asked to perform this test in ophthalmologists' offices, schools, industry,

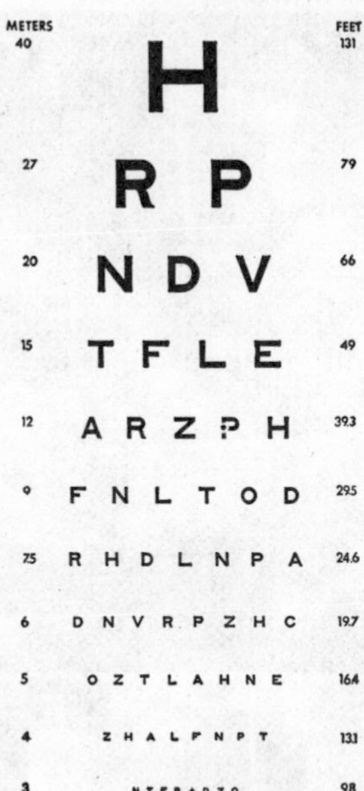

FIGURE 105-4. Snellen chart. (From Scheie, H. G., and Albert, D. M.: *Adler's Textbook of Ophthalmology.* 8th ed. 1969.)

or other settings. The chart is imprinted with a series of block letters (or other easily recognizable symbols if the patient is illiterate) in gradually decreasing sizes; the sizes are identified according to distances at which they are ordinarily visible, e.g., the largest letters can be read at a distance of 200 feet by persons with unimpaired vision. The chart is placed 20 feet from the patient and the examiner points to the line of letters he wishes the patient to read.

Visual acuity is recorded as a fraction. The fraction's numerator represents the distance to the chart; the denominator represents the distance at which a "normal eye" can read the line. For example, 20/30 means the patient is 20 feet away from the chart and can read the line that a normal eye should read at 30 feet. Thus, the larger the denominator, the poorer the patient's visual acuity.

Patients with vision so poor that they cannot see even the largest numbers on the Snellen chart are given additional tests to determine if they can see well enough to (a) count fingers (C.F.); (b) perceive hand movements (H.M.); or (c) perceive light (L.P.). An ophthalmologist does not consider a patient to be "*blind*" unless that patient cannot even perceive light. However, legally "blindness" is defined as vision (corrected by eyeglasses) of 20/200 or less, or less than 20 degrees of visual field in the better eye.

Near visual acuity is not routinely tested unless the patient is over 40 years of age or complains specifically of having difficulty reading. With increasing age *presbyopia* frequently occurs, i.e., the lens of the eye becomes less flexible. As a result the patient loses accommodation for near vision and therefore experiences difficulty with close reading unless he backs away from the material. Patients who cannot read newspaper print at one foot distance, with their own glasses on, should be advised to have an ophthalmologic examination and refraction.

Refraction. "Refraction" refers to the state of focus of the eye. When a patient is examined for refraction, the physician clinically measures the error of focus in the eye and then prescribes lenses to correct the error and thereby bring light rays into correct focus on the retina. Refraction is tested by the Snellen chart (previously discussed) and trial corrective lenses. Refraction is a common eye examination performed in the ophthalmologist's office. Correction of errors of refraction is discussed on

Ophthalmoscopic Examination. Examination of the fundus (posterior eye) is usually performed with an ophthalmoscope (Fig. 105-5). The ophthalmoscope has been of great value in clinical medicine. One professor of ophthalmology believes the ophthalmoscope is *the most valuable instrument used in medicine.* He comments: ". . . more different types of disease can be diagnosed with an ophthalmoscope than by any other single examining instrument except one – that one is the autopsy surgeon's scalpel."[40]

With an ophthalmoscope the blood vessels of the interior eye, as well as other structures, can be visualized and magnified. *The fundus is the only area of the body in which blood vessels can be directly observed.* Thus ophthalmoscopic examination not only is useful in diagnosing diseases of the eye and aberrations in the refractive mechanism, but also

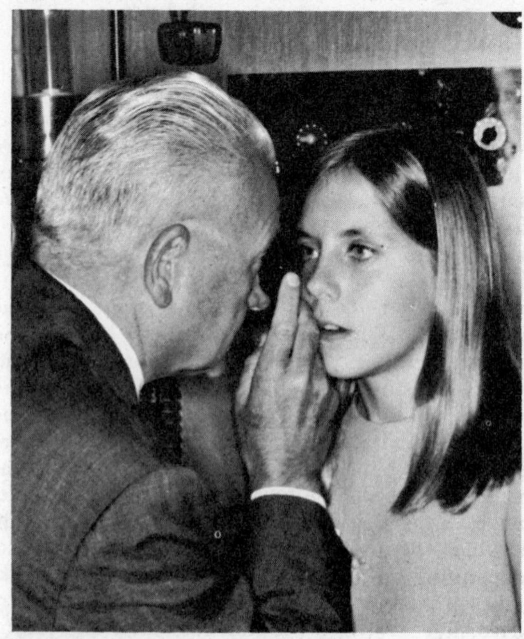

FIGURE 105-5. Ophthalmoscope. (From Scheie, H. G., and Albert, D. M.: *Adler's Textbook of Ophthalmology.* 8th ed. 1969.)

is extremely valuable in diagnosing many systemic and intracranial disorders. For example, arteriosclerosis, nephritis, brain tumor, and other disorders cause characteristic changes in the retina which can be recognized by the trained observer. Examination of the details of the posterior eye with an ophthalmoscope is part of every complete physical examination as well as ocular examination.

Ophthalmoscopic examination may be performed by either a *direct method* (as shown in Figure 105–5 and discussed above) or an *indirect method* (less common) in which a high plus lens is held in front of the patient's eye. In both methods a beam of light is focused upon the patient's retina. While the direct method gives an erect image which is highly magnified (about 15 times), only a relatively small portion of the field is visualized at a time. The direct method is thus useful in the detailed or minute examination of particular parts. The indirect method enables examination of the fundus with a stronger source of light and provides a larger field of view; however, the magnification is less (about four times), and the image is inverted. This method provides a general view or a larger portion of the background to be viewed at one time.[5] Details of the direct and indirect methods of ophthalmoscopy are presented in textbooks of ophthalmology.

With ophthalmoscopic experience the physican can often study the retina and optic nerve head without dilating the pupil. However, at times the physician may use a mydriatic to dilate the pupil so he can more clearly observe the retina (including the macula), blood vessels, and optic disk. After completing examination of the fundus, the physician can use the ophthalmoscope to visualize the vitreous body, lens, iris, aqueous humor, and cornea.

The ophthalmoscope should not be boiled, autoclaved, or soaked in solution but may be wiped off with benzalkonium chloride or alcohol. The instrument itself does not touch the patient's eye, but rather is held about 1 inch away from the eye. The nurse should see that the battery handle ophthalmoscope has fresh batteries and an operable bulb. A variety of self-luminous electric ophthalmoscopes are in use. The nurse darkens the room when the physician is ready to use the ophthalmoscope.

Other Procedures. Some additional procedures which are not routinely used in examination of the eye but are used as indicated are discussed in this section.

The *biomicroscope,* i.e., *slit lamp microscope,* is an instrument used in examining the *anterior* portion of the eye under high magnification and in optical section (obtained by a finely focused slit of brilliant light which may be focused in various ways) (Fig. 105–6). By combining intense illumination and magnification, the slit lamp and biomicroscope make it possible to study microscopic changes in the eyeball's anterior portion. By adding a strong concave lens to the slit lamp, the *posterior* vitreous and retina can be examined with the biomicroscope. The biomicroscope is used in a darkened room. The slit lamp is highly useful in determining the location of a foreign body or the depth of a corneal ulcer and in diagnosing inflammatory conditions of the eye.

We discussed on page 1463 the method of

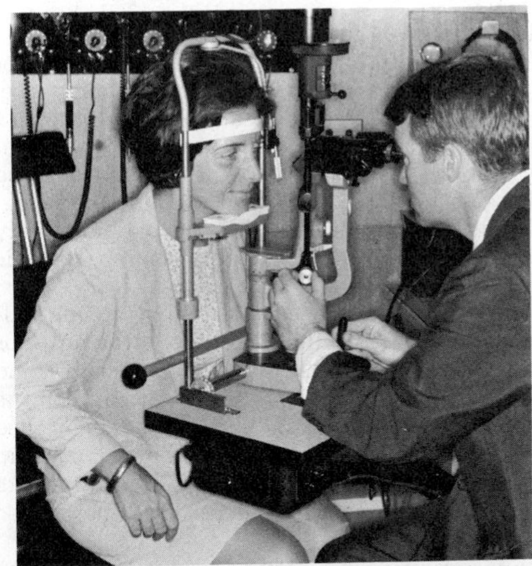

FIGURE 105–6. Bimicroscope and slit lamp. (From Scheie, H. G., and Albert, D. M.: *Adler's Textbook of Ophthalmology.* 8th ed. 1969.)

confrontation which serves to roughly determine peripheral visual fields. More precise methods of evaluation of the visual field may be used when additional investigation appears indicated. These methods may include use of a perimeter or tangent screen. A *perimeter* is a curved metallic device into which the patient looks. Inside, a test object is systematically moved along the inner surface of the arc, and the patient's peripheral vision is then outlined upon a diagram of a normal visual field. A similar principle is utilized with the *tangent screen.* In this procedure the test object is systematically moved across a large black curtain supported by a framework, and the visual field is mapped.

Precise evaluation of the peripheral and central visual fields is particularly important in examining patients with neurologic disorders, glaucoma, or retinal detachment and in making postoperative evaluations. A *scotoma* is an area of depressed vision or loss of vision within the visual field. There are various types of scotomas. Everyone has a normal physiologic scotoma which is often called the "blind spot." This is the area of the *optic disk.* In this area the optic nerve enters the eyeball, and there are no photosensitive receptors. The area of a scotoma may be plotted out, just as the normal visual field is mapped out.

The *color sense,* i.e., the faculty of distinguishing different colors, is tested by a variety of methods. The *central* perception of color is evaluated with color plates or samples of colored wool. The *peripheral* perception of color is tested in ways similar to those discussed for testing the visual field (e.g., confrontation, perimeter, tangent screen), except that the test objects are colored rather than white. The visual field for colors is smaller than that for white, but it has the same general shape. The visual field varies for different colors. The points measured in this test are those at which the colors are recognized, rather than those at which the patient merely perceives the moving test object coming into his visual field.

A *gonioscope* is a specialized kind of ophthalmoscope used to examine the angle of the anterior chamber and to demonstrate ocular motility and rotation. A special contact glass is placed upon the cornea in this procedure, and the cornea is magnified and brightly illuminated. Gonioscopy is used in evaluating patients with glaucoma or disorders of the ciliary body and iris. Gonioscopy is performed in a darkened room.

An *electroretinogram* (ERG) is a record of the changes in the retina's electric potential following stimulation by light. The ERG is clinically useful in some patients with retinal disease. An ERG is obtained by placing a contact lens electrode on the anesthetized cornea. The potential recorded on the cornea is identical with the response which would be obtained if the electrodes were placed directly upon the surface of the retina.

The *light sense,* i.e., ability to perceive gradations in the intensity or brightness of illumination, is tested by determining the patient's *light minimum,* i.e., lowest limit of illumination with which an object is visible, and his *light difference,* i.e., the smallest difference in illumination which can be perceived. Additionally, *adaptation* may be tested with a special apparatus called an *"adaptometer."* "Dark adaptation" is the ability of the eye to adjust from a brightly lit area to darkness; "light adaptation" is the ability of the eye to adjust to bright light after having been in darkness.

OCULAR SYMPTOMS AND THEIR SIGNIFICANCE

Some common ocular symptoms and their possible meanings are summarized below:

- *Pain:* Two serious eye disorders which cause pain are iritis and acute glaucoma. If these are not present, the patient may have an acute lid infection, corneal abrasion, or foreign body. The patient with a corneal ulcer or foreign body will note that his eye is more comfortable when he keeps it closed; blinking increases discomfort. Deep-seated pain occurs with intraocular inflammation; frequently the pain is referred to the trigeminal nerve's cutaneous distribution. This pain, like that of glaucoma, is often worse at night. Sinusitis often causes pain referred to the eyes.
- *Foreign body sensation:* may indicate superficial corneal erosions, e.g., staphylococcal conjunctivitis or actinic keratitis (inflammation of the cornea resulting from the action of ultraviolet light).
- *Subconjunctival hemorrhages* (gross extravasations of blood over the underlying sclera which are spontaneously absorbed within about two weeks): are asymptomatic, may occur at any age, generally following coughing, sneezing, and other straining efforts. Subconjunctival hemorrhages follow most types of ocular surgery; they are of no significance and clear within several weeks.
- *Retinal hemorrhages:* are always of importance, generally indicating such underlying systemic diseases as diabetes, blood dyscrasias, renal disease, or hypertension.
- *Vitreous hemorrhages* (extravasations of blood into the vitreous humor): commonly due to diabetes or rupture of a peripheral retinal vessel by a surrounding area of choroiditis.
- *Scotoma* (blind spot or area of loss of vision within visual field): when occurs in front of one eye is due to damage to optic nerve or retina, e.g., hemorrhage or choroiditis. When occurs in same area of both eyes, is commonly a quadratic defect due to a lesion involving the optic pathways.
- *Exophthalmos* (abnormal displacement of the eye forward out of the orbit in such a manner that the eye appears to be "bulging" forward) may be caused from thyroid disease or orbital disease.
- *Blurred vision:* may indicate refractive error, corneal opacities, cataract, retinal detachment, optic neuritis, optic atrophy, vitreous clouding, macular degeneration, central retinal vein thrombosis, or central retinal artery occlusion.
- *Photophobia* (abnormal intolerance of light): suggests keratitis, iritis, corneal ulcer, ocular albinism, or conjunctivitis, although usually photophobia is without significance. Blondes or lightly pigmented persons are often easily disturbed by glare or light.
- *Conjunctival discharge:* generally results from viral or bacterial conjunctivitis.
- *Nausea and vomiting:* may be presenting symptoms of acute glaucoma.
- *"Halos" or "rainbows" around lights:* may indicate acute glaucoma.
- *"Eyestrain" and headache:* these are common complaints. "Eyestrain" usually refers to eye discomfort associated with prolonged periods of close work or reading. Head pain related to the eye is discussed in Unit VIII. Causes of eyestrain and ocular headache include inadequate illumination; significant refractive error; early presbyopia; phoria, i.e., latent tendency to ocular deviation (usually exophoria with poor convergence).
- *Diplopia* (double vision): results from muscle imbalance or paralysis of an extraocular muscle, e.g., from infection of a nerve (6th cranial nerve commonly), hemorrhage, inflammation, or presence of a tumor.
- *"Spots" or "floaters":* "Spots before the eyes" or "floaters" in the visual field (accentuated in bright light) are vitreous opacities which generally have no clinical significance and come and go. They are more prevalent in highly myopic, i.e., "near-sighted," and older persons. Single spots or floaters are usually benign; however, the sudden appearance of multiple floaters may indicate posterior uveitis, impending retinal detachment, or intraocular hemorrhage (from diabetes or retinal detachment). *Frequently retinal detachment is preceded by a shower of "sparks"* in one quadrant of the visual field (diagnostically opposite to the tear in the retina), *followed by a sensation of a curtain moving across the eye.*

GENERAL EYE CARE AND PROTECTION OF VISION

NURSE'S ROLE

The nurse is in a key position to teach others about general eye care and the protection of vision. Also, the nurse may be the person called upon to administer first aid following ocular injuries or to offer advice concerning the need for referral of a patient to a physician. In schools and industrial settings the nurse may perform cursory procedures of visual testing to identify persons requiring further professional evaluation. Often it is the nurse who instills medication into the eyes of newborn infants to protect their vision. These are all important responsibilities which may ultimately prevent ocular disorders or improve or preserve vision. Foremost in the nurse's thoughts should be the remembrance that *blindness is often preventable* with proper care. With the appropriate application of medical knowledge, many ocular disorders can be prevented or successfully treated.

> *It is estimated that nearly one half of the present blindness could have been prevented if presently existing medical knowledge had been ideallly applied.*[40]

INCIDENCE OF IMPAIRED VISION

While the United States has the lowest incidence of blindness of all the major nations, there is much work still to be done if the goal of elimination of preventable blindness is to be attained. It is estimated* that more than 300,000 adults and children in the United States are legally blind, and that each year an additional 30,000 persons become blind. Also, an estimated 5 per cent of Americans experience an incorrectable loss of vision in one eye such that they cannot see the large "E" on the visual acuity chart (i.e., they have 20/200 vision).[40]

PROTECTION OF VISION

One means of preventing blindness and other less severe visual losses is through *teaching* the public proper general eye care, safety precautions, first-aid for eye injury, and the warning symptoms of eye disease.

Seven Eye Danger Signals. Seven eye danger signals which indicate the need for medical evaluation are: [40]

1. *Persistent redness* of the eye.
2. *Continuing pain or discomfort* around the eye or in the eye, particularly following injury.
3. *Visual disturbances,* such as difficulty seeing near or at a distance; fogginess or rainbow-colored halos around lights; sudden development of floating spots before the eyes; loss of side vision; or persistent double vision.
4. *Crossing of the eyes* (particularly in children).
5. *Growths* on the eye or eyelids or *opacities* noticeable in the normally transparent portions of the eye.
6. *Continuing discharge, crusting, or tearing* of the eyes.
7. *Pupil irregularities* (unequal size in the two pupils or distorted shape).

Self-treatment of ocular disorders may be disastrous! Unfortunately vision has been lost in many eyes through inappropriate self-treatment, e.g., instillation of contaminated or contraindicated drops or ointments. Encourage individuals with any of the above symptoms to seek professional care.

It is recommended that *the eyes should routinely be examined* at the following times: (a) at birth (to detect infections, injuries, or malformations); (b) between ages 4 and 5 (to detect "lazy eyes" which need correction prior to school entrance); (c) at age 10 and in early adolescence; (d) every five years during young adulthood; (e) every 2–5 years after age 40 (because the highest incidence of blindness is in older age groups and also because after age 40 the lens becomes less resilient); and (e) upon the appearance of ocular symptoms. When a history of glaucoma occurs in a patient's family, the patient's intraocular pressure should be examined annually.

Because the eyes' health is related to an individual's general state of health, regular total physical examinations (which include examination of the eyes) are important in eye care and visual protection. Blindness may be caused by such general disorders as hypertension, diabetes, poisoning, and disorders of the nervous system, e.g., brain tumors. Such conditions may *first* be recognized if the physician notes changes occurring in the patient's eyes at the time he performs a routine annual physical examination.

The eyes are more likely to be healthy if the total body is in a good nutritional state and is subjected to regular periods of exercise and rest.

Vision is also protected in the following ways:

> *Enforcement of safety regulations and standards,* e.g., shatterproof automobile glass and lenses in eyeglasses; safety goggles in industry; safety standards concerning protective sports equipment, e.g., face masks for hockey goalees and baseball catchers.
> *Outlawing dangerous toys, BB guns, arrows, fireworks.*
> *Early identification and treatment of strabismus in children.* This can prevent the blindness of disuse which occurs in the crossed eye of a cross-eyed child.
> *Routine programs of eye examinations in schools.*
> *Early consultation and treatment when eye symptoms occur.*
> *Instillation of silver nitrate drops in the eyes of every newborn infant.* This procedure is routinely carried out (by law) to prevent ophthalmia neonatorum (see p. 1483), an inflammatory condition of the eyes which has in the past blinded numerous unprotected infants.
> *Performance of blood tests required during pregnancy*

* It is difficult to obtain accurate statistics on the incidence of blindness because the definitions of "blindness" used vary.

to identify syphilis so it can be treated and thus prevent blindness.

> *Performance of vaccination against smallpox.* At one time smallpox was the leading cause of blindness because it produced blinding scars.
> *Performance of inoculation against rubella.* During pregnancy rubella can destroy the vision of the unborn infant.
> *Regulation of oxygen concentrations administered to premature infants.* If the oxygen concentration given to premature infants is too high, blindness results from the development of retrolental fibroplasia (see p. 1489). It is estimated that in the United States 5000 premature infants were blinded before the cause of this disorder was identified.
> *Prevention of ocular infections by properly treating injuries of the eye and other ocular disorders.*

DAILY GENERAL EYE CARE

Some factors of importance in the *daily general care of the eyes* are summarized below:

> *Do not habitually rub the eyes.* Rubbing may introduce bacteria or cause irritation of the eyes. The hands are generally best kept away from the face and eyes unless they are washed and brought up to the face for some specific purpose. Habits of rubbing and picking at the face and eyes, and having the hands up around the eyes, hair, and mouth should be broken; such habitual gestures are not only unsightly but are also unhealthy.
> *Supervise and instruct children regarding eye protection and eye care.* Children should be taught the dangers of (a) fireworks; (b) throwing rocks, dirt, and so forth; (c) poking, throwing, or running with sticks; (c) throwing or shooting paper wads, rubber bands, tin can lids, paper airplanes, sling shots, BB guns or other pellet guns, arrows, darts, and so forth; and (d) looking directly into the sun, eclipses, sun lamps, or other bright lights.
> *Reduce eyestrain.* While eyestrain (i.e., strain of the ciliary muscles when accommodation is difficult) does not permanently damage the eyes, it does cause discomfort and may slow down or impair performance of visual tasks. Eyestrain can be reduced by (a) having adequate lighting which is placed in such a manner that a shadow is not cast on the object being illuminated; and (b) periodically resting the eyes when engaging in prolonged periods of close work, reading, or television watching. The eyes may be rested by pausing occasionally to look at distant views, e.g., out the window or across the room, and by resting the head and closing the eyes occasionally. While prolonged television watching does not appear to damage vision, it is not advisable to sit too close to the set.
> *Reduce glare and wear protective goggles as indicated.* Shatterproof or unbreakable sunglasses should be worn in bright light, e.g., sunny days when snow is on the ground or when the sun is shining on a body of water. Ultraviolet rays can cause serious eye damage. Excessive exposure to sun lamps can be highly dangerous, producing not only serious skin burns but also eye injury.
> *Keep glasses clean, protected from scratching and breakage, and properly aligned.* If the glasses seem to tilt and not sit straight across the bridge of the nose and not at an even distance from both eyes, they should be readjusted by a specialist.
> *Do not use eyewashes, eyedrops, or any medications in the eyes unless they are prescribed by a physician.* The normal, healthy eye is bathed by protective conjunctival secretions which should not be washed off. *Eyecups* can spread infection or cause injury and thus should not be used.
> *Never use a soiled washcloth to wash around the eyes.* When cleaning matter from the eye's canthi, do not use the same tissue for both eyes.
> *Eat a well-balanced diet* with adequate vitamins A, B, and C. *Maintain a general state of good health.*
> *Exercise caution when using aerosol spray products.* Be certain the nozzle is pointing away from the eyes before pressing the spray button. Shut the eyes when using hair sprays.
> *Exercise caution when using solvents, lye solutions, ammonia, caustic solutions,* and so forth, to avoid splashing or spilling them into the eyes.

OCULAR EMERGENCIES AND OCULAR FIRST AID

Ocular emergencies include acute (angle closure) glaucoma; foreign bodies; corneal abrasions; contusions; actinic keratitis; corneal ulcer; chemical conjunctivitis and keratitis (e.g. chemical burns); gonococcic conjunctivitis; sympathetic ophthalmia; lacerations; orbital cellulitis; and vitreous hemorrhage. These conditions require immediate referral to an ophthalmologist. In some conditions appropriate first aid is indicated if vision is to be preserved.

Some general *first aid* considerations with reference to the eye are summarized below:

> Chemical burns of the eye, e.g., acids, poisons, caustics, need *immediate, prolonged irrigation.* Seconds may mean the difference between recovery of vision or blindness. Hold the patient's eyelids apart and pour plain water directly into the open eye. Irrigate the eye with water directly from the tap or any other source. *Continue to irrigate the eye for 15 minutes* at least before stopping to move the patient or to get a doctor. If water is not available use beer or a carbonated beverage. Following irrigation, have the patient close his eye and cover it with a protective dressing. The eye should similarly be immediately irrigated with water or sterile saline if an eyedrop is instilled into the wrong eye or if the wrong medication is instilled.
> *Do not touch* wounds penetrating into the eyeball. Do not attempt to withdraw any foreign object puncturing the eye. Leave the wound entirely alone. If possible cover the eye with a protective curved-out metal shield which will protect the eye from any accidental pressure. Obtain medical treatment immediately. Routinely, antibiotics are given to prevent endophthalmitis, and tetanus antitoxin or a toxoid booster is administered.
> If there is bleeding from the eye or eyelids, *let it bleed.* If you attempt to apply pressure to stop the bleeding, you may injure the eye.
> Do not rub the eye or pick at it if there is a scratch or foreign body on the cornea. Seek immediate medical attention so the eye can be treated with *sterile* instruments and protected against infection.

> Advise persons with a "black eye" to see a doctor. Perhaps the eyeball itself has been injured.
> Severe pain may be controlled with oral or parenteral narcotics and analgesics. Local (topical) anesthetics are not used except for diagnositic purposes. Topical anesthetics are used only in the physician's office and are not prescribed for home use in the injured eye. During anesthesia of the eye, the miotic and ameboid reparative activity of the corneal epithelium is completely prevented. Repeated instillation of anesthetics will even cause breakdown of the epithelium of a healthy undamaged cornea. Sedatives may be ordered for patients with severe eye pain.
> Never instill medications of any kind into the injured eye without a physician's order. Never use old drops in an injured eye, and do not use bottled solutions of fluorescein to stain the cornea. As discussed previously, bottled solutions are easily contaminated. If the physician wishes to stain the cornea (to look for corneal injury), he should be given dry fluorescein strips which are wetted for use.
> *Cover the injured eye with a sterile pad* or dressing but do not apply pressure on the eye with the dressing. In many cases sufficient first aid is provided by covering the eye and taking the patient to a physician. *Do not let the patient rub or touch the injured eye.* The irritation caused by the injury will prompt him to want to touch the eye. Children must be carefully watched and perhaps gently restrained, by being held, to prevent them from further injuring the eye by rubbing it before the physician evaluates the eye.

In general, when an eye injury is present it is advisable to "treat the patient but leave the eye alone."[4]

The exception to this rule is, of course, when a chemical injury has occurred and the eye itself must be *immediately* flushed with water. Following all eye injuries, seek medical attention as soon as possible.

Commonly a foreign particle blows into the eye and settles on the conjunctiva, i.e., "white of the eye," or a loose eyelash falls into the conjunctival sac. If you can easily see the particle and if the particle is truly on the conjunctiva and not the cornea, you may safely lift the particle out. This may be accomplished by carefully using a sterile applicator moistened in sterile saline (if available) or water. If the particle does not easily lift out, leave it alone and have the patient seen by a doctor. Sometimes foreign particles can be removed by irrigating the eye with sterile saline solution.

When removing foreign particles remember: do not touch the cornea! If the particle lies on the cornea a physician must remove it. Also, a physician should be consulted to remove any particles which have been in the eye for some time.

If the foreign body or eye lash settles in the lower fornix, it can be easily removed by having the patient look upward and pulling down the lower lid by applying pressure against the lower oribtal rim. If the particle lies beneath the upper lid, it scratches the cornea with each act of blinking and cannot be removed without everting the eyelid to expose its under surface. (Eversion of the eyelid is discussed on p. 1470.) Following removal of a foreign particle, the patient's eye may continue to feel uncomfortable for a few hours. If this persists for an abnormally long period of time, a physician should examine the eye.

When examining an injured eye, compare the injured eye with the normal eye using a small flashlight for focal illumination. Exercise extreme caution when examining an injured eye. *Do not press on the eye to examine it and do not press over the eye when trying to separate the eyelids.* Such pressure could destroy the eye. To open the eyelid, press instead over the portion of the lid which lies over the bony orbital rims. The pressure thus is placed on the hard bony skull rather than on the soft eye tissue. Always remember this when opening a patient's eyes. To elevate the upper lid press upward over the brow; to retract the lower lid pull down the skin overlying the cheekbone (Fig. 105–7). After elevating the upper lid, ask the patient to look up, down, right, and left. Practice this on one of your classmates.

Remember that you should *immediately stop* examination of any eye if you see that the eye has been penetrated, e.g., if it is lacerated, if the iris is prolapsed, if the vitreous humor protrudes, and so forth. Gently cover the eye with a *sterile* dressing and obtain professional medical help.

Injuries of the eye are discussed further on p. 1503.

GENERAL GUIDELINES, COMMON NURSING PROCEDURES, AND MEDICATIONS RELATED TO EYE CARE

GENERAL GUIDELINES RELATED TO EYE CARE

Summarized below are some general guidelines important in eye care. Some of these have been

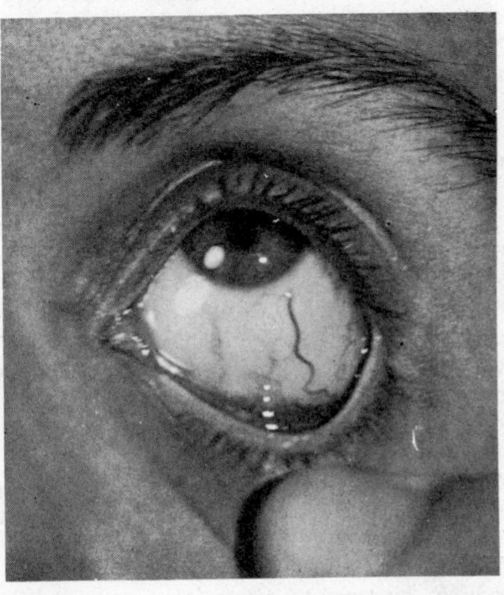

FIGURE 105–7. Method of exposing the eyeball. (From Scheie, H. G., and Albert, D. M.: *Adler's Textbook of Ophthalmology.* 8th ed. 1969.)

mentioned previously; others are discussed in the remainder of the chapter.

- Always wash before and after performing procedures related to the eye. If attending to both eyes, wash after caring for one and before approaching the other; treat the least infected eye first to minimize chances of accidentally infecting it from the other eye.
- Maintain aseptic technic to protect an unaffected eye from cross-contamination. Prevent cross-contamination between the two eyes not only by washing and treating the least infected eye first but also by having separate equipment for use on each eye, e.g., separate eye compress set-ups, if eye compresses are ordered for both eyes. When active infection is present, it is imperative to use separate medication droppers, ointment tubes, and so forth for each eye. Sometimes the physician orders the unaffected eye to be protectively covered with a shield or dressing if the other eye is seriously infected, e.g., with gonorrhea.
- Be gentle when giving eye care of any kind. Do not exert pressure over the eyeball when performing ocular procedures. A pressure dressing may be specifically used following removal of the eyeball, i.e., enucleation. However, a pressure dressing is never applied to a viable eyeball without a physician's order. Remember that the eye is a sensitive structure and that the patient has a natural tendency to protectively withdraw from ocular procedures. You can minimize this tendency if you tell the patient what you are going to do and how he can help you. At times you need to steady the patient's head to prevent him from pulling away as you treat his eye.
- Protect a patient's eyes as indicated. We have mentioned protection from cross-contamination and protection by holding the patient's head during ocular procedures. Other protective measures include prevention of corneal irritation if the patient's eyelid does not completely close. Do not touch the eyeball, e.g., with the tip of an eyedropper, ointment tube, irrigating syringe, or your fingers. Never direct forceful streams of solutions or ointments into the eye. Use low pressure for such procedures and do not direct the stream at the eyeball.
- Open the eyelids by pressing against the bony orbit rather than directly against the eyeball.
- Keep all strong solutions, which should *not* be used on the eye, away from the bedside of a patient with an ocular disorder and away from the area where ocular medications are stored.
- Find out from the partially sighted patient how well he can see and then provide appropriate care related to his level of vision. Make certain all staff members are aware of those patients with visual losses so appropriate care can be given.
- Post a sign on the patient's bed which clearly states any contraindicated activities, e.g., restricted positions or movements, activity limitations, dietary restrictions.
- Familiarize yourself with agencies which provide services for the blind and with other aspects of the rehabilitation of blind persons. Then make appropriate referrals for blind patients.
- Provide appropriate safety measures for the blind or partially sighted (including patients with eye dressings). For example, supervise smoking if it is allowed and assist the ambulatory patient to prevent bumps and falls. When the patient is in bed, keep siderails up, the bed in low position, and the call bell within easy reach and always located in the same place. Do not rearrange the patient's belongings or the furniture in his room; keep things orderly so he always knows where to find them. Maintain a safe environment around the patient's bed and chair, e.g., see that no electric cords run across the floor where the patient could fall over them. Keep footstools pushed under other furniture; keep casters locked on moveable furniture; keep the floor clean, picked up, and dry. Handrails are useful in bathrooms and along hallways.
- Place only sterile materials in the eye.
- Always have adequate light when performing ocular procedures; however, avoid directing light unnecessarily into the patient's eye. At times the patient's room is kept dimly lit, e.g., if the patient is photophobic.
- Familiarize yourself with general principles of daily eye care and protection of vision. Practice these yourself and teach others.
- Familiarize yourself with standard abbreviations used with reference to the eye. Particularly be certain you know that "O.D." (R. or R.E.) refers to oculus dexter or right eye; "O.S." (L. or L.E.) means oculus sinister or left eye; and "O.U." means oculus uterque or both eyes.
- Cleanse eyelids by moving in a direction from the inner to the outer canthus, unless an artificial eye is present.
- Encourage people to develop the habit of keeping their hands away from their eyes and faces. Rubbing the eyes may cause injury or introduce infection. Instruct patients to never touch their eyes, eye dressings, or eye shields. If the dressing needs adjusting, instruct the patient to call the nurse and have her attend to it.
- Familiarize yourself with general guidelines concerning ocular medications and with specific eye medications.
- Familiarize yourself with ocular first aid and teach basic principles to others.
- Teach patients how to correctly use contact lenses and eyeglasses.
- Attempt to prevent disorientation in the patient who has both eyes covered or in the newly blinded patient. Such patients experience sensory deprivation which may cause them to become disoriented, hallucinate, and so forth. Frequent drop-in visits, a radio softly playing for an hour or so (not steadily all day), and physical contact with the patient (e.g., holding his hand while talking to him) are all measures which help minimize the ill-effects of such sensory deprivation.
- Encourage persons with ocular disorders to seek professional evaluations and treatment.
- Familiarize yourself with basic ocular disorders, their symptoms and common treatments (medical and surgical).

COMMON NURSING PROCEDURES RELATED TO THE EYE

Common nursing procedures related to eye care include eversion of the upper eyelid; ocular irrigations; cleansing of the eyelids; instillation of eye drops and ocular ointments; application of hot and cold compresses; application and care of eye dressings; and removal and care of an artificial eye.

Eversion of the Upper Eyelid. Eversion of the

upper eyelid is necessary to inspect the palpebral conjunctiva and is accomplished as follows: (a) instruct the patient to look down (this relaxes the levator muscle, making eversion possible); (b) instruct the patient not to squeeze the lids shut but to relax his eyes; (c) lift the upper lid somewhat, hold the upper tarsal border (at least 1 cm. above the edge of the lid margin) with an applicator stick held horizontally or a tongue blade (be certain to push down and not to push in against the eye); and (e) as soon as the lid is everted, appose the fingers and hold the lashes up against the eyebrow. It may be necessary to evert the eyelid to remove foreign objects from the conjunctival region.

Ocular Irrigations. Cleansing and irrigating solutions of various kinds may be ordered to flush the conjunctival sac and remove secretions, e.g., preoperatively or in various inflammatory conditions, or to provide warmth to the eye. Examples of such solutions are sodium chloride in 1.4 per cent solution; alkaline eye drops; lactated Ringer's solution; mercuric chloride from 1:10,000 to 1:6,000; and methyl cellulose in 0.5 to 1 per cent solution. Cleansing and irrigating solutions should be bland and of lukewarm temperature when used. The solutions may be applied with (a) a commercial plastic irrigating bottle containing the sterile ophthalmic solution, e.g., Blinx, Dacriose; (b) a soft rubber bulb syringe; (c) an eye irrigator; or (d) they may be poured from an undine.

Prior to using any eyewash, cover the unaffected eye with sterile cotton and cleanse the eyelid and eyelashes with cotton wet with solution. The patient may be either sitting up with his head tilted slightly backward or lying flat in bed. By tilting the patient's head toward the side of the eye to be irrigated, the solution will flow away from the eye's inner canthus and will not flow across the bridge of the nose into the other eye. A piece of waterproof material and a clean towel are placed under the patient's head to protect the bedding if he is lying down. If the patient is sitting up, a towel is draped over his chest and shoulder on the side to be irrigated. A small curved basin is placed against the patient's cheek to catch the fluid running from the eye. Cotton balls or Cellucotton (cellulose) is pressed against the cheek below the lower lid to catch escaping fluid.

The nurse then holds the patient's eyelids apart with one hand (because the patient will instinctively try to close the eye) and asks the patient to look upward. With the other hand, resting lightly on the nasal bridge to prevent accidentally poking the eye, the nurse directs the flow of solution *away from the nose,* along the conjunctiva, and over the eyeball from the inner to the outer canthus. Do not direct the stream forcefully onto the eyeball itself and do not contaminate the irrigating apparatus by touching the eye's structures. The procedure is continued until obvious secretions are removed from the eye, and then the area around the eye is gently dried with cotton.

It is desirable for each patient to have his own irrigating equipment and irrigating solution. By using isotonic solutions, the necessary electrolytes are not removed from the eye's secretions.

Cleansing of the Eyelids. The nurse always cleanses a patient's eyelids before applying compresses, before removing or inserting an artificial eye, and before instilling medication into the eye. She may also cleanse the lids at other times, e.g., if the lid is crusted or has discharge on it following removal of dressings.

The eyelids are always cleansed *from the inner to the outer canthus* (except when an artificial eye is in place). Cotton balls moistened in sterile normal saline are used to cleanse the lids. A fresh cotton is used for each swipe. By gently pulling the skin of the outer orbital rim, the upper lid may be held taught and cleansed while the patient looks downward. The lower lid is cleansed while the patient looks upward. *Do not exert pressure on the eyeball.*

Instillation of Eyedrops and Ocular Ointments. First, be certain you have the *correct patient,* the *correct medication,* and the *correct eye.* Then tell the patient what you are going to do and what he can do to help. Cleanse the lid and lashes prior to instilling the medication. Position the patient with his head almost straight (yet turned slightly to the side so the solution will run away from the tear duct, i.e., away from the inner canthus) and tipped slightly backward (while lying in bed or sitting up in a chair).

Next, approach the eye from the side or from below, rather than straight on, so the patient doesn't watch your hand coming toward his eye. *Rest your hand* (holding the eyedropper, plastic squeeze bottle, or ointment tube) against the patient's forehead so you will not accidentally poke the patient's eye or touch his eyelids with the tip of the container. To do so not only contaminates the container (which must then be discarded) but also may injure the eye. With your other hand resting on the patient's face, gently evert the lower lid; in this hand hold a ball of cotton or gauze 2 inches × 2 inches to gently wipe off any excess solution or ointment.

Instruct the patient to look up at your hand holding the container. Then introduce the drop (one or two at most) into the center of the lower fornix; or, if an ointment is being used, express a ribbon of ointment long enough to cover the length of the fornix. Direct application of an ointment from the inner canthus to the outer canthus. Twist off the ribbon by turning the tube. As mentioned, do not touch the tip of the tube or the tip of the dropper to the eye or eyelid. Wipe the tip of the ointment tube clean with a sterile gauze pad before and after applying the ointment. Ointments are easiest to control if the tube is warmed for a few minutes in the hand before use. Do not drop the solution or place the ointment directly on the eyeball. By all means avoid the sensitive cornea.

Following instillation, direct the patient to gently close his eye and look down (if a solution was used) or roll his eyeball in various directions (if an ointment was used). If the patient tightly squeezes his eye shut it pushes out the solution or ointment; instruct the patient to avoid this tendency. Following application of an ointment, have the patient keep his eye shut for one minute to let the medication melt.

Many eye solutions will cause serious systemic symptoms if they are allowed to flow into the lacrimal system and to be absorbed from there into the general circulation. To prevent this, after instilling the eye drop, and after the patient closes his eye, press the inner angle of the eye gently against the nose to temporarily obstruct the lacrimal system's flow; do not press directly down against the eyeball. Wipe off excess solution or ointment with a sterile cotton or gauze. When not in use, keep tubes and bottles of ocular medications tightly capped. Take care not to contaminate the top of an ointment tube or the top of a dropper bottle by touching these areas with the unsterile outer edge of the cap. *Eye medications should be sterile.* If you contaminate them discard them; do not risk introducing a serious, perhaps blinding, infection into the eye.

It is desirable for each patient to have his individual bottle of medication, i.e., a plastic single-dose container, rather than to use stock solutions. Bottles of eye solutions should be warmed before instillation by holding the bottle in the hand for a few minutes. If eyedroppers are used, several factors are of importance: (a) blunt-edged droppers are safest; (b) cracked or jagged-edged droppers should be replaced (to see if the dropper edge is ragged, pull it gently across a sterile gauze pad and see if it catches); (c) keep the tip of the dropper pointing down so the solution does not flow back into the bulb where it can be contaminated; (d) withdraw only a small amount of solution into the dropper (enough for use at one time); (e) after instilling the ordered amount of medication into the eye, discard any solution remaining in the dropper (to avoid possible contamination of the rest of the solution in the bottle); (f) if the dropper itself has been contaminated, do not return it to the bottle until it has been sterilized (the glass part may be washed and sterilized); and (g) never use the same dropper for more than one solution without sterilizing it between solutions.

Application of Hot and Cold Eye Compresses. Wet compresses to the eye are a sterile procedure unless otherwise specified. When compresses are to be sterile, or if the eye has copious discharge, a new compress is used each time one is changed. If both eyes are to have compresses applied, use separate equipment for each eye and wash between the treatment of each eye to avoid cross-contamination.

Hot moist compresses may be applied to the eye to cleanse the eye, to relieve pain, and to increase circulation. This may reduce tension and increase absorption in the treatment of superficial infections and inflammation of the eye or eyelid, as well as such deep-seated disorders as iritis and acute glaucoma. Additionally, hot compresses may be useful following various types of eye surgery.

Cold compresses may be used to (a) relieve itching; (b) reduce swelling; (c) retard bacterial growth and prevent spread of infection; (d) reduce secretion; (e) relieve pain; (f) prevent or control edema; and (g) help control bleeding. Cold produces capillary constriction. Cold compresses are used in such conditions of the eye as inflammatory conjunctivitis and allergic conjunctivitis and following ocular injuries or ocular surgery. Cold compresses are contraindicated in deep-seated ocular inflammations because the cornea's nutrition is impaired when capillary constriction is produced.

To prepare the patient for the application of hot or cold compresses, move him to the side of the bed and place protective towels under his head and over his chest. Prior to applying moist heat or cold to the eye, apply a protective layer of sterile petroleum jelly to the eyelid (take care that it does not enter the eye). The best compresses are large enough to completely cover the eye and are composed of 7 to 8 thicknesses of gauze or cotton flannel. Hot compresses can be prepared by heating the compresses in a basin on an electric hot plate (set up on a bedside table). The solution used in the basin may be water or a prescribed solution. Excess moisture is wrung out of hot compresses by twisting them between two sterile forceps. The compresses are then carefully applied to the closed eye. Care is taken to lift the compress off at once if it feels too hot to the patient. If the compresses need not be sterile, the nurse can test their temperature by touching the outside of the pad to the back of her hand. Hot compresses are changed every 30–60 seconds, and the treatment is continued for 10–15 minutes. Compresses are applied as often as ordered. Warm compresses are typically ordered for 15 minutes four times a day. If the procedure need not be sterile, a clean washcloth may be used for a compress after it is placed in hot water and wrung out.

If the patient has impaired innervation to the eye, great care is taken to not burn him with the hot compress. It is recommended that the temperature of the solution in which the compresses are heated not exceed 120° F. (49° C.).

Cold sterile compresses are prepared by washing off chipped ice and then placing a small sterile bowl (containing sterile solution) within a larger basin containing the ice. If the procedure does not need to be sterile, the compresses or a clean washcloth may be placed directly on washed pieces of ice in a basin. It may be desirable to gently place a rubber glove containing some ice chips over the top of the compress once it is placed over the closed eye; if this is done, fewer compress changes are necessary. Cold compresses need not be changed as frequently as hot ones.

When applying any compress to the eye, be careful not to exert pressure on the eye. Following compresses, the eye is gently dried and another thin layer of Vaseline is applied.

Application and Care of Eye Dressings. Eye dressings may be applied for various reasons, e.g.,

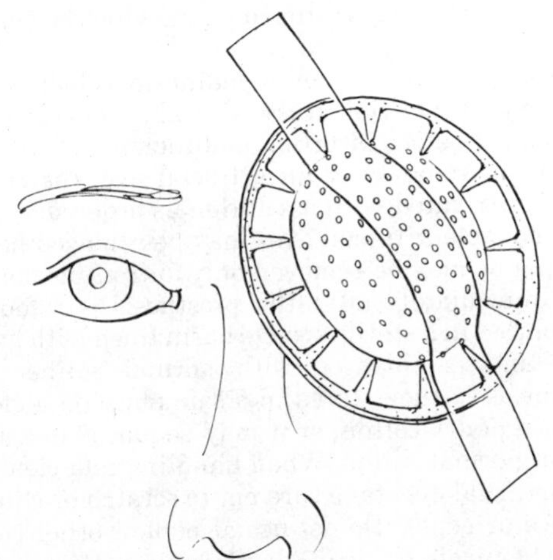

FIGURE 105–8. Metal eye shield. (From Sutton, A. L.: *Bedside Nursing Techniques.* 2nd ed. 1969.)

to apply pressure to the eye (following enucleation); to protect the eye from light, infection, or injury; to cover a deformity of the eye; to eliminate double vision; to limit movement of the eye and prevent usage of the eye (following surgery or trauma); and to absorb secretions and blood. *Unless specifically ordered to do so, do not apply pressure to the eye when applying an eye dressing.* However, do apply the dressing firmly enough to hold the eyelid fairly securely against the cornea. If pressure is desired, two or three eye pads are applied. Occasionally additional pressure is obtained with a wrap-around head dressing. *An eye with a surface bacterial infection should not be covered with a dressing because covering promotes bacterial growth.*

Eye pads are composed of a layer of absorbent cotton between two layers of gauze. The pads are oval and are held in place with three narrow strips of scotch tape or nonallergic plastic adhesive tape. If the eye does not completely close, a drop of lubricant, e.g., methylcellulose, may be ordered to be placed in the eye prior to applying the eye pad; this is done to prevent the gauze from scratching the cornea.

At times it is desirable, e.g., following surgery, to protect the eyeball from pressure or rubbing. To accomplish this protection a metal eye shield is bent so it rests upon the bony prominences of the brow, cheek, and nose without touching the underlying dressing. The shield is taped in place as shown in Figure 105–8.

Protective covering and care of the eyes of unconscious patients is discussed in Unit VIII.

As with other dressings, when removing an eye dressing loosen all the tape first by pulling the tape *toward* the wound, i.e., toward the eye. After all the tape is loosened, gently remove the dressing by lifting it straight up. Do not slide it across the eye. Do not change eye dressings unless the physician has instructed you to do so.

Removal, Insertion, and Care of an Artificial Eye; Care of Eye Socket. Artificial eyes are hollow or shell-shaped structures made of plastic or glass and painted to match the patient's normal eye. Shell-shaped prostheses are more common, but the type varies with the surgery performed. The artificial eye is generally fitted over a hollow plastic sphere, i.e., "implant," which remains in the eye socket to give movement to the artificial eye and to maintain the normal contour of the eyelids by filling the eye's socket. (See discussion of enucleation, p. 1507.)

While some implants are "exposed," others are "buried." *Exposed implants* are only incompletely covered with tissue in the eye's socket; eventually a prosthesis is attached postoperatively to the implant. Such a prosthesis is *always left in place.* To reduce the danger of infection, the eye socket must be routinely irrigated each morning with a solution such as Zephiran chloride, 1:1000. Additionally, some sources recommend nightly instillation of an antibiotic ointment into the socket. To irrigate the eye, an all-rubber ear syringe is placed beside the lower edge of the prosthesis, somewhat in the depth of the socket, and secretions are flushed out from behind the socket (see Fig. 105–9). Secretions normally continue only a week or two postoperatively. The patient is instructed never to touch the eyelids but rather to carry a small packet of sterile facial tissues with him to blot his eyelids if necessary. Additionally the patient is instructed not to let the socket get wet, e.g., when shampooing, showering, or swimming.[85]

Those artificial eyes which can be removed are *removed* by pulling down the lower lid and pressing under the eye with the fingers of one hand, while cupping the other hand under the eye to catch the prosthesis as it falls out of place (Fig. 105–10).

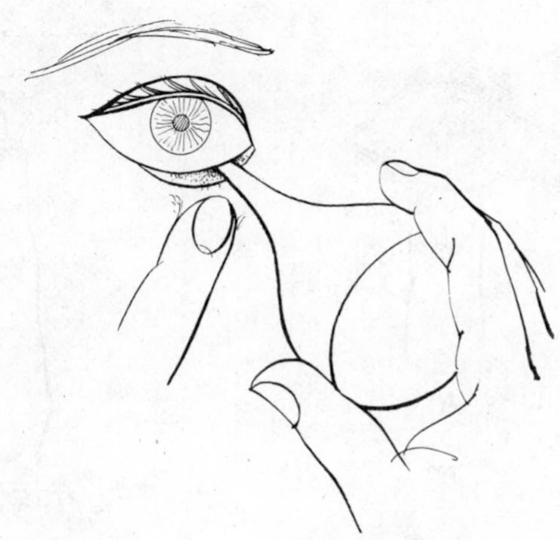

FIGURE 105–9. Irrigation of eye socket with all-rubber ear syringe. (From Sutton, A. L.; *Bedside Nursing Techniques.* 2nd ed. 1969.)

After slipping the lower edge of the shell-like prosthesis out over the edge of the lower eyelid, the fingers are placed on the upper eyelid and gently push down. This pushes the prosthesis down into the waiting hand below. It is advisable to remove the eye over a soft surface, e.g., a folded towel or pillow, so if you fail to catch the prosthesis as it drops out of place, it does not break as it falls.

To *insert* the artificial eye, the following steps are performed: (a) the eye is wetted; (b) the upper lid is lifted and pulled slightly outward; (c) the prosthesis is slipped as far as possible under the upper lid (with the point of the eye held toward the nose); and (d) the eye is held in the socket while the lower lid is pulled down until it slips over the bottom edge of the prosthesis. Before inserting an artificial eye, be certain you are holding the prosthesis in the correct position.

Frequently the patient who wears an artificial eye has a small rubber suction device which he uses to place and remove the prosthesis. To *remove* the eye, the suction cup is moistened, squeezed, placed against the iris of the artificial eye, and is twisted somewhat counterclockwise (after pulling the lower lid down with the index finger). After placing the eye on a soft surface, the suction is broken by squeezing the suction cup slightly. The device is then removed from the prosthesis. To *replace* the eye by using a suction device, first moisten the tip of the suction cup, squeeze it, and place it over the iris. Then retract the upper lid and place the eye as discussed in the preceding paragraph. Remove the suction device from the properly positioned eye by applying a small amount of pressure on the eye with one finger while squeezing and removing the suction cup.

Because it is important to maintain a clean socket and prevent infection, it is essential that one's hands be washed before insertion and removal of the eye. Following removal of an artificial eye, the socket may be irrigated with a solution as ordered.

Removable artificial eyes may be removed before retiring or may be removed only for routine cleansing. Immediately after the prosthesis is removed, it is placed in a sterile sponge basin lined with gauze pads and is cleansed with normal saline. The prosthesis is then stored in a safe place on a clean, soft bed of dry cotton, or it may be placed in a solution of normal saline. When handling and cleaning the artificial eye, take care not to scratch or chip its surface or edges. Do not use alcohol or other corrosive chemicals to clean plastic artificial eyes.

To minimize the formation of secretions in the socket, the prosthesis may be lubricated with a commercially prepared ophthalmic solution. If the patient develops sinusitis or a head cold, the amount of socket secretions may increase. When secretions are increased, it is desirable to more frequently remove the eye and cleanse the eye and socket.

The patient with an artificial eye requires instruction as follows:

- How to remove, cleanse, inspect and replace his prosthesis (if it is removable), and how to care for his socket. Daily the prosthesis's edges and surface should be inspected for rough places. If damaged, rough, or scratched, the eye should not be reinserted but should be taken to a prosthetist for possible repair.
- Always keep an extra prosthesis to use in event of loss or damage to the prosthesis being used.
- Do not vigorously rub the eye when the prosthesis is in place. Rubbing may displace the prosthesis (perhaps causing it to fall out); may injure the socket (by forcibly pushing the hard edge of the prosthesis against the socket rims); and may crack a glass eye.
- Do not wash the face with extremely hot or cold water

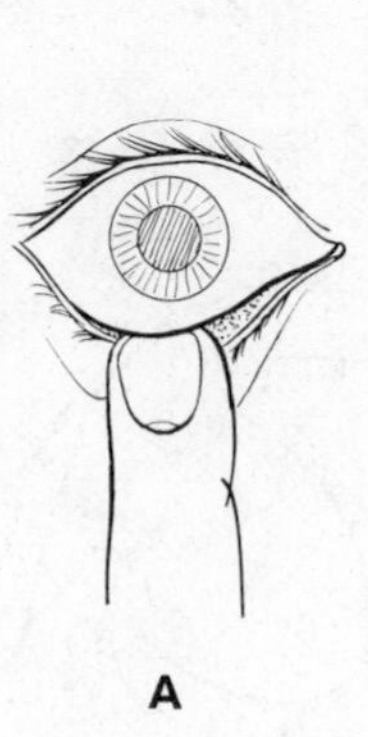

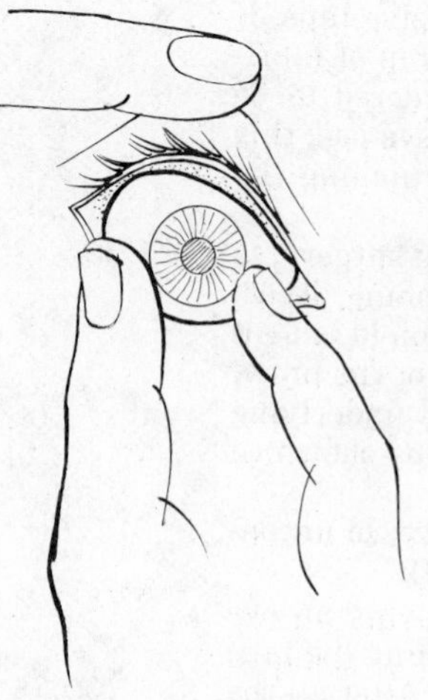

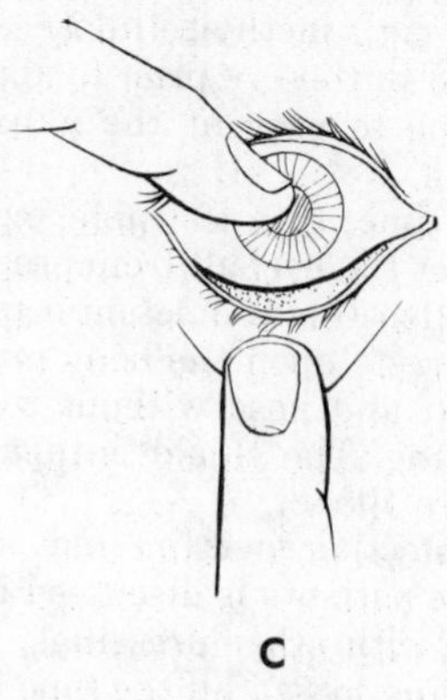

FIGURE 105-10. Removal and insertion of artificial eye. *A,* Lower lid is pulled down and finger inserted under eye for removal. *B,* Step No. 1: upper lid is held up and eye slipped under lid as far as possible (Note: point of eye is held toward nose). *C,* Step No. 2: eye is held in place and lower lid pulled down until it slips over lower edge of prosthesis. (From Sutton, A. L.: *Bedside Nursing Techniques.* 2nd ed. 1969.)

and do not apply ice packs or hot packs to the area of the eye when the prosthesis is in place. Temperature extremes may crack or break a glass eye. Glass eyes tend to become increasingly fragile with age.

> When the prosthesis is in place, if it is necessary to wipe the eyelid, do so in a direction *from the outer to the inner canthus.* You will observe that this is in a direction *opposite* that recommended for general eye care, e.g., this is in the direction opposite that which should be used when wiping a normal eye. If the eyelid over the artificial eye is wiped in a direction away from the inner canthus, the prosthesis tends to turn and be displaced in the socket.

In addition to instructing the patient concerning all the above points, the nurse of course practices these appropriate activities when she assumes care of a patient with a prosthesis who is unable to care for his eye or socket himself.

COMMON OCULAR MEDICATIONS

Numerous medications are used in ophthalmology. Some of the more common groups of these medications and some examples of specific medications in each group are briefly summarized in the following outline.

I. *Local anesthetics:* act to anesthetize the eye and thus prevent pain during various ocular procedures. Both topical and injectable anesthetics are available for use in ophthalmology.
   A. *Topical anesthetics:* proparacaine hydrochloride (Ophthaine, Ophthetic), 0.5 per cent; benoxinate hydrochloride (Dorsacaine), 0.4 per cent; tetracaine hydrochloride (Pontocaine), 0.5 per cent; cocaine hydrochloride, 2 to 10 per cent.
   B. *Injectable local anesthetics:* procaine hydrochloride (Novocaine), 1 and 2 per cent; lidocaine hydrochloride (Xylocaine), 1 to 2 per cent.

II. *Parasympathomimetic drugs,* i.e., drugs which produce effects resembling those of stimulation of parasympathetic nerves. Used as miotics to control intraocular pressure in glaucoma by widening filtration angle and permitting outflow of aqueous humor. Also used to treat certain types of strabismus.
   A. *Group I: Cholinergic drugs* which act directly on myoneural junction; produce strong contractions of iris (i.e., miosis) and ciliary body musculature (accommodation). Sympathomimetic agents will reverse the action of these drugs.
      1. *Examples* of cholinergic drugs: pilocarpine hydrochloride, 0.5 to 6 per cent; carbachol (Doryl), 1.5 to 3 per cent; acetylcholine chloride (Miochol), 1 per cent.
   B. *Group II: Cholinesterase inhibitors* (i.e., anticholinesterase drugs). Action of these drugs is difficult to reverse.
      1. *Examples* of cholinesterase inhibitors: echothiopate iodide (Phospholine iodide), 0.06 to 0.25 per cent; physostigmine salicylate (eserine), 0.25 and 0.5 per cent; isofluorophate (diisopropyl fluorophosphate, DFP, Floropryl), 0.25 per cent ophthalmic ointment and 0.1 per cent ophthalmic solution.

III. *Parasympathetic drugs* (anticholinergic drugs), i.e., those which produce effects resembling those of interruption of parasympathetic nerve supply to a part. Used to facilitate ophthalmoscopic examination and refraction; also used in treatment of uveitis (to rest eye in inflammatory conditions). Parasympatholytic medications cause smooth muscle of ciliary body and iris to relax, thus producing mydriasis (i.e., extreme pupillary dilatation) and cycloplegia (i.e., paralysis of ciliary muscle, resulting in paralysis of accommodation). *Note:* In predisposed persons pupillary dilatation can precipitate acute glaucoma, which can result in blindness if untreated.
   A. *Mydriatics:* e.g., eucatropine hydrochloride (Euphthalmine), 2 to 5 per cent.
   B. *Cycloplegics,* e.g., atropine sulfate, 0.5, 1, and 2 per cent; scopolamine hydrobromide (hyoscine), 0.25 to 5 per cent; homatropine hydrobromide, 1 to 5 per cent; cyclopentolate hydrochloride (Cyclogyl), 0.5 and 1 per cent; tropicamide (Mydriacyl), 1 per cent.

IV. *Sympathomimetic drugs (adrenergic drugs),* i.e., drugs which produce effects similar to those of impulses carried by adrenergic postganglionic fibers of sympathetic nervous system. Used in ophthalmology primarily to produce mydriasis and vasoconstriction; do not cause cycloplegia. Vasoconstriction appears to decrease rate of formation of aqueous humor. Also these drugs may increase outflow of aqueous humor, thus reducing intraocular pressure. Although used in treating some forms of glaucoma, adrenergic drugs are contraindicated in treatment of narrow angle glaucomas (dilation of pupil causes closure of anterior chamber angle and may markedly increase intraocular pressure).
   A. *Examples* of sympathomimetic drugs: epinephrine hydrochloride (Adrenaline), 1:1000; Epitrate, 2 per cent; phenylephrine hydrochloride (Neo-Synephrine), 0.125 to 10 per cent; hydroxyamphetamine hydrochloride ophthalmic solution (Paredrine), 1 per cent.

V. *Dyes:* Various dyes are used to stain cornea to identify corneal disorders, e.g., abrasions, ulcerations.
   A. *Examples* of dyes used in ophthalmology: sterile fluorescein sodium ophthalmic solution (sterile papers or single-dose containers of 2 per cent solution); merbromin (Mercurochrome), 2 per cent; rose bengal, 1 per cent.

VI. *Irrigating solutions:* Irrigating solutions used on an injured eye must be sterile and for single-patient use. If corneal epithelial tissues and sclera are intact, sterile nonirritating solutions may be used on more than one patient from same bottle.

VII. *Antibiotics:* May be used locally or systemically, depending upon disorder being treated.
   A. *Examples* of antibiotics: chloramphenicol (Chloromycetin), topically as 1 per cent ointment, or 0.25 to 0.5 per cent solution; neomycin sulfate (Mycifradin); Neosporin (combination of neomycin, polymyxin, and bacitracin); polymyxin B sulfate, topically as 0.25 per cent solution or 0.2 per cent ointment; bacitracin, ointment (1000 U./Gm.) or solution (250 U./ml.); penicillin; sodium methicillin (staphcillin); erythromycin, 1 per cent; streptomycin sulfate, 2.5 to 5 per cent.

VIII. *Sulfonamides:* Most commonly used medications in treating conjunctivitis.
   A. *Examples* of sulfonamides: sulfisoxazole (Gantrisin), 4 per cent ointment and 4 per cent solution; sulfacetamide sodium (sodium sulamyd), 10 per cent ointment and 30 per cent solution.

IX. *Adrenal corticosteroids:* Effective in treating nonpyogenic inflammations, allergic reactions, and severe ocular injuries. Useful in decreasing vascularization and scarring following chemical burns, trauma, and severe inflammation. May increase ocular susceptibility to fungus infection; prolonged ocular steroid therapy may cause open-angle glaucoma and cataracts. Corticosteroids come in various forms for ocular use and are available in various strengths and in combination with various antibiotics.

A. *Examples* of corticosteroids available for ocular use: cortisone acetate; hydrocortisone; methylprednisolone; prednisone; prednisolone; dexamethasone; betamethasone; triamcinolone acetonide; Medrysone; fludrocortisone acetate (Florinef, Alflorone, F-Cortef).

X. *Carbonic anhydrase inhibitors:* The enzyme carbonic anhydrase is one substance necessary for production of aqueous humor. Carbonic anhydrase inhibitors may be administered in treatment of glaucoma (where intraocular pressure is abnormally high) to reduce formation of aqueous humor and thus reduce intraocular pressure. Diuresis is produced.

A. *Examples* of carbonic anhydrase inhibitors: dichlorphenamide (Daranide, Oratrol); ethoxyzolamide (Cardrase, Ethamide); methazolamide (Neptazane); and acetazolamide (Diamox).

XI. *Other materials:*

A. *Silicone fluids:* Used to lubricate the eye socket when an artificial eye is worn. These fluids reduce irritation, increase comfort, prevent crusting on the lids, and give a lifelike effect to the prosthesis.

B. *Methylcellulose,* 0.5 to 2 per cent: This solution, sometimes called "artificial tears," provides moisture and lubrication to the eye when normal tear production is impaired or lid closure is incomplete.

Space does not permit detailed discussion of the various drugs used in ophthalmology. Familiarize yourself with details as necessary by refering to a textbook of pharmacology and watch for the development of side effects when caring for patients receiving these medications. Remember the importance of minimizing absorption of ocular medications through the lacrimal system during instillation of eye drops.

The following additional *guidelines* are important in the use of ophthalmic medications:

> *Never instill medication into the eye unless it is ordered by a physician.*

> *Do not use "old" medications,* i.e., those that have been on the shelf for a long while. Check the expiration date on the medication. Two weeks is a reasonable time to use a solution before discarding it. Date the bottle at the time it is procured from pharmacy.

> *Before using ocular solutions,* e.g., "eye drops," *inspect them,* e.g., for cloudiness, discoloration, and precipitation. If precipitate is present or if the solution is cloudy or discolored, do not use it.

> *Follow package instructions concerning proper storage of eye medications.*

> *Obtain new stock solutions weekly* Medications most likely to become contaminated are fluorescein, tetracaine (Pontocaine), proparacaine (Ophthaine, Ophthetic), and physostigmine.

> *Ophthalmic solutions must be sterile.* They are prepared and handled with the same degree of caution against contamination that is given to fluids intended for I.V. administration. Use sterile medications supplied in sterile, disposable, single-use eyedropper units if the eye has been injured (accidentally or surgically).

> *Use eyedroppers correctly.* Do not use the same eyedropper to instill two different medications. Do not allow medication in an eyedropper to flow back into the dropper's bulb, and do not return medication remaining in the eyedropper back into the bottle after instillation. Such practices cause contamination of the medication.

> *Check carefully which medication is to be inserted in which eye.* Different medications may be ordered for each of the two eyes.

> *Familiarize yourself with specific eye medications.* Certain medications are definitely contraindicated for certain eye disorders.

> *Never substitute a solution or medication of one strength for that of another strength without permission from the physician* Also, never substitute one eye medication for another without permission.

> *Carefully read instructions and labels for all ocular medications* (and any other ocular treatment). If labels are smeared or otherwise unreadable discard them or return them to pharmacy for relabeling.

> *Never use an unlabeled solution or ointment on the eye or around the eye.*

GENERAL FACTORS CONCERNING SURGERY ON THE EYE

INTRODUCTION

Eye surgery accounts for 15 per cent of the operations performed in the United States on persons over age 65. While some ocular surgeries (e.g., surgery on extraocular muscles) are performed under general anesthesia, most eye surgeries are performed under local anesthesia. Many ophthalmologists and anesthesiologists prefer anesthetizing procedures for ocular surgeries which include (a) large amounts of preoperative sedation; (b) topical eye medications; and (c) local anesthesia, including facial nerve blocks or retrobulbar injections. *Local anesthetics are preferred* to a general anesthetic for eye surgery when possible because restlessness may follow administration of general anesthesia; the restless patient may accidentally injure his eye. During local anesthesia the patient may be requested to keep his dentures in place to maintain his facial contour. During surgery the surgeon can enlist the help of the patient who has only had a local anesthetic. For example he can ask the patient to "look up," "look down," or follow other directions.

Strong solutions of germicides are not tolerated by the eye; otherwise the rules of asepsis and antisepsis which govern general surgery are also indicated for ophthalmic surgery. To prepare the operative area, the physician may preoperatively order prophylactic antibiotics (eyedrops or systemically), cleansing of the face, ocular irrigations, and cutting of the eyelashes. Many eye surgeons prefer to prepare the eye, e.g., irrigate it, cut lashes, and so forth in surgery rather than having these procedures performed on the ward.

Psychologic care is highly important for patients who are hospitalized for eye surgery. Fear and depression are common reactions. Many patients are apprehensive about having their eyes operated on while they are "awake." The possible loss of vision is of real concern. Older patients easily tend to become confused or disoriented.

The technics of ocular surgery have greatly improved over recent decades. Three major advances have been in the therapy of retinal detachment, the treatment of corneal scarring, and cataract extraction. The details of specific ocular surgeries have been discussed throughout the unit. Here we briefly discuss some general preoperative and postoperative considerations pertaining to eye surgery.

PREOPERATIVE CARE

Because the patient's vision may be absent or impaired following eye surgery (e.g., due to eye dressings and eye medications as well as the trauma of the operative procedure), it is particularly important to preoperatively orient the patient to his environment and to introduce him to other staff members as well as those patients in his room. Familiarizing the patient with his surroundings preoperatively not only makes the patient generally more comfortable psychologically but also may specifically lessen postoperative disorientation. This appears particularly true of elderly persons.

Before surgery attempt to identify and discuss the patient's operative concerns. Patients often are fearful of pain which may occur with operative procedures on the eye. Also, many patients are particularly tense about having any surgery performed on the eye because of emotional feelings about the eye and its importance. Tell the patient if his eyes will be bandaged after surgery so he will be prepared for this. Discuss with him ways in which you will help him during the time he has his eye (or eyes) bandaged. At an appropriate time before surgery, teach the patient about postoperative procedures and necessary restrictions. Be sure to tell the patient not to sit up in bed or not to lean over the edge of the bed after surgery because this increases intraocular pressure. Inform the patient that medication will be available for him after surgery for pain and that a medication may be ordered to prevent nausea if necessary. Additionally, medications may be ordered to suppress coughing and to facilitate bowel movements (to prevent straining). Emphasize to the patient that he should feel free to tell the nurse how he is feeling so she can give him medications and other appropriate care to keep him comfortable. If the patient is going to have a local anesthetic, instruct him to hold his head still during surgery and not to squeeze his eye shut. Tell the patient that his doctor will be talking to him during surgery and will be giving him directions.

Specific preoperative orders vary, depending upon the physician, hospital policies, the procedure to be performed, and the type of anesthetic to be used. Check orders carefully for each patient. Preoperative orders may specify for male patients to shave closely before surgery and for a shampoo to be given (to both male and female patients). Shaves, shampoos, and so forth may be ordered before eye surgery if these activities are going to be restricted for a time postoperatively to protect the eye. In some cases the condition of the patient's eye does not allow these activities even preoperatively. It may be adviseable to comb and braid the patient's hair if it is long. Cleansing enemas are usually not ordered before ocular surgery since local anesthetics are predominantly used. However, sometimes enemas are ordered preoperatively if straining is contraindicated after surgery. To rest the patient's eyes prior to surgery, keep the environment moderately darkened.

Give eye medications *at the precise time* they are ordered preoperatively, so the eye will be in a state of readiness at the time of surgery. Medications may be ordered to dilate the pupil. Other preoperative medications may include: pentobarbital sodium (Nembutal), chloral hydrate, or meperidine hydrochloride (Demerol). If a general anesthetic is to be given, atropine sulfate may be ordered. If a topical anesthetic is to be instilled on the ward before surgery, be certain to protectively cover the eye with an eye pad after instilling the drops. Do not apply adhesive tape to the patient's skin, but rather hold a sterile dressing in place with a 2-inch gauze roller dressing. As mentioned earlier, usually topical anesthetics are instilled in the operating room, and a local nerve block may also be administered.

If the surgeon wishes to cut off the eyelashes in preparation for surgery on the eye, he uses straight, short-bladed scissors. The blades are lubricated with petrolatum jelly so the cut lashes will adhere to the blade surface rather than falling into the eye. Before beginning surgery the eyebrows and area of the skin around the eye are cleaned, and the eye may be irrigated. Sometimes a mark is made on the forehead over the eye to be operated on so the correct eye is easily identified. At the time of surgery the operative team checks carefully to ensure that surgery is performed on the correct eye.

Preoperative charting should include comments concerning the patient's attitude toward the surgery to be performed, as well as charting regarding preparation of the patient for surgery.

POSTOPERATIVE CARE

As with preoperative orders, considerable variation exists concerning postoperative orders following ocular surgery. Usually few if any restrictions are placed on the activity of patients who have *not* had intraocular procedures. However, postoperative attempts are made to minimize the stress on the eye that has had intraocular surgery, because while the intact, healthy eye can tolerate numerous stresses upon it, the eye which is weakened or damaged by intraocular surgery is highly vulnerable. Following intraocular procedures, the eye is in a delicate condition for several weeks or months. Below are details relevant to postoperative care following *intraocular* surgical procedures.

> *Following intraocular surgery the major goals of care are to (a) prevent hemorrhage; (b) prevent stress on the suture line; (c) prevent increased intraocular pressure; (d) minimize movements of the patient's head and eyes; (e) prevent infection; (f) minimize sensory deprivation; and (g) prevent complications of immobility and anesthesia.*

Pressure on the eye must be prevented while the patient is being transferred from the operating table onto a bed or stretcher. The patient's body is lifted in horizontal alignment while one person supports and moves the patient's head. Once the patient is in bed, his head may or may not be held in a fixed position by placing rolled up towels or small pillows beside the head. (Sand bags are no longer used for this purpose.) The use of a "fixed-head position" and maintenance of complete immobilization following eye surgery are no longer common postoperative procedures. Today many surgeons do not want anything placed beside the patient's head (to remind the patient not to turn his head) because the patient may strike his eye against the rolled towel or the edge of the pillow. Also, today, some activity is recognized as being important for a more rapid recovery. Usually the patient is allowed restricted range of movement and is placed supine with a thin pillow under his head and the head of the bed slightly elevated for comfort.

Once the patient is correctly positioned in bed, put up the siderails and give the patient his call bell. Tell the patient who you are and reorient him to his surroundings and to the time of day. Avoid bumping the bed while giving care, and keep the immediate area free of bright lights. Keep a record of intake and output and observe for urinary retention and abdominal distention. Following ocular surgery the patient is *not* urged to routinely cough, but rather he is encouraged to frequently and regularly take deep breaths to expand his lungs and to keep his tracheobronchial tree clear of secretions. Coughing is contraindicated because it increases intraocular pressure. To improve the patient's circulation while in bed and to prevent fatigue, supervise the patient and see that he regularly performs active range of motion arm and leg exercises without moving his head. Some physicians prescribe muscle setting or isometric exercises.

Check the physician's orders before giving care to a patient following intraocular surgery to determine restrictions on activities. Are the following allowed: (a) head elevation (how much); (b) turning (both sides or one side); (c) a pillow (more than one); (d) shaving; (e) hair combing; (f) face washing; and (g) tooth brushing? Secure the physician's permission before allowing the patient to read, smoke, brush his teeth, shave, shampoo, or comb his hair.

Following intraocular surgery the patient must learn to prevent pressure upon the globe until the incision in the eye has healed and the eye can again tolerate the stresses of normal daily activities. The patient and family members are instructed concerning positions which he may and may not assume, and activities which are permitted or are contraindicated.

Following surgery on the eye, use restraints only as ordered; and then only as a last resort. Straining against restraints may dangerously elevate intraocular pressure. When used, explain to the patient why the restraint is being used ("to prevent you from hurting your eye") and tell the patient he will be restrained only for a short time. Carefully observe the restrained patient; do not assume the attitude that because he is restrained he is "O.K." Light wrist restraints made of gauze may serve as a reminder to prevent a patient from touching his dressing or rubbing his eyes when awakening. Frequent skin care and frequent position changes are important aspects of care for any restrained patient.

Usually to prevent putting pressure on the eye, the patient is initially allowed to *lie only on his unoperated side* or on his back with the head of the bed elevated to 30° for comfort. Lying on the unoperated side keeps the operated eye free from pressure and also prevents possible contamination of the dressing from vomitus if the patient has emesis. If the patient does vomit after intraocular surgery, do not raise his head, but rather hold his head toward the unoperated side and apply cold compresses to his throat.

Frequently patients are allowed out of bed on the first postoperative day, and time out of bed is then gradually increased. Generally activities which would increase venous pressure in the head and thus would increase intraocular pressure are restricted for several weeks. (The increase in venous blood in the head dilates blood vessels in the eye.) Also, an increase in the amount of aqueous humor secreted results from increased arterial or venous pressure. This increased secretion in turn increases intraocular pressure.

Activities which increase intraocular pressure, and are thus contraindicated, include excessive energy exertion, crying, extreme emotion, sudden movements, sneezing, blowing the nose, coughing, running, jumping, straining at bowel movements, bending, stooping over, lifting or pushing heavy objects, rubbing the eyes, squinting, and tightly closing the eyes. Intraocular pressure is also increased as a result of pulling the skin while shaving, washing the face, or brushing hair. Teach the patient to try to avoid coughing by deep breathing if he feels he needs to cough and to keep his mouth open while coughing if he must cough (this reduces pressure inside the head). Instruct the patient to immediately notify the nurse if he feels nauseated. Once told that the patient feels nauseated, the nurse immediately administers an antiemetic; she does not wait until the patient actually vomits before giving the medication. Also, tell the patient not to forcefully squeeze his eyelids shut or to rub or press on his eye or his eye dressing. Until toothbrushing can be resumed, frequently swab the mouth and teeth.

Because proper teaching is an important aspect of patient acceptance, be certain to *tell the patient the reasons why limitations are temporarily placed on his activities.* When emphasizing to the patient the need for postoperative restrictions, tell the patient that eye tissue requires more time to heal than other body tissues.

Observe sterile technic for all procedures performed on the eye following intraocular surgery. The development of intraocular infection is a serious complication.

Conveniently arrange items on the patient's bedside stand so he can easily reach them without straining. Then place the bedside stand on the patient's unoperated side so he is not tempted to turn onto his operated side. Give nursing care from the unoperated side whenever possible.

Keep the patient as comfortable as possible postoperatively by frequent slight position changes, by providing back and skin care, and by giving analgesics as indicated. Generally postoperative eye pain can be controlled with Demerol, 50–75 mg., Darvon, 32 mg., or aspirin, 0.6 Gm. Avoid opiates for pain control since they may cause vomiting.

Because sneezing and coughing are especially hazardous for patients following intraocular surgery, in some hospitals these patients are not allowed to have pepper on their trays (since it may make them sneeze or may cause them to choke and cough). The use of talcum powders or other similar products, which could cause sneezing and coughing, may also be prohibited. Care should be taken not to expose the patient to substances to which he is allergic, e.g., foods, drugs, plants. The nurse should be watchful for any indications of the development of an upper respiratory infection in a patient who has intraocular surgery. Indications of such a condition should be reported to the physician.

The dressings must never be removed from a patient's eye for inspection during the immediate postoperative period by anyone but the ophthalmologist, unless the physician has given specific orders for the nurse to do so. If an eye dressing comes loose, it should be gently replaced, including the protective metal shield. Normally a small amount of bleeding and serous drainage occurs postoperatively. Additionally the eyelid may be edematous for a few days, and subconjunctival hemorrhages may be present.

Notify the physician at once of any indications of complications. Prompt treatment may prevent serious eye injury. The physician should be informed of coughing, marked restlessness, sharp eye pain or eye pain which is not relieved by analgesics, disorientation, symptoms of an upper respiratory infection (e.g., rhinitis), obvious hemorrhage, disturbance of the dressing, and the patient assuming contraindicated postures or activities. Feelings of sharp pain or pressure in the eye suggest hemorrhage; sharp pain may also indicate possible infection.

Marked restlessness most often occurs when a patient has both eyes bandaged and when the patient is an older person. Since both eyes turn together, the surgeon may bandage both eyes to provide rest for the operated eye. Sometimes the physician leaves an order for the unoperated eye to be uncovered if the patient becomes quite restless. Usually removal of this one dressing helps the patient to become calmer and to become reoriented if he is disoriented. Minor mental symptoms which patients with bilateral eye patches may develop (as a result of sensory deprivation) include restlessness, mental clouding, perceptual disorientation, mood changes, and thinking disturbances. More serious mental symptoms include memory impairment, confusion, disorientation, and vivid hallucinations. These symptoms frequently increase in the evening when patients have bilateral eye patches. Patients experiencing these mental changes as a result of bilateral patching may also perform actions which they have been told are contraindicated, e.g., they may pull off their eye dressings and assume contraindicated postures. This special mental symptom is called "noncompliance" and is believed to result from states of reduced awareness (e.g., during sleep) in which normal vigilance controls are reduced, because of bilateral patching, thus allowing forbidden actions to occur.[32] It is obviously desirable to minimize sensory deprivation following intraocular surgery to prevent the above problems.

In an attempt to keep the patient oriented postoperatively and to combat sensory deprivation, the patient with bilateral eye dressings should (a) be placed in a room where he has the company of another oriented and active patient; (b) be observed closely for indications of disorientation (especially older persons); (c) be stimulated frequently verbally and physically (e.g., by frequently talking with the patient, and by touching the patient's hand or arm while talking with him); and (d) be visited frequently by nursing personnel and visitors to decrease isolation. If a general anesthetic is given, it is important to begin to reorient the patient as soon as he begins to recover from the anesthesia. Always tell the patient who has bilateral dressings (and thus cannot see) when you enter or leave his room and when you are going to touch him.

Following intraocular surgery, it is helpful if relaxing diversional activities are provided for the patient as he recovers. Such activities must be in keeping with the patient's interests and abilities.

The patient with impaired vision must be protected from accidental injury postoperatively. Keep siderails up on all patients with bilateral eye dressings and on all disoriented patients. Also be sure the patient's protective eye shield is properly positioned and secured in place. Following surgery observe the patient carefully to be certain he does not accidentally remove his eye patch and thus possibly injure his eye. Do not allow the patient to smoke without a physician's order (smoke is irritating to the eye), and then supervise the patient because it is easy for a lighted ash to fall unnoticed by the patient with impaired vision. Keep the patient's call bell in place at all times. Keep everything in its proper and familiar place so the patient will be less likely to have an accident while reaching for something or otherwise moving about. Once the patient can be out of bed, assist him with ambulation so he does not bump himself, fall, or otherwise injure himself. When assisting the patient with food or drink, be careful to prevent choking and aspiration.

Following intraocular surgery a liquid or soft diet may be ordered for a day or so to prevent possible nausea and vomiting and to prevent the stress of chewing. However, this is not always true. Sometimes a general diet is ordered. Some physicians believe that abdominal distention and discomfort are reduced if the patient receives a diet which requires moderate chewing. Sometimes iced beverages and other gas-forming foods are not permitted following ocular surgery.

When feeding a person who cannot see, be certain you first describe the food on the tray to the patient. Patients who cannot see what they are being fed frequently say that all food tastes the same to them. Descriptions of the food being fed helps to improve perceptions of that food. Attempt to make the meal time a pleasant, unhurried experience for the person who must be fed. Try to understand how difficult it is for the patient to eat when he cannot see and has to be fed. You might practice helping a sightless person to eat by blindfolding and feeding a classmate. Then reverse roles and take your turn as the patient.

If a patient must remain on *prolonged bedrest* following eye surgery, it is important that he continue frequently to perform isometric exercises and that other appropriate care be administered to prevent the complications of prolonged inactivity (see Unit V, Ch. 27). Frequent deep breathing sessions (not coughing) to clear the lungs and frequent position changes are also highly important (see also Unit VI). Of course, it is necessary to maintain the patient's fluid-electrolyte and nutritional status. Constipation due to inactivity must be prevented since straining at stool may cause a hazardous rise in intraocular pressure. Mineral oil or milk of magnesia may be ordered to minimize straining with bowel movements. Assist the patient on and off the bed pan so he does not raise his head up or strain during these maneuvers.

Family members can be very helpful following eye surgery. For example, they may be able to sit with the patient and watch to see that he stays properly positioned and that he does not disturb his eye dressing. Also, they may visit with and read to the patient and thus help keep him oriented. By being available to hand things to the patient, family members or friends may prevent him from lifting his head, reaching, straining, and possibly injuring his eye. Visitors can also help by feeding the patient.

Prior to discharge be sure the patient (and family) understands restrictions which are necessary to prevent elevation of intraocular pressure, and see that he is familiar with home care procedures, e.g., instillation of eye drops. Sponge baths may be necessary for a period of time at home, and it may be desirable for the patient to wear a metal eye shield at night or when lying down resting to protect his eye. Dark glasses may be worn for a while following removal of eye dressings to protect the eye from bright sunlight. All patients receiving atropine should wear dark glasses. Instruct the patient who will be wearing any type of glasses postoperatively that he should hold his glasses by the tips of their bows when putting them on to avoid accidentally poking his eye. Teach the patient how to properly care for eyeglasses or contact lenses or both. Instruct the patient to grasp both arms of a chair before sitting down, to prevent slipping and possibly falling. Emphasize to the patient that he should not rub his eyes with a soiled handkerchief. Be certain the patient realizes the importance of keeping follow-up appointments with his physician and the necessity for contacting the doctor whenever untoward symptoms develop. If enucleation has been performed, the patient must be instructed regarding the use and care of an artificial eye.

COMMON SPECIFIC DISORDERS OF THE EYE AND RELATED STRUCTURES AND THEIR CLINICAL MANAGEMENT

DISORDERS OF THE EYELIDS

Common disorders of the eyelids and their treatment are summarized below. The eyelids normally function to protect the eyes (from foreign bodies, external injury, undue exposure, excessive light) and to lubricate the eyeball by distributing secretions over the eyeball (thus washing away dust and keeping the cornea moist and transparent).

Blepharitis. Blepharitis is a common, chronic, bilateral inflammation of the lid margins, sometimes called "granulated eyelids." The patient experiences irritation, burning, and itching of the eyelids; the lid margins are "red-rimmed" in appearance and have scales or "granulations" clinging to them. In some cases the lid margins are ulcerated and the eyelashes tend to fall out. *Treatment* consists of (a) removal of scales from the lids daily with a damp cotton applicator; (b) cleanliness of the scalp, eyebrows, and lid margins; and (c) application of an antistaphylococcic antibiotic or sulfonamide eye ointment once daily to the lid margins with a cotton applicator.

Chalazion. Chalazion formation commonly occurs. A chalazion is a granulomatous enlargement of the meibomian gland resulting from occlusion of the gland's duct. Most frequently a chalazion points toward the lid's conjunctival side. The patient notices a painless, slow-growing, hard, nontender, round mass growing on the eyelid. The skin can be moved loosely over the growth; the conjunctiva in the region of the chalazion is elevated and red. Vision is distorted if the lesion is large enough to impress the cornea. *Treatment* consists of excision, or incision and curettage (performed in the physician's office or clinic) if the chalazion does not spontaneously absorb or recede following the application of hot compresses and topical steroid-antimicrobial therapy. After surgical removal, an eye pad may be worn for a day or two, and an antibacterial ointment, e.g., neomycin sulfate, may be applied to the conjunctiva.

Hordeolum (Sty). A hordeolum is a pustular inflammation of an eyelash follicle or sebaceous gland on the lid margin. Hordeola (styes) are common painful disorders of the eyelid. The intensity of the pain is directly related to the amount of swelling. Staphylococci are typically the causative organisms. Common in all age groups, styes often propagate a "crop" of infections along the lid margins which may last for long periods of time when the skin's resistance to staphylococci is reduced. Frequently styes are associated with blepharitis or a lowered state of health (e.g., from anemia, uncontrolled diabetes mellitus, infected tonsils and adenoids). Patients with styes should be instructed not to "squeeze" at the lesion, since this spreads the infection. The disorder typically begins with local irritation, redness, and swelling and progresses to an acutely tender abscess formation which points "outwards" from the lid margin. Usually styes discharge after 3–4 days. *Treatment* consists of application of warm, moist compresses to hasten suppuration. Usually if compresses are used the sty opens and drains without surgery. If resolution does not begin within 48 hours, incision is indicated. During the acute stage it is helpful to instill an antibiotic or sulfonamide into the conjunctival sac every 3 hours.

Virus Infections. *Herpes simplex* is an acute viral infection which produces superficial clear cutaneous vesicles that heal without scarring. When such vesicles occur on the eyelid, one must be cautious not to inoculate their contents onto the cornea. Such inoculation could produce a dendritic corneal ulcer. These corneal ulcers commonly occur. Corticosteroid treatment is *contraindicated* in the treatment of acute herpes simplex corneal infection, since it can cause spread of the infection (resulting in the formation of disabling corneal scar tissue).

Herpes zoster involving the eye typically has a unilateral trigeminal distribution (see Unit VIII). These skin lesions are deeper than those of the herpes simplex infection. Also, they are painful, tend to become secondarily infected, and often leave permanent scars. Ophthalmic herpes zoster is treated vigorously with mydriatic, antibiotic, and corticosteroid ointment. Skin lesions should be kept clean of infection and crusts by means of antibiotic ointment, mechanical cleansing, and hot soaks.

DISORDERS OF THE EXTRAOCULAR MUSCLES

Introduction. *Binocular vision,* i.e., the normal simultaneous use of both eyes which results in depth perception, was discussed briefly on page 1460 (see also pp. 1503 and 1504). In order to maintain binocular vision, simultaneous binocular movements of both eyes are necessary. Such movements require the coordinated use of the extraocular muscles. The eyes need to be properly aligned in order for corresponding retinal areas to be stimulated by the same object. Thus, convergence is necessary for near vision so that both macular areas can fixate on a single object. Normally anatomically corresponding areas in each retina have a common visual direction in space; the principal corresponding points of the retinas are the right and left *foveae.* The fovea is the central portion of the retina with the highest visual acuity.

The two pictures received from the eyes may be used within the brain in three different ways: (1) normal fusion may occur; (2) diplopia may occur; or (3) suppression may occur. In normal vision *fusion* occurs. "Fusion" refers to the cerebral synthesis of the two ocular pictures into a single mental image. Fusion occurs when the two eyes are perfectly aligned so that both foveae are aimed exactly at the same point. When disparate rather than corresponding retinal points are stimulated, the retinal images cannot be fused into a single mental impression. In such a situation *diplopia* results. "Diplopia" refers to double vision. Usually diplopia is caused from faulty alignment of the two eyes, e.g., with paralytic strabismus (to be discussed). *Suppression* may occur with nonparalytic strabismus. "Suppression" refers to the phenomenon of one mental image being ignored if the two eyes send two different mental images to the brain. If you are able to use a monocular microscope effectively with both eyes open you are practicing normal suppression; although the brain is receiving both the image of the table or surface upon which the microscope sits (from one open eye) and the image seen through the microscope (i.e., the magnified field), the brain focuses only on the image of the magnified field and suppresses the other image. If suppression is abnormally habitual, e.g., with nonparalytic strabismus, it seriously interferes with binocular vision and may irreversibly damage vision in the deviating eye. The latter visual loss is termed *"suppression amblyopia."*[40]

Strabismus. "Strabismus" refers to a deviation of an eye which the patient cannot overcome. Thus, the two eyes are not straight when fixing on an object, i.e., the visual axes do not remain parallel. While one eye (the fixing eye) looks directly at the object of attention, the other eye (the deviating eye) does not. Synonyms for strabismus include "squint," "tropia," and "heterotropia." Usually the various forms of strabismus are spoken of as "tropias," and their direction is indicated by an appropriate prefix, e.g., *esotropia* (inward or convergent deviation), *exotropia* (outward or divergent deviation), *hyper-*

tropia (upward), and *hypotropia* (downward). The preceding terms are listed in order of frequency. In all these forms, fusion is lacking.

Strabismus is easily observed and is a common symptom of ocular as well as central nervous and general systemic disorders. Strabismus may be paralytic or nonparalytic in origin. *Paralytic strabismus* usually is the result of nerve damage (e.g., cranial nerves III, IV, or VI); however, the lesion itself may be of the extraocular muscles. Paralytic strabismus occurs in such disorders as encephalitis, brain tumor, cerebral vascular accident, intracranial aneurysm, myasthenia gravis, orbital cellulitis, and thyrotoxic exophthalmos. *Nonparalytic strabismus* is not the result of a paralyzed extraocular muscle, but rather results from a defect of position of the two eyes relative to each other. Usually the tendency to develop nonparalytic strabismus is inherited; however, this type of ocular deviation may additionally be caused by serious disease of the brain or eye, e.g., retinoblastoma.

As discussed previously (see p. 1462), the effectiveness of the extraocular muscles is tested by having the patient rotate his eyes into the six cardinal positions of gaze. A "cardinal position" of the eye refers to a position which the eye cannot reach without the action of a specific extraocular muscle. If the eye fails to attain one of the cardinal positions of gaze, it means that that specific muscle is paralyzed. Paralytic strabismus is thus identified by this procedure. Paralysis of the ocular muscles, as occurs in paralytic strabismus, is termed "*ophthalmoplegia.*"

Nonparalytic strabismus is a positional defect of the two eyes relative to each other. This defect has been compared to that of a car with its front wheels out of alignment; the abnormal relationship of the front wheels to each other is not corrected no matter which way the steering wheel is turned. Thus, in nonparalytic strabismus the amount of crossing of the eyes does not change as the eyes are rotated through the six cardinal positions of gaze. When evaluating nonparalytic strabismus precise measurements of the amount of ocular deviation are made with prisms. Nonparalytic strabismus may be monocular or alternating. With monocular strabismus, the deviating eye is always the same one, while with alternating strabismus either eye may be used for fixation.

An estimated 5 per cent of children are born with or develop strabismus. Routine preschool examinations of visual acuity can detect almost all cases of amblyopia due to strabismus. Suppression amblyopia commonly occurs; *an estimated 0.5 per cent of patients have lost good vision in one eye because of suppression amblyopia. It is important for strabismus to be treated early in a child's life.* Generally by age six the brain has developed such severe suppression, when strabismus is present, that the condition will not respond readily to therapy.

As indicated earlier, esotropia, i.e., inward or convergent strabismus, is the most common form of strabismus. About one third of these patients have what is called "accommodative" esotropia, and the remaining two thirds have "nonaccommodative" esotropia. Patients in the first group may be successfully treated with the nightly instillation of parasympathomimetic drops, e.g., 0.025 per cent isoflurophate, either alone or in combination with the wearing of glasses.

In general, the treatment of all forms of nonparalytic strabismus is complex and requires the supervision of an ophthalmologist. While different combinations of treatment are used for the various specific disorders, some other aspects of treatment of strabismus are listed below:

- *Extensive evaluation* of the condition to rule out major cerebral and ocular disease. Such evaluation includes *cycloplegic refraction* to detect and correct refractive disorders.
- *Orthoptic evaluation and training.* The angle of strabismus is measured under various conditions; this is necessary to determine the method of surgical correction (if surgery is being considered) or to evaluate progress under nonsurgical management. Orthoptic training and eye exercises help restore fusion ability.
- *Occlusion* to restore good vision if suppression amblyopia has developed. Constant occlusion of the "good" eye often helps restore vision in the "bad" eye; however, after age 6 occlusion is useless.
- *Surgery* is necessary if the previous steps are insufficient. However, surgery does not help amblyopia. Surgery is performed to restore muscle balance.

The major types of surgeries performed on extraocular muscles to correct strabismus are (a) *tenotomy and recession,* and (b) *advancement, resection, and tucking.* These various procedures rotate the eye to a different position than it was preoperatively. The direction of rotation depends upon the procedure performed and the muscle or muscles which are the surgical target. "Tenotomy" refers to the cutting of a tendon. "Recession" consists of tenotomy and the suturing of the severed muscle back onto the sclera at a selected point *in back* of its original attachment (Fig. 105–11). The muscle is thus actually moved back further on the eyeball. With "advancing" procedures the opposite effect is obtained. In general, advancement refers to any surgical procedure which increases the action of a selected extraocular muscle. Three varieties of advancing procedures are (1) advancement, in which a muscle is reattached on the eyeball *ahead* of its original point of attachment; (2) resection, in which a muscle is shortened by actually cutting out a piece of the muscle (see Fig. 105–11); and (3) muscle tucking, in which the muscle is shortened by making a permanent fold in the muscle, i.e., by taking a "tuck" in the muscle.

Postoperatively following extraocular muscle surgery, the patient is typically cared for as follows:

- *Immediately:* (a) an antibiotic ointment is applied to the operated eye following closure of the conjunctiva; (b) no patch is used unless two or more muscles were cut on the same eye; then a patch may be applied on the operated eye only with adult patients; (c) the patient's wrists may be lightly attached to the side-

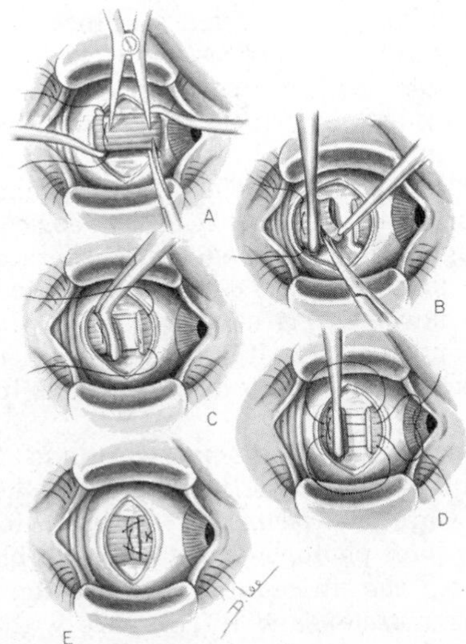

FIGURE 105-11. Resection of rectus muscle. This procedure generally is the same for each muscle. Operation on the right medial rectus muscle is illustrated. (From Dyer, J. A.; *Atlas of Extraocular Muscle Surgery*, 1970.)

rails with bandage to remind the patient not to rub his eyes; (d) the patient is ambulated as soon as possible; and (e) to prevent nausea and vomiting following general anesthetic, only carbonated beverages and soda crackers are permitted for the first 24 hours.

> *Post 24 hours:* (a) patch is removed if present and eyes are cleansed; (b) infants or children are discharged home and adults are dismissed if they feel well enough (orders are given for follow-up visits to physician); (c) dark glasses are prescribed for adults for a few days if required; (d) patient is permitted to use his eyes as tolerated; and (e) antibiotic-steroid drops may be prescribed for adults (t.i.d for 7–10 days), but no eye medication prescribed for children.

> *Later:* (a) patient is reexamined periodically until all reaction subsides and eyes attain a stable position; (b) hot packs and steroid drops are prescribed for 3–4 days if suture reaction occurs after 10 days to 4 weeks; and (c) antibiotic-steroid drops are stopped when the eye is healing well.

DISORDERS OF THE CONJUNCTIVA, SCLERA, AND CORNEA

Conjunctivitis. Inflammation of the conjunctiva is called "conjunctivitis" or "ophthalmia."

Conjunctivitis is the most common eye disease in the Western Hemisphere. It may be acute or chronic.

Generally conjunctivitis is exogenous and the result of bacterial or viral infection. Conjunctivitis may also result from endogenous inflammation, allergy (commonly associated with hay fever), chemical irritations, and fungal or parasitic infections. Regardless of the cause, the symptoms typically include redness, swelling, lacrimation, and pain. Discharge varies in amount and nature, depending upon the causative organism.

Acute bacterial conjunctivitis is a benign, self-limited disease commonly called *"pink eye."* This condition is *highly contagious,* particularly among children. Thus, precautions must be taken to prevent spreading the infection to other persons and to the patient's unaffected eye. Teach and practice thorough handwashing. Instruct the patient not to touch or rub his eyes and make certain he has his own clean towels and washcloths and does not share these with others.

Remember: all red eyes are not cases of "pink eye" or conjunctivitis. Thus, the nurse should refer all persons with red eyes to a physician for evaluation. A careful differential diagnosis is important to distinguish between acute conjunctivitis (generally a self-limited condition with no serious side effects) and such serious disorders as iritis, keratitis, or glaucoma (Table 105-2). One of the most common errors of diagnosis is that of conjunctivitis when the disorder is actually glaucoma or corneal ulcer.

Gonococcal conjunctivitis is not a self-limited, benign form of conjunctivitis. This condition constitutes a *medical emergency* which can cause serious complications, e.g., corneal ulceration, possibly resulting in blindness. Gonococcal conjunctivitis causes copious purulent secretions and is *highly contagious.* The gonococcus is one of the few pyogenic bacteria which is capable of attacking an intact corneal epithelium. This condition is easily transmitted to the eyes of nurses and others unless careful handwashing is practiced. The Credé method of instilling 1 per cent silver nitrate into the eyes of newborn infants was developed to destroy gonoccocci acquired during delivery. Such instillation must be carefully performed with the correct solution. Cases of permanent and severe eye injury are reported following the accidental substitution of ammoniacal silver nitrate solution (25–30 per cent) for the 1 per cent strength.[33]

The specific treatment of the various types of conjunctivitis depends upon the causative factor. However, generally the patient does best in a darkened room. The physian's orders may include orders for (a) specific antibacterial drugs locally and systemically; (b) eye irrigations; (c) hot moist compresses; and (d) eye drops or ointments. *Corticosteroids are contraindicated* in the presence of infectious conjunctivitis since they reduce ocular resistance to bacteria. Also, *eye dressings are contraindicated* since covering an eye which has a surface bacterial infection promotes bacterial growth. At times, e.g., with gonococcal conjunctivitis, the physician may order the "good" eye to be protectively dressed to prevent its becoming infected also. When the cause of conjunctivitis is allergic in origin (e.g., associated with hay fever, allergic rhinitis, or asthma) rather than bacterial, topical steroids may be ordered and may effectively relieve symptoms.

Ophthalmia Neonatorum (Conjunctivitis Neonatorum). This disorder is any purulent conjunctivitis of the newborn which is acquired from an infected birth canal. While most cases originally were due to gonococcal infections (discussed above), staphylococci, streptococci, pneumococci, and other bacteria and viruses may also be the causative organisms.

> *Trachoma causes more blindness throughout the* world *than any other condition.*

Trachoma. Although relatively rare in the United States (except among American Indians and Mexicans), trachoma has a worldwide distribution which is estimated to affect some 15 per cent of the world's population. This disease is especially prevalent in the Orient and Middle East, because of unsanitary conditions. Trachoma is a chronic infectious disease of the conjunctiva and cornea caused by an organism which appears to be an intermediate between the virus and the rickettsia. Trachoma is *highly communicable* and if untreated may result in *blindness.* Known cases must be isolated and treated. Teaching regarding personal cleanliness is also important in eliminating this disorder since it is spread by direct contact. The World Health Organization is helping eliminate trachoma throughout the world; however, much work remains. Vaccines are being developed. Trachoma responds well to treatment with local and systemic sulfonamides or local antibiotics (tetracyclines) or both. Corticosteroids activate trachoma viruses. (It is noteworthy that almost all fungi also grow better when corticosteroids are given, since these drugs inhibit host defenses. Since the advent and widespread use of corticosteroids, severe fungous eye infections are more common.) Figure 105-12 pictures an eye in which the cornea has been scarred from trachoma.

Scleritis. "Scleritis" refers to inflammation of the sclera. It may be superficial, i.e., *episcleritis,* or deep. Bulging and thinning of the sclera occur in the latter form. Scleritis causes the eye to be very red, and movement is usually painful. Generally iritis accompanies scleritis. Scleritis and ititis are treated similarly. (See discussion of iritis on p. 1488.)

Keratitis (Corneal Inflammation) and Corneal Ulcer. Inflammations of the cornea (i.e., keratitis) generally are characterized by the following symptoms: pain, photophobia, lacrimation, blepharospasm (i.e., the involuntary contraction of the orbicularis muscle), and interference with vision. Corneal inflammations may be divided into (a) superficial keratitis, (b) deep keratitis, and (c) corneal ulcer.

There are numerous different types of keratitis. Keratitis may be acute or chronic, superficial, or deep. *Dendritic keratitis* is a *superficial* corneal ulceration caused by the herpes simplex virus which can result in permanent corneal scarring unless properly treated. Idoxuridine (IDU) is almost the specific therapy for this condition. If this fails after 3–5 days, mechanical or chemical debridement is indicated. Topical adrenocortical steroids are contraindicated in the early stages of dendritic keratitis (unless covered with IDU). *Disciform keratitis* is a *deep,* disk-shaped corneal inflammation, with accompanying iritis, which often follows dendritic keratitis or trauma. Treatment consists of atropine, 1 per cent, to dilate the pupil, and topical or systemic adrenocorticosteroids, or both, with IDU to prevent recurrence of dendritic keratitis.

TABLE 105-2. DIFFERENTIAL DIAGNOSIS OF COMMON CAUSES OF INFLAMED EYE *

	Acute Conjunctivitis	Acute Iritis †	Acute Glaucoma ‡	Corneal Trauma or Infection
Incidence	Extremely common	Common	Uncommon	Common
Discharge	Moderate to copious	None	None	Watery or purulent
Vision	No effect on vision	Slightly blurred	Markedly blurred	Usually blurred
Pain	None	Moderate	Severe	Moderate to severe
Conjunctival injection	Diffuse; more toward fornices	Mainly circumcorneal	Diffuse	Diffuse
Cornea	Clear	Usually clear	Steamy	Clarity change related to cause
Pupil size	Normal	Small	Moderately dilated and fixed	Normal
Pupillary light response	Normal	Poor	None	Normal
Intraocular pressure	Normal	Normal	Elevated	Normal
Smear	Causative organisms	No organisms	No organisms	Organisms found only in corneal ulcers due to infection

* From Krupp, M. A., and Chatton, M. J.: Current Medical Diagnosis and Treatment. Los Altos, California, Lange Medical Publications, 1974.
† Acute anterior uveitis.
‡ Angle closure glaucoma.

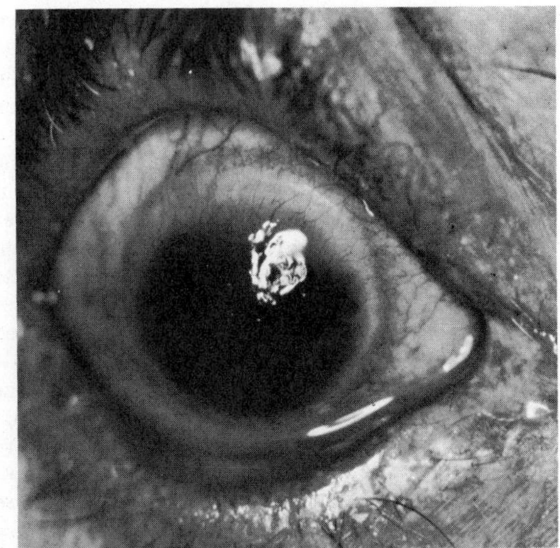

FIGURE 105-12. Corneal scarring from trachoma. (From Scheie, H. G., and Albert, D. M.: *Adler's Textbook of Ophthalmology.* 8th ed. 1969.)

Corneal ulcers constitute a medical emergency, because of the potential danger of perforation of the cornea, corneal scarring, or intraocular infection. Such complications can cause permanent visual impairment. Corneal ulcers may result from many causes, e.g., following exposure or trauma, or as a result of allergy, vitamin deficiency (avitaminosis A), lowered resistance (e.g., diabetes mellitus), or infections, e.g., bacterial, viral, or fungal. The commonest bacterial cause of corneal ulcer is the *Diplococcus pneumoniae* (producing the pneumococcic or "acute serpiginous" ulcer). Local therapy with sulfonamides and antibiotics is usually effective. Early, vigorous treatment is imperative to try to preserve vision. Treatment includes polymyxin locally plus streptomycin and a sulfonamide systemically. *Herpes simplex virus is a more common cause of corneal ulceration than any bacteria.* Herpes simplex has been discussed on page 1481.

The outline of a corneal ulcer may be visualized by using sterile fluorescein to stain the cornea. The specific treatment of a corneal ulcer depends upon its specific cause; however, some treatment measures which may be employed include (a) instillation of atropine sulfate or scopolamine to keep the pupil dilated (this puts the ciliary body and iris at rest, favors healing of the ulcer, provides sedation and minimizes pain); (b) antibiotics locally or systemically or both; (c) hot compresses to provide comfort and promote healing of the infection; (d) cortisone (unless contraindicated) to help control inflammation; (e) cleansing of the cornea with antiseptic solution; (f) cauterization (with heat or chemicals), scraping or treatment by thermophore* to limit spread of an infected ulcer by treating its advancing boarders; and (g) paracentesis of the anterior chamber (after topical anesthesia) to limit spread of an ulcer or prevent a threatened perforation.

Topical anesthetics should not be used more than absolutely necessary for pain relief and are not prescribed for home use due to their deleterious effects on the cornea. Ointments are not used on corneal ulcers or corneal abrasions because they delay healing and at times may cause recurrent corneal erosions. Dressings are not used on infectious suppurative lesions because they favor bacterial multiplication and prevent the free flow of discharge from the eye. However, with superficial epithelial erosions and clean corneal lesions, a dressing may be useful and may relieve pain.

Perforation of the cornea is a serious complication of corneal ulcer which may rapidly occur. Intraocular hemorrhage may follow sudden perforation and destroy vision. Perforation occurs spontaneously, or it may be caused from increased pressure (e.g., from blepharospasm, straining, or force exerted during examination). Following perforation the aqueous humor escapes (often prolapsing the iris and carrying it into the wound); the lens may become dislocated (occasionally it escapes); the eye feels soft; the anterior chamber is obliterated; and the pupil contracts (even though previously it may have been dilated with atropine). After spontaneous perforation of an ulcer, atropine is instilled, a firm dressing is applied, the patient is placed on *complete* rest, and he is instructed to avoid straining.

> *Corneal scarring or perforation of the cornea due to corneal ulceration is a major cause of blindness throughout the world, and causes about 10 per cent of blindness in the United States.*[88]

Because most forms of corneal ulceration are amenable to therapy, it is important that a patient with symptoms of corneal ulceration rapidly be given medical treatment.

Corneal Opacity. A perfectly smooth and transparent cornea is a necessary component of good vision. Normally the cornea is invisible except for reflections from its surface. "Corneal opacity" refers to a lack of transparency of the cornea resulting from inflammation, ulceration, or injury. Corneal opacities reduce vision when they encroach upon the pupil; disfigurement is caused from dense opacities.

In some patients, who have only superficial corneal opacity, vision may be improved by the surgical removal of the opaque corneal layers; this procedure is called "*superficial keratectomy.*" If the opacity entirely occludes the pupillary area, but there are still other regions of the cornea which are clear, *iridectomy* (i.e., excision of a part of the iris) may be performed to create an *artificial pupil.* The new opening (coloboma) is made opposite a clear part of the cornea. When the entire cornea is

**Thermophore* is a device with which a less intense but more accurately controlled application of heat can be made than with cautery. The instrument develops and maintains a set temperature below cauterization level at the tip of the instrument.

opaque and vision is greatly reduced, the surgical procedure of *corneal transplantation,* i.e., *keratoplasty,* may be performed in selected patients.

Corneal Transplantation (Keratoplasty). Keratoplasty may be performed not only to repair a corneal opacity but also to correct *keratoconus,* i.e., a condition in which there is a cone-shaped distortion of the central cornea. Additionally many ophthalmic surgeons now advocate corneal transplants when perforation of a corneal ulcer is imminent.

There are various types of corneal transplant procedures (Fig. 105-13). For example, a *lamellar keratoplasty* is a corneal graft which involves replacement of only some of the cornea's five layers, while a *penetrating keratoplasty* is a procedure in which all five layers of the cornea are replaced with a graft. A penetrating corneal transplant extends into the anterior chamber. Some transplants are *combination grafts* or *partial penetrating keratoplasties* in which a central penetrating area is surrounded with a peripheral lamellar area.

An eye graft for corneal transplantation is obtained from a fetus, a cadaver, or a patient whose eye has been removed surgically (provided that the cornea is normal). In working with cadavers, the donor's eye must be removed as soon after death as possible because the cornea begins to soften after death. At the time of death (when a patient is known to have donated his eyes), the cornea is preserved and protected by closing the eyelids over the cornea and placing on the lids pieces of gauze moistened with normal saline. Nothing is placed directly on the cornea itself.

Ideally a donated eye should be removed from the body within 2–4 hours following death; however, it may still be viable if removed up to 12 hours after death. Also, ideally the cornea should be transplanted into the recepient's eye immediately after it is removed from the donor. However, this is not always possible. The fresh eye may be transplanted up to 48 hours after death if it is kept in a sterile container (in an upright position on a piece of gauze soaked in normal saline) and placed in the cool part of a standard household refrigerator (a temperature of 4°C. is recommended for storage). Recently numerous successful *lamellar* transplants have been performed with corneas which have been stored for months in a frozen state or in glycerine. Until quite recently it was only possible to perform *penetrating* keratoplasties with fresh corneas (transplanted within 48 hours after removal from the donor); however, frozen grafts have now also been successfully transplanted with this procedure. Studies are underway to investigate the possibility of using artifical plastic corneas for replacement procedures; such procedures are called "*prosthokeratoplasties.*"[18]

Anyone wishing to do so can make arrangements (through his physician or by writing the national eye bank) to give legal permission for his eyes to be donated for use by a qualified ophthalmologist. To contact the eye bank write: Eye-Bank for Sight Restoration, Inc., 210 E. 64th St., New York, N.Y. 10021. Information may also be obtained by con-

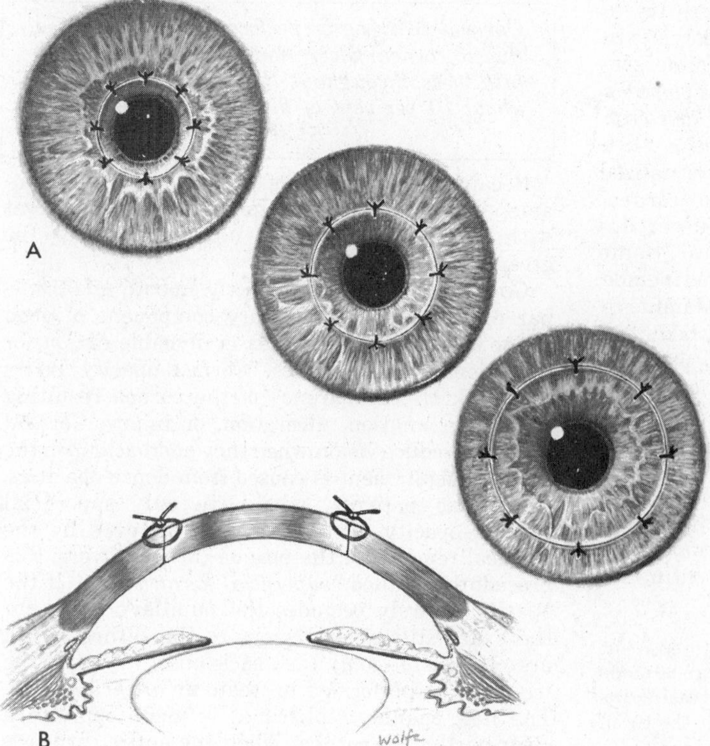

FIGURE 105-13. Corneal transplant. *A,* Grafts of three different sizes. Interrupted sutures. *B,* Sagittal section of cornea showing full-thickness graft. (From Scheie, H. G., and Albert, D. M.: *Adler's Textbook of Ophthalmology.* 8th ed. 1969.)

tacting your state's agency for the blind. Because eye banks cannot meet the demands of sightless persons wishing to have corneal transplants performed, there are currently lists of names of persons waiting to receive grafts.

Corneal transplantations are intraocular surgical procedures. Nursing care varies according to the type of transplant performed, but the general care of a patient preceding and following intraocular surgery is discussed on p. 1476. A partial lamellar graft requires less conservative postoperative care than a total penetrating transplant, which widely and completely opens the eyeball. Combination grafts, i.e., partial penetrating keratoplasties, may be performed in two stages or in one procedure.

Preoperative preparation of the patient varies, depending upon the anesthetizing procedure selected. Usually local anesthesia is preferred. Typically a miotic, e.g., pilocarpine, is preoperatively instilled to constrict the pupil. Miotics, by elongating and flattening the iris and extending it over the lens, help reduce the possibility of damage to these areas during the course of the operation. During surgery a round section of clear cornea is removed from the donor eye with a trephine (an instrument which has a structure and function similar to that of a cookie cutter). Next another trephine of exactly the same size (or the trephine used on the donor cornea) is used to remove the opaque area of the cornea from the recipient eye. The donor cornea is then carefully sutured into place.

Postoperatively, because the operated eye has been temporarily weakened and damaged, nursing care centers around preventing pressure increases upon or within the eye. Such pressure elevations could cause loss of aqueous humor through the suture line. Other postoperative nursing care goals include the promotion of healing by allowing the eye to completely rest and prevention of infection.[14]

Postoperative orders vary with the extent of the procedure and with the wishes of the physician. Following a penetrating graft transplant, the patient may wear bilateral eye dressings for 2–7 days. Until the unaffected eye is uncovered and the operated eye has begun to satisfactorily heal, the patient may be ordered to remain on a regimen of bedrest (similar to that of a patient with activity limitations due to a cardiac disorder), or he may be assisted to a chair several times each day, beginning on the second or third postoperative day. Such orders are determined by the type of transplant performed; the more restricted regimen is followed when a penetrating graft has been made. Dressing changes are performed daily, and the eye is inspected by the physician; he may then instill a miotic and an antibiotic. The patient who has had a combination graft may have both eyes bandaged and be kept very quiet for a minimum of 24 hours. Following a lamellar graft the patient may have only the operated eye dressed and may be allowed out of bed and to feed himself on the day of surgery.

Because the cornea is avascular, corneal grafts are slow to heal and may be easily infected. The cornea does not begin to heal firmly until at least 3 weeks have passed postoperatively. Because the cornea is weak during the interim, the danger remains of intraocular pressure pushing the healing graft forward. The patient must thus learn to protect his eye from sudden pressure increases.

The use of microsurgery and modern suture materials has reduced the postoperative period of hospitalization necessary following keratoplasty. While some suture materials need to be removed, others do not. If suture removal is necessary, the eye is anesthetized topically, e.g., with Pontocaine (tetracaine). Unabsorbable sutures (silk) are removed generally after 21–25 days.

The patient should be told that it takes about 4–6 weeks for the corneal graft to flatten and merge with the contour of the eyeball. Until this happens, irritation, e.g., photophobia, will occur due to the constant movement of the eyelids over the elevated edge of the donor cornea. Also, as the wound edema and inflammatory conditions gradually subside, vision will improve and photophobia will decrease. To protect the eye once the dressing is removed, the patient may be instructed to wear dark glasses (while convalescing and while photophobia is still present) and to wear a protective eye shield at night (to protect the healing eye from accidental injury). Care of the patient following intraocular surgery is discussed on p. 1477. Following corneal transplant, strong corrective lenses are not necessarily needed, e.g., like those needed after cataract surgery. The lens correction necessary before the corneal problem developed may be of adequate strength following the transplant.

Sometimes, unfortunately, after functioning for a while, a proportion of corneal grafts become opaque (from the immunologic process of rejection) (see Unit V). During the rejection process vascularization occurs in the normally avascular cornea. Such vascularization clouds the cornea, often making it necessary for a second grafting procedure to be undertaken. Attempts to prevent the complication of vascularization include steroid administration beginning 1 week after surgery (if given too early steroids delay healing), and the administration of beta irradiation to induce sclerosis.

Because corneal transplantation is an elective procedure, the patient must be in a state of general good health preoperatively, and the affected eye needs to be improved to its maximum. Corneal transplantation is usually not performed unless the physician believes there is a reasonable chance of success. However, in all cases there is the possibility that vision will only slightly improve (even though the procedure was technically excellent), or that the transplant will be rejected after several weeks or months. Follow-up visits are thus important after discharge. The feasibility of performing a second operation if the graft is rejected depends upon the condition of the patient's eye, as well as the availability of donor eyes.

DISORDERS OF THE UVEAL TRACT

Definitions. The *uveal tract* is composed of three parts: (1) the iris; (2) the ciliary body; and (3) the choroid. The uveal tract is the eye's middle vascular layer, contributing to the retina's blood supply. Externally the uveal tract is protected by the cornea and sclera. "*Uveitis*" is a general term referring to inflammatory disorders of the uveal tract. "*Anterior uveitis*" is the term generally used to refer to *iritis* and *iridocyclitis.* "Iritis" refers to inflammation of the iris; when the ciliary body is involved, the condition is called "iridocyclitis". "*Posterior uveitis*" is the term generally used to refer to *choroiditis* and *chorioretinitis,* i.e., inflammation of the choroid, and inflammation of the choroid and overlaying retina.

Uveitis. Inflammation of the uveal tract may be caused by numerous factors e.g., local or systemic disease, injury, or unidentified factors. The inflammation may involve only one portion of the tract or may simultaneously involve all three parts. *The most frequent form of uveitis is acute anterior uveitis* (*iritis*). Usually this is unilateral and is characterized by a history of pain, blurred vision, and photophobia. The pupil is typically small and the eye is red without purulent discharge. Uveitis may be either granulomatous (exogenous with acute onset) or nongranulomatous (endogenous with slow onset). The granulomatous form is most common.

Treatment of uveitis may involve such measures as:

- *Mydriatics,* e.g., atropine sulfate, 1 per cent, or 0.2 per cent scopolamine, to keep the pupil dilated. This prevents adhesion formation between the anterior capsule of the lens and the iris, relieves pain and photophobia, reduces congestion, and keeps the iris and ciliary body at rest.
- *Moist, hot compresses* several times each day to reduce pain and inflammation; applied for 10 minutes 3–4 times each day.
- *Local and systemic steroid therapy* is helpful in shortening the course of granulomatous uveitis by reducing inflammation.
- *Bedrest* may be prescribed during acute episodes.
- *Dark glasses* are worn to relieve photophobia.
- *Analgesics* are administered for pain relief, e.g., aspirin, morphine sulfate, as indicated.
- *Treatment of associated systemic disease* is important in the therapy for granulomatous uveitis.

Treatment is generally more satisfactory for nongranulomatous uveitis than for the granulomatous form; however, recurrences commonly occur. Serious complications can result from uveitis. Among these are glaucoma, cataract, and retinal detachment. Such complications can cause loss of vision. Obviously uveitis is a condition which must have the careful attention of an ophthalmologist.

When other measures fail in the treatment of uveitis, fever therapy may be employed using typhoid vaccine I.M. or I.V. Temperature elevations of 103° to 104° F. are desireable. Granulomatous uveitis may be highly resistant to treatment.

Sympathetic Ophthalmia (Sympathetic Uveitis). This is a rare, severe, bilateral, granulomatous uveitis of unknown etiology which occurs anytime from 10 days to as long as several years *following a penetrating injury near the ciliary body* (or following a retained foreign body). The injured eye (exciting eye) becomes inflamed first, then the other eye (sympathizing eye) also becomes red and photophobic, and vision becomes blurred. The *preventative* removal (enucleation) of any severely injured eye (with perforation of the sclera and ciliary body, with loss of vitreous humor and retinal damage) is the treatment of choice. (Enucleation is discussed on p. 1507.) However, such preventative treatment is difficult for some patients to accept. Ideally the severely injured eye should be enucleated within 10 days following injury. Once sympathetic ophthalmia begins, systemic and local steroid therapy may be useful, plus local atropine. Corticosteroids are continued for at least a year. Once inflammation is advanced in the sympathizing eye, it is not advisable to remove the exciting eye, since that eye may eventually prove to be the better of the two impaired eyes. *If untreated this devastating disorder slowly and relentlessly progresses until the patient is bilaterally blind.* Blindness occurs in a period of months or years. Very rarely sympathetic ophthalmia follows uncomplicated intraocular surgery for glaucoma or cataract.

DISORDERS OF THE RETINA

> The retina, the most essential part of the eye, is equivalent in function to the film in a camera; all the other structures of the eye exist only to nourish and protect the retina and to focus light rays upon it.[88]

The *retina,* the most complex of the ocular tissues, is a direct outgrowth of the central nervous system (an expansion of the optic nerve) and is thus not capable of regeneration. The rods and cones are the receptor cells of the retina. The retina is a thin, delicate, transparent membrane, which is said to have the highest rate of respiration (oxygen consumption per unit weight) of any of the body's tissues.[52] The retina is attached to the underlying choroid at the optic nerve border posteriorly and at the ora serrata anteriorly. Between these two points, the retina is in contact with the choroid but is not attached to it.

The "*fundus*" of the eye is the eye's internal surface, including the retina, the optic disk, and the choroidal or scleral details visible through the retina. A variety of systemic diseases are reflected in the appearance of the fundus, e.g., diabetes, hypertension, arteriosclerosis, and blood dyscrasias. Thus, by carefully studying the retina with an ophthalmoscope the physician can learn much of importance not only about the condition of the patient's eye, but also about the patient's general physical condition. A discussion of the eye and other bodily disorders, e.g., systemic disorders, is presented on p. 1507. Here we focus on specific disorders which primarily affect the retina.

Retinal disorders are diagnosed by history, testing visual acuity, ophthalmoscopy, and testing visual fields. The retina is designed to receive visual images and transmit them to the brain via the optic nerve. Thus, most disorders of the retina cause blurred vision. Because the retina contains no pain fibers, there is no pain with retinal disease. Also, the eye does not become red or inflamed.

Retinitis. "*Retinitis*" refers to inflammatory disease of the retina. However, inflammatory disease is seldom limited to the retina, but rather is commonly associated with disease of the choroid, i.e., "*chorioretinitis,*" and of the optic nerve head, i.e., "*neuroretinitis.*" Because retinitis is commonly dependent upon a constitutional factor, it is usually bilateral, lasting several weeks or months.

There are no external symptoms of retinitis, the typical retinal changes are observable only with an ophthalmoscope. The patient may notice diminution in visual acuity, changes in the visual field, alterations in the shape of objects, a feeling of discomfort in the eyes, and photophobia.

Retinitis may completely subside without impairing useful vision, or it may cause considerable visual loss or even blindness as a result of scarring and atrophy. Treatment of retinitis centers on treatment of the constitutional condition causing the retinal disorder. Local treatment includes providing *total rest for the eyes,* protection from light (smoked glasses may be worn), and frequently the use of atropine. Diaphoris is also useful, as are, at times, cathartics.

Retrolental Fibroplasia (Retinopathy of Prematurity). This condition is a *preventable* cause of blindness occurring in premature infants of low birth weight, before age 3 months. Bilateral retrolental fibroplasia is caused from exposure of the infant to an excessive concentration of oxygen while incubated in a premature nursery. Fortunately now this iatrogenic cause of loss of vision is extremely rare.

Retinal Detachment (Retinal Separation). The choroid and retina are not normally joined, but they are in close apposition. Normally the intraocular pressure of the vitreous helps hold the retina in contact with the choroid. "*Retinal detachment*" refers to the partial or complete detachment of the retina from the choroid. The detachment (or separation) is partial at first, but eventually becomes complete.

The retina is not firmly attached in position except at the optic nerve head and at the ora serrata. Thus, if the retina is torn or if a hole develops in it, fluid from the vitreous cavity (mixed with a transudate from the choroidal vessels) can seep through the opening, run behind the retina, and elevate the retina away from the choroid (Fig. 105–14). The portion of the retina which is thus separated from its choroidal nutrition becomes blind. *Early treatment is important* before irreparable damage occurs, resulting in irreversible blindness. If the condition is treated early enough, surgical repair may be able to successfully restore vision by reapproximating the retina and choroid.

Retinal detachment may occur as a *primary event* (from a break in the continuity of the retina, i.e., a hole or tear) or may occur *secondary* to various intraocular disorders. Traction phenomena can cause retinal tears which pull the retina away from its normal position. Retinal detachment may occur following surgery on the eye, e.g., cataract removal. Also it may occur following contrecoup injuries or following loss of vitreous humor, e.g., from perforating injuries. The most common predisposing causes of retinal datachment are aphakia (absence of lens)

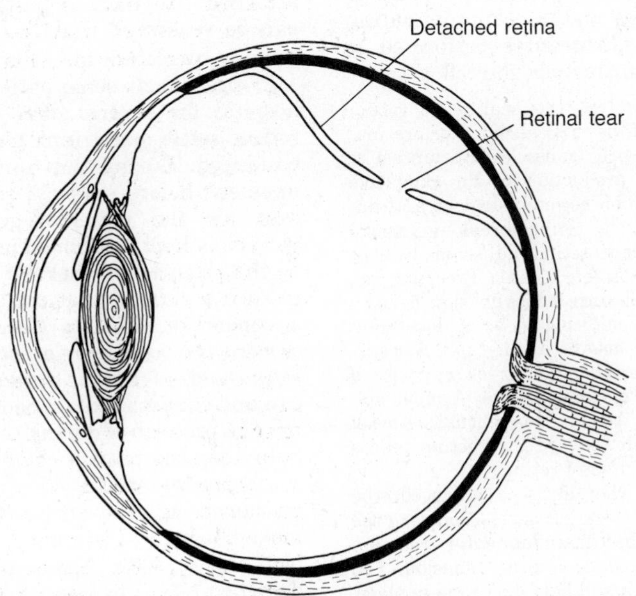

FIGURE 105–14. Detachment of retina caused by retinal tear.

and myopia. In the myopic eye (see p. 1503), a hole may develop in the retina because the retina does not stretch at the same rate as the scleral coat of the eyeball.

Retinal detachment most commonly occurs after age 40 and usually occurs spontaneously. Spontaneous detachments are ultimately bilateral in 20 to 25 per cent of cases. Unless treated, retinal detachment usually becomes total within 1–6 months. Retinal detachment may occur slowly or suddenly. The patient may notice the sudden appearance of flashes of light or floating spots before one eye, followed days or months later by the loss of a portion of the visual field, e.g., like a curtain descending over one of the eyes. The floating spots are caused from pigment or blood cells freed into the vitreous at the time the retina tears. The streaks and flashes of light are caused by vitreous traction on the retina. Vision is blurred in the affected eye and becomes progressively worse. No pain or redness occurs in the eye with retinal detachment. The area of visual loss depends upon the area of detachment, e.g., if the retina's upper portion is detached, the force of gravity pulls off the retina, creating the sensation of a descending curtain over the visual field. Ophthalmoscopic examination reveals a portion of the retina hanging like a gray cloud in the vitreous and one or more retinal tears (usually crescent-shaped and red or orange in color). The vitreous may appear cloudy. The physician may examine the eye by using a binocular indirect ophthalmoscope and a scleral depressor.

Surgery is necessary to reattach the retina. The surgical procedures by which retinal detachments are corrected are numerous and varied. However, these procedures all have in common the goals of closing the retinal breaks and of reapproximating the retina and choroid. Procedures performed to correct retinal detachment include the following:

> *Simple retinopexy:* Involves the sealing of retinal breaks by the production of localized chorioretinal adhesions associated with transscleral drainage of subretinal fluid. The production of an exudative sterile choroiditis may be accomplished at and immediately surrounding the retinal break in various ways. The making of chorioretinal adhesions by *electrical diathermy* is an obsolete technic. Freezing, i.e., *cryotherapy,* is preferable since it does not significantly damage the sclera. In addition to being less traumatic, cryotherapy can also be applied to a wet surface. The *photocoagulator* and *laser beam* incite a thermal inflammatory response in the pigment epithelium and choroid by focusing an external source of radiant energy through the eye's refracting media onto a relatively small area of retina.
>
> After an exudative choroiditis is produced, the retina must be brought back into apposition with the underlying choroid so that the inflammatory reaction will involve it and produce a firm adhesion, i.e., chorioretinal scar, which will hold the retina in place. Draining fluid from the subretinal space (by perforating the sclera and choroid) helps make it possible for the retina to return to its normal position. However, in addition to *subretinal fluid drainage,* other mechanical procedures may be performed.

> Various procedures have been designed to restore or support *mechanically* the contact of the retina with the pigment epithelium. Among these, various types of *"scleral buckling"* procedures can be implemented to depress or "buckle down" the area of sclera which lies over the retinal defect. By indenting the defect inward toward the vitreous, the retina and choroid are brought together. Either an *explant* or an *implant* may be used to depress the sclera. An elastic explant may be sutured over the outside of the sclera with external mattress suture; local intrascleral implants of various materials, e.g., dried fascia, may be placed within the scleral layers (within a surgically created scleral pocket), and the external layers are then sutured back in place over the implant. A similar result can be obtained with an infolded segment of sclera (*"scleral infolding technic"*), rather than an artificial implant, used to act as a tampon.
>
> *Circling procedures* are those in which the entire globe has a band of fascia "buckled" or tied around it so it tightly encircles the globe and indents it over the retinal defect. A circling strip of fascia is passed beneath the extraocular muscles and is fixed to the eye with anchoring sutures. The ends of the fascial band are then tied together and sewn under a scleral flap.
>
> In all the preceding mechanical procedures, the sclera is ultimately shortened, thereby pushing the choroid and retina into contact. *Intravitreal injections* push the retina up against the choroid by increasing the pressure within the globe. The falling retina is thus pushed back into place against the globe's wall, thereby ensuring the necessary contact between the retina and the induced inflammatory reaction. Injections of donor vitreous, saline solution, or air may be made into the vitreous cavity if the eye is hypotonic following surgery. In some cases liquefied silicone preparations are placed into the vitreous cavity.

Patients should always be told by the physician before surgery that there is a possibility that the surgery will not be successful. If the retina is still attached two months postoperatively, the patient can be reassured that the condition will probably remain corrected and that recurrence is unlikely.

Preoperatively some patients are admitted to the hospital for several days of bedrest, to help the retina settle back into place. Both eyes may be bandaged. During this period of tension and confinement before surgery, emotional care is important for the patient's general well-being. The patient is kept positioned preoperatively as ordered by the physician. Generally the patient is positioned in such a manner that the area of detachment is in a dependent position. *Carefully check orders concerning the position of a patient who has a detached retina* and inform the patient of positions which he can and cannot assume. Sedatives and tranquilizers may be prescribed during the preoperative period to help keep the patient comfortable and relaxed and to minimize strain on the eye. The patient is cautioned against straining and making sudden movements, e.g., sneezing, coughing, sitting up in bed, and so forth. Never allow the patient with a detached retina to lie with his face down or to stoop or bend over. Warn the patient not to rub or touch his eyes. Keep siderails up and the call bell within easy reach. When the patient's eyes are bandaged, be certain to speak when approaching him, visit the patient frequently and attempt to anticipate his needs. Feed the patient cautiously to avoid his choking, coughing, vomiting, and so forth. Such activities may cause further retinal detachment. Bowel care is given as ordered to prevent straining at stool. Small pillows or folded towels may be ordered placed by the patient's head to help remind him of the position in which he is to keep his head. Sometimes pinpoint glasses are worn instead of bandages to decrease eye movements. Such glasses have only a small circular opening in the center of the lens through which the patient can see.

Prior to surgery for retinal detachment the pupil is dilated widely with a mydriatic, phenylephrine (Neo-Synephrine), and a cycloplegic (Cyclogyl); this decreases movement of intraocular structures and facilitates visualization of the retina. Surgery is usually performed under general anesthesia.

Postoperatively, following buckling procedures, antibiotic ointment is instilled and a pressure dressing is applied with two eye pads and elastic plastic tape. Such a dressing greatly reduces postoperative lid conjunctival edema. Both eyes are usually padded for 1 to 2 days. The patient is positioned with the hole (retinal tear) dependent; however, he is usually allowed to turn into at least two positions (e.g., onto his back and onto his "hole" side). While in bed the patient is encouraged to perform isometric exercises (e.g., 5 minutes every half hour while awake). During such exercising the patient is instructed to take care not to violently agitate his head. Typically the patient is up on the second postoperative day with the unoperated eye uncovered. The patient is supervised and helped to get up slowly. Most patients are discharged to home care on the third or fourth postoperative day. To relieve discomfort, warm, moist compresses may be prescribed for 10 minutes at least three times each day. Shaving, hair care, bathing, dressing, and ambulation is permitted at home. Atropine, 1 per cent, is used once daily for 10–14 days. The dressing on the operated eye is no longer used once discharge and excessive swelling disappear. Television watching is permitted, but reading is not allowed for 2–3 weeks. No pinhole glasses or other occlusion is necessary. Light work is allowed after 3 weeks, and fully normal activity may be resumed within 6 weeks. The patient is told to be careful not to bump his head.[42]

The postoperative routine described in the preceding paragraph is that recommended by one authority.[42] Postoperative orders given by other physicians may differ from this recommended routine; thus orders are checked carefully for each patient, especially regarding the physician's orders concerning positioning allowed or forbidden activities. Some physicians recommend longer periods of postoperative bedrest; some prescribe the use of pinhole glasses after dressings are removed; and some tell their patients to avoid heavy lifting and deep bending or stooping forward for the remainder of their lives. Wearing of dark glasses may be advisable during the time mydriatics are used.

During the immediate postoperative period, it is generally advisable to remember to keep the patient's head and eyes at rest and to have him avoid straining (which increases venous pressure in the head). Antiemetics are frequently ordered to prevent emesis if the patient is nauseated, e.g., prochlorperazine, 10 mg. I.M. Medications to relieve pain are also ordered, as well as an antibiotic ointment for the eye and medications to dilate the pupil (dilation reduces intraocular inflammation and prevents adhesions between the iris and lens). Care of the patient with intraocular surgery is discussed further on p. 1476.

INCREASED INTRAOCULAR PRESSURE (GLAUCOMA)

Introduction. Glaucoma is not one disease but rather a complex of ocular disorders, all of which share the characteristic symptom of increased intraocular pressure. Over a period of time elevated intraocular pressure causes visual impairment, producing typical defects in the visual field due to atrophy of the retinal ganglion cells and atrophy of the optic nerve. If uncorrected, blindness may result.

Glaucoma is responsible for 12 per cent of blindness in the United States. This condition is often referred to as a "thief in the night" because in its most common form glaucoma steals away vision, unknown to the victim until he is almost blind. Glaucoma is the second most frequent cause of blindness. It is estimated that two persons in every 100 over age 40 now have glaucoma, but *do not realize they have it!* Routine tonometer measurements are thus important, since this is the only way to identify glaucoma before the eye is permanently damaged from the increased pressure within it. It is recommended that a tonometer reading be performed with every routine *general* physical examination, as well as with every routine *ocular* examination in persons over age 40. Because of the hereditary tendency associated with the most common forms of glaucoma, persons with a family history of glaucoma should have their intraocular pressures measured routinely every year.

Pathophysiology. Normally, the *aqueous humor* fills the anterior and posterior chambers and permeates the vitreous humor. Aqueous humor is mainly produced by the ciliary body and is crystal clear. In addition to serving as a refractive medium, the aqueous humor furnishes nutritional support to the avascular lens and cornea and contributes to the maintenance of intraocular pressure.

The *intraocular pressure* is determined by the rate of aqueous humor production and the resistance to outflow of aqueous humor from the eye. Normally an almost constant balance is maintained between the rate of formation and the rate of absorption of aqueous humor. From the posterior chamber, the aqueous humor passes between the iris and lens and leaves the posterior chamber through the pupil (Fig. 105–15). Emerging from the pupil into the anterior chamber, a portion of aqueous humor then passes through the trabecular meshwork of the chamber angle into the canal of Schlemm and out through the collector channels or aqueous veins into the anterior ciliary veins. This is the major direction of outflow of aqueous humor. Additionally, however, a portion of the aqueous humor is absorbed through the iris vessels, and some diffuses into the vitreous humor to leave the eye by posterior drainage routes.

Glaucoma (increased intraocular pressure) results from obstruction of the trabecular network and the canal of Schlemm, thus interfering with the mechanism of outflow in the angle of the anterior chamber. While many causes and types of obstruction exist (as we shall see), the *most common* is genetic loss of trabecular permeability, resulting in chronic simple glaucoma.

Types of Glaucoma. The various types of glaucoma can be broadly classified as follows:

A. Adult primary glaucoma
   1. Open angle (wide angle, simple, chronic simple, compensated) glaucoma
   2. Angle closure (narrow angle, closed angle, acute congestive, uncompensated) glaucoma
      a. Acute
      b. Chronic
B. Secondary glaucoma
C. Congenital glaucoma
D. Absolute glaucoma

Absolute glaucoma may be the end result of any form of glaucoma and refers to any blind eye (with no light perception) in which intraocular pressure is

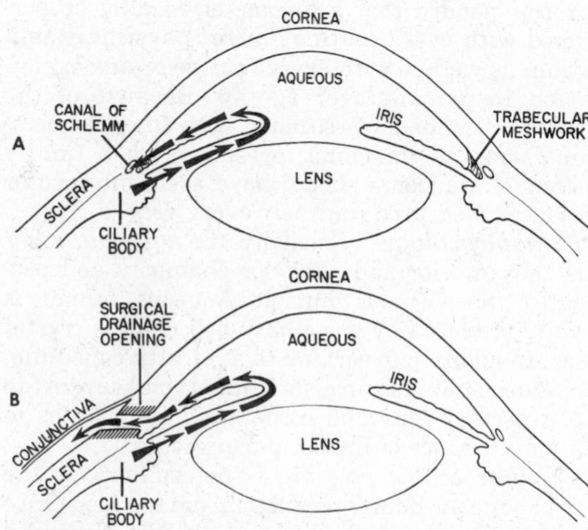

FIGURE 105–15. Normal flow of aqueous humor and creation of new channel with glaucoma surgery. (From Havener, W. H.: *Synopsis of Ophthalmology.* 3rd ed. St. Louis, The C. V. Mosby Co., 1971.)

elevated. To relieve the discomfort of the eye, enucleation is recommended. *Congenital glaucoma* occurs in an eye during its early period of growth and development and usually makes its appearance within the first 6 months of life. *Secondary glaucomas* may develop from numerous causes, e.g., uveitis, neovascular disorders, trauma, tumors, postoperatively, degenerative diseases of the eye. Our discussion focuses on adult primary glaucomas.

Hereditary factors appear to play an important role in *adult primary* glaucomas, particularly in *open angle glaucoma,* which is the most common of the primary glaucomas. Open angle glaucoma occurs in persons who appear to have normal "open" chamber angles but have a resistance to the flow of aqueous humor out of the chamber angle. This resistance may be in the meshwork, in Schlemm's canal, in the aqueous veins, or in the ciliary veins and usually results from degenerative changes. With *angle closure glaucoma* which is much less common, there is a forward displacement of the last roll and root of the iris against the cornea. This narrows (or perhaps entirely closes) the chamber angle, thus obstructing the outflow of aqueous humor. Complete closure of the angle, and thus complete obstruction to the outflow of aqueous, may occur in a person who has a narrowed angle as a result of sudden dilation of the pupil (administration of mydriatics is thus hazardous in the presence of a narrowed angle); swelling of the lens; swelling of the iris (from inflammation); or slight forward movement of the lens and iris. Mydriatic and cycloplegic medications should not be used until the anterior chamber angle has been evaluated by gonioscopy. Such precautionary practice can prevent accidental precipitation of an acute attack of glaucoma.

Open Angle (Chronic Simple) Glaucoma. This most common form of glaucoma is usually bilateral and may progress to complete blindness without ever producing an acute attack. Usually painless, open angle glaucoma occasionally causes a slight aching in the eyes. No symptoms appear in the early stages, and the disease progresses insidiously (usually in older persons).

There may be times when the patient notices foggy vision and diminished accommodation with open angle glaucoma. Other symptoms include disturbed dark adaptation and premature presbyopia. Symptoms are usually most apparent in the morning. Over a period of years peripheral vision is gradually, often unnoticeably, lost. Because central vision typically remains effective for a longer period of time, the patient may be unaware that he is losing the ability to see peripherally. The chronic elevation of intraocular pressure eventually destroys the eye's ability to function.

Late symptoms occur only after severe and irreversible eye damage has taken place: (a) visual field losses; (b) reduced visual acuity uncorrectible with glasses; (c) cupping and atrophy of the optic disk (as viewed by an ophthalmoscope); and (d) markedly elevated intraocular pressure which is detectable with a crude finger tension estimation. "Halos around lights" do not occur unless the intraocular tension is markedly elevated. Because these are late findings, it is obvious that case-finding of glaucoma is dependent upon careful specific measurements of intraocular pressure through the simple screening procedure of *tonometry.*

In addition to tonometry, other *diagnostic tests* which may be used to diagnose glaucoma include (a) *tonography* (an electric tonometer is allowed to rest on the patient's eye for 4 minutes while a record of the pressure is made on a moving drum); (b) various *provocative tests* to evaluate the effects of various conditions or agents upon intraocular pressure (such tests are explained in texts of ophthalmology and include procedures such as the water drinking test, the dark room test, mydriatic dilatation, and instillation of mydriatics); (c) *visual field* evaluation; (d) *ophthalmoscopy* (to evaluate the optic nerve head); and (e) *gonioscopy* (to examine the angle of the anterior chamber).

If untreated, chronic glaucoma which begins at age 40–45 will probably result in complete blindness by age 60–65. Useful vision can be preserved in most patients whose glaucoma is diagnosed early and controlled medically. It is important that the patient with glaucoma (of any type) realize that he has a condition which (like diabetes) requires *treatment for the rest of his life.* Periodic reevaluations of the patient's condition are important. Glaucoma is a condition which is controlled rather than cured; in this sense it is comparable to diabetes and tuberculosis.

The treatment of choice for open angle glaucoma is medical rather than surgical. However, surgery is necessary for some patients. The majority of patients with chronic, open angle glaucoma are treated with the following medications (in individualized combinations and dosages):

> *Miotics,* e.g., pilocarpine, 1–4 per cent. Miotics facilitate aqueous outflow by increasing the efficiency of the outflow channels. Thus by constricting the pupil intraocular pressure is controlled. Physostigmine (a *parasympathomimetic* drug) is sometimes used in combination with pilocarpine. Physostigmine ointment may be used at bedtime to supplement daytime drop medication. Miotics often cause a temporary dimness of vision for 1–2 hours following instillation. Stronger miotics, e.g., isoflurophate and echothiopate, can cause retinal detachment or insidious cataract formation or both. Periodic reevaluation is thus important for patients receiving anticholinesterase medications; at least every 6 months they should have their pupils carefully dilated and their lenses and fundi examined.

> *Carbonic anhydrase inhibitors,* e.g., acetazolamide (Diamox), ethoxyzolamide (Cardrase), decrease the rate of aqueous humor production. Epinephrine eyedrops (*sympathomimetic* drug) also decrease aqueous humor production.

Generally *surgical treatment* is delayed as long as possible in open angle glaucoma. If the tension is not maintained at an acceptable level with medical treatment and if there is progressive visual loss, filtering operations may be performed. *Filtering operations* create a fistula between the anterior chamber and the subconjunctival spaces. The aqueous humor can then bypass the trabecular block and flow out through the surgically created fistula. Iridencleisis and trephining are examples of filtering operations. With *iridencleisis* a wick of iris is used to maintain a scleral opening through which aqueous drains. *Trephining* is a procedure in which a small button of sclera is removed to permit aqueous outflow through the tunnel thus created. In both these procedures the aqueous humor flows out into the sub-Tenon's space. There, within the subconjunctival space, the aqueous drainage is absorbed. Other filtering operations are sclerectomy and cyclodialysis. *Sclerectomy* permits aqueous humor to escape through a notch cut from the sclera. *Cyclodialysis* is an operation which separates the ciliary body from the sclera, thus forming a new exit for the aqueous. *Cyclodiathermy* and *cyclocryosurgery* are also procedures used in the surgical treatment of glaucoma; these procedures directly reduce the amount of aqueous formation by damaging the ciliary body (by diathermy or cryosurgery).

Any of the antiglaucoma operations discussed above may speed up cataract formation. Thus, if lens opacity is present, *lens extraction* may be the first procedure performed in the treatment of glaucoma. Lens extraction is discussed later in this chapter. Frequently lens extraction alone favorably affects the course of glaucoma; miotics may control the intraocular pressure following cataract surgery when they have been unable to do so prior to the surgery. Postoperative nursing care following these procedures is similar to that following other intraocular surgery, except that following cyclodiathermy the patient may be ambulatory immediately following surgery. Relatively few restrictions on activity are necessary. Check the doctor's orders carefully.

Angle Closure (Narrow or Closed Angle) Glaucoma. *Acute* angle closure glaucoma is a medical emergency. Havener comments, "Acute glaucoma is one of the most dramatic and rapidly destructive diseases of the eye."[40] *The principal aim of the treatment of angle closure glaucoma (acute or chronic) is to open the closed chamber angle and thus permit outflow of aqueous humor.* While this goal may sometimes be achieved medically, *usually surgery is eventually required.* In some cases immediate surgery is necessary.

Angle closure glaucoma may produce *prodromal symptoms* in which the patient experiences transitory attacks characterized by diminished visual acuity, colored halos around lights, and some head and eye pain. These *transitory attacks* may last only a few hours, recurring at intervals of weeks or years before the patient experiences full-blown typical prolonged attacks of acute glaucoma.

Three basic mechanisms involved in the pathogenesis of an *acute* angle closure glaucoma attack are (1) the anatomically narrowed angle; (2) a relative pupil block (in which synechiae form between the lens and iris, obstructing the normal pathway of aqueous humor out from the posterior chamber); and (3) pupillary dilatation (which increases the thickness of the root of the iris, thus further blocking the angle and thwarting outflow of the aqueous humor).

When angle closure glaucoma occurs acutely, definite symptoms present themselves (unlike the asymptomatic picture of open angle glaucoma). A sudden rise in intraocular pressure results from closure of the angle, and this pressure elevation causes striking symptoms. Edema and congestion occur in the iris and ciliary process. Usually the patient with an *acute attack of glaucoma* rapidly seeks treatment. His eye is typically red, the cornea is steamy, the anterior chamber is shallow, the aqueous is turbid, the intraocular pressure is greatly elevated, and the pupil is moderately dilated and does not react to light. The patient also typically experiences blurred vision, halos around lights, or a rapid loss of vision. Excruciating pain (of a throbbing nature) occurs in the eye and radiates over the sensory distribution of the 5th cranial nerve. Nausea and vomiting also frequently occur. Usually attacks are unilateral. Following treatment the symptoms usually subside; however, after each acute attack the patient's vision and visual field worsen. Only surgery (peripheral iridectomy, to be discussed) will prevent further attacks.

Unless it is relieved, the excessive intraocular pressure which occurs with acute angle closure glaucoma will cause permanent damage to the eye, resulting in *absolute glaucoma*. Complete and permanent blindness will result within 3–5 days after symptoms appear. Emergency medical treatment is first given to reduce intraocular pressure, and then surgery is performed.

Medically the first objective is to establish miosis, since constriction of the pupil will pull the iris out of the chamber angle and thus open the outflow path for the aqueous. (Remember that with angle closure glaucoma the problem centers in the closure of the angle and not in the trabecular meshwork and Schlemm's canal. These structures will function normally once the angle is reopened.) Prior to surgery the intraocular pressure is lowered by (a) the local use of *miotics* (pilocarpine 1 per cent may be instilled as often as every 10–15 minutes until the pupil is constricted during an acute attack); (b) *osmotic agents* administered systemically (urea or mannitol may be given I.V.; glycerol is given orally in iced lemon juice); and (c) *carbonic anhydrase inhibitors* given systemically to restrict the action of the enzyme necessary to produce aqueous humor (in two to four times the normal dose). Medical treatment also directs itself at controlling nausea and relieving the intense pain associated with this acute eye disorder. Morphine or meperidine (Demerol) may be necessary to control pain. Because of nausea, and perhaps vomiting, give nothing by mouth unless ordered to do so.

If the above medical treatment regime reduces intraocular pressure within 4–6 hours, *surgery* is best deferred for a day or so until the eye is less inflamed. However, if the pressure is not reduced within 4–6 hours, emergency surgery is necessary before the high pressure causes death of nerve fibers. A *peripheral iridectomy* is the surgical procedure of choice once the acute episode has been relieved. A peripheral iridectomy can be performed without inserting any instruments into the anterior chamber. Thus some major complications of intraocular surgery are avoided, e.g., lens damage and cataract formation. In this procedure a small portion of the iris is excised, thus leaving a hole in the iris through which aqueous humor can bypass the pupil (Fig. 105–16). Iridectomy allows the iris to fall back and thus deepens the anterior chamber. The iridectomy is performed in the upper segment of the iris for cosmetic as well as functional reasons. Since the upper eye lid normally covers the upper segment of the cornea, it covers the iridectomy, thus occluding it and preventing the discomfort which accompanies an accessory pupil. Additionally, there is less likelihood of infection, since the flow of tears is gravitational, thereby carrying bacteria into the tear fluid which collects in the lower cul de sac.

If extensive peripheral anterior synechiae appear to have developed in the eye (and they will as a result of repeated glaucomatous attacks), a filtering operation may be indicated, preferably *iridencleisis.*

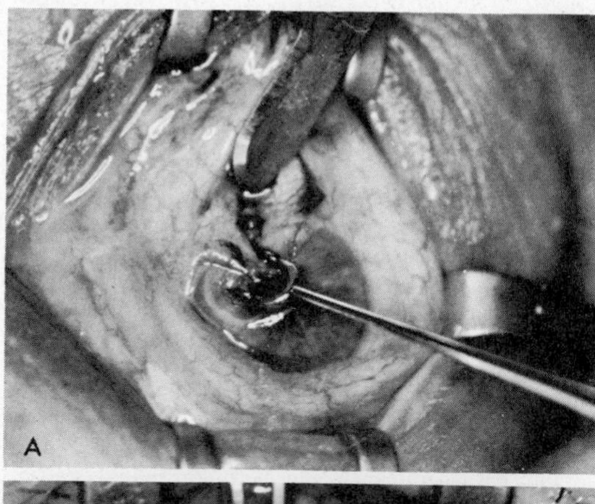

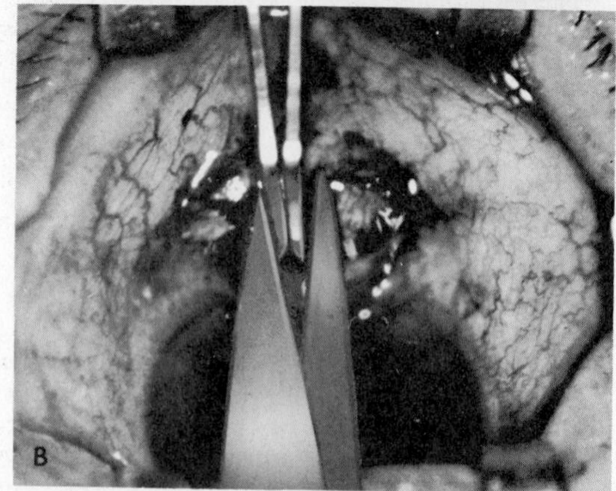

FIGURE 105–16. Peripheral iridectomy. *A,* Iris herniated through small scleral incision. *B,* Iris grasped by forceps and herniated portion excised. (From Scheie, H. G., and Albert, D. M.: *Adler's Textbook of Ophthalmology.* 8th ed. 1969).

Peripheral iridectomy is usually prophylactically performed on the fellow eye before the patient is discharged from the hospital (e.g., within a week after surgery on the originally operated eye). *Prophylactic peripheral iridectomy* is recommended because the glaucoma is a bilateral disorder, and thus an acute attack is likely to occur (or recur) in either eye. An acute attack occurs in the second eye in at least 50 per cent of cases, even though the patient may be conscientiously carrying out prophylactic miotic treatment. Peripheral iridectomy is thus desirable since well-controlled peripheral iridectomies have little operative risk and result in "true cure of angle-closure glaucoma if permanent anterior synechias have not formed."[88] Since permanent medical control of chronic angle closure glaucoma is generally impossible, it is desirable to have peripheral iridectomy performed as soon as possible. The earlier in the course of the disease that the surgery is performed the better the prognosis. Once the disease has progressed to the point that a filtration operation is necessary, the long-term visual prognosis becomes more greatly guarded.

Postoperatively following peripheral iridectomy the eye is bandaged for a week, with daily dressing changes. The pupil is kept dilated to prevent development of posterior synechiae. The patient may be ambulated on the second day. Postoperative care following iridencleisis is similar to that just described for peripheral iridectomy, except that some surgeons recommend daily massage at the iridencleisis site for 1–2 weeks postoperatively to help maintain patency of the filtering area.

Patient Teaching. Patient teaching is an important role for the nurse in caring for patients who have glaucoma. We have emphasized that case-finding and *early* diagnosis and treatment are highly important in preventing blindness from glaucoma. Also, we have stressed the importance of regular tonometry measurements on all persons with a family history of glaucoma. These are general facts of importance concerning protection of vision which nurses should emphasize to all persons whenever possible.

Now let us review some important areas which the nurse should plan to cover during planned teaching sessions with glaucoma patients and their relatives, when appropriate.

> *Follow your doctor's specific orders concerning your case.* Your doctor may advise you to (a) avoid excessive fluid intake; (b) attempt to remain reasonably calm and avoid highly upsetting situations which cause excessive worry, anger, excitement, or fear; (c) avoid wearing tight restrictive clothing, e.g., collars, neck scarves, tight belts, or girdles; (d) avoid heavy lifting or excessive straining; (d) seek prompt medical treatment of upper respiratory infections; and (e) attempt to avoid crying (it greatly increases intraocular pressure).

> *Take only those medications prescribed for you and faithfully use them as directed.* Do not substitute medications, do not use "old" medications, and do not miss even one instillation of eyedrops. Teach the patient important rules concerning ocular medications. Teach the patient how to properly instill medications into the eye (remember to teach him to occlude the tear duct to prevent excessive systemic absorption of very strong preparations). Teach him the important side effects of medications he is receiving and emphasize to him that he should contact his doctor at once if these symptoms develop. Instruct him to use eye medications *only* in the eye for which they are specifically ordered (accidental use of a mydriatic, e.g., atropine, in glaucomatous eye may precipitate an attack of acute glaucoma resulting in blindness).

> *Maintain regular contact with your physician, even though you may have had surgery performed on your eye.* Surgery does not necessarily correct glaucomatous conditions. Artificial pathways may become obstructed or closed, or other new problems may develop in the eye which require medical evaluation and treatment. Emphasize to the patient that he has a condition which will require medical supervision for the rest of his life. Tell the patient to contact his doctor at once if he develops ocular symptoms.

> *Inform others of your condition and emphasize to them that you need medication regularly* (if it is ordered for you). It is advisable to carry a card with you or wear an identification tag at all times which states that you have glaucoma. Thus, in case of accident, your condition will be recognized by persons caring for you and you will be given the medications necessary to preserve your vision. When you are admitted to a hospital for any reason, always inform your nurse at once that you have glaucoma, and tell her if you need medications regularly and the times of day when you are ordered to take your medication. It is usually advisable to continue this routine in the hospital unless the physician decides to change the pattern.

> *Keep an extra bottle of medication with you at all times* when away from home and keep an extra bottle at home.

> *Establish and maintain general health practices.* For example, protect your vision by having adequate light and by avoiding excessive, strenuous use of your eyes. Establish regular elimination habits which avoid constipation (straining at stool increases intraocular pressure). Exercise moderately to promote general circulation but avoid excessive exertion. Practice good habits of personal cleanliness.

> *Practice good safety habits.* Because mydriasis does not occur when miotics are being used, the patient will have difficulty seeing in dark places if he is using miotics. Instruct the patient to add extra lights in his home, as they are needed. Teach him to be particularly cautious when walking or driving in the dark. Instruct the patient to always use handrails when on stairs. Loss of accommodation makes added problems, e.g., the patient will have difficulty watching fast-moving objects.

As you plan your teaching sessions with a patient who has glaucoma (and with his family members), remember that during the few minutes you spend with the patient you will be teaching him how to live with a disorder which he will have for the remainder of his life. Your teaching may prevent future blindness for him. Your teaching may make it easier for him to adjust to his condition. Do not impose unnecessary restrictions on the patient. If you do so he may become uncooperative and not perform those activities which are essential to management of his glaucoma. Be certain to *individualize* your teaching plan. Base it on the doctor's suggestions for this particular patient. Encourage the patient to express his concerns and to ask questions which he may have about glaucoma and then plan accordingly to help him understand his condition.

OPACITY OF THE LENS (CATARACT)

Although a cataract may appear to be a growth over the eye, it is actually a clouding or opacity of the normally transparent crystalline lens. (Fig. 105-17). When the lens becomes opaque, it becomes milky or whitish in color; thus the *normally unobservable lens becomes noticeable.*

Normal Lens. The lens is a biconvex, colorless, and almost completely transparent structure which is suspended behind the iris by the zonular fibers (which connect it to the ciliary body). The aqueous humor is anterior to the lens; the vitreous body lies posterior to it. Devoid of blood vessels (except in fetal life), the lens derives its nourishment from the intraocular fluids. The lens capsule is a semipermeable membrane (slightly more permeable than a capillary wall) which admits water and electrolytes. The lens consists of about 65 per cent water, a trace of minerals, and about 35 per cent protein (the highest protein count of any body tissue). The lens has no pain fibers. With aging, subepithelial lamellar fibers are continuously produced; gradually the lens undergoes a loss of water and an increase in density, and it becomes larger and less elastic throughout life. The adult lens consists of a peripheral portion (cortex) and a central portion (nucleus). With advancing years, the nucleus increases in size and the cortex diminishes in proportion. In old age the entire lens is hard and unyielding. Thus, with aging, the lens undergoes a gradual reduction in its accommodative power. Accommodation, you will recall, is the focusing of near objects upon the retina by the lens. The only function of the lens is to focus light rays upon the retina. To accomplish such focusing the lens shape is altered by the actions of the ciliary muscles as they relax or contract.

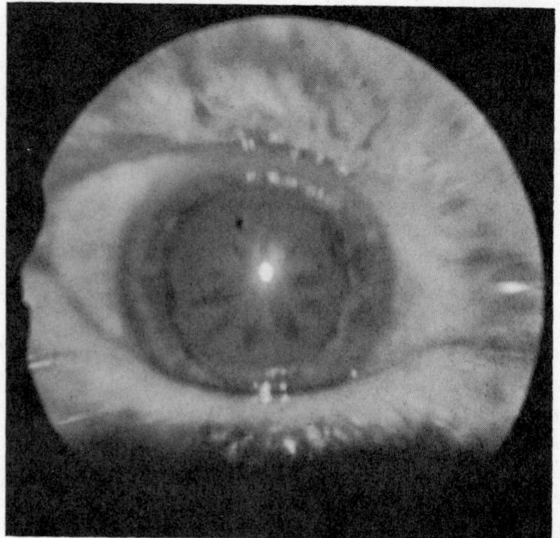

FIGURE 105-17. Flower-like cataract of ocular contusion. (From Scheie, H. G., and Albert, D. M.: *Adler's Textbook of Ophthalmology.* 8th ed. 1969.)

Cataract Formation. Some degree of cataract formation is expected in individuals over age 70. The precise cause of senile cataracts has not yet been identified; however, it appears to be a change in the metabolism of the lens and changes in the metabolism of the physical and chemical processes in its colloids. While senile cataract is the most common type, not all cataracts are associated with aging. In general there are two major groups of cataracts: (1) *developmental cataracts,* e.g., congenital and juvenile cataracts; and (2) *degenerative cataracts,* e.g., senile cataracts; toxic cataracts (resulting from ingestion of certain toxic substances or use of certain medications); radiation, lightning, electric, and heat ray cataracts; traumatic cataracts (most often due to a metallic intraocular foreign body striking the lens); complicated cataract (resulting from intraocular disease, e.g., severe recurrent uveitis); and cataract associated with systemic disease (e.g., diabetes). Senile cataracts pass through four stages: (1) incipient stage; (2) stage of swelling; (3) mature stage (cataract can easily be separated from lens capsule); and (4) hypermature stage. *Formerly it was necessary to wait until the mature stage was reached (the cataract was referred to as being "ripe") before surgery could be performed. This waiting period is no longer necessary.* Today the favorable time for extraction of senile cataracts is when the vision of the better-seeing eye has failed so greatly that it causes interference with the patient's comfort and normal daily activities. Cataract extraction can safely be performed on aged persons.

While cataracts are usually bilateral, they generally progress at different rates of speed in each eye. It is never advisable to perform bilateral surgery for cataract removal during one operation. If surgery is indicated, visual acuity improves in about 95 per cent of cases following lens extraction followed by corrective refraction to replace the removed lens. The remaining 5 per cent are not benefitted from surgery because they either have preexisting retinal damage or they develop postoperative complications, e.g., infection, retinal detachment, glaucoma, or hemorrhage.

The physician examines for disorders of the lens by testing visual acuity and by observing the lens with an ophthalmoscope, a hand flashlight, or a slit lamp or loupe. It is more helpful if the pupil can be dilated for examination. Cataracts vary markedly in their size, degree of density, and location. Cataracts are usually not noticeable externally until they reach the mature or hypermature stage and cause blindness. The retina becomes increasingly difficult to visualize as the cataract matures; ultimately the fundus reflection is absent, and the pupil is white when the cataract is mature. The patient with a cataract notices blurred vision which progressively worsens over months or years. The degree of visual loss corresponds to the opacity of the lens. No pain or redness of the eye is associated with cataract formation.

Cataract Surgery. Currently medical treatment is ineffective in stopping the changes which cause lens opacity. Thus, surgical treatment is the only available treatment. In cataract surgery the lens is removed from the eye, i.e., a lens extraction is performed. The two major methods of extracting the lens are (1) intracapsular extraction, and (2) extracapsular extraction. *Intracapsular extraction* has become the procedure of choice. In this procedure the lens is removed in toto, i.e., within its capsule. Figure 105–18 shows the lens capsule being grasped with a special lens capsule forceps and being slowly and gently pulled from the eye while counterpressure is applied on the limbus below with a blunt instrument.

The lens may also be delivered from the eye by means of *cryoextraction.* In this form of cryosurgery, a supercooled metal probe is applied to the lens to be removed. The probe then becomes firmly adherent to that area on the lens because an ice ball forms at the point of contact on the lens capsule and adjacent crystalline substance, i.e., the cold metal adheres to the wet, moist lens capsule. The bond forms in a matter of seconds, and the lens is then delivered from the eye by a gentle upward and then sideward pull. With cyroextraction the lens capsule is less likely to tear than with routine delivery with a forceps. Cryosurgery makes removal of a cataract safer and makes possible safe removal of immature lenses before they seriously interfere with vision.

During surgery, extraction of the lens may be made considerably easier by injecting some chymotrypsin (a fibrinolytic and proteolytic enzyme) into the eye's anterior chamber under the iris. This procedure is called *enzymatic zonulolysis.* The material is left in place 2–3 minutes before the lens is extracted. Then, because the material has a specific lytic action on the zonules, the lens can be lifted out more easily. Acetazolamide (Diamox) is given postoperatively following zonulolysis because it prevents secondary glaucoma (associated with prolapse of the iris and faulty wound healing) which chymotrypsin can cause.

Extracapsular extraction is still performed in the treatment of some types of congenital and traumatic cataract. In this procedure the capsule's anterior portion is first ruptured and removed, and then the lens cortex and nucleus are expressed from the eye. The posterior capsule of the lens is left in the eye. Although the extracapsular procedure is more conservative and is easier to perform than the intracapsular method, a secondary membrane develops in the eye which later requires severance (i.e., *discission*) in about one third of patients.

Cataract surgery is usually performed under local anesthesia. *Preoperative* medications may include secobarbital (Seconal) and meperidine (Demerol), given so the patient is drowsy upon coming to surgery, and sympathomimetic drugs (e.g., homatropine and Neo-Synephrine) instilled in the eye preoperatively to accomplish mydriasis and vasoconstriction. An important preoperative procedure is massage of the eye through the lid for 3 minutes prior to surgery; this reduces intraocular pressure. A "soft eye" is less likely to have loss of vitreous or dislocation of the lens.

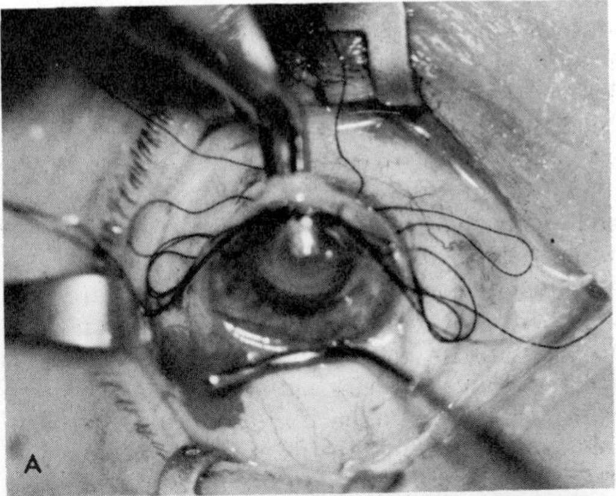

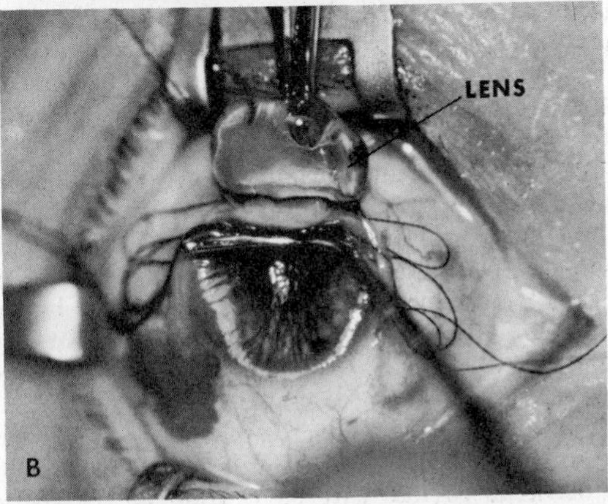

FIGURE 105–18. Intracapsular cataract extraction. *A,* Capsule forceps applied to lens. *B,* Delivery of lens through limbal incision. (From Scheie, H. G., and Albert, D. M.: *Adler's Textbook of Ophthalmology.* 8th ed. 1969.)

Postoperatively the patient's operated eye is patched and covered with a protective metal shield. This dressing may be changed by the physician after 24 hours and then daily. Usually the eye is kept covered for 10–14 days with a dressing and eye shield. The patient may be instructed to protectively cover his eye at night for a period of time after discharge home; the eye can easily be damaged during sleep from contact with bed linens. When it is time to remove the sutures from the eye, the eye is anesthetized, e.g., with Pontocaine, 1 per cent.

Postoperative restrictions on movement following cataract surgery are not as strict as they were previously because the wound is tightly sutured.

However, for the first 24–48 hours following cataract surgery, the patient is usually kept on bedrest. Check the physician's orders concerning positions which the patient can safely assume while on bedrest. Usually the patient can have a small, firm pillow and may have a 30° to 45° elevation of the head of the bed. The patient may be allowed to lie on his back or unoperated side. Instruct the patient not to lie on the operated side. Pain is usually easily controlled after lens extraction, since it is normally only of slight intensity. Generally the patient is up with assistance after 24 hours. Because the surgery performed was an intraocular procedure, the patient is cautioned to avoid placing strain on his eye and to move cautiously for at least 3 weeks. (Eye surgery is discussed on p. 1476.) Some limitations of activity may be advisable for up to 6 weeks postoperatively. It is thus important that the patient understand what he can and cannot do after he is discharged from the hospital.

Because the eye cannot function without a lens, the patient must be given a corrective lens to replace the defective lens which was surgically removed. During the period of healing a pair of temporary, thick convex *cataract glasses* may be prescribed for the patient (3–6 weeks following surgery). Temporary glasses are prescribed if the vision is poor in the other eye.

The patient must be prepared to spend several weeks learning to adjust to his new glasses. This adjustment period will be a time of frustration during which the patient will need the understanding and support of his physician and family. Great patience is necessary during the period of adjusting to cataract glasses. While the patient is still in the hospital, the nurse may be able to talk with him about how he can best use his glasses once he does receive them. Helpful hints concerning adjustment to cataract lenses include the following pointers:

> *Initially use the new glasses only while sitting down, because there is considerable distortion which must be adjusted to.* A cataract lens in glasses magnifies everything by one third. If surgery has been performed on only one eye, binocular vision is no longer possible with spectacles, and the patient must use only one eye at a time to prevent diplopia. If both eyes are aphakic, i.e., without a lens, binocular vision is possible since both eyes can be used simultaneously.

> *Practice looking through the center portion of the cataract corrective glasses' lenses; turn the head rather than only the eyes when looking to the side.* Clear vision is possible only through the center of the lens; a ring of a blind area occurs in the periphery of the visual field. Peripheral vision is poor due to the optical distortions created by strong lenses, e.g., curvature and distortion of detail occur. *New safety practices must be learned,* e.g., turning the head (not merely the eyes) in both directions before stepping off a curb.

> *Practice manual coordination with assistance initially until new spacial relationships become familiar.* Practice walking, going up and down steps, and so forth with assistance until these abilities are safely relearned. Teach the patient to always use handrails when they are available. The patient may practice finely coordinated movements by himself, e.g., practice picking up scattered buttons, practice pouring into and reaching for a cup or glass, practice writing.

> *Have your glasses checked if they are dropped, are bumped, or do not seem to be fitting your head correctly.* In order to effectively focus an image within the eye, the lenses must sit at the correct distance and at the correct angle with relation to the eye.

> *Wear your glasses at all times once you are accustomed to them.* Help the patient to understand that his glasses replace the lens removed from his eye and that without glasses he cannot effectively see.

> *Do not be surprised to find that the color of objects seen with the operated eye is slightly altered.*

Usually the patient learns to adjust to his new eyeglasses by the time the permanent expensive glasses are ordered; permanent glasses may be ordered from 2–12 months postoperatively (typically 3 months). Permanent lenses are not prescribed until the cornea's curvature stops changing (it changes continuously during healing). Loss of the lens (aphakia) causes the eye to have a high degree of hyperopia and usually to have a considerable astigmatism. Additionally the aphakic eye has loss of accommodation, a deep anterior chamber, and usually a tremulous iris.

It is now possible to obtain *plastic cataract eyeglass lenses* rather than the heavy glass lenses. The advent of these plastic lenses makes quite a change in the aphakic patient's postoperative care. Presently the cost of plastic lenses is about double that of the glass lenses. However, if patients can afford and use these plastic lenses, they are worth the investment. Advantages of the plastic eyeglass lenses are that they are two thirds lighter than glass, and they stay in focus longer and do not cause pressure lesions under the nose pads. Also, plastic lenses can be ground to the very edge, thus eliminating the peripheral distortion of vision and the tunnel vision which occurs with thick glass lenses. With plastic lenses the adjustment to the cataract lenses is no more difficult than the adjustment to regular prescription eyeglasses.

Some patients (mostly younger persons) wear a corrective *contact lens* rather than corrective eye glasses. Because a contact lens is worn closer to the retina than a lens in the eyeglass frame, the magnification is reduced to only about 5 per cent. Binocular vision is possible if the patient with a unilateral lens extraction is capable of wearing a contact lens. Older persons are sometimes unable to learn to adjust to contact lenses and to properly insert, remove, and care for such lenses. Thus, unfortunately some older persons cannot use contact lenses even though their vision would be greatly facilitated if they could do so. Corneal contact lenses allow almost normal vision without the degree of distortion or magnification, or the reduced peripheral vision attendant to the use of thick convex eyeglasses. Corneal contact lenses are especially helpful to those patients who have had cataract removal on only one eye, since the use of the contact lens makes binocular vision possible. (Contact lenses are discussed further on p. 1500.)

Recently it has become possible to insert a plastic (acrylic) lens *into* the eye at the time of surgery to replace the lens which is removed. Insertion of an *intraocular plastic lens* removes the need for either a contact lens or an eyeglass lens postoperatively. Use of acrylic intraocular lenses removes the self-consciousness which many people experience when wearing thick "cataract glasses." With intraocular lenses the patient may read and write without glasses and may indulge in sports and social activities which were not possible with the heavy glasses.

Before the patient is discharged home following cataract surgery he (and/or a family member) must be taught how to instill eyedrops. Limitations of activity which the doctor advises are also explained to the patient. Postoperatively and for a while at home atropine, 1 per cent, is instilled to paralyze the ciliary muscle and the iris sphincter, thus preventing the discomfort which would occur as a result of spasm of these muscles following intraocular surgery. The physician may permit the patient to perform light activities (e.g., reading, cooking) but may restrict bending, lifting, and any heavy work (usually for 4–6 weeks postoperatively). A pair of sunglasses or metal eye shield may be advisable to protect the eye from injury until permanent glasses are worn.

Complications. Various serious *postoperative complications* can follow cataract surgery. Early postoperative complications, which may be apparent at the first dressing change (24 hours following surgery), include prolapse of the iris and a flat anterior chamber. *Iris prolapse* occurs at a site of rupture in the cataract incision; usually *wound rupture* is the result of pressure exerted on the eye by the patient or those attending him. Bulging of the wound or a pear-shaped pupil are indicative of prolapse of the iris and should be reported if the nurse notices these at the time of dressing change. (Some physicians prefer to always change the dressing themselves so they can inspect the eye.) Wound rupture is a serious complication which may result in such problems as corneal opacity, infection, uveitis, or glaucoma. Prolapsed iris is thus immediately treated. The prolapsed portion of iris is incised, and the area of the wound where the prolapse occurred is carefully sutured. A *flat anterior chamber* is carefully evaluated to determine its cause and is treated according to the findings. If the chamber is allowed to remain flat for a prolonged period of time, adhesions tend to form between the peripheral iris and the cornea (since the iris is in contact with the cornea due to lack of fluid in the anterior chamber). Such adhesions obliterate the drainage angle and cause the subsequent development of *aphakic secondary angle closure glaucoma.*

Hemorrhage into the anterior chamber, i.e., *hyphema,* may occur about 5 days postoperatively. At this time the granulation tissue which is healing the wound is highly vascularized and the capillaries are fragile. Hemorrhage can injure the eye's

delicate structures by causing pressure on them. This is an ocular emergency. Notify the doctor immediately if the patient experiences sharp eye pain and instruct the patient to do the same if he develops such pain after discharge. Mild pain or aching of the eye is not uncommon postoperatively. Hyphema may be precipitated by strain on the eye (e.g., if the patient tightly squeezes his eye or otherwise exerts pressure on his eye), or it may occur for no apparent reason. Treatment consists of bedrest and keeping the pupil dilated. Usually the blood is rapidly reabsorbed. Severe hemorrhage may necessitate surgery to wash out the blood and debris. Diamox may be ordered if the angle is blocked by blood and debris and the intraocular pressure thus secondarily rises.

Postoperative infection, i.e., *endophthalmitis,* usually appears about 3–4 days postoperatively if it is going to develop. Vigorous treatment is necessary to save the eye. Treatment may include local administration of atropine, subconjunctival injection of antibiotics, parenteral antibiotics, parenteral steroids, and perhaps Diamox or related cholinesterase inhibitors.

Loss of vitreous is another possible complication of cataract surgery. Vitreous loss increases the likelihood of complications developing, such as glaucoma, uveitis, and retinal detachment. Vitreous strands may develop, and as these bands of scar tissue contract, they exert tension on the retina which will tear a retina undergoing degeneration.

Because of the *postoperative iritis* which usually occurs (mildly) following cataract surgery, there is a possibility that the eye may form *adhesions* between the iris and the vitreous face. The pupil is thus kept mobile postoperatively by alternate periods of dilatation and constriction or dilation of the pupil with atropine at the time of the first dressing change. Some sources recommend instillation of a cycloplegic drop daily for 1–2 months following cataract extraction. Keeping the pupil mobile is also prophylactic for the potential complication of *pupillary block glaucoma* following cataract surgery. At the time of surgery, iridectomy is usually performed as a prophylactic measure to prevent secondary pupillary block glaucoma and to minimize chances of the iris prolapsing postoperatively. Iridectomy prevents obstruction of the flow of aqueous humor, which could result from the forward movement of the vitreous humor in the globe (blocking the pupil and causing pressure against the iris).

TUMORS OF THE EYE AND RELATED STRUCTURES

The eye and its related structures may be the site of both benign and malignant tumors. Often such tumors can be visualized early in their development since they are readily apparent, displace the eyeball, or interfere with vision. Secondary (metastatic) ocular malignancies rarely occur. When they do, x-ray or other treatment may relieve the condition; however, it is hopeless to try to cure the metastatic cancer by enucleation.

The early diagnosis of tumors related to the eye is of importance and in some instances may mean the difference between cure or only palliation. Biopsies are taken of all suspicious accessible lesions. ^{125}I uptake studies may help detect intraocular tumors but may be unable to differentiate between benign or malignant neoplasms. Retinoblastomas and malignant melanomas are the most common ocular tumors. Cancer is discussed in detail in Unit VII.

ERRORS OF REFRACTION

> *Errors of refraction are the most common type of ocular disorder.*

General Considerations. "Refraction" refers clinically to an examination of the eye performed to determine the eye's refractive state. Refraction also refers to the bending of light as it passes through the eye's optical structures. The eye's refractive media include the cornea, the aqueous humor, the lens, and the vitreous body. The purpose of these structures is to bend light rays so they ultimately focus on the retina. The eye's refractive media are all normally transparent. When light obliquely strikes a transparent substance, while passing from one medium to another of different density, it is bent or deflected at the interface; this is the process of "refraction."

It is not possible to discuss in this text the precise technics of refraction. Such details are presented in specialized textbooks of ophthalmology. In general, the procedures of refraction may be classified as either being "cycloplegic" or "noncycloplegic."

Cycloplegic refraction determines the refractive state of the eye *at rest.* To obtain this state, various solutions may be instilled into the eye's conjunctival sac to produce cycloplegia, i.e., reduction of the accommodative power and weakening of the ciliary muscle. Coincidentally mydriasis occurs, i.e., pupillary dilation. This dilation makes ophthalmoscopic examination of the fundus easier. After leaving the physician's office, the patient should be told that his vision will be blurred temporarily and that he should wear sunglasses in bright light until the eye returns to its normal state.

During cycloplegic refraction, while the eye is in a state of rest, the eye may be examined objectively and/or subjectively. *Objective evaluation* includes performance of *retinoscopy.* In this procedure a beam of light is directed into the pupil (from a retinoscope) and the movement of a reflected light "shadow" in the fundus is neutralized by placing appropriate lenses before the eye. The observed patterns of movement emerging from the patient's eye are easily recognized by the trained observer as being characteristic of the various refractive errors, e.g., myopia, hyperopia, or astigmatism. *Subjective evaluation* includes having the patient look through various lenses and then asking him to identify the lens which best gives him visual sharpness. The patient thus chooses the best of a series of corrective lenses. Cycloplegic refraction is most frequently used on children and young adults. With aging, weakening of the power of accommodation occurs.

Noncycloplegic refraction is accomplished, as the name indicates, without the use of cycloplegics. Both objective and subjective evaluation of refraction are then made as described above, and allowances are made for the action of accommodation. Accommodation is highly active in youth and then diminishes with age as the eye becomes presbyopic.

Eyeglasses; Contact Lenses. Once the physician has completed his refractive examination, he knows whether or not the patient requires corrective lenses; if lenses are required, he knows the strength and type of lens necessary. The two major reasons for wearing corrective lenses are to improve visual acuity and to provide relief from the symptoms which refractive errors can cause. Refractive errors not only cause visual disorders but also cause many other associated symptoms, such as rubbing the eyes, blinking, frowning, closing one eye, photophobia, injection, tearing, head tilting, clumsiness, eyestrain, headache, dizziness, and occasionally nausea. Visual acuity is improved by selecting a lens which will correctly focus images on the retina. Corrective lenses may be either contact lenses or lenses worn in eyeglasses.

Prescription *eyeglasses* are available with case-hardened, shatterproof glass or plastic lenses. Plastic lenses are of lighter weight but scratch more easily and are more expensive. Persons who need to wear eyeglasses should use their glasses as prescribed and should keep the lenses clean and free from scratches. (The nurse should see that patients who need corrective glasses have them and that the glasses are clean.) When not in use, eyeglasses should be safely stored in a protective glass case.

It is advisable for persons needing prescription glasses to have an extra pair of glasses (in case of breakage or loss) and to have prescription sunglasses or dark lenses to clip over their regular prescription lenses. Because of the variety of ocular refractive disorders which exist, it is important that eyeglasses be individually prescribed. The practice of buying "dime-store glasses" or of borrowing other person's glasses should be discouraged.

Special bifocal or trifocal lenses may be prescribed to provide correction for vision at several different distances within one pair of lenses. *Bifocal lenses* are double lenses which are generally prescribed for persons with poor powers of accommodation, e.g., older persons; the lower portion of the lens provides correction for near vision while the upper portion enables focusing for distances. *Trifocal lenses* are triple lenses. Each lens is divided into three segments, the lower is for near vision, the middle for intermediate distance, and the upper is for distant vision. When a patient first is learning to adjust to bifocal lenses, it is helpful if you instruct him to be sure to drop his head down (by tucking his chin down and flexing his neck) when going down stairs or stepping off a curb. If he merely lowers his eyes, as he is accustomed to doing, he will look through the bottom portion of the lens (which is designed for near vision) and he will not be able to focus clearly on the stairs or curb.

Children, and all patients with severely limited vision or those following eye surgery, should learn how to safely put on their eyeglasses in a manner which reduces the likelihood of their eyes being poked by the bows of the glasses. This may be accomplished by picking up the glasses with both hands (one hand over the tip of each bow) and then guiding the bows past the eyes and along either side of the head to the ears.

A *contact lens* is essentially a small, thin, polished disk of plastic that is ground on the outer side to correct or improve vision while the inner side is designed to correspond to the surface shape of the eye. There are numerous sizes and shapes of contact lenses, but most are basically variations of two main types: (1) scleral lenses, and (2) corneal lenses. *Scleral lenses,* sometimes called "haptic" lenses, cover most of the visible portion of the eye. This type of lens is about 1 inch in diameter and rests on the sclera. Scleral lenses have been used for several types of eye disorders since they cover and protect the eye's entire anterior segment. For example, scleral lenses may be used immediately after thorough irrigation of the eye when chemical burns have occurred to the eye; the scleral lens prevents the lids from adhering to the cornea and conjunctiva. Scleral lenses will keep fluid in contact with the eye when the eye is dry from lack of tears. Also, if the cornea is severely ulcerated and has thin areas, the scleral lens acts as a splint, protecting the thin zone until it has healed.

The *corneal contact lens* is the type of contact lens most frequently used. This lens is usually tinted grey, light blue, light green, or brown. A corneal lens covers only the major area of the cornea and is about 1/3 inch in diameter. The corneal contact lens is held in place on the cornea by the surface tension of the eye's natural fluid or tears. Surface tension is the phenomenon which makes it difficult to pull two flat plates of glass apart if they are wet. Thus contact lenses actually tend to float on the eyeball's fluid layer. The capillary attraction of tears and the upper lid loosely hold the lens in place. The flow of tears over all surfaces not only provides the necessary lubricating fluid but also is important in refraction. Centered over the cornea, the lens moves with the eye.

Contact lenses are safe to wear if they are professionally prescribed, ground, and adjusted to the patient, and provided the patient uses the lenses as directed. Periodic check-ups are always of importance for the person who wears contact lenses, and he should see his physician if any problems occur between scheduled check-ups. Corneal lenses can now be worn comfortably for longer periods of time than formerly; however, they still should be worn only intermittently. The lenses should not be worn when the eye shows symptoms of marked inflammation or infection, or if the vision is blurred. If superficial scratches are present on the cornea and foreign bacteria are introduced with the lens, an infection may develop which requires immediate attention.

In recent years corneal contact lenses have become quite popular. Most frequently these lenses are fitted for cosmetic reasons (because the patient feels more attractive than with eyeglasses) or because they are better than eyeglasses for a patient's activities (corneal lenses do not "fog" from rain, steam, or perspiration). Other *advantages* of contact lenses are as follows: (a) improved peripheral vision; (b) safe for many athletic events (low incidence of breakage); (c) unobstructed vision when sighting through cameras, microscopes, binoculars; (d) less distortion and more realistic size of objects viewed; (e) usually require changing less often than eyeglasses; (f) automatically cleaned as the eye is blinked; (g) enable the eyes to more efficiently work together in some instances; and (h) greatly improve the postoperative status of patients with cataracts by replacing heavy cataract eyeglass lenses. Generally patients have reduced corneal sensation following cataract surgery and can wear the corneal contact lens all day.

In addition to being useful in unilateral aphakia (where the greater discrepancy in image size which occurs while wearing eyeglass lenses interferes with binocular vision), corneal contact lenses are also useful in (a) some types of astigmatism; (b) the presence of turned-in eyelashes; (c) absence of the iris (aniridia); (d) congenital absence of pigment; (e) treating hyperopia (near-vision is increased and visual field is larger); and (f) treating keratoconus. Keratoconus is a cone-shaped distortion of the central cornea; in this condition a satisfactory correction of the refractive error is impossible with eyeglasses. High myopics also benefit from contact lenses, because of increase in image size and visual field.

Some *disadvantages* of contact lenses are (a) they are relatively more expensive than eyeglasses; (b) they can be lost more easily than eyeglasses; (c) they require more care than eyeglasses; (d) they are more difficult to insert into the eye than eyeglasses are to place on the head; (e) several office visits are necessary for prescription and adjustments of the lens; (f) usually sensitivity to light increases while wearing contact lenses; (g) not all visual disorders can be corrected with contact lenses; (h) not all persons can adjust physically or psychologically to contact lenses; and (i) semiannual evaluations are necessary.

Not all ophthalmologists believe in the general use of contact lenses. All potential candidates for contact lenses should have a thorough evaluation of their visual problems by an ophthalmologist and should follow his recommendations. It is generally agreed that contact lenses should not be prescribed to persons who are not responsible, cooperative, and intelligent. Increasingly eyes are being damaged as a result of carelessly wearing contact lenses, e.g., wearing the lens when the eye is inflamed or infected. Contact lenses are contraindicated in the presence of inflammatory and allergic conditions, presbyopia, severe exophthalmos, abnormal overflow of tears (epiphora), local neoplasm, and pterygium. They cannot be worn if there is insufficient circulation of tears under the lenses. Contacts are hazardous during accidental chemical injury of the eye, since some of the chemical may seep under the lens and severely burn the cornea before the lens can be removed. Also, care must be taken by wearers of contacts to prevent dust or dirt from collecting behind the lens where it can cause corneal damage. Contact lenses are prohibited for workers in some occupations where these hazards are particularly great.

Because contact lenses are actually foreign bodies in the eye, it takes awhile for the eye to adjust to wearing corneal lenses. Definite metabolic changes occur in the cornea when contact lenses are initially introduced, e.g., edema, decreased corneal sensitivity. To facilitate adjustment of the eye to the lenses, the contact wearer is instructed to initially wear the lenses for only brief periods of time. Gradually the length of time is increased until the lenses are worn for the prescribed length of time. Contact lenses are worn maximally for 10–16 hours. They should never be worn during sleep. Contact of the cornea with the lens for excessive periods of time will cause corneal damage. Corneal abrasion is the most common complication from wearing contact lenses. However, the incidence of permanent eye damage from wearing contact lenses is low, considering the large number of persons wearing these lenses.

Patient teaching is an important part of preparing an individual for contact lenses. Once the patient's lenses have been properly fitted, it is the patient's responsibility to give the lenses and his eye the daily care which will ensure prevention of complications. The patient is taught the proper technic for applying and removing the lenses, in addition to the correct method of caring for the lenses. Unless cleaned, stored, and inserted in the recommended manner, the lenses may carry bacteria to the cornea. Before touching the lenses (for removal, insertion, or cleaning), the hands are washed. Lenses are cleaned prior to insertion with a recommended sterile, noncaustic solution. A wetting agent, e.g., methylcellulose, is applied to the lenses just before inserting them into the eye. Saliva should never be used as a wetting or cleaning agent; because the mouth contains pathogens, an infection can be introduced into the eye if there is a corneal abrasion present or if the person is passing through a period of low immunity. Stale, infected solutions, used to clean, wet, or store the lenses, must be discarded. After removal from the eye, the lenses are wiped dry of lid secretions and then stored in a dry, well-ventilated case or stored in a prescribed solution.[53] The lens case should be boiled weekly to sterilize it. If the storage case is moist, it fosters the growth of pathogenic bacteria. Because individual lenses are ground for each eye, the lenses should be stored in a labeled container, i.e., "right," "left."

It is necessary for the nurse to *know how to remove contact lenses from a helpless patient,* e.g., an accident victim. Persons wearing contact lenses should carry a card or wear an identification tag stating they wear contact lenses. Unconscious persons or persons suffering serious injury should be checked for such a card or medallion, and should also have their eyes checked for contact lenses. To look for a contact gently separate the eyelids and shine a small light into the eye from the side to obliquely view the cornea. If present, contacts must be removed so the cornea will not be damaged from prolonged contact with the lens. Always remove contact lenses before sending a patient to surgery. In an emergency situation if you suspect that contact lenses are in the patient's eyes, but you have not had the time to remove them or you believe it is unsafe for you to try to remove them (e.g., if the eye is injured), apply a strip of adhesive tape labeled "CONTACT LENSES" to the patient's forehead and inform the physician. Do not attempt to remove a contact lens without professional help if the cornea of the patient's eye is not visible upon opening the eyelids.

A corneal contact lens can usually be removed from a helpless person in the following manner:

- With clean hands, gently position one thumb on the upper eyelid and one thumb on the lower eyelid. Have the tips of the thumbs near the lids' margins but rest the thumbs themselves over the eye's bony orbit.
- Gently separate the eyelids. Do not apply pressure directly on the eye, but rather pull the lids (up or down) toward the orbital rim.
- A visible lens should slide easily with a gentle movement of the eyelid. A lens may be found correctly positioned over the cornea, on the sclera only, or on both the sclera and cornea. If the lens is not over the cornea, slide it to this position with an appropriate movement of the eyelids. The lens must be positioned over the cornea if it is to be safely removed.
- With the lens over the cornea, widen the opening of the eyelids beyond the top and bottom edges of the lens and maintain this opening.
- Press both eyelids gently but firmly against the eye.
- Move the lower eyelid margin to a position barely touching the bottom edge of the lens.
- Next bring the upper eyelid margin down to the top edge of the lens, while keeping both eyelids firmly pressed on the eye.
- By pressing slightly harder on the lower eyelid, move it underneath the bottom edge of the lens. This movement should cause the lens to tip outward from the eye by pivoting the top edge and flipping out on the bottom edge.

> Once the lens has tipped slightly, begin moving the eyelids toward one another. The lens should then slide out between the eyelids where it can safely be retrieved.

Remember: *Do not use force to remove a contact lens. If the lens can be seen but cannot be removed, gently slide it off the cornea, completely onto the sclera. It can safely remain on the sclera until the physician is available. Never try to remove a contact lens from an injured eye!*

The Nature of Refractive Error. Refractive errors types tend to be inherited, but in no definitely predictable manner. Numerous variables influence refraction, e.g., corneal curvature, depth of the anterior chamber, shape of the lens, and length of the eye. Upon entering the eye, a ray of light passes through the cornea, the aqueous humor, the anterior and posterior surfaces of the lens, and the vitreous to focus upon the retina's fovea.

The ideal refractive condition of the eye is called *emmetropia*. In this "ideal" condition the unaccommodated eye (with the lens perfectly at rest) focuses parallel light rays from a distant source (of 6 meters or more) into a sharp image on the fovea. This condition of emmetropia ("sight in proper measure") requires that there be no neural or retinal disorders; that there are no opacities of the cornea, lens, aqueous or vitreous; and that the eyeball be of normal size. As emphasized, this is actually an ideal rather than a normal condition, since most adults have some degree of refractive disorder. *Ametropia* ("sight not in proper measure") refers to all variations from the emmetropic state which are not due to opacities or disease. Among the variations of ametropia are *aniseikonia* (difference in image size in the two eyes) and *anisometropia* (variation in the refractive errors of the two eyes). The most commonly encountered variations of ametropia are discussed below (Fig. 105-19).

> *Hyperopia* (*hypermetropia, "farsightedness"*): In this condition parallel rays of light are brought to a *focus behind the retina* when accommodative powers are relaxed. Typically vision is normal beyond 20 feet, but near-vision is poor. Hyperopia may result from shortness of the anteroposterior dimension of the eyeball or weakness of the refractive power of the cornea or lens. Hyperopia may be corrected with the use of a *convex lens,* which increases the angle of incidence of the light rays entering the cornea and lens, thus focusing the light rays on the surface of the retina.

> *Myopia* (*"nearsightedness"*): In this condition parallel rays of light are brought to a *focus in front of the retina,* i.e., before reaching the retinal surface. Typically near vision is normal, but distant vision is defective. Myopia is caused by an abnormally long anteroposterior dimension of the eyeball or by an increase in the strength of the refractive power of the media. Heredity is highly important in myopia. The most common symptom is inability to distinguish objects clearly at a distance. The patient frequently frowns or squints in an effort to sharpen visual acuity by making the lid aperture smaller; a smaller opening eliminates peripheral rays of light from entering the eye and allows only the more axial rays to enter the eye. Myopia may be corrected with *concave* (minus) lenses which diverge the light rays so they will focus correctly on the retina. Myopia usually increases in the teens and levels off about age 25. In the 40's presbyopic symptoms develop, necessitating reading glasses or bifocals.

> *Presbyopia ("old sight"):* As discussed earlier, this is a disorder in which a *lessening of the effective powers of accommodation* occurs as a result of hardening of the lens due to the aging process. Loss of accommodation is manifested by blurring of near objects or visual fatigue when doing "close work." Presbyopia may be corrected with a lens which corrects any basic refractive error and which also has a proper *convex reading addition* for close work. This lens brings the near point within suitable range for focusing on the retina. Usually first reading lenses are necessary between ages 42–45. Presbyopia does not mean a worsening of hyperopia, but is merely a reduction of the powers of accommodation.

> *Astigmatism ("distorted vision")*: Astigmatism refers to vision which is "not at a point." Astigmatism is distorted vision caused by a *variation in refractive power along different meridians of the eye.* The optical distortion is most often caused by irregular corneal curvature, which prevents the clear focus of light from any point, i.e., rays in the horizontal and perpendicular planes do not focus at the same point. The lens may also cause astigmatism, e.g., in old age, due to cataractous changes. Astigmatism is identified according to the type of *cylindric lens* necessary to correct the condition, e.g., a concave cylinder is necessary for myopic astigmatism, while a convex cylindric lens is used for hyperopic astigmatism. The cylindric lens is oriented in a proper meridian (axis) to restore a spherical effect.

TRAUMA AFFECTING THE EYE AND RELATED STRUCTURES

Trauma to the eye or adjacent structures requires (a) careful evaluation to determine the extent and sites of injury, and (b) prompt treatment once the disorder is identified. *Many persons with serious injury of the eye can have useful vision salvaged if they receive immediate, correct treatment.* Gentle handling is imperative. As Havener notes: "Because of the thinness and delicacy of the eye structure, major damage may be caused by slight trauma that would be inconsequential elsewhere on the body." [40]

Previously we have discussed general eye care, the protection of vision, ocular emergencies, and ocular first aid. Here we briefly summarize some basic types of ocular trauma and some important principles concerning care of injured eyes.

The incidence of eye injuries remains high in spite of the protection which the eye can be given through the use of protective glasses and other protective devices, and in spite of the protection which the eye has anatomically, e.g., eyelashes, eyelids, bony orbit, and the cushioning effect of the retrobulbar fat.[88] The eye's deep structures or its outer surface may be traumatized, as well as the eye's adjacent structures, e.g., eyelids, bony orbit. For purposes of discussion, injuries of the eye may be divided into two groups: (1) penetrating, and (2) nonpenetrating. Both types of injuries are potentially dangerous.

Penetrating injuries to the eye include lacerations and intraocular foreign bodies. *Nonpenetrating injuries to the eye* include abrasions, contusions, rupture of the eyeball, superficial foreign bodies, and burns. Lacerations are a common *injury of the eyelid. Injuries to the bony orbit* include fractures of the walls of the orbit and an isolated orbital floor or "blowout" fracture occurring without concurrent orbital rim fracture. Some of these disorders have been discussed earlier in the unit. Summarized below are factors of importance concerning some of these various forms of trauma to the eye and related structures.

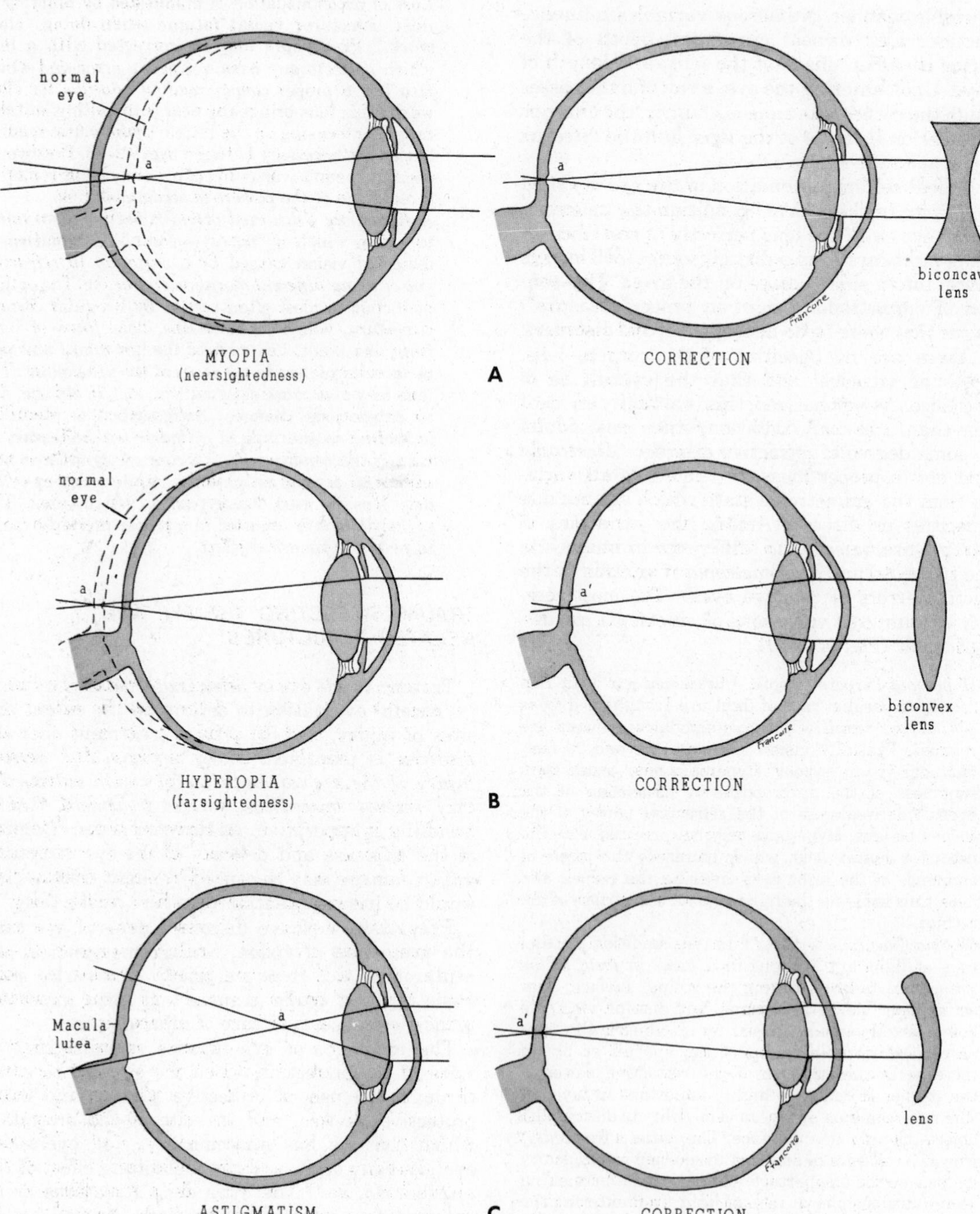

FIGURE 105-19. Common variations of ametropia and their correction. (From Jacob, S. W., and Francone, C. A.: *Structure and Function in Man.* 3rd ed. 1974.)

Penetrating Injuries of the Eye. In addition to possible loss of the contents of the eye, sympathetic ophthalmia is a serious potential complication of penetrating injuries. Either of these complications may ultimately necessitate enucleation of the eye. *Lacerations* of the eyeball are treated in different ways, depending upon whether or not prolapse of tissue has occurred. Generally a wound can be repaired surgically if the eyeball has been penetrated anteriorly, there is no obvious evidence of prolapse of intraocular contents, and the wound is clean and grossly free of contamination. The wound may also be surgically repaired if only a small portion of iris or only small amounts of uveal tissue have prolapsed. Following closure of such surgical repairs, a mydriatic is used, an antibiotic solution is instilled into the conjunctival sac, and the eyes are bilaterally bandaged. The patient is then usually kept on bedrest for several days, and systemic antibiotics are employed prophylactically. Enucleation is indicated when the wound is extensive and has resulted in significant loss of intraocular contents.

Intraocular foreign bodies lodged in the eyeball require immediate evaluation by an ophthalmologist. With delay, the ocular medium becomes progressively more cloudy, and the object may become impossible to visualize. The object may be localized in a variety of ways. Metal objects may be located with a special metal detector. Recently perfected ultrasonic probes reveal more information about the interior of an eye with an opaque medium than any other method. *Ultrasonography* projects (upon the front of a cathode ray tube) the echoes returning from interfaces of varying densities within the eye. In contrast to the oscilloscopic pattern of the contents of the normal eye, a prominent echo peak occurs as a result of the presence of a foreign body within the eye.[41]

Particles of iron or copper need to be removed to prevent later disorganization of ocular tissues from degenerative changes. If the object has magnetic properties, e.g., iron or steel, its removal may be facilitated by the use of the sterilized tip of a small portable electromagnet or the tip of a large, stationary electromagnet, e.g., the Müller giant eye magnet. Some of the newer metal alloys are more inert and may be tolerated by the eye.

The physician may try at once to remove pieces of glass, wood, lead, or copper by the use of delicate forceps introduced through the original wound or through an opening into the vitreous cavity made at the point at which the foreign body has been located. However, if the object cannot be easily removed, it is often best left in place rather than stirring up the vitreous. Not all nonmagnetic intraocular foreign bodies should be removed, since the removal of such objects from the eye cannot presently be accomplished in a satisfactory manner. Some inert substances are well tolerated by the eye. It is usually more hazardous and more destructive to try to surgically remove such foreign bodies than it is to allow the continued presence of such inert material in the eye. Dirty wood splinters often promote intraocular infection, and toxins are contained in many varieties of thorns.

If a foreign body causes a retinal hole in the far posterior portion, the hole may be sealed prophylactically by using a photocoagulator (providing the medium is clear). Retinal detachment is one of the most serious complications involving an intraocular foreign body. Usually such detachments occur several months following the injury. Visual prognosis is usually poor with intraocular foreign bodies.

Important practices when caring for patients with penetrating eye injuries include the following: (a) wash your hands thoroughly before approaching the eye; (b) refer the patient to an eye specialist immediately for care; (c) avoid applying pressure on the eye, and keep the patient from applying pressure to the eye; (d) penetrating injuries may be covered with a plastic or metal eye shield to protect the eye until the patient reaches the physician; (e) instruct the patient not to perform activities which will increase ocular pressure, e.g., not to bend his head down to get into a car and not to pull the car door closed (loss of intraocular contents could result); and (f) remember to use sterile medications and sterile technic whenever a penetrating injury has occurred. Tetanus prophylaxis is given routinely to all patients with penetrating eye injuries. Because surgical repairs of penetrating injuries are usually performed under general anesthesia, advise the patient not to eat or drink until the physician gives him permission to do so.

Nonpenetrating Injuries of the Eye. Abrasions of the lids, cornea, or conjunctiva may be treated with an antibiotic ointment prophylactically and an eye bandage applied with firm, gentle pressure. *Contusions* of the eyeball are carefully evaluated. Those contusions which are severe enough to cause intraocular hemorrhage may eventually cause intractable glaucoma and damage to the eyeball. Patients with intraocular hemorrhage may be put on complete bedrest for 6–7 days with both eyes bandaged in an attempt to prevent this complication. It may be necessary to administere acetazolamide (Diamox), mannitol, or other systemically administered agents to lower intraocular pressure. Also, a reversible cycloplegic, e.g., 5 per cent homatropine, may be administered. *Rupture of the eyeball* can be surgically repaired in some cases; in others, enucleation of the eye is necessary, followed by implantation of a plastic sphere (to act as a space-filler and to assist in movement of the artificial eye). *Corneal and conjunctival foreign bodies* have been discussed previously. Foreign bodies on the cornea must be removed by a physician. A sterile local anesthetic is instilled into the eye, and the object is removed with special spuds, a scalpel blade, or a hypodermic needle. After the object is removed, an antibiotic ointment is instilled in the eye three times daily. Untreated corneal infection is serious.

Foreign bodies and corneal abrasions are the most frequent causes of eye injury.

Thermal burns of ocular structures are treated essentially the same as burns of the skin structures elsewhere, as far as lid involvement is concerned. (Burns are discussed generally in Unit XVIII.) The lid surface is gently cleansed and greased thoroughly with an antibiotic ointment. If the lid is kept covered with ointment, dressings are not necessary. However, if lid closure is impaired (because of severity of the burn), the exposed cornea must be kept constantly covered with generous amounts of ointment, e.g., boric acid ointment. Gentle, mechanical swabbing or warm, moist compresses are used to remove crusting and discharge. If corneal tissue sloughs off, the eye is lost. *Infrared exposure* seldom causes an ocular reaction. However, permanent visual impairment can result from viewing the sun or an eclipse of the sun without an adequate filter. Excessive exposure to *nuclear devices* or *radiation* (x-ray) may cause cataractous changes which may not appear until several months have passed following exposure. Even moderate exposure to *ultraviolet radiation* (e.g., ultraviolet keratitis, actinic keratitis) produces a highly painful keratitis. Such exposure may come from exposure to a welding arc ("welder's flash"), excessive sunlight, sunlight on snow ("snow blindness"), or an artificial sunlamp. Pain typically occurs 6–12 hours after exposure. While such patients typically recover within 12–48 hours, cold compresses, local corticosteroids, systemic analgesics, and sedatives may provide comfort. Systemic sedations or narcotics are preferable to local anesthetics, although it may be necessary to use a sterile local anesthetic in order to examine the eye. (This is true of many types of eye injuries when pain or photophobia caused by the injury produces blepharospasm severe enough to prevent thorough examination of the eye.)

Chemical burns of the eye are treated *immediately by continuous irrigation of the eyes for 15–20 minutes* before this first aid treatment is stopped and an eye specialist is contacted. This important point has been emphasized before.

> *Regardless of the type of chemical, the emergency treatment is always the same: immediate, prolonged washing of the eye with plain water.*

Be certain to hold the lids widely apart during this irrigation. Do *not* attempt to neutralize an acid with an alkali or vice versa, because the heat generated by the reaction may cause further damage to the eye. While many compounds cause severe, often irreversible, damage to the cornea, those most highly destructive are acids, alkalies, alkylating agents, and other protein denaturants. Solvents and strong detergents may also cause disastrous damage. The numerous "spray products" (aerosols) available on the market are an additional source of chemical burns to the eye, e.g., insecticides, hair sprays. Household lye and ammonia are some of the most dangerous substances to the eye. Ammonia can penetrate the cornea so rapidly that even immediate treatment may fail to preserve vision. Acids usually produce only immediate damage to the eye. However, even mild alkali burns show progression of injury on subsequent days. Alkali injuries thus require prolonged irrigation, since alkalies are not precipitated by the proteins of the eye as acids are.

In the physician's office, the chemically burned eye is anesthetized with a local anesthetic and is again lavaged for a prolonged period of time (with normal saline). Next all particles of foreign matter are removed from under the everted upper eyelid. The pupil is dilated following chemical injury, and a combination corticosteroid and antibiotic solution or ointment is frequently instilled. Corticosteroids may minimize scarring and new blood vessel formation. Sedatives and narcotics are given because pain is intense. The burned surface must be frequently separated mechanically for the first few days following a chemical burn of the conjunctival cul de sac to prevent the eyelid and eyeball from healing together, forming thick bands of scar tissue.

Poisoning and the Eye. Lead, arsenic, carbon bisulphide, quinine, methyl alcohol, and tobacco are among the various toxins and chemical poisons which may affect the eye. *Ocular symptoms of poisoning* include:

- Miotic pupil (morphine addiction).
- Papilledema (vitamin A intoxication, lead poisoning).
- Reddened conjunctiva (alcoholic intoxication).
- Cataract formation (paradichlorobenzene poisoning, excessive corticosteroids, strong parasympathomimetic medications, excessive radiation exposure).
- "Yellow vision" (digitalis intoxication).

Posterior subcapsular lens opacities may develop if systemic corticosteroids are given for longer than 6 months in large or moderate doses. While these changes usually do not progress to cause an advanced cataract, they do cause some irreversible impairment of usual visual function.

Tobacco amblyopia may result from smoking of heavy tobacco in a pipe for many years. This condition results from disturbance of retinal ganglion cells and causes bilateral visual failure. Visual failure is typically first in color appreciation, especially the color red. Sometimes the condition is associated with excessive alcohol consumption (alcohol-tobacco amblyopia); it is more severe in patients who are also diabetic.

Injuries to the Eyelids. Eyelid lacerations should be treated by an ophthalmologist since he can evaluate possible damage to the eye. Lacerations may be sutured after foreign materials are removed and bleeding is controlled.

Injuries to the Bony Orbit. Concussion injuries to the orbital contents may produce hemorrhage or subsequent tissue atrophy, with enophthalmos.

Hemorrhage into the orbit often accompanies trauma to the eye or surrounding tissues. The result is a *hematoma* (*"black eye"*) of the lids and surrounding skin. Such bleeding generally stops spontaneously, but it is helpful to apply cold compresses initially to help reduce the bleeding and swelling.

Hot compresses may help to speed absorption of the blood after the initial 24 hours. Medications may also be given to help absorb the hematoma. All patients with ecchymosis around the eye and orbital structures are examined for possible skull fractures. When *traumatic subconjunctival hemorrhage* occurs, the pupil is usually dilated so a complete ophthalmoscopic examination can be performed.

THE EYE AND OTHER BODILY DISORDERS

Because the eye is intimately connected with the rest of the body, it provides large amounts of knowledge about the body as a whole. Since the eyes and their supporting structures are favorably exposed to easy inspection, the physician can learn a great deal about a patient's state of health by performing a thorough ocular examination.

The eye has been described as the body's "most important square inch"[40] in terms of its value during physical examination. More objective signs of abnormality can be found by examining the eye than by examining any other square inch of the body. Examination of the eye's portal can reveal not only disorders of the eye itself but also manifestations of many other disorders affecting the rest of the body. Ocular involvement occurs as part of the morbid process or as a complication of numerous disorders, which affect the body as a whole or which affect a particular system, e.g., nervous system, cardiovascular system, or endocrine system. Ocular symptoms may be the first manifestations of some of these diseases; in other instances, the ocular symptoms (by their evolution and course of resolution) are significant prognostic indications of the general disease.[5]

The nurse does not examine the eye's interior, e.g., with an ophthalmoscope, to look for ocular symptoms of disease. However, she should be aware that the following *external* ocular symptoms may indicate systemic or nervous system diseases: edema, conjunctival jaundice, xanthelasma (flattened, yellowish orange, slightly raised, lipoid plaques deposited in the lids' skin); bilateral subconjunctival hemorrhage; redness of the eyes; pupil disorders; paralysis of an extraocular muscle; and exophthalmos. Persons with these undiagnosed symptoms should be encouraged to seek a complete physical examination, which includes an ocular examination. The nurse can perform valuable health teaching by emphasizing that the general state of the body's health is reflected in the health of the eyes, and that because of this relationship general health practices (e.g., balanced nutrition, adequate rest and exercise, cleanliness) are important for eye health.

Space does not permit detailed discussion of the complex relationships between ocular findings and other bodily disorders. Such details are mainly of concern to the physician as he performs the physical examination and as he examines the *interior* as well as exterior of the eyes. Some systemic diseases cause very characteristic fundus pictures which the physician recognizes upon ophthalmoscopic examination. Common conditions which may be recognized in this way include hypertension, diabetes, blood dyscrasias, and arteriosclerosis.

REMOVAL OF THE EYEBALL (ENUCLEATION)

Some indications for *enucleation,* i.e., removal of the eyeball, are severe infections, malignant tumors, irritating foreign bodies which cannot be removed, management of severe pain in a blind eye, absolute glaucoma, cosmetic improvement of a blind and disfiguring eye, and extensive trauma to the eye. Prophylactically enucleation may be performed when sympathetic ophthalmia is likely to occur.

Enucleation may be performed under local or general anesthesia. During enucleation, when possible, the tendons of the rectus muscles are isolated and divided close to the globe. The muscles are then sutured to each other around an artificial globe or after they have been passed through special tunnels in an implant. This procedure results in a less sunken stump and produces improved appearance and motion when the artificial eye is eventually worn.

Implants are balls made of such materials as plastic, teflon, or gold. Later a prosthesis is fitted over the stump. Implants may be buried or exposed. With exposed implants a portion is left exposed to be fitted to the artificial eye. Following enucleation a "conformer" is placed in the socket until the patient receives his artificial eye. Usually the artificial eye is not placed until edema subsides, i.e., several days or weeks. Insertion, removal, and care of artificial eyes and care of the socket has been discussed previously. The physician discusses with the patient whether the eye should be removed or left in place at night.

Following enucleation a firm pressure dressing is applied for 48–72 hours. Usually the patient is allowed out of bed with no restrictions on his activity on the first postoperative day. Possible complications following enucleation include hemorrhage and infection. Infection may be indicated by pain and headache on the side of the enucleation. Occassionally infection results in abscess, thrombosis, or meningitis. Because the possibility of meningitis is increased if an actively suppurating eyeball is enucleated, panophthalmitis is a contraindication to enucleation. Usually panophthalmitis necessitates evisceration of the eyeball.

Evisceration is a surgical procedure in which the cornea and the entire contents of the eyeball are removed but the sclera remains. Recovery is less rapid following this procedure than it is following enucleation. Reaction and pain are greater. However, good support is left for use of an artificial eye following evisceration.

Exenteration is a procedure which is more radical than either enucleation or evisceration. With exenteration the eyelids, eyeball, and orbital contents are removed. Because of disfigurement it is usually necessary for a black patch to be worn rather than a prosthesis.

The patient who has had to have an eye surgically removed needs help in (a) understanding why it was necessary to remove the eye; (b) adjusting to his new body image (see Unit III, Ch. 14); (c) learning how to care for, insert, and remove an artificial eye if one is used; (d) learning how to care for the eye socket; (e) adjusting to vision with only one eye; and (f) learning how to protect vision in the remaining eye. The nurse may provide help in all these areas. A normal period of depression usually follows removal of an eye (see Unit III, Ch. 10). Typically satisfactory adjustment occurs to loss of the eye. The physician may recommend that the patient wear a safety glass over the remaining eye.

REHABILITATION OF THE BLIND INDIVIDUAL

Blindness may be present at birth or it may develop suddenly or slowly at any time during an individual's life. Because vision is highly important, its absence initially represents a great loss and presents a serious handicap.

The majority of blind persons lose their vision after 20 years of age. Thus they must make major adjustments in their adult years to learn to live without vision. Rehabilitation of the newly blinded person frequently begins in the hospital; however, extensive rehabilitation continues after the patient is discharged home or after he is transferred to a special rehabilitative facility for the blind. The patient's physician and a nurse or social worker help the patient and his family to contact appropriate agencies which will participate in the rehabilitative process.

It is important for the newly blinded person to be immediately introduced to the various national, state, and private agencies which will help him work toward successful rehabilitation before psychologic attitudes develop which could cause the patient unnecessary difficulties. Today rehabilitation is directed toward helping the blind to live as normal a life as possible. Blind persons are thus encouraged to live in their home community rather than in special settings where they associate primarily with other blind persons. Periods of stay at special schools for the blind may be helpful, but permanent residence in a facility for the blind is undesirable.

Lack of vision is all that blind persons have in common. Otherwise they differ from one another as greatly as the members of any heterogeneous group differ. If one emphasizes the loss, there is then the detrimental tendency to mentally lump all blind persons together as a group, and thus not to consider them as individuals. Also, emphasis on the loss of vision (rather than on the remaining capabilities of the blind) tends to foster dependence rather than independence for blind persons. Instead of assuming that the needs and problems of all blind persons are similar, the personalized problems of blind *individuals* need to be identified. Each blind person's uniqueness should be considered during the rehabilitative process, as well as during day-to-day contacts with blind persons.

REHABILITATIVE FACILITIES AND PROCEDURES

Government legislation provides many benefits for blind persons. The newly blinded person needs to be informed of these benefits and other services which are available to him. He thus should be referred when possible to a qualified social worker for appropriate counseling. When such a social worker is not available, it is often the nurse who helps the blind individual and his family to make appropriate contacts with federal and local agencies. All local and state agencies and their special services may be found listed in the *Directory of Agencies Serving Blind Persons in the United States* (available from the American Foundation for the Blind, Inc., 15 W. 16th St., New York, N.Y. 10011). This voluntary agency also distributes a catalogue of *Aids and Appliances* for blind persons which is distributed free of charge. A braille edition of the catalogue is also available on request.

The National Society for the Prevention of Blindness, 16 East 40th St., New York, N.Y. 10016, is a voluntary agency specializing in education, preventive services, and research. Pamphlets, films, and a quarterly publication (*The Sight Saving Review*) are available from this agency.

The newly blind individual may be advised to contact his State Welfare Department Division for the Blind. The federal government (through the Social and Rehabilitation Services Administration of the United States Department of Health, Education, and Welfare) allocates on a formula basis funds provided by Congress to be added to state funds for vocational rehabilitation programs within each state. These resources may be used by the blind to further their rehabilitation efforts and to obtain additional training.

Many blind persons benefit from contact with the closest library facility for the blind. These libraries provide numerous services, among which are books, magazines, and newspapers in braille, and "talking books," i.e., books, magazines, and so forth which have content read aloud and recorded for blind persons to listen to. Information concerning library resources for sightless persons can be obtained from the Library of Congress, Division for the Blind, Washington, D.C. Recordings of textbooks and educational materials, as well as the other recorded materials mentioned, are all available free of charge to blind persons. Talking book machines are loaned free of charge to the legally blind. Information may also be obtained from the national organizations for the blind mentioned previously, from public libraries, or from Recordings for the Blind, Inc., 215 East 58th St., New York, N.Y. 10022.

Blind children may be educated in special facilities, located in public or parochial schools, or in residential schools. Most states have a school for the blind. Students learn through the braille system and auditory instruction. Additionally the blind person can take a variety of correspondence courses with such schools as the Hadley Correspondence School for the Blind in Berwyn, Illinois. While older sightless persons may have difficulty learning braille (if they have some reduction in the ability to learn and in their tactile sense), many blind persons can be taught to read and write braille. Once this basic tool is learned, many avenues of study are open to the patient. Tape recorders are useful for the blind student to record lectures. Today it is not unusual for blind students to attend colleges and universities. There they may study with the help of braille notes, braille books, tape recorders, and readers.

Blind persons can learn numerous occupations and may become completely self-sufficient if given adequate rehabilitative help. Total rehabilitation may require the assistance of an occupational therapist, physical therapist, social worker, and psychiatrist in addition to the patient's personal physician and nurses in various agencies.

Appropriate timing is highly important for successful rehabilitation. The accomplishment of new performances may markedly improve the patient's spirits. Failure, however, may intensify depression. For example, if braille is introduced too early and the patient fails to learn the technic, he may become seriously depressed.

The first steps made by a blind individual in regaining self-sufficiency involve learning how to feed, dress, and groom himself and to walk about in a small area. When the blind person is learning to feed himself, he may find it helpful to practice once or twice with an empty spoon to gauge the distance from the plate to his mouth before he tries to handle food on the spoon. Practice with an empty cup and empty glass is also useful at first. Establishing a routine placement for the various table pieces, e.g., plate, utensils, glass, cup and saucer, helps the blind person to have a familiar orientation at every meal. It is important to always set up the blind individual's tray or table in the same pattern. If changes are made, the patient should be informed. Beverages should be served in vessels which are not easily overturned. The glass or cup should not be excessively full. If the patient mentally visualizes his plate as a clock or compass face, it is then possible to consistently place certain foods in the same location. For example, the patient may be told that his meat will always be located at "six o'clock" or "south" (i.e., on the portion of the plate closest to him). Other foods may then also be placed consistently in other areas which the patient can visualize, e.g., potatoes at "three o'clock" or "East." Privacy should be provided until the patient learns to feed himself reasonably well.

During the rehabilitation process, the blind individual learns to groom himself and learns in other ways not to call unnecessary attention to his lack of vision. For example, if the patient appears to be developing unnecessary postural attitudes or mannerisms, e.g., grimacing, he is kindly helped to become aware of these tendencies and to correct them.

If the blind individual is going to be independent and have a reasonable amount of privacy in his life, it is essential that he be able to get about by himself and not rely on another person to guide him. Through a mobility training program the blind individual can be taught to increase the usefulness of his remaining intact senses to help orient him to his surroundings. It is particularly helpful to increase the skillful use of hearing and object sense. The blind person may become quite sensitive to tones of voice; this helps him to communicate more effectively with others since he cannot see facial expression or other nonverbal cues.

The blind person may be trained to become more sensitive to *facial perception.* Facial perception is an echo interpretive factor which helps one to recognize the presence of such solid obstacles as high walls and fences. By becoming more sensitive to air currents in a room, the sightless person may obtain some idea about the placement of doors, windows, and so forth. By developing the sense of touch in his hands, it is possible for the blind person to more easily identify objects in his surroundings. The blind person benefits from learning to listen with greater acuity. Changes in the pitch of sounds may help him navigate by tapping a cane as he walks. A variety of canes are available and are usually selected according to the height of the blind individual. Specialists teach proper use of the cane during the rehabilitative process.

Some blind persons are suited to having a guide dog. Various guide dog schools are located throughout the country. Dogs are furnished free of charge to the blind. The sightless person who is selected to receive a dog lives in residence at the school for several weeks. At the school he and his dog learn to work with and care for one another.

Younger persons are especially suited to guide dog training. Canes are particularly useful for older persons or persons who for other reasons cannot walk rapidly enough to use a guide dog. When possible the blind person should use both cane and guide dog travel. The cane is useful when the dog is not in harness or when the blind person is temporarily without a dog. The individual who is properly trained to use a cane can become as mobile and independent as a person trained to use a dog.

By learning to use white canes, guide dogs, braille writing, and other helpful devices and by participating in appropriate training and educational programs, the blind individual can attain remarkable self-sufficiency if he is well motivated.

Regular physical examinations are encouraged for the blind individual (and for the individual's guide dog, if he has one). Hearing problems should be treated early, since hearing defects pose serious problems for the blind. The patient's general nutritional status and physical condition require periodic evaluation and correction to maintain the optimal state of health necessary to help the patient compensate for his visual loss.

COURTESIES TOWARD THE BLIND INDIVIDUAL

In the previous section we have discussed some of the compensatory technics which blind persons may learn to help themselves. Now let us consider some of the ways in which other persons can help the blind individual.

When blind persons are hospitalized they should have a call bell available at all times. Attempts should be made to keep the newly blinded patient oriented. He may be placed in a ward with other patients. It is helpful if you explain noises which the patient may wonder about. Show the patient around his room. Walk with him and have him touch various objects in the room, e.g., table, chair, window, door, sink, radio. Once the patient is able to walk about the halls, walk with him showing him where the nurses' station, elevator, visitors' lounge, telephone, rest rooms, and so forth are located. Try to help prevent the patient from feeling neglected, e.g., by frequently dropping in to visit briefly, by performing procedures on time.

Introductions are always important; this is particularly true with blind persons. Upon approaching the blind individual, speak to him so he knows someone is with him. When introduced to a blind person, speak to him, saying something about your relationship to him, e.g., "I am a student of nursing. I will be taking care of you this morning." If the patient extends his hand, shake hands with him. Speak clearly, yet quietly and calmly. When with a blind person do not try to avoid use of such words as "see" and do not avoid discussing the appearance of things. Do not apologize for the fact that you can see, e.g., "I feel guilty that I can see these lovely flowers and you cannot." When you are addressing a blind person in a group of people, call him by name so he will be aware that he is the person being spoken to. Always speak to the blind person when you approach him or enter or leave his room. Also, tell him when others enter or leave the room. Also, always tell him before you touch him. Prepare the blind person for what is going to happen next. This is particularly important when performing nursing procedures. Make smooth movements rather than sudden jerky ones. Attempt to appear relaxed and unhurried. Rushing the blind person may be confusing to him.

As emphasized previously, do not change the location of objects in the room or environment of a sightless person without telling him about the change. Keeping things in familiar places adds to the patient's independence and thus to his sense of security. The blind patient's environment should be kept well lit and pleasant. The patient should learn to put lights on when he is awake and moving about, even though he cannot benefit from them. This gives a more normal appearance to his life and prevents others from becoming startled when they encounter him.

In the hospital it is advisable to take special precautions to ensure the safety of a blind patient. For example, it is advisable to supervise smoking, keep siderails up, assist the patient when walking, and keep dangerous objects away from the bedside, e.g., hot plates. Restrictions may be greater for the newly blind than for the patient who has become accustomed to blindness. Never leave doors partially open, because the blind person may walk into them. Either completely open the door or completely shut it. Teach the patient to take hold of both armrests of a chair before sitting down.

The nurse should discuss safety factors with family members of the newly blinded patient. She may advise them how they can rearrange the home to make it possible for the patient to more easily and more safely move about. The visiting nurse may be helpful in this aspect of planning or in making home visits for other purposes. Family members must learn that an overprotective attitude toward the patient is harmful.

Do not rush up and offer help to a blind person unless he actually appears to want help. When you decide to offer help, don't sneak up on the blind person, but rather walk firmly up (approaching on the side opposite his cane or dog if he is walking) and ask in a clear, friendly voice if help is needed. Do not take hold of the person before speaking to him. This is most important if he has a guide dog. The guide dog is a disciplined worker, and when the dog is on duty he should not be disturbed. Do not try to touch or give directions to the guide dog while he is working. Do not touch him or speak to him until you have asked the dog's owner for permission to do so.

When walking with a sightless person, offer your arm rather than grasping the person's arm. The blind individual has a better sense of balance and direction of movement if he holds your arm and if you walk slightly ahead of him. Tell him when you are approaching stairs, a curb, an incline, and so forth. Then pause briefly before beginning to step up or down.

Visitors, friends, or family members may ask your advice about gifts for the blind patient. Suggest gifts which appeal to senses other than vision, e.g., a new record, scented flowers, cologne, or, if the patient is newly permanently blinded, objects which will help him to regain independence.

CHAPTER 106

Disorders of the Ear and Related Structures

BASIC ANATOMY AND PHYSIOLOGY OF THE EAR AND RELATED STRUCTURES

If you require an extenive review of these topics, consult an anatomy and physiology text. You should reacquaint yourself with the ear's basic anatomy; the path for sound; and the mechanism governing equilibrium. The following outline summarizes outstanding areas for review.

I. *Description:* The ears are a pair of sensory organs, located on either side of the head, which participate in both hearing and position sense. "Hearing" is the sense by which sounds are appreciated. "Position sense" includes orientation of the head in space and movement of the body through space: its balance and equilibrium. Each ear is divided into three main sections: (1) external ear; (2) middle ear; and (3) internal ear (Fig. 106–1)

II. *External ear:* Includes outer projection of ear, a canal, and tympanic membrane. Functions to receive sound waves and direct them to tympanic membrane.
   - A. *Pinna* or *auricle:* Projecting, visible part of ear composed of cartilage covered by skin.
   - B. *External auditory canal* or *meatus:* Opening in ear which extends inward, forward, and downward in adult for approximately 1–1½ inches. First part of canal contains *ceruminous glands* which form *cerumen,* i.e., wax. Normally cerumen is protective.
   - C. *Tympanic membrane* or *eardrum:* Located at end of auditory canal. Divides meatus and middle ear cavity. Normally eardrum vibrates with incoming sound waves.

III. *Middle ear:* Small, flattened space containing air and three small bones, i.e., ossicles.
   - A. *Ossicles:* Three bones joined in such a manner that they amplify sound waves received by tympanic membrane, then transmit the sound waves to fluid in inner ear. First bone, *malleus* ("hammer"), has handlelike portion attached to tympanic membrane and headlike portion which connects with second bone, *incus* ("anvil"). Incus connects with third bone, *stapes* ("stirrup"). Footplate of stapes fits into the *oval window* (also called *"vestibular window"*), which is a small opening in the wall between middle and inner ear. Oval window's membrane vibrates and conducts sound waves to fluid in inner ear. Normally ossicles have freely movable joints between them, thus forming a bony lever system.
   - B. *Eustachian tube* or *auditory tube:* Brings air into middle ear, thus equalizing pressure on both sides of tympanum. Middle ear's mucosal lining is continuous with that of nasopharynx via eustachian tube.
   - C. *Mastoid air cells:* Air-filled spaces in a portion of skull's temporal bone. Middle ear communicates posteriorly with mastoid air cells.

IV. *Inner ear* or *labyrinth:* Most complicated and important part of ear. Includes three separate spaces hollowed out inside temporal bone. Collectively these spaces are called *"bony labyrinth";* they contain fluid called *"perilymph."* Within bony labyrinth is *"membranous labyrinth,"* consisting of cochlear duct, utricle, saccule, and semicircular ducts; membranous labyrinth contains fluid called *"endolymph."*
   - A. *Vestibule:* Entrance space next to oval window; communicates with cochlea (toward front) and semicircular canals (toward back). In vestibule are vestibular receptors for position of head as it relates to pull of gravity.
   - B. *Cochlea:* Bony tube shaped like snail shell. Cochlear portion contains *organ of Corti,* the receptor end-organ of hearing.
   - C. *Semicircular canals:* Contain sensory organs related to equilibrium. These receptor end-organs are stimulated by changes in rate or direction of movement.
   - D. *Acoustic (8th cranial) nerve:* Cochlear nerve connects with receptors in cochlea. Nerve fibers from sacs in vestibule and from semicircular canals join cochlear nerve to form acoustic nerve. Acoustic nerve thus has an auditory and vestibular portion. Acoustic nerve forms sensory pathway to temporal lobe of cerebral cortex.

BASIC TYPES OF DISORDER OF THE EAR

The ear is subject to many of the same types of disorders that occur in other parts of the body. These include:

- *Obstructions:* of the external auditory canal or eustachian tube.
- *Trauma:* may affect all parts of the ear, or parts of the brain that connect or interpret auditory messages.
- *Inflammation and scarring:* of the tympanic membrane or ossicles
- *Skin disorders:* of the external auditory canal.
- *Infection:* of the external or middle ear or of the mastoid air cells.

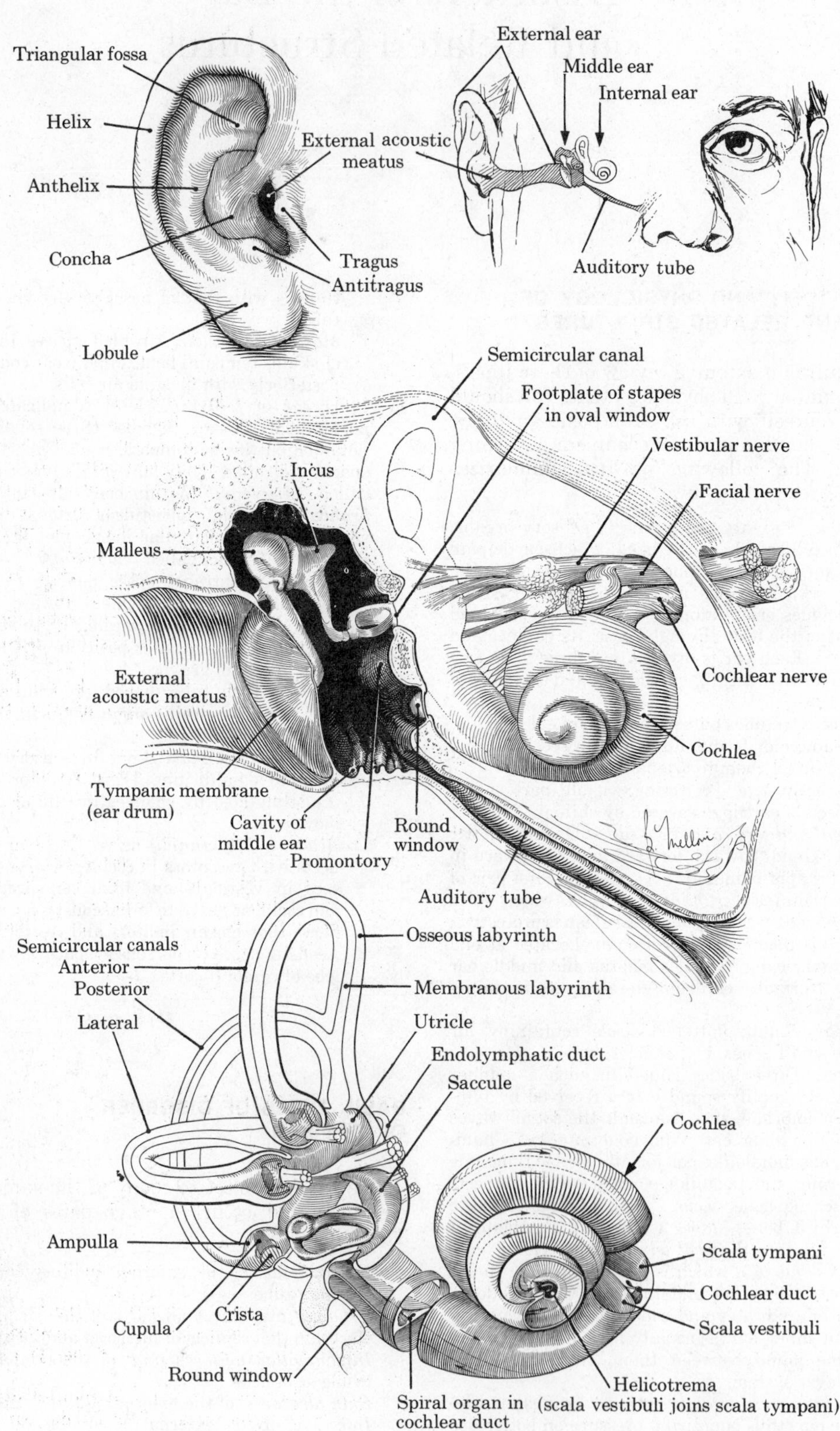

FIGURE 106–1. External and internal structures of the ear. (From *Dorland's Illustrated Medical Dictionary.* 25th ed. 1974.)

In addition, there are certain types of disorders peculiar to the ear:

> *Disturbances of balance:* Menière's syndrome and acute labyrinthitis (see below); dizziness; vertigo.
> *Disturbances of hearing:* conductive or transmission deafness; sensorineural or perceptive deafness; central deafness.
> *Tinnitus* (ringing in the ear): may be subjective or objective.

EXAMINATION OF THE EAR AND ASSESSMENT OF THE PATIENT WITH A DISORDER OF THE EAR

EXAMINATION OF THE EXTERNAL EAR

The external ear can be visualized directly; the middle ear and inner ear cannot be evaluated in this manner. In examining the external ear canal, the physician basically evaluates the condition of the ear's epithelium. Great care and gentleness are important in performing procedures in this area to prevent pain and bleeding. The first half of the ear canal is cartilaginous. About halfway to the eardrum, the cartilage stops and the supporting wall becomes osseous. Epithelium lining this bony portion of the canal is quite thin and *is highly sensitive.* One must be especially gentle in cleaning the inner half of the ear canal. This area is even more sensitive than the drumhead's outer surface. (*Note:* it is not advisable for anyone but the physician to perform cleaning of the inner half of the canal or of the drumhead. Cleaning of the ear is discussed further below.)

To look most easily into the ear, tip the patient's head sidewise (toward the opposite shoulder when sitting up) (see Fig. 106–2). This tipping is necessary because of the oblique direction of the ear canal.

Frequently the ear canal and drumhead are cleansed by the physician prior to examination of the ear. This cleansing is performed to remove accumulated cerumen, particulate matter, pus, and secretions which may otherwise impair visualization of the canal's epithelium and the drumhead. Cleansing may be accomplished with a cotton-tipped applicator, with a small angulated sucker tip, with a cerumen spoon, or by irrigation. (Irrigation is discussed on p. 1520.) When a cerumen spoon is used, it is inserted above the impacted wax and then is carefully withdrawn.

After cleansing of the ear, the auricle is inspected and palpated. Next the external auditory canal and tympanic membrane are visualized. The examination is started by *"straightening the ear canal,"* i.e., the auricle is pulled upward and backward and the tragus forward. The nurse should know how to straighten the canal, since she needs to do this before performing nursing procedures on the ear, such as instilling ear drops or performing ear irrigations. Straightening the canal makes it possible to see more easily into the canal. Also, straightening the canal enables solutions or medication to be introduced into the canal (see also p. 1520).

Various instruments may be used to inspect the

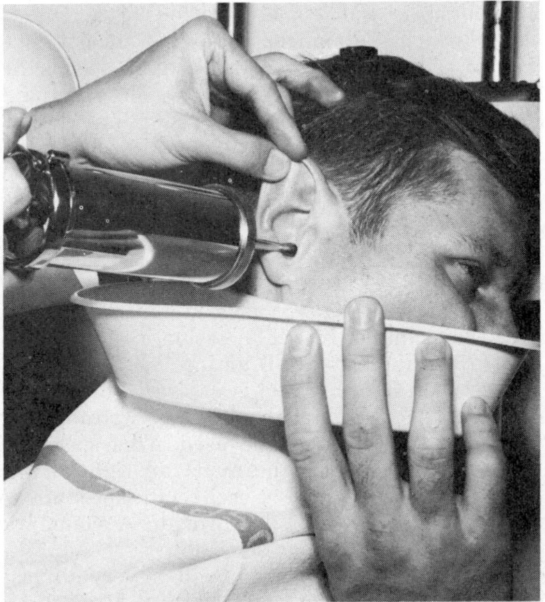

FIGURE 106–2. Irrigation to remove cerumen or other material in the ear canal blocking a view of the tympanic membrane. Be certain water is at approximate body temperature or vertigo may develop. (From Paparella, M. M., and Shumrick, D. A.: *Otolaryngology.* Vol. I. 1973.)

ear canal and drumhead. Among these are the (a) aural speculum, (b) otoscope, and (c) Zeiss operating microscope.

When an *aural speculum* is used to examine the eardrum, light is reflected into the ear from a *head mirror* (Fig. 106–3). Ear specula are plain, polished

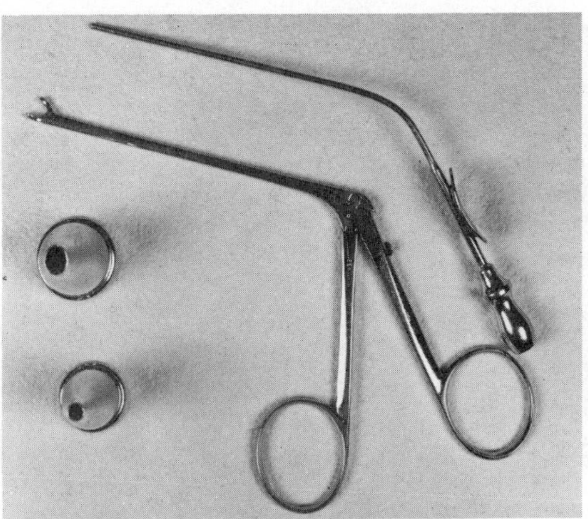

FIGURE 106–3. Two ear specula (always use the largest that will fit); an aural forceps and a small angulated sucker. (From Paparella, M. M., and Shumrick, D. A.: *Otolaryngology.* Vol. I. 1973.)

metal funnels which come in various sizes. One is selected which approximates the size of the patient's external auditory meatus. The speculum used is the largest which will fit the ear canal. The speculum is inserted to straighten and slightly dilate the cartilaginous ear canal.

The eardrum may be magnified for visualization by fitting a lens to the speculum or by using an operating microscope (Fig. 106-4) or an otoscope. Increasingly the Zeiss operating microscope is being used by otologists to examine the ear diagnostically (it is also used during ear surgery). This instrument gives the examiner binocular vision, magnification (4× to 25×), and brilliant illumination.

Sometimes the ear canal is aspirated during examination. To accomplish this an *aspirating* or *pneumatic speculum* can be used. This speculum has a window and can be made air-tight in the meatus. A bulb may then be used on the speculum to apply pressure or suction the eardrum. A pneumatic otoscope is also available (see below).

The normal, healthy drumhead is very slightly conical (with concavity externally), quite shiny, and pearly gray in color. With respect to the ear canal, the position of the drumhead is oblique. In the presence of disease, the drumhead's color changes. Blue indicates hemotympanum, a hemorrhagic exudation into the drum cavity of the ear; white pus in the middle ear; yellow or amber, serum in the middle ear; red or pink, myringitis infection of the middle ear.

Upon examination of the drumhead, the physician may discover not only changes in color, but also other abnormalities, such as (a) perforation or scars; (b) white plaques or flecks (usually indicative of old, healed disease); (c) bulging outward of the drumhead (indicative of pus in the middle ear); or (d) a retracted drumhead (resulting from reduced intratympanic pressures, e.g., from obstruction of the eustachian tube in association with too-rapid a descent in air travel).

DEMONSTRATION OF FUNCTION OF THE EUSTACHIAN TUBE

This special examination is performed to determine if the eustachian tube is patent. This procedure is important in evaluating patients with symptoms indicative of occlusion of the tube: tinnitus (a noise in the ears, e.g., ringing, buzzing, clicking, roaring, which may at times be heard by others than the patient), deafness, or dizziness. To perform the examination, the patient holds his nose and swallows while the drumhead is examined under magnification. Exactly when the patient swallows, the drumhead normally flicks outward and then inward again and the patient feels a sensation of pressure in his ears. Normally the eustachian tube opens during swallowing.

EXAMINATION WITH A PNEUMATIC OTOSCOPE

This instrument may be used to compress air in the ear canal and thus exert pressure against the drumhead; to suck out secretions from the mastoid antrum (in patients with chronic mastoiditis); or to remove fluid from the middle ear following myringotomy (Fig. 106-5). By exerting pressure against the drumhead, the physician can evaluate whether or not the drumhead is of normal flaccidity.

EXAMINATION OF THE NOSE AND THROAT

Examination of the ear is accompanied with examination of the nose and throat because infection

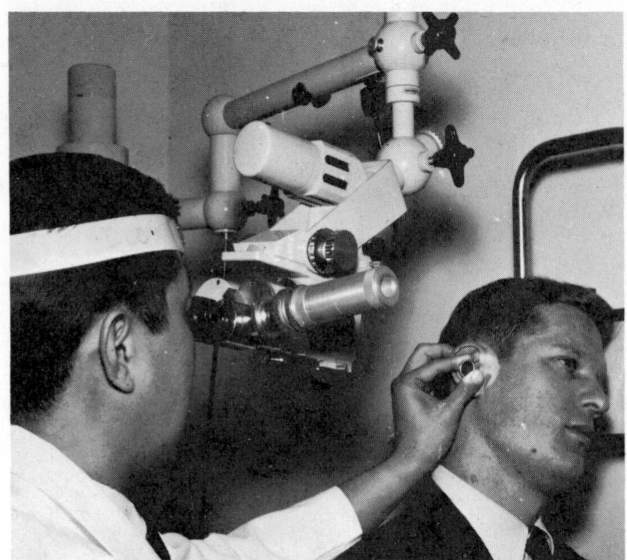

FIGURE 106-4. Operating microscope in use. The tube leading to one side is for a second observer. (From Paparella, M. M., and Shumrick, D. A.: *Otolaryngology.* Vol. I. 1973.)

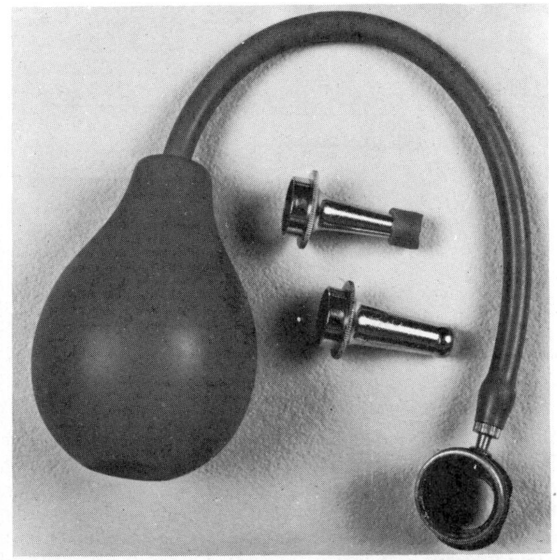

FIGURE 106-5. The Siegle or pneumatic otoscope. One of the specula can be fitted with a rubber tip if the special metal tip itself does not provide an airtight seal. (From Paparella, M. M., and Shumrick, D. A.: *Otolaryngology.* Vol. I. 1973.)

of these areas may be a contributing factor in ear disorders. Examination of the nose and throat is discussed in Unit XXII.

X-RAY EXAMINATION OF THE MASTOID

Patients who do not respond to treatment, who have acute otitis media, or who have chronic middle ear suppuration may have x-rays taken to further evaluate their conditions. X-ray examination of the temporal bone may be necessary to confirm the diagnosis of acute mastoiditis. In such a case the characteristic findings are clouding of the mastoid air cells and decalcification of the bony walls between the air cells. Most patients with chronic suppurative otitis media have a small, undeveloped, and acellular mastoid which can be demonstrated with roentgenograms of the mastoid. Also, cholesteatomas (see p. 1526) (a special type of chronic middle ear condition which is pathologically identical to epidermoid inclusion cysts) may enlarge, expand into the mastoid antrum, and eventually cause bony destruction with erosion into important adjacent structures. This erosion can be visualized by x-ray examination of the temporal bone.

EVALUATION OF HEARING

Classification of Types of Hearing Loss. Types of hearing losses may be classified in various ways. One classification is the following:

> *Conductive deafness* (transmission deafness): resulting from disturbances of the sound transmission mechanism of the external or middle ears, which prevents sound waves from reaching the inner ear.
> *Sensorineural deafness* (perceptive or "nerve" deafness): results from disturbances of the inner ear neural structures or nerve pathways leading to the brainstem.
> *Central deafness:* results from damage to the brain's auditory pathways or auditory center., e.g., from a cerebrovascular accident. (See Unit VIII.)
> *Mixed type deafness:* results from disturbances in both the conductive and nerve mechanisms.
> *Functional deafness* (psychogenic or nonorganic deafness): hearing loss for which no organic lesion can be detected.

Currently *conductive deafness* is the only type of organically caused deafness which can be effectively treated. If the basic disorder cannot be corrected, hearing aids which amplify sound are highly beneficial in conductive deafness, because the inner ear and organs which perceive sound are not damaged (see below).

Perceptive deafness commonly results from industrial noise and exposure to heavy gunfire. Recently this condition has appeared in teen-agers as a result of electric amplification of modern music; this condition is termed *"rock and roll" deafness. Presbycusis* refers to hearing loss due to aging. Presbycusis is a progressive, bilateral type of perceptive deafness. Since sensorineural forms of deafness cannot generally be effectively treated, prevention of such hearing losses is highly important, when possible, as discussed on p. 1518. Hearing aids are not as helpful with sensorineural deafness as they are with conductive deafness.

Deafness may also be classified as *congenital* (present at time of birth) or *acquired* (occurring at the time of birth or thereafter). So-called "congenital deafness" may be caused by such factors as ototoxic drugs, familial predisposition, or prenatal causes, such as exposure of the mother during the first trimester of pregnancy to viral diseases (German measles). "Neonatal" causes of perceptive deafness include anoxia during delivery, Rh incompatibility, and birth trauma (e.g., use of forceps during delivery).

Hearing acuity may be determined in various ways. A *gross evaluation* may be made by examining the patient's ability to hear a whispered or spoken voice or the ticking of a watch; a *precise evaluation* may be made by employing special equipment, such as an audiometer. Additional methods of evaluation include tuning fork tests, and a bevy of specialized evaluations.

Whispered or Spoken Voice Tests. During these tests the examiner uses one hand to shield the patient's eyes so he cannot lip-read. Then the examiner whispers or speaks to the patient, directing his voice toward the ear being evaluated. It is necessary to mask sound in the ear not being tested. Such masking may be achieved by using a Barany noisemaker at the ear not being tested. Masking is also necessary for other hearing tests to be discussed.

Watch Tick Test. The watch tick test is simply

a gross evaluation of the patient's ability to hear the tick of a watch, held at various distances from the ear being tested. Because the watch tick is a high-pitched sound, it is used in testing patients with high-frequency deafness. Many patients first discover their own hearing loss when they notice that they are unable to hear a watch tick.

Tuning Fork Tests. A tuning fork is a two-pronged forklike instrument of steel. When struck or stroked, the prongs give off a sound like a musical note. Testing hearing acuity by means of tuning fork tests is an important part of the otologic functional examination. Experts recommend use of tuning forks with vibrating frequencies of 512 and 1024 cycles per second; occasionally a fork is used which vibrates at 2048 cycles per second. To activate the fork, it is stroked between the thumb and index finger, or it is gently tapped (with a rubber reflex hammer or on a knuckle). Tuning forks are especially useful in differentiating between conductive and sensorineural hearing losses.

Normally when a vibrating tuning fork is placed in any midline position of the skull or over the maxillary incisors, sound waves travel through the bone of the skull, activate the cochlear fluids, and cause the sensation of hearing. The sound is heard at equal loudness in both ears.

Normally a tuning fork is heard twice as long by air conduction as by bone conduction. [*Air conduction* (AC) refers to the conduction of sound waves to the ear through the air. *Bone conduction* (BC) is conduction of sound waves to the inner ear through the bones of the skull.] When a vibrating fork is placed on one mastoid process, the sound is heard in that ear a certain length of time before it gradually fades away. (This hearing results from bone conduction.) Then, if the fork is moved immediately opposite the external auditory meatus without being reactivated, the sound should be heard again until it slowly dies down. (This hearing results from air conduction.)

In the *Weber test* the tuning fork is placed in the center of the forehead or on the maxillary incisors. As mentioned, normally the sound should be heard equally in both ears. If a patient has conductive hearing loss, the sound refers to the side of the defect. This is because ordinary room noise ("ambient noise") tends to mask hearing in the normal ear; the ear which has conductive loss does not hear such ambient noises and therefore has a better chance to hear the bone-conducted sound. When sensorineural loss is present in one ear, the sound from the fork is heard louder in the normal ear.

To perform the *Rinne test* (Fig. 106–6), the physician alternately places an activated tuning fork opposite one external auditory meatus and on the adjacent mastoid bone. As mentioned, the normal ear hears the sound from the fork about twice as long by air conduction as by bone conduction. The reverse findings occur in a patient with conductive hearing loss, i.e., he hears the sound longer by bone conduction than by air conduction. The Rinne test is called "positive" when the patient hears longer by air

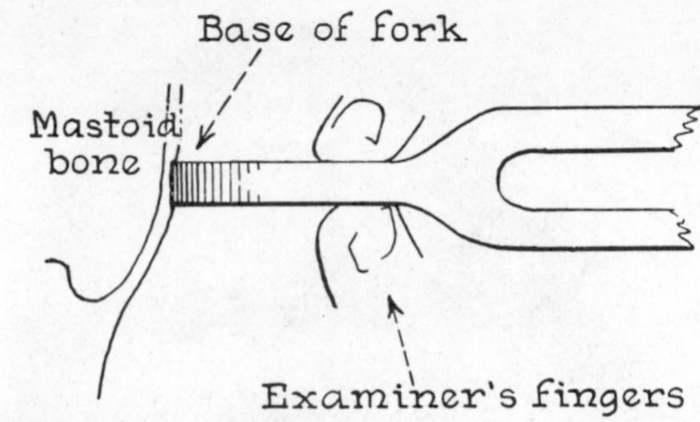

FIGURE 106–6. Rinne test. (From Williamson, P.: *Office Procedures.* 2nd ed. 1962.)

than by bone conduction (the normal pattern); the test is "negative" when the reverse findings occur. Patients who have sensorineural loss hear better by air conduction than by bone conduction, However, while they maintain the normal 2:1 ratio (of air conduction to bone conduction), their hearing *is typically reduced by both forms of conduction.*

In performing the *Schwabach test,* the physician compares his own normal hearing by bone conduction with the patient's hearing by bone conduction. To accomplish this, the vibrating fork is alternately placed on the patient's mastoid process and on the examiner's mastoid process. If the patient has sensorineural hearing loss, he will not hear the tone for as long a time as the physician does. If the patient has conductive hearing loss, he hears the tone for a longer time than the examiner. This is because the patient with conductive loss does not have the interference of ambient noise, while the examiner's normal ear is subjected to the masking effect of these normal environmental noises.

Audiometry. Most quantitative measurements of hearing are made with a *pure tone audiometer.* Occasionally a *speech audiometer* is used; this is basically the same instrument as the pure tone device except that it reproduces the spoken voice rather than pure tones.

The pure tone audiometer produces pure tones which can be varied according to frequency and intensity. Normally hearing is preserved in the lower intensities, and in the higher frequencies a drop occurs in the hearing. A chart is made of the patient's test results by plotting the intensity against the frequency. Frequency of vibration of sound waves is measured in cycles per second; intensity is measured in decibels. The greater the number of cycles per second, the higher the pitch of a sound.

The patient sits in a soundproof room for the audiometry test. He then listens to the sounds produced by the machine by listening through headpiece earphones. The patient is instructed to signal when he first hears each sound by pressing a button or raising a finger. Seven frequencies are tested (from 125 to 8000 cycles per second) by first presenting the tone loud enough for the patient to clearly hear it and then seeking the threshold for that frequency. The "threshold" is the lowest intensity at which the pure tone is heard. Each ear is tested, and both air and bone conduction measurements are made at the threshold levels. A bone oscillator, which produces mechanical vibrations of the skull, is placed against the head to test bone conduction. Hearing is normally most acute in the human ear at about 1000 cycles. Audiometers are equipped with a masking device which can be varied in intensity.

Specialized Tests. Additional tests to evaluate hearing acuity include (a) evaluation of such special auditory phenomena as *recruitment* (an abnormally rapid increase in loudness), *diplacusis* (the perception of a single auditory stimulus as two sounds), and *loss of aural discrimination* (ability to properly distinguish between speech sounds; a measurement of how meaningfully or accurately the patient hears, not how keenly he hears). There are a number of other specialized tests of hearing function described in textbooks of otology.

EVALUATION OF EQUILIBRIUM

When a patient is troubled by dizziness or vertigo, it is useful for the physician to determine if the labyrinths are functioning normally. This information can be obtained by *performing tests which artificially stimulate the semicircular canals. The Barany test and cold caloric tests are examples of tests used to evaluate labyrinthine reactions.* The findings of these tests are then compared with the known normal reaction. Normally stimulation of the utricle produces nystagmus, past pointing, and falling. (Nystagmus was discussed in Chapter 105.)

Nystagmus may be produced by ocular abnormalities and disturbances of the central nervous system, as well as disturbances of the labyrinth. In labyrinthine or central nystagmus, the movement of the eye is rhythmic, i.e., a slow movement of the eye in one direction is followed by a rapid compensatory movement in the opposite direction. In optic nystagmus, both excursions of the eye are of equal amplitude, the amplitude is greater, and the motion is of a wandering or pendulous nature rather than in the form of rhythmic excursions.

As mentioned, stimulation of the labyrinth also normally produces *past pointing* and *falling,* in addition to nystagmus. Both past pointing and falling always occur in the direction of flow of the endolymphatic fluid, as does the slow component of the nystagmus. Severe reactions to labyrinth stimulation include *dizziness* or *vertigo, nausea,* and *vomiting.* "Dizziness" refers to a disturbed sense of relationship to space in which the patient experiences a subjective sensation which is alarming and disturbing. Often the patient has difficulty describing exactly how he feels. He may have a feeling of turning or whirling or he may experience less clearly defined symptoms, such as weakness, giddiness, confusion, blankness, or unsteadiness. "True vertigo" is characterized by a sensation of true turning or whirling. For example, the patient may have an objective sense of the outside world turning or he may have a subjective sense that he himself is turning. With his eyes open the patient may feel that objects around him are moving, and with his eyes closed he may feel that he is in motion.

The nurse may care for patients experiencing dizziness or vertigo. Important *observations* for her to include in her charting include the following:

> Whether or not the patient experienced true whirling or turning sensations. The direction of the sense of turning and the influence of the position of the head on the sensations.
> Does the patient have paroxysmal attacks or is the sensation continuous? What time of day did the sensation occur? Is it related to a change in position? Is the patient's standing or walking affected? Is there an apparent relationship to occupation, menstrual periods, trauma, or medications?
> How severe is the sensation or attack? Did nausea or vomiting occur? Was there any associated hearing loss or tinnitus? If so, was it unilateral or bilateral? Was the episode followed by pallor,.slow pulse, and sweating?

Barany Test. This test of labyrinthine function was formerly widely used but is currently used only under special circumstances. The Barany test involves the use of a chair which is especially designed to (a) turn in a complete circle, and (b) hold the patient's head in different positions. To perform the test the chair is turned at a predetermined rate of speed, e.g., 10 turns in 20 seconds, and then is suddenly stopped. The endolymph continues to move (because of its momentum) even though the patient's body is stopped. The result is falling, past pointing, nystagmus, and subjective vertigo. This test stimulates both labyrinths simultaneously and is thus not as valuable as the caloric tests in which each labyrinth is separately tested.

Caloric Tests. The introduction of water or air (above or below body temperature) into the external auditory canal stimulates the semicircular canals. The most common caloric tests are those in which cold water or ice water are used. Cold caloric tests may be performed to induce either maximal or minimal stimulation.

Maximal stimulation is obtained by performing a cold caloric test *by douche.* A one-quart cannister is filled with cold water, the patient's head is tipped 30° forward, and the water (at 20° C.) is directed through a rubber tube into the ear canal. Water flowing out of the ear is caught in an emesis basin held under the patient's ear. Irrigation is terminated when nystagmus begins.

Minimal stimulation of the semicircular canals is obtained by directing ice water against the eardrum through an ear speculum. This procedure is called the "*Kobrak caloric test.*" The patient wears 20-diopter glasses over his eyes and sits with his head tipped forward at a 30° angle. A Luer-Lok syringe fitted with a 22-gauge needle is then used to direct 4–5 ml. of ice water against the eardrum for 15 seconds. Labyrinthine reactions typically begin after a short time. If they do not the test is repeated using 10 ml. of ice water. If a reaction still does not occur, the test is repeated using 15, 20, or 30 ml. of ice water. The *labyrinth is considered to be dead if no reaction occurs* with 30 ml.

Regardless of whether the maximal or minimal method of stimulation is used, the patient is allowed to rest for 10–15 minutes between the tests on the two ears. The expected reactions to both kinds of cold caloric test are (a) nystagmus in the direction opposite from the ear being stimulated; and (b) past-pointing and falling toward the ear stimulated. Thus, the physician observes the direction of the nystagmus and tests the patient for past-pointing following injection of the cold water. The nurse should be prepared to steady or catch the patient as he falls toward the ear being stimulated. Before the test, in addition to assembling equipment for the test, the nurse protectively drapes the patient's shoulders with a water repellant cover. Detailed explanations of what to expect during the test are not given to the patient, as they may foster false responses. However, the patient is briefly told that some cold water will be placed in his ear. Because maximal stimulation may precipitate vomiting, an emesis basin and tissues should be close at hand.

Warm caloric tests produce reactions which are opposite to those obtained by cold caloric tests. Regardless of whether cold or warm tests are being performed, both ears are tested separately, and stimulation of opposite ears gives opposite directions to the labyrinthine reactions.

CARE AND PROTECTION OF THE EAR

NURSE'S ROLE

A nurse has numerous opportunities to teach others how to care for and protect the valuable sensory apparatus located in the ear. Such teaching opportunities arise among the nurse's own family members, friends, and neighbors, as well as in the professional setting in which the nurse practices. In schools and industries nurses may participate in auditory screening programs directed at identifying persons with impaired hearing.

The nurse encourages persons with symptoms of auditory disorders to seek professional evaluation and care. For example, during home visits the community health nurse may observe a family member who is hard-of-hearing or a child with a draining ear. As a result of her counseling, these individuals may receive treatment.

In homes, hospitals, clinics, and physician's offices, nurses participate in the diagnosis and clinical care of persons with auditory disorders. When giving clinical care the nurse observes the general guidelines related to ear care to be discussed below.

INCIDENCE OF IMPAIRED HEARING

An estimated 12 million adults and 3 million children in the United States have some type of hearing disorder. Of these persons, 760,000 are totally deaf and 4 million are seriously handicapped.[40] Hearing problems most commonly occur among the elderly. However, only 35 per cent of persons over age 65 who have a hearing loss have had their condition checked by a doctor. The hard-of-hearing may not accept the fact that they have a hearing loss. Rehabilitation of the hard-of-hearing or deaf individual is discussed later in this chapter. It is important for deafness to be prevented, if possible, by adequate protection of the ear.

PROTECTION OF THE EAR

Protection of the ear involves five major activities: (1) proper general hygiene of the ear (discussed below); (2) prompt, adequate treatment of infections which could involve the ear (e.g., upper respiratory infections) or which already do involve the ear (e.g., acute purulent otitis media); (3) prevention of trauma to the ear; (4) early detection of hard-of-hearing individuals; and (5) periodic ear examinations.

Middle ear infection occurs more often in children than in adults because the eustachian tube is more horizontal in the child. In the adult the tube tends to slant toward the pharynx, thus making it somewhat more difficult for infected material to pass from the pharynx into the middle ear. Because many hearing defects begin in childhood, a child should receive prompt medical care if he develops respiratory infections or if he shows symptoms of ear discomfort or ear infection. Adequate clinical care at this time may prevent a hearing disorder. Middle ear infections are discussed further later in this chapter.

Prevention of trauma to the ear encompasses such activities as: (a) preventing children from injuring their ears with sharp objects or foreign bodies; (b) teaching children and adults never to poke into their ears with any small or sharp object, (c) preventing occupational hearing loss in industry or other occupations; and (d) preventing excessive environmental noise levels in all settings.

In the industrial setting the nurse may participate in teaching about the proper use of protective ear devices, e.g., ear plugs. Occupational hearing loss may result from loud noise, intense heat, explosions, or accidents involving the head. Trauma to the ear may result from concussion, hemorrhage, or tearing of the soft tissue of the cochlea or vestibule. As a result, the canal may be fractured, the eardrum may be destroyed, the ossicles may be disrupted, or the internal ear may be damaged or destroyed. The most common and most important type of occupational hearing loss is that caused by loud noise. Unions and individual workers have in recent years filed suits totaling millions of dollars for compensation for hearing loss caused by noise on job settings. Currently many industries require pre-employment audiometric examinations and periodic retesting.

Persons working in areas of high noise levels may wear protective ear plugs made of rubber or malleable plastic. Ear plugs come in several sizes or may be custom-made (molded to the individual's ear canal dimensions by impression technics). In settings with extremely high noise levels (e.g., jet engine factories), the workmen not only wear ear plugs but also ear muffs and a large shield over the entire head.

Sound *intensity,* i.e., the pressure exerted by sound, is measured in *decibels.* Ordinary speech is about 50 decibels; heavy traffic is about 70 decibels.

Above 80 decibels sound becomes quite uncomfortable to the human ear. Prolonged exposure (for months or years) to industrial noise levels greater than 85 to 90 decibels causes cochlear damage. In jet engine factories the sound level may reach 140 decibels.

Noise is often quite irritating to sick persons. The nurse strives to keep the environment of the ill quiet to enhance their rest and mental comfort.

The early detection of hard-of-hearing individuals is facilitated by *audiometric screening programs* in schools, industries, and other settings. Some nurseries test the hearing of newborn infants. Meconium may be sucked into the middle ear with the first breath of life, causing ear problems. Developmental defects may also be present. Early detection of hearing problems is then followed up by early evaluation and treatment.

Many communities have screening programs to test the hearing of preschool and school-aged children. Hearing defects seriously interfere with a child's ability to learn. Children who have difficulties learning to speak and who do not follow instructions properly may have hearing disorders which make it virtually impossible to learn. Periodic evaluation of hearing is also important in elderly persons because with aging degenerative changes frequently occur in the ear as well as in other body tissues. Persons of all ages should periodically have their ears examined by a physician. Examination of the ears is a routine part of a general complete examination. If a problem appears to be present, the patient is referred to a specialist for further evaluation and treatment.

GENERAL EAR CARE

Excessive cleaning of the ear is undesirable. Ear wax lubricates the ear's skin and entraps foreign material entering the canal. Because ear wax serves a protective function, attempts should not be made to clean all wax out of the canal. Excessive, repetitive cleaning of the ear canal results in loss of wax formation. In the absence of the protective wax, serious ear problems can develop. Too little cerumen may be more annoying than excessive cerumen. With an inadequate amount of cerumen the ear canal is dry and scaly, and itching may occur. While this disorder is not easily cured, the application of suitable ear ointments may improve the condition.

The following factors are important aspects of *routine, general ear care:*

> *It is generally recommended that the ear be cleansed only with a wet washcloth over the tip of a finger.* Nothing smaller than a finger should be inserted into the ear for routine care. Cotton tipped applicators should not be used. Items such as hairpins, matchsticks, or toothpicks should never be used to clean the ear since they may scratch the skin, thus creating a lesion which could become infected. *Nothing should be inserted into the ear canal beyond the extent of vision;* to do so could result in accidental puncture of the eardrum. When washing a patient's ears, observe for indications of irritation, infection, or other problems.

> *Protection of the ear from contamination from water when bathing, swimming, or diving is important if the patient has a history of ear infection.* This is particularly important if perforation of the drum has occurred. The ear should be plugged with lamb's wool or cotton which is saturated with petrolatum; additionally a swimming cap should be worn when swimming.

> *During acute upper respiratory infections ("colds") the nose should not be blown hard or douched.* Preferably the patient should blow his nose while keeping both nostrils open and his mouth open. Excessive pressure forces contaminated material into the eustachian tube.

GUIDELINES AND COMMON NURSING PROCEDURES IN EAR CARE

GENERAL GUIDELINES

The following are important guidelines to remember when caring for a patient with a disorder of the ear.

> Always wash your hands before and after caring for the patient's ear, and wash between caring for the two ears to prevent cross-contamination. If one ear is infected, care for the noninfected ear first.

> Observe strict asepsis when the middle ear or inner ear has been opened surgically or has been accidentally opened by trauma. The introduction of infection may cause suppurative labyrinthitis or meningitis.

> Have good light so you can see exactly what you are doing. An adjustable light is best.

> Straighten the ear canal as necessary for good visualization and so medications instilled will go into the ear canal. (See p. 1513 for discussion of how to straighten the adult ear canal.) In infants and young children the ear canal is straightened by pulling the auricle downward.

> Place nothing in a patient's ear without an order.

> Solutions used for irrigations of the ear (see below) and eardrop solutions should be at body temperature before they are instilled into the ear. Hot or cold temperatures easily stimulate the inner ear, causing vertigo and occasionally nausea and vomiting.

> Never insert objects (medication dropper, applicator, irrigation tip) into the ear canal beyond the extent of your vision.

> Avoid traumatizing the ear. Be sure glass-tipped medication droppers are not chipped on the tip.

> Be gentle. Some conditions make the ear extremely sensitive. Also, as discussed earlier, the inner ear canal is normally very tender.

> Never obstruct the ear canal during instillation of medications or during irrigations. Do not obstruct the ear canal with cotton or gauze unless ordered to do so. Obstruction may cause a dangerous pressure increase against the eardrum.

> Use every appropriate opportunity to teach the patient how to properly care for his own ears.

> When caring for a patient who has vertigo, instruct him to slow down his movements, and thereby reduce the possibility of precipitating an attack. Assist and protect the patient as necessary, as in getting up or

walking, and keep siderails on bed. Keep your movements slow and unhurried.

COMMON NURSING PROCEDURES RELATED TO EAR CARE

Routine cleansing of the ears, instillation of ear drops, softening and removal of wax deposits, irrigation of the ear, use of dry wipes, and insertion and removal of ear wicks are procedures which the nurse commonly performs. Remember to wash before and after each procedure; to identify the patient and which ear is to be treated before beginning; to explain to the patient what you are going to do and how he can help; and to chart after each procedure.

Instillation of Eardrops. Various eardrop solutions are instilled into the auditory canal to produce such local effects as anesthesia, destruction of microorganisms, destruction of an insect lodged in the ear canal, or to soften ear wax. (*Note:* As an emergency measure in the home, if an insect is in the ear canal, try holding a flashlight to the ear to see if this will attract the insect to the light. If this is unsuccessful, a few drops of mineral oil or olive oil can be placed in the ear canal to smother and immobilize the insect. The movements and wing-beating of an insect in the ear canal are very distressing. A physician must then remove the insect.)

> *Eardrops are instilled as follows:* (1) check glass eardropper to be sure it is not rough on the end, and warm correct solution to body temperature; (2) place patient on his side with ear to be treated uppermost; (3) direct light into ear and cleanse external ear with sponge; (4) place one hand on patient's head to straighten canal and steady head (this is most easily accomplished by gently placing the thumb on the ear lobe and grasping the auricle between the flat inner surfaces of the index and middle fingers, and then pulling the auricle up and back by extending and straightening the fingers); (5) instill the ordered number of drops (usually 3–4 gtts.) of the prescribed solution by directing the drops toward the *side* of the ear canal with the eardropper; (6) have the patient remain on his side for about 5–10 minutes so the medication will have prolonged contact with the inner surface of the external ear canal and drumhead; (7) insert loose cotton or gauze wick into canal *if ordered* so ear canal will have a continuous application of the solution instilled (see below); and (8) with a fresh sponge dry external ear of excessive liquid to prevent skin irritation.

Softening and Removal of Wax Deposits. Impacted, dry accumulations of ear wax may be softened for easy removal by daily instilling a few drops of hydrogen peroxide or warmed glycerine. Carbamide (urea) peroxide in glyceryl (Debrox) is another softening agent which may be instilled. After this is done for 2–3 days, the ear is irrigated to wash out the softened wax. This procedure should not be undertaken without the approval of the physician. The physician may use a cerumen spoon to remove ear wax plugs. Removal of wax with this instrument requires skill and the use of an ear speculum for direct vision.

Ear Irrigations. The ear may be irrigated to (a) cleanse the external auditory canal; (b) remove impacted wax; (c) apply heat to the ear; (d) apply antiseptic solutions for their local action; or (e) remove foreign bodies. (*Note:* Because moisture causes vegetable matter to swell, this procedure is never used to remove such foreign objects as beans, corn, and so forth.) The nurse does not irrigate a patient's ear unless a physician orders the treatment. Irrigations are typically not used if a patient's eardrum is punctured, since the irrigation could cause additional middle ear infection. The physician orders the solution to be used, e.g., tap water, normal saline, antiseptic solution, solution of bicarbonate of soda. The solution should be warmed to body temperature prior to instillation or else vertigo will occur due to vestibular stimulation. The irrigation may be performed with a rubber bulb syringe, a glass Asepto syringe, or a metal Pomeroy syringe (Fig. 106–7) Ear irrigations may also be performed with an irrigating can with tubing and an ear tip.*

> *To perform an ear irrigation:* (1) Protectively drape the patient, position him so his head is tilted slightly forward and toward the side of the affected ear (the procedure may be performed with the patient sitting up or lying down; sitting up is easiest), and position the light. (2) Have the patient hold a basin beneath his ear against his face to catch the irrigating solution. (3) Cleanse external ear with gauze wipes and some of the solution. (4) Fill syringe and expel air from the rubber tubing. (5) Straighten ear canal.

* A *glass ear tip* has two extensions; one for the solution to enter the ear, the other for it to leave the canal. Inspect tip for breakage prior to use.

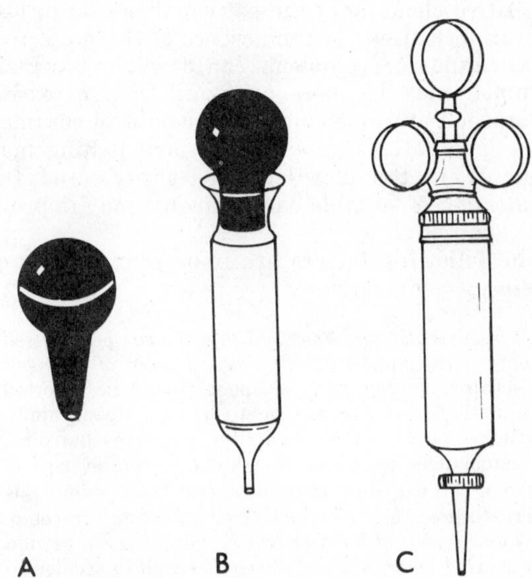

FIGURE 106–7. Three types of syringes used to irrigate the ear: *A*, rubber bulb syringe; *B*, glass Asepto syringe; and *C*, metal Pomeroy syringe.

(6) Place tip of syringe or tube just inside meatus and direct a slow, steady stream of solution against *roof* of auditory canal (directing the stream upward prevents forcing plugging materials further into the canal and prevents injury of tympanic membrane). (7) Do not use excessive force (if tubing is used do not elevate can higher than is necessary to remove the secretions). The least force results from use of a rubber bulb syringe; the Pomeroy syringe must be cautiously used because it can exert great pressure. (8) Do not occlude the auditory canal with the irrigating tip (the force of the stream will not damage the eardrum if space is left around the syringe to allow the fluid to escape). (9) Use approximately 500 ml. of irrigating liquid. (10) After the irrigation is completed, the ear canal should be carefully dried with a sterile cotton applicator (the physician may use a small length of cotton inserted with bayonet forceps). (11) Have the patient lie on the irrigated side for a few minutes after the treatment is complete so any remaining solution will drain out of the ear by gravity.

When charting following an ear irrigation, be certain to comment on the nature of the drainage, e.g., "Returning solution contained particles of brown wax."

Use of Dry Wipes. "Dry wipes" may be ordered to periodically clean the ear canal if a patient has ear discharge. The wipe is performed with a dry, sterile cotton-tipped applicator. Often applicators are especially prepared by hospital central services departments for use in the ear since commercial applicators are usually too stiff for such usage.

To perform the procedure: (1) position the patient on his side with the affected ear uppermost and position the light; (2) straighten the ear canal; (3) gently insert and rotate the applicator; (4) withdraw the applicator; and (5) note the appearance of discharge and discard the applicator. Generally it is necessary to use several applicators. Use a new, sterile applicator each time the canal is entered; never go repeatedly in and out with the same applicator.

Insertion and Removal of Ear Wicks. Wicks of small pieces of cotton or single pieces of gauze (picked up in the center, twisted, and sterilized) may be used as drains in the ear to encourage exudate drainage or following instillation of eardrops. The wick is gently inserted into the canal only as far as it is possible to see. The loose ends of the wick are left extending out of the canal. Wicks are changed frequently to prevent them from obstructing drainage flow or hardening or both.

GENERAL CARE OF THE PATIENT HAVING AURAL SURGERY

The following guidelines are important in the nursing care of any patient having ear surgery.

> *Preoperatively evaluate the patient's understanding* of the surgery he is going to have and the possible results of that surgery. Then provide appropriate answers to the patient's questions and see that he receives necessary explanations from you or his physician. If a procedure is being performed to improve hearing, inform the patient that improvement may not be noticeable for several weeks, until swelling leaves the operative area and dressings, packings, and so forth are removed.

> *Preoperatively review with the patient common postoperative restrictions.* For example: (a) discuss restrictions concerning positioning and movements; (b) tell the patient not to blow his nose, but rather to wipe off the end of the nose as necessary; (c) inform the patient not to sneeze or strenuously cough since such activities (including blowing the nose) may disrupt the delicate structures of the ear before healing occurs (e.g., may loosen the eardrum or dislocate a prosthesis) or may force air and possibly infected material into the eustachian tube; and (d) instruct the patient not to touch his ear or the ear dressing.

> *Prepare the ear for surgery as ordered.* The physician often prefers to clean the ear himself to prevent scratching or otherwise irritating the ear's tissues. A scratch could become infected. Prior to surgery topical and systemic antibiotic chemotherapy is ordered if a patient's ear has frequent or continuous discharge.

> *During surgery and postoperatively practice aseptic technic to prevent infection.* Infection is especially hazardous because of the ear's close proximity to the brain. Observe for symptoms of infection: temperature elevation, drainage from the ear, headache.

> *Administer antibiotics as ordered.* Assist with ear cultures if the physician takes them.

> *Postoperatively position the patient as ordered,* e.g., on side with operated ear up (to prevent displacement of grafts) or with operated ear down (to enhance drainage). In some cases the head of the bed is ordered flat or elevated 30°. Some orders state the patient may lie on whichever side causes less vertigo. Lying on the unoperated side sometimes minimizes nausea and vomiting. The patient may be on strict bedrest for 24–48 hours.

> *Provide pain relief as ordered.*

> *Reinforce external bandage if necessary,* but *do not disturb the inner ear dressing.*

> *Never apply pressure* to the ear or ear dressing. To do so could dislodge a graft or prosthesis.

> *Protect and help the patient with nausea and vertigo.* Vertigo and nausea commonly follow surgery on the ear (due to trauma and edema) and may be extremely uncomfortable as well as hazardous to the patient's safety. Discuss these symptoms with the patient, telling him they result from a *temporary* disturbance to the ear's balancing functions. Inform the patient that he can help minimize discomfort by (a) remaining positioned as ordered; (b) avoiding contraindicated activities or movements; (c) moving slowly; and (d) avoiding sudden turning. Keep siderails up while the patient is in bed and assist him when he does move about, e.g., get up. Also, encourage the patient to use handrails in the halls and bathrooms to help steady himself. Be careful not to bump or jar the patient or his bed when giving care. Do not rush the patient. The nauseated patient may obtain relief by taking slow, deep breaths through his open mouth. Give medications as ordered to minimize nausea and vertigo, e.g., Dramamine.

> *Provide nourishment as ordered.* A light or liquid diet may be ordered to prevent nausea or vomiting or to make it more comfortable for the patient to eat (if chewing is painful).

> *Observe for and report symptoms of postoperative complications.* Symptoms of infection have been discussed. Observe also for (a) fluctuations in hearing; (b) tinnitus; (c) vertigo; (d) gait disturbance; (e) bleeding (do not attempt to stop bleeding by applying pressure to the ear); or (f) indications of injury to the facial nerve, i.e., inability to frown, wrinkle the forehead, close the eyes, bare the teeth, or pucker the lips. During ear surgery the facial nerve may be injured temporarily (due to edema) or permanently. Paralysis resulting from edema may not appear for 12–24 hours postoperatively. The physician may loosen the ear dressing and order antiinflammatory medications in an attempt to relieve the pressure of edema. Protective eye care is sometimes indicated if the facial nerve is injured.

> *Prior to discharge tell the patient how to protect and care for his ear.* For example, the patient may be advised not to get his ear wet from showering, shampooing, or swimming. Infection could result from water in the ear. Contact with persons who have upper respiratory infections should be avoided because of the danger of the patient acquiring the infection and possibly developing a middle ear infection. Some patients, e.g., following stapedectomy (see p. 1529), are advised not to bend over, lift heavy objects, or fly until the physician says it is safe to do so.

> *Inform the patient of follow-up visits to the doctor's office or clinic.*

Specific aural surgical procedures are discussed later in the chapter.

COMMON DISORDERS OF THE EAR AND RELATED STRUCTURES AND THEIR CLINICAL MANAGEMENT

DISORDERS OF THE EXTERNAL EAR

Deformities. The external ear may be deformed as a result of trauma, ("cauliflower" ears associated with boxing), congenital malformation (atresia—absence or closure of the ear canal), or abnormal size or protrusion of the auricle. Often such disorders are amenable to corrective plastic surgery.

Foreign Bodies. As briefly mentioned earlier, foreign materials may become lodged in the ear canal. Poor technic in the removal of these objects can cause damage to the canal or tympanic membrane and possible middle ear infection, resulting in deafness. Thus, a physician should be consulted. Irrigation is contraindicated for substances which will swell when in contact with moisture and for pointed objects. Cautious removal by instrumentation is necessary in such cases. Removal of insects from the ear was discussed on p. 1520. Objects may be inserted into the ear by psychotic or mentally retarded individuals and by children.

Impacted Cerumen (Ear Wax). Some persons produce large quantities of cerumen. Impacted cerumen may cause conductive deafness. In addition to diminished hearing, other symptoms of impacted cerumen are itching or irritation of the ear canal; and feelings of plugging or discomfort in the ear. After examination of the ear the physician may advise that hard wax be softened and then removed by irrigation. If perforation of the eardrum is present, irrigation is contraindicated, and the physician must remove the wax with a curet. While accumulated earwax is usually hard, when mixed with water (as from swimming) it may soften and become a culture medium for bacteria, producing external otitis. The nurse should remember that accumulations of earwax are not necessarily indicative of poor personal hygiene. Patients who consider their condition as a sign of uncleanliness may be embarrassed to seek professional help.

External Otitis. "External otitis" is a general term used with reference to inflammatory disorders of the auricle and external auditory canal. These disorders may be caused by either infections or a dermatosis, or both. External otitis varies in severity from a diffuse mild eczematoid dermatitis to cellulitis or even furunculosis of the ear canal. In many cases there is no infection, and the reaction is a contact dermatitis (e.g., from earrings, earphones) or a variant of seborrheic dermatitis. Either bacteria or fungi may produce the infectious type. Usually infections of the ear canal are bacterial (staphylococcal and gram-negative rods); however, a few cases are caused by fungi (Aspergillus, Mucor, Penicillium). Predisposing factors include (a) moisture in the ear canal in a warm, moist climate or as a result of swimming; (b) trauma resulting from attempts to clean or scratch the itching ear; and (c) seborrheic and allergic dermatitis. Clinical findings include scaling, crusting, erythema, edema, and pustule formation. Major symptoms are itching and pain in a dry, scaling ear canal. Additional symptoms may include a watery or purulent (sticky yellow) discharge; intermittent deafness; adenopathy; and fever. Severe pain may occur if the ear canal becomes completely occluded with debris and edematous skin.

Treatment may include systemic analgesics for pain and systemic antibiotics if fever or lymphadenopathy are present. Local treatments may include (a) 70 per cent alcohol to control itching in a dry, scaling ear canal; (b) topical corticosteroids (to help control the underlying dermatitis and help decrease inflammatory edema); (c) topical antibiotic ointments and eardrops (e.g., neomycin, polymyxin, bacitracin) applied to ear canal with a cotton wick for 24 hours, followed by eardrops twice daily to help control infection; (d) compresses of Burow's solution (aluminum acetate solution) or 0.5 per cent acetic acid may be used with acute weeping infected eczema; and (e) use of glycerite of peroxide with urea drop eardrops t.i.d. to help remove debris. Debris may also be removed by gently wiping the ear canal with a cotton applicator, with suction, or occasionally by irrigation. During all local procedures be careful not to traumatize the area. Frequent gentle debridement is important to remove debris and to allow medicaments to reach the diseased tissue. Because the ear is often extremely sensitive, cool or warm compresses may be ordered to minimize discomfort. Touching or moving the auricle may produce intense pain, and thus patients may be naturally resistant to treatments which necessitate movement of the ear.

External otitis occurs in both acute and chronic forms. External otitis is often refractory to treatment and frequently recurrences occur. Thorough drying of the ear after swimming, bathing, or shampooing helps prevent infections. Persons having external otitis often are advised against swimming and are instructed to protect their ear canals from water when bathing or shampooing. Acute external otitis frequently follows swimming. With "swimmer's ear" the patient gets contaminated water in his ear; frequently the patient has wax in the ear which then absorbs the contaminated water, macerates the skin, and provides the basis for infection. In contrast to acute external otitis, with chronic otitis there is usually no pain when the auricle or tragus is manipulated. In chronic external otitis, itching rather than pain is the major discomfort, and the epithelium of the auricle, ear canal, and drum may become thickened, red, and quite insensitive. Frequently aural discharge is present.

Furunculosis. Furunculosis is a form of localized external otitis in the outer half of the ear canal. In this area glands and hair follicles may become infected and form furuncles (boils). Even a small furuncle causes *severe pain* until it either spontaneously breaks or is surgically drained. Furuncles on the canal floor cause pain upon mastication. Pain also occurs from movement of the auricle, and from pressure on the tragus. Onset may be acute. In addition to pain, the patient may notice a feeling of fullness in the ear, impaired hearing, adenopathy, and postauricular swelling. The area involved is red and may be severely swollen. At times the entire canal is obliterated.

Treatment generally includes insertion of a small gauze wick into the canal and wetting of this wick every few hours with 10 drops of halfstrength Burow's solution. This helps relieve pain. A piece of cotton saturated with the solution may also be applied to the external meatus. This therapy is continued for 48 hours. Usually local heat applications also help provide relief and hasten recovery. Once fluctuation is well developed the apex is incised. Pain may be controlled with codeine and APC. Systemic antibiotics are also given, especially in the presence of fever or cellulitis of adjacent tissues. Keeping the auditory canal dry, reasonably clean, and trauma-free are all important measures in the prevention of furuncles in this region.

Malignant Tumors. The external auditory meatus may be the site of both basal cell carcinomas and squamous cell carcinomas. Basal cell carcinomas invade the meatus and ear canal from the external ear. Squamous cell carcinomas may come from (a) the parotid gland; (b) skin of the auricle or epithelium of the external ear canal; (c) middle ear; or (d) mastoid. Symptoms include hearing loss, ear drainage, deep boring pain, and (late) peripheral facial paralysis. If the tumor is confined to the cartilaginous canal, the prognosis of carcinoma is reasonably good. Cure may result from wide local incision and skin grafting. The cure rate is greatly reduced if the osseous portion of the canal is invaded. Once the bone is involved, radical mastoidectomy and subsequent deep roentgenotherapy are usually employed in treatment of the cancer. (Cancer is also discussed in Unit VII.)

PERFORATION OF THE EARDRUM

The eardrum may be perforated as a result of infection (acute or chronic suppurative otitis media) or trauma (skull fracture, compression, burns, punctures). Usually accidental perforations spontaneously heal; sometimes corrective surgical procedures are necessary. While most traumatic perforations heal spontaneously in several days or weeks, some physicians give prophylactic antibiotics.

Some physicians advise patients with perforated eardrums not to dive, swim, or shower because of danger of water entering the middle ear and producing infection. In other cases the patient is advised to wear custom-molded ear plugs under a bathing cap to prevent water from entering the ear.

A perforated eardrum leaves a patient susceptible to chronic ear infections and their possible complications. Also, chronic perforations of the eardrum may cause conductive hearing loss. It is thus desirable for the eardrum to be repaired by plastic surgery, i.e., *myringoplasty,* if the tympanic membrane does not heal by itself. Various technics of myringoplasty may be employed. One method is to cauterize the edges of the wound and insert a piece of blood-soaked Gelfoam. New tissues then grow over the Gelfoam patch, filling in the hole. In other procedures the eardrum's opening is enlarged surgically, and a graft of skin, vein, or fascia is sutured over the hole. Gelfoam or clotted blood may be used to support the graft and keep it positioned (see also p. 1529).

The presence of an active infection or a history of chronic disease of the middle ear are obvious contraindications to the medical or surgical closure of perforations of the eardrum.

DISORDERS OF THE MIDDLE EAR

"Otitis media" refers to inflammation of the middle ear. There are several types of otitis media.

Serous (Catarrhal) Otitis Media. This condition may be acute or chronic, may occur at any age, and is characterized by the accumulation of sterile fluid (serous or mucoid) in the middle ear. Serous otitis media may be caused by[7] (a) an obstruction of the eustachian tube which prevents normal ventilation of the middle ear and subsequent transudation of serous fluid; (b) incomplete resolution of the exudate of purulent otitis media; or (c) an allergic exudate of serous fluid into the middle ear. Serous otitis media is distinguished from acute purulent otitis media by *absence of* fever, pain, and toxic symptoms. Symptoms of serous otitis media include a full plugged feeling in the ear; hearing loss; and an unnatural reverberation of the patient's voice.

Acute serous otitis media may occur spontaneously without symptoms of other disease, or it may accompany or follow virus diseases or episodes of allergy. Additionally, it may occur following sudden changes in atmospheric pressures, as during flying. Air moves out from the middle ear, through the eustachian tube, upon ascending from a high atmospheric pressure to a low atmospheric pressure. With descent, however, if the air is unable to pass back through the tube into the middle ear, feelings of discomfort develop. This condition is particularly likely to occur if the individual travels by air while he has an upper respiratory infection. It is advisable when flying to suck on hard candy, chew gum, or yawn several times during the plane's descent. These activities help open the eustachian tube and thus facilitate the entrance of air into the middle ear. Upon examination the patient displays a conductive hearing loss, and the eardrum is retracted. Air-fluid bubbles or a fluid level may be visible through the eardrum.

The *treatment* of acute serous otitis media may include such measures as (a) inflation of the eustachian tube; (b) myringotomy, i.e., incision of the tympanic membrane (eardrum), and sucking out of fluid in the middle ear; or (c) removal of fluid from the middle ear by needle aspiration (needle paracentesis of the eardrum with aspiration of middle ear contents). Additionally, such nasal decongestants as 0.25 per cent phenylephrine nasal spray or phenylpropanolamine, 25–50 mg. orally t.i.d., may be prescribed. If there are indications of contributing nasal allergy, antihistamines are given.

Chronic or recurrent serous otitis media can cause a serious threat to hearing. Chronic serous otitis media may be caused by (a) inadequate treatment of acute or subacute suppurative otitis media (inadequate chemotherapy with antibiotics has caused an increase in chronic serous otitis media); (b) allergy of the nose and nasopharynx; (c) overgrowth of lymphoid tissue in the nasopharynx; (d) chronic sinus infection; (e) hypometabolism; (f) lowered resistance to infection (evidenced by low gamma globulin in the blood plasma); or (g) carcinoma of the nasopharynx in the adult. Cancer of the nasopharynx must be ruled out in adult patients with persistent unilateral serous otitis media.

Chronic serous otitis media presents only minimal symptoms. There is no discharge from the ear. The most common symptom is hearing loss characterized by fluctuation. *Treatment* is directed at control of possible systemic disease and removal of fluid from the ear. Numerous myringotomies may be necessary. Sometimes a myringotomy is performed, and a polyethylene tube or a Teflon button is inserted through the eardrum and into the middle ear (Figs. 106–8 and 106–9). The tube makes it possible for secretions to drain out or be suctioned out over a period of several weeks. The tube also allows aeration of the middle ear and seems to hasten recovery of the eustachian tube obstruction. The myringotomy heals around the tube or button after a few hours. Tubes may be left in place for several months or until they extrude spontaneously from the ear.[10] In persistent cases local or systemic corticosteroids may be administered. Underlying factors must be corrected by tonsillectomy, adenoidectomy, control of nasal

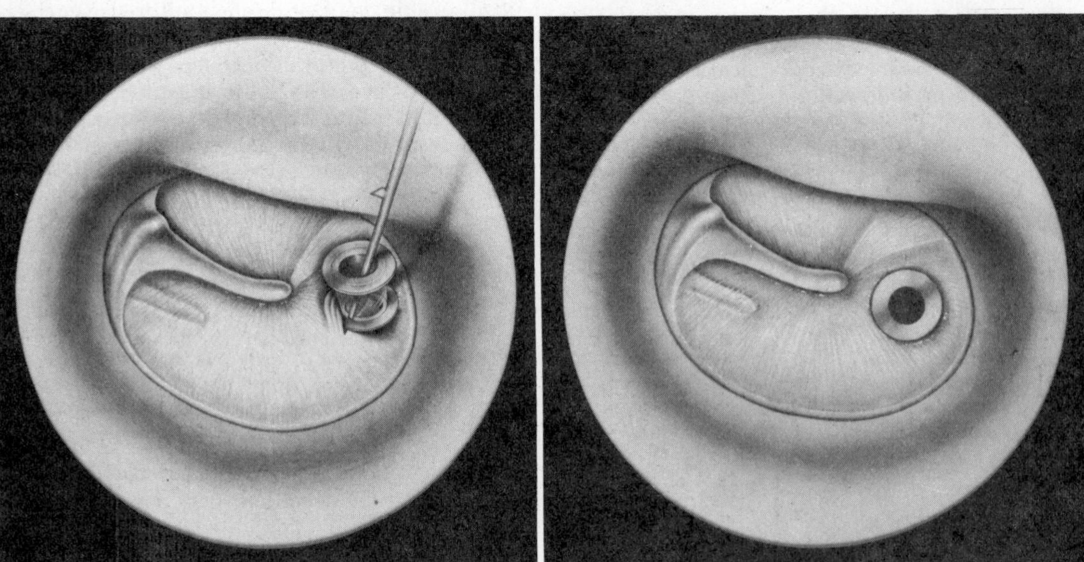

FIGURE 106–8. Insertion of Sheehy Button (left), and button in place (right). (From Paparella, M. M., and Shumrick, D. A.: *Otolaryngology.* Vol. II. 1973.)

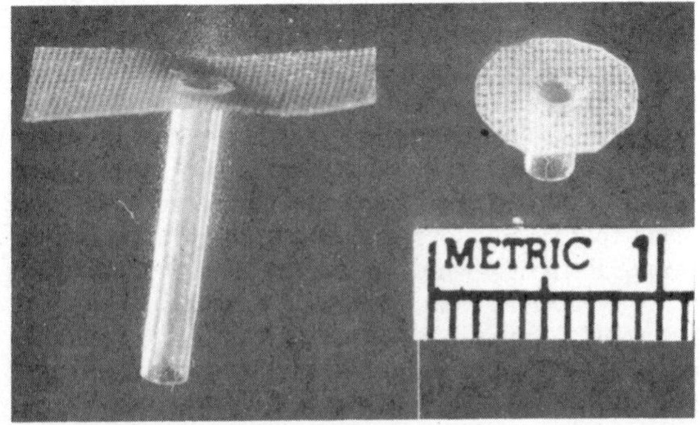

FIGURE 106-9. Silastic tube with siliconized Teflon mesh flange. The tube on the right has been trimmed for use. (Crabtree, J. A.: *Otolaryngologic Clinics of North America 3*:61-65, 1970.)

allergy, and treatment of nasal or sinus infections. Because hearing loss can result from untreated recurrent serous otitis media, the patient requires early treatment and follow-up supervison.

Suppurative (Purulent) Otitis Media. Normally the middle ear is sterile. An acute suppuration (pus formation) occurs when virulent bacteria enter the middle ear. Infections and inflammations of the middle ear are caused by spread of infection, via the eustachian tube, from the nose and nasopharynx. Occasionally the middle ear may become infected following traumatic perforation of the eardrum. Middle ear infection may follow measles, mumps, influenza, scarlet fever, pneumonia, or the common cold. Otitis media most commonly occurs in infants and young children because during the early stages of life the straight position of the eustachian tube favors the conduction of infection into the middle ear. Otitis media may also result from improper, forceful blowing of the nose (forcing infected material into the middle ear) and from swimming in contaminated water (if the water gains entrance to the middle ear.

Acute suppurative otitis media is characterized primarily by severe deep throbbing ear pain. Other symptoms include fever, deafness, chills, slight dizziness, nausea, vomiting, and a feeling of fullness and pressure in the ear. If unruptured, the tympanic membrane is fiery red and bulging. If the eardrum ruptures, discharge is found in the ear canal, and after the canal is cleaned a pulsing discharge may be seen coming from the perforation. Discharge from the ear is called "*otorrhea.*" ("Otorrhagia" refers to hemorrhage from the ear.) Usually the white count is increased. Culture of the drainage identifies the infecting organism. Hearing tests show a conductive hearing loss. Possible *complications* which can result from extension of the disease into adjacent structures include mastoiditis, periostitis, meningitis, lateral sinus thrombosis, brain abscess, labyrinthitis, and facial nerve paralysis.

Treatment of acute suppurative otitis media includes both local and systemic measures. Systemic treatment includes bedrest and systemic antibiotics. Antibiotics are given in full dosage, and the patient is instructed to take the prescribed medication for as long as it is ordered, even though the symptoms of the infection may have disappeared. Inadequate treatment results if the full course of antibiotics is not taken. Penicillin is the drug of choice. If sensitivity to penicillin is known to be present, the patient may be given sulfonamides, erythromycin, tetracyclines, or broad-spectrum antibiotics. Usually antibiotics are continued for at least 6 days to minimize the possibility of recurrence of an incompletely resolved infection after a latent period. Antibiotics are continued in full dosage until the ear is dry, the eardrum looks normal, and hearing is normal. Nasal decongestants (systemic and topical) help restore function of the eustachian tube. After rupture or myringotomy, sterile cotton is loosely placed in the outer ear to prevent the discharge from infecting the skin of the face and neck and the ear lobule. Usually medication for pain relief is not necessary once the eardrum has ruptured or has been lanced. However, if analgesics are required, codeine or acetylsalicylic acid may be ordered. Sometimes local cold applications relieve pain. Generally eardrops are of limited value. Local heat may be ordered to speed up resolution. Usually fluids are forced if the patient is febrile and is not vomiting or nauseated.

With modern chemotherapy, acute otitis media seldom reaches a highly painful stage. If it does, the condition usually resolves if it is adequately treated with antibiotics and myringotomy. Myringotomy is important when the infection does not promptly resolve or when bulging of the eardrum indicates that a discharge is present and is under pressure. Additional indications for myringotomy include continued pain or fever, increasing hearing loss, or vertigo. If complicating mastoiditis develops, it usually does so in cases which have received no treatment or in those inadequately treated. It is important to examine the ears and test hearing following otitis media to prevent persistent conductive hearing loss. Persistent conductive hearing loss (with or without fluid in the middle ear) may occur following incomplete resolution of the infection.

Chronic suppurative otitis media is usually preceded by neglected or recurrent acute otitis media and acute mastoiditis. *With chronic infection of the middle ear there is a permanent perforation of the eardrum.* Eventually a chronic change occurs in the mucosa of the ear, or the periosteum covering the ossicles is destroyed. Usually chronic suppurative ottitis media also produces a small, undeveloped, and acellular mastoid. Chronic suppurative middle ear infection occurs most commonly in persons who had ear disease in early childhood.

Chronic suppurative otitis media is characterized by recurrent painless discharge from the ear. The discharge may be foul-smelling or nearly odorless, and frequently worsens with upper respiratory infections. Hearing loss is always present. Pain or vertigo may indicate impending complications, e.g., pus under pressure, irritation of dura, brain abscess, irritation, or erosion of labyrinth.

A *cholesteatoma* is a special, chronic condition of the middle ear which is formed by squamous epithelium which has grown through the perforated ear drum. The epithelium grows into the middle ear from the external auditory canal. The cystic mass (which forms in the tympanum, epitympanum, and mastoid antrum) is lined with squamous epithelium and is filled with desquamating debris which frequently includes cholesterol. Over a period of years bony destruction can erode important adjacent structures.

Treatment of chronic suppurative otitis media may be medical or surgical or both. *Medical treatment* consists of such measures as (a) carefully cleaning the ear with cotton and the careful removal of granulation tissue, polyps, and visible cholesteatomas to allow medications to more effectively reach the areas of infection; (b) blowing various powders into the middle ear (performed by the physician); (c) instilling eardrops containing topical antibiotics and corticosteroids and urea peroxide to help eliminate fetid discharge, break up debris, and promote healing; (d) systemic administration of an appropriate antibiotic if the organism is known or if an acute exacerbation occurs in a chronically infected ear; and (e) instillation of dilute aluminum acetate solution into the ear as drops.

The *surgical treatment* of chronic suppurative otitis media may involve a *radical mastoidectomy* or a *modified radical mastoidectomy* if there is evidence of continued suppuration, mastoiditis, or other complications. If a cholesteatoma is present, it is surgically removed as is all diseased tissue. Frequently it is desirable to attempt to reconstruct the sound-conducting mechanism in an effort to restore the hearing loss. Examples of such reconstructive operations are *myringoplasty* (repair of defects such as perforation of the tympanic membrane), and *tympanoplasty* (rebuilding of the middle ear structures or replacement of these structures with prostheses).

The possible complications of chronic suppurative otitis media are similar to those mentioned earlier for the acute form of this middle ear disorder. In the absence of pain or symptoms of complications, the local medical therapy of chronic suppurative otitis media may continue for months or years. Generally systemic antibiotics are not helpful unless there is a superimposed acute process.

Serious infections of the middle ear are preventable with early medical treatment of ear disorders. *Ear aches should always be professionally treated* as should other symptoms of disorders of the ear. Fortunately severe ear infections and their serious complications occur less commonly today than previously. This reduced incidence is attributable to improved treatment of acute inections, e.g., with antibiotics, and improved methods of follow-up evaluation. Because antibiotic therapy may mask symptoms, the patient should be periodically evaluated by the otologist. All new symptoms should be promptly investigated. The virulence of the infecting organism, the patient's state of resistance, and the presence or absence of the organisms' resistance to chemotherapy are all factors influencing a patient's response to therapy.

Death from ear infections commonly occurred prior to the development of antimicrobial medications. Patients who did survive an ear infection often were left with extensive damage to the ear. Currently infections of the ear can usually be effectively treated before the ear is severly damaged. However, serious sequelae may develop if ear infections do not receive early, thorough treatment. Inadequate treatment with antibiotics results in the development of drug-resistant microorganisms which then make resolution of the infection problematical. Following some procedures, e.g., tympanoplasties, infection caused from resistant organisms may be treated by instilling topical antibiotics into a small catheter placed in the wound.

Mastoiditis. "Mastoiditis" refers to inflammation of the mastoid antrum and mastoid cells, usually by direct extension from a middle ear infection. *Acute* mastoiditis, a complication of acute suppurative otitis media, seldom occurs since chemotherapeutic treatment has become available for otitis media. When it does occur, however, bony necrosis of the mastoid process and breakdown of the bony intercellular structure occur in the second and third weeks of the acute suppurative otitis media infection. Drainage continues from the ear, and there is evidence of mastoid tenderness and of bone destruction on x-ray examination. Also, there are systemic manifestations of illness, such as fever and headache. If the ear ache is severe, analgesics and an ice bag may be ordered for pain relief. Possible *complications* include paralysis of facial muscles, meningitis, epidural or brain abscess, sigmoid sinus thrombosis, suppurative labyrinthitis, and subperiosteal abscess.

Before sulfonamides and antibiotics, the *treatment* of acute mastoiditis almost always was surgical. Currently the disease may be cured with wide myringotomy and massive doses of antibiotics if only clouding of the mastoid air cells and early decalcification of bone are visible. However, a *simple mastoidectomy* must be surgically performed if bone destruction is apparent.

Chronic mastoiditis is a complication of chronic suppurative otitis media. Usually antibiotics are of limited usefulness in clearing chronic infection of the mastoid, but they may help treat complications. The presence of a cholesteatoma in the middle ear or mastoid, paralysis of the facial nerve, and/or evidence of labyrinthine irritation are indications for radical or modified radical mastoidectomy or tympanoplasty. Other therapy is local cleansing of the ear and instillation of antibiotic powders or solutions, as previously discussed for chronic purulent otitis media.

Otosclerosis. Otosclerosis is the formation of spongy bone in the capsule of the labyrinth of the ear. Dystrophy occurs in the bony labyrinth, and normal bone is replaced by highly vascular otosclerotic bone which tends to grow over the normal bony labyrinth. As the otosclerotic bone advances in growth, it causes progressive *fixation of the footplate of the stapes,* eventually locking it in the oval window. Normally as the footplate of the stapes rocks in the oval window, sound pressure is transmitted directly to the perilymph of the inner ear. With obstruction of the oval window (by an ankylosed stapedial footplate), hearing by air condition is reduced, since there is ineffective displacement of the hair cells.

> *Otosclerosis is the most common cause of conductive deafness.*

While otosclerosis generally produces pure conductive hearing loss, it can cause a mixed hearing loss or a sensorineural hearing loss if the condition involves neural elements. The loss of hearing typically first occurs in the late teens or early twenties. Usually the patient notices difficulty hearing softly spoken tones. Tinnitus may occur. Otosclerosis appears to have hereditary tendency and affects women more than men. Five million persons in the United States are estimated to have otosclerosis.

Audiometric testing is used to diagnose otosclerosis. A tuning fork test demonstrates that bone conduction is greatly superior to air conduction.

Patients with otosclerotic deafness may be advised to try to improve their hearing by the use of a hearing aid or to undergo surgery on the ear. A hearing aid is least effective if there is sensorineural involvement. Surgical procedures may improve the patient's hearing in the presence of otosclerosis if cochlear function is normal. Surgical procedures used on the otosclerotic ear include fenestration, stapes mobilization, and stapedectomy (most common).

DISORDERS OF THE INNER EAR

Inner ear disorders are frequently due to circulatory problems. The following conditions may produce disturbances in the inner ear mechanism:[17] (a) suppurative labyrinthitis, arising primarily from acute or chronic otitis media; (b) cochlear otosclerosis; (c) trauma associated with brain concussion; (d) cardiovascular diseases, e.g., arteriosclerosis, vasomotor disturbances; (e) congenital malformations; (f) allergy (a possible cause of Ménière's disease): (g) endogenous or exogenous toxins, including ototoxic medications (e.g., kanamycin, neomycin, streptomycin, dihydrostreptomycin, nitrofurantoin, acetylsalicylic acid), and bacterial products from foci of infection; (h) blood dyscrasias; and (i) aging. Usually disorders of the inner ear are difficult to treat.

Typical symptoms of labyrinthine disease include deafness, tinnitus, vertigo, nausea, and vomiting. Other symptoms may include blurred vision, nystagmus, past-pointing, and a tendency to fall in a certain direction. *Ménière's disease* is a common labyrinthine disorder; it is discussed in Unit VIII. *Acute labyrinthitis* also is discussed in Unit VIII.

Inner ear deafness is of the sensorineural type.

As mentioned previously, this type of hearing loss typically cannot be improved with hearing aids or surgery. Many cases of nerve deafness result from intense noise, especially with high frequency components.

AURAL SURGICAL PROCEDURES

Included in this section are discussions of (a) paracentesis of the middle ear (needle aspiration, myringotomy); (b) mastoidectomies (simple, radical, modified radical); (c) tympanoplasties (including myringoplasty); (d) stapedectomy; (e) stapes mobilization; and (f) fenestration. The indications for these various procedures have been discussed throughout the chapter. Comments concerning the general care of the patient having aural surgery also have been presented; these aspects of clinical care are not repeated in this section.

Unfortunately, surgical procedures performed for the purpose of restoring or improving hearing are not always successful. Rarely the patient's hearing is even worsened by the surgical intervention. The physician preoperatively discusses with each patient the surgical risk.

PARACENTESIS

Draining fluid from the middle ear is called "paracentesis." This may be accomplished by needle aspiration or by an incision of the tympanic membrane (myringotomy).

Needle Aspiration. Needle paracentesis of the middle ear is performed with a 2-ml. syringe and a short-bevel 10-gauge needle. After the tympanic membrane is punctured with the needle, the fluid is withdrawn into the syringe.

Myringotomy. Myringotomy is in incision made in the tympanic membrane to relieve pressure and pus in the middle ear. Although still performed, this procedure is less commonly necessary now due to antibiotic therapy. Myringotomy is always performed if spontaneous rupture of the eardrum appears likely, because a ruptured eardrum may heal with scar tissue which can impair healing. Usually a myringotomy heals rapidly with only slight scarring and does not affect hearing. Lay persons often incorrectly believe myringotomy causes hearing loss.

To perform a myringotomy the physician needs good light, a head mirror, an aural speculum, and a myringotomy knife with a *very sharp* blade. The physician may elect to incise the eardrum under general anesthesia, local anesthesia, or no anesthesia. Local anesthesia may be obtained by moistening a small piece of cotton with Bonain's solution and placing it against the eardrum for 5 minutes. Myringotomy is carefully performed to avoid injuring the middle ear's medial wall. The incision is best made posteriorly and inferiorly, where no ossicles can be injured and the eardrum can be easily seen. A suction tip may be used to remove fluid from the middle ear after the incision is made. Cultures of the fluid may be taken. Following myringotomy drainage may continue for several days. Usually antibiotics are continued for several days following termination of drainage.

After myringotomy has been performed, the following aspects of care are important:

> *Maintain free drainage.* The physician may order eardrops to enhance drainage. Do not stuff plugs of cotton into the ear canal.
> *Keep external ear dry and clean.* A small piece of sterile cotton may be loosely placed in the external ear to absorb some drainage. Replace this cotton when it becomes moist to minimize possible secondary infection. Dry wipes may be ordered to remove excess drainage. Cleanse external ear frequently as ordered. To prevent excoriation of the skin from the drainage, apply petrolatum around the external ear.
> *Prevent contamination from the ear drainage.* Because the discharge may be infectious, wash after giving ear care.
> *Prevent infection of the wound.* Wash prior to caring for the ear and use only sterile cotton.
> *Observe for and report symptoms of complications,* e.g., headache, temperature elevation, disorientation, increasing ear pain (sometimes myringotomy must be performed again).

MASTOIDECTOMIES

Three types of mastoidectomy are simple, radical, and modified radical. These procedures are summarized below:

> *Simple mastoidectomy:* Performed through postaural (behind ear) or endaural (from ear canal) incision (Fig. 106–10). All necrotic mastoid cells are removed, but an inner table of bone is left intact over the dura. A small drain may be inserted. The middle ear is not disturbed except that a myringotomy is performed to drain the middle ear. Hearing is not affected. Usually complete healing occurs within 7–10 days. Postoperatively antibiotics are continued.
> *Radical mastoidectomy:* Performed through postaural or endaural incision. All mastoid air cells are removed, then the posterior wall of the external auditory canal is removed. Next the remnants of the eardrum, the ossicles (except the stapes), and all of the middle ear's mucosa are removed. The stapes is left in position to protect the entrance to the inner ear. The tensor tympani muscle is removed, and the middle ear orifice of the eustachian tube is cleaned of infected mucosa. Thus the middle ear and mastoid space are converted into one cavity. The cavity which results heals within 2–3 months by ingrowth of epithelium from the skin of the external canal. In some cases grafts of skin, fascia, or muscle are made to facilitate closure of the space. If a graft is used, the wound is packed to hold the graft in position and to ensure hemostasis and patency of the external meatus. Eventually the packing is removed postoperatively through the external ear. Following radical mastoidectomy some patients may be able to hear without a hearing aid; others permanently lose hearing in the operated ear.
> *Modified radical mastoidectomy:* Differs from radical mastoidectomy because eardrum and middle ear structures are preserved. Hearing is better than following a radical mastoidectomy. The eardrum is left attached posteriorly to the external auditory canal's skin. Thus the middle ear is sealed from the mastoid cavity.

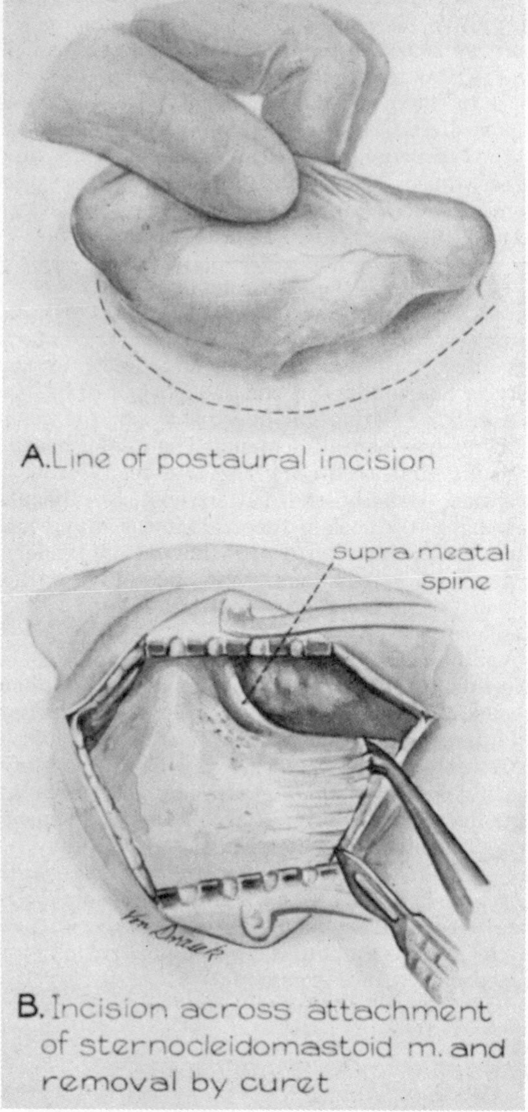

FIGURE 106–10. Incision and exposure for simple mastoidectomy. (From Shambaugh, G. E., Jr.: *Surgery of the Ear.* 2nd ed. 1967.)

Postoperatively following mastoidectomy a firm, bulky dressing is applied over the ear and a circling bandage is placed around the head to hold the ear dressing in place and thus provide hemostasis. Some serosanguineous drainage may seep through the dressing. If this happens, the dressing is reinforced with *sterile* dressings. Such reinforcement prevents contamination of the wound through the damp dressing.

Because mastoid surgery is performed close to the brain, meningitis is a serious possible complication. Sterile dressing technic is essential.

The nurse should not change a mastoid dressing. Usually the physician does this daily or every other day. Report at once the appearance of bright blood on the dressing or any symptoms of possible complications, e.g., stiff neck, excessively tight dressing (from edema), facial paralysis, vomiting, dizziness, disorientation, headache. Postoperative complications include facial nerve injury, meningitis, brain abscess, lateral sinus thrombosis, chronic purulent otitis media, hemorrhage, and wound infection.

Sedatives and analgesics may be ordered for a while postoperatively following mastoidectomy. After radical mastoidectomy, if a graft was taken from the arm or leg, be certain to check the donor site for indications of infection (e.g., temperature elevation, yellow or foul-smelling drainage through dressing) and reinforce the dressing as necessary. Packing may be removed entirely after 3–4 days. Fluids are forced postoperatively as tolerated. Usually the patient is allowed out of bed 24–48 hours after surgery. Vertigo may occur for several days as a disturbance to the inner ear.

Tympanoplasty may be performed with mastoidectomy or following mastoidectomy in an attempt to restore middle ear function. The ear must be free of infection before tympanoplasty is performed.

TYMPANOPLASTIES

"Tympanoplasty" is a term which collectively refers to a variety of reconstructive surgical procedures performed on deformed or diseased middle ear structures. Tympanoplasty may be useful in the presence of defects in the tympanic membrane, necrotic destruction of the ossicles, otosclerosis, stenosis, or the formation of deposits, fibrous or bony plaques, granulomas, or polyps.

Tympanoplastic procedures may include reconstruction of the eardrum, Type I tympanoplasty, also called "myringoplasty," utilization of grafts, removal of scar tissue interfering with ossicle function (see discussion of stapes mobilization); replacement of destroyed or malfunctioning ossicles with prostheses made of plastic or metal (see dis-discussion of stapedectomy; and the formation of "fenestra," i.e., windows or openings (see discussion of fenestration).

Myringoplasties and tympanoplasties involve precise work on minute, delicate structures. Thus, the surgeon requires effective illumination of the operative field and high magnification (obtained with an operating microscope). By reconstructing or preserving the middle ear's conductive mechanism, hearing may be improved or maintained.

Reconstructive procedures on the ear are highly individualized for each patient. A postauricular or an endaural approach may be used. After the middle ear has been exposed and the extent of mechanical derangement has been visualized, the surgeon decides on the method of reconstruction to be used. Materials which may be utilized in the reconstructive process may include grafts (of fascia, skin, or vein), cartilage, bone, perichondrium, silicones, Teflon, and stainless steel wire. The necessary tissues are obtained from the ear itself or from nearby sites. For example, at times a piece of vein from the hand or foot may be placed in the middle ear to create an air channel from the eustachian tube to the round window. In other cases, fresh tissue (a vein, a piece of perichondrium, or fascia) may be used to repair or replace the tympanic membrane and seal off a pocket of air in front of the round window. A sliding skin graft may be fashioned from the ear canal's inner part.

Some tympanoplasties are carried out in two stages. The first operation is performed to remove diseased tissue and to leave the middle ear dry and healed. Next, after the middle ear has been dry for 2–3 months, the reconstructive surgery is performed to restore the conductive mechanism necessary for hearing.

Myringoplasty (Type I Tympanoplasty). A myringoplasty is performed by grafting epithelium from the ear canal, fascia from the temporal muscle, or portions of vein from the hand or forearm to reconstruct the tympanic membrane. Gelfoam soaked in saline may be used to maintain the graft's position against the eardrum, and a gauze strip is placed in the ear canal. Hospitalization is a maximum of 3–4 days. One week after surgery the strip is removed. About 12 days postoperatively the Gelfoam and debris may be gently removed from the ear canal with capillary suction. To test the patency of the graft, gentle inflation may be performed.

Postoperative medications typically include antibiotics, Neosporin or Chloromycetin-boric powder topically (eardrops are never used), and an antihistamine medication with an ephedrine derivative. Postoperative care is directed at keeping the graft in place, promoting healing, preventing infection or contamination, e.g., from water, and preventing pressure on the healing drum.

Myringoplasty not only seals off the middle ear cavity (with a graft over the tear or hole in the eardrum) but also improves hearing by restoring the function of the eardrum in sound conduction. Closing the tympanic membrane prevents contamination of the middle ear with water.

Stapedectomy, Stapes Mobilization, Fenestration. Currently stapedectomy is the surgical procedure of choice in the treatment of otosclerosis. However, some physicians attempt a stapes mobilization before a stapedectomy is performed. Stapedectomy is performed, in such a situation, if stapes mobilization is not possible or is unsuccessful. Occasionally fenestration is still advisable.

Summarized below are the major characteristics of fenestration, stapes mobilization, and stapedectomy and some specific possible postoperative complications of each of these surgical procedures.

> *Fenestration:* Bypasses the fixed stapes and creates a new window which serves as a substitute for the immobile oval window. Thus a new pathway for sound is established. *Postoperative complications:* Some patients develop reduced hearing again 6–12 months postoperatively if sterile labyrinthitis develops or if fibrous or bony closure of the new window occurs.
> *Stapes mobilization:* Reestablishes the normal pathway of sound to the cochlea by freeing or remobilizing the fixed stapes. *Postoperative complications:* Approximately half the successful cases develop refixation of the stapes either by healing of the fractured footplate margin or new otosclerotic growth.
> *Stapedectomy:* Reestablishes the normal sound pathway by using various prostheses to replace the stapes (Fig. 106–11). *Postoperative complications:* External otitis, otitis media, or labyrinthitis may develop. Displacement or rejection of the graft or prosthesis is possible. Also, incomplete closure of the oval window may allow perilymph to leak around the prosthesis and into the middle ear. This may cause tinnitus, fluctuating hearing, and/or vertigo. (These are reportable postoperative symptoms.)

FENESTRATION. Although fenestration is seldom performed currently, it is still occasionally employed in an attempt to relieve deafness caused from otosclerosis. The fenestration operation does not alter the disease process but merely creates a new window into the labyrinth. The new window serves the function of the obstructed oval window and bypasses the fixed stapes and immobile oval window. In the fenestration procedure a window is surgically created in the horizontal semicircular canal. This new arrangement restores hearing because it again permits sound pressure to escape in such a manner that it displaces hair cells. (The hair cells must be stimulated by physical distortion or displacement for hearing to take place.)

The patient who is the best candidate for fenestration is one who has lost effective hearing in both ears and who requires hearing improvement to comfortably participate in daily life. A thorough audiometric examination is performed prior to fenestration. Following fenestration 99 per cent of properly selected patients again have serviceable hearing. Postoperative edema temporarily obscures the final possible benefits of the surgery. The patient is told to be prepared to wait 4–6 weeks before the effects of surgery can be determined.

Fenestration is a major surgical procedure usually performed under general anesthesia. During surgery asepsis is essential because the labyrinth's perilymphatic space and the perilymphatic fluid are in direct continuity with the spinal fluid.

Following fenestration *severe vertigo* may be present for 2–4 days, and the patient may be kept on bedrest for 3–4 days. Nausea may also occur, as well as pain upon moving the jaws. Analgesics may help the patient eat more comfortably. Postoperatively position the patient as ordered (usually on his back or operated side). If positioned on the unoperated side, drainage from the operative area may enter the ear. As the patient's vertigo lessens and as his condition otherwise improves, his activities are gradually increased. The cavity usually heals completely after 6–10 weeks.

STAPES MOBILIZATION. Under magnification the stapes may be mobilized in various ways during surgery. These methods include (a) applying pressure and manipulating various portions of the stapes; (b) prying or chiseling the otosclerotic bone around the footplate of the stapes; and (c) fracturing a portion of the stapes and cutting across the footplate to mobilize the posterior part of the footplate. Stapes mobilization may produce immediate, indeed dramatic, hearing improvement at the time of surgery if good mobilization is obtained. Stapes mobilization requires a briefer hospitalization than fenestration and only minimal postoperative care. Also, it may result in better hearing than that obtained following fenestration. Local anesthesia is usually used.

STAPEDECTOMY. In performing stapedectomy, a local anesthetic and operating microscope are used to remove the otosclerotic lesion at the footplate of the stapes and to insert a tissue implant and prosthesis. Prostheses used to replace the stapes may be fashioned of vein grafts and polyethylene tubes, wire and fat, wire and Gelfoam, or wire and Teflon. The opening in the oval window may be closed by the vein graft, fat, or Gelfoam. One end of the prosthesis is attached to the incus, the other to the graft or plug, to transmit sound to the inner ear. After surgery the ear is packed.

The success of stapedectomy cannot be determined during the immediate postoperative period. Following stapedectomy the patient's hearing is affected for a while due to postoperative edema and packing in the ear. Unless these reasons for diminished hearing are explained to the patient, he may be worried about why his hearing is not as effective immediately following surgery as it initially was in the operating room. Usually the ear packing is removed on the fifth or sixth day after surgery. Once the packing is removed the patient may be instructed to gently place a piece of cotton loosely in the meatus (not into the ear canal) to protect the ear for a few days. Be certain to tell the patient to change the cotton once or twice each day.

Usually the patient is off work for about 2 weeks and is hospitalized 4–5 days. The physician discusses postoperative restrictions with the patient. To prevent the prosthesis from moving out of place, the patient may be advised not to fly if he has an upper respiratory infection and not to engage in deep-water diving. With these exceptions, normal activities are usually permitted once the ear has healed, e.g., swimming and showering are allowed.

REHABILITATION OF THE HARD-OF-HEARING OR DEAF INDIVIDUAL

An estimated 10 per cent of our population has some degree of hearing loss.[5] Hearing impairments occur in varying degrees. Persons with slight or

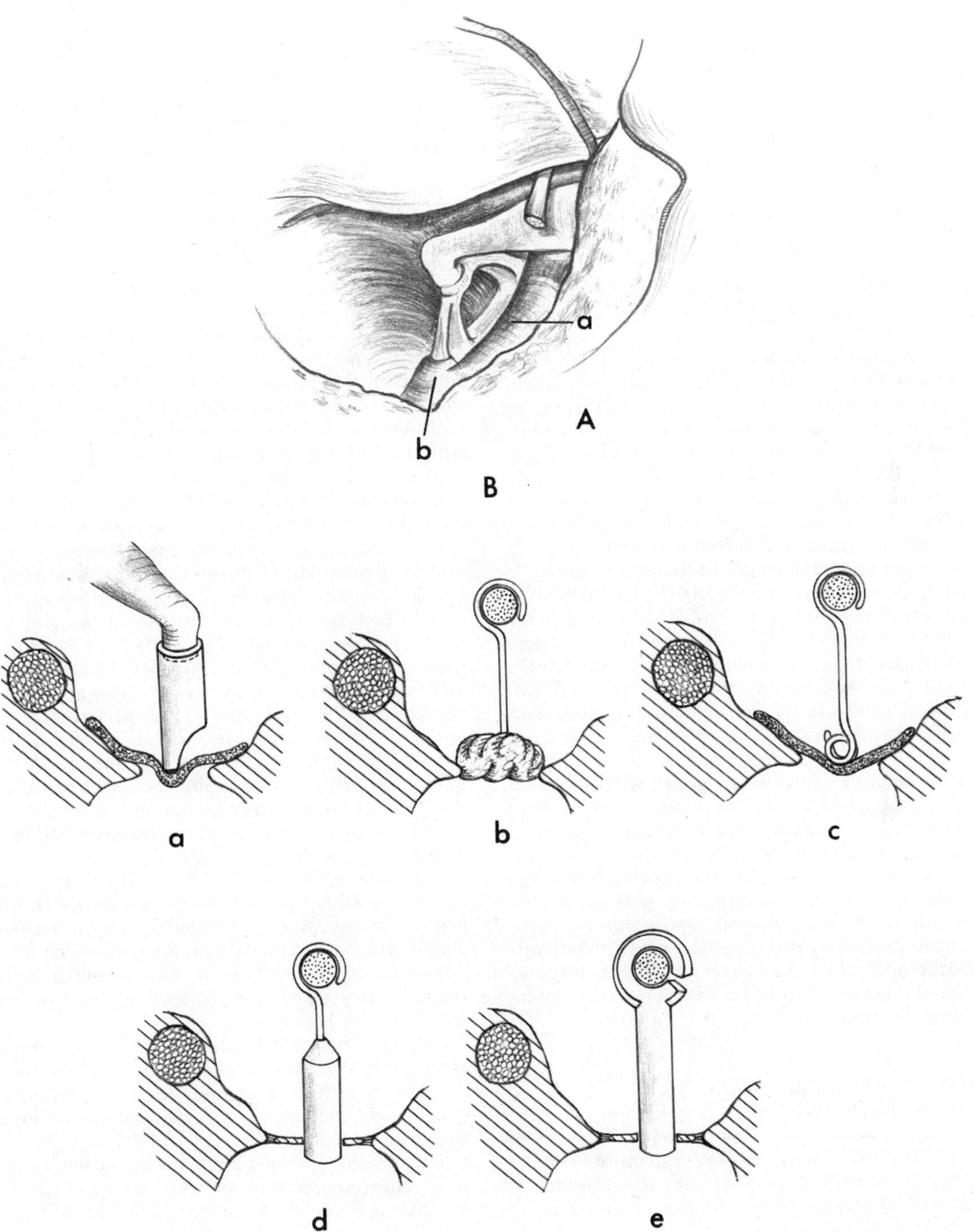

FIGURE 106–11. Stapedectomy. *A,* Adequate footplate exposure is achieved when (a) facial canal and (b) pyramidal process are seen. *B,* Stapedectomy prosthesis (a) vein-polyethylene strut (Shea); (b) wire fat (Schuknecht) (connective tissue preferred by author); (c) wire on compressed Gelfoam (House); (d) wire Teflon piston; (e) Teflon piston (Shea). (From Paparella, M. M., and Shumrick, D. A.: *Otolaryngology.* Vol. II. 1973.)

moderate hearing loss are often refered to as *"hard-of-hearing,"* while those with severe hearing loss are termed *"deaf."* Technically, "hard-of-hearing" persons are those whose hearing is defective but is serviceable with or without a hearing aid, while "deaf" persons have hearing which is nonfunctional for ordinary life.

RECOGNIZING THE NEED FOR HELP

The nurse can do much to identify persons with impaired hearing and to encourage them to seek professional diagnosis and treatment. Indications of impaired hearing include (a) excessive loudness or softness of speech; (b) abnormal awareness of sounds (dulled awareness or heightened awareness); (c) a strained facial expression or tilt of the head when listening; (d) the need for frequent clarification of conversation or inappropriate interpretation of the content of conversation; or (e) apparent inattentiveness or lack of response when spoken to.

Persons with hearing loss should not be falsely encouraged about the possible benefits of surgery or hearing aids. Professional evaluation of hearing loss is always necessary so that correct advice may be obtained about a person's individual disorder.

Often the person with difficulty in hearing tries to conceal his problem. He may refuse to acknowledge the need for professional help even when others mention that the need is obvious. Attempts at self-diagnosis and self-treatment may cause the hard-of-hearing person to try "quack cures" or fraudulent devices. The patient may buy a hearing aid without finding out the cause of his hearing loss or whether or not a hearing aid is necessary or will help. Perhaps the patient's reduction in hearing is merely caused by accumulated ear wax which is plugging the ear canal and can be easily removed; or perhaps the loss of hearing is the result of irreversible nerve damage and will not be improved with a hearing aid. Only the physician can diagnose the condition. We have previously discussed the medical and surgical methods which may be employed in some cases to improve hearing. Here we focus on other aspects of rehabilitation.

REHABILITATIVE FACILITIES AND PROCEDURES

> *Rehabilitation of the hard-of-hearing or deaf individual is directed at obtaining maximum use of any remaining hearing ability and teaching the patient more effective use of his senses of vision, touch, and vibrations.*

Rehabilitation is affected by a patient's age and the severity of his impairment. Rehabilitation is more difficult if the patient is older and has some visual reduction. Infants and children with hearing disorders require the rehabilitative efforts of specialists who help them to learn and to communicate. (Technically the process is one of *"habilitation"* rather than rehabilitation if the infant is born deaf or acquires deafness in early childhood and thus is unable to normally develop speech and language.) Rehabilitative or habilitative problems are compounded for the deaf-blind and deaf-retarded; however, if given appropriate help, the talents of these individuals can also be developed.

Special educational facilities are available for the deaf. Instructors are professional persons especially trained to work with the deaf. These settings have equipment designed to enhance communication with the deaf, e.g., earphones, microphones.

Successful rehabilitation of the adult requires the patient's acceptance of the fact that his hearing is impaired and that he needs help. As with other forms of rehabilitation, those patients who are the most successful are those who work diligently as directed and who have a high degree of motivation.

A careful, complete evaluation of the patient's abilities and disabilities is the first step in the rehabilitative process. Part of this evaluation is the administration of thorough audiometric studies, including a hearing aid evaluation. If useful, a suitable *hearing aid* is selected.

The deaf and hard-of-hearing must learn various compensatory technics to offset the effects of their disability. *Speech-reading* (also called "lip-reading") is one of these technics. Speech-reading is the ability to understand speech through observation of lip and tongue movements, facial expression, gestures, and body movements. *Sign language* is another tool which makes possible fluent communication by means of hand signals. The technic of sign language (e.g., the various hand signals which represent different letters of the alphabet, words, and so forth) is taught by specialists. Not all deaf persons are capable of learning sign language. However, it is highly rewarding for those who can. Sometimes the entire family learns sign language and communicates in this way in the presence of the deaf family member.

Patients with hearing disabilities may have speech problems which need correction through *speech therapy*. Speech problems develop when the deaf individual cannot hear his own voice or the voices of others (to mimic their sounds). Speech training may be directed at developing or conserving speech or both.

As mentioned, any hearing ability which remains is capitalized upon in the rehabilitative process. *Auditory training* is another aspect of rehabilitation which emphasizes speech discrimination and listening skills.

The employable person with impaired hearing may require *vocational training* as part of his rehabilitation. Some deaf persons have the additional problems of poor balance (resulting from damage to the inner ear's vestibular portion) and unusual sensitivity to noise (even though hearing is inadequate for normal conversation). Consideration is given to the presence of these problems in selecting appropriate work for a deaf individual.

The deaf individual may additionally benefit by having a *specially trained dog* which, in effect, serves as "ears" for his master (in the way that seeing-eye dogs serve as "eyes" for the blind). The dog is trained not to go forward or step off a curb if he hears an approaching sound (e.g., a car or siren). Also, in the home the dog gains his master's attention when someone knocks at the door or rings the doorbell or when the telephone rings.

Numerous *local and national agencies* are available which offer a variety of services for persons with impaired hearing. A social worker, the nurse, or the doctor may inform the patient of those agencies appropriate to help meet his needs. A few agencies concerned with hearing disorders are summarized below:

> *National Association of Hearing and Speech Agencies* (919 18th St. N.W., Washington, D.C. 20006): provides information and counseling.

> *The National Association for the Deaf* (2495 Shattuck Ave., Berkeley, California 94704): assists deaf individuals and groups of deaf persons with employment, education, and legislation. The *Silent Worker* is its monthly publication.

> *The Deafness Research Foundation* (366 Madison Ave., Suite 1010, New York, N.Y. 10017): conducts research of hearing impairments.

> *American Foundation of the Physically Handicapped, Inc.* (1370 National Press Bldg., Washington, D.C. 20004): provides information and counseling.

> *Alexander Graham Bell Association for the Deaf, Inc.* (1537 35th N.W., Washington, D.C. 20007): serves as information center for persons working with the deaf and promotes welfare of the deaf. The association has a "Volta Bureau" which has a large collection of books on deafness. The *Volta Review* is its monthly journal.

> *American Hearing Society* (919 18th St., N.W., Washington, D.C. 20036): has local chapters in many cities which provide educational literature and information, and have employment bureaus and social clubs. Assistance may also be given with speechreading and correct use of hearing aids. The *Hearing News* is its bimonthly periodical.

> *John Tracy Clinic* (807 West Adams Blvd., Los Angeles, California 90007): provides information and has correspondence classes for parents with deaf children.

> *The American Speech and Hearing Association* (930 Old Georgetown Road, Bethesda, MD. 20014): membership is of professional persons who teach individuals having speech and hearing disorders. Publishes *The Journal of Speech and Hearing Disorders* and *The Journal of Speech and Hearing Research.*

> *Veterans Administration* has audiology clinics in various cities for eligible veterans. Advise eligible veterans to contact their local Veterans Administration regional office for information on hearing rehabilitation.

> *State Offices of Vocational Rehabilitation* in the various states have employment and rehabilitation services which are helpful in vocational training and placement.

HEARING AIDS

The otologist determines whether a patient's hearing can be improved medically, surgically, or mechanically (with a hearing aid). Hearing aids can help some deaf or hard-of-hearing individuals to reestablish or maintain communication. A hearing aid is any kind of mechanical or electrical device which improves hearing. While hearing aids may improve a patient's hearing, they never restore hearing to a normal level; hearing aids amplify sound but do not improve the ear's ability to hear.

Patients with middle ear problems usually do well with a hearing aid. Patients with nerve damage, on the other hand, may be advised to rent a hearing aid for a month before purchasing one, to be certain that the hearing aid will actually be helpful. Amplification from a hearing aid may be uncomfortable in the presence of sensorineural hearing loss (i.e., nerve damage), because with this disorder there are typically intolerance for loud sounds, hearing loss in the higher frequencies, and difficulty in understanding speech. Frequently older persons have sensorineural hearing losses. With some types of hearing loss an *ear trumpet* actually provides the best type of amplification.

Speech audiometry is useful in prescribing an appropriate hearing aid. If the hearing aid selected is suitable for the patient's needs and is properly fitted, used, and maintained, it may add greatly to his pleasure.

The retail cost of hearing aids is a deterrent for some persons. The cost may exceed $600 if both ears require a hearing aid. Additionally there are maintenance costs.

Electric hearing aids have the following parts to properly amplify sound: (a) a microphone to convert sound waves into electric energy; (b) an amplifier; (c) a receiver to convert electric energy back into sound waves; and (d) a power source (batteries or transistors) to run the system.

While a variety of electric hearing aids are available, they are of two basic types: (1) *bone conduction receivers* (worn behind the ear against the skull); and (2) *air conduction receivers* (worn in a mold made to fit into the auditory canal). The design of hearing aids was formerly conspicuous and bulky. Today, hearing aids are frequently inconspicuous and small. Reductions in the size and weight of these instruments are possible due to the use of transistors in place of vacuum tubes. The size and design of a patient's hearing aid is determined by the nature of his specific disorder.[17]

Whatever type of hearing aid is prescribed, the patient needs instruction and psychologic preparation for its use. The patient is taught about his particular instrument: its use, maintenance, what to do if it doesn't work, and what it will and will not do. It may take several months for the patient to learn how to obtain maximum benefit from his aid.

Hearing aids have adjustable tone and volume controls. Several adjustments may be necessary before the aid is correctly set for the individual's needs. Initially the person wearing a hearing aid may find that amplified background noises are disturbing. The aid is not selective in amplifying sounds; it amplifies background noises as well as those sounds which the wearer wants to concentrate on. The problem of amplified background noise is alleviated somewhat by wearing hearing aids in both ears, i.e., *binaural aids.* Binaural hearing aids may be build into the stems of eyeglasses.

Some sources recommend that the patient initially wear his hearing aid for only short periods of time. By gradually lengthening the time the aid is worn, the patient can become accustomed to his "new world of sound."

Instruct the patient who wears a hearing aid to handle the instrument carefully. The ear mold should be washed daily in soap and water. A pipe cleaner or small applicator is used to clean the cannula. The mold is snapped into the receiver after it is thoroughly dry. It is advisable to carry an extra cord and battery.

If the hearing aid fails to work: (a) the on-off switch is checked; (b) the ear mold is cleaned; (c) the battery position is checked; (d) the cord plug-in is checked; (e) the cord is inspected for breaks; and (f) a new battery and new cord are tried. If these activities do not correct the mechanism, if must be taken to a local service agency.

It is not uncommon to meet people who are reluctant to wear a hearing aid because of cosmetic reasons. These persons require patient counseling about the benefits of the instrument and the fact that improved hearing will add to their social acceptance and pleasure. Wearing the hearing aid notifies others that difficulty in communicating is not necessarily due to an intellectual deficit. A hearing aid may serve the useful additional function of making others aware of the need to speak more clearly. A person's inability to hear may be a social detriment; this hearing impairment cannot be "covered up" by not wearing a hearing aid and "faking" an understanding. The patient needs to realize that a hearing aid actually makes others more comfortable in communicating with him than they are if he does not improve his hearing with the hearing aid. Of course, the patient himself will also be able to lead a more normal life if he takes advantage of the improved hearing which a hearing aid will give him.

The person who has a hearing disorder may find that speech-reading (lip-reading) is useful, even though he wears a hearing aid.

When a hospitalized patient has a hearing aid, it becomes the nurse's responsibility to store the instrument safely when it is not in use. Encourage family members to bring a patient's hearing aid to him if he does not have it with him.

"We could do much to ameliorate the tragedy of deafness if we changed some of our attitudes toward it. Blindness evokes our instant sympathy, and we go out of our way to help the blind person. But deafness often goes unrecognized. If a deaf person misunderstands what we say, we are apt to attribute it to a lack of intelligence instead of to faulty hearing. Very few people have the patience to help the deafened. To a deaf man the outside world appears unfriendly. He tries to hide his deafness, and this only brings on more problems."[45]

While blind people are often pitied, the deaf are frequently reacted to with ridicule and impatience. Perhaps one explanation for such reactions is the fact that generally deafness is not an obvious disability, while blindness is usually readily noticeable.

It is not surprising that the hard-of-hearing or deaf person frequently feels depressed, insecure, and removed from many of life's activities and pleasures. Additionally it is not unusual for him to feel that others are whispering or talking about him, when he observes people talking but cannot understand the conversation.

The individual with a hearing loss loses the multiple benefits of verbal communication and environmental sounds. Hearing loss in the infant and child removes valuable verbal learning clues. Because he cannot hear the speech of others, the deaf child cannot imitate speech patterns and learn to talk. At any age, hearing loss impairs the abilities to protect oneself and to communicate. Environmental sounds not only may be pleasant and help orient us to our surroundings but also may warn of impending danger, e.g., an approaching car.

Hearing helps maintain contact with reality and the environment. The inability to hear may cause disorientation and depression to a suicidal degree. In fact, *deafness may cause more serious emotional difficulties than blindness.* Persons with impaired hearing often tend to withdraw from social contacts. Sometimes this behavior is incorrectly interpreted as "aloofness." The patient may be increasingly excluded from conversation and social gatherings. The more this occurs, the more difficult it becomes for him to once again resume these activities. Friends and family often need help in understanding the feelings, behavior, and needs of a person who has a hearing impairment. The nurse may explain considerations which are important in communicating with such a person. Everyone (including the patient) must *accept the patient's disability* and make necessary adjustments.

In the hospital setting it is important to identify a patient who has difficulty hearing. The nurse then makes a special effort to clearly communicate with the patient. The patient requires additional attention to be certain that he understands important directions and that he understands procedures being performed on him. If he does not know what is happening or what is expected of him, the patient may appear to be uncooperative and resistant to care. Anxiety may reduce even further a patient's ability to hear.[25]

COURTESIES TOWARD THE INDIVIDUAL WITH HEARING LOSS

The following considerations are important in communicating with a person whose hearing is impaired:

- Do not rely on an intercommunication system, as from the nursing station in a hospital, to communicate with the patient. Rather, go to him in person. Then, before speaking gain the patient's attention if he has not seen you enter the room. Try to avoid startling the patient or giving the impression that you are "sneaking up" on him. If the patient wears a hearing aid, give him time to adjust it if necessary before you speak.
- Concentrate on communicating with the patient. Direct your complete attention to what you and the patient are saying and doing. Provide adequate light so the patient can see you clearly, and look directly at the patient when speaking. Speech-reading may help him understand you. Do not cover your mouth and do not eat, smoke, or chew gum when talking (these movements interfere with speech-reading).
- Employ nonverbal cues to help convey your meaning, e.g., facial expressions, hand gestures, writing, pointing.
- It may be helpful to slightly raise your voice. Do not drop your voice at the end of sentences. Speak slowly and distinctly rather than shouting. Excessive loudness distorts the voice and may actually impair understanding. If the patient wears a hearing aid, he is quite sensitive to loud noises and speaking loudly may be uncomfortable as well as ineffective. If necessary, rather than shouting at the patient try speaking to him through a rolled up newspaper or magazine. In some instances the patient may be given a stethoscope to wear while the nurse speaks into the amplifying end of it.
- When telling something to a person whose hearing is impaired, first state the major topic of discussion and then go ahead with the details. For example: "Breakfast. (pause) Do you want eggs or cereal?"
- Be calm and patient if the person cannot understand you. If he does not appear to understand you, use different words to restate your message. Some words are more easily understood than others. If it is necessary to introduce new or unfamiliar words, pronounce them carefully or write them out. Remember that many medical and nursing words are unfamiliar to patients. If you remain uncertain about whether your message is understood, always write out your statement. Keep paper and pen or a magic slate placed close to the patient for this purpose.
- If the patient speaks too loudly help him learn to properly modulate his voice. Tactfully tell him he is speaking too loudly and encourage him to try again.
- If the deaf person also has a speech disorder, attempt to understand the main message of what he is saying. After you have identified the main message, it then becomes easier to recognize associated details. If you do not understand the patient's communication, do not act as if you have understood. Ask for clarification. It may be necessary for him to write out his message.
- Encourage the patient's attempts to compensate for his hearing loss. Give appropriate praise.

References for Unit XXI

The Eye

1. A cataract is not necessarily a calamity. *Health 9*:10, March, 1972.
2. *A Glimpse of Vision.* (Pamphlet) Guide Dogs for the Blind, Inc., San Rafael, California, 94902.
3. Abrahamson, I.A., Jr.: Chalazion. *GP 38:*83, July, 1968.
4. Allen, H. F.: The eye. *In* Nardi, G. L., and Zuidema, G. D. (eds.): *Surgery.* 2nd ed. Boston; Little, Brown and Company, 1965.
5. Allen, J. H.: *May's Manual of the Diseases of the Eye.* 24th ed. Baltimore, Williams & Wilkins Company, 1968.
6. American Foundation for the Blind: *Directory of Agencies Serving Blind Persons in the United States.* 15th ed. New York; The William Byrd Press, Inc., 1967.
7. Barsam, P. C.: Specific prophylaxis of gonorrheal ophthalmia neonatorum: A review. *New England Journal of Medicine 274:*731, March 31, 1966.
8. Bartlett, R. E.: Plastic surgery for the enucleation patient. *American Journal of Ophthalmology 61*:68, 1966.
9. Bellows, J. G.: Understanding cataracts. *AORN Journal 7*:64, May, 1968.
10. Bergersen, B. S.: *Pharmacology in Nursing.* 12th ed. St. Louis; C. V. Mosby Co., 1973.
11. Bixler, D. P.: Bacterial decontamination and cleaning of contact lenses. *American Journal of Ophthalmology 62:*324, August, 1966.
12. Bledsoe, C. W., and Williams, R. C.: The vision needed to nurse the blind. *American Journal of Nursing 66:*2432, November, 1966.
13. Bonnett, K.: Adjusting to blindness. *Nursing Mirror 126:*21, February 2, 1968.
14. Bosanko, L.: Patients with corneal transplants. *In* Bergersen, B. S., et al.: *Current Concepts in Clinical Nursing.* St. Louis, C. V. Mosby Co., 1967.
15. Branson, H. K.: Caring for the blind patient. *American Journal of Nursing 63:*98, October, 1963.
16. Bronson, N. R., II: Management of intraocular foreign bodies. *American Journal of Ophthalmology 66:*279, 1968.
17. Buschman, W., and Hauff, D.: Results of diagnostic ultrasonography in ophthalmology. *American Journal of Ophthalmology 63:*926, May, 1967.
18. Cardona, H.: Restoring vision by prosthokeratoplasty. *Nursing Mirror 125*:iv, November 24, 1967.
19. Carr, R. E., and Gouras, P.: Clinical electroretinography. *Journal of the American Medical Association 198:*173, October 3, 1966.
20. Catford, G. V.: Glaucoma. *Nursing Times 63:*968, July 21, 1967.
21. Condl, E. D., et al.: Ophthalmic nursing. *Nursing Clinics of North America 5:*449, September, 1970.
22. Cullin, I. C.: Techniques for teaching patients with sensory defects. *Nursing Clinics of North America 5*:527, September, 1970.
23. Dallas, N. L.: Diseases of the eyelids. *Nursing Mirror 125*:v, July 7, 1967.

24. Delaney, W. V., Jr.: Preventable blindness. *GP 38:* 121, November, 1968.
25. Delaney, W. V., Jr.: Intravitreal saline in retinal detachment. *American Journal of Ophthalmology 74:*241, August, 1972.
26. De Roetth, A., Jr.: Cryosurgery for the treatment of advanced chronic simple glaucoma. *American Journal of Ophthalmology 66:*1034, 1968.
27. Dixon, J. M.: Ocular changes due to contact lenses. *American Journal of Ophthalmology 58:*424, September, 1964.
28. Dixon, J. M., et al.: Complications associated with the wearing of contact lenses. *Journal of the American Medical Association 195:*901, March 14, 1966.
29. Dyer, J. A.: *Atlas of Extraocular Muscle Surgery.* Philadelphia, W. B. Saunders Company, 1970.
30. Emery, J. M., von Noorden, G. K., and Schlernitzauer, D. A.: Management of orbital floor fractures. *American Journal of Ophthalmology 74:*299, August, 1972.
31. Epstein, D. L., and Paton, D.: Keratitis from misuse of corneal anesthetics. *New England Journal of Medicine 279:*396, August 22, 1968.
32. Fass, G. P.: Evaluation of complemental nursing care with cataract and stapedectomy patients. *In* Bergersen, B. S. (ed.): *Current Concepts in Clinical Nursing.* Vol. II. St. Louis, C. V. Mosby Co., 1969.
33. Giffin, R. B., Jr.: Eye damage in newborns from use of strong silver nitrate solutions. *California Medicine 107:*178, August, 1967.
34. Goldfarb, H. J., and Turtz, A. I.: A detergent-lubricant solution for artificial eyes. *American Journal of Ophthalmology 61:*1502, June, 1966.
35. Gordon, R. D.: Experience with a visually disabled mother. *American Journal of Nursing 68:*1943, September, 1968.
36. Grant, W. M.: Ocular complications of drugs: Glaucoma. *Journal of the American Medical Association 207:*2089, March 17, 1969.
37. Guyton, A. C.: *Textbook of Medical Physiology.* 4th ed. Philadelphia; W. B. Saunders Company, 1971, Chaps. 52 to 54.
38. Haddad, H. M.: Drugs for ophthalmic use. *American Journal of Nursing 68:*324, February, 1968.
39. Hamilton, M. J.: What the nurse should know about eye banks. *Nursing Clinics of North America 5:*483, September, 1970.
40. Havener, W. H.: *Synopsis of Ophthalmology.* 3rd. ed. St. Louis, C. V. Mosby Company, 1971.
41. Havener, W. H., and Gloeckner, S. L.: *Atlas of Diagnostic Techniques and Treatment of Retinal Detachment.* St. Louis, C. V. Mosby Company, 1967.
42. Havener, W. H., and Gloeckner, S. L.: *Atlas of Diagnostic Techniques and Treatment of Intraocular Foreign Bodies.* St. Louis, C. V. Mosby Company, 1969.
43. How to Remove Contact Lenses From an Unconscious Person. (Kit.) American Optometric Association, 7000 Chippewa St., St. Louis, Mo. 63119.
44. Hughes, W. F., and Hurt, A. C. Complications after corneal transplantation. *American Journal of Ophthalmology 61:*1171, May, 1966.
45. Jackson, C. R. S.: *The Eye in General Practice.* 5th ed. London; E. & S. Livingstone, Ltd., 1969.
46. Jacob, S. W., and Francone, C. A.: *Structure and Function in Man.* 3rd ed. Philadelphia, W. B. Saunders Company, 1974.
47. Jones, L. T.: The lacrimal secretory system and its treatment. *American Journal of Ophthalmology 62:*47, July, 1966.
48. Knapp, J. W.: Surgical techniques in retinal detachment repair. *Eye, Ear, Nose, Throat Monthly 47:* 584, November, 1968.
49. Knoblock, W. H., and Cibis, P. A.: Retinal detachment surgery with preserved human sclera. *American Journal of Ophthalmology 60:*191, August, 1965.
50. Kornzweig, A. L.: The eye in old age. *American Journal of Ophthalmology 60:*835, November, 1965.
51. Lebensohn, J. E.: Changes in the aging eye. *Postgraduate Medicine 40:*746, December, 1966.
52. Lerman, S.: *Basic Ophthalmology.* New York, McGraw-Hill Book Company, Inc., 1966.
53. Magoon, R. C., and Sexon; R.: Wet or dry contact lens storage. *Archives of Ophthalmology 77:*197, February, 1967.
54. McDonald, L. L.: Are you ready for contact lenses? *Family Health 4:*32, May, 1972.
55. McLean, J. M.: *Atlas of Glaucoma Surgery.* St. Louis, C. V. Mosby Company, 1967.
56. McLean, J. M.: Cryosurgery in ophthalmology. *Archives of Ophthalmology 77:*715, June, 1967.
57. Medical News: Frozen cornea: "A clinical success." *Journal of the American Medical Association 201:*27, August 21, 1967.
58. Medical News: System may let blind "see with their skins." *Journal of the American Medical Association 207:*2204, March 24, 1969.
59. Newell, F. W.: *Ophthalmology: Principles and Concepts.* 2nd ed. St. Louis, C. V. Mosby Company, 1969.
60. Nordstrom, W.: Adjusting to cataract glasses. *American Journal of Nursing 66:*1578, July, 1966.
61. Oerther, B.: The blind patient need not be helpless. *American Journal of Nursing 66:*2436, November, 1966.
62. Ohno, M. I.: The eye-patched patient. *American Journal of Nursing 71:*271, February, 1971.
63. Paton, D., and Goldberg, M. R.: *Injuries of the Eye, the Lids, and the Orbit: Diagnosis and Management.* W. B. Saunders Company, 1968.
64. Peczon, J. D., and Grant, W. M.: Diuretic drugs in glaucoma. *American Journal of Ophthalmology 66:* 680, October, 1968.
65. Rabb, M. F.: The present status of corneal transplantation. *Nursing Clinics of North America 5:*477, September, 1970.
66. Rakusin, W.: Traumatic hyphema. *American Journal of Ophthalmology 74:*284, August, 1972.
67. Riffenburgh, R. S.: The psychology of blindness. *Geriatrics 22:*127, October, 1967.
68. Riffenburgh, R. S.: The blind patient. *Archives of Ophthalmology 79:*361, April, 1968.
69. Rogers, C.: Nursing skills in ophthalmic surgery. *AORN Journal 6:*39, August, 1967.
70. Rosborough, J. F.: Ocular emergencies. *Hospital Medicine 7:*46, November, 1971.
71. Ruben, M.: Contact lenses today. *Nursing Mirror 127:*vi, January 19, 1968.
72. Rubenstein, K.: Ophthalmic cryosurgery. *Nursing Times 63:*1640, December 8, 1967.
73. Rubin, M. L.: Diagnosis and treatment of retinal detachment. *Geriatrics 23:*118, February, 1968.
74. Rycroft, P. V.: Modern trends of corneal grafting and its nursing management. *Nursing Mirror 127:*19, April 5, 1968.

75. Saunders, W. H., et al.: *Nursing Care in Eye, Ear, Nose and Throat Disorders*. 2nd ed. St. Louis, C. V. Mosby Company, 1968.
76. Scheie, H. G., and Albert, D. M.: *Adler's Textbook of Ophthalmology*. Philadelphia, W. B. Saunders Company, 1969.
77. Seaman, F. W.: Nursing care of glaucoma patients. *Nursing Clinics of North America 5:*489, September, 1970.
78. Sellors, P. J. H.: Senile cataract. *Nursing Times 64:* 1337, October, 4, 1968.
79. Shea, M., and Dickson, D.: Thermoelectric retinal cryosurgery. *Canadian Journal of Ophthalmology 1:*138, April, 1966.
80. Silva, D.: Orbital tumors. *American Journal of Ophthalmology 65:*318, March, 1968.
81. Simpson, N. L.: Acrylic implant: A new vision. *Nursing 64:*170 February 9, 1968.
82. Smith, J. F., and Nachazel, D.: Retinal detachment. *American Journal of Nursing 73:*1530, September, 1973.
83. Snyder, J.: Newer concepts in ophthalmic surgery. *Nursing Clinics of North America 3:*539, September, 1968.
84. Starin, I.: Need for routine glaucoma screening by hospitals and physicians. *Public Health Report 81:*12, January, 1966.
85. Sutton, A. L.: *Bedside Nursing Techniques in Medicine and Surgery.* 2nd ed. Philadelphia, W. B. Saunders Company, 1969.
86. Vaughan, D.: Common ocular disorders. *Hospital Medicine 7:*22, October, 1971.
87. Vaughan, D.: Eye. *In* Krupp, M. A., and Chatton, M. J. (eds.): *Current Diagnosis and Treatment.* Los Altos, California, Lange Medical Publications, 1972.
88. Vaughan, D., Cook, R., and Asbury, T.: *General Ophthalmology.* 5th ed. Los Altos, California, Lange Medical Publications, 1968.
89. Walter, J. R., and Fralich, F. B.: Use of Teflon in retinal detachment. *American Journal of Ophthalmology 63:*113, January, 1967.
90. Weinstock, F. J.: Emergency treatment of eye injuries. *American Journal of Nursing 71:*1928, October, 1971.
91. Whyte, D. K.: Blowout fractures of the orbit. *British Journal of Ophthalmology 52:*721, October, 1968.
92. Worthen, D. M., and Brubaker, R. F.: An evaluation of cataract cryoextraction. *Archives of Ophthalmology 79:*8, January, 1968.
93. Yanoff, M.: Ocular pathology of diabetes mellitus. *American Journal of Ophthalmology 67:*21, January, 1969.
94. Zimmerman, L. E.: Changing concepts concerning the malignancy of ocular tumors. *Archives of Ophthalmology 78:*166, August, 1967.
95. Zubek, J. P. (ed.): *Sensory Deprivation: Fifteen Years of Research.* New York, Appleton-Century-Crofts, Inc., 1969.

The Ear

1. Ballenger, J. J.: *Diseases of the Nose, Throat and Ear.* Philadelphia, Lea & Febiger, 1969.
2. Barber, H. O., et al.: The laboratory assessment of anti-motion sickness and anti-vertigo drugs. *Canadian Medical Association Journal 97:*1460, December, 1967.
3. Bender, R. E.: Communication with the deaf. *American Journal of Nursing 66:*757, April, 1966.
4. Brown, R. A.: Noise and urban man. *American Journal of Public Health 68:*2061, November, 1968.
5. Conover, M., and Cober, J.: Understanding and caring for the hearing impaired. *Nursing Clinics of North America 5:*497, September, 1970.
6. Cullin, I. C.: Techniques for teaching patients with sensory defects. *Nursing Clinics of North America 5:*527, September, 1970.
7. Deatsch, W. W.: Ear, nose, and throat. *In* Krupp, M. A., and Chatton, M. J. (eds.): *Current Diagnosis and Treatment.* Los Altos, California, Lange Medical Publications, 1972.
8. De Laney, R. E.: Stapedectomy. *American Journal of Nursing 69:*2406, November, 1969.
9. Denmark, J. C.: Mental illness and early profound deafness. *British Journal of Medical Psychology 39:*117, June, 1966.
10. De Weese, D. D., and Saunders, W. H.: *Textbook of Otolaryngology.* 3rd ed. Saint Louis, C. V. Mosby Company, 1968.
11. Dolowitz, D. A.: An appraisal of genetics in clinical otology. *Annals of Otology, Rhinology and Laryngology 80:*264, April, 1971.
12. Fredrickson, J. M., Kornhuber, H. H., and Goods, R. L.: Nystagmus: Diagnostic significance of recent observations. *Archives of Otolaryngology 89:*504, March, 1969.
13. Gerifacts. *Geriatrics 22:*66, August, 1967.
14. Glorig, A.: The effects of noise on hearing. *Journal of Laryngology and Otology 75:*447, May, 1961.
15. Glorig, A.: The effects of noise on man. *Journal of the American Medical Association 196:*832, June 6, 1966.
16. Hall, I. S., and Colman, B. H.: *Diseases of the Nose, Throat and Ear.* 9th ed. London; E. & S. Livingstone, Ltd., 1969.
17. Holvey, D. N. (ed.): *The Merck Manual.* 12th ed. Rahway, N. J., Merck, Sharp & Dohme Research Laboratories, 1972.
18. Hough, J. V. D.: Restoration of hearing loss after head trauma. *Annals of Otology, Rhinology and Laryngology 78:*210, April, 1969.
19. Hough, J. V. D., and Stuart, W. D.: Middle ear injuries in skull trauma. *Laryngoscope 78:*899, June, 1968.
20. Hughes, R. L.: Special devices for the hearing-handicapped patient. *Archives of Otolaryngology 86:*522, November, 1967.
21. Jaffe, B. F.: Sudden deafness: An otologic emergency. *Archives of Otolaryngology 86:*55, July, 1967.
22. Jerger, J.: Review of diagnostic audiometry. *Annals of Otology, Rhinology, and Laryngology 77:*1042, December, 1968.
23. Juers, A. L.: Non-organic hearing problems. *Laryngoscope 76:*1714, October, 1966.
24. Karmody, C. S.: Asymptomatic maternal rubella and congenital deafness. *Archives of Otolaryngology 89:*720, May, 1969.
25. Klotz, R. E., and Robinson, M.: Hard-of-hearing patients have special problems. *American Journal of Nursing 3:*88, May, 1963.
26. Konigsmark, B. W.: Hereditary congenital severe deafness syndromes. *Annals of Otology, Rhinology and Laryngology 80:*269, April, 1971.
27. Konopa, V. O., et al.: Noise—the challenge of the future. *Journal of School Health 42:*172, March, 1972.
28. Lebo, C. P., et al.: Acoustic trauma from rock-and-roll music. *California Medicine 107:*378, November, 1967.

29. Ludman, H.: Modern surgery of deafness. *Nursing Mirror 134:*36, May 12, 1972.
30. Meadow, K. P.: Self-image, family climate, and deafness. *Social Forces 47:*428, June, 1969.
31. Moore, M. V.: Diagnosis: Deafness. *American Journal of Nursing 69:*297, February, 1969.
32. Morrison, A. W.: Ultrasonic therapy in ear, nose and throat surgery. *Nursing Times 63:*1504, November, 1967.
33. Nilo, E. R.: Needs of the hearing impaired. *American Journal of Nursing 69:*114, January, 1969.
34. Palva, T., Palva, A., and Dammert, K.: Middle ear mucosa and chronic ear disease. *Archives of Otolaryngology 87:*3, January, 1968.
35. Patterson, M. E.: Temporalis fascia in tympanic membrane grafting. *Archives of Otolaryngology 85:*287, March, 1967.
36. Proctor, C. A., and Proctor, B.: Understanding hereditary nerve deafness. *Archives of Otolaryngology 85:*23, January, 1967.
37. Proud, G. O.: Surgery for chronic refractory otitis externa. *Archives of Otolaryngology 83:*436, May, 1966.
38. Sataloff, J.: *Hearing Loss.* Philadelphia, J. B. Lippincott Company, 1966.
39. Saunders, W. H., and Paparella, M. M.: *Atlas of Ear Surgery.* St. Louis, C. V. Mosby Company, 1968.
40. Saunders, W. H., et al.: *Nursing Care in Eye, Ear, Nose and Throat Disorders.* 2nd ed. S. Louis, C. V. Mosby Company, 1968.
41. Schlesinger, H. S.: Beyond the range of sound: The non-otological aspects of deafness. *California Medicine 110:*213, March, 1969.
42. Schuknecht, H. F.: Gelfoam as an implant in oval window following stapedectomy. *Annals of Otology, Rhinology and Laryngology 80:*415, June, 1971.
43. Shambaugh, G. E., Jr.: *Surgery of the Ear.* 2nd ed. Philadelphia, W. B. Saunders Company, 1967.
44. Taylor, G. D., and Williams, E.: Acoustic trauma in the sports hunter. *Laryngoscope 76:*863, May, 1966.
45. von Békésy, G.: The ear. *Scientific American,* August, 1957.
46. Wever, E. G.: The mechanics of hair-cell stimulation. *Annals of Otology, Rhinology and Laryngology. 80*:786, December, 1971.

UNIT XXII

Nursing Patients Experiencing Disturbances of the Nose, Sinuses, Pharynx, and Larynx

Introduction and Study Guide

This unit is divided into three chapters. *Chapter 107* focuses on disorders of the nose and sinuses; *Chapter 108* considers disorders of the pharynx; and *Chapter 109* discusses disorders of the larynx. Anatomy, physiology, and diagnostic procedures are discussed as appropriate in these chapters.

Two highly important areas of clinical care are considered in detail in this unit. These are (1) care of patients with cancer of the larynx; and (2) care of patients with tracheal intubation, i.e., intubation of the airway with a tracheostomy or endotracheal tube. Many of the disorders discussed in this unit occur quite frequently. Often the nurse is asked by friends to give advice about problems affecting these structures, or the nurse may be required to give emergency care in the presence of nosebleeds, aspirated foreign bodies, nasal fracture, or acute laryngeal edema.

Examples of some disorders affecting the nose, sinuses, pharynx (throat), and larynx are summarized below:

> *Disorders of the nose and sinuses:* rhinitis (simple acute rhinitis, allergic rhinitis, nonallergic vasomotor rhinitis); nasal polyps; hypertrophied turbinates; foreign bodies; epistaxis (nosebleed); deviated nasal septum; nasal fracture; infected and hypertrophied adenoids; and acute and chronic sinusitis.

> *Disorders of the pharynx:* acute pharyngitis; acute follicular pharyngitis; diphtheria; chronic pharyngitis; quinsy (peritonsillar abscess); tonsilitis; and aspirated foreign bodies.

> *Disorders of the larynx:* laryngeal spasm; laryngeal edema; laryngeal paralysis; laryngeal injury; laryngitis; and cancer of the larynx.

The following *study guides* may help the reader to more effectively understand disorders of the nose, sinuses, pharynx, and larynx and related aspects of clinical care. To facilitate usage of the study guides, they are divided into three sections: (1) study guide for disorders of the nose and sinuses; (2) study guide for disorders of the pharynx; and (3) study guide for disorders of the larynx.

I. *Study Guide for Disorders of the Nose and Sinuses*

A. *Answer the following questions:* What are the major functions of the nose? What purposes do the turbinate bones, vibrissae, and mucous blanket serve? Why is Kiesselbach's plexus ("Little's area") of clinical importance? What are some possible complications of the common cold? What is the common name for allergic rhinitis? Is nonallergic vasomotor rhinitis an acute or a chronic disorder? How are nasal polyps treated? What symptom most typically indicates the presence of a foreign object in the nose? What activities are of importance in giving first aid for nosebleeds? How is bleeding from the posterior nose treated? Why is prompt treatment important following nasal fracture? What information should be included in preoperative patient teaching prior to nasal surgery? Why is positioning of the patient important in the administration of nose drops? What is the "rebound effect" which can occur with nasal vasoconstricting medications? Is air conditioning helpful to persons with sinusitis? Why is early treatment of sinusitis important? How might surgery be helpful in treating chronic sinusitis?

B. *Define the following terms:* ozena, coryza, submucous resection, rhinoplasty, "mustache dressing," Proetz position, Parkinson position, multisinusitis, pansinusitis, Caldwell-Luc procedure.

C. *Perform the following activities:*

1. Identify actions of importance in the clinical care of patients with nasal packs and in postoperative care following nasal surgery.
2. Review instructions which should be given to a patient when teaching him how he should use a nasal atomizer or when preparing a patient for a nasal irrigation.
3. State the basic mechanical causes of sinusitis and some possible complications of acute and chronic sinusitis.
4. List the essentials of treatment of acute sinusitis and chronic sinusitis.

II. *Study Guide for Disorders of the Pharynx*

A. *Answer the following questions:* What microorganisms most commonly cause acute follicular pharyngitis? Tonsils are primarily composed of what type of tissue? What first aid should be given to a person who has aspirated a foreign object into his throat? Why is aspiration of organic foreign objects often more potentially serious than aspiration of nonorganic objects? What factors are of importance to ensure that a tracheostomy tube properly fits a patient? How is extubation accomplished in a patient with a tracheostomy? What aspects of patient teaching are emphasized to a patient with a permanent tracheostomy? How is mouth-to-neck resuscitation performed? How is endotracheal extubation accomplished? Why is it difficult or impossible for a patient with a tracheostomy to cough effectively? Is suctioning through a tracheal stoma a sterile procedure? Why is it important for cuffed tracheostomy and cuffed endotracheal tubes to periodically be deflated? Why should the upper airway be suctioned before the cuff is deflated?

B. *Define the following terms:* "Dick positive," tracheotomy, tracheostomy, tracheostoma, endotracheal tube.

C. *Perform the following activities:*

1. Name the microorganism which causes diphtheria.
2. Identify potential hazards associated with adenotonsillectomy and discuss important aspects of postoperative care following this procedure.
3. Review the procedures for throat sprays and throat irrigations.
4. List four purposes of tracheotomies.
5. Familiarize yourself with the parts of tracheostomy tubes and summarize nursing care associated with each piece of equipment, e.g., procedures for cleaning the tracheostomy tube and changing neck ties.
6. Review indications for tracheotomy and list groups of patients who may benefit from tracheotomy.
7. Familiarize yourself with the operative procedure for performing tracheotomy.
8. Summarize complications which may develop following tracheotomy. Identify symptoms of these complications and review appropriate clinical care.
9. State, in your own words, some advantages and disadvantages of tracheostomies and summarize essential aspects of clinical care for patients with tracheostomies.
10. Identify some advantages, disadvantages, and complications of endotracheal intubation with an orotracheal or nasotracheal tube.
11. Familiarize yourself with the procedure of suctioning through a tracheal stoma. Refer back to material on suctioning in Unit XIV as

necessary for review, e.g., review potential hazards associated with tracheal suctioning and the prevention of these hazards.

12. Summarize some advantages and disadvantages of cuffed tracheostomy and cuffed endotracheal tubes.

III. *Study Guide for Disorders of the Larynx*

A. *Answer the following questions:* What factors predispose to cancer of the larynx? What is a radical neck dissection? What postoperative complications may follow laryngectomy? What is esophageal speech?

B. *Define the following terms:* laryngoscopy, laryngoscope, laryngectomy, hemilaryngectomy, laryngectomee.

C. *Perform the following activities:*

1. State the functions of the larynx.
2. List symptoms of laryngeal disease.
3. Identify disorders which may produce acute laryngeal edema. Review appropriate emergency clinical care.
4. Summarize factors of importance in preoperative and postoperative clinical care with laryngectomy. Consider carefully the emotional trauma associated with this surgery.

CHAPTER 107

Disorders of the Nose and Sinuses

ANATOMY

Air enters the nose through two nostrils (nares), separated in the middle by the *nasal septum.* This septum is composed of both cartilage and bone. Usually it is not straight in adults but deviates from the midline and thus appears dislocated into one nasal vestibule. The *nasal cavities* are located between the roof of the mouth and the frontal, ethmoid, and sphenoid bones. The walls of the nasal cavities are composed of bone covered with mucous membrane. On the lateral walls of each nasal cavity are three projections (superior, middle, and inferior) called "*turbinate bones*" (or "conchae," meaning "shell-shaped" structures). These structures greatly increase the mucous membrane surface over which air travels as it passes through the nasal passages and into the *nasopharynx.* The turbinates also partially obstruct the air flow entering the body (see Fig. 107–1).

The *vestibule* of the nose is lined with skin which contains *nasal hairs* (*vibrissae*). The nose is lined with *respiratory mucosa* (except for the skin in the vestibule and olfactory epithelium far superiorly). *Mucus* secreted from this mucosa is carried back into the nasopharynx by *ciliary movements.* Nasal mucosa is normally redder in appearance than oral mucosa. This is because the lining of the nasal cavities is actually a *vascular membrane* which contains numerous blood vessels. The blood carries moisture and heat to the mucosa (the functions of these elements are discussed in the section on physiology). The blood supply to the nose comes from both the *external and internal carotid systems.* The blood and nerve supply of the nasal septum is illustrated in Figure 107–2.

The *paranasal sinuses* are small cavities, lined with mucous membrane, located in facial bones surrounding the nasal cavities. The sinuses drain into the nasal cavities through openings located in grooves between the turbinates. The sinuses are located in the frontal, sphenoid, ethmoid, and maxillary bones. The *maxillary sinuses* (or antra) are the largest and most accessible to treatment; they are located on either side of the nose in the maxillary bones. The *frontal sinuses* are located in the

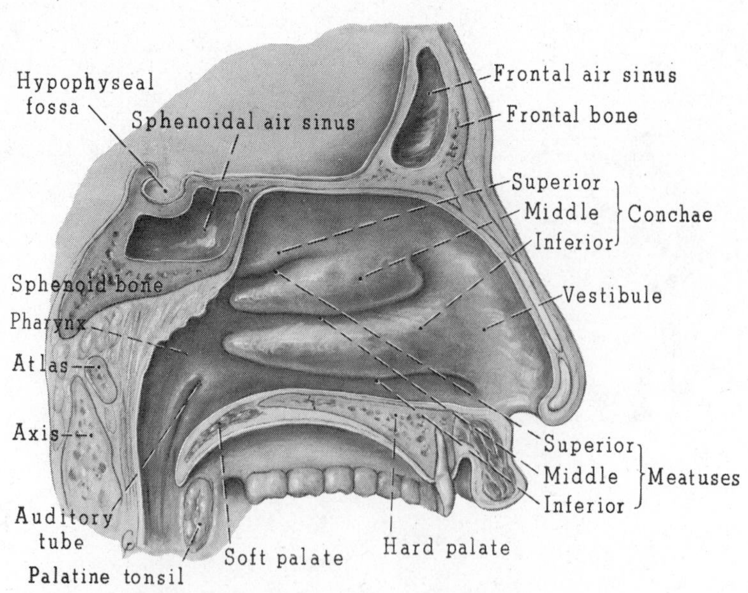

FIGURE 107–1. Nasal septum removed, showing lateral aspect of nasal cavity with conchae (turbinates). (From Jacob, S. W., and Francone, C. A.; *Structure and Function in Man.* 3rd ed. 1974.)

lower forehead between and above the eyes. The *sphenoid sinuses* are placed at the rear of the nasal cavity, and the *ethmoid sinuses* lie between the eyes over the roof of the nostrils. The sinuses function to lighten the weight of the skull and to give reasonance and timbre to the voice.

Olfactory sense organs (i.e., those associated with the sense of smell) are located in the olfactory membrane covering the roof of the nose and the floor of the anterior cranial fossa. The *nasolacrimal duct* is a small duct which communicates indirectly with the glands which produce tears. Hence, when tears flow the nose "runs."

PHYSIOLOGY

Major functions of the nose are *olfaction* (the act or process of smelling) and *air conditioning* (temperature control, humidity control, and particle removal in preparation for the air's entrance to the trachea, bronchi, and lungs). Of these two functions the air conditioning functions of inspired air are the most important. These activities are truly remarkable. Inspired atmospheric air varies widely in its temperature, humidity, and particulate matter content. For example, (a) atmospheric temperature may be below zero or above 100° F.; (b) humidity of atmospheric air may vary from less than 1 per cent to more than 90 per cent; and (c) the air may be relatively clean and free of particulate matter or may be heavily laden with it (as in a dust storm).

The inspired air reaches the nasopharynx in about one fourth of a second; during this brief period of time, the nose "conditions" the air for its inspiration into deeper respiratory structures. By the time the inspired air reaches the nasopharynx, its temperature will be adjusted to between 96.8 and 98.6° F., and it will have a constant relative humidity of 75–80 per cent. Temperature control is accomplished by enlargement or contraction of "blood spaces" or "swell spaces" located in the turbinates' erectile tissues. When inspired air is cold and dry, large amounts of water are absorbed by it from the nasal mucosa. A blanket of serum and mucus covers the surface of the nasal mucosa. As much as 1000 ml. of moisture can be evaporated from the nose during 24 hours of normal breathing. The submucosal glands replenish the moisture as it is evaporated.

Particle control is achieved by the *mucous blanket* which runs continuously throughout the nose, sinuses, pharynx, trachea, bronchi, and bronchioles. Airborne particles cling to this viscid blanket on contact with it. The blanket-secretion contains lysozyme, an enzyme which causes most bacteria to disintegrate on contact. The beating action of cilia carries the blanket (with its ensnared particulate matter) back toward the pharynx, where it is swallowed. Any residual bacteria are then destroyed by gastric juice and hydrochloric acid.[22]

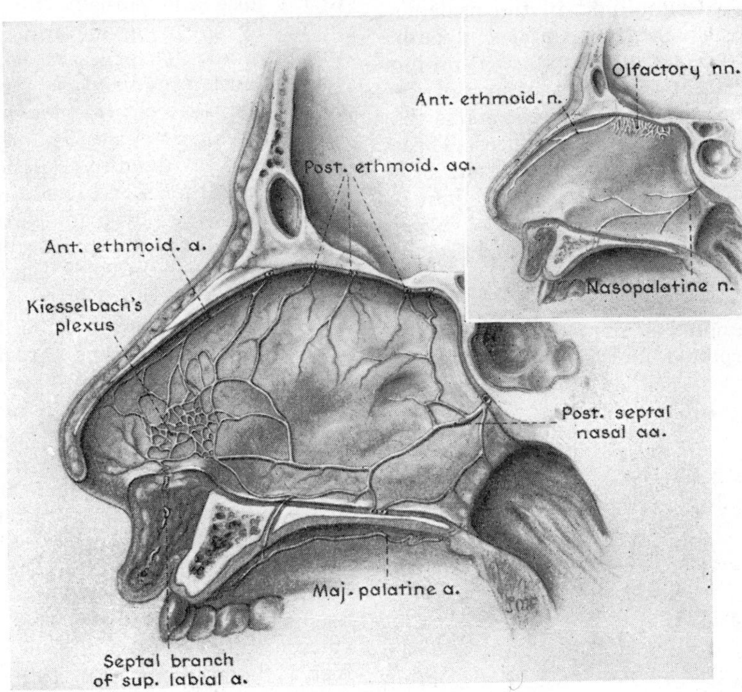

FIGURE 107–2. Blood and nerve supply of the nasal septum. (From Boies, L. R., Hilger, J. A., and Priest, R. E.: *Fundamentals of Otolaryngology*. 4th ed. 1964.)

DIAGNOSIS OF DISORDERS

EXAMINATION OF THE NOSE, NASOPHARYNX, AND PARANASAL SINUSES

Nasal chambers are examined anteriorly with a nasal speculum (see Fig. 107–3) and posteriorly with a postnasal mirror. Bright, well-focused light is important. Shrinkage of the nasal mucosa is frequently a necessary part of a complete intranasal inspection. This is accomplished by topical application of a vasoconstrictor, e.g., ephedrine, cocaine.

The *nasopharynx* is best examined with a postnasal mirror while the tongue is depressed with a tongue blade or gauze (Fig. 107–4). The mirror is warmed prior to placing it in the mouth. After it is cool the mirror is held next to one side of the uvula and light is focused on it. A small part of the nasopharynx can be observed with a nasal speculum. Specialists may use a nasopharyngoscope to examine the nasopharynx.

The *paranasal sinuses* are evaluated by (a) inspection and palpation of the soft overlying tissues; (b) observation of the location of purulent secretions in the nose (it is possible to determine which sinus is infected according to where purulent discharge appears in the nose); and (c) by transillumination of the maxillary and frontal sinuses. Transillumination of maxillary sinuses is performed by shining a bright light in the patient's mouth with the lips closed around a special bulb. The frontal sinuses are transilluminated by shining a shielded beam of light through the floor of the sinus, e.g., below the eyebrow. The light inside the closed mouth shines through the sinuses. These areas can be identified when the patient sits in a darkened room. If a sinus contains pus, the light is blacked in that region.

In order to more completely evaluate sinus conditions, the physician may also order *sinus x-rays.* The air which is normally present in the sinuses causes shadows to appear on the films; these shadows are then interpreted in the developed x-ray film.

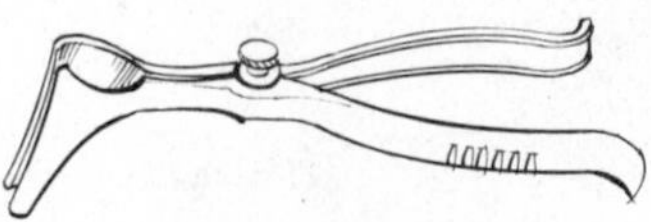

FIGURE 107–3. Nasal speculum. (From Sutton, A. L.: *Bedside Nursing Techniques in Medicine and Surgery.* 2nd ed. 1969.)

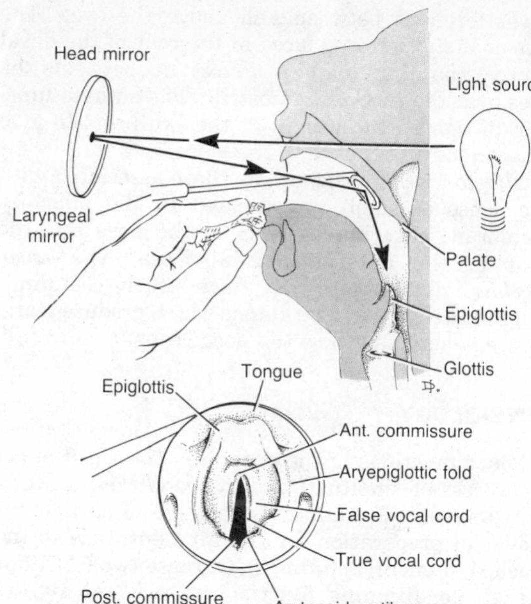

FIGURE 107–4. Nasopharyngeal examination is performed by inserting a warmed No. 1, 2, or 3 mirror into the oropharynx. With the tongue depressed, the mirror is inserted along the depressor behind the uvula and the nasopharynx inspected. The nasopharyngeal vault, the adenoid mass, the posterior ends of the middle and inferior turbinates, and the Eustachian tube orifices can be seen. (From Hill, G. J., II: *Outpatient Surgery.* 1973.)

NOSE AND THROAT CULTURES

Often it is diagnostically helpful for the physician to know which bacteria are present in a patient's nose and throat. This information is obtained by culturing material from the nose and throat. Many bacteria are normally present, including such organisms as streptococci, staphylococci, pneumococci, *Haemophilus influenzae,* and *Klebsiella pneumoniae.* The appearance of other organisms is definitely abnormal, e.g., those causing diphtheria or tuberculosis. In reading culture results, the physician considers other findings and decides if the appearance of certain organisms in the nose and throat is related to the patient's illness.

A sterile cotton swab is used for collecting material from the nose and throat for culture. After these areas have been swabbed, the swab is placed in a sterile culture tube. In some institutions the swab is suspended in a tube which contains 2 ml. of *broth* (to keep air in the tube moist and prevent evaporation and subsequent drying of the specimen); the broth is not a culture medium, and hence the swab should *not* touch the broth. (An exception, when the medium *should* touch the swab, is when a special culture tube containing Loeffler's medium is used, i.e., when diphtheria is suspected.) Sometimes culture tubes *without broth* are used if the specimen is taken immediately to the laboratory. In the laboratory the swab is streaked across a culture plate.

RHINITIS

"Rhinitis" refers to inflammation of the mucous membrane of the nose. Only the more common causes of this inflammation are considered here: simple acute rhinitis, allergic rhinitis, and nonallergic vasomotor rhinitis. Rhinitis may be an acute or chronic disorder. In acute cases the nasal mucous membrane becomes temporarily swollen, edematous, and congested. Chronic rhinitis causes the nasal mucous membrane to become thickened by connective tissue. Frequently nasal spurs and polyps develop. Some patients eventually develop an offensive-smelling nasal discharge, i.e., *ozena*.

Patients with rhinitis are instructed not to blow the nose too hard or unnecessarily. The nose should always be blown with the mouth open slightly and with both nostrils open. This prevents excessive pressure and the forcing of infected matter into the eustachian tubes.

Simple, acute rhinitis is also called "*coryza*" or the "*common cold*." The common cold is the most frequent cause of acute rhinitis. Caused by a filterable virus, the common cold is spread by droplet contact from sneezing. The condition is contagious for the first 2–3 days. Although the patient should avoid contact with others during this time, few people will remain in isolation. It is advisable for the person with a cold to avoid crowds, cover his nose and mouth when coughing and sneezing, and use disposable tissues.

Great diversity exists among agents known to cause the common cold. Among them are the rhinoviruses (30 different serologic types are currently identifiable); adenovirus; ECHO virus; Coxsackie virus; influenza viruses; parainfluenza viruses; and mycoplasmal organisms.[21]

A sore throat does *not* usually occur with a common cold. Symptoms which do occur include a feeling of burning and irritation in the nasopharynx; these symptoms are closely followed by sneezing, chilliness, copious nasal discharge, muscular aching, malaise, and mild fever. Headache may occur during the first 2 days, and as the condition progresses the nasal discharge becomes purulent and increasing nasal obstruction occurs.

If *uncomplicated*, the common cold is self-limited, and the patient is usually symptom-free after about 6–7 days. During this time treatment is symptomatic. The patient is advised to avoid chilling and to take bedrest, adequate fluids, a general diet, and aspirin if required. Warm salt water gargles and moist inhalations may also be helpful. There is no specific cure. Sometimes if antihistaminics are taken during the first day, some symptoms are alleviated. Antibiotics are not indicated.

Nose drops are recommended for *infrequent* use (e.g., every 4 hours for a few days) by some physicians; others do not recommend their use because they believe that closure of the nose during the period of acute symptoms and contagion may be a protective device which prevents spread of the infection elsewhere in the body. Examples of nose drops which may be used if the physician so recommends are naphazoline hydrochloride (Privine), 0.1 per cent; ephedrine sulfate, 1 per cent; or phenylephrine hydrochloride (Neo-Synephrine hydrochloride), 0.25 to 1 per cent. When applied locally these medications constrict capillaries and reduce hyperemia, thus relieving nasal congestion.

While antihistamines may minimize such symptoms of the common cold as tearing of the eyes and sneezing, they also produce drowsiness and should therefore be taken cautiously if the patient is attempting to work, drive a car, and so forth.

Secondary invasion of virulent bacteria may *complicate* the common cold, causing symptoms to persist and become worse. Possible complications are pneumonia, bronchitis, sinusitis, and otitis media.

Persons who have frequent colds should consult a doctor for a thorough physical examination. Additionally any person with a cold should be advised to see a physician if he has a temperature elevation or has symptoms lasting longer than a week.

Allergic rhinitis (frequently called "*hay fever*") may be seasonal and acute, or perennial and chronic. Common symptoms are sneezing, nasal obstruction, tearing, recurrent thin nasal discharge, frontal headache, and itching of the eyes and nose. Allergic rhinitis typically causes the turbinates to be pale and edematous. The posterior ends of the inferior turbinates can become so enlarged that they intrude into the nasopharynx. Nasal mucosa appears smooth and glistening.

Seasonal allergic rhinitis occurs as an acute episode lasting for several weeks before it disappears and recurs the next year. Usually the condition is caused by the pollens of grasses, flowers, or trees. *Perennial* allergic rhinitis may be constantly present all year or may occur intermittently without any set pattern over a period of many years. Frequently perennial allergic rhinitis is associated with allergic sinusitis. Generally perennial allergic rhinitis is caused from sensitivity to contacts which are constantly present in our environment, e.g., domestic animal hair and dandruff, mohair, newspaper, wool, house dust, foods, tobacco. The symptoms of this form of allergic rhinitis are less severe than those of seasonal allergic rhinitis; however, its treatment is more problematic since it is usually difficult to specifically identify the allergen.

The specific *treatment* for allergic rhinitis is to identify the specific allergen and then eliminate it, or desensitize the patient to his allergen. If skin tests are refused or cannot be performed, the patient is usually advised as follows: (a) eliminate or limit intake of chocolate, milk, and eggs; (b) cover mattress and pillows with plastic; (c) do not have domestic animals in the house; (d) use nonallergenic cosmetics; (e) cover overstuffed furniture; (f) use antihistaminics as directed; (g) install air conditioning in the house; and (h) avoid use of wool bedding. (Immunity, hypersensitivity, and allergy are discussed in Unit V, Chapter 23.)

Nonallergic vasomotor rhinitis is a condition in which the patient has *chronic,* intermittent nasal obstruction or nasal stuffiness accompanied frequently by nasal discharge. These nasal symptoms may result from stress, nervousness, tension, or some endocrine disturbances, e.g., hypothyroidism, hypometabolism. Deviation of the nasal septum commonly causes nasal obstruction. Occasionally severe obstruction develops during pregnancy and then clears shortly after delivery. Nasal stuffiness may result from overuse of nose drops (See below).

NASAL POLYPS

Nasal polyps gradually form from recurrent, localized swellings of the nasal or sinus mucosa. Once fully developed, they appear as smooth, pale tumors with pedunculated bases; the tumors themselves can be moved back and forth (see Fig. 107-5). Usually nasal polyps are multiple. They most frequently develop in patients who have allergic rhinitis. Symptoms of nasal obstruction occur when the polyps become large enough to obstruct the airway. Polyps must be surgically removed (polypectomy). Each polyp is avulsed with a wire snare. The procedure is performed under local anesthesia. If the underlying allergy cannot be well controlled, polyps tend to recur. Polyps may develop in the sinuses as well as in the nose. The most common site in the nose is the middle meatus. Occasionally it is necessary to remove polyps from the postnasal sinuses by an external operation. Sinus surgery is discussed later in this chapter.

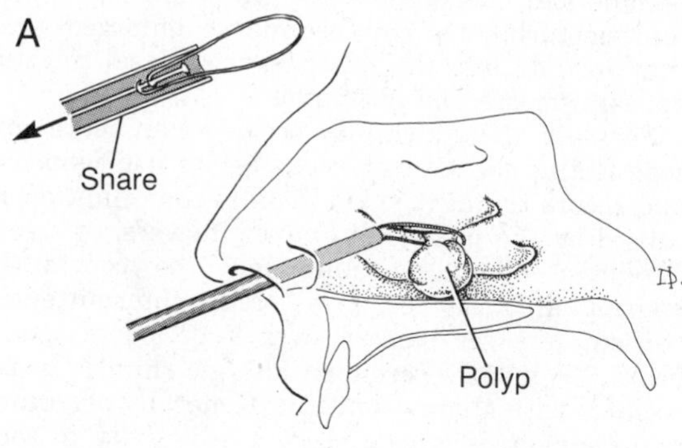

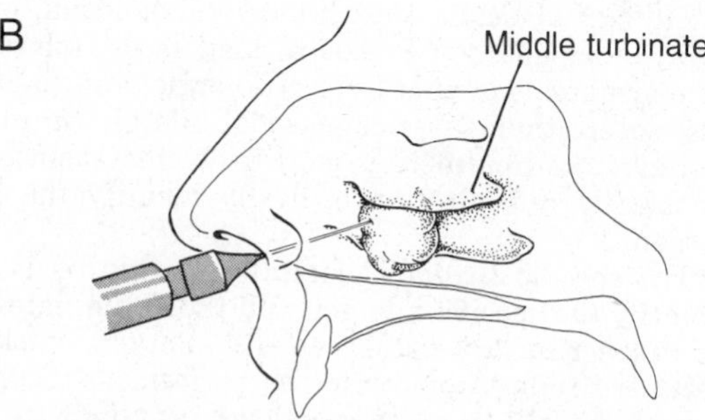

FIGURE 107-5. Removal of a nasal polyp. *A,* After anesthetizing the nose with tetracaine 2 per cent or cocaine 10 per cent, a nasal snare is slipped around the polyp and the polyp is transected. The polyp is then removed with a forceps. Usually more polyps will be seen after the initial ones have been removed. These should be excised in a similar fashion. *B,* The nasal polyp is visualized and a 25-gauge needle inserted into the polyp. A small amount of steroid solution (Depo-Medrol) is injected into the polyp. Usually 0.25–0.5 ml. is sufficient for this purpose. (From Hill, G. J., II: *Outpatient Surgery.* 1973.)

HYPERTROPHIED TURBINATES

Patients with chronic forms of rhinitis may develop enlarged turbinates in addition to nasal polyps. Astringent applications may be used to treat hypertrophied turbinates. These solutions act by shrinking the turbinates back against the side of the nose.

At times surgical correction of hypertrophied turbinates is indicated. An *anterior inferior turbinectomy* consists of removal of the anterior end of the inferior turbinate in order to restore respiration and proper drainage. It is performed preliminary to an antrum operation if the opening is to be made through the antral wall in the inferior meatus. ("Antrotomies" are discussed later in this chapter.) *Inferior turbinectomy* consists of the removal of the greater part of the lower border of the inferior turbinate. Hypertrophy of this structure causes pressure against the floor of the nose and interferes with drainage and respiration. *Anterior middle turbinectomy* consists of the removal of the anterior end of the middle turbinate body to restore proper drainage.

FOREIGN BODIES

Just as children often poke foreign objects into their ears, they likewise may poke them into their noses. Typically the presence of a foreign object in the nose causes unilateral purulent nasal discharge. Usually there is no pain, thus parents may be unaware of the accident. Objects most commonly poked into the nose are paper wads, rubber erasers, peas, beans, and pebbles. Sometimes a foreign body remains in the nose for years and eventually becomes encased in calcium. To remove a foreign body from the nose the physician may shrink the nose with a vasoconstrictor and then use a special grasping forceps or other instrument to dislodge it.

NOSEBLEED (EPISTAXIS)

Nosebleed may result from disease or trauma. Minor trauma, e.g., picking off crusts inside the nose, is the most common cause. More severe trauma, a deviated nasal septum, a perforated nasal septum, acute sinusitis, or local cancer may also cause nosebleed. Other more obscure causes include the presence of such diseases as arterial hypertension, sclerotic blood vessels, acute rheumatic fever, purpura, and leukemia. Patients who are not having bleeding from any other part of the body seldom have a nosebleed due to a hematologic disorder.

Severe epistaxis is a highly stressful condition for a patient to experience and for persons in attendance to observe. The patient's appearance is usually very bloody; his emotional state is generally anxiety ridden and fearful. In addition to blood flowing from the nares and being expectorated, occasionally blood appears in the auditory canal (as a result of passing up the eustachian tube and through a perforated ear drum) or in the corners of the patient's eyes (having passed through the lacrimal ducts).

An anterior plexus of blood vessels (Kiesselbach's plexus or Little's area) lies in the mucosa of the nasal septum; these small arteries and veins are a common source of epistaxis. Because almost 95 per cent of nosebleeds come from these very small vessels in the anterior part of the nose, *first aid* for nosebleeds usually consists of (a) pressing the soft tissues of the nose firmly against the nasal septum on the bleeding side (apply firm, steady pressure with a finger for 5–30 minutes); and (b) applying ice compresses to the nose. When pinching the end of the nose shut remember to tell the patient to mouth breathe. Other emergency measures important in treating nosebleed include (a) elevating the patient's trunk (have him sit up with his head tilted slightly forward over a basin); (b) instructing the patient not to talk; (c) having the patient breathe through his mouth; and (d) instilling a local vasoconstricting drug, e.g., Neo-Synephrine, to attempt to stop bleeding by producing vasoconstriction. Elevation of the patient's head reduces blood flow to the head. Instruct the patient not to blow his nose during, or for several hours following, nosebleed. Keep tissues and an emesis basin available for nosebleed, and tell the patient to gently expectorate any blood which accumulates in the nasopharynx. If the blood is swallowed, the severity of bleeding cannot be evaluated. Also, the blood in the patient's stomach may produce emesis. Keep the patient in a sitting position to minimize bleeding. Additionally this position keeps blood from dripping into his throat and causing gagging. If emergency measures fail to stop the bleeding, consult a physician.

In order to properly treat a nosebleed, the physician must look into the patient's nose and identify the exact site of the bleeding. This examination is best accomplished with the patient sitting up. As mentioned, the most common site of nosebleed is from Kiesselbach's plexus, a vascular network located in the anterior part of the nasal septum. Bleeding from the anterior portion of the nose is less severe than from the posterior part. This is because, in the posterior nose, bleeding may come from large vessels derived from either the external or internal carotid system. Typically bleeding is from only one side of the nose and is from only one spot. Bilateral nose bleed is uncommon but sometimes occurs following instrumentation in the nonbleeding side, following nasal fracture, or in the presence of blood dyscrasias.

Because the vessels are small and the site is

easily accessible, nosebleeds in the *anterior nose* are easiest to treat. Epistaxis in this area is controlled by applying aqueous epinephrine, 1:1000, to a cotton ball, inserting the ball in the bleeding nostril, and applying strong pressure for several minutes against the ala. Next the ball is removed and the site is cauterized electrically or chemically, e.g., with a silver nitrate stick, a chromic acid bead, or trichloroacetic acid. Local anesthesia is performed before intranasal cautery. Packing the nose is usually not necessary. The patient is instructed not to blow or pick his nose. After a week, mineral oil or petrolatum may be prescribed for application to the nasal septum.

Occasionally the physician decides the nose must be packed to treat an anterior epistaxis. Prior to packing, shrinkage of the mucosa is obtained with a decongestant, and the area is anesthetized with a topical anesthetic. The nose is then packed with ½-inch gauze lubricated with petrolatum or cod liver oil. (Nasal packs are discussed further below.)

As mentioned, bleeding from the *posterior nose* is frequently profuse. Point cautery is seldom possible; thus packing must be inserted to compress the vessel. The packing must be placed so it will remain in the correct location and will provide enough pressure to stop the bleeding. Although more comfortable for the patient, local packs tend to be inadequate, and thus conventional postnasal packs may need to be used (see below). Some physicians use an ointment containing oxytetracycline and polymyxin B in packs which are to be left in the nose for the treatment of nosebleed. (This preparation may also be used with sinus packs.)

Sometimes instead of using nasal packs the physician decides to use an alternative method of applying pressure and inserts an intranasal balloon. An intranasal balloon may be made by securing a finger cot around a rubber catheter. Once in place the balloon is inflated until the pressure holds it securely in the nose. Slow leaks of air are often a problem, but if they do not occur the inflated balloon may be left in place for up to 48 hours.[63]

Postnasal packs may be left in place 48–96 hours. They are replaced if the patient again bleeds severely following their removal. Arterial ligation may be necessary if proper packing fails to control severe nosebleed. Thus the patient is closely observed after the nose is packed for evidence of continued bleeding, and the doctor is notified as appropriate. Persistent bleeding from a site low in the nasal cavity may require external carotid artery ligation in the neck. Unmanageable epistaxis from an area high in the nose's vault may necessitate ligation of the anterior or posterior ethmoidal artery (or both) as it passes from the orbit into the ethmoidal labyrinth.

Some drugs are available for use in controlling epistaxis. However, *routine* reliance on medications to treat nosebleed is not advisable. Other treatment measures which may sometimes be used for epistaxis are (a) blood transfusion; (b) administration of vitamin K; (c) administration of vitamin C; (d) administration of Premarin; and (e) administration of carbazochrome (Andrenosem) if blood dyscrasias cause serious epistaxis. Occasionally patients require immediate blood transfusions if they have bled seriously enough to put them in a state of hemorrhagic shock. But usually, if a patient does bleed that much, the drop in his blood pressure as he goes into shock causes the bleeding to stop; the patient is thereby almost automatically protected from fatal exsanguination due to nosebleed. Sedation may be ordered since bleeding tends to be increased by apprehension and restlessness.

While most anterior nosebleeds are easily treated on an outpatient basis, complicated nosebleeds or posterior nosebleeds may require hospitalization.

DEVIATED NASAL SEPTUM

A deviated nasal septum inevitably causes nasal obstruction (see Fig. 107-6.) Other conditions which may or may not be present are headache, sinusitis, or nosebleeds. Inspection of the nose shows the septum to be bent or inclined towards one side (or sometimes both sides if an S-shaped curve is present). In addition to deviating from the midline, the nasal septum may contain rounded humps or sharp projections (ridges or spurs). If such deviations or irregularities interfere with respiration by obstructing the airway, they may require surgical correction by a procedure called "*submucous resection*" (SMR) or "*nasal septal reconstruction.*" These procedures are carried out in numerous different ways technically, but the goal of all of them is to straighten out the septum and thus relieve airway obstruction or other problems possibly related to deviation of the septum. During this surgery great care is taken not to perforate the septum and not to weaken the structure of the nose so much that the bridge will be deformed.

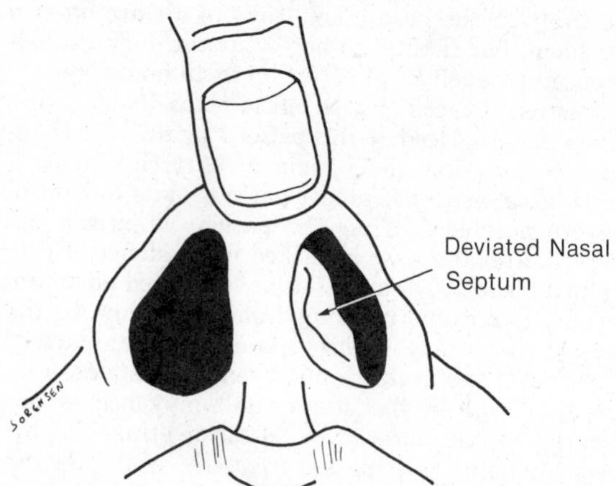

FIGURE 107-6. Deviated nasal septum, as viewed when tip of nose is pushed back. Dislocation of the columellar end of the septal cartilage has occurred, causing deflection of that portion of cartilage into left nostril. Note obstruction of nasal airway on that side.

Following local anesthesia an incision is made internally in the nose from the top to the bottom of the nasal septum on one side. After the mucous membrane is elevated, portions of bone and cartilage are removed, the mucous membrane is returned to its normal position, and plastic surgery is performed as necessary. Both sides of the nose are tightly packed postoperatively not only to prevent bleeding but also to serve as a splint and to hold the mucosa in place. The gauze packing used is usually soaked in liquid petrolatum to make its removal less traumatizing. Packing is typically removed after 24–36 hours. If a plastic procedure has been performed, an external protective dressing (adhesive tape) or splint (plastic or metal) is also applied. (Nasal surgery is discussed further below.)

NASAL FRACTURE

Injuries which result in nasal fracture usually produce copious bleeding from the nostrils and back into the nasopharynx. Soon after the injury, disfiguring edema of the soft tissues also occurs around the nose. Following a nasal injury apply an ice bag and try to control anterior bleeding by holding the nose tightly. Seek medical attention at once. If the doctor sees the patient before edema occurs, he may set the fracture at that time. Once edema is present it is necessary to wait 2–3 days for the edema to subside before setting the fracture. Usually the physician takes skull x-rays to rule out possible skull fracture and to identify the precise location of the fracture and bone fragments. If the nose is not set, it heals in improper alignment and may cause later disorders, e.g., facial deformity, nasal obstruction (deviated nasal septum), chronic rhinitis, chronic sinusitis.

A nasal fracture is reduced under intravenous anesthesia or local anesthesia. Once the displaced fragments of bone are pushed into proper alignment, they are held in place with intranasal packing and/or external dressings (adhesive tape) or nasal splints (see Fig. 107-7). If an external splint is worn, check the underlying skin periodically for indications of pressure. If observed, the physician needs to readjust the splint to prevent pressure necrosis. To minimize nasal swelling after reduction, have the patient sit with his head elevated in bed and apply ice compresses. Usually the physician removes the splint or dressing daily to again properly align the nose. Nasal fractures usually heal within about 10 days.

THERAPEUTIC PROCEDURES PERFORMED ON THE NOSE

NASAL PACKS

Local nasal packs consist of a small piece of petrolatum gauze or a small cotton ball soaked in

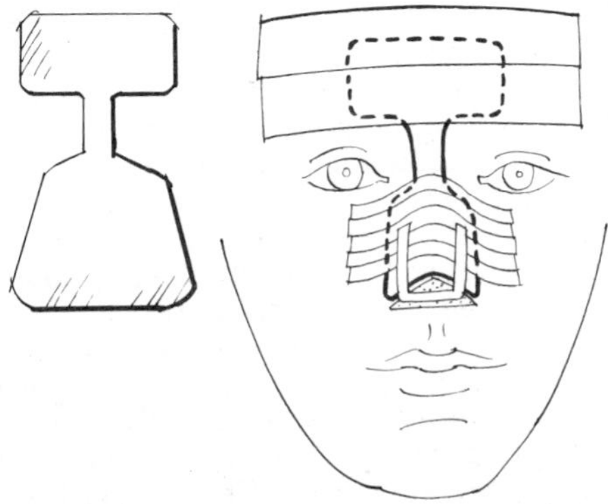

FIGURE 107–7. Nasal splint. (From Sutton, A. L.: *Bedside Nursing Techniques in Medicine and Surgery.* 2nd ed. 1969.)

epinephrine. The pack is placed with a small hemostat or bayonet forceps. After 1–2 days the physician removes the pack. *Conventional postnasal packs* are made of gauze which has strong silk sutures sewn through it to give it the desired shape and to provide traction (see Fig. 107–8). The pack may be impregnated with petrolatum or an antibiotic ointment. Sometimes a tampon may be used for a nasal pack. When this is used the string is taped to the patient's face to prevent the pack from slipping back into the throat and obstructing the airway.

To place a postnasal pack the physician first passes a soft rubber catheter through one nostril (the bleeding nostril in epistaxis) into the pharynx, and then he pulls it partially out of the mouth (see Fig. 107–9). Next he attaches two of the pack's strings onto the tip of the catheter coming out of the mouth. By pulling the catheter back out of the nose, he then pulls these two strings out of the nose and also pulls the postnasal pack into the mouth and then up into the nasopharynx and choana behind the soft palate. Care is taken not to roll the uvula upward beneath the pack. Once the pack is correctly positioned, the physician packs the anterior part of the nostril with a long strip of petrolatum gauze. He ties the two strings, brought out of the nostril from the pack, around the gauze or around a gauze bolster placed at the anterior nares. The third string (used later to pull the pack out) is left coming out of the mouth and is taped to the face, or it is cut about 4 inches long and is allowed to dangle in the pharynx.

Initially a patient may panic after nasal packing is placed because he feels unable to breathe. Quietly encourage the patient to breathe through his mouth. A patient with a nasal pack is told to gently expectorate any blood accumulating in the nasopharynx and not to swallow it. The position of a postnasal pack is periodically checked by the nurse with a flashlight directed into the patient's mouth.

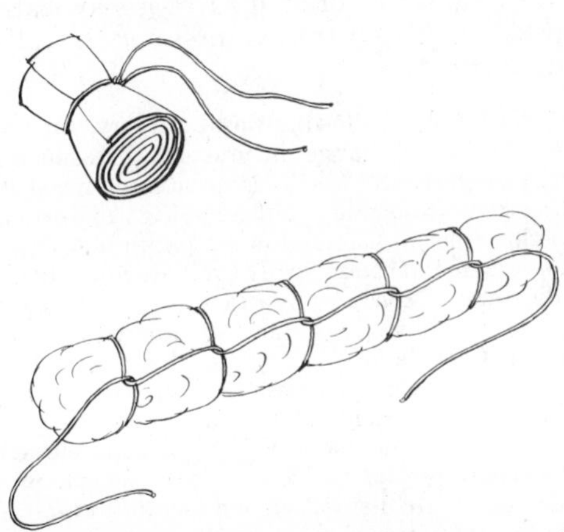

FIGURE 107–8. Postnasal packs. (From Sutton, A. L.: *Bedside Nursing Techniques in Medicine and Surgery.* 2nd ed. 1969.)

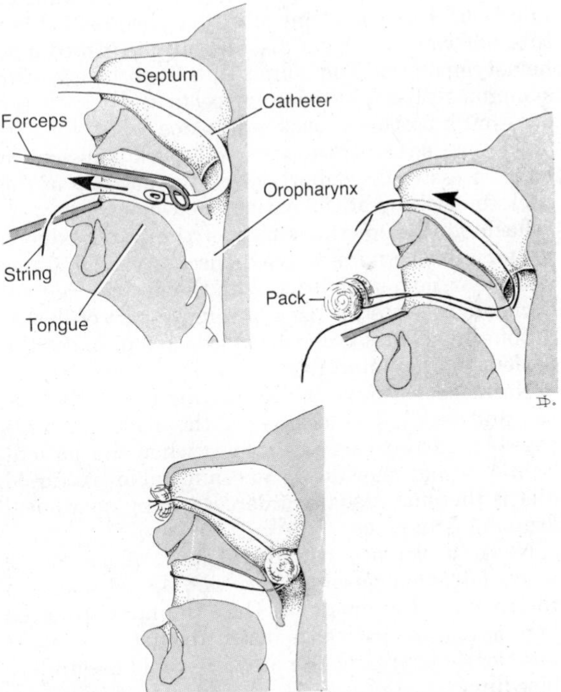

FIGURE 107–9. Posterior nasal pack. A pack is inserted after the nose has been anesthetized. A small rubber catheter (No. 10 French) is passed through the nose into the oropharynx where it is grasped and pulled through the mouth with a forceps (*A*). A pack is fashioned from a roll of gauze with three 18-inch lengths of string tied about it. The pack is then tied to the catheter with one of the strings, and the catheter and string are pulled through the nasopharynx, nasal cavity, and external naris. This procedure is repeated on the opposite side. With steady traction on the nasal strings and pressure from the index finger, the pack is directed into the nasopharynx (*B*). The third string is left hanging from the mouth and taped to the cheek to allow easy removal of the pack (*C*). (From Hill, G. J., II: *Outpatient Surgery.* 1973.)

Airway obstruction can occur if a postnasal pack accidentally slips back out of place.

In this emergency situation the nurse may save the patient's life by quickly cutting the strings on the pack and pulling it out of the patient's mouth with a hemostat. Always keep scissors, a flashlight and a hemostat available *at the bedside* for emergency care when a patient has a postnasal pack in place. Also, see that the patient's signal bell is at hand for him and is properly working so he can rapidly summon help if necessary. Of course, close observation of the patient is also important. Don't rely on him to call you, check him periodically yourself.

Rectal temperatures are taken whenever a patient has a nasal pack. Since he must rely on mouth breathing, the patient is unable to keep his mouth closed around an oral thermometer. Nasal packs usually cause a slight temperature elevation. However, fever generally subsides after packing is removed. Temperature elevations are always reported to the physician since they may also indicate infection. The pack may obstruct the eustachian tube and cause such ear disorders as otitis media or hemotympanum. The nurse thus reports any ear symptoms. The physician inspects the ear every day that a postnasal pack is in place.

If a patient with a postnasal pack appears to have excessive discomfort, check the position of the pack (by looking at the patient's nasopharynx with a flashlight). Sometimes part of the pack extends too far into the nasopharynx. Discuss your findings and the patient's condition with the doctor. He may decide to relocate the pack or remove part of it. Additionally he may prescribe a sedative to make the patient more comfortable.

Nasal packs make it difficult for the patient to eat and swallow. Blockage of the nasal airways causes a partial vacuum to form when the patient swallows and chewing is uncomfortable. A liquid diet is therefore usually ordered as long as a nasal dressing is in place.

Nasal packs are usually kept in place 24–48 hours following nasal surgery and 48–96 hours in the treatment of epistaxis. Once the nasal packing is removed, the patient is instructed not to blow his nose for 48 hours because pressure could precipitate bleeding.

NASAL SURGERY

Some details about various operative procedures performed on the nose have been previously discussed. Here we focus on aspects of general importance in the care of all patients undergoing nasal surgery.

Nasal surgery is typically performed with a local anesthesia, and the patient is premedicated with a sedative and narcotic. Remember to keep siderails up when a patient is sedated. Because nausea and vomiting can occur postoperatively, the patient usually is not allowed oral intake for 2 to 6 hours before surgery. Preoperatively an enema may be ordered to clear the lower bowel. This is done so that blood swallowed postoperatively can pass more rapidly through the gastrointestinal tract.

Preoperative teaching is an important aspect of nasal surgery. The patient will be less apprehensive and generally more comfortable during and after surgery if he is prepared for what to expect. *Preoperative teaching* should include (a) discussion of local anesthesia; (b) practice in breathing quietly through the mouth (since mouth breathing will be necessary for a few days following surgery); (c) discussion of nasal packs (inform the patient of their purpose and tell him you will be checking them after surgery); (d) instructions not to attempt to blow the nose and not to swallow secretions after surgery (tell him a basin and tissues will be available for him to "spit" into); (e) discussion of some postoperative reactions likely to occur, e.g., some postoperative bleeding, discoloration around the eyes, swelling of the operative area, and possible tarry stools; and (f) if nasal plastic surgery is going to be performed, discussion of the fact that the final cosmetic result may not be apparent for several weeks. Effective preoperative teaching may help minimize postoperative bleeding since anxiety tends to increase bleeding.

Local anesthesia of the nose is created by inserting into the nostrils cotton pledgets soaked in 10 per cent cocaine solution with Adrenaline. Patients are often highly anxious about having nasal surgery performed "while they are awake." Emotional support is thus important. During local anesthesia the patient may not be aware of the presence of blood trickling down the throat, i.e., he does not reflexly swallow. Thus it cannot be assumed that blood is not entering the stomach simply because the patient is conscious and is not swallowing. Of course with *general anesthesia* the patient is unconscious and thus does not have a swallow reflex.

The nostrils (one or both) are usually packed following nasal surgery. After the packing is in place, a folded piece of gauze is taped across the nostrils to catch any drainage which may leak past the packing. This external dressing is called a "*mustache dressing*."

> *Postoperatively* following nasal surgery, (a) observe for hemorrhage; (b) change the mustache dressing as necessary; (c) periodically check the position of nasal packs; (d) observe for respiratory difficulty (e.g., due to airway obstruction from a displaced nasal pack); (e) administer fluids as ordered; (f) periodically evaluate vital signs, e.g., for indications of shock or infection; (g) encourage relaxation and administer sedation as ordered and as indicated; (h) provide for frequent oral hygiene and mouth care; (i) provide ice compresses over the nose as ordered (to minimize pain, edema, discoloration, and bleeding; (j) position the conscious patient with his head elevated in mid–Fowler's position (to reduce local edema, promote drainage, minimize discomfort, and facilitate respiration); (k) observe for pressure areas on the skin if an external

nasal splint is present; (l) foster the patient's appetite (appetite is reduced due to inability to smell, difficulty swallowing, presence of postoperative blood and secretions, and the general discomfort of nasal packs); (m) reduce pain (e.g., by reducing the patient's anxiety, providing ice packs, promoting drainage, administering analgesics, and keeping the patient generally comfortable); and (n) administer a mild cathartic if ordered. Nasal surgery is usually not acutely painful.

Following nasal surgery *oral hygiene* is important to combat the offensive odor and taste in the mouth resulting from bleeding and postnasal discharges. Also, the mouth becomes dry owing to mouth breathing. Sometimes the throat is anesthetized with cocaine when nasal surgery is performed. Be certain such anesthesia is not still present (test the gag reflex) before giving oral hygiene or liquids postoperatively. If the gag reflex has not returned, serious aspiration of liquids may occur.

A cathartic may be ordered because the patient probably swallowed blood during the operative procedure and postoperatively. Because of the presence of this blood in the gastrointestinal tract, it is not unusual for stools to be tarry for a day or so following nasal surgery.

Postoperatively observe the patient closely for *indications of hemorrhage,* as mentioned. With a flashlight periodically look at the back of the patient's throat to see if blood is trickling down. Other indications of hemorrhage are (a) soaking with blood of the mustache dressing or nasal packing; (b) hemoptysis or hematemesis or both; (c) frequent swallowing; (d) belching (resulting from blood accumulating in the stomach); and (e) systemic symptoms of hemorrhage, e.g., rapid pulse. While some bleeding is expected following nasal surgery, unusual symptoms or excessive bleeding should not occur, and thus is reported immediately. It is not unusual for 2–3 mustache dressings to be saturated after nasal surgery.

Following surgery remind the patient not to try to blow his nose. Explain that the feeling of fullness in his nose results from swelling and packing, and therefore attempts to blow the nose will not relieve the condition.

Usually a liquid diet is given on the operative day and a general diet is ordered thereafter. Sedation may help keep the patient comfortable until the nasal packs are removed.

Self-care is encouraged once the patient is able. For example, the patient may take care of his own oral hygiene and ice compresses if the necessary equipment is placed at his bedside and he is given the necessary instructions. Remember to check, however, to be certain that the treatments ordered are actually carried out as scheduled. The patient may need your friendly reminder from time to time; your responsibility for the necessary treatments does not cease merely because the patient is assigned to self-care.

Plastic Surgery on the Nose (Rhinoplasty). Facial disfigurement resulting from gross nasal deformity may be a source of great unhappiness. Nasal deformity may be congenital in origin or acquired from disease or injury. "Rhinoplasty" refers to surgical formation of a new nose out of tissue derived from another part of the body or from various synthetic implantations. The results not only may cosmetically improve the patient's appearance, but also may make his nose function better if nasal airway obstruction was present.

Rhinoplasty is usually performed under local anesthesia. Incisions are made which are inconspicuous after healing. Many variations exist in rhinoplastic technics. In performing plastic surgery on the nose, the physician may add or remove tissue, and may lengthen or straighten the nose. Some individuals require grafting procedures. Silicone rubber (Silastic) is a synthetic substance used not only for rhinoplasty but also for surgical augmentation of the chin. This product causes very little postoperative reaction, and the prosthesis can be performed. Figure 107–10 shows some postoperative results following rhinoplasty.

NOSE DROPS

Oil base solutions are usually not used for nose drops, since they interfere with normal ciliary action and may cause pneumonitis if aspirated. Anesthetics and antiseptics may be used locally in the nose. However, *the medications most often instilled into the nose are vasoconstrictors,* e.g., epinephrine, used mainly to reduce nasal congestion. If such nose drops are used over a long period of time or if they are used too frequently or in excessive amounts, they become ineffective and, in fact, may actually worsen a patient's nasal congestion. A *rebound effect* occurs in which the stuffiness worsens after each successive dose. This occurs in the following way. The state of engorgement of the turbinates is controlled by the autonomic nervous system. Because vasoconstrictors stimulate the sympathetic nerves, a compensatory relaxation of the turbinal vessels occurs after the effect of the nose drop medication has stopped. Relaxation of these vessels is accompanied by nasal stuffiness. Thus, after a period of temporary relief from the nose drops, the nose becomes more stuffy than it was before. The only cure is for the patient to go without any type of vasoconstrictor for 2–3 weeks. During that interval the nose is stuffy, but eventually the normal reflexes should return, and the nose will again function properly.

Some nose drops contain drugs which may cause distressing symptoms, e.g., restlessness, heart palpitations, and tension. Patients need instructions so they will most effectively use nose drops and will not suffer rebound or side effects. Because vasoconstrictors can be systemically absorbed, they should be used by hypertensive patients *only* if prescribed by a physician.

Another word of caution! Various solutions are used in the examination and treatment of disorders of the nose and throat. Take care to accurately identify a solution before using it or before handing it to a physician for his use. For example, *distinguish between procaine and cocaine.* While procaine is an injectable local anesthetic, cocaine is highly toxic if injected and thus is used only by surface application. Additionally, be certain you are using a concentration of the correct strength of an ordered medication, e.g., Neo-Synephrine may be ordered in strengths of 0.5 or 0.25 per cent.

When possible direct nose drops toward the area of disease by positioning the patient in such a manner that the drops will flow toward the affected area once they are introduced into the nares.

For example, (a) place the patient flat on his back if the drops should reach the eustachian tube's opening; (b) place him with his head slightly over the edge of the bed and turned toward the affected side (Parkinson position) if the drops are to be directed toward the maximmary sinuses, the frontal sinuses, and nasal passages; and (c) place him with his head hanging straight back over the edge of the bed (Proetz position) to treat the ethmoid and sphenoid sinuses (see Fig. 107–11). If the patient is unable to hang his head over the edge of the bed to assume the Parkinson or Proetz position, instruct him to lie down with a *large* pillow under

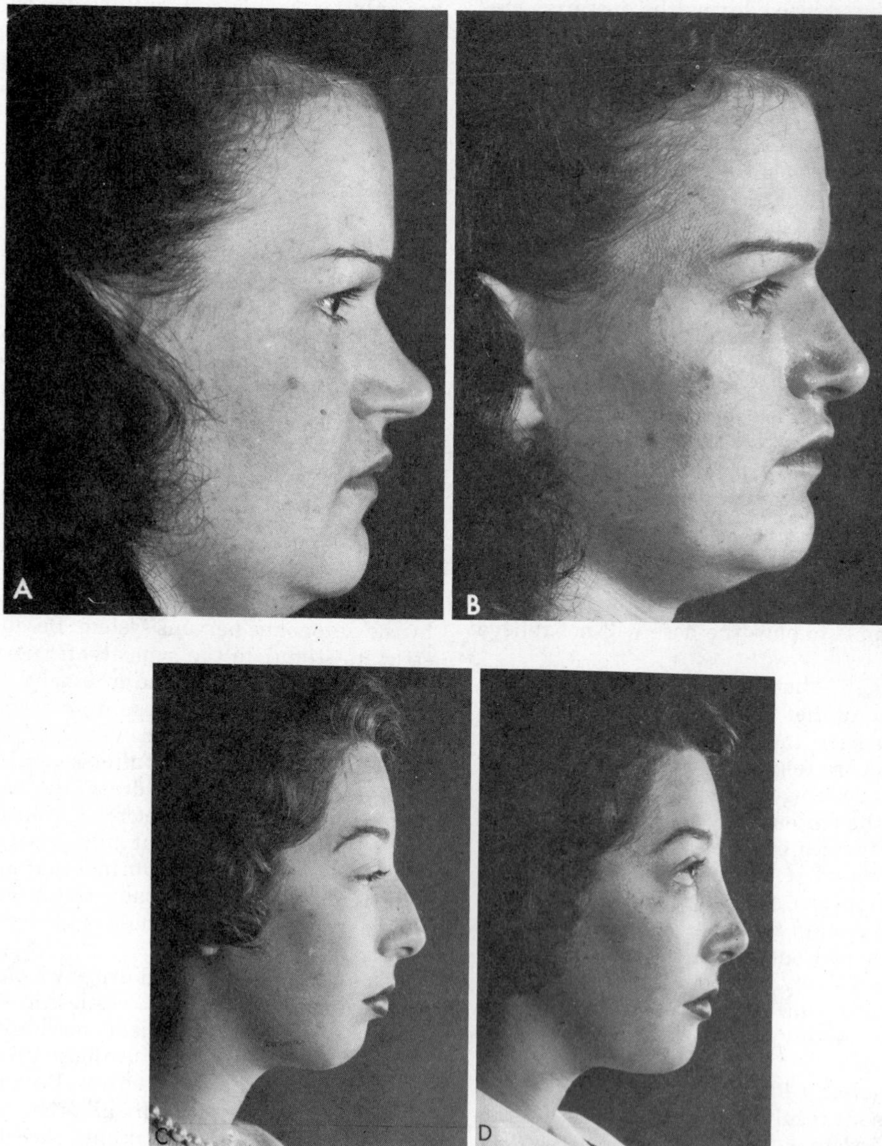

FIGURE 107–10. *A* and *B*, Moderate depression of nasal dorsum corrected by transplant of septal cartilage. *C* and *D*, Nasal convexity and chin retrusion corrected by plastic surgery. (From Paparella, M. M., and Shumrick, D. A.: *Otolaryngology.* Vol. 3. 1973.)

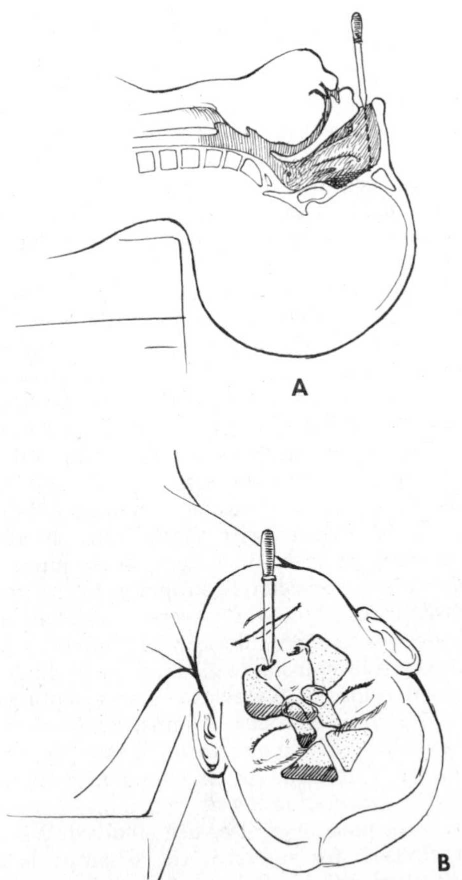

FIGURE 107-11. Two effective positions for administering nose drops. *A*, Proetz position, for treating ethmoid and sphenoid sinuses. *B*, Parkinson position, for treating frontal and maxillary sinuses and nasal passages. (From Sutton, A. L.: *Bedside Nursing Techniques in Medicine and Surgery.* 2nd ed. 1969.)

his shoulders so his head tips well back over his shoulders. Positioning the patient over the edge of the bed or over a pillow allows the solution to flow back into the nares. If the patient's head is merely tilted slightly back, the procedure is ineffective since the drops simply run down into the throat and are swallowed.

If a dropper is used, withdraw enough solution into it for instillation into both nostrils. Insert the tip of the dropper just inside the nares (about ⅓ inch) without touching the sides of the nostrils (to do so may cause sneezing). Instill no more than 3 drops of the prescribed solution into each nostril, unless the physician has specifically ordered a larger dose. Larger doses may be used in treating sinus disorders. Ask the patient to remain as positioned for at least 5 minutes after the drops are instilled. This prevents the escape of the solution from the anterior nares and gives the medication time to constrict the mucous membranes in the anterior portion of the nose. Then the solution can drain back into the posterior nose. Provide a basin for the patient to expectorate solution which runs into the oropharynx and mouth. Also have tissues available to wipe excess solution from the external nares and face.

NASAL SPRAYS OR INHALERS

Medications are ordered to be administered by nasal spray, e.g., nebulizer or hand atomizer, when the physician wishes them to be diffused over the nose's inner surface. Generally the patient is instructed how to administer his own treatments. Nebulization is most effective if the patient sits upright and tilts his head slightly backward. After the nebulizer is inserted into one nostril, the other nostril is held closed (by pressing against the side of the nose with one finger) and the patient inhales (breathes through his nose with his mouth open). Similar procedures are used with a hand atomizer or inhaler. To insert medication with an atomizer, the end of the nose is pushed slightly up and the tip of the nozzle is inserted just inside of the nostril and directed backward. The bulb is squeezed as the patient inhales. This may be repeated three times for each nostril. Excessive force is avoided in spraying medication into the nose since it may force contaminated matter into the eustachian tubes or sinuses or both. Medications used for nose drops may also be applied with a spray.

NASAL IRRIGATIONS

Occasionally nasal irrigations are ordered to cleanse the nose, e.g., of crusts blocking sinus drainage. Solutions (normal saline, antiseptic solutions) are used at body temperature. Normal saline is most commonly used. Patients with chronic atrophic rhinitis may be ordered to perform nasal irrigation at least once each day. At times the physician orders nasal irrigation with an alkaline solution (e.g., sodium bicarbonate) prior to the local application of an estrogenic compound. Patients are taught to do their own nasal irrigations if this procedure is used to treat chronic nasal conditions. However, nasal irrigations are not commonly ordered because of the potential danger of forcing infected matter into the patient's eustachian tubes or sinuses or both. Aspiration is also a potential hazard.

INFECTED AND HYPERTROPHIED ADENOIDS

The adenoid (pharyngeal tonsil) is a collection of lymphoid tissue which grows from the roof and posterior wall of the nasopharynx. This tissue is present in all children and in only a few adults. Normally adenoids atrophy during puberty. In children acute infections of the adenoids usually accompany acute tonsillitis. If repeated adenoid infection occurs, the tissue becomes hypertrophied.

Hypertrophied adenoids obstruct the eustachian tubes and posterior nares and cause changes in the eustachian tubes and ears. In children hypertrophied adenoids may cause conductive hearing loss (perhaps deafness), mastoid infections, earaches, draining ears, and middle ear infections (serous or purulent otitis media). (Disorders of the ear are discussed in Chapter 106.) Large adenoids may also cause nasal obstruction, noisy respirations, snoring, mouth breathing, difficulty swallowing, voice impairment ("nasal" voice), fetid breath, poor rest at night, bronchitis, and frequent head colds. The bone structure of a child's face may be altered if severe adenoid hypertrophy occurs during his formative years.

Adenoid hypertrophy indicates the need for surgical removal of the adenoid tissue. If indications of chronic infection of the tonsils is also present, the tonsils and adenoids are removed together. (Tonsillectomy and adenoidectomy are discussed on p. 1561).

SINUSITIS

As previously stated, the sinuses are cavities filled with air and lined with mucous membranes. "Sinusitis" refers specifically to inflammation of a sinus which produces an inflammatory change in the mucosa. Much of the head pain and mucoid nasal discharge commonly attributed to chronic sinusitis is actually caused by other disorders. Out of every 100 patients who consult an otolaryngologist because of "sinus trouble," fewer than 10 actually have sinusitis.[22]

Mechanically the basic causes of sinusitis are (a) spread of infection from the nasal passages to the sinuses; and (b) blockage of normal routes of sinus drainage. Normally the sinuses drain through openings (*ostia*) into the middle meatus (under the middle turbinate) (see Fig. 107–12). Obstructions cause a backup of secretions in the sinuses and produce pain in the region of the affected sinuses. Secretions trapped in the sinuses become foci for infections.

Blockage of sinus openings may result from disorders (e.g., a deviated nasal septum, nasal polyps resulting from allergy, edema of the turbinates) causing chronic nasal infections. Infection or allergy may cause swelling of the turbinates. Sinusitis is often caused by common colds and other respiratory infections, such as influenza. Infections easily spread from the nasal passages into the sinuses because the mucous membranes lining the nose are continuous with those lining the sinuses. If the openings remain patent, acute sinus infections usually subside quite rapidly. In the presence of obstruction, however, severe acute infection or prolonged secondary infection may occur.

Susceptible persons (e.g., those with an allergy, frequent colds, or a deviated nasal septum) may have recurrent episodes of sinusitis. Sinusitis may be *purulent* or *nonpurulent, acute* or *chronic.* Sinusitis is referred to as *ethmoid, frontal, maxillary, or sphenoid sinusitis,* depending upon which individual sinus or sinuses are involved. When several sinuses are infected, the disorder is called "*multisinusitis*"; if all are infected, "*pansinusitis.*"

The *anterior group of sinuses,* i.e., the maxillary, frontal, and anterior and middle ethmoid, all drain into the middle meatus of the nose. All these are affected to some degree by acute sinusitis. The maxillary sinus (antrum) is the sinus most frequently affected. In chronic antral sinusitis, the middle meatus may be bathed in pus, and, as a result, an

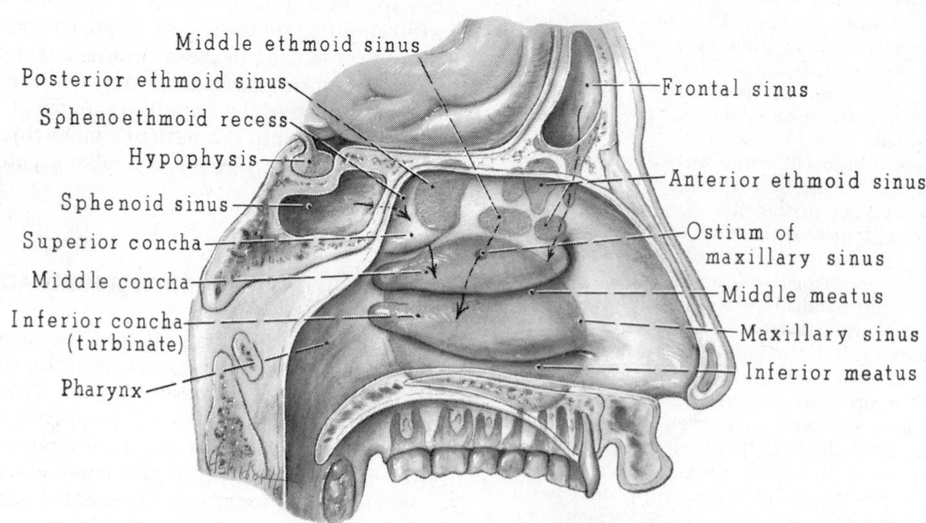

FIGURE 107–12. Sagittal section of the nasal cavity showing anatomy of the sinuses and direction of normal drainage. (From Jacob, S. W., and Francone, C. A.: *Structure and Function in Man.* 3rd ed. 1974.)

acute secondary infection may occur in the frontal and ethmoid sinuses. Likewise, nasal polyps in the ethmoid labyrinth may obstruct the openings of neighboring sinuses and thereby cause them to be secondarily infected. Often all sinuses in the anterior group are infected to varying degrees at the same time, but the symptoms are frequently localized to the one sinus most severely affected.

The posterior ethmoid and sphenoid sinuses form the *posterior group of sinuses.* These are seldom affected by acute sinusitis; however, they may be affected by chronic sinusitis accompanying infections in the anterior group of sinuses.

Complications of acute and chronic sinusitis occur with spread of the infection. Possible complications include orbital cellulitis; septicemia; periorbital abscess; cavernous sinus thrombosis; meningitis; epidural abscess; subdural abscess; brain abscess; osteitis; osteomyelitis; oroantral fistula (connecting the maxillary sinus with the oral cavity); choanal polyp; nasal obstruction; mucocele; pyocele; unilateral conductive deafness (due to edema of the eustachian tube); and bronchiectasis (resulting in part from chronic postnasal drip).

All persons with sinusitis, whether acute or chronic, benefit from (a) not smoking (smoking causes further irritation to the sinus mucous membranes); (b) avoidance of cold, damp conditions and chilling; and (c) a constant room temperature and room humidity of 40–50 per cent. Air conditioning tends to aggravate sinusitis. Some patients benefit from living in a warm, dry climate. Let us now consider acute and chronic sinusitis in greater detail.

ACUTE SINUSITIS

This inflammatory sinus condition is caused by infections (pneumonia, influenza, rhinitis) passing into the sinuses via the nasal passages. Frequently acute sinusitis accompanies or follows upper respiratory infections. Other causes of acute sinusitis are allergy, the presence of abscessed teeth, and tooth extraction. The *early treatment of acute sinusitis is important* to prevent chronic sinusitis or possible complications or both.

Symptoms of acute sinusitis include malaise; lack of appetite; nausea; nasal obstruction and congestion; purulent nasal discharge (if the duct remains open); cough and sore throat (from postnasal drainage); orbital edema or swelling over the sinuses involved; fever; feelings of pressure over the involved sinuses; and pain. Temperature elevations vary, according to the severity of the infection and whether the sinus remains open and draining or becomes occluded. Usually fever is low-grade. With complete sinus obstruction and a severe infection, the temperature may elevate to as high as 104° F. (40° C.).

Pain manifests itself in acute sinusitis as a severe, constant headache, as well as pain over the region of the infected sinuses. The location of pain is diagnostically important and thus is charted by the nurse. Pain increases with even slight pressure over the infected sinus, e.g., when the patient stoops over. Involvement of the *ethmoid* and *sphenoid* sinuses causes frontal headache with pain over the eyebrows. Infection of the *maxillary* sinuses causes pain in the cheek below the eyes and lateral to the nose; occasionally the upper teeth also ache on the affected side. Sometimes swelling and redness occur over the involved sinuses, causing the patient's face to appear asymmetrical and "puffy." The nasal mucosa may appear swollen and red upon examination, and pus may or may not be found in the nasal cavity or nasopharynx. Transillumination may demonstrate that a sinus contains pus; x-rays may be taken.

In general, *treatment* of acute sinusitis is directed at (a) relieving pain; (b) promoting sinus drainage; (c) controlling infection; and (d) strengthening resistance. Essentials of treatment include the following:

> *Pain may be relieved by the administration of such* analgesics as acetylsalicylic acid, codeine, meperidine (Demerol), or morphine sulfate. Pain relief may also be enhanced by the application of heat over the infected sinus, e.g., by heat lamp or hot, moist packs (see Unit IX).

> *Sinus drainage* is promoted by ensuring adequate fluid intake and by inhalation of moist steam; a room vaporizor may be used. Be certain windows are kept closed if a vaporizor is used. Drainage is also improved by the administration of medications which cause vasoconstriction and reduce hyperemia, e.g., ephedrine sulfate, 0.25 to 3 per cent; Otrivin, 0.1 per cent; or phenylephrine hydrochloride (Neo-Synephrine hydrochloride), 0.25 per cent. These medications are administered by inhalation or as nose drops, and may be ordered to be given as often as every 1–4 hours until drainage occurs. Care is taken, however, to avoid excessive use of nose drops because of possible rebound effects. Shrinkage of the edematous turbinates allows drainage through the openings beneath the middle turbinate. Mucolytic agents (e.g., plain normal saline or Alevaire) may be administered by inhalation. Mucolytic agents destroy or dissolve mucus.

> *Infection control* is obtained by giving the patient specific medications to which the infecting organism is sensitive, e.g., sulfonamides or antibiotics. Antibiotics may be given by inhalation. Chemotherapy is directed at speeding recovery and preventing complications.

> *Bedrest, intake of a nutritious diet,* and *mental rest* are advised to *heighten resistance.*

Very early in the course of sinusitis, an oral *antihistamine* may be prescribed (e.g., thenylpyramine furarate or Pyribenzamine) for symptomatic relief. However, these medications are given cautiously since (by thickening nasal secretions) they may prevent adequate sinus drainage.

Sometimes it is necessary for the physician to *manually irrigate the frontal or maxillary sinuses* to promote drainage and removal of purulent matter. Normal saline may be inserted through the sinuses' normal openings with a trocar and cannula. If insertion is not possible through the normal opening, the physician may perform trephination of the frontal sinus or an antrum puncture to irrigate the maxillary sinus. *Trephination of the frontal sinus* is accomplished by drilling a small hole into the frontal sinus and inserting a small tube into this hole to allow drainage and to provide a path by which medications can be directly instilled into the sinus.

An *antrum puncture* is accomplished by pushing a trocar through the *maxillary sinus* wall. Irrigation is then performed with warm, normal saline. The patient catches drainage from the puncture in a basin held under his nose. Antral puncture is not a dangerous procedure and is believed by some specialists to be the most beneficial method of treatment for subacute and early chronic suppurative sinusitis. This procedure can be repeated numerous times without permanently damaging the nose or maxillary sinus. Antral puncture may be performed for diagnosis as well as treatment. If pus is withdrawn, the presence of active infection is established.

Unlike the maxillary sinus, the *ethmoid and sphenoid sinuses* cannot be irrigated directly. Removal of retained purulent matter from these sinuses is accomplished by a procedure called the "*Proetz displacement method.*" Details of this procedure are discussed in textbooks of otolaryngology. Let us briefly say that the procedure utilizes the principle of gravity displacement of one fluid by another. Thick, purulent secretions are partially suctioned into the nose and a thinner fluid (isotonic saline solution containing a vasoconstrictor) is introduced into the sinus faster than the thick material can reenter.

CHRONIC SINUSITIS

Repeated or sustained sinus infections cause the mucous membrane lining a sinus to become thickened, and a chronic sinusitis develops which is difficult to treat effectively. In addition to the measures discussed above for the treatment of acute sinusitis, the treatment of chronic sinusitis is directed at correcting underlying disorders, e.g., removing polyps, eradicating dental infections, straightening a deviated nasal septum. If allergy is an underlying cause of chronic sinusitis, treatment is directed at that cause. The physician also investigates and treats general systemic conditions which adversely lower resistance to infection, e.g., anemia, malnutrition, hypometabolism, and lowered plasma gamma globulin. Nasal irrigations may be ordered as part of chronic sinusitis therapy, e.g., with sterile Ringer's solution. While a few patients may be cured by repeated irrigation or displacement and antihistaminics or antibiotics as indicated, most patients require surgical treatment.

Symptoms of chronic sinus infection include lethargy; difficulty sleeping; chronic cough (due to postnasal drip); chronic purulent nasal discharge; inability to smell (if nasal obstruction occurs); and a chronic sinus headache. Typically sinus headaches are dull head pains which are present upon awakening (due to the accumulation of secretions in the sinus during sleep). Movements during the day eventually help the sinus to drain so the headache typically is relieved after a while, only to reappear the following morning. Contrary to popular opinion, chronic infection of the paranasal sinuses is not a common cause of recurrent headache. Far more common causes of headache in the frontal region or between the eyes are allergic rhinitis and swelling of nasal tissue. Polyps commonly occur with allergic rhinitis. Also, with allergic rhinitis it is usual for the lining of the sinuses to undergo the same changes as those occurring in the nose.[22]

SINUS SURGERY

As mentioned, surgery may be part of the treatment for repeated episodes of sinusitis. Basically, this surgical treatment may be directed at (a) *correction of nasal deformities* which may be causing obstruction of sinus openings (correction of hypertrophied turbinated bones, submucous resection, or

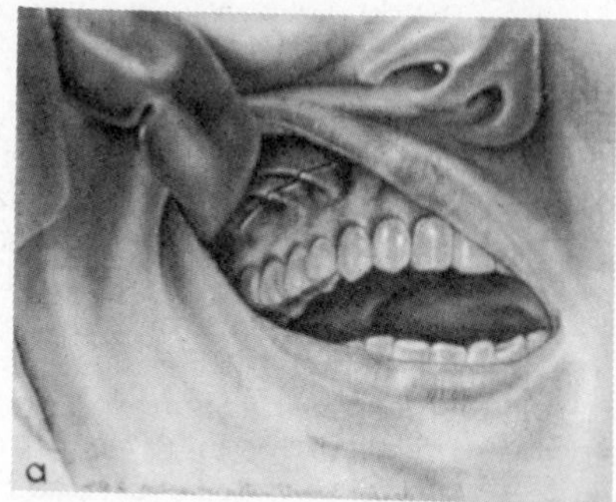

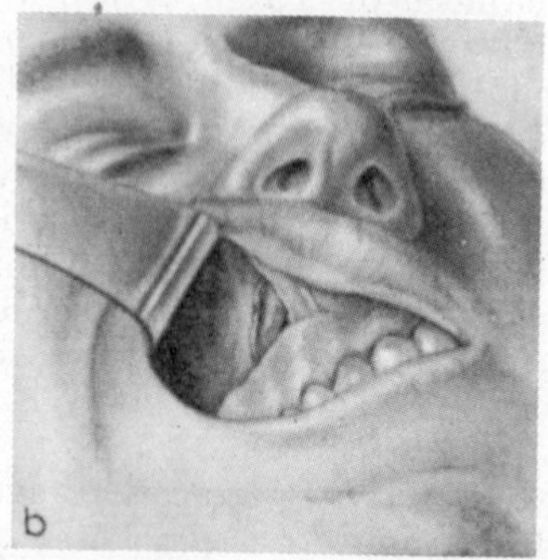

FIGURE 107–13. The purpose of the Caldwell-Luc ("radical antrum") operation is to clean out under direct vision the diseased tissue in the sinus. A horizontal incision (*A*) is made in the canine fossa, the soft tissue is elevated, the sinus is entered through its anterior wall, and enough of the wall is removed to provide adequate exposure. Then the diseased membrane in the sinus is removed and a large window made under the inferior turbinate (*B*). The incision in the canine fossa is then sutured. (From Boies, L. R., Hilger, J. A., and Priest, R. E.: *Fundamentals of Otolaryngology.* 4th ed. 1964.)

removal of nasal polyps; (b) *removal of diseased mucous membrane;* and/or (c) *enlargement of or creation of sinus openings to improve drainage.* The goal of every sinus operation is to eradicate the infection while leaving contiguous structures normal.

Generally sinus surgery is performed during the subacute stage of infection. Various surgical approaches are used under local or general anesthesia. The frontal, sphenoid, and ethmoid sinuses can be approached through a nostril (with local anesthesia); however, most often the surgeon prefers to make his surgical approach through an incision made from the upper half of the eyebrow and extending down along the side of the nose. Procedures performed through the nostril are called "*antrotomies.*"

The maxillary sinus can be approached through the nostril or by an incision made through the gum tissues under the upper lip (above the level of the roots of the maxillary teeth). This oral incision is called a *Caldwell-Luc procedure* or a *radical antrum operation* (see Fig. 107–13). The antrum may be packed with gauze after surgery to control bleeding. This packing is removed (after 24–48 hours) through the nose and the nasoantral window which has been created. It is not unusual for numbness of the upper lip and teeth to occur for several months postoperatively following a Caldwell-Luc procedure.

Sinus surgeries frequently cause a black eye and swelling of the operative area for a week or so postoperatively. Antibiotics may be administered prophylactically during the postoperative period. During this time the nurse reports indications of postoperative infection or insufficient sinus drainage, e.g., temperature elevation, tenderness, or pain in the area of the sinus.

Immediately after sinus surgery, if a general anesthetic was given, the patient is turned well over onto his side to prevent aspiration of bloody drainage before consciousness returns. Following return to consciousness or following local anesthesia, the patient is positioned with his head elevated 45° to encourage drainage and to minimize postoperative edema. Remind the patient to (a) breathe through his mouth (because of nasal packing); (b) not blow his nose (nasal packs are in place and also the pressure of blowing may traumatize the sinus); and (c) spit out drainage accumulating in the nasopharynx. Observe for indications of hemorrhage. If the patient swallows frequently, hemorrhage may be occurring and he may be swallowing the blood.

Postoperatively an ice bag or ice compresses may be ordered to relieve pain and constrict blood vessels (thus minimizing edema and bleeding). Cool or warm vapor inhalations may also be ordered. Mouth care is important during the postoperative period because nasal packing forces the patient to breathe through his mouth and because of the unpleasant taste of postoperative secretions. Oral hygiene also helps prevent infections. This is particularly true if an oral incision was made. Set up an oral hygiene tray at the patient's bedside and schedule the procedure as a treatment to be regularly performed. The tray should include not only refreshing aromatic solutions for rinsing the mouth but also petrolatum for application to the lips. Oral hygiene before meals improves the patient's appetite. Encourage fluid intake during the postoperative period. Following an oral incision the patient is usually given a liquid diet for 24 hours or so and then a soft diet for a few days to minimize oral trauma.

CHAPTER 108

Disorders of the Pharynx

"Pharynx" is the Greek word for "throat." The pharynx is the space behind the oral cavity which extends downward from the base of the skull to the larynx. The pharynx is subdivided into three sections: (1) *nasopharynx* (epipharynx), the area above the margin of the soft palate; (2) *oropharynx,* the area visible when the tongue is depressed with a tongue blade; and (3) *hypopharynx* (laryngopharynx), inferior to the base of the tongue.

ACUTE PHARYNGITIS

This disorder is the most common throat inflammation. Viral or bacterial in origin, acute pharyngitis may precede the common cold or other communicable diseases. Typical symptoms include mild fever, mild sore throat, hacking cough, and some difficulty swallowing. If uncomplicated, the symptoms remain mild and the throat returns to normal after 4–6 days.

Treatment for acute pharyngitis commonly includes rest, a liquid or soft diet, aspirin (orally or as Aspergum), and warm saline gargles or throat irrigations (see below). An ice collar may be worn and lozenges may be sucked which contain mild anesthetics. Moist inhalations may relieve the dry throat. Additionally the patient is encouraged to drink at least 2500 ml. per day. Oral hygiene and mouth care are refreshing for the patient and help prevent drying and cracking of the lips and oral pyoderma. If the patient has a distressing cough, an antitussive may be ordered, e.g., Toryn, Hycodan, or a codeine preparation.

ACUTE FOLLICULAR PHARYNGITIS

The throat is commonly afflicted with *streptococcal or staphylococcal infections.* Symptoms usually occur suddenly and may include temperature elevation (103° F. or more), chills, flushed face, headache, muscle and joint pain, general malaise, inflammation of the throat, and severe sore throat. The throat's mucous membrane appears acutely inflamed and is "studded" with white or yellow "follicles." Follicular exudate does not cover the tonsillar pillars or the soft palate. Possible serious complications may develop, e.g., cervical adenitis, sinusitis, otitis media, mastoiditis, acute rheumatic fever, and acute glomerulonephritis. In addition to being a severely distressing condition, acute follicular pharyngitis may be quite debilitating and highly dangerous. Some of the most serious infections are those caused by the Group A streptococci. The typical rash of scarlet fever may develop in persons infected with this organism who are "Dick-positive," i.e., are not immune to the organism's exotoxin. A blood leukocyte count exceeding 12,000 is also not unusual.

Treatment for acute follicular pharyngitis includes those measures discussed above for acute pharyngitis. In addition, antibiotics are prescribed as indicated by the findings of throat, nasal, and blood cultures. *Early antibiotic therapy* is especially important in treating hemolytic streptococcal infections, to prevent possible serious complications. While penicillin (I.M.) is the drug of choice, penicillin-sensitive patients may be treated with other antibiotics, e.g., tetracycline, oxytetracycline, erythromycin, and chlortetracycline. Antibiotics are continued for 24–48 hours after visible throat inflammation subsides, to prevent recurrence. Because the throat pain may be severe, codeine sulfate may be necessary as an analgesic. A barbiturate may be prescribed as a soporific at night, e.g., Nembutal.

Some patients require hospitalization for fluid therapy if their throats become too swollen and painful to permit them to swallow. Intravenous feedings are given until the acute inflammation subsides, e.g., 24–72 hours. In the hospital medical asepsis is carefully practiced to prevent spread of infection. Morning and evening temperatures are taken until the patient is completely recovered. Generally the patient is not allowed to resume full activity until he has been out of bed for as many days as he was on bedrest. Because complications may develop 2–3 weeks after the pharyngitis has apparently disappeared, the patient is advised to see his doctor promptly if indications of possible complications develop.

CHRONIC PHARYNGITIS

Chronic pharyngitis usually occurs in persons who (a) are habitual users of tobacco and alcohol;

(b) have a chronic cough; (c) are employed in or live in dusty environments; or (d) use their voices excessively. Chronic pharyngitis may cause relatively few symptoms (cough, dry throat, thick mucus in the throat which is expelled with difficulty, and an irritated, full feeling in the throat), or recurrent, more severe, acute episodes may occur, with sore throat, mild mucosal swelling, dull hyperemia, and thick, tenacious mucus in the hypopharynx.

Chronic pharyngitis is treated by (a) restricting irritants, e.g., tobacco, alcohol, spicy foods; (b) treatment of underlying disorders, e.g., infections of the nose, sinuses, or tonsils or other pulmonary or cardiac infections; (c) voice rest; (d) local removal of tenacious secretions with suction or saline irrigation and application of 2 per cent silver nitrate; (e) nasal sprays or instillations to relieve nasal congestion; and (f) in the early stages, administration of an antihistaminic. Some patients benefit from aspirin or acetophenetidin for malaise.

DIPHTHERIA

Diphtheria, a severe disease of the throat that most often affects children, is caused by the bacillus *Corynebacterium diphtheriae*. Because diphtheria is highly contagious, isolation technic is employed during treatment. (See discussion of prevention of spread of airborne organisms in Unit XIV.) Diphtheria may be transmitted directly via infected droplets of moisture (ejected from an infected person's throat, nose, or mouth) or via objects used by the patient, such as eating utensils, towels, handkerchiefs. Additionally, diphtheria may be spread by "carriers," i.e., healthy persons who carry the organisms even though they are not ill. An infected person may have bacilli in his throat 2–4 weeks following recovery from the acute effects of the infection.

Immunization programs have caused the incidence of diphtheria to decrease rapidly in the past 40–50 years. However, occasional infections occur, emphasizing the fact that preventative measures should not be relaxed. Artificial immunization is achieved by the administration of weakened toxins, given by injection in combination with pertussis ("whooping cough") and tetanus immunizing agents. These combined injections are commonly called "DPT" immunizations, i.e., diphtheria-pertussis-tetanus immunizations. Three separate injections are given (1 month apart), beginning when an infant is between $1\frac{1}{2}$ to 2 months of age.

The incubation period for diphtheria is typically 2–5 days, but may be longer. Diphtheria produces a white or gray membrane in the throat which advances rapidly and may cover all three sections of the pharynx and extend down into the trachea. A bleeding base becomes visible if one attempts to remove the membrane. The throat is swollen and breathing and swallowing may be impaired. (Emergency tracheostomy may be required to prevent asphyxiation).

Pseudomembranous inflammation develops on mucosal surfaces as an acute inflammatory response to a powerful necrotizing toxin, that is, the diphtheria exotoxin. The surface epithelial cells undergo necrosis and desquamation, and a fibrinosuppurative exudate pours forth. Robbins observes: "As the fibrin coagulates and traps the necrotic cellular debris, it produces a dirty gray-white, rubbery membrane which layers the inflamed, eroded surfaces."[82a]

The patient infected with diphtheria is severely ill and has a rapid, thready pulse. However, the body temperature seldom goes higher than 101° F. Early symptoms include sore throat, headache, nausea, and temperature elevation. Diagnosis is confirmed by culture of a specimen swabbed from a portion of bleeding base after a piece of membrane is lifted up (see Chapter 107). In addition to possible tracheostomy, treatment focuses on bedrest, large doses of penicillin, and intravenous and intramuscular injections of specific diphtheria antitoxin. Oxygen may be given to relieve cyanosis and dyspnea. Early treatment is important to prevent serious complications such as paralysis or cardiac complications. Permanent neurologic or cardiac damage may result from toxin produced by the diphtheria bacillus as this toxin spreads throughout the body. Prognosis is affected by the administration of antitoxin and the severity of the infection. It is desirable for the antitoxin to be administered *early* in the course of the illness. A prolonged period of recovery is often advisable.

PERITONSILLAR ABSCESS (QUINSY)

Acute streptococcal or staphylococcal tonsillitis (see below) may cause a peritonsillar abscess to form as a result of infection of tissue between the tonsil and the fascia covering the superior constrictor muscle (see Fig. 108–1). Typically the patient has tonsillitis for several days, appears to be improving, and then develops increasing pain on one side of his throat (and ear) and difficulty swallowing. Usually the patient's voice is described as a "hot potato voice" since his speech is muffled. Often he sits with his mouth partially open so he can drool rather than having to try to swallow. Thick secretions are "hawked" up with difficulty. A peritonsillar abscess causes extensive swelling of the soft palate. The uvula may be pushed to one side; half of the pharyngeal opening may be occluded by this swelling. The tonsil is pushed forward, downward, and toward the midline of the throat; this displacement is the result of pus forming in the fascial space.

A peritonsillar abscess may rupture spontaneously (causing pus to drain through the anterior pillar) or it may need to be surgically incised to provide good drainage (Fig. 108–1). Other therapeutic measures are topical anesthetic throat sprays or local anesthetic injections; narcotics; application of an ice collar; antibiotics; hot saline throat irrigations; or saline or alkaline mouthwashes or gargles (105–110° F.). The patient may be able to swallow more easily when drinking if someone stands behind him and pulls upward on the sides of his throat as he swallows.

If antibiotics, e.g., penicillin, are given early in the course of the infection, abscess formation (and possible surgical incision and drainage) may be avoided. However, if incision is necessary, the patient is positioned sitting up so he can expectorate pus and blood.

Usually it takes at least one month for the infection of a peritonsillar abscess to subside. Then a tonsillectomy is frequently advised to prevent recurrence.

TONSILLITIS

"Tonsillitis" means inflammation of a tonsil. The tonsils are masses of lymphatic tissue located on either side of the oropharynx. Normally the palatine (or faucial) tonsils do not project much beyond the limits of the tonsillar pillars, and they are approximately the same color as the rest of the oral mucosa. A pillar retractor may be used to withdraw the anterior pillar during examination. Each tonsil is a small, almond-shaped mass composed primarily of lymphoid tissue which is covered by mucous membrane. Within the tonsil are many crypts and lymph follicles which supply phagocytes to the mouth and pharynx.

Several decades ago undue emphasis was placed on sequelae which could possibly result from infected tonsils and adenoids. As a result, during the 1930's the removal of the tonsils and adenoids was the most common surgical procedure performed and represented almost 35 per cent of all operations. Currently fewer of these operations are performed, as it is realized that (a) the throat's lymphoid structures are important in immunity; (b) the incidence of upper respiratory disease is not lowered significantly by removal of tonsils and adenoids; and (c) a disservice may actually be given to the patient if tonsils and adenoids are indiscriminately removed in hopes of some future benefit.[22]

Acute tonsillitis begins as a sore throat accompanied by fever, anorexia, chills, muscular pain, and headache. Swollen, tender anterior cervical lymph glands are also usually present. The malaise and discomfort of uncomplicated tonsillitis increase for 24–72 hours before slowly subsiding over a period of 7–10 days. The tonsils appear enlarged and brightly inflamed. Pus or exudate is present on the tonsils or in the crypts. The tonsils are studded with yellow follicles if the infection is streptococcal. Throat cultures identify the infecting organism. Acute tonsillitis frequently elevates the white blood cell count and causes cervical lymph nodes to be swollen and tender.

The usual treatment for acute tonsillitis is bedrest, hot saline gargles or throat irrigations, and maintenance of adequate fluid intake. Severe cases may be given a sulfonamide or antibiotics. Once started, the antibiotics are continued for 24–28 hours after subsidence of symptoms. Pain may be relieved by an ice collar, acetylsalicylic acid, or codeine sulfate if necessary. Repeated acute attacks of tonsillitis are not indicative of the need to remove the tonsils surgically unless indications of persistent infection remain. Bedrest is recommended for 48 hours after the temperature returns to normal, to help prevent complications. Complications which may develop from streptococcal tonsillitis include pneumonia, nephritis, osteomyelitis, and rheumatic fever. Complications which can result from local extension of the infection are chronic tonsillitis, acute otitis media, acute rhinitis, acute sinusitis, and peritonsillar abscess or other deep neck abscesses.[21]

Acute tonsillitis is usually a bacterial infection and is most often due to streptococci. This contagious airborne or food-borne infection occurs most often in children but can occur at any age. If uncomplicated, acute tonsillitis typically resolves spontaneously after 5–7 days. Treatment is encouraged, since it not only makes the patient more comfortable and hastens recovery but also may prevent serious complications.

Chronic tonsillitis is not as common as formerly

A

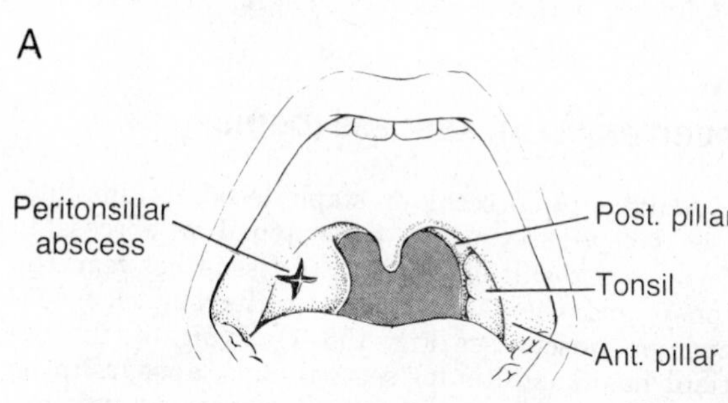

B

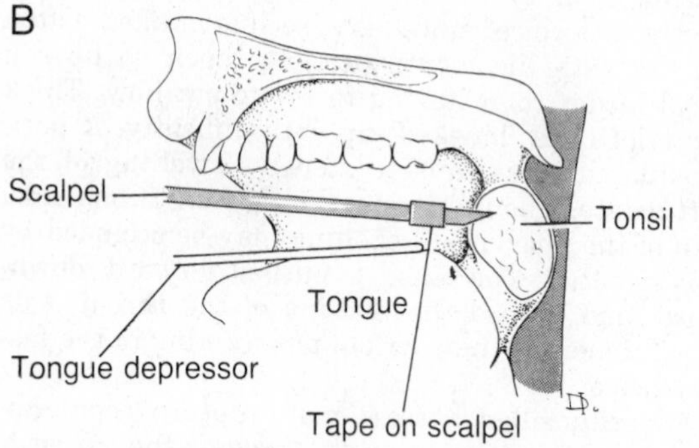

FIGURE 108–1. Peritonsillar abscess. The incision is made near the anterior pillar through the area of greatest fluctuance. Local anesthesia is usually quite adequate for this operation. (From Hill, G. J., II: *Outpatient Surgery.* 1973.)

believed. Recurrent sore throat is the most frequent symptom. Between episodes of acute tonsillitis the throat remains uncomfortable. The tonsils often appear enlarged and, if infected, a sharp line may be seen between the color of the buccal mucosa and the tonsillar pillar. The most reliable indication of chronic tonsillitis is the ability to express purulent material from the tonsil crypts with a wooden tongue blade. Once chronic tonsillitis is proved, surgical removal of the tonsils is the recommended treatment. Surgery is contraindicated during periods of acute tonsillar infection.

ADENOTONSILLECTOMY ("T & A")

Surgical removal of the tonsils ("tonsillectomy") and of the adenoids ("adenoidectomy") is collectively called "adenotonsillectomy" and is abbreviated "T & A." While the tonsils or adenoids may be removed in separate procedures, most often they are removed during one surgical operation. *Contraindications* for T & A are[22] (a) the presence of any acute infection (surgery is canceled if there is any indication that the patient may be developing an upper respiratory infection); (b) active tuberculosis; and (c) the presence of such disorders as hemophilia, aplastic anemia, purpura, or leukemia. *Potential hazards* associated with tonsillectomy and adenoidectomy include (a) failure to secure *obscure bleeding points;* (b) *airway obstruction* resulting from blood and secretions collecting in the airway during surgery (note: this can cause hypoxia, cardiac arrest, excessive bleeding); and (c) *aspiration.*

Because hemorrhage is a potential threat following T & A, the patient's hemostasis is evaluated *preoperatively.* In addition to checking bleeding and clotting times, urinalysis and blood count are performed. Preoperatively atropine is always given to reduce mucous secretions if a general anesthesia is to be administered.

During surgery the patient is placed in the dorsal position if general anesthesia is to be given. If local anesthesia is used, the patient is in a sitting position. Adults are usually given a local anesthetic, and the patient is typically premedicated with a barbiturate, a narcotic, and atropine, 1/150 Gr. General anesthesia is used for some adult T & A's. The most common operative method of removing the tonsils is by dissection and snare (see Fig. 108–2); however, some surgeons prefer the guillotine method. The main mass of adenoid tissue is removed with an adenotome or an adenoid curette. Remaining adenoid remnants are removed with a biting punch forceps.

During tonsillectomy, if the patient is under local anesthesia or is unconscious, blood often trickles down into his stomach; if the patient is conscious, he frequently swallows blood.

Postoperative care after adenotonsillectomy is as follows. If local anesthesia was used, the patient is positioned with his head elevated 45° for postoperative care. Following general anesthesia, to prevent aspiration the patient is placed so he lies with his face partially down and with a pillow under one shoulder, or he is placed prone with his head turned to one side. In these positions secretions are easily expelled from the mouth. The airway is left in place until the patient is able to handle his own secretions, i.e., is conscious enough to swallow. Have gauze wipes available to wipe the patient's nose and mouth and have a towel placed under his head. Keep the patient positioned well over onto his side with a towel and emesis basin under his mouth to catch secretions until he is fully conscious. Then position him with his head elevated 45°.

During the first postoperative hour take the patient's pulse and blood pressure every 15 minutes;

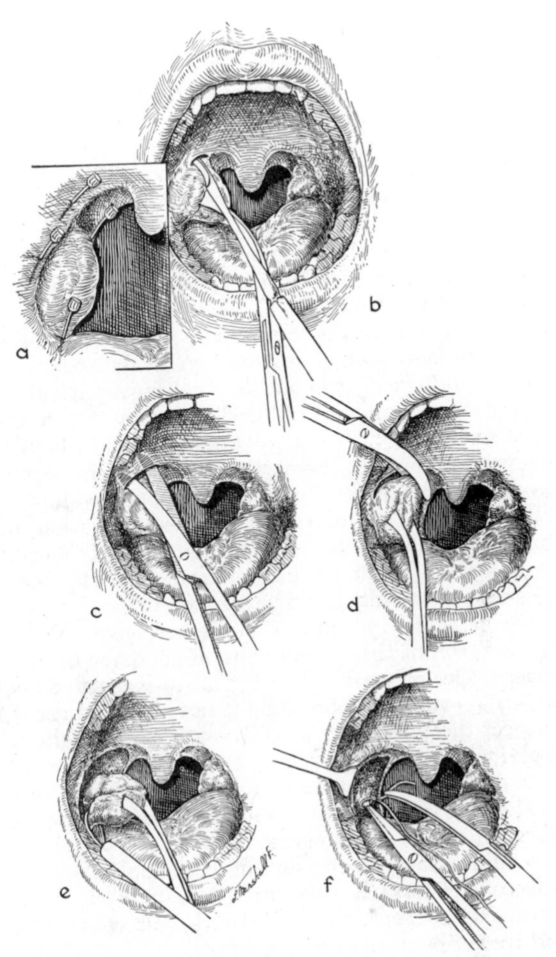

FIGURE 108–2. A method of dissection tonsillectomy. *A,* Points of infiltration for local anesthesia. *B,* Start of incision with tonsil knife at attachment of anterior pillar to the tonsil superiorly. *C,* Separation by scissor dissection of the superior pole of the tonsil. *D,* Continuation of dissection of tonsil from its attachment to pillars and bed of tonsillar fossa. *E,* Separation of the tonsil by snare at the lower pole, including the plica triangularis. *F,* Hemostasis. (From Boies, L. R., Hilger, J. A., and Priest, R. E.: *Fundamentals of Otolaryngology.* 4th ed. 1964.)

then every half hour for several hours. Take the temperature rectally (as with any patient who has oral surgery). A slight temperature elevation is not unusual for a day or so postoperatively.

Instruct the patient not to try to clear his throat or cough since these actions could precipitate bleeding. Also advise the patient to rest his throat by not talking excessively. Give aspirin or narcotics as ordered and apply an ice collar around the throat. An ice collar may provide some comfort for the patient and is believed by some to minimize postoperative bleeding.

The nurse observes the patient for possible postoperative hemorrhage because emergency treatment may be indicated. It is not unusual for a patient to vomit a *small* amount of blood following adenotonsillectomy or to have a *small* amount of dark bloody drainage. However, hemorrhage may be indicated by the vomiting of *large* amounts of swallowed blood (brown in color), by the expectoration of bright red colored blood, or large amounts of bloody drainage. A gradually increasing pulse rate, restlessness, a falling blood pressure, and pallor are other possible indications of hemorrhage. Notify the surgeon of these symptoms. Remember to save emesis specimens for the surgeon to inspect. Since external evidence of bleeding is not always present, inspect the throat periodically with a flashlight to look for blood trickling down the back of the throat; it is particularly important to do this if the patient is sleeping or is not fully conscious. Sometimes the surgeon can stop postoperative bleeding by simple procedures such as pressure of local applications of vasoconstrictors. If this fails, the patient is returned to surgery, reanesthetized, and vessels are sutured or cauterized as necessary.

Once full consciousness has returned and if there is no bleeding, the patient is allowed ice chips or liquids. Orange juice, grapefruit juice, and tomato juice are avoided because they cause burning sensations in the throat. Lukewarm water is less irritating than ice water to drink. Encourage the patient to take large swallows of fluid (rather than small swallows) because this causes less discomfort and also enables a greater fluid intake. The patient is *not* given a straw, since sucking can start bleeding, and also the careless or stuporous patient could injure his throat with a straw. Gradually the patient's diet progresses to include soft foods, e.g., custards, ice cream, mild-flavored cream soups, bland cereals, poached eggs. Hot liquids, spicy foods, and rough foods should be avoided for a week. If sutures were placed during tonsillectomy, a liquid or soft diet may be necessary until suture absorption has occurred because swallowing is more painful than if sutures are not in the throat.

Alkaline mouthwashes are offered to the patient. They are not only refreshing, but also they help clear away viscous mucous.

Usually following T & A the patient is kept on bedrest for 24 hours and is discharged on the first postoperative day. However, some patients are discharged the evening of surgery. All patients are kept hospitalized for at least a few hours because of the potential danger of postoperative bleeding. If serious bleeding occurs, it usually happens a few hours following surgery. Thus this dangerous period is over before the patient is discharged.

In preparation for the patient's discharge, he is told his doctor's orders and is given instructions for home care. He may be ordered to gargle every 2 hours during the day with warm salt water or other solutions, such as one half teaspoon of sodium bicarbonate and 5 grains (0.3 Gm.) of acetylsalicylic acid dissolved in half a glass of lukewarm water. The patient may also be advised to chew Aspergum before meals for 15 minutes and between meals if necessary to relieve soreness. Aspergum not only relieves pain in the throat and ears, but it also helps relax throat muscles. Dietary instructions, recommendations for rest, and follow-up appointments are given to the patient. Typically, following T & A the patient is advised to stay indoors for three days and to avoid strenuous exercise and sunbathing. Activities which are contraindicated because of the possibility of starting bleeding include sneezing, coughing, clearing the throat, and vigorous nose blowing.

Not all bleeding problems following T & A occur *immediately* after surgery; *sometimes bleeding problems are delayed and do not occur until the fifth to tenth postoperative day.* Delayed bleeding results from the premature separation of the white "scab" that forms postoperatively over the areas from which the tonsils and adenoids were removed. Between 5–10 days following surgery, the membrane which has formed over the operative area begins to slough off. As this occurs, the throat is usually quite sore, and there is danger of possible hemorrhage. Eating rough foods or the presence of infection may cause the scab to be removed; the surface vessels and small capillaries then begin to bleed.

Before discharge the patient is told that a very small percentage of patients have some bleeding after 5–6 days and that if this happens to him he should (a) remain calm, since the bleeding is usually only minor; (b) gently gargle the throat with ice water; (c) lie quietly down and gently spit the blood out; and (d) call his physician if the bleeding does not stop promptly. Although rarely dangerous, the physician's attention is required to remove a soft clot if one has formed. It takes about 3 weeks for the mucous membrane to completely heal.

The patient is also instructed before discharge to notify his doctor if he develops ear discomfort or temperature elevation lasting longer than 3 days.

Blood swallowed during surgery may cause the patient's stool to be tarry for a day or so following adenotonsillectomy. He is told that this is expected. Occasionally a mild laxative is necessary. Forcing fluids (e.g., 3000 ml. per day) helps relieve constipation and also the unpleasant mouth odor which follows oral surgery. Additionally, the fluid intake helps compensate for the slight temperature elevation which may occur for a few days.

ASPIRATED FOREIGN BODIES

Foreign bodies may be aspirated into the pharynx, larynx, or trachea. These objects may result in dyspnea or asphyxia (due to airway obstruction), and they may also cause serious tracheobronchial irritation if aspirated deeper into the tracheobronchial tree. If an aspirated foreign object lodges in the larynx, the patient should be placed in a position with his head and upper chest dependent and then be given sharp, vigorous slaps between the scapulae. (Unless the thorax is dependent, slapping the patient's back may merely cause the object to go lower into his airway.) If the object is not coughed up after this maneuver, emergency laryngoscopy or tracheotomy is indicated.

In addition to severe dyspnea and other symptoms of respiratory distress, the presence of a foreign body may be indicated by such symptoms as hemoptysis, mucous expectoration, or a croupy or whistling cough. In the presence of acute respiratory distress, the examiner attempts to remove a foreign body lodged in the pharynx with his finger. Emergency tracheotomy is indicated if the obstruction is lower in the airway (see below). When time permits, an x-ray is taken to confirm the presence of a foreign object and to localize the object. While nonorganic objects may sometimes be tolerated in the tracheobronchial tree for years without causing marked symptoms, organic matter, e.g., peanuts, may rapidly swell or cause serious infection, e.g., pneumonia. Foreign bodies may be removed in some cases by the use of special instruments inserted through a bronchoscope or laryngoscope.

THROAT SPRAYS AND IRRIGATIONS

Anesthetics and antiseptics may be applied to the throat by *spraying*. Medications commonly prescribed for use as throat sprays may come prepackaged in plastic, squeezable bottles attached to a spray tip. To properly spray the larynx, the patient is given the following instructions: (a) be certain the spray tip used turns down at the tip so the medication will be directed down into the throat rather than merely at the back of the throat; (b) open the mouth and gently place the spray tip at the back of the throat, behind the tongue; and (c) spray the medication down into the throat as you deeply inhale once or twice. Greater force is necessary when using a throat spray than when instilling a nasal spray.

The resolution of acute or chronic throat inflammations is often speeded up by periodic "bathing" of the throat with warm or hot normal saline. Other solutions which may be used are mild antiseptics or sodium bicarbonate. The latter is especially effective when secretions are tenacious. "Bathing" of the throat may be accomplished by *throat irrigations* or *gargling*. Throat irrigations are usually more effecive than gargling, since garling does not reach all the parts of the throat. Also, gargling is more uncomfortable, since it produces tension and stretching of the inflamed, painful throat tissues. However, either process not only provides comfort to the patient but also cleanses the throat (loosens and removes secretions) and increases surface blood supply by causing vasodilation. The degree of heat applied is important. Solutions are used as hot as a patient can tolerate them, but never hotter than 120° F. (48.8° C.).

Throat irrigations may be ordered 2 to 3 times daily or as often as every 1–2 hours while the patient is awake, depending upon the condition of the patient's throat. Throat irrigation is accomplished by attaching a rubber tube (with a clamp) and a plastic or glass irrigating tip onto an irrigating can or hot-water bottle. Before use, inspect the tip to be certain it is not chipped or cracked. The container is filled with the prescribed irrigating solution at the desired temperature. The container is then hung above the patient's head. Recommendations for the height at which the can should be hung vary from 2 to 3 feet [22] above the patient's head to only slightly above the level of the patient's mouth.[30] The patient leans over a washbasin or collecting basin so fluid will run back out of his mouth. He then opens his mouth and inserts the nozzle without touching the base of the tongue or uvula, since this could cause gagging. Then, while holding his breath to prevent aspiration, the patient directs the solution so that all parts of the throat are irrigated. Periodically it is, of course, necessary to clamp the tubing to breathe and rest. Approximately 1500 to 2000 ml. of irrigating fluid are used.

TRACHEOTOMY; TRACHEOSTOMY CARE

The trachea may be intubated in two basic ways: (1) by passing a tube through the nose or mouth into the trachea, i.e., *endotracheal intubation;* or (2) by making a surgical incision into the trachea via the throat, i.e., *tracheotomy,* and then inserting a tube through that incision into the trachea. Clinical care of the patient with tracheal intubation is considered in detail because this is an important aspect of modern nursing practice.

DEFINITION OF TERMS

A *tracheotomy* is an incision into the trachea through the second, third, or fourth tracheal ring. This surgical procedure is performed for such purposes as exploration, removal of a foreign body, removal of a local lesion (e.g., tumor), to obtain a biopsy specimen, or to gain access to the airway for purposes of assisting respirations.

The opening which results from a tracheotomy is called a "*tracheostomy.*" A tracheostomy may be a permanent or temporary opening. An indwelling tube (e.g., tracheostomy tube or laryngectomy tube) may be inserted through this opening to facilitate the removal of tracheobronchial secretions or to make the passage of air easier or both. Tracheostomies (a) facilitate prolonged artificial ventilation; (b) bypass serious upper respiratory obstructions (e.g., due to edema); (c) prevent aspiration of blood, secretions, or food into the lungs (e.g., when normal swallowing is impossible because of a reduced state of consciousness or muscular paralysis, or in the presence of hemorrhage); and (d) provide easier access to the lower airways than is possible through the nose or mouth.

TRACHEOSTOMY TUBES

As Figure 108–3 demonstrates, a variety of tracheostomy tubes are available. Space does not permit detailed discussion of the technics for using each of these tubes; consult specialized texts and equipment information for these details as necessary. Tracheostomy tubes may be made of various substances, e.g., disposable plastic, stainless steel, or sterling silver.

Tracheostomy tubes may consist of several separate pieces or only one piece. *Metal tubes* typically have three parts which are kept together as one set and are not interchangeable with other tube sets. These three parts are (1) an outer tube (also called "outer cannula"); (2) an inner tube ("inner cannula"); and (3) an olive-tipped "obturator." When tracheostomy tubes have three pieces, the *outer tube* remains held in place by a *ribbon* or *tie* which is passed through loops on either side of the tube's opening. (Tracheostomy neck ties or tapes are discussed further later in this section.)

The *obturator* is slipped into the outer tube before the tube is inserted into the trachea. The obturator's position in the outer tube is such that it extends beyond the tube's end and thus serves as a blunt, smooth guide while the tube is slipped into the trachea. Following insertion, the obturator is immediately removed, since it occludes the tube's lumen and thus prevents the exchange of air between the lungs and the atmosphere. *The obturator is kept at the patient's bedside in a place where it is easily seen in case the tube is expelled* and another sterile tube set is not available. In such a situation, the obturator is slipped into the expelled tube, and the tube may be immediately reinserted (see below). Because the obturator for a metal tracheostomy tube is part of a matched set, care is taken not to lose it or to separate it from the other pieces of the set. If one piece is lost, the entire set becomes useless.

The *inner tube* fits inside of the outer tube and is removed periodically for cleaning. Upon initial insertion of the outer tube, the inner tube is placed as soon as the obturator is removed. After it is slipped inside the outer tube, the inner tube is held in place by a small flip *lock* (located on the top part of the outer tube's face plate). *The inner tube is left out of place only during the period in which it is being cleaned.* If left out longer, secretions begin to form into crusts and other debris collects inside of the outer tube's lumen.

Silver tracheostomy tubes are carefully handled because silver is a soft metal which dents easily. Dents may cause trauma to the patient, a poor tracheal fit, or make it impossible for the various pieces of the matched set to fit together.

Tracheostomy tubes made of *synthetic materials* (e.g., nylon, plastic, polyethylene) are increasingly replacing the more traditional silver tubes. Some

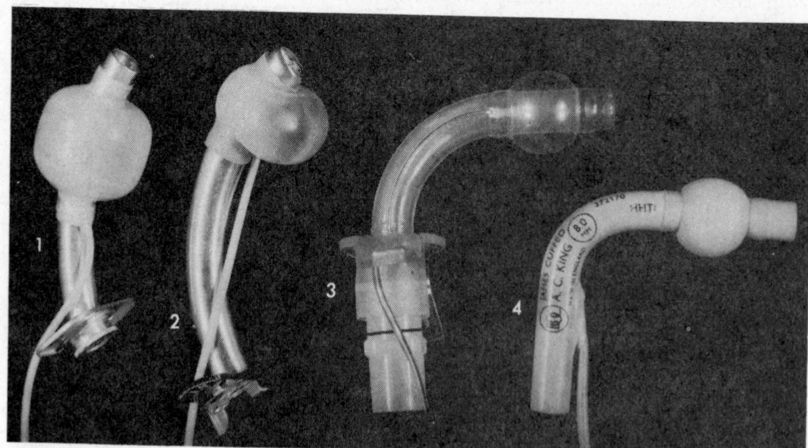

FIGURE 108–3. Tracheostomy tubes (from left to right): (1) The Hollinger tracheostomy tube with separately attached "Sof-Cuf" cuff. Note the relatively shallow curve of the tube and the evenly inflated (low-pressure) cuff; (2) The Jackson tracheostomy tube with separately attached cuff. Note the relatively sharp angle of the tube and the eccentrically inflated (high-pressure) cuff; (3) The Portex plastic tracheostomy tube with attached cuff which inflates evenly at relatively high pressure; and (4) The James tracheostomy tube with attached cuff which inflates evenly; this tube is occasionally used in short-necked patients. (From Sanderson, R. G. (ed.): *The Cardiac Patient*. 1972.)

synthetic tubes consist of a *single tube* which has one or two balloons affixed to the outer surface of the end of the tube which lies in the trachea. Some metal tracheostomy tubes also have balloons. Metal and plastic tracheostomy tubes (and endotracheal tubes) which have balloons of this sort are referred to as "cuffed" tubes (see below).

In addition to single tubes, plastic tracheostomy tubes are also available with an obturator ("pilot tube"), inner and outer cannula, and cork (used to plug the tube prior to extubation). Tracheostomy tubes with an inner removable cannula are sometimes called *"double-wall" tracheostomy tubes.*

Synthetic tubes (a) have interchangeable parts; (b) can be sterilized by boiling or autoclaving; (c) are of light weight; and (d) do not frost if exposed to cold air. The latter fact is of importance if a patient will be wearing a tracheostomy tube out-of-doors.

Tracheostomy tubes vary not only in their composition and number of separate parts but also in their *shapes* and *sizes.* The size and type to be used is carefully determined before the tracheotomy procedure is started. A tracheostomy tube's *diameter* should be sufficiently smaller than the trachea that it lies comfortably within the trachea's lumen. It should be possible for air to pass between the trachea's wall and the outer wall of the tube. Jackson tracheostomy tubes are available in 14 different sizes (from #00 through #12). Silver tubes #6 and #7 are most commonly used for adults; #00 is used for premature infants.

In addition to the tracheostomy tube's diameter, *its length* and *curve* are also of importance. Tracheostomy tubes may be long (e.g., the Hollinger tube) or short (end tracheostomy) and may be angulated from 50° to 90°. The most frequently used tracheostomy tubes are the shorter tubes with a 60° angle. Within the trachea the tube's length should be such that it prevents dislodging into the paratracheal areas as the patient turns his head or coughs; the tube's lower end should remain above the carina. The tracheostomy's curve should be such that, when in position, the inner opening of the tube points directly in line with the trachea and does not press against either the trachea's anterior or posterior walls. If the tube tilts against the posterior wall (or if the incision is made too low), injury and obstruction may result; if it tilts against the anterior wall, erosion of the innominate artery may occur. Frequently the position of the tube is checked by x-ray after insertion to prevent such complications.

Other criteria met to ensure a properly fitting tracheostomy tube are being certain that (a) the patient can breathe easily through the tube; (b) the tube's lumen is such that it can easily be suctioned with a catheter; and (c) the tube's faceplate does not cause pressure on the skin of the neck, yet is flush with the skin.

INDICATIONS FOR TRACHEOTOMY

Medical history cannot definitely document when someone first had the courage and foresight to attempt to improve respiration by cutting through the neck into the trachea. However, the life-saving value of this procedure is readily apparent to all persons involved in patient care.

Today tracheotomy is a procedure commonly performed. Tracheotomy trays are kept at hospital bedsides, readily available, as part of the routine care of numerous patients. Also, tracheotomies are routinely, often prophylactically, performed in a variety of conditions where easy access to the tracheobronchial tree is of importance. This situation is in contrast to that of the recent past. Conner et al. comment:[17] "The decision to do a tracheostomy was once dreaded, for it frequently was the death knell for the patient. It was, therefore, reserved for the desperately ill patient as a last resort."

As mentioned, a tracheostomy may be temporary or permanent. When tracheotomy is performed as the result of an emergency procedure, the stoma is usually closed later when normal respiration has been restored. Under certain circumstances, however, usually as the result of trauma or surgery, the stoma must remain open permanently to permit respiration to take place (see section on permanent tracheostomy below).

Because tracheotomy was once feared and indicated a serious prognosis, it is important that patients who are going to have tracheotomies performed (and their families) be told that the procedure will be of benefit and that it does not necessarily indicate worsening of physical condition. If the patient is unconscious and cannot be given such an explanation before the procedure, he is told as he regains consciousness that the tracheostomy will help him breathe more comfortably for awhile.

Apnea, respiratory obstruction, circulatory arrest, and exsanguinating hemorrhage are all medical emergencies which may require tracheotomy as part of their treatments.

Patients with any of the above conditions are *immediately* observed for indications of the possible need for tracheotomy. The patient's neck, thorax, and upper abdomen are uncovered and observed for retraction of the soft spots surrounding the thoracic cage. Such retraction serves as an index of the degree to which intrapleural pressure must be reduced in order to move air through an obstructed lumen. Simultaneously the patient's pulse is taken and is evaluated both qualitatively and quantitatively. The patient's facial expression is rapidly scanned for evidence of fatigue, anxiety, and apprehension. If it is determined that tracheotomy is not indicated, appropriate therapy is instituted, and the nurse is frequently left to continue evaluation of the patient's ability to satisfactorily maintain his ventilation. The nurse's vigilance must be constant during this period, because the patient's condition may worsen so rapidly that he is unable to summon help.[80]

Major indications of respiratory insufficiency include apprehension, restlessness, agitation, confusion, inability to sleep, increasing exhaustion, motor dysfunction, and a rising pulse or respiratory rate. Diaphoresis, headache, and flapping tremor may also occur. Even more serious symptoms of respiratory obstruction are chest wall retractions, stridor, and increasing tachycardia accompanied by a decreasing rate of respirations. Another late, ominous symptom is cyanosis due to impaired oxygenation of the blood. The physician is promptly notified if any of these symptoms begin to appear.

The nurse's complete evaluations and reports are highly important. The nurse must be a skilled observer if she is to summon the physician at the appropriate time. The trachea is intubated when doubt exists about the necessity for the procedure, rather than waiting until it is obvious that the procedure is unquestionably necessary.

In all situations in which tracheotomy may be indicated, attempts are made to perform the procedure before indications of the need for it become clear-cut. For example, the physician does not wait until cyanosis develops before he performs tracheotomy. In the presence of arterial unsaturation, the patient may die before tracheotomy can be performed. Proctor and Safar warn that ". . . cyanosis is a notoriously unreliable sign. Its apparent absence should never be counted as reliable evidence of adequate ventilation."[80] Likewise, in patients with upper airway obstruction, the decision to perform the tracheotomy is not postponed until the patient displays a lower arterial pO_2 or elevated pCO_2. It may be too late once such ventilatory failure has started. *Performance of an early tracheotomy is often the key to successful respiratory therapy.* When a tracheotomy is performed on this basis, the patient is ensured of greater comfort and safety.[80]

Types of patients who may benefit from tracheotomy include the following:

> *Patients requiring prophylactic tracheotomy.* As discussed, instead of waiting for patients to develop acute respiratory difficulties before performing tracheotomy, it is desirable to carry out this procedure prophylactically in various situations. For example, prophylactic tracheotomy is indicated preoperatively when a patient's ventilatory capacity is severely reduced, and postoperatively following some intrathoracic surgeries (e.g., cardiopulmonary procedures) and some neurosurgical procedures (e.g., those which could result in unconsciousness, impaired swallowing, or impaired respiration). Additionally, prophylactic tracheotomy is indicated in some patients with severe respiratory disease, critical illnesses (of various kinds), radical neck surgery, and in patients receiving irradiation therapy for laryngeal tumors encroaching on the airway. Most permanent stomas would of course be performed on a prophylactic, nonemergency basis.

> *Apneic patients.* Artificial respiration is indicated (see Unit X). If cardiac arrest is also present, tracheotomy is deferred until circulation is restored. In the interim, endotracheal intubation is employed. Tracheotomy is hazardous during external cardiac compression.

> *Unconscious patients with inadequate ventilation.* Attempts are rapidly made to determine the cause of the inadequate ventilation, e.g., obstruction of the airway, respiratory depression.

> *Patients in respiratory failure* who apparently will require respiratory assistance for periods longer than 1–2 days.

> *Patients with head, neck, or chest injuries.* Following throat trauma, airway obstruction may result from hemorrhage, unconsciousness, edema, muscular paralysis, or submucosal hematoma. Fracture of the larynx or trachea produces subcutaneous emphysema and may cause sudden airway obstruction. Following crushing chest injuries (resulting in "flail chest," i.e., an unstable chest wall), tracheotomy enables easier aspiration of blood and secretions and makes it possible to "splint" the chest from inside by using intermittent positive pressure ventilation. Other benefits are reduction of paradoxic movement (by decreasing airway resistance) and prevention of exhaustion from the effort of breathing in the presence of pain and an impaired respiratory system. (Chest injuries are discussed in Unit XIV.)

> *Patients with fulminating infections of the mouth, pharynx, or throat,* e.g., diphtheria, Ludwig's angina.

> *Conscious patients with upper airway obstruction.* In these patients tracheotomy is performed if there is evidence of severe obstruction or of the patient tiring in his attempts to overcome the obstruction to breathe. Emergency tracheotomy may be necessary if a foreign body is present in the hypopharynx or larynx.

> *Patients with accumulations of secretions in the lower tracheobronchial tree which could cause hypoxia or atelectasis or both.* Tracheotomy is commonly indicated when a patient cannot comfortably clear tracheobronchial secretions from his lower airways.

> *Patients with severe burns, especially around the head and face.* Laryngeal edema and pulmonary edema may develop, seriously jeopardizing patency of the airway. Tracheotomy helps overcome upper airway obstruction; it also helps assist ventilation and control secretions.

> *Patients who have had thyroidectomy or radical neck resection* may hemorrhage into the soft tissues of the neck. Pressure is then exerted on the trachea by the blood in the soft tissues. Tracheotomy may be indicated to prevent or relieve upper airway obstruction.

> *Patients with neurologic disorders* which impair respiratory muscles or the act of swallowing, e.g., head injuries, drug overdose, bulbar paralysis, cerebrovascular accidents. Also, patients with prolonged episodes of convulsive seizures.

> *Patients with severe pulmonary edema* who have poor gas transport across the alveolar capillary membrane.

> *Patients with severe emphysema* for whom it is desirable to reduce dead space because of impaired tidal volume.

> *Weak, feeble patients* for whom it is desirable to reduce the work of breathing. Tracheostomy reduces the work of breathing by reducing the volume of the anatomical dead space air by as much as 50 per cent. (A cuffed tube is employed when tracheotomy is performed to reduce dead space air.)

> *Postoperative patients with laryngeal edema due to prolonged intubation.* This emergency frequently occurs during recovery from anesthesia or following endotracheal extubation, and may cause airway obstruction. Before tracheotomy is resorted to, attempts may be made to correct the situation by using epinephrine, antihistamines, steroids, and high-humidity oxygen.

PERFORMING TRACHEOTOMY

A tracheotomy may be performed either as an emergency or as an elective surgical procedure. In emergency situations the incision may be made at the scene of an accident (if necessary with such crude instruments as a penknife) or at the patient's bedside (with an emergency tracheotomy set). The procedure for performing tracheotomy is discussed in detail, since nurses often assist with this procedure on wards and in emergency rooms as well as in surgery. In the hospital if an emergency tracheotomy is anticipated, a *basic emergency tracheotomy tray* is kept available at the patient's bedside. Usually these trays are preassembled and kept sterilized for immediate use. Items on the tray vary from hospital to hospital; basic items include the following: scalpel, dissecting scissors, hemostat, suture material, suction tip, syringes, needles, curved blunt bistoury (long, narrow surgical knife), two retractors, tracheal dilator, gauze sponges, sterile gloves, and tracheostomy tubes. Necessary antiseptic solutions and local anesthetics are also required.

Tracheotomies are less frequently employed as emergency measures now than formerly, owing to increasing use of emergency endotracheal intubation. Tracheotomy results are far superior when the procedure is performed electively in an operating room. In this setting, asepsis is more complete, and a general anesthetic may be administered if advisable. The procedure described in this section is that of a planned, orderly, elective tracheotomy.

Generally an orotracheal tube is passed before tracheotomy is performed. Passage of such a tube is desirable for the following reasons: (a) normal pulmonary ventilation may be rapidly restored; (b) time is obtained to perform tracheotomy more safely as an orderly surgical procedure; (c) after an adequate airway is established, a general anesthetic may be given (if indicated) to perform the tracheotomy; and (d) it is usually possible to eliminate the most common complications of tracheotomy, i.e., pneumothorax and mediastinal emphysema. In some cases orotracheal intubation may be impossible prior to tracheotomy. Some authorities feel that orotracheal intubation is contraindicated prior to tracheotomy because stimulation of the vagus nerves may result in the "vasovagal reflex," causing cardiac arrest.[80]

In preparation for tracheotomy, all necessary equipment is selected and made ready for use. A tracheostomy tube of the appropriate size and type is selected. If a cuffed tube is to be used, the cuff is checked for patency and uniformity of expansion when inflated. Adaptors are available for artificial ventilation, should it become necessary. During the procedure respiration is assisted as indicated (by mask or tracheal tube).

The patient is positioned on his back with his neck extended so the trachea becomes prominent. To accomplish this, a pillow or blanket roll is placed under the patient's shoulders. Following appropriate skin preparation and draping, a local or general anesthetic is administered and a skin incision is made. While some surgeons prefer a horizontal incision, most make a vertical incision midline in the throat, extending from the border of the cricoid cartilage downward about 5 cm. The resulting incision lies approximately 2 cm. above the suprasternal notch.

Dissection is carried out until the thyroid isthmus is identified. The isthmus is surgically divided over the trachea and is sutured back from the midline. Next the first tracheal ring is identified, and the trachea is incised through the second and third rings. A small window is cut in the trachea. If an orotracheal tube is in place during the procedure, it is partially withdrawn before the trachea is entered to prevent accidental cutting of the tube. (The tracheal tube is not completely removed until the tracheostomy tube is properly functioning.) Before the tracheostomy tube is inserted into the tracheotomy, the trachea is thoroughly aspirated to remove secretions and blood. Once properly positioned, the tube is secured in place with a tie around the neck.[80]

Some surgeons place two loose black silk sutures through the lateral tracheal edges and tape these sutures to the chest skin before completing the procedure; others suture a small flap of the tracheal edge to the neck skin. These actions may be taken so the trachea can easily be identified again if the tracheostomy tube becomes dislodged during the first few postoperative days (before an adequate tract has formed). Without such a flap or sutures, it may be difficult to find the trachea to replace the tube, because the trachea may become submerged as the various incised layers close over it. After a few days the path into the trachea becomes more clearly established and the tracheostomy tube can be more easily replaced. The sutures make it possible to pull the trachea up to the skin incision and thus ensure an airway until the tracheostomy tube can be properly reinserted.

If the tracheotomy is to be permanent, the margins of the entire tracheal opening are sutured to the skin so a permanent stoma will form. This facilitates replacing tubes. Eventually, once healing occurs, a tube may not be necessary to keep the stoma open.

Upon completion of tracheotomy, the incision is sealed with a plastic spray, or a sterile, dry dressing is placed over the incision around the tracheostomy tube to absorb secretions and protect the incision.

Recently a new emergency tracheostomy procedure has been developed which is performed *percutaneously* by inserting a small catheter into the trachea. The trachea is first punctured with a small needle, and then a special device is used to insert the catheter into the hole used to localize the trachea. The procedure can be rapidly performed. For details refer to Jacobs[46] and Toy and Weinstein.[113]

COMPLICATIONS OF TRACHEOTOMY

Possible complications to be aware of while giving post-tracheotomy care include subcutaneous emphysema, pneumothorax, or mediastinal emphysema (see Unit XIV); obstruction of the tracheostomy tube; respiratory insufficiency; displacement of the tube from its position in the trachea's lumen;

hemorrhage; pulmonary infection; atelectasis; and tracheoesophageal fistula. These complications may develop slowly or suddenly. Their *early detection* requires a nurse's vigilance. The nurse familiarizes herself with possible complications, systematically observes for their possible development, and institutes appropriate early action if complications develop.

Respiratory insufficiency may develop in the tracheotomized patient for various reasons, one of which is tracheobronchial obstruction occurring at a level lower than that of the tracheostomy tube. Evidences of such respiratory insufficiency include unequal respiratory movements on the two sides of the chest; marked respiratory effort; and retraction of all the soft spots surrounding the thoracic cage, e.g., supraclavicular, intercostal, and substernal retraction.

The airway may be obstructed (completely or partially) by such factors as external pressure; foreign bodies; swelling (edema) of the mucous membrane lining the tracheobronchial tree; or excessive secretions occluding respiratory lumina. A tracheostomy tube may be obstructed by accumulations of encrustations or by thick, dry secretions or by both.

> *If suctioning does not relieve obstruction of the tube, immediately call for the physician. In some cases the patient's life may be saved by removing the obstructed tube and holding the patient's trachea open with a tracheal dilator and hook.*

Ask the attending physician ahead of time whether you have his permission to remove the entire tracheostomy tube if the patient becomes obstructed and suctioning the tube does not relieve the obstruction. Make it clear that you will not do this if a physician is immediately available.

Accidental expulsion of a single cannula tracheostomy tube or the outer cannula of a double-walled tube occasionally occurs. When this happens, stay at the bedside and hold the tracheal incision open with a dilator (or hemostat) until help arrives and another tube is properly reinserted. A Trousseau tracheal dilator (or hemostat) and a tracheal hook are kept at the bedside of a tracheostomized patient at all times in case of this emergency (see Fig. 108–4). The nurse remembers during this emergency to reassure the patient and to act calmly.

Never try to forcefully push a "blown-out" tracheostomy tube back into place. Frantic attempts to do so may have tragic results due to compression of the trachea and misplacement of the tube. The tube may accidentally be pushed through the incision into soft tissues of the neck or mediastinum rather than into the trachea. Asphyxia may result because the trachea is compressed and any air being forced

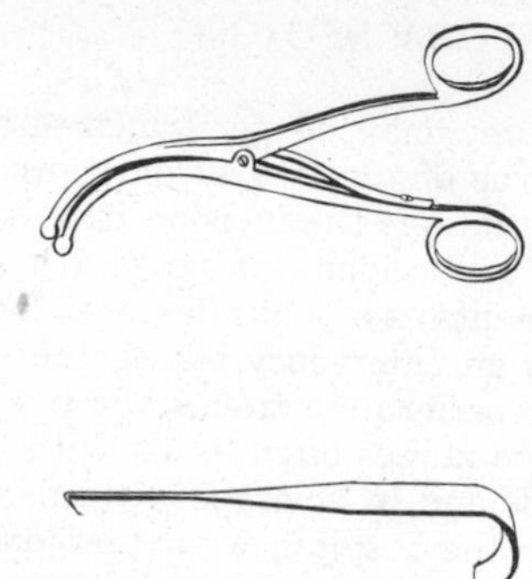

FIGURE 108–4. Tracheal dilator and hook. (From Sutton, A. L.: *Bedside Nursing Techniques in Medicine and Surgery.* 2nd ed. 1969.)

into the tracheostomy tube (e.g., by controlled ventilation) is forced into the soft tissue space. Attempts at reinsertion of a tracheostomy tube should be made only by persons qualified to do so and then only with adequate light, adequate retraction, and a tracheal hook and Trousseau dilator.

Accidental expulsion of the tube is rare, but it can happen as a result of neck ties not being properly secured or as a result of violent coughing. Caution is necessary when changing ties on a tracheostomy tube while the tube is in place to prevent accidental expulsion of the tube if the patient should suddenly cough or turn his head. As the wound heals, the possibility decreases of being unable to easily reinsert the tube if it is dislodged.

Inflammation and infection are other possible complications of tracheostomy. *Wound infection* can easily occur because of contact with tracheobronchial secretions. The wound is inspected frequently for indications of infection, and good preventative technic is used whenever tracheostomy care is given. The incision is kept as clean and dry as possible. *Tracheal perichondritis* may occur because some degree of local infection is usually present. "Tracheal perichondritis" refers to inflammation of the white, fibrous membrane (i.e., perichondrium) which covers the surface of tracheal cartilage. This inflammation may also involve the walls of such major blood vessels as the innominate and carotid arteries. This vessel erosion may result in exsanguinating hemorrhage.

Intubation (endotracheal or tracheostomy) causes reduction in a patient's ability to build up the intrapulmonary pressure necessary for an effective, expulsive cough. This *inability to cough up secretions* predisposes to *pulmonary infection* and *atelectasis.* A chest x-ray may be taken daily for several days following tracheostomy. For other measures for the detection of pulmonary complications, see Unit XIV.

Following tracheotomy *hemorrhage* may become manifest by bleeding around the tube at the incision site, by frank blood or bright blood-tinged tracheobronchial secretions, or by both. Other indications of hemorrhage are a rapid pulse rate and increasing restlessness. (Remember the latter two symptoms are also indicative of possible hypoxia.)

While it is not unusual for tracheostomy secretions to have some blood mixed with them immediately following tracheotomy, it is abnormal for frank blood to appear or for secretions tinged with bright blood to persist longer than 6–8 hours postoperatively. Notify the physician if these abnormal findings occur. Massive hemorrhage from the innominate artery can result from erosion of the trachea's anterior wall by a malpositioned tracheostomy cannula (see Fig. 108–5).

Sometimes a tracheotomized patient develops a *tracheoesophageal fistula* caused by erosion through the trachea's posterior wall. Important symptoms of the possible presence of a fistula of this nature include coughing or choking when eating or drinking, and aspiration of or leakage of food or liquids from the tracheostomy. Report these symptoms immediately.

The complications of tracheoesophageal fistula and hemorrhage may result from[111] (a) improper angulation of the tube; (b) improper cannula length; (c) improper fixation of the tube; and (d) an incorrect tracheostomy site (see Fig. 108–5).

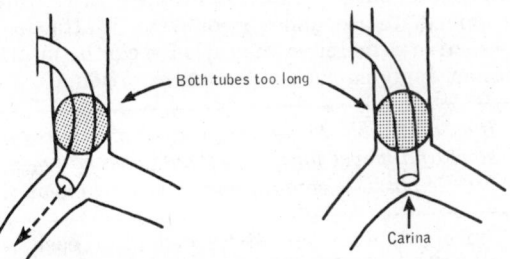

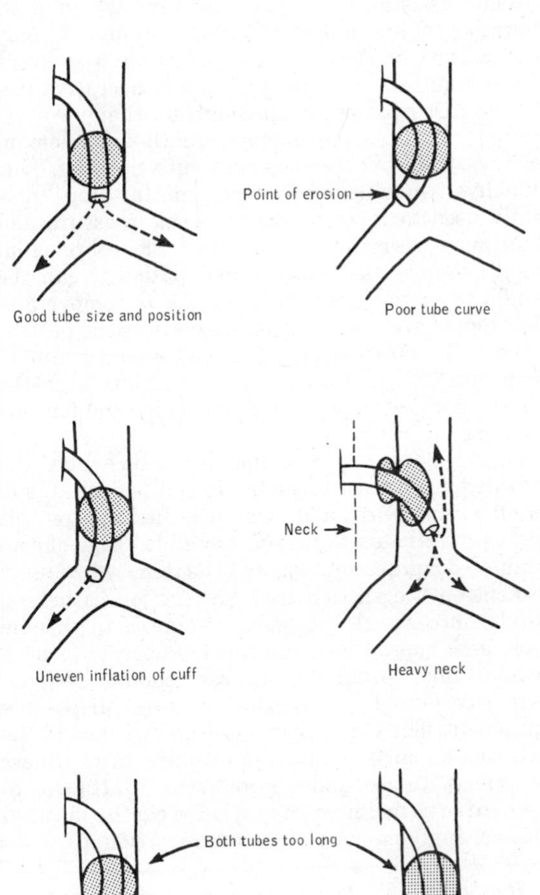

FIGURE 108–5. Tracheostomy tube positions and factors affecting them. (From Murphy, E. R.: Intensive nursing care in a respiratory unit. *Nursing Clinics of North America* 3:433, 1968.)

In addition to the possible development of the previously discussed complications, tracheostomy has certain inherent *disadvantages.* These include (a) loss of the cough reflex; (b) reduction or loss of the ability to speak normally; and (c) loss of the upper air passages' normal functions of warming, filtering, and humidifying inspired air. Loss of the latter three functions means that (a) microorganisms and foreign particles, e.g., dust, lint, may be directly inspired into the lungs; and (b) mucosa in the lower tract becomes irritated and dry, and tracheobronchial secretions become dry, tenacious, and difficult to raise (due to normal lack of warming and humidification of inspired air).

Obviously, nursing care must be directed at minimizing the effects of loss of the normal functions described above. Part of the nursing care of the tracheostomized patient therefore includes (a) recognition that the cough reflex cannot be relied upon to protect the tracheobronchial tree or to move secretions within that system; (b) provision for communication and instruction of the patient in communicating; (c) protection of the artificial tracheal opening to prevent introduction of microorganisms or foreign particles; and (d) ensuring humidification of inspired air. These aspects of clinical care, and others, are discussed more completely in the following section.

CLINICAL CARE OF THE TRACHEOSTOMIZED PATIENT

Important factors in the clinical care of any tracheostomized patient include those listed below. Some of these aspects of clinical care are discussed in detail in following sections.

> *Maintain an open airway.* Suction and clean the tube as indicated. Prevent aspiration, e.g., of water, solutions, and so forth, through the tracheostomy.

> *Observe the patient carefully for indications of respiratory difficulty,* e.g., alterations in respiratory rate, noisy respirations, restlessness, pallor, cyanosis, intercostal and substernal retraction, labored respirations.

> *Practice asepsis.* Fatal infection may be introduced directly into the tracheobronchial tree unless asepsis is maintained by *all* persons caring for the patient's tracheostomy.

> *Observe for complications of tracheostomy and take appropriate action should they develop.*

> *Ensure maximal humidification of inspired air and appropriately warm inspired air.*

> *Provide adequate hydration to help liquefy pulmonary secretions.* At least 3000 ml. of fluid intake is typically desirable daily. Intravenous fluids are ordered if adequate oral intake is not possible.

> *Maintain fluid-electrolyte balance.* Keep an accurate intake-output record and periodically evaluate the record.

> *Be gentle.* The tracheal mucosa can easily be traumatized, e.g., during suctioning. Also, because of ints sensitivity, procedures involving the trachea may be quite un-

comfortable for the patient, e.g., movement of the tube is extremely uncomfortable.

> *Keep appropriate equipment at the bedside.*

> *Prevent pressure trauma to the tracheobronchial tree.* If a cuffed tube is being used, see that the cuff is deflated as ordered to periodically relieve pressure on the trachea's wall.

> *Periodically inspect the tracheostomy for indications of trauma or infection.*

> *Ensure use of a fresh tracheostomy tube as needed.* Clean the inner cannula of mucus and encrustations as indicated. Assist with outer tube changes as scheduled or change the tube yourself *if* you are qualified to do so and you have the physician's permission.

> *Change dressing and tracheostomy ties as necessary.*

> *Provide appropriate skin care.* Keep skin clean and dry.

> *Provide frequent mouth care,* to minimize possible infection and to relieve halitosis. Set up an oral hygiene tray at the bedside and schedule mouth care as a treatment to be performed at definite times. Drinking large amounts of water is also important for oral hygiene.

> *Provide adequate nourishment.*

> *Administer medications as ordered.* Tracheostomy usually does not cause acute pain. Medications which depress the respiratory center, e.g., narcotics and sedatives, are usually avoided or given very cautiously if indicated. Mild tranquilizers or mild sedatives may initially be ordered if the patient is quite apprehensive.

> *Provide appropriate patient-family education,* preoperatively and predischarge.

> *Alleviate the patient's apprehension.* This may be accomplished in such ways as being readily available; closely observing the patient; providing care in a calm yet efficient manner; talking to the patient about what you are doing and how he can help; keeping the pateint's signal bell within reach; helping the patient communicate.

It is very important that you try to *anticipate* the needs of the tracheostomized patient. He is frequently under great stress as he attempts to adjust to his highly dependent situation. He should not be additionally subjected to the frustration of having to try to communicate obvious needs.

Bedside Tracheostomy Equipment. Equipment kept available in the room of a patient with a tracheostomy includes suction equipment; oral hygiene tray; respirator; self-inflating bag (Ambu bag); humidification equipment; extra sterile tracheotomy tray (complete with a sterile tracheostomy tube of proper size to replace the tube being used if necessary); sterile obturator of tube currently in use; sterile forceps, tracheal hook, and Trousseau tracheal dilator; sterile gauze squares appropriate for use on tracheostomy; sterile scissors; tracheostomy ties; appropriate solutions (clearly labeled) for cleansing the tube and for cleansing around the incision; roller gauze; small tube brush and pipe cleaners for cleansing the inner cannula; syringe and hemostat for inflating tube of cuffed tubes (see p. 1582).

Suctioning Through a Tracheal Stoma. Generally suctioning of a tracheostomy tube is performed only when secretions are audible, not just "routinely." It is, of course, desirable if the patient can cough and move bronchopulmonary secretions up into his trachea so the secretions either may be expelled from the tube by the force of the cough or can be removed by only superficial suctioning. Postural drainage with clapping (see Unit XIV) is useful to help move secretions into the trachea so they can easily be removed by suction. These technics of respiratory physical therapy can be used on patients being artificially ventilated, as well as on those with spontaneous respirations. Some positions of postural drainage are contraindicated in intubated patients, e.g., extreme head-low positions are contraindicated with tracheostomy.

An effective cough may be difficult or impossible with a treacheal stoma, because endotracheal pressure cannot be elevated by forcing expiration against a closed glottis. The nurse's encouragement to cough is often needed by the patient, since coughing requires energy which may be difficult for the patient to expend. Tracheostomized patients who are debilitated or have copious secretions often require suctioning, since they often are unable to clear their tracheobronchial trees of secretions without assistance. During the first 24–48 postoperative hours following tracheostomy, it may be necessary to suction a patient as often as every 15–30 minutes. Frequently strong, cooperative tracheostomized patients can cough up their own secretions if they take a deep breath and momentarily occlude the tracheostomy tube opening. This maneuver substitutes for the "glottal stop" normally used to increase intrathoracic pressure and thus move secretions up in the tracheobronchial tree.[116] Some tracheostomized patients can be taught to suction their own mouths, to remove oropharyngeal secretions. Self-care permits the patient to be more independent and also enables him to keep himself more comfortable than he might be when others attempt to anticipate his need for suctioning.

Various items are recommended to be kept at the bedside for purposes of suctioning. It is desirable to *set up a suction tray* and to change the items on this tray every 8 hours to prevent possible usage of contaminated equipment. Some *sterile* items which may be kept on the suction tray are suction catheters, towels, forceps, gloves, gauze squares, disposable cups, and appropriate solutions. Paper bags or a covered (foot pedal) waste can should be conveniently placed for disposal of used disposable equipment. The suction tube is kept attached to the wall suction outlet or suction machine in readiness for immediate use, and a Y-connector is attached to the suction catheter so the catheter can be inserted without applying suction during insertion.

> *It is advisable to use disposable sterile catheters and gloves for tracheal suctioning to minimize possible contamination of equipment.*

The above items are discarded after each suctioning. The ideal suction catheter is a disposable one with a thumb valve. If it is not possible to use disposable catheters, a catheter may be kept submerged in a basin of solution (e.g., 70 per cent alcohol, which is rinsed off the catheter with sterile normal saline or sterile water before use); this catheter is discarded when the tracheal care tray is changed.[17] Some sources recommend changing the tray and its contents (for a fresh supply of sterile equipment and solutions) every 4 hours when a catheter is kept stored in solution and is repeatedly used. Let us emphasize that the repeated use of a single catheter stored in a "sterile" solution is a procedure to be used *only* if it is *absolutely* impossible to use disposable catheters. Catheter storage solutions left at the bedside and believed to be "sterile" may actually introduce infection. Adaptors and introducers may be kept in an antiseptic noncorrosive solution, e.g., NP solution (neomycin, 1 mg./ml., plus polymyxin B, 0.1 mg./ml.[80]

Suction catheters for tracheostomies should (a) be smooth; (b) have a cone-shaped, noncollapsible proximal end for the adaptor; (c) have an opening at the tip and possibly a smaller opening 1–2 cm. above the tip on the side; and (d) have a slight curve at the tip. Unless the catheter is slightly curved, it has a tendency to pass into the right main bronchus. It is best for catheters of several sizes to be kept on the suctioning tray. The catheter size should be much smaller than the diameter of the tracheostomy tube, so that it passes easily into the lumen of the tube without completely obstructing it. For adults, a #14 or #16 (F) whistle tip catheter is frequently used.[65]

If the patient has tenacious sputum, which is difficult to remove, the physician may order a few ml.'s of sterile normal saline or sterile water to be inserted into the tube prior to suctioning. Sterile normal saline instilled into the trachea helps loosen secretions and stimulate coughing. This procedure should be used, however, only when indicated, since anything entering the tracheal tree is a potential source of infection. The normal saline may be obtained from a 30-ml. bottle or a 150-ml. I.V. bottle, depending upon how much may be required over an 8-hour period of time. Be certain to discard the bottle of solution at the end of each shift and use careful sterile technic when withdrawing solution from the bottle. Make every attempt to keep the solution sterile. Always remove the needle from the syringe before instilling the solution into the tube in the trachea. A needle not only is sharp but also may come loose and fall into the trachea.

It is important that the right and left mainstem bronchi each be suctioned separately. Position the patient with his head turned to the appropriate side to reach the desired bronchus, i.e., turn the head to the right to suction the left mainstem bronchus, vice versa for the right bronchus.

The suction procedure is essentially as follows:

> *Auscultate the chest* before and after suctioning to evaluate effectiveness.

> *Wash hands* and use sterile gloves or use a "no-touch" technic (i.e., with sterile forceps). Usually the catheter can be handled more easily with a gloved hand than with sterile forceps when suctioning.

> Place a sterile towel across the patient's chest, just below the tracheostomy tube.

> Clean the skin around the tube and the adaptors with a recommended antiseptic, noncorrosive solution, e.g., NP solution.

> Select catheter, attach it to the Y-connector (if one is necessary), lubricate the catheter with sterile normal saline in a disposable cup, and gently insert it into the tracheostomy tube. After it is inserted 6–8 inches, the obstruction created by the tracheal bifurcation (carina) may be felt. If deep suctioning is indicated, insert the tube as far as it can easily be inserted into one mainstem bronchus. Do not apply suction during insertion, i.e., keep the Y-vent open. Pull the catheter back slightly (1–2 cm.) to avoid completely blocking the bronchial lumen. Slowly withdraw the catheter while rotating or twirling it and intermittently apply suction by putting the thumb off and on the vent opening. Suctioning should generally not be continued for longer than 5 seconds at one time to prevent hypoxia and other complications. If necessary, suction again after oxygenating the patient. *Note:* successive reinsertions with the same catheter during one suctioning period are possible only if you have not contaminated the catheter. If in doubt, take another sterile catheter. *The tracheostomized patient is highly susceptible to infection; don't risk this complication.*

> After suctioning, discard the cup of saline rinsing solution as well as catheter and gloves. Do not leave a "sterile" bowl of normal saline at the bedside for repeated use to rinse or lubricate catheters. While rinsing the catheter to clear the tubing of secretions, note the amount and character of secretions aspirated.

> *Wash hands upon completion of procedure.*

If the suction catheter seems to be pulling or attaching to the tracheal wall when you are applying suction, immediately release the suction (i.e., open the vent) so you do not traumatize the tracheal wall. Begin to remove the catheter when it stimulates forceful coughing. If the catheter is not removed, the effects of the coughing are negated (since the tube obstructs the trachea or bronchus). Also, the patient must exert extra effort to create enough pressure to cough around the catheter. By suctioning as you remove the catheter, you will suction out some of the secretions being moved upward in the respiratory tree by the cough. Once the suction catheter is removed, be prepared to wipe away secretions which are coughed out of the tracheostomy tube opening. Plain gauze squares may be used to gently wipe away the expelled secretions. Be careful that threads in the gauze do not catch and pull on the tube's protruding pieces. *Never use facial tissues to wipe secretions away from the tube's orifice* because they contain lint which may be aspirated. Some cellulose tissues (e.g., Chix) may be used if they contain no lint. Mucus which is only partially expelled from the tube should be quickly wiped away before it can be drawn back into the trachea with the patient's next inspiration. Remember when the patient is coughing to keep your face away from the tube's opening as much as possible because of possible contagion.

Secretions may be ejected from the tracheal opening not only by coughing stimulated by suctioning but also during forceful expirations. Additionally some patients are able to cough up secretions through the tracheostomy tube by themselves, i.e., they do not require tracheal stimulation. If a patient has copious secretions, place a face-towel bib under the tracheostomy tube to protect the patient's gown and bedlinens. Teach the patient to hold either side of his tracheostomy tube during vigorous coughing to prevent possible accidental displacement or expulsion of the tube. If a patient cannot stabilize the tube, do so for him.

In addition to tracheal suction, nasopharyngeal suction is important in patients with tracheal stomas. *After* suctioning the trachea, you may use the catheter to suction the mouth and nose before discarding the catheter and other disposable equipment. If disposable catheters are not available, be certain to store the catheter used for nasopharyngeal suction in a clearly labeled container separate from that used for suction of the tracheal stoma.

Secretions should be cultured 2–3 times each week to evaluate the effectiveness of the sterile suctioning technic. The presence of *Pseudomonas* in the specimen does not by itself mean the patient is infected. Observations should also be made for clinical indications of infection, e.g., elevated white blood count, elevated temperature.[116]

Tracheal suctioning is associated with numerous potential hazards, some of which may be fatal. These hazards and their prevention (e.g., keeping the patient oxygenated prior to, during, and following the procedure if necessary) are discussed in Unit XIV. Factors of general importance in tracheal suctioning also are presented in that unit. For an excellent illustrated summary of suctioning tracheostomized patients, review Tyler and Synnestvedt.[116]

Cleansing the Inner Cannula. The tracheostomy tube is inspected frequently to determine the need for suctioning and cleaning. The inner cannula of a double-walled tracheostomy tube is removed and *cleaned as often as necessary* to keep it clear of secretions which cannot be removed by suctioning and encrustations of dried mucus. Sometimes crusts may be coughed out of the tube or may be removed with forceps. However, if this does not work, the tube is removed and cleaned. Immediately following the tracheotomy procedure, the inner tube may need cleaning approximately every half hour. While "routine" tracheostomy care (i.e., cleaning the inner cannula, changing dressings and ties as necessary) usually is *scheduled* every 2–4 hours, it is given oftener as indicated. Some patients need the tube cleaned hourly; others may need this done only every 6–8 hours.

Various procedures are reported for cleansing the inner cannula of a tracheostomy tube. Among these are (a) washing the inner cannula with a small test-tube brush and a cold solution of half-strength hydrogen peroxide sterile normal saline, or sterile 2 per cent sodium bicarbonate solution, then next washing with detergent; (b) simply using cold running water and gauze strips or pipe cleaners (pulled through the tube) to clean the inside of the tube; and (c) cleaning the inner cannula with soap and hot water. (Some sources recommend not using hot water to clean the tube because heat coagulates mucus, and not using pipe cleaners to clean the tube.) After cleaning the tube, hold it up and look through its lumen to be certain the lumen is clear. Next, sterilize the cannula by submerging it in boiling water for 3–5 minutes and then transfer it to sterile gauze with a sterile hemostat, so it can cool before being reinserted. If boiling is not possible (it damages some synthetic tubes), submerge the cannula in 70 per cent alcohol, then place it on a sterile gauze to dry; replace the cannula when the alcohol has evaporated. Wear sterile gloves when replacing the cannula.

Silver tubes must be cleaned carefully since they are easily bent or dented. Prior to sterilization, tarnish can be removed from silver tubes by using silver polish.

Before reinserting the inner cannula, suction and clean the outer cannula (without removing it). After reinserting the inner cannula be certain to lock it securely onto the outer cannula.

Do not leave the inner cannula out for longer than 5–10 minutes when removing it for cleaning. If left out longer, secretions and crusts begin to form in the outer cannula making it diffcult to reinsert the inner cannula.

Some tracheostomy tubes have two inner cannulas or identical interchangeable inner cannulas, so while one is removed for cleaning another can be inserted.

Some of the newer synthetic tracheostomy tubes, e.g., those made from Silastic and other synthetic substances, do not need an inner cannula since encrustations do not tend to form on them as easily as on metal tubes. Occasionally, however, crusts do form in them, e.g., due to insufficient humidification, and then the entire tube must be changed.

Connectors; Adaptors. Numerous types of adaptors are available for use with tracheostomy tubes. Some are part of the inner cannula; others are separate pieces which may or may not have accordion tubing. If the tracheostomy tube is to be connected to a mechanical respirator, a flexible swivel connector (e.g., Mörch swivel) is used to hook up the "trach" tube with the respirator's ventilatory tube. A connector of this sort minimizes the possibility of displacing the tube when turning or moving the patient. For example, use of a threaded swivel connector makes it possible to turn the patient into the semiprone position without dislodging the tube. By removing the threaded swivel cap, the nurse can suction the trachea without disconnecting the patient's oxygen supply. A connector is cleaned or replaced with a sterile one at the time routine tracheostomy care is given. If the patient is on a respirator, a sterile substitute inner cannula or adaptor is inserted into the outer cannula to continue ventilation while the tube or the connector removed or both are being cleaned.

Tracheostomy Tube Changes. Generally it

takes 4–5 days for a tracheostomy tract to be well established. During this interval, the outer (main) cannula should be changed only by a physician with the help of an assistant. Difficulty changing the tube is most likely to occur within 48 hours after tracheotomy. Problems also frequently occur in imperfectly performed tracheostomies and in apneic respirator patients. Ideally the outer tube should be changed every 24–48 hours.

Prior to tube removal, oxygen is administered. The nurse assembles the following *equipment for the tube change:* tracheal intubation equipment; bag-mask unit; sterile gloves; tracheal hook; retractor; Trousseau dilator; water-soluble lubricating jelly; tube ties; one replacement tube the same size as that currently in place; and another replacement tube one size smaller than that currently being used. Cuffs on replacement tubes are checked prior to their insertion. A spotlight is also essential equipment to have at the bedside.

If the channel from the skin to the tracheal opening is not clearly established as yet, the physician may insert a gloved finger into the incision and then slip a tracheal hook alongside his finger until he catches the trachea. Traction is then exerted on the edge of the tracheal incision, and the new tube is inserted. Sometimes the physician elects to intubate the patient from above the tracheostomy before the tracheostomy tube is changed. Then in case of difficulty, the patient's respirations can be maintained.

The nurse may be given permission to change outer tubes after approximately 10 postoperative days, or once the tract is established.

Skin Care; Dressing Changes. Keep the area around the tracheostomy clean and dry. Moisture encourages skin maceration and infection. Change dressings and ties as necessary to keep them clean and dry. *Skin* around the tracheostomy may be antiseptically cleansed with prescribed solutions, e.g., sterile normal saline, mild antiseptics, hydrogen peroxide, or a recommended soap solution. Be careful not to allow the solution to enter the stoma and be aspirated during the cleansing procedure. Generally it is not practically possible to mechanically cleanse the stoma itself. However the area is kept generally clean. Crusting may occur on the skin around the stoma. After these crusts are lubricated with a prescribed ointment, they are gently removed with a tweezers. Care is taken that the crusts are not aspirated. A small amount of antibiotic ointment may be prescribed for application when the tracheostomy tube is changed.

Report indications of irritation of the skin or stoma. Although it rarely happens, some patients develop allergic skin reactions to the composition of various types of tracheostomy tubes. This condition is usually relieved once a different kind of tube is used.

The *tracheostomy dressing* is most easily placed between the incision and the back of the tube's faceplate before the tapes are tied. When replacing the dressing be careful not to dislocate or unnecessarily move the tube. Normally wound drainage is minimal but the dressing may require changing owing to dampness or soilage from secretions.

Gauze squares may be used for tracheostomy dressings; these fit easily around the tube if they are cut halfway through, i.e., from the center of one edge into the center of the square (Fig. 108–6). The edges of these squares are bound to prevent loose strings being aspirated. Usually prepackaged, sterile tracheostomy dressings are available. In addition to not having loose strings, tracheostomy dressings must be made of gauze squares which do *not* have a layer of absorbent cotton; loose pieces of cotton could accidentally enter the tracheostomy tube. In some settings, cut 4 × 4's are not used for tracheostomy dressings because of the danger of loose threads. Instead the 4 × 4 is opened and folded into a long strip, and the strip is then folded over in the center and placed around the tracheostomy tube in the shape of an inverted "V."

If the tracheostomy tube is left open, e.g., is not connected to a respirator, the tube's opening may be protectively covered with a layer of gauze to reduce the risk of aspiration of foreign particles. Gauze used for this purpose should not have any absorbent or any loose threads. If dampened, this gauze layer helps humidify inspired air. The gauze should not be so wet, however, that drops could enter the tracheostomy. (Humidification is discussed in Unit XIV.) For cosmetic reasons, some patients like to keep a piece of gauze over their tracheostomies to somewhat conceal the tube or opening.

Tracheostomy Neck Ties or Tapes. Ties or tapes holding the tracheostomy tube in place are checked frequently to be certain they are clean and dry and neither too loose nor too tight. *Always keep scissors* at the bedside to cut the ties if they become too tight or if the tube must be removed. If the tube is partially coughed out, the tape is cut at once.

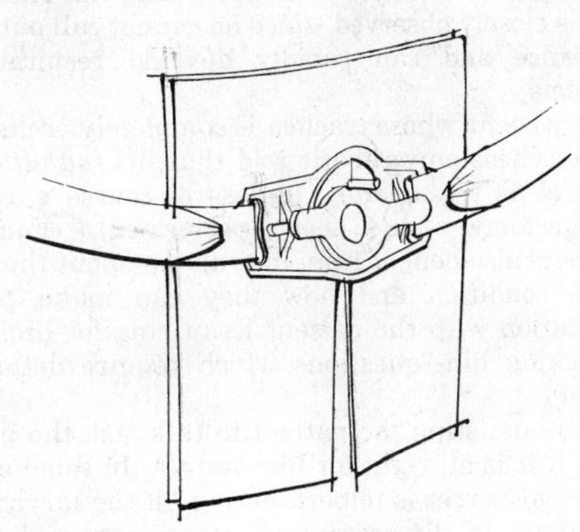

FIGURE 108–6. Gauze square cut to serve as tracheostomy dressing. (From Sutton, A. L.: *Bedside Nursing Techniques in Medicine and Surgery.* 2nd ed. 1969.)

Tracheostomy tie tapes may be made of 16-inch long pieces of 3/4-inch twill tape. One tie is fastened to each loop of the outer cannula. This is accomplished by making a horizontal cut through a portion of the tape about 1 inch from one end of the tape. Then this end of the tie is pulled through the tube's loop. Next, open the cut you have made in the tape, take the other end of the tape and pull it though the loop until the tie secures itself. This method of fastening the tie onto the faceplate's loops avoids the use of knots which could cause uncomfortable pressure on the patient's neck. The two ties are brought together and tied. The tie should be snug but not so uncomfortably tight that it obstructs veins. The tie is knotted on the side of the neck, not on the back of the neck where it would be uncomfortable and could not easily be observed. A secure knot is used (not a bow) to prevent the tube from accidentally being dislodged during coughing.

Two nurses are needed to safely adjust or change the ties on a tracheostomy tube while the tube is in place. One nurse gloves and holds the tube in place by placing the fingers of one hand on either side of the tube's faceplate. Then she places her other hand firmly behind the patient's neck. The other nurse then fixes the ties. The ties should be replaced as often as necessary.

If the patient is wearing a hospital gown, there is danger that the tracheal ties could accidentally be untied instead of the gown's ties. To prevent this possibility the gown is placed on the patient so it ties in front. The top tie is left open and the gown is secured by the second tie.

Communication. The tracheostomized patient should always have a signal light, tap bell, and pencil and paper or magic slate at hand so he can summon help and communicate as necessary. Some patients like to use picture charts, picture cards, or hand signals to make their needs known. The patient is closely observed, since he cannot call out for assistance and can rapidly develop respiratory problems.

The patient whose trachea is completely occluded by a tracheostomy tube is told that his *inability to speak is only temporary* (unless of course a total laryngectomy has been performed). Family members also benefit from instruction about the patient's condition and how they can make communication with the patient less tiring for him by not asking him questions which require detailed answers.

Before assisting the patient to talk, ask the physician if it is all right for him to talk. In some conditions voice rest is important, e.g., if the larynx is edematous, in the presence of other laryngeal disorders, or following laryngeal surgery. Some patients are allowed to use a cork to obstruct the tracheostomy opening for purposes of speaking. Other patients (without laryngectomy) can speak by taking a breath and then covering the tube with a finger while speaking. Only a word or two may be spoken before it is necessary to remove the finger to continue breathing. Speaking may fatigue the patient; thus the nurse makes every attempt to understand his communication and to anticipate his needs.

Oral Intake. An intake-output record is maintained for tracheostomized patients. Typically intravenous fluids are given for 24 hours following tracheotomy to ensure adequate hydration and nutrition; some patients may be allowed fluids orally a few hours after tracheotomy. Sometimes diet is ordered as tolerated, beginning the first postoperative day. It may be desirable for a few days to avoid serving foods which are hard to swallow.

When the tracheostomized patient first begins oral intake, he may cough and fear aspiration. However, he rapidly learns how to eat and drink safely with the tube in place. Nonetheless, the nurse remains prepared to suction as necessary because the patient may cough or aspirate while eating and drinking.

CARE OF THE NEWLY TRACHEOSTOMIZED PATIENT

Clinical care of the patient who has a tracheostomy requires scrupulous, uncompromising attention to detail 24 hours a day by all persons caring for the patient. Careless technic or the omission of necessary activities can seriously jeopardize the patient's chances of recovery. The newly tracheostomized patient is totally dependent upon others and thus requires constant supervision and alert care. The importance of excellent nursing care for the patient with a tracheostomy cannot be overemphasized.

Because the newly tracheostomized patient requires constant attendance, he is frequently cared for in an intensive care unit. The nurse carefully monitors the patient's general condition (pulse and respiratory rates, rhythms, and characters; blood pressure; skin and mucous membrane color), observing for indications of shock, respiratory insufficiency, hemorrhage, and other possible complications. As she carries out these activities, the nurse also works constantly to maintain the patency of the tracheostomy tube, to provide adequate humidification, and to protect the tracheotomy wound. The wound itself is periodically inspected. Aseptic technic is practiced when giving tracheostomy care.

Vital signs are checked at least every half hour for the first 24–48 postoperative hours. Additionally, during the postoperative period the patient's tidal and minute volumes are periodically evaluated. After the patient's pulse and blood pressure have stabilized and he is conscious, he is positioned with his head elevated approximately 45° to enhance comfortable breathing.

Frequent suctioning and cleaning of the inner cannula of double-walled tubes are usually necessary for the first 12–24 hours postoperatively owing to tracheobronchial hypersecretion. The trauma caused to the trachea by the surgical procedure of tracheotomy causes the trachea to react by producing increased secretions. While the newly tracheostomized patient may require suctioning every few minutes, eventually, as the amount of mucous subsides, he may need to be suctioned only every few hours.

In order to completely evaluate the patient's condition, the nurse listens to his chest with a stethoscope for sounds of pulmonary congestion, and she periodically uncovers his chest to look for such symptoms of respiratory distress as (a) uneven movements of the two sides of the chest; (b) exaggerated respiratory movements; and (c) retraction of tissues in the supraclavicular spaces and the suprasternal notch, intercostal soft tissues, and epigastric tissues. Cuffed tubes are cared for as ordered (see below).

Reportable situations during the postoperative period following tracheotomy include the : (a) tube displacement; (b) indications of shock, hemorrhage, respiratory insufficiency, hypoxia, and other possible complications (see earlier discussion); (c) respiratory obstruction (report immediately such symptoms as respiratory distress not relieved by suctioning, increasing respirations accompanied by rales, crowing, or wheezing); and (d) excessive restlessness or apprehension or both (these conditions influence cardiopulmonary actions in addition to serving as possible clues to other complications). Restlessness and apprehension are carefully evaluated as possible indications of hemorrhage or hypoxia.

The patient's mucous membranes and finger tips are closely observed for cyanosis. If *oxygen administration* is necessary, it may be given via a tent or via a clear plastic tracheal mask (or collar or funnel) into the tracheostomy tube. Because humidification of inspired air is essential, the oxygen device is connected to a humidity apparatus (see Fig. 108–7). A catheter is never used to administer oxygen into a tracheostomy, since it sends a jet of oxygen directly into the trachea and dries the mucosa and secretions. Obviously oxygen administered

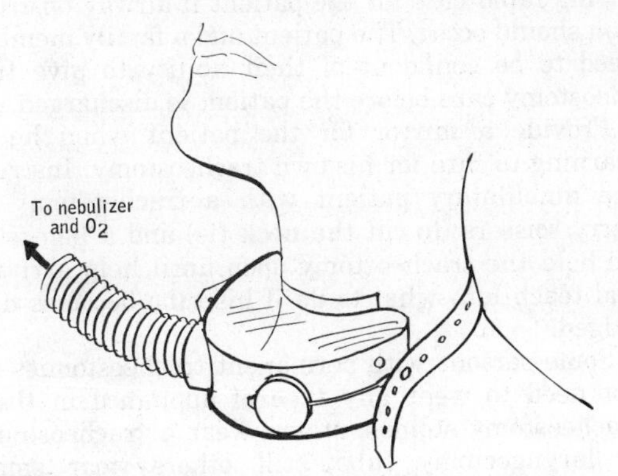

FIGURE 108–7. High-humidity collar. (From Sutton, A. L.: *Bedside Nursing Techniques in Medicine and Surgery.* 2nd ed. 1969.)

via nasal catheter does not help a patient who has a tracheostomy, since his upper airway does not effectively connect with his lower airway.

Complete charting is among the nurse's important contributions to the care of the newly tracheostomized patient. Remember to include comments about the character of secretions and the appearance of the incision and the skin around it.

The newly tracheostomized patient is often upset by frequent, brassy-sounding episodes of coughing which are productive of *mucus.* The patient is taught to wipe mucus away from the tracheostomy as he coughs it up and to protectively hold a piece of gauze (not tissue) in front of the opening (rather than in front of his mouth) when he coughs. The copious amounts of mucus initially present are due to the tracheobronchial tree's attempts to compensate for bypassage of the respiratory mucosa in the nose (which normally warms and humidifies inspired air). Increased tracheobronchial secretions and the noises they cause often make the patient fearful that his tube is obstructing and that he may drown in his own secretions. Gradually the tracheobronchial mucosa adapts to the upper respiratory tract bypassage, and the cough becomes less frequent and less productive.

Rhinorrhea also occurs with a tracheostomy, since air is not breathed through the nose to absorb nasal secretions. Rhinorrhea, the frequent tendency to cough, and the copious production of mucus all cause the newly tracheostomized patient to think that he may have a cold. Gentle suctioning is necessary to remove nasal secretions. Eventually rhinorrhea ceases as the body adjusts to its altered physiology.

Tracheostomy breathing differs from normal nasal-oral breathing in that the sensation of breathing is absent. Also there is loss of the Valsalva maneuver, making effective coughing impossible. These changes from normal physiologic experiences may also initially frighten the patient.

Often the newly tracheostomized patient needs *frequent reassurance* that his *tube is open* and that he *can breathe* through it. The patient may be afraid to go to sleep, for fear of suffocation. The nurse's verbal reassurance and constant attention are helpful in relieving this fear until the patient gains confidence in those caring for him and until he becomes less anxious about the tube.

EXTUBATION (DECANNULATION)

The process of removing the tracheostomy tube is called "extubation" or "decannulation." Patients with temporary tracheostomies are helped to *gradually* return to normal breathing before the tube is removed; the patient must learn again to breathe through his upper respiratory tract. Extubation is a time of fear and anxiety for many patients. They have learned that they can safely breathe through their tracheostomies and now they are concerned that independent respiratory function may no longer be possible.

When the physician believes that the patient is able to begin to breathe without respiratory assistance, he gives orders to begin to reduce the lumen of the tracheostomy tube for a day or so and then to partially obstruct the tracheostomy tube's outer opening for varying lengths of time. Eventually the patient is able to tolerate complete occlusion of the tracheostomy opening.

Occlusion of the tracheostomy tube (either partially or completely) is accomplished in various ways. For example, a special tube with a small opening may be inserted into the main tracheostomy tube; tape may be placed over the tube's opening; or corks of gradually increasing size may be inserted into the tube's opening until it is eventually completely occluded. Corks used are either plastic or pure rubber (natural cork could crumble and bits could be aspirated). The corks are secured to the tracheostomy tube with braided threads. *Remember, corking or other occlusion of the tracheostomy opening must be preceded by deflation of cuffed tubes and insertion of a fenestrated or smaller diameter tube.* If you fail to remember this and occlude the opening of the tracheostomy tube, you totally obstruct the patient's airway! During the "trial" periods of occlusion of the tracheostomy tube, the patient is closely observed and his tolerance of the procedure charted. Immediately remove the obstruction upon any evidence of respiratory difficulties. Once the patient has been able to comfortably tolerate complete plugging of the tube for 24 hours, the tracheostomy tube is removed.

Close nursing supervision continues following extubation, and pO_2 and pCO_2 levels are typically evaluated for several days. After tube removal, the incision is sutured closed, or the edges of the wound are pulled together with butterfly strips of adhesive tape for a few days until the wound heals. Following tube removal, an air leak occurs for a while at the area of the incision. This reduces the effectiveness of the patient's cough (because it makes it difficult to create high intrathoracic pressures) and can pose problems in maintaining a patent airway. (These problems do not occur following removal of an endotracheal tube since an incision was not made.) Teach the patient to hold a dressing firmly over the stoma's incision line when coughing until the incision is healed. Pressure of this sort can help the patient increase intrathoracic pressure, and hence he can cough more effectively. It takes several days for the tracheotomy wound to heal sufficiently enough to stop air from leaking through it.

Generally it is advisable for any patient who has had a tracheostomy to continue under medical supervision for at least a year following extubation. Tracheal scarring and tracheal stricture are problems which can develop and are watched for during this period.

A *Kistner button* is sometimes used as an intermediate step between use of a standard tracheostomy tube and complete extubation. This device is a short, straight tracheostomy tube which fits into the tracheostomy stoma but does not project down into the tracheal lumen. The Kistner button has a removable cap which has a one-way flap inside. Inhalation is possible through the cap's opening, but exhalation is not possible since the force of the air being exhaled pushes the flap over the cap's opening. When the cap is on the tube the patient can talk. The cap is removed for suctioning of the stoma. A Kistner button cannot be used with a ventilator, but may be used in place of a standard tracheostomy tube in patients with retained secretions who do not require ventilatory assistance. In these patients the button is substituted for the standard tube once a well-established tracheostomy tract has formed. Less airway resistance is created with a Kistner button than with a plugged standard tracheostomy tube. Breathing is therefore easier. Artificial humidification of inspired air is necessary with a Kistner button (as with any type of tracheostomy tube) since the natural airway is bypassed.

PERMANENT TRACHEOSTOMY

Some patients are not decannulated, but instead have a permanent tracheostomy. Most patients with permanent tracheostomies are laryngectomees. (See discussion of laryngectomy, Chapter 109.) A small percentage are victims of injury, burns, or infection.

Patient education regarding tracheostomy care is started early during the course of hospitalization if a patient is going to be discharged with a permanent tracheostomy. Instructions for self-care include care of the tracheostomy tube, skin care of the stoma, suctioning, and care of suction catheters. It is desirable to teach a family member as well as the patient. Supervise the patient's self-care until he is skilled enough to act without supervision. Teaching self-care early is the best means of assuring rapid care for the patient if airway obstruction should occur. The patient and a family member need to be confident of their ability to give tracheostomy care before the patient is discharged.

Provide a mirror for the patient when he is learning to care for his own tracheostomy. Instruct the ambulatory patient with a tracheostomy to carry scissors (to cut the neck tie) and a hemostat (to hold the tracheostomy open until help arrives) and teach him what to do if his tube becomes dislodged.

Some persons with permanent tracheostomies do not need to wear any type of appliance in their tracheostomy stomas; others wear a tracheostomy or laryngectomy tube; still others wear small plastic tracheostomy "buttons" which are hollow in the center and have a flange on each side to anchor the button just at the neck's skin surface.[22]

It is psychologically desirable for persons with permanent tracheostomies to cover the tracheostomy tube or stoma. Murphy and Ogura comment:[68] "Display of either the bib or . . . of the open stoma itself represents a public proclamation of 'difference' or disability not in keeping with the achievement of the most normal functioning possible." Shirts or blouses buttoned at the neck or scarves are means of effectively covering (and protecting) the tracheostomy opening and yet enabling easy accessibility to the stoma when necessary. Covering the opening helps warm and filter inspired air. High-necked, properly-fitted collars and neck scarves also help conceal the disfigurement resulting from unilateral or bilateral radical neck dissection when these procedures have been performed.

Teach patients with permanent tracheostomies that they must prevent accidental aspiration through the tracheostomy stoma, e.g., when washing hair, bathing, and so forth. Swimming is prohibited. When bathing in a tub, a towel should be placed around the neck to prevent water from entering the stoma. Likewise a mirror is always used when washing the face to prevent the accidental entrance of soap and water into the stoma. Tub baths should be taken with the drain open to prevent accidental drowning if the patient falls asleep. When showering the patient is told to direct the stream of water at chest height and to wear a special protective shower-shield to cover the stoma. If a shield is not available, he can hold a washcloth between his teeth with one end protectively hanging over the stoma. Special care is necessary when using aftershave lotions on the neck or any powder or spray (aerosol) product directed at the upper half of the body, e.g., aerosol shaving lathers, hair sprays, deodorants, to prevent accidentally directing them toward the stoma. When receiving haircuts, the patient needs to inform the operator to take care not to allow falling hair to enter the stoma, e.g., when shaking off the cape or brushing off the patient's shoulders. When aspiration does occur, it precipitates violent coughing which is not only uncomfortable but also frightening. Airway damage may occur, and, of course, at times aspiration may be fatal. (*Note:* these precautions are important for any patient with a tracheostomy, permanent or temporary.)

If suctioning is necessary, the patient is informed that many local chapters of the American Cancer Society have suction machines available for home use; machines can also be rented from hospital equipment rental firms. A list of necessary supplies for home care is given to the patient's family along with information about where the equipment can be purchased.

Instructions for home care also include emphasizing that the patient should not have contact with persons who have respiratory infections. Additionally, a family member should be taught how to give emergency mouth-to-neck resuscitation to the patient if the patient experiences respiratory depression or respiratory arrest.

MOUTH-TO-NECK RESUSCITATION

Emergency mouth-to-neck, i.e., "mouth-to-tracheostomy," resuscitation may be necessary if the tracheostomized patient experiences respiratory depression or respiratory arrest. Patients with tracheostomies are important exceptions to the standard emergency mouth-to-mouth artificial method. Cardiopulmonary resuscitation is discussed in detail in Unit X.

> *Immediately upon finding any unconscious person, check his neck to determine if he is a "neck-breather," i.e., if he has a tracheostomy.*

The nurse must be prepared to administer and to teach emergency resuscitation for neck-breathers and partial neck-breathers. This technic is discussed and illustrated in "First Aid for (Neck-Breathers) Laryngectomees," published by the American Cancer Society.[3]

It is possible to give emergency neck resuscitation mechanically with a rubber or plastic inflatable bag (e.g., Ambu bag) fitted with a baby-sized mask. However, mouth-to-neck breathing is more efficient and safer. Pressure of the mask on the neck's major blood vessels may interfere with circulation to the brain (cerebral circulation); also, it is difficult to maintain a tight seal over the tracheostomy with a mask.

ENDOTRACHEAL INTUBATION

An endotracheal tube is inserted by the physician into a patient's trachea through the nose or mouth. An *orotracheal tube* is passed through the mouth into the trachea; a *nasotracheal tube* is passed into the trachea via the nose.

Endotracheal intubation is used for reasons similar to those for tracheostomy, that is, to remove secretions and to facilitate ventilation.

ADVANTAGES AND DISADVANTAGES

Advantages of endotracheal intubation over tracheostomy are that (a) the intubation can be done rapidly, and (b) surgical trauma is avoided. Orotracheal or nasotracheal tubes may be used instead of a tracheostomy in patients whose conditions are expected to be *self-limited* within a day or so. Also, endotracheal intubation is preferred rather than tracheotomy in managing *emergency* situations. For example, a patient with exsanguinating pulmonary hemorrhage may have his life saved if it is possible to rapidly carry out orotracheal intubation and suctioning.[80] In most emergency situations orotracheal intubation is preferable to nasotracheal intubation or tracheostomy. *Orotracheal intubation is more advantageous than nasotracheal intubation* for the following reasons: (a) its results are more predictable; (b) it is less time-consuming to perform; (c) no nasal bacteria are introduced into the trachea; and (d) it is potentially less traumatic. (Nasotracheal intubation may precipitate epistaxis.)

Endotracheal tubes have several *disadvantages.* While it is possible to suction through an endotracheal tube, it is not as effective as suctioning through a tracheostomy. Usually frequent suctioning (with a sterile catheter) is necessary when an endotracheal tube is in place. An endotracheal tube cannot be passed in some conditions, e.g., severe burns, laryngeal edema. *Endotracheal tubes can be more damaging to the airway than tracheostomy tubes. Therefore, endotracheal tubes are not left in place for longer than 24–48 hours.* After this time, a tracheostomy is necessary if the patient cannot maintain adequate respiratory function. Nasotracheal or orotracheal tubes can cause extensive and permanent damage to the larynx and airway after 24 hours or more. Thus, when *long-term* airway care is necessary, tracheotomy becomes the procedure of choice because it is safer, it facilitates nursing care, and it is more comfortable for the conscious patient.

COMPLICATIONS

Complications which may be associated with usage of endotracheal tubes include (a) *vocal cord damage* (the tube keeps the cords open); (b) *laryngeal erosion* and eventual *stricture* (resulting from friction); (c) *pressure ulceration of the lip* (if an orotracheal tube is used); (d) *laryngeal edema* (following tube removal); and (e) *pulmonary infection* (resulting from inability to effectively cough or introduction of pathogens via the tube or both). Respiratory infection[111] may easily occur when endotracheal intubation removes the normal protective barrier against bacteria which the glottis usually provides for the airway. Additionally, bacterial exposure may be increased if contaminated ventilator equipment is used. Gram-negative organisms tend to grow easily in this equipment; therefore, all equipment must be changed daily, including the vaporizor, tubes, and valves. Infection of the respiratory tract may also be minimized by using isolation precautions to prevent cross-infection and employing an aseptic suctioning technic.

Other complications of endotracheal intubation include (a) *tracheal injuries;* (b) *hypoxia;* and (c) *cardiac arrhythmias.* Tracheal injuries, e.g., tracheoesophageal fistula, and tracheal stenosis, result from local tissue trauma. This trauma may result from such factors as (a) use of an excessively large tube; (b) prolonged inflation or overinflation of a cuff; (c) excessive movement of the endotracheal tube (e.g., due to improper fixation of the tube); (d) traumatic suctioning; and (e) "dragging" on the indwelling tube (e.g., due to lack of support of the cannula and its connecting tubes). Hypoxemic complications, e.g., cardiac arrhythmias, may result from prolonged endotracheal suctioning or dislodgment, plugging, or malposition of the endotracheal tube. Complications of endotracheal intubation can be fatal.[111]

Malfunctioning of an endotracheal tube can result from such problems as displacement or obstruction of the tube. *Malfunctioning of an endotracheal tube is a medical emergency, since asphyxiation can rapidly occur. Tube displacement* can occur into either the esophagus or the right mainstem bronchus. Any tube placed in the trachea has a tendency to enter the right mainstem bronchus, because this bronchus separates from the trachea at a smaller angle than in the left mainstem bronchus. If an endotracheal tube enters the right mainstem bronchus, only the right lung is intubated; consequently, the left lung is not ventilated. The inflated cuff of a cuffed tube placed too low in the trachea can completely block off a bronchus. Displacement of an endotracheal tube into the right mainstem bronchus may result in asphyxiation.

Displacement of the tube into the esophagus causes inflation of the stomach if a respirator is used. If the patient is capable of spontaneous respirations, he can continue to breathe if the tube is in his esophagus. However, if he must rely on a respirator, esophageal tube displacement results in asphyxiation.

Obstruction of an endotracheal tube may be detected not only by observable respiratory distress but also by auscultation of both lungs. Failure to hear breath sounds in either or both lungs can indicate obstruction. Endotracheal tube obstruction can result from such factors as (a) displacement of the inflated cuff over the tube's orifice; (b) tube kinkage; or (c) tube compression due to the patient biting the tube (prevent this by using "bite-block" or an oropharyngeal airway). Secretions are also a common cause of tube obstruction.

TYPES OF ENDOTRACHEAL TUBES

A wide variety of endotracheal tubes are available for orotracheal or nasotracheal intubation (see Fig. 108–8). All endotracheal tubes are available with inflatable cuffs near their tips. Because considerable variety exists in cuff design, the physician selects one which[111] (a) requires minimal cuff inflation pressure; (b) inflates evenly and uniformly over a broad area; and (c) is composed of material which is nonirritating to tissue and not subject to leakage. Before insertion into the trachea, the balloon or cuff of an endotracheal tube is tested for uniform inflation and for possible leakage. (Cuffed tubes are discussed further below.)

Orotracheal tubes are somewhat larger than nasotracheal tubes, and thus enable more effective suctioning. Of course, care is taken not to use a tube which is excessively large and will injure the larynx and mucosa. *While mucosal damage can result from an overinflated cuff, it most commonly results from use of too large a tube.* Generally it is most desirable to select a tube whose outside diameter is three fourths that of the inside diameter of the trachea.[80] Oral endotracheal tubes are commonly more uncomfortable than nasal endotracheal tubes.

Endotracheal tubes do not have inner cannulae which can be removed for cleaning (as do many tracheostomy tubes).

BEDSIDE ENDOTRACHEAL INTUBATION

Nurses often participate in bedside endotracheal intubation. Equipment necessary to insert a cuffed endotracheal tube includes (a) endotracheal tube; (b) syringe to inflate the cuff; (c) laryngoscope (to visualize the larynx, depress the tongue, and lift the jaw); (d) adequate bedside lighting; (e) a flexible copper stylet (may be employed to give the tube greater rigidity during insertion); and (f) syringes, needles, and medications. Sometimes a muscle relaxant medication is administered intravenously to facilitate intubation. Be certain to precheck the light in the laryngoscope to be certain it is properly functioning. Steps in endotracheal intubation are shown in Figure 108–9.

Because endotracheal intubation is difficult for the conscious patient to tolerate, carefully explain purposes of the procedure prior to intubation. Attempts to enlist the patient's cooperation make it easier for the patient to tolerate an uncomfortable but essential procedure.

If possible, prior to intubation topical anesthesia is applied between periods of assisted ventilation. If the patient is unconscious or if the airway must immediately be established, the orotracheal intubation is performed without the topical anesthesia. A nasopharyngeal airway should be lubricated with anesthetic jelly prior to insertion. The airway may then be left in place for up to a week. Orotracheal intubation is best performed by direct laryngoscopy with the patient supine. To obtain maximum laryngeal exposure in the supine patient, the patient's occiput is elevated and his head is tilted slightly backward at the atlanto-occipital joint so he appears to be in a "sniffing position."[80]

The physician can most effectively intubate a patient if he stands or sits on a stool directly behind the patient's head. If time permits, it is desirable for a patient in a standard hospital bed to be positioned with his head at the foot of the bed, so his head can more easily be reached.

During the intubation, an assistant can additionally facilitate exposure by retracting the right corner of the patient's mouth and pressing the patient's larynx backward or by raising further the occiput. The attending physician holds the laryngoscope in his left hand and inserts it into the right corner of the patient's mouth. Once he has positioned the scope so he can visualize the larynx, he passes the tube (with his right hand) while looking through the blade. A stylet is used to guide the tube's tip in difficult intubations; however, it is not "routinely" used because it can injure glottic structures.

Immediately after the tube is passed, its correct location is assured by observing the patient's breathing through it or by artificially inflating the patient's lungs. Auscultation of the chest may also be performed to rule out bronchial obstruction, and x-rays taken to ensure the tube's correct location. Finally the cuff is inflated (a cuffed tube is preferred in adults). The tube is firmly fixed to a bite-

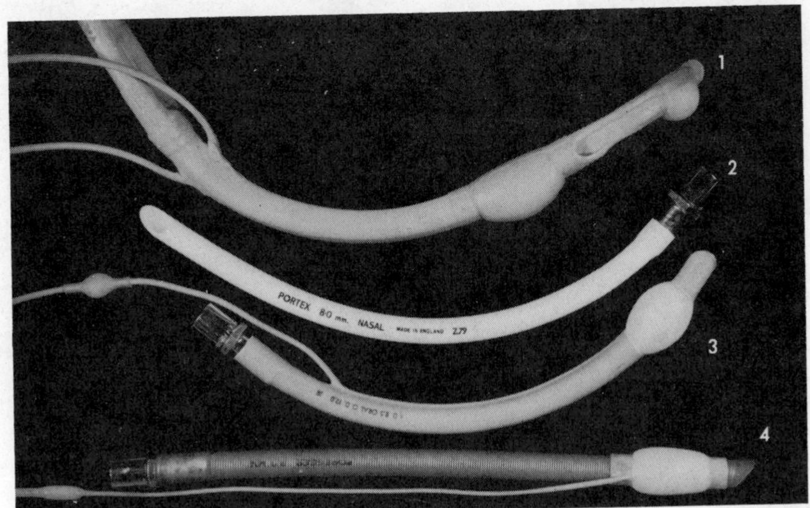

FIGURE 108–8. Endotracheal tubes (from top to bottom): (1) The Robert-Shaw double-lumen tube to isolate the flow to each lung. Note the individual inflatable cuffs for the trachea and the left bronchus; (2) The Portex nasotracheal tube, without attached cuff; (3) An orotracheal tube with attached inflatable cuff (very commonly used); and (4) The LA (Latex-Armored) tube. Note the spiral winding to prevent kinking. (From Sanderson, R. G. (ed.): *The Cardiac Patient.* 1972.)

block or pharyngeal tube and then to the patient's face. The patient is given continued ventilatory assistance as indicated.[80]

Frequently endotracheal tubes are used with a respirator, and the cuff is therefore inflated. To prevent pressure damage to the tracheal walls, a very slight air leak may be allowed, and the cuff is routinely deflated periodically (see discussion of cuffed tubes below). Ventilation therapy becomes inaccurate and ineffective if *uncontrolled air leaks* occur around endotracheal tubes, and alveolar ventilation may be inadequate. Air leaks make volume respirators particularly difficult to use with accuracy; thus these respirators are almost always used with cuffed tubes.

Following endotracheal intubation, care is taken to *provide adequate humidification* and to *prevent contamination of inhaled air.*

With proper endotracheal intubation, *both* sides of the thorax rise evenly during inspiration. Frequent observation of the intubated patient's chest is thus important in addition to using a stethoscope to listen for airflow in *both* lungs. To *prevent displacement,* the endotracheal tube must be anchored adequately exteriorly and care taken while giving care (e.g., turning the patient) not to exert traction on the tube. The position of the tube may be checked periodically with x-ray and is always checked immediately if displacement is suspected.

Secure oral endotracheal tubes to the patient's face in the following manner: (a) carefully apply tincture of benzoin to the patient's cheeks where the tape will be placed, cover the patient's eyes during this application; (b) wrap adhesive tape around the tube and extend the tape over the face on both sides; (c) tape the tube and slip-joint tightly

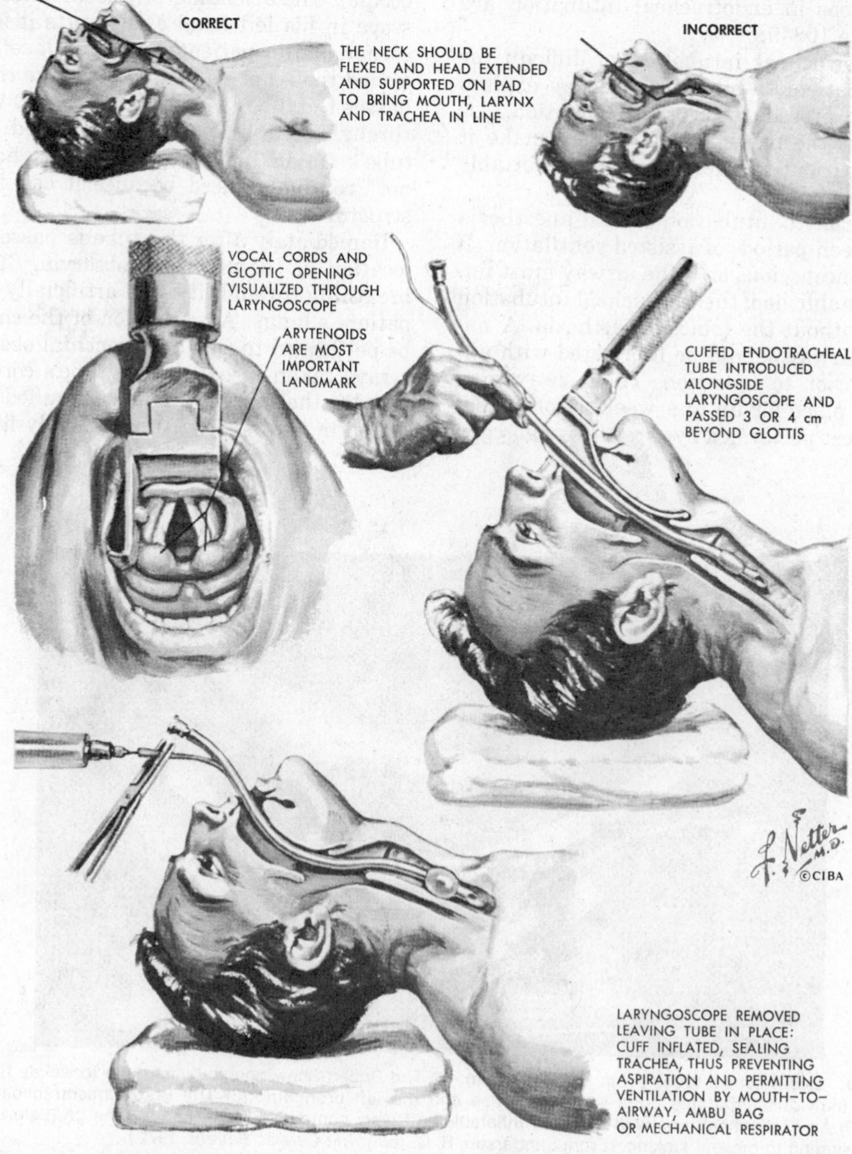
CORRECT
THE NECK SHOULD BE FLEXED AND HEAD EXTENDED AND SUPPORTED ON PAD TO BRING MOUTH, LARYNX AND TRACHEA IN LINE
INCORRECT
VOCAL CORDS AND GLOTTIC OPENING VISUALIZED THROUGH LARYNGOSCOPE
ARYTENOIDS ARE MOST IMPORTANT LANDMARK
CUFFED ENDOTRACHEAL TUBE INTRODUCED ALONGSIDE LARYNGOSCOPE AND PASSED 3 OR 4 cm BEYOND GLOTTIS
F. Netter M.D.
©CIBA
LARYNGOSCOPE REMOVED LEAVING TUBE IN PLACE: CUFF INFLATED, SEALING TRACHEA, THUS PREVENTING ASPIRATION AND PERMITTING VENTILATION BY MOUTH–TO–AIRWAY, AMBU BAG OR MECHANICAL RESPIRATOR

FIGURE 108–9. Endotracheal intubations. ©Copyright 1970 CIBA Pharmaceutical Company. Division of CIBA-GEIGY Corporation. Reproduced, with permission, from the CLINICAL SYMPOSIA illustrated by Frank H. Netter, M. D. All rights reserved.)

to the bite-block; and (d) if the patient is especially active, place the tape loosely around the patient's neck and place sand bags on either side of the patient's head to help immobilize his head. The patient's chest should be padded for protection, and the respiratory apparatus stabilized on the chest to prevent "dragging" or misplacement of the endotracheal tube.

Mild sedation may be necessary for the conscious patient who has endotracheal intubation because of discomfort, gagging, difficulty in swallowing, and so forth. Some conscious patients are unable to tolerate an endotracheal tube, even with mild sedation.

Give frequent mouth care to the patient who has an endotracheal tube in place, and suction as necessary. The tube may cause excessive oropharyngeal secretions which must be periodically removed by suctioning. *A catheter used for oropharyngeal suctioning is never used for tracheal suctioning,* since it could introduce pathogens into the tracheobronchial tree. (Suctioning is discussed in Ch. 70, Unit XIV.) When suctioning an endotracheal tube, make certain the suction catheter is long enough to reach beyond the length of the tube and touch the bronchial mucosa. This mucosal stimulation elicits coughing and thus helps the patient clear his tracheobronchial tree of secretions. Rubber suction catheters sometimes slide more easily in plastic endotracheal tubes than do plastic suction catheters. Periodically the endotracheal tube is repositioned (if it is an orotracheal tube) to prevent pressure necrosis on the lip. An emergency tracheostomy tray and an extra sterile endotracheal tube of correct size is always kept at the bedside of an intubated patient for emergency use. Inspect the nasal mucosa periodically for erosion when a nasal endotracheal tube is being used.

Patients with endotracheal tubes are not allowed anything orally; intravenous or nasogastric feedings are given.

"Crash Intubation."[84] "Crash intubation" procedures are often necessary in emergency rooms. In these settings patients often present numerous problems which are clinically challenging to the resuscitating team. For example, the patient may be head-injured, comatose, convulsing, cyanotic, vomiting, obstructed, and have trismus. Initially attempts may be made to suction quickly the patient's nose and mouth. If the patient does not have head injuries, this suctioning is best done with the patient supine and his head turned to one side. Then the patient is positioned with his head elevated about 45° (to counteract passive regurgitation and cerebral congestion) and with his legs elevated (to avoid postural hypotension). In this V-position, attempts may be made to start an intravenous infusion and to oxygenate the patient by use of bag and mask. If ventilation with bag and mask is inadequate, the immediate goal of care becomes intubation (of a well-oxygenated patient when possible) under full curarization, without vomiting, coughing, and straining.

In a patient with trismus (spasm of masticatory muscles producing difficulty opening the jaws, i.e., "lockjaw") and asphyxia, orotracheal intubation may be possible only after rapid curarization with succinylcholine. If the patient is unconscious, a fully paralyzing dose of succinylcholine or gallamine is administered intravenously. Full paralysis is necessary to prevent vomiting movements during intubation. As soon as full paralysis is obtained, the larynx is rapidly exposed (with suction ready), the trachea is intubated, and the cuff is inflated. If the patient's airway is open and if time permits, it is desirable *before* curarization to denitrogenate the lungs, e.g., by the spontaneous inhalation of 100 per cent oxygen (high flow) with bag and mask for at least 2 minutes. If the patient is conscious prior to paralysis, he is rapidly anesthetized lightly, e.g., with thiopental, halothane, or cyclopropane. If it has not been possible to carry out preliminary oxygenation under spontaneous breathing, positive pressure ventilation is instituted after paralysis is achieved. In the paralyzed patient, attempts at inflation may cause gastric insufflation and regurgitation.

ENDOTRACHEAL EXTUBATION

Accidental removal of an endotracheal tube can occur (a) if the tube is not properly secured in place; (b) from a confused patient pulling at the tube; or (c) from traction exerted on the tube when giving patient care. Accidental extubation is hazardous because of possible aspiration, tracheal trauma, laryngeal edema, laryngeal spasm, or respiratory arrest.

Prior to *planned endotracheal extubation,* some physicians order steroids intravenously in an attempt to prevent laryngeal edema. The physician performs the extubation after determining that the patient's respiratory status is satisfactory. In reaching this decision, the physician evaluates blood gas values, vital capacity, and other measurements of respiratory function. Before an endotracheal tube is removed the nurse checks the emergency respiratory equipment at the bedside. It may be necessary to reintubate the patient or to use resuscitory equipment, e.g., Ambu bag. Sometimes tracheotomy is required. If laryngospasm occurs, muscle relaxants may be administered. The pharynx is suctioned before the cuff is deflated on the endotracheal tube. Thus secretions which have accumulated above the cuff will not be aspirated when the cuff is deflated.

When possible the patient is placed in semi-Fowler's position for extubation. It is desirable to maintain this position or place the patient in high-Fowler's position after the tube is removed to improve alveolar ventilation and to encourage chest expansion. Following endotracheal intubation, the patient is generally given mist treatment (by mask or tent) and is *closely observed* for indications of *respiratory distress* or *laryngeal edema,* e.g., upper airway obstruction, laryngeal stridor. The nurse remains prepared to assist with reintubation or tracheotomy if necessary.

CUFFED TUBES

Previous sections have focused on tracheostomy and endotracheal tubes in general. Here our emphasis is on *cuffed* tracheostomy and endotracheal tubes. Inflation of the cuff with air (once the tube is properly positioned in the trachea) firmly fixes the tube in the trachea and forms a seal which prevents leakage of air around the tube or possible aspiration of food or secretions into the lungs (see Fig. 108–10). Most tubes are cuffed today. Some tubes have cuffs that are applied around the tube separately, but most have a cuff built into the tube, i.e., the tube and cuff are all-in-one.

Cuffed tubes are used for various reasons. As mentioned above, cuffed tubes help prevent aspiration of pharyngeal and regurgitated gastric contents by forming a seal between the tube and tracheal wall. Also, inflated cuffs are necessary for controlled positive pressure mechanical ventilation, since these cuffs prevent air leak around the tube. Thus, when controlled positive pressure ventilation cannot be given effectively by mask, endotracheal intubation or tracheostomy is performed with a cuffed tube, and the mechanical ventilator is attached to the tube. (Ventilators are discussed in Unit XIV.)

While cuffed tubes are advantageous in some situations, they also can cause serious *complications* unless properly used. (Many of these complications have been discussed in detail earlier in this chapter.) Pressure of the inflated cuff impairs blood supply to tracheal tissue; also, the presence of the cuff irritates the tracheal wall. After cuff inflation, tissue changes may begin as soon as 48 hours.[116] Complications which can result from *overinflation or prolonged inflation* of cuffs include tracheal necrosis, erosion, or ulceration; tracheo-innominate fistula; tracheoesophageal fistula; tracheomalacia; tracheal stenosis (from scarring and irritation); tracheitis above the site of the cuff (due to pooling of secretions there); and herniation of the tracheal wall over the distal portion of the tube (producing tube obstruction). *Misplacement* of a cuffed tube (such that the end of the tube is on the carina or in a mainstem bronchus) will produce airway obstruction, i.e., air will not flow in and out of the bronchus and lung opposite the side intubated. Following insertion of a cuffed tube, the chest is periodically auscultated (as previously mentioned) on both sides to make certain that airflow is occurring in both lungs.

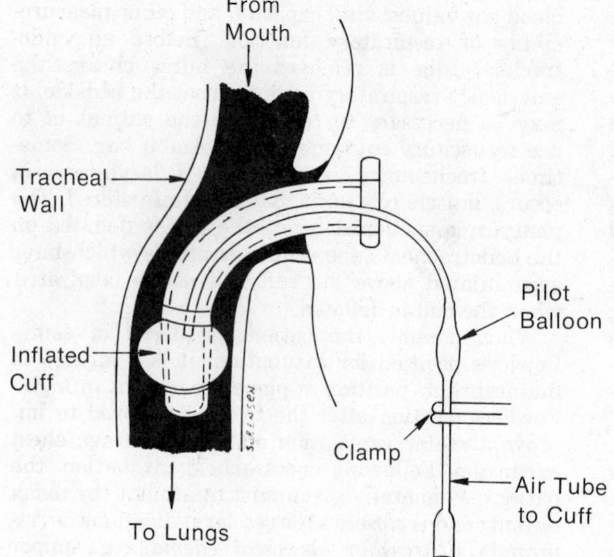

FIGURE 108–10. Cuffed tracheostomy tube with cuff inflated.

Soft *low-pressure cuffs* are now available which help minimize trauma. Also, some cuffs are now designed as an *elongated cuff* rather than the traditional more rounded cuff. Advocates of the elongated cuffs maintain that this type of cuff distributes pressure over a greater surface area, and thus minimizes pressure in any one place on the tracheal wall. Prestretching cuffs and periodically deflating them are technics used to help minimize cuff trauma. These procedures are discussed in following paragraphs.

> *Cuffed tubes may be* prestretched *and* periodically deflated *in an attempt to prevent tracheal complications associated with excessive cuff pressure.*

Prestretching an inflatable cuff makes the cuff more pliable. The cuff, therefore, conforms more readily to the rings of the trachea and does not excessively distort or compress the tracheal wall. A cuffed tracheostomy tube can be prestretched by[118] (a) placing the tube in 95° C. sterile water; (b) gently inflating the cuff with 20–30 ml. of air; and

(c) removing the tube from the water after 10 minutes and allowing it to cool.

A cuff should be inflated prior to insertion and examined to be certain it is uniformily rounded, i.e., does not have abnormal bulges or indentations. Discard the tube if its cuff is lopsided when inflated. A lopsided cuff is unsafe, since a bulged area may herniate over the distal end of the tube when in place in the trachea and obstruct the airway.

DEFLATION OF THE CUFF

The cuff of a cuffed tube is deflated periodically to allow blood to circulate through the affected area and thus prevent damage to the trachea caused by prolonged cuff pressure. Deflation routines vary with the doctor's orders and the patient's condition. Ideally the cuff should be deflated for 1 minute every 20–30 minutes.[118] However, in practice this is sometimes not possible because of the patient's condition. During periods of deflation the patient is constantly attended to prevent aspiration. Deflating the cuff for 5 minutes every hour is not adequate.[116]

If a patient with a cuffed tracheal tube develops sudden respiratory distress, the cuff should be immediately deflated until the problem has been identified. Also, the cuff should be deflated during suctioning (as described in the following paragraph). *If an acute airway emergency develops in an intubated patient,* Tyler and Synnestvedt recommend the following actions:[116] *first,* disconnect the mechanical ventilator and manually ventilate the patient (the problem may be in the ventilating machine); *second,* pass a catheter rapidly to clear any plugs from the lumen of the tube or from the tube's distal end (a plug at the end of a tube may permit inhalation but may obstruct the tube during exhalation—thus causing increasing trapping of air and distention of lung tissue); *third,* almost simultaneously deflate the cuff completely (a dislodged or herniated cuff may be obstructing the airway); and *finally,* remove the tube while summoning help *if* the preceding steps fail to immediately relieve the emergency. While waiting for help, continue ventilating with a self-inflating bag and mask. To prevent the escape of air through a tracheostomy stoma during ventilation, tightly cover the stoma.

Some important steps to remember when *deflating* cuffed tubes are:

> *Before deflating the cuff, suction the upper airway,* i.e., the nasal and oral pharynx, to remove secretions which have accumulated above the inflated cuff. Unless removed, these secretions may be aspirated when the cuff is deflated. *The tracheal tube is also suctioned before the cuff is deflated and again as the cuff is deflated* (to suction out any secretions which have accumulated on top of the inflated cuff).

> *Next, deflate the cuff.* Using a syringe, release the air slowly from the small tube leading to the pilot balloon and cuff. *While doing this maintain positive pressure* from an Ambu bag or ventilator. The positive pressure prevents pulmonary aspiration by forcing accumulated secretions in the upper trachea and larynx into the mouth (where they can be removed by suctioning).

> *After deflating the cuff, suction the lower airway* to remove secretions accumulated around the cuff and tube. Deflation of the cuff may cause the patient to cough and raise some secretions to a level from which they can be removed by suction.

> *Provide adequate ventilation and humidification during the time the cuff is deflated.*

> *Reinflate the cuff.* If the patient is on a respirator, inflate the cuff during inspiration, i.e., the positive pressure cycle. Reinflate with only enough air to prevent an obvious leak of air when positive pressure is reapplied to the airway. After the necessary amount of air has been inserted into the inflating tube, the tube is clamped shut with a small hemostat.

> *Check for air leaks* from the balloon and around the cuff.

Remember that positive pressure ventilation with a respirator is possible only when the cuff is inflated. Thus, if the patient cannot ventilate without assistance during the interval of cuff deflation, you need to have someone manually ventilate the patient with an anesthesia or self-inflating bag, e.g., Ambu bag. Some patients can ventilate themselves during the brief period of cuff deflation. It is necessary, however, to provide heated, humidified gas mixtures as ordered. If a patient has such high airway resistance that manual ventilation is impossible, he must be kept on a respirator and have his cuff frequently deflated for only a few seconds at a time, e.g., 30–60 seconds if the patient's condition permits. The apneic patient should not be kept off the respirator for longer than 15 seconds or he may develop cardiac arrhythmias or cardiac arrest.

If a patient is severely hypoxic and is on prolonged, controlled, ventilatory assistance, it is most desirable to deflate the cuff when the patient needs to be off the respirator for some other aspect of care, e.g., for endotracheal suctioning. The patient is hyperoxygenated prior to suctioning, i.e., the percentage of oxygen he receives from the respirator is increased for a few minutes. During this period of hyperoxygenation, the patient is given naso- or oropharyngeal suctioning. The cuff is then deflated, and simultaneously the trachea is suctioned. Two nurses work together to rapidly carry out hyperoxygenation, cuff deflation, endotracheal suctioning, and cuff reinflation. Another method is to leave the patient on the respirator while carrying out naso- or oropharyngeal and tracheal suctioning. Next, deflate the cuff and let oxygen from the respirator push any secretions pooled above the cuff up into the pharynx, where they can easily be removed by suctioning.[118]

Before adding more air to an inflated cuffed tube, be certain to suck out the air that is in the cuff. This is necessary to prevent excessively filling the cuff by adding air to the air which is left in the cuff. Air will not empty out of a stretched cuff by itself; it must be withdrawn.[116]

An *automatic intermittent cuff inflator* has been developed which can be used with either a pressure or volume controlled respirator. The volume to which the cuff is to be inflated is set on the machine. The machine is then connected to (a) an oxygen power source; (b) the cuff inflation tube; and (c) the respirator's exhalation valve. Then the cuff is automatically deflated with each expiration and is inflated to the preset volume with each inspiration. It is recommended that, if a patient is likely to aspirate or vomit, he have a nasal gastric tube in place as a precaution to prevent aspiration while the cuff is deflated.

The risk of tissue damage is especially great when a patient has both a tracheal tube and a nasogastric tube. The nurse closely observes for symptoms of tracheoesophageal fistula. If the nasogastric tube is to be used for tube feedings, prior to the feedings the patient is placed in semi-Fowler's position, and the cuff is inflated to prevent possible aspiration of regurgitated food. The patient is kept in the semi-Fowler's position during the feeding and for about 20 minutes after the feeding (to permit the contents of the feeding to pass through the stomach). (Tube feedings are discussed on p. 427 of Unit VIII.)

CUFFED TRACHEOSTOMY TUBES

In adults cuffed tracheostomy tubes are useful in the following situations: (a) in patients who are likely to aspirate (e.g., those who lack the swallowing reflex, those in coma and/or with bulbar paralysis, and those with upper airway bleeding or abdominal distention); (b) patients requiring assisted or controlled positive pressure ventilation (these two points have been discussed in the previous section); and (c) routinely for the first few hours after tracheostomy to prevent blood from leaking into the lungs.[80]

In some patients a cuffed tracheostomy tube is in place prophylactically, and the cuff is not inflated unless necessary. Therefore, always check the physician's orders concerning inflation of a cuff. If the cuff is to be inflated, this is accomplished by introducing air into the cuff via a syringe connected to a fine tube which leads into the cuff. Near the proximal end of this small inflating tube is a "pilot balloon" (see Figs. 108–3 and 108–10). The introduction of air into the airtube inflates both the cuff and the pilot balloon. If a leak occurs anywhere in the "tube-balloon-cuff" system, the pilot balloon becomes noticeably deflated. Thus the nurse frequently observes the pilot balloon to determine patency of the cuff seal. If the cuff is not inflating adequately and is to be inflated, the physician is notified and the tube is replaced. (*Note:* a nurse does not replace a tracheostomy tube unless she is trained to do so and has the physician's order.) It is also possible to detect a leak around a cuff by (a) briefly blocking off the tracheostomy tube and listening carefully for the sound of escaping air; (b) placing your hand in front of the patient's mouth or nose and having him blow against your hand (a leak is present if you can feel air moving); or (c) listening for a harsh oral sound during the inspiratory phase when the patient is on ventilatory assistance.

Check with the physician whether or not a patient's tracheostomy tube cuff is to be inflated or deflated while the patient eats or drinks. Some doctors prefer a deflated cuff at these times because they believe inflation of the cuff makes swallowing more difficult (owing to the pressure exerted on the esophagus by the inflated cuff). Other doctor's

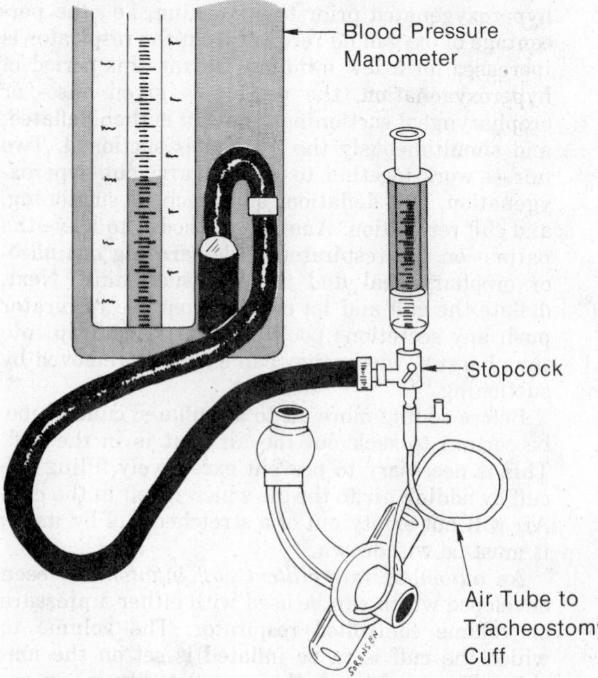

FIGURE 108–11. Method of measuring tracheostomy tube intracuff pressures by inserting stopcock between the air tube to the cuff and the blood pressure manometer tube.

prefer cuff inflation to prevent possible aspiration of oral intake.

With careful technic it is possible to use cuffed tracheostomy tubes for several months without causing tracheal trauma. Proctor and Safar[80] recommend observing the following precautions:*

> In managing patients who are in danger of aspirating, use a *"no-leak" or "full-seal" technic* which allows no air to leak around the tube or escape through the nose or mouth.

> In treating conscious respirator patients, employ a *"minimal-leak" technique* in which the cuff is slowly inflated until all audible leakage is abolished and then is deflated slowly.

> Never inflate the cuff without simultaneously applying positive pressure through the tube to prevent overinflation of the cuff.

> Practice asepsis and use optimal humidification. Increasing the moisture content of inspired air prevents drying of the tracheal mucosa and facilitates removal of secretions. Disposable rubber gloves and disposable suction catheters are used with aseptic technic during suctioning to protect the patient from foreign microorganisms.

Remember: A tracheostomy is a possible portal of entry for infectious microorganisms which may cause pulmonary infection. The minimal-leak inflation technic does not make it possible to obtain an accurate measurement of tidal volume; before this measurement is taken, the cuff must be fully inflated.

The *constant-leak* technic is one in which the cuff is deflated until a leak is detected during the inspiratory cycle. A clamp is then applied to prevent further deflation of the cuff. The constant-leak technic is used on patients being ventilated with volume ventilators. Also it may be possible with pressure ventilators which have terminal flow settings. This technic is useful when a tube has a cuff which is stiff (and is thus producing high intracuff pressures), but the tube cannot be immediately replaced. With constant-leak technic, it is important to frequently check the patient's exhaled tidal volume. A respirometer attached to the ventilator's exhalation manifold is used to obtain this measurement. Increases in the ventilator's volume or pressure may be necessary to compensate for air being leaked past the cuff. The constant-leak technic is helpful when indicated because it (a) minimizes lateral tracheal wall pressure; (b) enables some patients to talk with the leaked air; and (c) carries secretions out of the trachea on leaking air and thus prevents pooling of secretions above the cuff.[116]

The physician's orders serve as a guide for the pattern of periodically deflating and reinflating the cuff of a tracheostomy tube. These orders should specify the frequency with which the cuff is to be deflated, the interval of time it should remain deflated, and the amount of air to be reinserted to inflate the cuff. The nurse records the time of inflation of the tube, the interval of deflation, and the amount of air reintroduced. Generally insertion of 2–10 ml. of air inflates the cuff and produces a seal without creating a hazardous amount of pressure. The amount of air necessary to properly inflate a cuffed tube varies with the stiffness of the cuff, the tracheostomy tube size, and the size of the patient's trachea. Smaller tracheostomy tubes require more air than do larger tracheostomy tubes. Usually a leak-free closed system is obtained by inflating the cuff with from 2–5 ml. of air.[118]

The nurse evaluates serially the amounts of air recorded as necessary to inflate the cuff. A pattern of *decrease* in the amounts necessary may indicate that the trachea's lumen is being decreased owing to swelling and edema. A pattern of *increase* may indicate air leaking around the tube or tracheal damage. Increasing amounts of air necessary in the cuff may also indicate overdistention of the trachea. This situation produces tracheal necrosis and eventually tracheal stenosis. *Significant changes in the amounts of air required to inflate the cuff should be reported.*

> To check the intraluminal (intracuff) pressure of the cuff on a tracheostomy tube, put a stopcock in line between the cuff air-filling tube and a blood pressure manometer tube (see Fig. 108–11). Then push into the cuff the amount of air necessary to create a seal and turn the stopcock to open the line between the cuff and the manometer. Read the pressure. Refill the cuff after closing the stopcock and taking the reading. Currently the *maximum* acceptable intracuff pressure is 20 mm. Hg.[116]

Sometimes orders are given for a patient's tracheostomy opening to be obstructed during periods of deflation. This may be ordered when it is desirable for the patient to begin to breathe again through the upper airway, e.g., in preparation for extubation.

According to some sources, cuffed tracheostomy tubes which do not have inner cannulas may be used for days without changing. Others state that tracheostomy tubes should be changed every other day. Some physicians prefer use of cuffs inflated only by inspiratory positive pressure from the respirator or double cuffs. Double cuffs alternate the site of inflation. By inflating and deflating each balloon at predetermined intervals, the sites of tracheal irritation and pressure are alternated.

* This procedure is recommended for use with the silver tube with the Moerch modification (swivel adaptor) and a narrow, double-walled, seamless, slip-on cuff.

CHAPTER 109

Disorders of the Larynx

ANATOMY OF THE LARYNX

The larynx forms the upper extremity of the trachea. The entire *nerve supply* to the larynx is from the *vagus.* Most of the *blood supply* to the larynx comes from the *superior and inferior laryngeal arteries.* The larynx is composed of several cartilages which are connected below with the trachea and above with the hypopharynx through a wide opening (see Fig. 109–1). The cartilages are held together with muscles and ligaments. The larynx lies in front of the 4th, 5th, and 6th cervical vertebrae. In front of the larynx the *thyroid cartilage* protrudes, forming what is commonly called the "Adam's apple." The *cricoid cartilage* lies just below the thyroid cartilage. The *hyoid bone* lies just above

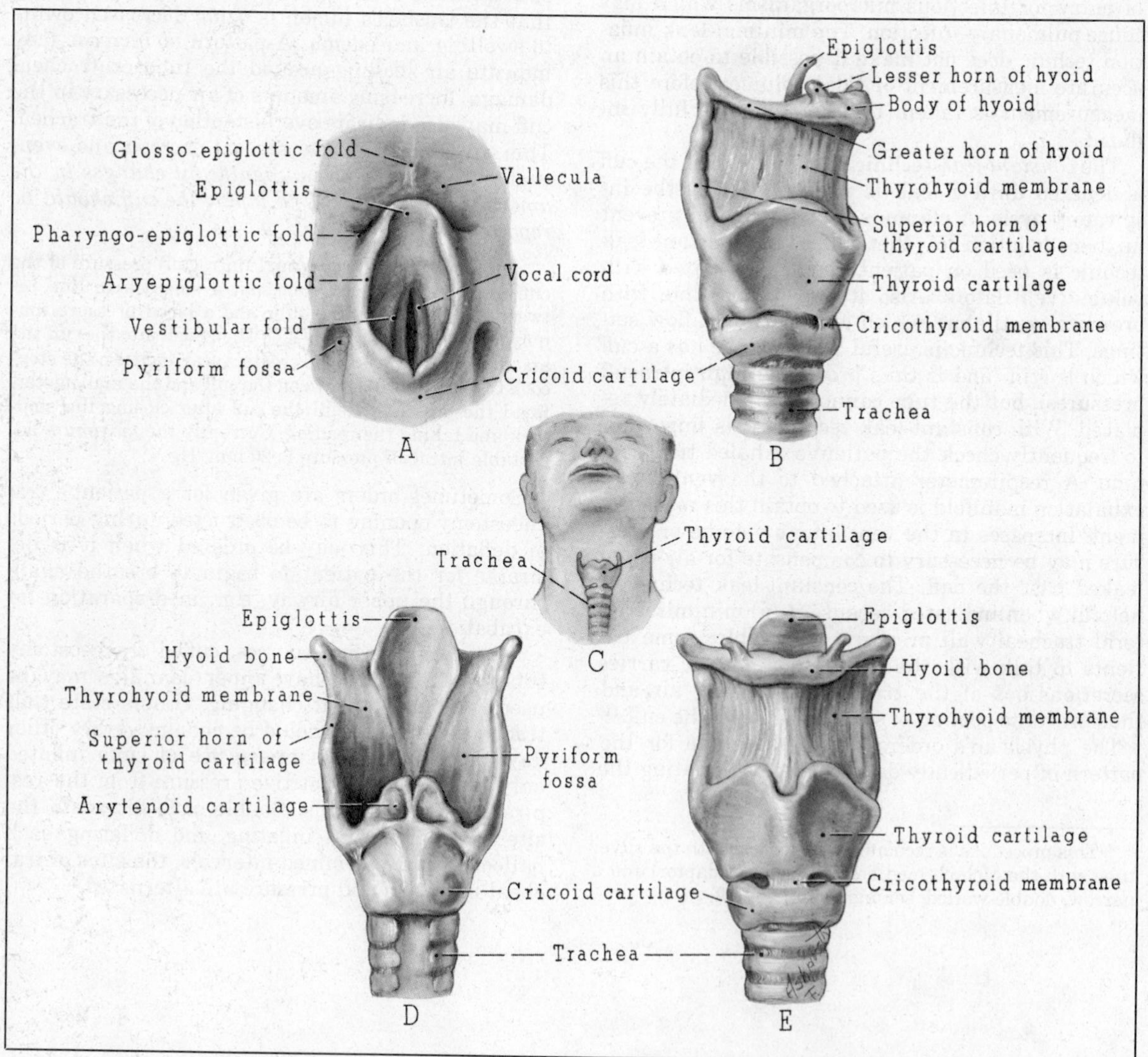

FIGURE 109–1. The larynx. (From Jacob, S. W., and Francone, C. A.: *Structure and Function in Man.* 3rd ed. 1974.)

the thyroid cartilage, forming an attachment for the larynx and for the tongue and other muscles. The hyoid bone can be excised surgically if necessary without causing any great deformity or physiologic problems.

The cricoid cartilage articulates not only with the thyroid but also with *arytenoid cartilages.* The latter swing in and out, opening and closing the *glottis,* i.e., the space between the vocal cords. The *epiglottis* is a cartilaginous structure attached to the base of the tongue and the thyroid and arytenoid cartilages.

FUNCTIONS OF THE LARYNX

The chief function of the larynx is *not* that of producing speech sounds, i.e., *phonation,* but rather it is to act efficiently as an *airway* between the trachea and pharynx. While the trachea is merely a tube (the walls of which have ciliary action), the larynx is an organ with important *sphincteric actions* which help to (a) *prevent aspiration;* and (b) *increase intrathoracic pressure.* Aspiration is prevented during swallowing because the larynx closes tightly to keep food out of the trachea. Likewise the glottis closes if a foreign body drops into the throat. The *cough reflex* (called "watchdog of the lungs") is triggered whenever a foreign body touches the highly sensitive laryngeal mucosa. By increasing intrathoracic pressure, the larynx assists during straining efforts, e.g., coughing, lifting. The increased pressure gives added advantage to the use of the muscles of the shoulders and thorax. The vocal cords are adducted for coughing as well as for speech.

Remember: *Following local anesthesia of the larynx, e.g., for laryngoscopy or bronchoscopy, the patient is not allowed to take anything orally for 2–3 hours because he may aspirate through the anesthetized larynx.*

Commonly called the "voice box," the larynx creates sounds as a result of vocal cord vibrations. The sounds are then formed into speech patterns by the pharynx, palate, tongue, teeth, and lips. Thus, words are not actually formed in the larynx. During phonation numerous changes occur within and around the larynx. For example, (a) the larynx moves up and down, changing the length of the air columns above and below the larynx; (b) the edges of the vocal cords are relaxed and firmed; and (c) the length of the cords varies. The air column and its vibrations are changed by these as well as other actions. As the vibrating column of air comes up from the larynx, the palate, tongue, and lips mold words.

EXAMINATION OF THE LARYNX

As part of a complete examination of the larynx, the neck is palpated externally, and the larynx is visualized internally, e.g., by direct or indirect laryngoscopy.

Direct laryngoscopy is performed with a laryngoscope, i.e., a hollow, rigid metal tube lighted at its distal end. The patient is given a preoperative sedative, and food and fluids are withheld for a specified number of hours before the procedure to prevent regurgitation and possible aspiration. The patient's eyeglasses and dentures are removed, and the patient is transported to the operating room. Laryngoscopy is usually performed with a local anesthesia, such as cocaine. While the patient lies motionless on his back, the laryngoscope is passed through the mouth and down to the larynx. The illuminated structures of the larynx are then directly observed. Minor surgical procedures may be performed through the laryngoscope, e.g., biopsy.

Following laryngoscopy the patient is allowed nothing to eat until the gag reflex returns. (The procedure by which the nurse tests the gag reflex is discussed in Unit VIII). After the gag reflex returns, allow the patient to drink water first, since it is least damaging if accidentally aspirated. Following laryngoscopy the patient is drowsy or asleep because of the preoperative sedation. The nurse therefore provides safeguards as necessary, e.g., siderails, and provides a restful environment. The patient is observed for any of the following reportable symptoms during the postoperative period: (a) apprehension (possibly due to bleeding or laryngeal edema); (b) coughing or spitting blood or blood-tinged mucus; (c) pain in the throat or chest; and (d) swelling in the throat and neck. Nursing care following laryngoscopy is similar to that given following bronchoscopy (see Ch. 68, Unit XIV).

With *indirect laryngoscopy* the larynx is viewed in a laryngeal mirror; light is directed onto the mirror as it is held in the pharynx (see Fig. 109–2).

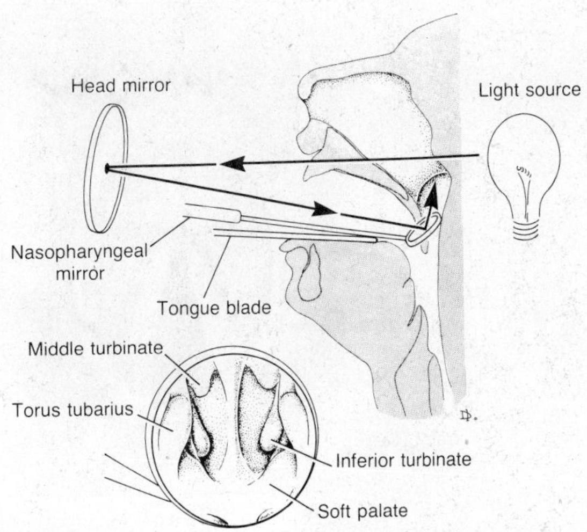

FIGURE 109–2. Indirect laryngoscopy. (From Hill, G. J., II: *Outpatient Surgery.* 1973.)

To prevent unnecessary "gagging" during inspection of the larynx, the patient is approached calmly and gently. The patient sits *very* erect for the examination with his chin drawn forward and both feet on the floor with knees drawn together. The tongue is protruded as far as possible and firmly grasped with a piece of gauze. A mirror (#5 for adults) is warmed over an alcohol lamp, tested on the back of the examiner's hand for heat, and inserted with its back side against the tip of the uvula. The patient is told to breathe quietly through the mouth, or "pant like a dog" to prevent gagging. If indicated, biopsy can be performed via indirect laryngoscopy.

The vocal cords are examined during quiet respiration and during phonation. Phonation causes adduction of the cords, and they can be seen to vibrate as sound is produced. Normally there is perfect approximation of the cords (see Fig. 109–3). In the aged, however, there is a small space which cannot be closed; thus older people may have quavering voices. With cord paralysis, the paralyzed cord (or cords) do not move.

SYMPTOMS OF LARYNGEAL DISORDERS

The larynx is easily examined. Thus, if a patient reports his symptoms soon after they occur, an early diagnosis of laryngeal disorders is generally possible. Among the symptoms of laryngeal disease are:

> *Hoarseness:* the most important and most common symptom. Usually caused from improper approximation of the vocal cords, inflammation of the larynx, or laryngeal paralysis. *The larynx should be carefully inspected whenever a patient is hoarse longer than two weeks.*

> *Cough:* a common symptom of laryngeal disorders.

> *Dyspnea:* an ominous symptom indicative of severe airway obstruction. Slowly developing laryngeal obstruction is tolerated far better than an equally severe sudden obstruction. Unlike the patient with asthma, the patient with laryngeal dyspnea can expire air easily. However, inspiration is difficult. *Tracheotomy or passage of an intracheal tube may be necessary to restore the airway in the presence of dyspnea or stridor or both.*

> *Stridor* (harsh respiration): an ominous symptom. Stridor associated with laryngeal disorder is usually inspiratory.

Encourage patients with dyspnea and stridor to try to relax and breathe quietly. Use of narcotics and sedatives is dangerous.

> *Dysphagia:* fairly uncommon symptom of laryngeal disorders. However, it may occur secondary to laryngeal inflammation or tumor obstruction. Tube feedings may be indicated.

> *Pain:* occurs occasionally as an early symptom of acute pharyngeal inflammatory disorders and as a late symptom of neoplasms. At times narcotics are indicated. Generally chronic laryngeal inflammatory disorders are not painful.

Laryngeal disorders are potentially serious because they may cause airway obstruction or constriction. *Symptoms of laryngeal obstruction* include dyspnea, stridor, cyanosis, and increased, ineffective inspiratory effort which produces retraction of soft tissues around the thoracic cage. *Sudden laryngeal obstruction* may result from trauma; an allergic response in a hypersensitive individual; serious inflammatory diseases (scarlet fever, diphtheria); laryngeal edema; laryngeal spasm; or aspiration of a foreign body. In these conditions emergency treatment (e.g., endotracheal intubation or tracheotomy) may be necessary to save the patient's life.

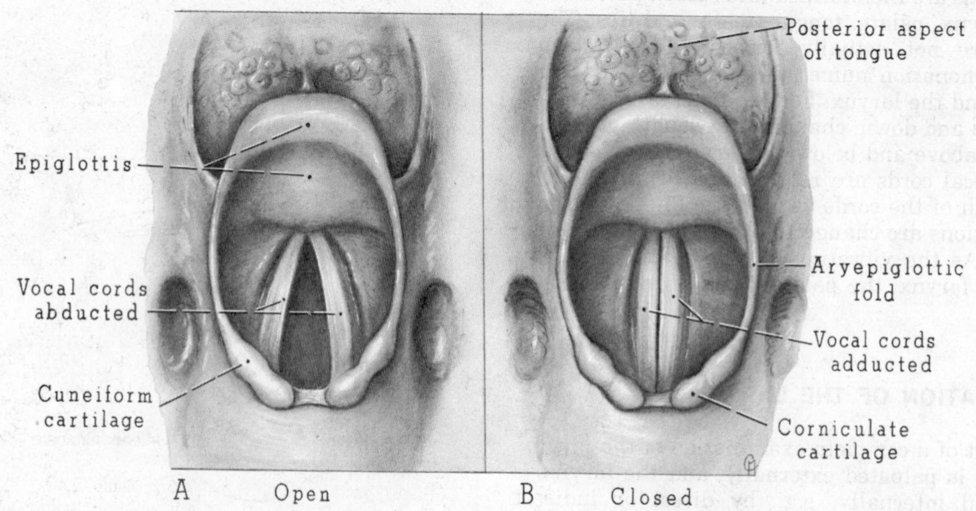

FIGURE 109–3. Superior view of vocal cords. (From Jacob, S. W., and Francone, C. A.: *Structure and Function in Man.* 3rd ed. 1974.)

LARYNGEAL SPASM

Occasionally following use of some general anesthetics, a spasm of laryngeal muscle tissue may occur, seriously jeopardizing the airway. Patients with low blood calcium levels also occasionally develop muscle tetany, which causes not only laryngeal spasm but also other skeletal muscle hyperirritability and spasm. In an attempt to relieve laryngeal muscle spasm, calcium chloride or calcium gluconate is given intravenously.

LARYNGEAL EDEMA

Because the larynx is a rigid structure, the airway size is reduced if edema occurs within the larynx (or glottis). *Acute* laryngeal edema requires immediate restoration of the airway. An endotracheal tube or tracheotomy may be necessary. Laryngeal edema is a potential medical emergency in the following disorders: anaphylaxis (i.e., angioneurotic edema); urticaria; acute laryngitis; direct injury to the larynx during surgery or intubation; and serious inflammatory conditions of the throat, such as erysipelas and scarlet fever. If laryngeal edema is caused by an allergic reaction, treatment may include (a) local application of ice to the neck; (b) administration of an adrenal corticosteroid; or (c) epinephrine (Adrenaline), 1:1,000 subcutaneously (see also Unit V, Ch. 23).

Chronic laryngeal edema is usually less of a medical emergency because the patient has adjusted somewhat to his breathing disorder. Tracheotomy may be necessary, however. Chronic laryngeal edema may result from irradiation treatment of the larynx; tumors of the neck; and infections obstructing the laryngeal lymphatics. In the presence of laryngeal edema, the larynx may be sprayed with vasoconstrictors and steroids prior to tracheal intubation. This procedure, in addition to the use of systemic steroids, may alleviate the need for tracheotomy.[80]

LARYNGEAL PARALYSIS

Generally laryngeal paralyses result from peripheral disorders, but they occasionally can also result from central nervous system disorders. Complete laryngeal paralysis rarely occurs. Among the peripheral causes of laryngeal paralysis are aortic aneurysm, mitral stenosis, carcinoma of the thyroid gland, neck injuries, tuberculosis, tumors (e.g., of bronchi, lungs, mediastinum); metallic poisons (lead); and infectious diseases (diphtheria). Trauma during thyroidectomy is one of the most common causes of laryngeal paralysis. These disorders cause paralysis by affecting the recurrent laryngeal nerve in a variety of ways (it may be stretched, eroded, crushed, or cut).

Either one or both vocal cords may be paralyzed. If only one cord is affected, the airway is adequate and the patient's only symptom may be hoarseness (sometimes not even this is present). With bilateral paralysis, the voice is weak (though adequate), and a poor airway causes incapacitating dyspnea and stridor upon exertion. If the paralyzed cords are bilaterally adducted, an emergency tracheotomy may be necessary. Numerous types of surgical procedures exist to open the glottis. One transoral procedure is called an *arytenoidectomy.*

LARYNGEAL INJURY

The larynx is seldom injured even though it appears to be relatively unprotected. Occasionally, however, fracture of the thyroid cartilage occurs, causing the mucosa and other soft tissues inside the larynx to be torn or causing hematoma formation. A tracheotomy may be necessary as a result of such airway damage. Before tracheotomy the patient may appear cyanotic, have a tender, swollen, and ecchymotic neck, and have stridor. Subcutaneous emphysema causes the swelling.

By themselves, tracheobronchial cartilages cannot effectively maintain the normal caliber of airways within the thorax. Such normal caliber is mainly dependent upon elastic fibers in the lungs which are kept stretched by the chest wall's elastic ability to expand. While these forces act within the thorax to maintain adequate tracheobronchial lumina, at the upper end of the airway an adequate tracheal lumen is maintained only by attachment of the trachea to the cricoid cartilage. This cartilage forms the only complete circle in the lower airway. Dangerous *tracheal stenosis* thus typically follows injury of the cricoid.[80]

Laryngeal (and tracheal) trauma may result from a patient's neck striking the steering wheel during an automobile accident. Severe trauma which completely cuts off the airway rapidly causes death unless tracheotomy is performed immediately. If the patient survives after tracheotomy, the larynx and tracheal airway must be surgically restored. In addition to fracture of the larynx, other laryngeal injuries include those resulting from inhalation of hot gases or the aspiration of caustic liquids.

LARYNGITIS

Acute laryngitis is a common laryngeal disorder which may occur (a) as an isolated infection involving only the vocal cords; (b) as part of a general upper respiratory infection; or (c) as a result of vocal abuse. No infection is present in the latter condition. Hoarseness is the main symptom of acute laryngitis and may progress to aphonia, i.e., complete voice loss. Other possible symptoms are cough, pain, and rough or tickling feelings in the throat. Patients with severe, acute laryngitis may develop stridor or dyspnea as a result of massive laryngeal edema. Hospitalization, even tracheotomy, may be necessary. Patients with laryngitis are advised not to smoke. Those with persistent cough, stridor, or fever are treated with steam or aerosol therapy, voice rest, and antibiotics if infection is present. Pain may be relieved with throat lozenges containing a topical anesthetic.

Chronic laryngitis refers to long-term inflammatory changes in laryngeal mucosa. Among the many causes of chronic laryngitis and factors contributing to this condition are constant use or misuse of the voice; repeated episodes of acute laryngitis; smoking; syphilis of the larynx; alcohol consumption; laryngeal tuberculosis (associated with far-advanced pulmonary tuberculosis); chronic sinusitis or bronchitis; chronic tonsillitis or adenoiditis; and allergic and hypometabolic states. Persons with chronic laryngitis should always have a laryngoscopic examination performed to rule out possible cancer of the larynx.

The main symptom of chronic laryngitis is hoarseness. Other symptoms are frequent cough; voice fatigue; and a tired, aching throat. Pain is usually only minimal or absent. When possible, treatment focuses on removing the cause. Treatment of chronic laryngitis is far more difficult than treatment of acute laryngitis. Often the cause is difficult to identify. Additionally, with chronic laryngitis tissue changes may be irreversible, and the causes of the disorder may be difficult to remove. Effective treatment measures include inhalation of unmedicated steam; stopping smoking; and *total* temporary voice rest (in which the patient does not speak at all). However, often patients who smoke will not stop, and total voice rest is difficult to maintain. Explain the term "voice rest" to the patient. Tell him that his doctor wants him not to speak or whisper for a while. Give the patient a writing pad and pencil or magic slate so he can communicate by writing. Also, provide a tap bell so he can attract attention as necessary.

The patient on total voice rest must rely on writing, hand signals, and so forth for communication. This is difficult for many patients. The nurse can help the patient who must maintain complete voice rest if she (a) posts a sign clearly on his bed stating he is to rest his voice and not speak; (b) keeps other means of communication close at hand for the patient; (c) instructs the family about the need for voice rest for the patient and ways in which they can help reduce the temptation for him to speak; and (d) anticipates the patient's needs.

CANCER OF THE LARYNX

"For thousands of years, man died as a result of cancer of the larynx and because of other laryngeal disorders and injuries. Today, the well-informed layman has some knowledge of the importance of the larynx in terms of its functions as a valve to protect the lungs and as a means of communication, but he is not always well enough informed to save his life or at best his voice from the ravages of cancer. We use the term *he* on purpose, for approximately ten men to one woman will have cancer of the larynx."[100]

Benign as well as malignant tumors of the larynx occur. As with carcinoma anywhere in the body, *early recognition is the key to the successful treatment of cancer of the larynx.* The longer the cancer remains undetected and untreated, the more radical surgical treatment needs to be and the greater the possibility of treatment failure. Radical surgery on the larynx (total laryngectomy) results in loss of important functions, e.g., loss of the ability to talk and breathe normally. (The effects of total laryngectomy are discussed more completely below.) Important improvements have been made in the surgical treatment of cancer of the larynx, however. Today, if recognized early, cancer of the larynx has an excellent chance for surgical cure while the patient is able to retain a good residual voice.

Cancer of the larynx is the most common upper respiratory malignancy; cancer of the tonsil is the second most common. Most laryngeal malignancies are squamous cell carcinomas. In 1972 an estimated 7000 new cases of cancer of the larynx were predicted to occur and 3000 deaths were estimated from this cancer.[2]

Approximately 30,000 persons with laryngectomies (called "laryngectomees") live in the United States, and more than 2000 laryngectomies are performed each year.[76] Predisposing factors in cancer of the larynx are irritants, e.g., alcohol, cigarette smoke, and other noxious fumes. Three out of four patients with cancer of the larynx are smokers. Relationships appear to exist between cancer of the larynx and a familial predisposition to cancer. The condition also appears to occur more often in persons who have chronic laryngitis, or frequently abuse their voices. Cancer of the larynx most often occurs in white males, at about age 60.

Cancer may develop within the larynx on the true vocal cord (intrinsic cancer) or in some other part of the larynx (extrinsic cancer).

Intrinsic cancer produces hoarseness very early; thus early diagnosis can be made if the patient promptly consults a physician and has his larynx examined. *With early treatment the prognosis is very good, and the treatment is not seriously disabling.* Unfortunately, however, the average patient who develops hoarseness sees three physicians and waits 8 months before a physician finally looks at his larynx and establishes diagnosis. The cancer is far advanced by then and has a poor prognosis.[22] Hoarseness occurs with tumors of the true cords because accurate approximation of the cords during phonation is not possible due to the space-occupying tumor.

In contrast to intrinsic cancer of the larynx, *tumors of the extrinsic larynx do not produce early symptoms.* One of the first symptoms of extrinsic cancer of the larynx is pain and burning of the throat when drinking hot liquids, orange juice, and so forth. A lump in the neck is another early symptom, frequently due to early metastasis. Late symptoms include dysphagia (difficulty swallowing), dyspnea, hoarseness, muffled voice, weight loss, general debility, and foul breath. Other symptoms of cancer of the larynx are cough and expectoration of blood.

If the cancer involves only the vocal cords, it grows slowly (because of limited blood supply) and metastasizes slowly (because of the area's paucity of lymph vessels). However, if the cancer involves other portions of the larynx, it typically grows and metastasizes rapidly. *Symptoms indicative of metastasis* include dysphagia and the sensation of a "lump" in the throat; dyspnea; cough; enlarged cervical lymph nodes; and pain radiating to the ear.

Cancer of the larynx is most easily *diagnosed* by mirror (indirect) laryngoscopy. Direct laryngoscopy may also be performed. A biopsy may be obtained by either method. Biopsy is performed with either local or general anesthesia. Staining the larynx with 2 per cent toluidine blue dye helps pinpoint the most likely area for a positive biopsy in early carcinoma. Carcinoma in situ takes up the dye which is applied to the larynx through a direct laryngoscope with fibroptic illumination.

Other diagnostic procedures which may be employed include special roentgenographic technics to help define the tumor's borders; e.g., after the larynx is cocainized, a radiopaque dye, such as Lipiodol, is instilled and an x-ray is taken. X-ray examination by tomography and routine barium esophagograms may also be helpful. Once the physician has determined the precise area of involvement, he recommends the form of treatment he believes will be most effective, i.e., surgery or radiation.

In *early intrinsic* cancer of the larynx, the cure rate is about the same whether the patient is treated surgically by partial laryngectomy or receives irradiation therapy. Surgery is usually the more effective treatment in more advanced cancer, e.g., with extrinsic involvement, neck involvement by metastases, and so forth. Preoperative irradiation may slightly increase cure rates in surgery for laryngeal cancer.[8]

Some cancers of the head and neck are too advanced for surgical therapy. Persons with these cancers may be treated palliatively by procedures such as intra-arterial infusion with methotrexate or vinblastine, followed by deep x-ray therapy. Soft lesions respond more readily to such treatment than do lesions involving bone.[40]

SURGICAL TREATMENT OF CANCER OF THE LARYNX

Basically there are three types of operations for carcinoma of the larynx. These are briefly summarized below. Many variations of these basic procedures are performed.

> *Partial laryngectomy:* useful in early, intrinsic lesions, e.g., a lesion on the true cord on one side may be excised along with a wide margin of normal tissue. Following surgery the patient is still able to talk and has a normal airway. Sometimes a *hemilaryngectomy* is performed, i.e., half of the thyroid cartilage is excised along with the soft tissue on the inside of the larynx. Some of the simpler partial laryngectomy procedures are *laryngofissure* or *thyrotomy,* in which the thyroid cartilage is split in the midline (to gain access to the interior of the larynx), and then the tumor-bearing portion is removed and the larynx closed.

> *Conservation laryngectomy:* useful in selected extrinsic tumors. Enough of the larynx remains to function, but the diseased part is removed and a *radical neck dissection* is performed on the involved side. Broadly speaking, a "radical neck dissection" means the surgical dissection and removal of lymph nodes and tissues adjacent to the larynx.

> *Total laryngectomy:* the best known operation related to cancer of the larynx. Necessary with far-advanced lesions; contraindicated in patients with distant metastases and in persons with unresectable local lesions. Along with the entire larynx, the hyoid bone, pre-epiglottic space, strap muscles, and one or more tracheal rings are removed. A total laryngectomy deprives the patient of two important factors necessary for speech: (1) a motor mechanism to blow a blast of air; and (2) a vibratory mechanism to vibrate the air wave into a sound wave.[104] After the necessary excision of tissue is made, the trachea's pharyngeal opening is closed, and the distal portion of the trachea is formed into a *permanent tracheostomy.* The latter opening becomes the patient's airway for the remainder of his life. A *radical neck dissection* may also be performed. The effects of total laryngectomy on the physiology of respiration and speech are pictured in Figure 109-4.

Let us briefly explain more completely what a *radical neck dissection* is and why this surgical procedure is performed. When cancer is believed to have spread beyond the lymphatics to the lymph nodes of the neck, all removable structures of the involved side of the neck (or both sides) are surgically excised. A radical neck dissection may be performed on the same side as the cancer, even though lymph nodes are not palpable and metastases cannot definitely be proved. This is done because as many as 35 per cent of patients with cancer of the larynx have had cervical lymph node metastases. When a total laryngectomy is performed with a radical neck dissection, in addition to removing the larynx and attached ribbon muscles, other structures are removed, e.g., the sternocleidomastoid and omohyoid muscles; the muscles of the floor of the mouth together with the stylohyoid and digastric muscles; the submaxillary gland; sometimes the ipsilateral half of the thyroid gland; the parathyroid glands of the affected side; the fat pad of the posterior triangle of the neck; the internal jugular vein and some of its branches; the external carotid artery and some of its branches; and the deep cervical chain of lymph nodes together with their lymphatic channels.

Following radical neck dissection, laryngectomees may experience paralysis of the trapezius muscle, shoulder pain, and sensory loss in a large area of the shoulder and into the chest and back.

When postoperative sensory loss occurs, it is important for the patient to be taught appropriate safety measures to prevent accidental trauma to the "numb" area, e.g., cutting while shaving. Occasionally the phrenic nerve is injured during radical neck surgery, producing paralysis of the hemidiaphragm. Often laryngectomees with radical neck dissections have more difficulty learning esophageal speech than those laryngectomees who did not require radical neck dissection.[50]

During laryngeal surgery it is essential for an adequate airway to be maintained. If endotracheal intubation is not possible, a tracheotomy is performed preoperatively so the anesthetist can intubate the patient through the stoma.[8]

Following total laryngectomy, the surgeon attempts to immediately reestablish continuity of the swallowing passages between the oral cavity and the upper esophagus. This is necessary because removal of the larynx leaves a hole in the lower pharynx. Until recently, almost all attempts to accomplish this closure at the time of the original operation were unsuccessful, and the patient had to be tube-fed for months while a new esophagus was laboriously fashioned through repeated surgeries.

Surgical research is constantly attempting to perfect operations for cancer of the larynx which permit more nearly normal speech than is possible following total laryngectomy. One new type of *total laryngectomy with laryngoplasty* has been developed which enables vocal rehabilitation of the laryngectomized patient. The procedure is a delicate three-stage operation called the *Asai operation* (named for the surgeon who developed the surgery).[97] Basically in this procedure a dermal tube is constructed from the upper end of the trachea into the hypopharynx. By closing the lower tracheal fistula (i.e., the permanent tracheostomy opening) with his finger, the patient can expire air up the dermal tube and into the pharyngeal cavity. The sound produced there is transformed into speech. The resultant voice is almost normal and is thus far superior to the esophageal speech which is usually practiced following removal of the larynx.

Increasingly the larynx is being viewed not as a single organ which must always be removed *in toto* simply because one section of it is the site of cancer, but rather as a structure composed of a number of parts, all of which need not be sacrificed. While the tumor-bearing portion is resected, many other parts can be preserved and surgically reformed into a new pseudolarynx. These are the goals of *partial* or *subtotal laryngectomies.* Pressman and Bailey[79] state that any subtotal laryngectomy should ideally fulfill the following five requirements: (1) remove the tumor-bearing area and an adequate margin of

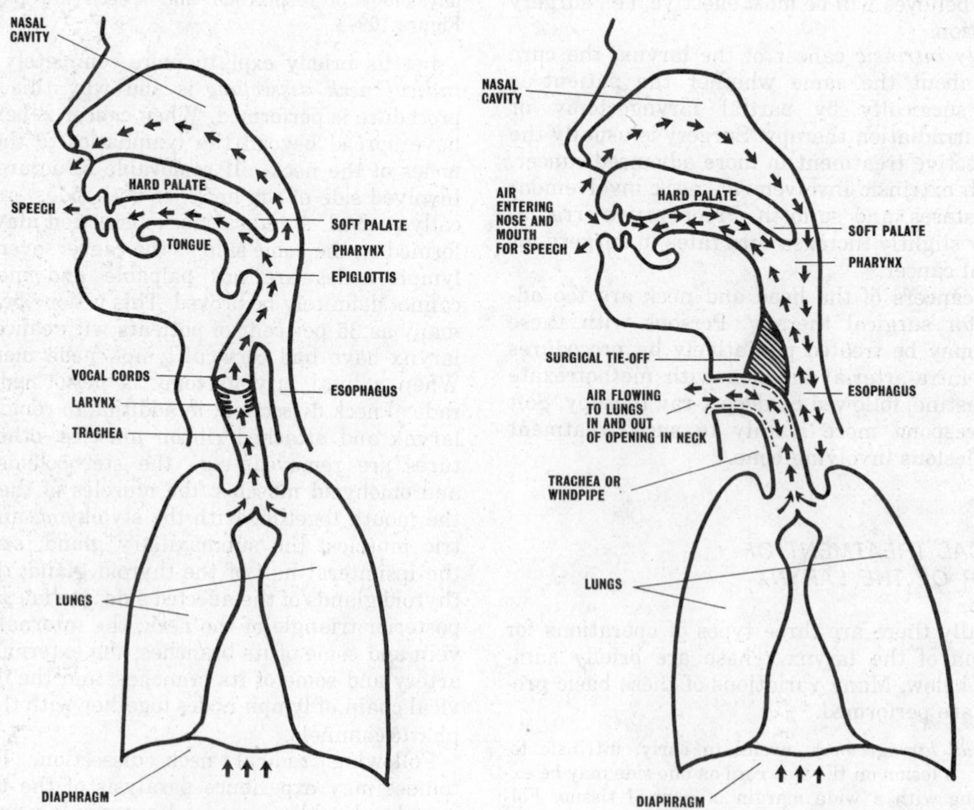

FIGURE 109–4. Total laryngectomy. (From *Rehabilitating Laryngectomies.* ©1960, American Cancer Society, Inc., 4R-50M-2/69-No. 4506-PS.)

uninvolved tissue around it; (2) provide opportunity at the time of surgery for the remaining larynx and corresponding lymph drainage areas of the neck to be inspected; (3) provide an airway which is well-lined, rigid, and adequate for both sound production and respiration; (4) preserve the "glottic valve" mechanism so the patient retains the ability to increase intrathoracic pressure for coughing, lifting, and bowel function; and (5) preserve the ability to swallow without aspiration. Numerous types of subtotal laryngectomy procedures are available to meet specific purposes.

Previously it was thought that subtotal laryngectomy procedures should always be limited to small unilateral carcinomas. More recently, however, some surgeons have been able to resect large tumors involving both sides of the larynx and leave sufficient parts of the larynx which can be reconstructed, resulting in adequate voices and adequate respiratory exchange. Significant surgical advances are being made, and many patients previously considered as requiring total laryngectomy have been spared the handicap of loss of the normal airway by less radical but more sophisticated technics. These accomplishments are being made without lessening the cure rate.

Some *postoperative complications* which may follow partial or total laryngectomies are[22] (a) *fistula formation,* between the reconstructed hypopharynx and the skin; (b) *carotid artery rupture* (occurs most often in patients who have had radical neck surgery or preoperative radiation therapy); and (c) *stenosis of the tracheostomy* (occurs weeks or months after surgery). The use of wound suction under the skin flaps postoperatively tends to prevent fistula formation. If they occur, fistulas are usually left to close by themselves, but a few are closed surgically. In the event of carotid artery hemorrhage, attempt to stop the bleeding by compressing the neck wound, suction as necessary, and get help *at once* so the patient can immediately be taken to surgery for carotid ligation. An immediate transfusion is given, and attempts are made to maintain blood pressure. Stoma stenosis may result from a fistula, fibrosis, or infection. Stenosis of the tracheostomy may be treated surgically (the opening is enlarged) or by fitting the patient with successively larger tracheostomy tubes (eventually a large one is left in place for many months or perhaps permanently).

Other possible complications are *atelectasis* and *pneumonia.* These complications can be warded off by careful nursing care during the immediate postoperative period and the first few postoperative days, e.g., suctioning, humidification, positioning, tracheostomy care.

Surgery on the larynx may be performed under general or local anesthesia.

*Preoperative Preparation for Total Laryngectomy.** Total laryngectomy is a radical surgical procedure which is naturally difficult for a patient to accept. Psychologic care of the patient with cancer of the larynx is therefore an important aspect of his total care. Pause to think for a moment about the many anxieties and fears which the patient may have as he thinks about his surgery, e.g., possible suffocation, choking, death, mutilation, recurrence of cancer, inability to speak or work, rejection by friends and loved ones. The patient, his family members and friends, all need the skilled emotional support and teaching which the nurse offers during the preoperative period and throughout the patient's hospitalization. The nurse is particularly careful to provide opportunities for the patient to discuss his concerns during the preoperative period. She realizes that it is especially important that this be accomplished *before* surgery, since it will be several weeks following surgery until the patient can learn to communicate verbally once again.

During the preoperative period the physician discusses with the patient what the postoperative results are expected to be, and the nurse discusses with the patient what will be happening to him during the immediate postoperative period, e.g., suctioning, care of the laryngectomy tube, feeding methods, vital sign measurements. When appropriate, family members are included in the preoperative teaching sessions. Both the physician and the nurse attempt before surgery to give the patient a realistic description of the sensations and apprehensions which the patient will experience upon awakening from anesthesia. Reassurance is also given at this time concerning the patient's safety and how he will be cared for. *Plentiful reassurance is one of the most necessary components of total care for the patient hospitalized for laryngectomy.*

It is important that the nurse and physician first discuss *together* what the results are expected to be following a patient's surgery. This is especially important when the larynx is going to be operated upon, since there are numerous surgical procedures producing various results. Obviously physician and nurse should both be describing the same expected results to a given patient, or he will be confused and frightened. For example, you would certainly not want to tell the patient he will lose his voice after surgery if he is not going to lose it.

If a *total* laryngectomy is to be performed, the physician tells the patient that the surgery will cause him to lose (a) normal speech (since the larynx is completely removed); (b) normal respiratory patterns through the nose and mouth; and (c) the ability to inspire and expire air through the nose and mouth. The patient is told how he will be able to breathe through a permanent tracheostomy and how he will learn to care for the tracheostomy by himself when he is able. The patient is also informed that there are other methods of speech which he will be helped to learn, i.e., he may learn esophageal speech, or he may use a mechanical or

* For a general discussion of preoperative care, refer to Unit VI.

electrical device. (Speech therapy is discussed more completely later in this chapter.) If the surgeon expects to perform radical neck dissection, he discusses this surgery with the patient.

Often it is difficult for a lay person to understand the new physiologic relationships which will result after a total laryngectomy. The patient may be unable to comprehend all of what the physician tells him and may ask the nurse for further clarification. It is therefore desirable for the nurse to be present when the physician talks preoperatively with the patient. As with any patient-education program, it is never assumed that a patient *understands* what he has been told merely because he "was told." Follow-up discussions are planned with the patient to explore further questions or concerns which he may have about information given him by the physician or nurse.

The patient's voice loss is referred to as a "temporary" voice loss when discussing it with him or with his family members, since he will learn new methods of speaking after surgery. Care is also taken not to discuss esophageal speech in terms which may be upsetting to some patients. For example the thought of "belching up air to speak with" is disgusting to some persons.[76]

Some physicians like to arrange for a laryngectomee who has been successfully rehabilitated to preoperatively visit a patient who is about to have a laryngectomy performed. Other physicians do not follow this practice. Some patients gain courage from meeting a person who can speak with an esophageal voice and who has successfully survived the procedure they are about to have performed on them. On the other hand, other patients are frightened by such a visit and may even cancel surgery after seeing what a tracheostomy stoma is like and after hearing an esophageal voice.[76] The nurse should therefore not take it upon herself to arrange a visit by a laryngectomee without the physician's approval. The physician may ask the nurse to arrange for a visitor to come from one of the clubs established for laryngectomees, e.g., a "New Voice Club" or a "Lost Chord Club." Lost Chord Club members distribute literature pertinent to laryngectomies; descriptions of their services and activities may be obtained by writing to the International Association of Laryngectomees in care of the American Cancer Society, Inc. (219 E. 42nd St., New York, N.Y., 10017).

Preoperatively some patients benefit by a visit from a speech therapist. The therapist may teach the patient how to take air into the esophagus so he can practice this before surgery, while he still has his voice to ask questions of the therapist. Not all patients are able to begin speech rehabilitation before surgery. Some are too anxious to learn effectively at this time.

If postoperative tube feedings will be used, an explanation of this procedure is given to the patient before surgery. Included is explanation of the fact that normal eating will be possible after removal of the tube. If tube feedings are used, they tend to be used for a much shorter interval of time now than formerly, perhaps only for a couple of days.

Be certain to establish with the patient preoperatively a means by which he can communicate with staff members after surgery. Inform him that a call bell will always be available to him in addition to writing materials. If the patient cannot write, discuss nonverbal communication, e.g., hand signals. Tell the patient that a nurse will be with him immediately following surgery and that he will not be left alone until he is able to again care for himself.

Preoperatively antibiotics may be ordered to minimize the possibility of infection. Oral hygiene is also important at this time. (General preoperative care is discussed in Unit VI.)

Postoperative Care Following Total Laryngectomy *

PSYCHOLOGIC CARE

> "However vivid one's imagination, it is difficult to prepare for the impact of finding oneself entirely voiceless. Upon awakening, the postoperative laryngectomy patient is suddenly confronted with the utter impossibility of making himself heard—of being unable to cry for help. It can be a profoundly frightening feeling. . . . Immediately upon awakening from surgical anesthesia, the patient discovers just how isolated he is without the ability to speak. His new way of breathing "through a hole in the neck" may also be alarming since the sensation of breathing is lacking."[68]

A total laryngectomy causes numerous "losses" of normal physiologic abilities. Sometimes socioeconomic losses also occur. All these losses result in profound disturbances in body image (see Unit III, Ch. 14). Men may associate loss of the larynx, i.e., "Adam's apple," with loss of masculinity. It is not unusual for loss of the larynx thus to be viewed by many as a form of castration. Loss of the voice means not only loss of a primary means of communicating thoughts but also loss of a highly individual characteristic. Human beings are recognized as individuals by others to a large extent by the personal qualities of their voices. Often we can identify who we are listening to if we can hear the other person speak only one or two words. Also, vocal abilities help to express emotions, e.g., a curt tone of voice indicates impatience while laughter is indicative of merriment. It is not unusual for a voice to be described as "sexy." Thus, loss of the voice may change an individual's sexual self-image and methods of sexual expression. A laryngectomy also causes loss of the normal means of breathing. Some patients are unable to continue with their presurgery means of employment following laryngectomy. In addition to losing the sense of smell, the laryngectomee can typically no longer blow his nose, blow air from his mouth, sip soup, suck on a straw, gargle, whistle or lift heavy ob-

* For a general discussion of postoperative care, see Unit VI. Prevention of complications of immobility is discussed in Unit V, Ch. 27.

jects. (The larynx makes it possible to lift and hold heavy objects by acting as a fixator factor for the thorax.)

The personal impact of the losses associated with the radical surgery of a total laryngectomy vary from individual to individual. However, postoperatively the patient normally experiences grief over loss of self and depression of varying degrees. The period of depression is commonly most intense about the third or fourth postoperative day. Severe, prolonged depression is not a "normal" reaction. Persons caring for the patient are alert to indications of severe depression (see Unit III, Ch. 10), and these symptoms are reported when observed. Remember that the severely depressed person may be suicidal. Professional skills are necessary in caring for the severely depressed patient, and he may benefit from psychiatric help.

Women usually react with greater despondency than do men when threatened with removal of the larynx. Appearance may be so shocking postoperatively that some patients faint. Some women are embarrassed at the low pitch of esophageal speech.

Postoperatively, even though the patient may know that his surgery was necessary, he may bitterly resent the changes that have been surgically performed on his body. It is not uncommon following total laryngectomy for a patient's moods to fluctuate from expressions of anger, bitterness, and fear to apathy, bewilderment, and depression. Family members also experience a gamut of emotions as they witness the effects of surgery on their loved one. The nurse draws on all resources available to her to provide skilled, effective emotional care during this period of psychologic suffering and intense feelings.

Because surgery on the larynx reduces or entirely removes a patient's ability to communicate orally (until new methods are learned or healing has taken place), *the patient requires constant attendance during the early postoperative period.* Life-threatening respiratory obstruction can rapidly develop. In addition to attentive nursing care (including frequent observations), the patient is given a tap bell and signal light to summon help and a magic slate or pad and pencil to write his requests upon. Remember not to start I.V.'s in the arm the patient needs to use for writing.

It is frustrating, tiresome, and time-consuming to a patient when he must write out everything he wishes to communicate. Naturally at times the patient appears obviously upset, perhaps angry, because he cannot speak. If the nurse can anticipate many of the patient's needs, she can greatly reduce his frustrations due to his inability to speak. Try to make it easier for the patient by carefully reading his written statements. To protect the privacy of the patient's communications with you, be certain to destroy his written notes in his presence before leaving the room. A magic slate reduces clutter and also helps to ensure privacy, since the patient can erase his statements whenever he wishes.[76]

Unknowingly staff members and visitors may add to a laryngectomee's communication problems in various ways. For example, (a) they may raise the tone of their voices as if the patient were hard-of-hearing; (b) they may be tempted to complete sentences verbally which the patient has started to write out (it is best to let the patient complete his own thought); and (c) they may talk nervously and excessively because of their own discomfort with the patient's silence.[76]

Some patients cannot read and write, and thus, following total laryngectomy, they are unable to communicate by writing. These patients are even more completely prisoners of silence than are literate patients until they learn esophageal speech or another method of artificial speech. Nonverbal communication, e.g., hand and facial gestures, is their only means of communication, and therefore they are closely observed by the nurse for indications of their needs.

If an intercom system exists between patient rooms and the nursing station, be certain to post a note on the control board to inform staff members that the patient cannot use the intercom following total laryngectomy because he cannot speak.

Postoperatively all clinical care and procedures, e.g., suctioning, changing the laryngectomy tube, and so forth, are carefully explained to the patient before care is started. This is helpful to the patient since he cannot speak to ask questions, and he may justifiably panic if he does not know what is going to be done to him.

CLINICAL CARE. Immediately following surgery the new laryngectomee is positioned on his side until consciousness is regained. Then, if his blood pressure is stable his head is elevated 30–45° to promote drainage, facilitate respirations, prevent uncomfortable strain on the suture lines, and minimize edema. When moving the patient about in bed or helping him to sit up, be certain to support the back of his neck with both hands. This gives him a feeling of security and prevents painful tension on the sutures. (When the patient begins to help himself, teach him to support his own head in this manner.[76]) Initially the patient is usually highly restless and anxious upon regaining consciousness. Positioning the patient with his head slightly flexed prevents tension on the suture line and possible wound dehiscence.

When the patient returns from surgery he may or may not have a tube in his tracheostomy and he may or may not have a neck dressing. If a tube is in place in the tracheostomy, it is a *laryngeal or laryngectomy tube* or a *cuffed tracheostomy tube.* A laryngectomy tube is shorter and slightly larger in diameter than a tracheostomy tube; however, the tube care is the same for either tube (see Ch. 108).

Suctioning is discussed in detail in Unit XIV and in Chapter 108. Here we mention only a few points of importance in suctioning the laryngectomized patient:[76] (a) the patient must be suctioned nasally as well as through the tracheostomy since he can no longer blow his nose (air can no longer be forced up through the nose to "blow" it); and (b) a size 14 catheter is usually appropriate for suctioning through a laryngectomy tube if one is in place. Do not use the same catheter to suction the nose and trachea. Suction the mouth gently. Do not attempt deep suction through the nose or mouth without permission; you could accidentally penetrate the suture line.

Because he cannot blow his nose, the laryngectomee must always resort to manual cleaning of his nose with a damp cloth or a handkerchief. It is advisable for him to *not* use paper tissues since they may contain irritating particles and also since pieces of them can tear off and be accidentally aspirated.

Artificial humidification must be provided for the patient with a permanent tracheostomy (see Unit XIV).

In giving postoperative care following laryngectomy, the nurse gives tracheostomy care as indicated and also observes for *indications of postoperative complications,* e.g., respiratory distress (cyanosis, dyspnea), hemorrhage, hemoptysis, excessive coughing, symptoms of shock. Vital signs are checked every 15 minutes until stable. Observe for hemorrhage from the wound and from the tracheostomy tube. (General postoperative care is discussed in Unit VI.)

Other nursing activities commonly performed during the early postoperative period following laryngectomy are (a) evaluation and recording of intake and output; (b) regulation of *intravenous feedings* or administration of *tube feedings;* (c) administration of medications, such as analgesics, vitamins, and antibiotics (postoperative wound contamination and infection may easily occur); and (d) administration of *frequent oral hygiene.* Oral hygiene is given frequently to prevent infection and to keep the patient more comfortable. Apply Vaseline to the patient's lips if they are dry. If diarrhea occurs, the patient is carefully evaluated to prevent fluid and electrolyte imbalances (see Unit V, Ch. 25).

Following surgery *drainage catheters* are usually inserted under the wound's skin flaps; they are then connected to *Gomco suction* or to a *Hemovac,* i.e., a small plastic device which creates its own suction. These drainage catheters are used to remove fluid from the potential dead space left after removal of the larynx and related structures. When wound suction is used, it is usually kept on constantly unless otherwise ordered; do not discontinue suction to measure contents without permission. Care is taken to maintain free drainage within the suction system. Wound drainage catheters are usually removed on about the third postoperative day. Dressings may not be present if wound drainage catheters are being used. If the catheters are not used, *pressure dressings* may be present to minimize serous fluid accumulation or hematoma formation under the skin flaps. Following radical neck dissection, drains may be left in the wound and pressure dressings applied. Check the dressings frequently for drainage and be certain they are not excessively interfering with the patient's respirations.

Narcotics are contraindicated for patients with head and neck surgery since they depress respirations and inhibit coughing.

Fortunately laryngectomy typically does not produce severe postoperative *pain.* Minimal postoperative pain occurs following laryngectomy because sensory nerve endings are cut by the skin flap incisions. Analgesics, such as buffered aspirin or dextropropoxyphene (Darvon), are usually adequate to relieve discomfort. These medications can be dissolved in water and given via the feeding tube or per rectum if the patient cannot take them orally. Occasionally small doses of opiates may be ordered. When they are given, the nurse watches carefully for indications of respiratory depression and immediately reports such findings if they occur. Hypoventilation and hypotension should be avoided.

Pain does occur during the immediate postoperative period following laryngectomy when the patient attempts to swallow. Gentle oral suctioning and allowing the patient to expectorate saliva rather than swallowing it are measures which give relief during this period of painful swallowing. While incisional pain is minimal, the patient may have a headache or other discomfort, e.g., sore throat due to the presence of a nasogastric tube.

A *nasogastric tube* may or may not be present postoperatively for *tube feedings.* Maintain patency of the tube. Some patients are given intravenous nourishment until the third postoperative day; then they may be allowed oral nourishment. Other patients are given oral fluids as early as the first postoperative day. Still other patients have a nasogastric feeding tube for several days following total laryngectomy. Gastric suction may be ordered if tube feedings cause nausea.

Possible advantages of tube feedings are (a) reduction of possible incision contamination; (b) prevention of fistula formation by relieving the tension which swallowing places on the pharyngeal suture line; and (c) enhancement of the healing process by avoiding the muscular activity necessary for swallowing. As discussed earlier, in some patients the anterior wall of the esophagus is reconstructed at the time laryngectomy is performed (this portion of esophagus connects with the posterior wall of the larynx). In such a situation, postoperative tube feedings minimize the esophageal irritation which swallowed food causes.

If a nasogastric tube is used for very long the patient may be instructed how to pass his own tube and give his own feedings. This is done with the physician's approval postoperatively. Nasogastric tube feedings should never be performed when the patient is reclining or the formula will be regurgitated. During feedings the patient should be awake and sitting erect with his feet over the side of the bed. If the tube is not in place when the patient returns from surgery, the doctor passes the tube the first time (usually he does this on the first postoperative day). A nurse should never attempt to reinsert a nasogastric tube following laryngeal surgery without the physician's permission, because of the potential danger of rupturing the internal suture line. Once the patient can safely swallow, the physician may permit him to take sips of water. The nasogastric tube is removed once the patient is able to satisfactorily take oral nourishment.

Following laryngectomy the patient's first attempts to take liquids orally are carefully supervised. Initial attempts to swallow may cause a choking feeling and severe coughing. Water is given until the patient can confidently swallow, then other fluids may be introduced. The nurse remains calm as the patient learns to swallow, and she is prepared to suction as necessary since coughing may raise secretions. Food inhalation is not possible orally following total laryngectomy because the food passage (esophagus) and breathing passage (trachea) are separate, i.e., the tracheal opening is sutured to the skin of the neck. Before oral feedings are started, the patient may be given some fluid to swallow which contains methylene blue dye if a fistula is suspected. Confirmation of a fistula usually means that tube feedings will be continued until the fistula is healed.

When the surgeon thinks it is advisable, the patient may begin to practice belching after oral feedings, e.g., an hour after eating. This is preliminary training for the explosive movement of air out of the esophagus which is necessary for esophageal speech.

SELF-CARE AND PATIENT TEACHING. *Self-care is started early in the postoperative course* following laryngectomy. As mentioned, if a nasogastric tube is in place the patient may be given instructions about how to give his own feedings as soon as he is able. On the first postoperative day the patient is usually taught to suction his own tracheostomy tube (be sure to provide a mirror for him to use). Normally the patient is also helped to get up for a while on this day, since early ambulation helps him improve faster. Within 4–5 days after surgery, the patient is typically ambulatory as desired, is able to feed and bathe himself, and is not only suctioning his laryngectomy tube but also removing and cleaning the inner cannula if one is present. Much of the nurse's time with the patient during these first few postoperative days is spent in teaching the patient self-care and in supervising the patient's early attempts at performing nursing procedures.

Because a considerable amount of the patient's care centers around teaching, it is necessary to *have a detailed care plan to be certain all aspects of patient education are covered.* Typically it is not possible for the same nurse to conduct all the necessary teaching sessions with one patient. A care plan makes it possible for several nurses to participate in the teaching process without duplicating their efforts and without overlooking some areas which should be covered.

As the patient begins to gain self-confidence, the nurse leaves his bedside for gradually longer periods of time. However, his call signal is always answered immediately, and the nurse continues to make frequent "drop-in" visits so the patient feels secure in the knowledge that he is being watched out for by a concerned person. Praise is freely given to the patient as he progresses in the difficult readjustments necessary for him to make. Remembering that a patient's self-esteem and self-image are dealt a severe blow by surgery as radical as that of a laryngectomy, the nurse utilizes every opportunity to show respect for the patient. If a speech therapist is visiting the patient, the nurse coordinates her plan of care with the goals of speech therapy.

Sometimes a patient's course of progress is slowed down by the development of an esophageal fistula during the postoperative period. This complication most often develops in those persons who have been treated with radiotherapy (see Unit VII).

Prior to *discharge* the patient and persons who will be with him at his home need detailed teaching about tracheostomy care and other aspects of care following surgery on the larynx. Humidification must be set up in the home before the patient's discharge. Air conditioning may provide air which is excessively cool or dry and thus is undesirable. The patient is instructed how to remove and replace the entire laryngectomy tube if one is still being worn. Generally suctioning is not necessary once the patient is ready for discharge. However, an occasional patient may need to have a suction machine placed in his home. (The local chapter of the American Cancer Society may help the patient obtain a suction machine.)

To insert his laryngectomy tube the patient breathes in, holds his breath, inserts the tube, and then resumes normal breathing. Tell the patient not to hyperextend his neck when inserting the tube since this is not helpful but will instead cause the stoma to become smaller. The laryngectomy tube is cleaned in a manner similar to cleaning a tracheostomy tube (see Ch. 108). The tube is cleaned at least once daily.

While an occasional patient needs to permanently wear a laryngectomy tube, most patients wear one only for the first 3 to 8 postoperative weeks until the stoma has permanently formed. A few patients are advised to wear the tube part of the time, e.g., at night if the stoma tends to collapse or does not provide adequate air exchange during sleeping.

The patient is taught precautions which he must take to prevent accidental cutting of his neck and to prevent aspiration through the tracheostomy stoma. Caution is necessary when shaving because it takes about 6 months for the sensory nerve endings which were cut at the time of surgery to regenerate. Accidental cutting can easily occur during this interval. Precautions necessary with a permanent tracheostomy were discussed in Chapter 108.

Before returning home the patient must be given *dietary instructions* appropriate for him. Usually the diet progresses from liquid to soft to general. Muscular tonus is important for esophageal speech. Often the entire muscular mechanism, necessary for esophageal speech, is weak and flaccid because of the soft and liquid foods which the patient's diet has been limited to before, during, and sometimes even after hospitalization. Some speech therapists will not begin to teach a laryngectomee esophageal speech until the patient is on a full and normal diet. While observing necessary dietary restrictions (as ordered by the physician), it is important as soon as possible for the patient to chew and swallow a normal diet so his throat and abdominal musculature will regain tonus. Desirable foods from this standpoint include raw vegetables, rough dry cereals, raisins, peanuts, and not-too-tender meats cut in moderately small pieces.[97]

REHABILITATION. Every attempt is made to minimize the patient's feelings of difference and to help him reestablish a life pattern which is normal for him. Family members are counseled not to treat the patient as an invalid and never to apologize to others for the patient's condition. Expressions of embarrassment accentuate the differences of the patient, cast him in the role of an invalid, and tender to foster reclusive and depressive tendencies.

It is desirable for the laryngectomee to return to employment as soon as possible, even before he has mastered esophageal speech. Steady employment is one of the strongest motivations for regaining speech and as such is important in speech rehabilitation as well as total rehabilitation. Following total laryngectomy a patient is often able to return to work within 4 to 8 weeks after hospitalization.

Occasionally it is necessary for a patient to change his mode of employment following laryngectomy, e.g., if his job is highly voice-dependent or is in a dusty environment. However, often patients are able to continue with their presurgery type of employment. Some patients manage quite well, even in sales positions which require quite a lot of talking.

Rehabilitation is the rule rather than the exception following laryngectomy. However, in spite of the generally good prospects for rehabilitation, about one fourth of laryngectomees fail to regain a good occupational or social adjustment, or the adjustment is delayed many months.[68]

Before hospital discharge the laryngectomee is informed of rehabilitative agencies which are available to help him. The *International Association of Laryngectomees* (IAL) is an autonomous agency, supported by the American Cancer Society, which has about 175 member clubs in the U.S. and various parts of the world. The IAL focuses on both social and educational aspects of cancer of the larynx. Bimonthly the *IAL News* is printed and distributed free of charge to more than 18,000 persons in 55 countries. While local *Lost Chord Clubs* and *New Voice Clubs* are now often affiliated with the IAL, they also continue to maintain their local autonomy and service to laryngectomees. The IAL publishes a "Directory of Sources of Supply for Items of Benefit to Laryngectomees." This directory lists such items as tracheostomy equipment, humidifiers, artificial larynxes, amplifiers for weak voices, films, exhibits, publications, and emergency instructions.

Other rehabilitation resources in the community which the patient should be made aware of are (a) a local or regional branch of the *American Cancer Society;* (b) a local, regional, or state university or college with a speech and hearing center; (c) the *American Speech and Hearing Association* (90030 Old Georgetown Road, Washington, D.C. 20014); and (d) the state office of vocational rehabilitation (helpful when a change of occupation is necessary). The American Speech and Hearing Association publishes a booklet listing persons especially qualified to teach esophageal speech. This association is active in speech research, therapy, and education.

Before discharge the laryngectomee is given an identification card which states that he has no vocal cords and also gives information for *artificial respiration* if needed. Because the laryngectomee breathes through a tracheostomy rather than through his nose and mouth, mouth-to-mouth resuscitation is ineffective. Effective first aid measures include mouth-to-neck resuscitation (see Ch. 108) and the administration of oxygen through the tracheostomy. The patient's head should not be turned to the side since this may obstruct the tracheostomy. On the back of his identification card the laryngectomee writes his name and the name of the person he wishes notified in case of emergency. Official laryngectomee identification cards are obtainable from the International Association of Laryngectomees.

Many postlaryngectomy patients benefit from associating with other persons who are laryngectomees. Membership in clubs like the Lost Chord Club helps give these persons social confidence and helps with their voice development. Other individuals who have had laryngectomies do not enjoy belonging to clubs of this nature, but rather they prefer dealing privately with the new situation.[68] Thus, the most desirable rehabilitation program is the one which meets the needs of a given patient and gives recognition to his individual pattern of best adapting to the changes imposed upon him as a result of his illness.

Although patients are usually advised not to smoke following laryngectomy, some continue to do so. Following total laryngectomy the smoke is no longer directly inhaled into the throat or lungs. Nonetheless the smoke-laden air is inhaled, to some extent, through the tracheostomy.

Postoperative Care Following Partial Laryngectomy. In the previous section we discussed at length clinical care given following *total* laryngectomy. Here let us briefly consider significant aspects of clinical care following *partial* laryngectomy.

During surgery a tracheostomy tube is placed. Postoperatively this tube is removed after tissue edema subsides. Following partial laryngectomy the patient is typically given nourishment by vein or nasogastric tube for the first two postoperative days. Oral fluids are usually then permitted.

A partial laryngectomy, e.g., laryngofissure, leaves the patient with a husky but useful voice. Postoperatively the patient is instructed not to attempt speaking until the doctor says he may do so. Voice rest is usually continued for the first two to three postoperative days. The patient may then be allowed to begin to whisper. Gradually, after further healing occurs, the patient is allowed to begin to use his voice again.

SPEECH REHABILITATION FOLLOWING LARYNGECTOMY

Following conservative or total laryngectomy, speech therapy is indicated to either (a) teach the patient how to correct speech problems resulting from his surgery (if he retains some ability to speak); or (b) teach him esophageal, i.e., alaryngeal, speech or other methods of artificial speech (if he is without the ability to speak).

As mentioned previously, preoperatively the physician, speech therapist, and nurse all reassure the patient that after his larynx is removed he will be able to use either esophageal speech or some type of artificial larynx as a new sound source. Nonetheless, the patient must accept the fact that his normal voice is lost forever. This loss causes noticeable reactions in others (as they listen to the patient's new voice) and in the patient's own self-image. The patient must adjust to the reactions of others and to the necessary change in his self-image. Initially the patient may seem "somewhat like a stranger" to himself and to persons who were familiar with his normal voice.

The physician gives orders for speech rehabilitation to begin. Speech therapy may begin while the patient is hospitalized and usually continues after the patient is discharged. Esophageal speech can best be learned by attending a speech clinic or working individually with a speech therapist. Some highly motivated patients are able to learn esophageal speech within 2 to 3 weeks of instruction. Because motivation is highly important in speech therapy, the patient benefits from enthusiastic encouragement from his family and friends as well as the speech therapist, physician, and nurse. Discouragement comes easily because of the repeated efforts necessary before esophageal speech can be effectively used. In addition to instruction, the patient needs opportunity to practice privately as well as in the presence of others. The patient is told that his new voice will continue to improve over many months of practice.

An estimated 80 per cent of laryngectomees are capable of learning esophageal speech if given good instruction.[98] In spite of being highly motivated, a few laryngectomees cannot learn esophageal speech. Advanced age prevents some patients from learning esophageal speech, e.g., hearing problems may be present which prevent effective learning. The aged man may also lack the motivation and strength necessary for esophageal speech. Occasionally esophageal speech is impossible because of other physical problems, e.g., esophageal stenosis, emphysema, asthma. Individuals who cannot learn esophageal speech may benefit from the use of an artificial larynx. Some laryngectomees learn to use both esophageal speech and an artificial larynx. Then they are able to use whichever method best meets their needs in various situations.

Esophageal Speech. "Esophageal speech" is a method of speaking in which the patient learns to take air in through his mouth, hold it in his upper esophagus, and then form words while expelling the air back out of the mouth in a controlled flow. In lay terms, esophageal speech is somewhat similar to a controlled belch. With practice, up to six to ten words may be spoken after each intake of air. Vibration at the top of the gullet replaces that from the lungs. (The "gullet" is the passage to the stomach including both the pharynx and the esophagus.)

When possible it is most desirable for a patient to begin to learn esophageal speech *before* he has surgery. This enables him to ask questions more readily during the learning process and also it helps to minimize the psychologic impact of losing his natural voice, i.e., he knows he will be able to communicate with esophageal speech postoperatively.

The basic act in learning esophageal speech is the "charging" and "releasing" of air from the upper portion of the esophagus. The esophagus has an elastic wall and thus can stretch with the intake of air. Most patients find it more difficult to take air into the esophagus, i.e., to "charge" the esophagus than it is to release the air. There are three well-established methods of charging air:[99] (1) the suction, "breathing," or inhalation method; (2) air injection by tongue and related structures; and (3) the glossopharyngeal press or plosive-injection method. Details of these methods are beyond the scope of this text. However, the goal of all of them is to rapidly take air into the esophagus so it can then be released and its force can be used to create the sounds of speech.

With practice the air-charge necessary for esophageal speech can be taken in in about one half to one fourth of a second. This is actually less time than that of a normal speaker inhaling for an intraphasal breath pause. Expert esophageal speakers speak relatively easily and are no more conscious of the "breathing" function than normal speakers, i.e., they are not consciously aware of the process of taking an air-charge.

Air is held only briefly in the top half or third of

the esophagus. The air intake should be immediately followed by the speech sound. Relaxation is necessary in order to get air into the top of the esophagus and to release it.

Diaphragmatic action and the exhalation of lung air facilitate expulsion of air from the esophagus. Pushing the head back when releasing air often helps improve loudness and quality. Voicing usually takes place in the cricopharyngeal area. A segment of the gullet and the top of the gullet vibrate. Esophageal voice sounds are somewhat hoarse and are more low-pitched than laryngeal voice sounds. However, the qualities of speech provided by the use of the nasopharynx are still present.

Practice enables the esophageal speaker to develop a speech which flows quite smoothly and is easily understood. Also, he learns to speak an increasing number of words with each swallow of air. Small amplifiers are available for the esophageal speaker to use when addressing conferences.

Temporary digestive problems may occur when a patient first begins to learn esophageal speech. These problems are related to nervous tension, tension placed on abdominal muscles, and air swallowing. Some persons are excessively troubled with flatulence as a result of air swallowing when using esophageal speech. Once efficient esophageal speech is learned, these disorders usually no longer occur.

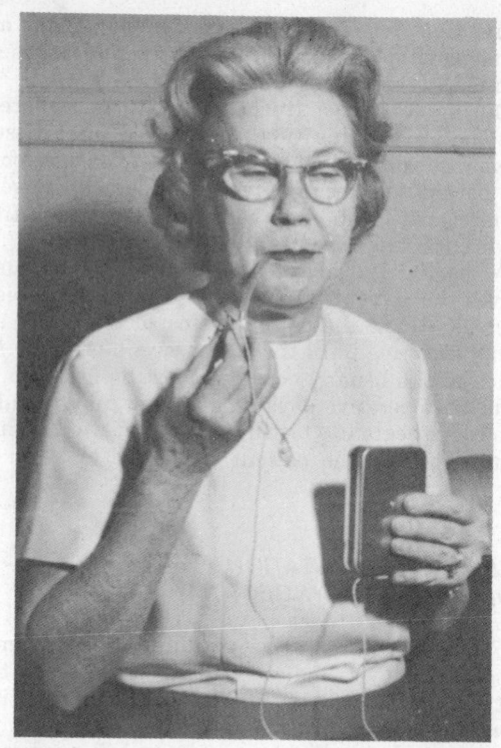
FIGURE 109–6. Cooper-Rand electronic speech aid. (From Flowers, A. M.: *Nursing Clinics of North America* 3:529, 1968.)

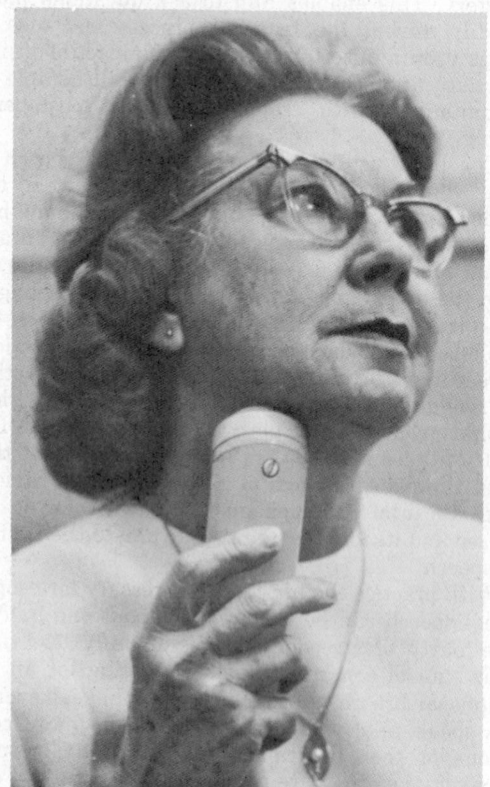
FIGURE 109–5. Western Electric artificial larynx. (From Flowers, A. M.: *Nursing Clinics of North America* 3:529, 1968.)

The person who speaks with an esophageal voice needs to avoid excessive fatigue; it is more difficult for him to speak when tired. Also, the laryngectomee's spouse should have his or her hearing evaluated. If the spouse is even a marginal candidate for a hearing aid, he or she should wear one. A hearing aid may make it easier for the spouse to understand the laryngectomee's esophageal speech. While the effective esophageal speaker has sufficient loudness for the normal listener, he cannot shout.

Artificial Larynx. If a patient has not been able to learn esophageal speech after 2 to 3 months of instruction and practice, or if he is initially obviously not a potential candidate for artificial speech, the speech therapist may recommend use of an artificial larynx. Also, many speech therapists advise use of an artificial larynx to get the patient communicating soon after surgery and thus to make the learning of esophageal speech easier. A wide variety of mechanical and electrical instruments are available to replace the phonation functions of the removed larynx. Basically three types of artificial larynxes are available: (1) the reed-type artificial larynx; (2) an electronic throat vibrator aid; and (3) an electronic aid which vibrates directly in the mouth.

The *reed-type artificial larynx* is perhaps best represented by the instruments developed by Western Electric. One of these instruments is powered by breath from the tracheal stoma; the air passes through a loop of tubing from the neck to the mouth. In the mouth the air is pushed out through a reed at the end of the tubing. Some believe the skilled user of this instrument can develop speech superior to that of esophageal speech. Others believe this instrument is superseded by newer instruments, e.g., the Western Electric Electronic Larynx *throat vibrator.* The latter instrument is an inexpensive, light-weight, transistorized device which is economic in its utilization of batteries. It is available in a model for the male voice and a model for the female voice. While the Western Electric Electronic Larynx is somewhat lacking in loudness, it has manual, continuous control of pitch modulation which provides some simulation of the complex changes in pitch which characterize the normal voice (see Fig. 109–5). Often a throat vibrator instrument cannot be used in the immediate postoperative period because the neck wounds are too sensitive at that time.

Two other throat vibrator electrolarynxes are (1) the Aurex larynx (highly favored by many laryngectomees); and (2) the Kett, Mark III larynx. Although somewhat heavy, the Kett, Mark III aid is rechargeable and is particularly useful when a loud voice is desirable.

Throat-vibrating artificial larynxes all are somewhat less favorable than superior esophageal speech, because even the newest and best of them are somewhat noisy. These devices all basically operate by a pulsating disk which sets the throat tissues vibrating.

Another type of aid is one that *vibrates directly in the mouth,* e.g., the Cooper-Rand Electronic Speech Aid (Fig. 109–6). This pipes sound into the mouth through a small plastic tube held in the corner of the mouth.

The design of artificial larynxes continues to improve. While some of the first models produced speech which sounded highly mechanized, monotonous, and artificial, modern artificial larynxes are capable of producing speech which more naturally fluctuates in volume and pitch.

Let us emphasize that the acquisition of an artificial larynx does not guarantee that clear and intelligible speech will automatically be possible. The patient needs to be properly instructed in the use of his particular instrument. Speech therapy is therefore desirable.

Space does not permit a detailed discussion of speech rehabilitation after laryngectomy. Nurses, patients, and other interested persons can obtain additional information about esophageal (alaryngeal) speech and artificial larynxes by contacting local chapters of the American Cancer Society, the International Association of Laryngectomees, or the American Speech and Hearing Association (addresses previously stated).

References for Unit XXII

1. Adler, S.: Speech after laryngectomy. *American Journal of Nursing 69:*2138, October, 1969.
2. *1973 Cancer Facts and Figures.* New York, American Cancer Society, 1973.
2a. *Cancer of the Larynx.* New York, American Cancer Society, 1968.
3. *First Aid for (Neck-Breathers) Laryngectomees.* New York, American Cancer Society, 1971.
4. *Rehabilitating Laryngectomees.* New York, American Cancer Society, 1960.
5. Arlen, H.: Microlaryngoscopy. *AORN Journal 16:*37, August, 1972.
6. Barton, R.: Life after laryngectomy. *Laryngoscope 75:*1408, September, 1965.
7. Beatrous, W. P.: Tracheostomy: Its expanded indications and present status. *Laryngoscope 78:*3, January, 1968.
8. Beattie, E. J., and Economou, S. G.: The current status of radical laryngectomy. *Nursing Clinics of North America 3:*515, September, 1968.
9. Beeson, P. B., and McDermott, W. (eds.): *Cecil-Loeb Textbook of Medicine.* 13th ed. Philadelphia, W. B. Saunders Company, 1971, pp. 865–946.
10. Beland, I. L.: *Clinical Nursing: Pathophysiological and Psychosocial Approaches.* 2nd ed. New York, The Macmillan Company, 1970.
11. Belinkoff, S.: *Introduction to Inhalation Therapy.* Boston, Little, Brown and Company, 1969.
12. Bendixen, H. H., et al.: *Respiratory Care.* St. Louis, C. V. Mosby Company, 1965.
13. Brown, E. B.: Hyposensitization therapy in respiratory allergy. *Modern Treatment 3:*845, July, 1966.
14. Brunner, L. S., et al.: *Textbook of Medical-Surgical Nursing.* 2nd ed. Philadelphia, J. B. Lippincott Company, 1970.
15. Bryce, D. P., Briant, T. D. R., and Pearson, F. G.: Laryngeal and tracheal complications of intubation. *Annals of Otology, Rhinology and Laryngology 77:*442, June, 1968.
16. Chiang, T. M., Sukis, A. E., and Ross, D. E.: Tonsillectomy performed on an outpatient basis. *Archives of Otolaryngology 88:*307, September, 1968.
17. Conner, G. H., et al.: Tracheostomy. *American Journal of Nursing 72:*68, January, 1972.
19. Davison, F. W.: Chronic sinus disease: Differential diagnosis. *Laryngoscope 78:*1738, October, 1968.
20. Dawes, J. D. K.: Diagnosis and treatment of sinusitis. *Nursing Mirror 125:*ix, 15 December, 1967.
21. Deatsch, W. W.: Ear, Nose and Throat, *In Current Diagnosis and Treatment.* Krupp, M. A., and Chatton, M. J. (eds.), Los Altos, Ca., Lange Medical Publications, 1972.
22. DeWeese, D. D., and Saunders, W. H.: *Textbook of Otolaryngology.* 3rd ed. St. Louis, C. V. Mosby Company, 1968.
23. Diedrich, W. M., and Youngstrom, K. A.: *Alaryngeal Speech.* Springfield, Ill., Charles C Thomas, Publisher, 1966.
24. Duguay, M.: Preoperative ideas of speech after

laryngectomy. *Archives of Otolaryngology 83:*237, March, 1966.
25. Egan, D.: *Fundamentals of Inhalation Therapy.* St. Louis, C. V. Mosby Company, 1969.
26. Feldman, S. A. (ed.): *Tracheostomy and Artificial Ventilation.* London, Edward Arnold (Publisher), Ltd., 1967.
27. Flowers, A. M.: Electronic mechanical aids for laryngectomized patient. *Nursing Clinics of North America 3:*529, September, 1968.
28. Frazell, E. L., Strong, E. W., and Newcombe, B.: Tumors of the parotid. *American Journal of Nursing 66:*2702, December, 1966.
29. Freedman, S. O. (ed.): Symposium on treatment of respiratory allergy. *Modern Treatment 3:*813, July, 1966.
30. Fuerst, E. V., and Wolff, L.: *Fundamentals of Nursing.* 4th ed. Philadelphia, J. B. Lippincott Company, 1969.
31. Gardner, W. H.: Adjustment problems of laryngectomized women. *Archives of Otolaryngology 83:*31, January, 1966.
32. Geffin, B., and Pontoppidan, H.: Reduction of tracheal damage by the prestretching of inflatable cuffs. *Anesthesiology 31:*462, November, 1969.
33. Goffe, W. F.: What to do when foreign bodies are inhaled or ingested. *Postgraduate Medicine 44:*135, October, 1968.
34. Grant, H., and Murray, R.: *Emergency Care.* Washington, D.C., Robert J. Brady Company, 1971.
35. Guyton, A. C.: *Function of the Human Body.* 4th ed. Philadelphia, W. B. Saunders Company, 1974.
36. Hall, I. S., and Colman, B. H.: *Diseases of the Nose, Throat and Ear.* 9th ed. London, E. and S. Livingstone, Ltd., 1969.
37. Harrison, T. R., et al. (eds.): *Principles of Internal Medicine.* 6th ed. New York, McGraw-Hill Book Company, 1970.
38. Hayes, T. P., Atkins, J. P., and Raventos, A.: Carcinoma of the larynx: Diagnosis and treatment by surgery or irradiation. *Annals of Otology, Rhinology and Laryngology 80:*627, October, 1971.
39. Hedden, M., et al.: Laryngotracheal damage after prolonged use of orotracheal tubes in adults. *Journal of the American Medical Association 207:*703, January 27, 1969.
40. Helman, P., et al.: Intra-arterial cytotoxic therapy and x-ray therapy for cancer of the head and neck. *American Journal of Surgery 112:*606, October, 1966.
41. Herzon, F. S.: Bacteremia and local infections with nasal packing. *Archives of Otolaryngology 94:*317, October, 1971.
42. Holinger, P. H.: Laryngoscopy, bronchoscopy, and esophagoscopy. *Journal American Operating Room Nurses 4:*61, May–June, 1966.
43. Holvey, D. N., et al. (eds.): *The Merck Manual.* 12th ed. Rahway, N.J., Merck Sharp & Dohme Research Laboratories, 1972.
44. *Helping Words for the Laryngectomee.* International Association of Laryngectomees, 1964. (Distributed by The American Cancer Society, Inc.)
45. Jacob, S. W., and Francone, C. A.: *Structure and Function in Man.* 3rd ed. Philadelphia, W. B. Saunders Company, 1974.
46. Jacobs, H. B.: Emergency percutaneous transtracheal catheter and ventilator. *Journal of Trauma 12:*50, January, 1972.
47. Jacquette, G.: To reduce hazards of tracheal suctioning. *American Journal of Nursing 71:*2362, December, 1971.
48. Jeffis, L., and Baker, C.: Nasopharyngeal and tracheal suctioning. *American Journal of Nursing 67:*2361, November, 1967.
49. Kearns, B.: Tracheostomy suctioning technique. *Canadian Nurse 66:*44, February, 1970.
50. King, P. S., et al.: Effect of radical neck dissection on total rehabilitation of the laryngectomee. *American Journal of Physical Medicine 52:*1, February, 1973.
51. Kolz, C.: Microlaryngoscopy: The nurse's role. *AORN Journal 16:*42, August, 1972.
52. Komorn, R. M.: Laryngectomy and surgical vocal rehabilitation. *AORN Journal 17:*73, June, 1973.
53. Kuner, J., and Goldman, A.: Prolonged nasotracheal intubation in adults versus tracheostomy. *Diseases of the Chest 51:*270, March, 1967.
54. Lambert, V.: Modern application of tracheostomy. *Nursing Mirror 126:*44, 19 April, 1968.
55. LeJeune, F. E., Jr.: Foreign bodies in the tracheobronchial tree and esophagus. *Surgical Clinics of North America 46:*1501, December, 1966.
56. Levin, N. M.: Rehabilitation after total laryngectomy. *Eye, Ear, Nose, and Throat Monthly 46:*756, June, 1967.
57. Loeb, W. J.: Experiences with a modified cuffed tracheostomy tube. *Annals of Otology, Rhinology and Laryngology 80:*549, August, 1971.
58. Ludman, H.: Tracheostomy. *Nursing Mirror 124:*i, 4 August, 1967.
59. Macbeth, P.: Chronic sinusitis. *Practitioner 197:*765, December, 1966.
60. Malcomson, K. G.: Tonsillitis: Acute and chronic. *Practitioner 199:*777, December, 1967.
61. McDevitt, T. J., Goh, A. S., and Acquarelli, M. J.: Epistaxis: Management and prevention. *Laryngoscope 77:*1109, July, 1967.
62. McGovern, F. H., et al.: The hazards of endotracheal intubation. *Annals of Otology, Rhinology and Laryngology 80:*556, August, 1971.
63. McNab Jones, R. F.: Treatment of epistaxis. *Nursing Mirror 124:*vi, August 18, 1967.
64. Medical news: Laryngeal staining highlights pathologic tissue. *Journal of the American Medical Association 208:*24, April 7, 1969.
65. Miller, B. F., and Keane, C. B.: *Encyclopedia and Dictionary of Medicine and Nursing.* Philadelphia, W. B. Saunders Company, 1972.
66. Mills, C. P.: Acute sinusitis. *Practitioner 197:*757, December, 1966.
67. Montgomery, W. W., and Toohill, R. J.: Voice rehabilitation after laryngectomy. *Archives of Otolaryngology 88:*499, November, 1968.
68. Murphy, G. E., and Ogura, J.: Rehabilitation following laryngectomy. *Geriatrics 22:*119, December, 1967.
69. Noakes, O., and Sykes, M. K.: Equipment for tracheostomy care. *Nursing Times 61:*1068, August 6, 1965.
70. Oliver, P.: Cancer of the nose and paranasal sinuses. *Surgical Clinics of North America 47:*595, June, 1967.
71. Olson, N. R., and Miles, W. K.: Treatment of acute blunt laryngeal injuries. *Annals of Otology, Rhinology and Laryngology 80:*704, October, 1971.
72. Parvulescu, N. F.: Care of the surgically speechless patient. *Nursing Clinics of North America 5:*517, September, 1970.

73. Pearson, F. G., et al.: Tracheal stenosis complicating tracheostomy with cuffed tubes. *Archives of Surgery 97:*380, September, 1968.
74. Peres, C. A., et al.: Irradiation of early carcinoma of the larynx. *Archives of Otolaryngology 93:*465, May, 1971.
75. Pilgrim, M. C., and Sands, D.: Reconstructive nasal surgery. *American Journal of Nursing 73:*451, March, 1973.
76. Pitorak, E.: Laryngectomy. *American Journal of Nursing 68:*780, April, 1968.
77. Pratt, L. W.: Complications of tracheotomy. *Eye, Ear, Nose and Throat Monthly 48:*119, February, 1969.
78. Pratt, L. W.: Tracheostomy or peroral endotracheal intubation. *Journal Maine Medical Association 59:*23, February, 1968.
79. Pressman, J. J., and Bailey, B. J.: The surgery of cancer of the larynx with especial reference to subtotal laryngectomy, *In Speech Rehabilitation of the Laryngectomized.* 2nd ed. Springfield, Ill., Charles C Thomas, Publisher, 1969.
80. Proctor, D. F., and Safar, P.: Management of airway obstruction, *In Respiratory Therapy.* Safar, P. (ed.), Philadelphia, F. A. Davis Company, 1965.
81. Rice, H.: Tracheostomy: General management and nursing care. *Nursing Mirror 124:*v, 4 August, 1967.
82. Ritter, F. N.: Tonsillectomy and adenoidectomy: Indications and complications. *Postgraduate Medicine 41:*342, April, 1967.
82a. Robbins, S. L.: *Pathology.* 3rd ed. Philadelphia, W. B. Saunders Company, 1967.
83. Rodman, T.: Management of tracheobronchial secretions. *American Journal of Nursing 66:*2474, November, 1966.
83a. Sabiston, D. C.: *Davis-Christopher Textbook of Surgery: The Biological Basis of Modern Surgical Practice.* 10th ed. Philadelphia, W. B. Saunders Company, 1972.
84. Safar, P.: Emergency resuscitation, *In Respiratory Therapy.* Safar, P. (ed.), Philadelphia, F. A. Davis Company, 1965.
85. Safar, P. (ed.): *Respiratory Therapy.* Philadelphia, F. A. Davis Company, 1965.
86. Saunders, W., et al.: *Nursing Care in Eye, Ear, Nose and Throat Disorders.* 2nd ed. St. Louis, C. V. Mosby Company, 1968.
87. Secor, J.: *Patient Care in Respiratory Problems.* Philadelphia, W. B. Saunders Company, 1969.
88. Sessions, R. B.: Cosmetic rhinoplasty today. *AORN Journal 15:*35, February, 1972.
89. Shafer, K. N., et al.: *Medical-Surgical Nursing.* 5th ed. St. Louis, C. V. Mosby Company, 1971.
90. Shan, N.: Epistaxis. *Nursing Mirror 134:*28, March 10, 1972.
91. Shan, N.: Foreign bodies in ENT. *Nursing Mirror 134:*39, March 17, 1972.
92. Shan, N.: Respiratory obstruction tracheostomy. *Nursing Mirror 134:*35, March 31, 1972.
93. Shaw, H. J.: Cancer of the larynx. *Practitioner 199:*785, December, 1967.
94. Shires, T.: Initial care of the injured patient. *The Journal of Trauma 10:*940, November, 1970.
95. Smith, C.: Infections of the mouth and pharynx. *Nursing Times 68:*566, May 11, 1972.
96. Smith, D. W., Hanley Germain, C. P., and Gips, C. D.: *Care of the Adult Patient.* 3rd ed. Philadelphia, J. B. Lippincott Company, 1971.
97. Snidecor, J. C.: Speech therapy for those with total laryngectomy, *In Speech Rehabilitation of the Laryngectomized.* 2nd ed. Springfield, Ill., Charles C Thomas, Publisher, 1969.
98. Snidecor, J. C.: The artificial larynx, *In Speech Rehabilitation of the Laryngectomized.* 2nd ed. Springfield, Ill., Charles C Thomas, Publisher, 1969.
99. Snidecor, J. C.: The charging and expulsion of esophageal air, *In Speech Rehabilitation of the Laryngectomized.* 2nd ed. Springfield, Ill., Charles C Thomas, Publisher, 1969.
100. Snidecor, J. C.: The nature of the problem, *In Speech Rehabilitation of the Laryngectomized.* 2nd ed. Springfield, Ill., Charles C Thomas, Publisher, 1969.
101. Snidecor, J. C., et al.: *Speech Rehabilitation of the Laryngectomized.* 2nd ed. Springfield, Ill., Charles C Thomas, Publisher, 1969.
102. Sovie, M., and Israel, J. S.: Use of the cuffed tracheostomy tube. *American Journal of Nursing 67:*1852, September, 1967.
103. Spencer, J. T.: Cancer of the larynx. *Laryngoscope 77:*962, June, 1967.
104. Stanley, L. M.: Meeting the psychologic needs of the laryngectomy patient. *Nursing Clinics of North America 3:*519, September, 1968.
105. Stivers, F. E., and Yarington, C. T., Jr.: Indications for tonsillectomy and adenoidectomy. *American Family Physician, 3:*72, March, 1971.
106. Sutton, A. L.: *Bedside Nursing Techniques.* 2nd ed. Philadelphia, W. B. Saunders Company, 1969.
107. Taub, S.: A different way of seeing the larynx and nasopharynx. *AORN Journal 16:*50, December, 1972.
108. Taylor, L.: Perennial nasal allergy. *Practitioner 197:*775, December, 1966.
109. Taylor, T. H.: Tracheostomy care. *Nursing Mirror 123:*i, February, 1967.
110. The bloody nose. *Emergency Medicine 4:*74, April, 1972.
111. Thomas, A. N.: Respiratory care, *In The Cardiac Patient.* Sanderson, R. G. (ed.), Philadelphia, W. B. Saunders Company, 1972.
112. Totman, L. E., and Lehman, R. H.: Tracheostomy care. *American Journal of Nursing 64:*96, March, 1964.
113. Toy, F. J., and Weinstein, J. D.: Percutaneous tracheostomy device. *Surgery 65:*384, February, 1969.
114. Tracheostomy is trauma. *Emergency Medicine 4:*169, May, 1972.
115. Trowbridge, J. E.: Caring for patients with facial or intraoral reconstruction. *American Journal of Nursing 73:*1930, November, 1973.
116. Tyler, M. L., and Synnestvedt, N.: Artificial airways. *Nursing '73 3:*21, February, 1973.
117. Watson, J. E.: *Medical-Surgical Nursing and Related Physiology.* Philadelphia, W. B. Saunders Company, 1972.
118. White, H. A.: Tracheostomy: Care with a cuffed tube. *American Journal of Nursing 72:*75, January, 1972.
119. Wilson, H. E.: Control of massive hemorrhage during bronchoscopy. *Diseases of the Chest 56:*412, November, 1969.
120. Zavertnick, J.: Emotional aspects of patients with head and neck surgery. *Nursing Clinics of North America 2:*503, 1967.

Index

Note: In this index, page numbers in *italics* refer to illustrations. Page numbers followed by (t) refer to tables.